Goodman & Gilman's

THE PHARMACOLOGICAL BASIS OF
THERAPEUTICS

THIRTEENTH EDITION

Goodman & Gilman's
THE PHARMACOLOGICAL BASIS OF
THERAPEUTICS

THIRTEENTH EDITION

Editor-in-chief

Laurence L. Brunton, PhD
Professor of Pharmacology and Medicine
School of Medicine, University of California, San Diego
La Jolla, California

Editors

Randa Hilal-Dandan, PhD
Lecturer in Pharmacology
School of Medicine, University of California, San Diego
La Jolla, California

Björn C. Knollmann, MD, PhD
William Stokes Professor of Medicine and Pharmacology
Director, Vanderbilt Center for Arrhythmia Research and Therapeutics
Division of Clinical Pharmacology
Vanderbilt University School of Medicine
Nashville, Tennessee

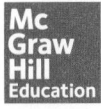

New York   Chicago   San Francisco   Athens   London   Madrid   Mexico City
Milan   New Delhi   Singapore   Sydney   Toronto

Goodman & Gilman's
The Pharmacological Basis of Therapeutics, Thirteenth Edition

Copyright © 2018 by McGraw-Hill Education. All rights reserved. Printed in the United States of America. Except as permitted under the United States Copyright Act of 1976, no part of this publication may be reproduced or distributed in any form or by any means, or stored in a database or retrieval system, without the prior written permission of the publisher.

1 2 3 4 5 6 7 8 9   LWI   22 21 20 19 18 17

ISBN 978-1-25-958473-2
MHID 1-25-958473-9

This book was set in Minion Pro by Cenveo® Publishers Services.
The editors were James F. Shanahan and Harriet Lebowitz.
The production manager was Jeffrey Herzich.
Project management was provided by Vastavikta Sharma, Cenveo Publisher Services.
The designer was Janice Bielawa.

Library of Congress Cataloging-in-Publication Data

Names: Brunton, Laurence L., editor. | Hilal-Dandan, Randa., editor. |
    Knollmann, Björn C., editor.
Title: Goodman & Gilman's the pharmacological basis of therapeutics / editor-in-chief,
    Laurence L. Brunton; editors, Randa Hilal-Dandan,
    Björn C. Knollmann.
Other titles: Goodman and Gilman's the pharmacological basis of therapeutics
    | Pharmacological basis of therapeutics
Description: Thirteenth edition. | New York : McGraw Hill Medical, [2018] |
    Includes bibliographical references and index.
Identifiers: LCCN 2017031869| ISBN 9781259584732 (hardcover) | ISBN
    1259584739 (hardcover)
Subjects: | MESH: Pharmacological Phenomena | Pharmaceutical Preparations |
    Pharmacokinetics | Drug Therapy
Classification: LCC RM300 | NLM QV 4 | DDC 615/.7—dc23 LC record available
at https://lccn.loc.gov/2017031869

McGraw-Hill books are available at special quantity discounts to use as premiums or sales promotions, or for use in corporate training programs. To contact a representative, please the Contact Us pages at www.mhprofessional.com.

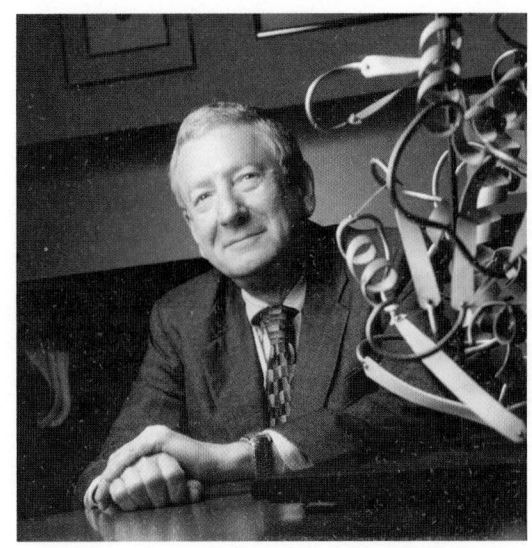

In Memoriam

Alfred Goodman Gilman

(1941-2015)

Mentor, teacher, researcher, Nobel laureate, raconteur, mensch,
and longtime editor of this book

Contents

Contributors

Edward P. Acosta, PharmD
Professor and Director, Division of Clinical Pharmacology
University of Alabama at Birmingham School of Medicine
Birmingham, Alabama

Susan G. Amara, PhD
Scientific Director
National Institute of Mental Health
National Institutes of Health
Bethesda, Maryland

Michael B. Atkins, MD
Professor of Oncology and Medicine
Georgetown University, School of Medicine
Washington DC

Jamil Azzi, MD, FAST
Assistant Professor of Medicine
Transplantation Research Center
Harvard Medical School
Boston, Massachusetts

Peter J. Barnes, DM, DSc, FRCP, FMedSci, FRS
Professor and Head of Respiratory Medicine
National Heart & Lung Institute
Imperial College, London

Robert R. Bies, PharmD, PhD
Associate Professor
School of Pharmacy and Pharmaceutical Sciences
University at Buffalo
The State University of New York
Buffalo, New York

Donald K. Blumenthal, PhD
Associate Professor of Pharmacology & Toxicology
College of Pharmacy
University of Utah
Salt Lake City, Utah

Katharina Brandl, PhD
Assistant Professor of Pharmacy
University of California San Diego
Skaggs School of Pharmacy and Pharmaceutical Sciences
La Jolla, California

Gregory A. Brent, MD
Professor of Medicine and Physiology
Geffen School of Medicine
University of California
Los Angeles, California

Joan Heller Brown, PhD
Professor and Chair of Pharmacology
University of California
San Diego, California

Craig N. Burkhart, MD
Associate Professor of Dermatology, School of Medicine
University of North Carolina
Chapel Hill, North Carolina

Iain L. O. Buxton, PharmD
Foundation Professor and Chair
Department of Pharmacology
University of Nevada, Reno School of Medicine
Reno, Nevada

Michael C. Byrns, PhD
Associate Professor of Environmental Health
Illinois State University
Normal, Illinois

William A. Catterall, PhD
Professor and Chair of Pharmacology
University of Washington School of Medicine
Seattle, Washington

Janet A. Clark, PhD
Director, Office of Fellowship Training
Intramural Research Program
National Institute of Mental Health
National Institutes of Health
Bethesda, Maryland

Michael W. H. Coughtrie, PhD
Professor and Dean
Faculty of Pharmaceutical Sciences
University of British Columbia
Vancouver, Canada

James E. Crowe, Jr.
Professor of Pediatrics, Pathology, Microbiology and Immunology
Director, Vanderbilt Vaccine Center
Vanderbilt University Medical Center
Nashville, Tennessee

David D'Alessio, MD
Professor, Department of Medicine
Director, Division of Endocrinology
Duke University Medical Center
Durham, North Carolina

Michael David, PharmD, PhD
Professor of Biology and Moores Cancer Center
University of California, San Diego
La Jolla, California

Ankit A. Desai, MD
Assistant Professor of Medicine
University of Arizona
Tucson, Arizona

Michelle Erickson, PhD
Research Assistant Professor of Gerontology and Geriatric
   Medicine, School of Medicine
University of Washington
Seattle, Washington

Thomas Eschenhagen, MD
Professor of Pharmacology and Toxicology
Chair of Pharmacology
University Medical Center Hamburg Eppendorf
Hamburg, Germany

Nancy Fares-Frederickson, PhD
Division of Biology and Moores Cancer Center
University of California, San Diego
La Jolla, California

Garret A. FitzGerald, MD
Professor of Medicine, Pharmacology and Translational Medicine
   and Therapeutics;
Chair of Pharmacology
University of Pennsylvania School of Medicine
Philadelphia, Pennsylvania

Charles W. Flexner, MD
Professor of Medicine, Pharmacology and Molecular
   Sciences, and International Health
The Johns Hopkins University School of Medicine and
   Bloomberg School of Public Health
Baltimore, Maryland

Dustin R. Fraidenburg, MD
Assistant Professor of Medicine
University of Illinois at Chicago
Chicago, Illinois

R. Benjamin Free, PhD
Staff Scientist, Molecular Neuropharmacology Section
National Institute of Neurological Disorders and Stroke
National Institutes of Health
Bethesda, Maryland

Peter A. Friedman, PhD
Professor of Pharmacology and Chemical Biology, and
   of Structural Biology
University of Pittsburgh School of Medicine
Pittsburgh, Pennsylvania

John W. Funder, AC, MD, BS, PhD, FRACP
Professor of Medicine, Prince Henry's Institute
Monash Medical Centre
Clayton, Victoria, Australia

Giuseppe Giaccone, MD, PhD
Professor of Medical Oncology and Pharmacology
Georgetown University
Washington DC

Kathleen M. Giacomini, PhD
Professor of Bioengineering and Therapeutic Sciences,
   School of Pharmacy
University of California
San Francisco, California

Alfred G. Gilman, MD, PhD (deceased)
Professor (Emeritus) of Pharmacology
University of Texas Southwestern Medical School
Dallas, Texas

Frank J. Gonzalez, PhD
Chief, Laboratory of Metabolism
Center for Cancer Research, National Cancer Institute
Bethesda, Maryland

Tilo Grosser, MD
Research Associate Professor of Pharmacology
Institute for Translational Medicine and Therapeutics
University of Pennsylvania
Philadelphia, Pennsylvania

Tawanda Gumbo, MD
Director, Center for Infectious Diseases Research and
   Experimental Therapeutics
Baylor Research Institute
Baylor University Medical Center
Dallas, Texas

Holly Gurgle, PharmD, BCACP, CDE
Assistant Professor (Clinical) of Pharmacotherapy
College of Pharmacy
University of Utah
Salt Lake City, Utah

David A. Hafler, MD
William S. and Lois Stiles Edgerly Professor of Neurology and
   Immunobiology
Chairman, Department of Neurology
Yale School of Medicine
New Haven, Connecticut

Stephen R. Hammes, MD, PhD
Professor of Medicine, Chief of Endocrinology and Metabolism
School of Medicine and Dentistry
University of Rochester
Rochester, New York

R. Adron Harris, PhD
Professor of Neuroscience and Pharmacology
Waggoner Center for Alcohol and Addiction Research
University of Texas
Austin, Texas

Lisa A. Hazelwood, PhD
Principal Research Scientist, Liver Disease and Fibrosis, AbbVie
North Chicago, Illinois

Jeffrey D. Henderer, MD
Professor of Ophthalmology
Dr. Edward Hagop Bedrossian Chair of Ophthalmology
Lewis Katz School of Medicine at Temple University
Philadelphia, Pennsylvania

Ryan E. Hibbs, PhD
Assistant Professor of Neuroscience
University of Texas Southwestern Medical School
Dallas, Texas

Randa Hilal-Dandan, PhD
Lecturer in Pharmacology
University of California
San Diego, California

Peter J. Hotez, MD, PhD
Professor of Pediatrics and Molecular Virology & Microbiology
Texas Children's Hospital Endowed Chair in Tropical Pediatrics
Dean, National School of Tropical Medicine
Baylor College of Medicine
Houston, Texas

Claudine Isaacs, MD, FRCPC
Professor of Medicine and Oncology
Georgetown University, School of Medicine
Washington DC

Nina Isoherranen, PhD
Professor of Pharmaceutics, School of Pharmacy
University of Washington
Seattle, Washington

Edwin K. Jackson, PhD
Professor of Pharmacology and Chemical Biology
University of Pittsburgh School of Medicine
Pittsburgh, Pennsylvania

Kenneth Kaushansky, MD
Dean, School of Medicine and Senior Vice President of Health Sciences
SUNY Stony Brook
New York, New York

Jennifer Keiser, PhD
Professor of Neglected Tropical Diseases
Swiss Tropical and Public Health Institute
Basel, Switzerland

Thomas J. Kipps, MD, PhD
Professor of Medicine, Moores Cancer Center
University of California
San Diego, California

Jennifer J. Kiser, PharmD
Associate Professor, Pharmaceutical Sciences
University of Colorado
Denver, Colorado

Ronald J. Koenig, MD, PhD
Professor of Metabolism, Endocrinology and Diabetes
Department of Internal Medicine
University of Michigan Health System
Ann Arbor, Michigan

George F. Koob, PhD
Director, National Institute on Alcohol Abuse and Alcoholism
National Institutes of Health
Rockville, Maryland

Alan M. Krensky, MD
Vice Dean
Professor of Pediatrics and Microbiology & Immunology
Feinberg School of Medicine
Northwestern University
Chicago, Illinois

Ellis R. Levin, MD
Professor of Medicine; Chief of Endocrinology
Diabetes and Metabolism
University of California, Irvine, and Long Beach
VA Medical Center
Long Beach, California

Heather Macarthur, PhD
Associate Professor of Pharmacology and Physiology
Saint Louis University School of Medicine
St. Louis, Missouri

Conan MacDougall, PharmD, MAS
Professor of Clinical Pharmacy
School of Pharmacy
University of California
San Francisco, California

Wallace K. MacNaughton, PhD
Professor and Head of Physiology and Pharmacology
Cumming School of Medicine,
University of Calgary
Calgary, Alberta, Canada

Kenneth P. Mackie, MD
Professor of Psychological and Brain Sciences
Indiana University
Bloomington, Indiana

Jody Mayfield, PhD
Science Writer and Editor
Waggoner Center for Alcohol and Addiction Research
University of Texas
Austin, Texas

James McCarthy, MD
Senior Scientist QIMR Berghofer Intitute of Medical Research
Department of Infectious Diseases, Royal Brisbane
  and Womens Hospital
Brisbane, Queensland, Australia

James O. McNamara, MD
Professor and Chair of Neurobiology
Director of Center for Translational Neuroscience
Duke University Medical Center
Durham, North Carolina

Cameron S. Metcalf, PhD
Research Assistant Professor
Associate Director, Anticonvulsant Drug Development Program
Department of Pharmacology & Toxicology
College of Pharmacy
University of Utah
Salt Lake City, Utah

Jonathan M. Meyer, MD
Psychopharmacology Consultant
California Department of State Hospitals
Assistant Clinical Professor of Psychiatry
University of California
San Diego, California

S. John Mihic, PhD
Professor of Neuroscience
Waggoner Center for Alcohol & Addiction Research
University of Texas
Austin, Texas

Mark E. Molitch, MD
Martha Leland Sherwin Professor of Endocrinology
Northwestern University
Chicago, Illinois

Dean S. Morrell, MD
Professor of Dermatology
University of North Carolina
Chapel Hill, North Carolina

Thomas D. Nolin, PharmD, PhD
Associate Professor of Pharmacy and Therapeutics, and of Medicine
University of Pittsburgh School of Pharmacy and School of Medicine
Pittsburgh, Pennsylvania

Charles P. O'Brien, MD, PhD
Professor of Psychiatry, School of Medicine
University of Pennsylvania
Philadelphia, Pennsylvania

James O'Donnell, PhD
Dean and Professor
School of Pharmacy & Pharmaceutical Sciences
University at Buffalo
The State University of New York
Buffalo, New York

Hemal H. Patel, PhD
Professor of Anesthesiology
University of California, San Diego
VA-San Diego Healthcare System
San Diego, California

Piyush M. Patel, MD, FRCPC
Professor of Anesthesiology
University of California, San Diego
VA-San Diego Healthcare System
San Diego, California

Matthew L. Pearn, MD
Associate Professor of Anesthesiology
University of California, San Diego
VA-San Diego Healthcare System
San Diego, California

Trevor M. Penning, PhD
Professor of Systems Pharmacology & Translational Therapeutics
Director, Center of Excellence in Environmental Toxicology
School of Medicine
University of Pennsylvania
Philadelphia, Pennsylvania

Margaret A. Phillips, PhD
Professor of Pharmacology
University of Texas Southwestern Medical School
Dallas, Texas

Alvin C. Powers, MD
Professor of Medicine, Molecular Physiology and Biophysics
Director, Vanderbilt Diabetes Center
Chief, Division of Diabetes, Endocrinology, and Metabolism
Vanderbilt University School of Medicine
Nashville, Tennessee

Christopher J. Rapuano, MD
Director, Cornea Service and Refractive Surgery
Wills Eye Hospital
Philadelphia, Pennsylvania

Anna T. Riegel, PhD
Professor of Oncology and Pharmacology
Georgetown University, School of Medicine
Washington DC

Suzanne M. Rivera, PhD, MSW
Assistant Professor of Bioethics
Case Western Reserve University
Cleveland, Ohio

Erik D. Roberson, MD, PhD
Associate Professor of Neurology and Neurobiology
Co-Director, Center for Neurodegeneration and
Experimental Therapeutics
University of Alabama at Birmingham
Birmingham, Alabama

Dan M. Roden, MD
Professor of Medicine, Pharmacology, and Biomedical Informatics
Senior Vice President for Personalized Medicine
Vanderbilt University Medical Center
Nashville, Tennessee

P. David Rogers, PharmD, PhD, FCCP
First Tennessee Endowed Chair of Excellence in Clinical Pharmacy
Vice-Chair for Research
Director, Clinical and Experimental Therapeutics
Co-Director, Center for Pediatric Pharmacokinetics and Therapeutics
Professor of Clinical Pharmacy and Pediatrics
University of Tennessee College of Pharmacy
Memphis, Tennessee

David M. Roth, MD, PhD
Professor of Anesthesiology
University of California, San Diego
VA-San Diego Healthcare System
San Diego, California

Edward A. Sausville, MD, PhD
Professor of Medicine; Adjunct Professor, Pharmacology &
Experimental Therapeutics
University of Maryland School of Medicine
Baltimore, Maryland

Matthew J. Sewell, MD
Pediatric Dermatology Fellow
Department of Dermatology
University of North Carolina
Chapel Hill, North Carolina

Bernard P. Schimmer, PhD
Professor (Emeritus) of Pharmacology and Toxicology
University of Toronto
Ontario, Canada

Keith A. Sharkey, PhD, CAGF, FCAHS
Professor of Physiology and Pharmacology
Cumming School of Medicine
University of Calgary
Calgary, Alberta, Canada

Richard C. Shelton, MD
Professor, Department of Psychiatry and Behavioral Neurobiology
The University of Alabama at Birmingham
Birmingham, Alabama

Danny Shen, PhD
Professor of Pharmaceutics, School of Pharmacy
University of Washington
Seattle, Washington

David R. Sibley, PhD
Senior Investigator, Molecular Neuropharmacology Section
National Institute of Neurological Disorders & Stroke
National Institutes of Health
Bethesda, Maryland

Randal A. Skidgel, PhD
Professor of Pharmacology
College of Medicine, University of Illinois-Chicago
Chicago, Illinois

Misty D. Smith, PhD
Research Assistant Professor, Department of
    Pharmacology & Toxicology;
Research Assistant Professor, School of Dentistry
Co-Investigator, Anticonvulsant Drug Development Program
University of Utah
Salt Lake City, Utah

Emer M. Smyth, PhD
Director, Cancer Research Alliances
Assistant Dean for Cancer Research
Assistant Professor, Pathology and Cell Biology
Herbert Irving Comprehensive Cancer Center
Columbia University Medical Center
New York, New York

Peter J. Snyder, MD
Professor of Medicine
University of Pennsylvania
Philadelphia, Pennsylvania

Yuichi Sugiyama, PhD
Head of Sugiyama Laboratory
RIKEN Innovation Center
RIKEN Yokohama
Yokohama, Japan

Palmer Taylor, PhD
Sandra & Monroe Trout Professor of Pharmacology,
    School of Medicine
Dean Emeritus, Skaggs School of Pharmacy and
    Pharmaceutical Sciences
University of California
San Diego, California

Kenneth E. Thummel, PhD
Professor and Chair, Department of Pharmaceutics
University of Washington
Seattle, Washington

Roberto Tinoco, PhD
Research Assistant Professor
Infectious and Inflammatory Diseases Center
Sanford Burnham Prebys Medical Discovery Institute
La Jolla, California

Robert H. Tukey, PhD
Professor of Pharmacology and Chemistry/Biochemistry
University of California
San Diego, California

Joseph M. Vinetz, MD
Professor of Medicine, Division of Infectious Diseases
University of California
San Diego, California

Wendy Vitek, MD
Assistant Professor of Obstetrics and Gynecology
University of Rochester School of Medicine and Dentistry
Rochester, New York

Mark S. Wallace, MD
Professor of Clinical Anesthesiology
University of California
San Diego, California

Jeffrey I. Weitz, MD, FRCP(C), FACP
Professor of Medicine
Biochemistry and Biomedical Sciences McMaster University
Executive Director, Thrombosis & Atherosclerosis
Research Institute
Hamilton, Ontario, Canada

Anton Wellstein, MD, PhD
Professor of Oncology and Pharmacology
Georgetown University, School of Medicine
Washington DC

Jürgen Wess, PhD
Chief, Molecular Signaling Section
Lab. of Bioorganic Chemistry
National Institute of Diabetes and Digestive and Kidney Diseases
Bethesda, Maryland

David P. Westfall, PhD
Professor (Emeritus) of Pharmacology
University of Nevada School of Medicine
Reno, Nevada

Thomas C. Westfall, PhD
Professor and Chair Emeritus, Department of Pharmacology
    and Physiology
Saint Louis University School of Medicine
St. Louis, Missouri

Dawn M. Wetzel, MD, PhD
Assistant Professor of Pediatrics (Division of Infectious Diseases)
    and Pharmacology
University of Texas Southwestern Medical Center
Dallas, Texas

Karen S. Wilcox, PhD
Professor and Chair, Department of Pharmacology
Director, Anticonvulsant Drug Development Program
University of Utah
Salt Lake City, Utah

Kerstin de Wit, MD
Department of Medicine
Divisions of Emergency and Haematology
McMaster University, Canada;
Thrombosis and Emergency Physician
Hamilton Health Sciences
Hamilton, Ontario, Canada

Tony L. Yaksh, PhD
Professor of Anesthesiology and Pharmacology
University of California, San Diego
La Jolla, California

Jason X.-J. Yuan, MD, PhD
Professor of Medicine and Physiology;
Chief, Division of Translational and Regenerative Medicine
University of Arizona
Tucson, Arizona

Alexander C. Zambon, PhD
Assistant Professor of Biopharmaceutical Sciences
Keck Graduate Institute
Claremont, California

Preface

The first edition of this book appeared in 1941, the product of a collaboration between two friends and professors at Yale, Louis Goodman and Alfred Gilman. Their purpose, stated in the preface to that edition, was to correlate pharmacology with related medical sciences, to reinterpret the actions and uses of drugs in light of advances in medicine and the basic biomedical sciences, to emphasize the applications of pharmacodynamics to therapeutics, and to create a book that would be useful to students of pharmacology and to physicians. We continue to follow these principles in the 13th edition.

The 1st edition was quite successful despite its high price, $12.50, and soon became known as the "blue bible of pharmacology." The book was evidence of the deep friendship between its authors, and when the Gilmans' son was born in 1941, he was named Alfred Goodman Gilman. World War II and the relocation of both authors—Goodman to Utah, Gilman to Columbia—postponed a second edition until 1955. The experience of writing the second edition during a period of accelerating basic research and drug development persuaded the authors to become editors, relying on experts whose scholarship they trusted to contribute individual chapters, a pattern that has been followed ever since.

Alfred G. Gilman, the son, served as an associate editor for the 5th edition (1975), became the principal editor for the 6th (1980), 7th (1985), and 8th (1990) editions, and consulting editor for the 9th and 10th editions that were edited by Lee Limbird and Joel Hardman. After an absence in the 11th edition, Al Gilman agreed to co-author the introductory chapter in the 12th edition. His final contribution to G&G, a revision of that chapter, is the first chapter in this edition, which we dedicate to his memory.

A multi-authored text of this sort grows by accretion, posing challenges to editors but also offering 75 years of wisdom, memorable pearls, and flashes of wit. Portions of prior editions persist in the current edition, and we have given credit to recent former contributors at the end of each chapter. Such a text also tends to grow in length with each edition, as contributors add to existing text and as pharmacotherapy advances. To keep the length manageable and in a single volume, Dr. Randa Hilal-Dandan and I prepared a shortened version of each chapter and then invited contributors to add back old material that was essential and to add new material. We also elected to discard the use of extract (very small) type and to use more figures to explain signaling pathways and mechanisms of drug action. Not wanting to favor one company's preparation of an agent over that of another, we have ceased to use trade names except as needed to refer to drug combinations or to distinguish multiple formulations of the same agent with distinctive pharmacokinetic or pharmacodynamic properties. Counter-balancing this shortening are five new chapters that reflect advances in the therapeutic manipulation of the immune system, the treatment of viral hepatitis, and the pharmacotherapy of cardiovascular disease and pulmonary artery hypertension.

Editing such a book brings into view a number of overarching issues: Over-prescribing of antibiotics and their excessive use in agricultural animal husbandry continues to promote the development of antimicrobial resistance; the application of CRISPR/cas9 will likely provide new therapeutic avenues; global warming and the sheer size of the human population require medical scientists and practitioners to promote remedial and preventive action based on data, not ideology.

A number of people have made invaluable contributions to the preparation of this edition. My thanks to Randa Hilal-Dandan and Bjorn Knollmann for their editorial work; to Harriet Lebowitz of McGraw-Hill, who guided our work, prescribed the updated style, and kept the project moving to completion; to Vastavikta Sharma of Cenveo Publishers Services, who oversaw the copy editing, typesetting, and preparation of the artwork; to Nelda Murri, our consulting pharmacist, whose familiarity with clinical pharmacy is evident throughout the book; to James Shanahan, publisher at McGraw-Hill, for supporting the project; and to the many readers who have written to critique the book and offer suggestions.

Laurence L. Brunton
San Diego, CA
1 September 2017

Acknowledgments

The editors appreciate the assistance of:

Harriet Lebowitz
Senior Project Development Editor
McGraw-Hill Education

Laura Libretti
Administrative Assistant
McGraw-Hill Education

Bryan Mott, PhD
Consulting Medicinal Chemist

Nelda Murri, PharmD, MBA
Consulting Pharmacist

Christie Naglieri
Senior Project Development Editor
McGraw-Hill Education

Joseph K. Prinsen, DO, PhD
Jason D. Morrow Chief Fellow in Clinical Pharmacology
Vanderbilt University School of Medicine

David Aaron Rice
Administrative Assistant
University of California, San Diego

James F. Shanahan
Publisher, Medical Textbooks
McGraw-Hill Education

Vastavikta Sharma
Lead Project Manager
Cenveo Publisher Services

Roberto Tinoco, PhD
Research Assistant Professor
Sanford-Burnham-Prebys Medical Discovery Institute

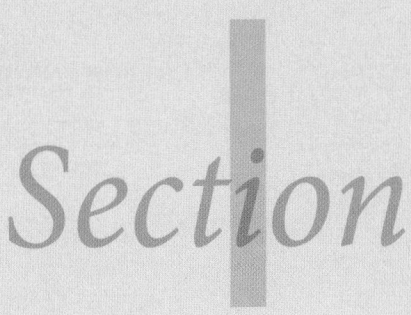

Section I

General Principles

Chapter 1

Drug Invention and the Pharmaceutical Industry

Suzanne M. Rivera and Alfred Goodman Gilman*

The first edition of *Goodman & Gilman*, published in 1941, helped to organize the field of pharmacology, giving it intellectual validity and an academic identity. That edition began: "The subject of pharmacology is a broad one and embraces the knowledge of the source, physical and chemical properties, compounding, physiological actions, absorption, fate, and excretion, and therapeutic uses of drugs. A *drug* may be broadly defined as any chemical agent that affects living protoplasm, and few substances would escape inclusion by this definition." This General Principles section provides the underpinnings for these definitions by exploring the processes of drug invention, development, and regulation, followed by the basic properties of the interactions between the drug and biological systems: *pharmacodynamics*, *pharmacokinetics* (including drug transport and metabolism), and *pharmacogenomics*, with a brief foray into *drug toxicity and poisoning*. Subsequent sections deal with the use of drugs as therapeutic agents in human subjects.

Use of the term *invention* to describe the process by which a new drug is identified and brought to medical practice, rather than the more conventional term *discovery,* is intentional. Today, useful drugs are rarely discovered hiding somewhere waiting to be found. The term *invention* emphasizes the process by which drugs are sculpted and brought into being based on experimentation and optimization of many independent properties; there is little serendipity.

From Early Experiences With Plants to Modern Chemistry

The human fascination—and sometimes infatuation—with chemicals that alter biological function is ancient and results from long experience with and dependence on plants. Because most plants are root bound, many of them produce harmful compounds for defense that animals have learned to avoid and humans to exploit (or abuse).

Earlier editions of this text described examples: the appreciation of coffee (caffeine) by the prior of an Arabian convent, who noted the behavior of goats that gamboled and frisked through the night after eating the berries of the coffee plant; the use of mushrooms and the deadly nightshade plant by professional poisoners; of belladonna ("beautiful lady") to dilate pupils; of the Chinese herb ma huang (containing ephedrine) as a circulatory stimulant; of curare by South American Indians to paralyze and kill animals hunted for food; and of poppy juice (opium) containing morphine (from the Greek *Morpheus*, the God of dreams) for pain relief and control of dysentery. Morphine, of course, has well-known addicting properties, mimicked in some ways by other problematic ("recreational") natural products—nicotine, cocaine, and ethanol.

Although terrestrial and marine organisms remain valuable sources of compounds with pharmacological activities, drug invention became more allied with synthetic organic chemistry as that discipline flourished over the past 150 years, beginning in the dye industry. Dyes are colored compounds with selective affinity for biological tissues. Study of these interactions stimulated Paul Ehrlich to postulate the existence of chemical receptors in tissues that interacted with and "fixed" the dyes. Similarly, Ehrlich thought that unique receptors on microorganisms or parasites might react specifically with certain dyes and that such selectivity could spare normal tissue. Ehrlich's work culminated in the invention of arsphenamine in 1907, which was patented as "salvarsan," suggestive of the hope that the chemical would be the salvation of humankind. This and other organic arsenicals were used for the chemotherapy of syphilis until the discovery of penicillin. The work of Gerhard Domagk demonstrated that another dye, prontosil (the first clinically useful sulfonamide), was dramatically effective in treating streptococcal infections, launching the era of antimicrobial chemotherapy.

The collaboration of pharmacology with chemistry on the one hand and with clinical medicine on the other has been a major contributor to the effective treatment of disease, especially since the middle of the 20th century.

Sources of Drugs

Small Molecules Are the Tradition

With the exception of a few naturally occurring hormones (e.g., insulin), most drugs were small organic molecules (typically <500 Da) until

*Deceased, December 23, 2015. AGG served on the Board of Directors of Regeneron Pharmaceuticals, Inc., a potential conflict of interest.

Abbreviations

ADME: absorption, distribution, metabolism, excretion
AHFS-DI: American Hospital Formulary Service-Drug Information
BLA: Biologics License Application
CDC: Centers for Disease Control and Prevention
CDER: Center for Drug Evaluation and Research
DHHS: U.S. Department of Health and Human Services
FDA: U.S. Food and Drug Administration
HCV: hepatitis C virus
HMG CoA: 3-hydroxy-3-methylglutaryl coenzyme A
IND: Investigational New Drug
LDL: low-density lipoprotein
NDA: New Drug Application
NIH: National Institutes of Health
NMEs: New Molecular Entities
NMR: nuclear magnetic resonance
PCSK9: proprotein convertase subtilisin/kexin type 9
PDUFA: Prescription Drug User Fee Act
PhRMA: Pharmaceutical Research and Manufacturers of America
R&D: research and development
SCHIP: State Children's Health Insurance Program
siRNAs: small interfering RNAs

recombinant DNA technology permitted synthesis of proteins by various organisms (bacteria, yeast) and mammalian cells. The usual approach to invention of a small-molecule drug is to screen a collection of chemicals ("library") for compounds with the desired features. An alternative is to synthesize and focus on close chemical relatives of a substance known to participate in a biological reaction of interest (e.g., congeners of a specific enzyme substrate chosen to be possible inhibitors of the enzymatic reaction), a particularly important strategy in the discovery of anticancer drugs.

Drug discovery in the past often resulted from serendipitous observations of the effects of plant extracts or individual chemicals on animals or humans; today's approach relies more on high-throughput screening of libraries containing hundreds of thousands or even millions of compounds for their capacity to interact with a specific molecular target or elicit a specific biological response. Ideally, the target molecules are of human origin, obtained by transcription and translation of the cloned human gene. The potential drugs that are identified in the screen ("hits") are thus known to react with the human protein and not just with its relative (ortholog) obtained from the mouse or another species.

Among the variables considered in screening are the "drugability" of the target and the stringency of the screen in terms of the concentrations of compounds that are tested. *Drugability* refers to the ease with which the function of a target can be altered in the desired fashion by a small organic molecule. If the protein target has a well-defined binding site for a small molecule (e.g., a catalytic or allosteric site), chances are excellent that hits will be obtained. If the goal is to employ a small molecule to mimic or disrupt the interaction between two proteins, the challenge is much greater.

From Hits to Leads

Initial hits in a screen are rarely marketable drugs, often having modest affinity for the target and lacking the desired specificity and pharmacological properties. Medicinal chemists synthesize derivatives of the hits, thereby defining the structure-activity relationship and optimizing parameters such as affinity for the target, agonist/antagonist activity, permeability across cell membranes, absorption and distribution in the body, metabolism, and unwanted effects.

This approach was driven largely by instinct and trial and error in the past; modern drug development frequently takes advantage of determination of a high-resolution structure of the putative drug bound to its target. X-ray crystallography offers the most detailed structural information if the target protein can be crystallized with the lead drug bound to it. Using techniques of molecular modeling and computational chemistry, the structure provides the chemist with information about substitutions likely to improve the "fit" of the drug with the target and thus enhance the affinity of the drug for its target. Nuclear magnetic resonance (NMR) studies of the drug-receptor complex also can provide useful information (albeit usually at lower resolution), with the advantage that the complex need not be crystallized.

The holy grail of this approach to drug invention is to achieve success entirely through computation. Imagine a database containing detailed chemical information about millions of chemicals and a second database containing detailed structural information about all human proteins. The computational approach is to "roll" all the chemicals over the protein of interest to find those with high-affinity interactions. The dream becomes bolder if we acquire the ability to roll the chemicals that bind to the target of interest over all other human proteins to discard compounds that have unwanted interactions. Finally, we also will want to predict the structural and functional consequences of a drug binding to its target (a huge challenge), as well as all relevant pharmacokinetic properties of the molecules of interest. Indeed, computational approaches have suggested new uses for old drugs and offered explanations for recent failures of drugs in the later stages of clinical development (e.g., torcetrapib; see Box 1-2) (Xie et al., 2007, 2009).

Large Molecules Are Increasingly Important

Protein therapeutics were uncommon before the advent of recombinant DNA technology. Insulin was introduced into clinical medicine for the treatment of diabetes following the experiments of Banting and Best in 1921. Insulins purified from porcine or bovine pancreas are active in humans, although antibodies to the foreign proteins are occasionally problematic. Growth hormone, used to treat pituitary dwarfism, exhibits more stringent species specificity. Only the human hormone could be used after purification from pituitary glands harvested during autopsy, and such use had its dangers—some patients who received the human hormone developed Creutzfeldt-Jakob disease (the human equivalent of mad cow disease), a fatal degenerative neurological disease caused by prion proteins that contaminated the drug preparation. Thanks to gene cloning and the production of large quantities of proteins by expressing the cloned gene in bacteria or eukaryotic cells, protein therapeutics now use highly purified preparations of human (or humanized) proteins. Rare proteins can be produced in quantity, and immunological reactions are minimized. Proteins can be designed, customized, and optimized using genetic engineering techniques. Other types of macromolecules may also be used therapeutically. For example, antisense oligonucleotides are used to block gene transcription or translation, as are siRNAs.

Proteins used therapeutically include hormones; growth factors (e.g., erythropoietin, granulocyte colony-stimulating factor); cytokines; and a number of monoclonal antibodies used in the treatment of cancer and autoimmune diseases (Chapters 34–36 and 67). Murine monoclonal antibodies can be "humanized" (by substituting human for mouse amino acid sequences). Alternatively, mice have been engineered by replacement of critical mouse genes with their human equivalents, such that they make completely human antibodies. Protein therapeutics are administered parenterally, and their receptors or targets must be accessible extracellularly.

Targets of Drug Action

Early drugs came from observation of the effects of plants after their ingestion by animals, with no knowledge of the drug's mechanism or site of action. Although this approach is still useful (e.g., in screening for the capacity of natural products to kill microorganisms or malignant cells), modern drug invention usually takes the opposite approach, starting with a statement (or hypothesis) that a certain protein or pathway plays a critical role in the pathogenesis of a certain disease, and that altering the protein's activity would be effective against that disease. Crucial questions arise:

- Can one find a drug that will have the desired effect against its target?
- Does modulation of the target protein affect the course of disease?
- Does this project make sense economically?

The effort expended to find the desired drug will be determined by the degree of confidence in the answers to the last two questions.

Is the Target Drugable?

The drugability of a target with a low-molecular-weight organic molecule relies on the presence of a binding site for the drug that exhibits considerable affinity and selectivity.

If the target is an enzyme or a receptor for a small ligand, one is encouraged. If the target is related to another protein that is known to have, for example, a binding site for a regulatory ligand, one is hopeful. However, if the known ligands are large peptides or proteins with an extensive set of contacts with their receptor, the challenge is much greater. If the goal is to disrupt interactions between two proteins, it may be necessary to find a "hot spot" that is crucial for the protein-protein interaction, and such a region may not be detected. Accessibility of the drug to its target also is critical. Extracellular targets are intrinsically easier to approach, and, in general, only extracellular targets are accessible to macromolecular drugs.

Has the Target Been Validated?

The question of whether the target has been validated is obviously a critical one. A negative answer, frequently obtained only retrospectively, is a common cause of failure in drug invention (Box 1–1). Modern techniques of molecular biology offer powerful tools for validation of potential drug targets, to the extent that the biology of model systems resembles human biology. Genes can be inserted, disrupted, and altered in mice. One can thereby create models of disease in animals or mimic the effects of long-term disruption or activation of a given biological process. If, for example, disruption of the gene encoding a specific enzyme or receptor has a beneficial effect in a valid murine model of a human disease, one may believe that the potential drug target has been validated. Mutations in humans also can provide extraordinarily valuable information.

For example, loss-of-function mutations in the *PCSK9* gene (encoding proprotein convertase subtilisin/kexin type 9) greatly lower concentrations of LDL cholesterol in blood and reduce the risk of myocardial infarction (Horton et al., 2009; Poirier and Mayer, 2013). Based on these findings, two companies now market antibodies that inhibit the action of *PCSK9*. These antibodies lower the concentration of LDL cholesterol in blood substantially and are essentially additive to the effects of statins; long-term outcome studies are in progress to determine whether the risk of significant cardiovascular events also is reduced. Additional molecules are in the queue.

BOX 1–1 ■ Target Validation: The Lesson of Leptin

Biological systems frequently contain redundant elements or can alter expression of drug-regulated elements to compensate for the effect of the drug. *In general, the more important the function, the greater the complexity of the system.* For example, many mechanisms control feeding and appetite, and drugs to control obesity have been notoriously difficult to find. The discovery of the hormone leptin, which suppresses appetite, was based on mutations in mice that cause loss of either leptin or its receptor; either kind of mutation results in enormous obesity in both mice and people. Leptin thus appeared to be a marvelous opportunity to treat obesity. However, on investigation, it was discovered that obese individuals have high circulating concentrations of leptin and appear insensitive to its action.

Is This Drug Invention Effort Economically Viable?

Drug invention and development is expensive (see Table 1-1), and economic realities influence the direction of pharmaceutical research. For example, investor-owned companies generally cannot afford to develop products for rare diseases or for diseases that are common only in economically underdeveloped parts of the world. Funds to invent drugs targeting rare diseases or diseases primarily affecting developing countries (especially parasitic diseases) often come from taxpayers or wealthy philanthropists.

Additional Preclinical Research

Following the path just described can yield a potential drug molecule that interacts with a validated target and alters its function in the desired fashion. Now, one must consider all aspects of the molecule in question—its affinity and selectivity for interaction with the target; its pharmacokinetic properties (ADME); issues of its large-scale synthesis or purification; its pharmaceutical properties (stability, solubility, questions of formulation); and its safety. One hopes to correct, to the extent possible, any obvious deficiencies by modification of the molecule itself or by changes in the way the molecule is presented for use.

Before being administered to people, potential drugs are tested for general toxicity by long-term monitoring of the activity of various systems in two species of animals, generally one rodent (usually the mouse) and one nonrodent (often the rabbit). Compounds also are evaluated for carcinogenicity, genotoxicity, and reproductive toxicity (see Chapter 4). In vitro and ex vivo assays are used when possible, both to spare animals and to minimize cost. If an unwanted effect is observed, an obvious question is whether it is mechanism based (i.e., caused by interaction of the drug with its intended target) or caused by an off-target effect of the drug, which might be minimized by further optimization of the molecule.

Before the drug candidate can be administered to human subjects in a clinical trial, the sponsor must file an IND application, a request to the U.S. FDA (see "Clinical Trials") for permission to use the drug for human research. The IND describes the rationale and preliminary evidence for efficacy in experimental systems, as well as pharmacology, toxicology, chemistry, manufacturing, and so forth. It also describes the plan (protocol) for investigating the drug in human subjects. The FDA has 30 days to review the IND application, by which time the agency may disapprove it, ask for more data, or allow initial clinical testing to proceed.

Clinical Trials

Role of the FDA

The FDA is a federal regulatory agency within the U.S. DHHS. It is responsible for protecting the public health by ensuring the safety, efficacy, and security of human and veterinary drugs, biological products, medical devices, our nation's food supply, cosmetics, and products that emit radiation (FDA, 2014). The FDA also is responsible for advancing public health by helping to speed innovations that make medicines and foods more effective, safer, and more affordable and by helping people obtain the accurate, science-based information they need to use medicines and foods to improve their health.

New governmental regulations often result from tragedies. The first drug-related legislation in the U.S., the Federal Food and Drug Act of 1906, was concerned only with the interstate transport of adulterated or misbranded foods and drugs. There were no obligations to establish drug efficacy or safety. This act was amended in 1938 after the deaths of over 100 children from "elixir sulfanilamide," a solution of sulfanilamide in diethylene glycol, an excellent but highly toxic solvent and an ingredient in antifreeze. The enforcement of the amended act was entrusted to the FDA, which began requiring toxicity studies as well as approval of an NDA (see "The Conduct of Clinical Trials") before a drug could be promoted and distributed. Although a new drug's safety had to be demonstrated, no proof of efficacy was required.

In the 1960s, thalidomide, a hypnotic drug with no obvious advantages over others, was introduced in Europe. Epidemiological research eventually established that this drug, taken early in pregnancy, was responsible for an epidemic of what otherwise is a relatively rare and severe birth defect, phocomelia, in which limbs are malformed. In reaction to this catastrophe, the U.S. Congress passed the Harris-Kefauver amendments to the Food, Drug, and Cosmetic Act in 1962. These amendments established the requirement for proof of efficacy as well as documentation of relative safety in terms of the risk-to-benefit ratio for the disease entity to be treated (the more serious the disease, the greater the acceptable risk).

Today, the FDA faces an enormous challenge, especially in view of the widely held belief that its mission cannot possibly be accomplished with the resources allocated by Congress. Moreover, harm from drugs that cause unanticipated adverse effects is not the only risk of an imperfect system; harm also occurs when the approval process delays the approval of a new drug with important beneficial effects.

The Conduct of Clinical Trials

Clinical trials of drugs are designed to acquire information about the pharmacokinetic and pharmacodynamic properties of a candidate drug in humans. Efficacy must be proven and an adequate margin of safety established for a drug to be approved for sale in the U.S.

The U.S. NIH identifies seven ethical principles that must be satisfied before a clinical trial can begin:

1. Social and clinical value
2. Scientific validity
3. Fair selection of subjects
4. Informed consent
5. Favorable risk-benefit ratio
6. Independent review
7. Respect for potential and enrolled subjects (NIH, 2011).

The FDA-regulated clinical trials typically are conducted in four phases. Phases I-III are designed to establish safety and efficacy, while phase IV postmarketing trials delineate additional information regarding new indications, risks, and optimal doses and schedules. Table 1–1 and Figure 1–1 summarize the important features of each phase of clinical trials; note the attrition at each successive stage over a relatively long and costly process. When initial phase III trials are complete, the sponsor (usually a pharmaceutical company) applies to the FDA for approval to market the drug; this application is called either an NDA or a BLA. These applications contain comprehensive information, including individual case report forms from the hundreds or thousands of individuals who have received the drug during its phase III testing. Applications are reviewed by teams of specialists, and the FDA may call on the help of panels of external experts in complex cases.

Under the provisions of the PDUFA (enacted in 1992 and renewed every 5 years, most recently in 2012), pharmaceutical companies now provide a significant portion of the FDA budget via user fees, a legislative effort to expedite the drug approval review process by providing increased resources. The PDUFA also broadened the FDA's drug safety program and increased resources for review of television drug advertising. Under the PDUFA, once an NDA is submitted to the FDA, review typically takes 6–10 months. During this time, numerous review functions are usually performed, including advisory committee meetings, amendments, manufacturing facility inspections, and proprietary name reviews (FDA, 2013a). Before a drug is approved for marketing, the company and the FDA must agree on the content of the "label" (package insert)—the official prescribing information. This label describes the approved indications for use of the drug and clinical pharmacological information, including dosage, adverse reactions, and special warnings and precautions (sometimes posted in a "black box").

Promotional materials used by pharmaceutical companies cannot deviate from information contained in the package insert. Importantly, the physician is not bound by the package insert; a physician in the U.S. *may* legally prescribe a drug for any purpose that he or she deems reasonable. However, third-party payers (insurance companies, Medicare, and so on) generally will not reimburse a patient for the cost of a drug used for an "off-label" indication unless the new use is supported by a statutorily named compendium (e.g., the AHFS-DI). Furthermore, a physician may be vulnerable to litigation if untoward effects result from an unapproved use of a drug.

Determining "Safe" and "Effective"

Demonstrating efficacy to the FDA requires performing "adequate and well-controlled investigations," generally interpreted to mean two replicate clinical trials that are usually, but not always, randomized, double blind, and placebo (or otherwise) controlled.

Is a placebo the proper control? The World Medical Association's *Declaration of Helsinki* (World Medical Association 2013) discourages use of placebo controls when an alternative treatment is available for comparison because of the concern that study participants randomized to placebo in such a circumstance would, in effect, be denied treatment during the conduct of the trial.

What must be measured in the trials? In a straightforward trial, a readily quantifiable parameter (a secondary or surrogate end point), thought to be predictive of relevant clinical outcomes, is measured in matched drug- and placebo-treated groups. Examples of surrogate end points include

TABLE 1–1 ■ TYPICAL CHARACTERISTICS OF THE VARIOUS PHASES OF THE CLINICAL TRIALS REQUIRED FOR MARKETING OF NEW DRUGS

PHASE I FIRST IN HUMAN	PHASE II FIRST IN PATIENT	PHASE III MULTISITE TRIAL	PHASE IV POSTMARKETING SURVEILLANCE
10–100 participants	50–500 participants	A few hundred to a few thousand participants	Many thousands of participants
Usually healthy volunteers; occasionally patients with advanced or rare disease	Patient-subjects receiving experimental drug	Patient-subjects receiving experimental drug	Patients in treatment with approved drug
Open label	Randomized and controlled (can be placebo controlled); may be blinded	Randomized and controlled (can be placebo controlled) or uncontrolled; may be blinded	Open label
Safety and tolerability	Efficacy and dose ranging	Confirm efficacy in larger population	Adverse events, compliance, drug-drug interactions
1–2 years	2–3 years	3–5 years	No fixed duration
U.S. $10 million	U.S. $20 million	U.S. $50–100 million	—
Success rate: 50%	Success rate: 30%	Success rate: 25%–50%	—

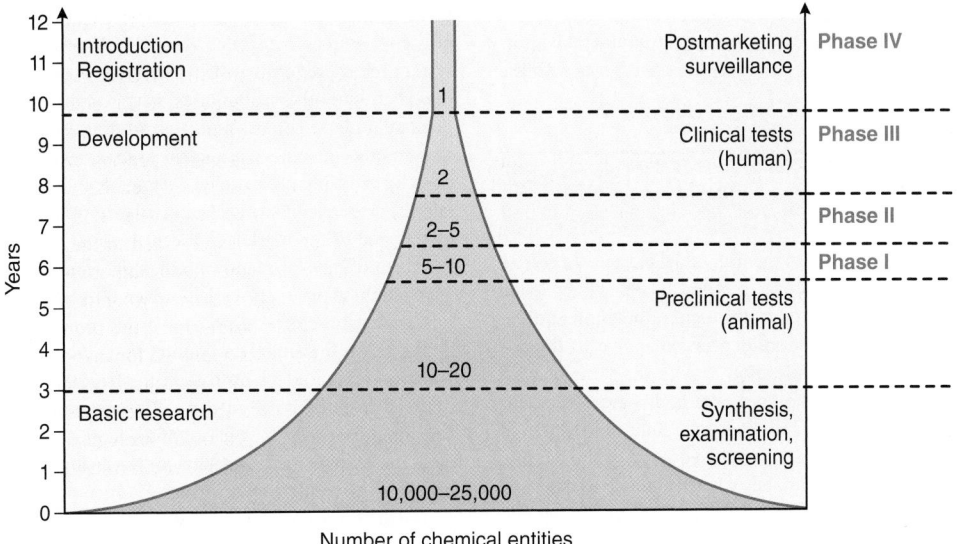

Figure 1–1 *The phases, time lines, and attrition that characterize the invention of new drugs.* See also Table 1–1.

LDL cholesterol as a predictor of myocardial infarction, bone mineral density as a predictor of fractures, or hemoglobin A_{1c} as a predictor of the complications of diabetes mellitus. More stringent trials would require demonstration of reduction of the incidence of myocardial infarction in patients taking a candidate drug in comparison with those taking an HMG CoA reductase inhibitor (statin) or other LDL cholesterol-lowering agent or reduction in the incidence of fractures in comparison with those taking a bisphosphonate. Use of surrogate end points significantly reduces cost and time required to complete trials, but there are many mitigating factors, including the significance of the surrogate end point to the disease that the candidate drug is intended to treat.

Some of the difficulties are well illustrated by experiences with ezetimibe, a drug that inhibits absorption of cholesterol from the gastrointestinal tract and lowers LDL cholesterol concentrations in blood, especially when used in combination with a statin. Lowering of LDL cholesterol was assumed to be an appropriate surrogate end point for the effectiveness of ezetimibe to reduce myocardial infarction and stroke, and the drug was approved based on such data. Surprisingly, a subsequent clinical trial (ENHANCE) demonstrated that the combination of ezetimibe and a statin did not reduce intima media thickness of carotid arteries (a more direct measure of subendothelial cholesterol accumulation) compared with the statin alone, despite the fact that the drug combination lowered LDL cholesterol concentrations substantially more than did either drug alone (Kastelein et al., 2008).

Critics of ENHANCE argued that the patients in the study had familial hypercholesterolemia, had been treated with statins for years, and did not have carotid artery thickening at the initiation of the study. Should ezetimibe have been approved? Must we return to measurement of true clinical end points (e.g., myocardial infarction) before approval of drugs that lower cholesterol by novel mechanisms? The costs involved in such extensive and expensive trials must be borne somehow (see below). A follow-up 7-year study involving over 18,000 patients (IMPROVE-IT) vindicated the decision to approve ezetimibe (Jarcho and Keaney, 2015). Taken in conjunction with a statin, the drug significantly reduced the incidence of myocardial infarction and stroke in high-risk patients (Box 1–2).

No drug is totally safe; all drugs produce unwanted effects in at least some people at some dose. Many unwanted and serious effects of drugs occur so infrequently, perhaps only once in several thousand patients, that they go undetected in the relatively small populations (a few thousand) in the standard phase III clinical trial (see Table 1–1). To detect and verify that such events are, in fact, drug-related would require administration of the drug to tens or hundreds of thousands of people during clinical trials, adding enormous expense and time to drug development and delaying access to potentially beneficial therapies. In general, the true spectrum and

incidence of untoward effects become known only after a drug is released to the broader market and used by a large number of people (phase IV, postmarketing surveillance). Drug development costs and drug prices could be reduced substantially if the public were willing to accept more risk. This would require changing the way we think about a pharmaceutical company's liability for damages from an unwanted effect of a drug that was not detected in clinical trials deemed adequate by the FDA. While the concept is obvious, many lose sight of the fact that extremely severe unwanted effects of a drug, including death, may be deemed acceptable if its therapeutic effect is sufficiently unique and valuable. Such dilemmas are not simple and can become issues for great debate.

Several strategies exist to detect adverse reactions after marketing of a drug. Formal approaches for estimation of the magnitude of an adverse drug response include the follow-up or "cohort" study of patients who are receiving a particular drug; the "case-control" study, in which the frequency of drug use in cases of adverse responses is compared to controls; and meta-analysis of pre- and postmarketing studies. Voluntary reporting of adverse events has proven to be an effective way to generate an early signal that a drug may be causing an adverse reaction (Aagard and Hansen, 2009). The primary sources for the reports are responsible, alert physicians; third-party payers (pharmacy benefit managers, insurance companies) and consumers also play important roles. Other useful sources are nurses, pharmacists, and students in these disciplines. In addition, hospital-based pharmacy and therapeutics committees and quality assurance committees frequently are charged with monitoring adverse drug reactions in hospitalized patients. In 2013, the reporting system in the U.S., called *MedWatch,* celebrated its 20th anniversary and announced improvements designed to encourage reporting by consumers (FDA, 2013b). The simple forms for reporting may be obtained 24 hours a day, 7 days a week, by calling 800-FDA-1088; alternatively, adverse reactions

---

BOX 1–2 ■ A Late Surprise in the Development of a Blockbuster

Torcetrapib elevates high-density lipoprotein (HDL) cholesterol (the "good cholesterol"), and higher levels of HDL cholesterol are statistically associated with (are a surrogate end point for) a lower incidence of myocardial infarction. Surprisingly, clinical administration of torcetrapib caused a significant *increase* in mortality from cardiovascular events, ending a development path of 15 years and $800 million. In this case, approval of the drug based on this secondary end point would have been a mistake (Cutler, 2007). A computational systems analysis suggested a mechanistic explanation of this failure (Xie et al., 2009).

can be reported directly using the Internet (http://www.fda.gov/Safety/MedWatch/default.htm). Health professionals also may contact the pharmaceutical manufacturer, who is legally obligated to file reports with the FDA.

Personalized (Individualized, Precision) Medicine

Drug inventors strive to "fit" the drug to the individual patient. To realize the full potential of this approach, however, requires intimate knowledge of the considerable heterogeneity of both the patient population and the targeted disease process. Why does one antidepressant appear to ameliorate depression in a given patient, while another with the same or very similar presumed mechanism of action does not? Is this a difference in the patient's response to the drug; in patient susceptibility to the drug's unwanted effects; in the drug's ADME; or in the etiology of the depression? By contrast, how much of this variability is attributable to environmental factors and possibly their interactions with patient-specific genetic variability? Recent advances, especially in genetics and genomics, provide powerful tools for understanding this heterogeneity. The single most powerful tool for unraveling these myriad mysteries is the ability to sequence DNA rapidly and economically. The cost of sequencing a human genome has fallen by six orders of magnitude since the turn of the 21st century, and the speed of the process has increased correspondingly. The current focus is on the extraordinarily complex analysis of the enormous amounts of data now being obtained from many thousands of individuals, ideally in conjunction with deep knowledge of their phenotypic characteristics, especially including their medical history.

Readily measured biomarkers of disease are powerful adjuncts to DNA sequence information. Simple blood or other tests can be developed to monitor real-time progress or failure of treatment, and many such examples already exist. Similarly, chemical, radiological, or genetic tests may be useful not only to monitor therapy but also to predict success or failure, anticipate unwanted effects of treatment, or appreciate pharmacokinetic variables that may require adjustments of dosage or choice of drugs. Such tests already play a significant role in the choice of drugs for cancer chemotherapy, and the list of drugs specifically designed to "hit" a mutated target in a specific cancer is growing. Such information is also becoming increasing useful in the choice of patients for clinical trials of specific agents—thereby reducing the time required for such trials and their cost, to say nothing of better defining the patient population who may benefit from the drug. These important subjects are discussed in detail in Chapter 7, Pharmacogenetics.

Public Policy Considerations and Criticisms of the Pharmaceutical Industry

Drugs can save lives, prolong lives, and improve the quality of people's lives. However, in a free-market economy, access to drugs is not equitable. Not surprisingly, there is tension between those who treat drugs as entitlements and those who view drugs as high-tech products of a capitalistic society. Supporters of the entitlement position argue that a constitutional right to life should guarantee access to drugs and other healthcare, and they are critical of pharmaceutical companies and others who profit from the business of making and selling drugs. Free-marketers point out that, without a profit motive, it would be difficult to generate the resources and innovation required for new drug development. Given the public interest in the pharmaceutical industry, drug development is both a scientific process and a political one in which attitudes can change quickly. Two decades ago, Merck was named as America's most admired company by *Fortune* magazine 7 years in a row—a record that still stands. In the 2015 survey of the most admired companies in the U.S., no pharmaceutical company ranked in the top 10.

Critics of the pharmaceutical industry frequently begin from the position that people (and animals) need to be protected from greedy and unscrupulous companies and scientists (Kassirer, 2005). In the absence of a government-controlled drug development enterprise, our current system relies predominantly on investor-owned pharmaceutical companies that, like other companies, have a profit motive and an obligation to shareholders. The price of prescription drugs causes great consternation among consumers, especially as many health insurers seek to control costs by choosing not to cover certain "brand-name" products (discussed later). Further, a few drugs (especially for treatment of cancer) have been introduced to the market in recent years at prices that greatly exceeded the costs of development, manufacture, and marketing of the product. Many of these products were discovered in government laboratories or in university laboratories supported by federal grants.

The U.S. is the only large country that places no controls on drug prices and where price plays no role in the drug approval process. Many U.S. drugs cost much more in the U.S. than overseas; thus, U.S. consumers subsidize drug costs for the rest of the world, and they are irritated by that fact. The example of new agents for the treatment of hepatitis C infection brings many conflicting priorities into perspective (Box 1–3).

The drug development process is long, expensive, and risky (see Figure 1–1 and Table 1–1). Consequently, drugs must be priced to recover the substantial costs of invention and development and to fund the marketing efforts needed to introduce new products to physicians and patients. Nevertheless, as U.S. healthcare spending continues to rise at an alarming pace, prescription drugs account for only about 10% of total U.S. healthcare expenditures (CDC, 2013), and a significant fraction of this drug cost is for low-priced, nonproprietary medicines. Although the increase in prices is significant in certain classes of drugs (e.g., anticancer agents), the total price of prescription drugs is growing at a slower rate than other healthcare costs. Even drastic reductions in drug prices that would

---

BOX 1–3 ■ The Cost of Treating Hepatitis C

Infection with hepatitis C virus (HCV) is a chronic disease afflicting millions of people. Some suffer little from this condition; many others eventually develop cirrhosis or hepatocellular carcinoma. Who should be treated? The answer is unknown. Until recently, the treatment of choice for people with genotype 1 HCV involved year-long administration of an interferon (by injection) in combination with ribavirin and a protease inhibitor. Unwanted effects of this regimen are frequent and severe (some say worse than the disease); cure rates range from 50% to 75%. A newer treatment involves an oral tablet containing a combination of sofosbuvir and ledipasvir (see Chapter 63). Treatment usually requires daily ingestion of one tablet, for 8–12 weeks; cure rates exceed 95%, and side effects are minimal.

Controversy surrounds the price of the treatment, about $1000/d. Some insurers refused to reimburse this high cost, relegating many patients to less-effective, more toxic, but less-expensive treatment. However, these third-party payers have negotiated substantial discounts of the price, based on the availability of a competing product. Is the cost exorbitant? Should insurers, rather than patients and their physicians, be making such important decisions?

Continued and excessive escalation of drug and other healthcare costs will bankrupt the healthcare system. The question of appropriate cost involves complex pharmacoeconomic considerations. What are the relative costs of the two treatment regimens? What are the savings from elimination of the serious sequelae of chronic HCV infection? How does one place value to the patient on the less-toxic and more effective and convenient regimen? What are the profit margins of the company involved? Who should make decisions about costs and choices of patients to receive various treatments? How should we consider cases (unlike that for HCV) for which the benefits are quite modest, such as when a very expensive cancer drug extends life only briefly? One astute observer (and an industry critic of many drug prices) summarized the situation as follows: "great, important problem; wrong example."

severely limit new drug invention would not lower the overall healthcare budget by more than a few percent.

Are profit margins excessive among the major pharmaceutical companies? There is no objective answer to this question. Pragmatic answers come from the markets and from company survival statistics. The U.S. free-market system provides greater rewards for particularly risky and important fields of endeavor, and many people agree that the rewards should be greater for those willing to take the risk. The pharmaceutical industry is clearly one of the more risky:

- The costs to bring products to market are enormous.
- The success rate is low (accounting for much of the cost).
- Accounting for the long development time, effective patent protection for marketing a new drug is only about a decade (see Intellectual Property and Patents), requiring every company to completely reinvent itself on roughly a 10-year cycle.
- Regulation is stringent.
- Product liability is great.
- Competition is fierce.
- With mergers and acquisitions, the number of companies in the pharmaceutical world is shrinking.

Many feel that drug prices should be driven more by their therapeutic impact and their medical need, rather than by simpler free-market considerations; there is movement in this direction. Difficulties involve estimation or measurement of value, and there are many elements in this equation (Schnipper et al., 2015). There is no well-accepted approach to answer the question of value.

Who Pays?

The cost of prescription drugs is borne by consumers ("out of pocket"), private insurers, and public insurance programs such as Medicare, Medicaid, and the SCHIP. Recent initiatives by major retailers and mail-order pharmacies run by private insurers to offer consumer incentives for purchase of generic drugs have helped to contain the portion of household expenses spent on pharmaceuticals; however, more than one-third of total retail drug costs in the U.S. are paid with public funds—tax dollars.

Healthcare in the U.S. is more expensive than everywhere else, but it is not, on average, demonstrably better than everywhere else. One way in which the U.S. system falls short is with regard to healthcare access. Although the Patient Protection and Affordable Care Act of 2010 has reduced the percentage of Americans without health insurance to a historic low, practical solutions to the challenge of providing healthcare for all who need it must recognize the importance of incentivizing innovation.

Intellectual Property and Patents

Drug invention produces intellectual property eligible for patent protection, protection that is enormously important for innovation. As noted in 1859 by Abraham Lincoln, the only U.S. president to ever hold a patent (for a device to lift boats over shoals), by giving the inventor exclusive use of his or her invention for a limited time, the patent system "added the fuel of interest to the fire of genius in the discovery and production of useful things (Lincoln, 1859)." The U.S. patent protection system provides protection for 20 years from the time the patent is filed. During this period, the patent owner has exclusive rights to market and sell the drug. When the patent expires, equivalent nonproprietary products can come on the market; a generic product must be therapeutically equivalent to the original, contain equal amounts of the same active chemical ingredient, and achieve equal concentrations in blood when administered by the same routes. These generic preparations are sold much more cheaply than the original drug and without the huge development costs borne by the original patent holder.

The long time course of drug development, usually more than 10 years (see Figure 1–1), reduces the time during which patent protection functions as intended. The Drug Price Competition and Patent Term Restoration Act of 1984 (Public Law 98-417, informally called the Hatch-Waxman Act) permits a patent holder to apply for extension of a patent term to compensate for delays in marketing caused by FDA approval processes;

nonetheless, the average new drug brought to market now enjoys only about 10–12 years of patent protection. Some argue that patent protection for drugs should be shortened, so that earlier generic competition will lower healthcare costs. The counterargument is that new drugs would have to bear even higher prices to provide adequate compensation to companies during a shorter period of protected time. If that is true, lengthening patent protection would actually permit lower prices. Recall that patent protection is worth little if a superior competitive product is invented and brought to market.

Bayh-Dole Act

The Bayh-Dole Act (35 U.S.C. § 200) of 1980 created strong incentives for federally funded scientists at academic medical centers to approach drug invention with an entrepreneurial spirit. The act transferred intellectual property rights to the researchers and their respective institutions (rather than to the government) to encourage partnerships with industry that would bring new products to market for the public's benefit. While the need to protect intellectual property is generally accepted, this encouragement of public-private research collaborations has given rise to concerns about conflicts of interest by scientists and universities (Kaiser, 2009).

Biosimilars

As noted previously, the path to approval of a chemically synthesized small molecule that is identical to an approved compound whose patent protection has expired is relatively straightforward. The same is not true for large molecules (usually proteins), which are generally derived from a living organism (e.g., eukaryotic cell or bacterial culture). Covalent modification of proteins (e.g., glycosylation) or conformational differences may influence pharmacokinetics, pharmacodynamics, immunogenicity, or other properties, and demonstration of therapeutic equivalence may be a complex process.

The Biologics Price Competition and Innovation Act was enacted as part of the Patient Protection and Affordable Care Act in 2010. The intent was to implement an abbreviated licensure pathway for certain "similar" biological products. *Biosimilarity* is defined to mean "that the biological product is highly similar to a reference product notwithstanding minor differences in clinically inactive components" and that "there are no clinically meaningful differences between the biological product and the reference product in terms of the safety, purity, and potency of the product." In general, an application for licensure of a biosimilar must provide satisfactory data from analytical studies, animal studies, and a clinical study or studies. The interpretation of this language has involved seemingly endless discussion, and hard-and-fast rules seem unlikely.

Drug Promotion

In an ideal world, physicians would learn all they need to know about drugs from the medical literature, and good drugs would thereby sell themselves. Instead, we have print advertising and visits from salespeople directed at physicians and extensive direct-to-consumer advertising aimed at the public (in print, on the radio, and especially on television). There are roughly 80,000 pharmaceutical sales representatives in the U.S. who target about 10 times that number of physicians. This figure is down from about 100,000 in 2010, and the decline is likely related to increased attention to real and actual conflicting interests caused by their practices. It has been noted that college cheerleading squads are attractive sources for recruitment of this sales force. The amount spent on promotion of drugs approximates or perhaps even exceeds that spent on research and development. Pharmaceutical companies have been especially vulnerable to criticism for some of their marketing practices.

Promotional materials used by pharmaceutical companies cannot deviate from information contained in the package insert. In addition, there must be an acceptable balance between presentation of therapeutic claims for a product and discussion of unwanted effects. Nevertheless, direct-to-consumer advertising of prescription drugs remains controversial and is permitted only in the U.S. and New Zealand. Canada allows a modified form of advertising in which either the product or the indication can be mentioned, but not both. Physicians frequently succumb with misgivings to patients' advertising-driven requests for specific medications.

The counterargument is that patients are educated by such marketing efforts and in many cases will then seek medical care, especially for conditions (e.g., depression) that they may have been denying (Avery et al., 2012).

The major criticism of drug marketing involves some of the unsavory approaches used to influence physician behavior. Gifts of value (e.g., sports tickets) are now forbidden, but dinners where drug-prescribing information is presented by non-sales representatives are widespread. Large numbers of physicians are paid as "consultants" to make presentations in such settings. The acceptance of any gift, no matter how small, from a drug company by a physician is now forbidden at many academic medical centers and by law in several states. In 2009, the board of directors of PhRMA adopted an enhanced Code on Interactions With Healthcare Professionals that prohibits the distribution of noneducational items, prohibits company sales representatives from providing restaurant meals to healthcare professionals (although exceptions are granted when a third-party speaker makes the presentation), and requires companies to ensure that their representatives are trained about laws and regulations that govern interactions with healthcare professionals.

Concerns About Global Injustice

Because development of new drugs is so expensive, private-sector investment in pharmaceutical innovation has focused on products that will have lucrative markets in wealthy countries such as the U.S., which combines patent protection with a free-market economy. Accordingly, there is concern about the degree to which U.S. and European patent protection laws have restricted access to potentially lifesaving drugs in developing countries.

To lower costs, pharmaceutical companies increasingly test their experimental drugs outside the U.S. and the E.U., in developing countries where there is less regulation and easier access to large numbers of patients. According to the U.S. DHHS, there has been a 2000% increase in foreign trials of U.S. drugs over the past 25 years. When these drugs are successful in obtaining marketing approval, consumers in the countries where the trials were conducted often cannot afford them. Some ethicists have argued that this practice violates the justice principle articulated in the Belmont Report (DHHS, 1979, p10), which states that "research should not unduly involve persons from groups unlikely to be among the beneficiaries of subsequent applications of the research." A counterargument is that the conduct of trials in developing nations also frequently brings needed medical attention to underserved populations. This is another controversial issue.

Product Liability

Product liability laws are intended to protect consumers from defective products. Pharmaceutical companies can be sued for faulty design or manufacturing, deceptive promotional practices, violation of regulatory requirements, or failure to warn consumers of known risks. So-called failure-to-warn claims can be made against drug makers even when the product is approved by the FDA. With greater frequency, courts are finding companies that market prescription drugs directly to consumers responsible when these advertisements fail to provide an adequate warning of potential adverse effects.

Although injured patients are entitled to pursue legal remedies, the negative effects of product liability lawsuits against pharmaceutical companies may be considerable. First, fear of liability may cause pharmaceutical companies to be overly cautious about testing, thereby delaying access to the drug. Second, the cost of drugs increases for consumers when pharmaceutical companies increase the length and number of trials they perform to identify even the smallest risks and when regulatory agencies increase the number or intensity of regulatory reviews. Third, excessive liability costs create disincentives for development of so-called orphan drugs, pharmaceuticals that benefit a small number of patients. Should pharmaceutical companies be liable for failure to warn when all of the rules were followed and the product was approved by the FDA but the unwanted effect was not detected because of its rarity or another confounding factor? The only way to find "all" of the unwanted effects that a drug may have is to market

it—to conduct a phase IV "clinical trial" or observational study. This basic friction between risk to patients and the financial risk of drug development does not seem likely to be resolved except on a case-by-case basis, in the courts.

The U.S. Supreme Court added further fuel to these fiery issues in 2009 in the case *Wyeth v. Levine*. A patient (Levine) suffered gangrene of an arm following inadvertent arterial administration of the antinausea drug promethazine. She subsequently lost her hand. The healthcare provider had intended to administer the drug by so-called intravenous push. The FDA-approved label for the drug *warned against*, but did not prohibit, administration by intravenous push. The state court and then the U.S. Supreme Court held both the healthcare provider *and the company* liable for damages. Specifically, the Vermont court found that Wyeth had inadequately labeled the drug. This means that FDA approval of the label does not protect a company from liability or prevent individual states from imposing regulations more stringent than those required by the federal government.

"Me Too" Versus True Innovation: The Pace of New Drug Development

Me-too drug is a term used to describe a pharmaceutical that is usually structurally similar to a drug already on the market. Other names used are *derivative medications*, *molecular modifications*, and *follow-up drugs*. In some cases, a me-too drug is a different molecule developed deliberately by a competitor company to take market share from the company with existing drugs on the market. When the market for a class of drugs is especially large, several companies can share the market and make a profit. Other me-too drugs result coincidentally from numerous companies developing products simultaneously without knowing which drugs will be approved for sale (Box 1–4).

There are valid criticisms of me-too drugs. First, an excessive emphasis on profit may stifle true innovation. Of the 487 drugs approved by the FDA between 1998 and 2003, only 67 (14%) were considered by the FDA to be NMEs. Between 1998 and 2011, on average only 24 NMEs were approved by the FDA's CDER. Second, some me-too drugs are more expensive than the older versions they seek to replace, increasing the costs of healthcare without corresponding benefit to patients. Nevertheless, for some patients, me-too drugs may have better efficacy or fewer side effects or promote compliance with the treatment regimen. For example, the me-too that can be taken once a day rather than more frequently is convenient and promotes compliance. Some me-too drugs add great value from a business and medical point of view. Atorvastatin was the seventh statin to be introduced to market; it subsequently became the best-selling drug in the world.

Critics argue that pharmaceutical companies are not innovative and do not take risks, and, further, that medical progress is actually slowed by their excessive concentration on me-too products. Figure 1–2 summarizes a few of the facts behind this and other arguments. Clearly, only a modest number of NMEs, about two dozen a year, achieved FDA approval in the years 1980 to 2011, with the exception of the several-year spike in approvals following the introduction of PDUFA. Yet, from 1980 to 2010, the industry's annual investment in research and development grew from

BOX 1–4 ■ A Not-So-New Drug

Some me-too drugs are only slightly altered formulations of a company's own drug, packaged and promoted as if really offering something new. An example is the heartburn medication esomeprazole, marketed by the same company that makes omeprazole. Omeprazole is a mixture of two stereoisomers; esomeprazole contains only one of the isomers and is eliminated less rapidly. Development of esomeprazole created a new period of market exclusivity, although generic versions of omeprazole are marketed, as are branded congeners of omeprazole/esomeprazole. Both omeprazole and esomeprazole are now available over the counter—narrowing the previous price difference.

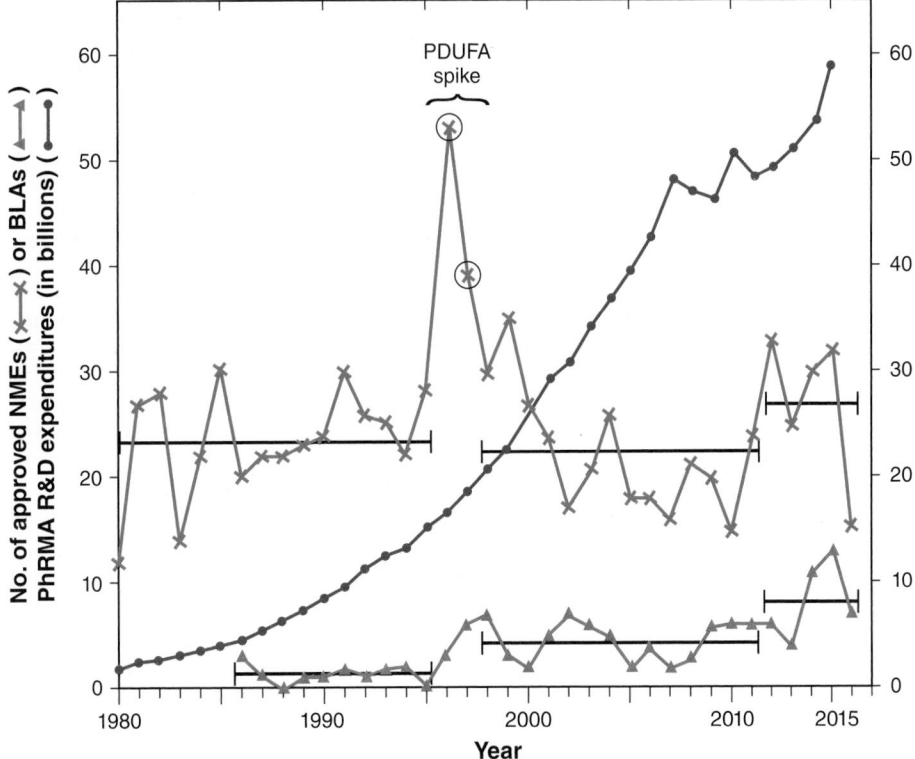

Figure 1–2 *The cost of drug invention is rising. Is productivity?* Each horizontal black line shows the average annual number of NMEs or BLAs for the time period bracketed by the line's length.

$2 billion to $50 billion. This disconnect between research and development investment and new drugs approved occurred at a time when combinatorial chemistry was blooming, the human genome was being sequenced, highly automated techniques of screening were being developed, and new techniques of molecular biology and genetics were offering novel insights into the pathophysiology of human disease.

In recent years, there has been a modest increase in approval of NMEs (inhibitors of a number of protein kinases) and new biologics (numerous therapeutic antibodies) (see Figure 1–2). A continued increase in productivity will be needed to sustain today's pharmaceutical companies as they face waves of patent expirations. There are strong arguments that development of much more targeted, individualized drugs, based on a new generation of molecular diagnostic techniques and improved understanding of disease in individual patients, will improve both medical care and the survival of pharmaceutical companies.

Finally, many of the advances in genetics and molecular biology are still new, particularly when measured in the time frame required for drug development. One can hope that modern molecular medicine will sustain the development of more efficacious and more specific pharmacological treatments for an ever-wider spectrum of human diseases.

Bibliography

Aagard L, Hansen EH. Information about ADRs explored by pharmacovigilance approaches: a qualitative review of studies on antibiotics, SSRIs and NSAIDs. *BMC Clin Pharmacol*, **2009**, 9:4.

Avery RJ, et al. The impact of direct-to-consumer television and magazine advertising on antidepressant use. *J Health Econ*, **2012**, *31*:705–718.

CDC. Health expenditures. **2013**. Available at: http://www.cdc.gov/nchs/fastats/health-expenditures.htm. Accessed July 8, 2015.

Cutler DM. The demise of a blockbuster? *N Engl J Med*, **2007**, *356*:1292–1293.

DHHS. The Belmont Report. Ethical Principles and Guidelines for the Protection of Human Subjects of Research. The National Commission for the Protection of Human Subjects of Biomedical and Behavioral Research, **1979**.

FDA. An evaluation of the PDUFA Workload Adjuster: Fiscal Years 2009–2013. **2013a**. Available at: http://www.fda.gov/downloads/

ForIndustry/UserFees/PrescriptionDrugUserFee/UCM350567.pdf. Accessed June 19, 2015.

FDA. MedWatch: Improving on 20 Years of Excellence. *FDA Voice*. **2013b**. Available at: http://blogs.fda.gov/fdavoice/index.php/2013/06/medwatch-improving-on-20-years-of-excellence/. Accessed May 11, 2017.

FDA. What we do. **2014**. Available at: http://www.fda.gov/AboutFDA/WhatWeDo/. Accessed June 19, 2015.

Horton JD, et al. PCSK9: a convertase that coordinates LDL catabolism. *Lipid Res*, **2009**, *50*:S172–S177.

Jarcho JA, Keaney JF Jr. Proof that lower is better—LDL cholesterol and IMPROVE-IT. *N Engl J Med*, **2015**, *372*:2448–2450.

Kaiser J. Private money, public disclosure. *Science*, **2009**, *325*:28–30.

Kassirer JP. *On the Take. How Medicine's Complicity With Big Business Can Endanger Your Health*. Oxford University Press, New York, **2005**.

Kastelein JJ, et al. Simvastatin with or without ezetimibe in familial hypercholesterolemia. *N Engl J Med*, **2008**, *358*:1421–1443.

Lincoln A. Second speech on discoveries and inventions. **1859**. Available at: http://quod.lib.umich.edu/l/lincoln/lincoln3/1:87?rgn=div1;view=fulltext. Accessed May 8, 2017.

NIH. Ethics in clinical research. **2011**. Available at: http://clinicalcenter.nih.gov/recruit/ethics.html. Accessed July 8, 2015.

Poirier S, Mayer G. The biology of PCSK9 from the endoplasmic reticulum to lysosomes: new and emerging therapeutics to control low-density lipoprotein cholesterol. *Drug Design Dev Ther*, **2013**, *7*:1135.

Schnipper LE, et al. American Society of Clinical Oncology Statement: a conceptual framework to assess the value of cancer treatment options. *J Clin Oncol*, **2015**, *33*:2563–2577.

World Medical Association. World Medical Association Declaration of Helsinki: ethical principles for medical research involving human subjects. *JAMA*, **2013**, *310*:2191–2194.

Xie L, et al. Drug discovery using chemical systems biology: identification of the protein-ligand binding network to explain the side effects of CETP inhibitors. *PLoS Comput Biol*, **2009**, *5*:e1000387.

Xie L, et al. In silico elucidation of the molecular mechanism defining the adverse effect of selective estrogen receptor modulators. *PLoS Comput Biol*, **2007**, *3*:e217.

Chapter 2

Pharmacokinetics: The Dynamics of Drug Absorption, Distribution, Metabolism, and Elimination

Iain L. O. Buxton

The human body restricts access to foreign molecules; therefore, to reach its target within the body and have a therapeutic effect, a drug molecule must cross a number of restrictive barriers en route to its target site. Following administration, the drug must be absorbed and then distributed, usually via vessels of the circulatory and lymphatic systems; in addition to crossing membrane barriers, the drug must survive metabolism (primarily hepatic) and elimination (by the kidney and liver and in the feces). ADME, the absorption, distribution, metabolism, and elimination of drugs, are the processes of *pharmacokinetics* (Figure 2–1). Understanding these processes and their interplay and employing pharmacokinetic principles increase the probability of therapeutic success and reduce the occurrence of adverse drug events.

The absorption, distribution, metabolism, and excretion of a drug involve its passage across numerous cell membranes. Mechanisms by which drugs cross membranes and the physicochemical properties of molecules and membranes that influence this transfer are critical to understanding the disposition of drugs in the human body. The characteristics of a drug that predict its movement and availability at sites of action are its molecular size and structural features, degree of ionization, relative lipid solubility of its ionized and nonionized forms, and its binding to serum and tissue proteins. Although physical barriers to drug movement may be a single layer of cells (e.g., intestinal epithelium) or several layers of cells and associated extracellular protein (e.g., skin), the plasma membrane is the basic barrier.

Passage of Drugs Across Membrane Barriers

The Plasma Membrane Is Selectively Permeable

The plasma membrane consists of a bilayer of amphipathic lipids with their hydrocarbon chains oriented inward to the center of the bilayer to form a continuous hydrophobic phase, with their hydrophilic heads oriented outward. Individual lipid molecules in the bilayer vary according to the particular membrane and can move laterally and organize themselves into microdomains (e.g., regions with sphingolipids and cholesterol, forming lipid rafts), endowing the membrane with fluidity, flexibility, organization, high electrical resistance, and relative impermeability to highly polar molecules. Membrane proteins embedded in the bilayer serve as structural anchors, receptors, ion channels, or transporters to transduce electrical or chemical signaling pathways and provide selective targets for drug actions. Far from being a sea of lipids with proteins floating randomly about, membranes are ordered and compartmented (Suetsugu et al., 2014), with structural scaffolding elements linking to the cell interior. Membrane proteins may be associated with caveolin and sequestered within caveolae, be excluded from caveolae, or be organized in signaling domains rich in cholesterol and sphingolipid not containing caveolin or other scaffolding proteins.

Modes of Permeation and Transport

Passive diffusion dominates transmembrane movement of most drugs. However, carrier-mediated mechanisms (*active transport* and *facilitated diffusion*) play important roles (Figure 2–2; Figure 5–4).

Passive Diffusion

In passive transport, the drug molecule usually penetrates by diffusion along a concentration gradient by virtue of its solubility in the lipid bilayer. Such transfer is directly proportional to the magnitude of the concentration gradient across the membrane, to the lipid:water partition coefficient of the drug, and to the membrane surface area exposed to the drug. At steady state, the concentration of the unbound drug is the same on both sides of the membrane if the drug is a nonelectrolyte. For ionic compounds, the steady-state concentrations depend on the electrochemical gradient for the ion and on differences in pH across the membrane, which will influence the state of ionization of the molecule disparately on either

Abbreviations

ABC: ATP-binding cassette
ACE: angiotensin-converting enzyme
AUC: area under the concentration-time curve of drug absorption and elimination
BBB: blood-brain barrier
CL: clearance
CNS: central nervous system
CNT1: concentrative nucleoside transporter 1
C_p: plasma concentration
CSF: cerebrospinal fluid
C_{ss}: steady-state concentration
CYP: cytochrome P450
F: bioavailability
GI: gastrointestinal
h: hours
k: a rate constant
MDR1: multidrug resistance protein
MEC: minimum effective concentration
min: minutes
SLC: solute carrier
T, t: time
$t_{1/2}$: half-life
V: volume of distribution
V_{ss}: volume of distribution at steady state

ionized form. The ratio of nonionized to ionized drug at any pH may be calculated from the Henderson-Hasselbalch equation:

$$\log \frac{[\text{protonated form}]}{[\text{unprotonated form}]} = pK_a - pH \qquad (\text{Equation 2-1})$$

Equation 2–1 relates the pH of the medium around the drug and the drug's acid dissociation constant (pK_a) to the ratio of the protonated (HA or BH$^+$) and unprotonated (A$^-$ or B) forms, where

$$HA \leftrightarrow A^- + H^+, \text{ where } K_a = \frac{[A^-][H^+]}{[HA]}$$

describes the dissociation of an acid, and

$$BH^+ \leftrightarrow B + H^+, \text{ where } K_a = \frac{[B][H^+]}{[BH^+]}$$

describes the dissociation of the protonated form of a base.

At steady state, an acidic drug will accumulate on the more basic side of the membrane and a basic drug on the more acidic side. This phenomenon, known as *ion trapping*, is an important process in drug distribution with potential therapeutic benefit (Perletti et al., 2009). Figure 2–3 illustrates this effect and shows the calculated values for the distribution of a weak acid between the plasma and gastric compartments.

One can take advantage of the effect of pH on transmembrane partitioning to alter drug excretion. In the kidney tubules, urine pH can vary over a wide range, from 4.5 to 8. As urine pH drops (as [H$^+$] increases), weak acids (A$^-$) and weak bases (B) will exist to a greater extent in their protonated forms (HA and BH$^+$); the reverse is true as pH rises, where A$^-$ and B will be favored. Thus, alkaline urine favors excretion of weak acids; acid urine favors excretion of weak bases. Elevation of urine pH (by giving sodium bicarbonate) will promote urinary excretion of weak acids such as aspirin ($pK_a \sim 3.5$) and urate ($pK_a \sim 5.8$). Another useful consequence of a drug's being ionized at physiological pH is illustrated by the relative lack of sedative effects of second-generation histamine H$_1$ antagonists (e.g., loratadine): Second-generation antihistamines are ionized molecules (less lipophilic, more hydrophilic) that cross the BBB poorly compared to first-generation agents such as diphenhydramine, which are now used as sleep aids.

side of the membrane and can effectively trap ionized drug on one side of the membrane.

Influence of pH on Ionizable Drugs

Many drugs are weak acids or bases that are present in solution as both the lipid-soluble, diffusible nonionized form and the ionized species that is relatively lipid insoluble and poorly diffusible across a membrane. Among the common ionizable groups are carboxylic acids and amino groups (primary, secondary, and tertiary; quaternary amines hold a permanent positive charge). The transmembrane distribution of a weak electrolyte is influenced by its pK_a and the pH gradient across the membrane. The pK_a is the pH at which half the drug (weak acid or base electrolyte) is in its

Carrier-Mediated Membrane Transport

Proteins in the plasma membrane mediate transmembrane movements of many physiological solutes; these proteins also mediate transmembrane movements of drugs and can be targets of drug action. Mediated transport

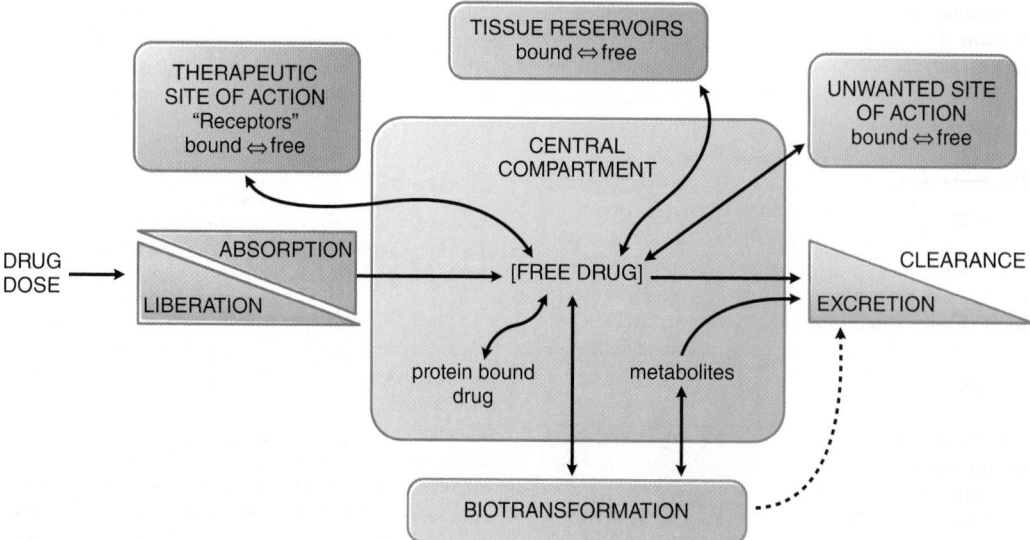

Figure 2–1 *The interrelationship of the absorption, distribution, binding, metabolism, and excretion of a drug and its concentration at its sites of action.* Possible distribution and binding of metabolites in relation to their potential actions at receptors are not depicted.

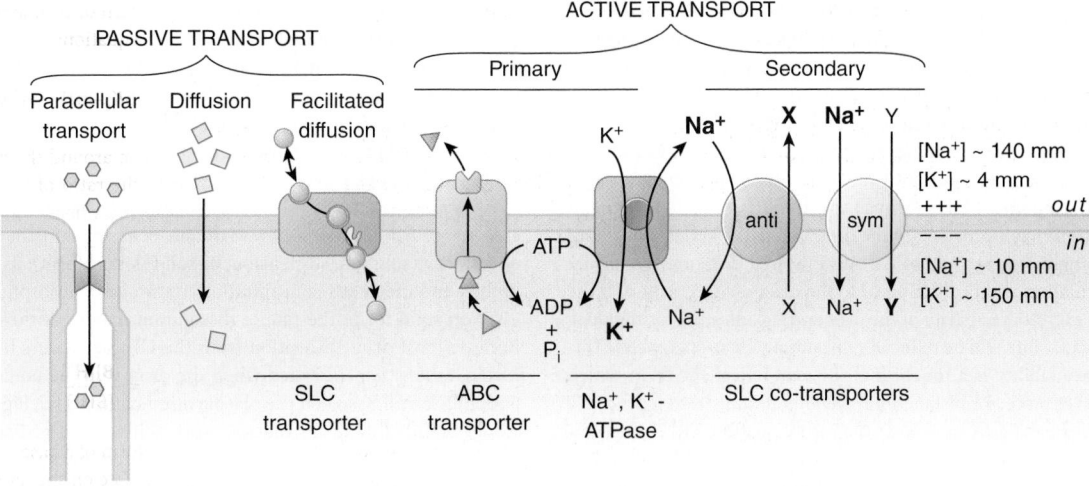

Figure 2–2 *Drugs move across membrane and cellular barriers in a variety of ways.* See details in Figures 5–1 through 5–5.

is broadly characterized as *facilitated diffusion* or *active transport* (see Figure 2–2; Figure 5–4). Membrane transporters and their roles in drug response are presented in detail in Chapter 5.

Facilitated Diffusion. *Facilitated diffusion* is a carrier-mediated transport process in which the driving force is simply the electrochemical gradient of the transported solute; thus, these carriers can facilitate solute movement either in or out of cells, depending on the direction of the electrochemical gradient. The carrier protein may be highly selective for a specific conformational structure of an endogenous solute or a drug whose rate of transport by passive diffusion through the membrane would otherwise be quite slow. For instance, the organic cation transporter OCT1 (SLC22A1) facilitates the movement of a physiologic solute, thiamine, and also of drugs, including metformin, which is used in treating type 2 diabetes. Chapter 5 describes OCT1 and other members of the human SLC superfamily of transporters.

Active Transport. *Active transport* is characterized by a direct requirement for energy, capacity to move solute against an electrochemical gradient, saturability, selectivity, and competitive inhibition by cotransported compounds. Na⁺,K⁺-ATPase is an important example of an active transport mechanism that is also a therapeutic target of digoxin in the treatment of heart failure (Chapter 29). A group of primary active transporters, the ABC family, hydrolyze ATP to export substrates across membranes. For example, the P-glycoprotein, also called ABCB1 and MDR1, exports bulky neutral or cationic compounds from cells; its physiologic substrates include steroid hormones such as testosterone and progesterone. MDR1 exports many drugs as well, including digoxin, and a great variety of other agents (see Table 5–4). P-glycoprotein in the enterocyte

limits the absorption of some orally administered drugs by exporting compounds into the lumen of the GI tract subsequent to their absorption. ABC transporters perform a similar function in the cells of the BBB, effectively reducing net accumulation of some compounds in the brain. By the same mechanism, P-glycoprotein also can confer resistance to some cancer chemotherapeutic agents (see Chapters 65–68).

Members of the SLC superfamily can mediate secondary active transport using the electrochemical energy stored in a gradient (usually Na⁺) to translocate both biological solutes and drugs across membranes. For instance, the Na⁺–Ca²⁺ exchange protein (SLC8) uses the energy stored in the Na⁺ gradient established by Na⁺,K⁺-ATPase to export cytosolic Ca²⁺ and maintain it at a low basal level, about 100 nM in most cells. SLC8 is thus an *antiporter*, using the inward flow of Na⁺ to drive an outward flow of Ca²⁺; SLC8 also helps to mediate the positive inotropic effects of digoxin and other cardiac glycosides that inhibit the activity of Na⁺,K⁺-ATPase and thereby reduce the driving force for the extrusion of Ca²⁺ from the ventricular cardiac myocyte. Other SLC cotransporters are *symporters*, in which driving force ion and solute move in the same direction. The CNT1 (SLC28A1), driven by the Na⁺ gradient, moves pyrimidine nucleosides and the cancer chemotherapeutic agents gemcitabine and cytarabine into cells. DAT, NET, and SERT, transporters for the neurotransmitters dopamine, norepinephrine, and serotonin, respectively, are secondary active transporters that also rely on the energy stored in the transmembrane Na⁺ gradient, symporters that coordinate movement of Na⁺ and neurotransmitter in the same direction (into the neuron); they are also the targets of CNS-active agents used in therapy of depression. Members of the SLC superfamily are active in drug transport in the GI tract, liver, and kidney, among other sites.

Paracellular Transport

In the vascular compartment, paracellular passage of solutes and fluid through intercellular gaps is sufficiently large that passive transfer across the endothelium of capillaries and postcapillary venules is generally limited by blood flow. Capillaries of the CNS and a variety of epithelial tissues have tight junctions that limit paracellular movement of drugs (Spector et al., 2015).

Drug Absorption, Bioavailability, and Routes of Administration

Absorption and Bioavailability

Absorption is the movement of a drug from its site of administration into the central compartment (see Figure 2–1). For solid dosage forms, absorption first requires dissolution of the tablet or capsule, thus liberating the drug. Except in cases of malabsorption syndromes, the clinician is concerned primarily with bioavailability rather than absorption (Tran et al., 2013).

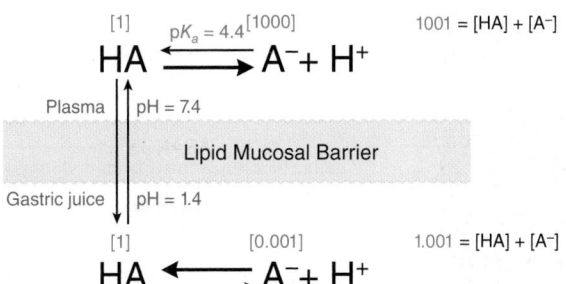

Figure 2–3 *Influence of pH on the distribution of a weak acid (pK$_a$ = 4.4) between plasma and gastric juice separated by a lipid barrier.* **A weak acid dissociates to different extents** in plasma (pH 7.4) and gastric acid (pH 1.4): The higher pH facilitates dissociation; the lower pH reduces dissociation. The uncharged form, HA, equilibrates across the membrane. Blue numbers in brackets show relative equilibrium concentrations of HA and A⁻, as calculated from Equation 2–1.

Bioavailability describes the fractional extent to which an administered dose of drug reaches its site of action or a biological fluid (usually the systemic circulation) from which the drug has access to its site of action. A drug given orally must be absorbed first from the GI tract, but net absorption may be limited by the characteristics of the dosage form, by the drug's physicochemical properties, by metabolic attack in the intestine, and by transport across the intestinal epithelium and into the portal circulation. The absorbed drug then passes through the liver, where metabolism and biliary excretion may occur before the drug enters the systemic circulation. Accordingly, less than all of the administered dose may reach the systemic circulation and be distributed to the drug's sites of action. If the metabolic or excretory capacity of the liver and the intestine for the drug is large, bioavailability will be reduced substantially (*first-pass effect*). This decrease in availability is a function of the anatomical site from which absorption takes place; for instance, intravenous administration generally permits all of the drug to enter the systemic circulation. Other anatomical, physiological, and pathological factors can influence bioavailability (described further in this chapter), and the choice of the route of drug administration must be based on an understanding of these conditions. We can define bioavailability F as:

$$F = \frac{\text{Quantity of drug reaching systemic circulation}}{\text{Quantity of drug administered}} \quad \text{(Equation 2–2)}$$

where $0 < F \leq 1$.

Factors modifying bioavailability apply as well to prodrugs that are activated by the liver, in which case availability results from metabolism that produces the form of the active drug.

Routes of Administration

Some characteristics of the major routes employed for systemic drug effect are compared in Table 2–1.

Oral Administration

Oral ingestion is the most common method of drug administration. It also is the safest, most convenient, and most economical. Its disadvantages include limited absorption of some drugs because of their physical characteristics (e.g., low water solubility or poor membrane permeability), emesis as a result of irritation to the GI mucosa, destruction of some drugs by digestive enzymes or low gastric pH, irregularities in absorption or propulsion in the presence of food or other drugs, and the need for cooperation on the part of the patient. In addition, drugs in the GI tract may be metabolized by the enzymes of the intestinal microbiome, mucosa, or liver before they gain access to the general circulation.

Absorption from the GI tract is governed by factors such as surface area for absorption; blood flow to the site of absorption; the physical state of the drug (solution, suspension, or solid dosage form); its aqueous solubility; and the drug's concentration at the site of absorption. For drugs given in solid form, the rate of dissolution may limit their absorption. Because most drug absorption from the GI tract occurs by passive diffusion, absorption is favored when the drug is in the nonionized, more lipophilic form. Based on the pH-partition concept (see Figure 2–3), one would predict that drugs that are weak acids would be better absorbed from the stomach (pH 1–2) than from the upper intestine (pH 3–6), and vice versa for weak bases. However, the surface area of the stomach is relatively small, and a mucus layer covers the gastric epithelium. By contrast, the villi of the upper intestine provide an extremely large surface area (~200 m²). Accordingly, the rate of absorption of a drug from the intestine will be greater than that from the stomach even if the drug is predominantly ionized in the intestine and largely nonionized in the stomach. Thus, any factor that accelerates gastric emptying (recumbent position right side) will generally increase the rate of drug absorption, whereas any factor that delays gastric emptying will have the opposite effect. The gastric emptying rate is influenced by numerous factors, including the caloric content of food; volume, osmolality, temperature, and pH of ingested fluid; diurnal and interindividual variation; metabolic state (rest or exercise); and the ambient temperature. Gastric emptying is influenced in women by the effects of estrogen (i.e., compared to men, emptying is slower for premenopausal women and those taking estrogen replacement therapy).

Drugs that are destroyed by gastric secretions and low pH or that cause gastric irritation sometimes are administered in dosage forms with an enteric coating that prevents dissolution in the acidic gastric contents. Enteric coatings are useful for drugs that can cause gastric irritation and for presenting a drug such as mesalamine to sites of action in the ileum and colon (see Figure 51–4).

TABLE 2–1 ■ SOME CHARACTERISTICS OF COMMON ROUTES OF DRUG ADMINISTRATION[a]

ROUTE AND BIOAVAILABILTY (F)	ABSORPTION PATTERN	SPECIAL UTILITY	LIMITATIONS AND PRECAUTIONS
Intravenous $F = 1$ by definition	Absorption circumvented	Valuable for emergency use	Increased risk of adverse effects
	Potentially immediate effects	Permits titration of dosage	Must inject solutions *slowly* as a rule
	Suitable for large volumes and for irritating substances, or complex mixtures, when diluted	Usually required for high-molecular-weight protein and peptide drugs	Not suitable for oily solutions or poorly soluble substances
Subcutaneous $0.75 < F < 1$	Prompt from aqueous solution	Suitable for some poorly soluble suspensions and for instillation of slow-release implants	Not suitable for large volumes
	Slow and sustained from repository preparations		Possible pain or necrosis from irritating substances
Intramuscular $0.75 < F < 1$	Prompt from aqueous solution	Suitable for moderate volumes, oily vehicles, and some irritating substances	Precluded during anticoagulant therapy
	Slow and sustained from repository preparations	Appropriate for self-administration (e.g., insulin)	May interfere with interpretation of certain diagnostic tests (e.g., creatine kinase)
Oral ingestion $.05 < F < 1$	Variable, depends on many factors (see text)	Most convenient and economical; usually safer	Requires patient compliance
			Bioavailability potentially erratic and incomplete

[a]See text for more complete discussion and for other routes.

Controlled-Release Preparations. The rate of absorption of a drug administered as a tablet or other solid oral dosage form is partly dependent on its rate of dissolution in GI fluids. This is the basis for *controlled-release, extended-release, sustained-release,* and *prolonged-action* pharmaceutical preparations that are designed to produce slow, uniform absorption of the drug for 8 h or longer. Potential advantages of such preparations are reduction in the frequency of administration compared with conventional dosage forms (often with improved compliance by the patient), maintenance of a therapeutic effect overnight, and decreased incidence and intensity of undesired effects (by dampening of the peaks in drug concentration) and nontherapeutic blood levels of the drug (by elimination of troughs in concentration) that often occur after administration of immediate-release dosage forms. Controlled-release dosage forms are most appropriate for drugs with short half-lives ($t_{1/2} < 4$ h) or in select patient groups, such as those receiving antiepileptic or antipsychotic agents (Bera, 2014).

Sublingual Administration. Absorption from the oral mucosa has special significance for certain drugs despite the fact that the surface area available is small. Venous drainage from the mouth is to the superior vena cava, thus bypassing the portal circulation. As a consequence, a drug held sublingually and absorbed from that site is protected from rapid intestinal and hepatic first-pass metabolism. For example, sublingual nitroglycerin (see Chapter 27) is rapidly effective because it is nonionic, has high lipid solubility, and is not subject to the first-pass effect prior to reaching the heart and arterial system.

Parenteral Injection

Parenteral (i.e., not via the GI tract) injection of drugs has distinct advantages over oral administration. In some instances, parenteral administration is essential for delivery of a drug in its active form, as in the case of monoclonal antibodies. Availability usually is more rapid, extensive, and predictable when a drug is given by injection; the effective dose can be delivered more accurately to a precise dose; this route is suitable for the loading dose of medications prior to initiation of oral maintenance dosing (e.g., digoxin). In emergency therapy and when a patient is unconscious, uncooperative, or unable to retain anything given by mouth, parenteral therapy may be necessary. Parenteral administration also has disadvantages: Asepsis must be maintained, especially when drugs are given over time (e.g., intravenous or intrathecal administration); pain may accompany the injection; and it is sometimes difficult for patients to perform the injections themselves if self-medication is necessary.

The major routes of parenteral administration are intravenous, subcutaneous, and intramuscular. Absorption from subcutaneous and intramuscular sites occurs by simple diffusion along the gradient from drug depot to plasma. The rate is limited by the area of the absorbing capillary membranes and by the solubility of the substance in the interstitial fluid. Relatively large aqueous channels in the endothelial layer account for the indiscriminate diffusion of molecules regardless of their lipid solubility. Larger molecules, such as proteins, slowly gain access to the circulation by way of lymphatic channels. Drugs administered into the systemic circulation by any route, excluding the intra-arterial route, are subject to possible first-pass elimination in the lung prior to distribution to the rest of the body. The lungs also serve as a filter for particulate matter that may be given intravenously and provide a route of elimination for volatile substances.

Intravenous. Factors limiting absorption are circumvented by intravenous injection of drugs in aqueous solution because bioavailability is complete ($F = 1.0$) and distribution is rapid. Also, drug delivery is controlled and achieved with an accuracy and immediacy not possible by any other procedures. Certain irritating solutions can be given only in this manner because the drug, when injected slowly, is greatly diluted by the blood.

There are advantages and disadvantages to intravenous administration. Unfavorable reactions can occur because high concentrations of drug may be attained rapidly in plasma and tissues. There are therapeutic circumstances for which it is advisable to administer a drug by bolus injection (e.g., tissue plasminogen activator) and other circumstances where slower or prolonged administration of drug is advisable (e.g., antibiotics).

Intravenous administration of drugs warrants careful determination of dose and close monitoring of the patient's response; once the drug is injected, there is often no retreat. Repeated intravenous injections depend on the ability to maintain a patent vein. Drugs in an oily vehicle, those that precipitate blood constituents or hemolyze erythrocytes, and drug combinations that cause precipitates to form *must not* be given intravenously.

Subcutaneous. Injection into a subcutaneous site can be done only with drugs that are not irritating to tissue; otherwise, severe pain, necrosis, and tissue sloughing may occur. The rate of absorption following subcutaneous injection of a drug often is sufficiently constant and slow to provide a sustained effect. Moreover, altering the period over which a drug is absorbed may be varied intentionally, as is accomplished with insulin for injection using particle size, protein complexation, and pH. The incorporation of a vasoconstrictor agent in a solution of a drug to be injected subcutaneously also retards absorption. Absorption of drugs implanted under the skin in a solid pellet form occurs slowly over a period of weeks or months; some hormones (e.g., contraceptives) are administered effectively in this manner.

Intramuscular. Absorption of drugs in aqueous solution after intramuscular injection depends on the rate of blood flow to the injection site and can be relatively rapid. Absorption may be modulated to some extent by local heating, massage, or exercise. Generally, the rate of absorption following injection of an aqueous preparation into the deltoid or vastus lateralis is faster than when the injection is made into the gluteus maximus. The rate is particularly slower for females after injection into the gluteus maximus, a feature attributed to the different distribution of subcutaneous fat in males and females and because fat is relatively poorly perfused. Slow, constant absorption from the intramuscular site results if the drug is injected in solution in oil or suspended in various other repository (depot) vehicles.

Intra-arterial. Occasionally, a drug is injected directly into an artery to localize its effect in a particular tissue or organ, such as in the treatment of liver tumors and head and neck cancers. Diagnostic agents sometimes are administered by this route (e.g., technetium-labeled human serum albumin). Inadvertent intra-arterial administration can cause serious complications and requires careful management (Sen et al., 2005).

Intrathecal. The BBB and the blood-CSF barrier often preclude or slow the entrance of drugs into the CNS, reflecting the activity of P-glycoprotein (MDR1) and other transporters to export xenobiotics from the CNS. Therefore, when local and rapid effects of drugs on the meninges or cerebrospinal axis are desired, as in spinal anesthesia, drugs sometimes are injected directly into the spinal subarachnoid space. Brain tumors (Calias et al., 2014) or serious CNS infections (Imberti et al., 2014) also may be treated by direct intraventricular drug administration, increasingly through the use of specialized long-term indwelling reservoir devices. Injections into the CSF and epidural space are covered in chapters on analgesia and local anesthesia (Chapters 20 and 22, respectively).

Pulmonary Absorption

Gaseous and volatile drugs may be inhaled and absorbed through the pulmonary epithelium and mucous membranes of the respiratory tract. Access to the circulation is rapid by this route because the lung's surface area is large. In addition, solutions of drugs can be atomized and the fine droplets in air (aerosol) inhaled. Advantages are the almost instantaneous absorption of a drug into the blood, avoidance of hepatic first-pass loss, and in the case of pulmonary disease, local application of the drug at the desired site of action (see Chapters 21 and 40), as in the use of inhaled nitric oxide for pulmonary hypertension in term and near-term infants and adults (see Chapter 31).

Topical Application

Mucous Membranes. Drugs are applied to the mucous membranes of the conjunctiva, nasopharynx, oropharynx, vagina, colon, urethra, and urinary bladder primarily for their local effects. Absorption from these sites is generally excellent and may provide advantages for immunotherapy because vaccination of mucosal surfaces using mucosal vaccines provides the basis for generating protective immunity in both the mucosal and systemic immune compartments.

Eye. Topically applied ophthalmic drugs are used primarily for their local effects (see Chapter 69). The use of drug-loaded contact lenses and ocular inserts allows drugs to be better placed where they are needed for direct delivery.

Skin: Transdermal Absorption. Absorption of drugs able to penetrate the intact skin is dependent on the surface area over which they are applied and their lipid solubility (see Chapter 70). Systemic absorption of drugs occurs much more readily through abraded, burned, or denuded skin. Toxic effects result from absorption through the skin of highly lipid-soluble substances (e.g., a lipid-soluble insecticide in an organic solvent). Absorption through the skin can be enhanced by suspending the drug in an oily vehicle and rubbing the resulting preparation into the skin. Hydration of the skin with an occlusive dressing may be used to facilitate absorption. Controlled-release topical patches are increasingly available, with nicotine for tobacco-smoking withdrawal, scopolamine for motion sickness, nitroglycerin for angina pectoris, testosterone and estrogen for replacement therapy, various estrogens and progestins for birth control, and fentanyl for pain relief.

Rectal Administration

Approximately 50% of the drug that is absorbed from the rectum will bypass the liver, thereby reducing hepatic first-pass metabolism. However, rectal absorption can be irregular and incomplete, and certain drugs can cause irritation of the rectal mucosa. Rectal administration may be desirable, as in the use of opioids in hospice care.

Novel Methods of Drug Delivery

Drug-eluting stents and other devices are being used to target drugs locally to maximize efficacy and minimize systemic exposure. Recent advances in drug delivery include the use of biocompatible polymers and nanoparticles for drug delivery (Yohan and Chithrani, 2014).

Bioequivalence

Drug products are considered to be pharmaceutical equivalents if they contain the same active ingredients and are identical in strength or concentration, dosage form, and route of administration. Two pharmaceutically equivalent drug products are considered to be *bioequivalent* when the rates and extents of bioavailability of the active ingredient in the two products are not significantly different under suitable and identical test conditions. Generic versus brand name prescribing is further discussed in connection with drug nomenclature and the choice of drug name in writing prescription orders (see Appendix I). Courts have not always found generic and brand name drugs to be legally equivalent (see Chapter 1).

Distribution of Drugs

Not All Tissues Are Equal

Following absorption or systemic administration into the bloodstream, a drug distributes into interstitial and intracellular fluids as functions of the physicochemical properties of the drug, the rate of drug delivery to individual organs and compartments, and the differing capacities of those regions to interact with the drug. Cardiac output, regional blood flow, capillary permeability, and tissue volume affect the rate of delivery and amount of drug distributed into tissues (Table 2–2 and Figure 2–4). Initially, liver, kidney, brain, and other well-perfused organs receive most of the drug; delivery to muscle, most viscera, skin, and fat is slower. This second distribution phase may require minutes to several hours before the concentration of drug in tissue is in equilibrium with that in blood. The second phase also involves a far larger fraction of body mass (e.g., muscle) than does the initial phase and generally accounts for most of the extravascular distribution. With exceptions such as the brain, diffusion of drug into the interstitial fluid occurs rapidly because of the highly permeable nature of the capillary endothelium. Thus, tissue distribution is determined by the partitioning of drug between blood and the particular tissue.

Binding to Plasma Proteins

Many drugs circulate in the bloodstream bound to plasma proteins. Albumin is a major carrier for acidic drugs; α_1-acid glycoprotein binds basic drugs. Nonspecific binding to other plasma proteins generally occurs to a much smaller extent. The binding is usually reversible. In addition, certain drugs may bind to proteins that function as specific hormone carrier proteins, such as the binding of estrogen or testosterone to sex hormone–binding globulin or the binding of thyroid hormone to thyroxin-binding globulin.

The fraction of total drug in plasma that is bound is determined by the drug concentration, the affinity of binding sites for the drug, and the concentration of available binding sites. For most drugs, the therapeutic range of plasma concentrations is limited; thus, the extent of binding and the unbound fraction are relatively constant. The extent of plasma protein binding also may be affected by disease-related factors (e.g., hypoalbuminemia). Conditions resulting in the acute-phase reaction response (e.g., cancer, arthritis, myocardial infarction, Crohn's disease) lead to elevated levels of α_1-acid glycoprotein and enhanced binding of basic drugs. Changes in protein binding caused by disease states and drug-drug interactions are clinically relevant mainly for a small subset of so-called high-clearance drugs of narrow therapeutic index that are administered intravenously, such as lidocaine. When changes in plasma protein binding occur in patients, unbound drug rapidly equilibrates throughout the body and only a transient significant change in unbound plasma concentration will occur. Only drugs that show an almost-instantaneous relationship between free plasma concentration and effect (e.g., antiarrhythmics) will show a measurable effect. Thus, unbound plasma drug concentrations will exhibit significant changes only when either drug input or clearance of unbound drug occurs as a consequence of metabolism or active transport. A more common problem resulting from competition of drugs for plasma protein-binding sites is misinterpretation of measured concentrations of drugs in plasma because most assays do not distinguish free drug from bound drug. Competition for plasma protein-binding sites may cause one drug to elevate the concentration of one bound less avidly.

Binding of a drug to plasma proteins limits its concentration in tissues and at its site of action because only unbound drug is in equilibrium across membranes. Accordingly, after distribution equilibrium is achieved, the concentration of unbound drug in intracellular water is the same as that in plasma except when carrier-mediated active transport is involved. Binding of a drug to plasma protein limits the drug's glomerular filtration and may also limit drug transport and metabolism.

TABLE 2–2 ■ DISTRIBUTION OF BLOOD FLOW IN 70-KG MALE AT REST								
	KIDNEYS	**HEART**	**LIVER**	**BRAIN**	**SKELETAL MUSCLE**	**FAT**	**REMAINDER**	**Σ**
Blood Flow (mL/min)	1100	250	1700	800	900	250	500	5500
Mass (kg)	0.3	0.3	2.6	1.3	34	10	21.5	70
Flow/Mass (mL/min/kg)	3667	833	654	615	26	25	23	
% Cardiac Output	20	4.5	31	14.5	16.4	4.5	9.1	100

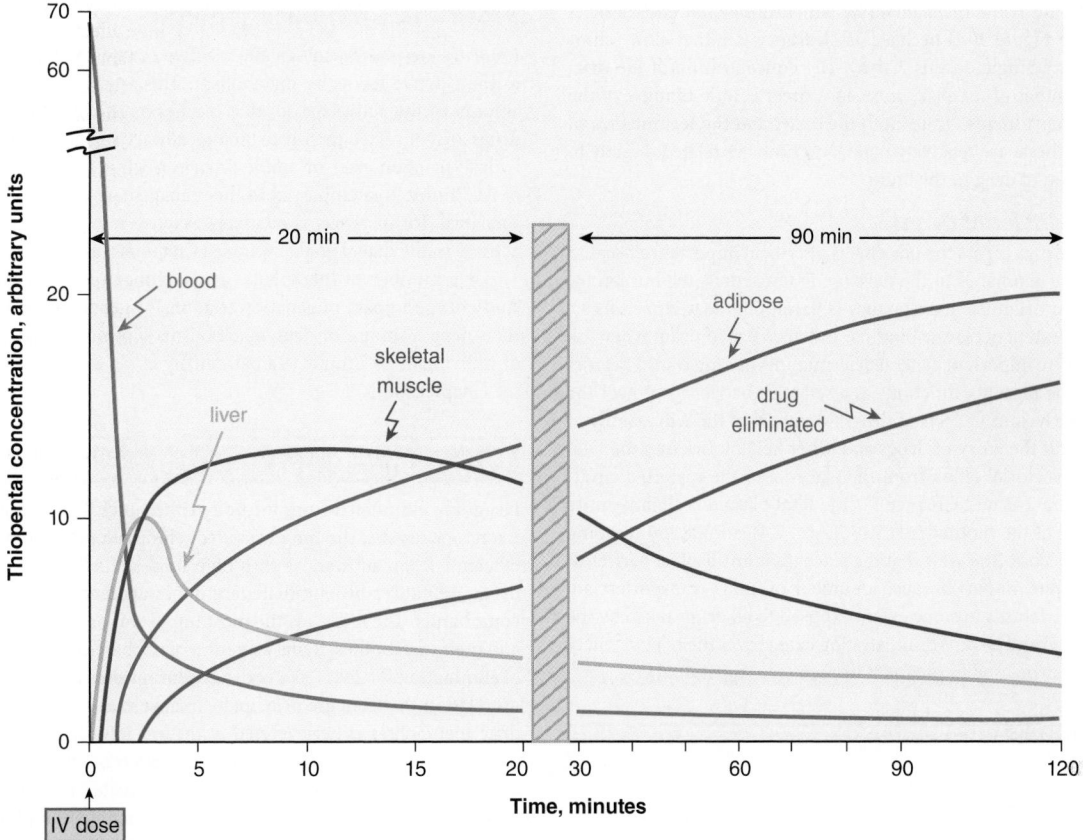

Figure 2–4 *Redistribution.* Curves depict the distribution of the barbiturate anesthetic thiopental into different body compartments following a single rapid intravenous dose. Note breaks and changes of scale on both axes. The drug level at thiopental's site of action in the brain closely mirrors the plasma level of the drug. The rate of accumulation in the various body compartments depends on regional blood flow; the extent of accumulation reflects the differing capacities of the compartments and the steady but slow effect of elimination to reduce the amount of drug available. Emergence from the anesthetic influence of this single dose of thiopental relies on redistribution, not on metabolism. The drug will partition out of tissue depots as metabolism and elimination take their course. Depletion of compartments will follow the same order as accumulation, as a function of their perfusion.

Tissue Binding

Many drugs accumulate in tissues at higher concentrations than those in the extracellular fluids and blood. Tissue binding of drugs usually occurs with cellular constituents such as proteins, phospholipids, or nuclear proteins and generally is reversible. A large fraction of drug in the body may be bound in this fashion and serve as a reservoir that prolongs drug action in that same tissue or at a distant site reached through the circulation. Such tissue binding and accumulation also can produce local toxicity (e.g., renal and ototoxicity associated with aminoglycoside antibiotics).

CNS, the BBB, and CSF

The brain capillary endothelial cells have continuous tight junctions; therefore, drug penetration into the brain depends on transcellular rather than paracellular transport. The unique characteristics of brain capillary endothelial cells and pericapillary glial cells constitute the BBB. At the choroid plexus, a similar blood-CSF barrier is present, formed by epithelial cells that are joined by tight junctions. The lipid solubility of the nonionized and unbound species of a drug is therefore an important determinant of its uptake by the brain; the more lipophilic a drug, the more likely it is to cross the BBB. In general, the BBB's function is well maintained; however, meningeal and encephalic inflammation increase local permeability. Drugs may also be imported to and exported from the CNS by specific transporters (see Chapter 5).

Bone

The tetracycline antibiotics (and other divalent metal-ion chelating agents) and heavy metals may accumulate in bone by adsorption onto the bone crystal surface and eventual incorporation into the crystal lattice. Bone can become a reservoir for the slow release of toxic agents such as lead or radium; their effects thus can persist long after exposure has ceased. Local destruction of the bone medulla also may result in reduced blood flow and prolongation of the reservoir effect as the toxic agent becomes sealed off from the circulation; this may further enhance the direct local damage to the bone. A vicious cycle results, whereby the greater the exposure to the toxic agent, the slower is its rate of elimination. The adsorption of drug onto the bone crystal surface and incorporation into the crystal lattice have therapeutic advantages for the treatment of osteoporosis.

Fat as a Reservoir

Many lipid-soluble drugs are stored by physical solution in the neutral fat. In obese persons, the fat content of the body may be as high as 50%, and even in lean individuals, fat constitutes 10% of body weight; hence, fat may serve as a reservoir for lipid-soluble drugs. Fat is a rather stable reservoir because it has a relatively low blood flow.

Redistribution

Termination of drug effect after withdrawal of a drug usually is by metabolism and excretion but also may result from redistribution of the drug from its site of action into other tissues or sites. Redistribution is a factor in terminating drug effect primarily when a highly lipid-soluble drug that acts on the brain or cardiovascular system is administered rapidly by intravenous injection or inhalation. Such is the case of the intravenous anesthetic thiopental, a lipid-soluble drug. Because blood flow to the brain is high and thiopental readily crosses the BBB, thiopental reaches its maximal concentration in brain rapidly after its intravenous injection. Subsequently, the plasma and brain concentrations decrease as thiopental redistributes to other tissues, such as muscle and, finally, adipose tissue.

This redistribution is the mechanism by which thiopental anesthesia is terminated (see Figure 2–4) because its clearance is rather slow (elimination $t_{1/2}$ after a single dose is 3–8 h). The concentration of the drug in brain follows that of the plasma because there is little binding of the drug to brain constituents. Thus, both the onset and the termination of thiopental anesthesia are relatively rapid, and both are related directly to the concentration of drug in the brain.

Placental Transfer of Drugs

The transfer of drugs across the placenta is of critical importance because drugs may cause anomalies in the developing fetus; thus, the burden for evidenced-based drug use in pregnancy is paramount (see Appendix I). Lipid solubility, extent of plasma binding, and degree of ionization of weak acids and bases are important general determinants in drug transfer across the placenta. The placenta functions as a selective barrier to protect the fetus against the harmful effects of drugs. Members of the ABC family of transporters limit the entry of drugs and other xenobiotics into the fetal circulation via vectorial efflux from the placenta to the maternal circulation (see Figure 2–2 and Chapter 5). The fetal plasma is slightly more acidic than that of the mother (pH 7.0–7.2 vs. 7.4), so that ion trapping of basic drugs occurs. The view that the placenta is an absolute barrier to drugs is inaccurate, in part because a number of influx transporters are also present. The fetus is to some extent exposed to all drugs taken by the mother. The Food and Drug Administration categorizes the relative safety of drugs that may be used in pregnant women (see Appendix I).

Metabolism of Drugs

A Few Principles of Metabolism and Elimination

The many therapeutic agents that are lipophilic do not pass readily into the aqueous environment of the urine. The metabolism of drugs and other xenobiotics into more hydrophilic metabolites is essential for their renal elimination from the body, as well as for termination of their biological and pharmacological activity.

From the point of view of pharmacokinetics, the following are the three essential aspects of drug metabolism:

- **First-order kinetics.** For most drugs in their therapeutic concentration ranges, the amount of drug metabolized per unit time is proportional to the plasma concentration of the drug (C_p) and *the fraction of drug removed by metabolism is constant (i.e., first-order kinetics).*
- **Zero-order kinetics.** For some drugs, such as ethanol and phenytoin, metabolic capacity is saturated at the concentrations usually employed, and drug metabolism becomes *zero order; that is, a constant amount of drug is metabolized per unit time.* Zero-order kinetics can also occur at high (toxic) concentrations as drug-metabolizing capacity becomes saturated.
- **Inducible biotransforming enzymes.** The major drug-metabolizing systems are inducible, broad-spectrum enzymes with some predictable genetic variations. Drugs that are substrates in common for a metabolizing enzyme may interfere with each other's metabolism, or a drug may induce or enhance metabolism of itself or other drugs.

In general, drug-metabolizing reactions generate more polar, inactive metabolites that are readily excreted from the body. However, in some cases, metabolites with potent biological activity or toxic properties are generated. Many of the enzyme systems that transform drugs to inactive metabolites also generate biologically active metabolites of endogenous compounds, as in steroid biosynthesis. The biotransformation of drugs occurs primarily in the liver and involves *phase 1 reactions* (oxidation, reduction, or hydrolytic reactions and the activities of CYPs) and *phase 2 reactions* (conjugations of the phase 1 product with a second molecule) and a few other reactions. Other organs with significant drug-metabolizing capacity include the GI tract, kidneys, and lungs. Drug-metabolizing enzymes, especially CYPs, are inducible by some drugs and inhibited by drugs and competing substrates. Chapter 6 covers drug metabolism at length. Knowing which CYP metabolizes a given drug and which other drugs may affect that metabolism is crucial to good drug therapy.

Prodrugs; Pharmacogenomics

Prodrugs are pharmacologically inactive compounds that are converted to their active forms by metabolism. This approach can maximize the amount of the active species that reaches its site of action. Inactive prodrugs are converted rapidly to biologically active metabolites, often by the hydrolysis of an ester or amide linkage. Such is the case with a number of ACE inhibitors employed in the management of high blood pressure. Enalapril, for instance, is relatively inactive until converted by esterase activity to the diacid enalaprilat (see Chapters 6 and 26).

For a number of therapeutic areas, clinical pharmacogenomics, the study of the impact of genetic variations or genotypes of individuals on their drug response or drug metabolism, allows for improved treatment of individuals or groups (Ramamoorthy et al., 2015; Zhang et al., 2015; see Chapter 7).

Excretion of Drugs

Drugs are eliminated from the body either unchanged or as metabolites. Excretory organs, the lung excluded, eliminate polar compounds more efficiently than substances with high lipid solubility. Thus, lipid-soluble drugs are not readily eliminated until they are metabolized to more polar compounds. The kidney is the most important organ for excreting drugs and their metabolites. Renal excretion of unchanged drug is a major route of elimination for 25%–30% of drugs administered to humans. Substances excreted in the feces are principally unabsorbed orally ingested drugs or drug metabolites either excreted in the bile or secreted directly into the intestinal tract and not reabsorbed. Excretion of drugs in breast milk is important not because of the amounts eliminated (which are small) but because the excreted drugs may affect the nursing infant (also small, and with poorly developed capacity to metabolize xenobiotics). Excretion from the lung is important mainly for the elimination of anesthetic gases (see Chapter 21).

Renal Excretion

Excretion of drugs and metabolites in the urine involves three distinct processes: glomerular filtration, active tubular secretion, and passive tubular reabsorption (Figure 2–5). The amount of drug entering the tubular lumen by filtration depends on the glomerular filtration rate and the extent of plasma binding of the drug; only unbound drug is filtered. In the proximal renal tubule, active, carrier-mediated tubular secretion also may add drug to the tubular fluid (see Chapters 5 and 25). Drug from the tubular lumen may be reabsorbed back into the systemic circulation. In the renal tubules, especially on the distal side, the nonionized forms of weak acids and bases undergo net passive reabsorption. Because the tubular cells are less permeable to the ionized forms of weak electrolytes, passive reabsorption of these substances depends on the pH. When the tubular urine is made more alkaline, weak acids are largely ionized and are excreted more rapidly and to a greater extent; conversely, acidification of the urine will reduce fractional ionization and excretion of weak acids. Effects of changing urine pH are opposite for weak bases. In the treatment of drug poisoning, the excretion of some drugs can be hastened by appropriate alkalinization or acidification of the urine (see Figure 2–3 and Chapter 4).

In neonates, renal function is low compared with body mass but matures rapidly within the first few months after birth. During adulthood, there is a slow decline in renal function, about 1% per year, so that in elderly patients a substantial degree of functional impairment may be present, and medication adjustments are often needed.

Biliary and Fecal Excretion

Transporters present in the canalicular membrane of the hepatocyte (see Figure 5–6) actively secrete drugs and metabolites into bile. Ultimately, drugs and metabolites present in bile are released into the GI tract during the digestive process. Subsequently, the drugs and metabolites can be reabsorbed into the body from the intestine, which, in the case of conjugated metabolites such as glucuronides, may require enzymatic hydrolysis

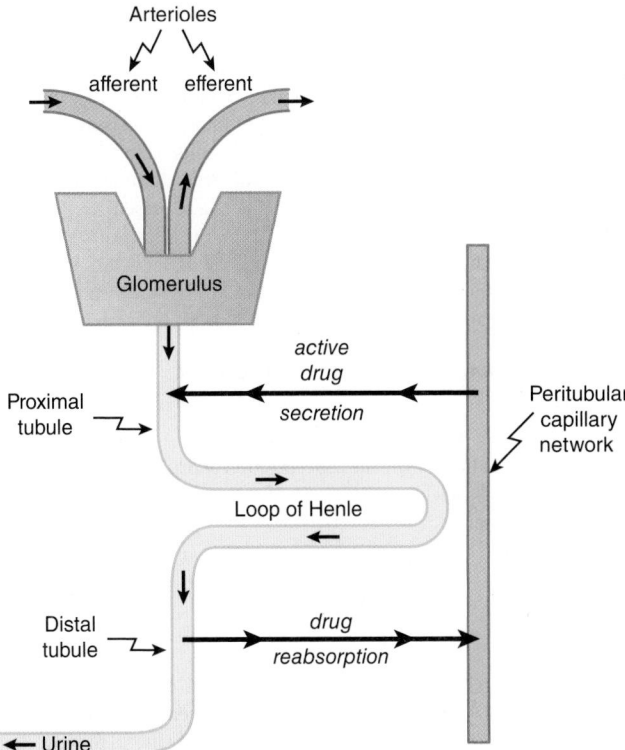

Figure 2–5 *Renal drug handling.* Drugs may be filtered from the blood in the renal glomerulus, secreted into the proximal tubule, reabsorbed from the distal tubular fluid back into the systemic circulation, and collected in the urine. Membrane transporters (OAT, OCT, MDR1, and MRP2, among others) mediate secretion into the proximal tubule (see Figures 5–12 and 5–13 for details). Reabsorption of compounds from the distal tubular fluid (generally acidic) is pH sensitive: Ionizable drugs are subject to ion trapping, and altering urinary pH to favor ionization can enhance excretion of charged species (see Figure 2–2).

by the intestinal microflora. Such *enterohepatic recycling,* if extensive, may prolong significantly the presence of a drug (or toxin) and its effects within the body prior to elimination by other pathways. To interrupt enterohepatic cycling, substances may be given orally to bind metabolites excreted in the bile (for instance, see bile acid sequestrants and ezetimibe, Chapter 33). Biliary excretions and unabsorbed drug are excreted in the feces.

Excretion by Other Routes

Excretion of drugs into sweat, saliva, and tears is quantitatively unimportant. Because milk is more acidic than plasma, basic compounds may be slightly concentrated in this fluid; conversely, the concentration of acidic compounds in the milk is lower than in plasma. Nonelectrolytes (e.g., ethanol and urea) readily enter breast milk and reach the same concentration as in plasma, independent of the pH of the milk (Rowe et al., 2015). Breast milk can also contain heavy metals from environmental exposures. The administration of drugs to breastfeeding women carries the general caution that the suckling infant will be exposed to some extent to the medication or its metabolites. Although excretion into hair and skin is quantitatively unimportant, sensitive methods of detection of drugs in these tissues have forensic significance.

Clinical Pharmacokinetics

Clinical pharmacokinetics relate the pharmacological effects of a drug and concentration of the drug in an accessible body compartment (e.g., in blood or plasma) as these change in time. In most cases, the concentration of drug at its sites of action will be related to the concentration of drug in the systemic circulation (see Figure 2–1). The pharmacological effect

that results may be the clinical effect desired or an adverse or toxic effect. Clinical pharmacokinetics attempts to provide

- a quantitative relationship between dose and effect, and
- a framework within which to interpret measurements of drug concentration in biological fluids and their adjustment through changes in dosing for the benefit of the patient.

The importance of pharmacokinetics in patient care is based on the improvement in therapeutic efficacy and the avoidance of unwanted effects that can be attained by application of its principles when dosage regimens are chosen and modified.

The following are the four most important parameters governing drug disposition:

1. *Bioavailability,* the fraction of drug absorbed as such into the systemic circulation.
2. *Volume of distribution,* a measure of the apparent space in the body available to contain the drug based on how much is given versus what is found in the systemic circulation.
3. *Clearance,* a measure of the body's efficiency in eliminating drug from the systemic circulation.
4. *Elimination* $t_{1/2}$, a measure of the rate of removal of drug from the systemic circulation.

Clearance

Clearance is the most important concept to consider when designing a rational regimen for long-term drug administration. The clinician usually wants to maintain steady-state concentrations of a drug within a *therapeutic window* or range associated with therapeutic efficacy and a minimum of toxicity for a given agent. Assuming complete bioavailability, the steady-state concentration of drug in the body will be achieved when the rate of drug elimination equals the rate of drug administration. Thus,

$$\textbf{Dosing rate} = CL \cdot C_{ss} \qquad \text{(Equation 2–3)}$$

where CL is clearance of drug from the systemic circulation, and C_{ss} is the steady-state concentration of drug. When the desired steady-state concentration of drug in plasma or blood is known, the rate of clearance of drug will dictate the rate at which the drug should be administered.

Knowing the clearance of a drug is useful because its value for a particular drug usually is constant over the range of concentrations encountered clinically. This is true because metabolizing enzymes and transporters usually are not saturated; thus, the absolute rate of elimination of the drug is essentially a linear function of its concentration in plasma (first-order kinetics), where a *constant fraction* of drug in the body is eliminated per unit of time. If mechanisms for elimination of a given drug become saturated, the kinetics approach zero order (the case for ethanol and high doses of phenytoin), in which case a *constant amount* of drug is eliminated per unit of time.

With first-order kinetics, clearance CL will vary with the concentration of drug (C), often according to Equation 2–4:

$$CL = \frac{v_m}{(K_m + C)} \qquad \text{(Equation 2–4)}$$

where K_m represents the concentration at which half the maximal rate of elimination is reached (in units of mass/volume), and v_m is equal to the maximal rate of elimination (in units of mass/time). Thus, clearance is derived in units of volume cleared of drug/time. This equation is analogous to the Michaelis-Menten equation for enzyme kinetics.

Clearance of a drug is its rate of elimination by all routes normalized to the concentration of drug C in some biological fluid where measurement can be made:

$$CL = \textbf{Rate of elimination}/C \qquad \text{(Equation 2–5)}$$

Thus, when clearance is constant, the rate of drug elimination is directly proportional to drug concentration. Clearance indicates the volume of biological fluid such as blood or plasma from which drug would have to be completely removed to account for the clearance per unit of body weight (e.g., mL/min per kg). Clearance can be defined further as blood clearance CL_b, plasma clearance CL_p, or clearance based on the concentration of unbound drug CL_u, depending on the measurement made (C_b, C_p, or C_u). Clearance of drug by several organs is additive. Elimination of drug from the systemic circulation may occur as a result of processes that occur in the kidney, liver, and other organs. Division of the rate of elimination by each organ by a concentration of drug (e.g., plasma concentration) will yield the respective clearance by that organ. Added together, these separate clearances will equal systemic clearance:

$$CL_{renal} + CL_{hepatic} + CL_{other} = CL \qquad \text{(Equation 2–6)}$$

Any significant alteration in renal or hepatic function can result in decreased clearance for those drugs with high renal or hepatic clearance. Systemic clearance may be determined at steady state by using Equation 2–3. For a single dose of a drug with complete bioavailability and first-order kinetics of elimination, systemic clearance may be determined from mass balance and the integration of Equation 2–5 over time:

$$CL = \text{Dose}/AUC \qquad \text{(Equation 2–7)}$$

AUC is the total area under the curve that describes the measured concentration of drug in the systemic circulation as a function of time (from zero to infinity), as in Figure 2–9.

Examples of Clearance

The plasma clearance for the antibiotic cephalexin is 4.3 mL/min/kg, with 90% of the drug excreted unchanged in the urine. For a 70-kg man, the clearance from plasma would be 301 mL/min, with renal clearance accounting for 90% of this elimination. In other words, the kidney is able to excrete cephalexin at a rate such that the drug is completely removed (cleared) from about 270 mL of plasma every minute (renal clearance = 90% of total clearance). Because clearance usually is assumed to remain constant in a medically stable patient (e.g., no acute decline in kidney function), the rate of elimination of cephalexin will depend on the concentration of drug in the plasma (see Equation 2–5).

The β adrenergic receptor antagonist propranolol is cleared from the blood at a rate of 16 mL/min/kg (or 1600 mL/min in a 100-kg man), almost exclusively by the liver. Thus, the liver is able to remove the amount of propranolol contained in 1600 mL of blood in 1 min, roughly equal to total hepatic blood (see Table 2–2). In fact, the plasma clearance of some drugs exceeds the rate of blood flow to this organ. Often, this is so because the drug partitions readily into and out of red blood cells (rbc), and the rate of drug delivered to the eliminating organ is considerably higher than expected from measurement of its concentration in plasma. The relationship between plasma clearance (subscript p) and blood clearance (subscript b; all components of blood) at steady state is given by

$$\frac{CL_p}{CL_b} = \frac{C_b}{C_p} = 1 + H\left[\frac{C_{rbc}}{C_p} - 1\right] \qquad \text{(Equation 2–8)}$$

Clearance from the blood therefore may be estimated by dividing the plasma clearance by the drug's blood-to-plasma concentration ratio, obtained from knowledge of the hematocrit (H = 0.45) and concentration ratio of red cells to plasma. In most instances, the blood clearance will be less than liver blood flow (1.5–1.7 L/min) or, if renal excretion also is involved, the sum of the blood flows to each eliminating organ. For example, the plasma clearance of the immunomodulator tacrolimus, about 2 L/min, is more than twice the hepatic plasma flow rate and even exceeds the organ's blood flow despite the fact that the liver is the predominant site of this drug's extensive metabolism. However, after taking into account the extensive distribution of tacrolimus into red cells, its clearance from the blood is only about 63 mL/min, and it is actually a drug with a rather low clearance, not a high-clearance agent as might be expected from the

plasma clearance value alone. Clearance from the blood by metabolism can exceed liver blood flow, and this indicates extrahepatic metabolism. In the case of the β_1 receptor antagonist esmolol, the blood clearance value (11.9 L/min) is greater than cardiac output (~5.5 L/min) because the drug is metabolized efficiently by esterases present in red blood cells.

A further definition of clearance is useful for understanding the effects of pathological and physiological variables on drug elimination, particularly with respect to an individual organ. The rate of presentation of drug to the organ is the product of blood flow Q and the arterial drug concentration C_A, and the rate of exit of drug from the organ is the product of blood flow and the venous drug concentration C_V. The difference between these rates at steady state is the rate of drug elimination by that organ:

$$\text{Rate of elimination} = Q \cdot C_A - Q \cdot C_V$$
$$= Q(C_A - C_V) \qquad \text{(Equation 2–9)}$$

Dividing Equation 2–8 by the concentration of drug entering the organ of elimination, C_A, yields an expression for clearance of the drug by the organ in question:

$$CL_{organ} = Q\left[\frac{C_A - C_V}{C_A}\right] = Q \cdot E \qquad \text{(Equation 2–10)}$$

The expression $(C_A - C_V)/C_A$ in Equation 2–10 can be referred to as the extraction ratio E of the drug. While not employed in general medical practice, calculations of a drug's extraction ratio(s) are useful for modeling the effects of disease of a given metabolizing organ on clearance and in the design of ideal therapeutic properties of drugs in development.

Hepatic Clearance

For a drug that is removed efficiently from the blood by hepatic processes (metabolism or excretion of drug into the bile), the concentration of drug in the blood leaving the liver will be low, the extraction ratio will approach unity, and the clearance of the drug from blood will become limited by hepatic blood flow. Drugs that are cleared efficiently by the liver (e.g., drugs with systemic clearances > 6 mL/min/kg, such as diltiazem, imipramine, lidocaine, morphine, and propranolol) are restricted in their rate of elimination not by intrahepatic processes but by the rate at which they can be transported in the blood to the liver.

Pharmacokinetic models indicate that when the capacity of the eliminating organ to metabolize the drug is large in comparison with the rate of presentation of drug to the organ, clearance will approximate the organ's blood flow. By contrast, when the drug-metabolizing capacity is small in comparison with the rate of drug presentation, clearance will be proportional to the unbound fraction of drug in blood and the drug's intrinsic clearance, where intrinsic clearance represents drug binding to components of blood and tissues or the intrinsic capacity of the liver to eliminate a drug in the absence of limitations imposed by blood flow (Guner and Bowen, 2013).

Renal Clearance

Renal clearance of a drug results in its appearance in the urine. In considering the clearance of a drug from the body by the kidney, glomerular filtration, secretion, reabsorption, and glomerular blood flow must be considered (see Figure 2–5). The rate of filtration of a drug depends on the volume of fluid that is filtered in the glomerulus and the concentration of unbound drug in plasma (because drug bound to protein is not filtered). The rate of secretion of drug into the tubular fluid will depend on the drug's intrinsic clearance by the transporters involved in active secretion as affected by the drug's binding to plasma proteins, the degree of saturation of these transporters, the rate of delivery of the drug to the secretory site, and the presence of drugs that can compete for these transporters. In addition, one must consider processes of drug reabsorption from the tubular fluid back into the bloodstream. The influences of changes in protein binding, blood flow, and the functional state of nephrons will affect renal clearance.

Aspirin demonstrates the interplay among these processes. Aspirin has a bimodal effect on the renal handling of uric acid: High doses of aspirin (>3 g/d) are uricosuric (probably by blocking urate reabsorption), while low dosages (1–2 g/d) cause uric acid retention (probably via inhibiting urate secretion). Low-dose aspirin, indicated for the prophylaxis of cardiovascular events, can cause changes in renal function and uric acid handling in elderly patients.

Distribution

Volume of Distribution

The volume of distribution V relates the amount of drug in the body to the concentration of drug C in the blood or plasma, depending on the fluid measured. This volume does not necessarily refer to an identifiable physiological volume but rather to the fluid volume that would be required to contain all of the drug in the body at the same concentration measured in the blood or plasma:

$$\text{Amount of drug in body}/V = C$$

or

$$V = \text{Amount of drug in body}/C \qquad \text{(Equation 2–11)}$$

View V as an imaginary volume because for many drugs V exceeds the known volume of any and all body compartments (Box 2–1). For example, the value of V for the highly lipophilic antimalarial chloroquine is some 15,000 L, whereas the volume of total-body water is about 42 L in a 70-kg male.

For drugs that are bound extensively to plasma proteins but are not bound to tissue components, the volume of distribution will approach that of the plasma volume because drug bound to plasma protein is measurable in the assay of most drugs. In contrast, certain drugs have high volumes of distribution even though most of the drug in the circulation is bound to albumin because these drugs are also sequestered elsewhere.

The volume of distribution defined in Equation 2–11 considers the body as a single homogeneous compartment. In this one-compartment model, all drug administration occurs directly into the central compartment, and distribution of drug is instantaneous throughout the volume V. Clearance of drug from this compartment occurs in a first-order fashion, as defined in Equation 2–5; that is, the amount of drug eliminated per unit of time depends on the amount (concentration) of drug in the body compartment at that time. Figure 2–6A and Equation 2–9 describe the decline of plasma concentration with time for a drug introduced into this central compartment:

$$C = \left[\frac{\text{Dose}}{V}\right][e^{-kt}] \qquad \text{(Equation 2–12)}$$

where k is the rate constant for elimination that reflects the fraction of drug removed from the compartment per unit of time. This rate constant is inversely related to the $t_{1/2}$ of the drug [$kt_{1/2} = \ln 2 = 0.693$]. The idealized one-compartment model does not describe the entire time course of the plasma concentration. Certain tissue reservoirs can be distinguished from the central compartment, and the drug concentration appears to decay in a manner that can be described by multiple exponential terms (Figure 2–6B).

Rates of Distribution

In many cases, groups of tissues with similar perfusion-to-partition ratios all equilibrate at essentially the same rate such that only one apparent phase of distribution is seen (rapid initial decrease in concentration of intravenously injected drug, as in Figure 2–6B). It is as though the drug starts in a "central" volume (see Figure 2–1), which consists of plasma and tissue reservoirs that are in rapid equilibrium, and distributes to a "final" volume, at which point concentrations in plasma decrease in a log-linear fashion with a rate constant of k (see Figure 2–6B). The multicompartment model of drug disposition can be viewed as though the blood and highly perfused lean organs such as heart, brain, liver, lung, and kidneys cluster as a single central compartment, whereas more slowly perfused tissues such as muscle, skin, fat, and bone behave as the final compartment (the tissue compartment).

If blood flow to certain tissues changes within an individual, rates of drug distribution to these tissues also will change. Changes in blood flow may cause some tissues that were originally in the "central" volume to equilibrate sufficiently more slowly so they appear only in the "final" volume. This means that central volumes will appear to vary with disease states that cause altered regional blood flow (such as would be seen in cirrhosis of the liver). After an intravenous bolus dose, drug concentrations in plasma may be higher in individuals with poor perfusion (e.g., shock) than they would be if perfusion were better. These higher systemic concentrations may in turn cause higher concentrations (and greater effects) in tissues such as brain and heart, whose usually high perfusion has not been reduced. Thus, the effect of a drug at various sites of action can vary depending on perfusion of these sites.

Multicompartment Volumes

In multicompartment kinetics, a volume of distribution term is useful especially when the effect of disease states on pharmacokinetics is to be determined. The volume of distribution at steady state V_{ss} represents the volume in which a drug would appear to be distributed during steady state if the drug existed throughout that volume at the same concentration as that in the measured fluid (plasma or blood). V_{ss} also may be appreciated as shown in Equation 2–13, where V_C is the volume of distribution of drug in the central compartment and V_T is the volume term for drug in the tissue compartment:

$$V_{ss} = V_C + V_T \qquad \text{(Equation 2–13)}$$

Steady-State Concentration

Equation 2–3 (Dosing rate = $CL \cdot C_{ss}$) indicates that a steady-state concentration eventually will be achieved when a drug is administered at a constant rate. At this point, drug elimination (the product of clearance and concentration; Equation 2–5) will equal the rate of drug availability. This concept also extends to regular intermittent dosage (e.g., 250 mg of drug every 8 h). During each interdose interval, the concentration of drug rises with absorption and falls by elimination. At steady state, the entire cycle is repeated identically in each interval (Figure 2–7). Equation 2–3 still applies for intermittent dosing, but it now describes the average

---

BOX 2–1 ■ V Values May Exceed Any Physiological Volume

For many drugs, Equation 2–11 will give V values that exceed any physiological volume. For example, if 500 μg of the cardiac glycoside digoxin were added into the body of a 70-kg subject, a plasma concentration of about 0.75 ng/mL would be observed. Dividing the amount of drug in the body by the plasma concentration yields a volume of distribution for digoxin of about 667 L, or a value about 15 times greater than the total-body volume of a 70-kg man. In fact, digoxin distributes preferentially to muscle and adipose tissue and binds to its specific receptors, the Na^+,K^+-ATPase, leaving a very small amount of drug in the plasma to be measured. A drug's volume of distribution therefore can reflect the extent to which it is present in extravascular tissues and not in the plasma.

Thus, V may vary widely depending on the relative degrees of binding to high-affinity receptor sites, plasma and tissue proteins, the partition coefficient of the drug in fat, and accumulation in poorly perfused tissues. The volume of distribution for a given drug can differ according to a patient's age, gender, body composition, and presence of disease. Total-body water of infants younger than 1 year of age, for example, is 75%–80% of body weight, whereas that of adult males is 60% and that of females is 55%.

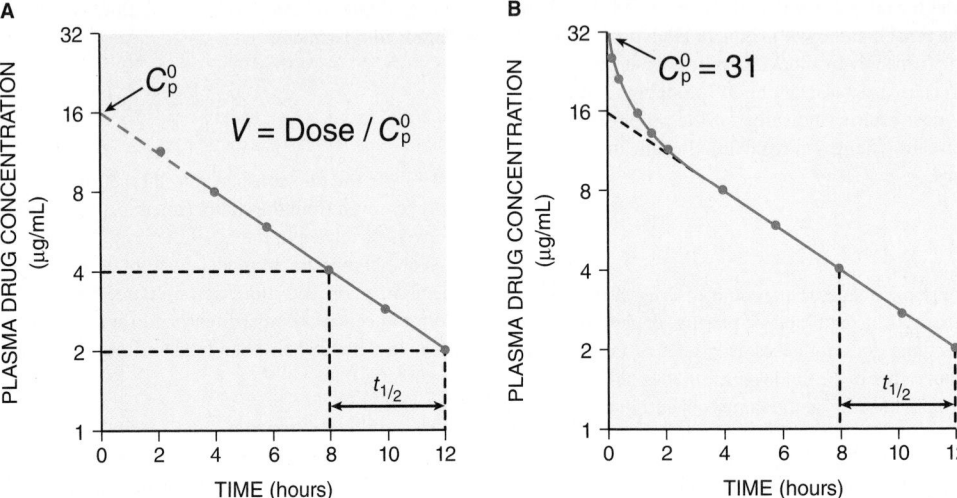

Figure 2–6 *Plasma concentration-time curves following intravenous administration of a drug (500 mg) to a 70-kg patient.* **A.** Drug concentrations are measured in plasma at 2-hour intervals following drug administration. The semilogarithmic plot of plasma concentration C_p versus time suggests that the drug is eliminated from a single compartment by a first-order process (see Equation 2–12) with a $t_{1/2}$ of 4 h ($k = 0.693/t_{1/2} = 0.173$ h^1). The volume of distribution V may be determined from the value of C_p obtained by extrapolation to zero-time. Volume of distribution (see Equation 2–11) for the one-compartment model is 31.3 L, or 0.45 L/kg ($V = \text{dose}/C_p^0$). The clearance for this drug is 90 mL/min; for a one-compartment model, $CL = kV$.
B. Sampling before 2 h indicates that the drug follows multiexponential kinetics. The terminal disposition $t_{1/2}$ is 4 h, clearance is 84 mL/min (see Equation 2–7), and V_{ss} is 26.8 L (see Equation 2–13). The initial or "central" distribution volume for the drug ($V = \text{dose}/C0p$) is 16.1 L. The example indicates that multicompartment kinetics may be overlooked when sampling at early times is neglected. In this particular case, there is only a 10% error in the estimate of clearance when the multicompartment characteristics are ignored. For many drugs, multicompartment kinetics may be observed for significant periods of time, and failure to consider the distribution phase can lead to significant errors in estimates of clearance and in predictions of appropriate dosage.

steady-state drug concentration during an interdose interval. Note the extension of this idea to derive $\bar{C}_{ss}$ during continuous intravenous drug infusion, as explained in the legend to Figure 2–7.

Half-Life

The $t_{1/2}$ is the time it takes for the plasma concentration to be reduced by 50%. For the one-compartment model of Figure 2–6A, $t_{1/2}$ may be determined readily by inspection of the data and used to make decisions about drug dosage. However, as indicated in Figure 2–6B, drug concentrations in plasma often follow a multicomponent pattern of decline.

Half-Life, Volume of Distribution, and Clearance

When using pharmacokinetics to calculate drug dosing in disease, note that $t_{1/2}$ changes as a function of both clearance and volume of distribution:

$$t_{1/2} \cong 0.693 \cdot V_{ss}/CL \qquad \text{(Equation 2–14)}$$

This $t_{1/2}$ reflects the decline of systemic drug concentrations during a dosing interval at steady state as depicted in Figure 2–7.

Terminal Half-Life

With prolonged dosing (or with high drug concentrations), a drug may penetrate beyond the central compartment into "deep" or secondary body compartments that equilibrate only slowly with the plasma. When the infusion or dosing stops, the drug will be initially cleared from plasma as expected but will eventually drop to a point at which net diffusion from the secondary compartments begins, and this slow equilibration will produce a prolongation of the half-life of the drug, referred to as the terminal half-life.

Steady-State $t_{1/2}$ and Terminal $t_{1/2}$ Compared

Examples of drugs with marked differences in terminal $t_{1/2}$ versus steady-state $t_{1/2}$ are gentamicin and indomethacin. Gentamicin has a $t_{1/2}$ of 2–3 h following a single administration, but a terminal $t_{1/2}$ of 53 h because drug accumulates in spaces such as kidney parenchyma (where this accumulation can result in toxicity). Biliary cycling probably is responsible for the 120-h terminal value for indomethacin (compared

to the steady-state value of 2.4 h). Intravenous anesthetics provide a good example; many have *context-sensitive* half-times; these agents, with short half-times after single intravenous doses, exhibit longer half-times in proportion to the duration of exposure when used in maintenance anesthesia (see Figure 21–2).

Clearance is the measure of the body's capacity to eliminate a drug; thus, as clearance decreases, owing to a disease process, for example, $t_{1/2}$ will increase as long as the volume of distribution remains unchanged; alternately, the volume of distribution may change but CL remains constant or a combination of the two changes. For example, the $t_{1/2}$ of diazepam increases with increasing age; however, this does not reflect a change in clearance but rather a change in the volume of distribution. Similarly, changes in protein binding of a drug (e.g., hypoalbuminemia) may affect its clearance as well as its volume of distribution, leading to unpredictable changes in $t_{1/2}$ as a function of disease. The $t_{1/2}$ defined in Equation 2–14 provides an approximation of the time required to reach steady state after a dosage regimen is initiated or changed (e.g., four half-lives to reach ~ 94% of a new steady state).

Extent and Rate of Absorption
Bioavailability

It is important to distinguish between the amount of drug that is administered and the quantity of drug that ultimately reaches the systemic circulation. Dissolution and absorption of drug may be incomplete; some drug may be destroyed prior to entering the systemic circulation, especially by hepatic first-pass metabolism. The first-pass effect is extensive for many oral medications that enter the portal vein and pass directly to the liver. The fraction of a dose F that is absorbed and escapes first-pass elimination measures the drug's *bioavailability*; thus, $0 < F \leq 1$ (see Equation 2–2).

For some drugs, extensive first-pass metabolism greatly reduces their effectiveness or precludes their use as oral agents (e.g., lidocaine, propranolol, naloxone, and glyceryl trinitrate). For other agents, the extent of absorption may be very low, thereby reducing bioavailability. When drugs are administered by a route that is subject to significant first-pass loss or incomplete absorption, the equations presented previously that contain

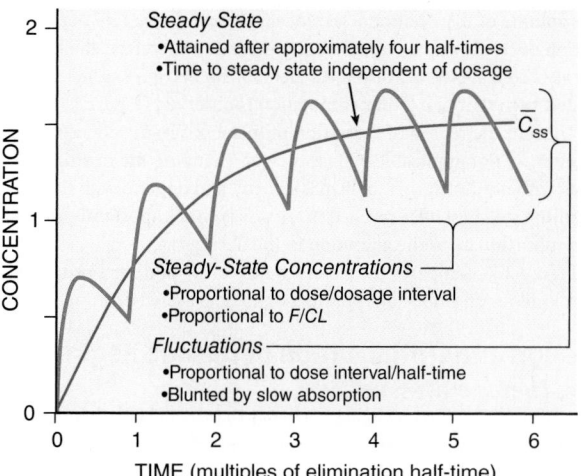

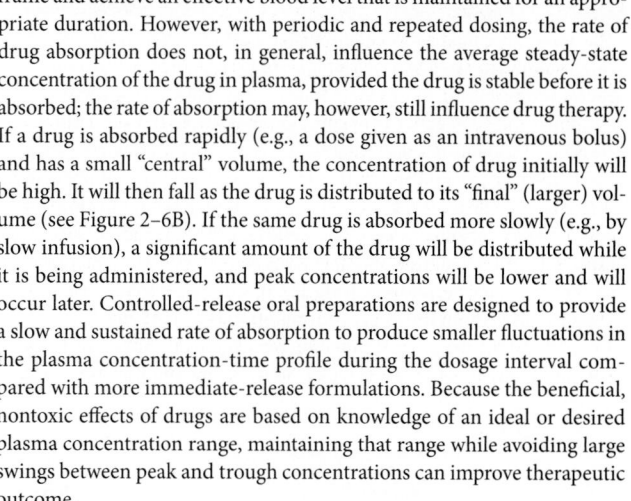

Figure 2–7 *Fundamental pharmacokinetic relationships for repeated administration of drugs.* The red line is the pattern of drug accumulation during repeated administration of a drug at intervals equal to its elimination half-time. With instantaneous absorption, each dose would add 1 concentration unit to C_p at the time of administration, and then half of that would be eliminated prior to administration of the next dose, resulting in the oscillation of C_p between 1 and 2 after four or five elimination half-times. However, this more realistic simulation uses a rate of drug absorption that is not instantaneous but is 10 times as rapid as elimination; drug is eliminated throughout the absorption process, blunting the maximal blood level achieved after each dose. With repeated administration, C_p achieves steady state, oscillating around the blue line at 1.5 units. The blue line depicts the pattern during administration of equivalent dosage by continuous intravenous infusion. Curves are based on the one-compartment model. Average drug concentration at steady state $\bar{C}_{ss}$ is:

$$C_{ss} = \frac{F \cdot dose}{CL \cdot T} = \frac{F \cdot dosing\ rate}{CL}$$

where the dosing rate is the dose per time interval and is dose/T, F is the fractional bioavailability, and CL is clearance. Note that substitution of infusion rate for [$F \cdot dose/T$] provides the concentration maintained at steady state during continuous intravenous infusion ($F = 1$ with intravenous administration).

the terms *dose* or *dosing rate* (see Equations 2–3, 2–7, and 2–12) also must include the bioavailability term F such that the available dose or dosing rate is used (Box 2–2). For example, Equation 2–2 is modified to

$$F \cdot \textbf{Dosing rate} = CL \cdot C_{ss} \qquad \text{(Equation 2–15)}$$

where the value of F is between 0 and 1.

Rate of Absorption

The rate of absorption can be important with a drug given as a single dose, such as a sleep-inducing medication that must act in a reasonable time

---

BOX 2–2 ■ Poor Absorption Notwithstanding, Some Agents With Low Bioavailability Are Effective Orally

The value of F varies widely for drugs administered by mouth, and successful therapy can still be achieved for some drugs with F values as low as 0.03 (e.g., etidronate and aliskiren). Aliskiren is the first orally applicable direct renin inhibitor approved for treatment of hypertension; its bioavailability is 2.6%. Etidronate, a bisphosphonate used to stabilize bone matrix in the treatment of Paget's disease and osteoporosis, has a similarly low bioavailability of 0.03, meaning that only 3% of the drug appears in the bloodstream following oral dosing. In these cases, therapy using oral administration is still useful, although the administered dose of the drug per kilogram is larger than would be given by injection.

---

frame and achieve an effective blood level that is maintained for an appropriate duration. However, with periodic and repeated dosing, the rate of drug absorption does not, in general, influence the average steady-state concentration of the drug in plasma, provided the drug is stable before it is absorbed; the rate of absorption may, however, still influence drug therapy. If a drug is absorbed rapidly (e.g., a dose given as an intravenous bolus) and has a small "central" volume, the concentration of drug initially will be high. It will then fall as the drug is distributed to its "final" (larger) volume (see Figure 2–6B). If the same drug is absorbed more slowly (e.g., by slow infusion), a significant amount of the drug will be distributed while it is being administered, and peak concentrations will be lower and will occur later. Controlled-release oral preparations are designed to provide a slow and sustained rate of absorption to produce smaller fluctuations in the plasma concentration-time profile during the dosage interval compared with more immediate-release formulations. Because the beneficial, nontoxic effects of drugs are based on knowledge of an ideal or desired plasma concentration range, maintaining that range while avoiding large swings between peak and trough concentrations can improve therapeutic outcome.

Nonlinear Pharmacokinetics

Nonlinearity in pharmacokinetics (i.e., changes in such parameters as clearance, volume of distribution, and $t_{1/2}$ as a function of dose or concentration of drug) is usually caused by saturation of protein binding, hepatic metabolism, or active renal transport of the drug.

Saturable Protein Binding

As the molar concentration of small drug molecules increases, the unbound fraction eventually also must increase (as all binding sites become saturated when drug concentrations in plasma are in the range of tens to hundreds of micrograms per milliliter). For a drug that is metabolized by the liver with a low intrinsic clearance-extraction ratio, saturation of plasma-protein binding will cause both V and CL to increase as drug concentrations increase; $t_{1/2}$ thus may remain constant (see Equation 2–14). For such a drug, C_{ss} will not increase linearly as the rate of drug administration is increased. For drugs that are cleared with high intrinsic clearance-extraction ratios, C_{ss} can remain linearly proportional to the rate of drug administration. In this case, hepatic clearance will not change, and the increase in V will increase the half-time of disappearance by reducing the fraction of the total drug in the body that is delivered to the liver per unit of time. Most drugs fall between these two extremes.

Saturable Elimination

In the case of saturable elimination, the Michaelis-Menten equation (see Equation 2–4) usually describes the nonlinearity. All active processes are undoubtedly saturable, but they will appear to be linear if values of drug concentrations encountered in practice are much less than K_m for that process (Box 2–3). When drug concentrations exceeds K_m, nonlinear kinetics are observed. Saturable metabolism causes oral first-pass metabolism to be less than expected (higher *fractional bioavailability*), resulting in a greater fractional increase in C_{ss} than the corresponding fractional increase in the rate of drug administration; basically, the rate of drug entry into the systemic circulation exceeds the maximum possible rate of drug metabolism, and elimination becomes zero order. The major consequences of saturation of metabolism or transport are the opposite of those for saturation of protein binding. Saturation of protein binding will lead to increased CL because CL increases as drug concentration increases, whereas saturation of metabolism or transport may decrease CL.

C_{ss} can be computed by substituting Equation 2–4 (with C = C_{ss}) into Equation 2–3 and solving for the steady-state concentration:

$$C_{ss} = \frac{Dosing\ rate \cdot K_m}{v_m - dosing\ rate} \qquad \text{(Equation 2–16)}$$

As the dosing rate approaches the maximal elimination rate v_m, the denominator of Equation 2–16 approaches zero, and C_{ss} increases disproportionately. Because saturation of metabolism should have no effect on

BOX 2–3 ■ Saturable Metabolism: Phenytoin

The antiseizure medication phenytoin is a drug for which metabolism can become saturated by levels of the drug in the therapeutic range. Factors contributing to this are phenytoin's variable half-life and clearance and an effective concentration that varies and can saturate clearance mechanisms, such that the C_{ss} may be saturating clearance mechanisms or be well above or below that value. The $t_{1/2}$ of phenytoin is 6–24 h. For clearance, K_m (5–10 mg/L) is typically near the lower end of the therapeutic range (10–20 mg/L). For some individuals, especially young children and newborns being treated for emergent seizures, K_m may be as low as 1 mg/L. Consider an extreme case of a 70kg adult in whom the target concentration (C_{ss}) is 15 mg/L, K_m = 1 mg/L, and the maximal elimination rate, v_m, (from Appendix II) is 5.9 mg/kg/day, or 413 mg/day/70kg. Substituting into Equation 2–16:

$$15\text{mg/L} = (\text{dosing rate})(1\text{mg/L})/(413\text{mg/day} - \text{dosing rate})$$

$$\text{dosing rate} = 387 \text{ mg/day}$$

In this case, the dosing rate is just below the elimination capacity. If the dosing rate were to vary upward by 10% (to 387 + 38.7 or ~426 mg/day), the dosing rate would exceed the elimination capacity by 13 mg/day and the C_p of phenytoin would begin a slow climb to toxic levels. Conversely, if the dosing rate were to vary downward by 10% (to 387-38.7 or ~348 mg/day), the C_{ss} achieved would be 5.4 mg/L, a drastic reduction to a level below the therapeutic range.

Consider a more common K_m, 8 mg/L, such that the desired C_{ss} of 15mg/L is farther from saturating the elimination capacity. In a 70 kg subject (v_m = 413 mg/day), these data require a dosing rate of only 269 mg/day. An increase in this rate by 10% (to 296 mg/day) would not saturate the elimination capacity but would lead to a C_{ss} = 20.2 mg/L. A 10% downward variance in the dosing rate (to 242 mg/day) will produce a C_{ss} = 11.3 mg/L, a much less drastic decrease than above and still in the therapeutic range.

Factoring in all the variables, predicting and controlling dosage so precisely (<10% error) can be difficult. Therefore, for patients in whom the target concentration for phenytoin is ≥10 times the K_m, alternating between inefficacious therapy and toxicity is common, careful monitoring is essential, and a pharmacokinetic consult to establish or revise dosing may be appropriate.

Other agents exhibiting saturated metabolism at or near the commonly employed concentrations include aspirin, fluoxetine, verapamil, and ethanol.

the volume of distribution, clearance and the relative rate of drug elimination decrease as the concentration increases; therefore, the log C_p time curve is concave-downward until metabolism becomes sufficiently desaturated such that first-order elimination is observed (Figure 2–8).

Thus, in the region of saturation of metabolism, the concept of a constant $t_{1/2}$ is not applicable. Consequently, changing the dosing rate for a drug with nonlinear metabolism is difficult and unpredictable because the resulting steady state is reached more slowly, and importantly, the effect is disproportionate to the alteration in the dosing rate.

Figure 2–8 compares the effects of first-order and zero-order elimination kinetics on important pharmacokinetic parameters.

Design and Optimization of Dosage Regimens
The Therapeutic Window

The intensity of a drug's effect is related to its concentration (usually C_p) above a minimum effective concentration, whereas the duration of the drug's effect reflects the length of time the drug level is above this value (Figure 2–9). These considerations, in general, apply to both desired and undesired (adverse) drug effects; as a result, a *therapeutic window* exists that reflects a concentration range that provides efficacy without unacceptable toxicity. Following administration of a single dose, a lag period precedes the onset of the drug effect, after which the magnitude of the effect increases to a maximum and then declines; if a subsequent dose is not administered, the effect eventually disappears as the drug is eliminated. This time course reflects changes in the drug's concentration as determined by the pharmacokinetics of its absorption, distribution, and elimination.

Similar considerations apply after multiple dosing associated with long-term therapy, and they determine the amount and frequency of drug administration to achieve an optimal therapeutic effect. *In general, the lower limit of a drug's therapeutic range is approximately equal to the drug concentration that produces about half the greatest possible therapeutic effect, and the upper limit of the therapeutic range is such that no more than 5%–10% of patients will experience a toxic effect.* For some drugs, this may mean that the upper limit of the range is no more than twice the lower limit. Of course, these figures can be highly variable, and some patients may benefit greatly from drug concentrations that exceed the therapeutic range, whereas others may suffer significant toxicity at much lower values (e.g., with digoxin).

For a limited number of drugs, some effect of the drug is easily measured (e.g., blood pressure, blood glucose) and can be used to optimize dosage using a trial-and-error approach. Even in an ideal case, certain

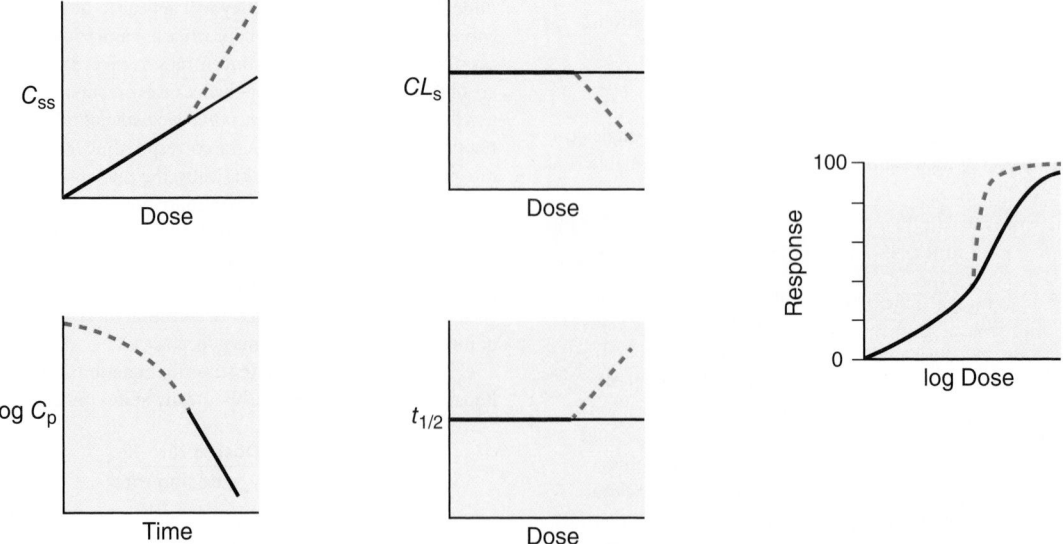

Figure 2–8 *Comparative pharmacokinetic parameters with first-order and zero-order elimination.* Black lines represent the relationships under first-order kinetics of elimination. Dashed red lines indicate the effects of transitioning to a region of saturated elimination (zero-order kinetics).

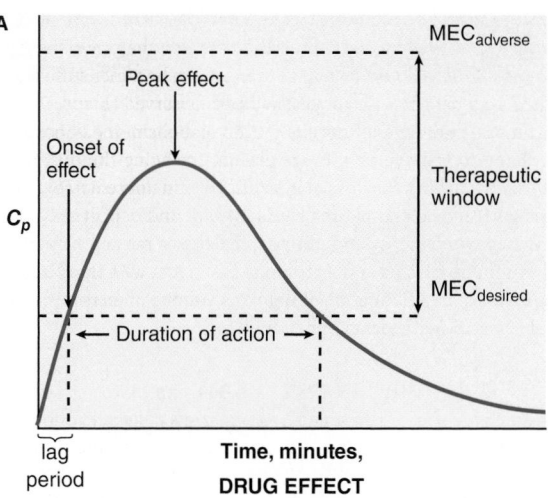

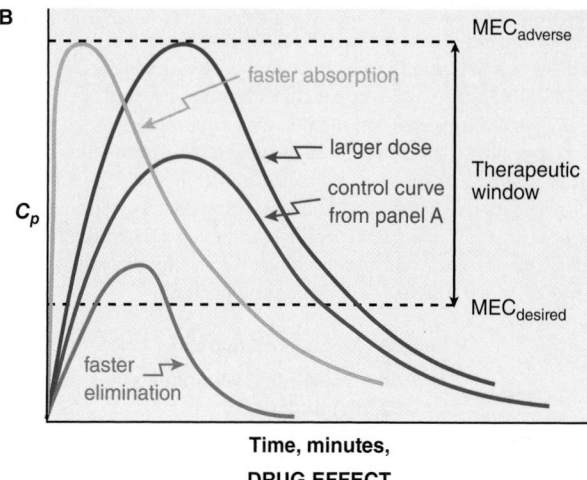

Figure 2–9 **A.** *Temporal characteristics of drug effect and relationship to the therapeutic window (e.g., single dose, oral administration).* A lag period is present before the plasma drug concentration C_p exceeds the MEC for the desired effect $MEC_{desired}$. Following onset of the response, the intensity of the effect increases as the drug continues to be absorbed and distributed. This reaches a peak, after which drug elimination results in a decline in C_p and in the effect's intensity. Effect disappears when the drug concentration falls below the $MEC_{desired}$. The duration of a drug's action is determined by the time period over which concentrations exceed the $MEC_{desired}$. An MEC also exists for each adverse response ($MEC_{adverse}$), and if the drug concentration exceeds this, toxicity will result. The therapeutic goal is to obtain and maintain concentrations within the therapeutic window for the desired response with a minimum of toxicity. Drug response *below* the $MEC_{desired}$ will be subtherapeutic; *above* the $MEC_{adverse}$, the probability of toxicity will increase. The AUC (pale red) can be used to calculate the clearance (see Equation 2–7) for first-order elimination. The AUC is also used as a measure of bioavailability (defined as 100% for an intravenously administered drug). Bioavailability is less than 100% for orally administered drugs, due mainly to incomplete absorption and first-pass metabolism and elimination. Changing drug dosage shifts the curve up or down the C_p scale and is used to modulate the drug's effect, as shown in panel B.
B. *Effects of altered absorption, elimination, and dosage and the temporal profile of a single dose administered orally.* The bold green curve is the same as that shown in panel A. Increasing the dose (blue line) decreases the lag period and prolongs the drug's duration of effectivess but at the risk of increasing the likelihood of adverse effects. Unless the drug is nontoxic (e.g., penicillins), increasing the dose is not a useful strategy for extending the duration of action if the increase puts the drug level near $MEC_{adverse}$. Instead, another dose of drug should be given, timed to maintain concentrations within the therapeutic window (see Figure 2–7). An increased rate of absorption of the dose (orange line) reduces the lag period, leads to a higher maximum C_p at an earlier time, but results in a shorter duration of action (time above $MEC_{desired}$). Increasing the rate of elimination of the dose decreases the maximum C_p and reduces the time of $C_p > MEC_{desired}$.

quantitative issues arise, such as how often to change dosage and by how much. These usually can be settled with simple rules of thumb based on the principles presented (e.g., change dosage by no more than 50% and no more often than every three or four half-lives). Alternatively, some drugs have little dose-related toxicity, and maximum efficacy usually is desired. In such cases, doses well in excess of the average required will ensure efficacy (if this is possible) and prolong drug action. Such a "maximal dose" strategy typically is used for penicillins. For many drugs, however, the effects are difficult to measure (or the drug is given for prophylaxis), toxicity and lack of efficacy are both potential dangers, or the therapeutic index is narrow. In these circumstances, doses must be titrated carefully, and drug dosage is limited by toxicity rather than efficacy.

Thus, the therapeutic goal is to maintain steady-state drug levels within the therapeutic window. When the concentrations associated with this desired range are not known, it is sufficient to understand that efficacy and toxicity depend on concentration and how drug dosage and frequency of administration affect the drug level. However, for a small number of drugs for which there is a small (2- to 3-fold) difference between concentrations resulting in efficacy and toxicity (e.g., digoxin, theophylline, lidocaine, aminoglycosides, cyclosporine, tacrolimus, sirolimus, warfarin, and some anticonvulsants), a plasma concentration range associated with effective therapy has been defined. In these cases, a desired (target) steady-state concentration of the drug (usually in plasma) associated with efficacy and minimal toxicity is chosen, and a dosage is computed that is expected to achieve this value. Drug concentrations are subsequently measured, and dosage is adjusted if necessary (described further in the chapter).

Maintenance Dose

In most clinical situations, drugs are administered in a series of repetitive doses or as a continuous infusion to maintain a steady-state concentration of drug associated with the therapeutic window. Calculation of the appropriate maintenance dosage is a primary goal. To maintain the chosen

steady-state or target concentration, the rate of drug administration is adjusted such that the rate of input equals the rate of loss. This relationship is expressed here in terms of the desired target concentration:

$$\text{Dosing rate} = \text{Target } C_p \cdot CL/F \qquad \text{(Equation 2–17)}$$

If the clinician chooses the desired concentration of drug in plasma and knows the clearance and bioavailability for that drug in a particular patient, the appropriate dose and dosing interval can be calculated (Box 2–4).

Dosing Interval for Intermittent Dosage

In general, marked fluctuations in drug concentrations between doses are not desirable. If absorption and distribution were instantaneous, fluctuations in drug concentrations between doses would be governed entirely by the drug's elimination $t_{1/2}$. If the dosing interval t were chosen to be equal to the $t_{1/2}$, then the total fluctuation would be 2-fold; this is often a tolerable variation. Pharmacodynamic considerations modify this. If a drug is relatively nontoxic such that a concentration many times that necessary for therapy can be tolerated easily, the maximal dose strategy can be used, and the dosing interval can be much longer than the elimination $t_{1/2}$ (for convenience). The $t_{1/2}$ of amoxicillin is about 2 h, but dosing every 2 h would be impractical. Instead, amoxicillin often is given in large doses every 8 or 12 h.

For some drugs with a narrow therapeutic range, it may be important to estimate the maximal and minimal concentrations that will occur for a particular dosing interval. The minimal steady-state concentration $C_{ss, min}$ may be reasonably determined by:

$$C_{ss, min} = \frac{F \cdot \text{dose}/V_{ss}}{1 - e^{-kT}} \cdot e^{-kT} \qquad \text{(Equation 2–18)}$$

where k equals 0.693 divided by the clinically relevant plasma $t_{1/2}$, and T is the dosing interval. The term e^{-kT} is the fraction of the last dose (corrected for bioavailability) that remains in the body at the end of a dosing interval.

BOX 2–4 ■ Calculating Dosage of Digoxin in Heart Failure

Oral digoxin is to be used as a maintenance dose to gradually "digitalize" a 63-year-old, 84-kg patient with congestive heart failure. A steady-state plasma concentration of 0.7–0.9 ng/mL is selected as a conservative target based on prior knowledge of the action of the drug in patients with heart failure to maintain levels at or below the 0.5- to 1.0-ng/mL range (Bauman et al., 2006). This patient's creatinine clearance CL_{Cr} is given as 56 mL/min/84 kg; knowing that digoxin's clearance may be estimated by consulting the entry for digoxin in Appendix II: $CL = 0.88\ CL_{Cr} + 0.33$ mL/min/kg. Thus,

$$CL = 0.88\ CL_{Cr} + 0.33 \text{ mL/min/kg}$$
$$= 0.88 \times 56/84 + 0.33 \text{ mL/min/kg}$$
$$= 0.92 \text{ mL/min/kg}$$

For this 84-kg patient:

$$CL = (84 \text{ kg})(0.92 \text{ mL/min/kg}) = 77 \text{ mL/min} = 4.6 \text{ L/h}$$

Knowing that the oral bioavailability of digoxin is 70% ($F = 0.7$) and with a target C_p of 0.75 ng/mL, one can use Equation 2–17 to calculate an appropriate dose rate for this 84-kg patient:

$$\textbf{Dosing rate} = \textbf{Target } C_p \cdot CL/F$$
$$= [0.75 \text{ ng/mL} \times 77 \text{ mL/min}] \div [0.7] = 82.5 \text{ ng/min}$$
$$\text{or } 82.5 \text{ ng/min} \times 60 \text{ min/h} \times 24 \text{ h/d} = 119 \text{ μg/d}$$

In practice, the dosing rate is rounded to the closest oral dosage size, 0.125 mg/d, which would result in a C_{ss} of 0.79 ng/mL (0.75 × 125/119, or using Equation 2–15). Digoxin is a well-characterized example of a drug that is difficult to dose, has a low therapeutic index (~2–3), and has a large coefficient of variation for the clearance equation in patients with heart failure (52%); the effective blood level in one patient may be toxic or ineffective in another. Thus, monitoring the clinical status of patients (new or increased ankle edema, inability to sleep in a recumbent position, decreased exercise tolerance), whether accomplished by home health follow-up or regular visits to the clinician, is essential to avoid untoward results (see Chapter 29).

BOX 2–5 ■ Estimating Maximal and Minimal Blood Levels of Digoxin

In the 84-kg patient with congestive heart failure discussed in Box 2–4, an oral maintenance dose of 0.125 mg digoxin per 24 h was calculated to achieve an average plasma concentration of 0.79 ng/mL during the dosage interval. Digoxin has a narrow therapeutic index, and plasma levels ≤ 1.0 ng/mL usually are associated with efficacy and minimal toxicity. What are the maximum and minimum plasma concentrations associated with this regimen? This first requires estimation of digoxin's volume of distribution based on pharmacokinetic data (Appendix II).

$$V_{ss} = 3.12\ CL_{Cr} + 3.84 \text{ L} \cdot \text{kg}^{-1}$$
$$= 3.12 \times (56/84) + 3.84 \text{ L} \cdot \text{kg}^{-1}$$
$$= 5.92 \text{ L/kg}$$

or 497 L in this 84-kg patient.

Combining this value with that of digoxin's clearance provides an estimate of digoxin's elimination $t_{1/2}$ in the patient (Equation 2–14).

$$t_{1/2} = 0.693\ V_{ss}/CL$$
$$= \frac{0.693 \times 497 \text{ L}}{4.6 \text{ L/h}} = 75 \text{ h} = 3.1 \text{ days}$$

Accordingly, the fractional rate constant of elimination k is equal to 0.22 day^{-1} (0.693/3.1 days). Maximum and minimum digoxin plasma concentrations then may be predicted depending on the dosage interval. With $T = 1$ day (i.e., 0.125 mg given every day),

$$C_{ss,max} = \frac{F \cdot dose/V_{ss}}{1 - e^{-kT}} \qquad \text{(Equation 2–19)}$$
$$= \frac{0.7 \times 0.125 \text{ mg}/497 \text{ L}}{0.2}$$
$$= 0.88 \text{ ng/mL} (\sim 0.9 \text{ ng/mL})$$

$$C_{ss,min} = C_{ss,max} \cdot e^{-kt} \qquad \text{(Equation 2–20)}$$
$$= (0.88 \text{ ng/mL})(0.8) = 0.7 \text{ ng/mL}$$

Thus, the plasma concentrations would fluctuate minimally about the steady-state concentration of 0.79 ng/mL, well within the recommended therapeutic range of 0.5–1.0 ng/mL.

For drugs that follow multiexponential kinetics (administered orally), estimation of the maximal steady-state concentration $C_{ss,max}$ involves a set of parameters for distribution and absorption (Box 2–5). If these terms are ignored for multiple oral dosing, one easily may estimate a maximal steady-state concentration by omitting the e^{-kT} term in the numerator of Equation 2–18 (see Equation 2–19 in Box 2–5). Because of the approximation, the predicted maximal concentration from Equation 2–19 will be greater than that actually observed.

Loading Dose

As noted, repeated administration of a drug more frequently than its complete elimination will result in accumulation of the drug to or around a steady-state level (see Figure 2–7). When a constant dosage is given, reaching a steady-state drug level (the desired therapeutic concentration) will take four to five elimination half-times. This period can be too long when treatment demands a more immediate therapeutic response. In such a case, one can employ a *loading dose*, one or a series of doses given at the onset of therapy with the aim of achieving the target concentration rapidly. The loading dose is calculated as

$$\textbf{Loading dose} = \textbf{Target } C_p \cdot V_{ss}/F \qquad \text{(Equation 2–21)}$$

Consider the case for treatment of arrhythmias with lidocaine, for example. The $t_{1/2}$ of lidocaine is usually 1–2 h. Arrhythmias encountered after myocardial infarction may be life threatening, and one cannot wait four half-times (4–8 h) to achieve a therapeutic concentration of lidocaine by infusion of the drug at the rate required to attain this concentration. Hence, use of a loading dose of lidocaine in the coronary care unit is standard.

The use of a loading dose also has significant disadvantages. First, the particularly sensitive individual may be exposed abruptly to a toxic concentration of a drug that may take a long time to decrease (i.e., long $t_{1/2}$). Loading doses tend to be large, and they are often given parenterally and rapidly; this can be particularly dangerous if toxic effects occur as a result of actions of the drug at sites that are in rapid equilibrium with plasma. This occurs because the loading dose calculated on the basis of V_{ss} subsequent to drug distribution is at first constrained within the initial and smaller "central" volume of distribution. It is therefore usually advisable to divide the loading dose into a number of smaller fractional doses that are administered over a period of time (Box 2–6). Alternatively, the loading dose should be administered as a continuous intravenous infusion over a period of time using computerized infusion pumps.

BOX 2–6 ■ A Loading Dose of Digoxin

In the 84-kg patient described previously, accumulation of digoxin to an effective steady-state level was gradual when a daily maintenance dose of 0.125 mg was administered (for at least 12.4 days, based on $t_{1/2} = 3.1$ days). A more rapid response could be obtained (if deemed necessary) by using a loading dose strategy and Equation 2–21. Choosing a target C_p of 0.9 ng/mL (the $C_{ss, max}$ calculated in Box 2–5 and below the recommended maximum of 1.0 ng/mL):

$$\text{Loading dose} = 0.9 \text{ ng} \cdot \text{mL}^{-1} \times 497 \text{ L}/0.7 = 639 \text{ μg}$$

Using standard dosage sizes, one would use a loading dose of 0.625 mg given in divided doses. To avoid toxicity, this oral loading dose would be given as an initial 0.25-mg dose followed by a 0.25-mg dose 6–8 h later, with careful monitoring of the patient, and the final 0.125-mg dose given another 6–8 h later.

Therapeutic Drug Monitoring

The major use of measured concentrations of drugs (at steady state) is to refine the estimate of CL/F for the patient being treated, using Equation 2–15 as rearranged:

$$CL/F_{patient} = \text{Dosing rate}/C_{ss}(\text{measured}) \qquad \text{(Equation 2–22)}$$

The new estimate of CL/F can be used in Equation 2–17 to adjust the maintenance dose to achieve the desired target concentration (Box 2–7).

Practical details associated with therapeutic drug monitoring should be kept in mind. The first of these relates to the time of sampling for measurement of the drug concentration.

The purpose of sampling during supposed steady state is to modify the estimate of CL/F and thus the choice of dosage. Early postabsorptive concentrations do not reflect clearance; they are determined primarily by the rate of absorption, the "central" (rather than the steady-state) volume of distribution, and the rate of distribution, all of which are pharmacokinetic features of virtually no relevance in choosing the long-term maintenance dosage. When the goal of measurement is adjustment of dosage, the sample should be taken just before the next planned dose, when the concentration is at its minimum.

If it is unclear whether efficacious concentrations of drug are being achieved, a sample taken shortly after a dose may be helpful. On the other hand, if a concern is whether low clearance (as in renal failure) may cause accumulation of drug, concentrations measured just before the next dose will reveal such accumulation and are considerably more useful for this purpose than is knowledge of the maximal concentration.

Determination of both maximal and minimal concentrations is recommended. These two values can offer a more complete picture of the behavior of the drug in a specific patient (particularly if obtained over more than one dosing period) and can better support pharmacokinetic modeling to adjust treatment.

When constant dosage is given, steady state is reached after four to five elimination half-times. If a sample is obtained too soon after dosage is begun, it will not reflect this state and the drug's clearance accurately. Yet, for toxic drugs, if sampling is delayed until steady state, the damage may have been done. In such cases, the first sample should be taken after two $t_{1/2}$ assuming that no loading dose has been given. If the concentration already exceeds 90% of the eventual expected mean steady-state concentration, the dosage rate should be halved, another sample obtained in another two (supposed) $t_{1/2}$, and the dosage halved again if this sample exceeds the target. If the first concentration is not too high, the initial rate of dosage is continued; even if the concentration is lower than expected, it is usually reasonable to await the attainment of steady state in another two estimated $t_{1/2}$ and then to proceed to adjust dosage as described in Box 2–7.

Acknowledgment: Grant R. Wilkinson, Leslie Z. Benet, Deanna L. Kroetz, and Lewis B. Sheiner contributed to this chapter in recent editions of this book. We have retained some of their text in the current edition.

BOX 2–7 ■ Adjusting the Dose at Steady State

If a drug follows first-order kinetics, the average, minimum, and maximum concentrations at steady state are linearly related to dose and dosing rate (see Equations 2–15, 2–18, and 2–19). Therefore, the ratio between the measured and desired concentrations can be used to adjust the dose, consistent with available dosage sizes:

$$\frac{C_{ss}(\text{measured})}{C_{ss}(\text{predicted})} = \frac{\text{Dose (previous)}}{\text{Dose (new)}} \qquad \text{(Equation 2–23)}$$

Consider the previously described patient given 0.125 mg digoxin every 24 h, for example. If the measured minimum (trough) steady-state concentration were found to be 0.35 ng/mL rather than the predicted level of 0.7 ng/mL, an appropriate, practical change in the dosage regimen would be to increase the daily dose by 0.125 mg to 0.25 mg digoxin daily.

Bibliography

Bauman JL, et al. A method of determining the dose of digoxin for heart failure in the modern era. *Arch Intern Med,* **2006,** 166:2539–2545.

Bera RB. Patient outcomes within schizophrenia treatment: a look at the role of long-acting injectable antipsychotics. *J Clin Psychiatry,* **2014,** 75(suppl 2):30–33.

Calias P, et al. Intrathecal delivery of protein therapeutics to the brain: a critical reassessment. *Pharmacol Ther,* **2014,** 144:114–122.

Guner OF, Bowen JP. Pharmacophore modeling for ADME. *Curr Top Med Chem,* **2013,** 13:1327–1342.

Imberti R, et al. Intraventricular or intrathecal colistin for the treatment of central nervous system infections caused by multidrug-resistant gram-negative bacteria. *Expert Rev Anti Infect Ther,* **2014,** 12:471–478.

Perletti G, et al. Enhanced distribution of fourth-generation fluoroquinolones in prostatic tissue. *Int J Antimicrob Agents,* **2009,** 33:206–210.

Ramamoorthy A, et al. Racial/ethnic differences in drug disposition and response: review of recently approved drugs. *Clin Pharmacol Ther,* **2015,** 97:263–273.

Rowe H, et al. Maternal medication, drug use, and breastfeeding. *Child Adolesc Psychiatr Clin N Am,* **2015,** 24:1–20.

Sen S, et al. Complications after unintentional intra-arterial injection of drugs: risks, outcomes, and management strategies. *Mayo Clin Proc,* **2005,** 80:783–795.

Spector R, et al. A balanced view of choroid plexus structure and function: focus on adult humans. *Exp Neurol,* **2015,** 267:78–86.

Suetsugu S, et al. Dynamic shaping of cellular membranes by phospholipids and membrane-deforming proteins. *Physiol Rev,* **2014,** 94:1219–1248.

Tran TH, et al. Drug absorption in celiac disease. *Am J Health Syst Pharm,* **2013,** 70:2199–2206.

Yohan D, Chithrani BD. Applications of nanoparticles in nanomedicine. *J Biomed Nanotechnol,* **2014,** 10:2371–2392.

Zhang G, et al. Web resources for pharmacogenomics. *Genomics Proteomics Bioinformatics,* **2015,** 13:51–54.

Chapter 3

Pharmacodynamics: Molecular Mechanisms of Drug Action

Donald K. Blumenthal

Pharmacodynamic Concepts

Pharmacodynamics is the study of the biochemical, cellular, and physiological effects of drugs and their mechanisms of action. The effects of most drugs result from their interaction with macromolecular components of the organism. The term drug *receptor* or drug *target* denotes the cellular macromolecule or macromolecular complex with which the drug interacts to elicit a cellular or systemic response. Drugs commonly alter the rate or magnitude of an intrinsic cellular or physiological response rather than create new responses. Drug receptors are often located on the surface of cells but may also be located in specific intracellular compartments, such as the nucleus, or in the extracellular compartment, as in the case of drugs that target coagulation factors and inflammatory mediators. Many drugs also interact with *acceptors* (e.g., serum albumin), which are entities that do not directly cause any change in biochemical or physiological response but can alter the pharmacokinetics of a drug's actions.

A large percentage of the new drugs approved in recent years are *therapeutic biologics*, including genetically engineered enzymes and monoclonal antibodies. Going far beyond the traditional concept of a drug are genetically modified viruses and microbes. One recently approved agent for treating melanoma is a genetically modified live oncolytic herpes virus that is injected into tumors that cannot be removed completely by surgery. *Gene therapy products* using viruses as vectors to replace genetic mutations that give rise to lethal and debilitating diseases have already been approved in China and Europe. The next generation of gene therapy products will be those capable of targeted genome editing using antisense oligonucleotides and RNAi and by delivering the CRISPR/Cas9 genome-editing system using viruses or genetically modified microorganisms. These new agents will have pharmacological properties that are distinctly different from traditional small-molecule drugs.

Physiological Receptors

Many drug receptors are proteins that normally serve as receptors for endogenous regulatory ligands. These drug targets are termed *physiological receptors*. Drugs that bind to physiological receptors and mimic the regulatory effects of the endogenous signaling compounds are termed *agonists*. If the drug binds to the same *recognition site* as the endogenous agonist, the drug is said to be a *primary agonist*. Allosteric (or *allotopic*) agonists bind to a different region on the receptor, referred to as an allosteric or allotopic site. Drugs that block or reduce the action of an agonist are termed *antagonists*. Antagonism generally results from competition with an agonist for the same or overlapping site on the receptor (a *syntopic interaction*), but can also occur by interacting with other sites on the receptor (*allosteric antagonism*), by combining with the agonist (*chemical antagonism*), or by *functional antagonism* by indirectly inhibiting the cellular or physiological effects of the agonist. Agents that are only partially as effective as agonists are termed *partial agonists*. Many receptors exhibit some constitutive activity in the absence of a regulatory ligand; drugs that stabilize such receptors in an inactive conformation are termed *inverse agonists* (Figure 3–1) (Kenakin, 2004; Milligan, 2003). In the presence of a full agonist, partial and inverse agonists will behave as competitive antagonists.

Specificity of Drug Responses

The strength of the reversible interaction between a drug and its receptor, as measured by the **dissociation constant**, is defined as the *affinity* of one for the other. (By tradition, only rarely will the inverse of the dissociation constant, the association constant, be used, even though both carry the same information.) Both the *affinity* of a drug for its receptor and its *intrinsic activity* are determined by its *chemical structure*. The chemical structure of a drug also contributes to the drug's *specificity*. A drug that interacts with a single type of receptor that is expressed on only a limited number of differentiated cells will exhibit high specificity. Conversely, a drug acting on a receptor expressed ubiquitously throughout the body will exhibit widespread effects.

Many clinically important drugs exhibit a broad (low) specificity because they interact with multiple receptors in different tissues. Such broad specificity might not only enhance the clinical utility of a drug but also contribute to a spectrum of adverse side effects because of off-target interactions. One example of a drug that interacts with multiple receptors is *amiodarone*, an agent used to treat cardiac arrhythmias. Amiodarone also has a number of serious toxicities, some of which are caused by the drug's structural similarity to thyroid hormone and, as a result, its capacity to interact with nuclear thyroid receptors. Amiodarone's salutary effects and toxicities may also be mediated through interactions with receptors that are poorly characterized or unknown.

Some drugs are administered as racemic mixtures of stereoisomers. The stereoisomers can exhibit different pharmacodynamic as well as pharmacokinetic properties. For example, the antiarrhythmic drug *sotalol* is prescribed as a racemic mixture; the D- and L-enantiomers are equipotent as K^+ channel blockers, but the L-enantiomer is a much more potent β adrenergic antagonist (see Chapter 30). A drug may have

Abbreviations

AAV: adeno-associated virus
AC: adenylyl cyclase
ACE: angiotensin-converting enzyme
ACh: acetylcholine
AChE: acetylcholinesterase
AKAP: A-kinase anchoring protein
AMPA: α-amino-3-hydroxy-5-methyl-4-isoxazole propionic acid
AngII: angiotensin II
ANP: atrial natriuretic peptide
Apaf-1: apoptotic activating protease factor 1
ASO: antisense oligonucleotide
ATG: autophagy gene
AT_1R: AT_1 receptor
BNP: brain natriuretic peptide
cAMP: cyclic adenosine monophosphate
cAMP-GEF: cAMP-guanine exchange factor
cGMP: cyclic guanosine monophosphate
CNG: cyclic nucleotide–gated channel
CNP: C-type natriuretic peptide
CREB: cAMP response element–binding protein
CRISPR/Cas9: clustered regularly interspersed short palindromic repeats/CRISPR-associated protein 9
DA: dopamine
DAG: diacylglycerol
DMD: Duchenne muscular dystrophy
DRAM: damage-regulated autophagy modulator
4EBP: eukaryotic initiation factor 4e (eif-4E)–binding protein
EC_{50}: half-maximally effective concentration
EGF: epidermal growth factor
eNOS: endothelial NOS (NOS3)
EPAC: exchange protein activated by cAMP
FADD: Fas-associated death domain
FGF: fibroblast growth factor
FKBP12: immunophilin target (binding protein) for tacrolimus (FK506)
FXR: farnesoid X receptor
GABA: γ-aminobutyric acid
GAP: GTPase-activating protein
GC: guanylyl cyclase
GEF: guanine nucleotide exchange factor
GI: gastrointestinal
GPCR: G protein–coupled receptor
GRK: GPCR kinase
HCN: hyperpolarization-activated, cyclic nucleotide–gated channel
HRE: hormone response element
5HT: serotonin
IGF1R: insulinlike growth factor 1 receptor
IKK: IκB kinase
iNOS: inducible NOS (NOS2)
IP_3: inositol 1,4,5-trisphosphate
IRAK: interleukin-1 receptor-associated kinase
Jak: Janus kinase
JNK: c-Jun N-terminal kinase
K_{ATP}: ATP-dependent K^+ channel

K_i: affinity of a competitive antagonist
LBD: ligand-binding domain
LDLR: low-density lipoprotein receptor
LXR: liver X receptor
MAO: monoamine oxidase
MAPK: mitogen-activated protein kinase
MHC: major histocompatibility complex
MLCK: myosin light chain kinase
mTOR: mammalian target of rapamycin
MyD88: myeloid differentiation protein 88
NE: norepinephrine
NF-κB: nuclear factor kappa B
NGF: nerve growth factor
NGG: 5′-(any Nucleotide)-Guanosine-Guanosine-3′
NMDA: N-methyl-D-aspartate
nmDMD: nonsense mutation Duchenne muscular dystrophy
nNOS: neuronal NOS (NOS1)
NO: nitric oxide
NOS: NO synthase
NPR-A: ANP receptor
NPR-B: natriuretic peptide B receptor
NPR-C: natriuretic peptide C receptor
NSAID: nonsteroidal anti-inflammatory drug
PDE: cyclic nucleotide phosphodiesterase
PAM: protospacer-adjacent motif
PDGF: platelet-derived growth factor
PDGF-R: PDGR receptor
PI3K: phosphatidylinositol 3-kinase
PIP_3: phosphatidylinositol 3,4,5-trisphosphate
PK_: protein kinase _ (e.g., PKA)
PKB: protein kinase B (also known as Akt)
PLC: phospholipase C
PPAR: peroxisome proliferator-activated receptor
RGS: regulator of G protein signaling
RIP1: receptor interacting protein 1
RISC: RNA-induced silencing complex
RNAi: RNA interference
RXR: retinoic acid receptor
SERCA: SR Ca^{2+}-ATPase
sGC: soluble guanylyl cyclase
sgRNA: single "guide" RNA
siRNA: small interfering RNA
S6K: S6 kinase
SMAC: second mitochondria-derived activator of caspase
SMC: smooth muscle cell
SR: sarcoplasmic reticulum
STAT: signal transducer and activator of transcription
TAK1: transforming growth factor β–activated kinase 1
TCR: T cell receptor
TGF-β: transforming growth factor β
TLR: Toll-like receptor
TNF-α: tumor necrosis factor α
TRADD: TNF receptor–associated death domain
TRAF: TNF receptor–associated factor
TRAIL: TNF-related apoptosis-inducing ligand
TRP: transient receptor potential
VEGF: vascular endothelial growth factor

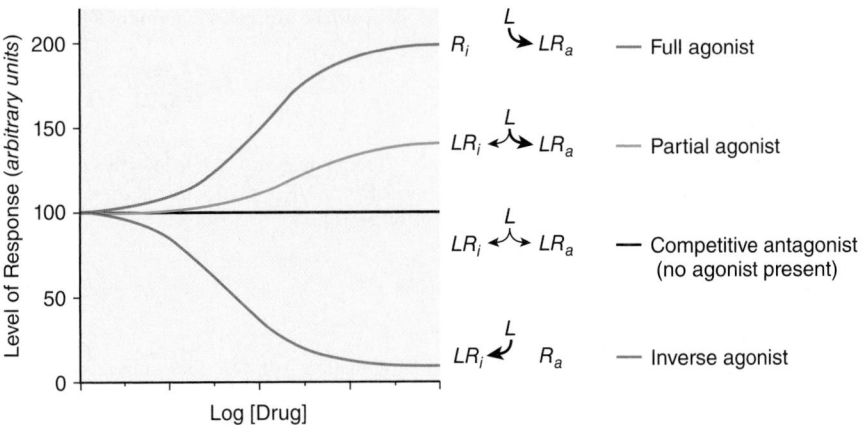

Figure 3–1 *Regulation of the activity of a receptor with conformation-selective drugs.* In this model, receptor R can exist in active (R_a) and inactive (R_i) conformations, and drugs binding to one, the other, or both states of R can influence the balance of the two forms of R and the net effect of receptor-controlled events. The ordinate is the activity of the receptor produced by R_a, the active receptor conformation (e.g., stimulation of AC by an activated β adrenergic receptor). If a drug L selectively binds to R_a, it will produce a maximal response. If L has equal affinity for R_i and R_a, it will not perturb the equilibrium between them and will have no effect on net activity; L would appear as a competitive antagonist if it blocks an agonist binding site (see Figure 3–4). If the drug selectively binds to R_i, then the net influence and amount of R_a will be diminished. If L can bind to receptor in an active conformation R_a but also bind to inactive receptor R_i with lower affinity, the drug will produce a partial response; L will be a partial agonist. If there is sufficient R_a to produce an elevated basal response in the absence of ligand (agonist-independent constitutive activity), and L binds to R_i, then that basal activity will be inhibited; L will then be an inverse agonist. Inverse agonists selectively bind to the inactive form of the receptor and shift the conformational equilibrium toward the inactive state. In systems that are not constitutively active, inverse agonists will behave like competitive antagonists, which helps explain that the properties of inverse agonists and the number of such agents previously described as competitive antagonists were only recently appreciated. Receptors that have constitutive activity and are sensitive to inverse agonists include benzodiazepine, histamine, opioid, cannabinoid, dopamine, bradykinin, and adenosine receptors.

multiple mechanisms of action that depend on receptor specificity, the tissue-specific expression of the receptor(s), drug access to target tissues, different drug concentrations in different tissues, pharmacogenetics, and interactions with other drugs.

Chronic administration of a drug may cause a *downregulation* of receptors or *desensitization* of response that can require dose adjustments to maintain adequate therapy. Chronic administration of nitrovasodilators to treat angina results in the rapid development of *complete tolerance*, a process known as *tachyphylaxis*. *Drug resistance* may also develop because of pharmacokinetic mechanisms (i.e., the drug is metabolized more rapidly with chronic exposure), the development of mechanisms that prevent the drug from reaching its receptor (i.e., increased expression of the multidrug resistance transporter in drug-resistant cancer cells; see Chapter 5), or the clonal expansion of cancer cells containing drug-resistant mutations in the drug receptor.

Some drug effects do not occur by means of macromolecular receptors. For instance, aluminum and magnesium hydroxides [$Al(OH)_3$ and $Mg(OH)_2$] reduce gastric acid chemically, neutralizing H^+ with OH^+ and raising gastric pH. Mannitol acts osmotically to cause changes in the distribution of water to promote diuresis, catharsis, expansion of circulating volume in the vascular compartment, or reduction of cerebral edema (see Chapter 25). Anti-infective drugs such as antibiotics, antivirals, and antiparasitics achieve specificity by targeting receptors or cell processes that are critical for the growth or survival of the infective agent but are nonessential or lacking in the host organism. Resistance to antibiotics, antivirals, and other drugs can occur through a variety of mechanisms, including mutation of the target receptor, increased expression of enzymes that degrade or increase efflux of the drug from the infective agent, and development of alternative biochemical pathways that circumvent the drug's effects on the infective agent.

Structure-Activity Relationships and Drug Design

The receptors responsible for the clinical effects of many drugs have yet to be identified. Conversely, sequencing of the entire human genome has identified novel genes related by sequence to known receptors, for which endogenous and exogenous ligands are unknown; these are called *orphan receptors*.

Both the affinity of a drug for its receptor and its intrinsic activity are determined by its chemical structure. This relationship frequently is stringent.

Relatively minor modifications in the drug molecule may result in major changes in its pharmacological properties based on altered affinity for one or more receptors. Exploitation of structure-activity relationships has frequently led to the synthesis of valuable therapeutic agents. Because changes in molecular configuration need not alter all actions and effects of a drug equally, it is sometimes possible to develop a congener with a more favorable ratio of therapeutic to adverse effects, enhanced selectivity amongst different cells or tissues, or more acceptable secondary characteristics than those of the parent drug. Therapeutically useful antagonists of hormones or neurotransmitters have been developed by chemical modification of the structure of the physiological agonist.

With information about the molecular structures and pharmacological activities of a relatively large group of congeners, it is possible to use computer analysis to identify the chemical properties (i.e., the *pharmacophore*) required for optimal action at the receptor: size, shape, position, and orientation of charged groups or hydrogen bond donors, and so on. Advances in molecular modeling of organic compounds and the methods for drug target (receptor) discovery and biochemical measurement of the primary actions of drugs at their receptors have enriched the quantitation of structure-activity relationships and its use in drug design (Carlson and McCammon, 2000). Such information increasingly is allowing the optimization or design of chemicals that can bind to a receptor with improved affinity, selectivity, or regulatory effect. Similar structure-based approaches also are used to improve pharmacokinetic properties of drugs, particularly if knowledge of their metabolism is known. Knowledge of the structures of receptors and of drug-receptor complexes, determined at atomic resolution by X-ray crystallography, is even more helpful in the design of ligands and in understanding the molecular basis of drug resistance and circumventing it. Emerging technology in the field of pharmacogenetics (see Chapter 7) is improving our understanding of the nature of and variation in receptors and their impact on pharmacotherapy (Jain, 2004).

Quantitative Aspects of Drug Interactions With Receptors

Receptor occupancy theory assumes that a drug's response emanates from a receptor occupied by the drug, a concept that has its basis in the law of mass action. The *dose-response curve* depicts the observed effect of a drug

34

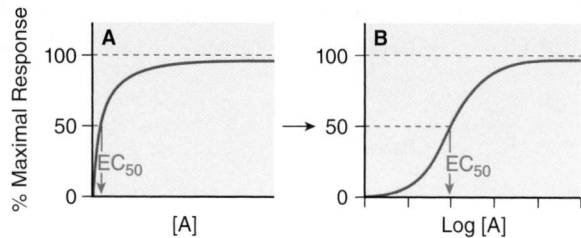

Figure 3–2 *Graded responses. On the* y *axis, the response is expressed as a percentage of maximal response plotted as a function of the concentration of drug A present at the receptor (x axis). The hyperbolic shape of the curve in panel* **A** *becomes sigmoid when plotted semilogarithmically, as in panel* **B**. The concentration of drug that produces 50% of the maximal response quantifies drug activity and is referred to as the EC$_{50}$ (effective concentration of agonist for 50% response). The range of concentrations needed to fully depict the dose-response relationship (~3 log$_{10}$ [10] units) is too wide to be useful in the linear format of Figure 3–2A; thus, most dose-response curves use log [Drug] on the x axis, as in Figure 3–2B. Dose-response curves presented in this way are sigmoidal in shape and have three noteworthy properties: threshold, slope, and maximal asymptote. These three parameters quantitate the activity of the drug.

as a function of its concentration in the receptor compartment. Figure 3–2 shows a typical dose-response curve, usually plotted as in Figure 3-2B.

Some drugs cause low-dose stimulation and high-dose inhibition. Such U-shaped relationships are said to display *hormesis*. Several drug-receptor systems can display this property (e.g., prostaglandins, endothelin, and purinergic and serotonergic agonists), which may be at the root of some drug toxicities (Calabrese and Baldwin, 2003).

Affinity, Efficacy, and Potency

In general, the drug-receptor interaction is characterized by (1) binding of drug to receptor and (2) generation of a response in a biological system, as illustrated in Equation 3–1, where the drug or ligand is denoted as *L* and the inactive receptor as *R*. The first reaction, the reversible formation of the ligand-receptor complex *LR*, is governed by the chemical property of *affinity*.

$$L+R \underset{k_{-1}}{\overset{k_{+1}}{\rightleftarrows}} LR \underset{k_{-2}}{\overset{k_{+2}}{\rightleftarrows}} LR^* \qquad \text{(Equation 3–1)}$$

LR* is produced in proportion to [*LR*] and leads to a *response*. This simple relationship illustrates the reliance of the affinity of the ligand (*L*) with receptor (*R*) on both the forward or *association rate* k_{+1} and the reverse or *dissociation rate* k_{-1}. At any given time, the concentration of ligand-receptor complex [*LR*] is equal to the product of $k_{+1}[L][R]$, the rate of formation of the bimolecular complex *LR*, minus the product $k_{-1}[LR]$, the rate of dissociation of *LR* into *L* and *R*. At equilibrium (i.e., when $\delta[LR]/\delta t = 0$), $k_{+1}[L][R] = k_{-1}[LR]$. The *equilibrium dissociation constant* K_D is then described by ratio of the off and on rate constants, k_{-1}/k_{+1}.

Thus, at equilibrium,

$$K_D = \frac{[L][R]}{[LR]} = \frac{k_{-1}}{k_{+1}} \qquad \text{(Equation 3–2)}$$

The *affinity constant* or *equilibrium association constant* K_A is the reciprocal of the equilibrium dissociation constant (i.e., $K_A = 1/K_D$); thus, *a high-affinity drug has a low K_D and will bind a greater number of a particular receptor at a low concentration than a low-affinity drug.* As a practical matter, the affinity of a drug is influenced most often by changes in its off rate (k_{-1}) rather than its on rate (k_{+1}).

Equation 3–2 permits us to describe the *fractional occupancy f* of receptors by agonist *L* as a function of [*R*] and [*LR*]:

$$f = \frac{[\text{ligand-receptor complexes}]}{[\text{total receptors}]} = \frac{[LR]}{[R]+[LR]} \qquad \text{(Equation 3–3)}$$

f can also be expressed in terms of K_A (or K_D) and [*L*]:

$$f = \frac{K_A[L]}{1+K_A[L]} = \frac{[L]}{1/K_A+[L]} = \frac{[L]}{K_D+[L]} \qquad \text{(Equation 3–4)}$$

From Equation 3–4, it follows that *when the concentration of drug equals the K_D (or $1/K_A$), f = 0.5, that is, the drug will occupy 50% of the receptors.* When [*L*] = K_D:

$$f = \frac{K_D}{K_D+K_D} = \frac{1}{2} \qquad \text{(Equation 3–4A)}$$

Equation 3–4 describes only receptor occupancy, not the eventual response that may be amplified by the cell. Because of downstream amplification, many signaling systems can reach a full biological response with only a fraction of receptors occupied.

Potency is defined by example in Figure 3–3. Basically, when two drugs produce equivalent responses, the drug whose dose-response curve (plotted as in Figure 3–3A) lies to the left of the other (i.e., the concentration producing a half-maximal effect [EC50] is smaller) is said to be the more potent.

Efficacy reflects the capacity of a drug to activate a receptor and generate a cellular response. Thus, a drug with high efficacy may be a full agonist, eliciting, at some concentration, a full response. A drug with a lower efficacy at the same receptor may not elicit a full response at any dose (see Figure 3–1). A drug with a low intrinsic efficacy will be a partial agonist. A drug that binds to a receptor and exhibits zero efficacy is an antagonist.

Quantifying Agonism

When the relative potency of two agonists of equal efficacy is measured in the same biological system and downstream signaling events are the same for both drugs, the comparison yields a relative measure of the affinity and efficacy of the two agonists (see Figure 3–3). We often describe agonist response by determining the *half-maximally effective concentration* (EC$_{50}$) for producing a given effect. We can also compare maximal

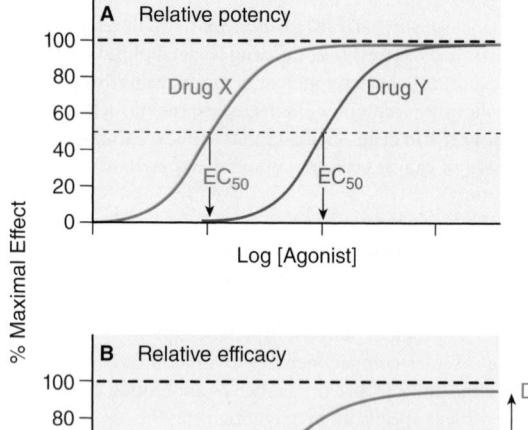

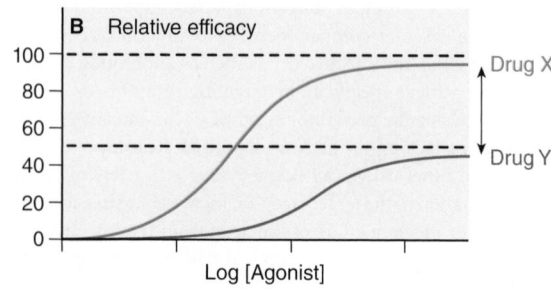

Figure 3–3 *Two ways of quantifying agonism.* **A.** The relative potency of two agonists (drug X, ____; *drug Y*, ____) obtained in the same tissue is a function of their relative affinities and intrinsic efficacies. The EC$_{50}$ of drug X occurs at a concentration that is one-tenth the EC$_{50}$ of drug Y. Thus, drug X is more potent than drug Y. **B.** In systems where the two drugs do not both produce the maximal response characteristic of the tissue, the observed maximal response is a nonlinear function of their relative intrinsic efficacies. Drug X is more efficacious than drug Y; their asymptotic fractional responses are 100% for drug X and 50% for drug Y.

asymptotes in systems where the agonists do not produce maximal response (Figure 3–3B). The advantage of using maxima is that this property depends solely on efficacy, whereas drug *potency* is a mixed function of both affinity and efficacy.

Quantifying Antagonism

Characteristic patterns of antagonism are associated with certain mechanisms of receptor blockade. One is straightforward *competitive antagonism*, whereby a drug with affinity for a receptor but lacking intrinsic efficacy (i.e., an antagonist) competes with the agonist for the primary binding site on the receptor (Ariens, 1954; Gaddum, 1957). *The characteristic pattern of such antagonism is the concentration-dependent production*

of a parallel shift to the right of the agonist dose-response curve with no change in the maximal response (Figure 3–4A). The magnitude of the rightward shift of the curve depends on the concentration of the antagonist and its affinity for the receptor (Schild, 1957). *A competitive antagonist will reduce the response to zero.*

A *partial agonist* similarly can compete with a "full" agonist for binding to the receptor. *However, increasing concentrations of a partial agonist will inhibit response to a finite level characteristic of the intrinsic efficacy of the partial agonist.* Partial agonists may be used therapeutically to buffer a response by inhibiting excessive receptor stimulation without totally abolishing receptor stimulation. For example, varenicline is a nicotinic receptor partial agonist used in smoking cessation therapy. Its utility

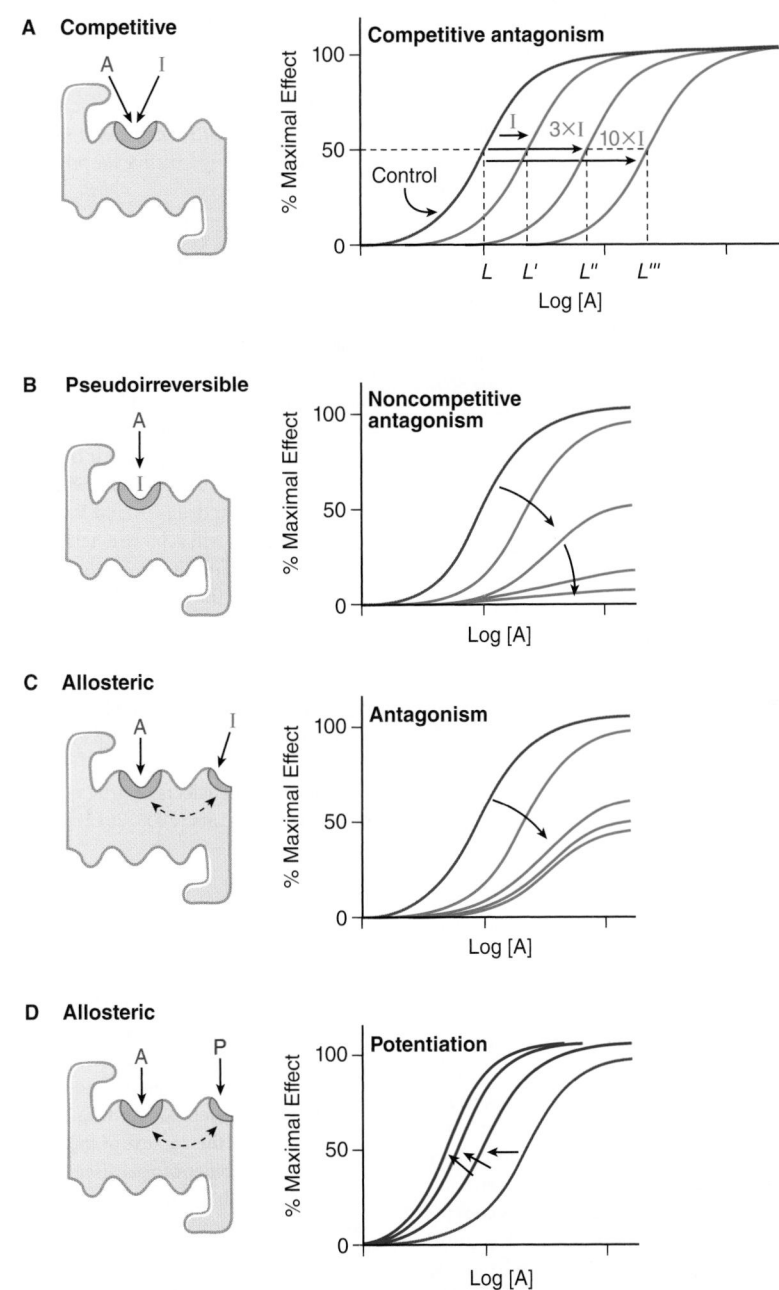

Figure 3–4 *Mechanisms of receptor antagonism.* In each set of curves, the green curve represents the effect of orthosteric agonist, unmodulated by any antagonist or potentiator. **A.** Competitive antagonism occurs when the agonist **A** and antagonist **I** compete for the same binding site on the receptor. Response curves for the agonist are shifted to the right in a concentration-related manner by the antagonist such that the EC$_{50}$ for the agonist increases (e.g., *L* versus *L′*, *L″*, and *L‴*) with the concentration of the antagonist. **B.** If the antagonist binds to the same site as the agonist but does so irreversibly or pseudoirreversibly (slow dissociation but no covalent bond), it causes a shift of the dose-response curve to the right, with progressive depression of the maximal response as [**I**] increases. Allosteric effects occur when an allosteric ligand **I** or **P** binds to a different site on the receptor to either inhibit (I) the response (panel **C**. Increasing concentrations of I shift the curves progressively to right and downward.) or potentiate (**P**) the response (panel **D**. Increasing concentrations of P shift the curves progressively to left.). This allosteric effect is saturable; inhibition or potentiation reaches a limiting value when the allosteric site is fully occupied.

derives from the fact that it activates brain nicotinic receptors sufficiently to prevent craving, but blocks the effects of high-dose nicotine delivered by smoking a cigarette.

An antagonist may dissociate so slowly from the receptor that its action is exceedingly prolonged. In the presence of a slowly dissociating antagonist, the maximal response to the agonist will be depressed at some antagonist concentrations (Figure 3–4B). Operationally, this is referred to as *noncompetitive antagonism*, although the molecular mechanism of action cannot be inferred unequivocally from the effect on the dose-response curve. An *irreversible antagonist* competing for the same binding site as the agonist can produce the same pattern of antagonism shown in Figure 3–4B. Noncompetitive antagonism can be produced by an *allosteric* or *allotopic antagonist*, which binds to a site on the receptor distinct from that of the primary agonist, thereby changing the affinity of the receptor for the agonist. *In the case of an allosteric antagonist, the affinity of the receptor for the agonist is decreased by the antagonist* (Figure 3–4C). In contrast, a drug binding at an allosteric site could potentiate the effects of primary agonists (Figure 3–4D); such a drug would be referred to as an *allosteric agonist* or *coagonist* (May et al., 2007).

The affinity of a competitive antagonist (K_i) *for its receptor can be determined in radioligand binding assays or by measuring the functional response of a system to a drug in the presence of the antagonist* (Cheng, 2004; Cheng and Prusoff, 1973; Limbird, 2005). Measuring a functional response, concentration curves are run with the agonist alone and with the agonist plus an effective concentration of the antagonist (see Figure 3–4A). As more antagonist (I) is added, a higher concentration of the agonist is needed to produce an equivalent response (the half-maximal, or 50%, response is a convenient and accurately determined level of response). *The extent of the rightward shift of the concentration-dependence curve is a measure of the affinity of the inhibitor, and a high-affinity inhibitor will cause a greater rightward shift than a low-affinity inhibitor at the same inhibitor concentration.*

Using Equations 3-3 and 3-4, one may write mathematical expressions of *fractional occupancy f* of the receptor R by an agonist ligand (L) for the agonist alone [$f_{control}$] and agonist in the presence of inhibitor [f_{+I}].

For the agonist drug alone, the fractional occupancy is given by Equations 3–3 and 3–4:

$$f_{control} = \frac{[L]}{[L] + K_D} \qquad \text{(Equation 3–5)}$$

For the case of agonist plus antagonist, the problem involves two equilibria:

$R + L \longleftrightarrow RL$ (fractional occupancy is expressed by Eq 3–5)

$$R + I \longleftrightarrow RI; \quad K_i = \frac{[R][I]}{[RI]} \text{ or } [RI] = \frac{[R][I]}{K_i} \qquad \text{(Equation 3–6)}$$

Fractional occupancy by the agonist L in the presence of I is:

$$f_{+I} = \frac{[RL]}{[RL] + [RI] + [R]} \qquad \text{(Equation 3–7)}$$

Equal fractional occupancies can occur in the absence and presence of a competitive inhibitor, but at different concentrations of agonist. The concentration of agonist needed to achieve a designated fractional occupancy in the presence of antagonist ([L']) will be greater than the concentration of agonist needed in the inhibitor's absence ([L]). Using the expressions for dissociation constants for the agonist and antagonist ligands (Equations 3-2 and 3-6) and applying a little algebraic tinkering to the righthand side of Equation 3-7, the fractional occupancy in the presence of the competitive inhibitor [f_{+I}] can be expressed in terms of L', K_D, K_i, and I:

$$f_{+I} = \frac{[L']}{[L'] + K_D \left(1 + \frac{[I]}{K_i}\right)} \qquad \text{(Equation 3–8)}$$

Assuming that equal responses result from equal fractional receptor occupancies in both the absence and presence of antagonist, one can set the fractional occupancies equal at experimentally determined agonist concentrations ([L] and [L']) that generate equivalent responses, as depicted in Figure 3–4A. Thus,

$$f_{control} = f_{+I} \qquad \text{(Equation 3–9)}$$

$$\frac{[L]}{[L] + K_D} = \frac{[L']}{[L'] + K_D \left(1 + \frac{[I]}{K_i}\right)} \qquad \text{(Equation 3–10)}$$

Simplifying, one obtains

$$\frac{[L']}{[L]} - 1 = \frac{[I]}{K_i} \qquad \text{(Equation 3–11)}$$

where all values are known except K_i. *Thus, one can determine the K_i for a reversible, competitive antagonist without knowing the K_D for the agonist and without needing to define the precise relationship between receptor and response.*

Additivity and Synergism: Isobolograms

Drugs with different mechanisms of action are often used in combination to achieve *additive* and *positive synergistic* effects (Figure 3–5). Such positive interactions of two agents may permit use of reduced concentrations of each drug, thereby reducing concentration-dependent adverse effects. *Positive synergism* refers to the *superadditive* effects of drugs used in combination. Drugs used in combination can also demonstrate *negative synergism* or *subadditive effects*, where the efficacy of the drug combination is less than would be expected if the effects were additive. Figure 3–5 is a plot known as an *isobologram*, which shows that a line connecting the EC_{50} values of two drugs, A and B, describes the relative concentrations of each drug that will achieve a half-maximal response *when A and B are used in combination, if the effects of A and B are additive*. Similar lines drawn parallel to the 50% additive line can be used to determine the relative concentrations of A and B required to achieve other responses (e.g., 10%, 20%, 80%, 90%, etc.). If A and B are superadditive (positive synergism), the relative concentrations of A and B needed to achieve a given response will fall below the additive response line. Conversely, if A and B are subadditive (negative synergism), their relative concentrations will lie above the additive response line. The basis for the use of isobolograms in characterizing the effects of drug combinations has been developed and reviewed by Tallarida (2006, 2012).

Pharmacodynamic Variability: Individual and Population Pharmacodynamics

Individuals vary in the magnitude of their response to the same concentration of a single drug, and a given individual may not always respond in the same way to the same drug concentration. Drug responsiveness may change because of disease, age, or previous drug administration. Receptors are dynamic, and their concentrations and functions may be up- or downregulated by endogenous and exogenous factors.

Data on the correlation of drug levels with efficacy and toxicity must be interpreted in the context of the pharmacodynamic variability in the population (e.g., genetics, age, disease, and the presence of coadministered drugs). The variability in pharmacodynamic response in the population may be analyzed by constructing a *quantal concentration-effect curve* (Figure 3–6A). The dose of a drug required to produce a specified effect in 50% of the population is the *median effective dose* (ED_{50}; see Figure 3–6A). In preclinical studies of drugs, the *median lethal dose* (LD_{50}) is determined in experimental animals (Figure 3–6B). The LD_{50}/ED_{50} ratio is an indication of the *therapeutic index*, a term that reflects how selective the drug is in producing its desired effects versus its adverse effects. A similar term, the *therapeutic window*, is the range of steady-state concentrations of drug that provides therapeutic efficacy with minimal toxicity (Figures 2–9 and 3–7). In clinical studies, the dose, or preferably the concentration, of a drug required to produce toxic effects can be compared with

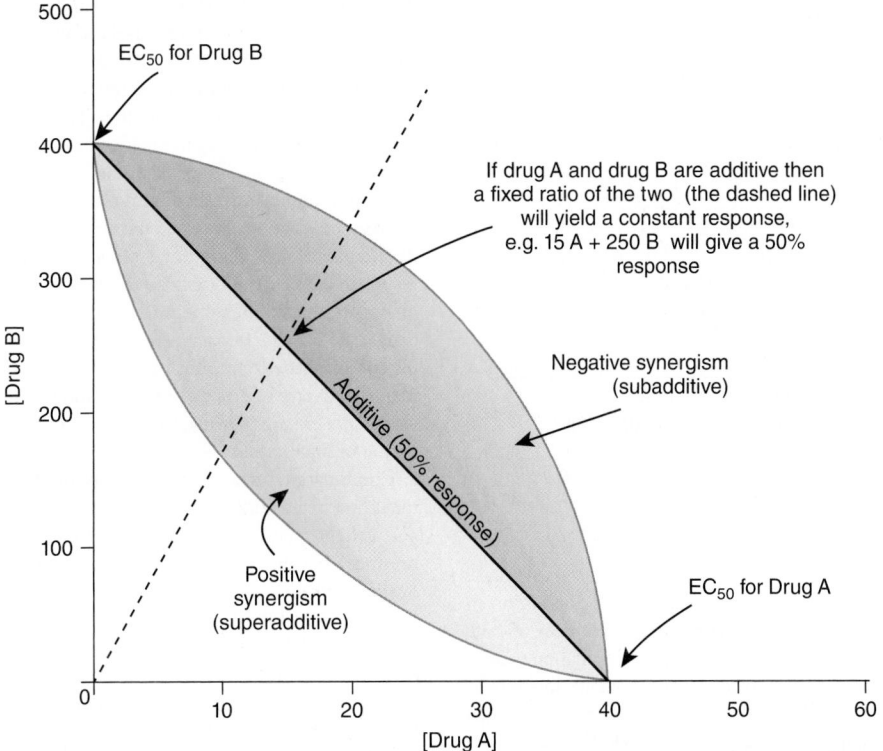

Figure 3–5 *Isobologram showing additivity and synergism of a drug combination.* The isobologram shows the line of additivity for a 50% effect obtained with a combination of two drugs (concentrations of drug A are on the *x* axis, concentrations of drug B are on the *y* axis) that have similar effects but different mechanisms of action. The intercept of the line of additivity (50% effect) with the *x* axis is the EC_{50} for A, while the intercept on the *y* axis is the EC_{50} for B. If the combination of A and B exhibits positive synergism (superadditivity), then the 50% effect with a combination of the two drugs will fall somewhere below the line of additivity, whereas negative synergism (subadditivity) will fall above the line of additivity. Lines of additivity for different percentage effects (e.g., 90% effect) are parallel to the 50% line of additivity. The isobologram can be used to estimate the concentrations of two drugs needed to obtain a given effect when used in combination. For a full explanation of the concept and utility of isoboles, consult Tallarida (2006, 2012).

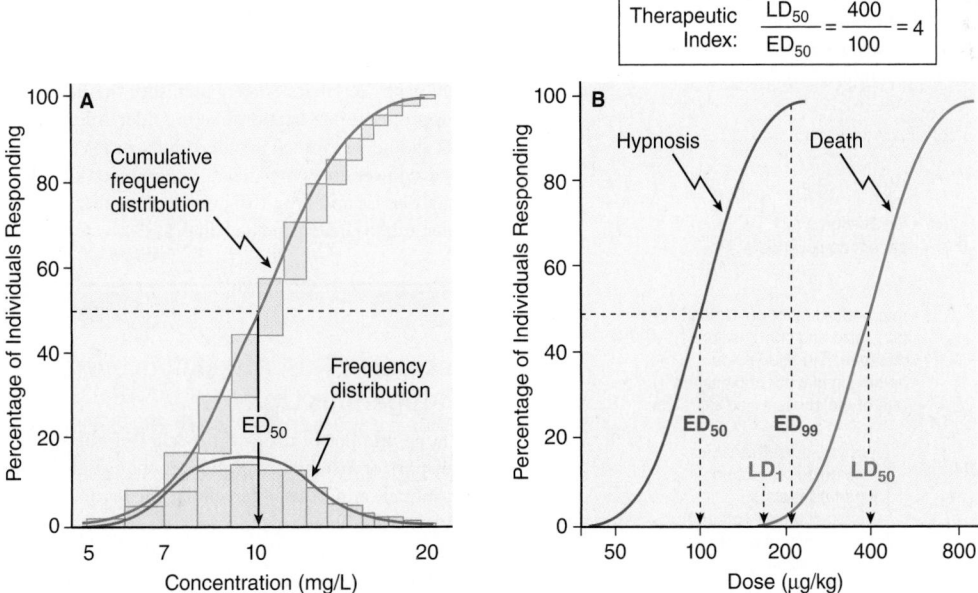

Figure 3–6 *Frequency distribution curves and quantal concentration-effect and dose-effect curves.* **A.** *Frequency distribution curves.* An experiment was performed on 100 subjects, and the effective plasma concentration that produced a quantal response was determined for each individual. The number of subjects who required each dose was plotted, giving a log-normal frequency distribution (**purple bars**). The normal frequency distribution, when summated, yields the cumulative frequency distribution—a sigmoidal curve that is a quantal concentration-effect curve (red bars, red line). **B.** *Quantal dose-effect curves.* Animals were injected with varying doses of a drug, and the responses were determined and plotted. The therapeutic index, the ratio of the LD_{50} to the ED_{50}, is an indication of how selective a drug is in producing its desired effects relative to its toxicity. See text for additional explanation.

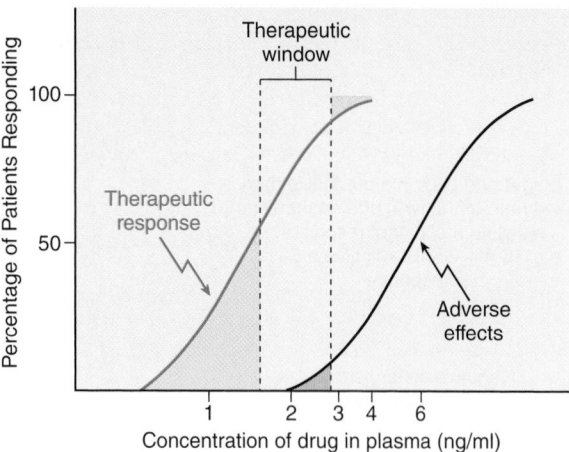

Figure 3–7 *Relation of the therapeutic window of drug concentrations to therapeutic and adverse effects in the population.* The ordinate is linear; the abscissa is logarithmic.

the concentration required for therapeutic effects in the population to evaluate the *clinical therapeutic index.* The concentration or dose of drug required to produce a therapeutic effect in most of the population usually will overlap the concentration required to produce toxicity in some of the population, even though the drug's therapeutic index in an individual patient may be large. Thus, a *population therapeutic window* expresses a range of concentrations at which the likelihood of efficacy is high and the probability of adverse effects is low (see Figure 3–7); it does not guarantee efficacy or safety. *Therefore, use of the population therapeutic window to optimize the dosage of a drug should be complemented by monitoring appropriate clinical and surrogate markers for drug effect(s) in a given patient.*

Factors Modifying Drug Action

Numerous factors contribute to the wide patient-to-patient variability in the dose required for optimal therapy observed with many drugs (Figure 3–8). The effects of these factors on variability of drug pharmacokinetics are described more thoroughly in Chapters 2, 5, 6, and 7.

Drug Interactions and Combination Therapy

Drugs are commonly used in combination with other drugs, sometimes to achieve an additive or synergistic effect, but more often because two or more drugs are needed to treat multiple conditions. When drugs are used

in combination, one cannot assume that their effects are the same as when each agent is administered by itself. Marked alterations in the effects of some drugs can result from coadministration with other agents, including prescription and nonprescription drugs, supplements, and nutraceuticals. Such interactions can cause toxicity or inhibit the drug effect and the therapeutic benefit. Drug interactions always should be considered when unexpected responses to drugs occur. Understanding the mechanisms of drug interactions provides a framework for preventing them.

Drug interactions may be pharmacokinetic (the delivery of a drug to its site of action is altered by a second drug) or pharmacodynamic (the response of the drug target is modified by a second drug). Examples of pharmacokinetic interactions that can enhance or diminish the delivery of drug to its site of action are provided in Chapter 2. In a patient with multiple comorbidities requiring a variety of medications, it may be difficult to identify adverse effects due to medication interactions and to determine whether these are pharmacokinetic, pharmacodynamic, or some combination of interactions.

Combination therapy constitutes optimal treatment of many conditions, including heart failure (see Chapter 29), hypertension (see Chapter 28), and cancer (see Chapters 65–68). However, some drug combinations produce pharmacodynamic interactions that result in adverse effects. For example, nitrovasodilators produce vasodilation via NO-dependent elevation of cGMP in vascular smooth muscle. The pharmacologic effects of sildenafil, tadalafil, and vardenafil result from inhibition of the PDE5 that hydrolyzes cGMP to 5′GMP in the vasculature. Thus, coadministration of an NO donor (e.g., nitroglycerin) with a PDE5 inhibitor can cause potentially catastrophic vasodilation and severe hypotension.

The oral anticoagulant warfarin has a narrow margin between therapeutic inhibition of clot formation and bleeding complications and is subject to numerous important pharmacokinetic and pharmacodynamic drug interactions. Alterations in dietary vitamin K intake may significantly affect the pharmacodynamics of warfarin and mandate altered dosing; antibiotics that alter the intestinal flora reduce the bacterial synthesis of vitamin K, thereby enhancing the effect of warfarin; concurrent administration of NSAIDs with warfarin increases the risk of GI bleeding almost 4-fold compared with warfarin alone. By inhibiting platelet aggregation, aspirin increases the incidence of bleeding in warfarin-treated patients.

Most drugs are evaluated in young and middle-aged adults, and data on their use in children and the elderly are sparse. At the extremes of age, drug pharmacokinetics and pharmacodynamics can be altered, possibly requiring avoidance of selected drugs or substantial alteration in the dose or dosing regimen to safely produce the desired clinical effect. The American Geriatrics Society publishes the Beers Criteria for Potentially Inappropriate Medication Use in Older Adults, an explicit list of drugs that should be avoided in older adults, drugs that should be avoided or be used at lower doses in patients with reduced kidney function, and specific drug-disease and drug-drug interactions that are known to be harmful in older adults (Beers Update Panel, 2015).

Mechanisms of Drug Action

Receptors That Affect Concentrations of Endogenous Ligands

A large number of drugs act by altering the synthesis, storage, release, transport, or metabolism of endogenous ligands such as neurotransmitters, hormones, and other intercellular mediators. For example, some of the drugs acting on adrenergic neurotransmission include *α-methyltyrosine* (inhibits synthesis of NE), *cocaine* (blocks NE reuptake), *amphetamine* (promotes NE release), and *selegiline* (inhibits NE breakdown by MAO) (see Chapters 8 and 12). There are similar examples for other neurotransmitter systems, including ACh (see Chapters 8 and 10), DA, and 5HT (see Chapters 13–16). Drugs that affect the synthesis and degradation of circulating mediators such as vasoactive peptides (e.g., ACE inhibitors; see Chapter 26) and lipid-derived autocoids (e.g., cyclooxygenase inhibitors; see Chapter 37) are also widely used in the treatment of hypertension, inflammation, myocardial ischemia, and heart failure.

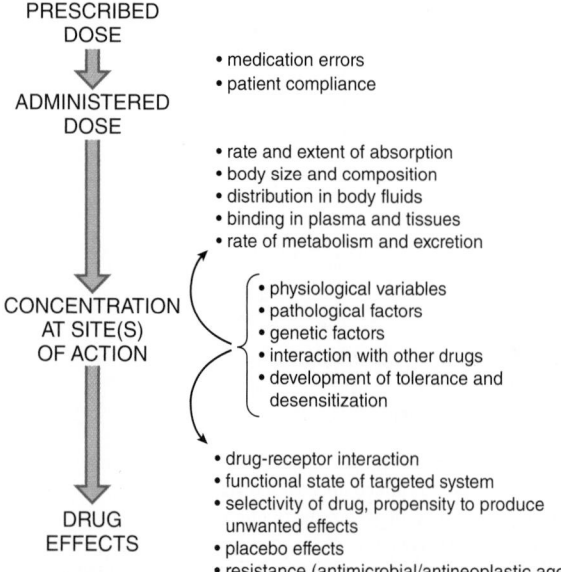

Figure 3–8 *Factors influencing the response to a prescribed drug dose.*

Drug Receptors Associated With Extracellular Processes

Many widely used drugs target enzymes and molecules that control extracellular processes such as thrombosis, inflammation, and immune responses. For instance, the coagulation system is highly regulated and has a number of drug targets that control the formation and degradation of clots, including several coagulation factors (thrombin and factor Xa), antithrombin, and glycoproteins on the surface of platelets that control platelet activation and aggregation (see Chapter 32).

Receptors Utilized by Anti-infective Agents

Anti-infective agents such as antibacterials, antivirals, antifungals, and antiparasitic agents target receptors that are microbial proteins. These proteins are key enzymes in biochemical pathways that are required by the infectious agent but are not critical for the host. Examples of the various mechanisms of action of antibiotics are described in Chapters 52 through 64. A novel approach to preventing infections such as that of the mosquito-borne malaria parasite is to genetically engineer the vector organism to be resistant to infection by the parasite using techniques such as the CRISPR-Cas9 system. Although this approach is just being tested outside the laboratory and must undergo numerous regulatory hurdles before being used on a wide scale, it provides proof of principle that interrupting the life cycle of a parasite in the vector could be as effective as treating the infected host (see Chapter 53).

Receptors That Regulate the Ionic Milieu

A relatively small number of drugs act by affecting the ionic milieu of blood, urine, and the GI tract. The receptors for these drugs are ion pumps and transporters, many of which are expressed only in specialized cells of the kidney and GI tract. Most of the diuretics (e.g., furosemide, chlorothiazide, amiloride) act by directly affecting ion pumps and transporters in epithelial cells of the nephron that increase the movement of Na^+ into the urine or by altering the expression of ion pumps in these cells (e.g., aldosterone). Another therapeutically important target is the H^+,K^+-ATPase (proton pump) of gastric parietal cells. Irreversible inhibition of this proton pump by drugs such as esomeprazole reduces gastric acid secretion by 80%–95% (see Chapter 49).

Intracellular Pathways Activated by Physiological Receptors

Signal Transduction Pathways

The largest number of drug receptors are physiological receptors expressed on the surface of cells that transduce extracellular signals to signals within cells that alter cellular processes. Physiological receptors on the surface of cells have two major functions, ligand binding and message propagation (i.e., transmembrane and intracellular signaling). These functions imply the existence of at least two functional domains within the receptor: a *LBD* and an *effector domain*.

The regulatory actions of a receptor may be exerted directly on its cellular target(s), on *effector protein(s)*, or on intermediary cellular signaling molecules called *transducers*. The receptor, its cellular target, and any intermediary molecules are referred to as a *receptor-effector system* or *signal transduction pathway*. Frequently, the proximal cellular effector protein is not the ultimate physiological target but rather is an enzyme, ion channel, or transport protein that creates, moves, or degrades a small molecule (e.g., a cyclic nucleotide, IP_3, or NO) or ion (e.g., Ca^{2+}) termed a *second messenger*. Second messengers can diffuse in the proximity of their synthesis or release and convey information to a variety of targets that may integrate multiple signals. Even though these second messengers originally were thought of as freely diffusible molecules within the cell, biochemical and imaging studies show that their diffusion and intracellular actions are constrained by *compartmentation*—selective localization of receptor/transducer/effector/signal/signal termination complexes—established by protein-lipid and protein-protein interactions (Baillie, 2009). All cells express multiple forms of proteins designed to localize signaling pathways

by protein-protein interactions; these proteins are termed *scaffolds* or *anchoring proteins* (Carnegie et al., 2009).

Receptors and their associated effector and transducer proteins also act as integrators of information as they coordinate signals from multiple ligands with each other and with the differentiated activity of the target cell. For example, signal transduction systems regulated by changes in cAMP and intracellular Ca^{2+} are integrated in many excitable tissues. In cardiac myocytes, an increase in cellular cAMP caused by activation of β adrenergic receptors enhances cardiac contractility by augmenting the rate and amount of Ca^{2+} delivered to the contractile apparatus; thus, cAMP and Ca^{2+} are positive contractile signals in cardiac myocytes. By contrast, cAMP and Ca^{2+} produce opposing effects on the contraction of SMCs: As usual, Ca^{2+} is a contractile signal; however, activation of β receptor-cAMP-PKA pathway in these cells leads to relaxation through the phosphorylation of proteins that mediate Ca^{2+} signaling, such as MLCK and ion channels that hyperpolarize the cell membrane.

Another important property of physiological receptors is their capacity to significantly amplify a physiological signal. Neurotransmitters, hormones, and other extracellular ligands are often present at the LBD of a receptor in very low concentrations (nanomolar to micromolar levels). However, the effector domain or the signal transduction pathway often contains enzymes and enzyme cascades that catalytically amplify the intended signal. These signaling systems are excellent targets for drugs.

Structural and Functional Families of Physiological Receptors

Receptors for physiological regulatory molecules can be assigned to functional families that share common molecular structures and biochemical mechanisms. Table 3–1 outlines six major families of receptors with examples of their physiological ligands, signal transduction systems, and drugs that affect these systems.

G Protein–Coupled Receptors

The GPCRs comprise a large family of transmembrane receptors (Figure 3–9) that span the plasma membrane as a bundle of seven α helices (Palczewski et al., 2000) (Figure 3–10). Amongst the ligands for GPCRs are neurotransmitters such as ACh, biogenic amines such as NE, all eicosanoids and other lipid-signaling molecules, peptide hormones, opioids, amino acids such as GABA, and many other peptide and protein ligands. GPCRs are important regulators of nerve activity in the CNS and are the receptors for the neurotransmitters of the peripheral autonomic nervous system (GPCR Network; Stevens et al., 2013). Because of their number and physiological importance, GPCRs are the targets for many drugs.

GPCR Subtypes.   There are multiple receptor subtypes within families of receptors. Ligand-binding studies initially identified receptor subtypes; molecular cloning has greatly accelerated the discovery and definition of additional receptor subtypes; their expression as recombinant proteins has facilitated the discovery of subtype-selective drugs. The distinction between classes and subtypes of receptors, however, is often arbitrary or historical. The $α_1$, $α_2$, and β adrenergic receptors differ from each other both in ligand selectivity and in coupling to G proteins (G_q, G_i, and G_s, respectively), yet α and β are considered receptor classes and $α_1$ and $α_2$ are considered subtypes. Pharmacological differences amongst receptor subtypes are exploited therapeutically through the development and use of receptor-selective drugs. For example, $β_2$ adrenergic agonists such as terbutaline are used for bronchodilation in the treatment of asthma in the hope of minimizing cardiac side effects caused by stimulation of the $β_1$ adrenergic receptor (see Chapter 12). Conversely, the use of $β_1$-selective antagonists minimizes the likelihood of bronchoconstriction in patients being treated for hypertension or angina (see Chapters 12, 27, and 28).

Receptor Dimerization.   GPCRs undergo both homo- and heterodimerization and possibly oligomerization. Dimerization of receptors may regulate the affinity and specificity of the complex for G proteins and the sensitivity of the receptor to phosphorylation by receptor kinases and the binding of arrestin, events important in termination of the action of agonists and removal of receptors from the cell surface. Dimerization also may permit binding of receptors to other regulatory proteins, such as transcription factors.

TABLE 3-1 ■ PHYSIOLOGICAL RECEPTORS

STRUCTURAL FAMILY	FUNCTIONAL FAMILY	PHYSIOLOGICAL LIGANDS	EFFECTORS AND TRANSDUCERS	EXAMPLE DRUGS
GPCR	β Adrenergic receptors	NE, EPI, DA	G_s; AC	Dobutamine, propranolol
	Muscarinic cholinergic receptors	ACh	G_i and G_q; AC, ion channels, PLC	Atropine
	Eicosanoid receptors	Prostaglandins, leukotrienes, thromboxanes	G_s, G_i, and G_q proteins	Misoprostol, montelukast
	Thrombin receptors (PAR)	Receptor peptide	$G_{12/13}$, GEFs	(In development)
Ion channels	Ligand gated	ACh (M_2), GABA, 5HT	Na^+, Ca^{2+}, K^+, Cl^-	Nicotine, gabapentin
	Voltage gated	None (activated by membrane depolarization)	Na^+, Ca^{2+}, K^+, other ions	Lidocaine, verapamil
Transmembrane enzymes	Receptor tyrosine kinases	Insulin, PDGF, EGF, VEGF, growth factors	SH2 domain and PTB-containing proteins	Herceptin, imatinib
	Membrane bound GC	Natriuretic peptides	cGMP	Nesiritide
	Tyrosine phosphatases	Pleiotrophin, contactins	Tyr-phosphorylated proteins	
Transmembrane, nonenzymes	Cytokine receptors	Interleukins and other cytokines	Jak/STAT, soluble tyrosine kinases	Interferons, anakinra
	Toll-like receptors	Lipopolysaccharide, bacterial products	MyD88, IRAKs, NF-kB	(In development)
Nuclear receptors	Steroid receptors	Estrogen, testosterone	Coactivators	Estrogens, androgens, cortisol
	Thyroid hormone receptors	Thyroid hormone		Thyroid hormone
	PPARγ	PPARγ		Thiazolidinediones
Intracellular enzymes	Soluble GC	NO, Ca^{2+}	cGMP	Nitrovasodilators

G Proteins. GPCRs couple to a family of heterotrimeric GTP-binding regulatory proteins termed *G proteins.* G proteins are signal transducers that convey the information from the agonist-bound receptor to one or more effector proteins. G protein–regulated effectors include enzymes such as AC, PLC, cGMP PDE6, and membrane ion channels selective for Ca^{2+} and K^+ (see Table 3–1 and Figure 3–10).

The G protein heterotrimer consists of a guanine nucleotide-binding α subunit, which confers specific recognition to both receptors and effectors, and an associated dimer of β and γ subunits that helps confer membrane localization of the G protein heterotrimer by prenylation of the γ subunit. In the basal state of the receptor-heterotrimer complex, the α subunit contains bound GDP, and the α-GDP:βγ complex is bound to the unliganded receptor (Gilman, 1987) (see Figure 3–9). The α subunits fall into four families (G_s, G_i, G_q, and $G_{12/13}$), which are responsible for coupling GPCRs to relatively distinct effectors. The G_sα subunit uniformly activates AC; the G_iα subunit inhibits certain isoforms of AC; the G_qα subunit activates all forms of PLCβ; and the $G_{12/13}$α subunits couple to GEFs, such as p115RhoGEF for the small GTP-binding proteins Rho and Rac (Etienne-Manneville and Hall, 2002). The signaling specificity of the large number of possible βγ combinations is not yet clear; nonetheless, it is known that K^+ channels, Ca^{2+} channels, and PI3K are some of the effectors of free βγ dimer. In the instance of cAMP signaling, endocytosis of GPCRs can prolong aspects of signaling and lend "spatial coding" to distal signaling and regulation of transcription (Irannejad et al., 2015). Figure 3–10 and its legend summarize the basic activation/inactivation scheme for GPCR-linked systems.

Second-Messenger Systems. *Cyclic AMP.* cAMP is synthesized by the enzyme AC; stimulation is mediated by the G_sα subunit, inhibition by the G_iα subunit. There are nine membrane-bound isoforms of AC and one soluble isoform found in mammals (Dessauer et al., 2017; Hanoune and Defer, 2001). cAMP generated by ACs has three major targets in most cells: the cAMP-dependent PKA; cAMP-regulated GEFs termed EPACs (Cheng et al., 2008; Roscioni et al., 2008); and, via PKA phosphorylation, a transcription factor termed CREB (Mayr and Montminy, 2001; Sands and Palmer, 2008). In cells with specialized functions, cAMP can have additional targets, such as CNG and HCN (Wahl-Schott and Biel, 2009), and cyclic nucleotide-regulated PDEs. For an overview of cyclic nucleotide action and a historical perspective, see Beavo and Brunton (2002).

- **PKA.** The PKA holoenzyme consists of two catalytic (C) subunits reversibly bound to a regulatory (R) subunit dimer to form a heterotetrameric complex (R_2C_2). When AC is activated and cAMP concentrations increase, four cAMP molecules bind to the R_2C_2 complex, two to each R subunit, causing a conformational change in the R subunits that lowers their affinity for the C subunits, resulting in their activation. The active C subunits phosphorylate serine and threonine residues on specific protein substrates. There are multiple isoforms of PKA; molecular cloning has revealed α and β isoforms of both the regulatory subunits (RI and RII), as well as three C subunit isoforms Cα, Cβ, and Cγ. The R subunits exhibit different subcellular localization and binding affinities for cAMP, giving rise to PKA holoenzymes with different thresholds for activation (Taylor et al., 2008). PKA function also is modulated by subcellular localization mediated by AKAPs (Carnegie et al., 2009).

- **PKG.** Stimulation of receptors that raise intracellular cGMP concentrations (see Figure 3–13) leads to the activation of the cGMP-dependent PKG that phosphorylates some of the same substrates as PKA and some that are PKG-specific. Unlike the heterotetramer (R_2C_2) structure of the PKA holoenzyme, the catalytic domain and cyclic nucleotide-binding domains of PKG are expressed as a single polypeptide, which dimerizes to form the PKG holoenzyme.

Protein kinase G exists in two homologous forms, PKG-I and PKG-II. PKG-I has an acetylated N terminus, is associated with the cytoplasm,

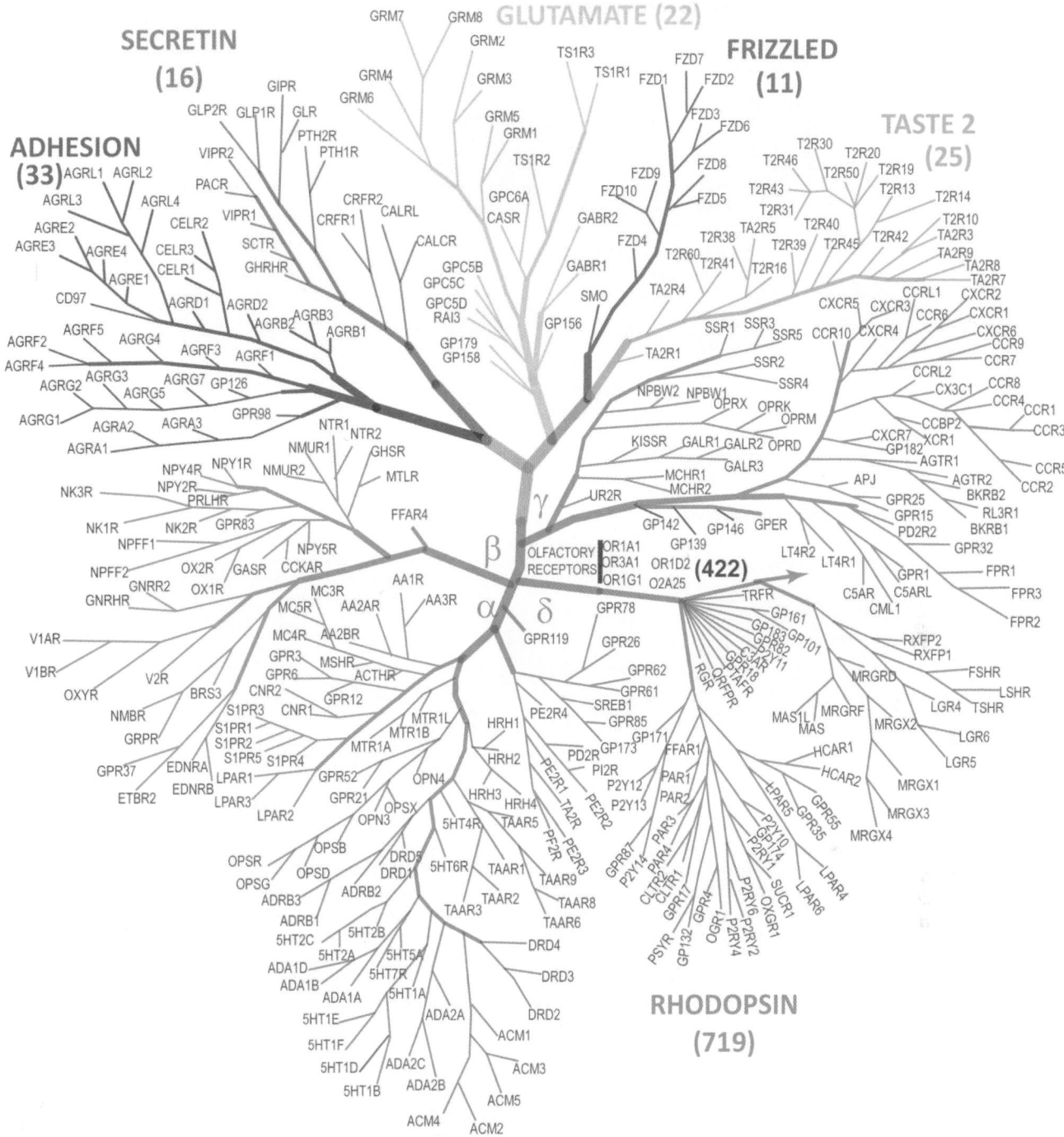

Figure 3–9 *The human GPCR superfamily.* Human GPCRs are targeted by about 30% of marketed drugs. This dendrogram, constructed using sequence similarities within the seven-transmembrane region, identifies GPCRs by their names in the UniProt database. There are over 825 human GPCRs, which can be subdivided into the color-coded groups named by the capitalized words on the outer edge of the dendrogram (number of group members in parentheses). These groups can be further subdivided on the basis of sequence similarity. The large Rhodopsin class is subdivided into four broad groups: α, β, δ, and γ. Olfactory receptors constitute the largest fraction of the Rhodopsin class of GPCRs, with 422 members. Receptors on the dendrogram that readers will frequently encounter include AA2AR, A$_{2A}$ adenosine receptor; ACM3, M$_3$ muscarinic acetylcholine receptor; ADRB1, β$_1$ adrenergic receptor; AGTR1, AT$_1$ angiotensin receptor; CNR1, CB$_1$ cannabinoid receptor; CXCR4, CXC$_4$ chemokine receptor; DRD2, D$_2$ dopamine receptor; EDNRA, ET$_A$ endothelin receptor; FPR1, f-Met-Leu-Phe receptor; GCGR, glucagon receptor; GRM1, mGluR$_1$ metabotropic glutamate receptor; HRH1, H$_1$ histamine receptor; 5HT2B, the 5HT$_{2B}$ serotonin receptor; OPRM, μ opioid receptor; RHO, rhodopsin; SMO, smoothened homolog; S1PR1, S1P$_1$ sphingosine-1-phosphate receptor, also known as EDG$_1$; TSHR, thyrotropin (TSH) receptor; and VIPR1, V$_1$ vasoactive intestinal peptide receptor. Details of entries on the dendrogram are available from the GPCR Network (http://gpcr.usc.edu). Additional information on GPCRs is available from the IUPHAR/BPS Guide to Pharmacology (http://www.guidetopharmacology.org). (Reproduced with permission from Angela Walker, Vsevolod Katrich, and Raymond Stevens of the GPCR Network at the University of Southern California, as created in the Stevens lab by Yekaterina Kadyshevskaya.)

A. Activation by Ligand Binding of GPCR

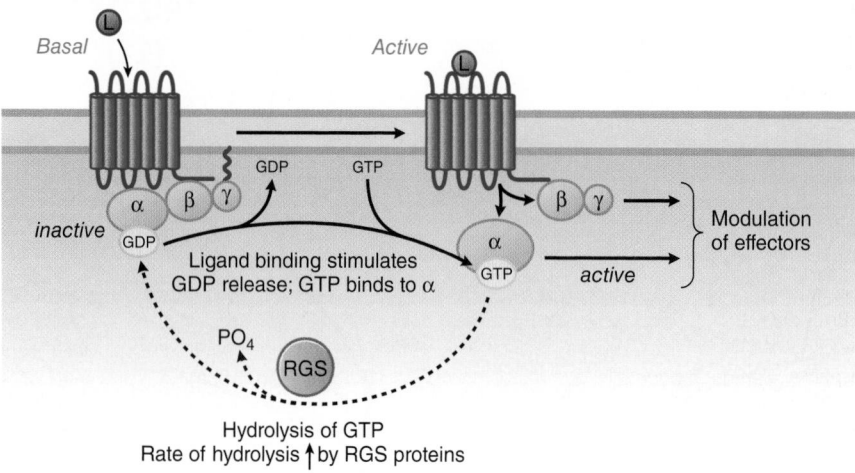

B. Modulation of Effectors

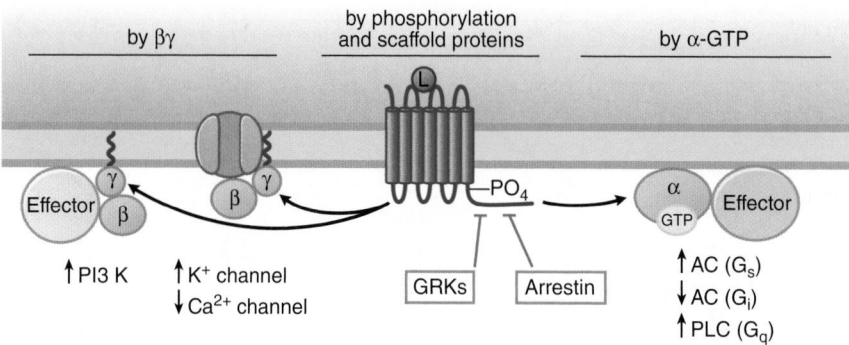

Figure 3–10 *The basic GPCR-G$_s$ protein-effector pathway.* In the absence of ligand, the GPCR and G protein heterotrimer form a complex in the membrane with the Gα subunit bound to GDP. Following binding of ligand, the receptor and G protein α subunit undergo a conformational change leading to release of GDP, binding of GTP, and dissociation of the complex. The activated GTP-bound Gα subunit and the freed βγ dimer bind to and regulate effectors. The system is returned to the basal state by hydrolysis of the GTP on the α subunit, a reaction that is markedly enhanced by the RGS proteins. Prolonged stimulation of the receptor can lead to downregulation of the receptor. This event is initiated by GRKs that phosphorylate the C-terminal tail of the receptor, leading to recruitment of proteins termed arrestins; arrestins bind to the receptor on the internal surface, displacing G proteins and inhibiting signaling. Detailed descriptions of these signaling pathways are given throughout the text in relation to the therapeutic actions of drugs affecting these pathways.

and has two isoforms (Iα and Iβ) that arise from alternate splicing. PKG-II has a myristylated N-terminus, is membrane-associated, and can be localized by PKG-anchoring proteins in a manner analogous to that for PKA, although the docking domains of PKA and PKG differ structurally. Pharmacologically important effects of elevated cGMP include modulation of platelet activation and relaxation of smooth muscle (Rybalkin et al., 2003). Receptors linked to cGMP synthesis are covered in a separate section that follows.

- **PDEs.** Cyclic nucleotide PDEs form another family of important signaling proteins whose activities are regulated via the rate of gene transcription as well as by second messengers (cyclic nucleotides or Ca^{2+}) and interactions with other signaling proteins such as β arrestin and PKs. PDEs hydrolyze the cyclic 3′,5′-phosphodiester bond in cAMP and cGMP, thereby terminating their action. The PDEs comprise a superfamily with more than 50 different proteins (Conti and Beavo, 2007). The substrate specificities of the different PDEs include those specific for cAMP hydrolysis and for cGMP hydrolysis and some that hydrolyze both cyclic nucleotides. PDEs (mainly PDE3 forms) are drug targets for treatment of diseases such as asthma, cardiovascular diseases such as heart failure, atherosclerotic coronary and peripheral arterial disease, and neurological disorders. PDE5 inhibitors (e.g., sildenafil)

are used in treating chronic obstructive pulmonary disease and erectile dysfunction (Mehats et al., 2002).

- **EPACs.** EPAC, also known as cAMP-GEF, is a novel cAMP-dependent signaling protein that plays unique roles in cAMP signaling. cAMP signaling through EPAC can occur in isolation or in concert with PKA signaling (Schmidt et al., 2013). EPAC serves as a cAMP-regulated GEF for the family of small Ras GTPases (especially the Rap small GTPases), catalyzing the exchange of GTP for GDP, thus activating the small GTPase by promoting formation of the GTP-bound form. Two isoforms of EPAC are known, EPAC1 and EPAC2; they differ in their architecture and tissue expression. Both EPAC isoforms are multidomain proteins that contain a regulatory cAMP-binding domain, a catalytic domain, and domains that determine the intracellular localization of EPAC. Compared to EPAC2, EPAC1 contains an additional N-terminal low-affinity cAMP-binding domain. The expression of EPAC1 and EPAC2 are differentially regulated during development and in a variety of disease states. EPAC2 can promote incretin-stimulated insulin secretion from pancreatic β cells through activation of Rap1 (Figure 47–3). Sulfonylureas, important oral drugs used to treat type II diabetes mellitus, may act in part by activating EPAC2 in β cells and increasing insulin release.

G*_q-*PLC-DAG/IP*₃-*Ca*²⁺ *Pathway. Calcium is an important messenger in all cells and can regulate diverse responses, including gene expression, contraction, secretion, metabolism, and electrical activity. Ca^{2+} can enter the cell through Ca^{2+} channels in the plasma membrane (see the Ion Channels section) or be released by hormones or growth factors from intracellular stores. In keeping with its role as a signal, the basal Ca^{2+} level in cells is maintained in the 100-nM range by membrane Ca^{2+} pumps that extrude Ca^{2+} to the extracellular space and a SERCA in the membrane of the ER that accumulates Ca^{2+} into its storage site in the ER/SR.

Hormones and growth factors release Ca^{2+} from its intracellular storage site, the ER, via a signaling pathway that begins with activation of PLC, of which there are two primary forms, PLCβ and PLCγ. GPCRs that couple to G_q or G_i activate PLCβ by activating the Gα subunit (see Figure 3–10) and releasing the βγ dimer. Both the active, G_q-GTP–bound α subunit and the βγ dimer can activate certain isoforms of PLCβ. PLCγ isoforms are activated by tyrosine phosphorylation, including phosphorylation by receptor and nonreceptor tyrosine kinases.

The PLCs are cytosolic enzymes that translocate to the plasma membrane on receptor stimulation. When activated, they hydrolyze a minor membrane phospholipid, phosphatidylinositol-4,5-bisphosphate, to generate two intracellular signals, IP_3 and the lipid DAG. DAG directly activates some members of the PKC family. IP_3 diffuses to the ER, where it activates the IP_3 receptor in the ER membrane, causing release of stored Ca^{2+} from the ER (Patterson et al., 2004). Release of Ca^{2+} from these intracellular stores raises Ca^{2+} levels in the cytoplasm many-fold within seconds and activates Ca^{2+}-dependent enzymes such as some of the PKCs and Ca^{2+}/calmodulin-sensitive enzymes such as one of the cAMP-hydrolyzing PDEs and a family of Ca^{2+}/calmodulin-sensitive PKs (e.g., phosphorylase kinase, MLCK, and CaM kinases II and IV) (Hudmon and Schulman, 2002). Depending on the cell's differentiated function, the Ca^{2+}/calmodulin kinases and PKC may regulate the bulk of the downstream events in the activated cells.

Ion Channels

Changes in the flux of ions across the plasma membrane are critical regulatory events in both excitable and nonexcitable cells. To establish the electrochemical gradients required to maintain a membrane potential, all cells express ion transporters for Na^+, K^+, Ca^{2+}, and Cl^-. For example, the Na^+,K^+-ATPase expends cellular ATP to pump Na^+ out of the cell and K^+ into the cell. The electrochemical gradients thus established are used by excitable tissues such as nerve and muscle to generate and transmit electrical impulses, by nonexcitable cells to trigger biochemical and secretory events, and by all cells to support a variety of secondary symport and antiport processes (see Figures 2–2 and 5–4).

Passive ion fluxes down cellular electrochemical gradients are regulated by a large family of ion channels located in the membrane. Humans express about 232 distinct ion channels to precisely regulate the flow of Na^+, K^+, Ca^{2+}, and Cl^- across the cell membrane (Jegla et al., 2009). Because of their roles as regulators of cell function, these proteins are important drug targets. The diverse ion channel family can be divided into subfamilies based on the mechanisms that open the channels, their architecture, and the ions they conduct. They can also be classified as *voltage-activated, ligand-activated, store-activated, stretch-activated,* and *temperature-activated channels.*

Voltage-Gated Channels.
Humans express multiple isoforms of voltage-gated channels for Na^+, K^+, Ca^{2+}, and Cl^- ions. In nerve and muscle cells, voltage-gated Na^+ channels are responsible for the generation of robust action potentials that depolarize the membrane from its resting potential of –70 mV up to a potential of +20 mV within a few milliseconds. These Na^+ channels are composed of three subunits, a pore-forming α subunit and two regulatory β subunits (Purves et al., 2011). The α subunit is a 260-kDa protein containing four domains that form a Na^+ ion–selective pore by arranging into a pseudotetramer shape. The β subunits are 36-kDa proteins that span the membrane once (Figure 3–11A). Each domain of the α subunit contains six membrane-spanning helices (S1–S6) with an extracellular loop between S5 and S6, termed the pore-forming or P loop; the P loop dips back into the pore and, combined

with residues from the corresponding P loops from the other domains, provides a selectivity filter for the Na^+ ion (see Figure 14–2). Four other helices surrounding the pore (one S4 helix from each of the domains) contain a set of charged amino acids that form the voltage sensor and cause a conformational change in the pore at more positive voltages, leading to opening of the pore and depolarization of the membrane (Figure 11–2). The voltage-activated Na^+ channels in pain neurons are targets for local anesthetics, such as lidocaine and tetracaine, which block the pore, inhibit depolarization, and thus block the sensation of pain (see Chapter 22). They are also the targets of the naturally occurring marine toxins *tetrodotoxin* and *saxitoxin*. Voltage-activated Na^+ channels are also important targets of many drugs used to treat cardiac arrhythmias (see Chapter 30).

Voltage-gated Ca^{2+} channels have a similar architecture to voltage-gated Na^+ channels with a large α subunit (four domains of five membrane-spanning helices) and three regulatory subunits (the β, δ, and γ subunits). Ca^{2+} channels can be responsible for initiating an action potential (as in the pacemaker cells of the heart) but are more commonly responsible for modifying the shape and duration of an action potential initiated by fast voltage-gated Na^+ channels. These channels initiate the influx of Ca^{2+} that stimulates the release of neurotransmitters in the central, enteric, and autonomic nervous systems and that control heart rate and impulse conduction in cardiac tissue (see Chapters 8, 14, and 30). The L-type voltage-gated Ca^{2+} channels are subject to additional regulation via phosphorylation by PKA. Voltage-gated Ca^{2+} channels expressed in smooth muscle regulate vascular tone; the intracellular concentration of Ca^{2+} is critical to regulating the phosphorylation state of the contractile apparatus via the activity of the Ca^{2+}/calmodulin-sensitive MLCK. Ca^{2+} channel antagonists such as nifedipine, diltiazem, and verapamil are effective vasodilators and are widely used to treat hypertension, angina, and certain cardiac arrhythmias (see Chapters 27, 28, and 30).

Voltage-gated K^+ channels are the most numerous and structurally diverse members of the voltage-gated channel family and include the voltage-gated K_v channels, the inwardly rectifying K^+ channel, and the tandem or two-pore domain "leak" K^+ channels (Jegla et al., 2009). The inwardly rectifying channels and the two-pore channels are voltage insensitive, regulated by G proteins and H^+ ions, and greatly stimulated by general anesthetics. Increasing K^+ conductance through these channels drives the membrane potential more negative (closer to the equilibrium potential for K^+); thus, these channels are important in regulating resting membrane potential and restoring the resting membrane at -70 to -90 mV following depolarization.

Ligand-Gated Channels.
Channels activated by the binding of a ligand to a specific site in the channel protein have a diverse architecture and set of ligands. Major ligand-gated channels in the nervous system are those that respond to excitatory neurotransmitters such as ACh (Figures 3–11B and 11–1) or glutamate (or agonists such as AMPA and NMDA) and inhibitory neurotransmitters such as glycine or GABA (Purves et al., 2011). Activation of these channels is responsible for the majority of synaptic transmission by neurons both in the CNS and in the periphery (see Chapters 8, 11, and 14). In addition, there are a variety of more specialized ion channels that are activated by intracellular small molecules and are structurally distinct from conventional ligand-gated ion channels. These include ion channels that are formally members of the K_v family, such as the HCN channel expressed in the heart that is responsible for the slow depolarization seen in phase 4 of atrioventricular and sinoatrial nodal cell action potentials (Wahl-Schott and Biel, 2009) (see Chapter 30) and the CNG channel that is important for vision (see Chapter 69). The intracellular small-molecule category of ion channels also includes the IP_3-sensitive Ca^{2+} channel responsible for release of Ca^{2+} from the ER and the sulfonylurea "receptor" (SUR1) that associates with the $K_{ir}6.2$ channel to regulate the K_{ATP} in pancreatic β cells. The K_{ATP} channel is the target of oral hypoglycemic drugs such as sulfonylureas and meglitinides that stimulate insulin release from pancreatic β cells and are used to treat type 2 diabetes (see Chapter 47).

The nicotinic ACh receptor is an instructive example of a ligand-gated ion channel. Isoforms of this channel are expressed in the CNS, in

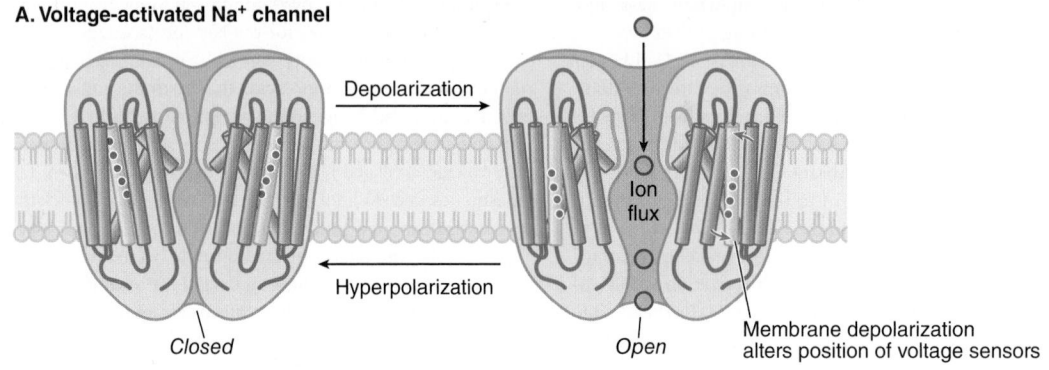

A. Voltage-activated Na⁺ channel

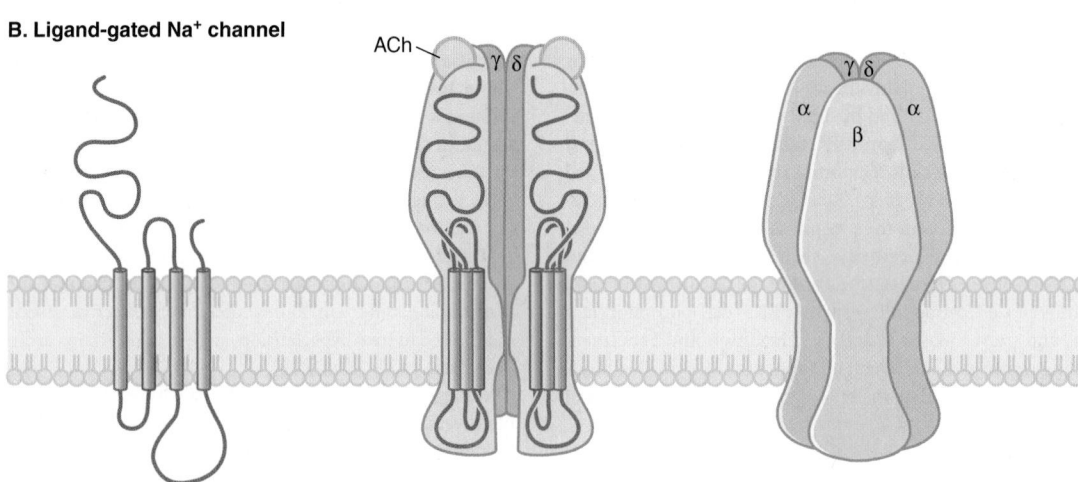

B. Ligand-gated Na⁺ channel

Figure 3–11 *Two types of ion channels regulated by receptors and drugs.* **A.** A voltage-activated Na⁺ channel with the pore in the closed and open states. The pore-forming P loops are shown in blue, angled into the pore to form the selectivity filter. The S4 helices forming the voltage sensor are shown in orange, with the positively charged amino acids displayed as red dots. **B.** Ligand-gated nicotinic ACh receptor expressed in the skeletal muscle neuromuscular junction. The pore is made up of five subunits, each with a large extracellular domain and four transmembrane helices (one of these subunits is shown at the left of panel **B**). The helix that lines the pore is shown in blue. The receptor is composed of two α subunits and β, γ, and δ subunits. See text for discussion of other ligand-gated ion channels. Detailed descriptions of specific channels are given throughout the text in relation to the therapeutic actions of drugs affecting these channels (see especially Chapters 11, 14, and 22). (Adapted with permission from Purves D et al., eds. *Neuroscience*. 5th ed. Sinauer Associates, Inc., Sunderland, MA, **2011**. By permission of Oxford University Press, USA.)

autonomic ganglia, and at the neuromuscular junction (Figures 3–11B and 11–2). The pentameric channel consists of four different subunits (2α, β, δ, γ) in the neuromuscular junction or two different subunits (2α, 3β) in autonomic ganglia (Purves et al., 2011). Each α subunit has an identical ACh binding site; the different compositions of the other three subunits between the neuronal and neuromuscular junction receptors account for the ability of competitive antagonists such as rocuronium to inhibit the receptor in the neuromuscular junction without effect on the ganglionic receptor. This property is exploited to provide muscle relaxation during surgery with minimal autonomic side effects (Chapter 11). Each subunit of the receptor contains a large, extracellular N-terminal domain, four membrane-spanning helices (one of which lines the pore in the assembled complex), and an internal loop between helices 3 and 4 that forms the intracellular domain of the channel. The pore opening in the channel measures about 3 nm, whereas the diameter of a Na⁺ or K⁺ ion is only 0.3 nm or less. Accordingly, ligand-gated ion channels do not possess the exquisite ion selectivity found in most voltage-activated channels, and activation of the nicotinic ACh receptor allows passage of both Na⁺ and K⁺ ions.

Transient Receptor Potential Channels. The TRP cation channels are involved in a variety of physiological and pathophysiological sensory processes, including nociception, heat and cold sensation, mechanosensation, and sensation of chemicals such as capsaicin and menthol. The TRP channel superfamily is diverse and consists of 28 channels in six families (Cao et al., 2013; Ramsey et al., 2006; Venkatachalam and Montell, 2007).

The typical TRP channel structure consists of monomers predicted to have six transmembrane helices (S1–S6) with a pore-forming loop between S5 and S6 and large intracellular regions at the amino and carboxyl termini. Most of the functional TRP channels are homotetramers, but heteromultimers are also formed. Genetic mutations in TRP channels are related to channelopathies that are associated with inherited pain syndrome, several different kidney and bladder diseases, and skeletal dysplasias. Agonists and antagonists are being developed and are in clinical trials for a wide variety of indications, including pain, gastroesophageal reflux disorder, respiratory disorders, osteoarthritis, skin disorders, and overactive bladder.

Transmembrane Receptors Linked to Intracellular Enzymes

Receptor Tyrosine Kinases. The receptor tyrosine kinases include receptors for hormones such as insulin; growth factors such EGF, PDGF, NGF, FGF, VEGF; and ephrins. With the exception of the insulin receptor, which has α and β chains (see Chapter 47), these macromolecules consist of single polypeptide chains with large, cysteine-rich extracellular domains, short transmembrane domains, and an intracellular region containing one or two protein tyrosine kinase domains. Activation of growth factor receptors leads to cell survival, cell proliferation, and differentiation. Activation of the ephrin receptors leads to neuronal angiogenesis, axonal migration, and guidance (Ferguson, 2008).

The inactive state of growth factor receptors is monomeric; binding of ligand induces dimerization of the receptor and cross-phosphorylation of the kinase domains on multiple tyrosine residues (Figure 3–12A). The phosphorylation of other tyrosine residues forms docking sites for the SH2 domains contained in a large number of signaling proteins. There

are over 100 proteins encoded in the human genome containing SH2 domains, and following receptor activation, large signaling complexes are formed on the receptor that eventually lead to cell proliferation.

Molecules recruited to phosphotyrosine-containing proteins by their SH2 domains include PLCγ, the activity of which raises intracellular levels

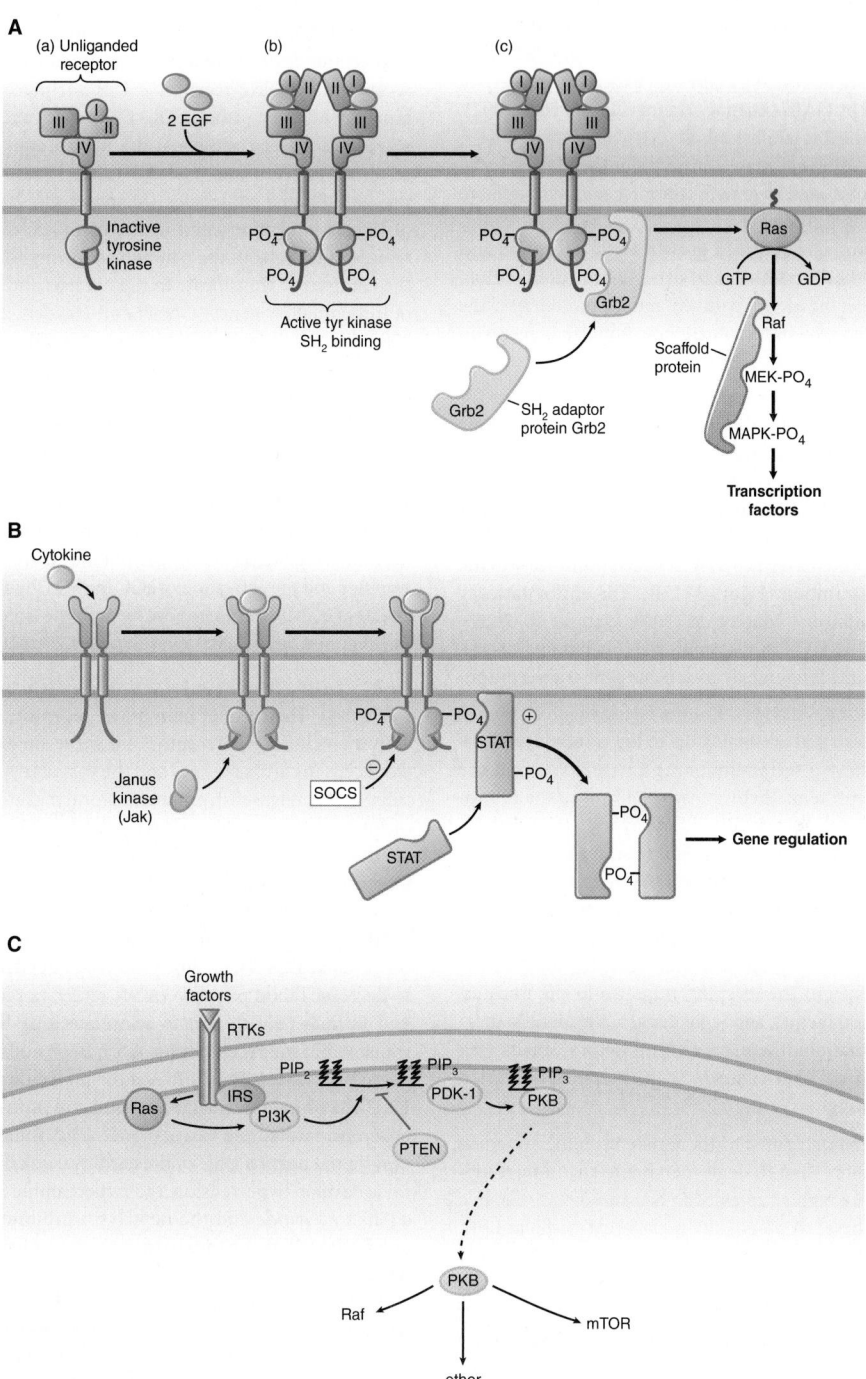

Figure 3–12 *Mechanism of activation of a receptor tyrosine kinase and a cytokine receptor.* **A.** *Activation of the EGF receptor.* The extracellular structure of the unliganded receptor (a) contains four domains (I–IV), which rearrange significantly on binding two EGF molecules. In (b), the conformational changes lead to activation of the cytoplasmic tyrosine kinase domains and tyrosine phosphorylation of intracellular regions to form SH2 binding sites. (c). The adapter molecule Grb2 binds to the phosphorylated tyrosine residues and activates the Ras-MAPK cascade. **B.** *Activation of a cytokine receptor.* Binding of the cytokine causes dimerization of the receptor and recruits the Jaks to the cytoplasmic tails of the receptor. Jaks transphosphorylate and lead to the phosphorylation of the STATs. The phosphorylated STATs translocate to the nucleus and regulate transcription. There are proteins termed SOCS (suppressors of cytokine signaling) that inhibit the Jak-STAT pathway. **C.** *Activation of the mTOR pathway.* Signaling via this pathway promotes growth, proliferation, and survival of cells via a complex web of signaling pathways (see Figures 35–2 and 67–4 and Guri and Hall, 2016). mTOR signaling is emerging as a major consideration in immunosuppression and cancer pharmacotherapy, and inhibitors of mTOR signaling are sometimes included as adjunct therapy.

of Ca^{2+} and activates PKC. The α and β isoforms of PI3K contain SH2 domains, dock at the phosphorylated receptor, are activated, and increase the level of PIP_3 and PKB (also known as Akt). PKB can regulate mTOR, which is upstream of various signaling pathways, and the *Bad* protein that is important in apoptosis.

In addition to recruiting enzymes, phosphotyrosine-presenting proteins can interact with SH2 domain-containing adaptor molecules without activity (e.g., Grb2), which in turn attract GEFs such as Sos that can activate the small GTP-binding protein Ras. The small GTP-binding proteins Ras and Rho belong to a large family of small monomeric GTPases. All of the small GTPases are activated by GEFs regulated by a variety of mechanisms and inhibited by GAPs (Etienne-Manneville and Hall, 2002). Activation of members of the Ras family leads in turn to activation of a PK cascade termed the Ras-MAPK pathway. Activation of the MAPK pathway is one of the major routes used by growth factor receptors to signal to the nucleus and stimulate cell growth (Figure 3–12A). Oncogenic mutations that result in constitutively activated growth factor receptors and Ras can also activate the MAPK pathway and drive tumor proliferation. Anticancer agents that target the MAPK pathway and the protein tyrosine kinase activity of oncogenic growth factors are now important agents in treating several forms of cancer (see Chapter 65 and 67).

Jak-STAT Receptor Pathway. Cells express a family of receptors for cytokines such as γ-interferon and hormones such as growth hormone and prolactin, which signal to the nucleus by a more direct manner than the receptor tyrosine kinases. These receptors have no intrinsic enzymatic activity; rather, the intracellular domain binds a separate, intracellular tyrosine kinase termed a Jak. On dimerization induced by ligand binding, Jaks phosphorylate other proteins termed STATs, which translocate to the nucleus and regulate transcription (Figure 3–12B). The entire pathway is termed the Jak-STAT pathway (Gough et al., 2008; Wang et al., 2009). There are four Jaks and six STATs in mammals that, depending on the cell type and signal, combine differentially to activate gene transcription.

Receptor Serine-Threonine Kinases. Protein ligands such as TGF-β activate a family of receptors that are analogous to the receptor tyrosine kinases except that they have a serine-threonine kinase domain in the cytoplasmic region of the protein. There are two isoforms of the monomeric receptor protein, type I (seven forms) and type II (five forms). In the basal state, these proteins exist as monomers; upon binding an agonist ligand, they dimerize, leading to phosphorylation of the kinase domain of the type I monomer, which activates the receptor. The activated receptor then phosphorylates a gene regulatory protein termed a *Smad*. Once phosphorylated by the activated receptor on a serine residue, Smad dissociates from the receptor, migrates to the nucleus, associates with transcription factors, and regulates genes leading to morphogenesis and transformation. There are also inhibitory Smads (the Smad6 and Smad7 isoforms) that compete with the phosphorylated Smads to terminate signaling.

Toll-like Receptors. Signaling related to the innate immune system is carried out by a family of more than 10 single membrane-spanning receptors termed TLRs, which are highly expressed in hematopoietic cells. In a single polypeptide chain, these receptors contain a large extracellular LBD, a short membrane-spanning domain, and a cytoplasmic region termed the TIR domain that lacks intrinsic enzymatic activity. *Ligands for TLRs comprise a multitude of pathogen products, including lipids, peptidoglycans, lipopeptides, and viruses.* Activation of TLRs produces an inflammatory response to the pathogenic microorganisms.

The first step in activation of TLRs by ligands is dimerization, which in turn causes signaling proteins to bind to the receptor to form a signaling complex. Ligand-induced dimerization recruits a series of adaptor proteins, including Mal and MyD88 to the intracellular TIR domain; these proteins in turn recruit the IRAKs. The IRAKs autophosphorylate in the complex and subsequently form a more stable complex with MyD88. The phosphorylation event also recruits TRAF6 to the complex, which facilitates interaction with a ubiquitin ligase that attaches a polyubiquitin molecule to TRAF6. This complex can now interact with TAK1 and the adaptor protein TAB1. TAK1 is a member of the

MAPK family, which activates the NF-κB kinases; phosphorylation of the NF-κB transcription factors causes their translocation to the nucleus and transcriptional activation of a variety of inflammatory genes (Gay and Gangloff, 2007).

TNF-α Receptors. The mechanism of action of TNF-α signaling to the NF-κB transcription factors is similar to that used by TLRs in that the intracellular domain of the receptor has no enzymatic activity. The TNF-α receptor is another membrane monospan protein with an extracellular LBD, a transmembrane domain, and a cytoplasmic domain termed the *death domain*. TNF-α binds a complex composed of TNF receptor 1 and TNF receptor 2. Upon trimerization, the death domains bind the adaptor protein TRADD, which recruits the RIP1 to form a receptor-adaptor complex at the membrane. RIP1 is polyubiquinated, resulting in recruitment of the TAK1 kinase and the IKK complex to the ubiquinated molecules (Skaug et al., 2009). The activation loop of IKK is phosphorylated in the complex, eventually resulting in the release of IκBα from the complex, allowing the p50/p65 heterodimer of the complex to translocate to the nucleus and activate the transcription of inflammatory genes (Ghosh and Hayden, 2008; Hayden and Ghosh, 2008; Kataoka, 2009). While there currently are no drugs that interdict the cytoplasmic portions of the TNF-α signaling pathway, humanized monoclonal antibodies to TNF-α itself, such as *infliximab* and *adalimumab*, are important for the treatment of rheumatoid arthritis and Crohn disease (see Chapters 34, 35, 37, and 51).

Receptors That Stimulate Synthesis of cGMP

The signaling pathways that regulate the synthesis of cGMP in cells include hormonal regulation of transmembrane guanylyl cyclases such as the ANP receptor and the activation of sGC by NO (Figure 3–13). The downstream effects of cGMP are carried out by multiple isoforms of PKG, cGMP-gated ion channels, and cGMP-modulated PDEs that degrade cAMP.

Natriuretic Peptide Receptors: Ligand-Activated Guanylyl Cyclases. The class of membrane receptors with intrinsic enzymatic activity includes the receptors for three small peptide ligands released from cells in cardiac tissues and the vascular system, the natriuretic peptides: ANP, released from atrial storage granules following expansion of intravascular volume or stimulation with pressor hormones; BNP, synthesized and released in large amounts from ventricular tissue in response to volume overload; and CNP, synthesized in the brain and endothelial cells. Like BNP, CNP is not stored in granules; rather, its synthesis and release are increased by growth factors and sheer stress on vascular ECs. The major physiological effects of these hormones are to decrease blood pressure (ANP, BNP), to reduce cardiac hypertrophy and fibrosis (BNP), and to stimulate long-bone growth (CNP). The transmembrane receptors for ANP, BNP, and CNP are ligand-activated guanylyl cyclases. The NPR-A is the molecule that responds to ANP and BNP. The protein is widely expressed and prominent in kidney, lung, adipose, and cardiac and vascular SMCs. ANP and BNP play a role in maintaining the normal state of the cardiovascular system; NPR-A knockout mice develop hypertension and hypertrophic hearts. The synthetic BNP agonist *nesiritide* and the neprilysin inhibitor *sacubitril* (blocks ANP and BNP breakdown) are used in the treatment of acute decompensated heart failure (Chapter 29).

The NPR-B receptor responds to CNP, is widely expressed, and has a physical structure similar to the NPR-A receptor. A role for CNP in bone is suggested by the observation that NPR-B knockout mice exhibit dwarfism. The NPR-C has an extracellular domain similar to those of NPR-A and NPR-B but does not contain the guanylyl cyclase domain. NPR-C has no enzymatic activity and is thought to function as a clearance receptor, removing excess natriuretic peptide from the circulation (Potter et al., 2009).

NO Synthase and Soluble Guanylyl Cyclase. NO is produced locally in cells by forms of the enzyme NOS. NO stimulates sGC to produce cGMP. There are three forms of NOS: nNOS (or NOS1), eNOS (or NOS3), and iNOS (or NOS2). All three forms are widely expressed but are especially important in the cardiovascular system, where they are found in myocytes, vascular smooth muscle cells, endothelial cells, hematopoietic

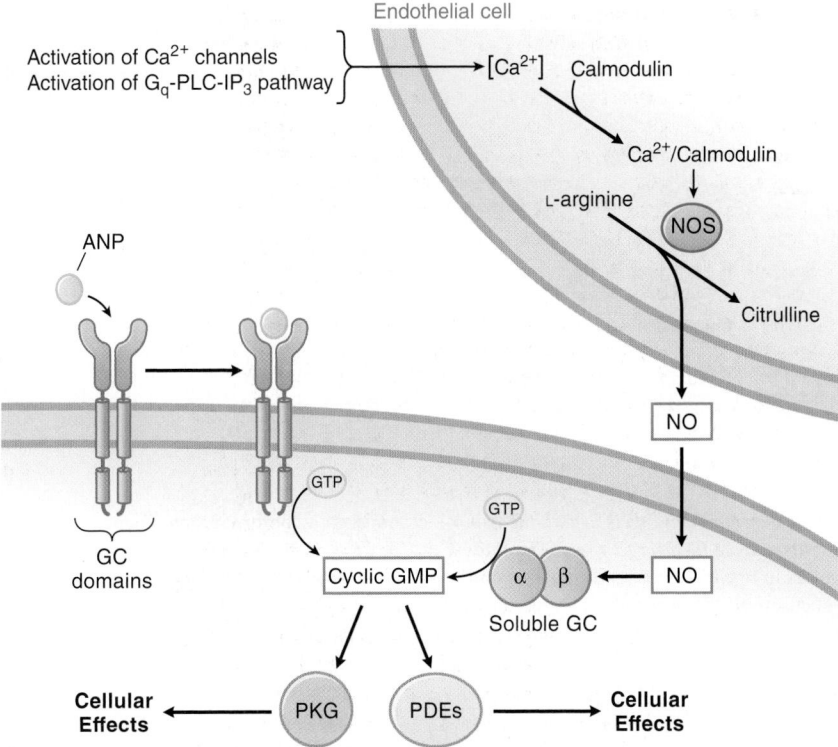

Figure 3–13 *Cyclic GMP signaling pathways.* Formation of cGMP is regulated by cell surface receptors with intrinsic GC activity and by soluble forms of GC. The cell surface receptors respond to natriuretic peptides such as ANP with an increase in cGMP. sGC responds to NO generated from L-arginine by NOS. Cellular effects of cGMP are carried out by PKG and cGMP-regulated PDEs. In this diagram, NO is produced by a Ca²⁺/calmodulin–dependent NOS in an adjacent endothelial cell. Detailed descriptions of these signaling pathways are given throughout the text in relation to the therapeutic actions of drugs affecting these pathways.

cells, and platelets. Elevated cell Ca²⁺, acting via calmodulin, markedly activates nNOS and eNOS; the inducible form is less sensitive to Ca²⁺, but synthesis of iNOS protein in cells can be induced more than 1000-fold by inflammatory stimuli such as endotoxin, TNF-α, interleukin 1β, and interferon γ.

Nitric oxide synthase produces NO by catalyzing the oxidation of the guanido nitrogen of L-arginine, producing L-citrulline and NO. NO activates sGC, a heterodimer that contains a protoporphyrin-IX heme domain. NO binds to this domain at low nanomolar concentrations and produces a 200- to 400-fold increase in the V_{max} of guanylyl cyclase, leading to an elevation of cellular cGMP (Tsai and Kass, 2009). The cellular effects of cGMP on the vascular system are mediated by a number of mechanisms, but especially by PKG. In vascular smooth muscle, activation of PKG leads to vasodilation by

- Inhibiting IP₃-mediated Ca²⁺ release from intracellular stores
- Phosphorylating voltage-gated Ca²⁺ channels to inhibit Ca²⁺ influx
- Phosphorylating phospholamban, a modulator of the sarcoplasmic Ca²⁺ pump, leading to a more rapid reuptake of Ca²⁺ into intracellular stores
- Phosphorylating and opening the Ca²⁺-activated K⁺ channel, leading to hyperpolarization of the cell membrane, which closes L-type Ca²⁺ channels and reduces the flux of Ca²⁺ into the cell

Nuclear Hormone Receptors and Transcription Factors

Nuclear hormone receptors comprise a superfamily of 48 receptors that respond to a diverse set of ligands. The nuclear receptor proteins are transcription factors able to regulate the expression of genes controlling numerous physiological processes, such as reproduction, development, and metabolism. Members of the family include receptors for circulating steroid hormones such as androgens, estrogens, glucocorticoids, thyroid hormone, and vitamin D. Other members of the family are receptors for a diverse group of fatty acids, bile acids, lipids, and lipid metabolites (McEwan, 2009).

Examples include the RXR; the LXR (the ligand is 22-OH cholesterol); the FXR (the ligand is chenodeoxycholic acid); and the PPARs α, β, and γ; 15-deoxy prostaglandin J2 is a possible ligand for PPARγ; the cholesterol-lowering fibrates bind to and regulate PPARγ. In the inactive state, receptors for steroids such as glucocorticoids reside in the cytoplasm and translocate to the nucleus on binding ligand. Other members of the family, such as the LXRs and FXRs reside in the nucleus and are activated by changes in the concentration of hydrophobic lipid molecules.

Nuclear hormone receptors contain four major domains in a single polypeptide chain. The N-terminal domain can contain an *activation region* (AF-1) essential for transcriptional regulation, followed by a very conserved region with two zinc fingers that bind to DNA (the *DNA-binding domain*). The N-terminal activation region (AF-1) is subject to regulation by phosphorylation and other mechanisms that stimulate or inhibit transcription. The C-terminal half of the molecule contains a *hinge region* (which can be involved in binding DNA), the domain responsible for binding the hormone or ligand (the LBD), and specific sets of amino acid residues for binding *coactivators* and *corepressors* in a second activation region (AF-2). The LBD is formed from a bundle of 12 helices; ligand binding induces a major conformational change in helix 12 that affects the binding of the coregulatory proteins essential for activation of the receptor-DNA complex (Figure 3–14) (Privalsky, 2004; Tontonoz and Spiegelman, 2008).

When binding to DNA, most of the nuclear hormone receptors act as dimers—some as homodimers, others as heterodimers. Steroid hormone receptors such as the glucocorticoid receptor are commonly homodimers, whereas those for lipids are heterodimers with the RXR receptor. The receptor dimers bind to repetitive DNA sequences, either direct repeat sequences or inverted repeats termed *HREs* that are specific for each type of receptor. The HREs in DNA are found upstream of the regulated genes or in some cases within the regulated genes. An agonist-bound nuclear hormone receptor often activates a large number of genes to carry out a program of cellular differentiation or metabolic regulation. *An important*

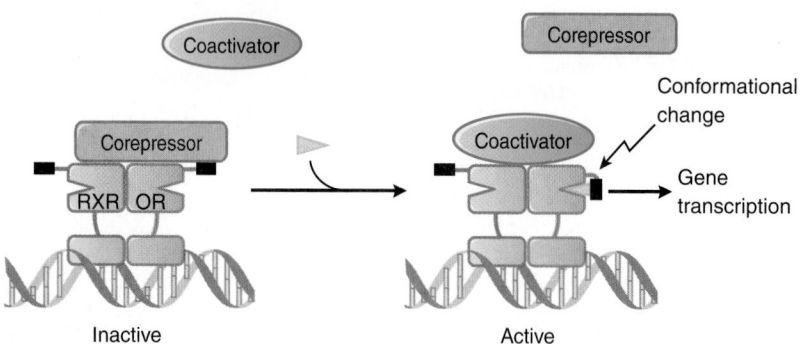

Figure 3–14 *Activation of nuclear hormone receptors.* A nuclear hormone receptor (OR) is shown in complex with the RXR. When an agonist (yellow triangle) and coactivator bind, a conformational change occurs in helix 12 (black bar), and gene transcription is stimulated. If corepressors are bound, activation does not occur. See text for details; see also Figure 6–12.

property of these receptors is that they must bind their ligand, the appropriate HRE, and a coregulator, to regulate their target genes. The activity of the nuclear hormone receptors in a given cell depends not only on the ligand but also on the ratio of coactivators and corepressors recruited to the complex. Coactivators recruit enzymes to the transcription complex that modify chromatin, such as histone acetylase that serves to unravel DNA for transcription. Corepressors recruit proteins such as histone deacetylase, which keeps DNA tightly packed and inhibits transcription.

Apoptosis and Autophagy Pathways

Organ development and renewal requires a balance between cell population survival and expansion versus cell death and removal. One process by which cells are genetically programmed for death is termed *apoptosis*. Defective apoptosis is an important characteristic of many cancers that contributes to both tumorigenesis and resistance to anticancer therapies. *Autophagy* an intracellular degradation pathway that may have evolved before apoptosis, can also lead to programmed cell death. The pharmacological perturbation of these processes could be of importance in many diseases.

Apoptosis

Apoptosis is a highly regulated program of biochemical reactions that leads to cell rounding, shrinking of the cytoplasm, condensation of the nucleus and nuclear material, and changes in the cell membrane that eventually lead to presentation of phosphatidylserine on the outer surface of the cell. Phosphatidylserine is recognized as a sign of apoptosis by macrophages, which engulf and phagocytize the dying cell. During this process, the membrane of the apoptotic cell remains intact, and the cell does not release its cytoplasm or nuclear material. Thus, unlike necrotic cell death, the apoptotic process does not initiate an inflammatory response. Alterations in apoptotic pathways are implicated in cancer, neurodegenerative diseases, autoimmune diseases. Thus, maintaining or restoring normal apoptotic pathways is the goal of major drug development efforts to treat diseases that involve dysregulated apoptotic pathways. Resistance to many cancer chemotherapies is associated with reduced function of apoptotic pathways.

Two major signaling pathways induce apoptosis. Apoptosis can be initiated by external signals that have features in common with those used by ligands such as TNF-α or by an internal pathway activated by DNA damage, improperly folded proteins, or withdrawal of cell survival factors (Figure 3–15). The apoptotic program is carried out by a large family of cysteine proteases termed *caspases*. The caspases are highly specific cytoplasmic proteases that are inactive in normal cells but become activated by apoptotic signals (Bremer et al., 2006; Ghavami et al., 2009).

The external apoptosis signaling pathway can be activated by ligands such as TNF, Fas (also called Apo-1), or TRAIL. The receptors for Fas and TRAIL are transmembrane receptors with no enzymatic activity, similar to the organization of the TNF receptor described previously. On binding TNF, Fas ligand, or TRAIL, these receptors form a receptor dimer,

undergo a conformational change, and recruit adapter proteins to the death domain. The adaptor proteins then recruit RIP1 and caspase 8 to form a complex that results in the activation of caspase 8. Activation of caspase 8 leads to the activation of caspase 3, which initiates the apoptotic program. The final steps of apoptosis are carried out by caspases 6 and 7, leading to degradation of enzymes, structural proteins, and DNA fragmentation characteristic of cell death (Danial and Korsmeyer, 2004; Wilson et al., 2009) (see Figure 3–15).

The internal apoptosis pathway can be activated by signals such as DNA damage, leading to increased transcription of the p53 gene, and involves damage to the mitochondria by proapoptotic members of the Bcl-2 family of proteins. This family includes proapoptotic members such as Bax, Bak, and Bad, which induce damage at the mitochondrial membrane. There are also antiapoptotic Bcl-2 members, such as Bcl-2, Bcl-X, and Bcl-W, which serve to inhibit mitochondrial damage and are negative regulators of the system (Rong and Distelhorst, 2008). When DNA damage occurs, p53 transcription is activated and holds the cell at a cell cycle checkpoint until the damage is repaired. If the damage cannot be repaired, apoptosis is initiated through the proapoptotic Bcl-2 members, such as Bax. Bax is activated, translocates to the mitochondria, overcomes the antiapoptotic proteins, and induces the release of cytochrome *c* and a protein termed the SMAC. SMAC binds to and inactivates the inhibitor of apoptosis proteins (IAPs) that normally prevent caspase activation. Cytochrome *c* combines in the cytosol with another protein, Apaf-1, and with caspase 9. This complex leads to activation of caspase 9 and ultimately to the activation of caspase 3 (Ghobrial et al., 2005; Wilson et al., 2009). Once activated, caspase 3 activates the same downstream pathways as the external pathway described previously, leading to the cleavage of proteins, cytoskeletal elements, and DNA repair proteins, with subsequent DNA condensation and membrane blebbing that eventually lead to cell death and engulfment by macrophages.

Autophagy

Autophagy is a highly regulated, multistep, catabolic pathway in which cellular contents (including aggregate-prone proteins, organelles such as mitochondria and peroxisomes, and infectious agents) are sequestered within double-membrane vesicles known as autophagosomes, then delivered to lysosomes, where fusion occurs and autophagosome contents are degraded by lysosomal proteases (Bento et al., 2016; Hurley and Young, 2017). The functions of autophagy are to remove cell contents that are damaged and provide cells with substrates for energy and biosynthesis under conditions of stress and starvation. Autophagy plays an important protective role in a number of diseases, including neurodegenerative diseases (e.g., Alzheimer, Parkinson, and Huntington diseases) caused by aggregate-prone proteins and certain infectious diseases (*Salmonella typhi* and *Mycobacterium tuberculosis*). Autophagy-related genes may also play a role in tumor suppression, and decreased autophagic capacity is correlated with poor prognosis in brain tumors. However, in breast, ovarian, and prostate cancers, autophagy can function as a tumor

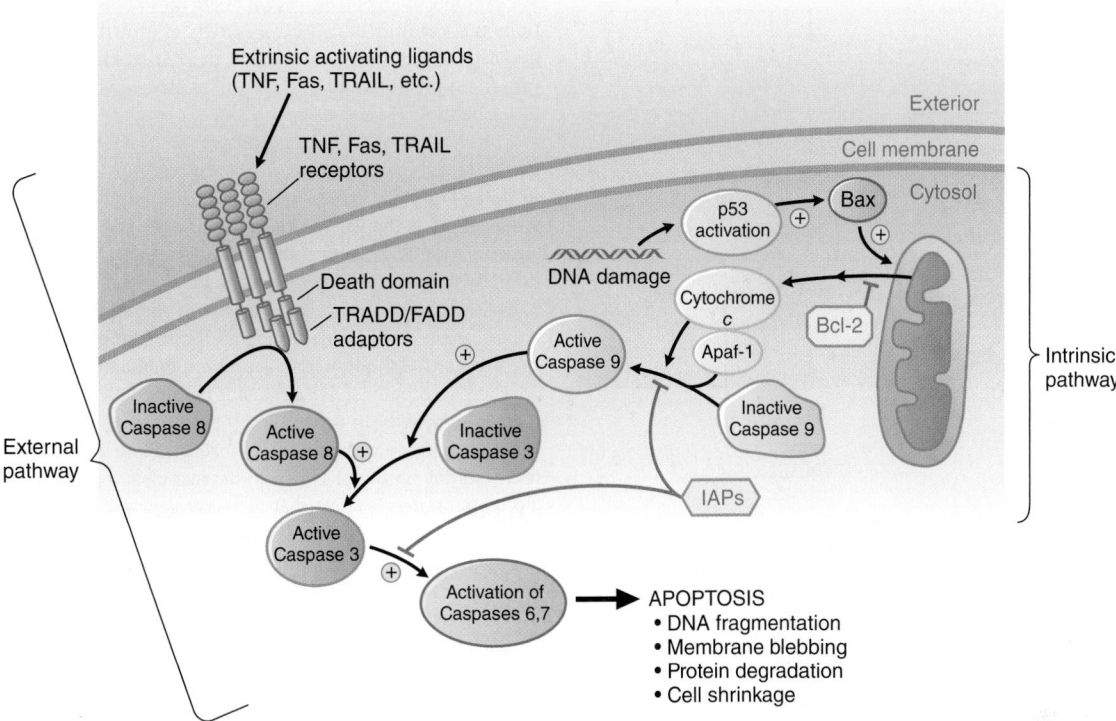

Figure 3–15 *Two pathways leading to apoptosis.* Apoptosis can be initiated by external ligands such as TNF, Fas, or TRAIL at specific transmembrane receptors (left half of figure). Activation leads to trimerization of the receptor, and binding of adaptor molecules such as TRADD, to the intracellular death domain. The adaptors recruit caspase 8 and activate it, leading to cleavage and activation of the effector caspase, caspase 3, which activates the caspase pathway, leading to apoptosis. Apoptosis can also be initiated by an *intrinsic pathway* regulated by Bcl-2 family members such as Bax and Bcl-2. Bax is activated by DNA damage or malformed proteins via p53 (right half of figure). Activation of this pathway leads to release of cytochrome *c* from the mitochondria, formation of a complex with Apaf-1 and caspase 9. Caspase 9 is activated in the complex and initiates apoptosis through activation of caspase 3. Either the extrinsic or the intrinsic pathway can overwhelm the inhibitor of apoptosis proteins (IAPs), which otherwise keep apoptosis in check.

promoter and may enhance the survival of metastatic cells at sites where nutrients are limited.

Autophagy is a highly conserved process controlled by autophagy-related genes (known as *ATGs*, AuTophaGy genes). More than 30 *ATGs* have been identified in eukaryotes, and the ATG proteins function at various steps in autophagy, including induction of cargo packaging, vesicle formation, vesicle fusion with lysosomes, and degradation of vesicular contents. Autophagy is primarily regulated by various cellular stress-mediated and growth factor signaling pathways that integrate signaling output via the PI3K-PKB-mTOR pathway (Figure 3–16). Activated mTORC1 inhibits autophagy. Another important regulator of autophagy is the antiapoptotic protein Bcl-2 through its interaction with Beclin-1, an ATG protein. The binding of Bcl-2 to Beclin-1 inhibits autophagy. Phosphorylation of Beclin-1 by JNK1 promotes the dissociation of Beclin-1 from Bcl-2, which promotes autophagy. The ubiquitin-proteasome system is a major protein degradation system that functionally complements autophagy and also regulates autophagy. Ubiquitination of Beclin-1 disrupts its interaction with Bcl-2 and initiates autophagy, but Beclin-1 degradation by the proteasome downregulates autophagy. The tumor suppressor p53 is also a regulator of autophagy through its inhibitory interactions with an ATG on the lysosomal membrane, DRAM.

Receptor Desensitization and Regulation of Receptors

Receptors are almost always subject to feedback regulation by their own signaling outputs. Continued stimulation of cells with agonists generally results in a state of *desensitization* (also referred to as *adaptation, refractoriness,* or *downregulation*) such that the effect of continued or repeated

exposure to the same concentration of drug is diminished. This phenomenon, called *tachyphylaxis*, occurs rapidly and is important therapeutically; an example is attenuated response to the repeated use of β adrenergic receptor agonists as bronchodilators for the treatment of asthma (see Chapters 12 and 40).

Desensitization can result from temporary inaccessibility of the receptor to agonist or from fewer receptors being synthesized (e.g., downregulation of receptor number). Phosphorylation of GPCRs by specific GRKs plays a key role in triggering rapid desensitization. Phosphorylation of agonist-occupied GPCRs by GRKs facilitates the binding of cytosolic proteins termed *arrestins* to the receptor, resulting in the uncoupling of G protein from the receptor. The β arrestins recruit proteins, such as PDE4, which limit cAMP signaling, and clathrin and β_2 adaptin, which promote sequestration of receptor from the membrane (*internalization*), thereby providing a scaffold that permits additional signaling steps.

Conversely, *supersensitivity* to agonists also frequently follows chronic reduction of receptor stimulation. As an example, supersensitivity can be noticeable following withdrawal from prolonged receptor blockade (e.g., the long-term administration of β adrenergic receptor antagonists such as metoprolol) or in the case where chronic denervation of a preganglionic fiber induces an increase in neurotransmitter release per pulse and to greater postsynaptic effect, indicating postganglionic neuronal supersensitivity.

Diseases Resulting From Receptor and Pathway Dysfunction

Alteration in receptors and their downstream signaling pathways can be the cause of disease. The loss of a receptor in a highly specialized

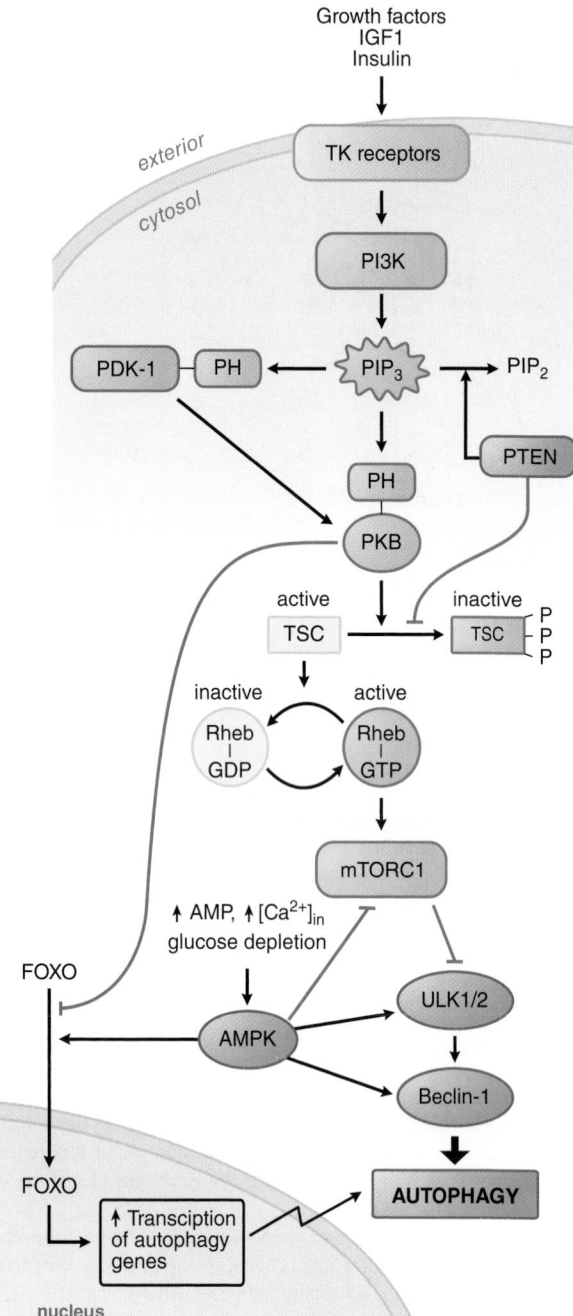

Figure 3–16 *Pathways regulating autophagy.* Two of the primary regulators of autophagy are growth factor signaling and cellular stress. Growth factor signaling pathways that lead to activation of mTORC1 (green boxes) inhibit autophagy, whereas cellular stress caused by nutrient starvation enhance autophagy through activation of AMPK (red boxes). These pathways not only interact with one another, but also with other pathways including apoptosis pathways as described in the text. See Figure 35–5 for the effect of mTOR inhibitors as immunosuppressants.

signaling system may cause a phenotypic disorder (e.g., deficiency of the androgen receptor and testicular feminization syndrome; see Chapter 45). Deficiencies in widely employed signaling pathways have broad effects, as are seen in myasthenia gravis (due to autoimmune disruption of nicotinic cholinergic receptor function; Chapter 11) and in some forms of insulin-resistant diabetes mellitus (as a result of autoimmune depletion of insulin and interference with insulin receptor function; Chapter 47). The expression of constitutively active, aberrant, or ectopic

receptors, effectors, and coupling proteins potentially can lead to *super-sensitivity, subsensitivity,* or *other untoward responses* (Smit et al., 2007). For example, many forms of cancer are now known to arise from mutations that result in constitutive activity of growth factor receptors and downstream signaling enzymes in the Ras-MAPK pathway, or loss of tumor suppressors and other proteins that regulate cell proliferation (see Chapter 67).

Common polymorphisms in receptors and proteins downstream of the receptor can also lead to variability in therapeutic responses in patient populations from different geographic and ethnic origins. An example is the variability in therapeutic response to β blockers in patients with heart failure. African American patients with heart failure do not respond as well to β blockade therapy as do patients of European and Asian descent, and at least part of the lower efficacy in African Americans is attributable to polymorphisms in several components of the myocardial β adrenergic receptor signaling pathway, including β_1 adrenergic receptor polymorphisms that increase its constitutive activity and sensitivity to activation by NE. Interestingly, a GRK5 gain-of-function polymorphism that is more common in African Americans increases the ability of GRK5 to desensitize β_1 receptors and provides a β_1 antiadrenergic effect that increases survival in patients with heart failure not receiving blocker therapy.

Pharmacotherapies That Modify Specific Genes and Their Transcription and Translation

Many hereditary diseases result from mutations in physiologically important proteins that are not receptors or proteins associated with downstream signaling. Until recently, it was difficult or impossible to treat many of these diseases except to provide supportive therapy. However, various gene therapies currently being tested in animal models and humans hold promise of curing or significantly ameliorating the effects of a mutation in a protein that is key to an important physiological process. Examples of diseases that might be treated or cured by gene therapies include DMD, cystic fibrosis, metabolic disorders, and various disorders of the eye.

Approximately 11% of genetic mutations in inherited disease are nonsense mutations that introduce a premature stop codon in the mRNA gene transcript. The first drug approved (in the E.U., but not yet in the U.S.) for the treatment of nmDMD is *ataluren*. This small-molecule drug is thought to act on the ribosome to override the premature stop (nonsense) codon in nonsense mutations, allowing the ribosome to "read through" the transcript and produce normal full-length protein. In the case of nmDMD, ataluren improves synthesis of functional dystrophin, a cytosolic socket protein that is a component of the complex that connects intracellular fibers of a muscle cell with the extracellular matrix. This effect of ataluren modestly improves the symptoms of patients. Ataluren is currently in clinical trials for treatment of other inherited diseases caused by nonsense mutations, including cystic fibrosis (nonsense mutation in the *CFTR* gene) and anaridia (nonsense mutation in the *PAX6* gene).

A different approach to treating diseases resulting from gene mutations is through the use of nucleic acids, including ASOs and RNAi. ASOs are synthetic nucleic acids that are complementary to the mRNA "sense" strand of the disease-causing gene and act by binding to the mRNA, preventing its translation. Examples of ASOs that have been approved include *fomivirsen* for treatment of cytomegalovirus retinitis viral infections of the eye (this agent has been discontinued in the U.S.) and *mipomersen* for treatment of homozygous familial hypercholesterolemia. The target gene for mipomersen is apolipoprotein B100.

Another way to selectively silence gene expression is using siRNA. RNAi is a ubiquitous cellular mechanism for small RNA-guided suppression of gene expression that uses the RISC. The antisense strand of the siRNA guides the RISC to destroy the target mRNA and is protected from degradation by the RISC, resulting in elimination of many copies of the target mRNA and gene knockdown effects that can persist for days to weeks. A number of clinical trials are in progress to treat cancer

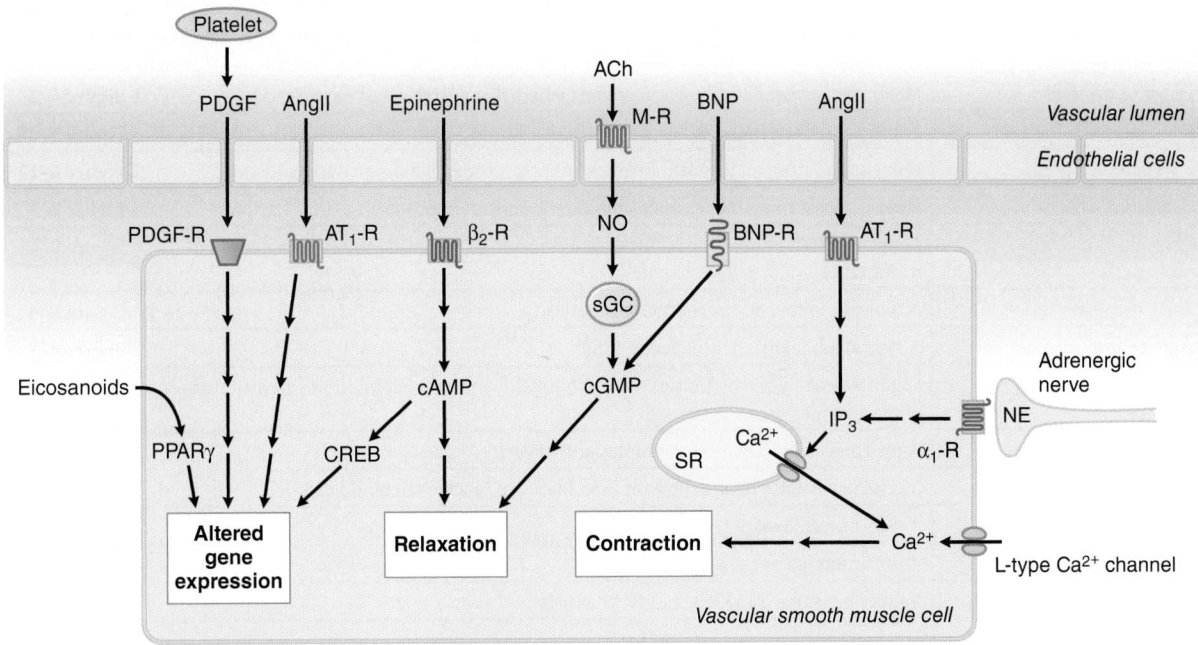

Figure 3–17 *Interaction of multiple signaling systems regulating vascular SMCs.* See text for explanation of signaling and contractile pathways and abbreviations.

using naked siRNAs as well as siRNA delivery systems using adenovirus, liposomes, polymers, and various kinds of nanoparticles.

Perhaps the therapeutic approach with the greatest potential to treat patients with a hereditary disease is the CRISPR/Cas9 genome-editing system using viruses or genetically modified microorganisms. The CRISPR/Cas9 system allows precise and imprecise editing of the genome using sgRNAs that target the Cas9 double-stranded DNA nuclease to specific sites in the genome that contain an adjacent NGG PAM sequence. The CRISPR/Cas9 system allows targeted replacement and modification of disease-causing genes. Recent proof-of-principle experiments in mouse models of DMD demonstrated that CRISPR/Cas9 delivered systemically using AAV vectors can correct disease-causing mutations in the dystrophin gene in young and adult mice. Although there are many technical, regulatory, and ethical hurdles to overcome before genome editing is approved for use in patients, the results of preclinical studies demonstrated the potential impact on treating and curing diseases that previously had no pharmacotherapeutic options.

Physiological Systems Integrate Multiple Signals

Consider the vascular wall of an arteriole (Figure 3–17). Several cell types interact at this site, including vascular smooth muscle cells, endothelial cells, platelets, and postganglionic sympathetic neurons. A variety of physiological receptors and ligands are present, including ligands that cause SMCs to contract (AngII, NE) and relax (NO, BNP, and epinephrine), as well as ligands that alter SMC gene expression (PDGF, AngII, NE, and eicosanoids).

Angiotensin II has both acute and chronic effects on SMCs. Interaction of AngII with AT_1Rs mobilizes stored Ca^{2+} via the G_q-PLC-IP_3-Ca^{2+} pathway. The Ca^{2+} binds and activates calmodulin and its target protein, MLCK. The activation of MLCK results in the phosphorylation of myosin, leading to SMC contraction. Activation of the sympathetic nervous system also regulates SMC tone through release of NE from postganglionic sympathetic neurons. NE binds α_1 adrenergic receptors, which also activate the G_q-PLC-IP_3-Ca^{2+} pathway, resulting in SMC contraction, an effect that is additive to that of AngII.

The contraction of SMCs is opposed by mediators that promote relaxation, including NO, BNP, and catecholamines acting at β_2 adrenergic receptors.

NO is formed in endothelial cells by eNOS when the G_q-PLC-IP_3-Ca^{2+} pathway is activated and by iNOS when that isoform is induced. The NO formed in the endothelium diffuses into SMCs and activates the sGC, which catalyzes the formation of cGMP, which leads to activation of PKG and phosphorylation of proteins in SMCs that reduce intracellular concentrations of Ca^{2+} and thereby promote relaxation. Intracellular concentrations of cGMP are also increased by activation of transmembrane BNP receptors (NPR-A, and to a lesser extent to NPR-B), whose guanylyl cyclase activity is increased when BNP binds.

As a consequence of the variety of pathways that affect arteriolar tone, a patient with hypertension may be treated with one or several drugs that alter signaling through these pathways. Drugs commonly used to treat hypertension include β_1 adrenergic receptor antagonists to reduce secretion of renin (the rate-limiting first step in AngII synthesis); a direct renin inhibitor (aliskiren) to block the rate-limiting step in AngII production; ACE inhibitors (e.g., enalapril) to reduce the concentrations of circulating AngII; AT_1R blockers (e.g., losartan) to block AngII binding to AT_1Rs on SMCs; α_1 adrenergic blockers to block NE binding to SMCs; sodium nitroprusside to increase the quantities of NO produced; or a Ca^{2+} channel blocker (e.g., nifedipine) to block Ca^{2+} entry into SMCs. The β_1 adrenergic receptor antagonists would also block the baroreceptor reflex increase in heart rate and blood pressure elicited by a drop in blood pressure induced by the therapy. ACE inhibitors also inhibit the degradation of a vasodilating peptide, bradykinin (see Chapter 26). Thus, the choices and mechanisms are complex, and the appropriate therapy in a given patient depends on many considerations, including the diagnosed causes of hypertension in the patient, possible side effects of the drug, efficacy in a given patient, and cost.

Signaling Pathways and Drug Action

Throughout this text, cellular signaling pathways figure prominently in explaining the actions of therapeutic agents. Not all pathways have been mentioned or fully explored in this chapter. To aid readers in finding more information on signaling and drug action, Table 3–2 lists relevant figures that appear in other chapters.

TABLE 3–2 ■ SUMMARY: RECEPTOR-SIGNALING PATHWAYS AS SITES OF DRUG ACTION

RECEPTOR/PATHWAY	FIGURE TITLE	FIGURE NUMBER
Drug transport proteins	Major mechanisms by which transporters mediate adverse drug responses	Figure 5–3
CYPs, drug metabolism	Location of CYPs in the cell	Figure 6–2
Nuclear receptors	Induction of drug metabolism by nuclear receptor–mediated signal transduction	Figure 6–13
General neurotransmission	Steps involved in excitatory and inhibitory neurotransmission	Figure 8–3
Exocytosis	Molecular basis of exocytosis: docking and fusion of synaptic vesicles with neuronal membranes	Figure 8–4
Cholinergic neurotransmission	A typical cholinergic neuroeffector junction	Figure 8–6
Adrenergic neurotransmission	A typical adrenergic neuroeffector junction	Figure 8–8
AChE and its inhibition	Steps involved in the hydrolysis of ACh by AChE and in the inhibition and reactivation of the enzyme	Figure 10–2
Transmission at the NMJ	A pharmacologist's view of the motor end plate	Figure 11–4
β Blockers and vasodilation	Mechanisms underlying actions of vasodilating β blockers in blood vessels	Figure 12–4
Serotonergic neurotransmission	A serotonergic synapse	Figure 13–4
Dopaminergic neurotransmission	A dopaminergic synapse	Figure 13–9
Voltage-sensitive cation channels	Voltage-sensitive Na^+, Ca^{2+}, and K^+ channels	Figure 14–2
Neurotransmission	Transmitter release, action, and inactivation	Figure 14–4
Ligand-gated ion channels	Pentameric ligand-gated ion channels	Figure 14–5
$GABA_A$ receptor	Pharmacologic binding sites on the $GABA_A$ receptor	Figure 14–11
NMDA receptor	Pharmacologic binding sites on the NMDA receptor	Figure 14–12
Glutamate toxicity	Mechanisms contributing to glutamate-induced cytotoxicity/neuronal injury during ischemia-reperfusion–induced glutamate release	Figure 14–13
Histamine signaling	Signal transduction pathways for histamine receptors	Figure 14–14
Cannabinoids in CNS	Anandamide synthesis and signaling	Figure 14–17
Neurotrophin signaling	Neurotrophic factor signaling in the CNS	Figure 14–18
Actions of antidepressants	Sites of action of antidepressants at noradrenergic and serotonergic nerve terminals	Figure 15–1
Na^+ channel	Antiseizure drug–enhanced Na^+ channel inactivation	Figure 17–2
$GABA_A$ receptor/channel	Some antiseizure drugs enhance GABA synaptic transmission	Figure 17–3
T-type Ca^{2+} channel	Antiseizure drug–induced reduction of current through T-type Ca^{2+} channels	Figure 17–4
Dopaminergic signaling	Dopaminergic nerve terminal	Figure 18–1
Endogenous opioid signaling	Receptor specificity of endogenous opioids; effects of receptor activation on neurons.	Figure 20–3
Biased opioid signaling	Biased signaling via opioid receptors	Figure 20–4
Cation signaling	Structure and function of voltage-gated Na^+ channels	Figure 22–2
Local anesthetic action on Na^+ channels	A pharmacologist's view of the interaction of a local anesthetic with a voltage-gated Na^+ channel	Figure 22–3
Aldosterone signaling	Effects of aldosterone on late distal tubule and collecting duct and diuretic mechanism of aldosterone antagonists	Figure 25–6
ANP signaling	Inter medullary collecting duct Na^+ transport and its regulation	Figure 25–7
V_1 receptor signaling	Mechanism of V_1 receptor-effector coupling	Figure 25–11
V_2 receptor signaling	Mechanism of V_2 receptor-effector coupling	Figure 25–12
Signals regulating renin release	Mechanisms by which the macula densa regulates renin release	Figure 26–4
Signals regulating blood pressure	Principles of blood pressure regulation and its modification by drugs	Figure 28–2
E-C coupling	Cardiac excitation-contraction coupling and its regulation by positive inotropic drugs	Figure 29–6
NO/cGMP signaling in pulmonary hypertension	Stimulators of NO/cGMP signaling	Figure 31–3
cAMP signaling in pulmonary hypertension	Membrane receptor agonists that increase cAMP	Figure 31–4
PLC signaling in pulmonary hypertension	Membrane receptor antagonists that inhibit activation of phospholipase C	Figure 31–5

(Continued)

TABLE 3–2 ■ SUMMARY: RECEPTOR-SIGNALING PATHWAYS AS SITES OF DRUG ACTION (*CONTINUED*)

RECEPTOR/PATHWAY	FIGURE TITLE	FIGURE NUMBER
Endothelium–smooth muscle signaling	Interactions between endothelium and vascular smooth muscle in pulmonary artery hypertension	Figure 31–7
Aggregatory signaling	Platelet adhesion and aggregation	Figure 32–1
Coagulatory signaling	Major reactions of blood coagulation	Figure 32–2
Fibrinolytic signaling	Fibrinolysis	Figure 32–3
Blood clotting and its prevention	Sites of action of antiplatelet drugs	Figure 32–7
LDLR and endocytosis	LDL catabolism: effects of PCSK9, antibody to PCSK9, and statins	Figure 33–4
T cell receptor (TCR) ligands	TCR signaling and its modulation by co-receptors and antibodies	Figure 34–4
MHC/antigen complexes leading to TCR signaling	Professional antigen-presenting cells (APCs)	Figure 34–5
T cell receptor signaling, immunophilins	T cell activation and sites of action of immunosuppressive agents	Figure 35–2
T cell activation	T cell activation: costimulation and coinhibitory checkpoints	Figure 35–4
Prostanoid receptors	Prostanoid receptors and their primary signaling pathways	Figure 37–4
Eicosanoid signaling	Human Eicosanoid Receptors	Table 37–2
Bradykinin/kallikrein signaling	Synthesis and receptor interactions of active peptides generated by the kallikrein-kinin and renin-angiotensin systems	Figure 39–4
Inflammatory signaling and glucocorticoid receptors	Mechanism of anti-inflammatory action of corticosteroids in asthma	Figure 40–7
Growth hormone receptor (GHR)	Mechanisms of GH and PRL action and of GHR antagonism	Figure 42–5
Oxytocin receptor signaling	Sites of action of oxytocin and tocolytic drugs in the uterine myometrium	Figure 42–8
Estrogen receptor (ER), nuclear signaling	Molecular mechanism of action of nuclear ER	Figure 44–4
Soluble guanylyl cyclase and PDE5	Mechanism of action of PDE5 inhibitors in the corpus cavernosum	Figure 45–6
Glucocorticoid receptor (GR)	Intracellular mechanism of action of the GR	Figure 46–5
Insulin secretion	Regulation of insulin secretion from a pancreatic β cell	Figure 47–3
Insulin receptor	Pathways of insulin signaling	Figure 47–4
FGF receptor	FGF23-FGFR-Klotho complex	Figure 48–4
H_2 and gastrin receptors; gastric secretion	Pharmacologist's view of gastric secretion and its regulation: the basis for therapy of acid-peptic disorders	Figure 49–1
EP_2 and EP_4 receptors; GI ion transporters; cAMP, cGMP	Mechanism of action of drugs that alter intestinal epithelial secretion and absorption	Figure 50–4
Emetic signaling	Pharmacologist's view of emetic stimuli	Figure 50–5
EGF receptor	Targeting the EGFR in cancer	Figure 67–1
Growth factor receptors	Cancer cell signaling pathway and drug targets	Figure 67–2
IGF1R	Caveat mTOR: effect of rapamycin on growth factor signaling	Figure 67–4
T cell/APC signaling	Targeting of immune checkpoints	Figure 67–5
IL-2 receptor	A pharmacologist's view of IL-2 receptors, their cellular signaling pathways, and their inhibition	Figure 67–6
Apoptotic signaling	BH3 mimetics enhance apoptosis	Figure 67–7
Rhodopsin	Pharmacologist's view of photoreceptor signaling	Figure 69–9

Acknowledgment: *Elliot M. Ross, Terry P. Kenakin, Iain L. O. Buxton, and James C. Garrison contributed to this chapter in recent editions of this book. We have retained some of their text in the current edition.*

Bibliography

Ariens EJ. Affinity and intrinsic activity in the theory of competitive inhibition. I. Problems and theory. *Arch Int Pharmacodyn Ther*, **1954**, 99:32–49.

Baillie GS. Compartmentalized signalling: spatial regulation of cAMP by the action of compartmentalized phosphodiesterases. *FEBS J*, **2009**, 276:1790–1799.

Beavo JA, Brunton LL. Cyclic nucleotide research—still expanding after half a century. *Nat Rev Mol Cell Biol*, **2002**, 3:710–718.

Beers Update Panel. American Geriatrics Society 2015 updated Beers Criteria for Potentially Inappropriate Medication Use in Older Adults. *J Am Geriatr Soc*, **2015**, 63:2227–2246.

Bento CF, et al. Mammalian autophagy: how does it work? *Annu Rev Biochem*, **2016**, 85:685–713.

Bremer E, et al. Targeted induction of apoptosis for cancer therapy: current progress and prospects. *Trends Mol Med*, **2006**, *12*: 382–393.

Calabrese EJ, Baldwin LA. Hormesis: the dose-response revolution. *Annu Rev Pharmacol Toxicol*, **2003**, 43:175–197.

Cao E, et al. TRPV1 structures in distinct conformations reveal activation mechanisms. *Nature*, **2013**, *504*:113–118.

Carlson HA, McCammon JA. Accommodating protein flexibility in computational drug design. *Mol Pharmacol*, **2000**, *57*:213–218.

Carnegie GK, et al. A-kinase anchoring proteins: from protein complexes to physiology and disease. *IUBMB Life*, **2009**, *61*:394–406.

Cheng HC. The influence of cooperativity on the determination of dissociation constants: examination of the Cheng-Prusoff equation, the Scatchard analysis, the Schild analysis and related power equations. *Pharmacol Res*, **2004**, *50*:21–40.

Cheng X, et al. Epac and PKA: a tale of two intracellular cAMP receptors. *Acta Biochim Biophys Sin (Shanghai)*, **2008**, *40*:651–662.

Cheng Y, Prusoff WH. Relationship between the inhibition constant (K_i) and the concentration of inhibitor which causes 50 per cent inhibition (I_{50}) of an enzymatic reaction. *Biochem Pharmacol*, **1973**, *22*: 3099–3108.

Conti M, Beavo J. Biochemistry and physiology of cyclic nucleotide phosphodiesterases: essential components in cyclic nucleotide signaling. *Annu Rev Biochem*, **2007**, *76*:481–511.

Danial NN, Korsmeyer SJ. Cell death: critical control points. *Cell*, **2004**, *116*:205–219.

Dessauer CW, et al. International Union of Basic and Clinical Pharmacology. CI. Structures and small molecule modulators of mammalian adenylyl cyclases. *Pharmacol Rev*, **2017**, *69*:93–139.

Etienne-Manneville S, Hall A. Rho GTPases in cell biology. *Nature*, **2002**, *420*:629–635.

Ferguson KM. Structure-based view of epidermal growth factor receptor regulation. *Annu Rev Biophys*, **2008**, *37*:353–373.

Gaddum JH. Theories of drug antagonism. *Pharmacol Rev*, **1957**, *9*:211–218.

Gay NJ, Gangloff M. Structure and function of toll receptors and their ligands. *Annu Rev Biochem*, **2007**, *76*:141–165.

Ghavami S, et al. Apoptosis and cancer: mutations within caspase genes. *J Med Genet*, **2009**, *46*:497–510.

Ghobrial IM, et al. Targeting apoptosis pathways in cancer therapy. *CA Cancer J Clin*, **2005**, *55*:178–194.

Ghosh S, Hayden MS. New regulators of NFκB in inflammation. *Nat Rev Immunol*, **2008**, *8*:837–848.

Gilman AG. G proteins: transducers of receptor-generated signals. *Annu Rev Biochem*, **1987**, *56*:615–649.

Gough DJ, et al. IFN-γ signaling—does it mean JAK-STAT? *Cytokine Growth Factor Rev*, **2008**, *19*:383–394.

GPCR Network. Understanding human GPCR biology. Home page. Available at: http://gpcr.usc.edu. Accessed March 15, 2017.

Hanoune J, Defer N. Regulation and role of adenylyl cyclase isoforms. *Annu Rev Pharmacol Toxicol*, **2001**, *41*:145–174.

Hayden MS, Ghosh S. Shared principles in NFκB signaling. *Cell*, **2008**, *132*:344–362.

Hudmon A, Schulman H. Structure-function of the multifunctional Ca^{2+}/calmodulin-dependent protein kinase II. *Biochem J*, **2002**, *364*:593–611.

Hurley JH, Young LN. Mechanisms of autophagy initiation. *Annu Rev Biochem*, **2017**, March 2017. doi:10.1146/annurev-biochem-061516-044820.

Irannejad R, et al. Effects of endocytosis on receptor-mediated signaling. *Curr Opin Cell Biol*, **2015**, *35*:137–114.

Jain KK. Role of pharmacoproteomics in the development of personalized medicine. *Pharmacogenomics*, **2004**, *5*:331–336.

Jegla TJ, et al. Evolution of the human ion channel set. *Comb Chem High Throughput Screen*, **2009**, *12*:2–23.

Kataoka T. Chemical biology of inflammatory cytokine signaling. *J Antibiot (Tokyo)*, **2009**, *62*:655–667.

Kenakin T. Efficacy as a vector: the relative prevalence and paucity of inverse agonism. *Mol Pharmacol*, **2004**, *65*:2–11.

Limbird LE. *Cell Surface Receptors: A Short Course on Theory and Methods*. Springer-Verlag, New York, **2005**.

May LT, et al. Allosteric modulation of G protein–coupled receptors. *Annu Rev Pharmacol Toxicol*, **2007**, 47:1–51.

Mayr B, Montminy M. Transcriptional regulation by the phosphorylation-dependent factor creb. *Nat Rev Mol Cell Biol*, **2001**, *2*: 599–609.

McEwan IJ. Nuclear receptors: one big family. *Methods Mol Biol*, **2009**, *505*:3–18.

Mehats C, et al. Cyclic nucleotide phosphodiesterases and their role in endocrine cell signaling. *Trends Endocrinol Metab*, **2002**, *13*: 29–35.

Milligan G. Constitutive activity and inverse agonists of G protein-coupled receptors: a current perspective. *Mol Pharmacol*, **2003**, *64*: 1271–1276.

Palczewski K, et al. Crystal structure of rhodopsin: a G protein-coupled receptor. *Science*, **2000**, *289*:739–745.

Patterson RL, et al. Inositol 1,4,5-trisphosphate receptors as signal integrators. *Annu Rev Biochem*, **2004**, *73*:437–465.

Potter LR, et al. Natriuretic peptides: their structures, receptors, physiologic functions and therapeutic applications. *Handb Exp Pharmacol*, **2009**, 341–366.

Privalsky ML. The role of corepressors in transcriptional regulation by nuclear hormone receptors. *Annu Rev Physiol*, **2004**, *66*: 315–360.

Purves D, et al. Channels and transporters. In: Purves D, et al., eds. *Neuroscience*. 5th ed. Sinauer, Sunderland, MA, **2011**, 61–84.

Ramsey IS, et al. An introduction to TRP channels. *Annu Rev Physiol*, **2006**, 68:619–647.

Rong Y, Distelhorst CW. Bcl-2 protein family members: versatile regulators of calcium signaling in cell survival and apoptosis. *Annu Rev Physiol*, **2008**, *70*:73–91.

Roscioni SS, et al. Epac: effectors and biological functions. *Naunyn Schmiedebergs Arch Pharmacol*, **2008**, *377*:345–357.

Rybalkin SD, et al. Cyclic GMP phosphodiesterases and regulation of smooth muscle function. *Circ Res*, **2003**, *93*:280–291.

Sands WA, Palmer TM. Regulating gene transcription in response to cyclic AMP elevation. *Cell Signal*, **2008**, *20*:460–466.

Schild HO. Drug antagonism and pA₂. *Pharmacol Rev*, **1957**, *9*: 242–246.

Schmidt M, et al. Exchange protein directly activated by cAMP (Epac): a multidomain cAMP mediator in the regulation of diverse biological functions. *Pharmacol Rev*, **2013**, *65*:670–709.

Skaug B, et al. The role of ubiquitin in NFκB regulatory pathways. *Annu Rev Biochem*, **2009**, *78*:769–796.

Smit MJ, et al. Pharmacogenomic and structural analysis of constitutive G protein-coupled receptor activity. *Annu Rev Pharmacol Toxicol*, **2007**, 47:53–87.

Stevens RC, et al. The GPCR Network: a large-scale collaboration to determine human GPCR structure and function. *Nat Rev Drug Discov*, **2013**, *12*:25–34.

Tallarida RJ. An overview of drug combination analysis with isobolograms. *J Pharmacol Exp Ther*, **2006**, *319*:1–7.

Tallarida RJ. Revisiting the isobole and related quantitative methods for assessing drug synergism. *J Pharmacol Exp Ther*, **2012**, *342*:2–8.

Taylor SS, et al. Signaling through cAMP and cAMP-dependent protein kinase: diverse strategies for drug design. *Biochim Biophys Acta*, **2008**, *1784*:16–26.

Tontonoz P, Spiegelman BM. Fat and beyond: the diverse biology of PPARγ. *Annu Rev Biochem*, **2008**, *77*:289–312.

Tsai EJ, Kass DA. Cyclic GMP signaling in cardiovascular pathophysiology and therapeutics. *Pharmacol Ther*, **2009**, *122*:216–238.

Venkatachalam K, Montell C. TRP channels. *Annu Rev Biochem*, **2007**, *76*:387–417.

Wahl-Schott C, Biel M. HCN channels: Structure, cellular regulation and physiological function. *Cell Mol Life Sci*, **2009**, *66*:470–494.

Wang X, et al. Structural biology of shared cytokine receptors. *Annu Rev Immunol*, **2009**, *27*:29–60.

Wilson NS, et al. Death receptor signal transducers: nodes of coordination in immune signaling networks. *Nat Immunol*, **2009**, *10*:348–355.

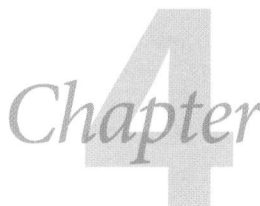

Chapter 4

Drug Toxicity and Poisoning

Michelle A. Erickson and Trevor M. Penning

Pharmacology intersects with *toxicology* when the physiological response to a drug is an *adverse effect*. A *poison* is any substance, including any drug, that has the capacity to harm a living organism. *Poisoning* generally implies that damaging physiological effects result from exposure to pharmaceuticals, illicit drugs, or chemicals.

Dose-Response

Conventional Dose-Response Curves

There is a graded dose-response relationship in an *individual* and a quantal dose-response relationship in the *population* (see Figures 3–2, 3–3, and 3–6). Graded doses of a drug given to an individual usually result in a greater magnitude of response as the dose increases. In a quantal dose-response relationship, the percentage of the population affected increases as the dose is increased; the relationship is quantal in that the effect is judged to be either present or absent in a given individual. This quantal dose-response phenomenon is used to determine the LD_{50} of drugs, as defined in Figure 4–1A.

One can also determine a quantal dose-response curve for the therapeutic effect of a drug to generate ED_{50}, the concentration of drug at which 50% of the population will have the desired response, and a quantal dose-response curve for lethality by the same agent (Figure 4–1B). These two curves can be used to generate a TI, which quantifies the relative safety of a drug:

$$TI = \frac{LD_{50}}{ED_{50}} \qquad \text{(Equation 4–1)}$$

Clearly, the higher the ratio, the safer the drug.

Values of TI vary widely, from 1–2 to more than 100. Drugs with a low TI must be administered with caution (e.g., the cardiac glycoside digoxin and cancer chemotherapeutic agents). Agents with very high TI (e.g., penicillin) are extremely safe in the absence of a known allergic response in a given patient. Note that use of median doses fails to consider that the slopes of the dose-response curves for therapeutic and lethal (toxic) effects may differ (Figure 4–1). As an alternative the ED_{99} for the therapeutic effect can be compared to the LD_1 for lethality (toxic effect), to yield a *margin of safety*.

$$\text{Margin of safety} = \frac{LD_1}{ED_{99}} \qquad \text{(Equation 4–2)}$$

Nonmonotonic Dose-Response Curves

Not all dose-response curves follow a typical sigmoidal shape. Three examples of these are shown in Figure 4–2. *U-shaped dose-response curves* can be observed for essential metals and vitamins (Figure 4–2A). At low dose, adverse effects are observed because there is a deficiency of these nutrients to maintain homeostasis. As dose increases, homeostasis is achieved, and the bottom of the U-shaped dose-response curve is reached. As dose increases to surpass the amount required to maintain homeostasis, overdose toxicity can ensue. Thus, adverse effects are seen at both low and high doses.

Some toxicants, such as formaldehyde, are also metabolic by-products for which cells have detoxifying mechanisms. Thus, very low doses of exogenous formaldehyde do not sufficiently exceed levels produced physiologically to elicit a significant adverse response, and do not saturate the detoxifying mechanisms, in this instance, alcohol dehydrogenase (ADH5/GSNOR; Pontel et al., 2015). When these endogenous protective mechanisms are overwhelmed, one will observe a toxic response. Toxicologists represent this type of response as a "hockey stick" (Figure 4–2B), a region of no response followed by an adverse response as the toxicant exceeds the endogenous protective mechanisms and rises sufficiently to cause an adverse response.

Inverted U-shaped dose response curves are observed when receptor downregulation/desensitization occurs following exposure to a ligand or when an additional and distinct negative effect occurs at a concentration beyond that which produces the primary positive effect.

For example, estrogen at high levels can have maximal effects. However, at supraphysiologic levels, the effects of estrogen are reduced, presumably due to downregulation of estrogen receptors. Many endocrine-disrupting chemicals are thought to have inverted U-shaped dose-response curves similar to that of estrogen. Indeed, multiphasic and U-shaped curves are

Abbreviations

ADEs: adverse drug events
ADME: absorption, distribution, metabolism, and elimination
CYP: cytochrome P450
ECG: electrocardiogram
ED$_{50}$: median effective dose
FDA: U.S. Food and Drug Administration
GI: gastrointestinal
Ig: immunoglobulin
IND: investigational new drug
IRB: institutional review board
LD$_{50}$: median lethal dose
SSRI: selective serotonin reuptake inhibitor
TI: therapeutic index
WBI: whole-bowel irrigation

common in complex systems in which an administered compound elicits multiple effects, first one effect and then another, possibly opposing, effect as the concentration increases. This phenomenon highlights a necessity for using an extensive dose range and a sufficient response time to ensure detection of the full spectrum of responsiveness and toxicity for a given substance.

Pharmacokinetics Versus Toxicokinetics

Alterations in ADME

Poisoning may significantly alter the functions of ADME (see Chapters 2, 5, and 6), and these alterations can profoundly alter treatment decisions and prognosis. The pharmacokinetics of a drug under circumstances that produce toxicity or excessive exposure are referred to as *toxicokinetics*. Ingesting larger-than-therapeutic doses of a pharmaceutical may prolong its absorption, alter its protein binding and apparent volume of distribution, and change its metabolic fate. When confronted with potential poisoning, two questions should be foremost in the clinician's mind:

- How long will an asymptomatic patient need to be monitored (drug absorption and dynamics)?
- How long will it take an intoxicated patient to get better (drug elimination and dynamics)?

Drug Absorption

Aspirin poisoning is a leading cause of overdose morbidity and mortality as reported to U.S. poison control centers (Bronstein et al., 2008). In therapeutic dosing, aspirin reaches peak plasma concentrations in about 1 h. However, aspirin overdose may cause spasm of the pyloric valve, delaying entry of the drug into the small intestine. Aspirin, especially enteric-coated forms, may coalesce into bezoars, reducing the effective surface area for absorption. Peak plasma salicylate concentrations from aspirin overdose may not be reached for 4–35 h after ingestion (Rivera et al., 2004).

Drug Elimination

Table 4–1 lists some pharmaceuticals notorious for their predilection to have initial symptoms develop *after* a typical 4- to 6-hour emergency medical observation period (Box 4–1).

Types of Therapeutic Drug Toxicity

In therapeutics, a drug typically produces numerous effects, but usually only one is sought as the primary goal of treatment; most of the other effects are undesirable effects for that therapeutic indication. *Side effects* of drugs usually are bothersome but not deleterious. Other undesirable effects may be characterized as toxic effects (Figure 4–3).

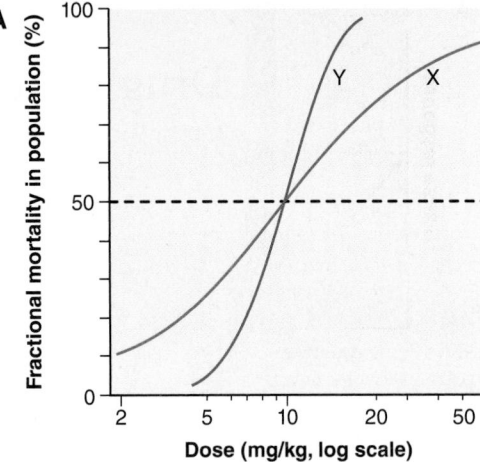

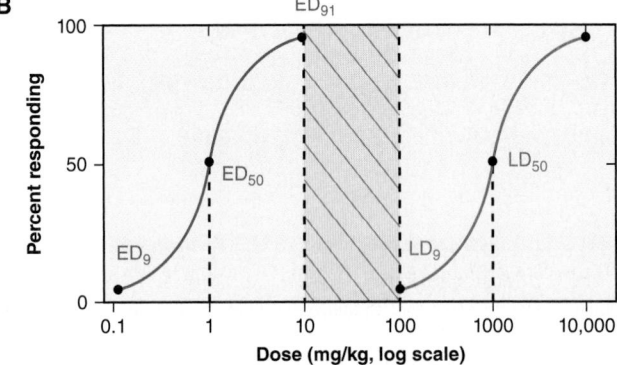

Figure 4–1 *Dose-response relationships.* **A.** The LD$_{50}$ of a compound is determined experimentally, usually by administration of the chemical to mice or rats (orally or intraperitoneally). The midpoint of the curve representing percentage of population responding (response here is death) versus dose (log scale) represents the LD$_{50}$, or the dose of drug that is lethal in 50% of the population. The LD$_{50}$ values for both compounds are the same (~10 mg/kg); however, the slopes of the dose-response curves are quite different. Thus, at a dose equal to one-half the LD$_{50}$ (5 mg/kg), fewer than 5% of the animals exposed to compound Y would die, but about 25% of the animals given compound X would die. **B.** Depiction of ED and LD. The crosshatched area between the ED$_{91}$ (10 mg/kg) and the LD$_9$ (100 mg/kg) gives an estimate of the margin of safety.

Dose-Dependent Reactions

Toxic effects of drugs may be classified as *pharmacological*, *pathological*, or *genotoxic*. Typically, the incidence and seriousness of the toxicity is proportionately related to the concentration of the drug in the body and to the duration of the exposure.

Pharmacological Toxicity. The CNS depression produced by barbiturates is largely predictable in a dose-dependent fashion. The progression of clinical effects goes from anxiolysis to sedation to somnolence to coma. Similarly, the degree of hypotension produced by nifedipine is related to the dose of the drug administered. Tardive dyskinesia (see Chapter 16), an extrapyramidal motor disorder associated with use of antipsychotic medications, seems to be dependent on duration of exposure. Pharmacological toxicity can also occur when the correct dose is given; for example, there is phototoxicity associated with exposure to sunlight in patients treated with tetracyclines, sulfonamides, chlorpromazine, and nalidixic acid.

Pathological Toxicity. Acetaminophen is metabolized to nontoxic glucuronide and sulfate conjugates and to a highly reactive metabolite NAPQI via CYP isoforms. At a therapeutic dose of acetaminophen, NAPQI binds

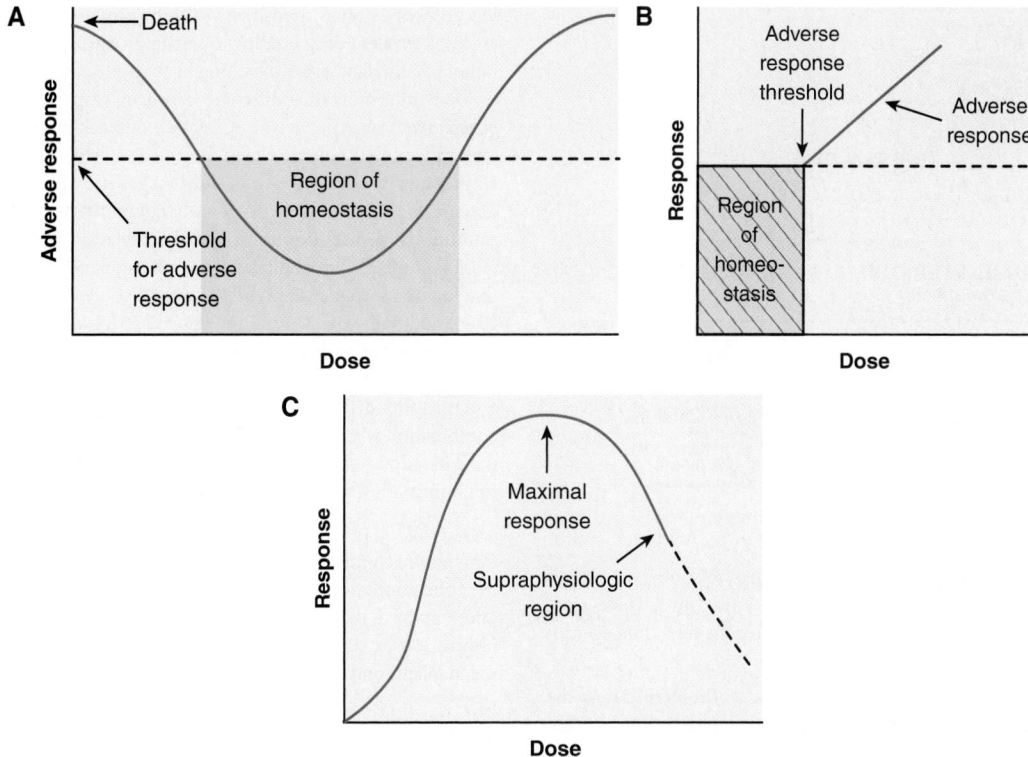

Figure 4–2 *Nonmonotonic dose-response relationships.* **A.** U-shaped dose-response curve for essential metals and vitamins. **B.** Hockey stick-shaped dose-response curve for toxicants that are also metabolic by-products. **C.** Inverted U-shaped dose-response curve for ligands that downregulate their receptors.

to nucleophilic glutathione, but in acetaminophen overdose, glutathione depletion may lead to the pathological finding of hepatic necrosis due to shunting of NAPQI toward interactions with nucleophilic cellular macromolecules (Figure 4–4).

Genotoxic Effects. Ionizing radiation and many environmental chemicals are known to injure DNA and may lead to mutagenic or carcinogenic toxicities. Many of the cancer chemotherapeutic agents (see Chapters 65–68) may be genotoxic (see Chapters 6 and 7).

Allergic Reactions

An *allergy* is an adverse reaction, mediated by the immune system, that results from previous sensitization to a particular chemical or to one that is structurally similar (see Chapter 34). Allergic responses have been divided into four general categories based on the mechanism of immunological involvement.

TABLE 4–1 ■ DRUGS THAT COMMONLY MANIFEST INITIAL SYMPTOMS MORE THAN 4–6 HOURS AFTER ORAL OVERDOSE[a]

Acetaminophen
Aspirin
Illicit drugs in rubber or plastic packages
Monoamine oxidase inhibitors
Sulfonylureas
Sustained-release formulation drugs
Thyroid hormones
Valproic acid
Warfarin-like anticoagulants

[a]Drugs coingested with agents having anticholinergic activity, as manifest by diminished GI motility, may also exhibit delayed onset of action.

Type I: Anaphylactic Reactions. Anaphylaxis is mediated by IgE antibodies. The Fc portion of IgE can bind to receptors on mast cells and basophils. If the Fab portion of the antibody molecule then binds an antigen, various mediators (e.g., histamine, leukotrienes, and prostaglandins) are released and cause vasodilation, edema, and an inflammatory response. The main targets of this type of reaction are the GI tract (food allergies), the skin (urticaria and atopic dermatitis), the respiratory system (rhinitis and asthma), and the vasculature (anaphylactic shock). These responses tend to occur quickly after challenge with an antigen to which the individual has been sensitized and are termed *immediate hypersensitivity reactions.*

Type II: Cytolytic Reactions. Type II allergies are mediated by both IgG and IgM antibodies and usually are attributed to their capacity to activate the complement system. The major target tissues for cytolytic reactions are the cells in the circulatory system. Examples of type II allergic responses include penicillin-induced hemolytic anemia, quinidine-induced thrombocytopenic purpura, and sulfonamide-induced granulocytopenia. These autoimmune reactions to drugs usually subside within several months after removal of the offending agent.

Type III: Arthus Reactions. Type III allergic reactions are mediated predominantly by IgG; the mechanism involves the generation of antigen-antibody complexes that subsequently fix complement. The complexes are deposited in the vascular endothelium, where a destructive inflammatory response called *serum sickness* occurs. The clinical symptoms of serum sickness include urticarial skin eruptions, arthralgia or

BOX 4–1 ■ Valproic Acid

After therapeutic dosing, valproic acid has an elimination $t_{1/2}$ of about 14 h. Valproic acid poisoning may lead to coma. In predicting the duration of the coma, it is important to consider that, after overdose, first-order metabolic processes for valproate appear to become saturated, and the apparent elimination $t_{1/2}$ may exceed 30–45 h (Sztajnkrycer, 2002), putting the patient at risk for a much longer time.

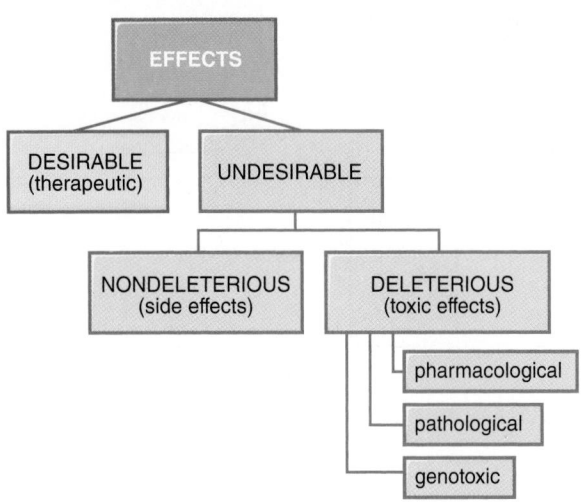

Figure 4–3 *Spectrum of the effects of pharmaceuticals.*

arthritis, lymphadenopathy, and fever. Several drugs, including commonly used antibiotics, can induce serum sickness-like reactions. These reactions usually last 6–12 days and then subside after the offending agent is eliminated.

Type IV: Delayed Hypersensitivity Reactions. These reactions are mediated by sensitized T lymphocytes and macrophages. When sensitized cells come in contact with antigen, an inflammatory reaction is generated by the production of lymphokines and the subsequent influx of neutrophils and macrophages. An example of type IV or delayed hypersensitivity is the contact dermatitis caused by poison ivy.

Idiosyncratic Reactions and Pharmacogenetic Contributions

Idiosyncrasy is an abnormal reactivity to a chemical that is peculiar to a given individual; the idiosyncratic response may be extreme sensitivity to

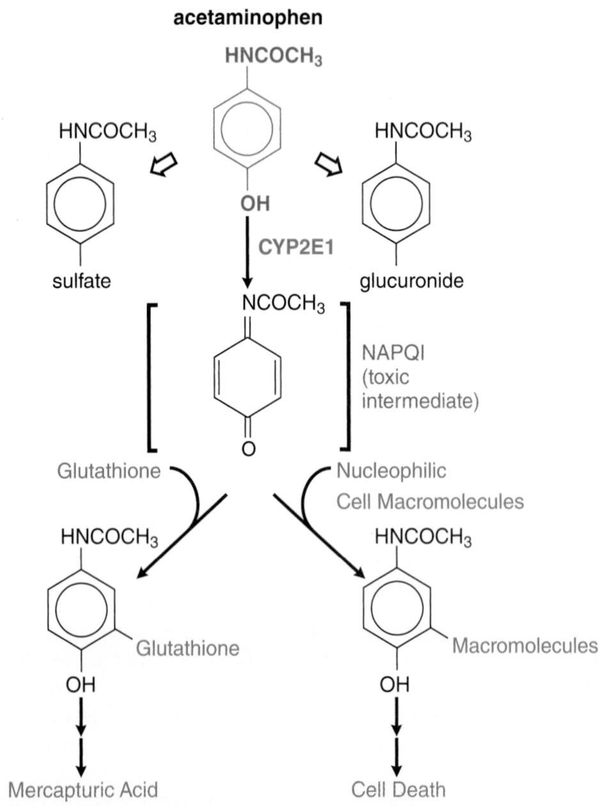

acetaminophen

HNCOCH₃

Figure 4–4 *Pathways of acetaminophen metabolism and toxicity.* The toxic intermediate NAPQI is *N*-acetyl-*p*-benzoquinoneimine.

low doses or extreme insensitivity to high doses of drugs. A common mechanism is covalent drug binding to serum proteins that leads to the presentation of a foreign hapten, resulting in an immunotoxicological response.

Many interindividual differences in drug responses have a *pharmacogenetic basis* (see Chapter 7). A fraction of black males (~10%) develop a serious hemolytic anemia when they receive primaquine as an antimalarial therapy; this development is due to a genetic deficiency of erythrocyte glucose-6-phosphate dehydrogenase. Polymorphisms in NAT2 lead to a multimodal distribution of isoniazid acetylation and clearance (Figures 60–3 and 60–4). Variability in the anticoagulant response to warfarin is due to polymorphisms in CYP2C9 and VKORC1 (see Figure 7–7, Figure 32–6, and Table 32–2). In addition, CYP3A4 and CYP2D6 metabolize a large number of drugs in the liver (see Figure 6–3). Single nucleotide polymorphic variants in CYP3A4 and CYP2D6 can affect enzyme activity and thus alter drug $t_{1/2}$. Administration of a drug that is a CYP substrate in combination with a drug that is an inhibitor of the same CYP can lead to drug overdose toxicity. Many package inserts for drugs provide prescribing information warning of these drug-drug interactions.

Drug-Drug Interactions

Patients are commonly treated with more than one drug may also be using over-the-counter medications, vitamins, and other "natural" supplements; and may have unusual diets. All of these factors can contribute to drug interactions, a failure of therapy, and toxicity. Figure 4–5 summarizes the mechanisms and types of interactions.

Interaction of Absorption. A drug may cause either an increase or a decrease in the absorption of another drug from the intestinal lumen. Ranitidine, an antagonist of histamine H_2 receptors, raises gastrointestinal pH and may increase the absorption of basic drugs such as triazolam (O'Connor-Semmes et al., 2001). Conversely, the bile acid sequestrant cholestyramine leads to significantly reduced serum concentrations of propranolol (Hibbard et al., 1984).

Interaction of Protein Binding. Many drugs, such as aspirin, barbiturates, phenytoin, sulfonamides, valproic acid, and warfarin, are highly protein bound in the plasma, and it is the free (unbound) drug that produces the clinical effects. These drugs may have enhanced toxicity in overdose if protein-binding sites become saturated in physiological states that lead to hypoalbuminemia, or when displaced from plasma proteins by other drugs (Guthrie et al., 1995).

Interaction of Metabolism. A drug can frequently influence the metabolism of one or several other drugs (see Chapter 6), especially when hepatic CYPs are involved. Acetaminophen is partially transformed by CYP2E1 to the toxic metabolite NAPQI (see Figure 4–4). Intake of ethanol, a potent inducer of CYP2E1, may lead to increased susceptibility to acetaminophen poisoning after overdose (Dart et al., 2006).

Interaction of Receptor Binding. Buprenorphine is an opioid with partial agonist and antagonist receptor activities, commonly used to treat opioid addiction. The drug binds to opiate receptors with high affinity and can prevent euphoria from concomitant use of narcotic drugs of abuse.

Interaction of Therapeutic Action. Aspirin is an inhibitor of platelet aggregation, heparin is an anticoagulant; given together, they may increase risk for bleeding. Sulfonylureas cause hypoglycemia by stimulating pancreatic insulin release, whereas biguanide drugs (e.g., metformin) lead to decreased hepatic glucose production, and these drugs can be used together to control diabetic hyperglycemia.

Such drug interactions are *additive* when the combined effect of two drugs equals the sum of the effect of each agent given alone and *synergistic* when the combined effect exceeds the sum of the effects of each drug given alone. *Potentiation of toxicity* describes the creation of a toxic effect from one drug due to the presence of another drug. *Antagonism* is the interference of one drug with the action of another. *Functional* or *physiological antagonism* occurs when two chemicals produce opposite effects on the same physiological function. *Chemical antagonism*, or *inactivation*, is a reaction between two chemicals to neutralize their effects, such as is seen with chelation therapy. *Dispositional antagonism* is the alteration of

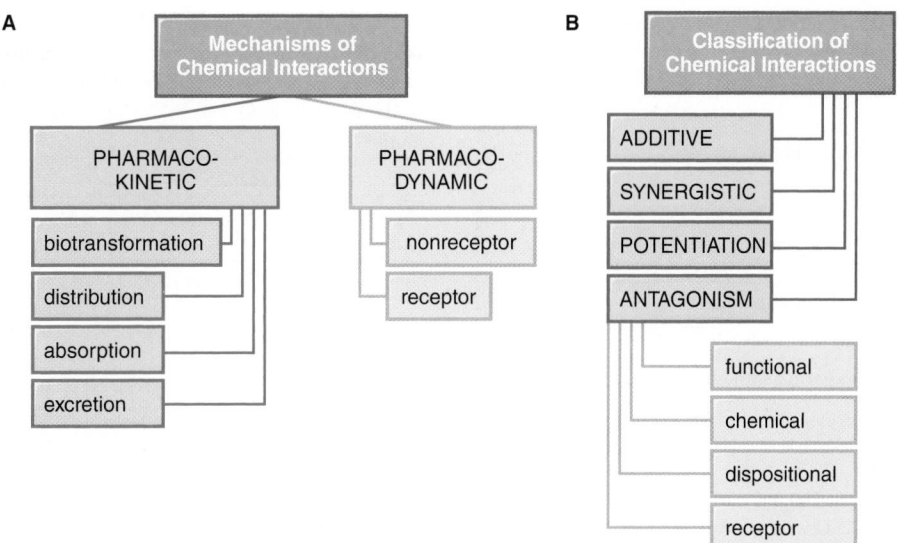

Figure 4–5 *Mechanisms and classification of drug interactions.*

the disposition of a substance (its absorption, biotransformation, distribution, or excretion) so that less of the agent reaches the target organ or its persistence in the target organ is reduced. *Receptor* (meaning receptor, enzyme, drug transporter, ion channel, etc.) *antagonism* is the blockade of the effect of one drug by another drug that competes at the receptor site.

Descriptive Toxicity Testing in Animals

Two main principles or assumptions underlie all descriptive toxicity tests performed in animals.

First, those effects of chemicals produced in laboratory animals, when properly qualified, apply to human toxicity. When calculated on the basis of dose per unit of body surface, toxic effects in human beings usually are encountered in the same range of concentrations as those in experimental animals. On the basis of body weight, human beings generally are more vulnerable than experimental animals.

Second, exposure of experimental animals to toxic agents in high doses is a necessary and valid method to discover possible hazards to human beings who are exposed to much lower doses. This principle is based on the quantal dose-response concept. As a matter of practicality, the number of animals used in experiments on toxic materials usually will be small compared with the size of human populations potentially at risk. For example, 0.01% incidence of a serious toxic effect (such as cancer) represents 25,000 people in a population of 250 million. Such an incidence is unacceptably high. Yet, detecting an incidence of 0.01% experimentally probably would require a minimum of 30,000 animals. To estimate risk at low dosage, large doses must be given to relatively small groups instead. *The validity of the necessary extrapolation is clearly a crucial question.*

Chemicals are first tested for toxicity by estimation of the LD_{50} in two animal species by two routes of administration; one of these is the expected route of exposure of human beings to the chemical being tested. The number of animals that die in a 14-day period after a single dose is recorded. The animals also are examined for signs of intoxication, lethargy, behavioral modification, and morbidity. The chemical is next tested for toxicity by repeat exposure, usually for 90 days. This study is performed most often in two species by the route of intended use or exposure with at least three doses. A number of parameters are monitored during this period, and at the end of the study, organs and tissues are examined by a pathologist.

Long-term or chronic studies are carried out in animals at the same time that clinical trials are undertaken. For drugs, the length of exposure depends somewhat on the intended clinical use. If the drug normally would be used for short periods under medical supervision, as would an antimicrobial agent, a chronic exposure of animals for 6 months might suffice. If the drug would be used in human beings for longer periods, a study of chronic use for 2 years may be required.

Studies of chronic exposure often are used to determine the carcinogenic potential of chemicals. These studies usually are performed in rats and mice for the average lifetime of the species. Other tests are designed to evaluate teratogenicity (congenital malformations), perinatal and postnatal toxicity, and effects on fertility. Teratogenicity studies usually are performed by administering drugs to pregnant rats and rabbits during the period of organogenesis. *In silico* computational methods of systems chemical biology may soon contribute to such studies.

Safety Pharmacology and Clinical Trials

Fewer than one-third of the drugs tested in clinical trials reach the marketplace. U.S. federal law and ethical considerations require that the study of new drugs in humans be conducted in accordance with stringent guidelines.

Once a drug is judged ready to be studied in humans, an IND application must be filed with the FDA. The IND includes (1) information on the composition and source of the drug; (2) chemical and manufacturing information; (3) all data from animal studies; (4) proposed clinical plans and protocols; (5) the names and credentials of physicians who will conduct the clinical trials; and (6) a compilation of the key data relevant to study the drug in humans made available to investigators and their IRBs.

Testing in humans begins only after sufficient acute and subacute animal toxicity studies have been completed. Chronic safety testing in animals, including carcinogenicity studies, is usually done concurrently with clinical trials. Accumulating and analyzing all necessary data often requires 4–6 years of clinical testing. In each of the three formal phases of clinical trials, volunteers or patients must be informed of the investigational status of the drug as well as the possible risks and must be allowed to decline or to consent to participate and receive the drug. These regulations are based on the ethical principles set forth in the Declaration of Helsinki. In addition, an interdisciplinary IRB at the facility where the clinical drug trial will be conducted must review and approve the scientific and ethical plans for testing in humans. The prescribed phases, time lines, and costs for developing a new drug are presented in Table 1–1 and Figure 1–1.

Epidemiology of Adverse Drug Responses and Pharmaceutical Poisoning

Poisoning can occur in many ways following therapeutic and nontherapeutic exposures to drugs or chemicals (Table 4–2). In the U.S., an estimated 2 million hospitalized patients have serious adverse drug

TABLE 4–2 ■ POTENTIAL SCENARIOS FOR THE OCCURRENCE OF POISONING

Therapeutic drug toxicity
Exploratory exposure by young children
Environmental exposure
Occupational exposure
Recreational abuse
Errors of prescribing, dispensing, or administering
Purposeful administration for self-harm
Purposeful administration to harm another

reactions each year, and about 100,000 suffer fatal adverse drug reactions (Lazarou et al., 1998). Use of good principles of prescribing, as described in Appendix I and Table 4–5, can aid in avoiding such adverse outcomes.

Some toxicities of pharmaceuticals can be predicted based on their known pharmacological mechanism; often, however, the therapeutic toxicity profile of a drug becomes apparent only during the postmarketing period. The Adverse Event Reporting System of the FDA relies on two signals to detect rarer ADEs. First, the FDA requires drug manufacturers to perform postmarketing surveillance of prescription drugs and nonprescription products. Second, the FDA operates a voluntary reporting system (MedWatch, at http://www.fda.gov/Safety/MedWatch) available to both health professionals and consumers. Hospitals may also support committees to investigate potential ADEs. Unfortunately, any national data set will likely underestimate the morbidity and mortality attributable to ADEs due to underreporting and the difficulty of estimating the denominator of total patient exposures.

Therapeutic drug toxicity is only a subset of poisoning, as noted in Table 4–2. Misuse and abuse of both prescription and illicit drugs are major public health problems. The incidence of unintentional, noniatrogenic poisoning is bimodal, primarily affecting exploratory young children, ages 1–5 years, and the elderly. *Intentional* overdose with pharmaceuticals is most common in adolescence and through adulthood. The substances most frequently involved in human exposures and fatalities are presented in Tables 4–3 and 4–4, respectively.

TABLE 4–3 ■ SUBSTANCES MOST FREQUENTLY INVOLVED IN HUMAN POISONING EXPOSURES

SUBSTANCE	%
Analgesics	11.3
Personal care products	7.7
Cleaning substances	7.7
Sedatives/hypnotics/antipsychotics	5.9
Antidepressants	4.4
Antihistamines	4.0
Cardiovascular drugs	4.0
Foreign bodies/toys/miscellaneous	3.9
Pesticides	3.2

In the subset of pediatric exposures (age < 5 years), cosmetic/personal care products and household cleaning products accounted for 25% of cases, followed by analgesics (9.3%), foreign bodies/toys (6.7%), topical preparations (5.8%), vitamins (4.5%), and antihistamines (4.3%).
Source: Data from Mowry et al., 2015.

TABLE 4–4 ■ POISONS ASSOCIATED WITH THE LARGEST NUMBER OF HUMAN FATALITIES

Sedatives/hypnotics/antipsychotics	Stimulants and street drugs
Cardiovascular drugs	Alcohols
Acetaminophen (alone and in combinations)	SSRIs
Opioids	

As reported in Mowry et al., 2015.

Prevention of Poisoning

Reduction of Medication Errors

Over the past decade, considerable attention has been given to the reduction of medication errors and ADEs. Medication errors can occur in any part of the medication prescribing or use process, whereas ADEs are injuries related to the use or nonuse of medications. It is believed that medication errors are 50–100 times more common than ADEs (Bates et al., 1995). The "five rights" noted in Box 4–2 can serve as a corrective.

In practice, accomplishing a reduction in medication errors involves scrutiny of the systems involved in prescribing, documenting, transcribing, dispensing, administering, and monitoring a therapy, as presented in Appendix I. Good medication use practices have mandatory and redundant checkpoints (Figure 4–6), such as having a pharmacist, a doctor, and a nurse, all review and confirm, prior to the drug's administration, that an ordered dose of a medication is appropriate for the patient. Several practical strategies can help to reduce medication errors within health care settings (Table 4–5).

Poisoning Prevention in the Home

There are several contexts into which poisoning prevention can be directed (Table 4–2). Depression and suicidal ideation need to be identified and treated. Exposure to hazards in the home, outdoor, and work environments need to be reduced to reasonably achievable levels. Poisoning prevention strategies may be categorized as *passive*, requiring no behavior change on the part of the individual, or *active*, requiring sustained adaptation to be successful. Passive prevention strategies are the most effective (Table 4–6). The incidence of poisoning in children has decreased dramatically over the past four decades, largely due to improved safety packaging of drugs, drain cleaners, turpentine, and other household chemicals; improved medical training and care; and increased public awareness of potential poisons.

Principles of Treatment of Poisoning

When toxicity is expected or occurs, the priorities of poisoning treatment are to

- *Maintain vital physiological functions*
- *Reduce or prevent absorption and enhance elimination to minimize the tissue concentration of the poison*
- *Combat the toxicological effects of the poison at the effector sites (Box 4–3)*

BOX 4–2 ■ Five Principles of Safe Medication

Following the "five rights" of safe medication administration can help practitioners avoid medication errors:

Right drug, right patient, right dose, right route, right time

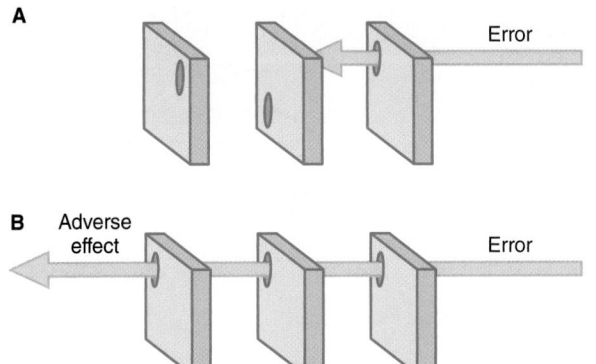

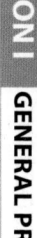

Figure 4–6 *The "Swiss cheese" model of medication error.* Several checkpoints typically exist to identify and prevent an adverse drug event, and that adverse event can only occur if holes in several systems align. **A.** One systematic error does not lead to an adverse event because it is prevented by another check in the system. **B.** Several systematic errors can align to allow an adverse event to occur. (Data from Reason J, *Br Med J*, 2000;320:768–770.)

Identification of Clinical Patterns of Toxicity

A medical history may allow for the creation of a list of available medications or chemicals implicated in a poisoning event. Often, an observation of physical symptoms and signs may be the only additional clues to a poisoning diagnosis. Groups of physical signs and symptoms associated with specific poisoning syndromes are known as *toxidromes* (Erickson et al., 2007; Osterhoudt, 2004) (Table 4–7).

The urine drug toxicology test is an immunoassay designed to detect common drugs of abuse, such as amphetamines, barbiturates, benzodiazepines, cannabis, cocaine, and opiates. Acute poisoning with these substances can usually be determined on clinical grounds, and the results of these assays are infrequently available fast enough to guide stabilization. In addition, detection of drugs or their metabolites on a urine immunoassay does not mean that the detected drug is responsible for the currently observed poisoning illness. When ingestion of acetaminophen or aspirin cannot clearly be excluded via the exposure history, serum quantification of these drugs is recommended. An ECG may be useful at detecting heart

blocks, Na^+ channel blockade, or K^+ channel blockade associated with specific medication classes (Table 4–8). Further laboratory analysis should be tailored to the individual poisoning circumstance.

Decontamination of the Poisoned Patient

Poisoning exposures may be by inhalation, by dermal or mucosal absorption, by injection, or by ingestion. The first step in preventing absorption of poison is to stop any ongoing exposure. If necessary, eyes and skin should be washed copiously. GI decontamination prevents or reduces absorption of a substance after it has been ingested. The strategies for GI decontamination are *gastric emptying, adsorption of poison, WBI, and catharsis.* Minimal indications for considering GI decontamination include

- The poison must be potentially dangerous.
- The poison must still be unabsorbed in the stomach or intestine, so it must be soon after ingestion.
- The procedure must be able to be performed safely and with proper technique.

Gastric emptying is rarely recommended anymore (Manoguerra and Cobaugh, 2005), but the administration of activated charcoal and the performance of WBI remain therapeutic options. Gastric emptying reduces drug absorption by about one-third under optimal conditions (American Academy of Clinical Toxicology, 2004; Tenenbein et al., 1987) (see Syrup of Ipecac section that follows).

Adsorption

Adsorption of a poison refers to the binding of a poison to the surface of another substance so that the poison is less available for absorption into

---

TABLE 4–6 ■ PASSIVE POISONING PREVENTION STRATEGIES AND EXAMPLES

Reduce manufacture/sale of poisons   *Withdrawal of phenformin from U.S. pharmaceutical market*
Decrease amount of poison in a consumer product   *Limiting number of pills in a single bottle of baby aspirin*
Prevent access to poison   *Using child-resistant packaging*
Change product formulation   *Removing ethanol from mouthwash*

TABLE 4–5 ■ BEST PRACTICE RECOMMENDATIONS TO REDUCE MEDICATION ADMINISTRATION ERRORS[a]

SHORT TERM

- Maintain unit-dose distribution systems for nonemergency medications
- Have pharmacies prepare intravenous solutions
- Remove inherently dangerous medications (e.g., concentrated KCl) from patient care areas
- Develop special procedures for high-risk drugs
- Improve drug-related clinical information resources
- Improve medication administration education for clinicians
- Educate patients about the safe and accurate use of medications
- Improve access of bedside clinicians to pharmacists

LONG TERM

Implement technology-based safeguards:

- Computerized order entry
- Computerized dose and allergy checking
- Computerized medication tracking
- Use of bar codes or electronic readers for medication preparation and administration

[a]See Massachusetts Coalition for the Prevention of Medical Errors, 2017.

BOX 4–3 ■ Initial Stabilization of the Poisoned Patient

The "ABCDE" mnemonic of emergency care applies to the treatment of acute poisoning:

Airway	Maintain patency
Breathing	Maintain adequate oxygenation and ventilation
Circulation	Maintain perfusion of vital organs
Disability	Assess for CNS dysfunction
	If neurological disability is noted, consider • O_2 *administration (check pulse oximetry)* • *Dextrose administration (check [glucose] in blood)* • *Naloxone administration (consider empiric trial)* • *Thiamine (for adult patients receiving dextrose)*
Exposure	Assess "toxidrome" (see Table 4–7)

In severe cases, endotracheal intubation, mechanical ventilation, pharmacological blood pressure support, or extracorporeal circulatory support may be necessary and appropriate.

TABLE 4–7 ■ COMMON TOXIDROMES

DRUG CLASS	EXAMPLE(S)	MENTAL STATUS	HR	BP	RR	T	PUPIL SIZE	OTHER
Sympathomimetic	Cocaine Amphetamine	Agitation	↑	↑		↑	↑	Tremor, diaphoresis
Anticholinergic	Diphenhydramine Atropine	Delirium	↑	↑		↑	↑	Ileus, flushing
Cholinergic	Organophosphates	Somnolence Coma			↑		↓	SLUDGE,[a] fasciculation
Opioid	Heroin Oxycodone	Somnolence Coma	↓		↓		↓	
Sedative-hypnotic	Benzodiazepines Barbiturates	Somnolence Coma		↓	↓			
Salicylate	Aspirin	Confusion	↑		↑	↑		Diaphoresis, vomiting
Ca^{2+} channel blocker	Verapamil		↓	↓				

BP, blood pressure; HR, heart rate; RR, respiratory rate; T, temperature.
[a]SLUDGE, muscarinic effects of salivation, lacrimation, urination, defecation, gastric cramping, and emesis.

the body. Fuller's earth has been suggested as an adsorbent for paraquat, Prussian blue binds thallium and cesium, and sodium polystyrene can adsorb lithium. The most common adsorbent used in the treatment of acute drug overdose is activated charcoal.

Activated Charcoal. Charcoal is created through controlled pyrolysis of organic matter and is *activated* through steam or chemical treatment, which increases its internal pore structure and adsorptive surface capacity. The surface of activated charcoal contains carbon moieties that are capable of binding poisons. The recommended dose is typically 0.5–2 g/kg of body weight, up to a maximum tolerated dose of about 75–100 g. As a rough estimate, 10 g of activated charcoal is expected to bind about 1 g of drug. Alcohols, corrosives, hydrocarbons, and metals are not well adsorbed by charcoal. Complications of activated charcoal therapy include vomiting, constipation, pulmonary aspiration, and death. Nasogastric administration of charcoal increases the incidence of vomiting (Osterhoudt et al., 2004) and may increase the risk for pulmonary aspiration. Charcoal should not be given to patients with suspected GI perforation or to patients who may be candidates for endoscopy. Use of activated charcoal in the treatment of poisoning has declined over the last 20 years to 2.1% of cases in 2014 (Mowry et al., 2015).

TABLE 4–8 ■ DIFFERENTIAL POISONING DIAGNOSIS (PARTIAL LISTING) FOR ELECTROCARDIOGRAPHIC MANIFESTATIONS OF TOXICITY

BRADYCARDIA/HEART BLOCK	QRS INTERVAL PROLONGATION	QTc INTERVAL PROLONGATION
Cholinergic agents Physostigmine Neostigmine Organophosphates, Carbamates *Sympatholytic agents* β Receptor antagonists Clonidine Opioids *Other* Digoxin Ca^{2+} channel blockers Lithium	Antiarrhythmia drugs Bupropion Chloroquine Diphenhydramine Lamotrigine Phenothiazines Propranolol Tricyclic antidepressants	See CredibleMeds® QTDrugs List: https://www.crediblemeds.org/new-drug-list/

Whole-Bowel Irrigation

Whole-bowel irrigation involves the enteral administration of large amounts of a high-molecular-weight, iso-osmotic polyethylene glycol electrolyte solution with the goal of passing poison by the rectum before it can be absorbed. Potential candidates for WBI include:

- "body packers" with intestinal packets of illicit drugs
- patients with iron overdose
- patients who have ingested patch pharmaceuticals
- patients with overdoses of sustained-release or bezoar-forming drugs

Polyethylene glycol electrolyte solution is typically administered at a rate of 25–40 mL/kg/h until the rectal effluent is clear and no more drug is being passed. To achieve these high administration rates, a nasogastric tube may be used. WBI is contraindicated in the presence of bowel obstruction or perforation and may be complicated by abdominal distention or pulmonary aspiration.

Cathartics. The two most common categories of simple cathartics are the Mg^{2+} salts, such as magnesium citrate and magnesium sulfate, and the nondigestible carbohydrates, such as sorbitol. The use of simple cathartics has been abandoned as a GI decontamination strategy.

Gastric Lavage. The procedure for gastric lavage involves passing an orogastric tube into the stomach with the patient in the left lateral decubitus position with head lower than feet. After withdrawing stomach contents, 10–15 mL/kg (up to 250 mL) of saline lavage fluid is administered and withdrawn. This process continues until the lavage fluid returns clear. Complications of the procedure include mechanical trauma to the stomach or esophagus, pulmonary aspiration of stomach contents, and vagus nerve stimulation.

Syrup of Ipecac. The alkaloids cephaeline and emetine within syrup of ipecac act as emetics because of both a local irritant effect on the enteric tract and a central effect on the chemoreceptor trigger zone in the area postrema of the medulla. *Based on review of existing evidence, the American Academy of Pediatrics no longer recommends syrup of ipecac as part of its childhood injury prevention program, and the American Academy of Clinical Toxicology dissuades routine use of gastric emptying in the poisoned patient.* As a result, ipecac was administered in only 0.006% of all human poisonings in the U.S. in 2014 (Mowry et al., 2015).

Enhancing the Elimination of Poisons

Once absorbed, the deleterious toxicodynamic effects of some drugs may be reduced by methods that hasten their elimination from the body, as described next.

Manipulating Urinary pH: Urinary Alkalinization

Drugs subject to renal clearance are excreted into the urine by glomerular filtration and active tubular secretion; nonionized compounds may be reabsorbed far more rapidly than ionized polar molecules (see Chapter 2). Weakly acidic drugs are susceptible to "ion trapping" in the urine. Aspirin is a weak acid with a pK_a = 3.0. As the pH of the urine increases, more salicylate is in its ionized form at equilibrium, and more salicylic acid diffuses into the tubular lumen of the kidney. Urinary alkalinization is also believed to speed clearance of phenobarbital, chlorpropamide, methotrexate, and chlorophenoxy herbicides. The American Academy of Clinical Toxicologists recommends urine alkalinization as first-line treatment only for moderately severe salicylate poisoning that does not meet criteria for hemodialysis (Proudfoot et al., 2004).

To achieve alkalinization of the urine, 100–150 mEq of sodium bicarbonate in 1 L of 5% dextrose in water (D5W) is infused intravenously at twice the maintenance fluid requirements and then titrated to effect. Hypokalemia should be treated because it will hamper efforts to alkalinize the urine due to H^+-K^+ exchange in the kidney. Urine alkalinization is contraindicated in renal failure or if fluid administration may worsen pulmonary edema or congestive heart failure. Acetazolamide is not used to alkalinize urine as it promotes acidemia.

Multiple-Dose Activated Charcoal

Activated charcoal adsorbs drug to its surface and promotes enteral elimination. Multiple doses of activated charcoal can speed elimination of absorbed drug by two mechanisms: Charcoal may interrupt enterohepatic circulation of hepatically metabolized drug excreted in the bile, and charcoal may create a diffusion gradient across the GI mucosa and promote movement of drug from the bloodstream onto the charcoal in the intestinal lumen. Activated charcoal may be administered in multiple doses, 12.5 g/h every 1, 2, or 4 h (smaller doses may be used for children). Charcoal enhances the clearance of many drugs of low molecular weight, small volume of distribution, and long elimination $t_{1/2}$. Multiple-dose activated charcoal is believed to have the highest potential utility in overdoses of carbamazepine, dapsone, phenobarbital, quinine, theophylline, and yellow oleander (American Academy of Clinical Toxicology, 1999; de Silva et al., 2003).

Extracorporeal Drug Removal

The ideal drug amenable to removal by hemodialysis has a low molecular weight, a low volume of distribution, high solubility in water, and minimal protein binding. Hemoperfusion involves passing blood through a cartridge containing adsorbent particles. The most common poisonings for which hemodialysis is sometimes used include salicylate, methanol, ethylene glycol, lithium, carbamazepine, and valproate.

Antidotal Therapies

Antidotal therapy involves antagonism or chemical inactivation of an absorbed poison. Among the most common specific antidotes used are *N*-acetyl-*L*-cysteine for acetaminophen poisoning, opioid antagonists for opioid overdose, and chelating agents for poisoning from certain metal ions. A list of antidotes used is presented in Table 4–9.

The pharmacodynamics of a poison can be altered by competition at a receptor, as in the antagonism provided by naloxone therapy in the setting of heroin overdose. A physiological antidote may use a different cellular mechanism to overcome the effects of a poison, as in the use of glucagon to circumvent a blocked β adrenergic receptor and increase cellular cyclic AMP in the setting of an overdose of a β adrenergic antagonist. Antivenoms and chelating agents bind and directly inactivate poisons. The biotransformation of a drug can also be altered by an antidote; for example, fomepizole will inhibit alcohol dehydrogenase and stop the formation of toxic acid metabolites from ethylene glycol and methanol. Many drugs used in the supportive care of a poisoned patient (anticonvulsants, vasoconstricting agents, etc.) may be considered nonspecific functional antidotes.

The mainstay of therapy for poisoning is good support of the airway, breathing, circulation, and vital metabolic processes of the poisoned patient until the poison is eliminated from the body.

TABLE 4–9 ■ COMMON ANTIDOTES AND THEIR INDICATIONS

ANTIDOTE	POISONING INDICATION(S)
Acetylcysteine	Acetaminophen
Atropine sulfate	Organophosphorus and carbamate pesticides
Benztropine	Drug-induced dystonia
Bicarbonate, sodium	Na^+ channel blocking drugs
Bromocriptine	Neuroleptic malignant syndrome
Calcium gluconate or chloride	Ca^{2+} channel blocking drugs, fluoride
Carnitine	Valproate hyperammonemia
Crotalidae polyvalent immune Fab	North American crotaline snake envenomation
Dantrolene	Malignant hyperthermia
Deferoxamine	Iron
Digoxin immune Fab	Cardiac glycosides
Diphenhydramine	Drug-induced dystonia
Dimercaprol (BAL)	Lead, mercury, arsenic
EDTA, CaNa$_2$	Lead
Ethanol	Methanol, ethylene glycol
Fomepizole	Methanol, ethylene glycol
Flumazenil	Benzodiazepines
Glucagon hydrochloride	β adrenergic antagonists
Hydroxocobalamin hydrochloride	Cyanide
Insulin (high dose)	Ca^{2+} channel blockers
Leucovorin calcium	Methotrexate
Methylene blue	Methemoglobinemia
Naloxone hydrochloride	Opioids
Octreotide acetate	Sulfonylurea-induced hypoglycemia
Oxygen, hyperbaric	Carbon monoxide
Penicillamine	Lead, mercury, copper
Physostigmine salicylate	Anticholinergic syndrome
Pralidoxime chloride (2-PAM)	Organophosphorus pesticides
Pyridoxine hydrochloride	Isoniazid seizures
Succimer (DMSA)	Lead, mercury, arsenic
Thiosulfate, sodium	Cyanide
Vitamin K$_1$ (phytonadione)	Coumarin, indanedione

Resources for Information on Drug Toxicity and Poisoning

Additional information on poisoning from drugs and chemicals can be found in many dedicated books of toxicology (Flomenbaum et al., 2006; Klaassen, 2013; Olson, 2011; Shannon et al., 2007). A popular computer database for information on toxic substances is POISINDEX® (Micromedex, Inc., Denver, CO). The National Library of Medicine offers information on toxicology and environmental health (http://sis.nlm.nih.gov/enviro.html), including a link to TOXNET® (http://toxnet.nlm.nih.gov/). Regional poison control centers are a resource for valuable poisoning information and may be contacted within the U.S. through the national Poison Help hotline: 1-800-222-1222.

Acknowledgment: *Curtis D. Klaassen and Kevin Osterhoudt contributed to this chapter in recent editions of this book. We have retained some of their text in the current edition.*

Bibliography

American Academy of Clinical Toxicology and the European Association of Poisons Centres and Clinical Toxicologists. Position paper: gastric lavage. *J Toxicol Clin Toxicol*, **2004**, *42*:933–943.

American Academy of Clinical Toxicology and the European Association of Poisons Centres and Clinical Toxicologists. Position statement and practice guidelines on the use of multi-dose activated charcoal in the treatment of acute poisoning. *Clin Toxicol*, **1999**, *37*:731–751.

Bates DW, et al. Relationship between medication errors and adverse drug events. *J Gen Intern Med*, **1995**, *10*:199–205.

Bronstein AC, et al. 2007 Annual report of the American Association of Poison Control Centers' National Poison Data System (NPDS): 25th annual report. *Clin Toxicol*, **2008**, *46*:927–1057.

CredibleMeds®. QTDrugs List. Available at: https://crediblemeds.org. Accessed May 24, 2017.

Dart RC, et al. Acetaminophen poisoning: an evidence-based consensus guideline for out-of-hospital management. *Clin Toxicol*, **2006**, *44*:1–18.

de Silva HA, et al. Multiple-dose activated charcoal for treatment of yellow oleander poisoning: a single-blind, randomized, placebo-controlled trial. *Lancet*, **2003**, *361*:1935–1938.

Erickson TE, et al. The approach to the patient with an unknown overdose. *Emerg Med Clin North Am*, **2007**, *25*:249–281.

Flomenbaum NE, et al., eds. *Goldfrank's Toxicologic Emergencies*, 8th ed. McGraw-Hill, New York, **2006**.

Guthrie SK, et al. Hypothesized interaction between valproic acid and warfarin. *J Clin Psychopharmacol*, **1995**, *15*:138–139.

Hibbard DM, et al. Effects of cholestyramine and colestipol on the plasma concentrations of propralolol. *Br J Clin Pharmacol*, **1984**, *18*:337–342.

Klaassen CD, ed. *Casarett and Doull's Toxicology: The Basic Science of Poisons*, 8th ed. McGraw-Hill, New York, **2013**.

Lazarou J, et al. Incidence of adverse drug reactions in hospitalized patients: a meta-analysis of prospective studies. *JAMA*, **1998**, *279*:1200–1205.

Manoguerra AS, Cobaugh DJ. Guidelines for the Management of Poisonings Consensus Panel. *Clin Toxicol*, **2005**, *43*:1–10.

Massachusetts Coalition for the Prevention of Medical Errors. **2017**. Available at: macoalition.org. Accessed May 24, 2017.

Mowry JB, et al. 2014 Annual report of the American Association of Poison Control Centers' National Poison Data System (NPDS): 32nd annual report. *Clin Toxicol*, **2015**, *53*:962–1147.

O'Connor-Semmes RL, et al. Effect of ranitidine on the pharmacokinetics of triazolam and alpha-hydroxytriazolam in both young and older people. *Clin Pharmacol Ther*, **2001**, *70*:126–131.

Olson KR, ed. *Poisoning & Drug Overdose*, 6th ed. McGraw-Hill, New York, **2011**.

Osterhoudt KC. No sympathy for a boy with obtundation. *Pediatr Emerg Care*, **2004**, *20*:403–406.

Osterhoudt KC, et al. Risk factors for emesis after therapeutic use of activated charcoal in acutely poisoned children. *Pediatrics*, **2004**, *113*:806–810.

Proudfoot AT, et al. Position paper on urine alkalinization. *J Toxicol Clin Toxicol*, **2004**, *42*:1–26.

Pontel LA, et al. Endogenous formaldehyde is a hematopoietic stem cell genotoxin and metabolic carcinogen. *Mol Cell*, **2015**, *60*:177–188.

Reason J. Human error: models and management. *Br Med J*, **2000**, *320*:768–770.

Rivera W, et al. Delayed salicylate toxicity at 35 hours without early manifestations following a single salicylate ingestion. *Ann Pharmacother*, **2004**, *38*:1186–1188.

Shannon MW, et al., eds. *Haddad and Winchester's Clinical Management of Poisoning and Drug Overdose*, 4th ed. Saunders/Elsevier, Philadelphia, **2007**.

Sztajnkrycer MD. Valproic acid toxicity: overview and management. *Clin Toxicol*, **2002**, *40*:789–801.

Tenenbein M, et al. Efficacy of ipecac-induced emesis, orogastric lavage, and activated charcoal for acute drug overdose. *Ann Emerg Med*, **1987**, *16*:838–841.

Membrane Transporters and Drug Response

Kathleen M. Giacomini and Yuichi Sugiyama

Membrane transport proteins are present in all organisms. These proteins control the influx of essential nutrients and ions and the efflux of cellular waste, environmental toxins, drugs, and other xenobiotics (Figure 5–1). Consistent with their critical roles in cellular homeostasis, about 2000 genes in the human genome, ~7% of the total number of genes, code for transporters or transporter-related proteins. The functions of membrane transporters may be facilitated (equilibrative, not requiring energy) or active (requiring energy). In considering the transport of drugs, pharmacologists generally focus on transporters from two major superfamilies, ABC and SLC transporters (Nigam, 2015).

Most ABC proteins are primary active transporters, which rely on ATP hydrolysis to actively pump their substrates across membranes. Among the best-recognized transporters in the ABC superfamily are Pgp (encoded by *ABCB1*, also termed *MDR1*) and CFTR (encoded by *ABCC7*).

The SLC superfamily includes genes that encode facilitated transporters and ion-coupled secondary active transporters. Fifty-two SLC families with about 395 transporters have been identified in the human genome (Hediger et al., 2013; Nigam et al., 2015). Many SLC transporters serve as drug targets or in drug absorption and disposition. Widely recognized SLC transporters include SERT and DAT, both targets for antidepressant medications.

Membrane Transporters in Therapeutic Drug Responses

Pharmacokinetics

Transporters important in pharmacokinetics generally are located in intestinal, renal, and hepatic epithelia, where they function in the selective absorption and elimination of endogenous substances and xenobiotics, including drugs. Transporters work in concert with drug-metabolizing enzymes to eliminate drugs and their metabolites (Figure 5–2). In addition, transporters in various cell types mediate tissue-specific drug distribution (drug targeting). Conversely, transporters also may serve as protective barriers to particular organs and cell types. For example, Pgp in the BBB protects the CNS from a variety of structurally diverse drugs through its efflux mechanisms.

Pharmacodynamics: Transporters as Drug Targets

Membrane transporters are the targets of many clinically used drugs. SERT (*SLC6A4*) is a target for a major class of antidepressant drugs, the SSRIs. Other neurotransmitter reuptake transporters serve as drug targets for the tricyclic antidepressants, various amphetamines (including amphetamine-like drugs used in the treatment of attention-deficit disorder in children), and anticonvulsants.

These transporters also may be involved in the pathogenesis of neuropsychiatric disorders, including Alzheimer and Parkinson diseases. An inhibitor of the vesicular monoamine transporter VMAT2 (SLC18A2), tetrabenazine, is approved for the symptomatic treatment of Huntington disease; the antichorea effect of tetrabenazine appears to relate to its capacity to deplete stores of biogenic amines by inhibiting their uptake into storage vesicles by VMAT2. Transporters that are nonneuronal also may be potential drug targets (e.g., cholesterol transporters in cardiovascular disease, nucleoside transporters in cancers, glucose transporters in metabolic syndromes, and Na⁺-Cl⁻ cotransporters in the SLC12 family in hypertension).

Recently, first-in-class drugs that inhibit Na^+-glucose transporters in the SLC5 family (SGLT1 and SGLT2) have been approved for the

Abbreviations

ABC: *ATP binding cassette*
ABCC: ATP binding cassette family C
ACE inhibitor: angiotensin-converting enzyme inhibitor
AUC: area under the concentration-time curve
BBB: blood-brain barrier
BCRP: breast cancer resistance protein
BSEP: *bile salt export pump*
CFTR: cystic fibrosis transmembrane regulator
$CL_{int,all}$: overall hepatic intrinsic clearance
CL_{met}: metabolic clearance
CPT-11: irinotecan hydrochloride
CSF: cerebrospinal fluid
DA: dopamine
DAT: dopamine transporter
FDA: U.S. Food and Drug Administration
GABA: γ-aminobutyric acid
GAT: GABA reuptake transporter
GSH, GSSG: reduced and oxidized glutathione
HIV: human immunodeficiency virus
HMG-CoA: 3-hydroxy-3-methylglutaryl coenzyme A
5HT: serotonin
α-KG: α-ketoglutarate
LAT: large amino acid transporter
MAO: monoamine oxidase
MATE1: multidrug and toxin extrusion protein 1
MDMA: 3,4-methylenedioxymethamphetamine
MRP: multidrug resistance protein
NBDs: nucleotide-binding domains
NE: norepinephrine
NET: NE transporter
NME: new molecular entity
NTCP: *Na⁺-taurocholate cotransporting polypeptide*
OAT1: organic anion transporter 1
OCT1: organic cation transporter 1
OCTN: novel organic cation transporter
PAH: *p-aminohippurate*
PGE₂: prostaglandin E₂
Pgp: P-glycoprotein
PPARα: peroxisome proliferator-activated receptor α
RAR: retinoic acid receptor
RXR: retinoid X receptor
SERT: serotonin transporter
SLC: *solute carrier*
SNP: single-nucleotide polymorphism
SXR: steroid X receptor
URAT1: uric acid transporter 1
XOI: xanthine oxidase inhibitor

both potentiators and correctors, compounds that enhance trafficking of mutant proteins to the plasma membrane.

Drug Resistance

Membrane transporters play critical roles in the development of resistance to anticancer drugs, antiviral agents, and anticonvulsants. *Decreased uptake of drugs,* such as folate antagonists, nucleoside analogues, and platinum complexes, is mediated by reduced expression of influx transporters required for these drugs to access the tumor. *Enhanced efflux of hydrophobic drugs* is one mechanism of antitumor resistance in cellular assays of resistance. The overexpression of MRP4 is associated with resistance to antiviral nucleoside analogues (Aceti et al., 2015). Pgp (MDR1, ABCB1) and BCRP (ABCG2) can be overexpressed in tumor cells after exposure to cytotoxic anticancer agents and are implicated in resistance to these agents, exporting anticancer drugs, reducing their intracellular concentration, and rendering cells resistant to the drugs' cytotoxic effects. Modulation of MDR1 expression and activity to regulate drug resistance could be a useful adjunct in pharmacotherapy (Gu and Manautou, 2010; He et al., 2011; Toyoda et al., 2008).

Membrane Transporters and Adverse Drug Responses

As controllers of import and export, transporters ultimately control the exposure of cells to chemical carcinogens, environmental toxins, and drugs. Thus, transporters play crucial roles in the cellular activities and toxicities of these agents. Transporter-mediated adverse drug responses generally can be classified into three categories (Figure 5–3):

- Decreased uptake or excretion at clearance organs
- Increased uptake or decreased efflux at target organs
- Altered transport of endogenous compounds at target organs

Transporters expressed in the liver and kidney, as well as metabolic enzymes, are key determinants of drug exposure in the systemic circulation, thereby affecting exposure, and hence toxicity, in all organs (Figure 5–3, top panel). For example, after oral administration of an HMG-CoA reductase inhibitor (e.g., pravastatin), the efficient first-pass hepatic uptake of the drug by the SLC OATP1B1 maximizes the effects of such drugs on hepatic HMG-CoA reductase. Uptake by OATP1B1 also minimizes the escape of these drugs into the systemic circulation, where they can cause adverse responses, such as skeletal muscle myopathy.

Transporters expressed in tissues that may be targets for drug toxicity (e.g., brain) or in barriers to such tissues (e.g., the BBB) can tightly control local drug concentrations and thus control the exposure of these tissues to the drug (Figure 5–3, middle panel). For example, endothelial cells in the BBB are linked by tight junctions, and some efflux transporters are expressed on the blood-facing (luminal) side, thereby restricting the penetration of compounds into the brain. The interactions of loperamide and quinidine are good examples of transporter control of drug exposure at this site. Loperamide is a peripheral opioid used in the treatment of diarrhea and is a substrate of Pgp, which prevents accumulation of loperamide in the CNS. Inhibition of Pgp–mediated efflux in the BBB would cause an increase in the concentration of loperamide in the CNS and potentiate adverse effects. Indeed, coadministration of loperamide and the potent Pgp inhibitor quinidine results in significant respiratory depression, an adverse response to loperamide. Pgp is also expressed in the intestine, where inhibition of Pgp will reduce intestinal efflux of loperamide, increase its systemic concentrations, and contribute to increased concentrations in the CNS.

Drug-induced toxicity sometimes is caused by the concentrative tissue distribution mediated by influx transporters. For example, biguanides (e.g., metformin), used for the treatment of type 2 diabetes mellitus, can produce lactic acidosis, a lethal side effect. Biguanides are substrates of the OCT1 (SLC22A1), which is highly expressed in the liver; of OCT2 (SLC22A2), expressed in the kidney; and of OCT3 (SLC22A3) in adipocytes and skeletal muscle. In experimental animals lacking OCT1,

treatment of type 2 diabetes. These drugs, which include canagliflozin, dapagliflozin, and empagliflozin, reduce renal reabsorption of glucose, thereby facilitating glucose elimination in the kidney. All three are prescribed as second-line therapy for treatment of inadequately controlled diabetes. In addition, lesinurad, a first-in-class drug that targets URAT1 (SLC22A12), was recently approved by the FDA for the treatment of gout when used with an XOI; other URAT1 inhibitors are in clinical trial. These drugs are uricosurics and act by selectively inhibiting uric acid reabsorption in the kidney.

Finally, a first-in-class drug, ivacaftor, was recently approved for the treatment of patients with cystic fibrosis who harbor a coding mutation in CFTR (ABCC7), CFTR-G551D. Ivacaftor, termed a potentiator, increases the probability that the mutant chloride channel, CFTR-G551D, remains in the open state. Other drugs in clinical trials for CFTR include

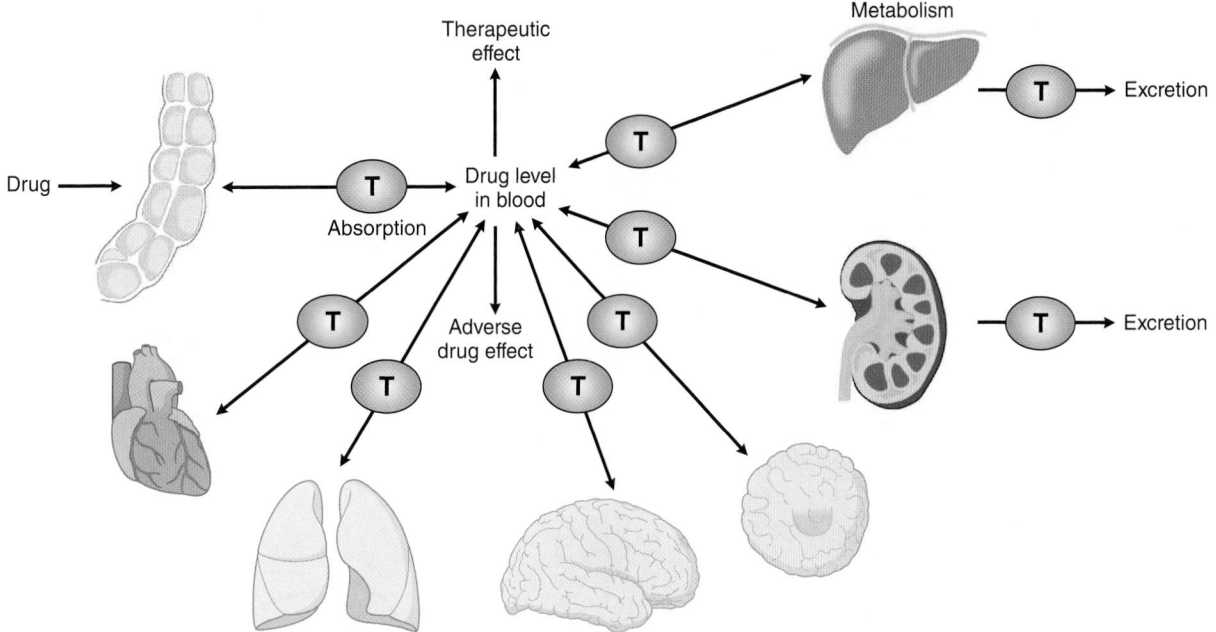

Figure 5–1 *Membrane transporters in pharmacokinetic pathways.* Membrane transporters (T) play roles in pharmacokinetic pathways (drug absorption, distribution, metabolism, and excretion), thereby setting systemic drug levels. Drug levels often drive therapeutic and adverse drug effects.

hepatic uptake of biguanides and development of lactic acidosis are greatly reduced. These results indicate that OCT1-mediated hepatic uptake of biguanides and uptake into tissues such as kidney and skeletal muscle mediated by other OCTs play an important role in facilitating tissue concentrations of biguanides and thus the development of lactic acidosis (Wang et al., 2003), which may result from biguanide-induced impairment of mitochondrial function and consequent increased glycolytic flux (Dykens et al., 2008). Biguanides are exported by the MATE1 transporter, and inhibition of this efflux by a variety of drugs, including tyrosine kinase inhibitors, enhances biguanide toxicity (DeCorter et al., 2012).

OAT1 (SLC22A1), OCT1, and OCT2 provide other examples of transporter-related toxicity. OAT1 is expressed mainly in the kidney and is responsible for the renal tubular secretion of anionic compounds. Substrates of OAT1, such as cephaloridine (a β-lactam antibiotic) and adefovir and cidofovir (antiviral drugs), reportedly cause nephrotoxicity.

Exogenous expression of OCT1 and OCT2 enhances the sensitivities of tumor cells to the cytotoxic effect of oxaliplatin for OCT1 and cisplatin and oxaliplatin for OCT2 (Zhang et al., 2006a). Renal toxicity of cisplatin is modulated by OCT2 present on the basolateral membrane of the proximal tubule as well as by transporters in the SLC47 family, MATE1 (SLC47A1) and MATE2 (SLC47A2), on the apical membrane (Harrach and Ciarimboli, 2015).

Drugs may modulate transporters for endogenous ligands and thereby exert adverse effects (Figure 5–3, bottom panel). For example, bile acids are taken up mainly by NTCP and excreted into the bile by BSEP (*ABCB11*). Bilirubin is taken up by OATP1B1 and conjugated with glucuronic acid; bilirubin glucuronide is excreted into the bile by the MRP2 (*ABCC2*) and transported into the blood by MRP3. Bilirubin glucuronide in the blood undergoes reuptake into the liver by OATP1B1. Inhibition of these transporters by drugs may cause cholestasis or hyperbilirubinemia.

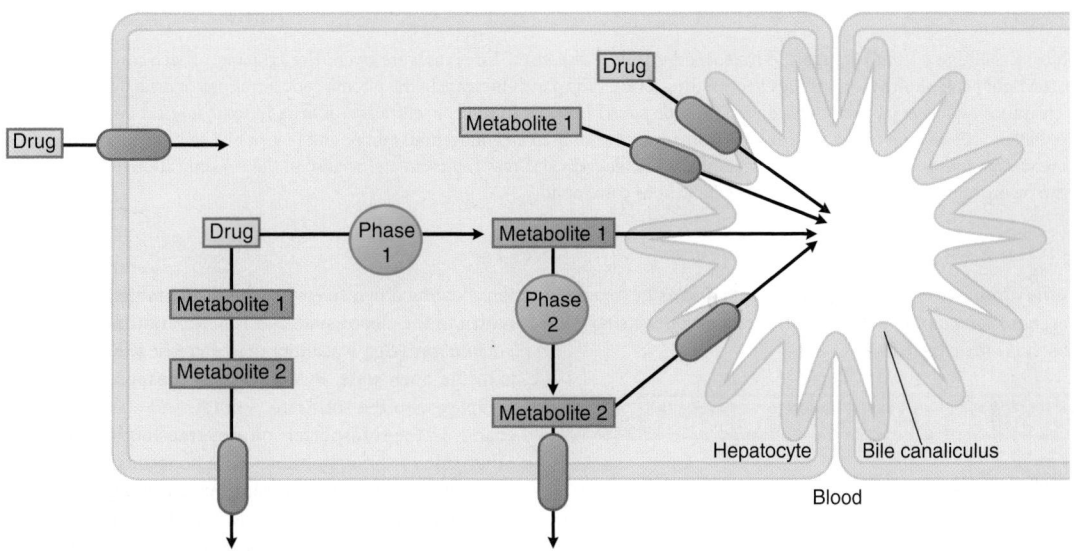

Figure 5–2 *Hepatic drug transporters.* Membrane transporters (red ovals with arrows) work in concert with phase 1 and phase 2 drug-metabolizing enzymes in the hepatocyte to mediate the uptake and efflux of drugs and their metabolites.

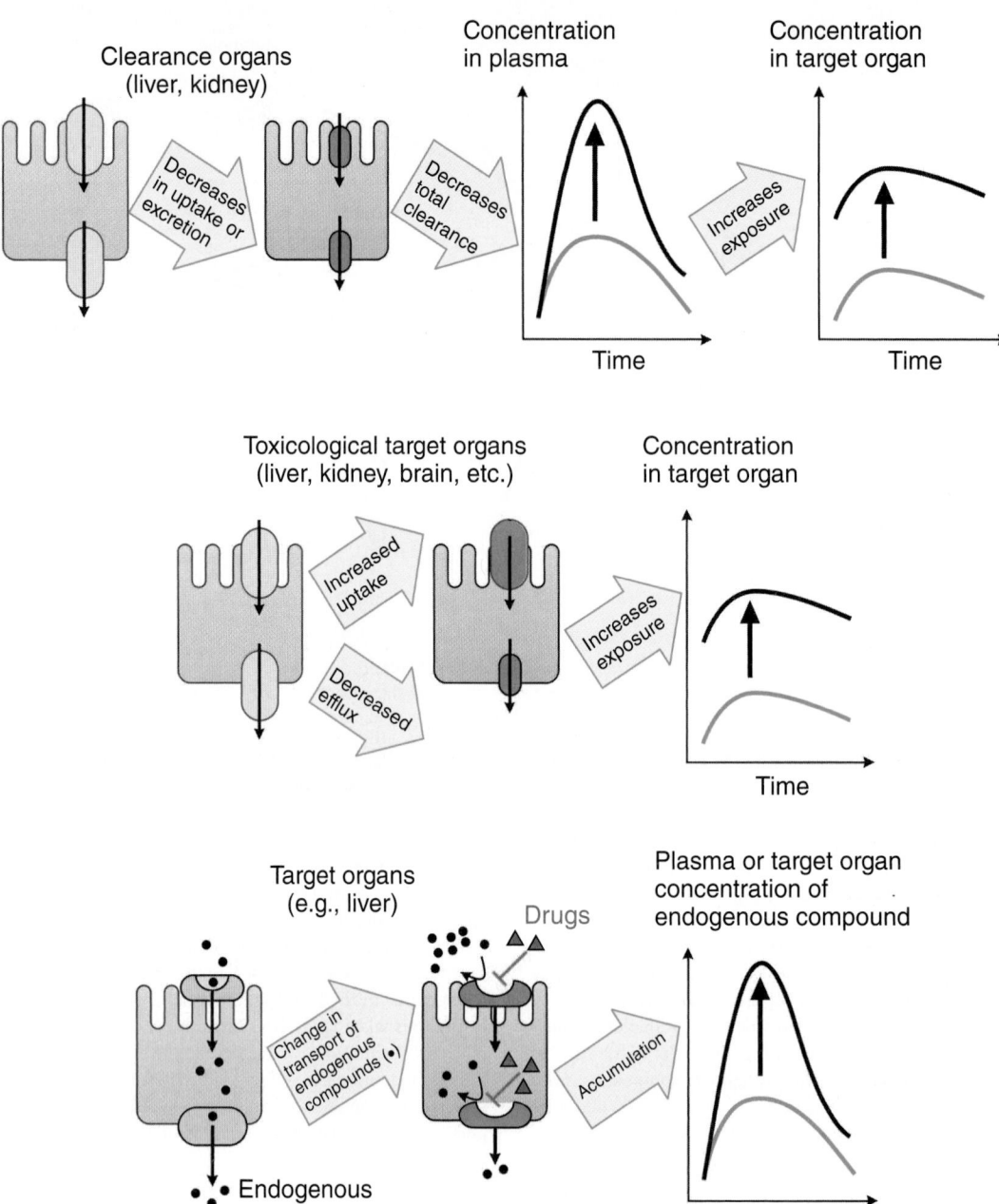

Figure 5–3 *Major mechanisms by which transporters mediate adverse drug responses.* Three cases are given. The left panel of each case provides a representation of the mechanism; the right panel shows the resulting effect on drug levels. (*Top panel*) Increase in the plasma concentrations of drug due to a decrease in the uptake or secretion in clearance organs (e.g., liver and kidney). (*Middle panel*) Increase in the concentration of drug in toxicological target organs due to enhanced uptake or reduced efflux. (*Bottom panel*) Increase in the plasma concentration of an endogenous compound (e.g., a bile acid) due to a drug inhibiting the influx of the endogenous compound in its eliminating or target organ. The diagram also may represent an increase in the concentration of the endogenous compound in the target organ owing to drug-inhibited efflux of the endogenous compound.

Uptake and efflux transporters determine the plasma and tissue concentrations of endogenous compounds and xenobiotics, thereby influencing the systemic or site-specific toxicity of drugs.

Basic Mechanisms of Membrane Transport

Transporters Versus Channels

Both channels and transporters facilitate the membrane permeation of inorganic ions and organic compounds. In general, channels have two primary states, open and closed, that are stochastic phenomena. Only in the open state do channels appear to act as pores for the selected ions flowing down an electrochemical gradient. After opening, channels return to the closed state as a function of time. As noted, drugs termed *potentiators* (e.g., ivacaftor) may increase the probability that a channel is in the open state. By contrast, a transporter forms an intermediate complex with the substrate (solute), and a subsequent conformational change in the transporter induces translocation of the substrate to the other side of the membrane. As a consequence, the kinetics of solute movement differ between transporters and channels. Typical turnover rate constants of channels are 10^6 to 10^8 s^{-1}; those of transporters are, at most, 10^1 to 10^3 s^{-1}. Because a particular transporter forms intermediate complexes with specific compounds (referred to as *substrates*), transporter-mediated membrane transport is characterized by saturability

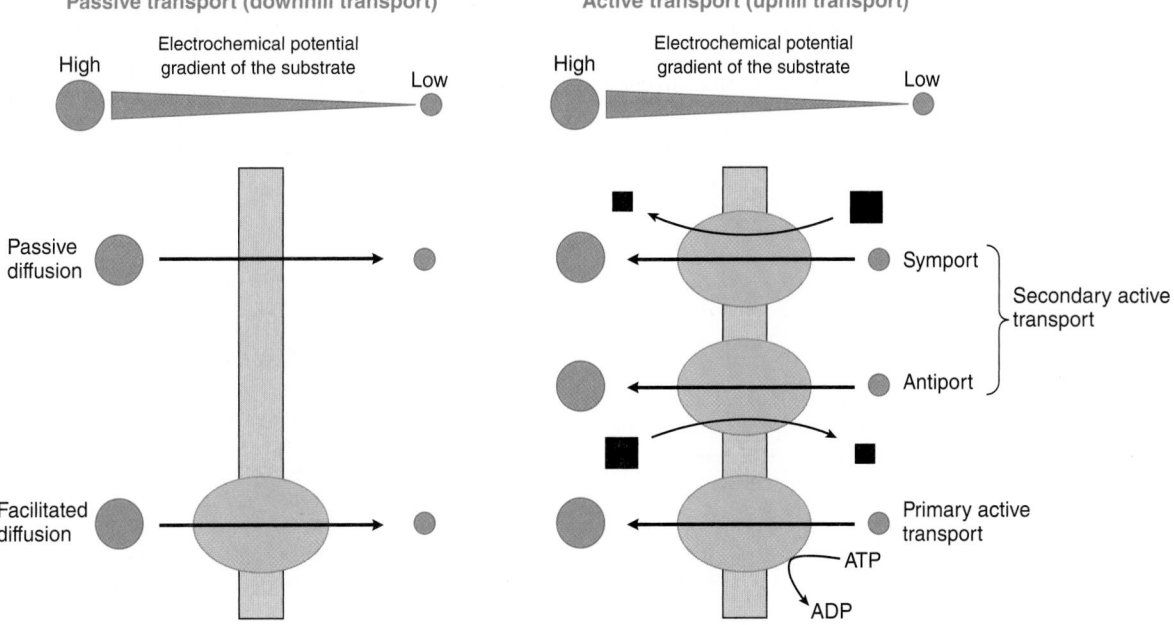

Figure 5–4 *Classification of membrane transport mechanisms.* Red circles depict the substrate. Size of the circles is proportional to the concentration of the substrate. Arrows show the direction of flux. Black squares represent the ion that supplies the driving force for transport (size is proportional to the concentration of the ion). Blue ovals depict transport proteins.

and inhibition by substrate analogues, as described in the section Kinetics of Transport.

The basic mechanisms involved in solute transport across biological membranes include passive diffusion, facilitated diffusion, and active transport. Active transport can be further subdivided into primary and secondary active transport. These mechanisms are depicted in Figure 5–4.

Passive Diffusion

Simple diffusion of a solute across the plasma membrane consists of three processes: partition from the aqueous to the lipid phase, diffusion across the lipid bilayer, and repartition into the aqueous phase on the opposite side. Passive diffusion of any solute (including drugs) occurs down an electrochemical potential gradient of the solute.

Facilitated Diffusion

Diffusion of ions and organic compounds across the plasma membrane may be facilitated by a membrane transporter. Facilitated diffusion is a form of transporter-mediated membrane transport that does not require energy input. Just as in passive diffusion, the transport of ionized and non-ionized compounds across the plasma membrane occurs down their electrochemical potential gradients. Therefore, steady state will be achieved when the electrochemical potentials of a compound on both sides of the membrane become equal.

Active Transport

Active transport is the form of membrane transport that requires the input of energy. It is the transport of solutes against their electrochemical gradients, leading to the concentration of solutes on one side of the plasma membrane and the creation of potential energy in the electrochemical gradient formed. Active transport plays an important role in the uptake and efflux of drugs and other solutes. Depending on the driving force, active transport can be subdivided into primary active transport in which ATP hydrolysis is coupled directly to solute transport, and secondary active transport, in which transport uses the energy in an existing electrochemical gradient established by an ATP-using process to move a solute uphill against its electrochemical gradient. Secondary active transport is further subdivided into symport and antiport. Symport describes movement of driving ion and transported solute in the same direction. Antiport occurs when the driving ion and the transported solute move in opposite directions, as when the

sodium/calcium exchanger (SLC8A1) transports $3Na^+$ *into* and $1Ca^{2+}$ *out of* a cardiac ventricular myocyte (see Figure 5–4).

Primary Active Transport

Membrane transport that directly couples with ATP hydrolysis is called *primary active transport*. ABC transporters are examples of primary active transporters. In mammalian cells, ABC transporters mediate the unidirectional efflux of solutes across biological membranes. Another example of primary active transport that establishes the inward Na^+ gradient and outward K^+ gradient across the plasma membrane, found in all mammalian cells, is the Na^+,K^+-ATPase.

Secondary Active Transport

In secondary active transport, the transport across a biological membrane of a solute S_1 against its concentration gradient is energetically driven by the transport of another solute S_2 in accordance with its electrochemical gradient. Depending on the transport direction of the solute, secondary active transporters are classified as either symporters or antiporters. For example, using the inwardly directed Na^+ concentration gradient across the plasma membrane that the Na^+,K^+-ATPase maintains, the inward movement of 3 Na^+ can drive the outward movement of 1 Ca^{++} via the Na^+/Ca^{++} exchanger, NCX. This is an example of antiport, or exchange transport, in which the transporter moves S_2 and S_1 in opposite directions. *Symporters*, also termed *cotransporters*, transport S_2 and S_1 in the same direction, as for glucose transport into the body from the lumen of the small intestine by the Na^+-glucose transporter SGLT1 (see Figure 5–4).

Kinetics of Transport

The flux of a substrate (rate of transport) across a biological membrane via a transporter-mediated process is characterized by saturability. The relationship between the flux v and substrate concentration C in a transporter-mediated process is given by the Michaelis-Menten equation:

$$v = \frac{V_{max}C}{K_m + C} \qquad \text{(Equation 5–1)}$$

where V_{max} is the maximum transport rate and is proportional to the density of transporters on the plasma membrane, and K_m is the Michaelis constant, which represents the substrate concentration at which the flux is half the V_{max} value. K_m is an approximation of the dissociation constant of the substrate from the intermediate complex. The K_m and V_{max} values can be determined by examining the flux at different substrate concentrations. Rearranging Equation 5–1 gives

$$v = -K_m \frac{v}{C} + V_{max} \qquad \text{(Equation 5–2)}$$

Plotting v versus v/C provides a convenient graphical method for determining the V_{max} and K_m values, the Eadie-Hofstee plot (Figure 5–5): The slope is $-K_m$ and the y intercept is V_{max}.

Transporter-mediated membrane transport of a substrate is also characterized by inhibition by other compounds. The manner of inhibition can be categorized as one of three types: *competitive, noncompetitive,* and *uncompetitive.* Competitive inhibition occurs when substrates and inhibitors share a common binding site on the transporter, resulting in an increase in the apparent K_m value in the presence of inhibitor. The flux of a substrate in the presence of a competitive inhibitor is

$$v = \frac{V_{max}C}{K_m(1+I/K_i)+C} \qquad \text{(Equation 5–3)}$$

where I is the concentration of inhibitor, and K_i is the inhibition constant. Noncompetitive inhibition assumes that the inhibitor has an allosteric effect on the transporter, does not inhibit the formation of an intermediate complex of substrate and transporter, but does inhibit the subsequent translocation process.

$$v = \frac{V_{max}C}{K_m(1+I/K_i)+C(1+I/K_i)} \qquad \text{(Equation 5–4)}$$

Uncompetitive inhibition assumes that inhibitors can form a complex only with an intermediate complex of the substrate and transporter and inhibit subsequent translocation.

$$v = \frac{V_{max}C}{K_m+C(1+I/K_i)} \qquad \text{(Equation 5–5)}$$

Transporter Structure and Mechanism

Predictions of secondary structure of membrane transport proteins based on hydropathy analysis indicate that membrane transporters in the SLC and ABC superfamilies are multimembrane-spanning proteins. Emerging crystals structures are adding to our ideas of the mechanisms of transport via these proteins.

ABC Transporters

The ABC superfamily includes 49 genes, each containing one or two conserved ABC regions. The core catalytic ABC regions of these proteins bind and hydrolyze ATP, using the energy for uphill transport of their substrates across the membrane. Most ABC transporters in eukaryotes move compounds from the cytoplasm to the cell exterior or into an intracellular compartment (endoplasmic reticulum, mitochondria, peroxisomes). ABC transporters also are found in prokaryotes, where they are involved predominantly in the import of essential compounds that cannot be obtained by passive diffusion (sugars, vitamins, metals, etc.).

ABC transporters have NBDs on the cytoplasmic side. The NBDs are considered the motor domains of ABC transporters and contain conserved motifs (e.g., Walker-A motif, ABC signature motif) that participate in binding and hydrolysis of ATP. Crystal structures of all four full ABC transporters show two NBDs, which are in contact with each other, and a conserved fold. The mechanism, shared by these ABC transporters, appears to involve binding of ATP to the NBDs, which subsequently triggers an outward-facing conformation of the transporters. Dissociation of the hydrolysis products of ATP appears to result in an inward-facing conformation. In the case of drug extrusion, when ATP binds, the transporters open to the outside, releasing their substrates to the extracellular media. On dissociation of the hydrolysis products, the transporters return to the inward-facing conformation, permitting the binding of ATP and substrate (Figure 5–6). Although some ABC superfamily transporters contain only a single ABC motif, they form homodimers (BCRP/ABCG2) or heterodimers (ABCG5 and ABCG8) that exhibit a transport function.

SLC Transporters

The SLC superfamily of transporters comprises a structurally diverse group that includes channels, facilitators, and secondary active

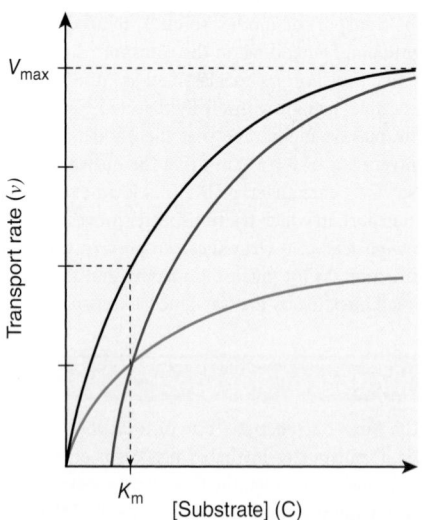
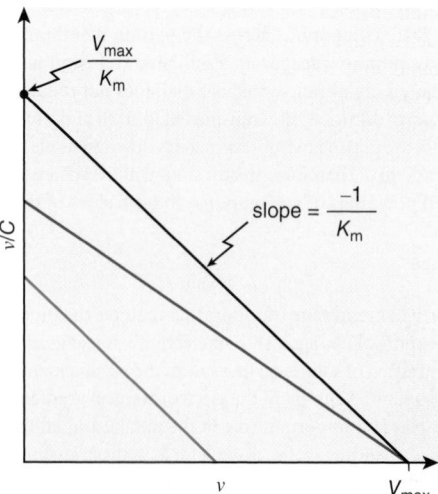

Figure 5–5 *Eadie-Hofstee plot of transport data.* The black lines show the hyperbolic concentration-dependence curve (v vs. C, left panel) and the Eadie-Hofstee transformation of the transport data (v/C vs. v, right panel) for a simple transport system. The blue lines depict transport in the presence of a competitive inhibitor (surmountable inhibition; achieves same V_{max}). The red lines depict the system in the presence of a noncompetitive inhibitor that effectively reduces the number of transporting sites but leaves the K_m of the functional sites unchanged. Involvement of multiple transporters with different K_m values gives an Eadie-Hofstee plot that is curved and can be resolved into multiple components. Algebraically, the Eadie-Hofstee plot of kinetic data is equivalent to the Scatchard plot of equilibrium binding data (see Chapter 3).

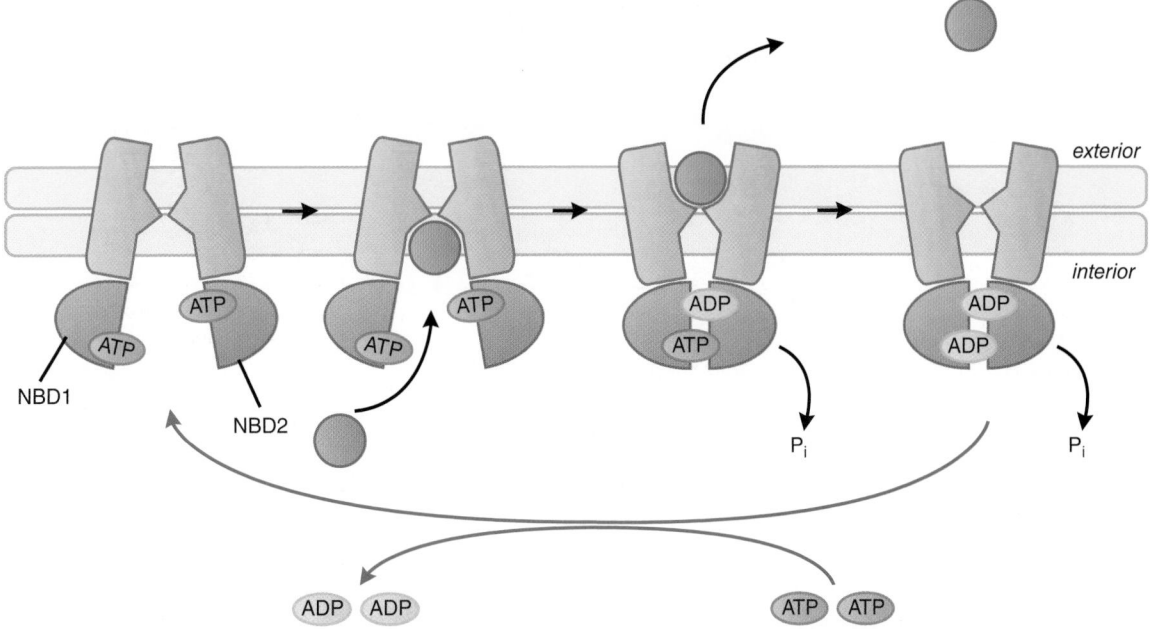

Figure 5–6 *Model of ABC transporter function.* The transporter accepts a solute molecule at the cytoplasmic membrane surface when its nucleotide NBDs are fully charged with ATP. Sequential hydrolysis of the ATP molecules produces steric change and leads to the translocation and release of the solute at the exterior membrane surface. Exchange of ADP for ATP on both NBDs completes the cycle and restores the system for readiness to transport another solute molecule.

transporters (Hediger et al., 2013). SLC substrates include ionic and nonionic species and a variety of xenobiotics and drugs. Nonetheless, for a number of SLC transporters that are important to pharmacokinetics and pharmacodynamics, there are a few common structural and mechanistic aspects. Human SLC transporters may use an alternating access, the gated pore mechanism, whereby the transporter exposes a single solute binding site interchangeably at either side of the membrane barrier (Figure 5–7).

In general terms, the transporter undergoes a reversible conformational change between the two sides of the membrane during the translocation process. The transport cycle would be as follows: The substrate accesses the substrate binding site on one side of the membrane; substrate binding induces structural changes in the carrier protein, reorienting the opening of the binding site to the opposite side. The substrate dissociates from the transport site, allowing another substrate to be bound and transported in the opposite direction. Such a mechanism requires that binding of different substrates (the "outbound" and "inbound" substrates) that is mutually exclusive; that is, there is a single reorienting binding site. Variations of the model are possible, and some are based on crystal structures of bacterial

homologs of human transporters, where two distinctive protomers are joined in the cytoplasmic side by a connecting loop, supporting a rocker switch mechanism (Figure 5–7).

Vectorial Transport

Asymmetrical transport across a monolayer of polarized cells, such as the epithelial and endothelial cells of brain capillaries, is called *vectorial transport* (Figure 5–8). Vectorial transport is important for the absorption of nutrients and bile acids in the intestine in the intestinal absorption of drugs (from lumen to blood). Vectorial transport also plays a major role in hepatobiliary and urinary excretion of drugs from the blood to the lumen. In addition, efflux of drugs from the brain via brain endothelial cells and brain choroid plexus epithelial cells involves vectorial transport. The ABC transporters mediate only unidirectional efflux, whereas SLC transporters mediate either drug uptake or drug efflux. For lipophilic compounds that have sufficient membrane permeability, ABC transporters alone are able to achieve vectorial transport without the help of influx transporters. For

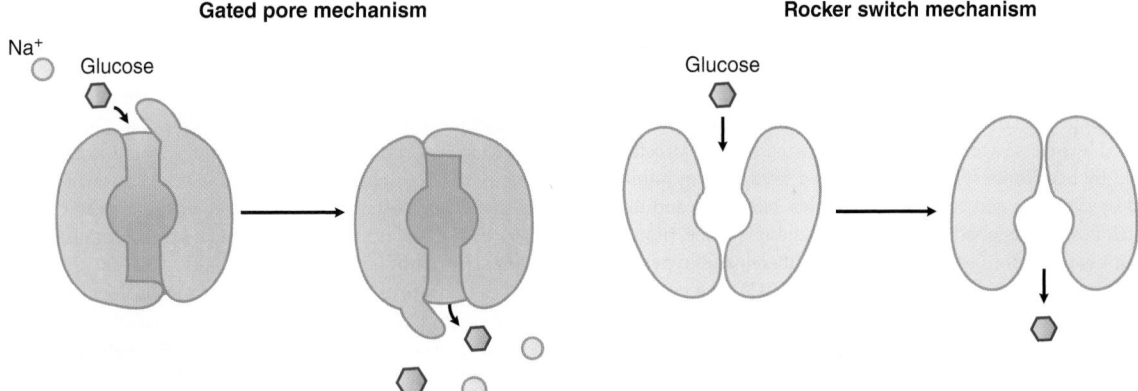

Figure 5–7 *Alternating access models of the transport of two transporters.* The gated pore represents the model for SGLT in which the rotation of two broken helices facilitates alternating access of substrates to the intracellular and extracellular sides of the plasma membrane. The rocker switch represents the model by which major facilitator superfamily (MFS) proteins, such as Lac Y, work. This example models a facilitated glucose transporter, GLUT2.

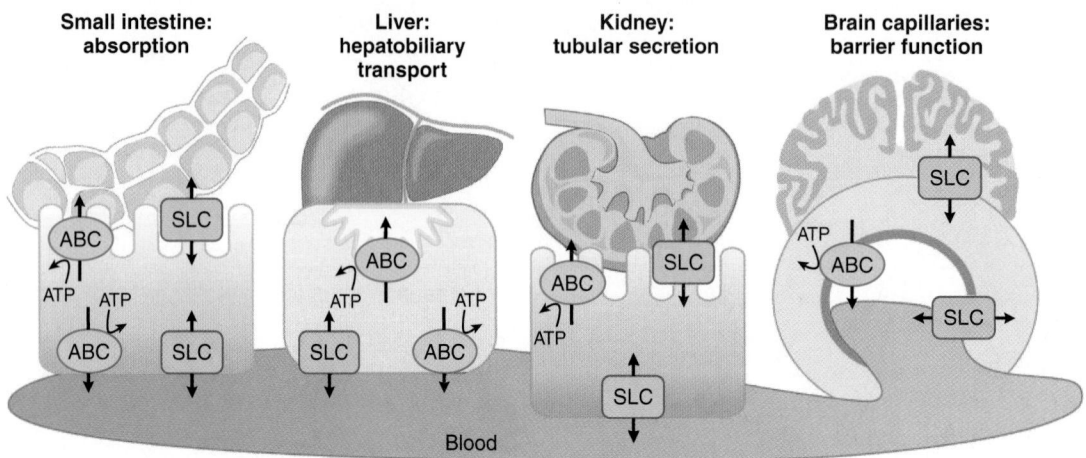

Figure 5–8 *Transepithelial and transendothelial flux.* Transepithelial or transendothelial flux of drugs requires distinct transporters at the two surfaces of the epithelial or endothelial barrier. These are depicted diagrammatically for transport across the small intestine (absorption), the kidney, liver (elimination), and brain capillary endothelial cells that comprise the BBB.

relatively hydrophilic organic anions and cations, coordinated uptake and efflux transporters in the polarized plasma membranes are necessary to achieve the vectorial movement of solutes across an epithelium. A typical configuration involves a primary or secondary active transporter at one membrane and a passive transporter at the other. In this way, common substrates of coordinated transporters are transferred efficiently across the epithelial barrier.

In the liver, a number of transporters with different substrate specificities are localized on the sinusoidal membrane (facing blood). These transporters are involved in the uptake of bile acids, amphipathic organic anions, and hydrophilic organic cations into the hepatocytes. Similarly, ABC transporters on the canalicular membrane (facing bile) export such compounds into the bile. Multiple combinations of uptake (OATP1B1, OATP1B3, OATP2B1) and efflux transporters (MDR1, MRP2, and BCRP) are involved in the efficient transcellular transport of a wide variety of compounds in the liver by using a system called "doubly transfected cells"; these cells express both uptake and efflux transporters on each side. In many cases, overlapping substrate specificities between the uptake transporters (OATP family) and efflux transporters (MRP family) make the vectorial transport of organic anions highly efficient. Similar transport systems also are present in the intestine, renal tubules, and endothelial cells of the brain capillaries (see Figure 5–8).

Transporter expression can be regulated transcriptionally in response to drug treatment and pathophysiological conditions, resulting in induction or downregulation of transporter mRNAs. Type II nuclear receptors, which form heterodimers with the 9-*cis*-retinoic acid receptor (RXR), can regulate transcription of genes for drug-metabolizing enzymes and transporters (see Table 6–4, Figure 6–8, and Urquhart et al., 2007). Such receptors include PXR (NR1I2), CAR (NR1I3), FXR (NR1H4), PPARα, and RAR. Except for CAR, these are ligand-activated nuclear receptors that, as heterodimers with RXR, bind specific elements in the enhancer regions of target genes. CAR has constitutive transcriptional activity that is antagonized by inverse agonists, such as androstenol and androstanol, and induced by barbiturates. PXR, also referred to as SXR in humans, is activated by synthetic and endogenous steroids, bile acids, and drugs such as clotrimazole, phenobarbital, rifampicin, sulfinpyrazone, ritonavir, carbamazepine, phenytoin, sulfadimidine, paclitaxel, and hyperforin (a constituent of St. John's wort) (Guo and Zhou, 2015). The potency of activators of PXR varies among species, such that rodents are not necessarily a model for effects in humans. There is an overlap of substrates between CYP3A4 and Pgp, and PXR mediates coinduction of CYP3A4 and Pgp, supporting their synergy in efficient detoxification. Recent studies in human hepatocytes treated with an activator of PXR suggested that the expression levels of enzymes in the CYP family are much more highly increased than the levels of transporters in the SLC or ABC families

(Smith et al., 2014). Table 5–1 summarizes the effects of drug activation of type II nuclear receptors on expression of transporters.

DNA methylation is one mechanism underlying the epigenetic control of gene expression. Reportedly, the tissue-selective expression of transporters is achieved by DNA methylation (silencing in the transporter-negative tissues) as well as by transactivation in the transporter-positive tissues. Transporters subjected to epigenetic control include OAT3, URAT1, OCT2, OATP1B2, NTCP, and PEPT2 in the SLC families and MDR1, BCRP, BSEP, and ABCG5/ABCG8 (Imai et al., 2009).

Transporter Superfamilies in the Human Genome

The SLC Superfamily

The SLC superfamily includes 52 families and represents about 395 genes in the human genome, the products of which are membrane-spanning proteins, some of which are associated with genetic diseases (Table 5–2). Myriad substrates, including inorganic and organic ions, interact with SLC transporters. There are highly selective transporters that interact with structurally similar molecules, such as transporters in the SLC18 family that interact with monoamines. On the other hand, there are transporters that accept a broad range of chemically diverse substrates, such as organic ion transporters in the SLC22 family. Unlike ABC transporters that rely on ATP hydrolysis to actively translocate their substrates, SLC transporters are mostly facilitative transporters, although some are secondary active transporters (see Figure 5–4). Knowledge of the superfamily continues to grow; in the past decade, about 100 new human SLC transporters have been identified (Lin et al., 2015).

The physiologic roles of SLC transporters are important and diverse. For example, transporters in the SLC1, SLC3, SLC6, SLC7, SLC25, and SLC36 families, which are expressed in the intestine and kidney, among other organs, transport an array of amino acids critical in protein synthesis and energy homeostasis. Glucose and other sugars interact with transporters in the SLC2, SLC5, and SLC50 families for absorption, elimination, and cellular distribution. Proteins in the SLC11, SLC30, SLC39, and SLC40 families transport zinc, iron, and other metals. Members of the SLC19, SLC46, and SLC52 families transport water-soluble vitamins. Transporters in the SLC6 family move neurotransmitters across the plasma membrane; SLC18 family members transport neurotransmitters into storage vesicles.

Pharmacologically, SLC transporters have been characterized for their role in drug absorption, elimination, and tissue distribution and importantly as mediators of drug-drug interactions. Notably, transporters in the solute carrier organic anion family, SLCO, interact with diverse substrates,

TABLE 5–1 ■ REGULATION OF TRANSPORTER EXPRESSION BY NUCLEAR RECEPTORS IN HUMANS

TRANSPORTER	TRANSCRIPTION FACTOR	LIGAND	EFFECT
MDR1 (Pgp)	PXR	Rifampin	↑ Transcription activity
			↑ Expression in duodenum
			↓ Oral bioavailability of digoxin
			↓ AUC of talinolol
			↑ Expression in primary hepatocyte
		St John's wort	↑ Expression in duodenum
			↓ Oral bioavailability of digoxin
	CAR	Phenobarbital	↑ Expression in primary hepatocyte
MRP2	PXR	Rifampin	↑ Expression in duodenum
		Rifampin/hyperforin	↑ Expression in primary hepatocyte
	FXR	GW4064/chenodeoxycholate	↑ Expression in HepG2-FXR
	CAR	Phenobarbital	↑ Expression in hepatocyte
BCR	PXR	Rifampin	↑ Expression in primary hepatocyte
	CAR	Phenobarbital	
MRP3	PXR	Rifampin	↑ Expression in hepatocyte
OATP1B1	SHP1	Cholic acid	Indirect effect on HNFiα expression
	PXR	Rifampin	↑ Expression in hepatocyte
OATP1B3	FXR	Chenodeoxycholate	↑ Expression in hepatoma cells
BSEP	FXR	Chenodeoxycholate	↑ Transcription activity
OSTα/β	FXR	Chenodeoxycholate/GW4064	↑ Transcription activity
		Chenodeoxycholate	↑ Expression in ileal biopsies

CAR, constitutive androstane receptor; FXR, farnesoid X receptor; HNF1a, hepatocyte nuclear factor 1a; PXR, pregnane X receptor; SHP1, small heterodimer partner 1.

including statins and antidiabetic drugs. Transporters in the SLC22 family interact with anionic and cationic drugs, including many antibiotics and antiviral agents, to mediate active renal secretion. SLC transporters are increasingly being targeted for treatment of human disease. Over 100 SLC transporters are associated with monogenic disorders and therefore may be usefully targeted in the treatment of rare diseases. Many SNPs in SLC transporters have reached a genome-wide level of significance in association studies of human disease. Notably, polymorphisms in *SLC30A8* are associated with type 1 diabetes mellitus, and polymorphisms in *SLC22A4* and *SLC22A5* are associated with inflammatory bowel disease.

The ABC Superfamily

The seven groups of ABC transporters are essential for many cellular processes, and mutations in at least 13 of the genes for ABC transporters cause or contribute to human genetic disorders (Table 5–3). In addition to conferring multidrug resistance, an important pharmacological aspect of these transporters is xenobiotic export from healthy tissues. In particular, MDR1/*ABCB1*, MRP2/*ABCC2*, and BCRP/*ABCG2* are involved in overall drug disposition.

Tissue Distribution of Drug-Related ABC Transporters

Table 5–4 summarizes the tissue distribution of drug-related ABC transporters in humans along with information about typical substrates. MDR1 (*ABCB1*), MRP2 (*ABCC2*), and BCRP (*ABCG2*) are all expressed in the apical side of the intestinal epithelia, where they serve to pump out xenobiotics, including many orally administered drugs. MRP3 (*ABCC3*) is expressed in the basal side of the epithelial cells.

Key to the vectorial excretion of drugs into urine or bile, ABC transporters are expressed in the polarized tissues of kidney and liver: MDR1, MRP2, BCRP, and MRP4 (*ABCC4*) on the brush border membrane of renal epithelia; MDR1, MRP2, and BCRP on the bile canalicular

membrane of hepatocytes; and MRP3 and MRP4 on the sinusoidal membrane of hepatocytes. Some ABC transporters are expressed specifically on the blood side of the endothelial or epithelial cells that form barriers to the free entrance of toxic compounds into tissues: the BBB (MDR1 and MRP4 on the luminal side of brain capillary endothelial cells), the blood-CSF barrier (MRP1 and MRP4 on the basolateral blood side of choroid plexus epithelia), the blood-testis barrier (MRP1 on the basolateral membrane of mouse Sertoli cells and MDR1 in several types of human testicular cells), and the blood-placenta barrier (MDR1, MRP2, and BCRP on the luminal maternal side and MRP1 on the antiluminal fetal side of placental trophoblasts).

MRP/ABCC Family

The substrates of transporters in the MRP/ABCC family are mostly organic anions. Both MRP1 and MRP2 accept glutathione and glucuronide conjugates, sulfated conjugates of bile salts, and nonconjugated organic anions of an amphipathic nature (at least one negative charge and some degree of hydrophobicity). They also transport neutral or cationic anticancer drugs, such as vinca alkaloids and anthracyclines, possibly by means of a cotransport or symport mechanism with GSH. MRP3 also has a substrate specificity that is similar to that of MRP2 but with a lower transport affinity for glutathione conjugates compared with MRP1 and MRP2. MRP3 is expressed on the sinusoidal side of hepatocytes and is induced under cholestatic conditions. MRP3 functions to return toxic bile salts and bilirubin glucuronides into the blood circulation. MRP4 accepts negatively charged molecules, including cytotoxic compounds (e.g., 6-mercaptopurine and methotrexate), cyclic nucleotides, antiviral drugs (e.g., adefovir and tenofovir), diuretics (e.g., furosemide and trichlormethiazide), and cephalosporins (e.g., ceftizoxime and cefazolin). Glutathione enables MRP4 to accept taurocholate and leukotriene B$_4$. MRP5 has a narrower substrate specificity and accepts nucleotide analogue and clinically

TABLE 5–2 ■ THE HUMAN SOLUTE CARRIER SUPERFAMILY

GENE	FAMILY	SELECTED DRUG SUBSTRATES	EXAMPLES OF LINKED HUMAN DISEASES
SLC1	Low-K_m glu/neutral aa T		Dicarboxylic aminoaciduria
SLC2	Facilitative GLUT		Fanconi-Bickel syndrome
SLC3	Heavy subunits, heteromeric aa Ts	Melphalan	Classic cystinuria type I
SLC4	Bicarbonate T		Distal renal tubule acidosis
SLC5	Na^+ glucose co-T	Dapagliflozin	Glucose-galactose malabsorption
SLC6	Na^+/Cl^--dependent neurotransmitter T	Paroxetine, fluoxetine	Cerebral creatine deficiency syndrome
SLC7	Cationic aa T	Melphalan	Lysinuric protein intolerance
SLC8	Na^+/Ca^{2+} Exch	Di-CH_3-arg	
SLC9	Na^+/H^+ Exch	Thiazide diuretics	Hypophosphatemic nephrolithiasis
SLC10	Na^+ bile salt co-T	Benzothiazepines (diltiazem)	Primary bile acid malabsorption
SLC11	H^+-coupled metal ion T		Hereditary hemochromatosis
SLC12	Electroneutral cation–Cl^- co-T		Gitelman syndrome
SLC13	Na^+–SO_4^-/COO^- co-T	SO_4^-/cys conjugates	
SLC14	Urea T		Kidd antigen blood group
SLC15	H^+–oligopeptide co-T	Valacyclovir	
SLC16	Monocarboxylate T	Salicylate, T_3/T_4, atorvastatin	Familial hyperinsulinemic hypoglycemia 7
SLC17	Vesicular glu T		Sialic acid storage disease
SLC18	Vesicular amine T	Reserpine	Myasthenic syndromes
SLC19	Folate/thiamine T	Methotrexate	Thiamine-responsive megaloblastic anemia
SLC20	Type III Na^+–PO_4^- co-T		
SLC21 (SLCO)	Organic anion T	Pravastatin	Rotor syndrome, hyperbilirubinemia
SLC22	Organic ion T	Pravastatin, metformin	Primary systemic carnitine deficiency
SLC23	Na^+-dependent ascorbate T	Vitamin C	
SLC24	$Na^+/(Ca^{2+}$-$K^+)$ Exch		Congenital stationary night blindness type 1D
SLC25	Mitochondrial carrier		Familial hypertrophic cardiomyopathy
SLC26	Multifunctional anion Exch	Salicylate, ciprofloxacin	Multiple epiphyseal dysplasia 4
SLC27	Fatty acid T		Ichthyosis prematurity syndrome
SLC28	Na^+-coupled nucleoside T	Gemcitabine, cladribine	
SLC29	Facilitative nucleoside T	Dipyridamole, gemcitabine	
SLC30	Zn efflux		Hypermanganesemia with dystonia
SLC31	Cu T	Cisplatin	
SLC32	Vesicular inhibitory aa T	Vigabatrin	
SLC33	Acetyl-CoA T		Congenital cataracts
SLC34	Type II Na^+–PO_4^-/ co-T		Hypercalciuric rickets
SLC35	Nucleoside-sugar T		Leukocyte adhesion deficiency II
SLC36	H^+-coupled aa T	D-Serine, cycloserine	Iminoglycinuria
SLC37	Sugar-phosphate/PO_4^- Exch		Glycogen storage disease
SLC38	Na^+-coupled neutral aa T		
SLC39	Metal ion T		Acrodermatitis enteropathica
SLC40	Basolateral Fe T		Hemochromatosis type IV
SLC41	MgtE-like Mg^{2+} T		
SLC42	Rh ammonium T		Rh-null regulator type disease
SLC43 SLC45 SLC52	Na^+-independent L-like aa T Unknown substrate Riboflavin transporter family	Riboflavin	Oculocutaneous albinism type 4 Riboflavin deficiency

aa, amino acid; Exch, exchanger; T, transporter T_3/T_4, thyroid hormone.

TABLE 5–3 ■ THE HUMAN ATP BINDING CASSETTE (ABC) SUPERFAMILY

GENE	FAMILY	NUMBER OF MEMBERS	EXAMPLES OF LINKED HUMAN DISEASES
ABCA	ABC A	12	Tangier disease (defect in cholesterol transport; ABCA1), Stargardt syndrome (defect in retinal metabolism; ABCA4)
ABCB	ABC B	11	Bare lymphocyte syndrome type 1 (defect in antigen presenting; ABCB3 and ABCB4), progressive familial intrahepatic cholestasis type 3 (defect in biliary lipid secretion; MDR3/ABCB4), X-linked sideroblastic anemia with ataxia (a possible defect in iron homeostasis in mitochondria; ABCB7), progressive familial intrahepatic cholestasis type 2 (defect in biliary bile acid excretion; BSEP/*ABCB11*)
ABCC	ABC C	13	Dubin-Johnson syndrome (defect in biliary bilirubin glucuronide excretion; MRP2/*ABCC2*), pseudoxanthoma (unknown mechanism; *ABCC6*), cystic fibrosis (defect in Cl⁻ channel regulation; *ABCC7*), persistent hyperinsulinemic hypoglycemia of infancy (defect in inwardly rectifying K⁺ conductance regulation in pancreatic B cells; SUR1/*ABCC8*)
ABCD	ABC D	4	Adrenoleukodystrophy (a possible defect in peroxisomal transport or catabolism of very long-chain fatty acids; ABCD1)
ABCE	ABC E	1	
ABCF	ABC F	3	
ABCG	ABC G	5	Sitosterolemia (defect in biliary and intestinal excretion of plant sterols; ABCG5 and ABCG8)

TABLE 5–4 ■ ABC TRANSPORTERS INVOLVED IN DRUG ABSORPTION, DISTRIBUTION, AND EXCRETION PROCESSES

NAME TISSUE DISTRIBUTION	SUBSTRATES
MDR1 (ABCB1) Liver, kidney, intestine, BBB, BTB, BPB	**Characteristics:** Bulky neutral or cationic compounds (many xenobiotics)—etoposide, doxorubicin, vincristine; diltiazem, verapamil; indinavir, ritonavir; erythromycin, ketoconazole; testosterone, progesterone; cyclosporine, tacrolimus; digoxin, quinidine, fexofenadine, loperamide
MRP1 (ABCC1) Ubiquitous	**Characteristics:** Negatively charged amphiphiles—vincristine (with GSH), methotrexate; GSH conjugate of LTC_4, ethacrynic acid; glucuronide of estradiol, bilirubin; estrone-3-sulfate; saquinavir; grepafloxacin; folate, GSH, GSSG
MRP2 (ABCC2) Liver, kidney, intestine, BPB	**Characteristics:** Negatively charged amphiphiles—methotrexate, vincristine; GSH conjugates of LTC_4, ethacrynic acid; glucuronides of estradiol, bilirubin; taurolithocholate sulfate; statins, AngII receptor antagonists, temocaprilat; indinavir, ritonavir; GSH, GSSG
MRP3 (ABCC3) Liver, kidney, intestine	**Characteristics:** Negatively charged amphiphiles—etoposide, methotrexate; GSH conjugates of LTC_4, PGJ_2; glucuronides of estradiol, etoposide, morphine, acetaminophen, hymecromone, harmol; sulfate conjugates of bile salts; glycocholate, taurocholate; folate, leucovorin
MRP4 (ABCC4) Ubiquitous, including BBB and BCSFB	**Characteristics:** Nucleotide analogues, 6-mercaptopurine, methotrexate; estradiol glucuronide; dehydroepiandrosterone sulfate; cyclic AMP/GMP; furosemide, trichlormethiazide; adefovir, tenofovir; cefazolin, ceftizoxime; folate, leucovorin, taurocholate (with GSH)
MRP5 (ABCC5) Ubiquitous	**Characteristics:** Nucleotide analogues 6-mercaptopurine; cyclic AMP/GMP; adefovir
MRP6 (ABCC6) Liver, kidney	**Characteristics:** Doxorubicin,[a] etoposide,[a] GSH conjugate of LTC_4; BQ-123 (cyclic penta peptide antagonist at the ETₐ endothelin receptor)
BCRP(MXR) (ABCG2) Liver, intestine, BBB	**Characteristics:** Neutral and anionic compounds—methotrexate, mitoxantrone, camptothecins, SN-38, topotecan, imatinib; glucuronides of 4-methylumbelliferone, estradiol; sulfate conjugates of dehydroepiandrosterone, estrone; nitrofurantoin, fluoroquinolones; pitavastatin, rosuvastatin; cholesterol, estradiol, dantrolene, prazosin, sulfasalazine, uric acid, allopurinol, oxypurinol
MDR3 (ABCB4) Liver	**Characteristics:** Phospholipids
BSEP (ABCB11) Liver	**Characteristics:** Bile salts
ABCG5, ABCG8 Liver, intestine	**Characteristics:** Plant sterols

BBB, blood-brain barrier; BTB, blood-testis barrier; BPB, blood-placenta barrier; BCSFB, blood-cerebrospinal fluid barrier; LTC, Leukotriene C; PGJ, prostaglandin J.

[a]Substrates and cytotoxic drugs with increased resistance (cytotoxicity with increased resistance is usually caused by the decreased accumulation of the drugs). Although MDR3 (ABCB4), BSEP (ABCB11), ABCG5, and ABCG8 are not directly involved in drug disposition, their inhibition will lead to unfavorable side effects.

important anti-HIV drugs. No substrates have been identified that explain the mechanism of the MRP6-associated disease pseudoxanthoma.

BCRP/ABCG2

BCRP accepts both neutral and negatively charged molecules, including cytotoxic compounds (e.g., topotecan, flavopiridol, and methotrexate); sulfated conjugates of therapeutic drugs and hormones (e.g., estrogen sulfate); antibiotics (e.g., nitrofurantoin and fluoroquinolones); statins (e.g., pitavastatin and rosuvastatin); and toxic compounds found in normal food [phytoestrogens, (2-amino-1-methyl-6-phenylimidazo[4,5-*b*] pyridine), and pheophorbide A, a chlorophyll catabolite]. In addition, genetic variants in the transporter have been implicated in hyperuricemia and gout and in the disposition of uric acid and the XOIs allopurinol and oxypurinol.

Physiological Roles of ABC Transporters

The physiological significance of the ABC transporters has been amply illustrated by studies involving knockout animals or patients with genetic defects in these transporters. For instance, mice deficient in MDR1 function are viable and fertile and do not display obvious phenotypic abnormalities other than hypersensitivity to the toxicity of drugs. There are equally remarkable data for MRP1, MRP4, BCRP, and BSEP. The lesson is this: Complete absence of these drug-related ABC transporters is not lethal and can remain unrecognized in the absence of exogenous perturbations due to food, drugs, or toxins. However, inhibition of physiologically important ABC transporters (especially those related directly to the genetic diseases described in Table 5–3) by drugs should be avoided to reduce the incidence of drug-induced side effects.

ABC Transporters in Drug Absorption and Elimination

With respect to clinical medicine, MDR1 is the most renowned ABC transporter yet identified. The systemic exposure to orally administered digoxin is decreased by coadministration of rifampin (an MDR1 inducer) and is negatively correlated with the MDR1 protein expression in the human intestine. MDR1 is also expressed on the brush border membrane of renal epithelia, and its function can be monitored using digoxin (> 70% excreted in the urine). MDR1 inhibitors (e.g., quinidine, verapamil, valspodar, spironolactone, clarithromycin, and ritonavir) all markedly reduce renal excretion of digoxin. Drugs with narrow therapeutic windows (e.g., digoxin, cyclosporine, tacrolimus) should be used with great care if MDR1-based drug-drug interactions are likely.

In the intestine, MRP3 can mediate intestinal absorption in conjunction with uptake transporters. MRP3 mediates sinusoidal efflux in the liver, decreasing the efficacy of the biliary excretion from the blood and excretion of intracellularly formed metabolites, particularly glucuronide conjugates. Thus, dysfunction of MRP3 results in shortening of the elimination $t_{1/2}$. MRP4 substrates also can be transported by OAT1 and OAT3 on the basolateral membrane of the epithelial cells in the kidney. The rate-limiting process in renal tubular secretion is likely the uptake process at the basolateral surface. Dysfunction of MRP4 enhances the renal concentration but has limited effect on the blood concentration.

Transporters Involved in Pharmacokinetics

Drug transporters play a prominent role in pharmacokinetics (see Figure 5–1 and Table 5–4). Transporters in the liver and kidney have important roles in removal of drugs from the blood and hence in metabolism and excretion.

Hepatic Transporters

Hepatic uptake of organic anions (e.g., drugs, leukotrienes, and bilirubin), cations, and bile salts is mediated by SLC-type transporters in the basolateral (sinusoidal) membrane of hepatocytes: OATPs (SLCO), OCTs (SLC22), and NTCP (SLC10A1), respectively. These transporters mediate uptake by either facilitated or secondary active mechanisms.

ABC transporters such as MRP2, MDR1, BCRP, BSEP, and MDR2 in the bile canalicular membrane of hepatocytes mediate the efflux (excretion) of drugs and their metabolites, bile salts, and phospholipids against a steep concentration gradient from liver to bile. This primary active transport is driven by ATP hydrolysis.

Vectorial transport of drugs from the circulating blood to the bile using an uptake transporter (OATP family) and an efflux transporter (MRP2, BCRP) is important for determining drug exposure in the circulating blood and liver. Moreover, there are many other uptake and efflux transporters in the liver (Figure 5–9).

The following examples illustrate the importance of vectorial transport in determining drug exposure in the circulating blood and liver and the role of transporters in drug-drug interactions.

HMG-CoA Reductase Inhibitors

Statins are cholesterol-lowering agents that reversibly inhibit HMG-CoA reductase, which catalyzes a rate-limiting step in cholesterol biosynthesis (see Chapter 33). Most of the statins in their acid form are substrates of hepatic uptake transporters and undergo enterohepatic recirculation (see Figure 5–6). In this process, hepatic uptake transporters such as OATP1B1 and efflux transporters such as MRP2 act cooperatively to produce *bisubstrate vectorial transcellular transport*. The efficient first-pass hepatic uptake of these statins by OATP1B1 helps concentrate them in the liver where they produce their pharmacological effects, thus minimizing their systemic levels and adverse effects in smooth muscle. Genetic polymorphisms of OATP1B1 also affect the function of this transporter (Meyer zu Schwabedissen et al., 2015).

Gemfibrozil

The cholesterol-lowering agent gemfibrozil, a PPARα activator, can enhance toxicity (myopathy) to several statins by a mechanism that involves transport. Gemfibrozil and its glucuronide inhibit the uptake of the active hydroxy forms of statins into hepatocytes by OATP1B1, resulting in an increase in the plasma concentration of the statin and a concomitant increase in toxicity.

Irinotecan

CPT-11 is a potent anticancer drug, but late-onset GI toxicities, such as severe diarrhea, make this a difficult agent to use safely. After intravenous administration of CPT-11, a carboxylesterase converts the drug to SN-38, an active metabolite. SN-38 is subsequently conjugated with glucuronic acid in the liver. SN-38 and SN-38 glucuronide are then excreted into the bile by MRP2, entering the GI tract and causing adverse effects. The inhibition of MRP2-mediated biliary excretion of SN-38 and its glucuronide by coadministration of probenecid reduces the drug-induced diarrhea in experimental systems and may prove useful in humans (Horikawa et al., 2002). For additional details, see Figures 6–6, 6–8, 6–9.

Bosentan

Bosentan is an endothelin antagonist used to treat pulmonary arterial hypertension. It is taken up in the liver by OATP1B1 and OATP1B3 and subsequently metabolized by CYP2C9 and CYP3A4. Transporter-mediated hepatic uptake can be a determinant of elimination of bosentan, and inhibition of its hepatic uptake by cyclosporine, rifampicin, and sildenafil can affect its pharmacokinetics.

Temocapril and other ACE inhibitors

Temocapril is an ACE inhibitor (see Chapter 26). Its active metabolite, temocaprilat, is excreted both in the bile and in the urine by the liver and kidney, respectively, whereas other ACE inhibitors are excreted mainly by the kidney. A special feature of temocapril among ACE inhibitors is that the plasma concentration of temocaprilat remains relatively unchanged even in patients with renal failure. However, the plasma AUC of enalaprilat and other ACE inhibitors is markedly increased in patients with renal disorders. Temocaprilat is a bisubstrate of the OATP family and MRP2, whereas other ACE inhibitors are not good substrates of MRP2 (although they are taken up into the liver by the OATP family). Taking these findings into consideration, the affinity for MRP2 may dominate in determining the biliary excretion of any series of ACE inhibitors. Drugs that are

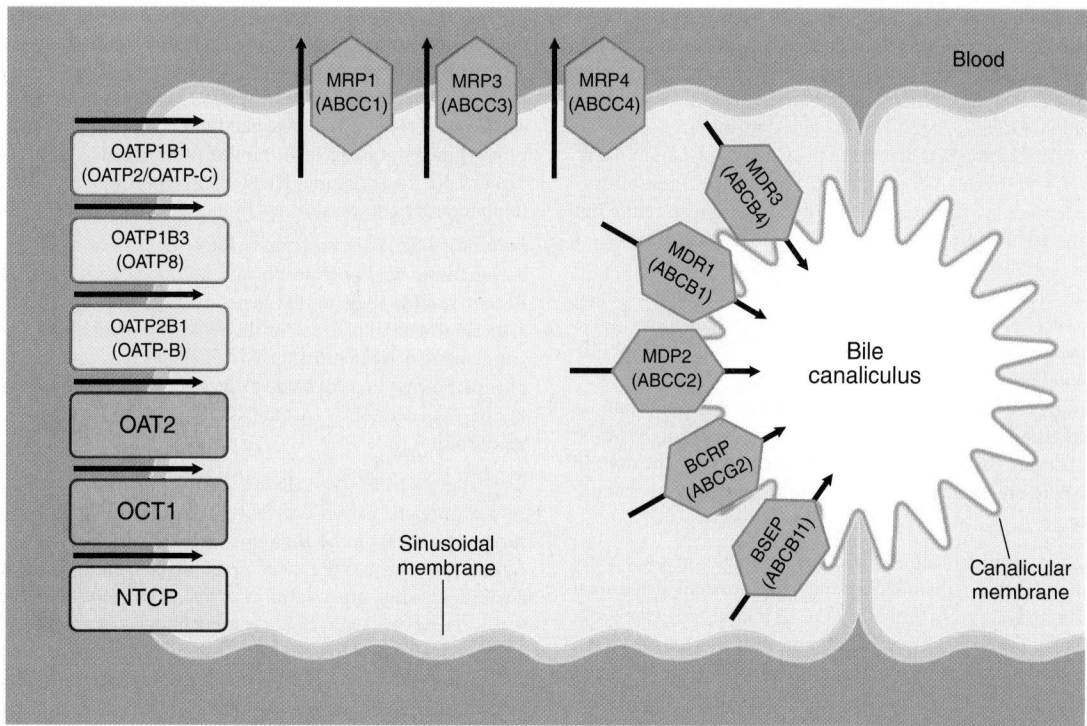

Figure 5–9 *Transporters in the hepatocyte that function in the uptake and efflux of drugs across the sinusoidal membrane and efflux of drugs into the bile across the canalicular membrane.* Arrows show the primary direction of transport. See text for details of the transporters pictured.

excreted into both the bile and urine to the same degree thus are expected to exhibit minimum interindividual differences in their pharmacokinetics.

Angiotensin II Receptor Antagonists

Angiotensin II receptor antagonists are used for the treatment of hypertension, acting on AT_1 receptors expressed in vascular smooth muscle, proximal tubule, adrenal medullary cells, and elsewhere. For most of these drugs, hepatic uptake and biliary excretion are important factors for their pharmacokinetics and pharmacological effects. Telmisartan is taken up into human hepatocytes in a saturable manner, predominantly via OATP1B3 (Ishiguro et al., 2006). On the other hand, both OATPs 1B1 and 1B3 are responsible for the hepatic uptake of valsartan and olmesartan, although the relative contributions of these transporters are unclear. Studies using doubly transfected cells with hepatic uptake transporters and biliary excretion transporters have clarified that MRP2 plays the most important role in the biliary excretion of valsartan and olmesartan.

Repaglinide and Nateglinide

Repaglinide is a meglitinide analogue antidiabetic drug. Although it is eliminated almost completely by the metabolism mediated by CYPs 2C8 and 3A4, transporter-mediated hepatic uptake is one of the determinants of its elimination rate. In subjects with the OATP1B1 (*SLCO1B1*) 521CC genotype, a significant change in the pharmacokinetics of repaglinide was observed (Niemi et al., 2005). Genetic polymorphism in *SLCO1B1* 521T>C results in altered pharmacokinetics of nateglinide, suggesting OATP1B1 is a determinant of its elimination, although it is subsequently metabolized by CYPs 2C9, 3A4, and 2D6 (Zhang et al., 2006b).

Renal Transporters

Organic Cation Transport

Structurally diverse organic cations are secreted in the proximal tubule. Many secreted organic cations are endogenous compounds (e.g., choline, *N*-methylnicotinamide, and DA), and renal secretion helps to eliminate excess concentrations of these substances. Another function of organic cation secretion is ridding the body of xenobiotics, including many positively charged drugs and their metabolites (e.g., cimetidine, ranitidine, metformin, varenicline, and trospium) and toxins from the environment

(e.g., nicotine and paraquat). Organic cations that are secreted by the kidney may be either hydrophobic or hydrophilic. Hydrophilic organic drug cations generally have molecular weights less than 400 Da; a current model for their secretion in the proximal tubule of the nephron is shown in Figure 5–10 involving the transporters described next.

For the transepithelial flux of a compound (e.g., secretion), the compound must traverse two membranes sequentially, the basolateral membrane facing the blood side and the apical membrane facing the tubular lumen. Organic cations appear to cross the basolateral membrane in the human proximal tubule by two distinct transporters in the SLC family 22 (SCL22): OCT2 (*SLC22A2*) and OCT3 (*SLCA22A3*). Organic cations are transported across this membrane down an electrochemical gradient.

Transport of organic cations from cell to tubular lumen across the apical membrane occurs through an electroneutral proton–organic cation

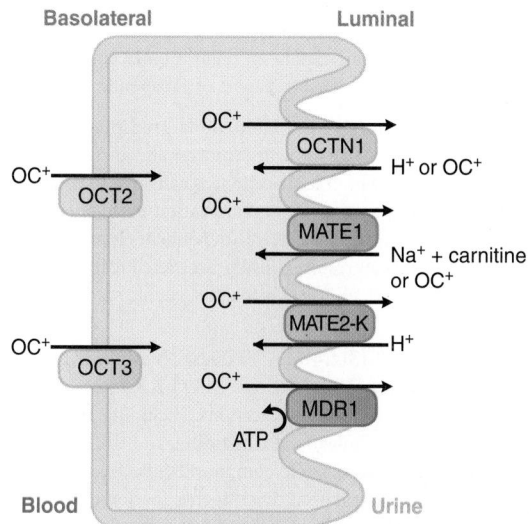

Figure 5–10 *Organic cation secretory transporters in the proximal tubule.* OC^+, organic cation. See text for details of the transporters pictured.

exchange, which is mediated by transporters in the SLC47 family, which comprises members of the MATE family. Transporters in the MATE family, assigned to the apical membrane of the proximal tubule, appear to play a key role in moving hydrophilic organic cations from tubule cell to lumen. In addition, OCTNs, located on the apical membrane, appear to contribute to organic cation flux across the proximal tubule. In humans, these include *OCTN1* (SLC22A4) and *OCTN2* (SLC22A5). These bifunctional transporters are involved not only in organic cation secretion but also in carnitine reabsorption. In the reuptake mode, the transporters function as Na^+ cotransporters, relying on the inwardly driven Na^+ gradient created by Na^+,K^+-ATPase to move carnitine from tubular lumen to cell. In the secretory mode, the transporters appear to function as proton–organic cation exchangers. That is, protons move from tubular lumen to cell interior in exchange for organic cations, which move from cytosol to tubular lumen. The inwardly directed proton gradient (tubular lumen → cytosol) is maintained by transporters in the SLC9 family, which are Na^+/K^+ exchangers (NHEs, antiporters). Of the two steps involved in secretory transport, transport across the luminal membrane appears to be rate limiting.

OCT2 (SLC22A2).

Human, mouse, and rat orthologs of OCT2 are expressed in abundance in human kidney and to some extent in neuronal tissue such as choroid plexus. In the kidney, OCT2 is localized in the proximal and distal tubules and collecting ducts. In the proximal tubule, OCT2 is restricted to the basolateral membrane. OCT2-mediated transport of model organic cations MPP^+ (1-methyl-4-phenylpyridinium) and TEA (tetraethylammonium) is electrogenic, and both OCT2 and OCT1 can support organic cation–organic cation exchange. OCT2 generally accepts a wide array of monovalent organic cations with molecular weights below 400 Da. OCT2 is also present in neuronal tissues; however, monoamine neurotransmitters have low affinities for OCT2.

OCT3 (SLC22A3).

The OCT3 gene is located in tandem with genes for OCT1 and OCT2 on chromosome 6. Tissue distribution studies suggest that human OCT3 is expressed in liver, kidney, intestine, placenta, skeletal muscle, and adipose tissue, although in the kidney it appears to be expressed in considerably less abundance than OCT2, and in the liver it is less abundant than OCT1. Like OCT1 and OCT2, OCT3 appears to support electrogenic potential-sensitive organic cation transport. OCT3 plays a role in both the renal elimination and the intestinal absorption of metformin.

OCTN1 (SLC22A4).

OCTN1 seems to operate as an organic cation–proton exchanger. OCTN1-mediated influx of model organic cations is enhanced at alkaline pH, whereas efflux is increased by an inwardly directed proton gradient. OCTN1 contains a nucleotide-binding sequence motif, and transport of its substrates appears to be stimulated by cellular ATP. OCTN1 also can function as an organic cation–organic cation exchanger. OCTN1 functions as a bidirectional pH- and ATP-dependent transporter at the apical membrane in renal tubular epithelial cells and appears to be important in renal transport of gabapentin.

OCTN2 (SLC22A5).

OCTN2 is a bifunctional transporter; it functions as both an Na^+-dependent carnitine transporter and an Na^+-independent OCT. OCTN2 transport of organic cations is sensitive to pH, suggesting that OCTN2 may function as an organic cation exchanger. The transport of *L*-carnitine by OCTN2 is an Na^+-dependent electrogenic process. Mutations in OCTN2 can result in insufficient renal reabsorption of carnitine and appear to be the cause of primary systemic carnitine deficiency (Tamai, 2013)

MATE1 and MATE2-K (SLC47A1, SLC47A2).

Multidrug and toxin extrusion family members MATE1 and MATE2-K interact with structurally diverse hydrophilic organic cations, including the antidiabetic drug metformin, the H_2 antagonist cimetidine, and the anticancer drug topotecan. In addition to cationic compounds, the transporters recognize some anions, including the antiviral agents acyclovir and ganciclovir. The zwitterions cephalexin and cephradine are specific substrates of MATE1. The herbicide paraquat, a bis-quaternary ammonium compound that is nephrotoxic in humans, is a high-affinity substrate of MATE1. Both

MATE1 and MATE2-K have been localized to the apical membrane of the proximal tubule. MATE1, but not MATE2-K, is also expressed on the canalicular membrane of the hepatocyte. These transporters appear to be the long-searched-for organic cation–proton antiporters on the apical membrane of the proximal tubule; that is, an oppositely directed proton gradient can drive the movement of organic cations via MATE1 or MATE2-K. The antibiotics levofloxacin and ciprofloxacin, though potent inhibitors, are not translocated by either MATE1 or MATE2-K.

Polymorphisms of OCTs and MATEs. OCT1 exhibits the greatest number of amino acid polymorphisms, followed by OCT2 and then OCT3. Recent studies suggest that genetic variants of OCT1 and OCT2 are associated with alterations in the renal elimination and response to the antidiabetic drug metformin. MATEs have fewer amino acid polymorphisms; however, recent studies suggested that noncoding region variants of SLC47A1 and SLC47A2 are associated with variation in response to metformin.

Organic Anion Transport

As with organic cation transport, a primary function of organic anion secretion appears to be the removal of xenobiotics from the body. The candidate substrates are structurally diverse and include many weakly acidic drugs (e.g., pravastatin, captopril, PAH, and penicillins) and toxins (e.g., ochratoxin). OATs not only move both hydrophobic and hydrophilic anions but also may interact with cations and neutral compounds.

Figure 5–11 shows a current model for the transepithelial flux of organic anions in the proximal tubule. Two primary transporters on the basolateral membrane mediate the flux of organic anions from interstitial fluid to tubule cell: OAT1 (*SLC22A6*) and OAT3 (*SLC22A8*). Energetically, hydrophilic organic anions are transported across the basolateral membrane against an electrochemical gradient, exchanging with intracellular α-ketoglutarate, which moves down its concentration gradient from cytosol to blood. The outwardly directed gradient of α-ketoglutarate is maintained at least in part by a basolateral Na^+-dicarboxylate transporter (NaDC3), using the Na^+ gradient established by Na^+,K^+-ATPase. Transport of low-molecular-weight organic anions by the cloned transporters OAT1 and OAT3 can be driven by α-ketoglutarate; coupled transport of α-ketoglutarate and low-molecular-weight organic anions (e.g., PAH)

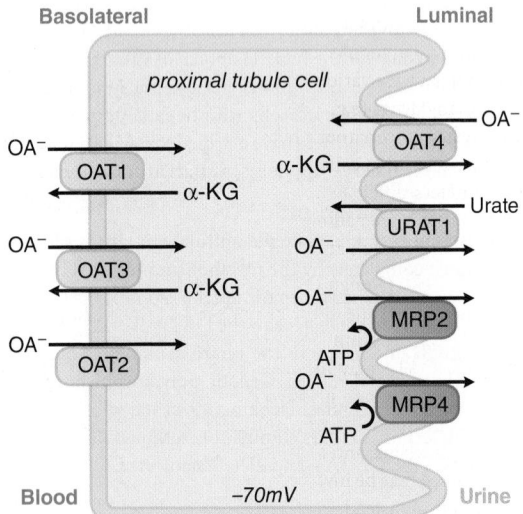

Figure 5–11 *Organic anion secretory transporters in the proximal tubule.* Two primary transporters on the basolateral membrane mediate the flux of OAs from interstitial fluid to tubule cell: OAT1 (*SLC22A6*) and OAT3 (*SLC22A8*). Hydrophilic OAs are transported across the basolateral membrane against an electrochemical gradient in exchange with intracellular α-ketoglutarate (α-KG), which moves down its concentration gradient from cytosol to blood. The outwardly directed gradient of α-KG is maintained at least in part by a basolateral Na^+-dicarboxylate uptake transporter (NaDC3). The Na^+ gradient that drives NaDC3 is maintained by Na^+,K^+-ATPase.

occurs in isolated basolateral membrane vesicles. The molecular pharmacology and molecular biology of OATs have recently been reviewed (Srimaroeng et al., 2008).

The mechanism responsible for the apical membrane transport of organic anions from tubule cell cytosol to tubular lumen remains controversial. OAT4 may serve as the luminal membrane transporter for organic anions, but the movement of substrates via this transporter can be driven by exchange with a α-ketoglutarate, suggesting that OAT4 may function in the reabsorptive, rather than secretory, flux of organic anions. NaPT1, originally cloned as a phosphate transporter, can support the low-affinity transport of hydrophilic organic anions such as PAH. MRP2 and MRP4, multidrug resistance transporters in the ABCC, can interact with some organic anions and may actively pump them from tubule cell cytosol to tubular lumen.

OAT1 (SLC22A6). Mammalian isoforms of OAT1 are expressed primarily in the kidney, with some expression in brain and skeletal muscle. Immunohistochemical studies suggest that OAT1 is expressed on the basolateral membrane of the proximal tubule in humans, with highest expression in the middle segment, S2 (see Figure 25-1). Based on quantitative PCR, OAT1 is expressed at a third of the level of OAT3. OAT1 exhibits saturable transport of organic anions such as PAH. This transport is transstimulated by other organic anions, including α-ketoglutarate. Thus, the inside negative-potential difference drives the efflux of the dicarboxylate α-ketoglutarate, which in turn supports the influx of monocarboxylates such as PAH. Sex steroids regulate expression of OAT1 in the kidney. OAT1 generally transports low-molecular-weight organic anions, either endogenous (e.g., PGE_2 and urate) or exogenous (ingested drugs and toxins). Some neutral compounds are also transported by OAT1 at a lower affinity (e.g., cimetidine).

OAT2 (SLC22A7). OAT2 is present in both kidney and liver; renal OAT2 is localized to the basolateral membrane of the proximal tubule. OAT2 functions as a transporter for nucleotides, particularly guanine nucleotides such as cyclic GMP, for which it is a bidirectional facilitative transporter (Cropp et al., 2008). Cellular studies indicate that OAT2 functions in both the influx and the efflux of guanine nucleotides. OAT2 transports organic anions such as PAH and methotrexate with low affinity, PGE_2 with high affinity, and some neutral compounds but with lower affinity (e.g., cimetidine).

OAT3 (SLC22A8). Human OAT3 is confined to the basolateral membrane of the proximal tubule. This protein consists of two variants, one of which transports a wide variety of organic anions, including PAH, estrone sulfate, and many drugs (e.g., pravastatin, cimetidine, 6-mercaptopurine, and methotrexate) (Srimaroeng et al., 2008). The longer variant does not support transport. The specificities of OAT3 and OAT1 overlap, although kinetic parameters differ: Estrone sulfate is transported by both but by OAT3 with a much higher affinity; OAT1 transports the H_2 receptor antagonist cimetidine with high affinity.

OAT4 (SLC22A11). Human OAT4 is expressed in placenta and kidney (on the luminal membrane of the proximal tubule). Organic anion transport by OAT4 can be stimulated by transgradients of α-ketoglutarate, suggesting that OAT4 may be involved in the reabsorption of organic anions from tubular lumen into cell (see Figure 5–11). The specificity of OAT4 includes the model compounds estrone sulfate and PAH, as well as zidovudine, tetracycline, and methotrexate. Collectively, emerging studies suggest that OAT4 may be involved not in secretory flux of organic anions but in reabsorption instead.

Other Anion Transporters. URAT1 (*SLC22A12*) is a kidney-specific transporter confined to the apical membrane of the proximal tubule. URAT1 is primarily responsible for urate reabsorption, mediating electroneutral urate transport that can be transstimulated by Cl⁻ gradients. NPT1, Na⁺-dependent phosphate transport protein 1 (SLC17A1), is expressed on the luminal membrane of the proximal tubule as well as in the brain. NPT1 transports PAH, probenecid, and penicillin G. It appears to be involved in organic anion efflux from tubule cell to lumen and interacts with uric acid.

MRP2 (*ABCC2*) is considered to be the primary transporter involved in efflux of many drug conjugates (such as GSH conjugates) across the canalicular membrane of the hepatocyte. MRP2 is also found on the apical membrane of the proximal tubule, where it is thought to play a role in the efflux of organic anions into the tubular lumen. In general, MRP2 transports larger, bulkier compounds than do most of the OATs in the SLC22 family. MRP4 (*ABCC4*), localized on the apical membrane of the proximal tubule, transports a wide array of conjugated anions, including glucuronides and GSH conjugates. MRP4 appears to interact with methotrexate, cyclic nucleotide analogues, and antiviral nucleoside analogues. BCRP (*ABCG2*) is localized to the apical membrane of the proximal tubule and duodenum and is involved in uric acid secretion and secretion of the XOIs allopurinol and oxypurinol.

Polymorphisms in OAT1 and OAT3 have been identified in ethnic human subpopulations (see https://www.pharmgkb.org). Notably, polymorphisms in ABCG2 have been associated with reduced response to allopurinol and oxypurinol.

Transporters and Pharmacodynamics: Drug Action in the Brain

Biogenic amine neurotransmitters are packaged in vesicles in presynaptic neurons, released in the synapse by fusion of the vesicles with the plasma membrane, and then taken back into the presynaptic neurons or postsynaptic cells (see Chapters 8 and 14). Transporters involved in the neuronal reuptake of the neurotransmitters and the regulation of their levels in the synaptic cleft belong to two major superfamilies, SLC1 and SLC6. Transporters in both families play roles in reuptake of GABA, glutamate, and the monoamine neurotransmitters NE, 5HT, and DA. These transporters may serve as pharmacologic targets for neuropsychiatric drugs. SLC6 family members localized in the brain and involved in the reuptake of neurotransmitters into presynaptic neurons include NET (*SLC6A2*), DAT (*SLC6A3*), SERT (*SLC6A4*), and several GATs (GAT1, GAT2, and GAT3). Each of these transporters appears to have 12 transmembrane (TM) regions and a large extracellular loop with glycosylation sites between TM3 and TM4.

SLC6 family members are secondary active transporters, depending on the Na⁺ gradient to transport their substrates into cells. Cl⁻ is also required, although to a variable extent depending on the family member. Through their reuptake mechanisms, the neurotransmitter transporters in the SLC6A family regulate the concentrations and dwell times of neurotransmitters in the synaptic cleft; the extent of transmitter uptake also influences subsequent vesicular storage of transmitters. Many of these transporters are present in other tissues (e.g., intestine, kidney, and platelets) and may serve other roles. Further, the transporters can function in the reverse direction; that is, the transporters can export neurotransmitters in a Na^{2+}-independent fashion.

GABA Uptake: GAT1 (*SLC6A1*), GAT3 (*SLC6A11*), GAT2 (*SLC6A13*), and BGT1 (*SLC6A12*)

GAT1 is the most important GABA transporter in the brain, expressed in GABAergic neurons and found largely on presynaptic neurons. GAT1 is abundant in the neocortex, cerebellum, basal ganglia, brainstem, spinal cord, retina, and olfactory bulb. GAT3 is found only in the brain, largely in glial cells. GAT2 is found in peripheral tissues, including the kidney and liver, and within the CNS in the choroid plexus and meninges. Physiologically, GAT1 appears to be responsible for regulating the interaction of GABA at receptors. The presence of GAT2 in the choroid plexus and its absence in presynaptic neurons suggest that this transporter may play a primary role in maintaining the homeostasis of GABA in the CSF. GAT1 is the target of the antiepileptic drug tiagabine (a nipecotic acid derivative), which presumably acts to prolong the dwell time of GABA in the synaptic cleft of GABAergic neurons by inhibiting the reuptake of GABA. A fourth GAT, BGT1, occurs in extrasynaptic regions of the hippocampus and cortex (Madsen et al., 2011).

Catecholamine Uptake: NET (*SLC6A2*)

NET is found in central and peripheral nervous tissues as well as in adrenal chromaffin tissue. NET colocalizes with neuronal markers, consistent with a role in reuptake of monoamine neurotransmitters. NET provides reuptake of NE (and DA) into neurons, thereby limiting the synaptic dwell time of NE and terminating its actions, salvaging NE for subsequent repackaging. NET serves as a drug target for the antidepressant desipramine, other tricyclic antidepressants, and cocaine. Orthostatic intolerance, a rare familial disorder characterized by an abnormal blood pressure and heart rate response to changes in posture, has been associated with a mutation in NET.

Dopamine Uptake: DAT (*SLC6A3*)

DAT is located primarily in the brain in dopaminergic neurons. The primary function of DAT is the reuptake of DA, terminating its actions. Although present on presynaptic neurons at the neurosynaptic junction, DAT is also present in abundance along the neurons, away from the synaptic cleft. Physiologically, DAT is involved in functions attributed to the dopaminergic system, including mood, behavior, reward, and cognition. Drugs that interact with DAT include cocaine and its analogues, amphetamines, and the neurotoxin MPTP (methylphenyltetrahydropyridine).

Serotonin Uptake: SERT (*SLC6A4*)

SERT is responsible for the reuptake and clearance of 5HT in the brain. Like the other SLC6A family members, SERT transports its substrates in a Na^+-dependent fashion and is dependent on Cl^- and possibly on the countertransport of K^+. Substrates of SERT include 5HT, various tryptamine derivatives, and neurotoxins such as MDMA (ecstasy) and fenfluramine. SERT is the specific target of the SSRI antidepressants (e.g., fluoxetine and paroxetine) and one of several targets of tricyclic antidepressants (e.g., amitriptyline). Genetic variants of SERT have been associated with an array of behavioral and neurological disorders. The precise mechanism by which reduced activity of SERT, caused by either a genetic variant or an antidepressant, ultimately affects behavior, including depression, is not known.

The Blood-Brain Barrier: A Pharmacological View

The CNS is well protected from circulating neurotransmitters, well supplied with necessary nutrients and ions, and able to exclude many toxins, bacteria, and xenobiotics. This careful set of conditions is achieved by a barrier called the BBB. This barrier results from the specialized properties of the microvasculature of the CNS. Functionally, the BBB is partly physical, partly a consequence of selective permeability (export of undesirable molecules and import of necessary molecules), and partly a consequence of the enzymatic destruction of certain permeants by enzymes in the barrier. There are some neurosensory and neurosecretory regions of the brain that lack the barrier: posterior pituitary, median eminence, area postrema, subfornical organ, subcommissural organ, and laminar terminalis.

The *physical part* of the BBB derives from the distinctive structure of the capillary endothelium in the brain and choroid plexus. Unlike the endothelial cells of peripheral microvasculature that have gaps between them that permit flow of water and small molecules to the interstitial space, endothelial cells in the CNS have tight junctions that limit paracellular flow and generally have very low rates of vesicular transport (transcytosis) compared to peripheral endothelium. Moreover, CNS endothelium is wrapped by basement membrane, pericytes, and the pseudopodial processes of astroglia. Lipophilic molecules and gases such as O_2 and CO_2 can readily diffuse across these layers from blood to brain. Hydrophilic molecules (nutrients, ions, charged molecules, many drugs) cannot cross these multiple membrane barriers by diffusion at sufficient rates.

Thus, the system relies on *selective permeability*. For instance, there are transport systems: for ions; for nutrients, many in the SLC family of transport proteins, such as SLC2A1/GLUT1 (glucose), SLC7A1

and SLC7A5/LAT1 (amino acids); for nucleosides; and for metabolic by-products such as lactate and pyruvate (SLC16A1). Members of the SLC22 family (OAT1 and OAT3) play a role in the efflux of xenobiotics from CSF to plasma. There are receptor-mediated transport systems for ferritin and insulin, and there is a low level of transcytosis (caveolin-dependent vesicle trafficking). The endothelial membranes also express exporters that basically prevent molecules such as drugs from crossing the endothelium. There are transporters such as Pgp (ABCB1/MDR1), the well-characterized efflux transporter that extrudes its substrates across the luminal membrane of the brain capillary endothelial cells into the blood, thereby limiting penetration into the brain. There is accumulating evidence for similar roles of BCRP and MRP4. The physiological compounds that need to cross the BBB are able to cross.

There is a *metabolic barrier* for some compounds. For instance, circulating catecholamines are inactivated by MAO in the endothelial cells and endothelial MAO and dopa decarboxylase (aromatic amino acid decarboxylase; see Chapter 8) metabolizes L-dopa to 3,4-dihydroxyphenylacetate (hence the necessity of including a dopa decarboxylase inhibitor when giving L-dopa to treat Parkinson disease). The metabolic barrier enzyme γ-glutamyl transpeptidase cleaves the leukotriene mediator produced by the 5-lipoxygenase pathway, LTC_4, and other glutathione adducts.

What about drug molecules? Once they reach the systemic circulation, delivery to the general region of the brain is not a problem: The brain receives about 15% of cardiac output (see Table 2–2). What about crossing the BBB? Small drugs can diffuse across the BBB as a function of their lipid solubility (oil/water partition coefficient). Thus, anesthetics such as nitrous oxide and thiopental move readily across the BBB. Some drugs may resemble substrates that are transported into the brain (e.g., amino acids, nucleosides) and thereby gain entry. LAT1 (SLC7A5) is involved in the influx of several drugs, such as L-dopa and gabapentin across the BBB. OAT1 and OAT3, which generally play a role in the efflux of drugs from the CSF, mediate the uptake of organic compounds such as β-lactam antibiotics, statins, and H_2 receptor antagonists. Charged and large drugs, on the other hand, generally do not penetrate so easily into the brain. The transport proteins, especially MDR1, BCRP, and MRP4, actively extrude many drugs; clearly, recognition by these transporters is a major disadvantage for a drug used to treat CNS disease.

There are methods of permeation under development: nanoparticles and liposomes containing drugs, drugs adducted to ferritin, and development of drug forms with suitable lipophilicity. Basic biomedical research is advancing our understanding of the role of nuclear receptors in the regulation of drug transporters in the BBB (Chan et al., 2013) and of the development of the BBB and the interaction of its cellular and subcellular components to maintain barrier function (Daneman and Prat, 2015). Kim and Bynoe (2015) reported that activation of the adenosine A_{2A} receptor in an in vitro human brain endothelial barrier model permeabilized the barrier sufficiently to permit passage of T cells and the chemotherapeutic agent gemcitabine. Such studies and techniques may provide progress in putting the control of BBB permeability into the hands of physicians.

The Extended Clearance Concept and Physiologically Based Pharmacokinetic (PBPK) Modeling

Based on the "extended clearance concept," hepatic clearance consists of some intrinsic processes, such as hepatic uptake PS_1, backflux from hepatocytes to blood PS_2, hepatic metabolism CL_{met}, and biliary sequestration PS_3 (Figure 5–12) (Shitara et al., 2006, 2013).

The overall hepatic intrinsic clearance $CL_{int,all}$ is expressed as

$$CL_{int,all} = PS_1 \cdot \frac{CL_{met} + PS_3}{PS_2 + CL_{met} + PS_3} \qquad \text{(Equation 5–6)}$$

If the sum of the intrinsic clearance of metabolism and biliary sequestration is much larger than the backflux clearance ($PS_2 << (CL_{met} + PS_3)$),

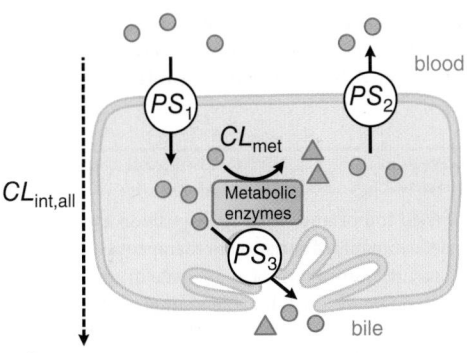

Figure 5–12 *Extended clearance concept: hepatic uptake, backflux into blood, metabolism, and efflux into bile.* The red circles represent parent drugs; the green triangles represent drug metabolites.

$CL_{int,all}$ approximates PS_1, and uptake is a rate-determining process of the overall hepatic intrinsic clearance. In general, many transporter substrates are efficiently excreted into bile or extensively metabolized rather than fluxed back into blood, so their uptake clearances often determine their overall intrinsic hepatic clearance. Assuming that an orally administered drug is completely absorbed from the small intestine and predominantly cleared by the liver, its blood AUC based on the "well-stirred model" can be described as

$$AUC_{blood} = \frac{Dose}{f_B \cdot CL_{int,all}} = \frac{Dose}{f_B \cdot PS_1 \cdot \dfrac{CL_{met} + PS_3}{PS_2 + CL_{met} + PS_3}} \qquad \text{(Equation 5–7)}$$

where f_B represents the unbound fraction in blood.

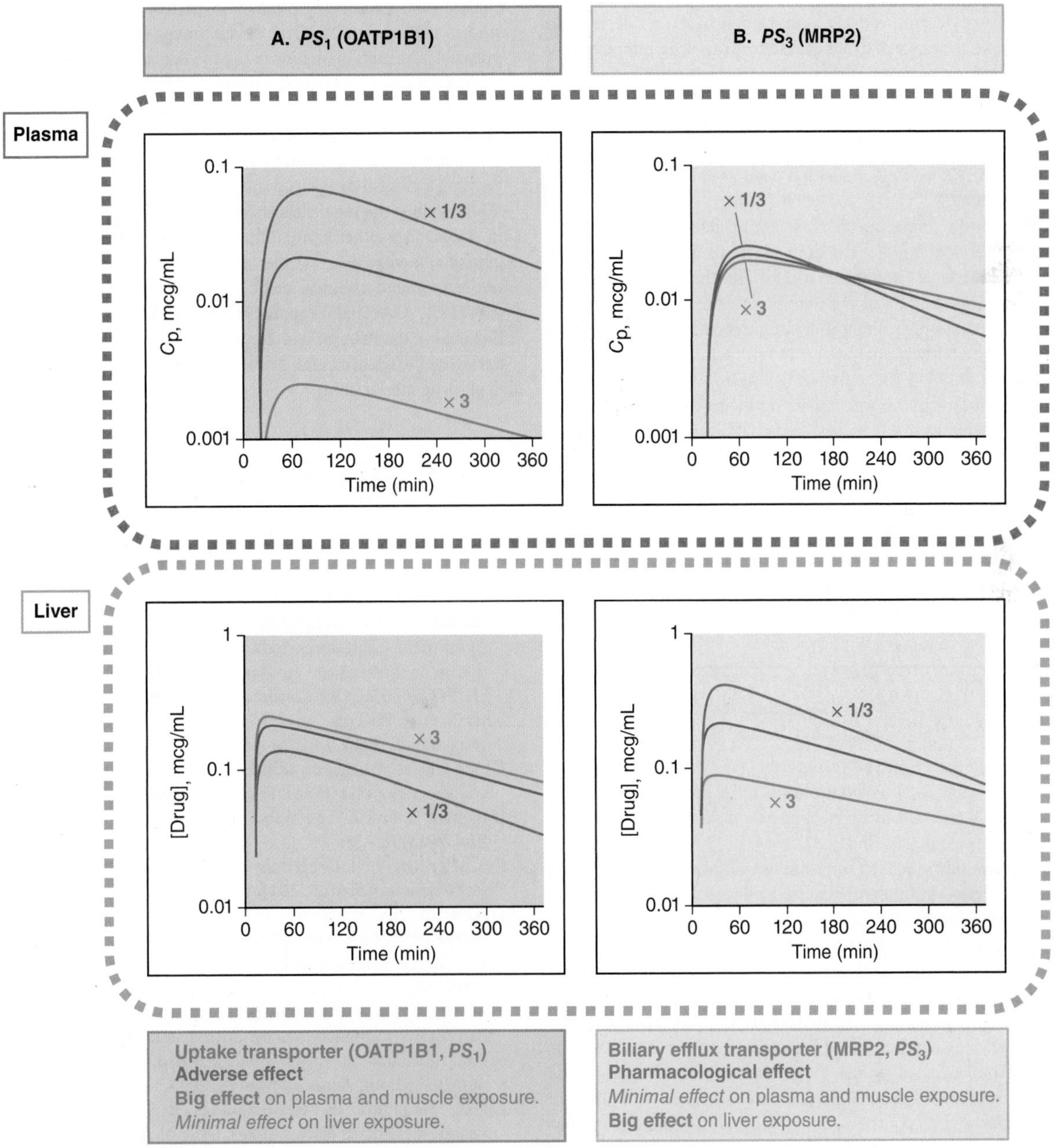

A. PS₁ (OATP1B1)

B. PS₃ (MRP2)

Plasma

Liver

× 1/3

× 3

× 1/3

× 3

× 3

× 1/3

× 1/3

× 3

Uptake transporter (OATP1B1, PS_1)
Adverse effect
Big effect on plasma and muscle exposure.
Minimal effect on liver exposure.

Biliary efflux transporter (MRP2, PS_3)
Pharmacological effect
Minimal effect on plasma and muscle exposure.
Big effect on liver exposure.

Figure 5–13 *Sensitivity analysis of the effect of functional changes of hepatic uptake clearance* $PS_1(A)$ *and biliary excretion clearance* $PS_3(B)$ *on the plasma and liver concentrations of pravastatin* (Watanabe et al., 2009). These sensitivity analyses were made based on the PBPK model, which connected five sequential liver compartments by blood flow so that this model can be used for drugs exhibiting transporter-mediated high clearance. Plasma and liver concentrations after oral administration (40 mg) were simulated with varying hepatic transport activities over a 1/3- to 3-fold range of the initial values.

The AUC_{liver} is described as (Shitara et al., 2013)

$$AUC_{liver} = \frac{PS_1}{PS_2 + CL_{met} + PS_3} \cdot AUC_{blood}$$

$$= \frac{PS_1}{PS_2 + CL_{met} + PS_3} \cdot \frac{Dose}{f_B \cdot PS_1 \cdot \dfrac{CL_{met} + PS_3}{PS_2 + CL_{met} + PS_3}}$$

$$= \frac{Dose}{f_B \cdot (CL_{met} + PS_3)} \qquad \text{(Equation 5–8)}$$

Equations 5–6 through 5–8 suggest that if the uptake clearance PS_1 is decreased, AUC_{blood} is increased in inverse proportion to PS_1, while AUC_{liver} is not affected. On the other hand, if drug uptake is a rate-determining process of the overall hepatic intrinsic clearance, the decrease in the function of metabolism or biliary sequestration causes the increase in AUC_{liver}, but not AUC_{blood}. Therefore, if the molecular targets of pharmacological effect and adverse effect induced by drugs are located inside and outside hepatocytes, respectively, as in the case of statins, decrease in the hepatic uptake clearance of drugs caused by drug-drug interaction or genetic polymorphism of transporters affect mainly adverse effect and not so much pharmacological effect.

To simulate the impact of variations in the transporter activities on the systemic and liver exposure of a statin, which is eliminated mainly via OATP1B1 and MRP2, a PBPK model has been used (Jamei et al., 2014; Watanabe et al., 2009).

In a PBPK model, compartments representing actual tissues are connected by blood flow to predict the time course of drug disposition in the body. A PBPK model allows deep insight into the factors governing the systemic exposure and tissue distribution of drugs and simulates the impact of variations in physiological or drug-dependent parameters on drug disposition. Sensitivity analyses based on the PBPK model indicate that the variation in OATP1B1 activities will have a minimal impact on the therapeutic efficacy but a large impact on the side effect (myopathy) of pravastatin; the opposite will be true for variations in MRP2 activities: a large impact on efficacy, a small impact on the side effect (Watanabe et al., 2009) (Figure 5–13). Such characteristics have been demonstrated for some statins (e.g., simvastatin and rosuvastatin): Pharmacogenomic variation of OATP1B1 activity is associated with the risk of adverse reactions, whereas variation of biliary excretion and intestinal absorption mechanisms result in variation in therapeutic response (Chasman et al., 2012; SEARCH Collaborative Group, 2008).

Genetic Variation in Membrane Transporters: Implications for Clinical Drug Response

There are inherited defects in SLC transporters (see Table 5–2) and ABC transporters (see Table 5–3). Polymorphisms in membrane transporters play roles in drug response and are yielding new insights in pharmacogenetics and pharmacology (see Chapter 7).

Clinical studies have focused on a limited number of transporters, relating genetic variation in membrane transporters to drug disposition and response. For example, two common SNPs in *SLCO1B1* (OATP1B1) are associated with elevated plasma levels of pravastatin (Niemi et al., 2011), a widely used drug for the treatment of hypercholesterolemia (see Chapter 33). Recent studies using genome-wide association methods show that genetic variants in *SLCO1B1* (OATP1B1) predispose patients to risk for muscle toxicity associated with use of simvastatin as well as altered response to selected statins. Other studies indicate that genetic variants in transporters in the SLC22A family are associated with variation in renal clearance and response to various drugs, including the antidiabetic drug metformin (Chen et al. 2013). Responses to the XOI allopurinol and to rosuvastatin have recently been associated with genetic variants in ABCG2 (BCRP) (Chasman et al., 2012; Wen et al., 2015). For both drugs, a pharmacokinetic mechanism is responsible for the altered pharmacodynamics. Likewise, genetic variants of MRP2 and MRP4 are associated with

drug-related phenotypes (Rungtivasuwan et al., 2015). For example, the disposition of tenofovir, an antiviral agent, has been associated with polymorphisms in both ABCC2 and ABCC4 (MRP2 and MRP4, respectively).

Transporters in Regulatory Sciences

Because of their importance in drug disposition and action, transporters are major determinants of variation in therapeutic and adverse drug reactions. As a result, transporters may mediate drug-drug interactions that result in drug safety issues. A notable example is the interaction between gemfibrozil and cerivastatin. Gemfibrozil glucuronide formed in hepatocytes reduces the hepatic uptake and metabolism of cerivastatin; the result is a high C_p for cerivastatin. Elevated statin levels result in statin-induced myopathies, including rhabdomyolysis, a life-threatening adverse effect. This interaction resulted in the removal of cerivastatin from the market because of deaths due to rhabdomyolysis. The U.S. FDA has issued a draft clinical pharmacology guidance on performing drug-drug interaction studies during clinical drug development (FDA, 2012). The guidance presents information on how to use in vitro data for transporter studies to make decisions about whether to conduct a clinical drug-drug interaction study. For example, if a new molecular entity (NME) inhibits the in vitro uptake of a canonical substrate of OCT2 at clinically relevant (unbound) concentrations, the guidance recommends that the sponsor consider performing a clinical drug-drug interaction study to determine whether the NME inhibits the renal clearance of an OCT2 substrate (e.g., metformin) in vivo. On the other hand, if the NME does not inhibit OCT2-mediated uptake in in vitro assays at therapeutic concentrations, the guidance does not recommend a clinical study. Although only a handful of transporters (OATP1B1, OATP1B3, Pgp, BCRP, OCT2, MATE1, OAT1, and OAT3) are included in the FDA guidance, an increasing number of studies are being performed to identify and characterize transporters that mediate clinical drug-drug interactions.

Bibliography

Aceti A, et al. Pharmacogenetics as a tool to tailor antiretroviral therapy: a review. *World J Virol*, **2015**, 4:198–208.

Chan GN, et al. Role of nuclear receptors in the regulation of drug transporters in the brain. *Trends Pharmacol Sci*, **2013**, 34:361–372.

Chasman DI, et al. Genetic determinants of statin-induced low-density lipoprotein cholesterol reduction: the Justification for the Use of Statins in Prevention: an Intervention Trial Evaluating Rosuvastatin (JUPITER) trial. *Circ Cardiovasc Genet*, **2012**, 5:257–264.

Chen S, et al. Pharmacogenetic variation and metformin response. *Curr Drug Metab*, **2013**, 14:1070–1082.

Cropp CD, et al. Organic anion transporter 2 (SLC22A7) is a facilitative transporter of cGMP. *Mol Pharmacol*, **2008**, 73:1151–1158.

Daneman R, Prat A. The blood-brain barrier. *Cold Spring Harb Perspect Biol*, **2015**, 7:1–23.

DeCorter MK, et al. Drug transporters in drug efficacy and toxicity. *Ann Rev Pharmacol Toxicol*, **2012**, 52:249–273.

Dykens JA, et al. Biguanide-induced mitochondrial dysfunction yields increased lactate production and cytotoxicity of aerobically-poised HepG2 cells and human hepatocytes in vitro. *Toxicol Appl Pharmacol*, **2008**, 233:203–210.

FDA. Draft guidance for industry: drug interaction studies—study design, data analysis, implications for dosing, and labeling recommendations, 2012. Available at: http://www.fda.gov/downloads/Drugs/Guidances/ucm292362.pdf. Accessed May 29, **2017**.

Gu X, Manautou JE. Regulation of hepatic ABC transporters by xenobiotics and in disease states. *Drug Metab Rev*, **2010**, 42:482–538.

Guo GL, Zhou H-P. Bile acids and nuclear receptors in the digestive system and therapy. *Acta Pharm Sin B*, **2015**, 5:89–168.

Harrach S, Ciarimboli G. Role of transporters in the distribution of platinum-based drugs. *Front Pharmacol*, **2015**, 6:85. doi:10.3389/fphar.2015.00085

He S-M, et al. Structural and functional properties of human multidrug resistance protein 1 (MRP1/ABCC1). *Curr Med Chem*, **2011**, *18*:439–481.

Hediger MA, et al. The ABCs of membrane transporters in health and disease (SLC series): introduction. *Mol Aspects Med*, **2013**, *34*:95–107.

Horikawa M, et al. The potential for an interaction between MRP2 (ABCC2) and various therapeutic agents: probenecid as a candidate inhibitor of the biliary excretion of irinotecan metabolites. *Drug Metab Pharmacokinet*, **2002**, *17*:23–33.

Imai S, et al. Analysis of DNA methylation and histone modification profiles of liver-specific transporters. *Mol Pharmacol*, **2009**, *75*:568–576.

Ishiguro N, et al. Predominant contribution of OATP1B3 to the hepatic uptake of telmisartan, an angiotensin II receptor antagonist, in humans. *Drug Metab Dispos*, **2006**, *34*:1109–1115.

Jamei M, et al. A mechanistic framework for in vitro–in vivo extrapolation of liver membrane transporters: prediction of drug–drug interaction between rosuvastatin and cyclosporine. *Clin Pharmacokinet*, **2014**, *53*:73–87.

Kim DG, Bynoe MS. A2A adenosine receptor regulates the human blood-brain barrier permeability. *Mol Neurobiol*, **2015**, *52*:664–678.

Lin L, et al. SLC transporters as therapeutic targets: emerging opportunities. *Nat Rev Drug Discov*, **2015**, *14*:543–560.

Madsen KK et al. Selective GABA transporter inhibitors Tiagabine and EF1502 exhibit mechanistic differences in their ability to modulate the ataxia and anticonvulsant action of the extrasynaptic GABAA receptor agonist Gaboxadol. *J Pharmacol Exp Therap*, **2011**, *338*:214–219.

Meyer zu Schwabedissen HE, et al. Function-impairing polymorphisms of the hepatic uptake transporter SLCO1B1 modify the therapeutic efficacy of statins in a population-based cohort. *Pharmacogenet Genomics*, **2015**, *25*:8–18.

Niemi M, et al. Organic anion transporting polypeptide 1B1: a genetically polymorphic transporter of major importance for hepatic drug uptake. *Pharmacol Rev*, **2011**, *63*:157–181.

Niemi M, et al. Polymorphic organic anion transporting polypeptide 1B1 is a major determinant of repaglinide pharmacokinetics. *Clin Pharmacol Ther*, **2005**, *77*:468–478.

Nigam S. What do drug transporters really do? *Nat Drug Discov*, **2015**, *14*:29–44.

Nigam S, et al. The organic anion transporter (OAT) family: a systems biology perspective. *Physiol Rev*, **2015**, *95*:83–123.

Rungtivasuwan K, et al. Influence of ABCC2 and ABCC4 polymorphisms on tenofovir plasma concentrations in Thai HIV-infected patients. *Antimicrob Agents Chemother*, **2015**, *59*:3240–3245.

SEARCH Collaborative Group. SLCO1B1 variants and statin-induced myopathy—a genomewide study. *N Engl J Med*, **2008**, *359*:789–799.

Shitara Y, et al. Transporters as a determinant of drug clearance and tissue distribution. *Eur J Pharm Sci*, **2006**, *27*:425–446.

Shitara Y, et al. Clinical significance of organic anion transporting polypeptides (OATPs) in drug disposition: their roles in hepatic clearance and intestinal absorption. *Biopharm Drug Dispos*, **2013**, *34*:45–78.

Srimaroeng C, et al. Physiology, structure, and regulation of the cloned organic anion transporters. *Xenobiotica*, **2008**, *38*:889–935.

Smith RP, et al. Genome-wide discovery of drug-dependent human liver regulatory elements. *PLoS Genet*, **2014**, *10*:e1004648.

Tamai I. Pharmacological and pathophysiological roles of carnitine/organic cation transporters (OCTNs: SLC22A4, SLC22A5 and Slc22a21). *Biopharm Drug Dispos*, **2013**, *34*:29–44.

Toyoda Y, et al. MRP class of human ATP binding cassette (ABC) transporters: historical background and new research directions. *Xenobiotica*, **2008**, *38*:833–862.

Urquhart BL, et al. Nuclear receptors and the regulation of drug-metabolizing enzymes and drug transporters: implications for interindividual variability in response to drugs. *J Clin Pharmacol*, **2007**, *47*:566–578.

Wang DS, et al. Involvement of organic cation transporter 1 in the lactic acidosis caused by metformin. *Mol Pharmacol*, **2003**, *63*:844–848.

Watanabe T, et al. Physiologically based pharmacokinetic modeling to predict transporter-mediated clearance and distribution of pravastatin in humans. *J Pharmacol Exp Ther*, **2009**, *328*:652–662.

Wen CC, et al. Genome-wide association study identifies ABCG2 (BCRP) as an allopurinol transporter and a determinant of drug response. *Clin Pharmacol Ther*, **2015**, *97*:518–525.

Zhang S, et al. Organic cation transporters are determinants of oxaliplatin cytotoxicity. *Cancer Res*, **2006a**, *66*:8847–8857.

Zhang W, et al. Effect of SLCO1B1 genetic polymorphism on the pharmacokinetics of nateglinide. *Br J Clin Pharmacol*, **2006b**, *62*:567–572.

Chapter 6

Drug Metabolism

Frank J. Gonzalez, Michael Coughtrie, and Robert H. Tukey

Coping With Xenobiotics

Humans come into contact with thousands of foreign chemicals or xenobiotics (substances foreign to the body) through diet and exposure to environmental contaminants. Fortunately, humans have developed a means to rapidly eliminate xenobiotics so that they do not accumulate in the tissues and cause harm. Plants are a common source of dietary xenobiotics, providing many structurally diverse chemicals, some of which are associated with pigment production and others that are actually toxins (called *phytoalexins*) that protect plants against predators. Poisonous mushrooms are a common example: They have many toxins that are lethal to mammals, including amanitin, gyromitrin, orellanine, muscarine, ibotenic acid, muscimol, psilocybin, and coprine. Animals must be able to metabolize and eliminate such chemicals to consume vegetation. While humans can now choose their dietary sources, a typical animal does not have this luxury and as a result is subject to its environment and the vegetation that exists in that environment. Thus, the ability to metabolize unusual chemicals in plants and other food sources is critical for adaptation to a changing environment and ultimately the survival of animals.

Enzymes that metabolize xenobiotics have historically been called drug-metabolizing enzymes; however, these enzymes are involved in the metabolism of many foreign chemicals to which humans are exposed and are more appropriately called *xenobiotic-metabolizing enzymes*. Myriad diverse enzymes have evolved in animals to metabolize foreign chemicals. Dietary differences among species during the course of evolution could account for the marked species variation in the complexity of the xenobiotic-metabolizing enzymes. Additional diversity within these enzyme systems has also derived from the necessity to "detoxify" a host of endogenous chemicals that would otherwise prove harmful to the organism, such as bilirubin, steroid hormones, and catecholamines. Many of these endogenous biochemicals are detoxified by the same or closely related xenobiotic-metabolizing enzymes.

Drugs are xenobiotics, and the capacity to metabolize and clear drugs involves the same enzymatic pathways and transport systems that are used for normal metabolism of dietary constituents. Indeed, many drugs are derived from chemicals found in plants, some of which have been used in Chinese herbal medicines for thousands of years. Of the prescription drugs in use today for cancer treatment, some are also derived from plants

(see Chapter 68); investigating folkloric claims led to the discovery of most of these drugs. The capacity to metabolize xenobiotics, although largely beneficial, has made development of drugs more time consuming and costly due in part to:

- species differences in expression of enzymes that metabolize drugs and thereby limit the utility of animal models to predict drug effects in humans
- interindividual variations in the capacity of humans to metabolize drugs
- drug-drug interactions involving xenobiotic metabolizing enzymes
- metabolic activation of chemicals to toxic and carcinogenic derivatives

Today, most xenobiotics to which humans are exposed come from sources that include environmental pollution, food additives, cosmetic products, agrochemicals, processed foods, and drugs.

In general, most xenobiotics are lipophilic chemicals; in the absence of metabolism, these would not be efficiently eliminated and thus would accumulate in the body, potentially resulting in toxicity. With few exceptions, all xenobiotics are subjected to one or multiple enzymatic pathways that constitute *phase 1 oxidation* and *phase 2 conjugation*. As a general paradigm, metabolism serves to convert these hydrophobic chemicals into more hydrophilic derivatives that can easily be eliminated from the body through the urine or the bile.

To enter cells and reach their sites of action, drugs generally must possess physical properties that allow them to move down a concentration gradient and across cell membranes. Many drugs are hydrophobic, a property that allows entry via diffusion across lipid bilayers into the systemic circulation and then into cells. With some compounds, transporters on the plasma membrane facilitate entry (see Chapter 5). This property of hydrophobicity renders drugs difficult to eliminate because, in the absence of metabolism, they accumulate in fat and cellular phospholipid bilayers. The xenobiotic-metabolizing enzymes convert drugs and other xenobiotics into derivatives that are more hydrophilic and thus easily eliminated via excretion into the aqueous compartments of the tissues and ultimately into the urine.

Metabolism of a drug can begin even before a drug is absorbed: Gut bacteria represent the first metabolic interface between orally administered drugs and the body. The microbiome of the GI tract can metabolize xenobiotics; interindividual differences in composition of the gut

Abbreviations

ADR: adverse drug reaction
AUC: area under the plasma concentration–time curve
AZA: azathioprine
CAR: constitutive androstane receptor
CES2: carboxylesterase 2
COMT: catechol-*O*-methyltransferase
CPT-11: irinotecan
CYP: cytochrome P450
DPYD: dihydropyrimidine dehydrogenase
EH: epoxide hydrolase
FMO: flavin-containing monooxygenase
GI: gastrointestinal
GSH and GSSG: reduced and oxidized glutathione
GST: glutathione-*S*-transferase
HGPRT: hypoxanthine guanine phosphoribosyl transferase
HIF: hypoxia-inducible factor
HIV: human immunodeficiency virus
HNMT: histamine *N*-methyltransferase
HPPH: 5-(-4-hydroxyphenyl)-5-phenylhydantoin
INH: isonicotinic acid hydrazide (isoniazid)
MAO: monoamine oxidase
MAPK: mitogen-activated protein kinase
mEH: microsomal epoxide hydrolase
6-MP: 6-mercaptopurine
MRP: multidrug resistance protein
MT: methyltransferase
NADPH: nicotinamide adenine dinucleotide phosphate
NAPQI: *N*-acetyl-*p*-benzoquinone imine
NAT: *N*-acetyltransferase
NNMT: nicotinamide *N*-methyltransferase
PAPS: 3′-phosphoadenosine-5′-phosphosulfate
Per: Period
Pgp: P-glycoprotein
PNMT: phenylethanolamine *N*-methyltransferase
POMT: phenol-*O*-methyltransferase
PPAR: peroxisome proliferator–activated receptor
PXR: pregnane X receptor
RXR: retinoid X receptor
SAM: *S*-adenosyl-methionine
sEH: soluble epoxide hydrolase
SULT: sulfotransferase
TBP: TATA box–binding protein
6-TGN: 6-thioguanine nucleotide
TMA: trimethylamine
TPMT: thiopurine methyltransferase
TPT: thiol methyltransferase
UDP-GA: uridine diphosphate–glucuronic acid
UGT: uridine diphosphate–glucuronosyltransferase

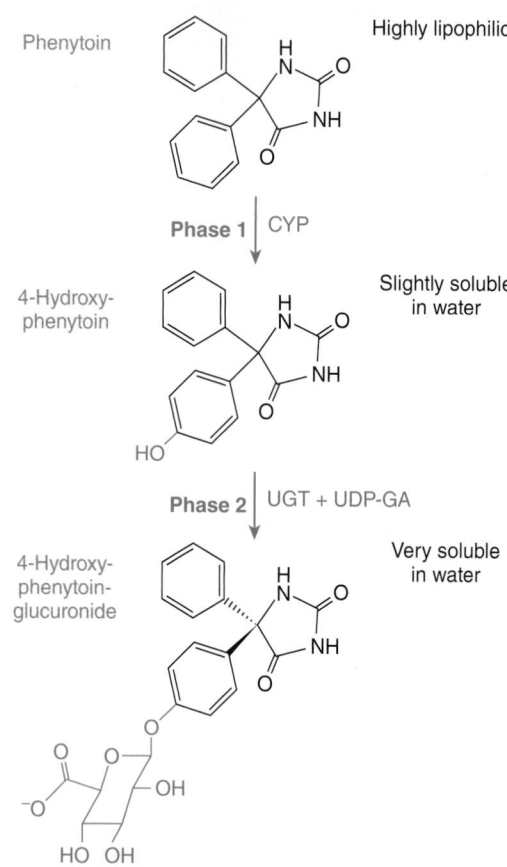

Figure 6–1 *Metabolism of phenytoin.* In phase 1, CYP facilitates 4-hydroxylation of phenytoin to yield HPPH. In phase 2, the hydroxy group serves as a substrate for UGT, which conjugates a molecule of glucuronic acid using UDP-GA as a cofactor. Together, phase 1 and phase 2 reactions convert a very hydrophobic molecule to a larger hydrophilic derivative that is eliminated via the bile.

flora could influence drug action and contribute to differences in drug response. Indeed, diurnal oscillations in GI bacteria and their metabolic capacity, superposed on host clock gene oscillations, appear to affect drug disposition and effect (FitzGerald et al., 2015).

The process of drug metabolism that leads to elimination also plays a major role in diminishing the biological activity of a drug. For example, *(S)-phenytoin*, an anticonvulsant used in the treatment of epilepsy, is virtually insoluble in water. Metabolism by the phase 1 CYPs followed by phase 2 UGT enzymes produces a metabolite that is highly water soluble and readily eliminated from the body (Figure 6–1). Metabolism also terminates the biological activity of the drug. Because conjugates are generally hydrophilic, elimination via the bile or urine is dependent on the

actions of many efflux transporters to facilitate transmembrane passage (see Chapter 5).

While xenobiotic-metabolizing enzymes facilitate the elimination of chemicals from the body, paradoxically these same enzymes can also convert certain chemicals to highly reactive, toxic, and carcinogenic metabolites. This occurs when an unstable intermediate is formed that has reactivity toward other compounds found in the cell. Chemicals that can be converted by xenobiotic metabolism to cancer-causing derivatives are called carcinogens. Depending on the structure of the chemical substrate, xenobiotic-metabolizing enzymes can produce electrophilic metabolites that react with nucleophilic cellular macromolecules such as DNA, RNA, and protein. This can cause cell death and organ toxicity. Most drugs and other xenobiotics that cause hepatotoxicity damage mitochondria and lead to hepatocyte death. Reaction of these electrophiles with DNA can sometimes result in cancer through the mutation of genes, such as oncogenes or tumor suppressor genes. It is generally believed that most human cancers are due to exposure to chemical carcinogens.

This potential for carcinogenic activity makes testing the safety of drug candidates of vital importance. Testing for cancer-causing potential is particularly critical for drugs that will be used for the treatment of chronic diseases. Because each species has evolved a unique combination of xenobiotic-metabolizing enzymes, nonprimate models (mostly rodents) cannot be solely used for testing the safety of new drug candidates targeted for human diseases. Nevertheless, testing in rodent models (e.g., mice and rats) can usually identify potential carcinogens. Fortunately, there are no instances of drugs that test negative in rodents but cause cancer in humans, albeit some rodent carcinogens are not associated with human cancer. However, many cytotoxic cancer drugs have the potential to cause cancer; this risk is minimized by their acute, rather than chronic, use in cancer therapy.

The Phases of Drug Metabolism

Xenobiotic-metabolizing enzymes have historically been categorized as

- *phase 1 reactions*, which include oxidation, reduction, or hydrolytic reactions; or
- *phase 2 reactions*, in which enzymes catalyze the conjugation of the substrate (the phase 1 product) with a second molecule.

The *phase 1 enzymes* lead to the introduction of what are called functional groups, such as –OH, –COOH, –SH, –O–, or NH_2 (Table 6-1). The addition of functional groups does little to increase the water solubility of the drug but can dramatically alter the biological properties of the drug. Reactions carried out by phase 1 enzymes usually lead to the inactivation of a drug. However, in certain instances, metabolism, usually the hydrolysis of an ester or amide linkage, results in bioactivation of a drug. Inactive drugs that undergo metabolism to an active drug are called prodrugs (Huttenen et al., 2011). Examples of prodrugs bioactivated by CYPs are the antitumor drug *cyclophosphamide*, which is bioactivated to a cell-killing electrophilic derivative (see Chapter 66), and the anti-thrombotic agent clopidogrel, which activated to 2-oxo-clopidogrel, which is further metabolized to an irreversible inhibitor of platelet ADP P2Y12 receptors. *Phase 2 enzymes* produce a metabolite with improved water solubility and thereby facilitate the elimination of the drug from the tissue, normally via efflux transporters described in Chapter 5. Thus, in general, phase 1 reactions result in biological inactivation of a drug, and phase 2 reactions facilitate the drug elimination and the inactivation of electrophilic and potentially toxic metabolites produced by oxidation.

Superfamilies of evolutionarily related enzymes and receptors are common in the mammalian genome; the enzyme systems responsible for drug metabolism are good examples. The phase 1 oxidation reactions are carried out by CYPs, FMOs, and EHs. The CYPs and FMOs are composed of superfamilies of enzymes. Each superfamily contains multiple genes. The phase 2 enzymes include several superfamilies of conjugating enzymes. Among the more important are the GSTs, UGTs, SULTs, NATs, and MTs (Table 6-1).

These conjugation reactions usually require the substrate to have oxygen (hydroxyl or epoxide groups), nitrogen, and sulfur atoms that serve as acceptor sites for a hydrophilic moiety, such as glutathione, glucuronic acid, sulfate, or an acetyl group, that is covalently conjugated to an acceptor site on the molecule. Examine the phase 1 and phase 2 metabolism of phenytoin (Figure 6-1). The oxidation by phase 1 enzymes either adds or exposes a functional group, permitting the products of phase 1 metabolism to serve as substrates for the phase 2 conjugating or synthetic enzymes. In the case of the UGTs, glucuronic acid is delivered to the functional group, forming a glucuronide metabolite that is more water soluble and is targeted for excretion in the urine or bile. When the substrate is a drug, these reactions usually convert the original drug to a form that is not able to bind to its target receptor, thus attenuating the biological response to the drug.

Sites of Drug Metabolism

Xenobiotic-metabolizing enzymes are found in most tissues in the body, with the highest levels located in the GI tract (liver, small and large intestines). The small intestine plays a crucial role in drug metabolism. Orally administered drugs first are exposed to the GI flora, which can metabolize some drugs. During absorption, drugs are exposed to xenobiotic-metabolizing enzymes in the epithelial cells of the GI tract; this is the initial site of drug metabolism. Once absorbed, drugs enter the portal circulation and are taken to the liver, where they can be extensively metabolized (the "first-pass effect"). The liver is the major "metabolic clearinghouse" for both endogenous chemicals (e.g., cholesterol, steroid hormones, fatty acids, and proteins) and xenobiotics. While a portion of active drug escapes metabolism in the GI tract and liver, subsequent passes through the liver result in more metabolism of the parent drug until the agent is eliminated. Thus, drugs that are poorly metabolized remain in the body for longer periods of time, and their pharmacokinetic profiles show much longer elimination half-lives than drugs that are rapidly metabolized.

During drug development, compounds are sought that have a favorable pharmacokinetic profile in which they are eliminated over the course of 24 h after administration. This allows the use of daily single dosing. If a compound with a favorable efficacy cannot be modified to improve its pharmacokinetic profile, twice-a-day or even three times-a-day dosing needs to be used. Other organs that contain significant xenobiotic-metabolizing enzymes include tissues of the nasal mucosa and lung, which play important roles in the metabolism of drugs that are administered through aerosol sprays. These tissues are also the first line of contact with hazardous chemicals that are airborne.

Within the cell, xenobiotic-metabolizing enzymes are found in the intracellular membranes and in the cytosol. The phase 1 CYPs, FMOs, and EHs and some phase 2 conjugating enzymes, notably the UGTs, are all located in the endoplasmic reticulum (ER) of the cell (Figure 6-2). The endoplasmic reticulum consists of phospholipid bilayers organized as tubes and sheets throughout the cytoplasm. This network has an inner lumen that is physically distinct from the rest of the cytosolic components of the cell and has connections to the plasma membrane and nuclear envelope. This membrane localization is ideally suited for the metabolic function of these enzymes: Hydrophobic molecules enter the cell and become embedded in the lipid bilayer, where they come into direct contact with the phase 1 enzymes. Once subjected to oxidation, drugs can be directly conjugated by the UGTs (in the lumen of the endoplasmic reticulum) or by the cytosolic transferases, such as GST and SULT. Glucuronide conjugates must be transported out of the endoplasmic reticulum. The metabolites are transported across the plasma membrane and into the bloodstream, then conveyed to the liver and into the bile through the bile canaliculus, from which they are deposited in the gut (see Figure 5-9).

TABLE 6-1 ■ XENOBIOTIC-METABOLIZING ENZYMES

ENZYMES	REACTIONS
Phase 1 enzymes (CYPs, FMOs, EHs)	
Cytochrome P450s (P450 or CYP)	C and O oxidation, dealkylation, others
Flavin-containing monooxygenases (FMOs)	N, S, and P oxidation
Epoxide hydrolases (EHs)	Hydrolysis of epoxides
Phase 2 "transferases"	
Sulfotransferases (SULT)	Addition of sulfate
UDP-glucuronosyltransferases (UGTs)	Addition of glucuronic acid
Glutathione-*S*-transferases (GSTs)	Addition of glutathione
N-Acetyltransferases (NATs)	Addition of acetyl group
Methyltransferases (MTs)	Addition of methyl group
Other enzymes	
Alcohol dehydrogenases	Reduction of alcohols
Aldehyde dehydrogenases	Reduction of aldehydes
NADPH-quinone oxidoreductase (NQO)	Reduction of quinones

mEH and sEH, microsomal and soluble epoxide hydrolase, respectively; NADPH, reduced nicotinamide adenine dinucleotide phosphate; UDP, uridine diphosphate.

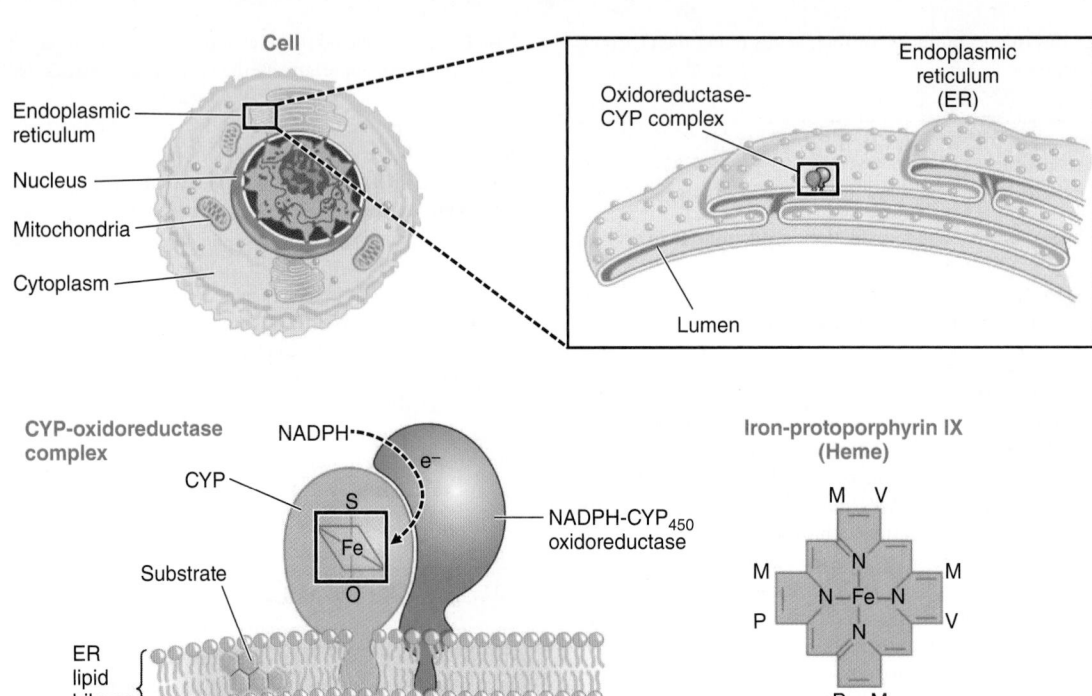

Figure 6–2 *Location of CYPs in the cell.* Increasingly microscopic levels of detail are shown, sequentially expanding the areas within the black boxes. CYPs are embedded in the phospholipid bilayer of the ER. Most of the enzyme is located on the cytosolic surface of the ER. A second enzyme, NADPH-CYP oxidoreductase, transfers electrons to the CYP where it can, in the presence of O_2, oxidize xenobiotic substrates, many of which are hydrophobic and dissolved in the ER. A single NADPH-CYP oxidoreductase species transfers electrons to all CYP isoforms in the ER. Each CYP contains a molecule of iron-protoporphyrin IX that functions to bind and activate O_2. Substituents on the porphyrin ring are methyl (M), propionyl (P), and vinyl (V) groups.

Phase 1 Reactions

CYPs: The Cytochrome P450 Superfamily

The CYPs are a superfamily of enzymes, each of which contains a molecule of heme bound noncovalently to the polypeptide chain (Figure 6–2). Many enzymes that use O_2 as a substrate for their reactions contain heme, and heme is the oxygen-binding moiety in hemoglobin. Heme contains one atom of iron in a hydrocarbon cage that functions to bind O_2 in the active site of the CYP as part of the catalytic cycle of these enzymes. CYPs use O_2, plus H^+ derived from the cofactor-reduced NADPH, to carry out the oxidation of substrates. The H^+ is supplied through the enzyme NADPH-CYP oxidoreductase. Metabolism of a substrate by a CYP consumes one molecule of O_2 and produces an oxidized substrate and a molecule of H_2O as a by-product. However, for most CYPs, depending on the nature of the substrate, the reaction is "uncoupled," consuming more O_2 than substrate metabolized and producing what is called activated oxygen or O_2^-. The O_2^- is usually converted to water by the enzyme superoxide dismutase. When elevated, O_2^-, also called a reactive oxygen species (ROS), can cause oxidative stress that is detrimental to cellular physiology and is associated with diseases such as hepatic cirrhosis.

Among the diverse reactions carried out by mammalian CYPs are *N*-dealkylation, *O*-dealkylation, aromatic hydroxylation, *N*-oxidation, *S*-oxidation, deamination, and dehalogenation (Table 6–2). More than 50 individual CYPs have been identified in humans. As a family of enzymes, CYPs are involved in the metabolism of dietary and xenobiotic chemicals, as well as the synthesis of endogenous compounds such as steroids and fatty acid signaling molecules such as epoxyeicosatrienoic acids. CYPs also participate in the production of bile acids from cholesterol.

In contrast to the drug-metabolizing CYPs, the CYPs that catalyze steroid and bile acid synthesis have specific substrate preferences. For example, the CYP that produces estrogen from testosterone, CYP19 or aromatase, can metabolize only testosterone or androstenedione and does not metabolize xenobiotics. Specific inhibitors for aromatase, such as *anastrozole*, have been developed for use in the treatment of estrogen-dependent tumors (see Chapters 44 and 66).

The synthesis of bile acids from cholesterol occurs in the liver, where, subsequent to CYP-catalyzed oxidation, the bile acids are conjugated with amino acids and transported through the bile duct and gallbladder into the small intestine. Bile acids are emulsifiers that facilitate the elimination of conjugated drugs from the liver and the absorption of fatty acids and vitamins from the diet. In this capacity, more than 90% of bile acids are reabsorbed by the gut and transported back to the hepatocytes. Similar to the steroid biosynthetic CYPs, CYPs involved in bile acid production have strict substrate requirements and do not participate in xenobiotic or drug metabolism.

The CYPs that carry out xenobiotic metabolism have a tremendous capacity to metabolize a large number of structurally diverse chemicals. This is due to multiple forms of CYPs and to the capacity of a single CYP to metabolize many structurally distinct chemicals. There is also significant overlapping substrate specificity among CYPs; a single compound may be metabolized, albeit at different rates, by different CYPs. In addition, CYPs can metabolize a single compound at different positions on the molecule. In contrast to enzymes in the body that carry out highly specific reactions in which there is a single substrate and one or more products or two simultaneous substrates, the CYPs are considered promiscuous in their capacity to bind and metabolize multiple substrates (Table 6–2).

This accommodating property, due to large and fluid substrate-binding sites in the CYP, sacrifices metabolic turnover rates: CYPs metabolize substrates at a fraction of the rate of more typical enzymes involved in intermediary metabolism and mitochondrial electron transfer. As a result, drugs generally have half-lives on the order of 3–30 h, while endogenous compounds have half-lives on the order of seconds or minutes (e.g., dopamine and insulin). Even though CYPs have slow catalytic rates, their activities are sufficient to metabolize drugs that are administered at high concentrations in the body.

This unusual feature of extensive overlapping substrate specificities by the CYPs is one of the underlying reasons for the predominance of

TABLE 6–2 ■ MAJOR REACTIONS INVOLVED IN DRUG METABOLISM

	REACTION	EXAMPLES
I. Oxidative reactions		
N-Dealkylation		Imipramine, diazepam, codeine, erythromycin, morphine, tamoxifen, theophylline, caffeine
O-Dealkylation		Codeine, indomethacin, dextromethorphan
Aliphatic hydroxylation		Tolbutamide, ibuprofen, phenobarbital, meprobamate, cyclosporine, midazolam
Aromatic hydroxylation		Phenytoin, phenobarbital, propanolol, ethinyl estradiol, amphetamine, warfarin
N-Oxidation		Chlorpheniramine, dapsone, meperidine
S-Oxidation		Cimetidine, chlorpromazine, thioridazine omeprazole
Deamination		Diazepam, amphetamine
II. Hydrolysis reactions		
		Carbamazepine (see Figure 6-4)
		Procaine, aspirin, clofibrate, meperidine, enalapril, cocaine
		Lidocaine, procainamide, indomethacin
III. Conjugation reactions		
Glucuronidation		Acetaminophen, morphine, oxazepam, lorazepam
Sulfation	PAPS + HO—R → HO₃S—O—R + PAP	Acetaminophen, steroids, methyldopa
Acetylation		Sulfonamides, isoniazid, dapsone, clonazepam
Methylation*	R—OH + AdoMet → R—O—CH₃ + AdoHomCys	L-dopa, methyldopa, mercaptopurine, captopril
Glutathionylation	GSH + R → R—GSH	Adriamycin, fosfomycin, busulfan

PAPS, 3′-phosphoadenosine-5′ phosphosulfate; PAP, 3′-phosphoadenosine-5′-phosphate; AdoMet, S-adenosylmethionine; AdoHomCys, S-adenosylhomocysteine.
*also for RS-, RN-.

drug-drug interactions. When two coadministered drugs are both metabolized by a single CYP, they compete for binding to the enzyme's active site. This can result in the inhibition of metabolism of one or both of the drugs, leading to elevated plasma levels. If there is a narrow therapeutic index for the drugs, the elevated serum levels may elicit unwanted toxicities. Drug-drug interactions are among the leading causes of ADRs.

The Naming of CYPs

The CYPs, responsible for metabolizing the vast majority of therapeutic drugs, are the most actively studied of the xenobiotic-metabolizing enzymes. CYPs are complex and diverse in their regulation and catalytic activities. Genome sequencing has revealed the existence of 102 putatively functional CYP genes and 88 pseudogenes in the mouse and 57 putatively functional genes and 58 pseudogenes in humans. These genes are grouped, based on amino acid sequence similarity, into a superfamily composed of families and subfamilies with increasing sequence similarity. CYPs are named with the root CYP followed by a number designating the family, a letter denoting the subfamily, and another number designating the CYP form. Thus, CYP3A4 is family 3, subfamily A, and gene number 4.

A Small Number of CYPs Metabolize the Majority of Drugs

A limited number of CYPs (15 in humans) that fall into families 1, 2, and 3 are primarily involved in xenobiotic metabolism. Because a single CYP can metabolize a large number of structurally diverse compounds, these enzymes can collectively metabolize scores of chemicals found in the diet, environment, and pharmaceuticals. In humans, 12 CYPs (CYP1A1, 1A2, 1B1, 2A6, 2B6, 2C8, 2C9, 2C19, 2D6, 2E1, 3A4, and 3A5) are important for metabolism of xenobiotics. The liver contains the greatest abundance of xenobiotic-metabolizing CYPs, thus ensuring efficient first-pass metabolism of drugs. CYPs are also expressed throughout the GI tract and in lower amounts in lung, kidney, and even in the CNS.

The expression of the different CYPs can differ markedly as a result of dietary and environmental exposure to inducers or through interindividual changes resulting from heritable polymorphic differences in gene structure, and tissue-specific expression patterns can affect overall drug metabolism and clearance. The most active CYPs for drug metabolism are those in the CYP2C, CYP2D, and CYP3A subfamilies. CYP3A4, the most abundantly expressed in liver, is involved in the metabolism of over 50% of clinically used drugs (Figure 6-3A). The CYP1A, CYP1B, CYP2A, CYP2B, and CYP2E subfamilies are not significantly involved in the metabolism of therapeutic drugs, but they do catalyze the metabolic activation of many protoxins and procarcinogens to their ultimate reactive metabolites.

There are large differences in levels of expression of each CYP between individuals as assessed by both clinical pharmacologic studies and analysis of expression in human liver samples. This large interindividual variability in CYP expression is due to the presence of genetic polymorphisms and differences in gene regulation (see discussion that follows). Several human CYP genes exhibit polymorphisms, including *CYP2A6*, *CYP2C9*, *CYP2C19*, and *CYP2D6*. Allelic variants have been found in the *CYP1B1* and *CYP3A4* genes, but they are present at low frequencies in humans and appear not to have a major role in interindividual levels of expression of these enzymes. However, homozygous mutations in the *CYP1B1* gene are associated with primary congenital glaucoma.

Drug-Drug Interactions

Differences in the rate of metabolism of a drug can be due to drug interactions. Most commonly, this occurs when two drugs (e.g., a statin and a macrolide antibiotic or antifungal agent) are coadministered and subjected to metabolism by the same enzyme. Because most of these drug-drug interactions are due to CYPs, it thus becomes important to determine the identity of the CYP that metabolizes a particular drug and to avoid coadministering drugs that are metabolized by the same enzyme. Some drugs can also inhibit CYPs independently of being substrates for a CYP. For example, the common antifungal agent *ketoconazole* is a potent inhibitor of CYP3A4 and other CYPs, and coadministration of ketoconazole with the anti-HIV viral protease inhibitors reduces the clearance of the protease inhibitor and increases its plasma concentration and the risk of toxicity.

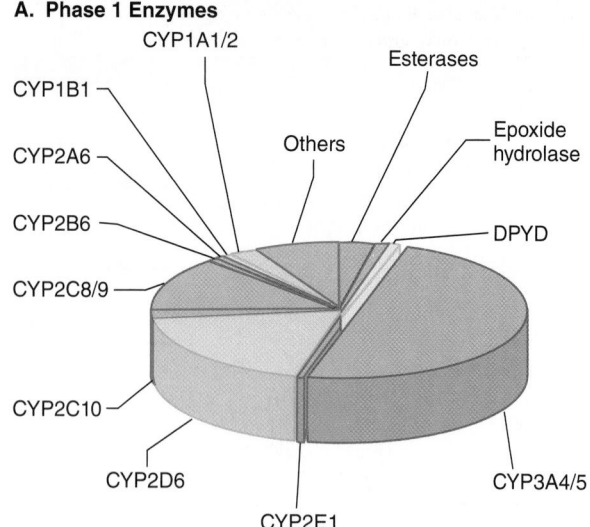

A. Phase 1 Enzymes

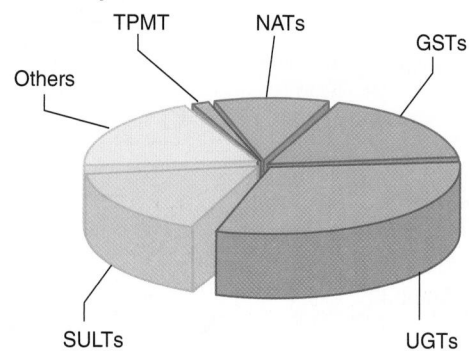

B. Phase 2 Enzymes

Figure 6-3 *The fraction of clinically used drugs metabolized by the major phase 1 and phase 2 enzymes.* The relative size of each pie section represents the estimated percentage of drugs metabolized by the major phase 1 (**A**) and phase 2 (**B**) enzymes, based on studies in the literature. In some cases, more than a single enzyme is responsible for metabolism of a single drug.

Some drugs are CYP inducers that not only can increase their own rates of metabolism but also can induce metabolism of other coadministered drugs (see the following discussion and Figure 6-12). Steroid hormones and herbal products such as St. John's wort can increase hepatic levels of CYP3A4, thereby increasing the metabolism of many orally administered drugs. Drug metabolism can also be influenced by diet. CYP inhibitors and inducers are commonly found in foods, and in some cases these can influence the toxicity and efficacy of a drug. For most drugs, descriptive information found on the package insert lists the CYP that carries out its metabolism and the potential for drug interactions. Components found in grapefruit juice (e.g., naringin, furanocoumarins) are potent inhibitors of CYP3A4, and thus some drug inserts recommend not taking medication with grapefruit juice because it could increase the bioavailability of a drug.

Terfenadine, a once-popular antihistamine, was removed from the market because its metabolism was inhibited by CYP3A4 substrates such as *erythromycin* and grapefruit juice. Terfenadine is actually a prodrug that requires oxidation by CYP3A4 to its active metabolite, and at high doses the parent compound caused arrhythmias. Elevated plasma levels of the parent drug resulting from CYP3A4 inhibition caused ventricular tachycardia in some individuals, which ultimately led to the withdrawal of terfenadine from the market.

Interindividual differences in drug metabolism are significantly influenced by polymorphisms in CYPs. The CYP2D6 polymorphism has led to the withdrawal of several clinically used drugs (e.g., *debrisoquine* and *perhexiline*) and the cautious use of others that are known CYP2D6 substrates (e.g., *encainide* and *flecainide* [antiarrhythmics], *desipramine* and *nortriptyline* [antidepressants], and *codeine*).

Flavin-Containing Monooxygenases

The FMOs are another superfamily of phase 1 enzymes involved in drug metabolism. Similar to CYPs, the FMOs are expressed at high levels in the liver and are bound to the endoplasmic reticulum, a site that favors interaction with and metabolism of hydrophobic drug substrates. There are six families of FMOs, with FMO3 the most abundant in liver. FMO3 is able to metabolize nicotine, as well as H_2-receptor antagonists (*cimetidine* and *ranitidine*), antipsychotics (*clozapine*), and antiemetics (*itopride*). Trimethylamine *N*-oxide (TMAO) occurs in high concentrations, up to 15% by weight, in marine animals, where it acts as an osmotic regulator. In humans, FMO3 normally metabolizes TMAO to TMA, but a genetic deficiency of FMO3 causes the fish-odor syndrome, in which unmetabolized TMAO accumulates in the body and causes a socially offensive fish odor.

FMOs are considered minor contributors to drug metabolism, and they almost always produce benign metabolites. In addition, FMOs are not readily inhibited and are not induced by any of the xenobiotic receptors (see discussion that follows); thus, in contrast to CYPs, FMOs would not be expected to be involved in drug-drug interactions. In fact, this has been demonstrated by comparing the pathways of metabolism of two drugs used in the control of gastric motility: itopride and cisapride. Itopride is metabolized by FMO3; cisapride is metabolized by CYP3A4. As predicted, itopride is less likely to be involved in drug-drug interactions than is cisapride. CYP3A4 participates in drug-drug interactions through induction and inhibition of metabolism, whereas FMO3 is not induced or inhibited by any clinically used drugs. It is possible that FMOs may be important in the development of new drugs. A candidate drug could be designed by introducing a site for FMO oxidation with the knowledge that selected metabolism and pharmacokinetic properties could be accurately calculated for efficient drug-based biological efficacy.

Hydrolytic Enzymes

Two forms of EH carry out hydrolysis of epoxides, most of which are produced by CYPs. The sEH is expressed in the cytosol; mEH is localized to the membrane of the endoplasmic reticulum. Epoxides are highly reactive electrophiles that can bind to cellular nucleophiles found in protein, RNA, and DNA, resulting in cell toxicity and transformation. Thus, EHs participate in the deactivation of potentially toxic metabolites generated by CYPs.

There are a few examples of the influence of mEH on drug metabolism. The antiepileptic drug *carbamazepine* is a prodrug that is converted to its pharmacologically active derivative carbamazepine-10,11-epoxide, by CYP. This metabolite is efficiently hydrolyzed to a dihydrodiol by mEH, resulting in inactivation of the drug (Figure 6–4). Inhibition of mEH can cause an elevation in plasma concentrations of the active metabolite and consequent side effects. The tranquilizer *valnoctamide* and anticonvulsant *valproate* inhibit mEH, resulting in clinically significant drug interactions with carbamazepine. This has led to efforts to develop new antiepileptic drugs, such as *gabapentin* and *levetiracetam*, that are metabolized by CYPs and not by EHs.

In general, the sEH complements the mEH in terms of substrate selectivity, with mEH degrading epoxides on cyclic systems and sEH having a high V_m and low K_m for fatty acid epoxides. Fatty acid epoxides are chemical mediators in the CYP branch of the arachidonic acid cascade. Simplistically, they can be thought of as balancing the generally pro-inflammatory and hypertensive prostaglandins, thromboxanes, and leukotrienes. The epoxides of arachidonic acid and docosahexaenoic acid reduce inflammation, hypertension, and pain but are normally degraded quickly by sEH to vicinal diols that are generally less biologically active (Figure 6–5). Thus, by inhibiting sEH, one can obtain dramatic biological effects. Recent work has focused on pain, where sEH inhibitors reduce both inflammatory and neuropathic pain and synergize with nonsteroidal anti-inflammatory drugs (Kodani and Hammock, 2015). In experimental systems, epoxides of dietary omega-3 and omega-6 fatty acids have anti-inflammatory

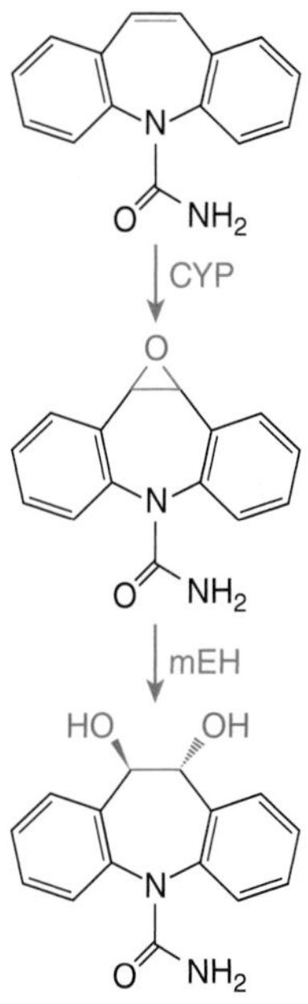

Figure 6–4 *Metabolism of carbamazepine by CYP and mEH.* Carbamazepine is oxidized to the pharmacologically active metabolite carbamazepine-10,11-epoxide by CYP. The epoxide is converted to a trans-dihydrodiol by mEH. This metabolite is biologically inactive and can be conjugated by phase 2 enzymes.

properties, moderating inflammation and autophagy in insulin-sensitive tissues, effects that inhibitors of sEH promote (Lopez-Vicario et al., 2015).

The *carboxylesterases* comprise a superfamily of enzymes that catalyze the hydrolysis of ester- and amide-containing chemicals. These enzymes are found in both the endoplasmic reticulum and the cytosol of many cell types and are involved in detoxification or metabolic activation of various drugs, environmental toxicants, and carcinogens. Carboxylesterases also catalyze the activation of prodrugs to their respective free acids. For example, the prodrug and cancer chemotherapeutic agent *irinotecan* is

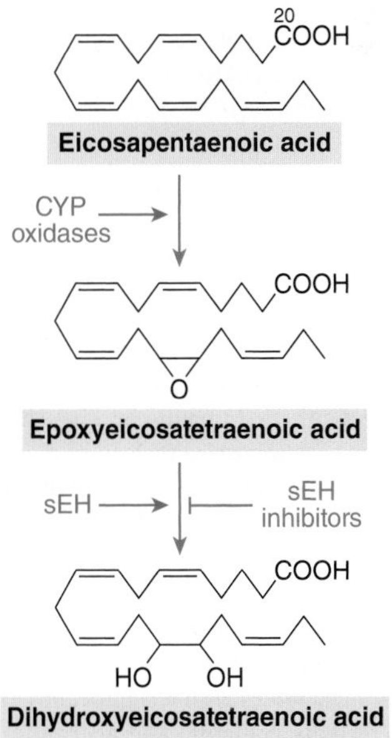

Figure 6–5 *Production and metabolism of an omega-3 fatty acid epoxide.* Fatty acid epoxides, such as the epoxide of the omega-3 fatty acid shown here, have a variety of anti-inflammatory and antinociceptive properties in test systems but are usually evanescent, metabolized to biologically less-active dihydroxy forms by sEH. Inhibition of sEH may promote the salutary effects of these epoxides.

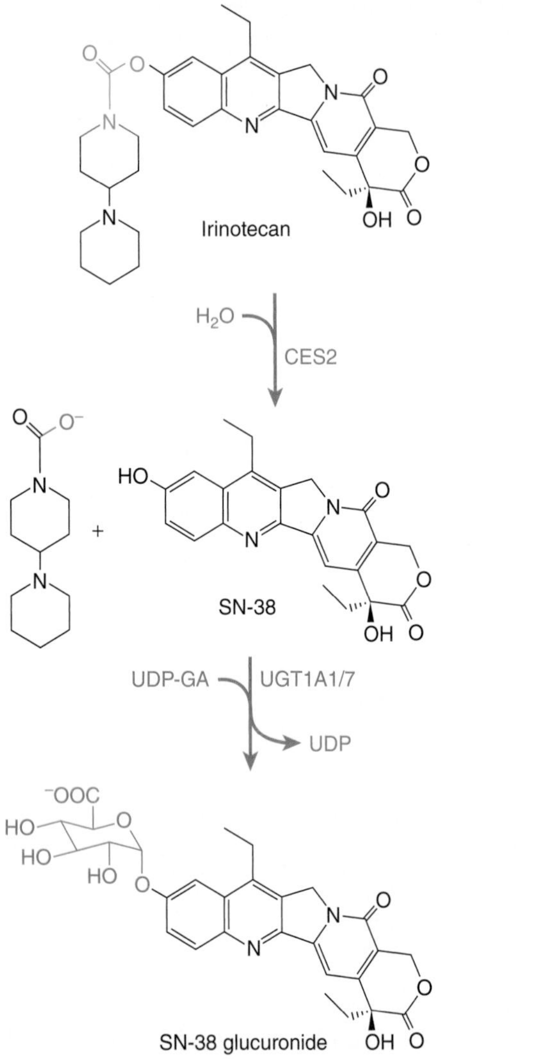

Figure 6–6 *Metabolism of irinotecan (CPT-11).* The prodrug CPT-11 is initially metabolized by a serum esterase (CES2) to the topoisomerase inhibitor SN-38, which is the active camptothecin analogue that slows tumor growth. SN-38 is then subject to glucuronidation, which results in loss of biological activity and facilitates elimination of SN-38 in the bile.

a camptothecin analogue that is bioactivated by intracellular carboxylesterases to the potent topoisomerase inhibitor SN-38 (Figure 6–6).

Phase 2 Reactions: Conjugating Enzymes

There are a large number of phase 2 conjugating enzymes, all of which are considered to be synthetic in nature because they result in the formation of metabolites with increased molecular mass. Phase 2 reactions also normally terminate the biological activity of the drug, although there are exceptions: For *morphine* and *minoxidil*, glucuronide and sulfate conjugates, respectively, are more pharmacologically active than the parent. The contributions of different phase 2 reactions to drug metabolism are shown in Figure 6–3B.

Two of the phase 2 reactions, glucuronidation and sulfation, result in the formation of metabolites with a significantly increased water-to-lipid partition coefficients. Sulfation and acetylation generally terminate the biological activity of drugs, and the minor change in overall charge increases the aqueous solubility of the metabolite. The enhanced hydrophilicity facilitates metabolite transport into the aqueous compartments of the cell and the body. Characteristic of the phase 2 reactions is the dependency on the catalytic reactions for cofactors (or, more correctly, cosubstrate): UDP-GA for UGT and PAPS for SULTs, which react

with available functional groups on the substrates. The reactive functional groups are often generated by the phase 1 CYPs, although there are many drugs (e.g., *acetaminophen*) for which glucuronidation and sulfation occur directly without prior oxidative metabolism. All of the phase 2 reactions are carried out in the cytosol of the cell, with the exception of glucuronidation, which is localized to the luminal side of the endoplasmic reticulum.

The catalytic rates of phase 2 reactions are significantly faster than the rates of the CYPs. Thus, if a drug is targeted for phase 1 oxidation through the CYPs, followed by a phase 2 conjugation reaction, usually the rate of elimination will depend on the initial (phase 1) oxidation reaction. Because the rate of conjugation is faster and the process leads to an increase in hydrophilicity of the drug, phase 2 reactions are generally considered to ensure efficient elimination and detoxification of most drugs.

Glucuronidation

Among the more important of the phase 2 reactions in drug metabolism is those catalyzed by UGTs (Figure 6–3B). These enzymes catalyze the transfer of glucuronic acid from the cofactor UDP-GA to a substrate to form β-d-glucopyranosiduronic acids (glucuronides), metabolites that are sensitive to cleavage by β-glucuronidase. Glucuronides can be formed via alcoholic and phenolic hydroxyl groups; carboxyl, sulfuryl, and carbonyl moieties; and primary, secondary, and tertiary amines. UGT substrates include many hundreds of chemically unique pharmaceuticals; dietary substances; environmental agents; humoral agents such as circulating hormones (androgens, estrogens, mineralocorticoids, glucocorticoids, thyroxine); bile acids; retinoids; and bilirubin, the end product of heme catabolism.

Examples of glucuronidation reactions are shown in Table 6–2 and Figures 6–1 and 6–6. The structural diversity of the drugs and other xenobiotics that are processed through glucuronidation ensures that most clinically efficacious therapeutic agents will be excreted as glucuronides.

The UGTs are expressed in a highly coordinated tissue-specific and often inducible fashion, with the highest concentration found in the GI tract and liver. Per tissue weight, there are a greater number and higher concentration of the UGTs in the small intestine compared to the liver, so efficient first-pass metabolism plays a role in predicting bioavailability of many orally administered medications. Formation of glucuronides and their increased polarity can result in their passage into the circulation, from which they are excreted into the urine. Alternatively, as xenobiotics enter the liver and are absorbed into hepatocytes, glucuronide formation provides substrates for active transport into the bile canaliculi and ultimate excretion with components of the bile (see Figure 5–9). Many of the glucuronides that are excreted into the bile eventually become substrates for soluble microbial β-glucuronidase in the large intestine, resulting in the formation of free glucuronic acid and the initial substrate. The colon actively absorbs water and a variety of other compounds (see Figure 50–3); depending on its solubility, the glucuronide or the original substrate may be reabsorbed via passive diffusion or by apical transporters in the colon and reenter the systemic circulation. This process, called *enterohepatic recirculation*, can extend the half-life of a xenobiotic that is conjugated in the liver because the compound's ultimate excretion is delayed (see Figures 6–8 and 6–9).

There are 19 human genes that encode the UGT proteins. Nine are encoded by the *UGT1A* locus on chromosome 2q37 (1A1, 1A3, 1A4, 1A5, 1A6, 1A7, 1A8, 1A9, and 1A10), while 10 genes are encoded by the *UGT2* family of genes on chromosome 4q13.2 (2B17, 2B15, 2B10, 2A3, 2B7, 2B11, 2B2, 2B4, 2A1, 2A2, and 2A3). Of these proteins, the major UGTs involved in drug metabolism are UGT1A1, 1A3, 1A4, 1A6, 1A9, and 2B7 (for a list of common UGT drug substrates, see Rowland et al., 2013). Although both families of proteins are associated with metabolism of drugs and xenobiotics, the UGT2 family of proteins appears to have greater specificity for the glucuronidation of endogenous substances.

The *UGT1* locus on chromosome 2 (Figure 6–7) spans nearly 200 kb, with over 150 kb of a tandem array of cassette exonic regions that encode approximately 280 amino acids of the amino terminal portion of the UGT1A proteins. Four exons are located at the 3′ end of the locus; these

UGT1 Locus

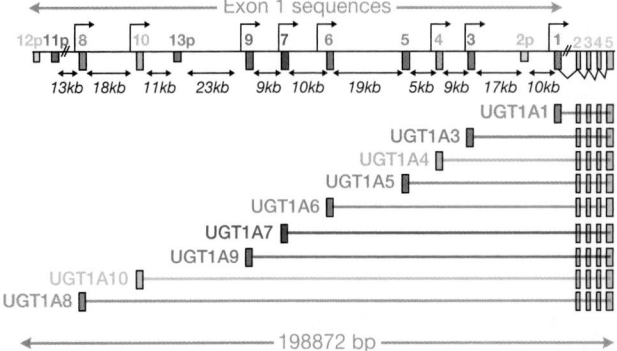

Figure 6–7 *Organization of the UGT1A locus.* Transcription of the *UGT1A* genes commences with the activation of PolII, which is controlled through tissue-specific events. Conserved exons 2 to 5 are spliced to each respective exon 1 sequence, resulting in the production of unique *UGT1A* sequences. The *UGT1A* locus encodes nine functional proteins.

encode the carboxyl 245 amino acids that combine with one of the consecutively numbered array of first exons to form the individual *UGT1A* gene products. Because exons 2 to 5 encode the same sequence for each UGT1A protein, the variability in substrate specificity for each of the UGT1A proteins results from the significant divergence in sequence encoded by the exon 1 regions. Reduced UGT activity resulting from allelic mutations in exons 2 to 5 affect all of the UGT1A proteins, whereas inactivating mutations in the exon 1 region lead to reduced glucuronidation by only the affected UGT1A protein. Over 100 allelic variants targeting the divergent exon 1 regions have been identified, many of which result in lowered UGT activity.

From a clinical perspective, the expression of UGT1A1 assumes an important role in drug metabolism because the glucuronidation of bilirubin by UGT1A1 is the rate-limiting step in ensuring efficient bilirubin clearance, and this rate can be affected by both genetic variation and competing substrates (drugs). Bilirubin is the breakdown product of heme, 80% of which originates from circulating hemoglobin and 20% from other heme-containing proteins, such as the CYPs. Bilirubin is hydrophobic, associates with serum albumin, and must be metabolized further by glucuronidation to ensure its elimination. The failure to efficiently metabolize bilirubin by glucuronidation leads to elevated serum levels and a clinical symptom called hyperbilirubinemia or jaundice. Delayed expression of the *UGT1A1* gene in newborns is the primary reason for neonatal hyperbilirubinemia.

There are more than 40 genetic lesions in the *UGT1A1* gene that can lead to inheritable unconjugated hyperbilirubinemia. Crigler-Najjar syndrome-type 1 (CN-1) is diagnosed as a complete lack of bilirubin glucuronidation and results from inactivating mutations in exon 1 or in the common exons of the *UGT1A1* gene. CN-2 is differentiated by the detection of low amounts of bilirubin glucuronides in duodenal secretions and is linked to promoter mutations or reading frame mutations in the *UGT1A1* gene that lead to greatly reduced glucuronide formation. The danger associated with CN-1 and CN-2 is the accumulation of toxic levels of unconjugated bilirubin, which can lead to CNS toxicity. Children diagnosed with CN-1 require immediate and extensive blue light therapy to break down circulating bilirubin; these patients eventually require liver transplantation. Agents that induce *UGT1A1* gene expression, such as phenobarbital, can improve bilirubin glucuronidation and its elimination in patients with CN-2. The *UGT1A1* gene is the only gene associated with xenobiotic metabolism that is essential for life because there is an absolute requirement for the daily elimination of serum bilirubin. Allelic variants associated with other xenobiotic-metabolizing genes (phase 1 and phase 2) can enhance disease and toxicity associated with drug use but show few or no phenotypic effects.

Gilbert syndrome is a generally benign condition that is present in 8%–23% of the population, based on ethnic diversity. It is diagnosed clinically by circulating bilirubin levels that are 100%–300% higher than normal. There is increasing epidemiological evidence to suggest that Gilbert syndrome may be protective against cardiovascular disease, potentially as a result of the antioxidant properties of bilirubin. The most common genetic polymorphism associated with Gilbert syndrome is a mutation in the *UGT1A1* gene promoter, identified as the *UGT1A1*28* allele, that leads to an $A(TA)_7TAA$ promoter sequence that differs from the more common $A(TA)_6TAA$ sequence. The elevated total serum bilirubin levels are associated with significantly reduced expression levels of hepatic UGT1A1.

Subjects diagnosed with Gilbert syndrome may be predisposed to ADRs (Table 6–3) resulting from a reduced capacity to metabolize drugs by UGT1A1. If a drug undergoes selective metabolism by UGT1A1, competition for drug metabolism with bilirubin glucuronidation will exist, resulting in pronounced hyperbilirubinemia as well as reduced clearance of the metabolized drug. *Tranilast* [*N*-(3′4′-demethoxycinnamoyl)-anthranilic acid] is an investigational drug used for the prevention of restenosis in patients who have undergone transluminal coronary revascularization (intracoronary stents). Tranilast therapy in patients with Gilbert syndrome can lead to hyperbilirubinemia, as well as potential hepatic complications resulting from elevated levels of tranilast.

Gilbert syndrome also alters patient responses to irinotecan. Irinotecan, a prodrug used in chemotherapy of solid tumors (see Chapter 66) is metabolized to its active form, SN-38, by tissue carboxylesterases (Figure 6–6). SN-38, a potent topoisomerase inhibitor, is inactivated by UGT1A1 and excreted in the bile (Figures 6–8 and 6–9). Once in the lumen of the intestine, the SN-38 glucuronide undergoes cleavage by bacterial β-glucuronidase and reenters the circulation through intestinal absorption. Elevated levels of SN-38 in the blood lead to hematological toxicities characterized by leukopenia and neutropenia, as well as damage to the intestinal epithelial cells, resulting in acute and life-threatening ileocolitis. Patients with Gilbert syndrome who are receiving irinotecan therapy are predisposed to the hematological and GI toxicities resulting from elevated serum levels of SN-38, the net result of insufficient UGT1A activity and the consequent accumulation of a toxic drug in the GI epithelium.

While most of the drugs that are metabolized by UGT1A1 compete for glucuronidation with bilirubin, patients with Gilbert syndrome who are HIV positive and on protease inhibitor therapy with atazanavir develop hyperbilirubinemia because atazanavir inhibits UGT1A1 function even though atazanavir is not a substrate for glucuronidation. Severe hyperbilirubinemia can develop in patients with Gilbert syndrome who have also been genotyped to contain inactivating mutations in the *UGT1A3* and *UGT1A7* genes. Clearly, drug-induced side effects attributed to the inhibition of the UGT enzymes can be a significant concern and can be complicated in the presence of gene-inactivating polymorphisms.

TABLE 6–3 ■ DRUG TOXICITY AND GILBERT SYNDROME	
PROBLEM	**FEATURE**
Gilbert syndrome	UGT1A1*28 (main variant in Caucasians)
Established toxicity reactions UGT1A1 substrates (potential risk?)	Irinotecan, atazanavir
	Gemfibrozil,[a] ezetimibe
	Simvastatin, atorvastatin, cerivastatin[a]
	Ethinylestradiol, buprenorphine, fulvestrant
	Ibuprofen, ketoprofen

[a] A severe drug reaction owing to the inhibition of glucuronidation (UGT1A1) and CYP2C8 and CYP2C9 when both drugs were combined led to the withdrawal of cerivastatin.

Source: Reproduced with permission from Strassburg CP. Pharmacogenetics of Gilbert's syndrome. *Pharmacogenomics*, **2008**, 9:703–715. Copyright © 2008 Future Medicine Ltd. All rights reserved.

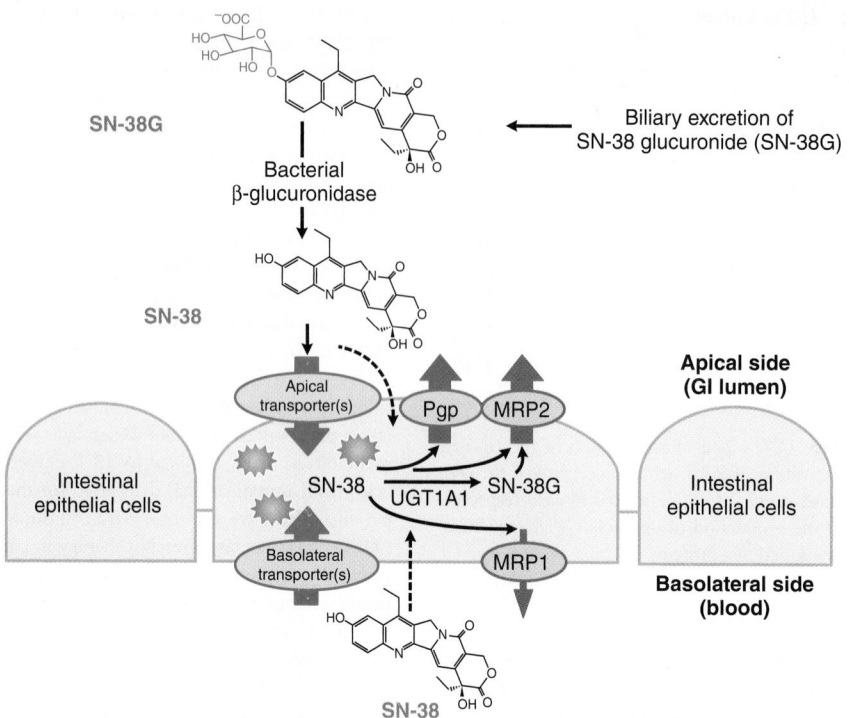

Figure 6–8 *Routes of SN-38 transport and exposure to intestinal epithelial cells.* SN-38 is transported into the bile following glucuronidation by liver UGT1A1 and extrahepatic UGT1A7. Following cleavage of luminal SN-38 glucuronide (SN-38G) by bacterial β-glucuronidase, reabsorption into epithelial cells can occur by passive diffusion (indicated by the dashed arrows entering the cell) as well as by apical transporters. Movement into epithelial cells may also occur from the blood by basolateral transporters. Intestinal SN-38 can efflux into the lumen through Pgp and MRP2 and into the blood via MRP1. Excessive accumulation of the SN-38 in intestinal epithelial cells, resulting from reduced glucuronidation, can lead to cellular damage and toxicity. (Modified and reproduced with permission from Tukey RH et al. Pharmacogenomics of human UDP-glucuronosyltransferases and irinotecan toxicity. *Mol Pharmacol*, **2002**, *62*:446–450. Copyright © 2002 The American Society for Pharmacology and Experimental Therapeutics.)

Sulfation

The SULTs, located in the cytosol, conjugate sulfate derived from PAPS to hydroxyl and, less frequently, amine groups of aromatic and aliphatic compounds. Like all of the xenobiotic-metabolizing enzymes, the SULTs metabolize a wide variety of endogenous and exogenous substrates. In humans, 13 SULT isoforms have been identified; based on sequence comparisons, they are classified into the SULT1 (SULT1A1, SULT1A2, SULT1A3/4, SULT1B1, SULT1C2, SULT1C3, SULT1C4, SULT1E1);

SULT2 (SULT2A1, SULT2B1a, SULT2B1b); SULT4 (SULT4A1); and SULT6 (SULT6A1) families. There are major interspecies differences in the expressed complement of SULTs, which makes extrapolation of data on xenobiotic sulfation in animals to humans particularly unreliable.

SULTs play an important role in normal human homeostasis. For example, SULT2B1b is a predominant form expressed in skin, carrying out the catalysis of cholesterol. Cholesterol sulfate is an essential metabolite in regulating keratinocyte differentiation and skin development. SULT2A1 is

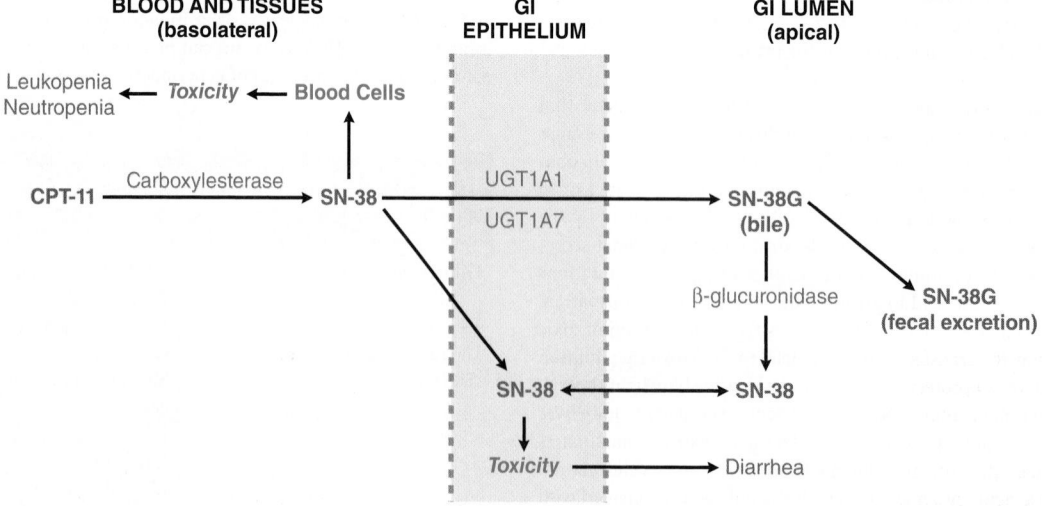

Figure 6–9 *Cellular targets of SN-38 in the blood and intestinal tissues.* Excessive accumulation of SN-38 can lead to blood toxicities, such as leukopenia and neutropenia, as well as damage to the intestinal epithelium. These toxicities are pronounced in individuals who have reduced capacity to form the SN-38 glucuronide, such as patients with Gilbert syndrome. Note the different body compartments and cell types involved. (Modified and reproduced with permission from Tukey RH et al. Pharmacogenomics of human UDP-glucuronosyltransferases and irinotecan toxicity. *Mol Pharmacol*, **2002**, *62*:446–450. Copyright © 2002 The American Society for Pharmacology and Experimental Therapeutics.)

highly expressed in the fetal adrenal gland, where it produces the large quantities of dehydroepiandrosterone sulfate that are required for placental estrogen biosynthesis during the second half of pregnancy. SULTs 1A3 and 1A4 are highly selective for catecholamines, while estrogens (in particular 17β-estradiol) are sulfated by SULT1E1. In humans, significant fractions of circulating catecholamines, estrogens, iodothyronines, and DHEA exist in the sulfated form.

Some human SULTs display unique substrate specificities, whereas others are promiscuous. Members of the SULT1 family are the major isoforms involved in xenobiotic metabolism, with SULT1A1 quantitatively and qualitatively the most important in the liver. SULT1A1 displays extensive diversity in its capacity to catalyze the sulfation of a broad variety of structurally heterogeneous xenobiotics with high affinity. The isoforms in the SULT1 family are recognized as phenol SULTs; they catalyze the sulfation of phenolic molecules such as *acetaminophen*, *minoxidil*, and *17α-ethinyl estradiol*. SULT1B1 is similar to SULT1A1 in its wide range of substrates, although it is much more abundant in the intestine than the liver. Three SULT1C isoforms exist in humans, but little is known of their substrate specificity. In rodents, SULT1C enzymes are capable of sulfating the hepatic carcinogen *N*-OH-2-acetylaminofluorene and are responsible for the bioactivation of this and related carcinogens. Their role in this pathway in humans is not clear. SULT1C enzymes are expressed abundantly in human fetal tissues, yet decline in abundance in adults. SULT1E catalyzes the sulfation of endogenous and exogenous steroids and is localized in liver and in hormone-responsive tissues such as the testis, breast, adrenal gland, and placenta. In the upper GI tract, SULT1A3/4 and SULT1B1 are particularly abundant.

The conjugation of drugs and xenobiotics is considered primarily a detoxification step, ensuring that the metabolites enter the aqueous compartments of the body and are targeted for elimination. However, drug metabolism through sulfation often leads to the generation of chemically reactive metabolites, wherein the sulfate is electron withdrawing and may be heterolytically cleaved, leading to the formation of an electrophilic cation. Most examples of the generation by sulfation of a carcinogenic or toxic response in animal or mutagenicity assays have been documented with chemicals derived from the environment or from heterocyclic arylamine food mutagens generated from well-cooked meat. Thus, it is important to understand whether genetic linkages can be made by associating known human SULT polymorphisms to cancers that are believed to originate from environmental sources. Because SULT1A1 is the most abundant SULT form in human tissues and displays broad substrate specificity, the polymorphic profiles associated with this gene and their associations with various human cancers are of considerable interest.

Gene copy number polymorphisms within the SULT1A1, SULT1A3, and SULT1A4 genes have been identified, which may help explain much of the interindividual variation in the expression and activity of these enzymes. Knowledge of the structure, activities, regulation, and polymorphisms of the SULT superfamily will aid in understanding the linkages between sulfation and cancer susceptibility, reproduction, and development. Structural data, the results of kinetic studies, and molecular dynamics simulations are beginning to provide a picture of the mechanisms by which the SULTs express their unique patterns of substrate specificity (Tibbs et al., 2015).

Glutathione Conjugation

The GSTs catalyze the transfer of glutathione to reactive electrophiles, a function that serves to protect cellular macromolecules from interacting with electrophiles that contain electrophilic heteroatoms (–O, –N, and –S) and in turn protects the cellular environment from damage (Hayes et al., 2005). The cosubstrate in the reaction is glutathione, a tripeptide consisting of γ-glutamic acid, cysteine, and glycine (Figure 6–10). Glutathione exists in the cell in oxidized (GSSG) and reduced (GSH) forms, and the GSH:GSSG ratio is critical in maintaining a cellular environment in the reduced state. In addition to affecting xenobiotic conjugation with GSH, a severe reduction in GSH content can predispose cells to oxidative damage, a state that has been linked to a number of human health issues.

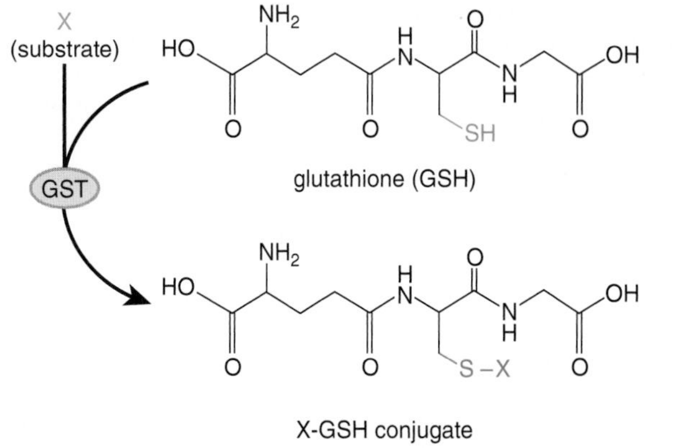

Figure 6–10 *Glutathione is a cosubstrate in the conjugation of a xenobiotic (X) by GST.*

In the formation of glutathione conjugates, the GST reaction generates a thioether linkage with drug or xenobiotic to the cysteine moiety of the tripeptide. Characteristically, all GST substrates contain an electrophilic atom and are hydrophobic; by nature, they will associate with cellular proteins. Because the concentration of glutathione in cells is usually high, typically 7 μmol/g of liver or in the 10-mM range, many drugs and xenobiotics can react nonenzymatically with glutathione. However, the GSTs have been found to occupy up to 10% of the total hepatocellular protein concentration, a property that ensures efficient conjugation of glutathione to reactive electrophiles. The high concentration of GSTs also provides the cells with a sink of cytosolic protein, a property that facilitates noncovalent and sometimes covalent interactions with compounds that are not substrates for glutathione conjugation. The cytosolic pool of GSTs, once identified as *ligandin*, binds steroids, bile acids, bilirubin, cellular hormones, and environmental toxicants, in addition to complexing with other cellular proteins.

There are in excess of 20 human GSTs, divided into two subfamilies: the *cytosolic* and the *microsomal* forms. The major differences in function between the microsomal and cytosolic GSTs reside in the selection of substrates for conjugation; the cytosolic forms have more importance in the metabolism of drugs and xenobiotics, whereas the microsomal GSTs are important in the endogenous metabolism of leukotrienes and prostaglandins. The cytosolic GSTs are divided into seven classes termed alpha (GSTA1 and 2), mu (GSTM1 through 5), omega (GSTO1), pi (GSTP1), sigma (GSTS1), theta (GSTT1 and GSTT2), and zeta (GSTZ1). Those in the alpha and mu classes can form heterodimers, allowing for a large number of active transferases to form. The cytosolic forms of GST catalyze conjugation, reduction, and isomerization reactions.

The high concentrations of GSH in the cell, as well as the overabundance of GSTs, means that few reactive molecules escape detoxification. Despite the appearance of overcapacity of enzyme and reducing equivalents, there is always concern that some reactive intermediates will escape detoxification and, by nature of their electrophilicity, will bind to cellular components and cause havoc. The potential for such an occurrence is heightened if GSH is depleted or if a specific form of GST is polymorphic and dysfunctional. While it is difficult to deplete cellular GSH levels, therapeutic agents that require large doses to be clinically efficacious have the greatest potential to lower cellular GSH levels.

Acetaminophen, normally metabolized by glucuronidation and sulfation, is also a substrate for oxidative metabolism by CYP2E1 and CYP3A4, which generate the toxic metabolite NAPQI, which, under normal dosing, is readily neutralized through conjugation with GSH. However, an overdose of acetaminophen can deplete cellular GSH levels and thereby increase the potential for NAPQI to interact with other cellular components, resulting in toxicity and cell death. Acetaminophen toxicity is associated with increased levels of NAPQI and hepatic necrosis, although it may be treated in a time- and drug concentration–dependent manner by administration of *N*-acetylcysteine (see Figure 4–4).

All of the GSTs are polymorphic. The mu (GSTM1*0) and theta (GSTT1*0) genotypes express a null phenotype; thus, individuals who are polymorphic at these loci are predisposed to toxicities by agents that are selective substrates for these GSTs. For example, the mutant GSTM1*0 allele is observed in 50% of the Caucasian population and links genetically to human malignancies of the lung, colon, and bladder. Null activity in the *GSTT1* gene associates with adverse side effects and toxicity in cancer chemotherapy with cytostatic drugs; the toxicities result from insufficient clearance of the drugs via GSH conjugation. Expression of the null genotype can be as high as 60% in Chinese and Korean populations. GST polymorphisms may influence efficacies and severity of adverse side effects of drugs.

While the GSTs play an important role in cellular detoxification, their activities in cancerous tissues have been linked to the development of drug resistance toward chemotherapeutic agents that are both substrates and nonsubstrates for the GSTs. Many anticancer drugs are effective because they initiate cell death or apoptosis, which is linked to the activation of MAPKs such as JNK and p38. Investigational studies demonstrated that overexpression of GSTs is associated with resistance to apoptosis and the inhibition of MAPK activity. In a variety of tumors, GSTs are overexpressed, leading to a reduction in MAPK activity and reduced efficacy of chemotherapy. Taking advantage of the relatively high levels of GST in tumor cells, inhibition of GST activity has been exploited as a therapeutic strategy to modulate drug resistance by sensitizing tumors to anticancer drugs. TLK199, a glutathione analogue, is a prodrug that plasma esterases convert to a GST inhibitor, TLK117, which potentiates the toxicity of different anticancer agents (Figure 6–11).

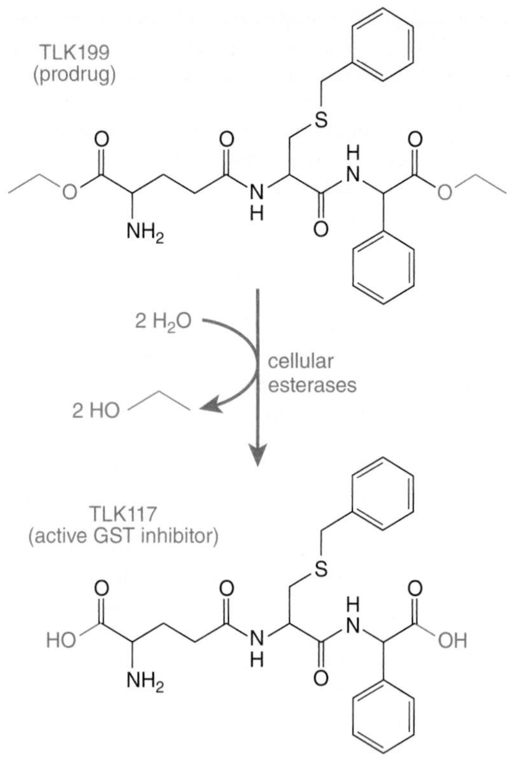

Alternatively, the elevated GST activity in cancer cells has been utilized to develop prodrugs that can be activated by the GSTs to form electrophilic intermediates. For example, TLK286 is a substrate for GST that undergoes a β-elimination reaction, forming a glutathione conjugate and a nitrogen mustard (Figure 6–12) that is capable of alkylating cellular nucleophiles and resulting in antitumor activity (Townsend and Tew, 2003).

N-Acetylation

The cytosolic NATs are responsible for the metabolism of drugs and environmental agents that contain an aromatic amine or hydrazine group. The addition of the acetyl group from the cofactor acetyl-coenzyme A

Figure 6–11 *Activation of TLK199 to TLK117, a GST inhibitor.*

often leads to a metabolite that is *less* water soluble because the potential ionizable amine is neutralized by the covalent addition of the acetyl group. NATs are among the most polymorphic of all the human xenobiotic drug-metabolizing enzymes.

The characterization of an acetylator phenotype in humans was one of the first hereditary traits identified and was responsible for the development of the field of pharmacogenetics (see Chapter 7). Following the discovery that isoniazid (isonicotinic acid hydrazide) could be used to treat

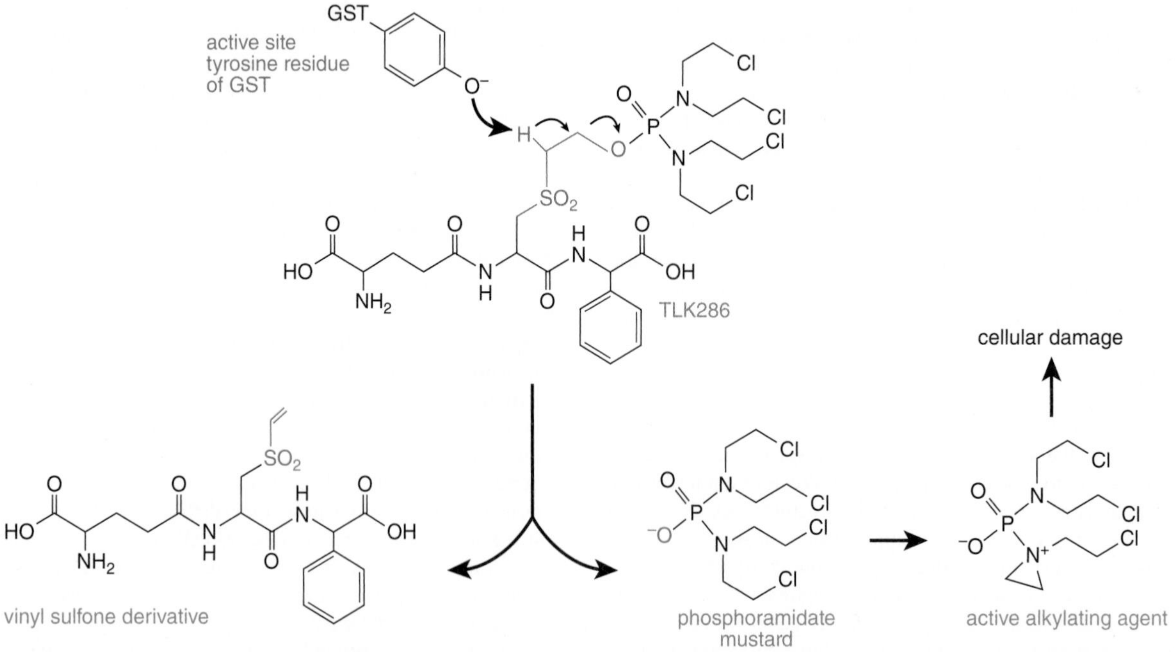

Figure 6–12 *Generation of the reactive alkylating agent following the conjugation of glutathione to TLK286.* GST interacts with the prodrug and GSH analogue TLK286 via a tyrosine in the active site of GST. The GSH portion is shown in blue. The interaction promotes β-elimination and cleavage of the prodrug to a vinyl sulfone and an active alkylating fragment.

tuberculosis, a significant proportion of the patients (5%–15%) experienced toxicities that ranged from numbness and tingling in their fingers to CNS damage. After finding that isoniazid was metabolized by acetylation and excreted in the urine, researchers noted that individuals who had the toxic effects of the drug excreted the largest amount of unchanged drug and the least amount of acetylated isoniazid. Pharmacogenetic studies led to the classification of "rapid" and "slow" acetylators, with the slow phenotype predisposed to toxicity (see Figure 60–4). Purification and characterization of NAT and the eventual cloning of its RNA provided sequence characterization of the gene for slow and fast acetylators, revealing polymorphisms that correspond to the slow acetylator phenotype.

There are two functional NAT genes in humans, *NAT1* and *NAT2*. Over 25 allelic variants of *NAT1* and *NAT2* have been characterized. In individuals in whom acetylation of drugs is compromised, homozygous genotypes for at least two variant alleles are required to predispose a patient to slower drug metabolism. Polymorphism in the *NAT2* gene and its association with the slow acetylation of isoniazid were one of the first completely characterized genotypes shown to affect drug metabolism, thereby linking pharmacogenetic phenotype to a genetic polymorphism. Although nearly as many mutations have been identified in the *NAT1* gene as the *NAT2* gene, the frequency of the slow acetylation patterns is attributed mostly to the polymorphism in the *NAT2* gene.

Some common drug substrates of NAT and their known toxicities are listed in Table 6–4 (see Meisel, 2002, for details). The therapeutic relevance of NAT polymorphisms is in avoiding drug-induced toxicities. The adverse drug response in a slow acetylator resembles a drug overdose; thus, reducing the dose or increasing the dosing interval is recommended. Aromatic amine or hydrazine groups exist in many classes of clinically used drugs, and if a drug is known to be subjected to metabolism through acetylation, determining an individual's phenotype can be important in maximizing a positive therapeutic outcome. For example, *hydralazine*, a once-popular orally active antihypertensive (vasodilator) drug, is metabolized by NAT2. The administration of therapeutic doses of hydralazine to a slow acetylator can result in extreme hypotension and tachycardia.

Several known targets for acetylation, such as the sulfonamides, have been implicated in idiosyncratic hypersensitivity reactions; in such instances, an appreciation of a patient's acetylation phenotype is particularly important. Sulfonamides are transformed into hydroxylamines that interact with cellular proteins, generating haptens that can elicit autoimmune responses, to which slow acetylators are predisposed.

Tissue-specific expression patterns of NAT1 and NAT2 have a significant impact on the fate of drug metabolism and the potential for eliciting a toxic episode. NAT1 is ubiquitously expressed among most human tissues, whereas NAT2 is found predominantly in liver and the GI tract. Characteristic of both NAT1 and NAT2 is the ability to form *N*-hydroxy–acetylated metabolites from bicyclic aromatic hydrocarbons, a reaction that leads to the nonenzymatic release of acetyl groups and the generation of highly reactive nitrenium ions. Thus, *N*-hydroxy acetylation is thought to activate certain environmental toxicants. In contrast, direct *N*-acetylation of bicyclic aromatic amines is stable and leads to detoxification. Individuals who are NAT2 fast acetylators are able to efficiently metabolize and detoxify bicyclic aromatic amines through liver-dependent acetylation. However, slow acetylators (NAT2 deficient) accumulate bicyclic aromatic amines that become substrates for CYP-dependent *N*-oxidation. These N-OH metabolites are eliminated in the urine. In tissues such as bladder epithelium, NAT1 is highly expressed and can efficiently catalyze the *N*-hydroxy acetylation of bicyclic aromatic amines, a process that leads to deacetylation and the formation of the mutagenic nitrenium ion, especially in NAT2-deficient subjects. Epidemiological studies have shown that slow acetylators are predisposed to bladder cancer if exposed environmentally to bicyclic aromatic amines.

Methylation

In humans, drugs and xenobiotics can undergo *O*-, *N*-, and *S*-methylation. Humans express two COMTs, three *N*-methyl transferases, a POMT, a TPMT, and a TMT. All of the MTs exist as monomers and use S-adenosylmethionine (AdoMet) as the methyl donor. With the exception of a signature sequence that is conserved among the MTs, there is limited conservation in sequence, indicating that each MT has evolved to display a unique catalytic function. Although the common theme among the MTs is the generation of a methylated product, substrate specificity is high and distinguishes the individual enzymes.

Among the *N*-methyl transferases, NNMT methylates serotonin and tryptophan as well as pyridine-containing compounds such as nicotinamide and nicotine. PNMT is responsible for the methylation of the neurotransmitter norepinephrine to form epinephrine; the HNMT metabolizes drugs containing an imidazole ring. COMT, which exists as two protein

TABLE 6–4 ■ THERAPEUTIC USES AND ADVERSE EFFECTS OF COMMON *N*-ACETYLTRANSFERASE SUBSTRATES

NAT SUBSTRATE	THERAPEUTIC USES	ADVERSE EFFECTS
Acebutolol	Adrenal cortex carcinoma, breast cancer	Drowsiness, weakness, insomnia
Aminoglutethimide	β Blockade, arrhythmias, hypertension	Clumsiness, nausea, dizziness, agranulocytosis
Aminosalicylic acid	Ulcerative colitis	Allergic fever, itching, leukopenia
Amrinone	Positive inotrope in heart failure	Thrombocytopenia, arrhythmias
Benzocaine	Local anesthesia	Dermatitis, itching, rash, methemoglobinemia
Caffeine	Neonatal respiratory distress syndrome	Dizziness, insomnia, tachycardia
Clonazepam	Seizures, anxiety	Drowsiness, ataxia, dizziness, slurred speech
Dapsone	Leprosy, dermatitis	Hemolysis, methemoglobinemia, nausea, dermatitis
Hydralazine	Hypertension (acts via vasodilation)	Hypotension, sympathetic baroreceptor reflex effects
Isoniazid	Tuberculosis	Peripheral neuritis, hepatotoxicity
Nitrazepam	Insomnia	Dizziness, somnolence
Phenelzine	Depression (acts via MAO inhibition)	Dizziness, CNS excitation, insomnia, orthostatic hypotension, hepatotoxicity
Procainamide	Ventricular tachyarrhythmia	Hypotension, bradycardia, lupus erythematosus
Sulfonamides	As bacteriostatic agents	Hypersensitivity, acute hemolytic anemia, reversible bone marrow suppression (with AIDS or myelosuppressive chemotherapy)

isoforms generated by alternate exon usage, methylates neurotransmitters containing a catechol moiety, such as dopamine and norepinephrine, as well as methyldopa and *ecstasy* (3,4-methylenedioxymethamphetamine, MDMA).

From a clinical perspective, the most important MT may be TPMT, which catalyzes the *S*-methylation of aromatic and heterocyclic sulfhydryl compounds, including the thiopurine drugs *AZA*, *6-MP*, and *thioguanine*. AZA and 6-MP are used for the management of inflammatory bowel disease (see Chapter 51), as well as autoimmune disorders such as systemic lupus erythematosus and rheumatoid arthritis. Thioguanine is used in the treatment of acute myeloid leukemia, and 6-MP is used worldwide for the treatment of childhood acute lymphoblastic leukemia (see Chapter 66). Because TPMT is responsible for the detoxification of 6-MP, a genetic deficiency in TPMT can result in severe toxicities in patients taking the drug (see metabolic scheme in Figure 51-5). When given orally at clinically established doses, 6-MP serves as a prodrug that is metabolized by HGPRT to 6-TGNs, which become incorporated into DNA and RNA, resulting in arrest of DNA replication and cytotoxicity.

Toxic side effects arise when a lack of 6-MP methylation by TPMT causes a buildup of 6-MP and the consequent generation of toxic levels of 6-TGNs. The identification of the inactive TPMT alleles and the development of a genotyping test to identify homozygous carriers of the defective allele permit identification of individuals who may be predisposed to the toxic side effects of 6-MP therapy. Simple adjustments in the patient's dosage regimen are a lifesaving intervention for those with TPMT deficiencies.

Role of Xenobiotic Metabolism in Safe and Effective Use of Drugs

Any xenobiotics entering the body must be eliminated through metabolism and excretion via the urine or bile/feces. Mechanisms of metabolism and excretion prevent foreign compounds from accumulating in the body and possibly causing toxicity. In the case of drugs, metabolism normally results in the inactivation of their therapeutic effectiveness and facilitates their elimination. The extent of metabolism can determine the efficacy and toxicity of a drug by controlling its biological half-life. Among the most serious considerations in the clinical use of drugs are ADRs. If a drug is metabolized too quickly, it rapidly loses its therapeutic efficacy. This can occur if specific enzymes involved in metabolism are overly active or are induced by dietary or environmental factors. If a drug is metabolized too slowly, the drug can accumulate in the bloodstream; as a consequence, the plasma clearance of the drug is decreased, the AUC (see Figure 5–3) is elevated, and exposure to the drug may exceed clinically appropriate levels. An increase in AUC often results when specific xenobiotic-metabolizing enzymes are inhibited, which can occur when an individual is taking a combination of different therapeutic agents and one of those drugs targets the enzyme involved in drug metabolism. For example, the consumption of grapefruit juice with drugs taken orally can inhibit intestinal CYP3A4, blocking the metabolism of many of these drugs. The inhibition of specific CYPs in the gut by dietary consumption of grapefruit juice alters the oral bioavailability of many classes of drugs, including certain antihypertensives, immunosuppressants, antidepressants, antihistamines, and the statins, to name a few. Among the components of grapefruit juice that inhibit CYP3A4 are *naringin* and *furanocoumarins*.

While environmental factors can alter the steady-state levels of specific enzymes or inhibit their catalytic potential, these phenotypic changes in drug metabolism are also observed clinically in groups of individuals who are genetically predisposed to ADRs because of pharmacogenetic differences in the expression of xenobiotic-metabolizing enzymes (see Chapter 7). Most of the xenobiotic-metabolizing enzymes display polymorphic differences in their expression, resulting from heritable changes in the structure of the genes. For example, hyperbilirubinemia can result from a reduction in the ability to glucuronidate circulating bilirubin due to a lowered expression of the *UGT1A1* gene (Gilbert syndrome). Drugs that are subject to glucuronidation by UGT1A1, such as the topoisomerase

inhibitor SN-38 (Figures 6–6, 6–8, and 6–9), will display an increased AUC in individuals with Gilbert syndrome because such patients cannot detoxify these drugs. Most cancer chemotherapeutic agents have a narrow therapeutic index, and increases in the circulating levels of the active form due to a deficiency in drug clearance can result in significant toxicities.

Nearly every class of therapeutic agent has been reported to initiate an ADR. In the United States, ADRs annually cost an estimated at $100 billion and cause over 100,000 deaths. An estimated 56% of drugs associated with ADRs are substrates for xenobiotic-metabolizing enzymes, notably CYPs and UGTs. Because many of the CYPs and UGTs are subject to induction as well as inhibition by drugs, dietary factors, and other environmental agents, these enzymes play an important role in most ADRs. Thus, prior to filing a New Drug Application (NDA), a new drug's route of metabolism must be known. Thus, it is routine practice in the pharmaceutical industry to establish which enzymes are involved in metabolism of a drug candidate and to identify the metabolites and determine their potential toxicity. In consideration of the major role of CYPs in the generation of ADRs, there is likely to be a move to avoid the major oxidative routes of metabolism when developing new small-molecule drugs.

Induction of Drug Metabolism

Xenobiotics can influence drug metabolism by activating transcription and inducing the expression of genes encoding drug-metabolizing enzymes. Thus, a foreign compound may induce its own metabolism, as may certain drugs. One potential consequence of this is a decrease in plasma drug concentration over the course of treatment, resulting in loss of efficacy, as the autoinduced metabolism of the drug exceeds the rate at which new drug enters the body. A list of ligands and the receptors through which they induce drug metabolism is shown in Table 6–5. A particular receptor, when activated by a ligand, can induce the transcription of a battery of target genes. Among these target genes are certain CYPs and drug transporters. Thus, any drug that is a ligand for a receptor that induces CYPs and transporters could lead to drug interactions. Figure 6–13 shows the scheme by which a drug may interact with nuclear receptors to induce its own metabolism.

The aryl hydrocarbon receptor (AHR) is a member of a superfamily of transcription factors with diverse roles in mammals, such as serving a regulatory role in the development of the mammalian CNS and modulating the response to chemical and oxidative stress. This superfamily of transcription factors includes (Period) and Sim (Simpleminded), two transcription factors involved in development of the CNS, and HIF1α, HIF2α, and their dimerization partner HIF1β, which activate genes in response to low cellular O_2 levels.

The AHR induces expression of genes encoding CYP1A1, CYP1A2, and CYP1B1, which are able to metabolically activate chemical carcinogens, including environmental contaminants and carcinogens derived from food. Many of these substances are inert unless metabolized by CYPs. Thus, induction of these CYPs by a drug could potentially result

TABLE 6–5 ■ NUCLEAR RECEPTORS THAT INDUCE DRUG METABOLISM

RECEPTOR	LIGANDS
Aryl hydrocarbon receptor (AHR)	Omeprazole
Constitutive androstane receptor (CAR)	Phenobarbital
Pregnane X receptor (PXR)	Rifampin
Farnesoid X receptor (FXR)	Bile acids
Vitamin D receptor (VDR)	Vitamin D
Peroxisome proliferator–activated receptor (PPARs)	Fibrates
Retinoic acid receptor (RAR)	*all-trans*-Retinoic acid
Retinoid X receptor (RXR)	*9-cis*-Retinoic acid

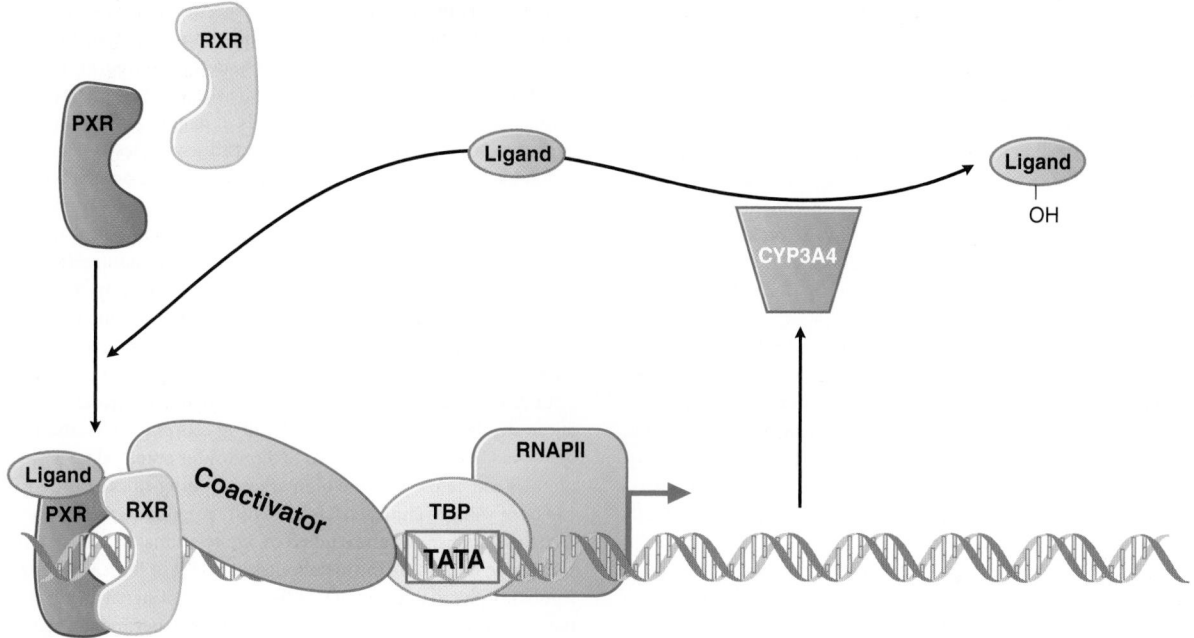

Figure 6–13 *Induction of drug metabolism by nuclear receptor–mediated signal transduction.* When a drug such as atorvastatin (Ligand) enters the cell, it can bind to a nuclear receptor such as the PXR. The PXR then forms a complex with the RXR, binds to DNA upstream of target genes, recruits coactivator (which binds to the TBP), and activates transcription. Among PXR target genes are *CYP3A4*, which can metabolize the atorvastatin and decrease its cellular concentration. Thus, atorvastatin induces its own metabolism. Atorvastatin undergoes both ortho- and parahydroxylation.

in an increase in the toxicity and carcinogenicity of procarcinogens. For example, *omeprazole*, a proton pump inhibitor used to treat gastric and duodenal ulcers (see Chapter 49), is a ligand for the AHR and can induce CYP1A1 and CYP1A2, with the possible consequences of toxin/carcinogen activation as well as drug-drug interactions in patients receiving agents that are substrates for either of these CYPs.

Another important induction mechanism is due to type 2 nuclear receptors that are in the same superfamily as the steroid hormone receptors. Many of these receptors, identified on the basis of their structural similarity to steroid hormone receptors, were originally termed *orphan receptors* because no endogenous ligands were known to interact with them. Subsequent studies revealed that some of these receptors are activated by xenobiotics, including drugs. The type 2 nuclear receptors of most importance to drug metabolism and drug therapy include PXR, CAR, and PPARs. PXR, discovered because it is activated by the synthetic steroid pregnenolone-16α-carbonitrile, is also activated by a number of other drugs, including antibiotics (*rifampicin* and *troleandomycin*), Ca^{2+} channel blockers (*nifedipine*), statins (*mevastatin*), antidiabetic drugs (*troglitazone*), HIV protease inhibitors (*ritonavir*), and anticancer drugs (*paclitaxel*).

Hyperforin, a component of St. John's wort, an over-the-counter herbal remedy used for depression, also activates PXR. This activation is thought to be the basis for the increase in failure of oral contraceptives in individuals taking St. John's wort: Activated PXR is an inducer of CYP3A4, which can metabolize steroids found in oral contraceptives. PXR also induces the expression of genes encoding certain drug transporters and phase 2 enzymes, including SULTs and UGTs. Thus, PXR facilitates the metabolism and elimination of xenobiotics, including drugs, with notable consequences.

The nuclear receptor CAR was discovered based on its ability to activate genes in the absence of ligand. Steroids such as *androstanol*, the antifungal agent *clotrimazole*, and the antiemetic *meclizine* are inverse agonists that inhibit gene activation by CAR, while the pesticide 1,4-bis[2-(3,5-dichloropyridyloxy)]benzene, the steroid 5-β-pregnane-3,20-dione, and probably other endogenous compounds are agonists that activate gene expression when bound to CAR. Genes induced by CAR include those encoding several CYPs (CYP2B6, CYP2C9, and CYP3A4); various phase 2 enzymes (including GSTs, UGTs, and SULTs); and drug and endobiotic

transporters. CYP3A4 is induced by both PXR and CAR; thus, its level is highly influenced by a number of drugs and other xenobiotics. In addition to a potential role in inducing the degradation of drugs, including the over-the-counter analgesic acetaminophen, this receptor may function in the control of bilirubin degradation, the process by which the liver decomposes heme.

Clearly, PXR and CAR can bind a great variety of ligands. As with the xenobiotic-metabolizing enzymes, species differences also exist in the ligand specificities of these receptors. For example, rifampicin activates human PXR, but not mouse or rat PXR, while pregnenolone-16α-carbonitrile preferentially activates the mouse and rat PXR. Paradoxically, meclizine activates mouse CAR but inhibits gene induction by human CAR. These findings further underscore that in some cases studies with rodent model systems do not reflect the response of humans to drugs.

The PPAR family is composed of three members: α, β, and γ. PPARα is the target for the fibrate class of hyperlipidemic drugs, including the widely prescribed *gemfibrozil* and *fenofibrate*. Activation of PPARα results in induction of target genes encoding fatty acid–metabolizing enzymes, resulting in lowering of serum triglycerides; in addition, activation of PPARα induces CYP4 enzymes that carry out the oxidation of fatty acids and drugs with fatty acid–containing side chains, such as *leukotriene* and arachidonate analogues. PPARγ is the target for the thiazolidinedione class of anti–type 2 diabetic drugs, including rosiglitazone and pioglitazone. PPARγ does not induce xenobiotic metabolism.

The UGT genes, in particular UGT1A1, are a target for AHR, PXR, CAR, PPARα, and Nrf2 (nuclear factor 2 (erythroid-derived 2-like factor), a major transcriptional regulator of cytoprotective genes induced by an antioxidant response). Because the UGTs are abundant in the GI tract and liver, regulation of the UGTs by drug-induced activation of these receptors would be expected to play a role concerning the pharmacokinetic parameters of many orally administered therapeutics.

Role of Drug Metabolism in Drug Development

There are two key elements associated with successful drug development: *efficacy* and *safety*. Both depend on drug metabolism. It is necessary to determine which enzymes metabolize a new drug candidate to predict whether the compound may cause drug-drug interactions or be susceptible to marked interindividual variation in metabolism due to genetic polymorphisms.

For determination of metabolism, the compound is subjected to analysis by human liver cells or extracts from these cells that contain the drug-metabolizing enzymes. Such studies determine how humans will metabolize a particular drug and, to a limited extent, predict the rate of metabolism. If a CYP is involved, a panel of recombinant CYPs can be used to determine which CYP predominates in the metabolism of the drug. If a single CYP, such as CYP3A4, is found to be the sole CYP that metabolizes a drug candidate, then a decision can be made about the likelihood of drug interactions.

Interactions become a problem when multiple drugs are simultaneously administered, for example, in elderly patients, who on a daily basis may take prescribed anti-inflammatory drugs, cholesterol-lowering drugs, blood pressure medications, a gastric acid suppressant, an anticoagulant, and a number of over-the-counter medications. Ideally, the best drug candidate would be metabolized by several CYPs so that variability in expression levels of one CYP or drug-drug interactions would not significantly affect its metabolism and pharmacokinetics.

Similar studies can be carried out with phase 2 enzymes and drug transporters to predict the metabolic fate of a drug. In addition to the use of recombinant human xenobiotic-metabolizing enzymes in predicting drug metabolism, human receptor-based (PXR and CAR) systems or cell lines expressing these receptors are used to determine whether a particular drug candidate could be a ligand or activator of PXR, CAR, or PPARα. For example, a drug that activates PXR may result in rapid clearance of other drugs that are CYP3A4 substrates, thus decreasing their bioavailability and efficacy.

Computer-based computational (in silico) prediction of drug metabolism is a prospect for the near future. The structures of several CYPs have been determined, including those of CYPs 2A6, 2C9, and 3A4. These structures may be used to predict metabolism of a drug candidate by fitting the compound to the enzyme's active site and determining oxidation potentials of sites on the molecule. However, the structures, determined by X-ray analysis of crystals of enzyme-substrate complexes, are static, whereas enzymes are flexible; this vital distinction may be limiting. The large size of the CYP active sites, which permits them to metabolize many different compounds, also renders them difficult to model. The potential for modeling ligand or activator interactions with nuclear receptors also exists with limitations similar to those discussed for the CYPs.

Determining the potential for a drug candidate to produce acute toxicity in preclinical studies is vital and routine in drug development. This is typically done by administering the drug candidate to rodents at escalating doses, usually above the predicted human therapeutic dose. For drug candidates proposed for chronic use in humans, such as for lowering serum triglycerides and cholesterol or for treatment of type 2 diabetes, long-term carcinogenicity studies are carried out in rodent models. Signs of toxicity are monitored and organ damage assessed by postmortem pathologies. This process is not high throughput and can be a bottleneck in development of lead compounds.

A new technology of high-throughput screening for biomarkers of toxicity is being adopted for drug development using *metabolomics*. Metabolomics is the systematic identification and quantification of all metabolites in a given organism or biological sample. Analytical platforms such as ^{1}H nuclear magnetic resonance and liquid chromatography or gas chromatography coupled to mass spectrometry, in conjunction with chemometric and multivariate data analysis, allow the simultaneous determination and comparison of thousands of chemicals in biological fluids such as serum and urine, as well as the chemical constituents of cells and tissues. This technology can be a screen for drug toxicity in whole-animal systems during preclinical drug development and can obviate the need for time-consuming and expensive necropsies and pathologies on thousands of animals.

Using metabolomics, animals, either treated or not treated with a drug candidate, can be analyzed for the presence of one or more metabolites in urine that correlate with drug efficacy or toxicity. Urine metabolites that are fingerprints for liver, kidney, and CNS toxicity have been identified using known chemical toxicants. Metabolic fingerprints of specific compounds that are elevated in urine can be used to determine, in dose escalation studies, whether a particular drug causes toxicity and can also be employed in early clinical trials to monitor for potential toxicities. Metabolomics can be used to find biomarkers for drug efficacy and toxicity that can be of value in clinical trials to identify responders and nonresponders. Drug metabolism can be studied in whole-animal model systems and in humans to determine the metabolites of a drug or indicate the presence of a polymorphism in drug metabolism that might signal an adverse clinical outcome. Finally, biomarkers developed from experimental metabolomics could eventually be developed for routine monitoring for signs of toxicity in patients receiving pharmacotherapy.

Bibliography

FitzGerald GA, et al. Molecular clocks and the human condition: approaching their characterization in human physiology and disease. *Diabetes Obes Metab*, **2015**, *17*:139–142.

Hayes JD, et al. Glutathione transferases. *Annu Rev Pharmacol Toxicol*, **2005**, *45*:51–88.

Huttenen KM, et al. Prodrugs-from serendipity to rational design. *Pharmacol Rev*, **2011**, *63*:750–71.

Kodani S, Hammock BD. Epoxide hydrolases: drug metabolism to therapeutics for chronic pain. *Drug Metab Dispos*, **2015**, *43*:788–802.

Lopez-Vicario C, et al. Inhibition of soluble epoxide hydrolase modulates inflammation and autophagy in obese adipose tissue and liver. Role for omega-3 epoxides. *Proc Natl Acad Sci USA*, **2015**, *112*:536–541.

Meisel P. Arylamine *N*-acetyltransferases and drug response. *Pharmacogenomics*, **2002**, *3*:349–366.

Rowland A, et al. The UDP-glucuronosyltransferases: their role in drug metabolism and detoxification. *Int J Biochem Cell Biol*, **2013**, *45*:1121–1132.

Strassburg CP. Pharmacogenetics of Gilbert's syndrome. *Pharmacogenomics*, **2008**, *9*:703–715.

Tibbs ZE, et al. Structural plasticity in the human cytosolic sulfotransferase dimer and its role in substrate selectivity and catalysis. *Drug Metab Pharmacokinet*, **2015**, *30*:3–20.

Townsend DM, Tew KD. The role of glutathione-*S*-transferase in anticancer drug resistance. *Oncogene*, **2003**, *22*:7369–7375.

Tukey RH, et al. Pharmacogenomics of human UDP-glucuronosyltransferases and irinotecan toxicity. *Mol Pharmacol*, **2002**, *62*:446–450.

Chapter 7

Pharmacogenetics

Dan M. Roden

It is a given that patients vary in their responses to drug therapy. Some patients derive striking and sustained benefits from drug administration; others may display no benefit, and still others display mild, severe, or even fatal adverse drug reactions (ADRs). Common sources of such variability include noncompliance, medication errors, drug interactions (see Chapter 4 and Appendix I), and genetic factors. *Pharmacogenetics* is the study of the genetic basis for variation in drug response and often implies large effects of a small number of DNA variants. *Pharmacogenomics*, on the other hand, studies larger numbers of variants, in an individual or across a population, to explain the genetic component of variable drug responses. Discovering which variants or combinations of variants have functional consequences for drug effects, validating those discoveries, and ultimately applying them to patient care and to drug discovery are the tasks of modern pharmacogenetics and pharmacogenomics.

Importance of Pharmacogenetics to Variability in Drug Response

An individual's response to a drug depends on the complex interplay among environmental factors (e.g., diet, age, infections, other drugs, exercise level, occupation, exposure to toxins, and tobacco and alcohol use) and genetic factors. Genetic variation may result in altered protein sequence and function or in altered protein levels through regulatory variation. Key genes involved in driving variable drug actions include those encoding drug-metabolizing enzymes, drug transport molecules, the molecular targets with which drugs interact, and a host of other genes that modulate the molecular context within which drugs act, notably genes dysregulated in the disease for which the drug is administered. In some situations, variation in nongermline genomes (e.g., in cancers or in infectious agents) can be critical determinants of variable drug responses.

Drug metabolism is highly heritable, as assessed using drug exposures in monozygotic versus fraternal twins, drug exposures in cell lines from related subjects, or analysis of very large data sets using technologies such as genome-wide genotyping, discussed further in this chapter. Twin studies suggested that up to 75% of the variability in elimination half-lives for metabolized drugs can be heritable. Some drug metabolism traits behave in a conventional "monogenic" fashion with three clearly definable (and separable) groups of drug response phenotypes: heterozygotes as well as major and minor allele homozygotes. The study of these types of responses has helped define key genetic variants that contribute to the striking variability in responses described in this chapter. However, large effect size single variants are the exception, and for many (most) drug responses, the genetic component of variable responses—although substantial—likely reflects interacting influences of many genetic variants. A major challenge to the field is to accrue large numbers of subjects with well-phenotyped drug responses to enable discovery, and subsequent replication and validation, of multigene effects or of interactions of gene(s) with environmental factors.

Principles of Pharmacogenetics

Phenotype-Driven Terminology

A trait (e.g., the CYP2D6 "poor metabolizer" [PM], as opposed to "extensive metabolizer" [EM]) may be apparent only with nonfunctional alleles on both the maternal and the paternal chromosomes. If the gene is on a nonsex chromosome, the trait is autosomal. The nonfunctional alleles may be the same; the trait is then termed *autosomal recessive*, or different, in which case the subject is a *compound heterozygote*. A trait is deemed *codominant* if heterozygotes exhibit a phenotype that is intermediate to that of homozygotes for the common allele and homozygotes for the variant allele. Many polymorphic traits (e.g., CYP2C19 metabolism of drugs such as clopidogrel and omeprazole) are now recognized to exhibit some degree of codominance; as a result, heterozygotes exhibit metabolizing activity that is intermediate between that of EM and PM subjects.

In some instances, such as clopidogrel, codeine, and irinotecan (described further in this chapter), variants in a single gene produce clearly defined and clinically important differences in drug response. However, these high effect size examples are the exception for two reasons. First, even within a single gene, a vast array of polymorphisms (promoter, coding, noncoding, completely inactivating, or modestly modifying) is possible. Each polymorphism may produce a different effect on gene function and therefore differentially affect a measured trait. Second, even if the designations of recessive, codominant, and dominant are informative for a given gene, their utility in describing the genetic variability that underlies variability in drug response phenotype is diminished because variability is often multigenic.

Types of Genetic Variants

The major types of sequence variation are *single-nucleotide polymorphisms* (SNPs, sometimes termed *single-nucleotide variants,* SNVs), and *insertions or deletions*, which can range in size from a single nucleotide to an entire

Abbreviations

ABCB1: multidrug resistance transporter (P-glycoprotein)
ACE: angiotensin-converting enzyme
ADR: adverse drug reaction
AUC: area under the curve
CBS: cystathionine β-synthase
CF: cystic fibrosis
CNV: copy number variation
cSNP: coding SNP
CYP: cytochrome P450
EGFR: epidermal growth factor receptor
EMR: electronic medical record
FDA: U.S. Food and Drug Administration
FH: familial hypercholesterolemia
GI: gastrointestinal
G6PD: glucose-6-phosphate dehydrogenase
GST: glutathione-*S*-transferase
GSTM1: glutathione-*S*-transferase M1
GWAS: genome-wide association study
HIV: human immunodeficiency virus
HMG-CoA: 3-hydroxy-3-methylglutaryl coenzyme A
5HT: 5-hydroxytryptamine, serotonin
indels: insertions or deletions
INR: international normalized ratio
iPSC: induced pluripotent stem cell
LDL: low-density lipoprotein
MAF: minor allele frequency
MDR1: multidrug resistance protein 1
mRNA: messenger RNA
MTHFR: methylenetetrahydrofolate reductase
nsSNP: nonsynonymous SNP
PharmGKB: Pharmacogenomics Knowledgebase
PheWAS: phenome-wide association study
PM: poor metabolizer
RCT: randomized clinical trial
SNP: single-nucleotide polymorphism
SNV: single-nucleotide variant
sSNP: synonymous or sense SNP
TPMT: thiopurine methyltransferase
TYMS: thymidylate synthase
UDP: uridine diphosphate
UGT: UDP-glucuronosyltransferase
UTR: untranslated region
VKORC1: vitamin K epoxide reductase

SNPs

Single-nucleotide polymorphisms

Coding, nonsynonymous
e.g., *TPMT*3A*

```
Pro
CCG
| • |
CAG
Gln
```

Coding, synonymous
e.g., *ABCB1 C3435T*

```
Pro
CCG
| | •
CCA
Pro
```

Noncoding (promoter, intronic)
e.g., *CYP3A5*3*

```
GAGCATTCT
| | • | | | | | |
GATCATTCT
```

Indels

Insertions/Deletions

e.g., 68 bp Insertion in *CBS*,   (TA)₇ TAA
e.g., TA repeat in *UGT1A1*   (TA)₆ TAA

CNVs

Copy number variations

Gene Duplications

e.g., *CYP2D6*, up to 13 copies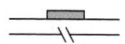

Large Deletions

e.g., entire *GSTT1* and *GSTM1*

Figure 7–1 *Molecular mechanisms of genetic polymorphisms.* The most common genetic variants are SNP substitutions. Coding nonsynonymous SNPs result in a nucleotide substitution that changes the amino acid codon (here proline to glutamine), which could change protein structure, stability, or substrate affinities or introduce a stop codon. Coding synonymous SNPs do not change the amino acid codon but may have functional consequences (transcript stability, splicing). Noncoding SNPs may be in promoters, introns, or other regulatory regions that may affect transcription factor binding, enhancers, transcript stability, or splicing. The second major type of polymorphism is indels. SNP indels can have any of the same effects as SNP substitutions: short repeats in the promoter (which can affect transcript amount) or indels that add or subtract amino acids. CNVs involve large segments of genomic DNA that may involve gene duplications (stably transmitted inherited germline gene replication that causes increased protein expression and activity), gene deletions that result in the complete lack of protein production, or inversions of genes that may disrupt gene function. All of these mechanisms have been implicated in common germline pharmacogenetic polymorphisms.

---

chromosome; smaller ones are generally termed *indels*, and larger ones are designated CNVs. SNPs are much more common than indels or CNVs (Figure 7–1). The term *polymorphism* was formerly applied to variants occurring at a frequency greater than 1%. However, the application of genome sequencing to large numbers of subjects has made it clear that each individual has more than 10 million sites across their genome at which they differ from some reference sequence (i.e., ~ 1 variant per 1000 base pairs). While some of these are "common" (>1% frequency), the vast majority are much rarer. For rare variants clearly associated with a genetic disease, the term *mutation* may also be used, but distinguishing between a very rare variant and a mutation may be difficult. Publically available web-based databases (e.g., http://gnomad.broadinstitute.org) aggregate sequence data in tens of thousands of subjects and highlight that MAFs may vary strikingly across ancestries (discussed later), and that for the vast majority of variants is much less than 1%.

The SNPs in the coding region are termed *cSNPs* and are further classified as *nonsynonymous* (changing the encoded amino acid sequence) or *synonymous* (or *sense*, with no amino acid change). A nucleotide substitution in an nsSNP that changes the amino acid codon (e.g., proline [CCG] to glutamine [CAG]) can as a result change protein structure, stability, or substrate affinities. There are 64 trinucleotide codons and only 20 amino acids, so multiple codons encode the same amino acid. Often, substitutions of the third base pair, termed the *wobble position*, in a codon with 3 base pairs, such as the G-to-A substitution in proline (CCG → CCA), do not alter the encoded amino acid. Up to about 10% of SNPs display more than two possible alleles (e.g., a C can be replaced by either an A or a G), so that the same polymorphic site can be associated with amino acid substitutions in some alleles but not others. As discussed in the material that follows, assessing the functional consequences of nsSNPs

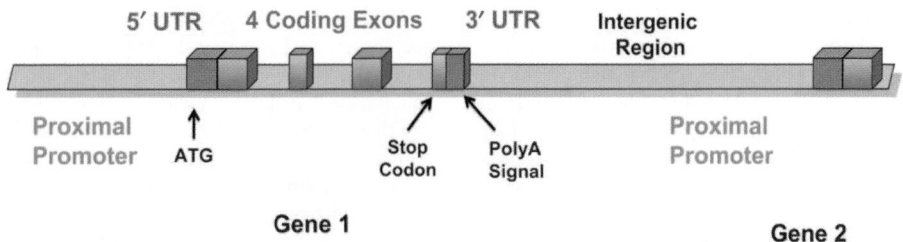

Figure 7–2 *Nomenclature of genomic regions.*

can be challenging. SNPs that introduce a premature stop codon, and small indels in a coding region that disrupt the open reading frame and thereby introduce abnormal 3′ protein sequences often with early stop codons, are termed *nonsense* variants, and these are thought to be most likely to display abnormal protein function.

Synonymous polymorphisms have been reported to contribute to a phenotypic trait. One example is a polymorphism in *ABCB1*, which encodes MDR1 (also termed P-glycoprotein), an efflux pump that interacts with many clinically used drugs. In *MDR1*, a synonymous polymorphism, C3435T, is associated with various phenotypes, and some evidence indicates that the one of the resulting mRNAs is translated at a slower rate, thereby altering folding of the protein, its insertion into the membrane, and thus its interaction with drugs (Kimchi-Sarfaty et al., 2007).

The vast majority (>97%–99%) of human DNA is noncoding, and the regulatory functions of noncoding sequences are only now being defined. Polymorphisms in noncoding regions may occur in the 3′ and 5′ untranslated regions, in promoter or enhancer regions, in intronic regions, or in large regions between genes, intergenic regions (for nomenclature guide, see Figure 7–2). Noncoding SNPs in promoter or enhancer sequences are thought to alter DNA binding by regulatory proteins to affect transcription. 3′ SNPs may alter binding of microRNAs that affect transcript stability. Noncoding SNPs may also create alternative intron-exon splicing sites, and the altered transcript may have fewer or more exons, or shorter or longer exons, than the wild-type transcript. Large consortia are defining the functions of noncoding DNA: The ENCODE project identifies functional elements (enhancers, promoters, etc.) in genome sequences; and GTEx relates genome sequence variation to tissue-specific variability in gene expression (ENCODE Project Consortium, 2012; GTEx Consortium, 2015).

Like SNPs, indels can be short repeats in the promoter (which can affect transcript amount) or insertions/deletions that add or subtract amino acids in the coding region. The number of TA repeats in the *UGT1A1* promoter affects the quantitative expression of this important glucuronosyltransferase in liver; the most common allele has six repeats and the seven-repeat variant (*UGT1A1*28*) decreases *UGT1A1* expression. The frequency of the *28 allele is up to 30%, with up to 10% of subjects (depending on ancestry) being homozygous. Decreased *UGT1A1* transcription can modulate drug actions as described further in the chapter and also accounts for a common form of mild hyperbilirubinemia (Gilbert syndrome; see Table 6–3 and Figure 6–7).

The CNVs appear to occur in about 10% of the human genome and in one study accounted for about 18% of the detected genetic variation in expression of about 15,000 genes in lymphoblastoid cell lines (Stranger et al., 2007). The ultrarapid CYP2D6 metabolizer phenotype arises as a result of *CYP2D6* duplication(s), and individuals with more than 10 functional copies of the gene have been described. A common *GSTM1* polymorphism is caused by a large (50-kb) deletion, and the null allele has a population frequency of 30%–50%. Biochemical studies indicated that livers from homozygous null individuals have only about 50% of the glutathione-conjugating capacity of those with at least one copy of the *GSTM1* gene.

A *haplotype*—a series of alleles found at a linked locus on a chromosome—specifies the DNA sequence variation in a gene or a gene region on one chromosome. For example, consider two SNPs in *ABCB1*. One SNP is a T-to-A base-pair substitution at position 3421, and the other is a C-to-T change at position 3435. Possible haplotypes would be $T_{3421}C_{3435}$, $T_{3421}T_{3435}$, $A_{3421}C_{3435}$, and $A_{3421}T_{3435}$. For any gene, individuals will have two haplotypes, one maternal and one paternal in origin. A haplotype represents the constellation of variants that occur together for the gene on each chromosome. In some cases, this constellation of variants, rather than the individual variant or allele, may be functionally important. In others, however, a single variant may be functionally important regardless of other linked variants within the haplotype(s).

Linkage disequilibrium is the term used to describe the situation in which genotypes at the two loci are not independent of one another. With complete linkage disequilibrium, genotype at one site is a perfect predictor of genotype at the linked site. Patterns of linkage disequilibrium are population specific, and as recombination occurs, linkage disequilibrium between two alleles will decay and linkage equilibrium will result. Linkage disequilibrium has been enabling for genome-wide association studies because genotyping at a small number of SNPs ("tag SNPs") in linkage disequilibrium with many others can capture common variation across regions.

Ancestral Diversity

Polymorphisms differ in their frequencies within human populations and have been classified as either cosmopolitan or population (or race and ethnic) specific. *Cosmopolitan polymorphisms* are those polymorphisms present in all ethnic groups and are likely to be ancient, having arisen before migrations of humans from Africa, although present-day frequencies may differ among ancestral groups. The presence of *ancestry-specific polymorphisms* is consistent with geographical isolation of human populations. These polymorphisms probably arose in isolated populations and then reached a certain frequency because they are either advantageous in some way (positive selection) or neutral to a population. Individuals descended from multiple ancestries may display haplotype structures and allele frequencies intermediate between their parents. In the U.S., African Americans have the highest number of population-specific polymorphisms (and the smallest haplotype blocks) in comparison to European Americans, Mexican Americans, and Asian Americans.

Pharmacogenetic Study Design Considerations

There are many important considerations for the conduct of an experiment designed to identify sources of genetic variation contributing to variable drug responses. These include material to be studied (e.g., cells, organs, human subjects); the subjects' genetic backgrounds; the presence of confounders such as diet or variable experimental conditions; the selection of variants to be studied (ranging from a single high-likelihood candidate SNP to "agnostic" approaches that interrogate the whole genome); the methods used for genotyping and quality control; statistical analysis considerations, including effect size estimates and consideration of ancestry; and replication of findings.

Pharmacogenetic Traits

A *pharmacogenetic trait* is any measurable or discernible trait associated with a drug. Some traits reflect the beneficial or adverse effect of a drug in a patient; lowering of blood pressure or reduction in tumor size are examples. These have the disadvantage that they reflect many genetic and nongenetic influences, but the advantage that they indicate a drug's clinical effects. Other traits represent drug response "endophenotypes," measures that may more directly reflect the action of a drug in a biologic system and thus be more amenable to genetic study but may be removed from the whole patient or a whole population. Examples of the latter include enzyme activity, drug or metabolite levels in plasma or urine, or drug-induced changes in gene expression patterns.

A variant drug metabolizer phenotype can be inferred from genotype data or in some cases directly measured by administering a "probe drug" (one thought to be metabolized by a single pathway) and measuring drug and metabolite concentrations. For example, one method to determine *CYP2D6* metabolizer status is to measure the urinary ratio of parent drug to metabolite after a single oral dose of the *CYP2D6* substrate dextromethorphan. Similarly, mephenytoin can be used as a probe drug for *CYP2C19* metabolizer phenotype. An important caveat is that other drugs can interfere with this assessment: If dextromethorphan is given with a potent inhibitor of CYP2D6, such as quinidine or fluoxetine, the phenotype may be consistent with or a "phenocopy of" the poor metabolizer genotype, even though the subject carries wild-type *CYP2D6* alleles. In this case, the assignment of a *CYP2D6* poor metabolizer phenotype would not be accurate. Another pharmacogenetic endophenotype, the erythromycin breath test (for CYP3A activity), can sometimes be unstable within a subject, indicating that the phenotype is highly influenced by nongenetic or multigenic factors. *Most pharmacogenetic traits are multigenic rather than monogenic* (Figure 7–3), and considerable effort is being made to identify the important polymorphisms that influence variability in drug response.

Genotyping

Most genotyping methods use DNA extracted from somatic, diploid cells, usually white blood cells or buccal cells. This "germline" DNA is extremely stable if appropriately extracted and stored, and the DNA sequence is generally (but likely not totally) invariant throughout an individual's lifetime. Any genotyping result should be subject to standard and rigorous quality control, which may include inspection of source genotyping experimental data, exclusion of SNPs with a high genotyping failure rate, exclusion of

subjects in which many SNP analyses failed, assessment of Hardy-Weinberg equilibrium, and ensuring the absence of important substructure (e.g., many related individuals) in a general population study. *Hardy-Weinberg* equilibrium is maintained when mating within a population is random and there is no natural selection effect on the variant. Such assumptions are described mathematically when the proportions of the population that are observed to be homozygous for the variant genotype (q^2), homozygous for the wild-type genotype (p^2), and heterozygous ($2*p*q$) are not significantly different from that predicted from the overall allele frequencies (p = frequency of wild-type allele; q = frequency of variant allele) in the population. A deviation from Hardy-Weinberg equilibrium (i.e., from the rule that $p^2 + 2pq + q^2 = 1$) suggests a specific survival disadvantage for a particular genotype or a genotyping or other experimental error.

Candidate Gene Versus Genome-Wide Approaches

A candidate gene study uses what is known about a drug (e.g., its metabolism, transport, or mechanism of action) to test the hypothesis that variants in the underlying genes account for variable drug response phenotypes. Variants may be chosen because they are common, known (or thought) to be functional, or tag haplotype blocks. After assays are developed for a set of such variants, statistical methods are used to relate genotype to phenotype. There are several databases that contain information on polymorphisms in human genes (Table 7–1); these databases allow the investigator to search by gene for reported polymorphisms. Some of the databases, such as PharmGKB, include phenotypic as well as genotypic data.

Large-Scale "Agnostic" Approaches

While the candidate gene approach has the intuitive appeal that known drug response pathways are studied, it has the drawback of looking only in regions of known biologic activity. Indeed, candidate genetic studies for susceptibility to common diseases have a remarkably high rate of failure to replicate, and this has been attributed to naïveté about the polygenic nature of most traits, small sizes with underpowering, and a "winner's curse" in which only positive results are published (Ioannidis et al., 2001). It has been argued that, unlike common disease studies, precedent has shown that drug responses may indeed reflect large effect sizes of a small

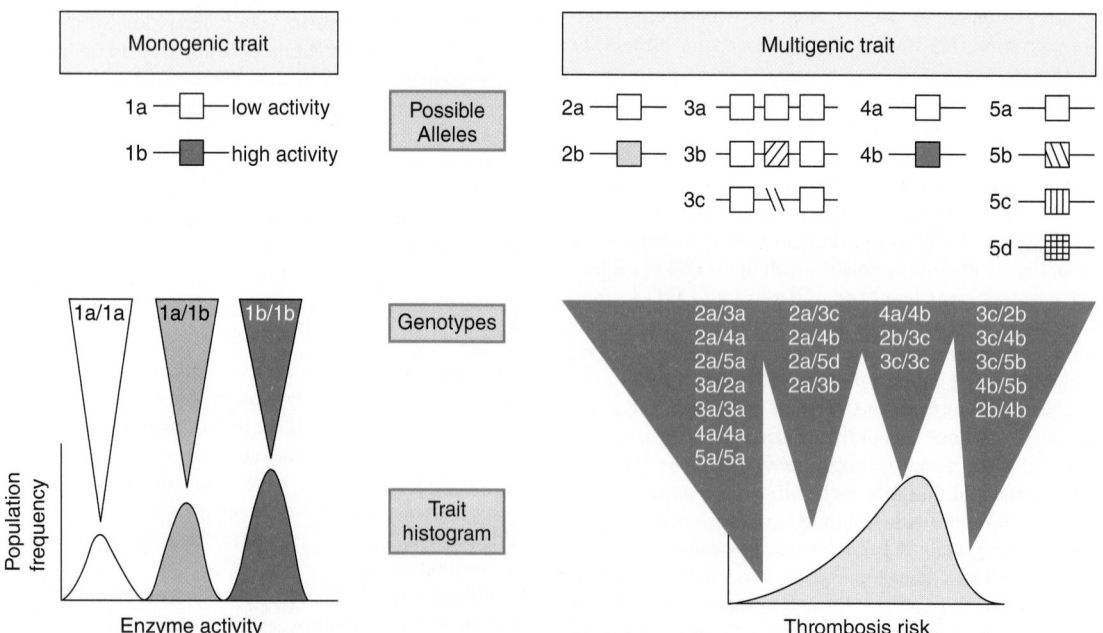

Figure 7–3 *Monogenic versus multigenic pharmacogenetic traits.* Possible alleles for a monogenic trait (*upper left*), in which a single gene has a low-activity (*1a*) and a high-activity (*1b*) allele. The population frequency distribution of a monogenic trait (*bottom left*), here depicted as enzyme activity, may exhibit a trimodal frequency distribution among low activity (homozygosity for *1a*), intermediate activity (heterozygote for *1a* and *1b*), and high activity (homozygosity for *1b*). This is contrasted with multigenic traits (e.g., an activity influenced by up to four different genes, genes 2 through 5), each of which has two, three, or four alleles (*a* through *d*). The population histogram for activity is unimodal skewed, with no distinct differences among the genotypic groups. Multiple combinations of alleles coding for low activity and high activity at several of the genes can translate into low-, medium-, and high-activity phenotypes.

TABLE 7–1 ■ DATABASES CONTAINING INFORMATION ON HUMAN GENETIC VARIATION

DATABASE NAME	URL (AGENCY)	DESCRIPTION OF CONTENTS
Pharmacogenomics Knowledgebase (PharmGKB)	www.pharmgkb.org (National Institutes of Health–sponsored research network and knowledge database)	Genotype and phenotype data related to drug response
dbSNP	www.ncbi.nlm.nih.gov/projects/SNP (National Center for Biotechnology Information [NCBI])	SNPs and frequencies
GWAS Central	www.gwascentral.org	Genotype/phenotype associations
Genome Aggregation Database	www.gnomad.broadinstitute.org	Variants identified by sequencing >120,000 exomes and >15,000 whole genomes
Online Mendelian Inheritance in Man (OMIM)	www.ncbi.nlm.nih.gov/omim	Human genes and genetic disorders
University of California Santa Cruz (UCSC) Genome Browser	http://genome.ucsc.edu	Sequence of the human genome; variant alleles
GTEx	www.gtexportal.org/home/	Genetics of gene expression
Broad Institute Software	www.broadinstitute.org/data-software-and-tools	Software tools for the analysis of genetic studies

number of genes, but these limitations should nevertheless be borne in mind in the conduct of these studies.

An alternate approach to the candidate gene approach is a GWAS, in which genotypes at more than 500,000 SNP sites (generally tagging haplotype blocks across the genome) are compared across a continuous trait or between cases and controls (e.g., those with or without a therapeutic response or an ADR). A GWAS requires large numbers of subjects, must consider the appropriate statistical approaches to minimize type I (false-positive) errors, and, if successful, identifies loci of interest that require further investigation to identify causative variants and the underlying biology. While associations identified by GWASs generally have modest effect sizes (odds ratios < 2), even with very low P values, pharmacogenetic GWASs provide some exceptions; for example, a GWAS in 51 cases of flucloxacillin-induced hepatotoxicity and 282 controls identified risk SNPs in the HLA-B locus with an odds ratio greater than 80 (Daly et al., 2009). Not all pharmacogenetic GWASs have successfully identified signals with this strength, but the approach has some promise and is increasingly used (Karnes et al., 2015; Mosley et al., 2015; Motsinger-Reif et al., 2013; Van Driest et al., 2015).

The GWAS analyses have also provided strong support for candidate gene studies that implicate variants in *CYP2C9* and *VKORC1* in warfarin dose requirement (Cooper et al., 2008; Takeuchi et al., 2009; see Figure 32–6 and Table 32–2) and variants in CYP2C19 in clopidogrel clinical response (Shuldiner et al., 2009). Newer genotyping platforms can capture both rare coding region variants and tags for common haplotype blocks, and the availability of increasing amounts of sequence data allows reasonable inferences (by a statistical method called imputation) of up to 10 million genotypes from a GWAS genotyping experiment.

While single experimental approaches can suggest a relationship between variable drug responses and a variant in a specific locus or gene, the use of multiple complementary approaches provides the strongest evidence supporting such relationships. One method is to establish that putative variants do in fact display altered function in an in vitro system, as discussed in the material that follows. Another approach is to integrate genotype data (by GWAS) with other large-scale measures of gene function, such as the abundance of mRNAs (transcriptomics) or proteins (proteomics). This has the advantage that the abundance of signal may itself directly reflect some of the relevant genetic variation. One such study identified six loci at which exposure to simvastatin in cell lines changed gene expression, and variants in one of these genes, glycine amidinotransferase, was associated with simvastatin myotoxicity in a clinical trial (Mangravite et al., 2013). However, both mRNA and protein expression are highly influenced by choice of tissue type, which may not be available; for example, it may not be feasible to obtain biopsies of brain tissue for studies of CNS toxicity. The GTEx project described previously couples whole-genome sequence to mRNA transcript levels across multiple tissues and should enable further such studies.

Large-scale coupling of genotypes to phenotypes in EMR systems with associated DNA biobanks represents another potential resource for pharmacogenomic studies. One interesting approach using such biobanks is to turn the GWAS paradigm "on its head" and to ask with what human phenotype is a particular genetic variant associated. This PheWAS can be used to replicate a GWAS result or to identify entirely new associations (Denny et al., 2013) and has been used to "repurpose" (suggest new indications for) marketed drugs (Rastegar-Mojarad et al., 2015).

Functional Studies of Polymorphisms

Once a gene or a locus modulating a drug response phenotype is identified, a major challenge is to establish which coding or regulatory variants contribute. Comparative genomics and functional studies of individual polymorphisms in vitro and in animal models are commonly used approaches. Precedents from Mendelian diseases suggest that the variants with the greatest potential effect sizes are rare nonsense variants or missense variants that drastically alter evolutionarily conserved residues. For example, studies of variants in membrane transporters and ion channels suggested that those conferring with the greatest change in function are at low allele frequencies and change an evolutionarily conserved amino acid residue. These data indicate that SNPs that alter evolutionarily conserved residues are most deleterious. For example, substitution of a charged amino acid (Arg) for a nonpolar, uncharged amino acid (Cys) is more likely to affect function than substitution of residues that are more chemically similar (e.g., Arg to Lys). The data also suggest that rare nsSNPs are more likely to alter function than common ones.

The link between Mendelian disease and variant drug responses is highlighted by the fact that one of the first pharmacogenetic examples to be discovered was G6PD deficiency, an X-linked monogenic trait that results in severe hemolytic anemia in individuals after ingestion of fava beans or various drugs, including many antimalarial agents. G6PD is normally present in red blood cells and regulates levels of the antioxidant glutathione. Antimalarials such as primaquine increase red blood cell fragility in individuals with G6PD deficiency, leading to profound hemolytic anemia; the trait is more common in African Americans. The severity of the deficiency syndrome varies among individuals and is related to the amino acid variant in G6PD. The severe form of G6PD deficiency is associated with changes at residues that are highly conserved across evolutionary history. *The information in* Table 7–2 *on genetic polymorphisms influencing drug response at the end of the chapter can be used as a guide for prioritizing polymorphisms in candidate gene association studies.*

With increasing application of exome or whole-genome sequencing in populations, millions of DNA variants are being identified, and methods to establish their function are evolving. One approach uses computational algorithms to identify potentially deleterious amino acid substitutions. Earlier methods (e.g., BLOSUM62, SIFT, and PolyPhen) use sequence comparisons across multiple species to identify and score substitutions, especially at highly conserved residues. More recent approaches use structural predictions (Kircher et al., 2014) or integrate multiple predictors (e.g., CADD). While these programs are becoming increasingly sophisticated, they have not yet reached the point that they can substitute for experimental verification.

The functional activity of amino acid variants for many proteins can be studied in isolation, in cellular assays, or in animal models. A traditional step in a cellular study of a nonsynonymous variant is to isolate the variant gene or to construct the variant by site-directed mutagenesis, express it in cells, and compare its functional activity (enzymatic activity, transport kinetics, ion channel gating, etc.) to that of the reference or most common form of the protein (Figure 7–4). Figure 7–5 shows an example of how the combination of population studies, in vitro functional assays, and in silico simulations can be integrated to identify a variant that modulates the risk of drug-induced arrhythmias.

The SNPs identified in GWASs as associated with clinical phenotypes, including drug response phenotypes, have largely been in noncoding regions. An example of profound functional effect of a noncoding SNP is provided by *CYP3A5*; a common noncoding intronic SNP in *CYP3A5* accounts for its polymorphic expression in humans. The SNP accounting for variation in CYP3A5 protein creates an alternative splice site, resulting

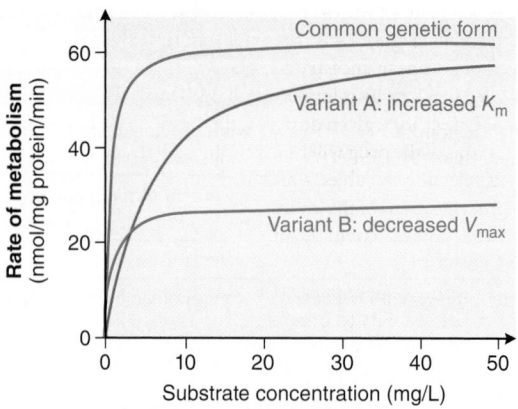

Figure 7–4 *Simulated concentration-dependence curves for the common genetic form of an enzyme and two nonsynonymous variants.* Compared to the common form of the enzyme, variant A exhibits an increased K_m, likely reflecting an altered substrate-binding site of the protein by the substituted amino acid. Variant B exhibits the same K_m as the common form but a reduced maximum rate of metabolism of the substrate (V_{max}). Because these measurements were made on cell extracts, the reduced V_{max} may be due to a reduced expression level of the enzyme. If similar data were obtained with purified protein, then the reduced activity of variant B could be ascribed to a structural alteration in the enzyme that affects its maximal catalytic rate but not its affinity for the substrate under these assay conditions.

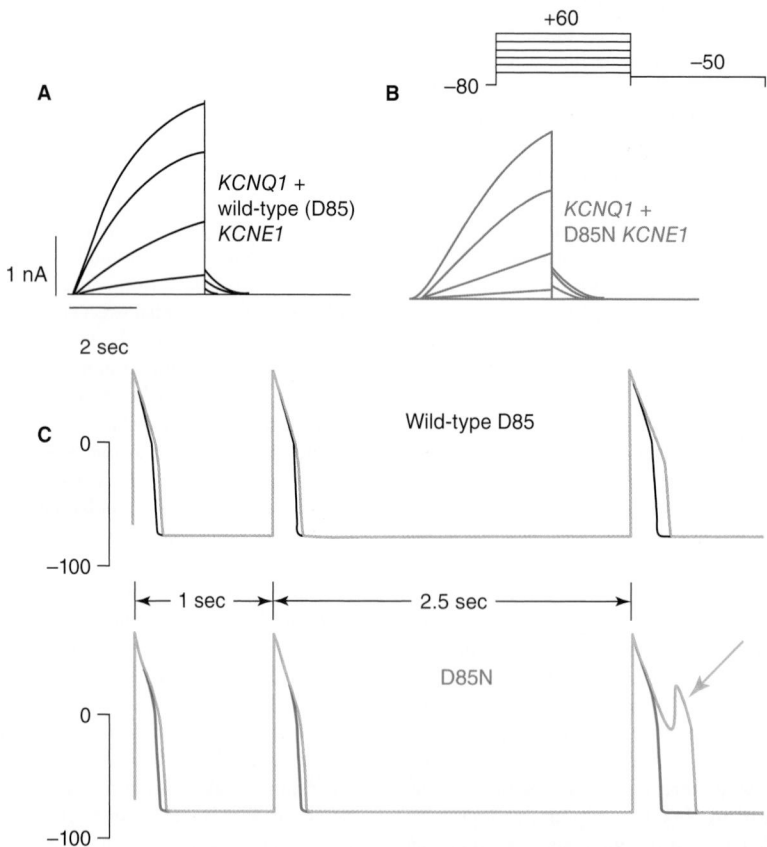

Figure 7–5 *Functional evaluation of an ion channel variant.* A population study implicated an nsSNP resulting in D85N in *KCNE1* as a modulator of the risk for arrhythmias when blockers of the KCNH2 K⁺ channel are administered to patients (Kääb et al., 2012). *KCNE1* encodes a function-modifying subunit for a different cardiac K⁺ channel (encoded by *KCNQ1*), and the ion currents generated at a range of voltages by heterologous coexpression of *KCNQ1* plus the wild-type or mutant *KCNE1* are shown in **A** and **B**, respectively. While there are subtle differences in activation kinetics and overall current amplitude, it is not clear whether these are functionally important. **C.** Results of numerical action potential simulations incorporating either the experimentally determined wild-type or variant K⁺ current. At baseline (black and green tracings), there is no difference in computed action potential duration. However, when drug block of the KCNH2 K⁺ channel is superimposed and the stimulation rate is slowed (orange tracings), an arrhythmogenic afterpotential (*arrow*) is seen with the mutant but not the wild-type *KCNE1*. Taken together, these functional data therefore provide support for the population study. (Data from Drs. Al George and Yoram Rudy.)

in not only a transcript with a larger exon 3 but also the introduction of an early stop codon (Figure 7–6). The nonfunctional allele is more common in subjects of European ancestry compared to those of African ancestry; as a result, CYP3A5 activity is lower in individuals expressing the noncoding intronic SNP (i.e., for a given dose of a drug that is a substrate of CYP3A5, concentrations of the drug will be higher in Europeans). Increased rates of transplant rejection in subjects of African descent may reflect decreased plasma concentrations of the antirejection drug tacrolimus, a substrate for CYP3A5 (the higher activity form lacking the noncoding intronic SNP) (Birdwell et al., 2012).

Two new technologies appear poised to revolutionize functional studies. The first is the ability to generate iPSCs from any individual and then use the cells to generate specific cell types (hepatocytes, cardiomyocytes, neurons, etc.), thereby enabling studies of that individual's cellular physiology. The second is rapid and efficient genome editing using CRISPR/cas9 in iPSCs or any other cell system (see Chapter 3). Multiple exciting applications of genome-editing technology, from rapid generation of genetically modified animals to curing genetic disease in humans, are being explored. Genome editing holds the promise that the function of individual coding or noncoding variants, alone or in combination, can be rapidly assessed in cellular systems.

Pharmacogenetic Phenotypes

Candidate genes for therapeutic and adverse response can be divided into three categories:

- those modifying drug disposition (*pharmacokinetic*)
- those altering the function of the molecules with which drugs interact to produce their beneficial or adverse effects (*receptor/target*)
- those altering the broad *biologic milieu* in which the drugs interact with target molecules, including the changes associated with the diseases for which the drug is being prescribed

This section summarizes important examples of each type but cannot be all inclusive. Web-based resources such as PharmGKB (Table 7–1) can be consulted for specific genes, variants, drugs, and diseases.

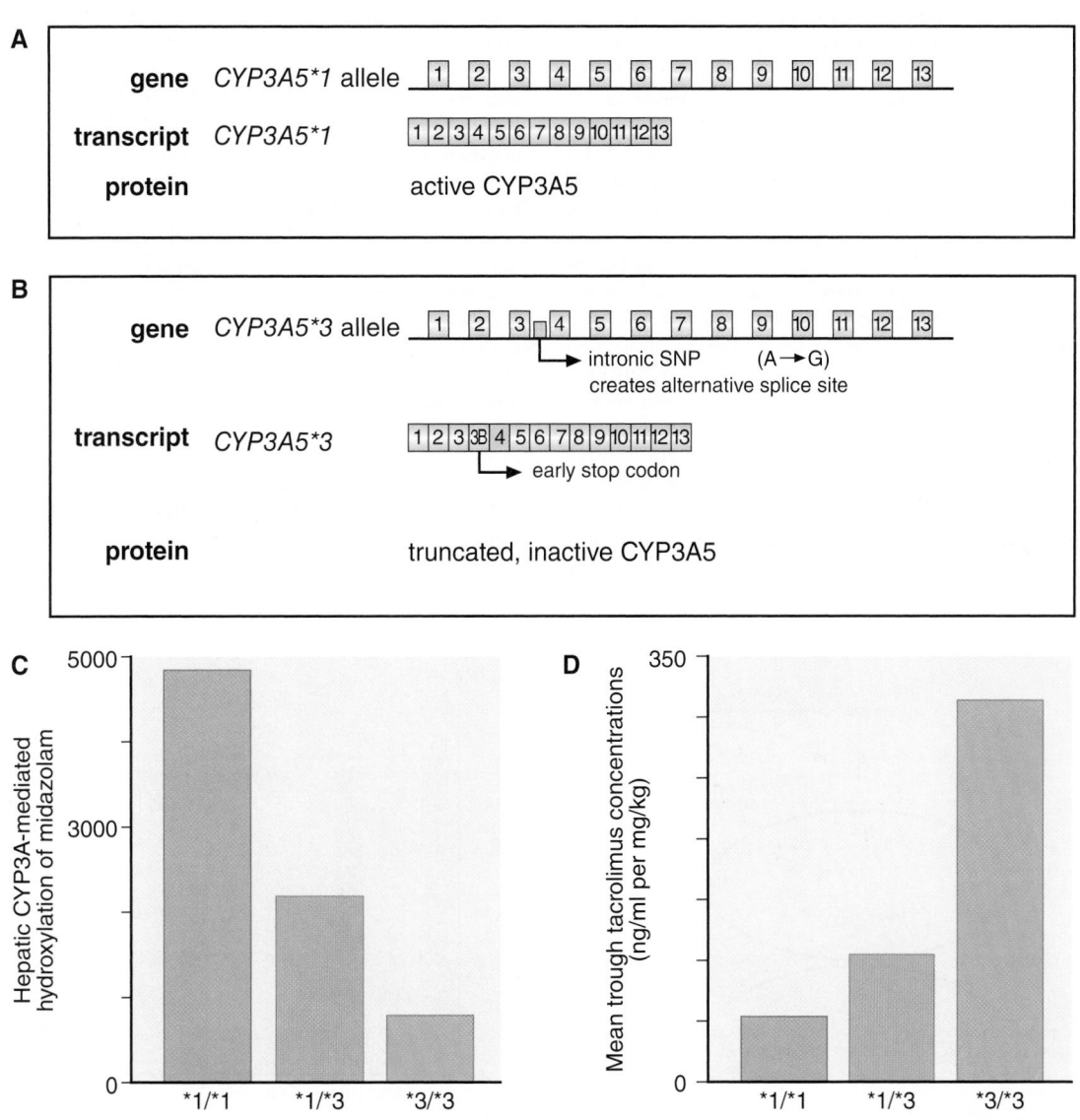

Figure 7–6 *An intronic SNP can affect splicing and account for polymorphic expression of CYP3A5.* A common polymorphism (A > G) in intron 3 of CYP3A5 defines the genotypes associated with the wild-type CYP3A5*1 allele or the variant nonfunctional CYP3A5*3 allele. This intronic SNP creates an alternative splice site that results in the production of an alternative CYP3A5 transcript carrying an additional intron 3B (**B**), with an early stop codon and truncated CYP3A5 protein. The wild-type gene (more common in African than Caucasian or Asian populations) results in production of active CYP3A5 protein (**A**); the *3 variant results in a truncated and inactive protein. Thus, metabolism of CYP3A5 substrates is diminished in vitro (**C**), and blood concentrations of such substrates (medications) are higher in vivo (**D**) for those with the *3 than the *1 allele. (Data from Haufroid et al., 2004; Kuehl et al., 2001; Lin et al., 2002.)

Pharmacokinetic Alterations

Germline variability in genes that encode determinants of the pharmacokinetics of a drug, in particular metabolizing enzymes and transporters, affect drug concentrations and are therefore major determinants of therapeutic and adverse drug response (at the end of the chapter, see Table 7–2 on genetic polymorphisms influencing drug response). A particularly high-risk situation is a drug with a narrow therapeutic margin eliminated by a single pathway: Loss of function in that pathway can lead to drastic increases in drug concentrations (and decreases in metabolite concentrations) with attendant loss of efficacy and an increased likelihood of ADRs (Roden and Stein, 2009). The loss of function can be genetic or can arise as a result of drug interactions or dysfunction of excretory organs (e.g., renal failure will elevate plasma concentrations of renally excreted drugs unless dosages are reduced).

CYP2C9-mediated metabolism of the more active *S*-enantiomer of warfarin is an example. Individuals with the loss of function *3 allele require lower steady-state warfarin dosages and are at increased risk of bleeding (Aithal et al., 1999; Kawai et al., 2014; see also Table 32–2). When multiple enzymes and transporters are involved in the pharmacokinetics of a drug, single variants are unlikely to produce large clinical effects.

Another high-risk situation is a drug that requires bioactivation to achieve pharmacological effect. Individuals with increased or decreased bioactivation, because of genetic variants or drug interactions, are at risk for variant drug responses. Clopidogrel, bioactivated by CYP2C19, and tamoxifen, bioactivated by CYP2D6, are examples (see Table 7–2 and Figure 6–3A). PM subjects homozygous for a common loss function variant in *CYP2C19* display decreased antiplatelet effects and increased stent thrombosis during clopidogrel treatment (Mega et al., 2010; Shuldiner et al., 2009). In heterozygotes (~20%) receiving clopidogrel, adequate antiplatelet effects can be achieved by increasing the dose, whereas in homozygotes (2%–3%) an alternate antiplatelet drug should be used because even large dose increases do not affect platelet function. Other loss-of-function variants (notably *3) are common in Chinese and Japanese populations. Several proton pump inhibitors, including omeprazole and lansoprazole, are inactivated by CYP2C19. Thus, PM patients have higher exposure to active parent drug, a greater pharmacodynamic effect (higher gastric pH), and a higher probability of ulcer cure than heterozygotes or homozygous wild-type individuals.

A variation on this theme is the use of codeine (a prodrug bioactivated to morphine by CYP2D6). In PMs, analgesia is absent. Perhaps more important, excess morphine is generated in ultrarapid metabolizers, and death due to respiratory arrest has been reported (Ciszkowski et al., 2009). A large number of medications (estimated at 15%–25% of all medicines in use) are substrates for CYP2D6.

The *UGT1A1*28* variant, encoding the 7-TA reduced function *UGT1A1* promoter mentioned previously, has been associated with higher levels of the active metabolite SN-38 of the cancer chemotherapeutic agent *irinotecan* (see Chapter 66), and this increased concentration has been associated with an increased risk of serious toxicities (see Figures 6–6, 6–8, and 6–9).

Drug Receptor/Target Alterations

Warfarin exerts its anticoagulant effect by interfering with the synthesis of vitamin K–dependent clotting factors, and the target molecule with which warfarin interacts to exert this effect is encoded by *VKORC1*, an enzyme in the vitamin K cycle (Figure 7–7). Rare coding region variants in the gene lead to partial or complete warfarin resistance; interestingly, these variants are common (5% allele frequency) in Ashkenazi patients and may account for high dosage requirements in carrier subjects. The *VKORC1* promoter includes common variants that strongly modulate its expression; in subjects with reduced expression, lower steady-state warfarin doses are required. These variants are more common in Asian subjects than in Caucasians or Africans. Inherited variation in *CYP2C9* and *VKORC1* account for more than 50% of the variability in warfarin doses needed to achieve the desired coagulation level. *VKORC1* is one example of how both rare and common variants in genes encoding drug targets can exert important effects on drug actions.

In some instances, highly penetrant variants with profound functional consequences may cause disease phenotypes that confer negative selective pressure; more subtle variations in the same genes can be maintained in the population without causing disease but nonetheless causing variation in drug response. For example, rare loss-of-function mutations in MTHFR cause severe mental retardation, cardiovascular disease, and a shortened life span. Conversely, the 677C→T SNP causes an amino acid substitution that is maintained in the population at a high frequency (40% allele frequency in most white populations) and is associated with modestly lower MTHFR activity (~30% less than the 677C allele) and modest but significantly elevated plasma homocysteine concentrations (~25% higher). This polymorphism does not alter drug pharmacokinetics but does appear to modulate pharmacodynamics by

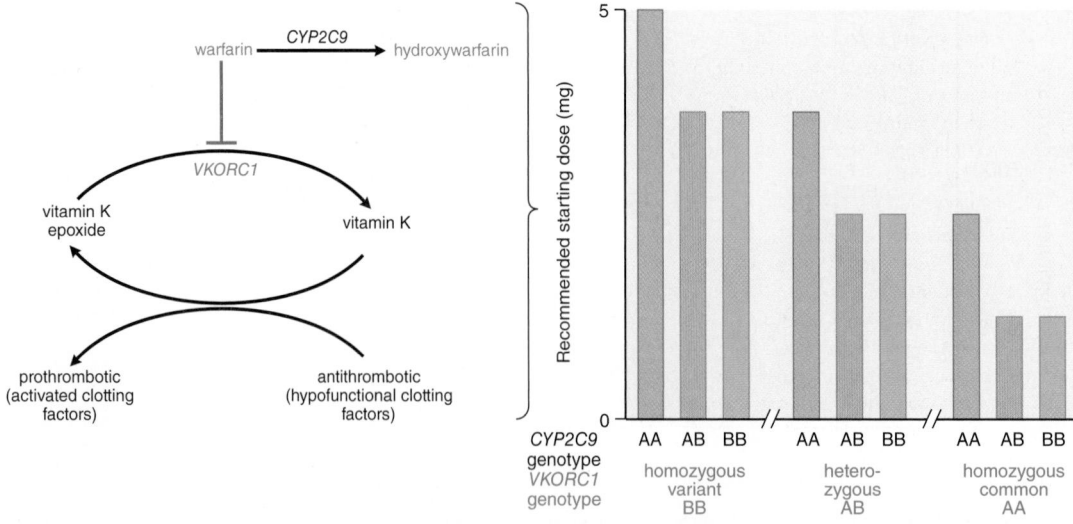

Figure 7–7 *Pharmacogenetics of warfarin dosing.* Warfarin is metabolized by *CYP2C9* to inactive metabolites and exerts its anticoagulant effect partly via inhibition of *VKORC1*, an enzyme necessary for reduction of inactive to active vitamin K. Common polymorphisms in both genes, *CYP2C9* and *VKORC1*, have an effect on warfarin pharmacokinetics and pharmacodynamics, respectively, to affect the population mean therapeutic doses of warfarin necessary to maintain the desired degree of anticoagulation (often measured by the INR blood test) and minimize the risk of too little anticoagulation (thrombosis) or too much anticoagulation (bleeding). See also Figure 32–6 and Table 32–2. (Data from Caraco et al., 2008; Schwarz et al., 2008; Wen et al., 2008.)

predisposing to GI toxicity to the antifolate drug methotrexate in stem cell transplant recipients.

Like warfarin, methotrexate's clinical effects are dependent on a number of polymorphisms affecting metabolism, transport, drug modifiers, and drug targets. Several of the direct targets (dihydrofolate reductase, purine transformylases, and TYMS) are also subject to common polymorphisms. A polymorphic indel in *TYMS* (two vs. three repeats of a 28–base pair sequence in the enhancer) affects the amount of enzyme expression in both normal and tumor cells. The *TYMS* polymorphism can affect both toxicity and efficacy of anticancer agents (e.g., fluorouracil and methotrexate) that target TYMS. Thus, the genetic contribution to variability in the pharmacokinetics and pharmacodynamics of methotrexate cannot be understood without assessing genotypes at a number of different loci.

Other examples of drug target variants affecting drug response are presented in Table 7–2 at the end of the chapter. Serotonin receptor polymorphisms have been implicated as predictors of responsiveness to antidepressants and of the overall risk of depression. β adrenergic receptor polymorphisms have been linked to asthma responsiveness, changes in renal function following ACE inhibitors, sinus heart rate following β blockers, and the incidence of atrial fibrillation during β blocker therapy. The degree of lowering of LDL by statins has been linked to polymorphisms in HMG-CoA reductase, the statin target (see Chapter 31). Ion channel polymorphisms have been linked by both candidate gene and exome sequencing approaches to a risk of cardiac arrhythmias in the presence and absence of drug triggers (Kääb et al., 2012; Weeke et al., 2014).

Modifiers of the Biologic Milieu

The *MTHFR* polymorphism is linked to homocysteinemia, which in turn affects thrombosis risk. The risk of drug-induced thrombosis is dependent not only on the use of prothrombotic drugs but also on environmental and genetic predisposition to thrombosis, which may be affected by germline polymorphisms in *MTHFR*, factor V, and prothrombin. These polymorphisms do not directly act on the pharmacokinetics or pharmacodynamics of prothrombotic drugs such as glucocorticoids, estrogens, and asparaginase but may modify the risk of the phenotypic event (thrombosis) in the presence of the drug. Likewise, polymorphisms in ion channels (e.g., *KCNQ1, KCNE1, KCNE2*) that are not themselves the targets of drugs that prolong QT intervals may affect the duration of the baseline QT interval and the overall risk of cardiac arrhythmias; this may in turn increase risk of long QT arrhythmias seen with antiarrhythmics and a number of other "noncardiovascular" drugs (e.g., macrolide antibiotics, antihistamines).

Cancer as a Special Case

Cancer appears to be a disease of genomic instability. In addition to the underlying variation in the germline of the host, tumor cells exhibit somatically acquired mutations, some of which generate mutant protein kinases that are drivers for the development of cancer. Thus, tumor sequencing is becoming standard of care for choosing among anticancer drugs in certain settings (see Chapters 65–68).

For example, patients with lung cancer with activating mutations in *EGFR*, encoding the epidermal growth factor receptor, display increased responses to the EGFR inhibitor gefitinib (Maemondo et al., 2010). Thus, the EGFR is altered, and patients with the activating mutation have, in treatment terms, a distinct pharmacogenetic category of lung cancer. The Her2 antibody trastuzumab can produce cardiomyopathy in all exposed patients. Patients with breast cancer whose tumors express the Her2 antigen may benefit from trastuzumab, whereas those whose tumors do not express Her2 do not benefit but are nevertheless susceptible to cardiomyopathy. Similarly, only patients with melanoma whose tumors express the mutant BRAF V600E respond to vemurafinib; interestingly, vemurafinib may also be effective in other tumors (thyroid cancer, hairy cell leukemia) that express BRAF V600E. Some genetic alterations affect both tumor and host: The presence of two instead of three copies of a *TYMS* enhancer repeat polymorphism not only increases the risk of host toxicity but also increases the chance of tumor susceptibility to TYMS inhibitors (Evans and McLeod, 2003).

Genomics as a Pathway to Identification of New Drug Targets

The identification of genetic pathways in normal physiology and in disease can provide important clues to new drug targets. Seminal studies of patients with the rare disease FH identified HMG-CoA reductase as the key rate-limiting enzyme in LDL cholesterol biosynthesis; now, inhibitors of that enzyme (the statins) are among the most effective and widely used medications in cardiovascular therapy (see Chapter 33). PCSK9 contributes to the degradation of LDL receptors, which are responsible for removing LDL cholesterol from the circulation; an increase in PCSK9 activity results in reduction of LDL receptor function and an increase in LDL cholesterol. One rare cause of FH is gain-of-function mutations in *PCSK9*. Conversely, work in the Dallas Heart Study showed that individuals carrying nonsense mutations in *PCSK9* had lower LDL cholesterol values and decreased risk for coronary artery disease compared to noncarriers (Cohen et al., 2006). This result, in turn, identified PCSK9 as a potential drug target. In 2015, two antibodies that target PCSK9, alirocumab and evolocumab, were approved by the FDA for clinical use in FH and other lipid disorders. These PCSK9 inhibitors prevent degradation of LDL receptors and enhance their recycling to the hepatocyte membrane, thereby facilitating removal of LDL cholesterol and lowering blood LDL cholesterol levels (see Figure 33–4).

In a similar fashion, new drug targets have been identified by work showing that rare loss-of-function variants in *APOC3* lower triglycerides and reduce the risk of coronary artery disease (Stitziel et al., 2014), and loss-of-function variants in *SLC30A8* reduce risk for type 2 diabetes (Flannick et al., 2014). Patients homozygous for *SCN9A* loss-of-function variants are pain insensitive (Cox et al., 2006); inhibitors of SCN9A might be useful analgesics. Hundreds of mutations in the chloride transporter encoded by CFTR cause CF, but through diverse mechanisms. Ivacaftor partially corrects abnormal gating of certain rare variants of CFTR (G551D and others), while lumacaftor improves cell surface expression of the most common variant, ΔF508. Ivacaftor (Ramsey et al., 2011) and the ivacaftor/lumacaftor combination (Wainwright et al., 2015) improve symptoms and outcomes in patients with CF; both agents have now been approved in genotyped patients.

Pharmacogenetics in Clinical Practice

The increasing understanding of genetic contributors to variable drug actions raises questions of how these data might be used by healthcare providers to choose among drugs, doses, and dosing regimens. One approach is point-of-care testing, in which genotyping is ordered at the time of drug prescription; platforms that reliably deliver relevant genotypes rapidly (often in less than an hour) now make such approaches feasible. However, one difficulty in this approach is that each drug requires a separate assay. An alternate approach envisions genotyping at multiple loci relevant for responses to large numbers of drugs, embedding this information in each patient's EMR, and using clinical decision support to advise on drug selection and dosing when a relevant drug is prescribed to a patient with a variant genotype. This approach is being tested in a number of "early adopter" sites (Pulley et al., 2012; Rasmussen-Torvik et al., 2014).

There are several barriers that must be addressed if such an approach is to become widely adopted. First, the evidence linking a variant to a variable drug response must be solid, the variable outcome must be clinically important, and some form of genetically guided advice should be provided (choose another drug, choose another dose, etc.). Drug gene pairs such as *CYP2C19*2*/clopidogrel or *CYP2C9*3*/warfarin may fall into this category; the Clinical Pharmacogenomics Implementation Consortium provides guidelines on such advice by genotype across multiple drugs (Relling and Klein, 2011). Second, the strength of the evidence supporting a genotype-specific prescribing strategy varies. The strongest level of evidence comes from RCTs, in which a clinically important, genotype-guided treatment strategy is compared to a standard of care. Using this approach, genotyping for HLA-B5701 has been shown to eliminate the risk for severe skin reactions (such as the Stevens-Johnson syndrome) during treatment with the antiretroviral agent abacavir (Mallal et al., 2008). A number of trials have studied the utility of genotyping for *CYP2C9* and *VKORC1* variants during warfarin therapy. The main outcome metric has been duration of drug exposure in therapeutic range during the first 30–90 days of therapy; the results have been inconsistent, with none showing a huge effect (Kimmel et al., 2013; Pirmohamed et al., 2013). These studies have few bleeding events, but EMR-based case-control studies looking at this problem have implicated variants in CYP2C9 or CYP4F2 as risk alleles (Kawai et al., 2014; Roth et al., 2014). Nonrandomized study designs are weaker than RCTs, but performing RCTs to target small subsets of patients carrying uncommon variants may not be feasible.

Acknowledgment: *Mary V. Relling and Kathleen M. Giacomini contributed to this chapter in recent editions of this book. We have retained some of their text in the current edition.*

TABLE 7–2 ■ EXAMPLES OF GENETIC POLYMORPHISMS INFLUENCING DRUG RESPONSE

GENE PRODUCT (*GENE*)	DRUGS[a]	RESPONSES AFFECTED
Drug metabolism and transport		
CYP2C9	Tolbutamide, warfarin,[a] phenytoin, nonsteroidal anti-inflammatory	Anticoagulant effect of warfarin
CYP2C19	Mephenytoin, omeprazole, voriconazole,[a] hexobarbital, mephobarbital, propranolol, proguanil, phenytoin, clopidogrel	Peptic ulcer response to omeprazole; cardiovascular events after clopidogrel
CYP2D6	β blockers, antidepressants, antipsychotics, codeine, debrisoquine, atomoxetine,[a] dextromethorphan, encainide, flecainide, fluoxetine, guanoxan, *N*-propylajmaline, perhexiline, phenacetin, phenformin, propafenone, sparteine, tamoxifen	Tardive dyskinesia from antipsychotics, narcotic side effects, codeine efficacy, imipramine dose requirement, β-blocker effect; breast cancer recurrence after tamoxifen
CYP3A4/3A5/3A7	Macrolides, cyclosporine, tacrolimus, Ca²⁺ channel blockers, midazolam, terfenadine, lidocaine, dapsone, quinidine, triazolam, etoposide, teniposide, lovastatin, alfentanil, tamoxifen, steroids	Efficacy of immunosuppressive effects of tacrolimus
Dihydropyrimidine dehydrogenase	Fluorouracil, capecitabine[a]	5-Fluorouracil toxicity
N-acetyltransferase (*NAT2*)	Isoniazid, hydralazine, sulfonamides, amonafide, procainamide, dapsone, caffeine	Hypersensitivity to sulfonamides, amonafide toxicity, hydralazine-induced lupus, isoniazid neurotoxicity
Glutathione transferases (*GSTM1, GSTT1, GSTP1*)	Several anticancer agents	Decreased response in breast cancer, more toxicity and worse response in acute myelogenous leukemia
Thiopurine methyltransferase (*TPMT*)	Mercaptopurine,[a] thioguanine,[a] azathioprine[a]	Thiopurine toxicity and efficacy, risk of second cancers
UDP-glucuronosyl-transferase (*UGT1A1*)	Irinotecan,[a] bilirubin	Irinotecan toxicity
P-glycoprotein (*ABCB1*)	Natural product anticancer drugs, HIV protease inhibitors, digoxin	Decreased CD4 response in HIV-infected patients, decreased digoxin AUC, drug resistance in epilepsy
UGT2B7	Morphine	Morphine plasma levels
Organic anion transporter (*SLCO1B1*)	Statins, methotrexate, ACE inhibitors	Statin plasma levels, myopathy; methotrexate plasma levels, mucositis
Catechol-*O*-methyltransferase	Levodopa	Enhanced drug effect
Organic cation transporter (*SLC22A1, OCT1*)	Metformin	Pharmacologic effect and pharmacokinetics
Organic cation transporter (*SLC22A2, OCT2*)	Metformin	Renal clearance
Novel organic cation transporter (*SLC22A4, OCTN1*)	Gabapentin	Renal clearance
CYP2B6	Cyclophosphamide	Ovarian failure

(Continued)

TABLE 7–2 ■ EXAMPLES OF GENETIC POLYMORPHISMS INFLUENCING DRUG RESPONSE (CONTINUED)

GENE PRODUCT (GENE)	DRUGS[a]	RESPONSES AFFECTED
Targets and receptors		
Angiotensin-converting enzyme (ACE)	ACE inhibitors (e.g., enalapril)	Renoprotective effects, hypotension, left ventricular mass reduction, cough
Thymidylate synthase	5-Fluorouracil	Colorectal cancer response
Chemokine receptor 5 (CCR5)	Antiretrovirals, interferon	Antiviral response
β_2 adrenergic receptor (ADBR2)	β_2-Antagonists (e.g., albuterol, terbutaline)	Bronchodilation, susceptibility to agonist-induced desensitization, cardiovascular effects (e.g., increased heart rate, cardiac index, peripheral vasodilation)
β_1 adrenergic receptor (ADBR1)	β_1-Antagonists	Blood pressure and heart rate after β_1 antagonists
5-Lipoxygenase (ALOX5)	Leukotriene receptor antagonists	Asthma response
Dopamine receptors (D_2, D_3, D_4)	Antipsychotics (e.g., haloperidol, clozapine, thioridazine, nemonapride)	Antipsychotic response (D_2, D_3 D_4), antipsychotic-induced tardive dyskinesia (D_3) and acute akathisia (D_3), hyperprolactinemia in females (D_2)
Estrogen receptor α	Estrogen hormone replacement therapy	High-density lipoprotein cholesterol
Serotonin transporter (5HTT)	Antidepressants (e.g., clomipramine, fluoxetine, paroxetine, fluvoxamine)	Clozapine effects, 5HT neurotransmission, antidepressant response
Serotonin receptor ($5HT_{2A}$)	Antipsychotics	Clozapine antipsychotic response, tardive dyskinesia, paroxetine antidepression response, drug discrimination
HMG-CoA reductase	Pravastatin	Reduction in serum cholesterol
Vitamin K oxidoreductase (VKORC1)	Warfarin[a]	Anticoagulant effect, bleeding risk
Corticotropin-releasing hormone receptor (CRHR1)	Glucocorticoids	Bronchodilation, osteopenia
Ryanodine receptor (RYR1)	General anesthetics	Malignant hyperthermia
Modifiers		
Adducin	Diuretics	Myocardial infarction or strokes, blood pressure
Apolipoprotein E	Statins (e.g., simvastatin), tacrine	Lipid lowering; clinical improvement in Alzheimer disease
Human leukocyte antigen	Abacavir, carbamazepine, phenytoin	Hypersensitivity reactions
G6PD deficiency	Rasburicase,[a] dapsone[a]	Methemoglobinemia
Cholesteryl ester transfer protein	Statins (e.g., pravastatin)	Slowing atherosclerosis progression
Ion channels (HERG, KvLQT1, Mink, MiRP1)	Erythromycin, cisapride, clarithromycin, quinidine	Increased risk of drug-induced torsades de pointes, increased QT interval (Roden, 2003, 2004)
Methylguanine-methyltransferase	DNA methylating agents	Response of glioma to chemotherapy
Parkin	Levodopa	Parkinson disease response
MTHFR	Methotrexate	GI toxicity (Ulrich et al., 2001)
Prothrombin, factor V	Oral contraceptives	Venous thrombosis risk
Stromelysin-1	Statins (e.g., pravastatin)	Reduction in cardiovascular events and in repeat angioplasty
Inosine triphosphatase	Azathioprine, mercaptopurine	Myelosuppression
Vitamin D receptor	Estrogen	Bone mineral density

[a]Information on genetics-based dosing, adverse events, or testing added to FDA-approved drug label (Grossman, 2007).

Bibliography

Aithal GP, et al. Association of polymorphisms in the cytochrome P450 CYP2C9 with warfarin dose requirement and risk of bleeding complications. *Lancet*, **1999**, *353*:717–719.

Birdwell KA, et al. The use of a DNA biobank linked to electronic medical records to characterize pharmacogenomic predictors of tacrolimus dose requirement in kidney transplant recipients. *Pharmacogenet Genomics*, **2012**, *22*:32–42.

Caraco Y, et al. CYP2C9 genotype-guided warfarin prescribing enhances the efficacy and safety of anticoagulation: a prospective randomized controlled study. *Clin Pharmacol Ther*, **2008**, *83*:460–470.

Ciszkowski C, et al. Codeine, ultrarapid-metabolism genotype, and postoperative death. *N Engl J Med*, **2009**, *361*:827–828.

Cohen JC, et al. Sequence variations in PCSK9, low LDL, and protection against coronary heart disease. *N Engl J Med*, **2006**, *354*:1264–1272.

Cooper GM, et al. A genome-wide scan for common genetic variants with a large influence on warfarin maintenance dose. *Blood*, **2008**, *112*:1022–1027.

Cox JJ, et al. An SCN9A channelopathy causes congenital inability to experience pain. *Nature*, **2006**, *444*:894–898.

Daly AK, et al. HLA-B*5701 genotype is a major determinant of drug-induced liver injury due to flucloxacillin. *Nat Genet*, **2009**, *41*:816–819.

Denny JC, et al. Systematic comparison of phenome-wide association study of electronic medical record data and genome-wide association study data. *Nat Biotechnol*, **2013**, *31*:1102–1111.

ENCODE Project Consortium. An integrated encyclopedia of DNA elements in the human genome. *Nature*, **2012**, *489*:57–74.

Evans WE, McLeod HL. Pharmacogenomics—drug disposition, drug targets, and side effects. *N Engl J Med*, **2003**, *348*:538–49.

Flannick J, et al. Loss-of-function mutations in SLC30A8 protect against type 2 diabetes. *Nat Genet*, **2014**, *46*:357–363.

GTEx Consortium. The Genotype-Tissue Expression (GTEx) pilot analysis: multitissue gene regulation in humans. *Science*, **2015**, *348*: 648–660.

Grossman I. Routine pharmacogenetic testing in clinical practice: Dream or reality? *Pharmacogenomics*, **2007**, *8*:1449–1459.

Haufroid V, et al. The effect of CYP3A5 and MDR1 (ABCB1) polymorphisms on cyclosporine and tacrolimus dose requirements and trough blood levels in stable renal transplant patients. *Pharmacogenetics*, **2004**, *14*:147–154.

Ioannidis JP, et al. Replication validity of genetic association studies. *Nat Genet*, **2001**, *29*:306–309.

Kääb S, et al. A large candidate gene survey identifies the KCNE1 D85N polymorphism as a possible modulator of drug-induced torsades de pointes. *Circ Cardiovasc Genet*, **2012**, *5*:91–99.

Karnes JH, et al. A genome-wide association study of heparin-induced thrombocytopenia using an electronic medical record. *Thromb Haemost*, **2015**, *113*:772–781.

Kawai VK, et al. Genotype and risk of major bleeding during warfarin treatment. *Pharmacogenomics*, **2014**, *15*:1973–1983.

Kimchi-Sarfaty C, et al. A "silent" polymorphism in the MDR1 gene changes substrate specificity. *Science*, **2007**, *315*:525–528.

Kimmel SE, et al. A pharmacogenetic versus a clinical algorithm for warfarin dosing. *N Engl J Med*, **2013**, *369*:2283–2293.

Kircher M, et al. A general framework for estimating the relative pathogenicity of human genetic variants. *Nat Genet*, **2014**, *46*:310–315.

Kuehl P, et al. Sequence diversity in CYP3A promoters and characterization of the genetic basis of polymorphic CYP3A5 expression. *Nat Genet*, **2001**, *27*:383–391.

Lin YS, et al. Co-regulation of CYP3A4 and CYP3A5 and contribution to hepatic and intestinal midazolam metabolism. *Mol Pharmacol*, **2002**, *62*:162–172.

Maemondo M, et al. Gefitinib or chemotherapy for non–small-cell lung cancer with mutated EGFR. *N Engl J Med*, **2010**, *362*:2380–2388.

Mallal S, et al. HLA-B*5701 screening for hypersensitivity to abacavir. *N Engl J Med*, **2008**, *358*:568–579.

Mangravite LM, et al. A statin-dependent QTL for GATM expression is associated with statin-induced myopathy. *Nature*, **2013**, *502*:377–380.

Mega JL, et al. Reduced-function CYP2C19 genotype and risk of adverse clinical outcomes among patients treated with clopidogrel predominantly for PCI: a meta-analysis. *JAMA*, **2010**, *304*:1821–1830.

Mosley JD, et al. A genome-wide association study identifies variants in KCNIP4 associated with ACE inhibitor-induced cough. *Pharmacogenomics J*, **2015**,

Motsinger-Reif AA, et al. Genome-wide association studies in pharmacogenomics: successes and lessons. *Pharmacogenet Genomics*, **2013**, *23*:383–394.

Pirmohamed M, et al. A randomized trial of genotype-guided dosing of warfarin. *N Engl J Med*, **2013**, *369*:2294–2303.

Pulley JM, et al. Operational implementation of prospective genotyping for personalized medicine: the design of the Vanderbilt PREDICT project. *Clin Pharmacol Ther*, **2012**, *92*:87–95.

Ramsey BW, et al. A CFTR potentiator in patients with cystic fibrosis and the G551D mutation. *N Engl J Med*, **2011**, *365*:1663–1672.

Rasmussen-Torvik LJ, et al. Design and anticipated outcomes of the eMERGE-PGx project: a multi-center pilot for pre-emptive pharmacogenomics in electronic health record systems. *Clin Pharmacol Ther*, **2014**, *96*:482–489.

Rastegar-Mojarad M, et al. Opportunities for drug repositioning from phenome-wide association studies. *Nat Biotechnol*, **2015**, *33*:342–345.

Relling MV, Klein TE. CPIC: Clinical Pharmacogenetics Implementation Consortium of the Pharmacogenomics Research Network. *Clin Pharmacol Ther*, **2011**, *89*:464–467.

Roden DM. Cardiovascular pharmacogenomics. *Circulation*, **2003**, *108*: 3071–3074.

Roden DM. Drug-induced prolongation of the QT interval. *N Engl J Med*, **2004**, *350*:1013–1022.

Roden DM, Stein CM. Clopidogrel and the concept of high-risk pharmacokinetics. *Circulation*, **2009**, *119*:2127–2130.

Roth JA, et al. Genetic risk factors for major bleeding in warfarin patients in a community setting. *Clin Pharmacol Ther*, **2014**, *95*:636–643.

Schwarz UI, et al. Genetic determinants of response to warfarin during initial anticoagulation. *N Engl J Med*, **2008**, *358*:999–1008.

Shuldiner AR, et al. Association of cytochrome P450 2C19 genotype with the antiplatelet effect and clinical efficacy of clopidogrel therapy. *JAMA*, **2009**, *302*:849–857.

Stitziel NO, et al. Inactivating mutations in NPC1L1 and protection from coronary heart disease. *N Engl J Med*, **2014**, *371*:2072–2082.

Stranger BE, et al. Relative impact of nucleotide and copy number variation on gene expression phenotypes. *Science*, **2007**, *315*:848–853.

Takeuchi F, et al. A genome-wide association study confirms VKORC1, CYP2C9, and CYP4F2 as principal genetic determinants of warfarin dose. *PLoS Genet*, **2009**, *5*:e1000433.

Ulrich CN, et al. Pharmacogenetics of methotrexate: toxicity among marrow transplantation patients varies with the methylenetetrahydrofolate reductase C677T polymorphism. *Blood*, **2001**, *9*:231–234.

Van Driest SL, et al. Genome-wide association study of serum creatinine levels during vancomycin therapy. *PLoS One*, **2015**, *10*:e0127791.

Wainwright CE, et al. Lumacaftor–ivacaftor in patients with cystic fibrosis homozygous for Phe508del CFTR. *N Engl J Med*, **2015**, *373*:220–231.

Weeke P, et al. Exome sequencing implicates an increased burden of rare potassium channel variants in the risk of drug-induced long QT interval syndrome. *J Am Coll Cardiol*, **2014**, *63*:1430–1437.

Wen MS, et al. Prospective study of warfarin dosage requirements based on CYP2C9 and VKORC1 genotypes. *Clin Pharmacol Ther*, **2008**, *84*:83–89.

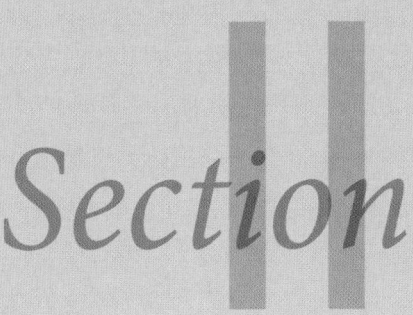

Section II

Neuropharmacology

Chapter 8

Neurotransmission: The Autonomic and Somatic Motor Nervous Systems

Thomas C. Westfall, Heather Macarthur, and David P. Westfall

Anatomy and General Functions

The autonomic nervous system, also called the *visceral, vegetative,* or *involuntary nervous system,* is distributed widely throughout the body and regulates autonomic functions that occur without conscious control. In the periphery, it consists of nerves, ganglia, and plexuses that innervate the heart, blood vessels, glands, other visceral organs, and smooth muscle in various tissues.

Differences Between Autonomic and Somatic Nerves

- The *efferent nerves* of the autonomic nervous system supply all innervated structures of the body except skeletal muscle, which is served by *somatic nerves.*
- The most distal synaptic junctions in the autonomic reflex arc occur in *ganglia* that are entirely *outside the cerebrospinal axis.* Somatic nerves contain no peripheral *ganglia,* and the synapses are located entirely *within the cerebrospinal axis.*
- Many autonomic nerves form extensive peripheral plexuses; such networks are absent from the somatic system.
- Postganglionic autonomic nerves generally are *nonmyelinated*; motor nerves to skeletal muscles are *myelinated.*
- When the spinal efferent nerves are interrupted, smooth muscles and glands generally retain some level of spontaneous activity, whereas the *denervated* skeletal muscles are paralyzed.

Sensory Information: Afferent Fibers and Reflex Arcs

Afferent fibers from visceral structures are the first link in the reflex arcs of the autonomic system. With certain exceptions, such as local axon reflexes, most visceral reflexes are mediated through the CNS.

Visceral Afferent Fibers. Information on the status of the visceral organs is transmitted to the CNS through two main sensory systems: the *cranial nerve (parasympathetic) visceral sensory system* and the *spinal (sympathetic) visceral afferent system.* The cranial visceral sensory system carries mainly mechanoreceptor and chemosensory information, whereas the afferents of the spinal visceral system principally convey sensations related to temperature and tissue injury of mechanical, chemical, or thermal origin.

Cranial visceral sensory information enters the CNS by four cranial nerves: the trigeminal (V), facial (VII), glossopharyngeal (IX), and vagus (X) nerves. These four cranial nerves transmit visceral sensory information from the internal face and head (V); tongue (taste, VII); hard palate and upper part of the oropharynx (IX); and carotid body, lower part of the oropharynx, larynx, trachea, esophagus, and thoracic and abdominal organs (X), with the exception of the pelvic viscera. The pelvic viscera are innervated by nerves from the second through fourth sacral spinal segments. The visceral afferents from these four cranial nerves terminate topographically in the STN (Altschuler et al., 1989).

Sensory afferents from visceral organs also enter the CNS from the spinal nerves. Those concerned with muscle chemosensation may arise at all spinal levels, whereas sympathetic visceral sensory afferents generally arise at the thoracic levels where sympathetic preganglionic neurons are found. Pelvic sensory afferents from spinal segments S2–S4 enter at that level and are important for the regulation of sacral parasympathetic outflow. In general, visceral afferents that enter the spinal nerves convey information concerned with temperature as well as nociceptive visceral inputs related to mechanical, chemical, and thermal stimulation. The primary pathways taken by ascending spinal visceral afferents are complex (Saper, 2002). An important feature of the ascending pathways is that they provide collaterals that converge with the cranial visceral sensory pathway at virtually every level (Saper, 2000).

The neurotransmitters that mediate transmission from sensory fibers have not been characterized unequivocally. Substance P and CGRP, present in afferent sensory fibers, dorsal root ganglia, and the dorsal horn of the spinal cord, likely communicate nociceptive stimuli from the periphery to the spinal cord and higher structures. SST, VIP, and CCK also occur in sensory neurons (Hökfelt et al., 2000). ATP appears to be a neurotransmitter in certain sensory neurons (e.g., the urinary bladder). Enkephalins, present in interneurons in the dorsal spinal cord (within the *substantia gelatinosa*), have antinociceptive effects both pre- and postsynaptically to inhibit the release of substance P and diminish the activity of cells that project from the spinal cord to higher centers in the CNS. The excitatory amino acids glutamate and aspartate also play major roles in transmission of sensory responses to the spinal cord. These transmitters and their signaling pathways are reviewed in Chapter 14.

Central Autonomic Connections

There probably are no purely autonomic or somatic centers of integration, and extensive overlap occurs. Somatic responses always are accompanied by visceral responses and vice versa. Autonomic reflexes

Abbreviations

AA: arachidonic acid
AAADC: aromatic L-amino acid decarboxylase
α-BTX: α-bungarotoxin
AC: adenylyl cyclase
ACh: acetylcholine
AChE: acetylcholinesterase
AD: aldehyde dehydrogenase
ADH: alcohol dehydrogenase
anti-ChE: anti-cholinesterase
AP: action potential
AR: aldehyde reductase
AV: atrioventricular
CaM: calmodulin
CCK: cholecystokinin
CGRP: calcitonin gene–related peptide
ChAT: choline acetyl transferase
CHT1: Choline transporter
CNS: central nervous system
COMT: catechol-O-methyltransferase
CSF: cerebrospinal fluid
DA: dopamine
DAG: diacylglycerol
DAT: DA transporter
DβH: dopamine β-hydroxylase
DOMA: 3,4-dihydroxymandelic acid
DOPEG: 3,4-dihydroxyphenyl glycol
DOPGAL: dihydroxyphenylglycolaldehyde
ENS: enteric nervous system
ENT: extraneuronal transporter
EPI: epinephrine
EPP: end-plate potential
EPSP: excitatory postsynaptic potential
ET: endothelin
GABA: γ-aminobutyric acid
GI: gastrointestinal
GRK: G protein-coupled receptor kinase
GPCR: G protein–coupled receptor
HR: heart rate
5HT: serotonin (5-hydroxytryptamine)
HVA: homovanillic acid
IP$_3$: inositol 1,4,5-trisphosphate
IPSP: inhibitory postsynaptic potential
KO: knockout
mAChR: muscarinic acetylcholine receptor
MAO: monoamine oxidase
MAPK: mitogen-activated protein kinase
mepps: miniature end-plate potentials
MOPEG: 3-methyl,4-hydroxyphenylglycol
MOPGAL: monohydroxyphenylglycolaldehyde
nAChR: nicotinic ACh receptor
NANC: nonadrenergic, noncholinergic
NE: norepinephrine (noradrenaline)
NET: norepinephrine transporter
NMJ: neuromuscular junction (of skeletal muscle)
NO: nitric oxide
NOS: nitric oxide synthase
NPY: neuropeptide Y
NSF: N-ethylmaleamide sensitive factor
PACAP: pituitary adenylyl cyclase–activating peptide
PG_: prostaglandin _, as in PGE$_2$
PK_: protein kinase _, as in PKA

PL_: phospholipase _, as in PLA$_2$, PLC, etc.
PNMT: phenylethanolamine-N-methyltransferase
PTX: pertussis toxin
rNTPase: releasable nucleotidase
SA: sinoatrial
SERT: serotonin transporter
SLC: solute carrier
SNAP: soluble NSF attachment protein, synaptosome-associated protein
SNARE: SNAP receptor
SST: somatostatin
STN: solitary tract nucleus
TH: tyrosine hydroxylase
VAChT: vesicular ACh transporter
VAT: vesicle-associated transporter
VIP: vasoactive intestinal polypeptide
VMA: vanillyl mandelic acid
VMAT2: vesicular uptake transporter

can be elicited at the level of the spinal cord. They clearly are demonstrable in experimental animals or humans with spinal cord transection and are manifested by sweating, blood pressure alterations, vasomotor responses to temperature changes, and reflex emptying of the urinary bladder, rectum, and seminal vesicles. Extensive central ramifications of the autonomic nervous system exist above the level of the spinal cord. For example, integration of the control of respiration in the medulla oblongata is well known. The hypothalamus and the STN generally are regarded as principal loci of integration of autonomic nervous system functions, which include regulation of body temperature, water balance, carbohydrate and fat metabolism, blood pressure, emotions, sleep, respiration, and reproduction. Signals are received through ascending spinobulbar pathways, the limbic system, neostriatum, cortex, and to a lesser extent other higher brain centers. Stimulation of the STN and the hypothalamus activates bulbospinal pathways and hormonal output to mediate autonomic and motor responses (Andresen and Kunze, 1994) (see Chapter 14). The hypothalamic nuclei that lie posteriorly and laterally are sympathetic in their main connections, whereas parasympathetic functions evidently are integrated by the midline nuclei in the region of the tuber cinereum and by nuclei lying anteriorly.

Highly integrated patterns of response generally are organized at a hypothalamic level and involve autonomic, endocrine, and behavioral components. More limited patterned responses are organized at other levels of basal forebrain, brainstem, and spinal cord.

Divisions of the Peripheral Autonomic System

On the efferent side, the autonomic nervous system consists of two large divisions: (1) the *sympathetic* or *thoracolumbar outflow* and (2) the *parasympathetic* or *craniosacral outflow*. Figure 8–1 schematically summarizes the arrangement of the principal parts of the peripheral autonomic nervous system.

The neurotransmitter of all preganglionic autonomic fibers, most postganglionic parasympathetic fibers, and a few postganglionic sympathetic fibers is ACh. Some postganglionic parasympathetic nerves use NO as a neurotransmitter and are termed *nitrergic* (Toda and Okamura, 2003). The majority of the postganglionic sympathetic fibers are *adrenergic*, in which the transmitter is NE (also called noradrenaline). The terms *cholinergic* and *adrenergic* describe neurons that liberate ACh or NE, respectively. Not all the transmitters of the primary afferent fibers, such as those from the mechano- and chemoreceptors of the carotid body and aortic arch, have been identified conclusively. Substance P and glutamate may mediate many afferent impulses; both are present in high concentrations in the dorsal spinal cord.

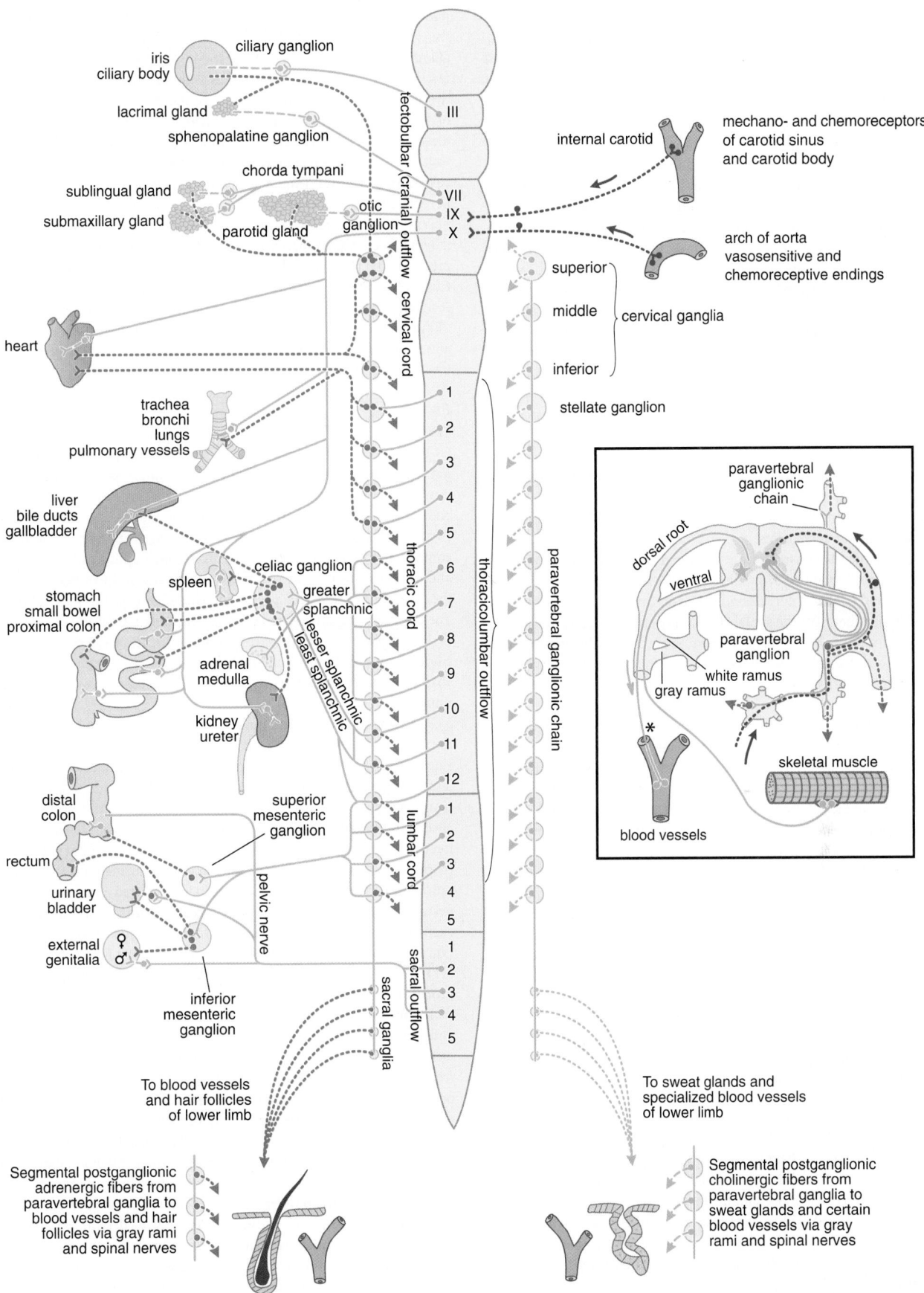

Figure 8–1 *The autonomic nervous system.* Schematic representation of the autonomic nerves and effector organs based on chemical mediation of nerve impulses. Yellow (———), cholinergic; red (———), adrenergic; dotted blue (– – – – –), visceral afferent; solid lines, preganglionic; broken lines, postganglionic. The rectangle at right shows the finer details of the ramifications of adrenergic fibers at any one segment of the spinal cord, the path of the visceral afferent nerves, the cholinergic nature of somatic motor nerves to skeletal muscle, and the presumed cholinergic nature of the vasodilator fibers in the dorsal roots of the spinal nerves. The asterisk (*) indicates that it is not known whether these vasodilator fibers are motor or sensory or where their cell bodies are situated.

Sympathetic Nervous System

The cells that give rise to the preganglionic fibers of the sympathetic nervous system division lie mainly in the intermediolateral columns of the spinal cord and extend from the first thoracic to the second or third lumbar segment. The axons from these cells are carried in the anterior (ventral) nerve roots and synapse, with neurons lying in sympathetic ganglia outside the cerebrospinal axis. Sympathetic ganglia are found in three locations: paravertebral, prevertebral, and terminal.

The 22 pairs of paravertebral sympathetic ganglia form the lateral chains on either side of the vertebral column. The ganglia are connected to each other by nerve trunks and to the spinal nerves by *rami communicantes*. The white rami are restricted to the segments of the thoracolumbar outflow; they carry the preganglionic myelinated fibers that exit the spinal cord by the anterior spinal roots. The gray rami arise from the ganglia and carry postganglionic fibers back to the spinal nerves for distribution to sweat glands and pilomotor muscles and to blood vessels of skeletal muscle and skin. The prevertebral ganglia lie in the abdomen and the pelvis near the ventral surface of the bony vertebral column and consist mainly of the celiac (solar), superior mesenteric, aorticorenal, and inferior mesenteric ganglia. The terminal ganglia are few in number, lie near the organs they innervate, and include ganglia connected with the urinary bladder and rectum and the cervical ganglia in the region of the neck. In addition, small intermediate ganglia lie outside the conventional vertebral chain, especially in the thoracolumbar region. They are variable in number and location but usually are in proximity to the communicating rami and the anterior spinal nerve roots.

Preganglionic fibers issuing from the spinal cord may synapse with the neurons of more than one sympathetic ganglion. Their principal ganglia of termination need not correspond to the original level from which the preganglionic fiber exits the spinal cord. Many of the preganglionic fibers from the fifth to the last thoracic segment pass through the paravertebral ganglia to form the splanchnic nerves. Most of the splanchnic nerve fibers do not synapse until they reach the celiac ganglion; others directly innervate the adrenal medulla.

Postganglionic fibers arising from sympathetic ganglia innervate visceral structures of the thorax, abdomen, head, and neck. The trunk and the limbs are supplied by the sympathetic fibers in spinal nerves. The prevertebral ganglia contain cell bodies whose axons innervate the glands and smooth muscles of the abdominal and the pelvic viscera. Many of the upper thoracic sympathetic fibers from the vertebral ganglia form terminal plexuses, such as the cardiac, esophageal, and pulmonary plexuses. The sympathetic distribution to the head and the neck (vasomotor, pupillodilator, secretory, and pilomotor) is by means of the cervical sympathetic chain and its three ganglia. All postganglionic fibers in this chain arise from cell bodies located in these three ganglia. All preganglionic fibers arise from the upper thoracic segments of the spinal cord, there being no sympathetic fibers that leave the CNS above the first thoracic level.

Pharmacologically, anatomically, and embryologically, the chromaffin cells of the adrenal medulla resemble a collection of postganglionic sympathetic nerve cells. Typical preganglionic fibers that release ACh innervate these chromaffin cells, stimulating the release of EPI (also called adrenaline), in distinction to the NE released by postganglionic sympathetic fibers.

Parasympathetic Nervous System

The parasympathetic nervous system consists of preganglionic fibers that originate in the CNS and their postganglionic connections. The regions of central origin are the midbrain, the medulla oblongata, and the sacral part of the spinal cord. The midbrain, or tectal, outflow consists of fibers arising from the Edinger-Westphal nucleus of the third cranial nerve and going to the ciliary ganglion in the orbit. The medullary outflow consists of the parasympathetic components of the VII, IX, and X cranial nerves.

The fibers in the VII (facial) cranial nerve form the chorda tympani, which innervates the ganglia lying on the submaxillary and sublingual glands. They also form the greater superficial petrosal nerve, which innervates the sphenopalatine ganglion. The autonomic components of the IX (glossopharyngeal) cranial nerve innervate the otic ganglia. Postganglionic

parasympathetic fibers from these ganglia supply the sphincter of the iris (pupillary constrictor muscle), the ciliary muscle, the salivary and lacrimal glands, and the mucous glands of the nose, mouth, and pharynx. These fibers also include vasodilator nerves to these same organs. Cranial nerve X (vagus) arises in the medulla and contains preganglionic fibers, most of which do not synapse until they reach the many small ganglia lying directly on or in the viscera of the thorax and abdomen. In the intestinal wall, the vagal fibers terminate around ganglion cells in the myenteric and submucosal plexuses. *Thus, in the parasympathetic branch of the autonomic nervous system, preganglionic fibers are very long, whereas postganglionic fibers are very short.* The vagus nerve also carries a far greater number of afferent fibers (but apparently no pain fibers) from the viscera into the medulla. The parasympathetic sacral outflow consists of axons that arise from cells in the second, third, and fourth segments of the sacral cord and proceed as preganglionic fibers to form the pelvic nerves (*nervi erigentes*). They synapse in terminal ganglia lying near or within the bladder, rectum, and sexual organs. The vagal and sacral outflows provide motor and secretory fibers to thoracic, abdominal, and pelvic organs (see Figure 8–1).

Enteric Nervous System

The processes of mixing, propulsion, and absorption of nutrients in the GI tract are controlled locally through a restricted part of the peripheral nervous system called the *ENS*. The ENS comprises components of the sympathetic and parasympathetic nervous systems and has sensory nerve connections through the spinal and nodose ganglia (see Chapter 46 and Furness et al., 2014). The ENS is involved in sensorimotor control and thus consists of both afferent sensory neurons and a number of motor nerves and interneurons that are organized principally into two nerve plexuses: the myenteric (Auerbach) plexus and the submucosal (Meissner) plexus. The myenteric plexus, located between the longitudinal and circular muscle layers, plays an important role in the contraction and relaxation of GI smooth muscle. The submucosal plexus is involved with secretory and absorptive functions of the GI epithelium, local blood flow, and neuroimmune activities.

Parasympathetic preganglionic inputs are provided to the GI tract via the vagus and pelvic nerves. ACh released from *preganglionic neurons* activates nAChRs on postganglionic neurons within the enteric ganglia. Excitatory preganglionic input activates both excitatory and inhibitory motor neurons that control processes such as muscle contraction and secretion/absorption. *Postganglionic sympathetic nerves* also synapse with intrinsic neurons and generally induce relaxation. Sympathetic input is excitatory (contractile) at some sphincters. Information from afferent and preganglionic neural inputs to the enteric ganglia is integrated and distributed by a network of interneurons. ACh is the primary neurotransmitter providing excitatory inputs between interneurons, but other substances, such as ATP (via postjunctional P2X receptors), substance P (by NK_3 receptors), and 5HT (via 5HT3 receptors) are also important in mediating integrative processing via interneurons.

The muscle layers of the GI tract are dually innervated by excitatory and inhibitory motor neurons, with cell bodies primarily in the myenteric ganglia. ACh is a primary excitatory motor neurotransmitter released from postganglionic neurons. ACh activates M_2 and M_3 receptors in postjunctional cells to elicit motor responses. Pharmacological blockade of mAChRs does not block all excitatory neurotransmission, however, because neurokinins (neurokinin A and substance P) are also coreleased by excitatory motor neurons and contribute to postjunctional excitation. Inhibitory motor neurons in the GI tract regulate motility events such as accommodation, sphincter relaxation, and descending receptive relaxation. Inhibitory responses are elicited by a purine derivative (either ATP or β-nicotinamide adenine dinucleotide) acting at postjunctional $P2Y_1$ receptors) and NO. Inhibitory neuropeptides, such as VIP and PACAP, may also be released from inhibitory motor neurons under conditions of strong stimulation.

In general, motor neurons do not directly innervate smooth muscle cells in the GI tract. Nerve terminals make synaptic connections with the interstitial cells of Cajal (ICCs), and these cells make electrical connections (gap junctions) with smooth muscle cells (Ward et al., 2000).

Thus, the ICCs are the receptive, postjunctional transducers of inputs from enteric motor neurons, and loss of these cells has been associated with conditions that appear to be neuropathies. ICCs have all of the major receptors and effectors necessary to transduce both excitatory and inhibitory neurotransmitters into postjunctional responses (Chen et al., 2007).

Comparison of Sympathetic, Parasympathetic, and Motor Nerves

Differences among somatic motor, sympathetic, and parasympathetic nerves are shown schematically in Figure 8–2. To summarize:

- The *sympathetic* system is distributed to effectors throughout the body, whereas *parasympathetic* distribution is much more limited.
- A *preganglionic sympathetic fiber* may traverse a considerable distance of the sympathetic chain and pass through several ganglia before it finally synapses with a postganglionic neuron; also, its terminals make contact with a large number of postganglionic neurons. The *parasympathetic*

system has terminal ganglia very near or within the organs innervated and is generally more circumscribed in its influences.

- The cell bodies of *somatic motor neurons* reside in the ventral horn of the spinal cord; the axon divides into many branches, each of which innervates a single muscle fiber; more than 100 muscle fibers may be supplied by one motor neuron to form a motor unit. At each NMJ, the axonal terminal loses its myelin sheath and forms a terminal arborization that lies in apposition to a specialized surface of the muscle membrane, termed the *motor end plate* (see Figure 11–3). Reciprocal trophic signals between muscle and nerve regulate the development of the NMJ (Witzemann, 2006).
- Ganglionic organization can differ among the different types of nerves and locales. In some organs innervated by the parasympathetic branch, a 1:1 relationship between the number of preganglionic and postganglionic fibers has been suggested. In sympathetic ganglia, one ganglion cell may be supplied by several preganglionic fibers, and the ratio of preganglionic axons to ganglion cells may be 1:20 or more; this organization

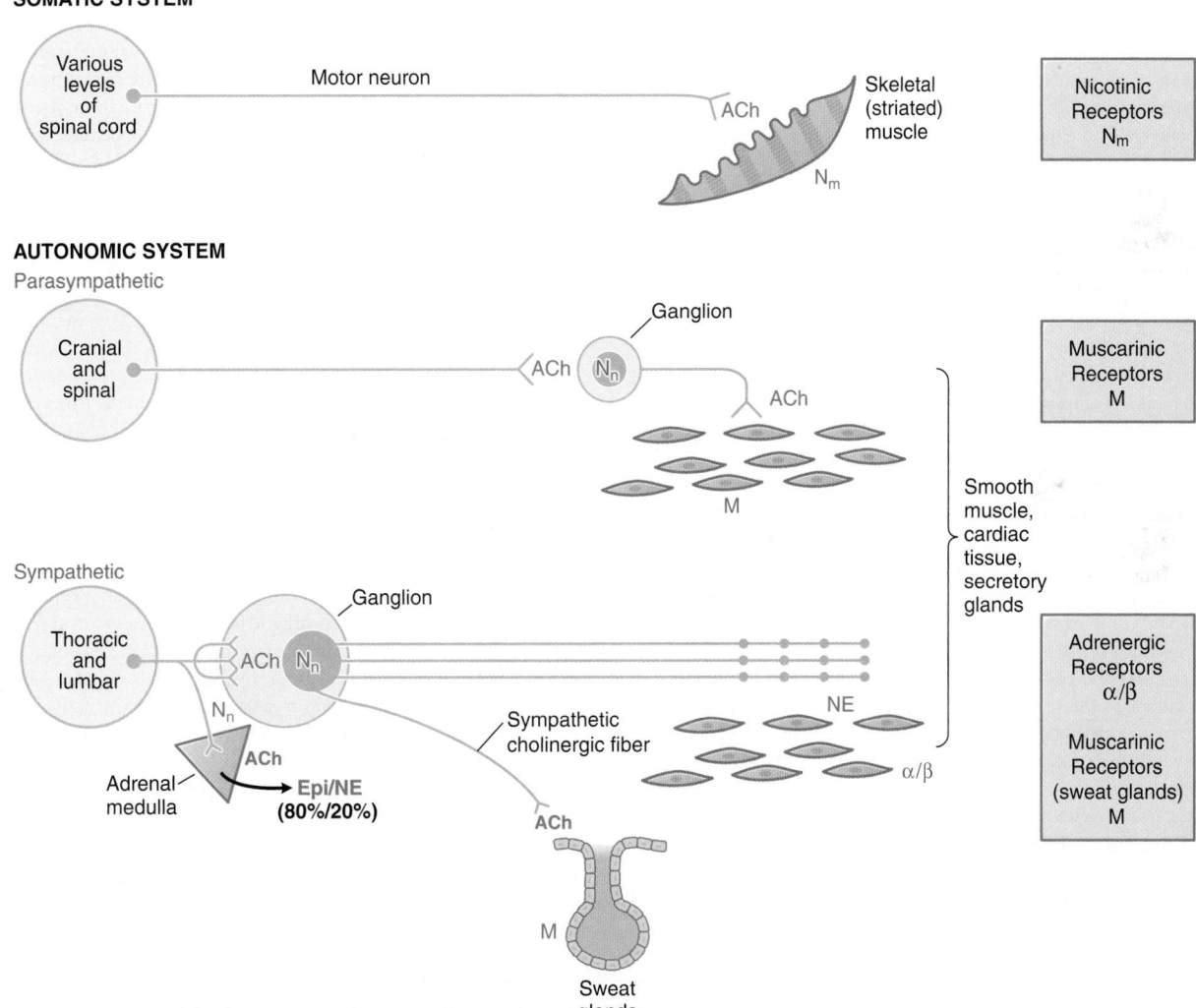

Figure 8–2 *Comparative features of somatic motor nerves and efferent nerves of the autonomic nervous system.* The principal neurotransmitters, ACh and NE, are shown in *red*. The receptors for these transmitters, nicotinic (N) and muscarinic (M) cholinergic receptors, α and β adrenergic receptors, are shown in *green*. Somatic nerves innervate skeletal muscle directly at a specialized synaptic junction, the motor end plate, where ACh activates N_m receptors. Autonomic nerves innervate smooth muscles, cardiac tissue, and glands. Both parasympathetic and sympathetic systems have ganglia, where ACh is released by the preganglionic fibers; ACh acts on N_n receptors on the postganglionic nerves. ACh is also the neurotransmitter at cells of the adrenal medulla, where it acts on N_n receptors to cause release of EPI and NE into the circulation. ACh is the dominant neurotransmitter released by postganglionic parasympathetic nerves and acts on muscarinic receptors. The ganglia in the parasympathetic system are near or within the organ being innervated, with generally a one-to-one relationship between pre- and postganglionic fibers. NE is the principal neurotransmitter of postganglionic sympathetic nerves, acting on α or β adrenergic receptors. Autonomic nerves form a diffuse pattern with multiple synaptic sites. In the sympathetic system, the ganglia are generally far from the effector cells (e.g., within the sympathetic chain ganglia). Preganglionic sympathetic fibers may make contact with a large number of postganglionic fibers.

permits diffuse discharge of the sympathetic system. The ratio of preganglionic vagal fibers to ganglion cells in the myenteric plexus has been estimated as 1:8000.

A Few Details About Innervation

The terminations of the postganglionic autonomic fibers in smooth muscle and glands form a rich plexus, or terminal reticulum. The terminal reticulum (sometimes called the *autonomic ground plexus*) consists of the final ramifications of the postganglionic sympathetic, parasympathetic, and visceral afferent fibers, all of which are enclosed within a frequently interrupted sheath of satellite or Schwann cells. At these interruptions, varicosities packed with vesicles are seen in the efferent fibers. Such varicosities occur repeatedly but at variable distances along the course of the ramifications of the axon.

"Protoplasmic bridges" occur between the smooth muscle fibers themselves at points of contact between their plasma membranes. They are believed to permit the direct conduction of impulses from cell to cell without the need for chemical transmission. These structures have been termed *nexuses*, or *tight junctions*, and they enable the smooth muscle fibers to function as a syncytial unit.

Sympathetic ganglia are extremely complex anatomically and pharmacologically (see Chapter 11). The preganglionic fibers lose their myelin sheaths and divide repeatedly into a vast number of end fibers with diameters ranging from 0.1 to 0.3 μm; except at points of synaptic contact, they retain their satellite cell sheaths. The vast majority of synapses are axodendritic. Apparently, a given axonal terminal may synapse with multiple dendritic processes.

Responses of Effector Organs to Autonomic Nerve Impulses. In many instances, the sympathetic and parasympathetic neurotransmitters can be viewed as physiological or functional antagonists (Table 8–1). Most viscera are innervated by both divisions of the autonomic nervous system, and their activities on specific structures may be either discrete and independent or integrated and interdependent. The effects of sympathetic and parasympathetic stimulation of the heart and the iris show a pattern of functional antagonism in controlling heart rate and pupillary aperture, respectively, whereas their actions on male sexual organs are complementary and are integrated to promote sexual function.

From the responses of the various effector organs to autonomic nerve impulses and the knowledge of the intrinsic autonomic tone, one can predict the actions of drugs that mimic or inhibit the actions of these nerves.

General Functions of the Autonomic Nervous System. The autonomic nervous system is the primary regulator of the constancy of the internal environment of the organism.

The *sympathetic system* and its associated adrenal medulla are not essential to life in a controlled environment, but the lack of sympathoadrenal functions becomes evident under circumstances of stress. In the absence of the sympathetic system, body temperature cannot be regulated when environmental temperature varies; the concentration of glucose in blood does not rise in response to urgent need; compensatory vascular

HISTORICAL PERSPECTIVE

The earliest concrete proposal of a neurohumoral mechanism was made shortly after the turn of the 20th century. Lewandowsky and Langley independently noted the similarity between the effects of injection of extracts of the adrenal gland and stimulation of sympathetic nerves. In 1905, T. R. Elliott, while a student with Langley at Cambridge, postulated that sympathetic nerve impulses release minute amounts of an EPI-like substance in immediate contact with effector cells. He considered this substance to be the chemical step in the process of transmission. He also noted that long after sympathetic nerves had degenerated, the effector organs still responded characteristically to the hormone of the adrenal medulla. Langley suggested that effector cells have excitatory and inhibitory "receptive substances," and that the response to EPI depended on which type of substance was present. In 1907, Dixon, impressed by the correspondence between the effects of the alkaloid muscarine and the responses to vagal stimulation, advanced the concept that the vagus nerve liberated a muscarine-like substance that acted as a chemical transmitter of its impulses. In the same year, Reid Hunt described the actions of ACh and other choline esters. In 1914, Dale investigated the pharmacological properties of ACh and other choline esters and distinguished its nicotine-like and muscarine-like actions. Intrigued with the remarkable fidelity with which this drug reproduced the responses to stimulation of parasympathetic nerves, he introduced the term *parasympathomimetic* to characterize its effects. Dale also noted the brief duration of action of this chemical and proposed that an esterase in the tissues rapidly splits ACh to acetic acid and choline, thereby terminating its action.

The studies of Loewi, begun in 1921, provided the first direct evidence for the chemical mediation of nerve impulses by the release of specific chemical agents. Loewi stimulated the vagus nerve of a perfused (donor) frog heart and allowed the perfusion fluid to come in contact with a second (recipient) frog heart used as a test object. The recipient frog heart was found to respond, after a short lag, in the same way as the donor heart. It thus was evident that a substance was liberated from the first organ that slowed the rate of the second. Loewi referred to this chemical substance as *Vagusstoff* ("vagus substance," "parasympathin");

subsequently, Loewi and Navratil presented evidence to identify it as ACh. Loewi also discovered that an accelerator substance similar to EPI and called *Acceleranstoff* was liberated into the perfusion fluid in summer, when the action of the sympathetic fibers in the frog's vagus, a mixed nerve, predominated over that of the inhibitory fibers. Feldberg and Krayer demonstrated in 1933 that the cardiac "vagus substance" also is ACh in mammals.

In the same year as Loewi's discovery, Cannon and Uridil reported that stimulation of the sympathetic hepatic nerves resulted in the release of an EPI-like substance that increased blood pressure and heart rate. Subsequent experiments firmly established that this substance is the chemical mediator liberated by sympathetic nerve impulses at neuroeffector junctions. Cannon called this substance "sympathin." In many of its pharmacological and chemical properties, sympathin closely resembled EPI, but also differed in certain important respects. As early as 1910, Barger and Dale noted that the effects of sympathetic nerve stimulation were reproduced more closely by the injection of sympathomimetic primary amines than by that of EPI or other secondary amines. The possibility that demethylated EPI (NE) might be sympathin had been advanced repeatedly, but definitive evidence for its being the sympathetic nerve mediator was not obtained until specific assays were developed for the determination of sympathomimetic amines in extracts of tissues and body fluids. In 1946, von Euler found that the sympathomimetic substance in highly purified extracts of bovine splenic nerve resembled NE by all criteria used (von Euler, 1946).

We now know that NE is the predominant sympathomimetic substance in the postganglionic sympathetic nerves of mammals and is the adrenergic mediator liberated by their stimulation. NE, its immediate precursor DA, and its *N*-methylated derivative EPI also are neurotransmitters in the CNS (see Chapter 14). As for ACh, in addition to its role as the transmitter of most postganglionic parasympathetic fibers and of a few postganglionic sympathetic fibers, ACh functions as a neurotransmitter in three additional classes of nerves: preganglionic fibers of both the sympathetic and the parasympathetic systems, motor nerves to skeletal muscle, and certain neurons within the CNS.

TABLE 8-1 ■ RESPONSES OF EFFECTOR ORGANS TO AUTONOMIC NERVE IMPULSES

ORGAN SYSTEM	SYMPATHETIC EFFECT[a]	ADRENERGIC RECEPTOR SUBTYPE[b]	PARASYMPATHETIC EFFECT[a]	CHOLINERGIC RECEPTOR SUBTYPE[b]
Eye				
Radial muscle, iris	Contraction (mydriasis)++	α_1		
Sphincter muscle, iris			Contraction (miosis)+++	M_3, M_2
Ciliary muscle	Relaxation for far vision+	β_2	Contraction for near vision+++	M_3, M_2
Lacrimal glands	Secretion+	α	Secretion+++	M_3, M_2
Heart[c]				
Sinoatrial node	↑ heart rate++	$\beta_1 > \beta_2$	↓ heart rate+++	$M_2 \gg M_3$
Atria	↑ contractility and conduction velocity++	$\beta_1 > \beta_2$	↓ contractility++ and shortened AP duration	$M_2 \gg M_3$
Atrioventricular node	↑ automaticity and conduction velocity++	$\beta_1 > \beta_2$	↓ conduction velocity; AV block+++	$M_2 \gg M_3$
His-Purkinje system	↑ automaticity and conduction velocity	$\beta_1 > \beta_2$	Little effect	$M_2 \gg M_3$
Ventricle	↑ contractility, conduction velocity, automaticity, and rate of idioventricular pacemakers+++	$\beta_1 > \beta_2$	Slight ↓ in contractility	$M_2 \gg M_3$
Blood vessels				
Arteries and arterioles[d]				
Coronary	Constriction+; dilation[e]++	α_1, α_2; β_2	No innervation[h]	—
Skin and mucosa	Constriction+++	α_1, α_2	No innervation[h]	—
Skeletal muscle	Constriction; dilation[e,f]++	α_1; β_2	Dilation[h] (?)	—
Cerebral	Constriction (slight)	α_1	No innervation[h]	—
Pulmonary	Constriction+; dilation	α_1; β_2	No innervation[h]	—
Abdominal viscera	Constriction+++; dilation+	α_1; β_2	No innervation[h]	—
Salivary glands	Constriction+++	α_1, α_2	Dilation[h]++	M_3
Renal	Constriction++; dilation++	α_1, α_2; β_1, β_2	No innervation[h]	
(Veins)[d]	Constriction; dilation	α_1, α_2; β_2		
Endothelium	—	—	↑ NO synthase[h]	M_3
Lung				
Tracheal and bronchial smooth muscle	Relaxation	β_2	Contraction	$M_2 = M_3$
Bronchial glands	↓ secretion, ↑ secretion	α_1	Stimulation	M_2, M_3
		β_2		
Stomach				
Motility and tone	↓ (usually)[i]+	α_1, α_2, β_1, β_2	↑[i]+++	$M_2 = M_3$
Sphincters	Contraction (usually)+	α_1	Relaxation (usually)+	M_3, M_2
Secretion	Inhibition	α_2	Stimulation++	M_3, M_2
Intestine				
Motility and tone	Decrease[h]+	α_1, α_2, β_1, β_2	↑[i]+++	M_3, M_2
Sphincters	Contraction+	α_1	Relaxation (usually)+	M_3, M_2
Secretion	↓	α_2	↑++	M_3, M_2
Gallbladder and ducts kidney	Relaxation+	β_2	Contraction+	M
Renin secretion	↓+; ↑++	α_1; β_1	No innervation	—
Urinary bladder				
Detrusor	Relaxation+	β_2	Contraction+++	$M_3 > M_2$
Trigone and sphincter	Contraction++	α_1	Relaxation++	$M_3 > M_2$

(Continued)

TABLE 8–1 ■ RESPONSES OF EFFECTOR ORGANS TO AUTONOMIC NERVE IMPULSES (CONTINUED)

ORGAN SYSTEM	SYMPATHETIC EFFECT[a]	ADRENERGIC RECEPTOR SUBTYPE[b]	PARASYMPATHETIC EFFECT[a]	CHOLINERGIC RECEPTOR SUBTYPE[b]
Ureter				
Motility and tone	↑	α_1	↑ (?)	M
Uterus	Pregnant contraction	α_1		
	Relaxation	β_2	Variable[j]	M
	Nonpregnant relaxation	β_2		
Sex organs, male skin	Ejaculation+++	α_1	Erection+++	M_3
Pilomotor muscles	Contraction++	α_1	—	
Sweat glands	Localized secretion[k]++	α_1	—	
	—		Generalized secretion+++	M_3, M_2
Spleen capsule	Contraction+++	α_1	—	—
	Relaxation+	β_2	—	
Adrenal medulla	—		Secretion of EPI and NE	N $(\alpha_3)_2(\beta_4)_3$; M (secondarily)
Skeletal muscle	Increased contractility; glycogenolysis; K+ uptake	β_2	—	
Liver	Glycogenolysis and gluconeogenesis+++	α_1	—	—
		β_2		
Pancreas				
Acini	↓ secretion+	α	Secretion++	M_3, M_2
Islets (β cells)	↓ secretion+++	α_2	—	
	↑ secretion+	β_2		
Fat cells[l]	Lipolysis+++; thermogenesis	$\alpha_1, \beta_1, \beta_2, \beta_3$	—	—
	Inhibition of lipolysis	α_2		
Salivary glands	K+ and water secretion+	α_1	K+ and water secretion+++	M_3, M_2
Nasopharyngeal glands	—		Secretion++	M_3, M_2
Pineal glands	Melatonin synthesis	β	—	
Posterior pituitary	ADH secretion	β_1	—	
Autonomic nerve endings				
Sympathetic terminal				
Autoreceptor	Inhibition of NE release	$\alpha_{2A} > \alpha_{2C} (\alpha_{2B})$		
Heteroreceptor	—		Inhibition of NE release	M_2, M_4
Parasympathetic terminal				
Autoreceptor	—	—	Inhibition of ACh release	M_2, M_4
Heteroreceptor	Inhibition ACh release	$\alpha_{2A} > \alpha_{2C}$	—	—

[a]Responses are designated + to +++ to provide an approximate indication of the importance of sympathetic and parasympathetic nerve activity in the control of the various organs and functions listed.

[b]Adrenergic receptors: α_1, α_2 and subtypes thereof; β_1, β_2, β_3. Cholinergic receptors: nicotinic (N); muscarinic (M), with subtypes 1–4. The receptor subtypes are described more fully in Chapters 9 and 12 and in Tables 8–2, 8–3, 8–6, and 8–7. When a designation of subtype is not provided, the nature of the subtype has not been determined unequivocally. Only the principal receptor subtypes are shown. Transmitters other than ACh and NE contribute to many of the responses.

[c]In the human heart, the ratio of β_1 to β_2 is about 3:2 in atria and 4:1 in ventricles. While M_2 receptors predominate, M_3 receptors are also present (Wang et al., 2004).

[d]The predominant α_1 receptor subtype in most blood vessels (both arteries and veins) is α_{1A}, although other α_1 subtypes are present in specific blood vessels. The α_{1D} is the predominant subtype in the aorta (Michelotti et al., 2000).

[e]Dilation predominates in situ owing to metabolic autoregulatory mechanisms.

[f]Over the usual concentration range of physiologically released circulating EPI, the β receptor response (vasodilation) predominates in blood vessels of skeletal muscle and liver; β receptor response (vasoconstriction) predominates in blood vessels of other abdominal viscera. The renal and mesenteric vessels also contain specific dopaminergic receptors whose activation causes dilation.

[g]Sympathetic cholinergic neurons cause vasodilation in skeletal muscle beds, but this is not involved in most physiological responses.

[h]The endothelium of most blood vessels releases NO, which causes vasodilation in response to muscarinic stimuli. However, unlike the receptors innervated by sympathetic cholinergic fibers in skeletal muscle blood vessels, these muscarinic receptors are not innervated and respond only to exogenously added muscarinic agonists in the circulation.

[i]While adrenergic fibers terminate at inhibitory β receptors on smooth muscle fibers and at inhibitory β receptors on parasympathetic (cholinergic) excitatory ganglion cells of the myenteric plexus, the primary inhibitory response is mediated via enteric neurons through NO, P2Y receptors, and peptide receptors.

[j]Uterine responses depend on stages of menstrual cycle, amount of circulating estrogen and progesterone, and other factors.

[k]Palms of hands and some other sites ("adrenergic sweating").

[l]There is significant variation among species in the receptor types that mediate certain metabolic responses. All three β adrenergic receptors have been found in human fat cells. Activation of β_3 receptors produces a vigorous thermogenic response as well as lipolysis. The significance is unclear. Activation of β receptors also inhibits leptin release from adipose tissue.

responses to hemorrhage, oxygen deprivation, excitement, and exercise are lacking; and resistance to fatigue is lessened. Sympathetic components of instinctive reactions to the external environment are lost, and other serious deficiencies in the protective forces of the body are discernible. The sympathetic system normally is continuously active, the degree of activity varying from moment to moment and from organ to organ, adjusting to a constantly changing environment. The sympathoadrenal system can discharge as a unit. Heart rate is accelerated; blood pressure rises; blood flow is shifted from the skin and splanchnic region to the skeletal muscles; blood glucose rises; the bronchioles and pupils dilate; and the organism is better prepared for "fight or flight." Many of these effects result primarily from or are reinforced by the actions of EPI secreted by the adrenal medulla.

The *parasympathetic system* is organized mainly for discrete and localized discharge. Although it is concerned primarily with conservation of energy and maintenance of organ function during periods of minimal activity, its elimination is not compatible with life. The parasympathetic system slows the heart rate, lowers the blood pressure, stimulates GI movements and secretions, aids absorption of nutrients, protects the retina from excessive light, and empties the urinary bladder and rectum.

Neurochemical Transmission

Nerve impulses elicit responses in smooth, cardiac, and skeletal muscles; exocrine glands; and postsynaptic neurons by liberating specific chemical neurotransmitters.

Evidence for Neurohumoral Transmission

The concept of neurohumoral transmission or chemical neurotransmission was developed primarily to explain observations relating to the transmission of impulses from postganglionic autonomic fibers to effector cells. Evidence supporting this concept includes the following:

- demonstration of the presence of a physiologically active compound and its biosynthetic enzymes at appropriate sites;
- recovery of the compound from the perfusate of an innervated structure during periods of nerve stimulation but not (or in greatly reduced amounts) in the absence of stimulation;
- demonstration that the compound is capable of producing responses identical to responses to nerve stimulation; and
- demonstration that the responses to nerve stimulation and to the administered compound are modified in the same manner by various drugs, usually competitive antagonists

While these criteria are applicable for most neurotransmitters, including NE and ACh, there are now exceptions to these general rules. For instance, NO has been found to be a neurotransmitter, in a few postganglionic parasympathetic nerves; in NANC neurons in the periphery; in the ENS; and in the CNS. However, NO is not stored in neurons and released by exocytosis. Rather, it is synthesized when needed and readily diffuses across membranes.

Neurotransmission in the peripheral nervous system and CNS once was believed to conform to the hypothesis that each neuron contains only one transmitter substance. However, we now find that synaptic transmission may be mediated by the release of more than one neurotransmitter. Additional peptides, such as enkephalin, substance P, NPY, VIP, and SST; purines such as ATP and adenosine; and small molecules such as NO have been found in nerve endings along with the "classical" biogenic amine neurotransmitters. These additional substances can depolarize or hyperpolarize nerve terminals or postsynaptic cells. For example, enkephalins are found in postganglionic sympathetic neurons and adrenal medullary chromaffin cells. VIP is localized selectively in peripheral cholinergic neurons that innervate exocrine glands, and NPY is found in sympathetic nerve endings. These observations suggest that synaptic transmission in many instances may be mediated by the release of more than one neurotransmitter (see the next section).

Steps Involved in Neurotransmission

The sequence of events involved in neurotransmission is of particular importance because pharmacologically active agents modulate the individual steps.

Axonal Conduction

Conduction refers to the passage of an electrical impulse along an axon or muscle fiber. At rest, the interior of the typical mammalian axon is about 70 mV negative to the exterior. In response to depolarization to a threshold level, an action potential is initiated at a local region of the membrane. The action potential consists of two phases. Following depolarization that induces an open conformation of the channel, the *initial phase* is caused by a rapid increase in the permeability and inward movement of Na^+ through voltage-sensitive Na^+ channels, and a rapid depolarization from the resting potential continues to a positive overshoot. The *second phase* results from the rapid inactivation of the Na^+ channel and the delayed opening of a K^+ channel, which permits outward movement of K^+ to terminate the depolarization. Although not important in axonal conduction, Ca^{2+} channels in other tissues (e.g., L-type Ca^{2+} channels in heart) contribute to the action potential by prolonging depolarization by an inward movement of Ca^{2+}. This influx of Ca^{2+} also serves as a stimulus to initiate intracellular events (Catterall, 2000), and Ca^{2+} influx is important in excitation-exocytosis coupling (transmitter release).

The transmembrane ionic currents produce local circuit currents such that adjacent resting channels in the axon are activated, and excitation of an adjacent portion of the axonal membrane occurs, leading to propagation of the action potential without decrement along the axon. The region that has undergone depolarization remains momentarily in a refractory state.

With the exception of the local anesthetics, few drugs modify axonal conduction in the doses employed therapeutically. The puffer fish poison, *tetrodotoxin*, and a close congener found in some shellfish, *saxitoxin*, selectively block axonal conduction by blocking the voltage-sensitive Na^+ channel and preventing the increase in Na^+ permeability associated with the rising phase of the action potential. In contrast, *batrachotoxin*, an extremely potent steroidal alkaloid secreted by a South American frog, produces paralysis through a selective increase in permeability of the Na^+ channel, which induces a persistent depolarization. Scorpion toxins are peptides that also cause persistent depolarization by inhibiting the inactivation process (Catterall, 2000). Na^+ and Ca^{2+} channels are discussed in more detail in Chapters 11, 14, and 22.

Junctional Transmission

The term *transmission* refers to the passage of an impulse across a synaptic or neuroeffector junction. The arrival of the action potential at the axonal terminals initiates a series of events that trigger transmission of an excitatory or inhibitory biochemical message across the synapse or neuroeffector junction. These events, diagrammed in Figures 8–3, 8–4, and 8–5, are the following:

1. *Storage and release of transmitter.* The nonpeptide (small-molecule) neurotransmitters, such as biogenic amines, are largely synthesized in the region of the axonal terminals and stored there in synaptic vesicles. Neurotransmitter transport into storage vesicles is driven by an electrochemical gradient generated by the vesicular proton pump (vesicular ATPase) (Figures 8–5 and 8–6). Synaptic vesicles cluster in discrete areas underlying the presynaptic plasma membrane, termed *active zones*, often aligning with the tips of postsynaptic folds. Proteins in the vesicular membrane (e.g., synapsin, synaptophysin, synaptogyrin) are involved in development and trafficking of the storage vesicle to the active zone. The processes of priming, docking, fusion, and exocytosis involve the interactions of proteins in the vesicular and plasma membranes and the rapid entry of extracellular Ca^{2+} and its binding to synaptotagmins (Figure 8–4).

Life Cycle of a Storage Vesicle; Molecular Mechanism of Exocytosis. Fusion of the storage vesicle and plasma membrane involves formation of a multiprotein complex that includes proteins in

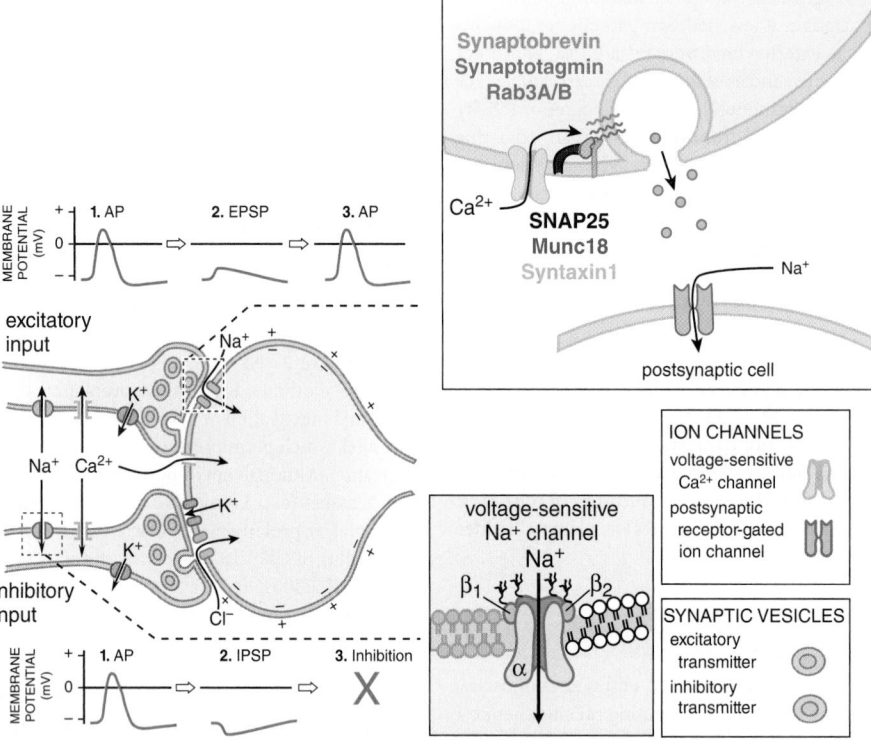

Figure 8–3 *Steps involved in excitatory and inhibitory neurotransmission.* **1.** The nerve AP consists of a transient self-propagated reversal of charge on the axonal membrane. (The internal potential E_i goes from a negative value, through zero potential, to a slightly positive value, primarily through increases in Na^+ permeability, and then returns to resting values by an increase in K^+ permeability.) When the AP arrives at the presynaptic terminal, it initiates release of the excitatory or inhibitory transmitter. Depolarization at the nerve ending and entry of Ca^{2+} initiate docking and then fusion of the synaptic vesicle with the membrane of the nerve ending. Some of the SNARE proteins involved in docking and fusion are shown. Figures 8–4 and 8–5 show some additional details of the life cycle of neurotransmitter storage vesicle and exocytosis. **2.** Interaction of the excitatory transmitter with postsynaptic receptors produces a localized depolarization, the EPSP, through an increase in permeability to cations, most notably Na^+. The inhibitory transmitter causes a selective increase in permeability to K^+ or Cl^-, resulting in a localized hyperpolarization, the IPSP. **3.** The EPSP initiates a conducted AP in the postsynaptic neuron; this can be prevented, however, by the hyperpolarization induced by a concurrent IPSP. The transmitter is dissipated by enzymatic destruction, by reuptake into the presynaptic terminal or adjacent glial cells, or by diffusion. Depolarization of the postsynaptic membrane can permit Ca^{2+} entry if voltage-gated Ca^{2+} channels are present.

the membrane of the synaptic vesicle, proteins embedded in the inner surface of the plasma membrane, and several cytosolic components. These proteins are referred to as SNARE proteins. Through the assembly of these proteins, vesicles draw near the membrane (priming, docking), spatially prepared for the next step, which the entry of Ca^{2+} initiates. When Ca^{2+} enters with the action potential, fusion and exocytosis occur rapidly. After fusion, the chaperone ATPase NSF and its SNAP adapters catalyze dissociation of the SNARE complex. Figures 8–4 and 8–5 depict this life cycle. Figure 8–4 shows some details of the assembly of the SNARE protein complex leading to fusion and exocytosis of neurotransmitter. The isoforms of the participating proteins may differ in different neurotransmitter systems, but the general mechanism seems to be conserved.

During the resting state, there is continual slow release of isolated quanta of the transmitter; this produces electrical responses (*miniature end-plate potentials* or *mepps*) at the postjunctional membrane that are associated with the maintenance of the physiological responsiveness of the effector organ. A low level of spontaneous activity within the motor units of skeletal muscle is particularly important because skeletal muscle lacks inherent tone.

The action potential causes the synchronous release of several hundred quanta of neurotransmitter. In the fusion/exocytosis process, the contents of the vesicles, including enzymes and other proteins, are discharged to the synaptic space. Synaptic vesicles may either fully exocytose with complete fusion or form a transient, nanometer-size pore that closes after transmitter has escaped, "kiss-and-run" exocytosis. In full-fusion exocytosis, the pit formed by the vesicle's fusing with the plasma membrane is clathrin-coated and retrieved from the membrane via endocytosis and transported to an endosome for full recycling. During kiss-and-run exocytosis, the

pore closes, and the vesicle is immediately and locally recycled for reuse in neurotransmitter repackaging (Alabi and Tsien, 2013; Südhof, 2014).

Modulation of Transmitter Release. A number of autocrine and paracrine factors may influence the exocytotic process, including the released neurotransmitter itself. Adenosine, DA, glutamate, GABA, prostaglandins, and enkephalins influence neurally mediated release of neurotransmitters. Receptors for these factors exist in the membranes of the soma, dendrites, and axons of neurons (Miller, 1998; Westfall, 2004): *Soma-dendritic receptors*, when activated, primarily modify functions of the soma-dendritic region, such as protein synthesis and generation of action potentials. *Presynaptic receptors*, when activated, modify functions of the terminal region, such as synthesis and release of transmitters.

Two main classes of presynaptic receptors have been identified on most neurons: *Heteroreceptors* are presynaptic receptors that respond to neurotransmitters, neuromodulators, or neurohormones released from adjacent neurons or cells. For example, NE can influence the release of ACh from parasympathetic neurons by acting on α_{2A}, α_{2B}, and α_{2C} receptors, whereas ACh can influence the release of NE from sympathetic neurons by acting on M_2 and M_4 receptors. *Autoreceptors* are receptors located on or close to axon terminals of a neuron through which the neuron's own transmitter can modify transmitter synthesis and release (see Figures 8–6 and 8–8). For example, NE released from sympathetic neurons may interact with α_{2A} and α_{2C} receptors to inhibit neurally released NE. Similarly, ACh released from parasympathetic neurons may interact with M_2 and M_4 receptors to inhibit neurally released ACh.

2. *Interaction of the transmitter with postjunctional receptors and production of the postjunctional potential.* The transmitter diffuses across the

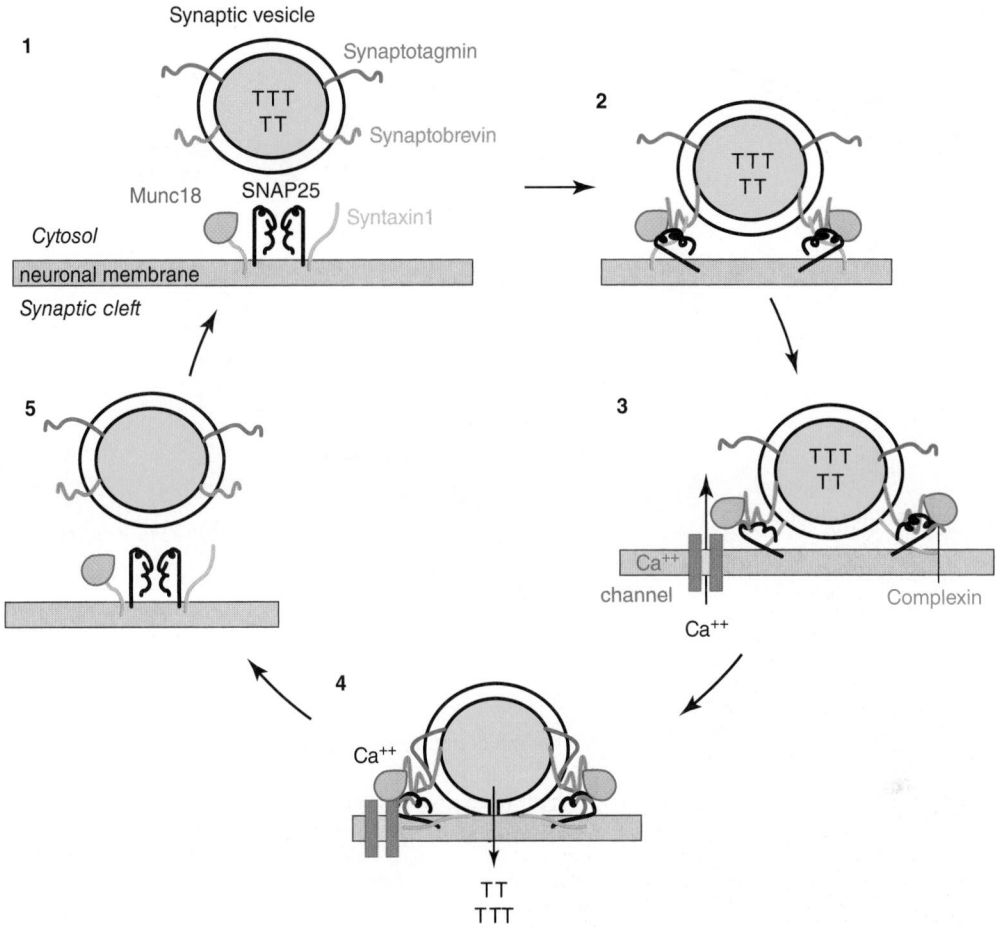

Figure 8–4 *Molecular basis of exocytosis: docking and fusion of synaptic vesicles with neuronal membranes.* **1.** *Vesicular docking in the active zone*: Munc18 binds to syntaxin 1, stabilizing the neuronal membrane SNARE proteins. **2.** *Priming I*: Syntaxin assembles with SNAP25, allowing for the vesicle SNARE protein synaptobrevin to bind to the complex. **3.** *Priming II*: Complexin binds to the SNARE complex and allows for the vesicular synaptotagmin to bind Ca^{2+} that drives the full fusion process. **4.** *Fusion pore opening*: Synaptotagmin interacts with the SNARE complex and binds Ca^{2+}, permitting pore fusion and exocytosis of neurotransmitter. Other components, not shown, are the vesicular GTP-binding Rab3/27; the linking proteins Munc13, RIM, and RIM-BP; and tethering to the Ca^{2+} channel. **5.** *Return to ground state*: After fusion, the chaperone ATPase NSF and its SNAP adapters catalyze dissociation of the SNARE-complex. For a more detailed view of this process, see Südhof (2014).

synaptic or junctional cleft and combines with specialized receptors on the postjunctional membrane; this often results in a localized increase in the ionic permeability, or conductance, of the membrane. With certain exceptions (noted in the following discussion), one of three types of permeability change can occur:

- Generalized increase in the permeability to cations (notably Na^+ but occasionally Ca^{2+}), resulting in a localized depolarization of the membrane, that is, an EPSP.
- Selective increase in permeability to anions, usually Cl^-, resulting in stabilization or actual hyperpolarization of the membrane, which constitutes an IPSP.
- Increased permeability to K^+. Because the K^+ gradient is directed out of the cell, hyperpolarization and stabilization of the membrane potential occur (an IPSP).

Electric potential changes associated with the EPSP and IPSP at most sites are the results of passive fluxes of ions down their concentration gradients. The changes in channel permeability that cause these potential changes are specifically regulated by the specialized postjunctional receptors for the neurotransmitter that initiates the response (see Figures 8–6, 8–8, and 11–4 and Chapter 14). These receptors may be clustered on the effector cell surface, as seen at the NMJs of skeletal muscle and other discrete synapses, or distributed more uniformly, as observed in smooth muscle. These *high-conductance, ligand-gated ion channels* usually permit

passage of Na^+ or Cl^-; K^+ and Ca^{2+} are involved less frequently. In the presence of an appropriate neurotransmitter, the channel opens rapidly to a high-conductance state, remains open for about a millisecond, and then closes. A short square-wave pulse of current is observed as a result of the channel's opening and closing. The summation of these microscopic events gives rise to the EPSP.

The ligand-gated channels belong to a superfamily of ionotropic receptor proteins that includes the nicotinic, glutamate, and certain 5HT3 and purine receptors, which conduct primarily Na^+, cause depolarization, and are excitatory; and GABA acid and glycine receptors, which conduct Cl^-, cause hyperpolarization, and are inhibitory. Neurotransmitters also can modulate the permeability of K^+ and Ca^{2+} channels indirectly. In these cases, the receptor and channel are separate proteins, and information is conveyed between them by G proteins (see Chapter 3).

The nicotinic, GABA, glycine, and 5HT3 receptors are closely related, whereas the glutamate and purinergic ionotropic receptors have distinct structures (see Figure 11–1 and Chapter 14). Neurotransmitters also can modulate the permeability of K^+ and Ca^{2+} channels indirectly. In these cases, the receptor and channel are separate proteins, and information is conveyed between them by G proteins. Other receptors for neurotransmitters act by influencing the synthesis of intracellular second messengers and do not necessarily cause a change in membrane potential. The most widely documented examples of receptor regulation of second-messenger systems are the activation or inhibition of adenylyl cyclase to modulate

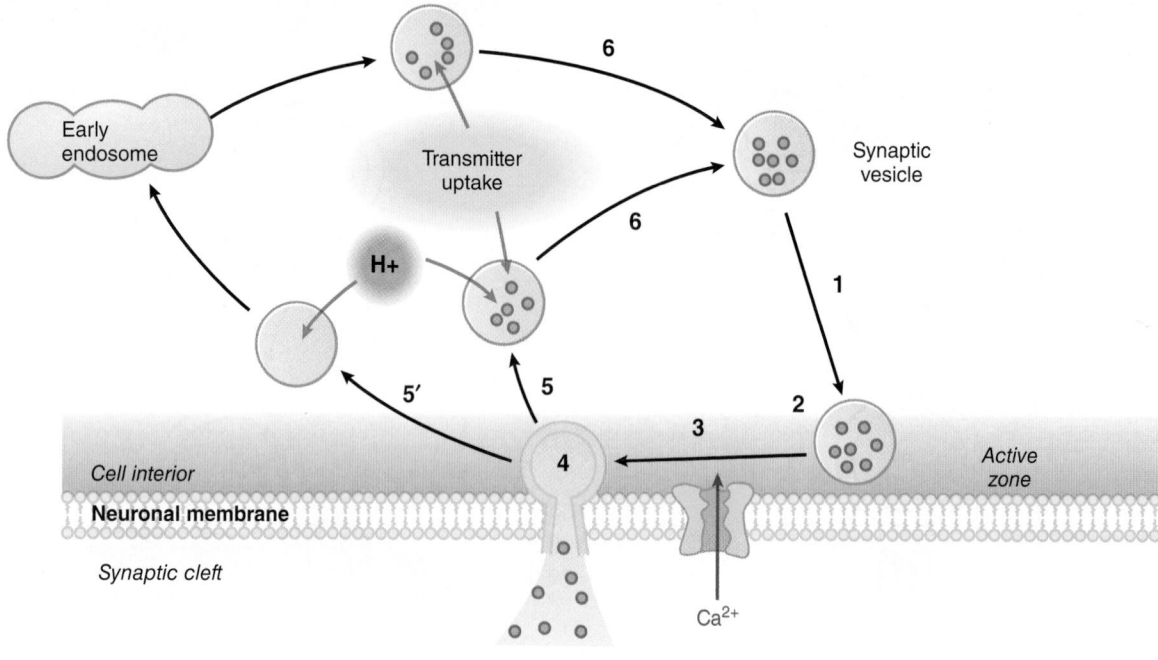

Figure 8–5 *Life cycle of a synaptic vesicle.* A mature storage vesicle, replete with transmitter, is translocated to the perimembrane space (*active zone*) (**1**). Once in the active zone (**2**), the vesicle undergoes docking and priming (see Figure 8–4), as proteins from the cytosol and the vesicular and plasma membranes (SNARE proteins) interact to tether the vesicle in a prefusion stage. The rapid entry of Ca^{2+} via voltage-sensitive channels located in the active zone (**3**) activates the calcium sensor synaptotagmin and initiates the process of fusion and exocytosis of the vesicular contents into the synaptic space (**4**). After transmitter release, the vesicle is endocytosed, the SNARE protein complex is disassembled by the action of the chaperone ATPase NSF and its SNAP adapters, and the empty vesicle is recycled, either trafficked directly back into use (**5**) or routed through an early endosomal pathway (**5′**). In either event, the vesicular ATPase is at work, promoting H^+ uptake to establish the gradient that drives transmitter uptake and repletion of the vesicle (**6**). For a more detailed view of the exocytotic process, see Südhof (2014). Secreted neuropeptides are stored in larger, dense core vesicles (see text). Their secretory process is similar; however, there are no uptake transporters for peptide neurotransmitters; rather, vesicles containing releasable peptides are formed in the trans-Golgi network of the nerve cell body and transported to the release site by molecular motors (kinesins, F-actin, etc.); nonsecreted vesicle components are recycled. Park and Loh (2008), Heaslip et al. (2014), and Salogiannis and Reck-Peterson (2016) have reviewed aspects of the transport of such vesicles.

cellular cAMP concentrations and the increase in cytosolic concentrations of Ca^{2+} that results from release of the ion from internal stores by inositol trisphosphate (see Chapter 3).

3. *Initiation of postjunctional activity.* If an EPSP exceeds a certain threshold value, it initiates a propagated action potential in a postsynaptic neuron or a muscle action potential in skeletal or cardiac muscle by activating voltage-sensitive channels in the immediate vicinity. In certain smooth muscle types in which propagated impulses are minimal, an EPSP may increase the rate of spontaneous depolarization, cause Ca^{2+} release, and enhance muscle tone; in gland cells, the EPSP initiates secretion through Ca^{2+} mobilization. An IPSP, which is found in neurons and smooth muscle but not in skeletal muscle, will tend to oppose excitatory potentials simultaneously initiated by other neuronal sources. Whether a propagated impulse or other response ensues depends on the summation of all the potentials.

4. *Destruction or dissipation of the transmitter.* When impulses can be transmitted across junctions at frequencies up to several hundred per second, there must be an efficient means of disposing of the transmitter following each impulse. At cholinergic synapses involved in rapid neurotransmission, high and localized concentrations of AChE are available for this purpose. When AChE activity is inhibited, removal of the transmitter is accomplished principally by diffusion. Under these circumstances, the effects of released ACh are potentiated and prolonged (see Chapter 10).

Rapid termination of NE occurs by a combination of simple diffusion and reuptake by the axonal terminals of most of the released

NE. Termination of the action of amino acid transmitters results from their active transport into neurons and surrounding glia. Peptide neurotransmitters are hydrolyzed by various peptidases and dissipated by diffusion.

5. *Nonelectrogenic functions.* The activity and turnover of enzymes involved in the synthesis and inactivation of neurotransmitters, the density of presynaptic and postsynaptic receptors, and other characteristics of synapses are controlled by trophic actions of neurotransmitters or other trophic factors released by the neuron or target cells.

Cholinergic Transmission

The neurochemical events that underlie cholinergic neurotransmission are summarized in Figure 8–6.

Synthesis and Storage of ACh

Two enzymes, choline acetyltransferase and AChE, are involved in ACh synthesis and degradation, respectively.

Choline Acetyltransferase. *Choline acetyltransferase* catalyzes the synthesis of ACh—the acetylation of choline with acetyl CoA. Choline acetyltransferase is synthesized within the perikaryon and then is transported along the length of the axon to its terminal. Axonal terminals contain a large number of mitochondria, where acetyl CoA is synthesized. Choline is taken up from the extracellular fluid into the axoplasm by active transport. The final step in the synthesis occurs within the cytoplasm, following which most of the ACh is sequestered within synaptic vesicles. Although moderately potent inhibitors of choline acetyltransferase exist, they have no

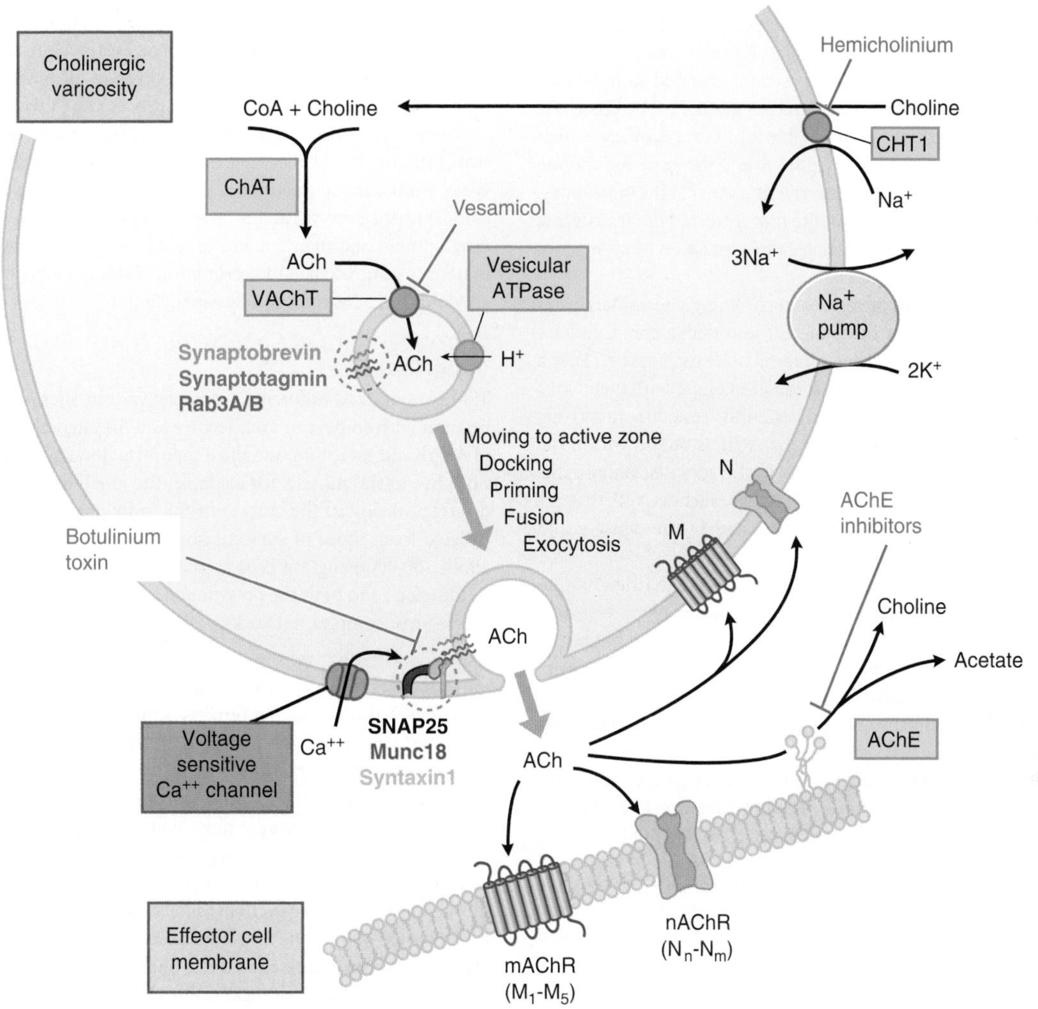

Figure 8–6 *A typical cholinergic neuroeffector junction.* The synthesis of ACh in the varicosity depends on the uptake of choline via a Na⁺-dependent carrier, CHT1, that hemicholinium can block. The enzyme ChAT catalyzes the synthesis of ACh from choline and the acetyl moiety of acetyl CoA. ACh is transported into the storage vesicle by VAChT, which can be inhibited by vesamicol. ACh is stored in vesicles (along with other potential cotransmitters, such as ATP and VIP, at certain neuroeffector junctions). Release of ACh and any cotransmitters occurs via exocytosis (the stages are itemized along the gray arrow), triggered by Ca^{2+} entry via a voltage-sensitive Ca^{2+} channel in response to membrane depolarization, as described in Figures 8–3, 8–4, and 8–5. Exocytotic release of ACh at the NMJ can be blocked by botulinum toxins, the active fragments of which are endopeptidases that cleave synaptobrevin, an essential member of the SNARE proteins that mediate docking/priming/exocytosis. Once released, ACh can interact with the muscarinic receptors (M), which are GPCRs, or nicotinic receptors (N), which are ligand-gated ion channels, to produce the characteristic response of the postsynaptic cell. ACh also can act on presynaptic mAChRs or nAChRs to modify its own release. The action of ACh is terminated by extracellular metabolism to choline and acetate by AChE, which is associated with synaptic membranes.

therapeutic utility, in part because the rate-limiting step in ACh biosynthesis is the uptake of choline.

Choline and Choline Transport. The availability of choline is critical to the synthesis of ACh. Choline must be derived primarily from the diet (there is little de novo synthesis of choline in cholinergic neurons) or, secondarily, from recycling of choline. Once ACh is released from cholinergic neurons in response to an action potential, ACh is hydrolyzed by AChE to acetate and choline. Much of the choline is taken up at cholinergic nerve terminals and reused for ACh synthesis. Under many circumstances, this reuptake and availability of choline appear to be rate limiting in ACh synthesis. There are three mammalian transport systems for choline; all three are transmembrane proteins with multiple TM segments; all are inhibited by hemicholinium but at distinct concentrations in the same order as their affinities for choline (Haga, 2014):

• The high-affinity (4-μM) choline transporter CHT1 (SLC5A7) present on presynaptic membranes of cholinergic neurons. This transporter is a member of the SLC5 family of solute carrier proteins that includes Na⁺-glucose cotransporters and shares about 25% homology with those transporters (Haga, 2014). Choline transport by CHT1 is Na⁺ and Cl⁻ dependent. This system provides choline for ACh synthesis and is the high-affinity hemicholinium-binding protein ($K_i = 0.05$ μM).

• A low-affinity (40-μM), Na⁺-independent transporter, CTL1 (SLC44A), which is widely distributed and appears to supply choline for phospholipid synthesis (e.g., phosphatidyl choline, sphigomyelin).

• A lower-affinity (100-μM) Na⁺-independent transporter, OCT2 (SLC22A2), a nonspecific organic cation secretory transporter found in renal proximal tubules (see Figures 5–8 and 5–9), hepatocytes, the choroid plexus, the lumenal membrane of brain endothelium, and synaptic vesicles from cholinergic neurons. Its role in neurons remains to be clarified.

In model systems, CHT1 localizes mainly to intracellular organelles, including transmitter storage vesicles; neural activity increases the fraction of CHT1 in the plasma membrane, and phosphorylation by PKC enhances internalization (Haga, 2014).

Storage of ACh. ACh is transported into synaptic vesicles by the VAChT (a solute carrier protein, SLC18A3) using the potential energy of a proton electrochemical gradient that a vacuolar ATPase establishes, such that the transport of protons out of the vesicle is coupled to uptake of ACh into the vesicle and against a concentration gradient. The process is inhibited by the noncompetitive and reversible inhibitor *vesamicol*, which does not affect the vesicular ATPase (Figure 8–6). The gene for choline acetyltransferase and the vesicular transporter are found at the same locus, with the transporter gene positioned in the first intron of the transferase gene. Hence, a common promoter regulates the expression of both genes (Eiden, 1998).

There appear to be two types of vesicles in cholinergic terminals: electron-lucent vesicles (40–50 nm in diameter) and dense-cored vesicles (80–150 nm). The core of the vesicles contains both ACh and ATP, at a ratio of about 11:1, which are dissolved in the fluid phase with metal ions (Ca^{2+} and Mg^{2+}) and a proteoglycan called vesiculin. Vesiculin, negatively charged and thought to sequester the Ca^{2+} or ACh, is bound within the vesicle, with the protein moiety anchoring it to the vesicular membrane. In some cholinergic terminals, there are peptides, such as VIP, that act as *cotransmitters*. The peptides usually are located in the dense-cored vesicles.

Estimates of the ACh content of synaptic vesicles range from 1000 to over 50,000 molecules per vesicle, with a single motor nerve terminal containing 300,000 or more vesicles. In addition, an uncertain but possibly significant amount of ACh is present in the extravesicular cytoplasm. Recording the electrical events associated with the opening of single channels at the motor end plate during continuous application of ACh has permitted estimation of the potential change induced by a single molecule of ACh (3×10^{-7} V); from such calculations, it is evident that even the lower estimate of the ACh content per vesicle (1000 molecules) is sufficient to account for the magnitude of the miniature end-plate potentials.

Release of ACh. Exocytotic release of ACh and cotransmitters (e.g., ATP, VIP) occurs on depolarization of the nerve terminals. Depolarization of the terminals allows the entry of Ca^{2+} through voltage-gated Ca^{2+} channels and promotes fusion of the vesicular membrane with the plasma membrane, allowing exocytosis to occur, as described previously and in Figure 8–6.

Two pools of ACh appear to exist. One pool, the "depot" or "readily releasable" pool, consists of vesicles located near the plasma membrane of the nerve terminals; these vesicles contain newly synthesized transmitter. Depolarization of the terminals causes these vesicles to release ACh rapidly or readily. The other pool, the "reserve pool," seems to replenish the readily releasable pool and may be required to sustain ACh release during periods of prolonged or intense nerve stimulation.

Botulinum toxin blocks ACh release by interfering with the machinery of transmitter release. The active fragments of botulinum toxins are endopeptidases; the SNARE proteins are their substrates. There are eight isotypes of botulinum toxin, each cleaving a specific site on SNARE proteins. Tetanus toxins act similarly, but in the CNS. The active fragments of these toxins cleave synaptobrevin and block exocytosis in specific sets of neurons (inhibitory neurons in the CNS for tetanus, the NMJ for botulinum).

Acetylcholinesterase. At the NMJ, immediate hydrolysis of ACh by AChE reduces lateral diffusion of the transmitter and activation of adjacent receptors. Rapid release of ACh onto the nAChRs of the motor end plate, followed by rapid hydrolysis of the neurotransmitter, spatially limits receptor activation and facilitates rapid control of responses. The time required for hydrolysis of ACh at the NMJ is less than a millisecond. Chapter 10 presents details of the structure, mechanism, and inhibition of AChE.

AChE is found in cholinergic neurons and is highly concentrated at the postsynaptic end plate of the NMJ. BuChE (butyrylcholinesterase, also called pseudocholinesterase) is virtually absent in neuronal elements of the central and peripheral nervous systems. BuChE is synthesized primarily in the liver and is found in liver and plasma; its likely physiological function is the hydrolysis of ingested esters from plant sources. AChE and BuChE typically are distinguished by the relative rates of ACh and butyrylcholine hydrolysis and by effects of selective inhibitors (see Chapter 10).

Almost all pharmacological effects of the anti-ChE agents are due to the inhibition of AChE, with the consequent accumulation of endogenous ACh in the vicinity of the nerve terminal. Distinct but single genes encode AChE and BuChE in mammals; the diversity of molecular structure of AChE arises from alternative mRNA processing (Taylor et al., 2000).

Numerous reports suggest that AChE plays roles in addition to its classical function in terminating impulse transmission at cholinergic synapses. Nonclassical functions of AChE might include hydrolysis of ACh in a nonsynaptic context, action as an adhesion protein involved in synaptic development and maintenance or as a bone matrix protein, involvement in neurite outgrowth, and acceleration of the assembly of Aβ peptide into amyloid fibrils (Silman and Sussman, 2005).

Characteristics of Cholinergic Transmission at Various Sites

There are marked differences amongst various sites of cholinergic transmission with respect to architecture and fine structure, the distributions of AChE and receptors, and the temporal factors involved in normal function. In skeletal muscle, for example, the junctional sites occupy a small, discrete portion of the surface of the individual fibers and are relatively isolated from those of adjacent fibers; in the superior cervical ganglion, about 100,000 ganglion cells are packed within a volume of a few cubic millimeters, and both the presynaptic and the postsynaptic neuronal processes form complex networks.

Skeletal Muscle. At the NMJ, ACh stimulates the nicotinic receptor's intrinsic channel, which opens for about 1 ms, admitting about 50,000 Na^+ ions. The channel-opening process is the basis for the localized depolarizing EPP within the end plate, which triggers the muscle action potential and leads to contraction. The amount of ACh (10^{-17} mol) required to elicit an EPP following its microiontophoretic application to the motor end plate of a rat diaphragm muscle fiber is equivalent to that recovered from each fiber following stimulation of the phrenic nerve.

Following sectioning and degeneration of the motor nerve to skeletal muscle or of the postganglionic fibers to autonomic effectors, there is a marked reduction in the threshold doses of the transmitters and of certain other drugs required to elicit a response; that is, denervation supersensitivity occurs. In skeletal muscle, this change is accompanied by a spread of the receptor molecules from the end-plate region to the adjacent portions of the sarcoplasmic membrane, which eventually involves the entire muscle surface. Embryonic muscle also exhibits this uniform sensitivity to ACh prior to innervation. Hence, innervation represses the expression of the receptor gene by the nuclei that lie in extrajunctional regions of the muscle fiber and directs the subsynaptic nuclei to express the structural and functional proteins of the synapse.

Autonomic Effector Cells. Stimulation or inhibition of autonomic effector cells occurs on activation of muscarinic ACh receptors (discussed below). In this case, the effector is coupled to the receptor by a G protein (Chapter 3). In contrast to skeletal muscle and neurons, smooth muscle and the cardiac conduction system sinoatrial (SA node, atrium, AV node, and the His-Purkinje system) normally exhibit intrinsic activity, both electrical and mechanical, that is modulated but not initiated by nerve impulses.

In the basal condition, unitary smooth muscle exhibits waves of depolarization or spikes that are propagated from cell to cell at rates considerably slower than the action potential of axons or skeletal muscle. The spikes apparently are initiated by rhythmic fluctuations in the membrane resting potential. Application of ACh (0.1 to 1 μM) to isolated intestinal muscle causes the membrane potential to become less negative and increases the frequency of spike production, accompanied by a rise in tension. A primary action of ACh in initiating these effects through muscarinic receptors is probably partial depolarization of the cell membrane brought about by an increase in Na^+ and, in some instances, Ca^{2+} conductance. ACh also can produce contraction of some smooth muscles when the membrane has been depolarized completely by high concentrations of K^+, provided that Ca^{2+} is present. Hence, ACh stimulates ion fluxes across membranes or mobilizes intracellular Ca^{2+} to cause contraction.

In the heart, spontaneous depolarizations normally arise from the SA node. In the cardiac conduction system, particularly in the SA and AV nodes, stimulation of the cholinergic innervation or the direct application of ACh causes inhibition, associated with hyperpolarization of the membrane and a marked decrease in the rate of depolarization. These effects are due, at least in part, to a selective increase in permeability to K^+.

Autonomic Ganglia. The primary pathway of cholinergic transmission in autonomic ganglia is similar to that at the NMJ of skeletal muscle. The initial depolarization is the result of activation of nAChRs, which are ligand-gated cation channels with properties similar to those found at the NMJ. Several secondary transmitters or modulators either enhance or diminish the sensitivity of the postganglionic cell to ACh (see Figure 11–5).

Prejunctional Sites. ACh release is subject to complex regulation by mediators, including ACh itself acting on M_2 and M_4 *autoreceptors*, and activation of *heteroreceptors* (e.g., NE acting on α_{2A} and α_{2C} adrenergic receptors) or substances produced locally in tissues (e.g., NO) (Philipp and Hein, 2004; Wess et al., 2007). ACh-mediated inhibition of ACh release following activation of M_2 and M_4 autoreceptors is a physiological negative-feedback control mechanism. At some neuroeffector junctions (e.g., the myenteric plexus in the GI tract or the cardiac SA node), sympathetic and parasympathetic nerve terminals often lie juxtaposed to each other. There, opposing effects of NE and ACh result not only from the opposite effects of the two neurotransmitters on the smooth muscle or cardiac cells but also from the inhibition of ACh release by NE or inhibition of NE release by ACh acting on heteroreceptors on parasympathetic or sympathetic terminals.

Inhibitory heteroreceptors on parasympathetic terminals include adenosine A_1 receptors, histamine H_3 receptors, opioid receptors, and α_{2A} and α_{2C} adrenergic receptors. The parasympathetic nerve terminal varicosities also may contain additional heteroreceptors that could respond by inhibition or enhancement of ACh release by locally formed autacoids, hormones, or administered drugs.

Extraneuronal Sites. All elements of the cholinergic system are functionally expressed independently of cholinergic innervation in numerous nonneuronal cells. These *nonneuronal cholinergic* systems can both modify and control phenotypic cell functions such as proliferation, differentiation, formation of physical barriers, migration, and ion and water movements.

The widespread synthesis of ACh in nonneuronal cells has changed the thinking that ACh acts only as a neurotransmitter. Each component of the cholinergic system in nonneuronal cells can be affected by pathophysiological conditions. Dysfunctions of nonneuronal cholinergic systems may be involved in the pathogenesis of diseases (e.g., inflammatory processes) (Wessler and Kirkpatrick, 2008).

HISTORICAL PERSPECTIVE

Sir Henry Dale noted that the various esters of choline elicited responses that were similar to those of either nicotine or muscarine depending on the pharmacological preparation. A similarity in response also was noted between muscarine and nerve stimulation in those organs innervated by the craniosacral divisions of the autonomic nervous system. Thus, Dale suggested that ACh or another ester of choline was a neurotransmitter in the autonomic nervous system; he also stated that the compound had dual actions, which he termed a "nicotine action" (*nicotinic*) and a "muscarine action" (*muscarinic*).

The capacities of tubocurarine and atropine to block nicotinic and muscarinic effects of ACh, respectively, provided further support for the proposal of two distinct types of cholinergic receptors. Although Dale had access only to crude plant alkaloids of then-unknown structure from *Amanita muscaria* and *Nicotiana tabacum*, this classification remains the primary subdivision of cholinergic receptors. Its utility has survived the discovery of several distinct subtypes of nicotinic and muscarinic receptors.

Cholinergic Receptors and Signal Transduction

Nicotinic receptors are ligand-gated ion channels whose activation always causes a rapid (millisecond) increase in cellular permeability to Na^+ and Ca^{2+}, depolarization, and excitation. *Muscarinic receptors* are GPCRs. Responses to muscarinic agonists are slower; they may be either excitatory or inhibitory, and they are not necessarily linked to changes in ion permeability. The muscarinic and nicotinic receptors for ACh belong to two different families whose features are described in Chapters 9 and 11, respectively.

Subtypes of nAChRs. The *nAChRs* exist at the skeletal NMJ, autonomic ganglia, adrenal medulla, and CNS and in nonneuronal tissues. The nAChRs are composed of five homologous subunits organized around a central pore (see Table 8–2 and Figure 11–2). In general, the nAChRs are further divided into two groups:

- *Muscle type* (N_m), found in the vertebrate skeletal muscle, where they mediate transmission at the NMJ
- *Neuronal type* (N_n), found mainly throughout the peripheral nervous system, CNS, and nonneuronal tissues

Neuronal nAChRs are widely distributed in the CNS and are found at presynaptic, perisynaptic, and postsynaptic sites. At pre- and perisynaptic sites, nAChRs appear to act as autoreceptors or heteroreceptors to regulate the release of several neurotransmitters (ACh, DA, NE, glutamate, and 5HT) at diverse sites in the brain (Albuquerque et al., 2009).

Muscle-Type nAChRs. In fetal muscle prior to innervation, in adult muscle after denervation, and in fish electric organs, the nAChR subunit stoichiometry is $(\alpha1)_2\beta1\gamma\delta$, whereas in adult muscle the γ subunit is replaced by ϵ to give the $(\alpha1)_2\beta1\epsilon\delta$ stoichiometry (Table 8–2). The γ/ϵ and δ subunits are involved together with the $\alpha1$ subunits in forming the ligand-binding sites and in the maintenance of cooperative interactions between the $\alpha1$ subunit. Different affinities to the two binding sites are conferred by the presence of different non-α subunits. Binding of ACh to the $\alpha\gamma$ and $\alpha\delta$ sites is thought to induce a conformational change predominantly in the $\alpha1$ subunits that interacts with the transmembrane region to cause channel opening.

Neuronal-Type nAChRs. Neuronal nAChRs are widely expressed in peripheral ganglia, the adrenal medulla, numerous areas of the brain, and nonneuronal cells, such as epithelial cells and cells of the immune system. To date, nine α ($\alpha2$–$\alpha10$) and three β ($\beta2$–$\beta4$) subunit genes have been cloned. The $\alpha7$–$\alpha10$ subunits are found either as homopentamers (of five $\alpha7$, $\alpha8$, and $\alpha9$ subunits) or as heteropentamers of $\alpha7$, $\alpha8$, and $\alpha9/\alpha10$. By contrast, the $\alpha2$–$\alpha6$ and $\beta2$–$\beta4$ subunits form heteropentamers usually with $(\alpha x)_2(\beta y)_3$ stoichiometry. The $\alpha5$ and $\beta3$ subunits do not appear to be able to form functional receptors when expressed alone or in paired combinations with α or β subunits, respectively (Kalamida et al., 2007).

The precise function of many of the neuronal nAChRs in the brain is not known; they appear to act more as synaptic modulators, the molecular diversity of the subunits putatively resulting in numerous nAChR subtypes with different physiological properties. Neuronal nAChRs are widely distributed in the CNS and are found at presynaptic, perisynaptic, and postsynaptic sites. At pre- and perisynaptic sites, nAChRs appear to act as autoreceptors or heteroreceptors to regulate the release of several neurotransmitters (ACh, DA, NE, glutamate, and 5HT) at sites throughout the brain (Exley and Cragg, 2008). The synaptic release of a particular neurotransmitter can be regulated by different neuronal-type nAChR subtypes in different CNS regions. For instance, DA release from striatal and thalamic DA neurons can be controlled by the $\alpha4\beta2$ subtype or both $\alpha4\beta2$ and $\alpha6\beta2\beta3$ subtypes, respectively. In contrast, glutametergic neurotransmission is regulated everywhere by $\alpha7$ nAChRs (Kalamida et al., 2007).

Subtypes of Muscarinic Receptors. In mammals, there are five distinct subtypes of mAChRs, each produced by a different gene. These variants have distinct anatomic locations in the periphery and CNS and differing chemical specificities. The mAChRs are GPCRs (see Table 8–3 and Chapter 9), present in virtually all organs, tissues, and cell types (Table 8–3

TABLE 8–2 ■ CHARACTERISTICS OF SUBTYPES OF NICOTINIC ACETYLCHOLINE RECEPTORS (NACHRS)

RECEPTOR (Primary Receptor Subtype)[a]	MAIN SYNAPTIC LOCATION	MEMBRANE RESPONSE	MOLECULAR MECHANISM	AGONISTS	ANTAGONISTS
Skeletal Muscle (N_m) $(\alpha 1)_2 \beta 1 \epsilon \delta$ adult $(\alpha 1)_2 \beta 1 \gamma \delta$ fetal	Skeletal neuromuscular junction (postjunctional)	Excitatory; end-plate depolarization; skeletal muscle contraction	Increased cation permeability (Na^+; K^+)	ACh Nicotine Succinylcholine	Atracurium Vecuronium d-Tubocurarine Pancuronium α-Conotoxin α-Bungarotoxin
Peripheral neuronal (N_n) $(\alpha 3)_2 (\beta 4)_3$	Autonomic ganglia; adrenal medulla	Excitatory; depolarization; firing of postganglion neuron; depolarization and secretion of catecholamines	Increased cation permeability (Na^+; K^+)	ACh Nicotine Epibatidine Dimethylphenyl-piperazinium	Trimethaphan Mecamylamine
CNS neuronal $(\alpha 4)_2 (\beta 4)_3$ *(α-BTX-insensitive)*	CNS; pre- and postjunctional	Pre- and postsynaptic excitation; prejunctional control of transmitter release	Increased cation permeability (Na^+; K^+)	Cytosine, epibatidine Anatoxin A	Mecamylamine DHbE Erysodine Lophotoxin
$(\alpha 7)_5$ *(α-BTX-sensitive)*	CNS; pre- and postsynaptic	Pre- and postsynaptic excitation; prejunctional control of transmitter release	Increased permeability (Ca^{2+})	Anatoxin A	Methyllycaconitine α-Bungarotoxin α-Conotoxin ImI

[a]Nine α (α2–α10) and three β (β2–β4) subunits have been identified and cloned in human brain, which combine in various conformations to form individual receptor subtypes. The structure of individual receptors and the subtype composition are incompletely understood. Only a finite number of naturally occurring functional nAChR constructs have been identified. DHbE, dihydro-β-erythroidine.

and Chapter 9). Most cell types have multiple mAChR subtypes, but certain subtypes often predominate in specific sites (Wess et al., 2007). For example, the M_2 receptor is the predominant subtype in the heart and in CNS neurons is mostly located presynaptically, whereas the M_3 receptor is the predominant subtype in the detrusor muscle of the bladder (Dhein et al., 2001; Fetscher et al., 2002).

In the periphery, mAChRs mediate the classical muscarinic actions of ACh in organs and tissues innervated by parasympathetic nerves, although receptors may be present at sites that lack parasympathetic innervation (e.g., most blood vessels). In the CNS, mAChRs are involved in regulating a large number of cognitive, behavioral, sensory, motor, and autonomic functions. Owing to the lack of specific muscarinic agonists and antagonists that demonstrate selectivity for individual mAChRs and the fact that most organs and tissues express multiple mAChRs, it has been a challenge to assign specific pharmacological functions to distinct mAChRs. The development of gene-targeting techniques in mice has been helpful in defining specific functions (Table 8–3) (Wess et al., 2007).

The functions of mAChRs are mediated by interactions with G proteins. The M_1, M_3, and M_5 subtypes couple through $G_{q/11}$ to stimulate the PLC-IP_3/DAG-Ca^{2+} pathway, leading to activation of PKC and Ca^{2+}-sensitive enzymes. Activation of M_1, M_3, and M_5 receptors can also cause the activation of PLA_2, leading to the release of arachidonic acid and consequent eicosanoid synthesis; these effects of M_1, M_3, and M_5 mAChRs are generally secondary to elevation of intracellular Ca^{2+}. Stimulated M_2 and M_4 cholinergic receptors couple to G_i and G_o, with resulting inhibition of adenylyl cyclase, leading to a decrease in cellular cAMP, activation of inwardly rectifying K^+ channels, and inhibition of voltage-gated Ca^{2+} channels (van Koppen and Kaiser, 2003). The functional consequences of these effects are hyperpolarization and inhibition of excitable membranes. In the myocardium, inhibition of adenylyl cyclase and activation of K^+ conductances account for the negative inotropic and chronotropic effects of ACh. In addition, heterologous systems may produce different receptor-transducer-effector interactions (Nathanson, 2008).

Following activation by classical or allosteric agonists, mAChRs can be phosphorylated by a variety of receptor kinases and second-messenger

regulated kinases; the phosphorylated mAChR subtypes then can interact with β-arrestin and possibly other adapter proteins. As a result, mAChR signaling pathways may be differentially altered. Agonist activation of mAChRs also may induce receptor internalization and downregulation (van Koppen and Kaiser, 2003). Muscarinic AChRs can also regulate other signal transduction pathways that have diverse effects on cell growth, survival, and physiology, such as MAPK, phosphoinositide-3-kinase, RhoA, and Rac1 (Nathanson, 2008).

Changes in mAChR levels and activity have been implicated in the pathophysiology of numerous major diseases in the CNS and in the autonomic nervous system (Table 8–3). Phenotypic analysis of mAChR-mutant mice as well as the development of selective agonists and antagonists has led to a wealth of new information regarding the physiological and potential pathophysiological roles of the individual mAChR subtype (Langmead et al., 2008; Wess et al., 2007).

Adrenergic Transmission

Norepinephrine (NE) is the principal transmitter of most sympathetic postganglionic fibers and of certain tracts in the CNS; DA is the predominant transmitter of the mammalian extrapyramidal system and of several mesocortical and mesolimbic neuronal pathways; and EPI is the major hormone of the adrenal medulla. Collectively, these three amines are called *catecholamines*. Drugs affecting these endogenous amines and their actions are used in the treatment of hypertension, mental disorders, and a variety of other conditions. The details of these interactions and of the pharmacology of the sympathomimetic amines themselves can be found in subsequent chapters. The basic physiological, biochemical, and pharmacological features are presented here.

Synthesis of Catecholamines

The steps in the synthesis of catecholamines and the characteristics of the enzymes involved are shown in Figure 8–7 and Table 8–4. Tyrosine is sequentially 3-hydroxylated and decarboxylated to form DA. DA is β-hydroxylated to yield NE, which is N-methylated in chromaffin tissue to give EPI. The enzymes involved have been identified, cloned, and characterized

TABLE 8–3 ■ CHARACTERISTICS OF MUSCARINIC ACETYLCHOLINE RECEPTOR (mAChRs) SUBTYPES

RECEPTOR	CELLULAR AND TISSUE LOCATION[a]	CELLULAR RESPONSE[b]	FUNCTIONAL RESPONSE[c]	DISEASE RELEVANCE
M_1	CNS; most abundant in cerebral cortex, hippocampus, striatum, and thalamus Autonomic ganglia Glands (gastric and salivary) Enteric nerves	Couples by $G_{q/11}$ to activate PLC-IP_3-Ca^{2+}-PKC pathway Depolarization and excitation ($\uparrow$ sEPSP) Activation of PLD_2, PLA_2; $\uparrow$AA	Increased cognitive function (learning and memory) Increased seizure activity Decrease in dopamine release and locomotion Increase in depolarization of autonomic ganglia Increase in secretions	Alzheimer disease Cognitive dysfunction Schizophrenia
M_2	Widely expressed in CNS, hindbrain, thalamus, cerebral cortex, hippocampus, striatum, heart, smooth muscle, autonomic nerve terminals	Couples by G_i/G_o (PTX sensitive) Inhibition of AC, $\downarrow$ cAMP Activation of inwardly rectifying K^+ channels Inhibition of voltage-gated Ca^{2+} channels Hyperpolarization and inhibition	**Heart:** SA node: slowed spontaneous depolarization; hyperpolarization, $\downarrow$ HR AV node: decrease in conduction velocity Atrium: $\downarrow$ refractory period, $\downarrow$ contraction Ventricle: slight $\downarrow$ contraction **Smooth muscle:** $\uparrow$ Contraction **Peripheral nerves:** Neural inhibition via autoreceptors and heteroreceptor $\downarrow$ Ganglionic transmission. **CNS:** Neural inhibition $\uparrow$ Tremors; hypothermia; analgesia	Alzheimer disease Cognitive dysfunction Pain
M_3	Widely expressed in CNS (<other mAChRs), cerebral cortex, hippocampus Abundant in smooth muscle and glands Heart	Couples by $G_{q/11}$ to activate PLC-IP_3/DAG-Ca^{2+}-PKC pathway Depolarization and excitation ($\uparrow$ sEPSP) Activation of PLD_2, PLA_2; $\uparrow$AA	**Smooth muscle:** $\uparrow$ Contraction (predominant in some, e.g., bladder) **Glands:** $\uparrow$ Secretion (predominant in salivary gland) Increases food intake, body weight, fat deposits Inhibition of DA release Synthesis of NO	Chronic obstructive pulmonary disease (COPD) Urinary incontinence Irritable bowel disease
M_4	Preferentially expressed in CNS, particularly forebrain, also striatum, cerebral cortex, hippocampus	Couples by G_i/G_o (PTX sensitive) Inhibition of AC, $\downarrow$ cAMP Activation of inwardly rectifying K^+ channels Inhibition of voltage-gated Ca^{2+} channels Hyperpolarization and inhibition	Autoreceptor- and heteroreceptor-mediated inhibition of transmitter release in CNS and periphery Analgesia; cataleptic activity Facilitation of DA release	Parkinson disease Schizophrenia Neuropathic pain
M_5	Substantia nigra Expressed in low levels in CNS and periphery Predominant mAchR in neurons in VTA and substantia nigra	Couples by $G_{q/11}$ to activate PLC-IP_3-Ca^{2+}-PKC pathway Depolarization and excitation ($\uparrow$ sEPSP) Activation of PLD_2, PLA_2; $\uparrow$AA	Mediator of dilation in cerebral arteries and arterioles (?) Facilitates DA release Augmentation of drug-seeking behavior and reward (e.g., opiates, cocaine)	Drug dependence Parkinson disease Schizophrenia

[a]Most organs, tissues, and cells express multiple mAChRs.
[b]M_1, M_3, and M_5 mAChRs appear to couple to the same G proteins and signal through similar pathways. Likewise, M_2 and M_4 mAChRs couple through similar G proteins and signal through similar pathways.
[c]Despite the fact that in many tissues, organs, and cells multiple subtypes of mAChRs coexist, one subtype may predominate in producing a particular function; in others, there may be equal predominance.
VTA, ventral tegmentum area.

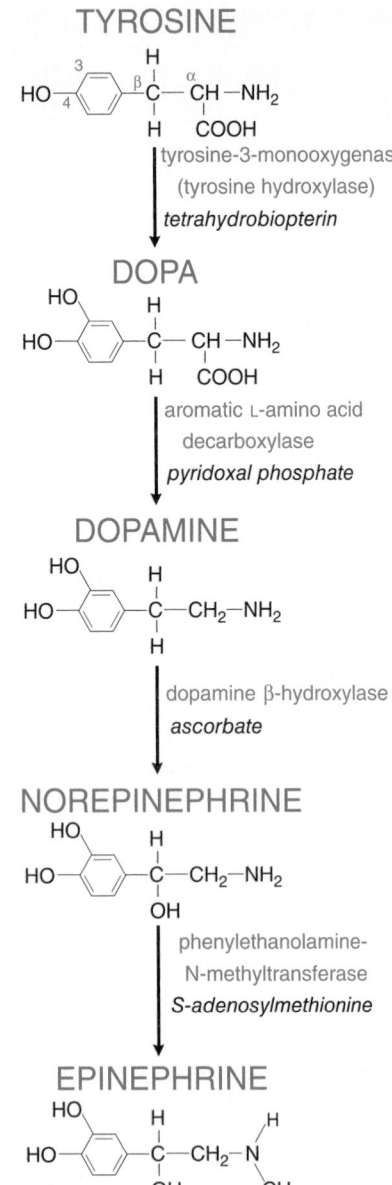

Figure 8–7 *Steps in the enzymatic synthesis of dopamine, norepinephrine and epinephrine.* The enzymes involved are shown in red; essential cofactors in italics. The final step occurs only in the adrenal medulla and in a few epinephrine-containing neuronal pathways in the brainstem.

(Nagatsu, 2006). Table 8–4 summarizes some of the important characteristics of the four enzymes. These enzymes are not completely specific; consequently, other endogenous substances, as well as certain drugs, are also substrates. For example, 5HT can be produced from 5-hydroxy-L-tryptophan by aromatic L-amino acid decarboxylase (or dopa decarboxylase). Dopa decarboxylase also converts dopa into DA (Chapter 13) and methyldopa to α-methyldopamine, which in turn is converted by DβH to methylnorepinephrine.

The hydroxylation of tyrosine by TH is the rate-limiting step in the biosynthesis of catecholamines (Zigmond et al., 1989). This enzyme is activated following stimulation of sympathetic nerves or the adrenal medulla. The enzyme is a substrate for PKA, PKC, and CaM kinase; phosphorylation is associated with increased hydroxylase activity. In addition, there is a delayed increase in TH gene expression after nerve stimulation. These mechanisms serve to maintain the content of catecholamines in response to increased transmitter release. TH also is subject to feedback inhibition by catechol compounds.

Deficiency of TH has been reported in humans and is characterized by generalized rigidity, hypokinesia, and low CSF levels of NE and DA metabolites HVA and 3-methoxy-4-hydroxyphenylethylene glycol (Wevers et al., 1999). TH knockout is embryonically lethal in mice, presumably because the loss of catecholamines results in altered cardiac function. Interestingly, residual levels of DA are present in these mice. Tyrosinase may be an alternate source for catecholamines, although tyrosinase-derived catecholamines are clearly not sufficient for survival (Carson and Robertson, 2002).

Deficiency of DβH in humans is characterized by orthostatic hypotension, ptosis of the eyelids, retrograde ejaculation, and elevated plasma levels of DA. In the case of DβH-deficient mice, there is about 90% embryonic mortality (Carson and Robertson, 2002).

Our understanding of the cellular sites and mechanisms of synthesis, storage, and release of catecholamines derives from studies of sympathetically innervated organs and the adrenal medulla. Nearly all the NE content of innervated organs is confined to the postganglionic sympathetic fibers; it disappears within a few days after section of the nerves. In the adrenal medulla, catecholamines are stored in chromaffin granules (Aunis, 1998). These vesicles contain extremely high concentrations of catecholamines (~21% dry weight), ascorbic acid, and ATP, as well as specific proteins, such as chromogranins, DβH, and peptides, including enkephalin and neuropeptide Y. Vasostatin 1, the *N*-terminal fragment of chromogranin A, has been found to have antibacterial and antifungal activity (Lugardon et al., 2000), as have other chromogranin A fragments, such as chromofungin, vasostatin II, prochromacin, and chromacins I and II (Taupenot et al., 2003). Two types of storage vesicles are found in sympathetic nerve terminals: large dense-core vesicles corresponding to chromaffin granules and small dense-core vesicles containing NE, ATP, and membrane-bound DβH.

The main features of the mechanisms of synthesis, storage, and release of catecholamines at an adrenergic neuroeffector junction and their modifications by drugs are summarized in Figure 8–8 and its legend. The *adrenal medulla* has two distinct catecholamine-containing cell types: those with NE and those with primarily EPI. The latter cell population contains the enzyme PNMT. In these cells, the NE formed in the granules leaves these structures and is methylated in the cytoplasm to EPI. EPI then reenters the chromaffin granules, where it is stored until released. EPI accounts for about 80% of the catecholamines of the adrenal medulla and NE about 20%.

A major factor that controls the rate of synthesis of EPI, and hence the size of the store available for release from the adrenal medulla, is the level of glucocorticoids secreted by the adrenal cortex. The intra-adrenal portal vascular system carries the corticosteroids directly to the adrenal medullary chromaffin cells, where they induce the synthesis of PNMT (Figure 8–7). The activities of both TH and DβH also are increased in the adrenal medulla when the secretion of glucocorticoids is stimulated (Viskupic et al., 1994). Thus, any stress that persists sufficiently to evoke an enhanced secretion of corticotropin mobilizes the appropriate hormones of both the adrenal cortex (predominantly cortisol in humans) and medulla (EPI). This remarkable relationship is present only in certain mammals, including humans, in which the adrenal chromaffin cells are enveloped entirely by steroid-secreting cortical cells. PMNT is expressed in mammalian tissues such as brain, heart, and lung, leading to extra-adrenal EPI synthesis (Ziegler et al., 2002).

In addition to de novo synthesis, NE stores in the terminal portions of the adrenergic fibers are replenished by reuptake and restorage of NE following its release (see discussion in the following material).

Storage, Release, and Reuptake of Catecholamines; Termination of Action

Storage. NE, ATP, and NPY are stored frequently in the same nerve endings.

Catecholamines. Catecholamines are stored in vesicles, thereby ensuring their regulated release, protecting them from metabolism by cellular enzymes, and preventing their leakage out of the neuron. The vesicular monoamine transporter VMAT2, a vesicular membrane protein, moves

TABLE 8–4 ■ ENZYMES FOR SYNTHESIS OF CATECHOLAMINES

ENZYME	OCCURRENCE	SUBCELLULAR DISTRIBUTION	COFACTORS	SUBSTRATE SPECIFICITY	COMMENTS
TH	Widespread	Cytoplasm	tetradrobiopterin (BH_4), O_2, Fe^{2+}	Specific for L-tyrosine	Rate-limiting step. Inhibition can deplete NE.
AAADC	Widespread	Cytoplasm	Pyridoxal PO_4	Nonspecific	Inhibition does not alter tissue NE and EPI appreciably.
DβH	Widespread	Synaptic vesicles	Ascorbate, O_2 (DβH contains Cu)	Nonspecific	Inhibition can ↓ NE and EPI levels.
PNMT	Largely in adrenal gland	Cytoplasm	S-adenosyl methionine (SAM) as (CH_3 donor)	Nonspecific	Inhibition can ↓ adrenal EPI/NE; regulated by glucocorticoids.

NE and other catecholamines from the cytosol into neuronal storage vesicles (Chaudhry et al., 2008). VMAT2 is driven by a pH gradient established by an ATP-dependent proton translocase in the vesicular membrane; for each molecule of amine taken up, two H^+ ions are extruded. VMAT2 is a member of the SLC protein superfamily and is designated SLC18A. Monoamine transporters in the SLC18 family are relatively promiscuous and transport DA, NE, EPI, and 5HT, as well as metaiodobenzylguanidine, which can be used to image chromaffin cell tumors (Schuldiner, 1994). *Reserpine* inhibits monoamine transport into storage vesicles and ultimately leads to depletion of catecholamine from sympathetic nerve endings and in the brain.

ATP. ATP is an essential component of catecholamine storage; the capacity of ATP and catecholamines to form relatively stable complexes apparently facilitates accumulation of high concentrations of neurotransmitter within the adrenergic storage granule. The granule accumulates ATP via another vesicular nucleotide carrier, VNUT, a member of the SLC superfamily. VNUT is a Na^+/anion cotransporter, designated as SLC17A9 (see Chapter 5). The frequency and quantal size of exocytotic release mirror VNUT activity (Estévez-Herrera et al., 2016). Thus, vesicular ATP has multiple actions beyond its role as a cellular energy source and energy storage molecule: Vesicular ATP facilitates vesicular storage of high concentrations of catecholamines and, when released with the vesicular contents, acts as a transmitter at purinergic receptors (Burnstock et al., 2015).

Neuropeptide Y. NPY, a peptide with 36 amino acids, is synthesized in the endoplasmic reticulum, first as a 97-amino-acid precursor, prepro-NPY, that is processed by three steps of proteolysis and a final C-terminal amidation; the resultant NPY_{1-36} is stored in large, dense-core vesicles that may also contain NE. NE and ATP are more generally stored in smaller dense-core vesicles, but NPY, ATP, and NE are often coreleased following nerve stimulation, albeit in proportions that change with the pattern and intensity of stimulation (Westfall, 2004). NPY is abundant in the brain and is a powerful orexigenic. In the peripheral nervous system, NPY occurs in sympathetic nerves and adrenal chromaffin cells; it can also be found in platelets, endothelium, and the GI tract and is inducible in the immune system (Hirsch et al., 2012).

Release. Details of excitation-secretion coupling in sympathetic neurons and adrenal medulla are becoming known and are summarized in Figures 8–3 and 8–8. The triggering event is the entry of Ca^{2+}, which results in the exocytosis of the granular contents, including the catecholamine, ATP, some neuroactive peptides (e.g., NPY) or their precursors, chromogranins, and DβH. The various SNARE proteins (e.g., SNAP-25, syntaxin, and synaptobrevin) described for exocytosis of ACh are also involved here (Figures 8–3 through 8–6).

Reuptake and Termination of Action. Following its release from a sympathetic nerve varicosity, NE interacts with presynaptic and postsynaptic membrane receptors. Adrenergic fibers can sustain the output of NE during prolonged periods of stimulation without exhausting their supply, provided that synthesis and reuptake of the transmitter are unimpaired. Acute regulation of transmitter synthesis involving activation of TH and DβH has been described previously in this chapter. Recycling of transmitter is also essential, and this is provided by reuptake, restorage, and reuse of transmitter. *The actions of catecholamines are terminated by reuptake into the nerve and postjunctional cells and to a smaller extent by diffusion out of the synaptic cleft.* Two distinct carrier-mediated transport systems are involved in reuptake (see Figure 8–8; Table 8–5):

- NET: This transporter, previously called *uptake 1*, moves NE across the neuronal membrane from the extracellular fluid to the cytoplasm. NET has a higher affinity for NE than for EPI (see Table 8–5). NET is a member of an SLC family of similar transporters and is designated as SLC6A2. This family of proteins transports amino acids and their derivatives into cells using cotransport of extracellular Na^+ as a driving force for substrate translocation against chemical gradients (see Chapter 5). The SLC6A monoamine transporters include NET, DAT (SLC6A3), and SERT (SLC6A4).
- ENT: This transporter, previously called *uptake 2,* is an organic cation transporter, OCT3, designated as SLC22A3. OCT3 facilitates passive transmembrane movement of organic anions down their electrochemical gradients, including the movement of catecholamines into nonneuronal cells. Compared to NET, it has a lower affinity for catecholamines, favors EPI over NE and DA, has a higher maximum uptake rate for catecholamines, is not Na^+ dependent, and has a different profile for pharmacological inhibition. The synthetic β adrenergic receptor agonist isoproterenol is not a substrate for this system. OCT3 activity is altered by MAPK and Ca^{2+}-CaM signaling (Roth et al., 2012). In addition to catecholamines, OCT3 can transport a wide variety of other organic cations, including 5HT, histamine, choline, spermine, guanidine, and creatinine, as can the closely related OCT1 and OCT2. The characteristics and locations of the nonneuronal transporters are summarized in Table 8–5.

For NE released by neurons, uptake by NET is more important than uptake by ENT. Sympathetic nerves as a whole remove about 87% of released NE by NET, compared with 5% by extraneuronal uptake (ENT) and 8% by diffusion to the circulation. In contrast, clearance of circulating catecholamines, such as those released from the adrenal medulla, is primarily by nonneuronal mechanisms, with liver and kidney accounting for over 60% of the clearance of circulating catecholamines. Because VMAT2 has a much higher affinity for NE than does MAO, over 70% of recaptured NE is resequestered into storage vesicles (Eisenhofer, 2001).

The NET is also present in the adrenal medulla, the liver, and the placenta, whereas DAT is present in the stomach, pancreas, and kidney (Eisenhofer, 2001). These plasma membrane transporters appear to have greater substrate specificity than does VMAT2. NET and DAT are targets for drugs such as cocaine and tricyclic antidepressants (e.g., imipramine); selective 5HT reuptake inhibitors such as fluoxetine inhibit SERT. Inhibitors of OCT3 include normetanephrine (an O-methylated metabolite of NE; see Figure 8–9), Pharmacological probes of OCT3 include corticosterone (an inhibitor), and the substrates metformin and cimetidine; the interaction of substrates and inhibitors at renal OCT3 can lead to adverse drug effects (see Chapter 5).

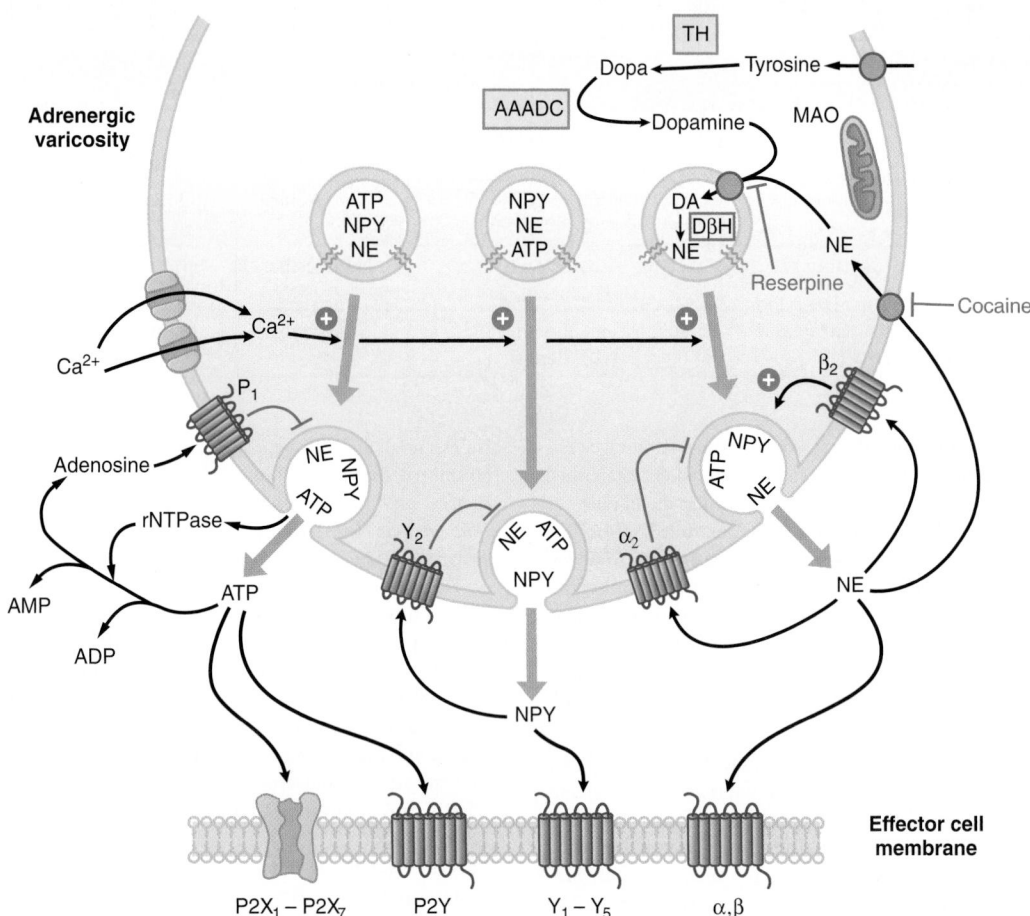

Figure 8–8 *A typical adrenergic neuroeffector junction.* Tyrosine is transported into the varicosity and is converted to DOPA by TH and DOPA to DA by the action of AAADC. DA is taken up into the vesicles of the varicosity by a transporter, VMAT2, that can be blocked by reserpine. Cytoplasmic NE also can be taken up by this transporter. DA is converted to NE within the vesicle via the action of DβH. NE is stored in vesicles along with other cotransmitters, NPY and ATP, depending on the particular neuroeffector junction. Release of the transmitters occurs via exocytosis, a process activated by depolarization of the varicosity, which allows entry of Ca^{2+} through voltage-dependent Ca^{2+} channels and the interaction of numerous docking and fusion proteins located in the vesicle and the neuronal cell membrane, as described in Figures 8–3, 8–4, and 8–5. In this schematic representation, NE, NPY, and ATP are stored in the same vesicles. Different populations of vesicles, however, may preferentially store different proportions of the cotransmitters. Once in the synapse, NE can interact with α and β adrenergic receptors (GPCRs) to produce the responses characteristic of the particular postsynaptic cell. The α and β receptors also can be located presynaptically, via which NE can either diminish ($α_2$) or facilitate (β) its own release and that of the cotransmitters. The principal mechanism by which NE is cleared from the synapse is via a cocaine-sensitive neuronal uptake transporter, NET. Once transported into the cytosol, NE can be re-stored in the vesicle or metabolized by MAO. NPY produces its effects by activating NPY receptors (also GCPRs), of which there are at least five types (Y_1 through Y_5). NPY can modify its own release and that of the other transmitters via presynaptic Y_2 receptors. NPY action is terminated by the actions of peptidases. ATP produces its effects by activating P2X receptors (ligand-gated ion channels) or P2Y receptors (GPCRs). There are multiple subtypes of both P2X and P2Y receptors. As with other cotransmitters, ATP can act prejunctionally to modify its own release via receptors for ATP or via its metabolic breakdown to adenosine that acts on P1 (adenosine) receptors. ATP is cleared from the synapse primarily by rNTPases and by cell-fixed ectonucleotidases.

The use of selective inhibitors of NET in animal and human studies and data from analysis of mice with targeted deletions (KO) of the NET and DAT genes reveal the impact of these uptake systems. The NET-KO and DAT-KO animals exhibit increased extracellular levels and decreased intracellular levels of NE despite increased or unaltered neurotransmitter synthesis (Xu et al., 2000; Gainetdinov and Caron, 2003). NET-KO mice also display marked behavioral alterations (Xu et al., 2000) and show characteristic hemodynamic changes (e.g., excessive tachycardia and increased blood pressure during sympathetic activation with wakefulness and activity), whereas resting mean arterial pressure and heart rate are maintained at nearly normal levels, most likely because of increased central sympathoinhibition (Keller et al., 2004). A coding mutation in humans (A457P in TM9) reduces NET activity and yields marked hemodynamic changes and orthostatic intolerance. When expressed in a heterologous cell line, the mutation resulted in a 98% loss of NET function compared with the wild-type transporter

(Shannon et al., 2000). Furthermore, when coexpressed with wild-type NET, the A457P mutant exerts a dominant negative effect on wild-type NET, likely reflecting transporter oligomerization (Hahn et al., 2003), providing an explanation for the phenotype observed in heterozygous carriers. Another human variant of NET with an F528C mutation displays increased membrane expression of NET associated with increased NE uptake compared with wild-type NET (Hahn et al., 2005); this variant may be associated with an increased incidence of depression (Haenisch et al., 2009).

Certain sympathomimetic drugs (e.g., ephedrine and tyramine) produce some of their effects indirectly by displacing NE from the nerve terminals to the extracellular fluid, where it then acts at receptor sites of the effector cells. The mechanisms by which these drugs release NE from nerve endings are complex. All such agents are substrates for NET. As a result of their uptake by NET, they make carrier available at the inner surface of the membrane for the outward transport of NE ("facilitated exchange diffusion"). In addition,

TABLE 8–5 ■ CHARACTERISTICS OF PLASMA MEMBRANE TRANSPORTERS FOR ENDOGENOUS CATECHOLAMINES

TYPE OF TRANSPORTER	SUBSTRATE SPECIFICITY	TISSUE	REGION/CELL TYPE	INHIBITORS
Neuronal				
NET	DA > NE > EPI	All sympathetically innervated tissue	Sympathetic nerves	Desipramine Cocaine Nisoxetine
		Adrenal medulla	Chromaffin cells	
		Liver	Capillary endothelial cells	
		Placenta	Syncytiotrophoblast	
DAT	DA > NE > EPI	Kidney	Endothelium	Cocaine Imazindol
		Stomach	Parietal and endothelial cells	
		Pancreas	Pancreatic duct	
Nonneuronal				
OCT1	DA > EPI >> NE	Liver	Hepatocytes	Isocyanines Corticosterone
		Intestine	Epithelial cells	
		Kidney (not human)	Distal tubule	
OCT2	DA >> NE > EPI	Kidney	Medullary proximal and distal tubules	Isocyanines Corticosterone
		Brain	Glial cells of DA-rich regions, some nonadrenergic neurons	
ENT (OCT3)	EPI >> NE > DA	Liver	Hepatocytes	Isocyanines Corticosterone *O*-methyl-isoproterenol
		Brain	Glial cells, others	
		Heart	Myocytes	
		Blood vessels	Endothelial cells	
		Kidney	Cortex, proximal and distal tubules	
		Placenta	Syncytiotrophoblasts (basal membrane)	
		Retina	Photoreceptors, ganglion amacrine cells	

these amines are able to mobilize NE stored in the vesicles by competing for the vesicular uptake process (VMAT2).

The actions of indirect-acting sympathomimetic amines are subject to *tachyphylaxis.* For example, repeated administration of tyramine results in rapidly decreasing effectiveness, whereas repeated administration of NE does not reduce effectiveness and, in fact, reverses the tachyphylaxis to tyramine. These phenomena have not been explained fully. One hypothesis is that the pool of neurotransmitter available for displacement by these drugs is small relative to the total amount stored in the sympathetic nerve ending. This pool is presumed to reside close to the plasma membrane, and the NE of such vesicles may be replaced by the less-potent amine following repeated administration of the latter substance. In any case, neurotransmitter release by displacement is not associated with the release of DβH and does not require extracellular Ca^{2+}; thus, it is presumed not to involve exocytosis.

Prejunctional Regulation of NE Release. The release of the three sympathetic cotransmitters can be modulated by prejunctional autoreceptors and heteroreceptors. Following their release from sympathetic terminals, all three cotransmitters—NE, NPY, and ATP—can feed back on prejunctional receptors to inhibit the release of each other (Westfall, 2004; Westfall et al., 2002). The most thoroughly studied have been prejunctional α_2 adrenergic receptors. The α_{2A} and α_{2C} adrenergic receptors are the principal prejunctional receptors that inhibit sympathetic neurotransmitter release, whereas the α_{2B} adrenergic receptors also may inhibit transmitter release at selected sites. Antagonists of this receptor, in turn, can enhance the electrically evoked release of sympathetic neurotransmitter. NPY, acting on Y_2 receptors, and ATP-derived adenosine, acting on P1 receptors, also can inhibit sympathetic neurotransmitter release. Activation of numerous heteroreceptors on sympathetic nerve varicosities can inhibit the release of sympathetic neurotransmitters; these include M_2

and M_4 muscarinic, 5HT, PGE_2, histamine, enkephalin, and DA receptors. Enhancement of sympathetic neurotransmitter release can be produced by activation of β_2 adrenergic receptors, angiotensin AT_2 receptors, and nAChRs. All of these receptors can be targets for agonists and antagonists (Kubista and Boehm, 2006).

Metabolism of Catecholamines. Uptake of released catecholamine terminates the neurotransmitter's effects at the synaptic junction. Following uptake, catecholamines can be metabolized (in neuronal and nonneuronal cells) or re-stored in vesicles (in neurons). Two enzymes are important in the initial steps of metabolic transformation of catecholamines—MAO and COMT.

MAO and COMT. MAO metabolizes transmitter that is released within the nerve terminal or that is in the cytosol as a result of reuptake and has not yet reached the safety of the storage vesicle. COMT, particularly in the liver, plays a major role in the metabolism of endogenous circulating and administered catecholamines. The importance of neuronal reuptake of catecholamines is shown by observations that inhibitors of uptake (e.g., cocaine and imipramine) potentiate the effects of the neurotransmitter; inhibitors of MAO and COMT have less effect.

Both MAO and COMT are distributed widely throughout the body, including the brain; their highest concentrations are in the liver and the kidney. However, little or no COMT is found in sympathetic neurons. In the brain, there is no significant COMT in presynaptic terminals, but it is found in some postsynaptic neurons and glial cells. In the kidney, COMT is localized in proximal tubular epithelial cells, where DA is synthesized and is thought to exert local diuretic and natriuretic effects.

There are distinct differences in the localizations of the two enzymes; MAO is associated chiefly with the outer surface of mitochondria,

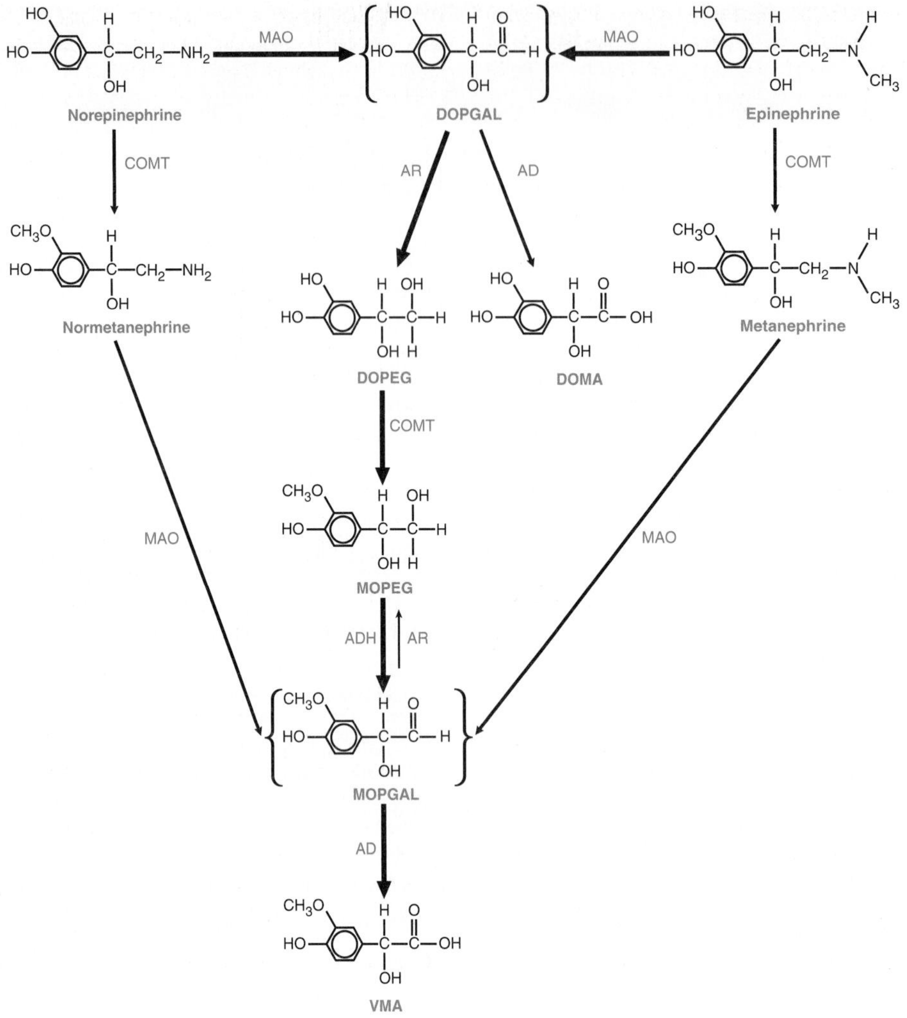

Figure 8–9 *Metabolism of catecholamines.* NE and EPI are first oxidatively deaminated to a short-lived intermediate (DOPGAL) by MAO. DOPGAL then undergoes further metabolism to more stable alcohol- or acid-deaminated metabolites. AD metabolizes DOPGAL to DOMA, while AR metabolizes DOPGAL to DOPEG. Under normal circumstances, DOMA is a minor metabolite, with DOPEG being the major metabolite produced from NE and EPI. Once DOPEG leaves the major sites of its formation (sympathetic nerves; adrenal medulla), it is converted to MOPEG by COMT. MOPEG is then converted to the unstable aldehyde (MOPGAL) by ADH and finally to VMA by AD. VMA is the major end product. Another route for the formation of VMA is conversion of NE or EPI into normetanephrine or metanephrine by COMT in either the adrenal medulla or extraneuronal sites, with subsequent metabolism to MOPGAL and thence to VMA. Catecholamines are also metabolized by *sulfotransferases*. AD, aldehyde dehydrogenase; ADH, alcohol dehydrogenase; AR, aldehyde reductase; COMT, catechol-*O*-methyltransferease; DOMA, 3,4-dihydroxymandelic acid; DOPEG, 3,4-dihydroxyphenyl glycol; DOPGAL, dihydroxyphenylglycolaldehyde; MAO, monoamine oxidase; MOPEG, 3-methyl,4-hydroxyphenylglycol; MOPGAL, monohydroxyphenylglycol aldehyde; VMA, vanillyl mandelic acid.

including those within the terminals of sympathetic or central noradrenergic neuronal fibers, whereas COMT is largely cytosolic, except in the chromaffin cells of the adrenal medulla, where COMT is membrane bound. These factors are of importance both in determining the primary metabolic pathways followed by catecholamines in various circumstances and in explaining the effects of certain drugs. The physiological substrates for COMT include L-dopa, all three endogenous catecholamines (DA, NE, and EPI), their hydroxylated metabolites, catecholestrogens, ascorbic acid, and dihydroxyindolic intermediates of melanin (Männistö and Kaakkola, 1999).

Two different isozymes of MAO (MAO-A and MAO-B) are found in widely varying proportions in different cells in the CNS and in peripheral tissues. In the periphery, MAO-A is located in the syncytiotrophoblast layer of term placenta and liver, whereas MAO-B is located in platelets, lymphocytes, and liver. In the brain, MAO-A is located in all regions containing catecholamines, with the highest abundance in the locus ceruleus. MAO-B, on the other hand, is found primarily in regions that are known to synthesize and store 5HT. MAO-B is most prominent not only in the nucleus raphe dorsalis but also in the posterior hypothalamus and in glial cells in regions known to contain nerve terminals. MAO-B is also present in osteocytes around blood vessels (Abell and Kwan, 2001).

Many MAO inhibitors are not selective for MAO-A or MAO-B, and these nonselective agents (e.g., phenelzine, tranylcypromine, and isocarboxazid) enhance the bioavailability of tyramine contained in many foods; tyramine-induced NE release from sympathetic neurons may lead to markedly increased blood pressure (hypertensive crisis). Drugs with selectivity for MAO-B (e.g., selegiline, rasagiline, pargyline) or reversible inhibitors of MAO-A (e.g., moclobemide) are less likely to cause this potential interaction (Volz and Gleiter, 1998; Wouters, 1998).

Inhibitors of MAO activity can cause an increase in the concentration of NE, DA, and 5HT in the brain and other tissues accompanied by a variety of pharmacological effects. No striking pharmacological action in the periphery can be attributed to the inhibition of COMT. However, the COMT inhibitors entacapone and tocapone are efficacious in the therapy of Parkinson disease (Chong and Mersfelder, 2000, and Chapter 18).

The Metabolic Pathway (Figure 8–9). There is ongoing passive leakage of catecholamines from vesicular storage granules of sympathetic neurons and adrenal medullary chromaffin cells. As a consequence, most metabolism of catecholamines takes place in the same cells where the amines are synthesized and stored. VMAT2 effectively sequesters about 90% of the amines leaking into the cytoplasm back into storage vesicles; about 10% escapes sequestration and is metabolized (Eisenhofer et al., 2004).

Sympathetic nerves contain MAO but not COMT, and this MAO catalyzes only the first step of a two-step reaction. MAO converts NE or EPI into a short-lived intermediate, DOPGAL, which undergoes further metabolism in a second step catalyzed by another group of enzymes forming more stable alcohol- or acid-deaminated metabolites. Aldehyde dehydrogenase metabolizes DOPGAL to DOMA, while aldehyde reductase metabolizes DOPGAL to DOPEG. In addition to aldehyde reductase, a related enzyme, aldose reductase, can reduce a catecholamine to its corresponding alcohol. This latter enzyme is present in sympathetic neurons and adrenal chromaffin cells. Under normal circumstances, DOMA is an insignificant metabolite of NE and EPI, with DOPEG being the main metabolite produced by deamination in sympathetic neurons and adrenal medullary chromaffin cells.

Once it leaves the sites of formation (sympathetic neurons, adrenal medulla), DOPEG is converted to MOPEG by COMT. Thus, most MOPEG comes from extraneuronal O-methylation of DOPEG produced in and diffusing rapidly from sympathetic neurons into the extracellular fluid. MOPEG is then converted to VMA by the sequential actions of alcohol and aldehyde dehydrogenases. MOPEG is first converted to the unstable aldehyde metabolite MOPGAL and then to VMA, with VMA being the major end product of NE and EPI metabolism. Another route for the formation of VMA is conversion by COMT of NE and EPI into normetanephrine and metanephrine, respectively, followed by deamination to MOPGAL and thence to VMA. This is now thought to be only a minor pathway, as indicated by the size of the arrows on Figure 8–9.

In contrast to sympathetic neurons, adrenal medullary chromaffin cells contain both MAO and COMT, the COMT mainly as the membrane-bound form. This isoform of COMT has a higher affinity for catecholamines than does the soluble form found in most other tissues (e.g., liver and kidney). In adrenal medullary chromaffin cells, leakage of NE and EPI from storage vesicles leads to substantial intracellular production of the O-methylated metabolites normetanephrine and metanephrine. In humans, over 90% of circulating metanephrine and 25%–40% of circulating normetanephrine are derived from catecholamines metabolized within adrenal chromaffin cells.

The sequence of cellular uptake and metabolism of catecholamines in extraneuronal tissues contributes only modestly (~25%) to the total metabolism of endogenously produced NE in sympathetic neurons or the adrenal medulla. However, extraneuronal metabolism is an important mechanism for the clearance of circulating and exogenously administered catecholamines.

Classification of Adrenergic Receptors

Adrenergic receptors are broadly classified as either α or β, with subtypes within each group (Table 8–6). The original subclassification was based on the rank order of agonist potency:

- EPI ≥ NE >> isoproterenol for α adrenergic receptors.
- Isoproterenol > EPI ≥ NE for β adrenergic receptors.

Elucidation of the characteristics of these receptors and the biochemical and physiological pathways they regulate has increased our understanding of the seemingly contradictory and variable effects of catecholamines on various organ systems. Although structurally related (discussed further in the chapter), different receptors regulate distinct physiological processes by controlling the synthesis or mobilization of a variety of second messengers.

Raymond Ahlquist and the Functional Definition of α and β Receptors.
Based on studies of the capacities of EPI, NE, and related agonists to regulate various physiological processes, Ahlquist (1948) proposed the existence of more than one adrenergic receptor. It was known that adrenergic agents could cause either contraction or relaxation of smooth

muscle depending on the site, the dose, and the agent chosen. For example, NE was known to have potent excitatory effects on smooth muscle and correspondingly low activity as an inhibitor; isoproterenol displayed the opposite pattern of activity. EPI could both excite and inhibit smooth muscle. Thus, Ahlquist proposed the designations α and β for receptors on smooth muscle where catecholamines produce excitatory and inhibitory responses, respectively (an exception was the gut, which generally is relaxed by activation of either α or β receptors). He developed the rank orders of potency that define α and β receptor–mediated responses, as noted above. This initial classification was corroborated by the finding that certain antagonists produced selective blockade of the effects of adrenergic nerve impulses and sympathomimetic agents at α receptors (e.g., phenoxybenzamine), whereas others produced selective β receptor blockade (e.g., propranolol).

α and β Receptor Subtypes.
Subsequent to Ahlquist's functional description of α and β receptors, adrenergic pharmacologists used increasingly sophisticated probes, tools, and methods to elucidate subtypes of α and β receptors. The β receptors were subclassified as β_1 (e.g., those in the myocardium) and β_2 (smooth muscle and most other sites), reflecting the finding that EPI and NE essentially are equipotent at β_1 sites, whereas EPI is 10–50 times more potent than NE at β_2 sites. Antagonists that discriminate between β_1 and β_2 receptors were subsequently developed (Chapter 12). Cloning confirmed that these β subtypes are products of different genes, and a human gene that encodes a third β receptor (designated β_3) was isolated (Emorine et al., 1989). Because the β_3 receptor is about 10-fold more sensitive to NE than to EPI and is relatively resistant to blockade by antagonists such as propranolol, the β_3 receptor may mediate responses to catecholamine at sites with "atypical" pharmacological characteristics (e.g., adipose tissue, which expresses all three β receptor subtypes). Animals treated with β_3 receptor agonists exhibit a vigorous thermogenic response as well as lipolysis (Robidoux et al., 2004). Polymorphisms in the β_3 receptor gene may be related to risk of obesity or type 2 diabetes in some populations (Arner and Hoffstedt, 1999), and Weyer and colleagues (1999) suggested that β_3 receptor–selective agonists may be beneficial in treating these disorders. The existence of a fourth β adrenergic receptor, β_4 was proposed but no such receptor has been cloned; rather, the "β_4 receptor" seems to be an affinity state of the β_1 adrenergic receptor rather than a distinct new protein (Gherbi et al., 2015; Hieble, 2007).

There is also heterogeneity among α adrenergic receptors. The initial distinction was based on functional and anatomic considerations: NE and other α adrenergic agonists profoundly inhibit the release of NE from neurons (Westfall, 1977) (Figure 8–8); conversely, certain α receptor antagonists markedly increase NE release when sympathetic nerves are stimulated. This feedback-inhibitory effect of NE on its release from nerve terminals is mediated by α receptors that are pharmacologically distinct from the classical postsynaptic α receptors. Accordingly, these presynaptic α adrenergic receptors were designated α_2, whereas the postsynaptic "excitatory" α receptors were designated α_1 (Langer, 1997). Compounds such as clonidine are more potent agonists at α_2 than at α_1 receptors; by contrast, phenylephrine and methoxamine selectively activate postsynaptic α_1 receptors.

Although there is little evidence to suggest that α_1 adrenergic receptors function presynaptically in the autonomic nervous system, α_2 receptors are present at postjunctional or nonjunctional sites in several tissues. For example, stimulation of postjunctional α_2 receptors in the brain is associated with reduced sympathetic outflow from the CNS and appears to be responsible for a significant component of the antihypertensive effect of drugs such as clonidine (Chapter 12). Thus, the anatomic concept of prejunctional α_2 and postjunctional α_1 adrenergic receptors has been abandoned in favor of a pharmacological and functional classification (Tables 8–6 and 8–7).

Cloning revealed additional heterogeneity of both α_1 and α_2 adrenergic receptors (Bylund, 1992). There are three pharmacologically defined α_1 receptors (α_{1A}, α_{1B}, and α_{1D}) with distinct sequences and tissue distributions and three cloned subtypes of α_2 receptors (α_{2A}, α_{2B}, and α_{2C}) (Table 8–6). A fourth type of α_1 receptor, α_{1L}, has been defined on the basis

TABLE 8–6 ■ CHARACTERISTICS FOR ADRENERGIC RECEPTOR SUBTYPES[a]

	G PROTEIN COUPLING	PRINCIPLE EFFECTORS	TISSUE LOCALIZATION	DOMINANT EFFECTS[b]
α_{1A}	$G\alpha_q$ ($\alpha_{11}/\alpha_{14}/\alpha_{16}$)	↑ PLC, ↑ PLA$_2$ ↑ Ca^{2+} channels ↑ Na$^+$/H$^+$ exchanger Modulation of K$^+$ channels ↑ MAPK Signaling	Heart, lung Liver Smooth muscle Blood vessels Vas deferens, prostate Cerebellum, cortex Hippocampus	• Dominant receptor for contraction of vascular smooth muscle • Promotes cardiac growth and structure • Vasoconstriction of large resistant arterioles in skeletal muscle
α_{1B}	$G\alpha_q$ ($\alpha_{11}/\alpha_{14}/\alpha_{16}$)	↑ PLC, ↑ PLA$_2$ ↑ Ca^{2+} channels ↑ Na$^+$/H$^+$ exchanger Modulation of K$^+$ channels ↑ MAPK signaling	Kidney, lung Spleen Blood vessels Cortex Brainstem	• Most abundant subtype in heart • Promotes cardiac growth and structure
α_{1D}	$G\alpha_q$ ($\alpha_{11}/\alpha_{14}/\alpha_{16}$)	↑ PLC, ↑ PLA$_2$ ↑ Ca^{2+} channels ↑ Na$^+$/H$^+$ exchanger Modulation of K$^+$ channels ↑ MAPK signaling	Platelets, aorta Coronary artery Prostate Cortex Hippocampus	• Dominant receptor for vasoconstriction in aorta and coronaries
α_{2A}	$G\alpha_i$ $G\alpha_o$ (α_{o1}/α_{o2})	↓ AC-cAMP-PKA pathway	Platelets Sympathetic neurons Autonomic ganglia Pancreas Coronary/CNS vessels Locus ceruleus Brainstem, spinal cord	• Dominant inhibitory receptor on sympathetic neurons • Vasoconstriction of precapillary vessels in skeletal muscle
α_{2B}	$G\alpha_i$ $G\alpha_o$ (α_{o1}/α_{o2})	↓ AC-cAMP-PKA pathway	Liver, kidney Blood vessels Coronary/CNS vessels Diencephalon Pancreas, platelets	• Dominant mediator of α_2 vasoconstriction
α_{2C}	$G\alpha_i$ ($\alpha_{11}/\alpha_{12}/\alpha_{13}$) $G\alpha_o$ (α_{o1}/α_{o2})	↓ AC-cAMP-PKA pathway	Basal ganglia Cortex, cerebellum Hippocampus	• Dominant receptor modulating DA neurotransmission • Dominant receptor inhibiting hormone release from adrenal medulla
β_1	$G\alpha_s$	↑ AC-cAMP-PKA pathway ↑ L-type Ca^{2+} channels	Heart, kidney Adipocytes Skeletal muscle Olfactory nucleus Cortex, brainstem Cerebellar nuclei Spinal cord	• Dominant mediator of positive inotropic and chronotropic effects in heart
β_2[c]	$G\alpha_s$	↑ AC-cAMP-PKA pathway ↑ Ca^{2+} channels	Heart, lung, kidney Blood vessels Bronchial smooth muscle GI smooth muscle Skeletal muscle Olfactory bulb Cortex, hippocampus	• Smooth muscle relaxation • Skeletal muscle hypertrophy
β_3[c,d]	$G\alpha_s$	↑ AC-cAMP-PKA pathway ↑ Ca^{2+} channels	Adipose tissue GI tract, heart	• Metabolic effects

[a]At least three subtypes each of α_1 and α_2 adrenergic receptors are known, but distinctions in their mechanisms of action have not been clearly defined.
[b]In some species (e.g., rat), metabolic responses in the liver are mediated by α_1 adrenergic receptors, whereas in others (e.g., dog) β_2 adrenergic receptors are predominantly involved. Both types of receptors appear to contribute to responses in human beings.
[c]β Receptor coupling to cell signaling can be more complex. In addition to coupling to G$_s$ to stimulate AC, β_2 receptors can activate signaling via a GRK/β-arrestin pathway. β_2 and β_3 receptors can couple to both G$_s$ and G$_i$ in a manner that may reflect agonist stereochemistry. See also Chapter 12.
[d]Metabolic responses in tissues with atypical pharmacological characteristics (e.g., adipocytes) may be mediated by β_3 receptors. Most β receptor antagonists (including propranolol) do not block these responses.

of a low affinity for the selective antagonists prazosin and 5-methyl urapidil but a high affinity for tamsulosin and silodosin. This phenotype could be of physiological significance; the α_{1L} profile has been identified in myriad tissues across a number of species, where it appears to regulate smooth muscle contractility in the vasculature and lower urinary tract. Despite intense efforts, the α_{1L} adrenergic receptor has not been cloned; currently, it is viewed as a second phenotype originating from the α_{1A} receptor gene (Hieble, 2007; Yoshiki et al., 2013). Distinct pharmacological phenotypes of the α_{1B} receptor have also been described (Yoshiki et al., 2014).

Owing to the lack of sufficiently subtype-selective ligands, the precise physiological function and therapeutic potential of the subtypes of adrenergic receptors have not been elucidated fully. Genetic approaches using transgenic and receptor knockout experiments in mice (discussed further in the chapter) have advanced our understanding. These mouse models have been used to identify and localize particular receptor subtypes and to describe the pathophysiological relevance of individual adrenergic receptor subtypes (Philipp and Hein, 2004; Tanoue et al., 2002a, 2002b; Xiao et al., 2006).

Molecular Basis of Adrenergic Receptor Function

Structural Features. All adrenergic receptors are GPCRs that link to heterotrimeric G proteins. Structurally, there are similarities in the regions for ligand binding and modulation by intracellular protein kinases (Figure 8–10). The coding region of each of the three β adrenergic receptor genes and the three α_2 adrenergic receptor genes is contained in a single exon, whereas each of the three α_1 adrenergic receptor genes has a single large intron separating regions that encode the body of the receptor from those that encode the seventh transmembrane domain and carboxy terminus (Dorn, 2010). Each major receptor type shows preference for a particular class of G proteins, that is, α_1 to G_q, α_2 to G_i, and β to G_s (see Table 8–6). The responses that follow receptor activation result from G protein–mediated effects on the generation of second messengers and on the activity of ion channels (see Chapter 3). The signaling pathways overlap broadly with those discussed for muscarinic ACh receptors.

α Adrenergic Receptors. The α_1 receptors (α_{1A}, α_{1B}, and α_{1D}) and the α_2 receptors (α_{2A}, α_{2B}, and α_{2C}) are heptahelical proteins that couple differentially to a variety of G proteins to regulate smooth muscle contraction, secretory pathways, and cell growth (see Table 8–6). Within the membrane-spanning domains, the three α_1 adrenergic receptors share about 75% identity in amino acid residues, as do the three α_2 receptors, but the α_1 and α_2 subtypes are no more similar than are the α and β subtypes (~30%–40%).

α_1 Adrenergic Receptors. Stimulation of α_1 receptors activates the G_q-PLC_β-IP_3/DAG-Ca^{2+} pathway and results in the activation of PKC and other Ca^{2+} and CaM-sensitive pathways, such as CaM kinases, with sequelae depending on cell differentiation (e.g., contraction of vascular smooth muscle, stimulation of growth in smooth muscles and hypertrophy in cardiac myocytes, and activation of endothelial NOS in vascular endothelium) (see Chapter 3). PKC phosphorylates many substrates, including membrane proteins such as channels, pumps, and ion exchange proteins (e.g., Ca^{2+}-transport ATPase). α_1 Receptor stimulation of PLA_2 leads to the release of free arachidonate, which is then metabolized by cyclooxygenase (yielding prostaglandins) and lipoxygenase (yielding leukotrienes) (see Chapter 37); PLD hydrolyzes phosphatidylcholine to yield phosphatidic acid, which can yield diacylglycerol, a cofactor for PKC activation. PLD is an effector for ADP-ribosylating factor, suggesting that PLD may play a role in membrane trafficking. In most smooth muscles, the increased concentration of intracellular Ca^{2+} causes contraction (see Figure 3–17). In contrast, the increased concentration of intracellular Ca^{2+} following α_1 stimulation of GI smooth muscle causes hyperpolarization and relaxation by activation of Ca^{2+}-dependent K^+ channels. Stimulation of α_1 receptors can activate p38/p42/p44, PI3K, JNK, and others to affect cell growth and proliferation, albeit in receptor subtype-specific and tissue-specific manners.

The α_{1A} receptor is the predominant receptor causing vasoconstriction in many vascular beds, including the following arteries: mammary, mesenteric, splenic, hepatic, omental, renal, pulmonary, and epicardial coronary. It is also the predominant subtype in the vena cava and the saphenous and pulmonary veins (Michelotti et al., 2000). Together with the α_{1B} receptor subtype, it promotes cardiac growth and structure. The α_{1B} receptor subtype is the most abundant subtype in the heart, whereas the α_{1D} receptor subtype is the predominant receptor causing vasoconstriction in the aorta. There is evidence to support the idea that α_{1B} receptors mediate behaviors such as reaction to novelty and exploration and are involved in behavioral sensitizations and in the vulnerability to addiction (see Chapter 24).

In addition to their traditional localization in the plasma membrane, α_1 receptors have nuclear localization signals (as do β receptors and receptors for endothelin and angiotensin) and have been found on the nuclear membrane of adult mouse cardiac myocytes, where they activate intranuclear signaling and appear to play a cardioprotective role (Wu and O'Connell, 2015).

α_2 Adrenergic Receptors. The α_2 receptors couple to a variety of effectors (Tan and Limbird, 2005). Inhibition of adenylyl cyclase activity was the first effect observed, but in some systems the enzyme actually is stimulated by G_i $\beta\gamma$ subunits or by weak direct stimulation of G_s. The physiological significance of these last processes is not currently clear. The α_2 receptors activate G protein–gated K^+ channels, resulting in membrane hyperpolarization. In some cases (e.g., cholinergic neurons in the myenteric plexus), this may be Ca^{2+} dependent, whereas in others (e.g., muscarinic ACh receptors in atrial myocytes) it results from direct interaction of $\beta\gamma$ subunits with K^+ channels. The α_2 receptors also can inhibit voltage-gated Ca^{2+} channels; this is mediated by G_o. Other second-messenger systems linked to α_2 receptor activation include acceleration of Na^+/H^+ exchange, stimulation of $PLC\beta_2$ activity and arachidonic

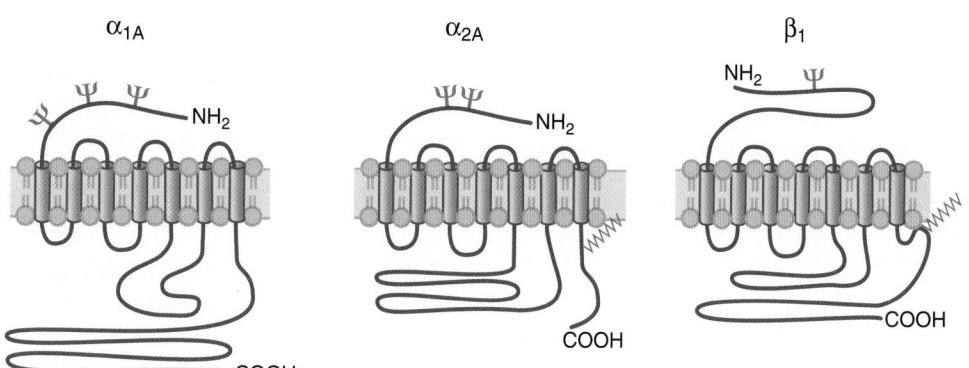

Figure 8–10 *Structural features of adrenergic receptor subtypes.* All of the adrenergic receptors are hepta-spanning GPCRs. A representative of each type is shown; each type has three subtypes: α_{1A}, α_{1B}, and α_{1D}; α_{2A}, α_{2B}, and α_{2C}; and β_1, β_2, and β_3. The principle effector systems affected by α_1, α_2 and β receptors are depicted in Table 8–6. ψ indicates a site for *N*-glycosylation.

acid mobilization, increased phosphoinositide hydrolysis, and increased intracellular availability of Ca^{2+}. The last is involved in the smooth muscle–contracting effect of α_2 adrenergic receptor agonists. In addition, the α_2 receptors activate MAPKs via mechanisms dependent on both the α and $\beta\gamma$ components of G_i, with involvement of protein tyrosine kinases and small GTPases (Goldsmith and Dhanasekaran, 2007). These pathways are reminiscent of pathways activated by tyrosine kinase activities of growth factor receptors. The α_{2A} and α_{2C} receptors play a major role in inhibiting NE release from sympathetic nerve endings and suppressing sympathetic outflow from the brain, leading to hypotension (Kable et al., 2000).

Thus, depending on subtype, the major biological effects of α_2 adrenergic receptors can be on platelet aggregation, regulation of sympathetic outflow from the CNS, reuptake of NE from within peripheral sympathetic nerve synapses, insulin secretion and lipolysis, or, to a limited extent, vasoconstriction (Gavras and Gavras, 2001). Similar studies with knockout mice have been carried out as was done with α_1 adrenergic receptors.

In the CNS, α_{2A} receptors, which appear to be the dominant adrenergic receptor, probably mediate the antinociceptive effects, sedation, hypothermia, hypotension, and behavioral actions of α_2 agonists (Lakhlani et al., 1997). The α_{2C} receptor occurs in the ventral and dorsal striatum and hippocampus. It appears to modulate DA neurotransmission and various behavioral responses. The α_{2B} receptor is the main receptor mediating α_2-induced vasoconstriction, whereas the α_{2C} receptor is the predominant receptor inhibiting the release of catecholamines from the adrenal medulla and modulating DA neurotransmission in the brain.

β Adrenergic Receptors

Subtypes. The three β receptor subtypes share about 60% amino acid sequence identity within the putative membrane-spanning domains where the ligand-binding pockets for EPI and NE are found. Based on results of site-directed mutagenesis, individual amino acids in the β_2 receptor that interact with each of the functional groups on the catecholamine agonist molecule have been identified. Figure 8–10 depicts the general hepta-spanning structure of adrenergic receptors and notes some differences in the sizes of the third and fourth intracellular loops.

The β receptors regulate numerous functional responses, including heart rate and contractility, smooth muscle relaxation, and myriad metabolic events in numerous tissues, including skeletal muscle, liver, and adipose tissue (Lynch and Ryall, 2008) (Table 8–1).

β Receptor Signaling. All three of the β receptor subtypes (β_1, β_2, and β_3) couple to G_s and activate adenylyl cyclase (Table 8–7). Stimulation of β adrenergic receptors leads to the accumulation of cAMP, activation of the PKA, and altered function of numerous cellular proteins as a result of their phosphorylation (Chapter 3). In addition, G_s subunits can enhance directly the activation of voltage-sensitive Ca^{2+} channels in the plasma membrane of skeletal and cardiac muscle cells.

The β_1, β_2, and β_3 receptors can differ in their intracellular signaling pathways and subcellular location (Brodde et al., 2006; Violin and Lefkowitz, 2007; Woo et al., 2009). While the positive chronotropic effects of β_1 receptor activation are clearly mediated by G_s in myocytes, dual coupling of β_2 receptors to G_s and G_i occurs in myocytes from newborn mice. Stimulation of β_2 receptors causes a transient increase in heart rate that is followed by a prolonged decrease. Following pretreatment with pertussis toxin, which prevents activation of G_i, the negative chronotropic effect of β_2 activation is abolished. These specific signaling properties of β receptor subtypes likely result from subtype-selective association with intracellular scaffolding and signaling proteins (Baillie and Houslay, 2005). The β_2 receptors normally are confined to caveolae in cardiac myocyte membranes. The activation of PKA by cAMP and the importance of compartmentation of components of the cAMP pathway are discussed in Chapter 3.

Refractoriness to Catecholamines. Exposure of catecholamine-sensitive cells and tissues to adrenergic agonists causes a progressive diminution in their capacity to respond to such agents. This phenomenon, variously termed *refractoriness, desensitization,* or *tachyphylaxis,* can limit the therapeutic efficacy and duration of action of catecholamines and other agents (Chapter 3). An understanding of the mechanisms involved in regulation of

GPCR desensitization and the roles of GRKs and β-arrestins has developed over the last two decades due to the efforts of Lefkowitz and colleagues (Violin and Lefkowitz, 2007) and Houslay and colleagues (Baillie and Houslay, 2005), among others. For a perspective on refractoriness and on the roles of GRKs and β-arrestins in biased agonism, see the discussion that follows.

Desensitization has functional correlates in human health. Long-term exposure to catecholamines can cause cardiac dysfunction and contribute to the course of deterioration in heart failure. Data support the idea that the β_1 receptor is the primary mediator of catecholamine cardiotoxicity (Communal et al., 1999). Studies in genetically manipulated mice indicate that β_1 receptor signaling has greater potential than β_2 receptor signaling to contribute to heart failure.

Desensitization, Downregulation, Sustained Signaling. Catecholamines promote β receptor feedback regulation, that is, desensitization, receptor downregulation, and internalization into endosomes. The β receptors differ in the extent to which they undergo such regulation, with the β_2 receptor being the most susceptible, as described in Chapter 3. Poststimulatory interactions of the agonist-liganded β_2 receptor with a GRK produces a phosphorylated receptor that readily interacts with β-arrestin, which blocks receptor access to the G protein and directs the receptor toward an endocytotic pathway, thereby reducing the number of receptors available at the cell surface. As a scaffolding protein, β-arrestin can also anchor proteins such as phosphodiesterase 4, which can modulate cAMP accumulation. The β receptor–β-arrestin complexes localize to coated pits and are subsequently internalized reversibly into endosomes (where the receptors may be dephosphorylated; such receptors can reenter the plasma membrane to aid resensitization), some complexes reaching lysosomes, where they are degraded (see Chapter 3). β-Arrestin also serves as an organizing center for the formation of a complex of a phospho-GPCR, a G protein, and β-arrestin, and this complex may provide sustained intracellular signaling from the internalized GPCR (Thomsen et al., 2016).

Biased Agonism and Selective Responsiveness. The original idea that a β adrenergic agonist activates just the G_s-AC-cAMP-PKA pathway is incomplete. Recent data demonstrate differences in downstream signals and events activated by the three β receptors and differences when various ligands activate a single receptor subtype. This concept, termed *biased agonism*, follows from four findings:

- signaling resulting from GPCR activation can be complex and involve a host of pathways
- ligand-activated GPCRs can adopt a multiplicity of conformations
- GRKs and β-arrestins are signal transducers, independently of G proteins
- distinct GRKs are recruited to and phosphorylate receptors based on specific ligand-induced receptor conformations, leading to specific signaling mediated by β-arrestin

A biased agonist stabilizes one or a subset of possible GPCR conformations and thereby activates a subset of all possible responses; these responses may involve signaling mechanisms mediated by β-arrestins through its myriad scaffolding partners. In work leading to the Nobel Prize in 2012, Lefkowitz and colleagues described this "pluridimensionality of β-arrestin–dependent signaling" at GPCRs (Reiter et al., 2012). This idea raises the possibility that one may design biased agonists that have unusually precise specificity. Biased agonism is discussed at greater length in Chapter 20 with regard to mu opioid agonists.

Adrenergic Receptor Polymorphism

Numerous polymorphisms and splice variants of adrenergic receptors continue to be identified. Such polymorphisms in adrenergic receptors could result in altered physiological responses to activation of the sympathetic nervous system, contribute to disease states, and alter the responses to adrenergic agonists or antagonists (Brodde, 2008). Knowledge of the functional consequences of specific polymorphisms could theoretically result in the individualization of drug therapy based on a patient's genetic makeup and could explain marked interindividual variability within the human population.

α₁ Adrenergic Receptor Polymorphisms. The α_1 adrenergic receptor is abundant in vascular smooth muscle and is implicated in regulating arterial resistance and blood pressure (Rokosh and Simpson, 2002). The α_1 adrenergic receptor polymorphism most often studied in human hypertension is α_{1A} Arg347Cys; the accumulated data so far suggest only a marginal effect of this polymorphism in cardiovascular responses to sympathetic stimulation or human hypertension. There are no functional phenotypes or cardiovascular disease associations reported for the α_{1B} and α_{1D} adrenergic receptors.

α₂A Adrenergic Receptor Polymorphisms. As with the α_{1A} adrenergic receptor, there is insufficient evidence supporting a major effect of α_2 receptor polymorphisms in hypertension. Likewise, although there are interesting and provocative studies suggesting an association between α_{2A}, α_{2BA}, and α_{2C} polymorphisms and coronary heart disease, heart failure, and sudden death, these linkages are not yet definitive. In contrast, a convincing role for α_{2A} adrenergic receptor polymorphisms in human type 2 diabetes has been elucidated. Moreover, in mice, deletion of the α_{2A} adrenergic receptor results in enhanced insulin secretion (Fagerholm et al., 2004) and β-cell–specific overexpression of $\alpha_{2A}R$ mimics diabetes (Devedjian et al., 2000).

β₁ Adrenergic Receptor Polymorphisms. Evidence does support the notion that increased cardiomyocyte β_1 receptor signaling by any means, including chronic agonist stimulation (Mobine et al., 2009), increased receptor expression (Dorn et al., 1999; Liggett et al., 2000), or enhanced receptor signaling (Mialet et al., 2003), can ultimately result in cardiac toxicity and contribute to heart failure. On the other hand, β_1 adrenergic receptor polymorphisms do not seem to be major risk factors in human hypertension.

Biochemical, functional, and structural studies in cultured cell expression systems and genetic mouse models indicate that the Gly389Arg β_1 adrenergic receptor exhibits a gain-of-signaling function that can initially improve cardiac contractility but ultimately predisposes to cardiomyopathic decompensation. This abnormally active Arg389 receptor is more sensitive to pharmacological blockade and exhibits distinctive pharmacological properties of different β blockers. This polymorphism may affect heart failure risk or progression, but the β blockers currently in use are sufficient to overcome the subtle differences that polymorphic receptor function may have on heart failure survival (Dorn, 2010).

β₂ Adrenergic Receptor Polymorphisms. Data supporting an interaction between β_2 adrenergic receptor polymorphisms and hypertension are inconclusive and suggest that effects of β_2 adrenergic receptor polymorphisms on blood pressure are modest. Similarly, there is no consensus about β_2 adrenergic receptor polymorphisms and heart disease (Dorn, 2010).

β₃ Adrenergic Receptor Polymorphisms. Polymorphisms of the β_3 adrenergic receptor appear to be associated with diabetes phenotypes, but there have been few clinical cardiac studies (Dorn, 2010).

Localization of Adrenergic Receptors

Presynaptic α_2 and β_2 receptors regulate neurotransmitter release from sympathetic nerve endings. Presynaptic α_2 receptors also may mediate inhibition of release of neurotransmitters other than NE in the central and peripheral nervous systems. Both α_2 and β_2 receptors are located at postsynaptic sites (Table 8–6), such as on many types of neurons in the brain. In peripheral tissues, postsynaptic α_2 receptors are found in vascular and other smooth muscle cells (where they mediate contraction), adipocytes, and various secretory epithelial cells (intestinal, renal, endocrine). Postsynaptic β_2 receptors can be found in the myocardium (where they mediate contraction) as well as on vascular and other smooth muscle cells (where they mediate relaxation), and skeletal muscle (where they can mediate hypertrophy). Indeed, most normal human cell types express β_2 receptors. Both α_2 and β_2 receptors may be situated at sites that are relatively remote from nerve terminals that release NE. Such extrajunctional receptors typically are found on vascular smooth muscle cells and blood elements (platelets and leukocytes) and may be activated preferentially by circulating catecholamines, particularly EPI.

In contrast, α_1 and β_1 receptors appear to be located mainly in the immediate vicinity of sympathetic adrenergic nerve terminals in peripheral target organs, strategically placed to be activated during stimulation of these nerves. These receptors also are distributed widely in the mammalian brain (Table 8–6).

The cellular distributions of the three α_1 and three α_2 receptor subtypes still are incompletely understood. Studies using in situ hybridization with receptor mRNA and receptor subtype-specific antibodies indicate that α_{2A} receptors in the brain may be both pre- and postsynaptic, suggesting that this receptor subtype may also function as a presynaptic autoreceptor in central noradrenergic neurons (Aantaa et al., 1995; Lakhlani et al., 1997). Using similar approaches, α_{1A} mRNA was found to be the dominant subtype message expressed in prostatic smooth muscle (Walden et al., 1997).

Pharmacological Considerations

Each step involved in neurotransmission is a potential point of pharmacological intervention. The diagrams of the cholinergic and adrenergic terminals and their postjunctional sites (Figure 8–6 and 8–8) show these points of intervention. Drugs that affect processes involved in the steps of transmission at both cholinergic and adrenergic junctions are summarized in Table 8–7, which lists representative agents that act through the mechanisms below.

Interference With the Synthesis or Release of the Transmitter

Cholinergic

Hemicholinium, a synthetic compound, blocks the transport system by which choline accumulates in the terminals of cholinergic fibers, thus limiting the synthesis of ACh. Vesamicol blocks the transport of ACh into its storage vesicles, thereby preventing repletion of ACh stores following transmitter release and thus reducing ACh available for subsequent release. The site on the presynaptic nerve terminal for block of ACh release by botulinum toxin was discussed previously; death usually results from respiratory paralysis unless patients with respiratory failure receive artificial ventilation. Injected locally, botulinum toxin type A is used in the treatment of certain ophthalmic conditions associated with spasms of ocular muscles (e.g., strabismus and blepharospasm) (Chapter 69) and for a wide variety of unlabeled uses, ranging from treatment of muscle dystonias and palsy (Chapter 11) to cosmetic erasure of facial lines and wrinkles (a modern medical testament to the vanity of human wishes; Chapter 70).

Adrenergic

α-Methyltyrosine (metyrosine) blocks the synthesis of NE by inhibiting TH, the enzyme that catalyzes the rate-limiting step in catecholamine synthesis. This drug occasionally may be useful in treating selected patients with pheochromocytoma. On the other hand, methyldopa, an inhibitor of aromatic *L*-amino acid decarboxylase, is—like dopa itself—successively decarboxylated and hydroxylated in its side chain to form the putative "false neurotransmitter" α-methylnorepinephrine. The use of methyldopa in the treatment of hypertension is discussed in Chapter 28. Bretylium, guanadrel, and guanethidine act by preventing the release of NE by the nerve impulse. However, such agents can transiently stimulate the release of NE because of their capacity to displace the amine from storage sites.

Promotion of Release of the Transmitter

Cholinergic

The ability of pharmacological agents to promote the release of ACh is limited. The latrotoxins from black widow spider venom and stonefish are known to promote neuroexocytosis by binding to receptors on the neuronal membrane.

TABLE 8–7 ■ REPRESENTATIVE AGENTS ACTING AT PERIPHERAL CHOLINERGIC AND ADRENERGIC NEUROEFFECTOR JUNCTIONS

MECHANISM OF ACTION	SYSTEM	AGENTS	EFFECT
1. Interference with synthesis of transmitter	Cholinergic	Choline acetyl transferase inhibitors	Minimal depletion of ACh
	Adrenergic	α-Methyltyrosine (inhibition of tyrosine hydroxylase)	Depletion of NE
2. Metabolic transformation by same pathway as precursor of transmitter	Adrenergic	Methyldopa	Displacement of NE by α-methyl-NE, which is an α_2 agonist, similar to clonidine, that reduces sympathetic outflow from CNS
3. Blockade of transport system at nerve terminal membrane	Cholinergic	Hemicholinium	Block of choline uptake with consequent depletion of ACh
	Adrenergic	Cocaine, imipramine	Accumulation of NE at receptors
4. Blockade of transport system of storage vesicle	Cholinergic	Vesamicol	Block of ACh storage
	Adrenergic	Reserpine	Destruction of NE by mitochondrial MAO and depletion from adrenergic terminals
5. Promotion of exocytosis or displacement of transmitter from storage sites	Cholinergic	Latrotoxins	Cholinomimetic followed by anticholinergic
	Adrenergic	Amphetamine, tyramine	Sympathomimetic
6. Prevention of release of transmitter	Cholinergic	Botulinum toxin (BTX, endopeptidase, acts on synaptobrevin)	Anticholinergic (prevents skeletal muscle contraction)
	Adrenergic	Bretylium, guanadrel	Antiadrenergic
7. Mimicry of transmitter at postjunctional sites	Cholinergic		
	Muscarinic[a]	Methacholine, bethanachol	Cholinomimetic
	Nicotinic[b]	Nicotine, epibatidine, cytisine	Cholinomimetic
	Adrenergic		
	α_1	Phenylephrine	Selective α_1 agonist
	α_2	Clonidine	Sympathomimetic (periphery); reduced sympathetic outflow (CNS)
	α_1, α_2	Oxymetazoline	Nonselective α adrenomimetic
	β_1	Dobutamine	Selective cardiac stimulation (also activates α_1 receptors)
	β_2	Terbutaline, albuterol metaproterenol	Selective β_2 receptor agonist (selective inhibition of smooth muscle contraction)
	β_1, β_2	Isoproterenol	Nonselective β agonist
8. Blockade of postsynaptic receptor	Cholinergic		
	Muscarinic[a]	Atropine	Muscarinic blockade
	Nicotinic (N_m)[b]	d-Tubucurarine, atracurium	Neuromuscular blockade
	Nicotinic (N_n)[b]	Trimethaphan	Ganglionic blockade
	Adrenergic		
	α_1, α_2	Phenoxybenzamine	Nonselective α receptor blockade (irreversible)
	α_1, α_2	Phentolamine	Nonselective α receptor blockade (reversible)
	α_1	Prazosin, terazosin, doxasozin	Selective α_1 receptor blockade (reversible)
	α_2	Yohimbine	Selective α_2 receptor blockade
	β_1, β_2	Propranolol	Nonselective β receptor blockade
	β_1	Metoprolol, atenolol	Selective β_1 receptor blockade (cardiomyocytes; renal j-g cells)
	β_2	—	Selective β_2 receptor blockade (smooth muscle)

(Continued)

TABLE 8-7 ■ REPRESENTATIVE AGENTS ACTING AT PERIPHERAL CHOLINERGIC AND ADRENERGIC NEUROEFFECTOR JUNCTIONS (CONTINUED)

MECHANISM OF ACTION	SYSTEM	AGENTS	EFFECT
9. Inhibition of enzymatic breakdown of transmitter	Cholinergic	AChE inhibitors edrophonium, neostigmine, pyridostigmine	Cholinomimetic (muscarinic sites) Depolarization blockade (nicotinic sites)
	Adrenergic	Nonselective MAO inhibitors: pargyline, nialamide	Little direct effect on NE or sympathetic response; potentiation of tyramine
		Selective MAO-B inhibitor: selegeline	Adjunct in Parkinson disease
		Peripheral COMT inhibitor: Entacapone	Adjunct in Parkinson disease
		COMT inhibitor: Tolcapone	

The j-g cells are renin-secreting cells in the juxtaglomerular complex of the kidney.
[a]At least five subtypes of muscarinic receptors exist (see Table 8-3). Agonists show little subtype selectivity; several antagonists show partial subtype selectivity (see Chapter 9).
[b]Two subtypes of muscle acetylcholine nicotinic receptors and several subtypes of neuronal receptors have been identified (see Table 8-2).

Adrenergic

Several drugs that promote the release of NE already have been discussed. On the basis of the rate and duration of the drug-induced release of NE from adrenergic terminals, one of two opposing effects can predominate. Tyramine, ephedrine, amphetamine, and related drugs cause a relatively rapid, brief liberation of the transmitter and produce a sympathomimetic effect. On the other hand, reserpine, by blocking the uptake of amines by VMAT2, produces a slow, prolonged depletion of the adrenergic transmitter from adrenergic storage vesicles, where it is largely metabolized by intraneuronal MAO. The resulting depletion of transmitter produces the equivalent of adrenergic blockade. Reserpine also causes the depletion of 5HT, DA, and possibly other, unidentified, amines from central and peripheral sites, and many of its major effects may be a consequence of the depletion of transmitters other than NE.

As discussed previously, deficiencies of TH in humans cause a neurologic disorder (Carson and Robertson, 2002) that can be treated by supplementation with the DA precursor levodopa.

A syndrome caused by congenital DβH deficiency is characterized by the absence of NE and EPI, elevated concentrations of DA, intact baroreceptor reflex afferent fibers and cholinergic innervation, and undetectable concentrations of plasma DβH activity (Carson and Robertson, 2002). Patients with this syndrome have severe orthostatic hypotension, ptosis of the eyelids, and retrograde ejaculations. Dihydroxyphenylserine (L-DOPS) improves postural hypotension in this rare disorder. This therapeutic approach takes advantage of the nonspecificity of aromatic L-amino acid decarboxylase, which synthesizes NE directly from this drug in the absence of DβH (Man in't Veld et al., 1988; Robertson et al., 1991). Despite the restoration of plasma NE in humans with L-DOPS, EPI levels are not restored, leading to speculation that PNMT may require DβH for appropriate functioning (Carson and Robertson, 2002).

Agonist and Antagonist Actions at Receptors

Cholinergic

The nicotinic receptors of autonomic ganglia and skeletal muscle are not identical; they respond differently to certain stimulating and blocking agents, and their pentameric structures contain different combinations of homologous subunits (Table 8-2). *Dimethylphenylpiperazinium* (DMPP) and phenyltrimethylammonium (PTMA) show some selectivity for stimulation of autonomic ganglion cells and muscle motor end plates. Trimethaphan and hexamethonium are relatively selective competitive and noncompetitive ganglionic blocking agents, respectively. Although tubocurarine effectively blocks transmission at both motor end plates and autonomic ganglia, its action at the former site predominates. Succinylcholine, a depolarizing agent, produces selective neuromuscular blockade. Transmission at autonomic ganglia and the adrenal medulla is complicated further by the presence of muscarinic receptors in addition to the principal nicotinic receptors (see Chapter 11).

Various toxins in snake venoms exhibit a high degree of specificity toward cholinergic receptors. The α-neurotoxins from the Elapidae family interact with the agonist-binding site on the nicotinic receptor. α-Bungarotoxin is selective for the muscle receptor and interacts with only certain neuronal receptors, such as those containing α7 through α9 subunits. Neuronal bungarotoxin shows a wider range of inhibition of neuronal receptors. A second group of toxins, called the *fasciculins*, inhibits AChE. A third group of toxins, termed the *muscarinic toxins* (MT_1 through MT_4), includes partial agonists and antagonists for muscarinic receptors. Venoms from the Viperidae family of snakes and the fish-hunting cone snails also have relatively selective toxins for nicotinic receptors.

Muscarinic ACh receptors, which mediate the effects of ACh at autonomic effector cells, now can be divided into five subclasses. Atropine blocks all the muscarinic responses to injected ACh and related cholinomimetic drugs whether they are excitatory, as in the intestine, or inhibitory, as in the heart. Newer muscarinic agonists, pirenzepine for M_1, tripitramine for M_2, and darifenacin for M_3, show selectivity as muscarinic-blocking agents. Several muscarinic antagonists show sufficient selectivity in the clinical setting to minimize the bothersome side effects seen with the nonselective agents at therapeutic doses (see Chapter 9).

Adrenergic

A vast number of synthetic compounds that bear structural resemblance to the naturally occurring catecholamines can interact with α and β adrenergic receptors to produce sympathomimetic effects (see Chapter 12). Phenylephrine acts selectively at α_1 receptors, whereas clonidine is a selective α_2 adrenergic agonist. Isoproterenol exhibits agonist activity at both β_1 and β_2 receptors. Preferential stimulation of cardiac β_1 receptors follows the administration of dobutamine. Terbutaline exerts relatively selective action on β_2 receptors; it produces effective bronchodilation with minimal effects on the heart. The main features of adrenergic blockade, including the selectivity of various blocking agents for α and β adrenergic receptors, are considered in detail in Chapter 12. Partial dissociation of effects at β_1 and β_2 receptors has been achieved by subtype-selective antagonists, as exemplified by the β_1 receptor antagonists metoprolol and atenolol, which antagonize the cardiac actions of catecholamines while causing somewhat less antagonism at bronchioles. Prazosin and yohimbine are representative of α_1 and α_2 receptor antagonists, respectively; prazosin has a relatively high affinity at α_{2B} and α_{2C} subtypes compared with α_{2A} receptors. Several important drugs that promote the release of NE (e.g., tyramine) or deplete the transmitter (e.g., reserpine) resemble, in their effects, activators or blockers of postjunctional receptors.

Interference With the Destruction of the Transmitter

Cholinergic

The anti-ChE agents (see Chapter 10) constitute a chemically diverse group of compounds, the primary action of which is inhibition of AChE, with the consequent accumulation of endogenous ACh. At the NMJ, accumulation of ACh produces depolarization of end plates and flaccid paralysis. At postganglionic muscarinic effector sites, the response is either excessive stimulation resulting in contraction and secretion or an inhibitory response mediated by hyperpolarization. At ganglia, depolarization and enhanced transmission are observed.

Adrenergic

The reuptake of NE by the adrenergic nerve terminals by means of NET is the major mechanism for terminating NE's transmitter action. Interference with this process is the basis of the potentiating effect of cocaine on responses to adrenergic impulses and injected catecholamines. The antidepressant actions and some of the adverse effects of imipramine and related drugs may be due to a similar action at adrenergic synapses in the CNS (Chapter 15).

Entacapone and tolcapone are nitro catechol-type COMT inhibitors. Entacapone is a peripherally acting COMT inhibitor, whereas tolcapone also inhibits COMT activity in the brain. COMT inhibition has been shown to attenuate levodopa toxicity on dopaminergic neurons and enhance DA's action in the brain of patients with Parkinson disease (Chapter 18). On the other hand, nonselective MAO inhibitors, such as tranylcypromine, potentiate the effects of tyramine and may potentiate effects of neurotransmitters. While most MAO inhibitors used as antidepressants inhibit both MAO-A and MAO-B, selective MAO-A and MAO-B inhibitors are available. Selegiline is a selective and irreversible MAO-B inhibitor that also has been used as an adjunct in the treatment of Parkinson disease.

Other Autonomic Neurotransmitters

ATP and ACh coexist in cholinergic vesicles (Dowdall et al., 1974), and ATP, NPY, and catecholamines are found within storage granules in nerves and the adrenal medulla (see previous discussion). ATP is released along with the transmitters, and it and its metabolites can play significant roles in synaptic transmission in some circumstances (see further discussion). Recently, attention has focused on the growing list of peptides that are found in the adrenal medulla, nerve fibers, or ganglia of the autonomic nervous system or in the structures that are innervated by the autonomic nervous system. This list includes enkephalins, substance P and other tachykinins, SST, gonadotropin-releasing hormone, CCK, CGRP, galanin, PACAP, VIP, chromogranins, and NPY (Hökfelt et al., 2000). Some of the orphan GPCRs discovered in the course of genome-sequencing projects may represent receptors for undiscovered peptides or other cotransmitters.

Cotransmission in the Autonomic Nervous System

There is a large body of literature on cotransmission in the autonomic nervous system. Much of the research in this area has focused on co-release of ATP by adrenergic and cholinergic nerves. Co-release of NPY, VIP, CGRP, substance P, and NO has also been studied. Whether these co-released factors act as neurotransmitters, neuromodulators, or trophic factors remains a topic of debate (Burnstock, 2013, 2015; Mutafova-Yambolieva et al., 2014).

The evidence is substantial that ATP plays a role in sympathetic nerves as a cotransmitter with NE (Silinsky et al., 1998; Westfall et al., 1991, 2002). For example, the rodent vas deferens is supplied with dense sympathetic innervation, and stimulation of the nerves results in a biphasic mechanical response that consists of an initial rapid twitch followed by a sustained contraction. The first phase of the response is mediated by ATP acting on postjunctional P2X receptors, whereas the second phase is mediated mainly by NE acting on α_1 receptors (Sneddon and Westfall,

1984). The cotransmitters apparently are released from the same types of nerves because pretreatment with 6-hydroxydopamine, an agent that specifically destroys adrenergic nerves, abolishes both phases of the neurogenically induced biphasic contraction. Whether ATP and NE originate from the same populations of vesicles within a nerve ending is still open to debate and experimentation (Todorov et al., 1996; Mutafova-Yambolieva et al, 2014; Burnstock, 2015).

Once ATP is released into the neuroeffector junction, some of it is metabolized by extracellularly directed membrane-bound nucleotidases to ADP, AMP, and adenosine (Gordon, 1986). However, the majority of its metabolism occurs by the actions of releasable nucleotidases. There is also evidence that ATP and its metabolites exert presynaptic modulatory effects on transmitter release by P2 receptors and receptors for adenosine. In addition to evidence showing that ATP is a cotransmitter with NE, there is evidence that ATP may be a cotransmitter with ACh in certain postganglionic parasympathetic nerves, such as those in the urinary bladder.

The NPY family of peptides is distributed widely in the central and peripheral nervous systems and consists of three members: NPY, pancreatic polypeptide, and peptide YY. NPY is colocalized and coreleased with NE and ATP in most sympathetic nerves in the peripheral nervous system, especially those innervating blood vessels (Westfall, 2004). There is also convincing evidence that NPY exerts prejunctional modulatory effects on transmitter release and synthesis. Moreover, there are numerous examples of postjunctional interactions that are consistent with a cotransmitter role for NPY at various sympathetic neuroeffector junctions. Thus, NPY, together with NE and ATP, qualifies as the third sympathetic cotransmitter of the sympathetic branch of the autonomic nervous system. Functions of NPY include

- direct postjunctional contractile effects
- potentiation of the contractile effects of the other sympathetic cotransmitters
- inhibitory modulation of the nerve stimulation–induced release of all three sympathetic cotransmitters, including actions on autoreceptors to inhibit its own release

Studies with selective NPY-Y_1 antagonists provided evidence that the principal postjunctional receptor is of the Y_1 subtype, although other receptors are also present at some sites and may exert physiological actions. Studies with selective NPY-Y_2 antagonists suggested that the principal prejunctional receptor is of the Y_2 subtype both in the periphery and in the CNS. There is evidence for a role for other NPY receptors, and clarification awaits the further development of selective antagonists. NPY also can act prejunctionally to inhibit the release of ACh, CGRP, and substance P. In the CNS, NPY exists as a cotransmitter with catecholamine in some neurons and with peptides and mediators in others. A prominent action of NPY is the presynaptic inhibition of the release of various neurotransmitters, including NE, DA, GABA, glutamate, and 5HT, as well as inhibition or stimulation of the release of neurohormones such as gonadotropin-releasing hormone, vasopressin, and oxytocin. Evidence also exists for stimulation of NE and DA release by NPY.

The NPY may use several mechanisms to produce its presynaptic effects, including inhibition of Ca^{2+} channels, activation of K^+ channels, and regulation of the vesicle release complex at some point distal to Ca^{2+} entry. NPY also may play a role in several pathophysiological conditions. The further development of selective NPY agonists and antagonists should enhance understanding about the physiological and pathophysiological roles of NPY.

The pioneering studies of Hökfelt and coworkers, which demonstrated the existence of VIP and ACh in peripheral autonomic neurons, initiated interest in the possibility of peptidergic cotransmission in the autonomic nervous system. Subsequent work has confirmed the frequent association of these two substances in autonomic fibers, including parasympathetic fibers that innervate smooth muscle and exocrine glands and cholinergic sympathetic neurons that innervate sweat glands (Hökfelt et al., 2000).

The role of VIP in parasympathetic transmission has been studied most extensively in the regulation of salivary secretion. The evidence for cotransmission includes the release of VIP following stimulation of the chorda lingual nerve and the incomplete blockade by atropine of vasodilation when the frequency of stimulation is raised; the last observation may indicate independent release of the two substances, which is consistent with histochemical evidence for storage of ACh and VIP in separate populations of vesicles. Synergism between ACh and VIP in stimulating vasodilation and secretion also has been described. VIP may be involved in parasympathetic responses in the trachea and in the GI tract, where it may facilitate sphincter relaxation.

Nonadrenergic, Noncholinergic (NANC) Transmission by Purines

The smooth muscle of many tissues that are innervated by the autonomic nervous system shows inhibitory junction potentials following stimulation by field electrodes. Because such responses frequently are undiminished in the presence of adrenergic and muscarinic cholinergic antagonists, these observations have been taken as evidence for the existence of NANC transmission in the autonomic nervous system.

Burnstock and colleagues have compiled compelling evidence for the existence of purinergic neurotransmission in the GI tract, genitourinary tract, and certain blood vessels; ATP fulfills all the criteria for a neurotransmitter. In at least some circumstances, primary sensory axons may be an important source of ATP (Burnstock et al., 2015). Although adenosine is generated from the released ATP by ectoenzymes and releasable nucleotidases, its primary function appears to be modulatory by causing feedback inhibition of transmitter release.

Adenosine can be transported from the cell cytoplasm to activate extracellular receptors on adjacent cells. The efficient uptake of adenosine by cellular transporters and its rapid metabolism to inosine or to adenine nucleotides contribute to its rapid turnover. Several inhibitors of adenosine transport and metabolism can influence concentrations of extracellular adenosine and ATP (Sneddon et al., 1999).

The purinergic receptors found on the cell surface may be divided into the adenosine (P1) receptors and the receptors for ATP (P2X and P2Y receptors) (Fredholm et al., 2000). Both P1 and P2 receptors have various subtypes. There are four adenosine receptors (A_1, A_{2A}, A_{2B}, and A_3) and multiple subtypes of P2X and P2Y receptors throughout the body. The adenosine receptors and the P2Y receptors mediate their responses via G proteins, whereas the P2X receptors are a subfamily of ligand-gated ion channels (Burnstock et al., 2015). Methylxanthines such as caffeine and theophylline preferentially block P1 adenosine receptors (Chapter 40).

Signal Integration and Modulation of Vascular Responses by Endothelium-Derived Factors: NO and Endothelin

The contents of adrenergic storage vesicles are not alone in regulating vascular tone. Many other factors modulate vascular contractility, including kinins, angiotensin, natriuretic peptides, substance P, VIP, CGRP, and eicosanoids, all described elsewhere in this volume. There are additional factors generated by the vascular endothelium that influence vascular reactivity: NO and endothelin.

Furchgott and colleagues demonstrated that an intact endothelium is necessary to achieve vascular relaxation in response to ACh (Furchgott, 1999). This inner cellular layer of the blood vessel now is known to modulate autonomic and hormonal effects on the contractility of blood vessels. In response to a variety of vasoactive agents and physical stimuli, endothelial cells release a short-lived vasodilator termed endothelium-derived relaxing factor, now identified as NO. Less commonly, an endothelium-derived hyperpolarizing factor and endothelium-derived contracting factor are released (Vanhoutte, 1996). Formation of endothelium-derived contracting factor depends on cyclooxygenase activity.

Products of inflammation and platelet aggregation (e.g., 5HT, histamine, bradykinin, purines, and thrombin) exert all or part of their action by stimulating the production of NO. Endothelium-dependent mechanisms of relaxation are important in a variety of vascular beds, including the coronary circulation (Hobbs et al., 1999). Activation of specific GPCRs linking to G_q and the mobilization of Ca^{2+} within endothelial cells promotes NO production. NO diffuses readily to the underlying smooth muscle and induces relaxation of vascular smooth muscle by activating the soluble form of guanylyl cyclase, which increases cyclic GMP concentrations (Figures 3–13 and 3–17). Nitrovasodilating drugs used to lower blood pressure or to treat ischemic heart disease probably act through conversion to or release of NO (Chapter 27). Certain nerves (termed *nitrergic*) innervating blood vessels and smooth muscles of the GI tract also release NO. NO has a negative inotropic action on the heart.

Alterations in the release or action of NO may affect a number of major clinical situations, such as atherosclerosis (Hobbs et al., 1999; Ignarro et al., 1999). Furthermore, there is evidence suggesting that the hypotension of endotoxemia or that induced by cytokines is mediated by induction of NOS2 (the inducible form of NOS) and the enhanced production NO; consequently, increased NO production may have pathological significance in septic shock.

Full contractile responses of cerebral arteries also require an intact endothelium. A family of peptides, termed *endothelins,* is stored in vascular endothelial cells. Endothelin contributes to the maintenance of vascular homeostasis by acting via multiple endothelin receptors that are GPCRs (Sokolovsky, 1995; Hilal-Dandan et al., 1997). The release of endothelin-1 (21 amino acids) onto smooth muscle promotes contraction by stimulation of the ET_A receptor. Endothelin antagonists are now employed in treating pulmonary artery hypertension (Chapter 31).

Bibliography

Aantaa R, et al. Molecular pharmacology of α_2-adrenoceptor subtypes. *Ann Med*, **1995**, 27:439–449.

Abell CW, Kwan SW. Molecular characterization of monoamine oxidases A and B. *Prog Nucleic Acid Res Mol Biol*, **2001**, 65:129–156.

Ahlquist RP. A study of the adrenotropic receptors. *Am J Physiol*, **1948**, 153:586–600.

Alabi AA, Tsien RW. Perspectives on kiss-and-run: role in exocytosis, endocytosis, and neurotransmission. *Annu Rev Physiol*, **2013**, 75:393–422.

Albuquerque EX, et al. Mammalian nicotinic acetylcholine receptors: from structure to function. *Physiol Rev*, **2009**, 89:73–120.

Altschuler SM, et al. Viscerotopic representation of the upper alimentary tract in the rat: sensory ganglia and nuclei of the solitary and spinal trigeminal tracts. *J Comp Neurol*, **1989**, 283:248–268.

Andresen MC, Kunze DL. Nucleus tractus solitarius: gateway to neural circulatory control. *Annu Rev Physiol*, **1994**, 56:93–116.

Arner P, Hoffstedt J. Adrenoceptor genes in human obesity. *J Intern Med*, **1999**, 245:667–672.

Aunis D. Exocytosis in chromaffin cells of the adrenal medulla. *Int Rev Cytol*, **1998**, 181:213–320.

Baillie G, Houslay M. Arrestin times for compartmentalized cAMP signalling and phosphodiesterase-4 enzymes. *Curr Opin Cell Biol*, **2005**, 17:129–134.

Brodde OE. β_1 and β_2 adrenoceptor polymorphisms: functional importance, impact on cardiovascular disease and drug responses. *Pharmacol Ther*, **2008**, 117:1–29.

Brodde OE, et al. Cardiac adrenoceptors: physiological and pathophysiological relevance. *J Pharmacol Sci*, **2006**, 100:323–337.

Burnstock G. Cotransmission in the autonomic nervous system. *Handb Clin Neurol*, **2013**, 117:23–35.

Burnstock G, et al. Purinergic signalling and the autonomic nervous system. *Autonomic Neurosci*, **2015**, 191:1–147.

Carson RP, Robertson D. Genetic manipulation of noradrenergic neurons. *J Pharmacol Exp Ther*, **2002**, 301:407–410.

Catterall WA. From ionic currents to molecular mechanisms: the structure and function of voltage-gated sodium channels. *Neuron*, **2000**, 26:13–25.

Chaudhry FA, et al. Vesicular neurotransmitter transporters as targets for endogenous and exogenous toxic substances. *Annu Rev Pharmacol Toxicol*, **2008**, 48:277–301.

Chen H, et al. Differential gene expression in functional classes of interstitial cells of Cajal in murine small intestine. *Physiol Genomics*, **2007**, 31:492–509.

Chong BS, Mersfelder TL. Entacapone. *Ann Pharmacother*, **2000**, *34*:1056–1065.

Communal C, et al. Opposing effects of beta(1)- and beta(2)-adrenergic receptors on cardiac myocyte apoptosis: role of a pertussis toxin-sensitive G protein. *Circulation*, **1999**, *100*:2210–2212.

Devedjian JC, et al. Transgenic mice overexpressing alpha2a-adrenoceptors in pancreatic beta-cells show altered regulation of glucose homeostasis. *Diabetologia*, **2000**, *43*:899–906.

Dhein S, et al. Muscarinic receptors in the mammalian heart. *Pharmacol Res*, **2001**, *44*:161–182.

Dorn GW. Adrenergic signaling polymorphisms and their impact on cardiovascular disease. *Phys Rev*, **2010**, *90*:1013–1062.

Dorn GW, et al. Low- and high-level transgenic expression of beta2-adrenergic receptors differentially affect cardiac hypertrophy and function in galphaq-overexpressing mice. *Proc Natl Acad Sci U S A*, **1999**, *96*:6400–6405.

Dowdall MJ, et al. Adenosine triphosphate, a constituent of cholinergic synaptic vesicles. *Biochem J*, **1974**, *140*:1–12.

Eiden LE. The cholinergic gene locus. *J Neurochem*, **1998**, *70*:2227–2240.

Eisenhofer G. The role of neuronal and extraneuronal plasma membrane transporters in the inactivation of peripheral catecholamine. *Pharmacol Ther*, **2001**, *91*:35–62.

Eisenhofer G, et al. Catecholamine metabolism: a contemporary view with implications for physiology and medicine. *Pharmacol Rev*, **2004**, *56*:331–349.

Emorine LJ, et al. Molecular characterization of the human β_3-adrenergic receptor. *Science*, **1989**, *245*:1118–1121.

Estévez-Herrera J, et al. ATP: the crucial component of secretory vesicles. *Proc Natl Acad Sci U S A*, **2016**, *113*:E4098–E4106.

Exley R, Cragg SJ. Presynaptic nicotinic receptors: a dynamic and diverse cholinergic filter of striatal dopamine neurotransmission. *Br J Pharmacol*, **2008**, *153*:5283–5297.

Fagerholm V, et al. Altered glucose homeostasis in alpha2a-adrenoceptor knockout mice. *Eur J Pharmacol*, **2004**, *505*:243–252.

Fetscher C, et al. M3 muscarinic receptors mediate contraction of human urinary bladder. *Br J Pharmacol*, **2002**, *136*:641–643.

Fredholm BB, et al. Adenosine receptors. In Girdleston D, ed. *The IUPHAR Compendium of Receptor Characterization and Classification*. IUPHAR Media, London; **2000**, 78–87.

Furchgott RF. Endothelium-derived relaxing factor: discovery, early studies, and identification as nitric oxide. *Biosci Rep*, **1999**, *19*:235–251.

Furness JB, et al. The enteric nervous system and gastrointestinal innervation: integrated local and central control. *Adv Exp Med Biol*, **2014**, *817*:39–71.

Gainetdinov RR, Caron MG. Monoamine transporters: from genes to behavior. *Ann Rev Pharmacol Toxicol*, **2003**, *43*:261–284.

Gavras I, Gavras H. Role of alpha2-adrenergic receptors in hypertension. *Am J Hyper*, **2001**, *14*:171S–177S.

Gherbi K, et al. Negative cooperativity across β_1-adrenoceptor homodimers provides insights into the nature of the secondary low-affinity CGP 12177 β_1-adrenoceptor binding conformation. *FASEB J*, **2015**, *29*:2859–2871.

Goldsmith ZG, Dhanasekaran DN. G protein regulation of MAPK networks. *Oncogene*, **2007**, *26*:3122–3142.

Gordon JL. Extracellular ATP: effects, sources and fate. *Biochem J*, **1986**, *233*:309–319.

Haenisch B, et al. Association of major depression with rare functional variants in norepinephrine transporter and serotonin1a receptor genes. *Am J Med Gen Pt B Neuropsych Gen*, **2009**, *150B*:1013–1016.

Haga T. Molecular properties of the high-affinity choline transporter CHT1. *J Biochem*, **2014**, *156*:181–194.

Hahn MK, et al. Single nucleotide polymorphisms in the human norepinephrine transporter gene affect expression, trafficking, antidepressant interaction, and protein kinase c regulation. *Mol Pharmacol*, **2005**, *68*:457–466.

Hahn MK, et al. A mutation in the human norepinephrine transporter gene (slc6a2) associated with orthostatic intolerance disrupts surface expression of mutant and wild-type transporters. *J Neurosci*, **2003**, *23*:4470–4478.

Heaslip AT, et al. Cytoskeletal dependence of insulin granule movement dynamics in INS-1 beta-cells in response to glucose. *PLoS One*, **2014**, *9*:e109082.

Hieble JP. Subclassification and nomenclature of α- and β-adrenoceptors. *Curr Top Med Chem*, **2007**, *7*:129–134.

Hilal-Dandan R, et al. The quasi-irreversible nature of endothelin binding and G protein-linked signaling in cardiac myocytes. *J Pharmacol Exp Ther*, **1997**, *281*:267–273.

Hirsch D, et al. NPY and stress 30 years later: the peripheral view. *Cell Mol Neurobiol*, **2012**, *32*:645–659.

Hobbs AJ, et al. Inhibition of nitric oxide synthase as a potential therapeutic target. *Annu Rev Pharmacol Toxicol*, **1999**, *39*:191–220.

Hökfelt T, et al. Neuropeptides: an overview. *Neuropharmacology*, **2000**, *39*:1337–1356.

Ignarro LJ, et al. Nitric oxide as a signaling molecule in the vascular system: an overview. *J Cardiovasc Pharmacol*, **1999**, *34*:879–886.

Kable JW, et al. In vivo gene modification elucidates subtype-specific functions of α_2-adrenergic receptors. *J Pharmacol Exp Ther*, **2000**, *293*:1–7.

Kalamida D, et al. Muscle and neuronal nicotinic acetylcholine receptors structure function and pathogenicity. *FEBS J*, **2007**, *274*:3799–3845.

Keller NR, et al. Norepinephrine transporter-deficient mice exhibit excessive tachycardia and elevated blood pressure with wakefulness and activity. *Circulation*, **2004**, *110*:1191–1196.

Kubista H, Boehm S. Molecular mechanisms underlying the modulation of exocytoxic noradrenaline release via presynaptic receptors. *Pharmacol Ther*, **2006**, *112*:213–242.

Lakhlani PP, et al. Substitution of a mutant α_{2A}-adrenergic receptor via "hit and run" gene targeting reveals the role of this subtype in sedative, analgesic, and anesthetic-sparing responses in vivo. *Proc Natl Acad Sci U S A*, **1997**, *94*:9950–9955.

Langer SZ. 25 years since the discovery of presynaptic receptors: present knowledge and future perspectives. *Trends Pharmacol Sci*, **1997**, *18*:95–99.

Langmead CJ, et al. Muscarinic acetylcholine receptors as CNS drug targets. *Pharmacol Ther*, **2008**, *117*:232–243.

Liggett SB, et al. Early and delayed consequences of beta(2)-adrenergic receptor overexpression in mouse hearts: critical role for expression level. *Circulation*, **2000**, *101*:1707–1714.

Lugardon K, et al. Antibacterial and anti-fungal activities of vasostatin-1, the N-terminal fragment of chromogranin A. *J Biol Chem*, **2000**, *275*:10745–10753.

Lynch GS, Ryall JG. Role of β-adrenoceptor signaling in skeletal muscle: implications for muscle wasting and disease. *Physiol Rev*, **2008**, *88*:729–767.

Man in't Veld A, et al. Patients with congenital dopamine β-hydroxylase deficiency: a lesson in catecholamine physiology. *Am J Hypertens*, **1988**, *1*:231–238.

Männistö PT, Kaakkola S. Catechol-*O*-methyltransferase (COMT): biochemistry, molecular biology, pharmacology, and clinical efficacy of the new selective COMT inhibitors. *Pharmacol Rev*, **1999**, *51*:593–628.

Mialet Perez J, et al. Beta 1-adrenergic receptor polymorphisms confer differential function and predisposition to heart failure. *Nat Med*, **2003**, *9*:1300–1305.

Michelotti GA, et al. α_1-Adrenergic receptor regulation: basic science and clinical implications. *Pharmacol Ther*, **2000**, *88*:281–309.

Miller RJ. Presynaptic receptors. *Annu Rev Pharmacol Toxicol*, **1998**, *38*:201–227.

Mobine HR, et al. Pheochromocytoma-induced cardiomyopathy is modulated by the synergistic effects of cell-secreted factors. *Circ Heart Fail*, **2009**, *2*:121–128.

Mutafova-Yambolieva VN, Durnin L. The purinergic neurotransmitter revisited: A single substance or multiple players? *Pharmacol Ther*, **2014**, *144*:162–191.

Nagatsu T. The catecholamine system in health and disease—relation to tyrosine 3-monooxygenase and other catecholamine-synthesizing enzymes. *Proc Jpn Acad Ser B Phys Biol Sci*, **2006**, *82*:388–415.

Nathanson NM. Synthesis, trafficking and localization of muscarinic acetylcholine receptors. *Pharmacol Ther*, **2008**, *119*:33–43.

Philipp M, Hein L. Adrenergic receptor knockout mice: distinct functions of 9 receptor subtypes. *Pharmacol Ther*, **2004**, *101*:65–74.

Reiter E, et al. Molecular mechanism of β-arrestin-biased agonism at seven-transmembrane receptors. *Annu Rev Pharmacol Toxicol*, **2012**, *52*:179–197.

Robertson D, et al. Dopamine β-hydroxylase deficiency: a genetic disorder of cardiovascular regulation. *Hypertension*, **1991**, *18*:1–8.

Robidoux J, et al. β-Adrenergic receptors and regulation of energy expenditure: a family affair. *Annu Rev Pharmacol Toxicol*, **2004**, *44*:297–323.

Rokosh DG, Simpson PC. Knockout of the alpha 1$_{a/c}$-adrenergic receptor subtype: the alpha 1a/c is expressed in resistance arteries and is required to maintain arterial blood pressure. *Proc Natl Acad Sci U S A*, **2002**, *99*:9474–9479.

Roth M, et al. OATPs, OATs and OCTs: the organic anion and cation transporters of the *SLCO* and *SLC22A* gene superfamilies. *Br J Pharmacol*, **2012**, *165*:1260–1287.

Salogiannis J, Reck-Peterson SL. Hitchhiking: a non-canonical mode of microtubule-based transport. *Trends Cell Biol*, **2016**. http://dx.doi.org/10.1016/j.tcb.2016.09.005.

Saper CB. Pain as a visceral sensation. *Prog Brain Res*, **2000**, *122*:237–243.

Saper CB. The central autonomic nervous system: conscious visceral perception and autonomic pattern generation. *Annu Rev Neurosci*, **2002**, *25*:433–469.

Schuldiner S. A molecular glimpse of vesicular monoamine transporters. *J Neurochem*, **1994**, *62*:2067–2078.

Shannon JR, et al. Orthostatic intolerance and tachycardia associated with norepinephrine-transporter deficiency. *N Engl J Med*, **2000**, *342*:541–549.

Silinsky EM, et al. Functions of extracellular nucleotides in peripheral and central neuronal tissues. In Turner JT, Weisman GA, Fedan JS, eds. *The P$_2$ Nucleotide Receptors*. Humana Press, Totowa, NJ, **1998**, 259–290.

Silman I, Sussman JL. Acetylcholinesterase: "classical and non-classical" functions and pharmacology. *Curr Opin Pharmacol*, **2005**, *5*:293–302.

Sneddon P, Westfall DP. Pharmacological evidence that adenosine trisphosphate and noradrenaline are co-transmitters in the guinea-pig vas deferens. *J Physiol*, **1984**, *347*:561–580.

Sneddon P, et al. Modulation of purinergic neurotransmission. *Prog Brain Res*, **1999**, *120*:11–20.

Sokolovsky M. Endothelin receptor subtypes and their role in transmembrane signaling mechanisms. *Pharmacol Ther*, **1995**, *68*:435–471.

Südhof TC. The molecular machine of neurotransmitter release. In Grandin K, ed. *The Nobel Prizes, 2013*. Nobel Foundation, Stockholm, **2014**.

Tan CM, Limbird LE. *The α$_2$-Adrenergic Receptors: Lessons From Knockouts*. Humana, Clifton, NJ, **2005**, 241–266.

Tanoue A, et al. Transgenic studies of α$_1$-adrenergic receptor subtype function. *Life Sci*, **2002a**, *71*:2207–2215.

Tanoue A, et al. The α$_{1D}$-adrenergic receptor directly regulates arterial blood pressure via vasoconstriction. *J Clin Invest*, **2002b**, *109*:765–775.

Taupenot L, et al. The chromogranin–secretogranin family. *N Engl J Med*, **2003**, *348*:1134–1149.

Taylor P, et al. The genes encoding the cholinesterases: structure, evolutionary relationships and regulation of their expression. In Giacobini E, ed. *Cholinesterase and Cholinesterase Inhibitors*. Martin Dunitz, London, **2000**, 63–80.

Thomsen AR, et al. GPCR-G protein-β-arrestin super-complex mediates sustained G protein signaling. *Cell*, **2016**, *166*:907–919.

Toda N, Okamura J. The pharmacology of nitric oxide in the peripheral nervous system of blood vessels. *Pharmacol Rev*, **2003**, *55*:271–324.

Todorov LD, et al. Evidence for the differential release of the cotransmitters ATP and noradrenaline from sympathetic nerves of the guinea-pig vas deferens. *J Physiol*, **1996**, *496*:731–748.

Vanhoutte PM. Endothelium-dependent responses in congestive heart failure. *J Mol Cell Cardiol*, **1996**, *28*:2233–2240.

van Koppen CJ, Kaiser B. Regulation of muscarinic acetylcholine signaling. *Pharmacol Ther*, **2003**, *98*:197–220.

Violin JD, Lefkowitz RJ. β-Arrestin-biased ligands at seven-transmembrane receptors. *Trends Pharmacol Sci*, **2007**, *28*:416–422.

Viskupic E, et al. Increase in rat adrenal phenylethanolamine *N*-methyltransferase mRNA level caused by immobilization stress depends on intact pituitary-adrenocortical axis. *J Neurochem*, **1994**, *63*:808–814.

Volz HP, Gleiter CH. Monoamine oxidase inhibitors: a perspective on their use in the elderly. *Drugs Aging*, **1998**, *13*:341–355.

Von Euler US. A substance with sympathin E properties in spleen extracts. *Nature*, **1946**, *157*:369.

Walden PD, et al. Localization of mRNA and receptor binding sites for the α$_{1A}$-adrenoceptor subtype in the rat, monkey and human urinary bladder and prostate. *J Urol*, **1997**, *157*:1032–1038.

Wang Z, et al. Functional M$_3$ muscarinic acetylcholine receptors in mammalian hearts. *Br J Pharmacol*, **2004**, *142*:395–408.

Ward SE, et al. Interstitial cells of cajal mediate cholinergic neurotransmission from enteric motor neurons *J Neurosci*, **2000**, *20*:1393–1403.

Wess J, et al. Muscarinic acetylcholine receptors: mutant mice provide new insights for drug development. *Nat Rev/Drug Discov*, **2007**, *6*:721–733.

Wessler I, Kirkpatrick CJ. Acetylcholine beyond neurons: the non-neuronal cholinergic system in humans. *Br J Pharmacol*, **2008**, *154*:1558–1571.

Westfall DP, et al. ATP as neurotransmitter, cotransmitter and neuromodulator. In Phillis T, ed. *Adenosine and Adenine Nucleotides as Regulators of Cellular Function*. CRC Press, Boca Raton, FL, **1991**, 295–305.

Westfall DP, et al. ATP as a cotransmitter in sympathetic nerves and its inactivation by releasable enzymes. *J Pharmacol Exp Ther*, **2002**, *303*:439–444.

Westfall TC. Local regulation of adrenergic neurotransmission. *Physiol Rev*, **1977**, *57*:659–728.

Westfall TC. Prejunctional effects of neuropeptide Y and its role as a cotransmitter. In Michel MC, ed. *Neuropeptide Y and Related Peptides, Handbook of Experimental Pharmacology*, vol. 162. Springer, Berlin, **2004**, 137–183.

Wevers RA, et al. A review of biochemical and molecular genetic aspects of tyrosine hydroxylase deficiency including a novel mutation (291delC). *J Inherit Metab Dis*, **1999**, *22*:364–373.

Weyer C, et al. Development of β$_3$-adrenoceptor agonists for the treatment of obesity and diabetes: an update. *Diabetes Metab*, **1999**, *25*:11–21.

Witzemann V. Development of the neuromuscular junction. *Cell Tissue Res*, **2006**, *326*:263–71.

Woo AY-H, et al. Stereochemistry of an agonist determines coupling preference of β$_2$-adrenoceptor to different G proteins in cardiomyocytes. *Mol Pharmacol*, **2009**, *75*:158–165.

Wouters J. Structural aspects of monoamine oxidase and its reversible inhibition. *Curr Med Chem*, **1998**, *5*:137–162.

Wu SC, O'Connell TD. Nuclear compartmentalization of α1-adrenergic receptor signaling in adult cardiac myocytes. *Cardiovasc Pharmacol*, **2015**, *65*:91–100.

Yoshiki H, et al. Agonist pharmacology at recombinant α1A- and α1L-adrenoceptors and in lower urinary tract α1-adrenoceptors. *Br J Pharmacol*, **2013**, *170*:1242–1252.

Yoshiki H, et al. Pharmacologically distinct phenotypes of α1B-adrenoceptors: variation in binding and functional affinities for antagonists. *Br J Pharmacol*, **2014**, *171*:4890–4901.

Xiao RP, et al. Sutype-specific α$_1$- and β-adrenoceptor signaling in the heart. *Trends Pharm Sci*, **2006**, *27*:330–337.

Xu F, et al. Mice lacking the norepinephrine transporter are supersensitive to psychostimulants. *Nat Neurosci*, **2000**, *3*:465–471.

Ziegler MG, et al. Location, development, control, and function of extraadrenal phenylethanolamine *N*-methyltransferase. *Ann N Y Acad Sci*, **2002**, *971*:76–82.

Zigmond RE, et al. Acute regulation of tyrosine hydroxylase by nerve activity and by neurotransmitters via phosphorylation. *Annu Rev Neurosci*, **1989**, *12*:415–461.

Chapter 9

Muscarinic Receptor Agonists and Antagonists

Joan Heller Brown, Katharina Brandl, and Jürgen Wess

Acetylcholine and Its Muscarinic Receptor Target

Muscarinic acetylcholine receptors in the peripheral nervous system are found primarily on autonomic effector cells innervated by postganglionic parasympathetic nerves. Muscarinic receptors are also present in autonomic ganglia and on some cells (e.g., vascular endothelial cells) that, paradoxically, receive little or no cholinergic innervation. Within the CNS, the hippocampus, cortex, and thalamus have high densities of muscarinic receptors.

Acetylcholine, the naturally occurring neurotransmitter for these receptors, has virtually no systemic therapeutic applications because its actions are diffuse, and its hydrolysis, catalyzed by both AChE and plasma butyrylcholinesterase, is rapid. Muscarinic agonists mimic the effects of ACh at these sites. These agonists typically are longer-acting congeners of ACh or natural alkaloids, some of which stimulate nicotinic as well as muscarinic receptors.

The mechanisms of action of endogenous ACh at the postjunctional membranes of the effector cells and neurons that represent different types of cholinergic synapses are discussed in Chapter 8. Cholinergic synapses occur at:

- autonomic effector sites innervated by postganglionic parasympathetic nerves (or, in the sweat glands, by postganglionic sympathetic nerves)
- sympathetic and parasympathetic ganglia and the adrenal medulla, innervated by preganglionic autonomic nerves
- motor end plates on skeletal muscle, innervated by somatic motor nerves
- certain synapses in the CNS (Krnjević, 2004) where ACh can have either pre- or postsynaptic actions

When ACh is administered systemically, it can potentially act at all of these sites; however, as a quaternary ammonium compound, its penetration to the CNS is limited, and the amount of ACh that reaches peripheral areas with low blood flow is limited due to hydrolysis by plasma butyrylcholinesterase.

The actions of ACh and related drugs at autonomic effector sites are referred to as *muscarinic*, based on the observation that the alkaloid muscarine acts selectively at those sites and produces the same qualitative effects as ACh. The muscarinic, or parasympathomimetic, actions of the drugs considered in this chapter are practically equivalent to the parasympathetic effects of ACh listed in Table 8–1. Muscarinic receptors are present in autonomic ganglia and the adrenal medulla but primarily function to modulate the nicotinic actions of ACh at these sites (Chapter 11). In the CNS, muscarinic receptors are widely distributed and have a role in mediating many important responses. The differences between the actions of ACh and other muscarinic agonists are largely quantitative, with limited selectivity for one organ system or another. All of the actions of ACh and its congeners at muscarinic receptors can be competitively inhibited by atropine.

Properties and Subtypes of Muscarinic Receptors

Muscarinic receptors were characterized initially by analysis of the responses of cells and organ systems in the periphery and the CNS. For example, differential effects of two muscarinic agonists, bethanechol and McN-A-343, on the tone of the lower esophageal sphincter led to the initial designation of muscarinic receptors as M_1 (ganglionic) and M_2 (effector cell) (Goyal and Rattan, 1978). Molecular cloning of muscarinic receptors has identified five distinct gene products (Bonner et al., 1987), now designated as M_1 through M_5 muscarinic receptors (Chapter 8). All of the known muscarinic receptors are G protein–coupled receptors that in turn couple to various cellular effectors (Chapter 3). Although selectivity is not absolute, stimulation of M_1, M_3, and M_5 receptors causes hydrolysis of polyphosphoinositides and mobilization of intracellular Ca^{2+} as a consequence of activation of the G_q-PLC pathway, resulting in a variety of Ca^{2+}-mediated responses. In contrast, M_2 and M_4 muscarinic receptors inhibit adenylyl cyclase and regulate specific ion channels via their coupling to the pertussis toxin–sensitive G proteins, G_i and G_o (Chapter 3).

Recent X-ray crystallographic studies convincingly demonstrated that the classical (*orthosteric*) binding site for muscarinic agonists and antagonists is highly conserved among muscarinic receptor subtypes (Haga et al., 2012; Kruse et al., 2012, 2013). The orthosteric binding site consists of a cleft deeply buried within the membrane, formed by conserved amino acid chains located on several of the receptors' seven TM helices (TM1–TM7). A key feature shared by other receptors for biogenic amine ligands is the presence of a charge-charge interaction between the tertiary or quaternary nitrogen of the orthosteric ligands and a conserved TM3 aspartic acid side chain. A feature unique to muscarinic receptors is hydrogen bond interactions between the orthosteric ligand and a TM6 asparagine residue. Agonist binding to the receptor leads to considerable contraction of the ligand-binding pocket, reflecting the relatively small size of muscarinic agonists, as compared to muscarinic antagonists. Because the residues that line the orthosteric binding site are highly conserved among all muscarinic receptors, developing

Abbreviations

ACh: acetylcholine
AChE: acetylcholinesterase
AV: atrioventricular
COPD: chronic obstructive pulmonary disease
eNOS: endothelial NO synthase
HCN: hyperpolarization-activated, cyclic nucleotide–gated (channels)
5HT: serotonin
I_{Ca-L}**:** L-type Ca^{2+} current
I_f**:** cardiac pacemaker current
I_{K-ACh}**:** ACh-activated K^+ current
M_1, M_2, M_3**:** muscarinic receptor subclasses
NO: nitric oxide

orthosteric muscarinic ligands endowed with a high degree of receptor subtype selectivity has proven difficult.

The five muscarinic receptor subtypes are widely distributed in both the CNS and peripheral tissues; most cells express at least two subtypes (Abrams et al., 2006; Wess, 1996; Wess et al., 2007). Identifying the role of a specific subtype in mediating a particular muscarinic response to ACh has been difficult due to the lack of subtype-specific agonists and antagonists. More recently, studies with M_1–M_5 receptor knockout mice have yielded novel information about the physiological roles of the individual muscarinic receptor subtypes (Kruse et al., 2014; Wess et al., 2007; Table 8–3); these studies demonstrated that multiple receptor subtypes are involved in mediating a specific muscarinic response in most cases. For example, abolition of cholinergic bronchoconstriction, salivation, pupillary constriction, and bladder contraction generally requires deletion of more than one receptor subtype.

Various lines of evidence suggest that muscarinic receptors possess one or more topographically distinct allosteric binding sites formed by amino acid side chains located within the extracellular loops or the outer segments of different transmembrane (TM) helices (Birdsall and Lazareno, 2005; May et al., 2007). Because these regions show a considerable degree of sequence variation among the M_1–M_5 receptors, considerable progress has been made in developing so-called allosteric modulators that show high selectivity for distinct muscarinic receptor subtypes (Conn et al., 2009, 2014; Gentry et al., 2015). These agents exert their pharmacological actions by altering the affinity or efficacy of orthosteric muscarinic ligands. Positive allosteric modulators (PAMs) enhance orthosteric activity, while negative allosteric modulators (NAMs) inhibit it. Allosteric agents that can directly activate muscarinic receptors are termed *allosteric agonists*. However, these designations are not absolute; they depend on the nature of the orthosteric ligand, receptor subtype under investigation, and assay system used. The remarkable progress that has been made recently in identifying subtype-selective muscarinic allosteric agents may lead to the development of new therapeutic agents with increased efficacy and reduced side effects. Currently, much research is focused on the potential of such agents for the treatment of several severe disorders of the CNS, including Alzheimer disease and schizophrenia.

A recent X-ray structure revealed the molecular details of a PAM–muscarinic receptor complex; the binding pocket for muscarinic PAMs is located just above the orthosteric binding crevice (Kruse et al., 2013). This new structure also illustrates that the bound PAM interferes with the dissociation of the bound orthosteric agonist from the receptor. Another potential strategy for achieving receptor subtype selectivity is the development of hybrid, bitopic orthosteric/allosteric ligands that interact with both the orthosteric binding cavity and an allosteric site (Lane et al., 2013; Mohr et al., 2010). By targeting orthosteric and allosteric sites simultaneously, bitopic ligands achieve both high affinity and receptor subtype selectivity.

Pharmacological Effects of Acetylcholine

The influence of ACh and parasympathetic innervation on various organs and tissues was introduced in Chapter 8; a more detailed description of the effects of ACh is presented here as background for understanding the physiological basis for the therapeutic uses of the muscarinic receptor agonists and antagonists.

Cardiovascular System

Acetylcholine has four primary effects on the cardiovascular system:

- vasodilation
- decrease in heart rate (negative chronotropic effect)
- decrease in the conduction velocity in the AV node (negative dromotropic effect)
- decrease in the force of cardiac contraction (negative inotropic effect)

The negative inotropic effect is of less significance in the ventricles than in the atria. In addition, some of these effects can be obscured by baroreceptor and other reflexes that dampen the direct responses to ACh.

Although ACh rarely is given systemically, its cardiac actions are important because the effects of cardiac glycosides, antiarrhythmic agents, and many other drugs are at least partly due to changes in parasympathetic (vagal) stimulation of the heart; in addition, afferent stimulation of the viscera during surgical interventions can reflexly increase the vagal stimulation of the heart.

The intravenous injection of a small dose of ACh produces a transient fall in blood pressure owing to generalized vasodilation (mediated by vascular endothelial NO), which is usually accompanied by reflex tachycardia. The generalized vasodilation produced by exogenously administered ACh is due to the stimulation of muscarinic receptors, primarily of the M_3 subtype located on vascular endothelial cells. Occupation of these receptors activates the G_q-PLC-IP_3 pathway, leading to Ca^{2+}-calmodulin–dependent activation of endothelial eNOS (NOS3) and production of NO (endothelium-derived relaxing factor) (Moncada and Higgs, 1995), which diffuses to adjacent vascular smooth muscle cells, where it stimulates guanylyl cyclase, thereby promoting relaxation via a cyclic GMP–dependent mechanism (see Figure 3-11; Furchgott, 1999; Ignarro et al., 1999). Baroreceptor or chemoreceptor reflexes or direct stimulation of the vagus can also elicit parasympathetic coronary vasodilation mediated by ACh and the consequent production of NO by the endothelium (Feigl, 1998). If the endothelium is damaged, however, as occurs under various pathophysiological conditions, ACh acts predominantly on M_3 receptors located on the underlying vascular smooth muscle cells, causing vasoconstriction. This capacity to both relax and constrict vessels is shared by many hormones that act via the G_q-PLC-IP_3-Ca^{2+} pathway and for which both endothelial cells and vascular smooth muscle cells express receptors. If the agonist can reach both cell types, each cell type will respond in its differentiated way to an elevation of intracellular Ca^{2+}, endothelium with a stimulation of NO synthase, smooth muscle with contraction.

Acetylcholine has direct effects on cardiac function at doses higher than those required for vasodilation. The cardiac effects of ACh are mediated primarily by M_2 muscarinic receptors (Stengel et al., 2000), which couple to G_i/G_o. Direct effects of ACh include an increase in the I_{K-ACh} due to activation of K-ACh channels, a decrease in the I_{Ca-L} due to inhibition of L-type Ca^{2+} channels, and a decrease in the I_f due to inhibition of HCN (pacemaker) channels (DiFrancesco and Tromba, 1987). ACh acting on M_2 receptors also leads to a G_i-mediated decrease in cyclic AMP, which opposes and counteracts the β_1 adrenergic/G_s–mediated increase in cyclic AMP, and an inhibition of the release of norepinephrine from sympathetic nerve terminals. The inhibition of norepinephrine release is mediated by presynaptic M_2 and M_3 receptors, which are activated by ACh released from adjacent parasympathetic postganglionic nerve terminals (Trendelenburg et al., 2005). There are also presynaptic M_2 receptors that inhibit ACh release from parasympathetic postganglionic nerve terminals in the human heart (Oberhauser et al., 2001).

In the SA node, each normal cardiac impulse is initiated by the spontaneous depolarization of the pacemaker cells (Chapter 30). At a critical level (the threshold potential), this depolarization initiates an action potential. ACh slows the heart rate primarily by decreasing the rate of spontaneous depolarization; attainment of the threshold potential and the succeeding events in the cardiac cycle are therefore delayed. Until recently, it was widely accepted that β_1 adrenergic and muscarinic cholinergic effects on heart rate resulted from regulation of the cardiac pacemaker current mentioned previously (I_f). Unexpected findings made through genetic deletion of HCN4 and pharmacological inhibition of I_f have generated an alternative theory involving a pace-making function for an intracellular Ca^{2+} "clock" (Lakatta and DiFrancesco, 2009) that might mediate effects of ACh on heart rate (Lyashkov et al., 2009).

In the atria, ACh causes hyperpolarization and decreased action potential duration by increasing $I_{K\text{-}ACh}$. ACh also inhibits cyclic AMP formation and norepinephrine release, decreasing atrial contractility. In the AV node, ACh slows conduction and increases the refractory period by inhibiting $I_{Ca\text{-}L}$; the decrement in AV conduction is responsible for the complete heart block that may be observed when large quantities of cholinergic agonists are administered systemically. When parasympathetic (vagal) tone to the resting heart is increased (e.g., by digoxin), the prolonged refractory period of the AV node can reduce the frequency with which aberrant atrial impulses are transmitted to the ventricles and thereby decrease the ventricular rate during atrial flutter or fibrillation.

The ventricular myocardium and His-Purkinje system receive only sparse cholinergic (vagal) innervation (Levy and Schwartz, 1994), and the effects of ACh are smaller than those observed in the atria and nodal tissues. The modest negative inotropic effect of ACh in the ventricle is most apparent when there is concomitant adrenergic stimulation or underlying sympathetic tone (Brodde and Michel, 1999; Levy and Schwartz, 1994; Lewis et al., 2001). Automaticity of Purkinje fibers is suppressed, and the threshold for ventricular fibrillation is increased.

Respiratory Tract

The parasympathetic nervous system plays a major role in regulating bronchomotor tone. A diverse set of stimuli cause reflex increases in parasympathetic activity that contributes to bronchoconstriction. The effects of ACh on the respiratory system include bronchoconstriction, increased tracheobronchial secretion, and stimulation of the chemoreceptors of the carotid and aortic bodies. These effects are mediated primarily by M_3 muscarinic receptors located on bronchial and tracheal smooth muscle (Eglen et al., 1996; Fisher et al., 2004).

Urinary Tract

Parasympathetic sacral innervation causes detrusor muscle contraction, increased voiding pressure, and ureteral peristalsis. These responses are difficult to observe with administered ACh because poor perfusion of visceral organs and rapid hydrolysis by plasma butyrylcholinesterase limit access of systemically administered ACh to visceral muscarinic receptors. Control of bladder contraction apparently is mediated by multiple muscarinic receptor subtypes. Muscarinic stimulation of bladder contraction is mediated primarily by M_3 receptors expressed by detrusor smooth muscle cells. Smooth muscle M_2 receptors also seem to make a small contribution to this response. M_2 receptors may also cause bladder contractions indirectly by reversing β receptor–cyclic AMP–mediated relaxation of the detrusor muscle (Hegde, 2006; Matsui et al, 2002).

GI Tract

Although stimulation of vagal input to the GI tract increases tone, amplitude of contractions, and secretory activity of the stomach and intestine, such responses are inconsistently seen with administered ACh for the same reasons that urinary tract responses are difficult to observe. As in the urinary tract, M_3 receptors appear to be primarily responsible for mediating cholinergic control of GI motility, but M_2 receptors also contribute to this activity (Matsui et al., 2002).

Secretory Effects

In addition to its stimulatory effects on the tracheobronchial and GI secretions, ACh stimulates secretion from other glands that receive parasympathetic or sympathetic cholinergic innervation, including the lacrimal, nasopharyngeal, salivary, and sweat glands. All of these effects are mediated primarily by M_3 muscarinic receptors (Caulfield and Birdsall, 1998); M_1 receptors also contribute significantly to the cholinergic stimulation of salivary secretion (Gautam et al., 2004).

Eye

When instilled into the eye, ACh produces miosis by contracting the pupillary sphincter muscle and accommodation for near vision by contracting the ciliary muscle; both of these effects are mediated primarily by M_3 muscarinic receptors, but other subtypes may contribute to the ocular effects of cholinergic stimulation.

CNS Effects

While systemically administered ACh has limited CNS penetration, muscarinic agonists that can cross the blood-brain barrier evoke a characteristic cortical arousal or activation response similar to that produced by injection of cholinesterase inhibitors or by electrical stimulation of the brainstem reticular formation. All five muscarinic receptor subtypes are expressed in the brain (Volpicelli and Levey, 2004), and recent studies suggest that muscarinic receptor–regulated pathways may have an important role in cognitive function, motor control, appetite regulation, nociception, and other processes (Wess et al., 2007).

Muscarinic Receptor Agonists

Muscarinic cholinergic receptor agonists can be divided into two groups:

- choline esters, including ACh and several synthetic esters
- the naturally occurring cholinomimetic alkaloids (particularly pilocarpine, muscarine, and arecoline) and their synthetic congeners

Of several hundred synthetic choline derivatives investigated, only methacholine, carbachol, and bethanechol (Figure 9–1) have had clinical applications.

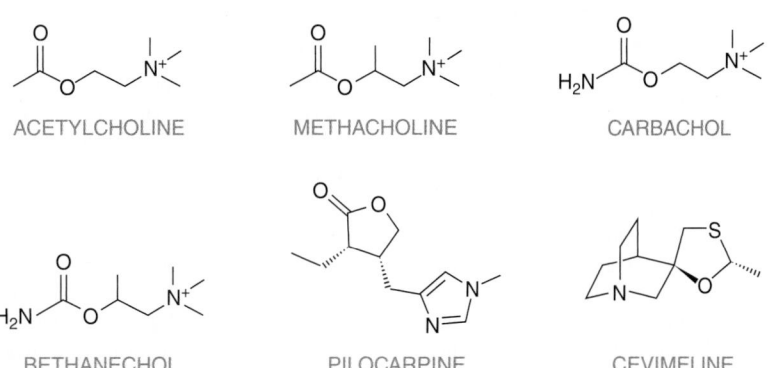

Figure 9–1 *Structural formulas of ACh, choline esters, and natural alkaloids that stimulate muscarinic receptors.*

TABLE 9–1 ■ PHARMACOLOGICAL PROPERTIES OF CHOLINE ESTERS AND NATURAL ALKALOIDS

	HYDROLYSIS BY AChE	NICOTINIC ACTIVITY
Acetylcholine	+++	++
Methacholine	+	+
Carbachol	–	+++
Bethanechol	–	–
Muscarine	–	–
Pilocarpine	–	–

Methacholine (acetyl-β-methylcholine), the β-methyl analogue of ACh, is a synthetic choline ester that differs from ACh chiefly in its greater duration and selectivity of action. Its action is more prolonged because the added methyl group increases its resistance to hydrolysis by cholinesterases. Its selectivity is reflected in a predominance of muscarinic with only minor nicotinic actions, the former manifest most clearly in the cardiovascular system (Table 9–1).

Carbachol, and its β-methyl analogue, bethanechol, are unsubstituted carbamoyl esters that are almost completely resistant to hydrolysis by cholinesterases; their $t_{1/2}$ values are thus sufficiently long that they become distributed to areas of low blood flow. Carbachol retains substantial nicotinic activity, particularly on autonomic ganglia. Bethanechol has mainly muscarinic actions, with prominent effects on motility of the GI tract and urinary bladder.

The major natural alkaloid muscarinic agonists—muscarine, pilocarpine, and arecoline—have the same principal sites of action as the choline esters. Muscarine acts almost exclusively at muscarinic receptor sites, and the classification of these receptors derives from the actions of this alkaloid. Pilocarpine has a dominant muscarinic action but is a partial rather than full agonist; the sweat glands are particularly sensitive to pilocarpine. Arecoline also acts at nicotinic receptors. Although these naturally occurring alkaloids are of great value as pharmacological tools and muscarine has toxicological significance (discussed further in the chapter), present clinical use is restricted largely to the employment of pilocarpine as a sialagogue and miotic agent (Chapter 69).

HISTORY AND SOURCES

The alkaloid muscarine was isolated from the mushroom *Amanita muscaria* by Schmiedeberg in 1869. Pilocarpine is the chief alkaloid obtained from the leaflets of South American shrubs of the genus *Pilocarpus*. Although the natives had long known that the chewing of leaves of *Pilocarpus* plants caused salivation, the active compound, pilocarpine, was isolated only in 1875 and shown to affect the pupil and sweat and salivary glands. Arecoline is the main alkaloid of areca or betel nuts, which are consumed as a euphoretic masticatory mixture by the natives of the Indian subcontinent and East Indies. Hunt and Taveau synthesized and studied methacholine as early as 1911. Carbachol and bethanechol were synthesized and investigated in the 1930s.

ADME

The absorption and distribution of these compounds may be predicted from their structures. Muscarine and the choline esters are quaternary amines; pilocarpine and arecoline are tertiary amines (see examples in Figure 9–1). The choline esters, as quaternary amines, are poorly absorbed following oral administration and have limited ability to cross the blood-brain barrier. Even though these drugs resist hydrolysis, the choline esters are short-acting agents due to rapid renal elimination. Pilocarpine and arecoline, as tertiary amines, are readily absorbed and can cross the

blood-brain barrier. While muscarine is a quaternary amine and is poorly absorbed, it can still be toxic when ingested and can even have CNS effects. The natural alkaloids are primarily eliminated by the kidneys; excretion of the tertiary amines can be accelerated by acidification of the urine to trap the cationic form in the urine.

Therapeutic Uses of Muscarinic Receptor Agonists

Muscarinic agonists are currently used in the treatment of urinary bladder disorders and xerostomia and in the diagnosis of bronchial hyperreactivity. They are also used in ophthalmology as miotic agents and for the treatment of glaucoma. There is growing interest in the use of M_1 agonists in treating the cognitive impairment associated with Alzheimer disease. Other receptor subtypes, including M_2 and M_5, also appear to be involved in the regulation of cognitive function, at least in animal models (Wess et al., 2007).

Acetylcholine

Although rarely given systemically, ACh is used topically for the induction of miosis during ophthalmologic surgery, instilled into the eye as a 1% solution (Chapter 69).

Methacholine

Methacholine is administered by inhalation for the diagnosis of bronchial airway hyperreactivity in patients who do not have clinically apparent asthma (Crapo et al., 2000). It is available as a powder that is diluted with 0.9% NaCl and administered via a nebulizer. While muscarinic agonists can cause bronchoconstriction and increased tracheobronchial secretions in all individuals, asthmatic patients respond with intense bronchoconstriction and a reduction in vital capacity. The response to methacholine may be exaggerated or prolonged in patients taking β adrenergic receptor antagonists. Contraindications to methacholine testing include severe airflow limitation, recent myocardial infarction or stroke, uncontrolled hypertension, or pregnancy. Emergency resuscitation equipment, oxygen, and medications to treat severe bronchospasm (e.g., $β_2$ adrenergic receptor agonists for inhalation) should be available during testing.

Bethanechol

Bethanechol primarily affects the urinary and GI tracts. In the urinary tract, bethanechol has utility in treating urinary retention and inadequate emptying of the bladder when organic obstruction is absent, as in postoperative urinary retention, diabetic autonomic neuropathy, and certain cases of chronic hypotonic, myogenic, or neurogenic bladder; catheterization can thus be avoided. When used chronically, 10–50 mg of the drug is given orally three to four times daily; the drug should be administered on an empty stomach (i.e., 1 h before or 2 h after a meal) to minimize nausea and vomiting.

In the GI tract, bethanechol stimulates peristalsis, increases motility, and increases resting lower esophageal sphincter pressure. Bethanechol formerly was used to treat postoperative abdominal distention, gastric atony, gastroparesis, adynamic ileus, and gastroesophageal reflux; more efficacious therapies for these disorders are now available (Chapters 49 and 50).

Carbachol

Carbachol is used topically in ophthalmology for the treatment of glaucoma and the induction of miosis during surgery; it is instilled into the eye as a 0.01%–3% solution (Chapter 69).

Pilocarpine

Pilocarpine hydrochloride is used for the treatment of xerostomia that follows head and neck radiation treatments or that is associated with Sjögren syndrome (Porter et al., 2004; Wiseman and Faulds, 1995), an autoimmune disorder occurring primarily in women in whom secretions, particularly salivary and lacrimal, are compromised. Treatment can enhance salivary secretion, ease of swallowing, and subjective improvement in hydration of the oral cavity provided salivary parenchyma maintains residual function. Side effects typify cholinergic stimulation, with sweating the most common complaint. The usual dose is 5–10 mg three times daily; the dose should be lowered in patients with hepatic impairment.

Pilocarpine is used topically in ophthalmology for the treatment of glaucoma and as a miotic agent; it is instilled in the eye as a 0.5%–6% solution and also can be delivered via an ocular insert (Chapter 69).

Cevimeline

Cevimeline is a muscarinic agonist that seems to preferentially activate M_1 and M_3 receptors on lacrimal and salivary gland epithelia. The drug has a long-lasting sialogogic action and may have fewer side effects and better patient compliance than pilocarpine (Noaiseh et al., 2014). The usual dose is 30 mg three times daily.

Contraindications, Precautions, and Adverse Effects

Most contraindications, precautions, and adverse effects are predictable consequences of muscarinic receptor stimulation. Thus, important contraindications to the use of muscarinic agonists include asthma, chronic obstructive pulmonary disease, urinary or GI tract obstruction, acid-peptic disease, cardiovascular disease accompanied by bradycardia, hypotension, and hyperthyroidism (muscarinic agonists may precipitate atrial fibrillation in hyperthyroid patients). Common adverse effects include diaphoresis; diarrhea, abdominal cramps, nausea/vomiting, and other GI side effects; a sensation of tightness in the urinary bladder; difficulty in visual accommodation; and hypotension, which can severely reduce coronary blood flow, especially if it is already compromised. These contraindications and adverse effects are generally of limited concern with topical administration for ophthalmic use.

Toxicology

Poisoning from the ingestion of plants containing pilocarpine, muscarine, or arecoline is characterized chiefly by exaggeration of their various parasympathomimetic effects. Treatment consists of the parenteral administration of atropine in doses sufficient to cross the blood-brain barrier and measures to support the respiratory and cardiovascular systems and to counteract pulmonary edema.

Muscarinic Receptor Antagonists

The muscarinic receptor antagonists include

- the naturally occurring alkaloids atropine and scopolamine
- semisynthetic derivatives of these alkaloids, which primarily differ from the parent compounds in their disposition in the body or their duration of action
- synthetic derivatives, some of which show a limited degree of selectivity for certain muscarinic receptor subtypes

Noteworthy agents among the last two categories are homatropine and tropicamide, which have a shorter duration of action than atropine, and methscopolamine, ipratropium, tiotropium, aclidinium, and umeclidinium, which are quaternary amines that do not cross the blood-brain barrier or readily cross membranes. The synthetic derivatives possessing some degree of receptor subtype selectivity include pirenzepine, an M_1 receptor–preferring antagonist, and darifenacin and solifenacin, two M_3 receptor–preferring agents.

Muscarinic antagonists prevent the effects of ACh by blocking its binding to muscarinic receptors on effector cells at parasympathetic (and sympathetic cholinergic) neuroeffector junctions in peripheral ganglia and the CNS. In general, muscarinic antagonists cause little blockade of nicotinic receptors. However, the quaternary ammonium antagonists generally exhibit a greater degree of nicotinic-blocking activity and therefore are more likely to interfere with ganglionic or neuromuscular transmission.

While many effects of muscarinic antagonists can be predicted from an understanding of the physiological responses mediated by muscarinic receptors at parasympathetic and sympathetic cholinergic neuroeffector junctions, paradoxical responses can occur. For example, presynaptic

TABLE 9–2 ■ EFFECTS OF ATROPINE IN RELATION TO DOSE

DOSE (mg)	EFFECTS
0.5	Slight cardiac slowing; some dryness of mouth; inhibition of sweating
1	Definite dryness of mouth; thirst; acceleration of heart, sometimes preceded by slowing; mild dilation of pupils
2	Rapid heart rate; palpitation; marked dryness of mouth; dilated pupils; some blurring of near vision
5	Previous symptoms marked; difficulty in speaking and swallowing; restlessness and fatigue; headache; dry, hot skin; difficulty in micturition; reduced intestinal peristalsis
≥10	Previous symptoms more marked; pulse rapid and weak; iris practically obliterated; vision very blurred; skin flushed, hot, dry, and scarlet; ataxia, restlessness, and excitement; hallucinations and delirium; coma

The clinical picture of a high (toxic) dose of atropine may be remembered by an old mnemonic device that summarizes the symptoms: *Red as a beet, Dry as a bone, Blind as a bat, Hot as firestone, and Mad as a hatter.*

muscarinic receptors of variable subtype are present on postganglionic parasympathetic nerve terminals. Because blockade of presynaptic receptors generally augments neurotransmitter release, the presynaptic effects of muscarinic antagonists may counteract their postsynaptic receptor blockade. Blockade of the modulatory muscarinic receptors in peripheral ganglia represents an additional mechanism for paradoxical responses.

An important consideration in the therapeutic use of muscarinic antagonists is the fact that physiological functions in different organs vary in their sensitivity to muscarinic receptor blockade (Table 9–2). Small doses of atropine depress salivary and bronchial secretion and sweating. With larger doses, the pupil dilates, accommodation of the lens to near vision is inhibited, and vagal effects on the heart are blocked so that the heart rate increases. Larger doses antagonize parasympathetic control of the urinary bladder and GI tract, thereby inhibiting micturition and decreasing intestinal tone and motility. Still larger doses are required to inhibit gastric motility and particularly secretion. Thus, doses of atropine and most related muscarinic antagonists that depress gastric secretion also almost invariably affect salivary secretion, ocular accommodation, micturition, and GI motility. This hierarchy of relative sensitivities is not a consequence of differences in the affinity of atropine for the muscarinic receptors at

HISTORY

The naturally occurring muscarinic receptor antagonists atropine and scopolamine are alkaloids of the belladonna (Solanaceae) plants. Preparations of belladonna were known to the ancient Hindus and have long been used by physicians. During the time of the Roman Empire and in the Middle Ages, the deadly nightshade shrub was frequently used to produce an obscure and often-prolonged poisoning, prompting Linnaeus to name the shrub *Atropa belladonna*, after Atropos, the oldest of the three Fates, who cuts the thread of life. The name *belladonna* derives from the alleged use of this preparation by Italian women to dilate their pupils; modern-day fashion models are known to use this same device for visual appeal. Atropine (D,L-hyoscyamine) also is found in *Datura stramonium* (Jamestown or jimson weed). Scopolamine (L-hyoscine) is found chiefly in *Hyoscyamus niger* (henbane). In India, the root and leaves of jimson weed were burned and the smoke inhaled to treat asthma. British colonists observed this ritual and introduced the belladonna alkaloids into Western medicine in the early 1800s. Atropine was isolated in pure form in 1831.

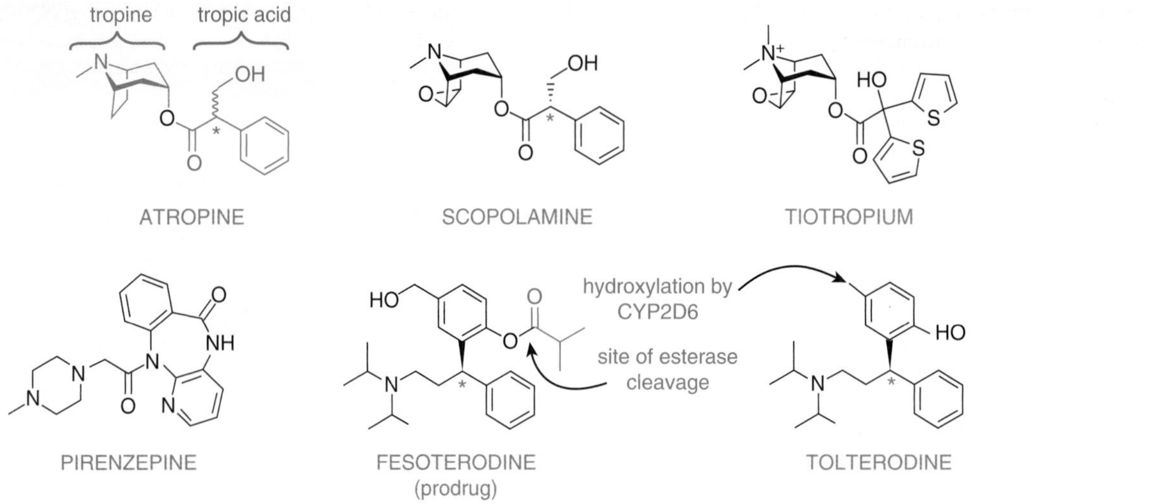

Figure 9–2 *Structural formulas of the belladonna alkaloids and semisynthetic and synthetic analogues.* Fesoterodine is converted to an active 5-hydroxymeythyl metabolite by esterase activity. CYP2D6 converts tolterodine to the same metabolite. Note that atropine, scopolamine, tolterodine, and fesoterodine each contain an asymmetric carbon atom (indicated by red asterisk); these compounds therefore exist as racemic mixtures. Clinically, only the (R)-enantiomers of tolterodine and fesoterodine are used.

these sites because atropine lacks selectivity toward different muscarinic receptor subtypes. More likely determinants include the degree to which the functions of various end organs are regulated by parasympathetic tone, the "spareness" of receptors and signaling mechanisms, the involvement of intramural neurons and reflexes, and the presence of other regulatory mechanisms.

Most clinically available muscarinic antagonists lack receptor subtype selectivity and their actions differ little from those of atropine, the prototype of the group. Notably, the clinical efficacy of some agents may actually depend on antagonistic actions on two or more receptor subtypes.

Structure-Activity Relationships

An intact ester of tropine and tropic acid (Figure 9–2) is essential for antimuscarinic action because neither the free acid nor the basic alcohol exhibits significant antimuscarinic activity. The presence of a free OH group in the acyl portion of the ester also is important for activity. Quaternary ammonium derivatives of atropine and scopolamine are generally more potent than their parent compounds in both muscarinic- and ganglionic- (nicotinic-) blocking activities when given parenterally. These derivatives are poorly and unreliably absorbed when given orally.

Mechanism of Action

Atropine and related compounds compete with ACh and other muscarinic agonists for the orthosteric ACh site on the muscarinic receptor. The antagonism by atropine is competitive; thus, it is surmountable by ACh if the concentration of ACh at muscarinic receptors is increased sufficiently. Muscarinic receptor antagonists inhibit responses to postganglionic cholinergic nerve stimulation less effectively than they inhibit responses to injected choline esters. The difference may be explained by the fact that release of ACh by cholinergic nerve terminals occurs in close proximity to the receptors, resulting in very high concentrations of the transmitter at the receptors.

Pharmacological Effects of Muscarinic Antagonists

The pharmacological effects of atropine, the prototypical muscarinic antagonist, provide a good background for understanding the therapeutic uses of the various muscarinic antagonists. The effects of other muscarinic antagonists will be mentioned only when they differ significantly from those of atropine. The major pharmacological effects of increasing doses of atropine, summarized in Table 9–2, offer a general guide to the problems associated with administration of this class of agents.

Cardiovascular System

Heart. The main effect of atropine on the heart is to alter the rate. Although the dominant response is tachycardia, there is often a transient bradycardia with average clinical doses (0.4–0.6 mg; Table 9–2). The slowing is modest (4–8 beats per min), occurs with no accompanying changes in blood pressure or cardiac output, and is usually absent after rapid intravenous injection. This unexpected effect has been attributed to the block of presynaptic M_1 muscarinic receptors on parasympathetic postganglionic nerve terminals in the SA node, which normally inhibit ACh release (Wellstein and Pitschner, 1988).

Larger doses of atropine cause progressive tachycardia by blocking M_2 receptors on the SA nodal pacemaker cells, thereby antagonizing parasympathetic (vagal) tone to the heart. The resting heart rate is increased by about 35–40 beats per min in young men given 2 mg of atropine intramuscularly. The maximal heart rate (e.g., in response to exercise) is not altered by atropine. The influence of atropine is most noticeable in healthy young adults, in whom vagal tone is considerable. In infants, the elderly, and patients with heart failure, even large doses of atropine may fail to accelerate the heart.

Atropine can abolish many types of reflex vagal cardiac slowing or asystole, such as that occurring from inhalation of irritant vapors, stimulation of the carotid sinus, pressure on the eyeballs, peritoneal stimulation, or injection of contrast dye during cardiac catheterization. Atropine also prevents or abruptly abolishes bradycardia or asystole caused by choline esters, acetylcholinesterase inhibitors, or other parasympathomimetic drugs, as well as cardiac arrest from electrical stimulation of the vagus.

The removal of vagal tone to the heart by atropine may facilitate AV conduction. Atropine shortens the functional refractory period of the AV node and can increase the ventricular rate in patients who have atrial fibrillation or flutter. In certain cases of second-degree AV block (e.g., Wenckebach AV block) in which vagal activity is an etiological factor (as with digoxin toxicity), atropine may lessen the degree of block. In some patients with complete AV block, the idioventricular rate may be accelerated by atropine; in others, it is stabilized. Atropine may improve the clinical condition of patients with inferior or posterior wall myocardial infarction by relieving severe sinus or nodal bradycardia or AV block.

Circulation. Atropine alone has little effect on blood pressure because most vessels lack significant cholinergic innervation. However, in clinical doses, atropine completely counteracts the peripheral vasodilation and sharp fall in blood pressure caused by choline esters. In toxic and occasionally in therapeutic doses, atropine can dilate cutaneous blood vessels, especially those in the blush area (atropine flush). This may be a compensatory reaction permitting the radiation of heat to offset the atropine-induced rise in temperature that can accompany inhibition of sweating.

Respiratory System

Although atropine can cause some bronchodilation and decrease in tracheobronchial secretion in normal individuals by blocking parasympathetic (vagal) tone to the lungs, its effects on the respiratory system are most significant in patients with respiratory disease. Atropine can inhibit the bronchoconstriction caused by histamine, bradykinin, and the eicosanoids, which presumably reflects the participation of reflex parasympathetic (vagal) activity in the bronchoconstriction elicited by these agents. The ability to block the indirect bronchoconstrictive effects of these mediators forms the basis for the use of muscarinic receptor antagonists, along with β adrenergic receptor agonists, in the treatment of asthma. Muscarinic antagonists also have an important role in the treatment of chronic obstructive pulmonary disease (Chapter 40).

Atropine inhibits the secretions of the nose, mouth, pharynx, and bronchi and thus dries the mucous membranes of the respiratory tract. This action is especially marked if secretion is excessive and formed the basis for the use of atropine and other muscarinic antagonists to prevent irritating inhalational anesthetics such as diethyl ether from increasing bronchial secretion; newer inhalational anesthetics are less irritating. Muscarinic antagonists are used to decrease the rhinorrhea ("runny nose") associated with the common cold or with allergic and nonallergic rhinitis. Reduction of mucous secretion and mucociliary clearance can, however, result in mucus plugs, a potentially undesirable side effect of muscarinic antagonists in patients with airway disease.

The quaternary ammonium compounds ipratropium, tiotropium, aclidinium, and umeclidinium are used exclusively for their effects on the respiratory tract. Dry mouth is the only frequently reported side effect, as the absorption of these drugs from the lungs or the GI tract is inefficient. In addition, aclidinium has been shown to undergo rapid hydrolysis in plasma to inactive metabolites, thus reducing systemic exposure to the drug (Gavalda et al., 2009). The degree of bronchodilation achieved by these agents is thought to reflect the level of basal parasympathetic tone, supplemented by reflex activation of cholinergic pathways brought about by various stimuli. A therapeutically important property of ipratropium and tiotropium is their minimal inhibitory effect on mucociliary clearance relative to atropine. Hence, the choice of these agents for use in patients with airway disease minimizes the increased accumulation of lower airway secretions encountered with atropine.

Eye

Muscarinic receptor antagonists block the cholinergic responses of the pupillary sphincter muscle of the iris and the ciliary muscle controlling lens curvature (Chapter 69). Thus, these agents dilate the pupil (mydriasis) and paralyze accommodation (cycloplegia). The wide pupillary dilation results in photophobia; the lens is fixed for far vision, near objects are blurred, and objects may appear smaller than they are. The normal pupillary reflex constriction to light or on convergence of the eyes is abolished. These effects are most evident when the agent is instilled into the eye but can also occur after systemic administration of the alkaloids.

Conventional systemic doses of atropine (0.6 mg) have little ocular effect, in contrast to equal doses of scopolamine, which cause evident mydriasis and loss of accommodation. Locally applied atropine produces ocular effects of considerable duration; accommodation and pupillary reflexes may not fully recover for 7–12 days. Other muscarinic receptor antagonists with shorter durations of action are therefore preferred as mydriatics in ophthalmologic practice. Pilocarpine and choline esters (e.g., carbachol) in sufficient concentrations can reverse the ocular effects of atropine.

Muscarinic receptor antagonists administered systemically have little effect on intraocular pressure except in patients predisposed to angle-closure glaucoma, in whom the pressure may occasionally rise dangerously. The rise in pressure occurs when the anterior chamber is narrow and the iris obstructs outflow of aqueous humor into the trabeculae. Muscarinic antagonists may precipitate a first attack in unrecognized cases of this relatively rare condition. In patients with open-angle glaucoma, an acute rise in pressure is unusual. Atropine-like drugs generally can be used safely in the latter condition, particularly if the glaucoma is being treated appropriately.

GI Tract

Knowledge of the actions of muscarinic receptor agonists on the stomach and intestine led to the use of muscarinic receptor antagonists as antispasmodic agents for GI disorders and to reduce gastric acid secretion in the treatment of peptic ulcer disease.

Motility. Parasympathetic nerves enhance GI tone and motility and relax sphincters, thereby favoring the passage of gastrointestinal contents. In normal subjects and in patients with GI disease, muscarinic antagonists produce prolonged inhibitory effects on the motor activity of the stomach, duodenum, jejunum, ileum, and colon, characterized by a reduction in tone and in amplitude and frequency of peristaltic contractions. Relatively large doses are needed to produce such inhibition, probably because the enteric nervous system can regulate motility independently of parasympathetic control; parasympathetic nerves serve only to modulate the effects of the enteric nervous system. Although atropine can completely abolish the effects of exogenous muscarinic agonists on GI motility and secretion, it does not completely inhibit the GI responses to vagal stimulation. This difference, particularly striking in the effects of atropine on gut motility, can be attributed to the fact that preganglionic vagal fibers innervating the GI tract synapse not only with postganglionic cholinergic fibers, but also with a network of noncholinergic intramural neurons that form the plexuses of the enteric nervous system and utilize neurotransmitters whose effects atropine does not block (e.g., 5HT, dopamine, and various peptides).

Gastric Acid Secretion. Similarly, atropine only partially inhibits the gastric acid secretory responses to vagal activity because vagal stimulation of gastrin secretion is mediated not by ACh but by peptidergic neurons in the vagal trunk that release gastrin-releasing peptide (GRP). GRP stimulates gastrin release from G cells; gastrin can act directly to promote acid secretion by parietal cells and to stimulate histamine release from enterochromaffin-like (ECL) cells (see Figure 49–1). Parietal cells (acid secretors) respond to at least three agonists: gastrin, histamine, and ACh. Atropine will inhibit only the components of acid secretion that result from muscarinic stimulation of parietal cells and from muscarinic stimulation of ECL cells that secrete histamine.

Secretions. Salivary secretion is particularly sensitive to inhibition by muscarinic receptor antagonists, which can completely abolish the copious, watery secretion induced by parasympathetic stimulation. The mouth becomes dry, and swallowing and talking may become difficult. The gastric cells that secrete mucin and proteolytic enzymes are more directly under vagal influence than are the acid-secreting cells, and atropine selectively decreases their secretory function. Although atropine can reduce gastric secretion, the doses required also affect salivary secretion, ocular accommodation, micturition, and GI motility (Table 9–2).

In contrast to most muscarinic receptor antagonists, pirenzepine, which shows some degree of selectivity for M_1 receptors, inhibits gastric acid secretion at doses that have little effect on salivation or heart rate. Because parietal cells primarily express M_3 receptors, perhaps M_1 receptors in intramural ganglia are the primary target of pirenzepine (Eglen et al., 1996). However, this concept has been questioned by the observation that pirenzepine is still able to inhibit carbachol-stimulated gastric acid secretion in M_1 receptor–deficient mice (Aihara et al., 2005). In general, histamine H_2 receptor antagonists and proton pump inhibitors have replaced muscarinic antagonists as inhibitors of acid secretion (Chapter 49).

Other Smooth Muscle

Urinary Tract. Muscarinic antagonists decrease the normal tone and amplitude of contractions of the ureter and bladder and often eliminate drug-induced enhancement of ureteral tone. However, this effect is usually accompanied by reduced salivation and lacrimation and blurred vision (Table 9–2).

Biliary Tract. Atropine exerts mild antispasmodic action on the gallbladder and bile ducts in humans. However, this effect usually is not sufficient to overcome or prevent the marked spasm and increase in biliary duct pressure induced by opioids. The nitrates are more effective than atropine in this respect.

Sweat Glands and Temperature

Small doses of atropine inhibit the activity of sweat glands innervated by sympathetic cholinergic fibers, and the skin becomes hot and dry. Sweating may be depressed enough to raise the body temperature, but only notably so after large doses or at high environmental temperatures.

CNS

Atropine has minimal effects on the CNS at therapeutic doses, although mild stimulation of the parasympathetic medullary centers may occur. With toxic doses of atropine, central excitation becomes more prominent, leading to restlessness, irritability, disorientation, hallucinations, or delirium (see the discussion of atropine poisoning further in the chapter). With still larger doses, stimulation is followed by depression, leading to circulatory collapse and respiratory failure after a period of paralysis and coma.

In contrast to atropine, scopolamine has prominent central effects at low therapeutic doses; atropine therefore is preferred over scopolamine for most purposes. The basis for this difference is probably the greater permeation of scopolamine across the blood-brain barrier. Scopolamine in therapeutic doses normally causes CNS depression, manifest as drowsiness, amnesia, fatigue, and dreamless sleep, with a reduction in REM sleep. It also causes euphoria and can therefore be subject to abuse. The depressant and amnesic effects formerly were sought when scopolamine was used as an adjunct to anesthetic agents or for preanesthetic medication. However, in the presence of severe pain, the same doses of scopolamine can occasionally cause excitement, restlessness, hallucinations, or delirium. These excitatory effects resemble those of toxic doses of atropine. Scopolamine also is effective in preventing motion sickness, probably by blocking neural pathways from the vestibular apparatus in the inner ear to the emetic center in the brainstem.

ADME

The belladonna alkaloids and the *tertiary* synthetic and semisynthetic derivatives are absorbed rapidly from the GI tract. They also enter the circulation when applied locally to the mucosal surfaces of the body. Absorption from intact skin is limited, although efficient absorption does occur in the postauricular region for some agents (e.g., scopolamine, allowing delivery by transdermal patch). Systemic absorption of inhaled or orally ingested *quaternary* muscarinic receptor antagonists is limited. The quaternary ammonium derivatives of the belladonna alkaloids also penetrate the conjunctiva of the eye less readily, and central effects are lacking because the quaternary agents do not cross the blood-brain barrier. Atropine has a $t_{1/2}$ of about 4 h; hepatic metabolism accounts for the elimination of about half of a dose, and the remainder is excreted unchanged in the urine.

Ipratropium is administered as an aerosol or solution for inhalation, whereas tiotropium is administered as a dry powder. As with most drugs administered by inhalation, about 90% of the dose is swallowed. When inhaled, their action is confined almost completely to the mouth and airways. Most of the swallowed drug appears in the feces. After inhalation, maximal responses usually develop over 30–90 min, with tiotropium having the slower onset. The effects of ipratropium last for 4–6 h; tiotropium's effects persist for 24 h, and the drug is amenable to once-daily dosing.

Therapeutic Uses of Muscarinic Receptor Antagonists

Muscarinic receptor antagonists have been used predominantly to inhibit effects of parasympathetic activity in the respiratory tract, urinary tract, GI tract, eye, and heart. Their CNS effects have resulted in their use in the treatment of Parkinson disease, the management of extrapyramidal side effects of antipsychotic drugs, and the prevention of motion sickness. The major limitation in the use of the nonselective drugs is often failure to obtain desired therapeutic responses without concomitant side effects. While these usually are not serious, they can be sufficiently disturbing to decrease patient compliance, particularly during long-term administration. To date, selectivity is mainly achieved by local administration (e.g., by pulmonary inhalation or instillation in the eye). The development of allosteric modulators that recognize sites unique to particular receptor subtypes is currently considered an important approach to obtain receptor subtype-selective drugs for the treatment of specific clinical conditions (Conn et al., 2009).

Respiratory Tract

Ipratropium, tiotropium, aclidinium, and umeclidinium are important agents in the treatment of chronic obstructive pulmonary disease; they are less effective in most patients with asthma (see Chapter 40). These agents often are used with inhaled long-acting β_2 adrenergic receptor agonists, although there is little evidence of true synergism.

Ipratropium appears to block all subtypes of muscarinic receptors and accordingly also antagonizes the inhibition of ACh release by presynaptic M_2 receptors on parasympathetic postganglionic nerve terminals in the lung; the resulting increase in ACh release may counteract the drug's blockade of M_3 receptor-mediated bronchoconstriction. In contrast, tiotropium shows some selectivity for M_1 and M_3 receptors. In addition, tiotropium and aclidinium have lower affinities for M_2 receptors and dissociate more slowly from M_3 than from M_2 receptors. This minimizes its presynaptic effect to enhance ACh release (Alagha et al., 2014).

Ipratropium is administered four times daily via a metered-dose inhaler or nebulizer; aclidinium is used twice daily via a dry powder inhaler. Tiotropium and umeclidinium are once-daily medications that can be used for maintenance therapy via a dry powder inhaler in patients with moderate-to-severe disease.

In normal individuals, inhalation of antimuscarinic drugs can provide virtually complete protection against the bronchoconstriction produced by the subsequent inhalation of such irritants as sulfur dioxide, ozone, or cigarette smoke. However, patients with atopic asthma or demonstrable bronchial hyperresponsiveness are less well protected. Although these drugs cause a marked reduction in sensitivity to methacholine in asthmatic subjects, more modest inhibition of responses to challenge with histamine, bradykinin, or PGF_{2a} is achieved, and little protection is afforded against the bronchoconstriction induced by 5HT or leukotrienes. The therapeutic uses of ipratropium and tiotropium are discussed further in Chapter 40.

Ipratropium also is approved by the FDA for use in nasal inhalers for the treatment of the rhinorrhea associated with the common cold or with allergic or nonallergic perennial rhinitis. Although the ability of muscarinic antagonists to reduce nasopharyngeal secretions may provide some symptomatic relief, such therapy does not affect the natural course of the condition. It is probable that the contribution of first-generation antihistamines employed in nonprescription cold medications is due primarily to their antimuscarinic properties, except in conditions with an allergic basis (see Chapters 34 and 39).

Genitourinary Tract

Overactive urinary bladder can be successfully treated with muscarinic receptor antagonists. These agents can lower intravesicular pressure, increase capacity, and reduce the frequency of contractions by antagonizing parasympathetic control of the bladder; they also may alter bladder sensation during filling (Chapple et al., 2005). Muscarinic antagonists can be used to treat enuresis in children, particularly when a progressive increase in bladder capacity is the objective, and to reduce urinary frequency and increase bladder capacity in spastic paraplegia.

The muscarinic receptor antagonists indicated for overactive bladder are oxybutynin, tolterodine, trospium chloride, darifenacin, solifenacin, and fesoterodine. Although some comparison trials have demonstrated small but statistically significant differences in efficacy between these agents (Chapple et al., 2008), the clinical relevance of these differences remains uncertain. The most important adverse reactions are consequences of muscarinic receptor blockade and include xerostomia, blurred vision, and GI side effects such as constipation and dyspepsia. CNS-related antimuscarinic effects, including drowsiness, dizziness, and confusion, can occur and are particularly problematic in elderly patients. CNS effects appear to be less likely with trospium, a quaternary amine, and with darifenacin and solifenacin; the last two agents show some preference for M_3 receptors and therefore seem to have minimal effects on M_1 receptors in the CNS, which appear to play an important role in memory and cognition (Kay et al., 2006). Adverse effects can limit the tolerability of these drugs with continued use, and patient acceptance declines. Xerostomia is the most common reason for discontinuation.

Oxybutynin, the oldest of the antimuscarinics currently used to treat overactive bladder disorders, is associated with a high incidence of antimuscarinic side effects, particularly xerostomia. In an attempt to increase patient acceptance, oxybutynin is marketed as a transdermal system that is associated with a lower incidence of side effects than the oral immediate- and extended-release formulations; a topical gel formulation of oxybutynin also appears to offer a more favorable side-effect profile. Because of the extensive metabolism of oral oxybutynin by enteric and hepatic CYP3A4, higher doses are used in oral than transdermal administration; the dose may need to be reduced in patients taking drugs that inhibit CYP3A4.

Tolterodine shows selectivity for the urinary bladder in animal models and in clinical studies, resulting in greater patient acceptance; however, the drug binds to all muscarinic receptors with similar affinity. Tolterodine is metabolized by CYP2D6 to 5-hydroxymethyltolterodine, a metabolite that possesses similar activity as the parent drug but differs pharmacokinetically. CYP2D6 is a polymorphic enzyme, with significant variability of expression; thus, the production of the 5-hydroxymethyl metabolite can vary, as can the half-life of the parent drug. In patients who poorly metabolize tolterodine via CYP2D6, the CYP3A4 pathway becomes important in tolterodine elimination. Because it is often difficult to assess which patients will be poor metabolizers, tolterodine doses may need to be reduced in patients taking drugs that inhibit CYP3A4 (dosage adjustments generally are not necessary in patients taking drugs that inhibit CYP2D6). Patients with significant renal or hepatic impairment also should receive lower doses of the drug. Fesoterodine is a prodrug that is rapidly hydrolyzed to the active metabolite of tolterodine by esterases (Figure 9-2) rather than CYP2D6, thereby providing a less variable source of the 5-hydroxymethyl metabolite of tolterodine regardless of CYP2D6 status.

Trospium, a quaternary amine, is as effective as oxybutynin and with better tolerability. It is the only antimuscarinic agent used for overactive bladder that is eliminated primarily by the kidneys; 60% of the absorbed trospium dose is excreted unchanged in the urine, and dosage adjustment is necessary for patients with impaired renal function.

Solifenacin shows some preference for M_3 receptors, giving it a favorable ratio of efficacy to side effect (Chapple et al., 2004). Solifenacin is significantly metabolized by CYP3A4; thus, patients taking drugs that inhibit CYP3A4 should receive lower doses.

Like solifenacin, darifenacin shows some degree of selectivity for M_3 receptors (Caulfield and Birdsall, 1998). It is metabolized by CYP2D6 and CYP3A4; as with tolterodine, the latter pathway becomes more important in patients who poorly metabolize the drug by CYP2D6. Darifenacin doses may need to be reduced in patients taking drugs that inhibit either of these CYPs.

GI Tract

Muscarinic receptor antagonists were once widely used for the management of peptic ulcer. Although they can reduce gastric motility and the secretion of gastric acid, antisecretory doses produce pronounced side effects, such as xerostomia, loss of visual accommodation, photophobia, and difficulty in urination (Table 9–2). As a consequence, patient compliance in the long-term management of symptoms of acid-peptic disease with these drugs is poor. H_2 receptor antagonists and proton pump inhibitors generally are considered to be the current drugs of choice to reduce gastric acid secretion (Chapter 49).

Pirenzepine, a tricyclic drug similar in structure to imipramine, displays a limited degree of selectivity for M_1 receptors (Caulfield and Birdsall, 1998). Telenzepine, an analogue of pirenzepine, has higher potency and similar selectivity for M_1 receptors. Both drugs are used in the treatment of acid-peptic disease in Europe, Japan, and Canada, but not currently in the U.S. At therapeutic doses of pirenzepine, the incidence of xerostomia, blurred vision, and central muscarinic disturbances is relatively low. Central effects are not seen because of the drug's limited penetration into the CNS.

Most studies indicate that pirenzepine (100–150 mg per day) produces about the same rate of healing of duodenal and gastric ulcers as the H_2 receptor antagonists cimetidine or ranitidine; pirenzepine also may be effective in preventing the recurrence of ulcers (Tryba and Cook, 1997). Side effects necessitate drug withdrawal in less than 1% of patients.

Myriad conditions known or supposed to involve increased tone (spasticity) or motility of the GI tract are treated with belladonna alkaloids (e.g., atropine, hyoscyamine sulfate, and scopolamine) alone or in combination with sedatives (e.g., phenobarbital) or antianxiety agents (e.g., chlordiazepoxide). The belladonna alkaloids and their synthetic substitutes can reduce tone and motility when administered in maximally tolerated doses. M_3-selective antagonists might achieve more selectivity but are unlikely to be better tolerated, as M_3 receptors also have an important role in the control of salivation, bronchial secretion and contraction, and bladder motility. Glycopyrrolate, a muscarinic antagonist that is structurally unrelated to the belladonna alkaloids, is used to reduce GI tone and motility; as a quaternary amine, it is less likely to cause adverse CNS effects than atropine, scopolamine, and other tertiary amines. Alternative agents for treatment of increased GI motility and its associated symptoms are discussed in Chapter 50.

Diarrhea associated with irritation of the lower bowel, such as mild dysenteries and diverticulitis, may respond to atropine-like drugs, an effect that likely involves actions on ion transport as well as motility. However, more severe conditions such as *Salmonella* dysentery, ulcerative colitis, and Crohn disease respond little, if at all, to muscarinic antagonists.

Dicyclomine hydrochloride is a weak muscarinic receptor antagonist that also has nonspecific direct spasmolytic effects on smooth muscle of the GI tract. It is occasionally used in the treatment of diarrhea-predominant irritable bowel syndrome.

Salivary Secretions

The belladonna alkaloids and synthetic substitutes are effective in reducing excessive salivation, such as drug-induced salivation and that associated with heavy-metal poisoning and Parkinson disease. Glycopyrrolate is a quaternary amine and as mentioned is less likely to penetrate the CNS. Glycopyrrolate (as oral solution) is indicated to reduce drooling (e.g., in patients with Parkinson disease).

Eye

Effects limited to the eye are obtained by topical administration of muscarinic receptor antagonists to produce mydriasis and cycloplegia. Cycloplegia is not attainable without mydriasis and requires higher concentrations or more prolonged application of a given agent. Mydriasis often is necessary for thorough examination of the retina and optic disc and in the therapy of iridocyclitis and keratitis. Homatropine hydrobromide, a semisynthetic derivative of atropine (Figure 9–2), cyclopentolate hydrochloride, and tropicamide are agents used in ophthalmological practice. These agents are preferred to topical atropine or scopolamine because of their shorter duration of action. Additional information on the ophthalmological properties and preparations of these and other drugs is provided in Chapter 69.

Cardiovascular System

The cardiovascular effects of muscarinic receptor antagonists are of limited clinical utility. Generally, these agents are used only in coronary care units for short-term interventions or in surgical settings. They are also sometimes used as an adjunct to stress testing to increase heart rate in the setting of chronotropic incompetence.

Atropine may be considered in the initial treatment of patients with acute myocardial infarction in whom excessive vagal tone causes sinus bradycardia or AV nodal block. Sinus bradycardia is the most common arrhythmia seen during acute myocardial infarction of the inferior or posterior wall. Atropine may prevent further clinical deterioration in cases of high vagal tone or AV block by restoring heart rate to a level sufficient to maintain adequate hemodynamic status and to eliminate AV nodal block. Dosing must be judicious; doses that are too low can cause a paradoxical bradycardia (described previously), while excessive doses will cause tachycardia that may extend the infarct by increasing the demand for O_2.

Atropine occasionally is useful in reducing the severe bradycardia and syncope associated with a hyperactive carotid sinus reflex. It has little effect on most ventricular rhythms. In some patients, atropine may eliminate premature ventricular contractions associated with a very slow atrial rate. It also may reduce the degree of AV block when increased vagal tone is a major factor in the conduction defect, such as the second-degree AV block that can be produced by digoxin. Selective M_2 receptor antagonists would be of potential utility in blocking ACh-mediated bradycardia or AV block; however, no such agents are currently available for clinical use.

Autonomic control of the heart is known to be abnormal in patients with cardiovascular disease, especially in heart failure. Patients with heart failure typically exhibit increased sympathetic tone accompanied by vagal withdrawal, both of which may contribute to the progression of disease. While β-blockers have now emerged as standard of care in heart failure, less is known about whether augmentation of vagal tone may be beneficial. Studies in animals suggest that augmenting vagal tone chronically decreases the inflammatory response and prevents adverse cardiac remodeling in heart failure, and early studies in humans support their use. However, the pivotal clinical trials of such therapy remain ongoing as of this writing (Dunlap et al., 2015; Schwartz and De Ferrari, 2011).

CNS

The belladonna alkaloids were among the first drugs to be used in the prevention of motion sickness. Scopolamine is the most effective of these agents for short (4- to 6-h) exposures to severe motion and probably for exposures of up to several days. All agents used to combat motion sickness should be given prophylactically; they are much less effective after severe nausea or vomiting has developed. A transdermal preparation of scopolamine has been shown to be highly effective when used prophylactically for the prevention of motion sickness. The drug, incorporated into a multilayer adhesive unit, is applied to the postauricular mastoid region, an area where transdermal absorption of the drug is especially efficient, resulting in the delivery of about 0.5 mg of scopolamine over 72 h. Xerostomia is common, drowsiness is not infrequent, and blurred vision occurs in some individuals using the scopolamine patch. Mydriasis and cycloplegia can occur by inadvertent transfer of the drug to the eye from the fingers after handling the patch. Rare but severe psychotic episodes have been reported.

Muscarinic receptor antagonists have long been used in the treatment of Parkinson disease, which is characterized by reduced dopaminergic input into the striatum, resulting in an imbalance between striatal muscarinic cholinergic and dopaminergic neurotransmission (see Chapter 18). The striatum, the major input area of the basal ganglia, contains multiple cell types, including cholinergic interneurons, all of which express one or more muscarinic receptor subtypes (Goldberg et al., 2012). Studies with muscarinic receptor mutant mice suggested that the beneficial effects of muscarinic antagonists in the treatment of Parkinson disease are primarily due to the blockade of M_1 and M_4 receptors, resulting in the activation or inhibition, respectively, of specific striatal neuronal subpopulations (Wess et al., 2007).

Muscarinic antagonists can be effective in the early stages of Parkinson disease if tremor is predominant, particularly in young patients. Muscarinic receptor antagonists also are used to treat the extrapyramidal symptoms that commonly occur as side effects of conventional antipsychotic drug therapy (Chapter 16). Certain antipsychotic drugs are relatively potent muscarinic receptor antagonists (Roth et al., 2004) and, perhaps for this reason, cause fewer extrapyramidal side effects.

The muscarinic antagonists used for Parkinson disease and drug-induced extrapyramidal symptoms include benztropine mesylate,

trihexyphenidyl hydrochloride, and biperiden; all are tertiary amines that readily gain access to the CNS.

Anesthesia

Atropine is commonly given to block responses to vagal reflexes induced by surgical manipulation of visceral organs. Atropine or glycopyrrolate are also used to block the parasympathomimetic effects of neostigmine when it is administered to reverse skeletal muscle relaxation after surgery. Serious cardiac arrhythmias have occasionally occurred, perhaps because of the initial bradycardia produced by atropine combined with the cholinomimetic effects of neostigmine.

Anticholinesterase Poisoning

The use of atropine in large doses for the treatment of poisoning by anticholinesterase organophosphorus insecticides is discussed in Chapter 10. Atropine also may be used to antagonize the parasympathomimetic effects of pyridostigmine or other anticholinesterases administered in the treatment of myasthenia gravis. It does not interfere with the salutary effects at the skeletal neuromuscular junction. It is most useful early in therapy, before tolerance to muscarinic side effects of anticholinesterases has developed.

Other Therapeutic Uses

Methscopolamine bromide is a quaternary ammonium derivative of scopolamine and therefore lacks the central actions of scopolamine. Although formerly used to treat peptic ulcer disease, at present it is primarily used in certain combination products for the temporary relief of symptoms of allergic rhinitis, sinusitis, and the common cold.

Homatropine methylbromide, the methyl derivative of homatropine, is less potent than atropine in antimuscarinic activity but four times more potent as a ganglionic blocking agent. Formerly used for the treatment of irritable bowel syndrome and peptic ulcer disease, at present it is primarily used with hydrocodone as an antitussive combination.

Contraindications and Adverse Effects

Most contraindications, precautions, and adverse effects are predictable consequences of muscarinic receptor blockade: xerostomia, constipation, blurred vision, dyspepsia, and cognitive impairment. Important contraindications to the use of muscarinic antagonists include urinary tract obstruction, GI obstruction, and uncontrolled (or susceptibility to attacks of) angle-closure glaucoma. Muscarinic receptor antagonists also are contraindicated (or should be used with extreme caution) in patients with benign prostatic hyperplasia. These adverse effects and contraindications generally are of more limited concern with muscarinic antagonists that are administered by inhalation or used topically in ophthalmology.

Toxicology of Drugs With Antimuscarinic Properties

The deliberate or accidental ingestion of natural belladonna alkaloids is a major cause of poisonings. Many histamine H_1 receptor antagonists, phenothiazines, and tricyclic antidepressants also block muscarinic receptors and, in sufficient dosage, produce syndromes that include features of atropine intoxication. Among the tricyclic antidepressants, protriptyline and amitriptyline are the most potent muscarinic receptor antagonists, with affinities for muscarinic receptors only an order of magnitude less than that of atropine. Because these drugs are administered in therapeutic doses considerably higher than the effective dose of atropine, antimuscarinic effects are often observed clinically (Chapter 15). In addition, overdose with suicidal intent is a danger in the population using antidepressants. Fortunately, most of the newer antidepressants and selective serotonin reuptake inhibitors have more limited anticholinergic properties.

Like the tricyclic antidepressants, many of the older antipsychotic drugs have antimuscarinic effects. These effects are most likely to be observed with the less-potent drugs (e.g., chlorpromazine and thioridazine), which must be given in higher doses. The newer antipsychotic drugs, classified as "atypical" and characterized by their low propensity for inducing extrapyramidal side effects, also include agents that are potent muscarinic receptor antagonists. In particular, clozapine binds to human brain muscarinic receptors with high affinity (10 nM, compared to 1–2 nM for atropine); olanzapine also is a potent muscarinic receptor antagonist (Roth et al., 2004). Accordingly, xerostomia is a prominent side effect of these drugs. A paradoxical side effect of clozapine is increased salivation and drooling, possibly the result of partial agonist properties of this drug.

Infants and young children are especially susceptible to the toxic effects of muscarinic antagonists. Indeed, cases of intoxication in children have resulted from conjunctival instillation for ophthalmic refraction and other ocular effects. Systemic absorption occurs either from the nasal mucosa after the drug has traversed the nasolacrimal duct or from the GI tract if the drug is swallowed. Poisoning with diphenoxylate-atropine, used to treat diarrhea, has been extensively reported in the pediatric literature. Transdermal preparations of scopolamine used for motion sickness have been noted to cause toxic psychoses, especially in children and in the elderly. Serious intoxication may occur in children who ingest berries or seeds containing belladonna alkaloids. Poisoning from ingestion and smoking of jimson weed is seen with some frequency today.

Table 9–2 shows the oral doses of atropine causing undesirable responses or symptoms of overdosage. These symptoms are predictable results of blockade of parasympathetic innervation. In cases of full-blown atropine poisoning, the syndrome may last 48 h or longer. Intravenous injection of the anticholinesterase agent physostigmine may be used for

confirmation. If physostigmine does not elicit the expected salivation, sweating, bradycardia, and intestinal hyperactivity, intoxication with atropine or a related agent is almost certain. Depression and circulatory collapse are evident only in cases of severe intoxication; the blood pressure declines, convulsions may ensue, respiration becomes inadequate, and death due to respiratory failure may follow after a period of paralysis and coma.

If the poison has been taken orally, begin measures to limit intestinal absorption without delay. For symptomatic treatment, slow intravenous injection of physostigmine rapidly abolishes the delirium and coma caused by large doses of atropine, but carries some risk of overdose in mild atropine intoxication. Because physostigmine is metabolized rapidly, the patient may again lapse into coma within 1–2 h, and repeated doses may be needed (Chapter 10). If marked excitement is present and more specific treatment is not available, a benzodiazepine is the most suitable agent for sedation and for control of convulsions. Phenothiazines or agents with antimuscarinic activity should not be used because their antimuscarinic action is likely to intensify toxicity. Support of respiration and control of hyperthermia may be necessary. Ice bags and alcohol sponges help to reduce fever, especially in children.

Acknowledgment: Nora Laiken and Palmer W. Taylor contributed to this chapter in recent editions of this book. We have retained some of their text in the current edition.

Drug Facts for Your Personal Formulary: *Muscarinic Receptor Agonists and Antagonists*

Drugs	Therapeutic Uses	Clinical Pharmacology and Tips
Muscarinic Receptor Agonists		
Methacholine	• Diagnosis of bronchial airway hyperreactivity	• Muscarinic effects: GI cramps, diarrhea, nausea, vomiting; lacrimation, salivation, sweating; urinary urgency; vision problems; bronchospasm • Do not use in patients with GI obstruction, urinary retention, asthma/COPD
Carbachol	• Glaucoma (topical administration)	• Systemic muscarinic effects minimal with proper topical application, otherwise similar to methacholine
Bethanechol	• Ileus (postoperative, neurogenic) • Urinary retention	• Similar to methacholine • Take on empty stomach to minimize nausea/vomiting

Pilocarpine	• Glaucoma (topical administration)
	• Xerostomia due to
	  • Sjögren syndrome
	  • Head and neck irradiation
		• Systemic muscarinic effects minimal with proper topical application, otherwise similar to methacholine

Cevimeline	• Xerostomia due to • Sjögren syndrome	• Similar to methacholine
Muscarinic Receptor Antagonists		
Atropine	• Acute symptomatic bradycardia (e.g., AV block) • Cholinesterase inhibitor intoxication • Aspiration prophylaxis	• Antimuscarinic adverse effects: xerostomia, constipation, blurred vision, dyspepsia, and cognitive impairment • Contraindicated in patients with urinary tract obstruction (especially in benign prostatic hyperplasia), GI obstruction, and angle-closure glaucoma
Scopolamine	• Motion sickness	• CNS effects (drowsiness, amnesia, fatigue)
Homatropine, cyclopentolate, tropicamide	• Ophthalmological examination (cycloplegia and mydriasis induction)	• Antimuscarinic adverse effects are minimal with proper topical application
Ipratropium, tiotropium, aclidinium, umeclidinium	• COPD • Rhinorrhea (ipratropium)	• Minimal absorption as quaternary amine ⇒ fewer antimuscarinic adverse effects, otherwise similar to atropine
Pirenzepine, telenzepine	• Peptic ulcer disease (not in U.S.)	• Antimuscarinic adverse effects and contraindications similar to atropine
Oxybutynin, trospium, darifenacin, solifenacin, tolterodine, fesoterodine	• Overactive bladder, enuresis, neurogenic bladder	• Antimuscarinic adverse effects and contraindications similar to atropine • CNS-related antimuscarinic effects less likely with trospium (quaternary amine), darifenacin and solifenacin (some selectivity for M_3 receptors), fesoterodine (prodrug of tolterodine), and tolterodine (preference for muscarinic receptors in the bladder)

Drug Facts for Your Personal Formulary: *Muscarinic Receptor Agonists and Antagonists* (*continued*)

Drugs	Therapeutic Uses	Clinical Pharmacology and Tips
Muscarinic Receptor Antagonists		
Glycopyrrolate	• Duodenal ulcer • Sialorrhea	• Antimuscarinic adverse effects and contraindications similar to atropine • Fewer CNS effects as glycopyrrolate is a quaternary amine and therefore unable to cross the blood-brain barrier
Dicyclomine, hyoscyamine	Diarrhea-predominant irritable bowel syndrome (IBS)	• Antimuscarinic adverse effects and contraindications similar to atropine (including constipation-dominant IBS) • Evidence for efficacy is limited
Trihexyphenidyl, benztropine	• Parkinson disease	• Antimuscarinic adverse effects and contraindications similar to atropine • Mainly used to treat the tremor in Parkinson disease • Not recommended for elderly or demented patients

Bibliography

Abrams P, et al. Muscarinic receptors: their distribution and function in body systems, and the implications for treating overactive bladder. *Br J Pharmacol*, **2006**, 148:565–578.

Aihara T, et al. Cholinergically stimulated gastric acid secretion is mediated by M_3 and M_5 but not M_1 muscarinic acetylcholine receptors in mice. *Am J Physiol*, **2005**, 288:G1199–G1207.

Alagha, et al. Long-acting muscarinic receptor antagonists for the treatment of chronic airways diseases. *Ther Adv Chronic Dis*, **2014**, 2:85–98.

Birdsall NJM, Lazareno S. Allosterism at muscarinic receptors: ligands and mechanisms. *Mini Rev Med Chem*, **2005**, 5:523–543.

Bonner TI, et al. Identification of a family of muscarinic acetylcholine receptor genes. *Science*, **1987**, 237:527–532.

Brodde OE, Michel MC. Adrenergic and muscarinic receptors in the human heart. *Pharmacol Rev*, **1999**, 51:651–690.

Caulfield MP, Birdsall NJ. International Union of Pharmacology, XVII. Classification of muscarinic acetylcholine receptors. *Pharmacol Rev*, **1998**, 50:279–290.

Chapple CR, et al. Randomized, double-blind placebo- and tolterodine-controlled trial of the once-daily antimuscarinic agent solifenacin in patients with symptomatic overactive bladder. *BJU Int*, **2004**, 93:303–310.

Chapple CR, et al. The effects of antimuscarinic treatments in overactive bladder: a systematic review and meta-analysis. *Eur Urol*, **2005**, 48:5–26.

Chapple CR, et al. The effects of antimuscarinic treatments in overactive bladder: an update of a systematic review and meta-analysis. *Eur Urol*, **2008**, 54(3):543–562.

Conn PJ, et al. Subtype-selective allosteric modulators of muscarinic receptors for the treatment of CNS disorders. *Trends Pharmacol Sci*, **2009**, 30:148–155.

Conn PJ, et al. Opportunities and challenges in the discovery of allosteric modulators of GPCRs for treating CNS disorders. *Nat Rev Drug Discov*, **2014**, 13:692–708.

Crapo RO, et al. Guidelines for methacholine and exercise challenge testing—1999. *Am J Respir Crit Care Med*, **2000**, 161:309–329.

DiFrancesco D, Tromba C. Acetylcholine inhibits activation of the cardiac hyperpolarizing-activated current, i_f. *Pflugers Arch*, **1987**, 410:139–142.

Dunlap ME, et al. Autonomic modulation in heart failure: ready for prime time? *Curr Cardiol Rep*, **2015**, 17:103.

Eglen RM, et al. Muscarinic receptor subtypes and smooth muscle function. *Pharmacol Rev*, **1996**, 48:531–565.

Feigl EO. Neural control of coronary blood flow. *J Vasc Res*, **1998**, 35:85–92.

Fisher JT, et al. Loss of vagally mediated bradycardia and bronchoconstriction in mice lacking M_2 or M_3 muscarinic acetylcholine receptors. *FASEB J*, **2004**, 18:711–713.

Furchgott RF. Endothelium-derived relaxing factor: discovery, early studies, and identification as nitric oxide. *Biosci Rep*, **1999**, 19:235–251.

Gautam D, et al. Cholinergic stimulation of salivary secretion studied with M_1 and M_3 muscarinic receptor single- and double-knockout mice. *Mol Pharmacol*, **2004**, 66:260–267.

Gavalda A, et al. Characterization of aclidinium bromide, a novel inhaled muscarinic antagonist, with long duration of action and a favorable pharmacological profile. *J Pharmacol Exp Ther*, **2009**, 331(2):740–751.

Gentry PR, et al. Novel allosteric modulators of G protein-coupled receptors. *J Biol Chem*, **2015**, 290:19478–19488.

Goldberg JA, et al. Muscarinic modulation of striatal function and circuitry. *Handb Exp Pharmacol*, **2012**, 208:223–241.

Goyal RK, Rattan S. Neurohumoral, hormonal, and drug receptors for the lower esophageal sphincter. *Gastroenterology*, **1978**, 74:598–619.

Haga K, et al. Structure of the human M_2 muscarinic acetylcholine receptor bound to an antagonist. *Nature*, **2012**, 482:547–551.

Hegde SS. Muscarinic receptors in the bladder: from basic research to therapeutics. *Br J Pharmacol*, **2006**, 147(suppl 2):S80–S87.

Ignarro LJ, et al. Nitric oxide as a signaling molecule in the vascular system: an overview. *J Cardiovasc Pharmacol*, **1999**, 34:879–886.

Kay G, et al. Differential effects of the antimuscarinic agents darifenacin and oxybutynin ER on memory in older subjects. *Eur Urol*, **2006**, 50:317–326.

Krnjević K. Synaptic mechanisms modulated by acetylcholine in cerebral cortex. *Prog Brain Res*, **2004**, 145:81–93.

Kruse AC, et al. Structure and dynamics of the M_3 muscarinic acetylcholine receptor. *Nature*, **2012**, 482:552–556.

Kruse AC, et al. Activation and allosteric modulation of a muscarinic acetylcholine receptor. *Nature*, **2013**, 504:101–106.

Kruse AC, et al. Muscarinic acetylcholine receptors: novel opportunities for drug development. *Nat Rev Drug Discov*, **2014**, 13:549–560.

Lakatta EG, DiFrancesco D. What keeps us ticking: a funny current, a calcium clock, or both? *J Mol Cell Cardiol*, **2009**, 47:157–170.

Lane JR, et al. Bridging the gap: bitopic ligands of G-protein-coupled receptors. *Trends Pharmacol Sci*, **2013**, 34:59–66.

Levy MN, Schwartz PJ, eds. *Vagal Control of the Heart: Experimental Basis and Clinical Implications*. Futura, Armonk, NY, **1994**.

Lewis ME, et al. Vagus nerve stimulation decreases left ventricular contractility in vivo in the human and pig heart. *J Physiol*, **2001**, 534:547–552.

Lyashkov AE, et al. Cholinergic receptor signaling modulates spontaneous firing of sinoatrial nodal cells via integrated effects on PKAH-dependent Ca^{2+} cycling and I_{KACh}. *Am J Physiol*, **2009**, 297:949–959.

Matsui M, et al. Mice lacking M_2 and M_3 muscarinic acetylcholine receptors are devoid of cholinergic smooth muscle contractions but still viable. *J Neurosci*, **2002**, 22:10627–10632.

May LT, et al. Allosteric modulation of G protein-coupled receptors. *Annu Rev Pharmacol Toxicol*, **2007**, 47:1–51.

Mohr K, et al. Rational design of dualsteric GPCR ligands: quests and promise. *Br J Pharmacol*, **2010**, 159:997–1008.

Moncada S, Higgs EA. Molecular mechanisms and therapeutic strategies related to nitric oxide. *FASEB J*, **1995**, 9:1319–1330.

Noiaseh G, et al. Comparison of the discontinuation rates and side-effect profiles of pilocarpine and cevimeline for xerostomia in primary Sjögren's syndrome. *Clin Exp Rheumatol*, **2014**, *32*:575–577.

Oberhauser V, et al. Acetylcholine release in human heart atrium: influence of muscarinic autoreceptors, diabetes, and age. *Circulation*, **2001**, *103*:1638–1643.

Porter SR, et al. An update of the etiology and management of xerostomia. *Oral Surg Oral Med Oral Pathol Oral Radiol Endod*, **2004**, *97*: 28–46.

Roth B, et al. Magic shotguns versus magic bullets: selectively non-selective drugs for mood disorders and schizophrenia. *Nat Rev Drug Discov*, **2004**, *3*:353–359.

Schwartz PJ, De Ferrari GM. Sympathetic—parasympathetic interaction in health and disease: abnormalities and relevance in heart failure. *Heart Fail Rev*, **2011**, *16*:101–107.

Stengel PW, et al. M_2 and M_4 receptor knockout mice: muscarinic receptor function in cardiac and smooth muscle in vitro. *J Pharmacol Exp Ther*, **2000**, *292*:877–885.

Trendelenburg AU, et al. Distinct mixtures of muscarinic receptor subtypes mediate inhibition of noradrenaline release in different mouse peripheral tissues, as studied with receptor knockout mice. *Br J Pharmacol*, **2005**, *145*:1153–1159.

Tryba M, Cook D. Current guidelines on stress ulcer prophylaxis. *Drugs*, **1997**, *54*:581–596.

Volpicelli LA, Levey AI. Muscarinic acetylcholine receptor sub-types in cerebral cortex and hippocampus. *Progr Brain Res*, **2004**, *145*:59–66.

Wellstein A, Pitschner HF. Complex dose-response curves of atropine in man explained by different functions of M_1- and M_2-cholinoceptors. *Naunyn Schmiedebergs Arch Pharmacol*, **1988**, *338*:19–27.

Wess J. Molecular biology of muscarinic acetylcholine receptors. *Crit Rev Neurobiol*, **1996**, *10*:69–99.

Wess J, et al. Muscarinic acetylcholine receptors: mutant mice provide new insights for drug development. *Nature Rev Drug Discov*, **2007**, *6*:721–733.

Wiseman LR, Faulds D. Oral pilocarpine: a review of its pharmacological properties and clinical potential in xerostomia. *Drugs*, **1995**, *49*:143–155.

Anticholinesterase Agents

Palmer Taylor

Acetylcholinesterase

The hydrolytic activity of AChE terminates the action of ACh at the junctions of the various cholinergic nerve endings with their effector organs or postsynaptic sites (Chapter 8). Drugs that inhibit AChE are called anti-ChEs, since they inhibit both AChE and BChE. BChE is not found in nerve ending synapses but in liver and plasma, where it metabolizes circulating esters. AChE inhibitors cause ACh to accumulate in the vicinity of cholinergic nerve terminals and thus are potentially capable of producing effects equivalent to excessive stimulation of cholinergic receptors throughout the central and peripheral nervous systems. In view of the widespread distribution of cholinergic neurons across animal species, it is not surprising that the anti-ChE agents have received extensive application as toxic agents, in the form of agricultural insecticides, pesticides, and potential chemical warfare "nerve gases." Moreover, several compounds of this class are used therapeutically; others that cross the blood-brain barrier have been approved or are in clinical trials for the treatment of Alzheimer disease.

Prior to World War II, only the "reversible" anti-ChE agents were generally known, of which physostigmine is the prototype (Box 10-1). Shortly before and during World War II, a new class of highly toxic chemicals, the organophosphates, was developed, first as agricultural insecticides and later as potential chemical warfare agents. The extreme toxicity of these compounds was found to be due to their "irreversible" inactivation of AChE, which resulted in prolonged enzyme inhibition. Because the pharmacological actions of both the reversible and irreversible anti-ChE agents are qualitatively similar, they are discussed here as a group. Interactions of anti-ChE agents with other drugs acting at peripheral autonomic synapses and the neuromuscular junction are described in Chapters 9 and 11.

Structure of Acetylcholinesterase

Acetylcholinesterase exists in two general classes of molecular forms: simple homomeric oligomers of catalytic subunits (monomers, dimers, and tetramers) and heteromeric associations of catalytic subunits with structural subunits (Massoulié, 2000; Taylor et al., 2000). The homomeric forms are found as soluble species in the cell, presumably destined for export or for association with the outer membrane of the cell, typically through an attached glycophospholipid. One heteromeric form, largely found in neuronal synapses, is a tetramer of catalytic subunits disulfide-linked to a 20-kDa lipid-linked subunit and localized to the outer surface of the cell membrane. The other heteromeric form consists of tetramers of catalytic subunits, linked by disulfide bonds to each of three strands of a collagen-like structural subunit. This molecular species, whose molecular mass approaches 10^6 Da, is associated with the basal lamina of neuromuscular junctional areas of skeletal muscle.

BOX 10–1 ■ History

Physostigmine, also called *eserine,* is an alkaloid obtained from the Calabar or ordeal bean, the dried, ripe seed of *Physostigma venenosum,* a perennial plant found in tropical West Africa. This Calabar bean once was used by native tribes of West Africa as an "ordeal poison" in trials for witchcraft, in which guilt was judged by death from the poison, innocence by survival after ingestion of a bean. A pure alkaloid was isolated by Jobst and Hesse in 1864 and named physostigmine. The first therapeutic use of the drug was in 1877 by Laqueur in the treatment of glaucoma, one of its clinical uses today. Karczmar (1970) and Holmstedt (2000) have presented accounts of the history of physostigmine.

After basic research elucidated the chemical basis of the activity of physostigmine, scientists began systematic investigations of a series of substituted aromatic esters of alkyl carbamic acids. Neostigmine was introduced in 1931 for its stimulant action on the GI tract and subsequently was reported to be effective in the symptomatic treatment of myasthenia gravis.

Following the synthesis of about 2000 compounds, Schrader defined the structural requirements for insecticidal activity (and, as learned subsequently, for anti-ChE activity). One compound in this early series, parathion (a phosphorothioate), later became the most widely used insecticide of this class. Malathion, which currently is used extensively, also contains the thionophosphorus bond found in parathion. Prior to and during World War II, the efforts of Schrader's group were directed toward the development of chemical warfare agents. The synthesis of several compounds of much greater toxicity than parathion, such as sarin, soman, and tabun, was kept secret by the German government. Investigators in the Allied countries also followed Lange and Krueger's lead in 1932 in the search for potentially toxic compounds; DFP, synthesized by McCombie and Saunders, was studied most extensively by British and American scientists (Giacobini, 2000).

Abbreviations

ACh: acetylcholine
AChE: acetylcholinesterase
anti-ChE: anticholinesterase
BChE: butyrylcholinesterase
ChE: cholinesterase
CNS: central nervous system
CYP: cytochrome P450
DFP: diisopropyl fluorophosphate (diisopropyl phosphorofluoridate)
EPA: Environmental Protection Agency
FDA: Food and Drug Administration
2-PAM: pralidoxime
PON1: paraoxonase isoform 1
TOCP: triorthocresyl phosphate

hydrolase activity, such as thyroglobulin and members of the tactin and neuroligin families (Taylor et al., 2000).

The three-dimensional structures of AChEs show the active center to be nearly centrosymmetric to each subunit, residing at the base of a narrow gorge about 20 Å in depth (Bourne et al., 1995; Sussman et al., 1991). At the base of the gorge lie the residues of the catalytic triad: Ser203, His447, and Glu334 in mammals (Figure 10–1). The catalytic mechanism resembles that of other hydrolases; the serine hydroxyl group is rendered highly nucleophilic through a charge-relay system involving the carboxylate anion from glutamate, the imidazole of histidine, and the hydroxyl of serine (Figure 10–2A).

During enzymatic attack of ACh, an ester with trigonal geometry, a tetrahedral intermediate between enzyme and substrate is formed (Figure 10–2A) that collapses to an acetyl enzyme conjugate with the concomitant release of choline. The acetyl enzyme is very labile to hydrolysis, which results in the formation of acetate and active enzyme (Froede and Wilson, 1971; Rosenberry, 1975). AChE is one of the most efficient enzymes known: One molecule of AChE can hydrolyze 6×10^5 ACh molecules per minute; this yields a turnover time of 100 μsec.

Is AChE Essential?

Knockout mice lacking the gene encoding AChE can survive under highly supportive conditions and with a special diet, but they exhibit continuous tremors and are stunted in growth (Xie et al., 2000). Mice that selectively lack AChE expression in skeletal muscle but have normal or near-normal expression in brain and organs innervated by the autonomic nervous system can reproduce but have tremors and severe compromise of skeletal muscle strength. By contrast, mice with selective reductions of CNS AChE by elimination of the exons encoding alternative spliced regions or expression of the structural subunits influencing expression in brain yield no obvious phenotype. This arises from large adaptive responses and compensatory reductions of ACh synthesis and storage and receptor responses (Camp et al., 2008; Dobbertin et al., 2009).

Molecular cloning revealed that a single gene encodes vertebrate AChEs (Schumacher et al., 1986; Taylor et al., 2000). However, multiple gene products arise from alternative processing of the mRNA that differ only in their carboxyl termini; the portion of the gene encoding the catalytic core of the enzyme is invariant. Hence, the individual AChE species can be expected to show identical substrate and inhibitor specificities.

A separate, structurally related, gene encodes butyrylcholinesterase, which is synthesized in the liver and is found primarily in plasma (Lockridge, 2015; Lockridge et al., 1987). The cholinesterases define a superfamily of proteins that share a common structural motif, the α,β-hydrolase fold (Cygler et al., 1993). The family includes several esterases, other hydrolases not found in the nervous system, and surprisingly, proteins without

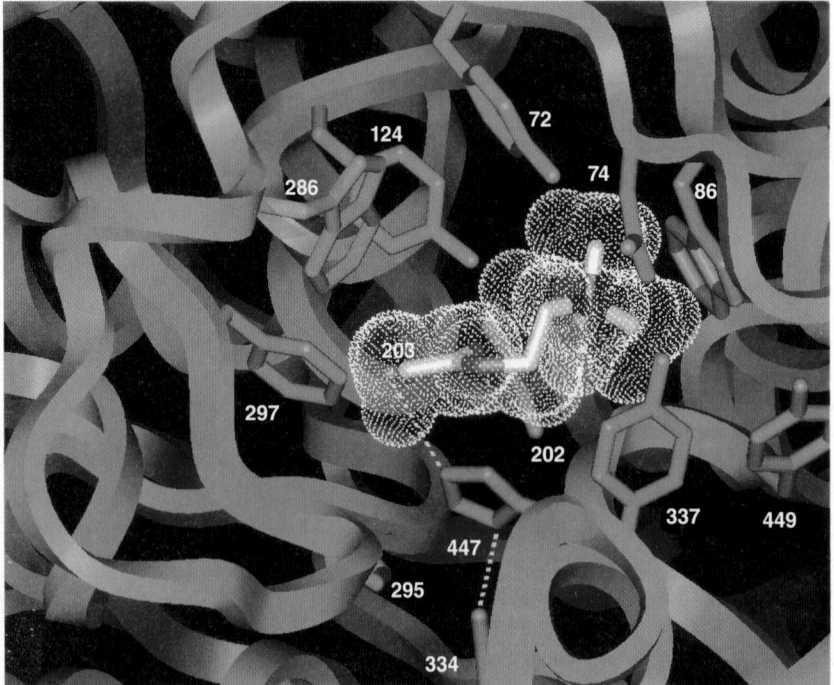

Figure 10–1 *The active center gorge of mammalian AChE, looking from the portal of substrate entry.* Bound ACh is shown by the dotted structure depicting its van der Waals radii. The crystal structure of mouse cholinesterase active center, which is virtually identical to human AChE, is shown (Bourne et al., 1995). Included are the side chains of (a) the catalytic triad: Glu334, His447, Ser203 (hydrogen bonds are denoted by the dotted lines); (b) acyl pocket: Phe295 and Phe297; (c) choline subsite: Trp86, Glu202, and Tyr337; and (d) the peripheral site: Trp286, Tyr72, Tyr124, and Asp74. Tyrosines 337 and 449 are further removed from the active center but likely contribute to stabilization of certain ligands. The catalytic triad, choline subsite, and acyl pocket are located at the base of the gorge, while the peripheral site is at the lip of the gorge. The gorge is 18- to 20-Å deep, with its base centrosymmetric to the subunit.

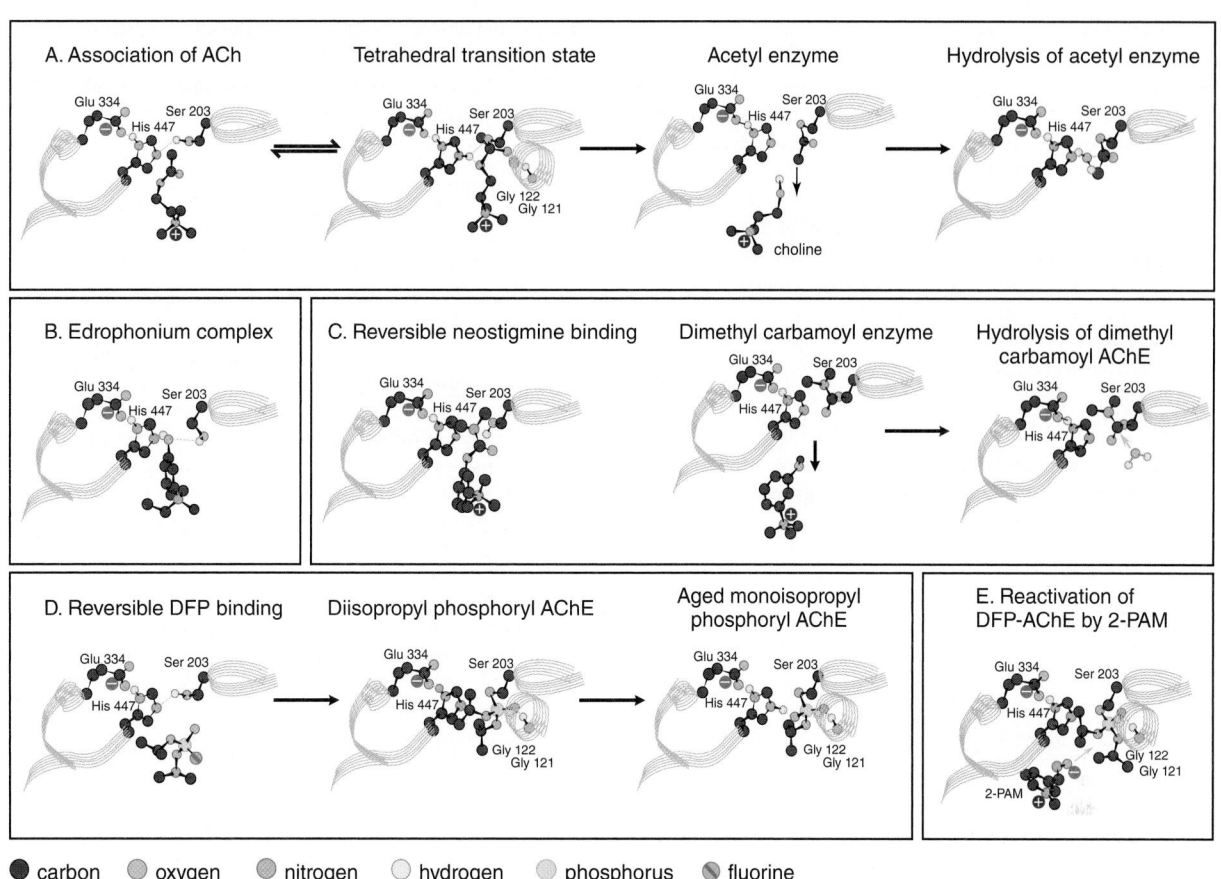

● carbon ● oxygen ● nitrogen ○ hydrogen ● phosphorus ● fluorine

Figure 10–2 *Steps involved in the hydrolysis of ACh by AChE and in the inhibition and reactivation of the enzyme.* Only the three residues of the catalytic triad shown in Figure 10–1 are depicted. Net charge in a region is represented by red and blue circles containing − or + signs, respectively. The associations and reactions shown are as follows: **A.** ACh catalysis: binding of ACh, formation of a tetrahedral transition state, formation of the acetyl enzyme with liberation of choline, rapid hydrolysis of the acetyl enzyme with return to the original state. **B.** Reversible binding and inhibition by edrophonium. **C.** Neostigmine reaction with and inhibition of AChE: reversible binding of neostigmine, formation of the dimethyl carbamoyl enzyme, slow hydrolysis of the dimethyl carbamoyl enzyme. **D.** DFP reaction and inhibition of AChE: reversible binding of DFP, formation of the diisopropyl phosphoryl enzyme, formation of the aged monoisopropyl phosphoryl enzyme. Hydrolysis of the diisopropyl enzyme is very slow and is not shown. The aged monoisopropyl phosphoryl enzyme is virtually resistant to hydrolysis and reactivation. The tetrahedral transition state of ACh hydrolysis resembles the conjugates formed by the tetrahedral phosphate inhibitors and accounts for their potency. Amide bond hydrogens from Gly121 and Gly122 stabilize the carbonyl and phosphoryl oxygens. **E.** Reactivation of the diisopropyl phosphoryl enzyme by 2-PAM. 2-PAM attack of the phosphorus on the phosphorylated enzyme will form a phospho-oxime with regeneration of active enzyme. The individual steps of phosphorylation reaction and oxime reaction have been characterized by mass spectrometry. (Data from Jennings et al, 2003).

Acetylcholinesterase Inhibitors

Molecular Mechanism of Action of AChE Inhibitors

The mechanisms of action of compounds that typify the three classes of anti-ChE agents are also shown in Figure 10–2.

Three distinct domains on AChE constitute binding sites for inhibitory ligands and form the basis for specificity differences between AChE and butyrylcholinesterase:

- the acyl pocket of the active center;
- the choline subsite of the active center; and
- the peripheral anionic site (Reiner and Radić, 2000; Taylor and Radić, 1994).

Reversible inhibitors, such as edrophonium and tacrine, bind to the choline subsite in the vicinity of Trp86 and Glu202 (Silman and Sussman, 2000) (Figure 10–2B). Edrophonium has a brief duration of action because its quaternary structure facilitates renal elimination, and it binds reversibly to the AChE active center. Additional reversible inhibitors, such as donepezil, bind with higher affinity to the active center gorge. Other reversible inhibitors, such as propidium and the snake peptidic toxin fasciculin, bind to the peripheral anionic site on AChE. This site

resides at the rim of the gorge and is defined by Try286 and Tyr72 and Tyr124 (Figure 10–1).

Drugs that have a carbamoyl ester linkage, such as physostigmine and neostigmine, are hydrolyzed by AChE, but much more slowly than is ACh. The quaternary amine neostigmine and the tertiary amine physostigmine exist as cations at physiological pH. By serving as alternate substrates to ACh (Figure 10–2C), their reaction with the active center serine progressively generates the carbamoylated enzyme. The conjugated carbamoyl moiety resides in the acyl pocket outlined by Phe295 and Phe297. In contrast to the acetyl enzyme, methylcarbamoyl AChE and dimethylcarbamoyl AChE are far more stable (the $t_{1/2}$ for hydrolysis of the dimethylcarbamoyl enzyme is 15–30 min). Sequestration of the enzyme in its carbamoylated form thus precludes the enzyme-catalyzed hydrolysis of ACh for extended periods of time. When administered systemically, the duration of inhibition by the carbamoylating agents is 3–4 h.

The organophosphate inhibitors, such as DFP, serve as true hemisubstrates; the resultant conjugate with the active center serine phosphorylated or phosphonylated is extremely stable (Figure 10–2D). The organophosphorus inhibitors are tetrahedral in configuration, a configuration that resembles the transition state formed in carboxyl ester hydrolysis. Similar to the carboxyl esters, the phosphoryl oxygen binds within the oxanion hole of the active center. If the alkyl groups in the phosphorylated enzyme are ethyl or methyl, spontaneous regeneration of active enzyme requires several hours. Secondary (as in DFP) or tertiary alkyl groups further enhance the stability of the phosphorylated enzyme, and significant regeneration of active enzyme usually is not observed. The stability of the phosphorylated enzyme is enhanced through "aging," which results from the loss of one of the alkyl groups. Hence, the return of AChE activity depends on biosynthesis of new AChE protein.

Thus, the terms *reversible* and *irreversible* as applied to the carbamoyl ester and organophosphate anti-ChE agents are relative terms, reflecting only quantitative differences in rates of decarbamoylation or dephosphorylation of the conjugated enzyme. Both chemical classes react covalently with the active center serine in essentially the same manner as does ACh in forming the transient acetyl enzyme.

Chemistry and Structure-Activity Relationships

Structure-activity relationships of anti-ChE agents have been extensively reviewed in the scientific literature. Only agents of general therapeutic or toxicological interest are considered here.

Noncovalent Inhibitors

While these agents interact by reversible and noncovalent association with the active site in AChE, they differ in their disposition in the body and their affinity for the enzyme. Edrophonium, a quaternary drug whose activity is limited to peripheral nervous system synapses, has a moderate affinity for AChE. Its volume of distribution is limited and renal elimination is rapid, accounting for its short duration of action. By contrast,

tacrine and donepezil (Figure 10–3) have higher affinities for AChE, are more hydrophobic, and readily cross the blood-brain barrier to inhibit AChE in the CNS. Partitioning into lipid and higher affinities for AChE account for their longer durations of action.

"Reversible" Carbamate Inhibitors

Drugs of this class that are of therapeutic interest are shown in Figure 10–3. Early studies showed that the essential moiety of the physostigmine molecule was the methylcarbmate of an amine-substituted phenol. The quaternary ammonium derivative neostigmine is a compound of equal or greater potency. Pyridostigmine is a close congener also used in myasthenia gravis patients.

Carbamoylating inhibitors with high lipid solubility (rivastigmine) have longer duration of action, cross the blood-brain barrier, and are used as an alternative in the treatment of Alzheimer disease (Cummings, 2004) (Chapter 18). The carbamate insecticides carbaryl, propoxur, and aldicarb, used extensively as garden insecticides, inhibit AChE with a mechanism identical to other carbamoylating agents. While more reversible and less toxic, symptoms parallel those of organophosphates (Eddleston and Clark, 2011; King and Aaron, 2015).

Organophosphorus Compound

The general formula for the organophosphorus compound class of ChE inhibitors is presented in Table 10–1. A great variety of substituents is possible: R_1 and R_2 may be alkyl, alkoxy, aryloxy, amido, mercaptan, or other groups; and X, the leaving group, typically a conjugate base of a weak acid, is a halide, cyanide, thiocyanate, phenoxy, thiophenoxy, phosphate,

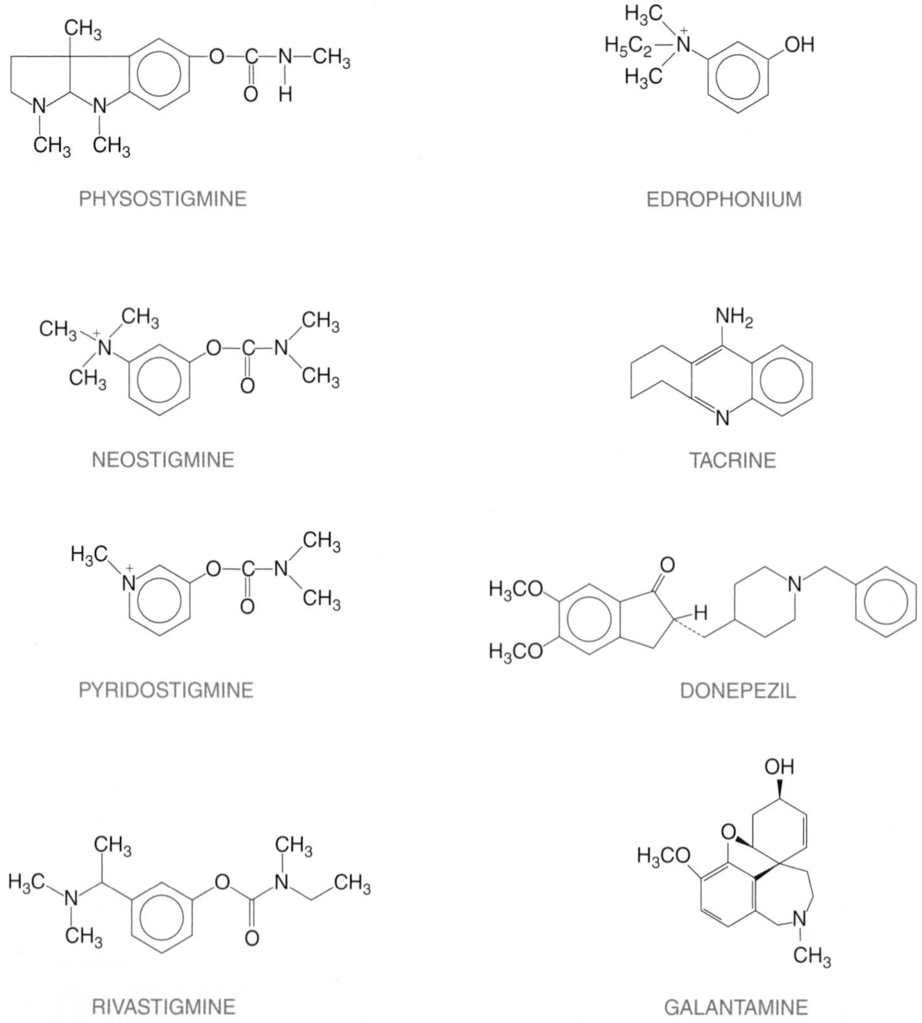

PHYSOSTIGMINE

EDROPHONIUM

NEOSTIGMINE

TACRINE

PYRIDOSTIGMINE

DONEPEZIL

RIVASTIGMINE

GALANTAMINE

Figure 10–3 *"Reversible" carbamate and noncovalent AChE inhibitors used clinically.*

TABLE 10-1 ■ CHEMICAL CLASSIFICATION OF REPRESENTATIVE ORGANOPHOSPHORUS AChE INHIBITORS

General formula

$$R_1 \diagdown \overset{O}{\underset{\displaystyle \diagup}{P}} \diagdown X \quad R_2$$

Group **A**, X = halogen, cyanide, or thiocyanate leaving group; group **B**, X = alkylthio, arylthio, alkoxy, or aryloxy leaving group; group **C**, thionophosphorus or thio-thionophosphorus compounds; group **D**, quaternary ammonium leaving group. R_1 can be an alkyl (phosphonates), alkoxy (phosphorates) or an alkylamino (phosphoramidates) group.

GROUP	STRUCTURAL FORMULA	COMMON, CHEMICAL, AND OTHER NAMES	COMMENTS
A	$i\text{-}C_3H_7O$, P(=O), F; $i\text{-}C_3H_7O$	DFP; Isoflurophate; diisopropyl fluorophosphate	Potent, irreversible inactivator
	$(CH_3)_2N$, P(=O), CN; C_2H_5O	Tabun Ethyl N-dimethylphosphoramidocyanidate	Extremely toxic "nerve gas"
	$i\text{-}C_3H_7O$, P(=O), F; CH_3	Sarin (GB) Isopropyl methylphosphonofluoridate	Extremely toxic "nerve gas"
	$CH_3\text{-}C(CH_3)\text{-}C(CH_3)H\text{-}O\text{-}P(=O)(CH_3)F$	Soman (GD) Pinacolyl methylphosphonofluoridate	Extremely toxic "nerve gas"; greatest potential for irreversible action/rapid aging
B	C_2H_5O, P(=O), $S\text{-}C_2H_4N(i\text{-}C_3H_7)_2$; H_3C	VX O-ethyl S [2-(diisopropylamino)ethyl] methyl phosponothioate	Potent, slower onset, skin-penetrating nerve agent
	CH_3O, P(=O), $S\text{-}CHCOOC_2H_5$; CH_3O, $CH_2COOC_2H_5$	Malaoxon O,O-Dimethyl S-(1,2-dicarboxyethyl)-phosphorothioate	Active metabolite of malathion
C	C_2H_5O, P(=S), $O\text{-}C_6H_4\text{-}NO_2$; C_2H_5O	Parathion O,O-Diethyl O-(4-nitrophenyl)-phosphorothioate	Agricultural insecticide, resulting in numerous cases of accidental poisoning; phased out in 2003.
	C_2H_5O, P(=S), O-pyrimidinyl; C_2H_5O	Diazinon, Dimpylate O,O-Diethyl O-(2-isopropyl-6-methyl-4-pyrimidinyl) phosphorothioate	Insecticide; use limited to non-residential agricultural settings
	H_5C_2O, P(=S), O-trichloropyridyl; H_5C_2O	Chlorpyrifos O,O-Diethyl O-(3,5,6-trichloro-2-pyridyl) phosphorothioate	Insecticide; use limited to non-residential agricultural settings
	CH_3O, P(=S), $S\text{-}CHCOOC_2H_5$; CH_3O, $CH_2COOC_2H_5$	Malathion O,O-Dimethyl S-(1,2-dicarbethoxyethyl) phosphorodithioate	Widely employed insecticide of greater safety than parathion or other agents because of rapid detoxification by higher organisms
D	C_2H_5O, P(=O), $SCH_2CH_2N^+(CH_3)_3$ I^-; C_2H_5O	Echothiophate (PHOSPHOLINE IODIDE), MI-217 Diethoxyphosphinylthiocholine iodide	Extremely potent choline derivative; administered locally in treatment of glaucoma; relatively stable in aqueous solution

thiocholine, or carboxylate group. For a compilation of the organophosphorus compounds and their toxicity, see Gallo and Lawryk (1991).

Diisopropyl fluorophosphate produces virtually irreversible inactivation of AChE and other esterases by alkylphosphorylation. Its high lipid solubility, low molecular weight, and volatility facilitate inhalation, transdermal absorption, and penetration into the CNS. After desulfuration, the insecticides in current use form the dimethoxy or diethoxyphosphoryl conjugate of AChE.

The "nerve gases"—tabun, sarin, soman, and VX—are among the most potent synthetic toxins known; they are lethal to laboratory animals in nanogram doses. Insidious employment of these agents occurred in the Matsumoto incident and Tokyo subway terrorism attacks in Japan and against civilians by despotic regimes in the Middle East (Council on Foreign Relations, 2013; Dolgin, 2013; King and Aaron, 2015; Nozaki and Aikawa, 1995). While estimates of lethality in Japan amounted to 8 and 10 people killed, in Syria estimates vary, ranging up to 1000 individuals, with over 3000 showing symptoms of organophosphate toxicity. Attacks continued into 2017 with release of sarin vapor from explosive devices. Toxicity results from inhalation and rapid distribution of sarin to the central and peripheral nervous systems. A assignation homicide also occurred in Malaysia in 2017 via slower dermal absorption of VX.

Parathion and methylparathion were widely used as insecticides because of their favorable properties of low volatility and stability in aqueous solution. Acute and chronic toxicity has limited their use, and potentially less-hazardous compounds have replaced them for home and garden use now largely throughout the world. These compounds are inactive in inhibiting AChE in vitro; paraoxon is the active metabolite. The phosphoryl oxygen for sulfur substitution is carried out predominantly by hepatic CYPs. This reaction also occurs in the insect, typically with more efficiency. Other insecticides possessing the phosphorothioate structure have been widely employed for agricultural use. These include *diazinon* and *chlorpyrifos*. Use of these agents is restricted because of evidence of chronic toxicity in the newborn animal. They have been banned from indoor and outdoor residential use since 2005.

Malathion also requires replacement of a sulfur atom with oxygen in vivo, conferring resistance to mammalian species. Also, this insecticide can be detoxified by hydrolysis of the carboxyl ester linkage by plasma carboxylesterases. Plasma carboxylesterase activity dictates species resistance to malathion: The detoxification reaction is much more rapid in mammals and birds than in insects (Costa et al., 2013). In recent years, malathion has been employed in aerial spraying of relatively populous areas for control of citrus orchard–destructive Mediterranean fruit flies and mosquitoes that harbor and transmit viruses harmful to human beings, such as the West Nile encephalitis virus.

Evidence of acute toxicity from malathion arises primarily with suicide attempts or deliberate poisoning. The lethal dose in mammals is about 1 g/kg. Exposure to the skin results in a small fraction (<10%) systemically absorbed. Malathion is used topically in the treatment of pediculosis (lice) infestations in cases of permethrin resistance (Centers for Disease Control and Prevention, 2015).

Among the quaternary ammonium organophosphorus compounds (group D in Table 10–1), only echothiophate is useful clinically, and its use is limited to ophthalmic administration. Being positively charged, it is not volatile and does not readily penetrate the skin.

Basis for the Pharmacological Effects of ChE Inhibitors

The characteristic pharmacological effects of the anti-ChE agents are due primarily to the prevention of hydrolysis of ACh by AChE at sites of cholinergic transmission. Transmitter thus accumulates, enhancing the response to ACh that is liberated by cholinergic impulses or that is spontaneously released from the nerve ending. Virtually all acute effects of moderate doses of organophosphates are attributable to this action. For example, the characteristic miosis that follows local application of DFP to the eye is not observed after chronic postganglionic denervation of the eye because there is no source from which to release endogenous ACh.

The consequences of enhanced concentrations of ACh at motor end plates are unique to these sites and are discussed below.

Generally, the pharmacological properties of anti-ChE agents can be predicted by knowing those loci where ACh is released physiologically by nerve impulses, the degree of nerve impulse activity, and the responses of the corresponding effector organs to ACh (see Chapter 8). The anti-ChE agents potentially can produce all the following effects:

- stimulation of muscarinic receptor responses at autonomic effector organs;
- stimulation, followed by depression or paralysis, of all autonomic ganglia and skeletal muscle (nicotinic actions); and
- stimulation, with occasional subsequent depression, of pre- and postsynaptic cholinergic receptor sites in the CNS.

At therapeutic doses, several modifying factors are significant. Compounds containing a quaternary ammonium group do not penetrate cell membranes readily; hence, anti-ChE agents in this category are absorbed poorly from the GI tract or across the skin and are excluded from the CNS by the blood-brain barrier after moderate doses. On the other hand, such compounds act preferentially at the neuromuscular junctions of skeletal muscle, exerting their action both as anti-ChE agents and as direct agonists. They have comparatively less effect at autonomic effector sites and ganglia. In contrast, the more lipid-soluble agents are well absorbed after oral administration, have ubiquitous effects at both peripheral and central cholinergic sites, and may be sequestered in lipids for long periods of time. Lipid-soluble organophosphorus agents, such as the chemical warfare agent VX, are well absorbed through the skin, whereas the volatile agents are transferred readily across the alveolar membranes in the lung (King and Aaron, 2015; Storm et al., 2000).

The actions of anti-ChE agents on autonomic effector cells and on cortical and subcortical sites in the CNS, where ACh receptors are largely of the muscarinic type, are blocked by atropine. Likewise, atropine blocks some of the excitatory actions of anti-ChE agents on autonomic ganglia because both nicotinic and muscarinic receptors are involved in ganglionic neurotransmission (Chapter 11).

Effects on Physiological Systems

The sites of action of anti-ChE agents of therapeutic importance are the CNS, eye, intestine, and neuromuscular junction of skeletal muscle; other actions are of toxicological consequence.

Eye

When applied locally to the conjunctiva, anti-ChE agents cause conjunctival hyperemia and constriction of the pupillary sphincter muscle around the pupillary margin of the iris (miosis) and the ciliary muscle (block of accommodation reflex with resultant focusing to near vision). Miosis is apparent in a few minutes and can last several hours to days. Although the pupil may be "pinpoint" in size, it generally contracts further when exposed to light. The block of accommodation is more transient and generally disappears before termination of miosis. Intraocular pressure, when elevated, usually falls as the result of facilitation of outflow of the aqueous humor (Chapter 69).

GI Tract

In humans, neostigmine enhances gastric contractions and increases the secretion of gastric acid. After bilateral vagotomy, the effects of neostigmine on gastric motility are greatly reduced. The lower portion of the esophagus is stimulated by neostigmine; in patients with marked achalasia and dilation of the esophagus, the drug can cause a salutary increase in tone and peristalsis.

Neostigmine also augments motor activity of the small and large bowel; the colon is particularly stimulated. Atony produced by muscarinic receptor antagonists or prior surgical intervention may be overcome, propulsive waves are increased in amplitude and frequency, and movement of intestinal contents is thus promoted. The total effect of anti-ChE agents on intestinal motility probably represents a combination of actions at the ganglion cells of the Auerbach plexus and at the smooth muscle fibers as a result of the preservation of ACh released by the cholinergic preganglionic and postganglionic fibers, respectively (Chapter 50).

Neuromuscular Junction

Most of the effects of potent anti-ChE drugs on skeletal muscle can be explained adequately on the basis of their inhibition of AChE at neuromuscular junctions. However, there is good evidence for an accessory direct action of neostigmine and other quaternary ammonium anti-ChE agents on skeletal muscle. For example, the intra-arterial injection of neostigmine into chronically denervated muscle, or muscle in which AChE has been inactivated by prior administration of DFP, evokes an immediate contraction, whereas physostigmine does not.

Normally, a single nerve impulse in a terminal motor-axon branch liberates enough ACh to produce a localized depolarization (end-plate potential) of sufficient magnitude to initiate a propagated muscle action potential. The ACh released is rapidly hydrolyzed by AChE, such that the lifetime of free ACh within the nerve-muscle synapse (~200 μsec) is shorter than the decay of the end-plate potential or the refractory period of the muscle. Therefore, each nerve impulse gives rise to a single wave of depolarization. After inhibition of AChE, the residence time of ACh in the synapse increases, allowing for lateral diffusion and rebinding of the transmitter to multiple receptors. Successive stimulation of neighboring receptors to the release site in the end plate results in a prolongation of the decay time of the end-plate potential. Quanta released by individual nerve impulses are no longer isolated. This action destroys the synchrony between end-plate depolarizations and the development of the muscle action potentials. Consequently, asynchronous excitation and fasciculations of muscle fibers occur. With sufficient inhibition of AChE, depolarization of the end-plate predominates, and blockade due to depolarization ensues (Chapter 11). When ACh persists in the synapse, it also may depolarize the axon terminal, resulting in antidromic firing of the motoneuron; this stimulation contributes to fasciculations that involve the entire motor unit.

Anti-ChE agents will reverse the antagonism caused by competitive neuromuscular blocking agents. By contrast, neostigmine is not effective against the skeletal muscle paralysis caused by succinylcholine, which produces neuromuscular blockade by depolarization; neostigmine will enhance depolarization and the resultant blockade.

Cardiopulmonary System

The cardiovascular actions of anti-ChE agents are complex because they reflect both ganglionic and postganglionic effects of accumulated ACh on the heart and blood vessels and actions in the CNS. The predominant effect on the heart from the peripheral action of accumulated ACh is bradycardia, resulting in a fall in cardiac output. Higher doses usually enhance the fall in blood pressure, as a consequence of effects of anti-ChE agents on the medullary vasomotor centers of the CNS.

Anti-ChE agents augment vagal influences on the heart. This shortens the effective refractory period of atrial muscle fibers and increases the refractory period and conduction time at the sinoatrial and atrioventricular nodes. At the ganglionic level, accumulating ACh initially is excitatory on nicotinic receptors, but at higher concentrations, ganglionic blockade ensues as a result of persistent depolarization of the postsynaptic nerve. The excitatory action on the parasympathetic ganglion cells would tend to reinforce the diminished cardiac output, whereas the opposite sequence results from the action of ACh on sympathetic ganglion cells. Excitation followed by inhibition also is elicited by ACh at the central medullary vasomotor and cardiac centers. All of these effects are complicated further by the hypoxemia resulting from the bronchoconstrictor and secretory actions of increased ACh on the respiratory system; hypoxemia, in turn, can reinforce both sympathetic tone and ACh-induced discharge of epinephrine from the adrenal medulla. Hence, it is not surprising that an increase in heart rate is seen with severe ChE inhibitor poisoning. Hypoxemia probably is a major factor in the CNS depression that appears after large doses of anti-ChE agents.

Actions at Other Sites

Secretory glands that are innervated by postganglionic cholinergic fibers include the bronchial, lacrimal, sweat, salivary, gastric (antral G cells and parietal cells), intestinal, and pancreatic acinar glands. Low doses of anti-ChE agents augment secretory responses to nerve stimulation, and higher doses actually produce an increase in the resting rate of secretion.

Anti-ChE agents increase contraction of smooth muscle fibers of the bronchioles and ureters, and the ureters may show increased peristaltic activity.

ADME

Physostigmine is absorbed readily from the GI tract, subcutaneous tissues, and mucous membranes. The conjunctival instillation of solutions of the drug may result in systemic effects if measures (e.g., pressure on the inner canthus) are not taken to prevent absorption from the nasal mucosa. Parenterally administered physostigmine is largely destroyed within 2–3 h, mainly by hydrolytic cleavage by plasma esterases.

Neostigmine and pyridostigmine are absorbed poorly after oral administration, such that much larger doses are needed than by the parenteral route. Whereas the effective parenteral dose of neostigmine is 0.5–2 mg, the equivalent oral dose may be 15–30 mg or more. Neostigmine and pyridostigmine are also destroyed by plasma esterases; the half-lives of these drugs are about 1–2 h (Cohan et al., 1976).

Organophosphate anti-ChE agents with the highest risk of toxicity are highly lipid-soluble liquids; others, such as sarin, have high vapor pressures, augmenting their dispersal. The less-volatile agents that are commonly used as agricultural insecticides (e.g., diazinon, malathion) generally are dispersed as aerosols or as dusts adsorbed to an inert, finely particulate material. Consequently, the compounds are absorbed rapidly through the skin and mucous membranes following contact with moisture, by the lungs after inhalation, and by the GI tract after ingestion (Storm et al., 2000).

Following their absorption, most organophosphates are excreted almost entirely as hydrolysis products in the urine. Plasma and liver esterases are responsible for hydrolysis to the corresponding phosphoric and phosphonic acids. However, CYPs are responsible for converting the inactive phosphorothioates containing a phosphorus-sulfur (thiono) bond to phosphorates with a phosphorus-oxygen bond, resulting in their activation. These enzymes also play a role in the inactivation of certain organophosphorus agents, and allelic differences are known to affect rates of metabolism (Furlong, 2007).

The organophosphate anti-ChE agents are hydrolyzed by two families of hepatic enzymes: the carboxylesterases and the paraoxonases (A-esterases). These enzymes are secreted into plasma and scavenge or hydrolyze a large number of organophosphates by cleaving the phosphoester, anhydride, phosphofluoridate, or phosphoryl cyanide bonds. Natural substrates of the paraoxonases appear to be lactones. In addition to catalyzing hydrolysis of organophosphates, the paraoxonase isozyme PON1 associates with high-density lipoproteins and appears to play a role in removing oxidized lipids, thereby exerting a protective effect in atherosclerosis and inflammation (Costa et al., 2013; Harel et al., 2004; Mackness and Mackness, 2015). Wide variations in paraoxonase activity exist among animal species. Young animals are deficient in carboxylesterases and paraoxonases, which may account for age-related toxicities seen in newborn animals and suspected to be a basis for organophosphate toxicity in humans (Padilla et al., 2004).

Plasma and hepatic carboxylesterases (aliesterases) and plasma butyrylcholinesterase are inhibited irreversibly by organophosphates (Costa et al., 2013; Lockridge 2015); their scavenging capacity for organophosphates can afford partial protection against inhibition of AChE in the nervous system. The carboxylesterases also catalyze hydrolysis of malathion and other organophosphates that contain carboxyl-ester linkages, rendering them less active or inactive. Because carboxylesterases are inhibited by organophosphates, toxicity from simultaneous exposure to two organophosphorus insecticides can prove synergistic.

Toxicology

Scope of the Problem

The toxicological aspects of the anti-ChE agents are of practical importance to clinicians. In addition to cases of accidental intoxication from the use and manufacture of organophosphorus compounds as agricultural insecticides, these agents have been used frequently for homicidal and suicidal purposes. Organophosphates account for as many as 80% of pesticide-related hospital admissions. The World Health Organization documents pesticide toxicity as a widespread global problem associated with over 300,000 deaths a year; most poisonings occur in Southeast Asia (Eddleston and Chowdhury, 2015; Eddleston and Clark, 2011). Occupational exposure occurs most commonly by the dermal and pulmonary routes, while oral ingestion is most common in cases of nonoccupational poisoning.

Sources of Information

In the U.S., the EPA, by virtue of revised risk assessments and the Food Quality Protection Act of 1996, has placed several organophosphate insecticides, including diazinon and chlorpyrifos, on restricted use and phased-out status in consumer products for home and garden use. A primary concern relates to exposure in pregnancy and to infants and children because the developing nervous system may be particularly susceptible to certain of these agents (Eaton et al., 2008). The National Pesticide Information Center (http://npic.orst.edu/) and the Office of Pesticide Programs of the EPA (https://www.epa.gov/pesticides) provide continuous reviews of the status of organophosphate pesticides, their tolerance reassessments, and revisions of risk assessments through their websites.

Acute Intoxication

Acute intoxication by anti-ChE agents is manifested by muscarinic and nicotinic signs and symptoms and, except for quaternary compounds of low lipid solubility, by signs referable to the CNS. Systemic effects appear within minutes after inhalation of vapors or aerosols, while onset of symptoms is delayed after GI and percutaneous absorption. The duration of toxic symptoms is determined largely by the properties of the compound: its lipid solubility, whether it must be activated to form the oxon, the stability of the organophosphate-AChE bond, and whether "aging" of the phosphorylated enzyme has occurred.

After local exposure to vapors or aerosols or after their inhalation, ocular and respiratory effects generally appear first. Ocular manifestations include marked miosis, ocular pain, conjunctival congestion, diminished vision, ciliary spasm, and brow ache. With acute systemic absorption, miosis may not be evident due to sympathetic discharge in response to hypotension. In addition to rhinorrhea and hyperemia of the upper respiratory tract, respiratory responses consist of tightness in the chest and wheezing caused by the combination of bronchoconstriction and increased bronchial secretion. GI symptoms occur earliest after ingestion and include anorexia, nausea and vomiting, abdominal cramps, and diarrhea. With percutaneous absorption of liquid, localized sweating and muscle fasciculations in the immediate vicinity are generally the earliest symptoms. Severe intoxication is manifested by extreme salivation, involuntary defecation and urination, sweating, lacrimation, penile erection, bradycardia, and hypotension.

Nicotinic actions at the neuromuscular junctions of skeletal muscle usually consist of fatigability and generalized weakness, involuntary twitchings, scattered fasciculations, and eventually severe weakness and paralysis. The most serious consequence is paralysis of the respiratory muscles.

A broad spectrum of effects of acute AChE inhibition on the CNS includes confusion, ataxia, slurred speech, loss of reflexes, Cheyne-Stokes respiration, generalized convulsions, coma, and central respiratory paralysis. Actions on the vasomotor and other cardiovascular centers in the medulla oblongata lead to hypotension.

The time of death after a single acute exposure may range from less than 5 min to nearly 24 h, depending on the dose, route, and agent. The cause of death primarily is respiratory failure, usually accompanied by a secondary cardiovascular component. Peripheral muscarinic and nicotinic as well as central actions all contribute to respiratory compromise; effects include laryngospasm, bronchoconstriction, increased tracheobronchial and salivary secretions, and compromised voluntary control of the diaphragm and intercostal muscles. Blood pressure may fall to alarmingly low levels, and cardiac arrhythmias may result from hypoxemia.

Delayed symptoms appearing after 1–4 days and marked by persistent low blood ChE and severe muscle weakness are termed the *intermediate syndrome* (Lotti, 2002). Delayed neurotoxicity and recurrent seizures also may be evident after severe intoxication (discussed below in "*Reactivation and Disposition*").

Diagnosis and Treatment

The diagnosis of severe, acute anti-ChE intoxication is made readily from the history of exposure and the characteristic signs and symptoms. In suspected cases of milder acute or chronic intoxication, determination of the ChE activities in erythrocytes and plasma generally will establish the diagnosis (Storm et al., 2000). Although these values vary considerably in the normal population, they usually are depressed well below the normal range before symptoms are evident.

Atropine in sufficient dosage (described further in the chapter) effectively antagonizes the actions at muscarinic receptor sites, including increased tracheobronchial and salivary secretion, bronchoconstriction, and bradycardia. Larger doses are required to get appreciable concentrations of atropine into the CNS. Atropine is virtually without effect against the peripheral neuromuscular compromise, which can be reversed by 2-PAM, a cholinesterase reactivator.

In moderate or severe intoxication with an organophosphorus anti-ChE agent, the recommended adult dose of 2-PAM is 1–2 g, slowly infused intravenously. If weakness is not relieved or if it recurs after 20–60 min, the dose should be repeated. Early treatment is important to ensure that the oxime reaches the phosphorylated AChE while the latter still can be reactivated. Many of the alkylphosphates are extremely lipid soluble, and if extensive partitioning into body fat has occurred and desulfuration is required for inhibition of AChE, toxicity will persist.

General supportive measures also are important, including

- termination of exposure, by removal of the patient or application of a gas mask if the atmosphere remains contaminated, removal and destruction of contaminated clothing, copious washing of contaminated skin or mucous membranes with water, or gastric lavage;
- maintenance of a patent airway, including endobronchial aspiration;
- artificial respiration; administration of O_2, if required;
- alleviation of persistent convulsions with diazepam (5–10 mg IV); and
- treatment of shock.

Atropine should be given in doses sufficient to cross the blood-brain barrier. Following an initial injection of 2–4 mg, given intravenously if possible, otherwise intramuscularly, 2 mg should be given every 5–10 min until muscarinic symptoms disappear, if they reappear, or until signs of atropine toxicity appear. More than 200 mg may be required on the first day. AChE reactivating agents and mild degree of atropine block then should be maintained for as long as symptoms are evident.

Although the phosphorylated esteratic site of AChE undergoes hydrolytic regeneration at a slow or negligible rate, nucleophilic agents, such as hydroxylamine (NH_2OH), hydroxamic acids (RCONH–OH), and oximes (RCH=NOH), reactivate the enzyme more rapidly than does spontaneous hydrolysis. Froede and Wilson (1971) reasoned that selective reactivation could be achieved by a site-directed nucleophile, wherein interaction of a quaternary nitrogen with the negative subsite of the active center would place the nucleophile in close apposition to the phosphorus. The oxime is oriented proximally to exert a nucleophilic attack on the phosphorus; a phosphoryloxime is formed, leaving the regenerated enzyme (Figure 10–2E).

Several *bis*-quaternary aldoximes are even more potent as reactivators for insecticide and nerve gas poisoning; examples are obidoxime and HI-6, which are used in Europe as antidotes (Worek and Thiermann, 2013; Steinritz et al., 2016). However, these compounds do not cross the blood-brain barrier, limiting their effectiveness to peripheral nervous system sites only.

Certain phosphorylated AChEs can undergo a fairly rapid process of "aging," so that within the course of minutes or hours they become completely resistant to the reactivators. Aging is due to the loss of one alkoxy group, leaving a much more stable monoalkyl- or monoalkoxy-phosphoryl-AChE (Figure 10–2D and 10–2E). Organophosphorus compounds containing tertiary alkoxy groups, such as soman, are more prone to aging than are congeners containing the secondary or primary alkoxy groups. The oximes are not effective in antagonizing the toxicity of the more rapidly hydrolyzing carbamoyl ester inhibitors; since 2-PAM itself has weak anti-ChE activity, it is not recommended for the treatment of overdosage with neostigmine or physostigmine or poisoning with carbamoylating insecticides such as carbaryl.

Reactivation and Disposition

The reactivating action of oximes in vivo is most marked at the skeletal neuromuscular junction. Antidotal effects are less striking at autonomic effector sites, and the quaternary ammonium group restricts entry into the CNS (Eddleston et al., 2008; Eddleston and Clark, 2011).

Although high doses or accumulation of oximes can inhibit AChE and cause neuromuscular blockade, they should be given until one can be assured of clearance of the offending organophosphate. Current antidotal therapy for organophosphate exposure resulting from warfare or terrorism includes parenteral atropine, an oxime (2-PAM, HI-6 or obidoxime), and diazepam or midazolam as anticonvulsants (King and Aaron, 2015; Worek and Thiermann, 2013). The oximes and their metabolites are readily eliminated by the kidney.

Parenterally administered human butyrylcholinesterase and recombinant DNA-expressed paraoxonases and phosphotriesterases with selected mutations are under development to scavenge the organophosphate at its portal of entry or plasma before it reaches peripheral and central tissue sites (Cerasoli et al., 2005; Mata et al., 2014; Worek et al., 2014). Because scavenging by butyrylcholinesterase is stoichiometric rather than catalytic, large quantities are required, so a broad spectrum of catalytic activities from other phosphoesterases is sought. Catalytic enzyme scavengers are limited by their slow distribution from intramuscular sites; rapid scavenging by enzymes requires intravenous administration.

Certain fluorine-containing organophosphorus anti-ChE agents (e.g., DFP, mipafox) have the property of inducing delayed neurotoxicity, a property they share with the triarylphosphates, of which TOCP is the classical example. This syndrome first received widespread attention following the demonstration that TOCP, an adulterant of Jamaica ginger, was responsible for an outbreak of thousands of cases of paralysis that occurred in the U.S. during Prohibition.

The clinical picture is that of severe polyneuropathy manifested initially by mild sensory disturbances, ataxia, weakness, muscle fatigue and twitching, reduced tendon reflexes, and tenderness to palpation. In severe cases, the weakness may progress to flaccid paralysis and muscle wasting. Recovery may require several years and may be incomplete.

Toxicity from this organophosphate-induced delayed polyneuropathy is not dependent on inhibition of cholinesterases; instead, a distinct esterase, termed *neurotoxic esterase,* is linked to the lesions (Johnson, 1993). This enzyme has a specificity for hydrophobic esters, but its natural substrate and function remain unknown (Glynn, 2006; Read et al., 2009). Myopathies that result in generalized necrotic lesions and changes in endplate cytostructure also are found in experimental animals after long-term exposure to organophosphates (De Bleecker et al., 1991).

Therapeutic Uses of AChE Inhibitors

Current use of anti-AChE agents is limited to four conditions in the periphery:

- atony of the smooth muscle of the intestinal tract and urinary bladder
- glaucoma
- myasthenia gravis
- reversal of the paralysis of competitive neuromuscular blocking drugs

Long-acting and hydrophobic ChE inhibitors are the only inhibitors with well-documented efficacy, albeit limited, in the treatment of dementia symptoms of Alzheimer disease. Physostigmine, with its shorter duration of action, is used to treat intoxication by atropine and several

drugs with anticholinergic side effects (discussed further in the chapter); it also is indicated for the treatment of Friedreich or other inherited ataxias. Edrophonium has been used for terminating attacks of paroxysmal supraventricular tachycardia.

Available Therapeutic Agents

The compounds described here are those commonly used as anti-ChE drugs and ChE reactivators in the U.S. Preparations used solely for ophthalmic purposes are described in Chapter 69. Conventional dosages and routes of administration are given in the further discussion of therapeutic applications.

Physostigmine salicylate is available for injection. Physostigmine sulfate ophthalmic ointment and physostigmine salicylate ophthalmic solution also are available. Pyridostigmine bromide is available for oral or parenteral use. Neostigmine bromide is available for oral use. Neostigmine methylsulfate is marketed for parenteral injection. Ambenonium chloride is available for oral use. Tacrine, donepezil, rivastigmine, and galantamine have been approved for the treatment of Alzheimer disease.

Pralidoxime chloride is the only AChE reactivator currently available in the U.S. and can be obtained in a parenteral formulation. HI-6 is available in several European and Near Eastern countries.

AMBENONIUM

PRALIDOXIME (2-PAM)

Paralytic Ileus and Atony of the Urinary Bladder

In the treatment of both paralytic ileus and urinary bladder atony, neostigmine generally is preferred among the anti-ChE agents. Directly acting muscarinic agonists (Chapter 9) are employed for the same purposes.

Neostigmine is used for the relief of abdominal distension and acute colonic pseudo-obstruction from a variety of medical and surgical causes (Ponec et al., 1999). The usual subcutaneous dose of neostigmine methylsulfate for postoperative paralytic ileus is 0.5 mg, given as needed. Peristaltic activity commences 10–30 min after parenteral administration, whereas 2–4 h are required after oral administration of neostigmine bromide (15–30 mg). It may be necessary to assist evacuation with a small low enema or gas with a rectal tube.

When neostigmine is used for the treatment of atony of the detrusor muscle of the urinary bladder, postoperative dysuria is relieved. The drug is used in a similar dose and manner as in the management of paralytic ileus. Neostigmine should not be used when the intestine or urinary bladder is obstructed, when peritonitis is present, when the viability of the bowel is doubtful, or when bowel dysfunction results from inflammatory bowel disease.

Glaucoma and Other Ophthalmologic Indications

Glaucoma is a complex disease characterized by an increase in intraocular pressure that, if sufficiently high and persistent, will damage the optic disc at the juncture of the optic nerve and the retina; irreversible blindness can result. Of the three types of glaucoma—primary, secondary, and congenital—anti-AChE agents are of value in the management of the primary as well as of certain categories of the secondary type (e.g., aphakic glaucoma, following cataract extraction); congenital glaucoma rarely responds to any therapy other than surgery. Primary glaucoma is subdivided into narrow-angle (acute congestive) and wide-angle (chronic simple) types, based on the configuration of the angle of the anterior chamber where the aqueous humor is reabsorbed.

Narrow-angle glaucoma is nearly always a medical emergency in which drugs are essential in controlling the acute attack, but the long-range management is often surgical (e.g., peripheral or complete iridectomy). Wide-angle glaucoma, on the other hand, has a gradual, insidious onset and is not generally amenable to surgical improvement; in this type, control of intraocular pressure usually is dependent on continuous drug therapy.

Because the cholinergic agonists and ChE inhibitors also block accommodation and induce myopia, these agents produce transient blurring of far vision, limited visual acuity in low light, and loss of vision at the margin when instilled in the eye. With long-term administration of the cholinergic agonists and anti-ChE agents, the compromise of vision diminishes. Nevertheless, other agents without these side effects, such as prostaglandin analogues, β adrenergic receptor antagonists, and carbonic anhydrase inhibitors, have become the primary topical therapies for open-angle glaucoma. AChE inhibitors are held in reserve for the chronic conditions when patients become refractory to the agents mentioned. Topical treatment with long-acting ChE inhibitors such as echothiophate give rise to symptoms characteristic of systemic ChE inhibition. (For a complete account of the use of anti-ChE agents in ocular therapy, see Chapter 69).

Myasthenia Gravis

Myasthenia gravis is a neuromuscular disease of complex genetic etiology characterized by exacerbations and remissions of weakness and marked fatigability of skeletal muscle (Drachman, 1994; Renton et al., 2015).

The relative importance of prejunctional and postjunctional defects in myasthenia gravis was unknown until Patrick and Lindstrom (1973) found that rabbits immunized with nicotinic receptor slowly developed muscular weakness and respiratory difficulties that resembled the symptoms of myasthenia gravis. This animal model prompted intense investigation into whether the natural disease represented an autoimmune response directed toward the ACh receptor. Antireceptor antibodies are detectable in sera of 90% of patients with the disease, although the clinical status of the patient does not correlate precisely with antibody titers (Drachman, 1994). Sequences and the structural location in the α_1 subunit constituting the main immunogenic region are well defined (Lindstrom, 2008).

The picture that emerges is that myasthenia gravis is caused by an autoimmune response primarily to the ACh receptor at the postjunctional end plate. These antibodies reduce the number of receptors detectable either by snake α-neurotoxin–binding assays (Fambrough et al., 1973) or by electrophysiological measurements of ACh sensitivity (Drachman, 1994). Immune complexes along with marked ultrastructural abnormalities appear in the synaptic cleft and enhance receptor degradation through complement-mediated lysis in the end plate.

In a subset of about 10% of patients presenting with a myasthenic syndrome, muscle weakness has a congenital rather than an autoimmune basis. Characterization of biochemical and genetic bases of the congenital condition has demonstrated mutations in the ACh receptor that affect ligand-binding, channel-opening kinetics and durations; receptor biosynthesis; and synaptic location of receptors (Engel et al., 2012; Sine and Engel, 2006). Other mutations occur as a deficiency in the form of AChE that contains the collagen-like tail unit, in presynaptic transporters involved in the uptake of choline, and in vesicular storage of ACh. In this group of patients, identification of the mutation is essential for ascertaining whether a specific pharmacologic treatment is warranted.

Diagnosis

Although the diagnosis of autoimmune myasthenia gravis usually can be made from the history, signs, and symptoms, its differentiation from certain neurasthenic, infectious, endocrine, congenital, neoplastic, and degenerative neuromuscular diseases can be challenging. However, in autoimmune myasthenia gravis, the aforementioned deficiencies and enhancement of muscle strength can be improved dramatically by anti-ChE medication. The edrophonium test for initial diagnosis relies on these responses. The edrophonium test is performed by rapid intravenous injection of 2 mg of edrophonium chloride, followed 45 sec later by an additional 8 mg if the first dose is without effect. A positive response consists of brief improvement in strength, unaccompanied by lingual fasciculation (which generally occurs in nonmyasthenic patients).

An excessive dose of an anti-ChE drug results in a *cholinergic crisis*. The condition is characterized by weakness resulting from generalized depolarization of the motor end plate; other features result from overstimulation of muscarinic receptors. The weakness resulting from depolarization blockade may resemble myasthenic weakness, which is manifest when anti-ChE medication is insufficient. The distinction is of obvious practical importance because the former is treated by withholding, and the latter by administering, the anti-ChE agent. Detection of antireceptor antibodies in muscle biopsies or plasma is now widely employed to establish the diagnosis.

Treatment of Myasthenia Gravis

Pyridostigmine, neostigmine, and ambenonium are the standard anti-ChE drugs used in the symptomatic treatment of myasthenia gravis. All can increase the response of myasthenic muscle to repetitive nerve impulses, primarily by the preservation of endogenous ACh. Following AChE inhibition, receptors over a greater cross-sectional area of the end plate presumably are exposed to concentrations of ACh that are sufficient for channel opening and production of a postsynaptic end-plate potential.

Unpredictable exacerbations and remissions of the myasthenic state may require adjustment of dosage. Pyridostigmine is available in sustained-release tablets containing a total of 180 mg, of which 60 mg are released immediately and 120 mg are released over several hours; this preparation is of value in maintaining patients for 6- to 8-h periods but should be limited to use at bedtime. Muscarinic cardiovascular and GI side effects of anti-ChE agents generally can be controlled by atropine or other anticholinergic drugs (Chapter 9). However, these anticholinergic drugs mask many side effects of an excessive dose of an anti-ChE agent. In most patients, tolerance develops eventually to the muscarinic effects. Several drugs, including curariform agents and certain antibiotics and general anesthetics, interfere with neuromuscular transmission (Chapter 11); their administration to patients with myasthenia gravis requires proper adjustment of anti-ChE dosage and other precautions.

Other therapeutic measures are essential elements in the management of this disease. Glucocorticoids promote clinical improvement in a high percentage of patients. However, when treatment with steroids is continued over prolonged periods, a high incidence of side effects may result (Chapter 46). Initiation of steroid treatment augments muscle weakness; however, as the patient improves with continued administration of steroids, doses of anti-ChE drugs can be reduced (Drachman, 1994). Other immunosuppressive agents, such as azathioprine and cyclosporine and high-dose cyclophosphamide (Drachman et al., 2008), have also been beneficial in more refractory cases (Chapter 35). Thymectomy should be considered in myasthenia associated with a thymoma or when the disease is not controlled adequately by anti-ChE agents and steroids. Because the thymus contains myoid cells with nicotinic receptors (Schluep et al., 1987), and a predominance of patients have thymic abnormalities, the thymus may be responsible for the initial pathogenesis. It also is the source of autoreactive T-helper cells.

Alzheimer Disease

A deficiency of intact cholinergic neurons, particularly those extending from subcortical areas such as the nucleus basalis, has been observed in patients with progressive dementia of the Alzheimer type (Chapter 18). Using a rationale similar to that in other CNS degenerative diseases, therapy for enhancing concentrations of cholinergic and other neurotransmitters in the CNS has been investigated.

In 1993, the FDA approved tacrine (tetrahydroaminoacridine) for use in mild-to-moderate Alzheimer disease, but a high incidence of enhanced alanine aminotransferase and hepatotoxicity limited the utility of this drug.

Subsequently, donepezil was approved for clinical use and has emerged as the primary agent for treatment in multiple countries (Lee et al., 2015).

Initially, 5-mg doses are administered daily, and if tolerated, doses are increased to 10 mg for mild-to-moderate conditions. Recent clinical trials in moderate-to-severe Alzheimer disease have confirmed benefits for a 23-mg/d sustained release form. Most studies are carried out for periods of 24 weeks, although treatment periods have been extended, usually extending the treatment baseline, but without further improvement or some decline after 6 months. Adverse side effects have been attributed to excessive peripheral cholinergic stimulation and include nasopharyngitis, diarrhea, nausea, and vomiting. Rhabdomyolysis reportedly occurs, requiring discontinuation of the drug. Cotreatment with memantine did not result in significant improvement over the higher-dose donepezil treatment (Howard et al., 2012).

Rivastigmine, a more lipid soluble, longer-acting carbamylating inhibitor, is approved for use in the U.S. and Europe in both oral and skin patch forms. While having similar side effects to other cholinesterase inhibitors, rivastigmine is reported to have shown a higher incidence of fatalities than other cholinesterase inhibitors used in Alzheimer dementias (Ali et al., 2015). It has not been determined whether the increase relates to misuse of the transdermal form of administration. Galantamine is another FDA-approved agent for Alzheimer dementias, acting as a reversible AChE inhibitor with a side-effect profile similar to that of donepezil.

These three cholinesterase inhibitors, which have the requisite affinity and hydrophobicity to cross the blood-brain barrier and exhibit a prolonged duration of action, along with an excitatory amino acid transmitter mimic, memantine, constitute current modes of therapy. These agents are not disease modifying and lack well-documented actions on the pathology of Alzheimer disease. However, the bulk of the evidence indicates that they slow the decline in cognitive function and behavioral manifestation for limited intervals of time (Chapter 18). Associated symptoms, such as depression, may be preferentially delayed (Lu et al., 2009). Current clinical research efforts are directed to synergistic actions of arresting inflammatory processes or neurodegeneration and combining cholinesterase inhibition with selective cholinergic receptor modulation.

Prophylaxis in Cholinesterase Inhibitor Poisoning

Studies in experimental animals have shown that pretreatment with pyridostigmine reduces the incapacitation and mortality associated with nerve agent poisoning, particularly for agents such as soman that show rapid aging. The first large-scale administration of pyridostigmine to humans occurred in 1990 in anticipation of nerve agent attack in the first Gulf War. At an oral dose of 30 mg every 8 h, the incidence of side effects was around 1%; fewer than 0.1% of the subjects had responses sufficient to warrant discontinuing the drug in the setting of military action (Keeler et al., 1991). Long-term follow-up indicates that veterans of the Gulf War who received pyridostigmine showed a low incidence of a neurologic syndrome, now termed the *Persian Gulf War syndrome*. It is characterized by impaired cognition, ataxia, confusion, myoneuropathy, adenopathy, weakness, and incontinence (Haley et al., 1997).

Controversy still surrounds the basis of Gulf War syndrome or illness, despite multiple reports and reviews by the U.S. Department of Veterans Affairs in 2008 and 2010 and the Institute of Medicine (Committee on Gulf War and Health, 2013; Institute of Medicine, 2013). Although several origins of the syndrome, such as pyridostigmine administration, have been ruled out as unlikely, the constellation of symptoms reflect an interplay of chemical toxicants and psychological factors, encompassing widespread pesticide use, and exposure from postwar demolition bombing of munitions facilities likely containing chemical warfare agents (sarin and mustards). Psychological factors, emerging as post-traumatic stress disorders, have been documented in prolonged wars since the early 20th century.

Intoxication by Anticholinergic Drugs

In addition to atropine and other muscarinic agents, many other drugs, such as the phenothiazines, antihistamines, and tricyclic antidepressants, have central and peripheral anticholinergic activity. Physostigmine is potentially useful in reversing the central anticholinergic syndrome produced by overdosage or an unusual reaction to these drugs (Nilsson, 1982). While the effectiveness of physostigmine in reversing anticholinergic side effects has been documented, other toxic effects of the tricyclic antidepressants and phenothiazines (Chapters 15 and 16), such as intraventricular conduction deficits and ventricular arrhythmias, are not reversed by physostigmine. In addition, physostigmine may precipitate seizures; hence, its usually small potential benefit must be weighed against this risk. The use of anti-ChE agents to reverse the effects of competitive neuromuscular blocking agents is discussed in Chapter 11.

Drug Facts for Your Personal Formulary: *Anticholinesterase Agents*

Drugs	Therapeutic Uses	Major Toxicity and Clinical Pearls
Noncovalent Reversible Inhibitors		
Edrophonium Tacrine Donepezil Propidium Fasciculin Galantamine	• Edrophonium can be used to diagnose myasthenia gravis • Tacrine, donepezil and galantamine used for Alzheimer disease	• Edrophonium and tacrine: bind reversibly to choline subsite near Trp86 and Glu202 • Edrophonium has a short duration of action because of rapid renal elimination; effects are limited to the peripheral nervous system. • Donepezil and tacrine: higher affinity for AChE, more hydrophobic, can cross BBB. • Tacrine: high incidence of hepatotoxicity • Donepezil binds with higher affinity to the active center gorge of AChE. • Propidium & fasciculin: bind peripheral anionic site on AChE
Carbamate Inhibitors		
"Reversible" Carbamate Inhibitors Physostigmine Neostigmine Pyridostigmine Ambenonium Rivastigmine	• Pyridostigmine, neostigmine and ambenonium are used for treatment of myasthenia gravis • Neostigmine is used for paralytic ileus and atony of the urinary bladder • Rivastigmine, a very lipid soluble alternative for treating Alzheimer disease • Pyridostigmine used prophylactically in nerve gas attacks	• Drugs with carbamoyl ester linkage: AChE substrates that block by carbamylation of AChE active center serine, are hydrolyzed slowly; regarded as hemi-substrate blockers • Neostigmine and pyridostigmine are poorly absorbed after oral administration • Pyridostigmine: available in sustained release tablets; oral dose much higher than parenteral dose • Rivastigmine can cross the BBB, has longer duration of action, and is available in oral and epidermal patch formulations

Drug Facts for Your Personal Formulary: *Anticholinesterase Agents (continued)*

Drugs	Therapeutic Uses	Major Toxicity and Clinical Pearls
Carbamate Inhibitors		
Carbamate insecticides Carbaryl Propoxur Aldicarb	• Garden insecticides	• Symptoms of poisoning resemble those of organophosphates but are more readily reversed and less toxic
Organophosphates		
Echothiophate	• Treatment of glaucoma	• Instilled locally in the eye • Stable in aqueous solution
Nerve Agents DFP Tabun Sarin Soman Cyclosarin VX	• Alkylphosphates are the most potent synthetic toxins • React covalently with the active site serine • Potent and irreversible inactivators of ChE • Recent documented use in terrorism	• Form a stable conjugate with the active site serine by phosphorylation/phosphonylation • Hydrolyzed by hepatic carboxyesterases and paraoxonases • Low MW, hydrophobic, rapidly penetrates into CNS from pulmonary inhalation • Tabun, sarin, and cyclosarin are volatile and extremely toxic "nerve gases" • VX is absorbed through the skin, has slower onset, but high toxicity • 2-PAM and related aldoximes are used to reactivate organophosphate-ChE conjugates • Resistance to organophosphate-AChE reactivation is enhanced through "aging" that results from loss of one alkyl group
Pesticides Parathion Methylparathion Malathion Diazonin Chlorpyrifos	• Insecticides largely agricultural • Malathion is used topically in the treatment of pediculosis in cases of permethrin resistance • Lethal dose of malathion in mammals is 1g/kg • Diazinon and chlorpyrifos are used widely in agriculture	• Metabolism of these *thion* pesticides to the corresponding *oxon* confers pesticide activity and toxicity, more rapid rate in insects • Malathion: detoxified by plasma carboxylesterases, a detoxification reaction that is more rapid in mammals and birds than insects, yielding a further margin of safety
Antidotal therapy for Organophosphate Exposure		
Cholinesterase reactivators 2-PAM HI-6 Obidoxime	• Quaternary pyridinium aldoxime reactivators indicated for insecticide and nerve gas poisoning • Improved agents in development	• Reactivates organophosphate-AChE conjugate by attacking the conjugated phosphorus to form phospho-oxime and regenerate the active enzyme • Dose is infused IV or IM with autoinjector; dosing should be repeated frequently • Early treatment helps insure that the oxime reaches the phosphorylated enzyme prior to complete "aging" • Reactivators do not cross the blood-brain barrier and do not reactivate CNS AChE
Anticholinergic agents Atropine	• Blocks symptoms mediated through muscarinic receptors	• Given by parenterally in 2-4mg doses every few min until muscarinic symptoms disappear
Benzodiazepines Diazepam Midazolam	• Minimize seizures and associated neuronal toxicity	• Administered parenterally post-exposure

Bibliography

Ali TB, et al. Adverse effects of cholinesterase inhibitors in dementia, according to pharmacovigilance data of the United States and Canada. *PLoS One*, **2015**, *10*:e0144337.

Bourne Y, et al. Acetylcholinesterase inhibition by fasciculin: crystal structure of the complex. *Cell*, **1995**, *83*:493–506.

Burkhart CG. Relationship of treatment resistant head lice to the safety and efficacy of pediculicides. *Mayo Clin Proc*, **2004**, *79*:661–666.

Camp S, et al. Acetylcholinesterase expression in muscle is specifically controlled by a promoter selective enhancesome in the first intron. *J Neurosci*, **2008**, *28*:2459–2470.

Centers for Disease Control and Prevention. Head lice: treatment. **2015**. http://www.cdc.gov/parasites/lice/head/treatment.html. Accessed March 12, 2016.

Cerasoli DM, et al. In vitro and in vivo characterization of recombinant human butyrylcholinesterase (Protexia) as a potential nerve agent scavenger. *Chem Biol Interactions*, **2005**, *157–158*:363–365.

Cohan SL, et al. The pharmacokinetics of pyridostigmine. *Neurology*, **1976**, *26*:536–539.

Committee on Gulf War and Health Reports, *Update of Health Effects of Serving in the Gulf War and Treatment of Chronic Multi-symptom Illness*. National Academies Press, Washington, DC, **2013**.

Costa LG, et al. Paraoxonase 1 (PON1) as a genetic determinant of susceptibility to organophosphate toxicity. *Toxicology*, **2013**, *307*:115–122.

Council on Foreign Relations. UN report on chemical weapons use in Syria. **2013**. http://www.cfr.org/syria/un-report-chemical-weapons-use-syria/p31404. Accessed March 12, 2016.

Cummings JL. Alzheimer's disease. *N Engl J Med*, **2004**, *351*:56–67.

Cygler M, et al. Relationship between sequence conservation and three dimensional structure in a large family of esterases, lipases and related proteins. *Protein Sci*, **1993**, *2*:366–382.

De Bleecker J, et al. Histological and histochemical study of paraoxon myopathy in the rat. *Acta Neurol Belg*, **1991**, *91*:255–270.

Dobbertin A, et al. Targeting acetylcholinesterase in neurons: a dual processing function for the proline-rich membrane anchor and the attachment domain of the catalytic subunit. *J Neurosci*, **2009**, *29*:4519–4530.

Dolgin E. Syrian gas attack reinforces need for better antisarin drugs. *Nat Med*, **2013**, *19*:1194–1195.

Drachman DB. Myasthenia gravis. *N Engl J Med*, **1994**, *330*:1797–1810.

Drachman DB, et al. Robooting the immune system with high-dose cyclophosphamide for treatment of refractory myasthenia gravis. *Ann N Y Acad Sci*, **2008**, *1132*:305–314.

Eaton DL, et al. Review of the toxicology of chlorpyrifos with an emphasis on human exposure and neurodevelopment. *Clin Rev Toxicol*, **2008**, *38*:1–125.

Eddleston M, Chowdhury FR. Pharmacological treatment of organo-phosphorus insecticide poisoning: the old and the (possible) new. *Brit J Clin Pharm*, **2015**, *81*:462–470.

Eddleston M, Clark R. Insecticides: organophosphorus compounds and carbamates. In Nelson LS, ed. *Goldfrank's Toxicologic Emergencies*. McGraw-Hill Medical, New York, **2011**, 150–166.

Engel AG, et al. New horizons for congenital myasthenic syndromes. *Ann N Y Acad Sci*, **2012**, *1275*:54–62.

Fambrough DM, et al. Neuromuscular junction in myasthenia gravis: decreased acetylcholine receptors. *Science*, **1973**, *182*:293–295.

Froede HC, Wilson IB. Acetylcholinesterase. In Boyer PD, ed. *The Enzymes*, vol. 5. Academic Press, New York, **1971**, 87–114.

Furlong CE. Genetic variability in the cytochrome P450–paraoxonase 1 pathway for detoxication of organophosphorus compounds. *J Biochem Molec Toxicol*, **2007**, *21*:197–205.

Gallo MA, Lawryk NJ. Organic phosphorus pesticides. In Hayes WJ Jr, Laws ER Jr, eds. *Handbook of Pesticide Toxicology*, vol. 2. Academic Press, San Diego, CA, **1991**, 917–1123.

Giacobini E. Cholinesterase inhibitors: from the Calabar bean to Alzheimer's therapy. In Giacobini E, ed. *Cholinesterases and Cholinesterase Inhibitors*. Martin Dunitz, London, **2000**, 181–227.

Glynn P. A mechanism for organophosphate-induced delayed neuropathy. *Toxicol Lett*, **2006**, *162*:94–97.

Haley RW, et al. Is there a Gulf War syndrome? *JAMA*, **1997**, *277*:215–222.

Harel M, et al. Structure and evolution of the serum paraoxonase family of detoxifying and anti-atherosclerotic enzymes. *Nat Struct Mol Biol*, **2004**, *11*:412–419.

Holmstedt B. Cholinesterase inhibitors: an introduction. In Giacobini E, ed. *Cholinesterases and Cholinesterase Inhibitors*. Martin Dunitz, London, **2000**, 1–8.

Institute of Medicine (National Academy of Science–USA). *Gulf War and Health*, vol. 2. National Academies Press, Washington, DC, **2013**.

Howard R, et al. Donepezil and memantine for moderate to severe Alzheimer's disease. *N Eng J Med*, **2012**, *366*:893–903.

Jennings LL, et al. Direct analysis of the kinetic profiles of organophosphate-acetylcholinesterase adducts by MALDI-TOF mass spectrometry. *Biochemistry*, **2003**, *42*:11083–11091.

Johnson MK. Symposium introduction: retrospect and prospects for neuropathy target esterase (NTE) and the delayed polyneuropathy (OPIDP) induced by some organophosphorus esters. *Chem Biol Interact*, **1993**, *87*:339–346.

Karczmar AG. History of the research with anticholinesterase agents. In Karczmar AG, ed. *Anticholinesterase Agents*, vol. 1, *International Encyclopedia of Pharmacology and Therapeutics*, section 13. Pergamon Press, Oxford, UK, **1970**, 1–44.

Keeler JR, et al. Pyridostigmine used as a nerve agent pretreatment under wartime conditions. *JAMA*, **1991**, *266*:693–695.

King AM, Aaron CK. Organophosphate and carbamate poisoning. *Emerg Med Clin N Am*, **2015**, *33*:133–151.

Lee J-H, et al. Donepezil across the spectrum of Alzheimer's disease: dose optimization and clinical relevance. *Acta Neurol Scand*, **2015**, *131*:259–267.

Lindstrom JM. Myasthenia gravis and the tops and bottoms of AChRs-antigenic structure of the MIR and specific immuno-suppression of EAMG using AChR cytoplasmic domains. *Ann N Y Acad Sci*, **2008**, *1132*:29–41.

Lockridge O. Review of human butyrylcholinesterase structure, function genetic variants history of use in the clinic and potential therapeutic uses. *Pharmacol Ther*, **2015**, *148*:34–46.

Lockridge O, et al. Complete amino acid sequence of human serum cholinesterase. *J Biol Chem*, **1987**, *262*:549–557.

Lotti M. Low-level exposures to organophosphorus esters and peripheral nerve function. *Muscle Nerve*, **2002**, *25*:492–504.

Lu PH, et al. Donepezil delays progression of A.D. in MCI subjects with depressive symptoms. *Neurology*, **2009**, *72*:2115–2212.

Mackness M, Mackness B. Human paraoxonase 1 (PON 1): gene structure and expression, promiscuous acitivties and multiple physiological roles. *Gene*, **2015**, *567*:12–21.

Massoulié J. Molecular forms and anchoring of acetylcholinesterase. In Giacobini E, ed. *Cholinesterases and Cholinesterase Inhibitors*. Martin Dunitz, London, **2000**, 81–103.

Mata DG, et al. Investigation of evolved paraoxonase-1 variants for prevention of organophosphate pesticide compound introxication. *J Pharmacol Exp Ther*, **2014**, *349*:549–558.

Nilsson E. Physostigmine treatment in various drug-induced intoxications. *Ann Clin Res*, **1982**, *14*:165–172.

Nozaki H, Aikawa N. Sarin poisoning in Tokyo subway. *Lancet*, **1995**, *346*:1446–1447.

Padilla S, et al. Further assessment of an in vitro screen that may help identify organophosphate insecticides that are more acutely toxic to the young. *J Toxicol Environ Health*, **2004**, *67*:1477–1489.

Patrick J, Lindstrom J. Autoimmune response to acetylcholine receptor. *Science*, **1973**, *180*:871–872.

Ponec RJ, et al. Neostigmine for the treatment of acute colonic pseudo-obstruction. *N Engl J Med*, **1999**, *341*:137–141.

Read DJ, et al. Neuropathy target esterase is required for adult vertebrate axon maintenance. *J Neurosci*, **2009**, *29*:11594–11600.

Reiner E, Radić Z. Mechanism of action of cholinesterase inhibitors. In Giacobini E, ed. *Cholinesterases and Cholinesterase Inhibitors*. Martin Dunitz, London, **2000**, 103–120.

Renton AE, et al. A genome-wide association study of myasthenia gravis. *JAMA Neurol*. **2015**, *72*:394–404.

Rosenberry TL. Acetylcholinesterase. *Adv Enzymol Relat Areas Mol Biol*, **1975**, *43*:103–218.

Schluep M, et al. Acetylcholine receptors in human thymic myoid cells in situ: an immunohistological study. *Ann Neurol*, **1987**, *22*: 212–222.

Schumacher M, et al. Primary structure of *Torpedo californica* acetyl-cholinesterase deduced from its cDNA sequence. *Nature*, **1986**, *319*: 407–409.

Silman I, Sussman JL. Structural studies on acetylcholinesterase. In Giacobini E, ed. *Cholinesterases and Cholinesterase Inhibitors*. Martin Dunitz, London, **2000**, 9–26.

Sine SM, Engel AG. Recent advances in Cys-loop receptor structure and function. *Nature (London)*, **2006**, *440*:448–455.

Steinritz D et al. Repetitive obidoxime treatment induced increase of red blood cell acetylcholinesterase activity even in a late phase of a severe methamidophos poisoning: A case report. *Toxicol Lett*, **2016**, *244*:121–123.

Storm JE, et al. Occupational exposure limits for 30 organophosphate pesticides based on inhibition of red blood cell acetylcholinesterase. *Toxicology*, **2000**, *150*:1–29.

Sussman JL, et al. Atomic structure of acetylcholinesterase from *Torpedo californica*: a prototypic acetylcholine-binding protein. *Science*, **1991**, *253*:872–879.

Taylor P, et al. The genes encoding the cholinesterases: structure, evolutionary relationships and regulation of their expression. In Giacobini E, ed. *Cholinesterases and Cholinesterase Inhibitors*. Martin Dunitz, London, **2000**, 63–80.

Taylor P, Radic Z. The cholinesterases: from genes to proteins. *Ann Rev Pharmacol*, **1994**, *34*:281–320.

Worek F, et al., Post-exposure treatment of VX poisoned guinea pigs with engineered phosphotriesterase mutant: a proof-of-concept study. *Toxicology Lett*, **2014**, *231*:45–54.

Worek F, Wille T, et al. Toxicology of organophosphorus compounds in view of an increasing terrorist threat. *Arch Toxicol*, **2016**, *90*:2131–2145.

Xie W, et al. Postnatal development delay and supersensitivity to organophosphate in gene-targeted mice lacking acetylcholinesterase. *J Pharmacol Exp Ther*, **2000**, *293*:892–902.

Chapter 11

Nicotine and Agents Acting at the Neuromuscular Junction and Autonomic Ganglia

Ryan E. Hibbs and Alexander C. Zambon

THE NICOTINIC ACETYLCHOLINE RECEPTOR
- Perspective
- Structure of Nicotinic Receptors

TRANSMISSION AT THE NEUROMUSCULAR JUNCTION
- Neuromuscular Blocking Agents
- Clinical Pharmacology

GANGLIONIC NEUROTRANSMISSION
- The Neural Nicotinic Receptor and Postsynaptic Potentials
- Ganglionic Stimulating Agents
- Ganglionic Blocking Agents

NICOTINE ADDICTION AND SMOKING CESSATION
- Nicotine Replacement Therapy
- Varenicline
- Cytisine

The Nicotinic Acetylcholine Receptor

The nicotinic ACh receptor mediates neurotransmission postsynaptically at the neuromuscular junction and peripheral autonomic ganglia; in the CNS, it largely modulates release of neurotransmitters from presynaptic sites. The receptor is called the *nicotinic ACh receptor* because both the alkaloid nicotine and the neurotransmitter ACh can stimulate the receptor. Distinct subtypes of nicotinic receptors exist at the neuromuscular junction (N_m), in autonomic ganglia, and in the CNS (the neuronal form, N_n). The binding of ACh to the nicotinic ACh receptor initiates an EPP in muscle or an EPSP in peripheral ganglia by directly mediating cation influx into the postsynaptic cell (see Chapter 8).

Perspective

Classical studies of the actions of curare and nicotine defined the concept of the nicotinic ACh receptor over a century ago and made this the prototypical pharmacological receptor. By taking advantage of specialized structures that have evolved to mediate cholinergic neurotransmission and of natural toxins that block motor activity, nicotinic receptors were isolated and characterized. These accomplishments represent landmarks in the development of molecular pharmacology.

Cholinergic neurotransmission mediates motor activity in marine vertebrates and mammals, and a large number of peptide, terpinoid, and alkaloid toxins that block the nicotinic receptors have evolved to enhance predation or protect plant and animal species from predation (Taylor et al., 2007). Among these toxins are the α-toxins: peptides of about 7 kDa from venoms of the krait, *Bungarus multicinctus*, and varieties of the cobra, *Naja naja*. These toxins potently inhibit neuromuscular transmission, are readily radiolabeled, and provide excellent probes for the nicotinic receptor.

The electrical organs from the aquatic species of *Electrophorus* and *Torpedo* provide rich sources of nicotinic receptor; up to 40% of the surface of the electric organ's membrane is excitable and contains cholinergic receptors, in contrast to vertebrate skeletal muscle, in which motor end plates occupy 0.1% or less of the cell surface. Using the α-toxin probes, the receptor from *Torpedo* was purified, the cDNAs of the subunits were isolated, and the genes were cloned for the multiple receptor subunits from mammalian neurons and muscle (Numa et al., 1983). By simultaneously expressing various permutations of the genes that encode the individual subunits in cellular systems and then measuring binding and the electrophysiological events that result from activation by agonists, researchers have been able to correlate functional properties with details of primary structures of the receptor subtypes (Changeux and Edelstein, 2005; Karlin, 2002; Sine et al., 2008).

Structure of Nicotinic Receptors

In vertebrates, the nicotinic receptors of skeletal muscle N_m are pentamers composed of four distinct subunits (α, β, γ, and δ) in a stoichiometric ratio of 2:1:1:1 (Changeux and Edelstein, 2005; Karlin, 2002; Unwin, 2005). In mature, innervated muscle end plates, the γ subunit is replaced by ε, a closely related subunit. The individual subunits are about 40% identical in their amino acid sequences. The nicotinic receptor is the prototype for other pentameric ligand-gated ion channels, which include the receptors for the inhibitory amino acids (GABA and glycine; Chapter 14) and $5HT_3$ receptors (Chapter 13). Each of the subunits in the pentameric receptor has a molecular mass of 40–60 kDa. In each subunit, the amino-terminal approximately 210 residues constitute a large extracellular domain. This is followed by four domains that span the membrane; the region between TM3 and TM4 forms most of the cytoplasmic component (Figure 11–1).

The five subunits of the nicotinic ACh receptor are arranged around a pseudoaxis of symmetry to circumscribe a channel. The resulting receptor is an asymmetrical molecule (16 × 8 nm) of 290 kDa, with the bulk of the non-membrane—spanning domain on the extracellular surface. The receptor is present at high densities ($10,000/\mu m^2$) in junctional areas (i.e., the motor end plate in skeletal muscle and the ventral surface of the *Torpedo* electrical organ). Agonist-binding sites occur at the subunit interfaces; in muscle, only two of the five subunit interfaces, αγ and αδ, bind ligands (Figure 11–2). Both of the subunits forming the subunit interface contribute to ligand specificity. Neuronal nicotinic N_n receptors found in ganglia and the CNS also exist as pentamers of one or more types of subunits. Subunit types α_2 through α_{10} and β_2 through β_4 are found in neuronal tissues. Although not all pentameric combinations of α and β subunits lead to functional receptors, the diversity in subunit composition is large and exceeds the capacity of ligands to distinguish subtypes on the basis of their selectivity.

Agonist-mediated changes in ion permeability occur through a cation channel intrinsic to the receptor structure. Measurements of membrane conductance demonstrate rates of ion translocation of 5×10^7 ions/s. The channel is generally nonselective among cations; while highly permeable to Na^+, K^+, and in some cases Ca^{2+}, the majority of the current is carried by Na^+ ions. The second of four TM α-helices in each subunit line the ion channel. The agonist-binding site is intimately coupled with the ion channel; in the N_m, simultaneous binding of two agonist molecules results in a rapid conformational change that opens the channel.

Abbreviations

ACh: acetylcholine
AChE: acetylcholinesterase
anti-ChE: anticholinesterase
CNS: central nervous system
EPP: end-plate potential
EPSP: excitatory postsynaptic potential
FDA: Food and Drug Administration
GABA: γ-aminobutyric acid
GI: gastrointestinal
5HT: 5-hydroxytryptamine (serotonin)
IPSP: inhibitory postsynaptic potential
M_x: muscarinic receptor subtype x (x = 1, 2, 3, 4, or 5)
N_m: nicotinic ACh receptor in skeletal muscle
N_n: nicotinic ACh receptor in neurons
NRT: nicotine replacement therapy
TM: transmembrane
VMAT2: vesicular monoamine transporter 2

Transmission at the Neuromuscular Junction

Neuromuscular Blocking Agents

Modern-day neuromuscular blocking agents fall generally into two classes, depolarizing and competitive/nondepolarizing. At present, only a single depolarizing agent, succinylcholine, is in general clinical use; multiple competitive or nondepolarizing agents are available (see Figure 11–3). Neuromuscular blocking agents are most commonly used for facilitating endotracheal intubation and to relax skeletal muscle during surgery.

Chemistry

Early structure-activity studies led to the development of the polymethylene bis-trimethyl-ammonium series (referred to as the methonium compounds, or depolarizing blockers). The most potent of these agents at the neuromuscular junction was the compound with 10 carbon atoms between the quaternary nitrogens: decamethonium (Figure 11–3). The compound with 6 carbon atoms in the chain, hexamethonium, was

HISTORY · Curare

In the mid-19th century, Claude Bernard demonstrated that the locus of action of curare was at or near the neuromuscular junction. Curare is a generic term for various South American arrow poisons. The drug has been used for centuries by Indians along the Amazon and Orinoco Rivers for immobilizing and paralyzing wild animals used for food; death results from paralysis of skeletal muscles. The preparation of curare was long shrouded in mystery and was entrusted only to tribal witch doctors. Soon after the discovery of the American continent, European explorers and botanists became interested in curare, and late in the 16th century, samples of the native preparations were brought to Europe. Following the pioneering work of scientist/explorer von Humboldt in 1805, the botanical sources of curare became the object of much field research. The curares from eastern Amazonia come from *Strychnos* species; these and other South American species of *Strychnos* contain chiefly quaternary neuromuscular blocking alkaloids. The Asiatic, African, and Australian species nearly all contain tertiary strychnine-like alkaloids.

Research on curare was accelerated by the work of Gill, who, after prolonged and intimate study of the native methods of preparing curare, brought to the U.S. a sufficient amount of the authentic drug to permit chemical and pharmacological investigations. The modern clinical use of curare apparently dates from 1932, when West employed highly purified fractions in patients with tetanus and spastic disorders. King established the essential structure of tubocurarine in 1935 (Figure 11–3). Griffith and Johnson reported the first trial of curare for promoting muscular relaxation in general anesthesia in 1942.

found to be essentially devoid of neuromuscular blocking activity but particularly effective as a ganglionic blocking agent (see following discussion).

Several structural features distinguish competitive and depolarizing neuromuscular blocking agents. The competitive agents (e.g., tubocurarine, the benzylisoquinolines, the amino steroids, and the asymmetric mixed-onium chlorofumarates) are relatively bulky, rigid molecules, whereas the depolarizing agents (e.g., decamethonium [no longer marketed in the U.S.] and succinylcholine) generally have more flexible structures that enable free bond rotations. While the distance between

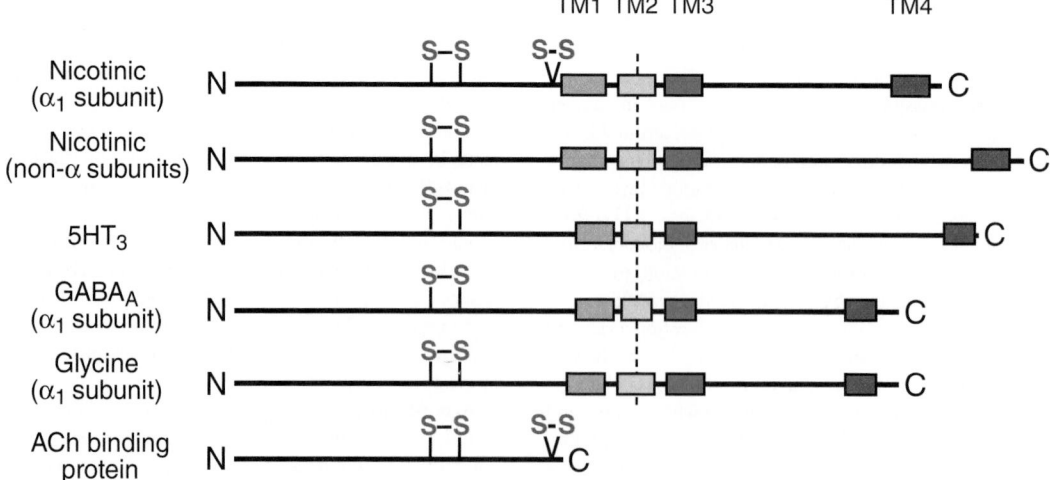

Figure 11–1 *Subunit organization of pentameric ligand-gated ion channels and the ACh-binding protein.* For each subunit of these pentameric receptors, the amino-terminal region of about 210 amino acids is found at the extracellular surface. It is then followed by four hydrophobic regions that span the membrane (TM1–TM4), leaving the small carboxyl terminus on the extracellular surface. The TM2 region is α-helical, and TM2 regions from each subunit of the pentameric receptor line the internal pore of the receptor. Two disulfide loops at positions 128–142 and 192–193 are found in the α subunit of the nicotinic receptor. The 128–142 motif is conserved in the family of receptors, whereas the vicinal cysteines at 192 and 193 distinguish α subunits and the ACh-binding protein from β, γ, δ, and ε in the nicotinic receptor.

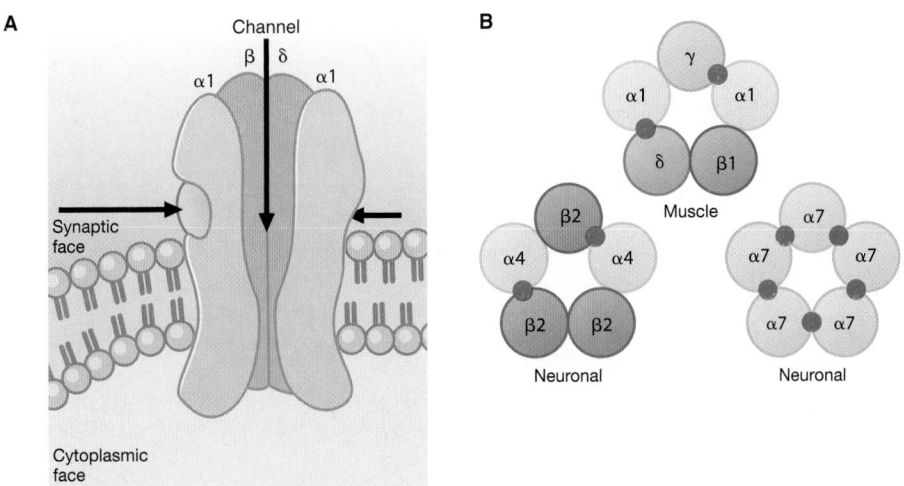

Figure 11–2 *Subunit arrangement and molecular structure of the nicotinic ACh receptor.* **A.** Longitudinal view of receptor schematic with the γ subunit removed. The remaining subunits, two copies of α, one of β, and one of δ, are shown to surround an internal channel with an outer vestibule and its constriction located deep in the membrane bilayer region. Spans of α-helices with slightly bowed structures form the perimeter of the channel and come from the TM2 region of the linear sequence (Figure 11–1). ACh-binding sites, indicated by red arrows, occur at the αγ and αδ (not visible) interfaces. **B.** Nicotinic receptor subunit arrangement, with examples of subunit assembly. Agonist binding sites (*red circles*) occur at α subunit–containing interfaces. A total of 17 functional receptor isoforms have been observed in vivo, with different ligand specificity, relative Ca^{2+}/Na^+ permeability, and physiological function as determined by their subunit composition. The only isoform found at the neuromuscular junction is that shown here. There are 16 neuronal receptor isoforms found at autonomic ganglia and in the CNS, homo- and heteropentamers of α (α2–α10) and β (β2–β4) subunits.

quaternary groups in the flexible depolarizing agents can vary up to the limit of the maximal bond distance (1.45 nm for decamethonium), the distance for the rigid competitive blockers is typically 1.0 ± 0.1 nm.

Mechanism of Action

Competitive antagonists bind the N_m and thereby competitively block the binding of ACh. The depolarizing agents, such as succinylcholine, depolarize the membrane by opening channels in the same manner as ACh. However, they persist longer at the neuromuscular junction primarily because of their resistance to AChE. The depolarization is thus longer lasting, resulting in a brief period of repetitive excitation that may elicit transient and repetitive muscle excitation (fasciculations), followed by blocking of neuromuscular transmission and flaccid paralysis (called *phase I block*). The block arises because, after an initial opening, perijunctional Na^+ channels close and will not reopen until the end plate is repolarized. At this point, neural release of ACh results in the binding of ACh to receptors on an already-depolarized end plate. These closed perijunctional channels keep the depolarization signal from affecting downstream channels and effectively shield the rest of the muscle from activity at the motor end plate. This sequence is influenced by such factors as the anesthetic agent used concurrently, the type of muscle, and the rate of drug administration. The characteristics of depolarization and competitive blockade are contrasted in Table 11–1.

Under clinical conditions, with increasing concentrations of succinylcholine and over time, the block may convert slowly from a depolarizing phase I block to a nondepolarizing *phase II block* (Durant and Katz, 1982). While the response to peripheral stimulation during phase II block resembles that of the competitive agents, reversal of phase II block by administration of anti-AChE agents (e.g., with neostigmine) is difficult to predict and should be undertaken cautiously. The characteristics of phase I and phase II blocks are shown in Table 11–2.

Many drugs and toxins block neuromuscular transmission by other mechanisms, such as interference with the synthesis or release of ACh (Figure 8-6), but most of these agents are not employed clinically for neuromuscular blockade. One exception is the group of botulinum toxins, which are administered locally into muscles of the orbit in the management of ocular blepharospasm and strabismus and have been used to control other muscle spasms and to facilitate facial muscle relaxation (Table 8–7 and Chapter 70). This toxin also has been injected into the lower esophageal sphincter to treat achalasia (Chapter 50). The sites of action and interrelationship of several agents that serve as pharmacological tools are shown in Figure 11–4.

Sequence and Characteristics of Paralysis

Following intravenous injection of an appropriate dose of a *competitive blocking agent*, motor weakness progresses to total flaccid paralysis. Small, rapidly moving muscles such as those of the eyes, jaw, and larynx relax before those of the limbs and trunk. Ultimately, the intercostal muscles and finally the diaphragm are paralyzed, and respiration then ceases. Recovery of muscles usually occurs in the reverse order to that of their paralysis, and thus the diaphragm ordinarily is the first muscle to regain function (Naguib et al., 2015).

After a single intravenous dose (10–30 mg) of the *depolarizing blocking agent* succinylcholine, muscle fasciculations, particularly over the chest and abdomen, occur briefly; then, relaxation occurs within 1 min, becomes maximal within 2 min, and generally disappears within 5 min. Transient apnea usually occurs at the time of maximal effect. Muscle relaxation of longer duration is achieved by continuous intravenous infusion. After infusion is discontinued, the effects of the drug usually disappear rapidly because of its efficient hydrolysis by plasma and hepatic butyrylcholinesterase. Muscle soreness may follow the administration of succinylcholine.

During prolonged depolarization, muscle cells may lose significant quantities of K^+ and gain Na^+, Cl^-, and Ca^{2+}. In patients with extensive injury to soft tissues, the efflux of K^+ following continued administration of succinylcholine can be life threatening. There are many conditions for which succinylcholine administration is contraindicated or should be undertaken with great caution. The change in the nature of the blockade produced by succinylcholine (from phase I to phase II) presents an additional complication with long-term infusions.

Effects in CNS and at Ganglia

Tubocurarine and other quaternary neuromuscular blocking agents are virtually devoid of central effects following ordinary clinical doses because of their inability to penetrate the blood-brain barrier.

Neuromuscular blocking agents show variable potencies in producing ganglionic blockade. Ganglionic blockade by tubocurarine and other stabilizing drugs is reversed or antagonized by anti-ChE agents (e.g., edrophonium, neostigmine, pyridostigmine, etc.).

Clinical doses of tubocurarine produce partial blockade both at autonomic ganglia and at the adrenal medulla, resulting in a fall in blood

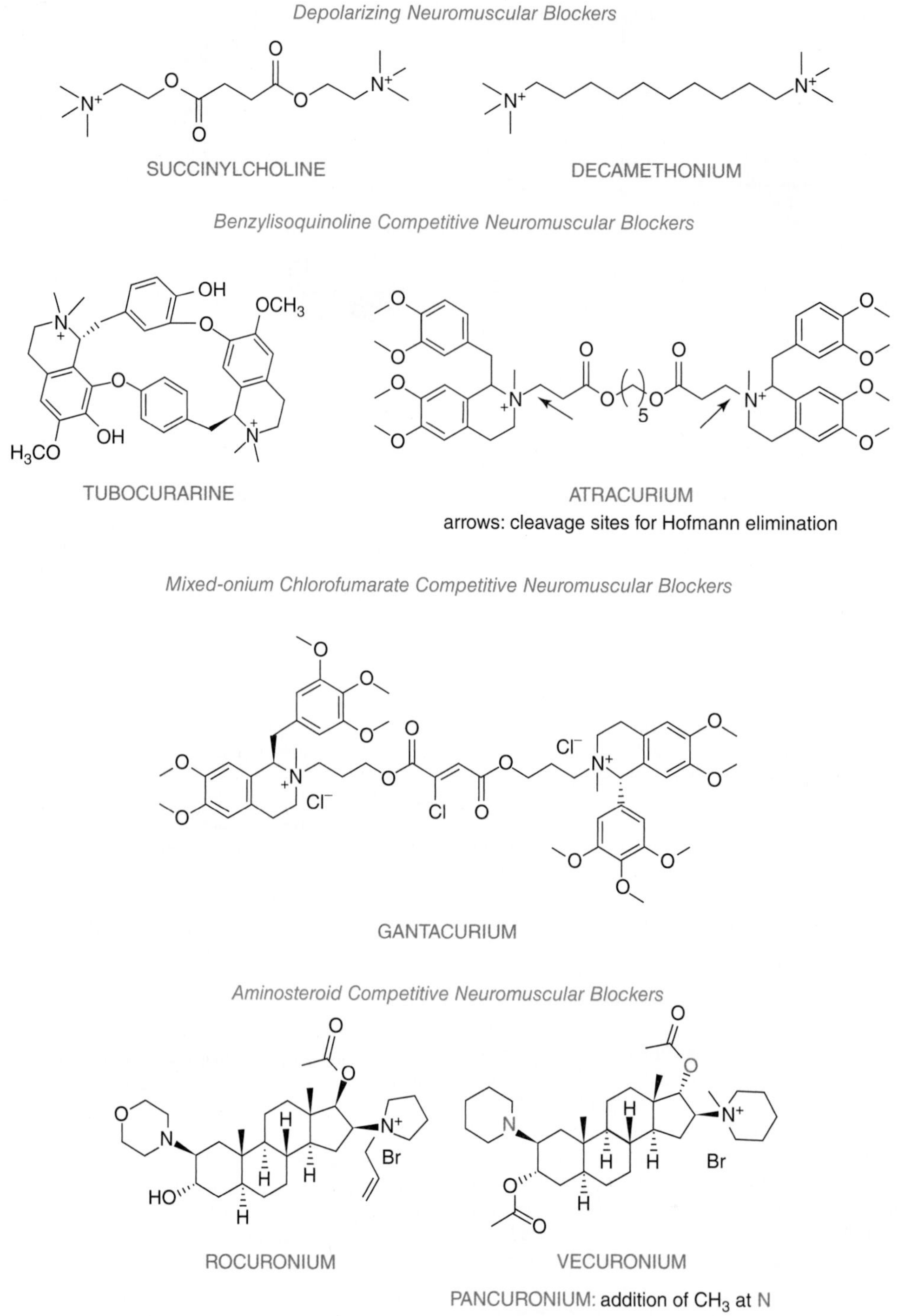

Figure 11–3 *Structural formulas of major neuromuscular blocking agents.*

pressure and tachycardia. Pancuronium shows less ganglionic blockade at common clinical doses. Atracurium, vecuronium, doxacurium, pipecuronium, mivacurium, and rocuronium are even more selective, showing less ganglionic blockade (Naguib et al., 2015). The maintenance of cardiovascular reflex responses usually is desired during anesthesia. Pancuronium has a vagolytic action, presumably from blockade of muscarinic receptors, which leads to tachycardia.

Of the depolarizing agents, succinylcholine at doses producing neuromuscular relaxation rarely causes effects attributable to ganglionic blockade. However, cardiovascular effects are sometimes observed, probably owing to the successive stimulation of vagal ganglia (manifested by

bradycardia) and sympathetic ganglia (resulting in hypertension and tachycardia).

ADME

Quaternary ammonium neuromuscular blocking agents are poorly absorbed from the GI tract. Absorption is adequate from intramuscular sites. Rapid onset is achieved with intravenous administration. The more potent agents must be given in lower concentrations, and diffusional requirements slow their rate of onset.

When long-acting competitive blocking agents such as D-tubocurarine and pancuronium are administered, blockade may diminish after 30 min

TABLE 11–1 ■ COMPARISON OF COMPETITIVE (D-TUBOCURARINE) AND DEPOLARIZING (DECAMETHONIUM) BLOCKING AGENTS

	D-TUBOCURARINE	DECAMETHONIUM
Effect of D-tubocurarine administered previously	Additive	Antagonistic
Effect of decamethonium administered previously	No effect or antagonistic	Some tachyphylaxis, but may be additive
Effect of anticholinesterase agents on block	Reversal of block	No reversal
Effect on motor end plate	Elevated threshold to acetylcholine; no depolarization	Partial, persisting depolarization
Initial excitatory effect on striated muscle	None	Transient fasciculations
Character of muscle response to indirect tetanic stimulation during *partial* block	Poorly sustained contraction	Well-sustained contraction

TABLE 11–2 ■ CLINICAL RESPONSES AND MONITORING OF PHASE I AND PHASE II NEUROMUSCULAR BLOCKADE BY SUCCINYLCHOLINE INFUSION

RESPONSE	PHASE I	PHASE II
End-plate membrane potential	Depolarized to –55 mV	Repolarization toward –80 mV
Onset	Immediate	Slow transition
Dose dependence	Lower	Usually higher or follows prolonged infusion
Recovery	Rapid	More prolonged
Train of four and tetanic stimulation	No fade	Fade[a]
Acetylcholinesterase inhibition	Augments	Reverses or antagonizes
Muscle response	Fasciculations → flaccid paralysis	Flaccid paralysis

[a]Posttetanic potentiation follows fade.

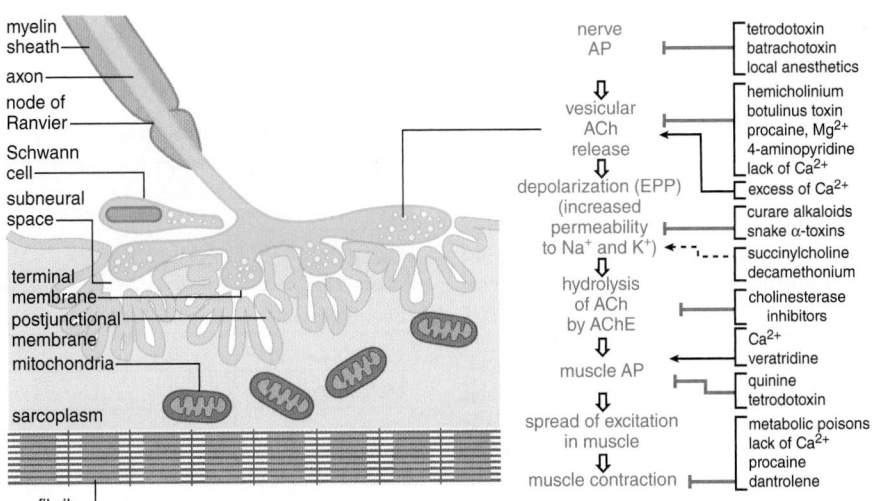

Figure 11–4 *A pharmacologist's view of the motor end plate.* The structures of the motor end plate (left side of figure) facilitate the series of physiological events leading from nerve action potential (AP) to skeletal muscle contraction (center column). Pharmacological agents can modify neurotransmission and excitation-contraction coupling at myriad sites (righthand column). ◄——, enhancement; ⊢——, blockade; ◄----, depolarization and phase II block.

TABLE 11–3 ■ NEUROMUSCULAR BLOCKING AGENTS

AGENT Chemical Class *Type of action*	ONSET (min)[a]	DURATION (min)[a]	MODE OF ELIMINATION
Ultrashort and short duration			
Succinylcholine DCE, *depolarizing*	0.8–1.4	6–11	Hydrolysis by plasma cholinesterases
Gantacurium[c] MOCF, *competitive*	1–2	5–10	Cysteine adduction, ester hydrolysis
Mivacurium BIQ, *competitive*	2–3	15–21	Hydrolysis by plasma cholinesterases
Intermediate duration			
Vecuronium AS, *competitive*	2–3	25–40	Hepatic and renal elimination
Atracurium BIQ, *competitive*	3	45	Hofmann elimination; ester hydrolysis
Rocuronium AS, *competitive*	0.5–2	36–73	Hepatic elimination
Cisatracurium BIQ, *competitive*	2–8	45–90	Hofmann elimination; renal elimination
Long duration			
Pipecuronium[b] AS, *competitive*	3–6	30–90	Renal elimination; hepatic metabolism/ clearance
D-Tubocurarine[b] CBI, *competitive*	6	80	Renal and hepatic elimination
Pancuronium AS, *competitive*	3–4	85–100	Renal and hepatic elimination
Metocurine[b] BIQ, *competitive*	4	110	Renal elimination
Doxacurium[b] BIQ, *competitive*	4–8	120	Renal elimination

[a]As achieved from dose ranges in Table 11–4.

[b]Not commercially available in the U.S.

[c]Gantacurium is in investigational status.

Abbreviations: AS, aminosteroid; BIQ, benzylisoquinoline; CBI (natural alkaloid), cyclic benzylisoquinoline; DCE, dicholine ester;

MOCF, assymetric mixed-onium chlorofumarate.

owing to redistribution of the drug, yet residual blockade and plasma levels of the drug persist. Subsequent doses show diminished redistribution *as tissues become saturated.* Long-acting agents may accumulate with multiple doses.

The amino steroids contain ester groups that are hydrolyzed in the liver. Typically, the metabolites have about one-half the activity of the parent compound and contribute to the total relaxation profile. Amino steroids of intermediate duration of action, such as vecuronium and rocuronium (Table 11–3), are cleared more rapidly by the liver than is pancuronium. The more rapid decay of neuromuscular blockade with compounds of intermediate duration argues for sequential dosing of these agents rather than administering a single dose of a long-duration neuromuscular blocking agent.

Atracurium is converted to less-active metabolites by plasma esterases and by spontaneous degradation in plasma and tissue (Hofmann elimination). Cisatracurium is also subject to this spontaneous degradation. Because of these alternative routes of metabolism, atracurium and cisatracurium do not exhibit an increased $t_{1/2}$ of elimination in patients with impaired renal function and therefore are good choices in this setting (Fisher et al., 1986; Naguib et al., 2015).

The extremely brief duration of action of succinylcholine is due largely to its rapid hydrolysis by the butyrylcholinesterase synthesized by the liver

and found in the plasma. Among the occasional patients who exhibit prolonged apnea following the administration of succinylcholine or mivacurium, most have an atypical plasma cholinesterase or a deficiency of the enzyme owing to allelic variations, hepatic or renal disease, or a nutritional disturbance; however, in some, the enzymatic activity in plasma is normal (Naguib et al., 2015).

Gantacurium is degraded by two chemical mechanisms, a rapid cysteine adduction and a slower hydrolysis of the ester bond adjacent to the chlorine. Both processes are purely chemical and hence not dependent on enzymatic activities. The adduction process has a $t_{1/2}$ of 1–2 min and is likely the basis for the ultrashort duration of action of gantacurium. Administration of exogenous cysteine, which may have excitotoxic side effects, can accelerate the antagonism of gantacurium-induced neuromuscular blockade (Naguib and Brull, 2009).

Clinical Pharmacology
Choice of Agent

Therapeutic selection of a neuromuscular blocking agent should be based on achieving a pharmacokinetic profile consistent with the duration of the interventional procedure and minimizing cardiovascular compromise or other side effects, with attention to drug-specific modes of elimination in patients with renal or hepatic failure (see Drug Facts Table).

Two characteristics are useful in distinguishing side effects and pharmacokinetic behavior of neuromuscular blocking agents:

- *The chemical nature of the agents (Figure 11–3 and Table 11–3).* Apart from a shorter duration of action, newer agents exhibit greatly diminished frequency of side effects, chiefly ganglionic blockade, block of vagal responses, and histamine release.
- *Duration of drug action.* These agents are categorized as long-, intermediate-, short-, or ultrashort-acting agents. Often, the long-acting agents are the more potent, requiring the use of low doses (Table 11–4). The necessity of administering potent agents at low concentrations delays their onset.

The prototypical amino steroid pancuronium induces virtually no histamine release; however, it blocks muscarinic receptors, an antagonism manifested primarily by vagal blockade and tachycardia. Tachycardia is eliminated in the newer amino steroids vecuronium and rocuronium. The benzylisoquinolines appear to be devoid of vagolytic and ganglionic blocking actions but show a slight propensity to cause histamine release. The unusual metabolism of the prototype compound atracurium and its

TABLE 11–4 ■ DOSING RANGES FOR NEUROMUSCULAR BLOCKING AGENTS

AGENT	INITIATION DOSE (mg/kg)	INTERMITTENT INJECTION (mg/kg)	CONTINUOUS INFUSION (µg/kg/min)
Succinylcholine	0.3–1	0.04–0.07	N/A
D-Tubocurarine[a]	0.6	0.25–0.5	2–3
Metocurine[a]	0.4	0.5–1	N/A
Atracurium	0.3–0.5	0.08–0.2	2–15
Cisatracurium	0.15–0.2	0.03	1–3
Mivacurium	0.15–0.25	0.1	9–10
Doxacurium[a]	0.03–0.06	0.005–0.01	N/A
Pancuronium	0.04–0.1	0.01	1[b]
Rocuronium	0.45–1.2	0.1–0.2	10–12
Vecuronium	0.04–0.28	0.01–0.015	0.8–1.2
Gantacurium[a]	0.2–0.5	N/A	N/A

[a]Not commercially available in the U.S.
[b]Off-label use.

congener mivacurium confers special indications for use of these compounds. For example, atracurium's disappearance from the body depends on hydrolysis of the ester moiety by plasma esterases and by a spontaneous or Hofmann degradation (cleavage of the *N*-alkyl portion in the benzylisoquinoline). Hence, two routes for termination of effect are available, both of which remain functional in renal failure. Mivacurium is extremely sensitive to catalysis by cholinesterase or other plasma hydrolases, accounting for its short duration of action. Side effects are not yet fully characterized for gantacurium, but transient adverse cardiovascular effects suggestive of histamine release have been observed at doses over three times the ED_{95} (Belmont et al., 2004).

Muscle Relaxation

The main clinical use of the neuromuscular blocking agents is as an adjuvant in surgical anesthesia to obtain relaxation of skeletal muscle, particularly of the abdominal wall, to facilitate operative manipulations. With muscle relaxation no longer dependent on the depth of general anesthesia, a much lighter level of anesthesia suffices. Thus, the risk of respiratory and cardiovascular depression is minimized, and postanesthetic recovery is shortened. Neuromuscular blocking agents of short duration often are used to facilitate endotracheal intubation and have been used to facilitate laryngoscopy, bronchoscopy, and esophagoscopy in combination with a general anesthetic agent. Neuromuscular blocking agents are administered parenterally, nearly always intravenously. These agents may be administered by continuous infusion in the intensive care setting for improving chest wall compliance and eliminating ventilator dyssynchrony.

Measurement of Neuromuscular Blockade in Humans

Assessment of neuromuscular block usually is performed by stimulation of the ulnar nerve (Naguib et al., 2015). Responses are monitored from compound action potentials or muscle tension developed in the adductor pollicis (thumb) muscle. Responses to repetitive or tetanic stimuli are most useful for evaluation of blockade of transmission. Rates of onset of blockade and recovery are more rapid in the airway musculature (jaw, larynx, and diaphragm) than in the thumb. Hence, tracheal intubation can be performed before onset of complete block at the adductor pollicis, whereas partial recovery of function of this muscle allows sufficient recovery of respiration for extubation.

Preventing Trauma During Electroshock Therapy

Electroconvulsive therapy of psychiatric disorders occasionally is complicated by trauma to the patient; the seizures induced may cause dislocations or fractures. Inasmuch as the muscular component of the convulsion is not essential for benefit from the procedure, neuromuscular blocking agents, usually succinylcholine, and a short-acting barbiturate, usually methohexital, are employed.

Control of Muscle Spasms and Rigidity

Botulinum toxins and dantrolene act peripherally to reduce muscle contraction; a variety of other agents act centrally to reduce skeletal muscle tone and spasm. IncobotulinumtoxinA, onabotulinumtoxinA, abobotulinumtoxinA, and rimabotulinumtoxinB, by blocking ACh release, produce flaccid paralysis of skeletal muscle and diminished activity of parasympathetic and sympathetic cholinergic synapses. Inhibition lasts from several weeks to 3–4 months, and restoration of function requires nerve sprouting.

Originally approved for the treatment of the ocular conditions of strabismus and blepharospasm and for hemifacial spasms, botulinum toxins have been used to treat spasms and dystonias and spasms associated with the lower esophageal sphincter and anal fissures. Botulinum toxin treatments also have become a popular cosmetic procedure for those seeking a wrinkle-free face. Like the bloom of youth, the reduction of wrinkles is temporary; unlike the bloom of youth, the effect of botulinum toxin can be renewed by readministration. The FDA has issued a safety alert, warning of respiratory paralysis from unexpected spread of the toxin from the site of injection (uses are described in Chapter 70).

Dantrolene inhibits Ca^{2+} release from the sarcoplasmic reticulum of skeletal muscle by limiting the capacity of Ca^{2+} and calmodulin to activate the ryanodine receptor, RYR1. Because of its efficacy in managing

an acute attack of malignant hyperthermia (described separately in the section Adverse Effects), dantrolene has been used experimentally in the treatment of muscle rigidity and hyperthermia in neuroleptic malignant syndrome. Dantrolene is also used in treatment of spasticity and hyperreflexia. With its peripheral action, it causes generalized weakness. Thus, its use should be reserved to nonambulatory patients with severe spasticity. Hepatotoxicity has been reported with chronic use, requiring frequent liver function tests and use of the lowest possible oral dose.

Several agents, many of limited efficacy, have been used to treat spasticity involving the α-motor neurons originating in the brainstem and spinal cord. Agents that act in the CNS at either higher centers or the spinal cord to block spasms, with the objective of increasing functional capacity and relieving discomfort, include baclofen, the benzodiazepines, tizanidine, and cyclobenzaprine. A number of other agents used as muscle relaxants seem to rely on sedative properties and blockade of nociceptive pathways; this group includes carisoprodol (which is metabolized to meprobamate; see Chapter 19); metaxalone; methocarbamol; and orphenadrine. Tetrabenazine is available for treatment of the chorea associated with Huntington disease; the drug is a VMAT2 inhibitor that depletes vesicular stores of dopamine in the CNS (Chapters 8 and 18).

Synergisms and Antagonisms

The comparison of interactions between competitive and depolarizing neuromuscular blocking agents is instructive (Table 11–1) and a good test of one's understanding of the drugs' actions. In addition, many other drugs affect transmission at the neuromuscular junction and thus can affect the choice and dosage of neuromuscular blocking agent used.

Because the anti-ChE agents neostigmine, pyridostigmine, and edrophonium preserve endogenous ACh and also act at the neuromuscular junction, they have been used in the treatment of overdosage with competitive blocking agents. Similarly, on completion of the surgical procedure, many anesthesiologists employ neostigmine or edrophonium to reverse and decrease the duration of competitive neuromuscular blockade. A muscarinic antagonist (atropine or glycopyrrolate) is used concomitantly to prevent stimulation of muscarinic receptors and thereby to avoid slowing of the heart rate. Anti-ChE agents will not reverse depolarizing neuromuscular blockade and, in fact, can enhance it.

Many inhalational anesthetics exert a stabilizing effect on the postjunctional membrane and therefore potentiate the activity of competitive blocking agents. Consequently, when such blocking drugs are used for muscle relaxation as adjuncts to these anesthetics, their doses should be reduced. The rank order of potentiation is desflurane > sevoflurane > isoflurane > halothane > nitrous oxide-barbiturate-opioid or propofol anesthesia (Naguib et al., 2015).

Aminoglycoside antibiotics produce neuromuscular blockade by inhibiting ACh release from the preganglionic terminal (through competition with Ca^{2+}) and to a lesser extent by noncompetitively blocking the receptor. The blockade is antagonized by Ca^{2+} salts but only inconsistently by anti-ChE agents (see Chapter 58). The tetracyclines also can produce neuromuscular blockade, possibly by chelation of Ca^{2+}. Additional antibiotics that have neuromuscular blocking action, through both presynaptic and postsynaptic actions, include polymyxin B, colistin, clindamycin, and lincomycin. Ca^{2+} channel blockers enhance neuromuscular blockade produced by both competitive and depolarizing antagonists. When neuromuscular blocking agents are administered to patients receiving these agents, dose adjustments should be considered.

Miscellaneous drugs that may have significant interactions with either competitive or depolarizing neuromuscular blocking agents include trimethaphan, lithium, opioid analgesics, procaine, lidocaine, quinidine, phenelzine, carbamazepine, phenytoin, propranolol, dantrolene, azathioprine, tamoxifen, magnesium salts, corticosteroids, digitalis glycosides, chloroquine, catecholamines, and diuretics.

Adverse Effects

The important untoward responses of the neuromuscular blocking agents include prolonged apnea, cardiovascular collapse, those resulting from histamine release, and, rarely, anaphylaxis. Related factors may include alterations in body temperature; electrolyte imbalance, particularly of K^+;

low plasma butyrylcholinesterase levels, resulting in a reduction in the rate of destruction of succinylcholine; the presence of latent myasthenia gravis or of malignant disease such as small cell carcinoma of the lung with Eaton-Lambert myasthenic syndrome; reduced blood flow to skeletal muscles, causing delayed removal of the blocking drugs; and decreased elimination of the muscle relaxants secondary to hepatic dysfunction (cisatracurium, rocuronium, vecuronium) or reduced renal function (pancuronium). Great care should be taken when administering neuromuscular blockers to dehydrated or severely ill patients. Depolarizing agents can cause rapid release of K^+ from intracellular sites; this may be a factor in production of the prolonged apnea in patients who receive these drugs while in electrolyte imbalance. Succinylcholine-induced hyperkalemia is a life-threatening complication of that drug.

Malignant Hyperthermia. Malignant hyperthermia is a potentially life-threatening event triggered by the administration of certain anesthetics and neuromuscular blocking agents. The clinical features include contracture, rigidity, and heat production from skeletal muscle, resulting in severe hyperthermia (increases of up to 1°C/5 min), accelerated muscle metabolism, metabolic acidosis, and tachycardia. Uncontrolled release of Ca^{2+} from the sarcoplasmic reticulum of skeletal muscle is the initiating event. Although the halogenated hydrocarbon anesthetics (e.g., halothane, isoflurane, and sevoflurane) and succinylcholine alone have been reported to precipitate the response, most of the incidents arise from the combination of depolarizing blocking agent and anesthetic. Susceptibility to malignant hyperthermia, an autosomal dominant trait, is associated with certain congenital myopathies, such as *central core disease*. In the majority of cases, however, no clinical signs are visible in the absence of anesthetic intervention.

Treatment entails intravenous administration of dantrolene, which blocks Ca^{2+} release from the sarcoplasmic reticulum of skeletal muscle (see previous discussion, Control of Muscle Spasms and Rigidity). Rapid cooling, inhalation of 100% O_2, and control of acidosis should be considered adjunct therapy in malignant hyperthermia.

Respiratory Paralysis. Treatment of respiratory paralysis arising from an adverse reaction or overdose of a neuromuscular blocking agent should be by positive-pressure artificial respiration with O_2 and maintenance of a patent airway until recovery of normal respiration is ensured. With the competitive blocking agents, this may be hastened by the administration of neostigmine methylsulfate (0.5–2 mg IV) or edrophonium (10 mg IV, repeated as required up to a total of 40 mg) (Watkins, 1994). In the case of overdose, a muscarinic cholinergic antagonist (atropine or glycopyrrolate) may be added to prevent undue slowing of the heart (see Synergisms and Antagonisms).

Histamine Release From Mast Cells. Some clinical responses to neuromuscular blocking agents (e.g., bronchospasm, hypotension, excessive bronchial and salivary secretion) appear to be caused by the release of histamine. Succinylcholine, mivacurium, and atracurium cause histamine release, but to a lesser extent than tubocurarine unless administered rapidly. The amino steroids pancuronium, vecuronium, pipecuronium, and rocuronium have even less tendency to release histamine after intradermal or systemic injection (Basta, 1992; Watkins, 1994). Histamine release typically is a direct action of the muscle relaxant on the mast cell rather than anaphylaxis mediated by immunoglobulin E.

Interventional Strategies for Toxic Effects

Neostigmine effectively antagonizes only the skeletal muscular blocking action of the competitive blocking agents and may aggravate such side effects as hypotension or induce bronchospasm. In such circumstances, sympathomimetic amines may be given to support the blood pressure. Atropine or glycopyrrolate is administered to counteract muscarinic stimulation. Antihistamines are definitely beneficial to counteract the responses that follow the release of histamine, particularly when administered before the neuromuscular blocking agent.

Reversal of Effects by Chelation Therapy. Sugammadex, a modified γ-cyclodextrin, is a chelating agent specific for rocuronium and vecuronium. Sugammadex at doses greater than 2 mg/kg is able to reverse neuromuscular blockade from rocuronium within 3 min. Sugammadex clearance is markedly reduced in patients with impaired renal function,

and use of this agent should be avoided. Sugammadex is approved for clinical use in Europe but not yet in the U.S. Side effects include dysgeusia and rare hypersensitivity.

Pediatric and Geriatric Indications and Problems

Because the neuromuscular junction is not fully developed at birth, additional care must be taken in administration of neuromuscular blocking agents to infants and children. Succinylcholine is not safe for routine use in pediatric patients, and its use must be reserved for extreme emergency situations where immediate securing of the airway is necessary and other options for neuromuscular blockade are not available. Competitive blocking agents, however, are commonly used in pediatric patients; generally, dosage is similar to adults but both rate of block onset and clearance are faster. Atracurium is an exception: The dosage and duration of action are not significantly different between children older than 2 years and adults, and the same dose (0.25 to 0.5 mg/kg) can be used among these populations for tracheal intubation. Vecuronium, cisatracurium, rocuronium, and mivacurium are also commonly administered to children for short procedures where only a single intubating dose is required.

There are normal changes at the neuromuscular junction in elderly patients that may affect pharmacodynamics of neuromuscular blocking agents. With aging, the distance between the terminus of the motor neuron and the end plate increases, the end-plate invaginations become flatter, the amount of transmitter per synaptic vesicle decreases, the vesicle release probability is lower, and the density of receptors at the end plate decreases. The end result of these changes is decreased efficiency of neuromuscular transmission. General physiological changes in aging patients, including decreases in body water and muscle, increases in total body fat, and decreases in renal and hepatic function, also contribute to the action of neuromuscular blockers. The dosing of succinylcholine is not significantly altered in the geriatric population. Among the competitive blocking agents, initial dose requirements are unchanged, however, the onset of blockade is delayed in an age-related manner, and block is prolonged. For compounds dependent on the kidney, liver, or both for clearance, such as pancuronium, vecuronium, and rocuronium, plasma clearance times are prolonged by 30%–50% (Naguib et al., 2015). For compounds such as atracurium that are not dependent on hepatic or renal blood flow for their elimination, pharmacodynamics and kinetics are largely unaltered.

Ganglionic Neurotransmission

The Neural Nicotinic Receptor and Postsynaptic Potentials

Neurotransmission in autonomic ganglia involves release of ACh by preganglionic fibers and the rapid depolarization of postsynaptic membranes via the activation of neuronal nicotinic (N_n) receptors by ACh. Unlike the neuromuscular junction, ganglia do not have discrete end plates with focal localization of receptors; rather, the dendrites and nerve cell bodies contain the receptors. The characteristics of nicotinic-receptor channels of the ganglia and the neuromuscular junction are similar. There are multiple nicotinic receptor subunits (e.g., α3, α5, α7, β2, and β4) in ganglia, with α3 and β4 most abundant and important. The ganglionic nicotinic ACh receptors are sensitive to classical blocking agents such as hexamethonium and trimethaphan (see discussion that follows). Measurements of single-channel conductances indicate that the characteristics of nicotinic receptor channels of the ganglia and the neuromuscular junction are similar.

Intracellular recordings from postganglionic neurons indicate that at least four different changes in postsynaptic membrane potential can be elicited by stimulation of the preganglionic nerve (Figure 11–5):

- An initial EPSP (via nicotinic receptors) that may result in an action potential
- An IPSP mediated by M_2 (G_i/G_o-coupled) muscarinic receptors
- A secondary slow EPSP mediated by M_1 (G_q/G_{11}-coupled) muscarinic receptors
- A late, slow EPSP mediated by myriad peptides

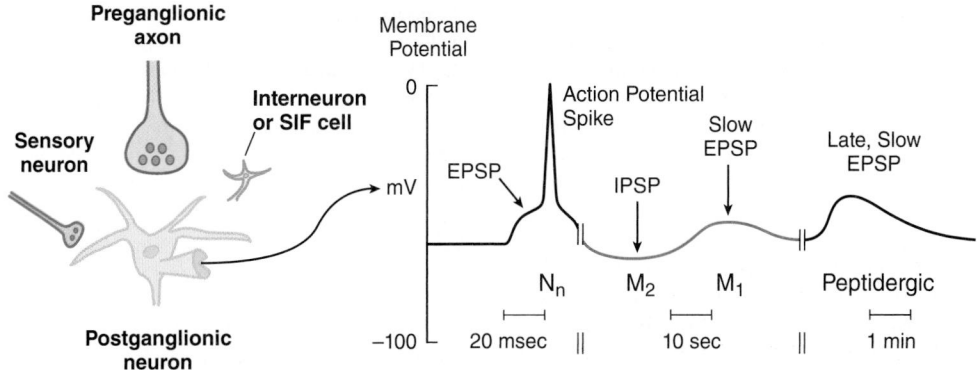

Figure 11–5 *Postsynaptic potentials recorded from an autonomic postganglionic nerve cell body after stimulation of the preganglionic nerve fiber.* The preganglionic nerve releases ACh onto postganglionic cells. The initial EPSP results from the inward Na⁺ current (and perhaps Ca²⁺ current) through the nicotinic receptor channel. If the EPSP is of sufficient magnitude, it triggers an action potential spike, which is followed by a slow IPSP, a slow EPSP, and a late, slow EPSP. The slow IPSP and slow EPSP are not seen in all ganglia. The electrical events subsequent to the initial EPSP are thought to modulate the probability that a subsequent EPSP will reach the threshold for triggering a spike. Other interneurons, such as catecholamine-containing SIF cells, and axon terminals from sensory, afferent neurons also release transmitters, which may influence the slow potentials of the postganglionic neuron. A number of cholinergic, peptidergic, adrenergic, and amino acid receptors are found on the dendrites and soma of the postganglionic neuron and the interneurons. The preganglionic fiber releases ACh and peptides; the interneurons store and release catecholamines, amino acids, and peptides; the sensory afferent nerve terminals release peptides. The initial EPSP is mediated through nicotinic (N_n) receptors, the slow IPSP and EPSP through M_2 and M_1 muscarinic receptors, and the late, slow EPSP through several types of peptidergic receptors.

An action potential is generated in the postganglionic neuron when the initial EPSP achieves a threshold potential. The events that follow the initial depolarization (IPSP; slow EPSP; late, slow EPSP) are insensitive to hexamethonium or other N_n antagonists. Electrophysiological and neurochemical evidence suggests that catecholamines participate in the generation of the IPSP. Dopamine and norepinephrine cause hyperpolarization of ganglia; however, in some ganglia IPSPs are mediated by M_2 muscarinic receptors.

The slow EPSP is generated by ACh activation of M_1 muscarinic receptors and is blocked by atropine and M_1-selective antagonists (see Chapter 9). The slow EPSP has a longer latency and greater duration (10–30 sec) than the initial EPSP. Slow EPSPs result from decreased K⁺ conductance, the *M current* that regulates the sensitivity of the cell to repetitive fast-depolarizing events. By contrast, the late, slow EPSP lasts for several minutes and is mediated by peptides released from presynaptic nerve endings or interneurons in specific ganglia (see next section). The peptides and ACh may be coreleased at the presynaptic nerve terminals; the relative stability of the peptides in the ganglion extends its sphere of influence to postsynaptic sites beyond those in the immediate proximity of the nerve ending.

Secondary synaptic events modulate the initial EPSP. A variety of peptides, including gonadotropin-releasing hormone, substance P, angiotensin, calcitonin gene–related peptide, vasoactive intestinal polypeptide, neuropeptide Y, and enkephalins, have been identified in ganglia by immunofluorescence. They appear localized to particular cell bodies, nerve fibers, or small, intensely fluorescent (SIF) cells; are released on nerve stimulation; and are presumed to mediate the late, slow EPSP. Other neurotransmitter substances (e.g., 5HT and GABA) can modify ganglionic transmission.

Ganglionic Stimulating Agents

Drugs that stimulate N_n cholinergic receptors on autonomic ganglia have been essential for analyzing the mechanism of ganglionic function; however, these ganglionic agonists have limited therapeutic use. They can be grouped into two categories. The first group consists of drugs with specificities similar to nicotine: lobeline, tetramethylammonium, and dimethylphenylpiperazinium. Nicotine's excitatory effects on ganglia are rapid in onset, are blocked by ganglionic nicotinic-receptor antagonists, and mimic the initial EPSP. The second group consists of muscarinic receptor agonists such as muscarine, McN-A-343, and methacholine (see Chapter 9); their excitatory effects on ganglia are delayed in onset, blocked by atropine-like drugs, and mimic the slow EPSP.

Nicotine

Nicotine is of considerable medical significance because of its toxicity, presence in tobacco, and propensity for conferring dependence on its users. The chronic effects of nicotine and the untoward effects of the chronic use of tobacco are considered in Chapter 24. Nicotine is one of the few natural liquid alkaloids. It is a colorless, volatile base (pK_a = 8.5) that turns brown and acquires the odor of tobacco on exposure to air.

NICOTINE

Mechanism of Action. In addition to the actions of nicotine on a variety of neuroeffector and chemosensitive sites, the alkaloid can both stimulate and desensitize receptors, making nicotine's effects complex and unpredictable. The ultimate response of any one system represents the summation of stimulatory and inhibitory effects of nicotine. Nicotine can increase heart rate by excitation of sympathetic ganglia or by paralysis of parasympathetic cardiac ganglia, and it can slow heart rate by paralysis of sympathetic or stimulation of parasympathetic cardiac ganglia. The effects of the drug on the chemoreceptors of the carotid and aortic bodies and on regions of the CNS also can influence heart rate, as can the compensatory baroreceptor reflexes resulting from changes in blood pressure caused by nicotine. Finally, nicotine can stimulate secretion of epinephrine from the adrenal medulla, which accelerates heart rate and raises blood pressure.

Effects on Physiological Systems

Peripheral Nervous System. The major action of nicotine consists initially of transient stimulation and then a more persistent depression of all autonomic ganglia. Small doses of nicotine stimulate the ganglion cells directly and may facilitate impulse transmission. Following larger doses, the initial stimulation is followed by a blockade of transmission. Whereas stimulation of the ganglion cells coincides with their depolarization, depression of transmission by adequate doses of nicotine occurs both during the depolarization and after it has subsided. Nicotine also possesses a biphasic action on the adrenal medulla: Small doses evoke the discharge of catecholamines; larger doses prevent their release in response to splanchnic nerve stimulation.

The effects of high doses of nicotine on the neuromuscular junction are similar to those on ganglia. However, the stimulant phase is obscured largely by the rapidly developing paralysis. In the latter stage, nicotine also produces neuromuscular blockade by receptor desensitization. At lower concentrations, such as those typically achieved by recreational tobacco use (~200 nM), nicotine's effects reflect its higher affinity for a neuronal nicotinic receptor ($\alpha 4 \beta 2$) than for the neuromuscular junction receptor ($\alpha_1 \beta_1 \gamma \delta$) (Xiu et al., 2009).

Nicotine, like ACh, stimulates a number of sensory receptors. These include mechanoreceptors that respond to stretch or pressure of the skin, mesentery, tongue, lung, and stomach; chemoreceptors of the carotid body; thermal receptors of the skin and tongue; and pain receptors. Prior administration of hexamethonium prevents stimulation of the sensory receptors by nicotine but has little, if any, effect on the activation of sensory receptors by physiological stimuli.

Central Nervous System. Nicotine markedly stimulates the CNS. Low doses produce weak analgesia; higher doses cause tremors, leading to convulsions at toxic doses. The excitation of respiration is a prominent action of nicotine: Large doses act directly on the medulla oblongata, whereas smaller doses augment respiration reflexly by excitation of the chemoreceptors of the carotid and aortic bodies. Stimulation of the CNS with large doses is followed by depression, and death results from failure of respiration owing to both central paralysis and peripheral blockade of the diaphragm and intercostal muscles that facilitate respiration.

Nicotine induces vomiting by both central and peripheral actions. The central component of the vomiting response is due to stimulation of the emetic chemoreceptor trigger zone in the area postrema of the medulla oblongata. In addition, nicotine activates vagal and spinal afferent nerves that form the sensory input of the reflex pathways involved in the act of vomiting. The primary sites of action of nicotine in the CNS are prejunctional, causing the release of other transmitters. The stimulatory and pleasure-reward actions of nicotine appear to result from release of excitatory amino acids, dopamine, and other biogenic amines from various CNS centers (Dorostkar and Boehm, 2008).

Chronic exposure to nicotine in several systems causes a marked increase in the density or number of nicotinic receptors, possibly contributing to tolerance and dependence. Nicotine is thought to act as an intracellular pharmacological chaperone; it is uncharged at physiological pH and readily permeates the plasma membrane. Inside the cell, it upregulates receptor expression by stabilizing nascent subunits in pentamers in the endoplasmic reticulum. Chronic low-dose exposure to nicotine also significantly increases the $t_{1/2}$ of nicotinic receptors on the cell surface (Kuryatov et al., 2005; Srinivasan et al., 2014).

Cardiovascular System. In general, the cardiovascular responses to nicotine are due to stimulation of sympathetic ganglia and the adrenal medulla, together with the discharge of catecholamines from sympathetic nerve endings. Contributing to the sympathomimetic response to nicotine is the activation of chemoreceptors of the aortic and carotid bodies, which reflexly results in vasoconstriction, tachycardia, and elevated blood pressure.

GI Tract. The combined activation of parasympathetic ganglia and cholinergic nerve endings by nicotine results in increased tone and motor activity of the bowel. Nausea, vomiting, and occasionally diarrhea are observed following systemic absorption of nicotine in an individual who has not been exposed to nicotine previously.

Exocrine Glands. Nicotine causes an initial stimulation of salivary and bronchial secretions that is followed by inhibition.

ADME. Nicotine is readily absorbed from the respiratory tract, buccal membranes, and skin. Severe poisoning has resulted from percutaneous absorption. As a relatively strong base, nicotine has limited absorption from the stomach. Intestinal absorption is far more efficient. Nicotine in chewing tobacco, because it is absorbed more slowly than inhaled nicotine, has a longer duration of effect. The average cigarette contains 6–11 mg nicotine and delivers about 1–3 mg nicotine systemically to the smoker; bioavailability can increase as much as 3-fold with the intensity of puffing and technique of the smoker (Benowitz, 1998).

Approximately 80%–90% of nicotine is altered in the body, mainly in the liver but also in the kidney and lung. Cotinine is the major metabolite. The $t_{1/2}$ of nicotine following inhalation is about 2 h. Nicotine and its metabolites are eliminated rapidly by the kidney. The rate of urinary excretion of nicotine diminishes when the urine is alkaline. Nicotine also is excreted in the milk of lactating women who smoke; the milk of heavy smokers may contain 0.5 mg/L.

Acute Adverse Effects. Poisoning from nicotine may occur from accidental ingestion of nicotine-containing insecticide sprays or in children from ingestion of tobacco products. The acutely fatal dose of nicotine for an adult is probably about 60 mg. Smoking tobacco usually contains 1%–2% nicotine. The gastric absorption of nicotine from tobacco taken by mouth is delayed because of slowed gastric emptying, so vomiting caused by the central effect of the initially absorbed fraction may remove much of the tobacco remaining in the GI tract.

The onset of symptoms of acute, severe nicotine poisoning is rapid; they include nausea, salivation, abdominal pain, vomiting, diarrhea, cold sweat, headache, dizziness, disturbed hearing and vision, mental confusion, and marked weakness. Faintness and prostration ensue; the blood pressure falls; breathing is difficult; the pulse is weak, rapid, and irregular; and collapse may be followed by terminal convulsions. Death may result within a few minutes from respiratory failure.

For treating nicotine poisoning, vomiting may be induced, or gastric lavage should be performed. Alkaline solutions should be avoided. A slurry of activated charcoal is then passed through the tube and left in the stomach. Respiratory assistance and treatment of shock may be necessary.

Ganglionic Blocking Agents

There are two categories of agents that block ganglionic nicotinic receptors. The prototype of the first group, nicotine, initially stimulates the ganglia by an ACh-like action and then blocks them by causing persistent depolarization (Volle, 1980). Compounds in the second category (e.g., *trimethaphan* and *hexamethonium*) impair transmission. Trimethaphan acts by competition with ACh, analogous to the mechanism of action of curare at the neuromuscular junction. Hexamethonium appears to block the channel after it opens; this action shortens the duration of current flow because the open channel either becomes occluded or closes. Thus, the initial EPSP is blocked, and ganglionic transmission is inhibited. Representative diverse chemicals that block autonomic ganglia without first causing stimulation are shown in Figure 11–6.

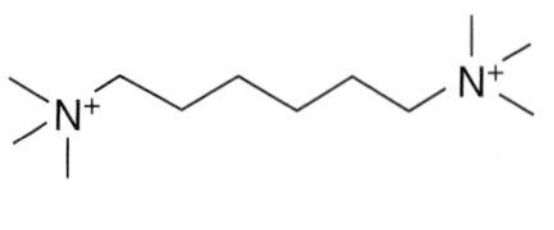

HEXAMETHONIUM (C6)

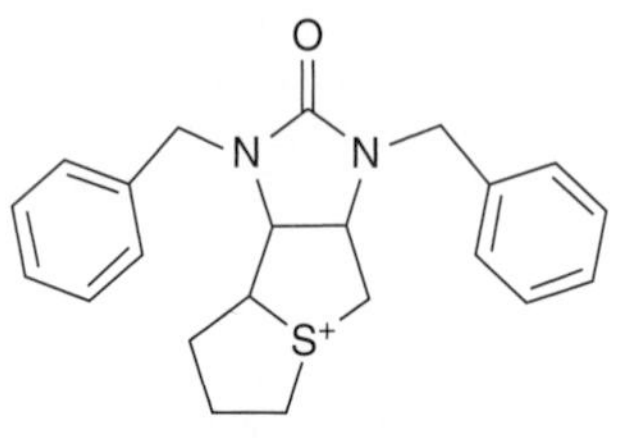

TRIMETHAPHAN

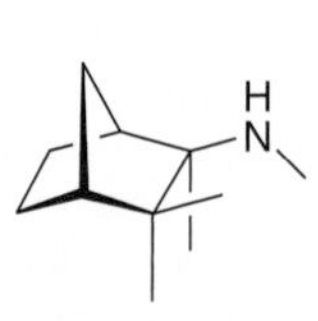

MECAMYLAMINE

Figure 11–6 *Ganglionic blocking agents.*

TABLE 11–5 ■ USUAL PREDOMINANCE OF SYMPATHETIC OR PARASYMPATHETIC TONE AT VARIOUS EFFECTOR SITES AND CONSEQUENCES OF AUTONOMIC GANGLIONIC BLOCKADE

SITE	PREDOMINANT TONE	EFFECT OF GANGLIONIC BLOCKADE
Arterioles	Sympathetic (adrenergic)	Vasodilation; increased peripheral blood flow; hypotension
Veins	Sympathetic (adrenergic)	Dilation: peripheral pooling of blood; decreased venous return; decreased cardiac output
Heart	Parasympathetic (cholinergic)	Tachycardia
Iris	Parasympathetic (cholinergic)	Mydriasis
Ciliary muscle	Parasympathetic (cholinergic)	Cycloplegia—focus to far vision
Gastrointestinal tract	Parasympathetic (cholinergic)	Reduced tone and motility; constipation; decreased gastric and pancreatic secretions
Urinary bladder	Parasympathetic (cholinergic)	Urinary retention
Salivary glands	Parasympathetic (cholinergic)	Xerostomia
Sweat glands	Sympathetic (cholinergic)	Anhidrosis
Genital tract	Sympathetic and parasympathetic	Decreased stimulation

Ganglionic blocking agents were the first effective therapy for the treatment of hypertension. However, due to the role of ganglionic transmission in both sympathetic and parasympathetic neurotransmission, the antihypertensive action of ganglionic blocking agents was accompanied by numerous undesirable side effects. Mecamylamine, a secondary amine with a channel block mechanism similar to hexamethonium, is available as an antihypertensive agent with good oral bioavailability.

Mechanism of Action

Nearly all the physiological alterations observed after the administration of ganglionic blocking agents can be anticipated with reasonable accuracy by a careful inspection of Figure 8–1 and Table 8–1, and by knowing which division of the autonomic nervous system exercises dominant control of various organs (Table 11–5). For example, blockade of sympathetic ganglia interrupts adrenergic control of arterioles and results in vasodilation, improved peripheral blood flow in some vascular beds, and a fall in blood pressure.

Generalized ganglionic blockade also may result in atony of the bladder and GI tract, cycloplegia, xerostomia, diminished perspiration, and, by abolishing circulatory reflex pathways, postural hypotension. These changes represent the generally undesirable features of ganglionic blockade that severely limit the therapeutic efficacy of ganglionic blocking agents.

Cardiovascular Effects

Existing sympathetic tone is a critical determinant of the degree ganglionic blockade will lower blood pressure. Thus, blood pressure may decrease only minimally in recumbent normotensive subjects but may fall markedly in sitting or standing subjects. Postural hypotension limits the use of ganglionic blockers in ambulatory patients. Changes in heart rate following ganglionic blockade depend largely on existing vagal tone. In humans, only mild tachycardia usually accompanies the hypotension, a sign that indicates fairly complete ganglionic blockade. However, a decrease may occur if the heart rate is high initially. Cardiac output often is reduced by ganglionic blocking drugs in patients with normal cardiac function, as a consequence of venodilation, peripheral pooling of blood, and the resulting decrease in venous return. In patients with cardiac failure, ganglionic blockade frequently results in increased cardiac output owing to a reduction in peripheral resistance. In hypertensive subjects, cardiac output, stroke volume, and left ventricular work are diminished. Although total systemic vascular resistance is decreased in patients who receive ganglionic blocking agents, changes in blood flow and vascular resistance of individual vascular beds are variable. Reduction of cerebral blood flow is small unless mean systemic blood pressure falls below 50–60 mm Hg. Skeletal muscle blood flow is unaltered, but splanchnic and renal blood flow decrease.

ADME

The absorption of quaternary ammonium and sulfonium compounds from the enteric tract is incomplete and unpredictable. This is due both to the limited ability of these ionized substances to penetrate cell membranes and to the depression of propulsive movements of the small intestine and gastric emptying. Although the absorption of mecamylamine is less erratic, reduced bowel activity and paralytic ileus are a danger. After absorption, the quaternary ammonium- and sulfonium-blocking agents are confined primarily to the extracellular space and are excreted mostly unchanged by the kidney. Mecamylamine concentrates in the liver and kidney and is excreted slowly in an unchanged form.

Therapeutic Uses; Adverse Effects

Trimethaphan was once used for the induction of controlled hypotension during surgery to reduce bleeding and for the rapid reduction of blood pressure in the treatment of hypertensive emergencies; however, the agent is no longer marketed in the U.S.

Among the milder untoward responses observed are visual disturbances, dry mouth, conjunctival suffusion, urinary hesitancy, decreased potency, subjective chilliness, moderate constipation, occasional diarrhea, abdominal discomfort, anorexia, heartburn, nausea, eructation, and bitter taste and the signs and symptoms of syncope caused by postural hypotension. More severe reactions include marked hypotension, constipation, syncope, paralytic ileus, urinary retention, and cycloplegia.

Nicotine Addiction and Smoking Cessation

As a therapeutic, nicotine is primarily used to aid in smoking cessation. Two goals of the pharmacotherapy of smoking cessation are the reduction of the craving for nicotine and inhibition of the reinforcing effects of smoking. Myriad approaches and drug regimens are used, including NRT, bupropion (a CNS-active nicotinic antagonist; see Chapter 15), and partial agonists of the nicotinic ACh receptor (e.g., varenicline).

Current consensus is that NRT, bupropion, and varenicline all help smokers to quit their smoking habit. Cytisine (not approved for use in Europe or the U.S.) also appears effective. The safety and efficacy of NRT are clear. The highest rates of smoking cessation (~30% success at maintaining abstinence from smoking for 6 months) result from the combination of NRT (e.g., patch plus inhaler) and varenicline (Cahill et al., 2013, 2014).

Nicotine Replacement Therapy

Nicotine replacement therapy is available in several dosage forms to help achieve abstinence from tobacco use. Nicotine is marketed for over-the-counter use as a gum or lozenge or transdermal patch and by prescription as a nasal spray or vapor inhaler. Different nicotine delivery systems produce different patterns of exposure (see Figure 24–2; St. Helen et al., 2016). The efficacy of these dosage forms in producing abstinence from smoking is enhanced when linked to counseling and motivational therapy (Frishman, 2009; Prochaska and Benowitz 2016).

Varenicline

Varenicline has been recently introduced as an aid to smoking cessation. The drug interacts with nicotinic ACh receptors. In model systems, varenicline is a partial agonist at $\alpha4\beta2$ receptors, which is thought to be the principal nicotinic receptor subtype involved in nicotine addiction. Varenicline is a full agonist at the $\alpha7$ subtype and exhibits weak activity toward $\alpha3\beta2$- and $\alpha6$-containing receptors. The drug is effective clinically; however, it is not benign: The FDA has issued a warning about mood and behavioral changes associated with its use, and there is some evidence of increased cardiovascular risk (Chelladurai and Singh, 2014; Singh et al., 2011).

Cytisine

Cytisine is a plant alkaloid and a partial agonist at nicotinic ACh receptors, with an affinity for the $\alpha4\beta2$ subtype. Cytisine is taken orally, has a half-life of about 5 h, and can produce mild GI side effects. In a recent small trial, cytisine was effective in producing effects similar to those of NRT and varenicline (Walker et al., 2014).

Drug Facts for Your Personal Formulary: *Agents Acting at the NMJ and Autonomic Ganglia; Antispasmodics; Nicotine*

Drug	Therapeutic Uses	Clinical Pharmacology and Tips
Nicotinic ACh Receptor Agonists		
Succinylcholine[US] (N_m agonist)	Induction of neuromuscular blockade in surgery and during intubation	• Induces rapid depolarization of motor end plate, inducing phase I block • Resistant to and augments AChE inhibition; induces fasciculations, then flaccid paralysis • Influenced by anesthetic agent, type of muscle, and rate of administration • Leads to phase II block after prolonged use • Metabolized by butyrylcholinesterase; not safe for infants and children • Contraindications: history of malignant hyperthermia, muscular dystrophy
Dexamethonium (depolarizer)	• Not used clinically in the U.S.	
Nicotine (N_n agonist)	• Smoking cessation	• Low dose induces postganglionic depolarization • High doses induce ganglionic transmission blockade
Varenicline (N_n [$\alpha4\beta2$ subtype])	• Smoking cessation • FDA warning about mood and behavioral changes	• Partial nicotinic receptor agonist preventing nicotine stimulation and decreasing craving • Potential for neuropsychiatric events, may cause seizures with alcohol use; excreted largely unchanged in urine
Competitive Nicotinic ACh Receptor Antagonists (Nondepolarizing Neuromuscular Blocking Agents)		
D-Tubocurarine[a,L]	• Induction of neuromuscular blockade in surgery and during intubation • All neuromuscular blocking agents are administered parenterally	• No longer used clinically in the U.S. or Canada • Produces partial blockade of ganglionic ACh transmission that can produce hypertension and reflex tachycardia • Can induce histamine release
Mivacurium[S]		• Short acting due to rapid hydrolysis by plasma cholinesterase • Use with caution in patients with renal or hepatic insufficiency
Pancuronium[L]		• Shows antimuscarinic receptor activity • Renal and hepatic elimination • Vagolytic activity may cause tachycardia, hypertension, and increased cardiac output
Rocuronium[I]		• Amino steroid • Stable in solution • More rapid onset than vecuronium and cisatracurium • Hepatic elimination
Vecuronium[I]		• Amino steroid • Not stable in solution • Hepatic and renal elimination
Metocurine[a,L]		• Three times more potent than tubocurarine • Less histamine release
Atracurium[I]	• Preferred agent for patients with renal failure	• Susceptible to Hofmann elimination and ester hydrolysis • Same dosage for infants > 1 month, children, and adults
Cisatracurium[I]		• More potent than atracurium, Hofmann elimination, no histamine release (unlike atracurium)
Doxacurium[a,L]		• Renal elimination
Pipecuronium[a,L]		• Hepatic metabolism; renal elimination

Competitive Nicotinic ACh Receptor Antagonists (Nondepolarizing Neuromuscular Blocking Agents) (continued)		
Gantacurium[b,US]		• New compound class; in clinical trial stage • Fastest onset and shortest acting • Metabolism: rapid cysteine adduction, slow ester hydrolysis
Hexamethonium	• Not used therapeutically	• N_n receptor antagonist; blocks ganglionic transmission
Trimethaphan	• Hypertensive crisis • No longer used	• N_n receptor antagonist; blocks ganglionic transmission
CNS-Active Agents		
Baclofen Benzodiazepines Tizanidine Cyclobenzaprine	• Control of muscle spasms	• See Chapter 22
Carisoprodol Metaxalone Methocarbamol Orphenadrine Tetrabenazine	• Muscle relaxants acting in CNS, having, in general, a depressant effect	• CYP2C19 metabolizes carisoprodol to largely to meprobamate • Tetrabenazine is a VCAT2 inhibitor and depletes neuronal monoamine stores
Agents That Block ACh Release		
AbobotulinumtoxinA	• Cervical dystonia • Glabellar lines (moderate to severe)	• Spread of toxin effect may induce paralysis of nontargeted muscle, rarely if administered carefully • Paralysis of swallowing and respiration can be life threatening
IncobotulinumtoxinA	• Blepharospasm, cervical dystonia • Glabellar lines (moderate to severe)	
OnabotulinumtoxinA	• Botox: axillary hyperhidrosis (severe) • Blepharospasm associated with dystonia; cervical dystonia; migraine (chronic) prophylaxis • Overactive bladder; strabismus; upper limb spasticity (severe); urinary incontinence (due to detrusor overactivity associated with a neurologic condition)	
RimabotulinumtoxinB	• Cervical dystonia	
Inhibitor of Release of Ca^{2+} From the SR		
Dantrolene	• Management and prevention of malignant hyperthermia • Treatment of spasticity associated with upper motor neuron disorders (e.g., spinal cord injury, stroke, cerebral palsy, or multiple sclerosis)	• Hepatic metabolism • Can cause significant hepatotoxicity

Duration of action: [L]long (> ~ 80 min), [i]intermediate (~20–80 min), [s]short (~15–20 min), [US]ultrashort (< ~ 15 min).

[a]Not available in the U.S.

[b]Gantacurium is in investigational status.

Bibliography

Basta SJ. Modulation of histamine release by neuromuscular blocking drugs. *Curr Opin Anaesthesiol*, **1992**, 5:512–566.

Belmont MR, et al. Clinical pharmacology of GW280430A in humans. *Anesthesiology*, **2004**, 100:768–773.

Benowitz NL. Nicotine and cardiovascular disease. In Benowitz NL, ed. *Nicotine Safety and Toxicity*. Oxford University Press, New York, **1998**, 3–28.

Cahill K, et al. Pharmacological interventions for smoking cessation: an overview and network meta-analysis. *Cochrane Database Syst Rev*, **2013**, 5:CD009329. doi:10.1002/14651858.CD009329.pub2. Accessed February 29, 2016.

Changeux JP, Edelstein SJ. *Nicotinic Acetylcholine Receptors*. Odile Jacob, New York, **2005**.

Chelladurai Y, Singh S. Varenicline and cardiovascular adverse events: a perspective review. *Ther Adv Drug Saf*, **2014**, 5:167–172.

Dorostkar MM, Boehm S. Presynaptic Ionotropic receptors. *Handb Exp Pharmacol*, **2008**, 184:479–527.

Durant NN, Katz RL. Suxamethonium. *Br J Anaesth*, **1982**, 54: 195–208.

Fisher DM, et al. Elimination of atracurium in humans: contribution of Hofmann elimination and ester hydrolysis versus organ-based elimination. *Anesthesiology*, **1986**, 65:6–12.

Frishman WH. Smoking cessation pharmacotherapy. *Ther Adv Cardiovasc Dis*, **2009**, 3:287–308.

Karlin A. Emerging structures of nicotinic acetylcholine receptors. *Nat Rev Neurosci*, **2002**, 3:102–114.

Kuryatov A, et al. Nicotine acts as a pharmacological chaperone to up-regulate human a4b2 acetylcholine receptors. *Mol Pharm*, **2005**, 68:1839–1851.

Naguib M, Brull SJ. Update on neuromuscular pharmacology. *Curr Opin Anaesthesiol*, **2009**, 22:483–490.

Naguib M, et al. Pharmacology of neuromuscular blocking drugs. In Miller RD, ed. *Miller's Anesthesia*. 8th ed. Saunders, an imprint of Elsevier, Philadelphia, **2015**, 958–994.

Prochaska JJ, Benowitz NL. The past, present, and future of nicotine addiction therapy. *Ann Rev Med*, **2016**, 67:467–486.

St. Helen G, et al. Nicotine delivery, retention and pharmacokinetics from various electronic cigarettes. *Addiction*, **2016**, *111*:534–544.

Singh S, et al. Risk of serious adverse cardiovascular events associated with varenicline: a systematic review and meta-analysis. *CMAJ*, **2011**, *183*:1359–1366.

Srinivasan R, et al. Pharmacological chaperoning of nAChRs: a therapeutic target for Parkinson's disease. *Pharmacol Res*, **2014**, *83*:20–29.

Unwin N. Refined structure of the nicotinic acetylcholine receptor at 4 Å resolution. *J Mol Biol*, **2005**, *346*:967–989.

Volle RL. Nicotinic ganglion-stimulating agents. In Kharkevich DA, ed. *Pharmacology of Ganglionic Transmission*. Springer-Verlag, Berlin, **1980**, 281–312.

Walker N, et al. Cytisine versus nicotine for smoking cessation. *N Engl J Med*, **2014**, *371*:2353–2362.

Watkins J. Adverse reaction to neuromuscular blockers: frequency, investigation, and epidemiology. *Acta Anaesthesiol Scand Suppl*, **1994**, *102*:6–10.

Xiu X, et al. Nicotine binding to brain receptors requires a strong cation-π interaction. *Nature*, **2009**, *458*:534–537.

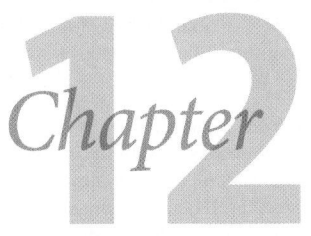
Chapter 12

Adrenergic Agonists and Antagonists
Thomas C. Westfall, Heather Macarthur, and David P. Westfall

Overview: Actions of Catecholamines and Sympathomimetic Drugs

Most of the actions of catecholamines and sympathomimetic agents can be classified into seven broad types:

1. *A peripheral excitatory action* on certain types of smooth muscle, such as those in blood vessels supplying skin, kidney, and mucous membranes; and on gland cells, such as those in salivary and sweat glands.
2. *A peripheral inhibitory action* on certain other types of smooth muscle, such as those in the wall of the gut, in the bronchial tree, and in blood vessels supplying skeletal muscle.
3. *A cardiac excitatory action* that increases heart rate and force of contraction.
4. *Metabolic actions*, such as an increase in the rate of glycogenolysis in liver and muscle and liberation of free fatty acids from adipose tissue.
5. *Endocrine actions*, such as modulation (increasing or decreasing) of the secretion of insulin, renin, and pituitary hormones.
6. *Actions in the CNS*, such as respiratory stimulation, an increase in wakefulness and psychomotor activity, and a reduction in appetite.
7. *Prejunctional actions* that either inhibit or facilitate the release of neurotransmitters, the inhibitory action being physiologically more important.

Many of these actions and the receptors that mediate them are summarized in Tables 8-1 and 8-6. Not all sympathomimetic drugs show each of the types of action to the same degree; however, many of the differences in their effects are only quantitative. The pharmacological properties of these drugs as a class are described in detail for the prototypical agent, epinephrine (EPI). Appreciation of the pharmacological properties of the drugs described in this chapter depends on an understanding of the classification, distribution, and mechanism of action of α and β adrenergic receptors (Chapter 8).

Classification of Sympathomimetic Drugs

Catecholamines and sympathomimetic drugs are classified as *direct-acting, indirect-acting, or mixed-acting sympathomimetics* (Figure 12–1). Direct-acting sympathomimetic drugs act directly on one or more of the adrenergic receptors. These agents may exhibit considerable selectivity for a specific receptor subtype (e.g., phenylephrine for α_1, terbutaline for β_2) or may have no or minimal selectivity and act on several receptor types (e.g., EPI for α_1, α_2, β_1, β_2, and β_3 receptors; NE for α_1, α_2, and β_1 receptors).

Indirect-acting drugs increase the availability of NE or EPI to stimulate adrenergic receptors by several mechanisms:

- By releasing or displacing NE from sympathetic nerve varicosities
- By inhibiting the transport of NE into sympathetic neurons (e.g., cocaine), thereby increasing the dwell time of the transmitter at the receptor
- By blocking the metabolizing enzymes, MAO (e.g., pargyline) or COMT (e.g., entacapone), effectively increasing transmitter supply

Drugs that indirectly release NE and also directly activate receptors are referred to as *mixed-acting sympathomimetic drugs* (e.g., ephedrine). A feature of *direct-acting sympathomimetic drugs* is that their responses are not reduced by prior treatment with reserpine or guanethidine, which deplete NE from sympathetic neurons. After transmitter depletion, the actions of direct-acting sympathomimetic drugs actually may increase because the loss of the neurotransmitter induces compensatory changes that upregulate receptors or enhance the signaling pathway. In contrast, the responses of indirect-acting sympathomimetic drugs (e.g., *amphetamine, tyramine*) are abolished by prior treatment with reserpine or guanethidine. The cardinal feature of mixed-acting sympathomimetic drugs is that their effects are blunted, but not abolished, by prior treatment with reserpine or guanethidine.

Abbreviations

AAAD: L-aromatic amino acid decarboxylase
ACEI: angiotensin-converting enzyme inhibitor
ADHD: attention-deficit/hyperactivity disorder
AV: atrioventricular
BPH: benign prostatic hyperplasia
CNS: central nervous system
COMT: catechol-*O*-methyltransferase
COPD: chronic obstructive pulmonary disease
DA: dopamine
ECG: electrocardiogram
EPI: epinephrine
FDA: Food and Drug Administration
GI: gastrointestinal
HDL: high-density lipoprotein
HMG CoA: 3-hydroxy-3-methylglutaryl coenzyme A
5HT: 5-hydroxytryptamine (serotonin)
INE: isoproterenol (Isopropyl NE)
LABA: long-acting β_2 adrenergic agonist
LDL: low-density lipoprotein
MAO: monoamine oxidase
NE: norepinephrine
NET: NE transporter
NPY: neuropeptide Y
PBZ: phenoxybenzamine
PDE: phosphodiesterase
PVR: peripheral vascular resistance
ROS: reactive oxygen species
SA: sinoatrial
VLABA: very long-acting β_2 adrenergic agonist

Because *the actions of NE are more pronounced on α and β_1 receptors than on β_2 receptors*, many noncatecholamines that release NE have predominantly α receptor–mediated and cardiac effects. However, certain noncatecholamines with both direct and indirect effects on adrenergic receptors show significant β_2 activity and are used clinically for these effects. Thus, ephedrine, although dependent on release of NE for some of its effects, relieves bronchospasm by its action on β_2 receptors in bronchial smooth muscle, an effect not seen with NE. Moreover, some noncatecholamines (e.g., phenylephrine) act primarily and directly on target cells. It therefore is impossible to predict precisely the effects of noncatecholamines solely on their ability to provoke NE release.

Structure-Activity Relationship of Sympathomimetic Amines

β-Phenylethylamine can be viewed as the parent compound of the sympathomimetic amines, *consisting of a benzene ring and an ethylamine side chain* (parent structure in Table 12–1). The structure permits substitutions to be made on the aromatic ring, the α- and β-carbon atoms, and the terminal amino group to yield a variety of compounds with sympathomimetic activity. *NE, EPI, DA, INE,* and a few other agents have hydroxyl groups substituted at positions 3 and 4 of the benzene ring. Because *o-dihydroxybenzene* is also known as *catechol*, sympathomimetic amines with these hydroxyl substitutions in the aromatic ring are termed *catecholamines*.

Many directly acting sympathomimetic drugs influence both α and β receptors, but the ratio of activities varies among drugs in a continuous spectrum from predominantly α activity (phenylephrine) to predominantly β activity (INE). Despite the multiplicity of the sites of action of sympathomimetic amines, several generalizations can be made (Table 12–1).

Separation of Aromatic Ring and Amino Group

By far the greatest sympathomimetic activity occurs when two carbon atoms separate the ring from the amino group. This rule applies with few exceptions to all types of action.

Substitution on the Amino Group

The effects of amino substitution are most readily seen in the actions of catecholamines on α and β receptors. *Increase in the size of the alkyl substituent increases β receptor activity (e.g., INE).* NE has, in general, rather feeble β_2 activity; this activity is greatly increased in EPI by the addition of a methyl group. A notable exception is phenylephrine, which has an *N*-methyl substituent but is an α-selective agonist. β_2-Selective compounds require a large amino substituent, but depend on other substitutions to define selectivity for β_2 rather than for β_1 receptors. *In general, the smaller the substitution on the amino group, the greater the selectivity for α activity, although N-methylation increases the potency of primary amines.* Thus, α activity is maximal in EPI, less in NE, and almost absent in INE.

Substitution on the Aromatic Nucleus

Maximal α and β activity depends on the presence of hydroxyl groups on positions 3 and 4. When one or both of these groups are absent, with no other aromatic substitution, the overall potency is reduced. Phenylephrine is thus less potent than EPI at both α and β receptors, with β_2 activity almost completely absent. Studies of the β adrenergic receptor suggest that the hydroxyl groups on serine residues 204 and 207 probably form hydrogen bonds with the catechol hydroxyl groups at positions 3 and 4, respectively. It also appears that aspartate 113 is a point of electrostatic interaction with the amine group on the ligand. Because the serines are in the fifth membrane-spanning region and the aspartate is in the third (Chapter 8), it is likely that catecholamines bind parallel to the plane of the membrane, forming a bridge between the two membrane spans. However, models involving DA receptors suggest alternative possibilities.

Hydroxyl groups in positions 3 and 5 confer β_2 receptor selectivity on compounds with large amino substituents. Thus, *terbutaline* and similar compounds relax the bronchial musculature in patients with asthma but cause less-direct cardiac stimulation than do the nonselective drugs. The response to noncatecholamines is partly determined by their capacity to release NE from storage sites. These agents thus cause effects that are mostly mediated by α and β_1 receptors because NE is a weak β_2 agonist. *Phenylethylamines that lack hydroxyl groups on the ring and the β-hydroxyl group on the side chain act almost exclusively by causing the release of NE from sympathetic nerve terminals.*

Because substitution of polar groups on the phenylethylamine structure makes the resultant compounds less lipophilic, *unsubstituted or alkyl-substituted compounds cross the blood-brain barrier more readily and have more central activity.* Thus, ephedrine, amphetamine, and methamphetamine exhibit considerable CNS activity. As noted, the absence of polar hydroxyl groups results in a loss of direct sympathomimetic activity.

Catecholamines have only a brief duration of action and are ineffective when administered orally because they are rapidly inactivated in the intestinal mucosa and in the liver before reaching the systemic circulation (Chapter 8). Compounds without one or both hydroxyl substituents are not acted on by COMT, and their oral effectiveness and duration of action are enhanced.

Groups other than hydroxyls have been substituted on the aromatic ring. In general, potency at α receptors is reduced, and β receptor activity is minimal; the compounds may even block β receptors. For example, methoxamine, with methoxy substituents at positions 2 and 5, has highly selective α stimulating activity and in large doses blocks β receptors. Albuterol, a β_2-selective agonist, has a substituent at position 3 and is an important exception to the general rule of low β receptor activity.

Substitution on the α-Carbon Atom

The substitution on the α-carbon atom blocks oxidation by MAO, greatly prolonging the duration of action of noncatecholamines because their degradation depends largely on the action of this enzyme. The duration of action of drugs such as ephedrine or amphetamine is thus measured in hours rather than in minutes. Similarly, compounds with an α-methyl

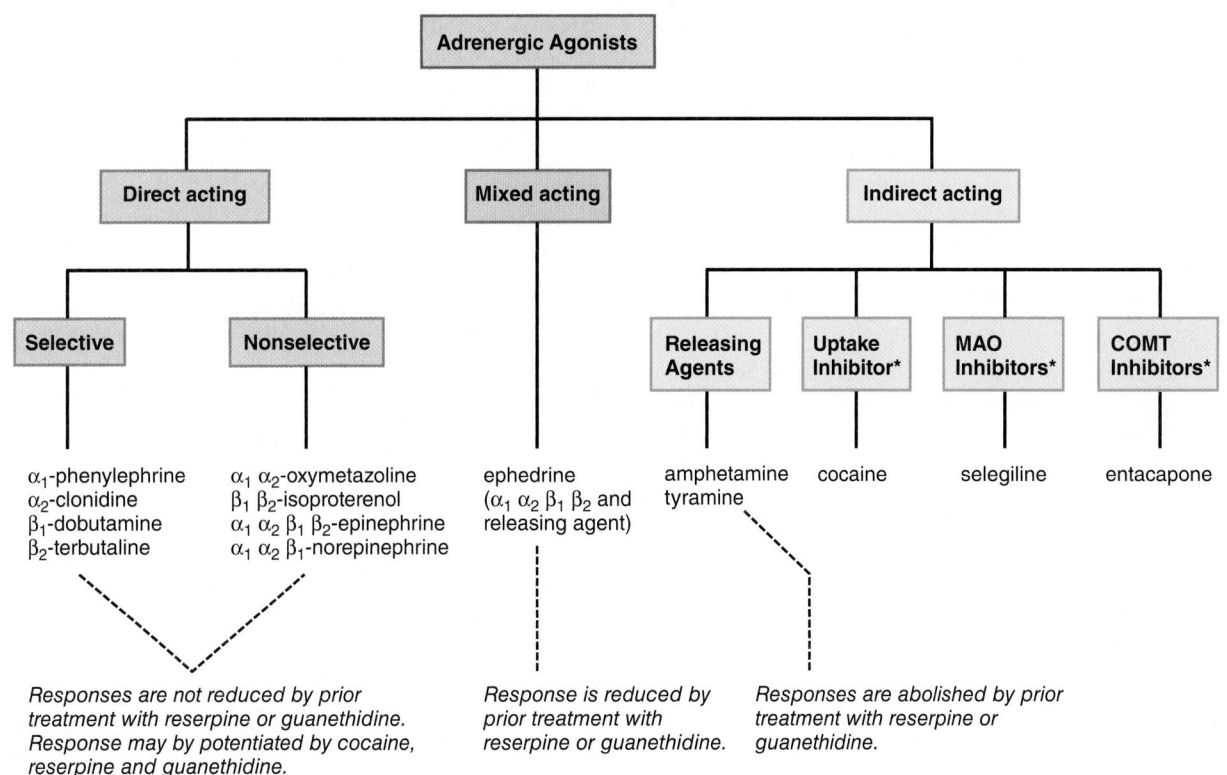

Figure 12–1 *Classification of adrenergic receptor agonists (sympathomimetic amines) or drugs that produce sympathomimetic-like effects.* For each category, a prototypical drug is shown. (*Not actually sympathetic drugs but produce sympathomimetic-like effects.)

TABLE 12–1 ■ STRUCTURES AND MAIN CLINICAL USES OF IMPORTANT SYMPATHOMIMETIC DRUGS

		CH	CH	NH	MAIN CLINICAL USES							
					α RECEPTOR				β RECEPTOR			
					A	N	P	V	B	C	U	CNS
Phenylethylamine		H	H	H								
Epinephrine	3-OH, 4-OH	OH	H	CH₃	A		P	V	B	C		
Norepinephrine	3-OH, 4-OH	OH	H	H			P			Cᵃ		
Dopamine	3-OH, 4-OH	H	H	H			P					
Droxidopa	3-OH, 4-OH	OH	COOH	H			P			Cᵃ		
Dobutamine	3-OH, 4-OH	H	H	X						C		
Isoproterenol	3-OH, 4-OH	OH	H	CH(CH₃)₂					B	C		
Terbutaline	3-OH, 5-OH	OH	H	C(CH₃)₃					B		U	
Metaraminol	3-OH	OH	CH₃	H			P					
Phenylephrine	3-OH	OH	H	CH₃		N	P					
Methoxamine	2-OCH₃, 5-OCH₃	OH	CH₃	H			P					
Albuterol	3-CH₂OH, 4-OH	OH	H	C(CH₃)₃					B		U	
Amphetamine		H	CH₃	H								++
Methamphetamine		H	CH₃	CH₃								++
Ephedrine		OH	CH₃	CH₃		N	P		B	C		

X: —CH—(CH₂)₂—⟨benzene ring⟩—OH
     |
     CH₃

α Activity: A, Allergic reactions (includes β action); N, Nasal decongestion; P, Pressor (may include β action); V, Other local vasoconstriction

β Activity: B, Bronchodilator; C, Cardiac; U, Uterus

ᵃDirect effects reduced by compensatory baroreceptor reflex.

substituent persist in the nerve terminals and are more likely to release NE from storage sites. Agents such as metaraminol exhibit a greater degree of indirect sympathomimetic activity.

Substitution on the β-Carbon Atom

Substitution of a hydroxyl group on the β-carbon generally decreases actions within the CNS, largely because it lowers lipid solubility. However, such substitution greatly enhances agonist activity at both α and β adrenergic receptors. Although ephedrine is less potent than methamphetamine as a central stimulant, it is more powerful in dilating bronchioles and increasing blood pressure and heart rate.

Optical Isomerism

Substitution on either α- or β-carbon yields optical isomers. Levorotatory substitution on the β-carbon confers the greater peripheral activity, so that the naturally occurring l-EPI and l-NE are at least 10 times more potent than their unnatural d-isomers. Dextrorotatory substitution on the α-carbon generally results in a more potent compound. d-Amphetamine is more potent than l-amphetamine in central but not peripheral activity.

Physiological Basis of Adrenergic Responsiveness

Important factors in the response of any cell or organ to sympathomimetic amines are the density and relative proportion of α and β adrenergic receptors. For example, NE has relatively little capacity to increase bronchial airflow because the receptors in bronchial smooth muscle are largely of the β_2 subtype. In contrast, INE and EPI are potent bronchodilators. Cutaneous blood vessels physiologically express almost exclusively α receptors; thus, NE and EPI cause constriction of such vessels, whereas INE has little effect. The smooth muscle of blood vessels that supply skeletal muscles has both β_2 and α receptors; activation of β_2 receptors causes vasodilation, and stimulation of α receptors constricts these vessels. In such vessels, the threshold concentration for activation of β_2 receptors by EPI is lower than that for α receptors, but when both types of receptors are activated at high concentrations of EPI, the response to α receptors predominates. Physiological concentrations of EPI primarily cause vasodilation.

The ultimate response of a target organ to sympathomimetic amines is dictated not only by the direct effects of the agents but also by the reflex homeostatic adjustments of the organism. One of the most striking effects of many sympathomimetic amines is a rise in arterial blood pressure caused by stimulation of vascular α adrenergic receptors. This stimulation elicits compensatory reflexes that are mediated by the carotid-aortic baroreceptor system. As a result, sympathetic tone is diminished and vagal tone is enhanced; each of these responses leads to slowing of the heart rate. Conversely, when a drug (e.g., a β_2 agonist) lowers mean blood pressure at the mechanoreceptors of the carotid sinus and aortic arch, the baroreceptor reflex works to restore pressure by reducing parasympathetic (vagal) outflow from the CNS to the heart and increasing sympathetic outflow to the heart and vessels. The baroreceptor reflex effect is of special importance for drugs that have little capacity to activate β receptors directly. With diseases such as atherosclerosis, which may impair baroreceptor mechanisms, the effects of sympathomimetic drugs may be magnified.

False-Transmitter Concept

Indirectly acting amines are taken up into sympathetic nerve terminals and storage vesicles, where they replace NE in the storage complex. Phenylethylamines that lack a β-hydroxyl group are retained there poorly, but β-hydroxylated phenylethylamines and compounds that subsequently become hydroxylated in the synaptic vesicle by DA β-hydroxylase are retained in the synaptic vesicle for relatively long periods of time. Such substances can produce a persistent diminution in the content of NE at functionally critical sites. When the nerve is stimulated, the contents of a relatively constant number of synaptic vesicles are released by exocytosis. If these vesicles contain phenylethylamines that are much less potent than NE, activation of postsynaptic α and β receptors will be diminished.

This hypothesis, known as the *false-transmitter concept*, is a possible explanation for some of the effects of MAO inhibitors. Phenylethylamines normally are synthesized in the GI tract as a result of the action of bacterial

tyrosine decarboxylase. The *tyramine* formed in this fashion usually is oxidatively deaminated in the GI tract and the liver, and the amine does not reach the systemic circulation in significant concentrations. However, when a MAO inhibitor is administered, tyramine may be absorbed systemically and transported into sympathetic nerve terminals, where its catabolism again is prevented because of the inhibition of MAO at this site; the tyramine then is β-hydroxylated to octopamine and stored in the vesicles in this form. As a consequence, NE gradually is displaced, and stimulation of the nerve terminal results in the release of a relatively small amount of NE along with a fraction of octopamine. The latter amine has relatively little ability to activate either α or β receptors. Thus, a functional impairment of sympathetic transmission parallels long-term administration of MAO inhibitors.

Despite such functional impairment, patients who have received MAO inhibitors may experience severe hypertensive crises if they ingest cheese, beer, or red wine. These and related foods, which are produced by fermentation, contain a large quantity of tyramine and, to a lesser degree, other phenylethylamines. When GI and hepatic MAO are inhibited, the large quantity of tyramine that is ingested is absorbed rapidly and reaches the systemic circulation in high concentration. A massive and precipitous release of NE can result, causing hypertension severe enough to precipitate a myocardial infarction or a stroke. The properties of various MAO inhibitors (reversible or irreversible; selective or nonselective at MAO-A and MAO-B) are discussed in Chapters 8 and 15.

Endogenous Catecholamines

Epinephrine

Epinephrine (adrenaline) is a potent stimulant of both α and β adrenergic receptors, and its effects on target organs are thus complex. Most of the responses listed in Table 8–1 are seen after injection of EPI, although the occurrence of sweating, piloerection, and mydriasis depends on the physiological state of the subject. Particularly prominent are the actions on the heart and on vascular and other smooth muscle.

Actions on Organ Systems

Effects on Blood Pressure. Epinephrine is one of the most potent vasopressor drugs known. If a pharmacological dose is given rapidly by an intravenous route, it evokes a characteristic effect on blood pressure, which rises rapidly to a peak that is proportional to the dose. The increase in systolic pressure is greater than the increase in diastolic pressure, so that the pulse pressure increases. As the response wanes, the mean pressure may fall below normal before returning to control levels.

The mechanism of the rise in blood pressure due to EPI is a triad of effects:

- a direct myocardial stimulation that increases the strength of ventricular contraction (*positive inotropic action*);
- an increased heart rate (*positive chronotropic action*); and
- vasoconstriction in many vascular beds—especially in the *precapillary resistance vessels* of skin, mucosa, and kidney—along with marked constriction of the veins.

The pulse rate, at first accelerated, may be slowed markedly at the height of the rise of blood pressure by compensatory vagal discharge (baroreceptor reflex). Small doses of EPI (0.1 µg/kg) may cause the blood pressure to fall. The depressor effect of small doses and the biphasic response to larger doses are due to greater sensitivity to EPI of vasodilator β_2 receptors than of constrictor α receptors.

Absorption of EPI after subcutaneous injection is slow due to local vasoconstrictor action; the effects of doses as large as 0.5–1.5 mg can be duplicated by intravenous infusion at a rate of 10–30 µg/min. There is a moderate increase in systolic pressure due to increased cardiac contractile force and a rise in cardiac output (Figure 12–2). Peripheral resistance decreases, owing to a dominant action on β_2 receptors of vessels in skeletal muscle, where blood flow is enhanced; as a consequence, diastolic pressure usually falls. Because the mean blood pressure is not, as a rule, greatly elevated, compensatory baroreceptor reflexes do not appreciably antagonize the direct cardiac

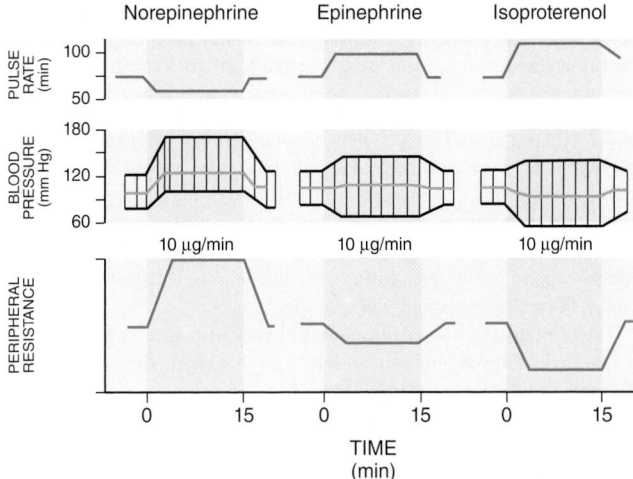

Figure 12–2 *Comparative effects of intravenous infusion of NE, EPI, and INE.* (Reproduced with permission from Allwood MJ, Cobbold AF, Ginsberg J. Peripheral vascular effects of noradrenaline, isopropyl-noradrenaline, and dopamine. *Br Med Bull.* **1963**;19:132–136. With permission from Oxford University Press.)

actions. Heart rate, cardiac output, stroke volume, and left ventricular work per beat are increased as a result of direct cardiac stimulation and increased venous return to the heart, which is reflected by an increase in right atrial pressure. At slightly higher rates of infusion, there may be no change or a slight rise in peripheral resistance and diastolic pressure, depending on the dose and the resultant ratio of α to β responses in the various vascular beds; compensatory reflexes also may come into play. The details of the effects of intravenous infusion of EPI, NE, and INE in humans are compared in Figure 12–2 and of EPI and NE in Table 12–2.

Vascular Effects. In the vasculature, *EPI acts chiefly on the smaller arterioles and precapillary sphincters,* although veins and large arteries also respond to the drug. Various vascular beds react differently, which results in a substantial redistribution of blood flow. *Injected EPI markedly decreases cutaneous blood flow, constricting precapillary vessels and small venules.* Cutaneous vasoconstriction accounts for a marked decrease in blood flow in the hands and feet. *Blood flow to skeletal muscles is increased by therapeutic doses in humans.* This is due in part to a powerful β_2-mediated vasodilator action that is only partially counterbalanced by a vasoconstrictor action on the α receptors that also are present in the vascular bed.

The effect of EPI on cerebral circulation is related to systemic blood pressure. In usual therapeutic doses, the drug has relatively little constrictor action on cerebral arterioles. Indeed, autoregulatory mechanisms tend to limit the increase in cerebral blood flow caused by increased blood pressure.

Doses of EPI that have little effect on mean arterial pressure consistently increase renal vascular resistance and reduce renal blood flow by as much as 40%. All segments of the renal vascular bed contribute to the increased resistance. Because the glomerular filtration rate is only slightly and variably altered, the filtration fraction is consistently increased. Excretion of Na^+, K^+, and Cl^- is decreased; urine volume may be increased, decreased, or unchanged. Maximal tubular reabsorptive and excretory capacities are unchanged. *The secretion of renin is increased as a consequence of a direct action of EPI on β_1 receptors in the juxtaglomerular apparatus.*

Arterial and venous pulmonary pressures are raised. Although direct pulmonary vasoconstriction occurs, redistribution of blood from the systemic to the pulmonary circulation, due to constriction of the more powerful musculature in the systemic great veins, doubtless plays an important part in the increase in pulmonary pressure. Very high concentrations of EPI may cause pulmonary edema precipitated by elevated pulmonary capillary filtration pressure and possibly by "leaky" capillaries.

Coronary blood flow is enhanced by EPI or by cardiac sympathetic stimulation under physiological conditions. The increased flow, which occurs even with doses that do not increase the aortic blood pressure, is the result

TABLE 12–2 ■ COMPARATIVE EFFECTS OF INFUSIONS OF EPINEPHRINE AND NOREPINEPHRINE IN HUMAN BEINGS[a]

EFFECT	EPI	NE
Cardiac		
Heart rate	+	–[b]
Stroke volume	++	++
Cardiac output	+++	0, –
Arrhythmias	++++	++++
Coronary blood flow	++	++
Blood pressure		
Systolic arterial	+++	+++
Mean arterial	+	++
Diastolic arterial	+, 0, –	++
Mean pulmonary	++	++
Peripheral circulation		
Total peripheral resistance	–	++
Cerebral blood flow	+	0, –
Muscle blood flow	+++	0, –
Cutaneous blood flow	–	–
Renal blood flow	–	–
Splanchnic blood flow	+++	0,+
Metabolic effects		
Oxygen consumption	++	0, +
Blood glucose	+++	0, +
Blood lactic acid	+++	0, +
Eosinopenic response	+	0
CNS		
Respiration	+	+
Subjective sensations	+	+

+, increase; 0, no change; –, decrease. Data from Goldenberg M, et al. *Arch Intern Med.* **1950**;86:823.
[a]0.1–0.4 µg/kg per minute.
[b]After atropine.

of two factors. The first is the increased relative duration of diastole at higher heart rates (described further in the chapter); this is partially offset by decreased blood flow during systole because of more forceful contraction of the surrounding myocardium and an increase in mechanical compression of the coronary vessels. The increased flow during diastole is further enhanced if aortic blood pressure is elevated by EPI; as a consequence, total coronary flow may be increased. The second factor is a metabolic dilator effect that results from the increased strength of contraction and myocardial O_2 consumption due to the direct effects of EPI on cardiac myocytes. This vasodilation is mediated in part by adenosine released from cardiac myocytes, which tends to override a direct vasoconstrictor effect of EPI that results from activation of α receptors in coronary vessels.

Cardiac Effects. Epinephrine is a powerful cardiac stimulant. It acts directly on the predominant β_1 receptors of the myocardium and of the cells of the pacemaker and conducting tissues; β_2, β_3, and α receptors also are present in the heart, although there are considerable species differences. The heart rate increases, and the rhythm often is altered. Cardiac systole is shorter and more powerful, cardiac output is enhanced, and the work of the heart and its oxygen consumption are markedly increased. Cardiac efficiency (work done relative to oxygen consumption) is lessened.

Direct responses to EPI include increases in contractile force, accelerated rate of rise of isometric tension, enhanced rate of relaxation, decreased time to peak tension, increased excitability, acceleration of the rate of spontaneous beating, and induction of automaticity in specialized regions of the heart.

In accelerating the heart, EPI preferentially shortens systole so that the duration of diastole usually is not reduced. Indeed, activation of β receptors increases the rate of relaxation of ventricular muscle. EPI speeds the heart by accelerating the slow depolarization of SA nodal cells that takes place during diastole, that is, during phase 4 of the action potential (Chapter 30). Consequently, the transmembrane potential of the pacemaker cells rises more rapidly to the threshold level of action potential initiation. The amplitude of the action potential and the maximal rate of depolarization (phase 0) also are increased. A shift in the location of the pacemaker within the SA node often occurs, owing to activation of latent pacemaker cells. In Purkinje fibers, EPI also accelerates diastolic depolarization and may activate latent pacemaker cells. These changes do not occur in atrial and ventricular muscle fibers, where EPI has little effect on the stable, phase 4 membrane potential after repolarization. If large doses of EPI are given, premature ventricular contractions occur and may herald more serious ventricular arrhythmias. This rarely is seen with conventional doses in humans, but ventricular extrasystoles, tachycardia, or even fibrillation may be precipitated by release of endogenous EPI when the heart has been sensitized to this action of EPI by certain anesthetics or by myocardial ischemia. The mechanism of induction of these cardiac arrhythmias is not clear.

Some effects of EPI on cardiac tissues are largely secondary to the increase in heart rate and are small or inconsistent when the heart rate is kept constant. For example, the effect of EPI on repolarization of atrial muscle, Purkinje fibers, or ventricular muscle is small if the heart rate is unchanged. When the heart rate is increased, the duration of the action potential is consistently shortened, and the refractory period is correspondingly decreased.

Conduction through the Purkinje system depends on the level of membrane potential at the time of excitation. Excessive reduction of this potential results in conduction disturbances, ranging from slowed conduction to complete block. EPI often increases the membrane potential and improves conduction in Purkinje fibers that have been excessively depolarized.

Epinephrine normally shortens the refractory period of the human AV node by direct effects on the heart, although doses of EPI that slow the heart through reflex vagal discharge may indirectly tend to prolong it. EPI also decreases the grade of AV block that occurs as a result of disease, drugs, or vagal stimulation. Supraventricular arrhythmias are apt to occur from the combination of EPI and cholinergic stimulation. Depression of sinus rate and AV conduction by vagal discharge probably plays a part in EPI-induced ventricular arrhythmias because various drugs that block the vagal effect confer some protection. The actions of EPI in enhancing cardiac automaticity and in causing arrhythmias are effectively antagonized by β receptor antagonists such as propranolol. However, α_1 receptors exist in most regions of the heart, and their activation prolongs the refractory period and strengthens myocardial contractions.

Cardiac arrhythmias have been seen in patients after inadvertent intravenous administration of conventional subcutaneous doses of EPI. Premature ventricular contractions can appear, which may be followed by multifocal ventricular tachycardia or ventricular fibrillation. Pulmonary edema also may occur.

Epinephrine decreases the amplitude of the T wave of the ECG in normal persons. In animals given relatively larger doses, additional effects are seen on the T wave and the ST segment. After decreasing in amplitude, the T wave may become biphasic, and the ST segment can deviate either above or below the isoelectric line. Such ST segment changes are similar to those seen in patients with angina pectoris during spontaneous or EPI-induced attacks of pain. These electrical changes therefore have been attributed to myocardial ischemia. Also, EPI as well as other catecholamines may cause myocardial cell death, particularly after intravenous infusions. Acute toxicity is associated with contraction band necrosis and other pathological changes. Recent interest has focused on the possibility that prolonged sympathetic stimulation of the heart, such as in congestive cardiomyopathy, may promote apoptosis of cardiomyocytes.

Effects on Smooth Muscles. The effects of EPI on the smooth muscles of different organs and systems depend on the type of adrenergic receptor in the muscle (Table 8–1). In general, EPI relaxes *GI smooth muscle* due to activation of both α and β receptors. Intestinal tone and the frequency and amplitude of spontaneous contractions are reduced. The stomach usually is relaxed and the pyloric and ileocecal sphincters are contracted, but these effects depend on the preexisting tone of the muscle. If tone already is high, EPI causes relaxation; if low, contraction.

The responses of *uterine muscle* to EPI vary with species, phase of the sexual cycle, state of gestation, and dose given. During the last month of pregnancy and at parturition, EPI inhibits uterine tone and contractions. Effects of adrenergic agents and other drugs on the uterus are discussed further in this chapter and in Chapter 44. *EPI relaxes the detrusor muscle of the bladder as a result of activation of β receptors and contracts the trigone and sphincter muscles owing to its α agonist activity.* This can result in hesitancy in urination and may contribute to retention of urine in the bladder. Activation of smooth muscle contraction in the prostate promotes urinary retention.

Respiratory Effects. *Epinephrine has a powerful bronchodilator action,* most evident when bronchial muscle is contracted because of disease, as in bronchial asthma, or in response to drugs or various autacoids. The beneficial effects of EPI in asthma also may arise from inhibition of antigen-induced release of inflammatory mediators from mast cells and to a lesser extent from diminution of bronchial secretions and congestion within the mucosa. *Inhibition of mast cell secretion is mediated by β_2 receptors, while the effects on the mucosa are mediated by α receptors;* however, other drugs, such as glucocorticoids and leukotriene receptor antagonists, have much more profound anti-inflammatory effects in asthma (Chapters 40 and 46).

Effects on the CNS. Because EPI is a polar compound, it penetrates poorly into the CNS and thus is not a powerful CNS stimulant. While the drug may cause restlessness, apprehension, headache, and tremor in many persons, these effects in part may be secondary to the effects of EPI on the cardiovascular system, skeletal muscles, and intermediary metabolism; that is, they may be the result of somatic manifestations of anxiety.

Metabolic Effects. Epinephrine elevates the concentrations of glucose and lactate in blood. *EPI inhibits secretion of insulin through an interaction with α_2 receptors, whereas activation of β_2 receptors enhances insulin secretions; the predominant effect of EPI is inhibition. Glucagon secretion is enhanced via activation of β receptors of the α cells of pancreatic islets.* EPI also decreases the uptake of glucose by peripheral tissues, at least in part not only because of its effects on the secretion of insulin, but also possibly due to direct effects on skeletal muscle. Glycosuria rarely occurs. The effect of EPI to stimulate glycogenolysis in most tissues and in most species involves β receptors. EPI raises the concentration of free fatty acids in blood by stimulating β receptors in adipocytes. The result is activation of triglyceride lipase, which accelerates the triglyceride breakdown to free fatty acids and glycerol. The calorigenic action of EPI (increase in metabolism) is reflected in humans by an increase of 20%–30% in O_2 consumption after conventional doses, an effect due mainly to enhanced breakdown of triglycerides in brown adipose tissue, providing an increase in oxidizable substrate (Chapter 8).

Miscellaneous Effects. Epinephrine reduces circulating plasma volume by loss of protein-free fluid to the extracellular space, thereby increasing hematocrit and plasma protein concentration. However, conventional doses of EPI do not significantly alter plasma volume or packed red cell volume under normal conditions, although such doses may have variable effects in the presence of shock, hemorrhage, hypotension, or anesthesia. EPI rapidly increases the number of circulating polymorphonuclear leukocytes, likely due to β receptor–mediated demargination of these cells. EPI accelerates blood coagulation and promotes fibrinolysis.

The effects of EPI on secretory glands are not marked; in most glands, secretion usually is inhibited, partly owing to the reduced blood flow caused by vasoconstriction. EPI stimulates lacrimation and scanty mucus secretion from salivary glands. Sweating and pilomotor activity are minimal after systemic administration of EPI, but occur after intradermal injection of very dilute solutions of either EPI or NE. Such effects are inhibited by α receptor antagonists.

Mydriasis occurs with physiological sympathetic stimulation but not when EPI is instilled into the conjunctival sac of normal eyes. However, EPI usually lowers intraocular pressure, possibly the result of reduced production of aqueous humor due to vasoconstriction and enhanced outflow (Chapter 69).

Although EPI does not directly excite *skeletal muscle, it facilitates neuromuscular transmission*, particularly that following prolonged rapid stimulation of motor nerves. In apparent contrast to the effects of α receptor activation at presynaptic nerve terminals in the autonomic nervous system (α_2 receptors), stimulation of α receptors causes a more rapid increase in transmitter release from the somatic motor neuron, perhaps as a result of enhanced influx of Ca^{2+}. These responses likely are mediated by α_1 receptors. These actions may explain in part the ability of EPI (given intra-arterially) to briefly increase strength of the injected limb of patients with myasthenia gravis. EPI also acts directly on white, fast-twitch muscle fibers to prolong the active state, thereby increasing peak tension. Of greater physiological and clinical importance is the capacity of EPI and selective β_2 agonists to increase physiological tremor, at least in part due to β receptor–mediated enhancement of discharge of muscle spindles.

Epinephrine promotes a fall in plasma K^+, largely due to stimulation of K^+ uptake into cells, particularly skeletal muscle, due to activation of β_2 receptors. This is associated with decreased renal K^+ excretion. These receptors have been exploited in the management of hyperkalemic familial periodic paralysis, which is characterized by episodic flaccid paralysis, hyperkalemia, and depolarization of skeletal muscle. The β_2-selective agonist albuterol apparently is able to ameliorate the impairment in the ability of the muscle to accumulate and retain K^+.

The administration of large or repeated doses of EPI or other sympathomimetic amines to experimental animals damages arterial walls and myocardium, even inducing necrosis in the heart that is indistinguishable from myocardial infarction. The mechanism of this injury is not yet clear, but α and β receptor antagonists and Ca^{2+} channel blockers may afford substantial protection against the damage. Similar lesions occur in many patients with pheochromocytoma or after prolonged infusions of NE.

ADME

Epinephrine is not effective after oral administration because it is rapidly conjugated and oxidized in the GI mucosa and liver. Absorption from subcutaneous tissues occurs relatively slowly because of local vasoconstriction. Absorption is more rapid after intramuscular injection. In emergencies, it may be necessary to administer EPI intravenously. When relatively concentrated solutions are nebulized and inhaled, the actions of the drug largely are restricted to the respiratory tract; however, systemic reactions such as arrhythmias may occur, particularly if larger amounts are used.

Epinephrine is rapidly inactivated in the liver by COMT and MAO (see Figure 8–9). Although only small amounts appear in the urine of normal persons, the urine of patients with pheochromocytoma may contain relatively large amounts of EPI, NE, and their metabolites.

Epinephrine is available in a variety of formulations geared for different clinical indications and routes of administration, including self-administration for anaphylactic reactions. EPI is unstable in alkaline solution; when exposed to air or light, it turns pink from oxidation to adrenochrome and then brown from formation of polymers. Injectable EPI is available in solutions of 1, 0.5, and 0.1 mg/mL. A subcutaneous dose ranges from 0.3 to 0.5 mg. The intravenous route is used cautiously if an immediate and reliable effect is mandatory. If the solution is given by vein, it must be adequately diluted and injected very slowly. The dose is seldom as much as 0.25 mg, except for cardiac arrest, when larger doses may be required.

Toxicity, Adverse Effects, and Contraindications

Epinephrine may cause restlessness, throbbing headache, tremor, and palpitations. The effects rapidly subside with rest, quiet, recumbency, and reassurance. More serious reactions include cerebral hemorrhage and cardiac arrhythmias. The use of large doses or the accidental, rapid intravenous injection of EPI may result in cerebral hemorrhage from the sharp rise in blood pressure. Ventricular arrhythmias may follow the administration of EPI. Angina may be induced by EPI in patients with coronary artery disease. *The use of EPI generally is contraindicated in patients who are receiving nonselective β receptor antagonists because its unopposed actions on vascular α_1 receptors may lead to severe hypertension and cerebral hemorrhage.*

Therapeutic Uses

A major use of EPI is to provide rapid, emergency relief of hypersensitivity reactions, including anaphylaxis, to drugs and other allergens. EPI also is used to prolong the action of local anesthetics, presumably by decreasing local blood flow and reducing systemic absorption. (Chapter 22). Its cardiac effects may be of use in restoring cardiac rhythm in patients with cardiac arrest due to various causes. It also is used as a topical hemostatic agent on bleeding surfaces, such as in the mouth or in bleeding peptic ulcers during endoscopy of the stomach and duodenum. Systemic absorption of the drug can occur with dental application. Inhalation of EPI may be useful in the treatment of postintubation and infectious croup.

Norepinephrine

Norepinephrine (levarterenol, *l*-noradrenaline, *l*-β-[3,4-dihydroxyphenyl]-α-aminoethanol) is a major chemical mediator liberated by mammalian *postganglionic sympathetic nerves*. It differs from EPI only by lacking the methyl substitution in the amino group (Table 12–1). NE constitutes 10%–20% of the catecholamine content of human adrenal medulla and as much as 97% in some pheochromocytomas, which may not express the enzyme phenylethanolamine-*N*-methyltransferase.

Pharmacological Properties

The pharmacological actions of NE and EPI are compared in Table 12–2. Both drugs are direct agonists on effector cells, and their actions differ mainly in the ratio of their effectiveness in stimulating α and β_2 receptors. *They are approximately equipotent in stimulating β_1 receptors. NE is a potent α agonist and has relatively little action on β_2 receptors*; however, it is somewhat less potent than EPI on the α receptors of most organs.

Cardiovascular Effects

In response to intravenous infusion of NE in humans (Figure 12–2), *systolic and diastolic pressures, and usually pulse pressure, are increased. Cardiac output is unchanged or decreased, and total peripheral resistance is raised. Compensatory vagal reflex activity slows the heart, overcoming a direct cardioaccelerator action, and stroke volume is increased. The peripheral vascular resistance increases in most vascular beds, and renal blood flow is reduced. NE constricts mesenteric vessels and reduces splanchnic and hepatic blood flow. Coronary flow usually is increased, probably owing both to indirectly induced coronary dilation, as with EPI, and to elevated blood pressure.* Although generally a poor β_2 receptor agonist, NE may increase coronary blood flow directly by stimulating β_2 receptors on coronary vessels. Patients with Prinzmetal variant angina may be supersensitive to the α adrenergic vasoconstrictor effects of NE.

Unlike EPI, NE in small doses does not cause vasodilation or lower blood pressure because the blood vessels of skeletal muscle constrict rather than dilate; α adrenergic receptor antagonists therefore abolish the pressor effects but do not cause significant reversal (i.e., hypotension).

Other Effects

Other responses to NE are not prominent in humans. The drug causes hyperglycemia and other metabolic effects similar to those produced by EPI, but these are observed only when large doses are given because NE is not as effective a "hormone" as EPI. Intradermal injection of suitable doses causes sweating that is not blocked by atropine.

Norepinephrine, like EPI, is ineffective when given orally and is absorbed poorly from sites of subcutaneous injection. It is rapidly inactivated in the body by the same enzymes that methylate (COMT) and oxidatively deaminate EPI (MAO). Small amounts normally are found in the urine. The excretion rate may be greatly increased in patients with pheochromocytoma.

Toxicity, Adverse Effects, and Precautions

The untoward effects of NE are similar to those of EPI, although there typically is greater elevation of blood pressure with NE. Excessive doses can cause severe hypertension.

Care must be taken that necrosis and sloughing do not occur at the site of intravenous injection owing to extravasation of the drug. The infusion should be made high in the limb, preferably through a long plastic cannula extending centrally. Impaired circulation at injection sites, with or without extravasation of NE, may be relieved by infiltrating the area with phentolamine, an α receptor antagonist. Blood pressure must be determined frequently during the infusion, particularly during adjustment of the rate of the infusion. Reduced blood flow to organs such as kidney and intestines is a constant danger with the use of NE.

Therapeutic Uses

Norepinephrine is used as a vasoconstrictor to raise or support blood pressure under certain intensive care conditions (discussed further in this chapter).

Droxidopa, a Synthetic Prodrug of Norepinephrine

Droxidopa (L-threo-3,4,-dihydroxyphenylserine) is a synthetic prodrug that is converted by AAAD into NE. It is FDA-approved for the treatment of orthostatic dizziness and light-headedness in adults with symptomatic neurogenic orthostatic hypotension associated with primary autonomic failure and impaired compensatory autonomic reflexes (Keating, 2014). The pharmacological effects of droxidopa are thought to be mediated through NE rather than through the parent drug or other metabolites. Droxidopa can cross the blood-brain barrier, presumably as the substrate of an amino acid transporter.

Dopamine

Dopamine (3,4-dihydroxyphenylethylamine) (Table 12–1) is the immediate metabolic precursor of NE and EPI; it is a central neurotransmitter particularly important in the regulation of movement (Chapters 14, 16, and 18) and possesses important intrinsic pharmacological properties. In the periphery, it is synthesized in epithelial cells of the proximal tubule and is thought to exert local diuretic and natriuretic effects. DA is a substrate for both MAO and COMT and thus is ineffective when administered orally. Classification of DA receptors is described in Chapter 13.

Pharmacological Properties Cardiovascular Effects

The cardiovascular effects of DA are mediated by several distinct types of receptors that vary in their affinity for DA (Chapter 13). At low concentrations, the primary interaction of DA is with vascular D_1 receptors, especially in the renal, mesenteric, and coronary beds. By activating adenylyl cyclase and raising intracellular concentrations of cAMP, D_1 receptor stimulation leads to vasodilation. Infusion of low doses of DA causes an increase in glomerular filtration rate, renal blood flow, and Na^+ excretion. Activation of D_1 receptors on renal tubular cells decreases Na^+ transport by cAMP-dependent and cAMP-independent mechanisms. Increasing cAMP production in the proximal tubular cells and the medullary part of the thick ascending limb of the loop of Henle inhibits the Na^+-H^+ exchanger and the Na^+,K^+-ATPase pump. The renal tubular actions of DA that cause natriuresis may be augmented by the increase in renal blood flow and the small increase in the glomerular filtration rate that follows its administration. The resulting increase in hydrostatic pressure in the peritubular capillaries and reduction in oncotic pressure may contribute to diminished reabsorption of Na^+ by the proximal tubular cells. As a consequence, DA has pharmacologically appropriate effects in the management of states of low cardiac output associated with compromised renal function, such as severe congestive heart failure.

At higher concentrations, DA exerts a positive inotropic effect on the myocardium, acting on β_1 adrenergic receptors. DA also causes the release of NE from nerve terminals, which contributes to its effects on the heart. Tachycardia is less prominent during infusion of DA than of INE (discussed further in the chapter). DA usually increases systolic blood pressure and pulse pressure and either has no effect on diastolic blood pressure or increases it slightly. Total peripheral resistance usually is unchanged when low or intermediate doses of DA are given, probably because of the ability of DA to reduce regional arterial resistance in some vascular beds, such as mesenteric and renal, while causing only minor increases in others. At high concentrations, DA activates vascular α_1 receptors, leading to more general vasoconstriction.

CNS Effects

Although there are specific DA receptors in the CNS, injected DA usually has no central effects because it does not readily cross the blood-brain barrier.

Precautions, Adverse Reactions, and Contraindications

Before DA is administered to patients in shock, hypovolemia should be corrected by transfusion of whole blood, plasma, or other appropriate fluid. Untoward effects due to overdosage generally are attributable to excessive sympathomimetic activity (although this also may be the response to worsening shock). Nausea, vomiting, tachycardia, anginal pain, arrhythmias, headache, hypertension, and peripheral vasoconstriction may be encountered during DA infusion. Extravasation of large amounts of DA during infusion may cause ischemic necrosis and sloughing. Rarely, gangrene of the fingers or toes has followed prolonged infusion of the drug. DA should be avoided or used at a much reduced dosage if the patient has received a MAO inhibitor. Careful adjustment of dosage also is necessary in patients who are taking tricyclic antidepressants.

Therapeutic Uses

Dopamine is used in the treatment of severe congestive heart failure, particularly in patients with oliguria and low or normal peripheral vascular resistance. The drug also may improve physiological parameters in the treatment of cardiogenic and septic shock. While DA may acutely improve cardiac and renal function in severely ill patients with chronic heart disease or renal failure, there is relatively little evidence supporting long-term benefit in clinical outcome (Marik and Iglesias, 1999).

Dopamine hydrochloride is used only intravenously, preferably into a large vein to prevent perivascular infiltration; extravasation may cause necrosis and sloughing of the surrounding tissue. The use of a calibrated infusion pump to control the rate of flow is necessary. The drug is administered at a rate of 2–5 µg/kg per min; this rate may be increased gradually up to 20–50 µg/kg per min or more as the clinical situation dictates. During the infusion, patients require clinical assessment of myocardial function, perfusion of vital organs such as the brain, and the production of urine. Reduction in urine flow, tachycardia, or the development of arrhythmias may be indications to slow or terminate the infusion. The duration of action of DA is brief, and hence the rate of administration can be used to control the intensity of effect.

Fenoldopam and Dopexamine.
Fenoldopam, a benzazepine derivative, is a rapidly acting vasodilator used for not more than 48 h for control of severe hypertension (e.g., malignant hypertension with end-organ damage) in hospitalized patients. Fenoldopam is an agonist for peripheral D_1 receptors and binds with moderate affinity to α_2 adrenergic receptors; it has no significant affinity for D_2 receptors or α_1 or β adrenergic receptors. Fenoldopam is a racemic mixture; the R-isomer is the active component. It dilates a variety of blood vessels, including coronary arteries, afferent and efferent arterioles in the kidney, and mesenteric arteries (Murphy et al., 2001). Fenoldopam must be administered using a calibrated infusion pump; the usual dose rate ranges from 0.01 to 1.6 µg/kg per min.

Less than 6% of an orally administered dose is absorbed because of extensive first-pass formation of sulfate, methyl, and glucuronide conjugates. The elimination $t_{1/2}$ of intravenously infused fenoldopam is about 10 min. Adverse effects are related to the vasodilation and include headache, flushing, dizziness, and tachycardia or bradycardia.

Dopexamine is a synthetic analogue related to DA with intrinsic activity at DA D_1 and D_2 receptors as well as at β_2 receptors; it may have other effects, such as inhibition of catecholamine uptake (Fitton and Benfield, 1990). It has favorable hemodynamic actions in patients with severe congestive heart failure, sepsis, and shock. In patients with low cardiac output, dopexamine infusion significantly increases stroke volume with a decrease in systemic vascular resistance. Tachycardia and hypotension can occur, but usually only at high infusion rates. Dopexamine is not currently available in the U.S.

β Adrenergic Receptor Agonists

β Adrenergic receptor agonists play a major role only in the treatment of bronchoconstriction in patients with asthma (reversible airway obstruction) or COPD. Minor uses include management of preterm labor, treatment of complete heart block in shock, and short-term treatment of cardiac decompensation after surgery or in patients with congestive heart failure or myocardial infarction. The development of β_2-selective agonists has resulted in drugs with even more valuable characteristics, including adequate oral bioavailability, lack of α adrenergic activity and relative lack of β_1 adrenergic activity, and thus diminished likelihood of adverse cardiovascular effects.

β Receptor agonists may be used to stimulate the rate and force of cardiac contraction. The chronotropic effect is useful in the emergency treatment of arrhythmias such as torsades de pointes, bradycardia, or heart block (Chapter 30), whereas the inotropic effect is useful when it is desirable to augment myocardial contractility.

Isoproterenol

Isoproterenol (INE, isopropyl norepinephrine, isoprenaline, isopropylarterenol, isopropyl noradrenaline, *d,l*-β-[3,4-dihydroxyphenyl]-α-isopropylaminoethanol) (Table 12–1) is a potent, nonselective β receptor agonist with very low affinity for α receptors. Consequently, INE has powerful effects on all β receptors and almost no action at α receptors.

Pharmacological Actions

The major cardiovascular effects of INE (compared with EPI and NE) are illustrated in Figure 12–2. *Intravenous infusion of INE lowers peripheral vascular resistance,* primarily in skeletal muscle but also in renal and mesenteric vascular beds. *Diastolic pressure falls. Systolic blood pressure may remain unchanged or rise, although mean arterial pressure typically falls. Cardiac output is increased because of the positive inotropic and chronotropic effects of the drug in the face of diminished peripheral vascular resistance.* The cardiac effects of INE may lead to palpitations, sinus tachycardia, and more serious arrhythmias; large doses of INE cause myocardial necrosis in experimental animals.

Isoproterenol relaxes almost all varieties of smooth muscle when the tone is high, an action that is most pronounced on bronchial and GI smooth muscle. INE prevents or relieves bronchoconstriction. Its effect in asthma may be due in part to an additional action to inhibit antigen-induced release of histamine and other mediators of inflammation, an action shared by β_2-selective stimulants.

ADME

Isoproterenol is readily absorbed when given parenterally or as an aerosol. *It is metabolized by COMT, primarily in the liver but also by other tissues.* INE is a relatively poor substrate for MAO and NET (SLC6A2) and is not taken up by sympathetic neurons to the same extent as are EPI and NE. The duration of action of INE therefore may be longer than that of EPI, but it still is relatively brief.

Therapeutic Uses

Isoproterenol may be used in emergencies to stimulate heart rate in patients with bradycardia or heart block, particularly in anticipation of inserting an artificial cardiac pacemaker or in patients with the ventricular arrhythmia torsades de pointes. In disorders such as asthma and shock, INE largely has been replaced by other sympathomimetic drugs (see further in this chapter and in Chapter 40).

Adverse Effects

Palpitations, tachycardia, headache, and flushing are common. Cardiac ischemia and arrhythmias may occur, particularly in patients with underlying coronary artery disease.

Dobutamine

Dobutamine resembles DA structurally but possesses a bulky aromatic substituent on the amino group (Table 12–1). The pharmacological effects of dobutamine are due to direct interactions with α and β receptors; its actions do not appear to result from release of NE from sympathetic nerve endings, and they are not exerted by dopaminergic receptors.

Dobutamine possesses a center of asymmetry; both enantiomeric forms are present in the racemate used clinically. The (–) isomer of dobutamine is a potent α_1 agonist and can cause marked pressor responses. In contrast, (+)-dobutamine is a potent α_1 receptor antagonist, which can block the effects of (–)-dobutamine. Both isomers are full agonists at β receptors; the (+) isomer is a more potent β agonist than the (–) isomer by about 10-fold.

Cardiovascular Effects

The cardiovascular effects of racemic dobutamine represent a composite of the distinct pharmacological properties of the (–) and (+) stereoisomers. Compared to INE, dobutamine has relatively more prominent inotropic than chronotropic effects on the heart. Although not completely understood, this useful selectivity may arise because peripheral resistance is relatively unchanged. Alternatively, cardiac α_1 receptors may contribute to the inotropic effect. At equivalent inotropic doses, dobutamine enhances automaticity of the sinus node to a lesser extent than does INE; however, enhancement of AV and intraventricular conduction is similar for both drugs.

In animals, infusion of dobutamine increases cardiac contractility and cardiac output without markedly changing total peripheral resistance; the relatively constant peripheral resistance presumably reflects counterbalancing of α_1 receptor–mediated vasoconstriction and β_2 receptor–mediated vasodilation. Heart rate increases only modestly when dobutamine is administered at less than 20 µg/kg per min. After administration of β receptor antagonists, infusion of dobutamine fails to increase cardiac output, but total peripheral resistance increases, confirming that dobutamine has modest direct effects on α adrenergic receptors in the vasculature.

ADME

Dobutamine has a $t_{1/2}$ of about 2 min; the major metabolites are conjugates of dobutamine and 3-O-methyldobutamine. The onset of effect is rapid. Steady-state concentrations generally are achieved within 10 min of initiation of the infusion by calibrated infusion pump. The rate of infusion required to increase cardiac output typically is between 2.5 and 10 µg/kg per min, although higher infusion rates occasionally are required. The rate and duration of the infusion are determined by the clinical and hemodynamic responses of the patient.

Therapeutic Uses

Dobutamine is indicated for the short-term treatment of cardiac decompensation that may occur after cardiac surgery or in patients with congestive heart failure or acute myocardial infarction. Dobutamine increases cardiac output and stroke volume in such patients, usually without a marked increase in heart rate. Alterations in blood pressure or peripheral resistance usually are minor, although some patients may have marked increases in blood pressure or heart rate. An infusion of dobutamine in combination with echocardiography is useful in the noninvasive assessment of patients with coronary artery disease.

Adverse Effects

Blood pressure and heart rate may increase significantly during dobutamine administration requiring reduction of infusion rate. Patients with a history of hypertension may exhibit an exaggerated pressor response more frequently. Because dobutamine facilitates AV conduction, patients with atrial fibrillation are at risk of marked increases in ventricular response rates; digoxin or other measures may be required to prevent this from occurring. Some patients may develop ventricular ectopic activity. Dobutamine may increase the size of a myocardial infarct by increasing myocardial O_2 demand, a property common to inotropic agents. The efficacy of dobutamine over a period of more than a few days is uncertain; there is evidence for the development of tolerance.

$β_2$-Selective Adrenergic Receptor Agonists

Some of the major adverse effects of β receptor agonists in the treatment of asthma or COPD are caused by stimulation of $β_1$ receptors in the heart. $β_2$-Selective agents have been developed to avoid these adverse effects. This selectivity, however, is not absolute and is lost at high concentrations of these drugs. Moreover, up to 40% of the β receptors in the human heart are $β_2$ receptors, activation of which can also cause cardiac stimulation (Brodde and Michel, 1999).

A second strategy that has increased the usefulness of several $β_2$-selective agonists in the treatment of asthma and COPD has been structural modification that results in lower rates of metabolism and enhanced oral bioavailability. Modifications have included placing the hydroxyl groups at positions 3 and 5 of the phenyl ring or substituting another moiety for the hydroxyl group at position 3. This has yielded drugs such as metaproterenol, terbutaline, and albuterol, which are not substrates for COMT. Bulky substituents on the amino group of catecholamines contribute to potency at β receptors with decreased activity at α receptors and decreased metabolism by MAO.

A final strategy to enhance preferential activation of pulmonary $β_2$ receptors is the administration by inhalation of small doses of the drug in aerosol form. This approach typically leads to effective activation of $β_2$ receptors in the bronchi but very low systemic drug concentrations. Consequently, there is less potential to activate cardiac $β_1$ or $β_2$ receptors or to stimulate $β_2$ receptors in skeletal muscle, which can cause tremor and thereby limit oral therapy.

Subcutaneous injection also causes prompt bronchodilation; for an orally administered agent, the peak effect may be delayed for several hours. Administration of β receptor agonists by aerosol (Chapter 40) typically leads to a very rapid therapeutic response, generally within minutes, although some agonists such as *salmeterol* have a delayed onset of action. Aerosol therapy depends on the delivery of drug to the distal airways. This, in turn, depends on the size of the particles in the aerosol and respiratory parameters such as inspiratory flow rate, tidal volume, breath-holding time, and airway diameter. Only about 10% of an inhaled dose actually enters the lungs; much of the remainder is swallowed and ultimately may be absorbed. Successful aerosol therapy requires that each patient master the technique of drug administration. In some patients, particularly children and the elderly, spacer devices may enhance the efficacy of inhalation therapy.

In the treatment of asthma and COPD, β receptor agonists are used to activate pulmonary receptors that relax bronchial smooth muscle and decrease airway resistance. β Receptor agonists also may suppress the release of leukotrienes and histamine from mast cells in lung tissue, enhance mucociliary function, decrease microvascular permeability, and possibly inhibit phospholipase A_2. Airway inflammation also contributes airway hyperresponsiveness; consequently, the use of anti-inflammatory drugs such as inhaled steroids has primary importance. Most authorities recommend that long-acting β agonists should not be used without concomitant anti-inflammatory therapy in the treatment of asthma (see Chapter 40; Drazen and O'Byrne, 2009; Fanta, 2009).

Short-Acting $β_2$ Adrenergic Agonists

Metaproterenol. Metaproterenol (called orciprenaline in Europe), along with *terbutaline* and *fenoterol*, belongs to the structural class of resorcinol bronchodilators that have hydroxyl groups at positions 3 and 5 of the phenyl ring (rather than at positions 3 and 4 as in catechols) (Table 12–1).

Consequently, metaproterenol is resistant to methylation by COMT, and a substantial fraction (40%) is absorbed in active form after oral administration. It is excreted primarily as glucuronic acid conjugates. Metaproterenol is considered to be $β_2$ selective, although it probably is less selective than albuterol or terbutaline and hence is more prone to cause cardiac stimulation. Effects occur within minutes of inhalation and persist for several hours. After oral administration, onset of action is slower, but effects last 3–4 h. Metaproterenol is used for the long-term treatment of obstructive airway diseases and asthma and for treatment of acute bronchospasm (Chapter 40). Side effects are similar to the short- and intermediate-acting sympathomimetic bronchodilators.

Albuterol. Albuterol is a selective $β_2$ receptor agonist with pharmacological properties and therapeutic indications similar to those of terbutaline. It can be administered by inhalation or orally for the symptomatic relief of bronchospasm.

When administered by inhalation, it produces significant bronchodilation within 15 min, and effects persist for 3–4 h. The cardiovascular effects of albuterol are much weaker than those of INE when doses that produce comparable bronchodilation are administered by inhalation. Oral albuterol has the potential to delay preterm labor. Although rare, CNS and respiratory side effects are sometimes observed.

Albuterol has been made available in a metered-dose inhaler free of CFCs (chlorofluorocarbons). The alternate propellant, HFA (hydrofluoroalkane), is inert in the human airway, but unlike CFCs, it does not deplete stratospheric ozone.

Levalbuterol. Levalbuterol is the *R*-enantiomer of albuterol, a racemate used to treat asthma and COPD. Although originally available only as a solution for a nebulizer, it is now available as a CFC-free metered-dose inhaler. Levalbuterol is $β_2$ selective and acts like other $β_2$ adrenergic agonists. In general, levalbuterol has similar pharmacokinetic and pharmacodynamics properties as albuterol.

Pirbuterol. Pirbuterol is a relatively selective $β_2$ agonist. Its structure differs from that of albuterol by the substitution of a pyridine ring for the benzene ring. Pirbuterol acetate is available for inhalation therapy; dosing is typically every 4–6 h. Pirbuterol is the only preparation available in a breath-activated metered-dose inhaler, a device meant to optimize medication delivery by releasing a spray of medication only on the patient's initiation of inspiration.

Terbutaline. Terbutaline is a $β_2$-selective bronchodilator. It contains a resorcinol ring and thus is not a substrate for COMT methylation. It is effective when taken orally or subcutaneously or by inhalation (not marketed for inhalation in the U.S.). Effects are observed rapidly after inhalation or parenteral administration; after inhalation, its action may persist 3–6 h. With oral administration, the onset of effect may be delayed 1–2 h. Terbutaline is used for the long-term treatment of obstructive airway diseases and for treatment of acute bronchospasm; it also is available for parenteral use for the emergency treatment of status asthmaticus (Chapter 40).

Isoetharine. Isoetharine is an older $β_2$-selective drug. Its selectivity for $β_2$ receptors does not approach that of some newer agents. Although resistant to metabolism by MAO, it is a catecholamine and thus is a good substrate for COMT. Consequently, it is used only by inhalation for the treatment of acute episodes of bronchoconstriction. Isoetharine is no longer marketed in the U.S.

Fenoterol. Fenoterol is a $β_2$-selective receptor agonist. After inhalation, it has a prompt onset of action, and its effect typically is sustained for 4–6 h. A possible association of fenoterol use with increased deaths from asthma, although controversial (Suissa and Ernst, 1997), has led to its withdrawal from the market. The dysrhythmias and cardiac effects associated with fenoterol are likely due to effects on $β_1$ adrenergic receptors.

Procaterol. Procaterol is a $β_2$-selective receptor agonist. After inhalation, it has a prompt onset of action that is sustained for about 5 h. Procaterol is not available in the U.S.

Long-Acting β₂ Adrenergic Agonists (LABAs)

Salmeterol

Mechanism of Action. Salmeterol is a lipophilic β_2-selective agonist with a prolonged duration of action (>12 h) and a selectivity for β_2 receptors about 50-fold greater than that of albuterol. Salmeterol provides symptomatic relief and improves lung function and quality of life in patients with COPD. It is as effective as the cholinergic antagonist ipratropium, more effective than theophylline, and has additive effects when used in combination with inhaled ipratropium or oral theophylline. Salmeterol also may have anti-inflammatory activity.

ADME. The onset of action of inhaled salmeterol is relatively slow, so it is not suitable monotherapy for acute attacks of bronchospasm. Salmeterol is metabolized by CYP3A4 to α-hydroxy-salmeterol, which is eliminated primarily in the feces.

Clinical Use, Precautions, and Adverse Effects. Salmeterol and formoterol are the agents of choice for nocturnal asthma in patients who remain symptomatic despite anti-inflammatory agents and other standard management.

Salmeterol generally is well tolerated but has the potential to increase heart rate and plasma glucose concentration, to produce tremors, and to decrease plasma K⁺ concentration through effects on extrapulmonary β_2 receptors. Salmeterol should not be used more than twice daily (morning and evening) and should not be used to treat acute asthma symptoms, which should be treated with a short-acting β_2 agonist (e.g., *albuterol*) when breakthrough symptoms occur despite twice-daily use of salmeterol (Redington, 2001).

Patients with moderate or severe persistent asthma or COPD benefit from the use of LABAs like salmeterol in combination with an inhaled corticosteroid. For that reason, salmeterol is available in a single formulate combination with the corticosteroid fluticasone. These benefits must be counterbalanced against data, oft-criticized, showing that the addition of a LABA to "usual therapy" was associated with an increased risk of fatal or near-fatal asthmatic attacks, as compared with usual therapy alone. On the other hand, there is a lack of reports of increased asthma mortality among patients taking both a LABA and an inhaled corticosteroid (Fanta, 2009). Nevertheless, the FDA has placed a **black-box warning** in the labeling information for *salmeterol, formoterol*, and *arformoterol*. Expert panels (Fanta, 2009) recommend the use of LABAs only for patients in whom inhaled corticosteroids alone either failed to achieve good asthma control or for initial therapy.

Formoterol.

Formoterol is a long-acting β_2-selective receptor agonist. Significant bronchodilation, which may persist for up to 12 h, occurs within minutes of inhalation of a therapeutic dose. It is highly lipophilic and has high affinity for β_2 receptors. Its major advantage over many other β_2-selective agonists is this prolonged duration of action, which may be particularly advantageous in settings such as nocturnal asthma. Formoterol's sustained action is due to its insertion into the lipid bilayer of the plasma membrane, from which it gradually diffuses to provide prolonged stimulation of β_2 receptors. It is FDA-approved for treatment of asthma and bronchospasm, prophylaxis of exercise-induced bronchospasm, and COPD. It can be used concomitantly with short-acting β_2 agonists, glucocorticoids (inhaled or systemic), and theophylline (Goldsmith and Keating, 2004). Formoterol is also available as a single formulaic combination with the glucocorticoids mometasone or budesonide for treatment of COPD.

Arformoterol.

Arformoterol, an enantiomer of formoterol, is a selective LABA that has twice the potency of racemic formoterol. It is FDA-approved for the long-term treatment of bronchoconstriction in patients with COPD, including chronic bronchitis and emphysema (Matera and Cazzola, 2007). It was the first LABA developed as inhalational therapy for use with a nebulizer (Abdelghany, 2007).

Systemic exposure to arformoterol is due to pulmonary absorption, with plasma levels reaching a peak in 0.25–1 h. It is primarily metabolized by direct conjugation to glucuronide or sulfate conjugates and secondarily by O-demethylation by CYP2D6 and CYP2C19. It does not inhibit any of the common CYPs (Fanta, 2009).

Very Long-Acting β₂ Adrenergic Agonists (VLABAs)

Very long-acting β_2 adrenergic agonists have been developed primarily for treating COPD. These drugs are not recommended for treating asthma.

Indacaterol, the first once-daily LABA approved for COPD, is a potent β_2 agonist with high intrinsic efficacy. It has a fast onset of action, appears well tolerated, and is effective in COPD with little tachyphylaxis on continued use. In contrast to salmeterol, indacaterol does not antagonize the bronchorelaxant effect of short-acting β_2 adrenergic agonists.

Olodaterol is also a once-daily, long-acting β_2 agonist approved for use in COPD. It is also offered in combination with tiotropium bromide, an antagonist at M_3 muscarinic receptors.

Vilanterol is a VLABA approved for use in combination with fluticasone. Vilanterol is available in Europe in combination with the long-acting muscarinic antagonist umeclidinium.

Other β₂-Selective Agonists

Ritodrine.

Ritodrine is a β_2-selective agonist that was developed specifically for use as a uterine relaxant. Its pharmacological properties closely resemble those of the other agents in this group. The pharmacokinetic properties of ritodrine are complex and incompletely defined, especially in pregnant women. Ritodrine is rapidly but incompletely (30%) absorbed following oral administration: The drug may be administered intravenously to selected patients to arrest premature labor. β_2-Selective agonists may not have clinically significant benefits on perinatal mortality and may actually increase maternal morbidity. Ritodrine is not available in the U.S. See Chapter 44 for the pharmacology of tocolytic agents.

Adverse Effects of β₂-Selective Agonists

The major adverse effects of β receptor agonists occur as a result of excessive activation of β receptors. Patients with underlying cardiovascular disease are particularly at risk for significant reactions. However, the likelihood of adverse effects can be greatly decreased in patients with lung disease by administering the drug by inhalation rather than orally or parenterally.

Tremor is a relatively common adverse effect of the β_2-selective receptor agonists. Tolerance generally develops to this effect; it is not clear whether tolerance reflects desensitization of the β_2 receptors of skeletal muscle or adaptation within the CNS. This adverse effect can be minimized by starting oral therapy with a low dose of drug and progressively increasing the dose as tolerance to the tremor develops. Feelings of restlessness, apprehension, and anxiety may limit therapy with these drugs, particularly oral or parenteral administration.

Tachycardia is a common adverse effect of systemically administered β receptor agonists. Stimulation of heart rate occurs primarily by means of β_1 receptors. It is uncertain to what extent the increase in heart rate also is due to activation of cardiac β_2 receptors or to reflex effects that stem from β_2 receptor–mediated peripheral vasodilation. During a severe asthma attack, heart rate actually may decrease during therapy with a β agonist, presumably because of improvement in pulmonary function with consequent reduction in endogenous cardiac sympathetic stimulation. In patients without cardiac disease, β agonists rarely cause significant arrhythmias or myocardial ischemia; however, patients with underlying coronary artery disease or preexisting arrhythmias are at greater risk. The risk of adverse cardiovascular effects also is increased in patients who are receiving MAO inhibitors. In general, at least 2 weeks should elapse between the use of MAO inhibitors and administration of β_2 agonists or other sympathomimetics.

When given parenterally, these drugs also may increase the concentrations of glucose, lactate, and free fatty acids in plasma and decrease the concentration of K⁺. The decrease in K⁺ concentration may be especially important in patients with cardiac disease, particularly those taking digoxin and diuretics. In some diabetic patients, hyperglycemia may be worsened by these drugs, and higher doses of insulin may be required. Side effects of LABAs and VLABAs include nasopharyngitis and increase in incidence of pneumonia. As a result of these side effects, postmarketing safety studies are under way.

Large doses of β receptor agonists cause myocardial necrosis in laboratory animals.

β3 Adrenergic Receptor Agonists

The existence of the β_3 adrenergic receptor subtype was first proposed in the 1970s but was not confirmed until the receptor was cloned in 1989 (Emorine et al., 1989). The β_3 receptor couples to the G_s-cAMP pathway and has a much stronger affinity for NE than EPI. The β_3 receptor displays much lower affinities for classic β antagonists (such as propranolol or atenolol) than do β_1 and β_2 receptors. In humans, the β_3 receptor is expressed in brown adipose tissue, gallbladder, and ileum and to a lesser extent in white adipose tissue and the detrusor muscle of the bladder; there is little expression elsewhere (Berkowitz et al., 1995). To date, the major therapeutic target that has emerged from this field has been the development of β_3 receptor agonists for use in urinary incontinence (Michel, 2016).

Mirabegron is a β_3 adrenergic receptor agonist approved for use against incontinence. Activation of this receptor in the bladder leads to detrusor muscle relaxation and increased bladder capacity. This action prevents voiding and provides relief for those with an overactive bladder and urinary incontinence. Side effects include increased blood pressure, increased incidence of urinary tract infection, and headache. Mirabegron is also a moderate CYP2D6 inhibitor, so care must be taken when prescribing with other drugs metabolized by CYP2D6, such as digoxin, metoprolol, and desipramine.

α Adrenergic Receptor Agonists

α1-Selective Adrenergic Receptor Agonists

The major effects of a number of sympathomimetic drugs are due to activation of α adrenergic receptors in vascular smooth muscle. As a result, peripheral vascular resistance is increased, and blood pressure is maintained or elevated. The clinical utility of these drugs is limited to the treatment of some patients with hypotension, including orthostatic hypotension, or shock. *Phenylephrine* and *methoxamine* (discontinued in the U.S.) are direct-acting vasoconstrictors and are selective activators of α_1 receptors. *Mephentermine* and *metaraminol* act both directly and indirectly. Midodrine is a prodrug that is converted, after oral administration, to *desglymidodrine*, a direct-acting α_1 agonist.

Phenylephrine

Phenylephrine is an α_1-selective agonist; it activates β receptors only at much higher concentrations. The pharmacological effects of phenylephrine are similar to those of methoxamine. The drug causes marked arterial vasoconstriction during intravenous infusion. Phenylephrine also is used as a nasal decongestant and as a mydriatic in various nasal and ophthalmic formulations (see Chapter 69).

Metaraminol

Metaraminol exerts *direct effects* on vascular α adrenergic receptors and acts *indirectly* by stimulating the release of NE. The drug has been used in the treatment of hypotensive states or off-label to relieve attacks of paroxysmal atrial tachycardia, particularly those associated with hypotension (see Chapter 30).

Midodrine

Midodrine is an orally effective α_1 receptor agonist. It is a prodrug, converted to an active metabolite, *desglymidodrine*, which achieves peak concentrations about 1 h after a dose of midodrine. The $t_{1/2}$ of desglymidodrine is about 3 h; its duration of action is about 4–6 h. Midodrine-induced rises in blood pressure are associated with contraction of both arterial and venous smooth muscle. This is advantageous in the treatment of patients with autonomic insufficiency and postural hypotension (McClellan et al., 1998). A frequent complication in these patients is supine hypertension. This can be minimized by administering the drug during periods when the patient will remain upright, avoiding dosing

within 4 h of bedtime, and elevating the head of the bed. Very cautious use of a short-acting antihypertensive drug at bedtime may be useful in some patients. Typical dosing, achieved by careful titration of blood pressure responses, varies between 2.5 and 10 mg three times daily.

α2-Selective Adrenergic Receptor Agonists

α_2-Selective adrenergic agonists are used primarily for the treatment of systemic hypertension. Their efficacy as antihypertensive agents is somewhat surprising, because many blood vessels contain postsynaptic α_2 adrenergic receptors that promote vasoconstriction (Chapter 8). Clonidine, an α_2-agonist, was developed as a vasoconstricting nasal decongestant; its lowers blood pressure by activating α_2 receptors in the CNS, thereby suppressing sympathetic outflow from the brain.

The α_2 agonists also reduce intraocular pressure by decreasing the production of aqueous humor. Two derivatives of clonidine, apraclonidine and brimonidine, applied topically to the eye, decrease intraocular pressure with little or no effect on systemic blood pressure.

Clonidine

Clonidine is an imidazoline derivative and an α_2 adrenergic agonist.

CLONIDINE

Mechanisms of Action and Pharmacological Effects. Intravenous infusion of clonidine causes an acute rise in blood pressure because of activation of postsynaptic α_2 receptors in vascular smooth muscle. This transient vasoconstriction (not usually seen with oral administration) is followed by a more prolonged hypotensive response that results from decreased sympathetic outflow from the CNS. The effect appears to result, at least in part, from activation of α_2 receptors in the lower brainstem region. Clonidine also stimulates parasympathetic outflow, which may contribute to the slowing of heart rate. In addition, some of the antihypertensive effects of clonidine may be mediated by activation of presynaptic α_2 receptors that suppress the release of NE, ATP, and NPY from postganglionic sympathetic nerves. Clonidine decreases the plasma concentration of NE and reduces its excretion in the urine.

Does Clonidine Act Via Imidazoline I1 Receptors?

Studies in knockout animals demonstrated the requirement for a functional α_2 receptor for the hypotensive effect of clonidine. Clonidine and its congeners, as imidazolines, also bind to imidazoline receptors, of which there are three subtypes (I_1, I_2, and I_3) that are widely distributed in the body, including the CNS. Activation of the I_1 receptor appears to reduce sympathetic outflow from the CNS. Whether activation of the CNS I_1 imidazoline receptor also plays a role in the hypotensive effects of clonidine and its congeners is a topic of ongoing research. The current hypothesis is that I_1 receptors are upstream from the hypotensive α_2 receptors in the CNS and work in tandem with them, such that activation of the I_1 receptors results in catecholamine release onto the α_2 receptors (Lowry and Brown, 2014; Nikolic and Agbaba 2012), thereby reducing sympathetic outflow and reducing blood pressure.

Clonidine decreases discharges in sympathetic preganglionic fibers in the splanchnic nerve and in postganglionic fibers of cardiac nerves. These effects are blocked by α_2-selective antagonists such as yohimbine. Clonidine also stimulates parasympathetic outflow, which may contribute to the slowing of heart rate as a consequence of increased vagal tone and diminished sympathetic drive. In addition, some of the antihypertensive effects of clonidine may be mediated by activation of presynaptic α_2 receptors that suppress the release of NE, ATP, and NPY from postganglionic sympathetic nerves. Clonidine decreases the plasma concentration of NE and reduces its excretion in the urine.

ADME. Clonidine is well absorbed after oral administration, with bioavailability about 100%. Peak concentration in plasma and the maximal hypotensive effect are observed 1–3 h after an oral dose. The elimination $t_{1/2}$ is 6–24 h (mean about 12 h). About half of an administered dose can be recovered unchanged in the urine; the $t_{1/2}$ of the drug may increase with renal failure. A transdermal delivery patch permits continuous administration of clonidine as an alternative to oral therapy. The drug is released at an approximately constant rate for a week; 3–4 days are required to reach steady-state concentrations in plasma. When the patch is removed, plasma concentrations remain stable for about 8 h and then decline gradually over a period of several days; this decrease is associated with a rise in blood pressure.

Therapeutic Uses. Clonidine is used mainly in the treatment of hypertension (see Chapter 27). Clonidine also has apparent efficacy in the off-label treatment of a range of other disorders: in reducing diarrhea in some diabetic patients with autonomic neuropathy; in treating and preparing addicted subjects for withdrawal from narcotics, alcohol, and tobacco (see Chapter 24) by ameliorating some of the adverse sympathetic nervous activity associated with withdrawal and decreasing craving for the drug; and in reducing the incidence of menopausal hot flashes (transdermal application). Acute administration of clonidine has been used in the differential diagnosis of patients with hypertension and suspected pheochromocytoma. Among the other off-label uses of clonidine are atrial fibrillation, ADHD, constitutional growth delay in children, cyclosporine-associated nephrotoxicity, Tourette syndrome, hyperhidrosis, mania, posthepatic neuralgia, psychosis, restless leg syndrome, ulcerative colitis, and allergy-induced inflammatory reactions in patients with extrinsic asthma.

Adverse Effects. The major adverse effects of clonidine are dry mouth and sedation, which may diminish in intensity after several weeks of therapy. Sexual dysfunction also may occur. Marked bradycardia is observed in some patients. These effects of clonidine frequently are related to dose, and their incidence may be lower with transdermal administration of clonidine. About 15%–20% of patients develop contact dermatitis when using the transdermal system. Withdrawal reactions follow abrupt discontinuation of long-term therapy with clonidine in some hypertensive patients (see Chapter 28).

Apraclonidine

Apraclonidine is a relatively selective α_2 receptor agonist that is used topically to reduce intraocular pressure with minimal systemic effects. This agent does not cross the blood-brain barrier and is more useful than clonidine for ophthalmic therapy. Apraclonidine is useful as short-term adjunctive therapy in patients with glaucoma whose intraocular pressure is not well controlled by other pharmacological agents. The drug also is used to control or prevent elevations in intraocular pressure that occur in patients after laser trabeculoplasty or iridotomy (see Chapter 69).

Brimonidine

Brimonidine is a clonidine derivative and α_2-selective agonist that is administered ocularly to lower intraocular pressure in patients with ocular hypertension or open-angle glaucoma. Unlike apraclonidine, brimonidine can cross the blood-brain barrier and can produce hypotension and sedation, although these CNS effects are slight compared to those of clonidine.

Guanfacine

Guanfacine is an α_2 receptor agonist that is more selective than clonidine for α_2 receptors. Like clonidine, guanfacine lowers blood pressure by activation of brainstem receptors with resultant suppression of sympathetic activity. A sustained-release form is FDA-approved for treatment of ADHD in children aged 6–17 years.

Clinical Use. The drug is well absorbed after oral administration. About 50% of guanfacine appears unchanged in the urine; the rest is metabolized.

The $t_{1/2}$ for elimination ranges from 12 to 24 h. Guanfacine and clonidine appear to have similar efficacy for the treatment of hypertension and a similar pattern of adverse effects. A withdrawal syndrome may occur after the abrupt discontinuation, but it is less frequent and milder than the syndrome that follows clonidine withdrawal; this difference may relate to the longer $t_{1/2}$ of guanfacine.

Guanabenz

Guanabenz is a centrally acting α_2-agonist that decreases blood pressure by a mechanism similar to those of clonidine and guanfacine. Guanabenz has a $t_{1/2}$ of 4–6 h and is extensively metabolized by the liver. Dosage adjustment may be necessary in patients with hepatic cirrhosis. The adverse effects caused by guanabenz (e.g., dry mouth and sedation) are similar to those seen with clonidine.

Methyldopa

Methyldopa (α-methyl-3,4-dihydroxyphenylalanine) is a centrally acting antihypertensive agent. It is metabolized to α-methylnorepinephrine in the brain, and this compound is thought to activate central α_2 receptors and lower blood pressure in a manner similar to that of clonidine (see Chapter 27).

Tizanidine

Tizanidine is a muscle relaxant used for the treatment of spasticity associated with cerebral and spinal disorders. It is also an α_2-agonist with some properties similar to those of clonidine.

Moxonidine

Moxonidine is a mixed α_2 receptor and imidazole I_1 receptor agonist. It acts to reduce sympathetic outflow from the CNS and thereby reduces blood pressure. Moxonidine also has analgesic activity, interacts synergistically with opioid agonists, and is used in treating neuropathic pain.

Miscellaneous Sympathomimetic Agonists

Amphetamine

Amphetamine, racemic β phenylisopropylamine (Table 12–1), has powerful CNS stimulant actions in addition to the peripheral α and β actions common to indirect-acting sympathomimetic drugs. Unlike EPI, it is effective after oral administration, and its effects last for several hours.

Cardiovascular System

Amphetamine given orally raises both systolic and diastolic blood pressure. Heart rate often is reflexly slowed; with large doses, cardiac arrhythmias may occur. Cardiac output is not enhanced by therapeutic doses, and cerebral blood flow does not change much. The *l*-isomer is slightly more potent than the *d*-isomer in its cardiovascular actions.

Other Smooth Muscles

In general, smooth muscles respond to amphetamine as they do to other sympathomimetic amines. The contractile effect on the sphincter of the urinary bladder is particularly marked, and for this reason amphetamine has been used in treating enuresis and incontinence. Pain and difficulty in micturition occasionally occur. The GI effects of amphetamine are unpredictable. If enteric activity is pronounced, amphetamine may cause relaxation and delay the movement of intestinal contents; if the gut already is relaxed, the opposite effect may occur. The response of the human uterus varies, but there usually is an increase in tone.

CNS

Amphetamine is one of the most potent sympathomimetic amines in stimulating the CNS. It stimulates the medullary respiratory center, lessens the degree of central depression caused by various drugs, and produces other signs of CNS stimulation. In eliciting CNS excitatory effects, the *d*-isomer (dextroamphetamine) is three to four times more potent than the *l*-isomer. The psychic effects depend on the dose and the mental state and personality of the individual. The main results of an oral dose of 10–30 mg include wakefulness, alertness, and a decreased sense of fatigue; elevation of mood, with increased initiative, self-confidence, and ability to concentrate; often, elation and euphoria; and increase in motor and speech activities. Performance of simple mental tasks is improved, but, although more work may be accomplished, the number of errors may increase. Physical performance (e.g., in athletes) is improved, and the drug often is abused for this purpose. These effects are variable and may be reversed by overdosage or repeated usage. Prolonged use or large doses are nearly always followed by depression and fatigue. Many individuals given amphetamine experience headache, palpitation, dizziness, vasomotor disturbances, agitation, confusion, dysphoria, apprehension, delirium, or fatigue.

Fatigue and Sleep. In general, amphetamine prolongs the duration of adequate performance before fatigue appears, and the effects of fatigue are at least partly reversed, most strikingly when performance has been reduced by fatigue and lack of sleep. Such improvement may be partly due to alteration of unfavorable attitudes toward the task. However, amphetamine reduces the frequency of attention lapses that impair performance after prolonged sleep deprivation and thus improves execution of tasks requiring sustained attention. The need for sleep may be postponed, but it cannot be avoided indefinitely. When the drug is discontinued after long use, the pattern of sleep may take as long as 2 months to return to normal.

Analgesia. Amphetamine and some other sympathomimetic amines have a small analgesic effect that is not sufficiently pronounced to be therapeutically useful. However, amphetamine can enhance the analgesia produced by opiates.

Respiration. Amphetamine stimulates the respiratory center, increasing the rate and depth of respiration. In normal individuals, usual doses of the drug do not appreciably increase respiratory rate or minute volume. Nevertheless, when respiration is depressed by centrally acting drugs, amphetamine may stimulate respiration.

Appetite. Amphetamine and similar drugs have been used for the treatment of obesity, although the wisdom of this use is at best questionable. Weight loss in obese humans treated with amphetamine is almost entirely due to reduced food intake and only in small measure to increased metabolism. The site of action probably is in the lateral hypothalamic feeding center; injection of amphetamine into this area, but not into the ventromedial region, suppresses food intake. Neurochemical mechanisms of action are unclear but may involve increased release of NE or DA. In humans, tolerance to the appetite suppression develops rapidly. Hence, continuous weight reduction usually is not observed in obese individuals without dietary restriction.

Mechanisms of Action in the CNS

Amphetamine exerts most or all of its effects in the CNS by releasing biogenic amines from their storage sites in nerve terminals. The neuronal DAT and the VMAT2 appear to be two of the principal targets of amphetamine's action (Fleckenstein, 2007; Sitte and Freissmuth, 2015). These mechanisms include amphetamine-induced exchange diffusion, reverse transport, channel-like transport phenomena, and effects resulting from the weakly basic properties of amphetamine. Amphetamine analogues affect monoamine transporters through phosphorylation, transporter trafficking, and the production of reactive oxygen and nitrogen species. These mechanisms may have potential implications for neurotoxicity as well as dopaminergic neurodegenerative diseases (discussed further in the chapter).

The alerting effect of amphetamine, its anorectic effect, and at least a component of its locomotor-stimulating action presumably are mediated by release of NE from central noradrenergic neurons. These effects can be prevented in experimental animals by inhibiting tyrosine hydroxylase and thus catecholamine synthesis. Some aspects of locomotor activity and the stereotyped behavior induced by amphetamine probably are a consequence of the release of DA from dopaminergic nerve terminals, particularly in the neostriatum. Higher doses are required to produce these behavioral effects, and this correlates with the higher concentrations of amphetamine required to release DA from brain slices or synaptosomes in vitro. With still higher doses of amphetamine, disturbances of perception and overt psychotic behavior occur. These effects may be due to release of 5HT from serotonergic neurons and of DA in the mesolimbic system.

In addition, amphetamine may exert direct effects on CNS receptors for 5HT (Chapter 13).

Toxicity and Adverse Effects

The acute toxic effects of amphetamine usually are extensions of its therapeutic actions and as a rule result from overdosage. CNS effects commonly include restlessness, dizziness, tremor, hyperactive reflexes, talkativeness, tenseness, irritability, weakness, insomnia, fever, and sometimes euphoria. Confusion, aggressiveness, changes in libido, anxiety, delirium, paranoid hallucinations, panic states, and suicidal or homicidal tendencies occur, especially in mentally ill patients. However, these psychotic effects can be elicited in any individual if sufficient quantities of amphetamine are ingested for a prolonged period. Fatigue and depression usually follow central stimulation. Cardiovascular effects are common and include headache, chilliness, pallor or flushing, palpitation, cardiac arrhythmias, anginal pain, hypertension or hypotension, and circulatory collapse. Excessive sweating occurs. GI symptoms include dry mouth, metallic taste, anorexia, nausea, vomiting, diarrhea, and abdominal cramps. Fatal poisoning usually terminates in convulsions and coma, and cerebral hemorrhages are the main pathological findings.

The toxic dose of amphetamine varies widely. Toxic manifestations occasionally occur as an idiosyncratic reaction after as little as 2 mg but are rare with doses less than 15 mg. Severe reactions have occurred with 30 mg, yet doses of 400–500 mg are not uniformly fatal. Larger doses can be tolerated after chronic use of the drug. Treatment of acute amphetamine intoxication may include acidification of the urine by administration of ammonium chloride; this enhances the rate of elimination. Sedatives may be required for the CNS symptoms. Severe hypertension may require administration of sodium nitroprusside or an α adrenergic receptor antagonist.

Chronic intoxication with amphetamine causes symptoms similar to those of acute overdosage, but abnormal mental conditions are more common. Weight loss may be marked. A psychotic reaction with vivid hallucinations and paranoid delusions, often mistaken for schizophrenia, is the most common serious effect. Recovery usually is rapid after withdrawal of the drug, but occasionally the condition becomes chronic. In these persons, amphetamine may act as a precipitating factor hastening the onset of incipient schizophrenia.

The abuse of amphetamine as a means of overcoming sleepiness and of increasing energy and alertness should be discouraged. The drug should be used only under medical supervision. The amphetamines are schedule II drugs under federal regulations. The additional contraindications and precautions for the use of amphetamine generally are similar to those described for EPI. Amphetamine use is inadvisable in patients with anorexia, insomnia, asthenia, psychopathic personality, or a history of homicidal or suicidal tendencies.

Dependence and Tolerance

Psychological dependence often occurs when amphetamine or dextroamphetamine is used chronically, as discussed in Chapter 24. Tolerance almost invariably develops to the anorexigenic effect of amphetamines and often is seen also in the need for increasing doses to maintain improvement of mood in psychiatric patients. Tolerance is striking in individuals who are dependent on the drug; a daily intake of 1.7 g without apparent ill effects has been reported. Development of tolerance is not invariable, and cases of narcolepsy have been treated for years without requiring an increase in the initially effective dose.

Therapeutic Uses

Amphetamine is used chiefly for its CNS effects. Dextroamphetamine, with greater CNS action and less peripheral action, is FDA-approved for the treatment of narcolepsy and ADHD (see discussion later in this chapter).

Methamphetamine

Methamphetamine is closely related chemically to amphetamine and ephedrine (Table 12–1). The drug acts centrally to release DA and other biogenic amines and to inhibit neuronal and VMATs as well as MAO.

Small doses have prominent central stimulant effects without significant peripheral actions; somewhat larger doses produce a sustained rise in systolic and diastolic blood pressures, due mainly to cardiac stimulation. Cardiac output is increased, although the heart rate may be reflexly slowed. Venous constriction causes peripheral venous pressure to increase. These factors tend to increase the venous return and thus cardiac output; pulmonary arterial pressure is raised.

Methamphetamine is a schedule II drug under federal regulations and has high potential for abuse (Chapter 24). It is widely abused as a cheap, accessible recreational drug. Illegal production of methamphetamine in clandestine laboratories throughout the U.S. is common. It is used principally for its central effects, which are more pronounced than those of amphetamine and are accompanied by less-prominent peripheral actions (see Therapeutic Uses of Sympathomimetic Drugs).

Methylphenidate

Methylphenidate is a piperidine derivative that is structurally related to amphetamine. Methylphenidate is a mild CNS stimulant with more prominent effects on mental than on motor activities. However, large doses produce signs of generalized CNS stimulation that may lead to convulsions.

The effects of methylphenidate resemble those of the amphetamines. Methylphenidate also shares the abuse potential of the amphetamines and is listed as a schedule II controlled substance in the U.S. Methylphenidate is effective in the treatment of narcolepsy and ADHD (described in the material that follows). Methylphenidate is readily absorbed after oral administration, reaching a peak C_p in about 2 h. The drug is a racemate; its more potent (+) enantiomer has a $t_{1/2}$ of about 6 h; the less-potent (−) enantiomer has a $t_{1/2}$ of approximately 4 h. Concentrations in the brain exceed those in plasma. The main urinary metabolite is a deesterified product, ritalinic acid, which accounts for 80% of the dose. The use of methylphenidate is contraindicated in patients with glaucoma.

Dexmethylphenidate

Dexmethylphenidate is the *d*-threo enantiomer of racemic methylphenidate. It is FDA-approved for the treatment of ADHD and is listed as a schedule II controlled substance in the U.S.

Pemoline

Pemoline is structurally dissimilar to methylphenidate but elicits similar changes in CNS function with minimal effects on the cardiovascular system. It is employed in treating ADHD. It can be given once daily because of its long $t_{1/2}$. Clinical improvement may require treatment for 3–4 weeks. Use of pemoline has been associated with severe hepatic failure. The drug was discontinued in the U.S. in 2006.

Lisdexamphetamine

Lisdexamphetamine is a therapeutically inactive prodrug that is converted primarily in the blood to lysine and D-amphetamine, the active component (Childress and Berry, 2012). It is approved for the treatment of ADHD in children, adolescents, and adults. The drug produces mild-to-moderate side effects, including decreased appetite, dizziness, dry mouth, fatigue, headache, insomnia, irritability, nasal congestion, nasal pharyngitis, upper respiratory infection, vomiting, and decreased weight.

Ephedrine

Ephedrine is an agonist at both α and β receptors; in addition, it enhances release of NE from sympathetic neurons and thus is a mixed-acting sympathomimetic (see Table 12–1 and Figure 12–1). Only *l*-ephedrine and racemic ephedrine are used clinically.

ADME and Pharmacological Actions

Ephedrine is effective after oral administration; effects may persist for several hours. Ephedrine is eliminated in the urine largely as unchanged drug, with a $t_{1/2}$ of 3–6 h. The drug stimulates heart rate and cardiac output and variably increases peripheral resistance; as a result, ephedrine usually increases blood pressure. Stimulation of the α receptors of smooth muscle cells in the bladder base may increase the resistance to the outflow of urine. Activation of β receptors in the lungs promotes bronchodilation. Ephedrine is a potent CNS stimulant.

Therapeutic Uses and Untoward Effects

The use of ephedrine as a bronchodilator in asthmatic patients is less common with the availability of β_2-selective agonists. Ephedrine has been used to promote urinary continence. Indeed, the drug may cause urinary retention, particularly in men with BPH. Ephedrine also has been used to treat the hypotension that may occur with spinal anesthesia.

Untoward effects of ephedrine include hypertension and insomnia. Tachyphylaxis may occur with repetitive dosing. Usual or higher-than-recommended doses may cause important adverse effects in susceptible individuals, especially in patients with underlying cardiovascular disease that might be unrecognized. Large amounts of herbal preparations containing ephedrine (ma huang, ephedra) are utilized around the world. There can be considerable variability in the content of ephedrine in these preparations, which may result in inadvertent consumption of higher-than-usual doses of ephedrine and its isomers, leading to significant toxicity and death. Thus, the FDA has banned the sale of dietary supplements containing ephedra. In addition, the Combat Methamphetamine Epidemic Act of 2005 regulates the sale of ephedrine, phenylpropanolamine, and pseudoephedrine, which can be used as precursors in the illicit manufacture of amphetamine and methamphetamine.

Other Sympathomimetic Agents

Several sympathomimetic drugs (e.g., propylhexedrine, naphazoline, oxymetazoline, and xylometazoline) are used primarily as vasoconstrictors for local application to the nasal mucous membrane or the eye.

Phenylephrine, pseudoephedrine (a stereoisomer of ephedrine), and phenylpropanolamine are the sympathomimetic drugs that have been used most commonly in oral preparations for the relief of nasal congestion. *Pseudoephedrine* is available without a prescription in a variety of solid and liquid dosage forms. *Phenylpropanolamine* shares the pharmacological properties of ephedrine and is approximately equal in potency except that it causes less CNS stimulation. Due to concern about the possibility that phenylpropanolamine increases the risk of hemorrhagic stroke, the drug is no longer licensed for marketing in the U.S.

Therapeutic Uses of Sympathomimetic Drugs

Shock

Shock is a clinical syndrome characterized by inadequate perfusion of tissues; it usually is associated with hypotension and ultimately with the failure of organ systems. Shock is an immediately life-threatening impairment of delivery of O_2 and nutrients to the organs of the body. Causes of shock include hypovolemia; cardiac failure; obstruction to cardiac output (due to pulmonary embolism, pericardial tamponade, or aortic dissection); and peripheral circulatory dysfunction (sepsis or anaphylaxis). Recent research on shock has focused on the accompanying increased permeability of the GI mucosa to pancreatic proteases, and on the role of these degradative enzymes on microvascular inflammation and multiorgan failure (Delano et al., 2013; Schmid-Schoenbein and Hugli, 2005). The treatment of shock consists of specific efforts to reverse the underlying pathogenesis as well as nonspecific measures aimed at correcting hemodynamic abnormalities. The accompanying fall in blood pressure generally leads to marked activation of the sympathetic nervous system. This, in turn, causes peripheral vasoconstriction and an increase in the rate and force of cardiac contraction. In the initial stages of shock, these mechanisms may maintain blood pressure and cerebral blood flow, although blood flow to the kidneys, skin, and other organs may be decreased, leading to impaired production of urine and metabolic acidosis.

The initial therapy of shock involves basic life support measures. It is essential to maintain blood volume, which often requires monitoring of hemodynamic parameters. Specific therapy (e.g., antibiotics for patients in septic shock) should be initiated immediately. If these measures do not lead to an adequate therapeutic response, it may be necessary to use vasoactive drugs in an effort to improve abnormalities in blood pressure and flow. Many of these pharmacological approaches, while apparently clinically reasonable, are of uncertain efficacy. Adrenergic receptor agonists may be used in an attempt to increase myocardial contractility or to modify peripheral vascular resistance. In general terms, β receptor agonists increase heart rate and force of contraction, α receptor agonists increase peripheral vascular resistance, and DA promotes dilation of renal and splanchnic vascular beds, in addition to activating β and α receptors (Breslow and Ligier, 1991).

Cardiogenic shock due to myocardial infarction has a poor prognosis; therapy is aimed at improving peripheral blood flow. Medical intervention is designed to optimize cardiac filling pressure (preload), myocardial contractility, and peripheral resistance (afterload). Preload may be increased by administration of intravenous fluids or reduced with drugs such as diuretics and nitrates. A number of sympathomimetic amines have been used to increase the force of contraction of the heart. Some of these drugs have disadvantages: INE is a powerful chronotropic agent and can greatly increase myocardial O_2 demand; NE intensifies peripheral vasoconstriction; and EPI increases heart rate and may predispose the heart to dangerous arrhythmias. DA is an effective inotropic agent that causes less increase in heart rate than does INE. DA also promotes renal arterial dilation; this may be useful in preserving renal function. When given in high doses (>10–20 μg/kg per min), DA activates α receptors, causing peripheral and renal vasoconstriction. Dobutamine has complex pharmacological actions that are mediated by its stereoisomers; the clinical effects of the drug are to increase myocardial contractility with little increase in heart rate or peripheral resistance.

In some patients in shock, hypotension is so severe that vasoconstricting drugs are required to maintain a blood pressure that is adequate for CNS perfusion. The α agonists such as NE, phenylephrine, metaraminol, mephentermine, midodrine, ephedrine, EPI, DA, and methoxamine all have been used for this purpose. This approach may be advantageous in patients with hypotension due to failure of the sympathetic nervous system (e.g., after spinal anesthesia or injury). However, in patients with other forms of shock, such as cardiogenic shock, reflex vasoconstriction generally is intense, and α receptor agonists may further compromise blood flow to organs such as the kidneys and gut and adversely increase the work of the heart. Indeed, vasodilating drugs such as nitroprusside are more likely to improve blood flow and decrease cardiac work in such patients by decreasing afterload if a minimally adequate blood pressure can be maintained.

The hemodynamic abnormalities in septic shock are complex and poorly understood. Most patients with septic shock initially have low or barely normal peripheral vascular resistance, possibly owing to excessive effects of endogenously produced NO as well as normal or increased cardiac output. If the syndrome progresses, myocardial depression, increased peripheral resistance, and impaired tissue oxygenation occur. The primary treatment of septic shock is antibiotics. Therapy with drugs such as DA or dobutamine is guided by hemodynamic monitoring.

Hypotension

Drugs with predominantly α agonist activity can be used to raise blood pressure in patients with decreased peripheral resistance in conditions such as spinal anesthesia or intoxication with antihypertensive medications. However, hypotension per se is not an indication for treatment with these agents unless there is inadequate perfusion of organs such as the brain, heart, or kidneys. Furthermore, adequate replacement of fluid or blood may be more appropriate than drug therapy for many patients with hypotension.

Patients with orthostatic hypotension (excessive fall in blood pressure with standing) often represent a pharmacological challenge. There are diverse causes for this disorder, including the Shy-Drager syndrome and idiopathic autonomic failure. Therapeutic approaches include physical maneuvers and a variety of drugs (fludrocortisone, prostaglandin synthesis inhibitors, somatostatin analogues, caffeine, vasopressin analogues, and DA antagonists). A number of sympathomimetic drugs also have been used in treating this disorder. The ideal agent would enhance venous constriction prominently and produce relatively little arterial constriction to avoid supine hypertension. No such agent currently is available. Drugs used in this disorder to activate α_1 receptors include both direct- and indirect-acting agents. Midodrine shows promise in treating this challenging disorder.

Hypertension

Centrally acting α_2 receptor agonists such as clonidine are useful in the treatment of hypertension. Drug therapy of hypertension is discussed in Chapter 28.

Cardiac Arrhythmias

Cardiopulmonary resuscitation in patients with cardiac arrest due to ventricular fibrillation, electromechanical dissociation, or asystole may be facilitated by drug treatment. EPI is an important therapeutic agent in patients with cardiac arrest; EPI and other α agonists increase diastolic pressure and improve coronary blood flow. The α agonists also help to preserve cerebral blood flow during resuscitation. Cerebral blood vessels are relatively insensitive to the vasoconstricting effects of catecholamines, and perfusion pressure is increased. Consequently, during external cardiac massage, EPI facilitates distribution of the limited cardiac output to the cerebral and coronary circulations. The optimal dose of EPI in patients with cardiac arrest is unclear. Once a cardiac rhythm has been restored, it may be necessary to treat arrhythmias, hypotension, or shock.

In patients with paroxysmal supraventricular tachycardias, particularly those associated with mild hypotension, careful infusion of an α agonist (e.g., phenylephrine) to raise blood pressure to about 160 mm Hg may end the arrhythmia by increasing vagal tone. However, this method of treatment has been replaced largely by Ca^{2+} channel blockers with clinically significant effects on the AV node, β antagonists, adenosine, and electrical cardioversion (Chapter 30). A β agonist such as INE may be used as adjunctive or temporizing therapy with atropine in patients with marked bradycardia who are compromised hemodynamically; if long-term therapy is required, a cardiac pacemaker usually is the treatment of choice.

Congestive Heart Failure

At first glance, sympathetic stimulation of β receptors in the heart would appear to be an important compensatory mechanism for maintenance of cardiac function in patients with congestive heart failure. However, the failing heart does not respond well to excess sympathetic stimulation. While β agonists may increase cardiac output in acute emergency settings such as shock, long-term therapy with β agonists as inotropic agents is not efficacious. Indeed, interest has grown in the use of β receptor antagonists in the treatment of patients with congestive heart failure, a topic covered in detail in Chapter 29.

Local Vascular Effects

Epinephrine is used in surgical procedures in the nose, throat, and larynx to shrink the mucosa and improve visualization by limiting hemorrhage. Simultaneous injection of EPI with local anesthetics retards their absorption and increases the duration of anesthesia (Chapter 22). Injection of α agonists into the penis may be useful in reversing priapism, a complication of the use of α receptor antagonists or PDE 5 inhibitors (e.g., sildenafil) in the treatment of erectile dysfunction. Both phenylephrine and oxymetazoline are efficacious vasoconstrictors when applied locally during sinus surgery.

Nasal Decongestion

α Receptor agonists are used as nasal decongestants in patients with allergic or vasomotor rhinitis and in acute rhinitis in patients with upper respiratory infections. These drugs probably decrease resistance to airflow by decreasing the volume of the nasal mucosa; this may occur by activation of α receptors in venous capacitance vessels in nasal tissues that have erectile characteristics. The receptors that mediate this effect appear to be α_1 receptors. α_2 Receptors may mediate contraction of arterioles that supply nutrition to the nasal mucosa. Intense constriction of these vessels may cause structural damage to the mucosa. A major limitation of therapy with nasal decongestants is loss of efficacy, "rebound" hyperemia, and worsening of symptoms with chronic use or when the drug is stopped. Although mechanisms are uncertain, possibilities include receptor desensitization and damage to the mucosa. Agonists that are selective for α_1 receptors may be less likely to induce mucosal damage.

The α agonists may be administered either orally or topically. Sympathomimetic decongestants should be used with great caution in patients with hypertension and in men with prostatic enlargement; these agents are contraindicated in patients who are taking MAO inhibitors. Topical decongestants are particularly useful in acute rhinitis because of their more selective site of action, but they are apt to be used excessively by patients, leading to rebound congestion. Oral decongestants are much less likely to cause rebound congestion but carry a greater risk of inducing adverse systemic effects. Patients with uncontrolled hypertension or ischemic heart disease generally should avoid the oral consumption of OTC products or herbal preparations containing sympathomimetic drugs.

Asthma

Use of β adrenergic agonists in the treatment of asthma and COPD is discussed in Chapter 40.

Allergic Reactions

Epinephrine is the drug of choice to reverse the manifestations of serious acute hypersensitivity reactions (e.g., from food, bee sting, or drug allergy). A subcutaneous injection of EPI rapidly relieves itching, hives, and swelling of lips, eyelids, and tongue. In some patients, careful intravenous infusion of EPI may be required to ensure prompt pharmacological effects. This treatment may be life-saving when edema of the glottis threatens airway patency or when there is hypotension or shock in patients with anaphylaxis. In addition to its cardiovascular effects, EPI is thought to activate β receptors that suppress the release from mast cells of mediators such as histamine and leukotrienes. Although glucocorticoids and antihistamines frequently are administered to patients with severe hypersensitivity reactions, EPI remains the mainstay. EPI autoinjectors are employed widely for the emergency self-treatment of anaphylaxis.

Ophthalmic Uses

Ophthalmic uses are discussed in Chapter 69.

Narcolepsy and Sleep/Wake Imbalance

Hypocretin neurons activate wake-promoting pathways in the CNS. A deficiency of hypocretin, likely due to autoimmune destruction of hypocretin neurons, produces narcolepsy, a condition of hypersomnia, including excessive daytime sleepiness and attacks of sleep that may occur suddenly under conditions that are not normally conducive to sleep. Hypocretin agonists will likely be available in the future. At present, treatment relies on the fact that monoamine pathways promote wakefulness; thus, current treatments utilize CNS stimulants, including those that enhance transmission in monoamine pathways (Black et al., 2015).

The CNS stimulants modafinil (a mixture of R- and S-enantiomers) and armodafinil (the R-enantiomer of modafinil) are first-line agents for narcolepsy. In the U.S., modafinil is a schedule IV controlled substance. Its mechanism of action in narcolepsy is unclear. Methylphenidate and amphetamines are also used. Therapy with amphetamines is complicated by the risk of abuse and the likelihood of the development of tolerance. Depression, irritability, and paranoia also may occur. Amphetamines may disturb nocturnal sleep, which increases the difficulty of avoiding daytime attacks of sleep in these patients. Armodafinil is also indicated to improve wakefulness in shift workers and to combat excessive sleepiness in patients with obstructive sleep apnea-hypopnea syndrome. See previous sections

for more details on these agents. Some patients respond to tricyclic antidepressants (Chapter 15) or MAO inhibitors (Chapter 8).

Sodium γ-hydroxybutyrate (Na$^+$-oxybate) is FDA-approved for treating the sleep/wake imbalance and cataplexy of narcolepsy. The mechanism of action of oxybate is unknown but likely relates to its structural similarity to glutamate and GABA and to actions on NE and DA neurons mediated by GABA$_B$ receptors. Oxybate is a schedule III controlled substance, available through a special program with the manufacturer. Oxybate carries an FDA black-box warning about severe CNS depressants and must be used with great caution (see FDA, 2012).

Weight Reduction

Amphetamine promotes weight loss by suppressing appetite rather than by increasing energy expenditure. Other anorexic drugs include methamphetamine, dextroamphetamine (and a prodrug form, lisdexamfetamine), phentermine, benzphetamine, phendimetrazine, phenmetrazine, diethylpropion, mazindol, phenylpropanolamine, and sibutramine (a mixed adrenergic/serotonergic drug). Phenmetrazine, mazindol, and phenylpropanolamine have been discontinued in the U.S. Available evidence does not support the isolated use of these drugs in the absence of a more comprehensive program that stresses exercise and modification of diet under medical supervision.

The β_3 receptor agonists have remarkable antiobesity and antidiabetic effects in rodents.

Mirabegron (see previous discussion) has some promising effects in humans (Cypess et al., 2015). Use of β_3 agonists in the treatment of obesity remains a possibility for the future (Arch, 2011).

Attention-Deficit/Hyperactivity Disorder

The ADHD syndrome, usually first evident in childhood, is characterized by excessive motor activity, difficulty in sustaining attention, and impulsiveness. Children with this disorder frequently are troubled by difficulties in school, impaired interpersonal relationships, and excitability. Academic underachievement is an important characteristic. A substantial number of children with this syndrome have characteristics that persist into adulthood. Behavioral therapy may be helpful in some patients.

Catecholamines may be involved in the control of attention at the level of the cerebral cortex. A variety of stimulant drugs have been utilized in the treatment of ADHD, and they are particularly indicated in moderate-to-severe cases. Dextroamphetamine has been demonstrated to be more effective than placebo. Methylphenidate is effective in children with ADHD and is the most common intervention (Swanson and Volkow, 2003). Treatment may start with a dose of 5 mg of methylphenidate in the morning and at lunch; the dose is increased gradually over a period of weeks depending on the response as judged by parents, teachers, and the clinician. The total daily dose generally should not exceed 60 mg; because of its short duration of action, most children require two or three doses of methylphenidate each day. The timing of doses is adjusted individually in accordance with rapidity of onset of effect and duration of action.

Methylphenidate, dextroamphetamine, and amphetamine probably have similar efficacy in ADHD and are the preferred drugs in this disorder. Sustained-release preparations of dextroamphetamine, methylphenidate, dexmethylphenidate, and amphetamine, Adderall may be used once daily in children and adults. Lisdexamfetamine can be administered once daily, and a transdermal formulation of methylphenidate is marketed for daytime use. Potential adverse effects of these medications include insomnia, abdominal pain, anorexia, and weight loss, which may be associated with suppression of growth in children. Minor symptoms may be transient or may respond to adjustment of dosage or administration of the drug with meals. Other drugs that have been utilized include tricyclic antidepressants, antipsychotic agents, and clonidine. A sustained-release formulation of guanfacine, an α_{2A} receptor agonist, has recently been approved for use in children (ages 6–17 years) in treating ADHD (May and Kratochvil, 2010).

Adrenergic Receptor Antagonists

Many types of drugs interfere with the function of the sympathetic nervous system and thus have profound effects on the physiology of sympathetically innervated organs. Several of these drugs are important in clinical medicine, particularly for the treatment of cardiovascular diseases.

The remainder of this chapter focuses on the pharmacology of adrenergic receptor *antagonists*, drugs that inhibit the interaction of NE, epinephrine, and other sympathomimetic drugs with α and β receptors (Figure 12–3). Most of these agents are competitive antagonists; an important exception is phenoxybenzamine, an irreversible antagonist that binds covalently to α receptors.

There are important structural differences amongst the various types of adrenergic receptors, differences that have permitted development of compounds with substantially different affinities for the various receptors. Thus, it is possible to interfere selectively with responses that result from stimulation of the sympathetic nervous system. The selectivity is relative, not absolute. Nonetheless, selective antagonists of β_1 receptors block *most* actions of epinephrine and NE on the heart, while having less effect on β_2 receptors in bronchial smooth muscle and no effect on responses mediated by α_1 or α_2 receptors.

Detailed knowledge of the autonomic nervous system and the sites of action of drugs that act on adrenergic receptors is essential for understanding the pharmacological properties and therapeutic uses of this important class of drugs. Additional background material is presented in Chapter 8. Agents that block DA receptors are considered in Chapter 13.

α Adrenergic Receptor Antagonists

The α adrenergic receptors mediate many of the important actions of endogenous catecholamines. The α_1 receptors mediate contraction of arterial, venous, and visceral smooth muscle, while the α_2 receptors are involved in suppressing sympathetic output, increasing vagal tone, facilitating platelet aggregation, inhibiting the release of NE and acetylcholine from nerve endings, and regulating metabolic effects (e.g., suppression of insulin secretion and inhibition of lipolysis). The α_2 receptors also mediate contraction of some arteries and veins.

Some of the most important effects of α receptor antagonists observed clinically are on the cardiovascular system. Actions in both the CNS and the periphery are involved; the outcome depends on the cardiovascular status of the patient at the time of drug administration and the relative selectivity of the agent for α_1 and α_2 receptors.

The α receptor antagonists have a wide spectrum of pharmacological specificities and are chemically heterogeneous. Some of these drugs have markedly different affinities for α_1 and α_2 receptors. For example, *prazosin* is much more potent in blocking α_1 than α_2 receptors (i.e., α_1 selective), whereas *yohimbine* is α_2 selective; *phentolamine* has similar affinities for both of these receptor subtypes. More recently, agents that discriminate among the various subtypes of a particular receptor have become available; for example, *tamsulosin* has higher potency at α_{1A} than at α_{1B} receptors. Prior editions of this textbook contain information about the chemistry of α receptor antagonists.

Catecholamines increase the output of glucose from the liver; in humans, this effect is mediated predominantly by β receptors, although α receptors may contribute. The α receptor antagonists therefore may reduce glucose release. Receptors of the α_{2A} subtype facilitate platelet aggregation; the effect of blockade of platelet α_2 receptors in vivo is not clear. Activation of α_2 receptors in the pancreatic islets suppresses insulin secretion; conversely, blockade of pancreatic α_2 receptors may facilitate insulin release (Chapter 47).

α_1 Adrenergic Receptor Antagonists

General Pharmacological Properties

Blockade of α_1 adrenergic receptors inhibits vasoconstriction induced by endogenous catecholamines; vasodilation may occur in both arteriolar resistance vessels and veins. The result is a fall in blood pressure due to decreased peripheral resistance.

The magnitude of such effects depends on the activity of the sympathetic nervous system at the time the antagonist is administered and thus is less in supine than in upright subjects and is particularly marked if there is hypovolemia. For most α receptor antagonists, the fall in blood pressure is opposed by *baroreceptor reflexes* that cause increases in heart rate and cardiac output, as well as fluid retention. These *reflexes* are exaggerated if the antagonist also blocks α_2 receptors on peripheral sympathetic nerve endings, leading to enhanced release of NE and increased stimulation of postsynaptic β_1 receptors in the heart and on juxtaglomerular cells (Chapter 8) (Starke et al., 1989). Although stimulation of α_1 receptors in the heart may cause an increased force of contraction, the importance of blockade at this site in humans is uncertain.

Blockade of α_1 receptors also inhibits vasoconstriction and the increase in blood pressure produced by the administration of a sympathomimetic amine. The pattern of effects depends on the adrenergic agonist that is administered: Pressor responses to phenylephrine can be completely suppressed; those to NE are only incompletely blocked because of residual

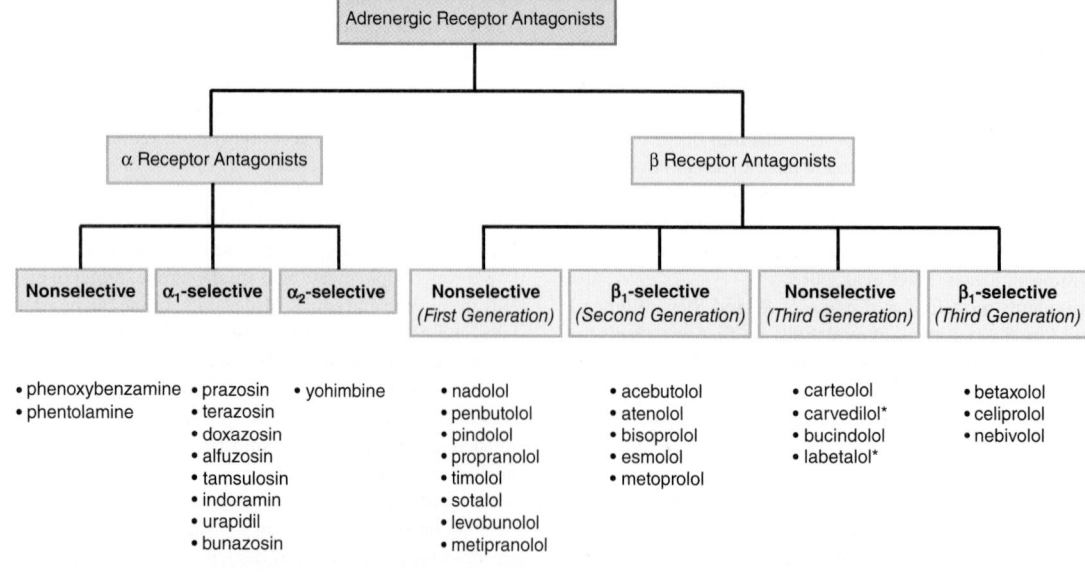

Figure 12-3 *Classification of adrenergic receptor antagonists.* Drugs marked by an asterisk (*) also block α_1 receptors.

stimulation of cardiac β_1 receptors; and pressor responses to EPI may be transformed to vasodepressor effects because of residual stimulation of β_2 receptors in the vasculature with resultant vasodilation.

Blockade of α_1 receptors can alleviate some of the symptoms of BPH. The symptoms of BPH include a resistance to urine outflow. This results from mechanical pressure on the urethra due to an increase in smooth muscle mass and an α adrenergic receptor–mediated increase in smooth muscle tone in the prostate and neck of the bladder. Antagonism of α_1 receptors permits relaxation of the smooth muscle and decreases the resistance to the outflow of urine. The prostate and lower urinary tract tissues exhibit a high proportion of α_{1A} receptors (Michel and Vrydag, 2006).

Available Agents

Prazosin. Due in part to its greater α_1 receptor selectivity, this class of α receptor antagonists exhibits greater clinical utility and has largely replaced the nonselective haloalkylamine (e.g., phenoxybenzamine) and imidazoline (e.g., phentolamine) α receptor antagonists.

Prazosin is the prototypical α_1-selective antagonist. The affinity of prazosin for α_1 adrenergic receptors is about 1000-fold greater than that for α_2 adrenergic receptors. Prazosin has similar potencies at α_{1A}, α_{1B}, and α_{1D} subtypes. Interestingly, the drug also is a relatively potent inhibitor of cyclic nucleotide PDEs, and it originally was synthesized for this purpose. *Prazosin* and the related α receptor antagonists *doxazosin* and *tamsulosin* frequently are used for the treatment of hypertension (Chapter 28).

Pharmacological Effects. The major effects of prazosin result from its blockade of α_1 receptors in arterioles and veins. This leads to a fall in peripheral vascular resistance and in venous return to the heart. Unlike other vasodilating drugs, administration of prazosin usually does not increase heart rate. Because prazosin has little or no α_2 receptor–blocking effect, it probably does not promote the release of NE from sympathetic nerve endings in the heart. Prazosin decreases cardiac preload and has little effect on cardiac output and rate, in contrast to vasodilators such as hydralazine that have minimal dilatory effects on veins. Although the combination of reduced preload and selective α_1 receptor blockade might be sufficient to account for the relative absence of reflex tachycardia, prazosin also may act in the CNS to suppress sympathetic outflow. Prazosin appears to depress baroreflex function in hypertensive patients. Prazosin and related drugs in this class decrease LDLs and triglycerides and increase concentrations of HDLs.

ADME. *Prazosin* is well absorbed after oral administration, and bioavailability is about 50%–70%. Peak concentrations of prazosin in plasma generally are reached 1–3 h after an oral dose. The drug is tightly bound to plasma proteins (primarily α_1-acid glycoprotein), and only 5% of the drug is free in the circulation; diseases that modify the concentration of this protein (e.g., inflammatory processes) may change the free fraction. Prazosin is extensively metabolized in the liver, and little unchanged drug is excreted by the kidneys. The plasma $t_{1/2}$ is about 3 h (may be prolonged to 6–8 h in congestive heart failure). The duration of action is approximately 7–10 h in the treatment of hypertension.

The initial dose should be 1 mg, usually given at bedtime so that the patient will remain recumbent for at least several hours to reduce the risk of syncopal reactions that may follow the first dose of prazosin. The dose is titrated upward depending on the blood pressure. A maximal effect generally is observed with a total daily dose of 20 mg in patients with hypertension. In the off-label treatment of BPH, doses from 1 to 5 mg twice daily typically are used.

Terazosin. *Terazosin,* a close structural analogue of prazosin, is less potent than prazosin but retains high specificity for α_1 receptors; terazosin does not discriminate among α_{1A}, α_{1B}, and α_{1D} receptors. The major distinction between the two drugs is in their pharmacokinetic properties.

Terazosin is more soluble in water than is prazosin, and its bioavailability is high (>90%). The $t_{1/2}$ of elimination of terazosin is about 12 h, and its duration of action usually extends beyond 18 h. Consequently, the drug may be taken once daily to treat hypertension and BPH in most patients. Terazosin has been found more effective than finasteride in treatment of BPH (Lepor et al., 1996). *Terazosin* and *doxazosin* induce apoptosis in prostate smooth muscle cells. This apoptosis may lessen the symptoms associated with chronic BPH by limiting cell proliferation. The apoptotic

effect of terazosin and doxazosin appears to be related to the quinazoline moiety rather than α_1 receptor antagonism; tamsulosin, a nonquinazoline α_1 receptor antagonist, does not produce apoptosis (Kyprianou, 2003). Only about 10% of terazosin is excreted unchanged in the urine. An initial first dose of 1 mg is recommended. Doses are slowly titrated upward depending on the therapeutic response. Doses of 10 mg/d may be required for maximal effect in BPH.

Doxazosin. *Doxazosin* is another congener of prazosin and a highly selective antagonist at α_1 receptors. It is nonselective among α_1 receptor subtypes and differs from prazosin in its pharmacokinetic profile.

The $t_{1/2}$ of doxazosin is about 20 h, and its duration of action may extend to 36 h. The bioavailability and extent of metabolism of doxazosin and prazosin are similar. Most doxazosin metabolites are eliminated in the feces. The hemodynamic effects of doxazosin appear to be similar to those of prazosin. Doxazosin should be given initially as a 1-mg dose in the treatment of hypertension or BPH. Doxazosin also may have beneficial actions in the long-term management of BPH related to apoptosis that are independent of α_1 receptor antagonism. Doxazosin is typically administered once daily. An extended-release formulation marketed for BPH is not recommended for the treatment of hypertension.

Alfuzosin. *Alfuzosin* is a quinazoline-based α_1 receptor antagonist with similar affinity at all of the α_1 receptor subtypes. It has been used extensively in treating BPH; it is not approved for treatment of hypertension. Alfuzosin has a $t_{1/2}$ of 3–5 h. Alfuzosin is a substrate of CYP3A4, and the concomitant administration of CPY3A4 inhibitors (e.g., ketoconazole, clarithromycin, itraconazole, ritonavir) is contraindicated. Alfuzosin should be avoided in patients at risk for prolonged QT syndrome. The recommended dosage is one 10-mg extended-release tablet daily to be taken after the same meal each day.

Tamsulosin. *Tamsulosin,* a benzenesulfonamide, is an α_1 receptor antagonist with some selectivity for α_{1A} (and α_{1D}) subtypes compared to the α_{1B} subtype (Kenny et al., 1996). This selectivity may favor blockade of α_{1A} receptors in prostate. Tamsulosin is efficacious in the treatment of BPH with little effect on blood pressure (Beduschi et al., 1998); tamsulosin is not approved for the treatment of hypertension. Tamsulosin is well absorbed and has a $t_{1/2}$ of 5–10 h. It is extensively metabolized by CYPs. Tamsulosin may be administered at a 0.4-mg starting dose; a dose of 0.8 mg ultimately will be more efficacious in some patients. Abnormal ejaculation is an adverse effect of tamsulosin, experienced by about 18% of patients receiving the higher dose.

Silodosin. *Silodosin* exhibits selectivity for the α_{1A}, over the α_{1B}, adrenergic receptor. The drug is metabolized by several pathways; the main metabolite is a glucuronide formed by UGT2B7; coadministration with inhibitors of this enzyme (e.g., probenecid, valproic acid, fluconazole) increases systemic exposure to silodosin. The drug is approved for the treatment of BPH and has lesser effects on blood pressure than the non–α_1-subtype selective antagonists. Nevertheless, dizziness and orthostatic hypotension can occur. The chief side effect of silodosin is retrograde ejaculation (in 28% of those treated). Silodosin is available as 4-mg and 8-mg capsules.

Adverse Effects

A major potential adverse effect of prazosin and its congeners is the first-dose effect; marked postural hypotension and syncope sometimes are seen 30–90 min after an initial dose of prazosin and 2–6 h after an initial dose of doxazosin.

Syncopal episodes also have occurred with a rapid increase in dosage or with the addition of a second antihypertensive drug to the regimen of a patient who already is taking a large dose of prazosin. The risk of the first-dose phenomenon is minimized by limiting the initial dose (e.g., 1 mg at bedtime), by increasing the dosage slowly, and by introducing additional antihypertensive drugs cautiously.

Because orthostatic hypotension may be a problem during long-term treatment with prazosin or its congeners, it is essential to check standing as well as recumbent blood pressure. Nonspecific adverse effects such as headache, dizziness, and asthenia rarely limit treatment with prazosin.

Therapeutic Uses

Hypertension. Prazosin and its congeners have been used successfully in the treatment of essential hypertension (Chapter 28). Pleotropic effects of these drugs improve lipid profiles and glucose-insulin metabolism in patients with hypertension who are at risk for atherosclerotic disease (Deano and Sorrentino, 2012). Catecholamines are also powerful stimulators of vascular smooth muscle hypertrophy, acting by α_1 receptors. To what extent these effects of α_1 antagonists have clinical significance in diminishing the risk of atherosclerosis is not known.

Congestive Heart Failure. α Receptor antagonists have been used in the treatment of congestive heart failure but are not the drugs of choice. Short-term effects of α receptor blockade in these patients are due to dilation of both arteries and veins, resulting in a reduction of preload and afterload, which increases cardiac output and reduces pulmonary congestion. In contrast to results obtained with inhibitors of angiotensin-converting enzyme or a combination of hydralazine and an organic nitrate, prazosin has not been found to prolong life in patients with congestive heart failure.

Benign Prostatic Hyperplasia. In a significant percentage of older men, BPH produces symptomatic urethral obstruction that leads to weak stream, increased urinary frequency, and nocturia. These symptoms are due to a combination of mechanical pressure on the urethra due to the increase in smooth muscle mass and the α_1 receptor–mediated increase in smooth muscle tone in the prostate and neck of the bladder (Kyprianou, 2003). α_1 Receptors in the trigone muscle of the bladder and urethra contribute to the resistance to outflow of urine. *Prazosin* reduces this resistance in some patients with impaired bladder emptying caused by prostatic obstruction or parasympathetic decentralization from spinal injury.

Finasteride and *dutasteride*, two drugs that inhibit conversion of testosterone to dihydrotestosterone (Chapter 45) and can reduce prostate volume in some patients, are approved as monotherapy and in combination with α receptor antagonists. α_1-Selective antagonists have efficacy in BPH owing to relaxation of smooth muscle in the bladder neck, prostate capsule, and prostatic urethra. α_1-Selective antagonists rapidly improve urinary flow, whereas the actions of finasteride are typically delayed for months. Combination therapy with doxazosin and finasteride reduces the risk of overall clinical progression of BPH significantly more than treatment with either drug alone (McConnell et al., 2003). Tamsulosin at the recommended dose of 0.4 mg daily and silodosin at 0.8 mg are less likely to cause orthostatic hypotension than are the other drugs. The predominant α_1 subtype expressed in the human prostate is the α_{1A} receptor (Michel and Vrydag, 2006). Developments in this area will provide the basis for the selection of α receptor antagonists with specificity for the relevant subtype of α_1 receptor. However, the possibility remains that some of the symptoms of BPH are due to α_1 receptors in other sites, such as bladder, spinal cord, or brain.

Other Disorders. Some studies indicated that prazosin can decrease the incidence of digital vasospasm in patients with Raynaud disease; however, its relative efficacy as compared with Ca^{2+} channel blockers is not known. Prazosin may have some benefit in patients with other vasospastic disorders. Prazosin may be useful for the treatment of patients with mitral or aortic valvular insufficiency, presumably by reducing afterload.

α_2 Adrenergic Receptor Antagonists

Activation of presynaptic α_2 receptors inhibits the release of NE and other cotransmitters from peripheral sympathetic nerve endings. Activation of α_2 receptors in the pontomedullary region of the CNS inhibits sympathetic nervous system activity and leads to a fall in blood pressure; these receptors are a site of action for drugs such as clonidine. *Blockade of α_2 receptors with selective antagonists such as yohimbine thus can increase sympathetic outflow and potentiate the release of NE from nerve endings, leading to activation of α_1 and β_1 receptors in the heart and peripheral vasculature with a consequent rise in blood pressure.* Antagonists that also block α_1 receptors give rise to similar effects on sympathetic outflow and release of NE, but the net increase in blood pressure is prevented by inhibition of vasoconstriction.

Although certain vascular beds contain α_2 receptors that promote contraction of smooth muscle, it is thought that these receptors are preferentially stimulated by circulating catecholamines, whereas α_1 receptors are activated by NE released from sympathetic nerve fibers. In other vascular beds, α_2 receptors reportedly promote vasodilation by stimulating the release of NO from endothelial cells. The physiological role of vascular α_2 receptors in the regulation of blood flow within various vascular beds is uncertain. The α_2 receptors contribute to smooth muscle contraction in the human saphenous vein, whereas α_1 receptors are more prominent in dorsal hand veins. The effects of α_2 receptor antagonists on the cardiovascular system are dominated by actions in the CNS and on sympathetic nerve endings.

Yohimbine

Yohimbine is a competitive antagonist that is selective for α_2 receptors. The compound is an indolealkylamine alkaloid and is found in the bark of the tree *Pausinystalia yohimbe* and in *Rauwolfia* root; its structure resembles that of *reserpine*. Yohimbine readily enters the CNS, where it acts to increase blood pressure and heart rate; it also enhances motor activity and produces tremors. These actions are opposite to those of clonidine, an α_2 agonist. Yohimbine also antagonizes effects of 5HT. In the past, it was used extensively to treat male sexual dysfunction (Tam et al., 2001). However, the efficacies of PDE5 inhibitors (e.g., *sildenafil*, *vardenafil*, and *tadalafil*) and *apomorphine* (off-label) have been much more conclusively demonstrated in oral treatment of erectile dysfunction. Some studies suggested that yohimbine may be useful for diabetic neuropathy and in the treatment of postural hypotension. In the U.S., yohimbine can be legally sold as a dietary supplement; however, labeling claims that it will arouse or increase sexual desire or improve sexual performance are prohibited. Yohimbine is approved in veterinary medicine for the reversal of xylazine anesthesia.

Nonselective α Adrenergic Antagonists

Phenoxybenzamine and Phentolamine

Phenoxybenzamine and *phentolamine* are nonselective α receptor antagonists. Phenoxybenzamine, a haloalkylamine compound, produces an irreversible antagonism, while phentolamine, an imidazaline, produces a competitive antagonism.

Phenoxybenzamine and *phentolamine* cause a progressive decrease in peripheral resistance due to antagonism of α receptors in the vasculature and an increase in cardiac output that is due in part to reflex sympathetic nerve stimulation. The cardiac stimulation is accentuated by enhanced release of NE from cardiac sympathetic nerve due to antagonism of presynaptic α_2 receptors by these nonselective α blockers. Postural hypotension is a prominent feature with these drugs, and this, accompanied by reflex tachycardia that can precipitate cardiac arrhythmias, severely limits the use of these drugs to treat essential hypertension. The α_1-selective antagonists, such as *prazosin*, have replaced the "classical" α-blockers in the management of essential hypertension. Phenoxybenzamine and phentolamine are still marketed for several specialized uses.

Therapeutic Uses. Phenoxybenzamine is used in the treatment of pheochromocytomas, tumors of the adrenal medulla and sympathetic neurons that secrete enormous quantities of catecholamines into the circulation. The usual result is hypertension, which may be episodic and severe. The vast majority of pheochromocytomas are treated surgically; phenoxybenzamine is often used in preparing the patient for surgery. The drug controls episodes of severe hypertension and minimizes other adverse effects of catecholamines, such as contraction of plasma volume and injury of the myocardium. A conservative approach is to initiate treatment with phenoxybenzamine (at a dosage of 10 mg twice daily) 1–3 weeks before the operation. The dose is increased every other day until the desired effect on blood pressure is achieved. The usual daily dose of phenoxybenzamine in patients with pheochromocytoma is 40–120 mg given in two or three divided portions. Prolonged treatment with phenoxybenzamine may be necessary in patients with inoperable or malignant pheochromocytoma. In some patients, particularly those with malignant disease, administration of *metyrosine*, a competitive inhibitor of tyrosine hydroxylase (the rate-limiting enzyme in the synthesis of catecholamines), may be a useful adjunct (Chapter 8). β Receptor antagonists also are used to treat pheochromocytoma, *but only after the administration of an α receptor antagonist* (described later in the chapter).

Phentolamine can also be used in short-term control of hypertension in patients with pheochromocytoma. Rapid infusions of phentolamine may cause severe hypotension, so the drug should be administered cautiously. Phentolamine also may be useful to relieve pseudo-obstruction of the bowel in patients with pheochromocytoma.

Phentolamine has been used locally to prevent dermal necrosis after the inadvertent extravasation of an α receptor agonist. The drug also may be useful for the treatment of hypertensive crises that follow the abrupt withdrawal of clonidine or that may result from the ingestion of tyramine-containing foods during the use of nonselective MAO inhibitors. Although excessive activation of α receptors is important in the development of severe hypertension in these settings, there is little information about the safety and efficacy of phentolamine compared with those of other antihypertensive agents in the treatment of such patients. Buccally or orally administered phentolamine may have efficacy in some men with sexual dysfunction.

Phentolamine is FDA-approved for reversing or limiting the duration of soft tissue anesthesia. Sympathomimetics are frequently administered with local anesthetics to slow the removal of the anesthetic by causing vasoconstriction. When the need for anesthesia is over, phentolamine can help reverse it by antagonizing the α receptor–induced vasoconstriction.

Phenoxybenzamine has been used off-label to control the manifestations of autonomic hyperreflexia in patients with spinal cord transection.

Toxicity and Adverse Effects. Hypotension is the major adverse effect of phenoxybenzamine and phentolamine. In addition, reflex cardiac stimulation may cause alarming tachycardia, cardiac arrhythmias, and ischemic cardiac events, including myocardial infarction. Reversible inhibition of ejaculation may occur due to impaired smooth muscle contraction in the vas deferens and ejaculatory ducts. Phentolamine stimulates GI smooth muscle, an effect antagonized by atropine, and also enhances gastric acid secretion due in part to histamine release. Thus, phentolamine should be used with caution in patients with a history of peptic ulcer. Phenoxybenzamine is mutagenic in the Ames test, and repeated administration of this drug to experimental animals causes peritoneal sarcomas and lung tumors.

Additional α Adrenergic Receptor Antagonists

Ergot Alkaloids

The ergot alkaloids were the first adrenergic receptor antagonists to be discovered. Ergot alkaloids exhibit a complex variety of pharmacological properties. To varying degrees, these agents act as partial agonists or antagonists at α receptors, DA receptors, and serotonin receptors. Additional information about the ergot alkaloids can be found in Chapter 13.

Indoramin

Indoramin is a selective, competitive α_1-selective receptor antagonist that also antagonizes H_1 and 5HT receptors. Indoramin lowers blood pressure with minimal tachycardia. The drug is not available in the U.S.; outside the U.S., indoramin is used for the treatment of hypertension and BPH and in the prophylaxis of migraine. The drug also decreases the incidence of attacks of Raynaud phenomenon. Some of the adverse effects of indoramin include sedation, dry mouth, and failure of ejaculation.

Ketanserin

Although developed as a 5HT receptor antagonist, ketanserin also blocks α_1 receptors. Ketanserin (not available in the U.S.) is discussed in Chapter 13.

Urapidil

Urapidil is a selective α_1 receptor antagonist that has a chemical structure distinct from those of prazosin and related compounds; the drug is not commercially available in the U.S. Blockade of peripheral α_1 receptors appears to be primarily responsible for the hypotension produced by urapidil, although it has actions in the CNS as well.

Bunazosin

Bunazosin is an α_1-selective antagonist of the quinazoline class that has been shown to lower blood pressure in patients with hypertension. Bunazosin is not available in the U.S.

Neuroleptic Agents

Chlorpromazine, haloperidol, and other neuroleptic drugs of the phenothiazine and butyrophenone types produce significant blockade of both α and D_2 receptors in humans.

β Adrenergic Receptor Antagonists

HISTORICAL PERSPECTIVE

Ahlquist's hypothesis that the effects of catecholamines were mediated by activation of distinct α and β receptors provided the initial impetus for the synthesis and pharmacological evaluation of β receptor antagonists (Chapter 8). The first such selective agent was dichloroisoproterenol, a partial agonist. Sir James Black and his colleagues initiated a program in the late 1950s to develop additional β blockers, with the resulting synthesis and characterization of propranolol.

Overview

Competitive antagonists of β adrenergic receptors, or β blockers, have received enormous clinical attention because of their efficacy in the treatment of hypertension, ischemic heart disease, congestive heart failure, and certain arrhythmias.

The myriad β antagonists can be distinguished by the following properties:

- Relative affinity for β_1 and β_2 receptors
- Intrinsic sympathomimetic activity
- Blockade of α receptors
- Differences in lipid solubility (CNS penetration)
- Capacity to induce vasodilation
- Pharmacokinetic parameters

Propranolol is a competitive β receptor antagonist and remains the prototype to which other β antagonists are compared. Propranolol is *a nonselective β adrenergic receptor antagonist* with equal affinity for β_1 and β_2 adrenergic receptors. Agents such as metoprolol, atenolol, acebutolol, bisoprolol, and esmolol have somewhat greater affinity for β_1 than for β_2 receptors; these are examples of *β_1-selective antagonists*, even though the selectivity is not absolute. Propranolol is a pure antagonist, and it has no capacity to activate β receptors. Several β blockers (e.g., pindolol and acebutolol) activate β receptors partially in the absence of catecholamines; however, the intrinsic activities of these drugs are less than that of a full agonist such as INE. These partial agonists have *intrinsic sympathomimetic activity*; this slight residual activity may prevent profound bradycardia or negative inotropy in a resting heart. The potential clinical advantage of this property, however, is unclear and may be disadvantageous in the context of secondary prevention of myocardial infarction. Other β receptor antagonists have the property of *inverse agonism* (Chapter 3); these drugs can decrease basal activity of β receptor signaling by shifting the equilibrium of spontaneously active receptors toward an inactive state (see Chapters 3 and 8).

Several β receptor antagonists also have local anesthetic or membrane-stabilizing activity, independent of β blockade. Such drugs include propranolol, acebutolol, and carvedilol. Pindolol, metoprolol, betaxolol, and labetalol have slight membrane-stabilizing effects. Although most β receptor antagonists do not block α adrenergic receptors, labetalol, carvedilol, and bucindolol block both α_1 and β adrenergic receptors. In addition to carvedilol, labetalol, and bucindolol, other β receptor antagonists have vasodilating properties due to mechanisms discussed in the following material. These include celiprolol, nebivolol, nipradilol, carteolol, betaxolol, bopindolol, and bevantolol (Toda, 2003).

Pharmacological Properties

The pharmacological properties of β receptor antagonists can be deduced and explained largely from knowledge of the responses elicited by the receptors in the various tissues and the activity of the sympathetic nerves that innervate these tissues (Table 8–1). For example, β receptor blockade has relatively little effect on the normal heart of an individual at rest but has profound effects when sympathetic control of the heart is dominant, as during exercise or stress.

The β adrenergic receptor antagonists are classified as non subtype-selective ("first generation"), β_1 selective ("second generation"), and non subtype- or subtype-selective *with additional cardiovascular actions* ("third generation"). These last drugs have additional cardiovascular properties (especially vasodilation) that seem unrelated to β blockade. Table 12–3 summarizes pharmacological and pharmacokinetic properties of β receptor antagonists.

Cardiovascular System. The major therapeutic effects of β receptor antagonists are on the cardiovascular system. It is important to distinguish these effects in normal subjects from those in subjects with cardiovascular disease such as hypertension or myocardial ischemia.

Catecholamines have positive chronotropic and inotropic actions. Conversely, β receptor antagonists slow the heart rate and decrease myocardial contractility, *if there are sympathetic stimuli to antagonize.* When tonic stimulation of β receptors is low, this effect is correspondingly modest. However, when the sympathetic nervous system is activated, as during exercise or stress, β receptor antagonists attenuate the expected rise in heart rate.

Short-term administration of β receptor antagonists decreases cardiac output; peripheral resistance increases in proportion to maintain blood pressure as a result of blockade of vascular β_2 receptors and compensatory reflexes, such as increased sympathetic nervous system activity, leading to activation of vascular α receptors. However, with long-term use of β antagonists, total peripheral resistance returns to initial values (Mimran and Ducailar, 1988) *or decreases in patients with hypertension* (Man in't Veld et al., 1988). With β antagonists that also are α_1 receptor antagonists, such as labetalol, carvedilol, and bucindolol, cardiac output is maintained with a greater fall in peripheral resistance. This also is seen with β receptor antagonists that are direct vasodilators.

The β receptor antagonists have significant effects on cardiac rhythm and automaticity. Although it had been thought that these effects were due exclusively to blockade of β_1 receptors, β_2 receptors likely also regulate heart rate in humans (Altschuld and Billman, 2000; Brodde and Michel, 1999). The β_3 receptors also have been identified in normal myocardial tissue (Moniotte et al., 2001). Signal transduction for β_3 receptors is complex and includes not only G_s but also G_i/G_o; stimulation of cardiac β_3 receptors inhibits cardiac contraction and relaxation. The physiological role of β_3 receptors in the heart remains to be established (Morimoto et al., 2004). β Receptor antagonists reduce the sinus rate, decrease the spontaneous rate of depolarization of ectopic pacemakers, slow conduction in the atria and in the AV node, and increase the functional refractory period of the AV node.

Although high concentrations of many β blockers exert a membrane-stabilizing activity, it is doubtful that this is significant at usual therapeutic doses. However, this effect may be important when there is overdosage. *d*-Propranolol may suppress ventricular arrhythmias independently of β receptor blockade.

The cardiovascular effects of β receptor antagonists are most evident during dynamic exercise. In the presence of β receptor blockade, exercise-induced increases in heart rate and myocardial contractility are attenuated. However, the exercise-induced increase in cardiac output is less

TABLE 12–3 ■ PHARMACOLOGICAL/PHARMACOKINETIC PROPERTIES OF β ADRENERGIC RECEPTOR BLOCKING AGENTS

DRUG	MEMBRANE STABILIZING ACTIVITY	INTRINSIC AGONIST ACTIVITY	LIPID SOLUBILITY	EXTENT OF ABSORPTION (%)	ORAL AVAILABILITY (%)	PLASMA $t_{1/2}$ (HOURS)	PROTEIN BINDING (%)
Classical nonselective β blockers: First generation							
Nadolol	0	0	Low	30	30–50	20–24	30
Penbutolol	0	+	High	~100	~100	~5	80–98
Pindolol	+	+++	Low	>95	~100	3–4	40
Propranolol	++	0	High	<90	30	3–5	90
Timolol	0	0	Low to moderate	90	75	4	<10
β_1 Selective blockers: Second generation							
Acebutolol	+	+	Low	90	20–60	3–4	26
Atenolol	0	0	Low	90	50–60	6–7	6–16
Bisoprolol	0	0	Low	≤90	80	9–12	~30
Esmolol	0	0	Low	NA	NA	0.15	55
Metoprolol	+[a]	0	Moderate	~100	40–50	3–7	12
Nonselective β blockers with additional actions: Third generation							
Carteolol	0	++	Low	85	85	6	23–30
Carvedilol	++	0	Moderate	>90	~30	7–10	98
Labetalol	+	+	Low	>90	~33	3–4	~50
β_1 selective blockers with additional actions: Third generation							
Betaxolol	+	0	Moderate	>90	~80	15	50
Celiprolol	0	+	Low	~74	30–70	5	4–5
Nebivolol	0	0	Low	NA	NA	11–30	98

[a]Detectable only at doses much greater than required for β blockade.

TABLE 12–4 ■ THIRD-GENERATION β RECEPTOR ANTAGONISTS WITH PUTATIVE ADDITIONAL MECHANISMS OF VASODILATION

NITRIC OXIDE PRODUCTION	β₂ RECEPTOR AGONISM	α₁ RECEPTOR ANTAGONISM	Ca²⁺ ENTRY BLOCKADE	K⁺ CHANNEL OPENING	ANTIOXIDANT ACTIVITY
Celiprolol[a]	Celiprolol[a]	Carvedilol	Carvedilol	Tilisolol[a]	Carvedilol
Nebivolol	Carteolol	Bucindolol[a]	Betaxolol		
Carteolol	Bopindolol[a]	Bevantolol[a]	Bevantolol[a]		
Bopindolol[a]		Nipradilol[a]			
Nipradilol[a]		Labetalol			

[a]Not currently available in the U.S., where most are under investigation for use.

affected because of an increase in stroke volume. The effects of β receptor antagonists on exercise are somewhat analogous to the changes that occur with normal aging. In healthy elderly persons, catecholamine-induced increases in heart rate are smaller than in younger individuals; however, the increase in cardiac output in older people may be preserved because of an increase in stroke volume during exercise. β Blockers tend to decrease work capacity, as assessed by their effects on intense short-term or more prolonged steady-state exertion. Exercise performance may be impaired to a lesser extent by β₁ selective agents than by nonselective antagonists. Blockade of β₂ receptors blunts the increase in blood flow to active skeletal muscle during submaximal exercise and also may attenuate catecholamine-induced activation of glucose metabolism and lipolysis.

Coronary artery blood flow increases during exercise or stress to meet the metabolic demands of the heart. By increasing heart rate, contractility, and systolic pressure, catecholamines increase myocardial O₂ demand. However, in patients with coronary artery disease, fixed narrowing of these vessels attenuates the expected increase in flow, leading to myocardial ischemia. β Receptor antagonists decrease the effects of catecholamines on the determinants of myocardial O₂ consumption. However, these agents may tend to increase the requirement for O₂ by increasing end-diastolic pressure and systolic ejection period. Usually, the net effect is to improve the relationship between cardiac O₂ supply and demand; exercise tolerance generally is improved in patients with angina, whose capacity to exercise is limited by the development of chest pain (Chapter 27).

Antihypertensive Activity. β Receptor antagonists generally do not reduce blood pressure in patients with normal blood pressure. However, these drugs lower blood pressure in patients with hypertension, but the mechanisms responsible for this important clinical effect are not fully understood. The release of *renin* from the juxtaglomerular cells is stimulated by the sympathetic nervous system by means of β₁ receptors, and this effect is blocked by β receptor antagonists (see Chapter 26). Some investigators have found that the antihypertensive effect of β blockade is most marked in patients with elevated concentrations of plasma renin, compared to patients with low or normal concentrations of renin. However, β receptor antagonists are effective even in patients with low plasma renin.

Presynaptic β receptors enhance the release of NE from sympathetic neurons, and diminished release of NE from β blockade is a possible response. Although β blockers would not be expected to decrease the contractility of vascular smooth muscle, long-term administration of these drugs to hypertensive patients ultimately leads to a fall in peripheral vascular resistance (Man in't Veld et al., 1988). The mechanism for this effect is not known, but this delayed fall in peripheral vascular resistance in the face of a persistent reduction of cardiac output appears to account for much of the antihypertensive effect of these drugs.

Some β receptor antagonists have additional effects that may contribute to their capacity to lower blood pressure. These drugs all produce peripheral vasodilation; at least six properties have been proposed to contribute to this effect, including production of NO, activation of β₂ receptors, blockade of α₁ receptors, blockade of Ca²⁺ entry, opening of K⁺ channels, and antioxidant activity (see Table 12–4 and Figure 12–4). These mechanisms appear to contribute to the antihypertensive effects by enhancing hypotension, increasing peripheral blood flow, and decreasing afterload.

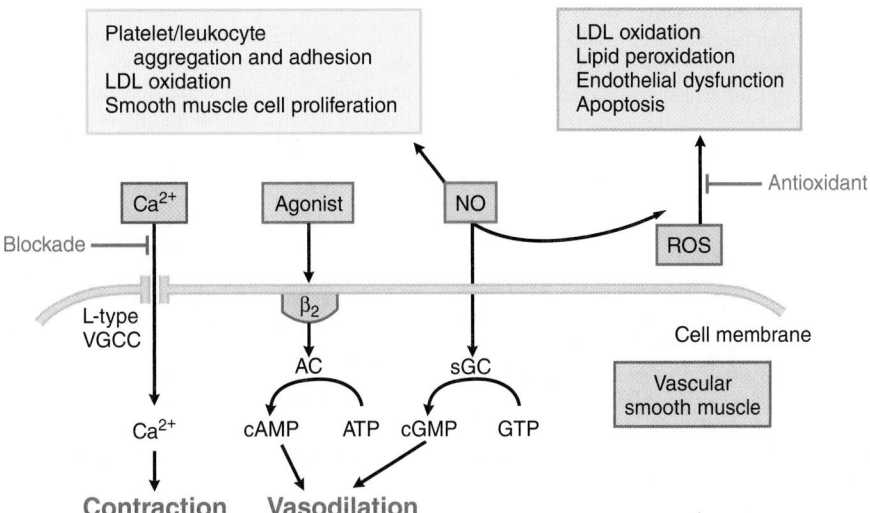

Figure 12-4 *Mechanisms underlying actions of vasodilating β blockers in blood vessels.* AC: adenylyl cyclase; sGC: soluble guanylyl cyclase; NO: nitric oxide; ROS: reactive oxygen species; VGCC: voltage-gated Ca²⁺ channel. (Modified with permission from Toda N. Vasodilating β adrenoceptor blockers as cardiovascular therapeutics. *Pharmacol Ther*, **2003**, 100:215–234. Copyright © Elsevier.)

Celiprolol and *nebivolol* also have been observed to produce vasodilation and thereby reduce preload.

Nonselective β receptor antagonists inhibit the vasodilation caused by INE and augment the pressor response to EPI. This is particularly significant in patients with pheochromocytoma, in whom β receptor antagonists should be used only after adequate α receptor blockade has been established. This avoids uncompensated α receptor–mediated vasoconstriction caused by EPI secreted from the tumor.

Pulmonary System. Nonselective β receptor antagonists such as propranolol block β_2 receptors in bronchial smooth muscle. This usually has little effect on pulmonary function in normal individuals. However, *in patients with COPD, such blockade can lead to life-threatening bronchoconstriction.* Although β_1-selective antagonists or antagonists with intrinsic sympathomimetic activity are less likely than propranolol to increase airway resistance in patients with asthma, these drugs should be used only with great caution, if at all, in patients with bronchospastic diseases. Drugs such as celiprolol, with β_1 receptor selectivity and β_2 receptor partial agonism, are of potential promise, although clinical experience is limited.

Metabolic Effects. The β receptor antagonists modify the metabolism of carbohydrates and lipids. Catecholamines promote glycogenolysis and mobilize glucose in response to hypoglycemia. Nonselective β blockers may delay recovery from hypoglycemia in type 1 (insulin-dependent) diabetes mellitus, but infrequently in type 2 diabetes mellitus. In addition to blocking glycogenolysis, β receptor antagonists can interfere with the counterregulatory effects of catecholamines secreted during hypoglycemia by blunting the perception of symptoms such as tremor, tachycardia, and nervousness. Thus, β adrenergic receptor antagonists should be used with great caution in patients with labile diabetes and frequent hypoglycemic reactions. If such a drug is indicated, a β_1-selective antagonist is preferred because these drugs are less likely to delay recovery from hypoglycemia (DiBari et al., 2003).

The β receptors mediate activation of hormone-sensitive lipase in fat cells, leading to release of free fatty acids into the circulation. This increased flux of fatty acids is an important source of energy for exercising muscle. β Receptor antagonists can attenuate the release of free fatty acids from adipose tissue. Nonselective β receptor antagonists consistently reduce HDL cholesterol, increase LDL cholesterol, and increase triglycerides. In contrast, β_1-selective antagonists, including celiprolol, carteolol, nebivolol, carvedilol, and bevantolol, reportedly improve the serum lipid profile of dyslipidemic patients. While drugs such as propranolol and atenolol increase triglycerides, plasma triglycerides are reduced with chronic celiprolol, carvedilol, and carteolol (Toda, 2003).

In contrast to classical β blockers, which decrease insulin sensitivity, the vasodilating β receptor antagonists (e.g., celiprolol, nipradilol, carteolol, carvedilol, and dilevalol) increase insulin sensitivity in patients with insulin resistance. Together with their cardioprotective effects, improvement in insulin sensitivity from vasodilating β receptor antagonists may partially counterbalance the hazard from worsened lipid abnormalities associated with diabetes.

When β blockers are required, β_1-selective or vasodilating β receptor antagonists are preferred. In addition, it may be necessary to use β receptor antagonists in conjunction with other drugs, (e.g., HMG CoA reductase inhibitors) to ameliorate adverse metabolic effects (Dunne et al., 2001).

The β receptor agonists decrease the plasma concentration of K^+ by promoting its uptake, predominantly into skeletal muscle. At rest, an infusion of EPI causes a decrease in the plasma concentration of K^+. The marked increase in the concentration of EPI that occurs with stress (such as myocardial infarction) may cause hypokalemia, which could predispose to cardiac arrhythmias. The hypokalemic effect of EPI is blocked by an experimental antagonist, ICI 118551, which has a high affinity for β_2 and, to a lesser degree, β_3 receptors. Exercise causes an increase in the efflux of K^+ from skeletal muscle. Catecholamines tend to buffer the rise in K^+ by increasing its influx into muscle. β Blockers negate this buffering effect.

Other Effects. The β receptor antagonists block catecholamine-induced tremor. They also block inhibition of mast cell degranulation by catecholamines.

Adverse Effects and Precautions

Cardiovascular System. β Receptor blockade may cause or exacerbate heart failure in patients with compensated heart failure, acute myocardial infarction, or cardiomegaly. It is not known whether β receptor antagonists that possess intrinsic sympathomimetic activity or peripheral vasodilating properties are safer in these settings. Nonetheless, there is convincing evidence that chronic administration of β receptor antagonists is efficacious in prolonging life in the therapy of heart failure in selected patients (discussed in Chapter 29).

Bradycardia is a normal response to β receptor blockade; however, in patients with partial or complete AV conduction defects, β antagonists may cause life-threatening *bradyarrhythmias*. Particular caution is indicated in patients who are taking other drugs, such as verapamil or various antiarrhythmic agents, which may impair sinus node function or AV conduction.

Some patients complain of cold extremities while taking β receptor antagonists. Symptoms of peripheral vascular disease may occasionally worsen, or Raynaud phenomenon may develop.

Abrupt discontinuation of β receptor antagonists after long-term treatment can exacerbate angina and may increase the risk of sudden death. There is enhanced sensitivity to β receptor agonists in patients who have undergone long-term treatment with certain β receptor antagonists after the blocker is withdrawn abruptly. This increased sensitivity is evident several days after stopping a β receptor antagonist and may persist for at least 1 week. Such enhanced sensitivity can be attenuated by tapering the dose of the β blocker for several weeks before discontinuation. Supersensitivity to INE also has been observed after abrupt discontinuation of metoprolol, but not of pindolol. This enhanced β responsiveness may result from upregulation of β receptors. The number of β receptors on circulating lymphocytes is increased in subjects who have received propranolol for long periods; pindolol has the opposite effect. For discontinuation of β blockers, it is prudent to decrease the dose gradually and to restrict exercise during this period.

Pulmonary Function. A major adverse effect of β receptor antagonists is caused by blockade of β_2 receptors in bronchial smooth muscle. These receptors are particularly important for promoting bronchodilation in patients with bronchospastic disease, and β_2 blockade may cause a life-threatening increase in airway resistance in such patients. Drugs with selectivity for β_1 receptors or those with intrinsic sympathomimetic activity at β_2 receptors seem less likely to induce bronchospasm. β Blocker drugs should be avoided if at all possible in patients with asthma. However, in selected patients with COPD and cardiovascular disease, the advantages of using β_1 receptor antagonists may outweigh the risk of worsening pulmonary function (Salpeter et al., 2005).

CNS. The adverse effects of β receptor antagonists that are referable to the CNS may include fatigue, sleep disturbances (including insomnia and nightmares), and depression. Interest has focused on the relationship between the incidence of the adverse effects of β receptor antagonists and their lipophilicity; however, no clear correlation has emerged.

Metabolism. β Adrenergic blockade may blunt recognition of hypoglycemia by patients; it also may delay recovery from insulin-induced hypoglycemia. β Receptor antagonists should be used with great caution in patients with diabetes who are prone to hypoglycemic reactions; β_1-selective agents may be preferable for these patients. The benefits of β receptor antagonists in type 1 diabetes with myocardial infarction may outweigh the risk in selected patients (Thompson, 2013).

Sexual Function and Reproduction. The incidence of sexual dysfunction in men with hypertension who are treated with β receptor antagonists is not clearly defined. Although experience with the use of β adrenergic receptor antagonists in pregnancy is increasing, information about the safety of these drugs during pregnancy still is limited.

Overdosage. The manifestations of poisoning with β receptor antagonists depend on the pharmacological properties of the ingested drug, particularly its β_1 selectivity, intrinsic sympathomimetic activity, and membrane-stabilizing properties. Hypotension, bradycardia, prolonged AV conduction times, and widened QRS complexes are common manifestations of overdosage. Seizures and depression may occur. Hypoglycemia and bronchospasm can occur. Significant bradycardia should be treated initially with atropine, but a cardiac pacemaker often is required. Large doses of INE or an α receptor agonist may be necessary to treat hypotension. Glucagon, acting through its own G protein–coupled receptor and independently of the β adrenergic receptor, has positive chronotropic and inotropic effects on the heart, and the drug has been useful in some patients who have an overdose of a β receptor antagonist.

Drug Interactions. Aluminum salts, cholestyramine, and colestipol may decrease the absorption of β blockers. Drugs such as phenytoin, rifampin, and phenobarbital, as well as smoking, induce hepatic biotransformation enzymes and may decrease plasma concentrations of β receptor antagonists that are metabolized extensively (e.g., propranolol). Cimetidine and hydralazine may increase the bioavailability of agents such as propranolol and metoprolol by affecting hepatic blood flow. β Receptor antagonists can impair the clearance of lidocaine.

Additive effects on blood pressure by β blockers and other antihypertensive agents often are employed to clinical advantage. However, the antihypertensive effects of β receptor antagonists can be opposed by indomethacin and other nonsteroidal anti-inflammatory drugs (see Chapter 38).

Therapeutic Uses

Cardiovascular Diseases. The β receptor antagonists are used extensively in the treatment of hypertension, angina and acute coronary syndromes, and congestive heart failure (Chapters 27–29). These drugs also are used frequently in the treatment of supraventricular and ventricular arrhythmias (Chapter 30). β Receptor antagonists are used in the treatment of hypertrophic obstructive cardiomyopathy, relieving angina, palpitations, and syncope in patients with this disorder. Efficacy probably is related to partial relief of the pressure gradient along the outflow tract. β Blockers also may attenuate catecholamine-induced cardiomyopathy in pheochromocytoma.

β Blockers are used frequently in the medical management of acute dissecting aortic aneurysm; their usefulness comes from reduction in the force of myocardial contraction and the rate of development of such force. Nitroprusside is an alternative, but when given in the absence of β receptor blockade, it causes an undesirable reflex tachycardia. Chronic treatment with β antagonists may be efficacious in slowing the progression of aortic dilation and its complications in patients with Marfan syndrome, although surgical aortic repair is still warranted as aortic diameter expands; losartan, an ACEI, is showing promise as a more effective treatment (Hiratzka et al., 2010).

Glaucoma. The β receptor antagonists are used in the treatment of chronic open-angle glaucoma (see Chapter 69). These agents decrease the production of aqueous humor, which appears to be the mechanism for their clinical effectiveness.

Other Uses. Many of the signs and symptoms of hyperthyroidism are reminiscent of the manifestations of increased sympathetic nervous system activity. β Receptor antagonists control many of the cardiovascular signs and symptoms of hyperthyroidism and are useful adjuncts to more definitive therapy. In addition, propranolol inhibits the peripheral conversion of thyroxine to triiodothyronine, an effect that may be independent of β receptor blockade (see Chapter 43).

Propranolol, timolol, and metoprolol are effective for the prophylaxis of migraine; these drugs are not useful for treatment of acute attacks of migraine.

Propranolol and other β blockers are effective in controlling acute panic symptoms in individuals who are required to perform in public or in other anxiety-provoking situations. Tachycardia, muscle tremors, and other evidence of increased sympathetic activity are reduced.

β Blockers may be of some value in the treatment of patients undergoing withdrawal from alcohol or those with akathisia. Propranolol and nadolol are efficacious in the primary prevention of variceal bleeding in patients with portal hypertension caused by cirrhosis of the liver (Bosch, 1998).

Clinical Selection of a β Receptor Antagonist

The various β receptor antagonists that are used for the treatment of hypertension and angina appear to have similar efficacies. Selection of the most appropriate drug for an individual patient should be based on pharmacokinetic and pharmacodynamic differences among the drugs, cost, and whether there are concurrent medical problems. β_1-Selective antagonists are preferable in patients with bronchospasm, diabetes, peripheral vascular disease, or Raynaud phenomenon. Although no clinical advantage of β receptor antagonists with intrinsic sympathomimetic activity has been clearly established, such drugs may be preferable in patients with bradycardia. In addition, third-generation β antagonists that block α_1 receptors, stimulate β_2 receptors, enhance NO production, block Ca^{2+} entry, open K^+ channels, or possess antioxidant properties may offer therapeutic advantages.

Nonselective β Adrenergic Receptor Antagonists

Propranolol

Propranolol (Table 12–5) interacts with β_1 and β_2 receptors with equal affinity, lacks intrinsic sympathomimetic activity, and does not block α receptors.

ADME. Propranolol is highly lipophilic and almost completely absorbed after oral administration. Much of the drug is metabolized by the liver during its first passage through the portal circulation; only about 25% reaches the systemic circulation. In addition, there is great interindividual variation in the presystemic clearance of propranolol by the liver; this contributes to enormous variability in plasma concentrations (~20-fold) after oral administration of the drug and to the wide dosage range for clinical efficacy. The degree of hepatic extraction of propranolol declines as the dose is increased. The bioavailability of propranolol may be increased by the concomitant ingestion of food and during long-term administration of the drug.

Propranolol readily enters the CNS. Approximately 90% of the drug in the circulation is bound to plasma proteins. It is extensively metabolized, with most metabolites appearing in the urine. One product of hepatic metabolism is 4-hydroxypropranolol, which has some β adrenergic antagonist activity.

Analysis of the distribution of propranolol, its clearance by the liver, and its activity is complicated by the stereospecificity of these processes (Walle et al., 1988). The (–) enantiomers of propranolol and other β-blockers are the active forms. The (–) enantiomer of propranolol appears to be cleared more slowly from the body than is the inactive enantiomer. The clearance of propranolol may vary with hepatic blood flow and liver disease and also may change during the administration of other drugs that affect hepatic metabolism.

Despite its short $t_{1/2}$ in plasma (~4 h), twice-daily administration suffices to produce the antihypertensive effect in some patients. Sustained-release formulations of propranolol maintain therapeutic concentrations of propranolol in plasma throughout a 24-h period. For the treatment of hypertension and angina, the initial oral dose of propranolol generally is 40–80 mg per day. The dose may then be titrated upward until the optimal response is obtained. For the treatment of angina, the dose may be increased at intervals of less than 1 week, as indicated clinically. In hypertension, the full blood pressure response may not develop for several weeks. Typically, doses are less than 320 mg/d. If propranolol is taken twice daily for hypertension, blood pressure should be measured just prior to a dose to ensure that the duration of effect is sufficiently prolonged. Adequacy of β adrenergic blockade can be assessed by measuring suppression of exercise-induced tachycardia (Table 12–5).

Propranolol may be administered intravenously for the management of life-threatening arrhythmias or to patients under anesthesia. Under these circumstances, the usual dose is 1–3 mg, administered slowly (<1 mg/min) with careful and frequent monitoring of blood pressure, ECG, and cardiac function. If an adequate response is not obtained, a second dose may be given after several minutes. If bradycardia is excessive, atropine should be administered to increase heart rate. A change to oral therapy should be initiated as soon as possible.

Nadolol

Nadolol is a long-acting antagonist with equal affinity for β_1 and β_2 receptors. It is devoid of both membrane-stabilizing and intrinsic sympathomimetic activity. A distinguishing characteristic of nadolol is its relatively long $t_{1/2}$. It can be used to treat hypertension and angina pectoris. Unlabeled uses have included migraine prophylaxis, parkinsonian tremors, and variceal bleeding in portal hypertension.

ADME. Nadolol is very soluble in water and is incompletely absorbed from the gut; its bioavailability is about 35%. Interindividual variability is less than with propranolol. The low lipid solubility of nadolol may result in lower concentrations of the drug in the brain. Nadolol is not extensively metabolized and is largely excreted intact in the urine. The $t_{1/2}$ of the drug in plasma is about 20 h; consequently, it generally is administered once daily. Nadolol may accumulate in patients with renal failure, and dosage should be reduced in such individuals.

Timolol

Timolol is a potent, nonselective β receptor antagonist with no intrinsic sympathomimetic or membrane-stabilizing activity. It is used for hypertension, congestive heart failure, acute myocardial infarction, and migraine prophylaxis. In ophthalmology, timolol has been used in the treatment of open-angle glaucoma and intraocular hypertension. The drug appears to reduce aqueous humor production through blockade of β receptors on the ciliary epithelium.

ADME. Timolol is well absorbed from the GI tract. It is metabolized extensively by CYP2D6 in the liver. Only a small amount of unchanged drug appears in the urine. The $t_{1/2}$ in plasma is about 4 h. The ocular formulation of timolol may be absorbed systemically (Chapter 69) and produce adverse effects in susceptible patients, such as those with asthma or congestive heart failure. The systemic administration of cimetidine with topical ocular timolol increases the degree of β blockade, resulting in a reduction of resting heart rate, intraocular pressure, and exercise tolerance (Ishii et al., 2000). For ophthalmic use, timolol is available combined with other medications (e.g., with dorzolamide or travoprost). Timolol also provides benefits to patients with coronary heart disease: In the acute period after myocardial infarction, timolol produced a 39% reduction in mortality in the Norwegian Multicenter Study.

Pindolol

Pindolol is a nonselective β receptor antagonist *with intrinsic sympathomimetic activity*. It has low membrane-stabilizing activity and low lipid solubility. It is used to treat angina pectoris and hypertension. β-Blockers with slight partial agonist activity may be preferred as antihypertensive agents in individuals with diminished cardiac reserve or a propensity for bradycardia. Nonetheless, the clinical significance of partial agonism has not been substantially demonstrated in controlled trials but may be of importance in individual patients.

ADME. Pindolol is almost completely absorbed after oral administration; the drug has a moderately high bioavailability and plasma $t_{1/2}$ of about 4 h. Approximately 50% of pindolol ultimately is metabolized in the liver; the remainder is excreted unchanged in the urine. Clearance is reduced in patients with renal failure.

β_1-Selective Adrenergic Receptor Antagonists

Metoprolol

Metoprolol is a β_1-selective receptor antagonist that is devoid of intrinsic sympathomimetic activity and membrane-stabilizing activity.

ADME. Metoprolol is almost completely absorbed after oral administration, but bioavailability is relatively low (~40%) due to first-pass metabolism. Plasma concentrations of the drug vary widely (up to 17-fold), possibly due to genetically determined differences in the rate of metabolism in the liver by CYP2D6. Only 10% of the administered drug is

recovered unchanged in the urine. The $t_{1/2}$ of metoprolol is 3–4 h, but can increase to 7–8 h in CYP2D6 poor metabolizers who have a 5-fold higher risk for developing adverse effects (Wuttke et al., 2002). An extended-release formulation is available for once-daily administration.

Therapeutic Uses. Metoprolol has been used to treat essential hypertension, angina pectoris, tachycardia, heart failure, and vasovagal syncope and as secondary prevention after myocardial infarction, an adjunct in treatment of hyperthyroidism, and for migraine prophylaxis. For the treatment of hypertension, the usual initial dose is 100 mg/d. The drug sometimes is effective when given once daily, although it frequently is used in two divided doses. Dosage may be increased at weekly intervals until optimal reduction of blood pressure is achieved. Metoprolol generally is used in two divided doses for the treatment of stable angina. For the initial treatment of patients with acute myocardial infarction, an intravenous formulation of metoprolol tartrate is available; oral dosing is initiated as soon as the clinical situation permits. Metoprolol generally is contraindicated for the treatment of acute myocardial infarction in patients with heart rates of less than 45 beats per min, heart block greater than first-degree (PR interval $\geq$ 0.24 sec), systolic blood pressure less than 100 mm Hg, or moderate-to-severe heart failure.

Atenolol

Atenolol is a β_1-selective antagonist that is devoid of intrinsic sympathomimetic and membrane-stabilizing activity. Atenolol is very hydrophilic and appears to penetrate the CNS only to a limited extent.

ADME. Atenolol is available in 25-, 50-, and 100-mg oral tablets (initial dose is 50 mg/d). It is incompletely absorbed (~50%) and is excreted largely unchanged in the urine, with elimination $t_{1/2}$ of 5–8 h. The drug accumulates in patients with renal failure, and dosage should be adjusted for patients whose creatinine clearance is less than 35 mL/min.

Therapeutic Uses. Atenolol can be used to treat hypertension, coronary heart disease, arrhythmias, and angina pectoris and to treat or reduce the risk of heart complications following myocardial infarction. Recent meta-analysis and clinical trials demonstrated a lack of benefit compared with placebo or other antihypertensive agents for reduction of stroke, cardiovascular and all-cause, in spite of similar blood pressure reduction compared to other antihypertensive agents (Ripley and Saseen, 2014). Compared with other active treatments, atenolol was associated with increased risk of all-cause mortality, cardiovascular mortality, and stroke and had a neutral effect on myocardial infarction. Atenolol is also used to treat Graves disease until antithyroid medication can take effect. The initial dose of atenolol for the treatment of hypertension usually is 50 mg/d, given once daily. If an adequate therapeutic response is not evident within several weeks, the daily dose may be increased to 100 mg. Atenolol has been shown to be efficacious, in combination with a diuretic, in elderly patients with isolated systolic hypertension. Atenolol causes fewer CNS side effects (depression, nightmares) than most β-blockers and few bronchospastic reactions due to its pharmacological and pharmacokinetic profile (Varon, 2008).

Esmolol

Esmolol is a β_1-selective antagonist with a rapid onset and a very short duration of action. It has little if any intrinsic sympathomimetic activity and lacks membrane-stabilizing actions. Esmolol is administered intravenously and is used when β blockade of short duration is desired or in critically ill patients in whom adverse effects of bradycardia, heart failure, or hypotension may necessitate rapid withdrawal of the drug. It is a class II antiarrhythmic agent (Chapter 30).

ADME. Esmolol is given by slow intravenous injection. Because esmolol is used in urgent settings where immediate onset of β blockade is warranted, a partial loading dose (500 µg/kg over 1 min) typically is administered, followed by a continuous infusion of the drug (maintenance dose of 50 µg/kg/min for 4 min). If an adequate therapeutic effect is not observed within 5 min, the same loading dose is repeated, followed by a maintenance infusion at a higher rate. This may need to be repeated until the desired end point (e.g., lowered heart rate or blood pressure) is approached. The drug is hydrolyzed rapidly by esterases in erythrocytes and has a $t_{1/2}$ of about 8 min. The $t_{1/2}$ of the carboxylic acid metabolite of esmolol is far longer (~4 h) and will accumulate during prolonged infusion of esmolol. However, this metabolite has very low potency as a β receptor antagonist (1/500 of the potency of esmolol); it is excreted in the urine.

Therapeutic Uses. Esmolol is commonly used in patients during surgery to prevent or treat tachycardia and in the treatment of supraventricular tachycardia. The onset and cessation of β receptor blockade with esmolol are rapid; peak hemodynamic effects occur within 6–10 min of administration of a loading dose, and there is substantial diminution of β-blockade within 20 min of stopping an infusion. Esmolol is particularly useful in severe postoperative hypertension and is a suitable agent in situations where cardiac output, heart rate, and blood pressure are increased. The American Heart Association/American College of Cardiology guidelines recommend against using esmolol in patients already on β blocker therapy, bradycardic patients, and patients with decompensated heart failure, as the drug may compromise their myocardial function (Varon, 2008). Esmolol is generally tolerated well, but it is associated with an increased risk of hypotension that is rapidly reversible (Garnock-Jones, 2012).

Acebutolol

Acebutolol is a β_1-selective antagonist with some intrinsic sympathomimetic and membrane-stabilizing activity.

ADME. Acebutolol is administered orally (starting dose 200 mg twice daily titrated up to 1200 mg/d). It is well absorbed and undergoes significant first-pass metabolism to an active metabolite, diacetolol, which accounts for most of the drug's activity. Overall bioavailability is 35%–50%. The elimination $t_{1/2}$ of acebutolol typically is about 3 h, but the $t_{1/2}$ of diacetolol is 8–12 h; it is excreted largely in the urine. Acebutolol has lipophilic properties and crosses the blood-brain barrier. It has no negative impact on serum lipids (cholesterol, triglycerides, or HDL).

Therapeutic Uses. Acebutol has been used to treat hypertension, ventricular and atrial cardiac arrhythmias, acute myocardial infarction in high-risk patients, and Smith-Magenis syndrome. The initial dose of acebutolol in hypertension usually is 400 mg/d; it may be given as a single dose, but two divided doses may be required for adequate control of blood pressure. Optimal responses usually occur with doses of 400–800 mg per day (range 200–1200 mg).

Bisoprolol

Bisoprolol is a highly selective β_1 receptor antagonist that lacks intrinsic sympathomimetic or membrane-stabilizing activity (McGavin and Keating, 2002). It has a higher degree of β_1-selective activity than atenolol, metoprolol, or betaxolol but less than nebivolol. It is approved for the treatment of hypertension.

Bisoprolol generally is well tolerated; side effects include dizziness, bradycardia, hypotension, and fatigue. Bisoprolol is well absorbed following oral administration, with bioavailability of about 90%. It is eliminated by renal excretion (50%) and liver metabolism to pharmacologically inactive metabolites (50%). Bisoprolol has a plasma $t_{1/2}$ of approximately 11–17 h. Bisoprolol can be considered a standard treatment option when selecting a β-blocker for use in combination with ACEIs and diuretics in patients with stable, moderate-to-severe chronic heart failure and in treating hypertension (McGavin and Keating, 2002; Simon et al., 2003). It has also been used to treat arrhythmias and ischemic heart disease. Bisoprolol was associated with a 34% mortality benefit in the CIBIS-II (Cardiac Insufficiency Bisoprolol Study-II).

Betaxolol

Betaxolol is a selective β_1 receptor antagonist with no partial agonist activity and slight membrane-stabilizing properties. Betaxolol is used to treat hypertension, angina pectoris, and glaucoma. The drug is well absorbed with high bioavailability; its elimination $t_{1/2}$ varies from 14 to 22 h. It is usually well tolerated; side effects are mild and transient.

β Adrenergic Receptor Antagonists With Additional Cardiovascular Effects ("Third-Generation" β-Blockers)

In addition to the classical nonselective and β_1 selective adrenergic receptor antagonists, there are drugs that possess vasodilating actions (Toda, 2003). These effects are produced through a variety of mechanisms, including the following:

- *α_1 adrenergic receptor blockade* (labetalol, carvedilol, bucindolol, bevantolol, nipradilol)
- *increased production of NO* (celiprolol, nebivolol, carteolol, bopindolol, nipradolol)
- *β_2 agonist properties* (celiprolol, carteolol, bopindolol)
- *Ca^{2+} entry blockade* (carvedilol, betaxolol, bevantolol)
- *opening of K^+ channels* (tilisolol)
- *antioxidant action* (carvedilol)

These actions are summarized in Table 12–4 and Figure 12–4. Some third-generation β receptor antagonists are not yet available in the U.S. but have undergone clinical trials and are available elsewhere.

Labetalol

Labetalol is representative of a class of drugs that act as competitive antagonists at both α_1 and β receptors. Labetalol has two optical centers, and the formulation used clinically contains equal amounts of the four diastereomers. The pharmacological properties of the drug are complex because each isomer displays different relative activities. The properties of the mixture include selective blockade of α_1 receptors (as compared with the α_2 subtype), blockade of β_1 and β_2 receptors, partial agonist activity at β_2 receptors, and inhibition of neuronal uptake of NE (cocaine-like effect) (Chapter 8). The potency of the mixture for β receptor blockade is 5- to 10-fold that for α_1 receptor blockade.

The pharmacological effects of labetalol have become clearer since the four isomers were separated and tested individually.

- *The R,R isomer* is about four times more potent as a β receptor antagonist than is racemic labetalol and accounts for much of the β blockade produced by the mixture of isomers. As an α_1 antagonist, this isomer is less than 20% as potent as the racemic mixture. The R,R isomer has some intrinsic sympathomimetic activity at β_2 adrenergic receptors; this may contribute to vasodilation.
- *The R,S isomer* is almost devoid of both α and β blocking effects.
- *The S,R isomer* has almost no β-blocking activity, yet is about five times more potent as an α_1 blocker than is racemic labetalol.
- *The S,S isomer* is devoid of β blocking activity and has a potency similar to that of racemic labetalol as an α_1 receptor antagonist.

The actions of labetalol on both α_1 and β receptors contribute to the fall in blood pressure observed in patients with hypertension. α_1 Receptor blockade leads to relaxation of arterial smooth muscle and vasodilation, particularly when the patient is upright. The β_1 blockade also contributes to a fall in blood pressure, in part by blocking reflex sympathetic stimulation of the heart. In addition, the intrinsic sympathomimetic activity of labetalol at β_2 receptors may contribute to vasodilation, and the drug may have some direct vasodilating capacity.

Labetalol is available in oral form for therapy of chronic hypertension and as an intravenous formulation for use in hypertensive emergencies. Labetalol has been associated with hepatic injury in a limited number of patients. Labetalol has been recommended as treatment of acute severe hypertension (hypertensive emergency). Its hypotensive action begins within 2–5 min after intravenous administration, reaching its peak at 5–15 min and lasting about 2–4 h. Heart rate is either maintained or slightly reduced, and cardiac output is maintained. Labetalol reduces systemic vascular resistance without reducing total peripheral blood flow. Cerebral, renal, and coronary blood flow is maintained. It can be used in the setting of pregnancy-induced hypertensive crisis because little placental transfer occurs due to the poor lipid solubility of labetalol.

ADME. Although labetalol is completely absorbed from the gut, there is extensive first-pass clearance; bioavailability is about 20%–40% but may be increased by food intake. The drug is rapidly metabolized in the liver; very little unchanged drug is found in the urine. The rate of metabolism of labetalol is sensitive to changes in hepatic blood flow. The elimination $t_{1/2}$ of the drug is about 8 h. The $t_{1/2}$ of the R,R isomer of labetalol is approximately 15 h.

Carvedilol

Carvedilol is a third-generation β receptor antagonist that has a unique pharmacological profile. *It blocks β_1, β_2, and α_1 receptors similarly to labetalol but also has antioxidant and anti-inflammatory properties* (Dandona et al., 2007). The antioxidant and anti-inflammatory properties may be beneficial in treating congestive heart failure. The drug has membrane-stabilizing activity but lacks intrinsic sympathomimetic activity.

Carvedilol reduces arterial blood pressure by decreasing vascular resistance and maintaining cardiac output while decreasing sympathetic vascular tone (DiNicolantonio et al., 2015; Zepeda et al., 2012). The hemodynamic effect exerted by carvedilol is similar to that of ACEIs and superior to that of traditional β blockers. Carvedilol is renoprotective and has favorable effects in patients with diabetes or metabolic syndrome. The drug is FDA-approved for use in hypertension, congestive heart failure, and left ventricular dysfunction following myocardial infarction.

Carvedilol possesses two distinct antioxidant properties: It is a chemical antioxidant that can bind to and scavenge ROS, and it can suppress the biosynthesis of ROS and oxygen radicals. Carvedilol is extremely lipophilic and protects cell membranes from lipid peroxidation. It prevents LDL oxidation, which in turn induces the uptake of LDL into the coronary vasculature. Carvedilol also inhibits ROS-mediated loss of myocardial contractility, stress-induced hypertrophy, apoptosis, and the accumulation and activation of neutrophils. *At high doses, carvedilol exerts Ca^{2+} channel-blocking activity.* Carvedilol does not increase β receptor density and does not show a high level of inverse agonist activity (Cheng et al., 2001; Dandona et al., 2007; Keating and Jarvis, 2003).

Carvedilol has been tested in numerous controlled trials (Cleland, 2003; Poole-Wilson et al., 2003). These trials showed that carvedilol improves ventricular function and reduces mortality and morbidity in patients with mild-to-severe congestive heart failure. Several experts recommend it as the standard treatment option in this setting. In addition, carvedilol combined with conventional therapy reduces mortality and attenuates myocardial infarction. In patients with chronic heart failure, carvedilol reduces cardiac sympathetic drive, but it is not clear if blockade of α_1 receptor–mediated vasodilation is maintained over long periods of time.

ADME. Carvedilol is rapidly absorbed following oral administration, with peak plasma concentrations occurring in 1–2 h. It is highly lipophilic and more than 95% protein bound. Hepatic CYPs 2D6 and 2C9 metabolized carvedilol, yielding a $t_{1/2}$ of 7–10 h. Stereoselective first-pass metabolism results in more rapid clearance of S(−)-carvedilol than R(+)-carvedilol. No significant changes in the pharmacokinetics of carvedilol are seen in elderly patients with hypertension, and no change in dosage is needed in patients with moderate-to-severe renal insufficiency (Cleland, 2003; Keating and Jarvis, 2003). Because of carvedilol's extensive oxidative metabolism by the liver, its pharmacokinetics can be profoundly affected by drugs that induce or inhibit oxidation. These include the inducer rifampin and inhibitors such as cimetidine, quinidine, fluoxetine, and paroxetine.

Bucindolol

Bucindolol is a third-generation *nonselective β adrenergic antagonist with weak α_1 adrenergic blocking properties.*

Bucindolol increases left ventricular systolic ejection fraction and decreases peripheral resistance, thereby reducing afterload. It increases plasma HDL cholesterol but does not affect plasma triglycerides. A large comprehensive clinical trial, the BEST (β Blocker Evaluation of Survival Trial), was terminated early because of a lack of a demonstrable survival benefit with bucindolol versus placebo. Further analysis has demonstrated that polymorphisms in β_1 and α_{2c} receptors predict the effect of bucindolol to prevent new-onset atrial fibrillation and ventricular arrhythmias (Cooper-DeHoff and Johnson, 2016; O'Connor et al., 2012).

Celiprolol

Celiprolol is a third-generation cardioselective β receptor antagonist. It has low lipid solubility and possesses weak vasodilating and bronchodilating effects attributed to *partial selective β_2-agonist* activity and possibly papaverine-like relaxant effects on smooth muscle (including bronchial). It also has been reported to *antagonize peripheral α_2 adrenergic receptor activity, to promote NO production, and to inhibit oxidative stress.* There is evidence for intrinsic sympathomimetic activity at the β_2 receptor. Celiprolol is devoid of membrane-stabilizing activity. Weak α_2 antagonistic properties are present but are not considered clinically significant at therapeutic doses (Toda, 2003).

Celiprolol reduces heart rate and blood pressure and can increase the functional refractory period of the AV node. Oral bioavailability ranges from 30% to 70%, and peak plasma levels are seen at 2–4 h. It is excreted largely unchanged in the urine and feces. The predominant mode of excretion is renal. Celiprolol is used for treatment of hypertension and angina (Witchitz et al., 2000).

Nebivolol

Nebivolol is a third-generation, long-acting, and highly selective β_1 adrenergic receptor antagonist that stimulates NO-mediated vasodilation via β_3 receptor agonism (Fongemia and Felix-Getzik, 2015). Nebivolol is devoid of intrinsic sympathomimetic effects as well as membrane-stabilizing activity and α_1 receptor blocking properties.

Therapeutic Uses. Nebivolol is approved for treatment of hypertension and has potential utility in the treatment of heart failure with reduced ejection traction. The drug lowers blood pressure by reducing peripheral vascular resistance and significantly increases stroke volume with preservation of cardiac output and maintains systemic flow and blood flow to target organs. Nebivolol also reduces oxidative stress and may have favorable effects on both carbohydrate and lipid metabolism. These benefits are also observed in the presence of metabolic syndrome, which often copresents with hypertension (Ignarro, 2008).

ADME. Nebivolol is administered as the racemate containing equal amounts of the *d*- and *l*-enantiomers. The *d*-isomer is the active β blocking component; the *l*-isomer is responsible for enhancing production of NO.

Nebivolol undergoes extensive first-pass metabolism, primarily by CYP2D6, yielding a mean terminal $t_{1/2}$ of about 10 h. Active metabolites (e.g., 4-OH nebivolol) contribute to the β-blocking effect of nebivolol. Polymorphisms in the CYP2D6 gene affect nebivolol's metabolism but not its efficacy due to the production of active hydroxylated metabolites (Lefebvre et al., 2007).

Nebivolol is lipophilic, and concomitant administration of chlorthalidone, hydrochlorothiazide, theophylline, or digoxin with nebivolol may reduce its extent of absorption. The NO-dependent vasodilating action of nebivolol and its high β_1 adrenergic receptor selectivity likely contribute to the drug's efficacy and comparative tolerability as an antihypertensive agent (e.g., less fatigue and sexual dysfunction) (Moen and Wagstaff, 2006).

TABLE 12–5 ■ SUMMARY OF ADRENERGIC AGONISTS AND ANTAGONISTS

SUB-CLASS	DRUGS	PROMINENT PRINCIPAL PHARMACOLOGICAL ACTIONS	THERAPEUTIC APPLICATIONS	UNTOWARD EFFECTS	COMMENTS
Direct-acting nonselective agonists					
	Epinephrine (α_1, α_2, β_1, β_2, β_3)	↑ Heart rate; ↑ blood pressure; ↑ contractility; slight ↓ in PVR; ↑ cardiac output; vasoconstriction (viscera); vasodilation (skeletal muscle); ↑ blood glucose and lactate	Open-angle glaucoma With local anesthetics to prolong action Anaphylactic shock Complete heart block or cardiac arrest Bronchodilator in asthma	Palpitation Cardiac arrhythmias Cerebral hemorrhage Headache Tremor Restlessness	Not given orally Life saving in anaphylaxis or cardiac arrest
	Norepinephrine (α_1, α_2, β_1 >> β_2)	↑ Systolic and diastolic blood pressure; vasoconstriction; ↑ PVR; direct ↑ in heart rate and contraction; reflex ↓ in heart rate	Hypotension	Similar to EPI Hypertension	Not absorbed orally
β Receptor agonists					
Nonselective ($\beta_1 + \beta_2$)	Isoproterenol	↓ PVR; ↑ cardiac output; bronchodilation	Bronchodilator in asthma Complete heart block or cardiac arrest Shock	Palpitations Tachycardia Tachyarrhythmias Headache Flushed skin Cardiac ischemia in patients with coronary artery disease	Intravenous administration Administered by inhalation in asthma
β_1 Selective	Dobutamine	↑ Contractility; some ↑ heart rate; ↑ AV conduction	Short-term treatment of cardiac decompensation after surgery or patients with congestive heart failure or myocardial infarction	↑ Blood pressure and heart rate	Intravenous only Use with caution in patients with hypertension or cardiac arrhythmias
β_2 Selective (intermediate acting)	Albuterol Bitolterol Fenoterol Isoetharine Levalbuterol Metaproterenol Pirbuterol Procaterol Terbutaline	Relaxation of bronchial smooth muscle Relaxation of uterine smooth muscle Activation of other β_2 receptors after systemic administration	Bronchodilators for treatment of asthma and COPD Short-/intermediate-acting drugs for acute bronchospasm	Skeletal muscle tremor Tachycardia and other cardiac effects seen after systemic administration (much less with inhalational use)	Use with caution in patients with cardiovascular disease (reduced by inhalational administration) Minimal side effects

(Continued)

TABLE 12–5 ■ SUMMARY OF ADRENERGIC AGONISTS AND ANTAGONISTS (CONTINUED)

SUB-CLASS	DRUGS	PROMINENT PRINCIPAL PHARMACOLOGICAL ACTIONS	THERAPEUTIC APPLICATIONS	UNTOWARD EFFECTS	COMMENTS
(Long acting)	Formoterol Salmeterol Arformoterol Carniterol Indacaterol Ritodrine	Relaxation of bronchial smooth muscle Relaxation of uterine smooth muscle	Bronchodilators for treatment of COPD Best choice for prophylaxis due to long action Ritodrine, to stop premature labor	Contraindicated in asthma	Long action, favored for prophylaxis
α Receptor agonists					
α₁ Selective	Methoxamine Phenylephrine Mephentermine Metaraminol Midodrine	Vasoconstriction	Nasal congestion (used topically) Postural hypotension	Hypertension Reflex bradycardia Dry mouth, sedation, rebound hypertension on abrupt withdrawal	Mephentermine and metaraminol also act indirectly to release NE Midodrine, a prodrug activated in vivo
α₂ Selective	Clonidine Apraclonidine Guanfacine Guanabenz Brimonidine α-Methyldopa	↓ Sympathetic outflow from brain to periphery resulting in ↓ PVR and blood pressure ↓ Nerve-evoked release of sympathetic transmitters ↓ Production of aqueous humor	Adjunctive therapy in shock Hypertension To reduce sympathetic response to withdrawal from narcotics, alcohol, and tobacco Glaucoma		Apraclonidine and brimonidine used topically for glaucoma and ocular hypertension Methyldopa is converted in CNS to α-methyl NE, an effective α₂ agonist
Indirect acting	Amphetamine Methamphetamine Methylphenidate (releases NE peripherally; NE, DA, 5HT centrally)	CNS stimulation ↑ Blood pressure Myocardial stimulation	Treatment of ADHD Narcolepsy Obesity (rarely)	Restlessness Tremor Insomnia Anxiety Tachycardia Hypertension Cardiac arrhythmias	Schedule II drugs Marked tolerance occurs Chronic use leads to dependence Can result in hemorrhagic stroke in patients with underlying disease Long-term use can cause paranoid schizophrenia
Mixed acting	Dopamine (α₁; α₂, β₁, D₁; releases NE)	Vasodilation (coronary, renal mesenteric beds) ↑ Glomerular filtration rate and natriuresis ↑ Heart rate and contractility ↑ Systolic blood pressure	Cardiogenic shock Congestive heart failure Treatment of acute renal failure	High doses lead to vasoconstriction Restlessness	Important for its ability to maintain renal blood flow Administered intravenously
	Ephedrine (α₁, α₂, β₁, β₂; releases NE)	Similar to epinephrine but longer lasting CNS stimulation	Bronchodilator for treatment of asthma Nasal congestion Treatment of hypotension and shock	Tremor Insomnia Anxiety Tachycardia Hypertension	Administered by all routes Not commonly used

α Blockers

Class	Drugs	Clinical applications	Pharmacologic effects	Adverse effects	Notes
Nonselective (classical α blockers)	PBZ, Phentolamine, Tolazoline	Treatment of catecholamine excess (e.g., pheochromocytoma)	↓ PVR and blood pressure; Venodilation	Postural hypotension; Failure of ejaculation	Cardiac stimulation due to initiation of reflexes and to enhanced release of NE via α_2 receptor blockade; PBZ produces long-lasting α receptor blockade, can block neuronal and extraneuronal uptake of amines
α_1 Selective	Prazosin, Terazosin, Doxazosin, Trimazosin, Alfuzosin, Tamsulosin, Silodosin	Primary hypertension; Increase urine flow in BPH	↓ PVR and blood pressure; Relax smooth muscles in neck of urinary bladder and in prostate	Postural hypotension when therapy instituted	Prazosin and related quinazolines are selective for α_1 receptors; Tamsulosin exhibits some selectivity for α_{1A} receptors

β Blockers

Class	Drugs	Clinical applications	Pharmacologic effects	Adverse effects	Notes
Nonselective (first generation)	Nadolol, Penbutolol, Pindolol, Propranolol, Timolol	Angina pectoris, Hypertension, Cardiac arrhythmias, Congestive heart failure, Pheochromocytoma, Glaucoma, Hypertrophic obstructive cardiomyopathy, Hyperthyroidism, Migraine prophylaxis, Acute panic symptoms, Substance abuse withdrawal, Variceal bleeding in portal hypertension	↓ Heart rate, ↓ Contractility, ↓ Cardiac output, Slow conduction in atria and AV node, ↑ Refractory period, AV node, Bronchoconstriction, Prolonged hypoglycemia, ↓ Plasma free fatty acids, ↓ HDL cholesterol, ↑ LDL cholesterol and triglycerides, Hypokalemia	Bradycardia, Negative inotropy, ↓ Cardiac output, Bradyarrhythmias, ↓ AV conduction, Bronchoconstriction, Fatigue, Sleep disturbances (insomnia, nightmares), Prolongation of hypoglycemia, Sexual dysfunction in men, Drug interactions	Effects depend on sympathoadrenal tone; Bronchoconstriction (do not use in asthma and COPD); Hypoglycemia (of concern in hypoglycemics and diabetics); Membrane-stabilizing effect (propranolol, and betaxolol); ISA (strong for pindolol; weak for penbutolol, carteolol, and betaxolol)
β_1 Selective (second generation)	Acebutolol, Atenolol, Bisoprolol, Betaxolol, Esmolol, Metoprolol	Similar to above	Similar to above but with less adverse effect on bronchial constriction	Similar to above	Effects depend on sympathoadrenal tone; Bronchoconstriction effect is less than for non-specific agents but use only with great caution in asthma and COPD
Nonselective (third-generation) vasodilators	Carteolol, Carvedilol, Bucindolol, Labetalol				Vasodilation seen in third-generation drugs; multiple mechanisms (see Figure 12–4); Weak ISA for labetalol
β_1 Selective (third-generation) vasodilators	Celiprolol, Nebivolol				Receptor polymorphisms affect response to bucindolol's anti-arrhythmic properties

See text. These agents affect multiple receptor types and signaling pathways. They are used to treat hypertension; carvedilol is also used to treat heart failure. Effects and applications generally resemble those of other β blockers with some α blocking properties:
- α_1 adrenergic receptor blockade (labetalol, carvedilol, bucindolol)
- increased production of NO (celiprolol, nebivolol, carteolol)
- β_2 agonist properties (celiprolol, carteolol)
- Ca^{2+} entry blockade (carvedilol)
- antioxidant action (carvedilol)

Bibliography

Abdelghany O. Arformoterol: the first nebulized long-acting beta$_2$-adrenergic agonist. *Formulary*, **2007**, *42*:99–109.

Altschuld RA, Billman GE. β$_2$-Adrenoceptors and ventricular fibrillation. *Pharmacol Ther*, **2000**, *88*:1–14.

Allwood MJ, et al. Peripheral vascular effects of noradrenaline, isopropylnoradrenaline, and dopamine. *Br Med Bull*, **1963**, *19*:132–136.

Arch JRS. Challenges in β$_3$-adrenoceptor agonist drug development. *Ther Adv Endocrinol Metab*, **2011**, *2*:59–64.

Beduschi MC, et al. α-Blockade therapy for benign prostatic hyperplasia: from a nonselective to a more selective α$_{1A}$-adrenergic antagonist. *Urology*, **1998**, *51*:861–872.

Berkowitz DE, et al. Distribution of beta 3-adrenoceptor mRNA in human tissues. *Eur J Pharmacol*, **1995**, *289*:223–228.

Black SW, et al. Challenges in the development of therapeutics for narcolepsy. *Prog Neurobiol*, **2015**, pii:S0301-0082(15)30023-X. doi:10.1016/j.pneurobio.2015.12.002.

Bosch J. Medical treatment of portal hypertension. *Digestion*, **1998**, *59*:547–555.

Breslow MJ, Ligier B. Hyperadrenergic states. *Crit Care Med*, **1991**, *19*:1566–1579.

Brodde OE, Michel MC. Adrenergic and muscarinic receptors in the human heart. *Pharmacol Rev*, **1999**, *51*:651–690.

Cheng J, et al. Carvedilol: molecular and cellular basis for its multifaceted therapeutic potential. *Cardiovasc Drug Rev*, **2001**, *19*:152–171.

Childress AC and Berry, SA. Pharmacotherapy of attention-deficit hyperactivity in adolescents. *Drugs*, **2012**, *72*:309–325.

Cleland JG. β-Blockers for heart failure: why, which, when, and where. *Med Clin North Am*, **2003**, *87*:339–371.

Cooper-DeHoff RM, Johnson JJ. Hypertension pharmacogenomics: in search of personalized treatment approaches. *Nat Rev Nephrol*, **2016**, *12*:110–122.

Cypess AM, et al. Activation of human brown adipose tissue by a β$_3$-adrenergic receptor agonist. *Cell Metab*, **2015**, *21*:33–38.

Dandona P, et al. Antioxidant activity of carvedilol in cardiovascular disease. *J Hypertension*, **2007**, *25*:731–741.

Deano R, Sorrentino M. Lipid effects of antihypertensive medications. *Curr Atheroscler Rep*, **2012**, *14*:70–77.

Delano FA, et al. Pancreatic digestive enzyme blockade in the intestine increases survival after experimental shock. *Sci Transl Med*, **2013**, *5*:169ra11.

DiBari M, et al. β-Blockers after acute myocardial infarction in elderly patients with diabetes mellitus: time to reassess. *Drugs Aging*, **2003**, *20*:13–22.

DiNicolantonio JJ, et al. β-Blockers in hypertension diabetes, heart failure and acute myocardial infarction. A review of the literature. *Open Heart*, **2015**, *2*:e000230.

Drazen JM, O'Byrne PM. Risks of long acting beta-agonists in achieving asthma control. *N Engl J Med*, **2009**, *360*:1671–1672.

Dunne F, et al. β-Blockers in the management of hypertension in patients with type 2 diabetes mellitus: is there a role? *Drugs*, **2001**, *61*:428–435.

Emorine LJ, et al. Molecular characterization of the human B$_3$ adrenergic receptor. *Science*, **1989**, *245*:1118–1121.

Fanta CH. Asthma. *N Engl J Med*, **2009**, *360*:1002–1014.

FDA. Full prescribing information, sodium oxybate. Revised **December 2012**. Available at: http://www.accessdata.fda.gov/drugsatfda_docs/label/2012/021196s013lbl.pdf. Accessed November 29, 2016.

Fitton A, Benfield P. Dopexamine hydrochloride. A review of its pharmacodynamic and pharmacokinetic properties and therapeutic potential in acute cardiac insufficiency. *Drugs*, **1990**, *39*:308–330.

Fleckenstein A. New insights into the mechanism of actions of amphetamines. *Annu Rev Pharmacol*, **2007**, *47*:691–698.

Fongemie J, Felix-Getzik E. A review of nebivolol pharmacology and clinical evidence. *Drugs*, **2015**, *75*:1349–1371. doi:1011007/s40265-015-0435-5.

Garnock-Jones KP. Esmolol. A review of its use in the short-term treatment of tachyarrhythmias and the short-term control of tachycardia and hypertension. *Drugs*, **2012**, *72*:109–132.

Goldsmith DR, Keating GM. Budesonide/fomoterol: a review of its use in asthma. *Drugs*, **2004**, *64*:1597–1618.

Hiratzka LF, et al. Guidelines for the diagnosis and management of patients with thoracic aortic disease. *Circulation*, **2010**, *121*:e266–e369. Available at: doi.org/10.1161/CIR.0b013e3181d4739e. Accessed June 26, 2017.

Ignarro LJ. Different pharmacological properties of two enantiomers in a unique β-blocker, nebivolol. *Cardiovasc Ther*, **2008**, *26*:115–134.

Ishii Y, et al. Drug interaction between cimetidine and timolol ophthalmic solution: effect on heart rate and intraocular pressure in healthy Japanese volunteers. *J Clin Pharmacol*, **2000**, *40*:193–199.

Keating GM. Droxidopa: a review of its use in symptomatic neurogenic orthostatic hypotension. *Adis Drug Evaluation*, **2014**, *10*:1007/S40265-019-0342. *Drugs*, **2015**, *75*:197–206.

Keating GM, Jarvis B. Carvedilol: a review of its use in chronic heart failure. *Drugs*, **2003**, *63*:1697–1741.

Kenny B, et al. Evaluation of the pharmacological selectivity profile of α$_1$ adrenoceptor antagonists at prostatic α$_1$ adrenoceptors: binding, functional and in vivo studies. *Br J Pharmacol*, **1996**, *118*:871–878.

Kyprianou N. Doxazosin and terazosin suppress prostate growth by inducing apoptosis. Clinical significance. *J Urol*, **2003**, *169*:1520–1525.

Lefebvre J, et al. The influence of CYP2D6 phenotype on the clinical response of nebivolol in patients with essential hypertension. *Br J Clin Pharmacol*, **2007**, *63*:575–582.

LePor H, et al. The efficacy of terazosin, finasteride, or both in benign prostatic hyperplasia. *N Eng J Med*, **1996**, *335*:533–539.

Lowry JA, Brown JT. Significance of the imidazoline receptors in toxicology. *J Clin Toxicol*, **2014**, *52*:454–469.

Man in't Veld AJ, et al. Do β blockers really increase peripheral vascular resistance? Review of the literature and new observations under basal conditions. *Am J Hypertens*, **1988**, *1*:91–96.

Marik PE, Iglesias J. Low-dose dopamine does not prevent acute renal failure in patients with septic shock and oliguria. NORASEPT II Study Investigators. *Am J Med*, **1999**, *107*:387–390.

Matera MG, Cazzola M. Ultra-long acting β$_2$-adrenoceptor agonist. An emerging therapeutic option for asthma and COPD. *Drugs*, **2007**, *67*:503–515.

May, DE, Kratochvil, CJ. Attention deficit hyperactivity disorder: recent advances in paediatric pharmacotherapy. *Drugs*, **2010**, *70*:15–40.

McClellan KJ, et al. Midodrine. A review of its therapeutic use in the management of orthostatic hypotension. *Drugs Aging*, **1998**, *12*:76–86.

McConnell JD, et al. The long-term effect of doxazosin, finasteride, and combination therapy on the clinical progression of benign prostatic hyperplasia. *N Engl J Med*, **2003**, *349*:2387–2398.

McGavin JK, Keating GM. Bisoprolol. A review of its use in chronic heart failure. *Drugs*, **2002**, *62*:2677–2696.

Michel MC. How β$_3$-adrenoceptor-selective is mirabegron? *Br J Pharmacol*, **2016**, *173*:429–430.

Michel MC, Vrydag W. α$_1$-, α$_2$- and β-Adrenoceptors in the urinary bladder urethra and prostate. *Br J Pharmacol*, **2006**, *147*:S88–S119.

Mimran A, Ducailar G. Systemic and regional haemodynamic profile of diuretics and α- and β-blockers. A review comparing acute and chronic effects. *Drugs*, **1988**, *35*(suppl 6):60–69.

Moen MD, Wagstaff AJ. Nebivolol: a review of its use in the management of hypertension and chronic heart failure. *Drugs*, **2006**, *66*:1389–1409.

Moniotte S, et al. Upregulation of β$_3$-adrenoceptors and altered contractile response to inotropic amines in human failing myocardium. *Circulation*, **2001**, *103*:1649–1655.

Morimoto A, et al. Endogenous β$_3$-adrenoceptor activation contributes to left ventricular and cardiomyocyte dysfunction in heart failure. *Am J Physiol Heart Circ Physiol*, **2004**, *286*:H2425–H2433.

Murphy MB, et al. Fenoldopam: a selective peripheral dopamine receptor agonist for the treatment of severe hypertension. *N Engl J Med*, **2001**, *345*:1548–1557.

Nikolic K, Agbaba D. Imidazoline antihypertensive drugs: selective I(1)-imidazoline receptors activation. *Cardiovasc Ther*, **2012**, *30*:209–216.

O'Connor CM, et al. Combinatorial pharmacogenetic interactions of bucindolol and β1, α2C adrenergic receptor polymorphisms. *PLoS One*, **2012**, *7*:e44324. Available at: doi.org/10.1371/journal.pone.0044324. Accessed June 27, 2017.

Poole-Wilson PA, et al. Comparison of carvedilol and metoprolol on clinical outcomes in patients with chronic heart failure in the Carvedilol

Or Metoprolol European Trial (COMET): randomised controlled trial. *Lancet*, **2003**, *362*:7–13.

Redington AE. Step one for asthma treatment: β_2-agonists or inhaled corticosteroids? *Drugs*, **2001**, *61*:1231–1238.

Ripley TL, Saseen JJ. β Blockers: a review of their pharmacological and physiological diversity. *Ann Pharmacother*, **2014**, *48*:723–733.

Salpeter SR, et al. Cardioselective beta-blockers for chronic obstructive pulmonary disease. *Cochrane Database Syst Rev*, **2005**, *(4)*:CD003566.

Schmid-Schoenbein G, Hugli T. A new hypothesis for microvascular inflammation in shock and multiorgan failure: self-digestion by pancreatic enzymes. *Microcirculation*, **2005**, *12*:71–82.

Simon T, et al. Bisoprolol dose-response relationship in patients with congestive heart failure: a subgroups analysis in the cardiac insufficiency bisoprolol study (CIBIS II). *Eur Heart J*, **2003**, *24*:552–559.

Sitte HH, Freissmuth M. Amphetamines, new psychoactive drugs, and the monoamine transporter cycle. *Trends Pharmacol Sci*, **2015**, *36*: 41–50.

Starke K, et al. Modulation of neurotransmitter release by presynaptic autoreceptors. *Physiol Rev*, **1989**, *69*:864–989.

Suissa S, Ernst P. Optical illusions from visual data analysis: example of the New Zealand asthma mortality epidemic. *J Clin Epidemiol*, **1997**, *50*:1079–1088.

Swanson JM, Volkow ND. Serum and brain concentrations of methylphenidate: implications for use and abuse. *Neurosci Biobehav Rev*, **2003**, *27*:615–621.

Tam SW, et al. Yohimbine: a clinical review. *Pharmacol Ther*, **2001**, *91*: 215–243.

Thompson PL. Should β-blockers still be routine after myocardial infarction? *Curr Opin Cardiol*, **2013**, *28*:399–404.

Toda N. Vasodilating β-adrenoceptor blockers as cardiovascular therapeutics. *Pharmacol Ther*, **2003**, *100*:215–234.

Varon J. Treatment of acute severe hypertension: current and newer agents. *Drugs*, **2008**, *68*:283–297.

Walle T, et al. Stereoselective delivery and actions of β receptor antagonists. *Biochem Pharmacol*, **1988**, *37*:115–124.

Witchitz S, et al. Treatment of heart failure with celiprolol, a cardioselective β blocker with β-2 agonist vasodilator properties. The CELICARD Group. *Am J Cardiol*, **2000**, *85*:1467–1471.

Wuttke H, et al. Increased frequency of cytochrome P450 2D6 poor metabolizers among patients with metoprolol-associated adverse effects. *Clin Pharmacol Ther*, **2002**, *72*:429–437.

Zependa RJ, et al. Carvedilol and nebivolol on oxidative stress-related parameters and endothelial function in patients with essential hypertension. *Basic Clin Pharmacol Toxicol*, **2012**, *111*:309–316.

Chapter 13

5-Hydroxytryptamine (Serotonin) and Dopamine

David R. Sibley, Lisa A. Hazelwood, and Susan G. Amara

Introduction

5-Hydroxytryptamine (5HT, serotonin) and DA are neurotransmitters in the CNS and also have prominent peripheral actions. 5HT is found in high concentrations in enterochromaffin cells throughout the GI tract, in storage granules in platelets, and throughout the CNS. The highest concentrations of DA are found in the brain; DA stores are also present peripherally in the adrenal medulla, in the plexuses of the GI, and in the enteric nervous system. Fourteen 5HT receptor subtypes and five DA receptor subtypes have been delineated by structural and pharmacological analyses. The identification of individual receptor subtypes has allowed for the development of subtype-selective drugs and the elucidation of actions of these neurotransmitters at a molecular level. Increasingly, therapeutic goals are being achieved by using drugs that selectively target one or more of the subtypes of 5HT or DA receptors, or that act on a combination of both 5HT and DA receptors.

5-Hydroxytryptamine

In the 1930s, Erspamer began to study the distribution of enterochromaffin cells, which were stained with a reagent for indoles. The highest concentrations of these cells were found in GI mucosa, followed by platelets and the CNS. Soon thereafter, Page and colleagues isolated and chemically characterized a vasoconstrictor substance released from platelets in clotting blood. This substance, named serotonin, was shown to be identical to the indole isolated by Erspamer. Subsequent discovery of the biosynthetic and degradative pathways for 5HT and clinical presentation of patients with carcinoid tumors of intestinal enterochromaffin cells spurred interest in 5HT. In the mid-1950s, the discovery that the pronounced behavioral effects of reserpine are accompanied by a profound decrease in brain 5HT led to the proposal that serotonin may function as a neurotransmitter in the mammalian CNS. Numerous synthetic or naturally occurring congeners of 5HT have pharmacological activity (see Figure 13–1 for chemical

structures). Many of the *N*- and *O*-methylated indoleamines, such as *N,N*-dimethyltryptamine, are hallucinogens. Another close relative of 5HT, melatonin (5-methoxy-*N*-acetyltryptamine), is formed by sequential *N*-acetylation and *O*-methylation (Figure 13–1). Melatonin, not to be confused with the pigment melanin, is the principal indoleamine in the pineal gland, where it serves a role in regulating circadian rhythms and shows promise in the treatment of jet lag and other sleep disturbances, such as insomnia. In that regard, melatonin could be thought of as a pigment of the imagination.

Synthesis and Metabolism of 5HT

Synthesis of 5HT is by a two-step pathway from the essential amino acid tryptophan (Figure 13–2). Tryptophan is actively transported into the brain by LAT1, a heteromeric carrier protein that also transports other large neutral and branched-chain amino acids and some drugs. Levels of tryptophan in the brain are influenced not only by its plasma concentration but also by the plasma concentrations of other amino acids that compete for the transporter. TPH, a mixed-function oxidase that requires molecular O_2 and a reduced pteridine cofactor for activity, is the rate-limiting enzyme in the synthetic pathway. TPH2, a brain-specific isoform of TPH, is entirely responsible for the synthesis of brain 5HT. Brain TPH is not generally saturated with substrate; consequently, the concentration of tryptophan in the brain influences the synthesis of 5HT.

L-5-hydroxytryptophan is converted to 5HT by AADC; AADC is widely distributed and has broad substrate specificity. The synthesized product, 5HT, is accumulated in secretory granules by VMAT2, which can be selectively inhibited by reserpine, thus depleting vesicular stores of monoamine transmitters. Based on its ability to deplete NE or DA, reserpine was once used an antihypertensive and antipsychotic agent. Stored vesicular 5HT is released by exocytosis from serotonergic neurons in response to an action potential. In the nervous system, the action of released 5HT is terminated via neuronal uptake by a specific SERT, localized in the membrane of serotonergic axon terminals and in the membranes of platelets.

Abbreviations

AADC: aromatic L-amino acid decarboxylase
AC: adenylyl cyclase
ACh: acetylcholine
ADD: attention-deficit disorder
ADHD: attention-deficit/hyperactivity disorder
ALDH: aldehyde dehydrogenase
BBB: blood-brain barrier
CNS: central nervous system
COMT: catechol-O-methyl transferase
CSF: cerebrospinal fluid
DA: dopamine
DAG: diacylglycerol
DAT: dopamine transporter
L-dopa: 3,4-dihydroxyphenylalanine
DOPAC: 3,4-dihydroxyphenylacetic acid
ENT: equilibrative nucleoside transporter
EPI: epinephrine
EPS: extrapyramidal symptoms
FDA: Food and Drug Administration
FSIAD: female sexual interest/arousal disorder
GABA: γ-aminobutyric acid
GI: gastrointestinal
GPCR: G protein–coupled receptor
GSK-3: glycogen synthase kinase 3
5-HIAA: 5-hydroxyindole acetic acid
HSDD: hypoactive sexual desire disorder
5HT: 5-hydroxytryptamine, serotonin
HVA: homovanillic acid
LAT1: L-type amino acid transporter 1
LSD: lysergic acid diethylamide
MAO: monoamine oxidase
MPP$^+$: 1-methyl-4-phenylpyridinium
MPTP: 1-methyl-4-phenyl-1,2,3,6-tetrahydropyridine
MSAA: multifunctional serotonin agonist and antagonist
NE: norepinephrine
NET: norepinephrine transporter
NMDA: N-methyl-D-aspartate
NO: nitric oxide
NSS: neurotransmitter–sodium symporter
OCT: organic cation transporter
6-OHDA: 6-hydroxydopamine
PCPA: para-chlorophenylalanine
PD: Parkinson disease
PFC: prefrontal cortex
PH: phenylalanine hydroxylase
PKC: protein kinase C
PL_: phospholipase _, as in PLC
RLS: restless leg syndrome
SERT: serotonin transporter
SNRI: serotonin-norepinephrine reuptake inhibitor
SSRI: selective serotonin reuptake inhibitor
TAAR1: trace amine-associated receptor 1
TCA: tricyclic antidepressant
TH: tyrosine hydroxylase
TPH: tryptophan hydroxylase
VMAT2: vesicular monoamine transporter
VNTR: variable number of tandem repeats

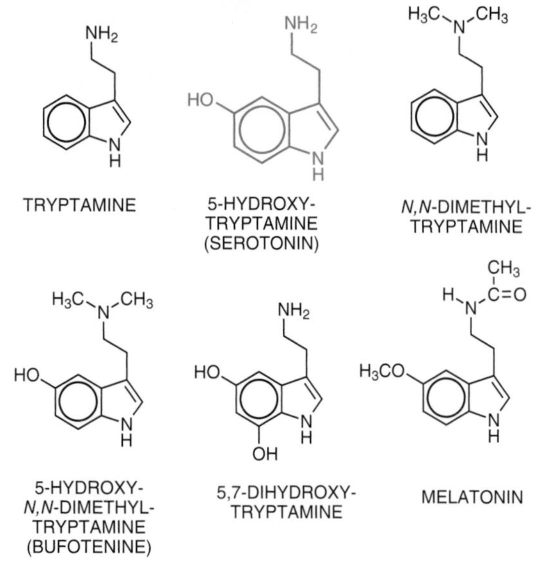

Figure 13–1 *Structures of representative indolealkylamines.*

a nonspecific amine carrier. SERT, the 5HT transporter or reuptake system is specific (see discussion that follows) and can be inhibited by SSRIs that are used to treat depression and other mood disorders.

The principal route of metabolism of 5HT involves oxidative deamination by MAO; the aldehyde intermediate thus formed is converted to 5-HIAA by aldehyde dehydrogenase (see Figure 13–2). An alternative route, reduction of the acetaldehyde to an alcohol, 5-hydroxytryptophol, is normally insignificant. 5-HIAA is actively transported out of the brain by a process that is sensitive to the nonspecific transport inhibitor probenecid. 5-HIAA from brain and peripheral sites of 5HT storage and metabolism is excreted in the urine along with small amounts of 5-hydroxytryptophol sulfate or glucuronide conjugates.

Of the two isoforms of MAO (see Chapter 8), MAO-A preferentially metabolizes 5HT and NE. Selective MAO-A inhibitors increase stores of 5HT and NE and are first-generation antidepressant agents (Chapter 15) MAO-B prefers β-phenylethylamine and benzylamine as substrates; low-dose selegiline is a relatively selective inhibitor of MAO-B. DA and tryptamine are metabolized equally well by both isoforms. Neurons contain both isoforms of MAO, localized primarily in the outer membrane of mitochondria. MAO-B is the principal isoform in platelets, which contain large amounts of 5HT.

Serotonergic Projection Pathways in the Brain

In the CNS, 5HT is almost entirely synthesized by cells located in the raphe nuclei in the brainstem. These neurons exhibit extensive projections throughout the brain and spinal cord. These projections are so extensive that it has been hypothesized that every neuron in the brain may be in synaptic contact with a serotonergic projection fiber (Figure 13–3).

A model of a serotonergic synapse is depicted in Figure 13–4. 5HT released from the nerve terminal activates cell-specific postsynaptic receptors, leading to signal transduction. Presynaptic 5HT receptors also exist on the nerve terminal where they can act to modulate 5HT release. Reuptake of 5HT by the 5HT transporter is the primary mechanism for termination of 5HT action and allows for either vesicular repackaging of transmitter or metabolism.

The 5HT Receptors

Multiple 5HT receptor subtypes mediate serotonin's diverse array of physiologic effects and comprise the largest known neurotransmitter-receptor family (Hoyer et al., 1994). The 5HT receptor subtypes are expressed in distinct but often overlapping patterns and are coupled to different transmembrane signaling mechanisms (Table 13–1). All of the 5HT receptor subtypes are GPCRs, with the exception of the 5HT$_3$ receptor, which is a ligand-gated ion channel (see Figures 3–11 and 11–1).

This uptake system is the means by which platelets acquire 5HT because they lack the enzymes required for 5HT synthesis. SERT is distinct from VMAT2, which concentrates amines in intracellular storage vesicles and is

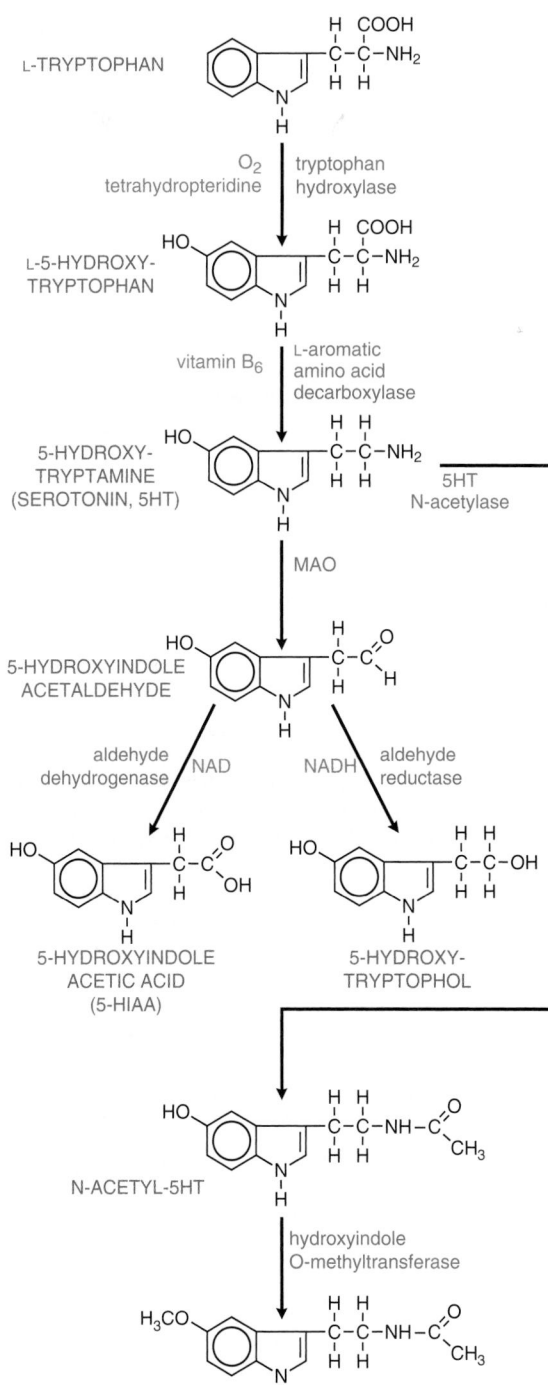

Figure 13–2 *Synthesis and inactivation of serotonin.* Enzymes are identified in red lettering, and cofactors are shown in *blue*.

The 5HT₁ Receptor Subfamily

- The 5HT$_1$ receptor family comprises five members, all of which preferentially couple to G$_{i/o}$ and inhibit adenylyl cyclase. 5HT$_1$ receptors are also known to modulate K$^+$ and Ca^{2+} channels.
- The 5HT$_{1A}$ and 5HT$_{1B/1D}$ receptors all act as autoreceptors, either on the cell bodies (5HT$_{1A}$) or on the axon terminals (5HT$_{1B/1D}$) (Figure 13–5). Antimigraine triptan drugs are 5HT$_{1B/1D}$ antagonists (see further discussion).
- In early literature, the 5HT$_{2C}$ receptor (see next section) was referred to as the 5HT$_{1C}$ receptor. To avoid confusion, the name 5HT$_{1C}$ is no longer in use (Hoyer et al., 1994).

- The 5HT$_{1D}$ receptors, abundantly expressed in the substantia nigra and basal ganglia, also regulate the firing rate of DA-containing cells and the release of DA at axonal terminals.
- The precise physiological roles of the 5HT$_{1E}$ and 5HT$_{1F}$ receptors are unclear at present.

The 5HT₂ Receptor Subfamily

- The three subtypes of 5HT$_2$ receptors couple to G$_q$/G$_{11}$ proteins and activate PLC-DAG/IP$_3$-Ca^{2+}-PKC pathways (Table 13–1). 5HT$_{2A}$ and 5HT$_{2C}$ receptors also activate phospholipase A$_2$, promoting the release of arachidonic acid.
- The 5HT$_{2A}$ receptors are broadly distributed in the CNS, primarily in serotonergic terminal areas. High densities are found in several brain structures, including prefrontal, parietal, and somatosensory cortex, as well as in blood platelets and smooth muscle cells. Many antipsychotic drugs inhibit 5HT$_{2A}$ receptors.
- The 5HT$_{2C}$ receptor is the only GPCR that is regulated by RNA editing. Multiple 5HT$_{2C}$ receptor isoforms are generated by RNA editing; extensively edited isoforms have modified G protein–coupling efficiencies (Burns et al., 1997). The 5HT$_{2C}$ receptor has been implicated in the control of CSF production and in feeding behavior and mood.

5HT₃ Receptors

- The 5HT$_3$ receptor is the only monoamine neurotransmitter receptor that functions as a ligand-gated ion channel.
- The functional 5HT$_3$ receptor forms pentameric complexes consisting of three distinct subunits; activation of these ligand-gated channels elicits a rapidly desensitizing depolarization, mediated by the gating of cations.
- The 5HT$_3$ receptors are located on parasympathetic terminals in the GI tract, including vagal and splanchnic afferents. In the CNS, a high density of 5HT$_3$ receptors occurs in the solitary tract nucleus and the area postrema. 5HT$_3$ receptors in both the GI tract and the CNS participate in the emetic response, providing a basis for the antiemetic property of the FDA-approved 5HT$_3$ receptor antagonists, including ondansetron and dolasetron.

5HT₄ Receptors

- The 5HT$_4$ receptor subtype couples to G$_s$ to activate AC and increase cAMP production.
- In the CNS, 5HT$_4$ receptors are found on neurons of the superior and inferior colliculi and in the hippocampus. In the GI tract, 5HT$_4$ receptors are located on neurons of the myenteric plexus and on smooth muscle and secretory cells. Stimulation of the 5HT$_4$ receptor is thought to evoke secretion and to facilitate the peristaltic reflex. The latter effect may explain the utility of prokinetic benzamides in GI disorders (see Chapter 50)
- Effects of pharmacological manipulation of 5HT$_4$ receptors on memory and feeding in animal models suggest possible clinical applications in the future.

5HT₅ Receptors

- The 5HT$_5$ subfamily couples to G$_{i/o}$ to inhibit AC.
- Humans only express a functional 5HT$_{5A}$ receptor, while rodents express both 5HT$_{5A}$ and 5HT$_{5B}$ receptors. The human 5HT$_{5B}$ gene is interrupted by a stop codon leading to a nonfunctional protein product.
- The 5HT$_{5A}$ receptor is expressed widely in the CNS, and its function is linked to circadian rhythms and cognition.

5HT₆ Receptors

- The 5HT$_6$ receptors couple to G$_s$ to activate AC and increase intracellular cAMP.
- The 5HT$_6$ receptor is almost exclusively found in the CNS; its abundance in cortical, limbic, and extrapyramidal regions suggests that it is important for motor control and cognition.
- Recent studies have focused on 5HT$_6$ receptor agonists as a therapeutic modality for cognitive decline in patients with Alzheimer disease.

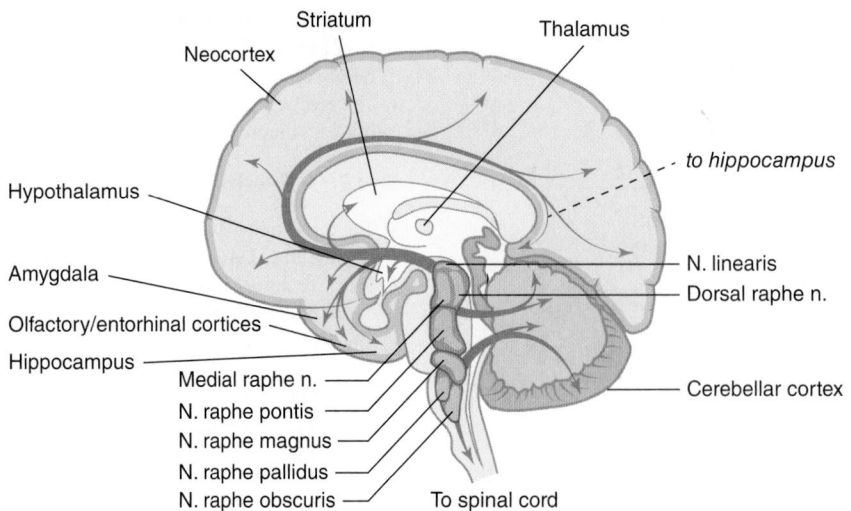

Figure 13–3 *Serotonergic pathways in the brain.* Serotonin is produced by several discrete brainstem nuclei, shown here in rostral and caudal clusters. The rostral nuclei, which include the nucleus, dorsal raphe, medial raphe, and raphe pontis, innervate most of the brain, including the cerebellum. The caudal nuclei, which comprise the raphe magnus, raphe pallidus, and raphe obscuris, have more limited projections that terminate in the cerebellum, brainstem, and spinal cord. Together, the rostral and caudal nuclei innervate most of the CNS. (Modified with permission from Nestler EJ et al., eds. *Molecular Neuropharmacology.* McGraw-Hill, New York, **2015**.)

5HT₇ Receptors

- The $5HT_7$ receptor couples to G_s to activate AC and increase intracellular cAMP. It is widely distributed throughout the CNS.
- Blockade of the $5HT_7$ receptor has recently been investigated as a putative therapeutic mechanism to treat depression. $5HT_7$ receptors may also play a role in the relaxation of smooth muscle in the GI tract and the vasculature.

The 5HT Transporter

- The actions of 5HT are primarily terminated by SERT, the transport protein responsible for the reuptake of 5HT into serotonergic neurons.
- Encoded by a single gene, SERT possesses 12 membrane-spanning domains and is a member of the NSS family that includes the carriers for DA, NE, GABA, and glycine. SERT is expressed prominently in central serotonin neurons that originate in the raphe nucleus, but is also found in platelets, placenta, lung, gut, enteric nervous system, and adrenal gland.
- SERT couples the transport of serotonin to the movement of Na^+ into the cell.
- SSRIs such as fluoxetine, paroxetine, citalopram, and sertraline bind to the SERT and inhibit serotonin transport. TCAs and a newer class of SNRIs that includes venlafaxine and duloxetine, block SERT, the NE transporter, or both with varying degrees of selectivity.
- SSRIs and SNRIs are prescribed for major depressive disorder, obsessive-compulsive disorder, panic disorder, generalized anxiety disorder, fibromyalgia and neuropathic pain.

Actions of 5HT in Physiological Systems

Platelets

Platelets differ from other formed elements of blood in expressing mechanisms for uptake, storage, and exocytotic release of 5HT. 5HT is not synthesized in platelets but is taken up from the circulation and stored in secretory granules by active transport, similar to the uptake and storage of serotonin by serotonergic nerve terminals. When platelets make contact with injured endothelium (see Chapter 32), they release substances that promote platelet aggregation; secondarily, they release 5HT (see Figure 13–6). 5HT binds to platelet $5HT_{2A}$ receptors and elicits a weak aggregation response that is markedly augmented by the presence of collagen. If the damaged blood vessel is injured to a depth where vascular smooth muscle is exposed, 5HT exerts a direct vasoconstrictor effect, thereby contributing to hemostasis, which is enhanced by locally released autocoids (thromboxane A_2 [TxA_2], kinins, and vasoactive peptides). Conversely, 5HT may interact with endothelial cells to stimulate production of NO and antagonize its own vasoconstrictor action, as well as the vasoconstriction produced by other locally released agents.

Cardiovascular System

The classical response of blood vessels to 5HT is contraction, particularly in the splanchnic, renal, pulmonary, and cerebral vasculatures. 5HT also induces a variety of responses in the heart that are the result of activation of multiple 5HT receptor subtypes, stimulation or inhibition of autonomic nerve activity, or dominance of reflex responses to 5HT. Thus, 5HT has positive inotropic and chronotropic actions on the heart that may be blunted by simultaneous stimulation of afferent nerves from baroreceptors and chemoreceptors. Activation of $5HT_3$ receptors on vagus nerve endings elicits the Bezold-Jarisch reflex, causing extreme bradycardia and hypotension. The local response of arterial blood vessels to 5HT also may be inhibitory, the result of the stimulation of endothelial NO production and prostaglandin synthesis and blockade of NE release from sympathetic nerves. Conversely, 5HT amplifies the local constrictor actions of NE, angII, and histamine, which reinforce the hemostatic response to 5HT.

Gastrointestinal Tract

Enterochromaffin cells in the gastric mucosa are the site of the synthesis and most of the storage of 5HT in the body and are the source of circulating 5HT. Motility of gastric and intestinal smooth muscle may be either enhanced or inhibited via signaling mediated by at least five subtypes of 5HT receptors (Table 13–2).

Mechanical stretching augments basal release of enteric 5HT, such as that caused by food and by efferent vagal stimulation. Released 5HT enters the portal vein and is metabolized by hepatic MAO-A. 5HT that survives hepatic oxidation may be captured by platelets or rapidly removed by the endothelium of lung capillaries and inactivated. 5HT released from enterochromaffin cells also acts locally to regulate GI function. $5HT_3$ receptors in the GI tract and the CNS participate in the emetic response, providing a basis for the antiemetic property of $5HT_3$ receptor antagonists (see Figure 50–5 and Table 50–6). A large series of selective $5HT_3$ receptor

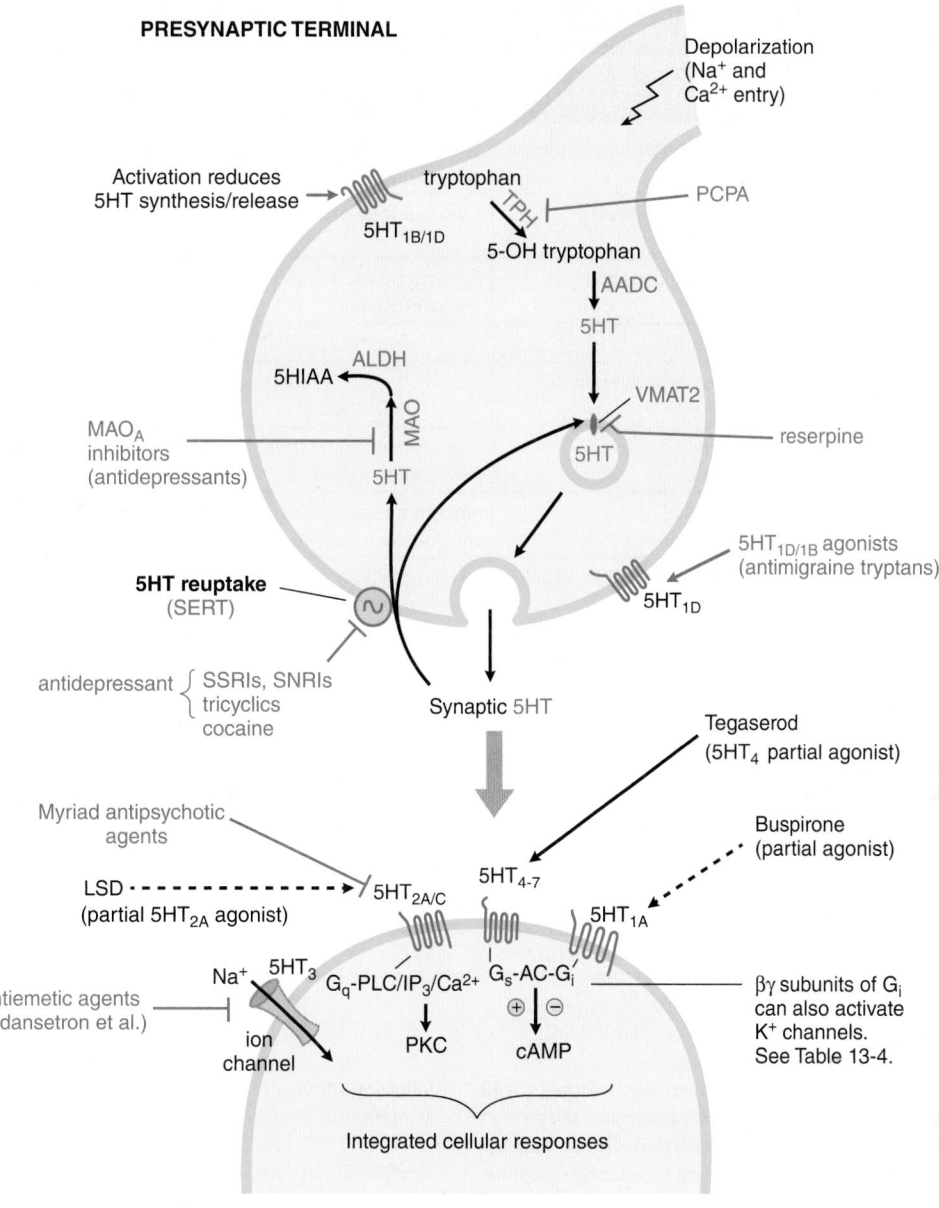

Figure 13–4 *A serotonergic synapse.* Presynaptic and postsynaptic molecular entities involved in the synthesis, release, signaling, and reuptake of serotonin are shown. MAO is shown extracellularly and in mitochondria within serotonergic nerve terminals.

antagonists, the "setrons," including ondansetron, dolasetron, granisetron, and palonosetron, are used in the treatment of various GI disturbances. All $5HT_3$ receptor antagonists are highly efficacious in the treatment of nausea, and alosetron and cilansetron are licensed for treating irritable bowel syndrome.

Inflammation

Acting via the $5HT_{2A}$ receptor, 5HT exerts a pro-inflammatory influence in acute inflammatory states, including models of airway inflammation and asthma (Nau et al., 2015). These preclinical findings agree with reports of higher expression of $5HT_{2A}$ receptors in peripheral blood mononuclear cells in patients with a history of asthma as compared to healthy volunteers (Ahangari et al., 2015). This research builds on several decades of analysis linking levels of plasma 5HT to incidents of asthma in human patients (Lechin et al., 2002). While this correlation between the $5HT_{2A}$ receptor and human inflammatory disease is still preliminary, the findings are compelling and merit additional investigation into the untapped role of 5HT and the $5HT_{2A}$ receptor in airway inflammation.

CNS

All 5HT receptor subtypes are expressed in the brain, where 5HT influences a multitude of functions, including sleep, cognition, sensory perception, motor activity, temperature regulation, nociception, mood, appetite, sexual behavior, and hormone secretion. The principal cell bodies of 5HT neurons are located in raphe nuclei of the brainstem and project throughout the brain and spinal cord (Figure 13–3). In addition to release at discrete synapses, serotonin release seems to occur at sites of axonal varicosities that do not form distinct synaptic contacts. 5HT released at nonsynaptic varicosities is thought to diffuse to outlying targets, rather than acting on discrete synaptic targets, perhaps acting as a neuromodulator as well as a neurotransmitter (see Chapter 14).

Sleep-Wake Cycle

Control of the sleep-wake cycle is one of the first behaviors in which a role for 5HT was identified. Depletion of 5HT with *p*-chlorophenylalanine, a tryptophan hydroxylase inhibitor, elicits insomnia that is reversed by

TABLE 13–1 ■ SEROTONIN RECEPTOR SUBTYPES[a]

SUBTYPE	SIGNALING EFFECTOR	LOCALIZATION	FUNCTION	AGONISTS	ANTAGONISTS
$5HT_{1A}$	↓ AC	Raphe nuclei, cortex, hippocampus	Somatodendritic autoreceptor	8-OH-DPAT, buspirone	WAY 100135
$5HT_{1B}$	↓ AC	Subiculum, globus pallidus, substantia nigra	Presynaptic autoreceptor	Sumatriptan, CP94253	GR-55562
$5HT_{1D}$	↓ AC	Cranial vessels, globus pallidus, substantia nigra	Presynaptic autoreceptor, vasoconstriction	Sumatriptan	SB 714786
$5HT_{1E}$	↓ AC	Cortex, striatum	—	—	—
$5HT_{1F}$	↓ AC	Dorsal raphe, hippocampus, periphery	—	LY334370	—
$5HT_{2A}$	↑ PLC, PLA_2	Platelets, smooth muscle, cerebral cortex	Aggregation, contraction, neuronal excitation	α-CH_3-5HT, DOI, MCPP	Ketanserin, LY53857
$5HT_{2B}$	↑ PLC	Stomach fundus	Smooth muscle contraction	α-CH_3-5HT, DOI	LY53857
$5HT_{2C}$	↑ PLC, PLA_2	Choroid plexus, substantia nigra, basal ganglia	CSF production, neuronal excitation	α-CH_3-5HT, DOI	LY53857, mesulergine
$5HT_3$	Cations	Parasympathetic nerves, solitary tract, area postrema, GI tract	Neuronal excitation	2-CH_3-5HT, quipazine	Ondansetron, tropisetron
$5HT_4$	↑ AC	Hippocampus, striatum, GI tract	Neuronal excitation	Renzapride	GR 113808
$5HT_{5A}$	↓ AC	Cortex, hippocampus	Unknown	—	SB-699551
$5HT_{5B}$	Unknown	—	Pseudogene in humans	—	—
$5HT_6$	↑ AC	Hippocampus, striatum, nucleus accumbens	Neuronal excitation	WAY-181187	SB-271046
$5HT_7$	↑ AC	Hypothalamus, hippocampus, GI tract	Smooth muscle relaxation	5-CT, LP-12	SB-269970

[a]For further information on the pharmacological properties of the 5HT subtypes, see IUPHAR/BPS Guide to Pharmacology: http://www.guidetopharmacology.org/index.jsp. Abbreviations: 5-CT, 5-carboxamino-tryptamine; DOI, 1-(2,5-dimethoxy-4-iodophenyl) isopropylamine; 8-OH-DPAT, 8-hydroxy-(2-N,N-dipropylamino)-tetraline; MCPP, metachlorphenylpiperazine; others are manufacturers' designations.

the 5HT precursor, 5-hydroxytryptophan. Conversely, treatment with L-tryptophan or with nonselective 5HT agonists accelerates sleep onset and prolongs total sleep time. 5HT antagonists reportedly can increase and decrease slow-wave sleep, probably reflecting interacting or opposing roles for subtypes of 5HT receptors. One relatively consistent finding in humans and in laboratory animals is an increase in slow-wave sleep

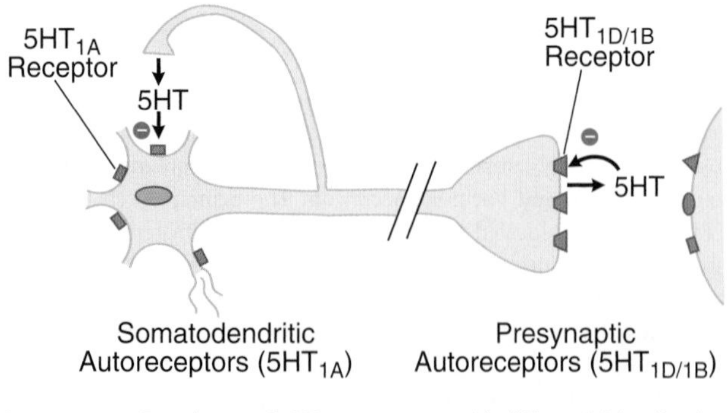

following administration of a selective $5HT_{2A/2C}$ receptor antagonist such as ritanserin.

Aggression and Impulsivity

Serotonin serves a critical role in aggression and impulsivity. Human studies reveal a correlation between low CSF 5-HIAA and violent impulsivity and aggression. Gene knockout mice lacking the $5HT_{1B}$ receptor exhibit extreme aggression, suggesting either a role for $5HT_{1B}$ receptors in the development of neuronal pathways important in aggression or a direct role in the mediation of aggressive behavior. A human genetic study identified a point mutation in the gene encoding MAO-A that was associated with extreme aggressiveness and mental retardation (Brunner et al., 1993); this has been confirmed in knockout mice lacking MAO-A (Cases et al., 1995).

Appetite and Obesity

Lorcaserin is a $5HT_{2C}$ receptor agonist approved for weight loss. The drug is thought to decrease food consumption and promote satiety by selectively activating $5HT_{2C}$ receptors on anorexigenic proopiomelanocortin neurons in the arcuate nucleus of the hypothalamus. Halogenated amphetamines, which are known to promote the release of 5HT and block its reuptake, are valuable experimental tools; two of them, fenfluramine and dexfenfluramine, were used clinically to reduce appetite; the once-popular diet drug regimen, "fen-phen," combined fenfluramine and phentermine. Fenfluramine and dexfenfluramine were withdrawn from the U.S. market in the late 1990s after reports of life-threatening heart valve disease and pulmonary hypertension associated with their use. This toxicity was the result of $5HT_{2B}$ receptor activation (Hutcheson et al., 2011).

Figure 13–5 *Two classes of 5HT autoreceptors with differential localizations.* Somatodendritic $5HT_{1A}$ autoreceptors decrease raphe cell firing when activated by 5HT released from axon collaterals of the same or adjacent neurons. The receptor subtype of the presynaptic autoreceptor on axon terminals in the forebrain has different pharmacological properties and has been classified as $5HT_{1D}$ (in humans) or $5HT_{1B}$ (in rodents). This receptor modulates the release of 5HT. Postsynaptic $5HT_1$ receptors are also indicated.

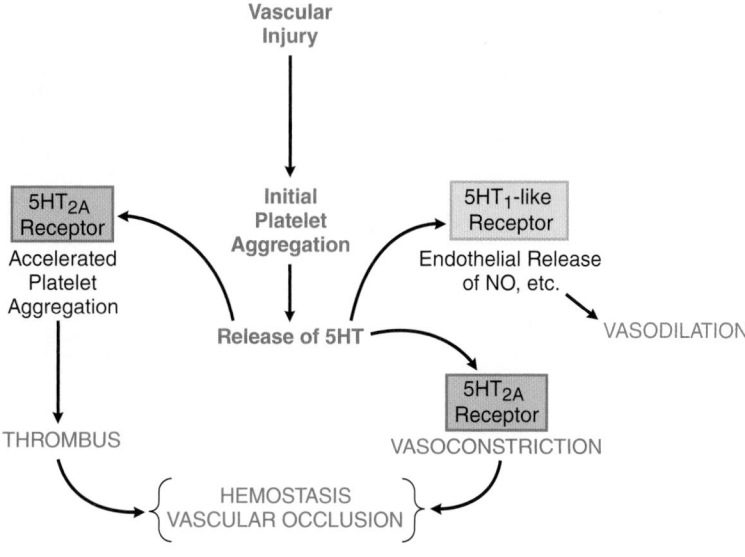

Figure 13–6 *The local influences of platelet 5HT.* The release of 5HT stored in platelets is triggered by aggregation. The local actions of 5HT include feedback actions on platelets (shape change and accelerated aggregation) mediated by interaction with platelet 5HT$_{2A}$ receptors, stimulation of NO production mediated by 5HT$_1$-like receptors on vascular endothelium, and contraction of vascular smooth muscle mediated by 5HT$_{2A}$ receptors. These influences act in concert with many other mediators to promote thrombus formation and hemostasis. See Chapter 32 for details of adhesion and aggregation of platelets and factors contributing to thrombus formation and blood clotting.

Drugs Affecting 5HT Signaling

Direct-acting 5HT receptor agonists have widely different chemical structures and diverse pharmacological properties and are used in the pharmacotherapy of a number of disorders (Table 13–3), including anxiety, depression, nausea, disorders of GI motility, and migraine. 5HT is a key mediator in the pathogenesis of migraine. Consistent with the 5HT hypothesis of migraine, 5HT receptor agonists are a mainstay for acute treatment of migraine headaches. The efficacy of antimigraine drugs varies with the absence or presence of aura, duration of the headache, its severity and intensity, and as yet undefined environmental and genetic factors.

TABLE 13–2 ■ ACTIONS OF 5HT IN THE GASTROINTESTINAL TRACT

SITE	RESPONSE	RECEPTOR
Enterochromaffin cells	Release of 5HT	5HT$_3$
	Inhibition of 5HT release	5HT$_4$
Enteric ganglion cells (presynaptic)	Release of ACh	5HT$_4$
	Inhibition of ACh release	5HT$_{1P}$[a] 5HT$_{1A}$
Enteric ganglion cells (postsynaptic)	Fast depolarization	5HT$_3$
	Slow depolarization	5HT$_{1P}$[a]
Smooth muscle, intestinal	Contraction	5HT$_{2A}$
Smooth muscle, stomach fundus	Contraction	5HT$_{2B}$
Smooth muscle, esophagus	Contraction	5HT$_4$

[a]5HT$_{1P}$ is an operationally defined serotoninergic response in the gut that does not correspond to any known monoamine receptor subtype. 5HT and certain 5HT derivatives are potent and selective agonists. The 5HT$_{1P}$ response may be due to receptor heteromerization resulting in a novel pharmacology.

5HT$_{1B/1D}$ Receptor Agonists: The Triptans

The triptans are indole derivatives that are effective, acute antimigraine agents. Their capacity to decrease the nausea and vomiting of migraine is an important advance in the treatment of the condition. Available compounds include almotriptan, eletriptan, frovatriptan, naratriptan, rizatriptan, sumatriptan, and zolmitriptan. Sumatriptan for migraine headaches is also marketed in a fixed-dose combination with naproxen. The triptans are effective in the acute treatment of migraine (with or without aura) but are not intended for use in prophylaxis of migraine. Treatment with triptans should begin as soon as possible after onset of a migraine attack. Oral dosage forms of the triptans are the most convenient to use, but they may not be practical in patients experiencing migraine-associated nausea and vomiting.

Sumatriptan

Serotonin

Migraine

Migraine headache afflicts 10%–20% of the population. Although migraine is a specific neurological syndrome, the manifestations vary widely. The principal types are migraine without aura (common migraine); migraine with aura (classic migraine, which includes subclasses of migraine with typical aura, migraine with prolonged aura, migraine aura without headache, and migraine with acute-onset aura), and several rarer types. Premonitory aura may begin as long as 24 h before the onset of pain and often is accompanied by photophobia, hyperacusis, polyuria, and diarrhea and by disturbances of mood and appetite. A migraine attack may last for hours or days and be followed by prolonged pain-free

TABLE 13–3 ■ SEROTONERGIC DRUGS: PRIMARY ACTIONS AND CLINICAL INDICATIONS

RECEPTOR	ACTION	DRUG EXAMPLES	CLINICAL DISORDER
$5HT_{1A}$	Partial agonist	Buspirone, ipsaperone	Anxiety, depression
$5HT_{1D}$	Agonist	Sumatriptan	Migraine
$5HT_{2A/2C}$	Antagonist	Methysergide, risperidone, ketanserin	Migraine, depression, schizophrenia
$5HT_3$	Antagonist	Ondansetron	Chemotherapy-induced emesis
$5HT_4$	Agonist	Cisapride	GI disorders
SERT (5HT transporter)	Inhibitor	Fluoxetine, sertraline	Depression, obsessive-compulsive disorder, panic disorder, social phobia, posttraumatic stress disorder

intervals. The frequency of migraine attacks is extremely variable. Therapy of migraine headaches is complicated by the variable responses among and within individual patients and by the lack of a firm understanding of the pathophysiology of the syndrome. The efficacy of antimigraine drugs varies with the absence or presence of aura, duration of the headache, its severity and intensity, and possibly undefined environmental and genetic factors.

The pathogenesis of migraine headache is complex, involving both neural and vascular elements. Evidence suggesting that 5HT is a key mediator in the pathogenesis of migraine includes the following:

- Plasma and platelet concentrations of 5HT vary with the different phases of the migraine attack.
- Urinary concentrations of 5HT and its metabolites are elevated during most migraine attacks.
- Migraine may be precipitated by agents (e.g., reserpine and fenfluramine) that release 5HT from intracellular storage sites.

Consistent with the 5HT hypothesis, 5HT receptor agonists have become a mainstay for *acute* treatment of migraine headaches. Treatments for the *prevention* of migraines, such as β adrenergic antagonists and newer antiepileptic drugs, have mechanisms of action that are, presumably, unrelated to 5HT (Mehrotra et al., 2008).

Mechanism of Action

The pharmacological effects of the triptans appear to be limited to the $5HT_1$ family of receptors, providing evidence that this receptor subclass plays an important role in the acute relief of a migraine attack. The triptans interact potently with $5HT_{1B}$ and $5HT_{1D}$ receptors and have a low or no affinity for other subtypes of 5HT receptors or for α_1 and α_2 adrenergic, β adrenergic, dopaminergic, muscarinic cholinergic, and benzodiazepine receptors. Clinically effective doses of the triptans correlate well with their affinities for both $5HT_{1B}$ and $5HT_{1D}$ receptors, supporting the hypothesis that $5HT_{1B}$ and $5HT_{1D}$ receptors are the most likely receptors involved in the mechanism of action of acute antimigraine drugs.

The mechanism of the efficacy of $5HT_{1B/1D}$ agonists in migraine is not resolved. One hypothesis of migraine suggests that unknown events lead to the abnormal dilation of carotid arteriovenous anastomoses in the head and shunting of carotid arterial blood flow, producing cerebral ischemia and hypoxia perceived as migraine pain; activation of $5HT_{1B/1D}$ receptors may cause constriction of intracranial blood vessels, including arteriovenous anastomoses, closing the shunts and restoring blood flow to the brain. An alternative hypothesis proposes that both $5HT_{1B}$ and $5HT_{1D}$ receptors serve as presynaptic autoreceptors that block the release of neurotransmitter or pro-inflammatory neuropeptides at nerve terminals in the perivascular space, which could account for the efficacy of agonists at those receptors in the acute treatment of migraine.

ADME

When given subcutaneously, sumatriptan reaches its peak plasma concentration in about 12 min, and an autoinjector with 6 mg of sumatriptan is available. Following oral administration of a tablet, sumatriptan has a bioavailability of about 15% and reaches a peak plasma concentration within 1–2 h; oral disintegrating tablets take advantage of sublingual absorption and produce more rapid effects; a nasal spray formulation of sumatriptan has an onset of action of about 15 min. A sumatriptan-naproxen combination tablet is available. An iontophoretic transdermal sumatriptan patch was recently withdrawn from the market. The other, newer triptans (see Drug Facts table) have higher oral bioavailabilities, and reach C_{Pmax} values within 1–3 h after ingestion of a tablet. The agents differ in their affinities for the $5HT_{1B}$ and $5HT_{1D}$ receptors, their half-lives and metabolic routes (usually CYP3A4 or MAO-A), and their reliance on the kidney for excretion. These differences, detailed in the Drug Facts table at the end of this chapter, define the likely drug interactions and precautions with age and reduced hepatic and renal function.

Clinical Use

The triptans are effective in the acute treatment of migraine (with or without aura) but are not intended for prophylaxis of migraine. Treatment with triptans should begin as soon as possible after onset of a migraine attack. Oral dosage forms of the triptans are the most convenient to use but may not be practical in patients experiencing migraine-associated nausea and vomiting, for whom injectable and nasal spray formulations are useful. Approximately 70% of individuals report significant headache relief from a 6-mg subcutaneous dose of sumatriptan, a dose that may be repeated once within a 24-h period if the first dose does not relieve the headache. The recommended oral dose of sumatriptan is 25–100 mg, repeatable after 2 h up to a total dose of 200 mg over a 24-h period. When administered by nasal spray, from 5 to 20 mg of sumatriptan is recommended, repeatable after 2 h up to a maximum dose of 40 mg over a 24-h period. The other triptans have distinct dosing requirements as summarized on their FDA-approved package inserts. A recent meta-analysis concluded that eletriptan is the most likely triptan to produce a favorable outcome at the 2-h and 24-h times after administration (Thorlund et al., 2014). The safety of treating more than three or four headaches over a 30-day period with triptans has not been established. No triptan should be used concurrently with (or within 24 h of) an ergot derivative (described in the next section) or another triptan.

Adverse Effects and Contraindications

In general, only minor side effects are seen with the triptans in the acute treatment of migraine. After subcutaneous injection of sumatriptan, patients often experience irritation at the site of injection (transient mild pain, stinging, or burning sensations). The most common side effect of sumatriptan nasal spray is a bitter taste. Triptans can cause paresthesias; asthenia and fatigue; flushing; feelings of pressure, tightness, or pain in the chest, neck, and jaw; drowsiness; dizziness; nausea; and sweating. In the extreme, these agents can cause serotonin syndrome, a consequence of a generalized excess of 5HT at 5HT receptors, especially when used in combination with SSRIs, SNRIs, TCAs, and MAO inhibitors.

Rare but serious cardiac events have been associated with the administration of $5HT_1$ agonists, including coronary artery vasospasm, transient myocardial ischemia, atrial and ventricular arrhythmias, and myocardial infarction, predominantly in patients with risk factors for coronary artery disease. The triptans are contraindicated in patients with a history of ischemic or vasospastic coronary artery disease (including history of stroke or transient ischemic attacks), cerebrovascular or peripheral vascular disease, hemiplegic or basilar migraines, other significant cardiovascular diseases, or ischemic bowel diseases. Because triptans may cause an acute, usually small, increase in blood pressure, they also are contraindicated in patients with uncontrolled hypertension. Naratriptan is contraindicated in patients with severe renal or hepatic impairment; rizatriptan should be used with caution in such patients. Eletriptan is contraindicated in hepatic disease. Almotriptan, rizatriptan, sumatriptan, and zolmitriptan are contraindicated in patients who have taken a MAO inhibitor within the preceding 2 weeks, and all triptans are contraindicated in patients with near-term prior exposure to ergot alkaloids, other triptans or 5HT agonists, SSRIs, and SNRIs. The triptans are classified as *pregnancy category C* (i.e., there are no adequate and well-controlled studies in pregnant women; use during pregnancy only if the potential benefit justifies a potential risk to the fetus) and should also be used with caution in nursing mothers; evidence of safety in pregnancy is best with sumatriptan. Källén and Reis (2016) have reviewed drugs for managing pain, including migraine, during pregnancy.

The Ergot Alkaloids

Ergot is the product of a fungus (*Claviceps purpurea*) that grows on rye and other grains. The elucidation of the constituents of ergot and their complex actions was an important chapter in the evolution of modern pharmacology, even though the very complexity of their actions limits their therapeutic uses. The pharmacological effects of the ergot alkaloids are varied and complex; in general, the effects result from their actions as partial agonists or antagonists at serotonergic, dopaminergic, and adrenergic receptors. All ergot alkaloids can all be considered to be derivatives of the tetracyclic compound 6-methylergoline (Table 13–4).

The natural alkaloids of therapeutic interest are amide derivatives of *d*-lysergic acid. Numerous semisynthetic derivatives of the ergot alkaloids have been prepared by catalytic hydrogenation of the natural alkaloids (e.g., dihydroergotamine). The synthetic derivative, bromocriptine (2-bromo-α-ergocryptine), is used to control the secretion of prolactin, a property derived from its DA agonist effect. Other products of this series include LSD, a potent hallucinogen, and methysergide, a serotonin antagonist. LSD interacts with most brain 5HT receptors as an agonist/partial agonist and elicits sensory distortions (especially visual) and hallucinations at doses as low as 1 µg/kg. Current hypotheses of the mechanism of action of LSD and other hallucinogens focus on $5HT_{2A}$ receptor-mediated disruption of thalamic gating with sensory overload of the cortex (Nichols, 2016). Of note, positron emission tomography imaging studies revealed that administration of the hallucinogen psilocybin (the active component of "'shrooms") mimics the pattern of brain activation found in schizophrenic patients experiencing hallucinations. This action of psilocybin is blocked by pretreatment with a $5HT_{2A/2C}$ antagonist. These and other studies have suggested that stimulation of the $5HT_{2A}$ receptor can lead to hallucinations (Nichols, 2016).

Ergots in the Treatment of Migraine

The multiple pharmacological effects of ergot alkaloids have complicated the determination of their precise mechanism of action in the acute treatment of migraine. The actions of ergot alkaloids at $5HT_{1B/1D}$ receptors

TABLE 13–4 ■ NATURAL AND SEMISYNTHETIC ERGOT ALKALOIDS

A. AMINE ALKALOIDS AND CONGENERS			B. AMINO ACID ALKALOIDS		

ALKALOID	X	Y	ALKALOID[b]	R(2')	R'(5')
d-Lysergic acid	—COOH	—H	Ergotamine	—CH₃	—CH₂—phenyl
d-Isolysergic acid	—H	—COOH	Ergosine	—CH₃	—CH₂CH(CH₃)₂
d-Lysergic acid diethylamide (LSD)	—C—N(CH₂CH₃)₂ (=O)	—H	Ergostine	—CH₂CH₃	—CH₂—phenyl
Ergonovine (ergometrine)	—C—NH—CHCH₂OH (=O) (CH₃)	—H	Ergotoxine group: Ergocornine	—CH(CH₃)₂	—CH(CH₃)₂
			Ergocristine	—CH(CH₃)₂	—CH₂—phenyl
Methylergonovine	—C—NH—CH (=O) (CH₂CH₃)(CH₂OH)	—H	α-Ergocryptine	—CH(CH₃)₂	—CH₂CH(CH₃)₂
			β-Ergocryptine	—CH(CH₃)₂	—CHCH₂CH₃ (CH₃)
Methysergide[a]	—C—NH—CH (=O) (CH₂CH₃)(CH₂OH)	—H	Bromocriptine[c]	—CH(CH₃)₂	—CH₂CH(CH₃)₂

[a]Contains methyl substitution at N1. [b]Dihydro derivatives contain hydrogen atoms at C9 and C10. [c]Contains bromine atom at C2.

likely mediate their *acute* antimigraine effects. The use of ergot alkaloids for migraine should be restricted to patients having frequent, moderate migraine or infrequent, severe migraine attacks. Ergot preparations should be administered as soon as possible after the onset of a headache. GI absorption of ergot alkaloids is erratic, perhaps contributing to the large variation in patient response to these drugs. Methysergide (1-methyl-*d*-lysergic acid butanolamide) is an ergot derivative but has very weak vasoconstrictor and oxytocic activity. It interacts with $5HT_1$ receptors, but its therapeutic effects appear primarily to reflect blockade of $5HT_{2A}$ and $5HT_{2C}$ receptors. Methysergide is used for the prophylactic treatment of migraine and other vascular headaches. A potentially serious complication of prolonged treatment is inflammatory fibrosis, giving rise to various syndromes that include pleuropulmonary fibrosis and coronary and endocardial fibrosis. Usually, the fibrosis regresses after drug withdrawal, although persistent cardiac valvular damage has been reported.

Use of Ergot Alkaloids in Postpartum Hemorrhage

All of the natural ergot alkaloids markedly increase the motor activity of the uterus; however, ergonovine and its semisynthetic derivative methylergonovine have primarily been used as uterine-stimulating agents in obstetrics. As the dose is increased, contractions become more forceful and prolonged, resting tone is dramatically increased, and sustained contracture can result. This characteristic is compatible with their use postpartum or after abortion to control bleeding and maintain uterine contraction. Oxytocin (see Chapter 44) is now the more prevalent agent in controlling postpartum hemorrhage.

Serotonin Receptor Partial Agonists, SSRIs, and MSAAs

Anxiolytic and Antidepressant Agents

Buspirone, gepirone, and ipsapirone are selective partial agonists at $5HT_{1A}$ receptors. Buspirone has been effective in the treatment of anxiety (see Chapter 15). Buspirone mimics the antianxiety properties of benzodiazepines but does not interact with $GABA_A$ receptors or display the sedative and anticonvulsant properties of benzodiazepines. The effects of 5HT–active drugs in anxiety and depressive disorders, like the effects of SSRIs, strongly suggest a role for 5HT in the neurochemical mediation of these disorders. Inhibition of neuronal reuptake of 5HT via the 5HT transporter prolongs the dwell time of 5HT in the synapse. SSRIs, such as fluoxetine, potentiate and prolong the action of 5HT released by neuronal activity. When coadministered with L-5-hydroxytryptophan, SSRIs elicit profound activation of serotonergic responses. However, the capacity to enhance serotonergic neurotransmission alone does not explain the antidepressant effectiveness: Uptake inhibition occurs immediately, whereas weeks of treatment are required to achieve clinical efficacy. This has led to the proposal that long-term homeostatic adaptations in brain function underlie the therapeutic effects of this class of antidepressants. SSRIs (citalopram, escitalopram, fluoxetine, fluvoxamine, paroxetine, and sertraline) are the most widely used treatment of major depressive disorder (see Chapter 15). Vilazadone is an SSRI and a partial agonist at the $5HT_{1A}$ receptor; it is FDA approved in adults for treatment of depression.

5HT and Sexual Dysfunction

One of the most common side effects of SSRIs and SNRIs is sexual dysfunction, such as anorgasmia, erectile dysfunction, diminished libido, and sexual anhedonia. Poor sexual function is one of the most common reasons that patients discontinue taking these medications. The mechanism by which SSRIs/SNRIs cause sexual side effects is not well understood. In contrast, the serotonergic drug flibanserin has recently been approved to treat hypoactive sexual desire disorder (HSDD) in premenopausal women. This disorder is also referred to as female sexual interest/arousal disorder (FSIAD). Flibanserin can increase the number of satisfying sexual events in some, but not all, women with this disorder. Flibanserin is a potent agonist of the $5HT_{1A}$ receptor and a moderately potent antagonist of the $5HT_2$ receptor subfamily; the drug is classified as a MSAA. Flibanserin is also a weak blocker of the D_4 DA receptor. Administration of flibanserin can decrease 5HT levels in the cortex while increasing DA and NE levels.

This redistribution of monoamine levels has been speculated to be the mechanism of the observed response of increased sexual function.

Clinical Manipulation of 5HT Levels: Serotonin Syndrome

Excessive elevation of 5HT levels in the body can cause *serotonin syndrome*, a constellation of symptoms sometimes observed in patients starting new or increased antidepressant therapy or combining an SSRI with an NE reuptake inhibitor or a triptan (for migraine). Symptoms may include restlessness, confusion, shivering, tachycardia, diarrhea, muscle twitches/rigidity, fever, seizures, loss of consciousness, and even death. Serotonin syndrome and its treatment are discussed in Chapter 15.

Dopamine

Dopamine consists of a catechol moiety linked to an ethyl amine, leading to its classification as a catecholamine (Figure 13–7). DA is a polar molecule that does not readily cross the BBB. It is closely related to melanin, a pigment that is formed by oxidation of DA, tyrosine, or L-dopa. Melanin exists in the skin and cuticle and gives the substantia nigra brain region its namesake dark color. Both DA and L-dopa are readily oxidized by nonenzymatic pathways to form cytotoxic reactive oxygen species and quinones. DA- and dopa-quinones form adducts with α-synuclein, a major constituent of Lewy bodies in PD (Chapter 22).

HISTORICAL PERSPECTIVE

Dopamine was first synthesized in 1910. Later that year, Henry Dale characterized the biological properties of DA in the periphery and described it as a weak, adrenaline-like substance. In the 1930s, DA was recognized as a transitional compound in the synthesis of NE and EPI but was believed to be little more than a biosynthetic intermediate. Not until the early 1950s were stores of DA identified in tissues, suggesting that DA had a signaling function of its own. Soon thereafter, Hornykiewicz discovered the DA deficit in Parkinsonian brains, fueling interest in the role of DA in neurological diseases and disorders (Hornykiewicz, 2002).

Synthesis and Metabolism

The biosynthesis and metabolism of DA are summarized in Figure 13–8. Phenylalanine and tyrosine are the precursors of DA. For the most part, mammals convert dietary phenylalanine to tyrosine by phenylalanine hydroxylase. Diminished levels of phenylalanine hydroxylase lead to high levels of phenylalanine, producing a condition known as phenylketonuria, which must be controlled by dietary restrictions to avoid intellectual impairment. Tyrosine crosses readily into the brain through uptake; normal brain levels of tyrosine are typically saturating. Conversion of tyrosine to L-dopa by the tyrosine hydroxylase is the rate-limiting step in the synthesis of DA (as in NE synthesis; see Chapter 8). Once generated, L-dopa is rapidly converted to DA by AADC, the same enzyme that generates 5HT from L-5-hydroxytryptophan. Unlike DA, L-dopa readily crosses the BBB and is converted to DA in the brain, which explains its utility in therapy for PD (see Chapter 18).

Metabolism of DA occurs primarily by MAO in both pre- and postsynaptic elements. MAO acts on DA to generate an inactive aldehyde derivative by oxidative deamination; the aldehyde is subsequently metabolized by

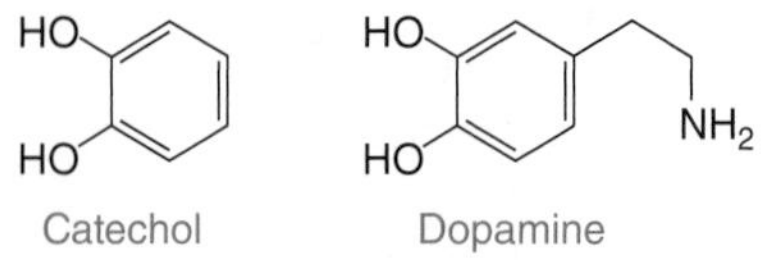

Figure 13–7 *The catechol nucleus of catecholamines.*

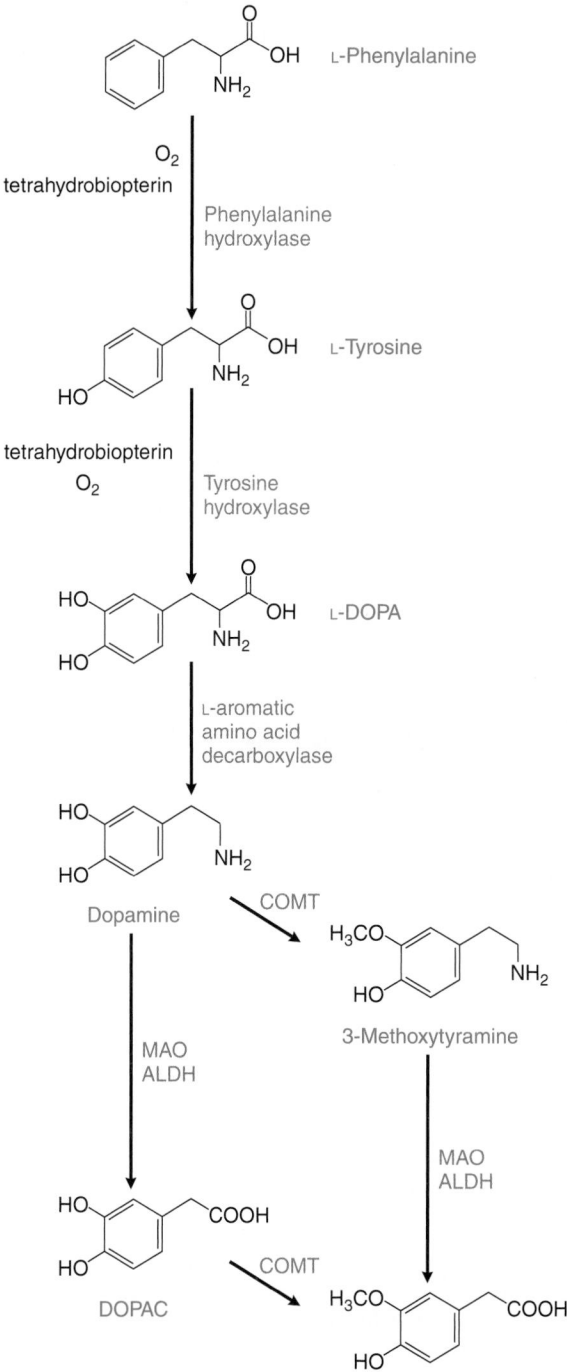

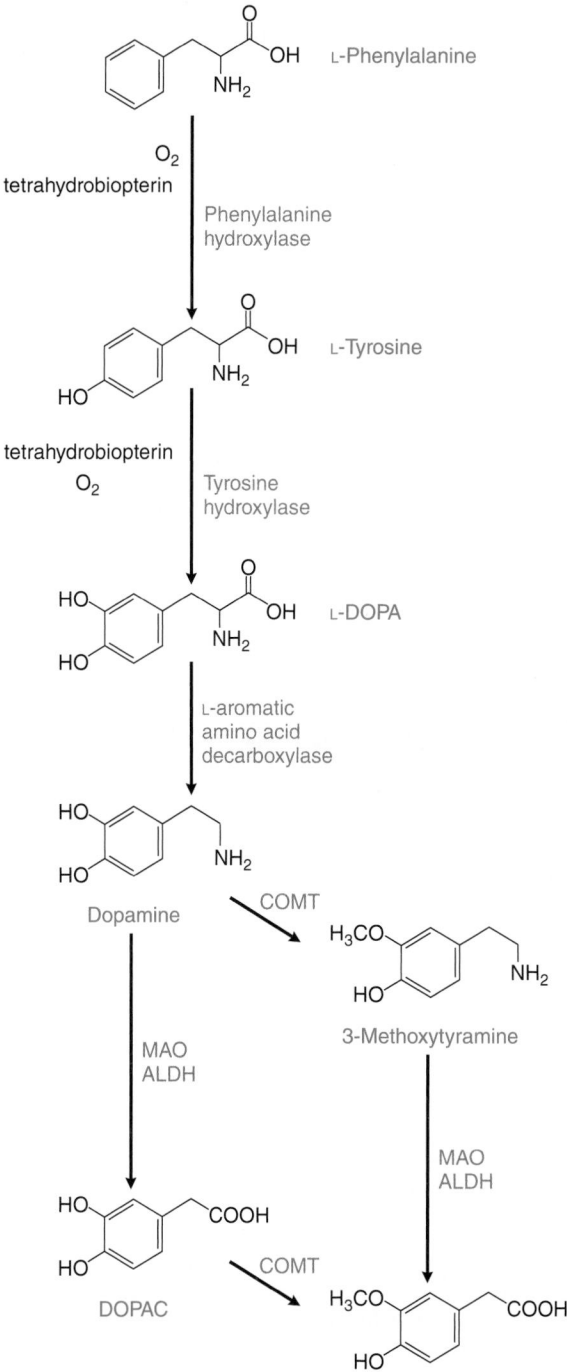

Figure 13–8 *Synthesis and inactivation of DA.* Enzymes are identified in blue lettering, and cofactors are shown in black letters.

aldehyde dehydrogenase to form DOPAC. DOPAC can be further metabolized by COMT to form HVA. In humans, HVA is the principal metabolite of DA. DOPAC, HVA, and DA are excreted in the urine, where they are readily measured. Levels of DOPAC and HVA are reliable indicators of DA turnover; ratios of these metabolites to DA in CSF serve as accurate representations of brain dopaminergic activity. In addition to metabolizing DOPAC, COMT acts on DA to generate 3-methoxytyramine, which is subsequently converted to HVA by MAO. MAO$_B$-selective inhibitors, such as selegiline and rasagiline, can increase DA levels and are currently used to treat PD (see Chapter 18). COMT in the periphery also metabolizes L-dopa to 3-*O*-methyldopa, which then competes with L-dopa for uptake into the CNS (see Figure 18–4). Consequently, L-dopa given in the

treatment of PD must be coadministered with peripheral COMT inhibitors, such as entacapone and tolcapone, to preserve L-dopa and allow sufficient entry into the CNS.

Figure 13–9 summarizes the neurochemical events that underlie DA neurotransmission. In dopaminergic neurons, synthesized DA is packaged into secretory vesicles by VMAT2. Drugs such as reserpine, which inhibit VMAT and deplete DA levels, were once used to treat psychosis. This packaging allows DA to be stored in readily releasable quanta and protects the transmitter from further anabolism or catabolism. By contrast, in adrenergic and noradrenergic cells, DA is not packaged; instead, it is converted to NE by DA β-hydroxylase and, in adrenergic cells, methylated to EPI in cells expressing phenylethanolamine *N*-methyltransferase (Chapter 8).

Synaptically released DA activates postsynaptic receptor subtypes, the expression of which is cell specific, leading to signal transduction via G protein–mediated pathways, although in some cases G protein–independent signaling is possible (see further discussion). DA receptor subtypes are also the targets of many therapeutically employed drugs and pharmacological tool compounds. Specific receptor subtypes of the D$_2$-like category can also be expressed on the presynaptic nerve terminal, where they regulate the release of DA. Reuptake of released DA by the DA transporter is the primary mechanism for termination of DA action and allows for either vesicular repackaging of transmitter or metabolism.

The DA transporter, DAT, localizes to dendrites, axons, and soma of mesencephalic DA neurons and is also found peripherally in the stomach, pancreas, and lymphocytes. Psychostimulants, such as cocaine, amphetamine, and methamphetamine, induce euphoria and hyperactivity by increasing extracellular DA. Cocaine potentiates DA signaling by acting as a nontransported antagonist of the plasma membrane DAT. However, the actions of amphetamines are more complex; amphetamines are competitive substrates for both the DATs and the VMATs. Amphetamines enter the cell through the DAT, where they displace DA from vesicular stores, causing an accumulation of DA within the neuronal cytoplasm. This resulting increase in cytosolic DA drives the release of DA by a nonvesicular mechanism that involves efflux through the DAT (Sitte et al., 2015). Newer studies also support the idea that amphetamines have additional targets within DA neurons that activate cellular signaling pathways, including G$_s$-dependent pathways coupled to increases in cAMP and G$_{12/13}$-dependent pathways coupled to the activation of the small GTPase, RhoA (Wheeler et al., 2015). The trace amine-associated receptor TAAR1, a predominantly intracellular GPCR, is activated by amphetamines, DA, and a variety of drugs and trace amines and has been proposed to mediate some of the intracellular actions of amphetamines (Miller, 2011).

The DA transporter can also serve as a molecular entryway for some neurotoxins, including 6-OHDA and MPP$^+$, the neurotoxic metabolite of MPTP. Following uptake into dopaminergic neurons, MPP$^+$ and 6-OHDA facilitate intra- and extracellular DA release and generate reactive oxygen species such as superoxide radicals (O$_2^-$) that cause neuronal death. This selective dopaminergic degeneration mimics PD and serves as an animal model for this disorder.

Dopamine Receptors

Early investigations found that DA increases cAMP levels in both the brain and retina, presumably by activating a DA-sensitive AC enzyme. Subsequent studies revealed the existence of DA receptors not linked to AC activation, suggesting multiple DA receptor subtypes. These were initially categorized as D$_1$ and D$_2$ receptors and could be distinguished on the basis of pharmacological properties and physiological function (Kebabian et al., 1979). Molecular biological studies have identified not only genes encoding the biochemically defined D$_1$ and D$_2$ receptor subtypes but also genes for additional DA receptors. We now recognize that there are five distinct DA receptors in mammals that are organized into two D$_1$-like and D$_2$-like subfamilies. The D$_1$-like subfamily consists of the D$_1$ and D$_5$ receptors; the D$_2$, D$_3$, and D$_4$ subtypes comprise the D$_2$-like subfamily. Receptors in the D$_1$-like subfamily (D$_1$ and D$_5$) couple to G$_s$ or G$_{olf}$ proteins to activate AC and increase cAMP levels; the D$_2$-like receptors (D$_2$, D$_3$, and D$_4$) couple to G$_i$ or G$_o$ proteins, which inhibit AC and diminish

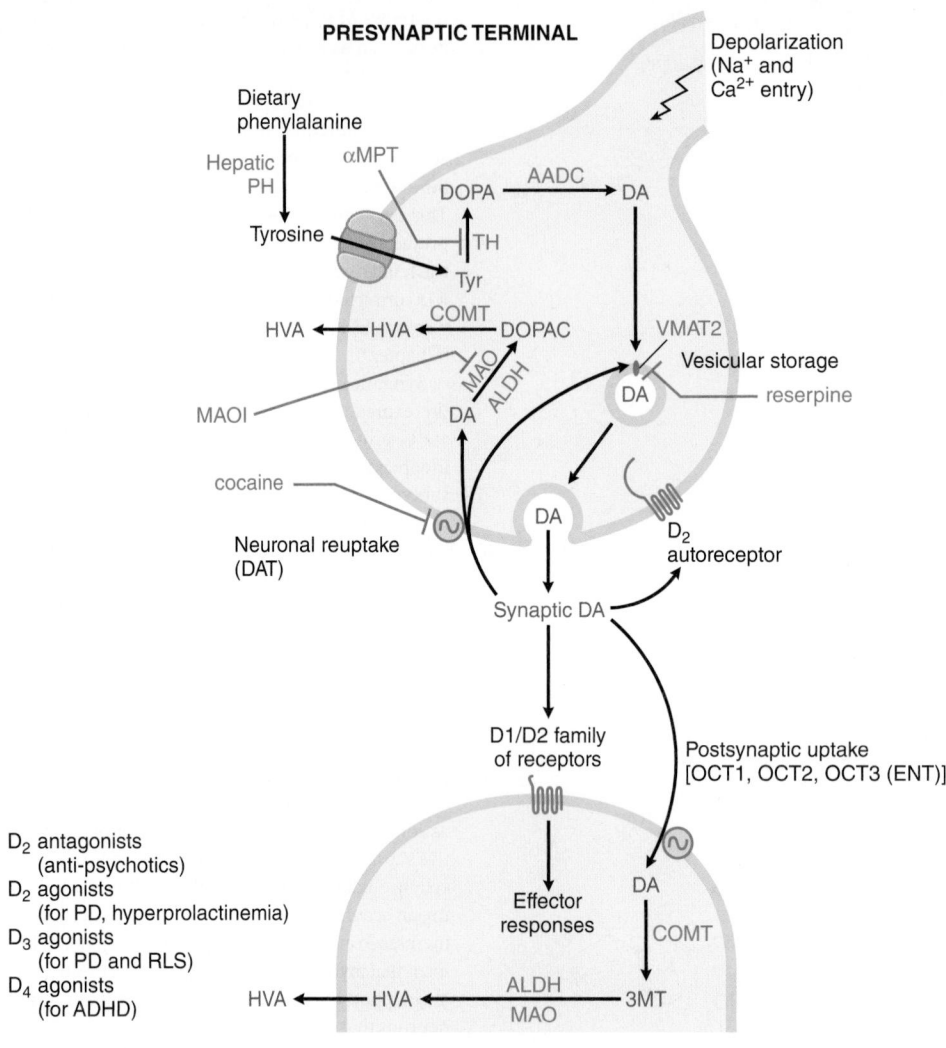

PRESYNAPTIC TERMINAL

POSTSYNAPTIC CELL

Figure 13–9 *A dopaminergic synapse.* Dopamine is synthesized from tyrosine in the nerve terminal by the sequential actions of TH and AADC. DA is sequestered by VMAT2 in storage granules and released by exocytosis. Synaptic DA activates presynaptic autoreceptors and postsynaptic D1 and D2 receptors. Synaptic DA may be taken up into the neuron via the DA transporter (DAT) or removed by postsynaptic uptake via OCT transporters. Cytosolic DA is subject to degradation by MAO/ALDH in the neuron, and by COMT in non-neuronal cells; the final metabolic product is HVA. See structures in Figure 13–8.

cyclic cAMP production. Activation of $G_{i/o}$ proteins can also directly modulate the activity of certain K^+ and Ca^{2+} channels (Figure 13–10). Signaling of D_2 receptors through β-arrestin–mediated pathways has also been postulated (see following discussion).

Pharmacological agents targeting DA receptors are used in the treatment of numerous neuropsychiatric disorders, including PD, schizophrenia, bipolar disorder, Huntington disease, ADHD, and Tourette syndrome. Like many GPCRs, DA receptors may form homo- and hetero-oligomers and also oligomerize with other GPCRs as well as ligand-gated ion channels (Fuxe et al., 2015). In most cases, the physiological significance of receptor oligomerization remains unclear. For recent in-depth reviews on DA receptor signaling, see the work of Beaulieu and Gainetdinov (2011) and Beaulieu et al. (2015).

The D₁ Receptor

- The D_1 receptor is the most highly expressed of the DA receptors; highest levels of D_1 receptor protein are found within the CNS, but it is also located in the kidney, retina, and cardiovascular system.
- The neostriatum expresses the highest levels of D_1 receptor in the CNS but does not express any detectable $G\alpha_s$. In this region, the D_1 receptor appears to couple to G_{olf} to increase levels of cAMP and its downstream effectors.

- The gene for the human D_1 receptor lacks introns.
- In addition to activating G proteins, the D_1 receptor can form hetero-oligomers with ionotropic NMDA glutamate receptors (Chapter 14) to modulate glutamatergic signaling.

The D₂ Receptor

- The D_2 receptor is the second most highly expressed DA receptor and consists of short (D_{2S}) and long (D_{2L}) isoforms that arise from alternative messenger RNA splicing. The D_{2S} isoform is missing 29 amino acids in the third intracellular loop that are present in the D_{2L} variant.
- The D_{2S} and D_{2L} receptors are pharmacologically identical; both couple to G_i or G_o to decrease cAMP production. The D_{2L} receptor is more prevalent and postulated to function postsynaptically. In contrast, the D_{2S} isoform functions as a putative presynaptic autoreceptor that regulates DA synthesis and release.
- The D_2 receptors can signal through $G_{\beta\gamma}$ subunits to regulate a variety of functions, including inwardly rectifying K^+ channels, N-type Ca^{2+} channels, and L-type Ca^{2+} channels.
- The D_2 receptor can signal through recruitment of the scaffolding protein, β-arrestin, thereby coupling to downstream signaling through the protein kinases PKB and GSK-3 (Beaulieu and Gainetdinov, 2011; Beaulieu et al., 2015).

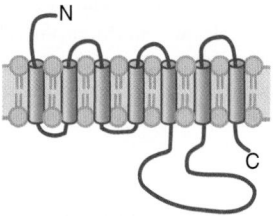

D1 receptor family

↑ cyclic AMP

D2 receptor family

↓ cyclic AMP
↑ K⁺ currents
↓ voltage-gated Ca²⁺ currents

Figure 13–10 *The two subfamilies of DA receptors and their major signaling pathways.*

The D$_3$ Receptor

- The D$_3$ receptor is less abundant than the D$_2$ receptor and is mainly expressed in the limbic regions of the brain. The highest levels of the D$_3$ receptor are found in the islands of Calleja, nucleus accumbens, substantia nigra pars compacta, and ventral tegmental area.
- The D$_3$ receptor signals through pertussis toxin–sensitive G$_{i/o}$ proteins, although not as effectively as the D$_2$ receptor.
- The D$_3$ receptor's tertiary structure has been determined by X-ray crystallography (Chien et al., 2010).

The D$_4$ Receptor

- The D$_4$ receptor is expressed in the retina, hypothalamus, PFC, amygdala, and hippocampus.
- The D$_4$ receptor is highly polymorphic, containing a VNTR encoding sequences within the third intracellular loop. In humans, the four-repeat variant is the most common. Association between a seven-repeat VNTR variant of the D$_4$ receptor and ADHD has been suggested.
- The D$_4$ receptor couples to G$_{i/o}$ to inhibit AC activity and depress intracellular cAMP levels.

The D$_5$ Receptor

- The D$_5$ receptor is most highly expressed in the hippocampus, but also is found in the substantia nigra, hypothalamus, striatum, cerebral cortex, nucleus accumbens, and olfactory tubercle.
- The D$_5$ receptor gene, like the D$_1$ receptor gene, is intronless.
- The D$_5$ receptor activates G$_s$ and G$_{olf}$ to increase cAMP production and can also modulate Na⁺ currents and N-, P-, and L-type Ca²⁺ currents via PKA-dependent pathways. The D$_5$ receptor can also directly interact with GABA$_A$ receptors to decrease Cl⁻ flux.

The Dopamine Transporter

- DAT (SLC6A3) clears extracellular DA released during neurotransmission and is a major target for both therapeutic and addictive psychostimulant drugs.
- Like SERT, the DAT is a member of the Neurotransmitter Sodium Symporter (NSS) family (see *Transporters and Pharmacodynamics: Drug Action in the Brain*, in Chapter 5), which couples neurotransmitter transport across the plasma membrane to the movement of Na⁺ ions into the cell.
- The DAT has 12 membrane-spanning domains; a recent high-resolution X-ray structure of a *Drosophila* DAT has been determined (Penmatsa et al., 2015).
- The DAT protein is abundantly expressed in mesostriatal, mesolimbic, and mesocortical DA pathways, where it can be found on cell bodies, dendrites, and axons of DA neurons (Ciliax et al., 1999).

However, the DAT is not readily detected within synapses, suggesting that rather than regulating synaptic neurotransmitter concentrations, it is poised to regulate spillover and diffusion of DA away from sites of release.

- The DAT is the therapeutic target of methylphenidate and amphetamine, the two major drugs used to treat attention-deficit disorders. The DAT inhibitor bupropion is used to treat depression and to support smoking cessation.

Actions of Dopamine in Physiological Systems

Heart and Vasculature

At low concentrations, circulating DA primarily stimulates vascular D$_1$ receptors (see discussion that follows), causing vasodilation and reducing cardiac load. The net result is a decrease in blood pressure and an increase in cardiac contractility. As circulating DA concentrations rise, DA is able to activate β adrenergic receptors to further increase cardiac contractility. At very high concentrations, circulating DA activates α adrenergic receptors in the vasculature, thereby causing vasoconstriction; thus, high concentrations of DA increase blood pressure. Clinically, DA administration is used to treat severe congestive heart failure, sepsis, or cardiogenic shock. It is only administered intravenously and is not considered a long-term treatment.

Kidney

Dopamine is a paracrine/autocrine transmitter in the kidney and binds to receptors of both the D$_1$ and D$_2$ subfamilies. Renal DA primarily serves to increase natriuresis, although it can also increase renal blood flow and glomerular filtration. Under basal sodium conditions, DA regulates Na⁺ excretion by inhibiting the activity of various Na⁺ transporters, including the apical Na⁺-H⁺ exchanger and the basolateral Na⁺,K⁺-ATPase. Activation of D$_1$ receptors increases renin secretion, whereas DA, acting on D$_3$ receptors, reduces renin secretion. Abnormalities in the DA system and its receptors have been implicated in human hypertension.

Pituitary Gland

Dopamine is the primary regulator of prolactin secretion from the pituitary gland. DA released from the hypothalamus into the hypophyseal portal blood supply acts on lactotroph D$_2$ receptors to decrease prolactin secretion (see Chapter 42). The ergot-based DA agonists bromocriptine and cabergoline are used in the treatment of hyperprolactinemia. Both have high affinity for D$_2$ receptors, with lower affinity for D$_1$, 5HT, and adrenergic receptors; both activate D$_2$ receptors in the pituitary to reduce prolactin secretion. The risk of valvular heart disease in ergot therapy is not associated with the lower doses used in treating hyperprolactinemia. The use of bromocriptine and cabergoline in the management of hyperprolactinemia is described in Chapter 42.

Catecholamine Release

Both D_1 and D_2 receptors modulate the release of NE and EPI. The D_2 receptor provides tonic inhibition of EPI release from chromaffin cells of the adrenal medulla and of NE release from sympathetic nerve terminals. In contrast, activation of the D_1 receptor promotes the release of catecholamines from the adrenal medulla.

CNS

There are three major groups of DA projections in the brain (Figure 13–11): mesocorticomesolimbic (originating in the ventral tegmental area), nigrostriatal (originating in the substantia nigra pars compacta), and tuberoinfundibular (originating in the hypothalamus). The physiological processes under dopaminergic control include reward, emotion, cognition, memory, and motor activity. Dysregulation of the dopaminergic system is critical in a number of disease states, including PD, Tourette syndrome, bipolar depression, schizophrenia, ADHD, and addiction/substance abuse.

The mesolimbic pathway is associated with reward and, less so, with learned behaviors. Dysfunction in this pathway is associated with addiction, schizophrenia, and psychoses (including bipolar depression) and learning deficits. The mesocortical projections are important for "higher-order" cognitive functions, including motivation, reward, emotion, and impulse control; they are also implicated in psychoses, including schizophrenia, and in ADHD. The nigrostriatal pathway is a key regulator of movement (see Chapter 18). Impairments in this pathway are involved in PD and underlie detrimental motor side effects associated with dopaminergic therapy, including tardive dyskinesia. As noted previously, DA released in the tuberoinfundibular pathway is carried by the hypophyseal blood supply to the pituitary, where it regulates prolactin secretion.

Dopaminergic neurons are strongly influenced by excitatory glutamate and inhibitory GABA input. In general, glutamate inputs enable burst-like firing of dopaminergic neurons, resulting in high concentrations of synaptic DA. GABA inhibition of DA neurons causes a tonic, basal level of DA release into the synapse. DA release also modulates GABA and glutamate neurons, thus providing an additional level of interaction between DA and other neurotransmitters.

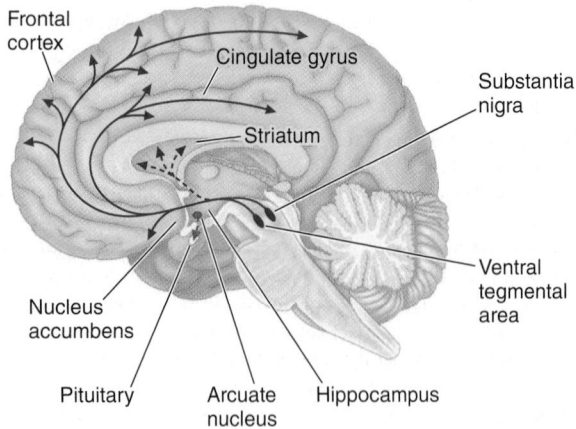

Figure 13–11   Major dopaminergic projections in the CNS.

- The nigrostriatal (or mesostriatal) pathway. Neurons in the substantia nigra compacta project to the dorsal striatum (*upward dashed blue arrows*); this is the pathway that degenerates in Parkinson disease.
- The mesocortico/mesolimbic pathway. Neurons in the ventral tegmental area project to the ventral striatum (nucleus accumbens), olfactory bulb, amygdala, hippocampus, orbital and medial prefrontal cortex, and cingulate gyrus (*solid blue arrows*).
- The tuberoinfundibular pathway. Neurons in the arcuate nucleus of the hypothalamus project by the tuberoinfundibular pathway in the hypothalamus, from which DA is delivered to the anterior pituitary (*red arrows*).

Motor Control and Parkinson Disease

In the early 1980s, several young people in California developed rapid-onset Parkinsonism. All of the affected individuals had injected a synthetic analogue of meperidine that was contaminated with MPTP. MPTP is metabolized by MAO-B to the neurotoxin MPP$^+$. Because of the high specificity of MPP$^+$ for the DA transporter, neuronal death is largely restricted to the substantia nigra and ventral tegmental area, resulting in a phenotype remarkably similar to PD. 6-OHDA is similar to MPTP in both mechanism of action and utility in animal models. Administration of MPTP or 6-OHDA to animals results in tremor, grossly diminished locomotor activity, and rigidity. As with PD, these motor deficits are alleviated with L-dopa therapy or dopaminergic agonists.

Other pharmacological agents that act on the DAT are known to potentiate locomotor activity via dopaminergic actions, including cocaine and amphetamine. The accumulation of extracellular DA increases stimulation of DA receptors and results in heightened locomotor activity. Mice lacking DAT are hyperactive and do not display increased locomotion in response to cocaine or amphetamine treatment.

Reward: Implications for Addiction

In general, drugs of abuse increase DA levels in the nucleus accumbens, an area critical for rewarded behaviors. This role for mesolimbic DA in addiction has led to numerous studies of abused drugs in DA receptor "knockout" mice in which the genes expressing specific receptors have been disrupted. Studies of D_1 receptor knockout mice showed a reduction in the rewarding properties of ethanol, suggesting that the rewarding and reinforcing properties of ethanol are dependent, at least in part, on the D_1 receptor. D_2 receptor knockout mice also display reduced preference for ethanol consumption. Morphine lacks rewarding properties in D_2 knockout mice when measured by conditioned place-preference or self-administration paradigms. However, mice lacking the D_2 receptor exhibit enhanced self-administration of high doses of cocaine. These data suggest a complex and drug-specific role for the D_2 receptor in rewarding and reinforcing behaviors. The D_3 receptor, highly expressed in the limbic system, has also been implicated in the rewarding properties of several drugs of abuse. However, D_3 knockout mice display drug-associated place preference similar to wild-type mice following amphetamine or morphine administration. Recently developed D_3 receptor-preferring ligands implicate a role for the D_3 receptor in motivation for drug seeking and in drug relapse, rather than in the direct reinforcing effects of the drugs (Heidbreder and Newman, 2010).

Cognition and Memory

Seminal work by Goldman-Rakic, Arnsten, and their colleagues (Vijayraghavan et al., 2007) showed that an optimum level of D_1 receptor activity in the PFC is required for optimum performance in learning and memory tasks. Either too little or too much D_1 receptor stimulation impairs PFC function in rats, monkeys, and humans. Thus, low doses of D_1 agonists improve working memory and attention, whereas high levels of DA release, such as during stress, impair PFC function. These observations have led to the "inverted U" hypothesis of the relationship between D_1 receptor stimulation and normal physiological functioning of the PFC (see Figure 4–2A). Interestingly, suboptimal levels of D_1 receptor stimulation have been suggested to underlie age-associated learning deficits and to contribute to the decreased cognition observed in various pathophysiological states, especially schizophrenia. Unsurprisingly, the D_1 receptor provides an attractive drug target for the treatment of a number of neuropsychiatric disorders.

Drugs Affecting Dopamine Signaling

Dopamine Receptor Agonists

Dopamine receptor agonists are mainly used in the treatment of PD, RLS, and hyperprolactinemia. One of the primary limitations to the therapeutic use of dopaminergic agonists is the lack of receptor subtype selectivity.

TABLE 13-5 ■ EXPERIMENTAL TOOLS AT DA RECEPTORS

RECEPTOR	AGONIST	ANTAGONIST
D_1-like[a]	SKF-81297 SKF-83959	SCH-23390 SCH-39166
D_2-like[b]	Quinpirole	Sulpiride
D_2	Sumanirole	L-741626 ML321
D_3	PD128907	SB-277011 SB-269652
D_4	PD168077	L-745870

[a]These compounds are selective for D_1-like versus D_2-like receptors. There are no useful tool compounds that can differentiate D_1 from D_5 receptors.
[b]These compounds are selective for D_2-like versus D_1-like receptors.

Recent advances in receptor-ligand structure-function relationships have enabled the development of drugs that can distinguish between D_1-like and D_2-like receptor subfamilies and, in some cases, show a preference for individual receptor subtypes. Many of these compounds have already proven to be useful experimental tools (Table 13–5), and this remains an active area of research.

Parkinson Disease
Dopamine does not cross the BBB; thus, the principal pharmacotherapy for PD is to administer the precursor to DA, L-dopa, which crosses the BBB and is converted to DA in the brain. Commonly, L-dopa is formulated with a decarboxylase inhibitor to prevent the peripheral conversion of L-dopa to DA, which can result in adverse side effects. While the response to L-dopa by patients with PD is usually quite favorable, longer-term treatment can result in a loss of effectiveness and the emergence of dyskinetic syndromes referred to as L-dopa–induced dyskinesias. These limitations to the therapeutic effects of L-dopa have generated interest in developing alternative therapies for PD, with the intent of either delaying the use of L-dopa or alleviating its side effects. DA receptor agonists can be used in conjunction with lower doses of L-dopa in a combined therapy approach or as monotherapy. Two general classes of dopaminergic agonists have been used in the treatment of PD: ergots and nonergots. The detailed use of these drugs in the management of PD is described in Chapter 18.

Ergot derivatives (see Table 13–4) act on several different neurotransmitter systems, including DA, 5HT, and adrenergic receptors. Bromocriptine and pergolide have been used for the treatment of PD; however, their use is associated with risk for serious cardiac complications, specifically, the promotion of valvular heart disease due to $5HT_{2B}$ serotonin receptor stimulation (Hutcheson et al., 2011). Bromocriptine is a potent D_2 receptor agonist and a weak D_1 antagonist. Pergolide is a partial agonist of D_1 receptors and a strong D_2 family agonist with high affinity for both D_2 and D_3 receptor subtypes. Ergot derivatives are commonly reported to cause unpleasant side effects, including nausea, dizziness, and hallucinations. Pergolide was removed from the U.S. market as therapy for PD after it was associated with an increased risk for valvular heart disease. Bromocriptine remains on the market primarily for the treatment of hyperprolactinemia or prolactin-secreting adenomas, where lower (D_2-selective) doses can be employed to avoid cardiac complications.

Several nonergot alkaloids are also employed in the management of PD. Apomorphine is a pan-DA receptor agonist most commonly used in the acute treatment of sudden "off" periods (bradykinesia, freezing) that can occur after long-term L-dopa treatment. Pramipexole and ropinirole are widely used in the treatment of PD, are agonists at all D_2-like receptors, but have the highest affinities for the D_3 receptor subtype. However, these agents are less effective than L-dopa in the early stages of PD treatment, and both are associated with the development of impulse control disorders, such as compulsive gambling or hypersexuality; notably, fewer drug-induced dyskinesias are observed.

The mechanisms underlying the impulse control disorders are currently unknown. Rotigotine is a DA agonist with preference for the D_2-like subfamily and is offered in a transdermal patch that is approved for the treatment of PD.

Hyperprolactinemia
Despite the contraindications for PD, ergot-based DA agonists are still used in the treatment of hyperprolactinemia. Like bromocriptine, cabergoline is a strong agonist at D_2 receptors and has lower affinity for D_1, 5HT, and α adrenergic receptors. The therapeutic utility of bromocriptine and cabergoline in hyperprolactinemia is derived from their properties as DA receptor agonists: They activate D_2 receptors in the pituitary to reduce prolactin secretion. The risk of valvular heart disease from ergot therapy is associated with higher doses of drug (necessary for PD treatment) but not with the lower doses used in treating hyperprolactinemia. The use of bromocriptine and cabergoline in the management of hyperprolactinemia is described in Chapter 42.

Restless Leg Syndrome
Restless leg syndrome is a neurological deficit characterized by abnormal sensations in the legs that are alleviated by movement. Decreased DA receptor expression and mild dopaminergic hypofunction are noted in patients with RLS. Rotigotine, ropinirole, and pramipexole are FDA-approved as pharmacotherapies for both PD and RLS.

Dopamine Receptor Antagonists

Just as enhancing DA neurotransmission can be clinically important, so can inhibiting dopaminergic signaling be useful in certain disease states. As with the DA receptor agonists, a lack of subtype-specific antagonists has limited the therapeutic utility of this group of ligands. Recent advances in elucidating GPCR structures and modeling ligand binding have advanced drug design, and subtype-selective antagonists are beginning to emerge as experimental tools (Table 13–5). Some receptor subtype-selective antagonists are in early stages of preclinical testing for therapeutic utility.

Schizophrenia
Dopamine receptor antagonists of the D_2-like subfamily are a mainstay in the pharmacotherapy of schizophrenia. While many neurotransmitter systems likely contribute to the complex pathology of schizophrenia (Chapter 16), modulating DA signaling is considered the basis of treatment. The DA hypothesis of schizophrenia has its origins in the characteristics of the drugs used to treat this disorder: All antipsychotic compounds used clinically have high affinity for DA receptors, especially with the D_2 receptor subtype. Moreover, psychostimulants that increase extracellular DA levels can induce or worsen psychotic symptoms in schizophrenic patients. The advent of neuroimaging techniques for visualization of DA in human brain regions has led to new insights in the role of specific DA systems. DA hyperfunction in subcortical regions, most notably the striatum, has been associated with the positive symptoms of schizophrenia, which respond well to antipsychotic treatment. In contrast, the PFC of schizophrenic patients exhibits dopaminergic hypofunction, which has been associated with the more treatment-refractory negative/cognitive symptoms. The drugs currently used to treat schizophrenia are classified as either typical (also referred to as first-generation) or atypical (second-generation) antipsychotics. This nomenclature stems from the fewer EPSs, or parkinsonian-like side effects, observed with atypical antipsychotics.

Typical Antipsychotics. The first antipsychotic drug used to treat schizophrenia was chlorpromazine. Its antipsychotic properties were attributed to its antagonism of DA receptors, especially the D_2 receptor. More D_2-selective ligands (e.g., haloperidol) were developed to improve the antipsychotic properties (see Chapter 16). Notably, drugs that are completely selective for the D_2 receptor subtype, without overlapping with affinity for the D_3 or D_4 receptor subtypes, are currently unavailable.

While all typical antipsychotics markedly improve positive symptoms (hallucinations, etc.), they are not very beneficial in the treatment of negative or cognitive symptoms of this disease.

CHLORPROMAZINE

ARIPIPRAZOLE

HALOPERIDOL

Atypical Antipsychotics. This class of antipsychotic drugs originated with clozapine and is distinguished by lower EPSs than typical antipsychotics. Atypical agents are also less likely to stimulate prolactin production. The lack of extrapyramidal side effects has been partly attributed to a much lower affinity for the D_2 receptor compared to typical antipsychotics. Most atypical antipsychotics are also high-affinity antagonists or inverse agonists at the $5HT_{2A}$ receptor. While the precise role of $5HT_{2A}$ receptor blockade in the atypical effects of antipsychotics remains unclear, dual DA–5HT receptor blockade has contributed to the development of antipsychotics for several decades (see Chapter 16).

Partial D_2-Like Receptor Agonists. Aripiprazole has even fewer side effects than earlier atypical antipsychotics. Aripiprazole diverges from the traditional atypical profile in several ways: First, it has higher affinity for D_2 receptors than for $5HT_{2A}$ receptors; second, it is a partial agonist at D_2 receptors. As a partial agonist, aripiprazole may diminish subcortical (striatal) DA hyperfunction by competing with DA for receptor binding, while simultaneously enhancing dopaminergic neurotransmission in the PFC by acting as an agonist. The dual mechanism afforded by a partial agonist may thus treat both the positive and negative symptoms associated with schizophrenia. Aripiprazole also exhibits functional selectivity at the D_2 receptor in that it exhibits higher efficacy for β-arrestin–mediated signaling than for G protein–mediated signaling. How this property may contribute to the unique effects of aripiprazole is not yet clear.

Recently, a derivative of aripiprazole, brexpiprazole, has been approved for the treatment of schizophrenia and as an adjunctive treatment of depression. The pharmacological properties of brexpiprazole are similar to those of aripiprazole except that brexpiprazole has lower D_2 receptor agonist efficacy and high partial agonist effects at the $5HT_{1A}$ receptor; perhaps this latter property underlies its effectiveness in treating depression.

Another partial agonist of the D_2 receptor, cariprazine, has recently been approved for treating schizophrenia and bipolar disorder. Interestingly, cariprazine is also a partial agonist at the D_3 receptor and actually exhibits higher affinity for the D_3 versus the D_2 receptor. In some studies, cariprazine has been shown to exhibit procognitive effects, suggesting that it may be useful for treating negative as well as positive symptoms of schizophrenia.

D_3 Receptor Antagonists and Drug Addiction

Although much work remains to determine their clinical utility, D_3-selective antagonists show promise in the treatment of addiction (Heidbreder and Newman, 2010; Newman et al., 2012). This interest stems from the high expression of the D_3 receptor in the limbic system, the reward center of the brain, and from animal studies of highly D_3-selective antagonists that suggest a role for the D_3 receptor in the motivation to abuse drugs and in the potential for drug-abuse relapse.

Acknowledgment: *Elaine Sanders-Bush and Steven E. Mayer contributed to this chapter in recent editions of this book. We have retained some of their text in the current edition.*

Drug Facts for Your Personal Formulary: *Serotonergic Ligands*

Drugs	Therapeutic Uses	Clinical Pharmacology and Tips
$5HT_3$ Receptor Antagonists · Antiemetic agents · Additional detail in Chapters 50 and 51		
Ondansetron Dolasetron Granisetron Palonosetron	• Antiemetics • Treatment of nausea	• Associated with asymptomatic electrocardiogram changes, including prolongation of PT and QTc intervals
Cilansetron Alosetron	• Antiemetics • Treatment of nausea • Irritable bowel syndrome	• Most useful in irritable bowel syndrome when diarrhea is the principal symptom
$5HT_{2C}$ Receptor Agonists · Weight loss		
Lorcarserin	• Promotes weight loss through decreased food consumption and increased satiety	• Hallucinogenic at supraclinical doses, likely caused by $5HT_{2A}$ agonist activity that can occur with higher doses • Hallucinogenic properties resulted in a class IV schedule designation
The Triptans: $5HT_{1B/1D}$ Receptor Agonists · Migraine		
Almotriptan[a] Eletriptan Frovatriptan Naratriptan Rizatriptan Sumatriptan[b] Zolmitriptan	• Acute treatment of migraine	• Most effective in acute settings; should be used as soon as possible after onset of attack • Usually dosed orally; onset, 1–3 h • Use with caution in patients with cardiovascular issues; contraindicated in patients with ischemic heart disease and coronary artery vasospasm • Drug interactions: CYP3A4 inhibitors ↑ C_p and $t_{1/2}$ of eletriptan, naratriptan; MAO inhibitors ↑levels of almo-, riza-, suma-, and zolmitriptan. • Side effects: dizziness, somnolence, neck and chest pain • May cause fetal harm; not recommended during pregnancy and nursing; reduce dose in renal and hepatic impairment; do not administer within 24 h of other triptans, ergots, SSRIs/SNRIs • Beware serotonin syndrome, especially in combination with SSRIs and SNRIs

The Ergot Alkaloids · Interact with multiple 5HT receptor isoforms · Broad therapeutic utility

LSD	• No longer employed clinically • Potent hallucinogen	• Positron emission tomographic imaging reveals similar activation patterns between schizophrenic patients experiencing hallucinations and LSD-induced hallucinations • $5HT_{2A}$ receptor activation is believed to mediate the hallucinogenic effect of LSD
Methysergide	• Acute treatment of migraine • Treatment of vascular headaches	• Restricted to use in patients with frequent, moderate, or infrequent, severe migraine attacks • Erratic drug absorption • Potential for inflammatory fibrosis with prolonged use, including pleuropulmonary and endocardial fibrosis
Ergonovine Methylergonovine	• Prevention of postpartum hemorrhage	• Increasing dose results in prolonged duration and increased force of uterine contraction • Sustained contracture can result at high doses

$5HT_{1A}$ Receptor Partial Agonists and SSRIs · Anxiolytics and antidepressants · Additional detail in Chapter 15

Buspirone	Treatment of anxiety	• Mimics antianxiety effects of benzodiazepines but does not interact with $GABA_A$ receptors • Partial agonist of the $5HT_{1A}$ receptor
Fluoxetine Fluvoxamine Paroxetine Citalopram Escitalopram Sertraline Vilazodone	• Antidepressants • Also used to treat anxiety, panic disorder, obsessive-compulsive disorder, fibromyalgia, and neuropathic pain	• Selectively inhibit the serotonin transporter (SSRIs) • Most widely used treatments for major depressive disorder • Sexual dysfunction is a common side effect with SSRIs • Precaution: serotonin syndrome

MSAAs · Treatment of sexual dysfunction · Activity at multiple receptor isoforms

Flibanserin	• Treatment of HSDD/FSIAD in premenopausal women	• Potent $5HT_{1A}$ receptor agonist and $5HT_2$ receptor family antagonist • Exerts both agonist and antagonist activity at 5HT receptors $\Rightarrow$ MSAA designation (multifunctional serotonin agonist and antagonist)

Dopamine Receptor Agonists · Little to no subtype specificity

Dopamine	• Congestive heart failure • Sepsis • Cardiogenic shock	• Only used acutely via intravenous administration
Bromocriptine Cabergoline	• PD (see Chapter 22) • Hyperprolactinemia	• Ergot derivatives with D_2 agonist activity and D_1 antagonist activity • Limited utility due to high potential for cardiac valvulopathies via $5HT_{2B}$ stimulation • Bromocriptine and cabergoline can be used at low doses to treat hyperprolactinemia
Apomorphine Pramipexole Ropinirole Rotigotine	• PD (see Chapter 22 for more details) • RLS	• Nonergot alkaloids with broader DA receptor agonist activity • Less efficacious than L-dopa in PD; often used as adjunct therapy in advanced PD • Use in early PD can lead to poor impulse control • Pramipexole, ropinirole, and rotigotine are used to treat RLS

Dopamine Receptor Antagonists · Antipsychotics · Emerging subtype specificity of ligands (Additional detail in Chapter 16)

Chlorpromazine Haloperidol	• Schizophrenia (see Chapter 16)	• Classified as typical antipsychotics • Agents block D_2 receptors but are not completely selective • Improvements are most notable in positive symptoms of schizophrenia
Clozapine	• Schizophrenia (see Chapter 16)	• Classified as atypical antipsychotics • Mixed $5HT_{2A}$–D_2 receptor blockade • Fewer extrapyramidal side effects than typical antipsychotics
Aripiprazole Brexpiprazole Cariprazine	• Schizophrenia (see Chapter 16)	• D_2 partial agonists with varied profiles at 5HT receptors • Improved side effect profile over many other antipsychotics

DAT Ligands · High potential for abuse · Interact with the dopamine transporter

Bupropion	• Depression • Smoking cessation	• Also inhibits NET • $\uparrow$ risk of suicidal ideation in pediatric/young adult patients taking this medication
Cocaine	• Rarely used therapeutically	• Schedule II classification • Limited clinical utility as a topical anesthetic in eye and nasal surgeries
Methylphenidate Methamphetamine Amphetamine	• ADHD, ADD • Narcolepsy • Obesity	• Can worsen psychosis; use with extreme caution in patients with bipolar disorder • Schedule II drug classification due to psychostimulant properties if misused

[a]Fewest side effects.
[b]Has best evidence for safety in pregnancy.

Bibliography

Ahangari G, et al. Investigation of 5HT2A gene expression in PBMCs of patients with allergic asthma. *Inflamm Allergy Drug Targets*, **2015**, *14*:60–64.

Beaulieu JM, Gainetdinov RR. The physiology, signaling, and pharmacology of dopamine receptors. *Pharmacol Rev*, **2011**, *63*:182–217.

Beaulieu JM, et al. Dopamine receptors—IUPHAR review 13. *Br J Pharmacol*, **2015**, *172*:1–23.

Brunner HG, et al. Abnormal behavior associated with a point mutation in the structural gene for monoamine oxidase A. *Science*, **1993**, *262*:578–580.

Burns CM, et al. Regulation of serotonin-2C receptor G-protein coupling by RNA editing. *Nature*, **1997**, *387*:303–308.

Cases O, et al. Aggressive behavior and altered amounts of brain serotonin and norepinephrine in mice lacking MAOA. *Science*, **1995**, *268*:1763–1766.

Chien EY, et al. Structure of the human dopamine D$_3$ receptor in complex with a D$_2$/D$_3$ selective antagonist. *Science*, **2010**, *330*:1091–1095.

Ciliax BJ, et al. Immunocytochemical localization of the dopamine transporter in human brain. *J Comp Neurol*, **1999**, *409*:38–56.

Fuxe K, et al. Dopamine heteroreceptor complexes as therapeutic targets in Parkinson's disease. *Expert Opin Ther Targets*, **2015**, *19*:377–398.

Heidbreder CA, Newman AH. Current perspectives on selective dopamine D(3) receptor antagonists as pharmacotherapeutics for addictions and related disorders. *Ann N Y Acad Sci*, **2010**, *1187*:4–34.

Hornykiewicz O. L-Dopa: from a biologically inactive amino acid to a successful therapeutic agent. *Amino Acids*, **2002**, *23*:65–70.

Hoyer D, et al. International Union of Pharmacology classification of receptors for 5-hydroxytryptamine (serotonin). *Pharmacol Rev*, **1994**, *46*:157–203.

Hutcheson JD, et al. Serotonin receptors and heart valve disease—it was meant 2B. *Pharmacol Ther*, **2011**, *132*:146–157.

Källén B, Reis M. Ongoing pharmacological management of chronic pain in pregnancy. *Drugs*, **2016**, *76*:915–924.

Kebabian JW, et al. Multiple receptors for dopamine. *Nature*, **1979**, *277*:93–96.

Lechin F, et al. Severe asthma and plasma serotonin. *Allergy*, **2002**, *57*:258–259.

Mehrotra S, et al. Current and prospective pharmacological targets in relation to antimigraine action. *N-S Arch Pharmacol*, **2008**, *378*:371–394.

Miller GM. The emerging role of trace amine-associated receptor 1 in the functional regulation of monoamine transporters and dopaminergic activity. *J Neurochem*, **2011**, *116*:164–176.

Nau F Jr, et al. Serotonin 5HT(2) receptor activation prevents allergic asthma in a mouse model. *Am J Physiol*, **2015**, *308*:L191–L198.

Newman AH, et al. Medication discovery for addiction: translating the dopamine D$_3$ receptor hypothesis. *Biochem Pharmacol*, **2012**, *84*:882–890.

Nichols DE. Psychedelics. *Pharmacol Rev*, **2016**, *68*:264–355.

Penmatsa A, et al. X-ray structures of *Drosophila* dopamine transporter in complex with nisoxetine and reboxetine. *Nat Struct Mol Biol*, **2015**, *22*:506–508.

Sitte H, et al. Amphetamines, new psychoactive drugs and the monoamine transporter cycle. *Trends Pharmacol Sci*, **2015**, *36*:41–50.

Thorlund K, et al. Comparative efficacy of triptans for the abortive treatment of migraine: a multiple treatment comparison meta-analysis. *Cephalalgia*, **2014**, *34*:258–267.

Vijayraghavan S, et al. Inverted-U dopamine D$_1$ receptor actions on prefrontal neurons engaged in working memory. *Nat Neurosci*, **2007**, *10*:376–384.

Wheeler DS, et al. Amphetamine activates Rho GTPase signaling to mediate dopamine transporter internalization and acute behavioral effects of amphetamine. *Proc Natl Acad Sci U S A*, **2015**, *112*:E7138–E7147.

Chapter 14

Neurotransmission in the Central Nervous System

R. Benjamin Free, Janet Clark, Susan Amara, and David R. Sibley

The brain is a complex assembly of interacting cells that regulate many of life's activities in a dynamic fashion, generally through the communication process of chemical neurotransmission. Because the CNS drives so many physiological responses, it stands to reason that centrally-acting drugs are invaluable for a plethora of conditions. CNS-acting drugs are used not only to treat anxiety, depression, mania, and schizophrenia, but also to target diverse pathophysiological conditions, such as pain, fever, movement disorders, insomnia, eating disorders, nausea, vomiting, and migraine. However, as the CNS dictates such diverse physiology, the recreational use of some CNS-acting drugs can lead to physical dependence (Chapter 24) with enormous societal impacts. The sheer breadth of physiological and pathological activities mediated by drug molecules acting in the CNS makes this class of therapeutics both wide-ranging and immeasurably important.

The identification of CNS targets, as well as the development of drug molecules for those targets, presents extraordinary scientific challenges. While years of investigation have begun to dissect the cellular and molecular bases for many aspects of neuronal signaling, complete understanding of the functions of the human brain remains in its infancy. Complicating the effort is the fact that a CNS-active drug may act at multiple sites with disparate and even opposing effects. Furthermore, many CNS disorders likely involve multiple brain regions and pathways, which can frustrate efforts focusing on a single therapeutic agent.

The pharmacology of CNS-acting drugs is primarily driven by two broad and overlapping goals:

- to develop/use drugs as probe compounds to both elucidate and manipulate the normal CNS; and
- to develop drugs to correct pathophysiological changes in the abnormal CNS.

Modern advances in molecular biology, neurophysiology, structural biology, epigenetics, biomarkers, immunity, and an array of other fields have facilitated both our understanding of the brain and the development of an ever-expanding repertoire of drugs that can selectively treat diseases of the CNS.

This chapter introduces fundamental principles and guidelines for the comprehensive study of drugs that affect the CNS. Specific therapeutic approaches to neurological and psychiatric disorders are discussed in subsequent chapters. For further detail, see specialized texts (Brady et al., 2012;

Kandel et al., 2013; Nestler et al., 2015; Sibley, 2007). Detailed information on nearly all specific receptors and ion channels can be found at the official databases of the IUPHAR/BPS Guide to Pharmacology (http://www.guidetopharmacology.org).

Cellular Organization of the Brain

The CNS is made up of several types of specialized cells that are physiologically integrated to form complex functional brain tissue. The primary communicating cell is the neuron, which is strongly influenced and sustained by a variety of important supporting cells. Specific connections between neurons, both within and across the macrodivisions of the brain, are essential for neurological function. Through patterns of neuronal circuitry, individual neurons form functional ensembles to regulate the flow of information within and between the regions of the brain. Under these guidelines, present understanding of the cellular organization of the CNS can be viewed from the perspective of the size, shape, location, and interconnections between neurons (Shepherd, 2004; Squire, 2013).

Neurons

Neurons are the highly polarized signaling cells of the brain and are subclassified into types based on a large number of factors, including function (sensory, motor, or interneuron); location; morphology; neurotransmitter phenotype; or the class(es) of receptor expressed. Neurons are electrically active cells that express a variety of ion channels and ion transport proteins that allow them to conduct nerve impulses or action potentials that ultimately trigger release of neurotransmitters during chemical neurotransmission. Neurons also exhibit the cytological characteristics of highly active secretory cells: large nuclei, large amounts of smooth and rough endoplasmic reticulum, and frequent clusters of specialized smooth endoplasmic reticulum (Golgi complex), in which secretory products of the cell are packaged into membrane-bound organelles for transport from the perikaryon to the axon or dendrites (Figure 14–1). The sites of interneuronal communication in the CNS are termed *synapses*. Although synapses are functionally analogous to "junctions" in the somatic motor and autonomic nervous systems, central synapses contain an array of specific proteins that comprise the active zone for transmitter release and response.

Abbreviations

AC: adenylyl cyclase
ACh: acetylcholine
ACTH: corticotropin (formerly adrenocorticotropic hormone)
ADHD: attention-deficit/hyperactivity disorder
AMPA: α-amino-3-hydroxy-5-methyl-4-isoxazole propionic acid
AP: action potential
BBB: blood-brain barrier
BDNF: brain-derived neurotrophic factor
cAMP: cyclic adenosine monophosphate
CFTR channel: cystic fibrosis transmembrane conductance regulated channel
CGRP: calcitonin gene–related peptide
CLC: chloride channel
CLIP: corticotropin-like intermediate lobe peptide
CNG channel: cyclic nucleotide–gated channel
CNS: central nervous system
CO: carbon monoxide
COX: cyclooxygenase
CSF: cerebrospinal fluid
CYP: cytochrome P450
DA: dopamine
DAG: diacylglycerol
DAT: dopamine transporter
DHEAS: dehydroepiandrosterone sulfate
EAAT: excitatory amino acid transporter
EPAC: exchange protein activated by cyclic AMP
EPI: epinephrine
ERK: extracellular signal-regulated kinase
GABA: γ-aminobutyric acid
GABA-T: GABA transaminase
GAD: glutamic acid decarboxylase
GAT: GABA transporter
GHB: γ-hydroxybutyric acid
GluR: AMPA/kainate type of glutamate receptor
GLYT: glycine transporter
GPCR: G protein–coupled receptor
GRK: G protein–coupled receptor kinase
HCN channel: hyperpolarization-activated, cyclic nucleotide-gated channel
HP loops: hairpin loop
5HT: serotonin
IL: interleukin
IFN: interferon
IP$_3$: inositol 1,4,5-trisphosphate
IPSP: inhibitory postsynaptic potential

IUPHAR/BPS: International Union of Basic and Clinical Pharmacology/British Pharmacological Society
KA: kainic acid
LOX: lipoxygenase
γ-LPH: γ-lipotrophic hormone
LTD: long-term depression
LTP: long-term potentiation
MAO: monoamine oxidase
MAPK: mitogen-activated protein kinase
mGluR: metabotropic glutamate receptor
MSH: melanocyte-stimulating hormone
mtPTP: mitochondrial permeability transition pore
NCX: Na$^+$/Ca^{2+} exchanger
NE: norepinephrine
NET: norepinephrine transporter
NGF: nerve growth factor
NMDA: N-methyl-D-aspartate
NMDA-R: NMDA receptor
NO: nitric oxide
NOS: nitric oxide synthase
NT: neurotrophin
O$_2^-$: superoxide radical
OCT: organic cation transporter
PC: phosphatidylcholine
PCP: phencyclidine
PDE: phosphodiesterase
PE: phosphatidylethanolamine
PEA: phenethylamine
PI3K: phosphoinositide 3-kinase
PIP$_2$: phosphatidylinositol 4,5-bisphosphate
PK_: protein kinase _, as in PKA, PKC
PL_: phospholipase _, as in PLA, PLD
POMC: pro-opiomelanocortin
SERT: serotonin transporter
SLC: solute carrier
TAAR: trace amine–associated receptor
TARPs: transmembrane AMPA receptor regulatory proteins
TAS2: taste receptor 2
THC: delta-9-tetrahydrocannabinol
TNF-α: tumor necrosis factor alpha
TRP channel: transient receptor potential channel
VAChT: vesicular acetylcholine transporter
VGAT: vesicular GABA and glycine transporter
VGLUT: vesicular glutamate transporter
VMAT: vesicular monoamine transporter
VSCC: voltage-sensitive Ca^{2+} channel

Like peripheral junctions, central synapses are denoted by accumulations of tiny (50- to 150-nm) *synaptic vesicles*. The proteins of these vesicles have specific roles in neurotransmitter storage, vesicle docking, and secretion and reaccumulation of neurotransmitter (see Figures 8–3 through Figures 8–6). The release of these neurotransmitters and their action on the neighboring cells via specific receptors, through mechanisms discussed in the material that follows, underlie the ability of these specialized cells to communicate with each other to dictate complex physiological actions.

Support Cells

A diverse cast of support cells outnumbers neurons in the CNS. These include neuroglia, vascular elements, the CSF-forming cells found within the intracerebral ventricular system, and the meninges that cover the surface of the brain and comprise the CSF-containing envelope. *Neuroglia* (sometimes referred to simply as *glia*) are the most abundant support cells. They are nonneuronal cells that maintain important brain functions, such as holding neurons in place, supplying oxygen and nutrients to neurons, insulating signaling between neurons, and destroying potential pathogens. Traditionally, it was thought that neuroglia acted only in a supporting role; however, newer studies have demonstrated that they may also be involved in some signaling processes.

Neuroglia are classified as either *micro-* or *macroglia*. In the CNS, the macroglia consist of astrocytes, oligodendroglia, ependymal cells, and radial glia. Astrocytes (cells interposed between the vasculature and the neurons) are the most abundant of these and often surround individual compartments of synaptic complexes. They play a variety of metabolic

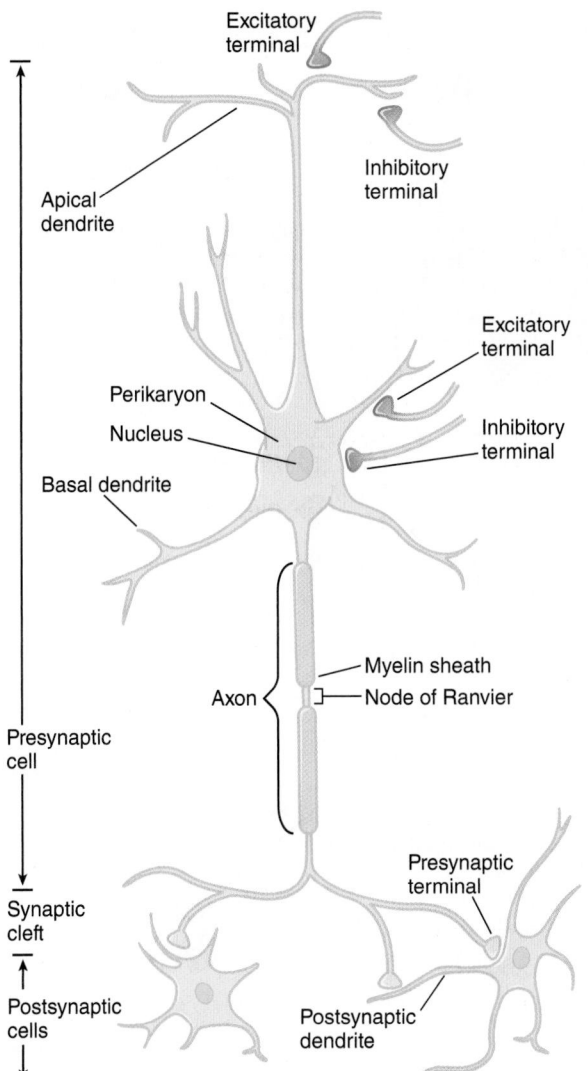

Figure 14–1 *Principal features of a neuron.* Dendrites, including apical dendrites, receive synapses from presynaptic terminals. The cell body (~50 μm in diameter) contains the nucleus and is the site of transcription and translation. The axon (0.2 to 20 μm wide, 100 μm to 2 m in length) carries information from the perikaryon to the presynaptic terminals, which form synapses (up to 1000) with the dendrites of other neurons. Axosomatic synapses also occur. Many CNS-active pharmacological agents act at the presynaptic and postsynaptic membranes of the synaptic clefts and at areas of transmitter storage near the synapses. (Adapted with permission from Kandel ER, et al., eds. *Principles of Neural Science.* 4th ed. McGraw-Hill, New York, **2000**, p. 22.)

support roles, including furnishing energy intermediates, anchoring neurons to their blood supply, and regulating the external environment of the neuron by active removal of neurotransmitters and excess ions following release. The oligodendroglia produce myelin, the multilayer, compacted membranes that electrically insulate segments of axons and permit nondecremental propagation of action potentials. Ependymal cells line the spinal cord and ventricular system and are involved in the creation of CSF, while radial cells act as neuroprogenitors and scaffolds. *Microglia* consist of specialized immune cells found within the CNS. Although the brain is immunologically protected by the BBB (see discussion that follows), these microglia act as macrophages to protect the neurons and are therefore mediators of immune response in the CNS. Microglia respond to neuronal damage and inflammation, and many diseases are associated with deficient microglia. In some instances, such as in chronic neuroinflammation, the balance between the numbers of

microglia and astrocytes can determine whether there will be resulting cell damage or protection. Thus, in addition to neurons, support cells such as glia are key players in facilitating most aspects of neuronal function and CNS signaling.

Blood-Brain Barrier

The *BBB* is an important boundary separating the periphery (capillaries carrying blood) from the CNS. This barrier consists of endothelial cells, astrocytes, and pericytes on a noncellular basement membrane. The BBB prevents or diminishes unencumbered access to the brain by circulating blood components. In terms of CNS therapeutics, the BBB represents a substantial obstacle to overcome for drug delivery to the site of action. An exception exists for lipophilic molecules, which diffuse fairly freely across the BBB and accumulate in the brain. In addition to its relative impermeability to small charged molecules such as neurotransmitters, the BBB can be viewed as a combination of the partitioning of solute across the vasculature (which governs passage by definable properties such as molecular weight, charge, and lipophilicity) and the presence or absence of energy-dependent transport systems (see Chapter 5). However, the cells within the barrier also have the capacity to actively transport molecules such as glucose and amino acids that are critical for brain function (see Chapter 5). One of these transport systems that is selective for large amino acids catalyzes the movement of L-dopa across the BBB and thus contributes to the therapeutic utility of L-dopa in the treatment of Parkinson disease. Furthermore, for some compounds, including neurotransmitter metabolites such as homovanillic acid and 5-hydroxyindoleacetic acid, the acid transport system of the choroid plexus provides an important route for clearance from the brain.

Substances that rarely gain access to the brain from the bloodstream can often reach the brain when injected directly into the CSF, and, under certain therapeutic conditions, bypassing the barrier may be beneficial to permit the entry of chemotherapeutic agents. Other clinical manifestations, such as cerebral ischemia and inflammation, can also modify the BBB, thereby increasing access to substances that ordinarily would not enter the brain. The barrier is nonexistent in the peripheral nervous system and is much less prominent in the hypothalamus and several small, specialized organs (the circumventricular organs) lining the third and fourth ventricles of the brain: the median eminence, area postrema, pineal gland, subfornical organ, and subcommissural organ. Although their structure and anatomical positioning may make these areas more accessible for physiological and pharmacological modulation, overall the BBB remains a constant consideration for pharmacological access to the CNS. For a pharmacologist's view of the BBB, see The Blood-Brain Barrier: A Pharmacological View in Chapter 5.

Neuronal Excitability and Ion Channels

As noted, neurons, the primary signaling cells of the brain, release neurotransmitters in response to a rapid rise and fall in membrane potential known as an action potential. Voltage-dependent ion channels within the plasma membrane open when the membrane potential increases to a threshold value, thus regulating the electrical excitability of neurons. Action potentials are the signals by which the brain and neurons receive and transmit information to one another through pathways determined by their connectivity.

We now understand in considerable detail how three major cations, Na^+, K^+, and Ca^{2+}, as well as Cl^- anion, are regulated via their flow through highly discriminative ion channels (Figures 14–2 and 14–3). The relatively high extracellular concentration of Na^+ (~140 mM) compared to its intracellular concentration (~14 mM) means that increases in permeability to Na^+ cause cellular depolarization, ultimately leading to the generation of an action potential. In contrast, the intracellular

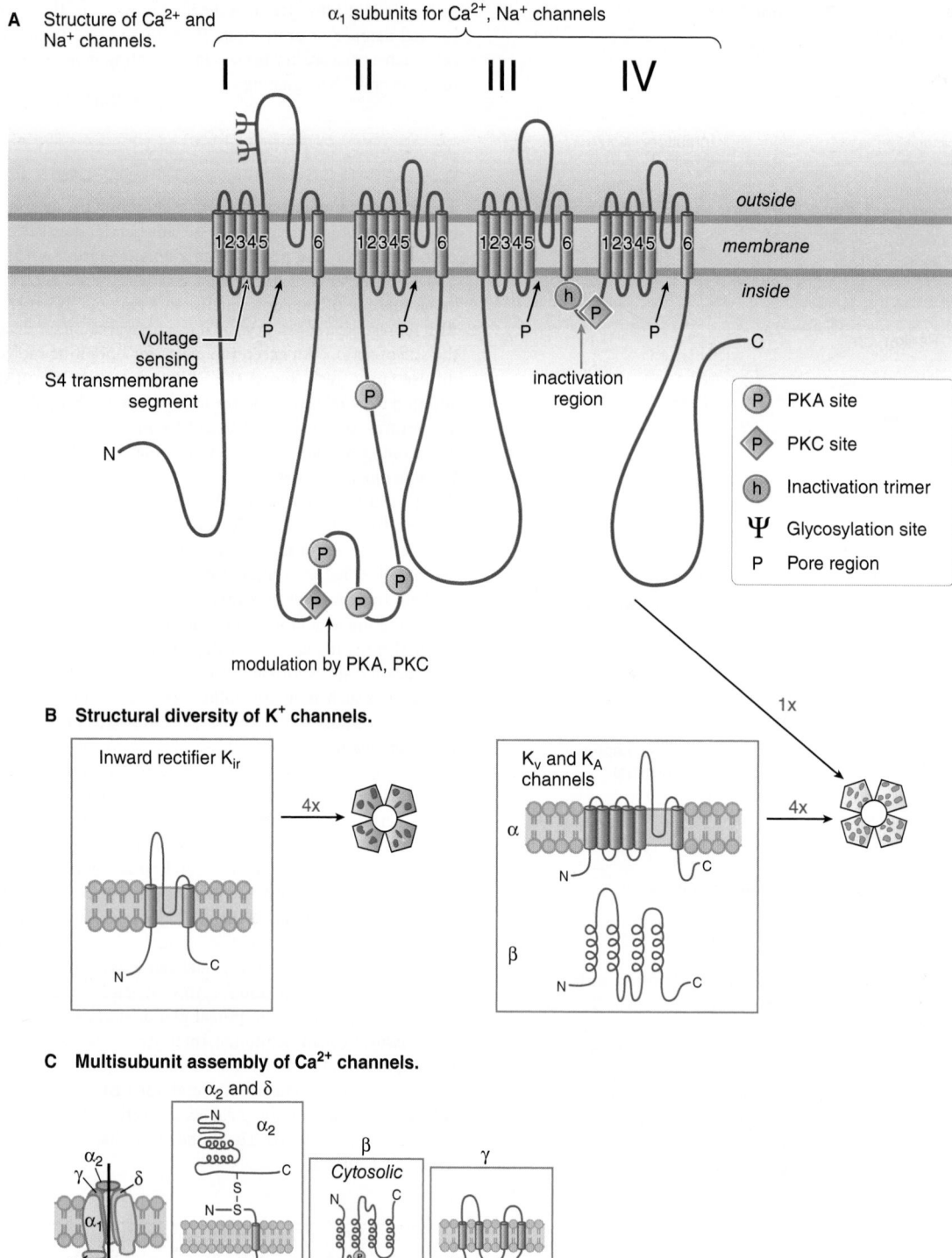

Figure 14–2 *Voltage-sensitive Na$^+$, Ca^{2+}, and K$^+$ channels.* Voltage-dependent channels provide for rapid changes in ion permeability along axons and within dendrites and for excitation-secretion coupling that releases neurotransmitters from presynaptic sites. The transmembrane Na$^+$ gradient (~140 mM outside vs. ~ 14 mM inside the cell) means that increases in permeability to Na$^+$ causes *depolarization*. In contrast, the K$^+$ gradient (~4 mM outside the cell vs. ~ 120 mM inside) is such that increased permeability to K$^+$ results in *hyperpolarization*. Changes in the concentration of intracellular Ca^{2+} (extracellular free Ca^{2+}: 1.25 mM; intracellular Ca^{2+}: resting ~ 100 nM, rising to ~ 1 μM when Ca^{2+} entry is stimulated) affects multiple processes in the cell and are critical in the release of neurotransmitters. **A.** *Structure of Ca^{2+} and Na$^+$ channels.* The α subunit in both Ca^{2+} and Na$^+$ channels consists of four sub-subunits or segments (labeled **I** through **IV**), each with six TM hydrophobic domains (blue cylinders). The hydrophobic regions that connect TM5 and TM6 in each segment associate to form the pore of the channel. Segment 4 in each domain includes the voltage sensor. (Adapted with permission from Catterall W. *Neuron* **2000**, *26*:13–25. © Elsevier.) **B.** *Structural diversity of K$^+$ channels. Inward rectifier, K$_{ir}$.* The basic subunit of the inwardly rectifying K$^+$ channel protein K$_{ir}$ has the general configuration of TM5 and TM6 of a segment of the α subunit shown in panel **A**. Four of these subunits assemble to create the pore. *Voltage-sensitive K$^+$ channel, K$_v$.* The α subunits of the voltage-sensitive K$^+$ channel K$_v$ and the rapidly activating K$^+$ channel K$_A$ share a putative hexaspanning structure resembling in overall configuration a single segment of the Na$^+$ and Ca^{2+} channel structure, with six TM domains. Four of these assemble to form the pore. Regulatory β subunits (cytosolic) can alter K$_v$ channel functions. **C.** *Multisubunit assembly of Ca^{2+} channels.* Ca^{2+} channels variably require several auxiliary small proteins (α$_2$, β, γ, and δ); α$_2$ and δ subunits are linked by a disulfide bond. Likewise, regulatory subunits also exist for Na$^+$ channels.

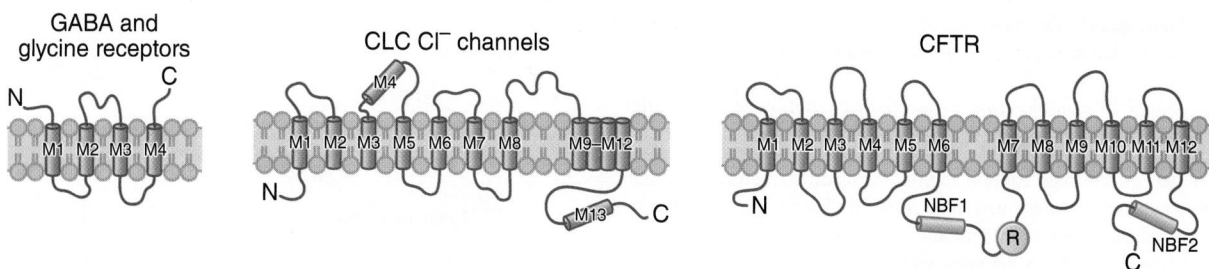

Figure 14–3 *Three families of Cl⁻ channels.* Due to the Cl⁻ gradient across the plasma membrane (~116 mM outside vs. 20 mM inside the cell), activation of Cl⁻ channels causes an IPSP that dampens neuronal excitability; inactivation of these channels can lead to hyperexcitability. There are three distinct types of Cl⁻ channel: *Ligand-gated channels* are linked to inhibitory transmitters, including GABA and glycine. *CLC Cl⁻ channels*, of which nine subtypes have been cloned, affect Cl flux, membrane potential, and the pH of intracellular vesicles. *CFTR channels* bind ATP and are regulated by phosphorylation of serine residues. M, transmembrane domains; NBF, nucleotide-binding fold; R, regulatory (phosphorylation) domain. (Reproduced with permission from Jentsch J. Chloride channels: a molecular perspective. *Curr Opin Neurobiol*, **1996**, 6:303–310. Copyright Elsevier.)

concentration of K⁺ is relatively high (~120 mM, vs. 4 mM outside the cell), and increased permeability to K⁺ results in hyperpolarization. Changes in the concentration of intracellular Ca^{2+} (100 nM to 1 μM) affects multiple processes in the cell and are critical in the release of neurotransmitters. Under basal conditions, cellular homeostatic mechanisms (Na^+,K^+-ATPase; Na^+,Ca^{2+} exchanger; Ca^{2+}-ATPases; etc.) and the sequestration of releasable Ca^{2+} in storage vesicles maintain the concentrations of these ions. Electrical excitability thus generates the action potential through changes in the distribution of charged ions across the neuronal cell membrane.

The Cl⁻ channels are a superfamily of ion channels that are important for maintaining resting potential and are also responsible for the IPSPs that dampen neuronal excitability. In most neurons, the Cl⁻ gradient across the plasma membrane is inwardly driven (~116 mM outside vs. 20 mM inside the cell), and, as a result, inactivation of these channels leads to hyperexcitability. There are several families of both voltage-gated and ligand-gated Cl⁻ channels (Figure 14–3). Ligand-gated Cl⁻ channels are linked to inhibitory transmitters, including GABA and glycine (discussed in detail in material that follows). A class of secondary active transporters, the cation-chloride cotransporters, plays an essential role in establishing the electrochemical Cl⁻ gradient that is required for the hyperpolarizing postsynaptic inhibition mediated by both GABA receptors and glycine receptors. In addition, during brain development, changes in the expression of neuronal cation-chloride cotransporter isoforms can result in shifts in the direction of the chloride gradient such that activation of a ligand-gated chloride channel becomes excitatory.

The CLC family of chloride channels comprises plasma membrane channels that affect Cl⁻ flux and membrane potential as well as channels that function as Cl⁻/H⁺ antiporters. CLC members can also influence the pH of intracellular vesicles. *CFTR channels* are gated by ATP and increase the conductance of certain anions. Overall, these channels are responsible for a variety of important neurophysiological roles, including regulation of membrane potential, volume homeostasis, and regulation of pH on internal extracellular compartments.

The *CNG channels* are nonselective cation channels that regulate ion flux in neurons. CNG channels are activated as a result of cyclic nucleotide binding, and their primary function involves sensory transduction, especially in the retina and olfactory neurons. Because CNG channels are nonselective and also allow alkali ions to flow, they can result in either depolarization or hyperpolarization. These channels consist of four subunits assembled around a central pore and are subclassified into α (four genes) and β (two genes) subunits. HCN channels are another type of cyclic nucleotide-gated channel; they are nonselective, ligand-gated, cation channels that are encoded by four genes and are widely expressed in the heart and throughout the CNS. These channels open with hyperpolarization and close with depolarization; the binding of cyclic AMP or cyclic GMP to the channels shifts their activation curves to more hyperpolarized potentials. These channels play essential roles in cardiac pacemaker cells and in rhythmic and oscillatory activity in the CNS.

The *TRP channels* are a large family of about 28 ion channels that are nonselectively permeable to cations, including Na^+, Ca^{2+}, and Mg^{2+}. They are broadly grouped into six receptor subfamilies possessing six transmembrane domains containing the cation-permeable pore. These channels can have diverse modes of activation and permeation. TRP channels respond to multiple stimuli and function in sensory physiology, including thermosensation, osmosensation, and taste. Importantly, some TRP channels are also mediators of pain as they function as detectors of thermal and chemical stimuli that activate sensory neurons. Spices such as garlic, chili powder, and wasabi activate certain subtypes. Others respond to such diverse chemicals as menthol, peppermint, and camphor. Mutations in TRP channels have been associated with neurodegenerative diseases as well as cancer. The diversity of their physiology has led to their investigation as important drug targets, particularly for the treatment of chronic pain, for which they play a central role in nociception associated with inflammation and neuropathy. In recent years, TRP channels have become novel and important targets for drug development (Nilius and Szallasi, 2014).

Chemical Communication in the CNS

A central concept of neuropsychopharmacology is that drugs that improve the functional status of patients with neurological or psychiatric diseases typically act by enhancing or blunting neurotransmission in the CNS. Therapeutic targets include *ion channels* (discussed previously), which mediate changes in excitability induced by neurotransmitters; *neurotransmitter receptors*, which physiologically respond to activation by neurotransmitters; and *transport proteins*, which reaccumulate released transmitter.

Identification of Central Neurotransmitters

Neurotransmitters are endogenous chemicals in the brain that act to enable signaling across a chemical synapse. They carry, boost, and modulate signals between neurons or other cell types and act on a variety of targets to elicit a host of biological functions. An essential step in understanding the functional properties of neurotransmitters within the context of the circuitry of the brain is to identify substances that are transmitters at specific interneuronal connections. The precise number of transmitters is unknown, but more than 100 chemical messengers have been identified to date. The criteria for identification of central transmitters is similar to that used to establish the transmitters of the autonomic nervous system (see Chapter 8):

- *The transmitter must be present in the presynaptic terminals of the synapse and in the neurons from which those presynaptic terminals arise.*
- *The transmitter must be released from the presynaptic nerve concomitantly with nerve activity, and in high enough quantity to have an effect.*
- *The effects of experimental application of the putative transmitter should mimic the effects of stimulating the presynaptic pathway.*

- *If available, specific pharmacological agonists and antagonists should stimulate and block, respectively, the measured functions of the putative transmitter.*
- *There should be a mechanism present (either reuptake or enzymatic degradation) that terminates the actions of the transmitter.*

Many nerve terminals contain multiple transmitter substances and coexisting substances (presumed to be released together) that either act jointly on the postsynaptic membrane or act presynaptically to affect release of transmitter from the presynaptic terminal. In these cases, the milieu of concurrently released signaling molecules makes mimicking or fully antagonizing the action of a given transmitter substance with a single drug compound difficult. This has emphasized complexity in identifying signaling molecules that has been partially overcome using defined in vitro cell culture systems, which can then be extrapolated back to the CNS.

Cell Signaling and Synaptic Transmission

Cellular signaling links neurotransmitter receptor activation to downstream biological effects. A number of mechanisms have been identified that can be broadly classified into two main types of signaling, fast and slow neurotransmission. The most commonly seen postreceptor events are fast transmission resulting from rapid changes in ion flux through ion channels. Slow neurotransmission is primarily the role of a second major group of receptors, the GPCRs, which interact with heterotrimeric GTP-binding proteins (Figure 3–10). There are additional and distinct mechanisms of signaling for growth factor receptors (Table 3–1; Figure 3–12) and for the nuclear receptors that transduce steroid hormone signaling (Figures 3–14 and 6–13). Because the majority of cell-to-cell communication in the CNS involves chemical transmission, neurons require specialized cellular functions to mediate these actions (Figure 14–4):

- *Neurotransmitter synthesis.* Small-molecule neurotransmitters are synthesized in nerve terminals, whereas others, such as peptides, are synthesized in cell bodies and transported to nerve terminals.
- *Neurotransmitter storage.* Synaptic vesicles store transmitters, often in association with various proteins and frequently with ATP.
- *Neurotransmitter release.* Release of stored transmitter from the storage vesicle into the synaptic cleft occurs by exocytosis. Depolarization of the presynaptic neuron results in a complex initiation of stimulus-secretion coupling, which involves vesicle docking at the plasma membrane, the formation of membrane fusion/release complexes, and the Ca^{2+}-dependent release of vesicular contents. Recycling of the transmitter storage vesicle generally follows. For details, see Figures 8–4 through 8–6.
- *Neurotransmitter recognition.* Neurotransmitters diffuse from sites of release and bind selectively to receptor proteins to initiate intracellular signal transduction events within the postsynaptic cell.
- *Termination of action.* A variety of mechanisms terminate the action of synaptically released transmitters, including diffusion from the synapse, enzymatic inactivation (for ACh and peptides), and uptake into neurons or glial cells by specific transporters.

Fast Neurotransmission

Responses to activation of receptors consisting of an ion channel as part of its structure tend to be rapid (milliseconds) because the effects are direct and generally do not require multiple steps leading to second-messenger generation and activation of a signaling pathway. In fast neurotransmission (also called directly gated transmission), neurotransmitters bind directly to ligand-gated ion channels on the postsynaptic membrane to rapidly open the channel and change the permeability of the postsynaptic site, leading to depolarization or hyperpolarization. Depolarization results in continuation of the nerve impulse, while hyperpolarization leads to diminished signaling (see Figure 11–5). Ligand-gated ion channels mediating fast transmission (also called ionotropic receptors) consist of multiple subunits, each usually having four transmembrane domains that associate to form pentameric receptors (Figure 14–5). Receptors with this structure include the receptors for the amino acids GABA, glycine, glutamate, and aspartate; the serotonin 5HT$_3$ receptor; and the nicotinic ACh

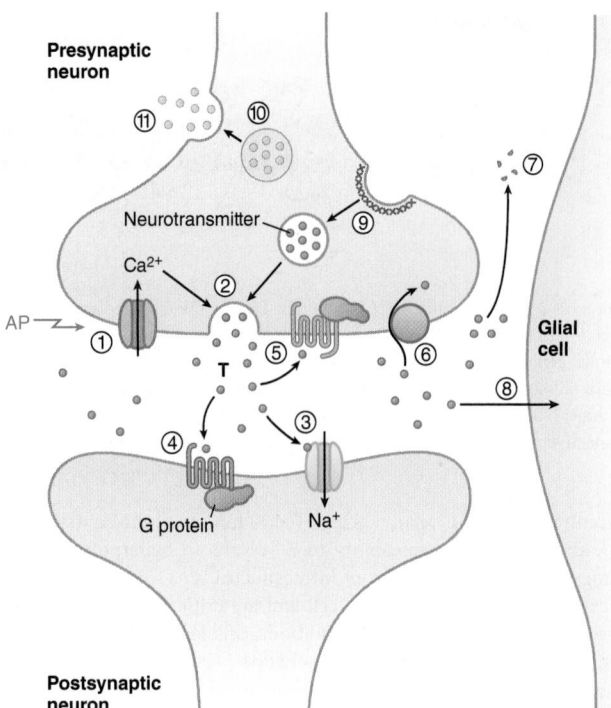

Figure 14–4 *Transmitter release, action, and inactivation.* Depolarization opens voltage-dependent Ca^{2+} channels in the presynaptic nerve terminal (1). The influx of Ca^{2+} during an action potential (AP) triggers (2) the exocytosis of small synaptic vesicles that store neurotransmitter (**T**). Released neurotransmitter interacts with receptors in the postsynaptic membranes that either couple directly with ion channels (3) or act through second messengers, such as GPCRs (4). Neurotransmitter receptors in the presynaptic nerve terminal membrane (5) can inhibit or enhance subsequent exocytosis. Released neurotransmitter is inactivated by reuptake into the nerve terminal by (6) a transport protein coupled to the Na$^+$ gradient (e.g., for DA, NE, or GABA); by (7) degradation (ACh, peptides); or by (8) uptake and metabolism by glial cells (glutamate). The synaptic vesicle membrane is recycled by (9) clathrin-mediated endocytosis. Neuropeptides and proteins are sometimes stored in (10) larger, dense core granules within the nerve terminal. These dense core granules can be released from sites (11) distinct from active zones after repetitive stimulation.

receptor. The nicotinic ACh receptor provides a good example of receptor structure and how subunit composition varies with anatomic location and affects function (Figure 14–6).

Slow Neurotransmission

Slower transmission (although still relatively fast, often on a time scale of seconds) is mediated by neurotransmitters that do not bind to ion channels but to receptors with a very different architecture called metabotropic receptors. Upon activation, these receptors generate second messengers. This major group of receptors consists of the membrane heptaspanning GPCRs (Figure 3–9). There are more than 825 human GPCRs, which can be classified into five major families: rhodopsin (class A); secretin (class B); adhesion; glutamate (class C); and frizzled. The GPCRs in the CNS are largely in the rhodopsin family. These receptors have sites for N-linked glycosylation on the extracellular amino tail and sometimes on the second extracellular loop. There are also multiple potential sites for phosphorylation on the third intracellular loop and the carboxyl tail, and some members of this class are palmitoylated on the carboxyl tail. Phosphorylation can regulate GPCR-G protein–effector coupling and provide docking sites for arrestins and other scaffolding proteins (see Chapter 3).

The GPCRs are associated with a broad spectrum of physiological effects, including activation of K$^+$ channels, activation of PLC-IP$_3$-Ca^{2+} pathways and regulation of adenylyl cyclase activity and downstream systems affected by cyclic AMP (multiple isoforms of PKA, EPAC, HCN,

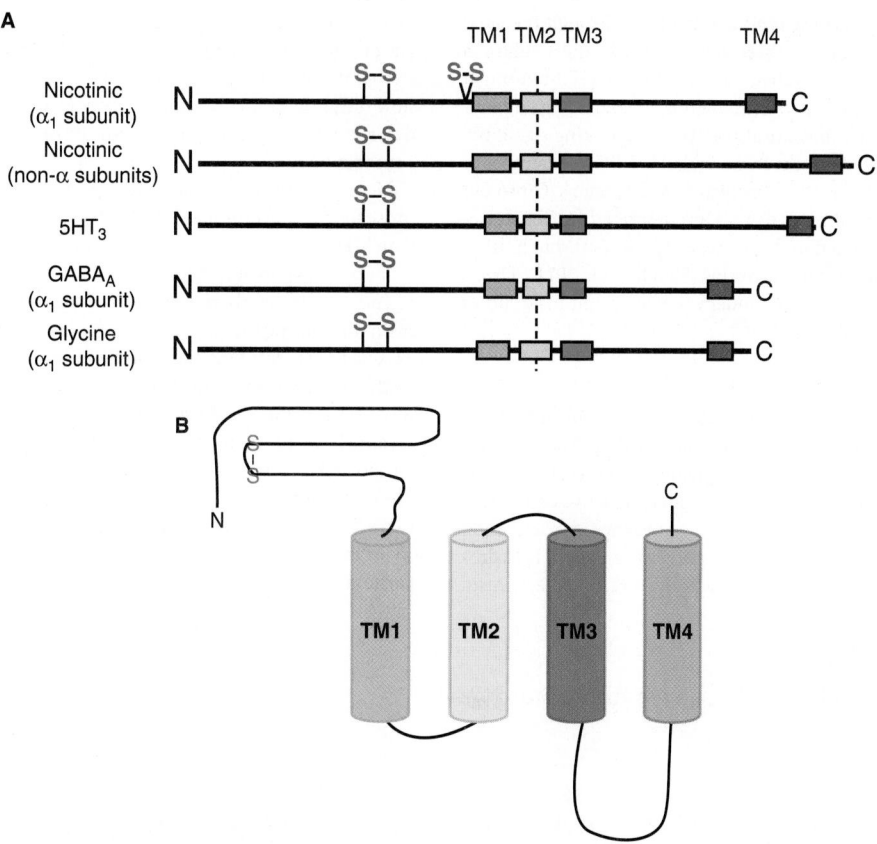

Figure 14–5 *Pentameric ligand-gated ion channels.* The subunits of these channels, which mediate fast synaptic transmission, are embedded in the plasma membrane to form a roughly cylindrical structure with a central pore. In response to binding of transmitter, the receptor proteins change conformation; the channel gate opens, and ions diffuse along their concentration gradient across the membrane through a hydrophilic opening in the otherwise-hydrophobic membrane. **A.** *Subunit organization.* For each subunit of these pentameric receptors, the amino terminal region of ~ 210 amino acids is extracellular. It is followed by four hydrophobic regions that span the membrane (TM1–TM4); a small carboxyl terminus is on the extracellular surface. The TM2 region is α helical, and TM2 regions from each subunit line the internal pore of the pentameric receptor. Two disulfide loops at positions 128–142 and 192–193 are found in the α subunit of the nicotinic receptor. The 128–142 motif is conserved in the family of pentameric receptors; the vicinal cysteines at 192–193 occur only in α subunit of the nicotinic receptor. **B.** *Schematic rendering of a nicotinic ACh non-α subunit.* Five such subunits form a pentameric receptor. See Figure 14–6 for an example.

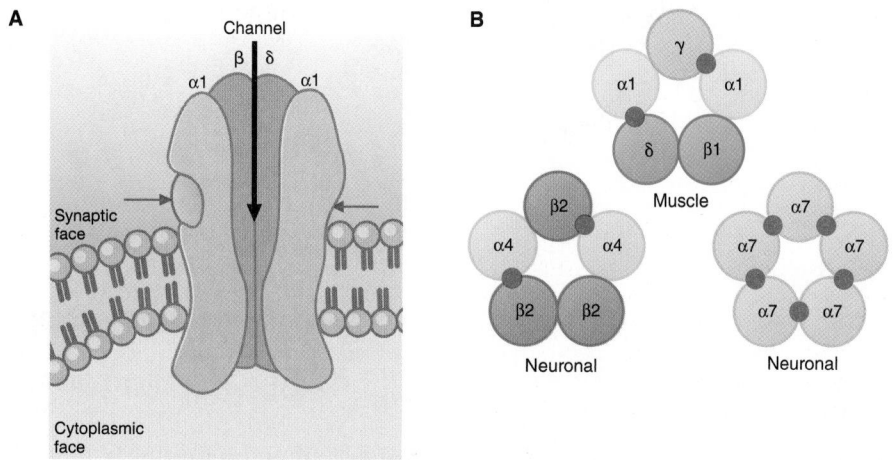

Figure 14–6 *Subunit arrangement: the nicotinic ACh receptor.* **A.** *Longitudinal view of receptor schematic with the γ subunit removed.* The remaining subunits, two copies of α, one of β, and one of δ, are shown to surround an internal channel with an outer vestibule and its constriction located deep in the membrane bilayer region. Spans of α helices with slightly bowed structures form the perimeter of the channel and come from the TM2 region of the linear sequence (Figure 14–5). ACh-binding sites, indicated by red arrows, occur at the $\alpha\gamma$ and $\alpha\delta$ (not visible) interfaces. **B.** *Nicotinic receptor subunit arrangements.* Agonist-binding sites (red circles) occur at α subunit–containing interfaces. At least 17 functional receptor isoforms have been observed in vivo, with different ligand specificity, relative Ca^{2+}/Na^+ permeability, and physiological function determined by their subunit composition. The only isoform found at the neuromuscular junction is shown for comparison. The neuronal receptor isoforms found at autonomic ganglia and in the CNS are homomeric or heteromeric pentamers of α ($\alpha2$–$\alpha10$) and β ($\beta2$–$\beta4$) subunits.

CNG, and PDE). These effects are typically mediated through the activation of specific G proteins, each a heterotrimer of α, β, and γ subunits where the β and γ units are constitutively associated. The GTP-binding α subunits can modulate the activities of numerous effectors (e.g., adenylyl cyclase, PLC). The βγ subunits are also active in mediating signaling, especially in the regulation of ion channels. Table 14–1 shows examples of the variety of physiological functions mediated by G proteins. G protein activation-inactivation signaling dynamics are described in Chapter 3. Notably, GPCRs can also signal to downstream pathways through other intermediary proteins, such as the β arrestins (Shukla et al., 2011). Drugs targeting GPCRs represent a core of modern medicine and make up as much as 40% of all pharmaceuticals.

Termination of Neurotransmitter Action

Mechanisms to terminate the actions of released neurotransmitters are essential for maintaining the balance of neuronal signaling. There are two primary mechanisms for terminating the signaling of released transmitters. One is the conversion of the transmitter into an inactive compound via an enzymatic reaction. The best example of enzymatic inactivation is for the transmitter ACh, which, after activating the receptor, is hydrolyzed by acetylcholinesterase to choline and acetate. A second mechanism

involves the clearance of the neurotransmitter by transport proteins present on presynaptic neurons, neighboring glial cells, and other neurons so that it can no longer act on the target receptors. In addition to these, slow diffusion of the transmitter away from the synapse and subsequent degradation also play a role for both conventional neurotransmitters and neuropeptides.

Neurons and glial cells express specific transporter proteins, such as those for the monoamines NE (NET), serotonin (SERT) and DA (DAT), which remove NE, 5HT, and DA, respectively, from the extracellular space by transporting it back into the presynaptic neuron (see Chapters 5, 8, and 13). These plasma membrane carriers serve as a major mechanism for limiting the extent and duration of neurotransmitter signaling. To accomplish this task, they couple the movement of neurotransmitters to the influx of Na$^+$, which provides a strong thermodynamic driving force for inward transport. The carriers for NE, 5HT, DA, GABA, and glycine have 12 hydrophobic membrane-spanning domains with their amino and carboxy termini located within the cytoplasm (Figure 14–8). These transporters are generally glycosylated along the large (second) extracellular loop and possess sites of phosphorylation and binding to intracellular regulatory proteins, primarily on their amino and carboxy tails.

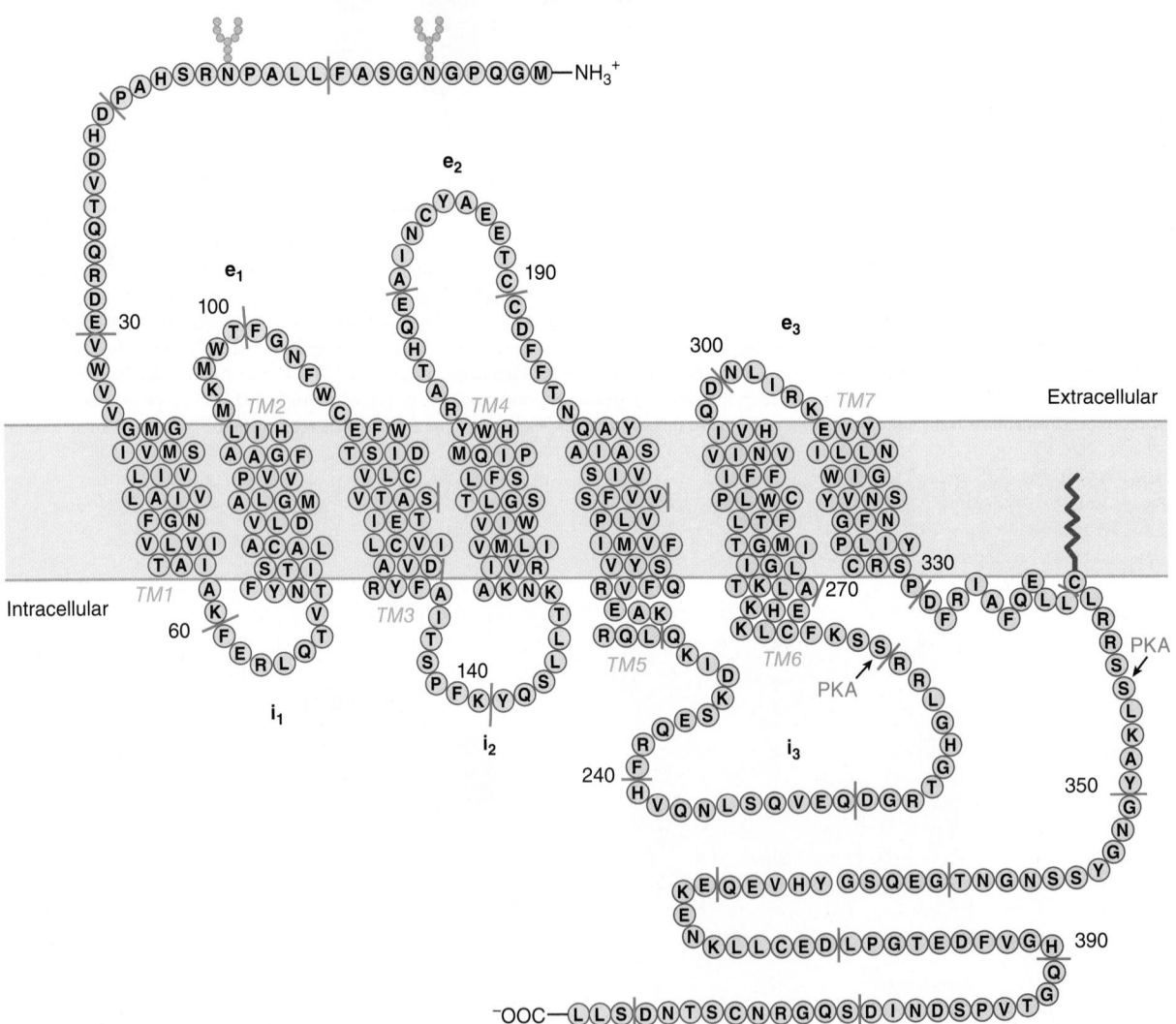

Figure 14–7 *The β adrenergic receptor as a model for GPCRs.* This two-dimensional model illustrates features common to most GPCRs. Red lines mark segments with 10 amino acids. The amino terminus (N) is extracellular, and the carboxyl terminus (C) is intracellular; in between are seven hydrophobic TM domains and alternating intracellular and extracellular loops (e$_{1–3}$ and i$_{1–3}$). Glycosylation sites are found near the N terminus; consensus sites for phosphorylation by PKA (arrows) are found in the i$_3$ loop and the carboxyl terminal tail. An aspartate residue in TM3 (asp^{113}) interacts with the nitrogen of catecholamine agonists while two serines (ser^{204}, ser^{207}) in TM5 interact with the hydroxyl groups on the phenyl ring of catecholamine agonists. A cysteine residue (cys^{341}) is a substrate for palmitoylation. Interaction of the palmitoyl group with membrane lipids reduces the flexibility of the carboxyl tail. (Reproduced with permission from Rasmussen SGF et al. Crystal structure of the human β2 adrenergic G-protein-coupled receptor. *Nature*, **2007**, *450*:383. Copyright © 2007.)

TABLE 14–1 ■ HETEROTRIMERIC G PROTEIN SUBUNITS

FAMILY	α SUBUNITS	SIGNALS TRANSDUCED
Family members		
G_s family		
G_s	α_s	Activation of AC
G_{olf}	α_{olf}	Activation of AC
G_i family		
G_i/G_o	α_i, α_o	Inhibition of AC
G_z	α_z	Inhibition of AC
G_{gust}	α_{gust}	Activation of PDE6
G_t	α_t	Activation of PDE6
G_q family		
G_q	α_q, α_{11}, α_{14}, α_{15}, α_{16}	Activation of PLC
$G_{12/13}$ family		
$G_{12/13}$	α_{12}, α_{13}	Activation of Rho GTPases
βγ Subunits[a] (acting as a heterodimer)		
G_β	β1, β2, β3, β4, β5	↓ AC, ↑ Ca^{2+} and K^+ channels, ↑ PI3K, ↑ PLC_β, ↑AC2 and AC4, ↑ Ras-dependent MAPK activation, ↑ recruitment of GRK2 and GRK3
G_γ	γ1, γ2, γ3, γ4, γ5, γ7, γ8, γ9, γ10, γ11, γ12, γ13	

[a]Khan and colleagues (2013) have reviewed the expanding roles of the βγ subunits.

A second family of plasma membrane neurotransmitter transporters mediates the clearance of glutamate and aspartate released during synaptic transmission. In humans, five subtypes of glutamate transporters (referred to as EAATs 1–5) clear glutamate into neurons and glial cells. The two glial carriers, EAATs 1 and 2, are responsible for the bulk of glutamate transport activity in the CNS and are critical for limiting the excitotoxic actions of glutamate described further in this chapter. These transporters have eight transmembrane domains (TM1–8) and two reentrant hairpin loops (HP1 and HP2) that appear to serve as intracellular and extracellular gates during the transport process (Figure 14–9). EAATs are members of the solute carrier family (SLC1A 1–3, 6, and 7) and are powered by Na^+ and other cations running down their electrochemical gradients.

There are also at least three distinct gene families of vesicular neurotransmitter transporters that sequester the neurotransmitters within synaptic vesicles for storage and, ultimately, for release during neuronal signaling. These include VMAT1, VMAT2, and VAChT (see Chapter 8), a vesicular carrier for both GABA and glycine (VGAT), and three vesicular glutamate carriers, VGLUT1, VGLUT2, and VGLUT3. These transporters ensure that vesicles fill rapidly during neurotransmission and provide a means for reducing cytoplasmic concentrations of neurotransmitter in areas where rates of reuptake are high. The driving force for vesicular uptake of neurotransmitter by these transporters is a proton electrochemical gradient across the membrane of the storage vesicle (vesicle interior more acidic than the cytosol).

The monoamine transporters DAT, NET, and SERT are well-established targets for therapeutic antidepressants and for addictive drugs, including cocaine and amphetamines. Selective inhibitors of these carriers can increase the duration and spatial extent of the actions of neurotransmitters. Inhibitors of the uptake of NE or 5HT are used to treat depression and other behavioral disorders, as described in Chapters 15 and 16. The psychostimulants methylphenidate and amphetamine are the major drugs used to treat ADHD in children and in adults. Although the two drugs have stimulant actions in healthy individuals, in patients with ADHD they reduce hyperactivity and increase attention by inhibiting DAT and NET and enhancing DA and NE neurotransmission. Transporters are discussed in further detail in Chapters 5, 8, and 13.

Central Neurotransmitters

Neurotransmitters can be classified by chemical structure into various categories, including *amino acids, ACh, monoamines, neuropeptides, purines, lipids*, and even *gases*. This section describes each category and examines some prominent members.

Amino Acids

The CNS contains high concentrations of certain amino acids, notably glutamate and GABA, that potently alter neuronal firing. They are ubiquitously distributed within the brain and produce rapid and readily reversible effects on neurons. The dicarboxylic amino acids glutamate and aspartate produce excitation, while the monocarboxylic amino acids GABA, glycine, β-alanine, and taurine cause inhibition. Following the emergence of selective agonists and antagonists, the identification of pharmacologically distinct amino acid receptor subtypes became possible (see discussion that follows). Figure 14–10 shows these amino acid transmitters and their drug congeners.

Gamma-Aminobutyric Acid

GABA is the main inhibitory neurotransmitter in the CNS. GABA is synthesized in the brain from the Krebs cycle intermediate α-ketoglutarate, which is transaminated to glutamate by GABA-T. GABA is subsequently formed from glutamate by the enzyme GAD; the presence of GAD in a neuron therefore delineates a neuron that uses GABA as a transmitter. Interestingly, intraneuronal GABA is also inactivated by GABA-T which converts it to succinic semialdehyde, but only in the presence of adequate α-ketoglutarate. This GABA shunt or cycle serves to maintain levels of GABA; thus, GABA-T is both a synthetic and a degradative enzyme (Brady et al., 2012). There is a vesicular GABA transporter (VGAT, SLC32A1, a member of the amino acid/polyamine transporter family) that is involved in storing GABA in vesicles for subsequent release into the synaptic cleft. The action of GABA is primarily terminated by reuptake by one of four different GATs present on both neurons and glia. GABA acts by binding to and activating specific ionotropic or metabotropic receptors on both pre- and postsynaptic membranes. *GABA_A receptors* (the most prominent GABA receptor subtype) are ionotropic, ligand-gated Cl⁻ channels. The *GABA_B receptors* are metabotropic GPCRs. One subtype formerly known as the *GABA_C receptor* is now classified as a type of GABA_A receptor.

The *GABA_A receptors* have been extensively characterized as important drug targets and are the site of action of many neuroactive drugs, notably benzodiazepines (such as valium), barbiturates, ethanol, anesthetic steroids, and volatile anesthetics, among others. These drugs are used to treat various neuropsychiatric disorders, including epilepsy, Huntington disease, addictions, sleep disorders, and more. As ligand-gated ion channels, GABA_A receptors are pentamers of subunits that each contain four transmembrane domains and assemble around a central anion-specific pore (Figures 14–5 and 14–6). The major forms of the GABA_A receptor contain at least three different types of subunits: α, β, and γ, with a likely stoichiometry of 2α, 2β, and 1γ. The IUPHAR/BPS recognizes 19 unique subunits that are known to form at least 11 native GABA_A receptors that can be pharmacologically differentiated. The particular combination of α and γ subunits can affect the efficacy of benzodiazepine binding and channel modulation. Many drugs, such as those noted, act as positive allosteric modulators of the GABA_A receptor, that is, act at sites distinct from the GABA-binding site to positively modulate the function of the receptor (Figure 14–11). The interaction of these drugs with the GABA_A receptor and their therapeutic use are discussed further in Chapter 17.

The *GABA_B receptors* are metabotropic GPCRs that function as obligate heterodimers of two subunits named GABA_B1 and GABA_B2. GABA_B receptors are widespread in the CNS and regulate both pre- and postsynaptic activity. These receptors interact with G_i to inhibit adenylyl cyclase,

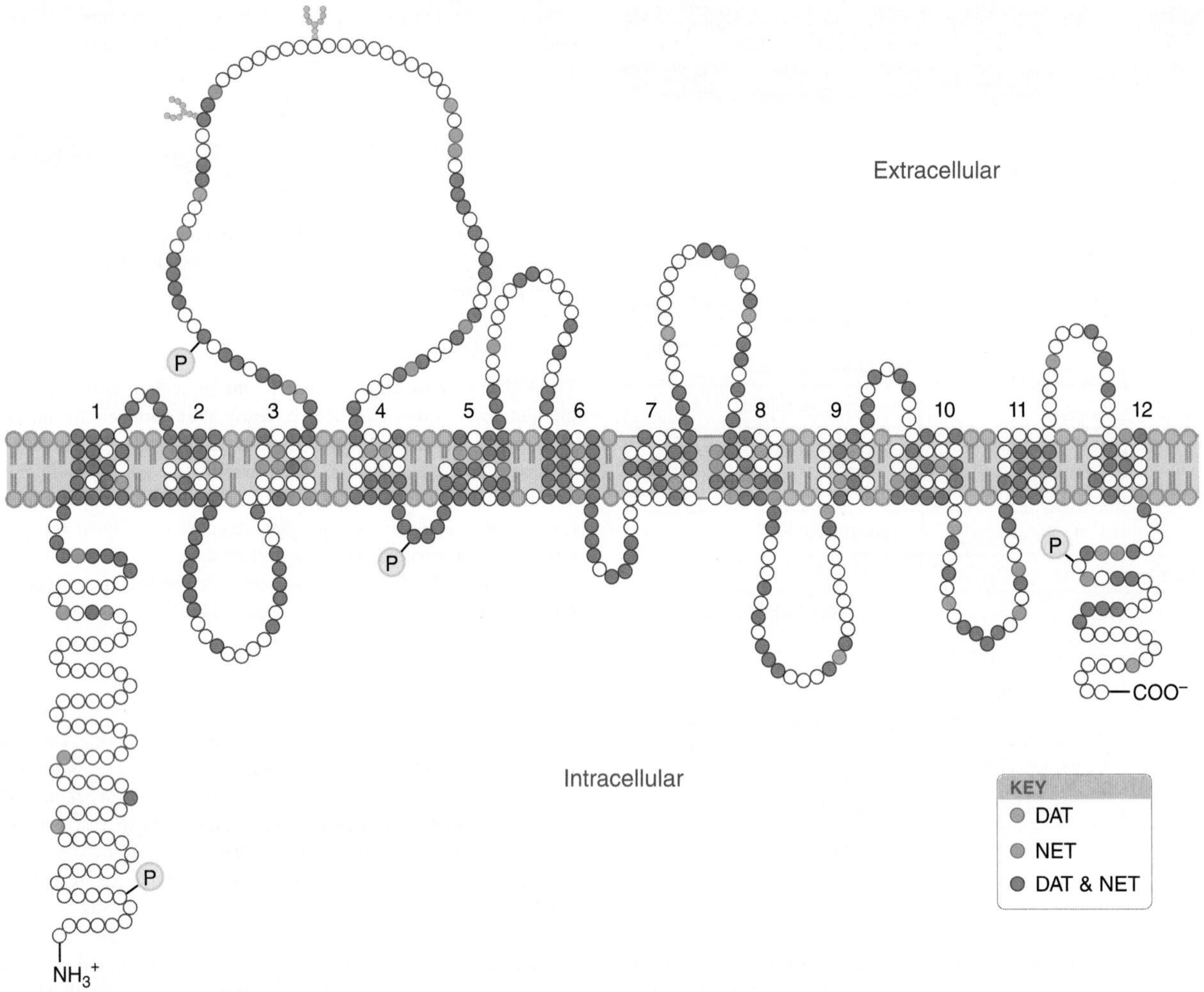

Extracellular

Intracellular

KEY
- DAT
- NET
- DAT & NET

Figure 14–8 *Structure of the rat 5HT transport protein.* Both the N terminus (NH_3^+) and C terminus (COO^-) are intracellular. These proteins typically have 12 hydrophobic, membrane-spanning domains with intervening extracellular and intracellular loops. The second extracellular loop is the largest and contains several potential glycosylation sites (indicated with tree-like symbols). Amino acid residues that are homologous to those in the DAT and the NET are colored, as noted. The most highly conserved regions of these transporters are located in the transmembrane domains; the most divergent areas occur in the N and C termini. (Used with permission from Dr. Beth J. Hoffman, Vertex Pharmaceuticals, San Diego, CA.)

activate K^+ channels, and reduce Ca^{2+} conductance and interact with G_q to enhance PLC activity. Presynaptic $GABA_B$ receptors function as autoreceptors, inhibiting GABA release, and may play the same role on neurons releasing other transmitters. A number of $GABA_B$ agonists have been

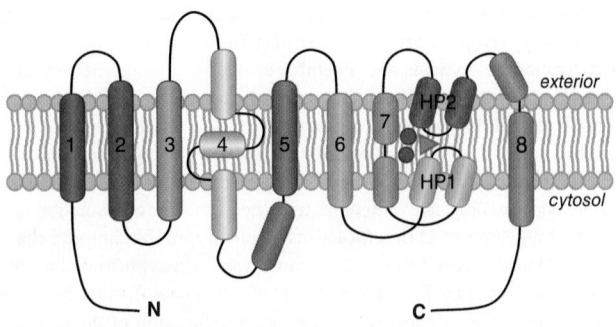

Figure 14–9 *General model of the mammalian EAATs.* The EAAT family includes the plasma membrane transporters EAAT1 to EAAT5. In this schematic model, transmembrane domains (colored oblongs) are labeled 1–8. Approximate binding sites occupied by Na^+ (blue dots) and substrate (green triangle) are formed by the nonhelical segments at the tips of two hairpin loops, HP1 and HP2.

identified, including baclofen (Figure 14–10), which is a skeletal muscle relaxant, and the psychoactive drug GHB, which is sometimes used to treat narcolepsy but is also used recreationally as an intoxicant.

Glycine

Glycine is an amino acid normally incorporated into proteins that can also act as an inhibitory neurotransmitter, particularly in the spinal cord and brainstem. Glycine is synthesized primarily from serine by serine hydroxymethyltransferase (SHMT). Glycine is imported into synaptic vesicles by a vesicular transport system identical to that used by GABA (VGAT). The action of glycine in the synaptic cleft is terminated by reuptake through specific transporters (GLYT1 and GLYT2) located on presynaptic nerve terminals and glia cells. These transporters can be distinguished pharmacologically and present attractive therapeutic targets for the modulation of glycine levels.

Actions of glycine are an active area of research, especially considering that there are glycine-binding sites on NMDA receptors. Glycine acts as a coagonist at NMDA receptors, such that both glutamate and glycine must be present for activation to occur (see discussion that follows). In addition to the NMDA receptor site, there are specific ionotropic glycine receptors that contain many of the structural features described for other ligand-gated ion channels (pentamers of subunits containing four transmembrane domains). These function as hyperpolarizing Cl^- channels and are prominent in the brainstem and spinal cord. Multiple subunits (currently four known

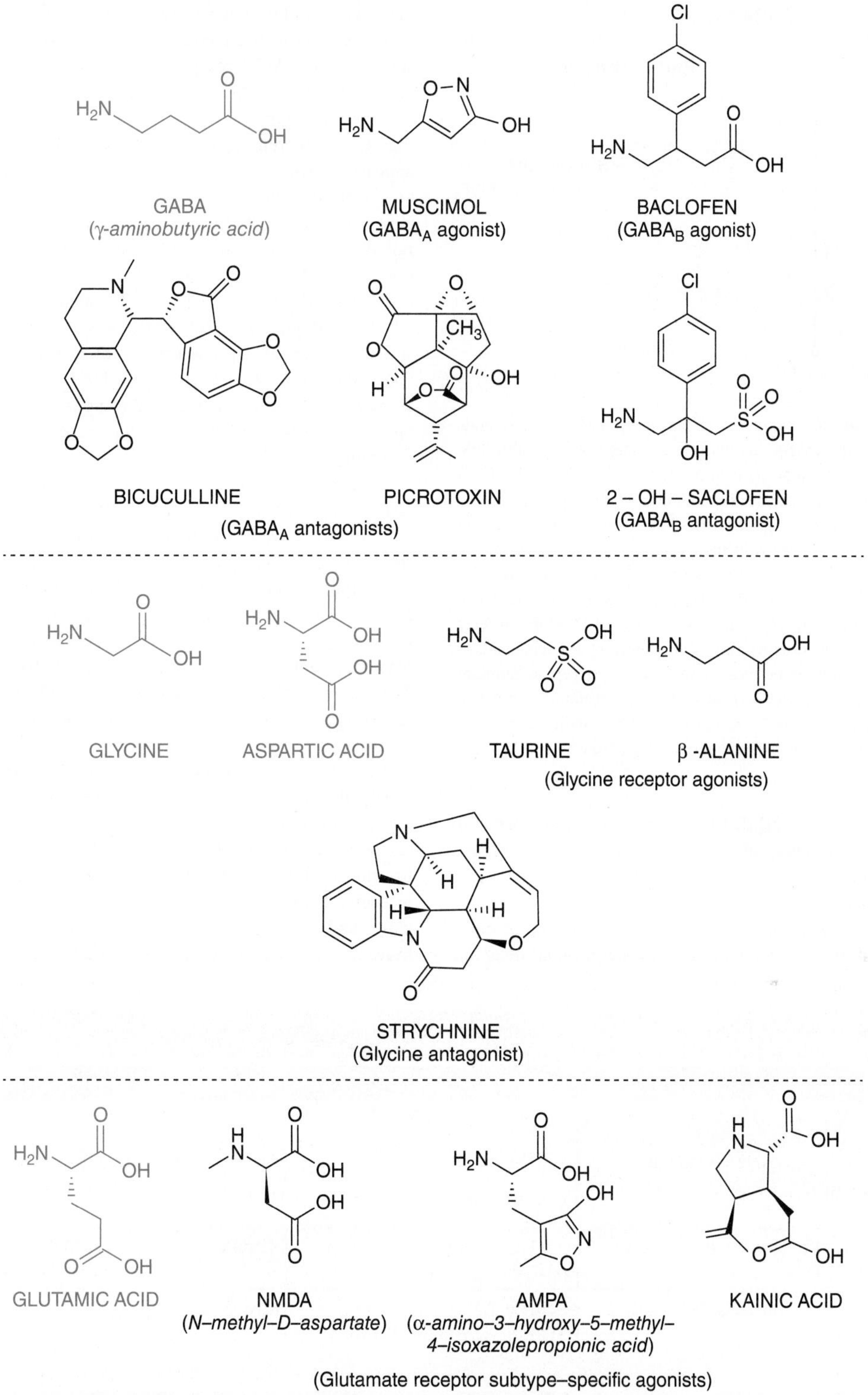

Figure 14–10 *Amino acid transmitters (red) and congeners (black).*

α subunits and a single β subunit) can assemble into a variety of glycine receptor subtypes. Taurine and β-alanine are agonists of glycine receptors; strychnine, a potent convulsant, is a selective antagonist (Figure 14–10).

Glutamate

Glutamate and aspartate are dicarboxylate amino acid neurotransmitters with excitatory actions in the CNS. Both amino acids are found in high concentrations in the brain and have powerful excitatory effects on neurons in virtually every region of the CNS. Glutamate is the most abundant

excitatory neurotransmitter and the principal fast excitatory neurotransmitter. Glutamate acts though receptors that are classified as either *ligand-gated ion channels (ionotropic)* or *metabotropic GPCRs* (Table 14–2). A well-characterized phenomenon involving glutamate transmission is the induction of LTP and its converse, LTD. These phenomena are known for strengthening and changing synapses and have long been hypothesized to be an important mechanism in learning and memory.

Ionotropic glutamate receptors are ligand-gated ion channels that were historically divided into three classes, each named for its preferred

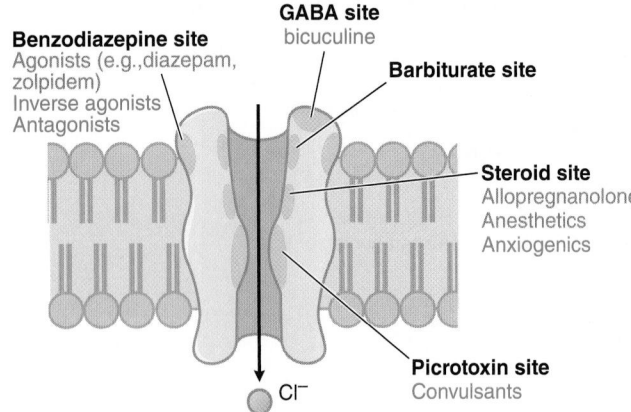

Figure 14–11 *Pharmacologic binding sites on the GABA$_A$ receptor.* GABA binds at the orthosteric site on the GABA$_A$ receptor. Other sites noted are allosteric sites at which agonists and antagonists may promote (green) or inhibit (red) receptor function. The GABA$_A$ receptor is a member of the Cys-loop family (Figure 11–1) but has a larger number of cavities in the transmembrane region and is susceptible to fewer natural toxins than several other family members. Miller and Smart (2010) have reviewed the features of this receptor and other Cys-loop receptors that contribute to orthosteric and allosteric modulation of receptor function. Hibbs and colleagues (Hibbs and Gouax, 2011; Morales-Perez et al, 2016) have recently provided structural data that suggest the mechanisms of activation, desensitization, and ion permeation in a Cys-loop receptor. Yamaura and colleagues (2016) have described a rapid screening procedure for putative allosteric modulators of the GABA$_A$ receptor.(Modified with permission from Nestler EJ et al., eds. *Molecular Neuropharmacology.* 3rd ed. McGraw-Hill, New York, **2015.**)

synthetic ligand (Figure 14–10): NMDA receptors, AMPA receptors, and KA receptors. With the discovery of an increasing number of subunits comprising these receptor categories, this classification has recently been refined (see Table 14–2).

The *NMDA receptors* consist of heteromers that are made up of multiple subunit combinations (termed GluNx) with the minimal receptor being a dimer of the GluN1 subunit and a GluN2 subunit. However, more complex heteromeric complexes are generated incorporating multiple subunits. The NMDA receptors have relatively high permeability to Ca^{2+} and are blocked by Mg^{2+} in a voltage-dependent manner. These receptors are unique in that their activation requires the simultaneous binding of two different agonists: In addition to glutamate, glycine binding appears necessary for activation (Figure 14–12). While NMDA receptors are involved in normal synaptic transmission, their activation is more closely associated with the induction of various forms of synaptic plasticity rather than fast point-to-point signaling in the brain. Aspartate is also a selective NMDA receptor agonist. Other NMDA receptor ligands include open-channel blockers such as PCP ("angel dust"); antagonists include 5,7-dichlorokynurenic acid, which acts at an allosteric glycine-binding site, and ifenprodil, which selectively inhibits NMDA receptors containing GluN2B subunits. The activity of NMDA receptors is sensitive to pH and to modulation by a variety of endogenous agents, including Zn^{2+}, some neurosteroids, arachidonic acid, redox reagents, and polyamines such as spermine.

The *AMPA receptors* exist predominantly as heterotetramers and contain multiple subunits (termed GluAx) as indicated in Table 14–2. In addition, there are TARPs that, together with a variety of scaffolding and regulatory proteins, modulate channel properties and alter the trafficking of receptors to and from perisynaptic and postsynaptic regions. AMPA receptors open and close rapidly, making them well suited to mediate the vast majority of excitatory synaptic transmission in the brain. Like NMDA receptors, AMPA receptors are involved in synaptic plasticity. They can be selectively antagonized by NBQX and CNQX, and similar antagonists are being explored as neuroprotective drugs for the treatment of stroke.

The *KA receptors* are composed of a distinct array of subunits (termed GluKx) that assemble as homo- or heterotetramers to form functional receptors. An important difference between KA and AMPA receptors is that KA receptors require extracellular Na$^+$ and Cl$^-$ for activation. KA receptors differ functionally from AMPA and NMDA receptors in other important ways. KA receptors do not reside predominantly within postsynaptic signaling complexes and are positioned to modulate neuronal excitability and synaptic transmission by altering the likelihood that the postsynaptic cell will fire in

TABLE 14–2 ■ CLASSIFICATION OF GLUTAMATE RECEPTORS

FAMILY	SUBTYPE	AGONISTS	ANTAGONISTS	
Ionotropic				
NMDA	GluN1, GluN2A, GluN2B, GluN2C, GluN2D, GluN3A, GluN3B	NMDA, aspartate	D-AP5, 2R-CPPene, MK-801, ketamine, phenycylidine, D-aspartate	
AMPA	GluA1, GluA2, GluA3, GluA4	AMPA, kainate, (s)-5-fluorowillardiine	CNQX, NBQX, GYK153655	
Kainate	GluK1, GluK2, GluK3, GluK4, GluK5	Kainate, ATPA, LY-339,434, SYM-2081, 5-iodowillardiine	CNQX, LY294486	
Metabotropic				
				SIGNALING
Group I	mGlu$_1$, mGlu$_5$	3,5-DHPG, quisqualate	AIDA S-(+)-CBPG	Activation of PLC (Gq)
Group II	mGlu$_2$, mGlu$_3$	APDC, MGS0028 DCG-IV, LY354740	EGLU PCCG-4	Inhibition of AC (Gi/Go)
Group III	mGlu$_4$, mGlu$_6$, mGlu$_7$, mGlu$_8$	L-AP4, (RS)-PPG	CPPG, MPPG, MSOP, LY341495	Inhibition of AC (Gi/Go)

AIDA, 1-aminoindan-1,5-dicarboxylic acid; AMPA, α-amino-3-hydroxy-5-methyl-4-isoxazolepropionic acid; L-AP4, L-2-amino-4-phosphonobutiric acid; ATPA, 2-amino-3(3-hydroxy-5-tert-butylisoxa-zol-4-yl)propanoic acid; CBPG, (S)-(+)-2-(3-carboxybicyclo(1.1.1)pentyl)-glycine; CNQX, 6-cyano-7-nitroquinoxaline-2,3-dione; D-AP5, D-2-amino-5-phosphonovaleric acid; DCG-IV, (2S,2'R,3'R)-2-(2',3'-Dicarboxycyclopropyl)glycine; (S)-3,4-DCPG, (S)-3,4-dicarboxyphenylglycine; 3,5-DHPG, 3,5-dihydroxyphenylglycine; EGLU, (2S)-α-ethylglutamic acid; MPPG, (RS)-α-methyl-4-phosphonophenylglycine; MSOP, (RS)-α-methylserine-O-phosphate; NBQX, 1,2,3,4-tetrahydro-6-nitro-2,3-dioxo-benzo[f]quinoxaline-7-sulfonamide; NMDA, *N*-methyl-D-aspartate; PCCG-4, phenylcarboxycyclopropylglycine; (RS)-PPG, (RS)-4-phosphonophenylglycine.

Glutamate is the principal agonist at both ionotropic and metabotropic receptors for glutamate and aspartate.

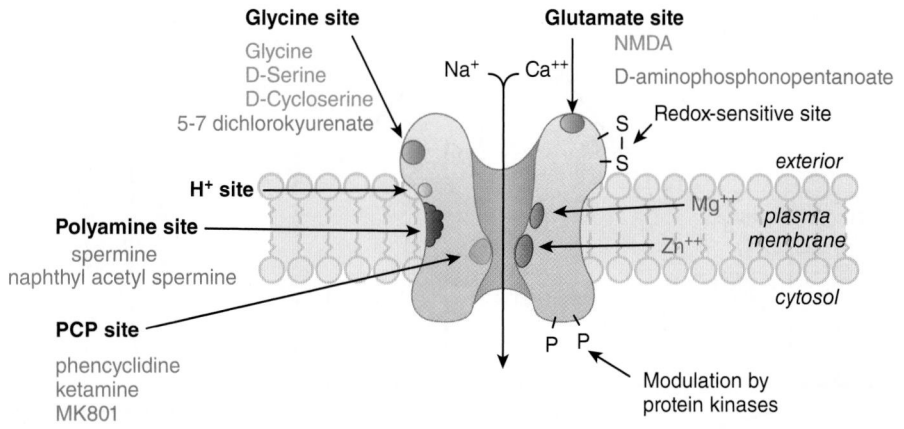

Figure 14–12 *Pharmacologic binding sites on the NMDA receptor.* Agents that promote receptor function are shown in ●. Those that inhibit receptor function appear in ●. Binding of both glutamate and glycine is necessary for activation.

response to subsequent stimulation. Presynaptic KA receptors have also been implicated in modulating GABA release through presynaptic mechanisms.

Glutamate-mediated excitotoxicity may underlie the damage that occurs when ischemia or hypoglycemia in the brain leads to a massive release and impaired reuptake of glutamate, resulting in excess stimulation of glutamate receptors and subsequent cell death. The cascade of events leading to neuronal death is thought to be triggered by excessive activation of NMDA or AMPA/KA receptors, allowing significant influx of Ca^{2+} into neurons (Figure 14–13). NMDA receptor antagonists can attenuate neuronal cell death induced by activation of these receptors. Glutamate receptors have become targets for diverse therapeutic interventions. For example, disordered glutamatergic transmission may play a role in the etiology of chronic neurodegenerative diseases (Chapter 18).

The *mGluRs* are GPCRs structurally defined by the presence of a large glutamate-binding N-terminal (extracellular) domain of about 560 amino acids. There are eight unique mGluRs organized into three subgroups (Table 14–2). mGluRs bind glutamate and function to "fine-tune" excitatory and inhibitory transmission by presynaptic, postsynaptic, and glial mechanisms, including the modulation of release and signaling of other neurotransmitters, among which are GABA, purines, DA, 5HT, and neuropeptides. Group I mGluRs couple to G_q, while groups II and III couple to G_i/G_o. mGluRs are located in a variety of brain regions and sometimes are linked to opposing functional responses. In general, group I receptors increase neuronal excitability, whereas both group II and group III suppress excitability. mGluRs play roles in the modulation of other receptors, function in synaptic plasticity, and are linked to several neurological diseases. They have recently become important drug targets, as subtype-selective agents are being discovered and investigated as potential therapies for various neuropsychiatric disorders.

Acetylcholine

Acetylcholine is present throughout the nervous system and functions as a neurotransmitter. It was the first neurotransmitter discovered and plays a primary role in the autonomic nervous system in ganglionic transmission as well as the peripheral nervous system, where it is the main neurotransmitter at the neuromuscular junction in vertebrates. ACh is synthesized by choline acetyltransferase and stored in the nerve endings. Following release and receptor activation, it is degraded by acetylcholinesterase (see Chapters 8–11). The effects of ACh result from interaction with two broad classes of receptors: ionotropic ligand-gated ion channels termed nicotinic receptors and metabotropic GPCRs called muscarinic receptors. In the CNS, ACh is found primarily in interneurons. The degeneration of particular cholinergic pathways is a hallmark of Alzheimer disease.

Nicotinic ACh receptors are found in skeletal muscle (see Figures 11–1 and 11–2) as well as in autonomic ganglia, the adrenal gland, and the CNS. Their activation by ACh results in a rapid increase in the influx of Na^+, depolarization, and the influx of Ca^{2+}. Nicotinic receptors are pentamers consisting of various combinations of 17 known subunits that can form the ion channel (Figure 14–6). In the CNS, nicotinic receptors are assembled as combinations of $\alpha(2-7)$ and $\beta(2-4)$ subunits. While pairwise combinations of α and β (e.g., α3β4 and α4β2), and in at least one case a homomeric α7 are sufficient to form a functional receptor in vitro, far more complex isoforms have been identified in vivo. The subunit composition strongly influences the biophysical and pharmacological properties of the receptor. Comprehensive listings of nicotinic receptor subunit combinations identified from recombinant expression systems, or in vivo, can be found in the work of Millar and Gotti (2009). Nicotinic cholinergic receptors have high therapeutic value, not only in the treatment of smoking cessation (they are the primary receptors for nicotine; see Chapter 11) but also for other neurological pathologies.

Muscarinic ACh receptors are GPCRs consisting of five subtypes, all of which are expressed in the brain. M_1, M_3, and M_5 couple to G_q, while the M_2 and M_4 receptors couple to G_i (Table 14–3). Chapter 9 presents detailed information on the physiology and pharmacology of muscarinic receptors.

Monoamines

Monoamines are neurotransmitters whose structure contains an amino group connected to an aromatic ring by a two-carbon chain. All are derived from aromatic amino acids and regulate neurotransmission that underlies cognitive processes, including emotion. Drugs that affect monoamine receptors and signaling are used to treat a variety of conditions, such as depression, schizophrenia, and anxiety, as well as movement disorders like Parkinson disease. Monoamines include DA, NE, EPI, histamine, 5HT, and the trace amines. Each system is anatomically distinct and serves separate, functional roles within its field of innervation.

Dopamine

Dopamine, NE, and EPI are catecholamine neurotransmitters (see Chapters 8 and 13). Notably, in contrast to the periphery, DA is the predominant catecholamine in the CNS. Its synthesis, degradation, and pharmacology are discussed in Chapter 13. There are several distinct pathways mediating DA signaling, including ones that play a role in motivation and reward (most drugs of abuse increase DA signaling), motor control, and the release of various hormones. These effects are mediated by five distinct GPCRs grouped into two subfamilies: D1-like receptors (D_1 and D_5) that stimulate adenylyl cyclase activity via coupling to G_s or G_{olf}, and D2-like receptors (D_2, D_3, and D_4) that couple to G_i/G_o to inhibit adenylyl

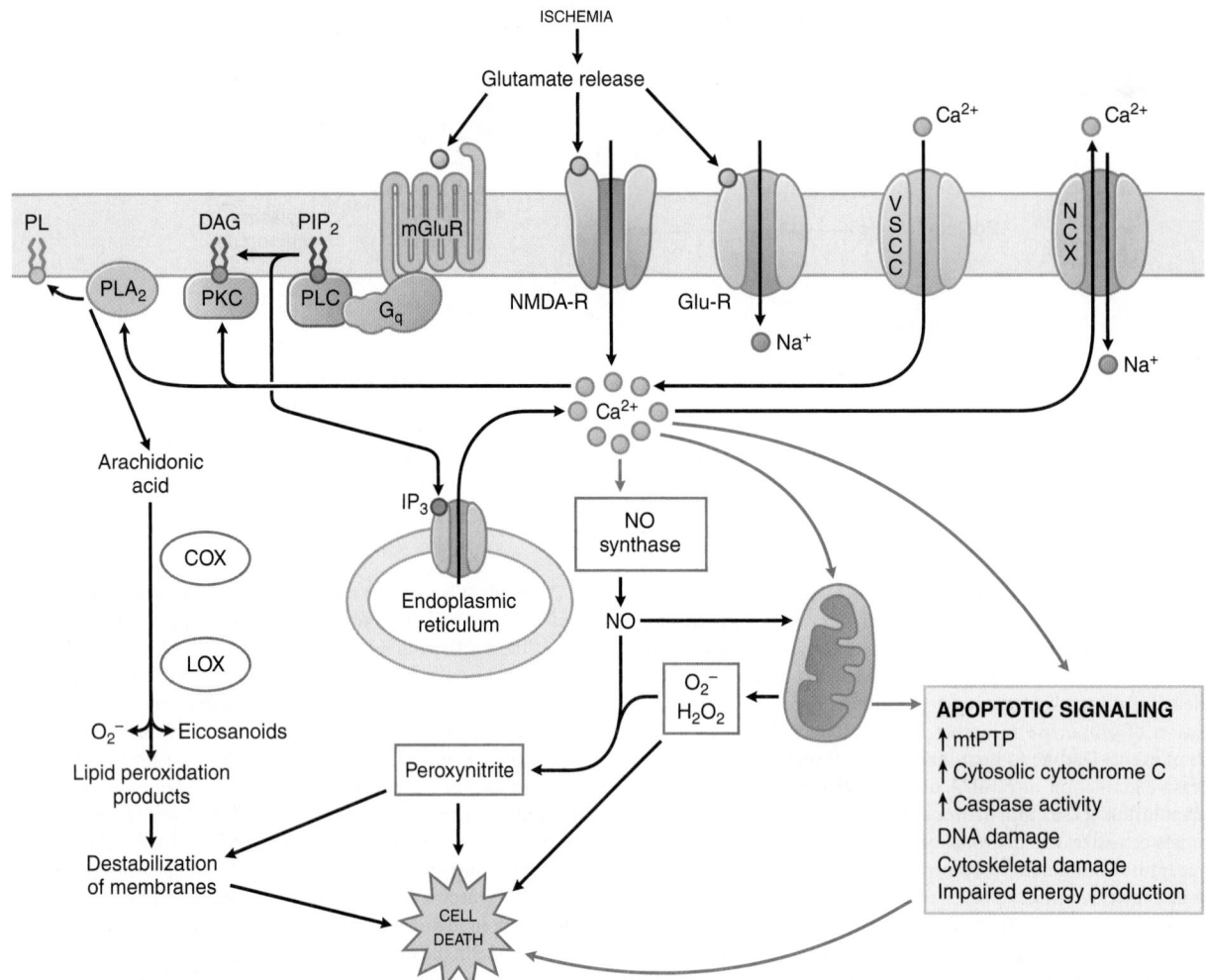

Figure 14–13 *Mechanisms contributing to glutamate-induced cytotoxicity/neuronal injury during ischemia-reperfusion–induced glutamate release.* Several pathways contribute to excitotoxic neuronal injury in ischemia, with excess cytosolic Ca²⁺ playing a precipitating role. (Reproduced with permission from Dugan LL, Kim-Han JS. Hypoxic-ischemic brain injury and oxidative stress. In: Siegel GS, et al., eds. *Basic Neurochemistry: Molecular, Cellular, and Medical Aspects.* 7th ed. Elsevier Academic Press, Burlington, MA, **2006**, 564. © 2006, American Society for Neurochemistry.) (See also Brady et al., 2012.)

cyclase activity and modulate various voltage-gated ion channels. DA receptor subtypes are discussed extensively in Chapter 13. DA-containing pathways and receptors have been implicated in the pathophysiology of schizophrenia and Parkinson disease and in the side effects following the pharmacotherapy of these disorders (see Chapters 16 and 18). There are three major DA-containing pathways in the CNS: the nigrostriatal, the mesocortical/mesolimbic, and the tuberoinfundibular, depicted in Figure 13–11.

TABLE 14–3 ■ SUBTYPES OF MUSCARINIC RECEPTORS IN THE CNS

SUBTYPE	TRANSDUCER EFFECTOR	AGONISTS (EXAMPLES)	ANTAGONISTS (EXAMPLES)
M₁	G_q Activation of PLC	Acetylcholine, carbachol, oxotremorine, pilocarpine, McN-A-343	Pirenzepine, telenzepine, 4-DAMP, xanomeline
M₂	G_iG_o Inhibition of AC	Acetylcholine, carbachol, oxotremorine	AF-DX 116, AF-DX 384, AQ-RA 741, tolterodine, (S)-(+)-dimethindene maleate, methoctramine
M₃	G_q Activation of PLC	Acetylcholine, carbachol, oxotremorine, pilocarpine, cevimeline	Darifenacin, 4-DAMP, DAU 5884, J-104129, tropicamide, tolterodine
M₄	G_iG_o Inhibition of AC	Acetylcholine, carbachol oxotremorine	AF-DX384, 4-DAMP, PD 102807, xanomeline
M₅	G_q Activation of PLC	Acetylcholine, carbachol, oxotremorine, pilocarpine	4-DAMP, xanomeline, VU-0488130 (ML381)

Acetylcholine is the endogenous transmitter for all muscarinic receptors. Nonselective antagonists include atropine, scopolamine, and ipratropium. 4-DAMP, 1,1-dimethyl-4-diphenylacetoxypiperidinium iodide.

TABLE 14–4 ■ ADRENERGIC RECEPTORS IN THE CNS

FAMILY	SUBTYPES	TRANSDUCER	AGONIST	ANTAGONIST
α_1 Adrenergic	α_{1A} α_{1B} α_{1D}	$G_{q/11}$	Epinephrine, phenylephrine, oxymetazoline, dabuzalgron (α_{1A}) A61603 (α_{1B})	Prazosin, doxazosin, terazosin, tamsulosin, alfuzosin, S(+)-niguldipine (α_{1A}), L-765314 (α_{1B}), BMY-7378 (α_{1D})
α_2 Adrenergic	α_{2A} α_{2B} α_{2C}	G_i/G_o	Epinephrine, norepinephrine, dexmedetomidine, clonidine, guanfacine	Yohimbine, rauwolscine
β Adrenergic	β_1 β_2 β_3	G_s	Epinephrine, norepinephrine, prenalterol (β_1), fenoterol (β_2), salbutamol (β_2), mirabegron (β_3), BRL37344 (β_3)	Carvedilol, bupranolol, levobunolol, metoprolol, propranolol, betaxolol (β_1), ICI118554 (β_2), SR 59230A (β_3)

Norepinephrine

NE is an endogenous neurotransmitter for the α and β adrenergic receptor subtypes that are present in the CNS; all are GPCRs (Table 14–4; see also Chapter 8). β adrenergic receptors couple to G_s to activate adenylyl cyclase. The α$_1$ adrenergic receptors couple to G_q, resulting in stimulation of the PLC-IP$_3$/DAG-Ca^{2+}-PKC pathway, and are associated predominantly with neurons. The interaction of NE with α$_1$ adrenergic receptors on noradrenergic target neurons causes a decrease in K$^+$ conductance, resulting in *depolarizing responses*. The α$_2$ adrenergic receptors are found on glial and vascular elements, as well as on neurons. They are prominent on noradrenergic neurons, where they couple to G_i, inhibit adenylyl cyclase, and mediate a *hyperpolarizing response* due to enhancement of an inwardly rectifying K$^+$ channel (via the βγ heterodimer). The α$_2$ adrenergic receptors are also located presynaptically, where they function as inhibitory autoreceptors to diminish the release of NE. The antihypertensive effects of clonidine may result from stimulation of such autoreceptors.

There are relatively large amounts of NE within the hypothalamus and in certain parts of the limbic system, such as the central nucleus of the amygdala and the dentate gyrus of the hippocampus. NE also is present in significant amounts in most brain regions. Mapping studies indicated that noradrenergic neurons of the locus ceruleus innervate specific target cells in a large number of cortical, subcortical, and spinomedullary fields.

Epinephrine

Most EPI in the brain is contained in vascular elements. Neurons in the CNS that contain EPI were recognized only after the development of sensitive enzymatic assays and immunocytochemical staining techniques for phenylethanolamine-*N*-methyltransferase, the enzyme that converts NE into EPI. EPI-containing neurons are found in the medullary reticular formation and make restricted connections to pontine and diencephalic nuclei, eventually coursing as far rostrally as the paraventricular nucleus of the thalamus. Their physiological properties have not been unequivocally identified.

Histamine

Histamine is a monoamine neurotransmitter in the CNS in addition to its well-known physiological function in immune and digestive responses in the periphery. Histaminergic neurons are located in the ventral posterior hypothalamus, where they give rise to long ascending and descending tracts that are typical of patterns characteristic of other monoaminergic systems. The histaminergic system is thought to affect arousal, body temperature, and vascular dynamics. The biosynthesis of histamine is described in Chapter 39. Histamine signals through four GPCR subtypes (H$_1$–H$_4$) that regulate either adenylyl cyclase or PLC (Figure 14–14). Interestingly, unlike other monoamine and amino acid transmitters, histamine does not appear to be a substrate for a unique reuptake transporter following its release, however, there are reports of its transport by NET and OCT3. Termination of its action likely involves its degradation by histamine-*N*-methyltransferase, a widely expressed cytosolic enzyme; diamine oxidase, which can oxidatively deaminate histamine, is lacking in the CNS. The histamine receptors, structure, signaling, functioning, and current understandings are reviewed in Chapter 39 and by Panula and colleagues (2015).

The H$_1$ receptors are widely distributed in the brain, where high densities are found in regions linked to neuroendocrine, behavioral, and nutritional state control. H$_1$ receptor activation excites neurons in most brain regions, and genetic knockout of the H$_1$ receptor results in behavioral abnormalities, consistent with the receptor's being a major player in cortical control of the sleep/wake cycle. This is evident in the well-known sedative actions of first-generation H$_1$ receptor blockers that are used in the treatment of allergies. The development of H$_1$ antagonists with low CNS penetration has reduced the incidence of sedation in the treatment of allergy-related disorders (see the table, Drug Facts for Your Personal Formulary: H$_1$ Antagonists, in Chapter 39), although, in some conditions the sedative effect of first-generation antihistamines can be beneficial in inducing sleep.

The H$_2$ receptors activate adenylyl cyclase and are primarily involved in gastric acid secretion and smooth muscle relaxation. H$_2$ receptor antagonists are a mainstay of treatment of dyspepsia and GI ulcers (see Chapter 49). H$_2$ receptors are also highly expressed in the brain, where they regulate neuronal physiology and plasticity. Mice lacking H$_2$ receptors show cognitive defects and impaired hippocampal LTP along with abnormalities in nociception. Difficulties in studying H$_2$ receptor signaling in the CNS are attributed to the fact that H$_2$ receptor ligands generally exhibit poor BBB penetration. However, there have been several clinical trials investigating H$_2$ receptor antagonists for treating supraspinal nociception; these trials have met with mixed results.

The H$_3$ receptors are also present in the CNS and can act as autoreceptors on histaminergic neurons to inhibit histamine synthesis and release. These receptors act to inhibit adenylyl cyclase and to modulate N-type voltage-gated Ca^{2+} channels. While it is known that H$_3$ receptors function as autoreceptors, they are not confined to histaminergic neurons and have been found to regulate serotonergic, cholinergic, noradrenergic, and dopaminergic neurotransmitter release. Exploiting the ability to modulate other neurotransmitters, the H$_3$ receptor has become a therapeutic target for treating conditions such as obesity, movement disorders, schizophrenia, ADHD, and wakefulness. A wide array of compounds have been developed that interact with the H$_3$ receptor, which have proved to be useful pharmacological tools both in vitro and in vivo. One compound, pitolisant, an inverse agonist at the H$_3$ receptor, has been granted orphan drug status for the treatment of narcolepsy and is currently in clinical trials for schizophrenia and Parkinson disease.

The H$_4$ receptors are expressed on cells of hematopoietic origin (eosinophils, T cells, mast cells, basophils, and dendritic cells) and are involved in eosinophil shape and mast cell chemotaxis. While some evidence has suggested that H$_4$ receptors are expressed in the CNS, this remains controversial and in need of further research. H$_4$ receptors have recently been demonstrated on microglia where they may indirectly affect neurons. Regardless, the vast majority of information about this subtype is related to allergy, asthma, and the antipruritic properties of H$_4$ antagonists.

Serotonin

The synthesis and degradation of 5HT are discussed in Chapter 13. There are diverse pathways mediating serotonin signaling that play a role in modulating mood, depression, anxiety, phobia, and GI effects. All but one

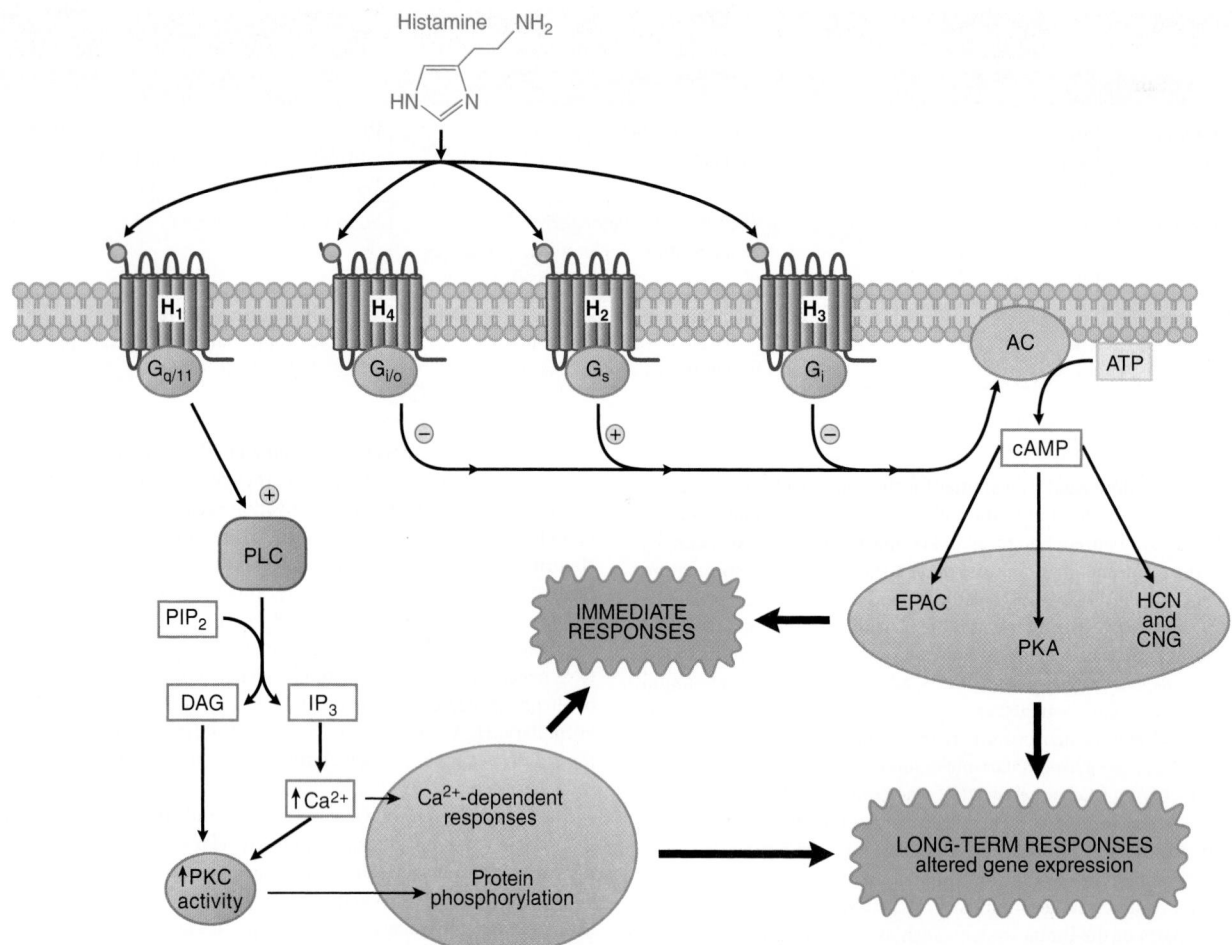

Figure 14–14 *Signal transduction pathways for histamine receptors.* Histamine can couple to a variety of G protein–linked signal transduction pathways via four different receptors. H_1 receptors activate phosphatidylinositol turnover via $G_{q/11}$. The other receptors couple either positively (H_2 receptor) or negatively (H_3 and H_4 receptor) to adenylyl cyclase activity via G_s and $G_{i/o}$, respectively. Signaling pathways affected by histamine provide both immediate and long-term regulation of cell function.

of the serotonin receptors are GPCRs and are targets for both therapeutic and recreational (hallucinogenic) drugs. These effects are mediated by 13 distinct GPCRs and 1 ligand-gated ion channel, which exhibit characteristic ligand-binding profiles, couple to different intracellular signaling systems, and exhibit subtype-specific distribution within the CNS. The 5HT receptors and their pharmacology are discussed in detail in Chapter 13.

Trace Amines

Trace amines, while discovered long ago, have only recently been appreciated as neurotransmitters. As the name implies, they are detected at trace levels (they have very short half-lives due to rapid metabolism by MAO). However, at least some trace amines act as neuromodulators/neurotransmitters at specific trace amine receptors. Trace amines are structurally related to catecholamines and consist of the PEAs (N-methylphenethylamine [an endogenous amphetamine isomer], phenylethanolamine, tyramine, tryptamine, N-methyltyramine, octopamine, synephrine, and 3-methoxytyramine). These trace amines are thought to act through GPCRs that were originally termed "trace amine receptors" but are now called TAARs because not all members have very high affinity for trace amines. The first receptor was identified in 2001 (Borowsky et al., 2001), and to date six TAAR genes (*TAAR1, TAAR2, TAAR5, TAAR6, TAAR8,* and *TAAR9*) have been identified in humans along with several potential pseudogenes. Multiple TAAR-related receptor genes have been identified in other species; several display prominent expression in the olfactory epithelium and are regarded as putative olfactory receptors for volatile amines. Only one TAAR (TAAR1) has been recognized

by IUPHAR as a trace amine receptor; it has been given the abbreviation TA₁. TA₁ has the highest affinity for the trace amines tyramine, β-phenylephrine, and octopamine. Emerging evidence suggests that TA₁ may modulate monoaminergic activity in the CNS. In addition to trace amines, TAARs can be activated by amphetamine-like psychostimulants and endogenous thyronamines such as thyronamine and 3-iodothyronamine.

Peptides

Neuropeptides typically behave as modulators in the CNS rather than causing direct excitation or inhibition. A growing number of neuropeptides have been described (Table 14–5) and are involved in a wide array of brain functions, ranging from analgesia to social behaviors, learning, and memory. In contrast to the biogenic amines or amino acids, peptide synthesis requires transcription of DNA to mRNA and translation of mRNA into protein. This takes place primarily in perikarya, and the resulting peptide is then transported to nerve terminals. Single genes can therefore, through transcriptional and posttranslational modifications, give rise to multiple neuropeptides. For example, proteolytic processing of POMC gives rise to, among other peptides, ACTH; α-, γ-, and β-MSHs; and β-endorphin (Figure 14–15). In addition, alternative splicing of RNA transcripts in different tissues may result in distinct mRNA species (e.g., calcitonin and CGRP). Furthermore, while some CNS peptides function independently, most are thought to act in concert with coexisting neurotransmitters. They are often packaged into vesicles and released along with other neurotransmitters to modulate their actions. While classical neurotransmitters generally signal to neurons by depolarizing or hyperpolarizing, neuropeptides

TABLE 14–5 ■ EXAMPLES OF NEUROPEPTIDES

Calcitonin Family	**Pituitary Hormones**
Calcitonin	Corticotropin (formerly adrenocorticotropic hormone; ACTH)
Calcitonin gene-related peptide (CGRP)	α-Melanocyte-stimulating hormone (α-MSH)
Hypothalamic Hormones	Growth hormone (GH)
Oxytocin, vasopressin	Follicle-stimulating hormone (FSH)
Hypothalamic Releasing and Inhibitory Hormones	β-Lipotropin (β-LPH), luteinizing hormone (LH)
Corticotropin-releasing factor (CRF or CRH)	**Tachykinins**
Gonadotropin-releasing hormone (GnRH)	Neurokinins A and B
Growth hormone-releasing hormone (GHRH)	Neuropeptide K, substance P
Somatostatin (SST)	**VIP-Glucagon Family**
Thyrotropin-releasing hormone (TRH)	Glucagon, glucagon-like peptide (GLP-1)
Neuropeptide Y Family	Pituitary adenylyl cyclase–activating peptide (PACAP)
Neuropeptide Y (NPY)	Vasoactive intestinal polypeptide (VIP)
Neuropeptide YY (PYY)	**Other Peptides**
Pancreatic polypeptide (PP)	Agouti-related peptide (ARP)
Opioid Peptides	Bombesin, bradykinin (BK)
β-Endorphin (also pituitary hormone)	Cholecystokinin (CCK)
Dynorphin peptides	Cocaine/amphetamine-regulated transcript (CART)
Leu-enkephalin	Galanin, ghrelin
Met-enkephalin	Melanin-concentrating hormone (MCH)
	Neurotensin, nerve growth factor (NGF)
	Orexins, orphanin FQ (nociceptin)
	Hemopressin (CB_1 inverse agonist)

Source: Modified with permission from Nestler EJ, et al., eds. *Molecular Neuropharmacology*. 2nd ed. McGraw-Hill, New York, **2009**.

have more diverse mechanisms of action and can also affect gene expression. Their action is not terminated by rapid reuptake into the presynaptic cell; rather, they are enzymatically inactivated by extracellular peptidases. As a result, their effects on neuronal signaling can be prolonged.

Neuropeptide Receptors

Most neuropeptide receptors are GPCRs, with the extracellular domains of the receptors playing primary roles in peptide-receptor interaction. As with other transmitter systems, there are often multiple receptor subtypes for the same peptide transmitter (Table 14–6). Neuropeptide receptors can exhibit different affinities for nascent neuropeptides and peptide analogues. Because peptides are typically inefficient as drugs, particularly at CNS targets due to difficulties permeating the BBB, major efforts have been made to develop small-molecule drugs that are effective as either agonists or antagonists at peptide receptors. Through a combination of structural biology, chemistry, high-throughput screening, and drug development, there are now small-molecule ligands for many neuropeptide receptors. Some of these compounds are listed in Table 14–6. Notably, natural products have not typically been good sources of drugs that affect peptidergic transmission. One exception is the plant alkaloid morphine, which acts selectively at opioid receptor subtypes (see Chapter 20).

Purines

Adenosine, ATP, UDP, and UTP have roles as extracellular signaling molecules. ATP is also a component of many neurotransmitter storage vesicles and is released along with transmitters. Intracellular nucleotides may reach the exterior cell surface by other means; for example, for example, extracellular adenosine can result from cellular release and metabolism of ATP. Released nucleotides can be hydrolyzed extracellularly by ectonucleotidases. Extracellular nucleotides and adenosine can act on a family of diverse purinergic receptors, which have been implicated in a variety of functions, including memory and learning, locomotor behavior, and feeding.

Purinergic Receptors

Purinergic receptors are divided into three classes: adenosine receptors (also called P1), P2Y, and P2X (Table 14–7). *Adenosine receptors* are GPCRs that consist of four subtypes (A_1, A_{2A}, A_{2B}, and A_3) activated endogenously by adenosine. A_1 and A_3 couple to G_i; A_2 receptors couple to G_s. Activation of A_1 receptors is associated with inhibition of adenylyl cyclase, activation of K^+ currents, and in some instances, activation of PLC; stimulation of A_2 receptors activates adenylyl cyclase. In the CNS, both A_1 and A_{2A} receptors are involved in regulating the release of other neurotransmitters, such as glutamate and DA, making the A_{2A} receptor a potential therapeutic target for disorders, including Parkinson disease.

The *P2Y receptors* are also GPCRs and are activated by ATP, ADP, UTP, UDP, and UDP-glucose. There are eight known subtypes of P2Y receptors that couple to a variety of G proteins (Table 14–7). The $P2Y_{14}$ receptor is expressed in the CNS, where it is stimulated by UDP-glucose and may play a role in neuroimmune functions. The $P2Y_{12}$ receptor is important clinically: Inhibition of this receptor in platelets inhibits platelet aggregation.

In contrast to the other two families, ATP-sensitive *P2X receptors* are ligand-gated cation channels that are expressed throughout the CNS on both presynaptic and postsynaptic nerve terminals and on glial cells. P2X receptors are found on nociceptive sensory neurons, where they primarily gate Na^+, K^+, and Ca^+ and are implicated in mediating sensory transduction. There are seven subtypes of P2X receptors with varying sensitivities to their endogenous agonist ATP (Table 14–7). Functional P2X receptors have a trimeric topology, existing as either homopolymers or heteropolymers with other P2X receptors, as confirmed by X-ray crystallography of a $P2X_4$ receptor (Kawate et al., 2009). The study of compounds that are selective for some P2X subtypes suggests that targeting these receptors may be useful in the therapy of neuropathic and inflammatory pain, thrombosis, arthritis, and depression.

Neuromodulatory Lipids

Cannabinoids

In the 1960s, THC (Figure 14–16) was identified as a psychoactive substance in marijuana. This led to the discovery and cloning of the two cannabinoid receptors and the identification of endogenous compounds that modulate them. The two receptor subtypes (CB_1 and CB_2) are GPCRs that couple to G_i/G_o to inhibit adenylyl cyclase and, in some

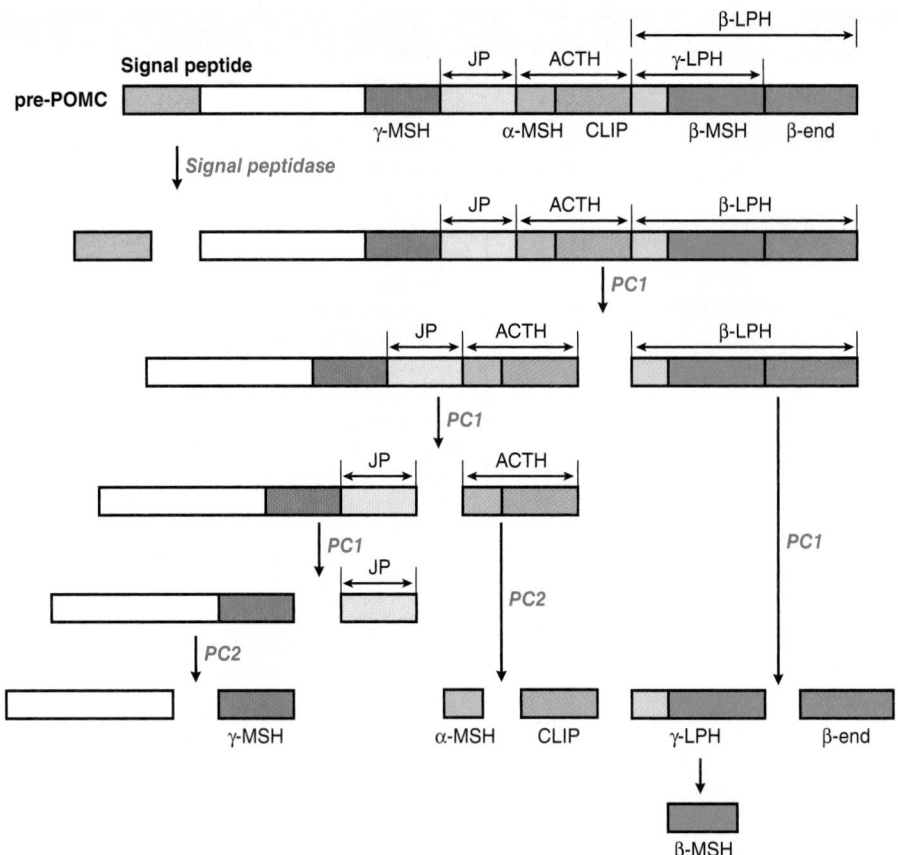

Figure 14–15 *Proteolytic processing of POMC.* After removal of the signal peptide from pre-POMC, the remaining propeptide undergoes endoproteolysis by prohormone convertases 1 and 2 (PC1 and PC2) at dibasic residues. PC1 liberates the bioactive peptides ACTH, β-endorphin (β-end), and γ-LPH. PC2 cleaves ACTH into CLIP and α-MSH and also releases γ-MSH from the N-terminal portion of the propeptide. The JP (joining peptide) is the region between ACTH and γ-MSH. β-MSH is formed by cleavage of γ-LPH. Some of the resulting peptides are amidated or acetylated before they become fully active.

TABLE 14–6 ■ PEPTIDE TRANSMITTERS AND RECEPTORS

FAMILY	SUBTYPE	TRANSDUCER	AGONISTS	ANTAGONISTS
Opioid	δ κ μ NOP	G_i/G_o	β-Endorphin, dynorphin, DPDPE (δ), salvinorin A(κ), hydromorphone (μ), fentanyl (μ), codeine (μ), methadone (μ), DAMGO (μ), etorphine Ro64-6198 (NOP)	Naltrexone, naloxone, SB612111
Somatostatin	sst_1, sst_2 sst_3, sst_4 sst_5	G_i	SST-14, SST-18, pasireotide, cortistatin, BIM23059, BIM23066, BIM23313, CGP23996, octreotide ($sst_{2,3,5}$)	SRA880 (sst_1), D-Tyr8-CYN154806 (sst_2), NVPACQ090 (sst_3)
Neurotensin	NTS_1 NTS_2	$G_{q/11}$	EISAI-1, JMV431, JMV449 (NTS_1), levocabastine (NTS_2)	SR142948A, meclinertant (NTS_1)
Orexin	OX_1 OX_2	$G_{q/11}$, G_s, G_i	Orexin-A, Orexin-B	Suvorexant, filorexant, SB-649868, almorexant, SB-410220, JNJ 10397049
Tachykinin	NK_1 NK_2 NK_3	$G_{q/11}$	Neurokinin A, neurokinin B, substance P, GR 73632 (NK_1), GR 64349 (NK_2), senktide	Aprepitant (NK_1), GR 159897 (NK_2), SB218795 (NK_3)
Cholecystokinin	CCK_1 CCK_2	$G_{q/11}$ (CCK_1), G_s	Cholecystokinin-8, CCK-33, CCK-58, gastrin, A-71623 (CCK_1)	Proglumide, FK-480, lintitript, PD-149164, devazepide (CCK_1), CL988 (CCK_2)
Neuropeptide Y	Y_1 Y_2 Y_4 Y_5	G_i/G_o	Neuropeptide Y, BWX 46	BIBO 3304 (Y_1), BIIE0246 (Y_2), UR-AK49, CGP 71683A GW438014A (Y_5)
Neuropeptide FF	NPFF1 NPFF2	$G_{q/11}$, G_i/G_o	Neuropeptide FF, RFRP-3 (NPFF1)	RF9

TABLE 14–7 ■ CHARACTERISTICS OF PURINERGIC RECEPTORS

CLASS	RECEPTOR			
Adenosine (P1)[a]	A_1	A_{2A}	A_{2B}	A_3
Transducer	$G_{i/o}$	G_s	G_s	$G_{i/o}$
Agonists	CPA	CGS21680	BAY 60-6583	1B-MECA
Antagonists	CPX	SCH58261	MRS1754	VUF5574

CLASS	RECEPTOR						
P2X (ionotropic)	$P2X_1$	$P2X_2$	$P2X_3$	$P2X_4$	$P2X_5$	$P2X_6$	$P2X_7$
Substrate specificity	ATP	ATP	ATP	ATP>CTP	ATP	ATP	ATP
Antagonist	NF449, TNP-ATP	NF770	TNP-ATP	5-BDBD, paroxetine	PPADS, suramin		AZ10606120

CLASS	RECEPTOR							
P2Y (metabotropic)	$P2Y_1$	$P2Y_2$	$P2Y_4$	$P2Y_6$	$P2Y_{11}$	$P2Y_{12}$	$P2Y_{13}$	$P2Y_{14}$
Transducer	$G_{q/11}$	$G_{q/11}$	$G_{q/11}$	$G_{q/11}$	$G_s, G_{q/11}$	$G_{i/o}$	$G_{i/o}$	$G_{i/o}$
Substrate specificity[b]	ADP>ATP	ATP>UTP	UTP>ATP	UDP>>UTP>ADP	ATP=UTP	ADP	ADP>>ATP	UDP-glucose[b]
Agonists	MRS2365	MRS2698, PSB1114	MRS4062	MRS2957	AR-C67085	2MeSADP	2MeSADP	MRS2690
Antagonists	MRS2279	ARC118925X		MRS2578	NF157	ticagrelor, clopidogrel	MRS2211, cangrelor	PPTN

CPA, N6-cyclopentyladenosine; CPX, 8-cyclopentyl-1,3-dipropylxanthine; 1B-MECA, N6-(3-iodobenzyl)-adenosine-5α-N-methylcarboxamide; NECA, 1-(6-amino-9H-purin-9-yl)-1-deoxy-N-ethyl-β-D-ribofuronamide; PPADS, pyridoxalphosphate-6-azophenyl-2',4'-disulfonic acid; TNP-ATP, 2',3'-O-(2,4,6-trinitrophenyl)adenosine-5'-triphosphate. For further details, consult information about the three classes of purinergic receptors at http://www.guidetopharmacology.org.

[a]NECA is a nonselective agonist of P1 receptors.

[b]$P2Y_{14}$ binds UDP-glucose, UDP-galactose, or UDP-acetylglucosamine.

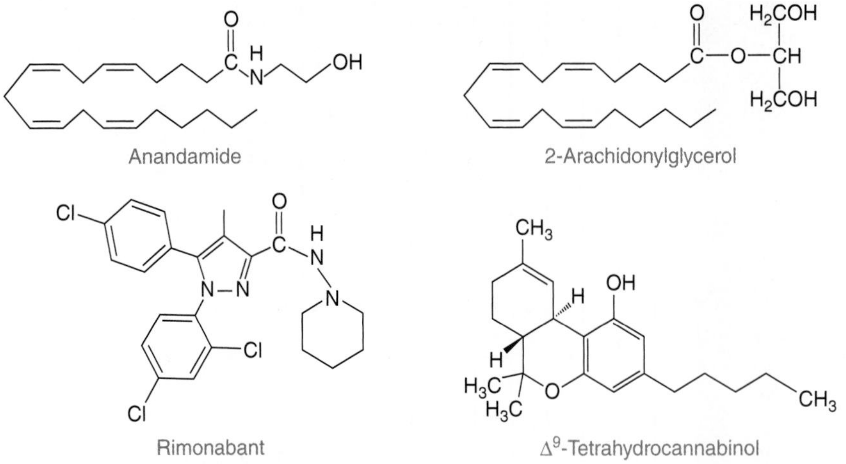

Figure 14–16 *Cannabinoid receptor ligands.* Anandamide and 2-arachidonylglycerol are endogenous agonists. Rimonabant is a synthetic CB receptor antagonist. Δ^9-tetrahydrocannabinol is a CB agonist derived from marijuana.

cell types, inhibit voltage-gated Ca^+ channels or stimulate K^+ channels. The receptors share relatively low overall homology and are found in differing locations, although both are found in the CNS. CB_1 receptors are found in high levels throughout the brain, whereas CB_2 receptors are prominent in immune cells. Within the CNS, CB_2 receptors are expressed less than CB_1 receptors and are thought to occur primarily on microglia. Several orphan GPCRs (GPCRs with no known endogenous agonist) have been implicated as being cannabinoid-like, and as such, more cannabinoid receptor subtypes may exist. The finding of endogenous cannabinoids responsible for signaling to these receptors, along with a host of clinical data from marijuana use, has fueled interest in this signaling system and has greatly expanded our understanding of its physiology.

The *ECS* (endogenous cannabinoid system) consists of the cannabinoid receptors, endogenous cannabinoids, and the enzymes that synthesize and degrade endocannabinoids. The endocannabinoids are lipid molecules and include anandamide (*N*-arachidonoylethanolamine) and 2-arachidonoylglycerol (2-AG), as well as other compounds that have been putatively identified to serve as endogenous endocannabinoids, including *O*-arachidonoylethanolamine (virodhamine), *N*-dihomo-γ-linolenoylethanolamine, *N*-docosatetraenoic-ethanolamine, oleamide, 2-arachidonyl-glyceryl-ether (2-AGE), N-arachidonoyl-dopamine (NADA), and *N*-oleoyl-dopamine. The actions of endocannabinoids are terminated by their uptake into cells, followed by hydrolysis. Two enzymes known to break down anandamide and 2-AG are fatty acid amide hydrolase (FAAH) and monoacylglycerol lipase (MGL), respectively. Although a few studies suggested the existence of a specific transport system for endocannabinoids, no molecular entity that mediates such a carrier-mediated process has been identified. Obviously, drugs that inhibit the transport or degradation of endocannabinoids would prolong their physiological actions.

There is now strong evidence that the ECS functions as a retrograde signaling messenger system, generally serving to inhibit the presynaptic release of neurotransmitters (Figure 14–17). Depending on the cell type, this action can last from seconds to hours, resulting in a large influence on neuronal circuit function. Endocannabinoids thus function as neuromodulators and have been linked to a variety of neuronal processes, including pain sensation, stress response, anxiety, appetite, and motor learning. The ECS has been targeted pharmacologically in a variety of ways, including compounds that act on the enzymes responsible for breaking down (FAAH inhibitors) or synthesizing endocannabinoids, compounds that target the transport mechanism (AM404, *N*-arachidonoylaminophenol), or drugs that directly stimulate or inhibit the CB receptors.

Marijuana is known to stimulate appetite via activation of the CB_1 receptor; thus, efforts have been undertaken to develop CB_1 antagonists for the treatment of obesity. Rimonabant, an inverse agonist of the CB_1 receptor, was initially approved in Europe as an anorectic, but subsequently was withdrawn due to adverse effects, including increased suicidality and depression. It currently remains unclear whether CB_1 receptor antagonism will prove useful for the treatment of appetitive or addictive disorders. However, CB_1 receptor agonists have a wide variety of effects that make them attractive candidates for drug discovery efforts. They stimulate appetite in patients with AIDS, reduce seizure frequency in epilepsy, decrease intraocular pressure in patients with glaucoma, treat nausea caused by cancer chemotherapy (dronabinol; see Table 50–4 and Figure 50–5), and reduce pain (nabilone). This wide range of potential therapeutic benefits has driven the medical marijuana movement such that, in some states, marijuana can be legally used as a therapeutic under a doctor's prescription.

Other Lipid Mediators

Arachidonic acid, normally stored within the cell membrane as a glycerol ester, can be liberated during phospholipid hydrolysis (by pathways involving phospholipases A_2, C, and D). Arachidonic acid can be converted to highly reactive modulators by three major enzymatic pathways (see Chapter 37: *cyclooxygenases* (leading to prostaglandins and thromboxane), *lipoxygenases* (leading to the leukotrienes and other transient catabolites of eicosatetraenoic acid), and *CYPs* (which are inducible and also expressed at low levels in brain). Arachidonic acid metabolites have been implicated as diffusible modulators in the CNS, possibly involved with the formation of LTP and other forms of neuronal plasticity.

Gases

Nitric Oxide and Carbon Monoxide

Both constitutive and inducible forms of NOS are expressed in the brain. The application of inhibitors of NOS (e.g., methylarginine) and of NO donors (such as nitroprusside) suggests the involvement of NO in a host of CNS phenomena, including LTP, activation of soluble guanylyl cyclase, neurotransmitter release, and enhancement of glutamate (NMDA)–mediated neurotoxicity. CO, generated in neurons or glia, is another diffusible gas that may act as an intracellular messenger stimulating soluble guanylyl cyclase through nonsynaptic actions. NO synthesis and signaling are presented in Chapter 3.

Regulatory Substances

Neurotrophins

The NTs constitute a family of proteins that include NGF, BDNF, NT-3, and NT-4/5, which regulate neuronal proliferation, differentiation, survival, migration, dendritic arborization, synaptogenesis, and activity-dependent

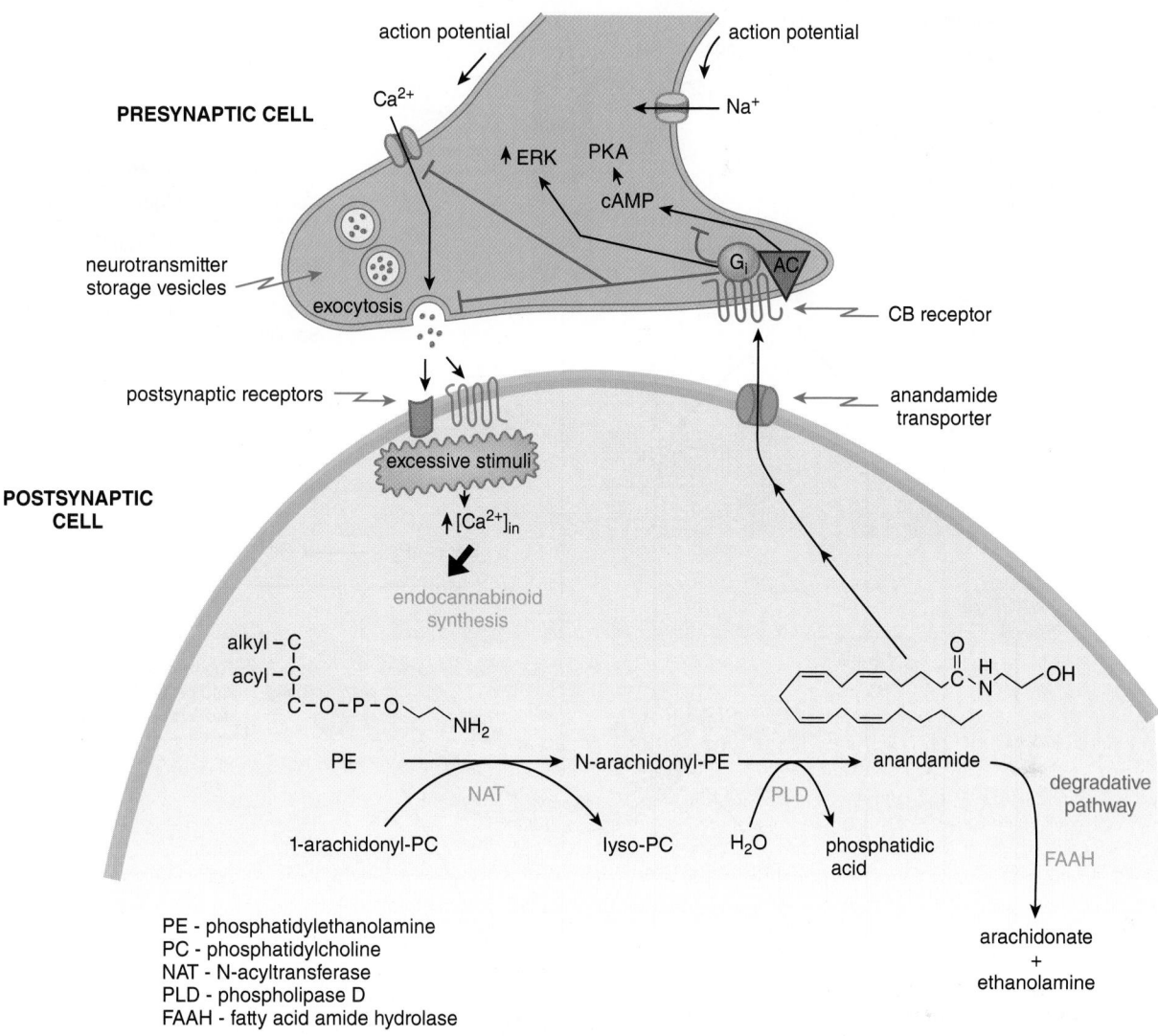

Figure 14–17 *Anandamide synthesis and signaling in the CNS.* Endocannabinoids, synthesized on demand in stimulated postsynaptic cells, appear to function as a negative feedback system to limit further presynaptic transmitter release.

forms of synaptic plasticity in the developing and mature CNS. NTs are synthesized as pro-NT precursors and processed to smaller, active NTs of about 13–26 kDa. Biological effects of NTs and pro-NTs are mediated by the Trk family of tyrosine kinase receptors and the p75 NT receptor through activation of complex signaling mechanisms summarized by Figure 14–18.

The function of BDNF has been most prominently studied; it modulates the establishment of neuronal circuits that regulate complex behaviors. Transcription and translation of the *Bdnf* gene are exquisitely regulated in the CNS with at least eight distinct promotors that initiate transcription of multiple distinct mRNA transcripts, each containing a full-length BDNF transcript after alternative splicing (Aid et al., 2007). In addition, *Bdnf* transcripts populate two different pools of mRNAs that are localized to distinct subcellular compartments in neurons (Timmusk et al., 1993). Finally, BDNF is initially synthesized as a precursor protein (preproBDNF) and, on cleavage of the signal peptide, is sorted into constitutive or regulated secretory vesicles. Conversion of the proBDNF to mature BDNF (mBDNF) occurs prior to release, and mBDNF is thought to be the main biologically active form, although proBDNF has biological activity at the sortilin-p75^{NTR} complex (Bothwell, 2016). There is strong evidence that BDNF plays a role in synaptic plasticity and cognitive function (Greenberg et al., 2009; Lu et al., 2008). As a consequence, dysregulation of BDNF function or expression is implicated in the pathophysiology of age-related neurodegenerative diseases (Pang and Lu, 2004) and susceptibility to

neuropsychiatric disorders such as anxiety and depression. Efforts to deliver NTs or modulate regulation of NT expression are being pursued as treatments for these CNS disorders. Despite these efforts, NTs are not yet used routinely in the clinic.

Neurosteroids

Neuroactive steroids that are synthesized in neuronal tissue are known as neurosteroids. Synthesis of neurosteroids occurs de novo from cholesterol or from circulating hormones (Reddy and Estes, 2016) by several key steroidogenic enzymes that are expressed throughout the vertebrate brain (Do Rego et al., 2009). Based on structural features, the neurosteroids can be categorized into three subtypes:

- pregnane neurosteroids such as allopregnanolone;
- androstane neurosteroids such as androstanediol; and
- sulfated neurosteroids such as DHEAS (Rahmani et al., 2015).

Neurosteroids can mediate an array of biological activities in the CNS through modulation of nuclear hormone receptors or through modulation of membrane receptor activity. More specifically, neurosteroids can allosterically modulate GABA$_A$ receptor complexes; glutamate receptors, including NMDA, AMPA, and KA; nicotinic and muscarinic ACh receptors; as well as sigma and glycine receptors (Do Rego et al., 2009). While little is known regarding the regulation of neurosteroid synthesis in the brain, in vivo studies indicate that these molecules can regulate a variety of

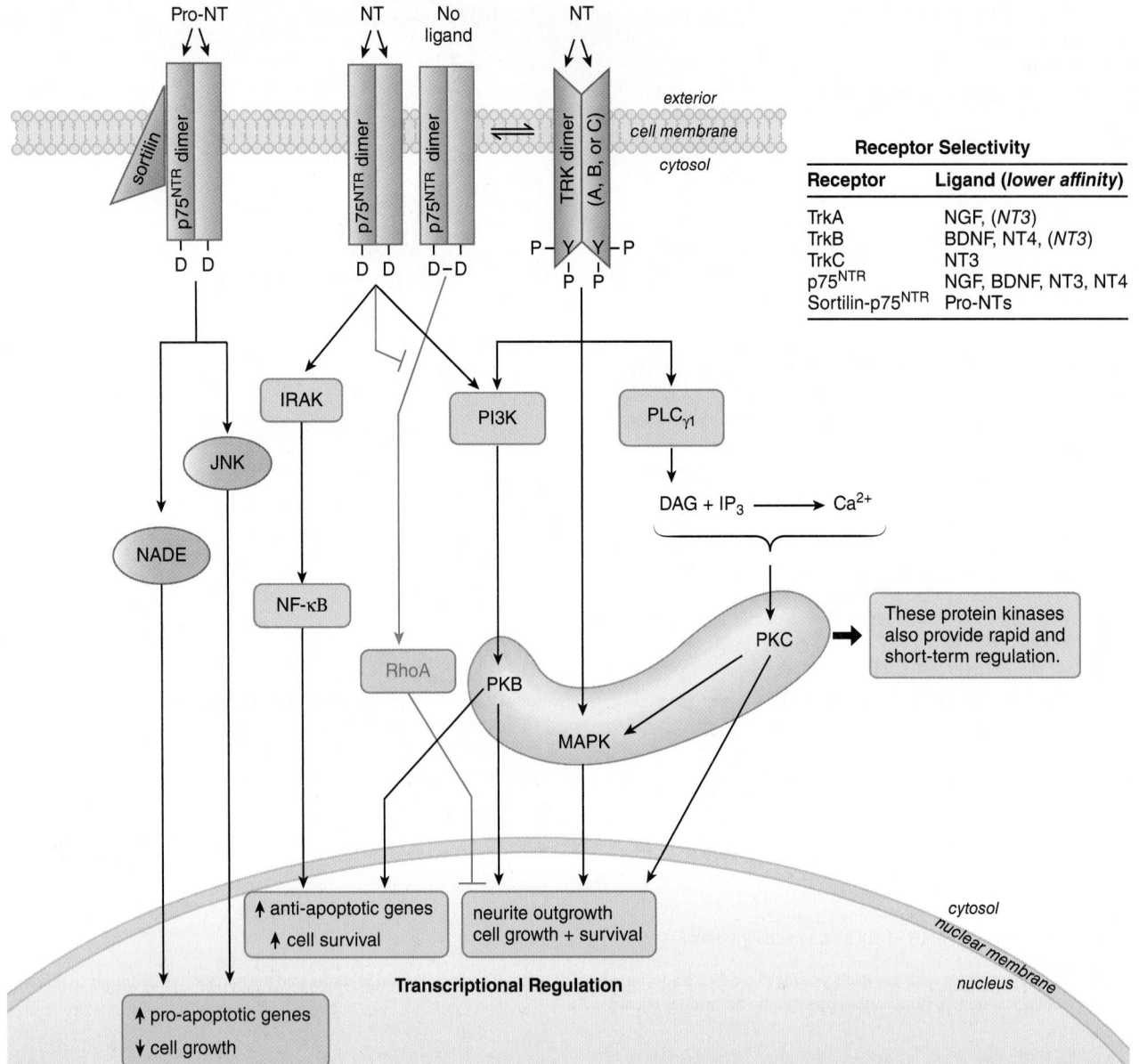

Figure 14–18 *Neurotrophic factor signaling in the CNS.* This schematic is a simplification of NT signaling pathways, which are complex and incompletely understood, with differential expression of NT receptors and NTs in different areas of the nervous system and a host of interacting systems that can affect signaling (Skaper, 2012; Bothwell, 2016). Pro-NTs and NTs interact with membrane receptor dimers of TRK receptors A, B, and C and of p75^{NTR} (a "death receptor" and member of the TNF receptor superfamily) with the specificities indicated by the table at the upper right. Ligand-receptor interactions stimulate signaling pathways that regulate transcription. Formation of an NT-TRK receptor dimer activates intracellular TRK receptor tyrosine kinase activities on the cytosolic tail of the receptor. Tyrosine phosphorylation (Y-P) provides binding sites for the adaptor proteins that lead to activation of the PI3K, MAPK, and PLCγ$_1$-PKC pathways (green boxes), which promote transcriptional regulation in support of neurite extension, cell growth, antiapoptosis, and cell survival. Unliganded p75^{NTR} may also modulate the activity of TRK receptor signaling. Unliganded p75^{NTR} dimers have a basal activity that results in activation of the RhoA pathway, leading to pro-apoptotic signaling (red boxes). NT binding to p75^{NTR} does not initiate intracellular signaling via activation of a receptor tyrosine kinase. Rather, NT binding to p75^{NTR} alters binding of various modulatory factors and causes proteolytic cleavages in the death domain region (DD); these perturbations of p75^{NTR} result in activation of the IRAK/NF-κB and PI3K pathways and inhibition of the RhoA pathway. The net result is neurite extension, cell growth, antiapoptosis, and cell survival. Pro-NT binding to p75^{NTR} in the presence of an accessory protein, sortilin, activates cellular events that permit binding/dimerization of death domain proteins (D), facilitating the activation of the NADE and JNK pathways, leading to inhibition of cell growth and an acceleration of pro-apoptotic events. A host of other signaling proteins can interact along the pathways sketched here. In addition, Trk receptors use signaling endosomes. Following activation near innervated tissues that produce NTs, Trk-NT complexes are endocytosed, and some receptors are recycled to the membrane, while others are destroyed in lysosomes. But, some other receptor-NT complexes (e.g., TrkA-NGF) are stable within the endosome and travel retrogradely along the neuron to the cell body as a signaling endosome. The cytoplasmic tail of an NT-p75^{NTR} complex may be cleaved and release into the cytosol, promoting signaling. IRAK, interleukin-associated kinase; JNK, c-Jun N-terminal kinase; NADE, p75NTR-associated death executor; NF-κB, nuclear factor kappa B; NT, neutrophin; NTR, neutrophin receptor; Trk, tropomyosin receptor kinase (tyrosine receptor kinase).

neurophysiological and behavioral processes, including cognition, stress, sleep, and arousal (Engel and Grant, 2001; Reddy and Estes, 2016). Neurosteroids are not currently used in the clinic, but there is evidence to suggest their utility for the treatment of psychiatric disorders, including cognitive deficits and negative symptoms in schizophrenia, anxiety and mood disorders, as well as mood-stabilizing agents in bipolar disorder (Vallee, 2016).

Cytokines

Cytokines are low-molecular-weight proteins that are secreted by many different cell types to modulate key cellular functions. The primary immune effector cells in the CNS are glia, microglia, and astrocytes. These cells can express and release a variety of cytokines, including the IL-1β and IL-6, TNF-α, and IFN-γ. Constitutive expression of cytokines is required for normal physiological functioning in the brain, particularly regarding the molecular and cellular mechanisms involved in neurite outgrowth, neurogenesis, neuronal survival, synaptic pruning during brain development, the strength of synaptic transmission, and synaptic plasticity. While glial cells are typically thought of as neuroprotective, overexpression or sustained stimulation can cause an elevation of pro-inflammatory cytokines in the brain, resulting in neuroinflammation, an innate immune response mediated by protein complexes known as inflammasomes (Singhal et al., 2014). Acute neuroinflammation involves the release of cytokines and chemokines, is the first line of defense against pathogens in the CNS, and is not likely to cause neuronal damage. Sustained chronic neuroinflammation accompanied by sustained brain exposure to pro-inflammatory cytokines is, however, a factor in the pathogenesis of neurodegenerative and psychiatric illnesses leading to cognitive and memory deficits and behavioral abnormalities (Furtado and Katzman, 2015; Heneka et al., 2015).

Acknowledgment: Floyd E. Bloom and Perry B. Molinoff contributed to this chapter in recent editions of this book. We have retained some of their text in the current edition.

Bibliography

Aid T, et al. Mouse and rat BDNF gene structure and expression revisited. *J Neurosci Res*, **2007**, *85*:525–535.

Borowsky B. et al. Trace amines: identification of a family of mammalian G protein-coupled receptors. *Proc Natl Acad Sci USA*, **2001**, *98*: 8966–8971.

Bothwell M. Recent advances in understanding neurotrophin signaling. *F1000Research* **2016** 5:F1000 Faculty Rev-1885. doi:10.12688/f1000research.8434.1. Accessed March 7, 2017.

Brady ST, et al. *Basic Neurochemistry: Principles of Molecular, Cellular, and Medical Neurobiology*. AElsevier/Academic Press, Boston, **2012.**

Catterall WA. From ionic currents to molecular mechanisms: the structure and function of voltage-gated sodium channels. *Neuron*, **2000**, *26*:13–25.

Do Rego JL, et al. Neurosteroid biosynthesis: enzymatic pathways and neuroendocrine regulation by neurotransmitters and neuropeptides. *Front Neuroendocrinol*, **2009**, *30*:259–301.

Engel SR, Grant KA. Neurosteroids and behavior. *Int Rev Neurobiol*, **2001**, *46*:321–348.

Furtado M, Katzman MA. Examining the role of neuroinflammation in major depression. *Psychiatry Res*, **2015**, *229*(1–2):27–36.

Greenberg ME, et al. New insights in the biology of BDNF synthesis and release: implications in CNS function. *J Neurosci*, **2009**, *29*:12764–12767.

Heneka MT, et al. Neuroinflammation in Alzheimer's disease. *Lancet Neurol*, **2015**, *14*:388–405.

Hibbs RE, Gouaux E. Principles of activation and permeation in an anion-selective Cys-loop receptor. *Nature*, **2011**, *474*:54–60.

Jentsch TJ. Chloride channels: a molecular perspective. *Curr Opin Neurobiol*, **1996**, *6*:303–310.

Kandel ER, et al. *Principles of Neural Science*. 5th ed. McGraw-Hill, Health Professions Division, New York, **2013.**

Kawate T, et al. Crystal structure of the ATP-gated P2X(4) ion channel in the closed state. *Nature*, **2009**, *460*:592–598.

Khan SM. The expanding roles of Gbg subunits in G protein–coupled receptor signaling and drug action. *Pharmacol Rev*, **2013**, *65*:545–577.

Lu Y, et al. BDNF: a key regulator for protein synthesis-dependent LTP and long-term memory? *Neurobiol Learn Mem*, **2008**, *89*:312–323.

Miller PS, Smart TG. Binding, activation, and modulation of Cys loop receptors. Trends Pharmacol Sci, **2010**, 31:161–174.

Millar NS, Gotti C. Diversity of vertebrate nicotinic acetylcholine receptors. *Neuropharmacology*, **2009**, *56*:237–246.

Morales-Perez CL, Noviello CM, Hibbs RE. X-ray structure of the human a4ß2 nicotinic receptor. *Nature*, **2016**, *538*:411–415.

Nestler EJ, et al. *Molecular Neuropharmacology: A Foundation for Clinical Neuroscience*. McGraw-Hill Companies, Inc., New York, **2015.**

Nilius B, Szallasi A. Transient receptor potential channels as drug targets: from the science of basic research to the art of medicine. *Pharmacol Rev*, **2014**, *66*:676–814.

Pang PT, Lu B. Regulation of late-phase LTP and long-term memory in normal and aging hippocampus: role of secreted proteins tPA and BDNF. *Ageing Res Rev*, **2004**, *3*:407–430.

Panula P, et al. International Union of Basic and Clinical Pharmacology. XCVIII. Histamine receptors. *Pharmacol Rev*, **2015**, *67*:601–655.

Rahmani B, et al. Neurosteroids; potential underpinning roles in maintaining homeostasis. *Gen Comp Endocrinol*, **2015**, *225*:242–250.

Reddy DS, Estes WA. Clinical potential of neurosteroids for CNS disorders. *Trends Pharmacol Sci*, **2016**, *37*:543–561.

Shepherd GM. *The Synaptic Organization of the Brain*. Oxford University Press, Oxford, U.K., **2004.**

Shukla AK, et al. Emerging paradigms of beta-arrestin-dependent seven transmembrane receptor signaling. *Trends Biochem Sci*, **2011**, *36*:457–469.

Sibley DR. *Handbook of Contemporary Neuropharmacology*. Wiley, Hoboken, NJ, **2007.**

Singhal G, et al. Inflammasomes in neuroinflammation and changes in brain function: a focused review. *Front Neurosci*, **2014**, *8*:315.

Skaper SD. The neurotrophin family of neurotrophic factors: an overview. *Methods Mol Biol*, **2012**, *846*:1–12.

Squire LR. *Fundamental Neuroscience*. Elsevier/Academic Press, Boston, **2013.**

Timmusk T, et al. Multiple promoters direct tissue-specific expression of the rat BDNF gene. *Neuron*, **1993**, *10*:475–489.

Vallee M. Neurosteroids and potential therapeutics: Focus on pregnenolone. *J Steroid Biochem Mol Biol*, **2016**, *160*:78–87.

Yamaura K, et al. Discovery of allosteric modulators for GABA$_A$ receptors by ligand-directed chemistry. *Nat Chem Biol*, **2016**, *12*:822–830.

Chapter 15

Drug Therapy of Depression and Anxiety Disorders

James M. O'Donnell, Robert R. Bies, and Richard C. Shelton

Depression and anxiety disorders are the most common mental illnesses, each affecting in excess of 15% of the population at some point in the life span. With the advent of more selective and safer drugs, the use of antidepressants and anxiolytics has moved from the exclusive domain of psychiatry to other medical specialties, including primary care. *The relative safety of the majority of commonly used antidepressants and anxiolytics notwithstanding, their optimal use requires a clear understanding of their mechanisms of action, pharmacokinetics, adverse effects, potential drug interactions, and the differential diagnosis of psychiatric illnesses* (Thronson and Pagalilauan, 2014).

Both depression and anxiety can affect an individual patient simultaneously; some of the drugs discussed here are effective in treating both types of disorders, suggesting common underlying mechanisms of pathophysiology and response to pharmacotherapy. In large measure, our current understanding of pathophysiological mechanisms underlying depression and anxiety has been inferred from the mechanisms of action of psychopharmacological compounds, notably their actions on neurotransmission involving serotonin (5HT), NE, and GABA (see Chapter 14). While depression and anxiety disorders comprise a wide range of symptoms, including changes in mood, behavior, somatic function, and cognition, some progress has been made in developing animal models that respond with some sensitivity and selectivity to antidepressant or anxiolytic drugs (Cryan and Holmes, 2005; Xu et al., 2012). The last half-century has seen notable advances in the discovery and development of drugs for treating depression and anxiety (Hillhouse and Porter, 2015).

Characterization of Depressive and Anxiety Disorders

Symptoms of Depression

Depression is classified as major depression (i.e., unipolar depression), persistent depressive disorder (dysthymia), or bipolar I and II disorders (i.e., manic-depressive illness). Bipolar depression and its treatment are discussed in Chapter 16. Lifetime risk of unipolar major depression is approximately 15%. Females are affected with major depression twice as frequently as males (Kessler et al., 1994). Depressive episodes are characterized by sad mood, pessimistic worry, diminished interest in normal activities, mental slowing and poor concentration, insomnia or increased sleep, significant weight loss or gain due to altered eating and activity patterns, psychomotor agitation or retardation, feelings of guilt and worthlessness, decreased energy and libido, and suicidal ideation. In depressive episodes, these symptoms occur most days for a period of at least 2 weeks. In some cases, the primary complaint of patients involves somatic pain or other physical symptoms and can present a diagnostic challenge for primary care physicians. Depressive symptoms also can occur secondary to

other illnesses, such as hypothyroidism, Parkinson disease, and inflammatory conditions. Further, depression often complicates the management of other medical conditions (e.g., severe trauma, cancer, diabetes, and cardiovascular disease, especially myocardial infarction) (Andrews and Nemeroff, 1994).

Depression is underdiagnosed and undertreated (Johansson et al., 2013; Suominen et al., 1998). Given that approximately 10%–15% of those with severe depression attempt suicide at some time (Chen and Dilsaver, 1996), it is important that symptoms of depression be recognized and treated in a timely manner. Furthermore, the response to treatment must be assessed and decisions made regarding continued treatment with the initial drug, dose adjustment, adjunctive therapy, or alternative medication.

Symptoms of Anxiety

Anxiety is a normal human emotion that serves an adaptive function from a psychobiological perspective. Anxiety disorders encompass a constellation of symptoms and include generalized anxiety disorder, obsessive-compulsive disorder, panic disorder, acute stress disorder, PTSD, separation anxiety disorder, social phobia, and specific phobias (Atack, 2003). In general, symptoms of anxiety that lead to pharmacological treatment are those that interfere significantly with normal function. In the psychiatric setting, feelings of fear or dread that are unfocused (e.g., generalized anxiety disorder) or out of scale with the perceived threat (e.g., specific phobias) often require treatment. All of these conditions, with the exception of specific phobias, can be treated with antidepressant medications, particularly SSRIs. Drug treatment includes acute drug administration to manage episodes of anxiety and chronic treatment to manage unrelieved and continuing anxiety disorders. Symptoms of anxiety also are often associated with depression and other medical conditions.

Pharmacotherapy for Depression and Anxiety

In general, antidepressants enhance serotonergic or noradrenergic transmission. Sites of interaction of antidepressant drugs with noradrenergic and serotonergic neurons are depicted in Figure 15–1. Table 15–1 summarizes the actions of the most widely used antidepressants. The most commonly used medications, often referred to as second-generation antidepressants, are the SSRIs and the SNRIs, which have less toxicity and improved safety compared to the first-generation drugs, which include MAOIs and TCAs (Millan, 2006; Rush et al., 2006).

In monoamine systems, neurotransmitter reuptake occurs via presynaptic high-affinity transporter proteins; inhibition of these transporters enhances neurotransmission, presumably by slowing clearance of the transmitter and prolonging its dwell time in the synapse (Shelton and Lester, 2006). Reuptake inhibitors block the neuronal SERT, the neuronal

Abbreviations

ACh: acetylcholine
ADHD: attention-deficit/hyperactivity disorder
α_2 AR: α_2 adrenergic receptor
BDNF: brain-derived neurotrophic factor
CNS: central nervous system
C_p: plasma concentration
CREB: cyclic AMP response element binding protein
CYP: cytochrome P450
DA: dopamine
DAT: dopamine transporter
EEG: electroencephalogram
FDA: Food and Drug Administration
GABA: γ-aminobutyric acid
GI: gastrointestinal
GPCR: G protein–coupled receptor
5HT: serotonin (5-hydroxytryptamine)
IP_3: inositol 1,4,5-trisphosphate
MAO: monoamine oxidase
MAOI: monoamine oxidase inhibitor
MDMA: methylenedioxymethamphetamine (Ecstasy)
NE: norepinephrine
NET: NE transporter
NMDA: *N*-methyl-D-aspartate
PTSD: posttraumatic stress disorder
SERT: 5HT transporter
SNRI: serotonin-norepinephrine reuptake inhibitor
SSRI: selective serotonin reuptake inhibitor
TCA: tricyclic antidepressant
VMAT2: vesicular monoamine transporter

NET, or both. Similarly, TCAs and MAOIs enhance monoaminergic neurotransmission—the TCAs by inhibiting 5HT and NE reuptake via SERT or NET and the MAOIs by inhibiting monoamine metabolism and thereby increasing the levels of neurotransmitter in storage granules available for later release.

Long-term effects of antidepressant drugs evoke regulatory mechanisms that might contribute to the effectiveness of therapy (Shelton, 2000). These responses include altered adrenergic or serotonergic receptor density or sensitivity, altered receptor–G protein coupling and cyclic nucleotide signaling, induction of neurotrophic factors, and increased neurogenesis in the hippocampus (Schmidt and Duman, 2007). Persistent antidepressant effects depend on the continued inhibition of SERT or NET or enhanced serotonergic or noradrenergic neurotransmission achieved by an alternative pharmacological mechanism (Delgado et al., 1991; Heninger et al., 1996). Compelling evidence suggests that sustained signaling via NE or 5HT increases the expression of specific downstream gene products, particularly BDNF, which appears to influence dendritic spine formation, synaptogenesis, and neurogenesis (Duman and Duman, 2015).

Genome-wide association studies have suggested novel pathways that might be exploited for the discovery of antidepressants (Cannon and Keller, 2006; Lin and Lane, 2015). One promising avenue of investigation is the targeting of NMDA glutamatergic receptors with ketamine; this results in a rapid and somewhat persistent antidepressant effect in patients (Abdallah et al., 2015). Other approaches involve enhancing neurogenesis (Pascual-Brazo et al., 2014) or cyclic nucleotide signaling (O'Donnell and Zhang, 2004), which may be impaired in depressed patients (Fujita et al, 2012).

Clinical Considerations With Antidepressant Drugs

The response to antidepressant drug treatment generally has a "therapeutic lag" lasting 3–4 weeks before a measurable therapeutic effect becomes evident; however, symptoms respond differentially, with sleep disturbances improving sooner and mood and cognitive deficits later (Katz et al., 2004). While some of the lag is pharmacokinetic in nature, it is likely that a component is related to delayed postsynaptic changes. After the successful initial treatment phase, a 6- to 12-month maintenance treatment phase is typical, after which the drug is gradually withdrawn. If a patient is chronically depressed (i.e., has been depressed for more than 2 years), lifelong treatment with an antidepressant is advisable. Approximately two-thirds of patients show a marked decrease in depressive symptoms with an initial course of treatment, with one-third showing complete remission (Rush et al., 2006).

Antidepressants are not recommended as monotherapy for bipolar disorder. These drugs, notably TCAs, SNRIs, and, to a lesser extent, SSRIs, can induce a switch from a depressed episode to a manic or hypomanic episode in some patients (Gijsman et al., 2004; Goldberg and Truman, 2003).

A controversial issue regarding the use of all antidepressants is their relationship to suicide (Mann et al., 2006). Data establishing a clear link between antidepressant treatment and suicide are lacking. However, the FDA has issued a "black-box" warning regarding the use of SSRIs and a number of other antidepressants in children and adolescents due to the possibility of an association between antidepressant treatment and suicide (Isacson and Rich, 2014). For seriously depressed patients, the risk of not being on an effective antidepressant drug outweighs the risk of being treated with one (Gibbons et al., 2007). However, it is important to monitor patients closely, particularly during initial treatment.

Classes of Antidepressant and Antianxiety Agents
Selective Serotonin Reuptake Inhibitors

The SSRIs are effective in treating major depression. SSRIs also are anxiolytics with demonstrated efficacy in the treatment of generalized anxiety, panic, social anxiety, and obsessive-compulsive disorders (Rush et al., 2006). Sertraline and paroxetine are approved for the treatment of PTSD. SSRIs also are used for treatment of premenstrual dysphoric syndrome and for preventing vasovagal symptoms in postmenopausal women.

The reuptake of 5HT into presynaptic terminals is mediated by SERT; neuronal uptake is the primary process by which neurotransmission via 5HT is terminated (see Figure 15–1). SSRIs block reuptake and enhance and prolong serotonergic neurotransmission. SSRIs used clinically are relatively selective for inhibition of SERT over NET (Table 15–2).

Treatment with an SSRI causes stimulation of $5HT_{1A}$ and $5HT_7$ autoreceptors on cell bodies in the raphe nucleus and of $5HT_{1D}$ autoreceptors on serotonergic terminals; this reduces 5HT synthesis and release. With repeated treatment with SSRIs, there is a gradual downregulation and desensitization of these autoreceptor mechanisms. In addition, downregulation of postsynaptic $5HT_{2A}$ receptors may contribute to antidepressant efficacy directly or by influencing the function of noradrenergic and other neurons via serotonergic heteroreceptors. Other postsynaptic 5HT receptors likely remain responsive to increased synaptic concentrations of 5HT and contribute to the therapeutic effects of the SSRIs.

Later-developing effects of SSRI treatment also may be important in mediating ultimate therapeutic responses. These include sustained increases in cyclic AMP signaling and phosphorylation of the nuclear transcription factor CREB, as well as increases in the expression of trophic factors such as BDNF and increases of neurogenesis from progenitor cells in the hippocampus and subventricular zone (Licznerski and Duman, 2013; Santarelli et al., 2003). Repeated treatment with SSRIs reduces the expression of SERT, resulting in reduced clearance of released 5HT and increased serotonergic neurotransmission (Benmansour et al., 1999).

Serotonin-Norepinephrine Reuptake Inhibitors

Five medications with a nontricyclic structure that inhibit the reuptake of both 5HT and NE have been approved for use in the U.S. for treatment of depression, anxiety disorders, pain, or other specific conditions: venlafaxine and its demethylated metabolite desvenlafaxine; duloxetine; milnacipran, and levomilnacipran.

The SNRIs inhibit both SERT and NET (see Table 15–2) and cause enhanced serotonergic or noradrenergic neurotransmission. Similar

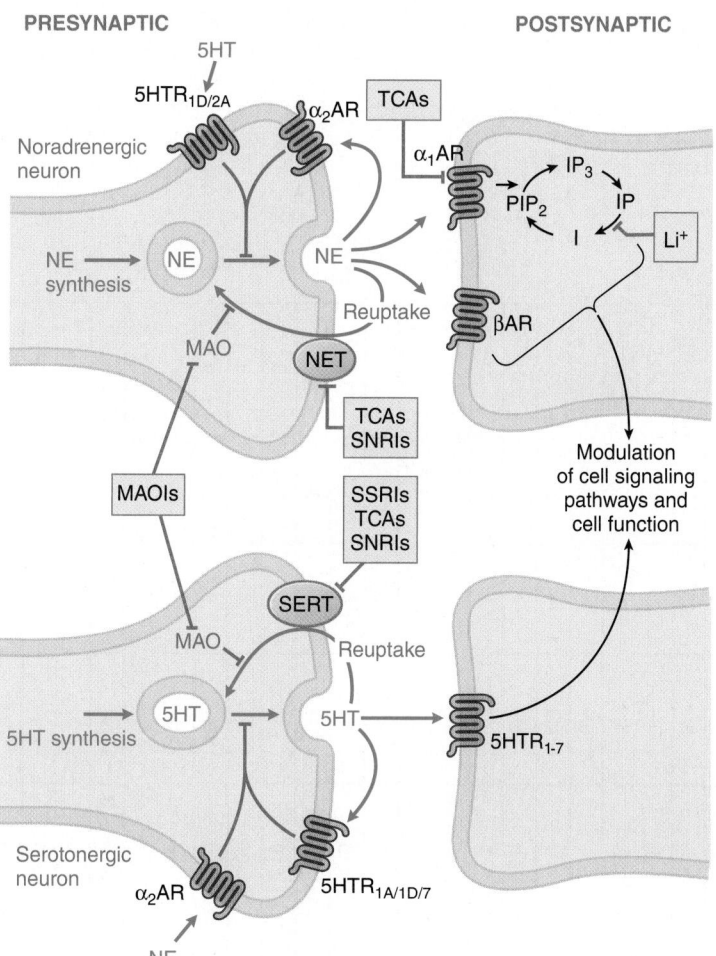

Figure 15-1 *Sites of action of antidepressants at noradrenergic (top) and serotonergic (bottom) nerve terminals.* SSRIs, SNRIs, and TCAs increase noradrenergic or serotonergic neurotransmission by blocking the NE or 5HT transporter (NET or SERT) at presynaptic terminals. MAOIs inhibit the catabolism of NE and 5HT. Trazodone and related drugs have direct effects on 5HT receptors (5HTRs) that contribute to their clinical effects. Chronic treatment with a number of antidepressants desensitizes presynaptic autoreceptors and heteroreceptors, producing long-lasting changes in monoaminergic neurotransmission. Postreceptor effects of antidepressant treatment, including modulation of GPCR signaling and activation of protein kinases and ion channels, are involved in the mediation of the long-term effects of antidepressant drugs. Li+ inhibits IP breakdown and thereby enhances its accumulation and sequelae (Ca++ mobilization, PKC activation, depletion of cellular I). Li+ may also alter release of neurotransmitters by a variety of putative mechanisms (see Chapter 16: Hypotheses for the Mechanism of Action of Lithium and Relationship to Anticonvulsants). Note that NE and 5HT may also affect each other's neurons by activating presynaptic receptors that couple to signaling pathways that reduce transmitter release. I, inositol; IP, inositol monophosphate; IP3, inositol 1,4,5-trisphosphate; PIP2, phosphatidylinositol 4,5-bisphosphate.

to the action of SSRIs, the initial inhibition of SERT induces activation of $5HT_{1A}$ and $5HT_{1D}$ autoreceptors, resulting in a decrease in serotonergic neurotransmission by a negative-feedback mechanism until these serotonergic autoreceptors are desensitized. Then, the enhanced 5HT concentration in the synapse can interact with postsynaptic 5HT receptors. The noradrenergic action of these drugs may contribute to downstream gene expression changes affecting BDNF, Trk-B (tyrosine receptor kinase B), and other neurotrophic factors and their signaling pathways (Shelton, 2000). Repeated treatment with SNRIs reduces the expression of SERT or NET, resulting in reduced neurotransmitter clearance and increased serotonergic or noradrenergic neurotransmission (Zhao et al., 2009).

The SNRIs were developed with the rationale that they might improve overall treatment response compared to SSRIs (Entsuah et al., 2001). The remission rate for venlafaxine appears slightly better than for SSRIs in head-to-head trials. Duloxetine, in addition to being approved for use in the treatment of depression and anxiety, is used for treatment of fibromyalgia and neuropathic pain associated with peripheral neuropathy (Finnerup et al., 2015). Off-label uses include stress urinary incontinence (duloxetine), autism, binge-eating disorders, hot flashes, pain syndromes, premenstrual dysphoric disorders, and PTSD (venlafaxine).

Serotonin Receptor Antagonists

Several antagonists of the $5HT_2$ family of receptors are effective antidepressants. These include two close structural analogues, trazodone and nefazodone, as well as mirtazapine and mianserin (not marketed in the U.S.).

The efficacy of trazodone may be somewhat more limited than that of the SSRIs; however, low doses of trazodone (50–200 mg) have been used widely, both alone and concurrently with SSRIs or SNRIs, to treat insomnia. Both mianserin and mirtazapine are quite sedating and are treatments of choice for some depressed patients with insomnia. Trazodone blocks $5HT_2$ and α_1 adrenergic receptors. Trazodone also inhibits SERT but is markedly less potent for this action relative to its blockade of $5HT_{2A}$ receptors. Similarly, the most potent pharmacological action of nefazodone also is the blockade of the $5HT_2$ receptors. Both mirtazapine and mianserin potently block histamine H_1 receptors. They also have some affinity for α_2 adrenergic receptors. Their affinities for $5HT_{2A}$, $5HT_{2C}$, and $5HT_3$ receptors are high, although less so than for histamine H_1 receptors. Both of these drugs increase the antidepressant response when combined with SSRIs compared to the action of the SSRIs alone. Vortioxetine is a potent SERT inhibitor and binds to a number of serotonergic receptors, resulting in complex mechanisms of action

TABLE 15-1 ■ PROFILES OF REPRESENTATIVE ANTIDEPRESSANTS

CLASS Agent	DOSE[a] mg/d	BIOGENIC AMINE	AGITATION	SEIZURES	SEDATION	HYPO-TENSION	ANTI-ACh EFFECTS	GI EFFECTS	WEIGHT GAIN	SEXUAL EFFECTS	CARDIAC EFFECTS
NE reuptake inhibitors: 3° amine tricyclics											
Amitriptyline	100–200	NE, 5HT	0	2+	3+	3+	3+	0/+	2+	2+	3+
Clomipramine	100–200	NE, 5HT	0	3+	2+	2+	3+	+	2+	3+	3+
Doxepin	100–200	NE, 5HT	0	2+	3+	2+	2+	0/+	2+	2+	3+
Imipramine	100–200	NE, 5HT	0/+	2+	2+	2+	2+	0/+	2+	2+	3+
(+)-Trimipramine	75–200	NE, 5HT	0	2+	3+	2+	3+	0/+	2+	2+	3+
NE reuptake inhibitors: 2° amine tricyclics											
Amoxapine	200–300	NE, DA	0	2+	+	2+	+	0/+	+	2+	2+
Desipramine	100–200	NE	+	+	0/+	+	+	0/+	+	2+	2+
Maprotiline	100–150	NE	0/+	3+	2+	2+	2+	0/+	+	2+	2+
Nortriptyline	75–150	NE	0	+	+	+	+	0/+	+	2+	2+
Protriptyline	15–40	NE	2+	2+	0/+	+	2+	0/+	+	2+	3+
SSRIs											
(±)-Citalopram	20–40	5HT	0/+	0	0/+	0	0	3+	0	3+	0
(±)-Escitalopram	10–20	5HT	0/+	0	0/+	0	0	3+	0	3+	0
(±)-Fluoxetine	20–80	5HT	+	0/+	0/+	0	0	3+	0/+	3+	0/+
Fluvoxamine	100–200	5HT	0	0	0/+	0	0	3+	0	3+	0
(−)-Paroxetine	20–40	5HT	+	0	0/+	0	0/+	3+	0	3+	0
(+)-Sertraline	100–150	5HT	+	0	0/+	0	0	3+	0	3+	0
(±)-Venlafaxine	75–225	5HT, NE	0/+	0	0	0	0	3+	0	3+	0/+
Atypical antidepressants											
(−)-Atomoxetine	40–80[b]	NE	0	0	0	0	0	0/+	0	0	0
Bupropion	200–300	DA, ?NE	3+	4+	0	0	0	2+	0	0	0
(+)-Duloxetine	80–100	NE, 5HT	+	0	0/+	0/+	0	0/+	0/+	0/+	0/+
(±)-Mirtazapine	15–45	5HT, NE	0	0	4+	0/+	0	0/+	0/+	0	0
Nefazodone	200–400	5HT	0	0	3+	0	0	2+	0/+	0/+	0/+
Trazodone	150–200	5HT	0	0	3+	0	0	2+	+	+	0/+
MAO inhibitors											
Phenelzine	30–60	NE, 5HT, DA	0/+	0	+	+	0	0/+	+	3+	0
Tranylcypromine	20–30	NE, 5HT, DA	2+	0	0	+	0	0/+	+	2+	0
(−)-Selegiline	10	DA, ?NE, ?5HT	0	0	0	0	0	0	+	+	0

SIDE EFFECTS

Imipramine

Desipramine

Fluoxetine

Bupropion

Selegiline

0, negligible; 0/+, minimal; +, mild; 2+, moderate; 3+, moderately severe; 4+, severe. Other significant side effects for individual drugs are described in the text. Selegiline transdermal patch approved for depression.
[a]Higher and lower doses are sometimes used, depending on patient's needs and response to the drug; see the literature and FDA recommendations.
[b]Children, 0.5–1 mg/kg, up to 70 kg; see black-box warning.

(Bang-Andersen et al., 2011). Vortioxetine is a partial agonist at $5HT_{1A}$ and $5HT_{1B}$ receptors and an antagonist at $5HT_{1D}$, $5HT_3$, and $5HT_7$ receptors.

Bupropion

Bupropion has the backbone of β-phenethylamine; it is discussed separately because it appears to act via multiple mechanisms that differ somewhat from the mechanisms of SSRIs and SNRIs (Foley et al., 2006; Gobbi et al., 2003). It enhances both noradrenergic and dopaminergic neurotransmission via inhibition of reuptake by NET and DAT (although its effects on DAT are not potent in animal studies) (see Table 15–2). Bupropion's mechanism of action also may involve the presynaptic release of NE and DA and effects on VMAT2 (see Figure 8–6). The hydroxybupropion metabolite may contribute to the therapeutic effects of the parent compound: This metabolite appears to have a similar pharmacology and is present at substantial levels. Bupropion is indicated for the treatment of depression, prevention of seasonal depressive disorder, and as a smoking cessation treatment (Carroll et al., 2014). Bupropion has effects on sleep EEGs that are opposite those of most antidepressant drugs. Bupropion may improve symptoms of ADHD and has been used off label for neuropathic pain and weight loss. Clinically, bupropion is widely used in combination with SSRIs with the intent of obtaining a greater antidepressant response; however, there are limited clinical data providing strong support for this practice.

Atypical Antipsychotics

In addition to their use in schizophrenia, bipolar depression, and major depression with psychotic disorders, atypical antipsychotics have gained further, off-label use for major depression without psychotic features (Jarema, 2007). The combination of aripiprazole or quetiapine with SSRIs and SNRIs and a combination of olanzapine and the SSRI fluoxetine have been FDA-approved for treatment-resistant major depression (i.e., following an inadequate response to at least two different antidepressants).

The olanzapine-fluoxetine combination is available in fixed-dose combinations of 3, 6, or 12 mg of olanzapine and 25 or 50 mg of fluoxetine. Quetiapine may have either primary antidepressant actions on its own or adjunctive benefit for treatment-resistant depression; it is used off label

for insomnia. The mechanism of action and adverse effects of the atypical antipsychotics are described in Chapter 16. The major risks of these agents are weight gain and metabolic syndrome, a greater problem for quetiapine and olanzapine than for aripiprazole.

Tricyclic Antidepressants

While TCAs have long-established efficacy, they exhibit serious side effects and generally are not used as first-line drugs for the treatment of depression (Hollister, 1981). TCAs and first-generation antipsychotics are synergistic for the treatment of psychotic depression. Tertiary amine TCAs (e.g., doxepin, amitriptyline) have been used for many years in relatively low doses for treating insomnia. In addition, because of the roles of NE and 5HT in nociception, these drugs are commonly used to treat a variety of pain conditions (Finnerup et al., 2015).

The pharmacological action of TCAs is antagonism of SERT and NET (see Table 15–2). In addition to inhibiting NET somewhat selectively (desipramine, nortriptyline, protriptyline, amoxapine) or both SERT and NET (imipramine, amitriptyline), these drugs block other receptors (H_1 histamine, $5HT_2$, $α_1$ adrenergic, and muscarinic cholinergic receptors). Given the comparable activities of clomipramine and SSRIs (see Tables 15–2 and 15–4; see also Decloedt and Stein, 2010), it is tempting to suggest that some combination of these additional pharmacological actions contributes to the therapeutic effects of TCAs and possibly SNRIs. One TCA, amoxapine, also is a DA receptor antagonist; its use, unlike that of other TCAs, poses some risk for the development of extrapyramidal side effects such as tardive dyskinesia.

Monoamine Oxidase Inhibitors

Monoamine oxidases A and B are widely distributed mitochondrial enzymes. MAO activities in the GI tract and liver, mainly MAO_A, protect the body from biogenic amines in the diet. In presynaptic nerve terminals, MAO metabolizes monoamine neurotransmitters via oxidative deamination. MAO_A preferentially metabolizes 5HT and NE and can metabolize DA; MAO_B is effective against 5HT and DA (see Chapters 8 and 13; see also Nestler et al., 2015). MAOIs have efficacy equivalent to that of the TCAs but are rarely used because of their toxicity and major interactions with some drugs (e.g., sympathomimetics and some opioids) and foods (those containing high amounts of tyramine) (Hollister, 1981). The MAOIs approved in the U.S. for treatment of depression include tranylcypromine, phenelzine, and isocarboxazid. These agents irreversibly inhibit both MAO_A and MAO_B, thereby inhibiting the body's capacity to metabolize not only endogenous monoamines such an NE and 5HT but also exogenous biogenic amines such as tyramine. Global inhibition of MAOs increases the bioavailability of dietary tyramine; tyramine-induced NE release can cause marked increases in blood pressure (hypertensive crisis) (see Chapter 8).

This potential to exacerbate the effects of indirectly acting sympathomimetic amines seems to relate mainly to inhibition of MAO_A. Selegiline is an irreversible MAO inhibitor but with specificity for MAO_B at low doses, thereby sparing MAO_A activity in the GI tract and elsewhere, and is less likely to cause this interaction (although at higher doses, selegiline will also inhibit MAO_A). Selegiline is available as a transdermal patch for the treatment of depression; transdermal delivery may reduce the risk for diet-associated hypertensive reactions. Some MAOIs are reversible competitive inhibitors of MAO_A. These agents such as moclobemide and eprobemide, permit tyramine to compete for MAO_A and thus exhibit reduced capacity to potentiate the effects of dietary tyramine; these agents are used elsewhere but are not approved for use in the U.S. (Finberg, 2014).

Pharmacokinetics

The metabolism of most antidepressants is mediated by hepatic CYPs (Table 15–3) (Probst-Schendzielorz et al., 2015). Some antidepressants inhibit the clearance of other drugs by the CYP system, and this possibility of drug interactions should be a significant factor in considering the choice of agents. Likewise, dose considerations have to include awareness of hepatic function (Mauri et al., 2014). While there are genetic polymorphisms that influence antidepressant metabolism, CYP genotyping

TABLE 15–2 ■ SELECTIVITY OF ANTIDEPRESSANTS AT THE HUMAN BIOGENIC AMINE TRANSPORTERS

DRUG	SELECTIVITY	DRUG	SELECTIVITY
NE SELECTIVE	NET vs. SERT	5HT SELECTIVE	SERT vs. NET
Oxaprotiline	800	S-Citalopram	7127
Maprotiline	532	R,S-Citalopram	3643
Viloxazine	109	Sertraline	1390
Nomifensine	64	Fluvoxamine	591
Desipramine	22	Paroxetine	400
Protriptyline	14	Fluoxetine	305
Atomoxetine	12	Clomipramine	123
Reboxetine	8.3	Venlafaxine	116
Nortriptyline	4.2	Zimelidine	60
Amoxapine	3.6	Trazodone	52
Doxepin	2.3	Imipramine	26
DA SELECTIVE	DAT vs. NET	Amitriptyline	8.0
Bupropion	1000	Duloxetine	7.0
		Dothiepin	5.5
		Milnacipran	1.6

Selectivity is defined as ratio of the relevant K_i values (SERT/NET, NET/SERT, NET/DAT). Bupropion is selective for the DAT relative to the NET and SERT.
Data from Frazer, 1997; Owens et al., 1997; and Leonard and Richelson, 2000.

TABLE 15–3 ■ DISPOSITION OF ANTIDEPRESSANTS

DRUG	ELIMINATION $t_{1/2}$ (h) OF PARENT DRUG ($t_{1/2}$ of active metabolite)	TYPICAL C_p (ng/mL)	PREDOMINANT CYP INVOLVED IN METABOLISM
Tricyclic antidepressants			
Amitriptyline	16 (30)	100–250	
Amoxapine	8 (30)	200–500	
Clomipramine	32 (70)	150–500	
Desipramine	30	125–300	
Doxepin	18 (30)	150–250	2D6, 2C19, 3A3/4, 1A2
Imipramine	12 (30)	175–300	
Maprotiline	48	200–400	
Nortriptyline	31	60–150	
Protriptyline	80	100–250	
Trimipramine	16 (30)	100–300	
Selective serotonin reuptake inhibitors			
R,S-Citalopram	36	75–150	3A4, 2C19
S-Citalopram	30	40–80	3A4, 2C19
Fluoxetine	53 (240)	100–500	2D6, 2C9
Fluvoxamine	18	100–200	2D6, 1A2, 3A4, 2C9
Paroxetine	17	30–100	2D6
Sertraline	23 (66)	25–50	2D6
Serotonin-norepinephrine reuptake inhibitors			
Duloxetine	11	—	2D6
Venlafaxine	5 (11)	—	2D6, 3A4
Other antidepressants			
Atomoxetine	5–20; child, 3	—	2D6, 3A3/4
Bupropion	11	75–100	2B6
Mirtazapine	16	—	2D6
Nefazodone	2–4	—	3A3/4
Reboxetine	12	—	—
Trazodone	6	800–1600	2D6

Values shown are elimination $t_{1/2}$ values for a number of clinically used antidepressant drugs; numbers in parentheses are $t_{1/2}$ values of active metabolites. Fluoxetine (2D6), fluvoxamine (1A2, 2C8, 3A3/4), paroxetine (2D6), and nefazodone (3A3/4) are potent inhibitors of CYPs; sertraline (2D6), citalopram (2C19), and venlafaxine are less-potent inhibitors. Plasma concentrations are those observed at typical clinical doses.
Information sources: FDA-approved package inserts and Appendix II of this book.

has not yet been shown to have a practical influence on choice of drug treatment in clinical settings (Dubovsky, 2015).

Selective Serotonin Reuptake Inhibitors

All of the SSRIs are orally active and possess elimination half-lives consistent with once-daily dosing (Hiemke and Hartter, 2000). In the case of fluoxetine, the combined action of the parent and the demethylated metabolite norfluoxetine allows for a once-weekly formulation. CYP2D6 is involved in the metabolism of most SSRIs, and the SSRIs are at least moderately potent inhibitors of this isoenzyme. This creates a significant potential for drug interaction for postmenopausal women taking the

breast cancer drug and estrogen antagonist tamoxifen (see Chapter 68). Because venlafaxine and desvenlafaxine are weak inhibitors of CYP2D6, these antidepressants are not contraindicated in this clinical situation. However, care should be used in combining SSRIs with drugs that are metabolized by CYPs. SSRIs such as escitalopram and citalopram that exhibit an age-dependent decrease in CYP2C19 metabolism should be dosed with care in elderly patients.

Serotonin-Norepinephrine Reuptake Inhibitors

Both immediate-release and extended-release (tablet or capsule) preparations of venlafaxine result in steady-state levels of drug in plasma within 3 days. The elimination half-lives for the parent venlafaxine and its active and major metabolite desmethylvenlafaxine are 5 and 11 h, respectively. Desmethylvenlafaxine is eliminated by hepatic metabolism and by renal excretion. Venlafaxine dose reductions are suggested for patients with renal or hepatic impairment. Duloxetine has a $t_{1/2}$ of 12 h. Duloxetine is not recommended for those with end-stage renal disease or hepatic insufficiency.

Serotonin Receptor Antagonists

Mirtazapine has an elimination $t_{1/2}$ of 16–30 h. Thus, dose changes are suggested no more often than 1–2 weeks. The recommended initial dosing of mirtazapine is 15 mg/d, with a maximal recommended dose of 45 mg/d. Clearance of mirtazapine is decreased in the elderly and in patients with moderate-to-severe renal or hepatic impairment. Pharmacokinetics and adverse effects of mirtazapine may have an enantiomer-selective component (Brockmöller et al., 2007). Steady-state trazodone is observed within 3 days following a dosing regimen. Trazodone typically is started at 150 mg/d in divided doses, with 50-mg increments every 3–4 days. The maximally recommended dose is 400 mg/d for outpatients and 600 mg/d for inpatients. Nefazodone has a $t_{1/2}$ of only 2–4 h; its major metabolite hydroxynefazodone has a $t_{1/2}$ of 1.5–4 h.

Bupropion

Bupropion elimination has a $t_{1/2}$ of 21 h and involves both hepatic and renal routes. Patients with severe hepatic cirrhosis should receive a maximum dose of 150 mg every other day; consideration for a decreased dose should also be made in cases of renal impairment.

Tricyclic Antidepressants

The TCAs, or their active metabolites, have plasma half-lives of 8–80 h; this makes once-daily dosing possible for most of the compounds (Rudorfer and Potter, 1999). Steady-state concentrations occur within several days to several weeks of beginning treatment, as a function of the $t_{1/2}$. TCAs are largely eliminated by hepatic CYPs (see Table 15–3). Dosage adjustments of TCAs are typically made according to a patient's clinical response, not based on plasma levels. Nonetheless, monitoring the plasma exposure has an important relationship to treatment response: There is a relatively narrow therapeutic window. About 7% of patients metabolize TCAs slowly due to a variant CYP2D6 isoenzyme, causing a 30-fold difference in plasma concentrations among different patients given the same TCA dose. To avoid toxicity in "slow metabolizers," plasma levels should be monitored and doses adjusted downward.

Monoamine Oxidase Inhibitors

The MAOIs are metabolized by acetylation. A significant portion of the population (50% of the Caucasian population and an even higher percentage among Asians) are "slow acetylators" (see Table 7–2 and Figure 60–4) and will exhibit elevated plasma levels. The nonselective MAOIs used in the treatment of depression are irreversible inhibitors; thus, it takes up to 2 weeks for MAO activity to recover, even though the parent drug is excreted within 24 h (Livingston and Livingston, 1996). Recovery of normal enzyme function is dependent on synthesis and transport of new MAO to monoaminergic nerve terminals.

Adverse Effects

Selective Serotonin Reuptake Inhibitors

The SSRIs have no major cardiovascular side effects. The SSRIs are generally free of antimuscarinic side effects (dry mouth, urinary retention, confusion) and do not block α adrenergic receptors; most SSRIs, with the exception of paroxetine, do not block histamine receptors and usually are not sedating (Table 15–4).

Adverse side effects of SSRIs from excessive stimulation of brain $5HT_2$ receptors may result in insomnia, increased anxiety, irritability, and decreased libido, effectively worsening prominent depressive symptoms. Excess activity at spinal $5HT_2$ receptors causes sexual side effects, including erectile dysfunction, anorgasmia, and ejaculatory delay (Clayton et al., 2014). These effects may be more prominent with paroxetine (Vaswani et al., 2003). Aspects of sexual dysfunction can be treated in both men and women with the phosphodiesterase 5 inhibitor sildenafil (Nurnberg, 2001; Nurnberg et al., 2008; see also Chapter 45). Stimulation of $5HT_3$ receptors in the CNS and periphery contributes to GI effects, which are usually limited to nausea but may include diarrhea and emesis. Some patients experience an increase in anxiety, especially with the initial dosing of SSRIs. With continued treatment, some patients also report a dullness of intellectual abilities and concentration. In general, there is not a strong relationship between SSRI serum concentrations and therapeutic efficacy. Thus, dosage adjustments are based more on evaluation of clinical response and management of side effects.

TABLE 15–4 ■ POTENCIES OF SELECTED ANTIDEPRESSANTS AT MUSCARINIC, HISTAMINE H_1, AND $α_1$ ADRENERGIC RECEPTORS

DRUG	RECEPTOR TYPE		
	MUSCARINIC CHOLINERGIC	HISTAMINE H_1	$α_1$ ADRENERGIC
Amitriptyline	18	1.1	27
Amoxapine	1000	25	50
Atomoxetine	≥1000	≥1000	≥1000
Bupropion	40,000	6700	4550
R,S-Citalopram	1800	380	1550
S-Citalopram	1240	1970	3870
Clomipramine	37	31.2	39
Desipramine	196	110	130
Doxepin	83.3	0.24	24
Duloxetine	3000	2300	8300
Fluoxetine	2000	6250	5900
Fluvoxamine	24,000	>100,000	7700
Imipramine	91	11.0	91
Maprotiline	560	2.0	91
Mirtazapine	670	0.1	500
Nefazodone	11,000	21	25.6
Nortriptyline	149	10	58.8
Paroxetine	108	22,000	>100,000
Protriptyline	25	25	130
Reboxetine	6700	312	11,900
Sertraline	625	24,000	370
Trazodone	>100,000	345	35.7
Trimipramine	59	0.3	23.8
Venlafaxine	>100,000	>100,000	>100,000

Values are experimentally determined potencies (K_i values, nM) for binding to receptors that contribute to common side effects of clinically used antidepressant drugs: muscarinic cholinergic receptors (e.g., dry mouth, urinary retention, confusion); histamine H_1 receptors (sedation); and $α_1$ adrenergic receptors (orthostatic hypotension, sedation).
Data from Leonard and Richelson, 2000.

Sudden withdrawal of antidepressants can precipitate a discontinuation syndrome (Harvey and Slabbert, 2014). For SSRIs or SNRIs, the symptoms of withdrawal may include dizziness, headache, nervousness, nausea, and insomnia. This withdrawal syndrome appears most intense for paroxetine and venlafaxine due to their relatively short half-lives and, in the case of paroxetine, lack of active metabolites. Conversely, the active metabolite of fluoxetine, norfluoxetine, has such a long $t_{1/2}$ (1–2 weeks) that few patients experience any withdrawal symptoms with discontinuation of fluoxetine.

Unlike the other SSRIs, paroxetine is associated with an increased risk of congenital cardiac malformations when administered in the first trimester of pregnancy (Gadot and Koren, 2015). Venlafaxine also is associated with an increased risk of perinatal complications.

Serotonin-Norepinephrine Reuptake Inhibitors

The SNRIs have a side-effect profile similar to that of the SSRIs, including nausea, constipation, insomnia, headaches, and sexual dysfunction. The immediate-release formulation of venlafaxine can induce sustained diastolic hypertension (diastolic blood pressure > 90 mm Hg at consecutive weekly visits) in 10%–15% of patients at higher doses; this risk is reduced with the extended-release form. This effect of venlafaxine may not be associated simply with inhibition of NET because duloxetine does not share this side effect.

Serotonin Receptor Antagonists

Regarding the serotonin receptor antagonists, the main side effects of mirtazapine, seen in more than 10% of the patients, are somnolence, increased appetite, and weight gain. A rare side effect of mirtazapine is agranulocytosis. Trazodone use is associated with priapism in rare instances. Nefazodone was voluntarily withdrawn from the market in several countries after rare cases of liver failure were associated with its use. In the U.S., nefazodone is marketed with a black-box warning regarding hepatotoxicity.

Bupropion

Typical side effects associated with bupropion include anxiety, mild tachycardia and hypertension, irritability, and tremor. Other side effects include headache, nausea, dry mouth, constipation, appetite suppression, insomnia, and, rarely, aggression, impulsivity, and agitation. Seizures are dependent on dose and C_p, with seizures occurring rarely within the recommended dose range. Bupropion should be avoided in patients with seizure disorders as well as those with bulimia due to an increased risk of seizures (Horne et al., 1988; Noe et al., 2011). At doses higher than that recommended for depression (450 mg/d), the risk of seizures increases significantly. The use of extended-release formulations often blunts the maximum concentration observed after dosing and minimizes the chance of reaching drug levels associated with an increased risk of seizures.

Tricyclic Antidepressants

The TCAs are potent antagonists at histamine H_1 receptors, and this antagonism contributes to the sedative effects of TCAs (see Table 15–4). Antagonism of muscarinic ACh receptors contributes to cognitive dulling as well as a range of adverse effects mediated by the parasympathetic nervous system (blurred vision, dry mouth, tachycardia, constipation, difficulty urinating). Some tolerance does occur for these anticholinergic effects. Antagonism of $α_1$ adrenergic receptors contributes to orthostatic hypotension and sedation. Weight gain is another side effect of this class of antidepressants.

The TCAs have quinidine-like effects on cardiac conduction that can be life threatening with overdose and limit the use of TCAs in patients with heart disease. This is the primary reason that only a limited supply should be available to the patient at any given time. Like other antidepressant drugs, TCAs also lower the seizure threshold.

Monoamine Oxidase Inhibitors

Hypertensive crisis resulting from food or drug interactions is one of the life-threatening toxicities associated with use of the MAOIs (Rapaport, 2007). Foods containing tyramine are a contributing factor. MAO_A within the intestinal wall and MAO_A and MAO_B in the liver normally degrade dietary tyramine. When MAO_A is inhibited, tyramine can enter the systemic circulation and be taken up into adrenergic nerve endings, where it causes release of catecholamines from storage vesicles. The released catecholamines stimulate postsynaptic receptors in the periphery, increasing blood pressure to dangerous levels. The concurrent use of MAOIs and medications that contain sympathomimetic compounds also results in a potentially life-threatening elevation of blood pressure. In comparison to tranylcypromine and isocarboxazid, the selegiline (selective for MAO_B) transdermal patch is better tolerated and safer, as are the reversible, competitive inhibitors moclobemide and eprobemide. Another serious, life-threatening issue with chronic administration of MAOIs is hepatotoxicity.

Drug Interactions

Many of these drugs are metabolized by hepatic CYPs, especially CYP2D6. Thus, other agents that are substrates or inhibitors of CYP2D6 can increase plasma concentrations of the primary drug. The combination of other classes of antidepressant agents with MAOIs is inadvisable and can lead to *serotonin syndrome*, a serious triad of abnormalities consisting of cognitive, autonomic, and somatic effects due to excess serotonin. Symptoms of the serotonin syndrome include hyperthermia, muscle rigidity, myoclonus, tremors, autonomic instability, confusion, irritability, and agitation; this can progress toward coma and death.

Selective Serotonin Reuptake Inhibitors

Paroxetine and, to a lesser degree, fluoxetine are potent inhibitors of CYP2D6 (Hiemke and Hartter, 2000). The other SSRIs, outside of fluvoxamine, are at least moderate inhibitors of CYP2D6. This inhibition can result in disproportionate increases in plasma concentrations of drugs metabolized by CYP2D6 when doses of these drugs are increased. Fluvoxamine directly inhibits CYP1A2 and CYP2C19; fluoxetine and fluvoxamine also inhibit CYP3A4. A prominent interaction is the increase in TCA exposure that may be observed during coadministration of TCAs and SSRIs.

The MAOIs enhance the effects of SSRIs due to inhibition of 5HT metabolism. Administration of these drugs together can produce synergistic increases in extracellular brain 5HT, leading to the serotonin syndrome (see previous discussion). Other drugs that may induce the serotonin syndrome include substituted amphetamines such as MDMA (Ecstasy), which directly releases 5HT from nerve terminals.

The SSRIs should not be started until at least 14 days following discontinuation of treatment with an MAOI; this allows for synthesis of the new MAO. For all SSRIs but fluoxetine, at least 14 days should pass prior to beginning treatment with an MAOI following the end of treatment with an SSRI. Because the active metabolite norfluoxetine has a $t_{1/2}$ of 1–2 weeks, at least 5 weeks should pass between stopping fluoxetine and beginning an MAOI.

Serotonin-Norepinephrine Reuptake Inhibitors

While a 14-day period is recommended between ending MAOI therapy and starting venlafaxine treatment, an interval of 7 days is considered safe. Duloxetine has a similar interval for initiation following MAOI therapy; conversely, only a 5-day waiting period is needed before beginning MAOI treatment after ending duloxetine. Failure to observe these required waiting periods can result in the serotonin syndrome.

Serotonin Receptor Antagonists

Trazodone dosing may need to be lowered when given together with drugs that inhibit CYP3A4. Mirtazapine is metabolized by CYPs 2D6, 1A2, and 3A4 and may interact with drugs that share these CYP pathways, requiring mutual dose reductions. Trazodone and nefazodone are weak inhibitors of 5HT uptake and should not be administered with MAOIs due to concerns about serotonin syndrome.

Bupropion

The major route of metabolism for bupropion is CYP2B6. Bupropion and its metabolite hydroxybupropion can inhibit CYP2D6, the CYP responsible for metabolism of several SSRIs (Table 15–3) as well as some β blockers

and haloperidol, among others. Thus, the potential for interactions of bupropion with SSRIs and other drugs metabolized by CYP2D6 should be kept in mind until the safety of the combination is firmly established.

Tricyclic Antidepressants

Drugs that inhibit CYP2D6, such as bupropion and SSRIs, may increase plasma exposures of TCAs. TCAs can potentiate the actions of sympathomimetic amines and should not be used concurrently with MAOIs or within 14 days of stopping MAOIs. A *number of other drugs have similar side-effect profiles as TCAs, and concurrent use risks enhanced side effects* (see previous discussion in Adverse Effects); this includes phenothiazine antipsychotic agents, type 1C antiarrhythmic agents, and other drugs with antimuscarinic, antihistaminic, and α adrenergic antagonistic effects.

Monoamine Oxidase Inhibitors

Serotonin syndrome is the most serious drug interaction for the MAOIs (see Adverse Effects). The most common cause of serotonin syndrome in patients taking MAOIs is the accidental coadministration of a 5HT reuptake-inhibiting antidepressant or tryptophan. Other serious drug interactions include those with meperidine and tramadol. MAOIs also interact with sympathomimetics such as pseudoephedrine, phenylephrine, oxymetazoline, phenylpropanolamine, and amphetamine; these are commonly found in cold and allergy medication and diet aids and should be avoided by patients taking MAOIs. Likewise, patients on MAOIs must avoid foods containing high levels of tyramine: soy products, dried meats and sausages, dried fruits, home-brewed and tap beers, red wine, pickled or fermented foods, and aged cheeses (FDA, 2010).

ANXIOLYTIC DRUGS

Primary treatments for anxiety-related disorders include the SSRIs, SNRIs, benzodiazepines, buspirone, and β adrenergic antagonists (Atack, 2003). The SSRIs and the SNRI venlafaxine are well tolerated with a reasonable side-effect profile; in addition to their documented antidepressant activity, they have anxiolytic activity with chronic treatment. The benzodiazepines are effective anxiolytics as both acute and chronic treatment. There is concern regarding their use because of their potential for dependence and abuse as well as negative effects on cognition and memory. Buspirone, like the SSRIs, is effective following chronic treatment. It acts, at least in part, via the serotonergic system, where it is a partial agonist at $5HT_{1A}$ receptors. Buspirone also has antagonistic effects at DA D_2 receptors, but the relationship between this effect and its clinical actions is uncertain. β Adrenergic antagonists, particularly those with higher lipophilicity (e.g., propranolol and nadolol), are occasionally used for performance anxiety such as fear of public speaking; their use is limited due to significant side effects, such as hypotension.

Antihistamines and sedative-hypnotic agents have been tried as anxiolytics but are generally not recommended because of their side-effect profiles and the availability of superior drugs. Hydroxyzine, which produces short-term sedation, is used in patients who cannot use other types of anxiolytics (e.g., those with a history of drug or alcohol abuse where benzodiazepines would be avoided). Chloral hydrate has been used for situational anxiety, but there is a narrow dose range where anxiolytic effects are observed in the absence of significant sedation; therefore, the use of chloral hydrate is not recommended.

Clinical Considerations With Anxiolytic Drugs

The choice of pharmacological treatment of anxiety is dictated by the specific anxiety-related disorders and the clinical need for acute anxiolytic effects (Millan, 2003). Among the commonly used anxiolytics, only the benzodiazepines and β adrenergic antagonists are effective acutely; the use of β adrenergic antagonists is generally limited to treatment of situational anxiety. Chronic treatment with SSRIs, SNRIs, and buspirone is required to produce and sustain anxiolytic effects. When an immediate anxiolytic effect is desired, benzodiazepines are typically selected.

Benzodiazepines, such as alprazolam, chlordiazepoxide, clonazepam, clorazepate, diazepam, lorazepam, and oxazepam, are effective in the treatment of generalized anxiety disorder, panic disorder, and situational anxiety. In addition to their anxiolytic effects, benzodiazepines produce sedative, hypnotic, anesthetic, anticonvulsant, and muscle relaxant effects. The benzodiazepines also impair cognitive performance and memory, adversely affect motor control, and potentiate the effects of other sedatives, including alcohol. The anxiolytic effects of this class of drugs are mediated by allosteric interactions with the pentameric benzodiazepine-GABA$_A$ receptor complex, in particular GABA$_A$ receptors comprising α2, α3, and α5 subunits (Chapters 14 and 19). The primary effect of the anxiolytic benzodiazepines is to enhance the inhibitory effects of the neurotransmitter GABA.

One area of concern regarding the use of benzodiazepines in the treatment of anxiety is the potential for habituation, dependence, and abuse. Patients with certain personality disorders or a history of drug or alcohol abuse are particularly susceptible. However, the risk of dependence must be balanced with the need for treatment because benzodiazepines are effective in both short- and long-term treatment of patients with sustained or recurring bouts of anxiety. Further, premature discontinuation of benzodiazepines, in the absence of other pharmacological treatment, results in a high rate of relapse. Withdrawal of benzodiazepines after chronic treatment, particularly with benzodiazepines with short durations of action, can include increased anxiety and seizures. For this reason, it is important that discontinuation be carried out in a gradual manner.

Benzodiazepines cause many adverse effects, including sedation, mild memory impairments, decreased alertness, and slowed reaction time (which may lead to accidents). Memory problems can include visual-spatial deficits but will manifest clinically in a variety of ways, including difficulty in word finding. Occasionally, paradoxical reactions can occur with benzodiazepines, such as increases in anxiety, sometimes reaching panic attack proportions. Other pathological reactions can include irritability, aggression, or behavioral disinhibition. Amnesic reactions (i.e., loss of memory for particular periods) can also occur. Benzodiazepines should not be used in pregnant women; there have been rare reports of craniofacial defects. In addition, benzodiazepines taken prior to delivery may result in sedated, underresponsive newborns and prolonged withdrawal reactions. In the elderly, benzodiazepines increase the risk for falls and must be used cautiously. These drugs are safer than classical sedative-hypnotics in overdosage and typically are fatal only if combined with other CNS depressants.

Benzodiazepines have some abuse potential, although their capacity for abuse is considerably below that of other classical sedative-hypnotic agents. When these agents are abused, it is generally in a multidrug abuse pattern, frequently connected with failed attempts to control anxiety.

Tolerance to the anxiolytic effects develops with chronic administration, with the result that some patients escalate the dose of benzodiazepines over time. Ideally, benzodiazepines should be used for short periods of time and in conjunction with other medications (e.g., SSRIs) or evidence-based psychotherapies (e.g., cognitive behavioral therapy for anxiety disorders).

The SSRIs and the SNRI venlafaxine are first-line treatments for most types of anxiety disorders, except when an acute drug effect is desired; fluvoxamine is approved only for obsessive-compulsive disorder. As for their antidepressant actions, the anxiolytic effects of these drugs become manifest following chronic treatment. Other drugs with actions on serotonergic neurotransmission, including trazodone, nefazodone, and mirtazapine, also are used in the treatment of anxiety disorders. Details regarding the pharmacology of these classes were presented previously in this chapter.

Both SSRIs and SNRIs are beneficial in specific anxiety conditions, such as generalized anxiety disorder, social phobias, obsessive-compulsive disorder, and panic disorder. These effects appear to be related to the capacity of serotonin to regulate the activity of brain structures, such as the amygdala and locus coeruleus, that are thought to be involved in the genesis of anxiety. Interestingly, the SSRIs and SNRIs often will produce some increases in anxiety in the short term that dissipate with time. Therefore, the maxim "start low and go slow" is indicated with anxious patients; however, many patients with anxiety disorders ultimately will require doses that are about the same as those required for the treatment of depression. Anxious patients appear to be particularly prone to severe discontinuation reactions with certain medications such as venlafaxine and paroxetine; therefore, slow off-tapering is required.

Buspirone is used in the treatment of generalized anxiety disorder (Goodman, 2004). Like the SSRIs, buspirone requires chronic treatment for effectiveness. Also, like the SSRIs, buspirone lacks many of the other pharmacological effects of the benzodiazepines: It is not an anticonvulsant, muscle relaxant, or sedative, and it does not impair psychomotor performance or result in dependence. Buspirone is primarily effective in the treatment of generalized anxiety disorder, but not for other anxiety disorders. In fact, patients with panic disorder often note an increase in anxiety acutely following initiation of buspirone treatment; this may be the result of the fact that buspirone causes increased firing rates of the locus coeruleus, which is thought to underlie part of the pathophysiology of panic disorder.

Acknowledgment: *Ross J. Baldessarini contributed to this chapter in recent editions of this book. We have retained some of his text in the current edition.*

Drug Facts for Your Personal Formulary: *Depression and Anxiety Disorders*

Drugs	Therapeutic Uses	Clinical Pharmacology and Tips
Selective Serotonin Reuptake Inhibitors		
Citalopram Escitalopram Fluoxetine Fluvoxamine Paroxetine Sertraline Vilazodone	• Anxiety and depression disorders • Obsessive-compulsive disorder, PTSD • SERT selective; little effect on NET • Vilazodone also acts as 5HT$_{1A}$ partial agonist	• Side effects include GI disturbances • May cause sexual dysfunctions • May increase risk of suicidal thoughts or behavior • Serotonin syndrome with MAOIs • Some CYP interactions • Vilazodone is not associated with sexual dysfunction or weight gain
Serotonin-Norepinephrine Reuptake Inhibitors		
Venlafaxine Desvenlafaxine Duloxetine Milnacipran Levomilnacipran	• Anxiety and depression, ADHD, autism, fibromyalgia, PTSD, menopause symptoms • Inhibitors of SERT and NET	• Side effects include nausea and dizziness • May increase risk of suicidal thoughts or behavior • May cause sexual dysfunctions • Duloxetine and milnacipran contraindicated in uncontrolled narrow-angle or angle-closure glaucoma

Drug Facts for Your Personal Formulary: *Depression and Anxiety Disorders* (*continued*)

Drugs	Therapeutic Uses	Clinical Pharmacology and Tips
Tricyclic Antidepressants		
Amitriptyline Clomipramine Doxepin Imipramine Trimipramine Nortriptyline Maprotiline Protriptyline Desipramine Amoxapine	• Block SERT, NET, α_1, H_1, and M_1 receptors • Major depression	• Generally replaced by newer antidepressants with fewer side effects • Numerous side effects: orthostatic hypertension, weight gain, GI disturbances, sexual dysfunction, seizures, irregular heart beats • Should not be used within 14 days of taking MAOIs • Suicidal thoughts or behavior
Atypical Antipsychotics		
Aripiprazole Brexpiprazole Lurasidone Olanzapine Quetiapine Risperidone	• Resistant major depression and psychotic disorders • Schizophrenia • Bipolar depression	• See Chapter 16 for details • Metabolic syndrome and weight gain
Monoamine Oxidase Inhibitors		
Isocarboxazid Phenelzine Selegiline Tranylcypromine	• Inhibit MAO_A and MAO_B to prevent NE, DA, and 5HT breakdown • Major depression disorders resistant to other antidepressants	• Many side effects, including weight gain and sexual dysfunction; replaced by newer antidepressants • Suicidal thoughts • Slow elimination • May cause hypertensive crisis if taken with tyramine-containing foods/beverages • Selegiline at lower doses is selective for MAO_B (found in serotonergic neurons) • Selegiline, as a transdermal patch, is approved for treatment of depression
Atypical Antidepressants		
Bupropion Trazodone Nefazodone Mirtazapine Mianserin (not marketed in the U.S.) Vortioxetine	• Depression • Smoking cessation (bupropion) • Insomnia (low-dose trazodone)	• Bupropion is a DAT inhibitor used to help quit smoking; no weight gain side effect • Mirtazapine, trazodone, and nefazodone are $5HT_2$ receptor antagonists • Mirtazapine and trazodone may cause drowsiness and should be taken at bedtime • Risk of hepatic failure with nefazodone • Vortioxetine: SERT inhibitor, $5HT_{1A}$ agonist, and $5HT_3$ antagonist • Suicidal thoughts or behavior • Do not use within 14 days of taking MAOI

Bibliography

Abdallah CG, et al. Ketamine as a promising prototype for a new generation of rapid-acting antidepressants. *Ann N Y Acad Sci*, **2015**, *1344*:66–77.

Andrews JM, Nemeroff CB. Contemporary management of depression. *Am J Med*, **1994**, *97*:24S–32S.

Atack JR. Anxioselective compounds acting at the GABA(A) receptor benzodiazepine binding site. *Curr Drug Targets CNS Neurol Disord*, **2003**, *2*:213–232.

Bang-Andersen B, et al. Discovery of 1-[2-(2,4-dimethylphenyl-sulfanyl) phenyl]piperazine (Lu AA21004): a novel multimodal compound for the treatment of major depressive disorder. *J Med Chem*, **2011**, *54*:3206–3221.

Benmansour S, et al. Effects of chronic antidepressant treatments on serotonin transporter function, density, and mRNA level. *J Neurosci*, **1999**, *19*:10494–10501.

Brockmöller J, et al. Pharmacokinetics of mirtazapine: enantioselective effects of the CYP2D6 ultra rapid metabolizer genotype and correlation with adverse effects. *Clin Pharmacol Ther*, **2007**, *81*:699–707.

Cannon TD, Keller MC. Endophenotypes in the genetic analyses of mental disorders. *Annu Rev Clin Psychol*, **2006**, *2*:267–290.

Carroll FI, et al. Bupropion and bupropion analogs as treatments for CNS disorders. *Adv Pharmacol*, **2014**, *69*:177–216.

Chen YW, Dilsaver SC. Lifetime rates of suicide attempts among subjects with bipolar and unipolar disorders relative to subjects with other axis I disorders. *Biol Psychiatry*, **1996**, *39*:896–899.

Clayton AH, et al. Antidepressants and sexual dysfunction: mechanisms and clinical implications. *Postgrad Med*, **2014**, *126*:91–99.

Cryan JF, Holmes, A. The ascent of mouse: advances in modelling human depression and anxiety. *Nat Rev*, **2005**, *4*:775–790.

Decloedt EH, Stein DJ. Current trends in drug treatment of obsessive-compulsive disorder. *Neuropsychiatr Dis Treat*, **2010**, *6*:233–242.

Delgado PL, et al. Rapid serotonin depletion as a provocative challenge test for patients with major depression: relevance to antidepressant action and the neurobiology of depression. *Psychopharmacol Bull*, **1991**, *27*:321–330.

Dubovsky SL. The usefulness of genotyping cytochrome P450 enzymes in the treatment of depression. *Expert Opin Drug Metab Toxicol*, **2015**, *11*:369–379.

Duman CH, Duman RS. Spine synapse remodeling in the pathophysiology and treatment of depression. *Neurosci Lett*, **2015**, *601*:20–29.

Entsuah AR, et al. Response and remission rates in different subpopulations with major depressive disorder administered venlafaxine, selective serotonin reuptake inhibitors, or placebo. *J Clin Psychiatry*, **2001**, *62*:869–877.

FDA. Avoid food-drug interactions. Publication no. (FDA) CDER 10-1933, **2010**, pp. 21–22. Available at: http://www.fda.gov/drugs. Accessed March 17, 2016.

Finberg JP. Update on the pharmacology of selective inhibitors of MAO-A and MAO-B: focus on modulation of CNS monoamine neurotransmitter release. *Pharmacol Ther*, **2014**, *143*:133–152.

Finnerup NB, et al. Pharmacotherapy for neuropathic pain in adults: a systematic review and meta-analysis. *Lancet Neurol*, **2015**, *14*:162–173.

Foley KF, et al. Bupropion: pharmacology and therapeutic applications. *Expert Rev Neurother*, **2006**, *6*:1249–1265.

Frazer A. Pharmacology of antidepressants. *J Clin Psychopharmacol*, **1997**, *17*(suppl 1):2S–18S.

Fujita M, et al. Downregulation of brain phosphodiesterase type IV measured with 11C-(R)-rolipram positron emission tomography in major depressive disorder. *Biol Psychiatry*, **2012**, *72*:548–554.

Gadot Y, Koren G. The use of antidepressants in pregnancy: focus on maternal risks. *J Obstet Gynaecol Can*, **2015**, *37*:56–63.

Gibbons RD, et al. Early evidence on the effects of regulators' suicidality warnings on SSRI prescriptions and suicide in children and adolescents. *Am J Psychiatry*, **2007**, *164*:1356–1363.

Gijsman HJ, et al. Antidepressants for bipolar depression: a systematic review of randomized, controlled trials. *Am J Psychiatry*, **2004**, *161*:1537–1547.

Gobbi G, et al. Neurochemical and psychotropic effects of bupropion in healthy male subjects. *J Clin Psychopharmacol*, **2003**, *23*:233–239.

Goldberg JF, Truman CJ. Antidepressant-induced mania: an overview of current controversies. *Bipolar Disord*, **2003**, *5*:407–420.

Goodman WK. Selecting pharmacotherapy for generalized anxiety disorder. *J Clin Psychiatry*, **2004**, *65*(suppl 13):8–13.

Harvey BH, Slabbert FN. New insights on the antidepressant discontinuation syndrome. *Hum Psychopharmacol*, **2014**, *29*:503–516.

Heninger GR, et al. The revised monoamine theory of depression: a modulatory role for monoamines, based on new findings from monoamine depletion experiments in humans. *Pharmacopsychiatry*, **1996**, *29*:2–11.

Hiemke C, Hartter S. Pharmacokinetics of selective serotonin reuptake inhibitors. *Pharmacol Ther*, **2000**, *85*:11–28.

Hillhouse TM, Porter JH. A brief history of the development of antidepressant drugs: from monoamines to glutamate. *Exp Clin Psychopharmacol*, **2015**, *23*:1–21.

Hollister LE. Current antidepressant drugs: their clinical use. *Drugs*, **1981**, *22*:129–152.

Horne RL, et al. Treatment of bulimia with bupropion: a multicenter controlled trial. *J Clin Psychiatry*, **1988**, *49*:262–266.

Isacsson G, Rich CL. Antidepressant drugs and the risk of suicide in children and adolescents. *Paediatr Drugs*, **2014**, *16*:115–122.

Jarema M. Atypical antipsychotics in the treatment of mood disorders. *Curr Opin Psychiatry*, **2007**, *20*:23–29.

Johansson R, et al. Depression, anxiety and their comorbidity in the Swedish general population: point prevalence and the effect on health-related quality of life. *Peer J*, **2013**, *1*:e98. doi:10.7717/peerj.98. Accessed March 16, 2016.

Katz MM, et al. Onset and early behavioral effects of pharmacologically different antidepressants and placebo in depression. *Neuropsychopharmacology*, **2004**, *29*:566–579.

Kessler RC, et al. Lifetime and 12-month prevalence of *DSM-III-R* psychiatric disorders in the United States. Results from the National Comorbidity Survey. *Arch Gen Psychiatry*, **1994**, *51*:8–19.

Leonard BE, Richelson E. Synaptic effects of anitdepressants. In: Buckley PF, Waddington JL, eds. *Schizophrenia and Mood Disorders: The New Drug Therapies in Clinical Practice*. Butterworth-Heinemann, Boston, **2000**, 67–84.

Licznerski P, Duman RS. Remodeling of axo-spinous synapses in the pathophysiology and treatment of depression. *Neuroscience*, **2013**, *251*:33–50.

Lin E, Lane HY. Genome-wide association studies in pharmacogenomics of antidepressants. *Pharmacogenomics*, **2015**, *6*:555–566.

Livingston MG, Livingston HM. Monoamine oxidase inhibitors. An update on drug interactions. *Drug Saf*, **1996**, *14*:219–227.

Mann JJ, et al. ACNP Task Force report on SSRIs and suicidal behavior in youth. *Neuropsychopharmacology*, **2006**, *31*:473–492.

Mauri MC, et al. Pharmacokinetics of antidepressants in patients with hepatic impairment. *Clin Pharmacokinet*, **2014**, *53*:1069–1081.

Millan MJ. The neurobiology and control of anxious states. *Prog Neurobiol*, **2003**, *70*:83–244.

Millan MJ. Multi-target strategies for the improved treatment of depressive states: conceptual foundations and neuronal substrates, drug discovery and therapeutic application. *Pharmacol Ther*, **2006**, *110*:135–370.

Nestler EJ, et al. *Molecular Neuropharmacology*. 3rd ed. McGraw-Hill, New York, **2015**.

Noe KH, et al. Treatment of depression in patients with epilepsy. *Curr Treat Options Neurol*, **2011**, *13*:371–379.

Nurnberg HG. Managing treatment-emergent sexual dysfunction associated with serotonergic antidepressants: before and after sildenafil. *J Psychiatr Pract*, **2001**, *7*:92–108.

Nurnberg HG, et al. Sildenafil treatment of women with antidepressant-associated sexual dysfunction: a randomized controlled trial. *JAMA*, **2008**, *300*:395–404.

O'Donnell JM, Zhang HT. Antidepressant effects of inhibitors of cAMP phosphodiesterase (PDE4). *Trends Pharmacol Sci*, **2004**, *25*:158–163.

Owens MJ, et al. Neurotransmitter receptor and transporter binding profile of antidepressants and their metabolites. *J Pharmacol Exp Ther*, **1997**, *283*:1305–1322.

Pascual-Brazo J, et al. Neurogenesis as a new target for the development of antidepressant drugs. *Curr Pharm Des*, **2014**, *20*:3763–3775.

Probst-Schendzielorz K, et al. Effect of cytochrome P450 polymorphism on the action and metabolism of selective serotonin reuptake inhibitors. *Expert Opin Drug Metab Toxicol*, **2015**, *11*:1219–1232.

Rapaport MH. Dietary restrictions and drug interactions with monoamine oxidase inhibitors: the state of the art. *J Clin Psychiatry*, **2007**, *68*(suppl 8):42–46.

Rudorfer MV, Potter WZ. Metabolism of tricyclic antidepressants. *Cell Mol Neurobiol*, **1999**, *19*:373–409.

Rush AJ, et al. Acute and longer-term outcomes in depressed outpatients requiring one or several treatment steps: a STAR*D report. *Am J Psychiatry*, **2006**, *163*:1905–1917.

Santarelli L, et al. Requirement of hippocampal neurogenesis for the behavioral effects of antidepressants. *Science*, **2003**, *301*:805–809.

Schmidt HD, Duman RS. The role of neurotrophic factors in adult hippocampal neurogenesis, antidepressant treatments and animal models of depressive-like behavior. *Behav Pharmacol*, **2007**, *18*:391–418.

Shelton RC. Cellular mechanisms in the vulnerability to depression and response to antidepressants. *Psychiatr Clin North Am*, **2000**, *23*:713–729.

Shelton RC, Lester N. SSRIs and newer antidepressants. In: Stein DJ, Kupfer DJ, Schatzburg AF, eds. *APA Textbook of Mood Disorders*. APA Press, Washington, DC, **2006**, Chapter 16.

Suominen KH, et al. Inadequate treatment for major depression both before and after attempted suicide. *Am J Psychiatry*, **1998**, *155*:1778–1780.

Thronson LR, Pagalilauan GL. Psychopharmacology. *Med Clin North Am*, **2014**, *98*:927–958.

Vaswani M, et al. Role of selective serotonin reuptake inhibitors in psychiatric disorders: a comprehensive review. *Prog Neuropsychopharmacol Biol Psychiatry*, **2003**, *27*:85–102.

Xu Y, et al. Animal models of depression and neuroplasticity: assessing drug action in relation to behavior and neurogenesis. *Methods Mol Biol*, **2012**, *829*:103–124.

Zhao Z, et al. Association of changes in norepinephrine and serotonin transporter expression with the long-term behavioral effects of antidepressant drugs. *Neuropsychopharmacology*, **2009**, *34*:1467–1481.

Pharmacotherapy of Psychosis and Mania
Jonathan M. Meyer

Treatment of Psychosis

Psychosis is a symptom of mental illnesses characterized by a distorted or nonexistent sense of reality. Psychotic disorders have different etiologies, each of which demands a unique treatment approach. Common psychotic disorders include mood disorders (major depression or mania) with psychotic features, substance-induced psychosis, dementia with psychotic features, delirium with psychotic features, brief psychotic disorder, delusional disorder, schizoaffective disorder, and schizophrenia.

Schizophrenia has a worldwide prevalence of 1% and is considered the prototypic disorder for understanding the phenomenology of psychosis and the impact of antipsychotic treatment, but patients with schizophrenia exhibit features that extend beyond those seen in other psychotic illnesses. Hallucinations, delusions, disorganized speech, and disorganized or agitated behavior are psychotic symptoms found individually, and occasionally together, in all psychotic disorders and are typically responsive to pharmacotherapy. In addition to *positive symptoms*, schizophrenia patients also suffer from *negative symptoms* (apathy, avolition, alogia) and *cognitive deficits*, with the latter the most disabling aspect of the disorder (Young and Geyer, 2015).

The Dopamine Hypothesis

The syntheses of chlorpromazine (1950) and haloperidol (1958) allowed Carlsson to deduce that postsynaptic DA receptor antagonism was their common mechanism. Carlsson's discovery informed the development of numerous *typical* or first-generation antipsychotic drugs that were found to act specifically at D_2 receptors (Seeman, 2013). The discovery of clozapine's unique clinical features and binding profile stimulated development of second-generation antipsychotics that potently antagonize the $5HT_{2A}$ receptor while possessing less affinity for D_2 receptors than typical antipsychotic agents, resulting in antipsychotic efficacy with lower potential for extrapyramidal side effects. Subsequent research led to the development of agents with D_2 partial agonist properties that act as modulators of dopaminergic neurotransmission (Meyer and Leckband, 2013).

The DA model of antipsychotic action has limitations: It does not explain the psychotomimetic effects of LSD (e.g., a potent $5HT_{2A}$ receptor agonist) or the effects of phencyclidine and ketamine, antagonists of the NMDA glutamate receptor. However, phencyclidine and ketamine indirectly act to stimulate DA availability by decreasing the glutamate-mediated tonic inhibition of DA release in the mesolimbic DA pathway (Howes et al., 2015). Exploration of nondopaminergic antipsychotic mechanisms led to approval of pimavanserin, a potent $5HT_{2A}$ inverse agonist for treatment

of Parkinson disease psychosis (PDP). Phase 3 trials of glutamate modulators have not been successful. Except for pimavanserin, all approved antipsychotic agents share a common mechanism of action: direct modulation of D_2 receptor activity (Figure 16–1).

Mechanism of Action of D_2 Receptors

Dopamine D_2 receptors share common properties with D_3 and D_4 receptors in that each is linked to inhibitory G protein G_i, and receptor stimulation results in decreased cyclic AMP production and thus a reduction in intracellular cyclic AMP (Figure 16–1), whereas agonists at D_1 and D_5 receptors stimulate the G_s–adenylyl cyclase–cyclic AMP pathway (Seeman, 2013). Antipsychotic actions at D_2 receptors are also mediated through non-G protein, particularly via modulation of the activity of GSK-3β through a β-arrestin-2/PKB/PP2A signaling complex (see Chapter 3). Atypical antipsychotics antagonize D_2 receptor/β-arrestin-2 interactions more than G protein–dependent signaling, but typical antipsychotics inhibit both pathways with similar efficacy (Urs et al., 2012).

Review of Relevant Pathophysiology

Not all psychosis is schizophrenia, and the pathophysiology relevant to effective schizophrenia treatment may not apply to other psychotic disorders. The effectiveness of dopamine D_2 antagonists for the positive symptoms of psychosis seen in most psychotic disorders suggests a common etiology related to excessive dopaminergic neurotransmission in mesolimbic DA pathways (i.e., the associative striatum) (Kuepper et al., 2012).

Delirium, Dementia, and Parkinson Disease Psychosis

The psychoses related to delirium and dementia, particularly dementia of the Alzheimer type, may share a common etiology: deficiency in muscarinic cholinergic neurotransmission due to medications, age- or disease-related neuronal loss (Koppel and Greenwald, 2014; Salahudeen et al., 2014). Delerium may have precipitants besides medication, such as infection, electrolyte imbalance, metabolic derangement, all of which require specific treatment, in addition to removal of anticholinergic medications (Khan et al., 2012). The development of PDP is due to Lewy body associated loss of serotonin raphe neurons and subsequent upregulation of cortical $5HT_{2A}$ receptors. The specific treatment for PDP is pimavanserin, a selective $5HT_{2A}$ inverse agonist devoid of DA receptor activity (Cummings et al., 2014).

Schizophrenia

Schizophrenia is a neurodevelopmental disorder with complex genetics and incompletely understood pathophysiology. In addition to environmental exposures such as fetal second-trimester infectious or nutritional

Abbreviations

ACEI: angiotensin-converting enzyme inhibitor
AUC: area under the curve
CBC: complete blood cell count
CNS: central nervous system
COX-2: cyclooxygenase 2
CV: cardiovascular
DA: dopamine
DAAO: D-amino acid oxidase
DAT: DA transporter
DM: diabetes mellitus
ECG: electrocardiogram
ECT: electroconvulsive therapy
eGFR: estimated glomerular filtration rate
EM: extensive metabolizer
ENaC: epithelial sodium channel
EPS: extrapyramidal symptom
FDA: Food and Drug Administration
G-CSF: granulocyte colony-stimulating factor
GFR: glomerular filtration rate
GlyT: glycine transporter
GSK: glycogen synthase kinase
5HT: serotonin
I_{kr}**:** inwardly rectifying K^+ channels
IM: intramuscular
LAI: long-acting injectable
MAO: monoamine oxidase
mGlu: metabotropic glutamate
NDI: nephrogenic diabetes insipidus
NE: norepinephrine
NMDA: N-methyl-D-aspartate
NMS: neuroleptic malignant syndrome
ODT: oral dissolving tablet
PDP: Parkinson disease psychosis
PET: positron emission tomography
PGP: P-glycoprotein
PK_: protein kinase _, as in PKA, PKC
PP2A: protein phosphatase 2A
SCD: sudden cardiac death
T_4**:** levorotatory thyroxine
TD: tardive dyskinesia
TH: tyrosine hydroxylase
TSH: thyrotropin (previously thyroid-stimulating hormone)
VMAT2: vesicular monoamine transporter 2

insults, birth complications, and substance abuse in the late teen or early adult years, over 150 genes appear to contribute to schizophrenia risk. Implicated are genes that regulate neuronal migration, synaptogenesis, cellular adhesion, and neurite outgrowth (*neuregulin 1, disrupted-in-schizophrenia-1*); synaptic DA availability (*Val [108/158]Met polymorphism of catechol-O-methyltransferase*, which increases DA catabolism); glutamate and DA neurotransmission (*dystrobrevin binding protein 1* or *dysbindin*); and nicotinic activity (*α7-receptor polymorphisms*) (Escudero and Johnstone, 2014). Patients with schizophrenia also have increased rates of genome-wide DNA microduplications, termed *copy number variants*, and *epigenetic* changes, including disruptions in DNA methylation patterns in various brain regions (Gavin and Floreani, 2014). This genetic variability is consistent with the heterogeneity of the clinical disease and suggests that any one specific mechanism is unlikely to account for large amounts of disease risk.

Review of Psychosis Pathology and the General Goals of Pharmacotherapy

Common to all psychotic disorders are positive symptoms, which may include hallucinatory behavior, disturbed thinking, and behavioral dyscontrol. Common to effective schizophrenia treatments is an impact on dopaminergic neurotransmission (Figure 16–1).

Short-Term Antipsychotic Treatment

For many psychotic disorders, the symptoms are transient, and antipsychotic drugs are only administered during and shortly after periods of symptom exacerbation. Patients with delirium, dementia, major depressive disorder or mania with psychotic features, substance-induced psychoses, and brief psychotic disorder will typically receive short-term antipsychotic treatment that is discontinued after resolution of psychotic symptoms, although the duration may vary considerably based on the etiology. Bipolar patients in particular may have antipsychotic treatment extended for several months after resolution of mania and psychosis because antipsychotic medications are effective in reducing mania relapse. Chronic psychotic symptoms in patients with dementia may also be amenable to drug therapy, but potential benefits must be balanced with the documented risk of mortality and cerebrovascular events associated with the use of antipsychotic medications in this patient population (Maust et al., 2015).

Long-Term Antipsychotic Treatment

Delusional disorder, schizophrenia, schizoaffective disorder, and PDP are chronic diseases that require long-term antipsychotic treatment. For schizophrenia and schizoaffective disorder in particular, the goal of antipsychotic treatment is to maximize functional recovery by decreasing the severity of positive symptoms and their behavioral influence and possibly improving negative symptoms and remediating cognitive dysfunction, although the impact on the last two symptom domains is modest at best. Continuous antipsychotic treatment reduces 1-year relapse rates from 80% among unmedicated patients to about 15% (Zipursky et al., 2014). Poor adherence to antipsychotic treatment increases relapse risk and is often related to adverse drug events, cognitive dysfunction, substance use, and limited illness insight (Remington et al., 2014).

Regardless of the underlying pathology, the immediate goal of antipsychotic treatment is a decrease in acute symptoms that induce patient distress, particularly behavioral symptoms (e.g., hostility, agitation) that may present a danger to the patient or others. The dosing, route of administration, and choice of antipsychotic depend on the underlying disease state, clinical acuity, drug-drug interactions with concomitant medications, and patient sensitivity to short- or long-term adverse effects. With the exception of pimavanserin for PDP, and clozapine's superior efficacy in treatment-refractory schizophrenia, neither the clinical presentation nor biomarkers predicts the likelihood of response to a specific antipsychotic class or agent. As a result, avoidance of adverse effects based on patient and drug characteristics and exploitation of certain medication properties (e.g., sedation related to histamine H_1 or muscarinic antagonism) are the principal determinants for choosing initial antipsychotic therapy (Leucht et al., 2013).

Short-Term Treatment

Delirium, Dementia, and Parkinson Disease Psychosis

Psychotic symptoms of delirium or dementia are generally treated with low medication doses, although doses may have to be repeated at frequent intervals initially to achieve adequate behavioral control. Despite widespread clinical use, no antipsychotic has received approval for dementia-related psychosis. Moreover, all antipsychotic drugs carry warnings that they may increase mortality in this setting (Maust et al., 2015). Because anticholinergic drug effects may worsen delirium and dementia, high-potency typical antipsychotic drugs (e.g., haloperidol) or atypical antipsychotic agents with limited antimuscarinic properties (e.g., risperidone) are often the drugs of choice (Khan et al., 2012).

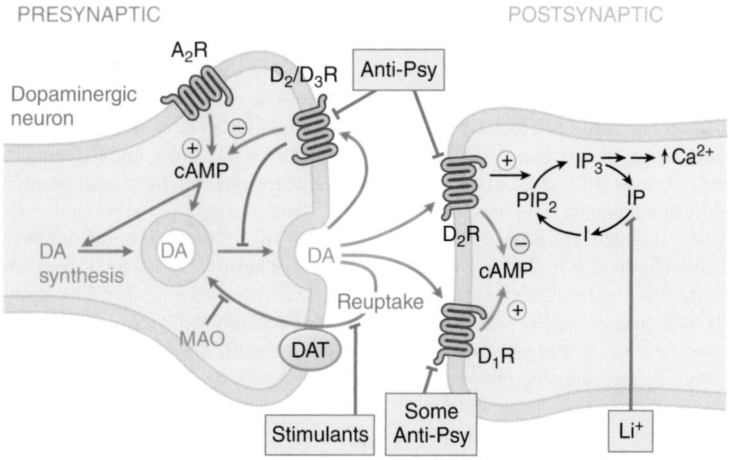

Figure 16–1 *Sites of action of antipsychotic agents and Li⁺.* Following exocytotic release, DA interacts with postsynaptic receptors (R) of D_1 and D_2 types and presynaptic D_2 and D_3 autoreceptors. Termination of DA action occurs primarily by active transport of DA into presynaptic terminals via the DAT, with secondary deamination by mitochondrial MAO. Stimulation of postsynaptic D_1 receptors activates the G_s–adenylyl cyclase–cAMP pathway. D_2 receptors couple through G_i to inhibit adenylyl cyclase and through G_q to activate the PLC-IP_3-Ca^{2+} pathway. Activation of the G_i pathway can also activate K^+ channels, leading to hyperpolarization. Li^+ inhibits IP breakdown and thereby enhances its accumulation and sequelae (Ca^{2+} mobilization, PKC activation, depletion of cellular I). Li^+ may also alter release of neurotransmitter by a variety of putative mechanisms (see text). D_2-like autoreceptors suppress synthesis of DA by diminishing phosphorylation of rate-limiting TH, and by limiting DA release. In contrast, presynaptic A_2Rs) activate the adenylyl cyclase–cAMP–PKA pathway and thence TH activity. All antipsychotic agents act at D_2 receptors and autoreceptors; some also block D_1 receptors (Table 16–2). Stimulant agents inhibit DA reuptake by DAT, thereby prolonging the dwell time of synaptic DA. Initially in antipsychotic treatment, DA neurons release more DA, but following repeated treatment, they enter a state of physiological depolarization inactivation, with diminished production and release of DA, in addition to continued receptor blockade. ——⊣, inhibition or blockade; ⊕, elevation of activity; ⊖, reduction of activity; cAMP, cyclic AMP; IP, inositol phosphate; IP3, inositol 1,4,5-trisphosphate; PIP2, phosphatidylinositol 4,5-bisphosphate.

The doses for patients with dementia are one-fourth of adult schizophrenia doses (e.g., risperidone 0.5–1.5 mg/d), as EPSs, orthostasis, and sedation are particularly problematic in this patient population (Chapter 18). In acute psychosis, significant antipsychotic benefits are usually seen within 60–120 min after drug administration. Delirious or demented patients may be reluctant or unable to swallow tablets, but ODT preparations or liquid concentrate forms are available. Intramuscular administration of ziprasidone or olanzapine represents an option for treating agitated and minimally cooperative patients and presents less risk for drug-induced parkinsonism than haloperidol. An inhaled form of loxapine 10 mg is available in the U.S., with a median T_{max} of less than 2 min. Following rapid distribution, levels drop 75% over the next 10 min and then follow typical kinetics with a $t_{1/2}$ of 7.6 h. Inhaled loxapine can be administered only in healthcare facilities that can provide advanced airway management in the rare event of acute bronchospasm. Pimavanserin for PDP has a $t_{1/2}$ of 57 h, and clinical effects are seen over 2-6 weeks. (See Use in Pediatric Populations and Use in Geriatric Populations later in the chapter.)

Mania

All atypical antipsychotics medications with the exception of clozapine, iloperidone, brexpiprazole, and lurasidone, have indications for acute mania, and doses are titrated rapidly close to or at the maximum FDA-approved dose over the first 24–72 h of treatment. Typical antipsychotic drugs are also effective in acute mania, but often are eschewed due to the risk for EPSs. Clinical response (decreased psychomotor agitation and irritability, increased sleep, and reduced or absent delusions and hallucinations) usually occurs within 7 days but may be apparent as early as day 2. Patients with mania may need to continue on antipsychotic treatment for many months after the resolution of psychotic and manic symptoms, typically in combination with a mood stabilizer such as lithium or valproic acid preparations (e.g., divalproex) (Malhi et al., 2012). Oral aripiprazole and olanzapine have indications as monotherapy for bipolar disorder maintenance treatment, but the use of olanzapine has decreased dramatically due to concerns over adverse metabolic effects (e.g., weight gain, hyperlipidemia, hyperglycemia). LAI risperidone also has indications for maintenance monotherapy (and adjunctively with lithium or valproate) in patients with bipolar I disorder.

Combining an antipsychotic agent with a mood stabilizer often improves control of manic symptoms and further reduces the risk of relapse. Weight gain from the additive effects of antipsychotic agents and mood stabilizers presents a significant clinical problem. Antipsychotic agents with greater weight-gain liabilities (e.g., olanzapine, clozapine) should be avoided unless patients are refractory to preferred treatments.

The recommended duration of treatment after resolution of bipolar mania varies considerably, but as symptoms permit, a gradual drug taper should be attempted after 6 months of treatment, to lessen weight gain when combined with a mood stabilizer (Yatham et al., 2016).

Major Depression

Patients with major depressive disorder with psychotic features require lower-than-average doses of antipsychotic drugs, given in combination with an antidepressant. Extended antipsychotic treatment is not usually required, but certain atypical antipsychotic agents provide adjunctive antidepressant benefit (Farahani and Correll, 2012). Most antipsychotic drugs show limited antidepressant benefit when used as monotherapy, with the exception of amisulpride, loxapine, lurasidone, and quetiapine. Some atypical antipsychotic agents are effective as adjunct therapy in treatment-resistant unipolar depression. The primary mechanisms of action include $5HT_{2C}$ antagonism (olanzapine and quetiapine's metabolite, norquetiapine), which facilitates DA and NE release, and DA D_3 partial agonism (aripiprazole, brexpiprazole, craiprazine), which may result in stimulation of reward centers. Quetiapine at doses of 300 mg/d is effective for bipolar depression, as is lurasidone in the dosage range of 20–120 mg/d administered with an evening meal of at least 350 kcal. One of lurasidone's postulated antidepressant mechanisms is potent $5HT_7$ antagonism (Turner et al., 2014; Wright et al., 2013).

Schizophrenia

The immediate goals of acute antipsychotic treatment are the reduction of agitated, disorganized, or hostile behavior, decreasing the impact of hallucinations, improvement in the organization of thought, and the reduction of social withdrawal. Doses used acutely may be higher than those required for maintenance treatment of stable patients. Aside from clozapine, which is uniquely efficacious in refractory schizophrenia, atypical antipsychotics are not more effective than typical agents but offer a better neurological side-effect profile than typical antipsychotic drugs. Excessive D_2 blockade, as is often the case with the use of high-potency typical agents (e.g., haloperidol), not only increases risk for neurological effects (e.g., muscular rigidity, bradykinesia, tremor, akathisia) but also slows mentation (bradyphrenia) and interferes with central reward pathways, resulting in patient complaints of anhedonia (loss of capacity to experience pleasure). Low-potency typical agents such as chlorpromazine are not commonly used due to the high affinities for H_1, M_1, and α_1 receptors that result in undesirable effects (sedation, anticholinergic properties, orthostasis). Concerns regarding QT_c prolongation further limit their clinical usefulness. In acute psychosis, sedation may be desirable, but the use of a sedating antipsychotic drug may interfere with cognitive function and assessment.

Because schizophrenia requires long-term treatment, antipsychotic agents with greater metabolic liabilities, especially weight gain (discussed further in this chapter), should be avoided as first-line therapies. Ziprasidone, aripiprazole, iloperidone, brexpiprazole, cariprazine, and lurasidone are the most weight and metabolically benign atypical agents (De Hert et al., 2012; Rummel-Kluge et al., 2010). Ziprasidone is available in acute intramuscular form, thus permitting continuation of the same drug treatment initiated parenterally in the emergency room. Patients with schizophrenia have a 2-fold higher prevalence of metabolic syndrome and type 2 DM and 2-fold greater CV-related mortality rates than the general population (Torniainen et al., 2015). For this reason, consensus guidelines recommend baseline determination of serum glucose, lipids, weight, blood pressure, and personal and family histories of metabolic and CV disease.

With the low EPS risk among atypical antipsychotic agents, prophylactic use of antiparkinsonian medications (e.g., benztropine, trihexyphenidyl) is not necessary. Drug-induced parkinsonism can occur at higher dosages or among elderly patients exposed to antipsychotic agents that have higher D_2 affinity; recommended doses are about 50% of those used in younger patients with schizophrenia. (See also Use in Pediatric Populations and Use in Geriatric Populations further in the chapter.)

Long-Term Treatment

The need for long-term treatment poses issues almost exclusively to the chronic psychotic illnesses, schizophrenia and schizoaffective disorder. However, long-term antipsychotic treatment is sometimes used for manic patients, for ongoing psychosis in patients with dementia, for PDP, and for adjunctive use in treatment-resistant depression. Safety concerns combined with limited long-term efficacy data have dampened enthusiasm for extended antipsychotic drug use in patients with dementia (Maust et al., 2015). Justification for ongoing use, based on documentation of patient response to tapering of antipsychotic medication, is often mandated in long-term care settings.

Antipsychotic Agents

The choice of antipsychotic agents for long-term schizophrenia treatment is based primarily on avoidance of adverse effects, prior history of patient response, and the need for a long-acting injectable formulation due to adherence issues. While concerns over EPSs and TD have abated with the introduction of the atypical antipsychotic agents, there has been increased concern over metabolic effects of antipsychotic treatment: weight gain, dyslipidemia (particularly hypertriglyceridemia), and an adverse impact on glucose-insulin homeostasis (Rummel-Kluge et al., 2010). Clozapine and olanzapine have the highest metabolic risk and are only used as last resort. Olanzapine is often used prior to clozapine after failure of more metabolically benign agents such as aripiprazole, ziprasidone, asenapine, iloperidone, and lurasidone.

Acutely psychotic patients usually respond within hours after drug administration, but weeks may be required to achieve maximal drug response, especially for negative symptoms. Analyses of symptom response in clinical trials indicate that the majority of response to any antipsychotic treatment in acute schizophrenia is seen by week 4 (Jager et al., 2010). Failure of response after 2 weeks should prompt clinical reassessment, including determination of medication adherence, before a decision is

made to increase the dose or consider switching to another agent (Kinon et al., 2010). Patients with first-episode schizophrenia often respond to lower doses, and chronic patients may require doses that exceed recommended ranges. While the acute behavioral impact of treatment is seen within hours to days, long-term studies indicate improvement may not plateau for 6 months, underscoring the importance of ongoing antipsychotic treatment in functional recovery for patients with schizophrenia.

Usual dosages for acute and maintenance treatment are noted in Table 16-1. Dosing should be adjusted based on clinically observable signs of antipsychotic benefit and adverse effects. For example, higher EPS risk is noted for risperidone doses that exceed 6 mg/d in nonelderly adult patients with schizophrenia. However, in the absence of EPSs, increasing the dose from 6 to 8 mg would be a reasonable approach in a patient with ongoing positive symptoms. Certain antipsychotic adverse effects, including weight gain, sedation, orthostasis, and EPSs, can be predicted based on potencies at neurotransmitter receptors (Table 16-2). The detection of dyslipidemia or hyperglycemia is based on laboratory monitoring (Table 16-1). Dose reduction often resolves hyperprolactinemia, EPSs, orthostasis, and sedation, but metabolic abnormalities improve only with discontinuation of the offending agent and a switch to a more metabolically benign medication. The decision to switch patients with stable schizophrenia and metabolic dysfunction solely for metabolic benefit must be individualized based on patient preferences, severity of the metabolic disturbance, likelihood of metabolic improvement with antipsychotic switching, and history of response to prior agents. Patients with refractory schizophrenia on clozapine are not good candidates for switching because they are resistant to other medications (see the definition of refractory schizophrenia further in this section).

Psychotic Relapse

There are many reasons for psychotic relapse or inadequate response to antipsychotic treatment in patients with schizophrenia; reasons include substance use, psychosocial stressors, inherent refractory illness, and poor medication adherence. The common problem of medication nonadherence among patients with schizophrenia has led to the development of LAI antipsychotic medications, often referred to as depot antipsychotics (Meyer, 2013). There are currently eight LAI forms available in the U.S.: decanoate esters of fluphenazine and haloperidol, risperidone-impregnated microspheres, 1-month and 3-month formulations of paliperidone palmitate, aripiprazole monohydrate, aripiprazole lauroxil, and olanzapine pamoate (Table 16-3). Patients receiving LAI antipsychotic medications show consistently lower relapse rates compared to patients receiving comparable oral forms and may have fewer adverse effects due to lower peak plasma levels.

Refractory Illness

Lack of response to adequate antipsychotic drug doses for adequate periods of time may indicate treatment-refractory illness. Use of antipsychotic plasma levels can help separate those who are nonadherent or are kinetic failures from those who are not responding to adequate medication exposure (Meyer, 2014). In treatment-refractory schizophrenia, response rates are 0% for typical antipsychotic agents, less than 10% for newer agents, but consistently about 60% for clozapine. Various studies have found correlations between trough plasma clozapine levels greater than 327–504 ng/mL and likelihood of clinical response (Rostami-Hodjegan et al., 2004). When therapeutic serum concentrations are reached, response to clozapine occurs within 8 weeks. Clozapine can have numerous adverse effects: risk of agranulocytosis (requires hematological monitoring), high metabolic burden, dose-dependent lowering of the seizure threshold, orthostasis, sedation, anticholinergic effects (especially constipation), and sialorrhea.

Electroconvulsive therapy also has proven efficacy for refractory schizophrenia.

Pharmacology of Antipsychotic Agents

Chemistry

Most early agents were derived from phenothiazine or butyrophenone structures. Presently, antipsychotic agents include many different chemical structures with a range of activities at different neurotransmitter receptors

TABLE 16–1 ■ DRUGS FOR PSYCHOSIS AND SCHIZOPHRENIA: DOSING AND METABOLIC RISK PROFILE

GENERIC NAME *Dosage Forms*	ORAL DOSAGE (mg/d)				METABOLIC SIDE EFFECTS		
	ACUTE PSYCHOSIS		MAINTENANCE				
	1ST EPISODE	CHRONIC	1ST EPISODE	CHRONIC	WEIGHT GAIN	LIPIDS	GLUCOSE
Phenothiazines							
Chlorpromazine *O, S, IM*	200–600	400–800	150–600	250–750	+++	+++	++
Perphenazine *O, S, IM*	12–50	24–48	12–48	24–60	+/–	–	–
Trifluoperazine *O, S, IM*	5–30	10–40	2.5–20	10–30	+/–	–	–
Fluphenazine *O, S, IM* decanoate *Depot IM*	2.5–15	5–20	2.5–10	5–15	+/–	–	–
	12.5–25 mg/wk (maximum 3 doses)		12.5–75 mg/2 wk		+/–	–	–
Selected other first-generation agents							
Loxapine *O, S, IM, Inhaled*	15–50	30–60	15–50	30–60	+	–	–
Thiothixene *O, S*	5–30	10–40	2.5–20	10–30	+/–	–	–
Haloperidol *O, S, IM* decanoate *Depot IM*	2.5–10	5–20	2.5–10	5–15	+/–	–	–
	100–200 mg/wk (max 3 loading doses)		100–400 mg/month		+/–	–	–
Second-generation agents							
Aripiprazole *O* monohydrate/lauroxil *Depot IM*	10–20	15–30	10–20	15–30	+/–	–	–
	Not for acute use		see note *a*	see note *a*	+/–	–	–
Amisulpride *O, S*[b]	200–800	400–1200	200–800	400–1200	+/–	–	–
Asenapine *ODT*	10	10–20	10	10–20	+/–	–	–
Brexpiprazole *O*	2–4	4	2–4	4	+/–	–	–
Cariprazine *O*	3–6	3–6	3–6	3–6	+/–	–	–
Clozapine *O, S, ODT*	200–600	400–900	200–600	300–900	++++	+++	+++
Iloperidone *O*		12–24[c]		8–16	+	+/–	+/–
Lurasidone *O*[d]	40–160	80–160	40–160	80–160	+	+/–	+/–
Olanzapine *O, ODT, IM* pamoate *Depot IM*[e]	7.5–20	10–30	7.5–15	15–30	++++	+++	+++
	Not for acute use		300–405	300–405	++++	+++	+++
Paliperidone palmitate *O Depot IM*[f]	6–9	6–12	3–9	6–15	+	+/–	+/–
	See note *f* on dosing				+	+/–	+/–
Quetiapine *O*	200–600	400–900	200–600	300–900	+	+	+/–
Risperidone *O, S, ODT* microspheres *Depot IM*	2–4	3–6	2–6	3–8	+	+/–	+/–
	Not for acute use		25–50 mg/2 wk		+	+/–	+/–
Sertindole *O*[b]	4–16	12–20	12–20	12–32	+/–	–	–
Ziprasidone *O, IM*[g]	120–160	120–200	80–160	120–200	+/–	–	–

Dosage Forms: IM, acute intramuscular; ODT, orally dissolving tablet; O, tablet; S, solution.

[a]Aripiprazole monohydrate dose: 300-400 mg IM/4 wks, with 14 days oral overlap. Aripiprazole lauroxil dose: 662-882 mg/4 wks or 882 mg/6 wks (equiv. to 662 mg/4 wks) with 21 days oral overlap. Dosages need to be adjusted for patients who are CYP2D6 poor metabolizers or those who are exposed to CYP2D6 or CYP3A4 inhibitors.

[b]Not available in the U.S.

[c]Due to orthostasis risk, dose titration of iloperidone is 1 mg twice daily on day 1, increasing to 2, 4, 6, 8, 10, and 12 mg twice daily on days 2–7 (as needed).

[d]Dose must be given with 350 kcal food to facilitate absorption. Administration with evening meal improves tolerability.

[e]Due to cases of postinjection delirium/sedation syndrome, patients must be observed after the injection for at least 3 h in a registered facility with ready access to emergency response services.

[f]Exists in two forms: 1-month and 3-month doses. In acute schizophrenia, deltoid intramuscular loading of 1-month form using doses of 234 mg at day 1 and 156 mg at day 8 to provide paliperidone levels equivalent to 6 mg oral paliperidone during the first week and peaking on day 15 at a level comparable to 12 mg oral paliperidone. No oral antipsychotic needed in first week. Maintenance intramuscular doses can be given every 4 weeks after day 8. Maintenance dose options for 1-month form: 39 to 234 mg every 4 weeks. Failure to give initiation doses (except for those switching from depot) will result in subtherapeutic levels for months. The 3-month form is only for those on 1-month dosing for at least 4 months. The 3-month dose is 3.5 times the stable monthly dose, administered every 12 weeks.

[g]Oral dose must be given with 500 kcal food to facilitate absorption.

TABLE 16–2 ■ POTENCIES OF ANTIPSYCHOTIC AGENTS AT NEUROTRANSMITTER RECEPTORS[a]

	DOPAMINE	SEROTONIN	MUSCARINIC	ADRENERGIC		HISTAMINE
	D_2	$5HT_{2A}$	M_1	A_{1A}	A_{1B}	H_1
First-generation agents						
Haloperidol	1.2	57	>10,000	12	7.6	1700
Fluphenazine	0.8	3.2	1100	6.5	13	14
Thiothixene	0.7	50	>10,000	12	35	8
Perphenazine	0.8	5.6	1500	10	—	8.0
Loxapine	11	4.4	120	42	53	4.9
Molindone[b]	20	>5000	>10,000	2600	—	2100
Thioridazine	8.0	28	13	3.2	2.4	16
Chlorpromazine	3.6	3.6	32	0.3	0.8	3.1
Second-generation agents						
Lurasidone	1.0	0.5	>1000	48	—	>1000
Aripiprazole	1.6[c]	8.7	6800	26	34	28
Brexpiprazole	0.4[c]	0.5	>1000	—	0.2	19
Cariprazine	0.6[c]	19	>1000	130	>1000	23
Asenapine	1.4	0.1	>10,000	1.2	3.9	1.0
Ziprasidone	6.8	0.6	>10,000	18	9.0	63
Sertindole[b]	2.7	0.4	>5000	1.8	—	130
Zotepine[b]	8.0	2.7	330	6.0	5.0	3.2
Risperidone	3.2	0.2	>10,000	5.0	9.0	20
Paliperidone	4.2	0.7	>10,000	2.5	0.7	19
Iloperidone	6.3	5.6	4900	0.3	—	12
Amisulpride[b]	2.2	8300	>10,000	>10,000	>10,000	>10,000
Olanzapine	31	3.7	2.5	110	260	2.2
Quetiapine	380	640	37	22	39	6.9
Clozapine	160	5.4	6.2	1.6	7.0	1.1

[a]Data are averaged K_i values (nM) from published sources determined by competition with radioligands for binding to the indicated cloned human receptors. Data derived from receptor binding to human or rat brain tissue were used when cloned human receptor data were lacking.
[b]Not available in the U.S.
[c]Partial agonist at D_2 receptor.
[d]Pimavanserin is a novel agent only indicated for PDP. Ki values: 5HT2A = 0.087 nM; 5HT2C = 0.44 nM. Affinity for DA, M1, H1 and other receptors > 300 nM

Source: PDSP K_i Database: https://kidbdev.med.unc.edu/databases/pdsp.php (Accessed June 1, 2015).

TABLE 16–3 ■ KINETIC PROPERTIES OF DEPOT ANTIPSYCHOTICS

PREPARATION	DILUENT	DOSAGE	T_{max} (days)	STEADY-STATE HALF-LIFE (days)
First-generation antipsychotics				
Fluphenazine decanoate	Sesame oil	12.5–100 mg/2 wk	0.3–1.5	14
Haloperidol decanoate	Sesame oil	25–400 mg/4 wk	3–9	21
Perphenazine decanoate[a]	Sesame oil	25–400 mg/4 wk	7	65
Zuclopenthixol decanoate[a]	Coconut oil (fractionated)	100–800 mg/4 wk	7	19
Atypical antipsychotics				
Aripiprazole monohydrate[b]	Water	300–400 mg/4 wk	6.5–7.1	30–46
Aripiprazole lauroxil[b]	Water	441–882 mg/4 wk	44–50	29–35
Olanzapine pamoate[c]	Water	150–300 mg/2 wk *or*, 300–405 mg/4 wk	7	30
Paliperidone palmitate monthly	Water	39–234 mg/4 wk	13	25–49
Paliperidone palmitate 3 months[d]	Water	273–819 mg/12 wk	30–33	84–95 (deltoid) 118–139 (gluteal)
Risperidone microspheres	Water	12.5–50 mg/2 wk	21	3–6

[a]Not available in the U.S.
[b]Dosages need to be adjusted for patients who are CYP2D6 poor metabolizers or those who are exposed to CYP2D6 or CYP3A4 inhibitors.
[c]Due to cases of postinjection delirium/sedation syndrome, patients must be observed after the injection for at least 3 h in a registered facility with ready access to emergency response services.
[d]Only indicated for patients who have been on paliperidone palmitate monthly injectable for at least 4 months.

(e.g., $5HT_{2A}$ antagonism, $5HT_{1A}$ partial agonism). As a result, structure-function relationships that were relied on in the past have become less important, while receptor binding and functional assays are more clinically relevant. Aripiprazole represents a good example of how an examination of the structure provides little insight into its mechanism, which is based on partial agonism at D_2 DA receptors (discussed further in this chapter). Detailed knowledge of receptor affinities (Table 16–2) and the functional effect at specific receptors (e.g., full, partial, or inverse agonism or antagonism) can provide important insight into the therapeutic and adverse effects of antipsychotic agents. Nevertheless, there are limits. For example, it is not known which properties are responsible for clozapine's unique effectiveness in refractory schizophrenia, although many hypotheses exist. Other notable antipsychotic properties not fully explained by receptor parameters include the reduced seizure threshold, the effects of antipsychotic agents on glucose and lipid metabolism, and the increased risk for cerebrovascular events and mortality among patients with dementia (see Adverse Effects and Drug Interactions further in the chapter).

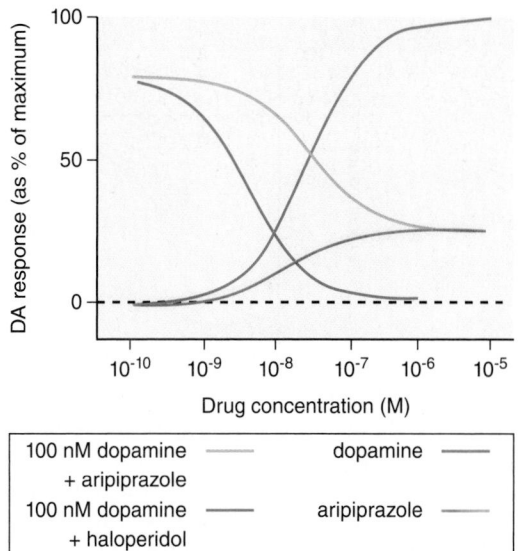

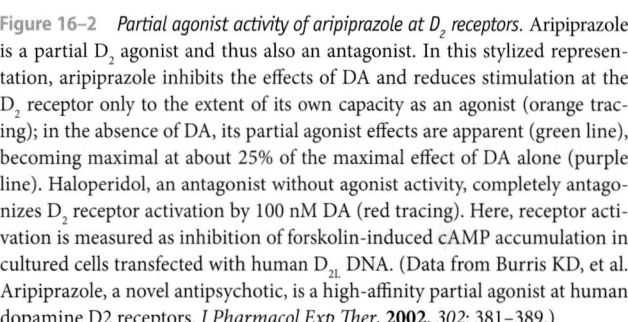

Figure 16–2 *Partial agonist activity of aripiprazole at D_2 receptors.* Aripiprazole is a partial D_2 agonist and thus also an antagonist. In this stylized representation, aripiprazole inhibits the effects of DA and reduces stimulation at the D_2 receptor only to the extent of its own capacity as an agonist (orange tracing); in the absence of DA, its partial agonist effects are apparent (green line), becoming maximal at about 25% of the maximal effect of DA alone (purple line). Haloperidol, an antagonist without agonist activity, completely antagonizes D_2 receptor activation by 100 nM DA (red tracing). Here, receptor activation is measured as inhibition of forskolin-induced cAMP accumulation in cultured cells transfected with human D_{2L} DNA. (Data from Burris KD, et al. Aripiprazole, a novel antipsychotic, is a high-affinity partial agonist at human dopamine D2 receptors. *J Pharmacol Exp Ther*, **2002**, *302*: 381–389.)

ARIPIPRAZOLE

CLOZAPINE

Mechanism of Action

With the exception of pimavanserin for PDP, no clinically available effective antipsychotic is devoid of D_2-modulating activity (Howes et al., 2015). This reduction in dopaminergic neurotransmission is presently achieved through one of two mechanisms: D_2 antagonism or partial D_2 agonism (aripiprazole, brexpiprazole, and cariprazine). The mechanism of action for partial agonist antipsychotics relies on intrinsic activity at D_2 receptors that is a fraction of the efficacy of DA (i.e., 20%–25% of DA's activity), as depicted in Figure 16–2 for aripiprazole. (Recall that a partial agonist will also occupy the receptor and antagonize the binding of full agonists; see Chapter 3). Unlike other antipsychotic agents, in which striatal D_2 occupancy (i.e., reduction in postsynaptic D_2 signal) greater than 78% increases risk for EPSs, partial agonist antipsychotics require significantly higher D_2 occupancy levels (80%–95%) (Sparshatt et al., 2010). However, the intrinsic dopaminergic agonism generates a sufficient postsynaptic signal to remain below the EPS threshold, although reports do exist, primarily in antipsychotic-naïve, younger patients.

Clozapine was not suspected to possess antipsychotic activity until experimental human use in the mid-1960s revealed it to be an effective treatment of schizophrenia, particularly in patients who had failed other antipsychotic medications, and with virtually absent EPS risk. Clozapine possesses weaker D_2 antagonism than existing antipsychotic agents, combined with potent $5HT_{2A}$ antagonism that facilitates DA release in mesocortical and nigrostriatal pathways. Clozapine, and its active metabolite *N*-desmethylclozapine, also possesses activity at numerous other receptors, including antagonism and agonism at various muscarinic receptor subtypes and antagonism at DA D_4 receptors (other D_4 antagonists that do not also have D_2 antagonism lack antipsychotic activity; Meyer and Leckband, 2013).

A search for the basis of clozapine's unique efficacy in refractory schizophrenia has recently pointed toward activity at glutamatergic sites, especially the NMDA receptor. The evolving NMDA hypofunction hypothesis

of schizophrenia led to clinical development of metabotropic glutamate $mGlu_2$ and $mGlu_3$ agonists and inhibitors of the type 1 glycine transporter. At present, however, it is unclear whether glutamate agonists that lack direct D_2 antagonist properties will be effective for schizophrenia treatment; agents with the mechanisms indicated have failed phase III studies (Howes et al., 2015).

Patients with schizophrenia also exhibit specific neurophysiological and cognitive abnormalities, including deficiencies in sensorimotor gating as assessed by prepulse inhibition (PPI) of the acoustic startle reflex. PPI is the automatic suppression of startle magnitude that occurs when the louder acoustic stimulus is preceded 30–500 milliseconds by a weaker prepulse (Javitt and Freedman 2015; Powell et al., 2012). In patients with schizophrenia, PPI is increased more robustly with atypical than typical antipsychotic agents, and in animal models, atypical antipsychotic agents are also more effective at opposing PPI disruption by NMDA antagonists.

Increased understanding of the pharmacological basis for neurophysiological deficits provides another means for developing antipsychotic treatments that are specifically effective for schizophrenia and may not necessarily apply to other forms of psychosis. Numerous agents have also been examined for remediating the cognitive deficits of schizophrenia, typically utilizing nicotinic and muscarinic agonism, but none has been approved (Prickaerts et al., 2012).

Dopamine Receptor Occupancy and Behavioral Effects

Dopaminergic projections from the midbrain terminate on septal nuclei, the olfactory tubercle and basal forebrain, the amygdala, and other structures within the temporal and prefrontal cerebral lobes and the hippocampus. Excessive dopaminergic neurotransmission in the associative striatum is central to the positive symptoms of psychosis. The behavioral effects and the time course of antipsychotic response parallel the decrease in postsynaptic D_2 activity in this region (Kuepper et al., 2012). Receptor occupancy predicts clinical efficacy, EPSs, and plasma level–clinical response relationships. Occupancy of greater than 78% of D_2 receptors in

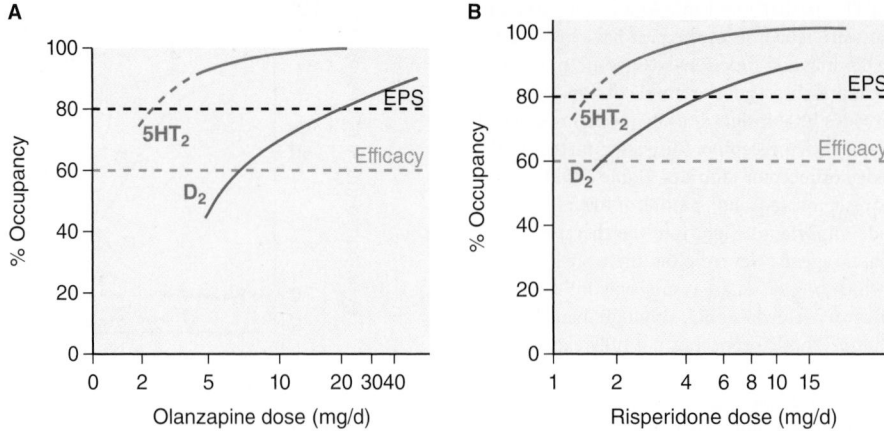

Figure 16–3 *Receptor occupancy and clinical response for antipsychotic agents.* Typically, in D_2 receptor occupancy by the drug more than 60% provides antipsychotic effects, receptor occupancy greater than 80% causes EPSs. Atypical agents combine weak D_2 receptor blockade with more potent $5HT_{2A}$ antagonism/inverse agonism. Inverse agonism at $5HT_2$ receptor subtypes may contribute to the reduced EPS risk of olanzapine (**A**) and risperidone (**B**) and efficacy at lower D_2 receptor occupancy (olanzapine, **A**). Aripiprazole is a partial D_2 agonist that can achieve only 75% functional blockade (see Figure 16–2).

the basal ganglia is associated with a risk of EPSs across all DA antagonist antipsychotic agents, while occupancies in the range of 60%–75% are associated with antipsychotic efficacy (Figure 16–3). With the exception of the D_2 partial agonists, all atypical antipsychotic drugs at low doses have much greater occupancy of $5HT_{2A}$ receptors (e.g., 75%–99%) than typical agents (Table 16–3). Given the large variations in drug metabolism, plasma levels of antipsychotic agents (rather than doses) are the best predictors of D_2 occupancy.

The Role of Nondopamine Receptors for Atypical Antipsychotic Agents.

The concept of atypicality was initially based on clozapine's absence of EPSs combined with potent $5HT_2$ receptor antagonism. $5HT_{2A}$ antagonism exerts its greatest effect on prefrontal and basal ganglia DA release, decreasing EPS risk in the context of nigrostriatal D_2 antagonism. The $5HT_{2C}$ antagonists stimulate midbrain noradrenergic outflow (Dremencov et al., 2006). Thus, $5HT_{2C}$ antagonist atypical agents exhibit a spectrum of antidepressant properties, although pure $5HT_{2C}$ agents are not, by themselves, effective antidepressants (Dremencov et al., 2006). Most atypical antipsychotics are partial agonists at $5HT_{1A}$ receptors, resulting in hyperpolarization of cortical pyramidal cells and clinically relevant anxiolytic effects. Pimavanserin is an inverse agonist at $5HT_{2A}$ receptors; its effectiveness in PDP may reflect on the unique pathology of PDP.

PIMAVANSERIN

Tolerance and Physical Dependence

As defined in Chapter 24, antipsychotic drugs are not addicting; however, tolerance to the α adrenergic, antihistaminic, and anticholinergic effects of antipsychotic agents usually develops over days or weeks. Loss of efficacy with prolonged treatment is not known to occur with antipsychotic agents; however, tolerance to antipsychotic drugs and cross-tolerance among the agents are demonstrable in behavioral and biochemical experiments in animals. One correlate of tolerance in striatal dopaminergic systems is the development of receptor supersensitivity (mediated by upregulation of supersensitive DA receptors), referred to as D_2^{High} receptors (Seeman, 2013). These changes may underlie the clinical phenomenon of withdrawal-emergent dyskinesias and may contribute to the pathophysiology of TD. These effects may also partly explain the ability of certain patients with chronic schizophrenia to tolerate high doses of potent DA antagonists with limited EPSs.

ADME

Absorption for most of these agents following oral administration is quite high, and concurrent administration of anticholinergic antiparkinsonian agents does not appreciably diminish intestinal absorption. Most ODTs and liquid preparations provide similar pharmacokinetics because there is little mucosal absorption and effects depend on swallowed drug. Asenapine is the only exception: it is available only as an ODT preparation administered sublingually; and absorption occurs via the oral mucosa with bioavailability of 35%. If asenapine is swallowed, the first-pass effect is greater than 98% and the drug is essentially not bioavailable. Intramuscular administration avoids much of the first-pass enteric metabolism and provides measurable concentrations in plasma within 15–30 min.

The pharmacokinetic constants and metabolic pathways for many atypical and typical antipsychotic drugs are listed in Table 16–4. Most antipsychotic drugs are highly lipophilic and accumulate in the brain, lung, and other tissues with a rich blood supply. Most antipsychotic agents are highly protein bound, primarily to acid glycoprotein, and do not significantly displace other medications bound to prealbumin or albumin. Antipsychotic agents also enter the fetal circulation and breast milk. Despite half-lives that may be short, the biological effects of single doses of most antipsychotic medications usually persist for at least 24 h, permitting once-daily dosing after the patient has adjusted to initial side effects. Due to accumulation in tissue stores, both parent compound and metabolites of LAI medications can been detected several months after discontinuation, a useful property for those who may miss injections (see Table 16–3).

Other Therapeutic Uses

Antipsychotic agents are also utilized in several nonpsychotic neurological disorders and as antiemetics.

Anxiety Disorders

Double-blind, placebo-controlled trials have shown the benefit of adjunctive treatment with antipsychotic drugs for obsessive-compulsive disorder, with a recent meta-analysis showing significant efficacy for risperidone but not for quetiapine and olanzapine (Dold et al., 2013). For generalized anxiety disorder, clinical trials demonstrated efficacy for quetiapine as monotherapy and for adjunctive low-dose risperidone. Recent data do not support routine use of risperidone for posttraumatic stress disorder (Krystal et al., 2011).

TABLE 16–4 ■ DRUG DISPOSITION AND EFFECTS OF CYP INHIBITION AND INDUCTION ON ORAL ANTIPSYCHOTIC LEVELS

	T_{max}, Oral Tablet Bioavailability	METABOLISM	EFFECT OF CYP INHIBITION	EFFECT OF CYP INDUCTION
Commonly used atypical antipsychotics				
Aripiprazole	Bioavailability: 87% T_{max}: 3–5 h	CYPs 2D6 and 3A4 produce active metabolite, dehydroaripiprazole. $t_{1/2}$: aripiprazole, 75h; dehydroaripiprazole, 94 h; Metabolite = 40% of AUC at steady state	In 2D6 PM: ↑ AUC of aripiprazole up to 80%, 30% ↓ AUC of metabolite. $t_{1/2}$: 146 h in PMs. Strong CYP2D6 inhibitors (e.g., ketoconazole) can double AUC of parent drug. Ketoconazole (a strong 3A4 inhibitor) increased the AUCs of aripiprazole and its active metabolite by 63% and 77%, respectively.	3A4 induction ↓ max concentration and AUC of aripiprazole and metabolite by 70%.
Asenapine	Bioavailability: Sublingual: 35% Oral: <2% T_{max}: 1 h	Primarily glucuronidation (UGT 1A4); limited oxidation via CYP 1A2 and to lesser extent 2D6 and 3A4. No active metabolites. $t_{1/2}$: 24h	Fluvoxamine, (25 mg twice daily for 8 days) ↑ C_{max} by 13% and AUC 29%. Paroxetine ↓ AUC and C_{max} (13%) Asenapine can double paroxetine exposure.	Smoking: no effect on clearance or other kinetic parameters. Carbamazepine, can ↓ C_{max} and AUC (16%).
Brexpiprazole	Bioavailability: 95% T_{max}: 4 h	CYPs 2D6 and 3A4 convert brexpiprazole to inactive metabolite (DM-3411). $t_{1/2}$: 91 h	Strong 2D6 or 3A4 inhibitor: ↑ AUC_{0-24h} by 2-fold. Strong 3A4 inhibitor with 2D6 inhibitor (or with 2D6 PM): ↑ AUC_{0-24h} by ~5 fold. ↓ dose by 50% with strong 2D6 or 3A4 inhibitor. ↓ dose by 75% with combined 2D6/3A4 inhibitors.	Inducers of CYP3A4 ↓ exposure AUC by ~70%. Do not use brexpiprazole with inducers.
Cariprazine	Bioavailability: 65% T_{max}: 3–6 h	CYP3A4 converts cariprazine to active metabolites DCAR and DDCAR. At steady state on 6 mg/d: cariprazine 28%, DCAR 9%, and DDCAR 63%. CYP2D6 is a minor pathway. Parent drug and DDCAR show good brain penetration; after oral cariprazine, brain-to-plasma ratios for both are ~9.8 $t_{1/2}$: 31.6–68.4 h; DCAR, 29.7–39.5 h; DDCAR, 314–446 h ≥50% of DDCAR present 1 week after discontinuation.	Ketoconazole 400 mg/d + cariprazine 0.5 mg/kg: ↑ AUCs of cariprazine (4×) and DDCAR (1.5), and ↑ DCAR AUC (~33%). Reduce dose by 50% with strong 3A4 inhibitors. No impact from 2D6 inhibitors.	Not studied. Impact unknown. Not recommended with 3A4 inducers.
Clozapine	Bioavailability: 60%–70% T_{max}: 2.5 h	Multiple CYPs (mainly 1A2, 2C19, 3A4) produce active desmethyl metabolite $t_{1/2}$: 12 h (up to 66 h with chronic dosing)	Fluvoxamine ↑ serum levels 5- to 10-fold. 2D6 inhibition may double Cp.	Loss of smoking-related 1A2 induction ⇒ 50% ↑ in clozapine serum levels. Carbamazepine decreases clozapine levels on average by 50%.

(Continued)

TABLE 16–4 ■ DRUG DISPOSITION AND EFFECTS OF CYP INHIBITION AND INDUCTION ON ORAL ANTIPSYCHOTIC LEVELS (CONTINUED)

	T_{max}; Oral Tablet Bioavailability	METABOLISM	EFFECT OF CYP INHIBITION	EFFECT OF CYP INDUCTION
Iloperidone	Bioavailability: well absorbed, no food effect on AUC T_{max} 2–4 h	2D6/3A4 produce active metabolites P88 & P95 Exposure to P88 and P95 can be significant P88 $t_{1/2}$: EM, 26 h; PM, 37 h P95 $t_{1/2}$: EM, 23h; PM, 31 h $t_{1/2}$: 18 h (CYP 2D6 EMs), 33 h (CYP 2D6 PMs)	Ketoconazole, fluoxetine, and paroxetine can ↑ AUC of iloperidone and metabolites by 50% to 300%, with similar effects on C_{max} at steady-state.	Impact of 3A4 inducers not documented.
Lurasidone	Bioavailability: 9%–19% Mean C_{max} and AUC increased 3-fold and 2-fold, respectively, when administered with food T_{max} 1–3 h	CYP 3A4 $t_{1/2}$: 18–36 h	DO NOT USE with strong 3A4 inhibitors (e.g., ketoconazole), which increase C_{max} 6.9-fold and AUC 9-fold. Moderate 3A4 inhibitors (diltiazem) increase C_{max} 2.1-fold and AUC 2.2-fold.	DO NOT USE with strong 3A4 inducers. Concurrent rifampin can decrease C_{max} to a seventh of prior levels and AUC by 80%.
Olanzapine	Bioavailability: 60% T_{max} 6 h	Direct glucuronidation or 1A2-mediated oxidation to N-desmethylolanzapine (inactive) $t_{1/2}$: 30 (21–54) h	Increase in olanzapine C_{max} following fluvoxamine is 54% in female nonsmokers and 77% in male smokers. Mean increases in olanzapine AUC are 52% and 108%, respectively.	Carbamazepine use increases clearance by 50%. Smokers have lower Cp and increased clearance.
Paliperidone	Bioavailability: 28% T_{max} 24 h	59% excreted unchanged in urine, 32% excreted as metabolites. Phase 2 metabolism accounts for no more than 10%.	Unlikely to have much of an effect	Carbamazepine use decreased steady-state C_{max} and AUC by 37%.
Quetiapine	Bioavailability: 9% T_{max} 1.5 h	3A4 mediated sulfoxidation to inactive metabolite $t_{1/2}$: 6 h (CNS half-life longer by neuroimaging)	Ketoconazole (200 mg once daily for 4 days) reduced oral clearance of quetiapine by 84%, ⇒ 335% increase in C_{max}.	Phenytoin increases clearance 5-fold.
Risperidone	Bioavailability: 66% in 2D6 EMs T_{max}: 1 h for risperidone, 3 h for 9-OH risperidone (paliperidone)	2D6 converts risperidone to, 9-OH risperidone (active). $t_{1/2}$: 3–4 h; 20–24 h (9-OH risperidone) In 2D6 PMs, half-lives are: risperidone, 20 h; 9-OH risperidone, 30 h.	SSRIs can increase plasma levels. Fluoxetine: ↑ [risperidone] ~2.6 fold Paroxetine: ↑ [risperidone] ~3–9 fold	Risperidone (6 mg/day for 3 weeks), followed by Carbamazepine (3 weeks), ⇒ 50% decrease in concentration (risperidone + 9-OH risperidone).

Ziprasidone	Bioavailability: 60% when given with food. A 500-kcal meal (of any composition) ↑ AUC of a 20-mg, 40-mg, and 80-mg capsule by 48%, 87% and 101%, respectively. T_{max} 6–8 h	Aldehyde oxidase (66%), CYP3A4 (34%) $t_{1/2}$: 7.5 h	35%–40% increase in ziprasidone AUC by concomitantly administered ketoconazole.	35% decrease in ziprasidone AUC by carbamazepine.
Typical antipsychotics			
Haloperidol	Bioavailability: 60% T_{max} 2–6 h	Multiple CYP pathways, particularly 2D6, 3A4. Most metabolites inactive, except reduced haloperidol formed by ketone reductase and transformed to haloperidol via CYP2D6. Therapeutic serum levels not well defined; 5–20 ng/mL used as a target for dosing. $t_{1/2}$: 24 h (12–36 h)[a]	In CYP2D6 PM: $t_{1/2}$ prolonged, [reduced haloperidol] increased significantly. Individuals with only one functional 2D6 gene experience 2-fold greater trough serum levels; those with no functioning alleles 3- to 4-fold higher.	Carbamazepine or phenytoin ↑ haloperidol clearance ~32%, with variable decrease in plasma levels (mean 47%). Discontinuation of carbamazepine results in 2.2- to 3.0-fold ↑ in serum levels.
Chlorpromazine	Bioavailability: 20–32% T_{max} 1–4 h	CYP2D6, over 10 identified human metabolites, most inactive. Chlorpromazine is a 2D6 inhibitor and induces its own metabolism. Levels drop ~30% during weeks 1–3 of treatment. $t_{1/2}$: 24 h (8–35 h with chronic dosing)	Case report of fluoxetine-chlorpromazine interaction, but no serum level data on extent of effect.	3A4/PGP inducers (e.g., phenobarbital, carbamazepine) ↓ chlorpromazine levels by ~35%. Carbamazepine discontinuation increases serum levels (~50%).

[a]May have multiphasic elimination with much longer terminal half-life.

Tourette Disorder

The ability of antipsychotic drugs to suppress tics in patients with Tourette disorder relates to reduced D_2 neurotransmission in basal ganglia sites. Aripiprazole is the only antipsychotic that is FDA-approved for the treatment of Tourette disorder; this agent is considered a first-line agent for this purpose, starting at doses of 2 mg/d and increasing if needed to a maximum of 10 mg/d for those weighing less than 50 kg or 20 mg/d if weighing 50 kg or more (Mogwitz et al., 2013).

In prior decades, low-dose, high-potency typical antipsychotic agents (e.g., haloperidol, pimozide) were treatments of choice, but these non-psychotic patients are extremely sensitive to the impact of DA blockade on cognitive processing speed and on reward centers. Moreover, safety concerns regarding pimozide's QT_c prolongation and increased risk for ventricular arrhythmias have largely ended its clinical use.

Huntington Disease

Huntington disease is another neuropsychiatric condition that, like tic disorders, is associated with basal ganglia pathology. DA blockade can suppress the severity of choreoathetotic movements but is not strongly endorsed due to the risks associated with excessive DA antagonism that outweigh the marginal benefit. Inhibition of the vesicular monoamine transporter 2 (VMAT2) with tetrabenazine compounds has replaced DA receptor blockade in the management of chorea (Chapter 18).

Autism

Autism is a disease whose neuropathology is incompletely understood, but in some patients is associated with explosive behavioral outbursts and aggressive or self-injurious behaviors that may be stereotypical. Risperidone and aripiprazole have FDA approval for irritability associated with autism in child and adolescent patients ages 5–16, with common use for disruptive behavior problems in autism and forms of mental retardation. Initial risperidone daily doses are 0.25 mg for patients weighing less than 20 kg and 0.5 mg for others, with a target dose of 0.5 mg/d in those weighing less than 20 kg and 1.0 mg/d for other patients, with a range of 0.5–3.0 mg/d. For aripiprazole, the starting dose is 2 mg/d, with a target range of 5–10 mg/d and maximum daily dose of 15 mg.

Antiemetic Use

Most antipsychotic drugs protect against the nausea- and emesis-inducing effects of DA agonists such as apomorphine that act at central DA receptors in the chemoreceptor trigger zone of the medulla. Drugs or other stimuli that cause emesis by an action on the nodose ganglion, or locally on the GI tract, are not antagonized by antipsychotic drugs, but potent piperazines and butyrophenones are sometimes effective against nausea caused by vestibular stimulation. The commonly used antiemetic phenothiazines are weak DA antagonists (e.g., prochlorperazine) without antipsychotic activity but can occasionally be associated with EPSs or akathisia. Emesis and antiemetic agents are discussed at length in Chapter 50.

Adverse Effects and Drug Interactions

Adverse Effects Predicted by Monoamine Receptor Affinities

Dopamine D_2 Receptors. With the exception of pimavanserin and the D_2 partial agonists (aripiprazole, brexpiprazole, cariprazine), all other antipsychotic agents possess D_2 antagonist properties, the strength of which determines the likelihood for EPSs, long-term TD risk, akathisia, NMS, and hyperprolactinemia.

Extrapyramidal Symptoms. The manifestations of EPSs are described in Table 16–5, along with the usual treatment approach. Acute dystonic reactions occur in the early hours and days of treatment, with highest risk among younger patients (peak incidence ages 10–19), especially antipsychotic, naïve individuals, in response to abrupt decreases in nigrostriatal D_2 neurotransmission. The dystonia typically involves head and neck muscles and the tongue and, in its severest form, the oculogyric crisis, extraocular muscles, and is frightening to the patient.

Parkinsonism resembling its idiopathic form may occur; it will respond to dose reduction or switching to an antipsychotic with weaker

TABLE 16–5 ■ NEUROLOGICAL SIDE EFFECTS OF ANTIPSYCHOTIC DRUGS

REACTION	FEATURES	TIME OF ONSET AND RISK INFO	PROPOSED MECHANISM	TREATMENT
Acute dystonia	Spasm of muscles of tongue, face, neck, back	Time: 1–5 days. Young, antipsychotic, naïve patients at highest risk	Acute DA antagonism	Antiparkinsonian agents are diagnostic and curative[a]
Akathisia	Subjective and objective restlessness; *not* anxiety or "agitation"	Time: 5–60 days	Unknown	Reduce dose or change drug; clonazepam, propranolol more effective than antiparkinsonian agents[b]
Parkinsonism	Bradykinesia, rigidity, variable tremor, mask facies, shuffling gait	Time: 5–30 days. Elderly at greatest risk	DA antagonism	Dose reduction; change medication; antiparkinsonian agents[c]
Neuroleptic malignant syndrome	Extreme rigidity, fever, unstable blood pressure, myoglobinemia; can be fatal	Time: weeks–months. Can persist for days after stopping antipsychotic	DA antagonism	Stop antipsychotic immediately; supportive care; dantrolene and bromocriptine[d]
Perioral tremor ("rabbit syndrome")	Perioral tremor (may be a late variant of parkinsonism)	Time: months or years of treatment	Unknown	Antiparkinsonian agents often help[c]
Tardive dyskinesia	Orofacial dyskinesia; rarely widespread choreoathetosis or dystonia	Time: months or years of treatment. Elderly at 5-fold greater risk. Risk proportional to potency of D_2 blockade	Postsynaptic DA receptor supersensitivity, upregulation	May be reversible with early recognition and drug discontinuation VMAT2 inhibitors valbenazine and deutetrabenazine are FDA-approved for TD

[a]Treatment: diphenhydramine 25–50 mg IM or benztropine 1–2 mg IM. Due to long antipsychotic $t_{1/2}$, may need to repeat or follow with oral medication.
[b]Propranolol often effective in relatively low doses (20–80 mg/d in divided doses). β_1-selective adrenergic receptor antagonists are less effective. Nonlipophilic β adrenergic antagonists have limited CNS penetration and are of no benefit (e.g., atenolol).
[c]Use of amantadine avoids anticholinergic effects of benztropine or diphenhydramine.
[d]Despite the response to dantrolene, there is no evidence of abnormal Ca^{2+} transport in skeletal muscle; with persistent antipsychotic effects (e.g., long-acting injectable agents) prolonged bromocriptine may be necessary in large doses (10–40 mg/d). Antiparkinsonian agents are not effective.

D_2 antagonism. If this is neither possible nor desirable, antiparkinsonian medication may be employed. Elderly patients are at greatest risk.

Muscarinic cholinergic receptors modulate nigrostriatal DA release, with blockade increasing synaptic DA availability. Important issues in the use of anticholinergics include the negative impact on cognition and memory; peripheral antimuscarinic adverse effects (e.g., urinary retention, dry mouth, cycloplegia, etc.); exacerbation of TD; and risk of cholinergic rebound following abrupt anticholinergic withdrawal. For parenteral administration, diphenhydramine (25–50 mg IM) and benztropine (1–2 mg IM) are the agents most commonly used. The antihistamine diphenhydramine also possesses anticholinergic properties. Benztropine combines a benzhydryl group with a tropane group to create a compound that is more anticholinergic than trihexyphenidyl but less antihistaminic than diphenhydramine. The clinical effect of a single dose lasts 5 h, thereby requiring two or three daily doses. Dosing usually starts at 0.5–1 mg twice daily, with a daily maximum of 6 mg, although slightly higher doses are used in rare circumstances. The piperidine compound trihexyphenidyl was one of the first synthetic anticholinergic agents available; it also inhibits the presynaptic DA reuptake transporter, which creates a higher risk of abuse than for the antihistamines or benztropine. Trihexyphenidyl has good GI absorption, achieving peak plasma levels in 1–2 h, with a serum $t_{1/2}$ of about 10–12 h generally necessitating multiple-daily dosing to achieve satisfactory clinical results. The total daily dosage range is 5–15 mg, given two or three times a day as divided doses. Biperiden is another drug in this class.

Amantadine, originally marketed as an antiviral agent for influenza A, is an alternative medication for antipsychotic-induced parkinsonism and avoids the adverse CNS and peripheral effects of anticholinergic medications (Ogino et al., 2014). Its mechanism of action is unclear but appears to involve presynaptic DA reuptake blockade, facilitation of DA release, postsynaptic DA agonism, and receptor modulation. Amantadine is well absorbed after oral administration, with peak levels achieved 1–4 h after ingestion; clearance is renal, with more than 90% recovered unmetabolized in the urine. The plasma $t_{1/2}$ is 12–18 h in healthy young adults but is longer in those with renal impairment, necessitating a 50% dose reduction. Starting dosage is 100 mg orally once daily in healthy adults, which may be increased to 100 mg twice daily. A dose of 100 mg twice daily yields peak plasma levels of 0.5–0.8 µg/mL and trough levels of 0.3 µg/mL. Toxicity is seen at serum levels between 1 and 5 µg/mL.

Tardive Dyskinesia. Tardive dyskinesia results from increased nigrostriatal dopaminergic activity as a consequence of postsynaptic receptor supersensitivity and upregulation from chronically high levels of postsynaptic D_2 blockade (and possible direct toxic effects of high-potency DA antagonists). TD occurs more frequently in older patients, and the risk may be somewhat greater in patients with mood disorders than in those with schizophrenia. Its prevalence averages 15%–25% in young adults treated with typical antipsychotic agents for more than a year; the risk is a third to a fifth of that with atypical agents.

Tardive dyskinesia is characterized by stereotyped, repetitive, painless, involuntary, quick choreiform (tic-like) movements of the face, eyelids (blinks or spasm), mouth (grimaces), tongue, extremities, or trunk, with varying degrees of slower athetosis (twisting movements); tardive dystonia and tardive akathisia are rare now that the use of high-dose, high-potency typical antipsychotic medications has abated. The movements disappear during sleep (as do many other extrapyramidal syndromes), vary in intensity over time, and are dependent on the level of arousal or emotional distress, sometimes reappearing during acute psychiatric illnesses following prolonged disappearance. The dyskinetic movements can be suppressed partially by use of a potent DA antagonist, but such interventions over time may worsen the severity, as this was part of the initial pharmacological insult. Switching patients from potent D_2 antagonists to weaker agents, especially clozapine, can be effective. When possible, drug discontinuation may be beneficial but is effective in less than 33% of cases.

The VMAT2 inhibitors valbenazine and deuterated-tetrabenazine (deutetrabenazine) were FDA-approved for TD in 2017. Both are derivatives of tetrabenazine and share mechanism and many of the adverse effects of tetrabenazine. Velbenazine is active and is metabolized to an active metabolite, dihydotetrabenazine. The clearance of valbenazine and its active metabolite involve CYPs 2D6 and 3A4. Thus, exposure to the parent drug and its active metabolite will be increased in CYP2D6 poor metabolizers, in the presence of strong inhibitors of 2D6 (e.g., paroxetine) or 3A4 (e.g., ketoconazole), or in patients with moderate-to-severe hepatic impairment. Use of valbenazine in the presence of strong inducers of 3A4 (e.g., rifampin) is not recommended; concomitant use of MAOIs should be avoided. Valbenazine inhibits P-glycoprotein and will increase digoxin exposure. Deutetrabenazine is also approved for treating the chorea of Huntington disease and is described in Chapter 18, as is tetrabenazine.

Akathisia. Unlike antipsychotic-induced parkinsonism and acute dystonia, the phenomenology and treatment of akathisia suggest involvement of structures outside the nigrostriatal pathway. Despite the association with D_2 blockade, akathisia does not have as robust a response to antiparkinsonian drugs, so other treatment strategies are often employed acutely, including high-potency benzodiazepines (e.g., clonazepam) and nonselective β blockers with good CNS penetration (e.g., propranolol). Over time, one should consider dose reduction or switching to another antipsychotic agent. That clonazepam and propranolol have significant cortical activity and are ineffective for other forms of EPSs points to an extrastriatal origin for akathisia symptoms.

Neuroleptic Malignant Syndrome. The rare NMS resembles a severe form of parkinsonism, with signs of autonomic instability (hyperthermia and labile pulse, blood pressure, and respiration rate), stupor, elevation of creatine kinase in serum, and sometimes myoglobinemia with potential nephrotoxicity. At its most severe, this syndrome may persist for more than a week after the offending agent is discontinued and is associated with mortality. This reaction has been associated with myriad antipsychotic agents, but its prevalence may be greater with relatively high doses of potent agents. Aside from cessation of antipsychotic treatment and provision of supportive care, including aggressive cooling measures, specific pharmacological treatment is unsatisfactory, although administration of dantrolene and the dopaminergic agonist bromocriptine may be helpful. While dantrolene also is used to manage the syndrome of malignant hyperthermia induced by general anesthetics, the neuroleptic-induced form of hyperthermia probably is not associated with a defect in Ca^{2+} metabolism in skeletal muscle. There are anecdotal reports of NMS with atypical antipsychotic agents, but this syndrome is now rarely seen in its full presentation (Gurrera et al., 2011).

Hyperprolactinemia. Hyperprolactinemia results from blockade of the pituitary actions of the tuberoinfundibular dopaminergic neurons; these neurons project from the arcuate nucleus of the hypothalamus to the median eminence, where they deliver DA to the anterior pituitary via the hypophyseoportal vessels. D_2 receptors on lactotropes in the anterior pituitary mediate the tonic prolactin-inhibiting action of DA. Correlations between the D_2 potency of antipsychotic drugs and prolactin elevations are excellent. With the exception of risperidone and paliperidone, atypical antipsychotic agents show limited effects (asenapine, iloperidone, olanzapine, quetiapine, ziprasidone) to almost no effects (clozapine, aripiprazole, brexpiprazole, cariprazine) on prolactin secretion.

Hyperprolactinemia can directly induce breast engorgement and galactorrhea and can cause amenorrhea in women and sexual dysfunction or infertility in women and men. Dose reduction can be tried to decrease serum prolactin levels, but caution must be exercised to keep treatment within the antipsychotic therapeutic range. When switching from offending antipsychotic agents is not feasible, bromocriptine can be employed. The hyperprolactinemia from antipsychotic drugs is rapidly reversed when the drugs are discontinued.

Histamine H_1 Receptors. Central antagonism of H_1 receptors is associated with two major adverse effects: sedation and weight gain via appetite stimulation (Kim et al., 2007), and certain antipsychotic agents cause these adverse effects.

Sedation. Examples of sedating antipsychotic drugs include low-potency typical agents such as chlorpromazine and the atypical agents clozapine and quetiapine. The sedating effect is predicted by their high H_1 receptor affinities (Table 16–2). Some tolerance to the sedative properties will develop, a helpful fact to remember when considering switching a patient to a nonsedating agent. Rapid discontinuation of sedating antihistaminic antipsychotic drugs is inevitably followed by significant complaints of rebound insomnia and sleep disturbance. If discontinuation of sedating antipsychotic treatment is deemed necessary, except for emergency cessation of clozapine for agranulocytosis, the medication should be tapered slowly over 4–12 weeks, and the clinician should be prepared to utilize a sedative at the end of the taper. Generous dosing of another antihistamine (hydroxyzine) or the anticholinergic antihistamine diphenhydramine are reasonable replacements. Sedation may be useful during acute psychosis, but excessive sedation can interfere with patient evaluation, may prolong emergency room and psychiatric hospital stays unnecessarily, and is poorly tolerated among elderly patients with dementia and delirium; thus, appropriate caution must be exercised with the choice of agent and the dose.

Weight Gain. Weight gain is a significant problem during long-term use of antipsychotic drugs and represents a major barrier to medication adherence, as well as a significant threat to the physical and emotional health of the patient. Weight gain has effectively replaced concerns over EPS as the adverse effect causing the most consternation among patients and clinicians alike. Appetite stimulation is the primary mechanism involved, with little evidence to suggest that decreased activity (due to sedation) is a main contributor to antipsychotic-related weight gain. Laboratory studies indicated that medications with significant H_1 antagonism induce appetite stimulation through effects at hypothalamic sites (Kim et al., 2007). The low-potency phenothiazine chlorpromazine and the atypical antipsychotic drugs olanzapine and clozapine are the agents of highest risk, but some weight gain occurs with nearly all antipsychotic drugs.

Acutely psychotic patients may lose weight; in placebo-controlled acute schizophrenia trials, the placebo cohort inevitably loses weight. Younger and antipsychotic drug-naïve patients are much more sensitive to the weight gain from all antipsychotic agents, including those that appear roughly weight neutral in adult studies, leading some to conjecture that DA blockade may also play a small additive role in weight gain (Correll et al., 2014). Antagonism at $5HT_{2C}$ receptors may play an additive role in promoting weight gain for medications that possess high H_1 affinities (e.g., clozapine, olanzapine) but appears to have no effect in the absence of significant H_1 blockade, as seen with ziprasidone, an antipsychotic with low weight gain risk but an extremely high $5HT_{2C}$ affinity.

Switching to more weight-neutral medications can achieve significant results; however, when changing medications is not feasible or unsuccessful, behavioral strategies must be employed, and should be considered for all chronically mentally ill patients given the prevalence of obesity in this patient population. There is also compelling data for the use of metformin to moderate the antipsychotic-induced weight gain from olanzapine and clozapine, particularly when commencing the antipsychotic (Praharaj et al., 2011).

Muscarinic M_1 Receptors.

Muscarinic antagonism is responsible for the central and peripheral anticholinergic effects of medications. The muscarinic receptor affinity and clinically relevant anticholinergic effects of the atypical antipsychotics are limited, whereas clozapine and low-potency phenothiazines have significant anticholinergic adverse effects (Table 16–2). Quetiapine has modest muscarinic affinity; its active metabolite norquetiapine is likely responsible for anticholinergic effects. Clozapine is particularly associated with significant constipation, perhaps due to anticholinergic properties, and possibly effects at sigma receptors. Routine use of stool softeners and repeated inquiry into bowel habits are necessary to prevent serious intestinal obstruction from undetected constipation. Medications with significant anticholinergic properties should be particularly avoided in elderly patients, especially those with dementia or delirium.

Adrenergic α_1 Receptors.

α_1 Adrenergic antagonism is associated with risk of orthostatic hypotension and can be particularly problematic for elderly patients who have poor vasomotor tone. The extent to which antipsychotic agents cause this effect in clinical practice is dependent on the doses employed and the rapidity of titration. Compared to high-potency typical agents, low-potency typical agents generally have greater affinities

for α_1 receptors and pose greater risk for orthostasis. Among newer medications, iloperidone carries a warning regarding minimization of orthostasis risk through slower titration. Clozapine can be associated with significant orthostasis, even when titrated slowly. Because clozapine-treated patients have few other antipsychotic options, the potent mineralocorticoid fludrocortisone is sometimes tried (0.1–0.3 mg/d) as a volume expander.

Adverse Effects Not Predicted by Monoamine Receptor Affinities

Adverse Metabolic Effects.

Metabolic effects are the area of greatest concern during long-term antipsychotic treatment, paralleling the overall concern for the high prevalence of prediabetic conditions, type 2 DM, and 2-fold greater CV mortality among patients with schizophrenia (Correll et al., 2014). Aside from weight gain, the two predominant metabolic adverse side effects seen with antipsychotic drugs are dyslipidemia, primarily elevated serum triglycerides, and impairments in glycemic control.

Low-potency phenothiazines elevate serum triglyceride values, an effect that is not seen with high-potency phenothiazines. Among atypical antipsychotic drugs, significant increases in fasting triglyceride levels are noted during clozapine and olanzapine exposure and, to a lesser extent, with quetiapine. Effects on total cholesterol and cholesterol fractions are significantly less but show expected associations related to agents of highest risk: clozapine, olanzapine, and quetiapine (Rummel-Kluge et al., 2010). Weight gain in general may induce deleterious lipid changes; the evidence indicates that antipsychotic-induced hypertriglyceridemia is a weight-independent adverse event that occurs within weeks of starting an offending medication and resolves within 6 weeks after medication discontinuation. In individuals not exposed to antipsychotic drugs, elevated fasting triglycerides are a direct consequence of insulin resistance because insulin-dependent lipases in fat cells are normally inhibited by insulin. As insulin resistance worsens, inappropriately high levels of lipolysis lead to the release of excess amounts of free fatty acids, which are transformed into triglyceride particles (Meyer and Stahl, 2009). Elevated fasting triglyceride levels thus become a sensitive marker of insulin resistance, leading to the hypothesis that the triglyceride increases seen during antipsychotic treatment are the result of derangements in glucose-insulin homeostasis.

The ability of antipsychotic drugs to induce hyperglycemia was first noted during low-potency phenothiazine treatment; indeed, chlorpromazine was occasionally exploited for this specific property as adjunctive presurgical treatment of insulinoma. As atypical antipsychotic drugs found widespread use, numerous case series documented the association of new-onset diabetes and diabetic ketoacidosis associated with treatment with atypical antipsychotic drugs, with most of cases observed during clozapine and olanzapine therapy (Meyer and Stahl, 2009). The mechanism by which antipsychotic drugs disrupt glucose-insulin homeostasis is not known, but in vivo animal experiments document immediate dose-dependent effects of clozapine and olanzapine on whole-body and hepatic insulin sensitivity (Meyer and Stahl, 2009).

There may also be inherent disease-related mechanisms that increase risk for metabolic disorders among patients with schizophrenia (Meyer and Stahl, 2009), but the medication itself is the primary risk factor, and all atypical antipsychotic drugs in the U.S. include a hyperglycemia warning on the drug label, although there is limited evidence that the newer medications asenapine, iloperidone, aripiprazole, brexpiprazole, cariprazine, and ziprasidone cause hyperglycemia. Use of metabolically more benign agents is recommended for the initial treatment of all patients for whom long-term treatment is expected. Clinicians should obtain baseline metabolic data, including a fasting glucose or hemoglobin A_{1c}, a fasting lipid panel, and weight and establish a plan for ongoing monitoring of these metabolic parameters. As with weight gain, the changes in fasting glucose and lipids should prompt reevaluation of ongoing treatment, institution of measures to improve metabolic health (diet, exercise, nutritional counseling), and consideration of switching antipsychotic agents.

Adverse Cardiac Effects.

Multiple ion channels are involved in the depolarization and repolarization of cardiac ventricular cells (Chapters 29 and 30). Some antipsychotic agents can interfere with the functioning of these channels, making the risk of ventricular arrhythmias and SCD a concern with the use of these drugs. While most of the older antipsychotic agents (e.g., thioridazine) significantly inhibited inwardly rectifying K⁺ channels (I_{kr}) in cardiac myocytes, this effect is much less pronounced for newer agents (Leucht et al., 2013). Chapters 29 and 30. Antagonism of voltage-gated Na⁺ channels causes QRS widening and an increase in the PR interval, with increased risk for ventricular arrhythmia. Thioridazine can inhibit Na⁺ channels at high dosages, but other antipsychotic medications do not (Nielsen et al., 2011). Myocyte repolarization is mediated in part by K⁺ current through two channels: the rapid I_{kr} and the slow I_{ks} channels. The α subunit of the I_{kr} channel, $K_v11.1$, is encoded by *hERG*, the human-ether-à-go-go related gene that codes for Kv11.1, the α subunit of the K⁺ channel that mediates the repolarizing I_{Kr} current of the cardiac action potential. Polymorphisms of *hERG* are involved in the congenital long QT syndrome associated with syncope and SCD. Antagonism of I_{kr} channels is responsible for most cases of drug-induced QT prolongation and is the suspected mechanism for the majority of antipsychotic-induced SCDs (Nielsen et al., 2011).

Aside from individual agents, for which anecdotal and pharmacosurveillance data indicate risk for torsade de pointes (e.g., thioridazine, pimozide), most of the commonly used newer antipsychotic agents are not associated with a known increased risk for ventricular arrhythmias, including ziprasidone in overdose up to 12,000 mg. One exception is sertindole, an agent not available in the U.S. that was withdrawn in 1998 based on anecdotal reports of torsade de pointes, but reintroduced in Europe in 2006 with strict ECG monitoring guidelines (Nielsen et al., 2011). Although in vitro data revealed sertindole's affinity for I_{kr}, several epidemiological studies published over the past decade were unable to confirm an increased risk of sudden death due to sertindole exposure, thereby providing justification for its reintroduction.

Currently, no data suggest a benefit of routine ECG monitoring for prevention of SCD among patients using antipsychotic drugs. Nonetheless, all antipsychotic medications marketed in the U.S. (with the exception of lurasidone) carry a class label warning regarding QT_c prolongation. A specific black-box warning exists for thioridazine, pimozide, intramuscular droperidol, and haloperidol (intravenous formulation but not oral or intramuscular) concerning torsade de pointes and subsequent fatal ventricular arrhythmias (discussed next and in Chapter 30).

Other Adverse Effects. In the U.S., there is a class label warning for seizure risk on all antipsychotic agents (except pimavanserin), with reported incidences well below 1%. Among commonly used newer antipsychotic drugs, only clozapine has a dose-dependent seizure risk, with a prevalence of 3%–5%. The structurally related olanzapine had an incidence of 0.9% in premarketing studies. Patients with seizure disorder who commence antipsychotic treatment must receive adequate prophylaxis, with consideration given to avoiding carbamazepine and phenytoin due to their capacity to induce CYPs and P-glycoprotein. Carbamazepine is also contraindicated during clozapine treatment due to its bone marrow effects. Valproate derivatives (e.g., divalproex sodium) are used for clozapine-associated seizures as they best cover the spectrum of generalized and myoclonic seizures (Meltzer, 2012).

Clozapine causes a host of other adverse effects, the most concerning of which is agranulocytosis, with an incidence of slightly under 1%; the highest risk occurs during the initial 6 months of treatment, peaking at months 2–3 and diminishing rapidly thereafter (Meltzer, 2012). The mechanism is immune mediated, and patients who have verifiable clozapine-related agranulocytosis are usually not rechallenged. An extensive algorithm guiding clinical response to agranulocytosis and lesser forms of neutropenia is available from manufacturer websites and must be followed, along with mandated CBC monitoring.

Other adverse effects include pigmentary retinopathy (thioridazine at daily doses ≥ 800 mg/d), photosensitivity (low-potency phenothiazines), and elevations of alkaline phosphatase and, rarely, hepatic transaminases (phenothiazines).

Increased Mortality in Patients With Dementia. Perhaps the least-understood adverse effect is the increased risk for cerebrovascular events and all-cause mortality among elderly patients with dementia exposed to antipsychotic medications (~1.7-fold increased mortality risk for drug vs. placebo) (Maust et al., 2015). Mortality is due to heart failure, sudden death, or pneumonia. The underlying etiology for antipsychotic-related cerebrovascular and mortality risk is unknown, but the finding of virtually equivalent mortality risk for typical agents compared to atypical antipsychotic drugs (including aripiprazole) suggests an impact of reduced D_2 signaling regardless of individual antipsychotic mechanisms.

Overdose with typical antipsychotic agents is of particular concern with *low*-potency agents (e.g., chlorpromazine) due to the risk of torsades de pointes, sedation, anticholinergic effects, and orthostasis. Patients who overdose on *high*-potency typical antipsychotic drugs (e.g., haloperidol) and the substituted benzamides are at greater risk for EPSs (due to the high D_2 affinity) and for ECG changes. Overdose experience with newer agents indicates a much lower risk for torsade de pointes ventricular arrhythmias compared to older antipsychotic medications; however, combinations of antipsychotic agents with other medications can lead to fatality, primarily through respiratory depression.

Drug-Drug Interactions

Antipsychotic agents are not significant inhibitors of CYPs, with a few notable exceptions: chlorpromazine, perphenazine, and thioridazine inhibit CYP2D6. The plasma half-lives of a number of these agents are altered by induction or inhibition of hepatic CYPs and by genetic polymorphisms that alter specific CYP activities (Table 16–4). While antipsychotic drugs are highly protein bound, there is no evidence of significant displacement of other protein-bound medications, so dosage adjustment is not required for anticonvulsants, warfarin, or other agents with narrow therapeutic indices.

With respect to drug-drug interactions, it is important to consider the effects of environmental exposures (smoking, nutraceuticals, grapefruit juice) and changes in these behaviors. Changes in smoking status can be especially problematic for clozapine-treated patients and will alter serum levels by 50% or more (Rostami-Hodjegan et al., 2004) due to the capacity of aromatic hydrocarbons in tobacco smoke to induce CYP1A2, the major metabolizer of clozapine. Thus, hospitalization of a smoker in a smoke-free environment results in decreased CYP1A2 activity and an elevation of clozapine plasma levels, with potentially toxic results. Conversely, a patient discharged from a nonsmoking ward who resumes smoking will experience an increase in CYP1A2 activity and a 50% decrease in plasma clozapine levels. Monitoring of plasma clozapine concentrations, anticipation of changes in smoking habits, and dosage adjustment can minimize development of subtherapeutic or supratherapeutic levels.

Use in Pediatric Populations

Aripiprazole, olanzapine, quetiapine, risperidone, lurasidone, and paliperidone have indications for adolescent schizophrenia (ages 13–17). Aripiprazole, quetiapine, and risperidone are approved in child and adolescent bipolar disorder (acute mania) for ages 10–17; risperidone and aripiprazole are also FDA-approved for irritability associated with autism in child and adolescent patients ages 5–16. As discussed in the sections on adverse effects, antipsychotic drug-naïve patients and younger patients are more susceptible than other patients to EPSs and weight gain (Correll et al., 2014; Peruzzolo et al., 2013). Use of the minimum effective dose can minimize EPS risk, and use of agents with lower weight gain liability is critical. The greater impact of risperidone and paliperidone on serum prolactin must be monitored by clinical inquiry. Delayed sexual maturation was not seen in adolescents in clinical trials with risperidone; nonetheless, the physician must be alert for such changes and for issues such as amenorrhea in girls and gynecomastia in boys and girls.

Use in Geriatric Populations

The increased sensitivity to EPSs, orthostasis, sedation, and anticholinergic effects are important for the geriatric population and often dictate the choice of antipsychotic medication. Avoidance of drug-drug interactions is also important, as older patients on numerous concomitant medications have multiple opportunities for interactions. Dose adjustment can offset known drug-drug interactions, but clinicians must be attentive to changes in concurrent medications and the potential pharmacokinetic consequences. Vigilance must also be maintained for the additive pharmacodynamic effects of α_1 adrenergic, antihistaminic, and anticholinergic properties of other agents.

Elderly patients have an increased risk for TD and parkinsonism, with TD rates about 5-fold higher than those seen with younger patients. With typical antipsychotics, the reported annual TD incidence among elderly patients is 20%–25% compared to 4%–5% for younger patients. With atypical antipsychotics, the annual TD rate in elderly patients is much lower (2%–3%). Increased risk for cerebrovascular events and all-cause mortality is also seen in elderly patients with dementia (see Increased Mortality in Patients With Dementia). Compared to younger patients, antipsychotic-induced weight gain is lower in elderly patients.

Use During Pregnancy and Lactation
Human data from large database studies do not show increased rates of major congenital malformations after first trimester exposure (Huybrechts et al., 2016). Nonetheless, the use of any medication during pregnancy must be balanced by concerns over fetal impact, especially first-trimester exposure, and the mental health of the mother. As antipsychotic drugs are designed to cross the blood-brain barrier, all have high rates of placental passage. Placental passage ratios are estimated to be highest for olanzapine (72%), followed by haloperidol (42%), risperidone (49%), and quetiapine (24%). Neonates exposed to olanzapine, the atypical agent with highest placental passage ratio, exhibit a trend toward greater neonatal intensive care unit admission. Use in nursing mothers raises a separate set of concerns due to the reduced capacity of the newborn to metabolize xenobiotics, thus presenting a significant risk for antipsychotic drug toxicity. Available data do not provide adequate guidance on choice of agent.

Major Drugs Available in the Class
Atypical antipsychotic drugs have largely replaced older agents, primarily due to their more favorable EPS profile. The older, typical agents are widely used when a higher level of D_2 antagonism is required. Table 16–1 describes the acute and maintenance doses for adult schizophrenia treatment based on consensus recommendations. There are numerous LAI formulations of typical antipsychotics (Table 16–3), but in the U.S., the only available LAI typical agents are fluphenazine and haloperidol (as decanoate esters) (Meyer, 2013), suitable for weekly injections. There are now six LAI atypical antipsychotics approved, including a 3-month form of LAI paliperidone. Pimavanserin is the only medication indicated for PDP, and does not worsen motor symptoms due to the lack of DA antagonism (Cummings et al., 2014).

Treatment of Mania

Mania is a period of elevated, expansive, or irritable mood with coexisting symptoms of increased energy and goal-directed activity and decreased need for sleep. Mania represents one pole of bipolar disorder (American Psychiatric Association, 2013). As with psychosis, mania may be induced by medications (e.g., DA agonists, antidepressants, stimulants) or substances of abuse, primarily cocaine and amphetamines, although periods of substance-induced mania should not be relied on solely to make a diagnosis of bipolar disorder. Nonetheless, there is recognition that patients who develop antidepressant-induced mania do have a bipolar diathesis even with no prior independent history of mania and should be followed carefully, especially if antidepressant treatment is again considered during periods of major depression.

Mania is distinguished from its less-severe form, hypomania, by the fact that hypomania, by definition, does not result in functional impairment or hospitalization and is not associated with psychotic symptoms. Patients who experience periods of hypomania and major depression have bipolar II disorder; those with mania at any time, bipolar I; and those with hypomania but less-severe forms of depression, cyclothymia (American Psychiatric Association, 2013). The prevalence of bipolar I disorder is roughly 1% of the population, and the prevalence of all forms of bipolar disorder is 3%–5%.

Genetics studies of bipolar disorder have yielded several loci of interest associated with disease risk and predictors of treatment response, but the data are not yet at the phase of clinical application. Unlike schizophrenia, for which the biological understanding of monoamine neurotransmission has permitted synthesis of numerous effective compounds, no medication has yet been designed to treat the full spectrum of bipolar disorder based on biological hypotheses of the illness. Lithium carbonate was introduced fortuitously in 1949 for the treatment of mania and approved for this purpose in the U.S. in 1970. While many classes of agents demonstrate efficacy in acute mania, including Li+, antipsychotic drugs, and certain anticonvulsants, no medication has surpassed lithium's efficacy for prophylaxis of future manic and depressive phases of bipolar disorder, and no other medication has demonstrated lithium's reduction in suicidality among bipolar patients (Geddes and Miklowitz, 2013).

Pharmacological Properties of Agents for Mania
Antipsychotic Agents
The chemistry and pharmacology of antipsychotic medications are addressed earlier in this chapter. When used for acute mania, the dosages are often at the high end of approved maximum dosing. Clozapine can be beneficial in patients with refractory mania as adjunctive therapy and as monotherapy (Geddes and Miklowitz, 2013). Certain antipsychotics have efficacy for adjunctive use (olanzapine) or as monotherapy (quetiapine, lurasidone) for bipolar depression, typically at much lower dosages than for acute mania.

Anticonvulsants
The pharmacology and chemistry of the anticonvulsants with significant use in treating acute mania (valproic acid compounds, carbamazepine) and for bipolar maintenance (lamotrigine) are covered extensively in Chapter 17. The therapeutic serum levels for the commonly used mood-stabilizing anticonvulsants and for Li+ are listed in Table 16–6.

TABLE 16–6 ■ COMPARATIVE EFFICACY AND TARGET SERUM LEVELS FOR MOOD STABILIZERS

	ACUTE MANIA	PROPHYLAXIS	BIPOLAR DEPRESSION
Lithium	+++ 1.0–1.5 mEq/L[a]	+++ 0.6–1.0 mEq/L	++ 0.6–1.0 mEq/L
Valproate	++++ 100–120 µg/mL[b]	+++ 60–100 µg/mL	—
Carbamazepine	+ 6–12 µg/mL	++ 6–12 µg/mL	+/− 6–12 µg/mL
Lamotrigine	−	++	++

[a]Lithium can be loaded with individual 10-mg/kg doses of an extended-release preparation administered at 4 PM, 6 PM, and 8 PM (Kook et al., 1985). Treatment should continue on day 2 with lithium carbonate given once nightly to minimize the risk of polyuria and renal insufficiency.
[b]Divalproex can be loaded at 30 mg/kg over 24 h, administered as a single dose or separated into two doses.

Lithium

Lithium is the lightest of the alkali metals (group Ia). Salts of Li^+ share some characteristics with those of Na^+ and K^+. Li^+ is readily assayed in biological fluids and can be detected in brain tissue by magnetic resonance spectroscopy. Traces of the ion occur normally in animal tissues, but it has no known physiological role. Lithium carbonate and lithium citrate are used therapeutically in the U.S.

Therapeutic concentrations of Li^+ have almost no discernible psychotropic effects in individuals without psychiatric symptoms. There are numerous molecular and cellular actions of Li^+, some of which overlap with identified properties of other mood-stabilizing agents (particularly valproate) and are discussed next. An important characteristic of Li^+ is that, unlike Na^+ and K^+, Li^+ develops a relatively small gradient across biological membranes. Although it can replace Na^+ in supporting a single action potential in a nerve cell, it is not a substrate for the Na^+ pump and therefore cannot maintain membrane potentials. It is uncertain whether therapeutic concentrations of Li^+ (0.5–1.0 mEq/L) affect the transport of other monovalent or divalent cations by nerve cells.

Hypotheses for the Mechanism of Action of Lithium and Relationship to Anticonvulsants

Plausible hypotheses for the mechanism of action focus on lithium's impact on monoamines implicated in the pathophysiology of mood disorders and on second-messenger and other intracellular molecular mechanisms involved in signal transduction, gene regulation, and cell survival. Li^+ has limited effects on catecholamine-sensitive adenylyl cyclase activity or on the binding of ligands to monoamine receptors in brain tissue, although it can influence response of 5HT autoreceptors to agonists (Grandjean and Aubry, 2009b). 5HT release from presynaptic terminals is regulated by $5HT_{1A}$ autoreceptors located on the cell body and $5HT_{1B}$ receptors on the nerve terminal. In vitro electrophysiological studies suggest that Li^+ facilitates 5HT release. Li^+ augments effects of antidepressants, and in animal models of depression, lithium's activity appears to be mediated through desensitizing actions at $5HT_{1B}$ sites; Li^+ also antagonizes mouse behaviors induced by administration of selective $5HT_{1B}$ agonists (Grandjean and Aubry, 2009b).

Li^+ inhibits inositol monophosphatase and interferes with the cycling of the PI pathway (Figure 16–1) (Grandjean and Aubry, 2009b). One result is an enhancement of IP_3 accumulation when the G_q-PLC-IP_3-Ca^{2+} pathway is activated. As a result, IP_3 signaling and consequent mobilization of Ca^{2+} from intracellular stores may also be enhanced acutely, along with the sequelae of those effects; Ca^{2+} mobilization, PKC activation, depletion of cellular inositol; another result is a decrease in available inositol for resynthesis/reincorporation into membrane PI phosphates. The uncompetitive inhibition of IP phosphatase by Li^+ occurs within the range of therapeutic Li^+ concentrations. A genome-wide association study implicated diacylglycerol kinase in the etiology of bipolar disorder, strengthening the association between Li^+ actions and PI metabolism. Further support for the role of inositol signaling in mania rests on the finding that valproate and its derivatives decrease intracellular inositol concentrations. Unlike Li^+, valproate decreases inositol through inhibition of *myo*-inositol-1-phosphate synthase. In cultured cell systems, carbamazepine appears to act via inositol depletion. Perhaps such a mechanism contributes to carbamazepine's mood-stabilizing properties (Rapoport et al., 2009).

Treatment with Li^+ ultimately leads to decreased activity of several protein kinases in brain tissue, including PKC, particularly isoforms α and β (Einat, 2014). Among other proposed antimanic or mood-stabilizing agents, this effect is also shared with valproate (particularly for PKC) but not with carbamazepine. Long-term treatment of rats with lithium carbonate or valproate decreases cytoplasm-to-membrane translocation of PKC and reduces PKC stimulation–induced release of 5HT from cerebral cortical and hippocampal tissue. Excessive PKC activation can disrupt prefrontal cortical regulation of behavior, but pretreatment of monkeys and rats with lithium carbonate or valproate blocks the impairment in working memory induced by activation of PKC in a manner also seen with the PKC inhibitor chelerythrine (Einat, 2014). A major substrate for cerebral PKC is the MARCKS protein, which is implicated in synaptic

and neuronal plasticity. The expression of MARCKS protein is reduced by treatment with both Li^+ and valproate but not by carbamazepine, antipsychotic medications, or antidepressants (Wang et al., 2001). This proposed mechanism of PKC inhibition has been the basis for therapeutic trials of tamoxifen, a selective estrogen receptor modulator that is also a potent centrally active PKC inhibitor. In acutely manic patients with bipolar I, tamoxifen has shown evidence of efficacy as adjunctive treatment (Einat, 2014). The impact of Li^+ or valproate on PKC activity may secondarily alter the activity of tyrosine hydroxylase. Li^+ may alter the release of neurotransmitters and hormones by a variety of putative mechanisms, and its acute effects may differ from its longterm effects (Sharp et al., 1991; Millienne-Petiot et al, 2017; Can et al, 2016; Fortin et al, 2016).

Both Li^+ and valproate treatment also inhibit the activity of GSK-3β (Williams et al., 2002). GSK-3 inhibition increases hippocampal levels of β-catenin, a function implicated in mood stabilization. In animal models, Li^+ induces molecular and behavioral effects comparable to that seen when one GSK-3β gene locus is inactivated (Urs et al., 2012). These lithium-sensitive behaviors are related to the impact of GSK-3β inhibition on the β-arrestin-2/PKB/PP2A signaling complex. Li^+ disrupts β-arrestin-2/PKB/PP2A complex formation by directly inhibiting GSK-3β.

Another proposed common mechanism for the actions of Li^+ and valproate relates to reduction in arachidonic acid turnover in brain membrane phospholipids. Rats fed Li^+ in amounts that achieve therapeutic CNS drug levels have reduced turnover of PI (↓83%) and phosphatidylcholine (↓73%); chronic intraperitoneal valproate achieves reductions of 34% and 36%, respectively. Li^+ also decreases gene expression of phospholipase A_2 and levels of COX-2 and its products (Rapoport et al., 2009).

ADME

Li^+ is almost completely absorbed from the GI tract. Peak plasma concentrations occur 2–4 h after an oral dose. Slow-release preparations of lithium carbonate minimize peak-to-trough ratios and permit once-daily dosing. Li^+ initially distributes to the extracellular fluid, does not bind appreciably to plasma proteins, and gradually accumulates in tissues, with a volume of distribution of 0.7–0.9 L/kg. The concentration gradient across plasma membranes is much smaller than those for Na^+ and K^+. Passage through the blood-brain barrier is slow, and when a steady state is achieved, the concentration of Li^+ in the cerebrospinal fluid and in brain tissue is about 40%–50% of the concentration in plasma. The kinetics of Li^+ can be monitored in human brain with magnetic resonance spectroscopy (Grandjean and Aubry, 2009b).

Approximately 95% of a single dose of Li^+ is eliminated in the urine, with a $t_{1/2}$ of about 24 h (varies with age and can be ~12 h in the young and ~36 h in the elderly [secondary to reduced GFR]). The $t_{1/2}$ generally supports once-daily dosing, which improves adherence and decreases risk for renal insufficiency by at least 20% (Castro et al., 2016). With repeated administration, Li^+ levels and excretion increase until a steady state is achieved (after four to five half-lives). When Li^+ is stopped, there is a rapid phase of renal excretion followed by a slow 10- to 14-day phase. Although the pharmacokinetics of Li^+ vary considerably among subjects, the volume of distribution and clearance are relatively stable in an individual patient.

Less than 1% of ingested Li^+ leaves the human body in the feces; 4%–5% is secreted in sweat (Grandjean and Aubry, 2009c). Li^+ is secreted in saliva in concentrations about twice those in plasma, while its concentration in tears is about equal to that in plasma. Li^+ is secreted in human milk, but serum levels in breast-fed infants are about 20% that of maternal levels and are not associated with notable behavioral effects (Diav-Citrin et al., 2014).

Li^+ competes with Na^+ for tubular reabsorption, and Li^+ retention can be increased by Na^+ loss related to diuretic use or diarrhea and other GI illness. Heavy sweating leads to a preferential secretion of Li^+ over Na^+; the repletion of excessive sweating using free water without electrolytes can cause hyponatremia and promote Li^+ retention (Grandjean and Aubry, 2009b).

Serum-Level Monitoring and Dose

Because of the low therapeutic index for Li^+, regular determination of serum concentrations is crucial. Concentrations considered to be effective and acceptably safe are between 0.6 and 1.5 mEq/L. The range of 1.0–1.5 mEq/L is favored for treatment of acutely manic patients. Somewhat lower values (0.6–1.0 mEq/L) are considered adequate and are safer for long-term prophylaxis. Serum concentrations of Li⁺ have been found to follow a clear dose-effect relationship between 0.4 and 1.0 mEq/L, but with a corresponding dose-dependent rise in polyuria and tremor as indices of adverse effects (Grandjean and Aubry, 2009b, 2009c). Nonetheless, patients who maintain trough levels of 0.8–1.0 mEq/L experience decreased relapse risk compared to those maintained at lower serum concentrations. There are patients who may do well with serum levels of 0.5–0.8 mEq/L, but there are no current clinical or biological predictors to permit a priori identification of these individuals. Individualization of serum levels is often necessary to obtain a favorable risk-benefit relationship.

By convention, the serum Li⁺ concentration is measured from samples obtained 10–12 h after the last oral dose of the day. When the peaks are reached, intoxication may result, even when concentrations in morning samples of plasma at the daily nadir are in the acceptable range of 0.6–1 mEq/L. Single daily doses generate relatively large oscillations of plasma Li⁺ concentration but lower mean trough levels than with multiple-daily dosing; moreover, single-nightly dosing means that peak serum levels occur during sleep, so complaints of CNS adverse effects are minimized (Grandjean and Aubry, 2009c). While relatively uncommon, GI complaints are a compelling reason for using delayed-release Li⁺ preparations, also given once daily.

Therapeutic Uses

Drug Treatment of Bipolar Disorder.
Treatment with Li⁺ ideally is conducted in patients with normal cardiac and renal function. Occasionally, patients with severe systemic illnesses are treated with Li⁺, provided that the indications are compelling, but the need for diuretics, nonsteroidal anti-inflammatory agents, or other medications that pose potential kinetic problems often precludes Li⁺ use in those with multiple medical problems. Treatment of acute mania and the prevention of recurrences of bipolar illness in adults or adolescents are uses approved by the FDA. Li⁺ is the mood stabilizer with the most robust data on suicide reduction in bipolar patients; Li⁺ is also efficacious for augmentation in unipolar depressive patients who respond inadequately to antidepressant therapy (Grandjean and Aubry, 2009a).

Pharmacotherapy of Mania.
The modern treatment of the manic, depressive, and mixed-mood phases of bipolar disorder was revolutionized by the introduction of Li⁺ in 1949, initially for acute mania only and later for prevention of recurrences of mania. While Li⁺, valproate, and carbamazepine have efficacy in acute mania, in clinical practice these are usually combined with atypical antipsychotic drugs, even in manic patients without psychotic features, due to their complementary modes of action. Li⁺, carbamazepine, and valproic acid preparations are effective only with daily dosing that maintains adequate serum levels (requires monitoring of serum levels). Patients with mania are often irritable and poorly cooperative with medication administration and phlebotomy; thus, atypical antipsychotic drugs may be the sole initial therapy, and they have proven efficacy as monotherapy. Moreover, acute intramuscular forms of olanzapine and ziprasidone can be used to achieve rapid control of psychosis and agitation. Benzodiazepines are often used adjunctively for agitation and sleep induction.

Li⁺ is effective in acute mania and can be loaded in those with normal renal function using three individual 10-mg/kg doses of a sustained-release preparation administered at 2-h intervals. The sustained-release form is used to minimize GI adverse effects (e.g., nausea, diarrhea); treatment may then be continued with Li⁺ carbonate. Acutely manic patients may require higher dosages to achieve therapeutic serum levels, and downward adjustment may be necessary once the patient is euthymic. Efficacy following loading can be achieved within 5 days. When adherence with oral capsules or tablets is an issue, the liquid Li⁺ citrate can be used.

The anticonvulsant sodium valproate also provides antimanic effects, with therapeutic benefit seen within 3–5 days (Cipriani et al., 2013). The most common form of valproate in use is divalproex sodium due to lower incidence of GI and other adverse effects. Divalproex is initiated at 30 mg/kg given as single or divided doses and titrated to effect based on the desired serum level. Serum concentrations of 90–120 μg/mL show the best response in clinical studies (Cipriani et al., 2013). With immediate-release forms of valproic acid and divalproex sodium, 12-h troughs are used to guide treatment. With the extended-release divalproex preparation, the true trough occurs 24 h after dosing. Obtaining serum levels at night may be difficult in outpatient settings, so 12-h troughs are commonly used, bearing in mind that 12-h trough levels are 18%–25% higher than the 24-h trough (Reed and Dutta, 2006).

Carbamazepine is effective for acute mania, but immediate-release forms of carbamazepine cannot be loaded or rapidly titrated over 24 h due to the development of adverse effects such as dizziness or ataxia, even within the therapeutic range (6–12 μg/mL) (Geddes and Miklowitz, 2013). An extended-release form of carbamazepine is effective as monotherapy with once-daily dosing. Carbamazepine response rates are lower than those for valproate compounds or for Li⁺, with mean rates of 45%–60% cited in the literature (Geddes and Miklowitz, 2013). Nevertheless, certain individuals respond to carbamazepine after failing Li⁺ and valproate. Initial doses are 400 mg/d in two divided doses. Titration proceeds by 200-mg increments every 24–48 h based on clinical response and serum trough levels, not to exceed 1600 mg/d.

The FDA has warned that serious and potentially fatal skin reactions (e.g., Stevens-Johnson syndrome and toxic epidermal necrolysis) may occur with the administration of carbamazepine in patients positive for the *HLA-B*1502* allele. Thus, the FDA recommends genetic screening for patients of Asian ancestry (among whom the prevalence of this allele exceeds 15%) before initiation of carbamazepine therapy and using alternative therapies in patients positive for the allele. See Chapter 17 for more information on carbamazepine.

Lamotrigine has no role in acute mania due to the slow, extended titration necessary to minimize risk of Stevens-Johnson syndrome and is used for bipolar maintenance (Rapoport et al., 2009; Selle et al., 2014).

Prophylactic Treatment of Bipolar Disorder.
The choice of ongoing prophylaxis is determined by the need for continued antipsychotic drug use and for use of a mood-stabilizing agent. Both aripiprazole and olanzapine are effective as monotherapy for mania prophylaxis, but olanzapine use is eschewed out of concern for metabolic effects, and aripiprazole shows no benefit for prevention of depressive relapse. LAI risperidone is approved for bipolar maintenance treatment as monotherapy or adjunctively with Li⁺ or valproate. If LAI risperidone is used as monotherapy, coverage with an oral antipsychotic is necessary for the first 4 weeks after the initial injection. When antipsychotic drugs have been employed as adjunctive agents, the optimal duration of treatment is unclear; recent data indicate no greater benefit beyond 6 months after remission from an acute manic episode (Yatham et al., 2016).

Overriding concerns guiding bipolar treatment are the high recurrence rate and the high risk of suicide. Individuals who experience mania have an 80%–90% lifetime risk of subsequent manic episodes. As with schizophrenia, lack of insight, poor psychosocial support, and substance abuse all interfere with treatment adherence. While the anticonvulsants lamotrigine, carbamazepine, and divalproex have data supporting their use in bipolar prophylaxis, only lithium has consistently been shown to reduce the risk of suicide compared to other treatments, specifically when compared to valproate acid derivatives (Goodwin et al., 2003).

A recent large trial comparing Li⁺ and valproate found no significant differences in time to relapse between the two agents (Cipriani et al., 2013). Lamotrigine has proven effective for bipolar patients whose most recent mood episode was manic or depressed, with greater effect on depressive relapse (Selle et al., 2014). The ability to provide prophylaxis for future depressive episodes combined with data in acute bipolar depression has made lamotrigine a useful choice for bipolar treatment, given that patients with bipolar I and II spend large amounts of time in depressive phases (Selle et al., 2014).

Bipolar disorder is a lifetime illness with high recurrence rates. Individuals who experience an episode of mania should be educated about the probable need for ongoing treatment. Stopping mood stabilizer therapy can be considered in patients who have experienced only one lifetime manic episode, particularly when there may have been a pharmacological precipitant (e.g., substance or antidepressant use), and who have been euthymic for extended periods. For patients with bipolar II, the impact of hypomania is relatively limited, so the decision to recommend prolonged maintenance treatment with a mood stabilizer is based on clinical response and risk:benefit ratio. Discontinuation of maintenance Li$^+$ treatment in patients with bipolar I carries a high risk of early recurrence and of suicidal behavior over a period of several months, even if the treatment had been successful for several years. Recurrence is much more rapid than is predicted by the natural history of untreated bipolar disorder, in which cycle lengths average about 1 year. This risk may be moderated by slow, gradual removal of Li$^+$; rapid discontinuation should be avoided unless dictated by medical emergencies.

Other Uses of Lithium. Li$^+$ is effective as adjunct therapy in treatment-resistant major depression (Grandjean and Aubry, 2009a). Clinical data also support Li$^+$ use as monotherapy for unipolar depression. Meta-analyses indicated that lithium's benefit on suicide reduction extends to patients with unipolar mood disorder (Baldessarini and Tondo, 2000). While maintenance Li$^+$ levels of 0.6–1.0 mEq/L are used for bipolar prophylaxis, a lower range (0.4–0.8 mEq/L) is recommended for antidepressant augmentation.

Based on its neuroprotective properties, Li$^+$ treatment has been suggested for conditions associated with excitotoxic and apoptotic cell death, such as stroke and spinal cord injury, and in neurodegenerative disorders, including dementia of the Alzheimer type, Parkinson disease, Huntington disease, amyotrophic lateral sclerosis, progressive supranuclear palsy, and spinocerebellar ataxia type I (Chiu et al., 2013).

Drug Interactions. Thiazide diuretics cause significant reductions in Li$^+$ clearance that result in toxic levels. The K$^+$-sparing diuretics have more modest effects on the excretion of Li$^+$, with concomitantly smaller increases in serum levels. Loop diuretics such as furosemide seem to have limited impact on Li$^+$ levels (Grandjean and Aubry, 2009b). Administration of osmotic diuretics or acetazolamide increases renal excretion of Li$^+$ but not sufficiently for the management of acute Li$^+$ intoxication. Through alteration of renal perfusion, some nonsteroidal anti-inflammatory agents can facilitate renal proximal tubular resorption of Li$^+$ and thereby increase serum concentrations (Grandjean and Aubry, 2009b). This interaction appears to be particularly prominent with indomethacin, but also may occur with ibuprofen, naproxen, and COX-2 inhibitors and possibly less so with sulindac and aspirin. ACEIs, particularly lisinopril, also cause Li$^+$ retention, with isolated reports of toxicity among stable Li$^+$-treated patients switched from fosinopril to lisinopril (Meyer et al., 2005).

Amiloride blocks entry of Li$^+$ into renal distal tubule ENaCs and has been used to safely manage NDI associated with Li$^+$ therapy (Bedford et al., 2008). The development of NDI is related to accumulation of Li$^+$ in distal tubular cells and subsequent inhibition of GSK-3β, leading to vasopressin insensitivity and downregulation of aquaporin-2 channels. The use of amiloride for this purpose requires electrolyte monitoring and Li$^+$ dosage adjustments to prevent toxicity (Bedford et al., 2008).

Adverse Effects of Lithium

CNS Effects. The most common effect of Li$^+$ in the therapeutic dose range is fine postural hand tremor, indistinguishable from essential tremor. Severity and risk for tremor are dose dependent, with incidence ranging from 15% to 70%. In addition to the avoidance of caffeine and other agents that increase tremor amplitude, therapeutic options include dose reduction (bearing in mind the increased relapse risk with lower serum Li$^+$ levels) and β adrenergic blockade (Grandjean and Aubry, 2009c); the approach to valproate-induced tremor is identical. At peak serum (and CNS) levels of Li$^+$, patients may complain of incoordination, ataxia, or slurred speech, all of which can be avoided by dosing Li$^+$ at bedtime. Patients may also complain of mental fatigue or cognitive dulling at higher serum Li$^+$ levels, but this should be carefully assessed to determine whether this reflects a true side effect or a desire to regain the mental high from hypomania.

Seizures have been reported in nonepileptic patients with therapeutic plasma concentrations of Li$^+$. Li$^+$ treatment has also been associated with increased risk of post-ECT confusion and is generally tapered off prior to a course of ECT (Grandjean and Aubry, 2009c). In some instances, addition of Li$^+$ to existing antipsychotics may increase the sensitivity to D$_2$ blockade, resulting in EPSs.

Li$^+$ treatment results in significant weight gain, a problem that is magnified by concurrent use of antipsychotic drugs. Mean weight change at 1 year in prospective Li$^+$ trials ranges from − 1 kg to + 4 kg, but the proportion of individuals who gain more than 5% of baseline weight is 13%–62%. Although the mechanism is unclear, central appetite stimulation at hypothalamic sites is the most plausible explanation (Grandjean and Aubry, 2009c).

Renal Effects. The kidney's ability to concentrate urine decreases during Li$^+$ therapy, and about 60% of individuals exposed to Li$^+$ experience some form of polyuria and compensatory polydipsia. The mechanism of polyuria is related to the fact that Li$^+$ has 1.5- to 2.0-fold greater affinity than Na$^+$ for ENaC present on the apical (i.e., luminal) surfaces of distal tubular cells. Once in the cell, Li$^+$ is a poor substrate for the Na$^+$-K$^+$-ATPase present on the basal membrane, leading to accumulation of Li$^+$ in these distal tubular cells (Grunfeld and Rossier, 2009). High intracellular Li$^+$ concentrations inhibit GSK-3β, leading to vasopressin insensitivity, downregulation of aquaporin-2 channels, and NDI. Mean 24-h urinary volumes of 3 L/d are common among long-term Li$^+$ users. Li$^+$ discontinuation or a switch to single-daily dosing may reverse the impact on renal concentrating ability in patients with less than 5 years of Li$^+$ exposure. Patients exposed to multiple-daily dosing are at greater risk for renal effects. Renal function should be monitored with semiannual serum blood urea nitrogen and creatinine levels and calculation of eGFR using standard formulas (Morriss and Benjamin, 2008). Spot urine osmolality measurements are used to determine the extent and development of problems with NDI and polyuria. Reassessment of Li$^+$ treatment should be considered when the eGFR is less than 60 mL/min on several periodic measurements, daily urinary volume exceeds 4 L, or serum creatinine continues to rise on three separate occasions (Morriss and Benjamin, 2008). With modern monitoring principles, no patient should develop chronic kidney disease to the extent of requiring renal dialysis (Aiff et al., 2014).

Thyroid and Endocrine Effects. A small number of patients on Li$^+$ develop a benign, diffuse, nontender thyroid enlargement suggestive of compromised thyroid function; many of these patients will have normal thyroid function. Measurable effects of Li$^+$ on thyroid indices are seen in a fraction of patients: 7%–10% develop overt hypothyroidism, and 23% have subclinical disease, with women at three to nine times greater risk (Grandjean and Aubry, 2009c). Ongoing monitoring of TSH and free T$_4$ is recommended throughout the course of Li$^+$ treatment. The development of hypothyroidism is easily treated through exogenous replacement and is not a reason to discontinue Li$^+$ therapy. Rare reports of hyperthyroidism during Li$^+$ treatment also exist (Persad et al., 1993). Hypercalcemia related to hyperparathyroidism has been reported in about ~10% of Li$^+$-treated patients. Routine monitoring of serum Ca^{2+} should be included with measurements of electrolytes, thyroid indices, renal function, and serum Li$^+$ levels (Shapiro and Davis, 2015).

ECG Effects. The prolonged use of Li$^+$ causes benign and reversible T-wave flattening in about 20% of patients. At therapeutic concentrations, there are rare reports of Li$^+$-induced effects on cardiac conduction and pacemaker automaticity, effects that become pronounced during overdose and lead to sinus bradycardia, A-V block, and possible CV compromise (Grandjean and Aubry, 2009c). Routine ECG monitoring may be considered in older patients, particularly those with a history of arrhythmia or coronary heart disease.

Skin Effects. Allergic reactions such as dermatitis, folliculitis, and vasculitis can occur with Li$^+$ administration. Worsening of acne vulgaris, psoriasis, and other dermatological conditions is a common problem that is usually treatable by topical measures but in a small number may improve only on discontinuation of Li⁺ (Grandjean and Aubry, 2009c). Some patients on Li⁺ (and valproate) may experience alopecia.

Pregnancy and Lactation. The use of Li⁺ in early pregnancy may be associated with an increase in the incidence of CV anomalies of the newborn, especially Ebstein malformation. The risk of Ebstein anomaly (about 1 per 20,000 live births in controls) may rise several-fold with first-trimester Li⁺ exposure; recent estimates indicate a risk of up to 1 per 2500 (Diav-Citrin et al., 2014). In balancing the risk versus benefit of using Li⁺ in pregnancy, it is important to evaluate the risk of inadequate prophylaxis for the patient with bipolar disorder patient and subsequent risk that mania poses for the patient and fetus. If there is a compelling need for Li⁺, screening ultrasonography for CV anomalies is recommended. In patients who choose to forgo medication exposure during the first trimester, potentially safer treatments for acute mania include antipsychotic drugs or ECT.

In pregnancy, maternal polyuria may be exacerbated by Li⁺. Concomitant use of Li⁺ with medications that waste Na⁺ or a low-Na⁺ diet during pregnancy can contribute to maternal and neonatal Li⁺ intoxication. Li⁺ freely crosses the placenta, and fetal or neonatal Li⁺ toxicity may develop when maternal blood levels are within the therapeutic range (Grandjean and Aubry, 2009c). Fetal Li⁺ exposure is associated with neonatal goiter, CNS depression, hypotonia ("floppy baby" syndrome), and cardiac murmur. Most experts recommend withholding Li⁺ therapy for 24–48 h before delivery, and this is considered standard practice to avoid the potentially toxic increases in maternal and fetal serum Li⁺ levels associated with postpartum diuresis. The physical and CNS sequelae of late-term neonatal Li⁺ exposure are reversible once Li⁺ exposure has ceased, and no long-term neurobehavioral consequences are observed (Diav-Citrin et al., 2014).

Other Effects. A benign, sustained increase in circulating polymorphonuclear leukocytes (12,000–15,000 cells/mm³) commonly occurs, related to Li⁺-induced increases in urinary levels of G-CSF and augmented production of G-CSF by peripheral blood mononuclear cells (Focosi et al., 2009). Li⁺ also directly stimulates the proliferation of pluripotent stem cells. Some patients may complain of a metallic taste, making food less palatable.

Acute Toxicity and Overdose. The occurrence of toxicity is related to the serum concentration of Li⁺ and its rate of rise following administration. Acute intoxication is characterized by vomiting, profuse diarrhea, coarse tremor, ataxia, coma, and convulsions. Symptoms of milder toxicity are most likely to occur at the absorptive peak of Li⁺ and include nausea, vomiting, abdominal pain, diarrhea, sedation, and fine tremor. The more serious effects involve the nervous system and include mental confusion, hyperreflexia, gross tremor, dysarthria, seizures, and cranial nerve and focal neurological signs, progressing to coma and death. Sometimes both cognitive and motor neurological damage may be irreversible, with persistent cerebellar tremor the most common (El-Mallakh, 1986). Other toxic effects are cardiac arrhythmias, hypotension, and albuminuria.

Treatment of Lithium Intoxication. There is no specific antidote for Li⁺ intoxication, and treatment is supportive, including intubation if indicated and continuous cardiac monitoring. Levels greater than 1.5 mEq/L are considered toxic, but inpatient medical admission is usually not indicated (in the absence of symptoms) until levels exceed 2 mEq/L. Care must be taken to ensure that the patient is not Na⁺ and water depleted (Grandjean and Aubry, 2009c). Dialysis is the most effective means of removing Li⁺ and is necessary in severe poisonings, that is, in patients exhibiting symptoms of toxicity or patients with serum Li⁺ concentrations of 3 mEq/L or greater in acute overdoses. Complete recovery occurs with an average maximal level of 2.5 mEq/L; permanent neurological symptoms result from mean levels of 3.2 mEq/L; death occurs with mean maximal levels of 4.2 mEq/L (El-Mallakh, 1986).

Use in Pediatric Populations. Li⁺ is FDA-approved for child/adolescent bipolar disorder for ages 12 years or older (Peruzzolo et al., 2013).

Aripiprazole, quetiapine, and risperidone are FDA approved for acute mania in children and adolescents aged 10–17 years. Children and adolescents have higher volumes of body water and higher eGFR than adults. The resulting shorter $t_{1/2}$ of Li⁺ demands dosing increases on a milligram/kilogram basis, and multiple-daily dosing is often required. In children ages 6–12 years, a dose of 30 mg/kg/d given in three divided doses will produce a Li⁺ concentration of 0.6–1.2 mEq/L in 5 days, although dosing is always guided by serum levels and clinical response (Peruzzolo et al., 2013). Use in children under 12 represents an off-label use for Li⁺, and caregivers should be alert to signs of toxicity. As with adults, ongoing monitoring of renal and thyroid function is important, along with clinical inquiry into extent of polyuria.

A limited number of controlled studies suggested that valproate has efficacy comparable to that of Li⁺ for mania in children or adolescents (Peruzzolo et al., 2013). As with Li⁺, weight gain and tremor can be problematic; moreover, there are reports of hyperammonemia in children with urea cycle disorders. Ongoing monitoring of platelets and liver function tests, in addition to serum drug levels, is recommended.

Use in Geriatric Populations. The majority of older patients on Li⁺ therapy are those maintained for years on the medication. Elderly patients frequently take numerous medications for other illnesses, and the potential for drug-drug interactions is substantial. Age-related reductions in total body water and creatinine clearance reduce the safety margin for Li⁺ treatment in older patients. Targeting lower maintenance serum levels (0.6–0.8 mEq/L) may reduce the risk of toxicity. As eGFR drops below 50 mL/min, strong consideration must be given to use of alternative agents, despite lithium's therapeutic advantages (Morriss and Benjamin, 2008). Li⁺ toxicity occurs more frequently in elderly patients, in part as the result of concurrent use of loop diuretics and ACEIs (Grandjean and Aubry, 2009c). Anticonvulsants, especially extended-release divalproex, are a reasonable alternative to Li⁺. Elderly patients who are drug naïve may be more sensitive to the CNS adverse effects of all types of medications used for acute mania, especially parkinsonism and TD from D_2 antagonism, confusion from antipsychotic medications with antimuscarinic properties, and ataxia or sedation from Li⁺ or anticonvulsants.

Clinical Summary: Treatment of Mania

Despite decades of data substantiating the superior efficacy of Li⁺ in patients with bipolar disorder, including suicide reduction, Li⁺ remains underutilized. Long-term studies spanning 10 or more years demonstrated that while polyuria may be relatively common, significant declines in renal function to the point of stage 4 chronic kidney disease are rare during Li⁺ treatment. Many agents are effective for acute mania, but long-term treatment requires careful consideration of extent and severity of prior depressive episodes, past history of treatment response, concurrent medical illness and medication use, patient preference, and concerns over particular adverse effects (e.g., weight gain). Combining mood stabilizers and antipsychotic agents shows greater benefit for acute mania than monotherapy of either agent class but may be associated with increased long-term weight gain. A realistic discussion with patients regarding long-term side effects for various treatments and clinical outcomes is paramount to improve adherence.

Serum-level monitoring is necessary for Li⁺, valproate acid compounds, and carbamazepine. Lamotrigine may be particularly useful in patients with type II bipolar disorder, for which mania prophylaxis is not a concern. The clinical data make a compelling argument for Li⁺ as the treatment of choice in bipolar I disorder. Ongoing research into lithium's mechanism of action may yield new agents without lithium's adverse effect profile, as well as genetic predictors of Li⁺ response.

Acknowledgment: *Ross J. Baldessarini and Frank I. Tarazi contributed to this chapter in recent editions of this book. We have retained some of their text in the current edition.*

Drug Facts for Your Personal Formulary: *Antipsychotic and Mood-Stabilizing Agents*

Drugs	Therapeutic Uses	Clinical Pharmacology and Tips
First-Generation Antipsychotics • Low-potency D$_2$ antagonists		
Chlorpromazine	• Schizophrenia • Acute mania	• High M$_1$, H$_1$, and α$_1$ adrenergic affinities increase rates of anticholinergic side effects, sedation and weight gain, and hypotension, respectively • Less QT$_c$ prolongation at high plasma levels than thioridazine • High risk of metabolic adverse effects • Photosensitivity
First-Generation Antipsychotics • Medium- and high-potency D$_2$ antagonists		
Haloperidol	• Schizophrenia • Acute mania	• Higher rates of EPSs, akathisia, hyperprolactinemia • Limited anticholinergic side effects, sedation, weight gain, and hypotension • Avoid intravenous use due to QT$_c$ prolongation • Chlorpromazine 100 mg oral equivalence: 2 mg
Fluphenazine	• Schizophrenia • Acute mania	• Higher rates of EPSs, akathisia, hyperprolactinemia • Limited anticholinergic side effects, sedation, weight gain, and hypotension • Chlorpromazine 100 mg oral equivalence: 2 mg
Trifluoperazine	• Schizophrenia • Acute mania	• Higher rates of EPSs, akathisia, hyperprolactinemia • Limited anticholinergic side effects, sedation, weight gain, and hypotension • Chlorpromazine 100 mg oral equivalence: 5 mg
Thiothixene	• Schizophrenia • Acute mania	• Higher rates of EPSs, akathisia, hyperprolactinemia • Limited anticholinergic side effects, sedation, weight gain, and hypotension • Chlorpromazine 100 mg oral equivalence: 5 mg
Perphenazine	• Schizophrenia • Acute mania	• Modest rates of EPSs, akathisia • Limited anticholinergic side effects, sedation, weight gain, and hypotension • Chlorpromazine 100 mg oral equivalence: 10 mg
Loxapine	• Schizophrenia • Acute mania	• Modest rates of EPS, akathisia • Limited anticholinergic side effects, sedation, weight gain, and hypotension • Chlorpromazine 100 mg oral equivalence: 10 mg
Second-Generation Antipsychotics • 5HT$_{2A}$ and D$_2$ antagonists		
Asenapine	• Schizophrenia • Acute mania	• Only available in ODT formulation due to 98% first-pass effect if swallowed • Administer sublingually: avoid water for 10 min to achieve maximum oral-buccal absorption (avoiding water for 2 min achieves 80% of maximum absorption) • Low risk of metabolic adverse effects
Clozapine	• Refractory schizophrenia • Refractory mania	• Must register patient and prescriber due to mandatory hematological monitoring • High M$_1$, H$_1$, and α$_1$ adrenergic affinity increases rates of anticholinergic side effects, sedation and weight gain, and hypotension, respectively • High risk of metabolic adverse effects • Significant constipation; avoid other anticholinergic agents, manage aggressively • Sialorrhea; manage with locally administered agents (sublingual atropine 1% drops or ipratropium 0.06% spray)
Iloperidone	• Schizophrenia	• High α$_1$ adrenergic affinity; titrate to minimize orthostasis • Low risk of metabolic adverse effects
Lurasidone	• Schizophrenia • Bipolar depression (monotherapy and adjunct)	• Low risk for anticholinergic side effects, sedation and weight gain, and hypotension, respectively • Low risk of metabolic adverse effects • Absorption increased 100% by administration with 350 kcal food
Olanzapine	• Schizophrenia • Acute mania • Bipolar depression (in combination with fluoxetine)	• High risk of metabolic adverse effects • Anticholinergic effects at high dosages
Paliperidone	• Schizophrenia	• Moderate risk of metabolic adverse effects • High rates of hyperprolactinemia
Quetiapine	• Schizophrenia • Acute mania • Bipolar depression (monotherapy) • Unipolar depression (adjunct)	• High risk of metabolic adverse effects at full therapeutic dosages for schizophrenia • High H$_1$ and α$_1$ adrenergic affinities increase rates of sedation and hypotension, respectively • Low rates of EPSs, akathisia, and hyperprolactinemia
Risperidone	• Schizophrenia • Acute mania	• Moderate risk of metabolic adverse effects • High rates of hyperprolactinemia

Drug Facts for Your Personal Formulary: *Antipsychotic and Mood-Stabilizing Agents (continued)*

Drugs	Therapeutic Uses	Clinical Pharmacology and Tips
Second-Generation Antipsychotics • 5HT$_{2A}$ and D$_2$ antagonists		
Sertindole	• Schizophrenia	• Not available in the U.S. • Restricted use in Europe, with extensive monitoring for QT$_c$ prolongation • Low risk of metabolic adverse effects
Ziprasidone	• Schizophrenia • Acute mania	• Low risk of metabolic adverse effects • Absorption increased 100% by administration with 500 kcal food • Improved tolerability at starting doses > 80 mg/d with food
Second-Generation Antipsychotics • D$_2$ partial agonists		
Aripiprazole	• Schizophrenia • Acute mania • Unipolar depression (adjunct)	• Low risk of metabolic adverse effects • Lowers serum prolactin • Akathisia noted in depression trials—can be lessened with starting dose of 2.0–2.5 mg at bedtime
Brexpiprazole	• Schizophrenia • Unipolar depression (adjunct)	• Low risk of metabolic adverse effects • Lowers serum prolactin
Cariprazine	• Schizophrenia • Acute mania	• Low risk of metabolic adverse effects • Lowers serum prolactin
Second-Generation Antipsychotics • D$_2$ and D$_3$ antagonists		
Amisulpride	• Schizophrenia • Unipolar depression (adjunct, at low dosages)	• Higher rates of EPSs • Higher rates of hyperprolactinemia • Low risk of metabolic adverse effects
5HT$_{2A}$ Inverse Agonist Without D$_2$ Binding		
Pimavanserin	Parkinson disease psychosis (PDP)	• Potent 5HT$_{2A}$ inverse agonist with no D2 affinity • Monotherapy efficacy data for psychosis available only for PDP • Only one dose available: 34 mg once daily, with or without food • ↓ dose by 50% with concurrent strong 3A4 inhibitors; may lose efficacy with strong 3A4 inducers • Clinical effects may not be seen for 2-6 weeks
Mood Stabilizers • Acute mania and/or bipolar maintenance		
Lithium	• Acute mania • Bipolar maintenance • Unipolar depression (adjunct)	• Reduces suicidality more than other treatments • Renally cleared • Higher risk for weight gain • Monitor TSH, renal function tests, levels • May cause tremor, hair loss • Therapeutic serum level: acute mania 1.0–1.5 mEq/mL • Therapeutic serum level: maintenance 0.6–1.0 mEq/mL
Valproate (divalproex)	• Acute mania • Bipolar maintenance	• Can be loaded in acute mania: 30 mg/kg over 24 h • Highly protein bound • Higher risk for weight gain • May cause thrombocytopenia, leukopenia, hyperammonemia, tremor, hair loss • Monitor CBC, liver function tests, levels • Therapeutic serum level: acute mania 100–120 µg/mL • Therapeutic serum level: maintenance 60–100 µg/mL
Carbamazepine	• Acute mania • Bipolar maintenance	• Less effective than lithium and valproic acid • Highly protein bound • HLA testing for those from east Asia to identify high risk of Stevens-Johnson syndrome • May cause hyponatremia, leukopenia • Strong inducer of CYP3A4 and P-glycoprotein • Avoid rapid titration to minimize risk of sedation, ataxia • Therapeutic serum level 6–12 µg/mL
Lamotrigine	• Bipolar maintenance	• Prolonged titration to minimize risk of Stevens-Johnson syndrome • 50% dosage reduction required if patient on valproic acid or divalproex

Bibliography

Aiff H, et al. The impact of modern treatment principles may have eliminated lithium-induced renal failure. *J Psychopharmacol*, **2014**, *28*:151–154.

American Psychiatric Association. (2013). *Diagnostic and Statistical Manual of Mental Disorders*. 5th ed. American Psychiatric Press, Washington, DC.

Baldessarini RJ, Tondo L. Does lithium treatment still work? Evidence of stable responses over three decades. *Arch Gen Psychiatry*, **2000**, *57*:187–190.

Bedford JJ, et al. Lithium-induced nephrogenic diabetes insipidus: renal effects of amiloride. *Clin J Am Soc Nephrol*, **2008**, *3*:1324–1331.

Burris KD, et al. Aripiprazole, a novel antipsychotic, is a high-affinity partial agonist at human dopamine D_2 receptors. *J Pharmacol Exp Ther*, **2002**, *302*:381–389.

Can A, et al. Chronic lithium treatment rectifies maladaptive dopamine release in the nucleus accumbens. *J Neurochem*, **2016**, *139*:576–585.

Castro VM, et al. Stratifying risk for renal insufficiency among lithium-treated patients: an electronic health record study. *Neuropsychopharmacol*, **2016**, *41*:1138–1143.

Chiu CT, et al. Therapeutic potential of mood stabilizers lithium and valproic acid: beyond bipolar disorder. *Pharmacol Rev*, **2013**, *65*:105–142.

Cipriani A, et al. Valproic acid, valproate and divalproex in the maintenance treatment of bipolar disorder. *Cochrane Database Syst Rev*, **2013**, *10*:CD003196.

Correll CU, et al. Cardiometabolic risk in patients with first-episode schizophrenia spectrum disorders: baseline results from the RAISE-ETP study. *JAMA Psychiatry*, **2014**, *71*:1350–1363.

Cummings J, et al. Pimavanserin for patients with Parkinson's disease psychosis: a randomised, placebo-controlled phase 3 trial. *Lancet*, **2014**, *383*:533–540.

De Hert M, et al. Body weight and metabolic adverse effects of asenapine, iloperidone, lurasidone and paliperidone in the treatment of schizophrenia and bipolar disorder: a systematic review and exploratory meta-analysis. *CNS Drugs*, **2012**, *26*:733–759.

Diav-Citrin O, et al. Pregnancy outcome following in utero exposure to lithium: a prospective, comparative, observational study. *Am J Psychiatry*, **2014**, *171*:785–794.

Dold M, et al. Antipsychotic augmentation of serotonin reuptake inhibitors in treatment-resistant obsessive-compulsive disorder: a meta-analysis of double-blind, randomized, placebo-controlled trials. *Int J Neuropsychopharmacol*, **2013**, *16*:557–574.

Dremencov E, et al. Modulation of dopamine transmission by 5-HT2C and 5-HT3 receptors: a role in the antidepressant response. *Current Drug Targets*, **2006**, *7*:165–175.

Einat H. Partial effects of the protein kinase C inhibitor chelerythrine in a battery of tests for manic-like behavior in black Swiss mice. *Pharmacol Rep*, **2014**, *66*:722–725.

El-Mallakh RS. Acute lithium neurotoxicity. *Psychiatr Dev*, **1986**, *4*:311–328.

Escudero I, Johnstone M. Genetics of schizophrenia. *Curr Psychiatry Rep*, **2014**, *16*:502.

Farahani A, Correll CU. Are antipsychotics or antidepressants needed for psychotic depression? A systematic review and meta-analysis of trials comparing antidepressant or antipsychotic monotherapy with combination treatment. *J Clin Psychiatry*, **2012**, *73*:486–496.

Focosi D, et al. Lithium and hematology: established and proposed uses. *J Leukocyte Biol*, **2009**, *85*:20–28.

Fortin SM, et al. The Aversive Agent Lithium Chloride Suppresses Phasic Dopamine Release Through Central GLP-1 Receptors. *Neuropsychopharmacol*, **2016**, *41*:906–915.

Gavin DP, Floreani C. Epigenetics of schizophrenia: an open and shut case. *Int Rev Neurobiol*, **2014**, *115*:155–201.

Geddes JR, Miklowitz DJ. Treatment of bipolar disorder. *Lancet*, **2013**, *381*:1672–1682.

Goodwin FK, et al. Suicide risk in bipolar disorder during treatment with lithium and divalproex. *JAMA*, **2003**, *290*:1467–1473.

Grandjean EM, Aubry JM. Lithium: updated human knowledge using an evidence-based approach: part I: clinical efficacy in bipolar disorder. *CNS Drugs*, **2009a**, *23*:225–240.

Grandjean EM, Aubry JM. Lithium: updated human knowledge using an evidence-based approach. Part II: clinical pharmacology and therapeutic monitoring. *CNS Drugs*, **2009b**, *23*:331–349.

Grandjean EM, Aubry JM. Lithium: updated human knowledge using an evidence-based approach: part III: clinical safety. *CNS Drugs*, **2009c**, *23*:397–418.

Grunfeld JP, Rossier BC. Lithium nephrotoxicity revisited. *Nat Rev Nephrol*, **2009**, *5*:270–276.

Gurrera RJ, et al. An international consensus study of neuroleptic malignant syndrome diagnostic criteria using the Delphi method. *J Clin Psychiatry*, **2011**, *72*:1222–1228.

Howes O, et al. Glutamate and dopamine in schizophrenia: an update for the 21st century. *J Psychopharmacol*, **2015**, *29*:97–115.

Huybrechts KF, et al. Antipsychotic use in pregnancy and the risk for congenital malformations. *JAMA Psychiatry*, **2016**, *73*:938–946.

Jager M, et al. Time course of antipsychotic treatment response in schizophrenia: results from a naturalistic study in 280 patients. *Schizophr Res*, **2010**, *118*:183–188.

Javitt DC, Freedman R. Sensory processing dysfunction in the personal experience and neuronal machinery of schizophrenia. *Am J Psychiatry*, **2015**, *172*:17–31.

Khan BA, et al. Delirium in hospitalized patients: implications of current evidence on clinical practice and future avenues for research—a systematic evidence review. *J Hosp Med*, **2012**, *7*:580–589.

Kim SF, et al. From the cover: antipsychotic drug-induced weight gain mediated by histamine H_1 receptor-linked activation of hypothalamic AMP-kinase. *Proc Natl Acad Sci U S A*, **2007**, *104*:3456–3459.

Kinon BJ, et al. Early response to antipsychotic drug therapy as a clinical marker of subsequent response in the treatment of schizophrenia. *Neuropsychopharmacology*, **2010**, *35*:581–590.

Kook KA, et al. Accuracy and safety of a priori lithium loading. *J Clin Psychiatry*, **1985**, *46*:49–51.

Koppel J, Greenwald BS. Optimal treatment of Alzheimer's disease psychosis: challenges and solutions. *Neuropsychiatr Dis Treat*, **2014**, *10*:2253–2262.

Krystal JH, et al. Adjunctive risperidone treatment for antidepressant-resistant symptoms of chronic military service-related PTSD: a randomized trial. *JAMA*, **2011**, *306*:493–502.

Kuepper R, et al. The dopamine dysfunction in schizophrenia revisited: new insights into topography and course. *Handb Exp Pharmacol*, **2012**, *212*:1–26.

Leucht S, et al. Comparative efficacy and tolerability of 15 antipsychotic drugs in schizophrenia: a multiple-treatments meta-analysis. *Lancet*, **2013**, *382*:951–962.

Malhi GS, et al. Mania: diagnosis and treatment recommendations. *Curr Psychiatry Rep*, **2012**, *14*:676–686.

Maust DT, et al. Antipsychotics, other psychotropics, and the risk of death in patients with dementia: number needed to harm. *JAMA Psychiatry*, **2015**, *72*:438–445.

Meltzer HY. Clozapine: balancing safety with superior antipsychotic efficacy. *Clin Schizophr Relat Psychoses*, **2012**, *6*:134–144.

Meyer JM. Understanding depot antipsychotics: an illustrated guide to kinetics. *CNS Spectr*, **2013**, *18*:55–68.

Meyer JM. A rational approach to employing high plasma levels of antipsychotics for violence associated with schizophrenia: case vignettes. *CNS Spectr*, **2014**, *19*:432–438.

Meyer JM, et al. Lithium toxicity after switch from fosinopril to lisinopril. *Int Clin Psychopharmacol*, **2005**, *20*:115–118.

Meyer JM, Leckband SG. A history of clozapine and concepts of atypicality. In: Domino EF, ed. *History of Psychopharmacology*. Vol. 2. Domemtech/NPP Books, Arlington, MA, **2013**, 95–106.

Meyer JM, Stahl SM. The metabolic syndrome and schizophrenia. *Acta Psychiatr Scand*, **2009**, *119*:4–14.

Millienne-Petiot M, et al. The effects of reduced dopamine transporter function and chronic lithium on motivation, probabilistic learning, and neurochemistry in mice: Modeling bipolar mania. *Neuropharmacology*, **2017**, 113, part A: 260–270.

Mogwitz S, et al. Clinical pharmacology of dopamine-modulating agents in Tourette's syndrome. *Int Rev Neurobiol*, **2013**, *112*:281–349.

Morriss R, Benjamin B. Lithium and eGFR: a new routinely available tool for the prevention of chronic kidney disease. *Br J Psychiatry*, **2008**, *193*:93–95.

Nielsen J, et al. Assessing QT prolongation of antipsychotic drugs. *CNS Drugs*, **2011**, *25*:473–490.

Ogino S, et al. Benefits and limits of anticholinergic use in schizophrenia: focusing on its effect on cognitive function. *Psychiatry Clin Neurosci*, **2014**, *68*:37–49.

Persad E, et al. Hyperthyroidism after treatment with lithium. *Can J Psychiatry* **1993**, *38*:599–602.

Peruzzolo TL, et al. Pharmacotherapy of bipolar disorder in children and adolescents: an update. *Rev Bras Psiquiatr*, **2013**, *35*:393–405.

Powell SB, et al. Genetic models of sensorimotor gating: relevance to neuropsychiatric disorders. *Curr Topics Behav Neurosci*, **2012**, *12*:251–318.

Praharaj SK, et al. Metformin for olanzapine-induced weight gain: a systematic review and meta-analysis. *Br J Clin Pharmacol*, **2011**, *71*:377–382.

Prickaerts J, et al. EVP-6124, a novel and selective alpha7 nicotinic acetylcholine receptor partial agonist, improves memory performance by potentiating the acetylcholine response of alpha7 nicotinic acetylcholine receptors. *Neuropharmacology*, **2012**, *62*:1099–1110.

Rapoport SI, et al. Bipolar disorder and mechanisms of action of mood stabilizers. *Brain Res Rev*, **2009**, *61*:185–209.

Reed RC, Dutta S. Does it really matter when a blood sample for valproic acid concentration is taken following once-daily administration of divalproex-ER? *Ther Drug Monitor*, **2006**, *28*:413–418.

Remington G, et al. The neurobiology of relapse in schizophrenia. *Schizophr Res*, **2014**, *152*:381–390.

Rostami-Hodjegan A, et al. Influence of dose, cigarette smoking, age, sex, and metabolic activity on plasma clozapine concentrations: a predictive model and nomograms to aid clozapine dose adjustment and to assess compliance in individual patients. *J Clin Psychopharmacol*, **2004**, *24*:70–78.

Rummel-Kluge C, et al. Head-to-head comparisons of metabolic side effects of second generation antipsychotics in the treatment of schizophrenia: a systematic review and meta-analysis. *Schizophr Res*, **2010**, *123*:225–233.

Salahudeen MS, et al. Impact of anticholinergic discontinuation on cognitive outcomes in older people: a systematic review. *Drugs Aging* **2014**, *31*:185–192.

Seeman P. Schizophrenia and dopamine receptors. *Eur Neuropsychopharmacol*, **2013**, *23*:999–1009.

Selle V, et al. Treatments for acute bipolar depression: meta-analyses of placebo-controlled, monotherapy trials of anticonvulsants, lithium and antipsychotics. *Pharmacopsychiatry*, **2014**, *47*:43–52.

Shapiro HI, Davis KA. Hypercalcemia and "primary" hyperparathyroidism during lithium therapy. *Am J Psychiatry*, **2015**, *172*:12–15.

Sharp T, et al. Effect of Short- and Long-Term Administration of Lithium on the Release of Endogenous 5-HT in the Hippocampus of the Rat *In Vivo* and *In Vitro*. *Neuropharmacology*, **1991**, *30*: 971–984.

Sparshatt A, et al. A systematic review of aripiprazole—dose, plasma concentration, receptor occupancy, and response: implications for therapeutic drug monitoring. *J Clin Psychiatry*, **2010**, *71*:1447–1456.

Torniainen M, et al. Antipsychotic treatment and mortality in schizophrenia. *Schizophr Bull*, **2015**, *41*:656–663. doi:10.1093/schbul/sbu164.

Turner P, et al. A systematic review and meta-analysis of the evidence base for add-on treatment for patients with major depressive disorder who have not responded to antidepressant treatment: a European perspective. *J Psychopharmacol*, **2014**, *28*:85–98.

Urs NM, et al. Deletion of GSK-3beta in D2R-expressing neurons reveals distinct roles for beta-arrestin signaling in antipsychotic and lithium action. *Proc Natl Acad Sci USA*, **2012**, *109*:20732–20737.

Wang L, et al. Transcriptional down-regulation of MARCKS gene expression in immortalized hippocampal cells by lithium. *J Neurochem*, **2001**, *79*:816–825.

Williams RS, et al. A common mechanism of action for three mood-stabilizing drugs. *Nature* **2002**, *417*:292–295.

Wright BM, et al. Augmentation with atypical antipsychotics for depression: a review of evidence-based support from the medical literature. *Pharmacotherapy*, **2013**, *33*:344–359.

Yatham LN et al. Optimal duration of risperidone or olanzapine adjunctive therapy to mood stabilizer following remission of a manic episode: A CANMAT randomized double-blind trial. *Molec Psychiatry*, **2016**, *21*:1050–1056.

Young JW, Geyer MA. Developing treatments for cognitive deficits in schizophrenia: the challenge of translation. *J Psychopharmacol*, **2015**, *29*:178–196.

Zipursky RB, et al. Risk of symptom recurrence with medication discontinuation in first-episode psychosis: a systematic review. *Schizophr Res*, **2014**, *152*:408–414.

Chapter 17

Pharmacotherapy of the Epilepsies

Misty D. Smith, Cameron S. Metcalf, and Karen S. Wilcox

Epilepsy and Antiseizure Therapy

The epilepsies are common and frequently devastating disorders, affecting about 2.5 million people in the U.S. alone. More than 40 distinct forms of epilepsy have been identified. Seizures often cause transient impairment of awareness, leaving the individual at risk of bodily harm and often interfering with education and employment. Current therapy is symptomatic: available ASDs inhibit seizures; neither effective prophylaxis nor cure is available. Adherence to prescribed treatment regimens is a major problem because of the need for long-term therapy together with unwanted effects of many drugs.

The mechanisms of action of ASDs fall into these major categories (see also Porter et al., 2012):

1. Modulation of cation channels (Na^+, K^+, Ca^{2+}). This can include prolongation of the inactivated state of voltage-gated Na^+ channels, positive modulation of K^+ channels, and inhibition of Ca^{2+} channels.
2. Enhancement of GABA neurotransmission through actions on $GABA_A$ receptors, modulation of GABA metabolism, and inhibition of GABA reuptake into the synaptic terminal.
3. Modulation of synaptic release through actions on the synaptic vesicle protein SV2A or Ca^{2+} channels containing the $\alpha2\delta$ subunit.
4. Diminishing synaptic excitation mediated by ionotropic glutamate receptors (e.g., AMPA receptors).

Beyond these broad classifications, many ASDs act through mechanisms distinct from the primary known mode of action. Furthermore, ASDs with similar mechanistic categories may have disparate clinical uses.

Much effort is devoted to elucidating the genetic causes and the cellular and molecular mechanisms by which a neural circuit becomes prone to seizure activity, with the goal of providing molecular targets for both symptomatic and preventive therapies.

Terminology and Seizure Classification

The term *seizure* refers to a transient alteration of behavior due to the disordered, synchronous, and rhythmic firing of populations of brain neurons. The term *epilepsy* refers to a disorder of brain function characterized by the periodic and unpredictable occurrence of seizures. Seizures can be provoked (i.e., by chemical agents or electrical stimulation) or unprovoked; the condition of

Abbreviations

AMPA: α-amino-3-hydroxy 5-methyl-4-isoxazolepropionic acid
ASD: antiseizure drug
CSF: cerebrospinal fluid
DS: depolarization shift
EEG: electroencephalogram
ETSP: Epilepsy Therapy Screening Project
GABA: γ-aminobutyric acid
JME: juvenile myoclonic epilepsy
NMDA: N-methyl-D-aspartate receptor
PEMA: phenylethylmalonamide
SV2A: synaptic vesicle glycoprotein 2A

epilepsy denotes the occurrence of spontaneous, unprovoked seizures. While agents in current clinical use inhibit seizures, whether any of these prevent the development of epilepsy (epileptogenesis) is uncertain.

This chapter employs the revised classification for seizures. Thus, seizures previously classified as *partial* seizures are referred to as *focal* seizures, whereas *generalized* seizures, those that involve both hemispheres widely from the outset, will still be referred to as generalized seizures (Fisher et al., 2017). In addition, the International League Against Epilepsy (ILAE) has added a classification for seizures with *unknown onset*, which includes such seizure types as tonic-clonic, atonic, and epileptic spasms.

From a network perspective, seizures arise from cortical, thalamocortical, limbic, or even brainstem circuits. The behavioral manifestations of a seizure are determined by the functions normally served by the brain region at which the seizure arises. For example, a seizure involving motor cortex is associated with clonic jerking of the body part controlled by this region of cortex. Thus, this type of focal seizure is associated with preservation of awareness. Focal seizures may also be associated with impairments of awareness. The majority of such focal seizures originate from the temporal lobe. Generalized seizures are now distinguished by the involvement of the motor system or those that lack motor involvement, for example, typical and atypical absence, eyelid myoclonic. The type of seizure is one determinant of the drug selected for therapy. Detailed information pertaining to seizure classifications is presented in Table 17–1.

Apart from this seizure classification, an additional classification specifies epilepsy syndromes, which refer to a cluster of symptoms frequently occurring together and include seizure types, etiology, age of onset, and other factors (Fisher RJ et al., 2017). More than 50 distinct epilepsy syndromes have been identified and categorized into focal versus generalized epilepsies. The focal epilepsies may consist of any of the focal seizure types (Table 17–1) and account for roughly 60% of all epilepsies. The etiology commonly consists of a cortical lesion, such as a tumor, developmental malformation, or damage due to trauma or stroke. Such lesions often are evident on brain MRI. Alternatively, the etiology may be genetic. The generalized epilepsies are characterized most commonly by one or more of the generalized seizure types listed in Table 17–1 and account for about 40% of all epilepsies; the etiology is usually genetic. The most common generalized epilepsy is referred to as juvenile myoclonic epilepsy (JME), accounting for about 10% of all epilepsy syndromes. The age of onset is in the early teens, and the condition is characterized by myoclonic, tonic-clonic, and often absence seizures. Like most of the generalized-onset epilepsies, JME is a complex genetic disorder that is probably due to inheritance of multiple susceptibility genes; there is a familial clustering of cases, but the pattern of inheritance is not Mendelian. The classification of epileptic syndromes guides clinical assessment and management and, in some instances, selection of ASDs.

TABLE 17–1 ■ CLASSIFICATION OF EPILEPTIC SEIZURES

SEIZURE TYPE	FEATURES	CONVENTIONAL ANTISEIZURE DRUGS	RECENTLY DEVELOPED ANTISEIZURE DRUGS
Focal seizures			
Focal Aware	Diverse manifestations determined by the region of cortex activated by the seizure (e.g., if motor cortex representing left thumb, clonic jerking of left thumb results; if somatosensory cortex representing left thumb, paresthesia of left thumb results), lasting approximating 20–60 sec. *Key feature is preservation of awareness.*	Carbamazepine, phenytoin, valproate	Brivaracetam, eslicarbazepine, ezogabine, gabapentin, lacosamide, lamotrigine, levetiracetam, perampanel, rufinamide, tiagabine, topiramate, zonisamide
Focal with Impaired Awareness	Impaired consciousness lasting 30 sec to 2 min, often associated with purposeless movements such as lip smacking or hand wringing.		
Focal to Bilateral Tonic-Clonic	Simple or complex focal seizure evolves into a tonic-clonic seizure with loss of awareness and sustained contractions (tonic) of muscles throughout the body, followed by periods of muscle contraction alternating with periods of relaxation (clonic), typically lasting 1–2 min.	Carbamazepine, phenobarbital, phenytoin, primidone, valproate	
Generalized seizures			
Generalized Absence	Abrupt onset of impaired consciousness associated with staring and cessation of ongoing activities, typically lasting less than 30 sec.	Ethosuximide, valproate, clonazepam	Lamotrigine
Generalized Myoclonic	A brief (perhaps a second), shock-like contraction of muscles that may be restricted to part of one extremity or may be generalized.	Valproate, clonazepam	Levetiracetam
Generalized Tonic-Clonic	As described above for partial with secondarily generalized tonic-clonic seizure except that it is not preceded by a partial seizure.	Carbamazepine, phenobarbital, phenytoin, primidone, valproate	Lamotrigine, levetiracetam, topiramate

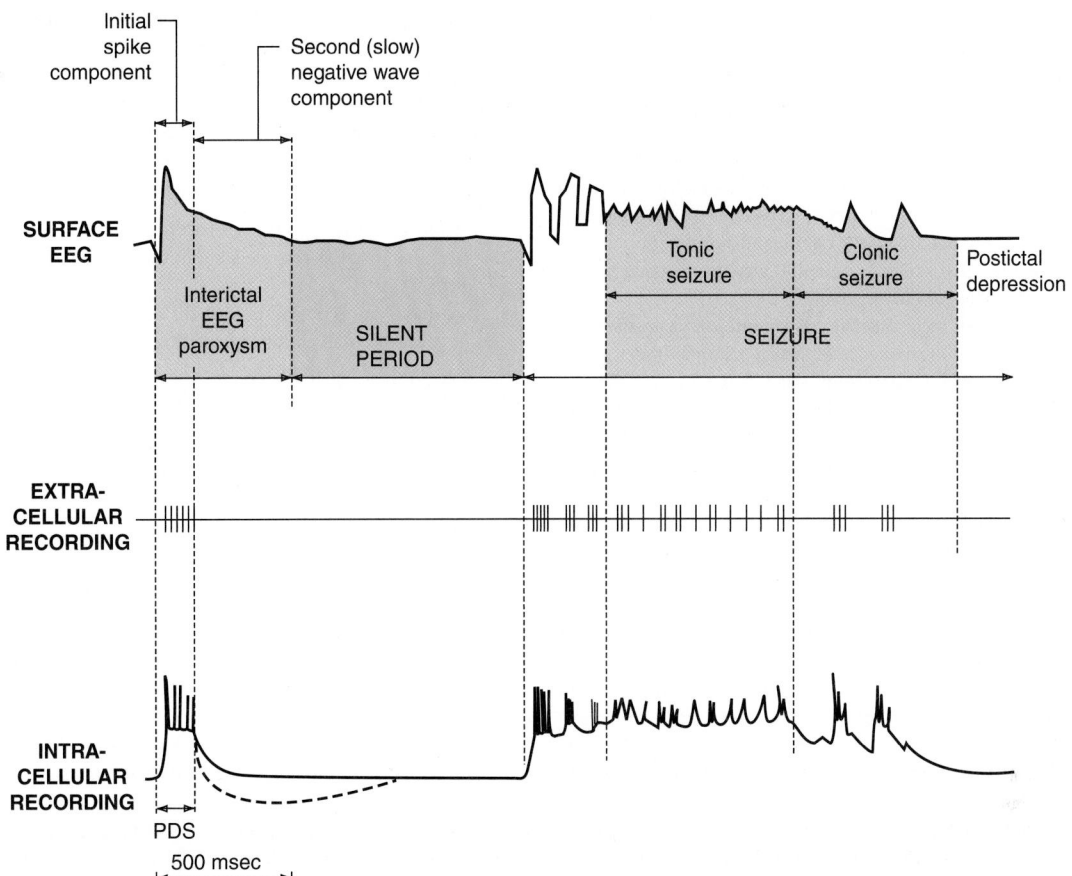

Figure 17–1 *Cortical EEG, extracellular, and intracellular recordings in a seizure focus induced by local application of a convulsant agent to mammalian cortex.* The extracellular recording was made through a high-pass filter. High-frequency firing of the neuron is evident in both extracellular and intracellular recording during the paroxysmal depolarization shift (PDS). (Modified with permission from Ayala GF *et al*. Genesis of epileptic interictal spikes. New knowledge of cortical feedback systems suggests a neurophysiological explanation of brief paroxysms. *Brain Res*, **1973**, *52*:1–17. © Elsevier.)

Nature and Mechanisms of Seizures and Antiseizure Drugs

Focal Epilepsies

More than a century ago, John Hughlings Jackson, the father of modern concepts of epilepsy, proposed that seizures were caused by "occasional, sudden, excessive, rapid and local discharges of gray matter," and that a generalized seizure resulted when normal brain tissue was invaded by the seizure activity initiated in the abnormal focus. This insightful proposal provided a framework for thinking about mechanisms of focal epilepsy. The advent of the EEG in the 1930s permitted the recording of electrical activity from the scalp of humans with epilepsy and demonstrated that the epilepsies are disorders of neuronal excitability.

The pivotal role of synapses in mediating communication amongst neurons in the mammalian brain suggested that defective synaptic function might lead to a seizure. That is, a reduction of inhibitory synaptic activity or enhancement of excitatory synaptic activity might be expected to trigger a seizure. Pharmacological studies of seizures support this notion. The neurotransmitters mediating the bulk of synaptic transmission in the mammalian brain are amino acids, with GABA and glutamate the principal inhibitory and excitatory neurotransmitters, respectively (Chapter 14). Pharmacological studies disclosed that *antagonists* of the GABA$_A$ receptor or *agonists* of different glutamate-receptor subtypes (NMDA, AMPA, or kainic acid) trigger seizures in experimental animals in vivo. Conversely, pharmacological agents that enhance GABA-mediated synaptic inhibition suppress seizures in diverse models. Glutamate-receptor antagonists also inhibit seizures in diverse models, including seizures evoked by electroshock and chemical convulsants (e.g., pentylenetetrazol).

These findings suggest pharmacological regulation of synaptic function can regulate the propensity for seizures and provide a framework for electrophysiological analyses aimed at elucidating the role of both synaptic and nonsynaptic mechanisms in seizures and epilepsy. Technical progress has fostered the progressive refinement of the analysis of seizure mechanisms from the EEG to populations of neurons (field potentials) to individual neurons to individual synapses and individual ion channels on individual neurons. Beginning in the mid-1960s, cellular electrophysiological studies of epilepsy focused on elucidating the mechanisms underlying the DS, the intracellular correlate of the "interictal spike" (Figure 17–1). The interictal (or between-seizures) spike is a sharp waveform recorded in the EEG of patients with epilepsy; it is asymptomatic, as it is not accompanied by overt change in the patient's behavior. However, the location of the interictal spike helps localize the brain region from which seizure activity originates in a given patient. The DS consists of a large depolarization of the neuronal membrane associated with a burst of action potentials. In most cortical neurons, the DS is generated by a large excitatory synaptic current that can be enhanced by activation of voltage-gated intrinsic membrane currents. Although the mechanisms generating the DS and whether the interictal spike triggers a seizure, inhibits a seizure, or is an epiphenomenon remains unclear, the study of the mechanisms underlying DS generation set the stage for inquiry into the cellular mechanisms of a seizure.

During the 1980s, various in vitro models of seizures were developed in isolated brain slice preparations in which many synaptic connections are preserved. Electrographic events with features similar to those recorded during seizures in vivo have been produced in hippocampal slices by multiple methods, including altering ionic constituents of media bathing the brain slices (McNamara, 1994), such as low Ca^{2+}, zero Mg^{2+}, or elevated K$^+$. The accessibility and experimental control provided by these in vitro preparations has permitted mechanistic investigations into the induction of seizures. Data from in vitro models confirmed the importance of synaptic function for initiating a seizure, demonstrating that subtle reductions (e.g., 20%) of inhibitory synaptic function could lead to epileptiform activity and that activation of excitatory synapses could be pivotal in seizure initiation. Other important factors include the volume of the extracellular space and intrinsic properties of a neuron, such as voltage-gated ion channels (e.g., K^+, Na^+, and Ca^{2+} channels) (Traynelis and Dingledine, 1988). Identification of these diverse synaptic and nonsynaptic factors controlling seizures in vitro provides potential pharmacological targets for regulating seizure susceptibility in vivo.

Some common forms of focal epilepsy arise months to years after cortical injury sustained as a consequence of stroke, trauma, infection, or other factors. Effective prophylaxis administered to patients at high risk would be highly desirable in the clinical setting. However, no effective antiepileptogenic agent has been identified. The drugs described in this chapter provide symptomatic therapy; that is, the drugs inhibit seizures in patients with epilepsy.

Understanding the mechanisms of epileptogenesis in cellular and molecular terms should provide a framework for development of novel therapeutic approaches. The availability of animal models provides an opportunity to investigate the underlying mechanisms and have also enabled the discovery of numerous ASDs that are proven safe and efficacious in humans.

One model, termed *kindling*, is induced by periodic administration of brief, low-intensity electrical stimulation of the amygdala or other limbic structures that evoke a brief electrical seizure recorded on the EEG without behavioral change. Repeated (e.g., 10–20) stimulations result in progressive intensification of seizures, culminating in tonic-clonic seizures that, once established, persist for the life of the animal. Additional models are produced by induction of continuous seizures that last for hours ("status epilepticus"). The inciting agent used in these models is typically either a chemoconvulsant, such as kainic acid or pilocarpine, or sustained electrical stimulation. The episode of status epilepticus is followed weeks later by the onset of spontaneous seizures, an intriguing parallel to the scenario of complicated febrile seizures in young children preceding the emergence of spontaneous seizures years later. In contrast to the limited or absent neuronal loss characteristic of the kindling model, overt destruction of hippocampal neurons occurs in models of status epilepticus, reflecting aspects of hippocampal sclerosis observed in humans with severe limbic seizures. Indeed, the discovery that complicated febrile seizures precede and presumably are the cause of hippocampal sclerosis in young children (VanLandingham et al., 1998) establishes yet another commonality between these preclinical models and the human condition.

Several questions arise with respect to these models. What transpires during the latent period between status epilepticus and emergence of spontaneous seizures that causes the epilepsy? Might an antiepileptogenic agent that was effective in one of these models demonstrate disease-modifying effects in other models and perhaps in patients?

Important insights into the mechanisms of action of drugs that are effective against focal seizures have emerged (Rogawski and Löscher, 2004), insights largely from electrophysiological studies of relatively simple in vitro models, such as neurons isolated from the mammalian CNS and maintained in primary culture. The experimental control and accessibility provided by these models—together with careful attention to clinically relevant concentrations of the drugs—led to clarification of their mechanisms. Although it is difficult to prove unequivocally that a given drug effect observed in vitro is both necessary and sufficient to inhibit a seizure in an animal or humans in vivo, there is an excellent likelihood that the putative mechanisms identified (Table 17–2) do in fact underlie the clinically relevant antiseizure effects. Electrophysiological analyses of individual neurons during a focal seizure demonstrate that the neurons undergo depolarization and fire action potentials at high frequencies (Figure 17–1). This pattern of neuronal firing is characteristic of a seizure and is uncommon during physiological neuronal activity. Thus, selective inhibition of this pattern of firing would be expected to reduce seizures with minimal adverse effects on neurons.

Carbamazepine, lamotrigine, phenytoin, lacosamide, and valproate inhibit high-frequency firing at concentrations known to be effective at limiting seizures in humans (Rogawski and Löscher, 2004). Inhibition of the high-frequency firing is thought to be mediated by reducing the ability of Na^+ channels to recover from inactivation (Figure 17–2). The rationale is as follows:

1. Depolarization-triggered opening of the Na^+ channels in the axonal membrane of a neuron is required for an action potential.
2. After opening, the channels spontaneously close, a process termed *inactivation.*
3. This inactivation period is thought to cause the refractory period, a short time after an action potential during which it is not possible to evoke another action potential.
4. On recovery from inactivation, the Na^+ channels are again poised to participate in another action potential.
5. Inactivation has little or no effect on low-frequency firing because firing at a slow rate permits sufficient time for Na^+ channels to recover from inactivation.
6. Reducing the rate of recovery of Na^+ channels from inactivation could limit the ability of a neuron to fire at high frequencies, an effect that likely underlies the effects of carbamazepine, lamotrigine, lacosamide, phenytoin, topiramate, valproate, and zonisamide against focal seizures.

Insights into mechanisms of seizures suggest that enhancing GABA-mediated synaptic inhibition would reduce neuronal excitability and raise the seizure threshold. Several drugs are thought to inhibit seizures by regulating GABA-mediated synaptic inhibition through an action at distinct sites of the synapse (Rogawski and Löscher, 2004). The principal postsynaptic receptor of synaptically released GABA is termed the GABA$_A$ receptor (Chapter 14). Activation of the GABA$_A$ receptor inhibits the postsynaptic cell by increasing the inflow of Cl^- ions into the cell, which tends to hyperpolarize the neuron. Clinically relevant concentrations of benzodiazepines and barbiturates enhance GABA$_A$ receptor–mediated inhibition through distinct actions on the GABA$_A$ receptor (Figure 17–3), and this enhanced inhibition probably underlies the effectiveness of these compounds against focal and tonic-clonic seizures in humans. At higher concentrations, such as might be used for status epilepticus, these drugs also can inhibit high-frequency firing of action potentials. A second mechanism of enhancing GABA-mediated synaptic inhibition is thought to underlie the antiseizure mechanism of tiagabine; tiagabine inhibits the GABA transporter GAT-1, reducing neuronal and glial uptake of GABA (Rogawski and Löscher, 2004), prolonging its dwell time in the synaptic cleft where it activates GABA$_A$ receptors. Finally, ASDs can decrease GABA metabolism GABA transaminase (i.e., valproate, vigabatrin) resulting in increased GABA concentrations (Ben-Menachem, 2011; Cai et al., 2012; Larsson et al., 1986) and increased signaling via the GABA$_A$ receptor.

Generalized-Onset Epilepsies: Absence Seizures

In contrast to focal seizures, which arise from localized regions of the brain, generalized-onset seizures arise from the reciprocal firing of the thalamus and cerebral cortex (Huguenard and McCormick, 2007). Amongst the diverse forms of generalized seizures, absence seizures have been studied most intensively. The striking synchrony in appearance of generalized seizure discharges in widespread areas of neocortex led to the idea that a structure in the thalamus or brainstem (the "centrencephalon") synchronized these seizure discharges. Focus on the thalamus emerged from the demonstration that low-frequency stimulation of midline thalamic structures triggered EEG rhythms in the cortex similar to spike-and-wave discharges characteristic of absence seizures. Intracerebral electrode recordings from humans subsequently demonstrated the presence of thalamic and neocortical involvement in the spike-and-wave discharge of absence seizures. Many of the structural and functional properties of the thalamus and neocortex that led to the generalized spike-and-wave discharges have been elucidated (Huguenard and McCormick, 2007).

TABLE 17–2 ■ PROPOSED MECHANISMS OF ACTION OF ANTISEIZURE DRUGS

MOLECULAR TARGET AND ACTIVITY	DRUG	CONSEQUENCES OF ACTION
Na⁺ channel modulators that: *Enhance fast inactivation*	PHT, CBZ, LTG, FBM, OxCBZ, TPM, VPA, ESL, RUF	• Block action potential propagation • Stabilize neuronal membranes • ↓ Neurotransmitter release, focal firing, and seizure spread
Enhance slow inactivation	LCM	• ↑ Spike frequency adaptation • ↓ Action potential bursts, focal firing, and seizure spread • Stabilize neuronal membrane
Ca²⁺ channel blockers	ESM, VPA, LTG	• ↓ Neurotransmitter release (N- and P- types) • ↓ Slow-depolarization (T-type) and spike-wave discharges
α2δ Ligands	GBP, PGB	• Modulate neurotransmitter release

GABA_A receptor allosteric modulators	BZDs, PB, FBM, PRM, TPM, CBZ, OxCBZ, STP, CLB	• ↑ Membrane hyperpolarization and seizure threshold
		• ↓ Focal firing
		  BZDs—attenuate spike-wave discharges
		  PB, CBZ, OxCBZ—aggravate spike-wave discharges

GABA uptake inhibitors/GABA-transaminase inhibitors	TGB, VGB	• ↑ Extrasynaptic GABA levels and membrane hyperpolarization • ↓ Focal firing • Aggravate spike-wave discharges
NMDA receptor antagonists	FBM	• ↓ Slow excitatory neurotransmission • ↓ Excitatory amino acid neurotoxicity • Delay epileptogenesis
AMPA/kainate receptor antagonists	PB, TPM, PER	• ↓ Fast excitatory neurotransmission and focal firing
Enhancers of HCN channel activity	LTG	• Buffers large hyperpolarizing and depolarizing inputs • Suppresses action potential initiation by dendritic inputs
Positive allosteric modulator of KCNQ2-5	**EZG**	• suppresses bursts of action potentials • hyperpolarizes membrane potentials
SV2A protein ligand	LEV, BRV	• Unknown; may decrease transmitter release
Inhibitors of brain carbonic anhydrase	ACZ, TPM, ZNS	• ↑ HCN-mediated currents • ↓ NMDA-mediated currents • ↑ GABA-mediated inhibition

ACZ, acetazolamide; BRV, brivaracetam; BZDs, benzodiazepines; CBZ, carbamazepine; CLB, clobazam; ESL, eslicarbazepine; EZG, ezogabine; FBM, felbamate; GBP, gabapentin; LEV, levetiracetam; LCM, lacosamide; LTG, lamotrigine; OxCBZ, oxcarbazepine; PER, perampanel; PB, phenobarbital; PGB, pregabalin; PHT, phenytoin; PRM, primidone; RUF, rufinamide; STP, stiripentol; TGB, tiagabine; TPM, topiramate; VGB, vigabatrin; VPA, valproate; ZNA, zonisamide.

Source: Modified with permission from Leppik IE, et al. Basic research in epilepsy and aging. *Epilepsy Res*, **2006**, *68*(suppl 1):21. Copyright © Elsevier.

The EEG hallmark of an absence seizure is generalized spike-and-wave discharges at a frequency of 3 Hz (3/s). These bilaterally synchronous spike-and-wave discharges, recorded locally from electrodes in both the thalamus and the neocortex, represent oscillations between the thalamus and neocortex. A comparison of EEG and intracellular recordings reveals that the EEG spikes are associated with the firing of action potentials and the following slow wave with prolonged inhibition. These reverberatory, low-frequency rhythms are made possible by a combination of factors, including reciprocal excitatory synaptic connections between the neocortex and thalamus as well as intrinsic properties of neurons in the thalamus (Huguenard and McCormick, 2007).

One intrinsic property of thalamic neurons that is involved in the generation of the 3-Hz spike-and-wave discharges is the low threshold ("T-type") Ca²⁺ current. T-type Ca²⁺ channels are activated at a much more negative membrane potential (hence, "low threshold") than most other voltage-gated Ca²⁺ channels expressed in the brain. T-type currents are much larger in many thalamic neurons than in neurons outside the thalamus. Indeed, bursts of action potentials in thalamic neurons are mediated by activation of the T-type currents. T-type currents amplify thalamic membrane potential oscillations, with one oscillation being the 3-Hz spike-and-wave discharge of the absence seizure. Importantly, the principal mechanism by which anti–absence seizure drugs (ethosuximide, valproate) are thought to act is by inhibition of the T-type Ca²⁺ channels (Figure 17–4) (Rogawski and Löscher, 2004). Thus, inhibiting voltage-gated ion channels is a common mechanism of action among ASDs, with anti–focal seizure drugs inhibiting voltage-activated Na⁺ channels and anti–absence seizure drugs inhibiting voltage-activated Ca²⁺ channels.

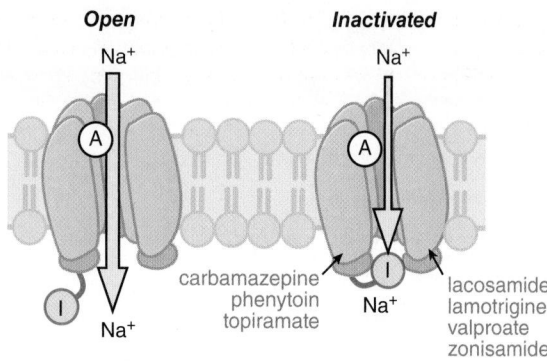

Figure 17–2 *Antiseizure drug–enhanced Na+ channel inactivation.* Some antiseizure drugs (noted in blue text) prolong the inactivation of the Na+ channels, thereby reducing the ability of neurons to fire at high frequencies. The inactivated channel itself appears to remain open but is blocked by the inactivation gate, **I**. Activation gate, **A**.

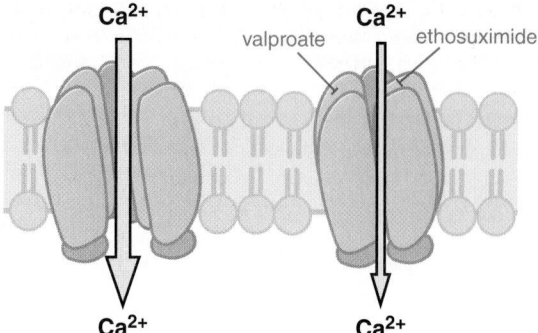

Figure 17–4 *Antiseizure drug–induced reduction of current through T-type Ca2+ channels.* Some antiseizure drugs (e.g., valproate and ethosuximide) reduce the flow of Ca^{2+} through T-type Ca^{2+} channels, thereby reducing the pacemaker current that underlies the thalamic rhythm in spikes and waves seen in generalized absence seizures.

Genetics of the Epilepsies

Genetic causes contribute to a wide diversity of human epilepsies. Genetic causes are solely responsible for rare forms inherited in an autosomal dominant or autosomal recessive manner. Genetic causes also are mainly responsible for more common forms such as Dravet syndrome, JME, or childhood absence epilepsy, the majority of which are likely due to inheritance of two or more susceptibility genes. Genetic determinants also may contribute some degree of risk to epilepsies caused by injury of the cerebral cortex.

Mutations in more than 70 genes are known to contribute to epilepsy. Not surprisingly, many of the identified epilepsy-conferring mutations

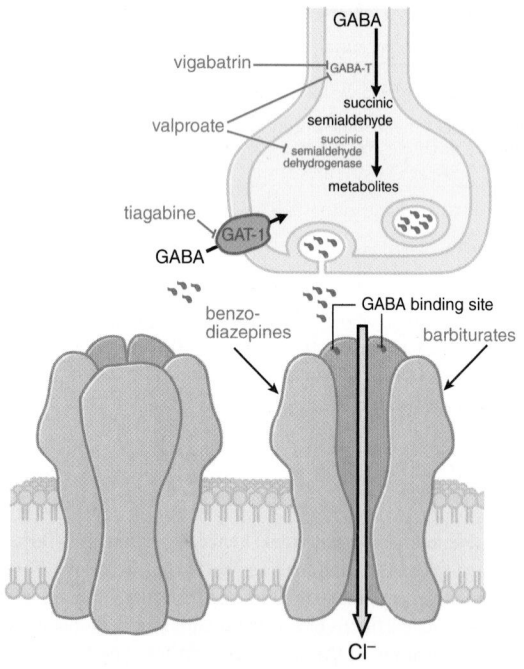

Figure 17–3 *Some antiseizure drugs enhance GABA synaptic transmission.* In the presence of GABA, the GABA$_A$ receptor (structure on bottom left) is opened, allowing an influx of Cl−, which in turn increases membrane polarization. Some ASDs (shown in blue text) act by reducing the metabolism of GABA. Others act at the GABA$_A$ receptor, enhancing Cl− influx in response to GABA or by prolonging its synaptic dwell time by inhibiting its reuptake by GAT-1. Gabapentin acts presynaptically to promote GABA release; its molecular target is currently under investigation. ↘ GABA molecules. GABA-T, GABA transaminase; GAT-1, neuronal GABA transporter (SLC6A1).

are in genes that encode voltage- or ligand-gated ion channels (Reid et al., 2009). However, mutations have also been identified in signaling pathways, transporters, and even synaptic vesicle proteins (EpiPM Consortium, 2015). Furthermore, many of the mutations arise de novo, thus complicating efforts in diagnoses. The genotype-phenotype correlations of these genetic syndromes are complex; the same mutation in one channel can be associated with divergent clinical syndromes, ranging from simple febrile seizures to intractable seizures with intellectual decline. Conversely, clinically indistinguishable epilepsy syndromes have been associated with mutation of distinct genes. The implication of genes encoding ion channels in familial epilepsy is particularly interesting because episodic disorders involving other organs also result from mutations of these genes. For example, episodic disorders of the heart (cardiac arrhythmias), skeletal muscle (periodic paralyses), cerebellum (episodic ataxia), vasculature (familial hemiplegic migraine), and other organs all have been linked to mutations in genes encoding components of voltage-gated ion channels (Ptacek and Fu, 2001).

The cellular electrophysiological consequences of these mutations can inform our understanding of the mechanisms of seizures and the actions of ASDs and allow for the determination of precise therapies for patients with specific mutations. For example, generalized epilepsy with febrile seizures is caused, in some cases, by a point mutation in the β subunit of a voltage-gated Na+ channel (*SCN1B*). Several ASDs act on Na+ channels to promote their inactivation; the phenotype of the mutated Na+ channel appears to involve defective inactivation (Wallace et al., 1998).

Spontaneous mutations in *SCN1A* (encoding the α subunit of the major voltage-gated Na+ channel in neurons) that result in truncations and presumed loss of Na+ channel function have been identified in a subset of infants with a catastrophic severe myoclonic epilepsy of infancy or Dravet syndrome. That these loss-of-function mutations in Na+ channels result in seizures is somewhat surprising. However, seizures may arise as a consequence of the cell types that express these channels within neural circuits that underlie seizure initiation. Interestingly, patients with these mutations are generally found to be refractory to ASDs that block Na+ channels.

Antiseizure Drugs: General Considerations

History of ASD Development

The first ASD was bromide, which was used in the late 19th century. Phenobarbital was the first synthetic organic agent recognized as having antiseizure activity. Its usefulness, however, was limited to generalized tonic-clonic seizures and, to a lesser degree, focal seizures. It had no effect on absence seizures. Merritt and Putnam developed the electroshock seizure test in experimental animals to screen chemical agents for antiseizure effectiveness; in the course of screening a variety of drugs, they discovered that diphenylhydantoin (later renamed phenytoin) suppressed seizures in the absence of sedative effects. The maximal electroshock seizure test is extremely valuable because drugs that are effective against the tonic hind limb extension induced by corneal electroshock generally have proven to be effective against focal and generalized tonic-clonic seizures in humans. In contrast, seizures induced by the chemoconvulsant pentylenetetrazol are most useful in the identification of ASDs that are effective against myoclonic seizures in humans. These screening tests and other phenotypically or etiologically relevant acute and chronic animal models are used in developing new ASDs.

The chemical structures of most of the drugs introduced before 1965 were closely related to phenobarbital. These included the hydantoins and the succinimides. Between 1965 and 1990, the chemically distinct structures of the benzodiazepines, an iminostilbene (carbamazepine), and a branched-chain carboxylic acid (valproate) were introduced, followed in the 1990s by a phenyltriazine (lamotrigine), a cyclic analogue of GABA (gabapentin), a sulfamate-substituted monosaccharide (topiramate), a nipecotic acid derivative (tiagabine), and a pyrrolidine derivative (levetiracetam). Since the 1970s, the National Institutes of Health has spurred development of ASDs via sponsorship of the Epilepsy Therapy Screening Program (ETSP), an ongoing partnership between government, private industry, and the University of Utah.

Therapeutic Aspects

The ideal ASD would suppress all seizures without causing any unwanted effects. Unfortunately, the drugs used currently not only fail to control seizure activity in approximately one-third of patients, but frequently cause unwanted adverse effects that range in severity from minimal impairment of the CNS to death from aplastic anemia or hepatic failure. In 2009, all manufacturers of ASDs were required by the FDA to update their product labeling to include a warning about an increased risk of suicidal thoughts or actions and to develop information targeted at helping patients understand this risk. The risk applies to all ASDs used for any indication. Details are available online at the FDA website.

The clinician who treats patients with epilepsy is faced with the task of selecting the appropriate drug or combination of drugs that best controls seizures in an individual patient at an acceptable level of untoward effects. As a general rule, complete control of seizures can be achieved in up to 50% of patients, while another 25% can be improved significantly. The degree of success varies as a function of seizure type, cause, and other factors.

To minimize toxicity, treatment with a single drug is preferred. If seizures are not controlled with the initial agent at adequate plasma concentrations, substitution of a second drug is preferred to the concurrent administration of another agent. However, multiple-drug therapy may be required, especially when two or more types of seizure occur in the same patient. With each concurrent add-on ASD, the likelihood of seizure freedom decreases (Kwan and Brodie, 2000).

Measurement of drug concentrations in plasma facilitates optimizing antiseizure medication, especially when therapy is initiated, after dosage adjustments, in the event of therapeutic failure, when toxic effects appear, or when multiple-drug therapy is instituted. However, clinical effects of some drugs do not correlate well with their concentrations in plasma, and recommended concentrations are only guidelines for therapy. *The ultimate therapeutic regimen must be determined by clinical assessment of effect and toxicity.*

The individual agents are introduced in the next sections, followed by a discussion of some general principles of the drug therapy of the epilepsies.

Hydantoins

Phenytoin

Phenytoin is effective against all types of focal and tonic-clonic seizures but not absence seizures. Oral phenytoin is indicated for the control of focal-to-bilateral tonic-clonic seizures and the prevention and treatment of seizures occurring during or following neurosurgery. Parenteral phenytoin is indicated for the control of generalized tonic-clonic status epilepticus and the treatment of seizures occurring during neurosurgery. Parenteral phenytoin should only be used when oral phenytoin administration is not possible.

Pharmacological Effects in the CNS

Phenytoin exerts antiseizure activity without causing general depression of the CNS. In toxic doses, it may produce excitatory signs and at lethal levels a type of decerebrate rigidity.

Mechanism of Action

Phenytoin limits the repetitive firing of action potentials evoked by a sustained depolarization of mouse spinal cord neurons maintained in vitro (McLean and Macdonald, 1986a). This effect is mediated by slowing of the rate of recovery of voltage-activated Na^+ channels from inactivation, an action that is both voltage (greater effect if membrane is depolarized) and use dependent. At therapeutic concentrations, the effects on Na^+ channels are selective, and no changes of spontaneous activity or responses to iontophoretically applied GABA or glutamate are detected. At concentrations 5- to 10-fold higher, multiple effects of phenytoin are evident, including reduction of spontaneous activity and enhancement of responses to GABA; these effects may underlie some of the unwanted toxicity associated with high levels of phenytoin.

ADME and Drug Interactions

Phenytoin is available in two types of oral formulations that differ in their pharmacokinetics: rapid-release and extended-release forms. Once-daily dosing is possible only with the extended-release formulations, and due to differences in dissolution and other formulation-dependent factors, the plasma phenytoin level may change when converting from one formulation to another. Confusion also can arise because different formulations can include either phenytoin or phenytoin sodium. Therefore, comparable doses can be approximated by considering "phenytoin equivalents," but serum-level monitoring is also necessary to ensure therapeutic safety. When changing routes of administration from oral to intramuscular (or vice versa), appropriate dose adjustments and blood level monitoring are recommended.

The pharmacokinetic characteristics of phenytoin are influenced markedly by its binding to serum proteins, by the nonlinearity of its elimination kinetics, and by its metabolism by hepatic CYPs (Table 17–3). Phenytoin is extensively bound (~90%) to serum proteins, mainly albumin. Small variations in the percentage of phenytoin that is bound dramatically affect the absolute amount of free (active) drug. Some agents can compete with phenytoin for binding sites on plasma proteins and increase free phenytoin at the time the new drug is added to the regimen. However, the effect on free phenytoin is only short-lived and usually does not cause clinical complications unless inhibition of phenytoin metabolism also occurs. For example, valproate competes for protein-binding sites and inhibits phenytoin metabolism, resulting in marked and sustained increases in free phenytoin. Measurement of free rather than total phenytoin permits direct assessment of this potential problem in patient management.

The rate of elimination of phenytoin varies as a function of its concentration (i.e., the rate is nonlinear). The plasma $t_{1/2}$ of phenytoin ranges between 6 and 24 h at plasma concentrations below 10 μg/mL. At low blood levels, metabolism follows first-order kinetics; as blood levels rise, the maximal limit of the liver to metabolize phenytoin is approached, and C_p increases disproportionately as dosage is increased, even with small adjustments for levels near the therapeutic range.

The majority (95%) of phenytoin is metabolized by CYP2C9 and to a lesser extent by CYP2C19 (Table 17–3). The principal metabolite, a parahydroxyphenyl derivative, is inactive. Because its metabolism is saturable, other drugs that are metabolized by these CYP enzymes can inhibit the metabolism of phenytoin and increase its plasma concentration. Conversely, the degradation rate of other drugs that serve as substrates for these enzymes can be inhibited by phenytoin; one such drug is warfarin, and addition of phenytoin to a patient receiving warfarin can lead to bleeding disorders (Chapter 32).

TABLE 17–3 ■ INTERACTIONS OF ANTI-SEIZURE DRUGS WITH HEPATIC MICROSOMAL ENZYMES

DRUG	INDUCES		INHIBITS		METABOLIZED BY	
	CYP	UGT	CYP	UGT	CYP	UGT
Brivaracatam	No	No	No	No	2C19/2C9	No
Carbamazepine	1A2/2C9/ 3A4	Yes	No	No	1A2/2C8/3A4	No
Clobazam	No	No	No	No	3A4	No
Clonazepam	No	No	No	No	3A4	No
Eslicarbazepine	3A4	No	No	No	No	Yes
Ethosuximide	No	No	No	No	3A4	No
Ezogabine	No	No	No	No	No	Yes
Felbamate	3A4	No	2C19	No	3A4/2E1	?
Gabapentin	No	No	No	No	No	No
Lacosamide	No	No	No	No	2C19	?
Lamotrigine	No	No	No	No	No	UGT1A4
Levetiracetam	No	No	No	No	No	No
Oxcarbazepine	3A4/5	UGT1A4	2C19	Weak	No	Yes
Perampanel	No	No	Weak	Weak	3A4/3A5	Yes
Phenobarbital	2C9/3A4/ 1A2	Yes	No	No	2C9/19/2E1	Yes
Phenytoin	2C9/3A4/ 1A2	Yes	2C9	No	2C9/19	No
Pregabalin	No	No	No	No	No	No
Primidone	2C/3A	Yes	Yes	No	2C9/19	No
Rufinamide	3A4 (weak)	No	2E1 (weak)	No	No	No
Stiripentol	No	No	1A2/3A4/ 2C19/2D6	No	No	No
Tiagabine	No	No	No	No	3A4	No
Topiramate	3A4 (>200 mg/day)	No	2C19	No	Yes	No
Valproate	No	No	2C9/3A4?	Yes	2C9/2C19/2A6/2B6	UGT1A3/2B7
Vigabatrin	No	No	No	No	No	No
Zonisamide	No	No	No	No	3A4	No

CYP, cytochrome P450; UGT, uridine diphosphate-glucuronosyltransferase. (Data modified from Johannessen and Johannessen, 2010 and Wheles and Vasquez, 2010, *Epilepsy Currents*, 10:1–6 and Cawello, 2015, *Clin Pharmacokinetic*, 54: 904–914.)

An alternative mechanism of drug interactions arises from phenytoin's ability to induce various CYPs (see discussion that follows and Chapter 6). Of particular note in this regard are oral contraceptives, which are metabolized by CYP3A4; treatment with phenytoin can enhance the metabolism of oral contraceptives and lead to unplanned pregnancy. The potential teratogenic effects of phenytoin underscore the importance of attention to this interaction. Carbamazepine, oxcarbazepine, phenobarbital, and primidone also induce CYP3A4 and likewise might increase degradation of oral contraceptives.

Concurrent administration of any drug metabolized by CYP2C9 can increase the plasma concentration of phenytoin by decreasing its rate of metabolism (Table 17–3). Conversely, the degradation rate of other drugs that are substrates for these enzymes can be inhibited by phenytoin. Carbamazepine, which may enhance the metabolism of phenytoin, causes a well-documented *decrease* in phenytoin concentration. Phenytoin can also induce expression of a number of different CYPs, leading to increased degradation of coadministered drugs, such as oral contraceptives. Conversely, phenytoin reduces the concentration of carbamazepine.

The low water solubility of phenytoin hindered its intravenous use and led to production of fosphenytoin, a water-soluble prodrug. Fosphenytoin is converted into phenytoin by phosphatases in liver and red blood cells with a $t_{1/2}$ of 8–15 min. Fosphenytoin is extensively bound (95%–99%) to human plasma proteins, primarily albumin. This binding is saturable and fosphenytoin displaces phenytoin from protein-binding sites. Fosphenytoin is useful for adults with focal or generalized seizures when either intravenous or intramuscular route of administration is indicated.

Adverse Effects and Toxicity

The toxic effects of phenytoin depend on the route of administration, the duration of exposure, and the dosage. When fosphenytoin, the water-soluble prodrug, is administered intravenously at an excessive rate in the emergency treatment of status epilepticus, the most notable toxic signs are cardiac arrhythmias with or without hypotension and CNS depression. Although cardiac toxicity occurs more frequently in older patients and in those with known cardiac disease, it also can develop in young, healthy patients. Because of the risk of adverse cardiovascular reactions with rapid administration, IV administartion should not exceed 50 mg per minute in adults. In pediatric patients, the drug should be administered at a rate not exceeding 1–3 mg/kg/min or 50 mg/min, whichever is slower. Acute oral overdosage results primarily in signs referable to the cerebellum and vestibular system; high doses have been associated with marked cerebellar atrophy.

Toxic effects associated with chronic treatment also are primarily dose-related cerebellar-vestibular effects but also include other CNS effects, behavioral changes, increased frequency of seizures, GI symptoms, gingival hyperplasia, osteomalacia, and megaloblastic anemia. Hirsutism is an annoying untoward effect in young females. Usually, these phenomena can be diminished by proper adjustment of dosage. Serious adverse effects, including those on the skin, bone marrow, and liver, probably are manifestations of drug allergy. Although rare, they necessitate withdrawal of the drug. Moderate transient elevation of the plasma concentrations of hepatic transaminases sometimes can also occur.

Gingival hyperplasia occurs in about 20% of all patients during chronic administration and can be minimized by good oral hygiene. Related to this, phenytoin can also produce coarsening of facial features. Inhibition of release of ADH has been observed. Hyperglycemia and glycosuria appear to be due to inhibition of insulin secretion. Osteomalacia, with hypocalcemia and elevated alkaline phosphatase activity, has been attributed to both altered metabolism of vitamin D and the attendant inhibition of intestinal absorption of Ca^{2+}. Phenytoin also increases the metabolism of vitamin K and reduces the concentration of vitamin K–dependent proteins that are important for normal Ca^{2+} metabolism in bone. This may explain why the osteomalacia is not always ameliorated by the administration of vitamin D.

Hypersensitivity reactions include morbilliform rash in 2%–5% of patients and occasionally more serious skin reactions, including Stevens-Johnson syndrome and toxic epidermal necrolysis. Drug-induced systemic lupus erythematosus; potentially fatal hepatic necrosis; hematological reactions, including neutropenia and leukopenia; red cell aplasia; agranulocytosis; and mild thrombocytopenia also have been reported. Hypoprothrombinemia and hemorrhage have occurred in the newborns of mothers who received phenytoin during pregnancy; vitamin K is effective treatment or prophylaxis.

Plasma Drug Concentrations

A good correlation usually is observed between the total concentration of phenytoin in plasma and its clinical effect. Thus, control of seizures generally is obtained with total concentrations above 10 µg/mL, while toxic effects such as nystagmus develop at total concentrations around 20 µg/mL. Control of seizures generally is obtained with free phenytoin concentrations of 0.75–1.25 µg/mL.

Therapeutic Uses

Epilepsy. Phenytoin is one of the more widely used ASDs; it is effective against focal and generalized tonic-clonic, focal-to-bilateral tonic-clonic, tonic-clonic of unknown onset (tonic-clonic), but not generalized absence seizures. The use of phenytoin and other agents in the therapy of epilepsies is discussed further at the end of this chapter. Phenytoin preparations differ significantly in bioavailability and rate of absorption. In general, patients should consistently be treated with the same drug from a single manufacturer. However, if it becomes necessary to temporarily switch between products, care should be taken to select a therapeutically equivalent product, and patients should be monitored for loss of seizure control or onset of new toxicities.

Other Uses. Trigeminal and related neuralgias occasionally respond to phenytoin, but carbamazepine may be preferable. The use of phenytoin in the treatment of cardiac arrhythmias is discussed in Chapter 30.

Benzodiazepines

The benzodiazepines are used primarily as sedative-antianxiety drugs; their pharmacology is described in Chapters 15 and 19. Discussion here is limited to their use in the therapy of the epilepsies. A large number of benzodiazepines have broad antiseizure properties. Clonazepam is FDA-approved alone or as an adjunctive treatment of Lennox-Gestaut syndrome, akinetic, and myoclonic seizures. It may also benefit patients with absence seizures which are inadequately responding to succinimides. Clorazepate is approved as an adjunct therapy for the management of focal seizures. Midazolam was designated an orphan drug in 2006 for intermittent treatment of bouts of increased seizure

activity in refractory patients with epilepsy who are on stable regimens of ASDs. More recently, midazolam was granted orphan drug designation in 2009 as a rescue treatment of seizures in patients who require control of intermittent bouts of increased seizure activity (i.e., acute repetitive seizure clusters), in 2012 for the treatment of nerve agent-induced seizures, and in 2016 for the treatment of status epilepticus and seizures induced by organophosporous poisoning. Diazepam and lorazepam have well-defined roles in the management of status epilepticus. Unlike other marketed 1,4-benzodiazepines, clobazam is a 1,5-benzodiazepine that is less lipophilic and less acidic and may be better tolerated than traditional 1,4-benzodiazepines (see benzodiazepine structure in Chapter 19). Clobazam is used in a variety of seizure phenotypes and is approved in the U.S. for the treatment of Lennox-Gastaut syndrome in patients aged 2 years or older.

Antiseizure Properties

In animal models, inhibition of pentylenetetrazol-induced seizures by the benzodiazepines is much more prominent than is their modification of the maximal electroshock seizure pattern. Clonazepam is unusually potent in antagonizing the effects of pentylenetetrazol, but it is almost without action on seizures induced by maximal electroshock. Benzodiazepines, including clonazepam, suppress the spread of kindled seizures and generalized seizures produced by stimulation of the amygdala, but do not abolish the abnormal discharge at the site of stimulation.

Mechanism of Action

The antiseizure actions of the benzodiazepines result in large part from their capacity to enhance GABA-mediated synaptic inhibition. Molecular cloning and study of recombinant receptors have demonstrated that the benzodiazepine receptor is an integral part of the $GABA_A$ receptor (see Figures 14–11 and 17–3). At therapeutically relevant concentrations, benzodiazepines act at subsets of $GABA_A$ receptors and increase the frequency, but not duration, of openings at GABA-activated Cl^- channels (Twyman et al., 1989). At higher concentrations, diazepam and many other benzodiazepines can reduce sustained high-frequency firing of neurons, similar to the effects of phenytoin, carbamazepine, and valproate. Although these concentrations correspond to concentrations achieved in patients during treatment of status epilepticus with diazepam, they are considerably higher than those associated with antiseizure or anxiolytic effects in ambulatory patients. Clobazam potentiates GABA-mediated neurotransmission in the same fashion as other benzodiazepines at $GABA_A$ receptors.

ADME

Benzodiazepines are well absorbed after oral administration, and concentrations in plasma are usually maximal within 1–4 h. After intravenous administration, they redistribute in a manner typical of that for highly lipid-soluble agents. Central effects develop promptly, but wane rapidly as the drugs move to other tissues. Diazepam is redistributed especially rapidly, with a $t_{1/2}$ of redistribution of about 1 h. The extent of binding of benzodiazepines to plasma proteins correlates with lipid solubility, ranging from about 99% for diazepam to about 85% for clonazepam.

Table 19–1 shows the scheme for metabolism of benzodiazepines, the major metabolite of diazepam, N-desmethyl-diazepam, is somewhat less active than the parent drug and may behave as a partial agonist. This metabolite also is produced by the rapid decarboxylation of clorazepate following its ingestion. Both diazepam and N-desmethyl-diazepam are slowly hydroxylated to other active metabolites, such as oxazepam. The $t_{1/2}$ of diazepam in plasma is ~43 h (see Table 19–2); that of N-desmethyl-diazepam is about 60 h. Clonazepam is metabolized principally by reduction of the nitro group to produce inactive 7-amino derivatives. Less than 1% of the drug is recovered unchanged in the urine. The $t_{1/2}$ of clonazepam in plasma is about 23 h. Lorazepam is metabolized chiefly by conjugation with glucuronic acid; its $t_{1/2}$ in plasma is about 14 h. Clobazam has a $t_{1/2}$ of 18 h and is effective at doses between 0.5 and 1 mg/kg daily, with limited development of tolerance. The active metabolite of clobazam is norclobazam.

Plasma Drug Concentrations

Because tolerance affects the relationship between drug concentration and drug antiseizure effect, plasma concentrations of benzodiazepines are of limited value.

Therapeutic Uses

Clonazepam is useful in the therapy of absence seizures as well as myoclonic seizures in children. However, tolerance to its antiseizure effects usually develops after 1–6 months of administration, after which some patients will no longer respond to clonazepam at any dosage. The initial dose of clonazepam for adults should not exceed 1.5 mg per day and for children 0.01–0.03 mg/kg per day. The dose-dependent side effects are reduced if two or three divided doses are given each day. The dose may be increased every 3 days in amounts of 0.25–0.5 mg per day in children and 0.5–1 mg per day in adults. The maximal recommended dose is 20 mg per day for adults and 0.2 mg/kg per day for children. Clonazepam intranasal spray is designated as an orphan drug for recurrent acute repetitive seizures.

While diazepam is an effective agent for treatment of status epilepticus, the effective duration of action of this lipid soluble agent is shortened by its rapid redistribution. Thus, lorazepam is more frequently used; it is less lipid soluble, is more effectively confined to the vascular compartment, and has a longer effective half-life after a single dose. Diazepam is not useful as an oral agent for the treatment of seizure disorders. Clorazepate is effective in combination with certain other drugs in the treatment of focal seizures. The maximal initial dose of clorazepate is 22.5 mg/d in three portions for adults and children older than 12 years and 15 mg/d in two divided doses in children 9–12 years of age. Clorazepate is not recommended for children under the age of 9. Clobazam is used in a variety of seizure phenotypes and is FDA-approved for the treatment of Lennox-Gastaut syndrome in patients aged 2 years or older. In patients weighing more than 30 kg, clobazam is initiated orally at 5 mg every 12 h and then titrated up to a maximum of 40 mg/d if tolerated. Dose escalation must be done gradually, not exceeding more than once per week.

Adverse Effects

The principal side effects of long-term oral therapy with clonazepam are drowsiness and lethargy. According to FDA-approved labeling, up to 30% of patients show a loss of anticonvulsant activity with continued administration of clonazepam, often within 3 months. In some cases, dose adjustment may reestablish efficacy. Muscular incoordination and ataxia are less frequent. Although these symptoms usually can be kept to tolerable levels by reducing the dosage or the rate at which it is increased, they sometimes force drug discontinuation.

Other side effects include hypotonia, dysarthria, and dizziness. Behavioral disturbances, especially in children, can be troublesome; these include aggression, hyperactivity, irritability, and difficulty in concentration. Both anorexia and hyperphagia have been reported. Increased salivary and bronchial secretions may cause difficulties in children. Seizures are sometimes exacerbated, and status epilepticus may be precipitated if the drug is discontinued abruptly. Other aspects of the toxicity of the benzodiazepines are discussed in Chapter 19. Cardiovascular and respiratory depression may occur after the intravenous administration of diazepam, clonazepam, or lorazepam, particularly if other ASDs or central depressants have been administered previously.

Antiseizure Barbiturates

While most barbiturates have antiseizure properties, only some barbiturates, such as phenobarbital, exert maximal antiseizure effects at doses below those that cause hypnosis. This therapeutic index determines a barbiturate's clinical utility as an antiseizure therapeutic drug. The pharmacology of the barbiturates as a class is described in Chapter 19; discussion in this chapter is limited to phenobarbital and primidone.

Phenobarbital

Phenobarbital was the first effective organic antiseizure agent. It has relatively low toxicity, is inexpensive, and is still one of the more effective and widely used antiseizure drugs.

Mechanism of Action

The mechanism by which phenobarbital inhibits seizures likely involves potentiation of synaptic inhibition through an action on the $GABA_A$ receptor. Phenobarbital enhances responses to iontophoretically applied GABA in mouse cortical and spinal neurons, effects that are observed at therapeutically relevant concentrations of phenobarbital; in patch-clamp studies, phenobarbital increases the $GABA_A$ receptor–mediated current by increasing the duration of bursts of $GABA_A$ receptor–mediated currents without changing the frequency of bursts (Twyman et al., 1989). At levels exceeding therapeutic concentrations, phenobarbital also limits sustained repetitive firing; this may underlie some of the antiseizure effects of higher concentrations of phenobarbital achieved during therapy of status epilepticus.

ADME

Oral absorption of phenobarbital is complete but somewhat slow; peak concentrations in plasma occur several hours after a single dose. It is 40%–60% bound to plasma proteins and bound to a similar extent in tissues, including brain. Up to 25% of a dose is eliminated by pH-dependent renal excretion of the unchanged drug; the remainder is inactivated by hepatic microsomal enzymes, principally CYP2C9, with minor metabolism by CYP2C19 and CYP2E1. Phenobarbital induces UGT enzymes as well as the CYP2C and CYP3A subfamilies. Drugs metabolized by these enzymes can be more rapidly degraded when coadministered with phenobarbital; importantly, oral contraceptives are metabolized by CYP3A4. The terminal $t_{1/2}$ of phenobarbital varies widely, 50–140 h in adults and 40–70 h in children younger than 5 years of age, often longer in neonates. Phenobarbital's duration of effect usually exceeds 6–12 h in nontolerant patients.

Plasma Drug Concentrations

During long-term therapy in adults, the plasma concentration of phenobarbital averages 10 μg/mL per daily dose of 1 mg/kg; in children, the value is 5–7 μg/mL per 1 mg/kg. Although a precise relationship between therapeutic results and concentration of drug in plasma does not exist, plasma concentrations of 10–35 μg/mL are usually recommended for control of seizures. The relationship between plasma concentration of phenobarbital and adverse effects varies with the development of tolerance. Sedation, nystagmus, and ataxia usually are absent at concentrations below 30 μg/mL during long-term therapy, but adverse effects may be apparent for several days at lower concentrations when therapy is initiated or whenever the dosage is increased. Concentrations more than 60 μg/mL may be associated with marked intoxication in the nontolerant individual. Because significant behavioral toxicity may be present despite the absence of overt signs of toxicity, the tendency to maintain patients, particularly children, on excessively high doses of phenobarbital should be resisted. The plasma phenobarbital concentration should be increased above 30–40 μg/mL only if the increment is adequately tolerated and only if it contributes significantly to control of seizures.

Therapeutic Uses

Phenobarbital is an effective agent for generalized tonic-clonic, focal-to-bilateral tonic-clonic, tonic-clonic of unknown onset (generalized tonic-clonic), and focal seizures. Its efficacy, low toxicity, and low cost make it an important agent for these types of epilepsy. However, its sedative effects and its tendency to disturb behavior in children have reduced its use as a primary agent. It is not effective for absence seizures.

Adverse Effects, Drug Interactions, and Toxicity

Sedation, the most frequent undesired effect of phenobarbital, is apparent to some extent in all patients on initiation of therapy, but tolerance develops during chronic medication. Nystagmus and ataxia occur at excessive dosage. Phenobarbital can produce irritability and hyperactivity in children and agitation and confusion in the elderly. Scarlatiniform or morbilliform rash, possibly with other manifestations of drug allergy, occurs in 1%–2% of patients. Exfoliative dermatitis is rare. Hypoprothrombinemia with hemorrhage has been observed in the newborns of mothers who have received phenobarbital during pregnancy; vitamin K is effective for treatment or prophylaxis. As with phenytoin, megaloblastic anemia that responds to folate and osteomalacia that responds to high doses of vitamin D occur during chronic phenobarbital therapy of epilepsy. Other adverse effects of phenobarbital are discussed in Chapter 19.

Interactions between phenobarbital and other drugs usually involve induction of the hepatic CYPs by phenobarbital. The interaction between phenytoin and phenobarbital is variable. Concentrations of phenobarbital in plasma may be elevated by as much as 40% during concurrent administration of valproate.

Primidone

Although primidone is indicated in the U.S. for patients with focal or generalized epilepsy, it has largely been replaced by carbamazepine and other newer ASDs that possess lower incidence of sedation.

Mechanism of Action

The exact mechanism of primidone's antiseizure effects is not fully understood. It is metabolized to two active metabolites: phenobarbital and phenylethylmalonamide (PEMA). Primidone and its two metabolites each have antiseizure effects on focal and generalized tonic-clonic seizures.

ADME

Primidone is completely absorbed and generally reaches peak plasma concentration within about 3 h of oral administration. Primidone is 30% protein bound in plasma and is rapidly metabolized to both phenobarbital and PEMA. Both primidone and phenobarbital undergo extensive conjugation prior to excretion. Primidone's $t_{1/2}$ is about 6–8 h. In contrast, the terminal $t_{1/2}$ of phenobarbital varies with age, with values ranging in adults from 50 to 140 h and in children less than 5 years of age from 40 to 70 h. Because of both slow accumulation and clearance, phenobarbital reaches therapeutic concentrations approximately two to three times higher than that of primidone. In fact, care should be taken and plasma closely monitored during titration of primidone doses because primidone may reach steady-state levels rapidly (1–2 days), whereas the metabolites phenobarbital and PEMA each attain steady state more slowly (20 days and 3–4 days, respectively).

Therapeutic Uses

Doses of 10–20 mg/kg/d reach clinically relevant steady-state plasma concentrations (8–12 µg/mL), although interpatient variability is common. In addition to its early use in patients with focal-onset or generalized epilepsy, primidone is still considered to be a first-line therapy for essential tremor with the β blocker propranolol.

Adverse Effects

The dose-dependent adverse effects of primidone are similar to those of phenobarbital, except that pronounced drowsiness is observed early after primidone administration. Common adverse effects include ataxia and vertigo, both of which diminish and may disappear with continued therapy. Primidone is contraindicated in patients with either porphyria or hypersensitivity to phenobarbital.

Iminostilbenes

Carbamazepine

Carbamazepine is considered to be a primary drug for the treatment of generalized tonic-clonic, focal-to-bilateral tonic-clonic, tonic-clonic of unknown onset (generalized tonic-clonic), and focal seizures. It is also used for the treatment of trigeminal neuralgia.

Carbamazepine is related chemically to the tricyclic antidepressants. It is a derivative of iminostilbene with a carbamyl group at the 5 position; this moiety is essential for potent antiseizure activity.

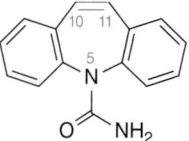

CARBAMAZEPINE

Mechanism of Action

Like phenytoin, carbamazepine limits the repetitive firing of action potentials evoked by a sustained depolarization of mouse spinal cord or cortical neurons maintained in vitro (McLean and Macdonald, 1986a). This appears to be mediated by slowing of the rate of recovery of voltage-activated Na+ channels from inactivation. These effects of carbamazepine are evident at concentrations in the range of therapeutic drug levels in CSF in humans and are relatively selective, producing no effects on spontaneous activity or on responses to iontophoretically applied GABA or glutamate. The carbamazepine metabolite 10,11-epoxycarbamazepine also limits sustained repetitive firing at therapeutically relevant concentrations, suggesting that this metabolite may contribute to the antiseizure efficacy of carbamazepine.

ADME

The pharmacokinetics of carbamazepine are complex. They are influenced by its limited aqueous solubility and by the capacity of many ASDs, including carbamazepine itself, to increase conversion to active metabolites by hepatic enzymes (Table 17–3). Carbamazepine is absorbed slowly and erratically after oral administration. Peak concentrations in plasma usually are observed 4–8 h after oral ingestion, but may be delayed by as much as 24 h, especially following the administration of a large dose. Once absorbed, the drug distributes rapidly into all tissues. Approximately 75% of carbamazepine binds to plasma proteins; concentrations in the CSF appear to correspond to the concentration of free drug in plasma. The predominant pathway of metabolism in humans involves conversion to the 10,11-epoxide, a metabolite as active as the parent compound; its concentrations in plasma and brain may reach 50% of those of carbamazepine, especially during the concurrent administration of phenytoin or phenobarbital. The 10,11-epoxide is metabolized further to inactive compounds that are excreted in the urine principally as glucuronides. Carbamazepine also is inactivated by conjugation and hydroxylation. Hepatic CYP3A4 is primarily responsible for the agent's biotransformation. Carbamazepine induces CYP2C, CYP3A, and UGT, thus enhancing the metabolism of drugs degraded by these enzymes. Of particular importance in this regard are oral contraceptives, which are also metabolized by CYP3A4.

Plasma Drug Concentrations

There is no simple relationship between the dose of carbamazepine and concentrations of the drug in plasma. Therapeutic concentrations are reported to be 6–12 µg/mL, although considerable variation occurs. Side effects referable to the CNS are frequent at concentrations above 9 µg/mL.

Therapeutic Uses

Carbamazepine is useful in patients with generalized tonic-clonic and both focal aware and focal with impaired awareness seizures (Table 17–1). When it is used, renal and hepatic function and hematological parameters should be monitored. The therapeutic use of carbamazepine is discussed further at the end of this chapter.

Carbamazepine can produce therapeutic responses in patients with bipolar disorder, including some for whom lithium carbonate is not effective. Further, carbamazepine has antidiuretic effects that are sometimes associated with increased concentrations of antidiuretic hormone (ADH) in plasma via mechanisms that are not clearly understood.

Carbamazepine is the primary agent for treatment of trigeminal and glossopharyngeal neuralgias. It is also effective for lightning-type ("tabetic") pain associated with bodily wasting. Carbamazepine is also used in the treatment of bipolar affective disorders, as discussed further in Chapter 16.

Adverse Effects, Drug Interactions, and Toxicity

Acute intoxication with carbamazepine can result in stupor or coma, hyperirritability, convulsions, and respiratory depression. During long-term therapy, the more frequent untoward effects of the drug include drowsiness, vertigo, ataxia, diplopia, and blurred vision. The frequency of seizures may increase, especially with overdose. Other adverse effects include nausea; vomiting; serious hematological toxicity (aplastic anemia, agranulocytosis); and hypersensitivity reactions (dangerous skin reactions, eosinophilia, lymphadenopathy, splenomegaly). A late complication of therapy with carbamazepine is retention of water, with decreased osmolality and concentration of Na^+ in plasma, especially in elderly patients with cardiac disease.

Some tolerance develops to the neurotoxic effects of carbamazepine, and they can be minimized by gradual increase in dosage or adjustment of maintenance dosage. Various hepatic or pancreatic abnormalities have been reported during therapy with carbamazepine, most commonly a transient elevation of hepatic transaminases in plasma in 5%–10% of patients. A transient, mild leukopenia occurs in about 10% of patients during initiation of therapy and usually resolves within the first 4 months of continued treatment; transient thrombocytopenia also has been noted. In about 2% of patients, a persistent leukopenia may develop that requires withdrawal of the drug. The initial concern that aplastic anemia might be a frequent complication of long-term therapy with carbamazepine has not materialized. In most cases, the administration of multiple drugs or the presence of another underlying disease has made it difficult to establish a causal relationship. The prevalence of aplastic anemia appears to be about 1 in 200,000 patients. It is not clear whether monitoring of hematological function can help to avert the development of irreversible aplastic anemia. Carbamazepine is not known to be carcinogenic in humans. Possible teratogenic effects are discussed later in the chapter.

Phenobarbital, phenytoin, and valproate may increase the metabolism of carbamazepine by inducing CYP3A4; carbamazepine may enhance the biotransformation of phenytoin. Concurrent administration of carbamazepine may lower concentrations of valproate, lamotrigine, tiagabine, and topiramate. Carbamazepine reduces both the plasma concentration and the therapeutic effect of haloperidol. The metabolism of carbamazepine may be inhibited by propoxyphene, erythromycin, cimetidine, fluoxetine, and isoniazid.

Oxcarbazepine

Oxcarbazepine is FDA-approved for monotherapy or adjunct therapy for focal seizures in adults, as monotherapy for focal seizures in children ages 4–16, and as adjunctive therapy in children aged 2–16 years. Oxcarbazepine (10,11-dihydro-10-oxocarbamazepine) is a keto analogue of carbamazepine and is a prodrug that is rapidly converted to its metabolite, eslicarbazepine. Eslicarbazepine is then extensively converted to its S(+) enantiomer, the active metabolite S-licarbazepine. Oxcarbazepine is inactivated by glucuronide conjugation, is eliminated by renal excretion, and has a short $t_{1/2}$ of only about 1–2 h.

Oxcarbazepine has a mechanism of action similar to that of carbamazepine but is a less-potent enzyme inducer than carbamazepine. Substitution of oxcarbazepine for carbamazepine is associated with increased levels of phenytoin and valproate, presumably because of reduced induction of hepatic enzymes. Oxcarbazepine does not induce the hepatic enzymes involved in its own degradation. Although oxcarbazepine does not appear to reduce the anticoagulant effect of warfarin, it does induce CYP3A and thus reduces plasma levels of steroid oral contraceptives. Fewer hypersensitivity reactions have been associated with oxcarbazepine, and cross-reactivity with carbamazepine does not always occur. Although most adverse effects are similar to that with carbamazepine, hyponatremia may occur more commonly with oxcarbazepine than with carbamazepine.

Eslicarbazepine Acetate

Eslicarbazepine acetate is a prodrug approved in the U.S. as a monotherapy and adjunctive treatment of focal-onset seizures. Eslicarbazepine is converted to its active metabolite S-licarbazepine faster than its prodrug,

oxcarbazepine; eslicarbazepine has a similar mechanism of action as oxcarbazepine because both are prodrugs that produce the same active metabolite, S-licarbazepine. Eslicarbazepine competitively inhibits fast voltage-gated sodium channels, stabilizing the inactivated state and the sodium-dependent release of neurotransmitters. Eslicarbazepine has a $t_{1/2}$ similar to that of carbamazepine, about 8–12 h, after which it is excreted as a glucuronide. Eslicarbazepine acetate in adults may be initiated at 400–1200 mg/d. Higher doses require careful titration based on patient response. Reduction in dosing is necessary in patients with renal impairment.

Succinimides

Ethosuximide

Ethosuximide is a primary agent for the treatment of generalized absence seizures.

Mechanism of Action

Ethosuximide reduces low threshold T-type Ca^{2+} currents in thalamic neurons (Coulter et al., 1989), and inhibition of T-type currents likely is the mechanism by which ethosuximide inhibits absence seizures. The thalamus plays an important role in generation of 3-Hz spike-and-wave rhythms typical of absence seizures (Huguenard and McCormick, 2007). Neurons in the thalamus exhibit large-amplitude T-type currents that underlie bursts of action potentials and likely play an important role in thalamic oscillatory activity, such as 3-Hz spike-and-wave activity. Ethosuximide reduces this current without modifying the voltage dependence of steady-state inactivation or the time course of recovery from inactivation. Ethosuximide does not inhibit sustained repetitive firing or enhance GABA responses at clinically relevant concentrations.

ADME

Absorption of ethosuximide appears to be complete, with peak C_p occurring within about 3 h after a single oral dose. Ethosuximide is not significantly bound to plasma proteins; during long-term therapy, its concentration in the CSF is similar to that in plasma. The apparent volume of distribution averages 0.7 L/kg.

Approximately 25% of the drug is excreted unchanged in the urine. The remainder is metabolized by hepatic microsomal enzymes, but whether CYPs are responsible is unknown. The major metabolite, the hydroxyethyl derivative, accounts for about 40% of ethosuximide metabolism, is inactive, and is excreted as such and as the glucuronide in the urine. The plasma $t_{1/2}$ of ethosuximide averages between 40 and 50 h in adults and about 30 h in children.

Plasma Drug Concentrations

During long-term therapy, the plasma concentration of ethosuximide averages about 2 µg/mL per daily dose of 1 mg/kg. A plasma concentration of 40–100 µg/mL usually is required for satisfactory control of absence seizures.

Therapeutic Uses

Ethosuximide is effective against absence seizures, but not tonic-clonic seizures. An initial daily dose of 250 mg in children (3–6 years old) and 500 mg in older children, and adult dosage is increased by 250-mg increments at weekly intervals until seizures are adequately controlled or toxicity intervenes. Divided dosage is required occasionally to prevent nausea or drowsiness associated with once-daily dosing. The usual maintenance dose is 20 mg/kg/d. Increased caution is required if the daily dose exceeds 1500 mg in adults or 750–1000 mg in children. The therapeutic use of ethosuximide is discussed further at the end of the chapter.

Adverse Effects and Toxicity

The most common dose-related side effects are GI complaints (nausea, vomiting, and anorexia) and CNS effects (drowsiness, lethargy, euphoria, dizziness, headache, and hiccough). Some tolerance to these effects develops. Parkinson-like symptoms and photophobia have been reported.

Restlessness, agitation, anxiety, aggressiveness, inability to concentrate, and other behavioral effects have occurred primarily in patients with a prior history of psychiatric disturbance.

Urticaria and other skin reactions, including Stevens-Johnson syndrome, systemic lupus erythematosus, eosinophilia, leukopenia, thrombocytopenia, pancytopenia, and aplastic anemia, also have been attributed to the drug. The leukopenia may be transient despite continuation of the drug, but several deaths have resulted from bone marrow depression. Renal and hepatic toxicity have not been reported.

Other Antiseizure Drugs

Acetazolamide

Acetazolamide, the prototype for the carbonic anhydrase inhibitors, is discussed in Chapter 25. Its antiseizure actions have been discussed in previous editions of this textbook. Although it is sometimes effective against absence seizures, its usefulness is limited by the rapid development of tolerance. Adverse effects are minimal when it is used in moderate dosage for limited periods.

Ezogabine

Mechanisms of Action

Ezogabine is a first-in-class K^+ channel opener, known as retigabine in the E.U. Ezogabine enhances transmembrane K^+ currents mediated by the KCNQ family of ion channels (i.e., Kv7.2–Kv7.5). Through its activation of the KCNQ channels, ezogabine may stabilize the resting membrane potential and reduce neuronal excitability. In vitro studies suggested that ezogabine may also enhance GABA-mediated currents.

ADME

Dosing in adults is typically initiated at 300 mg per day and gradually titrated to 600–1200 mg/d over several weeks. Ezogabine is rapidly absorbed after oral administration, and absorption is not affected by food. Ezogabine is approximately 80% protein bound in plasma. Ezogabine is metabolized by glucuronidation and acetylation and has a $t_{1/2}$ of 7–11 h; it and its metabolites are excreted in the urine. Thus, ezogabine generally requires dosing thrice daily. Concomitant administration of phenytoin or carbamazepine may reduce plasma concentrations of ezogabine; consequently, an increase in ezogabine dosage should be considered when adding phenytoin or carbamazepine.

Therapeutic Use

Ezogabine was approved in the U.S. as adjunctive treatment of focal-onset seizures in patients aged 18 years and older with inadequate response to alternative ASDs and for whom the benefits outweigh the risk of retinal abnormalities and potential visual acuity deficits. However, the FDA issued a warning for ezogabine citing safety concerns, including blue discoloration and retinal abnormalities. In response, the manufacturer announced that production of ezogabine would cease in June, 2017.

Adverse Effects and Toxicity

The most common adverse effects associated with ezogabine include dizziness, somnolence, fatigue, confusion, and blurred vision. Vertigo, diplopia, memory impairment, gait disturbance, aphasia, dysarthria, and balance problems also may occur. Serious side effects include skin discoloration, QT prolongation, and neuropsychiatric symptoms, including suicidal thoughts and behavior, psychosis, and hallucinations. Due to the presence of Kv7.2–Kv7.5 in the bladder uroepithelium, ezogabine is also associated with urinary retention. Blue pigmentation of skin and lips occurs in as many as one-third of patients maintained on long-term ezogabine therapy. Chronic treatment with ezogabine may cause retinal abnormalities, independent of changes in skin coloration. The FDA has changed the labeling of ezogabine to warn about the risks serious adverse effects, all of which may be permanent. Ezogabine should thus be discontinued if clinical benefit is not achieved after careful titration; however, the discontinuation of ezogabine should be done gradually, while under the care of a physician. In additon, the FDA recommends that all patients taking ezogabine should have baseline and periodic (every 6 months) systemic visual monitoring by an opthalmic professional, which includes both visual acuity and dilated fundus photography.

Felbamate

Felbamate is not indicated as a first-line therapy for any type of seizure activity. Rather, felbamate is FDA-approved for focal seizures in patients who have inadequately responded to alternative ASDs and in patients for whom the severity of their epilepsy outweighs the substantial risk of drug-induced aplastic anemia or liver failure. The potential for such serious and life-threatening adverse effects has limited the clinical utility of felbamate.

Mechanisms of Action

Clinically relevant concentrations of felbamate inhibit NMDA-evoked responses and potentiate GABA-evoked responses in whole-cell, voltage-clamp recordings of cultured rat hippocampal neurons (Rho et al., 1994). This dual action on excitatory and inhibitory transmitter responses may contribute to the wide spectrum of action of the drug in seizure models; however, the mechanism(s) by which felbamate exerts its anticonvulsant activity remain unknown.

Therapeutic Use

Despite the potential serious adverse effects, felbamate is used at doses ranging from 1 to 4 g/d. Clinical studies demonstrate the efficacy of felbamate in patients with poorly controlled focal and secondarily generalized seizures (Sachdeo et al., 1992) and in patients with Lennox-Gastaut syndrome (Felbamate Study Group in Lennox-Gastaut Syndrome, 1993). The clinical efficacy of this unique compound, which inhibits responses to NMDA while potentiating GABAergic neurotransmission, underscores the potential therapeutic value of identifying additional ASDs with novel mechanisms of action.

Gabapentin and Pregabalin

Gabapentin and pregabalin are ASDs that consist of a GABA molecule covalently bound to a lipophilic cyclohexane ring or isobutane, respectively. Gabapentin was designed to be a centrally active GABA agonist, with its high lipid solubility aimed at facilitating its transfer across the blood-brain barrier; the actual mechanism of action is notably different (see below).

Mechanisms of Action

Gabapentin inhibits tonic hind limb extension in the electroshock seizure model. Interestingly, gabapentin also inhibits clonic seizures induced by pentylenetetrazol. Its efficacy in both of these tests parallels that of valproate and distinguishes it from phenytoin and carbamazepine. Despite their design as GABA agonists, neither gabapentin nor pregabalin mimics GABA when iontophoretically applied to neurons in primary culture. Rather, these compounds bind with high affinity to a protein in cortical membranes with an amino acid sequence identical to that of the Ca^{2+} channel subunit α2δ-1 (Gee et al., 1996). This interaction with the α2δ-1 protein may mediate the anticonvulsant effects of gabapentin, but whether and how the binding of gabapentin to the α2δ-1 subunit regulates neuronal excitability remains unclear. Pregabalin binding is reduced but not eliminated in mice carrying a mutation in the α2δ-1 protein (Field et al., 2006). Analgesic efficacy of pregabalin is eliminated in these mice; whether the anticonvulsant effects of pregabalin are also eliminated was not reported.

ADME

Gabapentin and pregabalin are absorbed after oral administration and are not metabolized in humans. These compounds are not bound to plasma proteins and are excreted unchanged, mainly in the urine. Their half-lives, when used as monotherapy, approximate 6 h. These compounds have no known interactions with other ASDs.

Therapeutic Uses

Gabapentin and pregabalin are effective for focal onset seizures, with and without progression to bilateral tonic-clonic seizures, when used in addition to other ASDs. Gabapentin is also indicated for the management of the neuropathic pain associated with postherpetic neuralgia in adults.

Pregabalin is FDA-approved as an adjunctive therapy for adults with focal onset seizures. It is also indicated for the management of fibromyalgia and the neuropathic pain associated diabetic peripheral neuropathy, postherpetic neuralgia, or spinal cord injury.

In double-blind, placebo-controlled trials of adults with refractory focal seizures, addition of gabapentin or pregabalin to other ASDs is superior to placebo (French et al., 2003; Sivenius et al., 1991). Gabapentin monotherapy (900 or 1800 mg/d) is equivalent to carbamazepine (600 mg/d) for newly diagnosed focal or generalized epilepsy (Chadwick et al., 1998).

Gabapentin usually is effective in doses of 900–1800 mg daily in three doses, although 3600 mg may be required in some patients to achieve reasonable seizure control. Therapy usually is begun with a low dose (300 mg once on the first day), which is increased in daily increments of 300 mg until an effective dose is reached. In comparison, pregabalin is generally initiated at 50 mg three times a day (150 mg/day) and increase within 1 week to 300 mg/day based on efficacy and tolerability. Since both gabapentin and pregabalin are eliminated by renal excretion, appropriate dose adjustments are necessary in patients with reduced renal function.

Adverse Effects

Overall, gabapentin is well tolerated, with the most common adverse effects of somnolence, dizziness, ataxia, and fatigue. These effects usually are mild to moderate in severity but resolve within 2 weeks of onset during continued treatment. Gabapentin and pregabalin are both listed in pregnancy category C.

Lacosamide

Lacosamide is a stereoselective enantiomer of the amino acid, L-serine. This functionalized amino acid is FDA approved as adjunctive therapy for focal-onset seizures in patients older than 17 years. The FDA assigned lacosamide a Controlled Substance Act (CSA) schedule V designation, meaning it has a low potential for abuse.

Mechanisms of Action

Lacosamide is the first ASD to enhance (prolong) the slow inactivation of voltage-gated Na$^+$ channels and to limit sustained repetitive firing, the neuronal firing pattern characteristic of focal seizures. Lacosamide also binds collapsin response mediator protein-2 (CRMP-2), a phosphoprotein involved in neuronal differentiation and axon outgrowth, but the contribution of CRMP-2 to lacosamide's antiseizure efficacy remains unclear. Lacosamide was extensively evaluated by the ETSP and found to be highly effective in numerous preclinical animal models of seizures and epilepsy, including maximal electroshock, hippocampal kindling, Frings and 6-Hz models, giving lacosamide a unique preclinical profile compared to other Na$^+$ channel blockers.

ADME

Peak lacosamide plasma concentrations occur about 1–4 h after oral administration, and food consumption does not affect the absorption. Lacosamide has a $t_{1/2}$ of 12–16 h; 95% is excreted in the urine, about half of which is the unchanged parent compound. The major metabolite, O-desmethyl-lacosamide, is inactive.

Therapeutic Uses

Lacosamide is approved for both monotherapy and add-on therapy for focal-onset seizures in patients 17 years and older. As a monotherapy for the treatment of focal seizures, the initial recommended dose is 50–100 mg twice daily and, depending on patient response, may be increased at weekly intervals by 50 mg twice daily to a recommended maintenance dose of 100 mg to 200 mg twice daily, or 200–400 mg/d. The pharmacological profile is advantageous for hospitalized patients because it is available in an intravenous formulation, has minimal hepatic metabolism, and has no adverse respiratory effects. In addition, double-blind, placebo-controlled studies of adults with refractory focal seizures suggest that addition of lacosamide to other ASDs is superior to the addition of placebo.

Adverse Effects

Lacosamide is generally well tolerated. Although it has been associated with a brief (6-ms) prolongation of the PR interval, well-controlled studies in healthy patients suggested lacosamide does not prolong the QT interval. However, patients who are taking concomitant agents that prolong the PR internal should have a baseline electrocardiogram before starting lacosamide and be closely monitored due to a risk of AV block or bradycardia. Patients with renal impairment or hepatic impairment who are taking inhibitors of CYP3A4 or CYP2C9 may experience a significant increase in lacosamide exposure. No major adverse effects have been reported, although minor adverse effects include headache, dizziness, double vision, nausea, vomiting, fatigue, tremor, loss of balance, and somnolence. Like most currently available ASDs, lacosamide may contribute to suicidal ideations and suicide. As a consequence, the FDA has mandated a black-box warning for this agent.

Lamotrigine

Lamotrigine is a phenyltriazine derivative initially developed as an antifolate agent, based on the incorrect idea that reducing folate would effectively combat seizures. Structure-activity studies have since indicated that its effectiveness as an ASD is unrelated to its antifolate properties (Macdonald and Greenfield, 1997).

Mechanisms of Action

Lamotrigine suppresses tonic hind limb extension in the maximal electroshock model and focal and secondarily generalized seizures in the kindling model, but does not inhibit clonic motor seizures induced by pentylenetetrazol. Lamotrigine blocks sustained repetitive firing of mouse spinal cord neurons and delays the recovery from inactivation of recombinant Na$^+$ channels, mechanisms similar to those of phenytoin and carbamazepine (Xie et al., 1995). This may well explain lamotrigine's actions on focal and secondarily generalized seizures. However, as mentioned below, lamotrigine is effective against a broader spectrum of seizures than are phenytoin and carbamazepine, suggesting that lamotrigine may have actions in addition to regulating recovery from inactivation of Na$^+$ channels. One possibility, supported by basic research, is that lamotrigine inhibits synaptic release of glutamate by acting at Na$^+$ channels themselves.

ADME

Lamotrigine is completely absorbed from the GI tract. The drug is metabolized primarily by glucuronidation, yielding a plasma $t_{1/2}$ of a single dose of 24–30 h. Administration of phenytoin, carbamazepine, or phenobarbital reduces the $t_{1/2}$ and plasma concentrations of lamotrigine. Conversely, addition of valproate markedly increases plasma concentrations of lamotrigine, likely by inhibiting glucuronidation. Addition of lamotrigine to valproate produces a reduction of valproate concentrations by about 25% over a few weeks. Concurrent use of lamotrigine and carbamazepine is associated with increases of the 10,11-epoxide of carbamazepine and clinical toxicity in some patients.

Therapeutic Use

Lamotrigine is useful for monotherapy and add-on therapy of focal and secondarily generalized tonic-clonic seizures in adults and Lennox-Gastaut syndrome in both children and adults. Lennox-Gastaut syndrome is a disorder of childhood characterized by multiple seizure types, mental retardation, and refractoriness to antiseizure medication.

Lamotrigine monotherapy in newly diagnosed focal or generalized tonic-clonic seizures is equivalent to monotherapy with carbamazepine or phenytoin (Brodie et al., 1995; Steiner et al., 1999). Addition of lamotrigine to existing ASDs is effective against tonic-clonic seizures and drop attacks in children with the Lennox-Gastaut syndrome (Motte et al., 1997). Lamotrigine is also superior to placebo in children with newly diagnosed absence epilepsy (Frank et al., 1999).

Patients who are already taking a CYP-inducing ASD (e.g., carbamazepine, phenytoin, phenobarbital, or primidone, but not valproate) should be given lamotrigine initially at 50 mg/d for 2 weeks. The dose is increased to 50 mg twice per day for 2 weeks and then increased in increments of 100 mg/d each week up to a maintenance dose of 300–500 mg/d divided into two doses. For patients taking valproate in addition to an enzyme-inducing ASD, the initial dose should be 25 mg every other day for 2 weeks, followed by an increase to 25 mg/d for 2 weeks; the dose then can be increased by 25–50 mg/d every 1–2 weeks up to a maintenance dose of 100–150 mg/d divided into two doses.

Adverse Effects

The most common adverse effects are dizziness, ataxia, blurred or double vision, nausea, vomiting, and rash when lamotrigine is added to another ASD. A few cases of Stevens-Johnson syndrome and disseminated intravascular coagulation have been reported. The incidence of serious rash in pediatric patients (~0.8%) is higher than in the adult population (0.3%).

Levetiracetam and Brivaracetam

Levetiracetam is a pyrrolidine, the racemically pure *S*-enantiomer of α-ethyl-2-oxo-1-pyrrolidineacetamide, and is FDA-approved for adjunctive therapy for myoclonic, focal-onset, and generalized onset tonic-clonic seizures in adults and children as young as 4 years old. Brivaracetam, an analogue of levetiracetam, was FDA-approved in 2016 as an adjunctive therapy for focal-onset seizures in patients aged 16 years and older with epilepsy.

Mechanism of Action

Levetiracetam exhibits a novel pharmacological profile: It inhibits focal and secondarily generalized tonic-clonic seizures in the kindling model, yet is ineffective against maximum electroshock- and pentylenetetrazol-induced seizures, findings consistent with clinical effectiveness against focal and secondarily generalized tonic-clonic seizures. The mechanism by which levetiracetam exerts these antiseizure effects is not fully understood. However, the correlation between binding affinity of levetiracetam and its analogues and their potency toward audiogenic seizures suggests that the synaptic vesicle protein SV2A mediates the anticonvulsant effects of levetiracetam (Rogawski and Bazil, 2008). SV2A is an integral transmembrane glycoprotein; expression of human SV2A in hexose transport-deficient yeast shows that SV2A can function as a galactose transporter (Madeo et al, 2014). The neuronal function of the SV2A protein is not fully understood, but binding of levetiracetam to SV2A might affect neuronal excitability by modifying the release of glutamate and GABA through an action on vesicular function. In mice, a missense mutation in SV2A is reportedly associated with disruption of action-potential invoked GABA release in limbic regions (Ohno and Tokudome, 2017). Other workers have suggested that SV2A may play a role in vesicle recycling following exocytosis of neurotransmitter (Bartolome, et al., 2017). In addition, levetiracetam inhibits N-type Ca^{2+} channels and Ca^{2+} release from intracellular stores.

Brivaracetam binds with high affinity to SV2A and inhibits neuronal voltage-gated Na^+ channels (Kenda et al., 2004; Zona et al., 2010); preclinical studies suggested a broad spectrum of anticonvulsant protection (Matagne et al., 2008).

ADME

Levetiracetam is rapidly and almost completely absorbed after oral administration and is not bound to plasma proteins. The plasma $t_{1/2}$ is 6–8 h, but may be longer in elderly patients. Ninety-five percent of the drug and its inactive metabolite are excreted in the urine, 65% of which is unchanged drug; 24% of the drug is metabolized by hydrolysis of the acetamide group. Because levetiracetam neither induces nor is a high-affinity substrate for CYPs or glucuronidation enzymes, it is devoid of known interactions with other ASDs, oral contraceptives, or anticoagulants.

Brivaracetam is rapidly absorbed and well tolerated, with an elimination $t_{1/2}$ of approximately 7–8 h.

Therapeutic Use

Levetiracetam is marketed for the adjunctive treatment of focal seizures in adults and children, for primary onset tonic-clonic seizures, and for myoclonic seizures of JME. It is available in tablet (10, 25, 50, 75, or 100 mg), oral solution (10 mg/mL), or injectable form (50 mg/5 mL). Adult dosing is initiated at 500–1000 mg/d and increased every 2–4 weeks by 1000 mg to a maximum dose of 3000 mg/d. The drug is administered twice daily. In adults with either refractory focal seizures or uncontrolled generalized tonic-clonic seizures associated with idiopathic generalized epilepsy, addition of levetiracetam to other antiseizure medications is superior to

placebo. Levetiracetam also has efficacy as adjunctive therapy for refractory generalized myoclonic seizures (Andermann et al., 2005). Insufficient evidence is available about its use as monotherapy for focal or generalized epilepsy.

The recommended starting dose for brivaracetam is 50 mg twice daily, which may be adjusted to either 25 mg twice daily or 100 mg twice daily, based on patient response and tolerability.

Adverse Effects

Both levetiracetam and brivaracetam are well tolerated. The most frequently reported adverse effects associated with levetiracetam are somnolence, asthenia, ataxia, and dizziness. Behavioral and mood changes are serious, but less common. For brivaracetam, the most common adverse effects are similarly mild and include somnolence, sedation, dizziness, and GI upset. In patients with hepatic insufficiency, dose adjustment may be required with brivaracetam to 25 mg twice daily and a maximal dosage of 75 mg twice daily. Hypersensitivity reactions may occur.

Perampanel

Mechanisms of Action

Perampanel is a first-in class selective, noncompetitive antagonist of the AMPA-type ionotropic glutamate receptor (Bialer and White, 2010; Stephen and Brodie, 2011). Unlike NMDA antagonists, which shorten the duration of repetitive discharges, AMPA receptor antagonists prevent repetitive neuronal firing. Preclinical studies demonstrated a broad spectrum of activity in both acute and chronic seizure models, indicating that perampanel reduces fast excitatory signaling critical to the seizure generation (Tortorella et al., 1997) and spread (Namba et al., 1994; Rogawski and Donevan, 1999). Perampanel seems to have a greater inhibitory effect on seizure propagation than on seizure initiation (Hanada et al., 2011).

ADME and Drug Interactions

Perampanel is absorbed well after oral administration with a plasma $t_{1/2}$ of about 105 h, permitting once-daily administration. The drug is 95% bound to plasma protein, mainly albumin, and is metabolized by hepatic oxidation and glucuronidation. A linear relationship between perampanel dose and plasma concentration has been reported over the dose range of 2–12 mg/d.

Primary metabolism is mediated by hepatic CYP3A; thus, specific drug interactions and dose adjustments need to be considered. For example, perampanel may decrease the effectiveness of progesterone-containing hormone contraceptives, carbamazepine, clobazam, lamotrigine, and valproate, but it may increase the level of oxcarbazepine. Furthermore, serum perampanel may be decreased when taken with carbamazepine, oxcarbazepine, and topiramate.

Therapeutic Use

Perampanel is FDA-approved as an adjunctive therapy for the treatment of focal-onset seizures in patients 12 years and older with or without secondarily generalized seizures. The recommended oral starting dose is 2 mg once daily, titrated to a maximal dose of 4–12 mg/d at bedtime.

Adverse Effects

Common adverse effects include somnolence, anxiety, confusion, imbalance, double vision, dizziness, GI distress or nausea, and weight gain. Rare, but serious, adverse behavioral reactions, including hostility, aggression, and suicidal thoughts and behaviors, independent of clinical history of psychiatric disorder, have also been reported.

Rufinamide

Rufinamide, a triazole derivative, is structurally unrelated to other marketed ASDs. It is FDA-approved for adjunctive treatment of seizures related to Lennox-Gastaut syndrome in children more than 4 years old and adults.

Mechanism of Action

Rufinamide prolongs slow inactivation of voltage-gated Na^+ channels and limits sustained repetitive firing, the firing pattern characteristic of focal seizures. The complete mechanism of action of rufinamide remains unclear.

ADME

Rufinamide is well absorbed orally, binds minimally to plasma proteins, and reaches peak plasma concentrations about 4–6 h after oral administration. The $t_{1/2}$ is 6–10 h. Rufinamide is metabolized independent of CYPs and then excreted in the urine.

Therapeutic Use

Rufinamide has been shown to be effective against all seizure phenotypes in Lennox-Gastaut syndrome. In adults, 400–800 mg/d rufinamide is initially administered in two equal doses. Doses are then titrated upward every other day by 10 mg/kg to a maximum of the lesser of 45 mg/kg/d or 3200 mg/d. Children are initiated at 10 mg/kg/d divided into two equal daily doses, increasing to a maximum of the lesser of 45 mg/kg/d or 3200 mg/d.

Adverse Effects

Common adverse effects include headache, dizziness, somnolence, fatigue, and nausea.

Stiripentol

Stiripentol is an aromatic alcohol, structurally unrelated to any other ASDs. Stiripentol was granted orphan drug status for the treatment of Dravet syndrome in 2008 but has not received FDA approval due its complex pharmacokinetic and pharmacodynamic interactions with other drugs.

Mechanisms of Action

Although the exact nature of its antiseizure mechanism is not clear, stiripentol may increase CNS levels of the inhibitory transmitter GABA by inhibition of synaptosomal uptake of GABA or by inhibition of GABA transaminase. In model systems, stiripentol also enhances GABA$_A$ receptor–mediated neurotransmission and increases the mean open duration of GABA$_A$ receptor chloride channels in a barbiturate-like fashion (Fisher, 2011; Quilichini et al., 2006).

ADME and Drug Interactions

Stiripentol is quickly absorbed, reaching a peak C_p in about 1.5 h; the drug is highly bound to plasma proteins. Stiripentol's elimination kinetics are nonlinear, with a $t_{1/2}$ ranging from 4 to 13 h. Plasma clearance decreases markedly at high doses and after repeated administration, probably due to inhibition or saturation of the CYPs responsible for stiripentol metabolism. Metabolites are excreted in the urine.

Stiripentol has diverse pharmacokinetic and pharmacodynamic interactions with concomitantly administered drugs. It is a potent inhibitor of CYPs 3A4, 1A2, and 2C19. Thus, adjunctively administered ASDs, such as carbamazepine, valproate, phenytoin, phenobarbital, and benzodiazepines, may require dose adjustments due to the potent inhibition of CYPs involved in their hepatic metabolism. Concomitant stiripentol can increase clobazam and valproate concentrations by 2- to 3-fold, and dose reduction of either or both ASDs may be necessary to avoid toxicity.

Therapeutic Use

Stiripentol is used clinically in conjunction with clobazam and valproate as an adjunctive therapy for refractory generalized tonic-clonic seizures in patients with severe myoclonic epilepsy in infancy (Dravet syndrome) whose seizures are not adequately controlled with clobazam and valproate (Aneja and Sharma, 2013; Plosker, 2012). Adjunctive stiripentol in children with Dravet syndrome who fail to respond to valproate and clobazam have a 71% response rate (Chiron et al., 2000; Nabbout and Chiron, 2012). Stiripentol also reduces the frequency and severity of tonic-clonic seizures as well as status epilepticus in infants and children with a variety of epilepsy syndromes (Inoue et al., 2009; Perez et al., 1999; Rey et al., 1999).

Use of stiripentol is replete with potential drug interactions (see the section on ADME) that must be considered. Initiation of adjunctive therapy with stiripentol should be undertaken gradually, with frequent plasma monitoring for both the parent ASDs and their active metabolites. Plasma monitoring is important to inform reductions in concomitant ASDs as needed, based on patient response.

Adverse Effects

The most commonly reported adverse effects in patients on stiripentol include anorexia, weight loss, insomnia, drowsiness, ataxia, hypotonia, and dystonia.

Tiagabine

Tiagabine is a derivative of nipecotic acid and is FDA-approved as adjunct therapy for focal seizures in adults.

TIAGABINE
(nipecotic acid in black)

Mechanism of Action

Tiagabine inhibits the GABA transporter GAT-1 and thereby reduces GABA uptake into neurons and glia and prolongs the dwell time of GABA in the synaptic space. In CA1 neurons of the hippocampus, tiagabine increases the duration of inhibitory synaptic currents, findings consistent with prolonging the effect of GABA at inhibitory synapses through reducing its reuptake by GAT-1. Tiagabine inhibits maximum electroshock seizures and both limbic and secondarily generalized tonic-clonic seizures in the kindling model, results suggestive of clinical efficacy against focal and tonic-clonic seizures.

ADME

Tiagabine is rapidly absorbed after oral administration, extensively bound to serum proteins, and metabolized mainly in the liver, predominantly by CYP3A. Its $t_{1/2}$ of about 8 h is shortened by 2–3 h when coadministered with CYP-inducing drugs such as phenobarbital, phenytoin, or carbamazepine.

Therapeutic Use

Tiagabine is efficacious as add-on therapy for refractory focal seizures with or without secondary generalization. Its efficacy as monotherapy for newly diagnosed or refractory focal and generalized epilepsy has not been established.

Adverse Effects and Precautions

The principal adverse effects include dizziness, somnolence, and tremor; they are mild to moderate in severity and appear shortly after initiation of therapy. Tiagabine and other drugs that enhance effects of synaptically released GABA can facilitate spike-and-wave discharges in animal models of absence seizures. Case reports suggest that tiagabine treatment of patients with a history of spike-and-wave discharges causes exacerbations of their EEG abnormalities. Thus, tiagabine may be contraindicated in patients with generalized absence epilepsy. Paradoxically, tiagabine has been associated with the occurrence of seizures in patients without epilepsy; thus, off-label use of the drug is discouraged.

Topiramate

Topiramate is a sulfamate-substituted monosaccharide that is FDA-approved as initial monotherapy (in patients at least 10 years old) and as adjunctive therapy (for patients as young as 2 years) for focal-onset or primary generalized tonic-clonic seizures, for Lennox-Gastaut syndrome in patients 2 years of age and older, and for migraine headache prophylaxis in adults.

Mechanisms of Action

Topiramate reduces voltage-gated Na$^+$ currents in cerebellar granule cells and may act on the inactivated state of the channel similarly to phenytoin. In addition, topiramate activates a hyperpolarizing K$^+$ current, enhances postsynaptic GABA$_A$ receptor currents, and limits activation of the AMPA-kainate subtype(s) of glutamate receptors.

The drug is a weak inhibitor of carbonic anhydrase. Topiramate inhibits maximal electroshock and pentylenetetrazol-induced seizures as well as focal and secondarily generalized tonic-clonic seizures in the kindling model, findings predictive of a broad spectrum of antiseizure actions clinically.

ADME

Topiramate is rapidly absorbed after oral administration, exhibits little (10%–20%) binding to plasma proteins, and is excreted largely unchanged in the urine. A small fraction undergoes metabolism by hydroxylation, hydrolysis, and glucuronidation, with no single metabolite accounting for more than 5% of an oral dose. Its $t_{1/2}$ is about 1 day. Reduced estradiol plasma concentrations occur with concurrent topiramate, suggesting the need for higher doses of oral contraceptives when coadministered with topiramate.

Therapeutic Use

Topiramate is equivalent to valproate and carbamazepine in children and adults with newly diagnosed focal and primary generalized epilepsy (Privitera et al., 2003). The agent is effective as monotherapy for refractory focal epilepsy (Sachdeo et al., 1997) and refractory generalized tonic-clonic seizures (Biton et al., 1999). Topiramate is significantly more effective than placebo against both drop attacks and tonic-clonic seizures in patients with Lennox-Gastaut syndrome (Sachdeo et al., 1999).

Adverse Effects

Topiramate is well tolerated. The most common adverse effects are somnolence, fatigue, weight loss, and nervousness. It may precipitate renal calculi (kidney stones), probably due to inhibition of carbonic anhydrase. Topiramate has been associated with cognitive impairment, and patients may complain about a change in the taste of carbonated beverages.

Valproate

The antiseizure properties of valproic acid were discovered serendipitously when it was employed as a vehicle for other compounds that were being screened for antiseizure activity. Valproate (*n*-dipropylacetic acid) is a simple branched-chain carboxylic acid. Certain other branched-chain carboxylic acids have potencies similar to that of valproic acid in antagonizing pentylenetetrazol-induced seizures. However, increasing the number of carbon atoms to nine introduces marked sedative properties. Straight-chain carboxylic acids have little or no activity.

$$CH_3CH_2CH_2 \diagdown$$
$$CHCOO^-$$
$$CH_3CH_2CH_2 \diagup$$

VALPROATE

Pharmacological Effects

Valproate is strikingly different from phenytoin or ethosuximide in that it is effective in inhibiting seizures in a variety of models. Like phenytoin and carbamazepine, valproate inhibits tonic hind limb extension in maximal electroshock seizures and kindled seizures at nontoxic doses. Like ethosuximide, valproate at subtoxic doses inhibits clonic motor seizures induced by pentylenetetrazol. Its efficacy in diverse models parallels its efficacy against absence as well as focal and generalized tonic-clonic seizures in humans.

Mechanisms of Action

Valproate produces effects on isolated neurons similar to those of phenytoin and ethosuximide. At therapeutically relevant concentrations, valproate inhibits sustained repetitive firing induced by depolarization of mouse cortical or spinal cord neurons (McLean and Macdonald, 1986b). The action is similar to that of phenytoin and carbamazepine (Table 17–2) and appears to be mediated by a prolonged recovery of voltage-activated Na^+ channels from inactivation. Valproate does not modify neuronal responses to iontophoretically applied GABA. In neurons isolated from the nodose ganglion, valproate also produces small reductions of T-type

Ca^{2+} currents (Kelly et al., 1990) at clinically relevant concentrations that are slightly higher than those that limit sustained repetitive firing; this effect on T-type currents is similar to that of ethosuximide in thalamic neurons (Coulter et al., 1989). Together, these actions of limiting sustained repetitive firing and reducing T-type currents may contribute to the effectiveness of valproate against focal and tonic-clonic seizures and absence seizures, respectively.

In model systems, valproate can increase brain content of GABA, stimulate GABA synthesis (by glutamate decarboxylase), and inhibit GABA degradation (by GABA transaminase and succinic semialdehyde dehydrogenase). Such data notwithstanding, it has been difficult to relate the increased GABA levels to the antiseizure activity of valproate. Valproate is also a potent inhibitor of histone deacetylase. Thus, some of its antiseizure activity may be due to its ability to modulate gene expression through this mechanism.

ADME

Valproate is absorbed rapidly and completely after oral administration. Peak C_p occurs in 1 to 4 h, although this can be delayed for several hours if the drug is administered in enteric-coated tablets or is ingested with meals. Its extent of binding to plasma proteins is usually about 90%, but the fraction bound is reduced as the total concentration of valproate is increased through the therapeutic range. Although concentrations of valproate in CSF suggest equilibration with free drug in the blood, there is evidence for carrier-mediated transport of valproate both into and out of the CSF.

Valproate undergoes hepatic metabolism (95%), with less than 5% excreted unchanged in urine. Its hepatic metabolism occurs mainly by UGTs and β-oxidation. Valproate is a substrate for CYPs 2C9 and 2C19, but these enzymes account for a relatively minor portion of its elimination. Some of the drug's metabolites, notably 2-propyl-2-pentenoic acid and 2-propyl-4-pentenoic acid, are nearly as potent antiseizure agents as the parent compound; however, only the former accumulates in plasma and brain to a potentially significant extent. The $t_{1/2}$ of valproate is about 15 h but is reduced in patients taking other antiseizure drugs.

Plasma Drug Concentrations

Valproate plasma concentrations associated with therapeutic effects are about 30–100 μg/mL. However, there is a poor correlation between the plasma concentration and efficacy. There appears to be a threshold at about 30–50 μg/mL, the concentration at which binding sites on plasma albumin begin to become saturated.

Therapeutic Uses

Valproate is a broad-spectrum ASD effective in the treatment of absence, myoclonic, focal, and tonic-clonic seizures. The initial daily dose usually is 15 mg/kg, increased at weekly intervals by 5–10 mg/kg/d to a maximum daily dose of 60 mg/kg. Divided doses should be given when the total daily dose exceeds 250 mg. The therapeutic uses of valproate in epilepsy are discussed further at the end of this chapter.

Adverse Effects and Drug Interactions

The most frequent side effects are transient GI symptoms, including anorexia, nausea, and vomiting (~16%). Effects on the CNS include sedation, ataxia, and tremor; these symptoms occur infrequently and usually respond to a decrease in dosage. Rash, alopecia, and stimulation of appetite have been observed occasionally; weight gain has been seen with chronic valproate treatment in some patients. Elevation of hepatic transaminases in plasma is observed in up to 40% of patients and often occurs asymptomatically during the first several months of therapy.

A rare but frequently fatal complication is fulminant hepatitis. Children below 2 years of age with other medical conditions who were given multiple ASDs were especially likely to suffer fatal hepatic injury; there were no deaths reported for patients over the age of 10 years who received only valproate (Dreifuss et al., 1989). Acute pancreatitis and hyperammonemia have been frequently associated with the use of valproate. This agent can also produce teratogenic effects, such as neural tube defects.

Valproate inhibits the metabolism of drugs that are substrates for CYP2C9, including phenytoin and phenobarbital. Valproate also inhibits UGTs and thus inhibits the metabolism of lamotrigine and lorazepam. The high molar concentrations of valproate used clinically result in valproate's displacing phenytoin and other drugs from albumin. With respect to phenytoin in particular, valproate's inhibition of that drug's metabolism is exacerbated by displacement of phenytoin from albumin. The concurrent administration of valproate and clonazepam is associated with the development of absence status epilepticus; however, this complication appears to be rare.

Vigabatrin

Vigabatrin is FDA-approved as adjunct therapy of refractory focal seizures with impaired awareness in adults. In addition, vigabatrin is designated as an orphan drug for treatment of infantile spasms (described in the Therapeutic Use section that follows).

VIGABATRIN

Mechanism of Action

Vigabatrin, a structural analogue of GABA, irreversibly inhibits the major degradative enzyme for GABA, GABA transaminase, thereby leading to increased concentrations of GABA in the brain. This effect is hypothesized to result in increased extracellular GABA at its receptors and enhanced GABAergic transmission.

ADME

An oral dose is well absorbed, reaching a maximal C_p within 1 h; the presence of food prolongs absorption but does not reduce the area under the curve. Vigabatrin is excreted unmetabolized by the kidney, and the dose must be reduced for patients with renal impairment. Although vigabatrin has a $t_{1/2}$ of only 6–8 h, the pharmacodynamic effects are prolonged and do not correlate well with plasma $t_{1/2}$ or the C_p. Such kinetics would be expected due to the irreversible nature of the drug's inhibition of GABA transaminase and a recovery period that reflects the rate of enzyme resynthesis rather than the rate of drug elimination. Vigabatrin induces CYP2C9.

Therapeutic Use

Adult dosing is generally initiated orally at 500 mg twice daily and then increased in 500-mg increments weekly to 1.5 g twice daily.

A 2-week, randomized, single masked clinical trial of vigabatrin for infantile spasms in children younger than 2 years revealed time- and dose-dependent increases in responders, evident as freedom from spasms for 7 consecutive days. Children in whom infantile spasms were caused by tuberous sclerosis were particularly responsive to vigabatrin. As with other ASDs, vigabatrin should be withdrawn slowly, not stopped abruptly.

Toxicity, Adverse Effects, and Precautions

Due to progressive and permanent bilateral vision loss (FDA box warning), vigabatrin must be reserved for patients who have failed several alternative therapies. A patient's vision must be professionally monitored at the beginning of therapy and regularly throughout and after a therapeutic course. Due to this serious toxicity, vigabatrin is available only through SHARE (1-888-45-SHARE), a restricted distribution program.

The most common side effects (>10% patients) include weight gain, concentric visual field constriction, fatigue, somnolence, dizziness, hyperactivity, and seizures. Data in animal models suggest that vigabatrin may harm a developing fetus, and the drug is classified in pregnancy category C. Vigabatrin is excreted in the milk of nursing mothers.

Zonisamide

Zonisamide is FDA-approved as adjunctive therapy of focal seizures in adults 12 years or older.

Mechanism of Action

Zonisamide inhibits the sustained, repetitive firing of spinal cord neurons, presumably by prolonging the inactivated state of voltage-gated Na+ channels in a manner similar to actions of phenytoin and carbamazepine and by preventing neurotransmitter release. In addition, zonisamide inhibits T-type Ca²⁺ currents and reduces the influx of calcium. Zonisamide can also inhibit carbonic anhydrase and scavenge free radicals; whether and how these actions may contribute to the drug's neuroprotective effects are unknown.

ADME

Zonisamide is almost completely absorbed after oral administration, has a long $t_{1/2}$ (~60 h), is about 40% bound to plasma protein, and has linear kinetics at doses ranging from 100 to 400 mg. Approximately 85% of an oral dose is excreted in the urine, principally as unmetabolized zonisamide and a glucuronide of sulfamoylacetyl phenol, the product of metabolism by CYP3A4. Thus, phenobarbital, phenytoin, and carbamazepine will decrease the plasma concentration/dose ratio of zonisamide, whereas lamotrigine will increase this ratio. Zonisamide has little effect on the plasma concentrations of other ASDs.

Therapeutic Use

The addition of zonisamide to other drugs is superior to placebo. There is insufficient evidence for zonisamide's efficacy as monotherapy for newly diagnosed or refractory epilepsy.

Toxicity

Overall, zonisamide is well tolerated. The most common adverse effects include somnolence, dizziness, cognitive impairment, ataxia, anorexia, nervousness, and fatigue. Potentially serious skin rashes are rare but may occur. Approximately 1% of individuals develop renal calculi during treatment, which may relate to inhibition of carbonic anhydrase by zonisamide. As a carbonic anhydrase inhibitor, zonisamide may also cause metabolic acidosis. Thus, patients with predisposing conditions (e.g., renal disease, severe respiratory disorders, diarrhea, surgery, ketogenic diet) may be at greater risk for metabolic acidosis while taking zonisamide, a risk that appears to be more frequent and severe in younger patients. Measurement of serum bicarbonate prior to initiating therapy and periodically thereafter, even in the absence of symptoms, is recommended. Last, spontaneous abortions and congenital abnormalities have been reported at twice the rate (7%) of the healthy, control population (2%–3%) in female patients of childbearing age receiving polytherapy including zonisamide.

General Principles and Choice of Drugs for Therapy of the Epilepsies

Early diagnosis and treatment of seizure disorders with a single appropriate agent offers the best prospect of achieving prolonged seizure-free periods with the lowest risk of toxicity. An attempt should be made to determine the cause of the epilepsy with the hope of discovering a correctable lesion, either structural or metabolic. The drugs commonly used for distinct seizure types are listed in Table 17–1. The cost/benefit ratio of the efficacy and the adverse effects of a given drug should be considered in determining which drug is optimal for a given patient.

The first decision to make is whether and when to initiate treatment (French and Pedley, 2008). For example, it may not be necessary to initiate therapy after an isolated tonic-clonic seizure in a healthy young adult who lacks a family history of epilepsy and who has a normal neurological exam, a normal EEG, and a normal brain MRI scan. The odds of seizure recurrence in the next year (15%) are similar to the risk of a drug reaction sufficiently severe to warrant discontinuation of medication (Bazil and Pedley, 1998). On the other hand, a similar seizure occurring in an individual with a positive family history of epilepsy, an abnormal neurological exam, an abnormal EEG, and an abnormal MRI carries a risk of recurrence approximating 60%, odds that favor initiation of therapy.

Unless extenuating circumstances such as status epilepticus exist, only monotherapy should be initiated. Initial dosing should target a C_{pss} within the lower portion of the range associated with clinical efficacy to minimize dose-related adverse effects. Dosage is increased at appropriate intervals as required for control of seizures or as limited by toxicity, with monitoring of plasma drug concentrations. Compliance with a properly selected, single drug in maximal tolerated dosage results in complete control of seizures in about 50% of patients. If a seizure occurs despite optimal drug levels, the physician should assess the presence of potential precipitating factors such as sleep deprivation, a concurrent febrile illness, or drugs (e.g., large amounts of caffeine or over-the-counter medications that can lower the seizure threshold).

If compliance has been confirmed yet seizures persist, substitute another drug. Unless serious adverse effects of the drug dictate otherwise, always reduce dosage gradually to minimize risk of seizure recurrence. In the case of focal seizures in adults, the diversity of available drugs permits selection of a second drug that acts by a different mechanism (see Table 17–2). Among previously untreated patients, 47% became seizure free with the first drug and an additional 14% became seizure free with a second or third drug (Kwan and Brodie, 2000).

If therapy with a second single drug also is inadequate, combination therapy is warranted. This decision should not be taken lightly because most patients obtain optimal seizure control with the fewest adverse effects when taking a single drug. Nonetheless, some patients will not be controlled adequately without the simultaneous use of two or more ASDs. The chances of complete control with this approach are not high; according to Kwan and Brodie (2000), epilepsy is controlled by treatment with two drugs in only 3% of patients. It seems wise to select two drugs that act by distinct mechanisms (e.g., one that promotes Na⁺ channel inactivation and another that enhances GABA-mediated synaptic inhibition). Side effects of each drug and the potential drug interactions also should be considered. As specified in Table 17–3, many of these drugs induce expression of CYPs and thereby affect the metabolism of themselves or other drugs.

Essential to optimal management of epilepsy is the filling out of a seizure chart by the patient or a relative. Frequent visits to the physician may be necessary early in the period of treatment because hematological and other possible side effects may require a change in medication. Long-term follow-up with neurological examinations and possibly EEG and neuroimaging studies is appropriate. *Most crucial for successful management is patient adherence to the drug regimen; noncompliance is the most frequent cause for failure of therapy with ASDs.*

Measurement of plasma drug concentration at appropriate intervals facilitates the initial adjustment of dosage to minimize dose-related adverse effects without sacrificing seizure control. Periodic monitoring during maintenance therapy can also detect noncompliance. Knowledge of plasma drug concentrations can be especially helpful during multidrug therapy. If toxicity occurs, monitoring helps to identify the particular drug(s) responsible and can guide adjustment of dosage.

Duration of Therapy

Once initiated, ASDs are typically continued for at least 2 years. Tapering and discontinuing therapy should be considered if the patient is seizure free after 2 years; tapering should be done slowly over several months.

Factors associated with high risk for recurrent seizures following discontinuation of therapy include EEG abnormalities, known structural lesions, abnormalities on neurological exam, and history of frequent seizures or medically refractory seizures prior to control. Conversely, factors associated with low risk for recurrent seizures include idiopathic epilepsy, normal EEG, onset in childhood, and seizures easily controlled with a single drug. The risk of recurrent seizures ranges from 12% to 66% (French and Pedley, 2008). Typically, 80% of recurrences will occur within 4 months of discontinuing therapy. The clinician and patient must weigh the risk of recurrent seizure and the associated potential deleterious consequences (e.g., loss of driving privileges) against the implications of continuing medication, including cost, unwanted effects, implications of diagnosis of epilepsy, and so on.

Focal and Focal-to-Bilateral Tonic-Clonic Seizures

The efficacy and toxicity of carbamazepine, phenobarbital, and phenytoin for treatment of focal and secondarily generalized tonic-clonic seizures in adults have been examined (Mattson et al., 1985). Carbamazepine and phenytoin were the most effective agents. The choice between carbamazepine and phenytoin required assessment of toxic effects of each drug. Decreased libido and impotence were associated with all three drugs (carbamazepine 13%, phenobarbital 16%, and phenytoin 11%). In direct comparison with valproate, carbamazepine provided superior control of complex focal seizures (Mattson et al., 1992). With respect to adverse effects, carbamazepine was more commonly associated with skin rash, but valproate was more commonly associated with tremor and weight gain. Overall, carbamazepine and phenytoin are preferable for treatment of focal seizures, but phenobarbital and valproate are also efficacious.

Control of secondarily generalized tonic-clonic seizures does not differ significantly with carbamazepine, phenobarbital, or phenytoin (Mattson et al., 1985). Valproate was as effective as carbamazepine for control of secondarily generalized tonic-clonic seizures (Mattson et al., 1992). Because secondarily generalized tonic-clonic seizures usually coexist with focal seizures, these data indicate that among drugs introduced before 1990, carbamazepine and phenytoin are the first-line drugs for these conditions.

One key issue confronting the treating physician is choosing the optimal drug for initiating treatment in new-onset epilepsy. At first glance, this issue may appear unimportant because about 50% of newly diagnosed patients become seizure free with the first drug, whether old or new drugs are used (Kwan and Brodie, 2000). However, responsive patients typically receive the initial drug for several years, underscoring the importance of proper drug selection. Phenytoin, carbamazepine, and phenobarbital induce hepatic CYPs, thereby complicating use of multiple ASDs as well as affecting metabolism of oral contraceptives, warfarin, and many other drugs. Phenytoin, carbamazepine, and phenobarbital also enhance metabolism of endogenous compounds, including gonadal steroids and vitamin D, potentially affecting reproductive function and bone density. By contrast, most of the newer drugs have little, if any effect, on the CYPs. Factors arguing against use of recently introduced drugs include higher costs and less clinical experience with the compounds.

Ideally, a prospective study would systematically compare newly introduced ASDs with drugs available before 1990 in a study design adjusting dose as needed and observing responses for extended periods of time (e.g., 2 years or more), in much the same manner as that used when comparing the older ASDs with one another as described previously (Mattson et al., 1985). Unfortunately, such a study has not been performed. Many studies have compared a new ASD with an older ASD, but study design did not permit declaring a clearly superior drug; moreover, differences in study design and patient populations preclude comparing a new drug with multiple older drugs or with other new drugs.

The use of recently introduced ASDs for newly diagnosed epilepsy was analyzed by subcommittees of the American Academy of Neurology and the American Epilepsy Society (French et al., 2004a, 2004b); the authors concluded that available evidence supported the use of gabapentin, lamotrigine, and topiramate for newly diagnosed focal or mixed seizure disorders. None of these drugs, however, has been approved by the FDA for either of these indications. Insufficient evidence is available on the remaining newly introduced drugs to permit meaningful assessment of their effectiveness for this indication.

Generalized Absence Seizures

Ethosuximide and valproate are considered equally effective in the treatment of generalized absence seizures (Mikati and Browne, 1988). Between 50% and 75% of newly diagnosed patients are free of seizures following therapy with either drug. If tonic-clonic seizures are present or emerge during therapy, valproate is the agent of first choice. Available evidence also indicates that lamotrigine is effective for newly diagnosed absence epilepsy, but lamotrigine is not approved for this indication by the FDA (Ben-Menachem, 2011).

Myoclonic Seizures

Valproate is the drug of choice for myoclonic seizures in the syndrome of JME, in which myoclonic seizures often coexist with tonic-clonic and absence seizures. Levetiracetam also has demonstrated efficacy as adjunctive therapy for refractory generalized myoclonic seizures.

Febrile Convulsions

Between 2% and 4% of children experience a convulsion associated with a febrile illness; 25%–33% of these children will have another febrile convulsion. Only 2%–3% become epileptic in later years, a 6-fold increase in risk compared with the general population. Several factors are associated with an increased risk of developing epilepsy: preexisting neurological disorder or developmental delay, a family history of epilepsy, or a complicated febrile seizure (i.e., the febrile seizure lasted > 15 min, was one sided, or was followed by a second seizure in the same day). If all of these risk factors are present, the risk of developing epilepsy is about 10%.

The increased risk of developing epilepsy or other neurological sequelae led many physicians to prescribe ASDs prophylactically after a febrile seizure. Uncertainties regarding the efficacy of prophylaxis for reducing epilepsy combined with substantial side effects of phenobarbital prophylaxis (Farwell et al., 1990) argue against the use of chronic therapy for prophylactic purposes (Freeman, 1992). For children at high risk of developing recurrent febrile seizures and epilepsy, rectally administered diazepam at the time of fever may prevent recurrent seizures and avoid side effects of chronic therapy.

Seizures in Infants and Young Children

Infantile spasms with *hypsarrhythmia* (abnormal interictal high-amplitude slow waves and multifocal asynchronous spikes on EEG) are refractory to the usual ASD. Corticotropin or glucocorticoids are commonly used; repository corticotropin is designated as an orphan drug for this purpose. Vigabatrin (γ-vinyl GABA) is efficacious in comparison to placebo (Appleton et al., 1999); however, constriction of visual fields has been reported in a high percentage of patients treated with vigabatrin (Miller et al., 1999). To emphasize the potential for progressive and permanent vision loss, the FDA has instituted a black-box warning for vigabatrin, which is marketed under a restrictive distribution program. Vigabatrin has orphan drug status for the treatment of infantile spasms in the U.S. and is FDA-approved as adjunctive therapy for adults with refractory focal seizures with impaired awareness. Ganaxolone also has been designated as an orphan drug for the treatment of infantile spasms and completed a phase II clinical trial for uncontrolled focal-onset seizures in adults in 2009.

The Lennox-Gastaut syndrome is a severe form of epilepsy that usually begins in childhood and is characterized by cognitive impairments and multiple types of seizures, including tonic-clonic, tonic, atonic, myoclonic, and atypical absence seizures. Addition of lamotrigine to other ASDs improves seizure control in comparison to placebo in this treatment-resistant form of epilepsy (Motte et al., 1997). Felbamate also is effective for seizures in this syndrome, but the occasional occurrence of aplastic anemia and hepatic failure have limited its use (French et al., 1999). Topiramate is effective for Lennox-Gastaut syndrome (Sachdeo et al., 1999), and clobazam is approved for the adjunctive treatment in Lennox-Gastaut.

Status Epilepticus and Other Convulsive Emergencies

Status epilepticus is a neurological emergency. Mortality for adults approximates 20% (Lowenstein and Alldredge, 1998). The goal of treatment is rapid termination of behavioral and electrical seizure activity; the longer the episode of status epilepticus goes untreated, the more difficult it is to control and the greater the risk of permanent brain damage. Critical to the management are a clear plan, prompt treatment with effective drugs in adequate doses, and attention to hypoventilation and hypotension. Because hypoventilation may result from high doses of drugs used for treatment, it may be necessary to assist respiration temporarily.

To assess the optimal initial drug regimen, four intravenous treatments have been compared: diazepam followed by phenytoin; lorazepam; phenobarbital; and phenytoin alone (Treiman et al., 1998). The treatments had similar efficacies, with success rates ranging from 44% to 65%. Lorazepam alone was significantly better than phenytoin alone. No significant differences were found with respect to recurrences or adverse reactions. The more recent RAMPART trial indicated that midazolam (intramuscular) is as effective as intravenous lorazepam and was not associated with respiratory distress or seizure recurrence. Thus, emergency treatment with midazolam (intramuscular) may prove to be the preferred treatment prior to arrival to the hospital.

Antiseizure Therapy and Pregnancy

Use of ASDs has diverse implications of great importance for the health of women. Issues include interactions with oral contraceptives, potential teratogenic effects, and effects on vitamin K metabolism in pregnant women (Pack, 2006). Guidelines for the care of women with epilepsy have been published by the American Academy of Neurology (Morrell, 1998).

The effectiveness of oral contraceptives appears to be reduced by concomitant use of ASDs. The failure rate of oral contraceptives is 3.1/100 years in women receiving ASDs compared to a rate of 0.7/100 years in nonepileptic controls. One attractive explanation of the increased failure rate is the increased rate of oral contraceptive metabolism caused by ASDs that induce hepatic enzymes (Table 17–2); particular caution is needed with ASDs that induce CYP3A4.

Teratogenicity

Epidemiological evidence suggests that ASDs have teratogenic effects (Pack, 2006). These teratogenic effects add to the deleterious consequences of oral contraceptive failure. Infants of epileptic mothers are at 2-fold greater risk of major congenital malformations than offspring of nonepileptic mothers (4%–8% compared to 2%–4%). These malformations include congenital heart defects, neural tube defects, cleft lip, cleft palate, and others. Inferring causality from the associations found in large epidemiological studies with many uncontrolled variables can be hazardous, but a causal role for ASDs is suggested by association of congenital defects with higher concentrations of a drug or with polytherapy compared to monotherapy. Phenytoin, carbamazepine, valproate, lamotrigine, and phenobarbital all have been associated with teratogenic effects. Newer ASDs have teratogenic effects in animals, but whether such effects occur in humans is yet uncertain.

One consideration for a woman with epilepsy who wishes to become pregnant is a trial free of ASDs; monotherapy with careful attention to drug levels is another alternative. Polytherapy with toxic levels should be avoided. Folate supplementation (0.4 mg/d) has been recommended by the U.S. Public Health Service for all women of childbearing age to reduce the likelihood of neural tube defects, and this is appropriate for epileptic women as well.

The ASDs that induce CYPs have been associated with vitamin K deficiency in the newborn, which can result in a coagulopathy and intracerebral hemorrhage. Treatment with vitamin K_1, 10 mg/d during the last month of gestation, has been recommended for prophylaxis.

Drug Facts for Your Personal Formulary: *Antiseizure Agents*

Drugs	Therapeutic Uses (Seizure Types)	Clinical Pharmacology and Tips
Sodium Channel Modulators • Enhance fast inactivation		
Phenytoin	*Focal* • Aware • With impaired awareness *Generalized* • Tonic-clonic	• Once-daily dosing only available with extended-release formulation • Intravenous use with fosphenytoin • Nonlinear pharmacokinetics • May interfere with drugs metabolized by CYP2C9/19 • Induces CYPs (e.g., CYP3A4) • *Side effects*: gingival hyperplasia, facial coarsening; hypersensitivity (rare)
Carbamazepine	*Focal* • Aware • With impaired awareness • Focal to bilateral tonic-clonic *Generalized* • Tonic-clonic	• Induces CYP enzymes (e.g., CYP2C, CYP3A) and UGT • Active metabolite (10,11-epoxide) • *Side effects*: drowsiness, vertigo, ataxia, blurred vision, increased seizure frequency
Eslicarbazepine	*Focal* • Aware • With impaired awareness	
Lamotrigine	*Focal* • Aware • With impaired awareness *Generalized* • Absence • Tonic-clonic	• Reduced half-life in the presence of phenytoin, carbamazepine, or phenobarbital • Increased concentration in the presence of valproate • Also used in Lennox-Gastaut syndrome
Oxcarbazepine	*Focal* • Aware • With impaired awareness	• Prodrug, metabolized to eslicarbazepine • Short half-life • Less-potent enzyme induction (vs. carbamazepine) • *Side effects:* lower incidence of hypersensitivity reactions (vs. carbamazepine)
Rufinamide	*Focal* • Aware • With impaired awareness	• Can be used in Lennox-Gastaut syndrome
Sodium Channel Modulators • Enhance slow inactivation		
Lacosamide	*Focal* • Aware • With impaired awareness	
Calcium Channel Blockers • Block T-type calcium channels		
Ethosuximide	*Generalized* • Absence	• *Side effects*: gastrointestinal complaints, drowsiness, lethargy, dizziness, headache, hypersensitivity/skin reactions • Titration can reduce side-effect occurrence
Zonisamide	*Focal* • Aware • With impaired awareness	• *Side effects*: somnolence, ataxia, anorexia, fatigue
Calcium Channel Modulators • α2δ ligands		
Gabapentin	*Focal* • Aware • With impaired awareness	• *Side effects*: somnolence, dizziness, ataxia, fatigue
Pregabalin	*Focal* • Aware • With impaired awareness	• *Side effects: dizziness, somnolence* • Linear pharmacokinetics • Low potential for drug-drug interactions
GABA-Enhancing Drugs • GABA$_A$ receptor allosteric modulators (benzodiazepines, barbiturates)		
Clonazepam	*Generalized* • Absence • Myoclonic	• *Side effects*: drowsiness, lethargy, behavioral disturbances • Abrupt withdrawal can facilitate seizures • Tolerance to antiseizure effects
Clobazam	*Lennox-Gastaut syndrome* *Generalized* • Atonic • Tonic • Myoclonic	• *N*-Desmethyl-clobazam, clobazam's active metabolite, is increased in patients with poor CYP2C19 metabolism • *Side effects:* somnolence, sedation • Tapered withdrawal recommended

Drug Facts for Your Personal Formulary: *Antiseizure Agents (continued)*

Drugs	Therapeutic Uses (Seizure Types)	Clinical Pharmacology and Tips
GABA-Enhancing Drugs · GABA$_A$ receptor allosteric modulators (benzodiazepines, barbiturates) (continued)		
Diazepam	*Status epilepticus*	• Short duration of action • *Side effects*: drowsiness, lethargy, behavioral disturbances • Abrupt withdrawal can facilitate seizures • Tolerance to antiseizure effects
Phenobarbital	*Focal* • Focal to bilateral tonic-clonic *Generalized* • Tonic-clonic	• Induces CYPs (e.g., CYP3A4) and UGT • *Side effects*: sedation, nystagmus, ataxia; irritability and hyperactivity (children); agitation and confusion (elderly); allergy, hypersensitivity (rare)
Primidone	*Focal* • Focal to bilateral tonic-clonic *Generalized* • Tonic-clonic	• Induces CYP enzymes (e.g., CYP3A4) • Not commonly used
GABA-Enhancing Drugs · GABA uptake/GABA transaminase inhibitors		
Tiagabine	*Focal* • Aware • With impaired awareness	• Metabolized by CYP3A • *Side effects*: dizziness, somnolence, tremor
Stiripentol	*Generalized* • Tonic-clonic (Dravet syndrome)	• Used in Dravet syndrome • Inhibits CYP3A4/2C19
Vigabatrin	*Focal* • With impaired awareness	• Used in infantile spasms, especially when caused by tuberous sclerosis • *Side effects*: can cause progressive and bilateral vision loss
Glutamate Receptor Antagonists · AMPA receptor antagonists		
Perampanel	*Focal* • Aware • With impaired awareness	• Metabolized by CYP3A • *Side effects*: anxiety, confusion, imbalance, visual disturbance, aggressive behavior, suicidal thoughts
Potassium Channel Modulators · KCNQ2-5–positive allosteric modulator		
Ezogabine	*Focal* • Aware • With impaired awareness	• *Side effects*: blue pigmentation of skin and lips, dizziness, somnolence, fatigue, vertigo, tremor, attention disruption, memory impairment, retinal abnormalities, urinary retention, QT prolongation (rare)
Synaptic Vesicle 2A Modulators		
Levetiracetam	*Focal* • Aware • With impaired awareness *Generalized* • Myoclonic • Tonic-clonic	• *Side effects*: somnolence, asthenia, ataxia, dizziness, mood changes
Brivaracetam	*Focal* • Aware • With impaired awareness	
Mixed Mechanisms of Action		
Topiramate	*Focal* • Aware • With impaired awareness *Generalized* • Tonic-clonic	• Used in Lennox-Gastaut syndrome • *Side effects*: somnolence, fatigue, cognitive impairment
Valproate	*Focal* • Aware • With impaired awareness • Focal to bilateral tonic-clonic *Generalized* • Absence • Myoclonic • Tonic-clonic	• *Side effects*: transient gastrointestinal symptoms, sedation, ataxia, tremor, hepatitis (rare) • Inhibits CYP2C9, UGT

Acknowledgment: James O. McNamara contributed to this chapter in recent editions of this book. We have retained some of his text in the current edition.

Bibliography

Andermann E, et al. Seizure control with levetiracetam in juvenile myoclonic epilepsies. *Epilepsia*, **2005**, 46(suppl 8):205.

Aneja S, Sharma S. Newer anti-epileptic drugs. *Indian Pedatr*, **2013**, 50: 1033–1040.

Appleton RE, et al. Randomised, placebo-controlled study of vigabatrin as first-line treatment of infantile spasms. *Epilepsia*, **1999**, 40:1627–1633.

Bartholome O, et al. Puzzling out synaptic vesicle 2 family members functions. *Front Mol Neurosci*, **2017**, 10:148(1–15).

Bazil CW, Pedley TA. Advances in the medical treatment of epilepsy. *Annu Rev Med*, **1998**, 49:135–162.

Ben-Menachem E. Mechanism of action of vigabatrin: correcting misperceptions. *Acta Neurol Scand Suppl*, **2011**, 192:5–15.

Bialer M, White HS. Key factors in the discovery and development of new antiepileptic drugs. *Nat Rev Drug Disc*, **2010**, 9:68–82.

Biton V, et al. A randomized, placebo-controlled study of topiramate in primary generalized tonic-clonic seizures: Topiramate YTC Study Group. *Neurology*, **1999**, 52:1330–1337.

Brodie MJ, et al. Double-blind comparison of lamotrigine and carbamazepine in newly diagnosed epilepsy. UK Lamotrigine/ Carbamazepine Monotherapy Trial Group. *Lancet*, **1995**, 345:476–479.

Cai K, et al. The impact of gabapentin administration of brain GABA and glutamate concentrations: a 7T ^{1}H-MRS study. *Neuropsychopharmacology*, **2012**, 37:2764–2771.

Chadwick DW, et al. A double-blind trial of gabapentin monotherapy for newly diagnosed partial seizures: International Gabapentin Monotherapy Study Group 945–77. *Neurology*, **1998**, 51:1282–1288.

Chiron C, et al. Stiripentol in severe myoclonic epilepsy in infancy: a randomized placebo-controlled syndrome-dedicated trial, STICLO study group. *Lancet*, **2000**, 356:1638–1642.

Coulter DA, et al. Characterization of ethosuximide reduction of low-threshold calcium current in thalamic neurons. *Ann Neurol*, **1989**, 25:582–593.

Dreifuss FE, et al. Valproic acid hepatic fatalies. II. U.S. experience since 1984. *Neurology*, **1989**, 39:201–207.

EpiPM Consortium. A roadmap for precision medicine in the epilepsies. *Lancet Neurol*, **2015**, 14:1219–1228

Farwell JR, et al. Phenobarbital for febrile seizures—effects on intelligence and on seizure recurrence. *N Engl J Med*, **1990**, 322:364–369.

Felbamate Study Group in Lennox-Gastaut Syndrome. Efficacy of felbamate in childhood epileptic encephalopathy (Lennox-Gastaut Syndrome). *N Engl J Med*, **1993**, 328:29–33.

Field MJ, et al. Identification of the α_2-δ-1 subunit of voltage-dependent calcium channels as a molecular target for pain mediating the analgesic actions of pregabalin. *Proc Natl Acad Sci USA*, **2006**, 103: 17537–17542.

Fisher JL. The effects of stiripentol on GABA(A) receptors. *Epilepsia*, **2011**, 52(suppl 2):76–78.

Fisher RJ, et al. Operational classification of seizure types by the International League Against Epilepsy. *Epilepsia*, **2017**, 58:522–530.

Frank LM, et al. Lamictal (lamotrigine) monotherapy for typical absence seizure in children. *Epilepsia*, **1999**, 40:973–979.

Freeman JM. The best medicine for febrile seizures. *N Engl J Med*, **1992**, 327:1161–1163.

French JA, et al. Efficacy and tolerability of new antiepilepitic drugs. I. Treatment of new-onset epilepsy: report of the TTA and QSS subcommittees of the American Academy of Neurology and American Epilepsy Society. *Neurology*, **2004a**, 62:1252–1260.

French JA, et al. Efficacy and tolerability of the new antiepileptic drugs. II. Treatment of refractory epilepsy: report of the TTA and QSS subcommittees of the American Academy of Neurology and the American Epilepsy Society. *Neurology*, **2004b**, 62:1261–1273.

French JA, et al. Dose-response trial of pregabalin adjunctive therapy in patiens with partial seizures. *Neurology*, **2003**, 60:1631–1637.

French JA, Pedley TA. Initial management of epilepsy. *N Engl J Med*, **2008**, 359:166–176.

French J, et al. Practice advisory: the use of felbamate in the treatment of patients with intractable epilepsy. Report of the Quality Standards Subcommittee of the American Academy of Neurology and the American Epilepsy Society. *Neurology*, **1999**, 52:1540–1545.

Gee NS, et al. The novel anticonvulsant drug, gabapentin (Neurontin) binds to the 2 subunit of a calcium channel. *J Biol Chem*, **1996**, 271:5768–5776.

Hanada T, et al. Perampanel: a novel, orally active, noncompetitive AMPA-receptor antagonist that reduces seizure activity in rodent models of epilepsy. *Epilepsia*, **2011**, 52:1331–1340.

Huguenard JR, McCormick DA. Thalamic synchrony and dynamic regulation of global forebrain oscillations. *Trends Neurosci*, **2007**, 30:350–356.

Inoue Y, et al. Stiripentol open study in Japanese patients with Dravet syndrome. *Epilepsia*, **2009**, 50:2362–2368.

Kelly KM, et al. Valproic acid selectively reduces the low-threshold (T) calcium current in rat nodose neurons. *Neurosci Lett*, **1990**, 116:233–238.

Kenda BM, et al. Discovery of 4-substituted pyrrolidone butanamides as new agents with significant antiepileptic activity. *J Med Chem*, **2004**, 47:530–549.

Kwan P, Brodie MJ. Early identification of refractory epilepsy. *N Engl J Med*, **2000**, 342:314–319.

Larsson OM, et al. Mutual inhibition kinetic analysis of gamma-aminobutyric acid, taurine, and beta-alanine high-affinity transport into neurons and astrocytes: evidence for similarity between the taurine and beta-alanine carriers in both cell types. *J Neurochem*, **1986**, 47:426–432.

Lowenstein DH, Alldredge BK. Status epilepticus. *N Engl J Med*, **1998**, 338:970–976.

Macdonald RL, Greenfield LJ Jr. Mechanisms of action of new antiepileptic drugs. *Curr Opin Neurol*, **1997**, 10:121–128.

Madeo M, et al. The human synaptic vesicle protein, SV2A, functions as a galactose transporter in Saccharomyces cerevisiae. *J Biol Chem*, **2014**, 289:33066–33071.

Matagne A, et al. Anti-convulsive and anti-epileptic properties of brivaracetam (ucb 34714), a high-affinity ligand for the synaptic vesicle protein, SV2A. *Br J Pharmacol*, **2008**, 154:1662–1671.

Mattson RH, et al. A comparison of valproate with carbamazepine for the treatment of complex partial seizures and secondarily generalized tonic-clonic seizures in adults. The Department of Veterans Affairs Epilepsy Cooperative Study No. 264 Group. *N Engl J Med*, **1992**, 327:765–771.

Mattson RH, et al. Comparison of carbamazepine, phenobarbital, phenytoin, and primidone in partial and secondarily generalized tonic-clonic seizures. *N Engl J Med*, **1985**, 313:145–151.

McLean MJ, Macdonald RL. Carbamazepine and 10,11-epoxycarbamazepine produce use- and voltage-dependent limitation of rapidly firing action potentials of mouse central neurons in cell culture. *J Pharmacol Exp Ther*, **1986a**, 238:727–738.

McLean MJ, Macdonald RL. Sodium valproate, but not ethosuximide, produces use- and voltage-dependent limitation of high-frequency repetitive firing of action potentials of mouse central neurons in cell culture. *J Pharmacol Exp Ther*, **1986b**, 237:1001–1011.

McNamara JO. Cellular and molecular basis of epilepsy. *J Neurosci*, **1994**, 14:3413–3425.

Mikati MA, Browne TR. Comparative efficacy of antiepileptic drugs. *Clin Neuropharmacol*, **1988**, 11:130–140.

Miller NR, et al. Visual dysfunction in patients receiving vigabatrin: clinical and electrophysiologic findings. *Neurology*, **1999**, 53:2082–2087.

Morrell MJ. Guidelines for the care of women with epilepsy. *Neurology*, **1998**, 51:S21–S27.

Motte J, et al. Lamotrigine for generalized seizures associated with the Lennox-Gastaut syndrome. Lamictal Lennox-Gastaut Study Group. *N Engl J Med*, **1997**, 337:1807–1812.

Nabbout R, Chiron C. Stiripentol: an example of antiepileptic drug development in childhood epilepsies. *Eur J Pediatr Neurol*, **2012**, 16: S13–S17.

Namba T, et al. Antiepileptogenic and anticonvulsant effects of NBQX, a selective AMPA receptor antagonist, in the rat kindling model of epilepsy. *Brain Res*, **1994**, 638:36–44.

Ohno Y, Tokudome K. Therapeutic role of synaptic vesicle glycoprotein 2A (SV2A) in modulating epileptogenesis. *CNS Neurol Disord Drug Targets*, **2017**, DOI: 10.2174/1871527316666170404115027. Accessed July 14, 2017.

Pack AM. Therapy insight: clinical management of pregnant women with epilepsy. *Nat Clin Prac Neurol*, **2006**, 2:190–200.

Perez J, et al. Stiripentol: efficacy and tolerability in children with epilepsy. *Epilepsia*, **1999**, 40:1618–1626.

Plosker GL. Stiripentol: in severe myoclonic epilepsy of infancy (Dravet syndrome). *CNS Drugs*, **2012**, 26:993–1001.

Porter RJ, et al. Mechanisms of action of antiseizure drugs. *Handb Clin Neurol*, **2012**, 108:663–681.

Privitera MD, et al. Topiramate, carbamazepine and valproate monotherapy: double-blind comparison in newly diagnosed epilepsy. *Acta Neurol Scand*, **2003**, 107:165–175.

Ptacek LJ, Fu YH. Channelopathies: episodic disorders of the nervous system. *Epilepsia*, **2001**, 42(suppl 5):35–43.

Quilichini PP, et al. Stiripentol, a putative antiepileptic drug, enhances the duration of opening of GABA-A receptor channels. *Epilepsia*, **2006**, 47:704–716.

Reid CA, et al. Mechanisms of human inherited epilepsies. *Prog Neurobiol*, **2009**, 87:41–57.

Rey E, et al. Stiripentol potentiates clobazam in childhood epilepsy: a pharmacological study. *Epilepsia*, **1999**, 40:112–113.

Rho JM, et al. Mechanism of action of the anticonvulsant felbamate: opposing effects on N-methyl-D-aspartate and GABA$_A$ receptors. *Ann Neurol*, **1994**, 35:229–234.

Rogawski MA, Bazil CW. New molecular targets for antiepileptic drugs: alpha(2)delta, SV2A, and K$_v$7/KCNQ/M potassium channels. *Curr Neurol Neurosci Rep*, **2008**, 8:345–352.

Rogawski MA, Donevan SD. AMPA receptors in epilepsy and as targets for antiepileptic drugs. *Adv Neurol*, **1999**, 79:947–963.

Rogawski MA, Löscher W. The neurobiology of antiepileptic drugs. *Nat Rev Neurosci*, **2004**, 5:553–564.

Sachdeo RC, et al. A double-blind, randomized trial of topiramate in Lennox-Gastaut syndrome: Topiramate YL Study Group. *Neurology*, **1999**, 52:1882–1887.

Sachdeo RC, et al. Felbamate monotherapy: controlled trial in patients with partial onset seizures. *Ann Neurol*, **1992**, 32:386–392.

Sachdeo RC, et al. Tiagabine therapy for complex partial seizures: a dose-frequency study. The Tiagabine Study Group. *Arch Neurol*, **1997**, 54:595–601.

Sivenius J, et al. Double-blind study of gabapentin in the treatment of partial seizures. *Epilepsia*, **1991**, 32:539–542.

Steiner TJ, et al. Lamotrigine mono-therapy in newly diagnosed untreated epilepsy: a double-blind comparison with phenytoin. *Epilepsia*, **1999**, 40:601–607.

Stephen LJ, Brodie MJ. Pharmacotherapy of epilepsy: newly approved and developmental agents. *CNS Drugs*, **2011**, 25:89–107.

Tortorella A, et al. A crucial role of the alpha-amino-3-hydroxy-5-methylisoxazole-4-propionic acid subtype of glutamate receptors in piriform and perirhinal cortex for the initiation and propagation of limbic motor seizures. *J Pharmacol Exp Ther*, **1997**, 280:1401–1405.

Traynelis SF, Dingledine R. Potassium-induced spontaneous electrographic seizures in the rat hippocampal slice. *J Neurophysiol*, **1988**, 59:259–276.

Treiman DM, et al. A comparison of four treatments for generalized convulsive status epilepticus. Veterans Affairs Status Epilepticus Cooperative Study Group. *N Engl J Med*, **1998**, 339:792–798.

Twyman RE, et al. Differential regulation of γ-aminobutyric acid receptor channels by diazepam and phenobarbital. *Ann Neurol*, **1989**, 25:213–220.

VanLandingham KE, et al. Magnetic resonance imaging evidence of hippocampal injury after prolonged focal febrile convulsions. *Ann Neurol*, **1998**, 43:413–426.

Wallace RH, et al. Febrile seizures and generalized epilepsy associated with a mutation in the Na$^+$-channel β1 subunit gene *SCN1B*. *Nat Genet*, **1998**, 19:366–370.

Xie X, et al. Interaction of the antiepileptic drug lamotrigine with recombinant rat brain type IIA Na$^+$ channels and with native Na$^+$ channels in rat hippocampal neurons. *Pflugers Arch*, **1995**, 430:437–446.

Zona C1, et al. Brivaracetam (ucb 34714) inhibits Na(+) current in rat cortical neurons in culture. *Epilepsy Res*, **2010**, 88:46–54.

Chapter 18

Treatment of Central Nervous System Degenerative Disorders

Erik D. Roberson

Introduction to Neurodegenerative Disorders

Neurodegenerative disorders are characterized by progressive and irreversible loss of neurons from specific regions of the brain. Prototypical neurodegenerative disorders include PD and HD, where loss of neurons from structures of the basal ganglia results in abnormalities in the control of movement; AD, where the loss of hippocampal and cortical neurons leads to impairment of memory and cognitive ability; and ALS, where muscular weakness results from the degeneration of spinal, bulbar, and cortical motor neurons. Currently available therapies for neurodegenerative disorders alleviate the disease symptoms but do not alter the underlying neurodegenerative process.

Common Features of Neurodegenerative Disorders

Proteinopathies

Each of the major neurodegenerative disorders is characterized by accumulation of particular proteins in cellular aggregates: α-synuclein in PD; Aβ and the *microtubule-associated protein tau* in AD; *TDP-43* in most cases of ALS; and *huntingtin* in HD (Prusiner, 2013). The reason for accumulation of these proteins is unknown, and it is also unclear in most cases whether it is the large cellular aggregates or smaller soluble species of the proteins that most strongly drive pathogenesis.

Selective Vulnerability

A striking feature of neurodegenerative disorders is the exquisite specificity of the disease processes for particular types of neurons. For example, in PD there is extensive destruction of the dopaminergic neurons of the substantia nigra, whereas neurons in the cortex and many other areas of the brain are unaffected. In contrast, neural injury in AD is most severe in the hippocampus and neocortex, and even within the cortex, the loss of neurons is not uniform but varies dramatically in different brain networks. In HD, the mutant gene responsible for the disorder is expressed throughout the brain and in many other organs, yet the pathological changes are most prominent in the neostriatum. In ALS, there is loss of spinal motor neurons and the cortical neurons that provide their descending input. The diversity of these patterns of neural degeneration suggests that the process of neural injury results from the interaction of intrinsic properties of different neural circuits, genetics, and environmental influences. The intrinsic factors may include susceptibility to excitotoxic injury, regional variation in capacity for oxidative metabolism, and the production of toxic free radicals as by-products of cellular metabolism.

Genetics and Environment

Each of the major neurodegenerative disorders may be familial in nature. *HD is exclusively familial*; it is transmitted by autosomal dominant inheritance of an expanded repeat in the *huntingtin* gene. Nevertheless, environmental factors importantly influence the age of onset and rate of progression of HD symptoms. PD, AD, and ALS are usually sporadic, but for each there are well-recognized genetic forms. For example, there are both dominant (α-*synuclein, LRRK2*) and recessive (*parkin, DJ-1, PINK1*) gene mutations that may give rise to PD (Kumar et al., 2012; Singleton et al., 2013). In AD, mutations in the genes coding for APP and the *presenilins* (involved in APP processing) lead to inherited forms of the disease. About 10% of ALS cases are familial, most commonly due to mutations in the *C9ORF72* gene (Renton et al., 2014).

There are also genetic risk factors that influence the probability of disease onset and modify the phenotype. For example, the apoE genotype constitutes an important risk factor for AD. Three distinct isoforms of this protein exist, and individuals with even one copy of the high-risk allele, ε4, having several-fold higher risk of developing AD than those with the most common allele, ε3.

Environmental factors, including infectious agents, environmental toxins, and acquired brain injury, have been proposed in the etiology of neurodegenerative disorders. Traumatic brain injury has been suggested as a trigger for neurodegenerative disorders. At least one toxin, MPTP, can induce a condition closely resembling PD. More recently, evidence has linked pesticide exposure with PD. Exposure of soldiers to neurotoxic chemicals has been implicated in ALS (as part of "Gulf War syndrome").

Approaches to Therapy

Certain themes are apparent in the pharmacological approaches described in this chapter. Many of the existing therapies are *neurochemical*, aiming

Abbreviations

AADC: aromatic L-amino acid decarboxylase
Aβ: amyloid β
ACh: acetylcholine
AChE: acetylcholinesterase
AD: Alzheimer disease
ALDH: aldehyde dehydrogenase
ALS: amyotrophic lateral sclerosis
apoE: apolipoprotein E
APP: amyloid precursor protein
BuChE: butyrylcholinesterase
CNS: central nervous system
COMT: catechol-O-methyltransferase
DA: dopamine
DAT: DA transporter
DβH: dopamine-β-hydroxylase
DOPAC: 3,4-dihydroxyphenylacetic acid
GABA: γ-aminobutyric acid
Glu: glutamatergic
GPe: globus pallidus extern
GPi: globus pallidus interna
HD: Huntington disease
5HT: serotonin
HVA: homovanillic acid
MAO: monamine oxidase
MCI: mild cognitive impairment
MPTP: N-methyl-4-phenyl-1,2,3,6-tetrahydropyridine
3MT: 3-methoxyltyramine
NE: norepinephrine
NET: NE transporter
NMDA: N-methyl-D-aspartate
3-OMD: 3-O-methyl dopa
PD: Parkinson disease
PDD: Parkinson disease dementia
PET: positron emission tomography
PH: phenylalanine hydroxylase
REM: rapid eye movement
SNpc: substantia nigra pars compacta
SNpr: substantia nigra pars reticulate
SOD: superoxide dismutase
SSRI: selective serotonin reuptake inhibitor
STN: subthalamic nucleus
TAR: transactivation response element
TDP-43: TAR DNA-binding protein 43
TH: tyrosine hydrolase
VA/VL: ventroanterior and ventrolateral
VMAT2: vesicular monoamine transporter 2

to replace or compensate for damage to specific neurotransmitter systems that are selectively impaired. For example, dopaminergic therapy is a mainstay of PD therapy, and the primary agents used in AD aim to boost acetylcholinergic transmission. The goal of much current research is to identify therapies that are *neuroprotective* and can modify the underlying neurodegenerative process.

One target of neuroprotective therapies is *excitotoxicity, neural injury* that results from the presence of excess glutamate in the brain. *Glutamate* is used as a neurotransmitter to mediate most excitatory synaptic transmission in the mammalian brain. The presence of excessive amounts of glutamate can lead to excitotoxic cell death (see Figure 14–13). The destructive effects of glutamate are mediated by glutamate receptors, particularly those of the NMDA type (see Table 14–2). Excitotoxic injury

contributes to the neuronal death that occurs in acute processes such as stroke and head trauma. The role of excitotoxicity is less certain in the chronic neurodegenerative disorders; nevertheless, *glutamate antagonists* have been developed as neuroprotective therapies for neurodegeneration, with two such agents (*memantine* and *riluzole*, described later in the chapter) currently in clinical use.

Aging is the most important risk factor for all of the neurodegenerative diseases, and a likely contributor to the effect of age is the progressive impairment in the capacity of neurons for oxidative metabolism with consequent production of reactive compounds such as hydrogen peroxide and oxygen radicals. These reactive species can lead to DNA damage, peroxidation of membrane lipids, and neuronal death. This has led to pursuit of drugs that can enhance cellular metabolism (such as the mitochondrial cofactor coenzyme Q_{10}) and antioxidant strategies as treatments to prevent or retard degenerative diseases.

The discovery of specific proteins that accumulate and aggregate in each of the neurodegenerative disorders has opened the door to new therapeutic approaches. To date, there are no approved therapies that directly target the disease proteins (e.g., α-synuclein, Aβ, tau, TDP-43). However, there is intensive research to bring disease-modifying treatments that do directly target these proteins, such as passive immunotherapy with antibodies, into clinical care.

Parkinson Disease

Clinical Overview

Parkinsonism is a clinical syndrome with four cardinal features:

- Bradykinesia (slowness and poverty of movement)
- Muscular rigidity
- Resting tremor (which usually abates during voluntary movement)
- Impairment of postural balance, leading to disturbances of gait and to falling

The most common form of parkinsonism is idiopathic PD, first described by James Parkinson in 1817 as *paralysis agitans,* or the "shaking palsy." *The pathological hallmark of PD is the loss of the pigmented, dopaminergic neurons of the substantia nigra pars compacta, with the appearance of intracellular inclusions known as Lewy bodies.* The principal component of the Lewy bodies is aggregated α-synuclein (Goedert et al., 2013). A loss of 70%–80% of the DA-containing neurons accompanies symptomatic PD.

Without treatment, PD progresses over 5–10 years to a rigid, akinetic state in which patients are incapable of caring for themselves (Suchowersky et al., 2006). Death frequently results from complications of immobility, including aspiration pneumonia or pulmonary embolism. The availability of effective pharmacological treatment has radically altered the prognosis of PD; in most cases, good functional mobility can be maintained for many years. Life expectancy of adequately treated patients is increased substantially, but overall mortality remains higher than that of the general population.

While DA neuron loss is the most well-recognized feature of the disease, the disorder affects a wide range of other brain structures, including the brainstem, hippocampus, and cerebral cortex (Langston, 2006). There is increasing awareness of the "nonmotor" features of PD, which likely arise from pathology outside the DA system (Zesiewicz et al., 2010). Some nonmotor features may present before the characteristic motor symptoms: anosmia, or loss of the sense of smell; REM behavior disorder, a disorder of sleep with marked agitation and motion during periods of REM sleep; and disturbances of autonomic nervous system function, particularly constipation. Other nonmotor features are seen later in the disease and include depression, anxiety, and dementia.

Several disorders other than idiopathic PD also may produce parkinsonism, including some relatively rare neurodegenerative disorders, stroke, and intoxication with DA receptor antagonists. Drugs that may cause parkinsonism include antipsychotics such as haloperidol and chlorpromazine (see Chapter 16) and antiemetics such as prochlorperazine and metoclopramide (see Chapter 50). The distinction between idiopathic PD and other causes of parkinsonism is important because parkinsonism arising from other causes usually is refractory to all forms of treatment.

Pathophysiology

The dopaminergic deficit in PD arises from a loss of the neurons in the substantia nigra pars compacta that provide innervation to the striatum (caudate and putamen). The current understanding of the pathophysiology of PD is based on the finding that the striatal DA content is reduced in excess of 80%, with a parallel loss of neurons from the substantia nigra, suggesting that replacement of DA could restore function. We now have a model of the function of the basal ganglia that, while incomplete, is still useful.

Dopamine Synthesis, Metabolism, and Receptors

Dopamine, a catecholamine, is synthesized in the terminals of dopaminergic neurons from tyrosine and stored, released, reaccumulated, and metabolized by processes described in Chapter 13 and summarized in Figure 18–1. The actions of DA in the brain are mediated by the DA receptor, of which there are two broad classes, D1 and D2, with five distinct subtypes, D_1-D_5. All the DA receptors are GPCRs. Receptors of the **D1 group** (D_1 and D_5 subtypes) couple to G_s and thence to activation of the cyclic AMP pathway. The **D2 group** (D_2, D_3, and D_4 receptors) couple to G_i to reduce the adenylyl cyclase activity and voltage-gated Ca^{2+} currents while activating K^+ currents. Each of the five DA receptors has a distinct anatomical pattern of expression in the brain. D_1 and D_2 proteins are abundant in the striatum and are the most important receptor sites with regard to the causes and treatment of PD. The D_4 and D_5 proteins are largely extrastriatal, whereas D_3 expression is low in the caudate and putamen but more abundant in the nucleus accumbens and olfactory tubercle.

Neural Mechanism of Parkinsonism: A Model of Basal Ganglia Function

Considerable effort has been devoted to understanding how the loss of dopaminergic input to the neurons of the neostriatum gives rise to the clinical features of PD (Hornykiewicz, 1973). The basal ganglia can be viewed as a modulatory side loop that regulates the flow of information from the cerebral cortex to the motor neurons of the spinal cord (Albin et al., 1989) (Figure 18–2).

The neostriatum is the principal input structure of the basal ganglia and receives excitatory glutamatergic input from many areas of the cortex. Most neurons within the striatum are projection neurons that innervate other basal ganglia structures. A small but important subgroup of striatal neurons consists of interneurons that connect neurons within the striatum but do not project beyond its borders. ACh and neuropeptides are used as transmitters by these striatal interneurons.

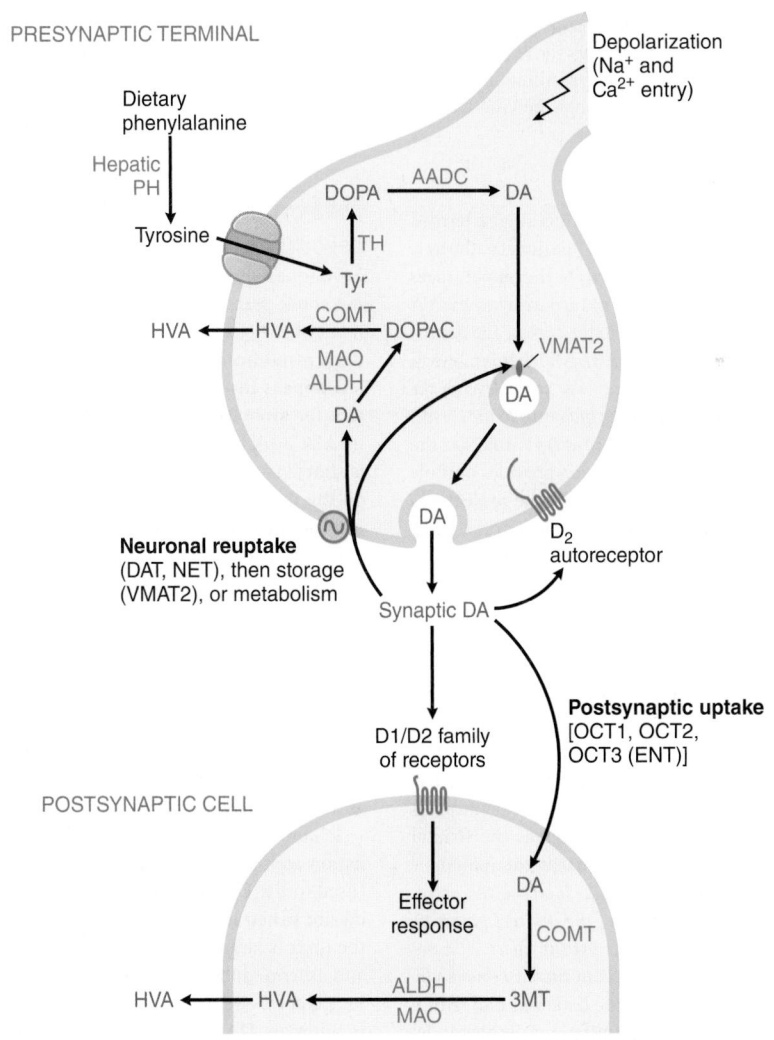

Figure 18–1 *Dopaminergic nerve terminal.* Dopamine is synthesized from tyrosine in the nerve terminal by the sequential actions of TH and AADC. DA is sequestered by VMAT2 in storage granules and released by exocytosis. Synaptic DA activates presynaptic autoreceptors and postsynaptic D1 and D2 receptors. Synaptic DA may be taken up into the neuron via the DA and NE transporters (DAT, NET) or removed by postsynaptic uptake via the organic cation transporter, OCT3 (see Chapter 5). Cytosolic DA is subject to degradation by MAO and ALDH in the neuron and by COMT and MAO/ALDH in nonneuronal cells; the final metabolic product is HVA. See structures in Figure 18–4.

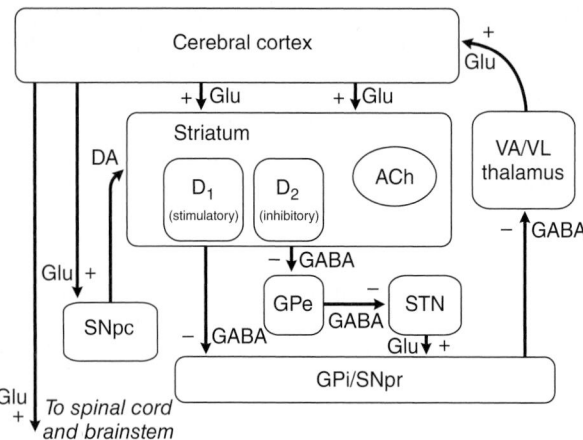

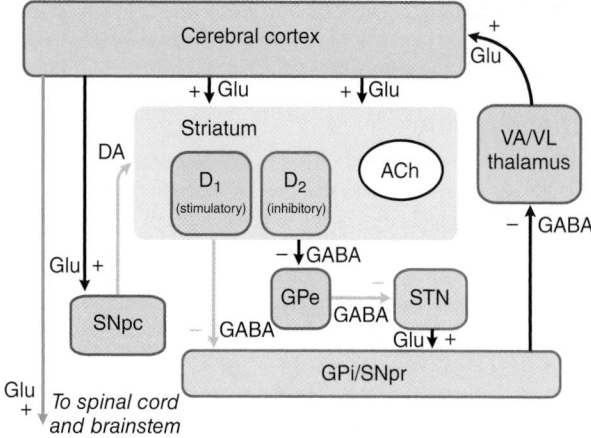

Figure 18–2 *Schematic wiring diagram of the basal ganglia.* The striatum is the principal input structure of the basal ganglia and receives excitatory glutamatergic input from many areas of cerebral cortex. The striatum contains projection neurons expressing predominantly D_1 or D_2 DA receptors, as well as interneurons that use ACh as a neurotransmitter. Outflow from the striatum proceeds along two routes. The direct pathway, from the striatum to the SNpr and GPi, uses the inhibitory transmitter GABA. The indirect pathway, from the striatum through the GPe and the STN to the SNpr and GPi, consists of two inhibitory GABA-ergic links and one excitatory Glu projection. The SNpc provides dopaminergic innervation to the striatal neurons, giving rise to both the direct and the indirect pathways, and it regulates the relative activity of these two paths. The SNpr and GPi are the output structures of the basal ganglia and provide feedback to the cerebral cortex through the VA/VL nuclei of the thalamus.

Figure 18–3 *The basal ganglia in PD.* The primary defect is destruction of the dopaminergic neurons of the SNpc. The striatal neurons that form the direct pathway from the striatum to the SNpr and GPi express primarily the *excitatory* D_1 DA receptor, whereas the striatal neurons that project to the GPe and form the indirect pathway express the *inhibitory* D_2 DA receptor. Thus, loss of the dopaminergic input to the striatum has a differential effect on the two outflow pathways; the direct pathway to the SNpr and GPi is less active (structures in purple), whereas the activity in the indirect pathway is increased (structures in red). The net effect is that neurons in the SNpr and GPi become more active. This leads to increased inhibition of the VA/VL thalamus and reduced excitatory input to the cortex. Light blue lines indicate primary pathways with reduced activity. (See Abbreviations list for definitions of anatomical abbreviations.)

The outflow of the striatum proceeds along two distinct routes, termed the *direct* and *indirect pathways* (Calabresi et al., 2014). The direct pathway is formed by neurons in the striatum that project directly to the output stages of the basal ganglia, the SNpr and the GPi; these, in turn, relay to the VA and VL thalamus, which provides excitatory input to the cortex. The neurotransmitter in both links of the direct pathway is GABA, which is inhibitory, so that *the net effect of stimulation of the direct pathway at the level of the striatum is to increase the excitatory outflow from the thalamus to the cortex.*

The indirect pathway is composed of striatal neurons that project to the GPe. This structure, in turn, innervates the STN, which provides outflow to the SNpr and GPi output stage. The first two links—the projections from striatum to GPe and GPe to STN—use the inhibitory transmitter GABA; however, the final link—the projection from STN to SNpr and GPi—is an excitatory glutamatergic pathway. Thus, *the net effect of stimulating the indirect pathway at the level of the striatum is to reduce the excitatory outflow from the thalamus to the cerebral cortex.* The key feature of this model of basal ganglia function, which accounts for the symptoms observed in PD as a result of loss of dopaminergic neurons, is the differential effect of DA on the direct and indirect pathways (Figure 18–3).

The dopaminergic neurons of the SNpc innervate all parts of the striatum; however, the target striatal neurons express distinct types of DA receptors. The striatal neurons giving rise to the direct pathway express primarily the *excitatory* D_1 DA receptor protein, whereas the striatal neurons forming the indirect pathway express primarily the *inhibitory* D_2 type. *Thus, DA released in the striatum tends to increase the activity of the direct pathway and reduce the activity of the indirect pathway, whereas the depletion that occurs in PD has the opposite effect. The net effect of the reduced dopaminergic input in PD is to increase markedly the inhibitory outflow from the SNpr and GPi to the thalamus and reduce excitation of the motor cortex.* There are several limitations of this model of basal ganglia function. The anatomical connections are considerably more complex, and many of the pathways involved use several neurotransmitters. Limitations notwithstanding, the model is useful and has important implications for the rational design and use of pharmacological agents in PD.

Treatment of Parkinson Disease

Levodopa

Levodopa (also called L-DOPA or L-3,4-dihydroxyphenylalanine), the metabolic precursor of DA, is the single most effective agent in the treatment of PD (Cotzias et al., 1969; Fahn et al., 2004). The effects of levodopa result from its decarboxylation to DA. When administered orally, levodopa is absorbed rapidly from the small bowel by the transport system for aromatic amino acids. Concentrations of the drug in plasma usually peak between 0.5 and 2 h after an oral dose. The $t_{1/2}$ in plasma is short (1–3 h). The rate and extent of absorption of levodopa depend on the rate of gastric emptying, the pH of gastric juice, and the length of time the drug is exposed to the degradative enzymes of the gastric and intestinal mucosa. Administration of levodopa with high-protein meals delays absorption and reduces peak plasma concentrations. *Entry of the drug into the CNS across the blood-brain barrier is mediated by a membrane transporter for aromatic amino acids.* In the brain, levodopa is converted to DA by decarboxylation primarily within the presynaptic terminals of dopaminergic neurons in the striatum. The DA produced is responsible for the therapeutic effectiveness of the drug in PD; after release, it is either transported back into dopaminergic terminals by the presynaptic uptake mechanism or metabolized by the actions of MAO and COMT (Figure 18–4).

In clinical practice, levodopa is almost always administered in combination with a peripherally acting inhibitor of AADC, such as *carbidopa* (used in the U.S.) or *benserazide* (available outside the U.S.), drugs that do not penetrate well into the CNS. If levodopa is administered alone, the drug is largely decarboxylated by enzymes in the intestinal mucosa and other peripheral sites so that relatively little unchanged drug reaches the cerebral circulation, and probably less than 1% penetrates the CNS. In addition, DA release into the circulation by peripheral conversion of levodopa produces undesirable effects, particularly nausea. Inhibition of peripheral decarboxylase markedly increases the fraction of administered levodopa that remains unmetabolized and available to cross the blood-brain barrier (Figure 18–5), and reduces the incidence of GI side effects and drug-induced orthostatic hypotension.

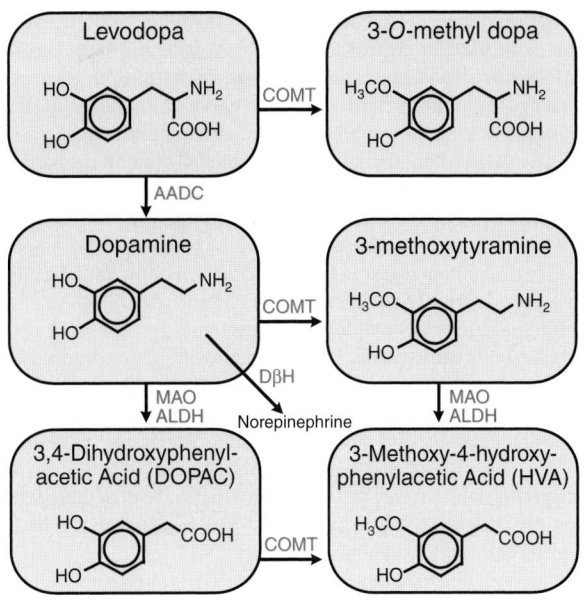

Figure 18–4 *Metabolism of levodopa (L-DOPA).*

A daily dose of 75 mg carbidopa is generally sufficient to prevent the development of nausea. For this reason, the most commonly prescribed form of carbidopa/levodopa is the 25/100 form, containing 25 mg carbidopa and 100 mg levodopa. With this formulation, dosage schedules of three or more tablets daily provide acceptable inhibition of decarboxylase in most individuals.

Levodopa therapy can have a dramatic effect on all the signs and symptoms of PD. Early in the course of the disease, the degree of improvement in tremor, rigidity, and bradykinesia produced by carbidopa/levodopa may be nearly complete. With long-term levodopa therapy, the "buffering" capacity is lost, and the patient's motor state may fluctuate dramatically with each dose of levodopa, producing the *motor complications* of levodopa (Pahwa et al., 2006).

A common problem is the development of the "wearing off" phenomenon: Each dose of levodopa effectively improves mobility for a period of time, perhaps 1–2 h, but rigidity and akinesia return rapidly at the end of the dosing interval. Increasing the dose and frequency of administration can improve this situation, but this often is limited by the development of dyskinesias, excessive and abnormal involuntary movements. In the later stages of PD, patients may fluctuate rapidly between being "off," having no beneficial effects from their medications, and being "on" but with disabling

dyskinesias (the *on/off phenomenon*). A sustained-release formulation consisting of carbidopa/levodopa in an erodable wax matrix is helpful in some cases, but absorption of this older sustained-release formulation is not entirely predictable.

Recently, two new formulations of levodopa intended to address wearing off have been approved. RYTARY carbidopa-levodopa extended-release capsules contain both immediate- and extended-release beads that provide reduced off time in patients with motor fluctuations (Hauser et al., 2013). DUOPA carbidopa-levodopa intestinal gel is administered through a gastrostomy tube into the jejunum using a pump and can have a dramatic effect on reducing "off" time (Olanow et al., 2014).

Does levodopa alter the course of the underlying disease or merely modify the symptoms? While the answer to this question is not entirely certain, a randomized trial has provided evidence that levodopa does not have an adverse effect on the course of the underlying disease, but has also confirmed that high doses of levodopa are associated with early onset of dyskinesias. Most practitioners have adopted a pragmatic approach, using levodopa only when the symptoms of PD cause functional impairment and other treatments are inadequate or not well tolerated.

A frequent and troubling adverse effect is the induction of hallucinations and confusion, especially in elderly patients or in patients with preexisting cognitive dysfunction. Conventional antipsychotic agents, such as the phenothiazines, are effective against levodopa-induced psychosis but may cause marked worsening of parkinsonism, probably through actions at the D_2 DA receptor, and should not be used in PD. An alternative approach has been to use "atypical" antipsychotic agents (see Chapter 16). The two drugs that are most effective and best tolerated in patients with advanced PD are clozapine and quetiapine. Both of these drugs, and others in the class, are associated with an increased rate of death due to stroke and other causes when used in the elderly. This risk needs to be weighed carefully against the risks created by hallucinations and psychosis.

Levodopa (and the DA agonists, described in the next section) may also lead to the development of "impulse control disorders" (Weintraub et al., 2015). These include compulsive behaviors, gambling, and hypersexuality and can be destructive socially. PD also appears to be associated with an increased risk of suicidality, but whether this is associated with the disease or a specific treatment is uncertain. Vigilance for signs of depression and suicidality should be practiced in all patients with PD.

Administration of levodopa with nonspecific inhibitors of MAO accentuates the actions of levodopa and may precipitate life-threatening hypertensive crisis and hyperpyrexia; nonspecific MAO inhibitors always should be discontinued at least 14 days before levodopa is administered (note that this prohibition does not include the MAO-B subtype-specific inhibitors selegiline and rasagiline). Abrupt withdrawal of levodopa or other dopaminergic medications may precipitate the *neuroleptic malignant syndrome* of confusion, rigidity, and hyperthermia, a potentially lethal adverse effect.

Dopamine Receptor Agonists

The DA receptor agonists in clinical use have durations of action substantially longer than that of levodopa; they are often used in the management of dose-related fluctuations in motor state and may be helpful in preventing motor complications (Parkinson Study Group, 2000). DA receptor agonists are proposed to have the potential to modify the course of PD by reducing endogenous release of DA as well as the need for exogenous levodopa, thereby reducing free-radical formation.

Two orally administered DA receptor agonists are commonly used for treatment of PD: *ropinirole* and *pramipexole*. Both are well absorbed orally and have similar therapeutic actions. There is also a transdermal formulation of the DA agonist *rotigotine* available. Ropinirole and pramipexole have selective activity at D2 class sites (specifically at the D_2 and D_3 receptor). Rotigotine acts at D2 sites and also has activity at D1 class sites. Like levodopa, these DA agonists can relieve the clinical symptoms of PD. The duration of action of the DA agonists (8–24 h) often is longer than that of levodopa (6–8 h), and they are particularly effective in the treatment of patients who have developed on/off phenomena. Both ropinirole and

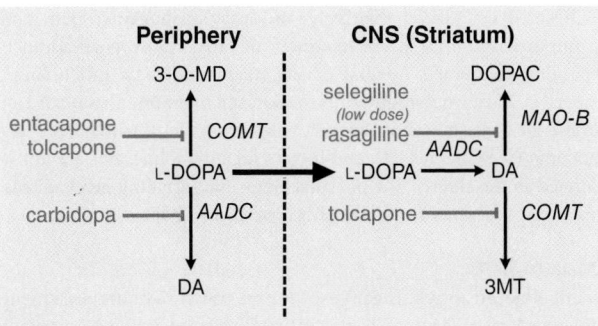

Figure 18–5 *Pharmacological preservation of levodopa (L-dopa) and striatal DA.* The principal site of action of inhibitors of COMT (e.g., tolcapone and entacapone) is in the peripheral circulation. They block the O-methylation of L-dopa and increase the fraction of the drug available for delivery to the brain. Tolcapone also has effects in the CNS. Inhibitors of MAO-B, such as low-dose selegiline and rasagiline, will act within the CNS to reduce oxidative deamination of DA, thereby enhancing vesicular stores.

pramipexole are also available in once-daily sustained-release formulations, which are more convenient and may reduce adverse effects related to intermittent dosing. The transdermal delivery of rotigotine produces stable plasma drug levels over 24 h.

Pramipexole, ropinirole, and rotigotine may produce hallucinosis or confusion, similar to that observed with levodopa, and may cause nausea and orthostatic hypotension. They should be initiated at low dose and titrated slowly to minimize these effects. The DA agonists, as well as levodopa itself, are also associated with fatigue and somnolence. Patients should be warned about the potential for sleepiness, especially while driving. Many practitioners prefer a DA agonist as initial therapy in younger patients to reduce the occurrence of motor complications. In older patients or those with substantial comorbidity, levodopa/carbidopa is generally better tolerated.

Apomorphine. Apomorphine is a dopaminergic agonist that can be administered by subcutaneous injection. It has high affinity for D_4 receptors; moderate affinity for D_2, D_3, D_5, and adrenergic α_{1D}, α_{2B}, and α_{2C} receptors; and low affinity for D_1 receptors. Apomorphine is FDA-approved as a "rescue therapy" for the acute intermittent treatment of "off" episodes in patients with a fluctuating response to dopaminergic therapy.

Apomorphine has the same side effects as the oral DA agonists. Apomorphine is highly emetogenic and requires pre- and posttreatment antiemetic therapy. Oral trimethobenzamide, at a dose of 300 mg, three times daily, should be started 3 days prior to the initial dose of apomorphine and continued at least during the first 2 months of therapy. Profound hypotension and loss of consciousness have occurred when apomorphine was administered with ondansetron; hence, the concomitant use of apomorphine with antiemetic drugs of the $5HT_3$ antagonist class is contraindicated. Other potentially serious side effects of apomorphine include QT prolongation, injection site reactions, and the development of a pattern of abuse characterized by increasingly frequent dosing leading to hallucinations, dyskinesia, and abnormal behavior.

Because of these potential adverse effects, use of apomorphine is appropriate only when other measures, such as oral DA agonists or COMT inhibitors, have failed to control the off episodes. Apomorphine therapy should be initiated with a 2-mg test dose in a setting where the patient can be monitored carefully. If tolerated, it can be titrated slowly up to a maximum dosage of 6 mg. For effective control of symptoms, patients may require three or more injections daily.

Catechol-O-Methyltransferase Inhibitors

Orally administered levodopa is largely converted by AADC to DA (see Figure 18–5), which causes nausea and hypotension. Addition of an AADC inhibitor such as carbidopa reduces the formation of DA but increases the fraction of levodopa that is methylated by COMT. COMT inhibitors block this peripheral conversion of levodopa to 3-O-methyl DOPA, increasing both the plasma $t_{1/2}$ of levodopa and the fraction of each dose that reaches the CNS.

The COMT inhibitors *tolcapone* and *entacapone* reduce significantly the "wearing off" symptoms in patients treated with levodopa/carbidopa (Parkinson Study Group, 1997). The two drugs differ in their pharmacokinetic properties and adverse effects: Tolcapone has a relatively long duration of action and appears to act by inhibition of both central and peripheral COMT. Entacapone has a short duration of action (2 h) and principally inhibits peripheral COMT. Common adverse effects of both agents include nausea, orthostatic hypotension, vivid dreams, confusion, and hallucinations. An important adverse effect associated with tolcapone is hepatotoxicity. At least three fatal cases of fulminant hepatic failure in patients taking tolcapone have been observed, leading to addition of a black-box warning to the label. Tolcapone should be used only in patients who have not responded to other therapies and with appropriate monitoring for hepatic injury.

Entacapone has not been associated with hepatotoxicity. Entacapone also is available in fixed-dose combinations with levodopa/carbidopa.

Selective MAO-B Inhibitors

Two isoenzymes of MAO oxidize catecholamines: MAO-A and MAO-B. MAO-B is the predominant form in the striatum and is responsible for most of the oxidative metabolism of DA in the brain. Selective MAO-B inhibitors are used for the treatment of PD: *selegiline* and *rasagiline*. These agents selectively and irreversibly inactivate MAO-B. Both agents exert modest beneficial effects on the symptoms of PD. The basis of this efficacy is, presumably, inhibition of breakdown of DA in the striatum.

Selective MAO-B inhibitors do not substantially inhibit the peripheral metabolism of catecholamines and can be taken safely with levodopa. These agents also do not exhibit the "cheese effect," the potentially lethal potentiation of catecholamine action observed when patients on nonspecific MAO inhibitors ingest indirectly acting sympathomimetic amines such as the tyramine found in certain cheeses and wine.

Selegiline is generally well tolerated in younger patients for symptomatic treatment of early or mild PD. In patients with more advanced PD or underlying cognitive impairment, selegiline may accentuate the adverse motor and cognitive effects of levodopa therapy. Metabolites of selegiline include amphetamine and methamphetamine, which may cause anxiety, insomnia, and other adverse symptoms. Selegiline is available in an orally disintegrating tablet as well as a transdermal patch. Both of these delivery routes are intended to reduce hepatic first-pass metabolism and limit the formation of the amphetamine metabolites.

Unlike selegiline, rasagiline does not give rise to undesirable amphetamine metabolites. Rasagiline monotherapy is effective in early PD. Adjunctive therapy with rasagiline significantly reduces levodopa-related wearing off symptoms in advanced PD (Olanow et al., 2008). Although selective MAO-B inhibitors are generally well tolerated, drug interactions can be troublesome. Similar to the nonspecific MAO inhibitors, selegiline can lead to the development of stupor, rigidity, agitation, and hyperthermia when administered with the analgesic meperidine. Although the mechanics of this interaction are uncertain, selegiline or rasagiline should not be given in combination with meperidine. Tramadol, methadone, propoxyphene dextromethorphan, St. John's wort, and cyclobenzaprine are also contraindicated with MAO-B inhibitors. Although development of the *serotonin syndrome* has been reported with coadministration of MAO-B inhibitors and antidepressants (tricyclic or serotonin reuptake inhibitors), this appears to be rare, and many patients are treated with this combination without difficulty. If concurrent treatment with MAO-B inhibitors and antidepressants is undertaken, close monitoring and use of low doses of the antidepressant are advisable (Panisset et al., 2014).

Muscarinic Receptor Antagonists

Antimuscarinic drugs currently used in the treatment of PD include *trihexyphenidyl* and *benztropine mesylate*, as well as the antihistaminic *diphenhydramine hydrochloride*, which also interacts at central muscarinic receptors. The biological basis for the therapeutic actions of muscarinic antagonists is not completely understood. They may act within the neostriatum through the receptors that normally mediate the response to intrinsic cholinergic innervation of this structure, which arises primarily from cholinergic striatal interneurons.

These drugs have relatively modest antiparkinsonian activity and are used only in the treatment of early PD or as an adjunct to dopamimetic therapy. Adverse effects result from their anticholinergic properties. Most troublesome are sedation and mental confusion. All anticholinergic drugs must be used with caution in patients with narrow-angle glaucoma (see Chapter 69), and in general anticholinergics are not well tolerated in the elderly. The pharmacology and signaling mechanisms of muscarinic receptors are thoroughly covered in Chapter 9.

Amantadine

Amantadine, an antiviral agent used for the prophylaxis and treatment of influenza A (see Chapter 62), has antiparkinsonian activity. Amantadine appears to alter DA release in the striatum, has anticholinergic properties, and blocks NMDA glutamate receptors. It is used as initial therapy of mild PD. It also may be helpful as an adjunct in patients on levodopa with dose-related fluctuations and dyskinesias. Amantadine is usually administered at a dose of 100 mg, twice per day, and is well tolerated. Dizziness, lethargy, anticholinergic effects, and sleep disturbance, as well as nausea and vomiting, side effects are mild and reversible.

Clinical Summary

Pharmacological treatment of PD should be tailored to the individual patient (Connolly and Lang, 2014). Drug therapy is not obligatory in early PD; many patients can be managed for a time with exercise and lifestyle interventions. For patients with mild symptoms, MAO-B inhibitors, amantadine, or (in younger patients) anticholinergics are reasonable choices. In most patients, treatment with a dopaminergic drug, either levodopa or a DA agonist, is eventually required. Many practitioners prefer a DA agonist as initial therapy in younger patients in an effort to reduce the occurrence of motor complications, although the evidence supporting this practice is inconclusive. In older patients or those with substantial comorbidity, levodopa/carbidopa is generally better tolerated.

Alzheimer Disease

Clinical Overview

The brain region most vulnerable to neuronal dysfunction and cell loss in AD is the medial temporal lobe, including entorhinal cortex and hippocampus. The proteins that accumulate in AD are Aβ and tau (Giacobini and Gold, 2013). AD has three major stages:

1. A "preclinical" stage during which accumulation of Aβ and tau begins, before any symptoms appear.
2. An MCI stage with episodic memory loss (repeated questions, misplaced items, etc.) that is not severe enough to impair daily function.
3. A dementia stage with progressive loss of functional abilities.

Death usually ensues within 6–12 years of onset, most often from a complication of immobility such as pneumonia or pulmonary embolism.

Diagnosis

Alzheimer disease remains a clinical diagnosis, based on the presence of memory impairment and other cognitive impairments that are insidious, progressive, and not well explained by another disorder. In recent years, there has been steady progress toward inclusion of biomarkers in the diagnostic criteria. This includes both *fluid biomarkers*, such as changes in Aβ and tau in the cerebrospinal fluid, and *imaging biomarkers*, such as hippocampal atrophy on structural magnetic resonance imaging and cortical hypometabolism on fluorodeoxyglucose PET scans. One of the most exciting advances is the ability to detect, using amyloid PET scans, Aβ deposition in patients. Three agents, *florbetapir, flutemetamol*, and *florbetaben*, are FDA-approved for determining whether individuals with cognitive impairment have Aβ deposition, which would suggest AD as a possible etiology. Similar agents for PET imaging of tau deposition are currently in development.

Genetics

Mutations in three genes have been identified as causes of autosomal dominant, early onset AD: *APP*, which encodes Aβ precursor protein, and *PSEN1* and *PSEN2*, encoding presenilin 1 and 2, respectively. All three genes are involved in the production of Aβ peptides. Aβ is generated by sequential proteolytic cleavage of APP by two enzymes, β-secretase and γ-secretase; the presenilins form the catalytic core of γ-secretase. The genetic evidence, combined with the fact that Aβ accumulates in the brain in the form of soluble oligomers and amyloid plaques and is toxic when applied to neurons, forms the basis for the amyloid hypothesis of AD pathogenesis. Many genes have been identified as having alleles that increase AD risk. By far the most important of these is *APOE*, which encodes the lipid carrier protein apoE. Individuals inheriting the ε4 allele of *APOE* have a 3-fold or more higher risk of developing AD. While these individuals make up less than one-fourth of the population, they account for more than half of all AD cases.

Pathophysiology

The pathological hallmarks of AD are amyloid plaques, which are extracellular accumulations of Aβ, and intracellular neurofibrillary tangles composed of the microtubule-associated protein tau. The development of amyloid plaques occurs earlier, and tangle burden accrues over time in a manner that correlates more closely with the development of cognitive impairment. In autosomal dominant AD, Aβ accumulates due to mutations that cause its overproduction. Aggregation of Aβ is an important event in AD pathogenesis. While plaques consist of highly ordered fibrils of Aβ, it appears that soluble Aβ oligomers, perhaps as small as dimers, are more highly pathogenic. Tau also aggregates to form the paired helical filaments that make up neurofibrillary tangles. Posttranslational modifications of tau, including phosphorylation, proteolysis, and other changes, increase tau's propensity to aggregate. Mechanisms by which Aβ and tau induce neuronal dysfunction and death may include direct impairment of synaptic transmission and plasticity, excitotoxicity, oxidative stress, and neuroinflammation.

Neurochemistry

The most striking neurochemical disturbance in AD is a *deficiency of ACh*. The anatomical basis of the cholinergic deficit is atrophy and degeneration of subcortical cholinergic neurons. The selective deficiency of ACh in AD and the observation that central cholinergic antagonists (e.g., atropine) can induce a confusional state resembling the dementia of AD have given rise to the "cholinergic hypothesis" that a deficiency of ACh is critical in the genesis of the symptoms of AD. AD, however, is complex and also involves multiple neurotransmitter systems, including glutamate, 5HT, and neuropeptides, and there is destruction of not only cholinergic neurons but also the cortical and hippocampal targets that receive cholinergic input.

Treatment

At present, no disease-modifying therapy for AD is available; current treatment is aimed at alleviating symptoms (Roberson and Mucke, 2006; Selkoe, 2013).

Treatment of Cognitive Symptoms

Augmentation of the cholinergic transmission is currently the mainstay of AD treatment. Three drugs, *donepezil, rivastigmine*, and *galantamine*, are widely used for this purpose (Table 18–1). All three are reversible antagonists of cholinesterases (see Chapter 10). Cholinesterase inhibitors are the usual first-line therapy for symptomatic treatment of cognitive impairments in mild or moderate AD. They are also widely used to treat other neurodegenerative diseases with cholinergic deficits, including dementia with Lewy bodies and vascular dementia. Their effect is generally modest, usually producing no dramatic improvement in symptoms but rather a 6- to 12-month delay in progression, after which clinical deterioration resumes. The drugs are usually well tolerated, with the most common side effects being GI distress, muscle cramping, and abnormal dreams. They should be used with caution in patients with bradycardia or syncope.

Memantine. Memantine is a noncompetitive antagonist of the NMDA-type glutamate receptor. It is used as either an adjunct or an alternative to cholinesterase inhibitors in AD, generally in later stages of dementia, as there is less evidence for its efficacy earlier. Memantine delays clinical deterioration in patients with moderate-to-severe AD dementia. Adverse effects of memantine include mild headache or dizziness. The drug is excreted by the kidneys, and dosage should be reduced in patients with severe renal impairment.

Treatment of Behavioral Symptoms

In addition to cognitive decline, behavioral and psychiatric symptoms in dementia (BPSD) are common, particularly in middle stages of the disease. These symptoms include irritability and agitation, paranoia and delusional thinking, wandering, anxiety, and depression. Treatment can be difficult, and nonpharmacological approaches should generally be first line.

A variety of pharmacological options are also available. Both cholinesterase inhibitors and memantine reduce some BPSD. However, their effects are modest, and they do not treat some of the most troublesome

TABLE 18–1 ■ CHOLINESTERASE INHIBITORS USED FOR THE TREATMENT OF ALZHEIMER DISEASE

	DONEPEZIL	RIVASTIGMINE	GALANTAMINE
Enzymes inhibited[a]	AChE	AChE, BuChE	AChE
Mechanism	Noncompetitive	Noncompetitive	Competitive
Typical maintenance dose[b]	10 mg once daily	9.5 mg/24 h (transdermal) 3–6 mg twice daily (oral)	8–12 mg twice daily (immediate release) 16–24 mg/d (extended release)
FDA-approved indications	Mild-severe AD	Mild-moderate AD Mild-moderate PDD	Mild-moderate AD
Metabolism[c]	CYP2D6, CYP3A4	Esterases	CYP2D6, CYP3A4

[a]AChE is the major cholinesterase in the brain; BuChE is a serum and hepatic cholinesterase that is upregulated in AD brain.
[b]Typical starting doses are one-half of the maintenance dose and are given for the first month of therapy.
[c]Drugs metabolized by CYP2D6 and CYP3A4 are subject to increased serum levels when coadministered with drugs known to inhibit these enzymes, such as ketoconazole and paroxetine.

symptoms, such as agitation. *Citalopram*, an SSRI (see Chapter 15), showed efficacy for agitation in a randomized clinical trial. Atypical antipsychotics, such as risperidone, olanzapine, and quetiapine (see Chapter 16) are perhaps even more efficacious for agitation and psychosis in AD, but their use is often limited by adverse effects, including parkinsonism, sedation, and falls. In addition, the use of atypical antipsychotics in elderly patients with dementia-related psychosis has been associated with a higher risk of stroke and overall mortality, leading to an FDA black-box warning (Schneider et al., 2005). Benzodiazepines (see Chapter 15) can be used for occasional control of acute agitation but are not recommended for long-term management because of their adverse effects on cognition and other risks in the elderly population. The typical antipsychotic haloperidol (see Chapter 16) may be useful for aggression, but sedation and extrapyramidal symptoms limit its use to control of acute episodes.

Clinical Summary

The typical patient with AD presenting in early stages of disease should probably be treated with a cholinesterase inhibitor. Patients and families should be counseled that a realistic goal of therapy is to induce a temporary reprieve from progression, or at least a reduction in the rate of decline, rather than long-term recovery of cognition. As the disease progresses, memantine can be added to the regimen. Behavioral symptoms are often treated with a serotonergic antidepressant or, if they are severe enough to warrant the risk of higher mortality, an atypical antipsychotic. Eliminating drugs likely to aggravate cognitive impairments, particularly anticholinergics, benzodiazepines, and other sedative/hypnotics, from the patient's regimen is another important aspect of AD pharmacotherapy.

Huntington Disease

Huntington disease is a dominantly inherited disorder characterized by the gradual onset of motor incoordination and cognitive decline in mid-life (Bates et al., 2015). Symptoms develop insidiously, as a movement disorder manifest by brief, jerk-like movements of the extremities, trunk, face, and neck (chorea), as personality changes, or both. Fine-motor incoordination and impairment of rapid eye movements are early features. As the disorder progresses, the involuntary movements become more severe, dysarthria and dysphagia develop, and balance is impaired. The cognitive disorder manifests first as slowness of mental processing and difficulty in organizing complex tasks. Memory is impaired, but affected persons rarely lose their memory of family, friends, and the immediate situation. Such persons often become irritable, anxious, and depressed. The outcome of HD is invariably fatal; over a course of 15–30 years, the affected person becomes totally disabled and unable to communicate, requiring full-time care; death ensues from the complications of immobility.

Pathology and Pathophysiology

Huntington disease is characterized by prominent neuronal loss in the striatum (caudate/putamen) of the brain. Atrophy of these structures proceeds in an orderly fashion, first affecting the tail of the caudate nucleus and then proceeding anteriorly from mediodorsal to VL. Other areas of the brain also are affected. Interneurons and afferent terminals are largely spared, whereas the striatal projection neurons (the medium spiny neurons) are severely affected. This leads to large decreases in striatal GABA concentrations, whereas somatostatin and DA concentrations are relatively preserved.

Selective vulnerability also appears to underlie the development of chorea. In most adult-onset cases, the medium spiny neurons that project to the GPi and SNpr (the indirect pathway) appear to be affected earlier than those projecting to the GPe (the direct pathway; see Figure 18–2). *The disproportionate impairment of the indirect pathway increases excitatory drive to the neocortex, producing involuntary choreiform movements* (Figure 18–6). In some individuals, rigidity rather than chorea is the predominant clinical feature; this is especially common in juvenile-onset

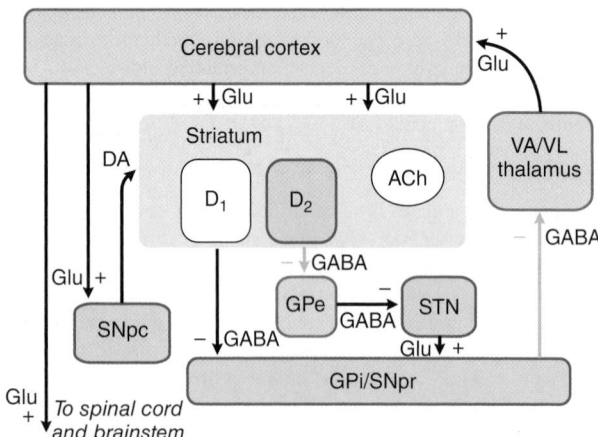

Figure 18–6 *The basal ganglia in Huntington disease.* HD is characterized by loss of neurons from the striatum. The neurons that project from the striatum to the GPe and form the indirect pathway are affected earlier in the course of the disease than those that project to the GPi. This leads to a loss of inhibition of the GPe. The increased activity in this structure, in turn, inhibits the STN, SNpr, and GPi, resulting in a loss of inhibition to the VA/VL thalamus and increased thalamocortical excitatory drive. Structures in purple have reduced activity in HD, whereas structures in red have increased activity. Light blue lines indicate primary pathways of reduced activity. (See Abbreviations list for definitions of anatomical abbreviations.)

cases. Here, the striatal neurons giving rise to both the direct and indirect pathways are impaired to a comparable degree.

Genetics

Huntington disease is an autosomal dominant disorder with nearly complete penetrance. The average age of onset is between 35 and 45 years, but the range varies from as early as age 2 to as late as the middle 80s. Although the disease is inherited equally from mother and father, more than 80% of those developing symptoms before age 20 inherit the defect from the father. Known homozygotes for HD show clinical characteristics identical to the typical HD heterozygote, indicating that the unaffected chromosome does not attenuate the disease symptomatology.

A region near the end of the short arm of chromosome 4 contains a polymorphic (CAG)$_n$ trinucleotide repeat that is significantly expanded in all individuals with HD. The expansion of this trinucleotide repeat is the genetic alteration responsible for HD. The range of CAG repeat length in normal individuals is between 9 and 34 triplets, with a median repeat length on normal chromosomes of 19. The repeat length in HD varies from 40 to over 100. Repeat length is correlated inversely with age of onset of HD. The younger the age of onset, the higher the probability of a large repeat number. The mechanism by which the expanded trinucleotide repeat leads to the clinical and pathological features of HD is unknown. The HD mutation lies within a large gene (10 kb) designated *HTT* (previously *IT15*) that encodes *huntingtin*, a protein of about 348,000 Da. The trinucleotide repeat, which encodes the amino acid glutamine, occurs at the 5′ end of HTT. Huntingtin does not resemble any other known protein.

Treatment

Symptomatic Treatment

None of the currently available medications slows the progression of the disease (Ross et al., 2014).

Tetrabenazine is used for the treatment of chorea associated with HD. Tetrabenazine and the related drug reserpine are inhibitors of VMAT2 and cause presynaptic depletion of catecholamines. Tetrabenazine is a reversible inhibitor; inhibition by reserpine is irreversible and may lead to long-lasting effects. Both drugs may cause hypotension and depression with suicidality; the shorter duration of effect of tetrabenazine simplifies clinical management. The recommended starting dose of tetrabenazine is 12.5 mg daily. Most patients can be managed with doses of 50 mg a day or less; however, tetrabenazine is extensively metabolized by CYP2D6. Genotyping for CYP2D6 may be needed to optimize therapy and is recommended for patients who require more than 50 mg daily. As might be expected with a drug that depletes DA stores, tetrabenazine can also cause parkinsonism. The recently approved deuterated tetrabenazine, *deutetrabenazine*, takes advantage of the stronger bonds that deuterium forms with carbon (the kinetic-isotope effect). The active deuterated dehydrometabolites are VMAT2 inhibitors with longer half-lives than the corresponding products of tetrabenazine metabolism. Deutetrabenazine has therapeutic uses and an adverse effect profile similar to those of tetrabenazine.

Symptomatic treatment is needed for patients who are depressed, irritable, paranoid, excessively anxious, or psychotic. Depression can be treated effectively with standard antidepressant drugs with the caveat that drugs with substantial anticholinergic profiles can exacerbate chorea. Fluoxetine (see Chapter 15) is effective treatment of both the depression and the irritability manifest in symptomatic HD. Carbamazepine (see Chapter 17) also has been found to be effective for the depression. Paranoia, delusional states, and psychosis are treated with antipsychotic drugs, usually at lower doses than those used in primary psychiatric disorders (see Chapter 16). These agents also reduce cognitive function and impair mobility and thus should be used in the lowest doses possible and should be discontinued when the psychiatric symptoms resolve. In individuals with predominantly rigid HD, clozapine, quetiapine (see Chapter 16), or carbamazepine may be more effective for treatment of paranoia and psychosis.

Many patients with HD exhibit worsening of involuntary movements as a result of anxiety or stress. In these situations, judicious use of sedative or anxiolytic benzodiazepines can be helpful. In juvenile-onset cases where rigidity rather than chorea predominates, DA agonists have had variable

success in the improvement of rigidity. These individuals also occasionally develop myoclonus and seizures that can be responsive to clonazepam, valproate, and other anticonvulsants (see Chapter 17).

Amyotrophic Lateral Sclerosis

Amyotrophic lateral sclerosis (ALS or Lou Gehrig disease) is a disorder of the motor neurons of the ventral horn of the spinal cord (lower motor neurons) and the cortical neurons that provide their afferent input (upper motor neurons) (Gordon, 2013). The disorder is characterized by rapidly progressive weakness, muscle atrophy and fasciculations, spasticity, dysarthria, dysphagia, and respiratory compromise. Many patients with ALS exhibit behavioral changes and cognitive dysfunction, and there is clinical, genetic, and neuropathological overlap between ALS and frontotemporal dementia spectrum disorders. ALS usually is progressive and fatal. Most patients die of respiratory compromise and pneumonia after 2–3 years, although some survive for many years.

Etiology

About 10% of ALS cases are familial (FALS), usually with an autosomal dominant pattern of inheritance. The most common genetic cause is a hexanucleotide repeat expansion in *C9ORF72*, which is responsible for up to 40% of FALS and around 5% of sporadic cases (Rohrer et al., 2015). Another 10% of FALS cases are due to mutations in the Cu/Zn SOD1. Mutations in the *TARDBP* gene encoding TDP-43 and in the *FUS/TLS* gene have been identified as causes of FALS. Both TDP-43 and FUS/TLS bind DNA and RNA and regulate transcription and alternative splicing. About 90% of ALS cases are sporadic. Of these, a few are caused by de novo mutations in *C9ORF72* (up to 7%), *SOD1*, *TDP-43*, *FUS/TLS*, or other genes, but for the majority of sporadic cases, the etiology remains unclear. The underlying pathophysiology remains under investigation, including roles for abnormal RNA processing, glutamate excitotoxicity, oxidative stress, and mitochondrial dysfunction.

Treatments

Riluzole

Riluzole (2-amino-6-[trifluoromethoxy] benzothiazole) is an agent with complex actions in the nervous system. Riluzole is absorbed orally and is highly protein bound. It undergoes extensive metabolism in the liver by CYP-mediated hydroxylation and glucuronidation. Its $t_{1/2}$ is about 12 h. In vitro studies showed that riluzole has both presynaptic and postsynaptic effects. It not only inhibits glutamate release, but also blocks postsynaptic NMDA- and kainate-type glutamate receptors and inhibits voltage-dependent Na$^+$ channels. The recommended dose is 50 mg twice daily, taken 1 h before or 2 h after a meal. Riluzole usually is well tolerated, although nausea or diarrhea may occur. Rarely, riluzole may produce hepatic injury with elevations of serum transaminases, and periodic monitoring of these is recommended. Meta-analyses of the available clinical trials indicated that riluzole extends survival by 2–3 months. Although the magnitude of the effect of riluzole on ALS is small, it represents a significant therapeutic milestone in the treatment of a disease refractory to all previous treatments (Miller et al., 2007).

Edaravone

Edaravone

Edaravone was approved by the FDA in 2017 for treatment of ALS, the first new drug approved for this indication since 1995. It is a small molecule with free radical scavenging properties that may reduce oxidative stress, although the exact mechanism of action is unknown. Edaravone has been used in Japan for acute stroke since 2001 and was approved by the FDA for ALS under an orphan drug designation. A phase 3 study showed no benefit, but after posthoc subgroup analyses suggested an effect in early ALS, a subsequent trial enrolling only early stage patients showed a smaller functional decline over 6 months in patients treated with edaravone. It is administered intravenously, with the first round daily for 14 days, followed by a 14 day holiday, then in subsequent cycles, 10 out of every 14 days followed by a 14-day holiday. The drug is metabolized to a glucuronide and a sulfate and excreted primarily in the urine as the glucuronide, yielding a terminal $t_{1/2}$ of 4.5-6 h. At clinical doses, edaravone is not expected to inhibit major CYPs, UGTs, or drug transporters, or to induce CYPs 1A2, 2B6, or 3A4; nor should inhibitors of these enzymes have substantial effects on the pharmacokinetics of edaravone. The infusion contains sodium bisulfite, which can cause hypersensitivity reactions. Other adverse effects include bruising, gait disorder, and headache.

Symptomatic Therapy of ALS: Spasticity

Spasticity is an important component of the clinical features of ALS and the feature most amenable to present forms of treatment. *Spasticity* is defined as an increase in muscle tone characterized by an initial resistance to passive movement of a joint, followed by a sudden relaxation (the so-called clasped-knife phenomenon). Spasticity results from loss of descending inputs to the spinal motor neurons, and the character of the spasticity depends on which nervous system pathways are affected.

Baclofen

The best agent for the symptomatic treatment of spasticity in ALS is baclofen, a $GABA_B$ receptor agonist (see Figure 14–10). Initial doses of 5–10 mg/d are recommended, which can be increased to as much as 200 mg/d, if necessary. Alternatively, baclofen can be delivered directly into the space around the spinal cord using a surgically implanted pump and an intrathecal catheter. This approach minimizes the adverse effects of the drug, especially sedation, but it carries the risk of potentially life-threatening CNS depression.

Tizanidine

Tizanidine is an agonist of α_2 adrenergic receptors in the CNS. It reduces muscle spasticity, probably by increasing presynaptic inhibition of motor neurons. Tizanidine is primarily used in the treatment of spasticity in multiple sclerosis or after stroke, but it also may be effective in patients with ALS. Treatment should be initiated at a low dose of 2–4 mg at bedtime and titrated upward gradually. Drowsiness, asthenia, and dizziness may limit the dose that can be administered.

Other Agents

Benzodiazepines (see Chapter 19) such as *clonazepam* are effective antispasticity agents, but they may contribute to respiratory depression in patients with advanced ALS.

Dantrolene, approved in the U.S. for the treatment of muscle spasm, *is not used* in ALS because it can exacerbate muscular weakness. Dantrolene acts directly on skeletal muscle fibers, impairing Ca^{2+} release from the sarcoplasmic reticulum. It is effective in treating spasticity associated with stroke or spinal cord injury and in treating malignant hyperthermia (see Chapter 11). Dantrolene may cause hepatotoxicity, so it is important to monitor liver-associated enzymes before and during therapy with the drug.

Acknowledgment: *David G. Standaert contributed to this chapter in recent editions of this book. We have retained some of his text in the current edition.*

Drug Facts for Your Personal Formulary: *Drugs for Neurodegenerative Disease*

Drugs	Therapeutic Uses	Clinical Pharmacology and Tips
Anti-Parkinson: L-DOPA (DA precursor); Carbidopa (inhibits AADC, reduces peripheral conversion of L-DOPA to DA)		
Carbidopa/levodopa	• Most effective symptomatic therapy for PD	• Therapeutic window narrows after several years of treatment: wearing off, dyskinesias, on/off phenomenon • Available as immediate-release tablets and orally disintegrated tablets
Carbidopa/levodopa sustained release	• Patients with PD with motor fluctuations on regular carbidopa/levodopa	• Bioavailability of immediate-release form, 75%
Carbidopa-levodopa extended-release capsules (RYTARY)	• Patients with PD with motor fluctuations on regular carbidopa/levodopa	• Mixture of immediate- and extended-release beads
Carbidopa-levodopa intestinal gel (DUOPA)	• Patients with PD with motor fluctuations on regular carbidopa/levodopa	• Requires placement of gastrostomy tube with jejunal extension • Useful for wearing off issues
Anti-Parkinson: DA agonists (longer acting than L-DOPA; can produce psychosis, impulse control disorder, sleepiness)		
Ropinirole	• PD • Restless legs syndrome	• Selective D2 receptor class agonist • Available in immediate release (3 times daily) and sustained release (once daily)
Pramipexole	• PD • Restless legs syndrome	• Selective D2 receptor class agonist • Available in immediate release (3 times daily) and sustained release (once daily)
Rotigotine	• PD • Restless legs syndrome	• D2 and D1 receptor class agonist • Transdermal formulation
Apomorphine	• Rescue therapy for acute intermittent treatment of off episodes	• Subcutaneous formulation • Emetogenic, requires concurrent antiemetic • Contraindicated with 5HT$_3$ antagonists
Anti-Parkinson: COMT Inhibitors (reduce peripheral conversion of levodopa, increasing $t_{1/2}$ and CNS dose)		
Entacapone	• Adjunctive PD therapy given with each dose of levodopa, for wearing off	• Short $t_{1/2}$, inhibits peripheral COMT
Tolcapone	• Adjunctive PD therapy given with each dose of levodopa, for wearing off	• Long $t_{1/2}$, inhibits central and peripheral COMT • May be hepatotoxic; use only in patients not responding satisfactorily to other treatments; monitor liver function
Carbidopa/levodopa/ entacapone	• PD, especially for wearing off on levodopa alone	• Fixed-dose combination formulation

Anti-Parkinson: MAO-B Inhibitors (reduce oxidative metabolism of dopamine in the CNS)

Rasagiline	• PD, either as initial monotherapy or adjunct to levodopa	• Adjunct to reduce wearing off • Many drug interactions • Should not be given with meperidine • When administered with CYP1A2 inhibitors, C_p of rasagiline may double • Risk of serotonin syndrome
Selegiline	• PD, as adjunctive therapy in patients with deteriorating response to levodopa	• Generates amphetamine metabolites, which can cause anxiety and insomnia • MAO-B selectivity lost at doses > 30–40 mg/d • Many drug interactions • Should not be given with meperidine • Risk of serotonin syndrome • Available in immediate release, orally disintegrating tablet, or transdermal patch

Anti-Parkinson: Other

Amantadine	• Early, mild PD • Levodopa-induced dyskinesias • Influenza	• Unclear mechanism of antiparkinsonian effects • Effective against dyskinesia
Trihexyphenidyl	• PD, as adjunctive therapy	• Muscarinic receptor antagonist • Anticholinergic side effects
Benztropine	• PD, as adjunctive therapy	• Muscarinic receptor antagonist

Anti-Alzheimer: Acetylcholinesterase Inhibitors (boost cholinergic neurotransmission; first line treatment)

Donepezil	• Mild, moderate, severe AD dementia	• GI symptoms: main dose-limiting side effect • Bradycardia/syncope less common
Rivastigmine	• Mild-moderate AD dementia • Mild-moderate PD dementia	• Transdermal formulation available, with lower risk of GI side effects • Also inhibits BuChE
Galantamine	• Mild-moderate AD dementia	• GI symptoms: main dose-limiting side effect • Bradycardia/syncope less common than GI side effects

Anti-Alzheimer: Low-Affinity Uncompetitive NMDA Antagonist

Memantine	• Moderate, severe AD dementia	• Reduces excitotoxicity through use-dependent blockade of NMDA receptors

Anti-Huntington

Tetrabenazine Deutetrabenazine	• Chorea in HD	• Reversible VMAT2 inhibitor: depletes presynaptic catecholamines • Adverse effects: hypotension, depression with suicidality • Adjust dose for CYP2D6 status; 2D6 inhibitors (e.g., paroxetine, fluoxetine, quinidine, bupropion) ↑ exposure ~3 fold • Contraindications: concurrent or recent MAO inhibitor or reserpine

Anti-ALS

Riluzole	Extends survival in ALS up to 3 months	• Uncertain mechanism of action: inhibits glutamate release, blocks sodium channels and glutamate receptors
Edaravone	Reduces progression in early stages of ALS	• Intensive intravenous administration regimen
Anti-Spastic Agents Baclofen	• GABA$_B$ receptor agonist	• Sedation and CNS depression
Tizanidine	• α_2 adrenergic receptor agonist	• Causes drowsiness; treatment is initiated with low dose and titrated upward
Benzodiazepines (e.g., clonazepam)	• See Chapter 19	• May contribute to respiratory depression
Dantrolene	• *Not used in ALS*, but for treating muscle spasm in stroke or spinal injury and for treating malignant hyperthermia	• May cause hepatotoxicity

Bibliography

Albin RL, et al. The functional anatomy of basal ganglia disorders. *Trends Neurosci*, **1989**, 12:366–375.

Bates GP, et al. Huntington disease. *Nat Rev Dis Primers*, **2015**, 1:15005.

Calabresi P, et al. Direct and indirect pathways of basal ganglia: a critical reappraisal. *Nat Neurosci*, **2014**, 17(8):1022–1030.

Connolly BS, Lang AE. Pharmacological treatment of Parkinson disease: a review. *JAMA*, **2014**, 311(16):1670–1683.

Cotzias GC, et al. Modification of Parkinsonism: chronic treatment with L-dopa. *N Engl J Med*, **1969**, 280:337–345.

Fahn S, et al. Levodopa and the progression of Parkinson's disease. *N Engl J Med*, **2004**, 351:2498–2508.

Giacobini E, Gold G. Alzheimer disease therapy—moving from amyloid-β to tau. *Nat Rev Neurol*, **2013**, 9:677–686.

Goedert M, et al. 100 years of Lewy pathology. *Nat Rev Neurol*, **2013**, 9(1):13–24.

Gordon PH. Amyotrophic lateral sclerosis: an update for 2013 clinical features, pathophysiology, management and therapeutic trials. *Aging Dis*, **2013**, 4(5):295–310.

Hauser RA, et al. Extended-release carbidopa-levodopa (IPX066) compared with immediate-release carbidopa-levodopa in patients with Parkinson's disease and motor fluctuations: a phase 3 randomised, double-blind trial. *Lancet Neurol*, **2013**, 12(4):346–356.

Hornykiewicz O. Dopamine in the basal ganglia: its role and therapeutic indications (including the clinical use of L-dopa). *Br Med Bull*, **1973**, 29:172–178.

Kumar KR, et al. Genetics of Parkinson disease and other movement disorders. *Curr Opin Neurol*, **2012**, *25*(4):466–474.

Langston JW. The Parkinson's complex: parkinsonism is just the tip of the iceberg. *Ann Neurol*, **2006**, *59*:591–596.

Miller RG, et al. Riluzole for amyotrophic lateral sclerosis (ALS)/motor neuron disease (MND). *Cochrane Database Syst Rev*, **2007**, (1):CD001447.

Olanow CW, et al. Continuous intrajejunal infusion of levodopa-carbidopa intestinal gel for patients with advanced Parkinson's disease: a randomised, controlled, double-blind, double-dummy study. *Lancet Neurol*, **2014**, *13*(2):141–149.

Olanow CW, et al. A randomized, double-blind, placebo-controlled, delayed start study to assess rasagiline as a disease modifying therapy in Parkinson's disease (the ADAGIO study): rationale, design, and baseline characteristics. *Mov Disord*, **2008**, *23*:2194–2201.

Pahwa R, et al. Practice parameter: treatment of Parkinson disease with motor fluctuations and dyskinesia (an evidence-based review): report of the Quality Standards Subcommittee of the American Academy of Neurology. *Neurology*, **2006**, *66*(7):983–995.

Panisset M, et al. Serotonin toxicity association with concomitant antidepressants and rasagiline treatment: retrospective study (STACCATO). *Pharmacotherapy*, **2014**, *34*(12):1250–1258.

Parkinson Study Group. Entacapone improves motor fluctuations in levodopa-treated Parkinson's disease patients. *Ann Neurol*, **1997**, *42*:747–755 (published erratum appears in *Ann Neurol*, **1998**, *44*:292).

Parkinson Study Group. Pramipexole vs. levodopa as initial treatment for Parkinson's disease: a randomized, controlled trial. *JAMA*, **2000**, *284*:1931–1938.

Prusiner SB. Biology and genetics of prions causing neurodegeneration. *Annu Rev Genet*, **2013**, *47*:601–623.

Renton AE, et al. State of play in amyotrophic lateral sclerosis genetics. *Nat Neurosci*, **2014**, *17*:17–23.

Roberson ED, Mucke L. 100 years and counting: prospects for defeating Alzheimer's disease. *Science*, **2006**, *314*:781–784.

Rohrer JD, et al. C9orf72 expansions in frontotemporal dementia and amyotrophic lateral sclerosis. *Lancet Neurol*, **2015**, *14*:291–301.

Ross CA, et al. Huntington disease: natural history, biomarkers and prospects for therapeutics. *Nat Rev Neurol*, **2014**, *10*:204–216.

Selkoe DJ. The therapeutics of Alzheimer's disease: where we stand and where we are heading. *Ann Neurol*, **2013**, *74*:328–336.

Schneider LS, et al. Risk of death with atypical antipsychotic drug treatment for dementia: meta-analysis of randomized placebo-controlled trials. *JAMA*, **2005**, *294*:1934–1943.

Singleton AB, et al. The genetics of Parkinson's disease: progress and therapeutic implications. *Mov Disord*, **2013**, *28*(1):14–23.

Suchowersky O, et al. Practice parameter: diagnosis and prognosis of new onset Parkinson disease (an evidence-based review): report of the Quality Standards Subcommittee of the American Academy of Neurology. *Neurology,* **2006**, *66*:968–975.

Weintraub D, et al. Clinical spectrum of impulse control disorders in Parkinson's disease. *Mov Disord*, **2015**, *30*(2):121–127.

Zesiewicz TA, et al. Practice parameter: treatment of nonmotor symptoms of Parkinson disease: report of the Quality Standards Subcommittee of the American Academy of Neurology. *Neurology,* **2010**, *74*:924–931.

Chapter 19

Hypnotics and Sedatives

S. John Mihic, Jody Mayfield, and R. Adron Harris

A *sedative* drug decreases activity, moderates excitement, and calms the recipient, whereas a *hypnotic* drug produces drowsiness and facilitates the onset and maintenance of a state of sleep that resembles natural sleep in its electroencephalographic characteristics and from which the recipient can be aroused easily. Sedation is a side effect of many drugs that are not considered general CNS depressants (e.g., antihistamines and antipsychotic agents). Although these and other agents can intensify the effects of CNS depressants, they usually produce their desired therapeutic effects at concentrations lower than those causing substantial CNS depression. For example, benzodiazepine sedative-hypnotics do not produce generalized CNS depression. Although coma may occur at very high doses, neither surgical anesthesia nor fatal intoxication is produced by benzodiazepines unless other drugs with CNS-depressant actions are concomitantly administered; an important exception is *midazolam*, which has been associated with decreased tidal volume and respiratory rate. Moreover, specific antagonists of benzodiazepines exist, such as *flumazenil*, which is used to treat cases of benzodiazepine overdose. This constellation of properties sets the benzodiazepine receptor agonists apart from other sedative-hypnotic drugs and imparts a measure of safety, such that benzodiazepines and the newer benzodiazepine receptor agonists (the "Z compounds") have largely displaced older agents for the treatment of insomnia and anxiety.

The CNS depressants discussed in this chapter include benzodiazepines, the Z compounds, barbiturates, as well as several sedative-hypnotic agents of diverse chemical structure. The sedative-hypnotic drugs that do not specifically target the benzodiazepine receptor belong to a group of older, less-safe, sedative-hypnotic drugs that depress the CNS in a dose-dependent fashion, progressively producing a spectrum of responses from mild sedation to coma and death. These older sedative-hypnotic compounds share these properties with a large number of chemicals, including general anesthetics (see Chapter 21) and alcohols, most notably ethanol (see Chapter 23). The newer sedative-hypnotic agents, such as benzodiazepines and Z drugs, are safer in this regard.

HISTORICAL PERSPECTIVE

Humans have long sought sleep unburdened by worry and, to this end, have consumed many potions. In the mid-19th century, bromide was introduced specifically as a sedative-hypnotic. Chloral hydrate, paraldehyde, urethane, and sulfonal were used before the introduction of barbiturates (barbital, 1903; phenobarbital, 1912), of which about 50 were distributed commercially. Barbiturates were so dominant that fewer than a dozen other sedative-hypnotics were marketed successfully before 1960.

The partial separation of sedative-hypnotic-anesthetic properties from anticonvulsant properties characteristic of phenobarbital led to searches for agents with more selective effects on CNS functions. As a result, relatively nonsedating anticonvulsants, notably phenytoin and trimethadione, were developed in the late 1930s and early 1940s (Chapter 17). The advent of chlorpromazine and meprobamate in the early 1950s, with their taming effects in animals, and the development of increasingly sophisticated methods for evaluating the behavioral effects of drugs, set the stage in the 1950s for the synthesis of chlordiazepoxide, the introduction of which into clinical medicine in 1961 ushered in the era of benzodiazepines. Most of the benzodiazepines in the marketplace were selected for high anxiolytic potency in relation to their depression of CNS function. However, all benzodiazepines possess sedative-hypnotic properties to varying degrees; these properties are exploited extensively clinically, especially to facilitate sleep. Mainly because of their remarkably low capacity to produce fatal CNS depression, the benzodiazepines displaced the barbiturates as sedative-hypnotic agents.

Abbreviations

ACh: acetylcholine
ALA: δ-aminolevulinic acid
AMPA: α-amino-3-hydroxy-5-methyl-4-isoxazole propionic acid
COPD: chronic obstructive pulmonary disease
CNS: central nervous system
CYP: cytochrome P450
EEG: electroencephalogram
FDA: Food and Drug Administration
GABA: γ-aminobutyric acid
GI: gastrointestinal
GPCR: G protein–coupled receptor
IM: intramuscular
IV: intravenous
MT: melatonin
OL: off-label use
OSA: obstructive sleep apnea
OTC: over the counter
REM: rapid eye movement
SSRI: selective serotonin reuptake inhibitor

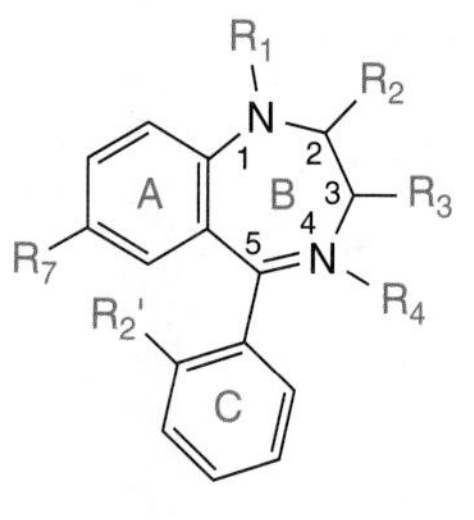

Figure 19–1 *Basic structure of benzodiazepines. Benzodiazepine* refers to the portion of this structure comprising the benzene ring (A) fused to a seven-member diazepine ring (B). Because all the important benzodiazepines contain a 5-aryl substituent (ring C) and a 1,4-diazepine ring, the term has come to mean the 5-aryl-1,4-benzodiazepines. Numerous modifications in the structure of the ring systems and substituents have yielded compounds with similar activities, including the benzodiazepine receptor antagonist flumazenil, in which ring C is replaced with a keto function at position 5 and a methyl substituent is added at position 4. A number of nonbenzodiazepine compounds (e.g., β-carbolines, zolpidem, eszopiclone) plus classic benzodiazepines and flumazenil bind to the benzodiazepine receptor, an allosteric site on the ionotropic $GABA_A$ receptor, a pentameric structure that forms a GABA-stimulated Cl^- channel.

Benzodiazepines

All benzodiazepines in clinical use promote the binding of the major inhibitory neurotransmitter GABA to the $GABA_A$ receptor, a pentameric ligand-gated, anion-conducting channel. Considerable heterogeneity exists among human $GABA_A$ receptors; this heterogeneity is thought to contribute to the myriad effects of these agents in vivo. Because receptor subunit composition appears to govern the interaction of various allosteric modulators with these channels, there has been a surge in efforts to find agents displaying different combinations of benzodiazepine-like properties that may reflect selective actions on one or more subtypes of $GABA_A$ receptors. A number of distinct mechanisms of action, reflecting involvement of specific subunits of the $GABA_A$ receptor, likely contribute to distinct effects of various benzodiazepines—the sedative-hypnotic, muscle-relaxant, anxiolytic, amnesic, and anticonvulsant effects.

Although the benzodiazepines exert qualitatively similar clinical effects, quantitative differences in their pharmacodynamic spectra and pharmacokinetic properties have led to varying patterns of therapeutic application. While only the benzodiazepines used primarily for hypnosis are discussed in detail, this chapter describes the general properties of the group and important differences amongst individual agents (Figure 19–1) (see also Chapters 15 and 17).

The Molecular Target for Benzodiazepines

Benzodiazepines act at $GABA_A$ receptors by binding directly to a specific site that is distinct from the GABA binding site.

The GABA$_A$ Receptor

The $GABA_A$ receptor is the major inhibitory receptor in the CNS. It is a transmembrane protein composed of five subunits that co-assemble around a central anion-conducting channel. Each subunit is composed of a large extracellular amino terminus, four transmembrane segments (M1-M4) and a short carboxy terminus. The M2 segment of each subunit contributes to the formation of the central anion-conducting pore. GABA binds at the interfaces of α and β classes of subunits, while benzodiazepines bind at α/γ interfaces. The five subunits come from 19 isoforms, so the number of possible pentameric combinations is large. The number of pentamers actually expressed in nature is uncertain, but likely numbers in the dozens. The $GABA_A$ receptor shares subunit organization with a number of other cys-loop ligand-gated ion channels and with the ACh binding protein (Figure 11–1).

The $GABA_A$ receptor pentamer contains a single benzodiazepine binding site, as well as other allosteric sites at which a variety of sedative-hypnotic-anesthetic agents exert modulatory effects on $GABA_A$ receptor function (Figure 14–11). The exact functional properties of the pentameric receptor depend on the subunit composition and arrangement of the individual subunits, and this heterogeneity likely contributes to the pharmacological diversity of benzodiazepine effects observed in behavioral, biochemical, and functional studies and to the selective effects of the Z compounds.

Effects of Benzodiazepines on GABA$_A$ Receptor–Mediated Events

Benzodiazepines are allosteric modulators of $GABA_A$ receptor function (Sieghart, 2015). They increase the affinity of the $GABA_A$ receptor for GABA and thereby enhance GABA-induced Cl^- currents. Thus, in terms of channel kinetics, benzodiazepines increase the frequency of opening of the $GABA_A$ receptor Cl^- channel in the presence of GABA (Nestler et al., 2015; Sigel and Steinmann, 2012). Inverse agonists do just the opposite, reducing GABA binding and the frequency of channel opening. Benzodiazepine antagonists (e.g., flumazenil) competitively block benzodiazepine binding and effect but do not independently alter channel function (Nestler et al., 2015; Sigel and Steinmann, 2012).

In pharmacodynamic terms, agonists at the benzodiazepine binding site shift the GABA concentration-response curve to the left, whereas inverse agonists shift the curve to the right. Both these effects are blocked by antagonists (e.g., flumazenil) that bind at the benzodiazepine binding site. Application of a benzodiazepine site antagonist, in the absence of either an agonist or antagonist at this same site, results in no change in $GABA_A$ receptor function. The behavioral and electrophysiological effects of benzodiazepines can also be reduced or prevented by prior treatment with antagonists of GABA binding (e.g., bicuculline).

The remarkable safety profile of the benzodiazepines likely relates to the fact that their effects in vivo depend on the presynaptic release of GABA; in the absence of GABA, benzodiazepines have no effects on $GABA_A$ receptor function.

The behavioral and sedative effects of benzodiazepines can be ascribed in part to potentiation of GABAergic pathways that serve to regulate the firing of monoamine-containing neurons known to promote behavioral arousal and to be important mediators of the inhibitory effects of fear and punishment on behavior. Inhibitory effects on muscular hypertonia or the spread of seizure activity can be attributed to potentiation of inhibitory GABAergic circuits at various levels of the neuraxis. The magnitude of the effects produced by benzodiazepines varies widely depending on such factors as the types of inhibitory circuits that are operating, the sources and intensity of excitatory input, and the manner in which experimental manipulations are performed and assessed. Accordingly, benzodiazepines markedly prolong the period after brief activation of recurrent GABAergic pathways during which neither spontaneous nor applied excitatory stimuli can evoke neuronal discharge; this effect is reversed by the GABA$_A$ receptor antagonist *bicuculline* (see Figure 14–10).

Benzodiazepines Versus Barbiturates at the GABA$_A$ Receptor

The two classes of agents, barbiturates and benzodiazepines, differ in their potencies: Barbiturates act to enhance GABA$_A$ receptor function at low micromolar concentrations; benzodiazepines bind with nanomolar affinity. Both benzodiazepines and barbiturates bind to allosteric sites on the GABA$_A$ receptor pentamer and thereby enhance GABA-stimulated Cl⁻ channel function. However, barbiturates also have an additional effect: Higher concentrations of barbiturates directly activate GABA$_A$ receptors. Furthermore, when tested using equieffective concentrations of GABA, maximally effective concentrations of barbiturates produce greater enhancement of GABA$_A$ receptor function than do benzodiazepines. This direct effect possibly contributes to the profound CNS depression that barbiturates can cause. The lack of direct channel activation by benzodiazepines and their dependence on the presynaptic release of GABA at the GABA$_A$ receptor likely contribute to the safety of these agents as compared to barbiturates.

Pharmacological Properties of Benzodiazepines

The therapeutic effects of the benzodiazepines result from their actions on the CNS. The most prominent of these effects are sedation, hypnosis, decreased anxiety, muscle relaxation, anterograde amnesia, and anticonvulsant activity. Only two effects of these drugs result from peripheral actions: coronary vasodilation, seen after intravenous administration of therapeutic doses of certain benzodiazepines, and neuromuscular blockade, seen only with very high doses.

CNS Effects

While benzodiazepines depress activity at all levels of the neuraxis, some structures are affected preferentially. The benzodiazepines do not produce the same magnitudes of neuronal depression produced by barbiturates and volatile anesthetics, likely because they have weaker enhancing effects at GABA$_A$ receptors than those compounds, even at saturating concentrations. All the benzodiazepines have similar pharmacological profiles. Nevertheless, the drugs differ in selectivity, and the clinical usefulness of individual benzodiazepines thus varies considerably. The vast majority of effects of benzodiazepine site agonists and inverse agonists can be reversed or prevented by flumazenil, which competes with agonists and inverse agonists at a common binding site at the GABA$_A$ receptor. As the dose of a benzodiazepine is increased, sedation progresses to hypnosis and then to stupor. Although the clinical literature often refers to the "anesthetic" effects and uses of certain benzodiazepines, these drugs do not cause a true general anesthesia; awareness usually persists, and a failure to respond to a noxious stimulus sufficient to allow surgery cannot be achieved. Nonetheless, at "preanesthetic" doses, there is amnesia for events occurring subsequent to administration of the drug. Although many attempts have been made to separate the anxiolytic actions of benzodiazepines from their sedative-hypnotic effects, distinguishing between these behaviors is problematic. Accurate measurements of anxiety and sedation are difficult in humans, and the validity of animal models for measuring anxiety and sedation is uncertain.

Although analgesic effects of benzodiazepines have been observed in experimental animals, only transient analgesia is apparent in humans after intravenous administration. Such effects actually may involve the production of amnesia. Unlike barbiturates, benzodiazepines do not cause hyperalgesia.

Tolerance. Although most patients who chronically ingest benzodiazepines report that drowsiness wanes over a few days, tolerance to the impairment seen in some measures of psychomotor performance (e.g.,

visual tracking) is not usually observed. Whether tolerance develops to the anxiolytic effects of benzodiazepines remains debatable. Many patients use a fairly constant maintenance dose; increases or decreases in dosage appear to correspond with changes in their perceived problems or stresses. Conversely, other patients either do not reduce their dosages when stress is relieved or steadily escalate dosing. Such behavior may be associated with the development of drug dependence (see Chapter 24).

Some benzodiazepines induce muscle hypotonia without interfering with normal locomotion and can decrease rigidity in patients with cerebral palsy. *Clonazepam* in nonsedating doses causes muscle relaxation, but *diazepam* and most other benzodiazepines do not. Tolerance occurs to the muscle relaxant and ataxic effects of these drugs.

Experimentally, benzodiazepines inhibit seizure activity induced by either pentylenetetrazol or picrotoxin, but suppress strychnine- and maximal electroshock-induced seizures only at doses that also severely impair locomotor activity. *Clonazepam, nitrazepam,* and *nordazepam* have greater selective anticonvulsant activity than do most other benzodiazepines. Benzodiazepines also suppress photic seizures in baboons and ethanol withdrawal seizures in humans. However, the development of tolerance to the anticonvulsant effects has limited the usefulness of benzodiazepines in the treatment of recurrent seizure disorders in humans (see Chapter 17).

Effects on the Electroencephalogram and Sleep Stages. The effects of benzodiazepines on the waking EEG resemble those of other sedative-hypnotic drugs. Alpha rhythm activity is decreased, but there is an increase in low-voltage fast activity. Tolerance also occurs to these effects. With respect to sleep, some differences in the patterns of effects exerted by the various benzodiazepines have been noted, but benzodiazepine users usually report a sense of deep or refreshing sleep. Benzodiazepines decrease sleep latency, especially when first used, and diminish the number of awakenings and the time spent in stage 0 (a stage of wakefulness). They also produce an increased arousal threshold from sleep. Time in stage 1 (descending drowsiness) usually is decreased, and there is a prominent decrease in the time spent in slow-wave sleep (stages 3 and 4). Most benzodiazepines increase the latency from onset of spindle sleep to the first burst of REM sleep. The time spent in REM sleep is usually shortened, but the number of cycles of REM sleep is typically increased, mostly late in the sleep time. *Zolpidem* and *zaleplon* suppress REM sleep less extensively than benzodiazepines and thus may be superior to benzodiazepines for use as hypnotics (Dujardin et al., 1998).

Despite the shortening of durations of stage 4 and REM sleep, benzodiazepine administration typically increases total sleep time, largely by increasing the time spent in stage 2, which is the major fraction of non-REM sleep. This effect is greatest in subjects with the shortest baseline total sleep time. In addition, despite the increased number of REM cycles, the number of shifts to lighter sleep stages (1 and 0) and the amount of body movement are diminished with benzodiazepine use. Nocturnal peaks in the secretion of growth hormone, prolactin, and luteinizing hormone are not affected. During chronic nocturnal use of benzodiazepines, the effects on the various stages of sleep usually decline within a few nights. When such use is discontinued, the pattern of drug-induced changes in sleep parameters may "rebound," and an increase in the amount and density of REM sleep may be especially prominent. If the dosage has not been excessive, patients usually will note only a shortening of sleep time rather than an exacerbation of insomnia.

Systemic Effects

Respiration. Hypnotic doses of benzodiazepines are without effect on respiration in normal subjects, but special care must be taken in the treatment of children and individuals with impaired hepatic or pulmonary function. At higher doses, such as those used for preanesthetic medication or for endoscopy, benzodiazepines slightly depress alveolar ventilation and cause respiratory acidosis as the result of a decrease in hypoxic rather than hypercapnic drive; these effects are exaggerated in patients with COPD, and alveolar hypoxia and CO_2 narcosis may result. These drugs can cause apnea during anesthesia or when given with opioids. Patients severely intoxicated with benzodiazepines only require respiratory assistance when they also have ingested another CNS depressant drug, most commonly ethanol.

Hypnotic doses of benzodiazepines may worsen sleep-related breathing disorders by adversely affecting control of the upper airway muscles or by decreasing the ventilatory response to CO_2. The latter effect may cause hypoventilation and hypoxemia in some patients with severe COPD. In patients with OSA, hypnotic doses of benzodiazepines may decrease muscle tone in the upper airway and exaggerate the impact of apneic episodes on alveolar hypoxia, pulmonary hypertension, and cardiac ventricular load. Benzodiazepines may promote the appearance of episodes of apnea during REM sleep (associated with decreases in O_2 saturation) in patients recovering from a myocardial infarction; however, no impact of these drugs on survival of patients with cardiac disease has been reported.

Cardiovascular System. The cardiovascular effects of benzodiazepines are minor in normal subjects except in cases of severe intoxication (see previous discussion for adverse effects in patients with obstructive sleep disorders or cardiac disease). At preanesthetic doses, all benzodiazepines decrease blood pressure and increase heart rate. With *midazolam*, the effects appear to be secondary to a decrease in peripheral resistance; however, with *diazepam*, the effects are secondary to a decrease in left ventricular work and cardiac output. *Diazepam* increases coronary flow, possibly by an action to increase interstitial concentrations of adenosine, and the accumulation of this cardiodepressant metabolite also may explain the negative inotropic effects of the drug. In large doses, *midazolam* considerably decreases cerebral blood flow and O_2 assimilation.

GI Tract. Benzodiazepines are thought by some gastroenterologists to improve a variety of "anxiety-related" GI disorders. There is a paucity of evidence for direct actions. Although diazepam markedly decreases nocturnal gastric secretion in humans, other drug classes are considerably more effective in acid-peptic disorders (see Chapter 49).

ADME

All benzodiazepines are absorbed completely except *clorazepate*. Clorazepate is decarboxylated rapidly in gastric juice to *N*-desmethyldiazepam (nordazepam), which subsequently is absorbed completely. Drugs active at the benzodiazepine receptor may be divided into four categories based on their elimination $t_{1/2}$:

- Ultrashort-acting benzodiazepines
- Short-acting agents ($t_{1/2}$ < 6 h), including midazolam, triazolam, the nonbenzodiazepine zolpidem ($t_{1/2}$ ~2 h), and eszopiclone ($t_{1/2}$, 5–6 h)
- Intermediate-acting agents ($t_{1/2}$, 6–24 h), including estazolam and temazepam
- Long-acting agents ($t_{1/2}$ > 24 h), including flurazepam, diazepam, and quazepam

Flurazepam itself has a short $t_{1/2}$ (~2.3 h), but a major active metabolite, *N*-des-alkyl-flurazepam, is long lived ($t_{1/2}$, 47–100 h); such features complicate the classification of certain benzodiazepines.

The benzodiazepines and their active metabolites bind to plasma proteins. The extent of binding correlates strongly with the oil:water partition coefficient and ranges from about 70% for alprazolam to nearly 99% for diazepam. The concentration in the cerebrospinal fluid is approximately equal to the concentration of free drug in plasma. Uptake of benzodiazepines occurs rapidly into the brain and other highly perfused organs after intravenous administration (or oral administration of a rapidly absorbed compound); rapid uptake is followed by a phase of redistribution into tissues that are less well perfused but capacious, especially muscle and fat (see Table 2–2 and Figure 2–4). Redistribution is most rapid for benzodiazepines with the highest oil:water partition coefficients. The kinetics of redistribution of diazepam and other lipophilic benzodiazepines are complicated by enterohepatic circulation. These drugs cross the placental barrier and are also secreted into breast milk.

Most benzodiazepines are metabolized extensively by hepatic CYPs, particularly CYP 3A4 and 2C19. Some benzodiazepines, such as *oxazepam*, are not metabolized by CYPs but are conjugated directly by phase 2 enzymes. Erythromycin, clarithromycin, ritonavir, itraconazole, ketoconazole, nefazodone, and grapefruit juice are examples of CYP3A4 inhibitors (see Chapter 6) that can affect the rate of metabolism of benzodiazepines. Benzodiazepines do not significantly induce hepatic CYPs, so their chronic administration does not usually affect metabolism of benzodiazepines or other drugs. Cimetidine and oral contraceptives inhibit *N*-dealkylation and 3-hydroxylation of benzodiazepines. Ethanol, isoniazid, and phenytoin are less effective in this regard. These phase 1 reactions usually are reduced to a greater extent in elderly patients and in patients with chronic liver disease than are those reactions involving conjugation.

The active metabolites of some benzodiazepines are biotransformed more slowly than are the parent compounds; thus, the durations of action of many benzodiazepines bear little relationship to the $t_{1/2}$ of elimination of the parent drug. Conversely, the rate of biotransformation of drugs that are inactivated by the initial metabolic reaction is an important determinant of their durations of action; examples include oxazepam, lorazepam, temazepam, triazolam, and midazolam.

Benzodiazepine metabolism can seem daunting but can be organized around a few basic principles. Metabolism of the benzodiazepines occurs in three major stages. These stages and the relationships between the drugs and their metabolites are shown in Table 19–1.

For benzodiazepines that bear a substituent at position 1 (or 2) of the diazepine ring, the *first phase* of metabolism involves modification or removal of the substituent. The eventual products are *N*-desalkylated compounds that are biologically active. Exceptions are triazolam, alprazolam, estazolam, and midazolam, which contain either a fused triazolo or an imidazolo ring and are α-hydroxylated.

The *second phase* of metabolism involves hydroxylation at position 3 and also usually yields an active derivative (e.g., oxazepam from nordazepam). The rates of these reactions are usually much slower than the first stage ($t_{1/2}$ > 40–50 h), such that appreciable accumulation of hydroxylated products with intact substituents at position 1 does not occur. (There are two significant exceptions to this rule: First, small amounts of temazepine accumulate during the chronic administration of diazepam; and second, following the replacement of S with O in quazepam, most of the resulting 2-oxoquazepam is hydroxylated slowly at position 3 without removal of the *N*-alkyl group. However, only small amounts of the 3-hydroxyl derivative accumulate during chronic administration of quazepam because this compound is conjugated at an unusually rapid rate. In contrast, the *N*-desalkylflurazepam that is formed by the "minor" metabolic pathway does accumulate during quazepam administration, and it contributes significantly to the overall clinical effect.)

The *third major phase* of metabolism is the conjugation of the 3-hydroxyl compounds, principally with glucuronic acid; the $t_{1/2}$ values of these reactions usually are about 6–12 h, and the products invariably are inactive. Conjugation is the only major route of metabolism for oxazepam and lorazepam and is the preferred pathway for temazepam because of the slower conversion of this compound to oxazepam. Triazolam and alprazolam are metabolized principally by initial hydroxylation of the methyl group on the fused triazolo ring; the absence of a chlorine residue in ring C of alprazolam slows this reaction significantly. The products, sometimes referred to as *α-hydroxylated compounds,* are quite active but are metabolized rapidly, primarily by conjugation with glucuronic acid, such that there is no appreciable accumulation of active metabolites. The fused triazolo ring in estazolam lacks a methyl group and is hydroxylated to only a limited extent; the major route of metabolism involves the formation of the 3-hydroxyl derivative. The corresponding hydroxyl derivatives of triazolam and alprazolam also are formed to a significant extent. Compared with compounds without the triazolo ring, the rate of this reaction for all three drugs is unusually swift, and the 3-hydroxyl compounds are rapidly conjugated or oxidized further to benzophenone derivatives before excretion.

Midazolam is metabolized rapidly, primarily by hydroxylation of the methyl group on the fused imidazo ring; only small amounts of 3-hydroxyl

TABLE 19–1 ■ STAGES AND RELATIONSHIPS AMONG SOME OF THE DIAZEPINES[a]

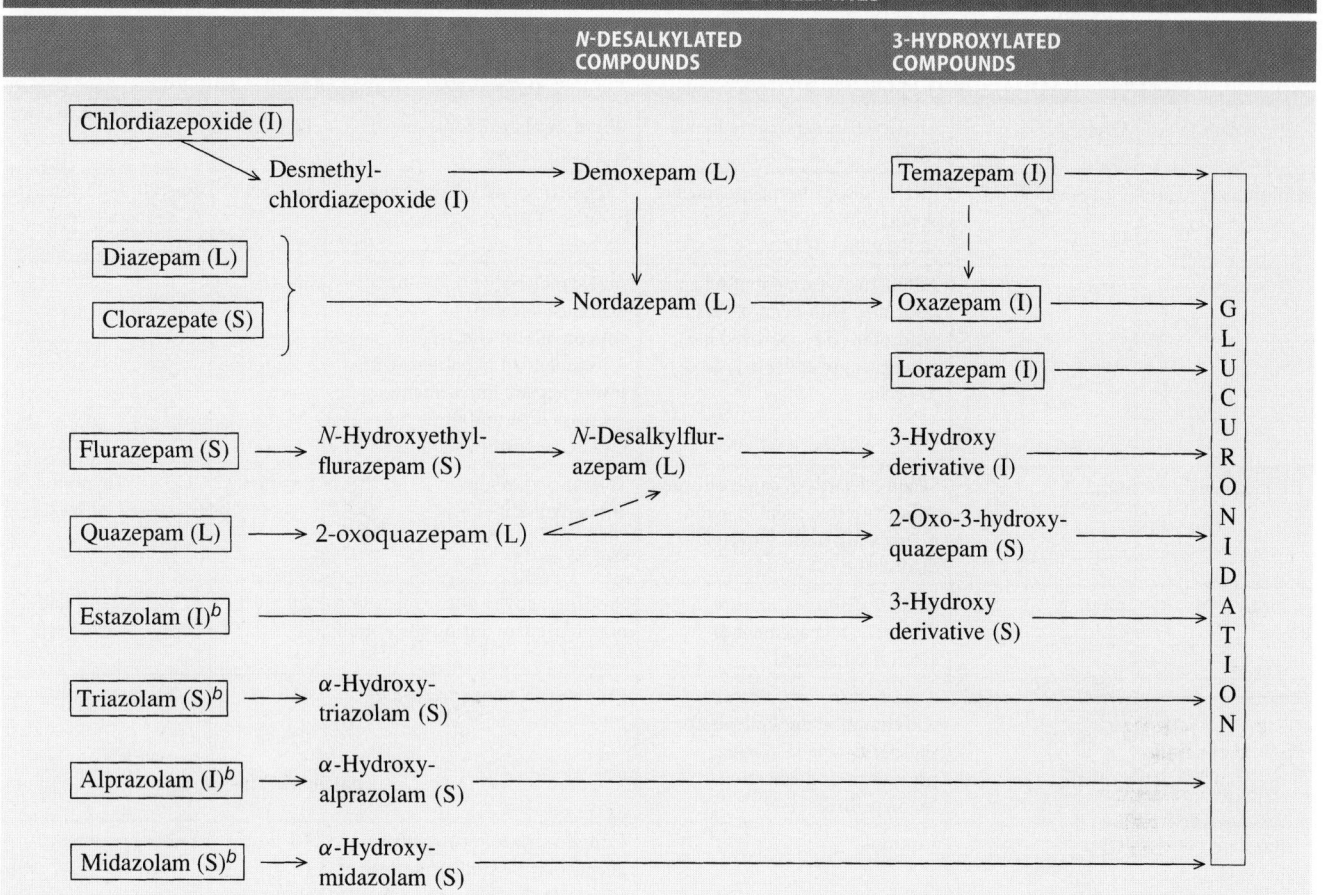

	N-DESALKYLATED COMPOUNDS	3-HYDROXYLATED COMPOUNDS

SECTION II NEUROPHARMACOLOGY

[a] Compounds enclosed in boxes are marketed in the U.S. The approximate half-lives of the various compounds are denoted in parentheses; S (short-acting), $t_{1/2}$ <6 h; I (intermediate-acting), $t_{1/2}$ = 6-24 h; L (long-acting), $t_{1/2}$ = >24 h. All compounds except clorazepate are biologically active; the activity of 3-hydroxydesalkylflurazepam has not been determined. Clonazepam (not shown) is an *N*-desalkyl compound, and it is metabolized primarily by reduction of the 7-NO$_2$ group to the corresponding amine (inactive), followed by acetylation; its $t_{1/2}$ is 20-40 h. [b] See text for discussion of other pathways of metabolism.

compounds are formed. The α-hydroxylated compound, which has appreciable biological activity, is eliminated with a $t_{1/2}$ of 1 h after conjugation with glucuronic acid. Variable and sometimes substantial accumulation of this metabolite has been noted during intravenous infusion (Oldenhof et al., 1988).

The aromatic rings (A and C) of the benzodiazepines are hydroxylated only to a small extent. The only important metabolism at these sites is reduction of the 7-nitro substituents of clonazepam, nitrazepam, and flunitrazepam; the $t_{1/2}$ of these reactions are usually 20–40 h. The resulting amines are inactive and are acetylated to varying degrees before excretion.

Therapeutic Uses

Table 19–2 summarizes the therapeutic uses and routes of administration of benzodiazepines that are marketed in the U.S. Most benzodiazepines can be used interchangeably. For example, diazepam can be used to treat alcohol withdrawal symptoms, and most benzodiazepines work as hypnotics. Benzodiazepines that are useful as anticonvulsants have a long $t_{1/2}$, and rapid entry into the brain is required for efficacy in treatment of status epilepticus. Antianxiety agents, in contrast, should have a long $t_{1/2}$ despite the drawback of the risk of neuropsychological deficits caused by drug accumulation. For a hypnotic sleep medication, one would want to have a rapid onset of action when taken at bedtime, a sufficiently sustained action to maintain sleep throughout the night, and no residual action by the following morning. In practice, there are some disadvantages to the use of agents that have a relatively rapid rate of disappearance, such as triazolam, including the early morning insomnia experienced by some patients and a greater likelihood of rebound insomnia on drug discontinuation. With

careful selection of dosage, flurazepam and other benzodiazepines with slower rates of elimination than triazolam's can be used effectively.

Untoward Effects

At peak concentrations in plasma, hypnotic doses of benzodiazepines cause varying degrees of light-headedness, lassitude, increased reaction time, motor incoordination, impairment of mental and motor functions, confusion, and anterograde amnesia. Cognition appears to be affected less than motor performance. *All of these effects can greatly impair driving and other psychomotor skills, especially if combined with ethanol.* When the drug is given at the intended time of sleep, persistence of these effects into the following waking hours is adverse. These dose-related residual effects can be insidious because most subjects underestimate the degree of their impairment. Residual daytime sleepiness also may occur, even though successful drug therapy can reduce the daytime sleepiness resulting from chronic insomnia. The intensity and incidence of CNS toxicity generally increase with age (Monane, 1992). Other common side effects of benzodiazepines are weakness, headache, blurred vision, vertigo, nausea and vomiting, epigastric distress, and diarrhea; joint pains, chest pains, and incontinence are much rarer. Anticonvulsant benzodiazepines sometimes increase the frequency of seizures in patients with epilepsy.

A wide variety of serious allergic, hepatotoxic, and hematologic reactions to the benzodiazepines may occur, but the incidence is low; these reactions have been associated with the use of *flurazepam*, *triazolam*, and *temazepam*. Large doses taken just before or during labor may cause hypothermia, hypotonia, and mild respiratory depression in the neonate. Abuse by the pregnant mother can result in a withdrawal syndrome in the newborn.

TABLE 19–2 ■ THERAPEUTIC USES OF BENZODIAZEPINES

COMPOUND	ROUTES OF ADMINISTRATION	THERAPEUTIC USES[a]	COMMENTS	$t_{1/2}$ (h)[b]	USUAL SEDATIVE-HYPNOTIC DOSE, mg[c]
Alprazolam	Oral	Anxiety disorders, agoraphobia (OL)	Withdrawal symptoms may be especially severe	12 ± 2	—
Chlordiazepoxide	Oral, IM, IV	Anxiety disorders, management of alcohol withdrawal, preanesthetic medication (OL)	Long-acting and self-tapering because of active metabolites	10 ± 3.4	50–100, 1–41× daily[d] (1 daily for sleep)
Clobazam	Oral	Adjunctive treatment of seizures associated with Lennox-Gastaut syndrome (U.S. approved use), other types of epilepsies, anxiety disorders	Active metabolite $t_{1/2}$ 71–82 h; tolerance develops to anticonvulsant effects; not recommended in patients with severe hepatic impairment; decrease dose and titrate in CYP2C19 poor metabolizers	36–42	—
Clonazepam	Oral	Seizure disorders, panic disorder, adjunctive treatment in acute mania and certain movement disorders (OL)	Tolerance develops to anticonvulsant effects	23 ± 5	0.25–0.5 (hypnotic)
Clorazepate	Oral	Anxiety disorders, seizure disorders, management of alcohol withdrawal	Prodrug; activity due to formation of nordazepam during absorption	2.0 ± 0.9	3.75–20, 2–4× daily[d]
Diazepam	Oral, IM, IV, rectal	Anxiety disorders, alcohol withdrawal, status epilepticus, skeletal muscle relaxation, preanesthetic medication, Meniere disease (OL)	Prototypical benzodiazepine	43 ± 13	5–10, every 4 h
Estazolam	Oral	Insomnia	Contains triazolo ring; adverse effects may be similar to those of triazolam	10–24	1–2
Flurazepam	Oral	Insomnia	Active metabolites accumulate with chronic use	74 ± 24	15–30
Lorazepam	Oral, IM, IV	Anxiety disorders, alcohol withdrawal, preanesthetic medication, seizure disorders	Metabolized solely by conjugation	14 ± 5	1–4
Midazolam	Oral, IV, IM	Preanesthetic and intraoperative medication, anxiety disorders (agitation, alcohol withdrawal, seizure disorders, OL)	Rapidly inactivated	1.9 ± 0.6	1–5[e]
Oxazepam	Oral	Anxiety disorders, alcohol withdrawal	Metabolized solely by conjugation	8.0 ± 2.4	15–30, 3–4× daily[d]
Quazepam	Oral	Insomnia	Active metabolites accumulate with chronic use	39	7.5–15
Temazepam	Oral	Insomnia	Metabolized mainly by conjugation	11 ± 6	7.5–30
Triazolam	Oral	Insomnia	Rapidly inactivated; may cause disturbing daytime side effects	2.9 ± 1.0	0.125–0.5

[a]The therapeutic uses are examples to emphasize that most benzodiazepines can be used interchangeably. In general, the therapeutic uses of a given benzodiazepine are related to its $t_{1/2}$ and may not match the marketed indications. The issue is addressed more extensively in the text.
[b]Half-life of active metabolite may differ. See Appendix II for additional information.
[c]For additional dosage information, see Chapter 21 (anesthesia), Chapter 15 (anxiety), and Chapter 17 (seizure disorders).
[d]Approved as a sedative-hypnotic only for management of alcohol withdrawal; doses in a nontolerant individual would be smaller.
[e]Recommended doses vary considerably depending on specific use, condition of patient, and concomitant administration of other drugs.

Adverse Psychological Effects

Benzodiazepines may at times cause paradoxical effects. *Flurazepam* occasionally increases the incidence of nightmares—especially during the first week of use—and sometimes causes garrulousness, anxiety, irritability, tachycardia, and sweating. Amnesia, euphoria, restlessness, hallucinations, sleep-walking, sleep-talking, other complex behaviors, and hypomanic behavior have been reported to occur during use of various benzodiazepines. Bizarre uninhibited behavior may occur in some users, hostility and rage in others; collectively, these are sometimes referred to as *disinhibition* or *dyscontrol reactions*. Paranoia, depression, and suicidal ideation also occasionally may accompany the use of these agents. Such paradoxical or disinhibition reactions are rare and appear to be dose related. Because of reports of an increased incidence of confusion and abnormal behaviors, triazolam has been banned in the U.K. The FDA declared triazolam to be safe and effective in low doses of 0.125–0.25 mg.

Chronic benzodiazepine use poses a risk for development of dependence and abuse (Woods et al., 1992). Mild dependence may develop in many patients who have taken therapeutic doses of benzodiazepines on a regular basis for prolonged periods, but not to the same extent as seen with older sedatives and other recognized drugs of abuse (Chapter 24; Uhlenhuth et al., 1999). Withdrawal symptoms may include temporary intensification of the problems that originally prompted their use (e.g., insomnia or anxiety). Dysphoria, irritability, sweating, unpleasant dreams, tremors, anorexia, and faintness or dizziness also may occur, especially when withdrawal of the benzodiazepine occurs abruptly. Hence, it is prudent to taper the dosage gradually when therapy is to be discontinued. Despite their adverse effects, benzodiazepines are relatively safe drugs, and fatalities are rare unless other drugs are taken concomitantly. Ethanol is a common contributor to deaths involving benzodiazepines, but true coma is uncommon in the absence of another CNS depressant. Although overdosage with a benzodiazepine rarely causes severe cardiovascular or respiratory depression, therapeutic doses of benzodiazepines can further compromise respiration in patients with COPD or OSA. Benzodiazepine abuse of a different sort includes the use of *flunitrazepam* (Rohypnol; not licensed for use in the U.S.) as a "date rape drug."

Drug Interactions

Except for additive effects with other sedative or hypnotic drugs, reports of clinically important pharmacodynamic interactions between benzodiazepines and other drugs have been infrequent. Ethanol increases both the rate of absorption of benzodiazepines and the associated CNS depression. Valproate and benzodiazepines used in combination may cause psychotic episodes.

Novel Benzodiazepine Receptor Agonists

Hypnotics in this class are commonly referred to as "Z compounds." They include zolpidem, zaleplon, zopiclone (not marketed in the U.S.), and eszopiclone, which is the S(+) enantiomer of zopiclone (Huedo-Medina et al., 2012). Although the Z compounds are structurally unrelated to each other and to benzodiazepines, their therapeutic efficacy as hypnotics is due to agonist effects at the benzodiazepine site of the $GABA_A$ receptor (Hanson et al., 2008). Compared to benzodiazepines, Z compounds are less effective as anticonvulsants or muscle relaxants, which may be related to their relative selectivity for $GABA_A$ receptors containing the α_1 subunit. Over the last decade, Z compounds have largely replaced benzodiazepines in the treatment of insomnia. Z compounds were initially promoted as having less potential for dependence and abuse than traditional benzodiazepines. However, based on postmarketing clinical experience with zopiclone and zolpidem, tolerance and physical dependence can be expected during long-term use of Z compounds, especially with higher doses. The Z drugs are classified as schedule IV drugs in the U.S. The clinical presentation of overdose with Z compounds is similar to that of benzodiazepine overdose and can be treated with the benzodiazepine antagonist flumazenil.

Zaleplon

Zaleplon is a member of the pyrazolopyrimidine class. Zaleplon preferentially binds to the benzodiazepine binding site on $GABA_A$ receptors containing the α_1 receptor subunit. It is absorbed rapidly and reaches peak plasma concentrations in about 1 h. Its bioavailability is about 30% because of presystemic metabolism. Zaleplon is metabolized largely by aldehyde oxidase and to a lesser extent by CYP3A4. Its $t_{1/2}$ is short, about 1 h. Zalepon's oxidative metabolites are converted to glucuronides and eliminated in urine. Less than 1% of zaleplon is excreted unchanged; none of zaleplon's metabolites is pharmacologically active. Zaleplon is usually administered in 5-, 10-, or 20-mg doses (Dooley and Plosker, 2000). Zaleplon-treated subjects with either chronic or transient insomnia experience shorter periods of sleep onset latency.

Zolpidem

Zolpidem is an imidazopyridine sedative-hypnotic. The actions of zolpidem are due to agonist effects at the benzodiazepine receptor site on $GABA_A$ receptors and generally resemble those of benzodiazepines. The drug has little effect on the stages of sleep in normal human subjects. It is effective in shortening sleep latency and prolonging total sleep time in patients with insomnia. After discontinuation of zolpidem, the beneficial effects on sleep reportedly persist for up to 1 week, but mild rebound insomnia on the first night of withdrawal may occur. Zolpidem is approved only for the short-term treatment of insomnia; however, tolerance and physical dependence are rare (Morselli, 1993). At therapeutic doses (5–10 mg), zolpidem infrequently produces residual daytime sedation or amnesia; the incidence of other adverse effects also is low. As with the benzodiazepines, large overdoses of zolpidem do not produce severe respiratory depression unless other agents (e.g., ethanol) also are ingested. Hypnotic doses increase the hypoxia and hypercarbia of patients with OSA.

Zolpidem is absorbed readily from the GI tract; first-pass hepatic metabolism results in an oral bioavailability of about 70% (lower when the drug is ingested with food). Zolpidem is eliminated almost entirely by conversion to inactive products in the liver, largely through oxidation of the methyl groups on the phenyl and imidazopyridine rings to the corresponding carboxylic acids. Its plasma $t_{1/2}$ is about 2 h in normal individuals, but this value may increase 2-fold or more in those with cirrhosis and also tends to be greater in older patients, requiring adjustment of dosage. Although little or no unchanged zolpidem is found in the urine, elimination of the drug is slower in patients with chronic renal insufficiency; the increased elimination time largely is due to an increase in its apparent volume of distribution.

Zaleplon and Zolpidem Compared

Zaleplon and zolpidem are effective in relieving sleep-onset insomnia. Both drugs are FDA-approved for use up to 7–10 days at a time. Zaleplon and zolpidem have sustained hypnotic efficacy without occurrence of rebound insomnia on abrupt discontinuation. Zolpidem has a $t_{1/2}$ of about 2 h, which is sufficient to cover most of a typical 8-h sleep period, and is presently approved for bedtime use only. Zaleplon has a shorter $t_{1/2}$ of about 1 h, which offers the possibility for safe dosing later in the night, within 4 h of the anticipated rising time. Zaleplon and zolpidem differ in residual side effects; late-night administration of zolpidem has been associated with morning sedation, delayed reaction time, and anterograde amnesia, whereas zaleplon does not differ from placebo.

Eszopiclone

Eszopiclone is the active S(+) enantiomer of zopiclone. It exerts its sleep-promoting effects by enhancing $GABA_A$ receptor function via the benzodiazepine binding site. Eszopiclone is used for the long-term (~12 months) treatment of insomnia, for sleep maintenance, and to decrease the latency to onset of sleep (Melton et al., 2005; Rosenberg et al., 2005). It is available in 1-, 2-, or 3-mg tablets. In clinical studies, no tolerance was observed, and no signs of serious withdrawal, such as seizures or rebound insomnia, were seen on discontinuation of the drug; however, there are such reports for *zopiclone*, the racemate used outside the U.S. Mild withdrawal consisting of abnormal dreams, anxiety, nausea, and upset stomach can occur (≤2%). A minor reported adverse effect of eszopiclone is a bitter taste. Eszopiclone is absorbed rapidly after oral administration, with a bioavailability of about 80%, and shows wide distribution throughout the body. It is 50%–60% bound to plasma proteins, is metabolized by CYPs 3A4 and 2E1, and has a $t_{1/2}$ of about 6 h.

Management of Patients After Long-Term Benzodiazepine Therapy

If a benzodiazepine has been used regularly for more than 2 weeks, its use should be tapered rather than discontinued abruptly. In some patients taking hypnotics with a short $t_{1/2}$, it is easier to switch first to a hypnotic with a long $t_{1/2}$ and then to taper. The onset of withdrawal symptoms from medications with a long $t_{1/2}$ may be delayed. Consequently, the patient should be warned about the symptoms associated with withdrawal effects.

Flumazenil: A Benzodiazepine Receptor Antagonist

Flumazenil is an imidazobenzodiazepine that binds with high affinity to the benzodiazepine binding site on the $GABA_A$ receptor, where it competitively antagonizes the binding and allosteric effects of benzodiazepines and other ligands (Hoffman and Warren, 1993). Flumazenil antagonizes both the electrophysiological and behavioral effects of agonist and inverse-agonist benzodiazepines and β-carbolines.

Flumazenil is available only for intravenous administration. Administration of a series of small injections is preferred to a single bolus injection. A total of 1 mg flumazenil given over 1–3 min usually is sufficient to abolish the effects of therapeutic doses of benzodiazepines. Additional courses of treatment with flumazenil may be needed within 20–30 min should sedation reappear. The duration of clinical effects usually is only 30–60 min. Although absorbed rapidly after oral administration, less than 25% of the drug reaches the systemic circulation owing to extensive first-pass hepatic metabolism. Flumazenil is eliminated almost entirely by hepatic metabolism to inactive products with a $t_{1/2}$ of about 1 h. Oral doses are apt to cause headache and dizziness.

The primary indications for the use of flumazenil are the management of suspected benzodiazepine overdose and the reversal of sedative effects produced by benzodiazepines administered during general anesthesia and diagnostic or therapeutic procedures. Flumazenil is not effective in single-drug overdoses with either barbiturates or tricyclic antidepressants. The administration of flumazenil in these settings may be associated with the onset of seizures, especially in patients poisoned with tricyclic antidepressants. Seizures or other withdrawal signs may be precipitated in patients taking benzodiazepines for protracted periods and in whom tolerance or dependence may have developed.

Melatonin Congeners

Melatonin is a circadian signaling molecule. In some fish and amphibians, melatonin modulates skin coloration through an action on melanin-containing pigment granules in melanophores. In humans, melatonin, not to be confused with the pigment melanin, is the principal indoleamine in the pineal gland, where it may be said to constitute a pigment of the imagination. The synthesis of melatonin in the pineal gland (by *N*-acetylation and *O*-methylation of serotonin; see Figure 13–2) is influenced by external factors, including environmental light. In mammals, melatonin induces pigment lightening in skin cells and suppresses ovarian functions; it also serves a role in regulating biological rhythms and has been studied as a treatment of jet lag and other sleep disturbances. Melatonin analogues have recently been approved for the treatment of insomnia.

MELATONIN   RAMELTEON

Ramelteon

Ramelteon is a synthetic tricyclic analogue of melatonin, approved in the U.S. for the treatment of insomnia, specifically difficulties of sleep onset (Spadoni et al., 2011).

Mechanism of Action

Melatonin levels in the suprachiasmatic nucleus rise and fall in a circadian fashion, with concentrations increasing in the evening as an individual prepares for sleep and then reaching a plateau and ultimately decreasing as the night progresses. Two GPCRs for melatonin, MT_1 and MT_2, in the suprachiasmatic nucleus, each play a different role in sleep. Binding of agonists such as melatonin to MT_1 receptors promotes the onset of sleep; melatonin binding to MT_2 receptors shifts the timing of the circadian system. Ramelteon binds to both MT_1 and MT_2 receptors with high affinity, but, unlike melatonin, it does not bind appreciably to quinone reductase 2, the structurally unrelated MT_3 receptor. Ramelteon is not known to bind to any other classes of receptors, such as nicotinic ACh, neuropeptide, dopamine, and opiate receptors, or the benzodiazepine binding site on $GABA_A$ receptors.

Clinical Pharmacology

Prescribing guidelines suggest that an 8-mg tablet be taken about 30 min before bedtime. Ramelteon is rapidly absorbed from the GI tract. Because of the significant first-pass metabolism that occurs after oral administration, ramelteon bioavailability is less than 2%. The drug is largely metabolized by hepatic CYPs 1A2, 2C, and 3A4, with a $t_{1/2}$ of about 2 h in humans. Of the four metabolites, M-II, acts as an agonist at MT_1 and MT_2 receptors and may contribute to the sleep-promoting effects of ramelteon.

Ramelteon is efficacious in combating both transient and chronic insomnia, with no tolerance occurring in its reduction of sleep onset latency even after 6 months of drug administration (Mayer et al., 2009). It is generally well tolerated by patients and does not impair next-day cognitive function. Sleep latency was consistently found to be shorter in patients given ramelteon compared to placebo controls. No evidence of rebound insomnia or withdrawal effects were noted on ramelteon withdrawal. Unlike most agents mentioned in this chapter, ramelteon is not a controlled substance.

Tasimelteon

Tasimelteon is a selective agonist for MT_1 and MT_2 receptors. It has been approved in the U.S. for treatment of non–24-h sleep-wake syndrome in totally blind patients experiencing circadian rhythm disorder (Johnsa and Neville, 2014).

Barbiturates

The barbiturates were once used extensively as sedative-hypnotic drugs. Except for a few specialized uses, they have been largely replaced by the much safer benzodiazepines and Z compounds. Table 19–3 lists the common barbiturates and their pharmacological properties.

Barbiturates are derivatives of this parent structure:

*O except in thiopental, where it is replaced by S.

Barbituric acid is 2,4,6-trioxohexahydropyrimidine. This compound lacks central depressant activity, but the presence of alkyl or aryl groups at position 5 confers sedative-hypnotic and sometimes other activities. Barbiturates in which the oxygen at C2 is replaced by sulfur are called *thiobarbiturates*. These compounds are more lipid soluble than the corresponding *oxybarbiturates*. In general, structural changes that increase lipid solubility decrease duration of action, decrease latency to onset of activity, accelerate metabolic degradation, and increase hypnotic potency.

Pharmacological Properties

The barbiturates reversibly depress the activity of all excitable tissues. The CNS is particularly sensitive, and even when barbiturates are given

TABLE 19–3 ■ THERAPEUTIC USES OF BARBITURATES

COMPOUND	ROUTES OF ADMINISTRATION	THERAPEUTIC USES	COMMENTS	$t_{1/2}$ (h)
Amobarbital	IM, IV	Insomnia, preoperative sedation, emergency management of seizures	Only Na$^+$ salt for injection is sold in the U.S.	10–40
Butabarbital	Oral	Insomnia, preoperative sedation, daytime sedation	Redistribution shortens duration of action of single dose to 8 h	35–50
Mephobarbital (not licensed for use in the U.S.)	Oral	Seizure disorders, daytime sedation	Second-line anticonvulsant	10–70
Methohexital	IV	Induction and maintenance of anesthesia	Only Na$^+$ salt available; single dose provides 5–7 min of anesthesia	3–5
Pentobarbital	Oral, IM, IV, rectal (only injectable form is marketed in the U.S.)	Insomnia, preoperative and procedural sedation, emergency management of seizures	Administer only Na$^+$ salt parenterally	15–50
Phenobarbital	Oral, IM, IV	Seizure disorders, status epilepticus, daytime sedation (hyperbilirubinemia, OL use)	First-line anticonvulsant; only Na$^+$ salt administered parenterally	80–120
Secobarbital	Oral	Insomnia, preoperative sedation	Only Na$^+$ salt available	15–40
Thiopental (not currently produced or marketed in the U.S.)	IV	Induction/maintenance of anesthesia, preoperative sedation, emergency management of seizures, intracranial pressure	Only Na$^+$ salt available; single dose provides brief period of anesthesia	8–10 ($t_{1/2}$ of anesthetic effects is short due to redistribution; see Figures 2–4 and 21–2)

in anesthetic concentrations, direct effects on peripheral excitable tissues are weak. However, serious deficits in cardiovascular and other peripheral functions occur in acute barbiturate intoxication.

ADME

For sedative-hypnotic use, the barbiturates usually are administered orally (see Table 19–2). Na$^+$ salts are absorbed more rapidly than the corresponding free acids, especially from liquid formulations. The onset of action varies from 10 to 60 min and is delayed by the presence of food. Intramuscular injections of solutions of the Na$^+$ salts should be placed deeply into large muscles to avoid the pain and possible necrosis that can result at more superficial sites. The intravenous route usually is reserved for the management of status epilepticus (phenobarbital sodium) or for the induction or maintenance of general anesthesia (e.g., thiopental or methohexital).

Barbiturates distribute widely in the body and readily cross the placenta. The highly lipid-soluble barbiturates such as *thiopental* and *methohexital*, used to induce anesthesia, undergo rapid redistribution after intravenous injection. Redistribution into less-vascular tissues, especially muscle and fat, leads to a decline in the concentration of barbiturate in the plasma and brain. With thiopental and methohexital, this results in the awakening of patients within 5–15 min of the injection of the usual anesthetic doses (see Figures 2–4 and 21–2).

Except for the less lipid-soluble *aprobarbital* and *phenobarbital*, nearly complete metabolism or conjugation of barbiturates in the liver precedes their renal excretion. The oxidation of radicals at C5 is the most important biotransformation that terminates biological activity. In some instances (e.g., phenobarbital), N-glycosylation is an important metabolic pathway. Other biotransformations include N-hydroxylation, desulfuration of thiobarbiturates to oxybarbiturates, opening of the barbituric acid ring, and N-dealkylation of N-alkyl barbiturates to active metabolites (e.g., mephobarbital to phenobarbital). About 25% of phenobarbital and nearly all of aprobarbital are excreted unchanged in the urine. Their renal excretion can be increased greatly by osmotic diuresis or alkalinization of the urine.

The metabolic elimination of barbiturates is more rapid in young people than in the elderly and infants, and half-lives are increased during pregnancy partly because of the expanded volume of distribution. Chronic liver disease, especially cirrhosis, often increases the $t_{1/2}$ of the biotransformable barbiturates. Repeated administration, especially of phenobarbital, shortens the $t_{1/2}$ of barbiturates that are metabolized as a result of the induction of microsomal enzymes.

The barbiturates commonly used as hypnotics in the U.S. have $t_{1/2}$ values such that the drugs are not fully eliminated in 24 h (see Table 19–3). Thus, these barbiturates will accumulate during repeated administration unless appropriate adjustments in dosage are made. Furthermore, the persistence of the drug in plasma during the day favors the development of tolerance and abuse.

CNS Effects

Actions on the GABA$_A$ Receptor

Enhancement of inhibition occurs primarily at synapses where neurotransmission is mediated by GABA acting at GABA$_A$ receptors. Barbiturates bind to a distinct allosteric site on the GABA$_A$ receptor (Figure 14–11); binding leads to an increase in the mean open time of the GABA-activated Cl$^-$ channel, with no effect on frequency. At higher concentrations, barbiturates directly activate channel opening, even in the absence of GABA (Nestler et al., 2015). Barbiturates also reportedly inhibit excitatory AMPA/kainate receptors (Marszalec and Narahashi, 1993) and inhibit glutamate release via an effect on voltage-activated Ca^{2+} channels. These multiple actions, especially the direct gating effect on the GABA$_A$ channel, may explain the potent CNS depressant effects of barbiturates as compared to benzodiazepines.

Effects in the CNS

Barbiturates enhance GABA-mediated inhibitory transmission throughout the CNS; nonanesthetic doses preferentially suppress polysynaptic responses. Facilitation is diminished, and inhibition usually is enhanced. The site of inhibition is either postsynaptic, as at *cortical and cerebellar pyramidal cells* and in the *cuneate nucleus, substantia nigra*, and *thalamic relay neurons*, or presynaptic, as in the *spinal cord*.

Barbiturates can produce all degrees of depression of the CNS, ranging from mild sedation to general anesthesia (see Chapter 21).

Certain barbiturates, particularly those containing a 5-phenyl substituent (e.g., phenobarbital and mephobarbital), have selective anticonvulsant activity (see Chapter 17). The antianxiety properties of the barbiturates are inferior to those exerted by the benzodiazepines.

Except for the anticonvulsant activities of phenobarbital and its congeners, the barbiturates possess a low degree of selectivity and a low therapeutic index. Pain perception and reaction are relatively unimpaired until the moment of unconsciousness, and in small doses, barbiturates increase reactions to painful stimuli. Hence, they cannot be relied on to produce sedation or sleep in the presence of even moderate pain.

Effects on Stages of Sleep

Hypnotic doses of barbiturates increase the total sleep time and alter the stages of sleep in a dose-dependent manner. Like the benzodiazepines, barbiturates decrease sleep latency, the number of awakenings, and the durations of REM and slow-wave sleep. During repetitive nightly administration, some tolerance to the effects on sleep occurs within a few days, and the effect on total sleep time may be reduced by as much as 50% after 2 weeks of use. Discontinuation leads to rebound increases in all the sleep parameters initially decreased by barbiturates.

Tolerance, Abuse, and Dependence

With chronic administration of gradually increasing doses, pharmacodynamic tolerance continues to develop over a period of weeks to months, depending on the dosage schedule, whereas pharmacokinetic tolerance reaches its peak in a few days to a week. Tolerance to the euphoric, sedative, and hypnotic effects occurs more readily and is greater than that to the anticonvulsant and lethal effects; thus, as tolerance increases, the therapeutic index decreases. Pharmacodynamic tolerance to barbiturates confers cross-tolerance to all general CNS depressant drugs, including ethanol. Like other CNS depressant drugs, barbiturates are abused, and some individuals develop physical dependence (see Chapter 24).

Effects on Peripheral Nerve Structures

Barbiturates selectively depress transmission in autonomic ganglia and reduce nicotinic excitation by choline esters. This effect may account, at least in part, for the fall in blood pressure produced by intravenous oxybarbiturates and by severe barbiturate intoxication. At skeletal neuromuscular junctions, the blocking effects of both *tubocurarine* and *decamethonium* are enhanced during barbiturate anesthesia. These actions probably result from the capacity of barbiturates at hypnotic or anesthetic concentrations to inhibit current flow through nicotinic ACh receptors. Several distinct mechanisms appear to be involved, and little stereoselectivity is evident.

Systemic Effects

Respiration

Barbiturates depress both the respiratory drive and the mechanisms responsible for the rhythmic character of respiration. The neurogenic drive is essentially eliminated by a dose three times greater than that used normally to induce sleep. Such doses also suppress the hypoxic drive and, to a lesser extent, the chemoreceptor drive. However, the margin between the lighter planes of surgical anesthesia and dangerous respiratory depression is sufficient to permit the ultrashort-acting barbiturates to be used, with suitable precautions, as anesthetic agents.

The barbiturates only slightly depress protective reflexes until the degree of intoxication is sufficient to produce severe respiratory depression. Coughing, sneezing, hiccoughing, and laryngospasm may occur when barbiturates are employed as intravenous anesthetic agents.

Cardiovascular System

When given orally in sedative or hypnotic doses, barbiturates do not produce significant overt cardiovascular effects. In general, the effects of thiopental anesthesia on the cardiovascular system are benign in comparison with those of the volatile anesthetic agents; there usually is either no change or a fall in mean arterial pressure (see Chapter 21). Barbiturates can blunt cardiovascular reflexes by partial inhibition of ganglionic transmission, most evident in patients with congestive heart failure or hypovolemic shock. Because barbiturates also impair reflex cardiovascular adjustments to inflation of the lung, positive-pressure respiration should be used cautiously and only when necessary to maintain adequate pulmonary ventilation in patients who are anesthetized or intoxicated with a barbiturate.

Other cardiovascular changes often noted when thiopental and other intravenous thiobarbiturates are administered after conventional preanesthetic medication include decreased renal and cerebral blood flow with a marked fall in CSF pressure. Although cardiac arrhythmias are observed only infrequently, intravenous anesthesia with barbiturates can increase the incidence of ventricular arrhythmias, especially when epinephrine and halothane also are present. Anesthetic concentrations of barbiturates depress the function of Na^+ channels and at least two types of K^+ channels. However, direct depression of cardiac contractility occurs only when doses several times those required to cause anesthesia are administered.

GI Tract

The oxybarbiturates tend to decrease the tone of the GI musculature and the amplitude of rhythmic contractions; the locus of action is partly peripheral and partly central. A hypnotic dose does not significantly delay gastric emptying in humans. The relief of various GI symptoms by sedative doses is probably largely due to the central depressant action.

Liver

The effects vary with the duration of exposure to the barbiturate. *Acutely,* the barbiturates interact with several CYPs and inhibit the biotransformation of a number of other drugs and endogenous substrates, such as steroids; other substrates may reciprocally inhibit barbiturate biotransformations (see Chapter 6).

Chronic administration of barbiturates markedly increases the protein and lipid content of the hepatic smooth endoplasmic reticulum, as well as the activities of glucuronyl transferase and CYPs 1A2, 2C9, 2C19, and 3A4. The induction of these enzymes increases the metabolism of a number of drugs (including barbiturates) and endogenous substances, including steroid hormones, cholesterol, bile salts, and vitamins K and D. The self-induced increase in barbiturate metabolism partly accounts for tolerance to barbiturates. The inducing effect is not limited to the microsomal enzymes; for example, there are increases in ALA synthetase, a mitochondrial enzyme, and aldehyde dehydrogenase, a cytosolic enzyme. The effect of barbiturates on ALA synthetase can cause dangerous disease exacerbations in persons with intermittent porphyria.

Kidney

Severe oliguria or anuria may occur in acute barbiturate poisoning largely as a result of the marked hypotension.

Therapeutic Uses

The major uses of individual barbiturates are listed in Table 19–3. As with the benzodiazepines, the selection of a particular barbiturate for a given therapeutic indication is based primarily on pharmacokinetic considerations. Benzodiazepines and other compounds have largely replaced barbiturates as sedatives.

Untoward Effects

Aftereffects

Drowsiness may last for only a few hours after a hypnotic dose of barbiturate, but residual CNS depression sometimes is evident the following day, and subtle distortions of mood and impairment of judgment and fine motor skills may be demonstrable. Residual effects also may take the form of vertigo, nausea, vomiting, or diarrhea or sometimes may be manifested as overt excitement.

Paradoxical Excitement

In some persons, barbiturates produce excitement rather than depression, and the patient may appear to be inebriated. This type of idiosyncrasy is relatively common among geriatric and debilitated patients and occurs most frequently with phenobarbital and *N*-methylbarbiturates.

Barbiturates may cause restlessness, excitement, and even delirium when given in the presence of pain and may worsen a patient's perception of pain.

Hypersensitivity

Allergic reactions occur, especially in persons with asthma, urticaria, angioedema, or similar conditions. Hypersensitivity reactions include localized swellings, particularly of the eyelids, cheeks, or lips, and erythematous dermatitis. Rarely, exfoliative dermatitis may be caused by phenobarbital and can prove fatal; the skin eruption may be associated with fever, delirium, and marked degenerative changes in the liver and other parenchymatous organs.

Other

Because barbiturates enhance porphyrin synthesis, they are absolutely contraindicated in patients with acute intermittent porphyria or porphyria variegata. Hypnotic doses in the presence of pulmonary insufficiency are contraindicated. Rapid intravenous injection of a barbiturate may cause cardiovascular collapse before anesthesia ensues. Blood pressure can fall to shock levels; even slow intravenous injection of barbiturates often produces apnea and occasionally laryngospasm, coughing, and other respiratory difficulties.

Drug Interactions

Barbiturates combine with other CNS depressants to cause severe depression; interactions with ethanol and with first-generation antihistamines are common. Isoniazid, methylphenidate, and monoamine oxidase inhibitors also increase the CNS depressant effects of barbiturates.

Barbiturates competitively inhibit the metabolism of certain other drugs; however, the greatest number of drug interactions results from induction of hepatic CYPs (as described previously) and the accelerated disappearance of many drugs and endogenous substances from the body. Hepatic enzyme induction enhances metabolism of endogenous steroid hormones, which may cause endocrine disturbances, and enhances metabolism of oral contraceptives, which may increase the likelihood of unwanted pregnancy. Barbiturates also induce the hepatic generation of toxic metabolites of chlorocarbons (chloroform, trichloroethylene, carbon tetrachloride) and consequently promote lipid peroxidation, which facilitates periportal necrosis of the liver caused by these agents.

Barbiturate Poisoning

The incidence of barbiturate poisoning has declined markedly, largely as a result of their decreased use as sedative-hypnotic agents. Most of the cases are the result of attempts at suicide, but some are from accidental poisonings in children or drug abusers. The lethal dose of barbiturate varies, but severe poisoning is likely to occur when more than 10 times the full hypnotic dose has been ingested at once. The lethal dose becomes lower if alcohol or other depressant drugs are present. In severe intoxication, the patient is comatose; respiration is affected early. Breathing may be either slow or rapid and shallow. Eventually, blood pressure falls because the effect of the drug and of hypoxia on medullary vasomotor centers; depression of cardiac contractility and sympathetic ganglia also contributes. Pulmonary complications (e.g., atelectasis, edema, and bronchopneumonia) and renal failure are likely to be the fatal complications of severe barbiturate poisoning.

The treatment of acute barbiturate intoxication is based on general supportive measures, which are applicable in most respects to poisoning by any CNS depressant. The use of CNS stimulants is contraindicated. If renal and cardiac functions are satisfactory and the patient is hydrated, forced diuresis and alkalinization of the urine will hasten the excretion of phenobarbital. See Chapter 4, Drug Toxicity and Poisoning.

Miscellaneous Sedative-Hypnotic Drugs

Many drugs with diverse structures have been used for their sedative-hypnotic properties, including *ramelteon, chloral hydrate, meprobamate,* and paraldehyde (no longer licensed in the U.S.). With the exception of ramelteon and meprobamate, the pharmacological actions of these drugs generally resemble those of the barbiturates:

- They all are general CNS depressants that can produce profound hypnosis with little or no analgesia.
- Their effects on the stages of sleep are similar to those of the barbiturates.
- Their therapeutic indices are low, and acute intoxication, which produces respiratory depression and hypotension, is managed similarly to barbiturate poisoning.
- Their chronic use can result in tolerance and physical dependence.
- The syndrome after chronic use can be severe and life threatening.

Chloral Hydrate

Chloral hydrate may be used to treat patients with paradoxical reactions to benzodiazepines. Chloral hydrate is reduced rapidly to the active compound trichloroethanol (CCl_3CH_2OH), largely by hepatic alcohol dehydrogenase. Its pharmacological effects probably are caused by trichloroethanol, which can exert barbiturate-like effects on $GABA_A$ receptor channels in vitro. Chloral hydrate is regulated as a schedule IV controlled substance.

In the U.S., chloral hydrate is best known as a literary poison, the "knockout drops" added to a strong alcoholic beverage to produce a "Mickey Finn" or "Mickey," a cocktail given to an unwitting imbiber to render the person malleable or unconscious, most famously Sam Spade in Dashiell Hammett's 1930 novel, *The Maltese Falcon.* Now that detectives drink wine rather than whiskey, this off-label use of chloral hydrate has waned.

Meprobamate

Meprobamate, a *bis*-carbamate ester, was introduced as an antianxiety agent, and this remains its only approved use in the U.S. However, it also became popular as a sedative-hypnotic agent. The pharmacological properties of meprobamate resemble those of the benzodiazepines in a number of ways. Meprobamate can release suppressed behaviors in experimental animals at doses that cause little impairment of locomotor activity, and although it can cause CNS depression, it cannot produce anesthesia. Large doses of meprobamate cause severe respiratory depression, hypotension, shock, and heart failure. Meprobamate appears to have a mild analgesic effect in patients with musculoskeletal pain, and it enhances the analgesic effects of other drugs.

Meprobamate is well absorbed when administered orally. Nevertheless, an important aspect of intoxication with meprobamate is the formation of gastric bezoars consisting of undissolved meprobamate tablets; treatment may require endoscopy, with mechanical removal of the bezoar. Most of the drug is metabolized in the liver by side-chain hydroxylation and glucuronidation; the kinetics of elimination may depend on dose. The $t_{1/2}$ of meprobamate may be prolonged during its chronic administration. The major unwanted effects of the usual sedative doses of meprobamate are drowsiness and ataxia; larger doses impair learning and motor coordination and prolong reaction time. Meprobamate enhances the CNS depression produced by other drugs. After long-term medication, abrupt discontinuation evokes a withdrawal syndrome usually characterized by anxiety, insomnia, tremors, and, frequently, hallucinations; generalized seizures occur in about 10% of cases.

Carisoprodol, a skeletal muscle relaxant whose active metabolite is meprobamate, also has abuse potential and has become a popular "street drug." Meprobamate and carisoprodol are designated as schedule IV controlled substances.

Other Agents

Etomidate is used in the U.S. and other countries as an intravenous anesthetic, often in combination with fentanyl. It is advantageous because it lacks pulmonary and vascular depressant activity, although it has a negative inotropic effect on the heart. Its pharmacology and anesthetic uses are described in Chapter 21.

Clomethiazole has sedative, muscle relaxant, and anticonvulsant properties. Given alone, its effects on respiration are slight, and the therapeutic index is high. However, deaths from adverse interactions with ethanol are relatively frequent.

Propofol is a rapidly acting and highly lipophilic diisopropylphenol used in the induction and maintenance of general anesthesia (see Chapter 21), as well as in the maintenance of long-term sedation. Propofol has found use in intensive care sedation in adults (McKeage and Perry, 2003), for sedation during GI endoscopy procedures, and during transvaginal oocyte retrieval.

Nonprescription Hypnotic Drugs

The antihistamines *diphenhydramine* and *doxylamine* are FDA-approved as ingredients in OTC nonprescription sleep aids. With elimination $t_{1/2}$ of about 9–10 h, these antihistamines can be associated with prominent residual sleepiness the morning after when taken as a sleep aid the night before.

New and Emerging Agents

Suvorexant

Suvorexant, an inhibitor of orexin 1 and 2 receptors, was approved by the FDA in late 2014 for the treatment of insomnia (Winrow and Renger, 2014). Orexins, produced by neurons in the lateral hypothalamus and projecting broadly throughout the CNS, play a major role in regulation of the sleep cycle. These neurons are quiescent during sleep but are active during wakefulness; thus, orexins promote wakefulness, while antagonists at orexin receptors enhance REM and non-REM sleep. Suvorexant decreases sleep onset latency and is superior to placebo in sleep maintenance. One 10-mg dose should be taken within 30 min of going to bed if at least 7 h remain until the projected time of awakening. The most common adverse reaction is daytime somnolence, and there is a possibility of the worsening of depression or suicidal ideation. Surorexant is a schedule IV controlled substance. A number of other orexin receptor antagonists are currently in clinical trials.

Doxepin

Doxepin, a tricyclic antidepressant, enhances subjective measures of sleep quality and is indicated for the treatment of difficulties with sleep maintenance (Yeung et al., 2015). It acts presumably via antagonism of H_1 receptor function when administered in low doses. Doxepin should be taken in initial doses of 6 mg (3 mg in the elderly) within 30 min of bedtime. Abnormal thinking and behavior have been observed following its use, and it can worsen suicidal ideation and depression. Doxepin was approved by the FDA in 2010 for the treatment of sleep maintenance insomnia.

Pregabalin

Pregabalin, an anxiolytic agent that binds to Ca^{2+} channel $\alpha_2\delta$ subunits, has proved useful in clinical trials (Holsboer-Trachsler and Prieto, 2013); pregabalin slightly decreased sleep onset latency and increased the proportion of time spent in slow-wave sleep. Pregabalin appears to be an effective treatment of the insomnia seen in patients suffering from a generalized anxiety disorder. Pregabalin is designated as a schedule V controlled substance.

Ritanserin

Ritanserin and other $5HT_{2A/2C}$ receptor antagonists show an ability to promote slow-wave sleep in patients with chronic primary insomnia or generalized anxiety disorder (Monti, 2010). Ritanserin is not licensed for use in the U.S.

Agomelatine

Agomelatine, a melatonin receptor agonist and a $5HT_{2C}$ receptor antagonist, is prescribed for the treatment of depression and may aid in ameliorating sleep disturbances often associated with depression. Agomelatine is not licensed for use in the U.S.

Management of Insomnia

Insomnia is one of the most common complaints in general medical practice. A number of pharmacological agents are available for the treatment of insomnia. The "perfect" hypnotic would allow sleep to occur with normal sleep architecture. It would not cause next-day effects, either of rebound anxiety or of continued sedation. It would not interact with other medications. It could be used chronically without causing dependence or rebound insomnia on discontinuation. Controversy in the management of insomnia revolves around two issues:

- Pharmacological versus nonpharmacological treatment
- Use of short-acting versus long-acting hypnotics

The side effects of hypnotic medications must be weighed against the sequelae of chronic insomnia, which include a 4-fold increase in serious accidents (Balter and Uhlenhuth, 1992). Regular moderate exercise or even small amounts of exercise often are effective in promoting sleep. In addition to appropriate pharmacological treatment, the management of insomnia should correct identifiable causes, address inadequate sleep hygiene, eliminate performance anxiety related to falling asleep, provide entrainment of the biological clock so that maximum sleepiness occurs at the hour of attempted sleep, and suppress the use of alcohol and OTC sleep medications.

Categories of Insomnia

- *Transient insomnia* lasts less than 3 days and usually is caused by a brief environmental or situational stressor. If hypnotics are prescribed, they should be used at the lowest dose and for only 2–3 nights. Note that benzodiazepines given acutely before important life events, such as examinations, may result in impaired performance.
- *Short-term insomnia* lasts from 3 days to 3 weeks and usually is caused by a personal stressor such as illness, grief, or job problems. Hypnotics may be used adjunctively for 7–10 nights and are best used intermittently during this time, with the patient skipping a dose after 1–2 nights of good sleep.
- *Long-term insomnia* lasts for more than 3 weeks; a specific stressor may not be identifiable.

Insomnia Accompanying Major Psychiatric Illnesses

The insomnia caused by major psychiatric illnesses often responds to specific pharmacological treatment of that illness. For example, in major depressive episodes with insomnia, SSRIs, which may cause insomnia as a side effect, usually will result in improved sleep because they treat the depressive syndrome. In a patient whose depression is responding to an SSRI but has persistent insomnia as a side effect of the medication, judicious use of evening trazodone may improve sleep, as well as augment the antidepressant effect of the reuptake inhibitor. However, the patient should be monitored for priapism, orthostatic hypotension, and arrhythmias.

Adequate control of anxiety disorders often produces adequate resolution of the accompanying insomnia. Sedative use in patients with anxiety disorders is decreasing because of a growing appreciation of the effectiveness of other agents, such as β adrenergic receptor antagonists (Chapter 12) for performance anxiety and SSRIs for obsessive-compulsive disorder and perhaps generalized anxiety disorder. The profound insomnia in patients with acute psychosis owing to schizophrenia or mania usually responds to dopamine receptor antagonists (see Chapters 13 and 16). Benzodiazepines often are used adjunctively in this situation to reduce agitation and improve sleep.

Insomnia Accompanying Other Medical Illnesses

For long-term insomnia owing to other medical illnesses, adequate treatment of the underlying disorder, such as congestive heart failure, asthma, or COPD, may resolve the insomnia. Adequate pain management in conditions of chronic pain will treat both the pain and the insomnia and may make hypnotics unnecessary. *Adequate attention to sleep hygiene, including reduced caffeine intake, avoidance of alcohol, adequate exercise, and regular sleep and wake times, often will reduce the insomnia.*

Conditioned (Learned) Insomnia

In those who have no major psychiatric or other medical illness and in whom attention to sleep hygiene is ineffective, attention should be directed to conditioned (learned) insomnia. These patients have associated the bedroom with activities consistent with wakefulness rather than sleep. In such patients, all other activities associated with waking, even such quiescent activities as reading and watching television, should be done outside the bedroom.

Sleep-State Misperception

Some patients complain of poor sleep but have been shown to have no objective polysomnographic evidence of insomnia. They are difficult to treat.

Long-Term Insomnia

Nonpharmacological treatments are important for all patients with long-term insomnia. These include education about sleep hygiene, relaxation training, and behavioral modification approaches, such as sleep restriction and stimulus-control therapies.

Long-term hypnotic use leads to a decrease in effectiveness and may produce rebound insomnia on discontinuance. Almost all hypnotics change sleep architecture. The barbiturates reduce REM sleep; the benzodiazepines reduce slow-wave non-REM sleep and, to a lesser extent, REM sleep. While the significance of these findings is not clear, there is an emerging consensus that slow-wave sleep is particularly important for physical restorative processes. REM sleep may aid in the consolidation of learning. The blockade of slow-wave sleep by benzodiazepines may partly account for their diminishing effectiveness over the long term, and it also may explain their effectiveness in blocking sleep terrors, a disorder of arousal from slow-wave sleep.

Long-acting benzodiazepines can cause next-day confusion, whereas shorter-acting agents can produce rebound next-day anxiety. Paradoxically, the acute amnestic effects of benzodiazepines may be responsible for the patient's subsequent report of restful sleep. Anterograde amnesia may be more common with triazolam. Hypnotics should not be given to patients with sleep apnea, especially the obstructive type, because these agents decrease upper airway muscle tone while also decreasing the arousal response to hypoxia.

Insomnia in Older Patients

The elderly, like the very young, tend to sleep in a *polyphasic* (multiple sleep episodes per day) pattern rather than the *monophasic* pattern characteristic of younger adults. This pattern makes assessment of adequate sleep time difficult.

Changes in the pharmacokinetic profiles of hypnotic agents occur in the elderly because of reduced body water, reduced renal function, and increased body fat, leading to a longer $t_{1/2}$ for benzodiazepines. A dose that produces pleasant sleep and adequate daytime wakefulness during week 1 may produce daytime confusion and amnesia by week 3 as the drug level continues to rise, particularly with long-acting hypnotics. For example, the benzodiazepine diazepam is highly lipid soluble and is excreted by the kidney. Because of the increase in body fat and the decrease in renal excretion that typically occur from age 20 to 80, the $t_{1/2}$ of the drug may increase 4-fold over this span.

Injudicious use of hypnotics in the elderly can produce daytime cognitive impairment and thereby impair overall quality of life. Once an older patient has been taking benzodiazepines for an extended period, whether for daytime anxiety or for nighttime sedation, terminating the drug can be a long, involved process. Attempts at drug withdrawal may not be successful, and it may be necessary to leave the patient on the medication, with adequate attention to daytime side effects.

Prescribing Guidelines for Managing Insomnia

Hypnotics that act at $GABA_A$ receptors—benzodiazepine hypnotics and the newer agents zolpidem, zopiclone, and zaleplon—are preferred to barbiturates; the $GABA_A$ receptor agents have a higher therapeutic index, smaller effects on sleep architecture, and less abuse potential. Compounds with a shorter $t_{1/2}$ are favored in patients with sleep-onset insomnia but without significant daytime anxiety who need to function at full effectiveness during the day. These compounds also are appropriate for the elderly because of a decreased risk of falls and respiratory depression. However, the patient and physician should be aware that early morning awakening, rebound daytime anxiety, and amnestic episodes also may occur. These undesirable side effects are more common at higher doses of the benzodiazepines.

Benzodiazepines with longer $t_{1/2}$ values are favored for patients who have significant daytime anxiety. These benzodiazepines also are appropriate for patients receiving treatment of major depressive episodes because the short-acting agents can worsen early morning awakening. However, longer-acting benzodiazepines can be associated with next-day cognitive impairment or delayed daytime cognitive impairment (after 2–4 weeks of treatment) as a result of drug accumulation with repeated administration.

Older agents—barbiturates, chloral hydrate, and meprobamate—should be avoided for the management of insomnia. They have high abuse potential and are dangerous in overdose.

Drug Facts for Your Personal Formulary: *Sedative-Hypnotic Agents*

Drug	Therapeutic Uses	Clinical Pharmacology and Tips
Benzodiazepines-synergistic with other CNS depressants, esp. ethanol; see Table 19–2.		
Alprazolam	Anxiety disorders, agoraphobia	Withdrawal symptoms may be especially severe
Chlordiazepoxide	Anxiety disorders, alcohol withdrawal, preanesthetic medication	Long-acting and self-tapering because of active metabolites
Clobazam	Adjunctive treatment of seizures associated with Lennox-Gastaut syndrome, other epilepsy and anxiety disorders	Active metabolite has long half-life Decrease dose and titrate in CYP2C19 poor metabolizers Tolerance develops to anticonvulsant effects
Clonazepam	Seizure disorders, adjunctive treatment in acute mania and certain movement disorders	Tolerance develops to anticonvulsant effects
Clorazepate	Anxiety disorders, seizure disorders	Prodrug; activity due to formation of nordazepam during absorption
Diazepam	Anxiety disorders, alcohol withdrawal, status epilepticus, skeletal muscle relaxation, preanesthetic medication	Prototypical benzodiazepine
Estazolam	Insomnia	Contains triazolo ring; adverse effects may be similar to those of triazolam

Drug Facts for Your Personal Formulary: *Sedative-Hypnotic Agents* (*continued*)

Drug	Therapeutic Uses	Clinical Pharmacology and Tips
Flurazepam	Insomnia	Active metabolites accumulate with chronic use
Lorazepam	Anxiety disorders, alcohol withdrawal, preanesthetic medication	Metabolized solely by conjugation
Midazolam	Preanesthetic and intraoperative medication	Rapidly inactivated
Oxazepam	Anxiety disorders, alcohol withdrawal	Metabolized solely by conjugation
Quazepam	Insomnia	Active metabolites accumulate with chronic use
Temazepam	Insomnia	Metabolized mainly by conjugation
Triazolam	Insomnia	Rapidly inactivated; may cause disturbing daytime side effects
"Z" Compounds-nonbenzodiazepines with agonist effects at the benzodiazepine site of GABA$_A$ receptors; have largely replaced benzodiazepines for treating insomnia.		
Zaleplon	Insomnia	Very short elimination half-life
Zolpidem	Insomnia	Short-term (2–6 week) treatment of insomnia
Eszopiclone	Insomnia	S(+) enantiomer of zopiclone
Benzodiazepine Antagonist		
Flumenazil	Benzodiazepine overdose (benzodiazepine and β-carboline antagonist	Headache, dizziness; do not use in tricyclic antidepressant poisoning (seizures!)
Miscellaneous and Emerging Agents		
Ramelteon	Insomnia	Melatonin receptor agonist; significant first-pass effect
Tasimelteon	Circadian rhythm disorder in blind patients	Melatonin receptor agonist
Suvorexant	Insomnia	Orexin receptor antagonist; needs at least 7 h after 10-mg dose before awakening
Doxepin	Depression, insomnia	Tricyclic antidepressant; sedating effects likely occur through H$_1$ receptor antagonism; beware of abnormal behavior, suicide ideation, depression; use half dose in the elderly
Propofol	Induction/maintenance of anesthesia, procedural sedation	Rapid recovery
Pregabalin (β-isobutyl–GABA)	Nerve/muscle pain, fibromyalgia, seizures	Schedule V substance, abuse potential; some concern for suicide ideation and angioedema
Barbiturates-synergistic with other CNS depressants, esp. ethanol; induce CYPs; respiratory depressants; see Table 19–3.		
Amobarbital	Insomnia, preoperative sedation, emergency management of seizures	• IM and IV • Short-acting (3-8 h)
Butabarbital	Insomnia, preoperative sedation, daytime sedation	• Oral • Fast onset of action • Short-acting (3-8 h)
Mephobarbital (not licensed for use in U.S.)	Seizure disorders, daytime sedation	• Oral • Short-acting (3-8 h)
Methohexital	Induction and maintenance of anesthesia	• IV • Ultra short-acting (5-15 min)
Pentobarbital	Insomnia, preoperative and procedural sedation, emergency management of seizures	• Oral, IM, IV, or rectal • Administer Na$^+$ salt parenterally • Short-acting (3-8 h)
Phenobarbital	Seizure disorders, status epilepticus, daytime sedation	• Oral, IM, IV • First-line anticonvulsant (see chapter 17); administer Na$^+$ salt parenterally • Long-acting (days)
Secobarbital	Insomnia, preoperative sedation	• Oral • Short-acting (3-8 h)
Thiopental	Induction and maintenance of anesthesia, preoperative sedation, emergency management of seizures, intracranial hypertension	• IV single dose provides brief period of anesthesia • Ultra short-acting (5-15 min)

Bibliography

Balter MB, Uhlenhuth EH. New epidemiologic findings about insomnia and its treatment. *J Clin Psychiatry,* **1992**, *53*(suppl):34–39.

Dooley M, Plosker GL. Zaleplon: a review of its use in the treatment of insomnia. *Drugs,* **2000**, *60*:413–445.

Dujardin K, et al. Comparison of the effects of zolpidem and flunitrazepam on sleep structure and daytime cognitive functions: a study of untreated insomniacs. *Pharmacopsychiatry,* **1998**, *31*:14–18.

Hanson SM, et al. Structural requirements for eszopiclone and zolpidem binding to the gamma-aminobutyric acid type-A (GABA$_A$) receptor are different. *J Med Chem,* **2008**, *51*:7243–7252.

Hoffman EJ, Warren EW. Flumazenil: a benzodiazepine antagonist. *Clin Pharmacol,* **1993**, *12*:641–656.

Holsboer-Trachsler E, Prieto R. Effects of pregabalin on sleep in generalized anxiety disorder. *Int J Neuropsychopharmacol,* **2013**, *16*:925–936.

Huedo-Medina TB, et al. Effectiveness of non-benzodiazepine hypnotics in treatment of adult insomnia: meta-analysis of data submitted to the Food and Drug Administration. *BMJ,* **2012**, *345*:e8343.

Johnsa JD, Neville MW. Tasimelteon: a melatonin receptor agonist for non-24-hour sleep-wake disorder. *Ann Pharmacother,* **2014**, *48*:1636–1641.

Marszalec W, Narahashi T. Use-dependent pentobarbital block of kainate and quisqualate currents. *Brain Res,* **1993**, *608*:7–15.

Mayer G, et al. Efficacy and safety of 6-month nightly ramelteon administration in adults with chronic primary insomnia. *Sleep,* **2009**, *32*:351–360.

McKeage K, Perry CM. Propofol: a review of its use in intensive care sedation of adults. *CNS Drugs,* **2003**, *17*:235–272.

Melton ST, et al. Eszopiclone for insomnia. *Ann Pharmacother,* **2005**, *39*:1659–1666.

Monane M. Insomnia in the elderly. *J Clin Psychiatry,* **1992**, *53*(suppl):23–28.

Monti JM. Serotonin 5-HT(2A) receptor antagonists in the treatment of insomnia: present status and future prospects. *Drugs Today (Barc),* **2010**, *46*:183–193.

Morselli PL. Zolpidem side effects. *Lancet,* **1993**, *342*:868–869.

Nestler EJ, et al. *Molecular Neuropharmacology.* 3rd ed. McGraw-Hill, New York, **2015**.

Oldenhof H, et al. Clinical pharmacokinetics of midazolam in intensive care patients, a wide interpatient variability? *Clin Pharmacol Ther,* **1988**, *43*:263–269.

Rosenberg R, et al. An assessment of the efficacy and safety of eszopiclone in the treatment of transient insomnia in healthy adults. *Sleep Med,* **2005**, *6*:15–22.

Sieghart W. Allosteric modulation of GABA$_A$ receptors via multiple drug-binding sites. *Adv Pharmacol,* **2015**, *72*:53–96.

Sigel E, Steinmann ME. Structure, function, and modulation of GABA$_A$ receptors. *J Biol Chem,* **2012**, *287*:40224–40231.

Spadoni G, et al. Melatonin receptor agonists: new options for insomnia and depression treatment. *CNS Neurosci Ther,* **2011**, *17*:733–741.

Uhlenhuth EH, et al. International study of expert judgment on therapeutic use of benzodiazepines and other psychotherapeutic medications: IV. Therapeutic dose dependence and abuse liability of benzodiazepines in the long-term treatment of anxiety disorders. *J Clin Psychopharmacol,* **1999**, *19*(suppl 2):23S–29S.

Winrow CJ, Renger JJ. Discovery and development of orexin receptor antagonists as therapeutics for insomnia. *Br J Pharmacol,* **2014**, *171*:283–293.

Woods JH, et al. Benzodiazepines: use, abuse, and consequences. *Pharmacol Rev,* **1992**, *44*:151–347.

Yeung WF, et al. Doxepin for insomnia: a systematic review of randomized placebo-controlled trials. *Sleep Med Rev,* **2015**, *19*:75–83.

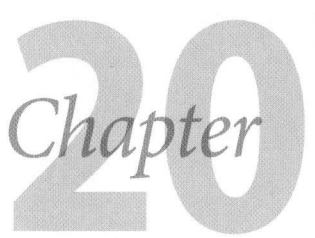

Chapter 20

Opioids, Analgesia, and Pain Management

Tony Yaksh and Mark Wallace

Pain

Pain is a component of virtually all clinical pathologies, and management of pain is a primary clinical imperative. Opioids are a mainstay of acute pain treatment, but in recent years, the efficacy and safety of long-term use of opioids to treat chronic pain has been questioned as instances of addiction and death from their misuse have mounted. Opioids are certainly no longer first-line treatment of chronic pain, and a more conservative approach may involve other drug classes, such as NSAIDs, anticonvulsants, and antidepressants.

The term *opiate* refers to compounds structurally related to products found in opium, a word derived from *opos*, the Greek word for "juice," natural opiates being derived from the resin of the opium poppy, *Papaver somniferum*. Opiates include the natural plant alkaloids, such as morphine, codeine, thebaine, and many semisynthetic derivatives. An *opioid* is any agent that has the functional and pharmacological properties of an opiate. Endogenous opioids are naturally occurring ligands for opioid receptors found in animals. The term *endorphin* not only is used synonymously with *endogenous opioid peptides* but also refers to a specific endogenous opioid, *β-endorphin*. The term *narcotic* was derived from the

Abbreviations

AAG: α_1-acid glycoprotein
AC: adenylyl cyclase
ACE: angiotensin-converting enzyme
ACh: acetylcholine
ACTH: corticotropin; formerly adrenocorticotropic hormone
ADH: antidiuretic hormone
ADME: absorption, distribution, metabolism, excretion
AT₁: angiotensin II receptor, type 1
ATC: around the clock
BBB: blood-brain barrier
CaMK: Ca^{2+}/calmodulin-dependent protein kinase
CDC: Centers for Disease Control and Prevention
CLIP: corticotropin-like intermediate lobe peptide
CNS: central nervous system
COPD: chronic obstructive pulmonary disease
COX: cyclooxygenase
CRH: corticotropin-releasing hormone
CSF: cerebrospinal fluid
CYP: cytochrome P450
DA: dopamine
DAMGO: [D-Ala²,MePhe⁴,Gly(ol)⁵]enkephalin
DHEA: dehydroepiandrosterone
DOR: δ opioid receptor
DYN: dynorphin
EEG: electroencephalogram
β-END: β-endorphin
L-ENK: Leu-enkephalin
ER/LA: extended-release/long-acting (a)
FDA: Food and Drug Administration
FSH: follicle-stimulating hormone
GABA: γ-aminobutyric acid
GI: gastrointestinal
GIRK: G protein–activated inwardly rectifying K^+ channel
GnRH: gonadotropin-releasing hormone
GPCR: G protein-coupled receptor
GRK: GPCR kinase
HPA: hypothalamic-pituitary-adrenal
5HT: serotonin
IM: intramuscular
IP₃: inositol triphosphate
IV: intravenous
JNK: c-Jun N-terminal kinase
KOR: κ opioid receptor
LH: luteinizing hormone
LPH: lipotropin
6-MAM: 6-monoacetylmorphine
MAO: monoamine oxidase
MAP: mitogen-activated protein
M-ENK: Met-enkephalin
MME: morphine milligram equivalent
MOR: μ opioid receptor
MSH: melanocyte-stimulating hormone
NAc: nucleus accumbens
NE: norepinephrine
α-NEO: α neoendorphin
NF-κB: nuclear factor kappa B
NMDA: N-methyl-D-aspartate
NOP: nociceptin/orphanin FQ (N/OFQ) receptor
NSAID: nonsteroidal anti-inflammatory drug
PAG: periaqueductal gray
PCA: patient-controlled anesthesia

PDMP: prescription drug monitoring program
PFC: prefrontal cortex
PI3K: phosphoinositide 3 kinase
PK: protein kinase
PLC: phospholipase C
POMC: pro-opiomelanocortin
pre-proDYN: pre-prodynorphin
pre-ProENK: pre-proenkephalin
SNRI: serotonin-norepinephrine reuptake inhibitor
SSRI: selective serotonin reuptake inhibitor
TM: transmembrane
VP: ventral pallidum
VTA: ventral tegmental area

Greek word *narkotikos,* for "benumbing" or "stupor." Although the term ***narcotic*** originally referred to any drug that induced narcosis or sleep, the word has become associated with opioids and is often used in a legal context to refer to substances with abuse or addictive potential.

Endogenous Opioid Peptides

A biological molecule found within the brain that acts through an opioid receptor is an endogenous opioid. The opioid peptide precursors are a protean family defined by the prohormone from which they are derived (Figure 20–1). Several distinct families of endogenous opioid peptides have been identified: principally the *enkephalins, endorphins,* and *dynorphins* (Table 20–1) (Höllt, 1986). These families have several common properties:

- Each derives from a distinct precursor protein, pre-POMC, *pre-proenkephalin*, and *preprodynorphin*, respectively, each encoded by a corresponding gene.
- Each precursor is subject to complex cleavages by distinct trypsin-like enzymes and to a variety of posttranslational modifications resulting in the synthesis of multiple peptides, some of which are active as opioids.
- Most opioid peptides with activity at a receptor share the common amino-terminal sequence of *Tyr-Gly-Gly-Phe-(Met or Leu),* followed by various C-terminal extensions yielding peptides of 5–31 residues; the endomorphins, with different terminal sequences, are exceptions.
- Not all cells that make a given opioid prohormone precursor store and release the same mixture of opioid peptides; this results from differential post-translational processing secondary to variations in the cellular complement of peptidases that produce and degrade the active opioid fragments.
- Processing of these peptides is altered by physiological demands, leading to the release of a different mix of post-translationally derived peptides by a given cell under different conditions.
- Opioid peptides are found in plasma and reflect release from secretory systems such as the pituitary and the adrenals and thus do not reflect neuraxial release. Conversely, levels of these peptides in brain/spinal cord and in CSF arise from neuraxial systems and not from peripheral systems.

Pro-opiomelanocortin

The major opioid peptide derived from *POMC* is *the potent opioid agonist β-endorphin.* The *POMC* sequence also is processed into a variety of nonopioid peptides, including ACTH, α-MSH, and β-LPH. Although β-endorphin contains the sequence for met-enkephalin at its amino terminus, it is not typically converted to this peptide.

Proenkephalin

The *prohormone* contains multiple copies of *met-enkephalin,* as well as a single copy of *leu-enkephalin. Proenkephalin peptides* are present in areas of the CNS believed to be related to the processing of pain information (e.g., spinal cord dorsal horn, the spinal trigeminal nucleus, and the PAG); to the modulation of affective behavior (e.g., amygdala, hippocampus,

HISTORICAL PERSPECTIVE

The first undisputed reference to opium is found in the writings of Theophrastus in the 3rd century BC. Arab physicians were well versed in the uses of opium. Arab traders introduced the opium concoction to the Orient, where it was employed mainly for the control of dysentery. Paracelsus named the product laudanum. By 1680, the utility of laudanum was so well appreciated that Thomas *Sydenham*, a 17th-century pioneer in English medicine noted that, "Among the remedies which it has pleased Almighty God to give to man to relieve his sufferings, none is so universal and so efficacious as opium," thereby, in his own way, connecting religion and opiates almost 200 years ahead of Marx.

Opium contains more than 20 distinct alkaloids. In 1806, Frederich Sertürner, a pharmacist's assistant, reported the isolation by crystallization of a pure substance in opium that he named morphine, after Morpheus, the Greek god of dreams (Booth, 1999). By the middle of the 19th century, the use of pure alkaloids in place of crude opium preparations began to spread throughout the medical world, an event that coincided with the development of the hypodermic syringe and hollow needle, permitting direct delivery of water-soluble formulations "under the skin" into the body.

In addition to the remarkable salutary benefits of opioids, the side effects and addictive potential of these drugs have been known for centuries. In the U.S. Civil War, the administration of "soldier's joy" often led to "soldier's disease," the opiate addiction brought about by medication of chronic pain states arising from war wounds. These problems stimulated a search for potent synthetic opioid analgesics free of addictive potential and other side effects. The early discovery of the synthetic product heroin by C.R. Alder Wright in 1874 was followed by its widespread utilization as a purportedly nonaddictive cough suppressant and sedative. Unfortunately, heroin and all subsequent synthetic opioids that have been introduced into clinical use share the liabilities of classical opioids, including their addictive properties. However, this search for new opioid agonists led to the synthesis of opioid antagonists and compounds with mixed agonist-antagonist properties, which expanded therapeutic options and provided important tools for exploring mechanisms of opioid actions.

Until the early 1970s, the effects of morphine, heroin, and other opioids as antinociceptive and addictive agents were well described, but mechanisms mediating the interaction of the opioid alkaloids with biological systems were unknown. Goldstein began a search for stereoselective binding sites in the CNS using radioligands (Goldstein et al., 1971), and Pert convincingly employed radioligands to demonstrate opiate-binding sites and an effect of Na⁺ that distinguished agonist from antagonist binding (Pert et al., 1973). In vivo and in vitro physiological studies of the pharmacology of opiate agonists, their antagonists, and cross-tolerance led to the hypothesis of three separate receptors: mu (μ), kappa (κ), and sigma (σ) (Martin et al., 1976). Efforts to isolate endogenous opioids led to the discovery of the molecules (see discussion that follows) that acted on a distinct receptor, the delta (δ) receptor. The μ, κ, and δ receptors, but not the σ receptor, shared the common property of being sensitive to blockade from agonist by agents such as naloxone. In concert with identification of these opioid receptors, Kostelitz and associates (Hughes et al., 1975) identified an endogenous opiate-like factor that they called *enkephalin* ("from the head"). Soon afterward, two more classes of endogenous opioid peptides were isolated, the endorphins and dynorphins (Akil et al., 1984).

In the early work by Martin, the σ receptor was thought to represent a site that accounted for paradoxical excitatory effects of opiates; this site is now thought to be the phencyclidine-binding site and is not, strictly speaking, an opiate receptor or an opiate site. Thus, three distinct receptors are now the basis of opioid pharmacology. The three-receptor hypothesis has been confirmed by cloning (Waldhoer et al., 2004). In 2000, the Committee on Receptor Nomenclature and Drug Classification of the International Union of Pharmacology adopted the terms MOP, DOP, and KOP receptors (**m**u **o**pioid **p**eptide receptor, etc.). This text uses MOR, DOR, and KOR to refer to both peptide and nonpeptide MORs, DORs, and KORs.

Attempts over at least half a century to dissociate the powerful analgesic effects of opioids from their undesirable effects have failed (Corbett et al., 2006). However, with our advancing understanding of biased agonism, prospects are looking up.

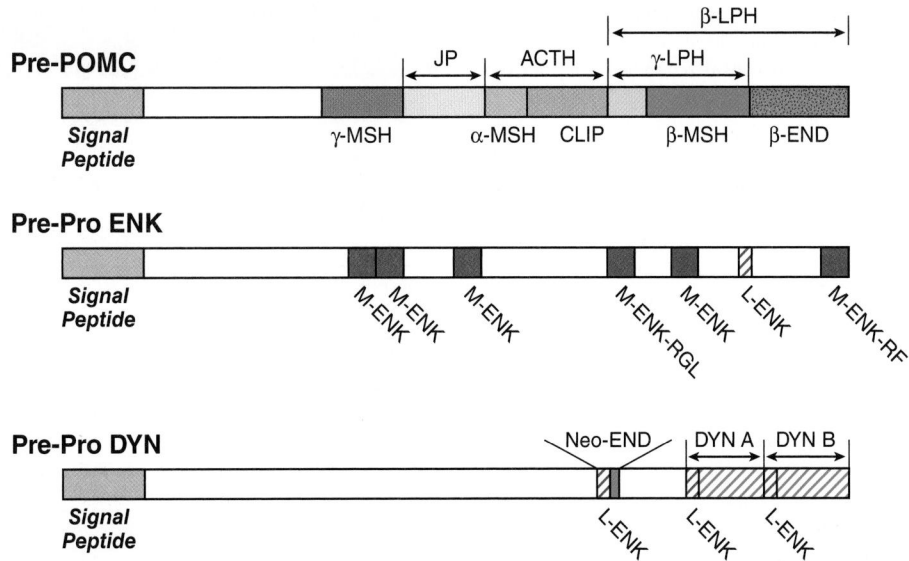

Figure 20–1 *Opioid peptide precursors.* Opioid peptides derive from precursor proteins that may also contain nonopioid peptides. *Pre-POMC* is a good example. Proteolytic processing of a pre-pro form by a signal peptidase removes the signal peptide; then, various prohormone convertases (endoproteases) attack at dibasic sequences, yielding α-, β-, and γ-MSH, ACTH, CLIP, β- and γ-LPH, and β-END. In similar manners, *Pre-ProENK* yields L-ENK and M-ENK and two relatives of M-ENK, M-ENK-RGL (Arg-Gly-Leu), and M-ENK-RF (Arg-Phe); and Pre-ProDYN yields α neoendorphin (α-NEO) and DYN A and DYN B, each of which contains an L-ENK sequence (Tyr-Gly-Gly-Phe-Leu) at its amino terminus. Figure 14–15 shows the processing of pre-POMC in greater detail. JF, joining peptide.

TABLE 20–1 ■ ENDOGENOUS OPIOID PEPTIDES

OPIOID LIGANDS	RECEPTOR SPECIFICITY		
	μ	δ	κ
Met-enkephalin	++	+++	
(Tyr-Gly-Gly-Phe-Met)			
Leu-enkephalin	++	+++	
(Tyr-Gly-Gly-Phe-Leu)			
β-Endorphin	+++	+++	
(Tyr-Gly-Gly-Phe-Met-Thr-Ser-Glu-Lys-Ser-Gln-Thr-Pro-Leu-Val-Thr-Leu-Phe-Lys-Asn-Ala-Ile-Ile-Lys-Asn-Ala-Tyr-Lys-Lys-Gly-Glu)			
Dynorphin A	++		+++
(Tyr-Gly-Gly-Phe-Leu-Arg-Arg-Ile-Arg-Pro-Lys-Leu-Lys-Trp-Asp-Asn-Gln)			
Dynorphin B	+	+	+++
(Tyr-Gly-Gly-Phe-Leu-Arg-Arg-Gln-Phe-Lys-Val-Val-Thr)			
α-Neoendorphin	+	+	+++
(Tyr-Gly-Gly-Phe-Leu-Arg-Lys-Tyr-Pro-Lys)			
Endomorphin 1	+++		
(Tyr-Pro-Trp-Phe-NH$_2$)			

+, agonist; + < ++ < +++ in potency.
Reproduced with permission from Raynor K, et al. Pharmacological characterization of the cloned kappa-, delta-, and mu-opioid receptors. *Mol Pharmacol*, **1994**, *45*:330–334.

locus ceruleus, and frontal cerebral cortex); to the modulation of motor control (e.g., caudate nucleus and globus pallidus); to the regulation of the autonomic nervous system (e.g., medulla oblongata); and to neuroendocrinological functions (e.g., median eminence). Peptides from proenkephalin also are found in chromaffin cells of the adrenal medulla and in nerve plexuses and exocrine glands of the stomach and intestine. Circulating proenkephalin products are considered to be largely derived from these sites.

Prodynorphin

Prodynorphin contains three peptides of differing lengths that all begin with the leu-enkephalin sequence: *dynorphin A, rimorphin (dynorphin B), and neoendorphin. Nociceptin peptide or orphanin FQ* (now termed N/OFQ) shares structural similarity with dynorphin A. The peptides derived from prodynorphin are distributed widely in neurons and to a lesser extent in astrocytes throughout the brain and spinal cord and are frequently found coexpressed with other opioid peptide precursors.

Endomorphins

The endomorphin peptides belong to a novel family of peptides that include *endomorphin 1 (Tyr-Pro-Trp-Phe-NH$_2$)* and *endomorphin 2 (Tyr-Pro-Phe-Phe-NH$_2$)*. Endomorphins have an atypical structure and display selectivity toward the MOR.

Opioid Receptors

Classes of Receptors

The three classes of opiate receptors—MOR, DOR, and KOR—share extensive sequence homologies (55%–58%) and belong to the rhodopsin family of GPCRs (see Figure 3–9). Opioid receptors appear early in vertebrate evolution (Stevens, 2009). Human opiate receptors have been mapped to chromosome 1p355–33 (DOR), chromosome 8q11.23–21 (KOR), and chromosome 6q25–26 (MOR) (Dreborg et al., 2008). Low-stringency hybridization procedures have identified no opioid receptor types other than these three cloned opioid receptors.

An opiate receptor-like protein (ORL$_1$ or NOP; chromosome 20q13.33) was cloned based on its structural homology (48%–49% identity) to other members of the opioid receptor family; it is G protein coupled, has an endogenous ligand (nociceptin [orphanin FQ]) but does not display an opioid pharmacology. As noted, a sigma (σ) receptor was early identified and was thought to represent a site that accounted for the paradoxical excitatory effects of opiates; agonist binding to the σ receptor is not antagonized by naloxone, and the receptor is not classified as an opiate receptor (Waldhoer et al., 2004).

Opioid Receptor Distribution

As defined by the distribution of receptor protein, message, ligand binding, and the pharmacological effects initiated by opiate molecules, all of the opioid receptors are widely distributed in the periphery and neuraxis on neuronal cell soma and terminals. Less well appreciated is the presence of opioid-binding sites on a variety of nonneuronal cells, including macrophage cell types (peripheral and central microglia) and astrocytes (Dannals, 2013; Yaksh, 1987), and in the enteric nervous system of the GI tract (Galligan and Akbarali, 2014).

Opioid Receptor Ligands

Opioid receptor ligands may be broadly defined by their functional properties as agonists and antagonists at the particular receptor.

Agonists

Highly selective agonists have been developed for the three binding sites (e.g., DAMGO for MOR; DPDPE for DOR; and U-50,488 for KOR) (Table 20–2). Virtually all of the clinically useful agonists are targeted at the μ receptor. Ligands that bind specifically but have limited intrinsic activity are referred to as partial agonists; for MOR, one such ligand is *buprenorphine*.

TABLE 20–2 ■ OPIOID AGONISTS

OPIOID LIGANDS	RECEPTOR TYPES		
	μ	δ	κ
Etorphine	+++	+++	+++
Fentanyl	+++		
Hydromorphone	+++		+
Levorphanol	+++		
Methadone	+++		
Morphine[a]	+++		+
Sufentanil	+++	+	+
DAMGO[a] ([D-Ala^2,MePhe^4,Gly(ol)^5] enkephalin)	+++		
Bremazocine[c]	+	+	+++
Buprenorphine	P		– –
Butorphanol[c]	P		+++
Nalbuphine	– –		++
DPDPE[b] ([D-Pen2,5]-Enkephalin])	+++		
U50,488[c]		++	

+, agonist; –, antagonist; P, partial agonist. In potency: + < ++ < +++
[a]Prototypical μ-preferring. [b]Prototypical δ-preferring. [c]Prototypical κ-preferring.
Source: Modified with permission from Raynor K et al. Pharmacological characterization of the cloned kappa-, delta-, and mu-opioid receptors. *Mol Pharmacol*, **1994**;*45*:330–334.

TABLE 20–3 ■ OPIOID ANTAGONISTS

OPIOID LIGANDS	RECEPTOR TYPES		
	μ	δ	κ
Naloxone[a]	– – –	–	– –
Naltrexone[a]	– – –	–	– – –
CTOP[b]	– – –		
Diprenorphine	– – –	– –	– – –
β-Funaltrexarnine[b,c]	– – –	–	++
Naloxonazine	– – –	–	–
nor-Binaltorphimine (nor-BNI)	–	–	– – –
Naltrindole[d]	–	– – –	–
Naloxone benzoylhydrazone	– – –	–	–

+, agonist; –, antagonist. – < – – < – – – in potency. CTOP, (D-Phe-Cys-Tyr-D-Trp-Orn-Thr-Pen-Thr-NH₂).
[a]Universal ligand.
[b]Prototypical μ preferring.
[c]Irreversible ligand.
[d]Prototypical δ preferring.
Reproduced with permission from Raynor K, et al. Pharmacological characterization of the cloned kappa-, delta-, and mu-opioid receptors. *Mol Pharmacol*, **1994**, 45:330–334.

Antagonists

Commonly used opiate antagonists, such as *naloxone* or *naltrexone,* are pan antagonists with affinity for all known opioid receptors. Antagonists for specific opiate receptors have been developed for research (Table 20–3) and include cyclic analogues of somatostatin, such as CTOP (D-Phe-Cys-Tyr-D-Trp-Orn-Thr-Pen-Thr-NH2) as an MOR antagonist, a derivative of naloxone called *naltrindole* as a DOR antagonist, and a bivalent derivative of naltrexone called nor-BNI as a KOR antagonist.

Opioid Receptor Structure

Each of the opiate receptors consists of an extracellular N-terminus, seven TM helices, three extra- and intracellular loops, and an intracellular C-terminus characteristic of the GPCRs (Figure 20–2). The opioid receptors also possess two conserved cysteine residues in the first and second extracellular loops, which form a disulfide bridge. Though there is significant complexity in opiate-receptor interactions (Kane et al., 2006), several general principles define binding and selectivity.

- All opioid receptors display a binding pocket formed by TM_3-TM_7.
- The pocket in the respective receptor is partially covered by the extracellular loops, which, together with the extracellular termini of the TM segments, provide a gate-conferring selectivity, allowing ligands, particularly peptides, to be differentially accessible to the different receptor types. Thus, alkaloids (e.g., morphine) bind in the core of the TM portion of the receptor, whereas large peptidyl ligands bind at the extracellular loops. As noted, it is the extracellular loops that show the greatest structural diversity across receptors.
- Selectivity has been attributed to extracellular loops: first and third for the MOR, second for the KOR, and third for the DOR. Alkaloid antagonists are thought to bind more deeply in the pocket, sterically hindering conformational changes and leading to a functional antagonism.
- In the membrane, opiate receptors can form both homo- and heterodimers, thereby altering the pharmacological properties of the receptors. Thus, the diversity of responses is increased beyond those of the basic MOR, DOR, and KOR monomers.
- Hetero- and homodimerization of opiate receptors and their postactivation trafficking are important in understanding the selectivity of several ligands and the physiological responses to them. The development of tolerance to opioids may involve mechanisms of receptor trafficking.
- Splice variants exist for the opioid receptors. For example, the gene for the human MOR has at least two promoters, multiple exons, with many exons generating at least 11 splice variants that encode multiple morphine-binding isoforms, varying largely at their carboxy termini. This alternative splicing is likely crucial to receptor and response diversity (Pan, 2005; Xu et al., 2017).

Opioid Receptor Signaling

The MOR, DOR, and KOR couple to pertussis toxin–sensitive, G_i/G_o proteins. On receptor activation, the G_i/G_o coupling results in a number

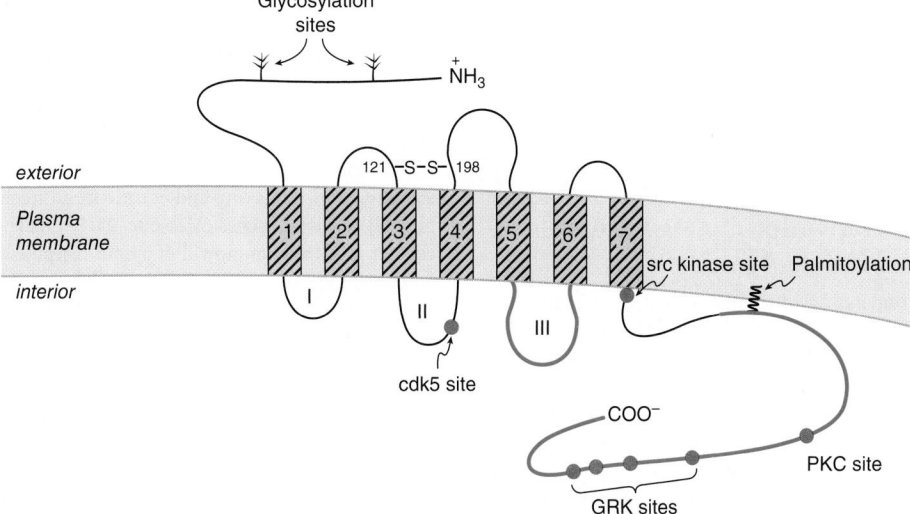

Figure 20–2 *General structure of an opioid receptor.* This schematic is based on the DOR (Gendron et al., 2016). The receptor has the characteristics of a GPCR: long external amino terminus with glycosylation sites, seven TM regions, a long intracellular carboxy tail, and phosphorylation sites in the areas where arrestins interact (portions of intracellular loop III and the carboxy tail, noted in green). The differential interaction of arrestins 1 and 2 with the phosphorylated sites may be a factor in the differential responses to different agonists (see Figure 20–4). An unusual feature is the extracellular disulfide linkage between Cys[121] and Cys[198]. Na⁺ affects receptor constitutive activity and ligand specificity of DOR, effects that have been localized to an allosteric site for Na⁺ in the core of the seven-TM bundle of DOR; changing Asn[131] in the Na⁺ site to Ala or Val alters the effect of naltrindole from DOR antagonist to a β-arrestin–biased agonist. The Na⁺-interacting residues seem to function as an "efficacy switch" (Fenalti et al., 2014).

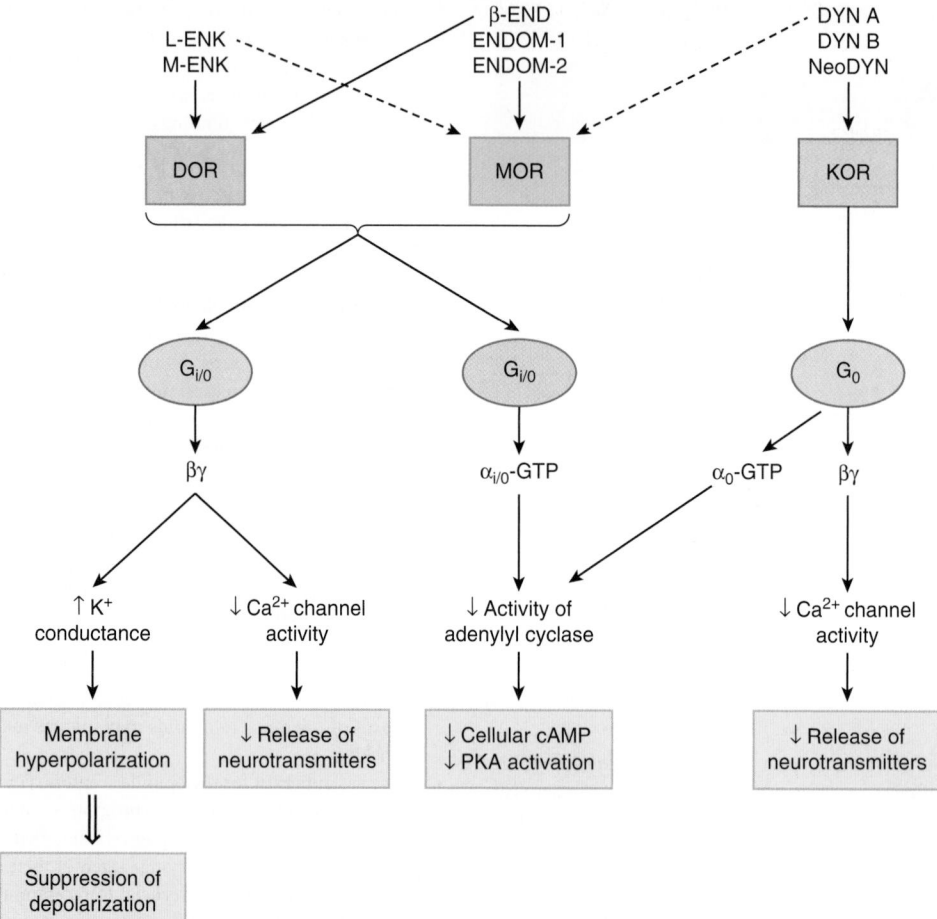

Figure 20–3 *Receptor specificity of endogenous opioids and effects of receptor activation on neurons.*

of intracellular events that are mediated by α and βγ subunits of these G proteins (see Figure 20–3), including the following:

- Inhibition of AC activity
- Reduced opening of voltage-gated Ca²⁺ channels (reduces neurotransmitter release from presynaptic terminals)
- Stimulation of K⁺ current through several channels, including GIRKs (hyperpolarizes and inhibits postsynaptic neurons)
- Activation of PKC and PLCβ (Shang and Filizola, 2015)

Regulation of Postactivation Opiate Receptor Trafficking; Biased Opioid Agonism

The MORs and DORs undergo rapid agonist-mediated internalization. MORs recycle to the membrane after internalization; DORs are degraded on internalization (Zhang et al., 2015). KORs do not internalize after prolonged agonist exposure (Williams et al., 2013).

Internalization of the MORs and DORs apparently occurs via partially distinct endocytic pathways, suggesting receptor-specific interactions with different mediators of intracellular trafficking. These processes may be induced differentially as a function of the structure of the ligand. For example, certain agonists, such as etorphine and enkephalins, cause rapid internalization of the receptor, whereas morphine does not cause MOR internalization, even though it decreases AC activity equally well. In addition, a truncated receptor with normal G protein coupling recycles constitutively from the membrane to the cytosol, suggesting that activation of signal transduction and internalization are controlled by distinct molecular mechanisms (von Zastrow et al., 2003). These studies support the assertion that different ligands induce different conformational changes in the receptor that result in divergent intracellular signaling, and they

may provide an explanation for differences in the spectrum of effects of various opioids and point to novel therapeutics (Violin et al., 2014). Figure 20–4 shows some of the receptor-effector-signaling pathways that may contribute to biased opioid agonism and the complexity of immediate and long-term responses (desensitization, tolerance, dependence, withdrawal).

As noted, more than a single type of opioid receptor may be expressed on a cell. Functional data suggest opioid receptors may interact, forming homo- and heterodimers, and that such complexes may alter receptor signaling and trafficking and contribute to tolerance to morphine and possibly to disease states (Massotte, 2015; Zhang et al., 2015). The intracellular loops and amino tail of opioid receptors have numerous known and potential sites of phosphorylation by several cellular protein kinases that can alter the receptor's signaling and interaction with intracellular scaffolds and signaling pathways (Figures 20–2 and 20–4).

Effects of Acute and Chronic Opiate Receptor Activation

In addition to the intended relief from pain, agonist occupancy of opiate receptors over both short- and long-term intervals leads to the loss of effect, with distinguishable properties relating to the development of tolerance and dependence.

Desensitization

In the face of a transient activation (minutes to hours), acute tolerance or desensitization occurs that is specific for that receptor and disappears with a time course parallel to the clearance of the agonist. Short-term desensitization probably involves phosphorylation of the receptors resulting in

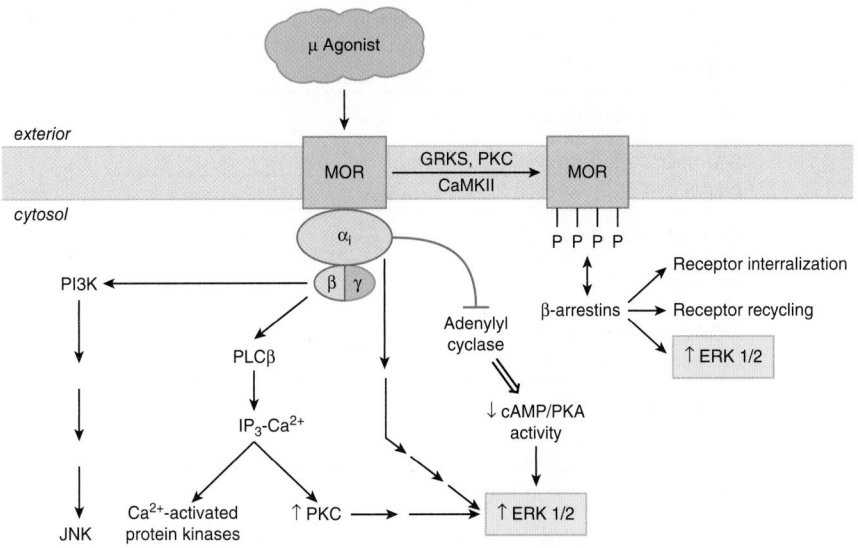

A. *Cell signaling pathways that may be differentially regulated opioid agonists.* Responses to opioid agonists may be biased toward β-arrestin signaling or toward G-protein signaling. ERK1/2 may be activated by either pathway, but possibly in distinct subcellular compartments with different sequelae. Activation of PI3K and PLCβ may lead to activation of additional protein kinases with numerous downstream effects. In addition to initiating signaling (e.g., ERK1/2), β-arrestins interact with phosphorylated receptors with consequences for desensitization and receptor trafficking. The differentiated state of the responding cell can affect what responses are possible, as can the properties of the agonist. Panel B shows some of the variables that can contribute to biased signaling in response to mu opioid agonists.

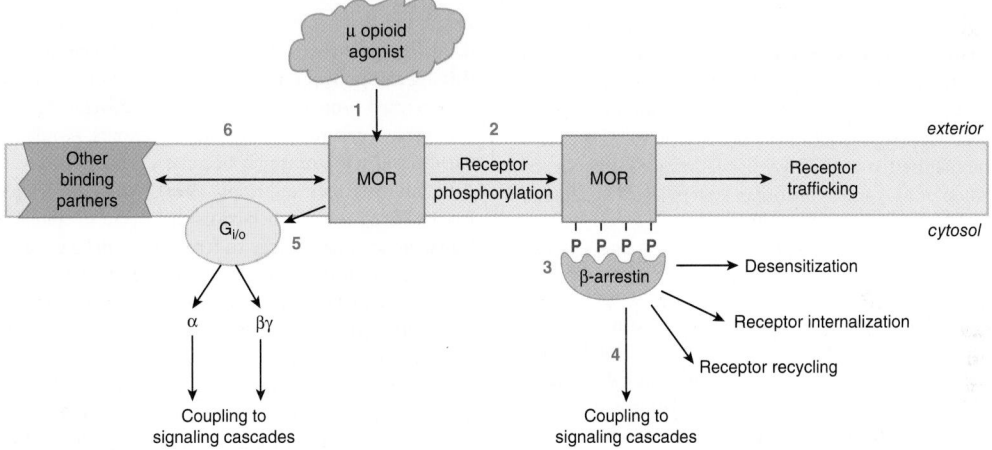

B. *Putative factors affecting the variable consequences of MOR activation.* The panoply of interactions that result from ligand binding to MOR is complex. As a consequence, biased activation of MOR may differentially affect multiple downstream pathways. A few possibilities are shown here, noted by number on the figure:

1. *Mu* agonists bind to MOR, a membrane GPCR. Biased responses could result from agonist preference for one of several forms of MOR that may result from alternative splicing. Biased responses could also result from interactions of *mu* agonists with MOR that stabilize conformations of the receptor that are agonist-specific and differ in their capacity to produce sequelae. In response to agonist, MOR interacts with a G-protein and is subject to phosphorylation, events that may also reflect a receptor isoform and the particular conformation stabilized by the agonist.

2. MOR has over a dozen phosphorylation sites accessible to various protein kinases. The pattern of phosphorylation may be determined by the receptor conformation that the agonist induces, mobilizing distinct protein kinases (e.g., GRKs, PKC, ERK1/2, CaMKII), or the receptor may fail to be phosphorylated. These protein kinases exist in multiple isoforms, lending additional variability/selectivity to the process. There are seven GRK isoforms (not uniformly expressed in all cells), and GRK-mediated phosphorylation may also be specific to agonist and receptor form (i.e., dependent on agonist-induced receptor conformation and heterogeneities [splice variants] in receptor structure).

3. MOR phosphorylation, largely by GRKs, facilitates β-arrestin binding, promotes uncoupling of MOR from G-proteins, and affects desensitization, receptor trafficking, and possibly tolerance. Two isoforms of β-arrestin can interact with phospho-MOR. These interactions appear to be agonist-specific (see **Panel C**). Interaction of phospho-MOR with β-arrestins initiates processes of receptor desensitization, internalization, and recycling. There is a strong correlation between MOR phosphorylation, recruitment of β-arrestin 2, and MOR internalization. The β-arrestin/phospho-MOR complex is recognized by clathrin. Phospho-MOR can be internalized to different fates depending on its participation in a clathrin-dependent or a clathrin-independent process.

4. The phospho-MOR/β-arrestin complexes can initiate cell signaling independently of G-proteins.

5. Agonist-liganded MOR interacts with the $G_{i/o}$ family to alter cell signaling pathways. The components of $G_{i/o}$ provide large possibilities for diversity of signaling (four α subunits; five β and twelve γ isoforms) and regulate proteins in the membrane and in various subcellular compartments (Khan et al, 2013).

6. Agonist-specific homo- and hetero-dimerization of receptor and its interaction with other proteins may also play roles in biased agonism.

Thus, a variety of ultimate responses are possible following the binding of a mu agonist to MOR. **Panel C** gives two examples.

Figure 20–4 *Biased Signaling via Opioid Receptors.*

SECTION II NEUROPHARMACOLOGY

Response		Morphine	Etorphine
G protein activation		+ + +	+ + +
MOR phosphorylation		+	+ + +
β-arrestin recruitment	β-arrestin 1	−	+ + +
	β-arrestin 2	+	+ + +
MOR internalization		+/−	+ + +
PKC$_\varepsilon$ activation		+ + +	−
MOR desensitization** (assessed as Ca^{2+} release)		+ + +	−
ERK 1/2 activation		+ + +	+ + +

* Responses assembled from literature data, mostly from cultured cell systems. See papers by Raehal et al. (2011) and Zheng et al. (2011).
** Result depends on response measured.

C. *Biased agonism: disparate effects of two MOR agonists*.*

Figure 20–4   (*Continued*).

an uncoupling of the receptor from its G protein or internalization of the receptor (Williams et al., 2013).

Tolerance

Tolerance to opioids refers to a decrease in the apparent effectiveness of the opioid agonist with continuous or repeated agonist administration (over days to weeks), that, following removal of the agonist, disappears over several weeks. This tolerance is reflected by a reduction in the maximum achievable effect or a right shift in the dose-response curve. This phenomenon can be manifested at the level of the intracellular cascade (e.g., reduced inhibition of AC) and at the organ system level (e.g., loss of sedative and analgesic effects) (Christie, 2008).

This loss of effect with persistent exposure to an opiate agonist has several key properties:

- Different physiological responses can develop tolerance at markedly different rates. Thus, at the organ system level, some end points show little or no tolerance development (pupillary miosis); some show moderate tolerance (constipation, emesis, analgesia, sedation); and some show rapid tolerance (euphoria). Accordingly, the chronic heroin abuser will continue to show pinpoint pupils and will require a rapid increase in dosing to achieve the drug-related euphoria.
- In general, opiate agonists of a given class will typically show a reduced response in a system rendered tolerant to another agent of that class (e.g., cross-tolerance between the MOR agonists, such as morphine and fentanyl). For reasons that are not clear, this cross-tolerance is neither absolute nor complete. This lack of complete cross-tolerance between agonists forms the basis for the clinical strategy of "opioid rotation" in pain therapy (Smith and Peppin, 2014).

Dependence

Dependence represents a state of adaptation manifested by a withdrawal syndrome produced by cessation of drug exposure (e.g., by drug abstinence) or administration of an antagonist (e.g., naloxone). Dependence is specific to the drug class and receptor involved. At the organ system level, opiate withdrawal is manifested by significant somatomotor and autonomic outflow (reflected by agitation, hyperalgesia, hyperthermia, hypertension, diarrhea, pupillary dilation, and release of virtually all pituitary and adrenomedullary hormones) and by affective symptoms (dysphoria, anxiety, and depression). The state of withdrawal is highly aversive and motivates the drug recipient to make robust efforts to avoid withdrawal, that is, to consume more of the drug. Consistent with the phenomenon of cross-tolerance, drugs interacting with the same opiate receptor will suppress the withdrawal observed in organisms tolerant to another drug acting on the same receptor (e.g., morphine and methadone).

Addiction

Addiction is a behavioral pattern characterized by compulsive use of a drug. The positive, rewarding effects of opiates are considered to be the driving component for initiating the recreational use of opiates. This positive reward property is subject to the development of tolerance. Given the aversive nature of withdrawal symptoms, avoidance and alleviation of withdrawal symptoms may become a primary motivation for compulsive drug taking (Kreek and Koob, 1998). When the drive to acquire the drug leads to drug-seeking behaviors that occur in spite of the physical, emotional, or societal damage suffered by the drug seeker, then the obsession or compulsion to acquire and use the drug is considered to reflect an addicted state. In animals, this may be manifest by willingness to tolerate stressful conditions to acquire drug delivery. Importantly, *drug dependence is not synonymous with drug addiction*. Tolerance and dependence are physiological responses seen in all patients but are not predictors of addiction (see Chapter 24). For example, cancer pain often requires prolonged treatment with high doses of opioids, leading to tolerance and dependence. Yet, such patients are not considered to be either addicts or abusers of the drug.

Mechanisms of Tolerance/Dependence/Withdrawal

The mechanisms underlying chronic tolerance and dependence/withdrawal are controversial. Several types of events may contribute.

Receptor Disposition

Acute desensitization or receptor internalization may play a role in the initiation of chronic tolerance but is not sufficient to explain the persistent changes observed. For instance, morphine, unlike other μ agonists, does not promote significant MOR internalization, receptor phosphorylation, or desensitization. Receptor desensitization and downregulation are agonist specific. Endocytosis and sequestration of receptors do not invariably lead to receptor degradation but can also result in receptor dephosphorylation and recycling to the surface of the cell. Accordingly, opioid tolerance may not be related to receptor desensitization but rather to a lack of desensitization. Agonists that cause rapid internalization of opioid receptors also rapidly desensitize signaling, but sensitivity can be at least partially restored by recycling of "reactivated" opioid receptors.

Adaptation of Intracellular Signaling Mechanisms

Assessment of the coupling of MOR to cellular effects, such as inhibition of AC, activation of inwardly rectifying K^+ channels, inhibition of Ca^{2+} currents, and inhibition of neurotransmitter release demonstrates functional uncoupling of receptor occupancy from effector function. Importantly, chronic application of opioids initiates adaptive counterregulatory change. A common example of such cellular counterregulatory processes is the rebound increase in cellular cyclic AMP levels produced by "superactivation" of AC and upregulation of the amount of enzyme as a result of long-term exposure to an opiate followed by its abrupt withdrawal (Williams et al., 2013).

System-Level Counteradaptation

The loss of antinociceptive effect with chronic opiate exposure may reflect an enhanced excitability of the regulated link. Thus, tolerance to the analgesic action of chronically administered μ opiates may result from an activation of *bulbospinal* pathways that increases the excitability of spinal dorsal horn pain transmission linkages. With chronic opiate exposure, opiate receptor occupancy will lead to the activation of PKC, which can phosphorylate and enhance the activation of local NMDA glutamate receptors. These receptors are considered to play an important role as an excitatory link in enhanced pain processing (see Chapter 14). Blockade of these receptors can at least partially attenuate the loss of analgesic efficacy with continued opiate exposure. Such system-level counteradaptation mechanisms may apply to specific systems (e.g., pain modulation) but not necessarily to others (e.g., sedation or miosis) (Christie, 2008). These changes may be mechanistically important in the phenomenon called opioid-induced hyperalgesia, by which higher doses of opiates may lead to a paradoxical increase in pain processing (Fletcher and Martinez, 2014).

Differential Tolerance Development and Fractional Occupancy Requirements

An interesting problem in explaining tolerance relates to the differential rates of the development of tolerance. It is unclear why responses such as miosis show no tolerance over extended exposure (indeed, miosis is considered symptomatic in drug overdose of highly tolerant patients), whereas analgesia and sedation are likely to show a reduction. One possibility is that tolerance represents a functional uncoupling of some fraction of the receptor population and that different physiological end points may require activation of different fractions of their coupled receptors to produce a given physiological effect.

Effects of Clinically Used Opioids

Opiates, depending on their receptor specificities, produce a variety of effects consistent with the roles played by the organ systems with which the receptors are associated. Although the primary clinical use of opioids is for their pain-relieving properties, opioids produce a host of other effects. This is not surprising in view of the wide distribution of opioid receptors in brain, spinal cord, and the periphery. Within the nervous system, these effects range from analgesia to effects on motivation and higher-order affect (euphoria), arousal, and a number of autonomic, hormonal, and motor processes. In the periphery, opiates can influence a variety of visceromotor systems, including those related to GI motility and smooth muscle tone.

Analgesia

Morphine-like drugs produce *analgesia*, *drowsiness*, and *euphoria* (changes in mood and mental clouding). When therapeutic doses of morphine are given to patients with pain, patients report the pain to be less intense or entirely gone. In addition to relief of distress, some patients may experience euphoria. Analgesia often occurs without loss of consciousness, although drowsiness commonly occurs. Morphine at these doses does not

have anticonvulsant activity and usually does not cause slurred speech, emotional lability, or significant impairment of motor coordination. When an analgesic dose of morphine is administered to normal, pain-free individuals, the patients may report the drug experience to be frankly unpleasant. They may experience drowsiness, difficulty in mentation, apathy, and lessened physical activity. As the dose is increased, the subjective, analgesic, and toxic effects, including respiratory depression, become more pronounced. The relief of pain by morphine-like opioids is selective in that other sensory modalities, such as light touch, proprioception, and the sense of moderate temperatures, are unaffected. Low doses of morphine can produce reductions in the affective response but not the perceived intensity of the pain experience; higher, clinically effective doses reduce both perceived intensity and affective responses to the pain (Price et al., 1985). Continuous dull pain (as generated by tissue injury and inflammation) is relieved more effectively than sharp intermittent (incident) pain, such as that associated with the movement of an inflamed joint. With sufficient amounts of opioid, it is possible to relieve even the severe piercing pain associated with, for example, acute renal or biliary colic.

Pain States and Mechanisms

Any meaningful discussion of the action of analgesic agents must include the appreciation that all pain is not the same, and that a number of variables contribute to the patient's pain report and therefore to the effect of the analgesic. Heuristically, one may think mechanistically of pain as several distinct sets of events, described in the next sections (Yaksh et al., 2015).

Acute Nociception. Acute activation of small, high-threshold sensory afferents (Aδ and C fibers) generates transient, stimulus-dependent input into the spinal cord, which in turn leads to activation of dorsal horn neurons that project contralaterally to the thalamus and thence to the somatosensory cortex. A parallel spinofugal projection runs through the medial thalamus and thence to portions of the limbic cortex, such as the anterior cingulate. The output produced by acutely activating these ascending systems is sufficient to evoke pain reports. Examples of such stimuli include a hot coffee cup, a needlestick, or an incision.

Tissue Injury. Following tissue injury or local inflammation (e.g., local skin burn, toothache, rheumatoid joint), an ongoing pain state arises that is characterized by burning, throbbing, or aching, and an abnormal pain response termed *hyperalgesia*, which can be evoked by otherwise innocuous or mildly aversive stimuli (tepid bathwater on a sunburn; moderate extension of an injured joint). This pain typically reflects the effects of active factors such as prostaglandins, bradykinin, cytokines, serine proteases, and H^+ ions, among many mediators. Such mediators are released locally into the injury site and have the capacity, through eponymous receptors on the terminals of small, high-threshold afferents (Aδ and C fibers), to activate these sensory afferents and to reduce the stimulus intensity required for their activation (e.g., peripheral sensitization). In addition, the ongoing afferent traffic initiated by the tissue injury and inflammation leads to activation of spinal facilitatory cascades, yielding a greater output to the brain for any given afferent input. This facilitation is thought to underlie hyperalgesic states (e.g., central sensitization). Such tissue injury/inflammation-evoked pain is often referred to as *nociceptive* pain (Figure 20–5) (Sorkin and Wallace, 1999). Examples of such states would be burn, postincision, abrasion of the skin, musculoskeletal injury, or inflammation of the joint.

Nerve Injury. Injury to a peripheral nerve yields complex anatomical and biochemical changes in the nerve and spinal cord that induce *spontaneous dysesthesias* (shooting, burning pain) and *allodynia* (hurt from a light touch). This nerve injury pain state may not depend on the activation of small afferents but may be initiated by low-threshold sensory afferents (e.g., Aβ fibers). Such nerve injuries result in the development of ectopic activity arising from neuromas formed by nerve injury and the dorsal root ganglia of the injured axons as well as changes in dorsal horn sensory processing. Such changes include activation of nonneuronal (glial) cells and loss of constitutive inhibitory circuits, such that low-threshold afferent input carried by Aβ fibers evokes a pain

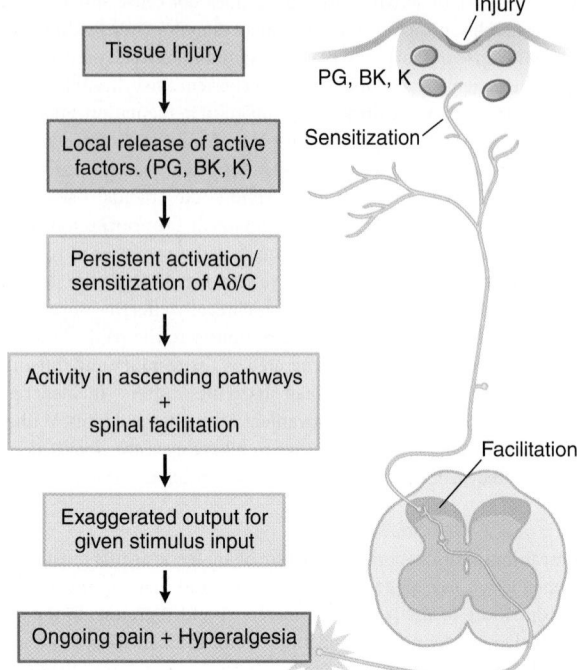

Figure 20–5 *Mechanisms of tissue injury–evoked nociception.* BK, bradykinin; K, potassium; PG, prostaglandins.

state (West et al., 2015). Examples of such nerve injury–inducing events include mononeuropathies secondary to nerve trauma or compression (carpal tunnel syndrome) and the postherpetic state (shingles). Polyneuropathies such as those occurring in diabetes or after chemotherapy (as for cancer) can also lead to ongoing dysesthesias and evoked hyperpathias. These pain states are said to be neuropathic (Figure 20–6). Many clinical pain syndromes, such as found in cancer, typically represent a combination of these inflammatory and neuropathic mechanisms. Although nociceptive pain usually is responsive to opioid analgesics, neuropathic pain is typically considered to respond less well to opioid analgesics. There is a growing perception that, in the face of chronic tissue injury or inflammation (e.g., arthritis), there can be a transition from an inflammatory to a neuropathic pain phenotype. Such a transition has important implications for analgesic drug efficacy.

Sensory Versus Affective Dimensions. Information generated by a high-intensity peripheral stimulus initiates activity in pathways activating higher-order systems that reflect the aversive magnitude of the stimulus.

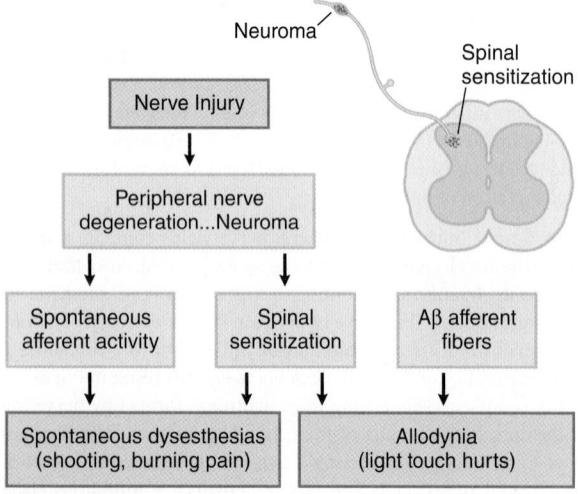

Figure 20–6 *Mechanisms of nerve injury–evoked nociception.*

Painful stimuli have the certain ability to generate strong emotional components that reflect a distinction between pain as a specific sensation subserved by distinct neurophysiological structures (the *sensory discriminative* dimension) and pain such as suffering (the original sensation plus the reactions evoked by the sensation: the *affective motivational* dimension of the pain experience) (Melzack and Casey, 1968). Opiates have potent effects on both components of the pain experience.

Mechanisms of Opioid-Induced Analgesia

The analgesic actions of opiates after systemic delivery represent actions in the brain, spinal cord, and in some instances the periphery.

Supraspinal Actions. Microinjections of morphine into a number of highly circumscribed brain regions will produce a potent analgesia that is reversible by naloxone, an MOR antagonist. The best characterized of these sites is the mesencephalic PAG region. Several mechanisms exist whereby opiates with an action limited to the PAG may act to alter nociceptive transmission. These are summarized in Figure 20–7. MOR agonists block release of the inhibitory transmitter GABA from tonically active PAG systems that regulate activity in projections to the medulla. PAG projections to the medulla activate medullospinal release of NE and 5HT at the level of the spinal dorsal horn. This release can attenuate dorsal horn excitability (Yaksh, 1997). Interestingly, this PAG organization can also serve to increase excitability of dorsal raphe and locus coeruleus, from which ascending serotonergic and noradrenergic projections to the limbic

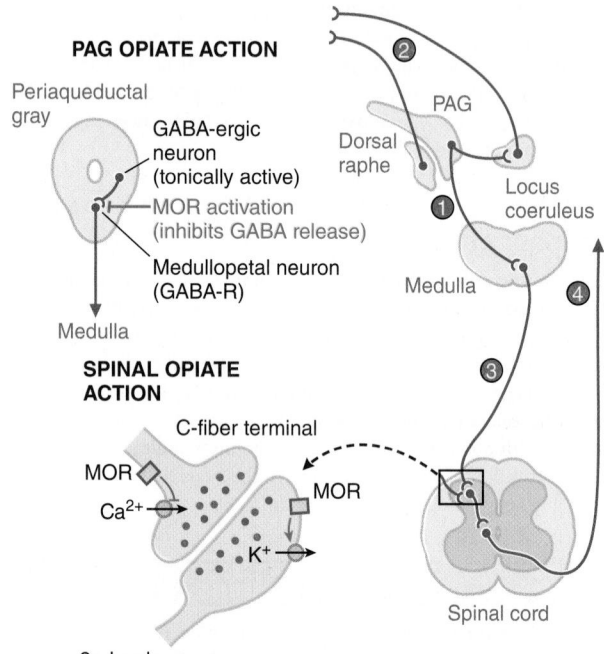

Figure 20–7 *Mechanisms of opiate action in producing analgesia.* **Top left:** Schematic of organization of opiate action in the PAG. **Top right:** Opiate-sensitive pathways in the PAG. Opiate actions via MOR block the release of GABA from tonically active systems that otherwise regulate the projections to the medulla (1), leading to an activation of PAG outflow that results in activation of forebrain (2) and spinal (3) monoamine receptors that regulate spinal cord projections (4), which provide sensory input to higher centers and mood. **Bottom left:** Schematic of primary afferent synapse with second-order dorsal horn spinal neuron, showing pre- and postsynaptic opiate receptors coupled to Ca^{2+} and K^+ channels, respectively. Opiate receptor binding is highly expressed in the superficial spinal dorsal horn (substantia gelatinosa). These receptors are located presynaptically on the terminals of small primary afferents (C fibers) and postsynaptically on second-order neurons. Presynaptically, activation of MOR blocks the opening of the voltage-sensitive Ca^{2+} channel, which otherwise initiates transmitter release. Postsynaptically, MOR activation enhances opening of K^+ channels, leading to hyperpolarization. Thus, an opiate agonist acting at these sites jointly serves to attenuate the afferent-evoked excitation of the second-order neuron.

forebrain, respectively, originate. Aside from direct supraspinal effects on forebrain structures, these limbic projections provide a mechanism for the effects of opiates on emotional tone (the role of forebrain 5HT and NE in mediating emotional tone is discussed in Chapter 15).

Spinal Opiate Action. A local action of opiates in the spinal cord will selectively depress the discharge of spinal dorsal horn neurons evoked by small (high-threshold) but not large (low-threshold) afferent nerve fibers. Intrathecal administration of opioids in animals ranging from mice to humans will reliably attenuate the response of the organism to a variety of somatic and visceral stimuli that otherwise evoke pain states. Specific opiate receptors are largely limited to the *substantia gelatinosa* of the superficial dorsal horn, the region in which small, high-threshold sensory afferents show their principal termination. A significant proportion of these opiate receptors are associated with small peptidergic primary afferent C fibers; the remainder are on local dorsal horn neurons.

Spinal opiates act on opiate receptors located presynaptically on small, high-threshold primary afferents to *prevent the opening of voltage-sensitive Ca²⁺ channels,* thereby preventing transmitter release from those afferents. A postsynaptic action is demonstrated by the ability of opiates to block excitation of dorsal horn neurons directly evoked by glutamate, reflecting a direct activation of dorsal horn projection neurons partly by *hyperpolarizing the neurons through the activation of K⁺ channels,* such that the membrane potential more closely approximates the equilibrium potential for K⁺. The joint capacity of spinal opiates to reduce the release of excitatory neurotransmitters from C fibers and to decrease the excitability of dorsal horn neurons is believed to account for the powerful and selective effect of opiates on spinal nociceptive processing. A variety of opiates delivered spinally (intrathecally or epidurally) can induce powerful analgesia that is reversed by low doses of systemic naloxone (Yaksh, 1997).

Peripheral Action. Direct application of high concentrations of opiates to a peripheral nerve can, in fact, produce a local anesthetic-like action, but this effect is not reversed by naloxone and is believed to reflect a "nonspecific" action. Conversely, at peripheral sites under conditions of inflammation where there is an increased terminal sensitivity leading to an exaggerated pain response (e.g., hyperalgesia), direct injection of opiates produces a local action that can exert a normalizing effect on the exaggerated thresholds. Whether the effects are uniquely on the peripheral afferent terminal or whether the opiate acts on inflammatory cells that release products that sensitize the nerve terminal, or both, is not known (Stein and Machelska, 2011).

Mood Alterations and Rewarding Properties

The mechanisms by which opioids produce euphoria, tranquility, and other alterations of mood (including rewarding properties) are complex and not entirely understood. Neural systems that mediate opioid reinforcement overlap with, but are distinct from, those involved in physical dependence and analgesia (Koob and Le Moal, 2008). Behavioral and pharmacological data point to a pivotal role of the mesocorticolimbic dopamine system that projects to the *NAc* in drug-induced reward and motivation (Figure 20–8). Increased dopamine release in this region is considered to underlie a positive reward state. In the NAc, MORs are present postsynaptically on GABAergic neurons. The reinforcing effects of opiates are thought to be mediated partly via inhibition of local GABAergic neuronal activity, which otherwise acts to inhibit DA outflow.

Respiratory Effects

Although effects of opiates on respiration are readily demonstrated, clinically significant respiratory depression rarely occurs with standard analgesic doses in the absence of other contributing variables (discussed in the next sections). It should be stressed, however, that *respiratory depression represents the primary cause of morbidity secondary to opiate therapy.* In humans, death from opiate poisoning is nearly always due to respiratory arrest or obstruction. Opiates depress all phases of respiratory activity (rate, minute volume, and tidal exchange) and produce irregular and aperiodic breathing. The diminished respiratory volume

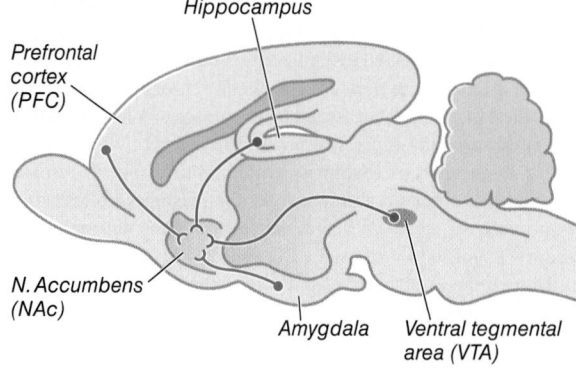

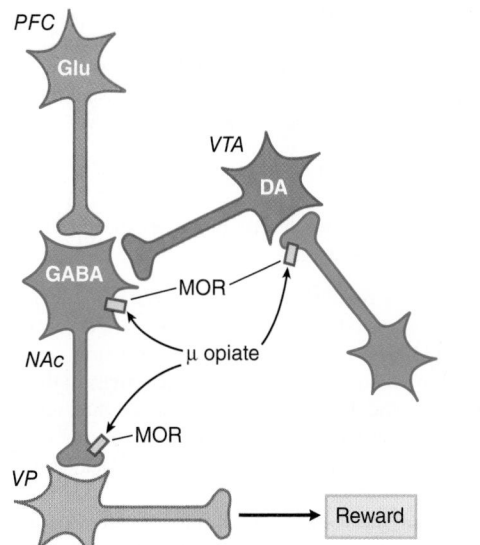

Figure 20–8 *Pathways underlying rewarding properties of opiates.* **Upper panel:** This sagittal section of rat brain shows DA and GABA inputs from the VTA and PFC, respectively, into the NAc. **Lower panel:** Neurons are labeled with their primary neurotransmitters. At a cellular level, MOR agonists reduce excitability and transmitter release at the sites indicated by inhibiting Ca²⁺ influx and enhancing K⁺ current (see Figure 20–7). Thus, opiate-induced inhibition in the VTA on GABAergic interneurons or in the NAc reduce GABA-mediated inhibition and increase outflow from the ventral pallidum (VP), which appears to correlate with a positive reinforcing state (enhanced reward).

is due primarily to a slower rate of breathing; with toxic amounts of opioids, the rate may fall to 3–4 breaths/min. Thus, to avoid apnea due to a decrease in respiratory drive coinciding with an increased airway resistance, opioids must be used with caution in patients with asthma, COPD, cor pulmonale, decreased respiratory reserve, preexisting respiratory depression, hypoxia, or hypercapnia. Although respiratory depression is not considered to be a favorable therapeutic effect of opiates, their ability to suppress respiratory drive is used as therapeutic advantage to treat dyspnea resulting, for example, in patients with COPD, where air hunger leads to extreme agitation, discomfort, and gasping; opiates will suppress the gasping and decease the panic of the patient. Similarly, opiates find use in patients who require artificial ventilation (Clemens and Klaschik, 2007).

Mechanisms Underlying Respiratory Depression
Morphine-like opioids depress respiration through MOR by several mechanisms:

- direct depressant effect on rhythm generation;
- depression of the ventilatory response to increased CO₂; and
- an effect on carotid and aortic body chemosensors that reduces ventilatory responses that are normally driven by hypoxia.

Respiratory rate and tidal volume depend on intrinsic rhythm generators located in the ventrolateral medulla. These systems generate a "respiratory" rhythm that is driven by afferent input reflecting the partial pressure of arterial O_2 as measured by chemosensors in the carotid and aortic bodies and CO_2 as measured by chemosensors in the brainstem. Morphine-like opioids depress respiration through MORs in part by a direct depressant effect on rhythm generation, with changes in respiratory pattern and rate observed at lower doses than changes in tidal volume. A key property of opiate effects on respiration is the depression of the ventilatory response to increased CO_2. This effect is mediated by opiate depression of the excitability of brainstem chemosensory neurons. In addition to the effects on the CO_2 response, opiates will depress ventilation otherwise driven by hypoxia though an effect on carotid and aortic body chemosensors. Importantly, with opiates, hypoxic stimulation of chemoreceptors still may be effective when opioids have decreased the responsiveness to CO_2, and inhalation of O_2 may remove the residual drive resulting from the elevated PO_2 and produce apnea (Pattinson, 2008). In addition to the effect on respiratory rhythm and chemosensitivity, opiates can have mechanical effects on airway function by increasing chest wall rigidity and diminishing upper airway patency (Lalley, 2008).

Factors Exacerbating Opiate-Induced Respiratory Depression

A number of factors can increase the risk of opiate-related respiratory depression even at therapeutic doses:

- *Other medications.* The combination of opiates with other depressant medications, such as general anesthetics, tranquilizers, alcohol, or sedative-hypnotics, produces additive depression of respiratory activity.
- *Sleep.* Natural sleep produces a decrease in the sensitivity of the medullary center to CO_2, and the depressant effects of morphine and sleep are at least additive. Obstructive sleep apnea is considered to be an important risk factor for increasing the likelihood of fatal respiratory depression.
- *Age.* Newborns can show significant respiratory depression and desaturation; this may be evident in lower Apgar scores if opioids are administered parenterally to women within 2–4 h of delivery because of transplacental passage of opioids. Elderly patients are at greater risk of depression because of reduced lung elasticity, chest wall stiffening, and decreased vital capacity.
- *Disease.* Opiates may cause a greater depressant action in patients with chronic cardiopulmonary or renal diseases because they can manifest a desensitization of their response to increased CO_2.
- *COPD.* Enhanced depression can also be noted in patients with COPD and sleep apnea secondary to diminished hypoxic drive.
- *Relief of pain.* Because pain stimulates respiration, removal of the painful condition (as with the analgesia resulting from the therapeutic use of the opiate) will reduce the ventilatory drive and lead to apparent respiratory depression.

Comparative Respiratory Effects of Different Opiates

Numerous studies have compared morphine and morphine-like opioids with respect to their ratios of analgesic to respiratory-depressant activities, and most have found that when equianalgesic doses are used, there is no significant difference. Maximal respiratory depression occurs within 5–10 min of intravenous administration of morphine or within 30–90 min of intramuscular or subcutaneous administration. Maximal respiratory depressant effects occur more rapidly with more lipid-soluble agents. After therapeutic doses, respiratory minute volume may be reduced for as long as 4–5 h. Agents that have persistent kinetics, such as methadone, must be carefully monitored, particularly after dose incrementation. Respiratory depression produced by any opiate agonist can be readily reversed by delivery of an opiate antagonist. Opiate antagonist reversal in the somnolent patient is considered to be indicative of an opiate-mediated depression. It is important to remember that most opiate antagonists have a relatively short duration of action compared to an agonist such as morphine or methadone, and fatal "renarcotization" can occur if vigilance is not exercised.

Opioid-Induced Hyperalgesia

A paradoxical increase in pain states has been observed in response to acute (hours to days) and chronic opiate exposure. This increase may be reflected by unexplained increases in pain reports, increased levels of pain with increasing opiate dosages, or a diffuse sensitivity unassociated with the original pain (Lee et al., 2011). The mechanisms of this increased pain profile is not understood, although an enhanced excitability of central systems with chronic opiate exposure is considered relevant. Other avenues have pointed to the stimulatory effects of opioids on innate immune signaling through Toll-like receptor 4 activation, leading to central sensitization (Grace et al., 2014).

Sedation

Opiates can produce drowsiness and cognitive impairment. Such depression can augment respiratory impairment. These effects are most typically noted following initiation of opiate therapy or after dose incrementation. Importantly, these effects on arousal resolve over a few days. As with respiratory depression, the degree of drug effect can be enhanced by a variety of predisposing patient factors, including dementia, encephalopathies, brain tumors, and other depressant medications, including sleep aids, antihistamines, antidepressants, and anxiolytics (Cherny, 1996).

Neuroendocrine Effects

The regulation of the release of hormones and factors from the pituitary is under complex regulation by opiate receptors in the HPA axis. Broadly considered, morphine-like opioids reduce the release of a large number of HPA hormones (Armario, 2010).

Sex Hormones

In males, acute opiate therapy reduces plasma cortisol, testosterone, and gonadotrophins. Inhibition of adrenal function is reflected by reduced cortisol production and reduced adrenal androgens (DHEA). In females, morphine will also result in lower LH and FSH release. In both males and females, chronic therapy can result in endocrinopathies, including hypogonadotrophic hypogonadism. In men, this may result in decreased libido and, with extended exposure, reduced secondary sex characteristics. In women, these exposures are associated with menstrual cycle irregularities. These changes are reversible with removal of the opiate.

Prolactin. Prolactin release from the anterior pituitary is under inhibitory control by DA released from neurons of the arcuate nucleus. MOR agonists act presynaptically on these DA-releasing terminals to inhibit DA release and thereby increase plasma prolactin.

Antidiuretic Hormone and Oxytocin. The effects of opiates on ADH and oxytocin release are complex. These hormones are synthesized in the perikarya of the magnocellular neurons in the paraventricular and supraoptic nuclei of the hypothalamus and released from the posterior pituitary (Chapter 42). KOR agonists inhibit the release of oxytocin and ADH and cause prominent diuresis. Note, however, that agents such as morphine may yield a hypotension secondary to histamine release; this would, by itself, promote ADH release.

Miosis

The MOR agonists induce pupillary constriction (miosis) in the awake state and block pupillary reflex dilation during anesthesia. The parasympathetic outflow from the *Edinger Westphal nucleus* activates parasympathetic outflow through the ciliary ganglion to the pupil, producing constriction. This outflow is locally regulated by GABAergic interneurons. Opiates block this GABAergic interneuron-mediated inhibition, leading to increased parasympathetic outflow (Larson, 2008). At high doses of agonists, the miosis is marked, and pinpoint pupils are pathognomonic; however, marked mydriasis will occur with the onset of asphyxia. While some tolerance to the miotic effect develops, addicts with high circulating concentrations of opioids continue to have constricted pupils. Therapeutic doses of morphine increase accommodative power and lower intraocular tension in normal and glaucomatous eyes (Larson, 2008).

Seizures and Convulsions

In older children and adults, moderately higher doses of opiates produce EEG slowing. In the newborn, morphine can produce epileptiform activity and occasionally seizure activity (Young and da Silva, 2000). Several mechanisms are likely involved in these excitatory actions:

- *Inhibition of inhibitory interneurons.* Morphine-like drugs indirectly excite certain groups of neurons, such as hippocampal pyramidal cells, by inhibiting the inhibition otherwise exerted by GABAergic interneurons (McGinty, 1988).
- *Direct stimulatory effects.* Opiates may interact with receptors coupled through both inhibitory and stimulatory G proteins, with the inhibitory coupling but not the excitatory coupling showing tolerance with continued exposures (King et al., 2005).
- *Actions mediated by nonopioid receptors.* The metabolites of several opiates (morphine-3-glucuronide, normeperidine) have been implicated in seizure activity (Seifert and Kennedy, 2004; Smith, 2000).

A special case is the withdrawal syndrome from an opiate-dependent state in the adult and in the infant born to an opiate-dependent mother. Withdrawal in these circumstances, either by antagonists or abstinence, can lead to prominent EEG activation, tremor, and rigidity. Approaches to the management of such activation are controversial. Anticonvulsant agents may not always be effective in suppressing opioid-induced seizures (see Chapter 17).

Cough

Cough is a protective reflex evoked by airway stimulation. It involves rapid expression of air against a transiently closed glottis. The reflex is complex, involving the central and peripheral nervous systems as well as the smooth muscle of the bronchial tree. Morphine and related opioids depress the cough reflex at least in part by a direct effect on a cough center in the medulla; this cough suppression can be achieved without altering the protective glottal function (Chung and Pavord, 2008). There is no obligatory relationship between depression of respiration and depression of coughing, and effective antitussive agents are available that do not depress respiration (antitussives are discussed further in the chapter).

Nauseant and Emetic Effects

Nausea and vomiting produced by morphine-like drugs are side effects caused by direct stimulation of the chemoreceptor trigger zone for emesis in the *area postrema* of the medulla (see Figure 50–5). All clinically useful agonists produce some degree of nausea and vomiting. Nausea and vomiting are relatively uncommon in recumbent patients given therapeutic doses of morphine, but nausea occurs in about 40% and vomiting in 15% of ambulatory patients given analgesic doses. Morphine and related synthetic analgesics produce an increase in vestibular sensitivity. A component of nausea is likely also due to the gastric stasis that occurs postoperatively and that is exacerbated by analgesic doses of morphine. (Greenwood-Van Meerveld, 2007).

Cardiovascular System

In the supine patient, therapeutic doses of morphine-like opioids have no major effect on blood pressure or cardiac rate and rhythm. Such doses can, however, produce peripheral vasodilation, reduced peripheral resistance, and an inhibition of baroreceptor reflexes. Thus, when supine patients assume the head-up position, orthostatic hypotension and fainting may occur. The peripheral arteriolar and venous dilation produced by morphine involves several mechanisms:

- Morphine induces *release of histamine* from mast cells, leading to vasodilation; this effect is reversed by naloxone but only partially blocked by H_1 antagonists.
- Morphine *blunts reflex vasoconstriction* caused by increased P_{CO_2}.

High doses of MOR agonists, such as fentanyl and sufentanil, used as anesthetic induction agents, have only modest effects on hemodynamic stability, in part because they do not cause release of histamine (Monk et al., 1988). Morphine may exert its therapeutic effect in the treatment

of angina pectoris and acute myocardial infarction by decreasing preload, inotropy, and chronotropy, thus favorably altering determinants of myocardial O_2 consumption. Morphine also produces cardioprotective effects. Morphine can mimic the phenomenon of ischemic preconditioning, whereby a short ischemic episode paradoxically protects the heart against further ischemia. This effect appears to be mediated through receptors signaling through a mitochondrial ATP-sensitive K^+ channel in cardiac myocytes; the effect also is produced by other GPCRs signaling through G_i. Morphine-like opioids should be used with caution in patients who have decreased blood volume because these agents can aggravate hypovolemic shock. Morphine should be used with great care in patients with cor pulmonale; deaths after ordinary therapeutic doses have been reported. Concurrent use of certain CNS depressants (phenothiazines, ethanol, benzodiazepines) may increase the risk of morphine-induced hypotension. Cerebral circulation is not affected directly by therapeutic doses of opiates. However, opioid-induced respiratory depression and CO_2 retention can result in cerebral vasodilation and an increase in CSF pressure. This pressure increase does not occur when P_{CO_2} is maintained at normal levels by artificial ventilation.

Skeletal Muscle Tone

At therapeutic doses required for analgesia, opiates have little effect on motor tone or function. However, high doses of opioids, as used for anesthetic induction, produce muscular rigidity. Myoclonus, ranging from mild twitching to generalized spasm, is an occasional side effect that has been reported with all clinically used opiate agonists and is particularly prevalent in patients receiving high doses. The increased muscle tone is mediated by a central effect, although the mechanisms of its effects are not clear. High doses of spinal opiates can increase motor tone, possibly through an inhibition of inhibitory interneurons in the ventral horn of the spinal cord. Alternately, intracranial delivery can initiate rigidity in animal models, possibly reflecting increased extrapyramidal activity. Increased motor tone and rigidity are reversed by opiate antagonists.

GI Tract

Opiates have important effects on all aspects of GI function. Between 40% and 95% of patients treated with opioids develop constipation and changes in bowel function (Benyamin et al., 2008). Opioid receptors are densely distributed in enteric neurons between the myenteric and submucosal plexuses and on a variety of secretory cells. The importance of these peripheral systems in altering GI motility is emphasized by the therapeutic efficacy of peripherally limited opiate agonists such as loperamide as antidiarrheals and the utility of peripherally limited opiate antagonists such as methylnaltrexone to reverse the constipatory actions of systemic opiate agonists.

Esophagus. The esophageal sphincter is under control by brainstem reflexes that activate cholinergic motor neurons originating in the esophageal myenteric plexus. This system regulates passage of material from the esophagus to the stomach and prevents regurgitation; conversely, it allows relaxation in the act of emesis. Morphine inhibits lower esophageal sphincter relaxation induced by swallowing and by esophageal distension; the effect is believed to be centrally mediated because peripherally restricted opiates such as loperamide do not alter esophageal sphincter tone (Sidhu and Triadafilopoulos, 2008).

Stomach. Morphine increases tonic contracture of the antral musculature and upper duodenum and reduces resting tone in the musculature of the gastric reservoir, thereby prolonging gastric emptying time and increasing the likelihood of esophageal reflux. Passage of the gastric contents through the duodenum may be delayed by as much as 12 h, and the absorption of orally administered drugs is retarded. Morphine and other opioid agonists usually decrease secretion of hydrochloric acid. Activation of opioid receptors on parietal cells enhances secretion, but indirect effects, including increased secretion of somatostatin from the pancreas and reduced release of ACh appear to be dominant in most circumstances (Kromer, 1988).

Intestine. Morphine reduces propulsive activity in the small and large intestines and diminishes intestinal secretions. Opiate agonists suppress rhythmic inhibition of muscle tone, leading to concurrent increases in basal tone in the circular muscle of the small and large intestines. This results in enhanced high-amplitude phasic contractions, which are *nonpropulsive* (Wood and Galligan, 2004). The upper part of the small intestine, particularly the duodenum, is affected more than the ileum. A period of relative atony may follow the period of elevated basal tone. The reduced rate of passage of the intestinal contents, along with reduced intestinal secretion, leads to increased water absorption, increasing viscosity of the bowel contents, and constipation. The tone of the anal sphincter is augmented greatly, and reflex relaxation in response to rectal distension is reduced. Patients who take opioids chronically remain constipated. Intestinal secretion arises from activation of enterocytes by local cholinergic submucosal plexus secretomotor neurons. Opioids act though μ/δ receptors on these secretomotor neurons to inhibit their excitatory output to the enterocytes and thereby reduce intestinal secretion (Kromer, 1988).

Biliary Tract. Morphine constricts the sphincter of Oddi, and the pressure in the common bile duct may rise more than 10-fold within 15 min. Fluid pressure also may increase in the gallbladder and produce symptoms that may vary from epigastric distress to typical biliary colic. All opioids can cause biliary spasm. Some patients with biliary colic experience exacerbation rather than relief of pain when given opioids. Spasm of the sphincter of Oddi probably is responsible for elevations of plasma amylase and lipase that sometimes occur after morphine administration. Atropine only partially prevents morphine-induced biliary spasm, but opioid antagonists prevent or relieve it.

Ureter and Urinary Bladder

Morphine inhibits the urinary voiding reflex and increases the tone of the external sphincter with a resultant increase in the volume of the bladder. Tolerance develops to these effects of opioids on the bladder. Clinically, opiate-mediated inhibition of micturition can be of such clinical severity that catheterization sometimes is required after therapeutic doses of morphine, particularly with spinal drug administration. Importantly, the inhibition of systemic opiate effects on micturition is reversed by peripherally restricted antagonists (Rosow et al., 2007).

Uterus

Morphine may prolong labor. If the uterus has been made hyperactive by oxytocics, morphine tends to restore the contractions to normal.

Skin

Therapeutic doses of morphine cause dilation of cutaneous blood vessels. The skin of the face, neck, and upper thorax frequently becomes flushed. Pruritus commonly follows systemic administration of morphine. Itching is readily seen with morphine and meperidine but to a much lesser extent with fentanyl or sufentanil. The systemic action is sensitive to antihistamines (diphenhydramine) and correlates with the mast cell degranulating properties of the opiate. Neither the pruritus nor the degranulation is reversed by opiate antagonists (Barke and Hough, 1993). This pruritus also can be caused by epidural or intrathecal opiate administration through a centrally mediated, naloxone-reversible mechanism (Kumar and Singh, 2013).

Immune System

Opioids modulate immune function by direct effects on cells of the immune system and indirectly through centrally mediated neuronal mechanisms (Vallejo et al., 2004). The acute central immunomodulatory effects of opioids may be mediated by activation of the sympathetic nervous system; the chronic effects of opioids may involve modulation of the HPA axis. Direct effects on immune cells may involve unique variants of the classical neuronal opioid receptors, with MOR variants being most prominent. A proposed mechanism for the immune-suppressive effects of morphine on neutrophils is through NO-dependent inhibition of NF-κB activation, or via activation of MAP kinases. Convincing data suggest that several opiates, including morphine, may interact with Toll-like receptor 4 to activate a variety of immunocytes independent of an opiate receptor (Hutchinson et al., 2007). Overall, however, opioids are modestly immunosuppressive, and increased susceptibility to infection and tumor spread have been observed. In some situations, immune effects appear more

prominent with acute administration than with chronic administration, which could have important implications for the care of the critically ill.

In addition to the effects of opiates on immune function, many opiate agonists evoke mast cell degranulation and histamine release. This action can cause bronchoconstriction and vasodilation. As a consequence, morphine has the potential to precipitate or exacerbate asthmatic attacks and should be avoided in patients with a history of asthma. The effect on mast cells is not prevented by opiate antagonists and appears to be independent of MORs. After potent opioids such as fentanyl, the incidence of mast cell degranulation is reduced compared to the effect of morphine. Through such mechanisms, opioid analgesics may evoke allergic phenomena that usually are manifested as urticaria, other types of skin rashes, and pruritus. The pruritus is often managed with antihistamines.

Temperature Regulation

Opioids alter the equilibrium point of the hypothalamic heat-regulatory mechanisms such that body temperature usually falls slightly. Agonists at the MOR (e.g., alfentanil and meperidine), acting in the CNS, result in slightly increased thresholds for sweating and significantly lower the threshold temperatures for evoking vasoconstriction and shivering.

Clinically Employed Opioid Drugs

Most of the clinically used opioid agonists presented in Table 20–4 are relatively selective for MORs. They produce analgesia, affect mood and rewarding behavior, and alter respiratory, cardiovascular, GI, and neuroendocrine function. KOR agonists, with few exceptions (e.g., butorphanol), are not typically employed for long-term therapy because they may produce dysphoric and psychotomimetic effects. DOR agonists, while analgesically active, have not found clinical utility, and NOP agonists lack analgesic effects. Opiates that are relatively receptor selective at lower doses may interact with additional receptor types when given at high doses, especially as doses are escalated to overcome tolerance.

The mixed agonist-antagonist agents frequently interact with more than one receptor type at usual clinical doses. A "ceiling effect" limiting the amount of analgesia attainable often is seen with these drugs, as is the case with buprenorphine, which is approved for the treatment of opioid dependence. Some mixed agonist-antagonist drugs, such as pentazocine and nalorphine (not available in the U.S.), can precipitate withdrawal in opioid-tolerant patients. For these reasons, except for the sanctioned use of buprenorphine to manage opioid addiction, the clinical use of mixed agonist-antagonist drugs is generally limited.

The dosing guidelines and duration of action for the numerous drugs that are part of opioid therapy are summarized in Table 20–4.

Morphine and Structurally Related Agonists

Sources of Opium

Two groups have recently reported the scalable biosynthesis of opiates in the laboratory using yeast (Galanie et al., 2015) or *Escherichia coli* (Nakagawa et al., 2016); thus, nonagricultural systems of opiate production may be at hand. Typically, however, morphine is obtained from opium or extracted from poppy straw. Opium is obtained from the unripe seed capsules of the poppy plant, *Papaver somniferum*. The milky juice is dried and powdered to make powdered opium. Powdered opium contains a number of alkaloids, only a few of which (morphine, codeine, and papaverine) have clinical utility. These opium alkaloids are divided into two distinct chemical classes, phenanthrenes and benzylisoquinolines. The principal phenanthrenes are morphine (10% of opium), codeine (0.5%), and thebaine (0.2%). The principal benzylisoquinolines are papaverine (1%) (a smooth muscle relaxant) and noscapine (6%).

Morphine and Its Congeners

Morphine remains the standard against which new analgesics are measured.

Chemistry. The structures of morphine and some of its surrogates and antagonists are shown in Figure 20–9. Many semisynthetic derivatives

TABLE 20–4 ■ DOSING DATA FOR CLINICALLY EMPLOYED OPIOID ANALGESICS

DRUG	APPROXIMATE EQUIANALGESIC ORAL DOSE	APPROXIMATE EQUIANALGESIC PARENTERAL DOSE	RECOMMENDED STARTING DOSE (Adults > 50 kg)		RECOMMENDED STARTING DOSE (Children and Adults < 50 kg)	
			ORAL	PARENTERAL	ORAL	PARENTERAL
Opioid Agonists						
Morphine	30 mg/3–4 h	10 mg/3–4 h	15 mg/3–4 h	5 mg/3–4 h	0.3 mg/kg/3–4 h	0.1 mg/kg/3–4 h
Codeine	130 mg/3–4 h	75 mg/3–4 h	30 mg/3–4 h	30 mg/2 h (IM/SC)	0.5 mg/kg/3–4 h	Not recommended
Hydromophone	6 mg/3–4 h	1.5 mg/3–4 h	2 mg/3–4 h	0.5 mg/3–4 h	0.03 mg/kg/3–4 h	0.005 mg/kg/3–4 h
Hydrocodone (typically with acetaminophen)	30 mg/3–4 h	Not available	5 mg/3–4 h	Not available	0.1 mg/kg/3–4 h	Not available
Levorphanol	4 mg/6–8 h	2 mg/6–8 h	4 mg/6–8 h	2 mg/6–8 h	0.04 mg/kg/6–8 h	0.02 mg/kg/6–8 h
Meperidine	300 mg/2–3 h	100 mg/3 h	Not recommended	50 mg/3 h	Not recommended	0.75 mg/kg/2–3 h
Methadone	10 mg/6–8 h	10 mg/6–8 h	5 mg/12 h	Not recommended	0.1 mg/kg/12 h	Not recommended
Oxycodone	20 mg/3–4 h	Not available	5 mg/3–4 h	Not available	0.1 mg/kg/3–4 h	Not available
Oxymorphone	10 mg/3–4 h	1 mg/3–4 h	5 mg/3–4 h	1 mg/3–4 h	0.1 mg/kg/3–4 h	Not recommended
Tramadol	100 mg	100 mg	50–100 mg/6 h	50–100 mg/6 h	Not recommended	Not recommended
Fentanyl	Transdermal 72-h patch (25 µg/h) = morphine 50 mg/24 h					
Opioid Agonist-Antagonists or Partial Agonists						
Buprenorphine	Not available	0.3–0.4 mg/6–8 h	Not available	0.4 mg/6–8 h	Not available	0.004 mg/kg/6–8 h
Butorphanol	Not available	2 mg/3–4 h	Not available	2 mg/3–4 h	Not available	Not recommended
Nalbuphine	Not available	10 mg/3–4 h	Not available	10 mg/3–4 h	Not available	0.1 mg/kg/3–4 h

These data are merely guidelines. Clinical response must be the guide for each patient, with consideration to hepatic and renal function, disease, age, concurrent medications (their effects and dose limitations [acetaminophen, 3 g/d for adults]), and other factors that could modify pharmacokinetics and drug response. Recommended start doses are approximately but not precisely equianalgesic and are driven by doses available from manufacturers. Transdermal fentanyl is contraindicated for acute pain and in patients receiving < 60 mg oral morphine equivalent per day. Use Table 20–8 for converting morphine to methadone dosing.

For morphine, hydromorphone, and oxymorphone, rectal administration is an alternate route for patients unable to take oral medications, but equianalgesic doses may differ from oral and parenteral doses because of pharmacokinetic differences.

Doses listed for patients with body weight less than 50 kg cannot be used as initial starting doses in babies less than 6 months of age; consult the *Clinical Practice Guideline #1, Acute Pain Management: Operative or Medical Procedures and Trauma* (cited below), section on neonates, for recommendations.

Source: Modified and updated from Agency for Healthcare Policy and Research, 1992. Acute Pain Management Guideline Panel. AHCPR Clinical Practice Guidelines, No. 1: Acute Pain Management: Operative or Medical Procedures and Trauma [Rockville (MD): Agency for Health Care Policy and Research (AHCPR); 1992].

are made by relatively simple modifications of morphine or thebaine. Codeine is methylmorphine, the methyl substitution being on the phenolic hydroxyl group. Thebaine differs from morphine only in that both hydroxyl groups are methylated and that the ring has two double bonds (6,7; 8,14). Thebaine has little analgesic action but is a precursor of several important 14-OH compounds, such as oxycodone and naloxone. Certain derivatives of thebaine are more than 1000 times as potent as morphine (e.g., etorphine). Diacetylmorphine, or heroin, is made from morphine by acetylation at the 3 and 6 positions. Apomorphine, which also can be prepared from morphine, is a potent emetic and dopaminergic agonist at D2- and D1-type receptors, does not interact with opiate receptors, and displays no analgesic actions (see Chapters 13, 18, and 50). Hydromorphone, oxymorphone, hydrocodone, and oxycodone also are made by modifying the morphine molecule.

Structure-Activity Relationship of the Morphine-Like Opioids. In addition to morphine, codeine, and the semisynthetic derivatives of the natural opium alkaloids, a number of other structurally distinct chemical classes of drugs have pharmacological actions similar to those of morphine. Clinically useful compounds include the morphinans, benzomorphans, methadones, phenylpiperidines, and propionanilides. Although the two-dimensional representations of these chemically diverse compounds appear to be quite different, molecular models show common

characteristics. Among the important properties of the opioids that can be altered by structural modification are their affinities for various types of opioid receptors, their activities as agonists versus antagonists, their lipid solubilities, and their resistance to metabolic breakdown. For example, blockade of the phenolic hydroxyl at position 3, as in codeine and heroin, drastically reduces binding to receptors; these compounds are converted in vivo to the potent analgesics morphine and 6-acetyl morphine, respectively.

ADME. Absorption. In general, the opioids are modestly well absorbed from the GI tract; absorption through the rectal mucosa is adequate, and a few agents (e.g., morphine, hydromorphone) are available in suppositories. The more lipophilic opioids are absorbed readily through the nasal or buccal mucosa. Those with the greatest lipid solubility also can be absorbed transdermally. Opioids, particularly morphine, have been widely used for spinal delivery to produce analgesia though a spinal action. These agents display useful transdural movement adequate to permit their use epidurally.

With most opioids, including morphine, the effect of a given dose is less after oral than after parenteral administration because of variable but significant first-pass metabolism in the liver. For example, the bioavailability of oral preparations of morphine is only about 25%. The shape of the time-effect curve also varies with the route of administration, so the duration of action often is somewhat longer with the oral route.

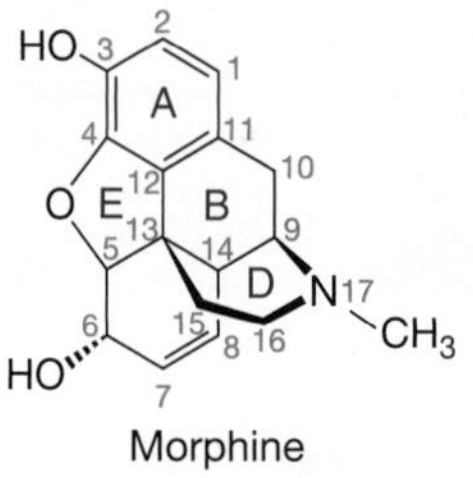

Nonproprietary name	Chemical radicals and position[a]			Other changes[†]
	3	6	17	
Morphine	—OH	—OH	—CH$_3$	—
Heroin	—OCOCH$_3$	—OCOCH$_3$	—CH$_3$	—
Hydromorphone	—OH	=O	—CH$_3$	(1)
Oxymorphone	—OH	=O	—CH$_3$	(1), (2)
Levorphanol	—OH	—H	—CH$_3$	(1), (3)
Levallorphan	—OH	—H	—CH$_2$CH=CH$_2$	(1), (3)
Codeine	—OCH$_3$	—OH	—CH$_3$	—
Hydrocodone	—OCH$_3$	=O	—CH$_3$	(1)
Oxycodone	—OCH$_3$	=O	—CH$_3$	(1), (2)
Nalmefene	—OH	=CH$_2$	—CH$_2$—▷	(1), (2)
Nalorphine	—OH	—OH	—CH$_2$CH=CH$_2$	—
Naloxone	—OH	=O	—CH$_2$CH=CH$_2$	(1), (2)
Naltrexone	—OH	=O	—CH$_2$—▷	(1), (2)
Buprenorphine	—OH	—OCH$_3$	—CH$_2$—▷	(1), (4)
Butorphanol	—OH	—H	—CH$_2$—◇	(1), (2), (3)
Nalbuphine	—OH	—OH	—CH$_2$—◇	(1), (2)
Methylnaltrexone	—OH	=O	—(N)—CH$_2$—▷ with CH$_3$	(1), (2)

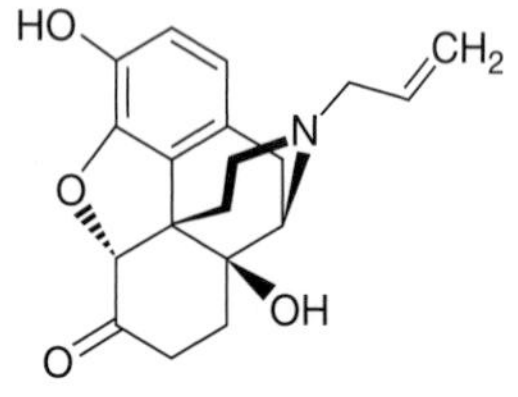

Naloxone 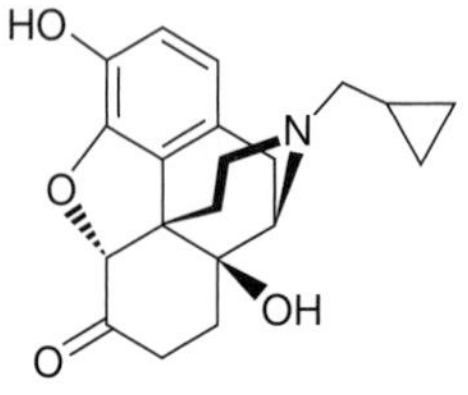 · Naltrexone 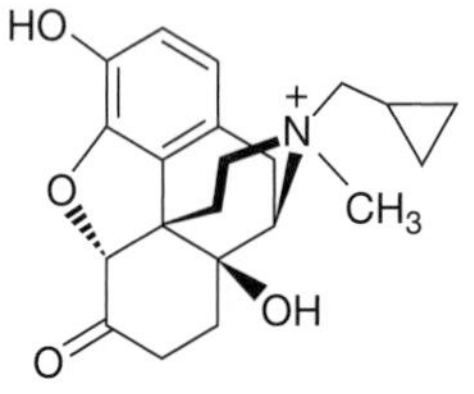 · Methylnaltrexone

[a]The numbers 3, 6, and 17 refer to positions in the morphine molecule, as shown above. †Other changes in the morphine molecule are (1) Single instead of double bond between C7 and C8; (2) OH added to C14; (3) No oxygen between C4 and C5; (4) Endoetheno bridge between C6 and C14; 1-hydroxy-1,2,2-trimethylpropyl substitution on C7.

Figure 20–9 *Structures of morphine-related opiate agonists and antagonists.*

If adjustment is made for variability of first-pass metabolism and clearance, adequate relief of pain can be achieved with oral administration of morphine. Satisfactory analgesia in patients with cancer is associated with a broad range of steady-state concentrations of morphine in plasma (16–364 ng/mL) (Neumann et al., 1982).

When morphine and most opioids are given intravenously, they act promptly. However, the more lipid-soluble compounds (e.g., fentanyl) act more rapidly than morphine after subcutaneous administration because of differences in the rates of absorption and entry into the CNS. Compared with more lipid-soluble opioids such as codeine, heroin, and methadone, morphine crosses the blood-brain barrier at a considerably lower rate.

Distribution and Metabolism. About one-third of morphine in the plasma is protein bound after a therapeutic dose. Morphine itself does not persist in tissues, and 24 h after the last dose, tissue concentrations are low.

The major pathway for the metabolism of morphine is conjugation with glucuronic acid. The two major metabolites formed are morphine-6-glucuronide and morphine-3-glucuronide. Small amounts of morphine-3,6-diglucuronide also may be formed. Although the 3-and 6-glucuronides are polar, both still can cross the blood-brain barrier to exert significant clinical effects (Christrup, 1997).

Morphine-6-glucuronide has pharmacological actions indistinguishable from those of morphine. Morphine-6-glucuronide given systemically is approximately twice as potent as morphine in animal models and in humans (Osborne et al., 1992). With chronic administration, the 6-glucuronide accounts for a significant portion of morphine's analgesic actions. Indeed, with chronic oral dosing, the blood levels of morphine-6-glucuronide typically exceed those of morphine. Given its greater MOR potency and its higher concentration, morphine-6-glucuronide may be responsible for most of morphine's analgesic activity in patients receiving chronic oral morphine. Morphine-6-glucuronide is excreted by the kidney. In renal failure, the levels of morphine-6-glucuronide can accumulate, perhaps explaining morphine's potency and long duration in patients with compromised renal function. In adults, the $t_{1/2}$ of morphine is about 2 h; the $t_{1/2}$ of morphine-6-glucuronide is somewhat longer. Children achieve adult renal function values by 6 months of age. In elderly patients, lower doses of morphine are recommended based on a smaller volume of distribution and the general decline in renal function in the elderly (Owens, et al, 1983).

Morphine-3-glucuronide, another important metabolite, has little affinity for opioid receptors but may contribute to excitatory effects of morphine (Smith, 2000). N-Demethylation of morphine to normorphine is a minor metabolic pathway in humans. N-Dealkylation also is important in the metabolism of some congeners of morphine.

Excretion. Morphine is eliminated by glomerular filtration, primarily as morphine-3-glucuronide; 90% of the total excretion takes place during the first day. Very little morphine is excreted unchanged. Enterohepatic circulation of morphine and its glucuronides occurs, which accounts for the presence of small amounts of morphine in feces and urine for several days after the last dose.

Morphine Congeners. **Codeine.** Codeine is an important natural product found in the poppy resin. It displays a modest affinity for the μ receptor, but its analgesic actions are considered by many to arise at least in part by its hepatic metabolism to morphine (see further discussion). Thus, in contrast to morphine, codeine is about 60% as effective orally as parenterally as an analgesic and as a respiratory depressant. Codeine is commonly employed for the management of cough, frequently in combination dose forms with acetaminophen or aspirin. The drug has an exceptionally low affinity for opioid receptors, and while the analgesic effect of codeine is likely due to its conversion to morphine, codeine's antitussive actions may involve distinct receptors that bind codeine itself.

Once absorbed, codeine is metabolized by the liver. Codeine analogues such as levorphanol, oxycodone, and methadone have a high ratio of oral-to-parenteral potency. The greater oral efficacy of these drugs reflects lower first-pass metabolism in the liver. Codeine's metabolites are excreted chiefly as inactive forms in the urine. A small fraction (~10%) of administered codeine is O-demethylated to morphine, and free and conjugated morphine can be found in the urine after therapeutic doses of codeine. The $t_{1/2}$ of codeine in plasma is 2–4 h. CYP2D6 catalyzes the conversion of codeine to morphine. Genetic polymorphisms in CYP2D6 lead to the inability to convert codeine to morphine, thus making codeine ineffective as an analgesic for about 10% of the Caucasian population (Eichelbaum and Evert, 1996). Other polymorphisms (e.g., the CYP2D6*2x2 genotype) can lead to ultrarapid metabolism and thus increased sensitivity to codeine's effects due to higher than expected serum morphine levels. Other variations in metabolic efficiency among ethnic groups are apparent. For example, Chinese produce less morphine from codeine than do Caucasians and also are less sensitive to morphine's effects. The reduced sensitivity to morphine may be due to decreased production of morphine-6-glucuronide (Caraco et al., 1999). Thus, it is important to consider the possibility of metabolic enzyme polymorphism in any patient who experiences toxicity or does not receive adequate analgesia from codeine or other opioid prodrugs (e.g., hydrocodone and oxycodone) (Johansson and Ingelman-Sundberg, 2011).

Heroin. Heroin (diacetylmorphine) is rapidly hydrolyzed to 6-MAM, which in turn is hydrolyzed to morphine. Heroin and 6-MAM are more lipid soluble than morphine and enter the brain more readily. Evidence suggests that morphine and 6-MAM are responsible for the pharmacological actions of heroin. Heroin is excreted mainly in the urine, largely as free and conjugated morphine (Rook et al., 2006).

Hydromorphone. Hydromorphone is a semisynthetic hydrogenated ketone derivative of morphine. It displays all of the opioid actions of morphine. It is commonly used as an intravenous medication. The drug is formulated in parenteral, rectal, subcutaneous, and oral preparations and as a nebulized formulation and is given off label by epidural or intrathecal routes. Hydromorphone has a higher lipid solubility than morphine, resulting in more rapid onset than morphine, and is considered to be several times more potent than morphine. Hydromorphone is metabolized in the liver to hydromorphone-3-glucuronide.

Oxycodone. Oxycodone is a semisynthetic opioid synthesized from the alkaloid thebaine. The molecule undergoes hepatic metabolism to the more potent μ opioid oxymorphone. Oxycodone is available as single-ingredient medication in immediate-release and controlled-release formulations. Parenteral formulations of 10 mg/mL and 50 mg/mL are available in the U.K. for intravenous or intramuscular administration. Combination products are also available as immediate-release formulations with non-narcotic ingredients such as NSAIDs. At present, oxycodone is one of the most commonly abused pharmaceutical drugs in the U.S.

Hydrocodone. Hydrocodone is synthesized from codeine. It is used orally for relief of moderate-to-severe pain and is employed in a liquid formulation as a cough suppressant. It is approximately equipotent to oxycodone, with an onset of action of 10–30 min and duration of 4–6 h. Hepatic CYPs 2D6 and 3A4 convert hydrocodone to hydromorphone and norhydrocodone, respectively. Hydrocodone shows a serum half-life of about 4 h.

Oxymorphone. Oxymorphone, a semisynthetic alkaloid, is produced from thebaine. Oxymorphone is a potent MOR agonist with an onset of analgesia after parenteral dosing of about 5–10 min and a duration of action of 3–4 h. Oxymorphone is extensively metabolized in liver and excreted as the 3- and 6-glucuronides.

Adverse Effects and Precautions

Morphine and related opioids, aside from their effects as analgesics, produce a wide spectrum of effects reflecting the distribution of opiate receptors across organ systems. These effects include respiratory depression, nausea, vomiting, dizziness, mental clouding, dysphoria, pruritus, constipation, increased pressure in the biliary tract, urinary retention, hypotension, and, rarely, delirium. Increased sensitivity to pain may occur after analgesia has worn off, and removal of opiate receptor occupancy (abstinence, antagonism) may lead to a highly aversive state of withdrawal.

Factors Affecting Patient Response to Morphine and Congeners

Beyond those mentioned, a number of other factors may alter a patient's response to opioid analgesics.

- *Blood-Brain Barrier.* Morphine is hydrophilic, so proportionately less morphine normally crosses into the CNS than with more lipophilic opioids. In neonates or when the blood-brain barrier is compromised, lipophilic opioids may give more predictable clinical results than morphine.
- *Age.* In adults, the duration of the analgesia produced by morphine increases progressively with age; however, the degree of analgesia that is obtained with a given dose changes little.
- *Pain State.* The patient with severe pain may tolerate larger doses of morphine. However, as the pain subsides, the patient may exhibit sedation and even respiratory depression as the stimulatory effects of pain are diminished.
- *Opioid Metabolism.* All opioid analgesics are metabolized by the liver and should be used with caution in patients with hepatic disease. Renal disease also significantly alters the pharmacokinetics of morphine, codeine, dihydrocodeine, and meperidine. Although single doses of morphine are well tolerated, the active metabolite, morphine-6-glucuronide, may accumulate with continued dosing, and symptoms of opioid overdose may result. This metabolite also may accumulate during repeated administration of codeine to patients with impaired renal function. When repeated doses of meperidine are given to such patients, the accumulation of normeperidine may cause tremor and seizures. Similarly, the repeated administration of propoxyphene

may lead to naloxone-insensitive cardiac toxicity caused by accumulation of the metabolite norpropoxyphene.

- *Sex.* There is a growing body of data that examines gender differences in the responses to pain and analgesics (Mogil, 2012). Females have the majority of chronic pain syndromes, and surveys examining sex differences in acute pain models report either no sex difference or greater sensitivity in females. Data on sex differences in opiate analgesia have thus far been inconsistent (Loyd and Murphy, 2014).

- *Respiratory Function.* Morphine and related opioids must be used cautiously in patients with compromised respiratory function (e.g., emphysema, kyphoscoliosis, severe obesity, or cor pulmonale). Although many patients with such conditions seem to be functioning within normal limits, they are already using compensatory mechanisms, such as increased respiratory rate. Many have chronically elevated levels of plasma CO_2 and may be less sensitive to the stimulating actions of CO_2. The further imposition of the depressant effects of opioids can be disastrous.

- *Head Injury.* The respiratory-depressant effects of opioids and the related capacity to elevate intracranial pressure must be considered in the presence of head injury or an already-elevated intracranial pressure. While head injury per se does not constitute an absolute contraindication to the use of opioids, the possibility of exaggerated depression of respiration and the potential need to control ventilation of the patient must be considered. Finally, because opioids may produce mental clouding and side effects such as miosis and vomiting, which are important signs in following the clinical course of patients with head injuries, the advisability of their use must be weighed carefully against these risks.

- *Hypovolemia; Hypotension.* Reduced blood volume causes patients to be considerably more susceptible to the vasodilating effects of morphine and related drugs, and these agents must be used cautiously in patients with hypotension from any cause.

- *Asthma; Allergic Responses; Histamine Release.* Morphine causes histamine release, which can cause bronchoconstriction and vasodilation. Morphine can precipitate or exacerbate asthmatic attacks and should be avoided in patients with a history of asthma. Other receptor agonists associated with a lower incidence of histamine release, such as the fentanyl derivatives, may be better choices for such patients.

Aside from their capacity to release histamine, opioid analgesics may evoke allergic phenomena, but a true allergic response is uncommon. The effects usually are manifested as urticaria and fixed eruptions; contact dermatitis in nurses and pharmaceutical workers also occurs. Wheals at the site of injection of morphine, codeine, and related drugs are likely secondary to histamine release. Anaphylactoid reactions have been reported after intravenous administration of codeine and morphine, but such reactions are rare. In addicts who use intravenous heroin, such reactions may contribute to sudden death, episodes of pulmonary edema, and other complications.

Other Morphinans

Levorphanol

Levorphanol is an opioid agonist of the morphinan series (Figure 20–9). Levorphanol has affinity at the MORs, KORs, and DORs and is available for intravenous, intramuscular, and oral administration. The pharmacological effects of levorphanol closely parallel those of morphine. Compared to morphine, this agent is about seven times more potent and may produce less nausea and vomiting. Levorphanol is metabolized less rapidly than morphine and has a $t_{1/2}$ of 12–16 h; repeated administration at short intervals may thus lead to accumulation of the drug in plasma (Prommer, 2014). The D-isomer (dextrorphan) is devoid of analgesic action but has inhibitory effects at NMDA receptors.

Piperidine and Phenylpiperidine Analgesics

Meperidine, Diphenoxylate, Loperamide

The agents meperidine, diphenoxylate, and loperamide are MOR agonists with principal pharmacological effects on the CNS and neural elements in the bowel.

Meperidine. Meperidine is predominantly an MOR agonist that produces a pattern of effects similar but not identical to those already described for morphine (Latta et al., 2002).

CNS Actions. Meperidine is a potent agonist at MORs in the CNS, yielding strong analgesic actions. Meperidine causes pupillary constriction, increases the sensitivity of the labyrinthine apparatus, and has effects on the secretion of pituitary hormones similar to those of morphine. Meperidine sometimes causes CNS excitation, characterized by tremors, muscle twitches, and seizures. These effects are due largely to accumulation of a metabolite, normeperidine. Meperidine has well-known local anesthetic properties, particularly noted after epidural administration. As with morphine, respiratory depression is responsible for an accumulation of CO_2, which in turn leads to cerebrovascular dilation, increased cerebral blood flow, and elevation of CSF pressure.

Cardiovascular Effects. The effects of meperidine on the cardiovascular system generally resemble those of morphine, including the release of histamine following parenteral administration. Intramuscular administration of therapeutic doses of meperidine does not affect heart rate significantly, but intravenous administration frequently produces a marked increase in heart rate.

Actions on Smooth Muscle, GI Tract, and Uterus. Meperidine does not cause as much constipation as morphine, even when given over prolonged periods; this may be related to its greater ability to enter the CNS, thereby producing analgesia at lower systemic concentrations. As with other opioids, clinical doses of meperidine slow gastric emptying sufficiently to delay absorption of other drugs significantly. The uterus of a nonpregnant woman usually is mildly stimulated by meperidine. Administered before an oxytocic, meperidine does not exert any antagonistic effect. Therapeutic doses given during active labor do not delay the birth process; in fact, frequency, duration, and amplitude of uterine contraction may be increased.

ADME. Meperidine is absorbed by all routes of administration. The peak plasma concentration usually occurs at about 45 min, but the range is wide. After oral administration, only about 50% of the drug escapes first-pass metabolism to enter the circulation, and peak concentrations in plasma occur in 1–2 h. Meperidine is metabolized chiefly in the liver, with a $t_{1/2}$ of about 3 h. Metabolites are the *N*-demethyl product, normeperidine, and the hydrolysis product, meperidinate, both of which may be conjugated. In patients with cirrhosis, the bioavailability of meperidine is increased to as much as 80%, and the $t_{1/2}$ of both meperidine and the metabolite normeperidine ($t_{1/2} \sim$ 15–20 h) are prolonged. Only a small amount of meperidine is excreted unchanged.

Therapeutic Use. The major use of meperidine is for analgesia. The analgesic effects of meperidine are detectable about 15 min after oral administration, peak in 1–2 h, and subside gradually. The onset of analgesic effect is faster (within 10 min) after subcutaneous or intramuscular administration, and the effect reaches a peak in about 1 h, corresponding closely to peak concentrations in plasma. In clinical use, the duration of effective analgesia is about 1.5–3 h. Peak respiratory depression is observed within 1 h of intramuscular administration, and there is a return toward normal starting at about 2 h. In general, 75–100 mg meperidine hydrochloride given parenterally is approximately equivalent to 10 mg morphine. In terms of total analgesic effect, meperidine is about one-third as effective when given orally as when administered parenterally.

Single doses of meperidine can be effective in the treatment of postanesthetic shivering. Meperidine, 25–50 mg, is used frequently with antihistamines, corticosteroids, acetaminophen, or NSAIDs to prevent or ameliorate infusion-related rigors and shaking chills that accompany the intravenous administration of agents such as amphotericin B, aldesleukin (interleukin 2), trastuzumab, and alemtuzumab. Meperidine crosses the placental barrier, and even in reasonable analgesic doses causes a significant increase in the percentage of babies who show delayed respiration, decreased respiratory minute volume, or decreased O_2 saturation or who require resuscitation. Fetal and maternal respiratory depression induced by meperidine can be treated with naloxone. Meperidine produces less respiratory depression in the newborn than does an equianalgesic dose of morphine or methadone (Fishburne, 1982).

Untoward Effects, Precautions, and Contraindications. The overall incidence of untoward effects is similar to those observed after equianalgesic doses of morphine, except that constipation and urinary retention and nausea may be less common. Patients who experience nausea and vomiting with morphine may not do so with meperidine; the converse also may be true. In patients or addicts who are tolerant to the depressant effects of meperidine, large doses repeated at short intervals may produce an excitatory syndrome that includes hallucinations, tremors, muscle twitches, dilated pupils, hyperactive reflexes, and convulsions. These excitatory symptoms are due to the accumulation of the long-lived metabolite normeperidine, which has a $t_{1/2}$ of 15–20 h, compared to 3 h for meperidine. Decreased renal or hepatic function increases the likelihood of toxicity. As a result of these properties, meperidine is not recommended for the treatment of chronic pain because of concerns over metabolite toxicity. It should not be used for longer than 48 h or in doses greater than 600 mg/d.

Interactions With Other Drugs. Severe reactions may follow the administration of meperidine to patients being treated with MAO inhibitors. There are two basic types of interaction. The more prominent is an excitatory reaction ("serotonin syndrome") with delirium, hyperthermia, headache, hyper- or hypotension, rigidity, convulsions, coma, and death. This reaction may be due to the capacity of meperidine to block neuronal reuptake of 5HT, resulting in serotonergic overactivity. Dextromethorphan (an analogue of levorphanol used as a nonnarcotic cough suppressant) also inhibits neuronal 5HT uptake and must be avoided in these patients. In the second type of interaction, several MAO inhibitors are substrates or inhibitors of hepatic CYPs and reduce meperidine metabolism, creating a condition resembling acute narcotic overdose. Therefore, meperidine and its congeners are contraindicated in patients taking MAO inhibitors or within 14 days after discontinuation of an MAO inhibitor.

Chlorpromazine increases the respiratory-depressant effects of meperidine, as do tricyclic antidepressants (but not diazepam). Concurrent administration of drugs such as promethazine or chlorpromazine also may greatly enhance meperidine-induced sedation without slowing clearance of the drug. Treatment with phenobarbital or phenytoin increases systemic clearance and decreases oral bioavailability of meperidine. As with morphine, concomitant administration of amphetamine has been reported to enhance the analgesic effects of meperidine and its congeners while counteracting sedation.

Diphenoxylate. Diphenoxylate is a meperidine congener that has a definite constipating effect in humans. Its only approved use is in the treatment of diarrhea. Diphenoxylate is unusual in that even its salts are virtually insoluble in aqueous solution, thus reducing the probability of abuse by the parenteral route. Diphenoxylate hydrochloride is available only in combination with atropine sulfate. The recommended daily dosage of diphenoxylate for the treatment of diarrhea in adults is 20 mg in divided doses. Difenoxin a metabolite of diphenoxylate and is marketed in a fixed dose with atropine for the management of diarrhea.

Loperamide. Loperamide, like diphenoxylate, is a piperidine derivative. It slows GI motility by effects on the circular and longitudinal muscles of the intestine (Kromer, 1988). Part of its antidiarrheal effect may be due to a reduction of GI secretory processes (see Chapter 50). In controlling chronic diarrhea, loperamide is as effective as diphenoxylate and little tolerance develops to its constipating effect. Concentrations of drug in plasma peak about 4 h after ingestion. The apparent elimination $t_{1/2}$ is 7–14 h. Loperamide is poorly absorbed after oral administration and, in addition, apparently does not penetrate well into the brain due to the exporting activity of P-glycoprotein, which is widely expressed in the brain endothelium. The usual dosage is 4–8 mg/d; the daily dose should not exceed 16 mg (Regnard et al., 2011). The most common side effect is abdominal cramps. Loperamide is unlikely to be abused parenterally because of its low solubility; large doses of loperamide given to human volunteers do not elicit pleasurable effects typical of opioids.

Fentanyl and Congeners

Fentanyl

Fentanyl is a synthetic opioid related to the phenylpiperidines. The actions of fentanyl and its congeners sufentanil, remifentanil, and alfentanil are similar to those of other MOR agonists. Fentanyl and sufentanil are important drugs in anesthetic practice because of their relatively short time to peak analgesic effect, rapid termination of effect after small bolus doses, cardiovascular safety, and capacity to significantly reduce the dosing requirement for the volatile agents (see Chapter 21). In addition to a role in anesthesia, fentanyl is used in the management of severe pain states delivered by several routes of administration (Willens and Myslinski, 1993).

ADME. These agents are highly lipid soluble and rapidly cross the blood-brain barrier. This is reflected in the $t_{1/2}$ for equilibration between the plasma and CSF of about 5 min for fentanyl and sufentanil. The levels in plasma and CSF decline rapidly owing to redistribution of fentanyl from highly perfused tissue groups to other tissues, such as muscle and fat. As saturation of less well-perfused tissue occurs, the duration of effect of fentanyl and sufentanil approaches the length of their elimination $t_{1/2}$, 3–4 h. Fentanyl and sufentanil undergo hepatic metabolism and renal excretion. With the use of higher doses or prolonged infusions, the drugs accumulate, these clearance mechanisms become progressively saturated, and fentanyl and sufentanil become longer acting.

Pharmacological Effects. ***CNS.*** Fentanyl and its congeners are all extremely potent analgesics and typically exhibit a very short duration of action when given parenterally. As with other opioids, nausea, vomiting, and itching can be observed. Muscle rigidity, while possible after all narcotics, appears to be more common after the high doses used in anesthetic induction. Rigidity can be treated with depolarizing or nondepolarizing neuromuscular-blocking agents, while controlling the patient's ventilation, but care must be taken to make sure that the patient is not simply immobilized and aware. Respiratory depression is similar to that observed with other MOR agonists, but onset is more rapid. As with analgesia, respiratory depression after small doses is of shorter duration than with morphine but of similar duration after large doses or long infusions. Delayed respiratory depression also can be seen after the use of fentanyl or sufentanil, possibly owing to enterohepatic circulation.

Cardiovascular System. Fentanyl and its derivatives decrease heart rate through vagal activation and may modestly decrease blood pressure. However, these drugs do not release histamine, and direct depressant effects on the myocardium are minimal. For this reason, high doses of fentanyl or sufentanil are commonly used as the primary anesthetic for patients undergoing cardiovascular surgery or for patients with poor cardiac function.

Therapeutic Uses. Fentanyl citrate and sufentanil citrate have widespread popularity as anesthetic adjuvants (see Chapter 21), administered intravenously and epidurally. After systemic delivery, fentanyl is about 100 times more potent than morphine; sufentanil is about 1000 times more potent than morphine. The time to peak analgesic effect after intravenous administration of fentanyl and sufentanil (~5 min) is notably less than that for morphine and meperidine (~15 min). Recovery from analgesic effects also occurs more quickly. However, with larger doses or prolonged infusions, the effects of these drugs become more lasting, with durations of action becoming similar to those of longer-acting opioids.

The use of fentanyl in chronic pain treatment has become more widespread. Transdermal patches that provide sustained release of fentanyl for 48–72 h are available. However, factors promoting increased absorption (e.g., fever) can lead to relative overdosage and increased side effects. Transbuccal absorption by the use of buccal tablets and lollipop-like lozenges permits rapid absorption and has found use in the management of acute incident pain and for the relief of breakthrough cancer pain. As fentanyl is poorly absorbed in the GI tract, the optimal absorption is through buccal administration. Fentanyl should only be used in opioid-tolerant patients, defined as consuming more than 60 mg of oral morphine equivalent. Epidural use of fentanyl and sufentanil for postoperative or labor analgesia is popular. A combination of epidural opioids with local anesthetics permits reduction in the dosage of both components. Illicit use (self-administration by chewing) of fentanyl patches can be deadly, and practitioners must be aware of this potential and keep careful control of fentanyl stocks.

Remifentanil

The pharmacological properties of remifentanil are similar to those of fentanyl and sufentanil. Remifentanil produces similar incidences of nausea, vomiting, and dose-dependent muscle rigidity.

ADME. Remifentanil has a more rapid onset of analgesic action than fentanyl or sufentanil. Analgesic effects occur within 1–1.5 min following intravenous administration. Peak respiratory depression after bolus doses of remifentanil occurs after 5 min. Remifentanil is metabolized by plasma esterases, with a $t_{1/2}$ of 8–20 min; thus, elimination is independent of hepatic metabolism or renal excretion. Age and weight can affect clearance of remifentanil. After 3- to 5-h infusions of remifentanil, recovery of respiratory function can be seen within 3–5 min; full recovery from all effects of remifentanil occurs within 15 min. The primary metabolite, remifentanil acid, has 0.05%–0.025% of the potency of the parent compound and is excreted renally.

Therapeutic Uses. Remifentanil hydrochloride is useful for short, painful procedures that require intense analgesia and blunting of stress responses; the drug is routinely given by continuous intravenous infusion because of its short duration of action. When postprocedural analgesia is required, remifentanil alone is a poor choice. In this situation, either a longer-acting opioid or another analgesic modality should be combined with remifentanil for prolonged analgesia, or another opioid should be used. Remifentanil is not used intraspinally (epidural or intrathecal administration) because of its formulation with glycine, an inhibitory neurotransmitter in the dorsal horn of the spinal cord (Stroumpos et al., 2010).

Methadone

Methadone is a long-acting MOR agonist with pharmacological properties qualitatively similar to those of morphine. The analgesic activity of methadone, a racemate, is almost entirely the result of its content of L-methadone, which is 8–50 times more potent than the D-isomer. D-Methadone also lacks significant respiratory depressant action and addiction liability but possesses antitussive activity (Fredheim et al., 2008).

Propoxyphene is a methadone analogue that was used to treat mild-to-moderate pain. The FDA removed the drug (trade name: DARVON) from the U.S. market in 2010 due to reports of cardiac toxicity.

Pharmacological Effects

The outstanding properties of methadone are its analgesic activity, its efficacy by the oral route, its extended duration of action in suppressing withdrawal symptoms in physically dependent individuals, and its tendency to show persistent effects with repeated administration. Miotic and respiratory-depressant effects can be detected for more than 24 h after a single dose; on repeated administration, marked sedation is seen in some patients. Effects on cough, bowel motility, biliary tone, and the secretion of pituitary hormones are qualitatively similar to those of morphine.

ADME

Methadone is absorbed well from the GI tract and can be detected in plasma within 30 min of oral ingestion; it reaches peak concentrations at about 4 h. Peak concentrations occur in brain within 1–2 h of subcutaneous or intramuscular administration, and this correlates well with the intensity and duration of analgesia. Methadone also can be absorbed from the buccal mucosa. Methadone undergoes extensive biotransformation in the liver. The major metabolites, pyrrolidine and pyrroline, result from N-demethylation and cyclization and are excreted in the urine and the bile along with small amounts of unchanged drug. The amount of methadone excreted in the urine is increased when the urine is acidified. The $t_{1/2}$ of methadone is long, 15–40 h. Methadone appears to be firmly bound to protein in various tissues, including brain. After repeated administration, there is gradual accumulation in tissues. When administration is discontinued, low concentrations are maintained in plasma by slow release from extravascular binding sites; this process probably accounts for the relatively mild but protracted withdrawal syndrome.

Therapeutic Uses

The primary use of methadone hydrochloride is detoxification and maintenance treatment of opioid addiction within certified treatment programs. Outside treatment programs, methadone is used for the management of chronic pain. The onset of analgesia occurs 10–20 min after parenteral administration and 30–60 min after oral medication. The typical oral dose is 2.5–10 mg repeated every 8–12 h as needed depending on the severity of the pain and the response of the patient. Care must be taken when increasing the dosage because of the prolonged $t_{1/2}$ of the drug and its tendency to accumulate over a period of several days with repeated dosing. The peak respiratory depressant effects of methadone typically occur later and persist longer than peak analgesia, so it is necessary to exercise vigilance and strongly caution patients against self-medicating with CNS depressants, particularly during treatment initiation and dose titration. Methadone should not be used in labor. Despite its longer plasma $t_{1/2}$, the duration of the analgesic action of single doses is essentially the same as that of morphine. With repeated use, cumulative effects are seen, so either lower dosages or longer intervals between doses become possible.

Because of its oral bioavailability and long $t_{1/2}$, methadone has been widely implemented as a replacement modality to treat heroin addiction. Figure 24-3 compares the time courses of response to heroin and methadone, emphasizing the favorable pharmacokinetics of oral methadone in treating addiction. Methadone, like other opiates, will produce tolerance and dependence. Thus, addicts who receive daily subcutaneous or oral therapy develop partial tolerance to the nauseant, anorectic, miotic, sedative, respiratory-depressant, and cardiovascular effects of methadone. Many former heroin users treated with oral methadone show virtually no overt behavioral effects. Development of physical dependence during the long-term administration of methadone can be demonstrated following abrupt drug withdrawal or by administration of an opioid antagonist. Likewise, subcutaneous administration of methadone to former opioid addicts produces euphoria equal in duration to that caused by morphine, and its overall abuse potential is comparable with that of morphine.

Adverse Effects

Side effects are similar to those described for morphine. Rifampin and phenytoin accelerate the metabolism of methadone and can precipitate withdrawal symptoms. Unlike other opioids, methadone is associated with the prolonged QT syndrome and is additive with agents known to prolong the QT interval.

Other Opioid Agonists

Tramadol

Tramadol is a synthetic codeine analogue that is a weak MOR agonist. Part of its analgesic effect is produced by inhibition of uptake of NE and 5HT. In the treatment of mild-to-moderate pain, tramadol is as effective as morphine or meperidine. However, for the treatment of severe or chronic pain, tramadol is less effective. Tramadol is as effective as meperidine in the treatment of labor pain and may cause less neonatal respiratory depression (Grond and Sablotzki, 2004). Tramadol is also available as a fixed-dose combination with acetaminophen.

ADME. Tramadol is 68% bioavailable after a single oral dose. Its affinity for the MOR is only 1/6000 that of morphine. The primary O-demethylated metabolite of tramadol is two to four times more potent than the parent drug and may account for part of the analgesic effect. Tramadol is supplied as a racemate that is more effective than either enantiomer alone. The (+)-enantiomer binds to the receptor and inhibits 5HT uptake. The (−)-enantiomer inhibits NE uptake and stimulates α_2 adrenergic receptors. Tramadol undergoes extensive hepatic metabolism by a number of pathways, including CYPs 2D6 and 3A4, and by conjugation with subsequent renal excretion. The elimination $t_{1/2}$ is 6 h for tramadol and 7.5 h for its active metabolite. Analgesia begins within an hour of oral dosing and peaks within 2–3 h. The duration of analgesia is about 6 h. The maximum recommended daily dose is 400 mg (300 mg in patients > 75 years old and for extended-release formulations; 200 mg is given for patients with low creatinine clearance).

Adverse Effects.
Side effects of tramadol include nausea, vomiting, dizziness, dry mouth, sedation, and headache. Respiratory depression appears to be less than with equianalgesic doses of morphine, and the degree of constipation is less than that seen after equivalent doses of codeine. Tramadol can cause seizures and possibly exacerbate seizures in patients with predisposing factors. Tramadol-induced respiratory depression is reversed by naloxone. Precipitation of withdrawal necessitates that tramadol be tapered prior to discontinuation. Tramadol should not be used in patients taking MAO inhibitors, SSRIs, or other drugs that lower the seizure threshold.

Tapentadol
Tapentadol is structurally and mechanistically similar to tramadol. It is a weak inhibitor of monoamine reuptake but has a significantly more potent activity at MORs, similar to oxycodone. Serotonin syndrome is a risk, especially when tapentadol is used concomitantly with SSRIs, SNRIs, tricyclic antidepressants, or MAO inhibitors that impair 5HT metabolism. Tapentadol is metabolized largely by glucuronidation. The drug is in pregnancy category C.

Opioid Partial Agonists

The drugs described in this section differ from clinically used MOR agonists. Drugs such as *nalbuphine* and *butorphanol* are competitive MOR antagonists but exert their analgesic actions by acting as agonists at KOR receptors. *Pentazocine* qualitatively resembles these drugs, but it may be a weaker MOR receptor antagonist or partial agonist while retaining its KOR agonist activity. *Buprenorphine* is a partial MOR agonist. The stimulus for the development of mixed agonist-antagonist drugs was a desire for analgesics with less respiratory depression and addictive potential. However, the clinical use of these compounds is often limited by undesirable side effects and limited analgesic effects.

Pentazocine
Pentazocine was synthesized as part of a deliberate effort to develop an effective analgesic with little or no abuse potential. It has agonistic actions and weak opioid antagonistic activity (Goldstein, 1985).

Pharmacological Actions and Side Effects.
The pattern of CNS effects produced by pentazocine generally is similar to that of the morphine-like opioids, including analgesia, sedation, and respiratory depression. The analgesic effects of pentazocine are due to agonistic actions at KORs. Higher doses of pentazocine (60–90 mg) elicit dysphoric and psychotomimetic effects; these effects may be reversible by naloxone. The cardiovascular responses to pentazocine differ from those seen with typical receptor agonists in that high doses cause an increase in blood pressure and heart rate. Pentazocine acts as a weak antagonist or partial agonist at MORs. Pentazocine does not antagonize the respiratory depression produced by morphine. However, when given to patients who are dependent on morphine or other MOR agonists, pentazocine may precipitate withdrawal. Ceiling effects for analgesia and respiratory depression are observed at doses above 50–100 mg of pentazocine.

Pentazocine lactate injection is indicated for the relief of mild-to-moderate pain and is also used as a preoperative medication and as a supplement to anesthesia. Pentazocine tablets for oral use are only available in fixed-dose combinations with acetaminophen or naloxone. Combination of pentazocine with naloxone reduces the potential misuse of tablets as a source of injectable pentazocine by producing undesirable effects in subjects dependent on opioids. An oral dose of about 50 mg pentazocine results in analgesia equivalent to that produced by a 60-mg oral dose of codeine.

Nalbuphine
Nalbuphine is a KOR agonist–MOR antagonist opioid with effects that qualitatively resemble those of pentazocine; however, nalbuphine produces fewer dysphoric side effects than pentazocine (Schmidt et al., 1985).

Pharmacological Actions and Side Effects.
An intramuscular dose of 10 mg nalbuphine is equianalgesic to 10 mg morphine, with similar onset and duration of analgesic and subjective effects. Nalbuphine depresses respiration as much as equianalgesic doses of morphine; however, nalbuphine exhibits a ceiling effect such that increases in dosage beyond 30 mg produce no further respiratory depression or analgesia. In contrast to pentazocine and butorphanol, 10 mg nalbuphine given to patients with stable coronary artery disease does not produce an increase in cardiac index, pulmonary arterial pressure, or cardiac work, and systemic blood pressure is not significantly altered; these indices also are relatively stable when nalbuphine is given to patients with acute myocardial infarction. Nalbuphine produces few side effects at doses of 10 mg or less; sedation, sweating, and headache are the most common. At much higher doses (70 mg), psychotomimetic side effects (e.g., dysphoria, racing thoughts, and distortions of body image) can occur. Nalbuphine is metabolized in the liver and has a plasma $t_{1/2}$ of 2–3 h. Nalbuphine is 20%–25% as potent when administered orally as when given intramuscularly. Prolonged administration of nalbuphine can produce physical dependence. The withdrawal syndrome is similar in intensity to that seen with pentazocine.

Therapeutic Use.
Nalbuphine is used to produce analgesia. Because it is an agonist-antagonist, administration to patients who have been receiving morphine-like opioids may create difficulties unless a brief drug-free interval is interposed. The usual adult dose is 10 mg parenterally every 3–6 h; this may be increased to 20 mg in nontolerant individuals. A caveat: Agents that act through the KORs are reportedly more effective in women than in men (Fillingim and Gear, 2004).

Butorphanol
Butorphanol is a morphinan congener with a profile of actions similar to those of pentazocine and nalbuphine: KOR agonist and MOR antagonist.

Pharmacological Actions and Side Effects.
In postoperative patients, a parenteral dose of 2–3 mg butorphanol produces analgesia and respiratory depression approximately equal to that produced by 10 mg morphine or 80–100 mg meperidine. The plasma $t_{1/2}$ of butorphanol is about 3 h. Like pentazocine, analgesic doses of butorphanol produce an increase in pulmonary arterial pressure and in the work of the heart; systemic arterial pressure is slightly decreased. The major side effects of butorphanol are drowsiness, weakness, sweating, feelings of floating, and nausea. While the incidence of psychotomimetic side effects is lower than that with equianalgesic doses of pentazocine, they are qualitatively similar. Nasal administration is associated with drowsiness and dizziness. Physical dependence can occur.

Therapeutic Use.
Butorphanol is used for the relief of acute pain (e.g., postoperative) and, because of its potential for antagonizing MOR agonists, should not be used in combination. Because of its side effects on the heart, it is less useful than morphine or meperidine in patients with congestive heart failure or myocardial infarction. The usual dose is 1–4 mg of the tartrate given intramuscularly, or 0.5–2 mg given intravenously, every 3–4 h. A nasal formulation is available and has proven to be effective in pain relief, including migraine pain (Gillis et al., 1995).

Buprenorphine
Buprenorphine is a highly lipophilic MOR partial agonist that is derived from thebaine and is 25–50 times more potent than morphine. As a partial MOR agonist, buprenorphine has limited intrinsic activity and accordingly can display antagonism when used in conjunction with a full agonist such as morphine. These properties have led it to have utility in managing opiate abuse and withdrawal (Elkader and Sproule, 2005).

ADME.
Buprenorphine is well absorbed by most routes and produces analgesia and other CNS effects that are qualitatively similar to those of morphine. The $t_{1/2}$ for dissociation from the receptor is 166 min for buprenorphine, as opposed to 7 min for fentanyl. Therefore, plasma levels of buprenorphine may not parallel clinical effects. Cardiovascular and other side effects (e.g., sedation, nausea, vomiting, dizziness, sweating, and headache) appear to be similar to those of morphine-like opioids. Administered sublingually, buprenorphine (0.4–0.8 mg) produces satisfactory analgesia in postoperative patients. Concentrations in blood peak within

5 min of intramuscular injection and within 1–2 h of oral or sublingual administration. While the plasma $t_{1/2}$ in plasma is about 3 h, this value bears little relationship to the rate of disappearance of effects. Buprenorphine is metabolized to norbuprenorphine by CYP3A4 and should not be taken with known inhibitors of CYP3A4 (e.g., azole antifungals, macrolide antibiotics, and HIV protease inhibitors) or drugs that induce CYP3A4 activity (e.g., certain anticonvulsants and rifampin). Both N-dealkylated and conjugated metabolites are detected in the urine, but most of the drug is excreted unchanged in the feces. When buprenorphine is discontinued, a withdrawal syndrome develops that is delayed in onset for 2–14 days and persists for 1–2 weeks.

Therapeutic Use. Buprenorphine injection and transdermal film are indicated for use as an analgesic. Sublingual/buccal formulations of buprenorphine alone and in fixed-dose combinations with naloxone are used for treatment of opioid dependence; the partial agonist properties of buprenorphine limit its utility in the treatment of addicts who require high maintenance doses of opioids; in the U.S., this use is limited by the Drug Addiction Treatment Act. The usual intramuscular or intravenous dose for analgesia is 0.3 mg given every 6 h.

About 0.3 mg IM buprenorphine is equianalgesic with 10 mg IM morphine. Some of the subjective and respiratory-depressant effects are unequivocally slower in onset and last longer than those of morphine. Buprenorphine is a partial MOR agonist; thus, it may cause symptoms of abstinence in patients who have been receiving MOR agonists for several weeks. It antagonizes the respiratory depression produced by anesthetic doses of fentanyl about as well as naloxone without completely reversing opioid pain relief. The respiratory depression and other effects of buprenorphine can be prevented by prior administration of naloxone, but they are not readily reversed by high doses of naloxone once the effects have been produced, probably due to slow dissociation of buprenorphine from opioid receptors.

Opioid Antagonists

A variety of agents bind competitively to one or more of the opioid receptors, display little or no intrinsic activity, and robustly antagonize the effects of receptor agonists. Relatively minor changes in the structure of an opioid can convert a drug that is primarily an agonist into one with antagonistic actions at one or more types of opioid receptors. Simple substitutions transform morphine to *nalorphine*, levorphanol to *levallorphan,* and oxymorphone to *naloxone* or naltrexone. In some cases, congeners are produced that are competitive antagonists at MOR but that also have agonistic actions at KORs; *nalorphine* and *levallorphan* have such properties. Other congeners, especially *naloxone* and *naltrexone*, appear to be devoid of agonistic actions and interact with all types of opioid receptors, albeit with somewhat different affinities. *Nalmefene* (not marketed in the U.S.) is a relatively pure MOR antagonist that is more potent than naloxone. The majority of these agents are relatively lipid soluble and have excellent CNS penetration after systemic delivery (Barnett et al., 2014). A recognition for antagonism limited to peripheral sites, as for example to manage opiate-induced constipation, led to the development of agents that have poor CNS bioavailability, such as *methylnaltrexone* (Becker et al., 2007).

Pharmacological Properties

Opioid antagonists have obvious therapeutic utility in the treatment of opioid overdose. Under ordinary circumstances, these opioid antagonists produce few effects in the absence of an exogenous agonist. However, under certain conditions (e.g., shock), when the endogenous opioid systems are activated, the administration of an opioid antagonist alone may have positive effects on hemodynamic changes.

Effects in the Absence of Opioid Agonist. Subcutaneous doses of naloxone up to 12 mg produce no discernible effects in humans, and 24 mg causes only slight drowsiness. Naltrexone also is a relatively pure antagonist but with higher oral efficacy and a longer duration of action. The effects of opiate receptor antagonists are usually both subtle and limited, likely reflecting the low levels of tonic activity and organizational

complexity of the opioid systems in various physiologic systems. Opiate antagonism in humans is associated with variable effects, ranging from no effect to mild hyperalgesia. A number of studies have suggested that agents such as naloxone may attenuate the analgesic effects of placebo medications and acupuncture.

Endogenous opioid peptides participate in the regulation of pituitary secretion apparently by exerting tonic inhibitory effects on the release of certain hypothalamic hormones (see Chapter 42). Thus, the administration of naloxone or naltrexone increases the secretion of GnRH and CRH and elevates the plasma concentrations of LH, FSH, and ACTH, as well as the steroid hormones produced by their target organs. Naloxone stimulates the release of prolactin in women. Endogenous opioid peptides probably have some role in the regulation of feeding or energy metabolism; however, naltrexone does not accelerate weight loss in very obese subjects, even though short-term administration of opioid antagonists reduces food intake in lean and obese individuals. Long-term administration of antagonists increases the density of opioid receptors in the brain and causes a temporary exaggeration of responses to the subsequent administration of opioid agonists.

Effects in the Presence of Opioid Agonists. *Antagonistic Effects.* Small doses (0.4–0.8 mg) of naloxone given intramuscularly or intravenously prevent or *promptly* reverse the effects of receptor agonists. In patients with respiratory depression, an increase in respiratory rate is seen within 1–2 min. Sedative effects are reversed, and blood pressure, if depressed, returns to normal. Higher doses of naloxone are required to antagonize the respiratory-depressant effects of buprenorphine; 1 mg naloxone intravenously completely blocks the effects of 25 mg heroin. Naloxone reverses the psychotomimetic and dysphoric effects of agonist-antagonist agents such as pentazocine, but much higher doses (10–15 mg) are required. The duration of antagonistic effects depends on the dose but usually is 1–4 h. Antagonism of opioid effects by naloxone often is accompanied by an "overshoot" phenomenon. For example, respiratory rates depressed by opioids transiently become higher than before the period of depression. Rebound release of catecholamines may cause hypertension, tachycardia, and ventricular arrhythmias. Pulmonary edema also has been reported after naloxone administration.

Effects in Opioid-Dependent Patients. In subjects who are dependent on morphine-like opioids, small subcutaneous doses of naloxone (0.5 mg) precipitate a moderate-to-severe withdrawal syndrome that is similar to that seen after abrupt withdrawal of opioids, except that the syndrome appears within minutes of administration and subsides in about 2 h. The severity and duration of the syndrome are related to the dose of the antagonist and to the degree and type of dependence. Higher doses of naloxone will precipitate a withdrawal syndrome in patients dependent on pentazocine, butorphanol, or nalbuphine. In dependent patients, peripheral side effects of opioids, notably reduced GI motility and constipation, can be reversed by methylnaltrexone, with subcutaneous doses (0.15 mg/kg) producing reliable bowel movements and no evidence of centrally mediated withdrawal signs (Thomas et al., 2008). Naloxone produces an *overshoot phenomenon* suggestive of early acute physical dependence 6–24 h after even a single dose of an MOR agonist.

ADME

Although absorbed readily from the GI tract, naloxone is almost completely metabolized by the liver (primarily by conjugation with glucuronic acid) before reaching the systemic circulation and thus must be administered parenterally. The $t_{1/2}$ of naloxone is about 1 h, but its clinically effective duration of action can be even less.

Compared with naloxone, naltrexone has more efficacy by the oral route, and its duration of action approaches 24 h after moderate oral doses. Peak concentrations in plasma are reached within 1–2 h and then decline with an apparent $t_{1/2}$ of about 3 h. Naltrexone is metabolized to 6-naltrexol, which is a weaker antagonist with longer $t_{1/2}$, about 13 h. Naltrexone is much more potent than naloxone, and 100-mg oral doses given to patients addicted to opioids produce concentrations in tissues sufficient to block the euphorigenic effects of 25-mg IV doses of heroin for 48 h. Methylnaltrexone is similar to naltrexone; it is converted to methyl-6-naltrexol isomers and eliminated primarily via active renal secretion. The $t_{1/2}$ of methylnaltrexone is about 8 h.

Therapeutic Uses

Treatment of Opioid Overdoses.
Opioid antagonists, particularly naloxone, have an established use in the treatment of opioid-induced toxicity, especially respiratory depression. Its specificity is such that reversal by naloxone is virtually diagnostic for the contribution of an opiate to the depression. Naloxone acts rapidly to reverse the respiratory depression associated with even high doses of opioids. It should be titrated cautiously as it will precipitate withdrawal in dependent subjects and cause undesirable cardiovascular side effects (hypertension/tachycardia). The duration of action of naloxone is relatively short, and it often must be given repeatedly or by continuous infusion to prevent renarcotization. In the home setting, 0.4 mg of naloxone can be administered via autoinjector every 2–3 min while awaiting emergency medical assistance. Opioid antagonists also have been employed effectively to decrease neonatal respiratory depression secondary to the intravenous or intramuscular administration of opioids to the mother. In the neonate, the initial dose is 10 μg/kg given intravenously, intramuscularly, or subcutaneously.

Management of Constipation.
The peripherally limited antagonists methylnaltrexone and naloxegol have important roles in the management of the constipation and the reduced GI motility present in the patient undergoing chronic opioid therapy (as for chronic pain or methadone maintenance). The use of the type 2 chloride channel activator lubiprostone and other strategies for the management of opioid-induced constipation are described in Chapter 50. An important application of the peripherally restricted opiate receptor antagonists is their use in managing ileus (disruption of normal propulsive activity in the GI tract) secondary to abdominal surgery. Treatment with such agents facilitates recovery of normal bowel function and leaves the analgesic (CNS) activity of the postoperative opiate intact (Vaughan-Shaw et al., 2012).

Alvimopan. Alvimopan is an MOR antagonist with quaternary amino group that restricts the distribution of the drug to the periphery. The drug has a high affinity for MOR of 0.4 nM. Following oral administration, a deamidated metabolite of alvimopam slowly and variably appears in the bloodstream and is attributed to activity of the intestinal microbiome. This metabolite is also an MOR antagonist (Ki = 0.8 nM). The parent drug appears to enter an enterohepatic cycle coupled to deamidation in the GI tract; both parent drug and metabolite have terminal half-lives of 10–18 h. The drug, as the deamidated metabolite, is excreted in the feces and urine. Alvimopan is FDA-approved for treatment of postoperative ileus in patients with less than 7 days of opioid exposure immediately prior to beginning alvimopan (usually 12 mg administered just prior to surgery and 12 mg twice daily for 7 days). This agent carries a black-box warning about increased incidence of myocardial infarction with prolonged use and thus is available only for short-term use (15 doses) through a restricted program.

Management of Abuse Syndromes.
There has been interest in the use of opiate antagonists such as naltrexone and nalmefene (not available in the U.S.) as adjuvants in treating a variety of nonopioid dependency syndromes, such as alcoholism (see Chapters 23 and 24), where an opiate antagonist may decrease the rate of relapse (Anton, 2008). Interestingly, patients with a single-nucleotide polymorphism in the MOR gene have significantly lower relapse rates to alcoholism when treated with naltrexone (Haile et al., 2008). Naltrexone is FDA-approved for treatment of alcohol dependence, to block the effects of exogenously administered opioids, and for the prevention of relapse to opioid dependence following detoxification. Naltrexone in combination with bupropion is also FDA-approved as an adjunct for weight management in patients with obesity.

Centrally Active Antitussives

Cough is a useful physiological mechanism that serves to clear the respiratory passages of foreign material and excess secretions; it should not be suppressed indiscriminately. There are, however, situations in which cough does not serve any useful purpose but may, instead, annoy the patient, prevent rest and sleep, or hinder adherence to otherwise-beneficial medication regimens (e.g., ACE inhibitor–induced cough). In such situations, the physician should try to substitute a drug with a different side-effect profile (e.g., an AT_1 antagonist in place of an ACE inhibitor) or add an antitussive agent that will reduce the frequency or intensity of the coughing. A number of drugs reduce cough as a result of their central actions, including opioid analgesics, of which codeine and hydrocodone are most commonly used. Cough suppression often occurs with lower doses of opioids than those needed for analgesia. A 10- or 20-mg oral dose of codeine, although ineffective for analgesia, produces a demonstrable antitussive effect, and higher doses produce even more suppression of chronic cough. A few other antitussive agents are noted next.

Dextromethorphan

Dextromethorphan (D-3-methoxy-*N*-methylmorphinan) is the D-isomer of the codeine analogue methorphan; however, unlike the L-isomer, it has no analgesic or addictive properties and does not act through opioid receptors. Rather, the drug acts centrally to elevate the threshold for coughing. Its effectiveness in patients with pathological cough has been demonstrated in controlled studies; its potency is nearly equal to that of codeine, but dextromethorphan produces fewer subjective and GI side effects. In therapeutic dosages, the drug does not inhibit ciliary activity, and its antitussive effects persist for 5–6 h. Its toxicity is low, but extremely high doses may produce CNS depression. The average adult dosage of dextromethorphan hydrobromide is 10–20 mg every 4 h or 30 mg every 6–8 h, not to exceed 120 mg daily. The drug is marketed for over-the-counter sale in liquids, syrups, capsules, soluble strips, lozenges, and freezer pops or in combinations with antihistamines, bronchodilators, expectorants, and decongestants. An extended-release dextromethorphan suspension is approved for twice-daily administration.

Although dextromethorphan is known to function as an NMDA receptor antagonist, the dextromethorphan binding sites are not limited to the known distribution of NMDA receptors. Naloxone antagonizes the antitussive effects of codeine but not those of dextromethorphan. Thus, the mechanisms by which dextromethorphan exerts its antitussive effects still are not clear. Pharmacological cough suppression can apparently be achieved by a variety of mechanisms.

Other Antitussives

Pholcodine [3-*O*-(2-morpholinoethyl) morphine] is used clinically in many countries outside the U.S. Although structurally related to the opioids, pholcodine has no opioid-like actions. Pholcodine is at least as effective as codeine as an antitussive; it has a long $t_{1/2}$ and can be given once or twice daily.

Benzonatate is a long-chain polyglycol derivative chemically related to procaine and believed to exert its antitussive action on stretch or cough receptors in the lung, as well as by a central mechanism. It is available in oral capsules. The dosage is 100 mg three times daily; doses as high as 600 mg daily have been used safely.

Routes of Analgesic Drug Administration

In addition to the traditional oral and parenteral formulations for opioids, many other methods of administration have been developed in an effort to improve therapeutic efficacy while minimizing side effects.

Patient-Controlled Analgesia

With PCA, the patient has limited control of the dosing of opioid from an infusion pump programmed within tightly mandated parameters. PCA can be used for intravenous, subcutaneous, epidural, or intrathecal administration of opioids. This technique avoids delays inherent in administration by a caregiver and generally permits better alignment between pain control and individual differences in pain perception and responsiveness to opioids. The PCA technique also gives the patient a greater sense of control over the pain. With shorter-acting opioids, serious toxicity or excessive use rarely occurs; however, caution is warranted due to the potential for serious medication errors associated with this delivery method. PCA is suitable for adults and children capable of understanding the principles involved. It is generally conceded that PCA is preferred over intramuscular injections for postoperative pain control.

Spinal Delivery

Administration of opioids into the epidural or intrathecal spaces provides more direct access to the first pain-processing synapse in the dorsal horn of the spinal cord. This permits the use of doses substantially lower than those required for oral or parenteral administration (Table 20–5). In postoperative pain management, sustained-release epidural injections are accomplished through the incorporation of morphine into a liposomal formulation, providing up to 48 h of pain relief (Hartrick and Hartrick, 2008). The management of chronic pain with spinal opiates has been addressed by the use of chronically implanted intrathecal catheters connected to subcutaneously implanted refillable pumps (Yaksh et al., 2017).

Epidural and intrathecal opioids have their own dose-dependent side effects, such as pruritus, nausea, vomiting, respiratory depression, and urinary retention. *Hydrophilic opioids* such as morphine have longer residence times in the CSF. As a consequence, after intrathecal or epidural morphine, respiratory depression can be delayed for as long as 24 h after a bolus dose. Given their more rapid clearance, the risk of *delayed* respiratory depression is reduced, *but not eliminated,* with *opioids that are more lipophilic.*

Extreme vigilance and appropriate monitoring are required for all opioid-naïve patients receiving intraspinal narcotics. Use of intraspinal opioids in the opioid-naïve patient is reserved for postoperative pain control in an inpatient monitored setting. Epidural administration of opioids has become popular in the management of postoperative pain and for providing analgesia during labor and delivery. Lower systemic opioid levels are achieved with epidural opioids, leading to less placental transfer and less potential for respiratory depression of the newborn. Many opioids and other adjuvants are commonly used for neuraxial administration in adults and children; however, the majority of agents employed have not undergone appropriate preclinical safety evaluation and approval for these clinical indications; thus, such uses are "off label." Thus, at this time, those agents approved for spinal delivery are certain preservative-free formulations of morphine sulfate and sufentanil. It is important to remember that the spinal route of delivery represents a novel environment wherein the neuraxis may be exposed to exceedingly high concentrations of an agent for an extended period of time and safety by another route (e.g., oral, intravenous) may not translate to safety after spinal delivery (Yaksh and Allen, 2004).

Patients on chronic spinal opioid therapy are less likely to experience respiratory depression. Selected patients who fail conservative therapies for chronic pain may receive intraspinal opioids chronically through an implanted programmable pump. Analogous to the relationship between systemic opioids and NSAIDs, intraspinal narcotics often are combined with other agents that include local anesthetics, N-type Ca^{2+} channel blockers (e.g., ziconotide), α_2 adrenergic agonists, and $GABA_B$ agonists. This permits synergy between drugs with different mechanisms, allowing the use of lower concentrations of both agents, minimizing side effects and the opioid-induced complications (Yaksh et al., 2017).

Use of intraspinal opioids in the opioid-naïve patient is reserved for postoperative pain control in an inpatient monitored setting. Epidural administration of opioids has become popular in the management of postoperative pain and for providing analgesia during labor and delivery. Lower systemic opioid levels are achieved with epidural opioids, leading to less placental transfer and less potential for respiratory depression of the newborn. Agents approved for spinal delivery are *specific preservative-free formulations* of morphine sulfate. A hydromorphone formulation is currently in clinical trials. The spinal route of delivery represents a novel environment wherein the neuraxis may be exposed to exceedingly high concentrations of an agent for an extended period of time. Safety as defined by another route of administration (e.g., oral, intravenous) may not translate temporally or dose-wise to safety after spinal delivery.

An important side effect associated with continued infusion of high concentrations of several opiates is formation of a space-occupying mass (a granuloma) at the catheter tip in the intrathecal space. These granulomas arise from meningeal mast cell degranulation and are the result of meningeal-derived fibroblast proliferation though an effect independent of an opioid receptor (Eddinger et al., 2016). The consequence of the spinal cord compression and neurologic sequelae may require discontinuation of spinal delivery and, in the extreme case, surgical removal of the mass (Deer, 2017).

Rectal Administration

The rectal route is an alternative for patients with difficulty swallowing or other oral pathology and who prefer a less invasive route than parenteral

TABLE 20–5 ■ EPIDURAL OR INTRATHECAL OPIOIDS FOR THE TREATMENT OF ACUTE (BOLUS) OR CHRONIC (INFUSION) PAIN

DRUG	SINGLE DOSE (mg)[a]	INFUSION RATE (mg/h)[b]	ONSET (min)	DURATION OF EFFECT OF SINGLE DOSE (h)[c]
Epidural				
Morphine	1–6	0.1–1.0	30	6–24
Meperidine	20–150	5–20	5	4–8
Methadone	1–10	0.3–0.5	10	6–10
Hydromorphone	1–2	0.1–0.2	15	10–16
Fentanyl	0.025–0.1	0.025–0.10	5	2–4
Sufentanil	0.01–0.06	0.01–0.05	5	2–4
Alfentanil	0.5–1	0.2	15	1–3
Subarachnoid (Intrathecal)				
Morphine	0.1–0.3		15	8–24+
Fentanyl	0.005–0.025		5	3–6

[a]Low doses may be effective when administered to the elderly or when injected in the thoracic region.

[b]If combining with a local anesthetic, consider using 0.0625% bupivacaine.

[c]Duration of analgesia varies widely; higher doses produce longer duration. With the exception of epidural/intrathecal morphine or epidural sufentanil, all other spinal opioid use is considered to be off label.

Source: Adapted and updated from Ready LB, Edwards WT, eds. *Management of Acute Pain: A Practical Guide.* International Association for Study of Pain, Seattle, **1992**.

administration. This route is not well tolerated by most children. Onset of action is within 10 min. In the U.S., only morphine, hydromorphone, and opium (in combination with belladonna) are available in rectal suppository formulations.

Oral Transmucosal Administration

Opioids can be absorbed through the oral mucosa more rapidly than through the stomach. Bioavailability is greater owing to avoidance of first-pass metabolism, and lipophilic opioids are absorbed better by this route than are hydrophilic compounds such as morphine. A variety of formulations of fentanyl are available for oral transmucosal use: Suspensions of fentanyl in a dissolvable sugar-based lollipop or rapidly dissolving buccal tablet, a buccal fentanyl "film," and a sublingual fentanyl tablet are approved for the treatment of cancer pain. In this setting, transmucosal fentanyl relieves pain within 15 min, and patients easily can titrate the appropriate dose.

Transnasal Administration

Butorphanol, a KOR agonist/MOR antagonist, has been employed intranasally. A transnasal, pectin-based, metered fentanyl spray is FDA-approved for the treatment of breakthrough cancer pain. Administration is well tolerated, and pain relief occurs within 10 min of delivery.

Transdermal Administration

Transdermal fentanyl patches are approved for use in sustained pain. The opioid permeates the skin, and a "depot" is established in the *stratum corneum* layer (see Figure 70–1). However, fever and external heat sources (heating pads, hot baths) can increase absorption of fentanyl and potentially lead to an overdose.

This modality is well suited for cancer pain treatment because of its ease of use, prolonged duration of action, and stable blood levels. It may take up to 12 h to develop analgesia and up to 16 h to observe full clinical effect. Plasma levels stabilize after two sequential patch applications, and the kinetics do not appear to change with repeated applications (Portenoy et al., 1993). However, there may be substantial variability in plasma levels after a given dose. The plasma $t_{1/2}$ after patch removal is about 17 h. If excessive sedation or respiratory depression occurs, antagonist infusions may need to be maintained for an extended period. Dermatological side effects from the patches, such as rash and itching, usually are mild. Opiate-addicted patients have been known to chew the patches and receive an overdose, sometimes with fatal outcomes, following rapid and efficient buccal and sublingual absorption.

Therapeutic Considerations in Pain Control

Given its profound impact on patient physiology and quality of life, the management of pain must be an important element in any therapeutic intervention. Failure to adequately manage pain can have important negative consequences on physiological function, such as autonomic hyperreactivity (increased blood pressure, heart rate, suppression of GI motility, reduced secretions); and reduced mobility, leading to deconditioning, muscle wasting, joint stiffening, and decalcification; and can contribute to deleterious changes in the psychological state (depression, helplessness syndromes, anxiety). By many hospital-accrediting organizations, and by law in many states, appropriate pain assessment and adequate pain management are considered to be standard of care, with pain considered the "fifth vital sign."

Acute Pain States

In acute pain states, opioids will reduce the intensity of pain. However, physical signs (such as abdominal rigidity with an acute abdomen) generally will remain. Relief of pain can facilitate history taking and examination in the emergency room and the patient's ability to tolerate diagnostic procedures. In most cases, analgesics should not be withheld for fear of obscuring the progression of underlying disease.

Chronic Pain States

The problems that arise in the relief of pain associated with chronic conditions are more complex. Repeated daily administration of opioid analgesics eventually will produce tolerance and some degree of physical dependence. The degree will depend on the particular drug, the frequency of administration, the quantity administered, the genetic predisposition, and the psychosocial status of the patient. The decision to control any chronic symptom, especially pain, by the repeated administration of an opioid must be made carefully. When pain is due to chronic nonmalignant disease, conservative measures using nonopioid drugs should be tried before resorting to the opioids. Such measures include the use of NSAIDs, local nerve blocks, antidepressant drugs, electrical stimulation, acupuncture, hypnosis, and behavioral modification. In end-of-life care, the analgesia, tranquility, and even euphoria afforded by the use of opioids can make the final days of life far less distressing for patient and family. Although physical dependence and tolerance may develop, this possibility should not prevent physicians from fulfilling their primary obligation to ease the patient's discomfort. The physician should not wait until the pain becomes agonizing; no patient should ever wish for death because of a physician's reluctance to use adequate amounts of effective opioids. This sometimes may entail the regular use of opioid analgesics in substantial doses. Such patients, while they may be physically dependent, are not "addicts" even though they may need large doses on a regular basis. As noted, physical dependence is not equivalent to addiction.

Guidelines for Opiate Dosing

The World Health Organization provides a three-step ladder as a guide to treat both cancer pain and chronic noncancer pain (Table 20–6). The three-step ladder encourages the use of more conservative therapies before initiating opioid therapy. Weaker opioids can be supplanted by stronger opioids in cases of moderate and severe pain. Antidepressants such as duloxetine and amitriptyline that are used in the treatment of chronic neuropathic pain have limited intrinsic analgesic actions in acute pain; however, antidepressants may enhance morphine-induced analgesia. In the presence of severe pain, the opioids should be considered sooner rather than later.

There has been a growing concern over the appropriate use of opiates in pain management. Since the last edition of this textbook, there has been increasing scrutiny of the use of opioids to treat chronic pain due to the high correlation between prescription opioids and opioid abuse. Drug overdose has become the leading cause of accidental death in the

TABLE 20–6 ■ WORLD HEALTH ORGANIZATION ANALGESIC LADDER

Step 1 Mild-to-Moderate Pain

Nonopioid ± adjuvant agent

- Acetaminophen or an NSAID should be used, unless contraindicated. Adjuvant agents are those that enhance analgesic efficacy, treat concurrent symptoms that exacerbate pain, or provide independent analgesic activity for specific types of pain.

Step 2 Mild-to-Moderate Pain or Pain Uncontrolled After Step 1

Short-acting opioid as required ± nonopioid ATC ± adjuvant agent

- Morphine, oxycodone, or hydromorphone should be added to acetaminophen or an NSAID for maximum flexibility of opioid dose.

Step 3 Moderate-to-Severe Pain or Pain Uncontrolled After Step 2

Sustained-release/long-acting opioid ATC or continuous infusion + short-acting opioid as required ± nonopioid ± adjuvant agent

- Sustained-release oxycodone, morphine, oxymorphone, or transdermal fentanyl is indicated.

Source: Adapted from http://www.who.int/cancer/palliative/painladder/en/.

U.S., driven by opioid addiction (NIDA, 2017; Rudd et al., 2016). These circumstances have led to several changes in the use of opioids in the U.S.:

- the rescheduling of hydrocodone to schedule II
- an FDA mandate that all ER/LA opioids fall under the Risk Evaluation and Mitigation Strategy, a classification reserved for "high-risk pharmaceuticals"
- the FDA's relabeling of all ER/LA opioids with a black-box warning that highlights the risks of addiction, abuse, misuse, overdose, and death; the risk of fatal respiratory depression on initiation or increase of dose; the necessity of swallowing, not chewing, an oral opioid formulation; the danger of accidental consumption, especially by children; for pregnant women who require opioids, possible requirement for treatment of neonatal opioid withdrawal syndrome and danger of life-threatening fetal opioid withdrawal syndrome with prolonged maternal use; and any adverse interactions with ethanol
- an updating by the FDA of postmarketing surveillance requirements for opioid analgesics, especially for ER/LA opioid analgesics
- the release by the CDC of new chronic opioid treatment guidelines (Dowell et al., 2016), as summarized by Table 20–7

The CDC guidelines were in response to an increasing number of deaths related to opioid overdose (of both prescription and illicit opioids), which exceeded 33,000 in 2015. The new guidelines are intended for primary care physicians who prescribe opioids to treat chronic pain. The guidelines stress the primary use of nonopioid pharmacotherapy, avoidance of ER/LA opioids in favor of immediate-release agents, and frequent and persistent follow-up by the prescribing physician. Methadone dosing is considered separately in Table 20–8. Suggestions for the oral and parenteral dosing of commonly used opioids (see Table 20–2) must be appreciated as representing only guidelines. Such guidelines are typically based on the use of these agents in the management of acute (e.g., postoperative) pain in opioid-naïve patients. A number of factors contribute to the dosing requirement (see the discussion that follows).

Variables Modifying the Therapeutic Use of Opiates

Patient Variability

There is substantial individual variability in the response to opioids. Thus, a standard intramuscular dose of 10 mg morphine sulfate will relieve severe pain adequately in two of three patients but will not suffice in one of three patients. Similarly, the minimal effective analgesic concentration for opioids, such as morphine, meperidine (pethidine), alfentanil, and sufentanil, varies among patients by factors of 5–10. Adjustments must be made based on clinical response. Appropriate therapeutics typically involve undertaking a treatment strategy that most efficiently addresses the pain state, minimizes the potential for undesired drug effects, and

---

TABLE 20–7 ■ SUMMARY OF CDC RECOMMENDATIONS FOR PRESCRIBING OPIOIDS FOR CHRONIC PAIN

Determining When to Initiate or Continue Opioids for Chronic Pain

- Nonpharmacological therapy and nonopioid pharmacologic therapy are preferred for chronic pain. Consider opioid therapy only if expected benefits for both pain and function are anticipated to outweigh risks to the patient. If opioids are used, combine them with nonpharmacological therapy and nonopioid pharmacotherapy, as appropriate.
- Before starting opioid therapy for chronic pain, establish treatment goals with the patient, including realistic goals for pain and function. Consider how therapy will be discontinued if benefits do not outweigh risks. Continue opioid therapy only if there is clinically meaningful improvement in pain and function that outweighs risks to patient safety.
- Before starting and periodically during opioid therapy, discuss with patient the known risks and realistic benefits of opioid therapy and patient and clinician responsibilities for managing therapy.

Opioid Selection, Dosage, Duration, Follow-Up, and Discontinuation

- When starting opioid therapy for chronic pain, prescribe immediate-release opioids instead of ER/LA opioids.
- When opioids are started, prescribe the lowest effective dosage. Use caution when prescribing opioids at any dosage. Reassess evidence of individual benefits and risks when increasing dosage to ≥ 50 MME/d. Avoid increasing dosage to ≥ 90 MME/d or carefully justify a decision to exceed this limit.
- Long-term opioid use often begins with treatment of acute pain. When opioids are used for acute pain, prescribe the lowest effective dose of immediate-release opioids and in no greater quantity than needed for the expected duration of pain severe enough to require opioids. Three days or less will often be sufficient; more than 7 days will rarely be needed.
- Reevaluate benefits and harms of opioids with the patient within 1 to 4 weeks of starting opioid therapy for chronic pain or of dose escalation and thereafter every 3 months or more frequently. If benefits do not outweigh harms of continued opioid therapy, optimize other therapies and work with the patient to taper opioids to lower dosages or to taper and discontinue opioids.

Assessing Risk and Addressing Harms of Opioid Use

- Incorporate into the management plan strategies to mitigate risk, including considering offering naloxone when factors that increase risk for opioid overdose, such as history of overdose, history of substance use disorder, higher opioid dosages (≥50 MME/d), or concurrent benzodiazepine use are present.
- Review the patient's history of controlled substance prescriptions using state PDMP data to determine whether the patient is receiving opioid dosages or dangerous combinations that carry high risk for overdose. Review PDMP data when starting opioid therapy for chronic pain and periodically during opioid therapy for chronic pain, ranging from every prescription to every 3 months.
- When prescribing opioids for chronic pain, use urine drug testing before starting opioid therapy and consider urine drug testing at least annually to assess for prescribed medications and other controlled prescription drugs and illicit drugs.
- Avoid prescribing opioid pain medication and benzodiazepines concurrently whenever possible.
- Offer or arrange evidence-based treatment (usually medication-assisted treatment with buprenorphine or methadone in combination with behavioral therapies) for a patient with opioid use disorder.

Note: Excluding active cancer, palliative, and end-of-life care.

Source: Adapted from Dowell D, et al. CDC guideline for prescribing opioids for chronic pain—United States, 2016. *MMWR Recomm Rep* **2016**, 65(RR-1):1–49. doi: http://dx.doi.org/10.15585/mmwr.rr6501e1. Accessed May 4, 2017.

TABLE 20–8 ■ MORPHINE MILLIGRAM EQUIVALENT (MME) DOSES FOR COMMONLY PRESCRIBED OPIOIDS

OPIOID	CONVERSION FACTOR[a]
Codeine	0.15
Fentanyl transdermal (in µg/h)	2.4
Hydrocodone	1
Hydromorphone	4
Methadone	
1–20 mg/d	4
21–40 mg/d	8
41–60 mg/d	10
≥61–80 mg/d	12
Morphine	1
Oxycodone	1.5
Oxymorphone	3

[a]Multiply the dose for each opioid by the conversion factor to determine the dose in MMEs. For example, tablets containing hydrocodone 5 mg and acetaminophen 300 mg taken four times a day would contain a total of 20 mg of hydrocodone daily, equivalent to 20 MME daily; extended-release tablets containing oxycodone 10 mg taken twice a day would contain a total of 20 mg of oxycodone daily, equivalent to 30 MME daily. Note the following precautions: (1) All doses are in milligrams/day except for fentanyl, which is micrograms/hour. (2) Equianalgesic dose conversions are only estimates and cannot account for individual variability in genetics and pharmacokinetics. (3) Do not use the calculated dose in MMEs to determine the doses to use when converting one opioid to another; when converting opioids, the new opioid is typically dosed at substantially lower than the calculated MME dose to avoid accidental overdose due to incomplete cross-tolerance and individual variability in opioid pharmacokinetics. (4) Use particular caution with methadone dose conversions because the conversion factor increases at higher doses. (5) Use particular caution with fentanyl because it is dosed in micrograms/hour instead of milligrams/day, and its absorption is affected by heat and other factors.

Source: Dowell D, et al. CDC guideline for prescribing opioids for chronic pain—United States, 2016. *MMWR Recomm Rep* **2016**, *65*(No. RR-1):1–49. doi:http://dx.doi.org/10.15585/mmwr.rr6501e1. Accessed May 4, 2017.

Adapted by the CDC from Von Korff M, et al. *Clin J Pain,* **2008**, *24*:521–527 and Washington State Interagency Guideline on Prescribing Opioids for Pain (http://www.agencymeddirectors.wa.gov/Files/2015AMDGOpioidGuideline.pdf).

accounts for the variables described next that can influence an individual patient's response to opiate analgesia.

Pain

Pain Intensity

Increased pain intensity may require titrating doses to produce acceptable analgesia with tolerable side effects.

Type of Pain State

Systems underlying a pain state may be broadly categorized as being mediated by events secondary to injury and inflammation and by injury to the sensory afferent or nervous system. Neuropathic conditions may be less efficaciously managed by opiates than pain secondary to tissue injury and inflammation. Such pain states are more efficiently managed by combination treatment modalities.

Acuity and Chronicity of Pain

In chronic pain states, the daily course of the pain may fluctuate, for example, being greater in the morning hours or on awakening. Arthritic states display flares that are associated with an exacerbated pain condition. Changes in the magnitude of pain occur during the daily routine, resulting in "breakthrough pain" during episodic events such as dressing changes (incident pain). These examples emphasize the need for individualized management of increased or decreased pain levels with baseline analgesic dosing supplemented with the use of short-acting "rescue" medications as required. In the face of ongoing severe pain, analgesics should be dosed

in continuous or "around-the-clock" fashion rather than on an as-needed basis. This provides more consistent analgesic levels and avoids unnecessary suffering.

Opioid Tolerance

Chronic exposure to one opiate agonist typically leads to a reduction in the efficacy of other opiate agonists. The degree of tolerance can be remarkable. For example, 10 mg of an oral opioid (such as morphine) is considered a high dose for a treatment-naïve individual, whereas 100 mg IV may produce only minor sedation in a severely tolerant individual.

Patient Physical State and Genetic Variables

Codeine, hydrocodone, and oxycodone are weak analgesic prodrugs that are metabolized into the much more effective analgesic drugs morphine, hydromorphone, and oxymorphone, respectively, by CYP2D6 (Supernaw, 2001). CYP2D6 activity is genetically diminished in 7% of whites, 3% of blacks, and 1% of Asians (Eichelbaum and Evert, 1996), rendering oxycodone, hydrocodone, and codeine relatively ineffective analgesics in these "poor metabolizers" and potentially toxic for "ultrarapid" metabolizers.

The activity of CYP2D6 is inhibited by SSRIs, which may render opioids less effective as analgesics in some patients. Whereas diminished activity of the CYP2D6 isoenzyme will lead to less efficacy of prodrug opioids, the opposite occurs with methadone. Although methadone is primarily metabolized by CYP3A4, other CYPs participate, and genetic polymorphisms involving deficiencies in the CYPs 2B6 and 2D6 may lead to high methadone C_p values (Zhou et al., 2009).

Opioids are highly protein bound, and factors such as plasma pH may dramatically change binding. In addition, AAG is an acute-phase reactant protein that is elevated in cancer patients and has a high affinity for basic drugs such as methadone and meperidine. Morphine and meperidine should be avoided in patients with renal impairment because morphine-6-glucuronide (a metabolite of morphine) and normeperidine (a metabolite of meperidine) are excreted by the kidney and will accumulate and lead to toxicity. Other states that may increase the risk of adverse effects of the opioids include COPD, sleep apnea, dementia, benign prostatic hypertrophy, unstable gait, and pretreatment constipation.

Routes of Administration

Typically, one chooses the least invasive routes, such as oral, buccal, or transdermal delivery, to facilitate patient compliance. Intravenous routes are more useful in pre- and post-operative in-hospital pain management and during end-of-life care. Patients with chronic pain states where side effects from systemic drug exposure are intolerable may be candidates for chronic spinal drug delivery, requiring surgery for indwelling catheterization and pump placement.

Dose Selection and Titration

The conservative approach to initiating chronic opioid therapy suggests starting with low doses that may be incremented on the basis of the pharmacokinetics of the drug. In chronic pain states, the aim would be to use long-acting medications to permit once- or twice-daily dosing (e.g., controlled-release formulations or methadone). Such agents reach steady state slowly. Rapid incrementation is to be avoided, and rescue medication should be made available for breakthrough pain during initial dosing titration.

Opioid Rotation

Changing to a different opioid, when the patient fails to achieve benefit or side effects become limiting before analgesia is sufficient, is widely employed. Failure or intolerance of one opioid cannot necessarily predict the patient's response or acceptance to another (Quang-Cantagrel et al., 2000). Practically, opioid rotation involves incrementing the dose of a given opioid (e.g., morphine) to a level limited by side effects and insufficient analgesia and then substituting an alternate opioid medication at an equieffective dose. Agents typically involved in such rotation sequences are various oral opioids (e.g., morphine, methadone, dilaudid, oxycodone)

TABLE 20–9 ■ SUMMARY OF DRUG TARGET AND SITE OF ACTION OF COMMON DRUG CLASSES AND RELATIVE EFFICACY BY PAIN STATE

DRUG CLASS (example)	DRUG ACTION	SITE OF ACTION[a]	RELATIVE EFFICACY IN PAIN STATES[a]
NSAIDs (ibuprofen, aspirin, acetaminophen)	Nonspecific COX inhibitors	Peripheral and spinal	Tissue injury >> acute stimuli = nerve injury = 0 (Chapter 38)
COX-2 inhibitor (celecoxib)	COX-2–selective inhibitor	Peripheral and spinal	Tissue injury >> acute stimuli = nerve injury = 0 (Chapter 38)
Opioids (morphine)	μ receptor agonist	Supraspinal and spinal	Tissue injury = acute stimuli ≥ nerve injury > 0 (see this chapter)
Anticonvulsants (gabapentin)	Na$^+$ channel block, $\alpha_2\delta$ subunit of Ca^{2+} channel	Supraspinal and spinal	Nerve injury > tissue injury = acute stimuli = 0 (Chapter 17)
Tricyclic antidepressants (amitryptiline)	Inhibit uptake of 5HT/NE	Supraspinal and spinal	Nerve injury ≥ tissue injury >> acute stimuli = 0 (Chapters 15 and 19)

[a]As defined by studies in preclinical models.

and the fentanyl patch systems. Care must be taken to titrate the doses and monitor the patient closely during such drug transitions.

Combination Therapy

In general, the use of combinations of drugs with the same pharmacological kinetic profile is not warranted (e.g., morphine plus methadone). The same holds if the drugs have overlapping targets and opposing effects (e.g., combining an MOR agonist with an agent having mixed agonist/antagonist properties). On the other hand, certain opiate combinations are useful. For example, in a chronic pain state with periodic incident or breakthrough pain, the patient might receive a slow-release formulation of morphine for baseline pain relief, and the acute incident (breakthrough) pain may be managed with a rapid-onset/short-lasting formulation such as buccal fentanyl. For inflammatory or nociceptive pain, opioids may be usefully combined with other analgesic agents, such as acetaminophen or other NSAIDs (Table 20–9). In some situations, NSAIDs can provide analgesia equal to that produced by 60 mg codeine. In the case of neuropathic pain, other drug classes may be useful alone or in combination with an opiate. For example, antidepressants that block amine reuptake, such as amitriptyline or duloxetine, and anticonvulsants such as gabapentin may enhance the analgesic effect and may be synergistic in some pain states.

Nonanalgesic Therapeutic Uses of Opioids

Dyspnea

Morphine is used to alleviate the dyspnea of acute left ventricular failure and pulmonary edema, and the patient's response to intravenous morphine may be dramatic. The mechanism underlying this pronounced relief is not clear. It may involve an alteration of the patient's reaction to impaired respiratory function and an indirect reduction of the work of the heart owing to reduced fear and apprehension. However, it is more probable that the major benefit is due to cardiovascular effects, such as decreased peripheral resistance secondary to histamine release and an increased capacity of the peripheral and splanchnic vascular compartments. Nitroglycerin, which also causes vasodilation, may be superior to morphine in this condition. In patients with normal blood gases but severe breathlessness owing to chronic obstruction of airflow ("pink puffers"), dihydrocodeine, 16 mg orally before exercise, reduces the feeling of breathlessness and increases exercise tolerance. Nonetheless, opioids generally are contraindicated in pulmonary edema unless severe pain is also present.

Anesthetic Adjuvants

High doses of opioids, notably fentanyl and sufentanil, are widely used as the primary anesthetic agents in many surgical procedures. They have powerful "MAC-sparing" effects; for example, they reduce the concentrations of volatile anesthetic otherwise required to produce an adequate anesthetic depth (see Chapter 21). Although respiration is so depressed that physical assistance is required, patients can retain consciousness. Therefore, when using an opioid as the primary anesthetic agent, it is used in conjunction with an agent that results in unconsciousness and produces amnesia, such as the benzodiazepines or lower concentrations of volatile anesthetics. High doses of opiate as employed in the operating room setting also result in prominent rigidity of the chest wall and masseters, requiring concurrent treatment with muscle relaxants to permit intubations and ventilation.

Acute Opioid Toxicity

Acute opioid toxicity may result from clinical overdosage, accidental overdosage, or attempts at suicide. Occasionally, a delayed type of toxicity may occur from the injection of an opioid into chilled skin areas or in patients with low blood pressure and shock. The drug is not fully absorbed; therefore, a subsequent dose may be given. When normal circulation is restored, an excessive amount may be absorbed suddenly. In nontolerant individuals, serious toxicity with methadone may follow the oral ingestion of 40–60 mg. In the case of morphine, a normal, pain-free adult is not likely to die after oral doses less than 120 mg or to have serious toxicity with less than 30 mg parenterally.

Symptoms and Diagnosis

The triad of coma, pinpoint pupils, and depressed respiration strongly suggests opioid poisoning. The patient who has taken an overdose of an opioid usually is stuporous or, if a large overdose has been taken, may be in a profound coma. The respiratory rate will be very low, or the patient may be apneic, and possibly cyanotic. If adequate oxygenation is restored early, the blood pressure will improve; if hypoxia persists untreated, there may be capillary damage, and measures to combat shock may be required. The pupils will be symmetrical and pinpoint in size; however, if hypoxia is severe, they may be dilated. Urine formation is depressed. Body temperature falls, and the skin becomes cold and clammy. The skeletal muscles are flaccid, the jaw is relaxed, and the tongue may fall back and block the airway. Frank convulsions occasionally may be noted in infants and children. When death occurs, it is nearly always from respiratory failure. Even if respiration is restored, death still may occur as a result of complications that develop during the period of coma, such as pneumonia or shock. Noncardiogenic pulmonary edema is seen commonly with opioid poisoning.

Treatment

The first step is to establish a patent airway and ventilate the patient. Opioid antagonists can produce dramatic reversal of the severe respiratory depression, and the antagonist naloxone is the treatment of choice. However, care should be taken to avoid precipitating withdrawal in dependent patients, who may be extremely sensitive to antagonists. The safest approach is to dilute the standard naloxone dose (0.4 mg) and slowly administer it intravenously, monitoring arousal and respiratory function. With care, it usually is possible to reverse the respiratory depression without precipitating a major withdrawal syndrome. If no response is seen with the first dose, additional doses can be given. Patients should be observed for rebound increases in sympathetic nervous system activity, which may result in cardiac arrhythmias and pulmonary edema. For reversing opioid poisoning in children, the initial dose of naloxone is 0.01 mg/kg. If no effect is seen after a total dose of 10 mg, one can reasonably question the role of an opiate in the diagnosis. Pulmonary edema sometimes associated with opioid overdosage may be countered by positive-pressure respiration. Tonic-clonic seizures, occasionally seen as part of the toxic syndrome with meperidine and tramadol, are ameliorated by treatment with naloxone.

The presence of general CNS depressants does not prevent the salutary effect of naloxone, and in cases of mixed intoxications, the situation will be improved largely owing to antagonism of the respiratory-depressant effects of the opioid (however, some evidence indicates that naloxone and naltrexone may also antagonize some of the depressant actions of sedative-hypnotics). One need not attempt to restore the patient to full consciousness. The duration of action of the available antagonists is shorter than that of many opioids; hence, patients can slip back into coma (e.g., renarcotization). This is particularly important when the overdosage is due to methadone. The depressant effects of these drugs may persist for 24–72 h, and fatalities have occurred as a result of premature discontinuation of naloxone. In cases of overdoses of these drugs, a continuous infusion of naloxone should be considered. Toxicity from overdose of pentazocine and other opioids with mixed actions may require higher doses of naloxone.

Novel Nonopioid Treatments for Pain

Myriad marine toxins target GPCRs, neurotransmitter transporters, and ion channels; a number (i.e., tetrodotoxin, saxitoxin, kainic acid, and various venoms from cone snails) have been useful to basic scientists (Sakai and Swanson 2014). One that has become an FDA-approved treatment of chronic pain is ziconotide.

Ziconotide

Ziconotide is a synthetic copy of a neuroactive cone snail toxin, a 25–amino acid basic polypeptide with three disulfide bridges. The molecule is hydrophilic and readily soluble in water and isotonic saline.

Mechanism of Action

Ziconotide binds to and blocks N-type Ca^{2+} channels on nociceptive afferents in the dorsal horn of the spinal cord. This leads to blockade of the release of excitatory neurotransmitter involved in nociception (Patel et al., 2017).

ADME

Ziconotide is administered intrathecally as a continuous infusion by a controlled microinfusion pump. The toxin's serum $t_{1/2}$ is 1.3 h; the $t_{1/2}$ in CSF is 4.6 h. The volume distribution in CSF approximates the total CSF volume, 140 mL. Ziconotide is stable in CSF but, following passage from the CSF into the systemic circulation, is metabolized by endo- and exopeptidases that are widely expressed in most tissues.

Therapeutic Use

Ziconotide is used to treat severe chronic pain in adults for whom intrathecal therapy is warranted and for whom other treatments have failed or are not suitable (allergy, etc.). The dosing should follow the FDA-approved schedule, titrating upward from 2.4 µg/d in increments of 2.4 µg no more than two or three times weekly to the maximum recommended intrathecal dose of 19.2 µg/d.

Adverse Effects and Precautions

Side effects include dizziness, nausea, confusion, nystagmus, anxiety, confusion, and blurred vision. Hallucinations and paranoia can occur; thus, ziconotide is contraindicated in patients with a preexisting history of psychosis. Inadvertent intravenous or epidural administration of ziconotide will cause hypotension. The analgesic effects of ziconotide appear to add with those of morphine; in laboratory experiments, intrathecal ziconotide potentiated the GI effects of morphine but not the respiratory depressant effects. Ziconotide is not an opiate, and its effects cannot be reversed by naloxone. Treatment of overdose is withdrawal of the agent and supportive care in a hospital. The agent is classified in pregnancy category C. The difficulties of long-term intrathecal delivery, the production of state-independent blockade, and the side-effect profile have been barriers to use of ziconotide (Patel et al., 2017).

Drug Facts for Your Personal Formulary: *Opioid Agonists and Antagonists*

Drug	Therapeutic Use	Clinical Pharmacology and Tips
Agonists: See Table 20-7 for CDC guidelines for prescribing opioids for chronic pain		
Morphine Hydromorphone Oxycodone Hydrocodone	• Potent μ agonists • Strong analgesic in moderate-to-severe pain states. • Morphine is a useful adjunct in pulmonary edema and general anesthesia.	• ↓ GI motility ⇒ constipation • Hydrocodone, oxycodone formulated with NSAIDs • Hydrocodone, oxycodone, and fentanyl are more potent than morphine • Among licit agents, LA/ER agents often preferred by abusers
Fentanyl	• Potent μ agonist • Administered orally (buccal tablet, sublingual tablet/spray, oral lozenge), intravenous (push/infusion), intramuscular, topical, topical iontophoretic, neuraxial	• Rapid onset, short duration of action • Slightly longer effective $t_{1/2}$ than sufentanil, alfentanil, and remifentanil
Sufentanil Alfentanil Remifentanil	• Similar to fentanyl • Rapid onset, short duration of action • Administered intravenously	• Sufentanil and alfentanil also given epidurally • Remifentanil: ultrashort acting
Meperidine	• Potent μ agonist • Rapid onset, intermediate duration of action	• Not for extended use due to accumulation of seizure-inducing metabolite
Methadone	• Potent MOR agonist • Rapid onset, long duration of action • Used in maintenance/rehab programs	• Long $t_{1/2}$, ~27 h ⇒ potential for accumulation with too frequent repeated delivery • Anticholinergic effects

Drug Facts for Your Personal Formulary: *Opioid Agonists and Antagonists* (*continued*)

Drug	Therapeutic Use	Clinical Pharmacology and Tips
Codeine	• Weak prodrug for morphine • Useful for mild-to-moderate pain • Less efficacious than morphine but will antagonize strong μ agonists • Administered orally	• Useful antitussive effects • Formulated with NSAIDs
Levorphanol	• Affinity at the MOR, KOR, and DOR • 5HT/NE reuptake inhibitor; NMDA receptor antagonist • Rapid onset, modest duration of analgesia • Administered orally	• Long elimination $t_{1/2}$ ~ 14h $\Rightarrow$ potential for accumulation with too frequent repeated delivery • Adverse effects: delirium, hallucinations
Peripherally Restricted Agonist		
Loperamide	• Mu opioid agonist • Effective antidiarrheal • Administered orally	• Loperamide crosses BBB poorly, can be formulated with simethicone
Agonist Restricted by Coformulation		
Diphenoxylate	• Mu opioid agonist • Effective antidiarrheal • Administered orally	• Diphenoxylate will cross the BBB, so it is formulated with atropine, the anticholinergic effects of which (weakness, nausea) discourage abuse.
Partial Agonists; Agonist/Antagonist Combinations		
Buprenorphine	• Partial agonist at MOR; KOR antagonist • Mild-to-moderate pain (ceiling effect) • Administered by intramuscular, intravenous, sublingual, transdermal, buccal film • Coformulated with naloxone for use in abuse management	• Delivery to a patient on a full opiate agonist may initiate withdrawal (may be done therapeutically in management of heroin addiction)
Butorphanol Nalbuphine Pentazocine	• KOR agonist/MOR antagonist • Analgesia to mild-to-moderate pain	• Delivery to patient on a full opiate agonist may initiate withdrawal • Ceiling effect • Pentazocine is also formulated with naloxone.
Other Agonists		
Tramadol	• Weak μ agonist and a 5HT/NE uptake inhibitor • Analgesia for moderate pain • Available as a fixed-dose combination with acetaminophen	• Potential for seizures • Serotonin syndrome risk • As an adjunct to other opioids for chronic pain
Tapentadol	• Weak μ agonist and a 5HT/NE uptake inhibitor • Analgesia for moderate pain	• Serotonin syndrome risk
Central Antitussives		
Dextromethorphan	• ↓ Cough reflex; receptor mechanisms unclear • Administered orally • Available as an extended-release formulation	• Serotonin syndrome risk • Has no analgesic or addictive properties
Codeine	• See codeine listing, above	• See codeine listing, above
Antagonists		
Naloxone	• Antagonist at MOR/DOR/KOR • Rapid onset, moderately short acting • Rapidly reverses central and peripheral opiate effects • Used in treating opioid overdose • Autoinjector available for emergency administration	• $t_{1/2}$ ~ 64 min • Renarcotization may occur with long-lasting agonists as naloxone is metabolized • May induce moderate hyperalgesia • Known as NARCAN; used by emergency medical technicians to revive comatose opioid abusers
Naltrexone Nalmefene	• Antagonist at MOR/DOR/KOR • Rapid onset, longer acting than naloxone • Reverses central and peripheral opiate effects • Used in treating alcohol and opiate dependence	• Naltrexone: formulated with bupropion for managing obesity and with morphine for severe pain; contraindicated in hepatitis and liver failure (*Black-Box Warning:* excessive doses cause hepatocellular injury) • Start naltrexone only after 7–10 days of abstinence from opioids • Long-term use of naltrexone $\Rightarrow$ hypersensitivity to opioids

Peripherally Restricted Antagonists		
Methylnaltrexone	• Antagonist at MOR/DOR/KOR • Reverses peripheral opiate effects (e.g., opiate-induced constipation) but not analgesia	• Does not cross BBB, thus not useful in treating addiction or reversing CNS effects of opioids
Alvimopan	• Antagonist at MOR/DOR/KOR • Penetrates poorly into CNS • FDA approved for ileus	• Reverses peripheral opiate effects

Bibliography

Akil H, et al. Endogenous opioids: biology and function. *Annu Rev Neurosci,* **1984,** 7:223–255.

Anton RF. Naltrexone for the management of alcohol dependence. *N Engl J Med,* **2008,** 359:715–721.

Armario A. Activation of the hypothalamic-pituitary-adrenal axis by addictive drugs: different pathways, common outcome. *Trends Pharmacol Sci,* **2010,** 31:318–325.

Barke KE, Hough LB. Opiates, mast cells and histamine release. *Life Sci,* **1993,** 53:1391–1399.

Barnett V, et al. Opioid antagonists. *J Pain Symptom Manage,* **2014,** 47:341–352.

Becker G, et al. Peripherally acting opioid antagonists in the treatment of opiate-related constipation: a systematic review. *J Pain Symptom Manage,* **2007,** 34:547–565.

Benyamin R, et al. Opioid complications and side effects. *Pain Physician,* **2008,** 11:S105–S120.

Booth M. *Opium: A History.* Macmillan, New York, **1999.**

Caraco Y, et al. Impact of ethnic origin and quinidine coadministration on codeine's disposition and pharmacodynamic effects. *J Pharmacol Exp Ther,* **1999,** 290:413–422.

Cherny NI. Opioid analgesics: comparative features and prescribing guidelines. *Drugs,* **1996,** 51:713–737.

Christie MJ. Cellular neuroadaptations to chronic opioids: tolerance, withdrawal and addiction. *Br J Pharmacol,* **2008,** 154:384–396.

Chung KF, Pavord ID. Prevalence, pathogenesis, and causes of chronic cough. *Lancet,* **2008,** 371:1364–1374.

Clemens KE, Klaschik E. Symptomatic therapy of dyspnea with strong opioids and its effect on ventilation in palliative care patients. *J Pain Symptom Manage,* **2007,** 33:473–481.

Corbett AD, et al. 75 years of opioid research: the exciting but vain quest for the Holy Grail. *Brit J Pharmacol,* **2006,** 147, S153–S162.

Dannals RF. Positron emission tomography radioligands for the opioid system. *J Labelled Comp Radiopharm,* **2013,** 56:187–195.

Deer TR, et al. The polyanalgesic consensus conference (PACC): recommendations for intrathecal drug delivery: guidance for improving safety and mitigating risks. *Neuromodulation,* **2017,** 20:155–176.

Dowell D, et al. CDC Guideline for prescribing opioids for chronic pain—United States, 2016. *MMWR Recomm Rep,* **2016,** 65:1–49. doi:http://dx.doi.org/10.15585/mmwr.rr6501e1. Accessed April 30, 2017.

Dreborg S, et al. Evolution of vertebrate opioid receptors. *Proc Natl Acad Sci U S A,* **2008,** 105:15487–15492.

Eddinger KA, et al. Intrathecal catheterization and drug delivery in Guinea pigs: a small-animal model for morphine-evoked granuloma formation. *Anesthesiology,* **2016,** 12:378–394.

Eichelbaum M, Evert B. Influence of pharmacogenetics on drug disposition and response. *Clin Exp Pharmacol Physiol,* **1996,** 23:983–985.

Elkader A, Sproule B. Buprenorphine: clinical pharmacokinetics in the treatment of opioid dependence. *Clin Pharmacokinet,* **2005,** 44:661–680.

Fenalti G, et al. Molecular control of δ-opioid receptor signaling. *Nature,* **2014,** 506:191–196.

Fillingim RB, Gear RW. Sex differences in opioid analgesia: clinical and experimental findings. *Eur J Pain,* **2004,** 8:413–425.

Fishburne JI. Systemic analgesia during labor. *Clin Perinatol,* **1982,** 9:29–53.

Fletcher D, Martinez V. Opioid-induced hyperalgesia in patients after surgery: a systematic review and a meta-analysis. *Br J Anaesth,* **2014,** 112:991–1004.

Fredheim OM, et al. Clinical pharmacology of methadone for pain. *Acta Anaesthesiol Scand,* **2008,** 52:879–889.

Galanie S, et al. Complete biosynthesis of opioids in yeast. *Science,* **2015,** 349:1095–1100.

Galligan JJ, Akbarali HI. Molecular physiology of enteric opioid receptors. *Am J Gastroenterol Suppl,* **2014,** 2:17–21.

Gendron L, et al. Molecular pharmacology of δ-opioid receptors. *Pharmacol Rev,* **2016,** 68:631–700.

Gillis JC, et al. Transnasal butorphanol. A review of its pharmacodynamic and pharmacokinetic properties, and therapeutic potential in acute pain management. *Drugs,* **1995,** 50:157–175.

Gintzler AR, Chakrabarti S. Post-opioid receptor adaptations to chronic morphine; altered functionality and associations of signaling molecules. *Life Sci,* **2006,** 79:717–722.

Goldstein A, et al. Stereospecific and nonspecific interactions of the morphine congener levorphanol in subcellular fractions of mouse brain. *Proc Natl Acad Sci U S A,* **1971,** 68:1742–1747.

Goldstein G. Pentazocine. *Drug Alcohol Depend,* **1985,** 14:313–323.

Grace PM, et al. Pathological pain and the neuroimmune interface. *Nat Rev Immunol,* **2014,** 14:217–231.

Greenwood-Van Meerveld B. Emerging drugs for postoperative ileus. *Expert Opin Emerg Drugs,* **2007,** 12:619–626.

Grond S, Sablotzki A. Clinical pharmacology of tramadol. *Clin Pharmacokinet,* **2004,** 43:879–923.

Haile CN, et al. Pharmacogenetic treatments for drug addiction: alcohol and opiates. *Am J Drug Alcohol Abuse,* **2008,** 34:355–381.

Höllt V. Opioid peptide processing and receptor selectivity. *Annu Rev Pharmacol Toxicol,* **1986,** 26:59–77.

Hughes J, et al. Identification of two related pentapeptides from the brain with potent opiate agonist activity. *Nature,* **1975,** 258:577–580.

Hutchinson MR, et al. Opioid-induced glial activation: mechanisms of activation and implications for opioid analgesia, dependence, and reward. *Scientific World J,* **2007,** 7:98–111.

Johansson I, Ingelman-Sundberg M. Genetic polymorphism and toxicology—with emphasis on cytochrome P450. *Toxicol Sci,* **2011,** 120:1–13.

Kane BE, et al. Molecular recognition of opioid receptor ligands. *AAPS J,* **2006,** 8:E126–E137.

Khan SM, et al. The expanding roles of Gβγ subunits in G Protein-coupled receptor signaling and drug action. *Pharmacol Rev,* **2013,** 65: 545–577.

Koob GF, Le Moal M. Neurobiological mechanisms for opponent motivational processes in addiction. *Philos Trans R Soc Lond B Biol Sci,* **2008,** 363:3113–3123.

Kreek MJ, Koob GF. Drug dependence: stress and dysregulation of brain reward pathways. *Drug Alcohol Depend,* **1998,** 51:23–47.

Kromer W. Endogenous and exogenous opioids in the control of gastrointestinal motility and secretion. *Pharmacol Rev,* **1988,** 40:121–162.

Kumar K, Singh SI. Neuraxial opioid-induced pruritus: an update. *J Anaesthesiol Clin Pharmacol,* **2013,** 29:303–307.

Lalley PM. Opioidergic and dopaminergic modulation of respiration. *Respir Physiol Neurobiol,* **2008,** 164:160–167.

Larson MD. Mechanism of opioid-induced pupillary effects. *Clin Neurophysiol,* **2008,** 119:1358–1364.

Latta KS, et al. Meperidine: a critical review. *Am J Ther,* **2002,** 9:53–68.

Lee M, et al. A comprehensive review of opioid-induced hyperalgesia. *Pain Physician,* **2011,** 14:145–161.

Loyd DR, Murphy AZ. The neuroanatomy of sexual dimorphism in opioid analgesia. *Exp Neurol,* **2014,** 259:57–63.

Martin WR, et al. The effects of morphine- and nalorphine-like drugs in the non-dependent and morphine-dependent chronic spinal dog. *J Pharmacol Exp Ther,* **1976,** *197:517–532.*

Massotte D. In vivo opioid receptor heteromerization: where do we stand? *Br J Pharmacol,* **2015,** *172:420–434.*

McGinty JF. What we know and still need to learn about opioids in the hippocampus. *NIDA Res Monogr,* **1988,** *82:1–11.*

Melzack R, Casey KL. Sensory, motivational, and central control determinants of chronic pain: A new conceptual model. In: The Skin Senses, [ed. D.L.Kenshalo] pp. 423–443. Springfield, Illinois. Thomas, 1968.

Mogil JS. Sex differences in pain and pain inhibition: multiple explanations of a controversial phenomenon *Nat Rev Neurosci,* **2012,** *13:859–866.*

Monk JP, et al. Sufentanil. A review of its pharmacological properties and therapeutic use. *Drugs,* **1988,** *36:286–313.*

Nakagawa A, et al. Total biosynthesis of opiates by stepwise fermentation using engineered *Escherichia coli. Nat Commun,* **2016,** *7:*10390. doi:10.1038/ncomms10390.

Neumann PB, et al. Plasma morphine concentrations during chronic oral administration in patients with cancer pain. *Pain,* **1982,** *13:247–252.*

NIDA. Overdose death rates. Revised January **2017.** https://www.drugabuse.gov/related-topics/trends-statistics/overdose-death-rates. Accessed April 30, 2017.

Osborne, R, et al. The analgesic activity of morphine-6-glucuronide. *Brit J Clin Pharmacol,* **1992,** *34:130–138.*

Owen JA, et al. Age-related morphine kinetics. *Clin Pharmacol Ther,* **1983,** *34:364–368.*

Pan YX. Diversity and complexity of the mu opioid receptor gene: alternative pre-mRNA splicing and promoters. *DNA Cell Biol,* **2005,** *24:736–750.*

Patel R, et al. Calcium channel modulation as a target in chronic pain control. *Br J Pharmacol,* **2017.** doi:10.1111/bph.13789.

Pattinson KT. Opioids and the control of respiration. *Br J Anaesth,* **2008,** *100:747–758.*

Pert CB, et al. Opiate agonists and antagonists discriminated by receptor binding in brain. *Science,* **1973,** *182:1359–1361.*

Portenoy RK, et al. Transdermal fentanyl for cancer pain. Repeated dose pharmacokinetics. *Anesthesiology,* **1993,** *78:36–43.*

Price DD, et al. A psychophysical analysis of morphine analgesia. *Pain,* **1985,** *22:261–269.*

Prommer E. Levorphanol: revisiting an underutilized analgesic. *Palliat Care,* **2014,** *8:7–10.*

Quang-Cantagrel ND, et al. Opioid substitution to improve the effectiveness of chronic non-cancer pain control: a chart review. *Anesth Analg,* **2000,** *90:933–937.*

Regnard C, et al. Loperamide. *J Pain Symptom Manage,* **2011,** *42:319–323.*

Rook EJ, et al. Pharmacokinetics and pharmacokinetic variability of heroin and its metabolites: review of the literature. *Curr Clin Pharmacol,* **2006,** *1:109–118.*

Rosow CE, et al. Reversal of opioid-induced bladder dysfunction by intravenous naloxone and methylnaltrexone. *Clin Pharmacol Ther,* **2007,** *82:48–53.*

Rudd RA, et al. Increases in drug and opioid-involved overdose deaths—United States, 2010-2015. *MMWR Morb Mortal Wkly Rep,* **2016,** *65:*1445–1452. doi:http://dx.doi.org/10.15585/mmwr.mm655051e1. Accessed April 30, 2017.

Sakai R, Swanson GT. Recent progress in neuroactive marine natural products. *Nat Prod Rep,* **2014,** *31:273–309.*

Schmidt WK, et al. Nalbuphine. *Drug Alcohol Depend,* **1985,** *14:339–362.*

Seifert CF, Kennedy S. Meperidine is alive and well in the new millennium: evaluation of meperidine usage patterns and frequency of adverse drug reactions. *Pharmacotherapy,* **2004,** *24:776–783.*

Shang Y, Filizola M. Opioid receptors: structural and mechanistic insights into pharmacology and signaling. *Eur J Pharmacol,* **2015,** *763:206–213.*

Sidhu AS, Triadafilopoulos G. Neuro-regulation of lower esophageal sphincter function as treatment for gastroesophageal reflux disease. *World J Gastroenterol,* **2008,** *14:985–990.*

Smith HS, Peppin JF. Toward a systematic approach to opioid rotation. *J Pain Res,* **2014,** *7:589–608.*

Smith MT. Neuroexcitatory effects of morphine and hydromorphone: evidence implicating the 3-glucuronide metabolites. *Clin Exp Pharmacol Physiol,* **2000,** *27:524–528.*

Sorkin LS, Wallace MS. Acute pain mechanisms. *Surg Clin North Am,* **1999,** *79:213–229.*

Stein C, Machelska H. Modulation of peripheral sensory neurons by the immune system: implications for pain therapy. *Pharmacol Rev,* **2011,** *63:860–881.*

Stevens CW. The evolution of vertebrate opioid receptors. *Front Biosci,* **2009,** *14:1247–1269.*

Stroumpos C, et al. Remifentanil, a different opioid: potential clinical applications and safety aspects. *Expert Opin Drug Saf,* **2010,** *9:355–364.*

Supernaw RB. CYP2D6 and the efficacy of codeine and codeine-like drugs. *Am J Pain Manage,* **2001,** *11:30–31.*

Thomas J, et al. Methylnaltrexone for opioid-induced constipation in advanced illness. *N Engl J Med,* **2008,** *358:* 2332–2343.

Vallejo R, et al. Opioid therapy and immunosuppression: a review. *Am J Ther,* **2004,** *11:354–365.*

Van Rijn RM, et al. Novel pharmaco-types and trafficking-types induced by opioid receptor heteromerization. *Curr Opin Pharmacol,* **2010,** *10:* 73–79.

Vaughan-Shaw PG, et al. A meta-analysis of the effectiveness of the opioid receptor antagonist alvimopan in reducing hospital length of stay and time to GI recovery in patients enrolled in a standardized accelerated recovery program after abdominal surgery. *Dis Colon Rectum,* **2012,** *55:611–620.*

Violin JD, et al. Biased ligands at G-protein-coupled receptors: promise and progress. *Trends Pharmacol Sci,* **2014,** *35:308–316.*

von Zastrow M, et al. Regulated endocytosis of opioid receptors: cellular mechanisms and proposed roles in physiological adaptation to opiate drugs. *Curr Opin Neurobiol,* **2003,** *13:348–353.*

Waldhoer M, et al. Opioid receptors. *Annu Rev Biochem,* **2004,** *73:* 953–990.

West SJ, et al. Circuitry and plasticity of the dorsal horn - Toward a better understanding of neuropathic pain. *Neuroscience,* **2015,** *300:254–275.*

Williams JT, et al. Regulation of μ-opioid receptors: desensitization, phosphorylation, internalization, and tolerance. *Pharmacol Rev,* **2013,** *65:223–254.*

Willens JS, Myslinski NR. Pharmacodynamics, pharmacokinetics, and clinical uses of fentanyl, sufentanil, and alfentanil. *Heart Lung,* **1993,** *22:239–251.*

Wood JD, Galligan JJ. Function of opioids in the enteric nervous system. *Neurogastroenterol Motil,* **2004,** 16(suppl 2):17–28.

Xu J, et al. Alternatively spliced mu opioid receptor C termini impact the diverse actions of morphine. *J Clin Invest,* **2017,** *127:1561–1573.*

Yaksh TL, et al. The search for novel analgesics: targets and mechanisms. *F1000Prime Rep,* **2015,** 7:56. doi:10.12703/P7-56. Accessed April 5, 2017.

Yaksh TL. Opioid receptor systems and the endorphins: a review of their spinal organization. *J Neurosurg,* **1987,** *67:157–176.*

Yaksh TL. Pharmacology and mechanisms of opioid analgesic activity. *Acta Anaesthesiol Scand,* **1997,** *41:94–111.*

Yaksh TL, et al. Current and future issues in the development of spinal agents for the management of pain. *Curr Neuropharmacol,* **2017,** *15:* 232–259.

Yaksh TL, Allen JW. Preclinical insights into the implementation of intrathecal midazolam: a cautionary tale. *Anesth Analg,* **2004,** *98:* 1509–1511.

Young GB, da Silva OP. Effects of morphine on the electroencephalograms of neonates: A prospective, observational study. *Clin Neurophysiol,* **2000,** *111:1955–1960.*

Zhang X, et al. Opioid receptor trafficking and interaction in nociceptors. *Brit J Pharmacol,* **2015,** *172:364–374.*

Zhou S-F et al. Polymorphism of human cytochrome P450 enzymes and its clinical impact. *Drug Metab Rev,* **2009,** *41:289–295.*

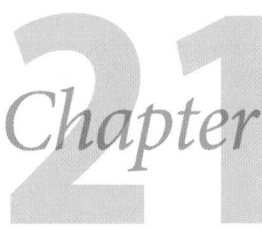

Chapter 21

General Anesthetics and Therapeutic Gases

Hemal H. Patel, Matthew L. Pearn, Piyush M. Patel, and David M. Roth

General anesthetics depress the CNS to a sufficient degree to permit the performance of surgery and unpleasant procedures. General anesthetics have low therapeutic indices and thus require great care in administration. The selection of specific drugs and routes of administration to produce general anesthesia is based on the pharmacokinetic properties and on the secondary effects of the various drugs. The practitioner should consider the context of the proposed diagnostic or surgical procedure and the individual patient's characteristics and associated medical conditions when choosing appropriate anesthetic agents.

General Principles of Surgical Anesthesia

The administration of general anesthesia is driven by three general objectives:

1. *Minimizing the potentially deleterious direct and indirect effects of anesthetic agents and techniques.*
2. *Sustaining physiologic homeostasis during surgical procedures* that may involve major blood loss, tissue ischemia, reperfusion of ischemic tissue, fluid shifts, exposure to a cold environment, and impaired coagulation.
3. *Improving postoperative outcomes* by choosing techniques that block or treat components of the surgical stress response that may lead to short- or long-term sequelae.

Hemodynamic Effects of General Anesthesia

The most prominent physiological effect of anesthesia induction is a decrease in systemic arterial blood pressure. The causes include direct vasodilation, myocardial depression, or both; a blunting of baroreceptor control; and a generalized decrease in central sympathetic tone. Agents vary in the magnitude of their specific effects, but in all cases the hypotensive response is enhanced by underlying volume depletion or preexisting myocardial dysfunction.

Respiratory Effects of General Anesthesia

Nearly all general anesthetics reduce or eliminate both ventilatory drive and the reflexes that maintain airway patency. Therefore, ventilation generally must be assisted or controlled for at least some period during surgery. The gag reflex is lost, and the stimulus to cough is blunted. Lower esophageal sphincter tone also is reduced, so both passive and active regurgitation may occur. Endotracheal intubation has been a major reason for a decline in the number of aspiration deaths during general anesthesia. Muscle relaxation is valuable during the induction of general anesthesia where it facilitates management of the airway, including endotracheal intubation. Neuromuscular blocking agents commonly are used to effect such relaxation (see Chapter 11). Alternatives to an endotracheal tube include a face mask and a laryngeal mask, an inflatable mask placed in the oropharynx forming a seal around the glottis. Airway management techniques are based on the anesthetic procedure, the need for neuromuscular relaxation, and the physical characteristics of the patient.

Hypothermia

Patients commonly develop hypothermia (body temperature < 36°C) during surgery. The reasons include low ambient temperature, exposed body cavities, cold intravenous fluids, altered thermoregulatory control, and reduced metabolic rate. Metabolic rate and total body O_2 consumption decrease with general anesthesia by about 30%, reducing heat generation. Hypothermia may lead to an increase in perioperative morbidity. Prevention of hypothermia is a major goal of anesthetic care.

Nausea and Vomiting

Nausea and vomiting continue to be significant problems following general anesthesia and are caused by an action of anesthetics on the chemoreceptor trigger zone and the brainstem vomiting center, which are modulated by 5HT, histamine, ACh, DA, and NK1. The $5HT_3$ receptor antagonists ondansetron, dolasetron, and palonosetron (see Chapters 13 and 50) are

Abbreviations

ACh: acetylcholine
AChE: acetylcholinesterase
ADME: absorption, distribution, metabolism, excretion
CBF: cerebral blood flow
CL: clearance
CMR: cerebral metabolic rate
CMR_{O_2}: cerebral metabolic rate of O_2 consumption
CNS: central nervous system
CO: cardiac output
DA: dopamine
ED_{50}: median effective dose
EEG: electroencephalogram
FDA: Food and Drug Administration
F_{IO_2}: inspired O_2 fraction
GABA: γ-aminobutyric acid
GFR: glomerular filtration rate
GPCR: G protein–coupled receptor
Hb: hemoglobin
HR: heart rate
5HT: 5-hydroxytryptamine: serotonin
ICP: intracranial pressure
IV: intravenous
LD_{50}: median lethal dose
MAC: minimum alveolar concentration
MAP: mean arterial pressure
MI: myocardial infarction
NE: norepinephrine
NK1: neurokinin 1
NMDA: *N*-methyl-D-aspartate
NSAID: nonsteroidal anti-inflammatory drug
Pa_{CO_2}: arterial CO_2 tension
P_{O_2}: partial pressure of O_2
PRIS: propofol infusion syndrome
RBF: renal blood flow
RR: respiratory rate
RT: room temperature
$t_{1/2}β$: β-phase (tissue elimination) half-life
TREK channel: mechanosensitive K^+ channel
$\dot{V}_E$: minute ventilation
VLPO: ventrolateral preoptic
V_{ss}: volume of distribution at steady state

effective in suppressing nausea and vomiting. Common preventive strategies include anesthetic induction with propofol; the combined use of droperidol, metoclopramide, and dexamethasone; and avoidance of nitrous oxide (N_2O). A new subclass of antiemetic drugs includes NK1 antagonists (e.g., aprepitant, rolapitant).

Other Emergent and Postoperative Phenomena

Hypertension and tachycardia are common during emergence from anesthesia as the sympathetic nervous system regains its tone and is enhanced by pain. Myocardial ischemia can appear or worsen during emergence in patients with coronary artery disease. Emergence excitement occurs in 5%–30% of patients and is characterized by tachycardia, restlessness, crying, moaning, and thrashing. Neurologic signs, including delirium, spasticity, hyperreflexia, and Babinski sign, are often manifest in the patient emerging from anesthesia. Postanesthesia shivering occurs frequently because of core hypothermia. A small dose of meperidine (12.5 mg) lowers the shivering trigger temperature and effectively stops the activity. The incidence of all of these emergence phenomena is greatly reduced with opioids and α₂ adrenergic agonists (dexmedetomidine).

Airway obstruction may occur during the postoperative period because of residual anesthetic effects. Pulmonary function is reduced following all types of anesthesia and surgery, and hypoxemia may occur. In the immediate postoperative period, pulmonary function reduction can be compounded by the respiratory suppression associated with opioids used for pain control. Regional anesthetic techniques are an important part of a perioperative approach that employs local anesthetic wound infiltration; epidural, spinal, and plexus blocks; and nonsteroidal anti-inflammatory drugs, opioids, α₂ adrenergic receptor agonists, and NMDA receptor antagonists.

Actions and Mechanisms of General Anesthetics

The Anesthetic State

The components of the anesthetic state include

- *Amnesia*
- *Analgesia*
- *Unconsciousness*
- *Immobility* in response to noxious stimulation
- *Attenuation of autonomic responses* to noxious stimulation

The potency of general anesthetic agents is measured by determining the concentration of general anesthetic that prevents movement in response to surgical stimulation. For inhalational anesthetics, anesthetic potency is measured in *MAC units*, with 1 MAC defined as the minimum alveolar concentration that prevents movement in response to surgical stimulation in 50% of subjects. The strengths of MAC as a measurement are the following:

- Alveolar concentrations can be monitored continuously by measuring end-tidal anesthetic concentration using infrared spectroscopy or mass spectrometry.
- MAC provides a direct correlate of the free concentration of the anesthetic at its site(s) of action in the CNS.
- MAC is a simple-to-measure end point that reflects an important clinical goal.

End points other than immobilization also can be used to measure anesthetic potency. For example, the ability to respond to verbal commands (MAC_{awake}) and the ability to form memories also have been correlated with alveolar anesthetic concentration. Verbal response and memory formation are suppressed at a fraction of MAC. The ratio of the anesthetic concentrations required to produce amnesia and immobility vary significantly among different inhalational anesthetic agents.

Generally, the potency of intravenous agents is defined as the free plasma concentration (at equilibrium) that produces loss of response to surgical incision (or other end points) in 50% of subjects.

Mechanisms of Anesthesia

The molecular and cellular mechanisms by which general anesthetics produce their effects have remained one of the great mysteries of pharmacology. The leading unitary theory was that anesthesia is produced by perturbation of the physical properties of cell membranes. This thinking was based largely on the observation that the anesthetic potency of a gas correlated with its solubility in olive oil. This correlation is referred to as the Meyer-Overton rule. Clear exceptions to the Meyer-Overton rule (Franks, 2006) suggest protein targets that may account for anesthetic effect. Increasing evidence supports the hypothesis that different anesthetic agents produce specific components of anesthesia by actions at different molecular targets. Given these insights, the unitary theory of anesthesia has been largely discarded.

Molecular Mechanisms of General Anesthetics

Most intravenous general anesthetics act predominantly through $GABA_A$ receptors and perhaps through some interactions with other ligand-gated ion channels such as NMDA receptors and two-pore K^+ channels.

Chloride channels gated by the inhibitory $GABA_A$ receptors (see Figures 14–5 and 14–11) are sensitive to a wide variety of anesthetics, including the halogenated inhalational agents, many intravenous agents (propofol, barbiturates, and etomidate), and neurosteroids. At clinical concentrations, general anesthetics increase the sensitivity of the $GABA_A$ receptor to GABA, thereby enhancing inhibitory neurotransmission and depressing nervous system activity. The action of anesthetics on the $GABA_A$ receptor probably is mediated by binding of the anesthetics to specific sites on the $GABA_A$ receptor protein (but they do not compete with GABA for its binding site). The capacity of propofol and etomidate to inhibit the response to noxious stimuli is mediated by a specific site on the β_3 subunit of the $GABA_A$ receptor, whereas the sedative effects of these anesthetics are mediated by on the β_2 subunit.

Structurally related to the $GABA_A$ receptors are other ligand-gated ion channels, including *glycine receptors* and neuronal *nicotinic ACh receptors* (see Figure 14–5). Glycine-gated Cl^- channels (glycine receptors) may play a role in mediating inhibition by anesthetics of responses to noxious stimuli. Inhalational anesthetics enhance the capacity of glycine to activate glycine receptors, which play an important role in inhibitory neurotransmission in the spinal cord and brainstem. Propofol, neurosteroids, and barbiturates also potentiate glycine-activated currents, whereas etomidate and ketamine do not. Subanesthetic concentrations of the inhalational anesthetics inhibit some classes of neuronal nicotinic ACh receptors, which seem to mediate other components of anesthesia such as analgesia or amnesia.

Ketamine, nitrous oxide, cyclopropane, and xenon are the only general anesthetics that do not have significant effects on $GABA_A$ or glycine receptors. These agents inhibit a different type of ligand-gated ion channel, the NMDA receptor (see Figure 14–12 and Table 14–2). NMDA receptors are glutamate-gated cation channels that are somewhat selective for Ca^{2+} and are involved in long-term modulation of synaptic responses (long-term potentiation) and glutamate-mediated neurotoxicity.

Halogenated inhalational anesthetics activate some members of a class of K^+ channels known as *two-pore domain channels*; other two-pore domain channel family members are activated by xenon, N_2O, and cyclopropane. These channels are located in both presynaptic and postsynaptic sites. The postsynaptic channels may be the molecular locus through which these agents hyperpolarize neurons.

Cellular Mechanisms of Anesthesia

General anesthetics produce two important physiologic effects at the cellular level:

1. Inhalational anesthetics can hyperpolarize neurons. Neuronal hyperpolarization may affect pacemaker activity and pattern-generating circuits.
2. Both inhalational and intravenous anesthetics have substantial effects on synaptic transmission and much smaller effects on action potential generation or propagation.

Inhalational anesthetics inhibit excitatory synapses and enhance inhibitory synapses in various preparations. The inhalational anesthetics inhibit neurotransmitter release. Inhalational anesthetics also can act postsynaptically, altering the response to released neurotransmitter. These actions are thought to be due to specific interactions of anesthetic agents with neurotransmitter receptors.

Intravenous anesthetics produce a narrower range of physiological effects. Their predominant actions are at the synapse, where they have profound and relatively specific effects on the postsynaptic response to released neurotransmitter. Most of the intravenous agents act predominantly by enhancing inhibitory neurotransmission, whereas ketamine predominantly inhibits excitatory neurotransmission at glutamatergic synapses.

Anatomic Sites of Anesthetic Action

In principle, general anesthetics could interrupt nervous system function at myriad levels, including peripheral sensory neurons, the spinal cord, the brainstem, and the cerebral cortex. Most anesthetics cause, with some

exceptions, a global reduction in CMR and in CBF. A consistent feature of general anesthesia is a suppression of metabolism in the thalamus (Alkire et al., 2008), which serves as a major relay by which sensory input from the periphery ascends to the cortex. Suppression of thalamic activity may serve as a switch between the awake and anesthetized states (Franks, 2008). General anesthesia also suppresses activity in specific regions of the cortex, including the mesial parietal cortex, posterior cingulate cortex, precuneus, and inferior parietal cortex.

Similarities between natural sleep and the anesthetized state suggest that anesthetics might also modulate endogenous sleep-regulating pathways, which include VLPO and tuberomammillary nuclei. VLPO projects inhibitory GABAergic fibers to ascending arousal nuclei, which in turn project to the cortex, forebrain, and subcortical areas; release histamine, 5HT, orexin, NE, and ACh; and mediate wakefulness. Intravenous and inhalational agents with activity at $GABA_A$ receptors can increase the inhibitory effects of VLPO, thereby suppressing consciousness. Dexmedetomidine, an α_2 adrenergic agonist, also increases VLPO-mediated inhibition by suppressing the inhibitory effect of locus ceruleus neurons on VLPO. Finally, both intravenous and inhalational anesthetics depress hippocampal neurotransmission, a probable locus for their amnestic effects.

Parenteral Anesthetics

Parenteral anesthetics are the most common drugs used for anesthetic induction of adults. Their lipophilicity, coupled with the relatively high perfusion of the brain and spinal cord, results in rapid onset and short duration after a single bolus dose. These drugs ultimately accumulate in fatty tissue. Each of these anesthetics has its own unique properties and side effects (Tables 21–1 and 21–2). Propofol is advantageous for procedures where rapid return to a preoperative mental status is desirable. Etomidate usually is reserved for patients at risk for hypotension or myocardial ischemia. Ketamine is best suited for patients with asthma or for children undergoing short, painful procedures. Thiopental has a long-established track record of safety; however, clinical use is limited currently by availability.

Pharmacokinetic Principles

Parenteral anesthetics are small, hydrophobic, substituted aromatic or heterocyclic compounds (Figure 21–1). Hydrophobicity is the key factor governing their pharmacokinetics. After a single intravenous bolus, these drugs preferentially partition into the highly perfused and lipophilic tissues of the brain and spinal cord, where they produce anesthesia within a single circulation time. Subsequently, blood levels fall rapidly, resulting in drug redistribution out of the CNS back into the blood. The anesthetic then diffuses into less-perfused tissues, such as muscle and viscera, and at a slower rate into the poorly perfused but very hydrophobic adipose tissue. Termination of anesthesia after single boluses of parenteral anesthetics primarily reflects redistribution out of the CNS rather than metabolism (see Figure 2–4).

After redistribution, anesthetic blood levels fall according to a complex interaction between the metabolic rate and the amount and lipophilicity of the drug stored in the peripheral compartments. Thus, parenteral anesthetic half-lives are "context sensitive," and the degree to which a $t_{1/2}$ is contextual varies greatly from drug to drug, as might be predicted based on their differing hydrophobicities and metabolic clearances (Figure 21–2; Table 21–1). For example, after a single bolus of thiopental, patients usually emerge from anesthesia within 10 min; however, a patient may require more than a day to awaken from a prolonged thiopental infusion. Most individual variability in sensitivity to parenteral anesthetics can be accounted for by pharmacokinetic factors. For example, in patients with lower cardiac output, the relative perfusion of the brain and the fraction of anesthetic dose delivered to the brain are higher; thus, patients in septic shock or with cardiomyopathy usually require lower doses of parenteral anesthetics. The elderly also typically require a smaller parenteral anesthetic dose, primarily because of a smaller initial volume of distribution.

TABLE 21–1 ■ PHARMACOLOGICAL PROPERTIES OF PARENTERAL ANESTHETICS

DRUG	IV INDUCTION DOSE (mg/kg)	MINIMAL HYPNOTIC LEVEL (µg/mL)	INDUCTION DOSE DURATION (min)	$t_{1/2}\beta$ (h)	CL (mL/min/kg)	PROTEIN BINDING (%)	V_{ss} (L/kg)
Propofol	1.5–2.5	1.1	4–8	1.8	30	98	2.3
Etomidate	0.2–0.4	0.3	4–8	2.9	17.9	76	2.5
Ketamine	1.0–4.5	1	5–10	2.5	19.1	27	3.1
Thiopental	3–5	15.6	5–8	12.1	3.4	85	2.3
Methohexital	1.0–1.5	10	4–7	3.9	10.9	85	2.2

Specific Parenteral Agents

Propofol, Fospropofol

Propofol is the most commonly used parenteral anesthetic in the U.S. Fospropofol is a prodrug form that is converted to propofol in vivo. The clinical pharmacological properties of propofol are summarized in Table 21–1.

The active ingredient in propofol, 2,6-diisopropylphenol, is an oil at room temperature and insoluble in aqueous solutions. Propofol is formulated for intravenous administration as a 1% (10-mg/mL) emulsion in 10% soybean oil, 2.25% glycerol, and 1.2% purified egg phosphatide. In the U.S., disodium EDTA (0.05 mg/mL) or sodium metabisulfite (0.25 mg/mL) is added to inhibit bacterial growth. Propofol should be administered within 4 h of its removal from sterile packaging; unused drug should be discarded. The lipid emulsion formulation of propofol is associated with significant pain on injection and hyperlipidemia.

A new aqueous formulation of propofol, fospropofol, which is not associated with these adverse effects, is available for use for sedation in patients undergoing diagnostic procedures (Fechner et al., 2008). Fospropofol, which itself is inactive, is a phosphate ester prodrug of propofol that is hydrolyzed by endothelial alkaline phosphatases to yield propofol, phosphate, and formaldehyde. The formaldehyde is rapidly converted to formic acid, which then is metabolized by tetrahydrofolate dehydrogenase to CO_2 and water.

Clinical Use and ADME. The induction dose of propofol in a healthy adult is 2–2.5 mg/kg. Dosages should be reduced in the elderly and in the presence of other sedatives and increased in young children. Because of its reasonably short elimination $t_{1/2}$, propofol often is used for maintenance of anesthesia as well as for induction. For short procedures, small boluses (10%–50% of the induction dose) every 5 min or as needed are effective. An infusion of propofol produces a more stable drug level (100–300 µg/kg/min) and is better suited for longer-term anesthetic maintenance. Sedating doses of propofol are 20%–50% of those required for general anesthesia.

Propofol has a context-sensitive $t_{1/2}$ of about 10 min with an infusion lasting 3 h and about 30 min for infusions lasting up to 8 h (see Figure 21–2). Propofol's shorter duration of action after infusion can be explained by its very high clearance, coupled with the slow diffusion of drug from the peripheral to the central compartment. Propofol is metabolized in the liver by conjugation to sulfate and glucuronide to less-active metabolites that are renally excreted. Propofol is highly protein bound, and its

pharmacokinetics, like those of the barbiturates, may be affected by conditions that alter serum protein levels. Clearance of propofol is reduced in the elderly. In neonates, propofol clearance is also reduced. By contrast, in young children, a more rapid clearance in combination with a larger central volume may necessitate larger doses of propofol for induction and maintenance of anesthesia.

Fospropofol produces dose-dependent sedation and can be administered in otherwise-healthy individuals at 2–8 mg/kg intravenously (delivered either as a bolus or by a short infusion over 5–10 min). The optimum dose for sedation is about 6.5 mg/kg. This results in a loss of consciousness in about 10 min. The duration of the sedative effect is approximately 45 min.

Side Effects

Nervous System. The sedation and hypnotic actions of propofol are mediated by its action on $GABA_A$ receptors; agonism at these receptors results in an increased Cl^- conduction and hyperpolarization of neurons. Propofol suppresses the EEG, and, in sufficient doses, can produce burst suppression of the EEG. Propofol decreases the $CMRo_2$, CBF, and intracranial and intraocular pressures by about the same amount as thiopental. Propofol can be used in patients at risk for cerebral ischemia; however, no human outcome studies have been performed to determine its efficacy as a neuroprotectant.

Cardiovascular System. Propofol produces a dose-dependent decrease in blood pressure that is significantly greater than that produced by thiopental. The fall in blood pressure can be explained by both vasodilation and possibly mild depression of myocardial contractility. Propofol appears to blunt the baroreceptor reflex and reduce sympathetic nerve activity. Propofol should be used with caution in patients at risk for, or intolerant of, decreases in blood pressure.

Respiratory System. Propofol produces a slightly greater degree of respiratory depression than thiopental. Patients given propofol should be monitored to ensure adequate oxygenation and ventilation. Propofol appears to be less likely than barbiturates to provoke bronchospasm and may be the induction agent of choice in patients with asthma. The bronchodilator properties of propofol may be attenuated by the metabisulfite preservative in some propofol formulations.

Other Side Effects. Propofol has a significant antiemetic action. Propofol elicits pain on injection that can be reduced with lidocaine and the use of larger arm and antecubital veins. A rare but potentially fatal complication, *PRIS*, has been described primarily in prolonged, higher-dose

TABLE 21–2 ■ SOME PHARMACOLOGICAL EFFECTS OF PARENTERAL ANESTHETICS[a]

DRUG	CBF	$CMRo_2$	ICP	MAP	HR	CO	RR	$\dot{V}_E$
Propofol	– – –	– – –	– – –	– –	+	–	– –	– – –
Etomidate	– – –	– – –	– – –	0	0	0	–	–
Ketamine	++	0	++	+	++	+	0	0
Thiopental	– – –	– – –	– – –	–	+	–	–	– –

[a]Typical effects of a single induction dose in humans; see text for references. Qualitative scale from – – – to +++ signifies slight, moderate, or large decrease or increase, respectively; 0 indicates no significant change.

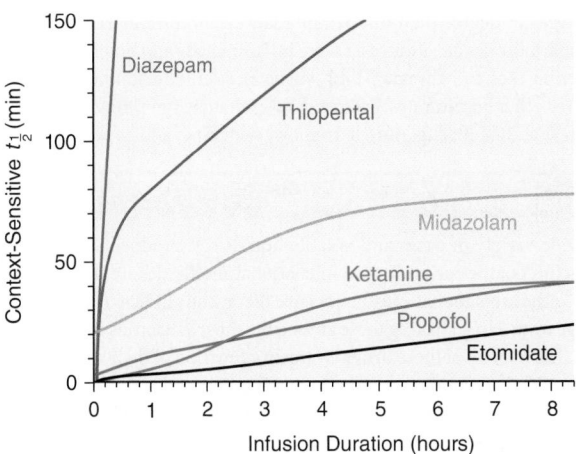

Figure 21–1 *Structures of some parenteral anesthetics.*

infusions of propofol in young or head-injured patients (Kam and Cardone, 2007). PRIS is characterized by metabolic acidosis, hyperlipidemia, rhabdomyolysis, and liver enlargement.

Etomidate

Etomidate is a substituted imidazole that is supplied as the active d-isomer. Etomidate is poorly soluble in water and is formulated as a 2-mg/mL solution in 35% propylene glycol. Unlike thiopental, etomidate does not induce precipitation of neuromuscular blockers or other drugs frequently given during anesthetic induction.

Clinical Use and ADME. Etomidate is primarily used for anesthetic induction of patients at risk for hypotension. Induction doses of etomidate (see Table 21–1) are accompanied by a high incidence of pain on injection and myoclonic movements. Lidocaine effectively reduces the pain of injection, while myoclonic movements can be reduced by premedication with either benzodiazepines or opiates. Etomidate is pharmacokinetically suitable for off-label infusion for anesthetic maintenance (10 μg/kg/min) or sedation (5 μg/kg/min); however, long-term infusions are not recommended because of side effects.

An induction dose of etomidate has a rapid onset; redistribution limits the duration of action. Metabolism occurs in the liver, primarily to inactive compounds. Elimination is both renal (78%) and biliary (22%). Compared to thiopental, the duration of action of etomidate increases less with repeated doses (see Figure 21–2).

Figure 21–2 *Context-sensitive half-time of general anesthetics.* The duration of action of single intravenous doses of anesthetic/hypnotic drugs is similarly short for all and is determined by redistribution of the drugs away from their active sites (see Figure 2–4). However, after prolonged infusions, drug half-lives and durations of action are dependent on a complex interaction between the rate of redistribution of the drug, the amount of drug accumulated in fat, and the drug's metabolic rate. This phenomenon has been termed the *context-sensitive half-time*; that is, the $t_{1/2}$ of a drug can be estimated only if one knows the context—the total dose and over what time period it has been given. Note that the half-times of some drugs such as etomidate, propofol, and ketamine increase only modestly with prolonged infusions; others (e.g., diazepam and thiopental) increase dramatically. (Reproduced with permission from Reves JG, Glass PSA, Lubarsky DA, et al. Intravenous anesthetics. In: Miller RD, et al., eds. *Miller's Anesthesia.* 7th ed. Churchill Livingstone, Philadelphia, **2010**, 718. Copyright © Elsevier.)

Side Effects

Nervous System. Etomidate produces hypnosis and has no analgesic effects. The effects of etomidate on CBF, metabolism, and intracranial and intraocular pressures are similar to those of thiopental (without dropping mean arterial blood pressure). Etomidate produces increased EEG activity in epileptogenic foci and has been associated with seizures.

Cardiovascular System. Cardiovascular stability after induction is a major advantage of etomidate over either propofol or barbiturates. Induction doses of etomidate typically produce a small increase in heart rate and little or no decrease in blood pressure or cardiac output. Etomidate has little effect on coronary perfusion pressure while reducing myocardial O_2 consumption.

Respiratory and Other Side Effects. The degree of respiratory depression due to etomidate appears to be less than that due to thiopental. Like methohexital, etomidate may induce hiccups; it does not significantly stimulate histamine release. Etomidate has been associated with nausea and vomiting. The drug also inhibits adrenal biosynthetic enzymes required for the production of cortisol and some other steroids. Although the hemodynamic profile of etomidate may be advantageous, potential negative effects on steroid synthesis raise concerns about its use in trauma and critically ill patients (van den Heuvel et al., 2013) and obviate etomidate use for long-term infusion. A rapidly metabolized and ultra-short-acting analogue, methoxycarbonyl-etomidate, retains the favorable pharmacological properties of etomidate but does not produce adrenocortical suppression after bolus dosing (Cotton and Claing, 2009).

Ketamine

Ketamine is an arylcyclohexylamine and congener of phencyclidine. Ketamine is supplied as a mixture of the R+ and S- isomers even though the S- isomers is more potent and has fewer side effects. Although more lipophilic than thiopental, ketamine is water soluble.

Clinical Use and ADME. Ketamine is useful for anesthetizing patients at risk for hypotension and bronchospasm and for certain pediatric procedures. However, significant side effects limit its routine use. Ketamine rapidly produces a hypnotic state quite distinct from that of other anesthetics. Patients have profound analgesia, unresponsiveness to commands, and amnesia but may have their eyes open, move their limbs involuntarily, and breathe spontaneously. This cataleptic state has been termed *dissociative anesthesia.* The administration of ketamine has been shown to reduce the development of tolerance to long-term opioid use. Ketamine typically is administered intravenously but also is effective by intramuscular, oral, and rectal routes. Ketamine does not elicit pain on injection or true excitatory behavior as described for methohexital, although involuntary movements produced by ketamine can be mistaken for anesthetic excitement. Low-dose ketamine has potential use in depression (Rasmussen et al., 2013).

The onset and duration of an induction dose of ketamine are determined by the same distribution/redistribution mechanisms operant for all the other parenteral anesthetics. Ketamine is metabolized to norketamine by hepatic CYPs (mainly by 3A4; less by 2B6 and 2D9). Norketamine, with ~20% of the activity of ketamine, is hydroxylated and excreted in urine and bile. Ketamine's large volume of distribution and rapid clearance make it suitable for continuous infusion (see Table 21–1 and Figure 21–2).

Side Effects

Nervous System. Ketamine has indirect sympathomimetic activity and produces distinct behavioral effects. The ketamine-induced cataleptic state is accompanied by nystagmus with pupillary dilation, salivation, lacrimation, and spontaneous limb movements with increased overall muscle tone. Patients are amnestic and unresponsive to painful stimuli. Ketamine produces profound analgesia, a distinct advantage over other parenteral anesthetics. Unlike other parenteral anesthetics, ketamine increases CBF and ICP with minimal alteration of cerebral metabolism. The effects of ketamine on CBF can be readily attenuated by the simultaneous administration of sedative-hypnotic agents.

Emergence delirium, characterized by hallucinations, vivid dreams, and delusions, is a frequent complication of ketamine that can result in serious patient dissatisfaction and can complicate postoperative management. Benzodiazepines reduce the incidence of emergence delirium.

Cardiovascular System. Unlike other anesthetics, induction doses of ketamine typically increase blood pressure, heart rate, and cardiac output. The cardiovascular effects are indirect and are most likely mediated by inhibition of both central and peripheral catecholamine reuptake. Ketamine has direct negative inotropic and vasodilating activity, but these effects usually are overwhelmed by the indirect sympathomimetic action. Thus, ketamine is a useful drug, along with etomidate, for patients at risk for hypotension during anesthesia. While not arrhythmogenic, ketamine increases myocardial O_2 consumption and is not an ideal drug for patients at risk for myocardial ischemia.

Respiratory System. The respiratory effects of ketamine are perhaps the best indication for its use. Induction doses of ketamine produce small and transient decreases in minute ventilation, but respiratory depression is less severe than with other parenteral anesthetics. Ketamine is a potent bronchodilator and is particularly well suited for anesthetizing patients at high risk for bronchospasm.

Barbiturates

Barbiturates are derivatives of barbituric acid with either an oxygen or a sulfur at the 2-position (see Figure 21–1 and Chapters 17 and 19). The three barbiturates most commonly used in clinical anesthesia are sodium *thiopental* (not currently marketed in the U.S.), *thiamylal* (currently licensed in the U.S. only for veterinary use), and *methohexital*. Sodium thiopental was used most frequently for inducing anesthesia.

Barbiturates are supplied as racemic mixtures despite enantioselectivity in their anesthetic potency. Barbiturates are formulated as the sodium salts with 6% sodium carbonate and reconstituted in water or isotonic saline to alkaline solutions, 10 < pH <11. *Mixing barbiturates with drugs in acidic solutions during anesthetic induction can result in precipitation of the barbiturate as the free acid; thus, standard practice is to delay the administration of other drugs until the barbiturate has cleared the intravenous tubing.*

The pharmacological properties and other therapeutic uses of the barbiturates are presented in Chapter 19. Table 19–3 lists the common barbiturates with their clinical pharmacological properties.

Clinical Use and ADME.
Recommended intravenous dosing for parenteral barbiturates in a healthy young adult is given in Table 21–1. The availability of thiopental is limited currently by the lack of an FDA-licensed product and the prohibition of its import due to controversy over its use in administration of the death penalty by lethal injection.

The principal mechanism limiting anesthetic duration after single doses is redistribution of these hydrophobic drugs from the brain to other tissues. However, after multiple doses or infusions, the duration of action of the barbiturates varies considerably depending on their clearances. See Table 21–1 for pharmacokinetic parameters.

Methohexital differs from the other two intravenous barbiturates in its much more rapid clearance; thus, it accumulates less during prolonged infusions. Because of their slow elimination and large volumes of distribution, prolonged infusions or very large doses of thiopental and thiamylal can produce unconsciousness lasting several days. All three barbiturates are primarily eliminated by hepatic metabolism and subsequent renal excretion of inactive metabolites; a small fraction of thiopental undergoes desulfuration to the longer-acting hypnotic pentobarbital. Hepatic disease or other conditions that reduce serum protein concentrations will increase the initial free concentration and hypnotic effect of an induction dose.

Side Effects

Nervous System. Barbiturates suppress the EEG and can produce EEG burst suppression. They reduce the CMR, as measured by CMR_{O_2}, in a dose-dependent manner. As a consequence of the decrease in CMR_{O_2}, CBF and ICP are similarly reduced. Presumably, their CNS depressant activity contributes to their anticonvulsant effects (see Chapter 17). Methohexital can increase ictal activity, and seizures have been described in patients who received doses sufficient to produce burst suppression of the EEG, properties that make methohexital a good choice for anesthesia in patients who undergo electroconvulsive therapy.

Cardiovascular System. The anesthetic barbiturates produce dose-dependent decreases in blood pressure. The effect is due primarily to vasodilation, particularly venodilation, and to a lesser degree to a direct decrease in cardiac contractility. Typically, heart rate increases as a compensatory response to a lower blood pressure, although barbiturates also blunt the baroreceptor reflex. Thiopental maintains the ratio of myocardial O_2 supply to demand in patients with coronary artery disease within a normal blood pressure range. Hypotension can be severe in patients with an impaired ability to compensate for venodilation, such as those with hypovolemia, cardiomyopathy, valvular heart disease, coronary artery disease, cardiac tamponade, or β adrenergic blockade. None of the barbiturates has been shown to be arrhythmogenic.

Respiratory System. Barbiturates are respiratory depressants. Induction doses of thiopental decrease minute ventilation and tidal volume, with a smaller and inconsistent decrease in respiratory rate. Reflex responses to hypercarbia and hypoxia are diminished by anesthetic barbiturates; at higher doses or in the presence of other respiratory depressants such as opiates, apnea can result. Compared to propofol, barbiturates produce a higher incidence of wheezing in asthmatics, attributed to histamine release from mast cells during induction of anesthesia.

Other Side Effects. Short-term administration of barbiturates has no clinically significant effect on the hepatic, renal, or endocrine systems. True allergies to barbiturates are rare; however, direct drug-induced histamine release is occasionally seen. Barbiturates can induce fatal attacks of porphyria in patients with acute intermittent or variegate porphyria and are contraindicated in such patients. Methohexital can produce pain on injection to a greater degree than thiopental. Inadvertent intra-arterial injection of thiobarbiturates can induce a severe inflammatory and potentially necrotic reaction that can threaten limb survival. Methohexital, and to a lesser degree other barbiturates, can produce excitatory symptoms on induction, such as cough, hiccup, muscle tremors, twitching, and hypertonus.

Inhalational Anesthetics

A wide variety of gases and volatile liquids can produce anesthesia. The structures of the currently used inhalational anesthetics are shown in Figure 21–3. The inhalational anesthetics have therapeutic indices (LD_{50}/ED_{50}) that range from 2 to 4, making these among the most dangerous drugs in clinical use. The toxicity of these drugs is largely a function of their side effects, and each of the inhalational anesthetics has a unique side-effect profile. Hence, the selection of an inhalational anesthetic often is based on balancing a patient's pathophysiology with drug side-effect profiles.

Table 21–3 lists the widely varying physical properties of the inhalational agents in clinical use. Ideally, an inhalational agent would produce rapid induction of anesthesia and rapid recovery following discontinuation.

Pharmacokinetic Principles

Inhalational agents behave as gases rather than as liquids and thus require different pharmacokinetic constructs to be used in analyzing their uptake and distribution. Inhalational anesthetics distribute between tissues (or between blood and gas) such that equilibrium is achieved when the partial pressure of anesthetic gas is equal in the two tissues. When a person has breathed an inhalational anesthetic for a sufficiently long time that all tissues are equilibrated with the anesthetic, the partial pressure of the anesthetic in all tissues will be equal to the partial pressure of the anesthetic in inspired gas. While the partial pressure of the anesthetic may be equal in all tissues, the concentration of anesthetic in each tissue will be different.

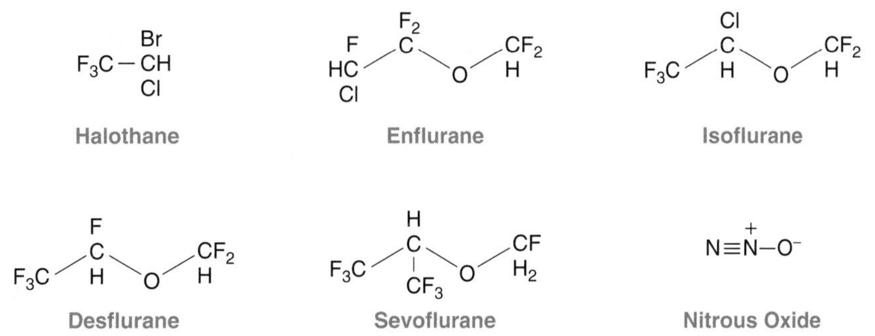

Figure 21–3 *Structures of inhalational general anesthetics*. Note that all inhalational general anesthetic agents except nitrous oxide and halothane are ethers, and that fluorine replaces chlorine in the development of the halogenated agents. All structural differences are associated with important differences in pharmacological properties.

Indeed, anesthetic partition coefficients are defined as the ratio of anesthetic concentration in two tissues when the partial pressures of anesthetic are equal in the two tissues. Blood:gas, brain:blood, and fat:blood partition coefficients for the various inhalational agents are listed in Table 21–3. These partition coefficients show that inhalational anesthetics are more soluble in some tissues (e.g., fat) than they are in others (e.g., blood). In clinical practice, equilibrium is achieved when the partial pressure in inspired gas is equal to the partial pressure in end-tidal (alveolar) gas. For inhalational agents that are not very soluble in blood or any other tissue, equilibrium is achieved quickly, as illustrated for nitrous oxide in Figure 21–4. If an agent is more soluble in a tissue such as fat, equilibrium may take many hours to reach. This occurs because fat represents a huge anesthetic reservoir that will be filled slowly because of the modest blood flow to fat. Anesthesia is produced when anesthetic partial pressure in brain is equal to or greater than MAC. Because the brain is well perfused, anesthetic partial pressure in brain becomes equal to the partial pressure in alveolar gas (and in blood) over the course of several minutes. Therefore, anesthesia is achieved shortly after alveolar partial pressure reaches MAC.

Elimination of inhalational anesthetics is largely a reversal of uptake. For inhalational agents with high blood and tissue solubility, recovery will be a function of the duration of anesthetic administration. This occurs because the accumulated amounts of anesthetic in the fat reservoir will prevent blood (and therefore alveolar) partial pressures from falling rapidly. Patients will be arousable when alveolar partial pressure reaches MAC$_{awake}$, a partial pressure somewhat lower than MAC (see Table 21–3).

Specific Inhalational Agents

Isoflurane

Isoflurane is a volatile liquid at room temperature and is neither flammable nor explosive in mixtures of air or O$_2$. Isoflurane is a commonly used inhalational anesthetic worldwide.

Clinical Use and ADME. Isoflurane is typically used for maintenance of anesthesia *after induction* with other agents because of its pungent odor. Induction of anesthesia can be achieved in less than 10 min with an inhaled concentration of 1.5%–3% isoflurane in O$_2$; this concentration is reduced to 1%–2% (~1–2 MAC) for maintenance of anesthesia. The use of adjunct agents such as opioids or nitrous oxide reduces the concentration of isoflurane required for surgical anesthesia.

Isoflurane has a blood:gas partition coefficient substantially lower than that of enflurane. Consequently, induction with isoflurane and recovery from isoflurane are relatively faster. More than 99% of inhaled isoflurane is excreted unchanged by the lungs. Isoflurane does not appear to be a mutagen, teratogen, or carcinogen.

Side Effects

Cardiovascular System. Isoflurane produces a concentration-dependent decrease in arterial blood pressure; cardiac output is well maintained; hypotension is the result of decreased systemic vascular resistance. Isoflurane produces vasodilation in most vascular beds, with pronounced effects in skin and muscle, and is a potent coronary vasodilator, simultaneously producing increased coronary blood flow and decreased myocardial O$_2$ consumption. Isoflurane significantly attenuates baroreceptor function. Patients anesthetized with isoflurane generally have mildly elevated heart rates as a compensatory response to reduced blood pressure; however, rapid changes in isoflurane concentration can produce both transient tachycardia and hypertension due to isoflurane-induced sympathetic stimulation.

Respiratory System. Isoflurane produces concentration-dependent depression of ventilation. This drug is particularly effective at depressing the ventilatory response to hypercapnia and hypoxia. Although isoflurane is a bronchodilator, it also is an airway irritant and can stimulate airway reflexes during induction of anesthesia, producing coughing and laryngospasm.

TABLE 21–3 ■ PROPERTIES OF INHALATIONAL ANESTHETIC AGENTS

AGENT	MAC^a (vol%)	MAC$_{AWAKE}$^{b} (vol%)	VAPOR PRESSURE (mm Hg, 20°C)	PARTITION COEFFICIENT AT 37°C			% RECOVERED AS METABOLITES
				BLOOD/GAS	BRAIN/BLOOD (Brain/Gas)	FAT/BLOOD (Fat/Gas)	
Isoflurane^c	1.05–1.28	0.4	238	1.43	2.6	45 (91)	0.17
Enflurane	1.68	0.4	175	1.91	1.4	36 (98)	2.4
Sevoflurane	1.4–3.3	0.6	157	0.63–0.69	1.7 (1.2)	48 (50)	3.5
Desflurane	5.2–9.2	2.4	669	0.424	1.3 (0.54)	27 (19)	<0.02
N$_2$O^c	105	60.0	Gas	0.47	1.1	2.3	0.004
Xe	55–71	32.6	Gas	0.115	—	(1.9)	0

^{a}MAC values are expressed as volume percent, the percentage of the atmosphere that is anesthetic. An MAC value greater than 100% means that hyperbaric conditions would be required.
^{b}MAC$_{AWAKE}$ is the concentration at which appropriate responses to commands are lost.
^{c}EC$_{50}$ for memory suppression (vol%): isoflurane, 0.24; N$_2$O, 52.5; values not available for other agents.

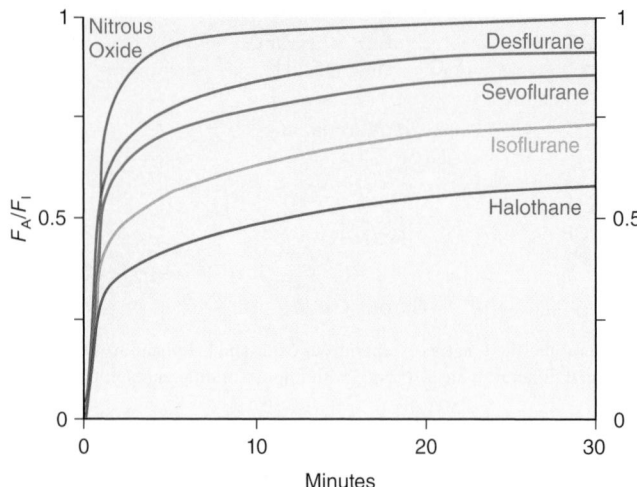

Figure 21–4 *Uptake of inhalational general anesthetics.* The rise in end-tidal alveolar F_A anesthetic concentration toward the inspired F_I concentration is most rapid with the least-soluble anesthetics (nitrous oxide and desflurane) and slowest with the most soluble anesthetic, halothane. All data are from human studies. (Reproduced with permission from Eger EI II. Inhaled anesthetics: uptake and distribution. In: Miller RD et al., eds. *Miller's Anesthesia.* 7th ed. Churchill Livingstone, Philadelphia, **2010**, 540. Copyright © Elsevier.)

Nervous System. Isoflurane dilates the cerebral vasculature, producing increased CBF (Drummond et al., 1983). There is a modest risk of an increase in ICP in patients with preexisting intracranial hypertension. Isoflurane reduces CMRo₂ in a dose-dependent manner.

Muscle. Isoflurane produces some relaxation of skeletal muscle by its central effects. It also enhances the effects of both depolarizing and nondepolarizing muscle relaxants. Like other halogenated inhalational anesthetics, isoflurane relaxes uterine smooth muscle and is not recommended for analgesia or anesthesia for labor and vaginal delivery.

Kidney. Isoflurane reduces renal blood flow and GFR, resulting in a small volume of concentrated urine.

Liver and GI Tract. Splanchnic and hepatic blood flows are reduced with increasing doses of isoflurane as systemic arterial pressure decreases. There are no reported incidences of hepatic toxicity.

Sevoflurane

Sevoflurane is a clear, colorless, volatile liquid at room temperature and must be stored in a sealed bottle. It is nonflammable and nonexplosive in mixtures of air or O₂. However, sevoflurane can undergo an exothermic reaction with desiccated CO₂ absorbent to produce airway burns or spontaneous ignition, explosion, and fire. *Sevoflurane must not be used with an anesthesia machine in which the CO₂ absorbent has been dried by prolonged gas flow through the absorbent. The reaction of sevoflurane with desiccated CO₂ absorbent also can produce CO, which can result in serious patient injury.*

Clinical Use and ADME. Sevoflurane is widely used for outpatient anesthesia because of its rapid recovery profile and because it is not irritating to the airway. Induction of anesthesia is rapidly achieved using inhaled concentrations of 2%–4% sevoflurane. Sevoflurane has properties that make it an ideal induction agent: pleasant smell, rapid onset, and lack of irritation to the airway. Thus, it has largely replaced halothane (not available in the U.S.) as the preferred agent for anesthetic induction in adult and pediatric patients.

The low solubility of sevoflurane in blood and other tissues provides for rapid induction of anesthesia and rapid changes in anesthetic depth following changes in delivered concentration. Approximately 5% of absorbed sevoflurane is metabolized by hepatic CYP2E1, with the predominant product being hexafluoroisopropanol. Hepatic metabolism of sevoflurane also produces inorganic fluoride. Interaction of sevoflurane with soda lime produces decomposition products that may be toxic, such

as compound A, pentafluoroisopropenyl fluoromethyl ether (see kidney discussion under Side Effects).

Side Effects

Cardiovascular System. Sevoflurane produces concentration-dependent decreases in arterial blood pressure (due to systemic vasodilation) and cardiac output. Sevoflurane does not produce tachycardia and thus may be a preferable agent in patients prone to myocardial ischemia.

Respiratory System. Sevoflurane produces a concentration-dependent reduction in tidal volume and increase in respiratory rate in spontaneously breathing patients. The increased respiratory frequency does not compensate for reduced tidal volume, with the net effect being a reduction in minute ventilation and an increase in Paco₂. Sevoflurane is not irritating to the airway and is a potent bronchodilator. As a result, sevoflurane is the most effective clinical bronchodilator of the inhalational anesthetics.

Nervous System. Sevoflurane produces effects on cerebral vascular resistance, CMRo₂, and CBF that are similar to those produced by isoflurane and desflurane. Sevoflurane can increase ICP in patients with poor intracranial compliance, the response to hypocapnia is preserved during sevoflurane anesthesia, and increases in ICP can be prevented by hyperventilation. In children, sevoflurane is associated with delirium on emergence from anesthesia. This delirium is short lived and without any reported adverse long-term sequelae.

Muscle. Sevoflurane produces skeletal muscle relaxation and enhances the effects of nondepolarizing and depolarizing neuromuscular blocking agents.

Kidney. Controversy has surrounded the potential nephrotoxicity of compound A, which is produced by interaction of sevoflurane with the CO₂ absorbent soda lime. Biochemical evidence of transient renal injury has been reported in human volunteers (Eger et al., 1997). Large clinical studies have shown no evidence of increased serum creatinine, blood urea nitrogen, or any other evidence of renal impairment following sevoflurane administration. *The FDA recommends that sevoflurane be administered with fresh gas flows of 1–2 L/min, with sevoflurane exposures not exceeding 2 MAC-hours to minimize exposure to compound A.*

Liver and GI Tract. Sevoflurane is not known to cause hepatotoxicity or alterations of hepatic function tests.

Desflurane

Desflurane is a highly volatile liquid at room temperature (vapor pressure = 669 mm Hg) and must be stored in tightly sealed bottles. Delivery of a precise concentration of desflurane requires the use of a specially heated vaporizer that delivers pure vapor that then is diluted appropriately with other gases (O₂, air, or N₂O). Desflurane is nonflammable and nonexplosive in mixtures of air or O₂.

Clinical Use and ADME. Desflurane is for outpatient surgery because of its rapid onset of action and rapid recovery time. The drug irritates the tracheobronchial tree and can provoke coughing, salivation, and bronchospasm. Anesthesia therefore usually is induced with an intravenous agent, with desflurane subsequently administered for maintenance of anesthesia. Maintenance of anesthesia usually requires inhaled concentrations of 6%–8% (~1 MAC). Lower concentrations of desflurane are required if it is coadministered with nitrous oxide or opioids.

Desflurane has a very low blood:gas partition coefficient (0.42) and also is not very soluble in fat or other peripheral tissues. Thus, the alveolar and blood concentrations rapidly rise to the level of inspired concentration, providing rapid induction of anesthesia and rapid changes in depth of anesthesia following changes in the inspired concentration. Emergence from desflurane anesthesia also is rapid. Desflurane is minimally metabolized; more than 99% of absorbed desflurane is eliminated unchanged through the lungs.

Side Effects

Cardiovascular System. Desflurane produces hypotension primarily by decreasing systemic vascular resistance. Cardiac output is well preserved, as is blood flow to the major organ beds (splanchnic, renal, cerebral, and coronary) (Eger, 1994). Transient tachycardia is often noted with abrupt increases in desflurane's delivered concentration, a result of this desflurane-induced stimulation of the sympathetic nervous system. The hypotensive effects of desflurane do not wane with increasing duration of administration.

Respiratory System. Desflurane causes a concentration-dependent increase in respiratory rate and a decrease in tidal volume. At low concentrations (<1 MAC), the net effect is to preserve minute ventilation. Desflurane concentrations greater than 1 MAC depress minute ventilation, resulting in elevated arterial CO_2 tension ($Paco_2$). Desflurane is a bronchodilator. However, it also is a strong airway irritant and can cause coughing, breath-holding, laryngospasm, and excessive respiratory secretions. *Because of its irritant properties, desflurane is not used as the primary anesthetic for induction of anesthesia.*

Nervous System. Desflurane decreases cerebral vascular resistance and $CMRo_2$. Burst suppression of the EEG is achieved with ~2 MAC; at this level, $CMRo_2$ is reduced by ~50%. Under conditions of normocapnia and normotension, desflurane produces an increase in CBF and can increase ICP in patients with poor intracranial compliance. The vasoconstrictive response to hypocapnia is preserved during desflurane anesthesia, and increases in ICP thus can be prevented by hyperventilation.

Muscle, Kidney, Liver, and GI Tract. Desflurane produces direct skeletal muscle relaxation as well as enhances the effects of nondepolarizing and depolarizing neuromuscular blocking agents. Consistent with its minimal metabolic degradation, desflurane has no reported nephrotoxicity or hepatotoxicity.

Desflurane and Carbon Monoxide. Inhaled anesthetics are administered via a system that permits unidirectional flow of gas and rebreathing of exhaled gases. To prevent rebreathing of CO_2 (which can lead to hypercarbia), CO_2 absorbers are incorporated into the anesthesia delivery circuits. With almost complete desiccation of the CO_2 absorbents, substantial quantities of carbon monoxide can be produced. This effect is greatest with desflurane and can be prevented by the use of well-hydrated, fresh CO_2 absorbent.

Halothane

Halothane is a volatile liquid at room temperature and must be stored in a sealed container. Because halothane is a light-sensitive compound, it is marketed in amber bottles with thymol added as a preservative. Mixtures of halothane with O_2 or air are neither flammable nor explosive.

Clinical Use and ADME. Halothane has been used for maintenance of anesthesia. Concerns over hepatic toxicity have limited its use in developed countries. Halothane can produce fulminant hepatic necrosis (*halothane hepatitis*) in ~1 in 10,000 patients receiving halothane and "is referred to as halothane *hepatitis*" ("Summary," 1966). This syndrome (with a 50% fatality rate) is characterized by fever, anorexia, nausea, and vomiting, developing several days after anesthesia, and can be accompanied by a rash and peripheral eosinophilia. Halothane hepatitis may be the result of an immune response to hepatic proteins that become trifluoroacetylated as a consequence of halothane metabolism. Halothane has a low cost and is still widely used in developing countries. Due to its side-effect profile and the availability of safer agents with more favorable pharmacokinetic profiles, halothane is no longer marketed in the U.S. Those interested in further information on halothane should consult previous recent editions of this book.

Enflurane

Enflurane is a clear, colorless liquid at room temperature and has a mild, sweet odor. Like other inhalational anesthetics, it is volatile and must be stored in a sealed bottle. It is nonflammable and nonexplosive in mixtures of air or oxygen.

Clinical Use and ADME. Enflurane is primarily utilized for maintenance rather than induction of anesthesia. Surgical anesthesia can be induced with enflurane in less than 10 min with an inhaled concentration of 2%–4.5% in oxygen and maintained with concentrations from 0.5% to 3%. Enflurane concentrations required to produce anesthesia are reduced when it is coadministered with nitrous oxide or opioids. Concerns over enflurane's ability to decrease seizure threshold and potentially produce nephrotoxicity have limited its clinical utility in developed countries (Mazze et al., 1977).

Because of its relatively high blood:gas partition coefficient, induction of anesthesia and recovery from enflurane are relatively slow. Enflurane is metabolized to a modest extent, with 2%–8% of absorbed enflurane undergoing oxidative metabolism by hepatic CYP2E1. Fluoride ions are a by-product of enflurane metabolism, but plasma fluoride levels are low and nontoxic. Patients taking isoniazid exhibit enhanced metabolism of enflurane with consequent elevation of serum fluoride.

Side Effects. Enflurane causes a decrease in arterial blood pressure, the result of vasodilation and depression of myocardial contractility, with minimal effects on heart rate. The drug is an effective bronchodilator and produces a pattern of rapid shallow breathing. Due to its actions as a cerebral vasodilator, enflurane can increase ICP. It can produce seizure activity and should not be used in patients with seizure disorders. Enflurane relaxes skeletal and uterine muscle. As with other anesthetic gases, enflurane reduces renal blood flow, GFR, and urinary output.

Nitrous Oxide

Nitrous oxide is a colorless, odorless gas at room temperature. N_2O is sold in steel cylinders and must be delivered through calibrated flowmeters provided on all anesthesia machines. N_2O is neither flammable nor explosive, but it does support combustion as actively as oxygen does when it is present in proper concentration with a flammable anesthetic or material.

Clinical Use and ADME. N_2O is a weak anesthetic agent that has significant analgesic effects. Surgical anesthetic depth is only achieved under hyperbaric conditions. By contrast, analgesia is produced at concentrations as low as 20%. The analgesic property of N_2O is a function of the activation of opioidergic neurons in the periaqueductal gray matter and the adrenergic neurons in the locus ceruleus. N_2O is frequently used in concentrations of ~50% to provide analgesia and mild sedation in outpatient dentistry. N_2O cannot be used at concentrations above 80% because this limits the delivery of adequate O_2. Because of this limitation, N_2O is used primarily as an adjunct to other inhalational or intravenous anesthetics.

Nitrous oxide is very insoluble in blood and other tissues. This results in rapid equilibration between delivered and alveolar anesthetic concentrations and provides for rapid induction of anesthesia and rapid emergence following discontinuation of administration. The rapid uptake of N_2O from alveolar gas serves to concentrate coadministered halogenated anesthetics; this effect (the "second gas effect") speeds induction of anesthesia. On discontinuation of N_2O administration, N_2O gas can diffuse from blood to the alveoli, diluting O_2 in the lung. This can produce an effect called *diffusional hypoxia. To avoid hypoxia, 100% O_2 rather than air should be administered when N_2O is discontinued.* Almost all (99.9%) of the absorbed N_2O is eliminated unchanged by the lungs.

Side Effects

Cardiovascular System. Although N_2O produces a negative inotropic effect on heart muscle in vitro, depressant effects on cardiac function generally are not observed in patients because of the stimulatory effects of N_2O on the sympathetic nervous system. The cardiovascular effects of N_2O also are heavily influenced by the concomitant administration of other anesthetic agents. When N_2O is coadministered with halogenated inhalational anesthetics, one observes increases in heart rate, arterial blood pressure, and cardiac output. In contrast, when N_2O is coadministered with an opioid, one generally sees decreases in arterial blood pressure and cardiac output. N_2O also increases venous tone in both the peripheral and the pulmonary vasculature. The effects of N_2O on pulmonary vascular resistance can be exaggerated in patients with preexisting pulmonary hypertension; thus, the drug generally is not used in these patients.

Respiratory System. N_2O causes modest increases in respiratory rate and decreases in tidal volume in spontaneously breathing patients. Even modest concentrations of N_2O markedly depress the ventilatory response to hypoxia. Thus, it is prudent to monitor arterial O_2 saturation directly in patients receiving or recovering from N_2O.

Nervous System. N_2O can significantly increase CBF and ICP. This cerebral vasodilatory capacity of N_2O is significantly attenuated by the simultaneous administration of intravenous agents such as opiates and propofol. By contrast, the combination of N_2O and inhaled agents results in greater vasodilation than the administration of the inhaled agent alone at equivalent anesthetic depth.

Muscle. N$_2$O does not relax skeletal muscle and does not enhance the effects of neuromuscular blocking drugs.

Kidney, Liver, and GI Tract. N$_2$O is not known to have nephrotoxic or hepatotoxic effects.

Other Adverse Effects. A major problem with N$_2$O is that it will exchange with N$_2$ in any air-containing cavity in the body. Moreover, because of their differential blood:gas partition coefficients, N$_2$O will enter the cavity faster than N$_2$ escapes, thereby increasing the volume or pressure in this cavity. Examples of air collections that can be expanded by N$_2$O include a pneumothorax, an obstructed middle ear, an air embolus, an obstructed loop of bowel, an intraocular air bubble, a pulmonary bulla, and intracranial air. N$_2$O should be avoided in these clinical settings.

Nitrous oxide interacts with the cobalt of vitamin B$_{12}$, thereby preventing vitamin B$_{12}$ from acting as a cofactor for methionine synthase (Sanders and Maze, 2007). Inactivation of methionine synthase can produce signs of vitamin B$_{12}$ deficiency, including megaloblastic anemia and peripheral neuropathy, a particular concern in patients with malnutrition, vitamin B$_{12}$ deficiency, or alcoholism. The clinical use of N$_2$O is controversial due to its potential metabolic effects related to increased homocysteine and changes in DNA and protein synthesis (Ko et al., 2014). For this reason, N$_2$O is not used as a chronic analgesic or as a sedative in critical care settings.

Xenon

Xenon, an inert gaseous element, is not approved for use in the U.S. and is unlikely to enjoy widespread use because it is a rare gas that cannot be manufactured and must be extracted from air; thus, xenon is expensive and available in limited quantities. Xenon, unlike other anesthetic agents, has minimal cardiorespiratory and other side effects.

Xenon exerts its analgesic and anesthetic effects at a number of receptor systems in the CNS. Of these, noncompetitive antagonism of the NMDA receptor and agonism at the TREK channel (a member of the two-pore K$^+$ channel family) are thought to be the central mechanisms of xenon action (Franks and Honore, 2004).

Xenon is extremely insoluble in blood and other tissues, providing for rapid induction and emergence from anesthesia. It is sufficiently potent to produce surgical anesthesia when administered with 30% oxygen. However, supplementation with an intravenous agent such as propofol appears to be required for clinical anesthesia. Xenon is well tolerated in patients of advanced age. No long-term side effects from xenon anesthesia have been reported.

Anesthetic Adjuncts

A general anesthetic is usually given with adjuncts to augment specific components of anesthesia, permitting lower doses of general anesthetics with fewer side effects.

Benzodiazepines

Benzodiazepines (see Chapters 15 and 19) can produce anesthesia similar to that of barbiturates; they are more commonly used for sedation rather than general anesthesia because prolonged amnesia and sedation may result from anesthetizing doses. As adjuncts, benzodiazepines are used for anxiolysis, amnesia, and sedation prior to induction of anesthesia or for sedation during procedures not requiring general anesthesia. The benzodiazepine most frequently used in the perioperative period is midazolam, followed distantly by diazepam and lorazepam.

Midazolam is water soluble and typically is administered intravenously but also can be given orally, intramuscularly, or rectally; oral midazolam is particularly useful for sedation of young children. Midazolam produces minimal venous irritation (as opposed to diazepam and lorazepam, which are formulated in propylene glycol and are painful on injection, sometimes producing thrombophlebitis). Midazolam has the pharmacokinetic advantage, particularly over lorazepam, of being more rapid in onset and shorter in duration of effect. Sedative doses of midazolam (0.01–0.05 mg/kg IV) reach peak effect in about 2 min and provide sedation for approximately 30 min. Elderly patients tend to be more sensitive to and have a

slower recovery from benzodiazepines. Midazolam is metabolized principally by hepatic CYP3A4, and drug interactions with inducers, inhibitors, and substrates of that CYP are predictable. Either for prolonged sedation or for general anesthetic maintenance, midazolam is more suitable than other benzodiazepines for infusion, although midazolam's duration of action ($t_{1/2}$) does significantly increase with prolonged infusions (see Figure 21–2). Benzodiazepines reduce CBF and cerebral metabolism, but at equianesthetic doses are less effective than barbiturates in this respect. Benzodiazepines modestly decrease blood pressure and respiratory drive, occasionally resulting in apnea.

α$_2$ Adrenergic Agonists

Dexmedetomidine is a selective α$_2$ adrenergic receptor agonist (Kamibayashi and Maze, 2000) used for short-term (<24 h) sedation of critically ill adults and for sedation prior to and during surgical or other medical procedures in nonintubated patients. Activation of the α$_{2A}$ adrenergic receptor by dexmedetomidine produces both sedation and analgesia.

The recommended loading dose is 1 μg/kg given over 10 min, followed by infusion at a rate of 0.2–0.7 μg/kg/h. Reduced doses should be considered in patients with risk factors for severe hypotension. Dexmedetomidine is highly protein bound and is metabolized primarily in the liver; the glucuronide and methyl conjugates are excreted in the urine. Common side effects of dexmedetomidine include hypotension and bradycardia, attributed to decreased catecholamine release by activation peripherally and in the CNS of the α$_{2A}$ receptor. Nausea and dry mouth also are common untoward reactions. At higher drug concentrations, the α$_{2B}$ subtype is activated, resulting in hypertension and a further decrease in heart rate and cardiac output. Dexmedetomidine provides sedation and analgesia with minimal respiratory depression. However, dexmedetomidine does not appear to provide reliable amnesia, and additional agents may be needed.

Analgesics

Analgesics typically are administered with general anesthetics to reduce anesthetic requirements and minimize hemodynamic changes produced by painful stimuli. Nonsteroidal anti-inflammatory drugs, cyclooxygenase 2 inhibitors, and acetaminophen (see Chapter 38) sometimes provide adequate analgesia for minor surgical procedures. However, opioids are the primary analgesics used during the perioperative period because of the rapid and profound analgesia they produce. Fentanyl, sufentanil, alfentanil, remifentanil, meperidine, and morphine are the major parenteral opioids used in the perioperative period. The primary analgesic activity of each of these drugs is produced by agonist activity at μ opioid receptors (see Chapter 20).

The choice of a perioperative opioid is based primarily on duration of action because, at appropriate doses, all produce similar analgesia and side effects. Remifentanil has an ultrashort duration of action (<10 min), accumulates minimally with repeated doses, and is particularly well suited for procedures that are briefly painful. Single doses of fentanyl, sufentanil, and alfentanil all have similar intermediate durations of action (30, 20, and 15 min, respectively), but recovery after prolonged administration varies considerably. Fentanyl's duration of action lengthens the most with infusion, sufentanil's much less so, and alfentanil's the least.

The frequency and severity of nausea, vomiting, and pruritus after emergence from anesthesia are increased by all opioids to about the same degree. A useful side effect of meperidine is its capacity to reduce shivering, a common problem during emergence from anesthesia; other opioids are not as efficacious against shivering, perhaps due to less κ receptor agonism. Finally, opioids often are administered intrathecally and epidurally for management of acute and chronic pain (see Chapter 20). Neuraxial opioids with or without local anesthetics can provide profound analgesia for many surgical procedures; however, respiratory depression and pruritus usually limit their use to major operations.

Neuromuscular Blocking Agents

The practical aspects of the use of neuromuscular blockers as anesthetic adjuncts are briefly described here. The detailed pharmacology of this drug class is presented in Chapter 11.

Depolarizing (e.g., succinylcholine) and nondepolarizing (e.g., vecuronium) muscle relaxants often are administered during the induction of anesthesia to relax muscles of the jaw, neck, and airway and thereby facilitate laryngoscopy and endotracheal intubation. Nondepolarizing muscle relaxants are generally better tolerated. Barbiturates will precipitate when mixed with muscle relaxants and should be allowed to clear from the intravenous line prior to injection of a muscle relaxant. The action of nondepolarizing muscle relaxants usually is antagonized, once muscle paralysis is no longer desired, with an acetylcholinesterase inhibitor such as neostigmine or edrophonium (see Chapter 10), in combination with a muscarinic receptor antagonist (e.g., glycopyrrolate or atropine; see Chapter 9) to offset the muscarinic activation resulting from esterase inhibition. Sugammadex, a first-in-class selective relaxant binding agent specific for reversal of rocuronium muscle-relaxing effect, is approved in Europe and awaits FDA approval in the U.S. (Ledowski, 2015).

Anesthetic Toxicity and Cytoprotection

The conventional view of general anesthesia is that anesthetics produce a reversible loss of consciousness and that CNS function returns to basal levels on termination of anesthesia and recovery of anesthesia. Recent data, however, cast doubt on this notion. Exposure of rodents to anesthetic agents during the period of synaptogenesis results in widespread neurodegeneration in the developing brain (Jevtovic-Todorovic et al., 2003). This neuronal injury resulted in disturbed electrophysiologic function and cognitive dysfunction in adolescent and adult rodents exposed to anesthetics during the neonatal period. The cognitive deficits attendant with neonatal anesthetic exposure have been attributed to neuronal apoptosis; however, recently published data have cast doubt on this premise. There is convincing data that exposure to anesthetics in the neonatal period leads to actin cytoskeleton dysregulation and profound synaptic loss; this may contribute to later cognitive and behavioral dysfunction. A variety of agents, including isoflurane, propofol, midazolam, nitrous oxide, and thiopental, manifest this toxicity (Patel and Sun, 2009). The underlying mechanism(s) in animal models are unclear, and the threat to humans is still uncertain.

By contrast, anesthetics reduce ischemic injury to a variety of tissues, including the heart and brain. This protective effect is robust and results in better functional outcomes in comparison to ischemic injury that occurs in the unanesthetized awake subjects. In the brain, several mechanisms for anesthetic-mediated protection have been proposed, including suppression of excitotoxicity from excess glutamate release, reduction in inflammation, and increased prosurvival signaling (Head and Patel, 2007). In the heart, the molecular mechanisms attendant to anesthetic-mediated protection include activation of "classical" preconditioning pathways, including GPCRs, endothelial NO synthase, survival protein kinases, PKC, reactive oxygen species, ATP-dependent K^+ channels, and the mitochondrial permeable transition pore (Kunst and Klein, 2015).

Therapeutic Gases

Oxygen

Oxygen is essential to life. Hypoxia is a life-threatening condition in which O_2 delivery is inadequate to meet the metabolic demands of the tissues. Hypoxia may result from alterations in tissue perfusion, decreased O_2 tension in the blood, or decreased O_2 carrying capacity. In addition, hypoxia may result from restricted O_2 transport from the microvasculature to cells or impaired utilization within the cell. An inadequate supply of O_2 ultimately results in the cessation of aerobic metabolism and oxidative phosphorylation, depletion of high-energy compounds, cellular dysfunction, and death.

Normal Oxygenation

Oxygen makes up 21% of air, which at sea level represents a partial pressure of 21 kPa (158 mm Hg). While the fraction (percentage) of O_2 remains constant regardless of atmospheric pressure, the Po_2 decreases

with lower atmospheric pressure. Ascent to elevated altitude reduces the uptake and delivery of O_2 to the tissues, whereas increases in atmospheric pressure (e.g., hyperbaric therapy or breathing at depth) raise the Po_2 in inspired air and increase gas uptake. As the air is delivered to the distal airways and alveoli, the Po_2 decreases by dilution with CO_2 and water vapor and by uptake into the blood.

Under ideal conditions, when ventilation and perfusion are well matched, the alveolar Po_2 will be about 14.6 kPa (110 mm Hg). The corresponding alveolar partial pressures of water and CO_2 are 6.2 kPa (47 mm Hg) and 5.3 kPa (40 mm Hg), respectively. Under normal conditions, there is complete equilibration of alveolar gas and lung capillary blood, and the Po_2 in end-capillary blood is typically within a fraction of a kilopascal of that in the alveoli. The Po_2 in arterial blood, however, is further reduced by venous admixture (shunt), the addition of mixed venous blood from the pulmonary artery, which has a Po_2 of about 5.3 kPa (40 mm Hg). Together, the diffusional barrier, ventilation-perfusion mismatches, and the shunt fraction are the major causes of the alveolar-to-arterial O_2 gradient, which is normally 1.3–1.6 kPa (10–12 mm Hg) when air is breathed and 4.0–6.6 kPa (30–50 mm Hg) when 100% O_2 is breathed. O_2 is delivered to the tissue capillary beds by the circulation and again follows a gradient out of the blood and into cells. Tissue extraction of O_2 typically reduces the Po_2 of venous blood by an additional 7.3 kPa (55 mm Hg). Although the Po_2 at the site of cellular O_2 utilization—the mitochondria—is not known, oxidative phosphorylation can continue at a Po_2 of only a few millimeters of mercury.

In the blood, O_2 is carried primarily in chemical combination with hemoglobin and is to a small extent dissolved in solution. The quantity of O_2 combined with hemoglobin depends on the Po_2, as illustrated by the sigmoidal oxyhemoglobin dissociation curve (Figure 21–5). Hemoglobin is about 98% saturated with O_2 when air is breathed under normal circumstances, and it binds 1.3 mL of O_2 per gram when fully saturated. The steep slope of this curve with falling Po_2 facilitates unloading of O_2 from hemoglobin at the tissue level and reloading when desaturated mixed venous blood arrives at the lung. Shifting of the curve to the right with increasing temperature, increasing Pco_2, and decreasing pH, as is found in metabolically active tissues, lowers the O_2 saturation for the same Po_2 and thus delivers additional O_2 where and when it is most needed. However, the flattening of the curve with higher Po_2 indicates that increasing blood Po_2 by inspiring O_2-enriched mixtures can increase the amount of O_2 carried by hemoglobin only minimally. Because of the low solubility of O_2 (0.226 mL/L per kPa or 0.03 mL/L per mm Hg at 37°C), breathing 100% O_2 can increase the amount of O_2 dissolved in blood by only 15 mL/L, less than one-third of normal metabolic demands. However, if the inspired Po_2 is increased to 3 atm (304 kPa) in a hyperbaric chamber, the amount of dissolved O_2 is sufficient to meet normal metabolic demands even in the absence of hemoglobin (Table 21–4).

Oxygen Deprivation. *Hypoxemia* generally implies a failure of the respiratory system to oxygenate arterial blood. Classically, there are five causes of hypoxemia:

- Low F_{IO_2}
- Hypoventilation
- Ventilation-perfusion mismatch
- Shunt or venous admixture
- Increased diffusion barrier

The term *hypoxia* denotes insufficient oxygenation of the tissues. In addition to failure of the respiratory system to oxygenate the blood adequately, a number of other factors can contribute to hypoxia at the tissue level. These may be divided into categories of O_2 delivery and O_2 utilization. O_2 delivery decreases globally when cardiac output falls or locally when regional blood flow is compromised, such as from a vascular occlusion (e.g., stenosis, thrombosis, or microvascular occlusion) or increased downstream pressure (e.g., compartment syndrome, venous stasis, or venous hypertension). Decreased O_2 carrying capacity of the blood likewise will reduce O_2 delivery, such as occurs with anemia, carbon monoxide poisoning, or hemoglobinopathy. Finally, hypoxia may occur when

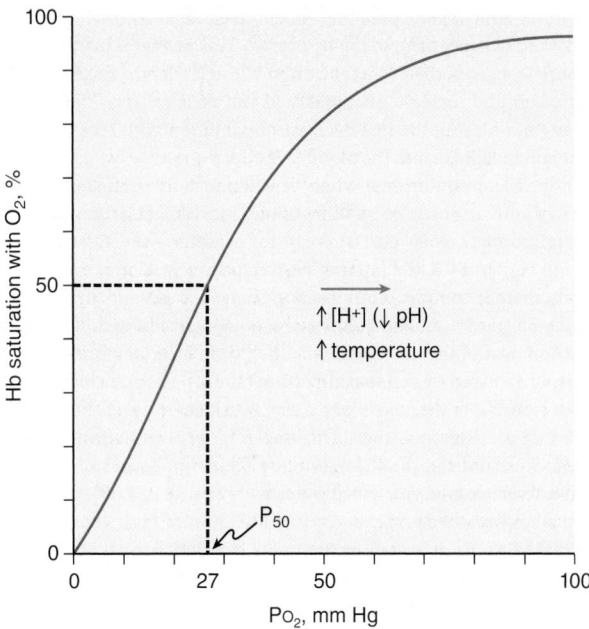

Figure 21-5 *Oxyhemoglobin dissociation curve for whole blood.* The relationship between P_{O_2} and Hb saturation is shown. The P_{50}, or the P_{O_2} resulting in 50% saturation, is indicated. An increase in temperature or a decrease in pH (as in working muscle) shifts this relationship to the right, reducing the hemoglobin saturation at the same P_{O_2} and thus aiding in the delivery of O_2 to the tissues.

transport of O_2 from the capillaries to the tissues is decreased (edema) or utilization of the O_2 by the cells is impaired (CN^- toxicity).

Effects of Hypoxia

Cellular and Metabolic Effects. At the molecular level, nonlethal hypoxia produces a marked alteration in gene expression, mediated in part by hypoxia inducible factor 1α (Guimarães-Camboa et al., 2015).

When the mitochondrial P_{O_2} falls below about 0.13 kPa (1 mm Hg), aerobic metabolism stops, and the less-efficient anaerobic pathways of glycolysis become responsible for the production of cellular energy. End products of anaerobic metabolism, such as lactic acid, are released into the circulation in measurable quantities. Energy-dependent ion pumps slow, and transmembrane ion gradients dissipate. Intracellular concentrations

of Na^+, Ca^{2+}, and H^+ increase, finally leading to cell death. The time course of cellular demise depends on the relative metabolic demands, oxygen storage capacity, and anaerobic capacity of the individual organs. Restoration of perfusion and oxygenation prior to hypoxic cell death paradoxically can result in an accelerated form of cell injury (ischemia-reperfusion syndrome), which is thought to result from the generation of highly reactive oxygen free radicals.

Cell and Organ Survival. Ultimately, hypoxia results in the cessation of aerobic metabolism, exhaustion of high-energy intracellular stores, cellular dysfunction, and death. The time course of cellular demise depends on the tissue's relative metabolic requirements, O_2 and energy stores, and anaerobic capacity. Survival times (the time from the onset of circulatory arrest to significant organ dysfunction) range from 1–2 min in the cerebral cortex to around 5 min in the heart and 10 min in the kidneys and liver, with the potential for some degree of recovery if reperfused. Revival times (the duration of hypoxia beyond which recovery is no longer possible) are about four to five times longer.

Organ System Effects. Less-severe degrees of hypoxia have progressive physiological effects on different organ systems (Nunn, 2005).

Respiratory System. Hypoxia stimulates the carotid and aortic baroreceptors to cause increases in both the rate and the depth of ventilation. Minute volume almost doubles when normal individuals inspire gas with a P_{O_2} of 6.6 kPa (50 mm Hg). Dyspnea is not always experienced with simple hypoxia but occurs when the respiratory minute volume approaches half the maximal breathing capacity; this may occur with minimum exertion in patients in whom maximal breathing capacity is reduced by lung disease. In general, little warning precedes the loss of consciousness resulting from hypoxia.

Cardiovascular System. Hypoxia causes reflex activation of the sympathetic nervous system by both autonomic and humoral mechanisms, resulting in tachycardia and increased cardiac output. Peripheral vascular resistance, however, decreases primarily through local autoregulatory mechanisms, with the net result that blood pressure generally is maintained unless hypoxia is prolonged or severe. In contrast to the systemic circulation, hypoxia causes pulmonary vasoconstriction and hypertension, an extension of the normal regional vascular response that matches perfusion with ventilation to optimize gas exchange in the lung (hypoxic pulmonary vasoconstriction).

CNS. The CNS is least able to tolerate hypoxia. Hypoxia is manifest initially by decreased intellectual capacity and impaired judgment and psychomotor ability. This state progresses to confusion and restlessness and ultimately to stupor, coma, and death as the arterial P_{O_2} decreases below 4–5.3 kPa (30–40 mm Hg). Victims often are unaware of this progression.

TABLE 21-4 ■ THE CARRIAGE OF OXYGEN IN BLOOD[a]

ARTERIAL P_{O_2} kPa (mm Hg)	ARTERIAL O_2 CONTENT (mL O_2/L)			MIXED VENOUS P_{O_2} kPa (mm Hg)	MIXED VENOUS O_2 CONTENT (mL O_2/L)			EXAMPLES
	DISSOLVED	BOUND TO Hb	TOTAL		DISSOLVED	BOUND TO Hb	TOTAL	
4.0 (30)	0.9	109	109.9	2.7 (20)	0.6	59	59.6	High altitude; respiratory failure breathing air
12.0 (90)	2.7	192	194.7	5.5 (41)	1.2	144	145.2	Normal person breathing air
39.9 (300)	9.0	195	204	5.9 (44)	1.3	153	154.3	Normal person breathing 50% O_2
79.7 (600)	18	196	214	6.5 (49)	1.5	163	164.5	Normal person breathing 100% O_2
239 (1800)	54	196	250	20.0 (150)	4.5	196	200.5	Normal person breathing hyperbaric O_2

[a]This table illustrates the carriage of oxygen in the blood under a variety of circumstances. As arterial O_2 tension increases, the amount of dissolved O_2 increases in direct proportion to the P_{O_2}, but the amount of oxygen bound to Hb reaches a maximum of 196 mL O_2/L (100% saturation of Hb at 15 g/dL). Further increases in O_2 content require increases in dissolved oxygen. At 100% inspired O_2, dissolved O_2 still provides only a small fraction of total demand. Hyperbaric oxygen therapy is required to increase the amount of dissolved oxygen to supply all or a large part of metabolic requirements. Note that, during hyperbaric oxygen therapy, the hemoglobin in the mixed venous blood remains fully saturated with O_2. The figures in this table are approximate and are based on the assumptions of 15 g/dL Hb, 50 mL O_2/L whole-body oxygen extraction, and constant cardiac output. When severe anemia is present, arterial P_{O_2} remains the same, but arterial content is lower; oxygen extraction continues, resulting in lower O_2 content and tension in mixed venous blood. Similarly, as cardiac output falls significantly, the same oxygen extraction occurs from a smaller volume of blood and results in lower mixed venous oxygen content and tension.

Adaptation to Hypoxia

Long-term hypoxia results in adaptive physiological changes; these have been studied most thoroughly in persons exposed to high altitude. Adaptations include increased numbers of pulmonary alveoli, increased concentrations of hemoglobin in blood and myoglobin in muscle, and a decreased ventilatory response to hypoxia. Short-term exposure to high altitude produces similar adaptive changes. In susceptible individuals, however, acute exposure to high altitude may produce *acute mountain sickness*, a syndrome characterized by headache, nausea, dyspnea, sleep disturbances, and impaired judgment progressing to pulmonary and cerebral edema. Mountain sickness is treated with rest and analgesics when mild or supplemental O_2, descent to lower altitude, or an increase in ambient pressure when more severe. Acetazolamide (a carbonic anhydrase inhibitor) and dexamethasone also may be helpful. The syndrome usually can be avoided by a slow ascent to altitude, adequate hydration, and prophylactic use of acetazolamide or dexamethasone.

Examples of "normal" hypoxia are widespread, and the comparative physiology of hypoxic tolerance offers clues to the mechanisms involved. Aspects of fetal and newborn physiology are strongly reminiscent of adaptation mechanisms found in hypoxia-tolerant animals (Guimarães-Camboa et al., 2015; Mortola, 1999), including shifts in the oxyhemoglobin dissociation curve (fetal hemoglobin), reductions in metabolic rate and body temperature (hibernation-like mode), reductions in heart rate and circulatory redistribution (as in diving mammals), and redirection of energy utilization from growth to maintenance metabolism. These adaptations probably account for the relative tolerance of the fetus and neonate to both chronic (uterine insufficiency) and short-term hypoxia.

Oxygen Inhalation

Physiological Effects. O_2 inhalation is used primarily to reverse or prevent the development of hypoxia. However, when O_2 is breathed in excessive amounts or for prolonged periods, secondary physiological changes and toxic effects can occur.

Respiratory System. Inhalation of O_2 at 1 atm or above causes a small degree of respiratory depression in normal subjects, presumably as a result of loss of tonic chemoreceptor activity. However, ventilation typically increases within a few minutes of O_2 inhalation because of a paradoxical increase in the tension of CO_2 in tissues. This increase results from the increased concentration of oxyhemoglobin in venous blood, which causes less-efficient removal of carbon dioxide from the tissues. Expansion of poorly ventilated alveoli is maintained in part by the nitrogen content of alveolar gas; nitrogen is poorly soluble and thus remains in the air spaces while O_2 is absorbed. High O_2 concentrations delivered to poorly ventilated lung regions dilute the nitrogen content and can promote absorption atelectasis (partial or complete collapse of the lung), occasionally resulting in an increase in shunt and a paradoxical worsening of hypoxemia after a period of O_2 administration.

Cardiovascular System. Heart rate and cardiac output are slightly reduced when 100% O_2 is breathed; blood pressure changes little. Elevated pulmonary artery pressures in patients living at high altitude who have chronic hypoxic pulmonary hypertension may reverse with O_2 therapy or return to sea level. In neonates with congenital heart disease and left-to-right shunting of cardiac output, O_2 supplementation must be regulated carefully because of the risk of further reducing pulmonary vascular resistance and increasing pulmonary blood flow.

Metabolism. Inhalation of 100% O_2 does not produce detectable changes in O_2 consumption, CO_2 production, respiratory quotient, or glucose utilization.

Oxygen Administration

Oxygen is supplied as a compressed gas in steel cylinders; purity of 99% is *medical grade*. For safety, O_2 cylinders and piping are color coded (green in the U.S.), and some form of mechanical indexing of valve connections is used to prevent the connection of other gases to O_2 systems.

Oxygen is delivered by inhalation except during extracorporeal circulation, when it is dissolved directly into the circulating blood. A closed delivery system with an endotracheal tube produces an airtight seal to the patient's airway, and complete separation of inspired from expired gases can precisely control F_{IO_2}. In all other systems, such as nasal cannulas and face masks, the actual delivered F_{IO_2} will depend on the ventilatory pattern (i.e., rate, tidal volume, inspiratory-expiratory time ratio, and inspiratory flow) and delivery system characteristics.

Monitoring of Oxygenation. Monitoring and titration are required to meet the therapeutic goal of O_2 therapy and to avoid complications and side effects. Although cyanosis is a physical finding of substantial clinical importance, it is not an early, sensitive, or reliable index of oxygenation. Noninvasive monitoring of arterial O_2 saturation can be achieved using transcutaneous pulse oximetry, in which O_2 saturation is measured from the differential absorption of light by oxyhemoglobin and deoxyhemoglobin and the arterial saturation determined from the pulsatile component of this signal. Pulse oximetry measures hemoglobin saturation and not P_{O_2}. It is not sensitive to increases in P_{O_2} that exceed levels required to saturate the blood fully. Pulse oximetry is useful for monitoring the adequacy of oxygenation during procedures requiring sedation or anesthesia, rapid evaluation and monitoring of potentially compromised patients, and titrating O_2 therapy in situations where toxicity from O_2 or side effects of excess O_2 are of concern. A specific tool for measuring cerebral oxygenation is near-infrared spectroscopy (Guarracino, 2008).

Complications of Oxygen Therapy. In addition to the potential to promote absorption atelectasis and depress ventilation, high flows of dry O_2 can dry out and irritate mucosal surfaces of the airway and the eyes, as well as decrease mucociliary transport and clearance of secretions. Humidified O_2 thus should be used when prolonged therapy (>1 h) is required. Finally, any O_2-enriched atmosphere constitutes a fire hazard, and appropriate precautions must be taken. Hypoxemia can occur despite the administration of supplemental O_2. Therefore, it is essential that both O_2 saturation and adequacy of ventilation be assessed frequently.

Therapeutic Uses of Oxygen

Correction of Hypoxia. The primary therapeutic use of O_2 is to correct hypoxia. Hypoxia is most commonly a manifestation of an underlying disease, and administration of O_2 thus should be viewed as temporizing therapy. Efforts must be directed at correcting the cause of the hypoxia. Hypoxia resulting from most pulmonary diseases can be alleviated at least partially by administration of O_2, allowing time for definitive therapy to reverse the primary process.

Reduction of Partial Pressure of an Inert Gas. Because nitrogen constitutes some 79% of ambient air, it also is the predominant gas in most gas-filled spaces in the body. In situations such as bowel distension from obstruction or ileus, intravascular air embolism, or pneumothorax, it is desirable to reduce the volume of air-filled spaces. Because nitrogen is relatively insoluble, inhalation of high concentrations of O_2 (and thus low concentrations of nitrogen) rapidly lowers the total-body partial pressure of nitrogen and provides a substantial gradient for the removal of nitrogen from gas spaces. Administration of O_2 for air embolism is also beneficial because it helps to relieve localized hypoxia distal to the vascular obstruction. In the case of *decompression sickness*, or *bends*, lowering the inert gas tension in blood and tissues by O_2 inhalation prior to or during barometric decompression reduces the supersaturation that occurs after decompression so that bubbles do not form.

Hyperbaric Oxygen Therapy. O_2 can be administered at greater than atmospheric pressure in hyperbaric chambers (Thom, 2009). Clinical uses of hyperbaric O_2 therapy include the treatment of trauma, burns, radiation damage, infections, nonhealing ulcers, skin grafts, spasticity, and other neurological conditions. Hyperbaric O_2 may be useful in generalized hypoxia. In carbon monoxide poisoning, hemoglobin and myoglobin become unavailable for O_2 binding because of the high affinity of these proteins for carbon monoxide. High P_{O_2} facilitates competition of O_2 for hemoglobin binding sites as carbon monoxide is exchanged in the alveoli. In addition, hyperbaric O_2 increases the availability of dissolved O_2 in the blood (see Table 21–4). Adverse effects of hyperbaric O_2 therapy include middle ear barotrauma, CNS toxicity, seizures, lung toxicity, and aspiration pneumonia.

Hyperbaric O_2 therapy has two components: increased hydrostatic pressure and increased O_2 pressure. Both factors are necessary for the treatment of decompression sickness and air embolism. The hydrostatic pressure reduces bubble volume, and the absence of inspired nitrogen increases the gradient for elimination of nitrogen and reduces hypoxia in downstream tissues. Increased O_2 pressure at the tissue is the primary therapeutic goal for other indications for hyperbaric O_2. A small increase in Po_2 in ischemic areas enhances the bactericidal activity of leukocytes and increases angiogenesis. Repetitive brief exposures to hyperbaric O_2 may enhance therapy for chronic refractory osteomyelitis, osteoradionecrosis, crush injury, or the recovery of compromised skin and tissue grafts. Increased O_2 tension can be bacteriostatic and useful in the treatment of the spread of infection with *Clostridium perfringens* and clostridial myonecrosis (gas gangrene).

Oxygen Toxicity

Oxygen can have deleterious actions at the cellular level. O_2 toxicity may result from increased production of hydrogen peroxide and reactive intermediates such as superoxide anion, singlet oxygen, and hydroxyl radicals that attack and damage lipids, proteins, and other macromolecules, especially those in biological membranes. A number of factors limit the toxicity of oxygen-derived reactive agents, including enzymes such as superoxide dismutase, glutathione peroxidase, and catalase, which scavenge toxic oxygen by-products, and reducing agents such as iron, glutathione, and ascorbate. These factors, however, are insufficient to limit the destructive actions of oxygen when patients are exposed to high concentrations over an extended time period. Tissues show differential sensitivity to oxygen toxicity, which is likely the result of differences in both their production of reactive compounds and their protective mechanisms.

Respiratory Tract. The pulmonary system is usually the first to exhibit toxicity, a function of its continuous exposure to the highest O_2 tensions in the body. Subtle changes in pulmonary function can occur within 8–12 h of exposure to 100% O_2. Increases in capillary permeability, which will increase the alveolar/arterial O_2 gradient and ultimately lead to further hypoxemia, and decreased pulmonary function can be seen after only 18 h of exposure. Serious injury and death, however, require much longer exposures. Pulmonary damage is directly related to the inspired O_2 tension, and concentrations of less than 0.5 atm appear to be safe over long time periods. The capillary endothelium is the most sensitive tissue of the lung. Endothelial injury results in loss of surface area from interstitial edema and leaks into the alveoli.

Nervous System. Retinopathy of prematurity is an eye disease in premature infants involving abnormal vascularization of the developing retina that can result from O_2 toxicity or relative hypoxia. CNS problems are rare, and toxicity occurs only under hyperbaric conditions where exposure exceeds 200 kPa (2 atm). Symptoms include seizures and visual changes, which resolve when O_2 tension is returned to normal. In premature neonates and those who have sustained in utero asphyxia, hyperoxia and hypocapnia are associated with worse neurologic outcomes.

Carbon Dioxide

Carbon dioxide is produced by metabolism at approximately the same rate as O_2 is consumed. At rest, this value is about 3 mL/kg/min, but it may increase dramatically with exercise. CO_2 diffuses readily from the cells into the blood, where it is carried partly as bicarbonate ion (HCO_3^-), partly in chemical combination with hemoglobin and plasma proteins, and partly in solution at a partial pressure of about 6 kPa (46 mm Hg) in mixed venous blood. CO_2 is transported to the lung, where it is normally exhaled at the rate it is produced, leaving a partial pressure of about 5.2 kPa (40 mm Hg) in the alveoli and in arterial blood. An increase in Pco_2 results in respiratory acidosis and may be due to decreased ventilation or the inhalation of CO_2, whereas an increase in ventilation results in decreased Pco_2 and respiratory alkalosis. Because CO_2 is freely diffusible, the changes in blood Pco_2 and pH soon are reflected by intracellular changes in Pco_2 and pH and by widespread effects in the body, especially on respiration, circulation, and the CNS.

Respiration

Carbon dioxide is a rapid, potent stimulus to ventilation in direct proportion to the inspired CO_2. CO_2 stimulates breathing by acidifying central chemoreceptors and the peripheral carotid bodies. Elevated Pco_2 causes bronchodilation, whereas hypocarbia causes constriction of airway smooth muscle; these responses may play a role in matching pulmonary ventilation and perfusion.

Circulation

The circulatory effects of CO_2 result from the combination of its direct local effects and its centrally mediated effects on the autonomic nervous system. The direct effect of CO_2 on the heart, diminished contractility, results from pH changes and a decreased myofilament Ca^{2+} responsiveness. The direct effect on systemic blood vessels results in vasodilation. CO_2 causes widespread activation of the sympathetic nervous system. The results of sympathetic nervous system activation generally are opposite to the local effects of carbon dioxide. The sympathetic effects consist of increases in cardiac contractility, heart rate, and vasoconstriction (see Chapter 12). The balance of opposing local and sympathetic effects, therefore, determines the total circulatory response to CO_2. The net effect of CO_2 inhalation is an increase in cardiac output, heart rate, and blood pressure. In blood vessels, however, the direct vasodilating actions of CO_2 appear more important, and total peripheral resistance decreases when the Pco_2 is increased. CO_2 also is a potent coronary vasodilator. Cardiac arrhythmias associated with increased Pco_2 are due to the release of catecholamines.

Hypocarbia results in opposite effects: decreased blood pressure and vasoconstriction in skin, intestine, brain, kidney, and heart. These actions are exploited clinically in the use of hyperventilation to diminish intracranial hypertension.

CNS

Hypercarbia depresses the excitability of the cerebral cortex and increases the cutaneous pain threshold through a central action. This central depression has therapeutic importance. For example, in patients who are hypoventilating from narcotics or anesthetics, increasing Pco_2 may result in further CNS depression, which in turn may worsen the respiratory depression. This positive-feedback cycle can have lethal consequences.

Methods of Administration

Carbon dioxide is marketed in gray metal cylinders as the pure gas or as CO_2 mixed with O_2. It usually is administered at a concentration of 5%–10% in combination with O_2 by means of a face mask. Another method for the temporary administration of CO_2 is by rebreathing, such as from an anesthesia breathing circuit or from something as simple as a paper bag.

Therapeutic Uses

Carbon dioxide is used for insufflation during endoscopic procedures (e.g., laparoscopic surgery) because it is highly soluble and does not support combustion. CO_2 can be used to flood the surgical field during cardiac surgery. Because of its density, CO_2 displaces the air surrounding the open heart so that any gas bubbles trapped in the heart are CO_2 rather than insoluble N_2. It is used to adjust pH during cardiopulmonary bypass procedures when a patient is cooled.

Hypocarbia still has some uses in anesthesia; it constricts cerebral vessels, decreasing brain size slightly, and thus may facilitate the performance of neurosurgical operations. While short-term hypocarbia is effective for this purpose, sustained hypocarbia has been associated with worse outcomes in patients with head injury. Hypocarbia should be instituted with a clearly defined indication and normocarbia should be reestablished as soon the indication for hypocarbia no longer applies.

Nitric Oxide

Nitric oxide is a free-radical gas now known as a critical endogenous cell-signaling molecule with an increasing number of potential therapeutic applications.

Endogenous NO is produced from L-arginine by NO synthases (neural, inducible, and endothelial) (see Chapter 3). In the vasculature, basal production of NO by endothelial cells is a primary determinant of resting vascular tone. NO causes vasodilation of smooth muscle cells and inhibition of platelet aggregation and adhesion. Impaired NO production is implicated in atherosclerosis, hypertension, cerebral and coronary vasospasm, ischemia-reperfusion injury, and inflammation and in mediating central nociceptive pathways. NO is rapidly inactivated in the circulation by oxyhemoglobin and by the reaction of NO with the heme iron, leading to the formation of nitrosyl-hemoglobin. Small quantities of methemoglobin are also produced, and these are converted to the ferrous form of heme iron by cytochrome b5 reductase. The majority of inhaled NO is excreted in the urine in the form of nitrate.

Therapeutic Uses

Inhaled NO selectively dilates the pulmonary vasculature (Cooper, 1999) and has potential as a therapy for numerous diseases associated with increased pulmonary vascular resistance. Inhaled NO is FDA-approved for only one indication, persistent pulmonary hypertension of the newborn.

Diagnostic Uses

Inhaled NO can be used during cardiac catheterization to evaluate the pulmonary vasodilating capacity of patients with heart failure and infants with congenital heart disease. Inhaled NO also is used to determine the diffusion capacity (D_L) across the alveolar-capillary unit. NO is more effective than CO_2 in this regard because of its greater affinity for hemoglobin and its higher water solubility at body temperature. NO is produced from the nasal passages and from the lungs of normal human subjects and can be detected in exhaled gas. The measurement of fractional exhaled NO is a noninvasive marker for airway inflammation with utility in the assessment of respiratory tract diseases, including asthma, respiratory tract infection, and chronic lung disease.

Toxicity

Administered at low concentrations (0.1–50 ppm), inhaled NO appears to be safe and without significant side effects. Pulmonary toxicity can occur with levels higher than 50–100 ppm. NO is an atmospheric pollutant; the Occupational Safety and Health Administration places the 7-hour exposure limit at 50 ppm. Part of the toxicity of NO may be related to its further oxidation to NO_2 in the presence of high concentrations of O_2.

The development of methemoglobinemia is a significant complication of inhaled NO at higher concentrations, and rare deaths have been reported with overdoses of NO. Methemoglobin concentrations should be monitored intermittently during NO inhalation. Inhaled NO can inhibit platelet function and has been shown to increase bleeding time in some clinical studies, although bleeding complications have not been reported. In patients with impaired function of the left ventricle, NO has a potential to further impair left ventricular performance by dilating the pulmonary circulation and increasing the blood flow to the left ventricle, thereby increasing left atrial pressure and promoting pulmonary edema formation.

The most important requirements for safe NO inhalation therapy include the following:

- Continuous measurement of NO and NO_2 concentrations using either chemiluminescence or electrochemical analyzers
- Frequent calibration of monitoring equipment
- Intermittent analysis of blood methemoglobin levels
- The use of certified tanks of NO
- Administration of the lowest NO concentration required for therapeutic effect

Methods of Administration

Courses of treatment of patients with inhaled NO are highly varied, extending from 0.1 to 40 ppm in dose and for periods of a few hours to several weeks in duration. The determination of a dose-response relationship on a frequent basis should assist in the titration of the optimum dose of NO. Commercial NO systems are available that will accurately deliver inspired NO concentrations between 0.1 and 80 ppm and simultaneously measure NO and NO_2 concentrations.

Helium

Helium is an inert gas whose low density, low solubility, and high thermal conductivity provide the basis for its medical and diagnostic uses. Helium can be mixed with O_2 and administered by mask or endotracheal tube. Under hyperbaric conditions, it can be substituted for the bulk of other gases, resulting in a mixture of much lower density that is easier to breathe.

The primary uses of helium are in pulmonary function testing, the treatment of respiratory obstruction, laser airway surgery, as a label in imaging studies, and for diving at depth. Helium is also suited for determinations of residual lung volume, functional residual capacity, and related lung volumes. These measurements require a highly diffusible nontoxic gas that is insoluble and does not leave the lung by the bloodstream so that, by dilution, the lung volume can be measured. Helium can be added to O_2 to reduce turbulence due to airway obstruction because the density of helium is less than that of air, and the viscosity of helium is greater than that of air. Mixtures of helium and O_2 reduce the work of breathing. Helium has high thermal conductivity, making it useful during laser surgery on the airway. Laser-polarized helium is used as an inhalational contrast agent for pulmonary magnetic resonance imaging. Helium also has potential as a cytoprotective agent (Smit et al., 2015).

Hydrogen Sulfide

Hydrogen sulfide, which has a characteristic rotten egg smell, is a colorless, flammable, water-soluble gas that is primarily considered as a toxin due to its capacity to inhibit mitochondrial respiration through blockade of cytochrome c oxidase. Inhibition of respiration can be toxic; however, if depression of respiration occurs in a controlled manner, it may allow nonhibernating species exposed to inhaled H_2S to enter a state akin to suspended animation (i.e., a slowing of cellular activity to a point at which metabolic processes are inhibited but not terminal) and thereby increase tolerance to stress. H_2S activates ATP-dependent K^+ channels, has vasodilating properties, and serves as a free-radical scavenger. H_2S can protect against whole-body hypoxia, lethal hemorrhage, and ischemia-reperfusion injury in various organs, including the kidney, lung, liver, and heart. Currently, effort is under way for development of gas-releasing molecules that could deliver H_2S and other therapeutic gases to diseased tissue. H_2S in low quantities may have the potential to limit cell death (Lefer, 2007).

Acknowledgment: Alex S. Evers, C. Michael Crowder, Jeffrey R. Balser, Brett A. Simon, Eric J. Moody, and Roger A. Johns contributed to this chapter in recent editions of this book. We have retained some of their text in the current edition.

Drug Facts for Your Personal Formulary: *General Anesthetics and Therapeutic Gases*

Drugs	Therapeutic Uses	Clinical Pharmacology and Tips
Parenteral Anesthetics		
Propofol Etomidate Ketamine Thiopental	• Anesthetic induction • Rapid-onset and short-duration anesthetics used in procedures for rapid return to preoperative mental status	• Highly lipophilic $\Rightarrow$ entry to brain and spinal cord, accumulation in fatty tissues • Propofol dosage: $\downarrow$ in elderly due to reduced clearance, $\uparrow$ in young children due to rapid clearance • PRIS: rare complication associated with prolonged and high-dose propofol infusion in young or head-injured patients • Etomidate: preferred for patients at risk of hypotension or MI; produces hypnosis, no analgesic effects; $\uparrow$ EEG activity, associated with seizures • Ketamine: suited for patients at risk for hypotension and asthma and for pediatric procedures; increases HR, BP, CO, CBF, and ICP; emergence delirium, hallucinations, vivid dreams limit use
Barbiturates Methohexital Thiopental	• Anesthetic induction	• Respiratory and EEG depressants • Methohexital: more rapid clearance than other barbiturates • Thiopental: action terminated by redistribution; good safety record; not available in the U.S. • Intra-arterial injection of thiobarbiturates $\Rightarrow$ severe inflammatory and potentially necrotic reaction
Inhalational Anesthetics		
Isoflurane	• Maintenance of anesthesia • Commonly used inhalational anesthetic	• Highly volatile at RT; not flammable in air or O_2 • $\downarrow$ Ventilation and RBF; $\uparrow$ CBF • Induces hypotension and $\uparrow$ coronary blood flow, thus $\downarrow$ myocardial O_2 consumption • $\downarrow$ Baroreceptor function • Excreted unchanged by the lungs
Enflurane	• Maintenance of anesthesia	• Volatile at RT; store in tightly sealed bottles • Slow induction and recovery • $\downarrow$ Arterial BP due to vasodilation and $\downarrow$ myocardial contractility • Possible effects: $\uparrow$ ICP, seizure activity
Sevoflurane	• Preferred agent for anesthetic induction • Used for outpatient anesthesia (not irritating airway; induction and recovery are rapid)	• Reacts exothermically with desiccated CO_2 absorbent • Ideal induction agent (pleasant smell, rapid onset) • $\downarrow$ AP pressure and CO; potent bronchodilator • Preferred for patients with myocardial ischemia • Compound A, product of interaction of sevoflurane with the CO_2-absorbent soda lime, is nephrotoxic
Desflurane	• Used for outpatient surgery (rapid onset, rapid recovery)	• Highly volatile at RT; store in tightly sealed bottles • Nonflammable in mixtures of air or O_2 • An airway irritant
Halothane	• Maintenance of anesthesia	• Highly volatile at RT, light sensitive; store in tightly sealed amber bottles with thymol (preservative) • Possible hepatic toxicity has limited its use and is no longer available in the U.S.
Nitrous oxide (N_2O)	• Weak anesthetic agent used for its significant analgesic effects	• Colorless and odorless gas at RT; used as adjunct to other anesthetics. • Will expand volume of air-containing cavities; thus, avoid use in obstructions of ear and bowel, and in intraocular and intracranial air bubbles, etc. • To avoid diffusional hypoxia, administer 100% O_2 rather than air when discontinuing N_2O • Can increase CBF and ICP • Clinical use of N_2O is controversial due to potential metabolic effects related to increased homocysteine and changes in DNA and protein synthesis
Xenon	• Analgesic and anesthetic effects	• Rapid induction and emergence from anesthesia • In CNS: NMDA receptor antagonist, TREK channel agonist • Well tolerated in older patients
Anesthetic Adjuncts • Augment anesthetic effects of general anesthesia		
Benzodiazepines Midazolam, diazepam, lorazepam	Used for anxiolysis, amnesia, preanesthetic sedation, and sedation during procedures not requiring general anesthesia	• Midazolam most commonly used, followed distantly by diazepam and lorazepam (see Chapters 15 and 19)
α_2 Adrenergic agonists Dexmedetomidine	• Short-term (<24 h) sedation of critically ill adults • Sedation prior to and during surgical or medical procedures in nonintubated patients	• Activation of the α_{2A} adrenergic receptor by dexmedetomidine $\Rightarrow$ sedation and analgesia • Side effects: hypotension and bradycardia due to decreased catecholamine release in the CNS; nausea and dry mouth

Anesthetic Adjuncts • Augment anesthetic effects of general anesthesia (continued)

Analgesics *Opioids* Fentanyl, Sufentanil, Alfentanil, Remifentanil, Meperidine, Morphine	• To reduce anesthetic requirement and minimize hemodynamic changes due to painful stimuli	• Opioids are the primary analgesics during perioperative period; the choice of opioid is based on duration of action (see Chapter 20) • Opioids often are administered intrathecally and epidurally for management of acute and chronic pain
NSAIDs Acetaminophen		• NSAIDs and acetaminophen are used for minor surgical procedures to control postoperative pain
Neuromuscular Blocking Agents Succinylcholine (Depolarizing) Atracurium, Vecuronium, et al. (Nondepolarizing, Competitive)	• Skeletal muscle relaxant	• Action of nondepolarizing muscle relaxants usually is antagonized, once muscle paralysis is no longer desired, with an AChE inhibitor (e.g., neostigmine or edrophonium; see Chapter 10), in combination with a muscarinic receptor antagonist

THERAPEUTIC GASES

Oxygen	• Used primarily to reverse or prevent the development of hypoxia	• Excessive $O_2 \downarrow$ ventilation • Monitoring and titration are required to avoid complications and side effects • HR and CO are slightly $\downarrow$ when 100% O_2 is breathed • High flows of dry O_2 can dry out and irritate mucosal surfaces of the airway and the eyes; humidified O_2 should be used with prolonged therapy (>1 h) • O_2-enriched atmosphere constitutes a fire hazard; take precautions
Carbon dioxide	• Insufflation during endoscopic procedures • Flooding the surgical field during cardiac surgery • Adjusting pH during cardiopulmonary bypass	• CO_2 is highly soluble, noncombustible, denser than air. • $\uparrow$ $P_{CO_2} \Rightarrow$ respiratory acidosis • Effects on CV system: combination of direct CNS and reflex sympathetic effects; net effect: $\uparrow$ in CO, HR, and BP
Nitric oxide	• Inhaled NO is used to dilate pulmonary vasculature in persistent pulmonary hypertension of the newborn	• Cell-signaling molecule; induces vasodilation • Pulmonary toxicity can occur with levels > 50-100 ppm • Use lowest NO concentration required for therapeutic effect • Monitor blood methemoglobin levels intermittently during inhalation therapy
Helium	• Pulmonary function testing, treatment of respiratory obstruction, laser airway surgery • As a label in imaging studies	• Mixtures of He and O_2 reduce the work of breathing • Potential as a cytoprotective agent • For diving at depth
Hydrogen sulfide	• Potential therapeutic use for protection against effects of hypoxia	

Bibliography

Alkire MT, et al. Consciousness and anesthesia. *Science*, **2008**, *322*:876–880.

Cooper CE. Nitric oxide and iron proteins. *Biochim Biophys Acta*, **1999**, *1411*:290–309.

Cotton M, Claing A. G protein-coupled receptors stimulation and the control of cell migration. *Cell Signal*, **2009**, *21*:1045–1053.

Drummond JC, et al. Brain surface protrusion during enflurane, halothane, and isoflurane anesthesia in cats. *Anesthesiology*, **1983**, *59*:288–293.

Eger EI II. New inhaled anesthetics. *Anesthesiology*, **1994**, *80*:906–922.

Eger EI II, et al. Nephrotoxicity of sevoflurane versus desflurane anesthesia in volunteers. *Anesth Analg*, **1997**, *84*:160–168.

Fechner J, et al. Pharmacokinetics and pharmacodynamics of GPI 15715 or fospropofol (Aquavan injection)—a water-soluble propofol prodrug. *Handb Exp Pharmacol*, **2008**, 253–266.

Franks NP. Molecular targets underlying general anaesthesia. *Br J Pharmacol*, **2006**, 147(suppl 1):S72–S81.

Franks NP. General anaesthesia: from molecular targets to neuronal pathways of sleep and arousal. *Nat Rev Neurosci*, **2008**, 9:370–386.

Franks NP, Honore E. The TREK K2P channels and their role in general anaesthesia and neuroprotection. *Trends Pharmacol Sci*, **2004**, *11*:601–608.

Guarracino F. Cerebral monitoring during cardiovascular surgery. *Curr Opin Anaesthesiol*, **2008**, *21*:50–54.

Guimarães-Camboa N, et al. HIF1α represses cell stress pathways to allow proliferation of hypoxic fetal cardiomyocytes. *Dev Cell*, **2015**, *33*:507–521.

Head BP, Patel P. Anesthetics and brain protection. *Curr Opin Anesthesiol*, **2007**, *20*:395–399.

Jevtovic-Todorovic V, et al. Prolonged exposure to inhalational anesthetic nitrous oxide kills neurons in adult rat brain. *Neuroscience*, **2003**, *122*:609–616.

Kam PC, Cardone D. Propofol infusion syndrome. *Anaesthesia*, **2007**, *62*:690–701.

Kamibayashi T, Maze M. Clinical uses of alpha2-adrenergic agonists. *Anesthesiology*, **2000**, *93*:1345–1349.

Ko H, et al. Nitrous oxide and perioperative outcomes. *J Anesthesia*, **2014**, *28*:420–428.

Kunst G, Klein AA. Peri-operative anaesthetic myocardial preconditioning and protection—cellular mechanisms and clinical relevance in cardiac anaesthesia. *Anaesthesia*, **2015**, *70*:467–482.

Ledowski T. Sugammadex: what do we know and what do we still need to know? A review of the recent (2013 to 2014) literature. *Anaesthes Intens Care*, **2015**, *43*:14–22.

Lefer DJ. A new gaseous signaling molecule emerges: cardioprotective role of hydrogen sulfide. *Proc Natl Acad Sci U S A*, **2007**, *104*:17907–17908.

Mazze RI, et al. Inorganic fluoride nephrotoxicity: prolonged enflurane and halothane anesthesia in volunteers. *Anesthesiology*, **1977**, *46*:265–271.

Mortola JP. How newborn mammals cope with hypoxia. *Respir Physiol*, **1999**, *116*:95–103.

Nunn JF. Hypoxia. In: *Nunn's Applied Respiratory Physiology.* Butterworth-Heineman, Oxford, UK, **2005**, 327–334.

Patel P, Sun L. Update on neonatal anesthetic neurotoxicity: insight into molecular mechanisms and relevance to humans. *Anesthesiology*, **2009**, *110*:703–708.

Rasmussen KG, et al. Serial infusions of low-dose ketamine for major depression. *J Psychopharmacol*, **2013**, *27*:444–450.

Sanders RD, Maze M. Alpha2-adrenoceptor agonists. *Curr Opin Invest Drugs*, **2007**, 8:25–33.

Smit KF, et al. Noble gases as cardioprotectants—translatability and mechanism. *Br J Pharmacol*, **2015**, *172*:2062–2073.

Summary of the National Halothane Study. Possible association between halothane anesthesia and postoperative hepatic necrosis. *JAMA*, **1966**, *197*:775–788.

Thom SR. Oxidative stress is fundamental to hyperbaric oxygen therapy. *J Appl Physiol*, **2009**, *106*:988–995.

van den Heuvel I, et al. Pros and cons of etomidate—more discussion than evidence? *Curr Opin Anaesthesiol*, **2013**, *26*:404–408.

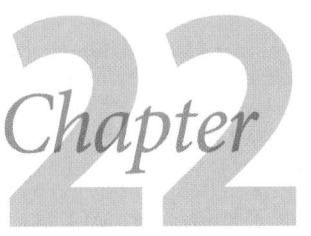

Local Anesthetics

William A. Catterall and Kenneth Mackie

Local anesthetics bind reversibly to a specific receptor site within the pore of the Na⁺ channels in nerves and block ion movement through this pore. When applied locally to nerve tissue in appropriate concentrations, local anesthetics can act on any part of the nervous system and on every type of nerve fiber, reversibly blocking the action potentials responsible for nerve conduction. Thus, a local anesthetic in contact with a nerve trunk can cause both sensory and motor paralysis in the area innervated. These effects of clinically relevant concentrations of local anesthetics are reversible with recovery of nerve function and no evidence of damage to nerve fibers or cells in most clinical applications.

History

The first local anesthetic, cocaine, was serendipitously discovered to have anesthetic properties in the late 19th century. Cocaine occurs in abundance in the leaves of the coca shrub (*Erythroxylon coca*). For centuries, Andean natives have chewed an alkali extract of these leaves for its stimulatory and euphoric actions. When, in 1860, Albert Niemann isolated cocaine, he tasted his newly isolated compound, noted that it numbed his tongue, and a new era began. Sigmund Freud studied cocaine's physiological actions, and Carl Koller introduced cocaine into clinical practice in 1884 as a topical anesthetic for ophthalmological surgery. Shortly thereafter, Halstead popularized its use in infiltration and conduction block anesthesia.

Chemistry and Structure-Activity Relationship

Cocaine is an ester of benzoic acid and the complex alcohol 2-carbomethoxy, 3-hydroxytropane (Figure 22–1). Because of its toxicity and addictive properties (Chapter 24), a search for synthetic substitutes

for cocaine began in 1892 with the work of Einhorn and colleagues, resulting in the synthesis of procaine, which became the prototype for local anesthetics for nearly half a century. The most widely used agents today are lidocaine, bupivacaine, and tetracaine.

Typical local anesthetics contain hydrophilic and hydrophobic moieties that are separated by an intermediate ester or amide linkage. A broad range of compounds containing these minimal structural features can satisfy the requirements for action as local anesthetics. The hydrophilic group usually is a tertiary amine but also may be a secondary amine; the hydrophobic moiety must be aromatic. The nature of the linking group determines some of the pharmacological properties of these agents. For example, plasma esterases readily hydrolyze local anesthetics with an ester link.

The structure-activity relationship and the physicochemical properties of local anesthetics have been well reviewed (Courtney and Strichartz, 1987). Hydrophobicity increases both the potency and the duration of action of the local anesthetics; association of the drug at hydrophobic sites enhances the partitioning of the drug to its sites of action and decreases the rate of metabolism by plasma esterases and hepatic enzymes. In addition, the receptor site for these drugs on Na⁺ channels is thought to be hydrophobic (see Mechanism of Action), so that receptor affinity for anesthetic agents is greater for the more hydrophobic drugs. Hydrophobicity also increases toxicity, so that the therapeutic index is decreased for more hydrophobic drugs.

Molecular size influences the rate of dissociation of local anesthetics from their receptor sites. Smaller drug molecules can escape from the receptor site more rapidly. This characteristic is important in rapidly firing cells, in which local anesthetics bind during action potentials and dissociate during the period of membrane repolarization. Rapid binding of local anesthetics during action potentials causes the frequency and voltage dependence of their action.

Abbreviations

ACh: acetylcholine
CSF: cerebrospinal fluid
CYP: cytochrome P450
EDTA: ethylenediaminetetraacetic acid
GI: gastrointestinal
IFM: isoleucine-phenylalanine-methionine
LA: local anesthetic
NE: norepinephrine
NET: norepinephrine transporter
PKA: protein kinase A, cyclic AMP-dependent protein kinase
PKC: protein kinase C
TRP: transient receptor potential
TRPV channel: TRP vanilloid subtype channel
TTX: tetrodotoxin

Mechanism of Action

Cellular Site of Action

Local anesthetics act at the cell membrane to prevent the generation and the conduction of nerve impulses. Conduction block can be demonstrated in squid giant axons from which the axoplasm has been removed.

Local anesthetics block conduction by decreasing or preventing the large transient increase in the permeability of excitable membranes to Na$^+$ that normally is produced by a slight depolarization of the membrane (Chapters 8, 11, and 14; Strichartz and Ritchie, 1987). This action of local anesthetics is due to their direct interaction with voltage-gated Na$^+$ channels. As the anesthetic action progressively develops in a nerve, the threshold for electrical excitability gradually increases, the rate of rise of the action potential declines, impulse conduction slows, and the safety factor for conduction decreases. These factors decrease the probability of propagation of the action potential, and nerve conduction eventually fails.

Local anesthetics can bind to other membrane proteins (Butterworth and Strichartz, 1990). In particular, they can block K$^+$ channels (Strichartz and Ritchie, 1987). However, because the interaction of local anesthetics with K$^+$ channels requires higher concentrations of drug, blockade of

conduction is not accompanied by any large or consistent change in resting membrane potential.

Quaternary analogues of local anesthetics block conduction when applied internally to perfused giant axons of squid but are relatively ineffective when applied externally. These observations suggest that the site at which local anesthetics act, at least in their charged form, is accessible only from the inner surface of the membrane (Narahashi and Frazier, 1971; Strichartz and Ritchie, 1987). Therefore, local anesthetics applied externally first must cross the membrane before they can exert a blocking action.

The Local Anesthetic Receptor Site on Na$^+$ Channels

The major mechanism of action of these drugs involves their interaction with one or more specific binding sites within the Na$^+$ channel (Butterworth and Strichartz, 1990). The Na$^+$ channels of the mammalian brain are complexes of glycosylated proteins with an aggregate molecular size in excess of 300,000 Da; the individual subunits are designated α (260,000 Da) and β$_1$ to β$_4$ (33,000–38,000 Da). The large α subunit of the Na$^+$ channel contains four homologous domains (I–IV); each domain is thought to consist of six transmembrane segments in α-helical conformation (S1–S6; Figure 22–2) and an additional, membrane-reentrant pore (*P*) loop. The Na$^+$-selective transmembrane pore of the channel resides in the center of a nearly symmetrical structure formed by the four homologous domains. The voltage dependence of channel opening is hypothesized to reflect conformational changes that result from the movement of "gating charges" within the voltage sensor module of the sodium channel in response to changes in the transmembrane potential. The gating charges are located in the S4 transmembrane helices, which are hydrophobic and positively charged, containing lysine or arginine residues at every third position. These residues are thought to move perpendicular to the plane of the membrane under the influence of the transmembrane potential, initiating a series of conformational changes in all four domains, which leads to the open state of the channel (Figure 22–2) (Catterall, 2000; Yu et al., 2005).

The transmembrane pore of the Na$^+$ channel is surrounded by the S5 and S6 transmembrane helices and the short membrane-associated segments between them that form the *P* loop. Amino acid residues in these short segments are the most critical determinants of the ion conductance and selectivity of the channel.

After it opens, the Na$^+$ channel inactivates within a few milliseconds due to closure of an inactivation gate. This functional gate is formed by the short intracellular loop of protein that connects homologous domains III

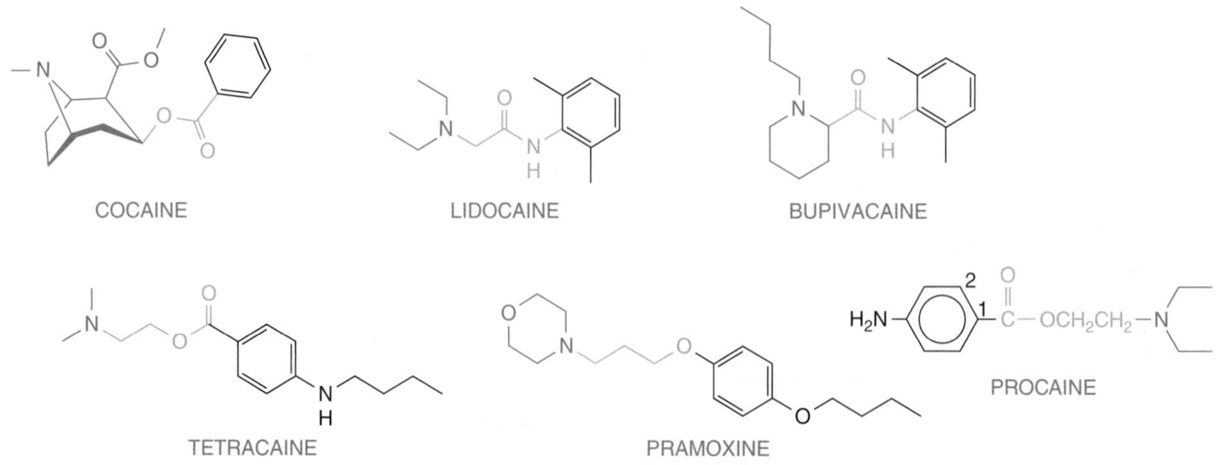

COCAINE   LIDOCAINE   BUPIVACAINE

TETRACAINE   PRAMOXINE   PROCAINE

Figure 22–1 *Structural formulas of selected local anesthetics.* Most local anesthetics consist of a hydrophobic (aromatic) moiety (black), a linker region (orange), and a substituted amine (hydrophilic region, red). The structures at the top are grouped by the nature of the linker region. Procaine is a prototypic ester-type local anesthetic; esters generally are rapidly hydrolyzed by plasma esterases, contributing to the relatively short duration of action of drugs in this group. Lidocaine is a prototypic amide-type local anesthetic; these structures generally are more resistant to clearance and have longer durations of action. There are exceptions, including benzocaine (poorly water soluble; used only topically) and the structures with a ketone, an amidine, and an ether linkage. Chloroprocaine has a chlorine atom on C2 of the aromatic ring of procaine.

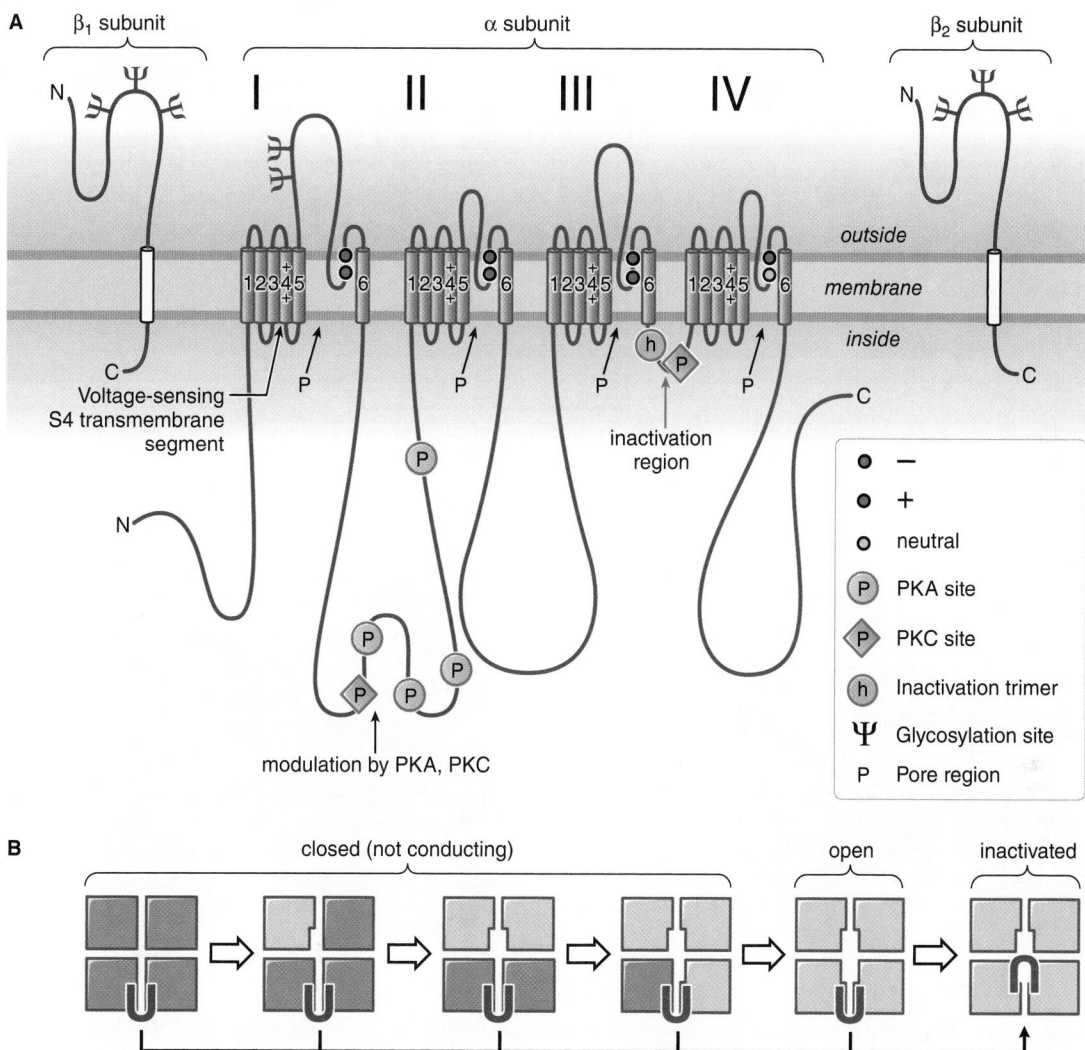

Figure 22–2 *Structure and function of voltage-gated Na⁺ channels.* **A.** A two-dimensional representation of the α (center), β₁ (left), and β₂ (right) subunits of the voltage-gated Na⁺ channel from mammalian brain. The polypeptide chains are represented by continuous lines with length approximately proportional to the actual length of each segment of the channel protein. Cylinders represent regions of transmembrane α helices. ψ indicates sites of demonstrated *N*-linked glycosylation. Note the repeated structure of the four homologous domains (I–IV) of the α subunit. **Voltage Sensing**. The S4 transmembrane segments in each homologous domain of the α subunit serve as voltage sensors. (+) represents the positively charged amino acid residues at every third position within these segments. Electrical field (negative inside) exerts a force on these charged amino acid residues, pulling them toward the intracellular side of the membrane; depolarization allows them to move outward and initiate a conformational change that opens the pore. **Pore**. The S5 and S6 transmembrane segments and the short membrane-associated loop between them (*P* loop) form the walls of the pore in the center of an approximately symmetrical square array of the four homologous domains (see **B**). The amino acid residues indicated by circles in the *P* loop are critical for determining the conductance and ion selectivity of the Na⁺ channel and its ability to bind the extracellular pore-blocking toxins TTX and saxitoxin. **Inactivation**. The short intracellular loop connecting homologous domains III and IV serves as the inactivation gate of the Na⁺ channel. It is thought to fold into the intracellular mouth of the pore and occlude it within a few milliseconds after the channel opens. Three hydrophobic residues (IFM) at the position marked **h** appear to serve as an inactivation particle, entering the intracellular mouth of the pore and binding therein to an inactivation gate receptor there. **Modulation**. The gating of the Na⁺ channel can be modulated by protein phosphorylation. Phosphorylation of the inactivation gate between homologous domains III and IV by PKC slows inactivation. Phosphorylation of sites in the intracellular loop between homologous domains I and II by either PKC or PKA reduces Na⁺ channel activation. (Adapted with permission from Catterall WA. From ionic currents to molecular mechanisms: the structure and function of voltage-gated sodium channels. *Neuron*, **2000**, *26*:13–25. Copyright © Elsevier). **B.** The four homologous domains of the Na⁺ channel α subunit are illustrated as a square array, as viewed looking down on the membrane. The sequence of conformational changes that the Na⁺ channel undergoes during activation and inactivation is diagrammed. On depolarization, each of the four homologous domains sequentially undergoes a conformational change to an activated state. After all four domains have activated, the Na⁺ channel can open. Within a few milliseconds after opening, the inactivation gate between domains III and IV closes over the intracellular mouth of the channel and occludes it, preventing further ion conductance (see Catterall, 2000).

and IV. This loop folds over the intracellular mouth of the transmembrane pore during the process of inactivation and binds to an inactivation gate "receptor" formed by the intracellular mouth of the pore.

Amino acid residues important for local anesthetic binding are found in the S6 segments in domains I, III, and IV (Ragsdale et al., 1994; Yarov-Yarovoy et al., 2002). Hydrophobic amino acid residues near the center and the intracellular end of the S6 segment may interact directly with

bound local anesthetics, locating the local anesthetic receptor site in the intracellular half of the transmembrane pore of the Na⁺ channel, with part of its structure contributed by amino acids in the S6 segments of domains I, III, and IV (Figure 22–3). Ancestral Na⁺ channels in bacteria comprise four identical subunits, each similar to one of the four domains of the mammalian Na⁺ channel α subunit and containing a similar voltage sensor and pore-lining segment. The three-dimensional structure of an ancestral

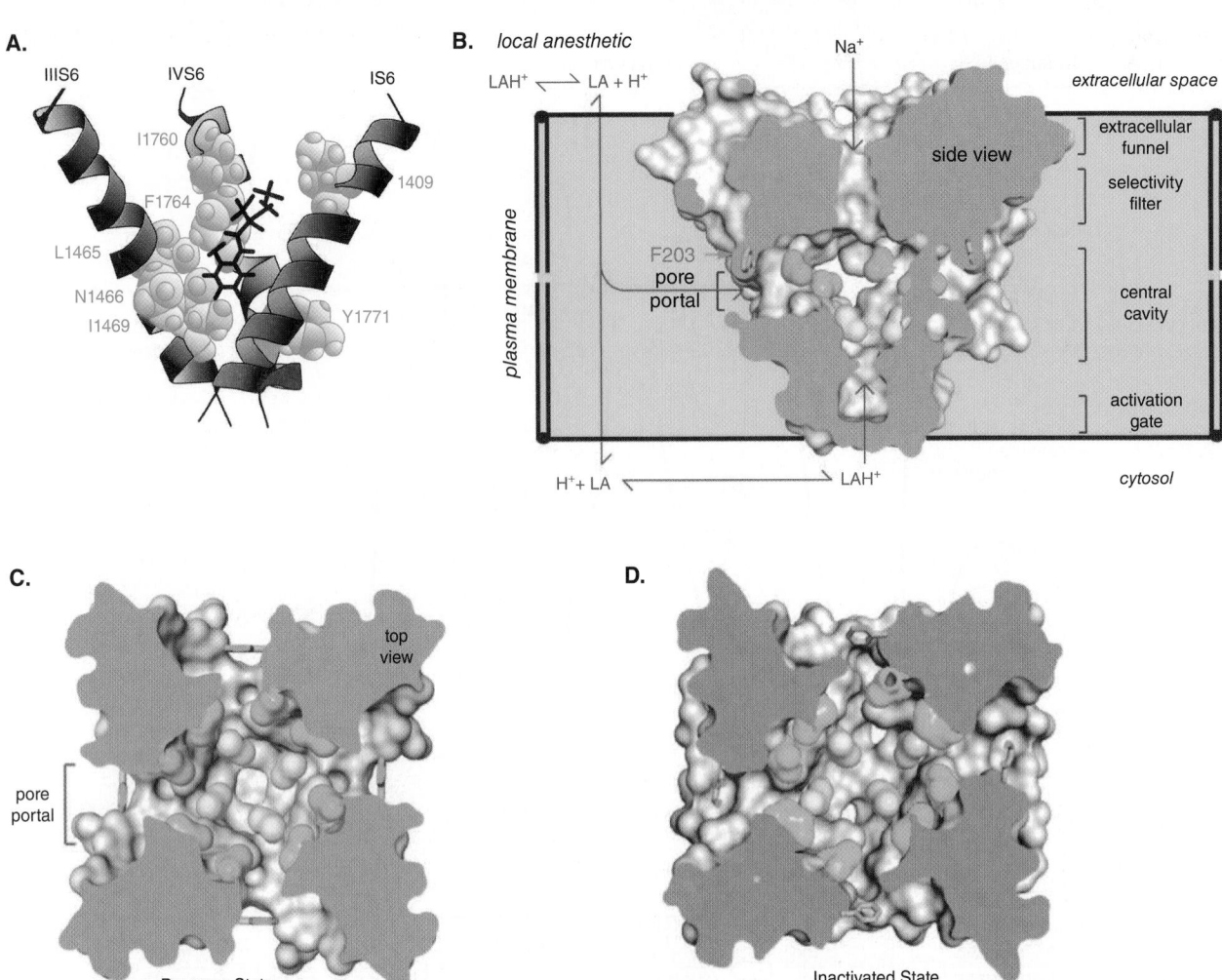

Figure 22–3 *A pharmacologist's view of the interaction of a local anesthetic with a voltage-gated Na⁺ channel.* A voltage-gated Na⁺ channel may be thought of as an antechamber (*extracellular funnel*) that feeds into a constricted area (*selectivity filter*), which opens onto a larger volume (*central cavity*) that has an exit door (*gate*). Functionally, the channel can exist in a cycle of multiple states, initiated by the local effects of an action potential on the S4 transmembrane segments of the α subunits of segments I–IV, shown in Figure 22–2A. These states are *resting/closed, intermediate/closed, open, inactivated*. LAs bind in the center of the region depicted by the light blue balls. LAs exist in charged and uncharged forms at physiological pH, in accordance with the Henderson-Hasselbalch relationship (Figure 2–2). The uncharged species, LA, can diffuse across the membrane, possibly interacting with the channel protein en route. Within the cell, LA equilibrates with H⁺; the charged form, LAH⁺, binds in the channel with greater affinity than does the uncharged species. The resting/closed conformation of the channel, in which the positive charges of the S4 segments are pulled toward the cell interior by the resting membrane potential, has a relatively low affinity for LA. The effect of an action potential is to initiate a conformational change in the selectivity funnel region of the channel, moving the positive charges outward and away from the pore interior. As a result, intermediate/closed, open, and inactivated states have a much higher affinity for LA. LAs prevent opening of the intermediate state, may block the channel in the open state, and extend the duration of the inactivated state. Ultimately, however, LA dissociates from its binding site (and the rate of LA's dissociation affects the extent of channel block), and the receptor returns to the resting state. Thus, stimulation of a nerve by an action potential enhances LA binding. With a low frequency of stimulation, LA has time to dissociate and the channels reliably return to their resting state (low affinity for LA). With a high frequency of stimulation, as in nociceptive sensory afferents after a wound, there is insufficient time for LA to fully dissociate; thus, the fraction of channels liganded by LA increases in the continued presence of LA, leading to greater and greater conduction blockade, as explained in the text. The marine neurotoxin TTX binds in the funnel with high affinity ($K_d = 10^{-10}$ nM), as does saxitoxin; both toxins block Na⁺ channel activity.

Na⁺ channel (Payandeh et al., 2011) revealed the arrangement of its transmembrane segments and the amino acid residues in the local anesthetic binding site in the pore.

Frequency and Voltage Dependence

The degree of block produced by a given concentration of local anesthetic depends on how the nerve has been stimulated and on its resting membrane potential. Thus, a resting nerve is much less sensitive to a local anesthetic than one that is repetitively stimulated; higher frequency of stimulation and more positive membrane potential cause a greater degree of anesthetic block. These frequency- and voltage-dependent effects of local anesthetics occur because the charged form of the local anesthetic molecule gains access to its binding site within the pore primarily when the Na⁺ channel is

open and because the local anesthetic binds more tightly to and stabilizes the inactivated state of the Na⁺ channel (Butterworth and Strichartz, 1990; Courtney and Strichartz, 1987; Hille, 1977). Remarkably, the conformation of the local anesthetic receptor site is changed considerably in the inactivated state (Payandeh et al., 2012; Figure 22–3D), revealing how preferential binding to inactivated Na⁺ channels may occur.

Local anesthetics exhibit frequency and voltage dependence to different extents depending on their pK_a, lipid solubility, molecular size, and binding to different channel states. In general, the frequency dependence of local anesthetic action depends critically on the rate of dissociation from the receptor site in the pore of the Na⁺ channel. A high frequency of stimulation is required for rapidly dissociating drugs so that drug binding during the action potential exceeds drug dissociation between action potentials. Dissociation of smaller and more hydrophobic drugs is more rapid, so a higher frequency of stimulation is required to yield frequency-dependent block. Frequency-dependent block of ion channels is also important for the actions of antiarrhythmic drugs (Chapter 30).

Differential Sensitivity of Nerve Fibers

For most patients, treatment with local anesthetics causes the sensation of pain to disappear first, followed by loss of the sensations of temperature, touch, deep pressure, and finally motor function (Table 22–1). Classical experiments with intact nerves showed that the δ wave in the compound action potential, which represents slowly conducting, small-diameter myelinated fibers, was reduced more rapidly and at lower concentrations of cocaine than was the α wave, which represents rapidly conducting, large-diameter fibers (Gasser and Erlanger, 1929). In general, autonomic fibers, small unmyelinated C fibers (mediating pain sensations), and small myelinated Aδ fibers (mediating pain and temperature sensations) are blocked before the larger myelinated Aγ, Aβ, and Aα fibers (mediating postural, touch, pressure, and motor information) (Raymond and Gissen, 1987). *The differential rate of block exhibited by fibers mediating different sensations is of considerable practical importance in the use of local anesthetics.*

The precise mechanisms responsible for this apparent specificity of local anesthetic action on pain fibers are not known, but several factors may contribute. The initial hypothesis was that sensitivity to local anesthetic block increases with decreasing fiber size, consistent with high sensitivity for pain sensation mediated by small fibers and low sensitivity for motor function mediated by large fibers (Gasser and Erlanger, 1929). However, when nerve fibers are dissected from nerves to allow direct measurement of action potential generation, no clear correlation of the concentration dependence of local anesthetic block with fiber diameter is observed (Fink and Cairns, 1984; Franz and Perry, 1974; Huang et al., 1997). Therefore, it is unlikely that the fiber size per se determines the sensitivity to local anesthetic block under steady-state conditions. However, the spacing of nodes of Ranvier increases with the size of nerve fibers. Because a fixed number of nodes must be blocked to prevent conduction, small fibers with closely spaced nodes of Ranvier may be blocked more rapidly during treatment of intact nerves because the local anesthetic reaches a critical length of nerve more rapidly. Differences in tissue barriers and location of smaller C fibers and Aδ fibers in nerves also may influence the rate of local anesthetic action. Different combinations of Na⁺ channel subtypes are also expressed in these nerve fibers, but all of these Na⁺ channels have similar affinity for block by local anesthetics.

Effect of pH

Local anesthetics tend to be only slightly soluble as unprotonated amines. Therefore, they generally are marketed as water-soluble salts, usually hydrochlorides. Because local anesthetics are weak bases (typical pK_a values range from 8 to 9), their hydrochloride salts are mildly acidic. This property increases the stability of the local anesthetic esters and the catecholamines added as vasoconstrictors. Under usual conditions of administration, the pH of the local anesthetic solution rapidly equilibrates to that of the extracellular fluids.

Although the unprotonated species of the local anesthetic is necessary for diffusion across cellular membranes, it is the cationic species that interacts preferentially with Na⁺ channels. The results of experiments on anesthetized mammalian nonmyelinated fibers support this conclusion (Ritchie and Greengard, 1966). In these experiments, conduction could be blocked or unblocked merely by adjusting the pH of the bathing medium to 7.2 or 9.6, respectively, without altering the amount of anesthetic present. The primary role of the cationic form also was demonstrated by Narahashi and Frazier, who perfused the extracellular and axoplasmic surface of the giant squid axon with tertiary and quaternary amine local anesthetics and found that the quaternary amines were active only when perfused intracellularly (Narahashi and Frazier, 1971). However, the unprotonated molecular forms also possess some anesthetic activity (Butterworth and Strichartz, 1990). Recent reports indicated that quaternary local anesthetics such as QX-314 can gain access to the cytoplasmic surface of the nerve cell membrane via TRPV1 channels (reviewed by Butterworth and Oxford, 2009). TRP channels, and possibly other ion channels, appear to lose selectivity and permit permeation of molecules like QX-314 in the face of prolonged or intense activation.

Prolongation of Action by Vasoconstrictors

The duration of action of a local anesthetic is proportional to the time of contact with nerve. Consequently, maneuvers that keep the drug at the nerve prolong the period of anesthesia. For example, cocaine inhibits the neuronal membrane transporters for catecholamines, thereby potentiating the effect of NE at α adrenergic receptors in the vasculature, resulting in vasoconstriction and reduced cocaine absorption in vascular beds where α adrenergic effects predominate (Chapters 8 and 12). In clinical practice,

TABLE 22–1 ■ SUSCEPTIBILITY OF NERVE TYPES TO LOCAL ANESTHETICS

CLASSIFICATION	ANATOMIC LOCATION	MYELIN	DIAMETER (μm)	CONDUCTION VELOCITY (m/s)	FUNCTION	CLINICAL SENSITIVITY TO BLOCK
A fibers						
A α	Afferent to and efferent from muscles and joints	Yes	6–22	10–85	Motor and proprioception	+
A β						++
A γ	Efferent to muscle spindles	Yes	3–6	15–35	Muscle tone	++
A δ	Sensory roots and afferent peripheral nerves	Yes	1–4	5–25	Pain, temperature, touch	+++
B fibers	Preganglionic sympathetic	Yes	<3	3–15	Vasomotor, visceromotor, sudomotor, pilomotor	++++
C fibers						
Sympathetic	Postganglionic sympathetic	No	0.3–1.3	0.7–1.3	Vasomotor, visceromotor, sudomotor, pilomotor	++++
Dorsal root	Sensory roots and afferent peripheral nerves	No	0.4–1.2	0.1–2	Pain, temperature, touch	++++

Adapted with permission from Carpenter RL, Mackey DC. Local anesthetics. In: Barash PG, Cullen BF, Stoelting RK, eds. *Clinical Anesthesia*. 2nd ed. Lippincott, Philadelphia, **1992**, 509–541. http://lww.com.

a vasoconstrictor, usually epinephrine, is often added to local anesthetics. The vasoconstrictor performs a dual service. By decreasing the rate of absorption, it localizes the anesthetic at the desired site and allows the drug's elimination to keep pace with its entry into the systemic circulation, thereby reducing the drug's systemic toxicity. Note, however, that epinephrine dilates skeletal muscle vascular beds via actions at β_2 adrenergic receptors and therefore has the potential to increase systemic toxicity of anesthetic deposited in muscle tissue.

Some of the vasoconstrictor agents may be absorbed systemically, occasionally to an extent sufficient to cause untoward reactions (see the next section). There also may be delayed wound healing, tissue edema, or necrosis after local anesthesia. These effects seem to occur partly because sympathomimetic amines increase the O_2 consumption of the tissue; this, together with the vasoconstriction, leads to hypoxia and local tissue damage. Thus, the use of vasoconstrictors in local anesthetic preparations for anatomical regions with limited collateral circulation is avoided.

Undesired Effects of Local Anesthetics

In addition to blocking conduction in nerve axons in the peripheral nervous system, local anesthetics interfere with the function of all organs in which conduction or transmission of impulses occurs. Thus, these agents affect the CNS, autonomic ganglia, neuromuscular junctions, and all forms of muscle (for a review, see Covino, 1987; Garfield and Gugino, 1987; Gintant and Hoffman, 1987). The danger of such adverse reactions is proportional to the concentration of local anesthetic achieved in the circulation. In general, in local anesthetics with chiral centers, the S-enantiomer is less toxic than the R-enantiomer (McClure, 1996).

CNS

Following absorption, local anesthetics may cause CNS stimulation, producing restlessness and tremor that may progress to clonic convulsions. In general, the more potent the anesthetic, the more readily convulsions may be produced. Alterations of CNS activity are thus predictable from the local anesthetic agent in question and the blood concentration achieved. Central stimulation is followed by depression; death usually is caused by respiratory failure.

The apparent stimulation and subsequent depression produced by applying local anesthetics to the CNS presumably is due solely to depression of neuronal activity; a selective depression of inhibitory neurons likely accounts for the excitatory phase in vivo. Rapid systemic administration of local anesthetics may produce death with no or only transient signs of CNS stimulation. Under these conditions, the concentration of the drug probably rises so rapidly that all neurons are depressed simultaneously. Airway control, along with ventilatory and circulatory support, are essential features of treatment in the late stage of intoxication. Intravenously administered benzodiazepines are the drugs of choice for both the prevention and the arrest of convulsions. Neither propofol nor a rapidly acting barbiturate is preferred; both are more likely to produce cardiovascular depression than a benzodiazepine (Chapter 19).

Although drowsiness is the most frequent complaint that results from the CNS actions of local anesthetics, lidocaine may produce dysphoria or euphoria and muscle twitching. Moreover, lidocaine may produce a loss of consciousness that is preceded only by symptoms of sedation (Covino, 1987). Whereas other local anesthetics also show the effect, cocaine has a particularly prominent effect on mood and behavior. These effects of cocaine and its potential for abuse are discussed in Chapter 24.

Cardiovascular System

Following systemic absorption, local anesthetics act on the cardiovascular system. The primary site of action is the myocardium, where decreases in electrical excitability, conduction rate, and force of contraction occur. In addition, most local anesthetics cause arteriolar dilation. Untoward cardiovascular effects usually are seen only after high systemic concentrations are attained and CNS symptoms are evident. However, on rare occasions, lower doses of some local anesthetics will cause cardiovascular collapse

and death, probably due to either an action on the pacemaker or the sudden onset of ventricular fibrillation. Ventricular tachycardia and fibrillation are relatively uncommon consequences of local anesthetics other than bupivacaine. The antiarrhythmic effects of local anesthetics such as lidocaine and procainamide are discussed in Chapter 30. Finally, it should be stressed that untoward cardiovascular effects of local anesthetic agents may result from their inadvertent intravascular administration, especially if epinephrine is also present.

Smooth Muscle

Local anesthetics depress contractions in the intact bowel and in strips of isolated intestine (Zipf and Dittmann, 1971). They also relax vascular and bronchial smooth muscle, although low concentrations initially may produce contraction (Covino, 1987). Spinal and epidural anesthesia, as well as instillation of local anesthetics into the peritoneal cavity, cause sympathetic nervous system paralysis, which can result in increased tone of GI musculature (described under Clinical Uses). Local anesthetics may increase the resting tone and decrease the contractions of isolated human uterine muscle; however, uterine contractions are seldom depressed directly during intrapartum regional anesthesia.

Neuromuscular Junction and Ganglia

Local anesthetics also affect transmission at the neuromuscular junction. At concentrations at which the muscle responds normally to direct electrical stimulation, procaine can block the response of skeletal muscle to maximal motor-nerve volleys and to ACh. Similar effects occur at autonomic ganglia. These effects are due to block of nicotinic ACh receptors by high concentrations of the local anesthetic (Charnet et al., 1990; Neher and Steinbach, 1978).

Hypersensitivity

Rare individuals are hypersensitive to local anesthetics. The reaction may manifest itself as an allergic dermatitis or a typical asthmatic attack (Covino, 1987). It is important to distinguish allergic reactions from toxic side effects and from the effects of coadministered vasoconstrictors. Hypersensitivity seems to occur more frequently with local anesthetics of the ester type and frequently extends to chemically related compounds. For example, individuals sensitive to procaine also may react to structurally similar compounds (e.g., tetracaine) through reaction to a common metabolite. Although allergic responses to agents of the amide type are uncommon, solutions of such agents may contain preservatives such as methylparaben that may provoke an allergic reaction (Covino, 1987). Local anesthetic preparations containing a vasoconstrictor also may elicit allergic responses due to the sulfite added as an antioxidant for the catecholamine/vasoconstrictor.

Metabolism

Local anesthetics of the ester type (e.g., tetracaine) are hydrolyzed and inactivated primarily by a plasma esterase, probably plasma cholinesterase. The liver also participates in hydrolysis of local anesthetics. Because spinal fluid contains little or no esterase, anesthesia produced by the intrathecal injection of an anesthetic agent will persist until the local anesthetic agent has been absorbed into the circulation. The amide-linked local anesthetics are, in general, degraded by the hepatic CYPs, with the initial reactions involving N-dealkylation and subsequent hydrolysis (Arthur, 1987). However, with prilocaine, the initial step is hydrolytic, forming o-toluidine metabolites that can cause methemoglobinemia. The extensive use of amide-linked local anesthetics in patients with severe hepatic disease requires caution.

Toxicity

The metabolic fate of local anesthetics is of great practical importance because toxicity can result from an imbalance between their rates of absorption and elimination. The rate of absorption of many local anesthetics into the systemic circulation can be considerably reduced by the incorporation of a vasoconstrictor agent in the anesthetic solution. However, the rate of degradation of local anesthetics varies greatly, and this is a major factor in determining the safety of a particular agent. Because toxicity is related to the concentration of free drug, binding of the anesthetic to proteins in the serum and to tissues reduces toxicity. For example, in intravenous regional anesthesia of an extremity, about half of the original anesthetic dose still is tissue bound 30 min after the restoration of normal blood flow (Arthur, 1987). Reversing the effects of local anesthetic systemic toxicity is a clinical challenge. One developing approach is promising and unusual: intravenous lipid emulsion therapy (Weinberg, 2012). Whether the lipids simply provide a favorable milieu of micelles into which lipophilic drugs can partition or the effect involves more complex biochemical pathways is not yet clear (Fettiplace et al., 2016).

Plasma binding sites serve to moderate local anesthetic levels on blood. The amide-linked local anesthetics bind extensively (55%–95%) to plasma proteins, particularly α_1-acid glycoprotein. Many factors increase (e.g., cancer, surgery, trauma, myocardial infarction, smoking, and uremia) or decrease (e.g., oral contraceptives) the level of this glycoprotein, thereby changing the amount of anesthetic delivered to the liver for metabolism and thus influencing systemic toxicity. Age-related changes in protein binding of local anesthetics also occur. The neonate is relatively deficient in plasma proteins that bind local anesthetics and thereby is more susceptible to toxicity. Plasma proteins are not the sole determinant of local anesthetic availability. Uptake by the lung also may play an important role in the distribution of amide-linked local anesthetics. Finally, reduced cardiac output slows delivery of the amide compounds to the liver, reducing their metabolism and prolonging their plasma half-lives.

Local Anesthetics and Related Agents

Cocaine

Chemistry
Cocaine, an ester of benzoic acid and methylecgonine, occurs in abundance in the leaves of the coca shrub. Ecgonine is an amino alcohol base closely related to tropine, the amino alcohol in atropine. It has the same fundamental structure as the synthetic local anesthetics (Figure 20–1).

Pharmacological Actions and Preparations
The clinically desired actions of cocaine are the blockade of nerve impulses as a consequence of its local anesthetic properties and local vasoconstriction secondary to inhibition of the NET (see Table 8–5). Toxicity and its potential for abuse have steadily decreased the clinical uses of cocaine. Its high toxicity is due to reduced catecholamine uptake in both the central and peripheral nervous systems and the resulting prolongation of transmitter dwell time in the synaptic cleft. Cocaine's euphoric properties are due primarily to inhibition of catecholamine uptake, particularly DA, in the CNS. Other local anesthetics do not block the uptake of NE and do not produce the sensitization to catecholamines, vasoconstriction, or mydriasis characteristic of cocaine. Currently, cocaine is used primarily for topical anesthesia of the upper respiratory tract, where its combination of both vasoconstrictor and local anesthetic properties provide anesthesia and shrinking of the mucosa. Cocaine hydrochloride is provided as a 1%, 4%, or 10% solution for topical application. For most applications, the 1% or 4% preparation is preferred to reduce toxicity. Because of its abuse potential, cocaine is listed as a schedule II controlled substance by the U.S. Drug Enforcement Agency.

Lidocaine

Lidocaine, an aminoethylamide (Figure 20–1), is the prototypical amide local anesthetic.

Pharmacological Actions and Preparations
Lidocaine produces faster, more intense, longer-lasting, and more extensive anesthesia than does an equal concentration of procaine. Lidocaine is an alternative choice for individuals sensitive to ester-type local anesthetics.

A lidocaine transdermal patch is used for relief of pain associated with postherpetic neuralgia. The combination of lidocaine (2.5%) and prilocaine (2.5%) under an occlusive dressing (EMLA, others) is used as an anesthetic prior to venipuncture, skin graft harvesting, and infiltration of anesthetics into genitalia. Lidocaine in combination with tetracaine in a formulation that generates a "peel" is approved for topical local analgesia prior to superficial dermatological procedures such as filler injections and laser-based treatments. Lidocaine in combination with tetracaine is also supplied in a formulation that generates heat on exposure to air, which is used prior to venous access and superficial dermatological procedures such as excision, electrodessication, and shave biopsy of skin lesions. The mild warming is intended to increase skin temperature by up to 5°C for the purpose of enhancing delivery of local anesthetic into the skin.

ADME
Lidocaine is absorbed rapidly after parenteral administration and from the GI and respiratory tracts. Although it is effective when used without any vasoconstrictor, epinephrine decreases the rate of absorption, thereby decreasing the probability of toxicity and prolonging the duration of action. In addition to preparations for injection, lidocaine is formulated for topical, ophthalmic, mucosal, and transdermal use.

Lidocaine is dealkylated in the liver by CYPs to monoethylglycine xylidide and glycine xylidide, which can be metabolized further to monoethylglycine and xylidide. Both monoethylglycine xylidide and glycine xylidide retain local anesthetic activity. In humans, about 75% of the xylidide is excreted in the urine as the further metabolite 4-hydroxy-2,6-dimethylaniline (Arthur, 1987).

Toxicity
The side effects of lidocaine seen with increasing dose include drowsiness, tinnitus, dysgeusia, dizziness, and twitching. As the dose increases, seizures, coma, and respiratory depression and arrest will occur. Clinically significant cardiovascular depression usually occurs at serum lidocaine levels that produce marked CNS effects. The metabolites monoethylglycine xylidide and glycine xylidide may contribute to some of these side effects.

Clinical Uses
Lidocaine has a wide range of clinical uses as a local anesthetic; it has utility in almost any application where a local anesthetic of intermediate duration is needed. Lidocaine also is used as an antiarrhythmic agent (Chapter 30).

Bupivacaine

Bupivacaine has a wide range of clinical uses as a local anesthetic; it has utility in almost any application where a local anesthetic of long duration is needed.

Pharmacological Actions and Preparations
Bupivacaine is a widely used amide local anesthetic; its structure is similar to that of lidocaine except that the amine-containing group is a butyl piperidine (Figure 20–1). Bupivacaine is a potent agent capable of producing prolonged anesthesia. Its long duration of action plus its tendency to provide more sensory than motor block has made it a popular drug for providing prolonged analgesia during labor or the postoperative period. By taking advantage of indwelling catheters and continuous infusions, bupivacaine can be used to provide several days of effective analgesia. Recently, a liposomal bupivacaine preparation has been FDA-approved. While safe and effective, its superiority over conventional bupivacaine and its ideal clinical applications remain to be determined (Uskova and O'Connor, 2015).

ADME
Bupivacaine is more slowly absorbed than lidocaine, so plasma levels increase more slowly following a bupivacaine nerve block or epidural. Conversely, bupivacaine levels fall more slowly following cessation of a continuous bupivacaine infusion than would be predicted from single-injection pharmacokinetics. Bupivacaine is primarily metabolized in the liver by CYP3A4 to pipecolylxylidide, which is then glucuronidated and excreted.

Toxicity

Bupivacaine is more cardiotoxic than equieffective doses of lidocaine. Clinically, this is manifested by severe ventricular arrhythmias and myocardial depression after inadvertent intravascular administration. Although lidocaine and bupivacaine both rapidly block cardiac Na^+ channels during systole, bupivacaine dissociates much more slowly than lidocaine during diastole, so a significant fraction of Na^+ channels at physiological heart rates remains blocked with bupivacaine at the end of diastole (Clarkson and Hondeghem, 1985). Thus, the block by bupivacaine is cumulative and substantially more than predicted by its local anesthetic potency. At least a portion of the cardiac toxicity of bupivacaine may be mediated centrally; direct injection of small quantities of bupivacaine into the medulla can produce malignant ventricular arrhythmias (Thomas et al., 1986). Bupivacaine-induced cardiac toxicity can be difficult to treat, and its severity is enhanced by coexisting acidosis, hypercarbia, and hypoxemia, emphasizing the importance of prompt airway control in resuscitation from bupivacaine overdose.

Local Anesthetics Suitable for Injection

The number of synthetic local anesthetics is so large that it is impractical to consider them all here. Some local anesthetic agents are too toxic to be given by injection. Their use is restricted to topical application to the eye (Chapter 69), the mucous membranes, or the skin (Chapter 70). Many local anesthetics are suitable, however, for infiltration or injection to produce nerve block; some of these also are useful for topical application. The discussion below presents the main categories of local anesthetics; agents are listed alphabetically.

Articaine

Articaine is approved in the U.S. for dental and periodontal procedures. Although it is an amide local anesthetic, it also contains an ester, whose hydrolysis terminates its action. Thus, articaine exhibits rapid onset (1–6 min) and duration of action of about 1 h.

Chloroprocaine

Chloroprocaine is a chlorinated derivative of procaine. Its major assets are its rapid onset and short duration of action and its reduced acute toxicity due to rapid metabolism (plasma $t_{1/2} \sim 25$ sec). Enthusiasm for its use has been tempered by reports of prolonged sensory and motor block after epidural or subarachnoid administration of large doses. This toxicity appears to have been a consequence of low pH and the use of sodium metabisulfite as a preservative in earlier formulations. There are no reports of neurotoxicity with newer preparations of chloroprocaine that contain calcium EDTA as the preservative, although these preparations are not recommended for intrathecal administration. A higher-than-expected incidence of muscular back pain following epidural anesthesia with 2-chloroprocaine has also been reported (Stevens et al., 1993). This back pain is thought to be due to tetany in the paraspinus muscles, which may be a consequence of Ca^{2+} binding by the EDTA included as a preservative; the incidence of back pain appears to be related to the volume of drug injected and its use for skin infiltration.

Mepivacaine

Mepivacaine is an intermediate-acting amino amide with pharmacological properties resembling those of lidocaine. Mepivacaine, however, is more toxic to the neonate and thus is not used in obstetrical anesthesia. The increased toxicity of mepivacaine in the neonate is related to ion trapping of this agent because of the lower pH of neonatal blood and the pK_a of mepivacaine, rather than to its slower metabolism in the neonate. Mepivacaine appears to have a slightly higher therapeutic index in adults than does lidocaine. Its onset of action is similar to, and its duration slightly longer (~20%) than, that of lidocaine in the absence of a coadministered vasoconstrictor. Mepivacaine is not effective as a topical anesthetic.

Prilocaine

Prilocaine is an intermediate-acting amino amide. It has a pharmacological profile similar to that of lidocaine. The primary differences are that it causes little vasodilation and thus can be used without a vasoconstrictor; its increased volume of distribution reduces its CNS toxicity, making it suitable for intravenous regional blocks (described further in the chapter).

The use of prilocaine is largely limited to dentistry because the drug is unique among the local anesthetics in its propensity to cause methemoglobinemia. This effect is a consequence of the metabolism of the aromatic ring to o-toluidine. Development of methemoglobinemia is dependent on the total dose administered, usually appearing after a dose of 8 mg/kg. If necessary, it can be treated by the intravenous administration of methylene blue (1–2 mg/kg).

Ropivacaine

The cardiac toxicity of bupivacaine stimulated interest in developing a less-toxic, long-lasting local anesthetic. One result of that search was the development of the amino ethylamide ropivacaine; the S-enantiomer was chosen because it has a lower toxicity than the R-isomer (McClure, 1996). Ropivacaine is slightly less potent than bupivacaine in producing anesthesia. Ropivacaine appears to be suitable for both epidural and regional anesthesia, with a duration of action similar to that of bupivacaine. Interestingly, it seems to be even more motor-sparing than bupivacaine.

Procaine

Procaine is no longer marketed in the U.S. as a single entity. It is an ingredient of some long-acting intramuscular formulations of penicillin.

Tetracaine

Tetracaine is a long-acting amino ester. It is significantly more potent and has a longer duration of action than procaine. Tetracaine may exhibit increased systemic toxicity because it is more slowly metabolized than the other commonly used ester local anesthetics. Currently, it is widely used in spinal anesthesia when a drug of long duration is needed. Tetracaine also is incorporated into several topical anesthetic preparations. With the introduction of bupivacaine, tetracaine is rarely used in peripheral nerve blocks because of the large doses often necessary, its slow onset, and its potential for toxicity.

Agents Used Primarily to Anesthetize Mucous Membranes and Skin

Some agents are useful as topical anesthetic agents on the skin or mucous membranes, although too irritating or too ineffective to be applied to the eye. These preparations are effective in the symptomatic relief of anal and genital pruritus, poison ivy rashes, and numerous other acute and chronic dermatoses. They sometimes are combined with a glucocorticoid or antihistamine and are available in a number of proprietary formulations.

Dibucaine

Dibucaine is a quinoline derivative. Its toxicity resulted in its removal from the U.S. market as an injectable preparation. It retains wide popularity outside the U.S. as a spinal anesthetic. It currently is available as an over-the-counter ointment for cutaneous use.

Dyclonine

Dyclonine hydrochloride is readily absorbed through the skin and mucous membranes. Its onset is rapid; its duration of action is short. Dyclonine is an active ingredient in a number of over-the-counter medications, including sore throat lozenges, a patch for cold sores, and a 0.75% solution.

Pramoxine

Pramoxine hydrochloride is a surface anesthetic agent that is not a benzoate ester. Its distinct chemical structure may help minimize the danger of cross-sensitivity reactions in patients allergic to other local anesthetics. Pramoxine produces satisfactory surface anesthesia and is reasonably well tolerated on the skin and mucous membranes. It is too irritating to be used on the eye or in the nose, but an otic solution containing chloroxylenol is marketed. Many preparations (currently 284 in the U.S.), including creams, lotions, sprays, gel, wipes, and foams, usually containing 1% pramoxine, are available for topical application.

Anesthetics With Low Aqueous Solubility

Some local anesthetics have low aqueous solubility and consequently are absorbed too slowly to cause classical local anesthetic toxicity. These compounds can be applied directly to wounds and ulcerated surfaces, where they remain localized for long periods of time, producing a sustained anesthetic action. Chemically, they are esters of para-aminobenzoic acid lacking the terminal amino group possessed by the previously described local anesthetics. The most important member of the series is benzocaine (ethyl aminobenzoate), which is incorporated into a large number of topical preparations. Benzocaine can cause methemoglobinemia (see the discussion of methemoglobinemia in the section on prilocaine); consequently, dosing recommendations must be followed carefully.

Agents for Ophthalmic Use

Anesthesia of the cornea and conjunctiva can be obtained readily by topical application of local anesthetics. However, most of the local anesthetics that have been described are too irritating for ophthalmological use. The two compounds used most frequently today are proparacaine and tetracaine. In addition to being less irritating during administration, proparacaine has the advantage of bearing little antigenic similarity to the other benzoate local anesthetics. Thus, it sometimes can be used in individuals sensitive to the amino ester local anesthetics.

For use in ophthalmology, these local anesthetics are instilled a single drop at a time. If anesthesia is incomplete, successive drops are applied until satisfactory conditions are obtained. The duration of anesthesia is determined chiefly by the vascularity of the tissue; thus, it is longest in normal cornea and shortest in inflamed conjunctiva. In the latter case, repeated instillations may be necessary to maintain adequate anesthesia. Long-term administration of topical anesthesia to the eye has been associated with retarded healing, pitting, and sloughing of the corneal epithelium and predisposition of the eye to inadvertent injury. Thus, these drugs should not be prescribed for self-administration. For issues of drug delivery, pharmacokinetics, and toxicity unique to drugs for ophthalmic use, see Chapter 69.

Biological Toxins: Tetrodotoxin and Saxitoxin

The two biological toxins, tetrodotoxin and saxitoxin, block the pore of the Na^+ channel. Tetrodotoxin is found in the gonads and other visceral tissues of some fish of the order Tetraodontiformes (to which the Japanese *fugu*, or puffer fish, belongs); it also occurs in the skin of some newts of the family Salamandridae and of the Costa Rican frog *Atelopus*. Saxitoxin is elaborated by the dinoflagellates *Gonyaulax catenella* and *G. tamarensis* and retained in the tissues of clams and other shellfish that eat these organisms. Given the right conditions of temperature and light, the *Gonyaulax* may multiply so rapidly as to discolor the ocean, causing the condition known as *red tide*. Shellfish feeding on *Gonyaulax* at this time become extremely toxic to humans and are responsible for periodic outbreaks of paralytic shellfish poisoning (Sakai and Swanson, 2014; Stommel and Watters, 2004). Although these toxins are chemically distinct, they have similar mechanisms of action. Both toxins, in nanomolar concentrations, specifically block the outer mouth of the pore of Na^+ channels in the membranes of excitable cells. As a result, the action potential is blocked. The receptor site for these toxins is formed by amino acid residues in the *P* loop of the Na^+ channel α subunit (Figure 22–2) in all four domains (Catterall, 2000; Terlau et al., 1991). Not all Na^+ channels are equally sensitive to tetrodotoxin; some Na^+ channels in cardiac myocytes and dorsal root ganglion neurons are resistant, and a tetrodotoxin-resistant Na^+ channel is expressed when skeletal muscle is denervated. Tetrodotoxin and saxitoxin are exceedingly potent; the minimal lethal dose of each in the mouse is about 8 µg/kg. Both toxins have caused fatal poisoning in humans due to paralysis of the respiratory muscles; therefore, the treatment of severe cases of poisoning requires support of respiration. Blockade of vasomotor nerves, together with a relaxation of vascular smooth muscle, seems to be responsible for the hypotension that is characteristic of tetrodotoxin poisoning. Early gastric lavage and pressor support also are indicated. If the patient survives paralytic shellfish poisoning for 24 h, the prognosis is good.

Clinical Uses of Local Anesthetics

Local anesthesia is the loss of sensation in a body part without the loss of consciousness or the impairment of central control of vital functions. It offers two major advantages over general anesthesia. First, physiological

perturbations associated with general anesthesia are avoided. Second, neurophysiological responses to pain and stress can be modified beneficially. However, local anesthetics have the potential to produce deleterious side effects. Proper choice of a local anesthetic and care in its use are the primary determinants in avoiding these problems.

There is a poor relationship between the amount of local anesthetic injected and peak plasma levels in adults. Furthermore, peak plasma levels vary widely depending on the area of injection. They are highest with interpleural or intercostal blocks and lowest with subcutaneous infiltration. Thus, recommended maximum doses serve only as general guidelines. This discussion summarizes the pharmacological and physiological consequences of the use of local anesthetics categorized by method of administration. A more comprehensive discussion of their use and administration is presented in textbooks on regional anesthesia (Cousins et al., 2008).

Topical Anesthesia

Anesthesia of mucous membranes of the nose, mouth, throat, tracheobronchial tree, esophagus, and genitourinary tract can be produced by direct application of aqueous solutions of salts of many local anesthetics or by suspension of the poorly soluble local anesthetics. Tetracaine (2%), lidocaine (2%–10%), and cocaine (1%–4%) typically are used. Cocaine is used only in the nose, nasopharynx, mouth, throat, and ear, where it uniquely produces vasoconstriction as well as anesthesia. The shrinking of mucous membranes decreases operative bleeding while improving surgical visualization. Comparable vasoconstriction can be achieved with other local anesthetics by the addition of a low concentration of a vasoconstrictor such as phenylephrine (0.005%). Epinephrine, topically applied, has no significant local effect and does not prolong the duration of action of local anesthetics applied to mucous membranes because of poor penetration. *Maximal safe total dosages* for topical anesthesia in a healthy 70-kg adult are 300 mg for lidocaine, 150 mg for cocaine, and 50 mg for tetracaine.

Peak anesthetic effect following topical application of cocaine or lidocaine occurs within 2–5 min (3–8 min with tetracaine), and anesthesia lasts for 30–45 min (30–60 min with tetracaine). Anesthesia is entirely superficial; it does not extend to submucosal structures. This technique does not alleviate joint pain or discomfort from subdermal inflammation or injury.

Local anesthetics are absorbed rapidly into the circulation following topical application to mucous membranes or denuded skin. Thus, topical anesthesia always carries the risk of systemic toxic reactions. Systemic toxicity has occurred even following the use of local anesthetics to control discomfort associated with severe diaper rash in infants. Absorption is particularly rapid when local anesthetics are applied to the tracheobronchial tree. Concentrations in blood after instillation of local anesthetics into the airway are nearly the same as those following intravenous injection. Surface anesthetics for the skin and cornea have been described earlier in the chapter.

Eutectic mixtures of local anesthetics lidocaine (2.5%)/prilocaine (2.5%) (EMLA) and lidocaine (7%)/tetracaine (7%) (Pliagis) bridge the gap between topical and infiltration anesthesia. The efficacy of each of these combinations lies in the fact that the mixture has a melting point less than that of either compound alone, existing at room temperature as an oil that can penetrate intact skin. These creams produce anesthesia to a maximum depth of 5 mm and are applied as a cream on intact skin under an occlusive dressing in advance (~30–60 min) of any procedure. These mixtures are effective for procedures involving skin and superficial subcutaneous structures (e.g., venipuncture and skin graft harvesting). Beware: the component local anesthetics will be absorbed into the systemic circulation, potentially producing toxic effects. Guidelines are available to calculate the maximum amount of cream that can be applied and area of skin covered. These mixtures must not be used on mucous membranes or abraded skin, as rapid absorption across these surfaces may result in systemic toxicity.

Infiltration Anesthesia

Infiltration anesthesia is the injection of local anesthetic directly into tissue without taking into consideration the course of cutaneous nerves.

Infiltration anesthesia can be so superficial as to include only the skin. It also can include deeper structures, including intra-abdominal organs, when these too are infiltrated.

The duration of infiltration anesthesia can be approximately doubled by the addition of epinephrine (5 μg/mL) to the injection solution; epinephrine also decreases peak concentrations of local anesthetics in blood. *Epinephrine-containing solutions are generally not injected into tissues supplied by end arteries—for example, fingers and toes, ears, the nose, and the penis—because of a concern that the resulting vasoconstriction may cause gangrene.* Similarly, epinephrine should be avoided in solutions injected intracutaneously. Because epinephrine also is absorbed into the circulation, its use should be avoided in those for whom adrenergic stimulation is undesirable.

The local anesthetics most frequently used for infiltration anesthesia are lidocaine (0.5%–1%) and bupivacaine (0.125%–0.25%). When used without epinephrine, up to 4.5 mg/kg of lidocaine or 2 mg/kg of bupivacaine can be employed in adults. When epinephrine is added, these amounts can be increased by one-third. Tumescent anesthesia is a special case of infiltration anesthesia for which large doses and volumes of lidocaine and epinephrine are administered (Lozinski and Huq, 2013).

Infiltration anesthesia and other regional anesthetic techniques have the advantage of providing satisfactory anesthesia without disrupting normal bodily functions. The chief disadvantage of infiltration anesthesia is that relatively large amounts of drug must be used to anesthetize relatively small areas. This is no problem with minor surgery. When major surgery is performed, however, the amount of local anesthetic that is required makes systemic toxic reactions likely. The amount of anesthetic required to anesthetize an area can be reduced significantly and the duration of anesthesia increased markedly by specifically blocking the nerves that innervate the area of interest. This can be done at one of several levels: subcutaneously, at major nerves, or at the level of the spinal roots.

Field Block Anesthesia

Field block anesthesia is produced by subcutaneous injection of a solution of local anesthetic to anesthetize the region distal to the injection. For example, subcutaneous infiltration of the proximal portion of the volar surface of the forearm results in an extensive area of cutaneous anesthesia that starts 2–3 cm distal to the site of injection. The same principle can be applied with particular benefit to the scalp, the anterior abdominal wall, and the lower extremity.

The drugs, concentrations, and doses recommended are the same as for infiltration anesthesia. The advantage of field block anesthesia is that less drug can be used to provide a greater area of anesthesia than when infiltration anesthesia is used. Knowledge of the relevant neuroanatomy obviously is essential for successful field block anesthesia.

Nerve Block Anesthesia

Injection of a solution of a local anesthetic into or about individual peripheral nerves or nerve plexuses produces even greater areas of anesthesia than do the techniques already described. Blockade of mixed peripheral nerves and nerve plexuses also usually anesthetizes somatic motor nerves, producing skeletal muscle relaxation, which is essential for some surgical procedures. The areas of sensory and motor block usually start several centimeters distal to the site of injection. Brachial plexus blocks are particularly useful for procedures on the upper extremity and shoulder. Intercostal nerve blocks are effective for anesthesia and relaxation of the anterior abdominal wall. Cervical plexus block is appropriate for surgery of the neck. Sciatic and femoral nerve blocks are useful for surgery distal to the knee. Other useful nerve blocks prior to surgical procedures include blocks of individual nerves at the wrist and at the ankle, blocks of individual nerves such as the median or ulnar at the elbow, and blocks of sensory cranial nerves.

There are four major determinants of the onset of sensory anesthesia following injection near a nerve: (1) proximity of the injection to the nerve; (2) concentration and volume of drug; (3) degree of ionization of the drug; and (4) time.

Local anesthetic is never intentionally injected into the nerve; this would be painful and could cause nerve damage. Instead, the anesthetic agent is deposited as close to the nerve as possible. Thus, the local anesthetic must diffuse from the site of injection into the nerve on which it acts. The rate of diffusion is determined chiefly by the concentration of the drug, its degree of ionization (ionized local anesthetic diffuses more slowly), its hydrophobicity, and the physical characteristics of the tissue surrounding the nerve. Higher concentrations of local anesthetic will provide a more rapid onset of peripheral nerve block. The utility of higher concentrations, however, is limited by systemic toxicity and by direct neural toxicity of concentrated local anesthetic solutions. For a given concentration, local anesthetics with lower pK_a values tend to have a more rapid onset of action because more drug is uncharged at neutral pH. For example, the onset of action of lidocaine occurs in about 3 min; 35% of lidocaine is in the basic form at pH 7.4. In contrast, the onset of action of bupivacaine requires about 15 min; only 5%–10% of bupivacaine is uncharged at this pH. Increased hydrophobicity might be expected to speed onset by increased penetration into nerve tissue. However, it also will increase binding in tissue lipids. Furthermore, the more hydrophobic local anesthetics also are more potent (and toxic) and thus must be used at lower concentrations, decreasing the concentration gradient for diffusion. Tissue factors also play a role in determining the rate of onset of anesthetic effects. The amount of connective tissue that must be penetrated can be significant in a nerve plexus compared to isolated nerves and can slow or even prevent adequate diffusion of local anesthetic to the nerve fibers.

Duration of nerve block anesthesia depends on the physical characteristics of the local anesthetic used and the presence or absence of vasoconstrictors. Especially important physical characteristics are lipid solubility and protein binding. Local anesthetics can be broadly divided into three categories:

- those with a short (20- to 45-min) duration of action in mixed peripheral nerves, such as procaine;
- those with an intermediate (60- to 120-min) duration of action, such as lidocaine and mepivacaine; and
- those with a long (400- to 450-min) duration of action, such as bupivacaine, ropivacaine, and tetracaine.

Block duration of the intermediate-acting local anesthetics such as lidocaine can be prolonged by the addition of epinephrine (5 μg/mL). The degree of block prolongation in peripheral nerves following the addition of epinephrine appears to be related to the intrinsic vasodilating properties of the local anesthetic and thus is most pronounced with lidocaine.

The types of nerve fibers that are blocked when a local anesthetic is injected about a mixed peripheral nerve depend on the concentration of drug used, nerve fiber size, internodal distance, and frequency and pattern of nerve impulse transmission (see the previous sections on Frequency and Voltage Dependence and Differential Sensitivity of Nerve Fibers). Anatomical factors are similarly important. A mixed peripheral nerve or nerve trunk consists of individual nerves surrounded by an investing epineurium. The vascular supply usually is centrally located. When a local anesthetic is deposited about a peripheral nerve, it diffuses from the outer surface toward the core along a concentration gradient. Consequently, nerves in the outer mantle of the mixed nerve are blocked first. These fibers usually are distributed to more proximal anatomical structures than are those situated near the core of the mixed nerve and often are motor. If the volume and concentration of local anesthetic solution deposited about the nerve are adequate, the local anesthetic eventually will diffuse inward in amounts adequate to block even the most centrally located fibers. Lesser amounts of drug will block only nerves in the mantle and the smaller and more sensitive central fibers. Furthermore, because removal of local anesthetics occurs primarily in the core of a mixed nerve or nerve trunk, where the vascular supply is located, the duration of blockade of centrally located nerves is shorter than that of more peripherally situated fibers.

The choice of local anesthetic and the amount and concentration administered are determined by the nerves and the types of fibers to be blocked, the required duration of anesthesia, and the size and health of the patient. For blocks of 2–4 h, lidocaine (1%–1.5%) can be used in the amounts recommended previously (see Infiltration Anesthesia). Mepivacaine (up to 7 mg/kg of a 1%–2% solution) provides anesthesia that lasts about as long as that from lidocaine. Bupivacaine (2–3 mg/kg of a 0.25%–0.375% solution) can be used when a longer duration of action is required. Addition of 5 μg/mL epinephrine slows systemic absorption and therefore prolongs duration and lowers the plasma concentration of the intermediate-acting local anesthetics.

Peak plasma concentrations of local anesthetics depend on the amount injected, the physical characteristics of the local anesthetic, whether epinephrine is used, the rate of blood flow to the site of injection, and the surface area exposed to local anesthetic. This is of particular importance in the safe application of nerve block anesthesia because the potential for systemic reactions is related to peak free serum concentrations. For example, peak concentrations of lidocaine in blood following injection of 400 mg without epinephrine for intercostal nerve blocks average 7 μg/mL; the same amount of lidocaine used for block of the brachial plexus results in peak concentrations in blood of about 3 μg/mL (Covino and Vassallo, 1976). Therefore, the amount of local anesthetic that can be injected must be adjusted according to the anatomical site of the nerve(s) to be blocked to minimize untoward effects. Addition of epinephrine can decrease peak plasma concentrations by 20%–30%. Multiple nerve blocks (e.g., intercostal block) or blocks performed in vascular regions require reduction in the amount of anesthetic that can be given safely because the surface area for absorption or the rate of absorption is increased.

Intravenous Regional Anesthesia (Bier Block)

The Bier block technique relies on using the vasculature to bring the local anesthetic solution to the nerve trunks and endings. In this technique, an extremity is exsanguinated with an Esmarch (elastic) bandage, and a proximally located tourniquet is inflated to 100–150 mm Hg above the systolic blood pressure. The Esmarch bandage is removed, and the local anesthetic is injected into a previously cannulated vein. Typically, complete anesthesia of the limb ensues within 5–10 min. Pain from the tourniquet and the potential for ischemic nerve injury limit tourniquet inflation to 2 h or less. However, the tourniquet should remain inflated for at least 15–30 min to prevent toxic amounts of local anesthetic from entering the circulation following deflation. Lidocaine, 40–50 mL (0.5 mL/kg in children) of a 0.5% solution without epinephrine, is the drug of choice for this technique. For intravenous regional anesthesia in adults using a 0.5% solution without epinephrine, the dose administered should not exceed 4 mg/kg. A few clinicians prefer prilocaine (0.5%) over lidocaine because of its higher therapeutic index.

The attractiveness of the Bier block lies in its simplicity. Its primary disadvantages are that it can be used only for a few anatomical regions, sensation (pain) returns quickly after tourniquet deflation, and premature release or failure of the tourniquet can produce toxic levels of local anesthetic (e.g., 50 mL of 0.5% lidocaine contains 250 mg of lidocaine). For the last reason and because its longer duration of action offers no advantage, the more cardiotoxic agent bupivacaine is not recommended for this technique. Intravenous regional anesthesia is used most often for surgery of the forearm and hand but can be adapted for the foot and distal leg.

Spinal Anesthesia

Spinal anesthesia follows the injection of local anesthetic into the CSF in the lumbar space. For a number of reasons, including the ability to produce anesthesia of a considerable fraction of the body with a dose of local anesthetic that produces negligible plasma levels, spinal anesthesia remains one of the most popular forms of anesthesia. In most adults, the spinal cord terminates above the second lumbar vertebra; between that point and the termination of the thecal sac in the sacrum, the lumbar and sacral roots are bathed in CSF. Thus, in this region there is a relatively large volume of CSF within which to inject drug, thereby minimizing the potential for direct nerve trauma.

The following is a brief discussion of the physiological effects of spinal anesthesia relating to the pharmacology of the local anesthetics. See more specialized texts (Cousins et al., 2008) for additional details.

Physiological Effects of Spinal Anesthesia

Most of the physiological side effects of spinal anesthesia are a consequence of the sympathetic blockade produced by local anesthetic block of the sympathetic fibers in the spinal nerve roots. A thorough understanding of these physiological effects is necessary for the safe and successful application of spinal anesthesia. Although some effects may be deleterious and require treatment, others can be beneficial for the patient or can improve operating conditions.

Most sympathetic fibers leave the spinal cord between T1 and L2 (see Figure 8–1). Although local anesthetic is injected below these levels in the lumbar portion of the dural sac, cephalad spread of the local anesthetic occurs with all but the smallest volumes injected. This cephalad spread is of considerable importance in the practice of spinal anesthesia and potentially is under the control of numerous variables, of which patient position and baricity (density of the drug relative to the density of the CSF) are the most important (Greene, 1983). The degree of sympathetic block is related to the height of sensory anesthesia; often, the level of sympathetic blockade is several spinal segments higher because the preganglionic sympathetic fibers are more sensitive to low concentrations of local anesthetic. The effects of sympathetic blockade involve both the actions (now partially unopposed) of the parasympathetic nervous system and the response of the unblocked portion of the sympathetic nervous system. Thus, as the level of sympathetic block ascends, the actions of the parasympathetic nervous system are increasingly dominant, and the compensatory mechanisms of the unblocked sympathetic nervous system are diminished. As most sympathetic nerve fibers leave the cord at T1 or below, few additional effects of sympathetic blockade are seen with cervical levels of spinal anesthesia. The consequences of sympathetic blockade will vary among patients as a function of age, physical conditioning, and disease state. Interestingly, sympathetic blockade during spinal anesthesia appears to be minimal in healthy children.

Clinically, the most important effects of sympathetic blockade during spinal anesthesia are on the cardiovascular system. At all but the lowest levels of spinal blockade, some vasodilation will occur. Vasodilation is more marked on the venous than on the arterial side of the circulation, resulting in blood pooling in the venous capacitance vessels. This reduction in circulating blood volume is well tolerated at low levels of spinal anesthesia in healthy patients. With an increasing level of block, this effect becomes more marked, and venous return becomes gravity dependent. If venous return decreases too much, cardiac output and organ perfusion decline precipitously. Venous return can be increased by a modest (10°–15°) head-down tilt or by elevating the legs.

At high levels of spinal blockade, the cardiac accelerator fibers, which exit the spinal cord at T1–T4, will be blocked. This is detrimental in patients dependent on elevated sympathetic tone to maintain cardiac output (e.g., during congestive heart failure or hypovolemia), and it also removes one of the compensatory mechanisms available to maintain organ perfusion during vasodilation. Thus, as the level of spinal block ascends, the rate of cardiovascular compromise can accelerate if not carefully observed and treated. Sudden asystole also can occur, presumably because of loss of sympathetic innervation in the continued presence of parasympathetic activity at the sinoatrial node (Caplan et al., 1988). In the usual clinical situation, blood pressure serves as a surrogate marker for cardiac output and organ perfusion. Treatment of hypotension usually is warranted when the blood pressure decreases to about 30% of *resting* values.

Therapy is aimed at maintaining brain and cardiac perfusion and oxygenation. To achieve these goals, administration of oxygen, fluid infusion, manipulation of patient position, and the administration of vasoactive drugs are all options. In practice, patients typically are administered a bolus (500–1000 mL) of fluid prior to the administration of spinal anesthesia in an attempt to prevent some of the deleterious effects of spinal blockade. Because the usual cause of hypotension is decreased venous return, possibly complicated by decreased heart rate, drugs with preferential venoconstrictive and chronotropic properties are preferred. For this reason, ephedrine, 5–10 mg intravenously, often is the drug of choice. In addition to the use of ephedrine to treat deleterious effects of sympathetic blockade, direct-acting α_1 adrenergic receptor agonists such as phenylephrine (Chapter 12) can be administered by either bolus or continuous infusion.

A beneficial effect of spinal anesthesia partially mediated by the sympathetic nervous system is on the intestine. Sympathetic fibers originating from T5 to L1 inhibit peristalsis; thus, their blockade produces a small, contracted intestine. This, together with flaccid abdominal musculature, produces excellent operating conditions for some types of bowel surgery. The consequences of spinal anesthesia on the respiratory system are mostly mediated by effects on the skeletal musculature. Paralysis of the intercostal muscles will reduce a patient's ability to cough and clear secretions, which may produce dyspnea in patients with bronchitis or emphysema. Respiratory arrest during spinal anesthesia seldom occurs due to paralysis of the phrenic nerves or to toxic levels of local anesthetic in the CSF of the fourth ventricle; it is much more likely to be due to medullary ischemia secondary to hypotension.

Pharmacology

Currently in the U.S., the drugs most commonly used in spinal anesthesia are lidocaine, tetracaine, and bupivacaine. The choice of local anesthetic is primarily determined by the desired duration of anesthesia. General guidelines are to use lidocaine for short procedures, bupivacaine for intermediate-to-long procedures, and tetracaine for long procedures. As mentioned, the factors contributing to the distribution of local anesthetics in the CSF have received much attention because of their importance in determining the height of block. The most important pharmacological factors include the amount, and possibly the volume, of drug injected and its baricity. The speed of injection of the local anesthesia solution also may affect the height of the block, just as the position of the patient can influence the rate of distribution of the anesthetic agent and the height of blockade achieved (described in the next section). For a given preparation of local anesthetic, administration of increasing amounts leads to a fairly predictable increase in the level of block attained. For example, 100 mg of lidocaine, 20 mg of bupivacaine, or 12 mg of tetracaine usually will result in a T4 sensory block. More complete tables of these relationships can be found in standard anesthesiology texts.

Epinephrine often is added to spinal anesthetics to increase the duration or intensity of block. Epinephrine's effect on duration of block is dependent on the technique used to measure duration. A commonly used measure of block duration is the length of time it takes for the block to recede by two dermatomes from the maximum height of the block, while a second is the duration of block at some specified level, typically L1. In most studies, addition of 200 μg of epinephrine to tetracaine solutions prolongs the duration of block by both measures. However, addition of epinephrine to lidocaine or bupivacaine does not affect the first measure of duration but does prolong the block at lower levels. In different clinical situations, one or the other measure of anesthesia duration may be more relevant, and this must be kept in mind when deciding whether to add epinephrine to spinal local anesthetics.

The mechanism of action of vasoconstrictors in prolonging spinal anesthesia is uncertain. It has been hypothesized that these agents decrease spinal cord blood flow, decreasing clearance of local anesthetic from the CSF, but this has not been convincingly demonstrated. Epinephrine and other α adrenergic agonists have been shown to decrease nociceptive transmission in the spinal cord, and studies in genetically modified mice suggested that α_{2A} adrenergic receptors play a principal role in this response (Stone et al., 1997). Such actions may contribute to the beneficial effects of epinephrine, clonidine, and dexmedetomidine when these agents are added to spinal local anesthetics.

Drug Baricity and Patient Position

The baricity of the local anesthetic injected will determine the direction of migration within the dural sac. Hyperbaric solutions will tend to settle in the dependent portions of the sac, while hypobaric solutions will tend to migrate in the opposite direction. Isobaric solutions usually will stay in the vicinity where they were injected, diffusing slowly in all directions. Consideration of the patient position during and after the performance of the block and the choice of a local anesthetic of the appropriate baricity is crucial for a successful block during some surgical procedures.

Lidocaine and bupivacaine are marketed in both isobaric and hyperbaric preparations and, if desired, can be diluted with sterile, preservative-free water to make them hypobaric.

Complications

Persistent neurological deficits following spinal anesthesia are extremely rare. Thorough evaluation of a suspected deficit should be performed in collaboration with a neurologist. Neurological sequelae can be both immediate and late. Possible causes include introduction of foreign substances (such as disinfectants, ultrasound gel, or talc) into the subarachnoid space, infection, hematoma, or direct mechanical trauma. Aside from drainage of an abscess or hematoma, treatment usually is ineffective; thus, avoidance and careful attention to detail while performing spinal anesthesia are necessary.

High concentrations of local anesthetic can cause irreversible block. After administration, local anesthetic solutions are diluted rapidly, quickly reaching nontoxic concentrations. However, there are several reports of transient or longer-lasting neurological deficits following lidocaine spinal anesthesia, particularly with 5% lidocaine HCl (i.e., ~ 180 mM) in 7.5% glucose (Zaric and Pace, 2009).

Spinal anesthesia sometimes is regarded as contraindicated in patients with preexisting disease of the spinal cord. No experimental evidence exists to support this hypothesis. Nonetheless, it is prudent to avoid spinal anesthesia in patients with progressive diseases of the spinal cord. However, spinal anesthesia may be useful in patients with a fixed, chronic spinal cord injury.

A more common sequela following any lumbar puncture, including spinal anesthesia, is a postural headache with classic features. The incidence of headache decreases with increasing age of the patient and decreasing needle diameter. Headache following lumbar puncture must be thoroughly evaluated to exclude serious complications such as meningitis. Treatment usually is conservative, with bed rest and analgesics. If this approach fails, an epidural blood patch with the injection of autologous blood can be performed; this procedure is usually successful in alleviating postdural puncture headaches, although a second blood patch may be necessary. If two epidural blood patches are ineffective in relieving the headache, the diagnosis of postdural puncture headache should be reconsidered. Intravenous caffeine (500 mg as the benzoate salt administered over 4 h) also has been advocated for the treatment of postdural puncture headache; however, the efficacy of caffeine is less than that of a blood patch, and relief usually is transient.

Evaluation of Spinal Anesthesia

Spinal anesthesia is a safe and effective technique, especially during surgery involving the lower abdomen, the lower extremities, and the perineum. It often is combined with intravenous medication to provide sedation and amnesia. The physiological perturbations associated with low spinal anesthesia often have less potential harm than those associated with general anesthesia. The same does not apply for high spinal anesthesia. The sympathetic blockade that accompanies levels of spinal anesthesia adequate for mid- or upper abdominal surgery, coupled with the difficulty in achieving visceral analgesia, is such that equally satisfactory and safer operating conditions can be realized by combining the spinal anesthetic with a "light" general anesthetic or by the administration of a general anesthetic and a neuromuscular blocking agent.

Epidural Anesthesia

Epidural anesthesia is administered by injecting local anesthetic into the epidural space—the space bounded by the ligamentum flavum posteriorly, the spinal periosteum laterally, and the dura anteriorly. Epidural anesthesia can be performed in the sacral hiatus (caudal anesthesia) or in the lumbar, thoracic, or cervical regions of the spine. Its current popularity arises from the development of catheters that can be placed into the epidural space, allowing either continuous infusions or repeated bolus administration of local anesthetics. The primary site of action of epidurally administered local anesthetics is on the spinal nerve roots. However, epidurally administered local anesthetics also may act on the spinal cord and on the paravertebral nerves.

The selection of drugs available for epidural anesthesia is similar to that for major nerve blocks. As for spinal anesthesia, the choice of drugs to be used during epidural anesthesia is dictated primarily by the duration of anesthesia desired. However, when an epidural catheter is placed, short-acting drugs can be administered repeatedly, providing more control over the duration of block. Bupivacaine, 0.5%–0.75%, is used when a long duration of surgical block is desired. Due to enhanced cardiotoxicity in pregnant patients, the 0.75% solution is not approved for obstetrical use. Lower concentrations—0.25%, 0.125%, or 0.0625%—of bupivacaine, often with 2 μg/mL of fentanyl added, frequently are used to provide analgesia during labor. They also are useful preparations for providing postoperative analgesia in certain clinical situations. Lidocaine 2% is the most frequently used intermediate-acting epidural local anesthetic. Chloroprocaine, 2% or 3%, provides rapid onset and a very short duration of anesthetic action. However, its use in epidural anesthesia has been clouded by controversy regarding its potential ability to cause neurological complications if the drug is accidentally injected into the subarachnoid space (discussed previously). The addition of epinephrine frequently prolongs the duration of action and reduces the toxicity of epidurally administered local anesthetics. Addition of epinephrine also makes inadvertent intravascular injection easier to detect and modifies the effect of sympathetic blockade during epidural anesthesia.

For each anesthetic agent, a relationship exists between the volume of local anesthetic injected epidurally and the segmental level of anesthesia achieved. For example, in 20- to 40-year-old, healthy, nonpregnant patients, each 1–1.5 mL of 2% lidocaine will give an additional segment of anesthesia. The amount needed decreases with increasing age and during pregnancy and in children. The concentration of local anesthetic used determines the type of nerve fibers blocked. The highest concentrations are used when sympathetic, somatic sensory, and somatic motor blockade are required. Intermediate concentrations allow somatic sensory anesthesia without muscle relaxation. Low concentrations will block only preganglionic sympathetic fibers. As an example, with bupivacaine these effects might be achieved with concentrations of 0.5%, 0.25%, and 0.0625%, respectively. The total amounts of drug that can be injected with safety at one time are approximately those mentioned in the sections Nerve Block Anesthesia and Infiltration Anesthesia. Performance of epidural anesthesia requires a greater degree of skill than does spinal anesthesia. The technique of epidural anesthesia and the volumes, concentrations, and types of drugs used are described in detail in standard texts on regional anesthesia (Cousins et al., 2008).

A significant difference between epidural and spinal anesthesia is that the dose of local anesthetic used can produce high concentrations in blood following absorption from the epidural space. Peak concentrations of lidocaine in blood following injection of 400 mg (without epinephrine) into the lumbar epidural space average 3–4 μg/mL; peak concentrations of bupivacaine in blood average 1 μg/mL after the lumbar epidural injection of 150 mg. Addition of epinephrine (5 μg/mL) decreases peak plasma concentrations by about 25%. Peak blood concentrations are a function of the total dose of drug administered rather than the concentration or volume of solution following epidural injection (Covino and Vassallo, 1976). The risk of inadvertent intravascular injection is increased in epidural anesthesia, as the epidural space contains a rich venous plexus.

Another major difference between epidural and spinal anesthesia is that there is no zone of differential sympathetic blockade with epidural anesthesia; thus, the level of sympathetic block is close to the level of sensory block. Because epidural anesthesia does not result in the zones of differential sympathetic blockade observed during spinal anesthesia, cardiovascular responses to epidural anesthesia might be expected to be less prominent. In practice, this is not the case; the potential advantage of epidural anesthesia is offset by the cardiovascular responses to the high concentration of anesthetic in blood that occurs during epidural anesthesia. This is most apparent when epinephrine is added to the epidural injection.

The resulting concentration of epinephrine in blood is sufficient to produce significant β_2 adrenergic receptor–mediated vasodilation. As a consequence, blood pressure decreases, even though cardiac output increases due to the positive inotropic and chronotropic effects of epinephrine (Chapter 12). The result is peripheral hyperperfusion and hypotension. Differences in cardiovascular responses to equal levels of spinal and epidural anesthesia also are observed when a local anesthetic such as lidocaine is used without epinephrine. This may be a consequence of the direct effects of high concentrations of lidocaine on vascular smooth muscle and the heart. The magnitude of the differences in responses to equal sensory levels of spinal and epidural anesthesia varies, however, with the local anesthetic used for the epidural injection (assuming no epinephrine is used). For example, local anesthetics such as bupivacaine, which are highly lipid soluble, are distributed less into the circulation than are less lipid-soluble agents such as lidocaine.

High concentrations of local anesthetics in blood during epidural anesthesia are of particular concern when this technique is used to control pain during labor and delivery. Local anesthetics cross the placenta, enter the fetal circulation, and at high concentrations may cause depression of the neonate. The extent to which they do so is determined by dosage, acid-base status, level of protein binding in both maternal and fetal blood, placental blood flow, and solubility of the agent in fetal tissue. These concerns have been lessened by the trend toward using more dilute solutions of bupivacaine for labor analgesia.

Epidural and Intrathecal Opiate Analgesia

Small quantities of opioid injected intrathecally or epidurally produce segmental analgesia (Yaksh and Rudy, 1976). This observation led to the clinical use of spinal and epidural opioids during surgical procedures and for the relief of postoperative and chronic pain (Cousins and Mather, 1984). As with local anesthesia, analgesia is confined to sensory nerves that enter the spinal cord dorsal horn in the vicinity of the injection. Presynaptic opioid receptors inhibit the release of substance P and other neurotransmitters from primary afferents, while postsynaptic opioid receptors decrease the activity of certain dorsal horn neurons in the spinothalamic tracts (Willcockson et al., 1986; see also Chapters 8 and 20). Because conduction in autonomic, sensory, and motor nerves is not affected by the opioids, blood pressure, motor function, and nonnociceptive sensory perception typically are not influenced by spinal opioids. The volume-evoked micturition reflex is inhibited, as manifested by urinary retention. Other side effects include pruritus, nausea, and vomiting in susceptible individuals. Delayed respiratory depression and sedation, presumably from cephalad spread of opioid within the CSF, occur infrequently with the doses of opioids currently used.

Spinally administered opioids by themselves do not provide satisfactory anesthesia for surgical procedures. Thus, opioids have found the greatest use in the treatment of postoperative and chronic pain, providing excellent analgesia following thoracic, abdominal, pelvic, or lower extremity surgery without the side effects associated with high doses of systemically administered opioids. For postoperative analgesia, spinally administered morphine, 0.2–0.5 mg, usually will provide 8–16 h of analgesia. Placement of an epidural catheter and repeated boluses or an infusion of opioid permits an increased duration of analgesia. Morphine, 2–6 mg every 6 h, commonly is used for bolus injections, while fentanyl, 20–50 μg/h, often combined with bupivacaine at 5–20 mg/h, is used for infusions. For cancer pain, repeated doses of epidural opioids can provide analgesia of several months' duration. The dose of epidural morphine is far less than the dose of systemically administered morphine that would be required to provide similar analgesia, thus reducing the complications that usually accompany the administration of high doses of systemic opioids, particularly sedation and constipation. Unfortunately, as with systemic opioids, tolerance will develop to the analgesic effects of epidural opioids, but this usually can be managed by increasing the dose.

Drug Facts for Your Personal Formulary: *Local Anesthetics*

Drugs	Therapeutic Uses or Duration	Clinical Pharmacology and Tips
Topical Anesthesia		
Lidocaine	• Superficial anesthesia of mucous membranes	• 2%–10% solution • ~30 min duration • Maximal healthy adult dose, ~4 mg/kg
Cocaine	• Superficial anesthesia of mucous membranes of nose, mouth, ear	• 1%–4% solution • ~30 min duration • Maximal healthy adult dose, ~1–3 mg/kg (maximum 400 mg); pediatric dose, < 1 mg/kg • Vasoconstriction + anesthesia
Eutectic mixtures, oil, or cream: Lidocaine (2.5%)/prilocaine (2.5%) (EMLA) or Lidocaine (7%)/tetracaine (7%) (PLIAGIS)	• Superficial anesthesia of cutaneous structures	• Effective to ~5-mm depth • Requires 30–60 min of contact to establish effective anesthesia • Should not be used on mucous membranes or abraded skin due to rapid absorption • Consult package insert for maximum dose
Infiltration Anesthesia		
Lidocaine	• Superficial anesthesia of cutaneous structures • Addition of dilute sodium bicarbonate (10:1—lidocaine: 8.4% sodium bicarbonate, ~0.75 mg/mL sodium bicarbonate) can lessen pain on injection	• 0.5%–1.0% solution • Maximal healthy adult dose, ~4 mg/kg • Addition of epinephrine (5 µg/mL) increases duration of action and maximal safe lidocaine dose
Bupivacaine	• Superficial anesthesia of cutaneous structures	• 0.125%–0.25% solution • Maximal healthy adult dose, ~2 mg/kg • Addition of epinephrine (5 µg/mL) increases duration of action and maximal safe bupivacaine dose
Nerve Block Anesthesia • Use with epinephrine-containing test dose • Risk of intravenous injection		
Articaine	• 1 h duration	• For dental and periodontal procedures • 4% solution, typically with epinephrine • Contains both an amide and ester, so degraded in both plasma and liver
Lidocaine, mepivacaine	• 1–2 h duration • Addition of epinephrine prolongs duration and increases maximal safe level of drug • Identification of blocked nerves (nerve stimulation or ultrasound) may increase safety and success of block	Safe doses depend on vascularity of tissue, generally: • Lidocaine: 1%–1.5%, maximal healthy adult dose, ~4 mg/kg • Mepivacaine: 1%–2%, maximal healthy adult dose, ~7 mg/kg (maximum 400 mg)
Bupivacaine, ropivacaine	• 6-8 h duration • Longer duration of sensory block with bupivacaine than with ropivacaine • Addition of epinephrine prolongs duration and increases maximal safe level of drug	Safe doses depend on vascularity of tissue, generally: • Bupivacaine: 0.25%–0.375%, maximal healthy adult dose, ~2–3 mg/kg (maximum 400 mg) • Ropivacaine: 0.5%–0.75%, maximal healthy adult dose, ~3–4 mg/kg (maximum 200 mg) • Infusions through a catheter placed adjacent to the nerve can provide sustained analgesia • Identification of blocked nerves (nerve stimulation or ultrasound) may increase safety and success of block
Epidural Anesthesia • Use with epinephrine-containing test dose • Risk of intravenous injection • Spread of block dependent on dose and volume injected • Epidural catheter allows repeated dosing • Consider coagulation status of patient		
Chloroprocaine	• Short duration • Epinephrine prolongs action	• 2%–3% solution • Possible increased incidence of postprocedure back pain
Lidocaine	• Intermediate duration • Epinephrine prolongs action	• 2% solution • Maximal healthy adult dose, ~4 mg/kg
Bupivacaine	• Long duration	• 0.5% solution • Maximal healthy adult dose, ~2–3 mg/kg
Ropivacaine	• Long duration	• 0.5%–1.0% solution • Maximal healthy adult dose, ~2–3 mg/kg • May have less toxicity than equiefficacious dose of bupivacaine
Spinal Anesthesia • Dose and baricity of anesthetic strongly influence spread • Addition of opioids can prolong analgesia • Consider coagulation status of patient		
Lidocaine	• Short duration (60–90 min)	• ~25–50 mg for perineal and lower extremity surgery • Association of spinal lidocaine with transient neurological symptoms
Tetracaine	• Long duration (210–240 min)	• Duration increased by epinephrine • ~5 mg for perineal surgery • ~10 mg for lower extremity surgery
Bupivacaine	• Long duration (210–240 min)	• ~10 mg for perineal and lower extremity surgery • 15–20 mg for abdominal surgery

Bibliography

Arthur GR. Pharmacokinetics. In: Strichartz GR, ed. *Local Anesthetics. Handbook of Experimental Pharmacology*, vol. 81. Springer-Verlag, Berlin, **1987**, 165–186.

Butterworth J, Oxford G. Local anesthetics: a new hydrophilic pathway for drug-receptor reaction. *Anesthesiology*, **2009**, *111*:12–14.

Butterworth JF IV, Strichartz GR. Molecular mechanisms of local anesthesia: a review. *Anesthesiology*, **1990**, *72*:711–734.

Caplan RA, et al. Unexpected cardiac arrest during spinal anesthesia: a closed claims analysis of predisposing factors. *Anesthesiology*, **1988**, *68*:5–11.

Carpenter RL, Mackey DC. Local anesthetics. In: Barash PG, Cullen BF, Stoelting RK, eds. *Clinical Anesthesia*. 2nd ed. Lippincott, Philadelphia, **1992**, 509–541.

Catterall WA. From ionic currents to molecular mechanisms: the structure and function of voltage-gated sodium channels. *Neuron*, **2000**, *26*:13–25.

Charnet P, et al. An open-channel blocker interacts with adjacent turns of α-helices in the nicotinic acetylcholine receptor. *Neuron*, **1990**, *4*:87–95.

Clarkson CW, Hondeghem LM. Mechanism for bupivacaine depression of cardiac conduction: fast block of sodium channels during the action potential with slow recovery from block during diastole. *Anesthesiology*, **1985**, *62*:396–405.

Courtney KR, Strichartz GR. Structural elements which determine local anesthetic activity. In: Strichartz GR, ed. *Local Anesthetics. Handbook of Experimental Pharmacology*, vol. 81. Springer-Verlag, Berlin, **1987**, 53–94.

Cousins MJ, Bridenbaugh PO, Carr DB, Horlocker TT, eds. *Neural Blockade in Clinical Anesthesia and Management of Pain*. 4th ed. Lippincott-Raven, Philadelphia, **2008**.

Cousins MJ, Mather LE. Intrathecal and epidural administration of opioids. *Anesthesiology*, **1984**, *61*:276–310.

Covino BG. Toxicity and systemic effects of local anesthetic agents. In: Strichartz GR, ed. *Local Anesthetics. Handbook of Experimental Pharmacology*, vol. 81. Springer-Verlag, Berlin, **1987**, 187–212.

Covino BG, Vassallo HG. *Local Anesthetics: Mechanisms of Action and Clinical Use*. Grune & Stratton, New York, **1976**.

Fettiplace MR, et al. Insulin signaling in bupivacaine-induced cardiac toxicity: sensitization during recovery and potentiation by lipid emulsion. *Anesthesiology*, **2016**, *124*: 428–442.

Fink BR, Cairns AM. Differential slowing and block of conduction by lidocaine in individual afferent myelinated and unmyelinated axons. *Anesthesiology*, **1984**, *60*:111–120.

Franz DN, Perry RS. Mechanisms for differential block among single myelinated and nonmyelinated axons by procaine. *J Physiol*, **1974**, *236*:193–210.

Garfield JM, Gugino L. Central effects of local anesthetics. In: Strichartz GR, ed. *Local Anesthetics. Handbook of Experimental Pharmacology*, vol. 81. Springer-Verlag, Berlin, **1987**, 253–284.

Gasser HS, Erlanger J. The role of fiber size in the establishment of a nerve block by pressure or cocaine. *Am J Physiol*, **1929**, *88*:581–591.

Gintant GA, Hoffman BF. The role of local anesthetic effects in the actions of antiarrhythmic drugs. In: Strichartz GR, ed. *Local Anesthetics. Handbook of Experimental Pharmacology*, vol. 81. Springer-Verlag, Berlin, **1987**, 213–251.

Greene NM. Uptake and elimination of local anesthetics during spinal anesthesia. *Anesth Analg*, **1983**, *62*:1013–1024.

Hille B. Local anesthetics: hydrophilic and hydrophobic pathways for the drug-receptor reaction. *J Gen Physiol*, **1977**, *69*:497–515.

Huang JH, et al. Susceptibility to lidocaine of impulses in different somatosensory fibers of rat sciatic nerve. *J Pharmacol Exp Ther*, **1997**, *292*:802–11.

Lozinski A, Huq NS. Tumescent liposuction. *Clin Plast Surg*, **2013**, *40*:593–613.

McClure JH. Ropivacaine. *Br J Anaesth*, **1996**, *76*:300–307.

Narahashi T, Frazier DT. Site of action and active form of local anesthetics. *Neurosci Res (NY)*, **1971**, *4*:65–99.

Neher E, Steinbach JH. Local anesthetics transiently block currents through single acetylcholine-receptor channels. *J Physiol*, **1978**, *277*:153–176.

Payandeh J, et al. The crystal structure of a voltage-gated sodium channel. *Nature*, **2011**, *475*:353–358.

Payandeh J, et al. Crystal structure of a voltage-gated sodium channel in two potentially inactivated states. *Nature*, **2012**, *486*:135–139.

Ragsdale DR, et al. Molecular determinants of state-dependent block of Na^+ channels by local anesthetics. *Science*, **1994**, *265*:1724–1728.

Raymond SA, Gissen AJ. Mechanism of differential nerve block. In: Strichartz GR, ed. *Local Anesthetics. Handbook of Experimental Pharmacology*, vol. 81. Springer-Verlag, Berlin, **1987**, 95–164.

Ritchie JM, Greengard P. On the mode of action of local anesthetics. *Annu Rev Pharmacol*, **1966**, *6*:405–430.

Sakai R, Swanson GT. Recent progress in neuroactive marine natural products. *Nat Prod Rep*, **2014**, *31*:273–309.

Stevens RA, et al. Back pain after epidural anesthesia with chloroprocaine. *Anesthesiology*, **1993**, *78*:492–497.

Stommel EW, Watters MR. Marine neurotoxins: ingestible toxins. *Curr Treat Options Neurol*, **2004**, *6*:105–114.

Stone LS, et al. The $α_{2a}$ adrenergic receptor subtype mediates spinal analgesia evoked by $α_2$ agonists and is necessary for spinal adrenergic-opioid synergy. *J Neurosci*, **1997**, *17*:7157–7165.

Strichartz GR, Ritchie JM. The action of local anesthetics on ion channels of excitable tissues. In: Strichartz GR, ed. *Local Anesthetics. Handbook of Experimental Pharmacology*, vol. 81. Springer-Verlag, Berlin, **1987**, 21–53.

Terlau H, et al. Mapping the site of block by tetrodotoxin and saxitoxin of sodium channel II. *FEBS Lett*, **1991**, *293*:93–96.

Thomas RD, et al. Cardiovascular toxicity of local anesthetics: an alternative hypothesis. *Anesth Analg*, **1986**, *65*:444–450.

Uskova A, O'Connor JE. Liposomal bupivacaine for regional anesthesia. *Curr Opin Anaesthesiol*, **2015**, *28*:593–597.

Weinberg GL. Lipid emulsion infusion: resuscitation for local anesthetic and other drug overdose. *Anesthesiology*, **2012**, *117*:180–187.

Willcockson WS, et al. Actions of opioid on primate spinothalamic tract neurons. *J Neurosci*, **1986**, *6*:2509–2520.

Yaksh TL, Rudy TA. Analgesia mediated by a direct spinal action of narcotics. *Science*, **1976**, *192*:1357–1358.

Yarov-Yarovoy V, et al. Role of amino acid residues in transmembrane segments IS6 and IIS6 of the sodium channel α subunit in voltage-dependent gating and drug block. *J Biol Chem*, **2002**, *277*: 35393–35401.

Yu F, et al. Overview of molecular relationships in the voltage-gated ion channel super-family. *Pharmacol Rev*, **2005**, *57*:387–395.

Zaric D, Pace NL. Transient neurological symptoms (TNS) following spinal anesthesia with lidocaine versus other local anesthetics. *Cochrane Database Syst Rev*, **2009**, *2*:CD003006.

Zipf HF, Dittmann EC. General pharmacological effects of local anesthetics. In: Lechat P, ed. *Local Anesthetics*, vol. 1. *International Encyclopedia of Pharmacology and Therapeutics*, Sect. 8. Pergamon Press, Oxford, UK, **1971**, 191–238.

Chapter 23

Ethanol

S. John Mihic, George F. Koob, Jody Mayfield,
and R. Adron Harris

Ethanol (CH_3CH_2OH), or beverage alcohol, is a two-carbon alcohol that directly affects many different types of neurochemical systems and signaling cascades and has rewarding and addictive properties. It is the oldest recreational drug and likely contributes to more morbidity, mortality, and public health costs than all illicit drugs combined. The current *Diagnostic and Statistical Manual of Mental Disorders* (*DSM-5*) integrates alcohol abuse and alcohol dependence into a single disorder called *alcohol use disorder* (AUD), with mild, moderate, and severe subclassifications (American Psychiatric Association, 2013). This chapter presents an overview of the effects of ethanol on various physiological systems, then focuses on the mechanisms of ethanol's effects in the CNS as the basis for understanding the rewards, disease processes, and treatments for ethanol-related conditions.

Human Consumption of Ethanol: A Brief History and Perspective

The use of alcoholic beverages has been documented as far back as 10,000 BC. By about 3000 BC, the Greeks, Romans, and inhabitants of Babylon were incorporating ethanol into religious festivals, while also using it for pleasure and in medicinal practice. Over the last 2000 years, alcoholic beverages have been identified in most cultures, including pre-Columbian America about AD 200 and the Islamic world in the 8th century.

The dangers of heavy consumption of alcohol have long been recognized by almost all cultures, with most stressing the importance of moderation; yet, problems with ethanol are as ancient as the use of this beverage itself. The increase in ethanol consumption in the 1800s, along with industrialization and the need for a more dependable work force, contributed to the development of more widespread organized efforts to discourage

drunkenness, including a constitutional ban on the sale of alcoholic beverages in the U.S. from 1920 to 1933.

Today, AUD is one of the most prevalent psychiatric disorders worldwide. In the U.S. among adults 18 years and older, AUD is associated with other substance use and psychiatric disorders; despite its prevalence and comorbidity, AUD often goes untreated (Grant et al., 2015). The highest quantities of ethanol intake per occasion are usually observed in the late teens to early 20s (CDC, 2012). Older adults drink more often but consume fewer total drinks each month (White et al., 2015). In the U.S., the per capita consumption of all alcoholic beverages for persons aged 14 and older is equivalent to 2.3 gallons (8.7 L) of absolute alcohol per year (NIAAA, 2015). Among drinkers, as many as half have experienced an alcohol-related problem, such as missing school or work, alcohol-related amnesia (blackouts), or operating a motor vehicle after consuming alcohol (Schuckit, 2009). Roughly one-third of men (36%) and one-quarter of women (23%) meet criteria for a mild, moderate, or severe AUD in their lifetimes (Grant et al, 2015). The CDC estimated that annually in the U.S. the excessive consumption of ethanol contributes to 10% of deaths of working adults 20–64 years old and to one-third of fatal traffic accidents and cost $249 billion in 2010 (CDC, 2014).

Ethanol Consumption

Compared with other drugs, surprisingly large amounts of ethanol are required for physiological effects. Ethanol is consumed in gram quantities. In contrast, most other drugs with affinities for specific proteins are taken in milligram or microgram doses. The alcohol content of beverages typically ranges from 4% to 6% (volume/volume) for beer, 10% to 15% for wine, and 40% and higher for distilled spirits (the proof of an alcoholic

Abbreviations

ACh: acetylcholine
ADH: alcohol dehydrogenase
ALDH: aldehyde dehydrogenase
ARBD: alcohol-related birth defect
ARND: alcohol-related neurodevelopmental disorder
AUD: alcohol use disorder
BEC: blood ethanol concentration
CHD: coronary heart disease
CYP: cytochrome P450
FAS: fetal alcohol syndrome
FASD: fetal alcohol spectrum disorder
GABA: γ-aminobutyric acid
HDL: high-density lipoprotein
5HT: serotonin
IHD: ischemic heart disease
LDL: low-density lipoprotein
LPS: lipopolysaccharide
nAChR: nicotinic acetylcholine receptor
NF-κB: nuclear factor kappa B
NMDA: *N*-methyl-D-aspartate
PTSD: post-traumatic stress disorder
SNP: single nucleotide polymorphism
SSRI: selective serotonin reuptake inhibitor
TLR: toll-like receptor

beverage is twice its percentage of alcohol; e.g., 40% alcohol is 80 proof). A 12-oz bottle of beer (355 mL), a 5-oz glass of wine (148 mL), and a 1.5-oz "shot" of 40% liquor (44 mL) each contain about 14 g ethanol (the density of ethanol is 0.79 g/mL at 25°C), and constitute what is defined as a "standard drink" in the U.S.

Because the ratio of ethanol in end-expiratory alveolar air and blood is relatively consistent, BECs in humans are readily estimated by the measurement of ethanol levels in expired air; the partition coefficient for ethanol between blood and alveolar air is about 2100:1. The legally allowed BEC for operating a motor vehicle is 80 mg% (80 mg ethanol per 100 mL blood; 0.08% w/v) in the United States, which is equivalent to a concentration of 17 mM ethanol in blood. The consumption of one standard drink (a 12-oz bottle of beer, a 5-oz glass of wine, or a 1.5-oz shot of 40% liquor) by a 70-kg person would produce a BEC of about 30 mg%. However, it is important to note that this is an estimation because the BEC is determined by several factors, including the rate of drinking, gender, body weight and water percentage, as well as the rates of metabolism and stomach emptying (see Acute Ethanol Intoxication further in the chapter).

Pharmacological Properties of Ethanol and Methanol

Ethanol

Absorption and Gastric Metabolism

After oral administration, ethanol is absorbed rapidly into the bloodstream from the stomach and small intestine and distributes into total body water (~0.65 L/kg body weight). Due to high surface area, absorption occurs more rapidly from the small intestine than from the stomach; delays in gastric emptying (e.g., due to the presence of food) slow ethanol absorption. Peak blood levels occur about 30 min after ingestion of ethanol when the stomach is empty. Because of first-pass metabolism by gastric and liver ADH, oral ingestion of ethanol leads to lower BECs than would be obtained if the same dose were administered intravenously. The rate of gastric metabolism of ethanol is lower in women than in men (Schuckit, 2006). Other factors also affect absorption and metabolism; for

example, aspirin (1 g) inhibits gastric ADH and increases the bioavailability of ethanol in men.

Liver Metabolism

Only small amounts of ethanol are excreted in urine, sweat, and breath. The main enzymes involved in ethanol metabolism are ADH and ALDH, followed by catalase and CYP2E1. CYPs 1A2 and 3A4 may also participate. Ethanol is metabolized primarily by sequential hepatic oxidation, first to acetaldehyde by ADH and then to acetic acid by ALDH (Figure 23–1). Each metabolic step requires NAD$^+$; thus, oxidation of 1 mol ethanol (46 g) to 1 mol acetic acid requires 2 mol NAD$^+$ (approximately 1.3 kg). This greatly exceeds the supply of NAD$^+$ in the liver; thus, the bioavailability of NAD$^+$ limits ethanol metabolism to about 8 g/h (10 mL/h, 170 mmol/h) in a 70-kg adult. Ethanol metabolism proceeds via zero-order kinetics at BECs greater than 10 mg% and by first-order kinetics at BECs less than 10 mg%.

In addition to limiting the rate of ethanol metabolism, the large increase in the hepatic NADH:NAD$^+$ ratio resulting from ethanol oxidation has profound consequences. The function of NAD$^+$-requiring enzymes is impaired, resulting in accumulation of lactate, reduced activity of the tricarboxylic acid cycle, and accumulation of acetyl-CoA (which is produced from ethanol-derived acetic acid; Figure 23–1). The combination of increased NADH and elevated acetyl-CoA supports fatty acid synthesis and the storage and accumulation of triacylglycerides; ketone bodies then accrue, exacerbating lactic acidosis.

Although ADH is responsible for the majority of ethanol metabolism, CYP2E1 accounts for about 10%. This constituent of the microsomal ethanol-oxidizing system can be altered by acute or chronic ethanol consumption. Competition between ethanol and other drugs (e.g., phenytoin and warfarin) that are metabolized by CYP2E1 is observed after acute consumption of ethanol. CYP2E1 is also induced by chronic consumption of ethanol, resulting in increased clearance of its substrates and increased susceptibility to certain toxins (e.g., CCl$_4$, which CYP2E1 metabolizes and thereby activates to the highly reactive trichloromethyl radical). Ethanol metabolism by the CYP2E1 pathway elevates NADP$^+$ and limits the availability of NADPH for the regeneration of reduced glutathione, thereby enhancing oxidative stress.

The mechanisms underlying hepatic disease resulting from heavy ethanol use probably reflect a complex combination of these metabolic factors, CYP2E1 induction (and enhanced activation of toxins and production of H$_2$O$_2$ and oxygen radicals), and possibly enhanced release of endotoxin as a consequence of ethanol's effect on gram-negative flora in the GI tract. The often-poor nutritional status of alcoholics (malabsorption and lack of vitamins A and D and thiamine), suppression of immune function, and a variety of other generalized effects likely compound the more direct adverse effects of excessive ethanol consumption. An overview of ethanol metabolism and how it can lead to tissue injury is found in the work of Molina et al. (2014).

Genetic Variation in Ethanol Metabolism

Genetic variations in metabolic enzymes for ethanol can alter its metabolism and susceptibility to its effects, thus influencing the risk for developing AUD and other pathology. Linkage analyses indicated that genes clustered in the *ADH* region affect risk for alcohol dependence (Edenberg et al., 2006). SNPs across the *ADH* region show strong evidence of association in and around the *ADH4* gene. In addition, a SNP in the *ADH1B* gene (*ADH1B*2*) is found in high frequencies in East Asians that may protect against AUD. This genetic variation produces faster metabolism of ethanol and a transient higher blood level of acetaldehyde, which are associated with a lower risk for heavy drinking and other ethanol-related problems, but a higher risk for esophageal cancer if one drinks. The *ALDH2*2* polymorphism (see discussion that follows) also leads to an increased incidence of esophageal cancer in those who consume alcohol. Another polymorphism (*ADH1B*3*) is protective in African Americans and is associated with lower risk of heavy drinking and ethanol-related problems.

Polymorphisms in the *ALDH2* gene are implicated in the development of AUD (Chen et al., 2014). ALDH2 is the most efficient ALDH isozyme in humans for the metabolism of ethanol-derived acetaldehyde. Low levels of acetaldehyde are rewarding and stimulating, while high blood

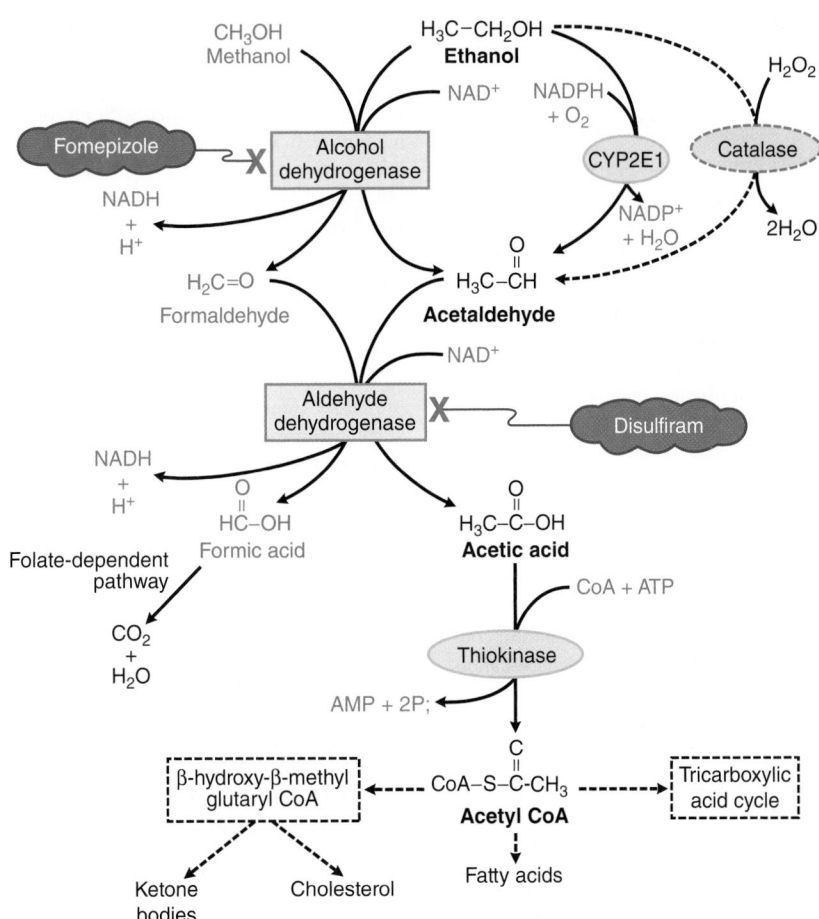

Figure 23–1 *Metabolism of ethanol and methanol.*

levels produce adverse reactions such as vomiting, diarrhea, and unstable blood pressure; thus, genetic variation in ALDH activity could affect the rewarding or aversive properties of ethanol. A mutation in the *ALDH2* gene (*ALDH2*2*) produces an enzyme that is incapable of metabolizing ethanol. Approximately 10% of Asians are homozygous for *ALDH2*2* and develop severe adverse reactions after the consumption of one drink or less. Similar adverse reactions occur if ethanol is consumed with the ALDH inhibitor disulfiram. Approximately 30%–40% of Asians are heterozygous for *ALDH2*2*, and these individuals experience facial flushing and enhanced sensitivity to alcohol but do not necessarily report an overall adverse response to the drug. Thus, several polymorphisms may decrease an individual's risk for developing AUD and other diseases that may be related to the toxic effects of aldehydes. The section Alcohol Use Disorder, Genetics, and Pharmacogenetics provides additional evidence for genetic determinants in AUD.

Methanol

Methanol (CH_3OH), also known as methyl or wood alcohol, is an important industrial reagent and solvent found in products such as paint removers, shellac, and antifreeze. Methanol is added to industrial use ethanol to make it unsafe for human consumption. Ingestion of as little as 10 mg of methanol produces toxicity ranging from blindness to death. The toxic effects of methanol take about 12 or more hours to manifest themselves and are dependent on methanol metabolism to formaldehyde and formic acid (Figure 23–1). Methanol poisoning consists of headache, GI distress, and pain (partially related to pancreatic necrosis), difficulty breathing, restlessness, and blurred vision. The visual disturbances occur from injury to ganglion cells of the retina and the optic nerve by formic acid, which produces inflammation, atrophy, and potential bilateral blindness. Severe metabolic acidosis can develop due to the accumulation of formic acid, and respiratory depression may be severe, resulting in coma or death.

ADME and Treatment of Poisoning

Methanol is rapidly absorbed via oral administration, inhalation, and through the skin, with the last two routes most relevant in industrial settings. Absorption of methanol taken orally typically occurs within 30–60 min. Methanol is metabolized by ADH to formaldehyde, which is then metabolized to formic acid by ALDH. Competition between methanol and ethanol for ADH is the basis for using ethanol to treat methanol poisoning because ethanol slows the rate of formic acid production, lessening the toxicity associated with accidental methanol consumption.

FOMEPIZOLE

Fomepizole (4-methylpyrazole), an ADH inhibitor (Figure 23–1), is also used to treat methanol or ethylene glycol poisoning, applied either alone or in combination with hemodialysis. Plasma levels of 0.8 mg/L are effective in inhibiting ADH. Fomepizole should not be used with ethanol because it prolongs the half-life of ethanol. Treatment of methanol poisoning also consists of treating patients with sodium bicarbonate to combat acidosis.

Effects of Ethanol on Physiological Systems

The Wisdom of Shakespeare

William Shakespeare described the acute pharmacological effects of imbibing ethanol in the Porter scene (act 2, scene 3) of *Macbeth*. The Porter, awakened from an alcohol-induced sleep by Macduff, explains three effects of alcohol and then wrestles with a fourth effect that combines the contradictory aspects of soaring overconfidence with physical impairment:

> **Porter:** … and drink, sir, is a great provoker of three things.
>
> **Macduff:** What three things does drink especially provoke?
>
> **Porter:** Marry, sir, nose-painting [*cutaneous vasodilation*], sleep [*CNS depression*], and urine [*a consequence of the inhibition of antidiuretic hormone (vasopressin) secretion, exacerbated by volume loading*]. Lechery, sir, it provokes and unprovokes: it provokes the desire but it takes away the performance. Therefore much drink may be said to be an equivocator with lechery: it makes him and it mars him; it sets him on and it takes him off; it persuades him and disheartens him, makes him stand to and not stand to [*the imagination desires what the corpus cavernosum cannot deliver*]; in conclusion, equivocates him in a sleep, and, giving him the lie, leaves him.

More recent research has added details to Shakespeare's enumeration—see the bracketed additions to the Porter's words in the preceding paragraph and the following sections on organ systems—but the most noticeable consequences of the recreational use of ethanol still are well summarized by the gregarious and garrulous Porter, whose delighted and devilish demeanor demonstrates a frequently observed influence of modest concentrations of ethanol on the CNS. The sections that follow detail ethanol's effects on physiological systems.

CNS

Ethanol is primarily a CNS depressant. Ingestion of moderate amounts of ethanol, like that of other sedative/hypnotics such as barbiturates and benzodiazepines, can have anxiolytic actions and produce behavioral disinhibition. Individual signs of intoxication vary from expansive and vivacious effects to uncontrolled mood swings and emotional outbursts that may have violent components. With more severe intoxication, CNS function becomes progressively more impaired, ultimately to the point of general anesthesia. Due to respiratory depression, there is little margin between the concentrations yielding the anesthetic and lethal effects of ethanol.

Acute Ethanol Intoxication

Many factors influence the BEC, including body weight, body composition, and the rate of absorption from the GI tract. In women with smaller body size and a lower body water percentage and, consequently, a lower volume of distribution for ethanol, BECs may be about 30%–50% higher than in men for the same quantity consumed.

Signs of intoxication typical of CNS depression are observed in most people after two or three drinks, with the most prominent effects seen at times of peak BEC, about 30–60 min following consumption on an empty stomach. These symptoms include an initial stimulatory effect (perhaps due to inhibition of CNS inhibitory systems), giddiness, muscle relaxation, and impaired judgment. Higher blood levels (~80 mg/dL or ~17 mM) are associated with slurred speech, incoordination, unsteady gait, and impaired attention; levels between 80 and 200 mg/dL are associated with more intense mood lability and greater cognitive deficits, potentially accompanied by aggressiveness, and anterograde amnesia (an "alcoholic blackout," i.e., loss of memory of events that transpired while intoxicated). BECs greater than 200 mg/dL can produce nystagmus and sedation, while levels of 300 mg/dL and higher produce failing vital signs, coma, and death. All of these symptoms are likely to be exacerbated and occur at a lower BEC if ethanol is taken along with other CNS depressants (e.g., benzodiazepines or barbiturates) or with any drug or medication that promotes sedation and incoordination (e.g., antihistamines).

The treatment of acute ethanol intoxication is based on the severity of respiratory and CNS depression. If respiratory depression is not severe, careful observation is the primary treatment. Patients with evidence of respiratory depression should be intubated to protect the airway and to provide ventilatory assistance; stomach lavage can also be considered if absorption is not yet complete. Because it is freely miscible with water, ethanol can be removed from the blood by hemodialysis. The usual protocol involves observing the patient in the emergency room for 4–6 h while the ingested ethanol is metabolized. The symptoms associated with diabetic coma, drug intoxication, cardiovascular accidents, and skull fractures are similar and may be confused with profound alcohol intoxication. Testing for breath odor in a case of suspected intoxication can be misleading because there can be other causes of breath odor similar to that of alcohol (e.g., diabetic ketoacidosis or other metabolic acidosis). Determining blood ethanol levels is necessary to confirm the absence or presence of alcohol intoxication, and diabetes or other underlying conditions should also be considered in patients with positive BECs.

Putative Mechanisms of Ethanol Action in the CNS

Ethanol produces distinct neuroadaptations that depend on acute versus chronic exposure. Ethanol perturbs the balance between excitatory and inhibitory transmission in the brain by either enhancing inhibitory or antagonizing excitatory neurotransmission (Table 23–1). The exact molecular sites responsible for ethanol action in vivo have yet to be resolved, although many ion channels have been implicated, including the ligand-gated NMDA and GABA$_A$ receptor-operated channels, as well as the large conductance Ca$^+$- and voltage-activated K$^+$ channel.

Advances in X-ray crystal structures of open and closed states of ion channels combined with structural modeling and site-directed mutagenesis have elucidated selective binding pockets for ethanol in different channel proteins (Howard et al., 2014; Trudell et al., 2014). Ethanol also alters ion channel function indirectly via receptor phosphorylation and trafficking mechanisms (Trudell et al., 2014). Mutant mouse models and genetic association studies in animals and humans further demonstrate a role for ligand-gated ion channels in alcohol dependence. To define the key sites of ethanol action, a combination of functional, structural, behavioral, and genomic approaches will be required.

Addiction, Tolerance, and Dependence

Alcohol use disorder is the chronically relapsing and compulsive use of alcohol, comprising three interacting stages that progressively worsen over time: binge-intoxication, withdrawal-negative affect, and preoccupation-anticipation ("craving"). The neurocircuitry of the basal ganglia is thought to mediate the neurobiological basis of the binge-intoxication stage, including the facilitation of incentive salience, a form of motivational salience associated with reward. The basal ganglia are associated with key functions, including voluntary motor control and procedural learning related to routine behaviors or habits. Release of dopamine and opioid peptides in the ventral striatum (nucleus accumbens) is associated with the reinforcing actions of alcohol (Volkow et al., 2007). Endocannabinoid signaling may also contribute to the motivational and reinforcing properties of ethanol, and ethanol drinking alters

TABLE 23–1 ■ ETHANOL TARGETS ION CHANNELS	
LIGAND- AND VOLTAGE-GATED ION CHANNELS	**EFFECTS OF ACUTE ETHANOL**
GABA$_A$ receptor-operated channels	Enhancement
Glycine receptor-operated channels	Enhancement
NMDA receptor-operated channels	Inhibition
Nicotinic ACh receptor-operated channels	Enhancement
5HT$_3$ receptor-operated channels	Enhancement
G protein–coupled inwardly rectifying K$^+$ channels	Enhancement
Voltage-gated Ca^{2+} channels	Inhibition
Large conductance, Ca^{2+}/voltage-activated K$^+$ channels (BK, slo1-containing subunits)	Enhancement

These ligand- and voltage-activated ion channels can be modulated by 50 mM ethanol or less. The enhancement or inhibition of channel function recorded here represents an overall consensus of the acute ethanol effects observed in multiple studies. Results depend on ethanol concentration, time of exposure, channel subunit composition, brain region, cell type, posttranslational modifications, and other factors.

endocannabinoid levels and cannabinoid receptor 1 expression in brain nuclei associated with addiction pathways (Pava and Woodward, 2012). Alcohol use facilitates incentive salience by imparting motivational properties to previously neutral stimuli. Activation of the ventral striatum leads to recruitment of basal ganglia–globus pallidus–thalamic–cortical loops that engage the dorsal striatum habit formation, hypothesized to be the beginning of compulsive-like responding for drugs.

Tolerance rapidly develops to the rewarding effects of alcohol and is defined as a reduced behavioral or physiological response to the same dose of drug, or the requirement of a higher dose to obtain the same effect (see Chapter 24). The major forms of tolerance are *acute* and *chronic*. Acute functional tolerance, also known as the Mellanby effect, occurs within hours of alcohol administration and is due to CNS adaptations to its effects. This is demonstrated by comparing behavioral impairment at the same BECs on the ascending limb of the absorption phase of the BEC–time curve and on the descending limb of the curve, as metabolism reduces the BEC. Behavioral impairment and subjective feelings of intoxication are much greater at a given BEC on the ascending than on the descending limb. Chronic tolerance also develops in the long-term heavy drinker. In contrast to acute tolerance, chronic tolerance has both pharmacodynamic and pharmacokinetic elements, the latter due to induction of alcohol-metabolizing enzymes. In general, the maximum pharmacokinetic tolerance attained would be a doubling of the normal metabolic rate.

Dependence is defined by a withdrawal syndrome observed several hours to days after alcohol consumption is terminated. The symptoms and severity are determined by the amount and duration of drinking and include major motivational changes, sleep disruption, autonomic nervous system (sympathetic) activation, tremors, and, in severe cases, seizures. In addition, two or more days after withdrawal, some individuals experience *delirium tremens*, characterized by hallucinations, delirium, tachycardia, and a potentially fatal fever. Individuals with AUD also show evidence of negative emotional states during acute withdrawal that persist into protracted abstinence; such states include symptoms related to anxiety, dysphoria, and depression. Persistent depression/anxiety-like symptoms may be relevant in the treatment considerations for AUD.

Two processes are thought to form the neurobiological basis for the withdrawal–negative affect stage: a decrease in functioning in reward systems in the ventral striatum and recruitment of the stress systems in the extended amygdala. As dependence develops, brain stress systems, involving corticotropin-releasing factor, norepinephrine, and dynorphin, are recruited (Koob, 2014), producing a powerful motivation for reengaging in drug seeking.

The preoccupation-anticipation ("craving") stage involves dysregulation of prefrontal cortex circuits, causing loss of executive control. The completion of complex tasks in the AUD brain may involve two opposing systems. A "go" system, consisting of the anterior cingulate cortex and dorsolateral prefrontal cortex, engages habits via the basal ganglia, while the "stop" system, consisting of the ventrolateral prefrontal cortex and orbitofrontal cortex, inhibits the basal ganglia incentive salience system and the extended amygdala stress system (Koob, 2015). Individuals with AUD present with impairments in decision-making, spatial information, and behavioral inhibition, all of which drive craving. Craving can be divided into "reward" craving (drug seeking induced by drugs or stimuli linked to drugs) and "relief" craving (drug seeking induced by an acute stressor or a state of stress) (Heinz et al., 2003). Thus, deficits in prefrontal cortical control of basal ganglia and extended amygdala function may represent a key mechanism to explain individual differences in the predisposition to and perpetuation of addiction. Residual dysregulation of the neurocircuits mediating incentive salience and stress responsivity help perpetuate compulsive drug taking and relapse.

Consequences of Ethanol Consumption on CNS Function

The transient CNS effects of heavy ethanol consumption that produce a "hangover"—the next-morning syndrome of headache, thirst, nausea, and cognitive impairment—may reflect mechanisms associated with ethanol withdrawal, dehydration, or mild acidosis. Insomnia is a common

and persistent problem in AUD, even after weeks of abstinence (Brower, 2015). Insomnia should be treated because it may be a factor contributing to relapse. Ethanol affects respiration and muscle relaxation, and heavy drinking can produce sleep apnea, especially in older alcohol-dependent subjects.

Alcohol use disorder causes shrinkage of the brain due to loss of both white and gray matter, and chronic heavy drinking increases the risk of developing *alcoholic dementia*. The cognitive deficits and brain atrophy observed soon after a heavy drinking period partially reverse over the subsequent weeks to months following abstinence. Furthermore, alcohol abuse reduces overall brain metabolism, which reverses during detoxification. The magnitude of the hypometabolic state is determined by the number of years of use and the patient's age.

Wernicke-Korsakoff syndrome consists of two neuropsychiatric disorders: Wernicke encephalopathy, which is largely reversible, and Korsakoff psychosis, which is generally not reversible. These syndromes are now considered a unitary disorder called *Wernicke-Korsakoff syndrome* that occurs subsequent to inadequate intake of thiamine, likely due to the poor dietary habits of patients with AUD. Thiamine deficiency, alone, can lead to Wernicke-Korsakoff syndrome (Scalzo et al., 2015).

Wernicke encephalopathy is characterized by a confusional state, ataxia, abnormal eye movements, blurred vision, double vision, nystagmus, and tremor. It is associated with a prolonged history of heavy drinking and an inadequate nutritional state. The neurological syndrome (ataxia, opthalmoplegia, and nystagmus) can be reversed in its early stages by high doses of thiamine, but the learning and memory impairments respond more slowly and incompletely. Untreated Wernicke encephalopathy leads to death in up to 20% of cases, and 85% of those who survive the encephalopathy go on to develop Korsakoff psychosis, characterized by severe anterograde and retrograde amnesia (Thomson et al., 2012) that is largely irreversible. Wernicke-Korsakoff syndrome is a medical emergency, and early treatment with intravenous thiamine (followed by oral maintenance treatment) is essential to reverse the Wernicke symptoms and prevent progression or reduce the severity of the Korsakoff state.

Neuroendocrine System

Both acute and chronic ethanol exposure alter endocrine regulation via the hypothalamo-pituitary-adrenal, hypothalamo-pituitary-gonadal, and hypothalamo-pituitary-thyroid axes (Molina et al., 2014). Some of the resulting endocrine-related disorders include hypothyroidism, growth retardation, diabetes, as well as hypogonadism and abnormal sexual function, discussed in the next section. Overall, alcohol abuse contributes to an impaired ability to respond to psychological and physical stressors and to maintain homeostasis.

Sexual Function

Many drugs of abuse, including ethanol, have disinhibiting effects that may initially increase libido. Despite the notion that ethanol enhances sexual function, the opposite effect generally prevails, as Shakespeare's Porter noted. Both acute and chronic ethanol use can lead to impotence in men. Increased BECs lead to decreased sexual arousal, increased ejaculatory latency, and decreased orgasmic pleasure. The incidence of sexual dysfunction may be as high as 70% in those with AUD. In addition, testicular atrophy and decreased fertility may occur. Many females with AUD complain of decreased libido, decreased vaginal lubrication, and menstrual cycle abnormalities. Their ovaries often are small and without follicular development; some data suggest that fertility rates are lower in women with AUD. Gynecomastia is associated with alcoholic liver disease and is related to an increased estrogen-to-testosterone ratio. Altered levels of reproductive hormones also affect bone metabolism.

Bone

Ethanol interferes with Ca^{2+} and bone metabolism by several processes. Acute ethanol exposure transiently decreases parathyroid hormone, resulting in increased loss of calcium. Chronic ethanol intake can disturb vitamin D metabolism and decrease Ca^{2+} absorption. Ethanol is also directly toxic to bone-forming cells and inhibits their activity. AUD is associated with decreased bone mineral density and mass and increased prevalence of osteoporosis, leading to increased risk of fractures. Anabolic hormones, particularly testosterone, are important in regulating bone remodeling and bone mass. The impaired hypothalamo-pituitary-gonadal axis and decreased testosterone levels observed in AUD further contribute to compromised bone health (Molina et al., 2014).

Body Temperature

Ingestion of ethanol causes a feeling of warmth due to enhanced cutaneous vasodilatation. Heat is transferred from the body core to the periphery and the core temperature falls due to an effect of ethanol on the central temperature-regulating mechanism in the hypothalamus. Intake of high ethanol doses may lead to pronounced decreases in body temperature, especially in cold ambient temperatures. Alcohol is a major risk factor contributing to deaths from hypothermia.

Diuresis

Ethanol inhibits the release of vasopressin (antidiuretic hormone) from the posterior pituitary gland, resulting in enhanced diuresis. Alcohol-dependent individuals in withdrawal exhibit increased vasopressin release and a consequential retention of water, as well as dilutional hyponatremia.

Cardiovascular System

There is a complex J-shaped relationship between ethanol consumption and heart disease, a leading cause of death and disability. In general, light-to-moderate ethanol intake decreases risks for coronary artery disease, congestive heart failure, and stroke, whereas high intake increases cardiovascular risk (O'Keefe et al., 2014). Epidemiological studies suggested that gender, ethanol consumption, and drinking patterns affect the association risk for IHD. AUD elevates the risk for IHD, but there is a beneficial association with IHD risk in people who consume less than 30 g per day without episodes of heavy drinking (Roerecke and Rehm, 2014). However, ethanol consumption recommendations from clinicians should remain guarded when judging the overall risk-benefit relationship given the wide range of effects and potential for other ethanol-related problems, presence of other disease states, and the lack of randomized controlled trials on ethanol's long-term effects. The risk-to-benefit ratio of drinking is also higher in younger individuals.

Serum Lipoproteins and Cardiovascular Effects

Epidemiological studies suggest that wine consumption (20–30 g ethanol per day) may confer a cardioprotective effect, resulting in decreased risk of CHD compared with abstainers. In contrast, daily consumption of greater amounts of ethanol leads to an increased incidence of arrhythmias, cardiomyopathy, and hemorrhagic stroke (Movva and Figueredo, 2013).

One possible mechanism by which ethanol could reduce the risk of CHD is through its effects on blood lipids. Changes in plasma lipoprotein levels, particularly increases in HDL (see Chapter 33), are linked with the protective effects of ethanol. HDL binds cholesterol and returns it to the liver for elimination or reprocessing, decreasing tissue cholesterol accumulation. Ethanol-induced increases in HDL cholesterol could thus decrease cholesterol accumulation in arterial walls, lessening the risk of infarction. HDL is found as two subfractions, HDL2 and HDL3. Increased levels of HDL2 (and possibly HDL3) are associated with reduced risk of myocardial infarction. Levels of both subfractions increase following ethanol consumption and decrease when consumption ceases. In addition to the antiatherogenic effects of low doses of ethanol, the flavonoids found in red wine (and purple grape juice) may play an additional role by protecting LDL from oxidative damage.

Hypertension

Heavy alcohol use can raise diastolic and systolic blood pressure. Consumption of 30 g of ethanol per day is associated with elevations in diastolic-systolic blood pressure, 1.5–2.3 mm Hg in men and 2.1–3.2 mm Hg in women.

Cardiac Arrhythmias and Cardiomyopathy

Ethanol-induced arrhythmias may be related to electrolyte abnormalities, prolongation of the QT interval, and hyperadrenergic states. Atrial arrhythmias associated with chronic alcohol use include supraventricular tachycardia, atrial fibrillation, and atrial flutter. Alcoholic cardiomyopathy is a specific disease that is classified among the acquired forms of dilated cardiomyopathy, causing left ventricular dysfunction and dilatation that may or may not be associated with right ventricular dysfunction. In general, studies suggest that consuming more than 80 g of alcohol per day over at least 5 years, in the absence of other causes of cardiomyopathy, constitutes a diagnosis of alcoholic cardiomyopathy (Guzzo-Merello et al., 2014). Women are more sensitive to alcohol than men and develop alcoholic cardiomyopathy at a lower total dose of ethanol. Lowering blood pressure with angiotensin-converting enzyme inhibitors, in particular, may be beneficial in alcoholic cardiomyopathy (Guzzo-Merello et al., 2014).

Stroke

A meta-analysis showed that low alcohol intake reduces risk of total stroke, ischemic stroke, and stroke mortality, while heavy intake increases risk of total stroke (Zhang et al., 2014). Clinical studies indicated an increased incidence of hemorrhagic and ischemic stroke in persons who drink more than 40–60 g alcohol per day. Proposed etiological factors include the following:

- Alcohol-induced cardiac arrhythmias and associated thrombus formation
- High blood pressure from chronic alcohol consumption and subsequent cerebral artery degeneration
- Acute increases in systolic blood pressure and alterations in cerebral artery tone
- Head trauma

Lungs

As in the heart and other organs, chronic alcohol abuse causes oxidative injury in the lungs. AUD increases risk of acute respiratory distress syndrome and pneumonia (Molina et al., 2014). Alcohol impairs the pulmonary response to injury, infection, and inflammation, resulting in an overall imbalance in the immune response.

Skeletal Muscle

Chronic ethanol abuse is associated with decreased muscle mass and strength, even when adjusted for other factors such as age, nicotine use, and chronic illness. Heavy doses of ethanol may irreversibly damage muscle, reflected by a marked increase in the activity of creatine kinase in plasma. Muscle biopsies from heavy drinkers also reveal decreased glycogen stores and reduced pyruvate kinase activity. Approximately 50% of chronic drinkers have skeletal muscle myopathy, which is much greater than the incidence of alcohol cirrhosis (Molina et al., 2014).

GI Tract and Digestive System

The GI system mediates ethanol absorption and metabolism and is a target for alcohol-induced pathophysiology, such as impaired esophageal and gastric motility, altered acid secretion, impaired nutrient absorption, and disrupted intestinal barrier function.

Esophagus

Alcohol is one of multiple factors associated with esophageal reflux, Barrett esophagus, traumatic rupture of the esophagus, Mallory-Weiss tears, and esophageal cancer. Either tobacco or alcohol use is associated with a 20%–30% increased likelihood of the development of esophageal squamous cell carcinoma; however, the concomitant use of both drugs increases the risk 3-fold. There is little change in esophageal function at low BECs, but at higher BECs peristalsis and lower esophageal sphincter pressure decrease. Patients with chronic reflux esophagitis may respond to proton pump inhibitors, as well as abstinence from alcohol.

Stomach

Heavy ethanol use can disrupt the gastric mucosal barrier and cause acute and chronic gastritis. Ethanol concentrations up to 5% stimulate gastric acid secretion, whereas concentrations above 5% have no effect. Alcohol concentrations above 15% inhibit gastric motility and retard emptying of stomach contents. Clinical symptoms of high concentrations of ethanol intake include acute epigastric pain that is relieved with antacids or histamine H_2 receptor antagonists.

Intestines

Many individuals with AUD have chronic diarrhea caused by malabsorption in the small intestine. The rectal fissures and pruritus ani that are associated with heavy drinking are likely related to chronic diarrhea. Diarrhea is caused by structural and functional changes in the small intestine; for example, the intestinal mucosa has flattened villi, and digestive enzyme levels often are decreased. These changes are usually reversible after a period of abstinence.

Pancreas

Heavy alcohol use is the most common cause of both acute and chronic pancreatitis in the U.S. Acute alcoholic pancreatitis, involving acinar cells, is characterized by the abrupt onset of abdominal pain, nausea, vomiting, and increased levels of serum or urine pancreatic enzymes. Treatment usually involves intravenous fluid replacement (often with nasogastric suction) and opioid pain medication. Similar to alcoholic cirrhosis, chronic pancreatitis results from progressive cellular destruction and fibrosis. Chronic pancreatitis is treated by replacing the resulting endocrine and exocrine deficiencies. Hyperglycemia can develop as a sequela of pancreatitis and often requires insulin to control blood sugar levels (see Chapter 47). Pancreatic enzyme capsules containing lipase, amylase, and proteases may be necessary to treat malabsorption (see Chapter 50). The alcohol-induced risk for chronic pancreatitis is increased in smokers, which further exacerbates the risk of pancreatic cancer (Molina et al., 2014).

Liver

As the main organ involved in ethanol metabolism, the liver is a primary target for the pathological effects of ethanol. Alcohol misuse is responsible for approximately 50% of liver disease in the U.S. Ethanol produces dose-dependent hepatic injuries that progress from fat accumulation (steatosis) and inflammation to collagen deposition (fibrosis) to loss of liver cells (cirrhosis). The clinical stages of alcoholic liver disease are hepatosteatosis, alcoholic hepatitis, and cirrhosis. Accumulation of fat in the liver is an early event and can occur in normal individuals after the ingestion of relatively small amounts of ethanol. The generation of excess NADH, via metabolism of ethanol and acetaldehyde by ADH and ALDH, inhibits the tricarboxylic acid cycle and the oxidation of fat, leading to steatosis (see Figure 23–1). Steatosis is usually reversible with abstinence.

Hepatic stellate cells play an important role in the development of alcohol-mediated liver fibrosis. Fibrosis, resulting from tissue necrosis and chronic inflammation, is the underlying cause of alcoholic cirrhosis. The histological hallmark of cirrhosis is the formation of intracytoplasmic bodies called Mallory bodies, which may be related to an altered intermediate filament cytoskeleton.

Patients with AUD and alcoholic liver disease show changes in the composition of their intestinal microbiomes, increased intestinal permeability, and increased levels of gut-derived microbial products (Hartmann et al., 2015). Chronic ethanol exposure in animals and humans increases the circulating concentration of LPS, and the severity of hepatic injury correlates with serum levels of LPS. LPS activates TLRs and induces a complex signaling cascade, causing release of reactive oxygen species, chemokines, and pro-inflammatory cytokines.

Treatment of alcoholic hepatitis involves abstinence from alcohol and administration of corticosteroids, but corticosteroids only reduce mortality in the short term (Louvet and Mathurin, 2015). Improved treatment options may come from compounds that target the gut microbiome (see previous discussion), liver inflammation/regeneration, and oxidative stress. Probiotics, antibiotics, anti-inflammatory agents, immunosuppressants, growth factors, and antioxidants are examples of some of the different compounds undergoing clinical trials.

Cancers

Ethanol consumption is strongly linked to cancers of the oral cavity, pharynx, larynx, esophagus, colorectum (especially in men), and breast (women); there is also some evidence for an increased risk of liver cancer (Roswall and Weiderpass, 2015). Alcohol dependence plays a role in approximately 3.6% of all cancer cases and a similar percentage of cancer-related deaths (Boffetta et al., 2006). Two- to three-fold increases in cancer susceptibility are seen in individuals who chronically consume 50 g of alcohol per day, and concomitant smoking has a synergistic effect. As mentioned, individuals deficient in ALDH2 activity are particularly vulnerable to esophageal cancer. A notable complication in the treatment of cancer patients with AUD is that ethanol can interfere in the metabolism of some chemotherapeutic agents. The effects of acetaldehyde, a demonstrated carcinogen in animal models, and oxidative stress are widely cited mechanisms for the increased rate of carcinogenesis among individuals with AUD. Evidence also points to a role for aberrant DNA methylation patterns and other epigenetic modifications that control genome activity as mechanisms in alcohol-induced cancer development and progression. Epigenetics refers to processes that affect gene expression without changes in DNA sequence.

Hematological and Immunological Effects

Chronic excessive ethanol use is associated with different anemias, including microcytic, macrocytic, normochromic, and sideroblastic anemias, the last of which may respond to vitamin B_6 supplementation. Ethanol use also is associated with reversible thrombocytopenia. Ethanol affects granulocytes and lymphocytes, causing leukopenia, alteration of lymphocyte subsets, decreased T-cell mitogenesis, and changes in immunoglobulin production. In some patients with AUD, depressed leukocyte migration into inflamed areas may contribute to poor resistance to some infections (e.g., *Klebsiella* pneumonia, listeriosis, and tuberculosis). Some effects of ethanol-induced innate immune mechanisms that spread from the periphery to brain are described in the inflammatory sequence of events depicted in the following section.

Neuroimmune Mechanisms

The interplay between brain, behavior, and immunity in the etiology and progression of drug abuse is a rapidly developing area of research. Chronic ethanol consumption increases the levels of innate immune signaling molecules that reach the brain, producing alterations in brain physiology and behavior (Mayfield et al., 2013). Binge drinking increases levels of LPS, disrupting tight junctions and contributing to a leaky gut that permits bacteria and endotoxins to enter the circulation and exacerbate liver inflammation (Crews and Vetreno, 2015). This in turn releases pro-inflammatory cytokines that are transported across the blood-brain barrier, eliciting long-lasting neuroimmune responses. Within brain microglia, the actions of innate immune cytokines, activated TLRs, etc., are amplified via complex signaling loops, one of which leads to activation of the transcription factor NF-κB. NF-κB then regulates transcription of pro-inflammatory immune-related genes. Ethanol-induced microglia activation and induction of neuroimmune genes can thus be initiated systemically, through blood-borne molecules, as well as locally in the brain through neuronal-glial signaling. Neuroimmune mechanisms appear to be involved in later stages of heavy drinking and may contribute to neuronal apoptosis. Ethanol-induced neuroimmune activation also occurs in the developing brain, which may be relevant in FASDs (Drew and Kane, 2014).

Teratogenic Effects: Fetal Alcohol Spectrum Disorders

Ethanol is the most common teratogen in humans. Children born to mothers who are heavy drinkers display mental deficits and a common pattern of distinct dysmorphology known as FAS. The diagnosis of FAS is typically based on the observance of a triad of abnormalities associated with a history of prenatal ethanol exposure (Dorrie et al., 2014):

- A cluster of craniofacial abnormalities
- CNS dysfunction (structural or functional)
- Pre- or postnatal growth deficiencies (weight or height)

Fetal alcohol spectrum disorder is not a diagnostic term used by clinicians but rather an umbrella term that encompasses all of the disabilities caused by prenatal alcohol exposure. For example, children who do not meet all of the criteria for a diagnosis of FAS may show physical or mental deficits consistent with partial phenotypes, including *partial FAS, ARND,* and *ARBD* (Dorrie et al., 2014). The incidence of FAS is about 0.5–2 per 1000 live births in the general U.S. population, while the incidence of FAS, ARND, and ARBD combined is at least 1%. Higher rates of FAS occur in African and Native American women. Children of binge-drinking mothers show severe mental and behavioral deficits, likely due to the high peak BECs (Dorrie et al., 2014).

The FAS craniofacial abnormalities associated with maternal drinking in the first trimester consist of microcephaly, shortened palpebral fissures, thin upper lip, smooth philtrum, and epicanthal folds. Magnetic resonance imaging studies demonstrate decreased volumes in the basal ganglia, corpus callosum, cerebrum, and cerebellum that correlate with the facial abnormalities. CNS dysfunction attributed to in utero ethanol exposure consists of hyperactivity; attention and mental deficits; learning disabilities; language, memory, and motor disorders; and psychiatric conditions. FAS is the number one preventable cause of cognitive and attention deficits in the Western world, with afflicted children consistently scoring lower than their peers on a variety of IQ tests. Although the evidence is not conclusive, it has been suggested that even moderate alcohol consumption (28 g per day) in the second trimester of pregnancy is correlated with impaired academic performance of children at age 6. Maternal age also may be a factor: Pregnant women over age 30 who drink alcohol create greater risks to their children than do younger women who consume similar amounts of alcohol. In addition, the intake of high amounts of alcohol, particularly during the first trimester, greatly increases the chances of spontaneous abortion. Current recommendations are to drink no alcohol during pregnancy.

Clinical Uses of Ethanol

As mentioned, systemically administered ethanol is confined to the treatment of poisoning by methanol or ethylene glycol. In addition, dehydrated alcohol is injected in close proximity to nerves or sympathetic ganglia to relieve the long-lasting pain related to trigeminal neuralgia, inoperable carcinoma, and other conditions. Epidural, subarachnoid, and lumbar paravertebral injections of ethanol are also administered for inoperable pain. For example, lumbar paravertebral ethanol injections destroy sympathetic ganglia and thereby cause vasodilation and pain relief and promote healing of lesions in patients with vascular disease of the lower extremities.

Drug Interactions

Due to synergistic effects, great care must be taken when using sedatives to treat patients who have ingested heavy doses of ethanol or other CNS depressants. Acute ethanol intoxication decreases general anesthetic requirements, and elective surgery should be postponed in intoxicated patients. In contrast, chronic ethanol exposure increases anesthetic requirements largely due to pharmacodynamic cross-tolerance. An additional complication is the use of neuromuscular blockers and sedative/anesthetic agents in patients with AUD presenting with compromised liver function. This is particularly true for patients administered succinylcholine and benzodiazepines.

Pharmacokinetic interactions between ethanol and other drugs also occur. *Acute administration* of ethanol inhibits the function of enzymes responsible for metabolizing a variety of different drugs, including codeine, morphine, phenytoin, some benzodiazepines, tolbutamide, and warfarin, among others. Because ethanol inhibits CYP2E1, any drug also metabolized by this CYP isozyme will be metabolized at a slower rate in the presence of ethanol. In contrast, the *chronic administration* of ethanol acts as an enzyme inducer, particularly of CYP2E1, increasing the rate of metabolism of phenytoin, warfarin, propranolol, and benzodiazepines.

Comorbidity of Alcohol Use Disorder With Other Diseases

Many systemic diseases are related to chronic alcohol abuse, such as cardiovascular and liver diseases, as well as several types of cancers. AUD appears to increase the risk for diabetes mellitus, hypertension, stroke, osteoporosis, pancreatitis, and many other diseases. In this section, we focus on comorbid mental health conditions that are often present in patients with AUD or other substance use disorders.

Psychiatric Diseases

Patients diagnosed with a mood or anxiety disorder are about twice as likely to suffer from a drug abuse disorder and vice versa. In addition, AUD or other drug abuse disorders often occur in people with schizophrenia, leading to increased social and medical problems and complicating the course and treatment of schizophrenia. Patients with AUD and comorbid psychiatric disorders require treatment strategies that address both conditions. Although SSRIs have not been shown to be effective treatments for AUD in patients without a comorbid mental disorder, SSRIs and other antidepressants may decrease intake when AUD and depression co-occur; if alcohol use occurs as a consequence of depression, treating the underlying problem can decrease drinking.

Post-Traumatic Stress Disorder

Post-traumatic stress disorder is characterized by extreme hyperarousal and hyperstress responsiveness that contributes in a major way to the classic symptom cluster of reexperiencing, avoidance, and arousal. The prevalence of AUD in individuals with PTSD may be as high as 30% (Ouimette et al., 2005). The study of PTSD neurocircuitry has evolved from animal work on fear circuits and shows significant overlap with the symptoms of hyperresponsiveness to stress observed during alcohol withdrawal. One attractive hypothesis of the functional neurocircuitry changes that occur in PTSD is that of a brain-state shift from mild stress, in which the prefrontal cortex inhibits the amygdala, to extreme stress, in which the amygdala dominates (Pitman et al., 2012). Relative cortical dominance conveys resilience, while relative amygdala dominance conveys vulnerability; similar arguments can be made for the resilience and vulnerability to alcoholism, as elaborated by studies of the neurobiology of the withdrawal–negative affect stage of the alcohol addiction cycle.

Alcohol Use Disorder, Genetics, and Pharmacogenetics

Similar to other complex trait disorders, the development and progression of AUD is influenced by the interaction of multiple genetic and environmental factors. Environmental and cultural factors include stress, drinking patterns within one's culture and peer group, availability of alcohol, and attitudes toward drunkenness. These influences contribute to the initial decision to drink and the transition from casual drinking to alcohol-related problems. The heritability of AUD is estimated to be 50%–60%, as judged by family and twin studies. Long-term alcohol abuse and dependence are linked to persistent changes in gene expression (Mayfield et al., 2008).

As discussed previously, SNPs of *ADH* and *ALDH* may explain why some populations have a lower risk for AUD. Genetic variants of *ADH* that exhibit high activity and variants of *ALDH* that exhibit low activity protect against heavy drinking, likely because ethanol consumption by individuals expressing these variants results in accumulation of acetaldehyde, producing a variety of unpleasant effects.

Many additional genes modulate responses to ethanol, including variants of the following: μ–opioid receptor (*OPRM1*), dopamine transporter (*SLC6A3*), serotonin transporter (*SLC6A4*), dopamine receptor D2 (*DRD2*), α_2 subunit of the GABA$_A$ receptor (*GABRA2*), and α_3 subunit of the glycine receptor (*GLRA3*) (Jones et al., 2015). Other candidate genes include corticotropin-releasing hormone receptor 1 (*CRHR1*) and corticotropin-releasing hormone binding protein (*CRHBP*), which are important in brain stress pathways. Ethanol also induces the expression of neuroimmune-related genes, producing increased levels of immune markers detectable in postmortem brains from individuals with AUD (e.g., high-mobility group box 1, interleukin 1β, and TLRs), which may mediate long-term changes in brain function and neurodegeneration. Polymorphisms of genes encoding interleukin 1β and other immune molecules are associated with susceptibility to alcohol dependence (Crews and Vetreno, 2015).

Some of the pharmacotherapies for AUD, discussed in the next section, may be more effective in individuals carrying particular genetic variants. Clinical advances through pharmacogenetic studies of AUD may make the goal of precision medicine a possibility, but this will require rigorous methodological and statistical analyses. Each individual has unique neurobiological, genetic, and environmental profiles that affect treatment outcome, making individualized strategies not only feasible, but also necessary to move treatment of AUD into mainstream medicine (Litten et al., 2015).

Because AUD involves multifactorial processes with genetic and environmental determinants, as well as neuroadaptations related to disease progression, moving beyond studying the significance of individual candidate genes must include a systems approach to identify the relevant gene and protein networks operating at different stages of the disease. (Gorini et al., 2014).

Pharmacotherapy of Alcohol Use Disorder

Currently, three drugs are FDA approved for the treatment of AUD: disulfiram, naltrexone, and acamprosate (Table 23–2). They have reasonable efficacy, with effect sizes similar to those of antidepressant drugs for depression; unfortunately, they are not routinely prescribed (Jonas et al., 2014). Their efficacies may be influenced by an individual's genetic makeup, and genotyping is likely to become important in future treatment strategies. Benzodiazepines are the treatment of choice for management of acute alcohol withdrawal and to prevent the progression from minor withdrawal symptoms to major ones, such as seizures and delirium tremens (see Chapter 24).

TABLE 23–2 ■ ORAL MEDICATIONS FOR TREATING ALCOHOL ABUSE

MEDICATION	USUAL DOSE	MECHANISM/EFFECT
Disulfiram	250 mg/d (range of 125–500 mg/d)	• Inhibits ALDH with resulting ↑ acetaldehyde after drinking. Abstinence is reinforced to avoid the resulting adverse reaction.
Naltrexone	50 mg/d	• μ-opioid receptor antagonist; may ↓ drinking through ↓ feelings of reward with alcohol or ↓ craving.
Acamprosate	666 mg three times daily	• Unknown mechanism, may block hyperglutamatergic state and may ↓ mild protracted abstinence syndromes with ↓ feelings of a "need" for alcohol.

Disulfiram

Disulfiram (tetraethylthiuram disulfide), the first drug approved to treat alcohol abuse, is relatively nontoxic when taken in the absence of ethanol. It inhibits ALDH activity and increases the blood acetaldehyde concentration by 5–10 times compared to the level measured when ethanol is administered alone. Disulfiram irreversibly inactivates cytosolic and mitochondrial forms of ALDH to varying degrees. It is unlikely that disulfiram itself is responsible for ALDH inactivation in vivo because several active metabolites of the drug, especially diethylthiomethylcarbamate, behave as suicide-substrate inhibitors of ALDH in vitro. These metabolites reach significant concentrations in plasma following the administration of disulfiram.

Alcohol consumption by individuals previously treated with disulfiram gives rise to marked signs and symptoms of acetaldehyde poisoning. At BECs of 5–10 mg%, mild effects are noted, increasing markedly in severity as the BEC reaches 50 mg%. If the patient attains a BEC of 125–150 mg%, loss of consciousness may occur. Within 5–10 min, the face feels hot and soon afterward becomes flushed and scarlet in appearance. As the vasodilation spreads over the whole body, intense throbbing is felt in the head and neck, and a pulsating headache may develop. Respiratory difficulties, nausea, copious vomiting, sweating, thirst, chest pain, considerable hypotension, orthostatic syncope, marked uneasiness, weakness, vertigo, blurred vision, and confusion are observed. The facial flush is then replaced by pallor, and blood pressure may fall to levels seen in shock. Thus, the use of disulfiram requires careful medical supervision and should only be attempted in motivated patients committed to maintaining abstinence. Patients must learn to avoid disguised forms of alcohol that may be present in sauces, fermented vinegar, cough syrups, and even aftershave lotions. Disulfiram treatment results in poor compliance, possibly because of the adverse effects that result if taken with ethanol.

Disulfiram should not be administered until the patient has abstained from alcohol for at least 12 h. In the initial phase of treatment, a maximal daily dose of 500 mg is given for 1–2 weeks. Maintenance dosage then ranges from 125 to 500 mg daily depending on tolerance to side effects. Unless sedation is prominent, the daily dose should be taken in the morning, the time when the resolve not to drink may be strongest. Sensitization to alcohol may last as long as 14 days after the last ingestion of disulfiram because of the slow rate of restoration of ALDH.

Disulfiram or its metabolites can inhibit many enzymes with sulfhydryl groups, producing a wide spectrum of biological effects. Hepatic CYPs are inhibited, thereby interfering with the metabolism of phenytoin, chlordiazepoxide, barbiturates, warfarin, and other drugs.

Naltrexone

Naltrexone, a μ-opioid receptor antagonist, is chemically related to naloxone but has higher oral bioavailability and a longer duration of action when administered orally. It is also approved for treatment of opioid overdose and dependence (see Chapters 18 and 24). There is evidence that naltrexone blocks activation of brain receptors by opioid peptides that are thought to be critical for the rewarding effects of drugs of abuse.

Naltrexone reduces craving and decreases relapse to heavy drinking. Meta-analyses indicated that naltrexone is better than placebo, especially in reducing risk of heavy drinking. It is typically administered after detoxification at a dose of 50 mg/d for several months. Adherence to this regimen is important to ensure the therapeutic value of naltrexone but is a problem for some patients. A long-acting depot formulation of naltrexone is available for monthly injection. Naltrexone implants lasting several months are available outside the U.S.

The most common side effect of naltrexone is nausea, which subsides if the patient abstains from alcohol. There is some evidence of dysphoria associated with administration of naltrexone, and it is contraindicated in patients with depressive disorders. Doses of naltrexone exceeding 300 mg can cause liver damage; the drug is contraindicated in patients with liver failure or acute hepatitis and should be used only after careful consideration in patients with active liver disease. Naltrexone cannot be given to patients taking opioids, but it is used following opioid detoxification for prevention of relapse to opioid dependence.

Acamprosate

Acamprosate (*N*-acetylhomotaurine) may work by blocking a hyperglutamatergic state in the alcoholic brain, but the exact molecular target has remained elusive. It is FDA-approved for the treatment of AUD and is generally well tolerated by patients, with mild diarrhea being the main side effect. Double-blind, placebo-controlled studies demonstrated that acamprosate decreases drinking frequency and reduces relapse drinking in abstinent individuals but may not be effective in those who are currently drinking or misusing other drugs. Meta-analyses of randomized clinical trials showed that acamprosate is associated with reduced relapse in drinking (Jonas et al., 2014). For dosing, see Table 23–2.

Other Agents

Baclofen (used in France) has shown positive results for the treatment of AUD in some studies but is not FDA-approved for this use. Three other drugs described next, although not FDA-approved for AUD, are either approved in Europe or may prove useful based on emerging evidence.

Nalmefene, an opioid receptor antagonist structurally similar to naltrexone, is used to treat opioid overdose and may also be used to manage addictive behaviors. It is approved in Europe for as-needed use (18 mg) to reduce heavy drinking. It has several advantages over naltrexone, including longer duration of action, lack of dose-dependent liver toxicity, and higher affinity of binding to μ– and κ–opioid receptors.

Nalmefene reduces the total amount of alcohol consumed and the number of heavy drinking days in alcohol-dependent patients (van den Brink et al., 2014). Nalmefene was used for opioid overdose in the U.S. but has been discontinued.

Gabapentin, which interacts with the α2δ subunit of neuronal voltage-gated Ca^{2+} channels, is primarily used to treat epileptic seizures and neuropathic pain. A clinical trial showed that gabapentin (particularly the daily 1800-mg dose) improved rates of abstinence and no heavy drinking days in alcohol-dependent adults, decreased the number of heavy drinking days and number of drinks consumed per week, and decreased the severity of craving, insomnia, and dysphoria (Mason et al., 2014). Additional studies are needed to determine if gabapentin or other agents can be repurposed to treat AUD. For additional information on gabapentin, see Chapter 17.

Varenicline, which is approved for smoking cessation, also reduces alcohol consumption in preclinical and clinical models (Rahman et al., 2014). Varenicline acts as a partial agonist at α3β4, α4β2, and α6β2 subtypes of nAChRs and as a high-efficacy agonist at α7 nAChRs. Given the role of nAChRs in mediating the rewarding properties of ethanol and drugs of abuse, their blockade may offer pharmacological targets for treating patients with AUD who are heavy smokers. For more information on varenicline, consult Chapter 11.

Acknowledgment: Marc A. Schuckit contributed to this chapter in a previous edition of this book, and some of his text has been retained in the current edition.

Drug Facts for Your Personal Formulary: *Drugs Used to Treat Alcohol Use Disorder*

Drugs	Therapeutic Uses	Clinical Pharmacology and Tips
Disulfiram	• AUD	ALDH inhibitor. Causes adverse effects from increased acetaldehyde when taken with alcohol. Poor patient compliance.
Naltrexone	• AUD • Opioid dependence after opioid detoxification	μ-opioid receptor antagonist. Nausea, liver damage at high doses. Available in oral and long-acting injectable formulations. Contraindicated in patients with liver disease or taking opioids concurrently.
Acamprosate	• AUD	Unknown mechanism, may block hyperglutamatergic state. May work best in abstinent alcoholics.
Benzodiazepines	• Management of alcohol withdrawal • Anxiety/panic/seizure disorders • Insomnia • Anesthetic premedication	↑ GABA binding at $GABA_A$ receptors. Chlordiazepoxide, lorazepam, diazepam, oxazepam, midazolam, and clorazepate are used in the U.S. to manage alcohol withdrawal symptoms.
Fomepizole	• Methanol poisoning	ADH inhibitor.
Drugs Not FDA Approved for Treatment of AUD But Approved Elsewhere or Found Clinically Useful		
Gabapentin	• AUD • Epileptic seizures and neuropathic pain	Blocks neuronal voltage-gated Ca^{2+} channels. Reduced alcohol cravings in a clinical trial.
Varenicline	• ↓ alcohol consumption in clinical trials • Smoking cessation	Partial or full agonist at some central nAChR subtypes.
Nalmefene	• AUD • Opioid overdose/dependence	μ- and κ-opioid receptor antagonist. Approved in Europe for as-needed use to decrease drinking. Advantages over naltrexone: no liver toxicity, longer duration of action, higher affinity. Approved for opioid overdose but was discontinued in the U.S.
Baclofen	• AUD • Spasticity	$GABA_B$ receptor agonist, skeletal muscle relaxant, and antispasmodic agent.

Bibliography

American Psychiatric Association. *Diagnostic and Statistical Manual of Mental Disorders*. 5th ed. American Psychiatric Association Publishing, Arlington, VA, **2013**.

Boffetta P, et al. The burden of cancer attributable to alcohol drinking. *Int J Cancer*, **2006**, *119*:884–887.

Brower KJ. Assessment and treatment of insomnia in adult patients with alcohol use disorders. *Alcohol*, **2015**, *49*:417–427.

CDC. Alcohol and public health, **2017**. Available at: http://www.cdc.gov/alcohol. Accessed May 13, 2017.

CDC. Vital Signs: Binge Drinking Prevalence, Frequency, and Intensity Among Adults—United States, 2010. *Morbidity and Mortality Weekly Report*, **2012**, *61*;14–19.

Chen CH, et al. Targeting aldehyde dehydrogenase 2: new therapeutic opportunities. *Physiol Rev*, **2014**, *94*:1–34.

Crews FT, Vetreno RP. Mechanisms of neuroimmune gene induction in alcoholism. *Psychopharmacology* (Berl), **2016**, *233*:1543–1557.

Dorrie N, et al. Fetal alcohol spectrum disorders. *Eur Child Adolesc Psychiatry*, **2014**, *23*:863–875.

Drew PD, Kane CJ. Fetal alcohol spectrum disorders and neuroimmune changes. *Int Rev Neurobiol*, **2014**, *118*:41–80.

Edenberg HJ, et al. Association of alcohol dehydrogenase genes with alcohol dependence: a comprehensive analysis. *Hum Mol Genet*, **2006**, *15*:1539–1549.

Gorini G, et al. Proteomic approaches and identification of novel therapeutic targets for alcoholism. *Neuropsychopharmacology*, **2014**, *39*:104–130.

Grant BF, et al. Epidemiology of DSM-5 Alcohol Use Disorder: Results From the National Epidemiologic Survey on Alcohol and Related Conditions III. *JAMA Psychiatry*, **2015**, *72*:757–766.

Guzzo-Merello G, et al. Alcoholic cardiomyopathy. *World J Cardiol*, **2014**, *6*:771–781.

Hartmann P, et al. Alcoholic liver disease: the gut microbiome and liver cross talk. *Alcohol Clin Exp Res*, **2015**, *39*:763–775.

Heinz A, et al. Reward craving and withdrawal relief craving: assessment of different motivational pathways to alcohol intake. *Alcohol Alcohol*, **2003**, *38*:35–39.

Howard RJ, et al. Seeking structural specificity: direct modulation of pentameric ligand-gated ion channels by alcohols and general anesthetics. *Pharmacol Rev*, **2014**, *66*:396–412.

Jonas DE, et al. Pharmacotherapy for adults with alcohol use disorders in outpatient settings: a systematic review and meta-analysis. *JAMA*, **2014**, *311*:1889–1900.

Jones JD, et al. The pharmacogenetics of alcohol use disorder. *Alcohol Clin Exp Res*, **2015**, *39*:391–402.

Koob GF. Neurocircuitry of alcohol addiction: synthesis from animal models. *Hand Clin Neurol*, **2014**, *125*:33–54.

Koob GF. Alcohol use disorders: tracts, twins, and trajectories. *Am J Psychiatry*, **2015**, *172*:499–501.

Litten RZ, et al. Heterogeneity of alcohol use disorder: understanding mechanisms to advance personalized treatment. *Alcohol Clin Exp Res*, **2015**, *39*:579–584.

Louvet A, Mathurin P. Alcoholic liver disease: mechanisms of injury and targeted treatment. *Nature Rev Gastroenterol Hepatol*, **2015**, *12*:231–242.

Mason BJ, et al. Gabapentin treatment for alcohol dependence: a randomized clinical trial. *JAMA Int Med*, **2014**, *174*:70–77.

Mayfield J, et al. Neuroimmune signaling: a key component of alcohol abuse. *Curr Opin Neurobiol*, **2013**, *23*:513–520.

Mayfield RD, et al. Genetic factors influencing alcohol dependence. *Br J Pharmacol*, **2008**, *154*:275–287.

Molina PE, et al. Alcohol abuse: critical pathophysiological processes and contribution to disease burden. *Physiology*, **2014**, *29*:203–215.

Movva R, Figueredo VM. Alcohol and the heart: to abstain or not to abstain? *Int J Cardiol*, **2013**, *164*:267–276.

NIAAA. Apparent Per Capita Alcohol Consumption: National, State, And Regional Trends, 1977–2013. *Surveillance Report #102*, **2015**. Available at: https://pubs.niaaa.nih.gov/publications/surveillance102/cons13.htm. Accessed May 13, 2017.

O'Keefe JH, et al. Alcohol and cardiovascular health: the dose makes the poison … or the remedy. *Mayo Clin Proc*, **2014**, *89*:382–393.

Ouimette P, et al. Consistency of retrospective reports of *DSM-IV* criterion A traumatic stressors among substance use disorder patients. *J Trauma Stress*, **2005**, *18*:43–51.

Pava MJ, Woodward JJ. A review of the interactions between alcohol and the endocannabinoid system: implications for alcohol dependence and future directions for research. *Alcohol*, **2012**, *46*:185–204.

Pitman RK, et al. Biological studies of post-traumatic stress disorder. *Nat Rev Neurosci*, **2012**, *13*:769–787.

Rahman S, et al. Nicotinic receptor modulation to treat alcohol and drug dependence. *Front Neurosci*, **2014**, *8*:426.

Roerecke M, Rehm J. Alcohol consumption, drinking patterns, and ischemic heart disease: a narrative review of meta-analyses and a systematic review and meta-analysis of the impact of heavy drinking occasions on risk for moderate drinkers. *BMC Med*, **2014**, *12*:182.

Roswall N, Weiderpass E. Alcohol as a risk factor for cancer: existing evidence in a global perspective. *J Prev Med Public Health*, **2015**, *48*:1–9.

Scalzo SJ, et al. Wernicke-Korsakoff syndrome not related to alcohol use: a systematic review. *J Neurol Neurosurg Pyschiatry*, **2015**, *86*:1362–1368.

Schuckit MA. Comorbidity between substance use disorders and psychiatric conditions. *Addiction*, **2006**, *101*:76–88.

Schuckit MA. Alcohol-use disorders. *Lancet*, **2009**, *373*:492–501.

Thomson AD, et al. The evolution and treatment of Korsakoff's syndrome: out of sight, out of mind? *Neuropsychol Rev*, **2012**, *22*:81–92.

Trudell JR, et al. Alcohol dependence: molecular and behavioral evidence. *Trends Pharmacol Sci*, **2014**, *35*:317–323.

van den Brink W, et al. Long-term efficacy, tolerability and safety of nalmefene as-needed in patients with alcohol dependence: a 1-year, randomised controlled study. *J Psychopharmacol*, **2014**, *28*:733–744.

Volkow ND, et al. Profound decreases in dopamine release in striatum in detoxified alcoholics: possible orbitofrontal involvement. *J Neurosci*, **2007**, *27*:12700–12706.

White AM, et al. Converging patterns of alcohol use and related outcomes among females and males in the United States, 2002 to 2012. *Alcohol Clin Exp Res*, **2015**, *39*:1712–1726.

Zhang C, et al. Alcohol intake and risk of stroke: a dose-response meta-analysis of prospective studies. *Int J Cardiol*, **2014**, *174*:669–677.

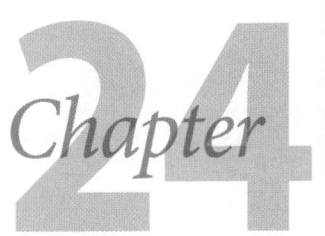

Chapter 24

Drug Use Disorders and Addiction

Charles P. O'Brien

THE CONFUSING TERMINOLOGY OF DRUG USE DISORDERS

ORIGINS OF SUBSTANCE USE DISORDERS
- Agent (Drug) Variables
- Host (User) Variables
- Environmental Variables

PHARMACOLOGICAL PHENOMENA
- Tolerance
- Physical Dependence
- Withdrawal Syndrome

CLINICAL ISSUES: CNS DEPRESSANTS
- Ethanol
- Benzodiazepines

- Barbiturates
- Nicotine
- Opioids

CLINICAL ISSUES: COCAINE AND OTHER PSYCHOSTIMULANTS
- Cocaine
- Amphetamine and Related Agents
- Caffeine
- Cannabinoids (Marijuana)
- Psychedelic Agents

The Confusing Terminology of Drug Use Disorders

The terminology of drug dependence, abuse, and addiction has long elicited confusion that stems from the fact that repeated use of certain prescribed medications can produce neuroplastic changes resulting in two distinctly abnormal states. The first state is *dependence*, or "physical" dependence, produced when there is progressive pharmacological adaptation to the drug resulting in tolerance. Tolerance is a normal reaction that is often mistaken for a sign of "addiction." In the tolerant state, repeating the same dose of a drug produces a smaller effect. If the drug is abruptly stopped, a withdrawal syndrome ensues in which the adaptive responses are now unopposed by the drug. The appearance of withdrawal symptoms is the cardinal sign of "physical" dependence. *Addiction*, the second abnormal state produced by repeated drug use, occurs in only a minority of those who initiate drug use; addiction leads progressively to compulsive, out-of-control drug use.

Addiction can be considered as a form of maladaptive memory. Addiction begins with the administration of substances (e.g., cocaine) or behaviors (e.g., the thrill of gambling) that directly and intensely activate brain reward circuits. Activation of these circuits motivates normal behavior, and most humans simply enjoy the experience without being compelled to repeat it. For some (~16% of those who try cocaine), the experience produces strong conditioned associations to environmental cues that signal the availability of the drug or the behavior. The individual becomes drawn into compulsive repetition of the experience, focusing on the immediate pleasure despite negative long-term consequences and neglect of important social responsibilities. The distinction between dependence and addiction is important because patients with pain sometimes are deprived of adequate opioid medication by their physician simply because they have shown evidence of tolerance or they exhibit withdrawal symptoms if the analgesic medication is stopped or reduced abruptly. The most recent revision of the classification system (*Diagnostic and Statistical Manual of Mental Disorders, Fifth Edition*; see American Psychiatric Association, 2013) makes a clear distinction between normal tolerance and a drug use disorder involving compulsive drug seeking.

Origins of Substance Use Disorders

Most of those who initiate use of a drug with addiction potential do not develop a drug use disorder. Many variables operate simultaneously to influence the likelihood that a beginning drug user will lose control and develop an addiction. These variables can be organized into three categories: agent (drug), host (user), and environment (Table 24–1).

Agent (Drug) Variables

Reinforcement refers to the capacity of drugs to produce effects that make the user wish to take them again. The more strongly reinforcing a drug is, the greater is the likelihood that the drug will be abused. Reinforcing properties of drugs are associated with their capacity to increase neuronal activity in brain reward areas (see Chapters 13 and 14). Cocaine, amphetamine, ethanol, opiates, cannabinoids, and nicotine reliably increase extracellular fluid DA levels in the ventral striatum, specifically the nucleus accumbens region. In contrast, drugs that block DA receptors generally produce bad feelings (i.e., *dysphoric effects*). Despite strong correlative findings, a precise causal relationship between DA and euphoria/dysphoria has not been established, and other findings emphasize additional roles of 5HT, glutamate, NE, endogenous opioids, and GABA in mediating the reinforcing effects of drugs.

The abuse liability of a drug is enhanced by rapidity of onset. When coca leaves are chewed, cocaine is absorbed slowly; this produces low cocaine levels in the blood and few, if any, behavioral problems. Crack cocaine, sold illegally and at a low price ($1–$3 per dose in 2016), is alkaloidal cocaine (free base) that can be readily vaporized by heating. Simply inhaling the vapors produces blood levels comparable to those resulting from intravenous cocaine owing to the large surface area for absorption into the pulmonary circulation following inhalation. Thus, inhalation of crack cocaine is much more addictive than chewing, drinking, or sniffing cocaine. The risk for developing addiction among those who try nicotine is about twice that for those who try cocaine (Table 24–2). This does not imply that the pharmacological addiction liability of nicotine is twice that of cocaine. Rather, there are other variables listed in Table 24–1 in the categories of Agent (e.g., mode of administration), Host, and Environment that influence the development of addiction.

Abbreviations

AIDS: acquired immune deficiency syndrome
CDC: U.S. Centers for Disease Control and Prevention
CNS: central nervous system
DA: dopamine
DAT: dopamine transporter
DEA: Drug Enforcement Agency
DMT: *N, N*-dimethyltryptamine
DOM: dimethoxymethylamphetamine
EEG: electroencephalogram
FDA: U.S. Food and Drug Administration
GABA: γ-aminobutyric acid
GI: gastrointestinal
GPCR: G protein–coupled receptor
5HT: serotonin
LSD: lysergic acid diethylamide
MDA: methylenedioxyamphetamine
MDMA: methylenedioxymethamphetamine
MOR: μ opioid receptor
NE: norepinephrine
NMDA: *N*-methyl-D-aspartate
PCP: phencyclidine
Δ-9-THC: Δ-9-tetrahydrocannabinol

TABLE 24–1 ■ MULTIPLE SIMULTANEOUS VARIABLES AFFECTING ONSET AND CONTINUATION OF DRUG ABUSE AND ADDICTION

Agent (drug)

Availability
Cost
Purity/potency
Mode of administration
   Chewing (absorption *via* oral mucous membranes)
   Gastrointestinal
   Intranasal
   Subcutaneous and intramuscular
   Intravenous
   Inhalation
Speed of onset and termination of effects (pharmacokinetics: combination of agent and host)

Host (user)

Heredity
   Innate tolerance
   Speed of developing acquired tolerance
   Likelihood of experiencing intoxication as pleasure
Metabolism of the drug (nicotine and alcohol data already available)
Psychiatric symptoms
Prior experiences/expectations
Propensity for risk-taking behavior

Environment

Social setting
Community attitudes
   Peer influence, role models
Availability of other reinforcers (sources of pleasure or recreation)
Employment or educational opportunities
Conditioned stimuli: environmental cues become associated with drugs after repeated use in the same environment

TABLE 24–2 ■ USE, ADDICTION, AND RISK AMONGST USERS OF TOBACCO, ETHANOL, AND ILLICIT DRUGS IN THE U.S., 1992–1994

AGENT	EVER USED[a] (%)	ADDICTION (%)	RISK OF ADDICTION (%)
Tobacco	75.6	24.1	31.9
Alcohol	91.5	14.1	15.4
Illicit drugs	51.0	7.5	14.7
Cannabis	46.3	4.2	9.1
Cocaine	16.2	2.7	16.7
Stimulants	15.3	1.7	11.2
Anxiolytics	12.7	1.2	9.2
Analgesics	9.7	0.7	7.5
Psychedelics	10.6	0.5	4.9
Heroin	1.5	0.4	23.1
Inhalants	6.8	0.3	3.7

[a]The ever-used and addiction percentages are those of the general population. The risk of addiction is specific to the drug indicated and refers to the percentage who met criteria for addiction among those who reported having used the agent at least once (i.e., each value in the rightmost column was obtained by expressing the number in the Addiction column as a percentage of the number in the Ever Used column, subject to errors of rounding).

Data source: Anthony JC, et al. Comparative epidemiology of dependence on tobacco, alcohol, controlled substances and the inhalants: basic findings from the National Comorbidity Survey. *Exp Clin Psychopharmacol*, **1994**, 2:244–268. This study was repeated in 2001–2003: Degenhardt L, et al. Epidemiological patterns of drug use in the United States: evidence from the National Comorbidity Survey Replication, 2001–2003. doi:10.1016/j.drugalcdep.2007.03.007. Accessed July 10, 2016. The National Institute on Drug Abuse conducted a related study in 2014: available at: https://www.drugabuse.gov/national-survey-drug-use-health. Accessed July 10, 2016.

Host (User) Variables

Effects of drugs vary among individuals. Polymorphism of genes that encode enzymes involved in absorption, metabolism, and excretion of a drug and its receptor-mediated responses may contribute to the effects of the drug across the addiction cycle (e.g., euphoria, reinforcement, etc.) (see Chapters 2 through 7). Innate tolerance to alcohol may represent a biological trait that contributes to the development of alcoholism. While innate tolerance increases vulnerability to alcoholism, impaired metabolism may *protect* against it (see Chapter 23). Similarly, individuals who inherit a gene associated with slow nicotine metabolism may experience unpleasant effects when beginning to smoke and reportedly have a lower probability of becoming nicotine dependent.

Psychiatric disorders constitute another category of host variables. People with anxiety, depression, insomnia, or even shyness may find that certain drugs give them relief. However, the apparent beneficial effects are transient, and repeated use of the drug may lead to tolerance and eventually compulsive, uncontrolled drug use. While psychiatric symptoms are seen commonly in drug abusers presenting for treatment, most of these symptoms begin *after* the person starts abusing drugs. Thus, drugs of abuse appear to produce more psychiatric symptoms than they relieve.

Environmental Variables

Initiating and continuing illegal drug use is influenced significantly by societal norms and peer pressure.

Pharmacological Phenomena

Tolerance

Tolerance, the most common response to repetitive use of the same drug, can be defined as the reduction in response to the drug after

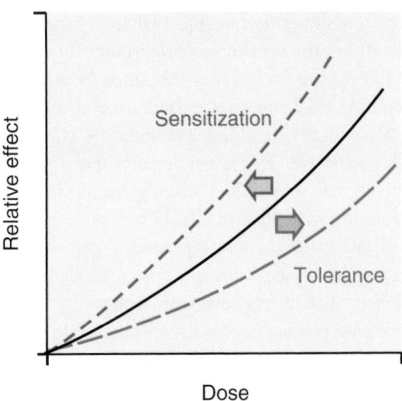

Figure 24–1 *Shifts in a dose-response curve with tolerance and sensitization.* The solid black curve describes the dose-response relationship to initial doses (the "control" curve). With tolerance, there is a shift of the curve to the right such that higher doses are required to achieve equivalent effects. With sensitization, the dose response shifts leftward, and a given dose produces a greater effect than in the control case.

repeated administrations. Consider an idealized drug dose-response curve (Figure 24–1). As the dose of the drug increases, the observed effect of the drug increases. With repeated use of the drug, however, the curve shifts to the right (tolerance). There are many forms of tolerance, likely arising through multiple mechanisms.

Tolerance to some drug effects develops much more rapidly than to other effects of the same drug. For example, tolerance develops rapidly to the euphoria produced by opioids such as heroin, and addicts tend to increase their dose to reexperience that elusive "high." In contrast, tolerance to the GI effects of opioids develops more slowly. The discrepancy between tolerance to euphorigenic effects (rapid) and tolerance to effects on vital functions such as respiration and blood pressure (slow) can lead to potentially fatal overdoses.

We can define multiple aspects of tolerance and give examples of some general mechanisms and dosing schedules that contribute:

- *Innate tolerance* refers to genetically determined lack of sensitivity to a drug the first time that it is experienced.
- *Acquired tolerance* can be divided into three major types—*pharmacokinetic*, *pharmacodynamic*, and *learned tolerance*—and includes acute, reverse, and cross-tolerance.
  1. *Pharmacokinetic* or *dispositional tolerance* refers to changes in the distribution or metabolism of a drug after repeated administrations, such that a given dose produces a lower blood concentration than the same dose did on initial exposure. The most common mechanism is an increase in the rate of metabolism of the drug. For example, chronic administration of barbiturates induces hepatic CYPs 1A2, 2C9, 2C19, and 3A4, thereby enhancing the metabolism of drugs that are substrates for these enzymes.
  2. *Pharmacodynamic tolerance* refers to adaptive changes that have taken place within systems affected by the drug so that response to a given concentration of the drug is altered (usually reduced). Examples include drug-induced changes in receptor density or efficiency of receptor coupling to signal transduction pathways (see Chapter 3).
  3. *Learned tolerance* refers to a reduction in the effects of a drug due to compensatory mechanisms that are acquired by past experiences. One type of learned tolerance is called *behavioral tolerance*. A common example is learning to walk a straight line despite the motor impairment produced by alcohol intoxication. At higher levels of intoxication, behavioral tolerance is overcome, and the behavioral deficits are obvious.
- *Conditioned tolerance* (situation-specific tolerance) develops when environmental cues or situations consistently are paired with the

administration of a drug. When a drug affects homeostatic balance by producing sedation and changes in blood pressure, pulse rate, gut activity, and so on, there is usually a reflexive counteraction or adaptation in the direction of maintaining the status quo. If a drug always is taken in the presence of specific environmental cues (e.g., smell of drug preparation and sight of syringe), these cues begin to predict the effects of the drug, and the adaptations begin to occur, which will prevent the full manifestation of the drug's effects (i.e., cause tolerance). This mechanism follows classical (Pavlovian) principles of learning and results in drug tolerance under circumstances where the drug is "expected."

- *Acute tolerance* refers to rapid tolerance developing with repeated use on a single occasion, such as in a "binge." For example, repeated doses of cocaine over several hours produce a decrease in response to subsequent doses of cocaine during the binge. This is the opposite of *sensitization*, observed with an intermittent-dosing schedule.
- *Sensitization* or *reverse tolerance* refers to an increase in response with repetition of the same dose of the drug. Sensitization results in a shift to the left of the dose-response curve (see Figure 24–1). Sensitization, in contrast to acute tolerance during a binge, requires a longer interval between doses, usually about 1 day. Sensitization can occur with stimulants such as cocaine or amphetamine.
- *Cross-tolerance* occurs when repeated use of a drug in a given category confers tolerance not only to that drug but also to other drugs in the same pharmacological category. Understanding cross-tolerance is important in the medical management of persons dependent on a drug.
- *Detoxification* is a form of treatment of drug dependence that involves giving gradually decreasing doses of the drug to prevent withdrawal symptoms, thereby weaning the patient from the drug of dependence. Detoxification can be accomplished with any medication in the same category as the initial drug of dependence. For example, users of heroin show cross-tolerance to other opioids. Thus, the detoxification of heroin-dependent patients can be accomplished with any medication that activates MORs.

These issues of tolerance, while straightforward, seem to produce a dangerous misunderstanding among self-medicating opioid users. Degrees of tolerance depend on the type of opioid, its half-life, and the route of administration. The typical addicted user is craving the "high" and seems willing to risk overdose by going beyond the safe level. This is especially dangerous when they have progressed to intravenous injection. Accidental overdose has become so common in the U.S. that death in this manner now exceeds the toll for traffic accidents in young people (Rudd et al., 2016).

Physical Dependence

Physical dependence is a state that develops as a result of the adaptation (tolerance) produced by a resetting of homeostatic mechanisms in response to repeated drug use. A person in this adapted or physically dependent state requires continued administration of the drug to maintain normal function. If administration of the drug is stopped abruptly, there is another imbalance, and the affected systems must readjust to a new equilibrium without the drug.

Withdrawal Syndrome

Withdrawal signs and symptoms occur when drug administration in a physically dependent person is terminated abruptly. The appearance of a withdrawal syndrome when administration of the drug is terminated is the only actual evidence of physical dependence. The type of withdrawal symptoms depends on the pharmacological category of the drug of dependence. Thus, withdrawal of a stimulant causes sedation during withdrawal. Withdrawal of an opioid produces craving for the opioid and physical symptoms, such as nausea, vomiting, and diarrhea, that are the opposite of the opioid's effects.

Pharmacokinetic variables are of considerable importance in the amplitude and duration of the withdrawal syndrome. Tolerance, physical dependence, and withdrawal are all biological phenomena. They are the natural consequences of drug use and can be produced in experimental animals and in any human being who takes certain medications repeatedly. These symptoms in themselves do not imply that the individual is involved in drug misuse or addiction. *Patients who take medicine for appropriate medical indications and in correct dosages still may show tolerance, physical dependence, and withdrawal symptoms* if the drug is stopped abruptly rather than gradually. A physician prescribing a medication that normally produces tolerance must understand the difference between dependence and addiction and be mindful of withdrawal symptoms if the dose is reduced.

Clinical Issues: CNS Depressants

Abuse of multiple drugs in combination is common. Alcohol is so widely available that it is combined with practically all other categories of drugs. Some combinations reportedly are taken because of their interactive effects. When confronted with a patient exhibiting signs of overdose or withdrawal, the physician must be aware of these possible combinations because each drug may require a different and specific treatment.

Ethanol

More than 90% of American adults report experience with ethanol (commonly called "alcohol"). Ethanol is classified as a depressant because it produces sedation and sleep. However, the initial effects of alcohol, particularly at lower doses, often are perceived as stimulation owing to a suppression of inhibitory systems (see Chapter 23). Heavy use of ethanol causes development of tolerance and physical dependence sufficient to produce an alcohol withdrawal syndrome when intake is stopped (Table 24–3).

Tolerance, Physical Dependence, and Withdrawal

The symptoms of mild intoxication by alcohol vary among individuals. Some experience motor incoordination and sleepiness. Others initially become stimulated. As the blood level increases, the sedating effects increase, with eventual coma and death occurring at high blood alcohol levels. The innate tolerance to alcohol varies greatly among individuals and is related to family history of alcoholism (Wilhelmsen et al., 2003). Experience with alcohol can produce greater tolerance (acquired tolerance) such that extremely high blood levels (300–400 mg/dL) can be found in alcoholics who do not appear grossly sedated. In these cases, the lethal dose does not increase proportionately to the sedating dose; thus, the margin of safety is decreased.

Heavy consumers of alcohol acquire tolerance and also develop a state of physical dependence. This often leads to drinking in the morning to restore blood alcohol levels diminished during the night. The alcohol withdrawal syndrome generally depends on the size of the average daily dose and usually is "treated" by resumption of alcohol ingestion. Withdrawal symptoms are experienced frequently but usually are not severe or life threatening until they occur in conjunction with other problems, such as

TABLE 24–3 ■ ALCOHOL WITHDRAWAL SYNDROME

Alcohol craving
Tremor, irritability
Nausea
Sleep disturbance
Tachycardia
Hypertension
Sweating
Perceptual distortion
Seizures (6–48 h after last drink)
Visual (and occasionally auditory or tactile) hallucinations
    (12–48 h after last drink)
Delirium tremens (48–96 h after last drink; rare in uncomplicated
    withdrawal)
    Severe agitation, confusion
    Fever, profuse sweating
    Tachycardia, dilated pupils
    Nausea, diarrhea

infection, trauma, malnutrition, or electrolyte imbalance. In the setting of such complications, the syndrome of *delirium tremens* becomes likely.

Alcohol addiction produces cross-tolerance to other sedatives, such as benzodiazepines. This tolerance is operative in abstinent alcoholics, but while the alcoholic is drinking, the sedating effects of alcohol add to those of other sedatives. This is particularly true for benzodiazepines, which are relatively safe in overdose when given alone but potentially are lethal in combination with alcohol. The chronic use of alcohol and other sedatives is associated with the development of depression and the risk of suicide. Cognitive deficits have been reported in alcoholics tested while sober. These deficits usually improve with abstinence. More severe recent memory impairment is associated with specific brain damage caused by nutritional deficiencies common in alcoholics (e.g., thiamine deficiency). Medical complications of alcohol abuse and dependence include liver disease, cardiovascular disease, endocrine and GI effects, and malnutrition, in addition to the CNS dysfunctions outlined previously. Ethanol readily crosses the placental barrier, producing the fetal alcohol syndrome, a major cause of mental retardation (see Chapter 23).

Pharmacological Interventions

Detoxification. Although most mild cases of alcohol withdrawal never come to medical attention, severe cases require general evaluation; attention to hydration and electrolytes; vitamins, especially high-dose thiamine; and a sedating medication that has cross-tolerance with alcohol. To block or diminish the symptoms described in Table 24–3, a short-acting benzodiazepine such as oxazepam can be used at a dose of 15–30 mg every 6–8 h according to the stage and severity of withdrawal; some authorities recommend a long-acting benzodiazepine unless there is demonstrated liver impairment. Anticonvulsants such as carbamazepine have been shown to be effective in alcohol withdrawal, but not as well as benzodiazepines.

Pharmacotherapy. Detoxification is the first step of treatment. Complete abstinence is the objective of long-term treatment, and this is best accomplished by a combination of relapse prevention, anticraving medication, and cognitive behavioral therapy. Disulfiram has been useful in some programs that focus behavioral efforts to promote ingestion of the medication. Disulfiram blocks aldehyde dehydrogenase, resulting in the accumulation of acetaldehyde (Figure 23–1), which produces an unpleasant flushing reaction and nausea when alcohol is ingested. Knowledge that this unpleasant reaction will ensue may help the patient to resist the urge to resume drinking alcohol. However, disulfiram has not proven to be effective in controlled clinical trials because so many patients choose to stop the medication rather than the alcohol.

Naltrexone is an opioid receptor antagonist that blocks the endorphin activation properties of alcohol. Chronic administration of naltrexone decreased the rate of relapse to heavy drinking in randomized clinical trials. The effect varied from strong to weak, but overall, reduction in heavy drinking was a consistent finding (Pettinati et al., 2006).

Naltrexone works best in combination with behavioral treatment programs that encourage adherence to medication and abstinence from alcohol. A depot preparation with a duration of 30 days is now available; it greatly improves medication adherence. Depot naltrexone can also be used in the prevention of relapse in opioid addiction (Lee et al., 2016).

Recent studies of alcohol detoxification have reported that gabapentin can aid in the transition to the abstinent state, possibly by improvement in sleep. Acamprosate, a competitive inhibitor of the NMDA-type glutamate receptor (see Table 23–2), appears to normalize the dysregulated neurotransmission associated with chronic ethanol intake and thereby to attenuate one of the mechanisms that lead to relapse.

Benzodiazepines

Benzodiazepines are used mainly for the treatment of anxiety disorders and insomnia (see Chapters 15 and 17). These agents are widely used, and abuse of prescription benzodiazepines is not uncommon. They may also be combined with alcohol or methadone in the treatment of opioid addiction. The proportion of patients who become tolerant and physically dependent on benzodiazepines increases after several months

TABLE 24-4 ■ BENZODIAZEPINE WITHDRAWAL SYMPTOMS

Following moderate-dose usage
  Anxiety, agitation
  Increased sensitivity to light and sound
  Paresthesias, strange sensations
  Muscle cramps
  Myoclonic jerks
  Sleep disturbance
  Dizziness

Following high-dose usage
  Seizures
  Delirium

of use, and abrupt reduction of the dose or stopping the medication produces withdrawal symptoms (Table 24–4).

It can be difficult to distinguish benzodiazepine withdrawal symptoms from the reappearance of the anxiety symptoms for which the benzodiazepine was originally prescribed. Some patients may increase their dose over time as tolerance develops to the sedative effects. Antianxiety benefits, however, seem to continue to occur long after tolerance to the sedating effects. Moreover, some patients continue to take the medication for years in appropriate doses according to medical directions and are able to function effectively as long as they take the medication. Patients with a history of alcohol or other drug abuse problems have an increased risk for the development of benzodiazepine abuse and should rarely, if ever, be treated with benzodiazepines on a chronic basis.

Pharmacological Interventions

If patients receiving long-term benzodiazepine treatment by prescription wish to stop their medication, the process may take months of gradual dose reduction. Withdrawal symptoms may occur during this outpatient detoxification, but in most cases the symptoms are mild. Patients who have been on low doses of benzodiazepines for years usually have no adverse effects. If anxiety symptoms return, a nonbenzodiazepine such as buspirone may be prescribed. Some authorities recommend transferring the patient to a benzodiazepine with a long $t_{1/2}$ during detoxification; others recommend the anticonvulsants carbamazepine and phenobarbital. The specific benzodiazepine receptor antagonist flumazenil is useful in the treatment of overdose and in reversing the effects of long-acting benzodiazepines used in anesthesia.

Abusers of high doses of benzodiazepines usually require inpatient detoxification. Frequently, benzodiazepine abuse is part of a combined dependence involving alcohol, opioids, and cocaine. Detoxification can be a complex clinical pharmacological challenge requiring knowledge of the pharmacokinetics of each drug. One approach to complex detoxification is to focus on the CNS depressant drug and temporarily hold the opioid component constant with a low dose of methadone or buprenorphine. A long-acting benzodiazepine such as diazepam or clorazepate or a long-acting barbiturate such as phenobarbital can be used to block the sedative withdrawal symptoms. After detoxification, the prevention of relapse requires a long-term outpatient rehabilitation program similar to the treatment of alcoholism. No specific medications have been found to be useful in the rehabilitation of sedative abusers, but specific psychiatric disorders such as depression or schizophrenia, if present, require appropriate medications.

Barbiturates

Abuse problems with barbiturates resemble those seen with benzodiazepines in many ways, and treatment of abuse and addiction to barbiturates should be handled similarly to interventions for the abuse of alcohol and benzodiazepines. Because drugs in this category frequently are prescribed as hypnotics for patients complaining of insomnia, physicians should be aware of the problems that can develop when the hypnotic

agent is withdrawn and of possible causes for insomnia that are treatable by other means. Insomnia often is a symptom of an underlying chronic problem, such as depression or respiratory dysfunction. Long-term prescription of sedative medications can change the physiology of sleep and should be avoided. When the sedative is stopped, there is a rebound effect with worsened insomnia. Whether from prescribed hypnotic or self-administered alcohol, medication-induced rebound insomnia requires detoxification by gradual dose reduction. Physicians should not recommend a bedtime drink of alcohol to relieve insomnia; the result is usually disordered sleep.

Nicotine

Nicotine and agents for smoking cessation are discussed in Chapter 11. Because nicotine provides the reinforcement for cigarette smoking, the most common cause of preventable death and disease in the U.S., it is arguably the most dangerous dependence-producing drug. Although more than 80% of smokers express a desire to quit, only 35% try to stop each year, and fewer than 5% are successful in unaided attempts to quit.

Tobacco (nicotine) addiction is influenced by multiple variables. Nicotine itself produces reinforcement; users compare nicotine to stimulants such as cocaine or amphetamine, although its effects are of lower magnitude. While there are many casual users of alcohol and cocaine, few individuals who smoke cigarettes smoke a small enough quantity (≤5 cigarettes per day) to avoid dependence. Nicotine is absorbed readily through the skin, mucous membranes, and lungs. The pulmonary route produces discernible CNS effects in as little as 7 sec. Thus, each puff produces some discrete reinforcement. With 10 puffs per cigarette, the 1-pack-per-day smoker reinforces the habit 200 times daily.

In dependent smokers, the urge to smoke correlates with a low blood nicotine level, as though smoking were a means to achieve a certain nicotine level and thus avoid nicotine withdrawal symptoms (Table 24–5). Depressed mood (dysthymic disorder, affective disorder) is associated with nicotine dependence, but it is not known whether depression can predispose one to begin smoking or whether depression develops secondarily during the course of nicotine dependence.

Pharmacological Interventions

The nicotine withdrawal syndrome can be alleviated by nicotine replacement therapy (e.g., nicotine inhaler and nasal spray, nicotine gum or lozenge, or nicotine transdermal patch). Different methods of nicotine delivery provide different blood nicotine levels over varying time courses (Figure 24–2). These methods suppress the symptoms of nicotine withdrawal. Although these treatments result in more smokers achieving abstinence, most resume smoking over the ensuing weeks or months. A sustained-release preparation of the antidepressant bupropion (see Chapter 15) improves abstinence rates among smokers and remains a useful option. The cannabinoid CB_1 receptor inverse agonist rimonabant improves abstinence rates and reduces the weight gain seen frequently in ex-smokers; unfortunately, rimonabant was found in clinical trials to be linked to depressive and neurologic symptoms and is not approved in the U.S.

Varenicline, a partial agonist at the α4β2 subtype of the nicotinic acetylcholine receptor, reduces cigarette craving and improves long-term abstinence rates. It has high receptor affinity, thus blocking access to nicotine, so if the treated smoker relapses, there is little reward, and abstinence is more likely to be maintained. In one clinical trial, the abstinence rate for

TABLE 24-5 ■ NICOTINE WITHDRAWAL SYMPTOMS

Irritability, impatience, hostility
Anxiety
Dysphoric or depressed mood
Difficulty in concentrating
Restlessness
Decreased heart rate
Increased appetite or weight gain

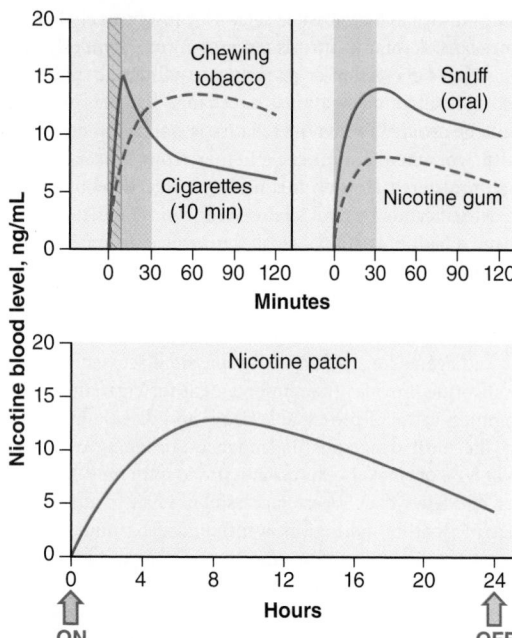

Figure 24–2 *Blood levels of nicotine resulting from different delivery systems.* In the upper panels, the shaded areas indicate the periods of nicotine delivery (30 min except for cigarettes, 10 min). In the lower panel, the arrows indicate the times of application and removal of a nicotine patch. These idealized curves are based on the findings of experiments by Benowitz et al., 1988, and Srivastava et al., 1991.

varenicline at 1 year was 36.7% versus 7.9% for placebo (Williams et al., 2007). There were initial reports of suicidal ideation in patients treated with this medication, but more recent studies in larger populations have failed to replicate these reports. See Chapter 11 for the pharmacology of varenicline.

Opioids

Opioid drugs are used primarily for the treatment of pain (see Chapter 20). Some of the CNS mechanisms that reduce the perception of pain also produce a state of well-being or euphoria. Thus, opioid drugs also are taken outside medical settings for the purpose of obtaining mood elevation or euphoria. Such use entails a high risk of overdose.

Death by Overdose

Heroin is the most frequently abused illicit opioid. Although there is no legal supply of heroin in the U.S., the drug is widely available on the illicit market. The purity of street heroin in the U.S. has increased over the past decade from about 4 mg heroin per 100-mg bag (range 0–8 mg/100 mg; the rest was nonopioid filler such as quinine) to a purity of 45%–75%, with some samples testing as high as 90%. This increase in purity has led to increased levels of physical dependence among heroin addicts. Users who interrupt regular dosing now develop more severe withdrawal symptoms. The more potent supplies can be smoked or administered nasally (snorted), making heroin use accessible to people who would not insert a needle into their veins. The increased potency of heroin has also contributed to more deaths by overdose.

Legal opioids are also abused. During early 21st century, there was increased interest among members of the medical profession in asking patients about pain, giving it a numerical rating, and treating it aggressively with prescription opioids as the agents of choice. In some cases, there was clear overprescribing, especially of extended-release forms of oxycodone, which have been linked to abuse, addiction, and overdose, and FDA approval of another long-acting formulation of oxycodone has provoked controversy (Manchikanti et al., 2014). Opioid overdose has become a common cause of death in many communities, and the latest

reports are worrisome, indicating that death from opioid overdose is now about 25,000 annually (DEA, 2015; Rudd et al., 2016). In response, the CDC announced more stringent guidelines for physicians to limit the prescription of opioids for chronic pain (Dowell et al., 2016; see Chapter 20).

Tolerance, Dependence, and Withdrawal

Injection of a heroin solution produces a variety of sensations, described as warmth, taste, or high and intense pleasure ("rush") often compared with sexual orgasm. There are some differences among the opioids in their acute effects; for instance, morphine produces a prominent histamine-releasing effect (causing itching), and meperidine is notable for producing excitation or confusion. Even experienced opioid addicts, however, cannot distinguish between heroin and the common opioid hydromorphone, often used for pain in hospitalized patients. The popularity of heroin may be due to its widespread availability on the illicit market and its rapid onset of effect.

After intravenous injection, the effects begin in less than a minute. Heroin has high lipid solubility, crosses the blood-brain barrier quickly, and is deacetylated to the active metabolites 6-monoacetyl morphine and morphine. After the intense euphoria, which lasts from 45 sec to several minutes, there is a period of sedation and tranquility ("on the nod") lasting up to an hour. The effects of heroin wear off in 3–5 h, depending on the dose. Experienced users may inject two to four times daily. Thus, the heroin addict is constantly oscillating between being "high" and feeling the sickness of early withdrawal (as depicted in Figure 24–3). This produces many problems in the homeostatic systems regulated at least in part by endogenous opioids.

Based on patient reports, tolerance develops early to the euphoria-producing effects of heroin and other opioids. There also is tolerance to the respiratory depressant, analgesic, sedative, and emetic properties. Heroin users tend to increase their daily dose, depending on their financial resources and the availability of the drug. Overdose is likely to occur when potency of the street sample is unexpectedly high or when the heroin is mixed with a far more potent opioid, such as fentanyl.

Addiction to heroin or other short-acting opioids produces behavioral disruptions and usually becomes incompatible with a productive life. Apart from the behavioral changes and the risk of overdose, chronic use of opioids is relatively nontoxic in and of itself. Nonetheless, the mortality rate for street heroin users is high. Heroin users commonly acquire bacterial infections producing skin abscesses, endocarditis; pulmonary infections, especially tuberculosis; and viral infections producing hepatitis C and AIDS.

Another factor is the use of opioids frequently in combination with other drugs, such as heroin and cocaine ("speedball"). Users report improved euphoria because of the combination, and there is evidence of

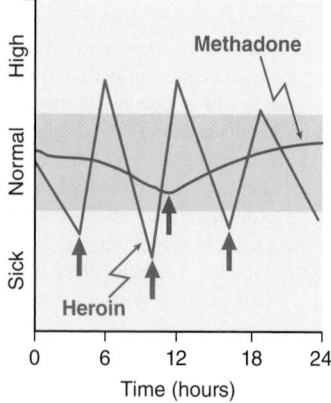

Figure 24–3 *Comparative time courses of response to heroin and methadone.* A person who injects heroin (↑) several times per day oscillates between being sick and being high (red line). In contrast, a methadone patient (purple line) remains in the "normal" range (blue band) with little fluctuation after dosing once per day. Ordinate values represent the subject's mental and physical state, not plasma levels of the drug.

TABLE 24–6 ■ CHARACTERISTICS OF OPIOID WITHDRAWAL

SYMPTOMS	SIGNS
Regular withdrawal	
Craving for opioids	Pupillary dilation
Restlessness, irritability	Sweating
Increased sensitivity to pain	Piloerection ("gooseflesh")
Nausea, cramps	Tachycardia
Muscle aches	Vomiting, diarrhea
Dysphoric mood	Increased blood pressure
Insomnia, anxiety	Yawning
	Fever
Protracted withdrawal	
Anxiety	Cyclic changes in weight, pupil
Insomnia	size, respiratory center sensitivity
Drug craving	

an interaction: Cocaine reduces the signs of opiate withdrawal, and heroin may reduce the irritability seen in chronic users of cocaine.

Pharmacological Interventions

Withdrawal and Detoxification. The first stage of treatment addresses physical dependence and consists of detoxification. The opioid withdrawal syndrome (Table 24–6) is unpleasant but not life threatening. It begins within 6–12 h after the last dose of a short-acting opioid and as long as 72–84 h after a long-acting opioid medication. The duration and intensity of the syndrome are related to the clearance of the individual drug. Heroin withdrawal is brief (5–10 days) and intense. Methadone withdrawal is slower in onset and lasts longer.

Opioid withdrawal signs and symptoms can be treated by three different approaches. *The first and most commonly used approach* consists of transfer to a prescription opioid medication and then gradual dose reduction. It is convenient to change the patient from a short-acting opioid such as heroin to a long-acting one such as methadone. The initial dose of methadone is typically 20–30 mg. The first day's total dose can be determined by the response and then reduced by 20% per day during the course of detoxification.

A second approach to detoxification involves the use of oral clonidine, an α_2 adrenergic agonist that decreases adrenergic neurotransmission from the locus ceruleus. This medication is approved for the treatment of hypertension but is commonly used off label to reduce symptoms of opioid withdrawal. Many of the autonomic symptoms of opioid withdrawal result from the loss of opioid suppression of the locus ceruleus system during the abstinence syndrome. Clonidine can alleviate many of these symptoms but not the generalized aches and opioid craving. Lofexidine, a similar medication, is FDA-approved for use as an opioid withdrawal suppressant. With clonidine and lofexidine, the dose must be titrated according to the stage and severity of withdrawal; postural hypotension is commonly a side effect.

A third method of treating opioid withdrawal involves activation of the endogenous opioid system without medication. The techniques proposed include acupuncture and several methods of CNS activation using transcutaneous electrical stimulation. While attractive theoretically, this method is not yet deemed practical.

Long-Term Management. If patients are simply discharged from the hospital after withdrawal from opioids, there is a high probability of a quick return to compulsive opioid use. Numerous factors influence relapse. The withdrawal syndrome does not end in 5–7 days; a *protracted withdrawal syndrome* (see Table 24–6) persists for up to 6 months. Physiological measures tend to oscillate as though a new set point were being established; during this phase, outpatient drug-free treatment has a low probability of success, even when the patient has received intensive prior treatment while protected from relapse in a residential program.

The most successful treatment of heroin addiction consists of stabilization on methadone in accordance with state and federal regulations. Patients who relapse repeatedly during drug-free treatment can be transferred directly to methadone without requiring detoxification. The dose of methadone must be sufficient to prevent withdrawal symptoms for at least 24 h.

The introduction of buprenorphine, a partial agonist at the MOR, represents a major change in the treatment of opiate addiction. This drug produces minimal withdrawal symptoms when discontinued and has a low potential for overdose, a long duration of action, and the ability to block heroin effects. Treatment can take place in a qualified physician's private office rather than in a special center, as required for methadone. When taken sublingually, buprenorphine is active; unfortunately, it also can be dissolved and injected (abused). As a solution to this problem, a buprenorphine-naloxone combination is available. When taken orally (sublingually), the naloxone moiety is not effective, but if the patient abuses the medication by injecting a solution of it, the naloxone will block or diminish the subjective high that could be produced by buprenorphine alone.

Antagonist Treatment. Naltrexone is an antagonist with a high affinity for MOR; it will competitively block the effects of heroin or MOR agonists. Naltrexone will not satisfy craving or relieve protracted withdrawal symptoms, but it can be used after detoxification for patients with high motivation to remain opioid free. Recently, an extended-release depot version of naltrexone has become available (Lee et al., 2016) .

Clinical Issues: Cocaine and Other Psychostimulants

Cocaine

In the U.S. in 2014–2015, the number of people aged 12 years or older who are regular users of cocaine (at least monthly) in 2009 was about 1.5 million (FDA, 2016). About 60% of these met the criteria for dependence or abuse defined by the *Diagnostic and Statistical Manual of Mental Disorders* (American Psychiatric Association, 2013). Cocaine abuse occurs about twice as frequently in men as in women. Not all users become addicts. A key factor in addiction is the widespread availability of relatively inexpensive cocaine in the alkaloidal form (free base, "crack"), suitable for smoking, and in the hydrochloride powder form, suitable for nasal or intravenous use.

The reinforcing effects of cocaine and cocaine analogues correlate best with their effectiveness in inhibiting DAT, the transporter that recovers DA from the synapse. This leads to increased DA concentrations at critical brain sites. However, cocaine also blocks both NE and 5HT reuptake, and chronic use of cocaine leads to changes in these neurotransmitter systems as well. Cocaine produces a dose-dependent increase in heart rate and blood pressure accompanied by increased arousal, improved performance on tasks of vigilance and alertness, and a sense of self-confidence and well-being. Higher doses produce euphoria, which has a brief duration and often is followed by a desire for more drug. Repeated doses of cocaine may lead to involuntary motor activity, stereotyped behavior, and paranoia. Irritability and increased risk of violence are found among heavy chronic users. The $t_{1/2}$ of cocaine in plasma is about 50 min, but inhalant (crack) users typically desire more cocaine after 10–30 min.

COCAINE

The major route for cocaine metabolism involves hydrolysis of its two ester groups. Tissue esterases and spontaneous hydrolysis remove the methyl ester to produce benzoylecgonine (30–40%); removal of the benzoyl moiety by butyrylcholinesterase yields ecgonine methyl ester (~50%). As a pharmacokinetic approach to treating cocaine toxicity and abuse, catalytic antibodies and mutations of human butyrylcholinesterase and a bacterial cocaine esterase have been developed that speed cocaine metabolism in animal models (Schindler and Goldberg, 2012).

Benzoylecgonine, produced on loss of the methyl group, represents the major urinary metabolite and can be found in the urine for 2–5 days after a binge. As a result, the benzoylecgonine test is a valid method for detecting cocaine use; the metabolite remains detectable in the urine of heavy users for up to 10 days. Ethanol is frequently abused with cocaine, as it reduces the irritability induced by cocaine. Dual addiction to alcohol and cocaine is common. When cocaine and alcohol are taken concurrently, cocaine may be transesterified to cocaethylene, which is equipotent to cocaine in blocking DA reuptake.

Addiction is the most common complication of cocaine abuse. In general, stimulants tend to be abused much more irregularly than opioids, nicotine, and alcohol. Binge use is common, and a binge may last hours to days, terminating only when supplies of the drug are exhausted.

Toxicity

Other risks of cocaine, beyond the potential for addiction, include cardiac arrhythmias, myocardial ischemia, myocarditis, aortic dissection, cerebral vasoconstriction, and seizures. Death from trauma also is associated with cocaine use. Cocaine may induce premature labor and abruptio placentae. Cocaine has been reported to produce a prolonged and intense orgasm if taken prior to intercourse, and users often indulge in compulsive and promiscuous sexual activity. However, chronic cocaine use reduces sexual drive. Chronic use is also associated with psychiatric disorders, including anxiety, depression, and psychosis.

Tolerance, Dependence, and Withdrawal

In intermittent users of cocaine, the euphoric effect typically is not subject to sensitization. On the contrary, most experienced users become desensitized and, over time, require more cocaine to obtain euphoria (i.e., tolerance develops). Because cocaine typically is used intermittently, even heavy users go through frequent periods of withdrawal or "crash." The symptoms of withdrawal seen in users admitted to hospitals are listed in Table 24–7. Careful studies of cocaine users during withdrawal showed gradual diminution of these symptoms over 1–3 weeks. Residual depression, often seen after cocaine withdrawal, should be treated with antidepressant agents if it persists (see Chapter 15).

Pharmacological Interventions

Because cocaine withdrawal is generally mild, treatment of withdrawal symptoms usually is not required. The major problem in treatment is not detoxification but helping the patient to resist the urge to resume compulsive cocaine use. Rehabilitation programs involving individual and group psychotherapy based on the principles of Alcoholics Anonymous and behavioral treatments based on reinforcing cocaine-free urine tests result in significant improvement in the majority of cocaine users.

Animal models suggest that enhancing GABAergic inhibition can reduce reinstatement of cocaine self-administration, and a controlled clinical trial of topiramate showed a significant reduction in cocaine use. Topiramate also reduced the relapse rate in alcoholics, prompting current studies in patients dually dependent on cocaine and alcohol. Baclofen, a $GABA_B$ agonist, was found in a single-site trial to reduce relapse in cocaine addicts but was not effective in a multisite trial. Modafinil is currently being tested in clinical trials of cocaine, methamphetamine, alcohol, and other substance abuse disorders. A mild stimulant approved for treating narcolepsy, modafinil has had several positive clinical trials for use in cocaine withdrawal (Morgan et al., 2016). The medication reduces the euphoria produced by cocaine and relieves cocaine withdrawal symptoms. It remains under investigation for this purpose.

A novel approach to cocaine addiction employs a vaccine that produces cocaine-binding antibodies. Cocaine itself is not antigenic in humans; however, a conjugate of the cocaine metabolite, nor-cocaine, with the B subunit of cholera toxin has been constituted as a vaccine, and it causes a vigorous immune response with the production of antibodies (immunoglobulin G) that neutralize cocaine in the bloodstream. Initial reports were promising, but in a recent trial the vaccine did not demonstrate the expected efficiency (Kosten et al., 2014). For now, behavioral therapy remains the treatment of choice, with medication indicated for specific coexisting disorders such as depression.

Amphetamine and Related Agents

Subjective effects similar to those of cocaine are produced by *amphetamine*, *dextroamphetamine*, *methamphetamine*, *phenmetrazine*, *methylphenidate*, and *diethylpropion*. Amphetamines increase synaptic DA, NE, and 5HT primarily by stimulating presynaptic release of stored neurotransmitter (see Chapter 8). Intravenous or smoked methamphetamine produces an abuse/dependence syndrome similar to that of cocaine, although clinical deterioration may progress more rapidly. Methamphetamine addiction has become a major public health problem in the U.S. Behavioral and medical treatments for methamphetamine addiction are similar to those used for cocaine.

Caffeine

Caffeine, a mild stimulant, is the most widely used psychoactive drug in the world. It is present in soft drinks, coffee, tea, cocoa, chocolate, and numerous prescription and over-the-counter drugs.

Caffeine can inhibit cyclic nucleotide phosphodiesterases, mildly increases NE and DA release, and enhances neural activity in numerous brain areas. Caffeine is absorbed from the digestive tract, is distributed rapidly throughout all tissues, and easily crosses the placental barrier. Caffeine is metabolized largely by CYP1A2, yielding a mean biological half-life of ~5 h, a number that can vary widely. For instance, tobacco smoking reduces it by ~40%; oral contraceptives double it; fluvoxamine increases caffeine's half-life tenfold. Many of caffeine's effects are believed to occur by means of competitive antagonism at adenosine receptors. Adenosine is a neuromodulator (see Chapter 14) that resembles caffeine structurally. The mild sedating effects that occur when adenosine activates particular adenosine receptor subtypes can be antagonized by caffeine. Tolerance occurs rapidly to the stimulating effects of caffeine. Thus, a mild withdrawal syndrome has been produced in controlled studies by abruptly discontinuing the intake of as little as one to two cups of coffee per day. Caffeine withdrawal consists of feelings of fatigue and sedation. With higher doses, headaches and nausea have been reported during withdrawal; vomiting is rare.

Cannabinoids (Marijuana)

The cannabis plant has been cultivated for centuries for its presumed medicinal and psychoactive properties. The smoke from burning cannabis contains many chemicals, including 61 different cannabinoids that have been identified. One of these, Δ9-THC, produces most of the characteristic pharmacological effects of smoked marijuana. In the U.S., marijuana use remains prohibited by federal law, but it is approved in thirteen states as medicine and in eight states for recreational purposes. This is leading to increased marijuana use and a greater number of marijuana-associated auto accidents. The issues of whether and how to control the use of marijuana have not been resolved. In addition, the potencies of available botanical forms have generally not been standardized, and the dangers inherent in inhaling a smoke replete with organic molecules have not been defined for marijuana smoke.

TABLE 24–7 ■ COCAINE WITHDRAWAL SYMPTOMS AND SIGNS
Dysphoria, depression
Sleepiness, fatigue
Cocaine craving
Bradycardia

The human cannabinoid endogenous ligand/receptor/signaling systems are described in Chapter 14 (see Figure 14–17). This system is stimulated by exogenous Δ9-THC. The pharmacological effects of Δ9-THC vary with the dose, route of administration, experience of the user, vulnerability to psychoactive effects, and setting of use. Intoxication with marijuana produces changes in mood, perception, and motivation, but the effects most frequently sought are a "high" and a "mellowing out." Effects vary with dose, but typically last about 2 h. During the high, cognitive functions, perception, reaction time, learning, and memory are impaired. Coordination and tracking behavior may be impaired for several hours beyond the perception of the high. Marijuana also produces complex behavioral changes such as giddiness and increased hunger. Unpleasant reactions such as panic or hallucinations and even acute psychosis may occur. These reactions are seen commonly with higher doses and with oral ingestion rather than smoked marijuana. Numerous clinical reports suggest that marijuana use may precipitate a recurrence of psychosis in people with a history of schizophrenia. One of the most controversial putative effects of marijuana is the production of an "amotivational syndrome." This syndrome is not an official diagnosis but has been used to describe young people who drop out of social activities and show little interest in school, work, or other goal-directed activity. At the cellular level, there is no evidence that marijuana damages brain cells or produces any permanent functional changes. There is evidence that the CB$_1$ receptor, a highly abundant GPCR in the mammalian brain, can deliver neuroprotective signals in animal models of striatal damage (Blázquez et al., 2015).

Marijuana has medicinal effects, including antiemetic properties that relieve side effects of anticancer chemotherapy. It also has muscle-relaxing effects, anticonvulsant properties, and the capacity to reduce the elevated intraocular pressure of glaucoma. These medical benefits come at the cost of the psychoactive effects that often impair normal activities. Dronabinol is an approved formulation of Δ9-THC (see Chapters 14 and 50).

Tolerance, Dependence, and Withdrawal

Tolerance to most of the effects of marijuana can develop rapidly after only a few doses, but also disappears rapidly. Withdrawal symptoms are not seen in clinical populations. Human subjects develop a withdrawal syndrome when they receive regular oral doses of the agent (Table 24–8). This syndrome, however, is only seen clinically in persons who use marijuana on a daily basis and then suddenly stop. Marijuana abuse and addiction have no specific treatments. Heavy users may suffer from accompanying depression and thus may respond to antidepressant medication.

Psychedelic Agents

There are two main categories of psychedelic compounds, indoleamines and phenethylamines. The indoleamine hallucinogens include LSD, DMT, and psilocybin. The phenethylamines include mescaline, DOM, MDA, and MDMA. Both groups have a relatively high affinity for 5HT$_2$ receptors (see Chapter 13), but they differ in their affinity for other subtypes of 5HT receptors. There is a good correlation between the relative affinity of these compounds for 5HT$_2$ receptors and their potency as hallucinogens in humans. LSD interacts with most brain 5HT receptors as an agonist/partial agonist and elicits sensory distortions (especially visual) and hallucinations at doses as low as 1 μg/kg. Current hypotheses of the mechanism of action of LSD and other hallucinogens focus on 5HT$_{2A}$ receptor–mediated disruption of thalamic gating with sensory overload of the cortex (Nichols, 2016).

TABLE 24–8 ■ MARIJUANA WITHDRAWAL SYNDROME
Restlessness
Irritability
Mild agitation
Insomnia
Sleep EEG disturbance
Nausea, cramping

LSD

LSD is the most potent hallucinogenic drug, more than 3000 times more potent than mescaline. LSD is sold on the illicit market in a variety of forms. A popular contemporary system involves postage stamp–size papers impregnated with varying doses of LSD (50–300 μg or more).

The effects of hallucinogenic drugs are variable, even in the same individual on different occasions. LSD is absorbed rapidly after oral administration, with effects beginning at 40–60 min, peaking at 2–4 h, and gradually returning to baseline over 6–8 h. At a dose of 100 μg, LSD produces perceptual distortions and sometimes hallucinations; mood changes, including elation, paranoia, or depression; intense arousal; and sometimes a feeling of panic. Signs of LSD ingestion include pupillary dilation, increased blood pressure and pulse, flushing, salivation, lacrimation, and hyperreflexia. Visual effects are prominent. Colors seem more intense, and shapes may appear altered. The subject may focus attention on unusual items, such as the pattern of hairs on the back of the hand.

A "bad trip" usually consists of severe anxiety, although at times it can be marked by intense depression and suicidal thoughts. Visual disturbances usually are prominent. There are no documented toxic fatalities from LSD use, but fatal accidents and suicides have occurred during or shortly after intoxication. Prolonged psychotic reactions lasting 2 days or more may occur after the ingestion of a hallucinogen. Schizophrenic episodes may be precipitated in susceptible individuals, and there is some evidence that chronic use of these drugs is associated with the development of persistent psychotic disorders. Claims about the potential of psychedelic drugs for enhancing psychotherapy and for treating addictions and other mental disorders are not supported by controlled studies; there is no generally accepted indication for these drugs as medications.

Tolerance, Physical Dependence, and Withdrawal. Frequent, repeated use of psychedelic drugs is unusual; thus, tolerance is not commonly seen. Tolerance does develop to the behavioral effects of LSD after three or four daily doses, but no withdrawal syndrome has been observed.

Pharmacological Intervention. Because of the unpredictability of psychedelic drug effects, any use carries some risk. Users may require medical attention because of bad trips. Severe agitation may respond to diazepam (20 mg orally). "Talking down" by reassurance also is effective and is the management of first choice. Antipsychotic medications (see Chapter 16) may intensify the experience and thus are contraindicated. A particularly troubling aftereffect of LSD and similar drugs is the occasional occurrence of episodic visual disturbances. These originally were called "flashbacks" and resembled the experiences of prior LSD trips. Flashbacks belong to an official diagnostic category called the *hallucinogen persisting perception disorder*. The symptoms include false fleeting perceptions in the peripheral fields, flashes of color, geometric pseudohallucinations, and positive afterimages. The visual disorder appears stable in half the cases and represents an apparently permanent alteration of the visual system. Precipitants include stress, fatigue, emergence into a dark environment, marijuana, antipsychotic agents, and anxiety states.

MDMA ("Ecstasy") and MDA

MDMA and MDA are phenylethylamines that have stimulant as well as psychedelic effects.

Acute effects are dose dependent and include feelings of energy, altered sense of time, and pleasant sensory experiences with enhanced perception. Negative effects include tachycardia, dry mouth, jaw clenching, and muscle aches. At higher doses, visual hallucinations, agitation, hyperthermia, and panic attacks have been reported. A typical oral dose is one or two 100-mg tablets, producing effects lasting 3–6 h, although dosage and potency of street samples are variable (~100 mg of active drug per tablet).

Phencyclidine

PCP was developed originally as an anesthetic in the 1950s and later was abandoned because of a high frequency of postoperative delirium with hallucinations. It was classified as a dissociative anesthetic because, in the anesthetized state, the patient remains conscious with staring gaze, flat facies, and rigid muscles. PCP became a drug of abuse in the 1970s, first in an oral form and then in a smoked version enabling a better regulation of the dose.

As little as 50 μg/kg produces emotional withdrawal, concrete thinking, and bizarre responses to projective testing. Catatonic posturing also is produced and resembles that of schizophrenia. Abusers taking higher doses may appear to be reacting to hallucinations and may exhibit hostile or assaultive behavior. Anesthetic effects increase with dosage; stupor or coma may occur with muscular rigidity, rhabdomyolysis, and hyperthermia. Intoxicated patients in the emergency room may progress from aggressive behavior to coma, with elevated blood pressure and enlarged, nonreactive pupils. PCP binds with high affinity to sites located in the cortex and limbic structures, blocking NMDA-type glutamate receptors (see Table 14–2 and Figures 14–12 and 14–13). There is evidence that NMDA receptors are involved in ischemic neuronal death caused by high levels of excitatory amino acids; as a result, there is interest in PCP analogues that block NMDA receptors but with fewer psychoactive effects. Both PCP and ketamine ("special K"), another "club drug," produce similar effects by altering the distribution of the neurotransmitter glutamate.

Medical Intervention. Overdose must be treated by life support; there is no antagonist of PCP effects and no proven way to enhance excretion, although acidification of the urine has been proposed. PCP coma may last 7–10 days. The agitated or psychotic state produced by PCP can be treated with diazepam. Prolonged psychotic behavior requires antipsychotic medication. Because of the anticholinergic activity of PCP, antipsychotic agents with significant anticholinergic effects such as chlorpromazine should be avoided.

Bibliography

American Psychiatric Association. *Diagnostic and Statistical Manual of Mental Disorders.* 5th ed. American Psychiatric Publishing, Arlington, VA, **2013**.

Benowitz NL, et al. Nicotine absorption and cardiovascular effects with smokeless tobacco use: comparison with cigarettes and nicotine gum. *Clin Pharmacol Ther*, **1988**, *44*:23–28.

Blázquez C, et al. The CB$_1$ cannabinoid receptor signals striatal neuroprotection via a PI3K/Akt/mTORC1/BDNF pathway. *Cell Death Differ*, **2015**, *22*:1618–1629.

DEA. 2015 National Drug Threat Assessment Summary. **2015**. Available at: https://www.dea.gov/docs/2015%20NDTA%20Report.pdf. Accessed July 13, 2016.

Dowell D, et al. CDC guideline for prescribing opioids for chronic pain—United-States, 2016. *MMWR Recomm Rep*, **2016**, *65*(No. RR-1):1–49. doi:http://dx.doi.org/10.15585/mmwr.rr6501e1. Accessed July 13, 2016.

FDA. What is the scope of cocaine use in the United States? **2016**. Available at: https://www.drugabuse.gov/publications/research-reports/cocaine/what-scope-cocaine-use-in-united-states. Accessed July 12, 2016.

Kosten TR, et al. Vaccine for cocaine dependence: a randomized double-blind placebo-controlled efficacy trial. *Drug Alcohol Depend*, **2014**, *140*:42–47.

Lee JD, et al. Extended-release naltrexone to prevent opioid relapse in criminal justice offenders. *N Engl J Med*, **2016**, *374*:1232–1242.

Manchikanti L, et al. Zohydro™ approval by Food and Drug Administration: controversial or frightening? A health policy review. *Pain Physician*, **2014**, *17*:E437–E450.

McLellan AT, et al. Drug dependence, a chronic medical illness: Implications for treatment, insurance, and outcomes evaluation. *JAMA*, **2000**, *13*:1689–1695.

Morgan PT, et al. Modafinil and sleep architecture in an inpatatient-outpatient treatment study of cocaine dependence. *Drug Alcohol Depend*, **2016**, *160*:49–56.

Nichols DE. Psychedelics. *Pharmacol Rev*, **2016**, *68*:264–355.

Pettinati HM, et al. The status of naltrexone in the treatment of alcohol dependence. *J Clin Psychopharmacol*, **2006**, *26*:610–625.

Rudd RA, et al. Increases in drug and opioid overdose deaths—United States, 2000–2014. *Am J Transplant*, **2016**, *16*:1323–1327.

Schindler CW, Goldberg SR. Accelerating cocaine metabolism as an approach to the treatment of cocaine abuse and toxicity. *Future Med Chem*, **2012**;*4*:163–175.

Srivastava ED, et al. Sensitivity and tolerance to nicotine in smokers and nonsmokers. *Psychopharmacology*, **1991**, *105*:63–68.

Wilhelmsen KC, et al. The search for genes related to a low-level response to alcohol determined by alcohol challenges. *Alcohol Clin Exp Res*, **2003**, *27*:1041–1047.

Williams KE, et al. A double-blind study evaluating the long-term safety of varenicline for smoking cessation. *Curr Med Res Opin*, **2007**, *23*:793–801.

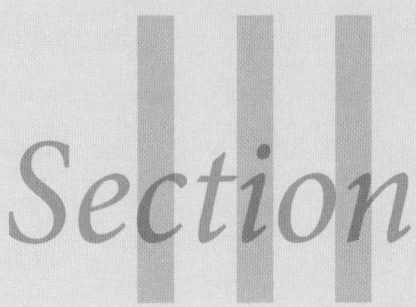

Section III

Modulation of Pulmonary, Renal, and Cardiovascular Function

Drugs Affecting Renal Excretory Function

Edwin K. Jackson

The kidney filters the extracellular fluid volume across the renal glomeruli an average of 12 times a day, and the renal nephrons precisely regulate the fluid volume of the body and its electrolyte content via processes of secretion and reabsorption. Disease states such as hypertension, heart failure, renal failure, nephrotic syndrome, and cirrhosis may disrupt this balance. Diuretics increase the rate of urine flow and Na⁺ excretion and are used to adjust the volume or composition of body fluids in these disorders. Precise regulation of body fluid osmolality is also essential. It is controlled by a finely tuned homeostatic mechanism that operates by adjusting both the rate of water intake and the rate of solute-free water excretion by the kidneys—that is, water balance. Abnormalities in this homeostatic system can result from genetic diseases, acquired diseases, or drugs and may cause serious and potentially life-threatening deviations in plasma osmolality.

Part I of this chapter first describes renal physiology, then introduces diuretics with regard to mechanism and site of action, effects on urinary composition, and effects on renal hemodynamics, and then integrates diuretic pharmacology with a discussion of mechanisms of edema formation and the role of diuretics in clinical medicine. Specific therapeutic applications of diuretics are presented in Chapters 28 (hypertension) and 29 (heart failure). *Part II* of this chapter describes the vasopressin system that regulates water homeostasis and plasma osmolality and factors that perturb those mechanisms and examines pharmacological approaches for treating disorders of water balance.

Part I: Renal Physiology and Diuretic Drug Action

Renal Anatomy and Physiology

The basic urine-forming unit of the kidney is the nephron. The initial part of the nephron, the renal (Malpighian) corpuscle, consists of a capsule (Bowman's capsule) and a tuft of capillaries (the glomerulus) residing within the capsule. The glomerulus receives blood from an afferent arteriole, and blood exits the glomerulus via an efferent arteriole. Ultrafiltrate produced by the glomerulus collects in the space between the glomerulus and capsule (Bowman's space) and enters a long tubular portion of the nephron, where the ultrafiltrate is reabsorbed and conditioned. Each human kidney is composed of about 1 million nephrons. Figure 25–1 illustrates subdivisions of the nephron.

Glomerular Filtration

In the glomerular capillaries, a portion of plasma water is forced through a filter that has three basic components: the fenestrated capillary endothelial cells, a basement membrane lying just beneath the endothelial cells, and the filtration slit diaphragms formed by epithelial cells that cover the basement membrane on its urinary space side. Solutes of small size flow with filtered water (solvent drag) into Bowman's space, whereas formed elements and macromolecules are retained by the filtration barrier.

Overview of Nephron Function

The kidney filters large quantities of plasma, reabsorbs substances that the body must conserve, and leaves behind or secretes substances that must be eliminated. The changing architecture and cellular differentiation along the length of a nephron are crucial to these functions (see Figure 25–1). The two kidneys in humans together produce about 120 mL of ultrafiltrate/min, yet only 1 mL of urine/min of urine; more than 99% of the glomerular ultrafiltrate is reabsorbed at a staggering energy cost. The kidneys consume 7% of total-body O_2 intake despite comprising only 0.5% of body weight.

The proximal tubule is contiguous with Bowman's capsule and takes a tortuous path until finally forming a straight portion that dives into the renal medulla. Normally, about 65% of filtered Na⁺ is reabsorbed in the proximal tubule, and because this part of the tubule is highly permeable to water, reabsorption is essentially isotonic. Between the outer and inner strips of the outer medulla, the tubule abruptly changes morphology to become the DTL, which penetrates the inner medulla, makes a hairpin turn, and then forms the ATL. At the juncture between the inner and outer medulla, the tubule once again changes morphology and becomes the TAL. Together, the proximal straight tubule, DTL, ATL, and TAL segments are known as the *loop of Henle*.

The DTL is highly permeable to water, yet its permeabilities to NaCl and urea are low. In contrast, the ATL is permeable to NaCl and urea but is impermeable to water. The TAL actively reabsorbs NaCl but is impermeable to water and urea. Approximately 25% of filtered Na⁺ is reabsorbed in the loop of Henle, mostly in the TAL, which has a large reabsorptive capacity. The TAL passes between the afferent and efferent arterioles and makes contact with the afferent arteriole by means of a cluster of specialized columnar epithelial cells known as the *macula densa*. The macula densa is strategically located to sense concentrations of NaCl leaving the loop of Henle. If the concentration of NaCl is too

Abbreviations

AA: arachidonic acid
ACTH: corticotropin (previously adrenocorticotropic hormone)
ADH: antidiuretic hormone
AIP: aldosterone-induced protein
Aldo: aldosterone
Ang: angiotensin
ANP: atrial natriuretic peptide
ATL: ascending thin limb
AVP: arginine vasopressin
BL: basolateral membrane
BNP: brain natriuretic peptide
CA: carbonic anhydrase
cGMP: cyclic guanosine monophosphate
CHF: congestive heart failure
CNGC: cyclic nucleotide-gated cation channel
CNP: C-type natriuretic peptide
CNT: connecting tubule
COX: cyclooxygenase
DAG: diacylgycerol
DCT: distal convoluted tubule
DDAVP: 1-deamino-8-D-AVP (desmopressin)
DI: diabetes insipidus
DTL: descending thin limb
ECFV: extracellular fluid volume
ENaC: epithelial Na^+ channel
ENCC1 or TSC: the absorptive Na^+-Cl^- symporter
ENCC2, NKCC2, or BSC1: the absorptive Na^+-K^+-$2Cl^-$
ENCC3, NKCC1, or BSC2: the secretory symporter
FDA: Food and Drug Administration
FF: filtration fraction
GFR: glomerular filtration rate
GPCR: G protein–coupled receptor
GTP: guanosine triphosphate
HCTZ: hydrochlorothiazide
HDL: high-density lipoprotein
HSD: 11-β-hydroxysteroid dehydrogenase
IMCD: inner medullary collecting duct
IP$_3$: inositol trisphosphate
LDL: low-density lipoprotein
LM: luminal membrane
LOX: lipoxygenase
LT: leukotriene
MR: mineralocorticoid receptor
MRA: mineralocorticoid receptor antagonist
mRNA: messenger RNA
NP: natriuretic peptide
NPA: asparagine-proline-alanine
NPR_: natriuretic peptide receptor _ (e.g., NPRA, B, or C)
NSAID: nonsteroidal anti-inflammatory drug
OAT: organic anion transporter
PA: phosphatidic acid
PG: prostaglandin
PK_: protein kinase _ (e.g. PKA, PKB, PKG)
PL_: phospholipase _ (e.g., PLC, PLD)
PTH: parathyroid hormone
PVN: paraventricular nucleus
RAAS: renin-angiotensin-aldosterone system
RAS: renin-angiotensin system
RBF: renal blood flow
SGK-1: serum and glucocorticoid-stimulated kinase 1
SIADH: syndrome of inappropriate secretion of ADH

SNS: sympathetic nervous system
SON: supraoptic nucleus
TAL: thick ascending limb
TGF: tubuloglomerular feedback
TX: thromboxane
VP: vasopressin
VRUT: vasopressin-regulated urea transporter
vWD: von Willebrand disease
WCV: water channel-containing vesicle

high, the macula densa sends a chemical signal (perhaps adenosine or ATP) to the afferent arteriole of the same nephron, causing it to constrict, thereby reducing the GFR. This homeostatic mechanism, known as *TGF*, protects the organism from salt and volume wasting. The macula densa also regulates renin release from the adjacent juxtaglomerular cells in the wall of the afferent arteriole.

Approximately 0.2 mm past the macula densa, the tubule changes morphology once again to become the DCT. Like the TAL, the DCT actively transports NaCl and is impermeable to water. Because these characteristics impart the capacity to produce dilute urine, the TAL and the DCT are collectively called the *diluting segment of the nephron*, and the tubular fluid in the DCT is hypotonic regardless of hydration status. However, unlike the TAL, the DCT does not contribute to the countercurrent-induced hypertonicity of the medullary interstitium (described in material that follows).

The collecting duct system (segments 10–14 in Figure 25–1) is an area of fine control of ultrafiltrate composition and volume. It is here that final adjustments in electrolyte composition are made, a process modulated by the adrenal steroid *aldosterone*. Vasopressin (also called ADH) modulates water permeability of this part of the nephron as well. The more distal portions of the collecting duct pass through the renal medulla, where the interstitial fluid is markedly hypertonic. In the absence of ADH, the collecting duct system is impermeable to water, and dilute urine is excreted. In the presence of ADH, the collecting duct system is permeable to water, and water is reabsorbed. The movement of water out of the tubule is driven by the steep concentration gradient that exists between tubular fluid and medullary interstitium.

The hypertonicity of the medullary interstitium plays a vital role in the capacity of mammals and birds to concentrate urine, which is accomplished by a combination of the unique topography of the loop of Henle and the specialized permeabilities of the loop's subsegments. The "passive countercurrent multiplier hypothesis" proposes that active transport in the TAL concentrates NaCl in the interstitium of the outer medulla. Because this segment of the nephron is impermeable to water, active transport in the ascending limb dilutes the tubular fluid. As the dilute fluid passes into the collecting duct system, water is extracted if, and only if, ADH is present. Because the cortical and outer medullary collecting ducts have low permeability to urea, urea is concentrated in the tubular fluid. The IMCD, however, is permeable to urea, so urea diffuses into the inner medulla, where it is trapped by countercurrent exchange in the vasa recta (medullary capillaries that run parallel to the loop of Henle). Because the DTL is impermeable to salt and urea, the high urea concentration in the inner medulla extracts water from the DTL and concentrates NaCl in the tubular fluid of the DTL. As the tubular fluid enters the ATL, NaCl diffuses out of the salt-permeable ATL, thus contributing to the hypertonicity of the medullary interstitium.

General Mechanism of Renal Epithelial Transport

There are multiple mechanisms by which solutes may cross cell membranes (see Figure 5–4). The kinds of transport achieved in a nephron segment depend mainly on which transporters are present and whether they are embedded in the luminal or basolateral membrane. Figure 25–2 presents a general model of renal tubular transport that be summarized as follows:

1. Na^+, K^+-ATPase (sodium pump) in the basolateral membrane transports Na^+ into the intercellular and interstitial spaces and K^+ into the cell,

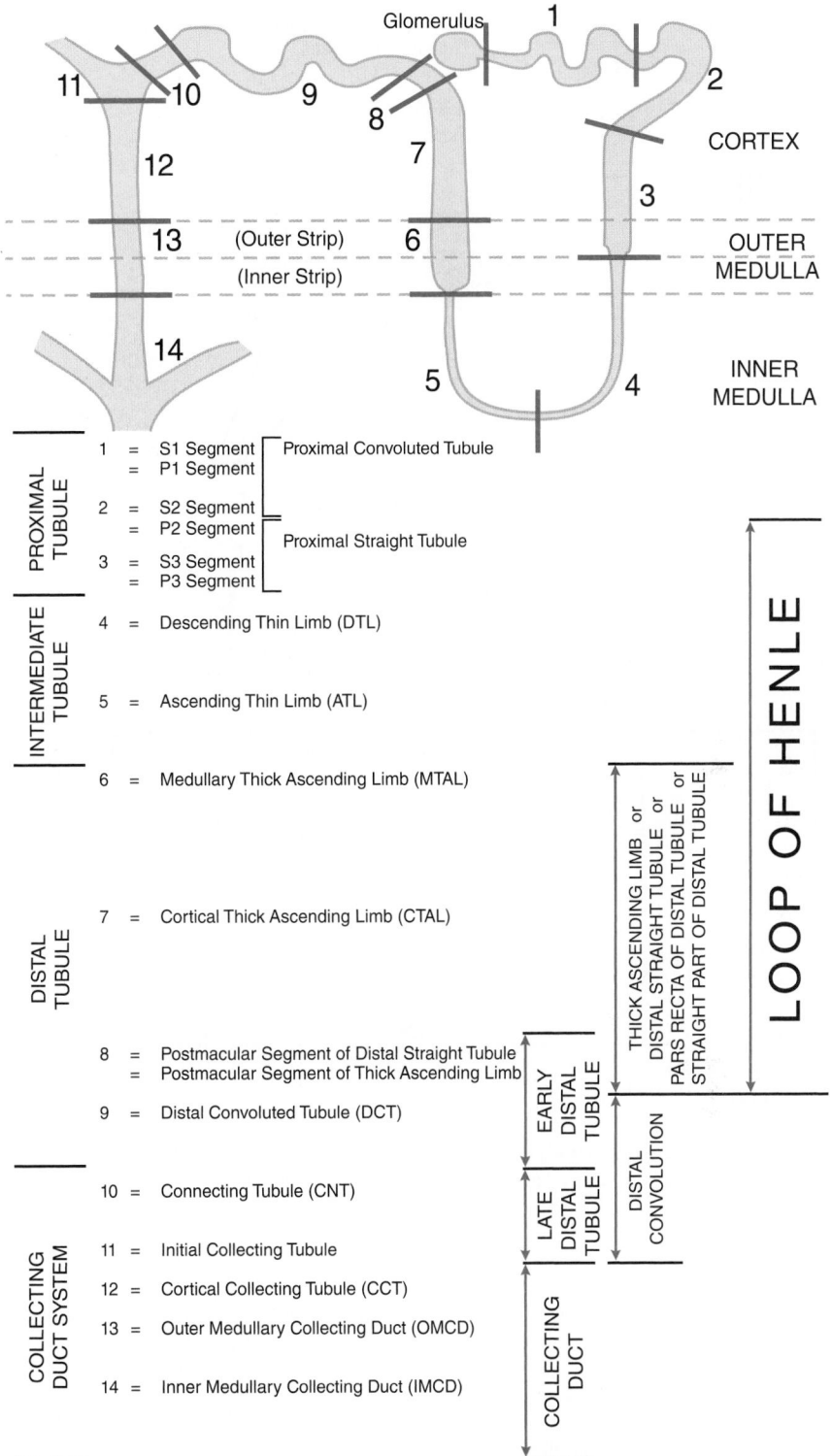

Figure 25–1 *Anatomy and nomenclature of the nephron.*

establishing an electrochemical gradient for Na^+ across the cell membrane directed inward.

2. Na^+ can diffuse down this Na^+ gradient across the luminal membrane via Na^+ channels and via membrane symporters that use the energy stored in the Na^+ gradient to transport solutes out of the tubular lumen and into the cell (e.g., Na^+-glucose, Na^+-$H_2PO_4^-$, and Na^+-amino acid) and antiporters (e.g., Na^+-H^+) that move solutes into the lumen as Na^+ moves down its gradient and into the cell.

3. Na^+ exits the basolateral membrane into intercellular and interstitial spaces via the Na^+ pump.

4. The action of Na^+-linked symporters in the luminal membrane causes the concentration of substrates for these symporters to rise in the epithelial cell. These substrate/solute gradients then permit simple diffusion or mediated transport (e.g., symporters, antiporters, uniporters, and channels) of solutes into the intercellular and interstitial spaces.

5. Accumulation of Na^+ and other solutes in the intercellular space creates a small osmotic pressure differential across the epithelial cell. In water-permeable epithelium, water moves into the intercellular spaces driven by the osmotic pressure differential. Water moves through aqueous pores in both the luminal and the basolateral cell membranes,

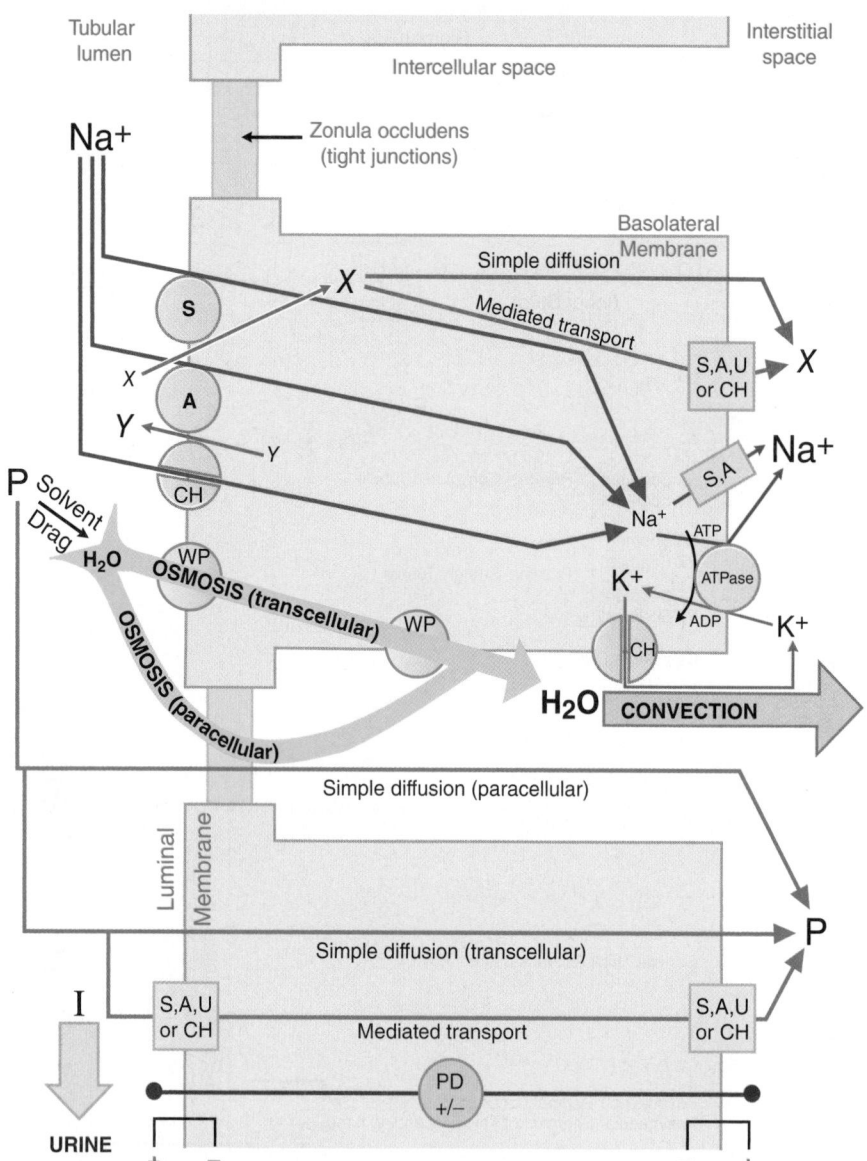

Figure 25–2 *Generic mechanism of renal epithelial cell transport* (see text for details). A, antiporter; ATPase, Na⁺, K⁺-ATPase (sodium pump); CH, ion channel; *I*, membrane-impermeable solutes; *P*, membrane-permeable solutes; PD, potential difference across indicated membrane or cell; S, symporter; U, uniporter; WP, water pore; *X* and *Y*, transported solutes.

as well as through tight junctions (paracellular pathway). Bulk water flow carries some solutes into the intercellular space by solvent drag.

6. Movement of water into the intercellular space concentrates other solutes in the tubular fluid, resulting in an electrochemical gradient for these substances across the epithelium. Membrane-permeable solutes then move down their electrochemical gradients into the intercellular space by both the transcellular (e.g., simple diffusion, symporters, antiporters, uniporters, and channels) and paracellular pathways. Membrane-impermeable solutes remain in the tubular lumen and are excreted in the urine with an obligatory amount of water.

7. As water and solutes accumulate in the intercellular space, hydrostatic pressure increases, thus providing a driving force for bulk water flow. Bulk water flow carries solute out of the intercellular space into the interstitial space and, finally, into the peritubular capillaries.

Organic Acid and Organic Base Secretion

The kidney is a major organ involved in the elimination of organic chemicals from the body. Organic molecules may enter the renal tubules by glomerular filtration or may be actively secreted directly into tubules. The proximal tubule has a highly efficient transport system for organic acids and an equally efficient but separate transport system for organic bases. Current models for these secretory systems are illustrated in Figure 25–3. Both systems are powered by the sodium pump in the basolateral membrane, involve secondary and tertiary active transport, and use a facilitated diffusion step. There are many organic acid and organic base transporters (see Chapter 5). A family of OATs links countertransport of organic anions with dicarboxylates (Figure 25–3A).

Renal Handling of Specific Anions and Cations

Reabsorption of Cl⁻ generally follows reabsorption of Na⁺. In segments of the tubule with low-resistance tight junctions (i.e., "leaky" epithelium), such as the proximal tubule and TAL, Cl⁻ movement can occur paracellularly. Cl⁻ crosses the luminal membrane by antiport with formate and oxalate (proximal tubule), symport with Na⁺/K⁺ (TAL), symport with Na⁺ (DCT), and antiport with HCO_3^- (collecting duct system). Cl⁻ crosses the basolateral membrane via symport with K⁺ (proximal tubule and TAL), antiport with Na⁺/HCO_3^- (proximal tubule), and Cl⁻ channels (TAL, DCT, collecting duct system).

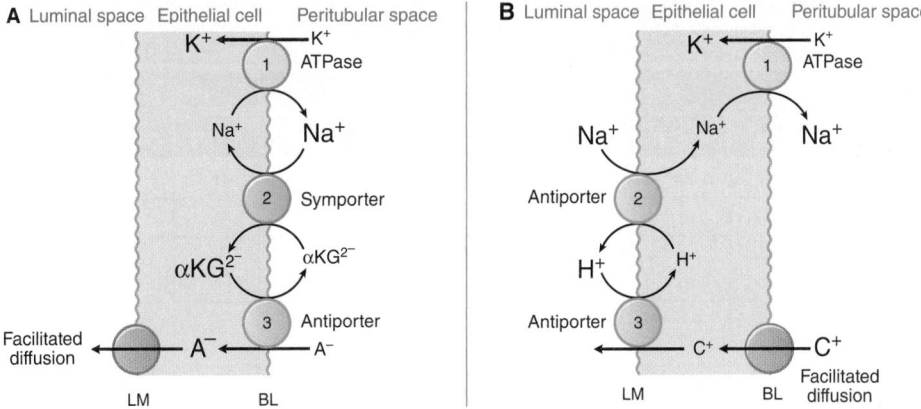

Figure 25–3 *Mechanisms of organic acid (**A**) and organic base (**B**) secretion in the proximal tubule.* The numbers 1, 2, and 3 refer to primary, secondary, and tertiary active transport, respectively. A^-, organic acid (anion); C^+, organic base (cation); αKG^{2-}, α-ketoglutarate but also other dicarboxylates. BL and LM indicate basolateral and luminal membranes, respectively.

Of filtered K^+, 80%–90% is reabsorbed in the proximal tubule (diffusion and solvent drag) and TAL (diffusion), largely through the paracellular pathway. The DCT and collecting duct system secrete variable amounts of K^+ by a channel-mediated pathway. Modulation of the rate of K^+ secretion in the collecting duct system, particularly by aldosterone, allows urinary K^+ excretion to be matched with dietary intake. The transepithelial potential difference V_T, lumen positive in the TAL and lumen negative in the collecting duct system, drives K^+ reabsorption and secretion, respectively.

Most of the filtered Ca^{2+} (~70%) is reabsorbed by the proximal tubule by passive diffusion through a paracellular route. Another 25% of filtered Ca^{2+} is reabsorbed by the TAL in part by a paracellular route driven by the lumen-positive V_T and in part by active transcellular Ca^{2+} reabsorption modulated by PTH (see Chapter 43). Most of the remaining Ca^{2+} is reabsorbed in DCT by a transcellular pathway. The transcellular pathway in the TAL and DCT involves passive Ca^{2+} influx across the luminal membrane through Ca^{2+} channels (TRPV5, **transient receptor potential cation channel V5**), followed by Ca^{2+} extrusion across the basolateral membrane by a Ca^{2+}-ATPase. Also, in DCT and CNT, Ca^{2+} crosses the basolateral membrane by Na^+-Ca^{2+} exchanger (antiport). P_i is largely reabsorbed (80% of filtered load) by the proximal tubule. The Na^+-P_i symporter uses the free energy of the Na^+ electrochemical gradient to transport P_i into the cell. The Na^+-P_i symporter is inhibited by PTH.

The renal tubules reabsorb HCO_3^- and secrete protons (tubular acidification), thereby participating in acid-base balance. These processes are described in the section on carbonic anhydrase inhibitors.

Principles of Diuretic Action

Diuretics are drugs that increase the rate of urine flow; clinically useful diuretics also increase the rate of Na^+ excretion (natriuresis) and of an accompanying anion, usually Cl^-. Most clinical applications of diuretics are directed toward reducing extracellular fluid volume by decreasing total-body NaCl content.

Although continued diuretic administration causes a sustained net deficit in total-body Na^+, the time course of natriuresis is finite because renal compensatory mechanisms bring Na^+ excretion in line with Na^+ intake, a phenomenon known as *diuretic braking*. These compensatory mechanisms include activation of the sympathetic nervous system, activation of the renin-angiotensin-aldosterone axis, decreased arterial blood pressure (which reduces pressure natriuresis), renal epithelial cell hypertrophy, increased renal epithelial transporter expression, and perhaps alterations in natriuretic hormones such as ANP. The net effects on extracellular volume and body weight are shown in Figure 25–4.

Diuretics may modify renal handling of other cations (e.g., K^+, H^+, Ca^{2+}, and Mg^{2+}), anions (e.g., Cl^-, HCO_3^-, and $H_2PO_4^-$), and uric acid. In addition, diuretics may alter renal hemodynamics indirectly. Table 25–1 compares the general effects of the major diuretic classes.

Inhibitors of Carbonic Anhydrase

There are three orally administered carbonic anhydrase inhibitors—*acetazolamide, dichlorphenamide,* and *methazolamide* (Table 25–2).

Mechanism and Site of Action

Proximal tubular epithelial cells are richly endowed with the zinc metalloenzyme carbonic anhydrase, which is found in the luminal and basolateral membranes (type IV carbonic anhydrase), as well as in the cytoplasm (type II carbonic anhydrase) (Figure 25–5). Carbonic anhydrase plays a role in $NaHCO_3$ reabsorption and acid secretion.

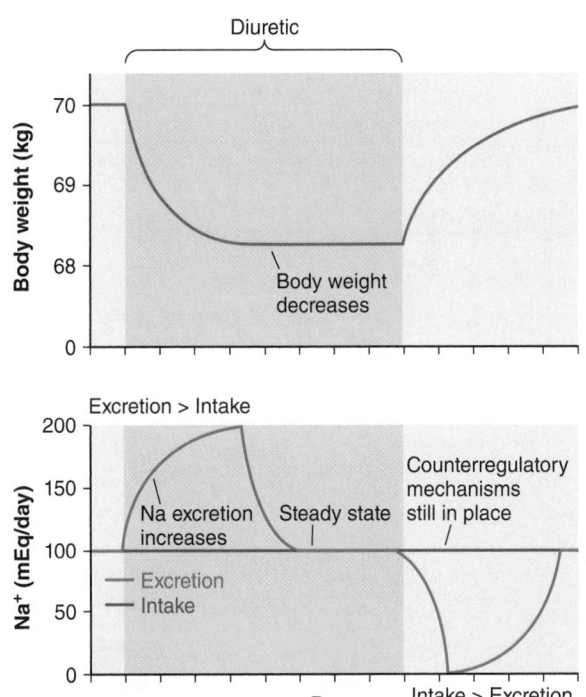

Figure 25–4 *Changes in extracellular fluid volume and weight with diuretic therapy.* The period of diuretic administration is shown in the shaded box along with its effects on body weight in the upper part of the figure and Na^{2+} excretion in the lower half of the figure. Initially, when Na^{2+} excretion exceeds intake, body weight and ECFV decrease. Subsequently, a new steady state is achieved where Na^+ intake and excretion are equal but at a lower ECFV and body weight. This results from activation of the RAAS and SNS, "the braking phenomenon." When the diuretic is discontinued, body weight and ECFV rise during a period when Na^{2+} intake exceeds excretion. A new steady state is then reached as stimulation of the RAAS and SNS wane.

TABLE 25–1 ■ EXCRETORY AND RENAL HEMODYNAMIC EFFECTS OF DIURETICS[a]

DIURETIC MECHANISM (Primary site of action)	CATIONS					ANIONS			URIC ACID		RENAL HEMODYNAMICS			
	Na$^+$	K$^+$	H^{+b}	Ca^{2+}	Mg^{2+}	Cl$^-$	HCO$_3$	H$_2$PO$_4^-$	*ACUTE*	*CHRONIC*	RBF	GFR	FF	TGF
Inhibitors of CA (proximal tubule)	+	++	−	NC	V	(+)	++	++	I	−	−	−	NC	+
Osmotic diuretics (loop of Henle)	++	+	I	+	++	+	+	+	+	I	+	NC	−	I
Inhibitors of Na$^+$-K$^+$-2Cl$^-$ symport (thick ascending limb)	++	++	+	++	++	++	+^{c}	+^{c}	+	−	V(+)	NC	V(−)	−
Inhibitors of Na$^+$-Cl$^-$ symport (distal convoluted tubule)	+	++	+	V(−)	V(+)	+	+^{c}	+^{c}	+	−	NC	V(−)	V(−)	NC
Inhibitors of renal epithelial Na$^+$ channels (late distal tubule, collecting duct)	+	−	−	−	−	+	(+)	NC	I	−	NC	NC	NC	NC
Antagonists of mineralocorticoid receptors (late distal tubule, collecting duct)	+	−	−	I		+	(+)	I	I	−	NC	NC	NC	NC

^{a}Except for uric acid, changes are for acute effects of diuretics in the absence of significant volume depletion, which would trigger complex physiological adjustments.
^{b}H$^+$ includes titratable acid and NH$_4^+$.
^{c}In general, these effects are restricted to those individual agents that inhibit carbonic anhydrase. However, there are notable exceptions in which symport inhibitors increase bicarbonate and phosphate (e.g., metolazone, bumetanide). ++, +, (+),−, NC, V, V(+), V(−) and I indicate marked increase, mild-to-moderate increase, slight increase, decrease, no change, variable effect, variable increase, variable decrease, and insufficient data, respectively. For cations and anions, the indicated effects refer to absolute changes in fractional excretion.

TABLE 25–2 ■ INHIBITORS OF CARBONIC ANHYDRASE

DRUG	RELATIVE POTENCY	ORAL AVAILABILITY	$t_{1/2}$ (hours)	ROUTE OF ELIMINATION
Acetazolamide	1	~100%	6–9	R
Dichlorphenamide	30	ID	ID	ID
Methazolamide	>1; <10	~100%	~14	~25% R, ~75% M

ID, insufficient data; M, metabolism; R, renal excretion of intact drug.

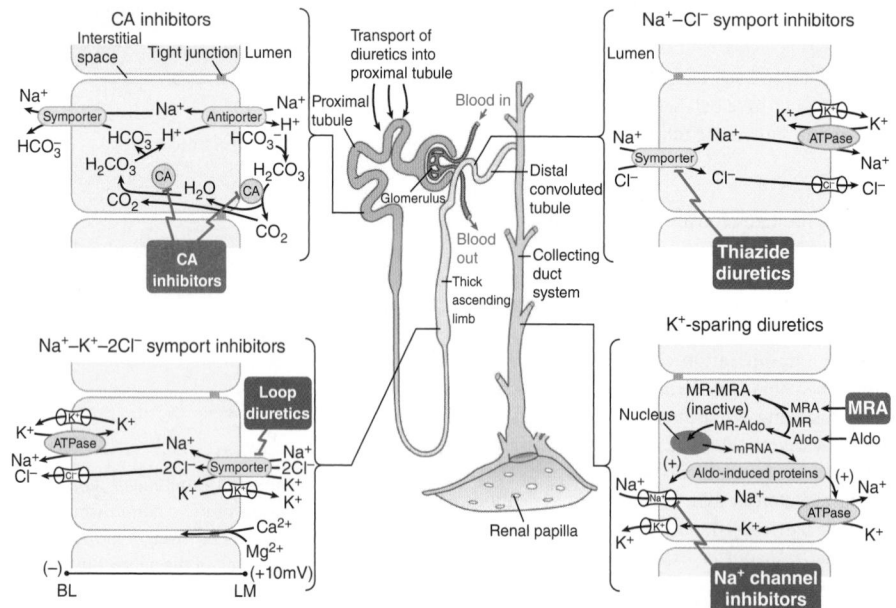

Figure 25–5 *Sites and mechanisms of action of diuretics.* Three important features are noteworthy: 1. Transport of solute across epithelial cells in all nephron segments involves highly specialized proteins, which for the most part are apical and basolateral membrane integral proteins. 2. Diuretics target and block the action of epithelial proteins involved in solute transport. 3. The site and mechanism of action of a given class of diuretics are determined by the specific protein inhibited by the diuretic.

In the proximal tubule, the free energy in the Na^+ gradient established by the basolateral Na^+ pump is used by a Na^+-H^+ antiporter (Na^+-H^+ exchanger type 3) in the luminal membrane to transport H^+ into the tubular lumen in exchange for Na^+. In the lumen, H^+ reacts with filtered HCO_3^- to form H_2CO_3, which decomposes rapidly to CO_2 and water in the presence of carbonic anhydrase in the brush border. Carbonic anhydrase reversibly accelerates this reaction several thousand fold. CO_2 is lipophilic and rapidly diffuses across the luminal membrane into the epithelial cell, where it reacts with water to form H_2CO_3, a reaction catalyzed by cytoplasmic carbonic anhydrase. Continued operation of the Na^+-H^+ antiporter maintains a low proton concentration in the cell, so H_2CO_3 ionizes spontaneously to form H^+ and HCO_3^-, creating an electrochemical gradient for HCO_3^- across the basolateral membrane. The electrochemical gradient for HCO_3^- is used by a Na^+-HCO_3^- symporter (also known as the Na^+-HCO_3^- cotransporter) in the basolateral membrane to transport $NaHCO_3$ into the interstitial space. The net effect of this process is transport of $NaHCO_3$ from the tubular lumen to the interstitial space, followed by movement of water (isotonic reabsorption). Removal of water concentrates Cl^- in the tubular lumen, and consequently, Cl^- diffuses down its concentration gradient into the interstitium by the paracellular pathway.

Carbonic anhydrase inhibitors potently inhibit both the membrane-bound and cytoplasmic forms of carbonic anhydrase, and can cause nearly complete abolition of $NaHCO_3$ reabsorption in the proximal tubule. However, due to the large excess of carbonic anhydrase activity in proximal tubules, a large fraction of the enzyme activity must be inhibited before an effect on electrolyte excretion is observed. Although the proximal tubule is the major site of action of carbonic anhydrase inhibitors, carbonic anhydrase also is involved in secretion of titratable acid in the collecting duct system, which is a secondary site of action for this class of drugs.

Effects on Urinary Excretion

Inhibition of carbonic anhydrase is associated with a rapid rise in urinary HCO_3^- excretion to about 35% of filtered load. This, along with inhibition of titratable acid and NH_4^+ secretion in the collecting duct system, results in an increase in urinary pH to about 8 and development of metabolic acidosis. However, even with a high degree of inhibition of carbonic anhydrase, 65% of HCO_3^- is rescued from excretion. The loop of Henle has large reabsorptive capacity and captures most of the Cl^- and a portion of the Na^+. Thus, only a small increase in Cl^- excretion occurs, HCO_3^- being the major anion excreted along with the cations Na^+ and K^+. The fractional excretion of Na^+ may be as much as 5%, and the fractional excretion of K^+ can be as much as 70%. The increased excretion of K^+ is in part secondary to increased delivery of Na^+ to the distal nephron, as described in the section on inhibitors of Na^+ channels. The effects of carbonic anhydrase inhibitors on renal excretion are self-limiting, probably because the resulting metabolic acidosis decreases the filtered load of HCO_3^- to the point that the uncatalyzed reaction between CO_2 and water is sufficient to achieve HCO_3^- reabsorption.

Effects on Renal Hemodynamics

By inhibiting proximal reabsorption, carbonic anhydrase inhibitors increase delivery of solutes to the macula densa. This triggers TGF, which increases afferent arteriolar resistance and reduces RBF and GFR.

Other Actions

These agents have extrarenal sites of action. Carbonic anhydrase in the ciliary processes of the eye mediates formation of HCO_3^- in aqueous humor. Inhibition of carbonic anhydrase decreases the rate of formation of aqueous humor and consequently reduces intraocular pressure. Acetazolamide frequently causes paresthesias and somnolence, suggesting an action of carbonic anhydrase inhibitors in the CNS. The efficacy of acetazolamide in epilepsy is due in part to the production of metabolic acidosis; however, direct actions of acetazolamide in the CNS also contribute to its anticonvulsant action. Owing to interference with carbonic anhydrase activity in erythrocytes, carbonic anhydrase inhibitors increase CO_2 levels in peripheral tissues and decrease CO_2 levels in expired gas. Acetazolamide causes vasodilation by opening vascular Ca^{2+}-activated K^+ channels; however, the clinical significance of this effect is unclear.

ADME

See Table 25–2 for pharmacokinetic data.

Therapeutic Uses

The efficacy of carbonic anhydrase inhibitors as single agents is low. The combination of acetazolamide with diuretics that block Na^+ reabsorption at more distal sites in the nephron causes a marked natriuretic response in patients with low basal fractional excretion of Na^+ (<0.2%) who are resistant to diuretic monotherapy. Even so, the long-term usefulness of carbonic anhydrase inhibitors often is compromised by the development of metabolic acidosis. The major indication for carbonic anhydrase inhibitors is open-angle glaucoma (Scozzafava and Supuran, 2014). Two products developed specifically for this use are dorzolamide and brinzolamide, which are available only as ophthalmic drops. Carbonic anhydrase inhibitors also may be employed for secondary glaucoma and preoperatively in acute-angle closure glaucoma to lower intraocular pressure before surgery (see Chapter 69). Orally administered acetazolamide also is used for the treatment of glaucoma (see Chapter 69) and absence seizures (see Chapter 21). Acetazolamide can provide symptomatic relief in patients with *high-altitude illness* or *mountain sickness* (Ritchie et al., 2012). Carbonic anhydrase inhibitors are also useful in patients with familial periodic paralysis. Dichlorphenamide is now approved for treating this syndrome. The mechanism for the beneficial effects of carbonic anhydrase inhibitors in altitude sickness and familial periodic paralysis may relate to the induction of a metabolic acidosis. Finally, carbonic anhydrase inhibitors can be useful for correcting metabolic alkalosis, especially one caused by diuretic-induced increases in H^+ excretion.

Toxicity, Adverse Effects, Contraindications, Drug Interactions

Serious toxic reactions to carbonic anhydrase inhibitors are infrequent; however, these drugs are sulfonamide derivatives and, like other sulfonamides, may cause bone marrow depression, skin toxicity, sulfonamide-like renal lesions, and allergic reactions. With large doses, many patients exhibit drowsiness and paresthesias. Most adverse effects, contraindications, and drug interactions are secondary to urinary alkalinization or metabolic acidosis, including (1) diversion of ammonia of renal origin from urine into the systemic circulation, a process that may induce or worsen hepatic encephalopathy (the drugs are contraindicated in patients with hepatic cirrhosis); (2) calculus formation and ureteral colic owing to precipitation of calcium phosphate salts in alkaline urine; (3) worsening of metabolic or respiratory acidosis (the drugs are contraindicated in patients with hyperchloremic acidosis or severe chronic obstructive pulmonary disease); and (4) reduction of the urinary excretion rate of weak organic bases.

Osmotic Diuretics

Osmotic diuretics (Table 25–3) are freely filtered at the glomerulus, undergo limited reabsorption by the renal tubule, and are relatively inert pharmacologically. Osmotic diuretics are administered in doses large enough to increase significantly the osmolality of plasma and tubular fluid. Of the osmotic diuretics listed, only glycerin and mannitol are currently available in the U.S.

TABLE 25–3 ■ OSMOTIC DIURETICS

DRUG	ORAL AVAILABILITY	$t_{1/2}$ (hours)	ROUTE OF ELIMINATION
Glycerin	Orally active	0.5–0.75	~80% M, ~20% U
Isosorbide[a]	Orally active	5–9.5	R
Mannitol	Negligible	0.25–1.7[b]	~80% R, ~20% M + B
Urea[a]	Negligible	1.2	R

B, excretion of intact drug into bile; M, metabolism; R, renal excretion of intact drug; U, unknown pathway of elimination.
[a]Not available in the U.S.
[b]In renal failure, 6–36 h.

Mechanism and Site of Action

Osmotic diuretics act in both the proximal tubule and the loop of Henle, with the latter the primary site of action. In the proximal tubule, osmotic diuretics act as nonreabsorbable solutes that limit the osmosis of water into the interstitial space and thereby reduce the luminal Na^+ concentration to the point that net Na^+ reabsorption ceases. By extracting water from intracellular compartments, osmotic diuretics expand extracellular fluid volume, decrease blood viscosity, and inhibit renin release. These effects increase RBF, and the increase in renal medullary blood flow removes NaCl and urea from the renal medulla, thus reducing medullary tonicity. A reduction in medullary tonicity causes a decrease in the extraction of water from the DTL, which in turn limits the concentration of NaCl in the tubular fluid entering the ATL. This latter effect diminishes the passive reabsorption of NaCl in the ATL. In addition, osmotic diuretics inhibit Mg^{2+} reabsorption in the TAL.

Effects on Urinary Excretion

Osmotic diuretics increase urinary excretion of nearly all electrolytes, including Na^+, K^+, Ca^{2+}, Mg^{2+}, Cl^-, HCO_3^-, and phosphate.

Effects on Renal Hemodynamics

Osmotic diuretics increase RBF by a variety of mechanisms, but total GFR is little changed.

ADME

Pharmacokinetic data on the osmotic diuretics are gathered in Table 25–3. Where available, glycerin and isosorbide can be given orally, whereas mannitol and urea must be administered intravenously (with the exception that mannitol powder is used by inhalation for diagnosis of bronchial hyperreactivity).

Therapeutic Uses

One use for mannitol is in the treatment of dialysis disequilibrium syndrome. Overly removing solutes from the extracellular fluid by hemodialysis results in a reduction in the osmolality of extracellular fluid. Consequently, water moves from the extracellular compartment into the intracellular compartment, causing hypotension and CNS symptoms (headache, nausea, muscle cramps, restlessness, CNS depression, and convulsions). Osmotic diuretics increase the osmolality of the extracellular fluid compartment and thereby shift water back into the extracellular compartment. By increasing the osmotic pressure of plasma, osmotic diuretics extract water from the eye and brain. Osmotic diuretics are used to control intraocular pressure during acute attacks of glaucoma and for short-term reductions in intraocular pressure both preoperatively and postoperatively in patients who require ocular surgery. Also, mannitol is used to reduce cerebral edema and brain mass before and after neurosurgery and to control intracranial pressure in patients with traumatic brain injury (Wakai et al., 2013). Mannitol is often used to treat or prevent acute kidney injury; however, it is questionable regarding whether mannitol improves renal outcomes (Nigwekar and Waikar, 2011). Other

FDA-approved uses of mannitol include enhancement of urinary excretion of salicylates, barbiturates, bromides, and lithium following overdose; for the diagnosis of bronchial hyperreactivity (by oral inhalation); and for antihemolytic urologic irrigation during transurethral procedures.

Toxicity, Adverse Effects, Contraindications, and Drug Interactions

Osmotic diuretics are distributed in the extracellular fluid and contribute to the extracellular osmolality. Thus, water is extracted from intracellular compartments, and the extracellular fluid volume becomes expanded. In patients with heart failure or pulmonary congestion, this may cause frank pulmonary edema. Extraction of water also causes hyponatremia, which may explain the common adverse effects, including headache, nausea, and vomiting. Conversely, loss of water in excess of electrolytes can cause hypernatremia and dehydration. Osmotic diuretics are contraindicated in patients who are anuric owing to severe renal disease. Urea may cause thrombosis or pain if extravasation occurs, and it should not be administered to patients with impaired liver function because of the risk of elevation of blood ammonia levels. Both mannitol and urea are contraindicated in patients with active cranial bleeding. Glycerin is metabolized and can cause hyperglycemia.

Inhibitors of Na^+-K^+-$2Cl^-$ Symport: Loop Diuretics, High-Ceiling Diuretics

The loop and high-ceiling diuretics inhibit activity of the Na^+-K^+-$2Cl^-$ symporter in the TAL of the loop of Henle, hence the moniker *loop diuretics*. Although the proximal tubule reabsorbs about 65% of filtered Na^+, diuretics acting only in the proximal tubule have limited efficacy because the TAL has the capacity to reabsorb most of the rejectate from the proximal tubule. In contrast, inhibitors of Na^+-K^+-$2Cl^-$ symport in the TAL, sometimes called *high-ceiling diuretics*, are highly efficacious because (1) about 25% of the filtered Na^+ load normally is reabsorbed by the TAL, and (2) nephron segments past the TAL do not possess the resorptive capacity to rescue the flood of rejectate exiting the TAL.

Of the inhibitors of Na^+-K^+-$2Cl^-$ symport (Table 25–4), only furosemide, bumetanide, ethacrynic acid, and torsemide are available in the U.S. Furosemide and bumetanide contain a sulfonamide moiety. Ethacrynic acid is a phenoxyacetic acid derivative; torsemide is a sulfonylurea. Furosemide and bumetanide are available as oral and injectable formulations. Torsemide is available as an oral formulation; ethacrynate sodium is available as an injectable solution and ethacrynic acid as an oral tablet.

Mechanism and Site of Action

These agents act primarily in the TAL, where the flux of Na^+, K^+, and Cl^- from the lumen into epithelial cells is mediated by a Na^+-K^+-$2Cl^-$ symporter (Figure 25–5). Inhibitors of this symporter block its function (Bernstein and Ellison, 2011; Wile, 2012), bringing salt transport in this segment of the nephron to a virtual standstill. There is evidence that these

TABLE 25–4 ■ INHIBITORS OF Na^+-K^+-$2Cl^-$ SYMPORT (LOOP DIURETICS, HIGH-CEILING DIURETICS)

DRUG	RELATIVE POTENCY	ORAL AVAILABILITY	$t_{1/2}$ (hours)	ROUTE OF ELIMINATION
Furosemide	1	~60%	~1.5	~65% R, ~35% M[a]
Bumetanide	40	~80%	~0.8	~62% R, ~38% M
Ethacrynic acid	0.7	~100%	~1	~67% R, ~33% M
Torsemide	3	~80%	~3.5	~20% R, ~80% M
Azosemide[b]	1	~12%	~2.5	~27% R, ~63% M
Piretanide[b]	3	~80%	0.6–1.5	~50% R, ~50% M

M, metabolism; R, renal excretion of intact drug.
[a]Metabolism of furosemide occurs predominantly in the kidney.
[b]Not available in the U.S.

drugs attach to the Cl⁻ binding site located in the symporter's transmembrane domain; however, more recent studies challenge this view. Inhibitors of Na^+-K^+-$2Cl^-$ symport also inhibit Ca^{2+} and Mg^{2+} reabsorption in the TAL by abolishing the transepithelial potential difference that is the dominant driving force for reabsorption of these cations.

Na^+-K^+-$2Cl^-$ symporters are found in many secretory and absorbing epithelia. There are two varieties of Na^+-K^+-$2Cl^-$ symporters. The "absorptive" symporter (called *ENCC2*, *NKCC2*, or *BSC1*) is expressed only in the kidney, is localized to the apical membrane and subapical intracellular vesicles of the TAL, and is regulated by the cyclic AMP/PKA pathway. The "secretory" symporter (called *ENCC3*, *NKCC1*, or *BSC2*) is a "housekeeping" protein that is expressed widely and, in epithelial cells, is localized to the basolateral membrane. The affinity of loop diuretics for the secretory symporter is somewhat less than for the absorptive symporter (e.g., 4-fold difference for bumetanide). Mutations in the Na^+-K^+-$2Cl^-$ symporter cause a form of inherited hypokalemic alkalosis called Bartter syndrome.

Effects on Urinary Excretion

Loop diuretics increase urinary Na^+ and Cl^- excretion profoundly (i.e., up to 25% of the filtered Na^+ load) and markedly increase Ca^{2+} and Mg^{2+} excretion. Furosemide has weak carbonic anhydrase–inhibiting activity and thus increases urinary excretion of HCO_3^- and phosphate. All inhibitors of Na^+-K^+-$2Cl^-$ symport increase urinary K^+ and titratable acid excretion. This effect is due in part to increased Na^+ delivery to the distal tubule (the mechanism by which increased distal Na^+ delivery enhances K^+ and H^+ excretion is discussed in the section on Na^+ channel inhibitors). Other mechanisms contributing to enhanced K^+ and H^+ excretion include flow-dependent enhancement of ion secretion by the collecting duct, nonosmotic vasopressin release, and activation of the RAS axis.

Acutely, loop diuretics increase uric acid excretion; their chronic administration results in reduced uric acid excretion. Chronic effects of loop diuretics on uric acid excretion may be due to enhanced proximal tubule transport or secondary to volume depletion or to competition between diuretic and uric acid for the organic acid secretory mechanism in the proximal tubule. Asymptomatic hyperuricemia is a common consequence of loop diuretics, but painful episodes of gout are rarely reported (Bruderer et al., 2014). By blocking active NaCl reabsorption in the TAL, inhibitors of Na^+-K^+-$2Cl^-$ symport interfere with a critical step in the mechanism that produces a hypertonic medullary interstitium. Therefore, loop diuretics block the kidney's ability to concentrate urine. Also, because the TAL is part of the diluting segment, inhibitors of Na^+-K^+-$2Cl^-$ symport markedly impair the kidney's ability to excrete a dilute urine during water diuresis.

Effects on Renal Hemodynamics

If volume depletion is prevented by replacing fluid losses, inhibitors of Na^+-K^+-$2Cl^-$ symport generally increase total RBF and redistribute RBF to the midcortex. The mechanism of the increase in RBF is not known but may involve PGs: NSAIDs attenuate the diuretic response to loop diuretics in part by preventing PG-mediated increases in RBF. Loop diuretics block TGF by inhibiting salt transport into the macula densa so that the macula densa no longer detects NaCl concentrations in the tubular fluid. Therefore, unlike carbonic anhydrase inhibitors, loop diuretics do not decrease the GFR by activating TGF. Loop diuretics are powerful stimulators of renin release. This effect is due to interference with NaCl transport by the macula densa and, if volume depletion occurs, to reflex activation of the sympathetic nervous system and stimulation of the intrarenal baroreceptor mechanism.

Other Actions

Loop diuretics, particularly furosemide, acutely increase systemic venous capacitance and thereby decrease left ventricular filling pressure. This effect, which may be mediated by PGs and requires intact kidneys, benefits patients with pulmonary edema even before diuresis ensues. High doses of inhibitors of Na^+-K^+-$2Cl^-$ symport can inhibit electrolyte transport in many tissues. This effect is clinically important in the inner ear and can result in ototoxicity, particularly in patients with preexisting hearing impairment.

ADME

Table 25–4 presents some pharmacokinetic properties of the agents. Because these drugs are bound extensively to plasma proteins, delivery of these drugs to tubules by filtration is limited. However, they are secreted efficiently by the organic acid transport system in the proximal tubule and thereby gain access to the Na^+-K^+-$2Cl^-$ symporter in the luminal membrane of the TAL. Approximately 65% of furosemide is excreted unchanged in urine, and the remainder is conjugated to glucuronic acid in the kidney. Thus, in patients with renal disease, the elimination $t_{1/2}$ of furosemide is prolonged. Bumetanide and torsemide have significant hepatic metabolism, so liver disease can prolong the elimination $t_{1/2}$ of these loop diuretics. Oral bioavailability of furosemide varies (10%–100%). In contrast, oral availabilities of bumetanide and torsemide are reliably high.

As a class, loop diuretics have short elimination half-lives; prolonged-release preparations are not available. Consequently, often the dosing interval is too short to maintain adequate levels of loop diuretics in the tubular lumen. Note that torsemide has a longer $t_{1/2}$ than other agents available in the U.S. As the concentration of loop diuretic in the tubular lumen declines, nephrons begin to avidly reabsorb Na^+, which often nullifies the overall effect of the loop diuretic on total-body Na^+. This phenomenon of "postdiuretic Na^+ retention" can be overcome by restricting dietary Na^+ intake or by more frequent administration of the loop diuretic.

Therapeutic Uses

A major use of loop diuretics is in the treatment of acute pulmonary edema. A rapid increase in venous capacitance in conjunction with brisk natriuresis reduces left ventricular filling pressures and thereby rapidly relieves pulmonary edema. Loop diuretics also are used widely for treatment of chronic CHF when diminution of extracellular fluid volume is desirable to minimize venous and pulmonary congestion (see Chapter 29). Diuretics cause a significant reduction in mortality and the risk of worsening heart failure, as well as an improvement in exercise capacity. Although furosemide is the most commonly used loop diuretic for the treatment of heart failure, patients with heart failure have fewer hospitalizations and better quality of life with torsemide than with furosemide, perhaps because of its more reliable absorption and due to other ancillary pharmacological effects (Buggey et al., 2015).

Although diuretics are used widely for treatment of hypertension (see Chapter 28), in patients with normal renal function, Na^+-K^+-$2Cl^-$ symport inhibitors are not considered first-line diuretics for the treatment of hypertension. This is due to the lower antihypertensive efficacy of loop diuretics in such patients and the lack of data demonstrating a reduction in cardiovascular events. However, in patients with a low GFR (<30 mL/min) or with resistant hypertension, loop diuretics are the diuretics of choice.

The edema of nephrotic syndrome often is refractory to less-potent diuretics, and loop diuretics often are the only drugs capable of reducing the massive edema associated with this renal disease. Loop diuretics also are employed in the treatment of edema and ascites of liver cirrhosis; however, care must be taken not to induce volume contraction. In patients with a drug overdose, loop diuretics can be used to induce forced diuresis to facilitate more rapid renal elimination of the offending drug. Loop diuretics, combined with isotonic saline administration to prevent volume depletion, are used to treat hypercalcemia. Loop diuretics interfere with the kidney's capacity to produce concentrated urine. Consequently, loop diuretics combined with hypertonic saline are useful for the treatment of life-threatening hyponatremia. Loop diuretics also are used to treat edema associated with chronic kidney disease, in which the dose-response curve may be right shifted, requiring higher doses of the loop diuretic.

Toxicity, Adverse Effects, Contraindications, Drug Interactions

Most adverse effects are due to abnormalities of fluid and electrolyte balance. Overzealous use of loop diuretics can cause serious depletion of total-body Na^+. This may manifest as hyponatremia or extracellular fluid volume depletion associated with hypotension, reduced GFR, circulatory collapse, thromboembolic episodes, and, in patients with liver disease, hepatic encephalopathy. Increased Na^+ delivery to the distal tubule, particularly when combined with activation of the renin–angiotensin system, leads to increased urinary K^+ and H^+ excretion, causing a hypochloremic alkalosis. If dietary K^+ intake is not sufficient, hypokalemia may develop, and this may induce cardiac arrhythmias, particularly in patients taking cardiac glycosides. Increased Mg^{2+} and Ca^{2+} excretion may result in hypomagnesemia (a risk factor for cardiac arrhythmias) and hypocalcemia (rarely leading to tetany). Loop diuretics should be avoided in postmenopausal osteopenic women, in whom increased Ca^{2+} excretion may have deleterious effects on bone metabolism.

Loop diuretics can cause ototoxicity that manifests as tinnitus, hearing impairment, deafness, vertigo, and a sense of fullness in the ears. Hearing impairment and deafness are usually, but not always, reversible. Ototoxicity occurs most frequently with rapid intravenous administration and least frequently with oral administration. To avoid ototoxicity, the rate of furosemide infusions should not exceed 4 mg/min. Ethacrynic acid appears to induce ototoxicity more often than do other loop diuretics and should be reserved for use only in patients who cannot tolerate other loop diuretics. Loop diuretics also can cause hyperuricemia (occasionally leading to gout) and hyperglycemia (infrequently precipitating diabetes mellitus) and can increase plasma levels of LDL cholesterol and triglycerides while decreasing plasma levels of HDL cholesterol. Other adverse effects include skin rashes, photosensitivity, paresthesias, bone marrow depression, and GI disturbances. Contraindications to the use of loop diuretics include severe Na^+ and volume depletion, hypersensitivity to sulfonamides (for sulfonamide-based loop diuretics), and anuria unresponsive to a trial dose of loop diuretic.

Drug interactions may occur when loop diuretics are coadministered with the following:

- Aminoglycosides, carboplatin, paclitaxel, and others (synergism of ototoxicity)
- Anticoagulants (increased anticoagulant activity)
- Digitalis glycosides (increased digitalis-induced arrhythmias)
- Lithium (increased plasma levels of Li^+)
- Propranolol (increased plasma levels of propranolol)
- Sulfonylureas (hyperglycemia)
- Cisplatin (increased risk of diuretic-induced ototoxicity)
- NSAIDs (blunted diuretic response and salicylate toxicity with high doses of salicylates)
- Probenecid (blunted diuretic response)
- Thiazide diuretics (synergism of diuretic activity of both drugs, leading to profound diuresis)
- Amphotericin B (increased potential for nephrotoxicity and intensification of electrolyte imbalance)

Inhibitors of Na^+-Cl^- Symport: Thiazide-Type and Thiazide-Like Diuretics

The term *thiazide diuretics* generally refers to all inhibitors of Na^+-Cl^- symport, so named because the original inhibitors of Na^+-Cl^- symport were benzothiadiazine derivatives. The class now includes diuretics that are benzothiadiazine derivatives (*thiazide* or *thiazide-type diuretics*) and drugs that are pharmacologically similar to thiazide diuretics but differ structurally (*thiazide-like diuretics*). Table 25–5 lists diuretics in this drug class that are currently available in the United States.

Mechanism and Site of Action

Thiazide diuretics inhibit NaCl transport in the DCT; the proximal tubule may represent a secondary site of action. Figure 25–5 illustrates the current model of electrolyte transport in the DCT. Transport is powered by a Na^+ pump in the basolateral membrane. Free energy in the electrochemical gradient for Na^+ is harnessed by a Na^+-Cl^- symporter in the luminal membrane that moves Cl^- into the epithelial cell against its electrochemical gradient. Cl^- then exits the basolateral membrane passively by a Cl^- channel. Thiazide diuretics inhibit the Na^+-Cl^- symporter (called *ENCC1* or *TSC*) that is expressed predominantly in kidney and localized to the apical membrane of DCT epithelial cells. Expression of the symporter is regulated by aldosterone. Mutations in the Na^+-Cl^- symporter cause a form of inherited hypokalemic alkalosis called Gitelman syndrome.

Effects on Urinary Excretion

Inhibitors of Na^+-Cl^- symport increase Na^+ and Cl^- excretion. However, thiazides are only moderately efficacious (i.e., maximum excretion of filtered Na^+ load is only 5%) because about 90% of the filtered Na^+ load is reabsorbed before reaching the DCT. Some thiazide diuretics also are weak inhibitors of carbonic anhydrase, an effect that increases HCO_3^- and phosphate excretion and probably accounts for their weak proximal tubular effects. Inhibitors of Na^+-Cl^- symport increase K^+ and titratable acid excretion by the same mechanisms discussed for loop diuresis. Acute thiazide administration increases uric acid excretion. However, uric acid excretion is reduced following chronic administration by similar mechanisms discussed for loop diuretics. In addition, thiazides may be transported from the basolateral compartment to the luminal compartment via the OAT4 antiporter in the apical membrane (Palmer, 2011; see Chapter 5). Acute effects of inhibitors of Na^+-Cl^- symport on Ca^{2+} excretion are variable; when administered chronically, thiazide diuretics decrease Ca^{2+} excretion. The mechanism involves increased proximal reabsorption owing to volume depletion, as well as direct effects of thiazides to increase Ca^{2+} reabsorption in the DCT. Thiazide diuretics may

TABLE 25–5 ■ INHIBITORS OF Na^+-Cl^- SYMPORT (THIAZIDE DIURETICS)

DRUG	RELATIVE POTENCY	ORAL AVAILABILITY	$t_{1/2}$ (hours)	ROUTE OF ELIMINATION
Thiazide diuretics				
Bendroflumethiazide	10	~100%	3–3.9	~30% R, ~70% M
Chlorothiazide	0.1	9%–56% (dose-dependent)	~1.5	R
Hydrochlorothiazide	1	~70%	~2.5	R
Methyclothiazide	10	ID	ID	M
Thiazide-like diuretics				
Chlorthalidone	1	~65%	~47	~65% R, ~10% B, ~25% U
Indapamide	20	~93%	~14	M
Metolazone	10	~65%	8–14	~80% R, ~10% B, ~10% M

B, excretion of intact drug into bile; ID, insufficient data; M, metabolism; R, renal excretion of intact drug; U, unknown pathway of elimination.

cause mild magnesuria; long-term use of thiazide diuretics may cause magnesium deficiency, particularly in the elderly. Because inhibitors of Na^+-Cl^- symport inhibit transport in the cortical diluting segment, thiazide diuretics attenuate the kidney's ability to excrete dilute urine during water diuresis. However, because the DCT is not involved in the mechanism that generates a hypertonic medullary interstitium, thiazide diuretics do not alter the kidney's ability to concentrate urine during hydropenia. In general, inhibitors of Na^+-Cl^- symport do not affect RBF and only variably reduce GFR owing to increases in intratubular pressure. Thiazides have little or no influence on TGF.

ADME

Table 25–5 lists pharmacokinetic parameters of Na^+-Cl^- symport inhibitors. Note the wide range of half-lives for these drugs. Sulfonamides, as organic acids, are secreted into the proximal tubule by the organic acid secretory pathway. Because thiazides must gain access to the tubular lumen to inhibit the Na^+-Cl^- symporter, drugs such as probenecid can attenuate the diuretic response to thiazides by competing for transport into the proximal tubule. However, plasma protein binding varies considerably among thiazide diuretics, and this parameter determines the contribution that filtration makes to tubular delivery of a specific thiazide.

Therapeutic Uses

Thiazide diuretics are used for the treatment of edema associated with diseases of the heart (CHF), liver (hepatic cirrhosis), and kidney (nephrotic syndrome, chronic renal failure, and acute glomerulonephritis). With the possible exceptions of metolazone and indapamide, most thiazide diuretics are ineffective when the GFR is less than 30–40 mL/min. Thiazide diuretics decrease blood pressure in hypertensive patients and are used widely for the treatment of hypertension in combination with other antihypertensive drugs (Tamargo et al., 2014) (see Chapter 28). Thiazide diuretics are inexpensive, as efficacious as other classes of antihypertensive agents, and well tolerated. Thiazides can be administered once daily, do not require dose titration, and have few contraindications. Moreover, thiazides have additive or synergistic effects when combined with other classes of antihypertensive agents. Although hydrochlorothiazide is the 10th most prescribed drug in the United States and is prescribed 20 times more often than chlorthalidone (Roush et al., 2014), there is strong evidence that chlorthalidone and other thiazide-like diuretics, such as indapamide, reduce blood pressure and cardiovascular events in hypertensive patients more so than does hydrochlorothiazide (Olde Engberink et al., 2015; Roush et al., 2014, 2015). This is likely due to the longer half-life of *thiazide-like* diuretics compared to hydrochlorothiazide, resulting in better 24-h control of arterial blood pressure by chlorthalidone.

Thiazide diuretics, which reduce urinary Ca^{2+} excretion, sometimes are employed to treat Ca^{2+} nephrolithiasis and may be useful for treatment of osteoporosis (see Chapter 44). Thiazide diuretics also are the mainstay for treatment of nephrogenic DI, reducing urine volume by up to 50%. Although it may seem counterintuitive to treat a disorder of increased urine volume with a diuretic, thiazides reduce the kidney's ability to excrete free water: They increase proximal tubular water reabsorption (secondary to volume contraction) and block the ability of the DCT to form dilute urine. This last effect results in an increase in urine osmolality. Because other halides are excreted by renal processes similar to those for Cl^-, thiazide diuretics may be useful for the management of Br^- intoxication.

Toxicity, Adverse Effects, Contraindications, Drug Interactions

Thiazide diuretics rarely cause CNS (e.g., vertigo, headache), GI, hematological, and dermatological (e.g., photosensitivity and skin rashes) disorders. The incidence of erectile dysfunction is greater with Na^+-Cl^- symport inhibitors than with several other antihypertensive agents (Grimm et al., 1997), but usually is tolerable. As with loop diuretics, most serious adverse effects of thiazides are related to abnormalities of fluid and electrolyte balance. These adverse effects include extracellular volume depletion, hypotension, hypokalemia, hyponatremia, hypochloremia, metabolic alkalosis, hypomagnesemia, hypercalcemia, and hyperuricemia (Palmer,

2011). Thiazide diuretics have caused fatal or near-fatal hyponatremia (Rodenburg et al., 2013), and some patients are at recurrent risk of hyponatremia when rechallenged with thiazides.

Thiazide diuretics also decrease glucose tolerance and unmask latent diabetes mellitus (Palmer, 2011). The mechanism of impaired glucose tolerance appears to involve reduced insulin secretion and alterations in glucose metabolism. Hyperglycemia is reduced when K^+ is given along with the diuretic. Importantly, thiazide-induced diabetes mellitus is not associated with the same cardiovascular disease risk as incident diabetes (Barzilay et al., 2012). Thiazide-induced hypokalemia also impairs the antihypertensive effect and cardiovascular protection afforded by thiazides in patients with hypertension. Thiazide diuretics also may increase plasma levels of LDL cholesterol, total cholesterol, and total triglycerides. Thiazide diuretics are contraindicated in individuals who are hypersensitive to sulfonamides. Thiazide diuretics may diminish the effects of anticoagulants, uricosuric agents used to treat gout, sulfonylureas, and insulin and may increase the effects of anesthetics, diazoxide, digitalis glycosides, lithium, loop diuretics, and vitamin D. The effectiveness of thiazide diuretics may be reduced by NSAIDs, nonselective or selective COX-2 inhibitors, and bile acid sequestrants (reduced absorption of thiazides). Amphotericin B and corticosteroids increase the risk of hypokalemia induced by thiazide diuretics.

In a potentially lethal interaction, thiazide diuretic–induced K^+ depletion may contribute to fatal ventricular arrhythmias associated with drugs that prolong the QT interval (i.e., quinidine, dofetilide, arsenic trioxide, see also Chapter 30).

Inhibitors of Renal Epithelial Na^+ Channels: K^+-Sparing Diuretics

Triamterene and amiloride are the only two drugs of this class in clinical use. Both drugs cause small increases in NaCl excretion and usually are employed for their antikaliuretic actions to offset the effects of other diuretics that increase K^+ excretion. Consequently, triamterene and amiloride, along with spironolactone and eplerenone (described in the next section), often are classified as *potassium* (K^+)–*sparing diuretics*.

Both drugs are organic bases, are transported by the organic base secretory mechanism in the proximal tubule, and have similar mechanisms of action (Figure 25–5). Principal cells in the late distal tubules and collecting ducts (particularly cortical collecting tubules) have, in their luminal membranes, ENaCs that provide a conductive pathway for Na^+ entry into the cell down the electrochemical gradient created by the basolateral Na^+ pump. The higher permeability of the luminal membrane for Na^+ depolarizes the luminal membrane but not the basolateral membrane, creating a lumen-negative transepithelial potential difference. This transepithelial voltage provides an important driving force for the secretion of K^+ into the lumen via K^+ channels (ROMK [Kir1.1] and BK channels) (Garcia and Kaczorowski, 2014) in the luminal membrane; however, the overall regulation of K^+ secretion in the late distal tubule and collecting duct involves multiple signaling mechanisms (Welling, 2013). Carbonic anhydrase inhibitors, loop diuretics, and thiazide diuretics increase Na^+ delivery to the late distal tubule and collecting duct, a situation that often is associated with increased K^+ and H^+ excretion.

Amiloride and triamterene block ENaCs in the luminal membrane of principal cells in late distal tubules and collecting ducts by binding to a site in the channel pore. ENaCs consist of three subunits (α, β, and γ) (Kellenberger and Schild, 2015). Although the α subunit is sufficient for channel activity, maximal Na^+ permeability is induced when all three subunits are coexpressed in the same cell, probably forming a tetrameric structure consisting of two α subunits, one β subunit, and one γ subunit. Incompletely understood, complex mechanisms, including proteolytic cleavage, regulate ENaC activation (Kellenberger and Schild, 2015).

Effects on Urinary Excretion

The late distal tubule and collecting duct have a limited capacity to reabsorb solutes; thus, Na^+ channel blockade in this part of the nephron increases Na^+ and Cl^- excretion rates only mildly (~2% of filtered load).

TABLE 25–6 ■ INHIBITORS OF RENAL EPITHELIAL Na⁺ CHANNELS (K⁺-SPARING DIURETICS)

DRUG	RELATIVE POTENCY	ORAL BIOAVAILABILITY	$t_{1/2}$ (hours)	ROUTE OF ELIMINATION
Amiloride	1	15%–25%	~21	R
Triamterene	0.1	~50%	~4	M

M, metabolism; R, renal excretion of intact drug; however, triamterene is transformed into an active metabolite that is excreted in the urine.

Blockade of Na⁺ channels hyperpolarizes the luminal membrane, reducing the lumen-negative transepithelial voltage. Because the lumen-negative potential difference normally opposes cation reabsorption and facilitates cation secretion, attenuation of the lumen-negative voltage decreases K⁺, H⁺, Ca²⁺, and Mg²⁺ excretion rates. Volume contraction may increase reabsorption of uric acid in the proximal tubule; hence, chronic administration of amiloride and triamterene may decrease uric acid excretion. Amiloride and triamterene have little or no effect on renal hemodynamics and do not alter TGF.

ADME

Table 25–6 lists pharmacokinetic data for amiloride and triamterene. Amiloride is eliminated predominantly by urinary excretion of intact drug. Triamterene is metabolized in the liver to an active metabolite, 4-hydroxytriamterene sulfate, and this metabolite is excreted in urine. Therefore, triamterene toxicity may be enhanced in both hepatic disease and renal failure.

Therapeutic Uses

Because of the mild natriuresis induced by Na⁺ channel inhibitors, these drugs seldom are used as sole agents in treatment of edema or hypertension; their major utility is in combination with other diuretics. Coadministration of a Na⁺ channel inhibitor augments the diuretic and antihypertensive response to thiazide and loop diuretics. More important, the ability of Na⁺ channel inhibitors to reduce K⁺ excretion tends to offset the kaliuretic effects of thiazide and loop diuretics and to result in normal plasma K⁺ values.

Liddle syndrome (described later in this chapter) can be treated effectively with Na⁺ channel inhibitors. Aerosolized amiloride has been shown to improve mucociliary clearance in patients with cystic fibrosis. By inhibiting Na⁺ absorption from the surfaces of airway epithelial cells, amiloride augments hydration of respiratory secretions and thereby improves mucociliary clearance. Amiloride also is useful for lithium-induced nephrogenic DI because it blocks Li⁺ transport into collecting tubule cells (Kortenoeven et al., 2009).

Toxicity, Adverse Effects, Contraindications, Drug Interactions

The most dangerous adverse effect of renal Na⁺ channel inhibitors is hyperkalemia, which can be life threatening. Consequently, amiloride and triamterene are contraindicated in patients with hyperkalemia, as well as in patients at increased risk of developing hyperkalemia (e.g., patients with renal failure, patients receiving other K⁺-sparing diuretics, patients taking angiotensin-converting enzyme inhibitors, or patients taking K⁺ supplements). Even NSAIDs can increase the likelihood of hyperkalemia in patients receiving Na⁺ channel inhibitors. Routine monitoring of the serum K⁺ level is essential in patients receiving K⁺-sparing diuretics. Cirrhotic patients are prone to megaloblastosis because of folic acid deficiency, and triamterene, a weak folic acid antagonist, may increase the likelihood of this adverse event. Triamterene also can reduce glucose tolerance and induce photosensitization and has been associated with interstitial nephritis and renal stones. Both drugs can cause CNS, GI, musculoskeletal, dermatological, and hematological adverse effects. The most common adverse effects of amiloride are nausea, vomiting, diarrhea, and headache; those of triamterene are nausea, vomiting, leg cramps, and dizziness.

Antagonists of Mineralocorticoid Receptors: Aldosterone Antagonists, K⁺-Sparing Diuretics

Mineralocorticoids cause salt and water retention and increase K⁺ and H⁺ excretion by binding to specific MRs. Two MR antagonists are available in the U.S., spironolactone and eplerenone (Table 25–7).

Mechanism and Site of Action

Epithelial cells in late distal tubule and collecting duct (particularly cortical collecting tubule) contain cytosolic MRs with high aldosterone affinity. When aldosterone binds to MRs, the MR-aldosterone complex translocates to the nucleus, where it regulates the expression of multiple gene products called aldosterone-induced proteins (AIPs) (Figure 25–6). AIPs affect the production, destruction, localization, and activation of multiple components of the system that mediates Na⁺ reabsorption in late distal tubules and collecting ducts (Figure 25–6A). Consequently, transepithelial NaCl transport is enhanced, and the lumen-negative transepithelial voltage is increased. The latter effect increases the driving force for K⁺ and H⁺ secretion into the tubular lumen.

Drugs such as spironolactone and eplerenone competitively inhibit the binding of aldosterone to the MR. Unlike the MR-aldosterone complex, the MR-spironolactone or MR-eplerenone complex is not able to induce the synthesis of AIPs. Because spironolactone and eplerenone block the biological effects of aldosterone, these agents also are referred to as *aldosterone antagonists*. MR antagonists are the only diuretics that do not require access to the tubular lumen to induce diuresis.

Both the β and β subunits of ENaC have a specific region in their C terminus called the PY motif. The PY motif interacts with the ubiquitin ligase Nedd4-2 (Figure 25–6B), a protein that ubiquitinates ENaC and targets it for destruction by the proteasome. Aldosterone increases the expression of SGK-1; SGK-1 phosphorylates and inactivates Nedd4-2. Thus, aldosterone results in attenuated internalization and proteasome-mediated degradation of ENaC, leading to increased expression of ENaC in the luminal membrane. Liddle syndrome, an autosomal-dominant, monogenic disease characterized by sodium retention and severe hypertension, is caused by mutations in the PY motif of either the β or γ subunit of ENaC, leading to MR-independent overexpression of ENaC. Thus, Liddle syndrome is responsive to ENaC inhibitors but not to MR antagonists.

TABLE 25–7 ■ MINERALOCORTICOID RECEPTOR ANTAGONISTS (ALDOSTERONE ANTAGONISTS, K⁺-SPARING DIURETICS)

DRUG	ORAL AVAILABILITY	$t_{1/2}$ (hours)	ROUTE OF ELIMINATION
Spironolactone	~65%	~1.6	M
Canrenone[a]	80%	3.7–22	M
Potassium canrenoate[a]	100%	3.7–22	M
Eplerenone	69%	~5	M

M, metabolism.
[a]Not available in U.S.

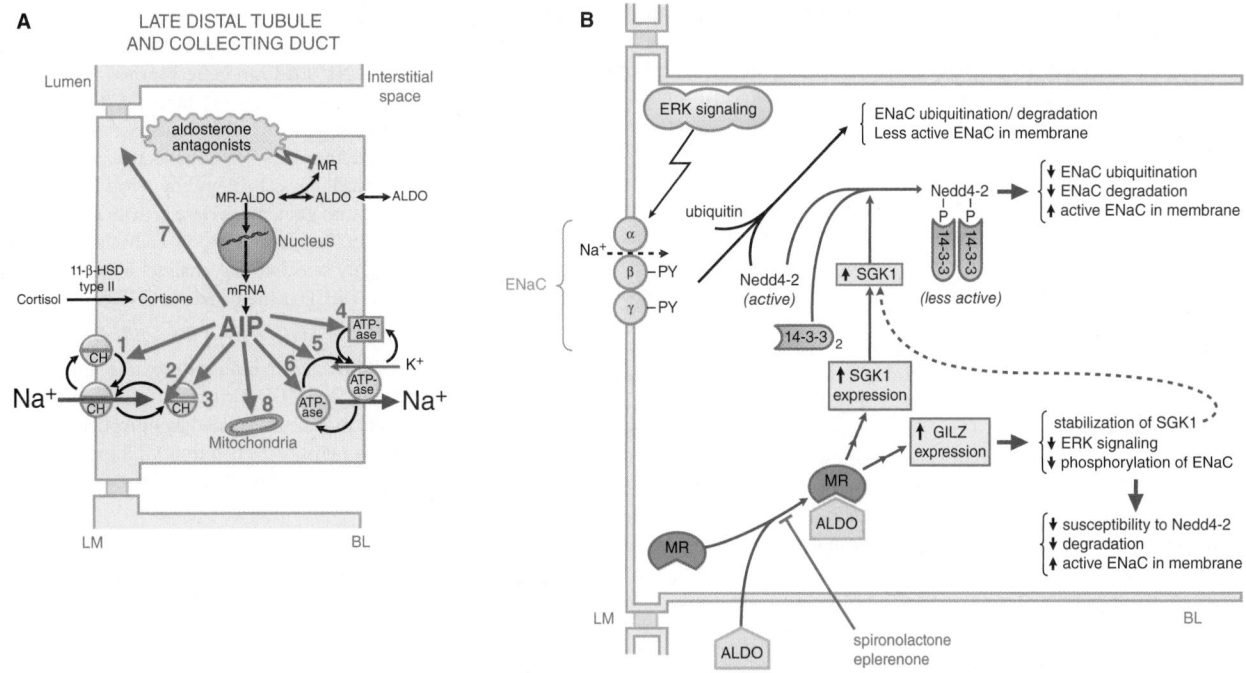

Figure 25–6 *Effects of aldosterone on late distal tubule and collecting duct and diuretic mechanism of aldosterone antagonists.*

A. *Overview of aldosterone's influences on Na⁺ retention.* Via interaction with the mineralocorticoid receptor (MR), aldosterone affects myriad renal pathways that handle Na⁺. Key to numbered items influenced by ALDO:

1. Activation of membrane-bound Na⁺ channels
2. Na⁺ channel (ENaC) removal from the membrane inhibited
3. *De novo* synthesis of Na⁺ channels
4. Activation of membrane-bound Na⁺,K⁺-ATPase
5. Redistribution of Na⁺,K⁺-ATPase from cytosol to membrane
6. *De novo* synthesis of Na⁺,K⁺-ATPase
7. Changes in permeability of tight junctions
8. Increased mitochondrial production of ATP

Cortisol also has affinity for the mineralocorticoid receptor but is inactivated in the cell by 11-β-hydroxysteroid dehydrogenase (HSD) type II.

B. *Details of aldosterone's influences on membrane ENaC.* ERK signaling phosphorylates components of ENaC, making them susceptible to interaction with Nedd4-2, a ubiquitin-protein ligase that ubiquitinates ENaC, leading to its degradation. The Nedd4-2 interaction with ENaC occurs via several proline-tyrosine-proline (PY) motifs of ENaC. ALDO enhances expression of the serum and glucocorticoid-regulated kinase-1 (SGK1) and the glucocorticoid-induced leucine zipper protein (GILZ; TSC22D3). SGK-1 phosphorylates and inactivates Nedd4-2; 14-3-3 dimers bind to the phosphorylated sites in Nedd4-2 and stabilize them. Phosphorylated Nedd4-2 no longer interacts well with the PY motifs of ENaC. As a result, ENaC is not ubiquitinated and remains in the membrane, leading to increased Na⁺ entry into the cell. GILZ stabilizes SGK1, enhancing its effects, and decreases ERK signaling and ENaC phosphorylation, events that prime ENaC for degradation; these effects all lead to less ubiquitination and more active ENaC in the cell membranes of the distal tubule and collecting duct. For details see Ronzaud and Staub (2014) and Ronchetti et al. (2015).

Abbreviations: AIP, aldosterone-induced proteins; ALDO, aldosterone; CH, ion channel; BL, basolateral membrane; LM, luminal membrane; MR, mineralocorticoid receptor.

Effects on Urinary Excretion

The effects of MR antagonists on urinary excretion are similar to those induced by renal ENaC inhibitors. However, unlike Na⁺ channel inhibitors, the clinical efficacy of MR antagonists is a function of endogenous aldosterone levels. The higher the endogenous aldosterone level, the greater the effects of MR antagonists on urinary excretion. MR antagonists have little or no effect on renal hemodynamics and do not alter TGF.

Other Actions

Spironolactone has some affinity toward progesterone and androgen receptors and thereby induces side effects such as gynecomastia, impotence, and menstrual irregularities. Owing to its 9,11-epoxide group, eplerenone has very low affinity for progesterone and androgen receptors (<1% and <0.1%, respectively) compared with spironolactone. High spironolactone concentrations can interfere with steroid biosynthesis by inhibiting steroid hydroxylases, but these effects have limited clinical relevance.

ADME

Spironolactone is absorbed partially (~65%), is metabolized extensively (even during its first passage through the liver), undergoes enterohepatic

recirculation, and is highly protein bound. Although spironolactone per se has a short $t_{1/2}$ (~1.6 h), it is metabolized to a number of active compounds (including canrenone; see discussion that follows) that have long half-lives. The $t_{1/2}$ of spironolactone is prolonged to 9 h in patients with cirrhosis. Eplerenone has good oral availability and is eliminated primarily by metabolism by CYP3A4 to inactive metabolites, with a $t_{1/2}$ of about 5 h. Canrenone and K⁺-canrenoate also are in clinical use (not available in the U.S.). Canrenoate is not active but is converted to canrenone.

Therapeutic Uses

The MR antagonists often are coadministered with thiazide or loop diuretics in the treatment of edema and hypertension. Such combinations result in increased mobilization of edema fluid while causing lesser perturbations of K⁺ homeostasis. MR antagonists are particularly useful in the treatment of resistant hypertension due to primary hyperaldosteronism (adrenal adenomas or bilateral adrenal hyperplasia) and of refractory edema associated with secondary aldosteronism (cardiac failure, hepatic cirrhosis, nephrotic syndrome, and severe ascites). MR antagonists are considered diuretics of choice in patients with hepatic cirrhosis. MR antagonists, added to standard therapy, substantially reduce morbidity and mortality in patients with heart failure with reduced ejection fraction (see Chapter 29) (D'Elia and Krum, 2014).

The MR antagonists may reduce mortality in patients with systolic dysfunction following a myocardial infarction if treated within 3 to 6 days (Roush et al., 2014). In patients with diastolic dysfunction with preserved ejection fraction, the use of MR antagonists is controversial. In such patients, MR antagonists improve left ventricular end-diastolic filling, left ventricular remodeling, and neurohumoral activation but do not improve maximal exercise capacity, quality of life, mortality, or hospitalization for heart failure (Edelmann et al., 2013; Pitt et al., 2014). MR antagonists also may reduce ventricular arrhythmias and sudden cardiac death.

The MR antagonists reduce proteinuria in patients with chronic kidney disease, and the use of these drugs in kidney diseases is under intense investigation (Bauersachs et al., 2015). Spironolactone, but not eplerenone, is widely considered to be an antiandrogenic compound and has been used to treat hirsutism and acne; however, evidence for efficacy is weak (Brown et al., 2009), and these uses are not FDA-approved. Biochemical studies suggested that spironolactone is a partial agonist of androgen receptors (Nirdé et al., 2001) and can exert antiandrogenic or androgenic effects depending on context (e.g., the prevailing levels of endogenous androgenic steroids). Indeed, a recent case report described spironolactone-induced worsening of prostate cancer attributed to androgen receptor stimulation (Sundar and Dickinson, 2012).

Toxicity, Adverse Effects, Contraindications, Drug Interactions

Hyperkalemia is the principal risk of MR antagonists. Therefore, these drugs are contraindicated in patients with hyperkalemia and in those at increased risk of developing hyperkalemia. MR antagonists also can induce metabolic acidosis in cirrhotic patients. Salicylates may reduce the tubular secretion of canrenone and decrease diuretic efficacy of spironolactone. Spironolactone may alter the clearance of cardiac glycosides. Owing to its affinity for other steroid receptors, spironolactone may cause gynecomastia, impotence, decreased libido, and menstrual irregularities. Spironolactone also may induce diarrhea, gastritis, gastric bleeding, and peptic ulcers (the drug is contraindicated in patients with peptic ulcers). CNS adverse effects include drowsiness, lethargy, ataxia, confusion, and headache. Spironolactone may cause skin rashes and, rarely, blood dyscrasias. Strong inhibitors of CYP3A4 may increase plasma levels of eplerenone, and such drugs should not be administered to patients taking eplerenone and vice versa. Other than hyperkalemia and GI disorders, the rate of adverse events for eplerenone is similar to that of placebo.

Inhibitors of the Nonspecific Cation Channel: Natriuretic Peptides

Four NPs are relevant with respect to human physiology: ANP, BNP, CNP, and urodilatin. The IMCD is a major site of action of NPs.

Three NPs—ANP, BNP, and CNP—share a common homologous 17-member amino acid ring formed by a disulfide bridge between cysteine residues, although they are products of different genes. Urodilatin, also structurally similar, arises from altered processing of the same precursor molecule as ANP and has four additional amino acids at the N terminus. ANP and BNP are produced by the heart in response to wall stretch, CNP is of endothelial and renal cell origin; urodilatin is found in the kidney and urine. NPRs, classified as types A, B, and C, are membrane monospans. NPRA (binds ANP and BNP) and NPRB (binds CNP) have intracellular domains with guanylate cyclase activity and a protein kinase element. NPRC (binds all NPs) has a truncated intracellular domain and may help with NP clearance. The various NPs have somewhat overlapping effects, causing natriuresis, inhibition of production of renin and aldosterone, and vasodilation (the result of cGMP elevation in vascular smooth muscle). A human recombinant BNP, nesiritide, with the same 32–amino acid structure as the endogenous peptide produced by the ventricular myocardium, is available for clinical use.

Mechanism and Site of Action

The IMCD is the final site along the nephron where Na^+ is reabsorbed. Up to 5% of the filtered Na^+ load can be reabsorbed here. The effects of nesiritide and other NPs are mediated via effects of cGMP on Na^+ transporters (Figure 25–7). Two types of Na^+ channels are expressed in IMCD. The *first* is a high conductance, 28-pS, nonselective, CNGC. This channel is inhibited by intracellular cGMP and by NPs via their capacity to stimulate membrane-bound guanylyl cyclase activity and elevate cellular cGMP. The *second* type of Na^+ channel expressed in the IMCD is the low-conductance, 4-pS, highly selective Na^+ channel ENaC. The majority of Na^+ reabsorption in the IMCD is mediated via CNGC.

Effects on Urinary Excretion and Renal Hemodynamics

Nesiritide inhibits Na^+ transport in both the proximal and distal nephron but its primary effect is in the IMCD. Urinary Na^+ excretion increases with nesiritide, but the effect may be attenuated by upregulation of Na^+ reabsorption in upstream segments of the nephron. GFR increases in response to nesiritide in normal subjects, but in treated patients with CHF, GFR may increase, decrease, or remain unchanged.

Other Actions

Administration of nesiritide decreases systemic and pulmonary resistances and left ventricular filling pressure and induces a secondary increase in cardiac output.

ADME

Natriuretic peptides are administered intravenously. Nesiritide has a distribution $t_{1/2}$ of 2 min and a mean terminal $t_{1/2}$ of 18 min. Clearance occurs via at least two mechanisms: internalization and subsequent degradation mediated by NPCR, and metabolism by extracellular proteases (Potter, 2011). There is no need to adjust the dose for renal insufficiency.

Therapeutic Uses

Human recombinant ANP (carperitide, available only in Japan) and BNP (nesiritide) are the available therapeutic agents of this class. Urodilatin (ularitide) is in development. Nesiritide is indicated for the management of acutely decompensated CHF. In patients who have dyspnea with minimal activity or at rest, nesiritide reduces pulmonary capillary wedge pressure and improves short-term symptoms of dyspnea. However, the ASCEND-HF trial found that nesiritide does not change mortality and

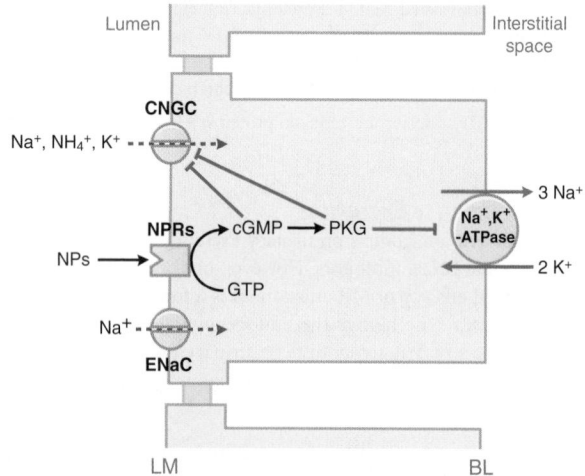

Figure 25–7 *The IMCD Na^+ transport and its regulation.* Na^+ enters the IMCD cell in one of two ways: via ENaC and through a CNGC that transports Na^+, K^+, and NH_4^+ and is gated by cGMP. Na^+ then exits the cell via the Na^+,K^+-ATPase. The CNGC is the primary pathway for Na^+ entry and is inhibited by NPs. NPs bind to cell surface NPRs A, B, and C. The A and B receptors are isoforms of particulate guanylyl cyclase that synthesize cGMP. The CNGC is inhibited by cGMP directly and indirectly through PKG. PKG activation also inhibits Na^+ exit via the Na^+,K^+-ATPase. ENaC is a low-conductance, 4-pS, highly selective Na^+ channel that plays a minor role in IMCD Na^+ transport (see Figure 25–6).

rehospitalization and has only a small effect on dyspnea (O'Connor et al., 2011). Thus, nesiritide is not recommended for routine use in the broad population of patients with acute heart failure (O'Connor et al., 2011).

Toxicity, Adverse Effects, Contraindications, Drug Interactions

Nesiritide can cause hypotension, and there are concerns about adverse renal effects. However, the ASCEND-HF trial did not demonstrate worsening of renal function in nesiritide-treated patients with heart failure (O'Connor et al., 2011).

Adenosine Receptor Antagonists

There are four adenosine receptor subtypes (A_1, A_{2A}, A_{2B}, and A_3). A_1, A_{2A}, and A_{2B} receptors regulate aspects of renal physiology. The A_1 receptor is expressed in the proximal tubule and stimulates reabsorption of Na^+. Consequently, antagonists of A_1 receptors cause diuresis/natriuresis, yet are K^+ sparing. Several naturally occurring methylxanthines (e.g., caffeine, theophylline, and theobromine) are A_1 receptor antagonists (albeit nonselective) and consequently cause diuresis. Pamabrom is a mild diuretic consisting of a one-to-one mixture of 8-bromotheophylline and 2-amino-2-methyl-1-propanol; 8-bromotheophylline, a methylxanthine, is the active component of pamabrom. Pamabrom is the diuretic ingredient in several over-the-counter products marketed for relief of premenstrual syndrome. Little is known regarding the pharmacology, diuretic mechanism of action, and efficacy of pamabrom. However, because 8-bromotheophylline is a methylxanthine, it is possible that the mild diuresis induced by pamabrom is related to blockade of renal A_1 receptors.

Clinical Use of Diuretics

Site and Mechanism of Diuretic Action

An understanding of the sites and mechanisms of action of diuretics enhances comprehension of the clinical aspects of diuretic pharmacology. Figure 25–5 provides a summary view of the sites and mechanisms of actions of diuretics.

The Role of Diuretics in Clinical Medicine

Figure 25–8 illustrates interrelationships among renal function, Na^+ intake, water homeostasis, distribution of extracellular fluid volume, and

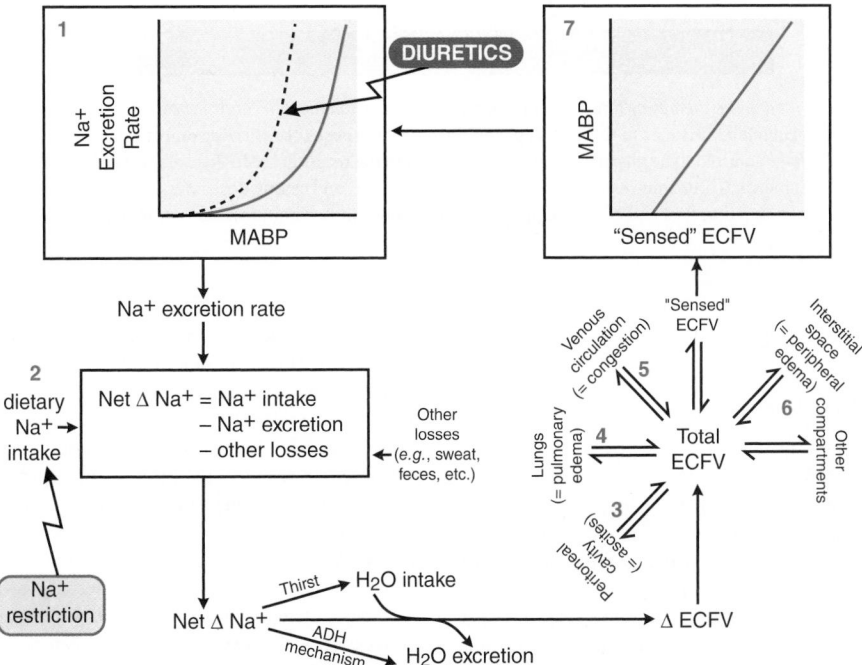

Figure 25–8 *Interrelationships amongst renal function, Na+ intake, water homeostasis, distribution of extracellular fluid volume, and mean arterial blood pressure.* Starting at upper left panel (#1), read this figure counterclockwise. Complex interrelationships exist amongst the cardiovascular system, kidneys, CNS, and capillary beds such that perturbations at one of these sites can affect all other sites. A primary law of the kidney is that Na^+ excretion is a steep function of mean arterial blood pressure (MABP) such that small increases in MABP cause marked increases in Na^+ excretion; this is known as the "pressure-natriuresis" relationship (upper left). Over any given time interval, the net change in total-body Na^+ is the dietary Na^+ intake minus the urinary excretion rate and other losses (lower left). If the pressure-natriuresis curve is right-shifted, a net positive Na^+ balance occurs, and the extracellular Na^+ concentration increases, thus stimulating water intake (thirst) and reducing urinary water output (via ADH release). These changes expand the extracellular fluid volume (ECFV), and the enlarged ECFV is distributed amongst many body compartments (lower right). ECFV on the arterial side of the circulation pressurizes the arterial tree ("sensed" ECFV), and increases MABP (upper right), thus increasing Na^+ excretion (and completing the loop). This loop cycles until net Na^+ accumulation is zero; i.e., in the long run, Na^+ intake must equal Na^+ loss.

These considerations explain the fundamental mechanisms of edema formation:

1. Rightward shift of renal pressure natriuresis curve.
2. Excessive dietary Na^+ intake.
3. Increased distribution of ECFV to peritoneal cavity (e.g., liver cirrhosis with increased hepatic sinusoidal hydrostatic pressure) leading to ascites formation.
4. Increased distribution of ECFV to lungs (e.g., left-sided heart failure with increased pulmonary capillary hydrostatic pressure) leading to pulmonary edema.
5. Increased distribution of ECFV to venous circulation (e.g., right-sided heart failure) leading to venous congestion.
6. Peripheral edema caused by altered Starling forces causing increased distribution of ECFV to interstitial space (e.g., diminished plasma proteins in nephrotic syndrome, severe burns, and liver disease).
7. Increased MABP resulting from "Sensed" ECFV on the arterial side of the heart.

These perturbations leading to edema can be addressed by: **A.** Correcting the underlying disease; **B.** Administering diuretics to left-shift the renal pressure-natriuresis relationship; **C.** Restricting dietary Na^+ intake.

ECFV, extracellular fluid volume; MABP, mean arterial blood pressure.

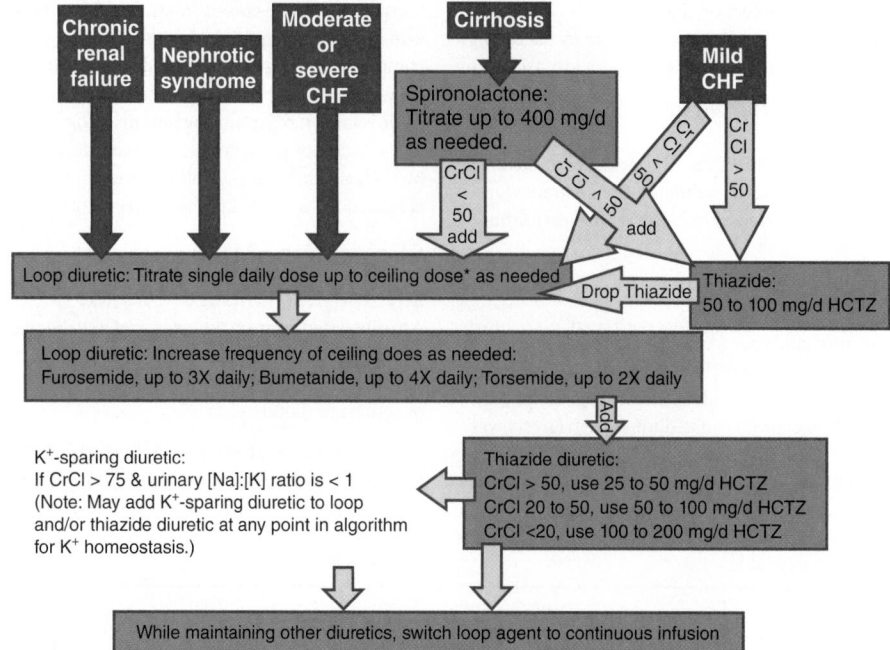

Figure 25–9 *"Brater's algorithm" for diuretic therapy of chronic renal failure, nephrotic syndrome, CHF, and cirrhosis.* Follow algorithm until adequate response is achieved. If adequate response is not obtained, advance to the next step. For illustrative purposes, the thiazide diuretic used is HCTZ. An alternative thiazide-type diuretic may be substituted with dosage adjusted to be pharmacologically equivalent to the recommended dose of HCTZ. *Do not combine two K$^+$-sparing diuretics due to the risk of hyperkalemia.* CrCl indicates creatinine clearance in milliliters per minute, and ceiling dose refers to the smallest dose of diuretic that produces a near-maximal effect. *Ceiling doses of loop diuretics and dosing regimens for continuous intravenous infusions of loop diuretics are disease-state specific. Doses are for adults only.

mean arterial blood pressure and suggests three fundamental strategies for mobilizing edema fluid:

- Correction of the underlying disease
- Restriction of Na$^+$ intake
- Administration of diuretics

Figure 25–9 presents a useful synthesis, Brater's algorithm, a logically compelling algorithm for diuretic therapy (specific recommendations for drug, dose, route, and drug combinations) in patients with edema caused by renal, hepatic, or cardiac disorders (Brater, 1998).

The clinical situation dictates whether a patient should receive diuretics and what therapeutic regimen should be used (type of diuretic, dose, route of administration, and speed of mobilization of edema fluid). Massive pulmonary edema in patients with acute left-sided heart failure is a medical emergency requiring rapid, aggressive therapy, including intravenous administration of a loop diuretic. In this setting, use of oral diuretics is inappropriate. Conversely, mild pulmonary and venous congestion associated with chronic heart failure is best treated with an oral loop or thiazide diuretic, the dosage of which should be titrated carefully to maximize the benefit-to-risk ratio. Loop and thiazide diuretics decrease morbidity and mortality in patients with heart failure (Faris et al., 2002): MR antagonists also demonstrate reduced morbidity and mortality in patients with heart failure receiving optimal therapy with other drugs (Roush et al., 2014).

Periodic administration of diuretics to cirrhotic patients with ascites may eliminate the necessity for or reduce the interval between paracenteses, adding to patient comfort and sparing protein reserves that are lost during paracenteses. Although diuretics can reduce edema associated with chronic renal failure, increased doses of more powerful loop diuretics usually are required. In nephrotic syndrome, diuretic response often is disappointing. In chronic renal failure and cirrhosis, edema will not pose an immediate health risk but can greatly reduce quality of life. In such cases, only partial removal of edema fluid should be attempted, and fluid should be mobilized slowly using a diuretic regimen that accomplishes the task with minimal perturbation of normal physiology.

Diuretic resistance refers to edema that is or has become refractory to a given diuretic. If diuretic resistance develops against a less-efficacious diuretic, a more efficacious diuretic should be substituted, such as a loop diuretic for a thiazide. However, resistance to loop diuretics can be due to several causes. NSAID coadministration is a common preventable cause of diuretic resistance. PG production, especially PGE$_2$, is an important counterregulatory mechanism in states of reduced renal perfusion such as volume contraction, CHF, and cirrhosis characterized by activation of the RAAS and sympathetic nervous system. NSAID administration can block PG-mediated effects that counterbalance the RAAS and sympathetic nervous system, resulting in salt and water retention. Diuretic resistance also occurs with COX-2–selective inhibitors.

In chronic renal failure, a reduction in RBF decreases delivery of diuretics to the kidney, and accumulation of endogenous organic acids competes with loop diuretics for transport at the proximal tubule. Consequently, diuretic concentration at the active site in the tubular lumen is diminished. In nephrotic syndrome, binding of diuretics to luminal albumin was postulated to limit response; however, the validity of this concept has been challenged. In hepatic cirrhosis, nephrotic syndrome, and heart failure, nephrons may have diminished diuretic responsiveness because of increased proximal tubular Na$^+$ reabsorption, leading to diminished Na$^+$ delivery to distal nephrons.

Faced with resistance to loop diuretics, the clinician has several options:

- Bed rest may restore drug responsiveness by improving the renal circulation.
- An increase in dose of loop diuretic may restore responsiveness; however, nothing is gained by increasing the dose above that which causes a near-maximal effect (the ceiling dose) of the diuretic.
- Administration of smaller doses more frequently or a continuous intravenous infusion of a loop diuretic will increase the length of time that an effective diuretic concentration is at the active site.
- Use of combination therapy to sequentially block more than one site in the nephron may result in a synergistic interaction between two diuretics. For example, a combination of a loop diuretic with a K$^+$-sparing or a

thiazide diuretic may improve therapeutic response; however, nothing is gained by the administration of two drugs of the same type. Thiazide diuretics with significant proximal tubular effects (e.g., metolazone) are particularly well suited for sequential blockade when coadministered with a loop diuretic.

- Reducing salt intake will diminish postdiuretic Na⁺ retention, which can nullify previous increases in Na⁺ excretion.
- Scheduling of diuretic administration shortly before food intake will provide effective diuretic concentration in the tubular lumen when salt load is highest.

Part II: Water Homeostasis and the Vasopressin System

Vasopressin Physiology

Arginine vasopressin (ADH in humans) is the main hormone that regulates body fluid osmolality. The hormone is released by the posterior pituitary whenever water deprivation causes an increased plasma osmolality or whenever the cardiovascular system is challenged by hypovolemia or hypotension. Vasopressin acts primarily in the renal collecting duct to increase the permeability of the cell membrane to water, thus permitting water to move passively down an osmotic gradient across the collecting duct into the extracellular compartment.

Vasopressin is a potent vasopressor/vasoconstrictor. It is also a neurotransmitter; among its actions in the CNS are apparent roles in the secretion of ACTH and in regulation of the cardiovascular system, temperature, and other visceral functions. Vasopressin also promotes release of coagulation factors by vascular endothelium and increases platelet aggregability.

Anatomy of the Vasopressin System

The antidiuretic mechanism in mammals involves two anatomical components: a CNS component for synthesis, transport, storage, and release of vasopressin and a renal collecting duct system composed of epithelial cells that respond to vasopressin by increasing their water permeability. The CNS component of the antidiuretic mechanism is called the *hypothalamoneurohypophyseal system* and consists of neurosecretory neurons with perikarya located predominantly in two specific hypothalamic nuclei, the SON and PVN. Long axons of magnocellular neurons in SON and PVN terminate in the neural lobe of the posterior pituitary (neurohypophysis), where they release vasopressin and oxytocin (see Figure 42–1).

Synthesis of Vasopressin

Vasopressin and oxytocin are synthesized mainly in the perikarya of magnocellular neurons in the SON and PVN. However, parvicellular neurons in the PVN also synthesize vasopressin, as do some non-CNS cells (see discussion that follows). Vasopressin synthesis appears to be regulated solely at the transcriptional level. In humans, a 168–amino acid preprohormone (Figure 25–10) is synthesized and then packaged into membrane-associated granules. The prohormone contains three domains: vasopressin (residues 1–9), vasopressin-neurophysin (residues 13–105), and vasopressin-glycopeptide (residues 107–145). The vasopressin domain is linked to the vasopressin-neurophysin domain through a GLY-LYS-ARG-processing signal, and the vasopressin-neurophysin is linked to the vasopressin-glycopeptide domain by an ARG-processing signal. In secretory granules, an endopeptidase, exopeptidase, monooxygenase, and lyase act sequentially on the prohormone to produce vasopressin, vasopressin-neurophysin (sometimes referred to as neurophysin II), and vasopressin-glycopeptide. The synthesis and transport of vasopressin depend on the preprohormone conformation. In particular, vasopressin-neurophysin binds vasopressin and is critical for correct processing, transport, and storage of vasopressin. Genetic mutations in either the signal peptide or vasopressin-neurophysin give rise to central DI.

Vasopressin also is synthesized by the heart and adrenal gland. In the heart, elevated wall stress increases vasopressin synthesis several-fold and may contribute to impaired ventricular relaxation and coronary vasoconstriction. Vasopressin synthesis in the adrenal medulla stimulates catecholamine secretion from chromaffin cells and may promote adrenal cortical growth and stimulate aldosterone synthesis.

Regulation of Vasopressin Secretion

Hyperosmolality. An increase in plasma osmolality is the principal physiological stimulus for vasopressin secretion by the posterior pituitary. The osmolality threshold for secretion is about 280 mOsm/kg. Below the

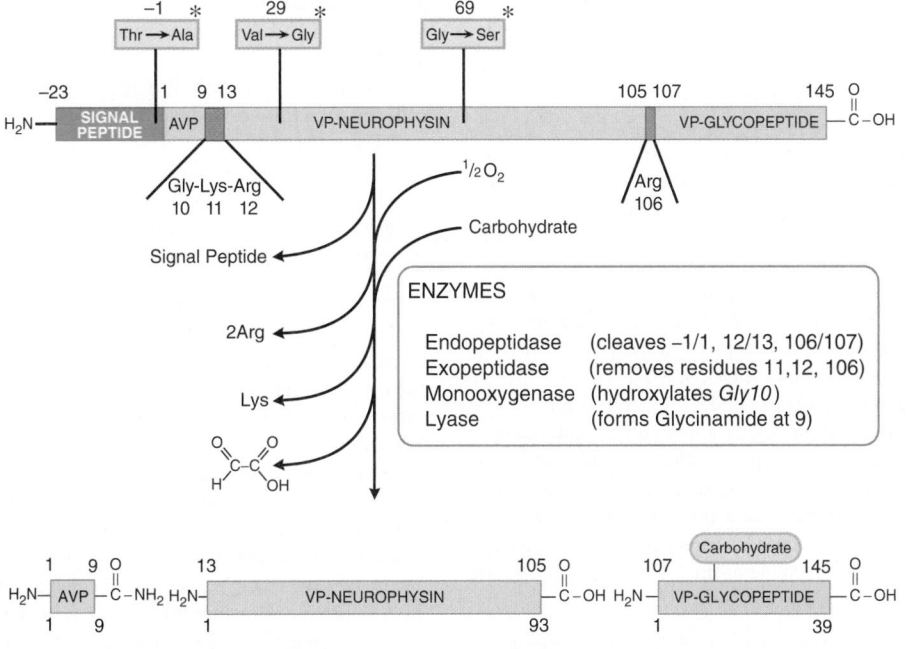

Figure 25–10 *Processing of human AVP preprohormone.* More than 40 mutations in the single gene on chromosome 20 that encodes AVP preprohormone give rise to central DI. *Boxes indicate mutations leading to central DI.

threshold, vasopressin is barely detectable in plasma, and above the threshold, vasopressin levels are a steep and relatively linear function of plasma osmolality. Indeed, a 2% elevation in plasma osmolality causes a 2- to 3-fold increase in plasma vasopressin levels, which in turn causes increased solute-free water reabsorption, with an increase in urine osmolality. Increases in plasma osmolality above 290 mOsm/kg lead to an intense desire for water (thirst). Thus, the vasopressin system affords the organism longer thirst-free periods and, in the event that water is unavailable, allows the organism to survive longer periods of water deprivation. Above a plasma osmolality of approximately 290 mOsm/kg, plasma vasopressin levels exceed 5 pM. Since urinary concentration is maximal (~1200 mOsm/kg) when vasopressin levels exceed 5 pM, further defense against hypertonicity depends entirely on water intake rather than on decreases in water loss.

Hepatic Portal Osmoreceptors. An oral salt load activates hepatic portal osmoreceptors, leading to increased vasopressin release. This mechanism augments plasma vasopressin levels even before the oral salt load increases plasma osmolality.

Hypovolemia and Hypotension. Vasopressin secretion is regulated hemodynamically by changes in effective blood volume or arterial blood pressure. Regardless of the cause (e.g., hemorrhage, Na^+ depletion, diuretics, heart failure, hepatic cirrhosis with ascites, adrenal insufficiency, or hypotensive drugs), reductions in effective blood volume or arterial blood pressure are associated with high circulating vasopressin concentrations. However, unlike osmoregulation, hemodynamic regulation of vasopressin secretion is exponential; that is, small decreases (5%) in blood volume or pressure have little effect on vasopressin secretion, whereas larger decreases (20%–30%) can increase vasopressin levels to 20–30 times normal (exceeding the vasopressin concentration required to induce maximal antidiuresis). Vasopressin is one of the most potent vasoconstrictors known, and the vasopressin response to hypovolemia or hypotension serves as a mechanism to stave off cardiovascular collapse during periods of severe blood loss or hypotension. Hemodynamic regulation of vasopressin secretion does not disrupt osmotic regulation; rather, hypovolemia/hypotension alters the set point and slope of the plasma osmolality-plasma vasopressin relationship.

Neuronal pathways that mediate hemodynamic regulation of vasopressin release are different from those involved in osmoregulation. Baroreceptors in the left atrium, left ventricle, and pulmonary veins sense blood volume (filling pressures), and baroreceptors in the carotid sinus and aorta monitor arterial blood pressure. Nerve impulses reach brainstem nuclei predominantly through the vagal trunk and glossopharyngeal nerve; these signals are ultimately relayed to the SON and PVN.

Hormones and Neurotransmitters. Vasopressin-synthesizing magnocellular neurons have a large array of receptors on both perikarya and nerve terminals; therefore, vasopressin release can be accentuated or attenuated by chemical agents acting at both ends of the magnocellular neuron (Iovino et al., 2014). Also, hormones and neurotransmitters can modulate vasopressin secretion by stimulating or inhibiting neurons in nuclei that project, either directly or indirectly, to the SON and PVN (Iovino et al., 2014). Because of these complexities, modulation of vasopressin secretion by most hormones or neurotransmitters is unclear. Several agents stimulate vasopressin secretion, including acetylcholine (by nicotinic receptors), histamine (by H_1 receptors), dopamine (by both D_1 and D_2 receptors), glutamine, aspartate, cholecystokinin, neuropeptide Y, substance P, vasoactive intestinal polypeptide, PGs, and AngII. Inhibitors of vasopressin secretion include ANP, γ-aminobutyric acid, and opioids (particularly dynorphin via κ receptors). The effects of AngII have received the most attention. AngII synthesized in the brain and circulating AngII may stimulate vasopressin release. Inhibition of the conversion of AngII to AngIII blocks AngII-induced vasopressin release, suggesting that AngIII is the main effector peptide of the brain renin-angiotensin system controlling vasopressin release.

Pharmacological Agents. A number of drugs alter urine osmolality by stimulating or inhibiting vasopressin secretion. In most cases, the mechanism is not known. Stimulators of vasopressin secretion include vincristine, cyclophosphamide, tricyclic antidepressants, nicotine, epinephrine, and high doses of morphine. Lithium, which inhibits the renal effects of vasopressin, also enhances vasopressin secretion. Inhibitors of vasopressin secretion include ethanol, phenytoin, low doses of morphine, glucocorticoids, fluphenazine, haloperidol, promethazine, oxilorphan, and butorphanol. Carbamazepine has a renal action to produce antidiuresis in patients with central DI but actually inhibits vasopressin secretion by a central action. Ethanol inhibits vasopressin secretion (see Chapter 23).

Vasopressin Receptors

Cellular vasopressin effects are mediated mainly by interactions of the hormone with the three types of receptors: V_{1a}, V_{1b}, and V_2. All are GPCRs. The V_{1a} receptor is the most widespread subtype of vasopressin receptor; it is found in vascular smooth muscle, adrenal gland, myometrium, bladder, adipocytes, hepatocytes, platelets, renal medullary interstitial cells, vasa recta in the renal microcirculation, epithelial cells in the renal cortical collecting duct, spleen, testis, and many CNS structures. V_{1b} receptors have a more limited distribution and are found in the anterior pituitary, several brain regions, pancreas, and adrenal medulla. V_2 receptors are located predominantly in principal cells of the renal collecting duct system but also are present on epithelial cells in TAL and on vascular endothelial cells.

Figure 25–11 summarizes the current model of V_1 receptor-effector coupling. Vasopressin binding to V_1 receptors activates the G_q-PLC-IP_3 pathway, thereby mobilizing intracellular Ca^{2+} and activating PKC, ultimately causing biological effects that include immediate responses (e.g., vasoconstriction, glycogenolysis, platelet aggregation, and ACTH release) and growth responses in smooth muscle cells.

Principal cells in renal collecting duct have V_2 receptors on their basolateral membranes that couple to G_s to stimulate adenylyl cyclase activity (Figure 25–12). The resulting activation of the cyclic AMP/PKA pathway triggers an increased rate of insertion of water channel-containing vesicles (WCVs) into the apical membrane and a decreased rate of endocytosis of WCVs from the apical membrane. Because WCVs contain preformed functional water channels (aquaporin 2), their net shift into apical membranes in response to V_2 receptor stimulation greatly increases water permeability of the apical membrane (Nejsum, 2005) (see Figures 25–12 and 25–13).

V_2 receptor activation also increases urea permeability by 400% in the terminal portions of the IMCD. V_2 receptors increase urea permeability by activating a vasopressin-regulated urea transporter (termed *VRUT*, *UT1*, or *UTA1*), most likely by PKA-induced phosphorylation. Kinetics of vasopressin-induced water and urea permeability differ, and vasopressin-induced regulation of VRUT does not entail vesicular trafficking to the plasma membrane.

V_2 receptor activation also increases Na^+ transport in TAL and collecting duct. Increased Na^+ transport in TAL is mediated by three mechanisms that affect the Na^+-K^+-$2Cl^-$ symporter: rapid phosphorylation of the symporter, translocation of the symporter into the luminal membrane, and increased expression of symporter protein. The multiple mechanisms by which vasopressin increases water reabsorption are summarized in Figure 25–14.

Renal Actions of Vasopressin

Several sites of vasopressin action in kidney involve both V_1 and V_2 receptors. V_1 receptors mediate contraction of mesangial cells in the glomerulus and contraction of vascular smooth muscle cells in vasa recta and efferent arterioles. V_1 receptor–mediated reduction of inner medullary blood flow contributes to the maximum concentrating capacity of the kidney. V_1 receptors also stimulate PG synthesis by medullary interstitial cells. Because PGE_2 inhibits adenylyl cyclase in collecting ducts, stimulation of PG synthesis by V_1 receptors may counterbalance V_2 receptor–mediated antidiuresis. V_1 receptors on principal cells in cortical collecting ducts may inhibit V_2 receptor–mediated water flux by activation of PKC. V_2 receptors mediate the most prominent response to vasopressin, which is increased water permeability of the collecting duct at concentrations as low as 50 fM. Thus, V_2 receptor–mediated effects of vasopressin occur at concentrations far lower than are required to engage

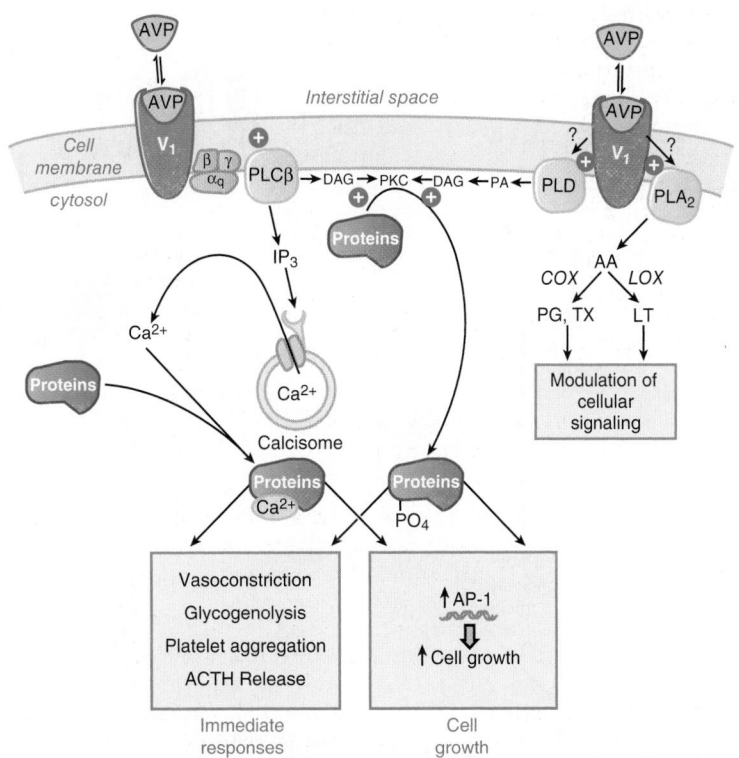

Figure 25–11 *Mechanism of V₁ receptor-effector coupling.* Binding of AVP to V₁ vasopressin receptors (V₁) stimulates membrane-bound phospholipases. Stimulation of G_q activates the PLCβ-IP₃/DAG-Ca²⁺-PKC pathway. Activation of V₁ receptors also causes influx of extracellular Ca²⁺ by an unknown mechanism. PKC and Ca²⁺/calmodulin-activated protein kinases phosphorylate cell-type–specific proteins, leading to cellular responses. A further component of the AVP response derives from the production of eicosanoids secondary to the activation of PLA₂; the resulting mobilization of AA provides substrate for eicosanoid synthesis by the COX and LOX pathways, leading to local production of PGs, TXs, and LT, which may activate myriad signaling pathways, including those linked to G_s and G_q.

V₁ receptor–mediated actions. Other renal actions mediated by V₂ receptors include increased urea transport in the IMCD and increased Na⁺ transport in the TAL; both effects contribute to the urine-concentrating ability of the kidney. V₂ receptors also increase Na⁺ transport in cortical collecting ducts, and this may synergize with aldosterone to enhance Na⁺ reabsorption during hypovolemia.

Pharmacological Modification of the Antidiuretic Response to Vasopressin

The NSAIDs, particularly indomethacin, enhance the antidiuretic response to vasopressin. Because PGs attenuate antidiuretic responses to vasopressin and NSAIDs inhibit PG synthesis, reduced PG production probably accounts for potentiation of vasopressin's antidiuretic response. Carbamazepine and chlorpropamide also enhance antidiuretic effects of vasopressin by unknown mechanisms. In rare instances, chlorpropamide can induce water intoxication. A number of drugs inhibit the antidiuretic actions of vasopressin. Lithium is of particular importance because of its use in the treatment of manic-depressive disorders (Kishore and Ecelbarger, 2013). Acutely, Li⁺ appears to reduce V₂ receptor–mediated stimulation of adenylyl cyclase. Also, Li⁺ increases plasma levels of PTH, a partial antagonist to vasopressin. In most patients, the antibiotic demeclocycline attenuates the antidiuretic effects of vasopressin, probably owing to decreased accumulation and action of cyclic AMP (Kortenoeven et al., 2013).

Nonrenal Actions of Vasopressin

Cardiovascular System. The cardiovascular effects of vasopressin are complex. Vasopressin is a potent vasoconstrictor (V₁ receptor mediated), and resistance vessels throughout the circulation may be affected. Vascular smooth muscle in the skin, skeletal muscle, fat, pancreas, and thyroid gland appears most sensitive, with significant vasoconstriction also occurring in the GI tract, coronary vessels, and brain. Despite the potency of vasopressin as a direct vasoconstrictor, vasopressin-induced pressor responses in vivo are minimal and occur only with vasopressin concentrations significantly higher than those required for maximal antidiuresis. To a large extent, this is due to circulating vasopressin actions on V₁ receptors to inhibit sympathetic efferents and potentiate baroreflexes. In addition, V₂ receptors cause vasodilation in some blood vessels.

Vasopressin helps to maintain arterial blood pressure during episodes of severe hypovolemia/hypotension. The effects of vasopressin on the heart (reduced cardiac output and heart rate) are largely indirect and result from coronary vasoconstriction, decreased coronary blood flow, and alterations in vagal and sympathetic tone. Some patients with coronary insufficiency experience angina even in response to the relatively small amounts of vasopressin required to control DI, and vasopressin-induced myocardial ischemia has led to severe reactions and even death.

CNS. Vasopressin likely plays a role as a neurotransmitter or neuromodulator. Although vasopressin can modulate CNS autonomic systems controlling heart rate, arterial blood pressure, respiration rate, and sleep patterns, the physiological significance of these actions is unclear. While vasopressin is not the principal corticotropin-releasing factor, vasopressin may provide for sustained activation of the hypothalamic-pituitary-adrenal axis during chronic stress. Studies in both laboratory animals and humans indicated that vasopressin and oxytocin are key regulators of social and emotional behaviors (Benarroch, 2013). CNS effects of vasopressin appear to be mediated predominantly by V₁ receptors.

Blood Coagulation. Activation of V₂ receptors by desmopressin or vasopressin increases circulating levels of procoagulant factor VIII and of von Willebrand factor. These effects are mediated by extrarenal V₂ receptors. Presumably, vasopressin stimulates secretion of von Willebrand factor and of factor VIII from storage sites in vascular endothelium. However, because release of von Willebrand factor does not occur when desmopressin is applied directly to cultured endothelial cells or to isolated blood vessels, intermediate factors are likely to be involved.

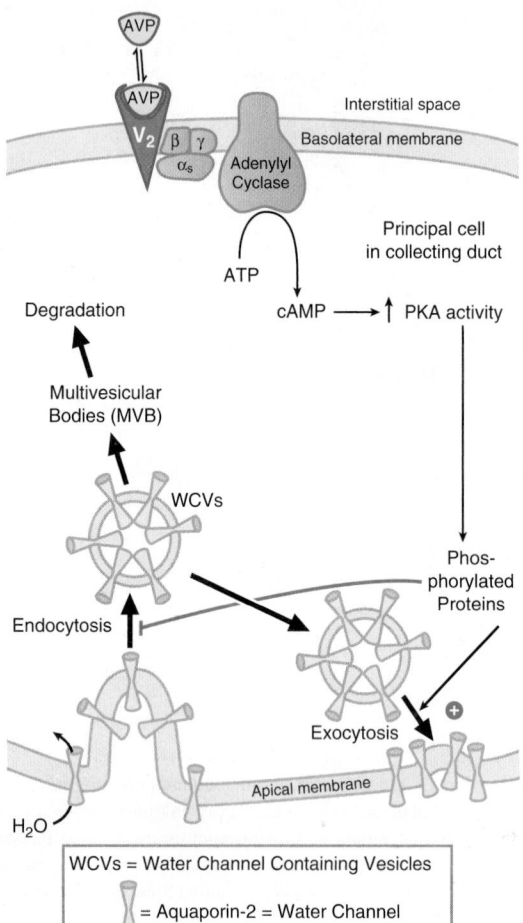

Figure 25–12 *Mechanism of V₂ receptor-effector coupling.* Binding of AVP to the V₂ receptor activates the Gₛ-adenylyl cyclase-cAMP-PKA pathway and shifts the balance of aquaporin 2 trafficking toward the apical membrane of the principal cell of the collecting duct, thus enhancing water permeability. Although phosphorylation of *Ser256* of aquaporin 2 is involved in V₂ receptor signaling, other proteins located in both the water channel–containing vesicles and the apical membrane of the cytoplasm also may be involved.

Other Nonrenal Effects. At high concentrations, vasopressin stimulates smooth muscle contraction in the uterus (by oxytocin receptors) and GI tract (by V₁ receptors). Vasopressin is stored in platelets, and activation of V₁ receptors stimulates platelet aggregation. Also, activation of V₁ receptors on hepatocytes stimulates glycogenolysis.

Vasopressin Receptor Agonists

A number of vasopressin-like peptides occur naturally across the animal kingdom (Table 25–8); all are nonapeptides. In all mammals except swine, the neurohypophyseal peptide is 8-arginine vasopressin, and the terms vasopressin, AVP, and ADH are used interchangeably. There are also a number of synthetic peptides with receptor-subtype specificity, and one nonpeptide agonist.

Many vasopressin analogues were synthesized with the goal of increasing duration of action and selectivity for vasopressin receptor subtypes (V₁ vs. V₂ receptors, which mediate pressor responses and antidiuretic responses, respectively). Thus, the antidiuretic-to-vasopressor ratio for the V₂–selective agonist, DDAVP, also called desmopressin, is about 3000 times greater than that for vasopressin; thus, desmopressin is the preferred drug for the treatment of central DI. Substitution of valine for glutamine in position 4 further increases the antidiuretic selectivity, and the anti-diuretic-to-vasopressor ratio for deamino [Val⁴, D-Arg⁸]AVP is about 11,000 times greater than that for vasopressin.

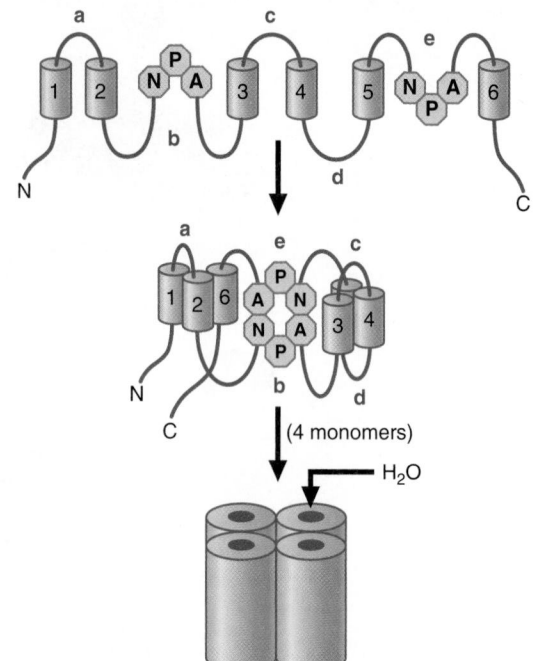

Figure 25–13 *Structure of aquaporins.* Aquaporins have six transmembrane domains, and the NH₂ and COOH termini are intracellular. Loops b and e each contain an NPA sequence. Aquaporins fold with transmembrane domains 1, 2, and 6 in close proximity and transmembrane domains 3, 4 and 5 in juxtaposition. The long b and e loops dip into the membrane, and the NPA sequences align to create a pore through which water can diffuse. Most likely, aquaporins form a tetrameric oligomer. At least seven aquaporins are expressed at distinct sites in the kidney. Aquaporin 1, abundant in the proximal tubule and DTL, is essential for concentration of urine. Aquaporin 2, exclusively expressed in the principal cells of the connecting tubule and collecting duct, is the major vaso-pressin-regulated water channel. Aquaporin 3 and aquaporin 4 are expressed in the basolateral membranes of collecting duct principal cells and provide exit pathways for water reabsorbed apically by aquaporin 2. Aquaporin 7 is in the apical brush border of the straight proximal tubule. Aquaporins 6–8 are also expressed in kidney; their functions remain to be clarified. Vasopressin regulates water permeability of the collecting duct by influencing the traffick-ing of aquaporin 2 from intracellular vesicles to the apical plasma membrane (Figure 25–12). AVP-induced activation of the cAMP-PKA pathway also enhances expression of aquaporin 2 mRNA and protein; chronic dehydration thus causes upregulation of aquaporin 2 and water transport in the collecting duct.

Increasing V₁ selectivity has proved more difficult than increasing V₂ selectivity. Vasopressin receptors in the adenohypophysis that mediate vasopressin-induced ACTH release are neither classical V₁ nor V₂ receptors. Because vasopressin receptors in the adenohypophysis appear to share a common signal-transduction mechanism with classical V₁ receptors, and because many vasopressin analogues with vasoconstrictor activity release ACTH, V₁ receptors have been subclassified into V₁ₐ (vascular/hepatic) and V₁ᵦ (pituitary) receptors (also called V₃ receptors). There are selective agonists for V₁ₐ and V₁ᵦ receptors.

The chemical structure of oxytocin is closely related to that of vaso-pressin: Oxytocin is [Ile³, Leu⁸]AVP. With such structural similarities, it is not surprising that vasopressin and oxytocin agonists and antagonists can bind to each other's receptors. Therefore, most of the available pep-tide vasopressin agonists and antagonists have some affinity for oxytocin receptors; at high doses, they may block or mimic the effects of oxytocin.

Diseases Affecting the Vasopressin System

Diabetes Insipidus

Diabetes insipidus is a disease of impaired renal water conservation owing either to inadequate vasopressin secretion from the neurohypophysis

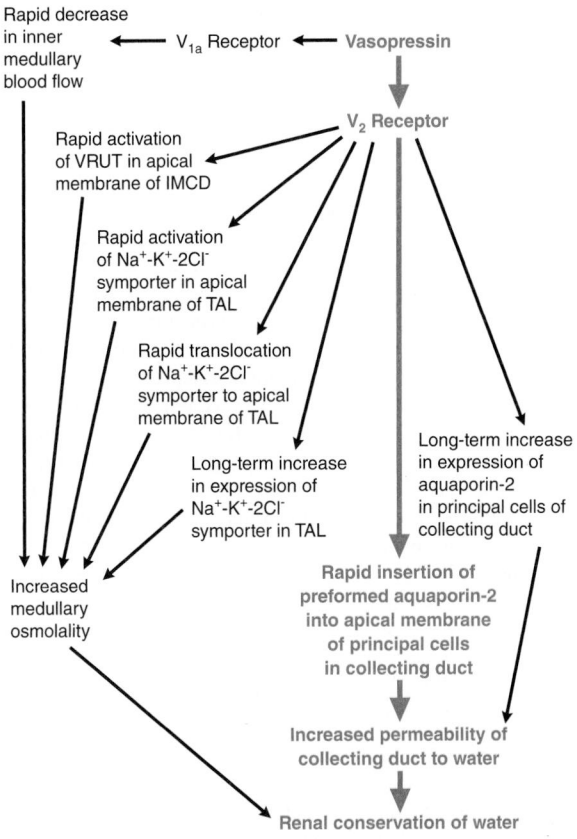

Figure 25–14 *Mechanisms by which vasopressin increases the renal conservation of water.* Red and black arrows denote major and minor pathways, respectively.

(central DI) or to insufficient renal vasopressin response (nephrogenic DI). Very rarely, DI can be caused by an abnormally high degradation rate of vasopressin by circulating vasopressinases. Pregnancy may accentuate or reveal central or nephrogenic DI by increasing plasma levels of vasopressinase and by reducing renal sensitivity to vasopressin. Patients with DI excrete large volumes (>30 mL/kg per day) of dilute (<200 mOsm/kg) urine and, if their thirst mechanism is functioning normally, are polydipsic. Central DI can be distinguished from nephrogenic DI by administration of desmopressin, which will increase urine osmolality in patients with central DI but have little or no effect in patients with nephrogenic DI. DI can be differentiated from primary polydipsia by measuring plasma osmolality, which will be low to low-normal in patients with primary polydipsia and high to high-normal in patients with DI.

Central DI. Head injury, either surgical or traumatic, in the region of the pituitary or hypothalamus may cause central DI. Postoperative central DI may be transient, permanent, or triphasic (recovery followed by permanent relapse). Other causes include hypothalamic or pituitary tumors, cerebral aneurysms, CNS ischemia, and brain infiltrations and infections. Central DI may also be idiopathic or familial. Familial central DI usually is autosomal dominant (chromosome 20), and vasopressin deficiency occurs several months or years after birth and worsens gradually. Autosomal dominant central DI is linked to mutations in the vasopressin preprohormone gene that cause the prohormone to misfold and oligomerize improperly. Accumulation of mutant vasopressin precursor causes neuronal death, hence the dominant mode of inheritance. Rarely, familial central DI is autosomal recessive owing to a mutation in the vasopressin peptide itself that gives rise to an inactive vasopressin mutant.

Antidiuretic peptides are the primary treatment of central DI, with desmopressin the peptide of choice. For patients with central DI who cannot tolerate antidiuretic peptides because of side effects or allergic reactions, other treatment options are available. Chlorpropamide, an oral sulfonylurea, potentiates the action of small or residual amounts of

TABLE 25–8 ■ VASOPRESSIN RECEPTOR AGONISTS

Naturally occurring vasopressin-like peptides	A	W	X	Y	Z
A. *Vertebrates*					
1. Mammals					
AVP[a] (humans and other mammals)	NH₂	Tyr	Phe	Gln	Arg
Lypressin[a] (pigs, marsupials)	NH₂	Tyr	Phe	Gln	Lys
Phenypressin (macropodids)	NH₂	Phe	Phe	Gln	Arg
2. Nonmammalian vertebrates					
Vasotocin	NH₂	Tyr	Ile	Gln	Arg
B. *Invertebrates*					
1. Arginine conopressin (*Conus striatus*)	NH₂	Ile	Ile	Arg	Arg
2. Lysine conopressin (*Conus geographicus*)	NH₂	Phe	Ile	Arg	Lys
3. Locust subesophageal ganglia peptide	NH₂	Leu	Ile	Thr	Arg
Synthetic vasopressin peptides					
A. *V₁-selective agonists*					
1. V₁ₐ-selective: [Phe², Ile³, Orn⁸] AVP	NH₂	Phe	Ile	Gln	Orn
2. V₁ᵦ-selective: Deamino [D-3-(3′-pyridyl)-Ala²] AVP	H	D-3-(3′-pyridyl)-Ala²	Phe	Gln	Arg
B. *V₂-selective agonists*					
1. Desmopressin[a] (DDAVP)	H	Tyr	Phe	Gln	D-Arg
2. Deamino [Val⁴, D-Arg⁸] AVP	H	Tyr	Phe	Val	D-Arg
Nonpeptide agonist					
A. *OPC-51803*					

[a]Available for clinical use.

circulating vasopressin and will reduce urine volume in more than half of all patients with central DI. Doses of 125–500 mg daily appear effective in patients with partial central DI. If polyuria is not controlled satisfactorily with chlorpropamide alone, addition of a thiazide diuretic to the regimen usually results in an adequate reduction in urine volume. Carbamazepine (800–1000 mg daily in divided doses) also reduces urine volume in patients with central DI. Long-term use may induce serious adverse effects; therefore, carbamazepine is used rarely to treat central DI. These agents are not effective in nephrogenic DI, which indicates that functional V_2 receptors are required for the antidiuretic effect. Because carbamazepine inhibits and chlorpropamide has little effect on vasopressin secretion, it is likely that carbamazepine and chlorpropamide act directly on the kidney to enhance V_2 receptor–mediated antidiuresis.

Nephrogenic DI. Nephrogenic DI may be congenital or acquired. Hypercalcemia, hypokalemia, postobstructive renal failure, Li^+, foscarnet, clozapine, demeclocycline, and other drugs can induce nephrogenic DI. As many as one in three patients treated with Li^+ may develop nephrogenic DI. X-linked nephrogenic DI is caused by mutations in the gene encoding the V_2 receptor, which maps to Xq28. Mutations in the V_2 receptor gene may cause impaired routing of the V_2 receptor to the cell surface, defective coupling of the receptor to G proteins, or decreased receptor affinity for vasopressin. Autosomal recessive and dominant nephrogenic DI result from inactivating mutations in aquaporin 2. These findings indicate that aquaporin 2 is essential for the antidiuretic effect of vasopressin in humans.

Although the mainstay of treatment of nephrogenic DI is assurance of an adequate water intake, drugs also can be used to reduce polyuria. Amiloride blocks Li^+ uptake by the Na^+ channel in the collecting duct system and may be effective in patients with mild-to-moderate concentrating defects. Thiazide *diuretics* reduce the polyuria of patients with DI and often are used to treat nephrogenic DI. In infants with nephrogenic DI, use of thiazides may be crucial because uncontrolled polyuria may exceed the child's capacity to imbibe and absorb fluids. It is possible that the natriuretic action of thiazides and resulting extracellular fluid volume depletion play an important role in thiazide-induced antidiuresis. The antidiuretic effects appear to parallel the thiazide's ability to cause natriuresis, and the drugs are given in doses similar to those used to mobilize edema fluid. In patients with DI, a 50% reduction of urine volume is a good response to thiazides. Moderate restriction of Na^+ intake can enhance the antidiuretic effectiveness of thiazides.

A number of case reports described the effectiveness of indomethacin in the treatment of nephrogenic DI; however, other PG synthase inhibitors (e.g., ibuprofen) appear to be less effective. The mechanism of the effect may involve a decrease in GFR, an increase in medullary solute concentration, or enhanced proximal fluid reabsorption. Also, because PGs attenuate vasopressin-induced antidiuresis in patients with at least a partially intact V_2 receptor system, some of the antidiuretic response to indomethacin may be due to diminution of the PG effect and enhancement of vasopressin effects on the principal cells of collecting duct.

Syndrome of Inappropriate Secretion of Antidiuretic Hormone

A disease of impaired water excretion with accompanying hyponatremia and hypoosmolality, SIADH caused by the *inappropriate* secretion of vasopressin. Clinical manifestations of plasma hypotonicity resulting from SIADH may include lethargy, anorexia, nausea and vomiting, muscle cramps, coma, convulsions, and death. A multitude of disorders can induce SIADH, including malignancies, pulmonary diseases, CNS injuries/diseases (e.g., head trauma, infections, and tumors), and general surgery.

Three drug classes are commonly implicated in drug-induced SIADH: psychotropic medications (e.g., selective serotonin reuptake inhibitors, haloperidol, and tricyclic antidepressants), sulfonylureas (e.g., chlorpropamide), and vinca alkaloids (e.g., vincristine and vinblastine). Other drugs strongly associated with SIADH include clonidine, cyclophosphamide, enalapril, felbamate, ifosfamide, methyldopa, pentamidine,

and vinorelbine. Many other drugs have been implicated. In a normal individual, an elevation in plasma vasopressin per se does not induce plasma hypotonicity because the person simply stops drinking owing to an osmotically induced aversion to fluids. Therefore, plasma hypotonicity only occurs when excessive fluid intake (oral or intravenous) accompanies inappropriate secretion of vasopressin.

Treatment of hypotonicity in the setting of SIADH includes water restriction, intravenous administration of hypertonic saline, loop diuretics (which interfere with kidney's concentrating ability), and drugs that inhibit the effect of vasopressin to increase water permeability in collecting ducts. To inhibit vasopressin's action in collecting ducts, demeclocycline, a tetracycline, has been the preferred drug, but tolvaptan and conivaptan, V_2 receptor antagonists, are now available (see next section and Table 25–9).

Although Li^+ can inhibit the renal actions of vasopressin, it is effective in only a minority of patients, may induce irreversible renal damage when used chronically, and has a low therapeutic index. Therefore, Li^+ should be considered for use only in patients with symptomatic SIADH who cannot be controlled by other means or in whom tetracyclines are contraindicated (e.g., patients with liver disease). It is important to stress that the majority of patients with SIADH do not require therapy because plasma Na^+ stabilizes in the range of 125–132 mM; such patients usually are asymptomatic. Only when symptomatic hypotonicity ensues, generally when plasma Na^+ levels drop below 120 mM, should therapy with demeclocycline be initiated. Because hypotonicity, which causes an influx of water into cells with resulting cerebral swelling, is the cause of symptoms, the goal of therapy is simply to increase plasma osmolality toward normal.

Other Water-Retaining States

In patients with CHF, cirrhosis, or nephrotic syndrome, *effective* blood volume often is reduced, and hypovolemia frequently is exacerbated by the liberal use of diuretics. Because hypovolemia stimulates vasopressin release, patients may become hyponatremic owing to vasopressin-mediated retention of water. The development of potent orally active V_2 receptor antagonists and specific inhibitors of water channels in the collecting duct has provided a new therapeutic strategy not only in patients with SIADH but also in the more common setting of hyponatremia in patients with heart failure, liver cirrhosis, and nephrotic syndrome.

Clinical Use of Vasopressin Agonists

Two antidiuretic peptides are available for clinical use in the U.S.:

- *Vasopressin* (synthetic 8-L-arginine vasopressin) is available as a sterile aqueous solution; it may be administered intravenously, subcutaneously, intramuscularly, intranasally, intraosseously (off label), intra-arterially, or endotracheally (off label; unreliable).
- *Desmopressin acetate* (synthetic DDAVP) is available as a sterile aqueous solution packaged for intravenous or subcutaneous injection, in a solution for intranasal administration with either a nasal spray pump or rhinal tube delivery system, and in tablets for oral administration.

Therapeutic Uses

The therapeutic uses of vasopressin and its congeners can be divided into two main categories according to the vasopressin receptor involved: V_1 receptor mediated and V_2 receptor mediated.

V_1 receptor–mediated therapeutic applications are based on the rationale that V_1 receptors cause GI and vascular smooth muscle contraction. *Vasopressin is the main agent used.* V_1 receptor–mediated GI smooth muscle contraction has been used to treat postoperative ileus and abdominal distension and to dispel intestinal gas before abdominal roentgenography to avoid interfering gas shadows. V_1 receptor–mediated vasoconstriction of the splanchnic arterial vessels reduces blood flow to the portal system and thereby attenuates pressure and bleeding in esophageal varices. Although endoscopic variceal banding ligation is the treatment of choice for bleeding esophageal varices, V_1 receptor agonists have been used in an emergency setting until endoscopy can be performed. Simultaneous administration of nitroglycerin with V_1 receptor agonists may attenuate the cardiotoxic effects of V_1 agonists while enhancing their beneficial

TABLE 25–9 ■ VASOPRESSIN RECEPTOR ANTAGONISTS

Peptide antagonists

	X	Y	Z
A. *V$_1$-selective antagonists*			
V$_{1a}$-selective antagonist d(CH$_2$)$_5$[Tyr(Me)^2] AVP	Tyr—OMe	Gln	Gly (NH$_2$)
V$_{1b}$-selective antagonist dP [Tyr(Me)^2] AVP[a,b]	Tyr—OMe	Gln	Gly (NH$_2$)
B. *V$_2$-selective antagonists*[a]			
1. des Gly-NH$_2$^{9}-d(CH$_2$)$_5$[D-Ile^2, Ile^4] AVP	D-Ile	Ile	—
2. d(CH$_2$)$_5$[D-Ile^2, Ile^4, Ala-NH$_2$^{9}] AVP	D-Ile	Ile	Ala(NH$_2$)

Nonpeptide antagonists

A. *V$_{1a}$-selective antagonists*
OPC-21268
SR 49059 (relcovaptan)

B. *V$_{1b}$-selective antagonists*
SSR 149415 (nelivaptan)

C. *V$_2$-selective antagonists*
SR 121463 (satavaptan)
VPA-985 (lixivaptan)
OPC-31260 (mozavaptan)
OPC-41061 (tolvaptan)[c]

D. *V$_{1a}$-/V$_2$-selective antagonists*
YM-471
YM 087 (conivaptan)[c]
JTV-605
CL-385004

[a]Also blocks V$_{1a}$ receptor.
[b]V$_2$ antagonistic activity in rats; however, antagonistic activity may be less or nonexistent in other species. Also, with prolonged infusion may exhibit significant agonist activity.
[c]Available for clinical use in United States.

splanchnic effects. Also, V$_1$ receptor agonists have been used during abdominal surgery in patients with portal hypertension to diminish the risk of hemorrhage during the procedure. V$_1$ receptor–mediated vasoconstriction has been used to reduce bleeding during acute hemorrhagic gastritis, burn wound excision, cyclophosphamide-induced hemorrhagic cystitis, liver transplant, cesarean section, and uterine myoma resection. Vasopressin levels in patients with vasodilatory shock are inappropriately low, and such patients are extraordinarily sensitive to the pressor actions of V$_1$ receptor agonists. Therefore, V$_1$ receptor agonists are indicated for the treatment of hypotension in patients with vasodilatory shock that responds insufficiently to therapy with fluids and catecholamines (Serpa Neto et al., 2012). Vasopressin combined with epinephrine and steroids showed improved outcomes after in-hospital cardiac arrest (Layek et al., 2014).

V$_2$ receptor–mediated therapeutic applications are based on the rationale that V$_2$ receptors cause water conservation and release of blood coagulation factors. *Desmopressin is the standard drug of choice.* Central, but not nephrogenic, DI can be treated with V$_2$ receptor agonists, and polyuria and polydipsia usually are well controlled by these agents. Some patients experience transient DI (e.g., in head injury or surgery in the area of the pituitary); however, therapy for most patients with DI is lifelong. Desmopressin is the drug of choice for the vast majority of patients. The duration of effect from a single intranasal dose is from 6 to 20 h; twice-daily administration is effective in most patients. The usual intranasal dosage in adults is 10–40 µg daily either as a single dose or divided into two or three doses. In view of the high cost of the drug and the importance of avoiding water intoxication, the schedule of administration should be adjusted to the minimal amount required. In some patients, chronic allergic rhinitis or other nasal pathology may preclude reliable peptide absorption following nasal administration. Oral administration of desmopressin in doses of 0.1–1.2 mg/d provides adequate desmopressin blood levels to control polyuria. Subcutaneous or intravenous administration of 2–4 µg daily of desmopressin also is effective in central DI.

Vasopressin has little, if any, place in the long-term therapy of DI because of its short duration of action and V$_1$ receptor–mediated side effects. Vasopressin can be used as an alternative to desmopressin in the initial diagnostic evaluation of patients with suspected DI and to control polyuria in patients with DI who recently have undergone surgery or experienced head trauma. Under these circumstances, polyuria may be transient, and long-acting agents may produce water intoxication.

Desmopressin is used in bleeding disorders. In most patients with type I vWD and in some with type IIn vWD, desmopressin will elevate von Willebrand factor and shorten bleeding time. However, desmopressin generally is ineffective in patients with types IIa, IIb, and III vWD. Desmopressin may cause a marked transient thrombocytopenia in individuals with type IIb vWD and is contraindicated in such patients. Desmopressin also increases factor VIII levels in patients with mild-to-moderate hemophilia A. Desmopressin is not indicated in patients with severe hemophilia A, those with hemophilia B, or those with factor VIII antibodies. In patients with renal insufficiency, desmopressin shortens bleeding time and increases circulating levels of factor VIII coagulant activity, factor VIII–related antigen, and ristocetin cofactor. It also induces the appearance of larger von Willebrand factor multimers. Desmopressin is effective in some patients with liver cirrhosis- or drug-induced (e.g., heparin, hirudin, and antiplatelet agents) bleeding disorders. Desmopressin, given intravenously at a dose of 0.3 µg/kg, increases factor VIII and von Willebrand factor for more than 6 h. Desmopressin can be given at intervals of 12–24 h depending on the clinical response and severity of bleeding. Tachyphylaxis to desmopressin usually occurs after several days (owing to depletion of factor VIII and von Willebrand factor storage sites) and limits its usefulness to preoperative preparation, postoperative bleeding, excessive menstrual bleeding, and emergency situations.

Another V$_2$ receptor–mediated therapeutic application is the use of desmopressin for primary nocturnal enuresis. Bedtime administration of desmopressin tablets provides a high response rate that is sustained with long-term use and that accelerates the cure rate. Intranasal desmopressin is no longer recommended for the treatment of primary nocturnal enuresis because of increased risk of hyponatremia. Desmopressin also relieves post–lumbar puncture headache, probably by causing water retention and thereby facilitating rapid fluid equilibration in the CNS.

SECTION III

MODULATION OF PULMONARY, RENAL, AND CARDIOVASCULAR FUNCTION

When vasopressin and desmopressin are given orally, they are inactivated quickly by trypsin. Inactivation by peptidases in various tissues (particularly liver and kidney) results in a plasma $t_{1/2}$ of vasopressin of 17–35 min. Following intramuscular or subcutaneous injection, antidiuretic effects of vasopressin last 2–8 h. The $t_{1/2}$ of desmopressin is 75 min to 3.5 h.

Toxicity, Adverse Effects, Contraindications, Drug Interactions

Most adverse effects are mediated through V_1 receptor activation on vascular and GI smooth muscle; such adverse effects are much less common and less severe with desmopressin than with vasopressin. After injection of large doses of vasopressin, marked facial pallor owing to cutaneous vasoconstriction is observed commonly. Increased intestinal activity is likely to cause nausea, belching, cramps, and an urge to defecate. Vasopressin should be administered with extreme caution in individuals suffering from vascular disease, especially coronary artery disease. Other cardiac complications include arrhythmia and decreased cardiac output. Peripheral vasoconstriction and gangrene were encountered in patients receiving large doses of vasopressin.

The major V_2 receptor–mediated adverse effect is water intoxication. Many drugs, including carbamazepine, chlorpropamide, morphine, tricyclic antidepressants, and NSAIDs, can potentiate the antidiuretic effects of these peptides. Several drugs, such as Li^+, demeclocycline, and ethanol, can attenuate the antidiuretic response to desmopressin. Desmopressin and vasopressin should be used cautiously in disease states in which a rapid increase in extracellular water may impose risks (e.g., in angina, hypertension, and heart failure) and should not be used in patients with acute renal failure. Patients receiving desmopressin to maintain hemostasis should be advised to reduce fluid intake. Also, it is imperative that these peptides not be administered to patients with primary or psychogenic polydipsia because severe hypotonic hyponatremia will ensue. Mild facial flushing and headache are the most common adverse effects. Allergic reactions ranging from urticaria to anaphylaxis may occur with desmopressin or vasopressin. Intranasal administration may cause local adverse effects in the nasal passages, such as edema, rhinorrhea, congestion, irritation, pruritus, and ulceration.

Clinical Use of Vasopressin Antagonists

Table 25–9 summarizes the selectivity of vasopressin receptor antagonists. Only tolvaptan and conivaptan are currently available in the United States.

Therapeutic Uses

When the kidney perceives the arterial blood volume to be low (as in the disease states of CHF, cirrhosis, and nephrosis), AVP perpetuates a state of total body salt and water excess. V_2 receptor antagonists or "aquaretics" may have a therapeutic role in these conditions, especially in patients with concomitant hyponatremia. They are also effective in hyponatremia associated with SIADH. Aquaretics increase renal free water excretion with little or no change in electrolyte excretion. Because they do not affect Na^+ reabsorption, they do not stimulate the TGF mechanism with its associated consequence of reducing GFR.

Tolvaptan is a selective oral V_2 receptor antagonist FDA-approved for clinically significant hypervolemic and euvolemic hyponatremia. Conivaptan is a nonselective V_{1a} receptor/V_2 receptor antagonist that is FDA-approved for the treatment of hospitalized patients with euvolemic and hypervolemic hyponatremia. Conivaptan is available only for intravenous infusion. Expert panels have yet to reach a consensus regarding the appropriate use of V_2 receptor antagonists (Berl, 2015).

ADME

Tolvaptan has a $t_{1/2}$ of 2.8–12 h and less than 1% is excreted in the urine. Tolvaptan is a substrate and inhibitor of P-glycoprotein and is eliminated entirely by CYP3A4 metabolism. Conivaptan is highly protein bound, has a terminal elimination $t_{1/2}$ of 5–12 h, is metabolized via CYP3A, and is partially excreted by the kidney.

Toxicity, Adverse Effects, Contraindications, Drug Interactions

The most dangerous adverse effect of V_2 receptor antagonists is due to their pharmacological action to increase free water excretion. This may correct hyponatremia too rapidly, resulting in serious and even fatal consequences (osmotic demyelination syndrome). Indeed, tolvaptan is labeled with a black-box warning against too rapid correction of hyponatremia and with the recommendation to initiate therapy in a hospital setting capable of close monitoring of serum Na^+. V_2 receptor antagonists should not be used with hypertonic saline. Antagonism of V_2 receptors can also cause polyuria, which likely explains the increased incidence of dehydration, hypotension, dizziness, pyrexia, increased thirst, and xerostomia with this class of drugs. Both tolvaptan and conivaptan can cause adverse GI adverse effects. Tolvaptan can cause liver damage; therefore, administration of tolvaptan generally should be limited to 30 days, and tolvaptan should not be used in patients with liver disease. Both tolvaptan and conivaptan can induce headaches, hypokalemia, and hyperglycemia, and both are contraindicated in anuria (no benefit) and in patients receiving drugs that inhibit CYP3A4 (e.g., clarithromycin, ketoconazole).

Acknowledgment: Robert F. Reilly contributed to this chapter in the prior edition of this book. We have retained some of his text in the current edition.

Drug Facts for Your Personal Formulary: *Diuretics and Agents Regulating Renal Excretion*

Drug	Major Therapeutic Uses	Clinical Pharmacology and Tips
Carbonic Anhydrase Inhibitors		
Acetazolamide Dichlorphenamide	• Glaucoma • Epilepsy • Altitude sickness • Diuretic resistance • Metabolic alkalosis • Familial periodic paralysis	• Ineffective as diuretic monotherapy because effects on renal excretion are self-limiting • Dichlorphenamide drug of choice for familial periodic paralysis
Osmotic Diuretics		
Mannitol	• Elevated intraocular pressure • Elevated intracranial pressure • Dialysis disequilibrium syndrome • Diagnosis of bronchial hyperreactivity • Urologic irrigation • Management of some overdoses	• Frequently used to treat or prevent acute kidney injuries, efficacy unclear • Expansion of extracellular fluid volume may cause pulmonary edema

Inhibitors of Na⁺-K⁺-2Cl⁻ Symport (Loop Diuretics; High-Ceiling Diuretics)

Bumetanide Ethacrynic acid Furosemide Torsemide	• Acute pulmonary edema • Edema associated with congestive heart failure, liver cirrhosis, chronic kidney disease, and nephrotic syndrome • Hyponatremia • Hypercalcemia • Hypertension	• Higher doses needed with impaired renal function • Torsemide may be superior to furosemide in heart failure • Increased risk of ototoxicity with ethacrynic acid compared to other loop diuretics • Risk for hypokalemia and arrhythmia when combined with QT-prolonging drugs

Inhibitors of Na⁺-Cl⁻ Symport (Thiazide Diuretics)

Thiazide type Chlorothiazide Hydrochlorothiazide Methyclothiazide **Thiazide-like** Chlorthalidone Indapamide Metolazone	• Hypertension • Edema associated with congestive heart failure, liver cirrhosis, chronic kidney disease, and nephrotic syndrome • Nephrogenic diabetes insipidus • Kidney stones caused by Ca²⁺ crystals	• Among first choice for treating hypertension • Thiazide-like have longer half-lives than thiazide-type and thus may be superior for hypertension • Higher doses needed for treating edema in patients with impaired renal function • Frequently combined with a loop diuretic to effect "sequential blockade" of tubular transport • Risk for hypokalemia and arrhythmia when combined with QT-prolonging drugs • Cause metabolic disturbances (e.g., elevate plasma glucose and LDL) • May cause severe hyponatremia in some patients

Inhibitors of Renal Epithelial Na⁺ Channels (K⁺-Sparing Diuretics)

Amiloride Triamterene	• Hypertension • Edema associated with congestive heart failure, liver cirrhosis, and chronic kidney disease • Liddle syndrome • Lithium-induced nephrogenic diabetes insipidus	• Low efficacy as monotherapy for edema • Frequently combined with loop or thiazide diuretics to prevent hypokalemia and increase diuresis • Risk of hyperkalemia in renal insufficiency or when combined with angiotensin-converting enzyme inhibitors or angiotensin-receptor antagonists

Mineralocorticoid Receptor Antagonists (Aldosterone Antagonists; K⁺-Sparing Diuretics)

Eplerenone Spironolactone	• Hypertension • Edema associated with congestive heart failure, liver cirrhosis, chronic kidney disease • Primary hyperaldosteronism • Acute myocardial infarction (eplerenone) • Heart failure (in combination with standard therapy) • Polycystic ovary disease	• Endogenous aldosterone levels determine therapeutic efficacy • Sometimes combined with loop or thiazide diuretics to prevent hypokalemia and increase diuresis • Diuretics of choice for treating resistant hypertension due to primary hyperaldosteronism and for refractory edema due to secondary aldosteronism (e.g., heart failure, hepatic cirrhosis). • High risk for hyperkalemia in chronic renal insufficiency • Eplerenone contraindicated with potent inhibitors of CYP3A4 (e.g., ketoconazole, itraconazole) • Spironolactone active metabolite has long half-life requiring slow dose adjustments (over days)

Inhibitors of the Nonspecific Cation Channel (Naturietic Peptide Analogues)

Nesiritide	• Hospitalized patients with acutely decompensated congestive heart failure (New York Heart Association class IV)	• Intravenous only • Clinical benefit remains questionable • High risk of serious hypotension

Vasopressin Receptor Agonist

V₁ receptor-agonist Vasopressin	• Postoperative abdominal distention • Abdominal roentgenography • Bleeding • Cardiac arrest • Hypovolemic shock	• Contraindicated in nephrogenic diabetes insipidus • Not for long-term therapy of central diabetes insipidus • Use with extreme caution in patients with vascular disease
V₂ receptor-agonist Desmopressin (DDAVP)	• Central diabetes insipidus • Primary nocturnal enuresis • Prevention of blood loss in patients with specific bleeding disorders	• Contraindicated in nephrogenic diabetes insipidus • Drug of choice for central diabetes insipidus • Can be administered orally at high doses • Major adverse effect is water intoxication

Vasopressin Receptor Antagonists

Conivaptan Tolvaptan	• Treatment of hypervolemic and euvolemic hyponatremia	• Risk of too rapid correction with serious consequences (osmotic demyelination syndrome) • Close monitoring of serum Na⁺ required

ACEI, angiotensin converting enzyme inhibitor; ARB, angiotensin receptor antagonist; DDAVP, Desmopressin; LDL, low density lipoprotein.

Bibliography

Barzilay JI, et al. Long-term effects of incident diabetes mellitus on cardiovascular outcomes in people treated for hypertension: the ALLHAT Diabetes Extension Study. *Circ Cardiovasc Qual Outcomes*, **2012**, *5*:153–162.

Bauersachs J, et al. Mineralocorticoid receptor activation and mineralocorticoid receptor antagonist treatment in cardiac and renal diseases. *Hypertension*, **2015**, *65*:257–263.

Benarroch EE. Oxytocin and vasopressin: social neuropeptides with complex neuromodulatory functions. *Neurology*, **2013**, *80*:1521–1528.

Berl T. Vasopressin antagonists. *N Engl J Med*, **2015**, *372*:2207–2216.

Bernstein PL, Ellison DH. Diuretics and salt transport along the nephron. *Semin Nephrol*, **2011**, *31*:475–482.

Brater DC. Diuretic therapy. *N Engl J Med*, **1998**, *339*:387–395.

Brown J, et al. Spironolactone versus placebo or in combination with steroids for hirsutism and/or acne. *Cochrane Database Syst Rev*, **2009**, (2):CD000194.

Bruderer S, et al. Use of diuretics and risk of incident gout: a population-based case-control study. *Arthritis Rheumatol*, **2014**, *66*:185–196.

Buggey J, et al. A reappraisal of loop diuretic choice in heart failure patients. *Am Heart J*, **2015**, *169*:323–333.

D'Elia E, Krum H. Mineralcorticoid antagonists in heart failure. *Heart Fail Clin*, **2014**, *10*:559–564.

Edelmann F, et al. Effect of spironolactone on diastolic function and exercise capacity in patients with heart failure with preserved ejection fraction: the Aldo-DHF randomized controlled trial. *JAMA*, **2013**, *309*:781–791.

Faris R, et al. Current evidence supporting the role of diuretics in heart failure: a meta analysis of randomised controlled trials. *Int J Cardiol*, **2002**, *82*:149–158.

Garcia ML, Kaczorowski GJ. Targeting the inward-rectifier potassium channel ROMK in cardiovascular disease. *Curr Opin Pharmacol*, **2014**, *15*:1–6.

Grimm RH Jr, et al. Long-term effects on sexual function of five antihypertensive drugs and nutritional hygienic treatment in hypertensive men and women. Treatment of Mild Hypertension Study (TOMHS). *Hypertension*, **1997**, *29*:8–14.

Iovino M, et al. Molecular mechanisms involved in the control of neurohypophyseal hormones secretion. *Curr Pharm Des*, **2014**, *20*:6702–6713.

Kellenberger S, Schild L. International Union of Basic and Clinical Pharmacology. XCI. Structure, function, and pharmacology of acid-sensing ion channels and the epithelial Na⁺ channel. *Pharmacol Rev*, **2015**, *67*:1–35.

Kishore BK, Ecelbarger CM. Lithium: a versatile tool for understanding renal physiology. *Am J Physiol Renal Physiol*, **2013**, *304*:F1139–F1149.

Kortenoeven MLA, et al. Amiloride blocks lithium entry through the sodium channel thereby attenuating the resultant nephrogenic diabetes insipidus. *Kidney Int*, **2009**, *76*:44–53.

Kortenoeven MLA, et al. Demeclocycline attenuates hyponatremia by reducing aquaporin-2 expression in the renal inner medulla. *Am J Physiol Renal Physiol*, **2013**, *305*:F1705–F1718.

Layek A, et al. Efficacy of vasopressin during cardio-pulmonary resuscitation in adult patients: a meta-analysis. *Resuscitation*, **2014**, *85*:855–863.

Nejsum LN. The renal plumbing system: aquaporin water channels. *Cell Mol Life Sci*, **2005**, *62*:1692–1706.

Nigwekar SU, Waikar SS. Diuretics in acute kidney injury. *Semin Nephrol*, **2011**, *31*:523–534.

Nirdé P, et al. Antimineralocorticoid 11β-substituted spirolactones exhibit androgen receptor agonistic activity: a structure function study. *Mol Pharmacol*, **2001**, *59*:1307–1313.

O'Connor CM, et al. Effect of nesiritide in patients with acute decompensated heart failure. *N Engl J Med*, **2011**, *365*:32–43.

Olde Engberink RHG, et al. Effects of thiazide-type and thiazide-like diuretics on cardiovascular events and mortality: systematic review and meta-analysis. *Hypertension*, **2015**, *65*:1033–1040.

Palmer BF. Metabolic complications associated with use of diuretics. *Semin Nephrol*, **2011**, *31*:542–552.

Pitt B, et al. Spironolactone for heart failure with preserved ejection fraction. *N Engl J Med*, **2014**, *370*:1383–1392.

Potter LR. Natriuretic peptide metabolism, clearance and degradation. *FEBS J*, **2011**, *278*:1808–1817.

Ritchie ND, et al. Acetazolamide for the prevention of acute mountain sickness—a systematic review and meta-analysis. *J Travel Med*, **2012**, *19*:298–307.

Rodenburg EM, et al. Thiazide-associated hyponatremia: a population-based study. *Am J Kidney Dis*, **2013**, *62*:67–72.

Ronchetti S, et al. GILZ as a mediator of the anti-inflammatory effects of glucocorticoids. Front Endocrinol (Lausanne) 2015, 6: article 170. doi: 10.3389/fendo.2015.00170, Accessed April 10, 2017.

Ronzaud C, Staub O. Ubiquitylation and control of renal Na+ balance and blood pressure. *Physiology*, **2014**, *29*:16–26.

Roush GC, et al. Diuretics: a review and update. *J Cardiovasc Pharmacol Ther*, **2014**, *19*:5–13.

Roush GC, et al. Head-to-head comparisons of hydrochlorothiazide with indapamide and chlorthalidone: antihypertensive and metabolic effects. *Hypertension*, **2015**, *65*:1041–1046.

Scozzafava A, Supuran CT. Glaucoma and the applications of carbonic anhydrase inhibitors. *Subcell Biochem*, **2014**, *75*:349–359.

Serpa Neto A, et al. Vasopressin and terlipressin in adult vasodilatory shock: a systematic review and meta-analysis of nine randomized controlled trials. *Crit Care*, **2012**, *16*:R154.

Sundar S, Dickinson PD. Spironolactone, a possible selective androgen receptor modulator, should be used with caution in patients with metastatic carcinoma of the prostate. *BMJ Case Rep*, **2012**, *25*:2012.

Tamargo J, et al. Diuretics in the treatment of hypertension. Part 1: thiazide and thiazide-like diuretics. *Expert Opin Pharmacother*, **2014**, *15*:527–547.

Wakai A, et al. Mannitol for acute traumatic brain injury. *Cochrane Database Syst Rev*, **2013**, (8):CD001049.

Welling PA. Regulation of renal potassium secretion: molecular mechanisms. *Semin Nephrol*, **2013**, *33*:215–228.

Wile D. Diuretics: a review. *Ann Clin Biochem*, **2012**, *49*:419–431.

Chapter 26

Renin and Angiotensin

Randa Hilal-Dandan

The Renin-Angiotensin System

The RAS participates in the pathophysiology of hypertension, congestive heart failure, myocardial infarction, and diabetic nephropathy. This realization has led to a thorough exploration of the RAS and the development of new approaches for inhibiting its actions. This chapter discusses the physiology, biochemistry, and cellular and molecular biology of the classical RAS and novel RAS components and pathways. The chapter also discusses the basic pharmacology of drugs that interrupt the RAS, and the clinical utility of inhibitors of the RAS. Therapeutic applications of drugs covered in this chapter are also discussed in Chapters 27–29.

History

In 1898, Tiegerstedt and Bergman found that crude saline extracts of the kidney contained a pressor substance that they named *renin*. In 1934, Goldblatt and his colleagues demonstrated that constriction of the renal arteries produced persistent hypertension in dogs. In 1940, Braun-Menéndez and his colleagues in Argentina and Page and Helmer in the U.S. reported that renin was an enzyme that acted on a plasma protein substrate to catalyze the formation of the actual pressor material, a peptide, that was named *hypertensin* by the former group and *angiotonin* by the latter. Ultimately, the pressor substance was renamed *angiotensin,* and the plasma substrate was called *angiotensinogen.*

In the mid-1950s, two forms of angiotensin were recognized, a decapeptide (AngI) and an octapeptide (AngII) formed by proteolytic cleavage of AngI by an enzyme termed *ACE*. The octapeptide was the more active form, and its synthesis in 1957 by Schwyzer and by Bumpus made the material available for intensive study. Later research showed that the kidneys are an important site of aldosterone action, and that angiotensin potently stimulates the production of aldosterone in humans. Moreover, renin secretion increased with depletion of Na$^+$. Thus, the RAS became recognized as a mechanism to stimulate aldosterone synthesis and secretion and an important homeostatic mechanism in the regulation of blood pressure and electrolyte composition.

In the early 1970s, polypeptides were discovered that either inhibited the formation of AngII or blocked AngII receptors. These inhibitors revealed important physiological and pathophysiological roles for the RAS and inspired the development of a new and broadly efficacious class of antihypertensive drugs: the orally active ACE inhibitors. Studies with ACE inhibitors uncovered roles for the RAS in the pathophysiology of hypertension, heart failure, vascular disease, and renal failure. Selective and competitive antagonists of AngII receptors were subsequently developed that yielded losartan, the first orally active, highly selective, and potent nonpeptide AngII receptor antagonist (Dell'Italia, 2011). Subsequently, many other AngII receptor antagonists have been developed; more recently, aliskiren, a direct renin inhibitor, was approved for antihypertensive therapy.

Classical RAS

Through the actions of AngII, the RAS participates in blood pressure regulation, aldosterone release, Na$^+$-reabsorption from renal tubules, electrolyte and fluid homeostasis, and cardiovascular remodeling. AngII is derived from angiotensinogen in two proteolytic steps. First, the enzyme renin, released into the circulation from the JG cells in the kidneys, cleaves the decapeptide AngI from the amino terminus of angiotensinogen (renin substrate). Then, an ACE, located on the endothelial cell lining of the vasculature, removes the carboxy-terminal dipeptide of AngI to produce the octapeptide AngII. These enzymatic steps are summarized in Figure 26–1. AngII acts by binding to two distinct heptaspanning GPCRs, AT$_1$ and AT$_2$.

New Paradigms in the RAS

The RAS has expanded from being solely an endocrine system to include a paracrine, autocrine/intracrine hormonal system with several new components and active pathways. The current understanding of the RAS involves local (tissue) RAS; alternative pathways for AngII synthesis (*ACE independent* and *renin independent*); an ACE2/Ang(1–7)/Mas receptor axis that opposes the vasoconstrictor effects of ACE/AngII/AT$_1$ receptor axis; an AngIV/AT$_4$ receptor axis that is important in brain functions and cognition; multiple biologically active angiotensin peptides such Ang(1–9), AngIII, Ang(3–7), angiotensin A, and alamandine; multiple receptors for angiotensin (AT$_1$, AT$_2$, AT$_4$; Mas; and MrgD); and

Abbreviations

ACE: angiotensin-converting enzyme
ACEI: angiotensin-converting enzyme inhibitor
Ac-SDKP: *N*-acetyl-seryl-aspartyl-lysyl-proline
ACTH: corticotropin (formerly adrenocorticotropic hormone)
Ang: angiotensin
ARB: angiotensin receptor blocker
ATR: angiotensin receptor
BP: blood pressure
cAMP: cyclic AMP
CNS: central nervous system
COX: cyclooxygenase
DRI: direct renin inhibitor
FDA: Food and Drug Administration
GFR: glomerular filtration rate
GI: gastrointestinal
GPCR: G protein–coupled receptor
HCTZ: hydrochlorothiazide
JG: juxtaglomerular
LDL: low-density lipoprotein
MrgD: Mas-related G protein–coupled receptor D
NE: norepinephrine
NO: nitric oxide
NOS: nitric oxide synthase
NSAID: nonsteroidal anti-inflammatory drug
PAI-1: plasminogen activator inhibitor type 1
PCP: prolylcarboxylpeptidase
PG: prostaglandin
PI$_3$K: phosphoinositide 3-kinase
PL: phospholipase
PRA: plasma renin activity
PRC: plasma renin concentration
(pro)renin: renin and prorenin
PRR: (pro)renin receptor
RAS: renin-angiotensin system
RBF: renal blood flow
ROS: reactive O_2 species
TGF: transforming growth factor
TPR: total peripheral resistance

the PRR. Differential activation of these multiple arms of the RAS may underlie the pathophysiological outcome in cardiovascular and renal disease (Campbell, 2014; Santos, 2014).

Components of the Renin-Angiotensin System

Renin

Renin is the major determinant of the rate of AngII production; its secretion is regulated by several mechanisms (Figures 26–1 through 26–3). Renin is synthesized, stored, and secreted by exocytosis into the renal arterial circulation by the granular JG cells located in the walls of the afferent arterioles that enter the glomeruli. Renin is an aspartyl protease that cleaves the bond between residues 10 and 11 at the amino terminus of angiotensinogen to generate AngI. The active form of renin is a glycoprotein that contains 340 amino acids. It is synthesized as a preproenzyme that is processed to prorenin.

Prorenin may be activated in two ways (Figure 26–2): *proteolytically,* by proconvertase 1 or cathepsin B enzymes that remove 43 amino acids (propeptide) from its amino terminus to uncover the active site of renin; and *nonproteolytically,* when prorenin binds to the PRR, resulting in

conformational changes that unfold the propeptide and expose the active catalytic site of the enzyme (Nguyen and Danser, 2008). Both renin and prorenin are stored in the JG cells and, when released, circulate in the blood. The concentration of prorenin in the circulation is about 10-fold greater than that of the active enzyme. The $t_{1/2}$ of circulating renin is about 15 min.

Control of Renin Secretion

Renin is secreted by the granular cells within the JG apparatus and is regulated by the following pathways (Figure 26–3):

1. The macula densa pathway
2. The intrarenal baroreceptor pathway
3. The β_1 adrenergic receptor pathway

The Macula Densa Pathway

The macula densa pathway provides an important function for salt and water regulation by the RAS. The macula densa lies adjacent to the JG cells and is composed of specialized columnar epithelial cells in the wall of that portion of the cortical thick ascending limb that passes between the afferent and efferent arterioles of the glomerulus. A change in NaCl reabsorption by the macula densa results in the transmission to nearby JG cells of chemical signals that modify renin release. Increases in NaCl flux across the macula densa inhibit renin release, whereas decreases in NaCl flux stimulate renin release.

Adenosine, ATP, and PGs modulate the macula densa pathway (Figure 26–4). ATP and adenosine *inhibit renin release* when NaCl transport *increases.* ATP acts via P2Y receptors to enhance Ca^{2+} release, and adenosine acts via the A_1 adenosine receptor to inhibit adenylyl cyclase activity and cyclic AMP production. PGE$_2$ and PGI$_2$ *stimulate renin release* when NaCl transport *decreases* through enhancing cyclic AMP formation. PG production is enhanced by inducible cyclooxygenase 2 (COX-2) and nNOS. The expression of COX-2 and nNOS is upregulated by chronic dietary Na^+ restriction; selective inhibition of either COX-2 or nNOS inhibits renin release (Peti-Peterdi et al., 2010).

Regulation of the macula densa pathway is more dependent on the luminal concentration of Cl^- than Na^+. NaCl transport into the macula densa is mediated by the Na^+-K^+-2Cl^- symporter (Figure 26–4), and the half-maximal concentrations of Na^+ and Cl^- required for transport via this symporter are 2–3 and 40 mEq/L, respectively. Because the luminal concentration of Na^+ at the macula densa usually is much greater than the level required for half-maximal transport, physiological variations in luminal Na^+ concentrations at the macula densa have little effect on renin release (i.e., the symporter remains saturated with respect to Na^+). Conversely, physiological changes in Cl^- concentrations (20–60 mEq/L) at the macula densa profoundly affect macula densa–mediated renin release.

The Intrarenal Baroreceptor Pathway

Increases and decreases in blood pressure or renal perfusion pressure in the preglomerular vessels inhibit and stimulate renin release, respectively. The immediate stimulus to secretion is believed to be reduced tension within the wall of the afferent arteriole. The release of renal PGs and biomechanical coupling via stretch-activated ion channels may mediate in part the intrarenal baroreceptor pathway.

The β_1 Adrenergic Receptor Pathway

The β_1 adrenergic receptor pathway is regulated by the release of NE from postganglionic sympathetic nerves; activation of β_1 receptors on JG cells increases cyclic AMP and enhances renin secretion. Treatment with β blockers reduces renin secretion and PRA.

Feedback Regulation

Renin release is subject to feedback regulation (Figure 26–3). Increased renin secretion enhances the formation of AngII, which stimulates AT_1 receptors on JG cells to inhibit renin release, an effect termed *short-loop negative feedback.* Inhibition of renin release due to AngII-dependent increase in blood pressure is termed *long-loop negative feedback.* AngII increases arterial blood pressure via AT_1 receptors; this effect inhibits renin release by the following:

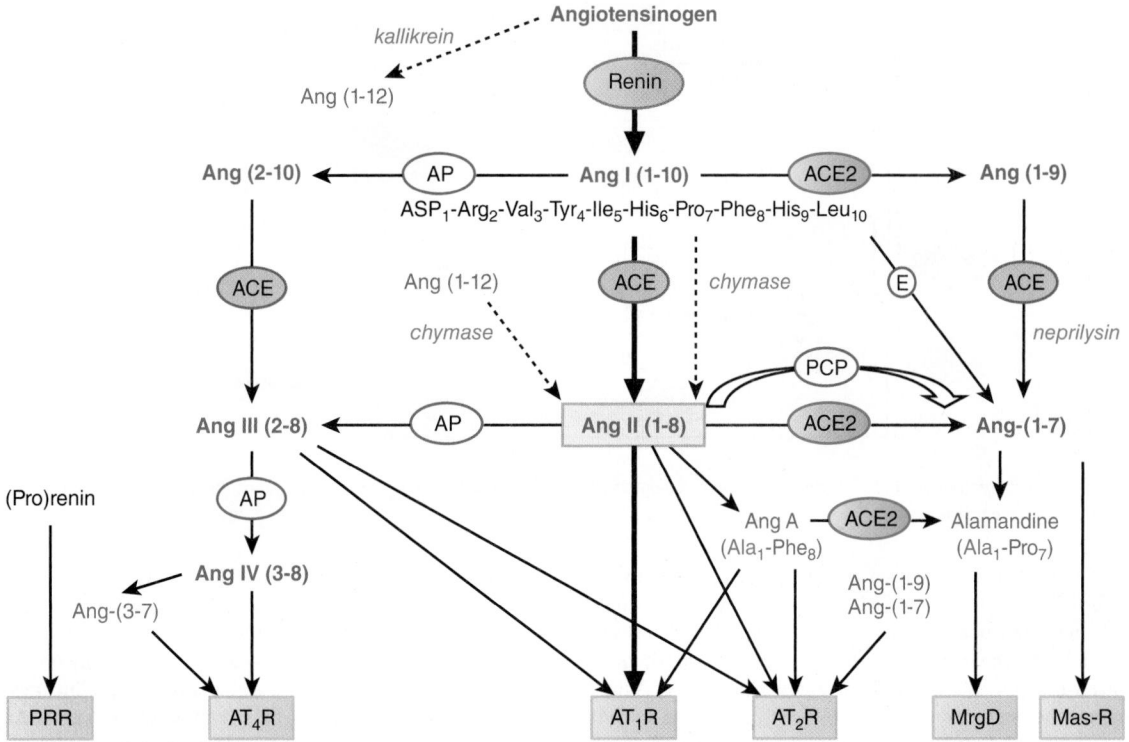

Figure 26–1 *Components of the RAS.* The heavy arrows show the classical pathway, and the light arrows indicate alternative pathways. Receptors involved: AT$_1$, AT$_2$, AT$_4$, Mas, MrgD, and PRR. AP, aminopeptidase; E, endopeptidases; PCP, prolylcarboxylpeptidase.

1. Activating high-pressure baroreceptors, thereby reducing renal sympathetic tone
2. Increasing pressure in the preglomerular vessels
3. Reducing NaCl reabsorption in the proximal tubule (pressure natriuresis), which increases tubular delivery of NaCl to the macula densa

Drugs That Affect Renin Secretion

Renin release is influenced by arterial blood pressure, dietary salt intake, and pharmacological agents (Figures 26–3 and 26–4). Loop diuretics stimulate renin release and increase PRC by decreasing arterial blood pressure and by blocking the reabsorption of NaCl at the macula densa. *NSAIDs* inhibit PG synthesis and thereby decrease renin release. ACE inhibitors, ARBs, and renin inhibitors interrupt both the short- and long-loop negative-feedback mechanisms and therefore increase renin release and PRC. Centrally acting sympatholytic drugs, as well as β_1 adrenergic

receptor antagonists, decrease renin secretion by reducing activation of β_1 adrenergic receptors on JG cells.

Angiotensinogen

The substrate for renin is angiotensinogen, an abundant globular glycoprotein. AngI is cleaved by renin from the amino terminus of angiotensinogen. Human angiotensinogen contains 452 amino acids and is synthesized as preangiotensinogen, which has a 24– or 33–amino acid signal peptide. Angiotensinogen is synthesized and secreted primarily by the liver, although angiotensinogen transcripts occur in many tissues, including the heart, kidneys, pancreas, adipocytes, and certain regions of the CNS. Biosynthesis of angiotensinogen is stimulated by inflammation, insulin, estrogens, glucocorticoids, thyroid hormone, and AngII. During pregnancy, plasma levels of angiotensinogen increase several-fold owing to increased estrogen.

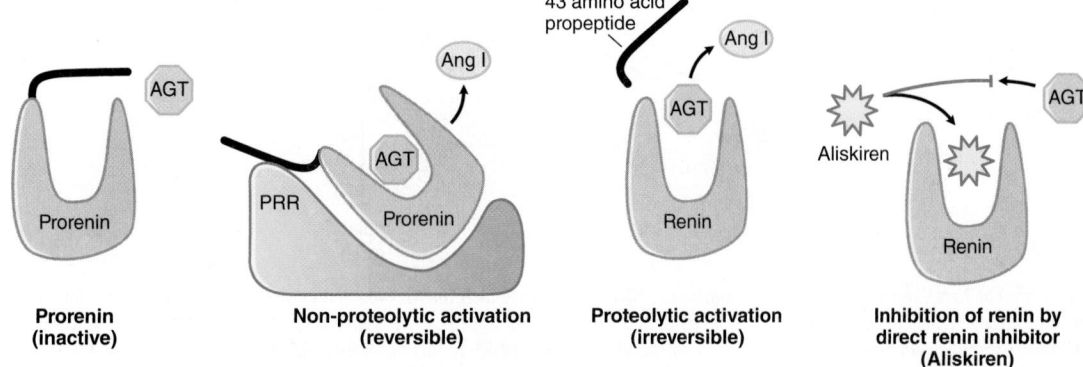

Figure 26–2 *Biological activation of prorenin and pharmacological inhibition of renin.* Prorenin is inactive; accessibility of AGT (angiotensinogen) to the catalytic site is blocked by the propeptide (black segment). The blocked catalytic site can be activated nonproteolytically by the binding of prorenin to the PRR or by proteolytic removal of the propeptide. The competitive renin inhibitor aliskiren has a higher affinity (~0.1 μm) for the active site of renin than does AGT (~1 μm).

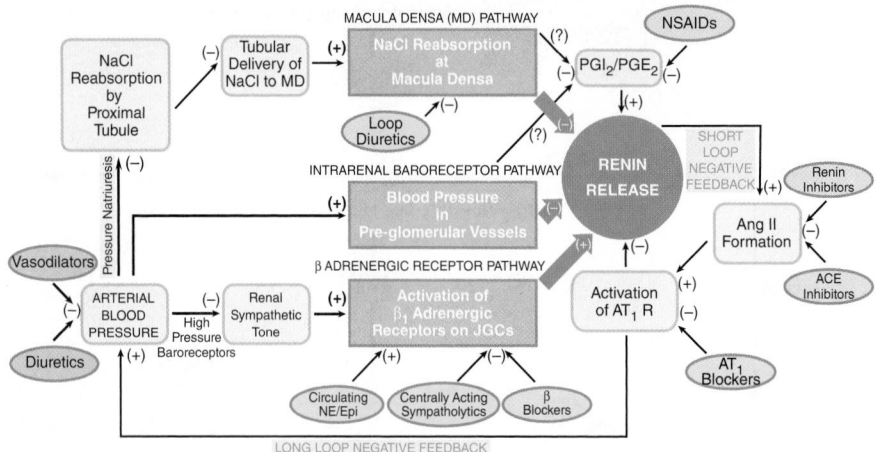

Figure 26–3 *Physiological pathways, feedback loops, and pharmacological regulation of the RAS.* Schematic portrayal of the three major physiological pathways regulating renin release. See text for details.

Circulating levels of angiotensinogen are approximately equal to the K_m of renin for its substrate (~1 μM). Consequently, the rate of AngII synthesis, and therefore blood pressure, can be influenced by changes in angiotensinogen levels. Oral contraceptives containing estrogen increase circulating levels of angiotensinogen and can induce hypertension. A missense mutation in the angiotensinogen gene (M235T in angiotensinogen) that increases plasma levels of angiotensinogen is associated with essential and pregnancy-induced hypertension (Sethi et al., 2003). Urinary angiotensinogen levels are considered an index for local intrarenal RAS activation and are elevated in patients with hypertension and progressive renal disease (Kobori and Urushihara, 2013).

Angiotensin-Converting Enzyme

Angiotensin-converting enzyme (ACE, kininase II, dipeptidyl carboxypeptidase) is an ectoenzyme and glycoprotein with an apparent molecular weight of 170 kDa. Human ACE contains 1277 amino acid residues and has two homologous domains, each with a catalytic site and a Zn^{2+}-binding region. ACE has a large amino-terminal extracellular domain, a short

carboxyl-terminal intracellular domain, and a 22–amino acid transmembrane hydrophobic region that anchors the ectoenzyme. ACE is rather nonspecific and cleaves dipeptide units from substrates with diverse amino acid sequences. Preferred substrates have only one free carboxyl group in the carboxyl-terminal amino acid, and proline must not be the penultimate amino acid; thus, the enzyme does not degrade AngII. ACE is identical to kininase II, the enzyme that inactivates bradykinin and other potent vasodilator peptides. Although slow conversion of AngI to AngII occurs in plasma, the very rapid metabolism that occurs in vivo is due largely to the activity of membrane-bound ACE present on the luminal surface of endothelial cells throughout the vascular system (Guang et al., 2012).

The *ACE* gene contains an insertion/deletion polymorphism in intron 16 that explains the large phenotypic variance in serum ACE levels. The deletion allele, associated with higher levels of serum ACE and increased metabolism of bradykinin, may confer an increased risk of hypertension, cardiac hypertrophy, atherosclerosis, and diabetic nephropathy (Sayed-Tabatabaei et al., 2006; Hadjadj et al., 2001).

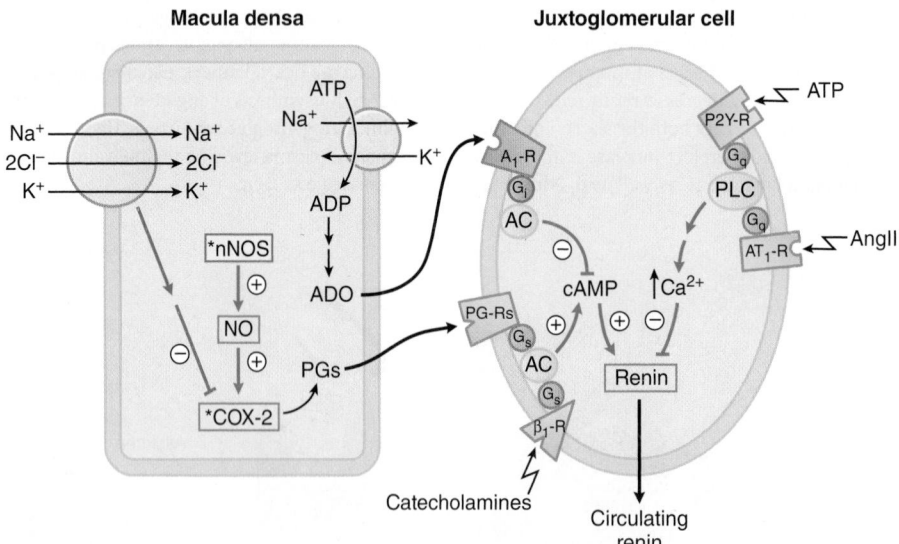

Figure 26–4 *Regulation of JG cell renin release by the macula densa.* Mechanisms by which the MD regulates renin release. Changes in tubular delivery of NaCl to the MD cause appropriate signals to be conveyed to the JG cells. Sodium depletion upregulates nNOS and COX-2 in the MD to enhance production of PGs. PGs and catecholamines stimulate adenylyl cyclase (AC) and cAMP production and thence renin release from the JG cells. Increased NaCl transport depletes ATP and increases adenosine (ADO) levels. Adenosine diffuses to the JG cells and inhibits cAMP production and renin release via G_i-coupled A_1 receptors. Increased NaCl transport in the MD augments the efflux of ATP, which may inhibit renin release directly by binding to P2Y receptors and activating the G_q-PLC-IP_3-Ca^{2+} pathway in JG cells. Circulating AngII also inhibits renin release on JG cells via G_q-coupled AT_1 receptors.
*Expression upregulated by chronic Na^+ depletion.

Angiotensin-Converting Enzyme 2

A carboxypeptidase, ACE2, cleaves one amino acid from the carboxyl terminal to convert AngII to Ang(1–7). ACE2 may also convert AngI to Ang(1–9), which is then converted to Ang(1–7) by ACE, neprilysin, and endopeptidases (Santos, 2014). ACE2 contains a single catalytic domain that is 42% identical to the two catalytic domains of ACE. AngII is the preferred substrate for ACE2, with 400-fold higher affinity than AngI (Guang et al., 2012).

The counterregulation of the actions of AngII by ACE2 occur in at least two ways:

1. It decreases AngII levels and limits its effects by metabolizing it to Ang(1–7).
2. It increases levels of Ang(1–7), which acts on Mas receptors to oppose AngII actions (Figure 26–5).

Angiotensin-converting enzyme 2 is not inhibited by the standard ACE inhibitors and has no effect on bradykinin. Reduced expression or deletion of ACE2 is associated with hypertension, defects in cardiac contractility, and elevated levels of AngII. Inhibition of AT$_1$ receptors by ARBs increases the expression of ACE2. Overexpression of the ACE2 gene decreases blood pressure and prevents AngII-induced cardiac hypertrophy in hypertensive rats. ACE2 is protective against diabetic nephropathy through the Ang(1–7)/Mas receptor pathway (Varagic et al., 2014). Ang(1–9), which is generated from AngI by ACE2, may also have vasodilating and protective effects by activating AT$_2$ receptors (Etelvino et al., 2014). In addition, ACE2 metabolizes Apelin peptides, serves as a receptor for the severe acute respiratory syndrome coronavirus (SARS), and has been reported to interact with and regulate amino acid transporters (Kuba et al., 2013).

Alternative Pathways for Angiotensin II Biosynthesis

Angiotensin II may be generated through ACE-independent pathways or "ACE escape." Angiotensinogen is converted to AngI, or directly to AngII

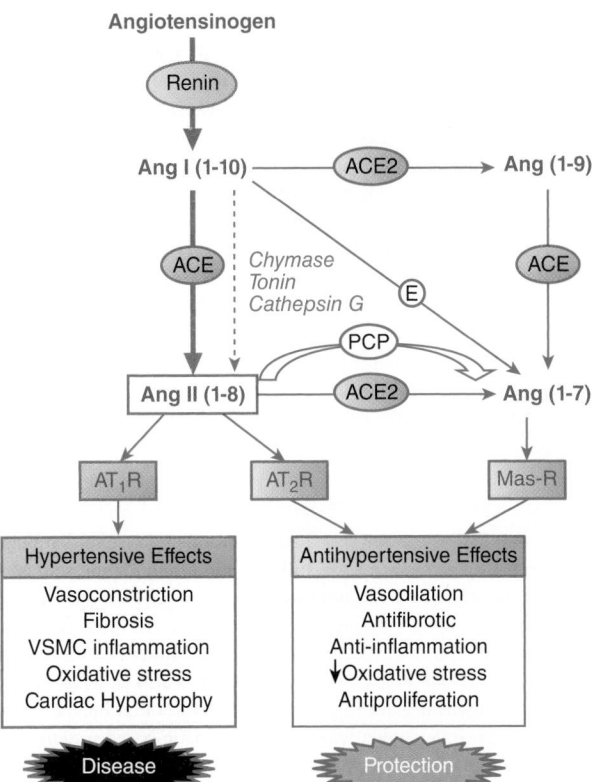

Figure 26–5 *Schematic diagram of opposing arms in the RAS.* Therapeutic interventions aim to inhibit the ACE/AngII/AT$_1$ receptor axis (red) and enhance ACE2/Ang(1–7)/Mas receptor axis (green). VSMC: vascular smooth muscle cells.

by cathepsin G and tonin. Enzymes that convert AngI to AngII include cathepsin G, chymostatin-sensitive AngII-generating enzyme, and chymase. Chymase contributes to tissue conversion of AngI and Ang(1–12) to AngII, particularly in the heart and kidneys. The major source of chymase is mast cells (Ferrario et al., 2014; Paul et al., 2006).

Angiotensinases

Angiotensinases include aminopeptidases, endopeptidases, carboxypeptidases, and other peptidases that metabolize angiotensin peptides; none is specific.

Angiotensin Peptides and Their Receptors

Table 26–1 shows the RAS peptides, their receptors, and overall effects of the receptor-peptide interactions.

AngII-AT$_1$ Receptor Axis

Angiotensin II binds to specific GPCRs, designated AT$_1$ and AT$_2$. The hypertensive, renal, and hypertrophic effects of AngII are mediated by activation of the AT$_1$ receptor (Dell'Italia, 2011). The AT$_1$ receptor gene contains a polymorphism (A1166C) associated with hypertension, hypertrophic cardiomyopathy, and coronary artery vasoconstriction. Moreover, the C allele synergizes with the ACE deletion allele with regard to increased risk of coronary artery disease (Álvarez et al., 1998). Preeclampsia is associated with the development of agonistic autoantibodies against the AT$_1$ receptor in some cases (Xia et al., 2013).

AngII-AT$_1$ Receptor-Effector Coupling. The AT$_1$ receptors link to a large array of signal transduction systems to produce effects that vary with cell type and that are a combination of primary and secondary responses. AT$_1$ receptors couple to several heterotrimeric G proteins, including G$_q$, G$_{12/13}$, and G$_i$, and the GPCR characteristics of being substrates for phosphorylation and desensitization by G protein-coupled receptor kinases (GRKs), interacting with β-arrestin, and being subsequently internalized.

In most cell types, AT$_1$ receptors couple to G$_q$ to activate the PLCβ-IP$_3$-Ca^{2+} pathway. Secondary to G$_q$ activation, activation of PKC, PLA$_2$, and PLD and eicosanoid production, Ca^{2+}-dependent and MAP kinases, Ca^{2+}-calmodulin–dependent activation of NOS may occur. Activation of G$_i$ may occur and will reduce the activity of adenylyl cyclase, lowering cellular cyclic AMP content; however, there also is evidence for G$_q$ → G$_s$ cross talk such that activation of the AT$_1$-G$_q$-PLC pathway enhances cyclic AMP production. The βγ subunits of G$_i$ and activation of G$_{12/13}$ lead to activation of tyrosine kinases and small G proteins such as Rho. Ultimately, the Jak/STAT pathway may be activated and a variety of transcriptional regulatory

TABLE 26–1 ■ RAS PEPTIDES AND THEIR IDENTIFIED RECEPTORS

RECEPTOR	RAS PEPTIDE	EFFECT
AT$_1$	AngII, AngIII, AngA, Ang(1–12)	Vasoconstriction hypertrophy Fibrosis, nephropathy
AT$_2$	AngII, AngIII, Ang(1–7), Ang(1–9), AngA	Vasodilation, antihypertrophy, antifibrosis Natriuresis
Mas	Ang(1–7)	Vasodilation, antihypertrophy, antifibrosis Natriuresis
MrgD	Alamandine	Vasodilation, antihypertrophy, antifibrosis
AT$_4$	AngIV, Ang(3–7)	Neuroprotection Cognition Renal vasodilation Natriuresis
PRR	Prorenin, renin	Hypertrophy, fibrosis Apoptosis

factors induced. By these mechanisms, angiotensin influences the expression of a host of gene products relating to cell growth and the production of components of the extracellular matrix. Through AT_1 receptors, AngII also stimulates the activity of a membrane-bound NADH/NADPH oxidase that generates ROS. ROS may contribute to some of the biochemical effects (activation of MAP kinase, tyrosine kinase, and phosphatases; inactivation of NO; and expression of monocyte chemoattractant protein-1) and physiological effects (acute effects on renal function, chronic effects on blood pressure, and vascular hypertrophy and inflammation) of AngII (Mehta and Griendling, 2007). The relative importance of these myriad signal transduction pathways in mediating biological responses to AngII is tissue specific. The AT_1 receptor is structurally flexible and may be activated, independently of AngII binding, by conformational changes such as mechanical stress (Kim et al., 2012). Functions of the AT_1 receptor may be modified by dimerization with AT_2 receptor, the bradykinin B_2 receptor, the β_2 adrenergic receptor, and the apelin receptor (Goupil et al., 2013).

AngII-AT₂ Receptor Axis

Activation of the AT_2 receptors counteracts many of the effects of the AT_1 receptors by having antiproliferative, anti-inflammatory, vasodilatory, natriuretic, and antihypertensive effects (Figure 26–5). The AT_2 receptors are distributed widely in fetal tissues, but their distribution is more restricted in adults. Expression of AT_2 receptors is upregulated in cardiovascular diseases, including heart failure, cardiac fibrosis, and ischemic heart disease (Jones et al., 2008). Signaling through the AT_2 receptor is mediated by G protein–dependent (G_{ia2} and G_{ia3}) and G protein–independent pathways. Consequences of AT_2 receptor activation include activation of phosphotyrosine phosphatases that inhibit MAP kinases and ERK 1/2; inhibition of Ca^{2+} channel functions; and enhancing NO, cyclic GMP, and bradykinin production. The AT_2 receptors can bind the AT_1 receptors to antagonize and reduce their expression; and the AT_2 receptors can form heterodimers with the bradykinin B_2 receptor to enhance NO production (Jones et al., 2008; Padia and Carey, 2013).

Angiotensin (1–7)/Mas Receptor Axis

The ACE2/Ang(1–7)/Mas receptor axis is a negative regulator of the pressor, profibrotic, and antinatriuretic effects of the ACE/AngII/AT_1 receptor axis of the RAS (Figure 26–5). Ang(1–7) is generated in several ways (Figure 26–1):

- from AngII by ACE2;
- from AngII by carboxypeptidases;
- from AngI by endopeptidases; and
- from AngI by a two-step conversion, by ACE2 to Ang(1–9) and then to Ang(1–7) by ACE or neprilysin.

The antihypertensive effects of Ang(1–7) are mediated through binding to the Mas receptors, although Ang(1–7) can bind and activate AT_2 receptors (Gironacci et al., 2014). Activation of the Mas receptor by Ang(1–7) induces vasodilation, stimulates PI_3K/Akt pathway that promotes NO production, potentiates the vasodilatory effects of bradykinin, and inhibits AngII-induced activation of ERK1/2 and NFκB; it has antiangiogenic, antiproliferative, and antithrombotic effects; and it is renoprotective and cardioprotective in cardiac ischemia and heart failure (Fraga-Silva et al., 2013; Varagic et al., 2014).

The *Mas* proto-oncogene encodes an orphan GPCR. Knockout of the *Mas* gene in mice causes increased vascular resistance and cardiac dysfunction (Santos, 2014; Varagic et al., 2014). The Mas receptor is present in the brain, and its activation is associated with improved memory and cognition (Gironacci et al., 2014).

The capacity of Ang(1–7) to counterbalance the actions of AngII may depend on the ratio of ACE-AngII-AT_1 receptor activity to ACE2-Ang(1–7)-Mas receptor activity (see Figure 26–5; Santos, 2014; Romero et al., 2015). Pharmacologically enhancing the ACE2-Ang(1–7)-Mas receptor pathway using ACE2 activators and specific Mas receptor agonists could provide new avenues for modulating RAS in cardiovascular and renal disease.

Angiotensin III

Angiotensin III, also called Ang(2–8), can be formed by the action of aminopeptidase A on AngII or by the action of ACE on Ang(2–10). AngIII binds to both AT_1 and AT_2 receptors, causing effects qualitatively similar to those of AngII. AngII and AngIII stimulate aldosterone secretion with equal potency; however, AngIII is less efficacious in elevating blood pressure (25%) and stimulating the adrenal medulla (10%). Data from model systems make clear that AngIII and the shorter angiotensin-derived peptides have significant activity, especially at the AT_2 receptor, and that there may be instances where AngIII is the active endogenous ligand (Bosnyak et al., 2011).

Angiotensin IV/AT₄ Receptor Axis

Angiotensin IV, also called Ang(3–8), is formed from AngIII through the catalytic action of aminopeptidase N. Central and peripheral actions of AngIV are mediated through a specific AT_4 receptor that was identified as IRAP (insulin-regulated aminopeptidase) (see Figure 26–1). This receptor is a single transmembrane protein (1025 amino acids) that colocalizes with the glucose transporter type 4. AT_4 receptors are detectable in a number of tissues, such as heart, vasculature, adrenal cortex, and brain regions processing sensory and motor functions. AngIV-dependent AT_4 receptor activation regulates cerebral blood flow, is neuroprotective, and facilitates long-term potentiation, memory consolidation, and cognition (Wright et al., 2013). AngIV binding to the AT_4 receptor inhibits the catalytic activity of IRAP and enables accumulation of various neuropeptides linked to memory potentiation. Other actions include renal vasodilation, natriuresis, neuronal differentiation, hypertrophy, inflammation, and extracellular matrix remodeling. Analogues of AngIV are being developed for their therapeutic potential in Alzheimer disease and head injury (Albiston et al., 2007; Wright et al., 2013).

New Physiologically Active Angiotensin Peptides

New biologically active angiotensin peptides and their receptors have been identified (Table 26–1). These peptides include Ang(1–9), AngA and alamandine, Ang(3–7), and proangiotensin/Ang(1–12) (Ferrario et al., 2014). Ang(1–9) is generated from AngI by the action of ACE2, carboxypeptidase A, and cathepsin. Ang(1–9) has cardioprotective and antipressor effects reportedly mediated through binding to AT_2 receptors and the release of NO (Etelvino et al., 2014). Alamandine is produced from Ang(1–7) by the decarboxylation of the Asp_1 residue into Ala_1 residue on the N-terminal. Alamandine acts through the *MrgD* to mediate vasodilatory and antifibrotic effects similar to Ang(1–7). Alamandine is an ACE substrate and may act as an ACE inhibitor. Alamandine is elevated in patients with chronic renal disease (Etelvino et al., 2014).

Angiotensin A is an octapeptide produced by decarboxylation of the Asp_1 residue of AngII into Ala_1. AngA binds to both AT_1 and AT_2 receptors and has effects similar to, but less potent than, AngII. AngA is reported to be elevated in patients with end-stage renal disease (Ferrario et al., 2014). Ang(3–7) is generated from AngIV and binds AT_4 receptors (Wright et al., 2013). Proangiotensin or Ang(1–12) is generated from angiotensinogen through a nonrenin pathway and can be converted to AngII through action of chymase. Ang(1–12) can bind to the AT_1 receptors and may be a precursor for autocrine/intracrine production of AngII (Ferrario et al., 2014).

Local (Tissue) Renin-Angiotensin System

Local (tissue) RAS is a tissue-based AngII-producing system that plays a role in hypertrophy, nephropathy, inflammation, remodeling, and apoptosis. ACE is present on the luminal face of vascular endothelial cells throughout the circulation; circulating (pro)renin can bind the PRR in the arterial wall and other tissues to mediate local generation of AngII (Campbell, 2014; Paul et al., 2016). Tissue RAS is also an autocrine and intracrine mechanism that can generate AngII and other bioactive angiotensin peptides independently of the renal/hepatic-based system. Many tissues—including the brain, pituitary, blood vessels, heart, kidney, and adrenal gland—produce renin, angiotensinogen, ACE and ACE2, chymase, PRR, and angiotensins I, II, III, IV, Ang(1–7) and the AT_1, AT_2, and Mas receptors (Campbell, 2014; Ferrario et al., 2014). Selective activation of the local RAS components is tissue specific and likely affects the pathophysiological outcomes in disease.

The (Pro) Renin Receptor

(Pro)renin/PRR binding enhances tissue-RAS activity and induces profibrotic intracellular signaling events that are independent of AngII production (Figure 26–6). The PRR is abundant in the heart, brain, eye, adrenals, placenta, adipose tissue, liver, and kidneys. The PRR gene is located in the locus p11.4 of the X chromosome and is named ATP6ap2 (ATPase-6 accessory protein 2). Knockout of the PRR gene is lethal, indicating an important role for PRR in development. In humans, mutations in the PRR gene are associated with mental retardation and epilepsy (Nguyen and Danser, 2008). Human PRR is a single transmembrane protein of 350 amino acids (~37 kDa). PRR is composed of N-terminal extracellular domain that binds (pro)renin, a transmembrane domain and a cytosolic domain that are associated with Vacuolar-H+-ATPase (V-ATPase) activity (Nguyen, 2011). Cleavage of the extracellular domain of PRR by furin or ADAM19 produces the N-terminal segment, soluble PRR, found in plasma and urine. Increased levels of urinary soluble PRR correlate with elevated urinary angiotensinogen levels, a biomarker of intrarenal RAS activity (Oshima et al., 2014).

(Pro)renin receptor binds (pro)renin with nanomolar affinity and high specificity to enhance the tissue-RAS. Binding of (pro)renin to PRR augments the catalytic activity of renin and induces nonproteolytic activation of prorenin by unfolding the 43 amino acid–prorenin prosegment and exposing the enzymatic cleft (Figure 26–2). Bound, activated (pro)renin catalyzes the conversion of angiotensinogen to AngI, with the consequent formation of AngII. The binding of (pro)renin to PRR also induces profibrotic signaling events that are *AngII independent* (Figure 26–6), including activation of ERK1/2, p38, tyrosine kinases, COX-2, TGF-β gene expression, and PAI-1 (Nguyen and Danser, 2008). These signaling pathways are not blocked by ACE inhibitors or AT_1 receptor antagonists and are reported to contribute to fibrosis, nephrosis, and end-organ damage (Kaneshiro et al., 2007). Overexpression of the human PRR in transgenic animals increases plasma aldosterone levels in the absence of changes in plasma renin levels and induces hypertension and nephropathy. Rats overexpressing PRR exhibit increased expression of COX-2 in the macula densa and develop proteinuria and glomerulosclerosis that increase with aging (Kaneshiro et al., 2007).

Circulating plasma concentrations of (pro)renin are elevated 100-fold in diabetic patients and are associated with increased risk of nephropathy, renal fibrosis, and retinopathy (Nguyen and Danser, 2008). The blockade of PRR by administration of a peptide antagonist, known as "handle region peptide" (HRP), was reported to be protective in animal models against diabetic nephropathy and retinopathy (Oshima et al, 2014); however, the efficacy and specificity of HRP was not strongly confirmed by other groups (reviewed by Binger and Muller, 2013; Nguyen, 2011). The pathophysiological significance of (pro)renin/PRR interaction outside the local tissue RAS is still unclear (Lu et al., 2016).

The PRR participates in many functions that are independent of (pro)renin binding. PRR functions as an accessory protein essential for V-ATPase activity, which is required for intracellular acidity, receptor-mediated endocytosis, and activation of lysosomal and autophagosomal enzymes (Oshima et al., 2014). Cardiomyocyte-specific PRR knockout mice and podocyte-specific PRR knockout mice develop lethal organ-specific failure due loss of V-ATPase and the dysregulation of intracellular acidification and autophagic functions (Binger and Muller, 2013). PRR also participates in the activation of Wnt/β-catenin and Wnt/planar cell polarity signaling pathways that are important in cell polarization in the plane of tissue (Nguyen, 2011). PRR reportedly can regulate LDL uptake and metabolism. In hepatocytes, silencing PRR expression decreased cellular LDL uptake by decreasing expression of LDL receptor and sortelin 1 protein, a regulator of LDL uptake and metabolism and a PRR-interacting protein (Lu et al., 2016). (Pro)renin also binds to mannose-6-phosphate receptor, an insulin-like growth factor II receptor that functions as a clearance receptor (Nguyen and Danser, 2008).

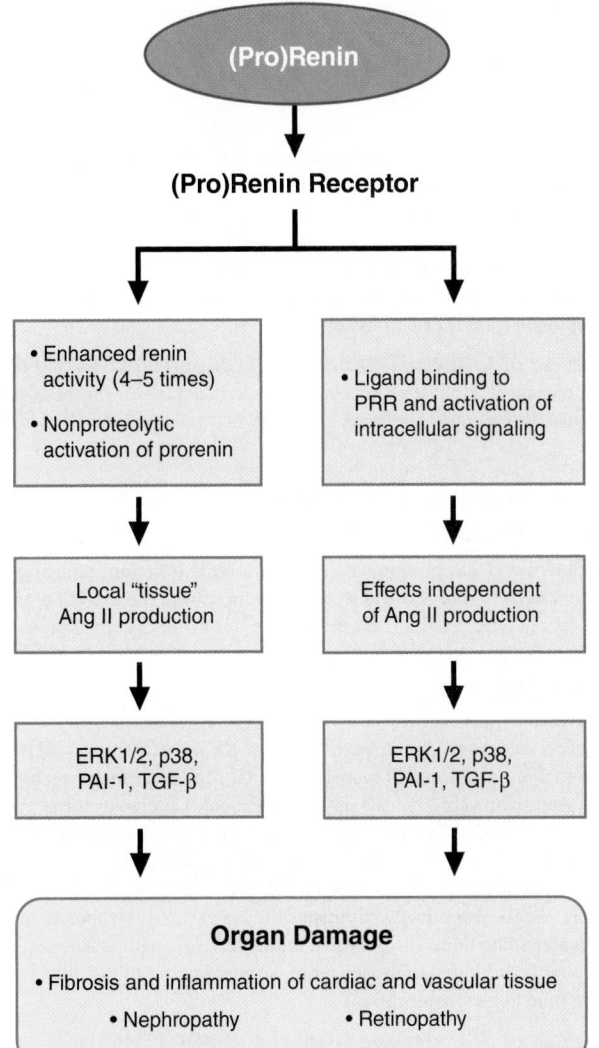

Figure 26–6 *(Pro)renin/PRR interaction activates AngII-dependent and AngII-independent signaling pathways.* See text for details.

Functions and Effects of Angiotensin II

Angiotensin II increases total peripheral resistance (TPR) and alters renal function and cardiovascular structure (Figure 26–7). Modest increases in plasma concentrations of AngII acutely raise blood pressure; on a molar basis, AngII is about 40 times more potent than NE; the EC_{50} of AngII for acutely raising arterial blood pressure is about 0.3 nM. When a single moderate dose of AngII is injected intravenously, systemic blood pressure begins to rise within seconds, peaks rapidly, and returns to normal within minutes (Figure 26–8). This *rapid pressor response* to AngII is due to a swift increase in TPR—a response that helps to maintain arterial blood pressure in the face of an acute hypotensive challenge (e.g., blood loss or vasodilation). Although AngII increases cardiac contractility directly (via opening voltage-gated Ca^{2+} channels in cardiac myocytes) and increases heart rate indirectly (via facilitation of sympathetic tone, enhancing adrenergic neurotransmission, and provoking adrenal catecholamine release), the rapid increase in arterial blood pressure activates a baroreceptor reflex that decreases sympathetic tone and increases vagal tone. Thus, depending on the physiological state, AngII may increase, decrease, or not change cardiac contractility, heart rate, and cardiac output. Changes in cardiac output therefore contribute little, if at all, to the rapid pressor response induced by AngII.

AngII also causes a *slow pressor response* that helps to stabilize arterial blood pressure over the long term. A continuous infusion of initially subpressor doses of AngII gradually increases arterial blood pressure, with

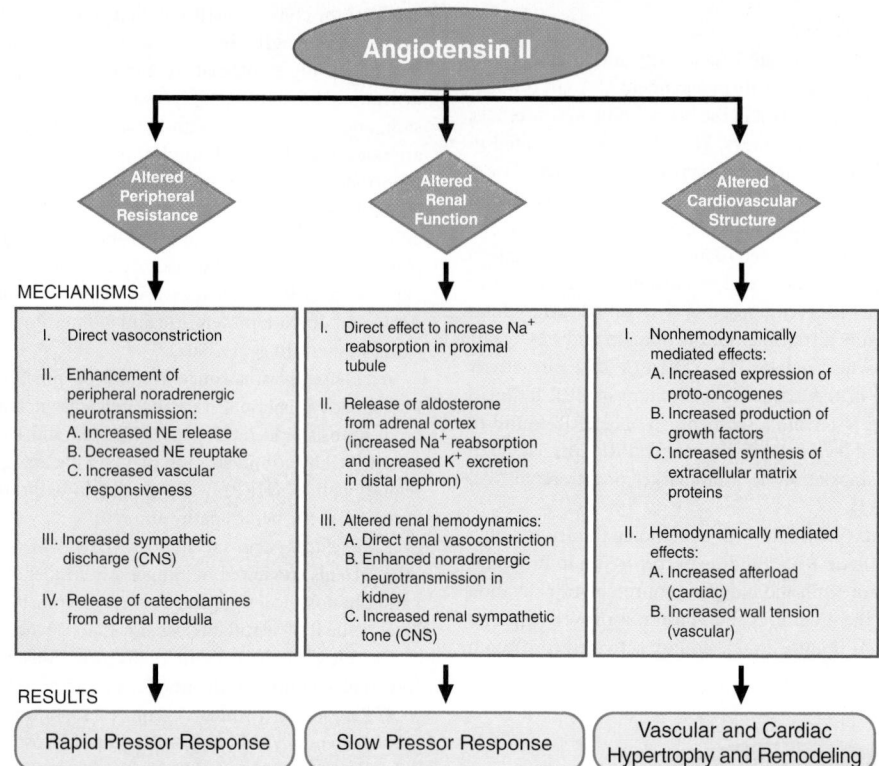

Figure 26–7 *Major physiological effects of AngII.*

the maximum effect requiring days to achieve. This slow pressor response probably is mediated by a decrement in renal excretory function that shifts the renal pressure–natriuresis curve to the right (see the next section). AngII stimulates the synthesis of endothelin 1 and superoxide anion, which may contribute to the slow pressor response.

In addition to its effects on arterial blood pressure, AngII stimulates remodeling of the cardiovascular system, causing hypertrophy of vascular and cardiac cells and increased synthesis and deposition of collagen by cardiac fibroblasts.

Mechanisms by Which Angiotensin II Increases Total Peripheral Resistance

Angiotensin II increases peripheral resistance via direct and indirect effects on blood vessels (Figure 26–7).

Direct Vasoconstriction

Angiotensin II constricts precapillary arterioles and, to a lesser extent, postcapillary venules by activating AT_1 receptors located on vascular smooth muscle cells and stimulating the G_q-PLC-IP_3-Ca^{2+} pathway. AngII has differential effects on vascular beds. Direct vasoconstriction is strongest in the kidneys (Figure 26–8) and somewhat less in the splanchnic bed. AngII-induced vasoconstriction is much less in vessels of the brain and still weaker in those of the lung and skeletal muscle. Nevertheless, high circulating concentrations of AngII may decrease cerebral and coronary blood flow.

Enhancement of Peripheral Noradrenergic Neurotransmission

Angiotensin II, binding to AT_1 receptors, augments NE release from sympathetic nerve terminals by inhibiting the reuptake of NE into nerve terminals and by enhancing the vascular response to NE in model systems (see Chapter 12). High concentrations of the peptide stimulate ganglion cells directly.

Effects on the CNS

Angiotensin II increases sympathetic tone. Small amounts of AngII infused into the vertebral arteries cause an increase in arterial blood pressure. This response reflects effects of the hormone on circumventricular nuclei that are not protected by a blood-brain barrier (e.g., area postrema,

subfornical organ, organum vasculosum of the lamina terminalis). Circulating AngII also attenuates baroreceptor-mediated reductions in sympathetic discharge, thereby increasing arterial pressure. The CNS is affected both by blood-borne AngII and by AngII formed within the brain. The brain contains all components of the RAS. AngII also causes a centrally mediated dipsogenic (thirst) effect and enhances the release of vasopressin from the neurohypophysis.

Release of Catecholamines From the Adrenal Medulla

Angiotensin II stimulates the release of catecholamines from the adrenal medulla by promoting Ca^{2+} entry secondary to depolarization of chromaffin cells.

Mechanisms by Which Angiotensin II Regulates Renal Function

Angiotensin II has pronounced effects on renal function, reducing the urinary excretion of Na^+ and water while increasing the excretion of K^+. The overall effect of AngII on the kidneys is to shift the renal pressure–natriuresis curve to the right (Figure 26–9).

Direct Effects of AngII on Na+ Reabsorption in the Renal Tubules

Very low concentrations of AngII stimulate Na^+/H^+ exchange in the proximal tubule—an effect that increases Na^+, Cl^-, and bicarbonate reabsorption. Approximately 20%–30% of the bicarbonate handled by the nephron may be affected by this mechanism. AngII also increases the expression of the Na^+–glucose symporter in the proximal tubule. Paradoxically, at high concentrations, AngII may inhibit Na^+ transport in the proximal tubule. AngII also directly stimulates the Na^+-K^+-$2Cl^-$ symporter in the thick ascending limb. The proximal tubule secretes angiotensinogen, and the connecting tubule releases renin, so a paracrine tubular RAS may contribute to Na^+ reabsorption.

Release of Aldosterone From the Adrenal Cortex

Angiotensin II stimulates the zona glomerulosa of the adrenal cortex to increase the synthesis and secretion of aldosterone and augments responses to other stimuli (e.g., ACTH, K^+). Increased output of aldosterone is

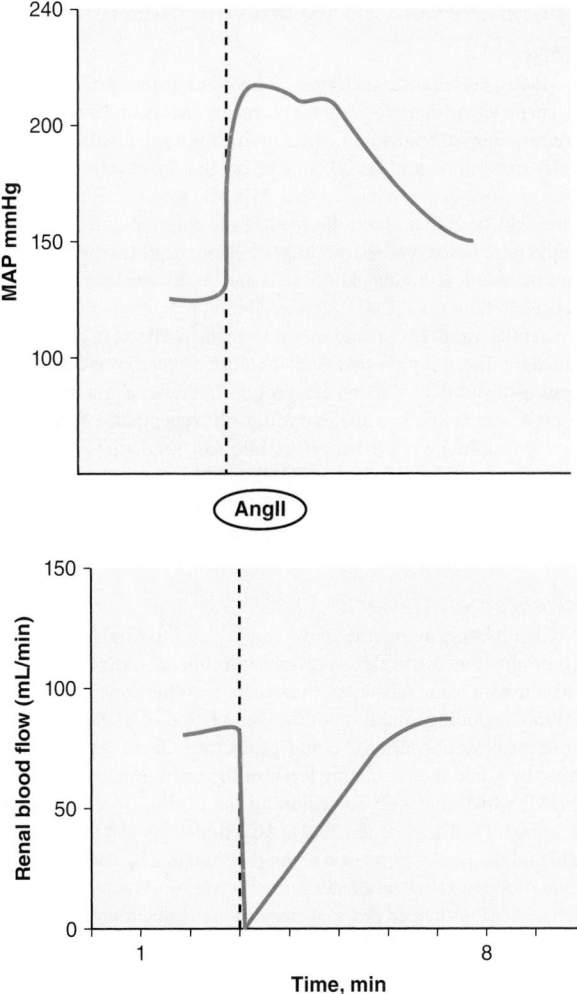

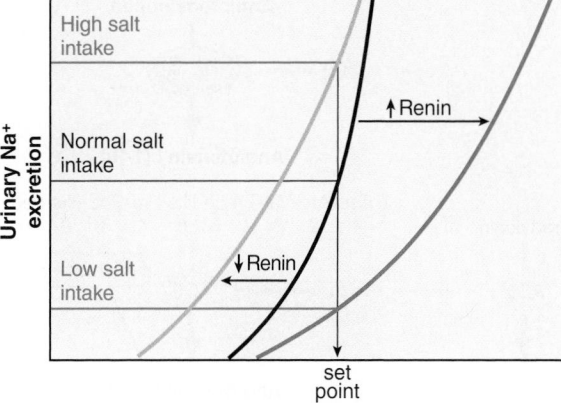

Figure 26–9 *Pressure-natriuresis curve: effects of Na+ intake on renin release (AngII formation) and arterial blood pressure.* Inhibition of the RAS will cause a large drop in blood pressure in Na+-depleted individuals. (Modified with permission from Jackson EK, Branch RA, Margolius HS, Oates JA. Physiological functions of the renal prostaglandin, renin, and kallikrein systems. In: Seldin DW, Giebisch GH, eds. *The Kidney: Physiology and Pathophysiology.* Vol 1. Lippincott Williams & Wilkins, Philadelphia, **1985**, 624.)

Figure 26–8 *Effect of an intravenous bolus of AngII on arterial BP and RBF.* Angiotensin was added at the time indicated by the dashed vertical line.

elicited by concentrations of AngII that have little or no acute effect on blood pressure. Aldosterone acts on the distal and collecting tubules to cause retention of Na+ and excretion of K+ and H+. The stimulant effect of AngII on aldosterone synthesis and release is enhanced under conditions of hyponatremia or hyperkalemia and is reduced when concentrations of Na+ and K+ in plasma are altered in the opposite directions.

Altered Renal Hemodynamics

Angiotensin II reduces renal blood flow and renal excretory function by directly constricting the renal vascular smooth muscle, by enhancing renal sympathetic tone (a CNS effect), and by facilitating renal adrenergic transmission (an intrarenal effect). AngII-induced vasoconstriction of preglomerular microvessels is enhanced by endogenous adenosine owing to signal transduction systems activated by AT_1 and the adenosine A_1 receptor.

Angiotensin II influences the GFR by several mechanisms:

- Constriction of the afferent arterioles, which reduces intraglomerular pressure and tends to reduce GFR
- Contraction of mesangial cells, which decreases the capillary surface area within the glomerulus available for filtration and also tends to decrease GFR
- Constriction of efferent arterioles, which increases intraglomerular pressure and tends to increase GFR

Normally, AngII slightly reduces GFR; however, with renal artery hypotension, the effects of AngII on the efferent arteriole predominate so that AngII increases GFR. Thus, blockade of the RAS may cause acute renal failure in patients with bilateral renal artery stenosis or in patients with unilateral stenosis who have only a single kidney.

Mechanisms by Which Angiotensin II Alters Cardiovascular Structure

Pathological alterations involving cardiovascular hypertrophy and remodeling increase morbidity and mortality. The cells involved include vascular smooth muscle cells, cardiac myocytes, and fibroblasts. AngII induces hypertrophy of cardiac myocytes; stimulates the migration, proliferation, and hypertrophy of vascular smooth muscle cells; increases extracellular matrix production by vascular smooth muscle cells; and increases extracellular matrix production by cardiac fibroblasts. In addition, AngII alters extracellular matrix formation and degradation indirectly by increasing aldosterone production and mineralocorticoid receptor activation. The adverse cardiovascular remodeling induced by AngII can be reduced but not entirely prevented by mineralocorticoid receptor antagonists.

Hemodynamically Mediated Effects of Angiotensin II on Cardiovascular Structure

In addition to the direct cellular effects of AngII on cardiovascular structure, changes in cardiac preload (volume expansion owing to Na+ retention) and afterload (increased arterial blood pressure) probably contribute to cardiac hypertrophy and remodeling. Arterial hypertension also contributes to hypertrophy and remodeling of blood vessels.

Role of the RAS in Long-Term Maintenance of Arterial Blood Pressure Despite Extremes in Dietary Na+ Intake

Arterial blood pressure is a major determinant of Na+ excretion. This is illustrated graphically by plotting urinary Na+ excretion versus mean arterial blood pressure (Figure 26–9), a plot known as the *renal pressure–natriuresis curve*. Over the long term, Na+ excretion must equal Na+ intake; therefore, the set point for long-term levels of arterial blood pressure can be obtained as the intersection of a horizontal line representing Na+ intake with the renal pressure–natriuresis curve. The RAS plays a major role in maintaining a constant set point for long-term levels of arterial blood pressure despite extreme changes in dietary Na+ intake. When dietary Na+ intake is low, renin release is stimulated, and AngII acts on the kidneys to shift the renal pressure–natriuresis curve to the right. Conversely, when dietary Na+ is high, renin release is inhibited, and the withdrawal of AngII shifts the renal pressure–natriuresis curve to the left. When modulation of the RAS is blocked by drugs, changes in salt intake markedly affect long-term levels of arterial blood pressure.

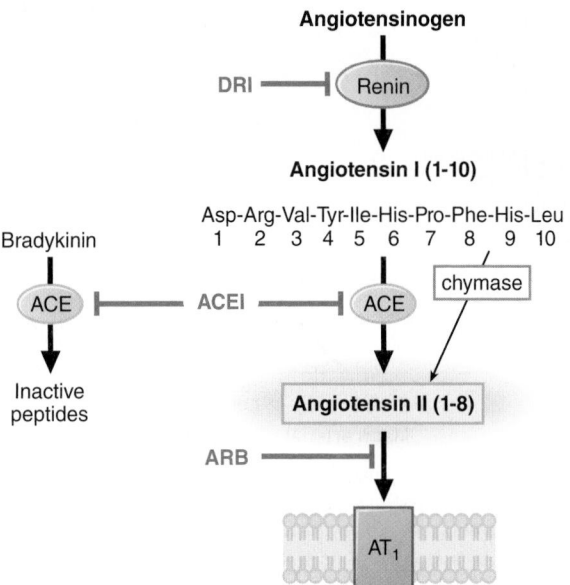

Figure 26–10 *Inhibitors of the RAS.*

Other Effects of the RAS

Expression of the RAS is required for the development of normal kidney morphology, particularly the maturational growth of the renal papilla. AngII causes a marked anorexigenic effect and weight loss, and high circulating levels of AngII may contribute to the anorexia, wasting, and cachexia of heart failure (Paul et al., 2006; Yoshida et al., 2013).

Inhibitors of the Renin-Angiotensin System

Drugs that interfere with the RAS play a prominent role in the treatment of cardiovascular disease. Besides β_1 blockers that inhibit renin release, the following three classes of inhibitors of the RAS are utilized therapeutically (Figure 26–10):

1. ACE inhibitors
2. Angiotensin receptor blockers
3. Direct renin inhibitors

All of these classes of agents will reduce the actions of AngII and lower blood pressure, but each has different effects on the individual components of the RAS (Table 26–2). Representative structures of agents inhibiting the RAS and reducing the effects of AngII are shown in Figure 26–11, near the end of the chapter.

Angiotensin-Converting Enzyme Inhibitors

History

In the 1960s, Ferreira and colleagues found that venom extract from the Brazilian pit viper (*Bothrops jararaca*) contains factors that intensify vasodilator responses to bradykinin. These bradykinin-potentiating factors are peptides that inhibit kininase II, an enzyme that inactivates bradykinin. Erdös and coworkers established that ACE and kininase II are the same enzyme, which catalyzes both the synthesis of AngII and the destruction of bradykinin. Based on these findings, the nonapeptide teprotide (snake venom peptide that inhibits kininase II and ACE) was later synthesized and tested in human subjects. It lowered blood pressure in many patients with essential hypertension and exerted beneficial effects in patients with heart failure. The orally effective ACE inhibitor *captopril* was developed by analysis of the inhibitory action of teprotide, inference about the action of ACE on its substrates, and analogy with carboxypeptidase A, which was known to be inhibited by D-benzylsuccinic acid. Ondetti, Cushman, and colleagues argued that inhibition of ACE might be produced by succinyl amino acids that corresponded in length to the dipeptide cleaved by ACE. This led to the synthesis of a series of carboxy alkanoyl and mercapto alkanoyl derivatives that are potent competitive inhibitors of ACE.

Pharmacological Effects

The ACE inhibitors inhibit the conversion of AngI to AngII. Inhibition of AngII production lowers blood pressure and enhances natriuresis. ACE is an enzyme with many substrates; thus, there are other consequences of its inhibition, including inhibition of the degradation of bradykinin, which has beneficial antihypertensive and protective effects. ACE inhibitors increase by 5-fold the circulating levels of the natural stem cell regulator Ac-SDKP, which may also contribute to the cardioprotective effects of ACE inhibitors (Rhaleb et al., 2001). ACE inhibitors will increase renin release and the rate of formation of AngI by interfering with both short- and long-loop negative feedbacks on renin release (Figure 26–3). Accumulating AngI is directed down alternative metabolic routes, resulting in the increased production of vasodilator peptides such as Ang(1–9) and Ang(1–7) (Figures 26–1 and 26–5).

Clinical Pharmacology

The ACE inhibitors can be classified into three broad groups based on chemical structure:

1. Sulfhydryl-containing ACE inhibitors structurally related to captopril
2. Dicarboxyl-containing ACE inhibitors structurally related to enalapril (e.g., lisinopril, benazepril, quinapril, moexipril, ramipril, trandolapril, perindopril, Figure 26–11)
3. Phosphorus-containing ACE inhibitors structurally related to fosinopril

Many ACE inhibitors are ester-containing prodrugs that are 100–1000 times less potent but have better oral bioavailability than the active molecules.

TABLE 26–2 ■ EFFECTS OF ANTIHYPERTENSIVE AGENTS ON COMPONENTS OF THE RAS

	DRIs	ACEIs	ARBs	DIURETICS	β_1-BLOCKERS
PRC	↑	↑	↑	↑	↓
PRA	↓	↑	↑	↑	↓
AngI	↓	↑	↑	↑	↓
AngII	↓	↓	↑	↑	↓
ACE activity	↔	Inhibition	↔		
Aldosterone	↓	↓	↓	↑	↓/↔
Bradykinin	↔	↑	↔		
AT$_1$R	↔	↔	Inhibition		
AT$_2$R	↔	↔	Stimulation		

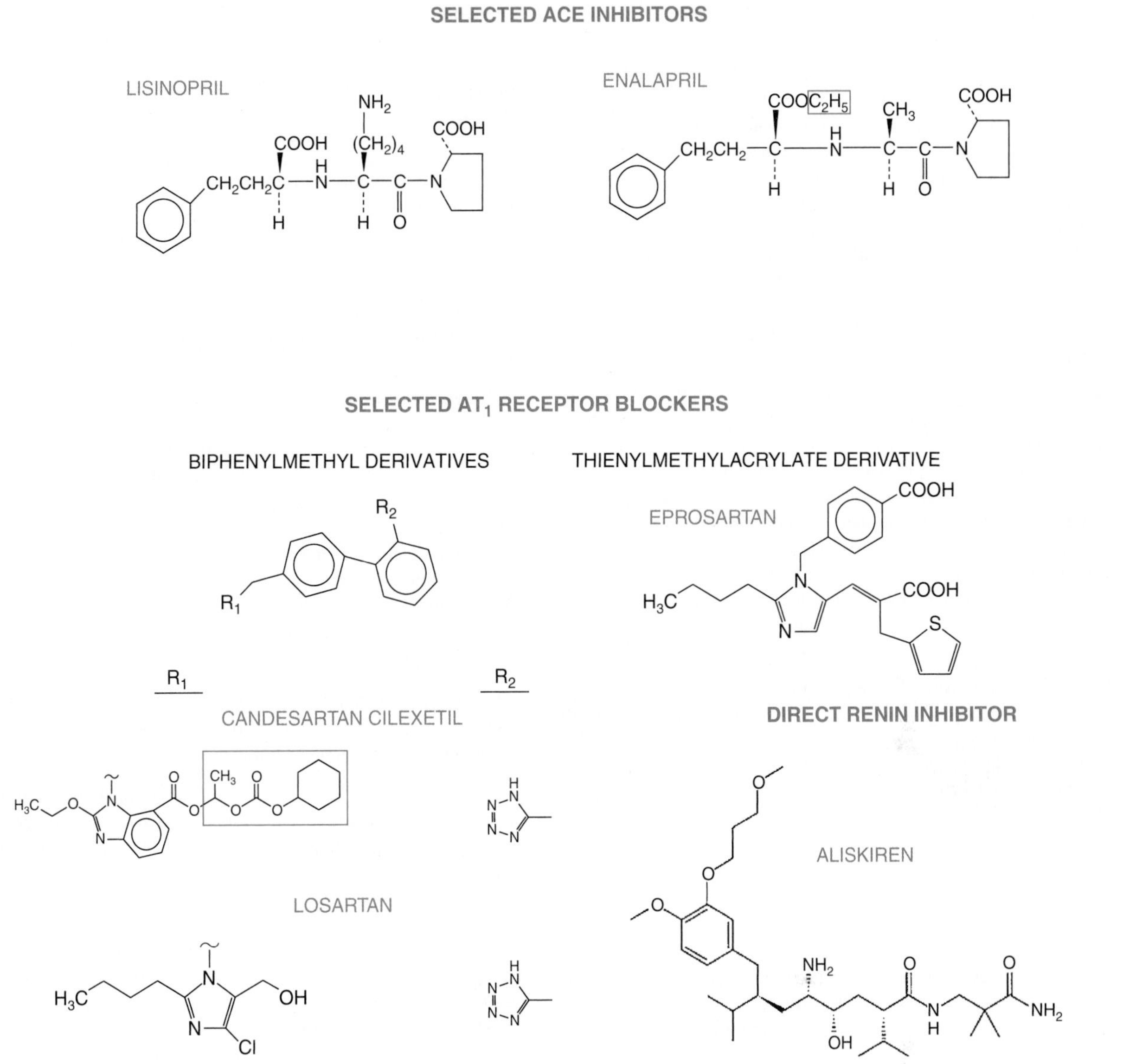

Figure 26–11 *Structures of representative RAS inhibitors.* Enalapril and candesartan cilexetil are pro-drugs, relatively inactive until in vivo esterases remove the region within the red box, replacing it with a hydrogen atom to form the active drug.

Currently, 11 ACE inhibitors are available for clinical use in the U.S. They differ with regard to potency, whether ACE inhibition is primarily a direct effect of the drug itself or the effect of an active metabolite, and pharmacokinetics.

All ACE inhibitors block the conversion of AngI to AngII and have similar therapeutic indications, adverse-effect profiles, and contraindications. Because hypertension usually requires lifelong treatment, quality-of-life issues are an important consideration in comparing antihypertensive drugs. With the exceptions of fosinopril, trandolapril, and quinapril (which display balanced elimination by the liver and kidneys), ACE inhibitors are cleared predominantly by the kidneys. Impaired renal function significantly diminishes the plasma clearance of most ACE inhibitors, and dosages of these drugs should be reduced in patients with renal impairment. *Elevated PRA renders patients hyperresponsive to ACE inhibitor–induced hypotension, and initial dosages of all ACE inhibitors should be reduced in patients with high plasma levels of renin (e.g., patients with heart failure and during salt depletion including diuretic use).* ACE inhibitors differ markedly in tissue distribution, and it is possible that this difference could be exploited to inhibit some local (tissue) RAS while leaving others relatively intact.

Captopril. Captopril is a potent ACE inhibitor with a K_i of 1.7 nM. Given orally, captopril is absorbed rapidly and has a bioavailability of about 75%.

Bioavailability is reduced by 25%–30% with food. Peak concentrations in plasma occur within an hour, and the drug is cleared rapidly, with a $t_{1/2}$ of about 2 h. Most of the drug is eliminated in urine, 40%–50% as captopril and the rest as captopril disulfide dimers and captopril–cysteine disulfide. The oral dose of captopril ranges from 6.25 to 150 mg 2–3 times daily, with 6.25 mg thrice daily or 25 mg twice daily appropriate for the initiation of therapy for heart failure or hypertension, respectively.

Enalapril. Enalapril maleate is a prodrug that is hydrolyzed by esterases in the liver to produce enalaprilat, the active dicarboxylic acid. Enalaprilat is a potent inhibitor of ACE with a K_i of 0.2 nM. Enalapril is absorbed rapidly when given orally and has an oral bioavailability of about 60% (not reduced by food). Although peak concentrations of enalapril in plasma occur within an hour, enalaprilat concentrations peak only after 3–4 h. Enalapril has a $t_{1/2}$ of about 1.3 h, but enalaprilat, because of tight binding to ACE, has a plasma $t_{1/2}$ of about 11 h. Elimination is by the kidneys as either intact enalapril or enalaprilat. The oral dosage of enalapril ranges from 2.5 to 40 mg daily, with 2.5 and 5 mg daily appropriate for the initiation of therapy for heart failure and hypertension, respectively.

Enalaprilat. Enalaprilat is not absorbed orally but is available for intravenous administration when oral therapy is not appropriate.

For hypertensive patients, the dosage is 0.625–1.25 mg given intravenously over 5 min. This dosage may be repeated every 6 h.

Lisinopril. Lisinopril is the lysine analogue of enalaprilat; unlike enalapril, lisinopril itself is active. In vitro, lisinopril is a slightly more potent ACE inhibitor than is enalaprilat. Lisinopril is absorbed slowly, variably, and incompletely (~30%) after oral administration (not reduced by food); peak concentrations in plasma are achieved in about 7 h. It is excreted unchanged by the kidney with a plasma $t_{1/2}$ of about 12 h. Lisinopril does not accumulate in tissues. The oral dosage of lisinopril ranges from 5 to 40 mg daily (single or divided dose), with 5 and 10 mg daily appropriate for the initiation of therapy for heart failure and hypertension, respectively. A daily dose of 2.5 mg with close medical supervision is recommended for patients with heart failure who are hyponatremic or have renal impairment.

Benazepril. Cleavage of the ester moiety by hepatic esterases transforms benazepril, a prodrug, into benazeprilat. Benazepril is absorbed rapidly but incompletely (37%) after oral administration (only slightly reduced by food). Benazepril is nearly completely metabolized to benazeprilat and to the glucuronide conjugates of benazepril and benazeprilat, which are excreted into the urine and bile; peak concentrations of benazepril and benazeprilat in plasma are achieved in 0.5–1 and 1–2 h, respectively. Benazeprilat has an effective plasma $t_{1/2}$ of 10–11 h. With the exception of the lungs, benazeprilat does not accumulate in tissues. The oral dosage of benazepril ranges from 5 to 80 mg daily (single or divided dose).

Fosinopril. Cleavage of the ester moiety by hepatic esterases transforms fosinopril into fosinoprilat. Fosinopril is absorbed slowly and incompletely (36%) after oral administration (rate but not extent reduced by food). Fosinopril is largely metabolized to fosinoprilat (75%) and to the glucuronide conjugate of fosinoprilat. These are excreted in both the urine and the bile; peak concentrations of fosinoprilat in plasma are achieved in about 3 h. Fosinoprilat has an effective plasma $t_{1/2}$ of about 11.5 h, a figure not significantly altered by renal impairment. The oral dosage of fosinopril ranges from 10 to 80 mg daily (single or divided dose). The initial dose is reduced to 5 mg daily in patients with Na$^+$ or water depletion or renal failure.

Trandolapril. An oral dose of trandolapril is absorbed without reduction by food and produces plasma levels of trandolapril (10% bioavailability) and trandolaprilat (70% bioavailability). Trandolaprilat is about 8 times more potent than trandolapril as an ACE inhibitor. Glucuronides of trandolapril and deesterification products are recovered in the urine (33%, mostly trandolaprilat) and feces (66%). Peak concentrations of trandolaprilat in plasma are achieved in 4–10 h.

Trandolaprilat displays biphasic elimination kinetics, with an initial $t_{1/2}$ of about 10 h (the major component of elimination), followed by a more prolonged $t_{1/2}$ (owing to slow dissociation of trandolaprilat from tissue ACE). Plasma clearance of trandolaprilat is reduced by both renal and hepatic insufficiency. The oral dosage ranges from 1 to 8 mg daily (single or divided dose). The initial dose is 0.5 mg in patients who are taking a diuretic or who have renal impairment.

Quinapril. Cleavage of the ester moiety by hepatic esterases transforms quinapril, a prodrug, into quinaprilat. Quinapril is absorbed rapidly (peak concentrations are achieved in 1 h), and the rate, but not extent, of oral absorption (60%) may be reduced by food (delayed peak). Quinaprilat and other minor metabolites of quinapril are excreted in the urine (61%) and feces (37%). Peak concentrations of quinaprilat in plasma are achieved in about 2 h. Conversion of quinapril to quinaprilat is reduced in patients with diminished liver function. The initial $t_{1/2}$ of quinaprilat is about 2 h; a prolonged terminal $t_{1/2}$ of about 25 h may be due to high-affinity binding of the drug to tissue ACE. The oral dosage of quinapril ranges from 5 to 80 mg daily.

Ramipril. Orally administered ramipril is absorbed rapidly (peak concentrations in 1 h; the rate but not extent of its oral absorption (50%–60%) is reduced by food. Ramipril is metabolized to ramiprilat by hepatic esterases and to inactive metabolites that are excreted predominantly by the kidneys. Peak concentrations of ramiprilat in plasma are achieved in about 3 h. Ramiprilat displays triphasic elimination kinetics ($t_{1/2}$ values: 2–4, 9–18, and more than 50 h) This triphasic elimination is due to extensive distribution to all tissues (initial $t_{1/2}$), clearance of free ramiprilat from plasma (intermediate $t_{1/2}$), and dissociation of ramiprilat from tissue ACE (long terminal $t_{1/2}$). The oral dosage of ramipril ranges from 1.25 to 20 mg daily (single or divided dose).

Moexipril. Moexipril's antihypertensive activity is due to its deesterified metabolite, moexiprilat. Moexipril is absorbed incompletely, with bioavailability as moexiprilat of about 13%. Bioavailability is markedly decreased by food. The time to peak plasma concentration of moexiprilat is almost 1.5 h; the elimination $t_{1/2}$ varies between 2 and 12 h. The recommended dosage range is 7.5–30 mg daily (single or divided doses). The dosage range is halved in patients who are taking diuretics or who have renal impairment.

Perindopril. Perindopril erbumine is a prodrug, and 30%–50% of systemically available perindopril is transformed to perindoprilat by hepatic esterases. Although the oral bioavailability of perindopril (75%) is not affected by food, the bioavailability of perindoprilat is reduced by about 35%. Perindopril is metabolized to perindoprilat and to inactive metabolites that are excreted predominantly by the kidneys. Peak concentrations of perindoprilat in plasma are achieved in 3–7 h. Perindoprilat displays biphasic elimination kinetics with half-lives of 3–10 h (the major component of elimination) and 30–120 h (owing to slow dissociation of perindoprilat from tissue ACE). The oral dosage ranges from 2 to 16 mg daily (single or divided dose).

Therapeutic Uses of ACE Inhibitors

The ACE inhibitors are effective in the treatment of cardiovascular disease, heart failure, and diabetic nephropathy.

ACE Inhibitors in Hypertension. Inhibition of ACE lowers systemic vascular resistance and mean, diastolic, and systolic blood pressures in various hypertensive states except when high blood pressure is due to primary aldosteronism (see Chapter 28). The initial change in blood pressure tends to be positively correlated with PRA and AngII plasma levels prior to treatment. However, some patients may show a sizable reduction in blood pressure that correlates poorly with pretreatment values of PRA. It is possible that increased local (tissue) production of AngII or increased responsiveness of tissues to normal levels of AngII makes some hypertensive patients sensitive to ACE inhibitors despite normal PRA.

The long-term fall in systemic blood pressure observed in hypertensive individuals treated with ACE inhibitors is accompanied by a leftward shift in the renal pressure–natriuresis curve (Figure 26–9) and a reduction in TPR in which there is variable participation by different vascular beds. The kidney is a notable exception: Because the renal vessels are extremely sensitive to the vasoconstrictor actions of AngII, ACE inhibitors increase renal blood flow via vasodilation of the afferent and efferent arterioles. Increased renal blood flow occurs without an increase in GFR; thus, the filtration fraction is reduced.

The ACE inhibitors cause systemic arteriolar dilation and increase the compliance of large arteries, which contributes to a reduction of systolic pressure. Cardiac function in patients with uncomplicated hypertension generally is little changed, although stroke volume and cardiac output may increase slightly with sustained treatment. Baroreceptor function and cardiovascular reflexes are not compromised, and responses to postural changes and exercise are little impaired. Even when substantial lowering of blood pressure is achieved, heart rate and concentrations of catecholamines in plasma generally increase only slightly, if at all. This perhaps reflects an alteration of baroreceptor function with increased arterial compliance and the loss of the normal tonic influence of AngII on the sympathetic nervous system.

Aldosterone secretion is reduced, but not seriously impaired, by ACE inhibitors. Aldosterone secretion is maintained at adequate levels by other steroidogenic stimuli, such as ACTH and K$^+$. The activity of these secretagogues on the zona glomerulosa of the adrenal cortex requires very small trophic or permissive amounts of AngII, which always are present because ACE inhibition never is complete. Excessive retention of K$^+$ is encountered in patients taking supplemental K$^+$, in patients with renal impairment, or in patients taking other medications that reduce K$^+$ excretion.

The ACE inhibitors alone normalize blood pressure in about 50% of patients with mild-to-moderate hypertension. Ninety percent of patients with mild-to-moderate hypertension will be controlled by the combination of an ACE inhibitor and a Ca^{2+} channel blocker, a β_1 adrenergic receptor blocker, or a diuretic. Diuretics augment the antihypertensive response to ACE inhibitors by rendering the patient's blood pressure renin dependent. Several ACE inhibitors are marketed in fixed-dose combinations with a thiazide diuretic or Ca^{2+} channel blocker for the management of hypertension.

ACE Inhibitors in Left Ventricular Systolic Dysfunction. Unless contraindicated, ACE inhibitors should be given to all patients with impaired left ventricular systolic function whether or not they have symptoms of overt heart failure (see Chapter 29). Several large clinical studies demonstrated that inhibition of ACE in patients with systolic dysfunction prevents or delays the progression of heart failure, decreases the incidence of sudden death and myocardial infarction, decreases hospitalization, and improves quality of life. Inhibition of ACE commonly reduces afterload and systolic wall stress, and both cardiac output and cardiac index increase, as do indices of stroke work and stroke volume. In systolic dysfunction, AngII decreases arterial compliance, and this is reversed by ACE inhibition. Heart rate generally is reduced. Systemic blood pressure falls, sometimes steeply at the outset, but tends to return toward initial levels. Renovascular resistance falls sharply, and renal blood flow increases. Natriuresis occurs as a result of the improved renal hemodynamics, the reduced stimulus to the secretion of aldosterone by AngII, and the diminished direct effects of AngII on the kidney. The excess volume of body fluids contracts, which reduces venous return to the right side of the heart. A further reduction results from venodilation and an increased capacity of the venous bed.

Although AngII has little acute venoconstrictor activity, long-term infusion of AngII increases venous tone, perhaps by central or peripheral interactions with the sympathetic nervous system. The response to ACE inhibitors also involves reductions of pulmonary arterial pressure, pulmonary capillary wedge pressure, and left atrial and left ventricular filling volumes and pressures. Consequently, preload and diastolic wall stress are diminished. The better hemodynamic performance results in increased exercise tolerance and suppression of the sympathetic nervous system. Cerebral and coronary blood flows usually are well maintained, even when systemic blood pressure is reduced. In heart failure, ACE inhibitors reduce ventricular dilation and tend to restore the heart to its normal elliptical shape. ACE inhibitors may reverse ventricular remodeling via changes in preload/afterload by preventing the growth effects of AngII on myocytes and by attenuating cardiac fibrosis induced by AngII and aldosterone.

ACE Inhibitors in Acute Myocardial Infarction. The beneficial effects of ACE inhibitors in acute myocardial infarction are particularly large in hypertensive and diabetic patients. Unless contraindicated (e.g., cardiogenic shock or severe hypotension), ACE inhibitors should be started immediately during the acute phase of myocardial infarction and can be administered along with thrombolytics, aspirin, and β adrenergic receptor antagonists (ACE Inhibitor Myocardial Infarction Collaborative Group, 1998). In high-risk patients (e.g., large infarct, systolic ventricular dysfunction), ACE inhibition should be continued long term (see Chapters 27 and 28).

ACE Inhibitors in Patients Who Are at High Risk of Cardiovascular Events. Patients at high risk of cardiovascular events benefit considerably from treatment with ACE inhibitors (Heart Outcomes Prevention Study Investigators, 2000). ACE inhibition significantly decreases the rate of myocardial infarction, stroke, and death in patients who do not have left ventricular dysfunction but have evidence of vascular disease or diabetes and one other risk factor for cardiovascular disease. In patients with coronary artery disease but without heart failure, ACE inhibition reduces cardiovascular disease death and myocardial infarction (European Trial, 2003).

ACE Inhibitors in Diabetes Mellitus and Renal Failure. Diabetes mellitus is the leading cause of renal disease. In patients with type 1 diabetes mellitus and diabetic nephropathy, ACE inhibitors prevent or delay the progression of renal disease, affording renoprotection, as defined by changes in albumin excretion. The renoprotective effects of ACE inhibitors in type 1 diabetes are in part independent of blood pressure reduction. In addition, ACE inhibitors may decrease retinopathy progression in type 1 diabetics and attenuate the progression of renal insufficiency in patients with a variety of nondiabetic nephropathies (Ruggenenti et al., 2010).

Several mechanisms participate in the renal protective effects of ACE inhibitors. Increased glomerular capillary pressure induces glomerular injury, and ACE inhibitors reduce this parameter by decreasing arterial blood pressure and by dilating renal efferent arterioles. ACE inhibitors increase the permeability selectivity of the filtering membrane, thereby diminishing exposure of the mesangium to proteinaceous factors that may stimulate mesangial cell proliferation and matrix production, two processes that contribute to expansion of the mesangium in diabetic nephropathy. Because AngII is a growth factor, reductions in the intrarenal levels of AngII may further attenuate mesangial cell growth and matrix production. ACE inhibitors increase Ang(1–7) levels by preventing its metabolism by ACE. Ang(1–7) binds to Mas receptors and has protective and antifibrotic effects (Santos, 2014). In the setting of diabetes, at the level of renal epithelial podocytes, activation of AT$_1$ receptors leads to activation of protein kinase signaling cascades, cytoskeletal rearrangements, retraction of podocyte processes, and a reduction in proteins of the slit diaphragm, all resulting in increased permeability of the renal epithelium to proteins (proteinuria). ACE inhibitors reduce these effects of AngII (Márquez et al., 2015).

ACE Inhibitors in Scleroderma Renal Crisis. The use of ACE inhibitors considerably improves survival of patients with scleroderma renal crisis.

Adverse Effects of ACE Inhibitors

In general, ACE inhibitors are well tolerated. The drugs do not alter plasma concentrations of uric acid or Ca^{2+} and may improve insulin sensitivity and glucose tolerance in patients with insulin resistance and decrease cholesterol and lipoprotein (a) levels in proteinuric renal disease.

Hypotension. A steep fall in blood pressure may occur following the first dose of an ACE inhibitor in patients with elevated PRA. Care should be exercised in patients who are salt depleted, are on multiple antihypertensive drugs, or have congestive heart failure.

Cough. In 5%–20% of patients, ACE inhibitors induce a bothersome, dry cough mediated by the accumulation in the lungs of bradykinin, substance P, or PGs. Thromboxane antagonism, aspirin, and iron supplementation reduce cough induced by ACE inhibitors. ACE dose reduction or switching to an ARB is sometimes effective. Once ACE inhibitors are stopped, the cough disappears, usually within 4 days.

Hyperkalemia. Significant K$^+$ retention is rarely encountered in patients with normal renal function. However, ACE inhibitors may cause hyperkalemia in patients with renal insufficiency or diabetes or in patients taking K$^+$-sparing diuretics, K$^+$ supplements, β receptor blockers, or NSAIDs.

Acute Renal Failure. Inhibition of ACE can induce acute renal insufficiency in patients with bilateral renal artery stenosis, stenosis of the artery to a single remaining kidney, heart failure, or volume depletion owing to diarrhea or diuretics.

Angioedema. In 0.1%–0.5% of patients, ACE inhibitors induce rapid swelling in the nose, throat, mouth, glottis, larynx, lips, or tongue. Once ACE inhibitors are stopped, angioedema disappears within hours; meanwhile, the patient's airway should be protected, and if necessary, epinephrine, an antihistamine, or a glucocorticoid should be administered. African Americans have a 4.5 times greater risk of ACE inhibitor–induced angioedema than Caucasians. Although rare, angioedema of the intestine (visceral angioedema) characterized by emesis, watery diarrhea, and abdominal pain also has been reported. ACE inhibitor-associated angioedema is a class effect, and patients who develop this adverse event should not be prescribed any other drugs within the ACE inhibitor class.

Fetopathic Potential. If a pregnancy is diagnosed, it is imperative that ACE inhibitors be discontinued as soon as possible. ACE inhibitors and ARBs have been associated with renal developmental defects when administered in the third trimester of pregnancy, and potentially earlier. The fetopathic effects may be due in part to fetal hypotension. This possible adverse effect should be discussed with any woman of childbearing potential, as should the necessity of appropriate birth control measures.

Skin Rash. The ACE inhibitors occasionally cause a maculopapular rash that may itch, but that may resolve spontaneously or with antihistamines.

Other Side Effects. Extremely rare but reversible side effects include *dysgeusia* (an alteration in or loss of taste), *neutropenia* (symptoms include sore throat and fever), *glycosuria* (spillage of glucose into the urine in the absence of hyperglycemia), *anemia,* and *hepatotoxicity.*

Drug Interactions. Antacids may reduce the bioavailability of ACE inhibitors; capsaicin may worsen ACE inhibitor–induced cough; NSAIDs, including aspirin, may reduce the antihypertensive response to ACE inhibitors; and K^+-sparing diuretics and K^+ supplements may exacerbate ACE inhibitor–induced hyperkalemia. ACE inhibitors may increase plasma levels of digoxin and lithium and hypersensitivity reactions to allopurinol.

Angiotensin II Receptor Blockers

HISTORY

Attempts to develop therapeutically useful AngII receptor antagonists date to the early 1970s. Initial endeavors concentrated on angiotensin peptide analogues. Saralasin, 1-sarcosine, 8-isoleucine AngII, and other 8-substituted angiotensins are potent AngII receptor antagonists but were of no clinical value because of lack of oral bioavailability and unacceptable partial agonist activity. A breakthrough came in the early 1980s with the synthesis and testing of a series of imidazole-5–acetic acid derivatives that attenuated pressor responses to AngII in rats. Two compounds, S-8307 and S-8308, proved to be highly specific, albeit very weak, nonpeptide AngII receptor antagonists that were devoid of partial agonist activity (Dell'Italia, 2011). Through a series of stepwise modifications, the orally active, potent, and selective nonpeptide AT_1 receptor antagonist losartan was developed and approved for clinical use in the U.S. in 1995. Since then, seven additional AT_1 receptor antagonists (see Drug Facts for Your Personal Formulary table) have been approved. Although these AT_1 receptor antagonists are devoid of partial agonist activity, structural modifications as minor as a methyl group can transform a potent antagonist into an agonist (Perlman et al., 1997).

Pharmacological Effects

The AngII receptor blockers bind to the AT_1 receptor with high affinity and are more than 10,000-fold selective for the AT_1 receptor over the AT_2 receptor. Although binding of ARBs to the AT_1 receptor is competitive, the inhibition by ARBs of biological responses to AngII often is functionally insurmountable. Insurmountable antagonism has the theoretical advantage of sustained receptor blockade even with increased levels of endogenous ligand and with missed doses of drug. ARBs inhibit most of the biological effects of AngII, which include AngII-induced (1) contraction of vascular smooth muscle; (2) rapid pressor responses; (3) slow pressor responses; (4) thirst; (5) vasopressin release; (6) aldosterone secretion; (7) release of adrenal catecholamines; (8) enhancement of noradrenergic neurotransmission; (9) increases in sympathetic tone; (10) changes in renal function; and (11) cellular hypertrophy and hyperplasia. ARBs reduce arterial blood pressure in animals with renovascular and genetic hypertension, as well as in transgenic animals overexpressing the renin gene. ARBs, however, have little effect on arterial blood pressure in animals with low-renin hypertension (e.g., rats with hypertension induced by NaCl and deoxycorticosterone) (Csajka et al., 1997).

Do ARBs Have Therapeutic Efficacy Equivalent to That of ACE Inhibitors?

Although both ARBs and ACE inhibitors of drugs block the RAS, they differ in several important aspects:

- *ARBs reduce activation of AT_1 receptors more effectively than do ACE inhibitors.* ACE inhibitors reduce the biosynthesis of AngII by the action of ACE, but do not inhibit AngII generation via chymase and other ACE-independent AngII-producing pathways. ARBs block the actions of AngII via the AT_1 receptor regardless of the biochemical pathway leading to AngII formation.
- In contrast to ACE inhibitors, *ARBs permit activation of AT_2 receptors.* ACE inhibitors increase renin release, but block the conversion of AngI to AngII. ARBs also stimulate renin release; however, with ARBs, this translates into a several-fold increase in circulating levels of AngII. Because ARBs block AT_1 receptors, this increased level of AngII is available to activate AT_2 receptors.
- *ACE inhibitors and ARBs increase Ang(1–7) levels by different mechanisms.* ACE is involved in the clearance of Ang(1–7), so inhibition of ACE increases Ang(1–7) levels. With ARBs, AngII, the preferred substrate of ACE2, is converted to Ang(1–7).
- *ACE inhibitors increase the levels of a number of ACE substrates, including bradykinin and Ac-SDKP.*

Whether the pharmacological differences between ARBs and ACE inhibitors result in significant differences in therapeutic outcomes is an open question.

Clinical Pharmacology

Oral bioavailability of ARBs generally is low (<50%) except for azilsartan (~60%) and irbesartan (~70%), and protein binding is high (>90%).

Candesartan Cilexetil. Candesartan cilexetil is an inactive ester prodrug that is completely hydrolyzed to the active form, candesartan, during absorption from the GI tract (Figure 26–11). Peak plasma levels are obtained 3–4 h after oral administration; the plasma $t_{1/2}$ is about 9 h. Plasma clearance of candesartan is due to renal elimination (33%) and biliary excretion (67%). The plasma clearance of candesartan is affected by renal insufficiency but not by mild-to-moderate hepatic insufficiency. Candesartan cilexetil should be administered orally once or twice daily for a total daily dose of 4–32 mg.

Eprosartan. Peak plasma levels are obtained 1–2 h after oral administration; the plasma $t_{1/2}$ is 5–9 h. Eprosartan is metabolized in part to the glucuronide conjugate. Clearance is by renal elimination and biliary excretion. The plasma clearance of eprosartan is affected by both renal insufficiency and hepatic insufficiency. The recommended dosage of eprosartan is 400–800 mg/d in one or two doses.

Irbesartan. Peak plasma levels are obtained about 1.5–2 h after oral administration; the plasma $t_{1/2}$ is 11–15 h. Irbesartan is metabolized in part to the glucuronide conjugate, and the parent compound and its glucuronide conjugate are cleared by renal elimination (20%) and biliary excretion (80%). The plasma clearance of irbesartan is unaffected by either renal or mild-to-moderate hepatic insufficiency. The oral dosage of irbesartan is 150–300 mg once daily.

Losartan. Approximately 14% of an oral dose of losartan is converted by CYP2C9 and CYP3A4 to the 5-carboxylic acid metabolite, EXP 3174, which is more potent than losartan as an AT_1 receptor antagonist. Peak plasma levels of losartan and EXP 3174 occur about 1–3 h after oral administration, and the plasma half-lives are 2.5 and 6–9 h, respectively. The plasma clearances of losartan and EXP 3174 are via the kidney and liver (metabolism and biliary excretion) and are affected by hepatic but not renal insufficiency. Losartan should be administered orally once or twice daily for a total daily dose of 25–100 mg. Losartan is a competitive antagonist of the thromboxane A_2 receptor and attenuates platelet aggregation. EXP 3179, another metabolite of losartan without angiotensin receptor effects, reduces COX-2 messenger RNA upregulation and COX-dependent PG generation (Krämer et al., 2002) (Figure 26–11).

Olmesartan Medoxomil. Olmesartan medoxomil is an inactive ester prodrug that is completely hydrolyzed to the active form, olmesartan, during absorption from the GI tract. Peak plasma levels are obtained 1.4–2.8 h after oral administration; the plasma $t_{1/2}$ is 10–15 h. Plasma clearance of olmesartan is due to both renal elimination and biliary excretion. Although renal impairment and hepatic disease decrease the plasma clearance of olmesartan, no dose adjustment is required in patients with mild-to-moderate renal or hepatic impairment. The oral dosage of olmesartan medoxomil is 20–40 mg once daily.

Telmisartan. Peak plasma levels are obtained 0.5–1 h after oral administration; the plasma $t_{1/2}$ is about 24 h. Telmisartan is cleared from the circulation mainly by biliary secretion of intact drug. The plasma clearance of telmisartan is affected by hepatic but not renal insufficiency. The recommended oral dosage of telmisartan is 40–80 mg once daily.

Valsartan. Peak plasma levels occur 2–4 h after oral administration; food markedly decreases absorption; the plasma $t_{1/2}$ is about 9 h. Valsartan is cleared from the circulation by the liver (~70% of total clearance), and hepatic insufficiency will reduce clearance. The oral dosage of valsartan is 80–320 mg once daily.

Azilsartan Medoxomil. The prodrug is hydrolyzed in the GI tract into the active form, azilsartan. The drug is available in 40- and 80-mg once-daily doses. At the recommended dose of 80 mg once a day, azilsartan medoxomil is superior to the maximal doses of valsartan and olmesartan in lowering blood pressure. Bioavailability of azilsartan is about 60% and is not affected by food. Peak plasma concentrations C_{max} are achieved within 1.5–3 h. The elimination $t_{1/2}$ is about 11 h. Azilsartan is metabolized mostly by CYP2C9 into inactive metabolites. Elimination of the drug is 55% in feces and 42% in urine. About 15% of the dose is eliminated as unchanged azilsartan in urine. Plasma clearance is not affected by renal or hepatic insufficiency.

Angiotensin Receptor–Neprilysin Inhibitor. A combination of sacubitril and valsartan, marketed as Entresto, is a first-in-class drug that combines the AT_1 receptor antagonistic moiety of valsartan with the neprilysin inhibitor moiety of sacubitril. The complex (sacubitril, valsartan, Na^+, and water [1:1:3:2.5]) dissociates into sacubitril and valsartan after oral administration. Sacubitril bioavailability is about 60%, and it is highly protein bound (94%–97%). Sacubitril is further metabolized by esterases into the active metabolite LBQ657, which has a $t_{1/2}$ of 11 h. The neprilysin inhibitor blocks the breakdown of natriuretic peptides ANP, BNP, and CNP, as well as AngI and bradykinin. The drug combination lowers vascular resistance and increases blood flow. In clinical trial, this combination agent was reported to be superior to enalapril in decreasing the risk of deaths from cardiovascular causes and heart failure by 20% (McMurray et al., 2014).

Entresto is approved for treatment of heart failure with reduced ejection fraction, with a recommended dose of 100–400 mg daily, divided into two doses. Because the ACE/neprilysin inhibitor omapatrilat demonstrated an increased risk of angioedema, use of Entresto is contraindicated in conjunction with an ACE inhibitor or in patients with a history of angioedema during ACE inhibitor or ARB use. The drug should not be used in conjunction with an ARB or ACE inhibitor, and in patients with diabetes should not be used in conjunction with aliskiren. Potential adverse effects discussed for valsartan also apply to this sacubutril-valsartan combination.

A New Class of ARBs in Development. A *β-arrestin-biased AT_1 receptor blocker,* TRV027 is a ligand that binds AT_1 receptor and blocks G protein–coupled signaling while engaging β-arrestin. β-Arrestin functions as an adaptor protein that participates in receptor desensitization and internalization. In animal models, β-arrestin–biased AT_1 receptor ligand increases myocyte contractility and protects against apoptosis (Kim et al., 2012). In phase II clinical studies, TRV027 decreased mean arterial pressure and was well tolerated. The safety and efficacy of TRV027 is being tested in the BLAST-HF study in patients with acute heart failure (Felker et al., 2015).

Therapeutic Uses of ARBs

All ARBs are approved for the treatment of hypertension. ARBs are renoprotective in type 2 diabetes mellitus, and many experts now consider them the drugs of choice for renoprotection in diabetic patients.

Irbesartan and losartan are approved for diabetic nephropathy, losartan is approved for stroke prophylaxis, and valsartan and candesartan are approved for heart failure and to reduce cardiovascular mortality in clinically stable patients with left ventricular failure or left ventricular dysfunction following myocardial infarction. The efficacy of ARBs in lowering blood pressure is comparable with that of ACE inhibitors and other established antihypertensive drugs, with a favorable adverse-effect profile. ARBs also are available as fixed-dose combinations with HCTZ or amlodipine (see Chapters 27–29).

The Losartan Intervention for Endpoint (LIFE) Reduction in Hypertension Study demonstrated the superiority of an ARB compared with a $β_1$ adrenergic receptor antagonist with regard to reducing stroke in hypertensive patients with left ventricular hypertrophy (Dahlöf et al., 2002). Also, irbesartan appears to maintain sinus rhythm in patients with persistent, long-standing atrial fibrillation (Madrid et al., 2002). Losartan is reported to be safe and highly effective in the treatment of portal hypertension in patients with cirrhosis and portal hypertension without compromising renal function (Schneider et al., 1999).

The ELITE (Evaluation of Losartan in the Elderly) study and a follow-up study (ELITE II) concluded that in elderly patients with heart failure, losartan is as effective as captopril in improving symptoms (Pitt et al., 2000). The VALIANT (Valsartan in Acute Myocardial Infarction) trial demonstrated that valsartan is as effective as captopril in patients with myocardial infarction complicated by left ventricular systolic dysfunction with regard to all-cause mortality (Pfeffer et al., 2003). Both valsartan and candesartan reduce mortality and morbidity in patients with heart failure (reviewed by Makani et al., 2013). Current recommendations are to use ACE inhibitors as first-line agents for the treatment of heart failure and to reserve ARBs for treatment of heart failure in patients who cannot tolerate or have an unsatisfactory response to ACE inhibitors.

The ARBs are renoprotective in type 2 diabetes mellitus, and many experts now consider them the drugs of choice for renoprotection in diabetic patients.

Dual Inhibition of the RAS. At present, there is contradictory evidence regarding the advisability of combining an ARB and an ACE inhibitor in patients with heart failure, with one study indicating that a combination of ARB and ACE inhibitors decreases morbidity and mortality in patients with heart failure, and another showing that combination therapy is associated with increased adverse effects and no added benefits (Dell'Italia, 2011; Makani et al., 2013; ONTARGET Investigators, 2008).

Adverse Effects

The ARBs are generally well tolerated. The incidence of angioedema and cough with ARBs is less than that with ACE inhibitors. As with ACE inhibitors, ARBs have teratogenic potential and should be discontinued in pregnancy. In patients whose arterial blood pressure or renal function is highly dependent on the RAS (e.g., renal artery stenosis), ARBs can cause hypotension, oliguria, progressive azotemia, or acute renal failure. ARBs may cause hyperkalemia in patients with renal disease or in patients taking K^+ supplements or K^+-sparing diuretics. ARBs enhance the blood pressure–lowering effect of other antihypertensive drugs, a desirable effect but one that may necessitate dosage adjustment. There are rare postmarketing reports of anaphylaxis, abnormal hepatic function, hepatitis, neutropenia, leukopenia, agranulocytosis, pruritus, urticaria, hyponatremia, alopecia, and vasculitis, including Henoch-Schönlein purpura.

Direct Renin Inhibitors

Angiotensinogen is the only specific substrate for renin. DRIs inhibit the cleavage of AngI from angiotensinogen by renin, an enzymatic reaction that is the rate-limiting step for the subsequent generation of AngII. Aliskiren is the only DRI approved for clinical use.

HISTORY

Earlier renin inhibitors were orally inactive peptide analogues of the prorenin propeptide or analogues of renin-substrate cleavage site. Orally active, first-generation renin inhibitors (*enalkiren, zankiren, CGP38560A, and remikiren*) were effective in reducing AngII levels, but none of them made it past clinical trials due to their low potency, poor bioavailability, and short $t_{1/2}$. Low-molecular-weight renin inhibitors were designed based on molecular modeling and crystallographic structural information of renin-substrate interaction (Wood et al., 2003). This led to the development of aliskiren, a second-generation renin inhibitor that is FDA approved for the treatment of hypertension. Aliskiren has blood pressure–lowering effects similar to those of ACE inhibitors and ARBs.

Pharmacological Effects

Aliskiren is a low-molecular-weight nonpeptide and a potent competitive inhibitor of renin. It binds the active site of renin to block conversion of angiotensinogen to AngI, thus reducing the consequent production of AngII. Aliskiren has a 10,000-fold higher affinity to renin ($IC_{50} \sim 0.6$ nM) than to any other aspartic peptidases. In healthy volunteers, aliskiren (40–640 mg/d) induces a dose-dependent decrease in blood pressure, reduces PRA and AngI and AngII levels, but increases PRC by 16- to 34-fold due to the loss of the short-loop negative feedback by AngII (Figure 26–3; Table 26–2). Aliskiren also decreases plasma and urinary aldosterone levels and enhances natriuresis (Nussberger et al., 2002).

Clinical Pharmacology

Aliskiren is recommended as a single oral dose of 150 or 300 mg/d. Bioavailability of aliskiren is low (~2.5%), but its high affinity and potency compensate for the low bioavailability. Peak plasma concentrations are reached within 3–6 h. The $t_{1/2}$ is 20–45 h. Steady state in plasma is achieved in 5–8 days. Plasma protein binding is 50% and is independent of concentration. Aliskiren is a substrate for P-glycoprotein, which contributes low bioavailability. Fatty meals significantly decrease the absorption of aliskiren. Hepatic metabolism by CYP3A4 is minimal. Elimination is mostly as unchanged drug in feces. About 25% of the absorbed dose appears in the urine as the parent drug.

Therapeutic Uses of Aliskiren

Therapeutic uses of aliskiren are discussed in Chapter 28.

Adverse Effects and Contraindications

Aliskiren is well tolerated, and adverse events are mild or comparable to placebo with no gender difference. Adverse effects include mild GI symptoms such as diarrhea at high doses (600 mg daily), abdominal pain, dyspepsia, and gastroesophageal reflux; headache; nasopharyngitis; dizziness; fatigue; upper respiratory tract infection; back pain; angioedema; and cough (much less common than with ACE inhibitors). Other adverse effects include rash, hypotension, hyperkalemia in diabetics on combination therapy, elevated uric acid, renal stones, and gout. Like other RAS inhibitors, aliskiren is not recommended in pregnancy.

Drug Interactions. Aliskiren does not interact with drugs that interact with CYPs. Aliskiren reduces absorption of furosemide by 50%. Irbesartan reduces the C_{max} of aliskiren by 50%. Aliskiren plasma levels are increased by drugs, such as ketoconazole, atorvastatin, and cyclosporine, that inhibit P-glycoprotein.

Effect of Pharmacological Blood Pressure Reduction on Function of the RAS

The RAS responds to alterations in blood pressure with compensatory changes (Figure 26–3). Thus, pharmacological agents that lower blood

Drug Facts for Your Personal Formulary: *Inhibitors of the RAS*

Drugs	Therapeutic Uses	Clinical Pharmacology and Tips
Angiotensin-Converting Enzyme Inhibitors • Inhibit the conversion of AngI to AngII		
Captopril Lisinopril Enalapril Benazepril Quinapril Ramipril Moexipril	• Inhibit AngII production, thus lowering arteriolar resistance • Hypertension • Acute myocardial infarction • Congestive heart failure • Diabetic nephropathy • Scleroderma renal crisis	• Antihypertensive effects potentiated by inhibition of ACE-catalyzed breakdown of bradykinin • Antihypertensive effects potentiated by increase in Ang(1–7) levels and activation of Ang(1–7)/Mas receptor pathway • Increase PRC and PRA • Adverse effects include cough in 5%–20% of patients, angioedema, hypotension, hyperkalemia, skin rash, neutropenia, anemia, fetopathic syndrome • Contraindicated in patients with renal artery stenosis and should be used with caution in patients with impaired renal function or hypovolemia • Should be stopped during pregnancy
Enalaprilat (IV)		• Intravenous administration
Fosinopril Trandolapril Perindopril		• Undergo both hepatic and renal elimination and should be used with caution in patients with renal or hepatic impairment
Angiotensin Receptor Blockers • Block AT$_1$ receptors		
Losartan Valsartan Eprosartan Irbesartan Candesartan Olmesartan Telmisartan Azilsartan	• Block the vasoconstrictor and profibrotic effects of AngII by inhibiting AT$_1$ receptors while permitting vasodilation through activation of AT$_2$ receptors • Hypertension • Congestive heart failure • Diabetic nephropathy	• Antihypertensive effects potentiated by activation of the AT$_2$ receptors • Antihypertensive effects potentiated by ACE2-dependent conversion of AngII to Ang(1–7) and activation of vasodilation via Ang(1–7)/Mas receptor pathway • Increase PRC and PRA • Adverse effects include hyperkalemia and hypotension • Contraindicated in patients with renal insufficiency • Should be stopped during pregnancy
Direct Renin Inhibitors • Inhibit renin and thus the conversion of angiotensinogen to AngI		
Aliskiren	• Decrease AngI and AngII levels • Hypertension	• Therapeutic value unclear; no evidence for superiority over ACEIs or ARBs • Increase PRC but decrease PRA • Contraindicated in diabetic nephropathy, pregnancy or renal insufficiency

pressure will alter the feedback loops that regulate the RAS and cause changes in the levels and activities of the system's components. These changes, summarized in Table 26–2, should be taken into account when interpreting laboratory evaluation of patients. Furthermore, during aliskiren treatment, the assay for PRA will be inhibited by persistence of aliskiren in this ex vivo reaction, whereas the renin concentration radioimmunoassay will not be inhibited.

Bibliography

ACE Inhibitor Myocardial Infarction Collaborative Group. Indications for ACE inhibitors in the early treatment of acute myocardial infarction: systematic overview of individual data from 100,000 patients in randomized trials. *Circulation*, **1998**, *97*:2202–2212.

Albiston AL, et al. Therapeutic targeting of insulin-regulated aminopeptidase: heads and tails? *Pharmacol Ther*, **2007**, *116*:417–427.

Álvarez R, et al. Angiotensin-converting enzyme and angiotensin II receptor 1 polymorphisms: association with early coronary disease. *Cardiovasc Res*, **1998**, *40*:375–379.

Binger KJ, Muller DN. Autopahgy and the (pro)renin receptor. *Front Endocrinol*, **2013**, *4*:155.

Bosnyak S, et al. Relative affinity of angiotensin peptides and novel ligands at AT$_1$ and AT$_2$ receptors. *Clin Sci* (Lond), **2011**, *121*:297–303.

Campbell DJ. Clinical relevance of local renin angiotensin systems. *Front Endocrinol*, **2014**, *5*:113.

Csajka C, et al. Pharmacokinetic–pharmacodynamic profile of angiotensin II receptor antagonists. *Clin Pharmacokinet*, **1997**, *32*:1–29.

Dahlöf B, et al., for the LIFE Study Group. Cardiovascular morbidity and mortality in the Losartan Intervention for Endpoint reduction in hypertension study (LIFE): a randomized trial against atenolol. *Lancet*, **2002**, *359*:995–1003.

Dell'Italia LJ. Translational success stories: angiotensin receptor 1 antagonists in heart failure. *Circ Res*, **2011**, *109*:437–452.

Etelvino GM, et al. New components of the renin-angiotensin system: alamandine and the MAS-related G protein coupled receptor D. *Curr Hypertens Rep*, **2014**, *16*:433.

EURopean trial On reduction of cardiac events with Perindopril in stable coronary Artery disease (EUROPA) Investigators. Efficacy of perindopril in reduction of cardiovascular events among patients with stable coronary artery disease: randomised, double-blind, placebo-controlled, multicentre trial (the EUROPA study). *Lancet*, **2003**, *362*:782–788.

Felker GM, et al. Heart failure therapeutics on the basis of a biased ligand of the angiotensin-2 type 1 receptor: rationale and design of the BLAST-AHF Study (Biased Ligand of the Angiotensin Receptor Study in Acute Heart Failure). *JACC Heart Fail*, **2015**, *3*:193–201.

Ferrario CM, et al. An evolving story of angiotensin-II-forming pathways in rodents and humans. *Clin Sci*, **2014**, *126*:461–469.

Fraga-Silva RA, et al. Opportunities for targeting the angiotensin-converting enzyme 2/angiotensin-(1–7)/Mas receptor pathway in hypertension. *Curr Hypertens Rep*, **2013**, *15*:31–38.

Gironacci MM, et al. Protective axis of the renin-angiotensin system in the brain. *Clin Sci*, **2014**, *127*:295–306.

Goupil E, et al. GPCR heterodimers: asymmetries in ligand binding and signaling output offer new targets for drug discovery. *Br J Pharmacol*, **2013**, *168*:1101–1103.

Guang C, et al. Three key proteases—angiotensin-I-converting enzyme (ACE), ACE2 and renin—within and beyond the renin-angiotensin system. *Arch Cardiovasc Dis*, **2012**, *105*:373–385.

Hadjadj S, et al. Prognostic value of angiotensin-I converting enzyme *I/D* polymorphism for nephropathy in type 1 diabetes mellitus: a prospective study. *J Am Soc Nephrol*, **2001**, *12*:541–549.

Heart Outcomes Prevention Study Investigators. Effects of an angiotensin-converting-enzyme inhibitor ramipril on cardiovascular events in high-risk patients. The Heart Outcomes Prevention Evaluation Study Investigators. *N Engl J Med*, **2000**, *342*:145–153 (published erratum appears in *N Engl J Med*, **2000**, *342*:478).

Jones E, Vinh A, et al. AT2 receptors: functional relevance in cardiovascular disease. *Pharmacol Ther*, **2008**, *120*:292–316.

Kaneshiro Y, et al. Slowly progressive, angiotensin II-independent glomerulosclerosis in human (pro)renin receptor-transgenic rats. *J Am Soc Nephrol*, **2007**, *18*:1789–1795.

Kim KS, et al. β-Arrestin-biased AT1R stimulation promotes cell survival during acute cardiac injury. *Am J Physiol Heart Circ Physiol*, **2012**, *303*:H1001–H1010.

Kobori H, Urushihara M. Augmented intrarenal and urinary angiotensinogen in hypertension and kidney disease. *Pflugers Arch*, **2013**, *465*:3–12.

Krämer C, et al. Angiotensin II receptor-independent antiinflammatory and angiaggregatory properties of losartan: role of the active metabolite EXP3179. *Circ Res*, **2002**, *90*:770–776.

Krum H, et al. Losing ALTITUDE? How should ASTRONAUT launch into ATMOSPHERE. *Eur J Heart Fail*, **2013**, *15*:1205–1207.

Kuba K, et al. Multiple functions of angiotensin-converting enzyme 2 and its relevance in cardiovascular diseases. *Circ J*, **2013**, *77*:301–308.

Lu X, et al. Identification of the (pro)renin receptor as a novel regulator of low-density lipoprotein metabolism. *Circ Res*, **2016**, *118*: 222–229.

Madrid AH, et al. Use of irbesartan to maintain sinus rhythm in patients with long-lasting persistent atrial fibrillation: a prospective and randomized study. *Circulation*, **2002**, *106*:331–336.

Makani H, et al. Efficacy and safety of dual blockade of the renin-angiotensin system: meta-analysis of randomized trials. *BMJ*, **2013**, *346*:1360.

Márquez E, et al. Renin-angiotensin system within the diabetic podocyte. *Am J Physiol Renal Physiol*, **2015**, *308*:1–10.

McMurray JJ, et al. Angiotensin-neprilysin inhibition versus enalapril in heart failure. *N Engl J Med*, **2014**, *371*:993–1004.

McMurray JJ, et al. Aliskiren, ALTITUDE, and the implications for ATMOSPHERE. *Eur J Heart Fail*, **2012**, *14*:341–343.

McMurray JJ, et al. Effects of the oral direct renin inhibitor aliskiren in patients with symptomatic heart failure. *Circ Heart Fail*, **2008**, *1*:17–24.

Mehta PK, Griendling KK. Angiotensin II cell signaling: physiological and pathological effects in the cardiovascular system. *Am J Physiol Cell Physiol*, **2007**, *292*:C82–C97.

Nguyen G. Renin and prorenin receptor in hypertension: what's new? *Curr Hypertens Rep*, **2011**, *13*:79–85.

Nguyen G, Danser AH. Prorenin and (pro)renin receptor: a review of available data from in vitro studies and experimental models in rodents. *Exp Physiol*, **2008**, *93*:557–563.

Nussberger J, et al. Angiotensin II suppression in humans by the orally active renin inhibitor aliskiren (SPP100): comparison with enalapril. *Hypertension*, **2002**, *39*:E1–E8.

Oh BH, et al. Aliskiren, an oral renin inhibitor, provides dose-dependent efficacy and sustained 24-hour blood pressure control in patients with hypertension. *J Am Coll Cardiol*, **2007**, *49*:1157–1163.

ONTARGET Investigators. Telmisartan, ramipril, or both in patients at high risk for vascular events. *N Engl J Med*, **2008**, *358*:1547–1559.

Oparil S, et al. Efficacy and safety of combined use of aliskiren and valsartan in patients with hypertension: a randomised, double-blind trial. *Lancet*, **2007**, *370*:221–229.

Oshima Y, et al. Roles of the (pro)renin receptor in the kidney. *World J Nephrol*, **2014**, *3*:302–307.

Padia SH, Carey RM. AT2 receptors: beneficial counter-regulatory role in cardiovascular and renal function. *Pflugers Arch*, **2013**, *465*:99–110.

Parving HH, et al., ALTITUDE Investigators. Cardiorenal end points in a trial of aliskiren for type 2 diabetes. *N Engl J Med*, **2012**, *367*:2204–2213.

Parving HH, et al. Aliskiren combined with losartan in type 2 diabetes and nephropathy. *N Engl J Med*, **2008**, *358*:2433–2246.

Paul M, et al. Physiology of local renin angiotensin systems. *Physiol Rev*, **2006**, *86*:747–803.

Perlman S, et al. Dual agonistic and antagonistic property of nonpeptide angiotensin AT$_1$ ligands: susceptibility to receptor mutations. *Mol Pharmacol*, **1997**, *51*:301–311.

Peti-Peterdi J, Harris RC. Macula densa sensing and signaling mechanisms of renin release. *J Am Soc Nephrol*, **2010**, *21*:1093–1096.

Pfeffer MA, et al., for the Valsartan in Acute Myocardial Infarction Trial Investigators. Valsartan, captopril, or both in myocardial infarction complicated by heart failure, left ventricular dysfunction, or both. *N Engl J Med*, **2003**, *349*:1893–1906.

Pitt B, et al., on behalf of the ELITE II investigators. Effect of losartan compared with captopril on mortality in patients with symptomatic heart failure: randomized trial—the Losartan Heart Failure Survival Study ELITE II. *Lancet*, **2000**, *355*:1582–1587.

Rhaleb N-E, et al. Long-term effect of *N*-acetyl-seryl-aspartyl-lysly-proline on left ventricular collagen deposition in rats with two-kidney, one-clip hypertension. *Circulation*, **2001**, *103*:3136–3141.

Ruggenenti P, et al. The RAAS in the pathogenesis and treatment of diabetic nephropathy. *Nat Rev Nephrol*, **2010**, *6*:319–330.

Sanoski CA. Aliskiren: an oral direct renin inhibitor for the treatment of hypertension. *Pharmacotherapy*, **2009**, *29*:193–212.

Santos RA. Angiotensin-(1–7). *Hypertension*, **2014**, *63*:1138–1134.

Sayed-Tabatabaei FA, et al. ACE polymorphisms. *Circ Res*, **2006**, *98*:1123–1133.

Schneider AW, et al. Effect of losartan, an angiotensin II receptor antagonist, on portal pressure in cirrhosis. *Hepatology*, **1999**, *29*:334–339.

Sethi AA, et al. Angiotensinogen single nucleotide polymorphisms, elevated blood pressure, and risk of cardiovascular disease. *Hypertension*, **2003**, *41*:1202–1211.

Solomon SD, et al. Effect of the direct renin inhibitor aliskiren, the angiotensin receptor blocker losartan, or both on left ventricular mass in patients with hypertension and left ventricular hypertrophy. *Circulation*, **2009**, *119*:530–537.

Solomon SD, et al. Effect of the direct renin inhibitor aliskiren on left ventricular remodelling following myocardial infarction with systolic dysfunction. *Eur Heart J*, **2011**, *32*:1227–1234.

Varagic J, et al. ACE2 AngiotenisnII/Angiotensin-(1–7) balance in cardiorenal injury. *Curr Hypertens Rep*, **2014**,*16*:420.

Wood JM, et al. Structure-based design of aliskiren, a novel orally effective renin inhibitor. *Biochem Biophys Res Commun,* **2003**, *308*:698–705.

Wright JW, et al. A role for the brain RAS in Alzheimer's and Parkinson's diseases. *Front Endocrinol*, **2013**,*4*:158.

Xia Y, Kellems RE. Angiotensin receptor agonistic autoantibodies and hypertension: preeclampsia and beyond. *Circ Res*, **2013**, *113*:78–87.

Yoshida et al. Molecular mechanisms and signaling pathways of angiotensin II-induced muscle wasting: potential therapeutic targets for cardiac cachexia. *Int J Biochem Cell Biol*, **2013**, *45*:2322–2232.

Chapter 27

Treatment of Ischemic Heart Disease

Thomas Eschenhagen

Pathophysiology of Ischemic Heart Disease

The pathophysiological understanding of ischemic heart disease has seen major changes over the past two decades—from a concept of localized calcification causing progressive constrictions of coronary arteries, ischemia, and exercise-induced angina pectoris to a systemic inflammatory disease of the arteries, including the coronaries (therefore the CAD name). A key finding in this change of paradigm was that most infarct-causing occlusions occur at small-to-medium plaques ("active plaques") by thrombosis rather than at hemodynamically relevant stenoses by progressive narrowing. Thus, in addition to the mere size of an obstructing plaque, the inflammatory activity of the atherosclerotic process, the stability of the plaque, and platelet reactivity appear to determine the prognosis (Libby et al., 2002).

Atherosclerosis encompasses increased lipid deposition in the subendothelial space (early plaque), endothelial dysfunction with decreased production of NO, less vasodilation and increased risk of platelet adhesion, influx of lipid scavenger cells (mainly macrophages), necrosis, sterile inflammation, proliferation of smooth muscle cells, and calcification and narrowing of the blood vessel by increasing plaque formation. If the endothelium covering of the plaque or the cell layer enclosing the necrotic core of the plaque disrupt, thrombogenic materials such as collagen are presented to the bloodstream, causing platelet adhesion, fibrin deposition, thrombus formation, and closure of the blood vessel.

Triggering factors can be not only acute inflammation (e.g., influenza), but also blood pressure peaks during physical exercise or emotional stress (e.g., demonstrated during a life-threatening emergency and in avid fans during football games). Importantly, the process is dynamic, and the net thrombus formation is the result of the balance between thrombosis and thrombolysis by the fibrinolytic system (plasminogen). The degree and the duration of coronary obstruction and thereby of the ischemia of downstream myocardium (and its size) determine the degree of necrosis of muscle tissue, that is, infarct size.

Taken together, important factors that determine the progress of CAD are the concentration of lipids in the blood, endothelial function, blood pressure (as a mechanical factor predisposing to plaque rupture), the activity of the inflammatory system, and the reactivity of pro- and antithrombotic systems. Patients with CAD should be advised not only to exercise regularly, stop smoking, and have blood pressure and body weight well controlled, but also to be treated with statins, aspirin, and β adrenergic receptor antagonists (β blockers) and have annual vaccinations

against influenza. The widespread implementation of this combination drug regimen and the considerably improved treatment of ACSs likely account for the continuous reduction in MIs and age-corrected cardiovascular lethality in Western countries (−42% between 2000 and 2011; Mozaffarian et al., 2015). Interestingly, the incidence of the classical large STEMI is declining as that of smaller non-STEMI increases. This raises the hypothesis that the dominant pathogenesis of acute coronary thrombosis may have changed from the rupture of lipid-rich, inflammatory plaques (in the prestatin era) to the erosion of stable plaques (Libby and Pasterkamp, 2015).

Antiplatelet agents, fibrinolytic drugs, anticoagulants, and statins (HMG-CoA reductase inhibitors) are systematically discussed in Chapters 32 and 33. This chapter concentrates on pharmacotherapy for angina pectoris and myocardial ischemia.

Pathophysiology of Angina Pectoris

Angina pectoris, the primary symptom of ischemic heart disease, is caused by transient episodes of myocardial ischemia that are due to an imbalance in the myocardial oxygen supply-demand relationship. This imbalance may be caused by an increase in myocardial oxygen demand (which is determined by heart rate, ventricular contractility, and ventricular wall tension) or by a decrease in myocardial oxygen supply (primarily determined by coronary blood flow, but occasionally modified by the oxygen-carrying capacity of the blood), or sometimes by both (Figure 27–1). Because blood flow is inversely proportional to the fourth power of the artery's luminal radius, the progressive decrease in vessel radius that characterizes coronary atherosclerosis can impair coronary blood flow and lead to symptoms of angina when myocardial O_2 demand increases, as with exertion (the so-called typical and most prevalent form of angina pectoris). In some patients, anginal symptoms may occur without any increase in myocardial O_2 demand, but rather as a consequence of an abrupt reduction in blood flow, as might result from coronary thrombosis (unstable angina or ACS) or localized vasospasm (variant or Prinzmetal angina). Regardless of the precipitating factors, the sensation of angina is similar in most patients. Typical angina is experienced as a heavy, pressing substernal discomfort (rarely described as a "pain"), often radiating to the left shoulder, flexor aspect of the left arm, jaw, or epigastrium. However, a significant minority of patients note discomfort in a different location or of a different character. Women, the elderly, and diabetics are more

Abbreviations

ACE: angiotensin-converting enzyme
ACEI: angiotensin-converting enzyme inhibitor
ACS: acute coronary syndrome
ALDH2: mitochondrial aldehyde dehydrogenase
ARB: angiotensin receptor blocker
AV: atrioventricular
CABG: coronary artery bypass grafting
CAD: coronary artery disease
COX-1: cyclooxygenase isoform 1
CYP: cytochrome P450
EC$_{50}$: half-maximal effective concentration
EMA: European Medicines Agency
eNOS: endothelial NOS
FDA: U.S. Food and Drug Administration
FFA: free fatty acid
GI: gastrointestinal
GTN: glyceryl trinitrate (nitroglycerin)
HCM: hypertrophic cardiomyopathy
HCN: hyperpolarization-activated cyclic nucleotide–gated
HMG-CoA: 3-hydroxy-3-methylglutaryl coenzyme A
iNOS: inducible NOS
IP$_3$: inositol 1,4,5-trisphosphate
ISDN: isosorbide dinitrate
ISMN: isosorbide-5-mononitrate
MI: myocardial infarction
nNOS: neuronal NOS
NO: nitric oxide
NOS: nitric oxide synthase
NSTEMI: non–ST-elevation myocardial infarction
PDE: cyclic nucleotide phosphodiesterase
Pgp: P-glycoprotein
PLC: phospholipase C
rTPA: recombinant tissue plasminogen activator
SA: sinoatrial
SNS: sympathetic nervous system
STEMI: ST-segment elevation myocardial infarction
Tn: troponin
TxA$_2$: thromboxane A$_2$

pattern over many years or may become unstable, increasing in frequency or severity and even occurring at rest. In typical stable angina, the pathological substrate is usually fixed atherosclerotic narrowing of an epicardial coronary artery, on which exertion or emotional stress superimposes an increase in myocardial O$_2$ demand. In variant angina, focal or diffuse coronary vasospasm episodically reduces coronary flow. Patients also may display a mixed pattern of angina with the addition of altered vessel tone on a background of atherosclerotic narrowing. In most patients with unstable angina, rupture of an atherosclerotic plaque, with consequent platelet adhesion and aggregation, decreases coronary blood flow. Superimposed thrombosis may lead to the complete abrogation of blood flow. Atherosclerotic plaques with thinner fibrous caps appear to be more "vulnerable" to rupture.

Myocardial ischemia also may be *silent*, with electrocardiographic, echocardiographic, or radionuclide evidence of ischemia appearing in the absence of symptoms. While some patients have only silent ischemia, most patients who have silent ischemia have symptomatic episodes as well. The precipitants of silent ischemia appear to be the same as those of symptomatic ischemia. We now know that the *ischemic burden* (i.e., the total time a patient is ischemic each day) is greater in many patients than was recognized previously. In most trials, the agents that are efficacious in typical angina also are efficacious in reducing silent ischemia. β Blockers appear to be more effective than the Ca^{2+} channel blockers in the prevention of episodes. Therapy directed at abolishing all silent ischemia has not been shown to be of additional benefit over conventional therapy.

Pharmacotherapy of Ischemic Heart Disease

The principal pharmacological agents used in the treatment of angina are nitrovasodilators, β blockers (see Chapter 12), and Ca^{2+} channel blockers. In patients with typical exercise-induced angina on the basis of CAD, these antianginal agents improve the balance of myocardial O$_2$ supply and O$_2$ demand principally by reducing myocardial O$_2$ demand by decreasing heart rate, myocardial contractility, or ventricular wall stress. Increased O$_2$ supply by dilating the coronary vasculature may play an additional role and is the major effect of nitrovasodilators and Ca^{2+} channel blockers in variant angina.

By contrast, the principal therapeutic goal in ACSs with unstable angina is to prevent or reduce coronary thrombus formation and increase myocardial blood flow; strategies include the use of antiplatelet agents and *heparin*, often accompanied by efforts to restore flow by mechanical means, including percutaneous coronary interventions using coronary stents, or (less commonly) emergency coronary bypass surgery. The principal therapeutic aim in variant or Prinzmetal angina is to prevent coronary vasospasm.

Antianginal agents may provide prophylactic or symptomatic treatment, but β blockers also reduce mortality, apparently by decreasing the incidence of sudden cardiac death associated with myocardial ischemia and infarction. The chronic use of organic nitrate vasodilators, which are highly efficacious in treatment of angina, is not associated with

likely to experience myocardial ischemia with atypical symptoms. In most patients with typical angina, whose symptoms are provoked by exertion, the symptoms are relieved by rest or by administration of sublingual nitroglycerin.

Angina pectoris is a common symptom, affecting 8 million Americans (Mozaffarian et al., 2015). Angina pectoris may occur in a stable

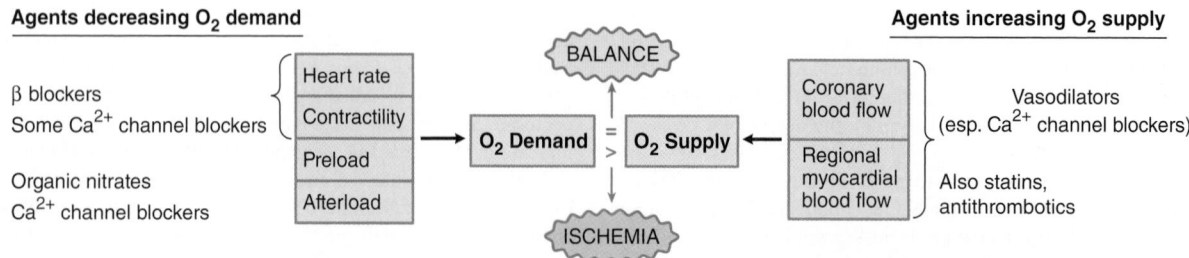

Figure 27–1 *Pharmacological modification of the major determinants of myocardial O$_2$ supply.* When myocardial O$_2$ requirements exceed O$_2$ supply, an ischemic episode results. This figure shows the primary hemodynamic sites of action of pharmacological agents that can reduce O$_2$ demand (left side) or enhance O$_2$ supply (right side). Some classes of agents have multiple effects. Stents, angioplasty, and coronary bypass surgery are mechanical interventions that increase O$_2$ supply. Both pharmacotherapy and mechanotherapy attempt to restore a dynamic balance between O$_2$ demand and O$_2$ supply.

improvements in cardiac mortality, and some investigators have suggested that chronic use of nitroglycerin may have adverse cardiovascular effects (Parker, 2004).

Besides symptomatic relief from angina pain conferred by antianginal drugs, patients with CAD should be treated with drugs that can reduce the progression of atherosclerosis and reduce the risk of coronary thrombosis and MI. *Aspirin* is used routinely in patients with myocardial ischemia, and daily aspirin at low doses reduces the incidence of clinical events (Fihn et al., 2012). The optimal dose appears to be between 75 and 150 mg/d (Montalescot et al., 2013), although most large studies have been done with a 325-mg dose. The oral ADP receptor antagonist clopidogrel was slightly superior to aspirin in patients with chronic atherosclerotic vascular disease and had a favorable safety profile (CAPRIE Steering Committee, 1996). When used in combination with aspirin in patients with ACS, clopidogrel reduced the cardiovascular death rate by 20%, but increased the incidence of major bleeding events by 38% (Yusuf et al., 2001). In patients with stable cardiovascular disease, clopidogrel conferred no benefit over aspirin and was associated with signs of harm in patients with multiple risk factors (Bhatt et al., 2006). Guidelines therefore recommend clopidogrel only as an alternative in patients with aspirin intolerance and advise against the routine use of dual platelet inhibition in patients with stable disease (Fihn et al., 2012; Montalescot et al., 2013). In contrast, dual platelet inhibition is routinely given in patients who underwent coronary artery stenting. The recommended time (1–12 months) varies depending on the intervention (e.g., bare metal vs. drug-eluting stent) and the risk profile of patients. The newer ADP receptor antagonists prasugrel and ticagrelor have a more useful pharmacokinetic profile and seem to have a better benefit/risk ratio than clopidogrel in the postintervention treatment phase (Cannon et al., 2010; Wiviott et al., 2007) but are not generally recommended as alternatives to clopidogrel in patients with stable CAD. Statins reduce mortality in patients with CAD. Although high-risk patients (including those with high plasma LDL cholesterol levels) have the greatest absolute benefit, the relative risk reduction of approximately 25% appears largely independent of baseline cholesterol blood levels. Statins should therefore be given to all patients with CAD. It is unclear whether ACEIs or angiotensin receptor blockers (see Chapter 26) reduce mortality or other end points in patients with CAD when given routinely in addition to aspirin, statins, and β blockers, but they are recommended for subgroups of patients with CAD with reduced left ventricular systolic function, hypertension, diabetes, or chronic kidney disease (Montalescot et al., 2013).

Coronary artery bypass surgery and percutaneous coronary interventions such as angioplasty and coronary artery stent deployment commonly complement pharmacological treatment. In some subsets of patients, percutaneous or surgical revascularization may have a survival advantage over medical treatment alone (Kappetein et al., 2011). Intracoronary drug delivery using drug-eluting coronary stents represents an intersection of mechanical and pharmacological approaches in the treatment of CAD.

Organic Nitrates

The organic nitrate agents are prodrugs that are sources of NO. NO activates the soluble isoform of guanylyl cyclase, thereby increasing intracellular levels of cGMP. In turn, cGMP promotes the dephosphorylation of the myosin light chain and the reduction of cytosolic Ca^{2+} and leads to the relaxation of smooth muscle cells in a broad range of tissues (see Figures 3-13, 3-17, and 44-7). The NO-dependent relaxation of vascular smooth muscle leads to vasodilation; NO-mediated guanylyl cyclase activation also inhibits platelet aggregation and relaxes smooth muscle in the bronchi and GI tract.

The broad biological response to nitrovasodilators reflects the existence of endogenous NO-modulated regulatory pathways. The endogenous synthesis of NO in humans is catalyzed by a family of NOSs that oxidize the amino acid L-arginine to form NO, plus L-citrulline as a coproduct. There are three distinct mammalian NOS isoforms: *nNOS*, *eNOS*, and *iNOS* (see Chapter 3), and they are involved in processes as diverse as neurotransmission, vasomotion, and immunomodulation. In several vascular disease

states, pathways of endogenous NO-dependent regulation appear to be deranged (reviewed in [Dudzinski et al., 2006]).

HISTORICAL PERSPECTIVE

Nitroglycerin was first synthesized in 1846 by Sobrero, who observed that a small quantity placed on the tongue elicited a severe headache. The explosive properties of nitroglycerin also were soon noted, and control of this unstable compound for military and industrial use was not realized until Alfred Nobel devised a process to stabilize the nitroglycerin and patented a specialized detonator in 1863. The vast fortune that Nobel accrued from the nitroglycerin detonator patent provided the funds later used to establish the Nobel prizes. In 1857, T. Lauder Brunton of Edinburgh (no relation to the editor of this volume) administered *amyl nitrite*, a known vasodepressor, by inhalation and noted that anginal pain was relieved within 30–60 sec. The action of amyl nitrite was transitory, however, and the dosage was difficult to adjust. Subsequently, William Murrell surmised that the action of nitroglycerin mimicked that of amyl nitrite and established the use of sublingual nitroglycerin for relief of the acute anginal attack and as a prophylactic agent to be taken prior to exertion. The empirical observation that organic nitrates could dramatically and safely alleviate the symptoms of angina pectoris led to their widespread acceptance by the medical profession. Indeed, Alfred Nobel himself was prescribed nitroglycerin by his physicians when he developed angina in 1890. Basic investigations defined the role of NO in both the vasodilation produced by nitrates and endogenous vasodilation. The importance of NO as a signaling molecule in the cardiovascular system and elsewhere was recognized by the awarding of the 1998 Nobel Prize in Medicine/Physiology to the pharmacologists Robert Furchgott, Louis Ignarro, and Ferid Murad.

Chemistry

Organic nitrates are polyol esters of nitric acid, whereas organic nitrites are esters of nitrous acid (Table 27–1). Nitrate esters ($-C-O-NO_2$) and nitrite esters ($-C-O-NO$) are characterized by a sequence of carbon-oxygen-nitrogen, whereas nitro compounds possess carbon-nitrogen bonds ($C-NO_2$). Thus, GTN is not a nitro compound, and it is erroneously called nitroglycerin; however, this nomenclature is both widespread and official. Amyl nitrite is a highly volatile liquid that must be administered by inhalation and is of limited therapeutic utility. Organic nitrates of low molecular mass (such as GTN) are moderately volatile, oily liquids, whereas the high-molecular-mass nitrate esters (e.g., erythrityl tetranitrate, ISDN, and isosorbide mononitrate) are solids. In the pure form (without an inert carrier such as lactose), nitroglycerin is explosive. The organic nitrates and nitrites, collectively termed *nitrovasodilators*, must be metabolized (reduced) to produce gaseous NO, which appears to be the active principle of this class of compounds. NO gas also can be directly administered by inhalation.

Pharmacological Properties

Mechanism of Action. Nitrites, organic nitrates, nitroso compounds, and a variety of other nitrogen oxide–containing substances (including *nitroprusside;* see further in the chapter) lead to the formation of the reactive gaseous free radical NO and related NO-containing compounds. NO gas also may be administered by inhalation. Surprisingly, more than 140 years after its introduction in the therapy of angina pectoris, the mode of action of organic nitrates is still incompletely understood (Mayer and Beretta, 2008). Established mechanisms of GTN bioactivation and action include a nonenzymatic reaction with L-cysteine, formation of nitrite and NO by ALDH2 (Chen et al., 2002), activation of soluble guanylyl cyclase, and generation of cGMP. The bioactivation of other nitrovasodilators such as ISDN and ISMN is ALDH2 independent, suggesting the involvement of other enzymes, such as CYPs, xanthine oxidoreductase, and cytosolic ALDH isoforms (Munzel et al., 2014). The action of NO on soluble

TABLE 27–1 ■ ORGANIC NITRATES AVAILABLE FOR CLINICAL USE

AGENT	PREPARATIONS, DOSES, ADMINISTRATION[a]	
Nitroglycerin (glyceryl trinitrate)	T: 0.3–0.6 mg as needed	O: 2.5–5 cm, topically every 4–8 h
	S: 0.4 mg per spray as needed	D: 1 disk (2.5–15 mg) for 12–16 h/d
	C: 2.5–9 mg 2–4 times daily	IV: 10–20 μg/min; ↑ 10 μg/min to max of 400 μg/min
	B: 1 mg every 3–5 h	
Isosorbide dinitrate	T: 2.5–10 mg every 2–3 h	T(O): 5–40 mg every 8 h
	T(C): 5–10 mg every 2–3 h	C: 40–80 mg every 12 h
Isosorbide-5-mononitrate	T: 10–40 mg twice daily	C: 60–120 mg daily

Nitroglycerin (glyceryl trinitrate, GTN)

Isosorbide dinitrate (ISDN)

Isosorbide-5-mononitrate (ISMN)

[a]B, buccal (transmucosal) tablet; C, sustained-release capsule or tablet; D, transdermal disk or patch; IV, intravenous injection; O, ointment; S, lingual spray; T, tablet for sublingual use; T(C), chewable tablet; T(O), oral tablet or capsule.

guanylyl cyclase seems to be elicited in substantial part by S-nitrosothiol. The different ALDH2 dependence of GTN and ISDN is clinically relevant because individuals of Asian origin carry an inactive ALDH2 variant and do not respond adequately to GTN but do respond to ISDN (Stamler, 2008).

The NO-stimulated elevation of cGMP activates PKG and modulates the activities of cyclic nucleotide PDEs (PDEs 2, 3, and 5) in a variety of cell types. In smooth muscle, the net result is reduced phosphorylation of myosin light chain, reduced Ca^{2+} concentration in the cytosol, and relaxation (Figure 44–7). Reduced phosphorylation of myosin light chain is the result of decreased myosin light-chain kinase activity and increased myosin light-chain phosphatase activity and promotes vasorelaxation and smooth muscle relaxation in many tissues. cGMP is a substrate for PDE 5, whose inhibition by sildenafil and related compounds potentiates the action of nitrovasodilators (see *Toxicity and Untoward Responses*).

Hemodynamic Effects. The nitrovasodilators promote relaxation of vascular smooth muscle. For reasons not understood, GTN dilates large blood vessels (>200-μm diameter) more potently than small vessels, explaining why low doses of GTN preferentially dilate veins and conductance arteries and leave the tone of the small-to-medium arterioles (that regulate resistance) unaffected. This profile has important consequences for the antianginal efficacy of nitrovasodilators. At low-to-medium doses, preferential venodilation decreases venous return, leading to a fall in left and right ventricular chamber size and end-diastolic pressures, reduced wall stress, and thereby reduced cardiac O_2 demand (see discussion that follows). Systemic vascular resistance and arterial pressure are not or only mildly decreased, leaving coronary perfusion pressure unaffected. Heart rate remains unchanged or may increase slightly in response to a decrease in blood pressure. Pulmonary vascular resistance and cardiac output are slightly reduced. Doses of GTN that do not alter systemic arterial pressure may still produce arteriolar dilation in the face and neck, resulting in a facial flush, or dilation of meningeal arterial vessels, causing headache.

Higher doses of organic nitrates cause further venous pooling and may decrease arteriolar resistance as well, thereby decreasing systolic and diastolic blood pressure and causing pallor, weakness, dizziness, and activation of compensatory sympathetic reflexes. This can happen to such an extent that coronary flow is compromised, and the sympathetic increase in myocardial O_2 demand overrides the beneficial action of the nitrovasodilators, leading to ischemia. In addition, sublingual nitroglycerin administration may produce bradycardia and hypotension, probably owing to activation of the Bezold-Jarisch reflex.

In patients with autonomic dysfunction and an inability to increase sympathetic outflow (multiple-system atrophy and pure autonomic failure are the most common forms, much less commonly seen in the autonomic dysfunction associated with diabetes), the fall in blood pressure consequent to the venodilation produced by nitrates cannot be compensated. In these clinical contexts, nitrates may reduce arterial pressure and coronary perfusion pressure significantly, producing potentially life-threatening hypotension and even aggravating angina.

ADME. As outlined previously, nitrovasodilators differ in their dependence on ALDH2 for bioactivation (note ALDH2 deficiency in many Asians). In addition, their pharmacokinetic profiles exhibit therapeutically relevant differences in sublingual resorption, onset of action, and half-life (Table 27–1).

Nitroglycerin. Peak concentrations of GTN are found in plasma within 4 min of sublingual administration; the drug has a $t_{1/2}$ of 1–3 min. The onset of action of GTN may be even more rapid if delivered as a sublingual spray rather than as a sublingual tablet. Glyceryl dinitrate metabolites, which have about one-tenth the vasodilator potency, appear to have half-lives of about 40 min.

Isosorbide Dinitrate. Sublingual administration of ISDN produces maximal plasma concentrations of the drug by 6 min, and the fall in concentration is rapid ($t_{1/2}$ of about 45 min). The primary initial metabolites, isosorbide-2-mononitrate and ISMN, have longer half-lives (3–6 h) and are presumed to contribute to the therapeutic efficacy of the drug. ISDN is therefore suitable both for standby and sustained therapy.

Isosorbide-5-Mononitrate. This agent is available in tablet form. ISMN does not undergo significant first-pass metabolism, so it has high bioavailability after oral administration, but its onset of action is too slow for acute treatment of angina.

Inhaled NO. Nitric oxide gas administered by inhalation appears to exert most of its therapeutic effects on the pulmonary vasculature because of the rapid inactivation of NO by hemoglobin in the blood. It is approved for the treatment of pulmonary hypertension in hypoxemic neonates, where it reduced morbidity and mortality (Bloch et al., 2007), and is currently tested in patients with pulmonary arterial hypertension.

Mechanisms of Antianginal Efficacy of Organic Nitrates

When GTN is injected directly into the coronary circulation of patients with CAD, anginal attacks (induced by electrical pacing) are not aborted even when coronary blood flow is increased. In contrast, sublingual administration of GTN does relieve anginal pain in the same patients, indicating that the major antianginal effect of nitrovasodilators is mediated by preload reduction rather than coronary artery dilation.

This interpretation is supported by studies in exercising patients showing that angina occurs at the same value of the *triple product* (Aortic pressure × Heart rate × Ejection time, which is roughly proportional to myocardial consumption of O_2) with or without nitroglycerin. Thus, the beneficial effect of nitroglycerin has to result from reduced cardiac O_2 demand rather than an increase in the delivery of O_2 to ischemic regions of myocardium. However, these results do not preclude the possibility that a favorable redistribution of blood flow to ischemic subendocardial myocardium may contribute to relief of pain in a typical anginal attack, and they do not preclude the possibility that direct coronary vasodilation may be the major effect of nitroglycerin in situations where vasospasm compromises myocardial blood flow.

Effects on Myocardial O_2 Requirements.
The major determinants of myocardial O_2 consumption are left ventricular wall tension, heart rate, and myocardial contractility (Figure 27–1). Ventricular wall tension is affected by preload and afterload. *Preload* is determined by the diastolic pressure that distends the ventricle (ventricular end-diastolic pressure). Increasing end-diastolic volume augments the ventricular wall tension (by the law of Laplace, tension is proportional to pressure times radius). Increasing venous capacitance with nitrates decreases venous return to the heart, decreases ventricular end-diastolic volume, and thereby decreases O_2 consumption. An additional benefit of reducing preload is that it increases the pressure gradient for perfusion across the ventricular wall, which favors subendocardial perfusion. *Afterload* is the impedance against which the ventricle must eject. In the absence of aortic valvular disease, afterload is related to peripheral resistance. Decreasing peripheral arteriolar resistance reduces afterload and thus myocardial work and O_2 consumption. The distensibility of the large conductance arteries such as the aorta may play an additional role.

Nitrovasodilators preferentially decrease preload by dilating venous capacitance vessels. The decrease in afterload is generally small and mainly observed at higher doses. The effect on aortic stiffness appears complex (Soma et al., 2000). NO and nitrovasodilators can directly modulate the inotropic or chronotropic state of the heart via cGMP and its stimulatory effect on PDE2 (thereby reducing cAMP) or an inhibitory effect on the cAMP-specific PDE3 (thereby increasing cAMP). An inotropic response depends on the extent to which the PDE isoforms are expressed in the appropriate cells and in the proper subcellular compartment (Steinberg and Brunton, 2001). Small NO concentrations favor a positive inotropic effect (Kojda et al., 1997); however, the effect size is small and its significance unclear. Because nitrates affect several of the primary determinants of myocardial O_2 demand, their net effect usually is to decrease myocardial O_2 consumption. In addition, an improvement in the lusitropic state of the heart may be seen with more rapid early diastolic filling. This may be secondary to the relief of ischemia rather than primary, or it may be due to a reflex increase in sympathetic activity. Nitrovasodilators also increase cGMP in platelets, with consequent inhibition of platelet function. While this may contribute to their antianginal efficacy, the effect appears to be modest and in some settings may be confounded by the potential of nitrates to alter the pharmacokinetics of heparin, reducing its antithrombotic effect.

Effects on Total and Regional Coronary Blood Flow.
When considering the effect of vasodilators in the ischemic heart, it is important to realize that myocardial ischemia itself is a powerful stimulus to coronary vasodilation and part of an autoregulatory mechanism. In the presence of atherosclerotic coronary artery narrowing, ischemia distal to the lesion stimulates vasodilation of downstream resistance arterioles and thereby helps maintain adequate perfusion of the ischemic area under rest. If the stenosis is severe, much of the capacity to dilate is used to maintain resting

blood flow. Further dilation may not be possible, neither under exercise nor with therapeutically applied vasodilators. In contrast, nonselective vasodilators such as adenosine or dipyridamole (which inhibits adenosine transmembrane transport and thereby increases extracellular concentrations) can worsen the perfusion of ischemic areas by dilating the relatively constricted arterioles of the healthy myocardium, leading to redistribution of blood flow away from the ischemic myocardium ("steal phenomenon"). Accordingly, dipyridamole is not used therapeutically but can be used as a stress test to provoke angina pectoris (Bodi et al., 2007).

Nitrovasodilators, in contrast, do not have a major effect on the smaller resistance arteries (and therefore do not cause steal phenomena) but can dilate the large, epicardial sections of the coronary arteries upstream of a stenosis and also in a stenosis (concept of the "dynamic stenosis"; Brown et al., 1981) and thereby increase blood flow distal to the narrowing. Collateral flow to ischemic regions also is increased. As outlined previously, GTN also reduces wall stress that opposes blood flow to the subendocardium, which is particularly sensitive to ischemia.

In patients with angina owing to coronary artery spasm, the capacity of nitrovasodilators to dilate epicardial coronary arteries, particularly regions affected by spasm, is the primary mechanism of their beneficial effect.

Other Effects.
The nitrovasodilators also relax smooth muscles of the bronchial tract, the gallbladder, biliary ducts, and sphincter of Oddi and the GI tract. Spontaneous motility decreased by nitrates both in vivo *and* in vitro. The effect may be transient and incomplete in vivo, but abnormal "spasm" frequently is reduced. Indeed, many incidences of atypical chest pain and "angina" are due to biliary or esophageal spasm, and these also can be relieved by nitrates. Nitrates can also relax ureteral and uterine smooth muscle, but these responses are of uncertain clinical significance.

Tolerance

Frequently repeated or continuous exposure to high doses of nitrovasodilators lead to tolerance, that is, marked attenuation in the magnitude of most of their pharmacological effects. The magnitude of tolerance is a function of dosage and frequency of use. Tolerance may result from a reduced capacity of the vascular smooth muscle to convert nitroglycerin to NO, *true vascular tolerance*, or to the activation of mechanisms extraneous to the vessel wall, *pseudotolerance* (Munzel et al., 1995). Multiple mechanisms have been proposed to account for nitrate tolerance, including volume expansion, neurohumoral activation, cellular depletion of sulfhydryl groups, and the generation of free radicals (Parker and Parker, 1998). A reactive intermediate formed during the generation of NO from organic nitrates may itself damage and inactivate the enzymes of the activation pathway (Munzel et al., 1995; Parker, 2004). Inactivation of ALDH2 (Sydow et al., 2004) and S-nitrosylation of soluble guanylyl cyclase (Sayed et al., 2008) are seen in models of nitrate tolerance and could explain cross-tolerance to different (nitro)vasodilators. Other changes observed in the setting of nitroglycerin tolerance include an enhanced response to vasoconstrictors such as angiotensin II, serotonin, and phenylephrine. Prolonged administration of GTN is associated with plasma volume expansion, which may be reflected by a decrease in hematocrit. Unfortunately, attempts to prevent nitrate tolerance based on these mechanisms (e.g., antioxidants, coapplication of vasodilators or diuretics) failed in clinical trials.

A clinically important lesson of research on nitrate tolerance is that prolonged treatment with nitrates may not only induce a loss of response to nitrates, but also actually decrease angina threshold in the interval (Parker et al., 1995). A special form of GTN tolerance is observed in individuals exposed to GTN in the manufacture of explosives. If protection is inadequate, workers may experience severe headaches, dizziness, and postural weakness during the first several days of employment ("Monday disease"). Tolerance then develops and can lead to organic nitrate dependence. Workers without demonstrable organic vascular disease have been reported to have an increase in the incidence of ACSs during the 24- to 72-h periods away from the work environment. It seems prudent not to withdraw nitrates abruptly from a patient who has received such therapy chronically.

Therapy should be designed to prevent tolerance. High doses should be avoided and therapy interrupted for 8–12 h daily, which allows the return of efficacy. In patients with exertional angina, it is usually most convenient to omit dosing at night either by adjusting dosing intervals of oral or buccal preparations or by removing cutaneous GTN. Patients whose anginal pattern suggests its precipitation by increased left ventricular filling pressures (e.g., in association with orthopnea or paroxysmal nocturnal dyspnea) may benefit from continuing nitrates at night and omitting them during a quiet period of the day. Some patients develop an increased frequency of nocturnal angina when a nitrate-free interval is employed using GTN patches; such patients may require another class of antianginal agent during this period. Continuous intravenous administration of GTN regularly induces tolerance and should therefore be avoided. Tolerance also has been seen with ISMN and ISDN; an eccentric twice-daily dosing schedule appears to maintain efficacy (Parker and Parker, 1998). Molsidomine, a direct NO donor, is approved in many European countries and is claimed to induce less tolerance than the organic nitrates, but the supporting evidence is weak. A recent study failed to demonstrate beneficial effects of molsidomine on endothelial dysfunction (Barbato et al., 2015).

Toxicity and Untoward Responses

Untoward responses to the therapeutic use of organic nitrates are almost all secondary to actions on the cardiovascular system. Headache is common and can be severe, usually decreasing over a few days if treatment is continued and often controlled by decreasing the dose. Transient episodes of dizziness, weakness, and other manifestations associated with postural hypotension may develop, particularly if the patient is standing immobile, and may progress occasionally to loss of consciousness, a reaction that appears to be accentuated by alcohol. It also may be seen with very low doses of nitrates in patients with autonomic dysfunction. Even in severe nitrate syncope, positioning and other measures that facilitate venous return are the only therapeutic measures required. All the organic nitrates occasionally can produce drug rash.

Interaction of Nitrates With PDE5 Inhibitors. Erectile dysfunction is a frequently encountered problem whose risk factors parallel those of CAD. Thus, many men desiring therapy for erectile dysfunction already may be receiving (or may require, especially if they increase physical activity) antianginal therapy. The combination of sildenafil and other PDE5 inhibitors with organic nitrate vasodilators can cause extreme hypotension.

Cells in the corpus cavernosum produce NO during sexual arousal in response to nonadrenergic, noncholinergic neurotransmission (Burnett et al., 1992). NO stimulates the formation of cGMP, which leads to relaxation of smooth muscle of penile arteries that fill the corpus cavernosum, leading to engorgement of the corpus cavernosum and erection. The accumulation of cGMP is enhanced by inhibition of the cGMP-specific PDE5 family. Sildenafil and congeners inhibit PDE5 and have been demonstrated to improve erectile function in patients with erectile dysfunction. Not surprisingly, PDE5 inhibitors have assumed the status of widely used recreational drugs. Sildenafil is also FDA and EMA approved in patients with pulmonary arterial hypertension in whom the drug decreased pulmonary vascular resistance and enhanced exercise capacity. PDE5 inhibitors also are being studied in patients with congestive heart failure, but a recent trial in patients with preserved ejection fraction failed (Redfield et al., 2013; Chapter 28). Tadalafil and vardenafil share similar therapeutic efficacy and side-effect profiles with sildenafil; tadalafil has a longer time to onset of action and a longer therapeutic $t_{1/2}$ than the other PDE5 inhibitors (Table 45–1). Sildenafil has been the most thoroughly characterized of these compounds, but all three PDE5 inhibitors are contraindicated for patients taking organic nitrate vasodilators, and the PDE5 inhibitors should be used with caution in patients taking α- or β blockers (see Chapter 12).

The side effects of sildenafil and other PDE5 inhibitors are largely predictable on the basis of their effects on PDE5. Headache, flushing, and rhinitis may be observed, as well as dyspepsia owing to relaxation of the lower esophageal sphincter. Sildenafil and vardenafil also weakly inhibit PDE6, the enzyme involved in photoreceptor signal transduction (Figure 69–9), and can produce visual disturbances, most notably changes in the perception of color hue or brightness. In addition to visual disturbances, sudden one-sided hearing loss has also been reported. Tadalafil inhibits PDE11, a widely distributed PDE isoform, but the clinical importance of this effect is not clear. The most important toxicity of all these PDE5 inhibitors is hemodynamic. When given alone to men with severe CAD, these drugs induce only a modest (<10%) decrease of blood pressure (Herrmann et al., 2000). However, PDE5 inhibitors and nitrates act synergistically to cause profound increases in cGMP and dramatic reductions in blood pressure (>25 mm Hg). *PDE5 inhibitors should therefore not be prescribed to patients receiving any form of nitrate* (Cheitlin et al., 1999); in prescribing nitrates, the physician should warn the patient that PDE5 inhibitors and nitrates must not be used concurrently, and that no PDE5 inhibitor should be used in the 24 h prior to initiating nitrate therapy. A period of longer than 24 h may be needed following administration of a PDE5 inhibitor for safe use of nitrates, especially with tadalafil, due to its prolonged $t_{1/2}$. In the event that patients develop significant hypotension following combined administration of sildenafil and a nitrate, fluids and α adrenergic receptor agonists, if needed, may be used for support.

Sildenafil, tadalafil, and vardenafil are metabolized via CYP3A4, and their toxicity may be enhanced in patients who receive inhibitors of this enzyme, including macrolide and imidazole antibiotics, and antiretroviral agents (see individual chapters and Chapter 6). PDE5 inhibitors also may prolong cardiac repolarization by blocking the I_{Kr}. Although these interactions and effects are important clinically, the overall incidence and profile of adverse events observed with PDE5 inhibitors, when used without nitrates, are consistent with the expected background frequency of the same events in the treated population. In patients with CAD whose exercise capacity indicates that sexual activity is unlikely to precipitate angina and who are not currently taking nitrates, the use of PDE5 inhibitors can be considered.

Therapeutic Uses

Stable Angina Pectoris. Diseases that predispose to CAD and angina should be treated as part of a comprehensive therapeutic program with the primary goal being to prolong life. Conditions such as hypertension, anemia, thyrotoxicosis, obesity, heart failure, cardiac arrhythmias, and acute emotional stress can precipitate anginal symptoms in many patients. Patients should be counseled to stop smoking, lose weight, and maintain a low-fat, high-fiber diet; hypertension and hyperlipidemia should be corrected; and daily aspirin (or clopidogrel if aspirin is not tolerated) and statins (see Chapter 33) should be prescribed. Exposure to sympathomimetic agents (e.g., those in nasal decongestants and other sources) and serotonin receptor agonists used in the treatment of migraine (sumatriptan and similar) should be avoided. The use of drugs that modify the perception of pain is a poor approach to the treatment of angina because the underlying myocardial ischemia is not relieved.

Table 27–1 lists the preparations and dosages of the nitrites and organic nitrates. The rapidity of onset, the duration of action, and the likelihood of developing tolerance are related to the method of administration.

Short-Acting Nitrates for Standby Therapy. GTN is the most commonly used drug for the rapid release of angina and can be applied as tablets, capsules, sublingual powder, spray, and aerosol. The onset of action is within 1–2 min (fastest with the spray), and the effects are undetectable by 1 h after administration. An initial dose of 0.3 mg GTN often relieves pain within 3 min. ISDN, but not ISMN, is an alternative to GTN. It has a slower onset of action (3–4 min), but a longer duration (>1 h). Anginal pain may be prevented when the drugs are used prophylactically immediately prior to exercise or stress. The smallest effective dose should be prescribed. Patients should be instructed to seek medical attention immediately if three tablets of GTN taken over a 15-min period do not relieve a sustained attack because this situation may be indicative of MI, unstable angina, or another cause of the pain.

Longer-Acting Nitrates for the Prophylaxis of Angina. Nitrates can also be used to provide prophylaxis against anginal episodes in patients who have more than occasional angina. However, such patients should be offered revascularizing therapy. Moreover, chronic treatment with nitrates is not associated with a prognostic benefit and may induce tolerance and endothelial dysfunction as discussed previously. Nitrates must therefore be considered a second choice compared to β blockers. Sustained-release oral preparations of ISDN, ISMN, and GTN are available. Sustained-release ISDN and ISMN are typically given in two doses administered 6–7 h apart, followed by a nitrate-free interval of at least 8 h.

Variant (Prinzmetal) Angina. The large coronary arteries normally contribute little to coronary resistance. However, in variant angina, coronary constriction results in reduced blood flow and ischemic pain. Multiple mechanisms have been proposed to initiate vasospasm, including endothelial cell injury. Whereas long-acting nitrates alone are occasionally efficacious in abolishing episodes of variant angina, additional therapy with Ca^{2+} channel blockers usually is required. Ca^{2+} channel blockers, but not nitrates, have been shown to influence mortality and the incidence of MI favorably in variant angina; they should generally be included in therapy.

Congestive Heart Failure. The utility of nitrovasodilators to relieve pulmonary congestion and to increase cardiac output in congestive heart failure is addressed in Chapter 28.

Unstable Angina Pectoris (Acute Coronary Syndromes, see discussion that follows). Resistance to nitrates classifies angina symptoms as "unstable" and is a characteristic feature of ACSs, typically caused by transient or permanent thrombotic occlusion of coronary vessels. Nitrates do not modify this process specifically and are second-line drugs.

Ca²⁺ Channel Blockers

Voltage-gated Ca^{2+} channels (L-type or slow channels) mediate the entry of extracellular Ca^{2+} into smooth muscle and cardiac myocytes and SA and AV nodal cells in response to electrical depolarization. In both smooth muscle and cardiac myocytes, Ca^{2+} is a trigger for contraction, albeit by different mechanisms. Ca^{2+} channel antagonists, also called *Ca^{2+} entry blockers* or *Ca^{2+} channel blockers*, inhibit Ca^{2+} influx. In vascular smooth muscle, this leads to relaxation, especially in arterial beds, in cardiac myocytes to negative inotropic effects. All Ca^{2+} channel blockers exert these two principal actions, but the ratio differs according to the class as does the presence of chronotropic and dromotropic effects.

Chemistry

The multiple Ca^{2+} channel blockers that are approved for clinical use in the U.S. have diverse chemical structures. Clinically used Ca^{2+} channel blockers include the phenylalkylamine verapamil, the benzothiazepine diltiazem, and numerous dihydropyridines, including amlodipine, clevidipine, felodipine, isradipine, lercanidine, nicardipine, nifedipine, nimodipine, and nisoldipine. The structures and relative specificities of representative drugs are shown in Table 27–2. Although these drugs are commonly grouped together as "calcium channel blockers," there are fundamental differences among verapamil, diltiazem, and the dihydropyridines with respect to pharmacodynamics, drug interactions, and toxicities.

Mechanisms of Action

An increased concentration of cytosolic Ca^{2+} causes increased contraction in both cardiac and vascular smooth muscle cells. In cardiac myocytes, the entry of extracellular Ca^{2+} causes a larger Ca^{2+} release from intracellular stores (Ca^{2+}-induced Ca^{2+} release) and thereby initiates the contraction twitch. In smooth muscle cells, entry of Ca^{2+} plays a dominant role, but the release of Ca^{2+} from intracellular storage sites also contributes

TABLE 27–2 ■ COMPARATIVE CV EFFECTS OF Ca²⁺ CHANNEL BLOCKERSª

DRUG CLASS: EXAMPLE	VASODILATION	↓ CARDIAC CONTRACTILITY	↓ AUTOMATICITY (SA NODE)	↓ CONDUCTION (AV NODE)
Phenylalkylamine: Verapamil	4	4	5	5
Benzothiazepine: Diltiazem	3	2	5	4
*Dihydropyridine*ᵇ: Amlodipine	5	1	1	0

Verapamil   Diltiazem   Amlodipine

ªRelative effects are ranked from *no effect* (0) to *prominent* (5).
ᵇSee text for individual characteristics of the numerous dihydropyridines.

to contraction of vascular smooth muscle, particularly in some vascular beds. In contrast to cardiac muscle, smooth muscles typically contract tonically. Cytosolic Ca^{2+} concentrations can be increased by diverse contractile stimuli in vascular smooth muscle cells. Many hormones and autocoids increase Ca^{2+} influx through so-called receptor-operated channels, whereas increases in external concentrations of K^+ and depolarizing electrical stimuli increase Ca^{2+} influx through voltage-gated, or "potential operated," channels. The Ca^{2+} channel blockers produce their effects by binding to the α_1 subunit of the L-type voltage-gated Ca^{2+} channels and reducing Ca^{2+} flux through the channel. The vascular and cardiac effects of some of the Ca^{2+} channel blockers are summarized in the next section and in Table 27–2.

Voltage-gated channels contain domains of homologous sequence that are arranged in tandem within a single large subunit. In addition to the major channel-forming subunit (termed α_1), Ca^{2+} channels contain several other associated subunits (termed α_2, β, γ, and δ) (Schwartz, 1992). Voltage-gated Ca^{2+} channels have been divided into at least three subtypes based on their conductances and sensitivities to voltage (Schwartz, 1992; Tsien et al., 1988). The channels best characterized to date are the L, N, and T subtypes. Only the L-type channel is sensitive to the dihydropyridine Ca^{2+} channel blockers. All approved Ca^{2+} channel blockers bind to the α_1 subunit of the L-type Ca^{2+} channel, which is the main pore-forming unit of the channel. This approximately 250,000-Da subunit is associated with a disulfide-linked $\alpha_2\delta$ subunit of about 140,000 Da and a smaller intracellular β subunit. The α_1 subunits share a common topology of four homologous domains, each of which is composed of six putative transmembrane segments (S1–S6). The α_2, δ, and β subunits modulate the α_1 subunit (see Figure 14–2). The phenylalkylamine Ca^{2+} channel blocker verapamil binds to transmembrane segment 6 of domain IV (IVS6), the benzothiazepine Ca^{2+} channel blocker diltiazem binds to the cytoplasmic bridge between domain III (IIIS) and domain IV (IVS), and the dihydropyridine Ca^{2+} channel blockers (nifedipine and several others) bind to transmembrane segments of both domains III and IV. These three separate receptor sites are linked allosterically.

Pharmacological Actions

Vascular Tissue. Depolarization of vascular smooth muscle cells depends primarily on the influx of Ca^{2+}. At least three distinct mechanisms may be responsible for contraction of vascular smooth muscle cells. First, voltage-gated Ca^{2+} channels open in response to depolarization of the membrane, and extracellular Ca^{2+} moves down its electrochemical gradient into the cell. After closure of Ca^{2+} channels, a finite period of time is required before the channels can open again in response to a stimulus. Second, agonist-induced contractions that occur without depolarization of the membrane result from stimulation of the G_q-PLC-IP_3 pathway, resulting in the release of intracellular Ca^{2+} from the sarcoplasmic reticulum (Chapter 3). Emptying of intracellular Ca^{2+} stores may trigger further influx of extracellular Ca^{2+} (store-operated Ca^{2+} entry), but its relevance in smooth muscle is unresolved. Third, receptor-operated Ca^{2+} channels allow the entry of extracellular Ca^{2+} in response to receptor occupancy. An increase in cytosolic Ca^{2+} results in enhanced binding of Ca^{2+} to calmodulin. The Ca^{2+}-calmodulin complex in turn activates myosin light-chain kinase, with resulting phosphorylation of the myosin light chain. Such phosphorylation promotes interaction between actin and myosin and leads to sustained contraction of smooth muscle. Ca^{2+} channel blockers inhibit the voltage-dependent Ca^{2+} channels in vascular smooth muscle and decrease Ca^{2+} entry. All Ca^{2+} channel antagonists relax arterial smooth muscle and thereby decrease arterial resistance, blood pressure, and cardiac afterload. Although experimentally large conductance veins of pig appear similarly or even more sensitive to Ca^{2+} channel blockers than arteries (Magnon et al., 1995), Ca^{2+} channel blockers do not affect cardiac preload significantly when given at normal doses in patients. This suggests that capacitance veins that determine venous return to the heart are resistant to the relaxing effect of Ca^{2+} channel antagonists.

Cardiac Cells. The mechanisms of excitation-contraction coupling in cardiac myocytes of the working myocardium differ from those in

vascular smooth muscle in that increases in intracellular Ca^{2+} are fast and transient (Chapter 28). They are initiated by a fast and short (<5 ms) Na^+ influx through voltage-gated Na^+ channels that causes depolarization of the membrane and opening of L-type Ca^{2+} channels. Repolarizing K^+ currents terminate the cardiac action potential and Ca^{2+} influx. Within the cardiac myocyte, Ca^{2+} binds to troponin C, relieving the inhibitory effect of the troponin complex on the contractile apparatus and permitting productive interaction of actin and myosin, leading to contraction. By inhibiting Ca^{2+} influx, Ca^{2+} channel blockers reduce the peak size of the systolic Ca^{2+} transient and thereby produce a negative inotropic effect. Although this is true of all classes of Ca^{2+} channel blockers, the greater degree of peripheral vasodilation seen with the dihydropyridines is accompanied by a baroreceptor reflex–mediated increase in sympathetic tone sufficient to overcome the negative inotropic effect.

In the SA and AV nodes, depolarization largely depends on the movement of Ca^{2+} through the slow channel. The effect of a Ca^{2+} channel blocker on AV conduction and on the rate of the sinus node pacemaker depends on whether the agent delays the recovery of the slow channel (Schwartz, 1992). Although nifedipine reduces the slow inward current in a dose-dependent manner, it does not affect the rate of recovery of the slow Ca^{2+} channel. Although nifedipine has clear negative chronotropic effects in isolated preparations (at ~ 5-fold higher concentrations than needed for negative inotropy), at doses used clinically, nifedipine does not directly affect pacemaking or conduction through the AV node. Rather, it stimulates the heart indirectly by eliciting reflex sympathetic activation in response to a lowering of blood pressure (Figure 27–2).

In contrast, verapamil not only reduces the magnitude of the Ca^{2+} current through the slow channel, but also decreases the rate of recovery of the channel. In addition, channel blockade caused by verapamil (and to a lesser extent by diltiazem) is enhanced as the frequency of stimulation increases, a phenomenon known as *frequency dependence* or *use dependence*. Verapamil and diltiazem depress the rate of the sinus node pacemaker and slow AV conduction at clinically used doses; the latter effect is the basis for their use in the treatment of supraventricular tachyarrhythmias (see Chapter 30). Verapamil also inhibits fast Na^+ and repolarizing K^+ currents (I_{Kr}). The contribution of these actions to the clinical profile is unclear, but note that verapamil, despite the effect on I_{Kr}, has not been associated with torsades des pointes arrhythmias as have other I_{Kr} blockers.

Integrated Cardiovascular Effects of Different Ca^{2+} Channel Antagonists. The hemodynamic profiles of the Ca^{2+} channel blockers approved for clinical use differ and depend mainly on the ratio of vasodilating and negative inotropic and chronotropic effects on the heart (Figure 27–2). The dihydropyridines dilate blood vessels at several-fold lower concentrations than those required for decreasing myocardial force; the ratio is close to one for diltiazem and verapamil. The published selectivity values differ widely, depending on the type of blood vessel and the mode of precontraction used for the comparison (Table 27–2 and Figure 27–3). The differences between the relatively vasoselective dihydropyridines and the much less-selective diltiazem and verapamil have important consequences because the decrease in arterial blood pressure elicits reflex sympathetic activation, resulting in the stimulation of heart rate, AV conduction velocity, and myocardial force, just the opposite of the direct effect of Ca^{2+} channel blockers. While direct and indirect effects normally balance each other in case of verapamil and diltiazem, sympathetic stimulation often prevails in dihydropyridines, causing an increase in heart rate and contractility. Cardiac depressant effects of dihydropyridines may be unmasked, though, in the presence of β blockers and in patients with heart failure.

The dihydropyridines in clinical use—amlodipine, clevidipine, felodipine, isradipine, lercanidipine, nicardipine, nifedipine, nimodipine, and nisoldipine—share most pharmacodynamic properties. Differences with regard to vascular selectivity or subvascular selectivity have been intensely addressed in the past, but claims of large vasoselectivity factors were based on indirect comparisons (Godfraind et al., 1992). Overall, the clinical relevance of vasoselectivity ratios appears questionable; actual differences are probably not great (Figure 27–3). In any event, the drugs exert their

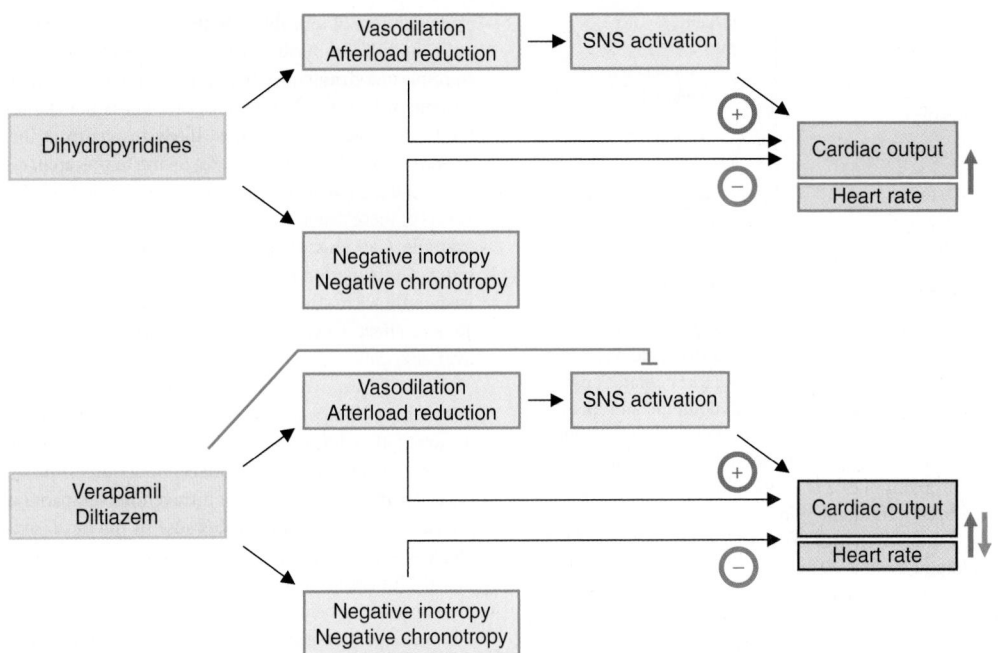

Figure 27–2 *Comparison of the integrated actions of Ca²⁺ channel blockers.* Due to different potencies and efficacies at various sites of action within the cardiovascular system, dihydropyridines produce integrated effects that are not identical to those of verapamil and diltiazem. Verapamil can have direct inhibitory effects on the SNS. The thickness of the arrow indicates the relative strength of the effect.

antianginal effect mainly by peripheral arterial vasodilation and afterload reduction and not by coronary artery dilation (exception in variant angina).

Verapamil, like the dihydropyridines, causes little effect on venous return and preload, but has more direct negative inotropic and chronotropic effects than the dihydropyridines at doses that produce arteriolar dilation and afterload reduction (Figure 27–2). Thus, the consequences of a reflex increase in adrenergic tone are generally offset by the direct cardiodepressant effects of the drug. In patients without heart failure, oral administration of verapamil reduces peripheral vascular resistance and blood pressure with minimal changes in heart rate. Ventricular performance is not impaired and actually may improve, especially if ischemia limits performance. In contrast, in patients with heart failure, intravenous verapamil can cause a marked decrease in contractility and left ventricular function. The antianginal effect of verapamil, like that of all Ca²⁺ channel blockers, is due primarily to a reduction in myocardial O_2 demand. The negative dromotropic effect has no relevance for the improvement of

exercise but can cause second-degree AV block, particularly when given in combination with β blockers (contraindicated). Diltiazem's effects lie in between those of dihydropyridines and verapamil.

The effects of Ca²⁺ channel blockers on diastolic ventricular relaxation (the lusitropic state of the ventricle) are complex. Nifedipine, diltiazem, and verapamil impaired parameters of ventricular relaxation in dogs, especially when given into the coronary arteries (Walsh and O'Rourke, 1985). However, reflex stimulation of sympathetic tone accelerates relaxation, which may outweigh a direct negative lusitropic effect. Likewise, a reduction in afterload will improve the lusitropic state. In addition, if ischemia is improved, the negative lusitropic effect will be reduced. The sum total of these effects in any given patient cannot be determined a priori.

ADME and Drug Interactions. Ca²⁺ channel blockers exhibit clinically relevant differences in pharmacokinetics (Figure 27–4). Immediate-release nifedipine is quickly absorbed after oral intake and produces only a briefly elevated blood level of the drug ($t_{1/2} \sim 1.8$ h) that is associated with an

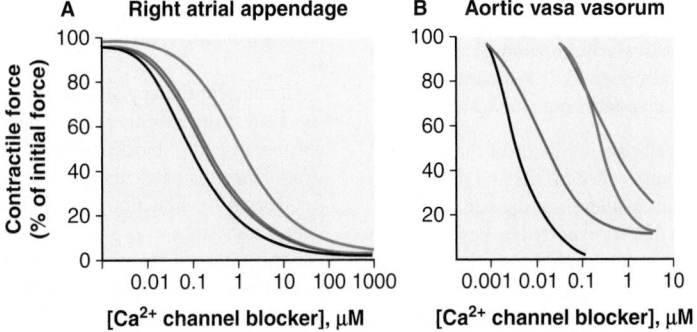

Figure 27–3 *Potency of Ca²⁺ channel blockers at different sites.* Effects were assessed on the contractile force of human right atrial appendages (**A**) and human arteries from aortic vasa vasorum precontracted with high-K⁺ concentrations (**B**). Felodipine (black), nifedipine (blue), amlodipine (green) are more potent on vascular muscle, inhibiting contraction of atrial muscle at concentrations about 10 times higher than those needed to reduce contraction in vascular tissue. Verapamil (red) inhibits atrial muscle force development at 20% of the concentration required to reduce contraction in vascular tissue. The vascular selectivities of the various Ca²⁺ channel blockers (EC₅₀ on atrial appendage/EC₅₀ on vasa vasorum) are as follows: felodipine, 12; nifedipine, 7; amlodipine, 5; verapamil, 0.2. (Figure is based on data of Angus et al., 2000.)

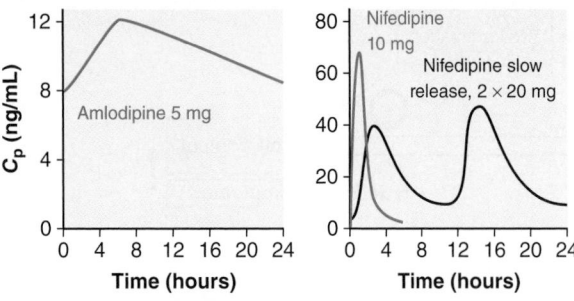

Figure 27–4 *Minimizing daily fluctuations in C_p values of Ca^{2+} channel blockers.* Graphs show plasma levels (C_p values) of amlodipine (left) and of nifedipine (right) in immediate-release (red) and slow-release (black) preparations; doses were administered at zero time. Plasma levels of amlodipine and nifedipine slow-release formulations were assessed after repeated application; thus, C_p values do not start at zero. Note the much smaller differences between trough and peak plasma concentrations in case of amlodipine compared to the rapid and brief pulse in plasma concentration of immediate-release nifedipine and the relatively large fluctuations even with the slow-release form of nifedipine. The plasma $t_{1/2}$ of amlodipine is about 39 h; that of nifedipine is about 1.8 h. A large fluctuation in C_p may result in adverse effects at the maximum and lack of efficacy at the minimum (see Figure 2–9A). (For original data, see Bainbridge et al., 1993; Debbas et al., 1986; and van Harten et al., 1987.)

abrupt decrease in blood pressure, reflex activation of the sympathetic nervous system, and tachycardia. This can cause a typical flush and can increase the risk of angina pectoris by abruptly decreasing coronary perfusion pressure concomitantly with tachycardia. Sustained-release preparations of nifedipine somewhat reduce fluctuations of plasma concentration. By contrast, amlodipine has slow absorption and a prolonged effect. With a plasma $t_{1/2}$ of 35–50 h, plasma levels and effect increase over 7–10 days of daily administration of a constant dose, resulting in a C_p with modest peaks and troughs. Such a profile allows the body to adapt and is associated with less reflex tachycardia. Felodipine, nitrendipine, lercanidipine, and isradipine have similar profiles for chronic treatment (Table 27–2). Clevidipine is available for intravenous administration and has a very rapid ($t_{1/2} \sim 2$ min) onset and offset of action. It is metabolized by esterases in blood. It may be useful in controlling blood pressure in severe or perioperative hypertension as an alternative to GTN, sodium nitroprusside, or nicardipine.

The bioavailability of all Ca^{2+} channel blockers is reduced, in some cases markedly, by first-pass metabolism by CYP3A4 enzymes in the intestinal epithelium and the liver. This has two consequences:

- The bioavailability of these drugs may be increased by strong inhibitors of CYP3A4, such as macrolide and imidazole antibiotics, antiretroviral agents, and grapefruit juice (see Chapter 6). Bioavailability is reduced by inducers of CYP3A4, such as rifampin, carbamazepine, and hypericum (St. John's wort).
- Some Ca^{2+} channel blockers (particularly verapamil) are strong CYP3A4 inhibitors and cause clinically relevant drug interactions with other CYP3A4 substrates, such as simvastatin and atorvastatin.

Moreover, verapamil is a relatively efficient inhibitor of the intestinal and renal ABC transport protein Pgp (also called MDR1 and ABCB1; see Chapter 5) and can thereby increase plasma levels of digoxin, cyclosporine, and loperamide and other agents that are exported by Pgp. This high potential of verapamil for drug-drug interactions is a clear disadvantage and one of the reasons for its declining use. In patients with hepatic cirrhosis, the bioavailabilities and half-lives of the Ca^{2+} channel blockers may be increased, and dosage should be decreased accordingly. The half-lives of these agents also may be longer in older patients.

Toxicity and Untoward Responses. The profile of adverse reactions to the Ca^{2+} channel blockers varies among the drugs in this class. Immediate-release capsules of nifedipine often cause headache, flushing, and dizziness and can actually worsen myocardial ischemia. Dizziness and flushing

are much less of a problem with the sustained-release formulations and with the dihydropyridines having a long $t_{1/2}$ and providing more constant plasma drug concentrations. Peripheral edema may occur in some patients with Ca^{2+} channel blockers but is not the result of generalized fluid retention; rather, it most likely results from increased hydrostatic pressure in the lower extremities owing to precapillary dilation and reflex postcapillary constriction (Epstein and Roberts, 2009). Other adverse effects of these drugs are due to actions in nonvascular smooth muscle. For example, Ca^{2+} channel blockers can cause or aggravate gastroesophageal reflux. Constipation is a common side effect of verapamil but occurs less frequently with other Ca^{2+} channel blockers. Urinary retention is a rare adverse effect. Uncommon adverse effects include rash and elevations of liver enzymes.

Although bradycardia, transient asystole, and exacerbation of heart failure have been reported with verapamil, these responses usually have occurred after intravenous administration of verapamil in patients with disease of the SA node, AV nodal conduction disturbances, or in the presence of β-blockade. The use of intravenous verapamil with an intravenous β blocker is contraindicated because of the increased propensity for AV block or severe depression of ventricular function. Patients with ventricular dysfunction, SA or AV nodal conduction disturbances, and systolic blood pressures below 90 mmHg should not be treated with verapamil or diltiazem, particularly intravenously. Verapamil may also exacerbate AV nodal conduction disturbances observed with digoxin, both for pharmacodynamic and pharmacokinetic reasons (Pgp inhibition; see previous discussion). When used with quinidine, verapamil may cause excessive hypotension, again due to pharmacodynamic and pharmacokinetic reasons (quinidine is CYP3A4 substrate and Pgp inhibitor).

Therapeutic Uses

Variant Angina. Variant angina results from reduced blood flow (a consequence of transient localized vasoconstriction) rather than increased O_2 demand. Drug-induced causes (e.g., cocaine, amphetamines, sumatriptan, and related antimigraine drugs) should be excluded. Ca^{2+} channel blockers are effective in about 90% of patients (Montalescot et al., 2013). These agents are considered first-line treatment and may be combined with nitrovasodilators (Amsterdam et al., 2014).

Exertional Angina. Ca^{2+} channel blockers also are effective in the treatment of exertional, or exercise-induced, angina. Numerous double-blind, placebo-controlled studies have shown that these drugs decrease the number of anginal attacks and attenuate exercise-induced ST-segment depression, but evidence for life-prolonging efficacy is lacking. They are therefore considered the drugs of choice if β blockers do not achieve sufficient symptomatic benefit or are not tolerated (Montalescot et al., 2013).

The Ca^{2+} channel blockers reduce the *double product*, Heart rate × Systolic blood pressure, an approximate index of myocardial O_2 demand. Because these agents reduce the level of the double product at a given external workload, and because the value of the double product at peak exercise is not altered, the beneficial effect of Ca^{2+} channel blockers likely derives from a decrease in O_2 demand rather than an increase in coronary flow.

Concurrent therapy of a dihydropyridine with a β blocker has proven more effective than either agent given alone in exertional angina, presumably because the β blocker suppresses reflex tachycardia. This concurrent drug therapy is particularly attractive because the dihydropyridines do not delay AV conduction and will not enhance the negative dromotropic effects associated with β receptor blockade. In contrast, the concurrent administration of verapamil or diltiazem with a β blocker is contraindicated for the potential for AV block, severe bradycardia, and decreased left ventricular function.

Unstable Angina (Acute Coronary Syndrome). In the past, Ca^{2+} channel blockers were routinely administered in patients presenting with unstable angina and ACS without persistent ST elevation. Reports about trends for harm with immediate-release nifedipine or nifedipine infusion in the absence of β blockers have led to the recommendation not to use dihydropyridines without concurrent therapy with β blockers.

Verapamil and diltiazem are recommended only for patients who continue to show signs of ischemia, do not tolerate β blockers, have no clinically significant left ventricular dysfunction, and show no signs of disturbed AV conduction (Amsterdam et al., 2014).

Other Uses. The use of verapamil and diltiazem (but not dihydropyridines) as antiarrhythmic agents in supraventricular tachyarrhythmias is discussed in Chapter 30; their use for the treatment of hypertension is discussed in Chapter 28. Ca^{2+} channel blockers are contraindicated in patients with heart failure with reduced ejection fraction, but amlodipine and felodipine did not worsen the prognosis and can therefore be administered if indicated for other reasons (Chapter 29). Verapamil improves left ventricular outflow obstruction and symptoms in patients with HCM. Diltiazem has shown early promising results in a clinical study in asymptomatic HCM mutation carriers (Ho et al., 2015). Verapamil also has been used in the prophylaxis of migraine headaches but is considered a second-choice drug. Nimodipine has been approved for use in patients with neurological deficits secondary to cerebral vasospasm after the rupture of a congenital intracranial aneurysm, but clinical evidence for greater effectiveness than verapamil or magnesium is sparse. Nifedipine, diltiazem, amlodipine, and felodipine appear to provide symptomatic relief in Raynaud disease. The Ca^{2+} channel blockers cause relaxation of the myometrium in vitro and may be effective in reducing preterm uterine contractions in preterm labor (see Chapter 44).

β Blockers

β blockers are the only drug class that is effective in reducing the severity and frequency of attacks of exertional angina and in improving survival in patients who have had an MI. They are therefore recommended as first-line treatment of patients with stable CAD (Montalescot et al., 2013) and unstable angina/ACS (Hamm et al., 2011). Recent meta-analyses raised doubts about the mortality-reducing effects of β blockers in the MI reperfusion era (Bangalore et al., 2014); however, some of the results, such as the slightly increased heart failure frequency in patients receiving β blockers, contradicted numerous well-controlled prospective trials (see Chapter 29) and raised doubts about the validity of the analysis. Thus, the issue has not been definitively resolved. β Blockers are not useful for vasospastic angina and, if used in isolation, may worsen that condition. β Blockers appear equally effective in the treatment of exertional angina (Fihn et al., 2012; Montalescot et al., 2013), but very short-acting agents or drug formulations giving rise to large fluctuations of plasma concentrations (e.g., unformulated metoprolol) should be avoided for treatment of chronic CAD.

The effectiveness of β blockers in the treatment of exertional angina is attributable primarily to a fall in myocardial O_2 consumption at rest and during exertion. The decrease in myocardial O_2 consumption is due to a negative chronotropic effect (particularly during exercise), a negative inotropic effect, and a reduction in arterial blood pressure (particularly systolic pressure) during exercise. A decrease in heart rate prolongs the time of myocardial perfusion during diastole. Moreover, there is evidence that β blockers can increase blood flow toward ischemic regions by increasing coronary collateral resistance and preventing blood from being shunted away from the ischemic myocardium during maximal coronary vasodilation (Billinger et al., 2001), a "reverse steal or Robin Hood phenomenon" (see previous discussion).

Not all actions of β blockers are beneficial in all patients. The decreases in heart rate and contractility cause increases in the systolic ejection period and left ventricular end-diastolic volume; these alterations tend to increase O_2 consumption. However, the net effect of β blockade usually is to decrease myocardial O_2 consumption, particularly during exercise. Nevertheless, in patients with limited cardiac reserve who are critically dependent on adrenergic stimulation, β blockade can result in profound decreases in left ventricular function. Despite this, several β blockers demonstrably reduce mortality in patients with congestive heart failure, and β blockers have become standard therapy for many such patients (see Chapters 12 and 29).

Numerous β blockers are approved for clinical use. Standard compounds for the treatment of angina are $β_1$-selective and without intrinsic

sympathomimetic activity (e.g., atenolol, bisoprolol, or metoprolol). Chapter 12 presents their pharmacology in detail.

Antiplatelet, Anti-integrin, and Antithrombotic Agents

Antiplatelet agents represent the cornerstone of therapy for ACS (Amsterdam et al., 2014; Roffi et al., 2015) and are systematically discussed in Chapter 32. They interfere either with two signaling pathways (TxA_2 and ADP) that cooperatively promote platelet aggregation in an auto- and paracrine manner or with a major common pathway of platelet aggregation, the GpIIb/IIIa fibrinogen receptor. Aspirin inhibits platelet aggregation by irreversibly inactivating the thromboxane-synthesizing COX-1 in platelets, thereby reducing production of TxA_2. Aspirin, given at doses of 160–325 mg at the onset of treatment of ACS, improves survival (Yeghiazarians et al., 2000). The thienopyridines are ADP receptor ($P2Y_{12}$ receptor) antagonists that block the proaggregatory effect of ADP, which is stored in vesicles within platelets and released when platelets adhere to prothrombotic structures. The proaggregatory synergism of TxA_2 and ADP on platelet aggregation and thrombus formation accounts for the potentiating effect of adding a thienopyridine to aspirin.

The addition of the thienopyridine clopidogrel to aspirin therapy reduces mortality in patients with ACS. Newer thienopyridines (prasugrel, ticagrelor, cangrelor) with favorable pharmacokinetic properties have been approved for the treatment of ACS. All three appear superior to clopidogrel in treating patients with ACS; contributing factors likely include faster onset of action and less-variable pharmacokinetics. Ticagrelor is a direct, reversible $P2Y_{12}$ receptor antagonist, while clopidogrel and prasugrel are both prodrugs. The hepatic activation of prasugrel is more stable and faster than that of clopidogrel. Cangrelor is the first $P2Y_{12}$ receptor antagonist for intravenous application, producing very rapid inhibition of platelet aggregation. Recent guidelines recommend ticagrelor and prasugrel as the primary choice in patients with ACS and clopidogrel as an alternative in patients who cannot receive the former or are on oral anticoagulation therapy (e.g., for stroke prevention in atrial fibrillation). The place of cangrelor is not yet fully defined (Roffi et al., 2015).

The optimal timing of the initiation of dual platelet treatment is controversial and depends on the likely clinical course. If conservative treatment is likely and the patient is not at an increased risk of bleeding, aspirin and a parenteral anticoagulant (see discussion that follows) should be given as soon as possible, with the addition of a $P2Y_{12}$ receptor antagonist as soon as the diagnosis of NSTEMI has been made. Dual platelet inhibition for 1 year is currently recommended for all patients after NSTEMI or STEMI and revascularization, independently of the type of revascularization and type of stent used (Roffi et al., 2015). Due to the irreversible (aspirin, clopidogrel, and prasugrel) or prolonged (ticagrelor) modes of action, the risk of bleeding remains increased for extended periods after withdrawal of these drugs. Nonemergency major noncardiac surgeries should therefore be postponed for 5 (ticagrelor, clopidogrel) or 7 days (prasugrel, aspirin) after intake of the last dose.

Anti-integrin agents directed against the platelet integrin GPIIb/IIIa (including abciximab, tirofiban, and eptifibatide) are highly effective by blocking the final effector pathway of platelet aggregation; however, these agents have a small therapeutic index and must be administered parenterally. Meta-analyses of studies in patients with ACS showed that the use of GpIIb/IIIa inhibitors in addition to heparin was associated with about a 10% reduction in mortality, but with an increase in bleeding. Because most of these trials were conducted before the widespread use of the newer and more effective thienopyridines prasugrel and ticagrelor, the current value of the GpIIb/IIIa antagonists is not clear. Guidelines recommend them in patients on prasugrel or ticagrelor only in bailout situations (Roffi et al., 2015).

Heparin, in its unfractionated form and as low-molecular-weight heparin (e.g., enoxaparin), also reduces symptoms and prevents infarction in unstable angina (Yeghiazarians et al., 2000). Fondaparinux, a heparinoid pentasaccharide, antithrombin III-dependent Factor Xa inhibitor has the best efficacy-safety profile of all anticoagulants and is therefore currently first choice. Thrombin inhibitors, such as hirudin or bivalirudin, directly inhibit even clot-bound thrombin, are not affected by circulating inhibitors, and function independently of antithrombin III. Bivalirudin provides no benefit over heparin in ACS (Valgimigli et al., 2015). Thrombolytic agents such as rTPA are of no benefit in unstable angina. The new oral anticoagulants (factor IIa inhibitor dabigatran and factor Xa inhibitors rivaroxaban, apixaban, and edoxaban) have no established place in the treatment of CAD.

Other Antianginal Agents

Ranolazine

Ranolazine is FDA and EMA approved as a second-line agent for the treatment of chronic angina. The drug may be used with a variety of other agents, including β blockers, Ca^{2+} channel blockers, ACEIs, ARBs, and therapeutic agents for lowering lipids and reducing platelet aggregation.

Mechanism of Action. The mechanism of ranolazine's therapeutic efficacy in angina is uncertain. Its anti-ischemic and antianginal effects occur independently of reductions in heart rate and arterial blood pressure or changes in coronary blood flow. Ranolazine inhibits several cardiac ion fluxes, including I_{Kr} and I_{Na}. Preferential inhibition of late I_{Na} may explain its cardiac effects (Hasenfuss and Maier, 2008). The late I_{Na} contributes to arrhythmias in patients with the rare long QT 3 syndrome (Chapter 30), and is increased in heart failure and ischemia. Reduction of the late I_{Na} could explain in part the elevated cytosolic Na^+ concentrations in cardiac myocytes in these conditions, leading to higher diastolic Ca^{2+} concentrations, Ca^{2+} overload, arrhythmias, and problems with diastolic relaxation. Inhibition of late I_{Na} by ranolazine could reduce $[Na^+]_i$-dependent Ca^{2+} overload and its detrimental effects on myocardial ATP hydrolysis and cardiac function.

Other mechanisms of action have been proposed. Ranolazine reduces cardiac fatty acid oxidation and stimulates glucose metabolism without inhibiting carnitine palmityl transferase 1, and on this basis ranolazine was initially categorized as a metabolic modulator (McCormack et al., 1998). However, the effect is small, occurs at ranolazine concentrations more than 5-fold higher than do therapeutic effects, and can be assessed in the absence of fatty acid oxidation (Belardinelli et al., 2006). Ranolazine has weak β receptor blocking activity (Letienne et al., 2001) that may contribute to its anti-anginal activity.

In a large prospective trial of patients with incomplete revascularization after percutaneous coronary intervention, anti-ischemic therapy with ranolazine did not improve the prognosis of these high-risk patients (Weisz et al., 2016). Clinical trials are currently testing ranolazine in HCM and heart failure with preserved ejection fraction.

ADME and Adverse Effects. Ranolazine, supplied as extended-release tablets, is administered without regard to meals at 500 to 1000 mg twice daily; higher doses are poorly tolerated. The drug's oral bioavailability is about 75%; inhibitors of Pgp (e.g., digoxin, cyclosporine; see Chapter 5) can increase absorption of ranolazine and increase exposure to both ranolazine and the competing drug. Ranolazine's terminal $t_{1/2}$ is about 7 h; with repeated dosing, a steady-state C_p is reached in 3 days. Ranolazine is metabolized mainly by CYP3A4 and to a lesser extent by CYP2D6; unchanged drug (5%) and metabolites are excreted in the urine. Ranolazine should not be used together with strong CYP3A4 inhibitors (e.g., macrolide and imidazole antibiotics, HIV protease inhibitors), and doses need to be limited when moderate CYP3A4 inhibitors such as verapamil, diltiazem, and erythromycin are used in combination. Inducers of CYP3A4 (e.g., rifampin, carbamazepine, and hypericum) can decrease ranolazine plasma levels, requiring dose adjustment. Ranolazine can affect plasma levels of other CYP3A4 substrates, including doubling levels of simvastatin and its active metabolite and requiring dose adjustment; dose reduction may be needed for other CYP3A4 substrates (e.g., lovastatin), especially for those with a narrow therapeutic range (e.g., cyclosporine, tacrolimus, sirolimus). Coadministration of ranolazine may increase exposure to other substrates of CYP2D6, such as tricyclic antidepressant drugs and antipsychotic agents.

The most frequent adverse effects are dizziness, headache, nausea, and constipation. Some CNS effects (e.g., dizziness, blurry vision, and confusional state) are reminiscent of class I antiarrhythmics. QT prolongations have to be considered, but no torsades des pointes arrhythmias or related events have been reported.

Ivabradine

Ivabradine is EMA approved for treating stable angina and heart failure in patients in whom β blockers are not tolerated or are insufficiently effective in reducing heart rate and FDA-approved only for the treatment of heart failure (Chapter 29). Ivabradine is a selective blocker of hyperpolarization-activated HCN ion channels involved in the generation of automaticity in the SA node. By reducing the pacemaker current I_f through HCN channels, the compound dose dependently reduces heart rate and, differently from β blockers, does not affect cardiac contractile force. The antianginal effect is explained solely by reduction of heart rate and thereby O_2 demand (Figure 27–1).

A typical, often transient, side effect are phosphenes, transient enhanced lightness in restricted areas of the visual field, that are explained by effects on retinal HCN channels (3%–5% of cases). In a recent study in patients with chronic angina and normal left ventricular function, the addition of ivabradine to β blockers did not confer benefit but was associated with a trend for more cardiovascular end points and an increase in symptomatic bradycardia, atrial fibrillation, and QT prolongation (Fox et al., 2014). The data raise doubts about the hypothesis that heart rate reduction per se is associated with better cardiovascular outcome and has led to restrictions on use of ivabradine (e.g., contraindication for concurrent therapy with verapamil or diltiazem).

Nicorandil

Nicorandil is a nitrate ester of nicotinamide developed as an antianginal agent and currently is approved in many Asian and European countries (but not in the U.S. and Germany) for the treatment of stable angina pectoris. Nicorandil is not available in the U.S.

Mechanism of Action and Pharmacological Effects. Nicorandil has nitrate-like (cGMP-dependent) properties and acts as an agonist at ATP-sensitive potassium (K_{ATP}) channels. Its vasodilating action is potentiated by PDE5 inhibitors and only partially blocked by inhibitors of K_{ATP} channels, such as glibenclamide, suggesting that both properties participate in nicorandil's effect. Nicorandil dilates both arterial and venous vascular beds, leading to decreases in afterload and preload of the heart. In the absence of direct effects on contractile force of the ventricles, the decrease in afterload causes cardiac output to increase. The last effect is stronger than that seen after administration of nitrovasodilators and partially explained by (reflex) tachycardia. Thus, the hemodynamic profile of nicorandil lies in between that of nitrovasodilators and dihydropyridine Ca^{2+} channel blockers. Its antianginal effect is described to be stable, but early studies reported a clear decrease or loss of antianginal effect after 2 weeks of oral treatment (Meany et al., 1989; Rajaratnam et al., 1999).

Experimental and clinical studies indicated that nicorandil has cardioprotective effects (Matsubara et al., 2000), mimicking that of ischemic preconditioning, a phenomenon that short periods of ischemia preceding prolonged stopping of perfusion (as in MI) reduce myocardial injury. While the exact mechanisms are not fully understood, a central role of mitochondrial K_{ATP} channels is assumed (Ardehali and O'Rourke, 2005; Sato et al., 2000). Retrospective studies indicated a survival-prolonging effect of chronic treatment with nicorandil in patients with stable CAD, but sufficiently powered prospective studies are lacking.

ADME and Adverse Effects. Nicorandil is rapidly absorbed after sublingual or oral administration and has a short $t_{1/2}$ (1 h), which does not provide relevant trough levels at the usual regimen of twice-daily dosing at 20 mg/dose. Besides nitrate-like headache and hypotension (note contraindication of concurrent PDE5 inhibitors), nicorandil has been associated with the appearance of ulcerations. They were first described in 1997 (Boulinguez et al., 1997) as large, painful buccal apthosis and seem to extend to a 40%–60% increased risk of GI ulcerations and perforations (Lee et al., 2015).

Trimetazidine

Trimetazidine was developed as an antianginal agent. Its effect is thought to be due to inhibition of long-chain 3-ketoacyl coenzyme A thiolase, the final enzyme in the FFA β-oxidation pathway. This leads to a partial shift from FFA to glucose oxidation in the heart, which provides less ATP but requires less O_2 and may therefore be beneficial in ischemia (Ussher et al., 2014). Numerous small studies provided evidence for the efficacy of the compound to reduce angina and increase exercise tolerance, particularly in patients with diabetes and heart failure (e.g., Tuunanen et al., 2008); as with nicorandil, large randomized studies to define the true therapeutic value of this compound are lacking.

Trimetazidine can cause GI upset, nausea, and vomiting, and, rarely, it has been associated with thrombocytopenia, agranulocytosis, and liver dysfunction. More important, trimetazidine may increase the risk of movement disorders such as Parkinson disease, particularly in older patients with decreased kidney function. This serious effect has led to use restrictions by the EMA and the recommendation to use trimetazidine only as second-line treatment of stable angina in patients inadequately controlled by or intolerant to first-line antianginal therapies. Trimetazidine is not available in the U.S.

Therapeutic Strategies

Stable Coronary Artery Disease

Guidelines

Task forces from the American College of Cardiology and the American Heart Association (Fihn et al., 2012) and the European Society of Cardiology (Montalescot et al., 2013) have published guidelines that are useful in the selection of appropriate initial therapy for patients with chronic stable angina pectoris. All patients with CAD should receive at least one drug for angina relief in addition to fast- and short-acting nitrovasodilators (GTN, ISDN) and, for event prevention, aspirin and a statin. ACEIs should be considered in patients with CAD who have left ventricular dysfunction or diabetes (Table 27–3).

The evidence for clinically relevant differences between the three main classes of antianginal drugs is not compelling. A meta-analysis of publications that compared two or more antianginal therapies concluded that β blockers are associated with fewer episodes of angina per week and a lower rate of withdrawal due to adverse events than is nifedipine. However, differences did not extend to Ca^{2+} channel blockers other than nifedipine. Of note, no significant differences were observed in outcome between *long-acting* nitrates, Ca^{2+} channel blockers, and β blockers. Nevertheless,

guidelines recommend that β blockers be considered first-line treatment of chronic angina relief; Ca^{2+} channel blockers with heart rate–lowering effects (diltiazem, verapamil) are alternatives. Dihydropyridines should be considered in patients who do not tolerate β blockers. In case of persistent angina, a combination of a dihydropyridine and a β blocker should be considered.

Second-Line Treatment

Longer-acting organic nitrates/nitrate formulation (e.g., cutaneous GTN) or ranolazine and, in non-U.S. countries, ivabradine, trimetazidine, and nicorandil may be considered as adjunct therapy in patients whose angina is not adequately controlled by first-line drugs. β Blockers can block the baroreceptor-mediated reflex tachycardia and positive inotropic effects that may occur with nitrates, whereas nitrates, by increasing venous capacitance, can attenuate the increase in left ventricular end-diastolic volume associated with β-blockade. Concurrent administration of nitrates also can alleviate the increase in coronary vascular resistance associated with blockade of β adrenergic receptors. Ranolazine and trimetazidine have a direct effect on the myocardium and likely act independently of hemodynamic effects. They can therefore be well combined with all other antianginal drugs where permitted. Ivabradine is a possible alternative to β blockers but is associated with toxicity when added to β blockers, verapamil, or diltiazem (Fox et al., 2014).

Ca^{2+} Channel Blockers and Nitrates. In severe exertional or vasospastic angina, the combination of a nitrate and a Ca^{2+} channel blocker may provide additional relief over that obtained with either type of agent alone. Because nitrates primarily reduce preload, whereas Ca^{2+} channel blockers reduce afterload, the net effect on reduction of O_2 demand should be additive; however, excessive vasodilation and hypotension can occur.

Acute Coronary Syndromes

The term *ACS* refers to chest pain with or without MI (i.e., myocardial necrosis). The latter diagnosis is essentially based on the presence or absence of increases in plasma levels of cardiac troponin (I or T). With tests becoming more and more sensitive, the number of MI diagnoses has increased, while that of unstable angina (i.e., chest pain without necrosis) has decreased. The term *unstable angina pectoris* is used for angina symptoms that present for the first time, change their usual pattern, occur at rest, or are resistant to nitrates.

Common to most clinical presentations of ACS is a disruption of a coronary plaque, leading to local platelet aggregation and thrombosis at the arterial wall, with subsequent partial or total occlusion of the vessel. Less commonly, vasospasm in minimally atherosclerotic coronary vessels

TABLE 27-3 ■ MANAGEMENT OF PATIENTS WITH STABLE CORONARY ARTERY DISEASE

TREATMENT LEVEL	ANGINA RELIEF	EVENT PREVENTION
All patients	Short-acting nitrates as standby medication	Education: Lifestyle management, control of risk factors
First-line treatment	β Blockers or diltiazem/verapamil	Aspirin + statins; consider ACEIs or ARBs
	Long-acting dihydropyridine if heart rate low or there are issues of intolerance/contraindications	
	β Blockers + dihydropyridines if angina persists	
	For vasospastic angina, consider dihydropyridines or long-acting nitrates; avoid β blockers	
Second-line treatment (first line in some cases, according to comorbidities and tolerance)	Add or switch to ivabradine, long-acting nitrates, nicorandil, ranolazine[a], or trimetazidine[a]	Consider clopidogrel in cases of aspirin intolerance
Invasive therapy	Consider angiography and stenting or CABG	

[a]In patients with diabetes mellitus.

Source: Adapted from the European Society for Cardiology Guidelines; for details, see Montalescot et al., **2013**.

may account for unstable angina. The pathophysiological principles that underlie therapy for exertional angina—which are directed at decreasing myocardial O_2 *demand*—have limited efficacy in the treatment of ACSs characterized by an insufficiency of myocardial O_2 (blood) *supply*. The most important interventions are as follows:

- Antiplatelet agents, including aspirin and thienopyridines (e.g., clopidogrel, prasugrel, or ticagrelor)
- Antithrombin agents such as heparin or fondaparinux
- Anti-integrin therapies that directly inhibit platelet aggregation mediated by glycoprotein GPIIb/IIIa
- Primary angioplasty with percutaneously deployed intracoronary stents or, if not possible for logistical reasons, fibrinolysis with rTPA
- Coronary bypass surgery for selected patients

The β blockers reduce O_2 consumption and arrhythmias and have been associated with a moderate reduction in mortality in ACS but should be avoided in patients with compromised ventricular function or decreased blood pressure (Roffi et al., 2015). Nitrates are useful in reducing vasospasm and in reducing myocardial O_2 consumption by decreasing ventricular wall stress. Intravenous administration of nitroglycerin allows high concentrations of drug to be attained rapidly. Because nitroglycerin is degraded rapidly, the dose can be titrated quickly and safely using intravenous administration. If coronary vasospasm is present, intravenous nitroglycerin is likely to be effective, although the addition of a Ca^{2+} channel blocker may be required to achieve complete control in some patients. If a patient has consumed a PDE5 inhibitor within the preceding 24 h, there is a risk of profound hypotension, and nitrates should be withheld in favor of an alternate antianginal therapy.

While these principles apply to the entire group of patients with ACS, specific treatment algorithms and the value of different drug classes in ACS depend on the exact diagnosis and should be chosen according to recent guidelines (Amsterdam et al., 2014; Roffi et al., 2015).

ST-elevation myocardial infarction is generally due to a complete obstruction of a large coronary artery. The mainstay in these patients is immediate reperfusion by primary angioplasty and stenting or, in the absence of invasive options, fibrinolytic therapy.

Non–ST-elevation myocardial infarction can present with variable symptoms and electrocardiographic signs and is likely due to transient obstruction of larger coronary arteries or occlusion of small branches, leading to disseminated myocardial necrosis. Primary angioplasty is also indicated in these patients.

Unstable angina is differentiated from NSTEMI by the absence of increased plasma troponin concentrations. These patients have a better long-term prognosis and benefit less from early invasive procedures and intensified antiplatelet therapy. Mainstays are β blockers and nitrovasodilators (in the absence of contraindications such as hypotension). Short-acting Ca^{2+} channel blockers (e.g., nifedipine; see Figure 27–4) should normally be avoided in ACS because of a strong reflex activation of the sympathetic nervous system, but they are the first choice if vasospasm is the underlying cause.

Claudication and Peripheral Vascular Disease

Most patients with peripheral vascular disease also have CAD, and the therapeutic approaches for peripheral and coronary arterial diseases overlap (Rooke et al., 2011). Mortality in patients with peripheral vascular disease is most commonly due to cardiovascular disease (Regensteiner and Hiatt, 2002), and treatment of CAD remains the central focus of therapy. Many patients with advanced peripheral arterial disease are more limited by the consequences of peripheral ischemia than by myocardial ischemia. In the cerebral circulation, arterial disease may be manifest as stroke or transient ischemic attacks. The painful symptoms of peripheral arterial disease in the lower extremities (claudication) typically are provoked by exertion, with increases in skeletal muscle O_2 demand exceeding blood flow that is impaired by proximal stenoses. When flow to the extremities becomes critically limiting, peripheral ulcers and rest pain from tissue ischemia can become debilitating.

Most of the therapies shown to be efficacious for treatment of CAD also have a salutary effect on progression of peripheral artery disease (Hirsch et al., 2006). Antiplatelet therapy using aspirin (75–325 mg) and clopidogrel (75 mg) are recommended, although the evidence for beneficial effects on cardiovascular or total mortality are mixed (Rooke et al., 2011). Oral anticoagulation is ineffective and increases bleeding risks. ACEIs and statins have been recommended for patients with peripheral artery disease (Hirsch et al., 2006), but the evidence for prognostic benefits is much weaker than in CAD. Interestingly, neither intensive treatment of diabetes mellitus nor antihypertensive therapy appears to alter the progression of symptoms of claudication. Other risk factor and lifestyle modifications remain cornerstones of therapy for patients with claudication; physical exercise, rehabilitation, and smoking cessation (possibly supported by drug treatment with varenicline or bupropion) have proven efficacy.

Drugs used specifically in the treatment of lower extremity claudication include pentoxifylline and cilostazol. Pentoxifylline is a methylxanthine derivative that is called a *rheologic modifier* for its effects on increasing the deformability of red blood cells. However, the effects of pentoxifylline on lower extremity claudication appear to be modest and not sufficiently supported by prospective evidence (Salhiyyah et al., 2015).

Cilostazol is an inhibitor of PDE3 and promotes accumulation of intracellular cAMP in many cells, including blood platelets. Cilostazol-mediated increases in cAMP inhibit platelet aggregation and promote vasodilation. The drug is metabolized by CYP3A4 and has important drug interactions with other drugs metabolized via this pathway (see Chapter 6). Cilostazol has been mainly studied in Asian populations and seems to improve symptoms of claudication, but the effect on cardiovascular mortality remains unclear (Bedenis et al., 2014). As a PDE3 inhibitor, cilostazol is in the same drug class as milrinone, which had been used orally as an inotropic agent for patients with heart failure. Milrinone therapy was associated with an increase in sudden cardiac death, and the oral form of the drug was withdrawn from the market. Concerns about several other inhibitors of PDE3 (inamrinone, flosequinan) followed. Cilostazol therefore is labeled as being contraindicated in patients with heart failure, although it is not clear that cilostazol itself leads to increased mortality in such patients. Cilostazol has been reported to increase nonsustained ventricular tachycardia; headache is the most common side effect.

Other treatments for claudication, including naftidrofuryl, propionyl levocarnitine, and prostaglandins, have been explored in clinical trials, and there is some evidence that some of these therapies may be efficacious.

Mechanopharmacological Therapy: Drug-Eluting Endovascular Stents

Intracoronary stents can ameliorate angina and reduce adverse events in patients with ACSs. However, the long-term efficacy of intracoronary stents is limited by subacute luminal restenosis within the stent, which, in bare metal stents, occurs in 20%–30% of patients during the first 6–9 months of follow-up (Montalescot et al., 2013). The pathways that lead to "in-stent restenosis" are complex, but smooth muscle proliferation within the lumen of the stented artery is a common pathological finding. Local antiproliferative therapies at the time of stenting have been explored over many years; several drug-eluting stents and, more recently, biodegradable stents have been introduced in the market. The drugs currently used in intravascular stents are paclitaxel, sirolimus (rapamycin), and the two sirolimus derivatives everolimus and zatarolimus. Paclitaxel is a tricyclic diterpene that inhibits cellular proliferation by binding to and stabilizing polymerized microtubules. Sirolimus is a hydrophobic macrolide that binds to the cytosolic immunophilin FKBP12; the FKBP12-sirolimus complex inhibits the protein kinase mTOR, the mammalian target of rapamycin (see Figure 35–2), thereby inhibiting cell cycle progression (Figure 65–2). Paclitaxel and sirolimus differ markedly in their mechanisms of action but share common chemical properties as hydrophobic small molecules. Stent-induced damage to the vascular endothelial cell layer can lead to thrombosis. The inhibition of cellular proliferation by paclitaxel and sirolimus or derivatives not only affects vascular smooth muscle cell proliferation but also attenuates the formation of an intact endothelial layer within the stented artery and thereby markedly reduces the rate of restenosis compared with bare metal stents. Dual antiplatelet therapy (aspirin, typically with clopidogrel) is recommended for one year after intracoronary stenting with drug-eluting stents, similar to bare metal stents. Evidence for the benefit of even longer periods is limited.

Acknowledgment: *Thomas Michel and Brian B. Hoffman contributed to this chapter in recent editions of this book. We have retained some of their text in the current edition.*

Drug Facts for Your Personal Formulary: *Coronary Artery Disease*

Drug	Therapeutic Uses	Major Toxicity and Clinical Pearls
Organic Nitrates		
Glyceryl trinitrate (GTN, nitroglycerin) Isosorbide dinitrate (ISDN) Isosorbide mononitrate (ISMN)	• Angina (sublingual) • Acute pulmonary edema (IV) • Acute hypertension (IV)	• NO-mediated vasodilation of large (venous, arterial) > small (resistance) vessels $\Rightarrow$ preferential preload reduction without steal effect • Short-acting formulations of GTN or ISDN are standby drugs for all patients with CAD • First choice for vasospastic angina, along with Ca^{2+} channel blockers • Second choice for the prevention of exertional angina (longer-acting formulations) • Adverse effects: headache, dizziness, postural hypotension, syncope • Tolerance after > 16 h (leave nitrate-free interval of > 8 h) • Do not use concurrently with PDE5 inhibitor
Molsidomine	• Angina	• Direct NO donor • Second choice for the prevention of angina • Adverse effects same as above • No documented advantage over GTN/ISDN/ISMN
Inhaled NO	• Pulmonary hypertension in neonates	• Relatively selective effect on pulmonary vascular bed
Ca^{2+} Channel Blockers		
Dihydropyridines Amlodipine Felodipine Lercanidipine Nifedipine Nitrendipine ***Others*** Diltiazem Verapamil	• Angina • Hypertension • Rate control in atrial fibrillation (verapamil, diltiazem)	• Preferential arterial vasodilation $\Rightarrow$ afterload reduction • First choice for vasospastic angina (dihydropyridines) • Second choice for preventing exertional angina • Immediate-release nifedipine and short-acting dihydropyridines can cause tachycardia and hypotension and trigger angina • Diltiazem and verapamil can $\downarrow$ heart rate and AV conduction; should not be used with β blockers • CYP3A4-mediated drug interactions with verapamil and diltiazem • Other unwanted effects: peripheral edema (dihydropyridines), obstipation (verapamil)
β Blockers		
Atenolol Bisoprolol Carvedilol Metoprolol Nadolol Nebivolol Many others	• Angina • Heart failure • Hypertension • Widely used for other indications (prevention of arrhythmias, rate control in atrial fibrillation, migraine, etc.)	• First choice for prevention of exertional angina • Only antianginal drug class with proven prognostic benefits in CAD • Adverse effects: bradycardia, AV block, bronchospasm, peripheral vasoconstriction, worsening of acute heart failure, depression, worsening of psoriasis • Polymorphic CYP2D6 metabolism (metoprolol) • Additional vasodilation (carvedilol, nebivolol)
Ranolazine		
	• Angina	• Inhibits late Na^+ and other cardiac ion currents • Has weak β blocking and metabolic effects • Second choice in the prevention of exertional angina • CYP3A4-dependent metabolism
Ivabradine		
	• Angina • Heart failure	• Selectively $\downarrow$ heart rate by inhibiting HCN currents in SA node • Second choice in the prevention of exertional angina; approved in patients not tolerating β blockers or having heart rate > 75 under β blockers • Unwanted effects: bradycardia, QT prolongation, atrial fibrillation, phosphenes • Contraindication: combination with diltiazem or verapamil
Nicorandil		
	• Angina	• Dual nitrate-like and I_{KATP}-stimulatory action • Hemodynamic profile between nitrates and dihydropyridines; $\downarrow$ afterload more than nitrates • Second choice in the prevention of exertional angina • Adverse effects: hypotension, headache, buccal and GI ulcers • Do not combine with PDE5 inhibitor

Drug Facts for Your Personal Formulary: *Coronary Artery Disease (continued)*

Drug	Therapeutic Uses	Major Toxicity and Clinical Pearls
Trimetazidine		
	• Angina	• Metabolic shift from fatty acid to glycolytic metabolism in the heart • Second choice in the prevention of exertional angina • May increase the incidence of Parkinson disease
Antiplatelet, Anti-integrin, and Antithrombotic Drugs		
Aspirin P2Y$_{12}$ receptor antagonists (clopidogrel, prasugrel, ticagrelor cangrelor [IV])	• Prevention of thrombotic events (MI, stroke) • Acute coronary syndromes • Prevention of stent thrombosis	• ↓ Platelet aggregation by inhibiting COX-1–mediated TxA$_2$ production (aspirin) or ADP receptors (P2Y$_{12}$ receptor antagonists) • Oral use only: clopidogrel, prasugrel, ticagrelor • Irreversible action: aspirin, clopidogrel, prasugrel • Prodrugs: clopidogrel, prasugrel • Variable, CYP2C9-dependent metabolism (clopidogrel) • Withdraw 5–7 days before surgery • First choice in NSTEMI and STEMI • Dual platelet inhibition after stenting
Abciximab Eptifibatide Tirofiban	• Percutaneous coronary interventions	• Antibody (abciximab) or small molecule antagonists at platelet GpIIb/IIIa receptor • Parenteral use only • Highly efficient platelet inhibition • Therapeutic value in the era of highly effective dual platelet inhibition unclear
Heparin Low-molecular-weight heparins (e.g., enoxaparine)	• Acute coronary syndromes • Percutaneous coronary interventions	• Endogenous polysaccharide, inhibits thrombin (factor IIa) and factor Xa in an antithrombin III–dependent manner • Parenteral use only • Heparin: short $t_{1/2}$, complex pharmacokinetics, low bioavailability after subcutaneous. injection • Low-molecular-weight heparin: longer half-life, renal excretion; accumulation in renal insufficiency • Heparin-induced thrombocytopenia
Fondaparinux	• Acute coronary syndromes • Percutaneous coronary interventions	• Synthetic pentasaccharide, antithrombin III-dependent, factor Xa inhibitor • Most favorable efficacy-safety ratio
Bivalirudin Lepirudin	• Percutaneous coronary interventions (bivalirudin) • Heparin-induced thrombocytopenia (HIT II) recombinant lepirudin	• Direct thrombin (factor IIa) inhibitors • Parenteral use only • Advantage of bivalirudin over heparin unclear

Bibliography

Amsterdam EA, et al. 2014 AHA/ACC guideline for the management of patients with non-ST-elevation acute coronary syndromes: a report of the American College of Cardiology/American Heart Association Task Force on Practice Guidelines. *J Am Coll Cardiol*, **2014**, *64*:e139–e228.

Angus JA, et al. Quantitative analysis of vascular to cardiac selectivity of L- and T-type voltage-operated calcium channel antagonists in human tissues. *Clin Exp Pharmacol Physiol*, **2000**, *27*:1019–1021.

Ardehali H, O'Rourke B. Mitochondrial K(ATP) channels in cell survival and death. *J Mol Cell Cardiol*, **2005**, *39*:7–16.

Bainbridge AD, et al. A comparative assessment of amlodipine and felodipine ER: pharmacokinetic and pharmacodynamic indices. *Eur J Clin Pharmacol*, **1993**, *45*:425–430.

Bangalore S, et al. Clinical outcomes with beta-blockers for myocardial infarction: a meta-analysis of randomized trials. *Am J Med*, **2014**, *127*:939–953.

Barbato E, et al. Long-term effect of molsidomine, a direct nitric oxide donor, as an add-on treatment, on endothelial dysfunction in patients with stable angina pectoris undergoing percutaneous coronary intervention: results of the MEDCOR trial. *Atherosclerosis*, **2015**, *240*:351–354.

Bedenis R, et al. Cilostazol for intermittent claudication. *Cochrane Database Syst Rev*, **2014**, (10):CD003748.

Belardinelli L, et al. Inhibition of the late sodium current as a potential cardioprotective principle: effects of the late sodium current inhibitor ranolazine. *Heart*, **2006**, *92*:iv6-iv14.

Bhatt DL, et al. Clopidogrel and aspirin versus aspirin alone for the prevention of atherothrombotic events. *N Engl J Med*, **2006**, *354*:1706–1717.

Billinger M, et al. Collateral and collateral-adjacent hyperemic vascular resistance changes and the ipsilateral coronary flow reserve. Documentation of a mechanism causing coronary steal in patients with coronary artery disease. *Cardiovasc Res*, **2001**, *49*:600–608.

Bloch KD, et al. Inhaled NO as a therapeutic agent. *Cardiovasc Res*, **2007**, *75*:339–348.

Bodi V, et al. Prognostic value of dipyridamole stress cardiovascular magnetic resonance imaging in patients with known or suspected coronary artery disease. *J Am Coll Cardiol*, **2007**, *50*:1174–1179.

Boulinguez S, et al. Giant buccal aphthosis caused by nicorandil [in French]. *Presse Med*, **1997**, *26*:558.

Brown BG, et al. The mechanisms of nitroglycerin action: stenosis vasodilatation as a major component of the drug response. *Circulation*, **1981**, *64*:1089–1097.

Burnett AL, et al. Nitric oxide: a physiologic mediator of penile erection. *Science*, **1992**, *257*:401–403.

Cannon CP, et al. Comparison of ticagrelor with clopidogrel in patients with a planned invasive strategy for acute coronary syndromes (PLATO): a randomised double-blind study. *Lancet*, **2010**, *375*:283–293.

CAPRIE Steering Committee. A randomised, blinded, trial of clopidogrel versus aspirin in patients at risk of ischaemic events (CAPRIE). CAPRIE Steering Committee. *Lancet*, **1996**, *348*:1329–1339.

Cheitlin MD, et al. ACC/AHA expert consensus document. Use of sildenafil (Viagra) in patients with cardiovascular disease. American

College of Cardiology/American Heart Association. *J Am Coll Cardiol*, **1999**, 33:273–282.

Chen Z, et al. Identification of the enzymatic mechanism of nitroglycerin bioactivation. *Proc Natl Acad Sci U S A*, **2002**, 99:8306–8311.

Debbas NM, et al. The bioavailability and pharmacokinetics of slow release nifedipine during chronic dosing in volunteers. *Br J Clin Pharmacol*, **1986**, 21:385–388.

Dudzinski DM, et al. The regulation and pharmacology of endothelial nitric oxide synthase. *Annu Rev Pharmacol Toxicol*, **2006**, 46:235–276.

Epstein BJ, Roberts ME. Managing peripheral edema in patients with arterial hypertension. *Am J Ther*, **2009**, 16:543–553.

Fihn SD, et al. 2012 ACCF/AHA/ACP/AATS/PCNA/SCAI/STS guideline for the diagnosis and management of patients with stable ischemic heart disease. *Circulation*, **2012**, 126:e354–e471.

Fleckenstein A, et al. Selective inhibition of myocardial contractility by competitive divalent Ca^{++} antagonists (iproveratril, D 600, prenylamine) [in German]. *Naunyn Schmiedebergs Arch Pharmakol*, **1969**, 264:227–228.

Fox K, et al. Ivabradine in stable coronary artery disease. *N Engl J Med*, **2014**, 371:2435.

Godfraind T, et al. Calcium antagonism and calcium entry blockade. *Pharmacol Rev*, **1986**, 38:321–416.

Godfraind T, et al. Selectivity scale of calcium antagonists in the human cardiovascular system based on in vitro studies. *J Cardiovasc Pharmacol*, **1992**, 20(suppl 5):S34–S41.

Hamm CW, et al. ESC guidelines for the management of acute coronary syndromes in patients presenting without persistent ST-segment elevation: the Task Force for the Management of Acute Coronary Syndromes (ACS) in Patients Presenting Without Persistent ST-Segment Elevation of the European Society of Cardiology (ESC). *Eur Heart J*, **2011**, 32:2999–3054.

Hasenfuss G, Maier LS. Mechanism of action of the new anti-ischemia drug ranolazine. *Clin Res Cardiol*, **2008**, 97:222–226.

Herrmann HC, et al. Hemodynamic effects of sildenafil in men with severe coronary artery disease. *N Engl J Med*, **2000**, 342:1622–1626.

Hirsch AT, et al. ACC/AHA 2005 Practice guidelines for the management of patients with peripheral arterial disease (lower extremity, renal, mesenteric, and abdominal aortic): a collaborative report. *Circulation*, **2006**, 113:e463–e654.

Ho CY, et al. Diltiazem treatment for pre-clinical hypertrophic cardiomyopathy sarcomere mutation carriers: a pilot randomized trial to modify disease expression. *JACC Heart Fail*, **2015**, 3:180–188.

Kappetein AP, et al. Comparison of coronary bypass surgery with drug-eluting stenting for the treatment of left main and/or three-vessel disease: 3-year follow-up of the SYNTAX trial. *Eur Heart J*, **2011**, 32:2125–2134.

Kojda G, et al. Positive inotropic effect of exogenous and endogenous NO in hypertrophic rat hearts. *Br J Pharmacol*, **1997**, 122: 813–820.

Lee CC, et al. Use of nicorandil is associated with increased risk for gastrointestinal ulceration and perforation—a nationally representative population-based study. *Sci Rep*, **2015**, 5:11495.

Letienne R, et al. Evidence that ranolazine behaves as a weak beta1- and beta2-adrenoceptor antagonist in the rat [correction of cat] cardiovascular system. *Naunyn Schmiedeberg's Arch Pharmacol*, **2001**, 363:464–471.

Libby P, Pasterkamp G. Requiem for the "vulnerable plaque." *Eur Heart J*, **2015**, 36:2984–2987.

Libby P, et al. Inflammation and atherosclerosis. *Circulation*, **2002**, 105:1135–1143.

Magnon M, et al. Intervessel (arteries and veins) and heart/vessel selectivities of therapeutically used calcium entry blockers: variable, vessel-dependent indexes. *J Pharmacol Exp Ther*, **1995**, 275:1157–1166.

Matsubara T, et al. Three minute, but not one minute, ischemia and nicorandil have a preconditioning effect in patients with coronary artery disease. *J Am Coll Cardiol*, **2000**, 35:345–351.

Mayer B, Beretta M. The enigma of nitroglycerin bioactivation and nitrate tolerance: news, views and troubles. *Br J Pharmacol*, **2008**, 155:170–184.

McCormack JG, et al. Ranolazine: a novel metabolic modulator for the treatment of angina. *Gen Pharmacol*, **1998**, 30:639–645.

Meany TB, et al. Exercise capacity after single and twice-daily doses of nicorandil in chronic stable angina pectoris. *Am J Cardiol*, **1989**, 63:66J–70J.

Montalescot G, et al. 2013 ESC guidelines on the management of stable coronary artery disease: the Task Force on the Management of Stable Coronary Artery Disease of the European Society of Cardiology. *Eur Heart J*, **2013**, 34:2949–3003.

Mozaffarian D, et al. Heart disease and stroke statistics—2015 update: a report from the American Heart Association. *Circulation*, **2015**, 131:e29–e322.

Munzel T, et al. Evidence for enhanced vascular superoxide anion production in nitrate tolerance. A novel mechanism underlying tolerance and cross-tolerance. *J Clin Invest*, **1995**, 95:187–194.

Munzel T, et al. Organic nitrates: update on mechanisms underlying vasodilation, tolerance and endothelial dysfunction. *Vascul Pharmacol*, **2014**, 63:105–113.

Parker JD. Nitrate tolerance, oxidative stress, and mitochondrial function: another worrisome chapter on the effects of organic nitrates. *J Clin Invest*, **2004**, 113:352–354.

Parker JD, et al. Intermittent transdermal nitroglycerin therapy. Decreased anginal threshold during the nitrate-free interval. *Circulation*, **1995**, 91:973–978.

Parker JD, Parker JO. Nitrate therapy for stable angina pectoris. *N Engl J Med*, **1998**, 338:520–531.

Rajaratnam R, et al. Attenuation of anti-ischemic efficacy during chronic therapy with nicorandil in patients with stable angina pectoris. *Am J Cardiol*, **1999**, 83:1120–1124, A1129.

Redfield MM, et al. Effect of phosphodiesterase-5 inhibition on exercise capacity and clinical status in heart failure with preserved ejection fraction: a randomized clinical trial. *JAMA*, **2013**, 309:1268–1277.

Regensteiner JG, Hiatt WR. Current medical therapies for patients with peripheral arterial disease: a critical review. *Am J Med*, **2002**, 112:49–57.

Roffi M, et al. 2015 ESC Guidelines for the management of acute coronary syndromes in patients presenting without persistent ST-segment elevation: Task Force for the Management of Acute Coronary Syndromes in Patients Presenting Without Persistent ST-Segment Elevation of the European Society of Cardiology (ESC). *Eur Heart J*, **2016**, 37:267–315.

Rooke TW, et al. 2011 ACCF/AHA focused update of the guideline for the management of patients with peripheral artery disease (updating the 2005 guideline): a report of the American College of Cardiology Foundation/American Heart Association Task Force on Practice Guidelines. *J Am Coll Cardiol*, **2011**, 58:2020–2045.

Salhiyyah K, et al. Pentoxifylline for intermittent claudication. *Cochrane Database Syst Rev*, **2015**, (9):CD005262.

Sato T, et al. Nicorandil, a potent cardioprotective agent, acts by opening mitochondrial ATP-dependent potassium channels. *J Am Coll Cardiol*, **2000**, 35:514–518.

Sayed N, et al. Nitroglycerin-induced S-nitrosylation and desensitization of soluble guanylyl cyclase contribute to nitrate tolerance. *Circ Res*, **2008**, 103:606–614.

Schwartz A. Molecular and cellular aspects of calcium channel antagonism. *Am J Cardiol*, **1992**, 70:6F–8F.

Soma J, et al. Sublingual nitroglycerin delays arterial wave reflections despite increased aortic "stiffness" in patients with hypertension: a Doppler echocardiography study. *J Am Soc Echocardiogr*, **2000**, 13:1100–1108.

Stamler JS. Nitroglycerin-mediated S-nitrosylation of proteins: a field comes full cycle. *Circ Res*, **2008**, 103:557–559.

Steinberg SF, Brunton LL. Compartmentation of G protein-coupled signaling pathways in cardiac myocytes. *Annu Rev Pharmacol Toxicol*, **2001**, 41:751–773.

Sydow K, et al. Central role of mitochondrial aldehyde dehydrogenase and reactive oxygen species in nitroglycerin tolerance and cross-tolerance. *J Clin Invest*, **2004**, 113:482–489.

Tsien RW, et al. Multiple types of neuronal calcium channels and their selective modulation. *Trends Neurosci*, **1988**, 11:431–438.

Tuunanen H, et al. Trimetazidine, a metabolic modulator, has cardiac and extracardiac benefits in idiopathic dilated cardiomyopathy. *Circulation*, **2008**, 118:1250–1258.

506 Ussher JR, et al. Treatment with the 3-ketoacyl-CoA thiolase inhibitor trimetazidine does not exacerbate whole-body insulin resistance in obese mice. *J Pharmacol Exp Ther*, **2014**, *349*:487–496.

Valgimigli M, et al. Bivalirudin or unfractionated heparin in acute coronary syndromes. *N Engl J Med*, **2015**, *373*:997–1009.

van Harten J, et al. Negligible sublingual absorption of nifedipine. *Lancet*, **1987**, *2*:1363–1365.

Walsh RA, O'Rourke RA. Direct and indirect effects of calcium entry blocking agents on isovolumic left ventricular relaxation in conscious dogs. *J Clin Invest*, **1985**, *75*:1426–1434.

Weisz G, et al. Ranolazine in Patients With Incomplete Revascularisation After Percutaneous Coronary Intervention (RIVER-PCI): a multicentre, randomised, double-blind, placebo-controlled trial. *Lancet*, **2016**, *387*:136–145.

Wiviott SD, et al. Prasugrel versus clopidogrel in patients with acute coronary syndromes. *N Engl J Med*, **2007**, *357*:2001–2015.

Yeghiazarians Y, et al. Unstable angina pectoris. *N Engl J Med*, **2000**, *342*:101–114.

Yusuf S, et al. Effects of clopidogrel in addition to aspirin in patients with acute coronary syndromes without ST-segment elevation. *N Engl J Med*, **2001**, *345*:494–502.

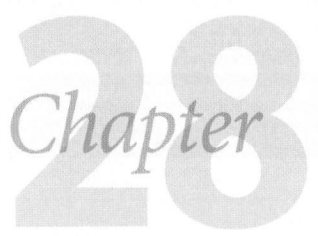

Chapter 28

Treatment of Hypertension

Thomas Eschenhagen

EPIDEMIOLOGY AND TREATMENT ALGORITHMS
- Principles of Antihypertensive Therapy

DIURETICS
- Benzothiadiazines and Related Compounds
- Other Diuretic Antihypertensive Agents
- K+-Sparing Diuretics
- Diuretic-Associated Drug Interactions

SYMPATHOLYTIC AGENTS
- β adrenergic receptor antagonist (β Blockers)
- α$_1$ adrenergic receptor antagonist (α$_1$ Blockers)
- Combined α$_1$ and β Blockers
- Centrally Acting Sympatholytic Drugs

Ca²⁺ CHANNEL BLOCKERS

INHIBITORS OF THE RENIN-ANGIOTENSIN SYSTEM
- Angiotensin-Converting Enzyme Inhibitors

- AT$_1$ Receptor Blockers
- Direct Renin Inhibitors

VASODILATORS
- Hydralazine
- K$_{ATP}$ Channel Openers: Minoxidil
- Sodium Nitroprusside
- Diazoxide

NONPHARMACOLOGICAL THERAPY OF HYPERTENSION

SELECTION OF ANTIHYPERTENSIVE DRUGS IN INDIVIDUAL PATIENTS

ACUTE ANTIHYPERTENSIVE TREATMENT

RESISTANT HYPERTENSION

Epidemiology and Treatment Algorithms

Hypertension is the most common cardiovascular disease. Elevated arterial pressure causes hypertrophy of the left ventricle and pathological changes in the vasculature. As a consequence, hypertension is the principal cause of stroke; a major risk factor for CAD and its attendant complications, MI and sudden cardiac death; and a major contributor to heart failure, renal insufficiency, and dissecting aneurysm of the aorta. The prevalence of hypertension increases with age; for example, about 50% of people between the ages of 60 and 69 years old have hypertension, and the prevalence further increases beyond age 70. According to a recent survey in the U.S., 81.5% of those with hypertension are aware they have it, 74.9% are being treated, yet only 52.5% are considered controlled (Go et al., 2014). The success of hypertension treatment programs, such as one organized in a large integrated healthcare delivery system in the U.S. (Jaffe et al., 2013), show that these figures can be substantially improved by electronic hypertension registries tracking hypertension control rates, regular feedback to providers, development and frequent updating of an evidence-based treatment guideline, promotion of single-pill combination therapies, and follow-up blood pressure checks. Between 2001 and 2009, this program increased the number of patients with a diagnosis of hypertension by 78%, as well as the proportion of subjects meeting target blood pressure goals from 44% to more than 84% (Jaffe et al., 2013).

Hypertension is defined as a sustained increase in blood pressure of 140/90 mmHg or higher, a criterion that characterizes a group of patients whose risk of hypertension-related cardiovascular disease is high enough to merit medical attention. Actually, the risk of both fatal and nonfatal cardiovascular disease in adults is lowest with systolic blood pressures of less than 120 mmHg and diastolic blood pressures less than 80 mmHg; these risks increase incrementally as systolic and diastolic blood pressures rise. Recognition of this continuously increasing risk prevents a simple definition of hypertension (Go et al., 2014) (Table 28–1). Although many of the clinical trials classified the severity of hypertension by diastolic pressure, progressive elevations of systolic pressure are similarly predictive of adverse cardiovascular events; at every level of diastolic pressure, risks are greater with higher levels of systolic blood pressure. Indeed, in patients more than 50 years old, systolic blood pressures predict adverse outcomes better than do diastolic pressures. Pulse pressure, defined as the difference between systolic and diastolic pressure, may add additional predictive value (Pastor-Barriuso et al., 2003). This may be at least in part due to higher-than-normal pulse pressure indicating adverse remodeling of blood vessels, representing an accelerated decrease in blood vessel compliance normally associated with aging and atherosclerosis. Isolated systolic hypertension (sometimes defined as systolic blood pressure greater than 140–160 mmHg with diastolic blood pressure less than 90 mmHg) is largely confined to people older than 60 years.

The presence of pathological changes in certain target organs heralds a worse prognosis than the same level of blood pressure in a patient lacking these findings. For instance, retinal hemorrhages, exudates, and papilledema in the eyes indicate a far worse short-term prognosis for a given level of blood pressure. Left ventricular hypertrophy defined by electrocardiogram, or more sensitively by echocardiography or cardiac magnetic resonance imaging, is associated with a substantially worse long-term outcome that includes a higher risk of sudden cardiac death. The risk of cardiovascular disease, disability, and death in hypertensive patients also is increased markedly by concomitant cigarette smoking, diabetes, or elevated LDL; the coexistence of hypertension with these risk factors increases cardiovascular morbidity and mortality to a degree that is compounded by each additional risk factor.

The purpose of treating hypertension is to decrease cardiovascular risk; thus, other dietary and pharmacological interventions may be required to treat these additional risk factors. Effective pharmacological treatment of patients with hypertension decreases morbidity and mortality from cardiovascular disease, reducing the risk of strokes, heart failure, and CAD (Rosendorff et al., 2015). The reduction in risk of MI may be less significant.

Abbreviations

ACE: angiotensin-converting enzyme
ACEI: angiotensin-converting enzyme inhibitor
Aldo: aldosterone
AngII: angiotensin II
ANP: atrial natriuretic peptide
ARB: angiotensin receptor blocker
AT$_1$: type 1 receptor for angiotensin II
ATPase: adenosine triphosphatase
AV: atrioventricular
BB: β blocker
β blocker: β adrenergic receptor antagonist
BNP: brain natriuretic peptide
BP: blood pressure
CAD: coronary artery disease
CCB: Ca^{2+} channel blocker
CNS: central nervous system
COX-2: cyclooxygenase 2
DOPA: 3,4-dihydroxyphenylalanine
DRI: direct renin inhibitor
ENaC: epithelial Na$^+$ channel
ESC: European Society of Cardiology
GI: gastrointestinal
GFR: glomerular filtration rate
HDL: high-density lipoprotein
HF: heart failure
HTN: hypertension
ISA: intrinsic sympathomimetic activity
ISDN: isosorbide dinitrate
JNC8: Eighth Joint National Committee
MI: myocardial infarction
MRA: mineralocorticoid receptor antagonist
NCC: NaCl cotransporter
NE: norepinephrine
NO: nitric oxide
NSAID: nonsteroidal anti-inflammatory drug
RAAS: renin-angiotensin-aldosterone system
RAS: renin-angiotensin system
SA: sinoatrial
SNS: sympathetic nervous system
VMAT2: vesicular catecholamine transporter 2

Principles of Antihypertensive Therapy

Nonpharmacological therapy, or lifestyle-related changes, is an important component of treatment of all patients with hypertension (James et al., 2014; Mancia et al., 2013). In some grade 1 hypertensives (Figure 28–1), blood pressure may be adequately controlled by a combination of weight loss (in overweight individuals), restricting sodium intake (to 5–6 g/d), increasing aerobic exercise (>30 min/d), moderating consumption of alcohol (ethanol/day ≤ 20–30 g in men [two drinks], ≤ 10–20 g in women [one drink]), smoking cessation, increased consumption of fruits, vegetables, and low-fat dairy products.

The majority of patients require drug therapy for adequate blood pressure control (Figure 28–1). Optimal blood pressure goals for drug therapy are still debated, and current guidelines from cardiovascular societies differ slightly (James et al., 2014). Recently, a large comparative study in nondiabetics with increased cardiovascular risk was prematurely stopped because the group of patients treated with antihypertensives to a systolic blood pressure target of 120 mmHg, with an average of 2.8 drugs, experienced a 25% lower rate of cardiovascular end points and total mortality than the group targeted to the current standard goal target of 140 mmHg

TABLE 28–1 ■ AMERICAN HEART ASSOCIATION CRITERIA FOR HYPERTENSION IN ADULTS

CLASSIFICATION	BLOOD PRESSURE (mmHg)	
	SYSTOLIC	DIASTOLIC
Normal	<120	and < 80
Prehypertension	120–139	or 80–89
Hypertension, stage 1	140–159	or 90–99
Hypertension, stage 2	≥160	or ≥ 100
Hypertensive crisis	>180	or > 110

(SPRINT Research Group, 2015). The rate of adverse effects such as hypotension and worsening of renal function were higher in the intensified treatment group, yet this did not translate to a signal for real harm. The data will likely lead to a reexamination of current guideline-recommended blood pressure targets.

Arterial pressure is the product of cardiac output and peripheral vascular resistance (Figure 28–2). Drugs lower blood pressure by actions on peripheral resistance, cardiac output, or both. Drugs may decrease the cardiac output by inhibiting myocardial contractility or by decreasing ventricular filling pressure. Reduction in ventricular filling pressure may be achieved by actions on the venous tone or on blood volume via renal effects. Drugs can decrease peripheral resistance by acting on smooth muscle to cause relaxation of resistance vessels or by interfering with the activity of systems that produce constriction of resistance vessels (e.g., the sympathetic nervous system, the RAS). In patients with isolated systolic hypertension, complex hemodynamics in a rigid arterial system contribute to increased blood pressure; drug effects may be mediated not only by changes in peripheral resistance but also via effects on large artery stiffness (Franklin, 2000).

Antihypertensive drugs can be classified according to their sites or mechanisms of action (Table 28–2, Figure 28–2). The hemodynamic consequences of long-term treatment with antihypertensive agents (Table 28–3) provide a rationale for potential complementary effects of concurrent therapy with two or more drugs. Concurrent use of drugs from different classes is a strategy for achieving effective control of blood pressure while minimizing dose-related adverse effects.

It generally is not possible to predict the responses of individuals with hypertension to any specific drug. For example, for some antihypertensive drugs, about two-thirds of patients will have a meaningful clinical response, whereas about one-third of patients will not respond to the same drug. Racial origin and age may have modest influence on the likelihood of a favorable response to a particular class of drugs. Polymorphisms in genes involved in the metabolism of antihypertensive drugs have been identified in the CYPs (phase I metabolism) and in phase II metabolism, such as catechol-O-methyltransferase (see Chapters 6 and 7). While these polymorphisms can change the pharmacokinetics of specific drugs quite markedly (e.g., five times higher plasma concentrations of metoprolol in CYP2D6 poor metabolizers), differences in efficacy are smaller (Rau et al., 2009) and of unknown clinical relevance. Polymorphisms that influence pharmacodynamic responses to antihypertensive drugs, including ACE inhibitors and diuretics, have also been identified, but evidence for clinically meaningful differences in drug response is sparse. Genome-wide scanning has identified several genetic variants associated with hypertension, but the effect sizes are much smaller than that of clinically established risk factors such as overweight.

Diuretics

An early strategy for the management of hypertension was to alter Na$^+$ balance by restriction of salt in the diet. Pharmacological alteration of Na$^+$ balance became practical with the development of the orally active thiazide diuretics (see Chapter 25). These and related diuretic agents have

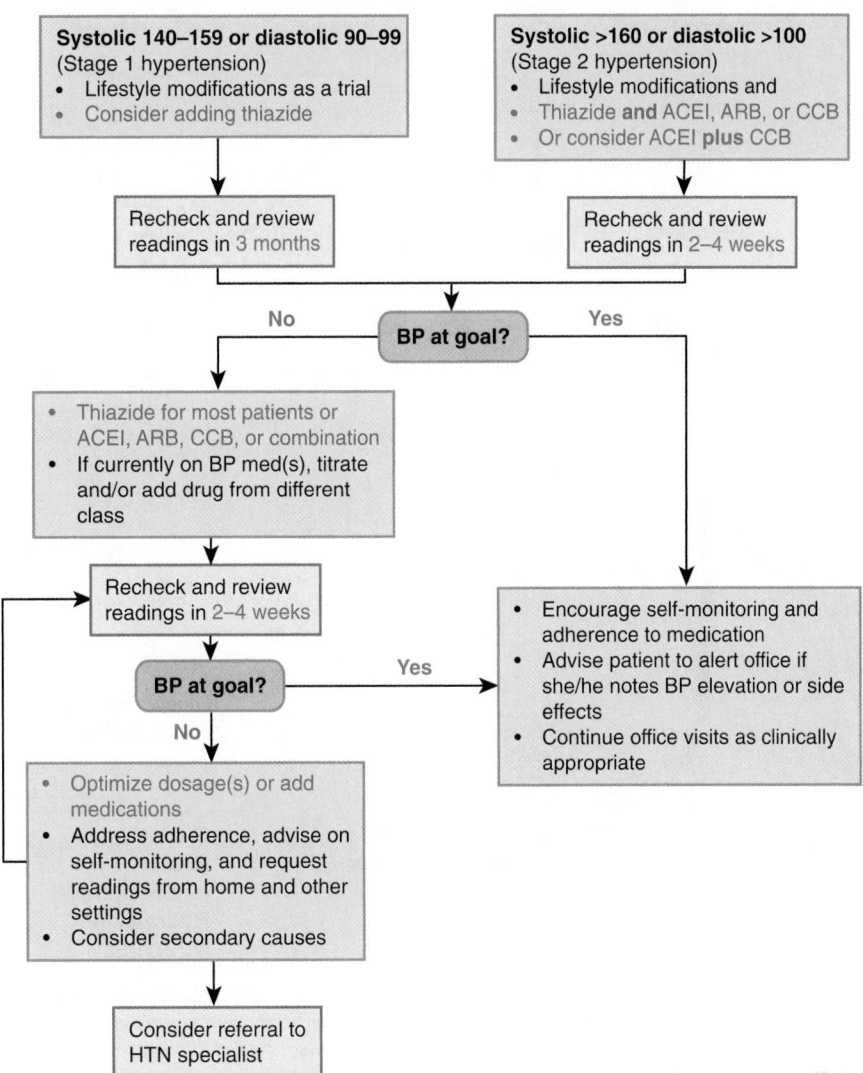

Figure 28–1 *Treatment algorithm for adults with hypertension.* Algorithm is based on recommendations of the American Heart Association and the American College of Cardiology (Go et al., 2013).

antihypertensive effects when used alone, and they enhance the efficacy of virtually all other antihypertensive drugs. Thus, this class of drugs remains important in the treatment of hypertension.

The exact mechanism for reduction of arterial blood pressure by diuretics is not certain. The initial action of thiazide diuretics decreases extracellular volume by interacting with a thiazide-sensitive NCC (*SLC12A3*) expressed in the distal convoluted tubule in the kidney, enhancing Na^+ excretion in the urine, and leading to a decrease in cardiac output. However, the hypotensive effect is maintained during long-term therapy due to decreased vascular resistance; cardiac output returns to pretreatment values, and extracellular volume returns to almost normal due to compensatory responses such as activation of the RAS. The explanation for the long-term vasodilation induced by thiazide diuretics is unknown. *Hydrochlorothiazide* may open Ca^{2+}-activated K^+ channels, leading to hyperpolarization of vascular smooth muscle cells, which leads in turn to closing of L-type Ca^{2+} channels and lower probability of opening, resulting in decreased Ca^{2+} entry and reduced vasoconstriction. Hydrochlorothiazide also inhibits vascular carbonic anhydrase, which, hypothetically, could alter smooth muscle cell systolic pH and thereby cause opening of Ca^{2+}-activated K^+ channels with the consequences noted previously.

The relevance of these findings—largely assessed in vitro—to the observed antihypertensive effects of thiazides is speculative. The major action of these drugs on SLC12A3—expressed predominantly in the distal convoluted tubules and not in vascular smooth muscle or the

heart—suggests that these drugs decrease peripheral resistance as an indirect effect of negative Na^+ balance. That thiazides lose efficacy in treating hypertension in patients with coexisting renal insufficiency is compatible with this hypothesis. Moreover, carriers of rare functional mutations in SLC12A3 that decrease renal Na^+ reabsorption have lower blood pressure than appropriate controls (Ji et al., 2008); in a sense, this is an experiment of nature that may mimic the therapeutic effect of thiazides.

Benzothiadiazines and Related Compounds

Benzothiadiazines ("thiazides") and related diuretics are the most frequently used class of antihypertensive agents in the U.S. Following the discovery of *chlorothiazide*, a number of oral diuretics were developed that have an arylsulfonamide structure and block the NCC. Some of these are not benzothiadiazines but have structural features and molecular functions that are similar to the original benzothiadiazine compounds; consequently, they are designated as members of the thiazide class of diuretics. For example, chlorthalidone (also written as chlortalidone), one of the nonbenzothiadiazines, is widely used in the treatment of hypertension, as is indapamide.

Regimen for Administration of the Thiazide-Class Diuretics in Hypertension

Because members of the thiazide class have similar pharmacological effects, they generally have been viewed as interchangeable with appropriate

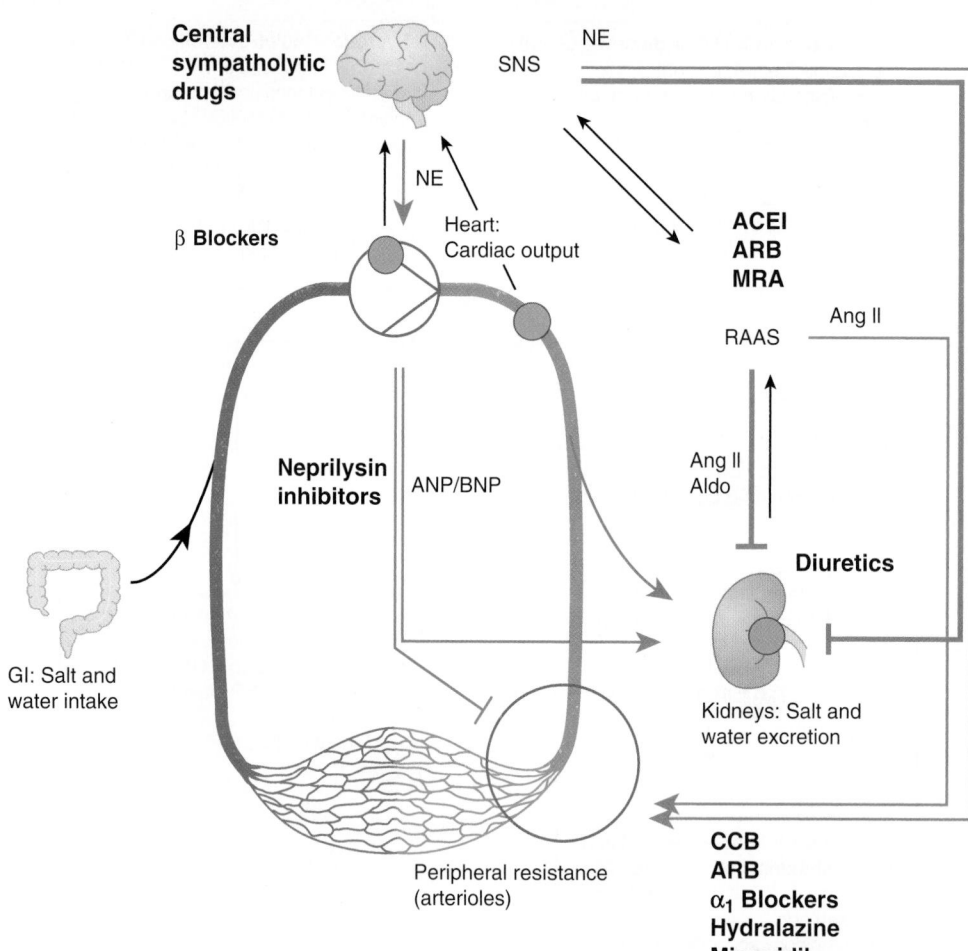

Figure 28–2 *Principles of blood pressure regulation and its modification by drugs.* Cardiac output and peripheral arteriolar resistance, the major determinants of arterial blood pressure, are regulated by myriad mechanisms, including the SNS (main peripheral neurotransmitter NE), the balance between salt intake by the intestine (GI) and salt excretion by the kidneys, the RAAS (main agonists AngII and Aldo), and natriuretic peptides produced in the heart (ANP and BNP). Sensors (green circles) provide afferent input on pressure in the heart and great vessels and on salt concentrations in the kidney. Note positive feedback between the SNS and RAAS via β_1-stimulated renin release and AngII-stimulated NE release. Drug classes are indicated in boldface type at their main site of action. Arrows indicate blood pressure-increasing (red) and -decreasing (green) effects. Neprilysin inhibitors (e.g., sacubitril) are in clinical testing for hypertension and have been approved for the treatment of heart failure (in combination with an ARB).

adjustment of dosage (see Chapter 25). However, the pharmacokinetics and pharmacodynamics of these drugs differ, so they may not necessarily have the same clinical efficacy in treating hypertension. In a direct comparison, the antihypertensive efficacy of chlorthalidone was greater than that of hydrochlorothiazide, particularly during the night (Ernst et al., 2006), suggesting the much longer $t_{1/2}$ of chlorthalidone (>24 h) compared to hydrochlorothiazide (several hours) gave more stable blood pressure reductions. In light of the considerable clinical trial data supporting the capacity of chlorthalidone to diminish adverse cardiovascular events—in comparison to that available for currently used low doses of hydrochlorothiazide—there is a growing concern that chlorthalidone may be an underutilized drug in hypertensive patients requiring a diuretic.

Antihypertensive effects can be achieved in many patients with as little as 12.5 mg daily of chlorthalidone or hydrochlorothiazide. Furthermore, when used as monotherapy, the maximal daily dose of thiazide-class diuretics usually should not exceed 25 mg of hydrochlorothiazide or chlorthalidone (or equivalent). Even though more diuresis can be achieved with higher doses, some evidence suggests that doses higher than this are not generally more efficacious in lowering blood pressure in patients with normal renal function. Low doses of either thiazide reduce the risk of adverse effects such as K^+ wasting and inhibition of uric acid excretion, indicating an improved risk-to-benefit ratio at low doses of a thiazide. However, other studies suggested that low doses of hydrochlorothiazide

have inadequate effects on blood pressure when monitored in a detailed manner (Lacourciere et al., 1995).

Clinical trials of antihypertensive therapy in the elderly demonstrated the best outcomes for cardiovascular morbidity and mortality when 25 mg of hydrochlorothiazide or chlorthalidone was the maximum dose given; if this dose did not achieve the target blood pressure reduction, a second drug was initiated (1991; Dahlof et al., 1991). A case-control study found a dose-dependent increase in the occurrence of sudden death at doses of hydrochlorothiazide greater than 25 mg daily (Siscovick et al., 1994), supporting the hypothesis that higher diuretic doses are associated with increased cardiovascular mortality as long as hypokalemia is not corrected. Thus, if adequate blood pressure reduction is not achieved with the 25-mg daily dose of hydrochlorothiazide or chlorthalidone, the addition of a second drug is indicated rather than an increase in the dose of diuretic.

Urinary K^+ loss can be a problem with thiazides. ACE inhibitors and ARBs will attenuate diuretic-induced loss of K^+ to some degree, and this is a consideration if a second drug is required to achieve further blood pressure reduction beyond that attained with the diuretic alone. Because the diuretic and hypotensive effects of these drugs are greatly enhanced when they are given in combination, care should be taken to initiate combination therapy with low doses of each of these drugs (Vlasses et al., 1983). Administration of ACE inhibitors or ARBs together with other

TABLE 28–2 ■ CLASSES OF ANTIHYPERTENSIVE DRUGS

Diuretics (Chapter 25)
- *Thiazides and related agents*: chlorothiazide, chlorthalidone, hydrochlorothiazide, indapamide
- *Loop diuretics*: bumetanide, furosemide, torsemide
- *K⁺-sparing diuretics*: amiloride, triamterene, MRA spironolactone

Sympatholytic drugs (Chapter 12)
- *β Blockers*: atenolol, bisoprolol, esmolol, metoprolol, nadolol, nebivolol, propranolol, timolol
- *α Blockers*: prazosin, terazosin, doxazosin, phenoxybenzamine
- *Mixed α/β blockers*: labetalol, carvedilol
- *Centrally acting sympatholytic agents*: clonidine, guanabenz, guanfacine, methyldopa, moxonidine, reserpine

Ca²⁺ channel blockers (Chapter 27): amlodipine, clevidipine, diltiazem, felodipine, isradipine, lercanidipine, nicardipine, nifedipine,[a] nisoldipine, verapamil

Renin-angiotensin antagonists **(Chapter 26)**
- *Angiotensin-converting enzyme inhibitors*: benazepril, captopril, enalapril, fosinopril, lisinopril, moexipril, perindopril, quinapril, ramipril, trandolapril
- *AngII receptor blockers*: candesartan, eprosartan, irbesartan, losartan, olmesartan, telmisartan, valsartan
- *Direct renin inhibitor*: aliskiren

Vasodilators **(Chapters 27 and 28)**
- *Arterial*: diazoxide, fenoldopam, hydralazine, minoxidil
- *Arterial and venous*: nitroprusside

[a]Only extended-release nifedipine is approved for hypertension.

K⁺-sparing agents or with K⁺ supplements requires great caution; combining K⁺-sparing agents with each other or with K⁺ supplementation can cause potentially dangerous hyperkalemia in some patients.

In contrast to the limitation on the dose of thiazide-class diuretics used as monotherapy, the treatment of severe hypertension that is unresponsive to three or more drugs may require larger doses of the thiazide-class diuretics. Indeed, hypertensive patients may become refractory to drugs that block the sympathetic nervous system or to vasodilator drugs,

because these drugs engender a state in which the blood pressure is very volume dependent. Therefore, it is appropriate to consider the use of thiazide-class diuretics in doses of 50 mg of daily hydrochlorothiazide equivalent when treatment with appropriate combinations and doses of three or more drugs fails to yield adequate control of the blood pressure. Alternatively, there may be a need to use higher-capacity diuretics such as furosemide, especially if renal function is not normal.

The effectiveness of thiazides as diuretics or antihypertensive agents is progressively diminished when the glomerular filtration rate falls below 30 mL/min. One exception is metolazone, which retains efficacy in patients with this degree of renal insufficiency.

Most patients will respond to thiazide diuretics with a reduction in blood pressure within about 4–6 weeks. Therefore, doses should not be increased more often than every 4–6 weeks. There is no way to predict the antihypertensive response from the duration or severity of the hypertension in a given patient, although diuretics are unlikely to be effective as sole therapy in patients with stage 2 hypertension (Table 28–1). Because the effect of thiazide diuretics is additive with that of other antihypertensive drugs, combination regimens that include these diuretics are common and rational. A wide range of fixed-dose combination products containing a thiazide are marketed for this purpose. Diuretics also have the advantage of minimizing the retention of salt and water that is commonly caused by vasodilators and some sympatholytic drugs. Omitting or underutilizing a diuretic is a frequent cause of "resistant hypertension."

Adverse Effects and Precautions

The adverse effects of diuretics are discussed in Chapter 25. Some of these determine whether a patient can tolerate and adhere to diuretic treatment.

The K⁺ depletion produced by thiazide-class diuretics is dose dependent and variable among individuals, such that a subset of patients may become substantially K⁺ depleted on diuretic drugs. Given chronically, even small doses lead to some K⁺ depletion, which is a well-known risk factor for ventricular arrhythmias by reducing cardiac repolarization reserve. The last has recently been used to explain that insults in a particular repolarization current do not necessarily result in QT interval prolongation, the principle clinical measure of repolarization (see Chapter 30). Hypokalemia directly reduces repolarization reserve by decreasing several K⁺ conductances (inward rectifier I_{K1}, delayed rectifier I_{Kr}, and the transient outward current I_{to}) and increases the binding activity of I_{Kr}-inhibiting drugs such as dofetilide (Yang and Roden, 1996). Hypokalemia also reduces

TABLE 28–3 ■ HEMODYNAMIC EFFECTS OF LONG-TERM ADMINISTRATION OF ANTIHYPERTENSIVE AGENTS

	HEART RATE	CARDIAC OUTPUT	TOTAL PERIPHERAL RESISTANCE	PLASMA VOLUME	PLASMA RENIN ACTIVITY
Diuretics	↔	↔	↓	–↓	↑
Sympatholytic agents					
Centrally acting	–↓	–↓	↓	–↑	–↓
α₁ Blockers	–↑	–↑	↓	–↑	↔
β Blockers					
No ISA	↓	↓	–↓	–↑	↓
ISA[a]	↓↑	↔	↓	–↑	–↓
Arteriolar vasodilators	↑	↑	↓	↑	↑
Ca²⁺ channel blockers	↓ or ↑	↓ or ↑	↓	–↑	–↑
ACEIs	↔	↔	↓	↔	↑
AT₁ receptor blockers	↔	↔	↓	↔	↑
Renin inhibitor	↔	↔	↓	↔	↓ (but renin ↑)

↑, increased; ↓, decreased; –↑, increased or no change; –↓, decreased or no change; ↔, unchanged.
[a]Heart rate can be increased at rest and decreased under exercise as a result of ISA. During rest, ISA may increase resting heart rate; during exercise, β adrenergic antagonism predominates, attenuating heart rate acceleration by NE.

the activity of the Na^+,K^+-ATPase (the Na^+ pump), causing intracellular accumulation of Na^+ and Ca^{2+}, further increasing the risk of afterdepolarizations (Pezhouman et al., 2015). Consequently, hypokalemia increases the risk of drug-induced polymorphic ventricular tachycardia (torsade de pointes; see Chapter 30) and the risk for ischemic ventricular fibrillation, the leading cause of sudden cardiac death and a major contributor to cardiovascular mortality in treated hypertensive patients. There is a positive correlation between diuretic dose and sudden cardiac death and an inverse correlation between the use of adjunctive K^+-sparing agents and sudden cardiac death (Siscovick et al., 1994). Thus, hypokalemia needs to be avoided by, for example, combining a thiazide with inhibitors of the RAS or with a K^+-sparing diuretic.

Thiazides have residual carbonic anhydrase–inhibiting activity, thereby reducing Na^+ reabsorption in the proximal tubule. The increased presentation of Na^+ at the macula densa leads to a reduced glomerular filtration rate via tubuloglomerular feedback. While this effect is clinically not meaningful in patients with normal renal function, it reduces diuretic effectiveness and may gain importance in patients with reduced kidney function. RAS inhibitors and Ca^{2+} channel blockers interfere with tubuloglomerular feedback, providing one explanation for the synergistic effect on blood pressure. Erectile dysfunction is a troublesome adverse effect of the thiazide-class diuretics, and physicians should inquire specifically regarding its occurrence in conjunction with treatment with these drugs. Gout may be a consequence of the hyperuricemia induced by these diuretics. The occurrence of either of these adverse effects is a reason for considering alternative approaches to therapy. However, precipitation of acute gout is relatively uncommon with low doses of diuretics. Hydrochlorothiazide may cause rapidly developing, severe hyponatremia in some patients. Thiazides inhibit renal Ca^{2+} excretion, occasionally leading to hypercalcemia; although generally mild, this can be more severe in patients subject to hypercalcemia, such as those with primary hyperparathyroidism. The thiazide-induced decreased Ca^{2+} excretion may be used therapeutically in patients with osteoporosis or hypercalciuria.

Thiazide diuretics have also been associated with changes in plasma lipids and glucose tolerance that have led to some concern. The clinical significance of the changes has been disputed because the clinical studies demonstrated comparable efficacy of the thiazide diuretic chlortalidone in reducing cardiovascular risk (ALLHAT Officers, 2002).

All thiazide-like drugs cross the placenta. While they have no direct adverse effects on the fetus, administration of a thiazide during pregnancy increases a risk of transient volume depletion that may result in placental hypoperfusion. Because the thiazides appear in breast milk, they should be avoided by nursing mothers.

Other Diuretic Antihypertensive Agents

The thiazide diuretics are more effective antihypertensive agents than are the loop diuretics, such as furosemide and bumetanide, in patients who have normal renal function. This differential effect is most likely related to the short duration of action of loop diuretics. In fact, a single daily dose of loop diuretics does not cause a significant net loss of Na^+ for an entire 24-h period because the strong initial diuretic effect is followed by a rebound mediated by activation of the RAS. Unfortunately, loop diuretics are frequently and inappropriately prescribed as a once-a-day medication in the treatment not only of hypertension, but also of congestive heart failure and ascites. The high efficacy of loop diuretics to produce a rapid and profound natriuresis can be detrimental for the treatment of hypertension. When a loop diuretic is given twice daily, the acute diuresis can be excessive and lead to more side effects than occur with a slower-acting, milder thiazide diuretic. Loop diuretics may be particularly useful in patients with azotemia or with severe edema associated with a vasodilator such as minoxidil.

K^+-Sparing Diuretics

Amiloride and triamterene are K^+-sparing diuretics that have little value as antihypertensive monotherapy but are important in combination with thiazides to antagonize urinary K^+ loss and the concomitant risk of ventricular arrhythmias. They act by reversibly inhibiting the ENaC in the distal tubule membrane, the transporter responsible for the reabsorption of Na^+ in exchange for K^+. The importance of ENaC for hypertension is illustrated by the fact that an inherited form of hypertension, Liddle syndrome, is due to hyperactivity of ENaC. Gene expression of ENaC is mineralocorticoid sensitive, explaining the antihypertensive and K^+-sparing effect of another class of K^+-sparing diuretics, the MRAs spironolactone and eplerenone. In contrast to the immediate and short-term inhibition of ENaC by amiloride and triamterene, the action of MRAs is delayed for about 3 days and is long lasting because MRAs regulate the density of the channel protein in the tubule membrane.

The MRAs have a particular role in hypertension and heart failure (see Chapter 27) because small doses of spironolactone are often highly effective in patients with "resistant hypertension." First described decades ago (Ramsay et al., 1980), the concept was recently validated in a prospective, placebo-controlled trial comparing spironolactone (25–50 mg) with bisoprolol or doxazosin as add-ons in patients with uncontrolled hypertension despite triple standard antihypertensive therapy (Williams et al., 2015). Spironolactone had about a 2-fold larger blood pressure–lowering effect (8.7 vs. 4.8 and 4 mmHg, respectively). The efficacy of the MRA spironolactone in resistant hypertension supports a primary role of Na^+ retention in this condition. Some of the effect may be related to the so-called aldosterone-escape phenomenon, or a return to pre-RAS-inhibitor plasma aldosterone levels with extended time of treatment, observed under treatment with RAS inhibitors. Primary hyperaldosteronism occurs in a significant fraction of patients with resistant hypertension (Calhoun et al., 2002).

Spironolactone has some significant adverse effects, especially in men (e.g., erectile dysfunction, gynecomastia, benign prostatic hyperplasia). Eplerenone is a more specific, though less-potent, MRA with reduced side effects.

All K^+-sparing diuretics should be used cautiously, with frequent measurements of plasma K^+ concentrations in patients predisposed to hyperkalemia. Patients should be cautioned regarding the possibility that concurrent use of K^+-containing salt substitutes could produce hyperkalemia. Renal insufficiency is a relative contraindication to the use of K^+-sparing diuretics. Concomitant use of an ACE inhibitor or an ARB magnifies the risk of hyperkalemia with these agents.

Diuretic-Associated Drug Interactions

Because the antihypertensive effects of diuretics are additive with those of other antihypertensive agents, a diuretic commonly is used in combination with other drugs. The K^+- and Mg^{2+}-depleting effects of the thiazides and loop diuretics can potentiate arrhythmias that arise from digitalis toxicity. Corticosteroids can amplify the hypokalemia produced by the diuretics. NSAIDs (see Chapter 38) that inhibit the synthesis of prostaglandins reduce the antihypertensive effects of diuretics and all other antihypertensives. The renal effects of selective COX-2 inhibitors are similar to those of the traditional NSAIDs. NSAIDs and RAS inhibitors reduce plasma concentrations of aldosterone and can potentiate the hyperkalemic effects of a K^+-sparing diuretic. All diuretics can decrease the clearance of Li^+, resulting in increased plasma concentrations of Li^+ and potential toxicity.

Sympatholytic Agents

With the demonstration in 1940 that bilateral excision of the thoracic sympathetic chain could lower blood pressure, there was a search for effective chemical sympatholytic agents. Many of the early sympatholytic drugs were poorly tolerated and had limiting adverse side effects, particularly on mood. A number of sympatholytic agents are currently in use (Table 28–2). Antagonists of α and β adrenergic receptors have been mainstays of antihypertensive therapy.

β Blockers

β Adrenergic receptor antagonists (β blockers) were not expected to have antihypertensive effects when they were first investigated in patients with angina, their primary indication. However, *pronethalol*, a drug that was never marketed, was found to reduce arterial blood pressure in hypertensive patients with angina pectoris. This antihypertensive effect was subsequently demonstrated for *propranolol* and all other β blockers. The basic pharmacology of these drugs is discussed in Chapter 12; characteristics relevant to their use in hypertension are described here.

Locus and Mechanism of Action

Antagonism of β adrenergic receptors affects the regulation of the circulation through a number of mechanisms, including a reduction in myocardial contractility and heart rate (i.e., cardiac output; see Figure 27–1). Antagonism of β_1 receptors of the juxtaglomerular complex reduces renin secretion and RAS activity. This action likely contributes to the antihypertensive action. Some members of this large, heterogeneous class of drugs have additional effects unrelated to their capacity to bind to β adrenergic receptors. For example, labetalol and carvedilol are also α_1 blockers, and nebivolol promotes endothelial cell–dependent vasodilation via activation of NO production (Pedersen and Cockcroft, 2006) (see Figure 12–4).

Pharmacodynamic Differences

The β blockers vary in their selectivity for the β_1 receptor subtype, presence of partial agonist or intrinsic sympathomimetic activity, and vasodilating capacity. While all of the β blockers are effective as antihypertensive agents, these differences influence the clinical pharmacology and spectrum of adverse effects of the various drugs. The antihypertensive effect resides in antagonism of the β_1 receptor, while major unwanted effects result from antagonism of β_2 receptors (e.g., peripheral vasoconstriction, bronchoconstriction, hypoglycemia). Standard therapies are β_1 blockers without intrinsic sympathomimetic activity (e.g., atenolol, bisoprolol, metoprolol). They produce an initial reduction in cardiac output (mainly β_1) and a reflex-induced rise in peripheral resistance, with little or no acute change in arterial pressure. In patients who respond with a reduction in blood pressure, peripheral resistance gradually returns to pretreatment values or less. Generally, persistently reduced cardiac output and possibly decreased peripheral resistance account for the reduction in arterial pressure. Nonselective β blockers (e.g., propranolol) have stronger adverse effects on peripheral vascular resistance by also blocking β_2 receptors that normally mediate vasodilation. Vasodilating β blockers (e.g., carvedilol, nebivolol) may be preferred in patients with peripheral artery disease. Drugs with intrinsic sympathomimetic activity (e.g., pindolol, xamoterol) are not recommended for the treatment of hypertension or any other cardiovascular disease because they actually increase nighttime mean heart rate due to their direct partial agonistic activity.

Pharmacokinetic Differences

Lipophilic β blockers (metoprolol, bisoprolol, carvedilol, propranolol) appear to have more antiarrhythmic efficacy than the hydrophilic compounds (atenolol, nadolol, labetalol), possibly related to a central mode of action. Many β blockers have relatively short plasma half-lives and require more than once-daily dosing (metoprolol, propranolol, carvedilol), a significant disadvantage in the treatment of hypertension. They should generally be prescribed in sustained-release forms. Bisoprolol and nebivolol have $t_{1/2}$ values of 10–12 h and thus achieve sufficient trough levels at once-daily dosing. Hepatic metabolism of metoprolol, carvedilol, and nebivolol is CYP2D6 dependent. The relevance is probably greatest in case of metoprolol, for which CYP2D6 poor metabolizers (~7% of the Caucasian population) show 5-fold higher drug exposure and 2-fold higher heart rate decreases than the majority of extensive metabolizers (Rau et al., 2009).

Effectiveness in Hypertension

Meta-analyses have suggested that β blockers reduce the incidence of MI similar to other antihypertensives but are only be about half as effective in preventing stroke (Lindholm et al., 2005). This has led to downgrading of this class of drugs in certain national guidelines (e.g., U.K. standards); however, many of the studies supporting this conclusion were conducted with atenolol, which may not be the ideal β blocker. Atenolol may not lower central (aortic) blood pressure as effectively as it appears when conventionally measured in the brachial artery using a standard arm cuff (Williams et al., 2006). Indeed, atenolol, in contrast to bisoprolol, carvedilol, metoprolol, or nebivolol, has not been positively tested in heart failure trials. Prospective studies of hypertensive agents have not compared different β blockers head to head; therefore, the clinical relevance of pharmacological differences in this heterogeneous drug class remains unclear. Results of a detailed meta-analysis of 147 randomized trials of blood pressure reduction showed that, regardless of blood pressure before treatment, lowering systolic blood pressure by 10 mmHg or diastolic blood pressure by 5 mmHg using any of the main classes of antihypertensive drugs significantly reduced coronary events and stroke without an increase in nonvascular mortality (Law et al., 2009).

Adverse Effects and Precautions

The adverse effects of β blockers are discussed in Chapter 12. These drugs should be avoided in patients with reactive airway disease (e.g., asthma) or with SA or AV nodal dysfunction or in combination with other drugs that inhibit AV conduction, such as verapamil. The risk of hypoglycemic reactions may be increased in diabetics taking insulin, but type 2 diabetes is not a contraindication. β Blockers increase concentrations of triglycerides in plasma and lower those of HDL cholesterol without changing total cholesterol concentrations. The long-term consequences of these effects are unknown.

Sudden discontinuation of β blockers can produce a withdrawal syndrome that is likely due to upregulation of β receptors during blockade, causing enhanced tissue sensitivity to endogenous catecholamines—potentially exacerbating the symptoms of CAD. The result, especially in active patients, can be rebound hypertension. Thus, β blockers should not be discontinued abruptly, except under close observation; dosage should be tapered gradually over 10–14 days prior to discontinuation.

Epinephrine can produce severe hypertension and bradycardia when a nonselective β blocker is present. The hypertension is due to the unopposed stimulation of α adrenergic receptors when vascular β_2 receptors are blocked. The bradycardia is the result of reflex vagal stimulation. Such paradoxical hypertensive responses to β blockers have been observed in patients with hypoglycemia or pheochromocytoma, during withdrawal from *clonidine*, following administration of epinephrine as a therapeutic agent, or in association with the illicit use of cocaine.

Therapeutic Uses

The β blockers provide effective therapy for all grades of hypertension. Marked differences in their pharmacokinetic properties should be considered; once-daily dosing is preferred for better compliance. Populations that tend to have a lesser antihypertensive response to β blockers include the elderly and African Americans. However, intraindividual differences in antihypertensive efficacy are generally much larger than statistical evidence of differences between racial or age-related groups. Consequently, these observations should not discourage the use of these drugs in individual patients in groups reported to be less responsive.

The β blockers usually do not cause retention of salt and water, and administration of a diuretic is not necessary to avoid edema or the development of tolerance. However, diuretics do have additive antihypertensive effects when combined with β blockers. The combination of a β blocker, a diuretic, and a vasodilator is effective for patients who require a third antihypertensive drug. β Blockers (i.e., bisoprolol, carvedilol, metoprolol, or nebivolol) are highly preferred drugs for hypertensive patients with conditions such as MI, ischemic heart disease, or congestive heart failure and may be preferred for younger patients with signs of increased sympathetic drive. However, for other hypertensive patients, particularly older patients with a high risk for stroke, enthusiasm for their early use in treatment has diminished.

α_1 Blockers

The availability of drugs that selectively block α_1 adrenergic receptors without affecting α_2 adrenergic receptors adds another group of antihypertensive agents. The pharmacology of these drugs is discussed in detail in Chapter 12. Prazosin, terazosin, and doxazosin are the agents available for the treatment of hypertension. Phenoxybenzamine, an irreversible α blocker ($\alpha_1 > \alpha_2$), is used in the treatment of catecholamine-producing tumors (pheochromocytoma).

Pharmacological Effects

Initially, α_1 blockers reduce arteriolar resistance and increase venous capacitance; this causes a sympathetically mediated reflex increase in heart rate and plasma renin activity. During long-term therapy, vasodilation persists, but cardiac output, heart rate, and plasma renin activity return to normal. Renal blood flow is unchanged during therapy with an α_1 blocker. The α_1 blockers cause a variable amount of postural hypotension, depending on the plasma volume. Retention of salt and water occurs in many patients during continued administration, and this attenuates the postural hypotension. The α_1 blockers reduce plasma concentrations of triglycerides and total LDL cholesterol and increase HDL cholesterol. These potentially favorable effects on lipids persist when a thiazide-type diuretic is given concurrently. The long-term consequences of these small, drug-induced changes in lipids are unknown.

Therapeutic Uses

α_1 Blockers are not recommended as monotherapy for hypertensive patients, primarily as a consequence of the ALLHAT study (see further discussion). Consequently, they are used primarily in conjunction with diuretics, β blockers, and other antihypertensive agents. β Blockers enhance the efficacy of α_1 blockers. α_1 Blockers are not the drugs of choice in patients with pheochromocytoma because a vasoconstrictor response to epinephrine can still result from activation of unblocked vascular α_2 adrenergic receptors. α_1 Blockers are attractive drugs for hypertensive patients with benign prostatic hyperplasia because they also improve urinary symptoms.

Adverse Effects

The use of doxazosin as monotherapy for hypertension increases the risk for developing congestive heart failure (ALLHAT Officers, 2002). This may be a class effect that represents an adverse effect of all of the α_1 blockers and has led to recommendations not to use this class of drugs in patients with heart failure. Interpretation of the outcome of the ALLHAT study is controversial, but the commonly held belief that the higher rate of apparent heart failure development in the groups of patients treated with a nondiuretic was caused by withdrawal of prestudy diuretics has not been substantiated (Davis et al., 2006).

A major precaution regarding the use of the α_1 blockers for hypertension is the so-called first-dose phenomenon, in which symptomatic orthostatic hypotension occurs within 30–90 min (or longer) of the initial dose of the drug or after a dosage increase. This effect may occur in up to 50% of patients, especially in patients who are already receiving a diuretic. After the first few doses, patients develop a tolerance to this marked hypotensive response.

Combined α_1 and β Blockers

Carvedilol (see Chapter 12) is a nonselective β blocker with α_1-antagonist activity. Carvedilol is approved for the treatment of hypertension and symptomatic heart failure. The ratio of α_1- to β-antagonist potency for carvedilol is approximately 1:10. The drug dissociates slowly from its receptor, explaining why the duration of action is longer than the short $t_{1/2}$ (2.2 h) and why its effect can hardly be overcome by catecholamines. Carvedilol undergoes oxidative metabolism and glucuronidation in the liver; the oxidative metabolism occurs via CYP2D6. As with labetalol, the long-term efficacy and side effects of carvedilol in hypertension are predictable based on its properties as a β and α_1 blocker. Carvedilol reduces mortality in patients with congestive heart failure (Chapter 29). Due to the vasodilating effect, it is a β blocker of choice in patients with peripheral artery disease.

Labetalol (see Chapter 12) is an equimolar mixture of four stereoisomers. One isomer is an α_1 blocker, another is a nonselective β blocker with partial agonist activity, and the other two isomers are inactive. Labetalol has efficacy and adverse effects that would be expected with any combination of an α_1 and a β blocker. It has the disadvantages that are inherent

in fixed-dose combination products: The extent of α_1- to β-blockade is somewhat unpredictable and varies from patient to patient. Labetalol is FDA-approved for eclampsia, preeclampsia, hypertension, and hypertensive emergencies. The main indication for labetalol is hypertension in pregnancy, for which it is one of the few compounds known to be safe (Magee et al., 2016).

Centrally Acting Sympatholytic Drugs

Methyldopa

Methyldopa, a centrally acting antihypertensive agent, is a prodrug that exerts its antihypertensive action via an active metabolite. Although used frequently as an antihypertensive agent in the past, methyldopa's adverse effect profile limits its current use largely to treatment of hypertension in pregnancy, where it has a record for safety.

Methyldopa (α-methyl-3,4-dihydroxy-L-phenylalanine), an analogue of DOPA, is metabolized by the L-aromatic amino acid decarboxylase in adrenergic neurons to α-methyldopamine, which then is converted to α-methylnorepinephrine, the pharmacologically active metabolite. α-Methylnorepinephrine is stored in the secretory vesicles of adrenergic neurons, substituting for NE, such that the stimulated adrenergic neuron now discharges α-methylnorepinephrine instead of NE. α-Methylnorepinephrine acts in the CNS to inhibit adrenergic neuronal outflow from the brainstem, probably via acting as an agonist at presynaptic α_2 adrenergic receptors in the brainstem, attenuating NE release and thereby reducing the output of vasoconstrictor adrenergic signals to the peripheral sympathetic nervous system.

ADME. Because methyldopa is a prodrug that is metabolized in the brain to the active form, its C_p has less relevance for its effects than that for many other drugs. C_{pmax} occurs 2–3 h following an oral dose. The drug is eliminated with a $t_{1/2}$ of about 2 h. Methyldopa is excreted in the urine primarily as the sulfate conjugate (50%–70%) and as the parent drug (25%). Other minor metabolites include methyldopamine, methylnorepinephrine, and their O-methylated products. The $t_{1/2}$ of methyldopa is prolonged to 4–6 h in patients with renal failure.

Despite its rapid absorption and short $t_{1/2}$, the peak effect of methyldopa is delayed for 6–8 h, even after intravenous administration, and the duration of action of a single dose is usually about 24 h; this permits once- or twice-daily dosing. The discrepancy between the effects of methyldopa and the measured concentrations of the drug in plasma is most likely related to the time required for transport into the CNS, conversion to the active metabolite storage of α-methyl NE, and its subsequent release in the vicinity of relevant α_2 receptors in the CNS. Methyldopa is a good example of a complex relationship between a drug's pharmacokinetics and its pharmacodynamics. Patients with renal failure are more sensitive to the antihypertensive effect of methyldopa, but it is not known if this is due to alteration in excretion of the drug or to an increase in transport into the CNS.

Therapeutic Uses. Methyldopa is a preferred drug for treatment of hypertension during pregnancy based on its effectiveness and safety for both mother and fetus (Magee et al., 2016). The usual initial dose of methyldopa is 250 mg twice daily; there is little additional effect with doses greater than 2 g/d. Administration of a single daily dose of methyldopa at bedtime minimizes sedative effects, but administration twice daily is required for some patients.

Adverse Effects and Precautions. Methyldopa produces sedation that is largely transient. A diminution in psychic energy may persist in some patients, and depression occurs occasionally. Methyldopa may produce dryness of the mouth. Other adverse effects include diminished libido, parkinsonian signs, and hyperprolactinemia that may become sufficiently pronounced to cause gynecomastia and galactorrhea. Methyldopa may precipitate severe bradycardia and sinus arrest.

Methyldopa also produces some adverse effects that are not related to its therapeutic action in the CNS. Hepatotoxicity, sometimes associated with fever, is an uncommon but potentially serious toxic effect of methyldopa. At least 20% of patients who receive methyldopa for a year develop a positive Coombs test (antiglobulin test) that is due to autoantibodies directed against the Rh antigen on erythrocytes. The development of a positive Coombs test is not necessarily an indication to stop treatment with methyldopa; however, 1%–5% of these patients will develop a hemolytic anemia that requires prompt discontinuation of the drug. The Coombs test may remain positive for as long as a year after discontinuation of methyldopa, but the hemolytic anemia usually resolves within a matter of weeks. Severe hemolysis may be attenuated by treatment with glucocorticoids. Adverse effects that are even rarer include leukopenia, thrombocytopenia, red cell aplasia, lupus erythematosus–like syndrome, lichenoid and granulomatous skin eruptions, myocarditis, retroperitoneal fibrosis, pancreatitis, diarrhea, and malabsorption.

Clonidine and Moxonidine

The detailed pharmacology of the α_2 adrenergic agonists clonidine and moxonidine is discussed in Chapter 12. These drugs stimulate α_{2A} adrenergic receptors in the brainstem, resulting in a reduction in sympathetic outflow from the CNS (MacMillan et al., 1996). The hypotensive effect correlates directly with the decrease in plasma concentrations of NE. Patients who have had a spinal cord transection above the level of the sympathetic outflow tracts do not display a hypotensive response to clonidine. At doses higher than those required to stimulate central α_{2A} receptors, these drugs can activate α_{2B} receptors on vascular smooth muscle cells (MacMillan et al., 1996). This effect accounts for the initial vasoconstriction that is seen when overdoses of these drugs are taken and may be responsible for the loss of therapeutic effect that is observed with high doses. A major limitation in the use of these drugs is the paucity of information about their efficacy in reducing the risk of cardiovascular consequences of hypertension.

Pharmacological Effects. The α_2 adrenergic agonists lower arterial pressure by effects on both cardiac output and peripheral resistance. In the supine position, when the sympathetic tone to the vasculature is low, the major effect is a reduction in heart rate and stroke volume; however, in the upright position, when sympathetic outflow to the vasculature is normally increased, these drugs reduce vascular resistance. This action may lead to postural hypotension. The decrease in cardiac sympathetic tone leads to a reduction in myocardial contractility and heart rate that could promote congestive heart failure in susceptible patients.

Therapeutic Uses. The CNS effects are such that this class of drugs is not a leading option for monotherapy of hypertension. Indeed, there is no fixed place for these drugs in the treatment of hypertension. They effectively lower blood pressure in some patients who have not responded adequately to combinations of other agents. The greater clinical experience exists with clonidine. A recent study with moxonidine in patients with hypertension and paroxysmal atrial fibrillation indicated that the drug reduced the incidence of atrial fibrillation (Giannopoulos et al., 2014). Clonidine may be effective in reducing early morning hypertension in patients treated with standard antihypertensives. Overall, enthusiasm for α_2 receptor antagonists is diminished by the relative absence of evidence demonstrating reduction in risk of adverse cardiovascular events.

Clonidine has been used in hypertensive patients for the diagnosis of pheochromocytoma. The failure of clonidine to suppress the plasma concentration of NE to less than 500 pg/mL 3 h after an oral dose of 0.3 mg of clonidine suggests the presence of such a tumor. A modification of this test, wherein overnight urinary excretion of NE and epinephrine is measured after administration of a 0.3-mg dose of clonidine at bedtime, may be useful when results based on plasma NE concentrations are equivocal.

Adverse Effects and Precautions. Many patients experience persistent and sometimes intolerable adverse effects with these drugs. Sedation and xerostomia are prominent adverse effects. The xerostomia may be accompanied by dry nasal mucosa, dry eyes, and swelling and pain of the parotid gland. Postural hypotension and erectile dysfunction may be prominent in some patients. Clonidine may produce a lower incidence of dry mouth and sedation when given transdermally, perhaps because high peak concentrations are avoided. Moxonidine has additional activity at central imidazoline receptors and may produce less sedation than clonidine, but

direct comparisons are lacking. Less-common CNS side effects include sleep disturbances with vivid dreams or nightmares, restlessness, and depression. Cardiac effects related to the sympatholytic action of these drugs include symptomatic bradycardia and sinus arrest in patients with dysfunction of the SA node and AV block in patients with AV nodal disease or in patients taking other drugs that depress AV conduction. Some 15%–20% of patients who receive transdermal clonidine may develop contact dermatitis.

Sudden discontinuation of clonidine and related α_2 adrenergic agonists may cause a withdrawal syndrome consisting of headache, apprehension, tremors, abdominal pain, sweating, and tachycardia. Arterial blood pressure may rise to levels above those present prior to treatment, but the withdrawal syndrome may occur in the absence of an overshoot in pressure. Symptoms typically occur 18–36 h after the drug is stopped and are associated with increased sympathetic discharge, as evidenced by elevated plasma and urine concentrations of catecholamines and metabolites. The frequency of occurrence of the withdrawal syndrome is not known, but withdrawal symptoms are likely dose related and more dangerous in patients with poorly controlled hypertension. Rebound hypertension also has been seen after discontinuation of transdermal administration of clonidine (Metz et al., 1987).

Treatment of the withdrawal syndrome depends on the urgency of reducing the arterial blood pressure. In the absence of life-threatening target organ damage, patients can be treated by restoring the use of clonidine. If a more rapid effect is required, *sodium nitroprusside* or a combination of an α and β blocker is appropriate. β Blockers should not be used alone in this setting because they may accentuate the hypertension by allowing unopposed α adrenergic vasoconstriction caused by activation of the sympathetic nervous system and elevated circulating catecholamines.

Because perioperative hypertension has been described in patients in whom clonidine was withdrawn the night before surgery, surgical patients who are being treated with an α_2 adrenergic agonist either should be switched to another drug prior to elective surgery or should receive their morning dose or transdermal clonidine prior to the procedure. All patients who receive one of these drugs should be warned of the potential danger of discontinuing the drug abruptly, and patients suspected of being noncompliant with medications should not be given α_2 adrenergic agonists for hypertension.

Adverse drug interactions with α_2 adrenergic agonists are rare. Diuretics predictably potentiate the hypotensive effect of these drugs. Tricyclic antidepressants may inhibit the antihypertensive effect of clonidine, but the mechanism of this interaction is not known.

Reserpine

Reserpine is an alkaloid extracted from the root of *Rauwolfia serpentina*, a climbing shrub indigenous to India. Ancient Hindu Ayurvedic writings describe medicinal uses of the plant; Sen and Bose described its use in the Indian biomedical literature. However, rauwolfia alkaloids were not used in Western medicine until the mid-1950s. Reserpine was the first drug found to interfere with the function of the sympathetic nervous system in humans, and its use began the modern era of effective pharmacotherapy of hypertension.

Mechanism of Action. Reserpine binds tightly to adrenergic storage vesicles in central and peripheral adrenergic neurons and remains bound for prolonged periods of time. The interaction inhibits the vesicular catecholamine transporter VMAT2, so that nerve endings lose their capacity to concentrate and store NE and dopamine. Catecholamines leak into the cytoplasm, where they are metabolized. Consequently, little or no active transmitter is released from nerve endings, resulting in a pharmacological sympathectomy. Recovery of sympathetic function requires synthesis of new storage vesicles, which takes days to weeks after discontinuation of the drug. Because reserpine depletes amines in the CNS as well as in the peripheral adrenergic neuron, it is probable that its antihypertensive effects are related to both central and peripheral actions.

Pharmacological Effects. Both cardiac output and peripheral vascular resistance are reduced during long-term therapy with reserpine.

ADME. Few data are available on the pharmacokinetic properties of reserpine because of the lack of an assay capable of detecting low concentrations of the drug or its metabolites. Reserpine that is bound to isolated storage vesicles cannot be removed by dialysis, indicating that the binding is not in equilibrium with the surrounding medium. Because of the irreversible nature of reserpine binding, the amount of drug in plasma is unlikely to bear any consistent relationship to drug concentration at the site of action. Free reserpine is entirely metabolized; therefore, none of the parent drug is excreted unchanged.

Toxicity and Precautions. Most adverse effects of reserpine are due to its effect on the CNS. Sedation and inability to concentrate or perform complex tasks are the most common adverse effects. More serious is the occasional psychotic depression that can lead to suicide. Depression usually appears insidiously over many weeks or months and may not be attributed to the drug because of the delayed and gradual onset of symptoms. Reserpine must be discontinued at the first sign of depression. Reserpine-induced depression may last several months after the drug is discontinued. The risk of depression is likely dose related. Depression is uncommon, but not unknown, with doses of 0.25 mg/d or less. The drug should never be given to patients with a history of depression. Other adverse effects include nasal stuffiness and exacerbation of peptic ulcer disease, which is uncommon with small oral doses.

Therapeutic Uses. Reserpine at low doses, in combination with diuretics, is effective in the treatment of hypertension, especially in the elderly. Several weeks are necessary to achieve maximum effect. In elderly patients with isolated systolic hypertension, reserpine (at 0.05 mg/d) was used as an alternative to atenolol together with a diuretic (Perry et al., 2000; SHEP Cooperative Research Group, 1991). However, with the availability of newer drugs that have proven life-prolonging effects and are well tolerated, the use of reserpine has largely diminished, and it is no longer recommended for the treatment of hypertension (Mancia et al., 2013).

Ca²⁺ Channel Blockers

The Ca²⁺ channel–blocking agents are an important group of drugs for the treatment of hypertension. The general pharmacology of these drugs is presented in Chapter 27. The basis for their use in hypertension comes from the understanding that hypertension generally is the result of increased peripheral vascular resistance. Because contraction of vascular smooth muscle is dependent on the free intracellular concentration of Ca²⁺, inhibition of transmembrane movement of Ca²⁺ through voltage-sensitive Ca²⁺ channels can decrease the total amount of Ca²⁺ that reaches intracellular sites. Indeed, all of the Ca²⁺ channel blockers lower blood pressure by relaxing arteriolar smooth muscle and decreasing peripheral vascular resistance. As a consequence of a decrease in peripheral vascular resistance, the Ca²⁺ channel blockers evoke a baroreceptor reflex–mediated sympathetic discharge. In the case of the dihydropyridines, tachycardia may occur from the adrenergic stimulation of the SA node; this response is generally quite modest except when the drug is administered rapidly. Tachycardia is typically minimal or absent with verapamil and diltiazem because of the direct negative chronotropic effect of these two drugs. Indeed, the concurrent use of a β blocker may magnify negative chronotropic effects of these drugs or cause heart block in susceptible patients. Consequently, the concurrent use of β blockers with either verapamil or diltiazem should be avoided.

The Ca²⁺ channel blockers are among the preferred drugs for the treatment of hypertension, both as monotherapy and in combination with other antihypertensives, because they have a well-documented effect on cardiovascular end points and total mortality. The combination of amlodipine and the ACE inhibitors perindopril proved superior to the combination of the β blocker atenolol and hydrochlorothiazide (Dahlof et al., 2005), and amlodipine was superior to hydrochlorothiazide as the combination partner for the ACEI benazepril (Jamerson et al., 2008).

The Ca²⁺ channel blockers most studied and used for the treatment of hypertension are long-acting dihydropyridines with sufficient 24-h

efficacy at once-daily dosing (e.g., amlodipine, felodipine, lercanidipine, and sustained-release formulations of others). Peripheral edema (ankle edema) are the main unwanted effects. Fewer patients appear to experience this harmless, but possibly distracting, side effect with newer compounds such as lercanidipine (Makarounas-Kirchmann et al., 2009), but the commonly used combination with RAS inhibitors has the same effect (Messerli et al., 2000). Immediate-release nifedipine and other short-acting dihydropyridines have no place in the treatment of hypertension. Verapamil and diltiazem also have short half-lives, more cardiac side effects, and a high drug interaction potential (verapamil > diltiazem) and are therefore not first-line antihypertensives.

Compared with other classes of antihypertensive agents, there may be a greater frequency of achieving blood pressure control with Ca²⁺ channel blockers as monotherapy in elderly subjects and in African Americans, population groups in which the low renin status is more prevalent. However, intrasubject variability is more important than relatively small differences between population groups. Ca²⁺ channel blockers are effective in lowering blood pressure and decreasing cardiovascular events in the elderly with isolated systolic hypertension (Staessen et al., 1997) and may be a preferred treatment in these patients.

Inhibitors of the Renin-Angiotensin System

Angiotensin II is an important regulator of cardiovascular function (see Chapter 26). The capacity to reduce the effects of AngII with pharmacological agents has been an important advance in the treatment of hypertension and its sequelae. Chapter 26 presents the basic physiology of the RAS and the pharmacology of inhibitors of the RAS. Table 26–2 summarizes the effects of a variety of antihypertensive agents on components of the RAS and warrants careful study.

Angiotensin-Converting Enzyme Inhibitors

The ability to reduce levels of AngII with orally effective ACE inhibitors represents an important advance in the treatment of hypertension. Captopril was the first such agent to be developed for the treatment of hypertension. Since then, enalapril, lisinopril, quinapril, ramipril, benazepril, moexipril, fosinopril, trandolapril, and perindopril have become available. These drugs are useful for the treatment of hypertension because of their efficacy and a favorable adverse effect profile that enhances patient adherence. Chapter 26 presents the pharmacology of ACE inhibitors in detail.

The ACE inhibitors appear to confer a special advantage in the treatment of patients with diabetes, slowing the development and progression of diabetic glomerulopathy. They also are effective in slowing the progression of other forms of chronic renal disease, such as glomerulosclerosis, which coexists with hypertension in many patients. An ACE inhibitor is the preferred initial agent in these patients. Patients with hypertension and ischemic heart disease are candidates for treatment with ACE inhibitors. Administration of ACE inhibitors in the immediate post-MI period has been shown to improve ventricular function and reduce morbidity and mortality (see Chapter 27).

The endocrine consequences of inhibiting the biosynthesis of AngII are of importance in a number of facets of hypertension treatment. Because ACE inhibitors blunt the rise in aldosterone concentrations in response to Na⁺ loss, the normal role of aldosterone to oppose diuretic-induced natriuresis is diminished. Consequently, ACE inhibitors tend to enhance the efficacy of diuretic drugs. This means that even very small doses of diuretics may substantially improve the antihypertensive efficacy of ACE inhibitors; conversely, the use of high doses of diuretics together with ACE inhibitors may lead to excessive reduction in blood pressure and to Na⁺ loss in some patients.

Attenuation of aldosterone production by ACE inhibitors also influences K⁺ homeostasis; there is a small and clinically unimportant rise in serum K⁺ when these agents are used alone in patients with normal renal function. However, substantial retention of K⁺ can occur in some patients with renal insufficiency. Furthermore, the potential for developing hyperkalemia should be considered when ACE inhibitors are used with other drugs that can cause K⁺ retention, including the K⁺-sparing diuretics (amiloride, triamterene, and the MRAs spironolactone and eplerenone), NSAIDs, K^+ supplements, and β blockers. Some patients with diabetic nephropathy may be at greater risk of hyperkalemia.

There are several cautions in the use of ACE inhibitors in patients with hypertension. Cough is a common (~5%) adverse effect and a reason to switch to AT_1 receptor blockers. Angioedema is a rare but serious and potentially fatal adverse effect of the ACE inhibitors. Patients starting treatment with these drugs should be explicitly warned to discontinue their use with the advent of any signs of angioedema. Due to the risk of severe fetal adverse effects, ACE inhibitors are contraindicated during pregnancy, a fact that should be communicated to women of childbearing age.

In most patients, there is little or no appreciable change in glomerular filtration rate following the administration of ACE inhibitors. However, in renovascular hypertension, the glomerular filtration rate is generally maintained as the result of increased resistance in the postglomerular arteriole caused by AngII. Accordingly, in patients with bilateral renal artery stenosis or stenosis in a sole kidney, the administration of an ACE inhibitor will reduce the filtration fraction and cause a substantial reduction in glomerular filtration rate. In some patients with preexisting renal disease, the glomerular filtration may decrease with an ACE inhibitor. Thus, it should be kept in mind that ACE inhibitors, while inhibiting the progression of chronic kidney disease, carry a risk of reversible drug-induced impairment of glomerular filtration. Serum creatinine levels and K^+ should therefore be monitored in the first weeks after establishing therapy. Increases of serum creatinine of greater than 20% predict the presence of renal artery stenosis (van de Ven et al., 1998) and are a reason to discontinue the treatment with ACE inhibitors.

The ACE inhibitors lower the blood pressure to some extent in most patients with hypertension. Following the initial dose of an ACE inhibitor, there may be a considerable fall in blood pressure in some patients; this response to the initial dose is a function of plasma renin activity prior to treatment. The potential for a large initial drop in blood pressure is the reason for using a low dose to initiate therapy, especially in patients who may have a very active RAS supporting blood pressure, such as patients with diuretic-induced volume contraction or congestive heart failure. It should also be realized that, generally, no reason exists for normalizing blood pressure in a few days in patients with a lifelong disease. Attempts to do so increase the frequency of side effects and decrease compliance. With continuing treatment, there usually is a progressive fall in blood pressure that in most patients does not reach a maximum for several weeks. The blood pressure seen during chronic treatment is not strongly correlated with the pretreatment plasma renin activity. Young and middle-aged Caucasian patients have a higher probability of responding to ACE inhibitors; elderly African American patients as a group are more resistant to the hypotensive effect of these drugs. While most ACE inhibitors are approved for once-daily dosing for hypertension, a significant fraction of patients has a response that lasts less than 24 h and may require twice-daily dosing for adequate control of blood pressure (e.g., enalapril, ramipril). Captopril, with its very short duration of action, is not a good choice in the treatment of hypertension.

AT_1 Receptor Blockers

The importance of AngII in regulating cardiovascular function has led to the development of nonpeptide antagonists of the AT_1 subtype of AngII receptor. Losartan, candesartan, irbesartan, valsartan, telmisartan, olmesartan, and eprosartan have been approved for the treatment of hypertension. The pharmacology of AT_1 receptor blockers is presented in detail in Chapter 26. By antagonizing the effects of AngII, these agents relax smooth muscle and thereby promote vasodilation, increase renal salt and water excretion, reduce plasma volume, and decrease cellular hypertrophy. Given the central role of AT_1 receptors for the action of AngII, it is not surprising that AT_1 receptor blockers have the same pharmacological profile as ACE inhibitors with one notable exception. AT_1 receptor blockers do not inhibit the ACE-mediated degradation of bradykinin and substance P and thereby cause no cough.

Initial hopes for superiority of AT_1 receptor blockers over ACE inhibitors have not been fulfilled. They were based on the idea that the AT_2 subtype elicits beneficial effects of AngII (e.g., antigrowth and antiproliferative responses). Because the AT_1 receptor mediates feedback inhibition of renin release, renin and AngII concentrations are increased during AT_1 receptor antagonism, leading to increased stimulation of uninhibited AT_2 receptors. Despite considerable interest, not much evidence supports any extra benefit from AT_1 blockade versus ACE inhibition, and attempts to show greater reductions in cardiovascular events by AT_1 receptor blockers or by the combination of an AT_1 receptor blocker plus an ACE inhibitor over ACE inhibitor alone failed. ON-TARGET, one of the largest studies to date in patients with high vascular risk (70% hypertension) showed that telmisartan caused less cough and angioedema than ramipril (1.1% vs. 4.2%, and 0.1% vs. 0.3%) but had identical efficacy. The combination, although not more efficacious, was associated with greater worsening of renal function (13.5% vs. 10.2%), hypotension, and syncope (Yusuf et al., 2008).

Therapeutic Uses

The AT_1 receptor blockers have a sufficient 24-h effect at once-daily dosing (except losartan). The full effect of AT_1 receptor blockers on blood pressure typically is not observed until about 4 weeks after the initiation of therapy. If blood pressure is not controlled by an AT_1 receptor blocker alone, a second drug acting by a different mechanism (e.g., a diuretic or Ca^{2+} channel blocker) may be added. The combination of an ACE inhibitor and an AT_1 receptor blocker is not recommended for the treatment of hypertension.

Adverse Effects and Precautions

Adverse effects of ACE inhibitors that result from inhibiting AngII-related functions (see previous discussion and Chapter 26) also occur with AT_1 receptor blockers. These include hypotension, hyperkalemia, and reduced renal function, including that associated with bilateral renal artery stenosis and stenosis in the artery of a solitary kidney. Hypotension is most likely to occur in patients in whom the blood pressure is highly dependent on AngII, including those with volume depletion (e.g., with diuretics), renovascular hypertension, cardiac failure, and cirrhosis; in such patients, initiation of treatment with low doses and attention to blood volume are essential. Hyperkalemia may occur in conjunction with other factors that alter K^+ homeostasis, such as renal insufficiency, ingestion of excess K^+, and the use of drugs that promote K^+ retention. Cough and angioedema occur rarely. ACE inhibitors and AT_1 receptor blockers should not be administered during pregnancy and should be discontinued as soon as pregnancy is detected.

Direct Renin Inhibitors

Aliskiren, the first orally effective direct renin inhibitor is FDA-approved for the treatment of hypertension. The detailed pharmacology of aliskiren is covered in Chapter 26. Aliskiren is an effective antihypertensive drug but has not been studied sufficiently in monotherapy of hypertension. A large study comparing a placebo or aliskiren added to a background of an ARB or an ACE inhibitor was stopped prematurely for a trend toward increased cardiovascular events in the aliskiren treatment group (McMurray et al., 2012). The combination also induced more renal worsening, hypotension, and hyperkalemia. This mirrors previous studies with ARB/ACE inhibitor combinations and indicates that complete blockade of the RAS system achieves more harm than benefit.

Pharmacology

The initial renin inhibitors were peptide analogues of sequences either in renin itself or included the renin cleavage site in angiotensinogen. While effective in inhibiting renin and lowering blood pressure, these peptide analogues were effective only parenterally. However, aliskiren is effective following oral administration; it directly and competitively inhibits the catalytic activity of renin, leading to diminished production of AngI, AngII, and aldosterone—with a resulting fall in blood pressure. Aliskiren along with ACE inhibitors and AT_1 receptor blockers lead to an adaptive increase in the plasma concentrations of renin; however, because aliskiren inhibits renin activity, plasma renin activity does not increase as occurs with these other classes of drugs (Table 26–2). Nevertheless, the aldosterone escape known from ACE inhibitors and AT_1 receptor blockers has also been observed under continuous treatment with aliskiren (Bomback et al., 2012).

ADME

Aliskiren is poorly absorbed, with an oral bioavailability of less than 3%. Taking the drug with a high-fat meal may substantially decrease plasma concentrations. Aliskiren has an elimination $t_{1/2}$ of at least 24 h. Elimination of the drug may be primarily through hepatobiliary excretion with limited metabolism via CYP3A4.

Therapeutic Uses

Given the unclear effectiveness and safety of aliskiren monotherapy, the place of this drug in the treatment of hypertension remains clouded. The combination of aliskiren with other RAS inhibitors is contraindicated, and the European Society of Cardiology guideline does not recommend its use (Mancia et al., 2013).

Toxicity and Precautions

Aliskiren is generally well tolerated. Diarrhea may occur, especially at higher-than-recommended doses. The incidence of cough may be higher than for placebo but substantially less than found with ACE inhibitors. Aliskiren has been associated with several cases of angioedema in clinical trials (Frampton and Curran, 2007). Drugs acting on the RAS may damage the fetus and should not be used in pregnant women.

Vasodilators

Hydralazine

Hydralazine (1-hydrazinophthalazine) was one of the first orally active antihypertensive drugs to be marketed in the U.S.; however, the drug initially was used infrequently because of tachycardia and tachyphylaxis. With a better understanding of the compensatory cardiovascular responses that accompany use of arteriolar vasodilators, hydralazine was combined with sympatholytic agents and diuretics with greater therapeutic success. Nonetheless, its role in the treatment of hypertension has markedly diminished with the introduction of new classes of antihypertensive agents.

Mechanism of Action

Hydralazine directly relaxes arteriolar smooth muscle with little effect on venous smooth muscle. The molecular mechanisms mediating this action are not clear but may ultimately involve a reduction in intracellular Ca^{2+} concentrations. While a variety of changes in cellular signaling pathways are influenced by hydralazine, precise molecular targets that explain its capacity to dilate arteries remain uncertain. Potential mechanisms include inhibition of inositol trisphosphate–induced release of Ca^{2+} from intracellular storage sites, opening of high-conductance Ca^{2+}-activated K^+ channels in smooth muscle cells, and activation of an arachidonic acid, COX, and prostacyclin pathway that would explain sensitivity to NSAIDs (Maille et al., 2016).

Hydralazine-induced vasodilation is associated with powerful stimulation of the sympathetic nervous system, likely due to baroreceptor-mediated reflexes, resulting in increased heart rate and contractility, increased plasma renin activity, and fluid retention. These effects tend to counteract the antihypertensive effect of hydralazine.

Pharmacological Effects

Most of the effects of hydralazine are confined to the cardiovascular system. The decrease in blood pressure after administration of hydralazine is associated with a selective decrease in vascular resistance in the coronary, cerebral, and renal circulations, with a smaller effect in skin and muscle. Because of preferential dilation of arterioles over veins, postural hypotension is not a common problem; hydralazine lowers blood pressure similarly in the supine and upright positions.

ADME

Following oral administration, hydralazine is well absorbed via the GI tract. Hydralazine is N-acetylated in the bowel and the liver, contributing to the drug's low bioavailability (16% in fast acetylators and 35% in slow acetylators). The rate of acetylation is genetically determined; about half of the U.S. population acetylates rapidly, and half does so slowly. The acetylated compound is inactive; thus, the dose necessary to produce a systemic effect is larger in fast acetylators. Because the systemic clearance exceeds hepatic blood flow, extrahepatic metabolism must occur. Indeed, hydralazine rapidly combines with circulating α-keto acids to form hydrazones, and the major metabolite recovered from the plasma is hydralazine pyruvic acid hydrazone. This metabolite has a longer $t_{1/2}$ than hydralazine but appears to be relatively inactive. Although the rate of acetylation is an important determinant of the bioavailability of hydralazine, it does not play a role in the systemic elimination of the drug, probably because hepatic clearance is so high that systemic elimination is principally a function of hepatic blood flow. The peak concentration of hydralazine in plasma and the peak hypotensive effect of the drug occur within 30–120 min of ingestion. Although its $t_{1/2}$ in plasma is about 1 h, the hypotensive effect of hydralazine can last as long as 12 h. There is no clear explanation for this discrepancy.

Therapeutic Uses

Hydralazine is no longer a first-line drug in the treatment of hypertension on account of its relatively unfavorable adverse-effect profile. The drug has a role as a combination pill containing isosorbide dinitrate (BiDil) in the treatment of heart failure (see Chapter 29). Hydralazine may have utility in the treatment of some patients with severe hypertension, can be part of evidence-based therapy in patients with congestive heart failure (in combination with nitrates for patients who cannot tolerate ACE inhibitors or AT_1 receptor blockers), and may be useful in the treatment of hypertensive emergencies, especially preeclampsia, in pregnant women. Hydralazine should be used with great caution in elderly patients and in hypertensive patients with CAD because of the possibility of precipitating myocardial ischemia due to reflex tachycardia. The usual oral dosage of hydralazine is 25–100 mg twice daily. Off-label twice-daily administration is as effective as administration four times a day for control of blood pressure, regardless of acetylator phenotype. The maximum recommended dose of hydralazine is 200 mg/d to minimize the risk of drug-induced lupus syndrome.

Toxicity and Precautions

Two types of adverse effects occur after the use of hydralazine. The first, which are extensions of the pharmacological effects of the drug, include headache, nausea, flushing, hypotension, palpitations, tachycardia, dizziness, and angina pectoris. Myocardial ischemia can occur on account of increased O_2 demand induced by the baroreceptor reflex–induced stimulation of the sympathetic nervous system. Following parenteral administration to patients with CAD, the myocardial ischemia may be sufficiently severe and protracted to cause frank MI. For this reason, parenteral administration of hydralazine is not advisable in hypertensive patients with CAD, hypertensive patients with multiple cardiovascular risk factors, or older patients. In addition, if the drug is used alone, there may be salt retention with development of high-output congestive heart failure. When combined with a β blocker and a diuretic, hydralazine is better tolerated, although adverse effects such as headache are still commonly described and may necessitate discontinuation of the drug.

The second type of adverse effect is caused by immunological reactions, of which the drug-induced lupus syndrome is the most common. Administration of hydralazine also can result in an illness that resembles serum sickness, hemolytic anemia, vasculitis, and rapidly progressive glomerulonephritis. The mechanism of these autoimmune reactions is unknown, although it may involve the drug's capacity to inhibit DNA methylation (Arce et al., 2006). The drug-induced lupus syndrome usually occurs after at least 6 months of continuous treatment with hydralazine, and its incidence is related to dose, gender, acetylator phenotype, and race. In one study, after 3 years of treatment with hydralazine, drug-induced lupus occurred in 10% of patients who received 200 mg daily, 5% who received 100 mg daily, and none who received 50 mg daily (Cameron and Ramsay, 1984). The incidence is four times higher in women than in men, and the syndrome is seen more commonly in Caucasians than in African Americans. The rate of conversion to a positive antinuclear antibody test is faster in slow acetylators than in rapid acetylators, suggesting that the native drug or a nonacetylated metabolite is responsible. However, the majority of patients with positive antinuclear antibody tests do not develop the drug-induced lupus syndrome, and hydralazine need not be discontinued unless clinical features (arthralgia, arthritis, and fever) of the syndrome appear. Discontinuation of the drug is all that is necessary for most patients with the hydralazine-induced lupus syndrome, but symptoms may persist in a few patients, and administration of corticosteroids may be necessary.

Hydralazine also can produce a pyridoxine-responsive polyneuropathy. The mechanism appears to be related to the ability of hydralazine to combine with pyridoxine to form a hydrazone. This side effect is unusual with doses of 200 mg/d or less.

K$_{ATP}$ Channel Openers: Minoxidil

The discovery in 1965 of the hypotensive action of minoxidil was a significant advance in the treatment of hypertension; the drug has proven to be efficacious in patients with the most severe and drug-resistant forms of hypertension.

Locus and Mechanism of Action

Minoxidil is not active in vitro but must be metabolized by hepatic sulfotransferase to the active molecule, minoxidil N-O sulfate; the formation of this active metabolite is a minor pathway in the metabolic disposition of minoxidil. Minoxidil sulfate relaxes vascular smooth muscle in isolated systems where the parent drug is inactive. Minoxidil sulfate activates the ATP-modulated K$^+$ channel permitting K$^+$ efflux, and causes hyperpolarization and relaxation of smooth muscle.

Pharmacological Effects

Minoxidil produces arteriolar vasodilation with essentially no effect on the capacitance vessels; the drug resembles hydralazine and diazoxide in this regard. Minoxidil increases blood flow to skin, skeletal muscle, the GI tract, and the heart more than to the CNS. The disproportionate increase in blood flow to the heart may have a metabolic basis in that administration of minoxidil is associated with a reflex increase in myocardial contractility and in cardiac output. The cardiac output can increase markedly, as much as 3- to 4-fold. The principal determinant of the elevation in cardiac output is the action of minoxidil on peripheral vascular resistance to enhance venous return to the heart; by inference from studies with other drugs, the increased venous return probably results from enhancement of flow in the regional vascular beds, with a fast time constant for venous return to the heart (Ogilvie, 1985). The adrenergically mediated increase in myocardial contractility contributes to the increased cardiac output but is not the predominant causal factor.

The effects of minoxidil on the kidney are complex. Minoxidil is a renal artery vasodilator, but systemic hypotension produced by the drug occasionally can decrease renal blood flow. Renal function usually improves in patients who take minoxidil for the treatment of hypertension, especially if renal dysfunction is secondary to hypertension. Minoxidil is a potent stimulator of renin secretion. This effect is mediated by a combination of renal sympathetic stimulation and activation of the intrinsic renal mechanisms for regulation of renin release.

Discovery of K$^+_{ATP}$ channels in a variety of cell types and in mitochondria is prompting consideration of K$^+_{ATP}$ channel modulators as therapeutic agents in many cardiovascular diseases (Pollesello and Mebazaa, 2004). Minoxidil, similar to other K$^+_{ATP}$ channel openers such as diazoxide, pinacidil, and nicorandil, may have protective effects on the heart during ischemia/reperfusion (Sato et al., 2004). It also promotes the synthesis of vascular elastin in rats (Slove et al., 2013), a potentially interesting therapeutic effect.

ADME

Minoxidil is well absorbed from the GI tract. Although peak concentrations of minoxidil in blood occur 1 h after oral administration, the maximal hypotensive effect of the drug occurs later, possibly because formation of the active metabolite is delayed.

The bulk of the absorbed drug is eliminated as a glucuronide; about 20% is excreted unchanged in the urine. The extent of biotransformation of minoxidil to its active metabolite, minoxidil N-O sulfate, has not been evaluated in humans. Minoxidil has a plasma $t_{1/2}$ of 3–4 h, but its duration of action is 24 h and occasionally even longer. It has been proposed that persistence of minoxidil in vascular smooth muscle is responsible for this discrepancy, but without knowledge of the pharmacokinetic properties of the active metabolite, an explanation for the prolonged duration of action cannot be given.

Therapeutic Uses

Systemic minoxidil is best reserved for the treatment of severe hypertension that responds poorly to other antihypertensive medications, especially in male patients with renal insufficiency. Minoxidil has been used successfully in the treatment of hypertension in both adults and children. Minoxidil should never be used alone; it must be given concurrently with a diuretic to avoid fluid retention, with a sympatholytic drug (e.g., β blocker) to control reflex cardiovascular effects and an inhibitor of the RAS to prevent remodeling effects on the heart. The drug usually is administered either once or twice a day, but some patients may require more frequent dosing for adequate control of blood pressure. The initial daily dose of minoxidil may be as little as 1.25 mg, which can be increased gradually to 40 mg in one or two daily doses.

Adverse Effects and Precautions

The adverse effects of minoxidil, which can be severe, fall into three major categories: fluid and salt retention, cardiovascular effects, and hypertrichosis. Retention of salt and water results from increased proximal renal tubular reabsorption, which is secondary to reduced renal perfusion pressure and to reflex stimulation of renal tubular α adrenergic receptors. Similar antinatriuretic effects can be observed with the other arteriolar dilators (e.g., diazoxide and hydralazine). Although administration of minoxidil causes increased secretion of renin and aldosterone, this is not an important mechanism for retention of salt and water in this case. Fluid retention usually can be controlled by the administration of a diuretic. However, thiazides may not be sufficiently efficacious, and it may be necessary to use a loop diuretic, especially if the patient has any degree of renal dysfunction.

The cardiac consequences of the baroreceptor-mediated activation of the sympathetic nervous system during minoxidil therapy are similar to those seen with hydralazine; there is an increase in heart rate, myocardial contractility, and myocardial O$_2$ consumption. Thus, myocardial ischemia can be induced by minoxidil in patients with CAD. The cardiac sympathetic responses are attenuated by concurrent administration of a β blocker. The adrenergically induced increase in renin secretion also can be ameliorated by a β blocker or an ACE inhibitor, with enhancement of blood pressure control.

The increased cardiac output evoked by minoxidil has particularly adverse consequences in those hypertensive patients who have left ventricular hypertrophy and diastolic dysfunction. Such poorly compliant ventricles respond suboptimally to increased volume loads, with a resulting increase in left ventricular filling pressure. This probably is a major contributor to the increased pulmonary artery pressure seen with minoxidil (and hydralazine) therapy in hypertensive patients and is compounded by the retention of salt and water caused by minoxidil. Cardiac failure can result from minoxidil therapy in such patients; the potential for this complication can be reduced but not prevented by effective diuretic therapy. Pericardial effusion is an uncommon but serious complication of minoxidil. Mild and asymptomatic pericardial effusion is not an indication for discontinuing minoxidil, but the situation should be monitored closely to avoid progression to tamponade. Effusions usually clear when the drug is discontinued but can recur if treatment with minoxidil is resumed.

Flattened and inverted T waves frequently are observed in the electrocardiogram following the initiation of minoxidil treatment. These are not ischemic in origin and are seen with other drugs that activate K$^+$ channels. In model systems, pinacidil is associated with a lowered ventricular fibrillation threshold and increased spontaneous ventricular fibrillation in the ischemic canine heart, and minoxidil causes cardiac antiarrhythmias in the rabbit; whether such findings translate to events in humans is unknown.

Excess hair growth occurs in patients who receive minoxidil for an extended period and is probably a consequence of K^+ channel activation. Growth of hair occurs on the face, back, arms, and legs and is particularly offensive to women. Frequent shaving or depilatory agents can be used to manage this problem. Topical minoxidil is marketed over the counter for the treatment of male pattern baldness and hair thinning and loss on the top of the head in women. The topical use of minoxidil also can cause measurable cardiovascular effects in some individuals.

Other side effects of the drug are rare and include rashes, Stevens-Johnson syndrome, glucose intolerance, serosanguineous bullae, formation of antinuclear antibodies, and thrombocytopenia.

Sodium Nitroprusside

Although sodium nitroprusside has been known since 1850 and its hypotensive effect in humans was described in 1929, its safety and usefulness for the short-term control of severe hypertension were not demonstrated until the mid-1950s. Several investigators subsequently demonstrated that sodium nitroprusside also was effective in improving cardiac function in patients with left ventricular failure (see Chapter 29).

Sodium nitroprusside

Mechanism of Action

Nitroprusside is a nitrovasodilator that acts by releasing NO. NO activates the guanylyl cyclase–cyclic guanosine monophosphate–protein kinase G pathway, leading to vasodilation, mimicking the production of NO by vascular endothelial cells, which is impaired in many hypertensive patients. The mechanism of release of NO from nitroprusside is not clear and likely involves both enzymatic and nonenzymatic pathways. Tolerance develops to *nitroglycerin* but not to nitroprusside. The pharmacology of the organic nitrates, including nitroglycerin, is presented in Chapter 27.

Pharmacological Effects

Nitroprusside dilates both arterioles and venules, and the hemodynamic response to its administration results from a combination of venous pooling and reduced arterial impedance. In subjects with normal left ventricular function, venous pooling affects cardiac output more than does the reduction of afterload; cardiac output tends to fall. In contrast, in patients with severely impaired left ventricular function and diastolic ventricular distention, the reduction of arterial impedance is the predominant effect, leading to a rise in cardiac output (see Chapter 29).

Sodium nitroprusside is a nonselective vasodilator, and regional distribution of blood flow is little affected by the drug. In general, renal blood flow and glomerular filtration are maintained, and plasma renin activity increases. Unlike minoxidil, hydralazine, diazoxide, and other arteriolar vasodilators, sodium nitroprusside usually causes only a modest increase in heart rate and an overall reduction in myocardial O_2 demand.

ADME

Sodium nitroprusside is an unstable molecule that decomposes under strongly alkaline conditions or when exposed to light. The drug must be protected from light and given by continuous intravenous infusion to be effective. Its onset of action is within 30 sec; the peak hypotensive effect occurs within 2 min, and when the infusion of the drug is stopped, the effect disappears within 3 min.

Sodium nitroprusside is available in vials that contain 50 mg. The contents of the vial should be dissolved in 2–3 mL of 5% dextrose in water. Because the compound decomposes in light, only fresh solutions should be used, and the bottle should be covered with an opaque wrapping. The drug must be administered as a controlled continuous infusion, and the patient must be closely observed. The majority of hypertensive patients respond to an infusion of 0.25–1.5 µg/kg/min. Higher infusion rates are necessary to produce controlled hypotension in normotensive patients under surgical anesthesia. Patients who are receiving other antihypertensive medications usually require less nitroprusside to lower blood pressure. If infusion rates of 10 µg/kg/min do not produce adequate reduction of blood pressure within 10 min, the rate of administration of nitroprusside should be reduced to minimize potential toxicity.

The metabolism of nitroprusside by smooth muscle is initiated by its reduction, which is followed by the release of cyanide and then NO. Cyanide is further metabolized by hepatic rhodanase to form thiocyanate, which is eliminated almost entirely in the urine. The mean elimination $t_{1/2}$ for thiocyanate is 3 days in patients with normal renal function and much longer in patients with renal insufficiency.

Therapeutic Uses

Sodium nitroprusside is used primarily to treat hypertensive emergencies but also can be used in situations when short-term reduction of cardiac preload or afterload is desired. Nitroprusside has been used to lower blood pressure during acute aortic dissection; to improve cardiac output in congestive heart failure, especially in hypertensive patients with pulmonary edema that does not respond to other treatment (see Chapter 29); and to decrease myocardial O_2 demand after acute MI. In addition, nitroprusside is used to induce controlled hypotension during anesthesia to reduce bleeding in surgical procedures. In the treatment of acute aortic dissection, it is important to administer a β blocker with nitroprusside because reduction of blood pressure with nitroprusside alone can increase the rate of rise in pressure in the aorta as a result of increased myocardial contractility, thereby enhancing propagation of the dissection.

Toxicity and Precautions

The short-term adverse effects of nitroprusside are due to excessive vasodilation, with hypotension and its consequences. Close monitoring of blood pressure and the use of a continuous variable-rate infusion pump will prevent an excessive hemodynamic response to the drug in the majority of cases.

Less commonly, toxicity may result from conversion of nitroprusside to cyanide and thiocyanate. Toxic accumulation of cyanide leading to severe lactic acidosis usually occurs when sodium nitroprusside is infused at a rate greater than 5 µg/kg/min but also can occur in some patients receiving doses on the order of 2 µg/kg/min for a prolonged period. The limiting factor in the metabolism of cyanide appears to be the availability of sulfur-containing substrates in the body (i.e., mainly thiosulfate). The concomitant administration of sodium thiosulfate can prevent accumulation of cyanide in patients who are receiving higher-than-usual doses of sodium nitroprusside; the efficacy of the drug is unchanged. The risk of thiocyanate toxicity increases when sodium nitroprusside is infused for more than 24–48 h, especially if renal function is impaired. Signs and symptoms of thiocyanate toxicity include anorexia, nausea, fatigue, disorientation, and toxic psychosis. The plasma concentration of thiocyanate should be monitored during prolonged infusions of nitroprusside and should not be allowed to exceed 0.1 mg/mL. Rarely, excessive concentrations of thiocyanate may cause hypothyroidism by inhibiting iodine uptake by the thyroid gland. In patients with renal failure, thiocyanate can be removed readily by hemodialysis.

Nitroprusside can worsen arterial hypoxemia in patients with chronic obstructive pulmonary disease because the drug interferes with hypoxic pulmonary vasoconstriction and therefore promotes mismatching of ventilation with perfusion.

Diazoxide

Diazoxide was used in the treatment of hypertensive emergencies but fell out of favor at least in part due to the risk of marked falls in blood pressure when large bolus doses of the drug were used. Other drugs are now preferred for parenteral administration in the control of hypertension. Diazoxide also is administered orally to treat patients with various forms of hypoglycemia (see Chapter 47).

Nonpharmacological Therapy of Hypertension

Nonpharmacological approaches to the treatment of hypertension may suffice in patients with modestly elevated blood pressure. Such approaches also can augment the effects of antihypertensive drugs in patients with more marked initial elevations in blood pressure. The indications and efficacy of various lifestyle modifications in hypertension were reviewed in recent guidelines (James et al., 2014; Mancia et al., 2013).

- Reduction in body weight for people who are modestly overweight or frankly obese may be useful (Goodpaster et al., 2010).
- Restricting sodium consumption lowers blood pressure in some patients.
- Restriction of ethanol intake to modest levels (daily consumption < 20 g in women, < 40 g in men) may lower blood pressure.
- Increased physical activity improves control of hypertension.
- Renal denervation may be effective in patients with well-defined resistant hypertension (Azizi et al., 2015).
- Bariatric surgery in grossly overweight individuals may normalize blood pressure and increase life expectancy (Sjostrom et al., 2007).

Selection of Antihypertensive Drugs in Individual Patients

Choice of antihypertensive drugs for individual patients may be complex; there are many sources of influence that modify therapeutic decisions. While results derived from randomized, controlled clinical trials are the optimal foundation for rational therapeutics, sorting through the multiplicity of those results and addressing how to apply them to an individual patient can be vexing. While therapeutic guidelines can be useful in reaching appropriate therapeutic decisions, it often is difficult for clinicians to apply guidelines at the point of care, and guidelines often do not provide enough information about recommended drugs. In addition, intense marketing of specific drugs to both clinicians and patients may confound optimal decision-making. Moreover, persuading patients to continue taking drugs that may be expensive for an asymptomatic disease is a challenge. Clinicians may be reluctant to prescribe and patients reluctant to consume the number of drugs that may be necessary to adequately control blood pressure. For these and other reasons, perhaps one-half of patients being treated for hypertension have not achieved therapeutic goals in blood pressure lowering.

Choice of an antihypertensive drug should be driven by the likely benefit in an individual patient, taking into account concomitant diseases such as diabetes mellitus, problematic adverse effects of specific drugs, and cost. The last factor is losing relevance as the most important antihypertensive drug classes (diuretics, Ca^{2+} channel blockers, ACE inhibitors/AT_1 receptor blockers, and β blockers) are out of patent protection and available as low-cost generics.

After a long debate about blood pressure–independent effects of certain antihypertensive drug classes, there is a consensus that blood pressure lowering per se is the most important goal of antihypertensive treatment. This conclusion is based on a number of large comparative prospective trials that, overall, did not show major differences in outcome depending on drug class (reviewed by Mancia et al., 2013). The JNC8 guidelines formulated a preference for an initial therapy with thiazide diuretics, Ca^{2+} channel blockers, and ACE inhibitor/ARB in the general non-black population (including diabetics) and a preference for thiazides and Ca^{2+} channel blockers in black patients (James et al., 2014). The ESC guidelines state that "although meta-analyses occasionally appear, claiming superiority of one class of agents over another for some outcomes, this largely depends on the selection bias of trials, and the largest meta-analyses available do not show clinically relevant differences between drug classes." They conclude "that diuretics (including thiazides, chlorthalidone and indapamide), β blockers, calcium channel blockers, ACE inhibitors and AT_1-receptor blockers are all suitable for the initiation and maintenance of antihypertensive treatment, either as monotherapy or in some

combinations" (Mancia et al., 2013). Major guideline recommendations around the world have been recently compared (Kjeldsen et al., 2014) and are the basis of recommendations for a compilation of drug choices in Table 28–4.

A number of pharmacological principles should be considered for optimizing the antihypertensive drug regimen.

1. **Pharmacokinetics:** Hypertension is a chronic, often lifelong disease without major symptoms but with serious complications, making compliance to antihypertensive drugs a factor of utmost prognostic importance. Antihypertensives should be chosen that exhibit relatively even plasma concentrations at once-daily dosing, achieving sufficient 24-h control of blood pressure and trough-peak effect ratios greater than 50%. The longer the half-life, the less the variation of plasma concentrations (e.g., chlorthalidone vs. hydrochlorothiazide). Drugs with stable pharmacokinetics, that is, low drug interaction potential and no pharmacogenetic influence, are preferred (e.g., bisoprolol vs. metoprolol).
2. **Drug combinations:** Two-thirds of patients with hypertension require two or more antihypertensives for sufficient blood pressure control (<140/90 mmHg). It is therefore reasonable to start combining drugs at low-to-medium doses instead of increasing the dose of a single drug. Prescribing fixed drug combinations (e.g., a Ca^{2+} channel blocker + ACE inhibitor or an ACE inhibitor + diuretic) improves compliance.
3. **Strength of scientific evidence:** Data from large prospective trials provide a high level of confidence for a beneficial risk-benefit ratio and are a reason to use one drug over another.

TABLE 28–4 ■ ANTIHYPERTENSIVE AGENTS PREFERRED IN SPECIFIC PATIENT POPULATIONS

MEDICAL CONDITION	PREFERRED ANTIHYPERTENSIVE AGENTS
Left ventricular hypertrophy	ACEI, ARB, CCB
Asymptomatic atherosclerosis	CCB
Microalbuminuria	ACEI, ARB
Renal dysfunction	ACEI, ARB
Previous stroke	ACEI, ARB, diuretics
Previous myocardial infarction	ACEI, ARB, BB
Coronary artery disease	ACEI, ARB, BB
Angina pectoris	BB, CCB
Heart failure	ACEI, ARB, BB, diuretics, MRA
Aortic aneurysm	BB
Atrial fibrillation, prevention	ACEI, ARB, BB
Atrial fibrillation, rate control	BB, CCB (nondihydropyridines)
End-stage renal disease, proteinuria	ACEI
Peripheral artery disease	ACEI, CCB
Isolated systolic hypertension	ACEI, ARB, CCB, diuretics
Metabolic syndrome	ACEI, ARB, CCB
Diabetes mellitus	ACEI, ARB, CCB, diuretics
Diabetes mellitus with proteinuria	ACEI, ARB
Hyperaldosteronism	MRA
Pregnancy	BB, CCB, α-methyldopa
Black ethnicity	CCB, diuretics

The drug choices depicted represent a combined view from nine guidelines that differ; thus, the table is, necessarily, a didactic simplification (for details, consult Kjeldsen et al., 2014).

4. **Pharmacodynamic considerations:** Although not formally tested in prospective trials, certain drug combinations make more sense than others. Thiazide diuretics increase the antihypertensive actions of all other classes, but their combination with RAS inhibitors makes particular sense as their K^+-sparing effect and thus their main risk are reduced by members of this class.

5. **Adverse drug effects and contraindications:** The major classes of antihypertensives are generally well tolerated and, in placebo-controlled trials, showed rates of adverse effects in the range of placebo with some notable exceptions that need to be taken into consideration when choosing a specific drug for a specific patient (Table 28–5). The rate of adverse effects such as hypotension or bradycardia can be largely reduced by starting antihypertensives at low doses and employing a slow dose-escalation strategy.

6. **Compelling indications:** A number of compelling indications exist for specific antihypertensive agents on account of other serious, underlying cardiovascular disease (Table 28–4). These include heart failure, CAD, post-MI, chronic kidney disease, or diabetes. For example, a hypertensive patient with congestive heart failure ideally should be treated with a diuretic, β blocker, ACE inhibitor/AT_1 receptor blocker, and, in selected patients, spironolactone because of the benefit of these drugs in congestive heart failure, even in the absence of hypertension (see Chapter 29). Similarly, ACE inhibitors/AT_1 receptor blockers should be first-line drugs in the treatment of diabetics with hypertension in view of these drugs' well-established benefits in diabetic nephropathy.

7. **Comorbidities:** Some patients have other diseases that could influence the choice of antihypertensive drugs. For example, a hypertensive patient with symptomatic benign prostatic hyperplasia might benefit from having an α_1 blocker as part of his therapeutic program because α_1 blockers are efficacious in both diseases. Similarly, a patient with recurrent migraine attacks might particularly benefit from use of a β blocker because a number of drugs in this class are efficacious in preventing migraine attacks. Women with a high risk of osteoporosis may benefit from the Ca^{2+}-increasing effect of thiazide diuretics. On the other hand, in pregnant hypertensives, some drugs that are otherwise little used (e.g., methyldopa) may be preferred and popular drugs (e.g., ACE inhibitors) need to be avoided on account of concerns about safety.

8. **Second- and third-line hypertensives:** In the vast majority of cases, hypertension can well be controlled by antihypertensives of the five major classes with or without spironolactone at low doses. However, patients with chronic kidney disease often require the additional use of drugs such as hydralazine or minoxidil. The place of clonidine/moxonidine or α_1 blockers in the treatment of hypertension is not well defined.

Acute Antihypertensive Treatment

The considerations mentioned apply to patients with hypertension who need treatment to reduce long-term risk, not patients in immediately life-threatening settings due to hypertension. While there are limited

TABLE 28–5 ■ COMPELLING AND POSSIBLE CONTRAINDICATIONS[a] TO ANTIHYPERTENSIVE DRUGS

DRUG CLASS	COMPELLING	POSSIBLE CONTRAINDICATION/PRECAUTION
Diuretics (thiazides)	Gout	Metabolic syndrome Glucose intolerance Pregnancy Hypercalcemia Hypokalemia Erectile dysfunction
Mineralocorticoid receptor antagonists (MRA)	Hyperkalemia Serum creatinine >2.5 mg/dL in men, >2.0 mg/dL in women)	Situations associated with higher risk of hyperkalemia (ACEI, ARB, diabetes)
ACE inhibitors	Pregnancy Angioneurotic edema Hyperkalemia Bilateral renal artery stenosis	Women with child-bearing potential
Angiotensin receptor blockers	Pregnancy Hyperkalemia Bilateral renal artery stenosis	Women with child-bearing potential
Ca^{2+} channel blockers (dihydropyridines)		Tachycardia/arrhythmia Heart failure
Ca^{2+} channel blockers (verapamil, diltiazem)	AV block (grade 2-3) Severe LV dysfunction Heart failure	Co-medication with CYP3A4- or Pgp–dependent drugs (e.g. statins, digoxin)
β Blockers	Asthma AV block (grade 2-3)	Metabolic syndrome Glucose intolerance Athletes and physically active patients Chronic obstructive lung disease Psoriasis Depression
α Blockers	Heart failure	
Central sympatholytic drugs	Depression AV block (grade 2-3)	Erectile dysfunction Xerostomia

[a]*Possible contraindications and precautions* noted in column 3 are not formal contraindications, but rather patient characteristics that should be considered on an individual basis and that may mitigate against use of a class of drugs (e.g., metabolic syndrome and glucose intolerance for diuretics and β blockers). Similarly, some patients with chronic obstructive lung disease can be treated with β_1 blockers without deterioration of lung function, whereas other patients may experience significant bronchoconstriction with β blockers.

clinical trial data, clinical judgment favors rapidly lowering blood pressure in patients with life-threatening complications of hypertension, such as encephalopathy or pulmonary edema due to severe hypertension. However, rapid reduction in blood pressure has considerable risks for the patients; if blood pressure is decreased too quickly or extensively, cerebral blood flow may diminish due to adaptations in the cerebral circulation that protect the brain from the sequelae of very high blood pressures. The temptation to treat patients merely on the basis of increased blood pressure should be resisted. Appropriate therapeutic decisions need to encompass how well a patient's major organs are reacting to the very high blood pressures. While many drugs have been used parenterally to rapidly decrease blood pressure in emergencies (including nitroprusside, enalaprilat, esmolol, fenoldopam, labetalol, clevidipine and nicardipine, hydralazine, and phentolamine), the clinical significance of differing actions of many of these drugs in this setting is largely unknown (Perez et al., 2009).

Resistant Hypertension

Some patients with hypertension fail to respond to recommended antihypertensive treatments. There are many potential explanations. To achieve stringent control of hypertension, many patients require two, three, or four appropriately selected drugs used at optimal doses. Exhibiting *an abundance of caution* and *therapeutic inertia*, clinicians may be reluctant to prescribe sufficient numbers of medications that exploit the drugs' full dose-response curves; conversely, patients may not adhere to the recommended pharmacological regimen. Sometimes, multiple drugs in the same therapeutic class that act by the same mechanism are combined; that is generally not a rational approach. Excess salt intake and the tendency of some antihypertensive drugs, especially vasodilators, to promote salt retention may mitigate falls in blood pressure; consequently, inadequate diuretic treatment commonly is found in patients with resistant hypertension. A relevant fraction of patients with resistant hypertension has primary hyperaldosteronism and benefits from the addition of daily spironolactone at 25–50 mg (Williams et al., 2015). Patients may take prescription drugs, over-the-counter drugs, or herbal preparations that oppose the actions of antihypertensive drugs (e.g., NSAIDs, sympathomimetic decongestants, cyclosporine, erythropoietin, ephedra [also called ma huang], or licorice). Illicit drugs such as cocaine and amphetamines may raise blood pressure. The physician must inquire about a patient's other medications and supplements and individualize the antihypertensive regimen.

Acknowledgment: Thomas Michel and Brian B. Hoffman contributed to this chapter in recent editions of this book. We have retained some of their text in the current edition.

Drug Facts for Your Personal Formulary: *Antihypertensives*

Antihypertensive Drug	Therapeutic Uses	Major Toxicity and Clinical Pearls
Diuretics		
Thiazide type Chlorothiazide Hydrochlorothiazide **Thiazide-like** Chlorthalidone Indapamide Metolazone	• Hypertension • Edema associated with HF, liver cirrhosis, chronic kidney disease, nephrotic syndrome • Nephrogenic diabetes insipidus • Kidney stones caused by Ca^{2+} crystals	• First choice for treating HTN • Chlorthalidone may be superior to hydrochlorothiazide in HTN • Lose efficacy at GFR < 30–40 mL/min (exceptions: indapamide, metolazone) • Potentiate effect of loop diuretics in HF (sequential tubular blockade) • Risk of hypokalemia and arrhythmia when combined with QT-prolonging drugs • Combine with ACEI/ARB or K+-sparing diuretic/MRA to prevent hypokalemia
Loop diuretics Bumetanide Furosemide Torsemide	• Acute pulmonary edema • Edema associated with HF, liver cirrhosis, chronic kidney disease, nephrotic syndrome • Hyponatremia • Hypercalcemia • Hypertension	• Not first choice for treating HTN with normal renal function: action too short and followed by rebound • Indicated acutely in malignant HTN and GFR < 30–40 mL/min • Torsemide may be superior to furosemide in HF • Risk of hypokalemia and arrhythmia when combined with QT-prolonging drugs
Sympatholytic Drugs		
β₁ Blockers Atenolol Bisoprolol Metoprolol Nebivolol Many others	• Hypertension • Heart failure (bisoprolol, metoprolol, nebivolol) • Widely used for other indications (angina, prevention of arrhythmias, rate control in atrial fibrillation, migraine, etc.)	• Role as first choice in the treatment of HTN debated; clear indication for angina, HF, atrial fibrillation, etc. • Bradycardia and AV block • Bronchospasm, peripheral vasoconstriction • Worsening of *acute* heart failure • Depression • Worsening of psoriasis • Polymorphic CYP2D6 metabolism (metoprolol) • Nebivolol NO-mediated vasodilation
Nonselective β blocker Propranolol	• Hypertension • Migraine	• Not first choice for treating HTN • Unwanted effects via blockade of β₂ receptors
α₁ Blockers Alfuzosin Doxazosin Prazosin Tamsulosin Silodosin	• Benign prostate hyperplasia • Hypertension	• Not first choice for treating HTN • Higher rate of HF development (?) • Tachyphylaxis • Phenoxybenzamine (irreversible α₁/α₂ blockade) used in pheochromocytoma
α₁ and β blockers Carvedilol Labetalol	• Hypertension • Heart failure (carvedilol)	• β blocker of choice in patients with peripheral artery disease • Among first choices for treating HF • Labetalol first choice for HTN in pregnancy

Drug Facts for Your Personal Formulary: *Antihypertensives* (*continued*)

Antihypertensive Drug	Therapeutic Uses	Major Toxicity and Clinical Pearls
Sympatholytic Drugs		
Central sympatholytic drugs Methyldopa Clonidine/moxonidine Reserpine Guanfacine	• Hypertension	• Not first choice in treating HTN • Fatigue, depression • Nasal congestion
Ca²⁺ Channel Blockers		
Dihydropyridines Amlodipine, felodipine Nifedipine Clevidipine, isradipine Lercanidipine, nitrendipine **Others** Diltiazem, verapamil	• Hypertension • Angina • Rate control in atrial fibrillation (verapamil, diltiazem)	• Extended-release, long-acting dihydropyridines among first choice in HTN • Diltiazem and verapamil: only if effects on heart rate and AV conduction are wanted, not in combination with β blockers; beware CYP3A4-mediated drug interactions
Inhibitors of the Renin-Angiotensin System		
ACE inhibitors Benazepril Captopril Enalapril Lisinopril Quinapril Ramipril Moexipril Fosinopril Trandolapril Perindopril	• Hypertension • Heart failure • Diabetic nephropathy	• Among first choice for treating HTN • Short-acting captopril only for initiation of therapy; enalapril and ramipril twice daily • Cough in 5%–10% of patients, angioedema • Hypotension, hyperkalemia, skin rash, neutropenia, anemia, fetopathic syndrome • Contraindications: pregnancy, renal artery stenosis; caution in patients with impaired renal function or hypovolemia • Fosinopril: hepatic and renal elimination, thus eliminated in patients with HF and low renal perfusion
Angiotensin receptor blockers Candesartan Eprosartan Irbesartan Losartan Olmesartan Telmisartan Valsartan Azilsartan	• Hypertension • Heart failure • Diabetic nephropathy	• Same as ACEI, less cough or angioedema • No evidence for superiority over ACEI • In combination with ACEI, more harm than benefit • Contraindicated in pregnancy
Direct renin inhibitors Aliskiren	• Hypertension	• Therapeutic value unclear; no evidence for superiority over ACEIs or ARBs • Combination with RAS inhibitors contraindicated
Vasodilators		
Hydralazine	• Hypertension • Heart failure in African Americans (fixed combination with ISDN)	• Not first choice in treating HTN • Adverse effects: headache, nausea, flushing, hypotension, palpitations, tachycardia, dizziness, and angina pectoris; generally combined with β blocker to reduce baroreceptor reflex effects • Use cautiously in patients with CAD • Lupus syndrome at high doses
Minoxidil	• Hypertension • Alopecia	• Reserve antihypertensive in patients with renal insufficiency • Water retention, tachycardia, angina, pericardial effusion • Use in combination with diuretic, β blocker, and RAS inhibitor • Hypertrichosis
Sodium nitroprusside	• Hypertensive emergencies	• Only short-term intravenously • Adverse effect: hypotension • Cyanide intoxication

Bibliography

ALLHAT Officers. Major outcomes in high-risk hypertensive patients randomized to angiotensin-converting enzyme inhibitor or calcium channel blocker vs. diuretic: the Antihypertensive and Lipid-Lowering Treatment to Prevent Heart Attack Trial (ALLHAT). *JAMA*, **2002**, *288*:2981–2997.

Arce C, et al. Hydralazine target: from blood vessels to the epigenome. *J Transl Med*, **2006**, *4*:10.

Azizi M, et al. Optimum and stepped care standardised antihypertensive treatment with or without renal denervation for resistant hypertension (DENERHTN): a multicentre, open-label, randomised controlled trial. *Lancet*, **2015**, *385*:1957–1965.

Bomback AS, et al. Aldosterone breakthrough during aliskiren, valsartan, and combination (aliskiren + valsartan) therapy. *J Am Soc Hypertens*, **2012**, *6*:338–345.

Calhoun DA, et al. Hyperaldosteronism among black and white subjects with resistant hypertension. *Hypertension*, **2002**, *40*:892–896.

Cameron HA, Ramsay LE. The lupus syndrome induced by hydralazine: a common complication with low dose treatment. *Br Med J (Clin Res Ed)*, **1984**, *289*:410–412.

Dahlof B, et al. Morbidity and mortality in the Swedish Trial in Old Patients with Hypertension (STOP-Hypertension). *Lancet*, **1991**, *338*:1281–1285.

Dahlof B, et al. Prevention of cardiovascular events with an antihypertensive regimen of amlodipine adding perindopril as required versus atenolol adding bendroflumethiazide as required, in the Anglo-Scandinavian Cardiac Outcomes Trial-Blood Pressure Lowering Arm (ASCOT-BPLA): a multicentre randomised controlled trial. *Lancet*, **2005**, *366*:895–906.

Davis BR, et al. Role of diuretics in the prevention of heart failure: the Antihypertensive and Lipid-Lowering Treatment to Prevent Heart Attack Trial. *Circulation*, **2006**, *113*:2201–2210.

Ernst ME, et al. Comparative antihypertensive effects of hydrochlorothiazide and chlorthalidone on ambulatory and office blood pressure. *Hypertension*, **2006**, *47*:352–358.

Frampton JE, Curran MP. Aliskiren: a review of its use in the management of hypertension. *Drugs*, **2007**, *67*:1767–1792.

Franklin SS. Is there a preferred antihypertensive therapy for isolated systolic hypertension and reduced arterial compliance? *Curr Hypertens Rep*, **2000**, *2*:253–259.

Giannopoulos G, et al. Central sympathetic inhibition to reduce postablation atrial fibrillation recurrences in hypertensive patients: a randomized, controlled study. *Circulation*, **2014**, *130*:1346–1352.

Go AS, et al. An effective approach to high blood pressure control: a science advisory from the American Heart Association, the American College of Cardiology, and the Centers for Disease Control and Prevention. *Hypertension*, **2014**, *63*:878–885.

Goodpaster BH, et al. Effects of diet and physical activity interventions on weight loss and cardiometabolic risk factors in severely obese adults: a randomized trial. *JAMA*, **2010**, *304*:1795–1802.

Jaffe MG, et al. Improved blood pressure control associated with a large-scale hypertension program. *JAMA*, **2013**, *310*:699–705.

Jamerson K, et al. Benazepril plus amlodipine or hydrochlorothiazide for hypertension in high-risk patients. *N Engl J Med*, **2008**, *359*:2417–2428.

James PA, et al. 2014 evidence-based guideline for the management of high blood pressure in adults: report from the panel members appointed to the Eighth Joint National Committee (JNC 8). *JAMA*, **2014**, *311*:507–520.

Ji W, et al. Rare independent mutations in renal salt handling genes contribute to blood pressure variation. *Nat Genet*, **2008**, *40*:592–599.

Kjeldsen S, et al. Updated national and international hypertension guidelines: a review of current recommendations. *Drugs*, **2014**, *74*:2033–2051.

Lacourciere Y, et al. Antihypertensive effects of amlodipine and hydrochlorothiazide in elderly patients with ambulatory hypertension. *Am J Hypertens*, **1995**, *8*:1154–1159.

Law MR, et al. Use of blood pressure lowering drugs in the prevention of cardiovascular disease: meta-analysis of 147 randomised trials in the context of expectations from prospective epidemiological studies. *Brit Med J*, *338*:b1665.

Lindholm LH, et al. Should beta blockers remain first choice in the treatment of primary hypertension? A meta-analysis. *Lancet*, **2005**, *366*:1545–1553.

MacMillan LB, et al. Central hypotensive effects of the alpha2a-adrenergic receptor subtype. *Science*, **1996**, *273*:801–803.

Magee LA, et al. Do labetalol and methyldopa have different effects on pregnancy outcome? Analysis of data from the Control of Hypertension In Pregnancy Study (CHIPS) trial. *BJOG*, **2016**, *123*:1143–1151.

Maille N, et al. Mechanism of hydralazine-induced relaxation in resistance arteries during pregnancy: hydralazine induces vasodilation via a prostacyclin pathway. *Vascul Pharmacol*, **2016**, *78*:36–42.

Makarounas-Kirchmann K, et al. Results of a meta-analysis comparing the tolerability of lercanidipine and other dihydropyridine calcium channel blockers. *Clin Ther*, **2009**, *31*:1652–1663.

Mancia G, et al. 2013 ESH/ESC guidelines for the management of arterial hypertension: the Task Force for the Management of Arterial Hypertension of the European Society of Hypertension (ESH) and of the European Society of Cardiology (ESC). *Eur Heart J*, **2013**, *34*:2159–2219.

McMurray JJ, et al. Aliskiren, ALTITUDE, and the implications for ATMOSPHERE. *Eur J Heart Fail*, **2012**, *14*:341–343.

Messerli FH, et al. Comparison of efficacy and side effects of combination therapy of angiotensin-converting enzyme inhibitor (benazepril) with calcium antagonist (either nifedipine or amlodipine) versus high-dose calcium antagonist monotherapy for systemic hypertension. *Am J Cardiol*, **2000**, *86*:1182–1187.

Metz S, et al. Rebound hypertension after discontinuation of transdermal clonidine therapy. *Am J Med*, **1987**, *82*:17–19.

Ogilvie RI. Comparative effects of vasodilator drugs on flow distribution and venous return. *Can J Physiol Pharmacol*, **1985**, *63*:1345–1355.

Pastor-Barriuso R, et al. Systolic blood pressure, diastolic blood pressure, and pulse pressure: an evaluation of their joint effect on mortality. *Ann Intern Med*, **2003**, *139*:731–739.

Pedersen ME, Cockcroft JR. The latest generation of beta-blockers: new pharmacologic properties. *Curr Hypertens Rep*, **2006**, *8*:279–286.

Perez MI, et al. Effect of early treatment with anti-hypertensive drugs on short and long-term mortality in patients with an acute cardiovascular event. *Cochrane Database Syst Rev*, **2009**, (4):CD006743.

Perry HM Jr, et al. Effect of treating isolated systolic hypertension on the risk of developing various types and subtypes of stroke: the Systolic Hypertension in the Elderly Program (SHEP). *JAMA*, **2000**, *284*:465–471.

Pezhouman A, et al. Molecular basis of hypokalemia-induced ventricular fibrillation. *Circulation*, **2015**, *132*:1528–1537.

Pollesello P, Mebazza A. ATP-dependent potassium channels as key targets for the treatment of myocardial and vascular dysfunction. *Curr Opin Crit Care*, **2004**, *10*:436–441.

Ramsay LE, et al. Diuretic treatment of resistant hypertension. *Br Med J*, **1980**, *281*:1101–1103.

Rau T, et al. Impact of the CYP2D6 genotype on the clinical effects of metoprolol: a prospective longitudinal study. *Clin Pharmacol Ther*, **2009**, *85*:269–272.

Rosendorff C, et al. Treatment of hypertension with coronary artery disease: a scientific statement from the American Heart Association, American College of Cardiology, and American Society of Hypertension. *Circulation*, *131*:e435–e470.

Sato T, et al. Minoxidil opens mitochondrial K(ATP) channels and confers cardioprotection. *Br J Pharmacol*, **2004**, *141*:360–366.

SHEP Cooperative Research Group. Prevention of stroke by antihypertensive drug treatment in older persons with isolated systolic hypertension. Final results of the Systolic Hypertension in the Elderly Program (SHEP). *JAMA*, **1991**, *265*:3255–3264.

Siscovick DS, et al. Diuretic therapy for hypertension and the risk of primary cardiac arrest. *N Engl J Med*, **1994**, *330*:1852–1857.

Sjostrom L, et al. Effects of bariatric surgery on mortality in Swedish obese subjects. *N Engl J Med*, **2007**, *357*:741–752.

Slove S, et al. Potassium channel openers increase aortic elastic fiber formation and reverse the genetically determined elastin deficit in the BN rat. *Hypertension*, **2013**, *62*:794–801.

SPRINT Research group. A randomized trial of intensive versus standard blood-pressure control. *N Engl J Med*, **2015**, *373*:2103–2116.

Staessen JA, et al. Randomised double-blind comparison of placebo and active treatment for older patients with isolated systolic hypertension. The Systolic Hypertension in Europe (Syst-Eur) Trial Investigators. *Lancet*, **1997**, *350*:757–764.

van de Ven PJ, et al. Angiotensin converting enzyme inhibitor-induced renal dysfunction in atherosclerotic renovascular disease. *Kidney Int*, **1998**, *53*:986–993.

Vlasses PH, et al. Comparative antihypertensive effects of enalapril maleate and hydrochlorothiazide, alone and in combination. *J Clin Pharmacol*, **1983**, *23*:227–233.

Williams B, et al. Differential impact of blood pressure-lowering drugs on central aortic pressure and clinical outcomes: principal results of the Conduit Artery Function Evaluation (CAFE) study. *Circulation*, **2006**, *113*:1213–1225.

Williams B, et al. Spironolactone versus placebo, bisoprolol, and doxazosin to determine the optimal treatment for drug-resistant hypertension (PATHWAY-2): a randomised, double-blind, crossover trial. *Lancet*, **2015**, *386*:2059–2068.

Yang T, Roden DM. Extracellular potassium modulation of drug block of IKr. Implications for torsade de pointes and reverse use-dependence. *Circulation*, **1996**, *93*:407–411.

Yusuf S, et al. Telmisartan, ramipril, or both in patients at high risk for vascular events. *N Engl J Med*, **2008**, *358*:1547–1559.

Therapy of Heart Failure

Thomas Eschenhagen

Heart failure is responsible for more than half a million deaths annually in the U.S. Its prevalence is increasing worldwide, likely due to improved survival of those who have had an acute myocardial infarction and an aging population. Median survival rates after the first hospitalization associated with heart failure are worse than those of most cancers, but have improved over the past 30 years (1.3 to 2.3 years in men and 1.3 to 1.7 years in women) (Jhund et al., 2009). This positive trend was associated with a 2- to 3-fold higher prescription rate of ACEIs and ARBs, β receptor antagonists (β blockers), and MRAs, suggesting that improved drug therapy has contributed to enhanced survival of heart failure.

Pathophysiology of Heart Failure

Definitions

Heart failure is a state in which the heart is unable to pump blood at a rate commensurate with the requirements of the body's tissues or can do so only at elevated filling pressure. This leads to symptoms that define the heart failure syndrome clinically. Low output (forward failure) causes fatigue, dizziness, muscle weakness, and shortness of breath, which is aggravated by physical exercise. Increased filling pressure leads to congestion of the organs upstream of the heart (backward failure), clinically apparent as peripheral or pulmonary edema, maldigestion, and ascites.

Most patients with heart failure are diagnosed exclusively on the basis of symptoms; that is, their heart function has never been directly measured (e.g., by echocardiography). Under these circumstances, it is not possible to differentiate between HFrEF (or systolic heart failure) and HFpEF (or diastolic heart failure, see discussion that follows). Other diseases associated with similar symptoms can therefore be wrongly categorized as heart failure (e.g., chronic obstructive pulmonary disease).

Common Final Pathway of Multiple Cardiac Diseases

Heart failure is not a single disease entity but a clinical syndrome that represents the final pathway of multiple cardiac diseases. The most common reason for systolic heart failure today is ischemic heart disease causing either acute (myocardial infarction) or chronic loss of viable heart muscle mass. Other reasons include chronic arterial hypertension and valvular diseases (both are decreasing in incidence due to improved therapy), genetically determined primary heart muscle defects (cardiomyopathies), viral infections (cytomegalovirus and possibly parvovirus), and toxins. The last encompass excessive alcohol, cocaine, amphetamines, and cancer drugs such as doxorubicin or trastuzumab, the monoclonal antibody directed against the growth factor receptor Her-2/Erb-B2 (see Chapter 67).

Pathophysiological Mechanisms

The pathophysiology of systolic heart failure is relatively well understood. The mechanisms of HFpEF are much less clear, but surely differ and are discussed further in this chapter. The pathophysiology of heart failure is complex and involves four major interrelated systems (Figure 29–1):

- the heart itself
- the vasculature
- the kidney
- neurohumoral regulatory circuits

The Heart Itself: Cardiomyopathy of the Overload

Any overload of the myocardium—loss of relevant muscle mass, which overloads the remaining healthy myocardium; chronic hypertension; or valvular defects—will eventually lead to the organ's failure to produce sufficient cardiac output. This concept can be extended to the genetically determined cardiomyopathies in which essentially any defect in an organelle of cardiac myocytes can lead to primary myocyte contractile dysfunction and then, secondarily, to the picture commonly seen in the cardiomyopathy of the overload. Not surprisingly, the most common cardiomyopathies (HCM, DCM) are due to mutations in genes encoding proteins of the contractile machinery, the sarcomere, proteins anchoring the sarcomere to the plasma membrane, or proteins mediating and maintaining cell-cell contact.

The overload (or the primary contractile defect) leads to alterations of the heart that can partially compensate but that come at a price. Because cardiac myocytes essentially stop replicating in the early postnatal period,

Abbreviations

ACC: American College of Cardiology
ACE: angiotensin-converting enzyme
ACEI: angiotensin-converting enzyme inhibitor
ACh: acetylcholine
ADH: antidiuretic hormone (vasopressin)
ADR: adverse drug reaction
AF: atrial fibrillation
AHA: American Heart Association
AngII: angiotensin II
ANP: atrial natriuretic peptide
ARB: AT$_1$ angiotensin receptor antagonist (blocker)
ARNI: angiotensin receptor/neprilysin inhibitor
AV: atrioventricular
AVP: arginine vasopressin
BB: β blocker
BNP: brain-type natriuretic peptide
CAD: coronary artery disease
CCB: calcium channel blocker
CG: cardiac glycoside
CHF: congestive heart failure
CM: cardiomyopathy
CNP: C-type natriuretic peptide
COX: cyclooxygenase
CPT1: Carnitine palmitoyltransferase 1
CRT: cardiac resynchronization therapy
CYP: cytochrome P450
DCM: dilated cardiomyopathy
DM: diabetes mellitus
ECG: electrocardiogram
EF: ejection fraction
EMA: European Medicines Agency
eNOS: endothelial nitric oxide synthase
EPI: epinephrine
ESC: European Society of Cardiology
ET: endothelin
FDA: Food and Drug Administration
GC: guanylyl cyclase
GDMT: guideline-directed medical therapy
GFR: glomerular filtration rate
GI: gastrointestinal
GPCR: G protein–coupled receptor
GTN: glycerol trinitrate
HCM: hypertrophic cardiomyopathy
HCN: hyperpolarization-activated, cyclic nucleotide–gated cation channel
HF: heart failure
HFpEF: heart failure with preserved ejection fraction (diastolic heart failure)
HFrEF: heart failure with reduced ejection fraction (systolic heart failure)
HMG CoA: 3-hydroxy-3-methylglutaryl coenzyme A
HRQOL: health-related quality of life
HTN: hypertension
ICD: implantable cardioverter-defibrillator
ISDN: isosorbide 2,5′-dinitrate
ISMN: isosorbide 5′-mononitrate
LV: left ventricular
LVH: left ventricular hypertrophy
MCS: mechanical circulatory support
MI: myocardial infarction
MRA: mineralocorticoid receptor antagonist

NCX: Na$^+$/Ca^{2+} exchanger
NE: norepinephrine
NO: nitric oxide
NSAID: nonsteroidal anti-inflammatory drug
NYHA: New York Heart Association
PD: pharmacodynamic
PDE: cyclic nucleotide phosphodiesterase
PKA: protein kinase A
PLB: phospholamban
PLM: phospholemman
RAAS: renin-angiotensin-aldosterone system
ROS: reactive oxygen species
RyR: ryanodine receptor
SERCA: sarco/endoplasmic reticulum Ca^{2+} ATPase
sGC: soluble guanylyl cyclase
SL: sarcolemma
SNS: sympathetic nervous system
SR: sarcoplasmic reticulum
TnC: troponin C
TNF: tumor necrosis factor
TnI: inhibitory subunit of troponin

the usual response to overload is not myocyte division but rather hypertrophy, growing in size and assembling more sarcomeres that can contribute to contractile force development. Whereas hypertrophy is principally a normal response to physiological needs such as body growth, pregnancy, and physical exercise ("physiological hypertrophy"), hypertrophy in response to chronic overload comes with features that make it a major risk factor for the development of heart failure ("pathological hypertrophy"). A direct consequence of cardiac myocyte hypertrophy is a reduced capillary/myocyte ratio (i.e., less O_2 and nutrient supply per myocyte), causing an energy deficit and metabolic reprogramming. Altered gene expression of ion channels, Ca^{2+}-regulating proteins, and contractile proteins can be interpreted as partially beneficial, energy-saving adaptations; on the other hand, the adaptations also aggravate contractile failure and favor arrhythmias. Concurrently, fibroblasts proliferate and deposit increased amounts of extracellular matrix (e.g., collagen). This fibrosis in heart failure also favors arrhythmias, increases the stiffness of the heart, and interrupts myocyte-to-myocyte communication (coordinated conduction and force transmission). Finally, overload leads to cardiac myocyte death by apoptosis or necrosis. Collectively, these adverse adaptations are called *pathological remodeling*.

Some of these alterations are direct, heart-intrinsic consequences of overload (e.g., hypertrophy, altered gene expression); others are secondary to neurohumoral activation and thereby susceptible to neurohumoral blocking agents (see discussion that follows and Figure 29–1).

The Vasculature

A critical parameter of cardiac function is the stiffness of the vasculature. It determines the resistance against which the heart has to expel the blood and increases with aging. Heart failure may be the consequence of premature aging of the vasculature (Strait and Lakatta, 2012). Aging-induced loss of elasticity of the great blood vessels reduces their compliance, that is, the elasticity that permits vessels to extend in systole and contract in diastole. Good compliance reduces peak systolic pressure and increases diastolic pressure, which favors perfusion in diastole. It is negatively correlated with pulse pressure, that is, the difference between systolic and diastolic blood pressure, which is low in children and high in the elderly. Arterial hypertension and diabetes mellitus are the major reasons for premature stiffening of blood vessels, which imposes increased afterload to the heart and contributes to heart failure. Theoretically, stiffening and loss of compliance could be directly tackled by drugs (see section Recent Developments; Novel Approaches).

Another critical aspect of vascular function is the ability to adapt the vessel diameter to hemodynamic and neurohumoral stimuli, a function

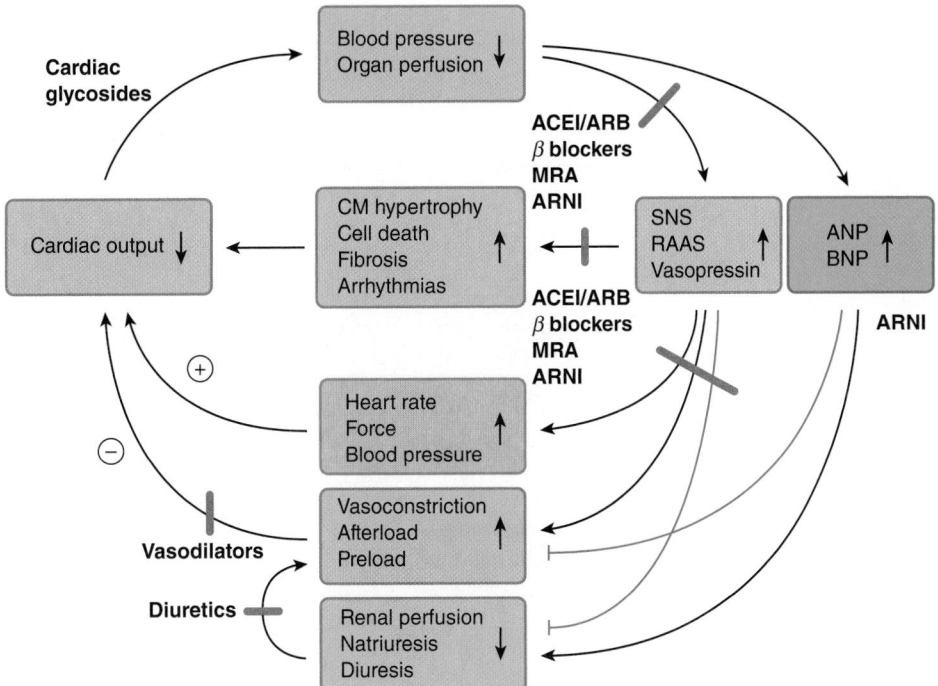

Figure 29–1 *Pathophysiologic mechanisms of systolic heart failure (HFrEF) and therapeutic interventions.* Any major decrease in cardiac contractile function leads to activation of neurohumoral systems, including the SNS, the RAAS, and vasopressin (ADH) secretion, which acutely stabilize blood pressure and organ perfusion by stimulating cardiac output, constricting resistance vessels, decreasing kidney perfusion, and increasing Na⁺ and H₂O retention. Unfortunately, these responses are maladaptive, causing chronic overloading and overstimulation of the failing heart. Direct hypertrophic, pro-apoptotic, fibrotic, and arrhythmogenic effects of NE and AngII further accelerate the deleterious process. Note that the concomitant activation of the ANP/BNP system is the consequence of stretch and increased wall stress in the heart and has opposite and beneficial effects. See Abbreviations list at beginning of chapter.

that is governed by cross talk between luminal endothelial and underlying smooth muscle cells (Chapter 28). The main signaling pathway involves receptors that increase intracellular Ca²⁺ levels in endothelial cells, which activates eNOS to produce NO. This gaseous transmitter diffuses into smooth muscle cells and activates sGC to produce cGMP, which causes relaxation of vascular smooth muscle. Heart failure is always accompanied by endothelial dysfunction, which is a disturbed balance between vasodilating NO and proconstrictor ROS. ROS, by inactivating the two critical enzymes eNOS and sGC and converting NO in peroxynitrite, a strong ROS, favor vasoconstriction. Several common cardiovascular drugs (ACEIs/ARBs, MRAs, statins) improve endothelial function by reducing ROS production. PDE5 inhibitors have similar consequences by inhibiting cGMP degradation in smooth muscle cells and thereby promoting relaxation.

The Kidney

The kidney regulates Na⁺ and H₂O excretion and thereby intravascular volume. Under normal conditions, autoregulatory and neurohumoral mechanisms ensure an adequate GFR and diuresis over a wide range of renal perfusion pressures. Prominent mechanisms with relevance for heart failure are (1) the AngII-mediated regulation of filtration rate by regulating the diameter of efferent glomerular arteriole; (2) the regulation of kidney perfusion by a balance between constrictor-promoting effects of AngII (via AT₁ receptors) and vasopressin (AVP, via V₁ receptors) and the vasodilating influence of prostaglandins (hence the deleterious effects of NSAIDs); (3) the aldosterone-mediated regulation of Na⁺ reabsorption in the distal tubule; and (4) AVP-regulated water transport in the collecting ducts (via V₂ receptors). In heart failure, all mechanisms are dysregulated and constitute therapeutic targets of ACEIs/ARBs, MRAs, and diuretics. Newer agents, such as adenosine A₁ receptor antagonists and AVP receptor antagonists, have failed to exert therapeutic benefit in clinical studies.

Neurohumoral Regulation and HFrEF

The decrease in cardiac output in heart failure leads to the activation of the SNS and the RAAS and increases in plasma levels of AVP and ET

(Figure 29–1). This concerted response ensures the perfusion of centrally important organs such as the brain and the heart (at the expense of kidney, liver, and skeletal muscle perfusion) in situations of acute blood loss. These responses are components of the "fight-or-flight response" and provide useful short-term physiological responses to alarm and danger. Chronically, however, neurohumoral activation exerts deleterious effects that constitute a vicious cycle in heart failure. Vasoconstriction initially not only stabilizes blood pressure but also increases afterload, which is the resistance against which the heart works to expel blood (see Figures 29–4 and 27–1). Because of the decreased contractile reserve, the failing heart is particularly sensitive to increases in afterload (see Figure 29–4); such increases further decrease cardiac output. Decreased kidney perfusion and increased aldosterone production reduce diuresis and promote volume overload, which increases cardiac preload, dilation, and ventricular wall stress, a major determinant of cardiac O₂ consumption. Tachycardic and positive inotropic actions of catecholamines not only acutely increase cardiac output but also promote arrhythmias and increase O₂ consumption in a failing, energy-depleted heart. AngII, NE, and ET accelerate pathological cardiac remodeling (hypertrophy, fibrosis, and cell death). Aldosterone has prominent profibrotic actions. This spectrum of adverse consequences of chronic neurohumoral activation explains why inhibitors of these systems (ACEIs/ARBs, β blockers, and MRAs) exert long-term, life-prolonging effects in heart failure and are the cornerstones of current therapy.

Unexpectedly, ET and AVP receptor antagonists provide no beneficial effect in patients with heart failure, despite promising results in preclinical studies. Clinical trials suggested that neurohumoral activation in response to altered cardiac function may be sufficiently inhibited by the standard combination therapy, leaving no room for improvement from the addition of ET and AVP antagonists; however, recent data indicate that additional benefit may accrue via another therapeutic route: a drug combination called ARNIs. The FDA has approved a fixed-dose combination of the ARB valsartan with the neprilysin inhibitor sacubitril. Valsartan blocks AT₁ receptors, reducing the deleterious effects of AngII.

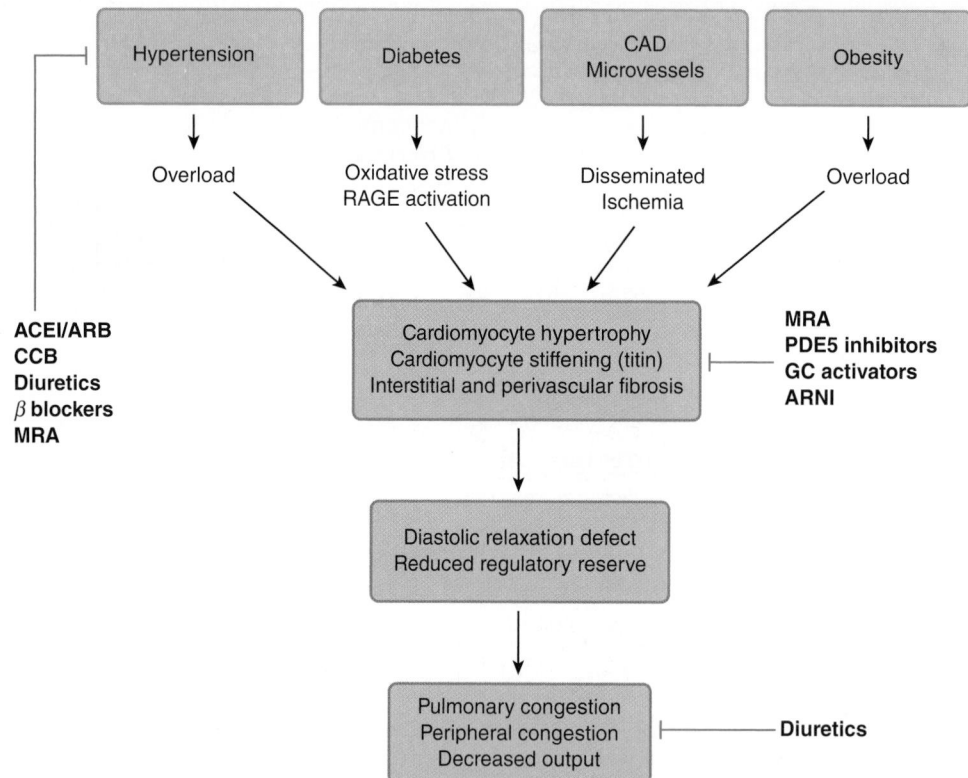

Figure 29–2 *Pathophysiological mechanisms of diastolic heart failure HFpEF and possible therapeutic interventions.* Unlike the case with HFrEF, the pharmacological agents shown have not been proven to have clinical efficacy toward HFpEF, although these agents can help to control underlying diseases, such as hypertension, diabetes, and obesity. Only exercise training has proven effective in increasing maximal exercise capacity. RAGE; receptor for advanced glycosylation end-products.

Sacubitril inhibits the degradation of the natriuretic peptides ANP and BNP. The valsartan-sacubitril combination appears superior to the ACEI enalapril, reducing the rates of hospitalization and death from all cardiovascular causes in patients with HFrEF (Hubers and Brown, 2016).

This finding reflects the fact that neurohumoral activation in heart failure includes one system that exerts beneficial effects: the natriuretic peptides. Normally, ANP and BNP are expressed in the atria and released on increased preload (stretch). During heart failure, ANP and BNP are also produced by the ventricles, such that plasma levels are elevated. Indeed, BNP is used as a biomarker of heart failure. ANP and BNP stimulate the plasma membrane guanylyl cyclase. In the kidney, elevated cGMP has diuretic effects. Elevated cellular cGMP mediates vasodilation in the vasculature and, in the heart, antihypertrophic, antifibrotic, and compliance-increasing effects related to phosphorylation of titin. Enhancing these effects by inhibiting the degradation of ANP/BNP likely explains the clinical benefits of sacubitril-valsartan.

Heart Failure With Preserved Ejection Fraction

Systematic echocardiographic determination of left ventricular EF in thousands of patients with heart failure revealed that about 50% had no reduction; that is, they exhibited EF values greater than 50%. Still, patients had typical heart failure symptoms, including acute decompensation with pulmonary edema and a survival prognosis not much better or even identical to patients with reduced EF (systolic heart failure or HFrEF). These data point to a different pathophysiology in which abnormalities of the diastolic and not the systolic component of cardiac function prevail. Due to difficulties in defining diastolic function by standard techniques, the term *HFpEF* has been introduced and applies to patients with typical heart failure symptoms and "normal" (>50%) or only mildly reduced EF.

Even more than HFrEF, HFpEF is a multifactorial disease (Figure 29–2). HFpEF is typically associated with arterial hypertension, ischemic heart disease, diabetes mellitus, and obesity (metabolic syndrome); it is more frequent in women than men and shows a strong increase in prevalence with age. Hearts of patients with HFpEF are generally not dilated, wall thickness is enlarged (hypertrophy), and left atrial size often is enlarged as a sign of chronically elevated end-diastolic pressures. Central to the pathophysiology of HFpEF is, presumably, compromised diastolic relaxation of the left ventricle, which causes congestion of the lung, shortness of breath, or pulmonary edema. Clinical decompensation is often associated with strongly elevated blood pressure.

Molecular alterations include increased myocardial fibrosis (causing a permanent relaxation deficit) as well as more dynamic changes, such as reduced phosphorylation of titin, the sarcomeric protein that spans the large region from the Z to the M band. Titin contains several molecular spring domains whose elastic modulus determines the passive tension of cardiomyocytes, particularly at low-to-medium levels of stretch. At higher levels of stretch, the extracellular matrix becomes involved. Titin stiffness is determined by its isoforms and by cGMP-dependent phosphorylation, suggesting that agents that increase cellular cGMP might be beneficial in HFpEF. However, the PDE5 inhibitor sildenafil, which preserves and elevates cellular cGMP in some cells (see Chapters 3, 31, and 45), failed to show benefit (Redfield et al., 2013). This lack of efficacy is, unfortunately, also true for all other pharmacological interventions in HFpEF, including ACEIs, ARBs, and spironolactone. Exercise training is presently the only intervention that significantly increases maximal physical activity in HFpEF patients. In the absence of evidence-based clinical trial data, current therapy recommendations concentrate on optimal treatment of the underlying diseases, such as hypertension, diabetes, and obesity.

Heart Failure Staging

Heart failure was one of the first diseases for which guidelines described specific therapies for each stage of the disease. An early classification of the stages of heart failure was that of the NYHA, a classification still in use: class I (left ventricular dysfunction, no symptoms); class II (symptoms at medium-to-high levels of physical exercise); class III (symptoms at low levels of physical exercise); and class IV (symptoms at rest or daily life physical activities such as brushing teeth). The more recent guidelines of the AHA and ACC extended this classification by taking into account that

- heart failure is part of the cardiovascular continuum with preventable risk factors (stage A)
- an asymptomatic stage exists that requires treatment to delay transition to symptomatic heart failure (stage B)
- patients oscillate between different degrees of symptoms and therefore between class II and III (class C, which generally includes NYHA class II/III patients)
- a final stage of the disease requires different treatment and special considerations, such as heart transplantation and left ventricular assist device implantation (stage D).

This chapter uses the AHA/ACC classification (Yancey et al., 2013) but also considers the recent guidelines of the European Society of Cardiology (Ponikowski et al., 2016), which provide more specific treatment algorithms, and the 2016 AHA/ACC update (Yancy et al., 2016). Treatment guidelines are summarized in Figure 29–3.

Prevention and Treatment

Ischemic heart disease, hypertension, and valvular diseases are the most prevalent causes of heart failure. People at high risk (stage A) should therefore be consequently treated with drugs with an established effect on the natural course of these diseases, in conjunction with appropriate lifestyle changes. Studies in thousands of patients have reproducibly shown that blood pressure lowering in hypertensive patients and lipid-lowering with statins in dyslipidemic patients reduce not only the incidence of myocardial infarction and death but also the incidence of heart failure. The data are weaker for antidiabetic drugs, but consensus exists that blood glucose should be controlled with a hemoglobin A_{1C} goal of 7%–7.5%.

Treatment of heart failure has seen a dramatic change over the past decades. Until the late 1980s, drugs and drug dosing were symptom oriented and based on pathophysiological considerations of *acute* systolic heart failure. Treatment was mainly directed toward symptom relief and short-term improvement of hemodynamic function. With the era of

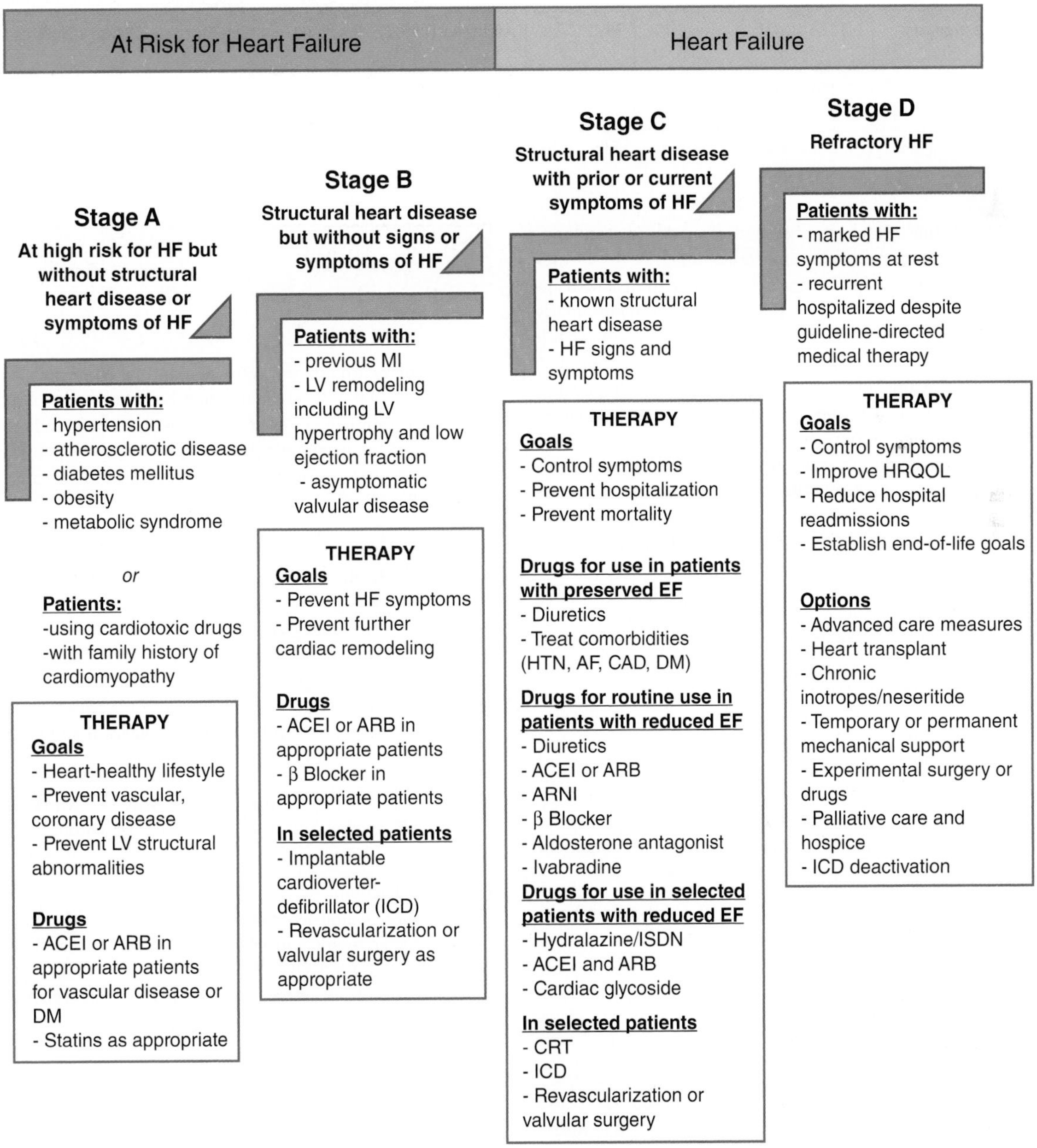

Figure 29–3   *AHA/ACC 2013 Heart Failure Treatment Guidelines: stages in the development of HF and recommended therapy by stage.* (See Yancey et al., 2013 and 2016, for details.)

SECTION III MODULATION OF PULMONARY, RENAL, AND CARDIOVASCULAR FUNCTION

TABLE 29–1 ■ LANDMARK STUDIES IN THE TREATMENT OF PATIENTS WITH CHRONIC HEART FAILURE WITH REDUCED EJECTION FRACTION

STUDY (as cited in Bibliography)	STUDY POPULATION	NO. OF SUBJECTS	BASELINE DRUGS (% of patients on each)	DRUG EFFECT (on all-cause mortality)
Cohn et al., 1986	Men, impaired cardiac function and exercise capacity	642	CG, D	ISDN/hydralazine ↓ 34% Prazosin +/– vs. placebo
CONSENSUS Trial Study Group, 1987	Severe HF, NYHA class IV	253	D 100, CG 93, BB 2, spironolactone 52, vasodilators ~ 50	Enalapril ↓ 40% vs. placebo
SOLVD Investigators, 1991	NYHA II–III, left EF < 35%	2569	D 86, CG 67, BB 7.5, vasodilators 51	Enalapril ↓ 16% vs. placebo
SOLVD Investigators, 1992	NYHA I, left EF < 35%	4228	Vasodilators 46, D 17, CG 13	Enalapril ↓ 8% (n.s.) vs. placebo (heart failure development ↓ 20%)
Digitalis Investigation Group, 1997	NYHA II–III	6800	D 81, ACE 95, nitrates 43	Digoxin +/– (HF hospitalizations ↓ 27%)
RALES (Pitt et al., 1999)	Severe HF, left EF < 35%	1663	D 100, ACEI 94, CG 72, BB 10	Spironolactone ↓ 30% vs. placebo
MERIT-HF Investigators, 1999	NYHA II–IV	3991	ACEI/ARB 95, D 90, CG 63	Metoprolol CR/XL ↓ 34% vs. placebo
PARADIGM-HF (McMurray et al., 2014)	NYHA II–IV	8442	BB 93, MRA 56, CG 30, ICD 15, CRT 7, D 80	Sacubitril/valsartan ↓ 16% vs. enalapril

D, diuretics; n.s., nonsignificant; NYHA indicates classification of HF according to the NYHA.

randomized clinical trials, which mainly tested effects of drugs on long-term morbidity (hospitalizations) and mortality, much of the former beliefs have proven to be wrong. For example, positive inotropic drugs (sympathomimetics and PDE inhibitors) that exert acute symptomatic benefit reduce life expectancy when given chronically. In contrast, β blockers decrease cardiac output acutely and may make people feel weak at the start of therapy but prolong life expectancy when given in increasing doses for extended periods. Vasodilators once seemed a logical choice for heart failure, but pure vasodilators such as the α_1 receptor antagonist prazosin or the nitrate ISDN, in combination with the vasodilator hydralazine, do not positively affect the prognosis in Caucasians (see further discussion). Thus, clinical trials have established important principles for assessing efficacy of therapies for heart failure:

1. Drugs for the treatment of chronic heart failure should reduce the patient morbidity and mortality.
2. Short-term drug effects poorly predict the outcome of randomized clinical trials and optimal therapies for heart failure.
3. Considerations of stage of disease are critical.
4. New drugs for heart failure should be compared to the most effective current combination therapy, a principle often ignored in preclinical animal work.
5. Nonpharmacological treatment options such as cardiac resynchronization devices and intracardiac defibrillator/cardioverters are important for their documented lifesaving effect in selected patient populations.

Attention to these principles for assessing long-term efficacy of heart failure therapies has provided evidence-based principles of treatment.

HISTORICAL PERSPECTIVE

A series of landmark studies over three decades has established the current thinking on the treatment of patients with chronic HFrEF. These studies are not reviewed here, but interested readers may wish to consult the evidence that supports current therapies. These studies, often indicated by an acronym, are summarized in Table 29–1.

Drug Treatment of Chronic Systolic Heart Failure (Stages B and C)

Treatment Principle I: Neurohumoral Modulation

Dampening neurohumoral activation and its deleterious consequences on the heart, blood vessels, and kidney is the cornerstone of heart failure therapy. Therapy consists of ACEIs/ARBs, β blockers, and MRAs. Further activation of the natriuretic peptide system adds benefit (Figure 29–1). A systematic discussion of the drugs is found in Chapters 12, 25, 26, 27, and 28.

Angiotensin-Converting Enzyme Inhibitors

Angiotensin II, the most active angiotensin peptide, is largely derived from angiotensinogen in two proteolytic steps. First, *renin*, an enzyme released from the kidneys, cleaves the decapeptide AngI from the amino terminus of angiotensinogen (renin substrate). Then, ACE removes a carboxy-terminal dipeptide (His⁹-Leu¹⁰) from AngI, yielding the active octapeptide, AngII (Figure 26–1). Thus, ACEIs reduce circulating levels of AngII. All patients with heart failure (stages B and C; NYHA I–IV) should receive an ACEI.

Mechanism of Action. AngII interacts with two heptahelical GPCRs, AT_1 and AT_2, and has four major cardiovascular actions that are all mediated by the AT_1 receptor:

- vasoconstriction
- stimulation of aldosterone release from the adrenal glands
- direct hypertrophic and proliferative effects on cardiomyocytes and fibroblasts, respectively
- stimulation of NE release from sympathetic nerve endings and the adrenal medulla

Physiological Effects. The ACEIs lower the circulating level of AngII and thereby reduce its deleterious effects. Thus, ACEIs not only act as vasodilators but also reduce aldosterone levels and thereby act as an indirect diuretic, have direct antiremodeling effects on the heart, and produce sympatholytic effects (thus moderating the reflex tachycardia that accompanies vasodilation and the lowering of blood pressure).

The ACEIs have important renal effects. When renal perfusion pressure is reduced, AngII constricts renal efferent arterioles, and this serves to maintain glomerular filtration pressure and GFR. Thus, under circumstances in which renal perfusion pressure is compromised, inhibition of the RAAS may induce a sudden and marked decrease in GFR. For this reason, ACEIs are contraindicated in bilateral renal artery stenosis. Likewise, because patients with heart failure often have low renal perfusion pressures, aggressive treatment with ACEIs may induce acute renal failure. To avoid this, for patients with heart failure patients, ACEIs should be initiated at very low doses; blood pressure, blood creatinine, and K^+ levels should be monitored; and the ACEI dose slowly increased over weeks toward target levels (for agents that have been carefully evaluated in clinical trials; Table 29–2). The potentially dangerous acute effects become beneficial with long-term use of ACEIs because the (small) chronic lowering of glomerular pressures protects the glomerulus from fibrotic degeneration.

The ACEI-induced lowering of aldosterone levels causes reduced expression of the aldosterone-dependent epithelial Na^+ channel (ENaC) in the distal tubule (see Figure 25-6). This target of K^+-sparing diuretics (see discussion that follows) normally mediates Na^+ reabsorption and K^+ excretion. Lower levels of ENaC lead to less absorption of Na^+ and less excretion of K^+. Thus, ACEIs favor hyperkalemia, which can be detrimental in patients with renal insufficiency but is normally beneficial for patients with heart failure who more often present with hypokalemia, a condition that promotes cardiac arrhythmias. ACEIs shift the balance of vascular smooth muscle tone toward vasodilation and thereby increase renal blood flow, another reason for their chronic protective effects on the kidney. This effect also explains why NSAIDs, which reduce the production of vasodilating prostaglandins, antagonize effects of ACEIs and should be avoided in patients with heart failure.

Other Actions, Good and Adverse. Angiotensin-converting enzyme has other actions, including the inactivation of bradykinin and substance P. ACEIs increase bradykinin and substance P levels, with two prominent consequences: cough, the most frequent ADR (~5%); and angioedema, a rare (~0.7%), but life-threatening condition presenting with swelling of the skin and mucous membranes of the throat and asphyxia (three times more common amongst African Americans). Experimental evidence suggests that increases in bradykinin contribute to the therapeutic efficacy of ACEIs and may explain why ARBs, which do not increase bradykinin (and therefore cause no cough), have not been consistently associated with improved survival in patients with HFrEF (Ponikowski et al., 2016).

The ACEIs are generally well tolerated in the majority of patients. Important ADRs are the following:

- dry cough, necessitating a change to ARBs;
- creatinine plasma concentration increase (<20%, normal; 20%–50%: careful observation and reduction of ACEI dosage; > 50%, stop ACEI and consult specialist for diagnosis of renal artery);
- hyperkalemia (small increase normal, but requires careful observation in patients with diabetes, renal insufficiency, or comedication with MRAs, K^+-sparing diuretics, or NSAIDs);
- angioedema (stop drug immediately, treat with antihistamines, corticosteroids, or, in severe case, EPI); and
- allergic skin reactions.

Angiotensin Receptor Antagonists

The ARBs are systematically discussed in Chapter 26. They are highly selective, competitive receptor antagonists at the AT_1 receptor, which mediates the major effects of AngII. They are therapeutic alternatives to ACEIs and second choice in all stages of heart failure in patients who do not tolerate ACEIs. Given the central role of the AT_1 receptor for the actions of AngII, it is not surprising that ARBs show the same pharmacological profile as ACEIs with the exception of not inducing cough. The unopposed activity of AT_2 receptor pathways in the presence of AT_1 blockade by an ARB seems to confer no therapeutic advantage to ARBs over ACEIs. Moreover, the addition of an ARB to therapy with an ACEI does not affect the prognosis of patients with heart failure but does increase hypotension, hyperkalemia, and renal dysfunction. A negative interaction between ACEIs and ARBs appears to extend to patients with higher renal risk. There is, therefore, no routine indication for this combination.

β Adrenergic Receptor Antagonists

Major Effects of β Adrenergic Antagonists. The sympathetic neurotransmitters NE (released at adrenergic nerve varicosities) and EPI (secreted by the adrenal medulla) are strong stimuli of heart function. They increase heart rate (positive chronotropic effect) and force of contraction (positive inotropic effect) and thereby augment cardiac output. They quicken the rate of force development (increased +dP/dt, positive clinotropy) and accelerate cardiac muscle relaxation (greater –dP/dt, positive lusitropic effect, which aids ventricular filling during diastole). Acceleration of the atrial-ventricular conduction rate (positive dromotropic effect) shortens the heart cycle and allows higher beating rates. Catecholamines enhance cardiac myocyte automaticity and lower the

TABLE 29–2 ■ PROPERTIES AND THERAPEUTIC DAILY DOSES OF ACEIs AND ARBs APPROVED AND CLINICALLY EVALUATED FOR THE THERAPY OF HFrEF[a]

CLASS/ Drug	HALF-LIFE (h)	STARTING DOSE (mg)	TARGET DOSE (mg)	IMPORTANT ADVERSE EFFECTS, INTERACTIONS, AND CONTRAINDICATIONS
ACE inhibitors				
Captopril	1.7	3 × 6.25	3 × 50	**Adverse effects:** Cough (~5%), ↑ serum creatinine (<25% is normal; if > 50%, possibility of renal artery stenosis), hyperkalemia, hypotension, angioedema
Enalapril	11	2 × 2.5	2 × 20	
Lisinopril	13	1 × 2.5–5	1 × 20–35	**Interactions:** Increased rate of hyperkalemia in combination with K^+-sparing diuretics, K^+ supplements, cyclosporine, NSAIDs (PD), reduced efficacy in combination with NSAIDs (PD), ↑ [Li^+] in serum (PK), ↑ hypoglycemic risk in combination with insulin or oral antidiabetics; increased effect in renal insufficiency (PK)
Ramipril	13–17	1 × 2.5	1 × 10	
Trandolapril	15–23	1 × 0.5	1 × 4	**Contraindications:** Bilateral renal artery stenosis
Angiotensin receptor blockers				
Candesartan	9	1 × 4–8	1 × 32	**Adverse effects:** Similar to ACE, but no cough
Losartan	6–9	1 × 50	1 × 150	**Interactions and contraindications:** As ACEI
Valsartan	6	2 × 40	2 × 160	

[a]Plasma half-lives partially apply to active metabolites (e.g., losartan). PD, pharmacodynamic; PK, pharmacokinetic.

threshold for arrhythmias (positive bathmotropic effect). All these acute effects are mediated by β_1 receptors and, to a smaller extent, β_2 receptors. Extracardiac effects include bronchodilation (β_2), vasodilation (β_2) as well as vasoconstriction (α_1 receptors, which dominate at higher concentrations of catecholamines), stimulation of hepatic glycogen metabolism and gluconeogenesis (β_2), and, importantly, stimulation of renin release from the macula densa (β_1). Thus, activation of the SNS coactivates the RAAS, and, as outlined previously, activation of the RAAS activates the SNS by stimulation of NE release (see Chapters 12 and 26).

The β blockers competitively reduce β receptor–mediated actions of catecholamines and thus, depending on the activation level of the SNS, reduce heart rate and force, slow relaxation, slow AV conduction, suppress arrhythmias, lower renin levels, and, depending on their selectivity for the β_1 receptor, permit more or less bronchoconstriction, vasoconstriction, and lowering of hepatic glucose production.

Why Use β Blockers in Heart Failure? In light of the above actions, the efficacy of β blockers in heart failure came as a surprise and had to overcome resistance in the medical community. How can a drug with cardiodepressant actions on heart function be beneficial in a clinical situation in which the heart is already dysfunctional and depending on catecholamines to maintain cardiac output? The first therapeutic application of β blockers at low doses was to a Swedish cohort of patients with heart failure with cardiac decompensation and heart rate greater than 120 beats/min; the goal was to reduce heart rate and cardiac energy consumption (Waagstein et al., 1975). The success of the experiment led to large clinical trials that showed an impressive 35% prolongation of life expectancy in patients treated with β blockers (Table 29–1), on top of effects of ACEIs, diuretics, and digoxin.

Key to the understanding of the success of β blockers in heart failure were two lessons. *First*, therapy must be initiated in a clinically stable condition and at very low doses (1/8 of target), and dose escalation requires time (e.g., doubling every 4 weeks in ambulatory settings; "start low, go slow"). Under these conditions, the heart has time to adapt to decreasing stimulation by catecholamines and to find a new equilibrium at a lower adrenergic drive. Importantly, β blockers do not fully block the receptors; rather, they are competitive antagonists that shift the concentration-response curve of catecholamines to the right (see Figure 3–4).

Second, although the acute effects of catecholamines can be lifesaving, that level of β adrenergic stimulation applied chronically, as the SNS does in response to heart failure, is deleterious. Positive chronotropic, inotropic, and lusitropic effects all come at the price of overproportional increase in energy consumption. This is irrelevant in situations of acute blood loss or other stresses, but critical if persistent. The heart reacts to chronic sympathetic stimulation by a heart failure–specific gene program (e.g., downregulation of β adrenergic receptor density; upregulation of inhibitory G proteins; and decreases of SR Ca^{2+}-ATPase, the fast isoform of myosin heavy chain, and repolarizing K^+ currents), changes that come at the price of decreased dynamic range and increased propensity for arrhythmias. Reversal of the heart failure gene program by β blockers (Lowes et al., 2002) likely contributes to the paradoxical increase in left ventricular EF after 3–6 months of therapy and to the reduced rate of arrhythmogenic sudden cardiac death noted in the large studies. In a simple view, β blockers protect the heart from the adverse long-term consequences

of adrenergic overstimulation, for example, increased energy consumption, fibrosis, arrhythmias, and cell death. Lower heart rates not only save energy but also improve contractile function because the failing heart, in contrast to the healthy human heart, has a negative force-frequency relation (Pieske et al., 1995). In addition, β blockers improve perfusion of the myocardium by prolonging diastole, thereby reducing ischemia.

Available Agents. Four β blockers have been successfully tested in randomized clinical trials (Table 29–1): the β_1-selective agents metoprolol (MERIT-HF Investigators, 1999) and bisoprolol (CIBIS-II Investigators, 1999) and the third-generation agents with additional actions, carvedilol and nebivolol. Carvedilol is a nonselective β blocker and an α_1 receptor antagonist. Nebivolol (Flather et al., 2005) is β_1 selective and has additional vasodilatory actions that may be NO mediated (Figure 12–4; Table 12–4). Early evidence of superiority of carvedilol over metoprolol (Poole-Wilson et al., 2003) has not been confirmed.

Pharmacokinetic Considerations. There are important pharmacokinetic differences amongst these β blockers (Table 29–3), distinctions that are relevant because successful therapy of heart failure (and most other chronic cardiovascular diseases) requires stable plasma concentrations over the entire day (trough levels before next dose application > 50% of maximum).

Metoprolol has a too short $t_{1/2}$ (3–5 h) and should be prescribed only as the zero-order prolonged-release formulation used by all successful clinical studies. Standard extended-release formulations likely do not suffice. A further disadvantage of metoprolol is its dependency on the polymorphic CYP2D6 for its metabolism. CYP2D6 "poor metabolizers," about 8% of the Caucasian population, exhibit C_{Pmax} levels of metoprolol 5-fold higher than those of standard metabolizers; in a prospective longitudinal study, that difference correlated with 2-fold differences in heart rate responses (Rau et al., 2009). Bisoprolol has a sufficiently long plasma $t_{1/2}$ (10–12 h) for once-daily dosing and is not metabolized by CYP2D6. Carvedilol has a shorter $t_{1/2}$ (6–10 h) and requires twice-daily dosing. An advantageous peculiarity of carvedilol is that it dissociates only slowly from β receptors and therefore acts longer than its plasma $t_{1/2}$ suggests. Carvedilol metabolism depends on CYP2D6, but less so than metoprolol. Nebivolol plasma concentrations are 10- to 15-fold higher in CYP2D6 poor metabolizers, but this is without clinical consequence, likely because the first metabolite is similarly active as the parent compound. Nebivolol is not approved in the U.S. for the treatment of heart failure, but it is approved in 71 countries worldwide, including Europe (patients > 70 years of age).

Clinical Use. All patients with symptomatic heart failure (stage C, NYHA II–IV) and all patients with left ventricular dysfunction (stage B, NYHA I) after myocardial infarction should be treated with a β blocker. The therapy with β blockers should be initiated only in clinically stable patients at very low doses, generally 1/8 of the final target dose, and titrated upward every 4 weeks. Even when initiated properly, a tendency to retain fluid exists that may require diuretic dose adjustment. The improvement of left ventricular function generally takes 3–6 months, and in this period, patients should be carefully monitored.

The β blockers should not be administered in new-onset or acutely decompensated heart failure. If patients are hospitalized with acute decompensation under current therapy with β blockers, doses often have to be

TABLE 29–3 ■ PROPERTIES AND THERAPEUTIC DOSES OF β BLOCKERS APPROVED AS THERAPY OF HFrEF

β BLOCKER	β₁ SELECTIVE	VASODILATION	HALF-LIFE (h)	START DOSE (mg)	TARGET DOSE (mg)	METABOLISM BY CYPs[a]
Bisoprolol	Yes	No	10–12	1 × 1.25	1 × 10	None
Carvedilol	No	Yes	6–10	2 × 3.125	2 × 25	CYP2D6
Metoprolol succinate[a]	Yes	No	>12[b]	1 × 12.5[a]	1 × 200	CYP2D6
Nebivolol	Yes	Yes	10	1 × 1.25	1 × 10	CYP2D6

[a]CYP2D6 indicates dependence on polymorphic CYP2D6 metabolism, likely less relevant for nebivolol because the first metabolite is active.
[b]Clinical studies in heart failure have mainly used metoprolol succinate in a slow-release formulation (zero order of kinetics); metoprolol, itself, has a $t_{1/2}$ of 3–5 h.

reduced or the drug discontinued until clinical stabilization, after which therapy should again be initiated.

Precautions. Formally, β blockers have long lists of adverse drug responses and contraindications. Practically, however, they are generally well tolerated if properly initiated. If doses are increased too rapidly, fall of blood pressure, fluid retention, and dizziness are common and require dose reduction.

The major cardiovascular responses associated with use of β blockers are the following:

- *Heart rate lowering,* a desirable effect that indicates proper dosing (no decrease indicates insufficient dosing). A reasonable target resting heart rate is 60–70/min.
- *AV block* (beware preexisting conduction disturbance; consider pacemaker implantation).
- *Bronchoconstriction.* Allergic asthma is a contraindication for all β blocker use; however, chronic obstructive lung disease is not, because the $β_2$ receptor–dependent dynamic range is low in these patients, and studies have documented safety. Nonetheless, only $β_1$-selective compounds should be used in patients with chronic obstructive pulmonary disease.
- *Peripheral vasoconstriction (cold extremities).* Initial vasoconstriction turns into vasodilation under chronic therapy with β blockers. Cold extremities are generally not a problem in patients with heart failure. Yet, patients with peripheral artery disease or symptoms of claudication or Raynaud disease should be carefully monitored and treated with carvedilol if a β blocker is employed.

Mineralocorticoid Receptor Antagonists

The third group of drugs with a documented life-prolonging effect in patients with heart failure is MRAs. They should be given in low doses to all patients in stage C (NYHA class II–IV), that is, with symptomatic HFrEF, despite the fact that the combination of ACEIs/ARBs, and MRA is formally contraindicated due to the risk of hyperkalemia. The safety of a low-dose MRA (25 mg vs. a standard of 100 mg spironolactone) was demonstrated in a large randomized trial in a patient cohort with severe heart failure (NYHA III–IV), with the MRA added to ACEIs, diuretics, and digoxin (Pitt, 2004). Later studies with eplerenone in less-severe heart failure essentially confirmed the efficacy of this class of drugs.

Mechanism of Action. The MRAs act as antagonists of nuclear receptors of aldosterone (Figure 25-6). They are K^+-sparing diuretics (see discussion that follows) but gained more importance in the treatment of heart failure for their additional efficacy in suppressing the consequences of neurohumoral activation. Aldosterone, as the second major actor of the RAAS, promotes Na^+ and fluid retention, loss of K^+ and Mg^{2+}, sympathetic activation, parasympathetic inhibition, myocardial and vascular fibrosis, baroreceptor dysfunction, and vascular damage, all adverse effects in the setting of heart failure. Aldosterone plasma levels decrease under therapy with ACEIs or ARBs, but quickly increase again, a phenomenon called *aldosterone escape.* It is likely explained by incomplete blockade of the RAAS (e.g., AngI can be converted to AngII by chymase, in addition to ACE; see Figure 26–1) and by the fact that aldosterone secretion is regulated not only by AngII but also by sodium and potassium plasma Na^+ and K^+. MRAs inhibit all the effects of aldosterone, of which the reduction in fibrosis is most pronounced in animal models.

Clinical Use; Adverse Responses. Currently, two MRAs are available, spironolactone and eplerenone. Only eplerenone is FDA-approved for the therapy of heart failure because no economic interest exists for the approval of spironolactone, which is free of patent protection. Nevertheless, guidelines recommend both. Spironolactone is a nonspecific steroid hormone receptor antagonist with similar affinity for progesterone and androgen receptors; it causes gynecomastia (painful breast swelling, 10% of patients) in men and dysmenorrhea in women. Eplerenone is selective for the mineralocorticoid receptor and therefore does not cause gynecomastia.

The most important ADR of both MRAs is hyperkalemia. Under the well-controlled conditions of clinical trials, serious hyperkalemia (>5.5 mmol/L) occurred in 12% in the eplerenone group and in 7% in

the placebo group (Zannad et al., 2011). Rates may be higher in clinical practice when risk conditions, comedication, and dose restrictions are not well controlled (Juurlink et al., 2004). Guidelines for the use of MRAs in patients with heart failure are:

- Administer no more than 50 mg/d.
- Do not use if the GFR is less than 30 mL/min (creatinine ~ 2 mg/dL).
- Be careful with elderly patients, in whom improvement in prognosis may be less relevant than prevention of serious side effects.
- Be careful with diabetics, who carry a higher risk of hyperkalemia.
- Do not combine with NSAIDs, which are contraindicated in heart failure but are frequently prescribed for chronic degenerative diseases of the musculoskeletal system.
- Do not combine with other K^+-sparing diuretics.

Angiotensin Receptor and Neprilysin Inhibitors

The latest addition to standard combination therapy of heart failure is sacubitril/valsartan. It is made by cocrystallizing the well-known ARB valsartan with sacubritril, a prodrug that, after deesterization, inhibits neprilysin, a peptidase mediating the enzymatic degradation and inactivation of natriuretic peptides (ANP, BNP, CNP), bradykinin, and substance P. Thus, the drug combines inhibition of the RAAS with activation of a beneficial axis of neurohumoral activation, the natriuretic peptides. Consequently, the ARNI is expected to promote the beneficial effects natriuresis, diuresis, and vasodilation of arterial and venous blood vessels and to inhibit thrombosis, fibrosis, cardiac myocyte hypertrophy, and renin release. Augmentation of ANP/BNP levels by inhibiting degradation is probably a better pharmacological principle than giving the agonist BNP (neseritide; see under acute heart failure) directly because it enhances *endogenous* regulation of plasma and tissue levels. Sacubitril/valsartan causes smaller increases in bradykinin and substance P than omapatrilat, an earlier drug combining a neprilysin inhibitor and an ACEI. This difference may explain why sacubitril/valsartan is not associated with an increased rate of angioedema, the adverse effect that stopped the development of omapatrilat. A large head-to-head comparison study in patients with stable heart failure showed superiority of sacubitril/valsartan over enalapril (McMurray et al., 2014).

Treatment Principle II: Preload Reduction

Fluid overload with increased filling pressures (increased preload) and dilation of the ventricles in heart failure is the consequence of decreased kidney perfusion and activation of the RAAS. Normally, increased preload and stretch of the myofilaments increase contractile force in an autoregulatory manner, the positive force-length relationship or Frank-Starling mechanism. However, the failing heart in congestion operates at the flat portion of this relationship (Figure 29–4) and cannot generate sufficient force with increasing preload, leading to edema in the lungs and the periphery.

Diuretics increase Na^+ and water excretion by inhibiting transporters in the kidney and thereby improve symptoms of CHF by moving patients to lower cardiac filling pressures along the same ventricular function curve. Diuretics are an integral part of the combination therapy of symptomatic forms of heart failure. Prognostic efficacy of diuretics in heart failure will remain an academic question, simply because randomization for a trial of diuretics would be ethically impermissible. Diuretics should *not* be given to patients without congestion because they activate the RAAS and may accelerate a vicious downward spiral. On the other hand, in severe heart failure, diuretic resistance may occur for various reasons and cause clinical deterioration (Table 29–4).

Loop Diuretics

Loop diuretics (furosemide, torasemide, bumetanide; Table 29–5) inhibit the Na^+-K^+-2Cl symporter in the ascending limb of the loop of Henle, where up to 15% of the primary filtrate (~150 L/d) is reabsorbed, explaining their strong diuretic action. The increase in Na^+ and fluid delivery to distal nephron segments has two consequences:

- It is sensed in the macula densa and normally activates tubuloglomerular feedback to decrease GFR. This autoregulation explains the quick

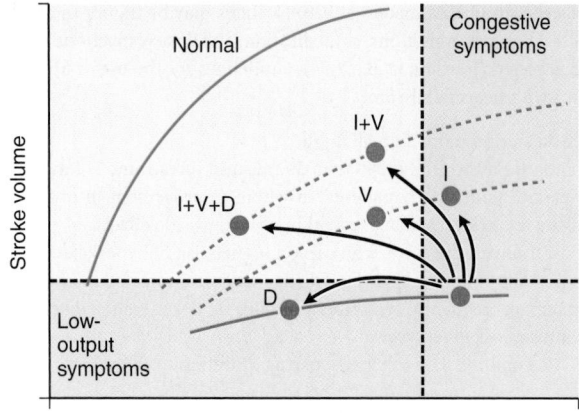

Figure 29–4 *Hemodynamic responses to pharmacologic interventions in heart failure.* The relationships between diastolic filling pressure (preload) and stroke volume (ventricular performance) are illustrated for a normal heart (green line; the Frank-Starling relationship) and for a patient with heart failure with systolic dysfunction (red line). Note that positive inotropic agents (I), such as CGs or dobutamine, move patients to a higher ventricular function curve (lower dashed line), resulting in greater cardiac work for a given level of ventricular filling pressure. Vasodilators (V), such as ACEIs or nitroprusside, also move patients to improved ventricular function curves while reducing cardiac filling pressures. Diuretics (D) improve symptoms of CHF by moving patients to lower cardiac filling pressures along the same ventricular function curve.

loss of efficacy of older diuretics of the carbonic anhydrase inhibitor class (e.g., acetazolamide), acting in the proximal tubule. Thiazides (see discussion that follows) are derived from this class and cause a small decrease in the GFR. Loop diuretics inhibit the feedback mechanism because it is mediated by the Na^+-K^+-$2Cl^-$ symporter; they exhibit stable action and do not affect the GFR.

- It leads to increased ENaC-mediated reabsorption of Na^+ and, in exchange, to more K^+ excretion in the distal tubule, explaining the main side effect, hypokalemia.

The bioavailability of orally administered furosemide ranges from 40% to 70%. High drug doses are often required to initiate diuresis in patients with worsening symptoms or in those with impaired GI absorption, as may occur in severely hypervolemic patients with CHF-induced GI edema. Oral bioavailabilities of bumetanide and torasemide are greater than 80%, and as a result, these agents are more consistently absorbed than furosemide. Furosemide and bumetanide are short-acting drugs.

TABLE 29–4 ■ CAUSES OF DIURETIC RESISTANCE IN HEART FAILURE

Noncompliance with medical regimen; excess dietary Na^+ intake
Decreased renal perfusion and glomerular filtration rate due to
Excessive vascular volume depletion and hypotension due to aggressive diuretic or vasodilator therapy
Decline in cardiac output due to worsening heart failure, arrhythmias, or other primary cardiac causes
Selective reduction in glomerular perfusion pressure following initiation (or dose increase) of ACEI therapy
Nonsteroidal anti-inflammatory drugs
Primary renal pathology (e.g., cholesterol emboli, renal artery stenosis, drug-induced interstitial nephritis, obstructive uropathy)
Reduced or impaired diuretic absorption due to gut wall edema and reduced splanchnic blood flow

The $t_{1/2}$ of furosemide in normal kidney function is about 1 h (increases in terminal kidney failure to > 24 h), and rebound Na^+ retention normally requires dosing twice a day or more. Bumetanide reaches maximal plasma concentrations in 0.5–2 h and has a $t_{1/2}$ of 1–1.5 h. Torasemide has a slower onset of action (maximal effect 1–2 h after ingestion) and a plasma $t_{1/2}$ of 3–4 h. Kidney failure does not critically affect the elimination of bumetanide or torasemide.

Thiazide Diuretics

Thiazide diuretics (hydrochlorothiazide, chlorthalidone; Table 29–5) have a limited role in heart failure for their low maximal diuretic effect and loss of efficacy at a GFR below 30 mL/min. However, combination therapy with loop diuretics is often effective in those refractory to loop diuretics alone, as refractoriness is often caused by upregulation of the Na^+-Cl^- cotransporter in the distal convoluted tubule, the main target of thiazide diuretics (see Chapter 25). Thiazides are associated with a greater degree of K^+ wasting per fluid volume reduction than loop diuretics, and combination therapy requires careful monitoring of K^+ loss.

K⁺-Sparing Diuretics

K^+-Sparing diuretics (see Chapter 25) inhibit apical Na^+ channels in distal segments of the tubulus directly (ENaC; e.g., amiloride, triamterene) or reduce its gene expression (MRAs spironolactone and eplerenone). These agents are weak diuretics, but they are often used in the treatment of hypertension in combination with thiazides or loop diuretics to reduce K^+ and Mg^{2+} wasting. The prognostic efficacy of MRAs, which is at least partially independent of its K^+-sparing activity, make amiloride and triamteren largely dispensable in the therapy of heart failure. They should not be combined with ACEIs and MRAs.

Treatment Principle III: Afterload Reduction

The failing heart is exquisitely sensitive to increased arterial resistance (i.e., afterload) (Figure 29–5). Vasodilators, therefore, should have beneficial effects on patients with heart failure by reducing afterload and allowing the heart to expel blood against lower resistance. However, clinical trials with pure vasodilators were mainly disappointing, whereas inhibitors of the RAAS, vasodilators with a broader mode of action, were successful. Likely reasons include reflex tachycardia and tachyphylaxis (prazosin, ISDN) and negative inotropic effects (dihydropyridine calcium channel antagonists).

Hydralazine–Isosorbide Dinitrate

A remarkable exception is the therapeutic effect of a fixed combination of hydralazine and ISDN. In a pioneering trial, Cohn and colleagues showed moderate efficacy of this combination in patients with heart failure (Cohn et al., 1986). The benefit was restricted to improvement in the cohort of African Americans. In a second trial in African Americans only, the combination conferred a 43% survival benefit (Taylor et al., 2004). It was FDA-approved in 2006, the first ethnically restricted approval.

As an orally available organic nitrate, ISDN, similar to GTN and ISMN, preferentially dilates large blood vessels, for instance, venous capacitance and arterial conductance vessels (Chapter 27). The main effect is "venous pooling" and reduction of diastolic filling pressure (preload) with little effect on systemic vascular resistance (which is regulated by small-to-medium arterioles). Sustained monotherapy is compromised by nitrate tolerance (i.e., loss of effect and induction of a pro-constrictory state with high levels of ROS). Hydralazine is a direct vasodilator whose mechanism of action remains unresolved (Chapter 28). It was suggested that hydralazine prevents nitrate tolerance by reducing ROS-mediated inactivation of NO (Munzel et al., 2005), an action that could explain the efficacy of this drug combination in heart failure amongst African Americans. A test of this hypothesis in patients with NYHA class II–III heart failure (Chirkov et al., 2010) failed to confirm the hypothesis. The relevant differences in responsiveness between African American and Caucasian patients with heart failure have not been explained.

The fixed-combination formulation in use contains 37.5 mg hydralazine and 20 mg ISDN and is uptitrated to a target dose of 2 tablets, thrice

TABLE 29–5 ■ PROPERTIES AND THERAPEUTIC DOSES OF DIURETICS FOR THE THERAPY OF HFrEJ[a]

DIURETIC	START DOSE (mg)	COMMON DAILY DOSE (mg)	TIME TO START OF EFFECT (h)	HALF-LIFE (h)	ADVERSE EFFECTS AND INTERACTIONS
Loop diuretics					
Bumetanide	0.5–1	1–5	0.5	1–1.5	**Adverse effects**: Hypokalemia, hyponatremia, hypomagnesemia, hyperuricemia, hypocalcemia (loop diuretics, hypercalcemia (thiazides), glucose intolerance
					Interactions: ↑[Li+] in serum (PK) and cardiac glycoside toxicity (PD, hypokalemia), anion exchanger resins (PK), non-steroidal anti-inflammatory drugs (NSAID), and glucocorticoids (PD) can ↓ effect of diuretics.
Furosemide	20–40	40–240	0.5	1	
Torasemide	5–10	10–20	1	3–4	
Thiazides					
Chlorthalidone	50	50–100	2	50	
Hydrochlorothiazide	25	12.5–100	1–2	6–8	
Potassium-sparing diuretics					
Eplerenone, spironolactone	50[b]	100–200[b]	2–6	24–36	**Adverse effects**: Hyperkalemia (all), gynecomasty, erectile dysfunction, and menstrual bleeding disorders (spironolactone)
Amiloride	5[b]	10–20[b]	2	10–24	**Interactions**: ↑ Risk of hyperkalemia when given with ACE or ARB (use 50% lower dose), also with cyclosporine and NSAIDs
Triamterene	50[b]	200[b]	2	8–16	**Contraindication**: Renal insufficiency with creatinine clearance < 30 mL/min

[a]Dosing recommendations were adapted from ESC guidelines (Ponikowski et al., 2016). [b]50% dose reduction when co-administered with RAS blocker.

daily. Patients will also generally be taking a β blocker. Hypotension may be dose limiting. Frequent adverse effects include dizziness and headache. Adherence to the thrice-daily dosing regimen may impose practical problems (Cohn et al., 1986), and hydralazine doses greater than 200 mg have been associated with lupus erythematosus.

Treatment Principle IV: Increasing Cardiac Contractility

The failing heart is unable to generate force sufficient to meet the needs of the body for perfusion of oxygenated blood (Figure 29-1). Historically, physicians attempted to stimulate force generation with positive inotropic drugs. Unfortunately, when used chronically, these agents do not improve life expectancy or cardiac performance. Rather, chronic use of positive inotropes is associated with excess mortality. Of the available inotropic agents, only CGs are used in the treatment of chronic heart failure; this is for two reasons: history and one large trial in patients with NYHA class II–III heart failure showing that digoxin reduced the rate of heart failure–associated hospitalizations without increasing mortality (Table 29–1).

Inotropic Agents and the Regulation of Cardiac Contractility

Cardiac myocytes contract and develop force in response to membrane depolarization and subsequent increases in intracellular Ca^{2+} concentrations (Figure 29-6). The mechanisms of this *excitation-contraction coupling* are the basis for understanding the mode of action of positive inotropic drugs and cardiac myocyte function in general. Most currently employed positive inotropes and novel compounds in development act by increasing the concentration of free intracellular Ca^{2+} ($[Ca^{2+}]_i$). Ca^{2+} "sensitizers" (e.g., levosimendan) sensitize myofilaments to Ca^{2+}; that is, they shift the sigmoidal relationship between free Ca^{2+} concentration and force to the left.

Na+/K+ ATPase Inhibitors. Cardiac glycosides inhibit the plasma membrane Na^+/K^+ ATPase, a key enzyme that actively pumps Na^+ out and K^+ into the cell and thereby maintains the steep concentration gradients of Na^+ and K^+ across the plasma membrane. Inhibition of this enzyme slightly reduces the Na^+ gradient across the myocyte membrane, reducing the driving force for Ca^{2+} extrusion by the NCX, thereby providing more Ca^{2+} for storage in the SR and subsequent release to activate contraction. The details are explained by Figure 29–6 and its legend.

cAMP-Dependent Inotropes. The strongest stimulation of the heart is achieved by receptor-mediated stimulation of adenylyl cyclase. This explains the use of dobutamine, EPI, and NE in cardiogenic shock (see discussion that follows). Inhibition of cAMP degradation by PDE inhibitors such as milrinone or enoximone elevates cellular cAMP concentrations and activates the cAMP-PKA pathway and other cAMP-responsive systems (see Chapter 3). This concerted action results in higher peak Ca^{2+} concentrations in systole and thereby peak force (Figure 29–6). All cAMP-dependent inotropes hasten contraction (positive clinotropic effect) and relaxation (positive lusitropic effect), allowing sufficient perfusion of the ventricles in diastole under catecholamine stimulation and with the concomitant tachycardia. On the downside, acceleration of contraction during catecholamine stimulation, by promoting net Ca^{2+} entry per unit of time, increases the utilization of ATP for Ca^{2+} reuptake into the SR via the SERCA and to restore the membrane potential by the activity of the Na^+/K^+ ATPase.

Myofilament Ca^{2+} Sensitizers. Calcium sensitizers increase the affinity of the myofilaments for Ca^{2+}, for example, by inducing a conformational change in TnC. They enhance force for a given $[Ca^{2+}]_i$ and do not elevate $[Ca^{2+}]_i$ with its potentially deleterious pro-arrhythmic and energy-increasing consequences. But, increased myofilament Ca^{2+} sensitivity also causes reduced dissociation of Ca^{2+} from the myofilaments in

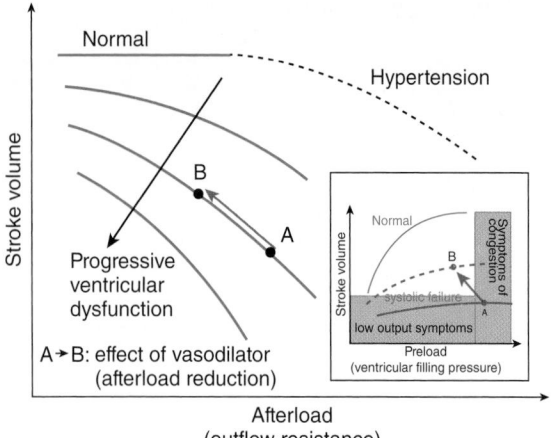

Figure 29–5 *Stroke volume versus afterload (outflow resistance): effects of heart failure. Increasing the resistance to ventricular outflow, a basic determinant of afterload, has little effect on stroke volume in normal hearts until high levels of outflow resistance (top curve).* However, in patients with systolic ventricular dysfunction (lower curves), an increase in outflow resistance elicits a noticeable decrease in cardiac performance (= stroke volume) that is progressive with increasing failure. Such an increase in outflow resistance can occur as a compensatory response by the SNS and RAAS to decreased cardiac function and depressed arterial pressure as a result of heart failure. A higher resistance to ventricular outflow increases peak pressure development in the left ventricle in opening the aortic valve, thereby increasing ventricular wall stress and end-systolic volume. This can cause end-diastolic volume to increase. In the normal heart, increasing ventricular stretch enhances cardiac contractile performance (stroke volume); this is the Frank-Starling effect (inset). However, in the failing heart, the positive contractile response embodied in the Frank-Starling effect is poor and provides only a small increase in stroke volume. Reducing outflow resistance with agents that reduce systemic vascular resistance, such as arterial vasodilators, can shift cardiac performance to a larger stroke volume in patients with myocardial dysfunction (from A to B). Such an increase in stroke volume may provide sufficient output and compensate for the decrease in systemic vascular resistance and moderate the fall in systemic arterial pressure due to the vasodilator. For details, see Figure 29–4 and the work of Klabunde (2015).

diastole and prolongation of relaxation ("negative lusitropic effect"). This effect can aggravate the already-compromised diastolic function in heart failure. It could also lead to delayed Ca^{2+} release from myofilaments in diastole and arrhythmias (Schober et al., 2012). Calcium sensitizers failed to improve prognosis in clinical trials of patients with chronic heart failure. However, levosimendan is approved in some countries for the treatment of acute heart failure. It has additional selective and potent inhibitory effects on PDE III, whose positive lusitropic consequence appears to antagonize the negative lusitropic effect of Ca^{2+} sensitization. Agonists of G_q-coupled receptors (α_1, AT_1, ET_A) also increase myofilament Ca^{2+} sensitivity, likely due to increased myosin light chain phosphorylation. The positive inotropic effect is smaller than that of β receptor stimulation, develops more slowly, and is independent of cAMP.

Cardiac Glycosides

Actions and Therapeutic Use of Digoxin. *Positive Inotropic Effect.*
CGs at therapeutic concentrations mildly inhibit the cardiac Na^+/K^+ ATPase, causing an increase in intracellular $[Na^+]$. Increased $[Na^+]_i$ inhibits Ca^{2+} extrusion via the NCX resulting in higher intracellular $[Ca^{2+}]$ and enhanced contractility (Figure 29–6). The increased contractility and hence cardiac output provides symptomatic relief in patients with heart failure (Figure 29–1). With the main trigger for neurohumoral activation removed, sympathetic nerve tone and, consequently, heart rate and peripheral vascular resistance drop. These decreases in preload and afterload reduce chamber dilation and thereby wall stress, a strong determinant of myocardial O_2 consumption. Increased renal perfusion lowers renin production and increases diuresis, further decreasing preload.

HISTORICAL PERSPECTIVE

The British botanist William Withering (1741–1799) systematically described the actions of *Digitalis purpurea* in patients with heart failure ("dropsy") and gave exact dosing recommendations (Skou 1986). Oswald Schmiedeberg (1833–1921), working in Strasbourg, France, isolated the first chemical entities from foxglove leaves; one of these entities was digitoxin. Until diuretics became available, CGs were the only heart failure drugs. CGs encompass many chemical entities, but only digoxin, its derivatives β-acetyl digoxin, methyldigoxin, and digitoxin are in clinical use in most countries. Until the 1980s, CGs were dosed according to therapeutic effects (e.g., improved diuresis [Withering considered CGs as diuretics], reduction of heart size [verifiable by X-ray], or alterations of the surface ECG) and to symptoms of overdosing, such as nausea and altered color perception (yellow-green). Now, serum digoxin concentrations can be measured by radioimmunoassay. Digoxin has therapeutic efficacy (including a small survival benefit) only at serum concentrations between 0.5 and 0.8 ng/mL (Rathore et al., 2003). Concentrations greater than 1.2 ng/mL are associated with increased mortality. Serum digoxin concentrations greater than 0.8 ng/mL should be avoided.

Electrophysiological Actions. CGs at therapeutic concentrations shorten action potentials by accelerating the inactivation of L-type Ca^{2+} channels due to higher $[Ca^{2+}]_i$. Shorter action potentials (= refractory period) favor reentry arrhythmias, a reason that CGs promote atrial fibrillation. With the loss of intracellular K^+ and increase in intracellular Na^+, the resting membrane potential (determined largely by the K^+ current, now diminished) moves to less-negative values with two consequences. Diastolic depolarization and automaticity are enhanced, and, due to partial inactivation of Na^+ channels, impulse propagation is strongly reduced. Both phenomena promote reentry arrhythmias. At even higher CG concentrations, SR Ca^{2+} overload reaches a point at which Ca^{2+} is spontaneously released at amounts large enough to initiate Ca^{2+} waves and, via the NCX, depolarization of the cell (Figure 29–6). The typical ECG signs at this stage of CG intoxication are extrasystoles and bigeminies with a high risk of ventricular fibrillation.

Extracardiac Effects. CGs also inhibit Na^+/K^+ ATPase in other excitable tissues. (1) At low plasma concentrations, CGs stimulate vagal efferents and sensitize baroreceptor reflex mechanisms, causing increased parasympathetic and decreased sympathetic tone. The beneficial effect of digoxin at low plasma concentrations (Rathore et al., 2003), at which positive inotropic effects are minor, suggests that the neurohumoral actions of CGs may be therapeutically more relevant than the direct positive inotropic effects. (2) CGs at higher plasma concentrations increase Ca^{2+} concentrations in vascular smooth muscle cells and cause vasoconstriction. In patients with heart failure, vasodilation normally prevails due to the decrease in sympathetic nervous tone, but the direct vascular effect explains mesenteric artery ischemia or occlusion, a rare but severe adverse effect of CGs.

Indirect Actions. The vagotonic and sympatholytic effects of CGs cause bradycardia and AV prolongation (negative dromotropic effect) and can promote atrial flutter and fibrillation. Fibrillation is explained by the ACh-induced shortening of atrial action potentials, which is further enhanced by the direct CG effect described previously. On the other hand, CGs are therapeutically used for frequency control of permanent atrial fibrillation because of their negative dromotropic effects.

Interactions With K^+, Ca^{2+}, and Mg^{2+}. Hyperkalemia reduces and hypokalemia increases the binding affinity of CG to the Na^+/K^+ ATPase. In addition, hypokalemia reduces repolarizing K^+ currents, with the consequence of increased spontaneous diastolic depolarization and automaticity. Hypokalemia is therefore a major risk factor for arrhythmogenic effects of CGs. Hypercalcemia as well as hypomagnesemia favor SR Ca^{2+} overload and spontaneous Ca^{2+} release events. Control of serum electrolytes is therefore mandatory.

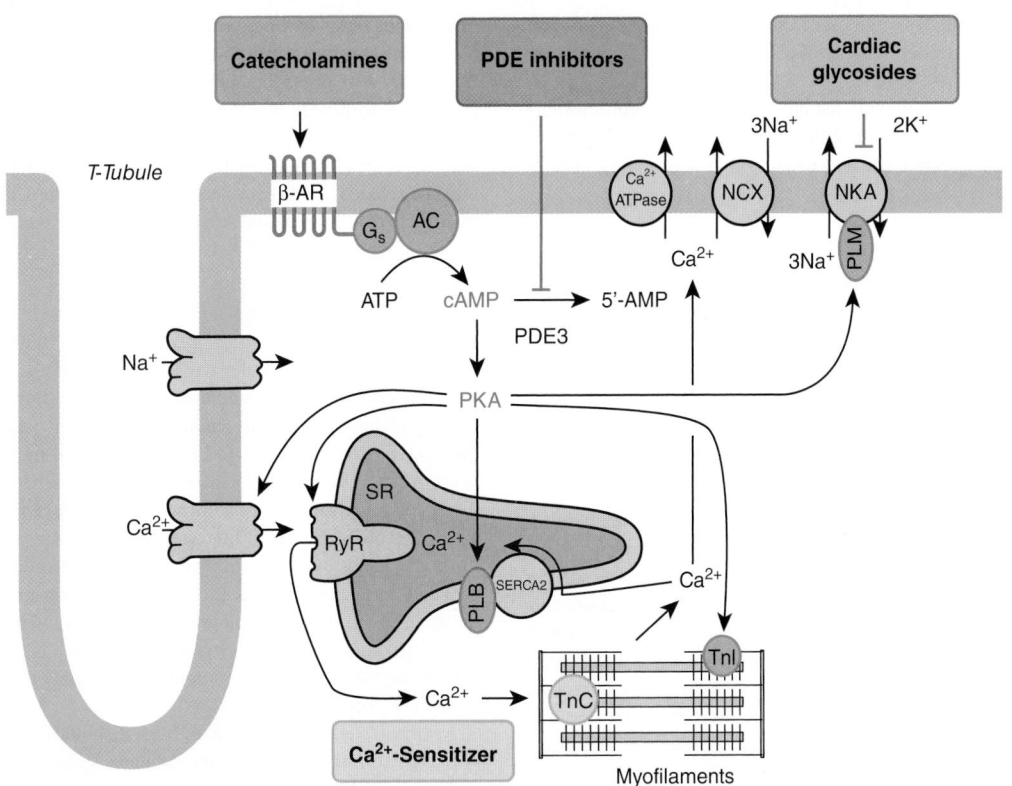

Figure 29–6 *Cardiac excitation-contraction coupling and its regulation by positive inotropic drugs.* The cardiac cycle is initiated by membrane depolarization, which causes the opening of voltage-dependent Na⁺ and L-type Ca²⁺ channels, permitting Na⁺ and Ca²⁺ flow down their electrochemical gradients into the myocyte. Thus, Na⁺ and Ca²⁺ enter the cardiac myocyte during each cycle of membrane depolarization, triggering the release, through the RyR, of larger amounts of Ca²⁺ from internal stores in the SR. The resulting increase in intracellular Ca²⁺ interacts with troponin C and activates interactions between actin and myosin that result in sarcomere shortening. The electrochemical gradient for Na⁺ across the sarcolemma is maintained by active transport of Na⁺ out of the cell by the sarcolemmal Na⁺/K⁺ ATPase (NKA). The bulk of cytosolic Ca²⁺ (70%) is pumped back into the SR by a Ca²⁺-ATPase, SERCA2. The remainder is removed from the cell by either a sarcolemmal Ca²⁺-ATPase or a high-capacity NCX. The NCX exchanges three Na⁺ for a Ca²⁺, using the electrochemical potential of Na⁺ to drive Ca²⁺ extrusion. The β adrenergic agonists (acting at βAR, the β adrenergic receptor) and PDE inhibitors, by increasing intracellular cAMP levels, activate PKA, which phosphorylates PLB in the SR, the α subunit of the L-type Ca²⁺ channel, and regulatory components of the RyR, as well as TnI. As a result, the probabilities of opening of the L-type Ca²⁺ channel and the RyR2 Ca²⁺ channel are increased; SERCA2 inhibition by PLB is released, with the result that SERCA2 accumulates Ca²⁺ into the SR faster, more avidly, and to a higher concentration; and relaxation occurs at slightly higher [Ca²⁺]ᵢ due to slightly reduced sensitivity of the troponin complex to Ca²⁺. The net effect of these phosphorylations is a positive inotropic effect: a faster rate of tension development to a higher level of tension, followed by a faster rate of relaxation. CGs, by inhibiting the Na⁺/K⁺ ATPase, reduce Na⁺ extrusion from the cell, thereby permitting [Na⁺]ᵢₙ to rise, reducing the inward gradient for Na⁺ that drives Ca²⁺ extrusion by NCX. As a consequence, Ca²⁺ accumulates in the SR, and a positive inotropic effect follows, as noted previously for the effect of increased cellular cAMP. See the text for details of additional effects of CGs. Note that, under steady-state conditions, the amount of Ca²⁺ leaving the cell exactly matches the amount entering it. As NCX exchanges three Na⁺ for every Ca²⁺, it creates a depolarizing current. This makes not only the direction of transport dependent on the chemical gradients of Na⁺ and Ca²⁺ across the membrane but also the membrane potential. Thus, the direction of Na⁺-Ca²⁺ exchange may briefly reverse during depolarization, when the electrical gradient across the sarcolemma is transiently reversed. PLM is an tonic inhibitor of the Na⁺/K⁺ ATPase, which supplies the driving force (an appropriately low [Na⁺]ᵢₙ) for maintaining low diastolic Ca²⁺. Phosphorylation of PLM by PKA removes this inhibitory influence, thereby stimulating the activity of the Na⁺/K⁺ ATPase and limiting [Na⁺]ᵢₙ and [Ca²⁺]ᵢₙ. This may reduce the tendency toward arrhythmias during adrenergic stimulation (see Pavlovic et al., 2013).

Adverse Effects. The therapeutic index of CG is extremely narrow, about 2, as documented in the DIG trial: plasma concentrations between 0.5 and 0.8 ng/mL are associated with beneficial effects, and concentrations of 1.2 ng/mL and greater are associated with a tendency toward increased mortality (Rathore et al., 2003). The most frequent and most serious adverse effects are arrhythmias. In CG overdosing, patients exhibit arrhythmias (90%), GI symptoms (~55%), and neurotoxic symptoms (~12%). The most frequent causes of toxicity are renal insufficiency and overdosing.

Cardiac toxicity in healthy persons presents as extreme bradycardia, atrial fibrillation, and AV block, whereas ventricular arrhythmias are rare. In patients with structural heart disease, frequent signs of CG toxicity are ventricular extrasystoles, bigeminy, ventricular tachycardia, and fibrillation. In principle, however, every type of arrhythmia can be CG induced. GI adverse effects are anorexia, nausea, and vomiting, mainly as a result of CG effects on chemosensors in the area postrema. Spastic contraction of the mesenteric artery can rarely lead to severe diarrhea and life-threatening necrosis of the intestine. Headache, fatigue, and sleeplessness can be early symptoms of CG toxicity.

Typical, albeit not too common (10%), are visual effects: altered color perception and coronas (halos). Some have speculated that the visual effects of digitalis intoxication contributed to the qualities of late paintings by Vincent van Gogh, who may have been treated for neurological complaints with foxglove by Dr. Paul Gachet, whose portraits by van Gogh (painted in June 1890) show the doctor seated next to a sprig of the plant, a natural source of CGs and used widely in the 19th century (Lee, 1981).

Therapy of CG Toxicity. Cessation of CG medication normally suffices as therapy of CG toxicity. However, severe arrhythmias, such as extreme bradycardia or complex ventricular arrhythmias, require active therapy.

• Extreme sinus bradycardia, sinoatrial block, or AV block grade II or III: Atropine (0.5–1 mg) IV. If not successful, a temporary pacemaker may be necessary.

- Tachycardic ventricular arrhythmias and hypokalemia: K⁺ infusion (40–60 mmol/d). Consider that high K+ can aggravate AV conduction defects.
- An effective antidote for digoxin toxicity is antidigoxin immunotherapy. Purified Fab fragments from ovine antidigoxin antisera (Digibind) are usually dosed by the estimated total dose of digoxin ingested to achieve a fully neutralizing effect.

Treatment Principle V: Heart Rate Reduction

Heart rate is a strong determinant of cardiac energy consumption, and higher heart rates in patients with heart failure are associated with poor prognosis (Bohm et al., 2010). Partial agonists at β receptors such as xamoterol increase nocturnal heart rate (i.e., they prevent the physiological dip) and are associated with excess mortality in patients with heart failure (Xamoterol Study Group, 1990). Conversely, β blockers lower heart rate and improve survival prognosis.

Ivabradine

The circumstantial evidence for beneficial effects of heart rate lowering led to the development of ivabradine, a selective inhibitor of cardiac pacemaker channels (HCNs). The compound is approved in Europe for the treatment of heart failure and stable angina pectoris in patients not tolerating β blockers or in whom β blockers did not sufficiently lower heart rate (<75/min). Approval was based on a study showing a decrease in hospitalization and heart failure mortality, but not total or cardiovascular mortality (Swedberg et al., 2010). Of note, the effect of ivabradine was not superior to that of digoxin in an earlier study (Digitalis Investigation Group, 1997). In a recent large study in patients with stable angina (85% on β blockers), ivabradine conferred no benefit but led to phosphenes (typical transient enhanced brightness in a restricted area of the visual field) and increased the rate of bradycardia, atrial fibrillation, and QT prolongation (Fox et al., 2014), casting doubts about the role of the compound in ischemic heart disease. Ivabradine is not approved in the U.S.

Drug Treatment of Acutely Decompensated Heart Failure

Acutely decompensated heart failure is a leading cause of hospitalization in patients older than 65 and represents a sentinel prognostic event in the natural course of the disease, with a high recurrence rate and a 1-year mortality rate of about 30%. Even in decompensated heart failure, about 50% of patients exhibit preserved left ventricular function (HFpEF). The HFpEF cohort is older, more likely to be female and hypertensive, and with less coronary artery disease than the HFrEF cohort. Therapeutically, it is important to quickly identify and treat specific reasons for decompensation. These include, besides acute myocardial ischemia, uncorrected high blood pressure, atrial fibrillation and other arrhythmias, pulmonary embolism, and kidney failure, as well as several pharmacological reasons: nonadherence to heart failure medication and Na⁺/fluid restriction, negative inotropic drugs (e.g., verapamil, diltiazem, nifedipine, β blockers), and NSAIDs and COX-2 inhibitors.

The therapy of acutely decompensated heart failure aims at fast symptom relief, short-term survival, fast recompensation, and reduction of readmission rates. It is less evidence-based than the therapy of chronic heart failure, and no single drug given to patients experiencing acute decompensation has yet been shown to improve the long-term prognosis. The main principles (besides nonpharmacological treatment modalities such as O₂ and noninvasive or [rarely] invasive ventilatory support) are diuretics and vasodilators, with positive inotropes in selected cases and mechanical support systems as an ultimate step.

Diuretics

Patients with dyspnea and signs of fluid overload/congestion should be promptly treated with an intravenous loop diuretic such as furosemide that exerts an acute vasodilator and slightly delayed but still fast diuretic effect. Optimal doses and regimens need to be adapted to the clinical picture. An

intravenous bolus of 40–80 mg furosemide is a common starting dose, often continued by an infusion of furosemide at a daily dose equal to the (oral) daily dose prescribed before hospitalization. Doses may need to be escalated according to symptoms and diuresis. Additional use of a thiazide diuretic in small doses can break a relative resistance to loop diuretics but requires careful monitoring of K⁺ losses. Excessive doses of furosemide must be avoided because they can cause hypotension, a reduction in GFR, electrolyte disturbance, and further neurohumoral activation.

Vasodilators

Vasodilators such as *nitroglycerin* and *nitroprusside* reduce preload and afterload. The reduction in preload (= diastolic filling pressure) moves the patient to the left on the stroke volume-preload relationship, similar to the effect of diuretic-induced volume reduction (Figure 29–3). The accompanying reduction in chamber dimension reduces wall stress and thus O₂ consumption. The additional reduction in afterload allows the heart to expel blood against a lower output resistance (Figure 29–4). These mechanisms explain why vasodilators (which have no inotropic efficacy and lower blood pressure) increase stroke volume. Yet, robust evidence for symptomatic benefit or improved clinical outcome is lacking. They are probably best suited for patients with hypertension and should be avoided in patients with systolic blood pressure less than 110 mm Hg (Ponikowski et al., 2016). The main risk is hypotension, which is negatively associated with favorable outcomes in patients with acutely decompensated heart failure (Patel et al., 2014).

Neseritide, recombinant human BNP, dilates arterial and venous blood vessels by stimulating the membrane-bound guanylyl cyclase to produce more cGMP. By this mechanism, it decreases preload and afterload and reduces pulmonary capillary wedge pressure. It is approved for the treatment of acutely decompensated heart failure in the U.S., but not in several European countries. Early clinical studies and a meta-analysis raised concerns that the use of neseritide was associated with an increased risk for renal failure and death when compared to a noninotrope control therapy (Sackner-Bernstein et al., 2005). This risk was not confirmed in a more recent study (O'Connor et al., 2011), but beneficial effects (dyspnea relief) were also modest.

Positive Inotropic Agents

Stimulating the heart's force of contraction in a situation of critically diminished cardiac output may appear to be the most intuitive intervention. Yet, inotropes in acutely decompensated heart failure are associated with worse outcome and should therefore be restricted to patients with critically low cardiac output and perfusion of vital organs. Hypotension less than 85 mm Hg has been suggested as a practical limit (Ponikowski et al., 2016). Reasons for the adverse consequences of positive inotropes are probably complex. All inotropic agents increase cardiac energy expenditure (greater and faster force development ⇒ more ATP consumption ⇒ greater O₂ demand), which carries the risk of diffuse cardiac myocyte death. In acutely decompensated heart failure, the risk is exaggerated by the low perfusion pressure, any preexisting coronary artery disease, and the likely presence of cardiac myocyte hypertrophy and myocyte-endothelial cell mismatch. Tachycardia, aggravated by many inotropes, adds to the problem by strongly increasing energy expenditure and reducing the time for coronary perfusion in diastole. All positive inotropes increase the risk of arrhythmias.

Dobutamine

Dobutamine is the β adrenergic agonist of choice for the management of patients with acute CHF with systolic dysfunction. Dobutamine has relatively well-balanced cardiac and vascular actions: stimulation of cardiac output with less tachycardia than EPI and with a concomitant decrease in pulmonary artery wedge pressure. Dobutamine is a racemic mixture of (–) and (+) enantiomers. The (–) enantiomer is a potent agonist at α₁ adrenergic receptors and a weak agonist at β₁ and β₂ receptors. The (+) enantiomer is a potent β₁ and β₂ agonist without much activity at α₁ adrenergic receptors. Dobutamine has no activity at dopamine receptors. At infusion rates that result in a positive inotropic effect in humans, the β₁ adrenergic effect in the myocardium predominates. In the vasculature, the α_1 adrenergic agonist effect of the (−) enantiomer appears to be offset by the vasodilating effects of the (+) enantiomer at β_2 receptors. Thus, the principal hemodynamic effect of dobutamine is an increase in stroke volume from positive inotropy, augmented by a small decrease in systemic vascular resistance and, therefore, afterload. Lowering of pulmonary artery capillary pressure is considered an advantage compared to other catecholamines, as is the smaller chronotropic effect (reasons for which are not clear).

Continuous dobutamine infusions are typically initiated at 2–3 µg/kg/min and uptitrated until the desired hemodynamic response is achieved. Pharmacologic tolerance may limit infusion efficacy beyond 4 days; therefore, addition or substitution a PDE3 inhibitor may be necessary to maintain adequate circulatory support. The major side effects of dobutamine are tachycardia and supraventricular/ventricular arrhythmias, which may require a reduction in dosage. The concurrent use of β blockers is a common cause of blunted clinical responsiveness to dobutamine. It can be overcome by higher doses in case of bisoprolol and metoprolol, but not as easily for carvedilol, which has a very slow dissociation rate.

Epinephrine

The natural sympathetic agonist is mainly produced by the adrenal gland and systemically released. It is a balanced β_1, β_2, and α_1 adrenergic agonist and has a similar net hemodynamic effect as dobutamine, but with a stronger tachycardic effect, which makes it a second-choice inotrope in acutely decompensated heart failure.

Norepinephrine

The main sympathetic neurotransmitter released from sympathetic nerve endings is a potent β_1 and α_1 agonist and weak β_2 receptor agonist. This profile causes the positive inotropism accompanied by prominent vasoconstriction and increased afterload. Vasoconstriction of coronary blood vessels promotes ischemia; increased afterload may impede cardiac output (Figure 29–4). However, the stronger blood pressure–increasing effect of NE may be needed in persistent hypotension despite adequate cardiac filling pressures. Moreover, the increase in mean blood pressure leads to a reflex increase in parasympathetic nervous tone that can antagonize the direct tachycardic effect of NE and actually cause bradycardia.

Dopamine

The pharmacologic and hemodynamic effects of DA vary with concentration. Low doses (≤2 µg/kg lean body mass/min) induce cAMP-dependent vascular smooth muscle vasodilation by direct stimulation of D2 receptors. Activation of D2 receptors on sympathetic nerves in the peripheral circulation also inhibits NE release and reduces α adrenergic stimulation of vascular smooth muscle, particularly in splanchnic and renal arterial beds. This is the pharmacological basis for the "low-dose DA infusion" historically used to increase renal blood flow and maintain an adequate GFR and diuresis in hospitalized patients with CHF with impaired renal function refractory to diuretics. However, mainly negative clinical studies argue against the validity of this concept (Chen et al., 2013; Vargo et al., 1996). At intermediate infusion rates (2–5 µg/kg/min), dopamine directly stimulates cardiac β receptors to enhance myocardial contractility. At higher infusion rates (5–15 µg/kg/min), α adrenergic receptor stimulation–mediated peripheral arterial and venous constriction occurs. The complex profile and negative clinical data on low-dose infusion make DA a second or third choice in the treatment of heart failure.

Phosphodiesterase Inhibitors

The cAMP-PDE inhibitors decrease cellular cAMP degradation, resulting in elevated levels of cAMP. This results in positive inotropic and chronotropic effects in the heart and dilation of resistance and capacitance vessels, effectively decreasing preload and afterload (thus the term *inodilator*). PDE inhibitors may be more advantageous than catecholamines in patients on β blockers and in patients with high systemic or pulmonary artery resistance. Hypotension is often dose limiting; tachycardic and arrhythmogenic effects are similar to those of catecholamines.

Milrinone and Enoximone. Parenteral formulations of milrinone and enoximone are used for short-term circulation support in advanced CHF.

Enoximone (not available in the U.S.) is a relative selective inhibitor of PDE3, the cGMP-inhibited cAMP PDE and main isoform involved in inotropic control in human heart. Milrinone inhibits human heart PDE3 and PDE4 with similar potency (Bethke et al., 1992). By increasing intracellular cAMP concentrations, they have similar actions as the β receptor agonists dobutamine and EPI, but tend to lower systemic and pulmonary vascular resistance more than do the catecholamines. It should be kept in mind that PDE inhibitors potentiate the actions of β receptor agonists, both beneficial and detrimental. The loading dose of milrinone is ordinarily 25–75 µg/kg, and the continuous infusion rate ranges from 0.375 to 0.75 µg/kg/min. Bolus doses of enoximone at 0.5–1.0 mg/kg over 5–10 min are followed by an infusion of 5–20 µg/kg/min. The elimination half-lives of milrinone and enoximone in normal individuals are 0.5–1 h and 2–3 h, respectively, but can be increased in patients with severe CHF.

Myofilament Calcium Sensitizers (Levosimendan, Pimobendan)

In some countries but not in the U.S., calcium sensitizers are approved for the short-term treatment of acutely decompensated heart failure (e.g., levosimendan in Sweden, pimobendan in Japan). Calcium sensitizers increase the sensitivity of contractile myofilaments to Ca^{2+} by binding to and inducing a conformational change in the thin-filament regulatory protein troponin C. This causes an increased force for a given cytosolic Ca^{2+} concentration, theoretically without raising the $[Ca^{2+}]_{cytosol}$. However, a variety of other effects has been ascribed to pimobendan and levosimendan, including inhibition of PDEs, inhibition of the production of pro-inflammatory cytokines, and opening of ATP-dependent potassium channels. Clinical data provide evidence for symptomatic benefit and reductions in the length of stay in the hospital but do not support a better safety profile of levosimendan compared to catecholamines or classical PDE inhibitors (Mebazaa et al., 2007). Increased rates of arrhythmia and death are likely related to the PDE3 inhibitor activity of these compounds.

Other Drugs Used in Heart Failure

The vasopressin receptor antagonist tolvaptan is FDA-approved for the treatment of therapy-resistant hyponatremia, a common and difficult-to-treat complication in decompensated heart failure. Studies in a more general cohort of patients with heart failure failed to show convincing beneficial effects of this compound. Severe thirst and dehydration are common side effects. Heparin or other anticoagulants are routinely used in hospitalized patients with heart failure to prevent thromboembolism.

Role of Standard Combination Therapy

The majority of patients hospitalized with acutely decompensated heart failure have preexisting heart failure and respective maintenance therapy. Guidelines suggest reviewing a patient's existing therapy on admission to determine whether recent changes in the medication could be causally related to an exacerbation of cardiac disease. If not, the standard heart failure medication (ACEI, β blocker, MRA, diuretic) should be continued in the absence of hemodynamic instability or contraindications (Yancey et al., 2013).

Lessons From Heart Failure Drug Development

Heart failure is an attractive but difficult indication for drug development. The number of drug development failures over the past two decades largely exceeded that of successes, indicating our incomplete understanding of the pathophysiology of heart failure, but sometimes also signaling problematic trial design. Even negative trials have helped to better understand the disease. Examples of drugs that have been tested in large prospective trials and failed are listed in Table 29–6.

Lessons From Failed Drugs

The failure of *positive inotropic agents* (PDE inhibitors, catecholamines, calcium sensitizers, mixed-acting compounds such as flosequinan or

TABLE 29–6 ■ FAILURES IN DRUG DEVELOPMENT FOR HEART FAILURE

DRUG (type)	YEAR OF PUBLICATION	REASON FOR FAILURE
Milrinone (PDE inhibitor)	1991	Increased mortality
Pimobendan (PDE inhibitor)	1996	Trend toward increased mortality
Flosequinan (unclear)	1993	Increased mortality
Vesnarinone (unclear)	1998	Increased mortality, arrhythmias
Moxonidine (central antisympathetic)	1998	Increased mortality
Infliximab (TNFα blocker)	2003	Increased mortality
Etanercept (TNFα blocker)	2004	Trend toward increased mortality
Bosentan (ET receptor blocker)	2005	Liver toxicity, trend toward benefit over time (?)
Etomoxir (CPT1 blocker)	2007	Liver toxicity
Omapatrilat (dual ACEI and neprilysin inhibitor)	2002	Angioedema, no clear benefit
ARB + ACEI	2003 and 2008	No benefit, more angioedema and renal side effects
Rosuvastatin (HMG CoA reductase inhibitor)	2007	No benefit
Tolvaptan (vasopressin V2 receptor blocker)	2009	No benefit
Rolophylline (adenosine A_1 receptor blocker)	2009	No benefit, seizures

vesnarinone; Cohn et al., 1998) to improve long-term outcome of patients with heart failure has induced a paradigm shift toward drugs that unload the heart and reduce neurohumoral activation, the current standard. It demonstrated that further stimulating the failing heart may transiently improve symptoms but increase mortality. But, simply reducing the load without protecting the heart from the adverse consequences of the activated SNS and RAAS also seems inefficient, as exemplified by the neutral effect of the α_1 receptor antagonist *prazosin* in the VeHeFT-I trial (Cohn et al., 1986). *Moxonidine*, a centrally acting α_2/imidazole agonist with similar sympatholytic actions as clonidine, should have had efficacy similar to that of β blockers, but moxonidine increased mortality in a larger prospective trial (Cohn et al., 2003). It is unclear whether doses and dose titration were too aggressive or whether the principle of central sympatholysis is unsafe in heart failure. Multiple lines of laboratory and clinical evidence suggested that heart failure has an important inflammatory component; yet, two blockers of TNF, *infliximab* and *etanercept,* induced harm rather

than benefit in patients with chronic heart failure (Chung et al., 2003; Mann et al., 2004).

Endothelin 1, a potent vasoconstrictor, is upregulated in heart failure and could play an adverse role in heart failure, similar to that of AngII. Nonselective ET receptor antagonists such as *bosentan* had striking efficacy in postinfarct rodent models and are successfully used in pulmonary hypertension (Chapter 31). However, bosentan showed no efficacy in patients with chronic heart failure (Packer et al., 2005). *Omapatrilat*, a dual inhibitor of ACE and neprilysin, can decrease AngII and increase ANP/BNP, conditions promoting vasodilation, diuresis, and antihypertrophic effects; however, expectations that omapatrilat would be more efficacious than an ACEI in heart failure were not confirmed in a prospective study (Packer et al., 2002).

Numerous clinical trials have tested the idea that adding an ARB or the renin inhibitor *aliskiren* to standard therapy that includes an ACEI would be beneficial by more completely inhibiting the RAAS. With the exception of one trial (McMurray et al., 2003), studies of these combinations consistently showed a lack of benefit and an increase in adverse effects, particularly decreased renal function and hyperkalemia. The premise was that if some inhibition of the RAAS is good, more would be better; perhaps the premise was wrong.

Statins were proposed to have anti-inflammatory, antihypertrophic, and pro-angiogenic effects independent of their cholesterol-lowering effect (Liao and Laufs, 2005). Trials testing this hypothesis by adding statins to standard treatment of chronic heart failure demonstrated that the combination was safe but had no added beneficial effect on mortality (Kjekshus et al., 2007). An antagonist of the V_2 vasopressin receptor tolvaptan was ineffective in patients with chronic stable heart failure (Udelson et al., 2007). The discrepancy to several positive preclinical and early clinical studies suggests that the vasopressin axis of the neurohumoral activation program in heart failure may be sufficiently addressed by standard combination therapy, leaving no room for further improvement.

Lessons From Treating Acute Heart Failure

The drugs currently recommended (furosemide, nitroglycerin, dobutamine) for the treatment of acutely decompensated heart failure have never been tested in adequately powered prospective clinical trials. All novel drugs tested either in comparison to standard inotropes or noninotropes or as an add-on have failed to show convincing superiority or benefit in terms of symptoms, duration of hospitalization, and 30-day mortality. The A_1 adenosine receptor antagonist *rolophylline* should produce several beneficial effects on the kidney, including inhibition of tubular reabsorption of Na$^+$ and water, dilation of the afferent arteriole, and inhibition of tubular-glomerular feedback, but its addition to standard therapy in patients with acute heart failure with impaired kidney function produced no salutary renal or cardiac effects and caused unacceptable adverse effects such as seizures, a typical side effect of central A_1 adenosine antagonism known also from theophylline (Massie et al., 2010).

Recent Developments; Novel Approaches

Numerous pharmacological and nonpharmacological treatment options are being tested in preclinical and clinical studies (https://www.clinicaltrials.gov). They range from cell and gene therapies to food supplements (vitamins, polyunsaturated fatty acid) and intravenous iron to classical small molecules. In the CUPID2 trial, gene therapy, in the form of an intracoronary infusion of adeno-associated virus 1/SERCA2, did not provide any benefit in HFrEF (Greenberg et al., 2016). *Serelaxin*, recombinant human *relaxin 2*, is a naturally occurring peptide with 53 amino acids discovered in 1926 as an ovarian hormone inducing relaxation of the uterus during pregnancy. Its actions on the cardiovascular system include increased arterial compliance, cardiac output, and renal blood flow, characteristics of a promising drug for the treatment of acutely decompensated heart failure. However, the promising results of an earlier study (Teerlink et al., 2013) were not confirmed in a larger phase III trial (announced online March 2017).

Guanylyl cyclases are established targets for natriuretic peptides (the membrane form, mGC) and NO and organic nitrates (the soluble form, sGC). *Riociguat* is a direct, heme-dependent stimulator of sGC; *cinaciguat* is a heme-independent activator of sGC. Oxidative inactivation of sGC is believed to be a common pathology in cardiovascular disease and a reason for endothelial dysfunction. sGC activators have maintained (or even enhanced) effects at sGC enzymes inactivated by oxidation. Riociguat is approved for the treatment of pulmonary artery hypertension and chronic thromboembolic pulmonary hypertension (see Chapter 31). A prospective study with cinaciguat was prematurely stopped because the drug not only lowered pulmonary wedge pressure and increased cardiac output, but also markedly increased the rate of symptomatic hypotension (Erdmann et al., 2013), a classical problem of vasodilator therapy in acute heart failure.

Heart failure is often associated with anemia, a predictor of a poor prognosis. Yet, correction of anemia by an erythropoietin derivative, darbapoetin alpha, did not affect any clinical end point but increased the rate of thromboembolic events and ischemic strokes in patients with heart failure and mild-to-moderate anemia (Swedberg et al., 2013). However, intravenous iron, added to standard therapy in patients with NYHA class II–III heart failure, iron deficiency, and hemoglobin levels of 9.5–13.5 g/dL, improved quality of life, NYHA class, and physical exercise capacity (Anker et al., 2009). The beneficial effects seemed to be independent of the presence of anemia and may be related to other roles of iron in the body. Larger prospective studies are needed to confirm the effects.

Acknowledgment: *Henry Ooi, Wilson Colucci, Bradley A. Maron, James C. Fang, and Thomas P. Rocco have contributed to this chapter in recent editions of this book. We have retained some of their text in the current edition.*

Drug Facts for Your Personal Formulary: *Heart Failure Drugs*

Drug	Therapeutic Uses	Major Toxicity and Clinical Pearls
Inhibitors of the Renin-Angiotensin System		
ACE Inhibitors Benazepril Captopril Enalapril Lisinopril Quinapril Ramipril	• Heart failure • Hypertension • Diabetic nephropathy	• First choice in treating heart failure • Short-acting captopril only for initiation of therapy; enalapril requires twice-daily dosing • Cough in 5%–10% of patients, angioedema • Hypotension, hyperkalemia, skin rash, neutropenia, anemia, fetopathic syndrome • Contraindicated in patients with renal artery stenosis; caution in patients with impaired renal function or hypovolemia
Fosinopril Trandolapril Perindopril		• Both hepatic and renal elimination, caution in patients with renal or hepatic impairment
Angiotensin Receptor Blockers Candesartan Eprosartan Irbesartan Losartan Olmesartan Telmisartan Valsartan	• Hypertension • Heart failure • Diabetic nephropathy	• Only in cases of intolerance to ACEI • Unwanted effects as ACEI, but no cough or angioedema • No evidence for superiority over ACEI • In combination with ACEI more harm than benefit
β Blockers		
Bisoprolol Carvedilol Metoprolol Nebivolol	• Heart failure • Hypertension • Widely used for angina, prevention of arrhythmias, rate control in atrial fibrillation, migraine	• First choice in the treatment of heart failure • Start low (1/10 target dose), go slow (2- to 4-weekly doubling) • Adverse effects: bradycardia, AV block, bronchospasm, peripheral vasoconstriction, worsening of acute heart failure, depression, worsening of psorias • Polymorphic CYP2D6 metabolism (metoprolol)
Mineralocorticoid Receptor Antagonists		
Eplerenone Spironolactone	• Heart failure • Hypertension • Hyperaldosteronism, hypokalemia, ascites	• First choice in treating symptomatic heart failure • Low doses (25–50 mg) • Most serious side effect is hyperkalemia • Spironolactone causes painful breast swelling and impotence in men, dysmenorrhea in women due to nonselective binding to sex hormone receptors
Neprilysin Inhibitor/Angiotensin Receptor Blocker		
Sacubitril/valsartan	• Heart failure	• Superior to the ACEI enalapril • May become first choice in treating heart failure • ↓ Degradation of natriuretic peptides, ↑ their beneficial actions • Hypotension
Diuretics		
Thiazide Type Chlorothiazide Hydrochlorothiazide **Thiazide-like** Chlorthalidone Indapamide Metolazone	• Edema associated with congestive heart failure, liver cirrhosis, chronic kidney disease, and nephrotic syndrome • Hypertension • Nephrogenic diabetes insipidus • Kidney stones caused by Ca^{2+} crystals	• Symptomatic treatment of milder forms of heart failure • Loose efficacy at GFR < 30–40 mL/min (exception indapamide and metolazone) • Potentiate effect of loop diuretics in severe heart failure (sequential tubulus blockade) • Risk for hypokalemia and arrhythmia when combined with QT-prolonging drugs

Drug Facts for Your Personal Formulary: *Heart Failure Drugs (continued)*

Drug	Therapeutic Uses	Major Toxicity and Clinical Pearls
Loop Diuretics Bumetanide Furosemide Torasemide	• Acute pulmonary edema (intravenous) • Edema associated with congestive heart failure, liver cirrhosis, chronic kidney disease, and nephrotic syndrome • Hyponatremia • Hypercalcemia • Hypertension with renal insufficiency	• Symptomatic treatment of severe heart failure and acute decompensation • Often required in treating severe chronic heart failure, twice-daily dosing or more • Torasemide may be superior to furosemide in heart failure • Risk for hypokalemia and arrhythmia when combined with QT-prolonging drugs
Vasodilators		
ISDN/hydralazine	• Heart failure in African Americans	• Approved only for African Americans • Adverse effects: headache, nausea, flushing, hypotension, palpitations, tachycardia, dizziness, angina pectoris; ⇒ use in combination with β blocker • Compliance problems • Lupus syndrome
Positive Inotropes		
Digoxin Digitoxin	• Heart failure	• Not first choice in treating heart failure • May exert benefits in heart failure and atrial fibrillation • Low therapeutic index: proarrhythmic, nausea, diarrhea, visual disturbances • Digoxin kidney dependent, digitoxin not • Half-life 1.5 (digoxin) or 7 days (digitoxin) • Plasma concentration: 0.5–0.8 ng/mL (digoxin) or 10–25 ng/mL (digitoxin)
Heart Rate Reduction		
Ivabradine	• Heart failure	• Not first choice in treating heart failure • May exert benefits in patients not tolerating β blockers or having heart rate > 75 under β blockers • Unwanted effects: bradycardia, QT prolongation, atrial fibrillation, phosphenes
Intravenous Vasodilators: Acute decompensated heart failure		
Nitroglycerin Sodium nitroprusside	• Acute decompensated heart failure	• May ↑ cardiac output in acute congestion (↑ filling pressure and dilation) via ↓ preload and afterload • NO releaser, stimulates soluble guanylyl cyclase • Avoid if systolic blood pressure < 110 mmHg • Prognostic benefit unclear
Neseritide	• Acute decompensated heart failure	• Recombinant human BNP • Stimulates membrane-bound guanylyl cyclase • May ↑ cardiac output via ↓ preload and afterload • Therapeutic benefit unclear
Intravenous Positive Inotropes: Acutely decompensated heart failure		
Dobutamine Dopamine Epinephrine Norepinephrine	• Acute decompensated heart failure	• β_1 receptor-mediated stimulation of cardiac output and, depending on drug, complex vascular actions • Last option in patients with systolic blood pressure <85 mmHg • ↑ Cardiac energy consumption and risk of arrhythmia • Use of catecholamines correlates with poor prognosis; use lowest possible doses for shortest possible time • Dobutamine causes less tachycardia than EPI and less afterload increase than NE • Role of low-dose dopamine unclear
Enoximone Milrinone	• Acute decompensated heart failure	• PDE3/4 inhibitors, ↑ cellular cAMP • ↑ Cardiac output and dilate blood vessels ("inodilator") • May be used in patients on β blockers and with high peripheral and pulmonary arterial resistance • Blood pressure decrease is dose limiting • Risks and prognostic effects: same as catecholamines (above)
Levosimendan	• Acute decompensated heart failure	• Combined Ca^{2+} sensitizer (troponin C binding) and PDE3 inhibitor • ↑ Cardiac output and ↓ vascular resistance ("inodilator") • Advantages over catecholamines or simple PDE inhibitors unclear

Anker SD, et al. Ferric carboxymaltose in patients with heart failure and iron deficiency. *N Engl J Med*, **2009**, *361*:2436–2448.

Bethke T, et al. Phosphodiesterase inhibition by enoximone in preparations from nonfailing and failing human hearts. *Arzneimittelforschung*, **1992**, *42*:437–445.

Bohm M, et al. Heart rate as a risk factor in chronic heart failure (SHIFT): the association between heart rate and outcomes in a randomised placebo-controlled trial. *Lancet*, **2010**, *376*:886–894.

Chen HH, et al. Low-dose dopamine or low-dose nesiritide in acute heart failure with renal dysfunction: the ROSE acute heart failure randomized trial. *JAMA*, **2013**, *310*:2533–2543.

Chirkov YY, et al. Hydralazine does not ameliorate nitric oxide resistance in chronic heart failure. *Cardiovasc Drugs Ther*, **2010**, *24*:131–137.

Chung ES, et al. Randomized, double-blind, placebo-controlled, pilot trial of infliximab, a chimeric monoclonal antibody to tumor necrosis factor-alpha, in patients with moderate-to-severe heart failure: results of the anti-TNF Therapy Against Congestive Heart Failure (ATTACH) trial. *Circulation*, **2003**, *107*:3133–3140.

CIBIS-II Investigators. The Cardiac Insufficiency Bisoprolol Study II (CIBIS-II): a randomised trial. *Lancet*, **1999**, *353*:9–13.

Cohn JN, et al. Effect of vasodilator therapy on mortality in chronic congestive heart failure. Results of a Veterans Administration Cooperative Study. *N Engl J Med*, **1986**, *314*:1547–1552.

Cohn JN, et al. A dose-dependent increase in mortality with vesnarinone among patients with severe heart failure. Vesnarinone Trial Investigators. *N Engl J Med*, **1998**, *339*:1810–1816.

Cohn JN, et al. Adverse mortality effect of central sympathetic inhibition with sustained-release moxonidine in patients with heart failure (MOXCON). *Eur J Heart Fail*, **2003**, *5*:659–667.

CONSENSUS Trial Study Group. Effects of enalapril on mortality in severe congestive heart failure. Results of the Cooperative North Scandinavian Enalapril Survival Study (CONSENSUS). *N Engl J Med*, **1987**, *316*:1429–1435.

Digitalis Investigation Group. The effect of digoxin on mortality and morbidity in patients with heart failure. *N Engl J Med*, **1997**, *336*:525–533.

Erdmann E, et al. Cinaciguat, a soluble guanylate cyclase activator, unloads the heart but also causes hypotension in acute decompensated heart failure. *Eur Heart J*, **2013**, *34*:57–67.

Flather MD, et al. Randomized trial to determine the effect of nebivolol on mortality and cardiovascular hospital admission in elderly patients with heart failure (SENIORS). *Eur Heart J*, **2005**, *26*:215–225.

Fox K, et al. Ivabradine in stable coronary artery disease. *N Engl J Med*, **2014**, *371*:2435.

Greenberg B, et al. Calcium Upregulation by Percutaneous Administration of Gene Therapy in Patients With Cardiac Disease (CUPID 2): a randomised, multinational, double-blind, placebo-controlled, phase 2b trial. *Lancet*, **2016**, *387*:1178–1186.

Hubers SA, Brown NJ. Combined angiotensin receptor antagonism and neprilysin inhibition. *Circulation*, **2016**, *133*:1115–1124.

Jhund PS, et al. Long-term trends in first hospitalization for heart failure and subsequent survival between 1986 and 2003: a population study of 5.1 million people. *Circulation*, **2009**, *119*:515–523.

Juurlink D, et al. Rates of hyperkalemia after publication of the Randomized Aldactone Evaluation Study. *N Engl J Med*, **2004**, *351*:543–551.

Kjekshus J, et al. Rosuvastatin in older patients with systolic heart failure. *N Engl J Med*, **2007**, *357*:2248–2261.

Klabunde RE. Cardiovascular physiology concepts: ventricular systolic dysfunctions. **2015**. Available at: http://www.cvphysiology.com/Heart%20Failure/HF005. Accessed February 26, 2017.

Lee TC. Van Gogh's vision: digitalis intoxication? *JAMA*, **1981**, *245*:727–729.

Liao JK, Laufs U. Pleiotropic effects of statins. *Annu Rev Pharmacol Toxicol*, **2005**, *45*:89–118.

Lowes BD, et al. Myocardial gene expression in dilated cardiomyopathy treated with beta-blocking agents. *N Engl J Med*, **2002**, *346*:1357–1365.

Mann DL, et al. Targeted anticytokine therapy in patients with chronic heart failure: results of the Randomized Etanercept Worldwide Evaluation (RENEWAL). *Circulation*, **2004**, *109*:1594–1602.

Massie BM, et al. Rolofylline, an adenosine A_1-receptor antagonist, in acute heart failure. *N Engl J Med*, **2010**, *363*:1419–1428.

McMurray JJ, et al. Effects of candesartan in patients with chronic heart failure and reduced left-ventricular systolic function taking angiotensin-converting-enzyme inhibitors: the CHARM-Added trial. *Lancet*, **2003**, *362*:767–771.

McMurray JJ, et al. Angiotensin-neprilysin inhibition versus enalapril in heart failure. *N Engl J Med*, **2014**, *371*:993–1004.

Mebazaa A, et al. Levosimendan vs dobutamine for patients with acute decompensated heart failure: the SURVIVE Randomized Trial. *JAMA*, **2007**, *297*:1883–1891.

MERIT-HF Investigators. Effect of metoprolol CR/XL in chronic heart failure: Metoprolol CR/XL Randomised Intervention Trial in Congestive Heart Failure (MERIT-HF). *Lancet*, **1999**, *353*:2001–2007.

Munzel T, et al. Explaining the phenomenon of nitrate tolerance. *Circ Res*, **2005**, *97*:618–628.

O'Connor CM, et al. Effect of nesiritide in patients with acute decompensated heart failure. *N Engl J Med*, **2011**, *365*:32–43.

Packer M, et al. Comparison of omapatrilat and enalapril in patients with chronic heart failure: the Omapatrilat Versus Enalapril Randomized Trial of Utility in Reducing Events (OVERTURE). *Circulation*, **2002**, *106*:920–926.

Packer M, et al. Clinical effects of endothelin receptor antagonism with bosentan in patients with severe chronic heart failure: results of a pilot study. *J Card Fail*, **2005**, *11*:12–20.

Patel PA, et al. Hypotension during hospitalization for acute heart failure is independently associated with 30-day mortality: findings from ASCEND-HF. *Circ Heart Fail*, **2014**, *7*:918–925.

Pavlovic D, et al. Novel regulation of cardiac Na pump via phospholemman. *J Mol Cell Cardiol*, **2013**, *61*:83–93.

Pieske B, et al. Alterations in intracellular calcium handling associated with the inverse force-frequency relation in human dilated cardiomyopathy. *Circulation*, **1995**, *92*:1169–1178.

Pitt B. Effect of aldosterone blockade in patients with systolic left ventricular dysfunction: implications of the RALES and EPHESUS studies. *Mol Cell Endocrinol*, **2004**, *217*:53–58.

Pitt B, et al. The effect of spironolactone on morbidity and mortality in patients with severe heart failure. *N Engl J Med*, **1999**, *341*:709–717.

Ponikowski P, et al. 2016 European Society of Cardiology Guidelines for the diagnosis and treatment of acute and chronic heart failure. *Eur Heart J*, **2016**, *37*:2129–2200.

Poole-Wilson PA, et al. Comparison of carvedilol and metoprolol on clinical outcomes in patients with chronic heart failure in the Carvedilol Or Metoprolol European Trial (COMET): randomised controlled trial. *Lancet*, **2003**, *362*:7–13.

Rathore SS, et al. Association of serum digoxin concentration and outcomes in patients with heart failure. *JAMA*, **2003**, *289*:871–878.

Rau T, et al. Impact of the CYP2D6 genotype on the clinical effects of metoprolol: a prospective longitudinal study. *Clin Pharmacol Ther*, **2009**, *85*:269–272.

Redfield MM, et al. Effect of phosphodiesterase-5 inhibition on exercise capacity and clinical status in heart failure with preserved ejection fraction: a randomized clinical trial. *JAMA*, **2013**, *309*:1268–1277.

Sackner-Bernstein JD, et al. Short-term risk of death after treatment with nesiritide for decompensated heart failure: a pooled analysis of randomized controlled trials. *JAMA*, **2005**, *293*:1900–1905.

Schober T, et al. Myofilament Ca sensitization increases cytosolic Ca binding affinity, alters intracellular Ca homeostasis, and causes pause-dependent Ca-triggered arrhythmia. *Circ Res*, **2012**, *111*:170–179.

Skou JC. William Withering—the man and his work. In: Erdmann E, Greeff K, Skou JC, eds. *Cardiac Glycosides 1785–1985*. Springer-Verlag, Berlin, **1986**, 1–10.

SOLVD Investigators. Effect of enalapril on survival in patients with reduced left ventricular ejection fractions and congestive heart failure. *N Engl J Med*, **1991**, *325*:293–302.

SOLVD Investigators. Effect of enalapril on mortality and the development of heart failure in asymptomatic patients with reduced left ventricular ejection fractions. *N Engl J Med,* **1992,** 327:685–691.

Strait JB, Lakatta EG. Aging-associated cardiovascular changes and their relationship to heart failure. *Heart Fail Clin,* **2012,** 8:143–164.

Swedberg K, et al. Ivabradine and outcomes in chronic heart failure (SHIFT): a randomised placebo-controlled study. *Lancet,* **2010,** *376*: 875–885.

Swedberg K, , et al. Treatment of anemia with darbepoetin alfa in systolic heart failure. *N Engl J Med,* **2013,** 368:1210–1219.

Taylor AL, et al. Combination of isosorbide dinitrate and hydralazine in blacks with heart failure. *N Engl J Med,* **2004,** 351:2049–2057.

Teerlink JR, et al. Serelaxin, recombinant human relaxin-2, for treatment of acute heart failure (RELAX-AHF): a randomised, placebo-controlled trial. *Lancet,* **2013,** *381*:29–39.

Udelson JE, et al. Multicenter, randomized, double-blind, placebo-controlled study on the effect of oral tolvaptan on left ventricular dilation and function in patients with heart failure and systolic dysfunction. *J Am Coll Cardiol,* **2007,** *49*:2151–2159.

Vargo DL, et al. Dopamine does not enhance furosemide-induced natriuresis in patients with congestive heart failure. *J Am Soc Nephrol,* **1996,** *7*:1032–1037.

Waagstein F, et al. Effect of chronic beta-adrenergic receptor blockade in congestive cardiomyopathy. *Br Heart J,* **1975,** *37*:1022–1036.

Xamoterol Study Group. Xamoterol in severe heart failure. *Lancet,* **1990,** *336*:1–6.

Yancy CW, et al. 2013 ACCF/AHA guideline for the management of heart failure: a report of the American College of Cardiology Foundation/ American Heart Association Task Force on practice guidelines. *Circulation,* **2013,** *128*:e240–e327. doi:10.1161/CIR.0b013e31829e8776. Accessed March 7, 2017.

Yancy CW, et al. 2016 ACCF/AHA/HFSA focused update on new pharmcological therapy for heart failure: an update of the 2013 guideline for the management of heart failure. *Circulation,* **2016,** *135*:e282–e293. doi:10.1161/CIR.0000000000000435. http://circ. ahajournals.org/content/early/2016/05/18/CIR.0000000000000435. Accessed March 7, 2017.

Zannad F, et al. Eplerenone in patients with systolic heart failure and mild symptoms. *N Engl J Med,* **2011,** *364*:11–21.

Antiarrhythmic Drugs

Bjorn C. Knollmann and Dan M. Roden

Cardiac cells undergo depolarization and repolarization about 60 times per minute to form and propagate cardiac action potentials. The shape and duration of each action potential are determined by the activity of ion channel protein complexes in the membranes of individual cells, and the genes encoding most of these proteins and their regulators now have been identified. Action potentials in turn provide the primary signals to release Ca²⁺ from intracellular stores and to thereby initiate contraction. Thus, each normal heartbeat results from the highly integrated electrophysiological behavior of multiple proteins on the surface and within multiple cardiac cells. Disordered cardiac rhythm can arise from influences such as inherited variation in ion channel or other genes, ischemia, sympathetic stimulation, or myocardial scarring. Available antiarrhythmic drugs suppress arrhythmias by blocking flow through specific ion channels or by altering autonomic function. An increasingly sophisticated understanding of the molecular basis of normal and abnormal cardiac rhythm may lead to identification of new targets for antiarrhythmic drugs and perhaps improved therapies (Dobrev et al., 2012; Van Wagoner et al., 2015).

Arrhythmias can range from incidental, asymptomatic clinical findings to life-threatening abnormalities. Mechanisms underlying cardiac arrhythmias have been identified in cellular and animal experiments. For some human arrhythmias, precise mechanisms are known, and treatment can be targeted specifically to those mechanisms. In other cases, mechanisms can be only inferred, and the choice of drugs is based largely on results of prior experience. Antiarrhythmic drug therapy has two goals: termination of an ongoing arrhythmia or prevention of an arrhythmia. Unfortunately, antiarrhythmic drugs may not only help control arrhythmias but also can cause them, even during long-term therapy. Thus, prescribing antiarrhythmic drugs requires that precipitating factors be excluded or minimized, that a precise diagnosis of the type of arrhythmia (and its possible mechanisms) be made, that the prescriber has reason to believe that drug therapy will be beneficial, and that the risks of drug therapy can be minimized.

Principles of Cardiac Electrophysiology

The flow of ions across cell membranes generates the currents that make up cardiac action potentials. Factors that determine the magnitude of individual currents and their modulation by drugs include transmembrane potential, time since depolarization, or the presence of specific ligands (Nerbonne and Kass, 2005; Priori et al., 1999). Further, because the function of many channels is time and voltage dependent, even a drug that targets a single ion channel may, by altering the trajectory of the action potential, alter the function of other channels. Most antiarrhythmic drugs affect more than one ion current, and many exert ancillary effects, such as modification of cardiac contractility or autonomic nervous system function. Thus, antiarrhythmic drugs usually exert multiple actions and can be beneficial or harmful in individual patients (Priori et al., 1999; Roden, 1994).

The Cardiac Cell at Rest: a K⁺-Permeable Membrane

Ions move across cell membranes in response to electrical and concentration gradients, not through the lipid bilayer but through specific ion channels or transporters. The normal cardiac cell at rest maintains a transmembrane potential approximately 80 to 90 mV negative to the exterior; this gradient is established by pumps, especially the Na⁺, K⁺–ATPase, and fixed anionic charges within cells. There are both an electrical and a

Abbreviations

AF: atrial fibrillation/flutter
4-AP: 4-aminopyridine
AV: atrioventricular
β blocker: β adrenergic receptor antagonist
CPVT: catecholaminergic polymorphic ventricular tachycardia
DAD: delayed afterdepolarization
DC: direct current
EAD: early afterdepolarization
ECG: electrocardiogram
ERP: effective refractory period
GX: glycine xylidide
HERG: human ether-a-go-go related gene
ICD: implantable cardioverter-defibrillator
IV: intravenous
LQTS: long QT syndrome
LV: left ventricle
NCX: Na+-Ca2+ exchanger
PSVT: paroxysmal supraventricular tachycardia
RV: right ventricle
RyR2: ryanodine receptor type 2
SA: sinoatrial
SERCA2: SR-Ca2+ ATPase
SR: sarcoplasmic reticulum
VF: ventricular fibrillation
VT: ventricular tachycardia
WPW: Wolff-Parkinson-White

concentration gradient that would move Na+ ions into resting cells (Figure 30–1). However, Na+ channels, which allow Na+ to move along this gradient, are closed in the cardiac cell at rest, so Na+ does not enter normal resting cardiac cells. In contrast, a specific type of K+ channel protein (the inward rectifier channel) remains open at negative resting

potentials. Hence, K+ can move through these channels across the cell membrane at negative potentials in response to either electrical or concentration gradients (Figure 30–1). For each individual ion, there is an equilibrium potential E_x at which there is no net driving force for the ion to move across the membrane. E_x can be calculated using the Nernst equation:

$$E_x = -(RT/FZx) \ln([x]_i/[x]_o) \tag{30-1}$$

where Zx is the valence of the ion, T is the absolute temperature, R is the gas constant, F is Faraday's constant, $[x]_o$ is the extracellular concentration of the ion, and $[x]_i$ is the intracellular concentration. For typical values for K+, $[K]_o = 4$ mM and $[K]_i = 150$ mM, the calculated K+ equilibrium potential E_K is –96 mV. There is thus no net force driving K+ ions into or out of a cell when the transmembrane potential is –96 mV, which is close to the resting potential. If $[K]_o$ is elevated to 10 mM, as might occur in diseases such as renal failure or myocardial ischemia, the calculated E_K rises to –70 mV. In this situation, there is excellent agreement between changes in theoretical E_K owing to changes in $[K]_o$ and the actual measured transmembrane potential, indicating that the normal cardiac cell at rest is permeable to K+ (because inward rectifier channels are open) and that $[K]_o$ is the major determinant of resting potential.

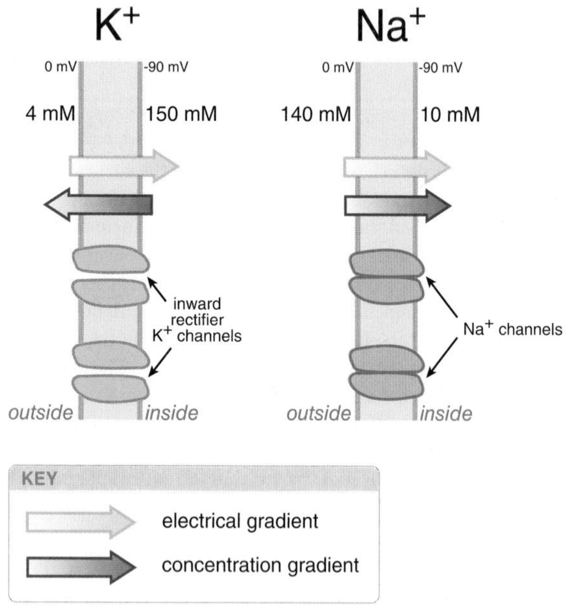

The Cardiac Action Potential

Transmembrane current through voltage-gated ion channels is the primary determinant of cardiac action potential morphology and duration. Channels are macromolecular complexes consisting of a pore-forming transmembrane structure (which may be a single protein, often termed an α subunit, or a multimer), as well as function-modifying β subunits and other accessory proteins. Common features of the pore-forming structure include a voltage-sensing domain, a selectivity filter, a conducting pore, and an inactivating particle (Figure 30–2; see also Figure 22–2). In response to changes in local transmembrane potential, ion channels undergo conformational changes, allowing for, or preventing, the flow of ions through the conducting pore along their electrochemical gradient, generally in time-, voltage-, or ligand-dependent fashion.

To initiate an action potential, a cardiac myocyte at rest is depolarized above a threshold potential, usually via gap junctions by a neighboring myocyte. On membrane depolarization, Na+ channel proteins change conformation from the "closed" (resting) state to the "open" (conducting) state (Figure 30–2), allowing up to 10^7 Na+ ions/s to enter each cell and moving the transmembrane potential toward E_{Na} (+65 mV). This surge of Na+ ions lasts only about a millisecond, after which the Na+ channel protein rapidly changes conformation from the open state to an "inactivated," nonconducting state (Figure 30–2). The maximum upstroke slope of phase 0 (dV/dt_{max}, or V_{max}) of the action potential (Figure 30–3) is largely governed by

Figure 30–1 *Electrical and chemical gradients for K+ and for Na+ in a resting cardiac cell.* Inward rectifier K+ channels are open (left), allowing K+ ions to move across the membrane and the transmembrane potential to approach E_K. In contrast, Na+ does not enter the cell despite a large net driving force because Na+ channel proteins are in the closed conformation (right) in resting cells.

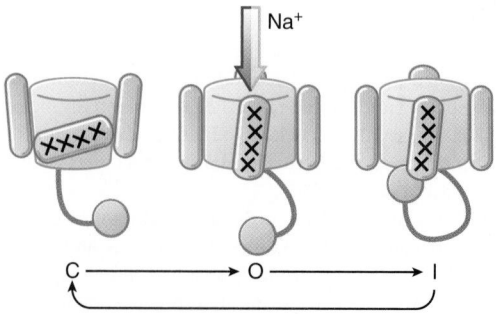

Figure 30–2 *Voltage-dependent conformational changes determine current flow through Na+ channels.* At hyperpolarized potentials, the channel is in a closed conformation, and no current can flow (left). As depolarization begins, the voltage sensor (indicated here as ++++) moves, thus altering channel conformation and opening the pore, allowing conduction (middle). As depolarization is maintained, an intracellular particle blocks current flow, making the channel nonconducting in this inactivated state (right).

Na$^+$ current and is a major determinant of conduction velocity of a propagating action potential. Under normal conditions, Na$^+$ channels, once inactivated, cannot reopen until they reassume the closed conformation. However, a small population of Na$^+$ channels may continue to open during the action potential plateau in some cells (Figure 30–3), providing further inward current, often termed a "late" Na$^+$ current. As the cell membrane repolarizes, the negative membrane potential moves Na$^+$ channel proteins from inactivated to closed conformations, from which they are again available to open and depolarize the cell. The relationship between Na$^+$ channel availability and transmembrane potential is an important determinant of conduction and refractoriness in many cells, as discussed in the material that follows.

The changes in transmembrane potential generated by the inward Na$^+$ current produce, in turn, a series of openings (and in some cases subsequent inactivation) of other channels (Figure 30–3). For example, when a cell is depolarized by the Na$^+$ current, "transient outward" K$^+$ channels quickly change conformation to enter an open, or conducting, state; because the transmembrane potential at the end of phase 0 is positive to E_K, the opening of transient outward channels results in an outward, or repolarizing, K$^+$ current (termed I_{TO}), which contributes to the phase 1 "notch" seen in some action potentials (e.g., more prominent in epicardium than in endocardium). Transient outward K$^+$ channels, like Na$^+$ channels, inactivate rapidly. During the phase 2 plateau of a normal cardiac action potential, inward, depolarizing currents, primarily through L-type Ca^{2+} channels, are balanced by outward, repolarizing currents primarily through K$^+$ ("delayed rectifier") channels. Delayed rectifier currents (collectively termed I_K) increase with time, whereas Ca^{2+} currents inactivate (and so decrease with time); as a result, cardiac cells repolarize (phase 3) several hundred milliseconds after the initial Na$^+$ channel opening.

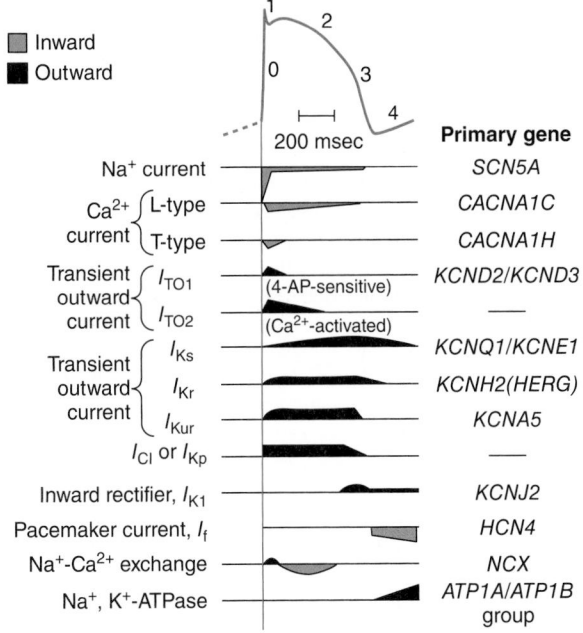

Figure 30–3 *The relationship between an action potential from the conducting system and the time course of the currents that generate it.* The current magnitudes are not to scale; the Na$^+$ current is ordinarily 50 times larger than any other current, although the portion that persists into the plateau (phase 2) is small. Multiple types of Ca^{2+} current, transient outward current I_{TO}, and delayed rectifier I_K have been identified. Each represents a different channel protein, usually associated with ancillary (function-modifying) subunits. 4-AP is a widely used in vitro blocker of K$^+$ channels. I_{TO2} may be a Cl$^-$ current in some species. Components of I_K have been separated on the basis of how rapidly they activate: slowly (I_{Ks}), rapidly (I_{Kr}), or ultrarapidly (I_{Kur}). The voltage-activated, time-independent current may be carried by Cl$^-$ (I_{Cl}) or K$^+$ (I_{Kp}, p for plateau). The genes encoding the major pore-forming proteins have been cloned for most of the channels shown here and are listed in the right-hand column.

A common mechanism whereby drugs prolong cardiac action potentials and provoke arrhythmias is inhibition of a specific delayed rectifier current, I_{Kr}, generated by expression of *KCNH2* (formerly termed the *HERG*). The ion channel protein generated by *KCNH2* expression differs from other ion channels in important structural features that make it much more susceptible to drug block; understanding these structural constraints is an important first step to designing drugs lacking I_{Kr}-blocking properties (Mitcheson et al., 2000). Avoiding I_{Kr}/*KCNH2* channel block has become a major issue in drug development (Roden, 2004).

Maintenance of Intracellular Ion Homeostasis

With each action potential, the cell interior gains Na$^+$ ions and loses K$^+$ ions. An ATP-requiring Na$^+$-K$^+$ exchange mechanism, or pump, is activated in most cells to maintain intracellular homeostasis. This Na$^+$, K$^+$-ATPase extrudes three Na$^+$ ions for every two K$^+$ ions shuttled from the exterior of the cell to the interior; as a result, the act of pumping itself is electrogenic, generating a net outward (repolarizing) current.

Normally, intracellular Ca^{2+} is maintained at very low levels (<100 nM). In cardiac myocytes, the entry of Ca^{2+} during each action potential through L-type Ca^{2+} channels is a signal to the SR to release its Ca^{2+} stores, and thus initiate Ca^{2+}-dependent contraction, a process termed excitation-contraction coupling. The efflux of Ca^{2+} from the SR occurs through ryanodine receptor release channels (RyR2) and subsequent removal of intracellular Ca^{2+} occurs by both SERCA2, which moves Ca^{2+} ions back into the SR, and an electrogenic NCX on the cell surface, which exchanges three Na$^+$ ions from the exterior for each Ca^{2+} ion extruded.

Genetic Arrhythmia Diseases

Rare congenital arrhythmia diseases such as the LQTS and CPVT can cause sudden death due to fatal arrhythmias, often in young subjects. The identification of disease genes not only has resulted in improved care of affected patients and their families but also has contributed importantly to our understanding of the normal action potential, arrhythmia mechanisms, and potential antiarrhythmic drug targets (Keating and Sanguinetti, 2001). For example, mutations in the cardiac Na$^+$ channel gene *SCN5A* can cause one form of LQTS by destabilizing fast inactivation, increasing late Na$^+$ current, thereby prolonging action potentials, and thus the QT interval (as discussed in material that follows). Drugs inhibiting this abnormal current may be antiarrhythmic in this form of LQTS (Remme and Wilde, 2013), and drugs increasing late Na$^+$ current may cause arrhythmias (Yang et al., 2014). Inhibitors may include not only antiarrhythmics such as mexiletine or flecainide discussed in this chapter, but also the antianginal agent ranolazine (see Chapter 28), which appears to be a late Na$^+$ current blocker.

Similarly, mutations in the *RyR2* gene encoding an intracellular Ca^{2+} release channel (or less commonly in other genes regulating RyR2 function) cause CPVT by generating "leaky" RyR2 channels, perturbing intracellular Ca^{2+} homeostasis and causing DAD-dependent arrhythmias described further in this chapter. Drugs such as flecainide and propafenone that inhibit these abnormal RyR2 channels appear to prevent CPVT in mouse models and in humans (Watanabe et al., 2009). Intriguingly, some arrhythmias in acquired heart disease have been attributed to increased late Na$^+$ current or leaky RyR2 channels. Thus, studies in the rare congenital arrhythmia syndromes may point to new avenues for drug development in more common arrhythmias in acquired heart disease (Knollmann and Roden, 2008 Priori et al., 1999).

Action Potential Heterogeneity in the Heart

The general description of the action potential and the currents that underlie it must be modified for certain cell types (Figure 30–4), primarily due to variability in the expression of ion channels and electrogenic ion transport pumps. The resultant diversity of action potentials in different regions of the heart plays a role in understanding the pharmacological profiles of antiarrhythmic drugs. In the ventricle, action potential duration varies across the wall of each chamber, as well as apicobasally, largely as a consequence of varying densities of repolarizing currents. In the

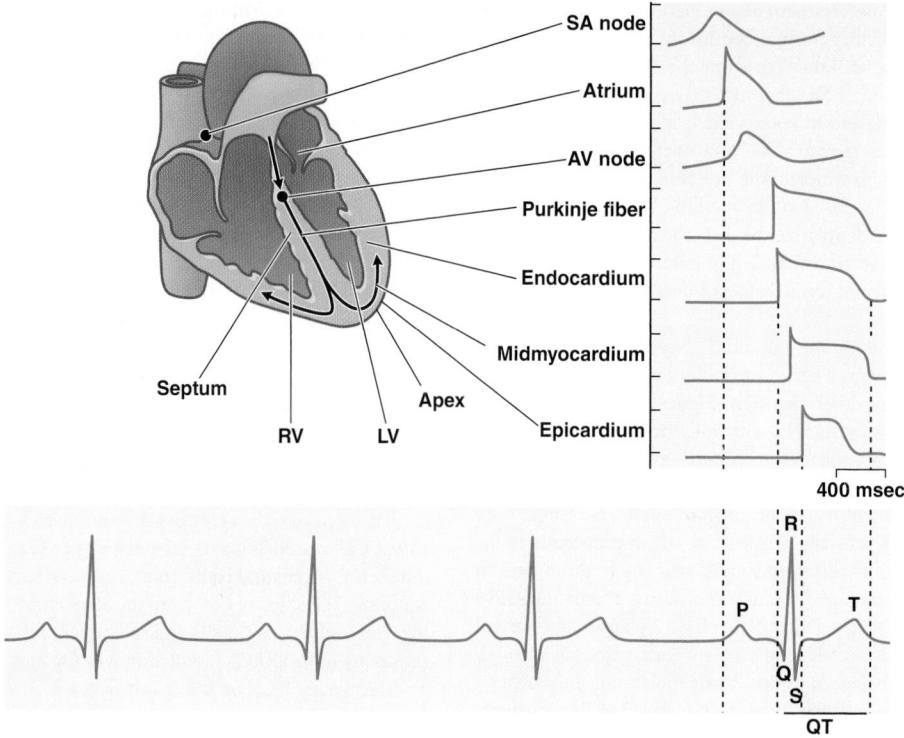

Figure 30–4 *Normal impulse propagation.* A schematic of the human heart with example action potentials from different regions of the heart (top) for a normal beat and their corresponding contributions to the macroscopic ECG (bottom). (Reproduced with permission from Nerbonne JM, Kass RS. Molecular physiology of cardiac repolarization. *Physiol Rev*, **2005**, 85:1205–1253. Used with permission of the American Physiological Society.)

neighboring His-Purkinje conduction system, action potentials are longer, probably due to decreased K⁺ currents, increased "late" Na⁺ currents, and differences in intercellular Ca²⁺ handling (Dun and Boyden, 2008).

Atrial cells have shorter action potentials than ventricular cells because of larger early repolarization currents such as I_{TO}. Atrial cells also express an additional repolarizing K⁺ channel that is activated by the neurotransmitter acetylcholine and accounts for action potential shortening with vagal stimulation. Cells of the sinus and AV nodes lack substantial Na⁺ currents, and depolarization is achieved by inward current generated by opening of Ca²⁺ channels. In addition, these cells, as well as cells from the conducting system, normally display the phenomenon of spontaneous diastolic, or phase 4, depolarization and thus spontaneously reach threshold for regeneration of action potentials. The rate of spontaneous firing usually is fastest in sinus node cells, which therefore serve as the natural pacemaker of the heart. The slow diastolic depolarization that underlies pacemaker activity is generated by a nonselective channel that conducts both Na⁺ and K⁺ and is activated at hyperpolarized membrane potentials (Cohen and Robinson, 2006). In diseased cells, pacemaker-like activity can arise from spontaneous Ca²⁺ release from the SR, followed by membrane depolarization due to activation of NCX.

Certain ion channels are expressed only in some tissues or become active only under specific pathophysiologic conditions. For example, the T-type Ca²⁺ channel may be important in diseases such as hypertension and play a role in pacemaker activity (Ono and Iijima, 2010). A T-type-selective Ca²⁺ channel antagonist, *mibefradil* was commercially available briefly in the late 1990s but was withdrawn because of concerns over potentially life-threatening pharmacokinetic interactions with many other drugs. A second example is a channel that transports Cl⁻ ions and results in repolarizing currents (I_{Cl}) (Duan, 2013); some of these are observed only in association with pathophysiological conditions. A third example is the K⁺ channel that are quiescent when intracellular ATP stores are normal and become active when these stores are depleted. Such ATP-inhibited K⁺ channel may become particularly important in repolarizing cells during states of metabolic stress such as myocardial ischemia (Tamargo et al., 2004).

Impulse Propagation and the Electrocardiogram

Normal cardiac impulses originate in the sinus node. Impulse propagation in the heart depends on the magnitude of the depolarizing current (usually Na⁺ current) and the geometry and density of cell-cell electrical connections (Kleber and Saffitz, 2014). Cardiac cells are relatively long and thin and well coupled through specialized gap junction proteins at their ends, whereas lateral ("transverse") gap junctions are sparser. As a result, impulses spread along cells two to three times faster than across cells. This "anisotropic" (direction-dependent) conduction may be a factor in the genesis of certain arrhythmias described in the material that follows (Priori et al., 1999).

Once impulses leave the sinus node, they propagate rapidly throughout the atria, resulting in atrial systole and the P wave of the surface ECG (Figure 30–4). Propagation slows markedly through the AV node, where the inward current (through Ca²⁺ channels) is much smaller than the Na⁺ current in atria, ventricles, or the subendocardial conducting system. This conduction delay, represented as the PR interval on the ECG, allows the atrial contraction to propel blood into the ventricle, thereby optimizing cardiac output.

Once impulses exit the AV node, they enter the conducting system, where Na⁺ currents are larger than in any other tissue, and propagation is correspondingly faster, up to 0.75 m/s longitudinally. Activation spreads from the His-Purkinje system on the endocardium of the ventricles throughout the rest of the ventricles, stimulating coordinated ventricular contraction. This electrical activation manifests itself as the QRS complex on the ECG. Ventricular repolarization is presented on the surface ECG as the T wave. The time from initial depolarization in the ventricle until the end of repolarization is termed the QT interval. Lengthening of ventricular action potentials prolongs the QT interval and may be associated with arrhythmias in LQTS and other settings.

Refractoriness and Conduction Failure

In atrial, ventricular, and His-Purkinje cells, if a restimulation occurs very early during the plateau of an action potential, no Na⁺ channels are available to open, so no inward current results, and no new action potential is generated: At this point, the cell is termed *refractory* (Figure 30–5). On the other hand, if a stimulus occurs after the cell has repolarized completely, Na⁺ channels have recovered from inactivation, and a normal Na⁺ channel–dependent upstroke results with the same amplitude as the previous upstroke (Figure 30–5A). When a stimulus occurs during phase 3 of the action potential, the upstroke of the premature action potential is slower and of smaller magnitude. The magnitude depends on the number of Na⁺ channels that have recovered from inactivation (Figure 30–5A), which in turn is dependent on the membrane potential. Thus, refractoriness is determined by the voltage-dependent recovery of Na⁺ channels from inactivation.

Refractoriness frequently is measured by assessing whether premature stimuli applied to tissue preparations (or the whole heart) result in propagated impulses. While the magnitude of the Na⁺ current is one major determinant of propagation of premature beats, cellular geometry also is important in multicellular preparations. Propagation from cell to cell requires current flow from the first site of activation and consequently can fail if inward current is insufficient to drive activation in many neighboring cells. The *ERP* is the longest interval at which a premature stimulus fails to generate a propagated response and often is used to describe drug effects in intact tissue.

The situation is different in tissue whose depolarization is largely controlled by Ca²⁺ channel current, such as the AV node. Because Ca²⁺ channels have a slower recovery from inactivation, these tissues are often referred to as *slow response* (Figure 30–5C), in contrast to *fast response* in the remaining cardiac tissues. Even after a Ca²⁺ channel–dependent action potential has repolarized to its initial resting potential, not all Ca²⁺ channels are available for reexcitation. Therefore, an extra stimulus applied shortly after repolarization is complete generates a reduced Ca²⁺ current, which may propagate slowly to adjacent cells prior to extinction. An extra stimulus applied later will result in a larger Ca²⁺ current

and faster propagation. Thus, in Ca²⁺ channel–dependent tissues, which include not only the AV node but also tissues whose underlying characteristics have been altered by factors such as myocardial ischemia, refractoriness is prolonged, and propagation occurs slowly. Conduction that exhibits such dependence on the timing of premature stimuli is termed *decremental*. Slow conduction in the heart, a critical factor in the genesis of reentrant arrhythmias (see further discussion), also can occur when Na⁺ currents are depressed by disease or membrane depolarization (e.g., elevated [K]ₒ), resulting in decreased steady-state Na⁺ channel availability (Figure 30–5B).

Mechanisms of Cardiac Arrhythmias

An arrhythmia is by definition a perturbation of the normal sequence of impulse initiation and propagation. Failure of impulse initiation, in the sinus node, may result in slow heart rates (bradyarrhythmias), whereas failure in the normal propagation of action potentials from atrium to ventricle results in dropped beats (commonly referred to as heart block) and usually reflects an abnormality in either the AV node or the His-Purkinje system. These abnormalities may be caused by drugs (Table 30–1) or by structural heart disease; in the latter case, permanent cardiac pacing may be required.

Abnormally rapid heart rhythms (tachyarrhythmias) are common clinical problems that may be treated with antiarrhythmic drugs. Three major underlying mechanisms have been identified: enhanced automaticity, triggered automaticity, and reentry. These are often interrelated mechanisms as abnormal beats arising from one mechanism can elicit a second; for example, a triggered automatic beat can initiate reentry.

Enhanced Automaticity

Enhanced automaticity may occur in cells that normally display spontaneous diastolic depolarization—the sinus and AV nodes and the His-Purkinje system. β Adrenergic stimulation, hypokalemia, and mechanical stretch of cardiac muscle cells increase phase 4 slope and so accelerate pacemaker rate, whereas *acetylcholine* reduces pacemaker rate both by decreasing phase 4 slope and by hyperpolarization (making the maximum diastolic potential more negative). In addition, automatic behavior may occur in sites that ordinarily lack spontaneous pacemaker activity; for example, depolarization of ventricular cells (e.g., by ischemia) may produce "abnormal" automaticity. When impulses propagate from a region of enhanced normal or abnormal automaticity to excite the rest of the heart, more complex arrhythmias may result from the induction of reentry.

Afterdepolarizations and Triggered Automaticity

Under some pathophysiological conditions, a normal cardiac action potential may be interrupted or followed by an abnormal depolarization (Figure 30–6). If this abnormal depolarization reaches threshold, it may, in turn, give rise to secondary upstrokes that can propagate and create abnormal rhythms. These abnormal secondary upstrokes occur only after an initial normal, or "triggering," upstroke and thus are termed *triggered rhythms*.

Two major forms of triggered rhythms are recognized. In the first case, under conditions of intracellular or SR Ca²⁺ overload (e.g., myocardial ischemia, adrenergic stress, digitalis intoxication, or CPVT), a normal action potential may be followed by a *DAD* (Figure 30–6A); as discussed previously, enhanced NCX current is thought to be a common mechanism underlying DADs. If this afterdepolarization reaches threshold, a secondary triggered beat or beats may occur. DAD amplitude is increased in vitro by rapid pacing, and clinical arrhythmias thought to correspond to DAD-mediated triggered beats are more frequent when the underlying cardiac rate is rapid (Priori et al., 1999).

In the second type of triggered activity, the key abnormality is marked prolongation of the cardiac action potential. When this occurs, phase 3 repolarization may be interrupted by an EAD (Figure 30–6B). EAD-mediated triggering in vitro and clinical arrhythmias are most common when the

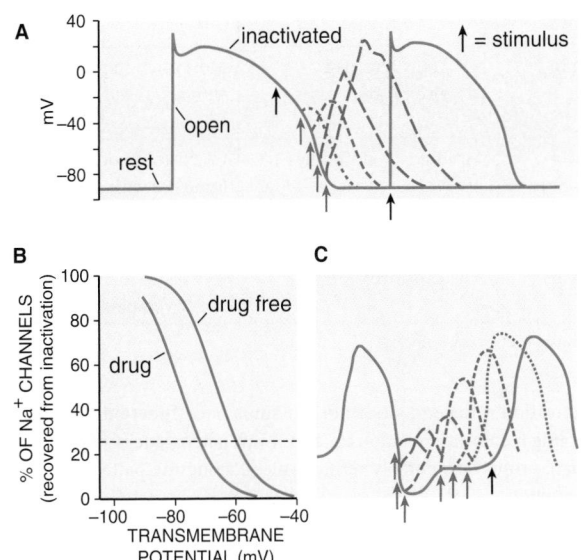

Figure 30–5 *Qualitative differences in responses of nodal and conducting tissues to premature stimuli.* **A.** With a very early premature stimulus (black arrow) in ventricular myocardium, all Na⁺ channels still are in the inactivated state, and no upstroke results. As the action potential repolarizes, Na⁺ channels recover from the inactivated to the resting state, from which opening can occur. The phase 0 upstroke slopes of the premature action potentials (purple) are greater with later stimuli because recovery from inactivation is voltage-dependent. **B.** The relationship between transmembrane potential and degree of recovery of Na⁺ channels from inactivation. The dotted line indicates 25% recovery. Most Na⁺ channel–blocking drugs shift this relationship to the left. **C.** In Ca²⁺-dependent slow-response tissues such as the AV node, premature stimuli delivered even after full repolarization of the action potential are depressed; recovery from inactivation is time-dependent.

TABLE 30–1 ■ DRUG-INDUCED CARDIAC ARRHYTHMIAS

ARRHYTHMIA	DRUG	LIKELY MECHANISM	TREATMENT*	CLINICAL FEATURES
Sinus bradycardia, AV block	Digoxin	↑Vagal tone	Antidigoxin antibodies, temporary pacing	Atrial tachycardia may also be present
Sinus bradycardia, AV block	Verapamil, diltiazem	Ca^{2+} channel block	Ca^{2+}, temporary pacing	
Sinus bradycardia	β Blockers	Sympatholytic	Isoproterenol	
AV block	Clonidine Methyldopa		Temporary pacing	
Sinus tachycardia Any other tachycardia	β Blocker withdrawal	Upregulation of β receptors with chronic therapy; β blocker withdrawal →↑β effects	β Blockade	Hypertension, angina also possible
↑Ventricular rate in atrial flutter	Quinidine Flecainide Propafenone	Conduction slowing in atrium, with enhanced (quinidine) or unaltered AV conduction	AV nodal blockers	QRS complexes often widened at fast rates
↑Ventricular rate in atrial fibrillation in patients with WPW syndrome	Digoxin Verapamil	↓ Accessory pathway refractoriness	IV procainamide DC cardioversion	Ventricular rate can exceed 300 beats/min
Multifocal atrial tachycardia	Theophylline	↑Intracellular Ca^{2+} and DADs	Withdraw theophylline ?Verapamil	Often in advanced lung disease
Polymorphic VT with ↑QT interval (torsades de pointes)	Quinidine Sotalol Procainamide Disopyramide Dofetilide Ibutilide "Noncardioactive" drugs (see text) Amiodarone (rare)	EAD-related triggered activity	Cardiac pacing Isoproterenol Magnesium	Hypokalemia, bradycardia frequent Related to ↑ plasma concentrations, except for quinidine
Frequent or difficult to terminate VT ("incessant" VT)	Flecainide Propafenone Quinidine (rarer)	Conduction slowing in reentrant circuits	Na^+ bolus reported effective in some cases	Most often in patients with advanced myocardial scarring
Atrial tachycardia with AV block; ventricular bigeminy, others	Digoxin	DAD-related triggered activity (± ↑ vagal tone)	Antidigoxin antibodies	Coexistence of abnormal impulses with abnormal sinus or AV nodal function
Ventricular fibrillation	Inappropriate use of IV verapamil	Severe hypotension and/or myocardial ischemia	Cardiac resuscitation (DC cardioversion)	Misdiagnosis of VT as PSVT and inappropriate use of verapamil

*In each of these cases, recognition and withdrawal of the offending drug(s) are mandatory ↑, increase; ↓, decrease; ?, unclear.

underlying heart rate is slow, extracellular K^+ is low, and certain drugs that prolong action potential duration (antiarrhythmics and others) are present. EAD-related triggered upstrokes probably reflect inward current through Na^+ or Ca^{2+} channels. Due to their intrinsically longer action potential, EADs are induced more readily in Purkinje cells and in endocardial than in epicardial cells.

When cardiac repolarization is markedly prolonged, polymorphic ventricular tachycardia with a long QT interval, termed *torsades de pointes*, may occur. This arrhythmia is thought to be caused by EADs, which trigger functional reentry (discussed next) owing to heterogeneity of action potential durations across the ventricular wall (Priori et al., 1999). Congenital LQTS, a disease in which *torsades de pointes* causes syncope or death, is most often caused by mutations in the genes encoding the Na^+ channels (10%) or the channels underlying the repolarizing currents I_{Kr} and I_{Ks} (80-90%) (Nerbonne and Kass, 2005).

Reentry

Reentry occurs when a cardiac impulse travels in a path such as to return to its original site and reactivate the original site, thus perpetuating rapid reactivation independent of normal sinus node function. Key features enabling reentrant excitation are a pathway; heterogeneity of electrophysiologic properties, notably refractoriness, along the pathway; and slow conduction.

Anatomically Defined Reentry

The prototypical example of reentry is the WPW syndrome in which patients have an accessory connection between the atrium and ventricle (Figure 30–7). With each sinus node depolarization, impulses can excite the ventricle via the normal structures (AV node) or the accessory pathway, and this often results in an unusual and characteristic QRS complex in normal sinus rhythm. Importantly, the electrophysiological properties of the AV node and accessory pathways are different: Accessory pathways usually consist of nonnodal tissue with longer refractory periods and without decremental conduction. Thus, with a premature atrial beat (e.g., from abnormal automaticity), conduction may fail in the accessory pathway but continue, albeit slowly, in the AV node and then through the His-Purkinje system; there the propagating impulse may encounter the ventricular end of the accessory pathway when it is no longer refractory. The likelihood

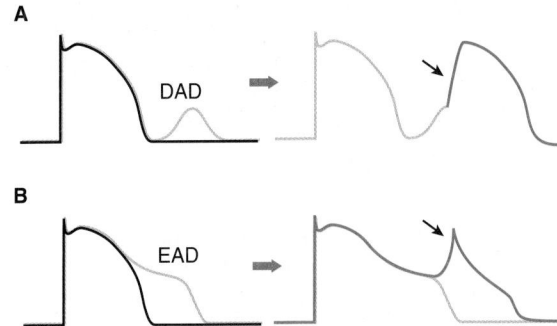

A

DAD

B

EAD

Figure 30–6 *Afterdepolarizations and triggered activity.* **A.** Delayed after-depolarization arising after full repolarization. DADs are typically caused by spontaneous Ca^{2+} release from the SR under conditions of Ca^{2+} overload. The extracytosolic Ca^{2+} is removed from the cytosol by the electrogenic Na-Ca exchanger, which produces Na^+ influx and causes a cell membrane depolarization in the form of a DAD. A DAD that reaches threshold results in a triggered upstroke (black arrow, right). **B.** Early afterdepolarization interrupting phase 3 repolarization. Multiple ion channels and transporters can contribute to EADs (e.g., Na^+ channel, L-type Ca^{2+} channel, Na-Ca exchanger). Under some conditions, triggered beat(s) can arise from an EAD (black arrow, right).

that the accessory pathway is no longer refractory increases as AV nodal conduction slows, demonstrating how slow conduction enables reentry. When the impulse reenters the atrium, it then can reenter the ventricle via the AV node, reenter the atrium via the accessory pathway, and so on (Figure 30–7).

Reentry of this type, referred to as *AV reentrant tachycardia*, is determined by the following:

1. The presence of an anatomically defined circuit
2. Heterogeneity in refractoriness among regions in the circuit
3. Slow conduction in one part of the circuit

Similar "anatomically defined" reentry commonly occurs in the region of the AV node (*AV nodal reentrant tachycardia*), in the atrium (*atrial flutter*), and in scarred ventricle (*ventricular tachycardia*). The term *PSVT* includes both AV reentry and AV nodal reentry, which share many clinical features.

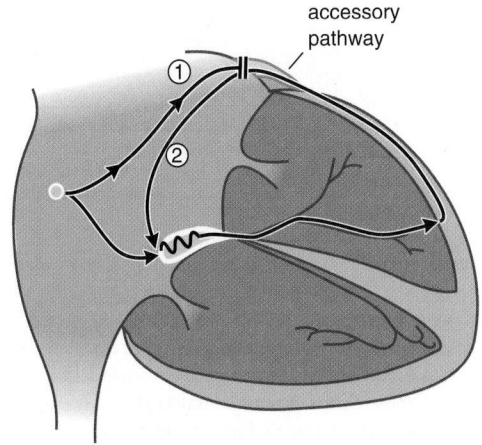

accessory
pathway

① ②

Figure 30–7 *Atrioventricular reentrant tachycardia in the WPW syndrome.* In these patients, an accessory AV connection is present (light blue). A premature atrial impulse blocks in the accessory pathway (1) and propagates slowly through the AV node and conducting system. On reaching the accessory pathway (by now no longer refractory), the impulse reenters the atrium (2), where it then can reenter the ventricle via the AV node and become self-sustaining (see Figure 30–9C). AV nodal blocking drugs readily terminate this tachycardia. Recurrences can be prevented by drugs that prevent atrial premature beats, by drugs that alter the electrophysiological characteristics of tissue in the circuit (e.g., they prolong AV nodal refractoriness), and by nonpharmacological ablation techniques that selectively destroy the accessory pathway.

While antiarrhythmic drugs or electrical cardioversion are used to terminate reentry acutely (discussed further in the chapter and Table 30–2), the primary therapy for anatomically defined reentry is radio-frequency ablation because its consistent pathway often makes it possible to identify and ablate critical segments of this pathway effectively, curing the patient and obviating the need for long-term drug therapy. Radio-frequency ablation is carried out through a catheter advanced to the interior of the heart and requires minimal convalescence.

Functionally Defined Reentry

Reentry also may occur in the absence of a distinct, anatomically defined pathway (Figure 30–8). For example, a premature beat from within the ventricular wall may encounter refractory tissue in only one direction, allowing for conduction throughout the rest of the wall until the originally refractory area recovers, reexcites, and then propagates back through the original location of the premature beat. Another example is localized ischemia or other electrophysiological perturbations that result in an area of sufficiently slow conduction in the ventricle that impulses exiting from that area find the rest of the myocardium reexcitable, in which case reentry may ensue. Atrial fibrillation and VF are extreme examples of "functionally defined" reentry: Cells are reexcited as soon as they are repolarized sufficiently to allow enough Na^+ channels to recover from inactivation. The abnormal activation pathway subsequently provides abnormal spatial heterogeneity of repolarization that can cause other reentrant circuits to form. In atrial fibrillation, these can persist for years, and rotor-like activity can sometimes be recorded, presumably reflecting reentrant circuits that can be transiently stable or meander around the atrium.

Common Arrhythmias and Their Mechanisms

The primary tool for diagnosis of arrhythmias is the ECG. More sophisticated approaches sometimes are used, such as recording from specific regions of the heart during artificial induction of arrhythmias by specialized pacing techniques. Table 30–2 lists common arrhythmias, their likely mechanisms, and approaches that should be considered for their acute termination and for long-term therapy to prevent recurrence. Examples of some arrhythmias discussed here are shown in Figure 30–9. Some arrhythmias, notably VF, are treated not pharmacologically but with DC cardioversion—the application of a large electric current across the chest. This technique also can be used to immediately restore normal rhythm in less-serious cases; if the patient is conscious, a brief period of general anesthesia is required. ICDs, devices that are capable of detecting VF and automatically delivering a defibrillating shock, are used increasingly in patients judged to be at high risk for VF. Often, drugs are used with these devices if defibrillating shocks, which are painful, occur frequently.

Mechanisms of Antiarrhythmic Drug Action

Antiarrhythmic drugs almost invariably have multiple effects in patients, and their effects on arrhythmias can be complex. A drug can modulate other targets in addition to its primary site of action. At the same time, a single arrhythmia may result from multiple underlying mechanisms (e.g., torsades de pointes [Figure 30–9H] can result either from increased Na^+ channel late currents or decreased inward rectifier currents). Thus, antiarrhythmic therapy should be tailored to target the most relevant underlying arrhythmia mechanism, where it is known. Drugs may be antiarrhythmic by suppressing the initiating mechanism or by altering reentrant circuits. In some cases, drugs may suppress an initiator but nonetheless promote reentry (see discussion that follows).

Drugs may slow automatic rhythms by altering any of the four determinants of spontaneous pacemaker discharge (Figure 30–10): (1) increase maximum diastolic potential, (2) decrease phase 4 slope, (3) increase threshold potential, or (4) increase action potential duration. *Adenosine* and acetylcholine may increase maximum diastolic potential, and β blockers (see Chapter 12) may decrease phase 4 slope. Blockade of Na^+ or Ca^{2+} channels usually results in altered threshold, and blockade of cardiac K^+ channels prolongs the action potential.

TABLE 30–2 ■ A MECHANISTIC APPROACH TO ANTIARRHYTHMIC THERAPY

ARRHYTHMIA	COMMON MECHANISM	ACUTE THERAPY[a]	CHRONIC THERAPY[a]
Premature atrial, nodal, or ventricular depolarizations	Unknown	None indicated	None indicated
Atrial fibrillation	Disorganized "functional" reentry Continual AV node stimulation and irregular, often rapid, ventricular rate	1. Control ventricular response: AV node block[b] 2. Restore sinus rhythm: DC cardioversion	1. Control ventricular response: AV nodal block[b] 2. Maintain normal rhythm: K$^+$ channel block, Na$^+$ channel block, Na$^+$ channel block with $\tau_{recovery}$ >1 sec
Atrial flutter	Stable reentrant circuit in the right atrium Ventricular rate often rapid and irregular	Same as atrial fibrillation Same as atrial fibrillation	Same as atrial fibrillation AV nodal blocking drugs especially desirable to avoid ↑ ventricular rate Ablation in selected cases[c]
Atrial tachycardia	Enhanced automaticity, DAD-related automaticity, or reentry in atrium	Adenosine sometimes effective Same as atrial fibrillation	Same as atrial fibrillation Ablation of tachycardia "focus"[c]
AV nodal reentrant tachycardia (PSVT)	Reentrant circuit within or near AV node	AV nodal block[b] Less commonly: ↑ vagal tone (digitalis, edrophonium, phenylephrine)	*AV nodal block Flecainide Propafenone *Ablation[c]
Arrhythmias associated with WPW syndrome: 1. AV reentry (PSVT)	Reentry (Figure 30–7)	Same as AV nodal reentry *DC cardioversion	K$^+$ channel block Na$^+$ channel block with $\tau_{recovery}$ >1 sec *Ablation[c]
2. Atrial fibrillation with atrioventricular conduction via accessory pathway	Very rapid rate due to nondecremental properties of accessory pathway	*Procainamide Lidocaine	K$^+$ channel block Na$^+$ channel block with $\tau_{recovery}$ >1 sec (AV nodal blockers can be harmful)
VT in patients with remote myocardial infarction	Reentry near the rim of the healed myocardial infarction	Amiodarone Procainamide DC cardioversion Adenosine[e]	*ICD[d] Amiodarone K$^+$ channel block Na$^+$ channel block
VT in patients without structural heart disease	DADs triggered by ↑ sympathetic tone	Verapamil[e] β Blockers[e] *DC cardioversion	Verapamil[e] β Blockers[e]
VF	Disorganized reentry	Lidocaine Amiodarone Procainamide Pacing	*ICD[d] Amiodarone K$^+$ channel block Na$^+$ channel block
Torsades de pointes, congenital or acquired; (often drug related)	EAD-related triggered activity	Magnesium Isoproterenol	β Blockade Pacing

*Indicates treatment of choice. [a]Acute drug therapy is administered intravenously; chronic therapy implies long-term oral use. [b]AV nodal block can be achieved clinically by adenosine, Ca^{2+} channel block, β adrenergic receptor blockade, or increased vagal tone (a major antiarrhythmic effect of digitalis glycosides). [c]Ablation is a procedure in which tissue responsible for the maintenance of a tachycardia is identified by specialized recording techniques and then selectively destroyed, usually by high-frequency radio waves delivered through a catheter placed in the heart. [d]ICD, implanted cardioverter–defibrillator: a device that can sense VT or VF and deliver pacing and/or cardioverting shocks to restore normal rhythm. [e]These may be harmful in reentrant VT and so should be used for acute therapy only if the diagnosis is secure.

Antiarrhythmic drugs may suppress arrhythmias owing to DADs or EADs by two major mechanisms:

1. inhibition of the development of afterdepolarizations; and
2. interference with the inward current (usually through Na$^+$ or Ca^{2+} channels), which is responsible for the upstroke

Thus, arrhythmias owing to DADs (i.e., due to *digitalis* toxicity or CPVT) may be inhibited by *verapamil* (which blocks the development of DAD by reducing Ca^{2+} influx into the cell, thereby decreasing SR Ca^{2+} load and the likelihood of spontaneous Ca^{2+} release from the SR) or by Na$^+$ channel–blocking drugs, which elevate the threshold required to produce the abnormal upstroke. In CPVT, more effective than *verapamil* is combined RyR2 and Na$^+$ channel block by agents such as *flecainide* or *propafenone*. Similarly, two approaches are used in arrhythmias related to EAD-triggered beats (Tables 30–1 and 30–2). EADs can be inhibited by shortening action potential duration; in practice, heart rate is

accelerated by *isoproterenol* infusion or by pacing. Triggered beats arising from EADs can be inhibited by Mg^{2+} without normalizing repolarization in vitro or QT interval through mechanisms that are not well understood. In most forms of congenital LQTS, torsades de pointes occurs with adrenergic stress; therapy includes β adrenergic blockade (which does not shorten the QT interval but may prevent EADs) as well as pacing to shorten action potentials.

In anatomically determined reentry, drugs may terminate the arrhythmia by blocking propagation of the action potential. Conduction usually fails in a "weak link" in the circuit. In the example of the WPW-related arrhythmia described previously, the weak link is the AV node, and drugs that prolong AV nodal refractoriness and slow AV nodal conduction, such as Ca^{2+} channel blockers, β blockers, or adenosine, are likely to be effective. On the other hand, slowing conduction in functionally determined reentrant circuits may change the pathway without extinguishing the circuit. In fact, slow conduction generally promotes the development of reentrant

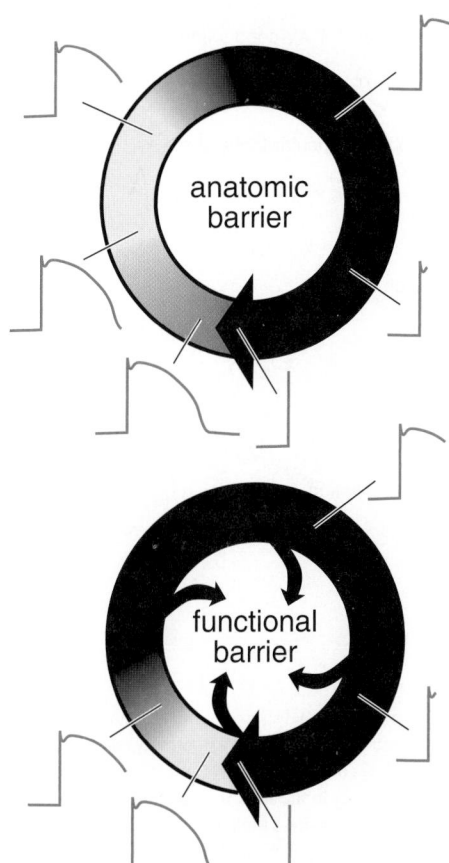

Figure 30–8 *Two types of reentry.* The border of a propagating wavefront is denoted by a heavy black arrowhead. In anatomically defined reentry (top), a fixed pathway is present (e.g., Figure 30–7). The black area denotes tissue in the reentrant circuit that is completely refractory because of the recent passage of the propagating wavefront; the gray area denotes tissue in which depressed upstrokes can be elicited (see Figure 30–5A), and the dark red area represents tissue in which restimulation would result in action potentials with normal upstrokes. The dark red area is termed an *excitable gap.* In functionally defined, or "leading circle," reentry (bottom), there is no anatomic pathway and no excitable gap. Rather, the circulating wavefront creates an area of inexcitable tissue at its core. In this type of reentry, the circuit does not necessarily remain in the same anatomic position during consecutive beats. During mapping of excitation sequences in the heart, this type of activity may be manifest as one or more "rotors."

arrhythmias, whereas the most likely approach for terminating functionally determined reentry is prolongation of refractoriness (Knollmann and Roden, 2008; Priori et al., 1999; Task Force, 1991). In atrial and ventricular myocytes, refractoriness can be prolonged by delaying the recovery of Na⁺ channels from inactivation. Drugs that act by blocking Na⁺ channels generally shift the voltage dependence of recovery from block (Figure 30–5B) and so prolong refractoriness (Figure 30–11).

Drugs that increase action potential duration without direct action on Na⁺ channels (e.g., by blocking delayed rectifier currents) also will prolong refractoriness (Figure 30–11). Particularly in SA or AV nodal tissues, Ca²⁺ channel blockade prolongs refractoriness. Drugs that interfere with cell-cell coupling also theoretically should increase refractoriness in multicellular preparations; *amiodarone*, a drug with a multiplicity of electrophysiologic actions that may be antiarrhythmic, may exert this effect in diseased tissue. Acceleration of conduction in an area of slow conduction also could inhibit reentry; *lidocaine* may exert such an effect, and peptides that suppress experimental arrhythmias by increasing gap junction conductance have been described. Arrhythmia-prone hearts often display abnormal anatomy and histology, notably enhanced fibrosis, and some evidence suggests anti-inflammatory or antifibrotic

State-Dependent Ion Channel Block

Knowing the structural and molecular determinants of ion channel permeation and drug block has provided key information for analyzing the actions of available and new antiarrhythmic compounds (MacKinnon, 2003). A key concept is that ion channel–blocking drugs bind to specific sites on the ion channel proteins to modify function (e.g., decrease current). The affinity of the ion channel protein for the drug on its target site generally varies as the ion channel protein shuttles among functional conformations (or ion channel "states"; see Figure 30–2). Physicochemical characteristics, such as molecular weight and lipid solubility, are important determinants of this state-dependent binding. State-dependent binding has been studied most extensively in the case of Na⁺ channel–blocking drugs. Most useful agents of this type block open or inactivated Na⁺ channels and have little affinity for channels in the resting state. Most Na⁺ channel blockers bind to a local anesthetic binding site in the pore of Nav1.5 (Fozzard et al., 2005). Thus, during each action potential, drugs bind to Na⁺ channels and block them, and with each diastolic interval, drugs dissociate, and the block is released. Allosteric mechanisms have also been described whereby drug binding to a site distant from the pore nevertheless alters channel conformation and thus permeation though the pore.

As illustrated in Figure 30–12, the dissociation rate is a key determinant of steady-state block of Na⁺ channels. When heart rate increases, the time available for dissociation decreases, and steady-state Na⁺ channel block increases. The rate of recovery from block also slows as cells are depolarized, as in ischemia. This explains the finding that Na⁺ channel blockers depress Na⁺ current, and hence conduction, to a greater extent in ischemic tissues than in normal tissues. Open- versus inactivated-state block also may be important in determining the effects of some drugs. Increased action potential duration, which results in a relative increase in time spent in the inactivated state, may increase block by drugs that bind to inactivated channels, such as lidocaine or amiodarone.

The rate of recovery from block often is expressed as a time constant ($\tau_{recovery}$, the time required to complete approximately 63% of an exponentially determined process to be complete). In the case of drugs such as lidocaine, $\tau_{recovery}$ is so short (<<1 sec) that recovery from block is very rapid, and substantial Na⁺ channel block occurs only in rapidly driven tissues, particularly in ischemia. Conversely, drugs such as *flecainide* have such long $\tau_{recovery}$ values (>10 sec) that roughly the same numbers of Na⁺ channels are blocked during systole and diastole. As a result, slowing of conduction occurs even in normal tissues at normal rates.

Classifying Antiarrhythmic Drugs

Classifying drugs by common electrophysiological properties emphasizes the connection between basic electrophysiological actions and antiarrhythmic effects (Vaughan Williams, 1992). To the extent that the clinical actions of drugs can be predicted from their basic electrophysiological properties, such classification schemes have merit. However, as each compound is better characterized in a range of in vitro and in vivo test systems, it becomes apparent that differences in pharmacological effects occur even among drugs that share the same classification, some of which may be responsible for the observed clinical differences in responses to drugs of the same broad "class" (Table 30–3).

An alternative way of approaching antiarrhythmic therapy is to attempt to classify arrhythmia mechanisms and then to target drug therapy to the electrophysiological mechanism most likely to terminate or prevent the arrhythmia (Priori et al., 1999; Task Force, 1991) (Table 30–2). This approach has been further enhanced by an increasing understanding of arrhythmia mechanisms in genetic diseases such as LQTS and CPVT, so a genetic framework represents a complementary approach for improving antiarrhythmic drug development and therapy (Knollmann and Roden, 2008).

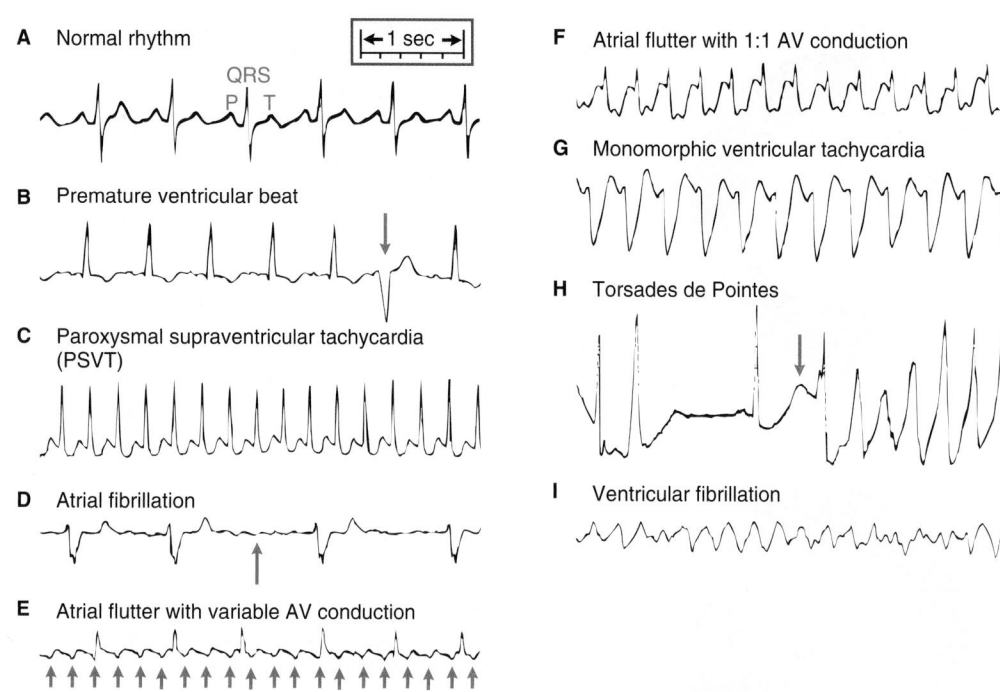

Figure 30–9 *Electrocardiograms showing normal and abnormal cardiac rhythms.* The P, QRS, and T waves in normal sinus rhythm are shown in panel **A**. Panel **B** shows a premature beat arising in the ventricle (arrow). PSVT is shown in panel **C**; this is most likely reentry using an accessory pathway (see Figure 30–7) or reentry within or near the AV node. In atrial fibrillation (panel **D**), there are no P waves, and the QRS complexes occur irregularly (and at a slow rate in this example); electrical activity between QRS complexes shows small undulations (arrow) corresponding to fibrillatory activity in the atria. In atrial flutter (panel **E**), the atria beat rapidly, approximately 250 beats/min (arrows) in this example, and the ventricular rate is variable. If a drug that slows the rate of atrial flutter is administered, 1:1 AV conduction (panel **F**) can occur. In monomorphic VT (panel **G**), identical wide QRS complexes occur at a regular rate, 180 beats per min. The electrocardiographic features of the torsades de pointes syndrome (panel **H**) include a very long QT interval (>600 ms in this example, arrow) and VT in which each successive beat has a different morphology (polymorphic VT). Panel **I** shows the disorganized electrical activity characteristic of VF.

Na⁺ Channel Block

The extent of Na⁺ channel block depends critically on heart rate and membrane potential, as well as on drug-specific physicochemical characteristics that determine $\tau_{recovery}$ (Figure 30–12). The description that follows applies when Na⁺ channels are blocked, that is, at rapid heart rates in diseased tissue with a rapid-recovery drug such as *lidocaine* or even at normal rates in normal tissues with a slow-recovery drug such as *flecainide*. When Na⁺ channels are blocked, threshold for excitability is decreased; that is, greater membrane depolarization is required to open enough Na⁺ channels to overcome K⁺ currents at the resting membrane potential and elicit an action potential. This change in threshold probably contributes to the clinical finding that Na⁺ channel blockers tend to increase both pacing threshold and the energy required to defibrillate the fibrillating heart. These deleterious effects may be important if antiarrhythmic drugs are used in patients with pacemakers or implanted defibrillators. Na⁺ channel block decreases conduction velocity in nonnodal tissue and increases QRS duration. Usual doses of flecainide prolong QRS intervals by 25% or more during normal rhythm, whereas lidocaine increases QRS intervals only at very fast heart rates. Drugs with $\tau_{recovery}$ values greater than 10 sec (e.g., *flecainide*) also tend to prolong the PR interval; it is not known whether this represents additional Ca²⁺ channel block (see discussion that follows) or block of fast-response tissue in the region of the AV node. Drug effects on the PR interval also are highly modified by autonomic effects. For example, *quinidine* actually tends to shorten the PR interval largely as a result of its vagolytic properties. Action potential duration is either unaffected or is shortened by Na⁺ channel block; some Na⁺ channel–blocking drugs do prolong cardiac action potentials but by other mechanisms, usually K⁺ channel block (Table 30–3).

By increasing threshold, Na⁺ channel block decreases automaticity (Figure 30–10B) and can inhibit triggered activity arising from DADs or EADs. Many Na⁺ channel blockers also decrease phase 4 slope (Figure 30–10A). In anatomically defined reentry, Na⁺ channel blockers may decrease conduction sufficiently to extinguish the propagating reentrant wavefront. However, as described previously, conduction slowing owing to Na⁺ channel block may exacerbate reentry. Block of Na⁺ channels also shifts the voltage dependence of recovery from inactivation (Figure 30–5B) to more negative potentials, thereby tending to increase refractoriness. Thus, whether a given drug exacerbates or suppresses reentrant arrhythmias depends on the balance between its effects on refractoriness and on conduction in a particular reentrant circuit. *Lidocaine* and *mexiletine* have short $\tau_{recovery}$ values and are not useful in atrial fibrillation or flutter, whereas *quinidine, flecainide, propafenone*, and similar agents are effective in some patients. Many of these agents owe part of their antiarrhythmic activity to blockade of K⁺ channels.

Na⁺ Channel Blocker Toxicity

Conduction slowing in potential reentrant circuits can account for toxicity of drugs that block the Na⁺ channel (Table 30–1). For example, Na⁺ channel block decreases conduction velocity and hence slows atrial flutter rate. Normal AV nodal function permits a greater number of impulses to penetrate the ventricle, and heart rate actually may increase (Figure 30–9). Thus, with Na⁺ channel blocker therapy, atrial flutter rate may drop from 300 per min, with 2:1 or 4:1 AV conduction (i.e., a heart rate of 150 or 75 beats per min), to 220 per min, but with 1:1 transmission to the ventricle (i.e., a heart rate of 220 beats per min), with potentially disastrous consequences. This form of drug-induced arrhythmia is especially common during treatment with quinidine because the drug also increases AV nodal conduction through its vagolytic properties; flecainide, propafenone, and occasionally amiodarone also have been implicated. Therapy with Na⁺ channel blockers in patients with reentrant ventricular tachycardia after a myocardial infarction can increase the frequency and severity of arrhythmic episodes. Although the mechanism is unclear, slowed conduction allows the reentrant wavefront to persist within the tachycardia circuit. Such drug-exacerbated arrhythmia can be difficult to

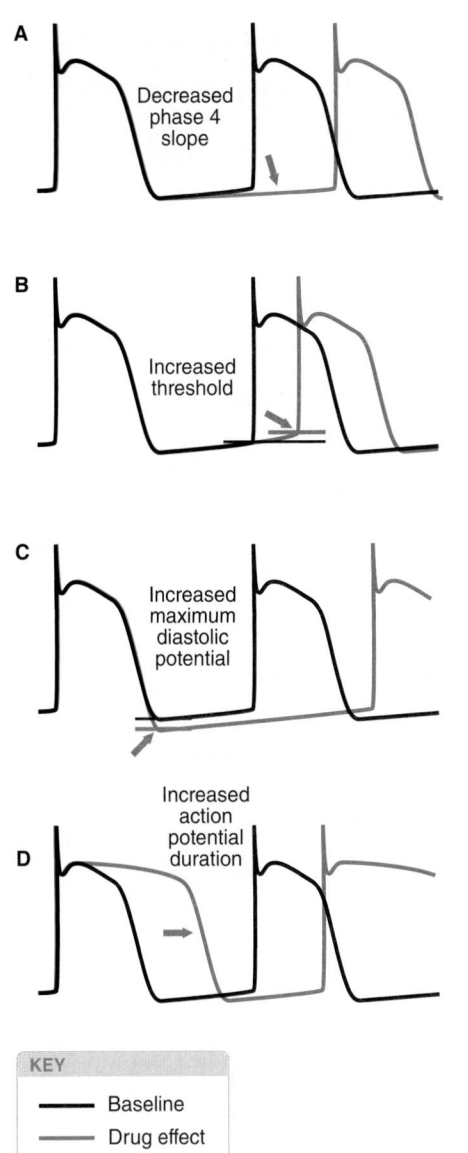

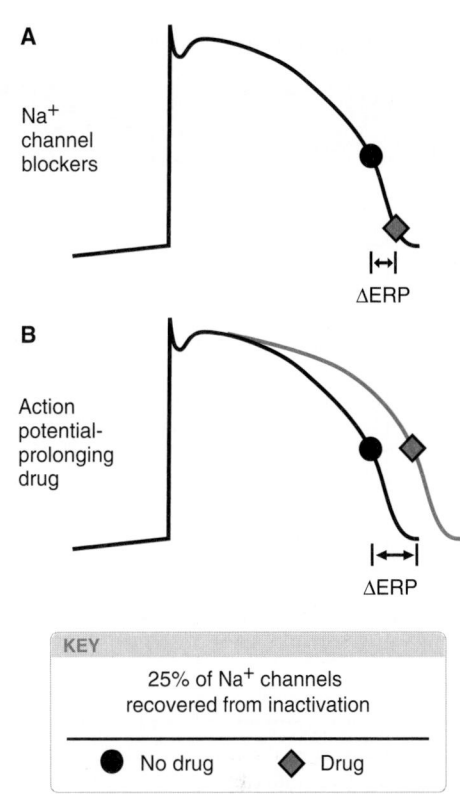

Figure 30–11 *Two ways to increase refractoriness.* In this figure, the black dot indicates the point at which a sufficient number of Na⁺ channels (an arbitrary 25%; see Figure 30–5B) have recovered from inactivation to allow a premature stimulus to produce a propagated response in the absence of a drug. Block of Na⁺ channels (**A**) shifts voltage dependence of recovery (see Figure 30–5B) and so delays the point at which 25% of channels have recovered (red diamond), prolonging the ERP. Note that if the drug also dissociates slowly from the channel (see Figure 30–12), refractoriness in fast-response tissues actually can extend beyond full repolarization ("postrepolarization refractoriness"). Drugs that prolong the action potential (**B**) also will extend the point at which an arbitrary percentage of Na⁺ channels have recovered from inactivation, even without directly interacting with Na⁺ channels.

Figure 30–10 *Four ways to reduce the rate of spontaneous discharge.* The horizontal lines in panels **B** and **C** mark the threshold potentials for triggering an action potential before and after drug application.

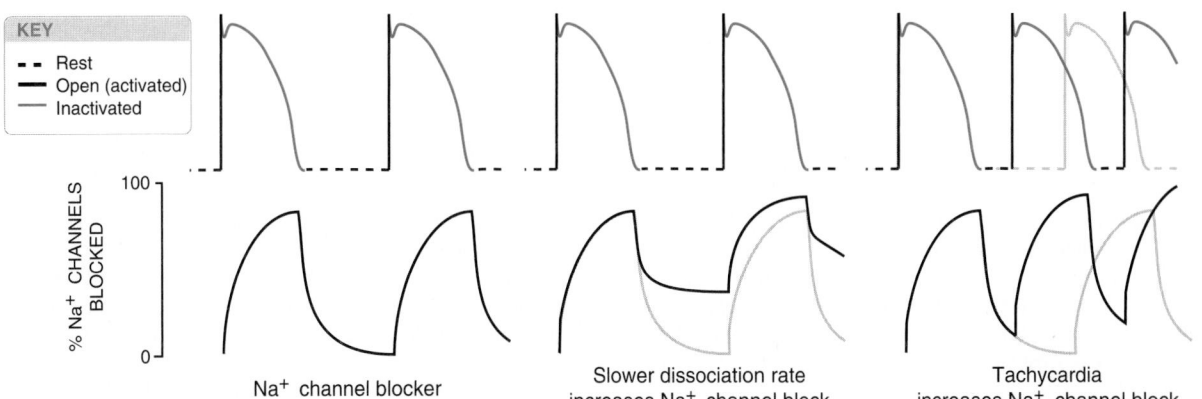

Figure 30–12 *Recovery from block of Na⁺ channels during diastole.* This recovery is the critical factor determining extent of steady-state Na⁺ channel block. Na⁺ channel blockers bind to (and block) Na⁺ channels in the open or inactivated states, resulting in phasic changes in the extent of block during the action potential. As shown in the middle panel, a decrease in the rate of recovery from block increases the extent of block. Different drugs have different rates of recovery, and depolarization reduces the rate of recovery. The right panel shows that increasing heart rate, which results in relatively less time spent in the rest state and also increases the extent of block. (Reproduced with permission from Roden DM, et al. Clinical pharmacology of antiarrhythmic agents. In: Josephson ME, ed. *Sudden Cardiac Death*. Blackwell Scientific, London, **1993**, 182–185.)

SECTION III MODULATION OF PULMONARY, RENAL, AND CARDIOVASCULAR FUNCTION

TABLE 30–3 ■ MAJOR ELECTROPHYSIOLOGIC ACTIONS OF ANTIARRHYTHMIC DRUGS

DRUG	Na⁺ CHANNEL BLOCK		↑APD	Ca²⁺ CHANNEL BLOCK	AUTONOMIC EFFECTS	OTHER EFFECTS
	$\tau_{RECOVERY}$[1], SECONDS	STATE DEPENDENCE[1]				
Lidocaine	0.1	I > O				
Phenytoin	0.2	I				
Mexiletine[a]	0.3					
Procainamide	1.8	O	√		Ganglionic blockade (especially intravenous)	√: Metabolite prolongs APD
Quinidine	3	O	√	(x)	α Blockade, vagolytic Anticholinergic	
Disopyramide[b]	9	O	√		Anticholinergic	
Propafenone[b]	11	O ≈ I	√		β Blockade (variable clinical effect)	√ RyR2 channel block
Flecainide[a]	11	O	(x)	(x)		
β Blockers: Propanolol[b]					β Blockade	Na⁺ channel block in vitro
Sotalol[b]			√		β Blockade	
Amiodarone, dronedarone	1.6	I	√	(x)	Noncompetitive β blockade	Antithyroid action
Dofetilide			√			
Ibutilide			√			
Verapamil[a]				√		
Diltiazem[a]				√		
Digoxin					√: Vagal stimulation	√: Inhibition of Na⁺, K⁺-ATPase
Adenosine					√: Adenosine receptor activation	√: Activation of outward K⁺ current
Magnesium				?√		Mechanism not well understood

√Indicates an effect that is important in mediating the clinical action of a drug. (x)Indicates a demonstrable effect whose relationship to drug action in patients is less well established. [a]Indicates drugs prescribed as racemates, and the enantiomers are thought to exert similar electrophysiologic effects. [b]Indicates racemates for which clinically relevant differences in the electrophysiologic properties of individual enantiomers have been reported (see text). One approach to classifying drugs is:

Class	Major action
I	Na⁺ channel block
II	β blockade
III	action potential prolongation (usually by K⁺ channel block)
IV	Ca²⁺ channel block

Drugs are listed here according to this scheme. It is important to bear in mind, however, that many drugs exert multiple effects that contribute to their clinical actions. It is occasionally clinically useful to subclassify Na⁺ channel blockers by their rates of recovery from drug-induced block ($\tau_{recovery}$) under physiologic conditions. Because this is a continuous variable and can be modulated by factors such as depolarization of the resting potential, these distinctions can become blurred: class Ib, $\tau_{recovery}$ <1 s; class Ia, $\tau_{recovery}$ 1–10 s; class Ic, $\tau_{recovery}$ >10 s. These class and subclass effects are associated with distinctive ECG changes, characteristic "class" toxicities, and efficacy in specific arrhythmia syndromes (see text). [1]These data are dependent on experimental conditions, including species and temperature. The $\tau_{recovery}$ values cited here are from Courtney (1987). O, open-state blocker; I, inactivated-state blocker.

manage, and deaths owing to intractable drug-induced ventricular tachycardia have been reported. In this setting, Na⁺ infusion may be beneficial. Drug-exacerbated ventricular tachycardia or VF also likely accounts for increased mortality with Na⁺ channel blockers compared to placebo in patients convalescing from acute myocardial infarction in the CAST (Echt et al., 1991). Several Na⁺ channel blockers (e.g., *procainamide* and *quinidine*) have been reported to exacerbate neuromuscular paralysis by D-tubocurarine (see Chapter 11).

Action Potential Prolongation

Most drugs that prolong the action potential do so by blocking I_Kr (Roden et al., 1993), although increased late Na⁺ current also produces this effect (Lu et al., 2012; Yang et al., 2014). Both drug effects increase action potential duration and reduce normal automaticity (Figure 30–10D). Increased action potential duration, seen as an increase in QT interval, increases refractoriness (Figure 30–11) and therefore should be an effective way

of treating reentry (Task Force, 1991). Experimentally, K⁺ channel block produces a series of desirable effects: reduced defibrillation energy requirement, inhibition of VF owing to acute ischemia, and increased contractility (Roden, 1993; Singh, 1993). As shown in Table 30–3, many K⁺ channel–blocking drugs also interact with β adrenergic receptors (sotalol) or other channels (e.g., amiodarone and quinidine). Amiodarone and sotalol appear to be at least as effective as drugs with predominant Na⁺ channel–blocking properties in both atrial and ventricular arrhythmias. "Pure" action potential–prolonging drugs (e.g., dofetilide and ibutilide) also are available (Murray, 1998; Torp-Pedersen et al., 1999).

Toxicity of Drugs That Prolong the Action Potential

Most of these agents disproportionately prolong cardiac action potentials and the QT interval when underlying heart rate is slow and can cause torsades de pointes (Table 30–1, Figure 30–9). While this effect usually is seen with QT-prolonging antiarrhythmic drugs, it can occur more rarely with drugs that are used for noncardiac indications. For such agents, the risk of torsades de pointes may become apparent only after widespread use postmarketing, and recognition of this risk has been a common cause for drug withdrawal (Roden, 2004). Sex hormones modify cardiac ion channels and help account for the clinically observed increased incidence of drug-induced torsades de pointes in women (Tadros et al., 2014).

Ca²⁺ Channel Block

The major electrophysiological effects resulting from block of cardiac Ca^{2+} channels are in nodal tissues. Dihydropyridines, such as nifedipine, which are used commonly in angina and hypertension (see Chapters 27 and 28), preferentially block Ca^{2+} channels in vascular smooth muscle; their cardiac electrophysiological effects, such as heart rate acceleration, result principally from reflex sympathetic activation secondary to peripheral vasodilation. Only verapamil, diltiazem, and bepridil (no longer available in the U.S.) block Ca^{2+} channels in cardiac cells at clinically used doses. These drugs generally slow heart rate (Figure 30–10A), although hypotension, if marked, can cause reflex sympathetic activation and tachycardia. The velocity of AV nodal conduction decreases, so the PR interval increases. AV nodal block occurs as a result of decremental conduction, as well as increased AV nodal refractoriness. These effects form the basis of the antiarrhythmic actions of Ca^{2+} channel blockers in reentrant arrhythmias whose circuit involves the AV node, such as AV reentrant tachycardia (Figure 30–7).

Another important indication for antiarrhythmic therapy is to reduce the ventricular rate in atrial flutter or fibrillation. Parenteral verapamil and diltiazem are approved for temporary control of rapid ventricular rate in atrial flutter or fibrillation and for rapid conversion of PSVT to sinus rhythm (where their use has largely been supplanted by adenosine). Oral verapamil or diltiazem may be used to control the ventricular rate in chronic atrial flutter or fibrillation and for prophylaxis of repetitive PSVT. Unlike β blockers, Ca^{2+} channel blockers have not been shown to reduce mortality after myocardial infarction (Singh, 1990). In contrast to other Ca^{2+} channel blockers, bepridil increases action potential duration in many tissues and can exert an antiarrhythmic effect in atria and ventricles. However, because bepridil can cause torsades de pointes, it is not prescribed widely and has been discontinued in the U.S.

Verapamil and Diltiazem

The major adverse effect of intravenous verapamil or diltiazem is hypotension, particularly with bolus administration. This was a particular problem when the drugs were used mistakenly in patients with ventricular tachycardia (in which Ca^{2+} channel blockers usually are not effective) misdiagnosed as PSVT; the drugs are now rarely used for this indication. Hypotension also is frequent in patients receiving other vasodilators and in patients with underlying left ventricular dysfunction, which the drugs can exacerbate. Severe sinus bradycardia or AV block also occurs, especially in susceptible patients, such as those also receiving β blockers. With oral therapy, these adverse effects tend to be less severe. Constipation can occur with oral verapamil.

Verapamil is prescribed as a racemate. L-Verapamil is the more potent Ca^{2+} channel blocker. However, with oral therapy, the L-enantiomer undergoes more extensive first-pass hepatic metabolism. For this reason, a given concentration of verapamil prolongs the PR interval to a greater extent when administered intravenously (where concentrations of the L- and D-enantiomers are equivalent) than when administered orally. Diltiazem also undergoes extensive first-pass hepatic metabolism, and both drugs have metabolites that exert Ca^{2+} channel–blocking actions. In clinical practice, adverse effects during therapy with verapamil or diltiazem are determined largely by underlying heart disease and concomitant therapy; plasma concentrations of these agents are not measured routinely. Both drugs can increase serum digoxin concentration, although the magnitude of this effect is variable; excess slowing of ventricular response may occur in patients with atrial fibrillation.

Blockade of β Adrenergic Receptors

β Adrenergic stimulation increases the magnitude of the Ca^{2+} current and slows its inactivation; increases the magnitude of the repolarizing current I_{Ks}; increases pacemaker current (thereby increasing sinus rate; DiFrancesco, 1993); increases the Ca^{2+} stored in the SR (thereby increasing likelihood of spontaneous Ca^{2+} release and DADs); and under pathophysiological conditions, can increase both DAD- and EAD-mediated arrhythmias. The increases in plasma epinephrine associated with severe stress (e.g., acute myocardial infarction or resuscitation after cardiac arrest) lower serum K^+, especially in patients receiving chronic diuretic therapy. β blockers inhibit these effects and can be antiarrhythmic by reducing heart rate, decreasing intracellular Ca^{2+} overload, and inhibiting afterdepolarization-mediated automaticity. Epinephrine-induced hypokalemia appears to be mediated by β_2 adrenergic receptors and is blocked by "noncardioselective" antagonists such as propranolol (see Chapter 12). In acutely ischemic tissue, β blockers increase the energy required to fibrillate the heart, an antiarrhythmic action. These effects may contribute to the reduced short-term and long-term mortality observed in trials of chronic therapy with β blockers—after myocardial infarction (Singh, 1990).

As with Ca^{2+} channel blockers and digitalis, β blockers increase AV nodal conduction time (increased PR interval) and prolong AV nodal refractoriness; hence, they are useful in terminating reentrant arrhythmias that involve the AV node and in controlling ventricular response in atrial fibrillation or flutter. In many (but not all) patients with the congenital LQTS, in all patients with the CPVT syndrome, as well as in many other patients, arrhythmias are triggered by physical or emotional stress; β blockers may be useful in these cases (Roden and Spooner, 1999; Schwartz et al., 2000). β blockers also reportedly are effective in controlling arrhythmias owing to Na^+ channel blockers; this effect may be due in part to slowing of the heart rate, which then decreases the extent of rate-dependent conduction slowing by Na^+ channel block.

Adverse effects of β blockade include fatigue, bronchospasm, hypotension, impotence, depression, aggravation of heart failure, worsening of symptoms owing to peripheral vascular disease, and masking of the symptoms of hypoglycemia in diabetic patients (see Chapter 12). In patients with arrhythmias owing to excess sympathetic stimulation (e.g., pheochromocytoma or *clonidine* withdrawal), β blockers can result in unopposed α adrenergic stimulation, with resulting severe hypertension or α adrenergic–mediated arrhythmias. In such patients, arrhythmias should be treated with both α and β blockers or with a drug such as labetalol that combines α- and β-blocking properties. Abrupt discontinuation of chronic β-blocker therapy can lead to "rebound" symptoms, including hypertension, increased angina, and arrhythmias; thus, β blockers are tapered over 2 weeks prior to discontinuation of chronic therapy (see Chapters 12 and 27–29).

Selected β Blockers

It is likely that most β blockers share antiarrhythmic properties. Some, such as propranolol, also exert Na^+ channel–blocking effects at high concentrations. Similarly, drugs with intrinsic sympathomimetic activity may be less useful as antiarrhythmics (Singh, 1990). Acebutolol is as effective as quinidine in suppressing ventricular ectopic beats, an arrhythmia that many clinicians no longer treat. Sotalol (see its discussion in a separate section) is more effective for many arrhythmias than other β blockers, probably because of its K^+ channel–blocking actions. Esmolol (see separate discussion that follows) is a β_1-selective agent that has a very short elimination half-life. Intravenous esmolol is useful in clinical situations in which immediate β adrenergic blockade is desired. Some β blockers (e.g., propranolol) are CYP2D6 substrates; thus, efficacy may vary across individuals (Chapter 7). Many clinicians now favor nadolol when β blockade is needed in congenital arrhythmias (CPVT, LQTS).

Principles in the Clinical Use of Antiarrhythmic Drugs

Drugs that modify cardiac electrophysiology often have a very narrow margin between the doses required to produce a desired effect and those associated with adverse effects. Moreover, antiarrhythmic drugs can induce new arrhythmias with possibly fatal consequences. Nonpharmacological treatments, such as cardiac pacing, electrical defibrillation, or ablation of targeted regions, are indicated for some arrhythmias; in other cases, no therapy is required, even though an arrhythmia is detected. Therefore, the fundamental principles of therapeutics described here must be applied to optimize antiarrhythmic therapy.

1. Identify and Remove Precipitating Factors

Factors that commonly precipitate cardiac arrhythmias include hypoxia, electrolyte disturbances (especially hypokalemia), myocardial ischemia, and certain drugs. Antiarrhythmics, including cardiac glycosides, are not the only drugs that can precipitate arrhythmias (Table 30–1). For example, *theophylline* can cause multifocal atrial tachycardia, which sometimes can be managed simply by reducing the dose of theophylline. Torsades de pointes can arise during therapy not only with action potential–prolonging antiarrhythmics but also with other "noncardiovascular" drugs not ordinarily classified as having effects on ion channels (Roden, 2004). The incidence can vary from 1% to 3% in patients receiving sotalol or dofetilide to very rare (<1/50,000) with some noncardiovascular drugs. Drugs with a very wide range of clinical indications have been implicated: These include some antibiotics (including antibacterials, antiprotozoals, antivirals, and antifungals), antipsychotics, antihistamines, antidepressants, and methadone. The website https://crediblemeds.org maintains a list of drugs (and levels of evidence) that have been implicated in this adverse effect.

2. Establish the Goals of Treatment

Some Arrhythmias Should Not Be Treated: The CAST Example

Abnormalities of cardiac rhythm are readily detectable by a variety of recording methods. However, the mere detection of an abnormality does not equate with the need for therapy. This was illustrated in CAST. The presence of asymptomatic ventricular ectopic beats is a known marker for increased risk of sudden death owing to VF in patients convalescing from myocardial infarction. In CAST, patients whose ventricular ectopic beats were suppressed by the potent Na$^+$ channel blocker encainide (no longer marketed) or flecainide were randomly assigned to receive those drugs or placebo. Unexpectedly, the mortality rate was 2- to 3-fold higher among patients treated with the drugs than those treated with placebo (Echt et al., 1991). While the explanation for this effect is not known, several lines of evidence suggest that, in the presence of these drugs, transient episodes of myocardial ischemia or sinus tachycardia can cause marked conduction slowing (because these drugs have a very long $\tau_{recovery}$), resulting in fatal reentrant ventricular tachyarrhythmias.

One consequence of this pivotal clinical trial was to reemphasize the concept that therapy should be initiated only when a clear benefit to the patient can be identified. When symptoms are obviously attributable to an ongoing arrhythmia, there usually is little doubt that termination of the arrhythmia will be beneficial; when chronic therapy is used to prevent recurrence of an arrhythmia, the risks may be greater (Roden, 1994). *Among the antiarrhythmic drugs discussed here, only β adrenergic blockers and, to a lesser extent, amiodarone* (Connolly, 1999) *demonstrably reduce mortality during long-term therapy.*

Symptoms Due to Arrhythmias

Some patients with an arrhythmia may be asymptomatic; in this case, establishing any benefit for treatment will be difficult. Some patients may present with presyncope, syncope, or even cardiac arrest, which may be due to brady- or tachyarrhythmias. Other patients may present with a sensation of irregular heartbeats (i.e., palpitations) that can be minimally symptomatic in some individuals and incapacitating in others. The irregular heartbeats may be due to intermittent premature contractions or to sustained arrhythmias such as atrial fibrillation (which results in an irregular ventricular rate) (Figure 30–9). Finally, patients may present with symptoms owing to decreased cardiac output attributable to arrhythmias. The most common symptom is breathlessness either at rest or on exertion. Occasionally, sustained or frequent tachycardias may produce no "arrhythmia" symptoms (such as palpitations) but will depress contractile function; these patients may present with heart failure due to "tachycardia-induced cardiomyopathy", a condition that can be controlled by treating the arrhythmia.

Choosing Among Therapeutic Approaches

In choosing among available therapeutic options, it is important to establish clear therapeutic goals. For example, three options are available in patients with atrial fibrillation: (1) reduce the ventricular response using AV nodal-blocking agents such as digitalis, verapamil, diltiazem, or β blockers (Table 30–1); (2) restore and maintain normal rhythm using drugs such as flecainide or amiodarone; or (3) decide not to implement antiarrhythmic therapy, especially if the patient truly is asymptomatic. Most patients with atrial fibrillation also benefit from anticoagulation to reduce stroke incidence regardless of symptoms (Dzeshka and Lip, 2015) (see Chapter 32).

Factors that contribute to choice of therapy include not only symptoms but also the type and extent of structural heart disease, the QT interval prior to drug therapy, the coexistence of conduction system disease, and the presence of noncardiac diseases (Table 30–4). In the rare patient with the WPW syndrome and atrial fibrillation, the ventricular response can be extremely rapid and can be accelerated paradoxically with digitalis or Ca^{2+} channel blockers; deaths owing to drug therapy have been reported under these circumstances.

The frequency and reproducibility of arrhythmia should be established prior to initiating therapy because inherent variability in the occurrence of arrhythmias can be confused with a beneficial or adverse drug effect. Techniques for this assessment include recording cardiac rhythm for prolonged periods or evaluating the response of the heart to artificially induced premature beats. It is important to recognize that drug therapy may be only partially effective. A marked decrease in the duration

TABLE 30–4 ■ PATIENT-SPECIFIC ANTIARRHYTHMIC DRUG CONTRAINDICATIONS

CONDITION	EXCLUDE/USE WITH CAUTION
Cardiac	
Heart failure	Disopyramide, flecainide
Sinus or AV node dysfunction	Digoxin, verapamil, diltiazem, β blockers, amiodarone
Wolff–Parkinson–White syndrome (risk of extremely rapid rate if atrial fibrillation develops)	Digoxin, verapamil, diltiazem
Infranodal conduction disease	Na$^+$ channel blockers, amiodarone
Aortic/subaortic stenosis	Bretylium
History of myocardial infarction	Flecainide
Prolonged QT interval	Quinidine, procainamide, disopyramide, sotalol, dofetilide, ibutilide, amiodarone
Cardiac transplant	Adenosine
Noncardiac	
Diarrhea	Quinidine
Prostatism, glaucoma	Disopyramide
Arthritis	Chronic procainamide
Lung disease	Amiodarone
Tremor	Mexiletine
Constipation	Verapamil
Asthma, peripheral vascular disease, hypoglycemia	β blockers, propafenone

of paroxysms of atrial fibrillation may be sufficient to render a patient asymptomatic even if an occasional episode still can be detected.

3. Minimize Risks

Antiarrhythmic Drugs Can Cause Arrhythmias

One well-recognized risk of antiarrhythmic therapy is the possibility of provoking new arrhythmias, with potentially life-threatening consequences. Antiarrhythmic drugs can provoke arrhythmias by different mechanisms (Table 30–1). These drug-provoked arrhythmias must be recognized because further treatment with antiarrhythmic drugs often exacerbates the problem, whereas withdrawal of the causative agent is curative. Thus, establishing a precise diagnosis is critical, and targeting therapies at underlying mechanisms of the arrhythmias may be required. For example, treating a ventricular tachycardia with verapamil not only may be ineffective but also can cause catastrophic cardiovascular collapse.

Monitoring of Plasma Concentration

Some adverse effects of antiarrhythmic drugs result from excessive plasma drug concentrations. Measuring plasma concentration and adjusting the dose to maintain the concentration within a prescribed therapeutic range may minimize some adverse effects. In many patients, serious adverse reactions relate to interactions involving antiarrhythmic drugs (often at usual plasma concentrations), transient factors such as electrolyte disturbances or myocardial ischemia, and the type and extent of the underlying heart disease (Roden, 1994). Factors such as generation of unmeasured active metabolites, variability in elimination of enantiomers (which may exert differing pharmacological effects), and disease- or enantiomer-specific abnormalities in drug binding to plasma proteins can complicate the interpretation of plasma drug concentrations.

Patient-Specific Contraindications

Another way to minimize the adverse effects of antiarrhythmic drugs is to avoid certain drugs in certain patient subsets altogether. For example, patients with a history of congestive heart failure are particularly prone to develop heart failure during *disopyramide* therapy. In other cases, adverse effects of drugs may be difficult to distinguish from exacerbations of underlying disease. Amiodarone may cause interstitial lung disease; its use therefore is undesirable in a patient with advanced pulmonary disease in whom the development of this potentially fatal adverse effect would be difficult to detect. Specific diseases that constitute relative or absolute contraindications to specific drugs are listed in Table 30–4.

4. Consider the Electrophysiology of the Heart as a "Moving Target"

Cardiac electrophysiology varies dynamically in response to external influences such as changing autonomic tone, myocardial ischemia, and myocardial stretch (Priori et al., 1999). For example, myocardial ischemia results in changes in extracellular K^+ that make the resting potential less negative, inactivate Na^+ channels, decrease Na^+ current, and slow conduction. In addition, myocardial ischemia can result in the formation and release of metabolites such as lysophosphatidylcholine, which can alter ion channel function; ischemia also may activate channels that otherwise are quiescent, such as the ATP-inhibited K^+ channels. Thus, in response to myocardial ischemia, a normal heart may display changes in resting potential, conduction velocity, intracellular Ca^{2+} concentrations, and repolarization, any one of which then may create arrhythmias or alter response to antiarrhythmic therapy.

Antiarrhythmic Drugs

Summaries of important electrophysiological and pharmacokinetic features of the drugs considered here are presented in Tables 30–3 and 30–5. Ca^{2+} channel blockers and β blockers are discussed in Chapters 12 and 27 to 29. The drugs are presented in alphabetical order. Prescribing patterns have changed over the past several decades in part because fewer suppliers market older drugs, such as quinidine or procainamide, which are therefore increasingly difficult to obtain, a problem for a small number of patients who may still benefit from treatment (Inama et al., 2010; Viskin et al., 2013).

Adenosine

Adenosine is a naturally occurring nucleoside that is administered as a rapid intravenous bolus for the acute termination of reentrant supraventricular arrhythmias (Link, 2012). Rare cases of ventricular tachycardia in patients with otherwise-normal hearts are thought to be DAD mediated and can be terminated by adenosine. Adenosine also has been used to produce controlled hypotension during some surgical procedures and in the diagnosis of coronary artery disease. Intravenous ATP appears to produce effects similar to those of adenosine.

ADENOSINE

Pharmacological Effects

The effects of adenosine are mediated by its interaction with specific G protein–coupled adenosine receptors. Adenosine activates acetylcholine-sensitive K^+ current in the atrium and sinus and AV nodes, resulting in shortening of action potential duration, hyperpolarization, and slowing of normal automaticity (Figure 30–10C). Adenosine also inhibits the electrophysiological effects of increased intracellular cyclic AMP that occur with sympathetic stimulation. Because adenosine thereby reduces Ca^{2+} currents, it can be antiarrhythmic by increasing AV nodal refractoriness and by inhibiting DADs elicited by sympathetic stimulation.

Administration of an intravenous bolus of adenosine to humans transiently slows sinus rate and AV nodal conduction velocity and increases AV nodal refractoriness. A bolus of adenosine can produce transient sympathetic activation by interacting with carotid baroreceptors; a continuous infusion can cause hypotension.

Adverse Effects

A major advantage of adenosine therapy is that adverse effects are short-lived because the drug is transported into cells and deaminated so rapidly. Transient asystole (lack of any cardiac rhythm whatsoever) is common but usually lasts less than 5 sec and is in fact the therapeutic goal. Most patients feel a sense of chest fullness and dyspnea when therapeutic doses (6 to 12 mg) of adenosine are administered. Rarely, an adenosine bolus can precipitate atrial fibrillation, presumably by heterogeneously shortening atrial action potentials, or bronchospasm.

Clinical Pharmacokinetics

Adenosine is eliminated with a half-life of seconds by carrier-mediated uptake, which occurs in most cell types, including the endothelium, followed by metabolism by adenosine deaminase. Adenosine probably is the only drug whose efficacy requires a rapid bolus dose, preferably through a large central intravenous line; slow administration results in elimination of the drug prior to its arrival at the heart.

The effects of adenosine are potentiated in patients receiving *dipyridamole*, an adenosine-uptake inhibitor, and in patients with cardiac transplants owing to denervation hypersensitivity. Methylxanthines (see Tables 14-7, 40-2, and 40-3, and Figure 40-5) such as theophylline and caffeine block adenosine receptors; therefore, larger-than-usual doses are required to produce an antiarrhythmic effect in patients who have consumed these agents in beverages or as therapy.

Amiodarone

Amiodarone exerts a multiplicity of pharmacological effects, none of which is clearly linked to its arrhythmia-suppressing properties. Amiodarone is a structural analogue of thyroid hormone, and some of its antiarrhythmic

TABLE 30-5 ■ PHARMACOKINETIC CHARACTERISTICS AND DOSES OF ANTIARRHYTHMIC DRUGS

DRUG	BIOAVAILABILITY REDUCED FIRST-PASS METABOLISM	PROTEIN BINDING >80%	RENAL	HEPATIC	OTHER	ELIMINATION[a] $t_{1/2}$	ACTIVE METABOLITE(S)	THERAPEUTIC[b] PLASMA CONCENTRATION	LOADING DOSES	MAINTENANCE DOSES
Adenosine[d]					√	<10 s	√		6-12 mg (IV only)	
Amiodarone		√		√		wk	√	0.5-2 µg/mL	800-1600 mg/d × 1-3 wk (IV: 1000 mg over 24 h)	100-200 mg/day IV: 0.5 mg/min
Digoxin	~80%		√			36 h		0.5-2.0 ng/mL	0.6-1 mg over 12-24 h	0.0625-0.5 mg/24 h
Diltiazem	√			√		4 h	(x)		0.25 mg/kg over 10 min (IV)	5-15 mg/h (IV); 180-360 mg/d in 3-4 divided doses (immediate release); 120-180 mg/24 h (extended release)[e]
Disopyramide	>80%		√	√		4-10 h	(x)	2-5 µg/mL		150 mg/6 h (immediate release); 300 mg (controlled release)[f]
Dofetilide	>80%		√	(x)		7-10 h				0.5 mg/12 h
Dronedarone	√	>98%	√			13-19 h	√			400 mg/12 h
Esmolol					√	5-10 min			0.5 mg/kg over 1 min (IV)	0.05-0.3 mg/kg/min for 4 min (IV)
Flecainide	>80%			√		10-18 h		0.2-1 µg/mL		50-100 mg/12 h
Ibutilide	√						(x)		1 mg (IV) over 10 min; may repeat once 10 min later	
Lidocaine	√	√		√		120 min		1.5-5 µg/mL	50-100 mg administered at a rate of 25-50 mg/min (IV)	1-4 mg/min (IV)
Mexiletine	>80%			√		9-15 h		0.5-2 µg/mL	400 mg	200 mg/8 h
Procainamide	>80%		√	√		3-4 h	√	4-8 µg/mL	500-600 mg (IV), given at 20 mg/min	2-6 mg/min (IV); 250 mg q3h; 500-1000 mg q6h
(N-Acetyl procainamide)	(>80%)		(√)			(6-10 h)		(10-20 µg/mL)		

Drug		Bioavailability			Half-life ($t_{1/2}$)	IV/Acute dosing	Therapeutic range	Oral dosing
Propafenone	√			√	2-32 h		<1 µg/mL	150 mg/8h (immediate release); 225 mg/12h (extended release)
Propranolol	√		√	√	4 h	1-3 mg administered no faster than 1 mg/min, may repeat after 2 min (IV)		10-30 mg q6-8h (immediate release)
Quinidine	>80%	−80%	(x)	√	4-10 h		2-5 µg/mL	648 mg (gluconate) every 8h
Sotalol	>80%		√	√	8 h		<5 µg/mL (?)	80-160 mg/12h
Verapamil	√		√	√	3-7 h	5-10 mg given over 2 min or more (IV)		40-120 mg/6-8h (immediate release)

√ Indicates an effect that affects the clinical action of the drug. (x): metabolite or route of elimination probably of minor clinical importance. aThe elimination $t_{1/2}$ is one, but not the only, determinant of how frequently a drug must be administered to maintain a therapeutic effect and avoid toxicity (Chapter 2). For some drugs with short elimination half-lives, infrequent dosing is nevertheless possible, e.g., verapamil. Formulations that allow slow release into the GI tract of a rapidly eliminated compound (available for many drugs, including procainamide, disopyramide, verapamil, diltiazem, and propranolol) also allow infrequent dosing. bThe therapeutic range is bounded by a plasma concentration below which no therapeutic effect is likely, and an upper concentration above which the risk of adverse effects increases. Many serious adverse reactions to antiarrhythmic drugs can occur at "therapeutic" concentrations in susceptible individuals. When only an upper limit is cited, a lower limit has not been well defined. Variable generation of active metabolites may further complicate the interpretation of plasma concentration data (Chapter 2). cOral doses are presented unless otherwise indicated. Doses are presented as suggested ranges in adults of average build; lower doses are less likely to produce toxicity. Lower maintenance dosages may be required in patients with renal or hepatic disease. Loading doses are only indicated when a therapeutic effect is desired before maintenance therapy would bring drug concentrations into a therapeutic range—that is, for acute therapy (e.g., lidocaine, verapamil, adenosine) or when the elimination $t_{1/2}$ is extremely long (amiodarone). dBioavailability reduced by incomplete absorption. eIndicates suggested dosage using slow-release formulation. IV, intravenous.

actions and its toxicity may be attributable to interaction with nuclear thyroid hormone receptors. Amiodarone is highly lipophilic, is concentrated in many tissues, and is eliminated extremely slowly; consequently, adverse effects may resolve very slowly. In the U.S., the drug is indicated for oral therapy in patients with recurrent ventricular tachycardia or VF resistant to other drugs. In addition, the intravenous form is a first-line drug for management of ventricular tachycardia or VF causing cardiac arrest (Dorian et al., 2002). Trials of oral amiodarone have shown a modest beneficial effect on mortality after acute myocardial infarction (Amiodarone Trials Meta-Analysis Investigators, 1997). Despite uncertainties about its mechanisms of action and the potential for serious toxicity, amiodarone is used widely in the treatment of common arrhythmias such as atrial fibrillation (Roy et al., 2000).

AMIODARONE

Pharmacological Effects

Studies of the acute effects of amiodarone in in vitro systems are complicated by its insolubility in water, necessitating the use of solvents such as dimethyl sulfoxide, which can have electrophysiological effects on its own. Amiodarone's effects may be mediated by perturbation of the lipid environment of the ion channels. Amiodarone blocks inactivated Na^+ channels and has a relatively rapid rate of recovery (time constant ≈ 1.6 sec) from block. It also decreases Ca^{2+} current and transient outward delayed rectifier and inward rectifier K^+ currents and exerts a noncompetitive adrenergic-blocking effect. Amiodarone potently inhibits abnormal automaticity and, in most tissues, prolongs action potential duration. Amiodarone decreases conduction velocity by Na^+ channel block and by a poorly understood effect on cell-cell coupling that may be especially important in diseased tissue. Prolongations of the PR, QRS, and QT intervals and sinus bradycardia are frequent during chronic therapy. Amiodarone prolongs refractoriness in all cardiac tissues; Na^+ channel block, delayed repolarization owing to K^+ channel block, and inhibition of cell-cell coupling all may contribute to this effect.

Adverse Effects

Hypotension owing to vasodilation and depressed myocardial performance are frequent with the intravenous form of amiodarone and may be due in part to the solvent. While depressed contractility can occur during long-term oral therapy, it is unusual. Despite administration of high doses that would cause serious toxicity if continued long term, adverse effects are unusual during oral drug-loading regimens, which typically require several weeks. Occasional patients develop nausea during the loading phase, which responds to a decrease in daily dose.

Adverse effects during long-term therapy reflect both the size of daily maintenance doses and the cumulative dose, suggesting that tissue accumulation may be responsible. The most serious adverse effect during chronic amiodarone therapy is pulmonary fibrosis, which can be rapidly progressive and fatal. Underlying lung disease, doses of 400 mg/d or more, and recent pulmonary insults such as pneumonia appear to be risk factors. Serial chest X-rays or pulmonary function studies may detect early amiodarone toxicity, but monitoring plasma concentrations has not been useful. With low doses, such as 200 mg/d or less as used in atrial fibrillation, pulmonary toxicity is less common (Zimetbaum, 2007). Other adverse effects during long-term therapy include corneal microdeposits (which often are asymptomatic), hepatic dysfunction, neuromuscular symptoms (most commonly peripheral neuropathy or proximal muscle weakness), photosensitivity, and hypo- or hyperthyroidism. The multiple effects of amiodarone on thyroid function are discussed further in Chapter 43. Treatment consists of withdrawal of the drug and supportive measures, including corticosteroids, for life-threatening pulmonary toxicity; reduction of dosage may be sufficient if the drug is deemed necessary and the adverse effect is not life threatening. Despite the marked QT prolongation and bradycardia typical of chronic amiodarone therapy, torsades de pointes and other drug-induced tachyarrhythmias are unusual.

Clinical Pharmacokinetics

Amiodarone's oral bioavailability is about 30%, presumably due to poor absorption. This incomplete bioavailability is important in calculating equivalent dosing regimens when converting from intravenous to oral therapy. The drug distributes into lipid; heart tissue-to-plasma concentration ratios of greater than 20:1 and lipid-to-plasma ratios of greater than 300:1 have been reported. After the initiation of amiodarone therapy, increases in refractoriness, a marker of pharmacological effect, require several weeks to develop. Amiodarone undergoes hepatic metabolism by CYP3A4 to desethyl-amiodarone, a metabolite with pharmacological effects similar to those of the parent drug. When amiodarone therapy is withdrawn from a patient who has been receiving therapy for several years, plasma concentrations decline with a half-life of weeks to months. The mechanisms of amiodarone and desethyl-amiodarone elimination are not well established.

A therapeutic plasma amiodarone concentration range of 0.5 to 2 μg/mL has been proposed. However, efficacy apparently depends as much on duration of therapy as on plasma concentration, and elevated plasma concentrations do not predict toxicity. Because of amiodarone's slow accumulation in tissue, a high-dose oral loading regimen (e.g., 800 to 1600 mg/d) usually is administered for several weeks before maintenance therapy is started. The maintenance dose is adjusted based on adverse effects and the arrhythmias being treated. If the presenting arrhythmia is life threatening, dosages of more than 300 mg/d normally are used unless unequivocal toxicity occurs. On the other hand, maintenance doses of 200 mg/d or less are used if recurrence of an arrhythmia would be tolerated, as in patients with atrial fibrillation, because amiodarone slows the ventricular rate during atrial fibrillation.

Dosage adjustments are not required in hepatic, renal, or cardiac dysfunction. Amiodarone potently inhibits the hepatic metabolism or renal elimination of many compounds. Mechanisms identified to date include inhibition of CYP3A4, CYP2C9, and P-glycoprotein (see Chapters 5 and 6). Dosages of warfarin, other antiarrhythmics (e.g., flecainide, procainamide, and quinidine), or digoxin usually require reduction during amiodarone therapy.

Bretylium

Bretylium is a quaternary ammonium compound that prolongs cardiac action potentials and interferes with reuptake of norepinephrine by sympathetic neurons. In the past, bretylium was used to treat VF and prevent its recurrence; the drug is currently not available in the U.S.

Digoxin

DIGOXIN

Pharmacological Effects

Digitalis glycosides exert positive inotropic effects and have been used in heart failure; now, they are rarely prescribed (see Chapter 29). Their inotropic action results from increased intracellular Ca^{2+}, which also forms the basis for arrhythmias related to cardiac glycoside intoxication. Cardiac glycosides increase phase 4 slope (i.e., increase the rate of automaticity), especially if $[K]_o$ is low. These drugs (e.g., digoxin) also exert prominent vagotonic actions, resulting in inhibition of Ca^{2+} currents in the AV node and activation of acetylcholine-mediated K^+ currents in the atrium. Thus, the major "indirect" electrophysiological effects of cardiac glycosides are hyperpolarization, shortening of atrial action potentials, and increases in AV nodal refractoriness. The last action accounts for the utility of digoxin in terminating reentrant arrhythmias involving the AV node and in controlling ventricular response in patients with atrial fibrillation. Cardiac glycosides may be especially useful in the last situation because many such patients have heart failure, which can be exacerbated by other AV nodal–blocking drugs such as Ca^{2+} channel blockers or β blockers. However, sympathetic drive is increased markedly in many patients with advanced heart failure, so digitalis is not very effective in decreasing the rate; on the other hand, even a modest decrease in rate can ameliorate heart failure.

Similarly, in other conditions in which high sympathetic tone drives rapid AV conduction (e.g., chronic lung disease and thyrotoxicosis), digitalis therapy may be only marginally effective in slowing the rate. In heart transplant patients, in whom innervation has been ablated, cardiac glycosides are ineffective for rate control. Increased sympathetic activity and hypoxia can potentiate digitalis-induced changes in automaticity and DADs, thus increasing the risk of digitalis toxicity. A further complicating feature in thyrotoxicosis is increased digoxin clearance.

The major ECG effects of cardiac glycosides are PR prolongation and a nonspecific alteration in ventricular repolarization (manifested by depression of the ST segment), whose underlying mechanism is not well understood.

Adverse Effects

Because of the low therapeutic index of cardiac glycosides, their toxicity is a common clinical problem (see Chapter 29). Arrhythmias, nausea, disturbances of cognitive function, and blurred or yellow vision are the usual manifestations. Elevated serum concentrations of digitalis, hypoxia (e.g., owing to chronic lung disease), and electrolyte abnormalities (e.g., hypokalemia, hypomagnesemia, and hypercalcemia) predispose patients to digitalis-induced arrhythmias. While digitalis intoxication can cause virtually any arrhythmia, certain types of arrhythmias are characteristic. Arrhythmias that should raise a strong suspicion of digitalis intoxication are those in which DAD-related tachycardias occur along with impairment of sinus node or AV nodal function. Atrial tachycardia with AV block is classic, but ventricular bigeminy (sinus beats alternating with beats of ventricular origin), "bidirectional" ventricular tachycardia (a rare entity), AV junctional tachycardias, and various degrees of AV block also can occur. With severe intoxication (e.g., with suicidal ingestion), severe hyperkalemia owing to poisoning of Na^+, K^+–ATPase and profound bradyarrhythmias, which may be unresponsive to pacing therapy, are seen. In patients with elevated serum digitalis levels, the risk of precipitating VF by DC cardioversion probably is increased; in those with therapeutic blood levels, DC cardioversion can be used safely.

Minor forms of cardiac glycoside intoxication may require no specific therapy beyond monitoring cardiac rhythm until symptoms and signs of toxicity resolve. Sinus bradycardia and AV block often respond to intravenous atropine, but the effect is transient. Mg^{2+} has been used successfully in some cases of digitalis-induced tachycardia. Any serious arrhythmia should be treated with antidigoxin Fab fragments (Digibind, Digifab), which are highly effective in binding digoxin and digitoxin and greatly enhance their renal excretion (see Chapter 29). Serum glycoside concentrations rise markedly with antidigitalis antibodies, but these represent bound (pharmacologically inactive) drug. Temporary cardiac pacing may be required for advanced sinus node or AV node dysfunction. Digitalis exerts direct arterial vasoconstrictor effects, which can be especially deleterious in patients with advanced atherosclerosis who receive intravenous drug; mesenteric and coronary ischemia have been reported.

Clinical Pharmacokinetics

The only digitalis glycoside used in the U.S. is digoxin. Digitoxin (various generic preparations) also is used for chronic oral therapy outside the U.S. Digoxin tablets are incompletely (75%) bioavailable. In some patients, intestinal microflora may metabolize digoxin, markedly reducing bioavailability. In these patients, higher-than-usual doses are required for clinical efficacy; toxicity is a serious risk if antibiotics are administered that destroy intestinal microflora. Inhibition of P-glycoprotein (see further discussion) also may play a role in cases of toxicity. Digoxin is 20% to 30% protein bound.

The antiarrhythmic effects of digoxin can be achieved with intravenous or oral therapy. However, digoxin undergoes relatively slow distribution to effector site(s); therefore, even with intravenous therapy, there is a lag of several hours between drug administration and the development of measurable antiarrhythmic effects such as PR interval prolongation or slowing of the ventricular rate in atrial fibrillation. To avoid intoxication, a loading dose of approximately 0.6 to 1 mg digoxin is administered over 24 h. Measurement of postdistribution serum digoxin concentration and adjustment of the daily dose (0.0625 to 0.5 mg) to maintain concentrations of 0.5 to 2 ng/mL are useful during chronic digoxin therapy (Table 30–5). Some patients may require and tolerate higher concentrations, but with an increased risk of adverse effects.

The elimination half-life of digoxin ordinarily is about 36 h, so maintenance doses are administered once daily. Renal elimination of unchanged drug accounts for about 80% of digoxin elimination. Digoxin doses should be reduced (or dosing interval increased) and serum concentrations monitored closely in patients with impaired excretion owing to renal failure or in patients who are hypothyroid. Digitoxin undergoes primarily hepatic metabolism and may be useful in patients with fluctuating or advanced renal dysfunction. Digitoxin metabolism is accelerated by drugs such as phenytoin and rifampin that induce hepatic metabolism. Digitoxin's elimination half-life is even longer than that of digoxin (about 7 days); it is highly protein bound, and its therapeutic range is 10 to 30 ng/mL.

Amiodarone, quinidine, verapamil, diltiazem, cyclosporine, itraconazole, propafenone, and flecainide decrease digoxin clearance, likely by inhibiting P-glycoprotein, the major route of digoxin elimination (Fromm et al., 1999). New steady-state digoxin concentrations are approached after four to five half-lives (i.e., in about a week). Digitalis toxicity results so often with quinidine or amiodarone that it is routine to decrease the dose of digoxin if these drugs are started. In all cases, digoxin concentrations should be measured regularly and the dose adjusted if necessary. Hypokalemia, which can be caused by many drugs (e.g., diuretics, amphotericin B, and corticosteroids), will potentiate digitalis-induced arrhythmias.

Disopyramide

Disopyramide exerts electrophysiological effects very similar to those of quinidine, but the drugs have different adverse effect profiles. Disopyramide can be used to maintain sinus rhythm in patients with atrial flutter or atrial fibrillation and to prevent recurrence of ventricular tachycardia or VF. Because of its negative inotropic effects, it is sometimes used in hypertrophic cardiomyopathy. Disopyramide is prescribed as a racemate.

Pharmacological Actions and Adverse Effects

The in vitro electrophysiological actions of S-(+)-disopyramide are similar to those of quinidine. The R-(−)-enantiomer produces similar Na^+ channel block but does not prolong cardiac action potentials. Unlike quinidine, racemic disopyramide does not antagonize α adrenergic receptors, but does exert prominent anticholinergic actions that account for many of its adverse effects. These include precipitation of glaucoma, constipation, dry mouth, and urinary retention; the last is most common in males with prostatism but also can occur in females. Disopyramide can cause torsades de pointes and also commonly depresses contractility, which can precipitate heart failure. In patients with hypertrophic cardiomyopathy, this depression contractility may be exploited to therapeutic advantage to decrease dynamic outflow tract obstruction (Sherrid and Arabadjian, 2012).

Clinical Pharmacokinetics

Disopyramide is well absorbed. Binding to plasma proteins is concentration dependent, so a small increase in total concentration may represent a disproportionately larger increase in free drug concentration. Disopyramide is eliminated by both hepatic metabolism (to a weakly active metabolite) and renal excretion of unchanged drug. The dose should be reduced in patients with renal dysfunction. Higher-than-usual dosages may be required in patients receiving drugs that induce hepatic metabolism, such as phenytoin.

Dofetilide

Dofetilide prolongs action potentials and the QT interval by potently blocking the I_{Kr} channel. Increased late Na^+ current, likely due to inhibition of phosphoinositide 3–kinase (Yang et al., 2014), may also contribute. The drug has virtually no extracardiac pharmacological effects. Dofetilide is effective in maintaining sinus rhythm in patients with atrial fibrillation. In the DIAMOND studies (Torp-Pedersen et al., 1999), dofetilide did not affect mortality in patients with advanced heart failure or in those convalescing from acute myocardial infarction. Dofetilide currently is available through a restricted distribution system that includes only physicians, hospitals, and other institutions that have received special educational programs covering proper dosing and in-hospital treatment initiation.

Adverse Effects

Torsades de pointes occurred in 1%–3% of patients in clinical trials where strict exclusion criteria (e.g., hypokalemia) were applied and continuous ECG monitoring was used to detect marked QT prolongation in the hospital. Other adverse effects were no more common than with placebo during premarketing clinical trials.

Clinical Pharmacokinetics

Most of a dose of dofetilide is excreted unchanged by the kidneys. In patients with mild-to-moderate renal failure, decreases in dosage based on creatinine clearance are required to minimize the risk of torsades de pointes. The drug should not be used in patients with advanced renal failure or with inhibitors of renal cation transport. Dofetilide also undergoes minor hepatic metabolism.

Dronedarone

Dronedarone is a noniodinated benzofuran derivative of amiodarone that is FDA-approved for the treatment of atrial fibrillation and atrial flutter. In randomized placebo-controlled trials, it was effective in maintaining sinus rhythm and reducing the ventricular response rate during episodes of atrial fibrillation (Patel et al., 2009). Compared to amiodarone, dronedarone treatment is associated with significantly fewer adverse events, but it is also significantly less effective in maintaining sinus rhythm. Dronedarone decreased hospital admissions compared to placebo in patients with a history of atrial fibrillation (Hohnloser et al., 2009). In other studies, however, the drug increased mortality in patients with permanent atrial fibrillation (Connolly et al., 2011) and in those with severe heart failure (Kober et al., 2008).

Pharmacological Effects

Like amiodarone, dronedarone is a blocker of multiple ion currents, including the rapidly activating delayed-rectifier K^+ current (I_{Kr}), the slowly activating delayed-rectifier K^+ current (I_{Ks}), the inward rectifier K^+ current (I_{K1}), the acetylcholine-activated K^+ current, the peak Na^+ current, and the L-type Ca^{2+} current. It has stronger antiadrenergic effects than amiodarone.

Adverse Effects and Drug Interactions

The most common adverse reactions are diarrhea, nausea, abdominal pain, vomiting, and asthenia. Dronedarone causes dose-dependent prolongation of the QTc interval, but torsades de pointes is rare. Dronedarone is metabolized by CYP3A and is a moderate inhibitor of CYP3A, CYP2D6, and P-glycoprotein. Potent CYP3A4 inhibitors such as ketoconazole may increase dronedarone exposure by as much as 25-fold. Consequently, dronedarone should not be coadministered with potent CYP3A4 inhibitors (e.g., antifungals, macrolide antibiotics). Coadministration with other drugs metabolized by CYP2D6 (e.g., metoprolol) or P-glycoprotein (e.g., digoxin) may result in increased drug concentrations. Dronedarone may cause severe liver injury; the FDA recommends monitoring of hepatic enzymes.

Esmolol

Esmolol is a β_1-selective agent that is metabolized by erythrocyte esterases and so has a very short elimination half-life (9 min). Intravenous esmolol is useful in clinical situations in which immediate β adrenergic blockade is desired (e.g., for rate control of rapidly conducted atrial fibrillation). Because of esmolol's very rapid elimination, adverse effects due to β adrenergic blockade—should they occur—dissipate rapidly when the drug is stopped. Although methanol is a metabolite of esmolol, methanol intoxication has not been a clinical problem. The pharmacology of esmolol is described in further detail in Chapter 12.

Flecainide

The effects of flecainide therapy are thought to be attributable to the drug's very long $\tau_{recovery}$ from Na^+ channel block. Suppression of DADs triggered by RyR2 Ca^{2+} release may also contribute to flecainide's antiarrhythmic effect. In CAST, flecainide increased mortality in patients convalescing from myocardial infarction (Echt et al., 1991). However, it continues to be approved for certain arrhythmias in patients in whom structural heart disease is absent (Henthorn et al., 1991); this includes the maintenance of sinus rhythm in patients with supraventricular arrhythmias, including atrial fibrillation, as well as life-threatening ventricular arrhythmias, such as sustained ventricular tachycardia. Clinical case series suggested long-term flecainide efficacy in two congenital ventricular arrhythmia syndromes: type 3 LQTS due to mutations that cause late Na^+ currents and CPVT due to mutations that cause "leaky" RyR2 SR Ca^{2+} release channels. Supported by data from a recent randomized clinical trial (Kannankeril et al. 2017), flecainide has become the drug of choice for preventing arrhythmias in CPVT patients uncontrolled by β blockers.

Pharmacological Effects

Flecainide blocks Na^+ current and delayed rectifier K^+ current (I_{Kr}) in vitro at similar concentrations, 1 to 2 μM. It also blocks Ca^{2+} currents in vitro. Action potential duration is shortened in Purkinje cells, probably owing to block of late-opening Na^+ channels, but is prolonged in ventricular cells, probably owing to block of delayed rectifier current. Flecainide does not cause EADs in vitro but has been associated with rare cases of torsades de pointes. In atrial tissue, flecainide disproportionately prolongs action potentials at fast rates, an especially desirable antiarrhythmic drug effect; this effect contrasts with that of quinidine, which prolongs atrial action potentials to a greater extent at slower rates. Flecainide prolongs the duration of PR, QRS, and QT intervals even at normal heart rates. Flecainide is also an open channel blocker of RyR2 Ca^{2+} release channels and prevents arrhythmogenic Ca^{2+} release from the SR and hence DADs in isolated myocytes (Hilliard et al., 2010). The RyR2 channel block by flecainide targets directly the underlying molecular defect in patients with mutations in the RyR2 gene and the cardiac calsequestrin gene, which may explain why flecainide suppresses ventricular arrhythmias in patients with CPVT refractory to β blocker therapy (Watanabe et al., 2009; Kannankeril et al, 2017).

Adverse Effects

Flecainide produces few subjective complaints in most patients; dose-related blurred vision is the most common noncardiac adverse effect. It can exacerbate congestive heart failure in patients with depressed left ventricular performance. The most serious adverse effects are provocation or exacerbation of potentially lethal arrhythmias. These include acceleration of ventricular rate in patients with atrial flutter, increased frequency of episodes of reentrant ventricular tachycardia, and increased mortality in patients convalescing from myocardial infarction. As discussed previously, it is likely that all these effects can be attributed to Na^+

channel block. Flecainide also can cause heart block in patients with conduction system disease.

Clinical Pharmacokinetics

Flecainide is well absorbed. The elimination $t_{1/2}$ is shorter with urinary acidification (10 h) than with urinary alkalinization (17 h), but it is nevertheless sufficiently long to allow dosing twice daily (Table 30–5). Elimination occurs by both renal excretion of unchanged drug and hepatic metabolism to inactive metabolites. The latter is mediated by the polymorphically distributed enzyme CYP2D6. However, even in patients in whom this pathway is absent because of genetic polymorphism or inhibition by other drugs (e.g., quinidine or fluoxetine), renal excretion ordinarily is sufficient to prevent drug accumulation. In the rare patient with renal dysfunction and lack of active CYP2D6, flecainide may accumulate to toxic plasma concentrations. Flecainide is a racemate, but there are no differences in the electrophysiological effects or disposition kinetics of its enantiomers. Some reports have suggested that plasma flecainide concentrations greater than 1 μg/mL should be avoided to minimize the risk of flecainide toxicity; however, in susceptible patients, the adverse electrophysiological effects of flecainide therapy can occur at therapeutic plasma concentrations.

Ibutilide

Ibutilide is an I_{Kr} blocker that in some systems also activates an inward Na^+ current (Murray, 1998). The action potential–prolonging effect of the drug may arise from either mechanism. Ibutilide is administered as a rapid infusion (1 mg over 10 min) for the immediate conversion of atrial fibrillation or flutter to sinus rhythm. The drug's efficacy rate is higher in patients with atrial flutter (50%-70%) than in those with atrial fibrillation (30%–50%). In atrial fibrillation, the conversion rate is lower in those in whom the arrhythmia has been present for weeks or months compared with those in whom it has been present for days. The major toxicity with ibutilide is torsades de pointes, which occurs in up to 6% of patients and requires immediate cardioversion in up to one-third of these. The drug undergoes extensive first-pass metabolism, so it is not used orally. It is eliminated by hepatic metabolism and has a $t_{1/2}$ of 2–12 h (average 6 h).

Lidocaine

Lidocaine is a local anesthetic that also is useful in the acute intravenous therapy of ventricular arrhythmias. When lidocaine was administered to all patients with suspected myocardial infarction, the incidence of VF was reduced. However, survival to hospital discharge tended to be decreased, perhaps because of lidocaine-exacerbated heart block or congestive heart failure. Therefore, lidocaine no longer is administered routinely to all patients in coronary care units.

Pharmacological Effects

Lidocaine blocks both open and inactivated cardiac Na^+ channels. In vitro studies suggested that lidocaine-induced block reflects an increased likelihood that the Na^+ channel protein assumes a nonconducting conformation in the presence of drug (Balser et al., 1996). Recovery from block is rapid, so lidocaine exerts greater effects in depolarized (e.g., ischemic) or rapidly driven tissues. Lidocaine is not useful in atrial arrhythmias, possibly because atrial action potentials are so short that the Na^+ channel is in the inactivated state only briefly compared with diastolic (recovery) times, which are relatively long. In some studies, lidocaine increased current through inward rectifier channels, but the clinical significance of this effect is not known. Lidocaine can hyperpolarize Purkinje fibers depolarized by low $[K]_o$ or stretch; the resulting increased conduction velocity may be antiarrhythmic in reentry.

Lidocaine decreases automaticity by reducing the slope of phase 4 and altering the threshold for excitability. Action potential duration usually is unaffected or is shortened; such shortening may be due to block of the few Na^+ channels that inactivate late during the cardiac action potential. Lidocaine usually exerts no significant effect on PR or QRS duration; QT is unaltered or slightly shortened. The drug exerts little effect

on hemodynamic function, although rare cases of lidocaine-associated exacerbations of heart failure have been reported, especially in patients with very poor left ventricular function. For additional information on lidocaine, see Chapter 22 on local anesthetics.

Adverse Effects

When a large intravenous dose of lidocaine is administered rapidly, seizures can occur. When plasma concentrations of the drug rise slowly above the therapeutic range, as may occur during maintenance therapy, tremor, dysarthria, and altered levels of consciousness are more common. Nystagmus is an early sign of lidocaine toxicity.

Clinical Pharmacokinetics

Lidocaine is well absorbed but undergoes extensive though variable first-pass hepatic metabolism; thus, oral use of the drug is inappropriate. In theory, therapeutic plasma concentrations of lidocaine may be maintained by intermittent intramuscular administration, but the intravenous route is preferred (Table 30–5). Lidocaine's metabolites, GX and monoethyl GX, are less potent as Na^+ channel blockers than the parent drug. GX and lidocaine appear to compete for access to the Na^+ channel, suggesting that with infusions during which GX accumulates, lidocaine's efficacy may be diminished. With infusions lasting longer than 24 h, the clearance of lidocaine falls—an effect that may result from competition between parent drug and metabolites for access to hepatic drug-metabolizing enzymes.

Plasma concentrations of lidocaine decline biexponentially after a single intravenous dose, indicating that a multicompartment model is necessary to analyze lidocaine disposition. The initial drop in plasma lidocaine following intravenous administration occurs rapidly, with a $t_{1/2}$ of about 8 min, and represents distribution from the central compartment to peripheral tissues. The terminal elimination $t_{1/2}$ of about 2 h represents drug elimination by hepatic metabolism. Lidocaine's efficacy depends on maintenance of therapeutic plasma concentrations in the central compartment. Therefore, the administration of a single bolus dose of lidocaine can result in transient arrhythmia suppression that dissipates rapidly as the drug is distributed and concentrations in the central compartment fall. To avoid this distribution-related loss of efficacy, a loading regimen of 3 to 4 mg/kg over 20–30 min is used (e.g., an initial 100 mg followed by 50 mg every 8 min for three doses). Subsequently, stable concentrations can be maintained in plasma with an infusion of 1 to 4 mg/min, which replaces drug removed by hepatic metabolism. The time to steady-state lidocaine concentrations is approximately 8–10 h. If the maintenance infusion rate is too low, arrhythmias may recur hours after the institution of apparently successful therapy. On the other hand, if the rate is too high, toxicity may result. In either case, routine measurement of plasma lidocaine concentration at the time of expected steady state is useful in adjusting maintenance infusion rate.

In heart failure, the central volume of distribution is decreased, so the total loading dose should be decreased. Because lidocaine clearance also is decreased, the rate of the maintenance infusion should be decreased. Lidocaine clearance also is reduced in hepatic disease, during treatment with *cimetidine* or β blockers, and during prolonged infusions. Frequent measurement of plasma lidocaine concentration and dose adjustment to ensure that plasma concentrations remain within the therapeutic range (1.5 to 5 μg/mL) are necessary to minimize toxicity in these settings. Lidocaine is bound to the acute-phase reactant $α_1$-acid glycoprotein. Diseases such as acute myocardial infarction are associated with increases in $α_1$-acid glycoprotein and protein binding and hence a decreased proportion of free drug. These findings may explain why some patients require and tolerate higher-than-usual total plasma lidocaine concentrations to maintain antiarrhythmic efficacy.

Magnesium

The intravenous administration of 1 to 2 g $MgSO_4$ reportedly is effective in preventing recurrent episodes of torsades de pointes, even if the serum Mg^{2+} concentration is normal (Brugada, 2000). However, controlled studies of this effect have not been performed. The mechanism of action is unknown because the QT interval is not shortened; an effect on the inward current, possibly a Ca^{2+} current, responsible for the triggered upstroke arising from EADs (black arrow, Figure 30–6B) is possible. Intravenous Mg^{2+} also has been used successfully in arrhythmias related to digitalis intoxication.

Large placebo-controlled trials of intravenous Mg^{2+} to improve outcome in acute myocardial infarction have yielded conflicting results (ISIS-4 Collaborative Group, 1995; Woods and Fletcher, 1994). While oral Mg^{2+} supplements may be useful in preventing hypomagnesemia, there is no evidence that chronic Mg^{2+} ingestion exerts a direct antiarrhythmic action.

Mexiletine

Mexiletine is an analogue of lidocaine that has been modified to reduce first-pass hepatic metabolism and permit chronic oral therapy. The electrophysiological actions are similar to those of lidocaine. Tremor and nausea, the major dose-related adverse effects, can be minimized by taking the drugs with food.

Mexiletine undergoes hepatic metabolism, which is inducible by drugs such as phenytoin. Mexiletine is approved for treating ventricular arrhythmias; combinations of mexiletine with quinidine or sotalol may increase efficacy while reducing adverse effects. In vitro studies and clinical case series have suggested a role for mexiletine (or flecainide; see previous discussion) in correcting the aberrant late inward Na^+ current in type 3 congenital LQTS (Napolitano et al., 2006).

Procainamide

Procainamide is an analogue of the local anesthetic procaine (see Figure 22–1). It exerts electrophysiological effects similar to those of quinidine but lacks quinidine's vagolytic and α adrenergic blocking activity. Procainamide is better tolerated than quinidine when given intravenously. Loading and maintenance intravenous infusions are used in the acute therapy of many supraventricular and ventricular arrhythmias. However, long-term oral treatment is poorly tolerated and often is stopped owing to adverse effects.

Pharmacological Effects

Procainamide is a blocker of open Na^+ channels with an intermediate $\tau_{recovery}$ from block. It also prolongs cardiac action potentials in most tissues, probably by blocking outward K^+ current(s). Procainamide decreases automaticity, increases refractory periods, and slows conduction. The major metabolite, *N*-acetyl procainamide, lacks the Na^+ channel–blocking activity of the parent drug but is equipotent in prolonging action potentials. Because the plasma concentrations of *N*-acetyl procainamide often exceed those of procainamide, increased refractoriness and QT prolongation during chronic procainamide therapy may be partly attributable to the metabolite. However, it is the parent drug that slows conduction and produces QRS interval prolongation. Although hypotension may occur at high plasma concentrations, this effect usually is attributable to ganglionic blockade rather than to any negative inotropic effect, which is minimal.

Adverse Effects

Hypotension and marked slowing of conduction are major adverse effects of high concentrations (>10 μg/mL) of procainamide, especially during intravenous use. Dose-related nausea is frequent during oral therapy and may be attributable in part to high plasma concentrations of *N*-acetyl procainamide. Torsades de pointes can occur, particularly when plasma concentrations of *N*-acetyl procainamide rise to greater than 30 μg/mL. Procainamide produces potentially fatal bone marrow aplasia in 0.2% of patients; the mechanism is not known, but high plasma drug concentrations are not suspected.

During long-term therapy, most patients will develop biochemical evidence of the drug-induced lupus syndrome, such as circulating antinuclear antibodies. Therapy need not be interrupted merely because of the presence of antinuclear antibodies. However, 25%–50% of patients eventually develop symptoms of the lupus syndrome; common early symptoms are rash and small-joint arthralgias. Other symptoms of lupus, including pericarditis with tamponade, can occur, although renal involvement is unusual. The lupus-like symptoms resolve on cessation of therapy or during treatment with *N*-acetyl procainamide (see discussion that follows).

Clinical Pharmacokinetics

Procainamide is eliminated rapidly ($t_{1/2} \sim$ 3–4 h) by both renal excretion of unchanged drug and hepatic metabolism. The major pathway for hepatic metabolism is conjugation by *N*-acetyl transferase, whose activity is determined genetically, to form *N*-acetyl procainamide. *N*-Acetyl procainamide is eliminated by renal excretion ($t_{1/2} \sim$ 6–10 h) and is not significantly converted back to procainamide. Because of the relatively rapid elimination rates of both the parent drug and its major metabolite, oral procainamide usually is administered as a slow-release formulation. In patients with renal failure, procainamide or *N*-acetyl procainamide can accumulate to potentially toxic plasma concentrations. Reduction of procainamide dose and dosing frequency and monitoring of plasma concentrations of both compounds are required in this situation. Because the parent drug and metabolite exert different pharmacological effects, the past practice of using the sum of their concentrations to guide therapy is inappropriate.

In individuals who are "slow acetylators," the procainamide-induced lupus syndrome develops more often and earlier during treatment than among rapid acetylators. In addition, the symptoms of procainamide-induced lupus resolve during treatment with *N*-acetyl procainamide. Both these findings support results of in vitro studies suggesting that it is chronic exposure to the parent drug (or an oxidative metabolite) that results in the lupus syndrome; these findings also provided one rationale for the further development of *N*-acetyl procainamide and its analogues as antiarrhythmic agents (Roden, 1993).

Propafenone

Propafenone is a Na^+ channel blocker with a relatively slow time constant for recovery from block (Funck-Brentano et al., 1990). Some data suggest that, like flecainide, propafenone also blocks K^+ channels. Its major electrophysiological effect is to slow conduction in fast-response tissues. The drug is prescribed as a racemate; while the enantiomers do not differ in their Na^+ channel–blocking properties, *S*-(+)-propafenone is a β adrenergic receptor antagonist in vitro and in some patients. Propafenone prolongs PR and QRS durations. Chronic therapy with oral propafenone is used to maintain sinus rhythm in patients with supraventricular tachycardias, including atrial fibrillation; like other Na^+ channel blockers, it also can be used in ventricular arrhythmias, but with only modest efficacy. *R*-(−) propafenone blocks RyR2 channels and may be an alternative to flecainide in CPVT (Hwang et al, 2011).

Adverse Effects

Adverse effects during propafenone therapy include acceleration of ventricular response in patients with atrial flutter, increased frequency or severity of episodes of reentrant ventricular tachycardia, exacerbation of heart failure, and the adverse effects of β adrenergic blockade, such as sinus bradycardia and bronchospasm (see previous discussion and Chapter 12).

Clinical Pharmacokinetics

Propafenone is well absorbed and is eliminated primarily by CYP2D6-mediated hepatic metabolism (see Chapter 6). In most subjects ("extensive metabolizers"), propafenone undergoes extensive first-pass hepatic metabolism to 5-hydroxy propafenone, a metabolite equipotent to propafenone as a Na^+ channel blocker but much less potent as a β adrenergic receptor antagonist. A second metabolite, *N*-desalkyl propafenone, is formed by non-CYP2D6–mediated metabolism and is a less-potent blocker of Na^+ channels and β adrenergic receptors. CYP2D6-mediated metabolism of propafenone is saturable, so small increases in dose can increase plasma propafenone concentration disproportionately. In "poor metabolizer" subjects, in whom CYP2D6 activity is low or absent, first-pass hepatic metabolism is much less than in extensive metabolizers, and plasma propafenone concentrations will be much higher after an equal dose. The incidence of adverse effects during propafenone therapy is significantly higher in poor metabolizers.

CYP2D6 activity can be inhibited markedly by a number of drugs, including quinidine and fluoxetine. In extensive metabolizer subjects receiving such drugs or in poor metabolizer subjects, plasma propafenone concentrations of more than 1 μg/mL are associated with clinical effects of β adrenergic receptor blockade, such as reduction of exercise heart rate. It is recommended that dosage in patients with moderate-to-severe liver disease should be reduced to approximately 20%–30% of the usual dose, with careful monitoring. It is not known if propafenone doses must be decreased in patients with renal disease. A slow-release formulation allows twice-daily dosing.

Quinidine

As early as the 18th century, the bark of the cinchona plant was used to treat "rebellious palpitations" (Levy and Azoulay, 1994). Studies in the early 20th century identified quinidine, a diastereomer of the antimalarial quinine, as the most potent of the antiarrhythmic substances extracted from the cinchona plant, and by the 1920s, quinidine was used as an antiarrhythmic agent. Quinidine is used to maintain sinus rhythm in patients with atrial flutter or atrial fibrillation and to prevent recurrence of ventricular tachycardia or VF (Grace and Camm, 1998). Quinidine may be especially useful in preventing recurrent VF in unusual congenital arrhythmias syndromes such as Brugada syndrome or short QT syndrome (Inama et al., 2010; Viskin et al., 2013).

QUINIDINE

Pharmacological Effects

Quinidine blocks Na^+ current and multiple cardiac K^+ currents. It is an open-state blocker of Na^+ channels, with a $\tau_{recovery}$ in the intermediate (~3-sec) range; as a consequence, QRS duration increases modestly, usually by 10%–20%, at therapeutic dosages. At therapeutic concentrations, quinidine commonly prolongs the QT interval up to 25%, but the effect is highly variable. At concentrations as low as 1 μM, quinidine blocks Na^+ current and the rapid component of delayed rectifier (I_{Kr}); higher concentrations block the slow component of delayed rectifier, inward rectifier, transient outward current, and L-type Ca^{2+} current.

Quinidine's Na^+ channel–blocking properties result in an increased threshold for excitability and decreased automaticity. As a consequence of its K^+ channel–blocking actions, quinidine prolongs action potentials in most cardiac cells, most prominently at slow heart rates. In some cells, such as midmyocardial cells and Purkinje cells, quinidine consistently elicits EADs at slow heart rates, particularly when $[K]_o$ is low (Priori et al., 1999). Quinidine prolongs refractoriness in most tissues, probably as a result of both prolongation of action potential duration and Na^+ channel blockade.

In intact animals and humans, quinidine also produces α adrenergic receptor blockade and vagal inhibition. Thus, the intravenous use of quinidine is associated with marked hypotension and sinus tachycardia. Quinidine's vagolytic effects tend to inhibit its direct depressant effect on AV nodal conduction, so the effect of drug on the PR interval is variable. Moreover, quinidine's vagolytic effect can result in increased AV nodal transmission of atrial tachycardias such as atrial flutter (Table 30–1).

Adverse Effects

Noncardiac. Diarrhea is the most common adverse effect during quinidine therapy, occurring in 30%–50% of patients; the mechanism is not known. Diarrhea usually occurs within the first several days of quinidine therapy but can occur later. Diarrhea-induced hypokalemia may potentiate torsades de pointes due to quinidine.

A number of immunological reactions can occur during quinidine therapy. The most common is thrombocytopenia, which can be severe but which resolves rapidly with discontinuation of the drug. Hepatitis, bone marrow depression, and lupus syndrome occur rarely. None of these effects is related to elevated plasma quinidine concentrations.

Quinidine also can produce cinchonism, a syndrome that includes headache and tinnitus. In contrast to other adverse responses to quinidine therapy, cinchonism usually is related to elevated plasma quinidine concentrations and can be managed by dose reduction.

Cardiac. Of patients receiving quinidine therapy, 2%–8% will develop marked QT interval prolongation and torsades de pointes. In contrast to effects of sotalol, N-acetyl procainamide, and many other drugs, quinidine-associated torsades de pointes generally occurs at therapeutic or even subtherapeutic plasma concentrations. The reasons for individual susceptibility to this adverse effect are not known.

At high plasma concentrations of quinidine, marked Na^+ channel block can occur, with resulting ventricular tachycardia. This adverse effect occurs when very high doses of quinidine are used to try to convert atrial fibrillation to normal rhythm; this aggressive approach to quinidine dosing has been abandoned, and quinidine-induced ventricular tachycardia is unusual.

Quinidine can exacerbate heart failure or conduction system disease. However, in most patients with congestive heart failure, quinidine is well tolerated, perhaps because of its vasodilating actions.

Clinical Pharmacokinetics

Quinidine is well absorbed and is 80% bound to plasma proteins, including albumin and, like lidocaine, the acute-phase reactant α_1-acid glycoprotein. As with lidocaine, greater-than-usual doses (and total plasma quinidine concentrations) may be required to maintain therapeutic concentrations of free quinidine in high-stress states such as acute myocardial infarction. Quinidine undergoes extensive hepatic oxidative metabolism, and approximately 20% is excreted unchanged by the kidneys. One metabolite, 3-hydroxyquinidine, is nearly as potent as quinidine in blocking cardiac Na^+ channels and prolonging cardiac action potentials. Concentrations of unbound 3-hydroxyquinidine equal to or exceeding those of quinidine are tolerated by some patients. Other metabolites are less potent than quinidine, and their plasma concentrations are lower; thus, they are unlikely to contribute significantly to the clinical effects of quinidine.

There is substantial individual variability in the range of dosages required to achieve therapeutic plasma concentrations of 2 to 5 μg/mL. Some of this variability may be assay dependent because not all assays exclude quinidine metabolites. In patients with advanced renal disease or congestive heart failure, quinidine clearance is decreased only modestly. Thus, dosage requirements in these patients are similar to those in other patients.

Drug Interactions

Quinidine is a potent inhibitor of CYP2D6. As a result, the administration of quinidine to patients receiving drugs that undergo extensive CYP2D6-mediated metabolism may result in altered drug effects owing to accumulation of parent drug and failure of metabolite formation. For example, inhibition of CYP2D6-mediated metabolism of *codeine* to its active metabolite *morphine* results in decreased analgesia. On the other hand, inhibition of CYP2D6-mediated metabolism of propafenone results in elevated plasma propafenone concentrations and increased β adrenergic receptor blockade. Quinidine reduces the clearance of digoxin; inhibition of P-glycoprotein–mediated digoxin transport has been implicated (Fromm et al., 1999). Dextromethorphan, a CYP2D6 substrate that undergoes extensive first-pass bioinactivation, has shown promise in treatment of various neurological disorders, notably pseudobulbar affect. A combination of dextromethorphan and very low-dose quinidine (30 mg) inhibits the first-pass metabolism, achieves higher systemic concentrations than monotherapy, and is now approved for use in pseudobulbar affect (Olney and Rosen, 2010).

Quinidine metabolism is induced by drugs such as *phenobarbital* and phenytoin. In patients receiving these agents, very high doses of quinidine may be required to achieve therapeutic concentrations. If therapy with the inducing agent is then stopped, quinidine concentrations may rise to very high levels, and its dosage must be adjusted downward. Cimetidine and verapamil also elevate plasma quinidine concentrations, but these effects usually are modest.

Sotalol

Sotalol is a nonselective β adrenergic receptor antagonist that also prolongs cardiac action potentials by inhibiting delayed rectifier and possibly other K[+] currents (Hohnloser and Woosley, 1994). Sotalol is prescribed as a racemate; the L-enantiomer is a much more potent β adrenergic receptor antagonist than the D-enantiomer, but the two are equipotent as K[+] channel blockers. In the U.S., sotalol is approved for use in patients with both ventricular tachyarrhythmias and atrial fibrillation or flutter. Clinical trials suggest that it is at least as effective as most Na[+] channel blockers in ventricular arrhythmias.

Sotalol prolongs action potential duration throughout the heart and QT interval on the ECG. It decreases automaticity, slows AV nodal conduction, and prolongs AV refractoriness by blocking both K[+] channels and β adrenergic receptors, but it exerts no effect on conduction velocity in fast-response tissue. Sotalol causes EADs and triggered activity in vitro and can cause torsades de pointes, especially when the serum K[+] concentration is low. Unlike the situation with quinidine, the incidence of torsades de pointes (1.5%–2% incidence) seems to depend on the dose of sotalol; indeed, torsades de pointes is the major toxicity with sotalol overdose. Occasional cases occur at low dosages, often in patients with renal dysfunction, because sotalol is eliminated by renal excretion of unchanged drug. The other adverse effects of sotalol therapy are those associated with β adrenergic receptor blockade (see previous discussion and Chapter 12).

Vernakalant

Vernakalant is an inhibitor of multiple ion channels and prolongs atrial refractory periods without significantly affecting ventricular refractoriness. Intravenous vernakalant has modest efficacy in terminating atrial fibrillation (Roy et al., 2008) and is available for this indication in several European countries, but not the U.S. Consult the 12th edition of this text for more information on this drug.

Acknowledgment: *Kevin J Simpson and Robert S. Kass contributed to this chapter in the previous edition of this book. We have retained some of their text in the current edition.*

Drug Facts for Your Personal Formulary: *Antiarrhythmic Agents*

Antiarrhythmic Drug	Therapeutic Uses	Major Toxicity and Clinical Pearls
Class IA: Na[+] Channel Blockers · Slow to intermediate off rate · Concomitant class III action (prolong QT)		
Procainamide	• Acute treatment of AF, VT, and VF • Chronic treatment to prevent AF, VT, and VF	• 40% of patients discontinue within 6 months of therapy due to side effects: hypotension (especially from intravenous use), nausea • QT prolongation and torsades de pointes due to accumulation of active *N*-acetyl metabolite • Lupus-like syndrome (25%–50% with chronic use), especially in genetic slow acetylators • Oral drug no longer widely available
Quinidine	• Chronic treatment to prevent AF, VT, and VF	• Diarrhea (30%–50% of patients); diarrhea-induced hypokalemia may potentiate torsades de pointes • Marked QT prolongation and high risk (~1%–5%) of torsades de pointes at therapeutic or subtherapeutic concentrations • Immune thrombocytopenia (~1%) • Cinchonism: tinnitus, flushing, blurred vision, dizziness, diarrhea • Potent inhibitor of *CYP2D6* and *ABCB1*: altered effects of digitalis, many antidepressants, and others
Disopyramide	• Chronic treatment to prevent AF, VT, and VF	• Anticholinergic effects (dry eyes, urinary retention, constipation) • Long QT (torsades de pointes) • Depression of contractility can precipitate or worsen heart failure; paradoxically, this can be useful in hypertrophic cardiomyopathy to reduce outflow tract obstruction
Class IB: Na[+] Channel Blockers · Fast off rate · Little effect on ECG		
Lidocaine	• Acute treatment of VT and VF	• CNS: seizures and tinnitus • CNS: tremor, hallucinations, drowsiness, coma
Mexiletine	• Chronic treatment to prevent VT and VF	• Tremor and nausea
Class IC: Na[+] Channel Blockers · Slow off rate · Prolong PR and broaden QRS intervals		
Flecainide	• Chronic treatment to prevent PSVT, AF, VT, and VF in the absence of structural heart disease • Available in some countries for intravenous use in PSVT, AF • Useful in CPVT uncontrolled by β-blockers	• Much better tolerated than class IA or IB agents • Risk of severe proarrhythmia in patients with structural heart disease; increased mortality in patients with myocardial infarction (CAST) • Blurred vision • Can worsen heart failure

Class IC: Na⁺ Channel Blockers · Slow off rate · Prolong PR and broaden QRS intervals (continued)

Propafenone	• Chronic treatment to prevent PSVT, AF, VT, and VF in the absence of structural heart disease • Available in some countries for intravenous use in PSVT, AF • Alternative to flecainide for CPVT	• Also has β adrenergic blocking effects (worsening of heart failure and bronchospasm), especially prominent in *CYP2D6* poor metabolizers • Risk of severe proarrhythmia in patients with structural heart disease

Class II: β Blockers

Nadolol Propranolol Metoprolol Many others	• Chronic treatment to prevent arrhythmias in congenital LQTS and CPVT • Rate control in AF • Widely used for other indications (angina, hypertension, migraine, etc.)	• β Adrenergic blocking effects (worsening of heart failure, bradycardia, bronchospasm) • Nadolol preferred by many for LQTS and CPVT
Esmolol	• Acute treatment to control rate in AF	• Ultrashort $t_{1/2}$, intravenous use only

Class III: K⁺ Channel Blocker · Increase refractory period (prolong QT)

Amiodarone	• Drug of choice for acute treatment of VT and VF and to slow ventricular rate and convert AF • Chronic treatment to prevent AF, VT, and VF	• Hypotension, depressed ventricular function and torsades de pointes (*rare*) with intravenous administration • Pulmonary fibrosis with chronic therapy, which can be fatal (requires periodic monitoring of lung function) • Many other adverse effects: corneal microdeposits, hepatotoxicity, neuropathies, photosensitivity, thyroid dysfunction • Note: tissue half-life of several months • Inhibitor of many drug-metabolizing and transport systems, with high potential for drug interactions
Dronedarone	• Chronic treatment to prevent AF	• Amiodarone analogue with lower efficacy than amiodarone • GI disturbances, risk for fatal hepatotoxicity • Increases mortality in patients with severe heart failure
Sotalol	• Chronic treatment to prevent AF, VT, and VF	• Also has β adrenergic blocking effects • High risk (~1%–5%) of torsades de pointes
Dofetilide	• Chronic treatment to prevent AF	• Few adverse effects except high risk (~1%–5%) of torsades de pointes
Ibutilide	• Acute treatment to convert AF	• High risk (~1%–5%) of torsades de pointes

Class IV: Ca²⁺ Channel Blockers · Nondihydropyridine · Inhibit SA and AV nodes · Prolong PR

Diltiazem, Verapamil	• Acute intravenous use to convert PSVT and for rate control in AF • Chronic treatment to prevent PSVT and control rate in AF	• Hypotension (intravenous) • Sinus bradycardia or AV block especially in combination with β-blockers • Constipation • Worsening of heart failure

Antiarrhythmic Drugs With Miscellaneous Mechanisms

Adenosine (activates A receptors)	Drug of choice for acute treatment PSVT	• Short $t_{1/2}$ (<5 sec) • Transient asystole • Transient dyspnea • Transient atrial fibrillation (rare)
MgSO₄	• Acute treatment of torsades de pointes	
Digoxin (Na⁺-K⁺–ATPase inhibitor)	• Ventricular rate control in atrial fibrillation • Modest positive inotropic effect	• Adverse effects common and include GI symptoms, visual/cognitive dysfunction, and arrhythmias, typically supraventricular arrhythmias with heart block or atrial or ventricular extrasystoles • Severe toxicities (e.g., with overdose) can be treated with antibody • Probably mortality neutral

Bibliography

Amiodarone Trials Meta-Analysis Investigators. Effect of prophylactic amiodarone on mortality after acute myocardial infarction and in congestive heart failure—meta-analysis of individual data from 6500 patients in randomised trials. *Lancet*, **1997**, *350*:1417–1424.

Balser JR, et al. Local anesthetics as effectors of allosteric gating: lidocaine effects on inactivation-deficient rat skeletal muscle Na channels. *J Clin Invest*, **1996**, *98*:2874–2886.

Brugada P. Magnesium: an antiarrhythmic drug, but only against very specific arrhythmias. *Eur Heart J*, **2000**, *21*:1116.

Cohen IS, Robinson RB. Pacemaker currents and automatic rhythms: toward a molecular understanding. *Handb Exp Pharmacol*, **2006**, *171*:41–71.

Connolly SJ. Evidence-based analysis of amiodarone efficacy and safety. *Circulation*, **1999**, *100*:2025–2034.

Connolly SJ, et al. Dronedarone in high-risk permanent atrial fibrillation. *N Engl J Med*, **2011**, *365*:2268–2276.

Courtney, KR. Progress and prospects for optimum antiarrhythmic drug design. *Cardiovasc Drug Ther*, **1987**, *1*:117–123.

DiFrancesco D. Pacemaker mechanisms in cardiac tissue. *Annu Rev Physiol*, **1993**, *55*:455–472.

Dobrev D, et al. Novel molecular targets for atrial fibrillation therapy. *Nat Rev Drug Discov*, **2012**, 11(4):275–291.

Dorian P, et al. Amiodarone as compared with lidocaine for shock-resistant ventricular fibrillation. *N Engl J Med*, **2002**, 346:884–890.

Duan DD. Phenomics of cardiac chloride channels. *Compr Physiol*, **2013**, 3:667–692.

Dun W, Boyden PA. The purkinje cell; 2008 style. *J Mol Cell Cardiol*, **2008**, 45(5):617–624.

Dzeshka MS, Lip GY. Non-vitamin K oral anticoagulants in atrial fibrillation: where are we now? *Trends Cardiovasc Med*, **2015**, 25: 315–336.

Echt DS, et al. Mortality and morbidity in patients receiving encainide, flecainide, or placebo. *N Engl J Med*, **1991**, 324:781–788.

Fozzard HA, et al. Mechanism of local anesthetic drug action on voltage-gated sodium channels. *Curr Pharm Des*, **2005**, 11(21):2671–2686.

Fromm MF, et al. Inhibition of P-glycoprotein-mediated drug transport: a unifying mechanism to explain the interaction between digoxin and quinidine. *Circulation*, **1999**, 99: 552–557.

Funck-Brentano C, et al. Propafenone. *N Engl J Med*, **1990**, 322:518–525.

Grace AA, Camm J. Quinidine. *N Engl J Med*, **1998**, 338:35–45.

Henthorn RW, et al. Flecainide acetate prevents recurrence of symptomatic paroxysmal supraventricular tachycardia. The Flecainide Supraventricular Tachycardia Study Group. *Circulation*, **1991**, 83: 119–125.

Hilliard FA, et al. Flecainide inhibits arrhythmogenic Ca(2+) waves by open state block of ryanodine receptor Ca(2+) release channels and reduction of Ca(2+) spark mass. *J Mol Cell Cardiol*, **2010**, 48:293–301.

Hohnloser SH, et al. Effect of dronedarone on cardiovascular events in atrial fibrillation. *N Engl J Med*, **2009**, 360:668–678.

Hohnloser SH, Woosley RL. Sotalol. *N Engl J Med*, **1994**, 331:31–38.

Hwang HS, et al. Inhibition of cardiac Ca^{2+} release channels (RyR2) determines efficacy of class I antiarrhythmic drugs in catecholaminergic polymorphic ventricular tachycardia. *Circ Arrhythm Electrophysiol*, **2011**, 4:128–135.

Inama G, et al. "Orphan drugs" in cardiology: nadolol and quinidine. *J Cardiovasc Med*, **2010**, 11:143–144.

ISIS-4 Collaborative Group. ISIS-4: a randomised factorial trial assessing early oral captopril, oral mononitrate, and intravenous magnesium sulphate in 58,050 patients with suspected acute myocardial infarction. ISIS-4 (Fourth International Study of Infarct Survival) Collaborative Group. *Lancet*, **1995**, 345:669–685.

Kannankeril PJ, et al. Efficacy of flecainide in the treatment of catecholaminergic polymorphic ventricular tachycardia: a randomized clinical trial. *JAMA Cardiol*. Published online May 10, 2017. doi:10.1001/jamacardio.2017.1320

Keating MT, Sanguinetti MC. Molecular and cellular mechanisms of cardiac arrhythmias. *Cell*, **2001**, 104:569–580.

Kleber AG, Saffitz JE. Role of the intercalated disc in cardiac propagation and arrhythmogenesis. *Front Physiol*, **2014**, 5:404.

Knollmann BC, Roden DM. A genetic framework for improving arrhythmia therapy. *Nature*, **2008**, 451:929–936.

Kober L, et al. Increased mortality after dronedarone therapy for severe heart failure. *N Engl J Med*, **2008**, 358:2678–2687.

Levy S, Azoulay S. Stories about the origin of quinquina and quinidine. *J Cardiovasc Electrophysiol*, **1994**, 5:635–636.

Link MS. Clinical practice. Evaluation and initial treatment of supraventricular tachycardia. *N Engl J Med*, **2012**, 367:1438–1448.

Lu Z, et al. Suppression of phosphoinositide 3-kinase signaling and alteration of multiple ion currents in drug-induced long QT syndrome. *Sci Transl Med*, **2012**, 4:131.

MacKinnon R. Potassium channels. *FEBS Lett*, **2003**, 555:62–65.

Mitcheson JS, et al. A structural basis for drug-induced long QT syndrome. *Proc Natl Acad Sci U S A*, **2000**, 97:12329–12333.

Murray KT. Ibutilide. *Circulation*, **1998**, 97:493–497.

Napolitano C, et al. Gene-specific therapy for inherited arrhythmogenic diseases. *Pharmacol Ther*, **2006**, 100:1–13.

Nerbonne JM, Kass RS. Molecular physiology of cardiac repolarization. *Physiol Rev*, **2005**, 85:1205–1253.

Olney N, Rosen H. AVP-923, a combination of dextromethorphan hydrobromide and quinidine sulfate for the treatment of pseudobulbar affect and neuropathic pain. *IDrugs*, **2010**, 13:254–265.

Ono K, Iijima T. Cardiac T-type Ca(2+) channels in the heart. *J Mol Cell Cardiol*, **2010**, 48:65–70.

Patel C, et al. Dronedarone. *Circulation*, **2009**, 120:636–644.

Priori SG, et al. Genetic and molecular basis of cardiac arrhythmias: impact on clinical management. Study group on molecular basis of arrhythmias of the Working Group on Arrhythmias of the European Society of Cardiology. *Eur Heart J*, **1999**, 20:174–195.

Remme CA, Wilde AA. Late sodium current inhibition in acquired and inherited ventricular (dys)function and arrhythmias. *Cardiovasc Drugs Ther*, **2013**, 27:91–101.

Roden DM. Current status of class III antiarrhythmic drug therapy. *Am J Cardiol*, **1993**, 72:44B–49B.

Roden DM. Drug-induced prolongation of the QT interval. *N Engl J Med*, **2004**, 350:1013–1022.

Roden DM. Risks and benefits of antiarrhythmic therapy. *N Engl J Med*, **1994**, 331:785–791.

Roden DM, et al. Clinical pharmacology of antiarrhythmic agents. In: Josephson ME, ed. *Sudden Cardiac Death*. Blackwell Scientific, London, **1993**, 182–185.

Roden DM, Spooner PM. Inherited long QT syndromes: a paradigm for understanding arrhythmogenesis. *J Cardiovasc Electrophysiol*, **1999**, 10:1664–1683.

Roy D, et al. Vernakalant hydrochloride for rapid conversion of atrial fibrillation: a phase 3, randomized, placebo-controlled trial. *Circulation*, **2008**, 117:1518–1525.

Roy D, et al. Amiodarone to prevent recurrence of atrial fibrillation. Canadian Trial of Atrial Fibrillation Investigators. *N Engl J Med*, **2000**, 342:913–920.

Schwartz PJ, et al. Long QT syndrome. In: Zipes DP, Jalife J, eds. *Cardiac Electrophysiology: From Cell to Bedside*. 3rd ed. Saunders, Philadelphia, **2000**, 615–640.

Sherrid MV, Arabadjian M. A primer of disopyramide treatment of obstructive hypertrophic cardiomyopathy. *Prog Cardiovas Dis*, **2012**, 54:483–492.

Singh BN. Advantages of beta blockers versus antiarrhythmic agents and calcium antagonists in secondary prevention after myocardial infarction. *Am J Cardiol*, **1990**, 66:9C–20C.

Singh BN. Arrhythmia control by prolonging repolarization: the concept and its potential therapeutic impact. *Eur Heart J*, **1993**, 14(suppl H):14–23.

Tadros R, et al. Sex differences in cardiac electrophysiology and clinical arrhythmias: epidemiology, therapeutics, and mechanisms. *Can J Cardiol*, **2014**, 30:783–792. Erratum in: *Can J Cardiol*, **2014**, 30:1244.

Tamargo J, et al. Pharmacology of cardiac potassium channels. *Cardiovasc Res*, **2004**, 62:9–33.

Task Force of the Working Group on Arrhythmias of the European Society of Cardiology. The Sicilian gambit: a new approach to the classification of antiarrhythmic drugs based on their actions on arrhythmogenic mechanisms. *Circulation*, **1991**, 84:1831–1851.

Torp-Pedersen C, et al. Dofetilide in patients with congestive heart failure and left ventricular dysfunction. Danish Investigations of Arrhythmia and Mortality on Dofetilide Study Group. *N Engl J Med*, **1999**, 341:857–865.

Van Wagoner DR, et al. Progress toward the prevention and treatment of atrial fibrillation: a summary of the Heart Rhythm Society Research Forum on the Treatment and Prevention of Atrial Fibrillation, Washington, DC, December 9–10, 2013. *Heart Rhythm*, **2015**, 12:e5–e29.

Vaughan Williams EM. Classifying antiarrhythmic actions: by facts or speculation. *J Clin Pharmacol*, **1992**, 32:964–977.

Viskin S, et al. Quinidine, a life-saving medication for Brugada syndrome, is inaccessible in many countries. *J Am Coll Cardiol*, **2013**, 61:2383–2387.

Watanabe H, et al. Flecainide prevents catecholaminergic polymorphic ventricular tachycardia in mice and humans. *Nat Med*, **2009**, 15:380–383.

Woods KL, Fletcher S. Long-term outcome after intravenous magnesium sulphate in suspected acute myocardial infarction: the second Leicester Intravenous Magnesium Intervention Trial (LIMIT-2). *Lancet*, **1994**, 343:816–819.

Yang T, et al. Screening for acute IKr block is insufficient to detect torsades de pointes liability: role of late sodium current. *Circulation*, **2014**, 130:224–234.

Zimetbaum P. Amiodarone for atrial fibrillation. *N Engl J Med*, **2007**, 356:935–941.

Chapter 31

Treatment of Pulmonary Arterial Hypertension

Dustin R. Fraidenburg, Ankit A. Desai, and Jason X.-J. Yuan

Introduction to Pulmonary Hypertension

The pulmonary circulation plays a unique and essential role in gas exchange and, in particular, oxygenation of venous blood. It is a low-resistance and low-pressure circulatory system; the mean PAP in a healthy man is about 12 mm Hg. PAP is a function of CO and PVR. PH is defined as the mean PAP of 25 mm Hg or greater at rest. In patients with PH, pressure overload (i.e., increased afterload) places additional stress on the RV, leading to RV dysfunction and hypertrophy, and in some cases right heart failure. Patients present with a range of symptoms, including dyspnea, fatigue, chest pain, and syncope. PH is a complication of many chronic diseases and is estimated to affect as much as 10%–20% of the general population (McLaughlin et al., 2009).

Pulmonary Hypertension Classification

Pulmonary hypertension is a primary disorder of the pulmonary vasculature and a complication of other cardiopulmonary, vascular, and inflammatory diseases. Based on shared pathophysiological and pathological characteristics as well as response to therapies, PH can be classified into five groups (Simonneau et al., 2013):

1. PAH
2. PH owing to left heart disease
3. PH owing to lung diseases or hypoxia
4. Chronic thromboembolic PH
5. PH with unclear multifactorial mechanisms

Pulmonary Arterial Hypertension

Pulmonary arterial hypertension is a rare, progressive, and fatal disease in which vascular changes in the small arteries and arterioles lead to progressive increases in PVR, resulting in increased PAP (McLaughlin et al., 2009). In patients with PAH, elevated afterload increases stress on the RV, leading to right heart dysfunction and failure, the major cause of morbidity and mortality in this population. The disease is defined clinically by hemodynamic parameters measured during a right heart catheterization: mean PAP 25 mm Hg or greater, accompanied by normal pulmonary venous pressure measured as pulmonary artery occlusion pressure or left ventricular end-diastolic pressure of 15 mm Hg or less. The median survival in untreated disease is 2.8 years, yet with modern therapies, the median survival has been estimated to be about 9 years (Benza et al., 2012). This group of patients is the most well-studied subset and the primary target of available therapeutics (Frumkin, 2012).

Pulmonary Hypertension Associated With Other Disease States

Other PH groups represent the majority of recognized cases of PH. The presence of PH in these more common diseases portends a much poorer prognosis, often identifying people with multiple comorbidities, late-stage presentations, or more severe disease. While recognition of PH in heart and lung disease carries important prognostic implications, to date there are no approved targeted therapies for PH in these other disease states, with the exception of CTEPH. While surgical pulmonary thromboendarterectomy is the treatment of choice in CTEPH, nonsurgical patients or those with persistent PH following surgery respond to pulmonary vasodilator therapy (Fedullo et al., 2011; Ghofrani, et al., 2013).

Routes of Drug Delivery to the Pulmonary Circulation

The pulmonary circulation permits delivery of drugs through multiple routes. The pulmonary circulation runs in series with the systemic circulation, receiving the entire CO in each cardiac cycle. Thus, exposure of pulmonary tissue to drugs is excellent and reliable. Continuous intravenous infusion is used to deliver high concentrations of drugs that exhibit short half-lives to the pulmonary circulation while avoiding first-pass metabolism. Alternatively, drug administration by subcutaneous pump may be used to lower risk of adverse effects. Oral delivery remains a safe, effective, and reliable route for many classes of drugs used to treat PAH. The small pulmonary arteries and precapillary arterioles are also unique in their close proximity to the alveoli and lower airways. Hence, inhalational delivery of therapeutic compounds can directly target the lung vasculature and pulmonary circulation, limit systemic side effects, and preferentially affect well-ventilated parts of the lung to improve ventilation-perfusion matching (see Chapter 40).

Mechanisms of Pulmonary Arterial Hypertension

Pulmonary arterial hypertension is thought to arise from pathophysiological changes in the small pulmonary arteries and arterioles. Regardless of the initial etiological trigger, the putative mechanisms contributing to elevated PVR and PAP include the following:

- pulmonary vascular remodeling
- sustained pulmonary vasoconstriction
- in situ thrombosis
- pulmonary vascular wall stiffening

Abbreviations

ATPase: adenosine triphosphatase
BMPR2: bone morphogenetic protein receptor type 2
$[Ca^{2+}]_{cyt}$: cytosolic free Ca^{2+} concentration
CCB: calcium channel blocker
COPD: chronic obstructive pulmonary disease
CTEPH: chronic thromboembolic pulmonary hypertension
CYP: cytochrome P450
DAG: diacylglycerol
EC: endothelial cell
ECE: endothelin-converting enzyme
EGF: epidermal growth factor
ERA: endothelin receptor antagonist
ET: endothelin-1
FDA: Food and Drug Administration
HCN: hyperpolarization-activated cyclic nucleotide–gated
HIV: human immunodeficiency virus
HPAP: heritable pulmonary arterial hypertension
HPV: hypoxic pulmonary vasoconstriction
5HT: serotonin
IP_3: inositol triphosphate
IPAH: idiopathic pulmonary arterial hypertension
IPR: prostacyclin receptor
LV: left ventricle
mGC: membrane guanylate cyclase
6MWT: six-minute walk testing
NO: nitric oxide
NO_2: nitric dioxide
NYHA: New York Heart Association
PA: pulmonary artery
PAEC: pulmonary arterial endothelial cell
PAH: pulmonary arterial hypertension
Pao_2: partial pressure of arterial O_2
PAOP: pulmonary artery occlusion pressure
PAP: pulmonary arterial pressure
PASMC: pulmonary artery smooth muscle cell
PDE: phosphodiesterase
PDGF: platelet-derived growth factor
PGI_2: prostacyclin, prostaglandin I_2
PH: pulmonary hypertension
PIP_2: phosphatidylinositol 4,5-biphosphate
PKA: protein kinase A
PKG: protein kinase G
PLC: phospholipase C
PVR: pulmonary vascular resistance
RAP: right atrial pressure
ROC: receptor-operated Ca^{2+} channel
RV: right ventricle
RVF: right ventricular failure
RVH: right ventricular hypertrophy
RVSP: right ventricular systolic pressure
sGC: soluble guanylate cyclase
SR: sarcoplasmic reticulum
SVR: systemic vascular resistance
TKR: tyrosine kinase receptor
TxA_2: thromboxane A_2
VDCC: voltage-dependent Ca^{2+} channel
VEGF: vascular endothelial growth factors
VIP: vasoactive intestinal peptide
VSM: vascular smooth muscle

Each of these mechanisms (Figure 31–1) can contribute to the development and progression of PAH and forms the basis for drug therapy for this disease. Accordingly, an effective therapy for PAH would (1) cause pulmonary vasodilation; (2) exert antiproliferative or proapoptotic effects on highly proliferative cells in the pulmonary vascular wall (e.g., fibroblasts, myofibroblasts, and smooth muscle cells); (3) prevent or resolve in situ thrombosis in small arteries and precapillary arterioles; (4) exert antifibrotic effects to attenuate extracellular matrix stiffness; and (5) reduce pulmonary vascular wall stiffness due to myogenic tone and cholesterol-associated membrane stiffness (Mandegar et al., 2004; Morrell et al., 2009).

Although the cellular and molecular mechanisms leading to these changes in the pulmonary vasculature are complex, an imbalance of vasoactive mediators, mitogenic and angiogenic factors, and pro- and antiapoptotic proteins plays an important role in PAH development. Relative deficiencies of vasodilators (e.g., NO and prostacyclin) deleteriously accompany an excess of vasoconstrictors (e.g., ET-1 and TxA_2). NO released by the vascular ECs normally promotes the production of cyclic GMP in the PASMCs, resulting in PASMC relaxation and pulmonary vasodilation. PGI_2, also released from the vascular endothelium, promotes the synthesis of cAMP, causing PASMC relaxation and pulmonary vasodilation. In addition, NO and PGI_2 both have antiproliferative and anticoagulant effects that inhibit concentric pulmonary vascular wall thickening and in situ thrombosis. ET-1 is a potent vasoconstrictor secreted by ECs; it exerts vasoconstrictive and proliferative effects on PASMCs. Other vasoactive mediators such as TxA_2, 5HT, and VIP appear to play a role in the development of PAH, but the therapeutic potential of targeting these substances has not been well established. Table 31–1 summarizes the changes in these vasoactive mediators and the likely contributions of those changes to the development of PAH.

Sustained vasoconstriction and pulmonary vascular remodeling also result from functional and transcriptional changes in membrane receptors and ion channels on the surface of PASMCs. Several GPCRs and TKRs are implicated in the development and progression of PAH. Increased cytosolic $[Ca^{2+}]$ is an important common pathway by which receptor activation and downstream cellular signaling cascades exert their effects in the pulmonary vasculature. A rise in $[Ca^{2+}]_{cyt}$ in PASMCs is a major trigger for PASMC contraction and an important mediator for PASMC proliferation, migration, and vascular remodeling. In addition, ion channels, particularly Ca^{2+}-permeable cation channels and K^+-permeable channels (e.g., KCNA5 and KCNK3) in the plasma membrane of PASMCs, can directly influence $[Ca^{2+}]_{cyt}$ (Mandegar et al., 2004). Ion channels and transporters, such as VDCCs, ROCs, store-operated Ca^{2+} channels, and the Na^+-Ca^{2+} exchanger, are implicated in the development of PAH; all are potential therapeutic targets. Downregulation of K^+-permeable channels in PASMCs leads to membrane depolarization and opening of VDCCs, enhancing Ca^{2+} influx, with a consequent increase in $[Ca^{2+}]_{cyt}$ and further sustained vasoconstriction and vascular remodeling (Kuhr et al., 2012).

Clinical Use of Drugs for Pulmonary Hypertension

Treatment of PAH must include a proper assessment of symptoms, functional classification, and RV performance for optimal selection of appropriate agents. The most widely used criterion for initiating treatment is the presence of symptoms and impairments in functional capacity, as measured by functional classification. This classification measures the physical limitations imposed on a particular patient from the disease, progressing from class I through class IV (from no impairment through mounting functional limitation to inability to perform physical activity). Clinical trials suggested that class II patients may benefit from therapy, with greater benefit seen in class III. While overall number of patients is low, patients with the most severe functional impairments, class IV, fare far worse. RV dysfunction results from increased PVR, in part, and is the major contributor to morbidity and mortality in this population; therefore, assessment of the RV often is used in conjunction with functional assessment to guide therapy (Figure 31–2).

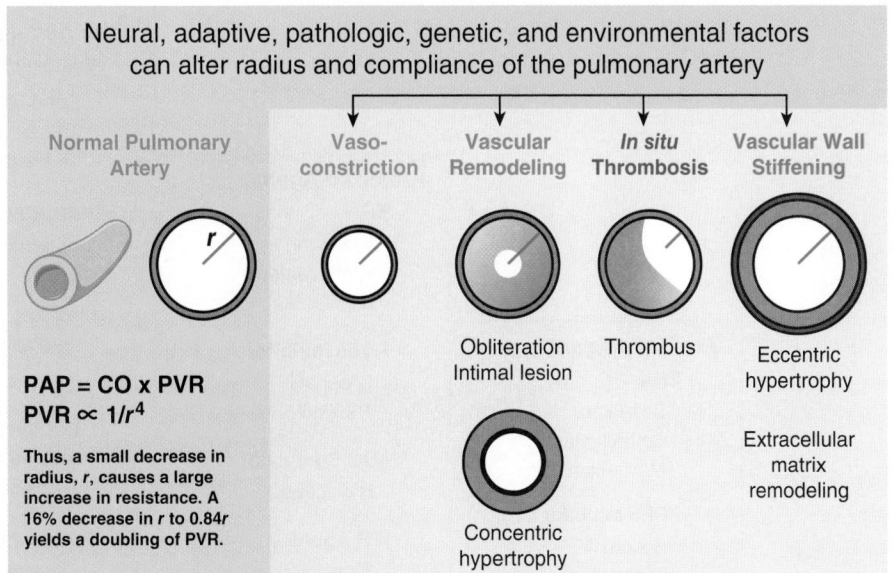

Neural, adaptive, pathologic, genetic, and environmental factors can alter radius and compliance of the pulmonary artery

Normal Pulmonary Artery

Vasoconstriction

Vascular Remodeling

Obliteration Intimal lesion

Concentric hypertrophy

In situ Thrombosis

Thrombus

Vascular Wall Stiffening

Eccentric hypertrophy

Extracellular matrix remodeling

$$PAP = CO \times PVR$$
$$PVR \propto 1/r^4$$

Thus, a small decrease in radius, r, causes a large increase in resistance. A 16% decrease in r to $0.84r$ yields a doubling of PVR.

Figure 31–1 *Major pathogenic components in the development of PAH.* Vascular remodeling occurs as changes in the intraluminal radius with or without changes in the vascular wall thickness. Changes in intraluminal radius of small pulmonary arteries and arterioles have dramatic effects on the PVR. Pathogenic factors contributing to the development and progression of PAH include sustained vasoconstriction, pulmonary vascular remodeling, in situ thrombosis, and vascular wall stiffening.

Goals of treatment include improvement in symptoms, such as dyspnea, fatigue, chest pain, or syncope; improved functional capacity, including 6-min walk distance; and improvement in pulmonary and RV hemodynamics. Oral formulations, either ERAs, PDE5 inhibitors, or sGC stimulators, are usually employed as first-line agents due to ease of use. Treatment of the most severe PAH patients generally involves parenteral therapy with epoprostenol or treprostinil, the most potent pulmonary vasodilators, yet controversy exists on the initial treatment of patients with moderate-to-severe functional limitations. Sequential combination therapy with the addition of separate classes of medications is often utilized for severe or progressive disease (Ghofrani and Humbert, 2014). Modest effects with single agents may be enhanced with the use of up-front combinations and could lead to more dramatic improvements in both symptoms and hemodynamics (Sitbon et al., 2014; Galie et al., 2015).

Pulmonary hypertension is a complex disease process often complicating common diseases of the heart and lungs and heralding poor outcomes. Despite this, PAH, and more recently CTEPH, are the only two subtypes of PH with safe and effective pharmacotherapy. Supportive care therapies described in other chapters include volume management with diuretics (e.g., furosemide), anticoagulants (e.g., warfarin) for patients at high risk for thrombotic disease, supplemental oxygen therapy for hypoxic patients,

and inotropic therapy (e.g., digoxin) to improve cardiac contractility in patients with RV dysfunction.

Pharmacotherapy for Pulmonary Hypertension

Pharmacotherapy for PH targets the major pathogenic mechanisms of the disease—pulmonary vascular remodeling (e.g., concentric pulmonary vascular thickening and intraluminal obliteration), sustained pulmonary vasoconstriction, in situ thrombosis, and pulmonary vascular wall stiffening—with the goals of attenuating the development and progression of PAH and reversing these pathologic changes in patients with established PAH. Currently available PAH therapeutics are classified based on their cellular and molecular mechanisms (see Humbert and Ghofrani, 2016):

- NO and stimulators of cGMP and PKG signaling
- membrane receptor agonists
- membrane receptor antagonists
- ion channel blockers and openers

Stimulators of cGMP and PKG Signaling

Nitric oxide is synthesized mainly in vascular ECs and diffuses into vascular smooth muscle cells (PASMCs) to activate sGC. Activated sGC generates cGMP, which in turn is inactivated by cyclic nucleotide PDE5 to 5′-GMP (Figure 31–3). cGMP is an important intracellular second messenger that signals through (1) cGMP-dependent PKG, the principal downstream mediator of cGMP, and (2) cyclic nucleotide–gated and hyperpolarization-activated cyclic nucleotide–gated (HCN) channels (Craven and Zagotta, 2006). Increased cellular cGMP exerts relaxant and antiproliferative effects on PASMCs and myofibroblasts through activation of cGMP-gated K^+ channels, inhibition of Ca^{2+}-permeable channels (e.g., L-type VDCCs, transient receptor potential cation channels), and attenuation of several specific intracellular signaling cascades that are related to cell proliferation, growth, and migration (cAMP [via activated PKA] has similar effects). The drugs currently available for the treatment of PAH in this category include inhaled NO, stimulators and activators of sGC, and inhibitors of PDE5.

The enzymic catalysts of cGMP formation in tissues are sGC and particulate (plasma membrane) mGC. NO stimulates sGC, while the natriuretic peptides stimulate mGC (see Chapter 3 for information on the structure and mechanisms of activation of these enzymes). The sGC is

TABLE 31–1 ■ ROLES OF VASOACTIVE MEDIATORS IN PAH

EFFECTOR	Δ IN PAH	CONSEQUENCE OF ALTERED [EFFECTOR] ON		
		VASCULAR CONTRACTION	THROMBUS FORMATION	CELL PROLIFERATION
NO	↓	↑	↑	–/↑
PGI$_2$	↓	↑	↑	↑
TxA$_2$	↑	↑	↑	↑
VIP	↓	↑	↑	↑
5HT	↑	↑	↑	↑
ET	↑	↑	–[a]	↑

↑, increased; ↓, decreased; -, no change.
[a] ↓ in plexiform lesions.

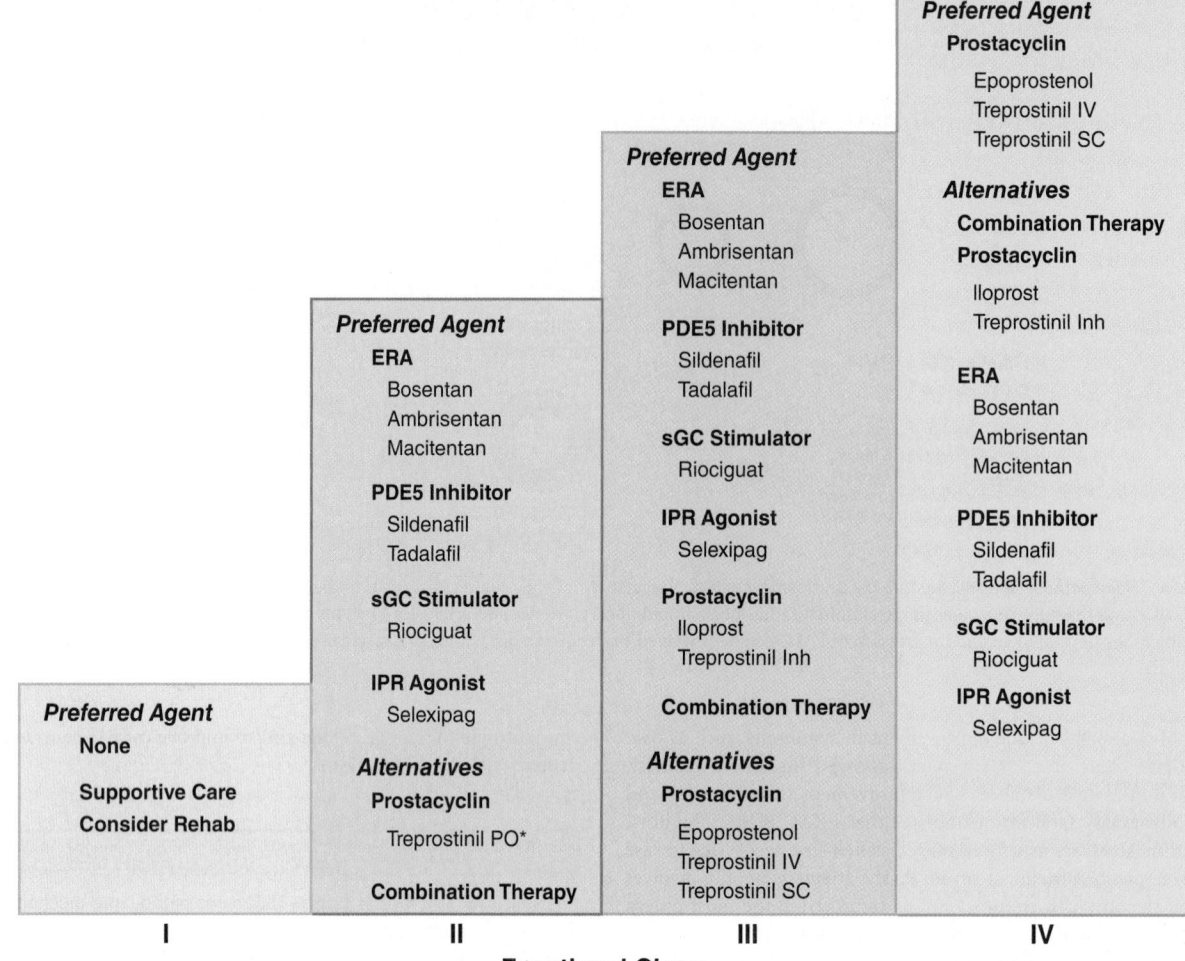

Figure 31–2 *Clinical use of PAH drugs based on functional class.* Treatment of PAH is generally based on the patient's functional classification at the time of presentation. Four functional classes have been defined for PAH: (I) no symptoms or functional limitation; (II) slight limitation of physical activity; (III) marked limitation of physical activity; and (IV) symptoms with any activity or at rest. In patients with no functional limitation, there is no specific therapy that has shown benefit in clinical trials. Expert guidelines recommend only supportive care and physical rehabilitation in this group. Patients with symptoms consistent with functional classes II and III have the best evidence for therapeutic benefits. First-line therapeutics include oral agents such as ERAs, PDE5 inhibitors, sGC stimulators, and the IPR antagonist selexipag. Inhaled PGI_2 analogues can also be considered. The oral formulation of treprostinil has been approved for use in minimally symptomatic individuals but should be reserved for use only as monotherapy. The most severely limited patients, those in functional class IV, or those with evidence of right heart dysfunction should be started on the most potent vasodilators, which include the intravenous and subcutaneous formulations of PGI_2 analogues. Alternatively, combination therapy using multiple agents has been shown to be effective in small clinical trials and one phase 3 clinical trial combining ambrisentan and tadalafil. *approved for monotherapy only.

the source of cGMP synthesis on which therapeutics agents for PAH rely. In the lung, activation of the cGMP-PKG pathway causes relaxation of smooth muscle, inhibits proliferation of bronchial smooth muscle and vascular smooth muscle cells, and has an antiproliferative effect (and can induce apoptosis) in pulmonary vascular smooth muscle cells and ECs (Figure 31–3).

Nitric Oxide

Nitric oxide is biosynthesized from the terminal nitrogen of L-arginine by the enzyme nitric oxide synthase (see Chapter 3) Endogenous NO levels are reduced in patients with PAH, PH associated with connective tissue disease, COPD, and interstitial lung disease (Girgis et al., 2005; Kawaguchi et al., 2006).

ADME. NO is a soluble gas. *Inhaled NO* is a gaseous blend of NO and N_2 (0.01% and 99.99%, respectively, for 100 ppm NO). NO must be compressed and stored with an inert gas such as N_2 to minimize the exposure to O_2, decreasing the risk of the accumulation of NO_2. Inhaled NO increases the PaO_2 by preferentially vasodilating better-ventilated lung regions from poorly inflated lung areas (i.e., with low ventilation/perfusion [V/Q]

ratios). Inhaled NO is generally administered continuously or with a pulsing device that is rapidly triggered with the onset of inspiration; careful monitoring of response is warranted (Griffiths and Evans, 2005). Inhaled NO is a selective pulmonary vasodilator. Its acute and relatively specific effects on PAP and PVR are due to its route of administration and short half-life (2–6 sec), which is primarily a result of the rapid inactivation of NO by hemoglobin binding and oxidation to nitrite; the nitrite interacts with oxyhemoglobin, leading to the formation of nitrate and met-hemoglobin (Bueno et al., 2013). Nitrate has been identified as the predominant NO metabolite excreted in the urine, accounting for more than 70% of the NO dose inhaled (Ichinose et al., 2004).

Clinical Use. NO can acutely lower PAP and PVR without altering systemic arterial pressure. Inhaled NO is used for the treatment of term and near-term neonates with persistent pulmonary hypertension of the newborn and acute hypoxemic respiratory failure (Abman, 2013). Acute vasodilator testing is another well-established but off-label use of inhaled NO in adult patients with PAH. Vasodilator testing is performed in the course of deciding whether a patient might derive clinical benefit from

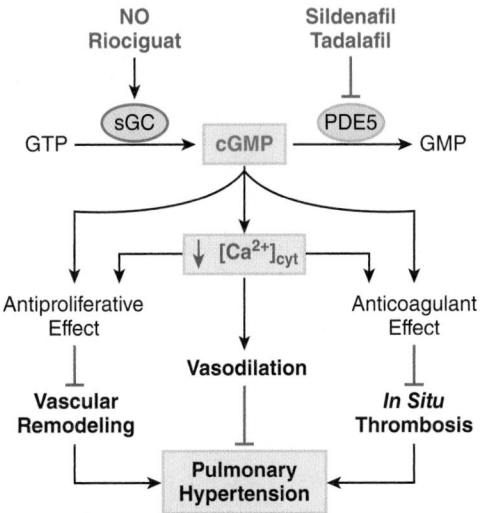

Figure 31–3 *Stimulators of NO/cGMP signaling.* NO stimulates sGC to produce cGMP, which has vasodilating effects through decreased $[Ca^{2+}]_{cyt}$ as well as anticoagulant and antiproliferative effects that are both dependent and independent of $[Ca^{2+}]_{cyt}$. cGMP is degraded primarily by PDE5 in PASMCs, which is targeted by the PDE5 inhibitors sildenafil and tadalafil.

Ca²⁺ channel blockade therapy (e.g., *nifedipine*) (Abman, 2013). In the treatment of PH, a 30% decrease in PVR during the inhalation of NO (10 ppm for 10 min) has been used to identify an association with vascular responsiveness and a favorable response to CCBs in a small cohort of patients with primary PH (McLaughlin et al., 2009).

Adverse Effects and Precautions.

High doses of inhaled NO (500–1000 ppm) are lethal. However, NO doses of less than 40 ppm are well tolerated chronically for up to 6 months and do not cause methemoglobinemia in adults who have normal methemoglobin reductase activity (Griffiths and Evans, 2005). In neonates, methemoglobin accumulation has been investigated during the first 12 h of exposure to 0, 5, 20, and 80 ppm of inhaled NO (Abman, 2013). Methemoglobin concentrations increased during the first 8 h of NO exposure. The mean methemoglobin level remained below 1% in the placebo group and in the 5- and 20-ppm groups, but reached approximately 5% in the 80-ppm inhaled NO group.

Drug interactions between properly dosed NO and other medications are not expected, but side effects may include noisy breathing, hematuria, or possibly atelectasis. Overdosage with inhaled NO manifests as elevations in methemoglobin and pulmonary toxicities associated with inspired NO₂, including acute respiratory distress syndrome. Elevations in methemoglobin reduce the O₂ delivery capacity of the circulation. Based on clinical studies, NO₂ levels greater than 3 ppm or methemoglobin levels greater than 7% are treated by reducing the dose of, or discontinuing, inhaled NO therapy (Abman, 2013). Methemoglobinemia that does not resolve after reduction or discontinuation of inhaled NO therapy can be treated with intravenous vitamin C, intravenous methylene blue, or blood transfusion, based on the clinical situation.

Inhaled NO gas has limitations: Dosing must be individualized and frequently adjusted; delivery is cumbersome and expensive; off-target effects from reactive nitrogen species are possible; and rebound PH may appear when the NO administration is interrupted. The oxidative product of NO metabolism, the inorganic anion nitrite NO_2^- is relatively stable compared to NO ($t_{1/2} = 51$ min); NO_2^- can be reduced back to NO under physiological and pathological hypoxia by enzymatic and nonenzymatic processes and thus can serve as an intravascular endocrine reservoir of potential NO bioactivity (Bueno et al., 2013). Other NO donor drugs such as sodium nitroprusside and nitroglycerin offer protective benefits in PVR or remodeling, but when administered intravenously, however, these drugs have limited use given their significant systemic vasodilating effects.

Riociguat

In patients with NO deficiency due to dysfunctional endothelial nitric oxide synthase or arginine insufficiency, activation of sGC increases signaling through the cGMP-PKG pathway and exerts a therapeutic effect (Stasch and Evgenov, 2013). Riociguat, a direct activator of sGC, has recently been approved.

Mechanism of Action. Riociguat is the first-in-class stimulator of sGC. The agent exhibits a dual mode of action; it sensitizes sGC to endogenous NO, and it also directly stimulates sGC independently of NO.

ADME. The drug has excellent oral absorption, and the plasma concentration peaks approximately 1.5 h after oral intake (Stasch and Evgenov, 2013). Food does not affect the bioavailability of riociguat; its volume of distribution is about 30 L. Riociguat is metabolized by CYPs 1A1, 3A, 2C8, and 2J2. The action of CYP1A1 forms the major and active metabolite, M1, which is converted to an inactive *N*-glucuronide. The terminal elimination half-life is about 12 h in patients with PAH (7 h in healthy subjects) (Stasch and Evgenov, 2013).

Clinical Use. Riociguat at doses up to 2.5 mg given three times daily for 12 weeks increased walking distance and significantly delayed time to clinical worsening for patients with PAH (Ghofrani, 2013). Riociguat was also effective in patients with CTEPH, for whom improvements in walking distance were apparent from week 2 onward (Ghofrani, et al., 2013).

Adverse Reactions and Precautions. Concurrent use of riociguat with nitroglycerin or PDE5 inhibitors can cause severe hypotension and syncope (Stasch and Evgenov, 2013). Serious adverse effects include embryo-fetal toxicity, hypotension, and bleeding. Other common adverse reactions include headache, dyspepsia, dizziness, nausea, diarrhea, vomiting, anemia, reflux, constipation, palpitations, nasal congestion, epistaxis, dysphagia, abdominal distension, and peripheral edema (Ghofrani, et al., 2013; Ghofrani, et al., 2013; Stasch and Evgenov, 2013).

PDE5 Inhibitors

Cyclic nucleotide PDEs comprise a superfamily of enzymes that hydrolyze 3′-5′ cyclic nucleotides to their cognate 5′ monophosphates (Omori and Kotera, 2007). PDE5, an isoform that is relatively specific for cGMP, is abundant in PASMCs (Kass et al., 2007). The physiological importance of PDE5 in the regulation of smooth muscle tone has been most effectively demonstrated by the successful clinical use of its specific inhibitors in the treatment of erectile dysfunction and PAH (Galiè et al., 2005; Ravipati et al., 2007).

Sildenafil. Mechanism of Action. Sildenafil, which structurally mimics the purine ring of cGMP, is a competitive and selective inhibitor of PDE5. Sildenafil has a relatively high selectivity (>1000-fold) for human PDE5 over other PDEs. By inhibiting cGMP hydrolysis, sildenafil elevates cellular levels of cGMP and augments signaling through the cGMP-PKG pathway, *provided guanylyl cyclase is active.*

ADME. The drug is rapidly absorbed and reaches a peak plasma concentration 1 h after oral administration. Sildenafil is cleared by the hepatic CYP3A (major route) and CYP2C9 (minor). Sildenafil and its major active metabolite, *N*-desmethyl sildenafil, have terminal half-lives of about 4 h. Both the parent compound and the major metabolite are highly bound to plasma proteins (96%) (Cockrill and Waxman, 2013). Metabolites are predominantly excreted into the feces (73%–88%) and to a lesser extent into the urine; unmetabolized drug is not detected in urine or feces (Muirhead et al., 2002). Clearance is reduced in the elderly (>65 years), leading to an increase in area-under-the-curve values for the parent drug and the *N*-desmethyl metabolite.

Clinical Use and Adverse Effects and Precautions. Sildenafil, 5 to 20 mg three times per day improves exercise capacity, functional class, and hemodynamics. In addition to improved exercise capacity and hemodynamic parameters, sildenafil (initiated at 20 mg three times daily, titrated to 40–80 mg three times daily) plus long-term epoprostenol therapy also resulted in delayed time to clinical worsening of PAH in clinical studies.

Dose adjustments for reduced renal and hepatic function are usually not necessary except for severe hepatic and renal impairment (Cockrill and Waxman, 2013). Concomitant administration of potent CYP3A inducers (e.g., bosentan) will generally cause substantial decreases in plasma levels of sildenafil. The mean reduction in the bioavailability of sildenafil (80 mg three times a day) when coadministered with epoprostenol was 28% (Cockrill and Waxman, 2013). CYP3A inhibitors (e.g., protease inhibitors used in HIV therapy, erythromycin, and cimetidine) inhibit sildenafil metabolism, thereby prolonging the $t_{1/2}$ and elevating blood levels of sildenafil. Consistent with its mechanism of action, potentiation of cGMP signaling, sildenafil and other PDE5 inhibitors potentiate the hypotensive effects of nitrate vasodilators, producing dangerously low blood pressure. Thus, the administration of PDE5 inhibitors to patients receiving organic nitrates is contraindicated. In any event, the patient's underlying cardiovascular status and concurrent use of hypotensive agents (e.g., nitrate vasodilators, α adrenergic antagonists) must be considered prior to use of this class of drugs.

Headache (16%) and flushing (10%) are the most frequently reported side effects. Patients taking sildenafil or vardenafil may notice a transient blue-green tinting of vision due to inhibition of retinal PDE6, which is involved in phototransduction (see Figure 69-9).

Other PDE5 Inhibitors. *Vardenafil* is structurally similar to sildenafil and a potent inhibitor of PDE5. Although not FDA-approved for PAH in the U.S., its clinical efficacy in PAH appears similar to that of sildenafil (Cockrill and Waxman, 2013). *Tadalafil*, another PDE5 inhibitor used for the treatment of PAH, differs structurally from sildenafil and has a longer half-life (Cockrill and Waxman, 2013). See Table 45–2 for comparative pharmacokinetic data of PDE5 inhibitors.

Prostacyclin Receptor Agonists

Prostacyclin is mainly synthesized in and released from vascular ECs and exerts relaxant and antiproliferative effects on vascular smooth muscle cells. Similar to NO, endogenous PGI_2 is considered an endothelium-derived relaxing factor. Decreased PGI_2 synthesis occurs in patients with idiopathic PAH, a finding that provided the rationale for using PGI_2 and its analogues for treatment of PAH (Christman et al., 1992).

Mechanism of Action. Prostacyclin binds to the IPR in the plasma membrane of PASMCs and activates the G_s-AC-cAMP-PKA pathway (Figure 31–4). PKA continues the signaling cascade by (1) decreasing $[Ca^{2+}]_{cyt}$ via activating K^+ channels (which causes membrane hyperpolarization and repolarization, leading to closure of VDCCs) and (2) inhibiting myosin light chain kinase, thereby causing smooth muscle relaxation and vasodilation (Olschewski et al., 2004). Activated PKA can also exert an antiproliferative effect on PASMCs by inhibiting the signaling cascades of hedgehog, ERK/p21, and Akt/mTOR. Inhibition of cyclic nucleotide PDEs, mainly PDE3 and PDE4, enhances the cAMP-PKA–mediated relaxant and antiproliferative effects on vascular smooth muscle cells.

Epoprostenol (Prostacyclin)

Clinical Use, Adverse Effects and Precautions. The first synthetic PGI_2, epoprostenol, has dose-dependent inhibitory effects on both SVR and PVR, paired with increases in cardiac output, for patients with PAH (Rubin et al., 1982). Epoprostenol's short half-life (3–5 min) requires the use of a drug delivery pump system for continuous intravenous infusion to achieve long-term efficacy in the treatment of PAH. In a clinical trial, epoprostenol treatment caused significant improvements in pulmonary hemodynamics, patient symptoms, and survival over a 12-week period (Barst et al., 1996).

Epoprostenol is light and temperature sensitive, although a more recent thermostable formulation is now available that permits its use at room temperature (20°C–25°C). This agent remains a mainstay of PAH treatment, particularly in advanced stages of the disease. Adverse effects of epoprostenol are similar for the entire class of PGI_2 analogues and include myalgias and pain in the extremities, jaw pain, nausea, headaches, abdominal discomfort, diarrhea, flushing, dizziness, and systemic hypotension. Side effects are generally dose dependent, and slow titration is required for the drug to be sufficiently tolerated.

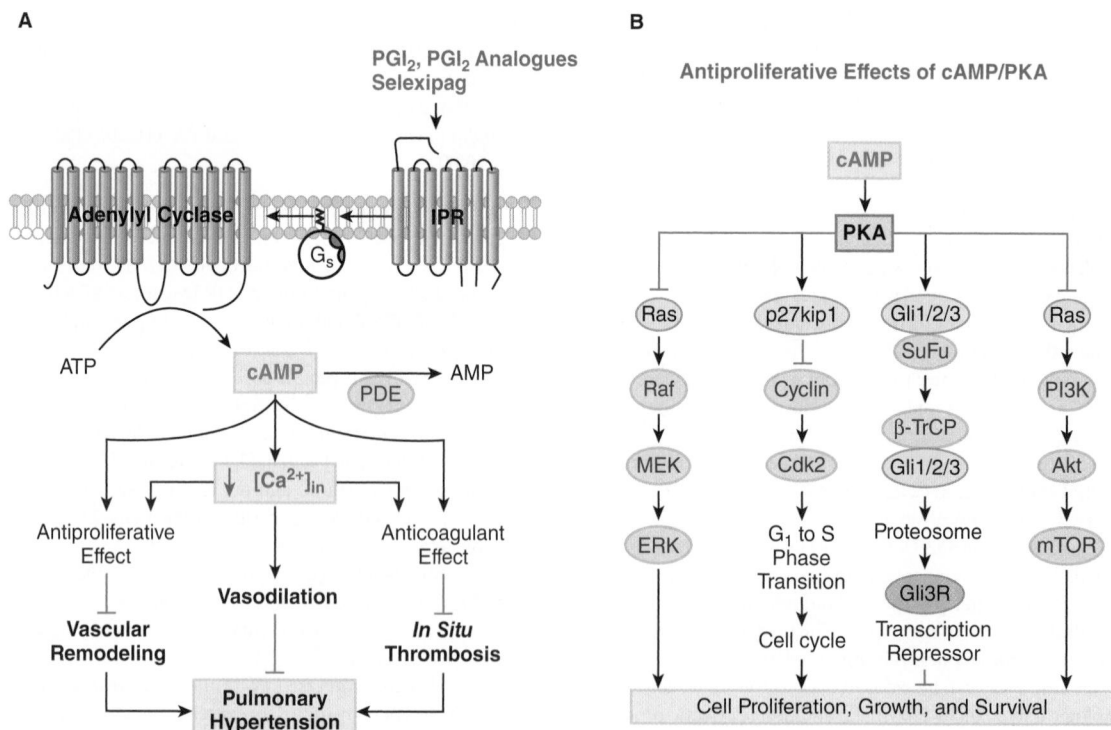

Figure 31–4 *Membrane receptor agonists that increase cAMP.* Therapies targeting the IPR, including PGI_2, PGI_2 analogues, and selexipag, increase cAMP through stimulation of its production by AC. The vasodilating properties of cAMP are produced through decreased $[Ca^{2+}]_{cyt}$ as well as anticoagulant and antiproliferative effects that are both dependent and independent of $[Ca^{2+}]_{cyt}$. The antiproliferative effects of cAMP (panel **B**) are shown through numerous distinct pathways, many of which are currently under investigation as novel therapies.

Treprostinil

Clinical Use. Treprostinil, a PGI$_2$ analogue with longer half-life than that of epoprostenol, is available for continuous intravenous infusion, subcutaneous infusion, inhalation, and oral delivery. The risk of bacteremia or other catheter-related complications can be reduced by subcutaneous delivery. Subcutaneous treprostinil has similar efficacy to intravenous formulations of epoprostenol and treprostinil (Simonneau et al., 2002). Adverse effects related to delivery into the subcutaneous tissue of the lower abdomen are common, including pain and erythema in a majority of patients; these effects subside over time.

Compared to intravenous treprostinil, the inhaled formulation has more potent pulmonary vasodilating effects, but patients find the dosing scheme complex: Multiple breaths are taken through a nebulizer or inhaler four times a day and slowly titrated up to a maximum of nine breaths four times a day. Inhaled treprostinil has comparable hemodynamic effects to inhaled iloprost with a longer duration of effect in patients with PAH. The most common adverse effect related to inhalation is transient coughing.

Monotherapy with extended-release oral formulations of treprostinil are effective in patients with PAH with moderate functional impairments (Jing et al., 2013). The dose is given twice a day, starting at 0.25 mg and titrating up every 3 days to a maximum of 21 mg twice a day. Serum concentrations at a steady dose of 3.5 mg twice daily are thought to approximate therapeutic levels of intravenous treprostinil. Oral treprostinil fails to show any significant improvement in 6-min walk distance for patients on baseline treatment with either an ERA or PDE5 inhibitor and is therefore not recommended in patients already treated (Tapson et al., 2012).

Iloprost

Clinical Use, Adverse Effects and Precautions. The first PGI$_2$ analogue available in an inhaled formulation, iloprost was designed to target the pulmonary vasculature with minimal systemic side effects. Inhalation has potent vasodilative effects on the pulmonary circulation, with less systemic vasodilation than intravenous PGI$_2$ (Olschewski et al., 1996). The effects of a single inhalation decline to baseline over 60–120 min, and current dosing strategies suggest 6–9 inhalations daily. The dose is generally titrated from 2.5 mg/inhalation to 5 mg after the first 2–4 weeks. Minor side effects common to the PGI$_2$ class include headache and jaw pain. Side effects specific to the inhaled formulation are cough, although this appears to resolve over time.

Beraprost

The first orally available PGI$_2$ analogue, beraprost, showed promise in early trials, but long-term trials showed no benefit over 12 months of therapy (Barst et al., 2003). As a result, beraprost is not approved for use in the U.S. or E.U.

Selexipag

Selexipag is an orally active, selective IPR agonist that is chemically distinct and has different kinetic properties compared to other PGI$_2$ analogues.

ADME. Selexipag is rapidly absorbed and hydrolyzed in the liver ($t_{1/2}$ = 1–2 h) to an active metabolite, ACT-333679 (Kaufmann et al., 2015). The active metabolite has a longer half-life, 10–14 h, allowing twice-daily dosing.

Clinical Use, Adverse Effects, and Precautions. The drug is taken at a starting dose of 200 μg and titrated upward weekly to a maximum dose of 1600 μg twice daily. In phase 3 clinical trials, selexipag reduced the risk of morbidity and mortality in patients with PAH (Simonneau et al., 2012; Sitbon et al., 2015). Selexipag was added to existing pulmonary vasodilator therapy in a majority of patients in the clinical trials for this agent. Adverse effects of selexipag are similar to those of PGI$_2$ analogues and include headache, jaw pain, nausea, dizziness, flushing, nasopharyngitis, and vomiting. Adverse effects appear to be more common when the drug is taken while fasting and wane over time.

Endothelin 1

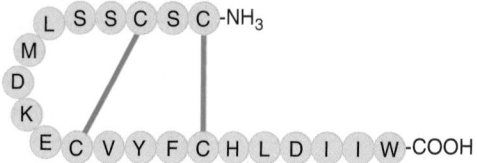

Amino Acid Sequence of Human Endothelin 1

Biosynthesis. Endothelins are a trio of 21 amino acid peptides, each the product of a different gene, produced through a pre-pro and pro-peptide sequence by ECE activities (ECE-1, ECE-2). ECE-1 is the rate-limiting step in ET-1 synthesis. Each mature ET peptide contains two disulfide bridges. ET-1, the predominant form, is encoded by the *EDN1* gene and produced in vascular ECs, although other cell types can also produce endothelin. A variety of cytokines, angiotensin II, and mechanical stress enhance ET-1 production. NO and PGI$_2$ reduce *EDN1* gene expression. ETs interact with two GPCRs, the ET$_A$ and ET$_B$ receptors, as described in the material that follows. ET-1 is cleared by interaction with the ET$_B$ receptor and via proteolytic degradation by neutral endopeptidase NEP24.11. Davenport and colleagues (2016) have reviewed key concepts of the biosynthesis, signaling, and pharmacology of ETs.

Endothelin Signaling. Endothelin 1 was discovered as a potent, endothelium-derived, constricting factor (Yanagisawa et al., 1988). The constrictor response is mediated by the ET$_A$ receptor, which is localized on PASMCs. The ET$_B$ receptor is present on both PASMCs and PAEC. Binding of ET-1 to ET$_A$ receptor on PASMCs activates the G$_q$-PLC-IP$_3$-Ca^{2+} and DAG-Ca^{2+}-PKC pathways (Figure 31–5 and Chapter 3). IP$_3$ activates the Ca^{2+} release channel on intracellular Ca^{2+} storage organelles, thereby

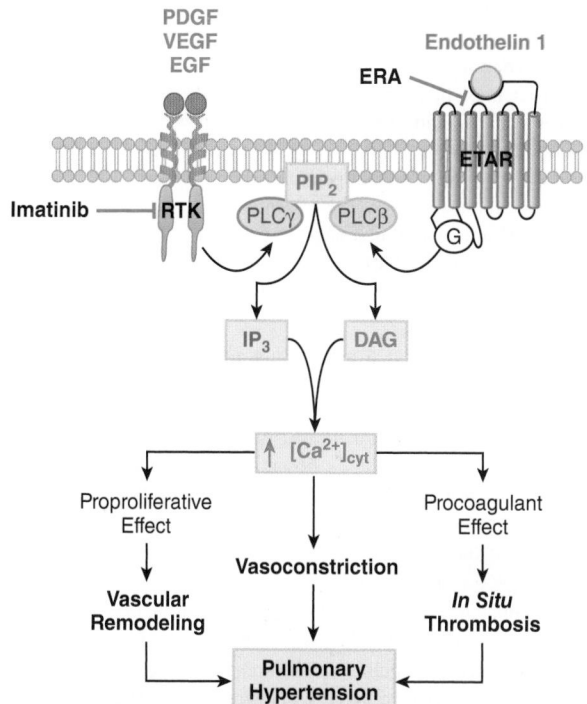

Figure 31–5 *Agents that inhibit receptor-mediated activation of phospholipase C.* The potent vasoconstricting agent ET-1 exerts effect on PASMCs primarily through the endothelin receptor ET$_A$, a GPCR. Stimulation of the receptor leads to activation of PLC and production of IP$_3$ and DAG, both of which lead to increased [Ca^{2+}]$_{cyt}$. Similarly, distinct receptor tyrosine kinases, such as PDGF, VEGF, and EGF, can lead to increased IP$_3$ and DAG and subsequent increases in [Ca^{2+}]$_{cyt}$ through a similar, yet distinct, pathway.

mobilizing Ca^{2+} and increasing $[Ca^{-+}]_{cyt}$. DAG can reportedly activate ROCs on the plasma membrane, enhance Ca^{2+} influx, and contribute to the increased $[Ca^{2+}]_{cyt}$. The elevated cytosolic Ca^{2+} produces vasoconstriction (Figure 3–14). ET-1 is also a mitogenic factor that exerts proliferative effects on many types of cells, including vascular smooth muscle cells and myofibroblasts via intracellular signaling cascades (e.g., PI3K/Akt/mTOR and Ras/ERK/p21 pathways) (Davenport et al., 2016). The activation of ET_B receptors on ECs mediates vasodilation by increasing production of NO and PGI_2 and can inhibit ET-1 production.

Rationale for Antagonizing ET's Effects in PAH. Endothelin 1 is implicated as a contributory factor in idiopathic PAH (Giaid et al., 1993): Plasma ET-1 levels are increased up to 10-fold in patients with PAH and correlate well with severity of disease and the elevation of right atrial pressure. There are no clinically available specific inhibitors of ECE-1, the rate-limiting step in ET-1 synthesis, but a number of orally effective small molecule antagonists of ET receptors have been developed. Despite the opposing effects of ET_A and ET_B receptor activation, pharmacological targeting of specific ET_A receptors has not led to significantly altered clinical responses compared to dual antagonism (e.g., antagonism of ET-1 binding to both ET_A and ET_B receptors) in treating PAH.

Endothelin Receptor Antagonists

Available ET receptor antagonists (ERAs) are bosentan, macitentan, and ambrisentan.

Commonalities. Endothelin antagonists generally share adverse effects. Common side effects of the class include headache, pulmonary edema, and nasal congestion/pharyngitis, with a risk of testicular atrophy and infertility. Bosentan and ambrisentan may increase liver transaminases, which should be monitored closely, and the drugs are contraindicated in patients with moderate-to-severe liver disease; the elevation of liver enzymes generally resolves after discontinuation of treatment.

The three available ET antagonists are metabolized by CYP3A4 and to some extent by CYPs 2C9 and 2C19. Repeated bosentan dosing elicits induction of CYPs 3A4 and 2C9, reducing exposure to drugs that are also metabolized by these CYPs (contraceptives, warfarin, some statins; coadministration with cyclosporine and glyburide is contraindicated); likewise, coadministration of bosentan or macitentan with a CYP inducer such as rifampin should be avoided. Inhibitors of these CYPs (e.g., ketoconazole and ritonavir) can increase bosentan and macitentan exposure (O'Callaghan et al., 2011).

The ERAs are potent teratogens and should be used with caution in women of childbearing age. These agents must not be used in pregnant patients. Documentation of a negative pregnancy test prior to initiation of therapy and a clear contraceptive plan are recommended, and fertile women must use two acceptable methods of birth control while taking ET antagonists.

Bosentan. Bosentan is a nonpeptide, orally effective, competitive antagonist of ET_A and ET_B receptors. In patients with PAH with mild-to-severe functional impairment (functional classes II–IV), bosentan improves symptoms, functional capacity, and pulmonary hemodynamic parameters (Rubin et al., 2002). Bosentan is usually started at 62.5 mg twice daily, increasing to 125 mg twice daily after 4 weeks. Bosentan is metabolized by hepatic CYPs 2C9 and 3A4 with a $t_{1/2}$ of about 5 h, with excretion of metabolites in the bile.

Macitentan. Macitentan is an orally active, competitive ET_A and ET_B receptor antagonist. At a dose of 10 mg daily, macitentan improves the time to disease progression or death in PAH and improves symptoms, functional capacity, and pulmonary hemodynamic measurements (Pulido et al., 2013). The drug is relatively well tolerated and has thus far not been associated with elevation of liver-associated enzymes, but caution is recommended. Macitentan is metabolized by CYPs to an active metabolite; the $t_{1/2}$ of the parent compound is about 16 h, that of the active metabolite about 48 h, such that the metabolite contributes about 40% of the total pharmacologic activity over time.

Ambrisentan. Unlike bosentan and macitentan, ambrisentan is a relatively selective ET_A antagonist (approximately 4000 times greater affinity

for ET_A than ET_B). Ambrisentan is initiated at a dose of 5 mg daily and increased to a maximum of 10 mg daily. The $t_{1/2}$ is 9 h at steady state. Liver-associated enzyme abnormalities are much less common than with bosentan, yet monitoring of liver function tests is still recommended. Elimination is largely via nonrenal pathways that have not been extensively characterized. There is some metabolism by CYPs 3A4 and 2C19, followed by glucuronidation; thus, drug interactions might be expected, although clinically relevant interactions have not been reported.

Receptor Tyrosine Kinase Inhibitors

Many growth factors and mitogenic factors are reportedly upregulated in tissues of patients with PAH. Elevations of ET-1, ATP, VIP, PDGF, VEGFs, EGF, fibroblast growth factor, and insulin-like growth factor in lung tissue, vascular smooth muscle cells, and peripheral blood have been assessed in PAH (Budhiraja et al., 2004; Du et al., 2003; Schermuly et al., 2005). These myriad mitogenic factors can activate TKRs, such as PDGF and EGF receptors. Activation of these receptors induces cell proliferation, growth, migration, and contraction in PASMCs, PAECs, and pulmonary vascular fibroblasts. With these actions as a rationale, antagonists of TKRs have been tried as therapeutics for PAH (Moreno-Vinasco et al, 2008; Gomberg-Maitland et al, 2010).

Imatinib

Imatinib was initially developed as targeted treatment of chronic myelogenous leukemia by targeting the ABL TKR; the compound is now known to have many other targets, one of which is the PDGF receptor that has been linked to vascular smooth muscle hypertrophy in the development of PAH (Humbert et al., 1998). Imatinib as add-on therapy for refractory PAH has shown efficacy in both case reports and a clinical trial, although serious adverse reactions, particularly subdural hematoma, are of concern (Hoeper et al., 2013). Larger clinical trials are needed before imatinib can be used in PAH treatment regimens.

Calcium Channels and Their Blockers

An increase in $[Ca^{2+}]_{cyt}$ in PASMCs causes pulmonary vasoconstriction and is an important stimulant of proliferation, migration, and vascular remodeling. $[Ca^{2+}]_{cyt}$ in PASMCs can be increased by Ca^{2+} influx through membrane Ca^{2+} channels and Ca^{2+} mobilization through the Ca^{2+} release channels/IP_3 receptors in the SR membrane. $[Ca^{2+}]_{cyt}$ can be decreased in three ways: by Ca^{2+} extrusion via the Ca^{2+}/Mg^{2+} ATPase (the Ca^{2+} pump

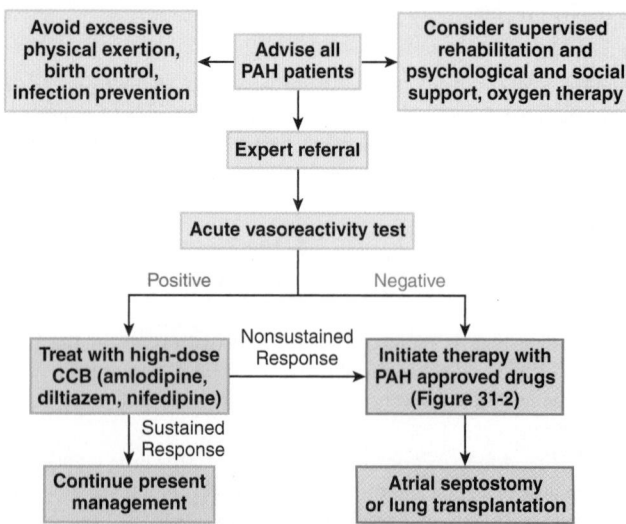

Figure 31–6 *Treatment algorithm for use of CCBs in PAH.* Vasoreactivity testing is used to identify the minority of patients who may have a substantial benefit from high-dose CCB therapy. These individuals must be monitored closely to ensure a sustained response. Patients without a positive vasodilator response should potentially be started on therapies approved for PAH based on symptoms at presentation. The patients with the most severe disease who fail to respond to therapy may need referral for surgical intervention to treat their disease.

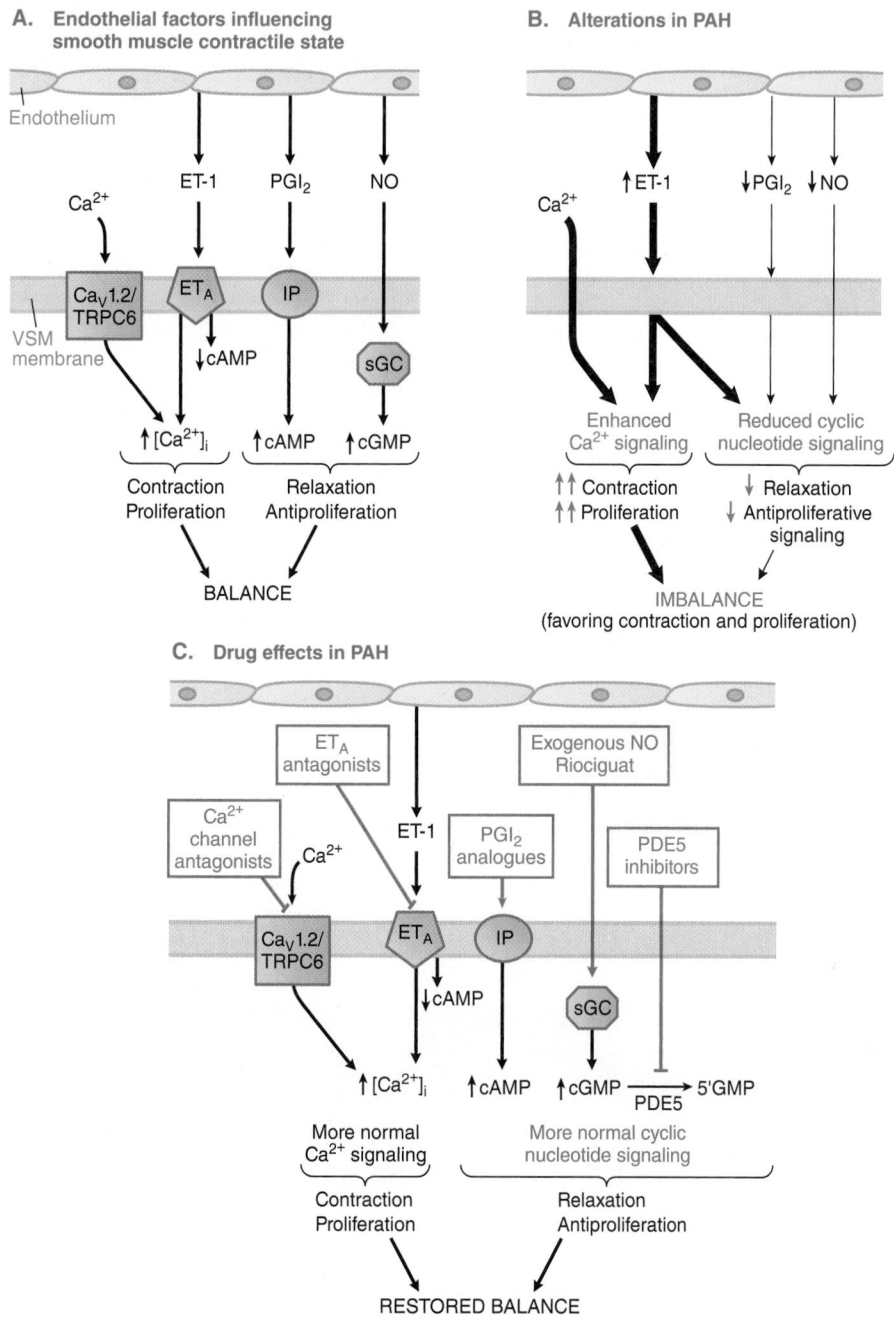

A. Endothelial factors influencing smooth muscle contractile state

B. Alterations in PAH

C. Drug effects in PAH

Figure 31–7 *Interactions between endothelium and vascular smooth muscle in PAH.* **A. Balance.** In normal pulmonary artery, there is a balance between constrictor and relaxant influences that may be viewed as competition between Ca^{2+} signaling pathways and cyclic nucleotide signaling pathways in VSM. ET-1 binds to the ET_A receptor on VSM cells and activates the G_q-PLC-IP_3 pathway to increase cytosolic Ca^{2+}; ET-1 may also couple to G_i to inhibit cAMP production. As VSM cells depolarize, Ca^{2+} may enter via the L-type Ca^{2+} channel ($Ca_v1.2$) or transient receptor potential cation channel (TRPC6). ECs also produce relaxant factors, PGI_2, and NO. NO stimulates the sGC, causing accumulation of cGMP in VSM cells; PGI_2 binds to the IPR and stimulates cAMP production; elevation of these cyclic nucleotides promotes VSM relaxation (see Figures 31-3, 40-4 and 45-6). **B. Imbalance.** In PAH, ET-1 production is enhanced, production of PGI_2 and NO is reduced, and the balance is shifted toward constriction and proliferation of VSM. **C. Restored balance.** In treating PAH, ET_A receptor antagonists can reduce the constrictor effects of ET-1, and Ca^{2+} channel antagonists can further reduce Ca^{2+}-dependent contraction. Exogenous PGI_2 and NO can be supplied to promote vasodilation (relaxation of VSM); the sGC can be activated pharmacologically (riociguat); inhibition of PDE5 can enhance the relaxant effect of elevated cGMP by inhibiting the degradation of cGMP. Thus, these drugs can reduce Ca^{2+} signaling and enhance cyclic nucleotide signaling, restoring the balance between the forces of contraction/proliferation and relaxation/antiproliferation. Remodeling and deposition of extracellular matrix by adjacent fibroblasts is influenced positively and negatively by the same contractile and relaxant signaling pathways, respectively. Effects of pharmacological agonists are noted by green arrows, effects of antagonists by red T-bars.

in the plasma membrane), export of Ca^{2+} by the Na^+/Ca^{2+} exchanger, and by sequestration of cytosolic Ca^{2+} into the SR by SR Ca^{2+}-ATPase. There are three classes of Ca^{2+}-permeable channels functionally expressed in the plasma membrane of PASMCs: (1) VDCCs, (2) ROCs, and (3) store-operated Ca^{2+} channels. These are targets in the current therapy of PAH and putative targets for therapeutics of the future.

Voltage-Gated Ca²⁺ Channel Blockers

A rare subset of patients (typically less than 5%–15% of all group I PAH confirmed by right heart catheterization) is considered vasoreactive, which is defined as a significant decrease in mean PAP (>10 mm Hg drop to absolute mean PAP < 40 mm Hg) while preserving cardiac output during the administration of inhaled NO or intravenous injection of PGI_2 or adenosine (Rich and Brundage, 1987). Vasoreactive patients can achieve prolonged survival, sustained functional improvement, and hemodynamic improvement with CCB therapy (Hemnes et al., 2015; Rich and Brundage, 1987). The utility of CCB therapy in patients with vasoreactive PAH was supported by a series of well-designed observational studies (Hemnes et al., 2015; Rich and Brundage, 1987; Sitbon et al., 2005).

Clinical Use. Therapy with CCB can be initiated with a low dose of long-acting nifedipine, amlodipine, diltiazem, or verapamil. The dose is then increased to the maximal tolerated dose. Systemic blood pressure, heart rate, and oxygen saturation should be carefully monitored during titration. Sustained-release preparations of nifedipine, verapamil, and diltiazem are available that minimize the adverse effects of therapy, especially systemic hypotension. Patients who respond (defined as asymptomatic or minimal symptoms) to CCB therapy with a dihydropyridine or diltiazem are typically reassessed for sustaining the response (Figure 31–6).

Adverse Effects and Precautions. Adverse effects are common with CCB therapy. Systemic vasodilation may cause hypotension, while pulmonary vasodilation may reduce HPV. Loss or inhibition of HPV can worsen V/Q mismatch and cause hypoxemia. CCBs may also be associated with deterioration of RV function because of their inhibitory effect on VDCC in cardiomyocytes. The pharmacology of CCBs is discussed in detail in Chapter 27.

PAH Drugs in Development

In addition to the PAH drugs in clinical use, there are many repurposed drugs and newly developed drugs that have therapeutic benefits in experimental models of PH. These agents have potential as future therapies for PAH:

- antagonists of $5HT_{2B}$ receptors and transporters (e.g., LY393558);
- allosteric antagonists of Ca^{2+}-sensing receptors (e.g., NPS2143 and calhex 231);
- openers or activators of Ca^{2+}-activated and voltage-gated K^+ channels and ATP-sensitive K^+ channels (e.g., cromakalim);
- inhibitors of the PI3K/Akt1/mTOR signaling cascades (e.g., perifosine, ipatasertib, and rapamycin derivatives sirolimus, temsirolimus, everolimus, deforolimus);
- inhibitors of the Notch signaling pathway (e.g., DAPT and MK-0752);
- VIP;
- blockers of transient receptor potential cation channels (e.g., 2-APB, ML204, aniline-thiazoles);
- extracellular elastase inhibitors (e.g., elafin and sivelestat);
- Rho kinase inhibitors (e.g., fasudil); and
- angiopoietin 1 inhibitors (e.g., trebananib).

Some of these drugs are already in phase 3 clinical trials; others are still in preclinical development.

A Pharmacologist's View of Signal Integration in PAH

As noted, an imbalance of vasoactive mediators, mitogenic and angiogenic factors, and pro- and antiapoptotic proteins plays an important role in PAH development. The pharmacological agents employed in PAH are focused on restoring the balance between contraction and proliferation on the one hand and relaxation and antiproliferation on the other, as summarized in Figure 31–7.

Drug Facts for Your Personal Formulary: *Pulmonary Hypertension Therapeutics*

Drug	Indication	Clinical Pharmacology and Tips
cGMP Signaling Modulators: PDE5 Inhibitors		
Sildenafil Tadalafil Vardenafil	• First-line therapy for moderate PAH (functional class II-III)	• Oral administration • Avoid nitrates and α adrenergic antagonists due to hypotension • Major side effects: epistaxis, headache, dyspepsia, vision or hearing loss (not sildenafil), flushing, insomnia, dyspnea, priapism • Vardenafil, currently not recommended due to limited evidence for efficacy in PAH
cGMP Signaling Modulators: sGC Stimulator		
Riociguat	• First-line therapy for moderate PAH (functional class II-III)	• Oral administration • Efficacy confirmed in PAH patients and CTEPH patients • Side effects: headache, dyspepsia, edema, nausea, dizziness, syncope
IP Receptor Agonists: Prostacyclin and Prostacyclin Analogs		
Epoprostenol	• First-line therapy for severe PAH (functional class IV)	• Administration by continuous IV infusion • Major side effects: jaw pain, hypotension, myalgia, flushing, nausea, vomiting, dizziness • Short half-life requires immediate medical attention to pump failure
Treprostinil	• Same as epoprostenol	• Available as IV, SC, inhaled and oral preps • Longer half-life than epoprostenol with similar side effects • Local adverse effects of SC dose may improve over time • Oral administration to be used as monotherapy only

IP Receptor Agonists: Prostacyclin and Prostacyclin Analogs (continued)		
Iloprost	• Alternative for epoprostenol in combination therapy for severe PAH (function class IV)	• Inhaled administration, at least 2 h apart • Side effects include flushing, hypotension, headache, nausea, throat irritation, cough, insomnia
Selexipag	• Alternative for eprostenol in combination therapy for severe PAH (functional class IV)	• Oral administration • Selective PGI_2 receptor agonist • Side effects include headache, jaw pain, nausea, diarrhea
Endothelin Receptor Antagonists: Oral administration, teratogenic		
Bosentan	• First-line therapy for moderate PAH (functional class II-III)	• Monitor liver function and hemoglobin levels • Metabolized by CYP2C9 and CYP3A4 • Side effects: liver impairment, palpitations, itching, edema, anemia, respiratory infections
Ambrisentan	• First-line therapy for moderate PAH (functional class II-III)	• Side effects: edema, nasal congestion, constipation, flushing, palpitations, abdominal pain • Cyclosporin coadministration increases drug levels • Low risk for liver toxicity
Macitentan	• First-line therapy for moderate PAH (functional class II-III)	• Metabolized by CYP3A4 • Side effects include nasopharyngitis, headache, anemia • Liver function and hemoglobin testing recommended prior to therapy
L-type Ca^{2+} Channel Blockers		
Nifedipine (long acting) Amlodipine Diltiazem	• Use only in PAH patients with positive vasodilator testing	• Oral administration • Side effects include edema, fatigue, hypotension • Diltiazem: significant negative chronotropic and inotropic effects; avoid in bradycardia

Abbreviations: PAH, Pulmonary Arterial Hypertension; ERA, Endothelin Receptor Antagonist; CTEPH, Chronic Thromboembolic Pulmonary Hypertension; IV, intravenous; SC, subcutaneous.

Bibliography

Abman SH. Inhaled nitric oxide for the treatment of pulmonary arterial hypertension. *Handb Exp Pharmacol*, **2013**, *218*:257–276.

Barst RJ, Beraprost Study Group. Beraprost therapy for pulmonary arterial hypertension. *J Am Coll Cardiol*, **2003**, *41*:2119–2125.

Barst RJ, Primary Pulmonary Hypertension Study Group. A comparison of continuous intravenous epoprostenol (prostacyclin) with conventional therapy for primary pulmonary hypertension. *N Engl J Med*, **1996**, *334*:296–301.

Benza RL, et al. An evaluation of long-term survival from time of diagnosis in pulmonary arterial hypertension from the REVEAL Registry. *Chest*, **2012**, *142*:448–456.

Budhiraja R. Endothelial dysfunction in pulmonary hypertension. *Circulation*, **2004**, *109*:159–165.

Bueno M, et al. Nitrite signaling in pulmonary hypertension: mechanisms of bioactivation, signaling, and therapeutics. *Antioxid Redox Signal*, **2013**, *18*:1797–1809.

Christman BW, et al. An imbalance between the excretion of thromboxane and prostacyclin metabolites in pulmonary hypertension. *N Engl J Med*, **1992**, *327*:70–75.

Cockrill BA, Waxman AB. Phosphodiesterase-5 inhibitors. *Handb Exp Pharmacol*, **2013**, *218*:229–255.

Craven KB, Zagotta WN. CNG and HCN channels: two peas, one pod. *Annu Rev Physiol*, **2006**, *68*:375–401.

Davenport AP, et al. Endothelin. *Pharmacol Rev*, **2016**, *68*:357–418.

Du L, et al. Signaling molecules in nonfamilial pulmonary hypertension. *N Engl J Med*, **2003**, *348*:500–509.

Fedullo P, et al. Chronic thromboembolic pulmonary hypertension. *Am J Respir Crit Care Med*, **2011**, *183*:1605–1613.

Frumkin LR. The pharmacological treatment of pulmonary arterial hypertension. *Pharmacol Rev*, **2012**, *64*:583–620.

Galiè N, Sildenafil Use in Pulmonary Arterial Hypertension Study Group. Sildenafil citrate therapy for pulmonary arterial hypertension. *N Engl J Med*, **2005**, *353*:2148–2157.

Galie, N, et al. Initial use of ambrisentan plus tadalafil in pulmonary arterial hypertension. *N Engl J Med*, **2015**, *373*:834–844.

Ghofrani HA, et al. Riociguat for the treatment of chronic thromboembolic pulmonary hypertension. *N Engl J Med*, **2013**, *369*:319–329.

Ghofrani HA, et al. Riociguat for the treatment of pulmonary arterial hypertension. *N Engl J Med*, **2013**, *369*:330–340.

Ghofrani HA, Humbert M. The role of combination therapy in managing pulmonary arterial hypertension. *Eur Respir Rev*, **2014**, *23*:469–475.

Giaid A, et al. Expression of endothelin-1 in the lungs of patients with pulmonary hypertension. *N Engl J Med*, **1993**, *328*:1732–1739.

Girgis RE, et al. Decreased exhaled nitric oxide in pulmonary arterial hypertension: response to bosentan therapy. *Am J Respir Crit Care Med*, **2005**, *172*:352–357.

Gomberg-Maitland M, et al. A dosing/cross-development study of the multikinase inhibitor sorafenib in patients with pulmonary arterial hypertension. *Clin Pharmacol Ther*, **2010**, *87*:303-310.

Griffiths MJ, Evans TW. Inhaled nitric oxide therapy in adults. *N Engl J Med*, **2005**, *353*:2683–2695.

Hemnes AR, et al. Peripheral blood signature of vasodilator-responsive pulmonary arterial hypertension. *Circulation*, **2015**, *131*:401–409.

Hoeper MM, et al. Imatinib mesylate as add-on therapy for pulmonary arterial hypertension: results of the randomized IMPRES study. *Circulation*, **2013**, *127*:1128–1138.

Humbert M, et al. Platelet-derived growth factor expression in primary pulmonary hypertension: comparison of HIV seropositive and HIV seronegative patients. *Eur Respir J*, **1998**, *11*:554–559.

Humbert M, Ghofrani H-A. The molecular targets of approved treatments for pulmonary arterial hypertension. *Thorax*, **2016**, *71*:73–83.

Ichinose F, et al. Inhaled nitric oxide: a selective pulmonary vasodilator: current uses and therapeutic potential. *Circulation*, **2004**, *109*: 3106–3111.

Jing ZC, et al. Efficacy and safety of oral treprostinil monotherapy for the treatment of pulmonary arterial hypertension: a randomized, controlled trial. *Circulation*, **2013**, *127*:624–633.

Kaufmann P, et al. Pharmacokinetics and tolerability of the novel oral prostacyclin IP receptor agonist selexipag. *Am J Cardiovasc Drugs*, **2015**, *15*:195–203.

Kawaguchi Y, et al. NOS2 polymorphisms associated with the susceptibility to pulmonary arterial hypertension with systemic sclerosis: contribution to the transcriptional activity. *Arthritis Res Ther,* **2006**, 8:R104.

Kass DA, et al. Phosphodiesterase type 5: expanding roles in cardiovascular regulation. *Circ Res,* **2007**, *101*:1084–1095.

Kuhr FK, et al. New mechanisms of pulmonary arterial hypertension: role of Ca^{2+} signaling. *Am J Physiol Heart Circ Physiol,* **2012**, *302*: H1546–H1562.

Mandegar M, et al. Cellular and molecular mechanisms of pulmonary vascular remodeling: role in the development of pulmonary hypertension. *Microvasc Res,* **2004**, *68*:75–103.

McLaughlin VV, et al. ACCF/AHA 2009 expert consensus document on pulmonary hypertension. *J Am Coll Cardiol,* **2009**, *53*:1573–1619.

Moreno-Vinasco L, et al. Genomic assessment of a multikinase inhibitor, sorafenib, in a rodent model of pulmonary hypertension. *Physiol Genomics,* **2008**, *33*:278-291.

Morrell NW, et al. Cellular and molecular basis of pulmonary arterial hypertension. *J Am Coll Cardiol,* **2009**, *54*(suppl):S20–S31.

Muirhead GJ, et al. Comparative human pharmacokinetics and metabolism of single-dose oral and intravenous sildenafil. *Br J Clin Pharmacol,* **2002**, *53*(suppl 1):13S–20S.

O'Callaghan DS, et al. Endothelin receptor antagonists for the treatment of pulmonary arterial hypertension. *Expert Opin Pharmacother,* **2011**, *12*:1585–1596.

Olschewski H, et al. Prostacyclin and its analogues in the treatment of pulmonary hypertension. *Pharmacol Ther,* **2004**, *102*:139–153.

Olschewski H, et al. Aerosolized prostacyclin and iloprost in severe pulmonary hypertension. *Ann Intern Med,* **1996**, *124*:820–824.

Omori K, Kotera J. Overview of PDEs and their regulation. *Circ Res,* **2007**, *100*:309–327.

Pulido T, Seraphin Investigators. Macitentan and morbidity and mortality in pulmonary arterial hypertension. *N Engl J Med,* **2013**, *369*:809–818.

Ravipati G, et al. Type 5 phosphodiesterase inhibitors in the treatment of erectile dysfunction and cardiovascular disease. *Cardiol Rev,* **2007**, *15*:76–86.

Rich S, Brundage BH. High-dose calcium channel-blocking therapy for primary pulmonary hypertension: evidence for long-term reduction in pulmonary arterial pressure and regression of right ventricular hypertrophy. *Circulation,* **1987**, *76*:135–141.

Rossaint R, et al. Inhaled nitric oxide for the adult respiratory distress syndrome. *N Engl J Med,* **1993**, *328*:399–405.

Rubin LJ, et al. Bosentan therapy for pulmonary arterial hypertension. *N Engl J Med,* **2002**, *346*:896–903.

Rubin LJ, et al. Frosolono M, Handel F, Cato AE. Prostacyclin-induced acute pulmonary vasodilation in primary pulmonary hypertension. *Circulation,* **1982**, *66*:334–338.

Schermuly RT, et al. Reversal of experimental pulmonary hypertension by PDGF inhibition. *J Clin Invest,* **2005**, *115*:2811–2821.

Simonneau G, et al. Updated clinical classification of pulmonary hypertension. *J Am Coll Cardiol,* **2013**, *62*:D34–D41.

Simonneau G, et al. Selexipag: an oral, selective prostacyclin receptor agonist for the treatment of pulmonary arterial hypertension. *Eur Respir J,* **2012**, *40*:874–880.

Simonneau G, Treprostinil Study Group. Continuous subcutaneous infusion of treprostinil, a prostacyclin analogue, in patients with pulmonary arterial hypertension: a double-blind, randomized, placebo-controlled trial. *Am J Respir Crit Care Med,* **2002**, *165*: 800–804.

Sitbon O, Griphon Investigators. Selexipag for the treatment of pulmonary arterial hypertension. *N Engl J Med,* **2015**, *373*:2522–2533.

Sitbon O, et al. Long-term response to calcium channel blockers in idiopathic pulmonary arterial hypertension. *Circulation,* **2005**, *111*:3105–3111.

Sitbon O, et al. Upfront triple combination therapy in pulmonary arterial hypertension: a pilot study. *Eur Respir J,* **2014**, *43*:1691–1697.

Stasch JP, Evgenov OV. Soluble guanylate cyclase stimulators in pulmonary hypertension. *Handb Exp Pharmacol,* **2013**, *218*: 279–313.

Tapson VF, et al. Oral treprostinil for the treatment of pulmonary arterial hypertension in patients on background endothelin receptor antagonist and/or phosphodiesterase type 5 inhibitor therapy (the FREEDOM-C study): a randomized controlled trial. *Chest,* **2012**, *142*:1383–1390.

Yanagisawa M, et al. A novel potent vasoconstrictor peptide produced by vascular endothelial cells. *Nature,* **1988**, *332*:411–415.

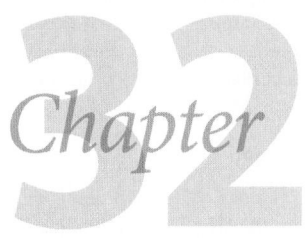

Chapter 32

Blood Coagulation and Anticoagulant, Fibrinolytic, and Antiplatelet Drugs

Kerstin Hogg and Jeffrey I. Weitz

Blood must remain fluid within the vasculature and yet clot quickly when exposed to subendothelial surfaces at sites of vascular injury. Under normal circumstances, a delicate balance between coagulation and fibrinolysis prevents both thrombosis and hemorrhage. Alteration of this balance in favor of coagulation results in thrombosis. Thrombi, composed of platelet aggregates, fibrin, and trapped red blood cells, can form in arteries or veins. Antithrombotic drugs used to treat thrombosis include antiplatelet drugs, which inhibit platelet activation or aggregation; anticoagulants, which attenuate fibrin formation; and fibrinolytic agents, which degrade fibrin. All antithrombotic drugs increase the risk of bleeding.

This chapter reviews the agents commonly used for controlling blood fluidity, including

- the parenteral anticoagulant heparin and its derivatives, which activate antithrombin, a natural inhibitor of coagulant proteases;
- the coumarin anticoagulants, which block multiple steps in the coagulation cascade;
- the direct oral anticoagulants, which inhibit factor Xa or thrombin;
- fibrinolytic agents, which degrade fibrin;
- antiplatelet agents, which attenuate platelet activation (aspirin, clopidogrel, prasugrel, ticagrelor, and vorapaxar) or aggregation (glycoprotein IIb/IIIa inhibitors); and
- vitamin K, which is required for the biosynthesis of key coagulation factors.

Overview of Hemostasis: Platelet Function, Blood Coagulation, and Fibrinolysis

Hemostasis is the cessation of blood loss from a damaged vessel. Platelets first adhere to macromolecules in the subendothelial regions of the injured blood vessel, where they become activated. Adherent platelets release substances that activate nearby platelets, thereby recruiting them to the site of injury. Activated platelets then aggregate to form the primary hemostatic plug.

Vessel wall injury also exposes tissue factor (*TF*), which initiates the coagulation system. Activated platelets enhance activation of the coagulation system by providing a surface onto which clotting factors assemble and by releasing stored clotting factors. This results in a burst of *thrombin* (*factor IIa*) generation. Thrombin converts soluble fibrinogen to fibrin, activates platelets, and feeds back to promote additional thrombin generation. The fibrin strands tie the platelet aggregates together to form a stable clot.

The processes of platelet activation and aggregation and blood coagulation are summarized in Figures 32–1 and 32–2 (see also the animation on the Goodman & Gilman site on *AccessMedicine.com*). Coagulation involves a series of zymogen activation reactions, as shown in Figure 32–2. At each stage, a precursor protein, or *zymogen*, is converted to an active protease by cleavage of one or more peptide bonds in the precursor molecule. The final protease generated is thrombin. Later, as wound healing occurs, the fibrin clot is degraded. The pathway of clot removal, fibrinolysis, is shown in Figure 32–3, along with sites of action of fibrinolytic agents.

Conversion of Fibrinogen to Fibrin

Fibrinogen, a 340,000-Da protein, is a dimer, each half of which consists of three pairs of polypeptide chains (designated Aα, Bβ, and γ). Disulfide bonds covalently link the chains and the two halves of the molecule. Thrombin converts fibrinogen to fibrin monomers by releasing fibrinopeptide A (a 16–amino acid fragment) and fibrinopeptide B (a 14–amino acid fragment) from the amino termini of the Aα and Bβ chains, respectively.

Abbreviations

ACT: activated clotting time
ADP: adenosine diphosphate
α$_2$-AP: α$_2$-antiplasmin
aPTT: activated partial thromboplastin time
CNS: central nervous system
COX: cyclooxygenase
CPR: cardiopulmonary resuscitation
CrCL: creatinine clearance
CYP: cytochrome P450
EDTA: ethylenediaminetetraacetic acid
EPCR: endothelial protein C receptor
GI: gastrointestinal
Gla: γ-carboxyglutamic acid
Glu: glutamic acid
GP: glycoprotein
INR: international normalized ratio
IP$_3$: inositol 1,4,5-trisphosphate
KGD: lysine-glycine-aspartate
LMWH: low-molecular-weight heparin
NO: nitric oxide
PAI: plasminogen activator inhibitor
PAR: protease-activated receptor
PGI$_2$: prostaglandin I$_2$ or prostacyclin
PLC: phospholipase C
PT: prothrombin time
RGD: arginine-glycine-aspartate
TF: tissue factor
TFPI: tissue factor pathway inhibitor
t-PA: tissue plasminogen activator
TxA$_2$: thromboxane A$_2$
u-PA: urokinase plasminogen activator
USP: U.S. Pharmacopeia
VKOR: vitamin K epoxide reductase
VKORC1: C1 subunit of vitamin K epoxide reductase
vWF: von Willebrand factor

Removal of the fibrinopeptides creates new amino termini, which form knobs that fit into preformed holes on other fibrin monomers to form a fibrin gel, which is the end point of in vitro tests of coagulation (see Coagulation In Vitro). Initially, the fibrin monomers are bound to each other noncovalently. Subsequently, factor XIII, a transglutaminase that is activated by thrombin, catalyzes interchain covalent cross-links between adjacent fibrin monomers, which strengthen the clot.

Structure of Coagulation Factors

In addition to factor XIII, the coagulation factors include factors II (prothrombin), VII, IX, X, XI, XII, high-molecular-weight kininogen and prekallikrein. A stretch of about 200 amino acid residues at the carboxyl termini of each of these zymogens exhibits homology to trypsin and contains the active site of the proteases. In addition, 9–12 Glu residues near the amino termini of factors II, VII, IX, and X are converted to Gla residues in a vitamin K–dependent posttranslational step. The Gla residues bind Ca^{2+} and are essential for the coagulant activities of these proteins by enabling their interaction with the anionic phospholipid membrane of activated platelets.

Nonenzymatic Protein Cofactors

TF, factor V, and factor VIII are critical cofactors in coagulation. A nonenzymatic lipoprotein cofactor, TF is not normally present on blood-contacting cells. TF is constitutively expressed on the surface of subendothelial smooth muscle cells and fibroblasts, which are exposed when the vessel wall is damaged. TF binds factor VIIa and enhances its catalytic efficiency. The TF/factor VIIa complex initiates coagulation by activating factors IX and X.

Factor VIII and Factor V Are Procofactors

Factor VIII circulates in plasma bound to *von Willebrand factor*, which serves to stabilize it. Factor V circulates in plasma, is stored in platelets in a partially activated form, and is released when platelets are activated. Thrombin releases von Willebrand factor from factor VIII and activates factors V and VIII to yield factor Va and VIIIa, respectively. Once activated, the cofactors bind to the surface of activated platelets and serve as receptors; factor VIIIa serves as the receptor for factor IXa, while factor Va serves as the receptor for factor Xa. In addition to binding factors IXa and Xa, factors VIIIa and Va bind their substrates, factors X and prothrombin (factor II), respectively.

Activation of Prothrombin

By cleaving two peptide bonds on prothrombin, factor Xa converts it to thrombin. In the presence of factor Va, a negatively charged phospholipid surface, and Ca^{2+} (the so-called prothrombinase complex), factor Xa activates prothrombin with 10^9-fold greater efficiency. This maximal rate of activation only occurs when prothrombin and factor Xa contain Gla residues at their amino terminals, which endows them with the capacity to bind calcium and interact with the anionic phospholipid surface.

Initiation of Coagulation

TF exposed at sites of vessel wall injury initiates coagulation via the *extrinsic pathway*. The small amount of factor VIIa circulating in plasma binds subendothelial TF and the TF–factor VIIa complex, then activates factors X and IX (see Figure 32–2). When bound to TF in the presence of anionic phospholipids and Ca^{2+} (extrinsic tenase), factor VIIa activity is increased 30,000-fold over that of factor VIIa alone.

The *intrinsic pathway* is initiated in vitro when factor XII, prekallikrein, and high-molecular-weight kininogen interact with kaolin, glass, or another negatively charged surface to generate small amounts of factor XIIa. Factor XII can be activated in vivo by contact of the blood with medical devices, such as mechanical heart valves or extracorporeal circuits, or by cell-free DNA, neutrophil extracellular traps, which are web-like structures composed of DNA and histones extruded from activated neutrophils, or inorganic polyphosphates released from activated platelets. Factor XIIa activates factor XI and the resultant factor XIa, then activates factor IX. Factor IXa activates factor X in a reaction accelerated by factor VIIIa, anionic phospholipids, and Ca^{2+}. Optimal thrombin generation depends on the formation of this factor IXa complex (intrinsic tenase) because it activates factor X more efficiently than the TF–factor VIIa complex.

Activation of factor XII is not essential for hemostasis, as evidenced by the fact that patients deficient in factor XII, prekallikrein, or high-molecular-weight kininogen do not have excessive bleeding. Factor XI deficiency is associated with a variable and usually mild bleeding disorder. In contrast, congenital deficiency of factor VIII or IX results in hemophilia A or B, respectively, and is associated with spontaneous bleeding, which can be fatal.

Fibrinolysis

The fibrinolysis pathway is summarized in Figure 32–3. The fibrinolytic system dissolves intravascular *fibrin* through the action of *plasmin*. To initiate fibrinolysis, plasminogen activators convert single-chain plasminogen, an inactive precursor, into two-chain *plasmin* by cleavage of a specific peptide bond. There are two distinct plasminogen activators: *t-PA* and *u-PA*, which is also known as urokinase. Although both activators are synthesized by endothelial cells, t-PA predominates under most conditions and drives intravascular fibrinolysis, while synthesis of u-PA mainly

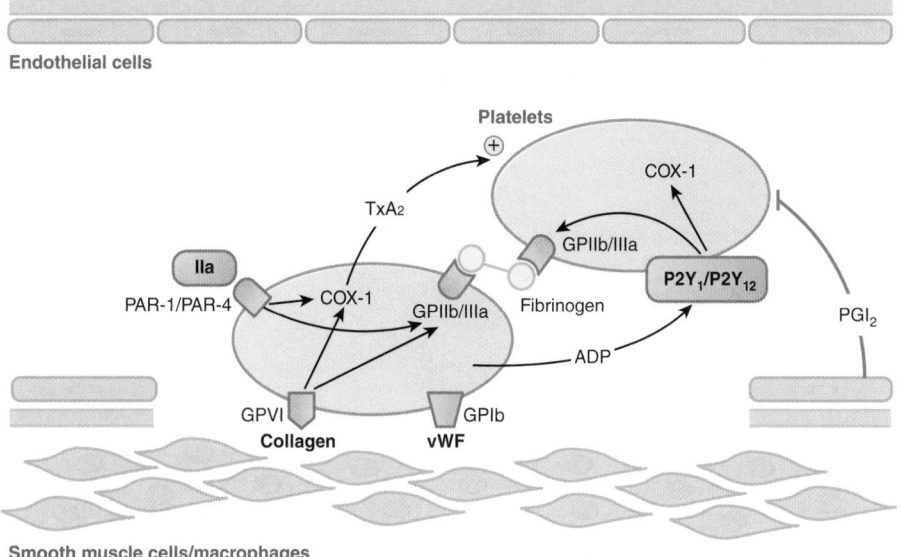

Figure 32–1 *Platelet adhesion and aggregation.* GPVI and GPIb are platelet receptors that bind to collagen and vWF, causing platelets to adhere to the subendothelium of a damaged blood vessel. PAR-1 and PAR-4 are PARs that respond to thrombin (IIa); P2Y$_1$ and P2Y$_{12}$ are receptors for ADP; when stimulated by agonists, these receptors activate the fibrinogen-binding protein GPIIb/IIIa and COX-1 to promote platelet aggregation and secretion. TxA$_2$ is the major product of COX-1 involved in platelet activation. Prostacyclin (PGI$_2$), synthesized by endothelial cells, inhibits platelet activation.

occurs in response to inflammatory stimuli and promotes extravascular fibrinolysis.

The fibrinolytic system is regulated such that unwanted fibrin thrombi are removed, while fibrin in wounds is preserved to maintain hemostasis. t-PA is released from endothelial cells in response to various stimuli. Released t-PA is rapidly cleared from blood or inhibited by *PAI-1* and, to a lesser extent, by *PAI-2*. Therefore, t-PA exerts little effect on circulating plasminogen in the absence of fibrin, and circulating α$_2$-*antiplasmin* rapidly inhibits any plasmin that is generated. The catalytic efficiency of t-PA activation of plasminogen increases more than 300-fold in the presence of fibrin, which promotes plasmin generation on its surface.

Plasminogen and plasmin bind to lysine residues on fibrin via five loop-like regions near their amino termini, which are known as *kringle domains*. To inactivate plasmin, α$_2$-antiplasmin binds to the first of these kringle domains and then blocks the active site of plasmin. Because the kringle

domains are occupied when plasmin binds to fibrin, plasmin on the fibrin surface is protected from inhibition by α$_2$-antiplasmin and can digest the fibrin. Once the fibrin clot undergoes degradation, α$_2$-antiplasmin rapidly inhibits any plasmin that escapes from this local milieu. To prevent premature clot lysis, factor XIIIa mediates covalent cross-linking of small amounts of α$_2$-antiplasmin onto fibrin.

When thrombi occlude major arteries or veins, therapeutic doses of plasminogen activators are sometimes administered to rapidly degrade the fibrin and restore blood flow. In high doses, these plasminogen activators promote the generation of so much plasmin that the inhibitory controls are overwhelmed. Plasmin is a relatively nonspecific protease; in addition to degrading fibrin, it degrades several coagulation factors. Reduction in the levels of these coagulation proteins impairs the capacity for thrombin generation, which can contribute to bleeding. In addition, unopposed plasmin tends to dissolve fibrin in hemostatic plugs as well as

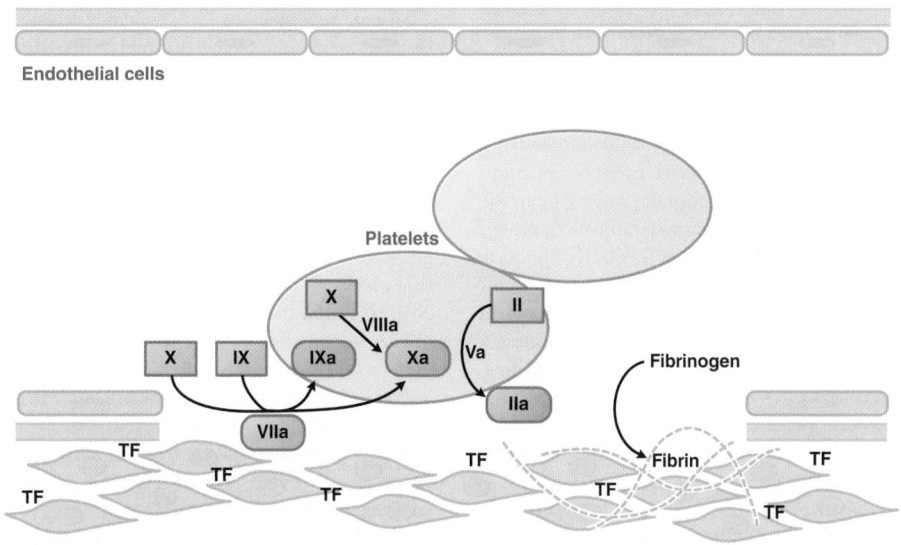

Figure 32–2 *Major reactions of blood coagulation.* Shown are interactions among proteins of the "extrinsic" (TF and factor VII), "intrinsic" (factors IX and VIII), and "common" (factors X, V, and II) coagulation pathways that are important in vivo. Boxes enclose the coagulation factor zymogens (indicated by Roman numerals); the rounded boxes represent the active proteases. Activated coagulation factors are followed by the letter *a*: II, prothrombin; IIa, thrombin.

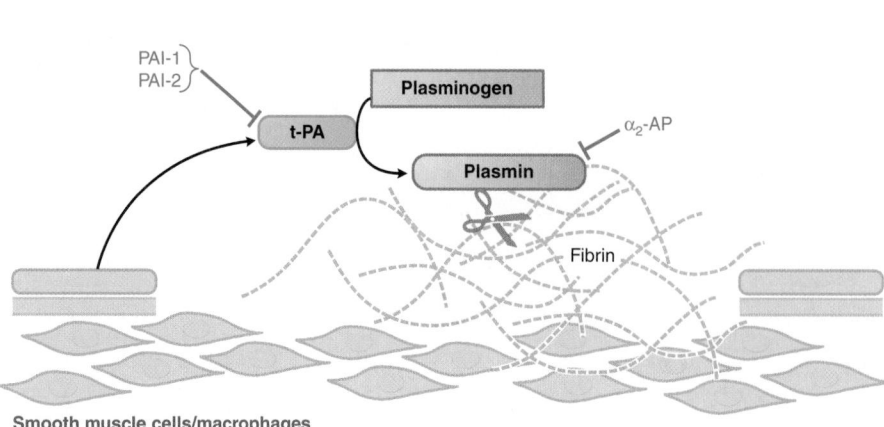

Endothelial cells

Smooth muscle cells/macrophages

Figure 32–3 *Fibrinolysis*. Endothelial cells secrete t-PA at sites of injury. t-PA binds to fibrin and converts plasminogen to plasmin, which digests fibrin. PAI-1 and PAI-2 inactivate t-PA; α_2-AP inactivates plasmin.

that in pathological thrombi, a phenomenon that also increases the risk of bleeding. Therefore, fibrinolytic drugs can produce hemorrhage as their major side effect.

Coagulation In Vitro

Whole blood normally clots in 4–8 min when placed in a glass tube. Under these conditions, contact of the blood with glass activates factor XII, thereby initiating coagulation via the *intrinsic pathway*. Clotting is prevented if a chelating agent such as EDTA or citrate is added to bind Ca^{2+}. Recalcified plasma normally clots in 2–4 min. The clotting time after recalcification is shortened to 26–33 sec by the addition of negatively charged phospholipids and particulate substances, such as kaolin (aluminum silicate) or celite (diatomaceous earth), which activate factor XII; the measurement of this is termed the *aPTT*. Alternatively, recalcified plasma clots in 12–14 sec after addition of "thromboplastin" (a mixture of TF and phospholipid) and calcium; the measurement of this is termed the *PT*.

Natural Anticoagulant Mechanisms

Platelet activation and coagulation do not normally occur within an intact blood vessel. Thrombosis is prevented by several regulatory mechanisms that require healthy vascular endothelium. Nitric oxide and prostacyclin synthesized by endothelial cells inhibit platelet activation (see Chapter 37).

Antithrombin is a plasma protein that inhibits coagulation enzymes of the extrinsic, intrinsic, and common pathways. Heparan sulfate proteoglycans synthesized by endothelial cells enhance the activity of antithrombin by about 1000-fold. Another regulatory system involves protein C, a plasma zymogen that is homologous to factors II, VII, IX, and X; its activity depends on the binding of Ca^{2+} to Gla residues within its amino terminal domain. Protein C binds to EPCR, which presents it to the thrombin-thrombomodulin complex for activation. Activated protein C then dissociates from EPCR, and, in combination with protein S, its nonenzymatic Gla-containing cofactor, activated protein C degrades factors Va and VIIIa. Without these activated cofactors, the rates of activation of prothrombin and factor X are greatly diminished, and thrombin generation is attenuated. Congenital or acquired deficiency of protein C or protein S is associated with an increased risk of venous thrombosis.

Tissue factor pathway inhibitor is a natural anticoagulant found in the lipoprotein fraction of plasma or bound to endothelial cell surface. TFPI first binds and inhibits factor Xa, and this binary complex then inhibits factor VIIa bound to TF. By this mechanism, factor Xa regulates its own generation.

Parenteral Anticoagulants: Heparin, LMWHs, Fondaparinux

Heparin and Its Standardization

Heparin, a glycosaminoglycan found in the secretory granules of mast cells, is synthesized from UDP-sugar precursors as a polymer of alternating D-glucuronic acid and N-acetyl-D-glucosamine residues. Heparin is commonly extracted from porcine intestinal mucosa, which is rich in mast cells, and preparations may contain small amounts of other glycosaminoglycans. Various commercial heparin preparations have similar biological activity (~150 USP units/mg). A USP unit reflects the quantity of heparin that prevents 1 mL of citrated sheep plasma from clotting for 1 h after calcium addition. European manufacturers measure potency with an anti–factor Xa assay. To determine heparin potency, residual factor Xa activity in the sample is compared with that detected in controls containing known concentrations of an international heparin standard. When assessed this way, heparin potency is expressed in international units per milligram. Effective October 1, 2009, the new USP unit dose was harmonized with the international unit dose. As a result, the new USP unit dose is about 10% less potent than the old one, which results in a requirement for somewhat higher heparin doses to achieve the same level of anticoagulation.

Heparin Derivatives

Derivatives of heparin in current use include LMWH and fondaparinux (see their comparison in Table 32–1).

Mechanism of Action. Heparin, LMWHs, and fondaparinux have no intrinsic anticoagulant activity; rather, these agents bind to antithrombin and accelerate the rate at which it inhibits various coagulation proteases. Synthesized in the liver, antithrombin circulates in plasma at an approximate concentration of 2.5 μM. Antithrombin inhibits activated coagulation factors, particularly thrombin and factor Xa, by serving as a "suicide substrate." Thus, inhibition occurs when the protease attacks a specific Arg–Ser peptide bond in the reactive center loop of antithrombin and becomes trapped as a stable 1:1 complex. Heparin binds to antithrombin via a specific pentasaccharide sequence that contains a 3-O-sulfated glucosamine residue (Figure 32–4).

Pentasaccharide binding to antithrombin induces a conformational change in antithrombin that renders its reactive site more accessible to the target protease (Figure 32–5). This conformational change accelerates the rate of factor Xa inhibition by at least two orders of magnitude but has no effect on the rate of thrombin inhibition. To enhance the rate of thrombin

TABLE 32–1 ■ COMPARISON OF THE FEATURES OF SUBCUTANEOUS HEPARIN, LOW-MOLECULAR-WEIGHT HEPARIN, AND FONDAPARINUX

FEATURES	HEPARIN	LMWH	FONDAPARINUX
Source	Biological	Biological	Synthetic
Mean molecular weight (Da)	15,000	5000	1500
Target	Xa and IIa	Xa and IIa	Xa
Subcutaneous			
Bioavailability (%)	30 (at low doses)	90	100
$t_{1/2}$ (h)	1–8[a]	4	17
Renal excretion	No	Yes	Yes
Antidote effect	Complete	Partial	None
Thrombocytopenia	<5%	<1%	<0.1%

[a]Half-life $t_{1/2}$ is dose dependent; half-life is 1 h with 5000 units given subcutaneously and can extend to 8 h with higher doses.

inhibition by antithrombin, heparin serves as a catalytic template to which both the inhibitor and the protease bind. Only heparin molecules composed of 18 or more saccharide units (molecular weight > 5400) are of sufficient length to bridge antithrombin and thrombin together. Consequently, by definition, heparin catalyzes the rates of factor Xa and thrombin inhibition to a similar extent, as expressed by an anti–factor Xa to anti–factor IIa (thrombin) ratio of 1:1 (Figure 32–5A). In contrast, at least half of LMWH molecules (mean molecular weight of 5000, which corresponds with about 17 saccharide units) are too short to provide this bridging function and have no effect on the rate of thrombin inhibition by antithrombin (Figure 32–5B). Because these shorter molecules still induce the conformational change in antithrombin that accelerates inhibition of factor Xa, LMWH has greater anti–factor Xa activity than anti–factor IIa activity, and the ratio ranges from 3:1 to 2:1 depending on the preparation. Fondaparinux, a synthetic analogue of the pentasaccharide sequence in heparin or LMWH that mediates their interaction with antithrombin, has only anti–factor Xa activity because it is too short to bridge antithrombin to thrombin (Figure 32–5C).

Heparin, LMWH, and fondaparinux act in a catalytic fashion. After binding to antithrombin and promoting the formation of covalent complexes between antithrombin and target proteases, the heparin, LMWH, or fondaparinux dissociates from the complex and can then catalyze other antithrombin molecules.

Platelet factor 4, a cationic protein released from α-granules during platelet activation, binds heparin and prevents it from interacting with antithrombin. This phenomenon may limit the activity of heparin in the vicinity of platelet-rich thrombi. Because LMWH and fondaparinux have a lower affinity for platelet factor 4, these agents may retain their activity in the vicinity of such thrombi to a greater extent than heparin.

Miscellaneous Pharmacological Effects. High doses of heparin can interfere with platelet aggregation and prolong the bleeding time. In contrast, LMWH and fondaparinux have little effect on platelets. Heparin "clears" lipemic plasma in vivo by causing the release of lipoprotein lipase into the circulation. Lipoprotein lipase hydrolyzes triglycerides to glycerol and free fatty acids. The clearing of lipemic plasma may occur at concentrations of heparin below those necessary to produce an anticoagulant effect.

Clinical Use. Heparin, LMWH, or fondaparinux can be used to initiate treatment of deep vein thrombosis and pulmonary embolism. They also can be used for the initial management of patients with unstable angina or acute myocardial infarction (Gara et al., 2013; Roffi et al., 2015). For most of these indications, LMWH or fondaparinux has replaced continuous heparin infusions because of their pharmacokinetic advantages, which permit subcutaneous administration once or twice daily in fixed or weight-adjusted doses without coagulation monitoring. Thus, LMWH or fondaparinux can be used for out-of-hospital management of patients with deep vein thrombosis or pulmonary embolism.

Heparin or LMWH is used during coronary balloon angioplasty with or without stent placement to prevent thrombosis. Fondaparinux is not used in this setting because of the risk of catheter thrombosis, a complication caused by catheter-induced activation of factor XII; longer heparin molecules are better than shorter ones for blocking this process. Cardiopulmonary bypass circuits also activate factor XII, which can cause clotting of the oxygenator. Heparin remains the agent of choice for surgery requiring cardiopulmonary bypass. Heparin or LMWH also is used to treat selected patients with disseminated intravascular coagulation. Subcutaneous administration of low-dose heparin or LMWH is often used for thromboprophylaxis in immobilized medically ill patients (Kahn et al., 2012) or in those who have undergone major surgery (Falck-Ytter et al., 2012; Gould et al., 2012).

Unlike the oral anticoagulants, heparin, LMWH, and fondaparinux do not cross the placenta and have not been associated with fetal malformations, making them the drugs of choice for anticoagulation during pregnancy. Heparin, LMWH, and fondaparinux do not appear to increase fetal mortality or prematurity. If possible, the drugs should be discontinued 24 h before delivery to minimize the risk of postpartum bleeding.

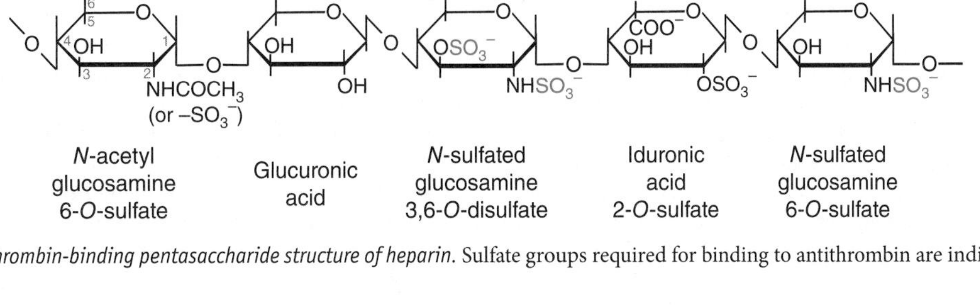

Figure 32–4 *The antithrombin-binding pentasaccharide structure of heparin.* Sulfate groups required for binding to antithrombin are indicated in red.

A

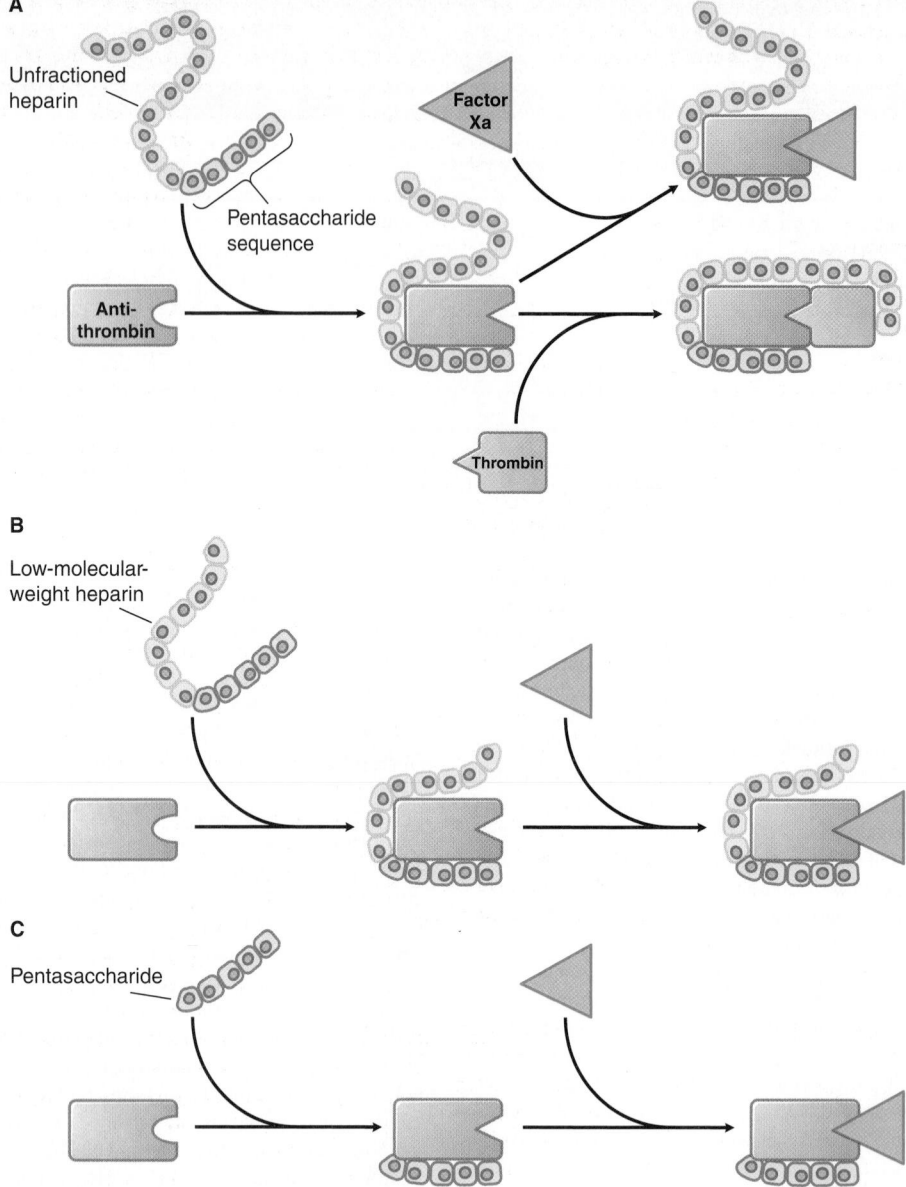

Figure 32–5 *Mechanism of action of heparin, LMWH, and fondaparinux, a synthetic pentasaccharide.* **A.** Heparin binds to antithrombin via its pentasaccharide sequence. This induces a conformational change in the reactive center loop of antithrombin that accelerates its interaction with factor Xa. To potentiate thrombin inhibition, heparin must simultaneously bind to antithrombin and thrombin. Only heparin chains composed of at least 18 saccharide units (MW ~ 5400 Da) are of sufficient length to perform this bridging function. With a mean MW of approximately 15,000 Da, virtually all of the heparin chains are long enough to do this. **B.** LMWH has greater capacity to potentiate factor Xa inhibition by antithrombin than thrombin because at least half of the LMWH chains (mean MW ~ 4500–5000 Da) are too short to bridge antithrombin to thrombin. **C.** The pentasaccharide accelerates only factor Xa inhibition by antithrombin; the pentasaccharide is too short to bridge antithrombin to thrombin.

ADME. Heparin, LMWH, and fondaparinux are not absorbed through the GI mucosa and must be given parenterally. Heparin is given by continuous intravenous infusion, intermittent infusion every 4–6 h, or subcutaneous injection every 8–12 h. Heparin has an immediate onset of action when given intravenously. In contrast, there is considerable variation in the bioavailability of heparin given subcutaneously, and the onset of action is delayed by 1–2 h. LMWH and fondaparinux are absorbed more uniformly after subcutaneous injection. The $t_{1/2}$ of heparin in plasma depends on the dose administered. When doses of 100, 400, or 800 units/kg of heparin are injected intravenously, the half-lives are about 1, 2.5, and 5 h, respectively. Heparin appears to be cleared and degraded primarily by the reticuloendothelial system; a small amount of intact heparin appears in the urine.

Both LMWH and fondaparinux have longer biological half-lives than heparin, 4–6 and 17 h, respectively. Because these smaller heparin fragments are cleared almost exclusively by the kidneys, the drugs can accumulate in patients with renal impairment and lead to bleeding. Both LMWH and fondaparinux are contraindicated in patients with a creatinine clearance below 30 mL/min. In addition, thromboprophylaxis with fondaparinux is contraindicated in patients undergoing hip fracture, hip replacement, knee replacement, or abdominal surgery who have a body weight less than 50 kg.

Administration and Monitoring. Full-dose heparin usually is administered by continuous intravenous infusion. Treatment of venous thromboembolism is initiated with a fixed-dose bolus injection of 5000 units or with a weight-adjusted bolus, followed by 800–1600 units/h delivered by an infusion pump. Therapy is monitored by measuring the aPTT. The therapeutic range for heparin is considered to be that which is equivalent to a plasma heparin level of 0.3–0.7 units/mL, as determined with an anti–factor Xa assay. An aPTT that is two or three times the normal mean aPTT value generally is assumed to be therapeutic. The aPTT should be measured initially and the infusion rate adjusted every 6 h. Once a steady dosage schedule has been established, daily aPTT monitoring usually is sufficient. Very high doses of heparin are required to prevent clotting in patients undergoing percutaneous coronary intervention or cardiac surgery with cardiopulmonary bypass. The aPTT is infinitely prolonged with these high doses of heparin, so a less-sensitive coagulation test, the ACT, is employed to monitor therapy in this situation.

For therapeutic purposes, heparin also can be administered subcutaneously on a twice-daily basis. A total daily dose of about 35,000 units administered as divided doses every 8–12 h usually is sufficient to achieve an aPTT of twice the control value (measured midway between doses). For low-dose heparin therapy (to prevent venous thromboembolism in hospitalized medical or surgical patients), a subcutaneous dose of 5000 units is given two or three times daily.

Heparin Resistance. Patients who fail to achieve a therapeutic aPTT with daily doses of heparin of 35,000 units or more are considered to have heparin resistance, which may reflect pseudo- or true resistance. Concomitant measurement of the aPTT and the anti–factor Xa level distinguishes between these two possibilities. With heparin pseudoresistance, the anti–factor Xa level is therapeutic despite the subtherapeutic aPTT, whereas with true heparin resistance both the anti–factor Xa level and the aPTT are subtherapeutic. Pseudoresistance to heparin occurs if the aPTT is shorter than the control value prior to initiating heparin treatment because of high concentrations of factor VIII and fibrinogen. True heparin resistance occurs because of high plasma levels of proteins that compete with antithrombin for heparin binding or because of antithrombin deficiency. Heparin does not require dose adjustment in patients with pseudoresistance because the anti–factor Xa level is therapeutic. In contrast, with true resistance, heparin doses need to be increased until a therapeutic aPTT or anti-factor Xa level is achieved. Patients with severe antithrombin deficiency may require antithrombin concentrate to achieve therapeutic anticoagulation with heparin.

LMWH Preparations

Enoxaparin and dalteparin are the LMWH preparations marketed in the U.S.; tinzaparin is available in other countries. The composition of these agents differs, as do their dosing regimens. Because LMWH produces a relatively predictable anticoagulant response, monitoring is not done routinely. Patients with renal impairment may require monitoring with an anti–factor Xa assay because this condition can prolong the $t_{1/2}$ and slow the elimination of LMWH. Obese patients, pregnant women, and children given LMWH also may require monitoring.

Fondaparinux

Fondaparinux, a synthetic pentasaccharide, is administered by subcutaneous injection, reaches peak plasma levels in 2 h, has a $t_{1/2}$ of 17 h, and is excreted in the urine. Because of the risk of accumulation and subsequent bleeding, fondaparinux should not be used in patients with a creatinine clearance less than 30 mL/min. Fondaparinux can be given subcutaneously once a day at a fixed or weight-adjusted dose without coagulation monitoring. Fondaparinux is much less likely than heparin or LMWH to trigger heparin-induced thrombocytopenia, and the drug has been used successfully to treat patients with this condition. Fondaparinux is approved for thromboprophylaxis in patients undergoing hip or knee surgery or surgery for hip fracture and for initial therapy of patients with deep vein thrombosis or pulmonary embolism. In some countries, but not the U.S., fondaparinux also is licensed as an alternative to heparin or LMWH in patients with acute coronary syndrome. For this indication and for thromboprophylaxis, fondaparinux is administered subcutaneously once daily at a dose of 2.5 mg.

Bleeding. The major untoward effect of heparin, LMWH, and fondaparinux is bleeding. Major bleeding occurs in 1%–5% of patients treated with intravenous heparin for venous thromboembolism. The incidence of bleeding is somewhat less in patients treated with LMWH for this

indication. Often, an underlying cause for bleeding is present, such as recent surgery, trauma, peptic ulcer disease, or platelet dysfunction due to concomitant administration of aspirin or other antiplatelet drugs.

The anticoagulant effect of heparin disappears within hours of discontinuation of the drug. Mild bleeding due to heparin usually can be controlled without administration of an antagonist. If life-threatening hemorrhage occurs, heparin can rapidly be reversed by the intravenous infusion of *protamine sulfate* (a mixture of basic polypeptides isolated from salmon sperm), which binds tightly to heparin and neutralizes its anticoagulant effect. Protamine also interacts with platelets, fibrinogen, and other plasma proteins and may cause an anticoagulant effect of its own. Therefore, one should give the minimal amount of protamine required to neutralize the heparin present in the plasma. This amount is 1 mg of protamine for every 100 units of heparin remaining in the patient; protamine is given intravenously at a slow rate (up to a maximum of 50 mg over 10 min). Protamine binds only long heparin molecules. Therefore, protamine only partially reverses the anticoagulant activity of LMWH and has no effect on that of fondaparinux.

Heparin-Induced Thrombocytopenia. Heparin-induced thrombocytopenia (platelet count < 150,000/mL or a 50% decrease from the pretreatment value) occurs in about 0.5% of medical patients 5–10 days after initiation of therapy with heparin. Although the incidence is lower, thrombocytopenia also occurs with LMWH and rarely with fondaparinux. Life-threatening thrombotic complications that can lead to limb amputation, which occurs in up to one-half of the affected heparin-treated patients and may precede the onset of thrombocytopenia. Women are twice as likely as men to develop this condition, and heparin-induced thrombocytopenia is more common in surgical patients than medical patients.

Venous thromboembolism occurs most commonly, but arterial thrombosis causing limb ischemia, myocardial infarction, or stroke also occurs. Bilateral adrenal hemorrhage, skin lesions at the site of subcutaneous heparin injection, and a variety of systemic reactions may accompany heparin-induced thrombocytopenia. The development of immunoglobulin G antibodies against complexes of heparin with platelet factor 4 (or, rarely, other chemokines) causes most of these reactions.

Heparin or LMWH should be discontinued immediately if unexplained thrombocytopenia or any of the clinical manifestations mentioned occur 5 or more days after beginning therapy, regardless of the dose or route of administration. The diagnosis of heparin-induced thrombocytopenia can be confirmed with a heparin-dependent platelet activation assay or an immunoassay for antibodies that react with heparin–platelet factor 4 complexes. Because thrombotic complications may occur after cessation of therapy, an alternative anticoagulant such as bivalirudin or argatroban (see the next section) or fondaparinux should be administered to patients with heparin-induced thrombocytopenia. LMWH should be avoided because it cross-reacts with heparin antibodies. *Warfarin may precipitate venous limb gangrene or skin necrosis in patients with heparin-induced thrombocytopenia and should not be used until the platelet count returns to normal.*

Other Toxicities. Abnormalities of hepatic function tests occur frequently in patients who are receiving heparin or LMWH. Osteoporosis occurs occasionally in patients who have received therapeutic doses of heparin (>20,000 units/d) for extended periods (e.g., 3–6 months). The risk of osteoporosis is lower with LMWH or fondaparinux than it is with heparin. Heparin can inhibit the synthesis of aldosterone by the adrenal glands and occasionally causes hyperkalemia.

Other Parenteral Anticoagulants

Desirudin and Lepirudin

Desirudin and lepirudin (not available in the U.S.) are recombinant forms of hirudin. Desirudin is indicated for thromboprophylaxis in patients undergoing elective hip replacement surgery. Both desirudin and lepirudin are also used for treating thrombosis in the setting of heparin-induced thrombocytopenia (Kelton et al., 2013). Desirudin and lepirudin are eliminated by the kidneys; the $t_{1/2}$ is about 2 h after subcutaneous administration and about 10 min after intravenous infusion. Both drugs should be used cautiously in patients with decreased renal function, and serum creatinine and aPTT should be monitored daily.

Bivalirudin

Bivalirudin is a synthetic 20–amino acid polypeptide that directly inhibits thrombin. Bivalirudin is administered intravenously and is used as an alternative to heparin in patients undergoing coronary angioplasty or cardiopulmonary bypass surgery (Barria Perez et al. 2016). Patients with heparin-induced thrombocytopenia or a history of this disorder also can be given bivalirudin instead of heparin during coronary angioplasty. The $t_{1/2}$ of bivalirudin is 25 min; dosage reductions are recommended for patients with renal impairment.

Argatroban

Argatroban, a synthetic compound based on the structure of L-arginine, binds reversibly to the active site of thrombin. Argatroban is administered intravenously and has a $t_{1/2}$ of 40–50 min. It is metabolized in the liver and excreted in the bile. Therefore, argatroban can be used in patients with renal impairment, but dose reduction is required for patients with hepatic insufficiency. Argatroban is licensed for the prophylaxis or treatment of patients with, or at risk of developing, heparin-induced thrombocytopenia (Grouzi, 2014). In addition to prolonging the aPTT, argatroban prolongs the PT, which can complicate the transitioning of patients from argatroban to warfarin. A factor X assay can be used instead of the PT to monitor warfarin in these patients.

Vitamin K Antagonist

Warfarin

Warfarin or other vitamin K antagonists are commonly used oral anticoagulants.

Mechanism of Action

Coagulation factors II, VII, IX, and X and proteins C and S are synthesized in the liver and are biologically inactive unless 9–13 of the amino-terminal Glu residues are γ-carboxylated to form the Ca^{2+}-binding Gla domain. This carboxylation reaction requires CO_2, O_2, and reduced vitamin K and is catalyzed by γ-glutamyl carboxylase (Figure 32–6). Carboxylation is coupled to the oxidation of vitamin K to its corresponding epoxide form. Reduced vitamin K must be regenerated from the epoxide form for sustained carboxylation and synthesis of functional proteins. The enzyme that catalyzes this reaction, VKOR is inhibited by therapeutic doses of warfarin.

At therapeutic doses, warfarin decreases the functional amount of each vitamin K–dependent coagulation factor made by the liver by 30%–70%. Warfarin has no effect on the activity of fully γ-carboxylated factors already in the circulation, and these must be cleared before it can produce an anticoagulant effect. The approximate $t_{1/2}$ values of factors VII, IX, X, and II are 6, 24, 36, and 50 h, respectively, while the $t_{1/2}$ values of protein C and protein S are 8 and 24 h, respectively. Because of the long $t_{1/2}$ of some of the coagulation factors, in particular factor II, the full antithrombotic effect of warfarin is not achieved for 4 to 5 days. For this reason, warfarin must be overlapped with a rapidly acting parenteral anticoagulant, such as heparin, LMWH, or fondaparinux, in patients with thrombosis or at high risk for thrombosis.

ADME

The bioavailability of warfarin is nearly complete when the drug is administered orally, intravenously, or rectally. Generic warfarin tablets may vary in their rate of dissolution, and this may cause some variation in the rate and extent of absorption. Food in the GI tract also can decrease the rate of absorption. Plasma warfarin concentrations peak in 2–8 h. Warfarin is administered as a racemic mixture of *S*- and *R*-warfarin. *S*-Warfarin is 3- to 5-fold more potent than *R*-warfarin and is mainly metabolized by CYP2C9. Inactive metabolites of warfarin are excreted

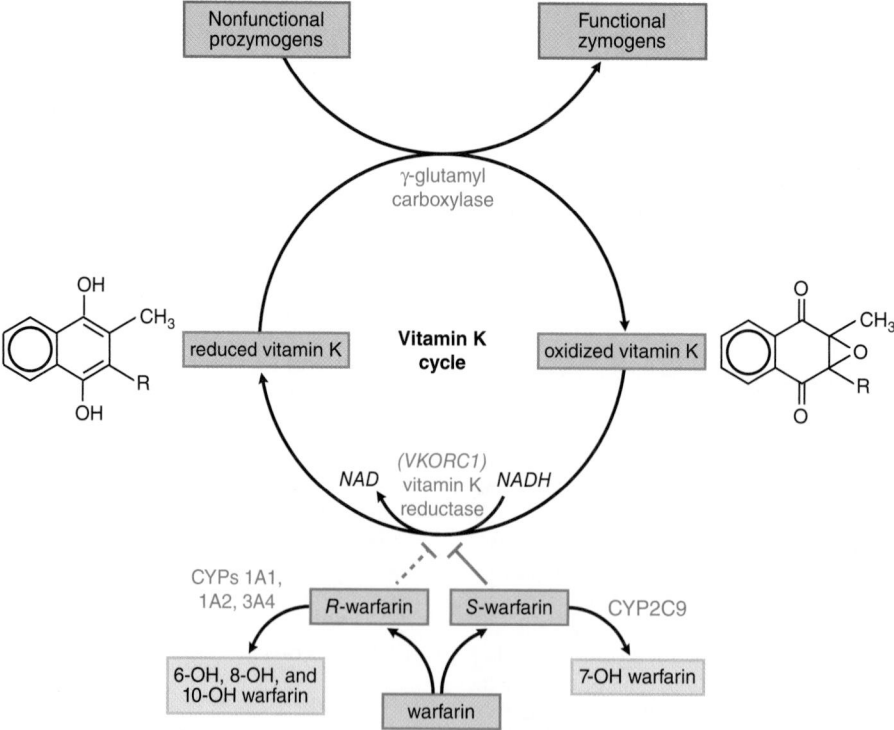

Figure 32–6 *The vitamin K cycle and mechanism of action of warfarin.* In the racemic mixture of *S*- and *R*-enantiomers, *S*-warfarin is more active. By blocking VKOR encoded by the *VKORC1* gene, warfarin inhibits the conversion of oxidized vitamin K epoxide into its reduced form, vitamin K hydroquinone. This inhibits vitamin K–dependent γ-carboxylation of factors II, VII, IX, and X because reduced vitamin K serves as a cofactor for a γ-glutamyl carboxylase that catalyzes the γ-carboxylation process whereby prozymogens are converted to zymogens capable of binding Ca^{2+} and interacting with anionic phospholipids. *S*-Warfarin is metabolized by *CYP2C9*; common genetic polymorphisms in this enzyme increase warfarin metabolism. Polymorphisms in the VKORC1 increase the susceptibility of the enzyme to warfarin-induced inhibition. Thus, patients expressing polymorphisms in these two enzymes require reduction of warfarin dosage (see Table 32–2).

TABLE 32–2 ■ EFFECT OF *CYP2C9* GENOTYPES AND *VKORC1* HAPLOTYPES ON WARFARIN DOSING

GENOTYPE/HAPLOTYPE	FREQUENCY (%)			DOSE REDUCTION COMPARED WITH WILD TYPE (%)
	CAUCASIANS	AFRICAN AMERICANS	ASIANS	
CYP2C9				
*1/*1	70	90	95	—
*1/*2	17	2	0	22
*1/*3	9	3	4	34
*2/*2	2	0	0	43
*2/*3	1	0	0	53
*3/*3	0	0	1	76
VKORC1				
Non-A/non-A	37	82	7	—
Non-A/A	45	12	30	26
A/A	18	6	63	50

Polymorphisms in two genes, *CYP2C9* and *VKORC1*, largely account for the genetic contribution to the variability in warfarin response. *CYP2C9* variants affect warfarin pharmacokinetics. *CYP2C9* metabolizes warfarin, and the non-*1/*1 variants are less active than *CYP2C9*1/*1, necessitating a reduction in dose. *VKORC1* variants affect warfarin pharmacodynamics. *VKORC1* is the target of coumarin anticoagulants such as warfarin. The non-A/A and A/A forms have decreased requirements for warfarin.

Source: Ghimire LV, Stein CM. Warfarin pharmacogenetics. Goodman and Gilman Online.

in urine and stool. The $t_{1/2}$ varies (25–60 h), but the duration of action of warfarin is 2–5 days.

Table 32–2 summarizes the effects of known genetic factors on warfarin dose requirements. Polymorphisms in two genes, *CYP2C9* and *VKORC1* account for most of the genetic contribution to variability in warfarin response (International Warfarin Pharmacogenetics Consortium, 2009; McClain et al., 2008). *CYP2C9* variants affect warfarin pharmacokinetics, whereas *VKORC1* variants affect warfarin pharmacodynamics. Common variations in the *CYP2C9* gene (designated *CYP2C9*2* and *3*), encode an enzyme with decreased activity and thus are associated with higher drug concentrations and reduced warfarin dose requirements. *VKORC1* variants are more prevalent than those of *CYP2C9*, particularly in Asians, followed by European Americans and African Americans (Limdi et al., 2015). The warfarin dose requirement is decreased in patients with these variants (Shi et al., 2015). Point-of-care methods for *CYP2C9* and *VKORC1* genotyping and algorithms that incorporate genotype information have been developed to facilitate precision dosing of warfarin. It remains uncertain, however, whether precision dosing improves clinical outcome compared with usual warfarin management.

Clinical Use

Vitamin K antagonists are used to prevent the progression or recurrence of acute deep vein thrombosis or pulmonary embolism following an initial course of heparin, LMWH, or fondaparinux (Kearon et al., 2016). They also are effective in preventing stroke or systemic embolization in patients with atrial fibrillation, mechanical heart valves, or ventricular assist devices.

Prior to initiation of therapy, laboratory tests are used in conjunction with the history and physical examination to uncover hemostatic defects that might make the use of warfarin more dangerous (e.g., congenital coagulation factor deficiency, thrombocytopenia, hepatic or renal insufficiency, vascular abnormalities). Thereafter, the INR calculated from the patient's PT is used to monitor the extent of anticoagulation and compliance. Therapeutic INR ranges for various clinical indications have been established and reflect the extent of anticoagulation that reduces the morbidity from thromboembolic disease while minimally increasing the risk of serious hemorrhage. For most indications, an INR range of 2–3 is used. A higher INR range (2.5–3.5) is recommended for patients with mechanical heart valves in the mitral position or for patients with mechanical valves in another position who have concomitant atrial fibrillation or a prior history of stroke.

For treatment of acute venous thromboembolism, heparin, LMWH, or fondaparinux usually is continued for at least 5 days after warfarin therapy is begun. The parenteral agent is stopped when the INR is in the therapeutic range on 2 consecutive days. This overlap allows for adequate depletion of vitamin K–dependent coagulation factors with long half-lives, especially factor II. Frequent INR measurements are indicated at the onset of therapy to ensure that a therapeutic effect is obtained. Once a stable dose of warfarin has been identified, the INR can be monitored every 3 to 4 weeks.

Dosage

The usual adult dosage of warfarin is 2–5 mg/d for 2–4 days, followed by 1–10 mg/d as indicated by measurements of the INR (see the functional definition of INR in the section on clinical use). A lower initial dose should be given to patients with an increased risk of bleeding, including the elderly.

Interactions

Warfarin interactions can be caused by drugs, foods, or genetic factors that alter (1) uptake or metabolism of warfarin or vitamin K; (2) synthesis, function, or clearance of clotting factors; or (3), the integrity of any epithelial surface. Reduced warfarin efficacy can occur because of reduced absorption (e.g., binding to cholestyramine in the GI tract) or increased hepatic clearance from induction of hepatic enzymes (e.g., *CYP2C9* induction by barbiturates, carbamazepine, or rifampin). Warfarin has a decreased volume of distribution and a short $t_{1/2}$ with hypoproteinemia, such as occurs with nephrotic syndrome. Relative warfarin resistance can also be caused by ingestion of large amounts of vitamin K–rich foods or supplements or by increased levels of coagulation factors during pregnancy.

Drug interactions that enhance the risk of hemorrhage in patients taking warfarin include decreased metabolism due to *CYP2C9* inhibition by amiodarone, azole antifungals, cimetidine, clopidogrel, cotrimoxazole, disulfiram, fluoxetine, isoniazid, metronidazole, sulfinpyrazone, tolcapone, or zafirlukast. Relative deficiency of vitamin K may result from inadequate diet (e.g., postoperative patients on parenteral fluids), especially when coupled with the elimination of intestinal flora by antimicrobial agents. Gut bacteria synthesize vitamin K and are an important source of this vitamin. Consequently, antibiotics can cause an increase in the INR in patients on warfarin. Low concentrations of coagulation factors may result from impaired hepatic function, congestive heart failure, or hypermetabolic states, such as hyperthyroidism; generally, these conditions enhance the effect of warfarin on the INR. Serious interactions that do not alter the

INR include inhibition of platelet function by agents such as *aspirin* and gastritis or frank ulceration induced by anti-inflammatory drugs. Agents may have more than one effect (e.g., clofibrate increases the rate of turnover of coagulation factors and inhibits platelet function).

Hypersensitivity to Warfarin

About 10% of patients require less than 1.5 mg/d of warfarin to achieve an INR of 2–3. These patients often possess variants of *CYP2C9* or *VKORC1*; these affect the pharmacokinetics or pharmacodynamics of warfarin, respectively. Supplementation with low daily doses of vitamin K renders these patients less sensitive to warfarin and may result in more stable dosing.

Adverse Effects

Bleeding. The most common side effect of warfarin is bleeding. The risk of bleeding increases with the intensity and duration of anticoagulant therapy, the use of other medications that interfere with hemostasis, and the presence of an anatomical source of bleeding. The incidence of major bleeding episodes is generally less than 3% per year in patients treated to a target INR of 2–3. The risk of intracranial hemorrhage increases dramatically with an INR greater than 4, although up to two-thirds of intracranial bleeds on warfarin occur when the INR is therapeutic.

If the INR is above the therapeutic range and the patient is not bleeding or in need of a surgical procedure, warfarin can be held temporarily and restarted at a lower dose once the INR is within the therapeutic range. If the INR is 10 or greater, vitamin K_1 can be given orally at a dose of 2.5 to 5 mg. These doses of oral vitamin K_1 generally cause the INR to decrease substantially within 24–48 h without rendering the patient resistant to further warfarin therapy. Higher doses or parenteral administration may be required if more rapid correction of the INR is necessary. The effect of vitamin K_1 is delayed for at least several hours because reversal of anticoagulation requires synthesis of fully carboxylated coagulation factors. If immediate hemostatic competence is necessary because of serious bleeding or profound warfarin overdosage, adequate concentrations of vitamin K–dependent coagulation factors can be restored by transfusion of four-factor prothrombin complex concentrate, supplemented with 10 mg of vitamin K_1, given by slow intravenous infusion. Vitamin K_1 administered intravenously carries the risk of anaphylactoid reactions. Patients who receive high doses of vitamin K_1 may become unresponsive to warfarin for several days, but heparin or LMWH can be given if continued anticoagulation is required.

Birth Defects. Administration of warfarin during pregnancy causes birth defects and abortion. CNS abnormalities have been reported following exposure during the second and third trimesters. Fetal or neonatal hemorrhage and intrauterine death may occur, even when maternal INR values are within the therapeutic range. Vitamin K antagonists should not be used during pregnancy, but heparin or LMWH can be used safely.

Skin Necrosis. Warfarin-induced skin necrosis is a rare complication characterized by the appearance of skin lesions 3–10 days after treatment is initiated. The lesions typically are on the extremities, but adipose tissue, the penis, and the female breast also may be involved. Skin necrosis occurs in patients with protein C or S deficiency or in those with heparin-induced thrombocytopenia.

Other Toxicities. A reversible, sometimes painful, blue-tinged discoloration of the plantar surfaces and sides of the toes that blanches with pressure and fades with elevation of the legs (purple toe syndrome) may develop 3–8 weeks after initiation of therapy with warfarin; cholesterol emboli released from atheromatous plaques have been implicated as the cause. Other infrequent reactions include alopecia, urticaria, dermatitis, fever, nausea, diarrhea, abdominal cramps, and anorexia.

Direct Oral Anticoagulants

Direct Oral Thrombin Inhibitor

Dabigatran

Dabigatran etexilate is a synthetic prodrug with a molecular weight of 628 Da.

Mechanism of Action. Dabigatran etexilate is rapidly converted to dabigatran by plasma esterases. Dabigatran competitively and reversibly blocks the active site of free and clot-bound thrombin. In turn, this blocks thrombin-mediated conversion of fibrinogen to fibrin, feedback activation of coagulation, and platelet activation.

ADME. Dabigatran has oral bioavailability of about 6%, a peak onset of action in 2 h, and a plasma $t_{1/2}$ of 12–14 h. Dabigatran is given twice a day in capsule form. The bioavailability of the drug is altered if capsules are chewed or broken prior to ingestion. Therefore, the capsules should be swallowed whole. Circulating dabigatran is 35% bound to plasma proteins. Around 80% of absorbed dabigatran is excreted unchanged by the kidneys. A dosage reduction is required when dabigatran is administered to patients with severe renal impairment (creatinine clearance 15 to 30 mL/min). Dosage recommendations are not available for patients with a creatinine clearance below 15 mL/min.

When given in fixed doses, dabigatran etexilate produces such a predictable anticoagulant response that routine coagulation monitoring is unnecessary. Although dabigatran prolongs the aPTT, the values plateau with higher drug levels. Dabigatran has an unreliable effect on the INR. The thrombin time is too sensitive to use to monitor dabigatran therapy because the test is markedly prolonged with even low levels of drug. To circumvent this problem, a diluted thrombin time assay has been developed. By comparing the results with those obtained with dabigatran calibrators, this test can be used to quantify plasma dabigatran concentrations.

Therapeutic Uses. Dabigatran is licensed for treatment of acute venous thromboembolism after at least 5 days of parenteral anticoagulation with heparin, LMWH, or fondaparinux (Schulman et al., 2009) and for secondary prevention of venous thromboembolism (Beyer-Westendorf and Ageno, 2015; Gomez-Outes et al., 2015). Dabigatran also is licensed for stroke prevention in patients with nonvalvular atrial fibrillation (Connolly et al., 2009). It is contraindicated in patients with mechanical heart valves (Eikelboom et al., 2013). In some countries, lower-dose regimens of once-daily dabigatran are licensed for thromboprophylaxis after knee or hip arthroplasty. Dabigatran is contraindicated for stroke prevention in patients with mechanical heart valves.

Adverse Effects. Bleeding is the major side effect of dabigatran. In elderly patients with atrial fibrillation, the annual risk of major bleeding with dabigatran 150 mg twice daily is similar to that with warfarin, about 3.0%. However, the risk of intracranial bleeding is reduced by 70% with dabigatran compared with warfarin. In contrast, the risk of GI bleeding is higher with dabigatran, particularly in those over 75 years of age. Additional risks for bleeding with dabigatran include renal impairment and concurrent use of antiplatelet agents or nonsteroidal anti-inflammatory drugs.

Drug Interactions. Dabigatran is a substrate for P-glycoprotein, so drugs that inhibit or induce P-glycoprotein have the potential to increase or decrease plasma dabigatran concentrations, respectively. Verapamil, dronedarone, quinidine, ketoconazole, and clarithromycin can increase dabigatran concentrations, while rifampicin may decrease the concentration.

Direct Oral Factor Xa Inhibitors

Rivaroxaban, Apixaban, and Edoxban

Mechanism of Action. Rivaroxaban, apixaban, and edoxaban inhibit free and clot-associated factor Xa, which results in reduced thrombin generation. In turn, platelet aggregation and fibrin formation are suppressed.

ADME. Rivaroxaban has 80% oral bioavailability, a peak onset of action in 3 h, and a plasma $t_{1/2}$ of 7–11 h. Maximum absorption of rivaroxaban occurs in the stomach, and when given in therapeutic doses, the drug should be administered with a meal to enhance absorption. Rivaroxaban is provided in tablet form; the tablet can be crushed and delivered via nasogastric tube. Rivaroxaban is 95% plasma protein bound. About one-third of the drug is excreted unchanged in the urine; the remainder is metabolized by the hepatic CYP3A4 system, and inactive metabolites are excreted equally in the urine and feces. Rivaroxaban exposure is increased in patients with renal impairment or severe hepatic dysfunction. The therapeutic dose of rivaroxaban is reduced from 20 mg once daily to 15 mg once daily if the creatinine clearance is 15–50 mL/min. The drug should not be used in those with a lower creatinine clearance.

The bioavailability of apixaban is around 50%, and peak concentrations are achieved 1 to 3 h after ingestion. Food does not affect absorption, and the drug can be administered as a whole tablet or the tablet can be crushed in water and delivered via a nasogastric tube. Apixaban is 87% plasma protein bound, and about 27% of the drug is cleared unchanged via the kidneys. Apixaban is metabolized by the hepatic CYP3A4 system, and metabolites are excreted in the bile, intestines, and urine. The usual dose of apixaban is 5 mg twice daily. The dose is reduced to 2.5 mg twice daily in patients who have two of the following three characteristics: age over 80 years, body weight of 60 kg or less, or serum creatinine concentration of 1.5 mg/dL or higher. In patients with acute venous thromboembolism, patients start apixaban at a dose of 10 mg twice daily for 7 days, and the dose is then decreased to 5 mg twice daily thereafter. For those requiring treatment beyond 6 to 12 months, the apixaban dose can be decreased to 2.5 mg twice daily.

The bioavailability of edoxaban is 62%, and peak drug concentrations are achieved 1 to 2 h after ingestion. Food does not affect absorption. Edoxaban is 55% protein bound. Of the absorbed edoxaban, about 50% is eliminated as unchanged drug in the urine. There is minimal hepatic metabolism, and liver disease does not affect drug pharmacodynamics. Drug exposure is increased by renal impairment, low body weight, and concomitant intake of potent P-glycoprotein inhibitors. Therefore, the dose of edoxaban should be reduced from 60 to 30 mg once daily in patients with a creatinine clearance between 15 and 50 mL/min, in those with a body weight of 60 kg or less, or in those taking quinidine, dronedarone, rifampin, erythromycin, ketoconazole, or cyclosporine. Edoxaban is contraindicated in those with a creatinine clearance below 15 mL/min. Edoxaban is also not recommended in patients with a high creatinine clearance over 95 mL/min because of increased risk of ischemic stroke compared with warfarin.

Rivaroxaban, apixaban, and edoxaban are given in fixed doses and do not require routine coagulation monitoring. The drugs affect the PT more than the aPTT, but they prolong the PT to a variable extent, and this test does not provide a reliable measure of their anticoagulant activity. Anti–factor Xa assays using specific drug calibrators can be used to measure drug levels. Renal function should be assessed at least yearly in patients taking oral factor Xa inhibitors or more frequently in patients with renal dysfunction.

Therapeutic Uses. Rivaroxaban, apixaban, and edoxaban are licensed for stroke prevention in patients with atrial fibrillation (Giugliano et al., 2013; Granger et al., 2011; Patel et al., 2011) and for treatment of acute deep vein thrombosis or pulmonary embolism (Beyer-Westendorf and Ageno, 2015; Gomez-Outes et al., 2015). For the last indication, edoxaban is only started after a minimum 5-day course of treatment with heparin, LMWH, or fondaparinux (Hokusai VTE Investigators, 2013). In contrast, rivaroxaban and apixaban can be started immediately without the need for heparin bridging (EINSTEIN investigators, 2010, 2012; Granziera et al., 2016). Rivaroxaban and apixaban are also licensed for postoperative thromboprophylaxis in patients undergoing hip or knee arthroplasty (Falck-Ytter et al., 2012); for this indication, the drugs are given at doses of 10 mg once daily and 2.5 mg twice daily, respectively. All three drugs are contraindicated for stroke prevention in patients with mechanical heart valves.

Adverse Effects. As with all anticoagulants, the major adverse effect is bleeding. Rates of intracranial bleeding with rivaroxaban, apixaban, and edoxaban are at least 50% lower than that with warfarin. Rates of bleeding in other sites are similar or lower than those with warfarin. The sole exception is the GI tract; rates of GI bleeding with rivaroxaban and edoxaban, but not apixaban, are higher than that with warfarin. The explanation for this difference is uncertain, but it may reflect the capacity of unabsorbed anticoagulant in the gut to promote bleeding from preexisting lesions. Despite the increased risk of GI bleeding, rates of life-threatening and fatal bleeding are lower with all of the oral factor Xa inhibitors than with warfarin. Like with other anticoagulants, the risk of bleeding with rivaroxaban, apixaban, or edoxaban is increased in patients taking concomitant antiplatelet agents or nonsteroidal anti-inflammatory agents.

Drug Interactions. All of the oral factor Xa inhibitors are substrates for P-glycoprotein. Consequently, potent inhibitors or inducers of P-glycoprotein will increase or decrease drug concentrations, respectively. Rivaroxaban and apixaban are metabolized by CYP3A4, whereas edoxaban undergoes only minimal CYP3A4-mediated metabolism. Plasma levels of rivaroxaban and apixaban are reduced by potent inducers of both P-glycoprotein and CYP3A4, such as carbamazepine, phenytoin, rifampin, and St. John's wort and increased by potent inhibitors, such as dronedarone, ketoconazole, itraconazole, ritonavir, clarithromycin, erythromycin, and cyclosporine.

Reversal Agents for Direct Oral Anticoagulants

Life-threatening bleeding can occur with the direct oral anticoagulants, and patients taking these drugs may require urgent surgery or interventions. Therefore, the availability of specific reversal agents streamlines the management of such patients. Idarucizumab, the reversal agent for dabigatran, is licensed. Andexanet alfa, a reversal agent for rivaroxaban, apixaban, and edoxaban, is in advanced phase 3 evaluation, while ciraparantag, a potential reversal agent for all of the direct anticoagulants, is at an earlier stage of development.

If specific reversal agents are not available, prothrombin complex concentrate, activated prothrombin complex concentrate, or recombinant factor VIIa have been recommended to manage patients taking dabigatran, rivaroxaban, apixaban, or edoxaban who present with life-threatening bleeding, such as intracranial or pericardial bleeding. In patients taking dabigatran who present with serious bleeding in the setting of acute renal failure, hemodialysis can be used to remove dabigatran from the circulation. Dialysis is of no value for removal of rivaroxaban, apixaban or edoxaban because of their higher protein binding.

Idarucizumab

A specific reversal agent for dabigatran, idarucizumab is a humanized mouse monoclonal antibody fragment directed against dabigatran. The antibody binds dabigatran with an affinity 350-fold higher than that of dabigatran for thrombin, and the essentially irreversible idarucizumab-dabigatran complex is cleared by the kidneys. Idarucizumab is infused as two intravenous boluses, each of 2.5 g. It rapidly reverses the anticoagulant effects of dabigatran, and patients have then safely undergone major surgery (Pollack et al., 2015).

Andexanet Alfa

Designed as a decoy for the oral factor Xa inhibitors, andexanet alfa is a recombinant analogue of factor Xa that has the active site serine residue replaced with an alanine residue to eliminate catalytic activity and the Gla domain removed to preclude its incorporation in the prothrombinase complex. Andexanet is administered as an intravenous bolus followed by a 2-h infusion. By sequestering circulating factor Xa inhibitors, andexanet rapidly reverses the anti–factor Xa activity produced by these agents and restores thrombin generation (Siegal et al., 2015). Higher doses of andexanet are needed to reverse rivaroxaban or edoxaban than apixaban. An ongoing phase 3 study is evaluating the effect of andexanet in patients taking these agents who present with serious bleeding.

Ciraparantag

Ciraparantag is a synthetic, small cationic molecule that is reported to bind dabigatran, rivaroxaban, apixaban, and edoxaban, as well as heparin and LMWH. In healthy volunteers given edoxaban, an intravenous bolus of ciraparantag restored the whole-blood clotting time to normal. Ciraparantag has yet to be evaluated in patients.

Fibrinolytic Drugs

Fibrinolytic drugs initiate the fibrinolytic pathway, which is summarized in Figure 32–3. These agents include recombinant t-PA and its variants, urokinase and streptokinase, although the latter are rarely used.

Tissue Plasminogen Activator

Tissue plasminogen activator is a serine protease and a poor plasminogen activator in the absence of fibrin. When bound to fibrin, t-PA activates fibrin-bound plasminogen several 100-fold more rapidly than it activates plasminogen in the circulation. Because it has little activity except in the presence of fibrin, physiological t-PA concentrations of 5–10 ng/mL do not induce systemic plasmin generation. With therapeutic infusion of recombinant t-PA, the concentrations rise to 300–3000 ng/mL, which can induce systemic fibrinogen degradation. Clearance of t-PA primarily occurs via hepatic metabolism, and its $t_{1/2}$ is about 5 min. t-PA is effective for treatment of acute myocardial infarction (Gara et al., 2013), acute ischemic stroke, and life-threatening pulmonary embolism (Meyer et al., 2014).

For coronary thrombolysis, t-PA is given as a 15-mg intravenous bolus, followed by 0.75 mg/kg over 30 min (not to exceed 50 mg) and 0.5 mg/kg (up to 35 mg accumulated dose) over the following hour. Recombinant variants of t-PA include *reteplase* and *tenecteplase*. They differ from native t-PA by having longer plasma half-lives that allow convenient bolus dosing. In addition, in contrast to t-PA, tenecteplase is relatively resistant to inhibition by PAI-1. Despite these apparent advantages, these agents are similar to t-PA in efficacy and toxicity.

Hemorrhagic Toxicity of Thrombolytic Therapy

The major toxicity of all thrombolytic agents is hemorrhage. It is due to (1) degradation of fibrin in hemostatic plugs at sites of vascular injury or (2) the systemic lytic state that results from the systemic generation of plasmin, which degrades fibrinogen and other coagulation factors, especially factors V and VIII. Contraindications to fibrinolytic therapy are listed in Table 32–3.

If heparin is used concurrently with t-PA, serious hemorrhage will occur in 2%–4% of patients. Intracranial hemorrhage is the most serious problem and can occur in up to 1% of patients. For this reason, mechanical reperfusion is preferred over systemic thrombolysis in patients with acute myocardial infarction with ST-segment elevation. In patients with acute ischemic stroke, the current standard of care is mechanical thrombus extraction, which can be done with or without adjunctive t-PA or tenecteplase.

TABLE 32–3 ■ ABSOLUTE AND RELATIVE CONTRAINDICATIONS TO FIBRINOLYTIC THERAPY

Absolute Contraindications

- Prior intracranial hemorrhage
- Known structural cerebral vascular lesion
- Known malignant intracranial neoplasm
- Ischemic stroke within 3 months
- Suspected aortic dissection
- Active bleeding or bleeding diathesis (excluding menses)
- Significant closed-head trauma or facial trauma within 3 months

Relative Contraindications

- Uncontrolled hypertension (systolic blood pressure > 180 mm Hg or diastolic blood pressure > 110 mm Hg)
- Traumatic or prolonged CPR or major surgery within 3 weeks
- Recent (within 2–4 weeks) internal bleeding
- Noncompressible vascular punctures
- For streptokinase: prior exposure (more than 5 days ago) or prior allergic reaction to streptokinase
- Pregnancy
- Active peptic ulcer
- Current use of warfarin and INR > 1.7

Inhibitors of Fibrinolysis

ε-Aminocaproic Acid and Tranexamic Acid

ε-Aminocaproic acid and tranexamic acid are lysine analogues that compete for lysine binding sites on plasminogen and plasmin, thereby blocking their interaction with fibrin. Therefore, these agents inhibit fibrinolysis and can reverse states that are associated with excessive fibrinolysis.

The main problem with their use is that thrombi that form during treatment are not degraded. For example, in patients with hematuria, ureteral obstruction by clots may lead to renal failure after treatment with ε-aminocaproic acid or tranexamic acid. ε-Aminocaproic acid has been used intravenously to reduce bleeding after prostatic surgery and orally to reduce bleeding after tooth extractions in hemophiliacs. ε-Aminocaproic acid is absorbed rapidly after oral administration, and 50% is excreted unchanged in the urine within 12 h. For intravenous use, a loading dose of 4–5 g is given over 1 h, followed by an infusion of 1–1.25 g/h until bleeding is controlled. No more than 30 g should be given in a 24-h period. Rarely, the drug causes myopathy and muscle necrosis.

Tranexamic acid is given intravenously in trauma resuscitation and in patients with massive hemorrhage (CRASH2 trial investigators, 2010). It is also used to reduce operative bleeding in patients undergoing hip or knee arthroplasty or cardiac surgery. There appears to be little or no increased risk of thrombosis. Tranexamic acid is excreted in the urine; therefore, dose reduction is necessary in patients with renal impairment. Oral tranexamic acid is approved for treatment of heavy menstrual bleeding, usually given at a dose of 1 g four times daily for 4 days.

Antiplatelet Drugs

Platelet aggregates form the initial hemostatic plug at sites of vascular injury. Platelets also contribute to the pathological thrombi that lead to myocardial infarction, stroke, and peripheral arterial thrombosis. Potent inhibitors of platelet function have been developed in recent years. These drugs act by discrete mechanisms (Figure 32–7); thus, in combination, their effects are additive or even synergistic.

Aspirin

In platelets, the major COX-1 product is TxA_2, a labile inducer of platelet aggregation and a potent vasoconstrictor. Aspirin blocks production of TxA_2 by acetylating a serine residue near the active site of platelet COX-1. Because platelets do not synthesize new proteins, the action of aspirin on platelet COX-1 is permanent, lasting for the lifetime of the platelet (7–10 days). Thus, repeated doses of aspirin produce a cumulative effect on platelet function.

Complete inactivation of platelet COX-1 is achieved with a daily aspirin dose of 75 mg. Therefore, aspirin is maximally effective as an antithrombotic agent at doses much lower than those required for other actions of the drug. Numerous trials indicated that aspirin, when used as an antithrombotic drug, is maximally effective at doses of 50–325 mg/d. Higher doses do not improve efficacy and potentially are less efficacious because of inhibition of prostacyclin production, which can be largely spared by using lower doses of aspirin. Higher doses also increase toxicity, especially bleeding. Therefore, daily aspirin doses of 100 mg or less are used for most indications (Cohen et al., 2015; Ittaman et al., 2014). Nonsteroidal anti-inflammatory drugs that are reversible inhibitors of COX-1 have not been shown to have antithrombotic efficacy and in fact may even interfere with low-dose aspirin regimens (see Chapters 37 and 38).

Dipyridamole

Dipyridamole interferes with platelet function by increasing the intracellular concentration of cyclic AMP. This effect is mediated by inhibition of phosphodiesterase or by blockade of uptake of adenosine, thereby increasing the dwell time of adenosine at cell surface adenosine A_2 receptors that link to the stimulation of platelet adenylyl cyclase. Dipyridamole is a vasodilator that, in combination with warfarin, inhibits embolization

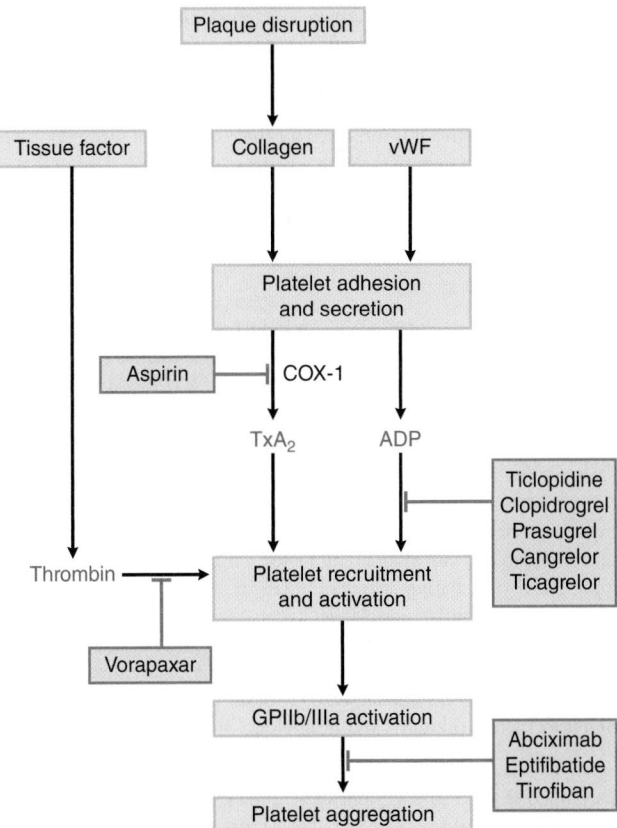

Figure 32–7 *Sites of action of antiplatelet drugs.* Aspirin inhibits TxA$_2$ synthesis by irreversibly acetylating COX-1. Reduced TxA$_2$ release attenuates platelet activation and recruitment to the site of vascular injury. Ticlopidine, clopidogrel, and prasugrel irreversibly block P2Y$_{12}$, a key ADP receptor on the platelet surface; cangrelor and ticagrelor are reversible inhibitors of P2Y$_{12}$. Abciximab, eptifibatide, and tirofiban inhibit the final common pathway of platelet aggregation by blocking fibrinogen and vWF from binding to activated GPIIb/IIIa. Vorapaxar inhibits thrombin-mediated platelet activation by targeting PAR-1, the major thrombin receptor on platelets.

from prosthetic heart valves. Dipyridamole is approved for secondary prevention of stroke when it is combined with low-dose aspirin.

P2Y$_{12}$ Receptor Antagonists

Clopidogrel

Clopidogrel is a thienopyridine prodrug that inhibits the P2Y$_{12}$ receptor. Platelets contain two purinergic receptors, P2Y$_1$ and P2Y$_{12}$; both are G protein–coupled receptors for ADP. The ADP-activated platelet P2Y$_1$ receptor couples to the G$_q$-PLC-IP$_3$–Ca^{2+} pathway and induces a shape change and aggregation. The P2Y$_{12}$ receptor couples to G$_i$ and, when activated by ADP, inhibits adenylyl cyclase, resulting in lower levels of intracellular cyclic AMP and thereby less cyclic AMP–dependent inhibition of platelet activation. Both receptors must be stimulated to result in maximal platelet activation.

Clopidogrel is an irreversible inhibitor of P2Y$_{12}$. It has largely replaced ticlopidine because clopidogrel is more potent and less toxic, with thrombocytopenia and leukopenia occurring only rarely. Clopidogrel is a prodrug that requires metabolic activation in the liver. Therefore, it has a slow onset of action. It also has a slow offset of action because of its irreversible effect on P2Y$_{12}$. Metabolic activation of clopidogrel can be affected by polymorphisms in *CYP2C19* that result in reduced or absent CYP2C19 activity. These polymorphisms contribute to the variable effect of clopidogrel on ADP-induced platelet aggregation. Inhibition of platelet activation is seen 2 h postingestion of a loading dose of clopidogrel, and platelets are affected for the remainder of their life span.

Therapeutic Uses. Clopidogrel is somewhat better than aspirin for secondary prevention of stroke, and the combination of clopidogrel plus aspirin is superior to aspirin alone for prevention of recurrent ischemia in patients with unstable angina. The FDA-approved indications for clopidogrel are to reduce the rate of stroke, myocardial infarction, and death in patients with recent myocardial infarction or stroke, established peripheral artery disease, or acute coronary syndrome (Amsterdam et al., 2014; Gara et al., 2013; Park et al., 2016; Roffi et al., 2015; Zhang et al., 2015). Clopidogrel is often used in combination with aspirin after coronary stent implantation.

Adverse Effects. Clopidogrel increases the risk of bleeding, particularly when combined with aspirin or an anticoagulant. Thrombotic thrombocytopenic purpura can occur but is rare.

Drug Interactions. CYP219 inhibition by proton pump inhibitors (e.g., omeprazole, lansoprazole, deslansprazole, and pantoprazole) may reduce conversion to the active metabolite of clopidogrel, which may contribute to the lower efficacy of clopidogrel when coadministered with proton pump inhibitors.

Prasugrel

The newest member of the thienopyridine class, prasugrel is a prodrug that requires metabolic activation in the liver. However, because the activation of prasugrel is more efficient than that of clopidogrel, prasugrel has a more rapid onset of action, and it produces greater and more predictable inhibition of ADP-induced platelet aggregation.

Prasugrel is rapidly and completely absorbed from the gut. It is hydrolyzed in the intestine to a thiolactone, which is then converted to the active metabolite in the liver. Virtually all of the absorbed prasugrel undergoes activation; by comparison, only 15% of absorbed clopidogrel undergoes metabolic activation. Because the active metabolites of prasugrel bind irreversibly to the P2Y$_{12}$ receptor, its effect lasts the lifetime of the platelets. This slow offset of action can be problematic if patients require urgent surgery. Prasugrel is inactivated by methylation or conjugation with cysteine. Moderate renal or hepatic impairment does not appear to change the drug pharmacodynamics.

Therapeutic Uses. Prasugrel is indicated to reduce the rate of thrombotic cardiovascular events (including stent thrombosis) in patients with acute coronary syndrome who are managed with percutaneous coronary intervention (Gara et al., 2013; Guimaraúes and Tricoci, 2015; Lhermusier and Waksman, 2015). The incidence of cardiovascular death, myocardial infarction, and stroke is significantly lower with prasugrel than with clopidogrel, mainly reflecting a reduction in the incidence of nonfatal myocardial infarction. The incidence of stent thrombosis is also lower with prasugrel than with clopidogrel.

Adverse Effects. Prasugrel is associated with higher rates of fatal and life-threatening bleeding than clopidogrel. Because patients with a history of a prior stroke or transient ischemic attack are at particularly high risk of intracranial bleeding, the drug is contraindicated in such patients. Patients over 75 years of age should not be prescribed prasugrel because of the increased bleeding risk. After a loading dose of 60 mg, prasugrel is given once daily at a dose of 10 mg. The daily dose should be reduced to 5 mg in patients weighing less than 60 kg. No dose adjustment is required in patients with hepatic or renal impairment. If patients present with serious bleeding, platelet transfusion may be beneficial. Prasugrel has been reported to cause thrombotic thrombocytopenic purpura.

Drug Interactions. Concomitant administration of prasugrel with an anticoagulant or nonsteroidal anti-inflammatory drugs increases the risk of bleeding.

Ticagrelor

Ticagrelor is an orally active, reversible inhibitor of P2Y$_{12}$. The drug is given twice daily and not only has a more rapid onset and offset of action than clopidogrel, but also produces greater and more predictable inhibition of ADP-induced platelet aggregation. The bioavailability of ticagrelor is about 36%. It can be given as a whole tablet or crushed in water and administered via a nasogastric tube. Ticagrelor is metabolized by hepatic CYP3A4.

Therapeutic Uses. Ticagrelor is FDA-approved for reduction in the risk of cardiovascular death, myocardial infarction, and stroke in patients with acute coronary syndrome (Gara et al., 2013) or a history of myocardial infarction (Dobesh and Oestreich, 2014). In contrast to prasugrel in patients with acute coronary syndrome, which is only indicated in those undergoing percutaneous intervention, ticagrelor is indicated in those undergoing intervention and in those managed medically.

Adverse Effects. Dyspnea is reported in 17% of patients. This is often transient and not associated with pulmonary disease. Ticagrelor is associated with a higher risk of intracranial bleeding than clopidogrel and is contraindicated in patients with a history of prior intracranial bleeding. Platelet transfusion is ineffective in patients taking ticagrelor who present with serious bleeding, and a neutralizing antibody is under investigation for urgent reversal.

Drug Interactions. Concomitant aspirin at a dose greater than 100 mg daily may reduce the effectiveness of ticagrelor. Potent inhibitors of CYP3A (such as ketoconazole, itraconazole, voriconazole, clarithromycin, nefazodone, ritonavir, saquinavir, nelfinavir, indinavir, atazanavir, and telithromycin) and strong inducers of CYP3A (such as rifampin, phenytoin, carbamazepine, and phenobarbital) should be avoided. Ticagrelor increases serum concentrations of simvastatin and lovastatin and may affect digoxin metabolism.

Cangrelor

Cangrelor is a parenteral reversible inhibitor of $P2Y_{12}$. When administered intravenously as a bolus followed by an infusion, cangrelor inhibits ADP-induced platelet aggregation within minutes, and its effect on platelet aggregation disappears within 1 h of discontinuation of the drug. Cangrelor has a short half-life because it is rapidly dephosphorylated in the circulation to an inactive metabolite.

Therapeutic Use. Cangrelor is indicated for reduction in the risk of periprocedural myocardial infarction, repeat coronary revascularization, and stent thrombosis in patients undergoing percutaneous coronary intervention who have not been treated with an oral $P2Y_{12}$ inhibitor and are not given a glycoprotein IIb/IIIa antagonist (Keating et al., 2015).

Adverse Effects. The risk of bleeding with cangrelor is greater than that with clopidogrel during the coronary intervention.

Drug Interactions. Coadministered clopidogrel or prasugrel will have no antiplatelet effect. Administration of ticagrelor, prasugrel, or clopidogrel should be delayed until the cangrelor infusion is stopped.

Thrombin Receptor Inhibitor

There are two major thrombin receptors on the platelet surface, PAR-1 and PAR-4, respectively. Thrombin binds to these G protein–coupled receptors and cleaves them at their amino terminals. The newly created amino terminals then serve as tethered ligands to activate the receptors. PAR-1 is activated by lower concentrations of thrombin than are required to activate PAR-4.

Vorapaxar

Vorapaxar is a competitive antagonist of PAR-1 and inhibits thrombin-induced platelet aggregation. The drug is 90% bioavailable and has a rapid onset of action and a circulating half-life of 3 or 4 days. However, because vorapaxar remains tightly bound to PAR-1 on platelets, its effect on thrombin-induced platelet aggregation can persist for up to 4 weeks after the drug is stopped. Vorapaxar is metabolized in the liver by CYP3A4.

Therapeutic Uses. Vorapaxar is given orally in combination with either aspirin or clopidogrel. It is indicated for the reduction of thrombotic cardiovascular events in patients with a history of myocardial infarction or peripheral artery disease (Arif et al., 2015; Moschonas et al., 2015).

Adverse Effects. Vorapaxar increases the risk of bleeding and is contraindicated in patients with a history of intracranial bleeding, stroke, or transient ischemic attack.

Drug Interactions. Potent CYP3A4 inducers, such as rifampin, reduce drug exposure, while strong CYP3A4 inhibitors, such as ketoconazole, increase drug exposure. Antacids and pantoprazole reduce drug exposure.

Glycoprotein IIb/IIIa Inhibitors

Glycoprotein IIb/IIIa is a platelet-surface integrin, designated $\alpha_{IIb}\beta_3$ by the integrin nomenclature. This dimeric glycoprotein undergoes a conformational transformation when platelets are activated to serve as a receptor for fibrinogen and von Willebrand factor, which anchor platelets to each other, thereby mediating aggregation (Figure 32-1). Thus, inhibitors of this receptor are potent antiplatelet agents that act by a mechanism distinct from that of aspirin or $P2Y_{12}$ or PAR-1 inhibitors. Three agents are approved for use at present; their features are highlighted in Table 32–4. The use of these agents has decreased with the availability of potent $P2Y_{12}$ inhibitors such as prasugrel and ticagrelor.

Abciximab

Abciximab is the Fab fragment of a humanized monoclonal antibody directed against the $\alpha_{IIb}\beta_3$ receptor. It also binds to the vitronectin receptor on platelets, vascular endothelial cells, and smooth muscle cells.

The antibody is administered to patients undergoing percutaneous coronary intervention and, when used in conjunction with aspirin and heparin, has been shown to prevent recurrent myocardial infarction and death (Gara et al., 2013; Roffi et al., 2015). The $t_{1/2}$ of the circulating antibody is about 30 min, but antibody remains bound to the $\alpha_{IIb}\beta_3$ receptor and inhibits platelet aggregation as measured in vitro for 18–24 h after infusion. It is given as a 0.25-mg/kg bolus followed by an infusion of 0.125 µg/kg/min (maximum 10 µg/kg/min) for 12 to 24 h.

Adverse Effects. The major side effect of abciximab is bleeding, and the contraindications to its use are similar to those for the fibrinolytic agents listed in Table 32–4. The frequency of major hemorrhage in clinical trials varies from 1% to 10%, depending on the intensity of concomitant anticoagulation with heparin. Thrombocytopenia with a platelet count below 50,000 occurs in about 2% of patients and may be due the formation of antibodies directed against neoepitopes induced by bound antibody. Because the duration of action is long, if major bleeding occurs, platelet transfusion may reverse the aggregation defect because free antibody concentrations fall rapidly after cessation of infusion.

Eptifibatide

Eptifibatide is a cyclic peptide inhibitor of the fibrinogen binding site on $\alpha_{IIb}\beta_3$. It is administered intravenously and blocks platelet aggregation. In patients undergoing percutaneous coronary intervention,

TABLE 32–4 ■ FEATURES OF GPIIb/IIIa ANTAGONISTS			
FEATURE	**ABCIXIMAB**	**EPTIFIBATIDE**	**TIROFIBAN**
Description	Fab fragment of humanized mouse monoclonal antibody	Cyclical KGD-containing heptapeptide	Nonpeptidic RGD-mimetic
Specific for GPIIb/IIIa	No	Yes	Yes
Plasma $t_{1/2}$	Short (minutes)	Long (2.5 h)	Long (2.0 h)
Platelet-bound $t_{1/2}$	Long (days)	Short (seconds)	Short (seconds)
Renal clearance	No	Yes	Yes

eptifibatide is typically given as a double intravenous bolus of 180 µg/kg (spaced 10 min apart), followed by an infusion of 2 µg/kg/min for 18 to 24 h. The drug is cleared by the kidneys and has a short plasma half-life of 10 to 15 min. Like abciximab, eptifibatide is mainly used in patients undergoing primary percutaneous coronary intervention for acute ST-segment elevation myocardial infarction, although it also can be used in patients with unstable angina.

Adverse Effects. The major side effect is bleeding. Thrombocytopenia occurs in 0.5%–1% of patients and is less frequent than with abciximab.

Tirofiban

Tirofiban is an intravenously administered nonpeptide, small-molecule inhibitor of $\alpha_{IIb}\beta_3$. It has a short duration of action and is used for management of patients with non–ST-segment elevation acute coronary syndrome. Tirofiban is administered as an intravenously bolus of 25 µg/kg followed by an infusion of 0.15 µg/kg/min for up to 18 h. The infusion dose is reduced by half in patients with a creatinine clearance below 60 mL/min. Like the other agents in this class, the major side effect of tirofiban is bleeding, and it may induce thrombocytopenia.

The Role of Vitamin K

Green plants are a nutritional source of vitamin K for humans, in whom vitamin K is an essential cofactor in the γ-carboxylation of multiple glutamate residues of several clotting factors and anticoagulant proteins. The vitamin K–dependent formation of Gla residues permits the appropriate interactions of clotting factors, Ca^{2+}, and membrane phospholipids and modulator proteins (see Figures 32–1, 32–2, and 32–3). Vitamin K antagonists (coumarin derivatives) block Gla formation and thereby inhibit clotting; excess vitamin K_1 can reverse the effects.

Vitamin K activity is associated with at least two distinct natural substances, designated as vitamin K_1 and vitamin K_2. Vitamin K_1, or *phytonadione* (also referred to as *phylloquinone*), is 2-methyl-3-phytyl-1,4-naphthoquinone; it is found in plants and is the only natural vitamin K available for therapeutic use. Vitamin K_2 actually is a series of compounds (the *menaquinones*) in which the phytyl side chain of phytonadione has been replaced by a side chain built up of 2–13 prenyl units. Considerable synthesis of menaquinones occurs in gram-positive bacteria; indeed, intestinal flora synthesizes the large amounts of vitamin K contained in human and animal feces. Menadione is at least as active on a molar basis as phytonadione.

PHYTONADIONE (vitamin K_1, phylloquinone)

Physiological Functions and Pharmacological Actions

Phytonadione and menaquinones promote the biosynthesis of the clotting factors II (prothrombin), VII, IX, and X as well as the anticoagulant proteins C and S and protein Z (a cofactor to the inhibitor of Xa).

Figure 32–6 summarizes the coupling of the vitamin K cycle with glutamate carboxylation. The γ-glutamyl carboxylase and epoxide reductase are integral membrane proteins of the endoplasmic reticulum and function as a multicomponent complex. With respect to proteins affecting blood coagulation, these reactions occur in the liver, but γ-carboxylation of glutamate also occurs in lung, bone, and other cell types. Mutations in γ-glutamyl carboxylase lead to bleeding disorders.

Human Requirements

In patients rendered vitamin K deficient by a starvation diet and antibiotic therapy for 3–4 weeks, the minimum daily requirement is estimated to be 0.03 µg/kg of body weight and possibly as high as 1 µg/kg, which is approximately the recommended intake for adults (70 µg/d).

Symptoms of Deficiency

The major clinical manifestation of vitamin K deficiency is bleeding. Ecchymoses, epistaxis, hematuria, GI bleeding, and postoperative hemorrhage are common; intracranial hemorrhage may occur. Hemoptysis is uncommon. The presence of vitamin K–dependent proteins in bone such as osteocalcin and matrix Gla protein may explain why fetal bone abnormalities can occur with maternal warfarin administration in the first trimester of pregnancy. Vitamin K plays a role in adult skeletal maintenance and the prevention of osteoporosis. Low concentrations of the vitamin are associated with decreased bone mineral density and subsequent fractures; vitamin K supplementation increases the carboxylation state of osteocalcin and improves bone mineral density, but the relationship between these effects is unclear. Bone mineral density in adults does not appear to be changed with long-term warfarin therapy, but new bone formation may be affected.

Toxicity

Phytonadione and the menaquinones are nontoxic. Menadione and its derivatives (synthetic forms of vitamin K) may produce hemolytic anemia and kernicterus in neonates and should not be used as therapeutic forms of vitamin K.

ADME

The mechanism of intestinal absorption of compounds with vitamin K activity varies depending on their solubility. In the presence of bile salts, phytonadione and the menaquinones are adequately absorbed from the intestine, phytonadione by an energy-dependent, saturable process in proximal portions of the small intestine and menaquinones by diffusion in the distal small intestine and the colon. After absorption, phytonadione is incorporated into chylomicrons in close association with triglycerides and lipoproteins. The low phytonadione levels in newborns may partly reflect the low plasma lipoprotein concentrations at birth and may lead to an underestimation of vitamin K tissue stores. After absorption, phytonadione and menaquinones are concentrated in the liver, but the concentration of phytonadione declines rapidly. Menaquinones, produced in the distal bowel, are less biologically active because of their long side chain. Very little vitamin K accumulates in other tissues. There is only modest storage of vitamin K in the body. Consequently, when lack of bile interferes with absorption of vitamin K, there is progressive reduction in the levels of the vitamin K–dependent clotting factors over the course of several weeks.

Therapeutic Uses

Vitamin K is used therapeutically to correct the bleeding tendency or hemorrhage associated with its deficiency. Vitamin K deficiency can result from inadequate intake, absorption, or utilization of the vitamin or as a consequence of the action of warfarin.

Phytonadione is available in tablet form and in a dispersion with buffered polysorbate and propylene glycol or polyoxyethylated fatty acid derivatives and dextrose. Phytonadione may be given by any route; however, the subcutaneous route should be avoided in patients with a coagulopathy because of the risk of bleeding. The oral route is preferred, but if more rapid reversal is required, phytonadione can be given by slow intravenous infusion; it should not be given rapidly because severe reactions resembling anaphylaxis can occur.

Inadequate Intake

After infancy, hypoprothrombinemia due to dietary deficiency of vitamin K is extremely rare. The vitamin is present in many foods and is synthesized by intestinal bacteria. Occasionally, the use of a broad-spectrum antibiotic may itself produce hypoprothrombinemia that responds readily to small doses of vitamin K and reestablishment of normal bowel flora. Hypoprothrombinemia can occur in patients receiving prolonged intravenous alimentation; to prevent this, it is recommended that such patients receive 1 mg of phytonadione per week (the equivalent of about 150 µg/day).

Hypoprothrombinemia of the Newborn

Healthy newborn infants have decreased plasma concentrations of vitamin K–dependent clotting factors for a few days after birth, the time required for adequate dietary intake of the vitamin and for establishment of normal intestinal flora. Measurements of non-γ-carboxylated prothrombin suggest that vitamin K deficiency occurs in about 3% of live births.

Hemorrhagic disease of the newborn has been associated with breastfeeding; human milk has low concentrations of vitamin K. In addition, the microbiome of breast-fed infants may lack microorganisms that synthesize the vitamin. Commercial infant formulas are supplemented with vitamin K. In the neonate with hemorrhagic disease of the newborn, administration of vitamin K raises the concentration of these clotting factors to levels normal for newborns and controls the bleeding tendency within about 6 h. Routine administration of 1 mg phytonadione intramuscularly at birth is required by law in the U.S. The dose may have to be increased or repeated if the mother has received warfarin or anticonvulsant drug therapy or if the infant develops a bleeding diathesis. Alternatively, some clinicians treat mothers who are receiving anticonvulsants with oral vitamin K prior to delivery (20 mg/d for 2 weeks).

Inadequate Absorption

Vitamin K is poorly absorbed in the absence of bile. Thus, hypoprothrombinemia may be associated with intrahepatic or extrahepatic biliary obstruction or with defective intestinal absorption of fat from other causes.

Biliary Obstruction or Fistula

Bleeding that accompanies obstructive jaundice or a biliary fistula responds promptly to the administration of vitamin K. Oral phytonadione administered with bile salts is both safe and effective and should be used in the care of the jaundiced patient, both preoperatively and postoperatively. In the absence of significant hepatocellular disease, the prothrombin level rapidly returns to normal. If oral administration is not feasible, a parenteral preparation should be used. The usual daily dose of vitamin K is 10 mg.

Malabsorption Syndromes

Among the disorders that result in inadequate absorption of vitamin K from the intestinal tract are cystic fibrosis, celiac disease, Crohn disease, ulcerative colitis, dysentery, and extensive resection of bowel. Because drugs that reduce the bacterial population of the bowel are used frequently in many of these disorders, the availability of the vitamin may be further reduced. For immediate correction of the deficiency, parenteral vitamin K should be given.

Inadequate Utilization

Hepatocellular disease or long-standing biliary obstruction may be accompanied or followed by hypoprothrombinemia. If inadequate secretion of bile salts is contributing to the syndrome, some benefit may be obtained from the parenteral administration of 10 mg of phytonadione daily. Paradoxically, administration of large doses of vitamin K or its analogues in an attempt to correct the hypoprothrombinemia can be associated with severe hepatitis or cirrhosis, which may contribute to a further reduction in the level of prothrombin.

Drug- and Venom-Induced Hypoprothrombinemia

Warfarin and its congeners act as competitive antagonists of vitamin K and interfere with the hepatic biosynthesis of Gla-containing clotting factors. The treatment of bleeding caused by oral anticoagulants was described previously. Vitamin K may be of help in combating the bleeding and hypoprothrombinemia that follow the bite of the tropical American pit viper or other species whose venom degrades or inactivates prothrombin.

Drug Facts for Your Personal Formulary: *Agents That Modify Blood Coagulation*

Drugs	Therapeutic Uses	Clinical Pharmacology and Tips
Unfractionated Heparin		
Heparin	• Prophylaxis/treatment of venous thromboembolism • Acute coronary syndrome • Percutaneous coronary intervention • Cardiopulmonary bypass surgery • Disseminated intravascular coagulation	• Administered SC 2–3 times daily for thromboprophylaxis • Administered IV for immediate onset of action with aPTT monitoring • Can be used in renal impairment • Can be used in pregnancy
Low-Molecular-Weight Heparin		
Enoxaparin Dalteparin Tinzaparin (not in the U.S.)	• Prophylaxis against venous thrombosis • Initial treatment of venous thromboembolism • Maintenance treatment in patients with cancer-associated venous thromboembolism • Acute coronary syndrome	• Administered SC once or twice daily • Routine anti-factor Xa monitoring not required • Dosage adjustment required when CrCL < 30 mL/min • Can be used in pregnancy
Fondaparinux		
Fondaparinux	• Prophylaxis against venous thromboembolism • Initial treatment of venous thromboembolism • Heparin-induced thrombocytopenia • Acute coronary syndrome in some countries	• Once-daily SC injection • Lower dose used for thromboprophylaxis and in acute coronary syndrome • Contraindicated if CrCL < 30 mL/min • Use in pregnancy less established than for low-molecular-weight heparin • Routine anti-factor Xa monitoring not required
Other Anticoagulants		
Desirudin	• Thromboprophylaxis after hip arthroplasty	• Twice-daily SC injection • Dosage adjustment required with renal impairment
Bivalirudin	• Percutaneous coronary intervention • Heparin-induced thrombocytopenia	• Administered IV • ACT or aPTT monitoring • Requires dose reduction with renal impairment
Argatroban	• Heparin-induced thrombocytopenia	• Hepatic metabolism • Can be used in renal impairment • Increases INR, which can complicate transition to warfarin

Vitamin K Antagonist

Warfarin	• Treatment of venous thromboembolism in tandem with parenteral anticoagulation • Secondary prevention of venous thromboembolism • Prevention of stroke in atrial fibrillation • Prevention of stroke in patient with mechanical heart valves or ventricular assist devices	• Oral vitamin K antagonist • Narrow therapeutic index • Requires regular INR monitoring • Multiple drug interactions • Dietary vitamin K interactions • Can be used in renal failure • Contraindicated in pregnancy

Direct Oral Thrombin Inhibitor

Dabigatran etexilate	• Treatment of acute venous thromboembolism after at least 5 days of parenteral anticoagulation • Secondary prevention of venous thromboembolism • Prevention of stroke in atrial fibrillation • Thromboprophylaxis after hip or knee arthroplasty	• Fixed twice-daily oral dosing (once daily if used for thromboprophylaxis) • Reduce the dose with CrCL 15–30 mL/min • Contraindicated if CrCL < 15 mL/min • Use with caution in patients with recent bleeding, especially GI bleeding • Can be reversed with idarucizumab

Direct Oral Factor Xa Inhibitors

Rivaroxaban	• Treatment of acute venous thromboembolism • Secondary prevention of venous thromboembolism • Prevention of stroke in atrial fibrillation • Thromboprophylaxis after hip or knee arthroplasty • Prevention of recurrent ischemia in stabilized acute coronary syndrome patients (not in North America)	• Fixed oral dosing (once daily with the exception of initial treatment of venous thromboembolism, which starts with twice-daily dosing for 21 days and once daily thereafter, or secondary prevention after acute coronary syndrome where the drug is given twice daily) • Avoid in patients with renal/hepatic dysfunction • Use with caution in patients with recent bleeding, especially GI bleeding
Apixaban	• Treatment of acute venous thromboembolism • Secondary prevention of venous thromboembolism • Prevention of stroke in atrial fibrillation • Thromboprophylaxis after hip or knee arthroplasty	• Fixed oral dosing (twice daily, higher dose for the first 7 days for acute venous thromboembolism) • Reduce dose for stroke prophylaxis if any two of age > 80 years, body weight < 60 kg, or serum creatinine ≥ 1.5 mg/dL • Use with caution in patients with recent bleeding, especially GI bleeding
Edoxaban	• Treatment of acute venous thromboembolism after at least 5 days of parenteral anticoagulation • Secondary prevention of venous thromboembolism • Prevention of stroke in atrial fibrillation	• Fixed once-daily dosing • Reduce the dose if any of CrCL 15–50 mL/min, body weight < 60 kg, or concomitant potent P-glycoprotein inhibitor • Not recommended for patients with CrCL < 15 mL/min • Contraindicated if CrCL > 95 mL/min • Use with caution in patients with recent bleeding, especially GI bleeding

Reversal Agents for Direct Oral Anticoagulants

Idarucizumab	• Reversal of dabigatran	• Humanized Fab fragment against dabigatran • Bolus IV administration • Rapid and complete reversal
Andexanet alfa	• Reversal of rivaroxaban, apixaban, or edoxaban	• Recombinant analogue of factor Xa • Acts as a decoy for oral factor Xa inhibitors • Given as IV bolus followed by 2-h IV infusion • In phase 3 evaluation
Ciraparantag	• Reversal of dabigatran, rivaroxaban, apixaban, or edoxaban	• Synthetic small molecule • Binds target drugs • In phase 2 evaluation

Fibrinolytic Drugs

Alteplase	• Thrombolysis in acute ischemic stroke, massive pulmonary embolism, or myocardial infarction	• IV bolus followed by an infusion • Risk of major bleeding, including intracranial bleeding
Reteplase	• Thrombolysis in myocardial infarction	• Two IV boluses • Risk of major bleeding, including intracranial bleeding
Tenecteplase	• Thrombolysis in pulmonary embolism and myocardial infarction	• Single IV bolus • Risk of major bleeding, including intracranial bleeding

Inhibitors of Fibrinolysis

ε-Aminocaproic acid	• Reduce intraoperative bleeding	• Inhibits plasmin-mediated degradation of fibrin • IV infusion
Tranexamic acid	• Major head injury • Major trauma resuscitation • Reduce intraoperative bleeding • Topical application for dental bleeding and epistaxis • Menorrhagia	• Inhibits plasmin-mediated degradation of fibrin • Available in oral or IV form • Given orally in patients undergoing dental procedures or in women with menorrhagia and IV in patients with major trauma or undergoing major orthopedic surgery

SECTION III — MODULATION OF PULMONARY, RENAL, AND CARDIOVASCULAR FUNCTION

Drug Facts for Your Personal Formulary: *Agents That Modify Blood Coagulation (continued)*

Drugs	Therapeutic Uses	Clinical Pharmacology and Tips
Antiplatelet Drugs		
Aspirin	• Acute myocardial infarction or acute ischemic stroke • Secondary prevention in patients with stroke, coronary artery disease, or peripheral artery disease	• COX-1 inhibitor (selectivity > 100x over COX-2) • Antithrombotic effect achieved with low doses (<100 mg daily) • Reduced toxicity with lower doses
Dipyridamole	• Secondary prevention of stroke when combined with aspirin	• Available as a fixed-dose combined tablet with aspirin
Clopidogrel	• Acute coronary syndrome • Secondary prevention in patients with myocardial infarction, stroke, or peripheral artery disease	• Irreversible inhibitor of $P2Y_{12}$ • Given once daily • Variable response because common genetic polymorphisms attenuate metabolic activation • Proton pump inhibitors reduce conversion to active metabolite
Prasugrel	• After coronary intervention for acute coronary syndrome	• Irreversible inhibitor of $P2Y_{12}$ • Given once daily • More predictable inhibition of ADP-induced platelet activation than clopidogrel because of more efficient metabolic activation • Contraindicated in patients with cerebrovascular disease, prior intracranial bleed, or > 75 years of age • Reduce dose in patients weighing < 60 kg • Higher bleeding risk than clopidogrel
Ticagrelor	• Acute coronary syndrome with or without coronary intervention	• Reversible inhibitor of $P2Y_{12}$ • Given twice daily • Does not require metabolic activation • Higher bleeding risk than clopidogrel • Contraindicated in patients with a history of intracranial bleeding
Cangrelor	• Percutaneous coronary intervention	• $P2Y_{12}$ inhibitor • Rapid onset and offset IV agent • Higher bleeding risk than clopidogrel • Coadministration of clopidogrel or prasugrel with cangrelor will have no antiplatelet effect
Vorapaxar	• Secondary prevention in patients with a history of myocardial infarction or peripheral artery disease	• PAR-1 antagonist • Contraindicated in patients with cerebrovascular disease or prior intracranial bleed
Abciximab	• Coronary intervention for acute coronary syndrome	• Glycoprotein IIb/IIIa antagonist • Up to 10% bleeding risk • Can cause thrombocytopenia
Eptifibatide	• Coronary intervention for acute coronary syndrome	• Glycoprotein IIb/IIIa antagonist • Up to 10% bleeding risk • Can cause thrombocytopenia • Contraindicated in renal failure
Tirofiban	• Coronary intervention for acute coronary syndrome	• Glycoprotein IIb/IIIa antagonist • Up to 10% bleeding risk • Reduce dose if CrCL ≤ 60 mL/min
Vitamin Supplementation		
Vitamin K	• Reversal of warfarin • Hypoproteinemia of the newborn • Biliary obstruction • Malnutrition	• Oral or SC administration preferred • Can be given by slow IV infusion but high risk of adverse events

Bibliography

Amsterdam EA, et al. 2014 AHA/ACC guideline for the management of patients with non-ST-elevation acute coronary syndromes. A report of the American College of Cardiology/American Heart Association Task Force on Practice Guidelines. *J Am Coll Cardiol*, **2014**, *64*:e139–e228.

Arif SA, et al. Vorapaxar for reduction of thrombotic cardiovascular events in myocardial infarction and peripheral artery disease. *Am J Health Syst Pharm*, **2015**, *72*:1615–1622.

Barria Perez AE, et al. Meta-analysis of effects of bivalirudin versus heparin on myocardial ischemic and bleeding outcomes after percutaneous coronary intervention. *Am J Cardiol*, **2016**, *117*:1256–1266.

Beyer-Westendorf J, Ageno W. Benefit-risk profile of non-vitamin K antagonist oral anticoagulants in the management of venous thromboembolism. *Thromb Haemost*, **2015**, *113*:231–246.

Cohen AT, et al. The use of aspirin for primary and secondary prevention in venous thromboembolism and other cardiovascular disorders. *Thromb Res*, **2015**, *135*:217–225.

Connolly SJ, et al. Dabigatran versus warfarin in patients with atrial fibrillation. *N Engl J Med*, **2009**, *361*:1139–1151.

CRASH2 trial investigators. Effects of tranexamic acid on death, vascular occlusive events, and blood transfusion in trauma patients with significant haemorrhage (CRASH-2): a randomised, placebo-controlled trial. *Lancet*, **2010**, *376*:23–32.

Dobesh PP, Oestreich JH. Ticagrelor: pharmacokinetics, pharmacodynamics, clinical efficacy, and safety. *Pharmacotherapy*, **2014**, *34*:1077–1090.

Eikelboom JW, et al. Dabigatran versus warfarin in patients with mechanical heart valves. *N Engl J Med*, **2013**, *369*:1206–1214.

EINSTEIN investigators. Oral rivaroxaban for symptomatic venous thromboembolism. *N Engl J Med*, **2010**, *363*:2499–2510.

EINSTEIN investigators. Oral rivaroxaban for the treatment of symptomatic pulmonary embolism. *N Engl J Med*, **2012**, *366*:1287–1297.

Falck-Ytter Y, et al. Prevention of venous thromboembolism in orthopedic surgery patients: antithrombotic therapy and prevention of thrombosis, 9th ed: American College of Chest Physicians evidence-based clinical practice guidelines. *Chest*, **2012**, *141*:e278S–e325S.

Gara PT, et al. 2013 ACCF/AHA guideline for the management of ST-elevation myocardial infarction: a report of the American College of Cardiology Foundation/American Heart Association Task Force on Practice Guidelines. *Circulation*, **2013**, *127*:e362–e425.

Giugliano RP, et al. Edoxaban versus warfarin in patients with atrial fibrillation. *N Engl J Med*, **2013**, *369*:2093–2104.

Gomez-Outes A, et al. Direct-acting oral anticoagulants: pharmacology, indications, management, and future perspectives. *Eur J Haematol*, **2015**, *95*:389–404.

Gould MK, et al. Prevention of venous thromboembolism in nonorthopedic surgical patients: antithrombotic therapy and prevention of thrombosis, 9th ed: American College of Chest Physicians evidence-based clinical practice guidelines. *Chest*, **2012**, *141*:e227S–e277S.

Granger CB, et al. Apixaban versus warfarin in patients with atrial fibrillation. *N Engl J Med*, **2011**, *365*:981–992.

Granziera S, et al. Direct oral anticoagulants and their use in treatment and secondary prevention of acute symptomatic venous thromboembolism. *Clin Appl Thromb Hemost*, **2016**, *22*:209–221.

Grouzi E. Update on argatroban for the prophylaxis and treatment of heparin-induced thrombocytopenia type II. *J Blood Med*, **2014**, *5*:131–141.

Guimaraúes PO, Tricoci P. Ticagrelor, prasugrel, or clopidogrel in ST-segment elevation myocardial infarction: which one to choose? *Expert Opin Pharmacother*, **2015**, *16*:1983–1995.

Hokusai VTE investigators. Edoxaban versus warfarin for the treatment of symptomatic venous thromboembolism. *N Engl J Med*, **2013**, *369*:1406–1415.

International Warfarin Pharmacogenetics Consortium. Estimation of the warfarin dose with clinical and pharmacogenetic data. *N Engl J Med*, **2009**, *360*:753–764.

Ittaman SV, et al. The role of aspirin in the prevention of cardiovascular disease. *Clin Med Res*, **2014**, *12*:147–154.

Kahn SR, et al. Prevention of VTE in nonsurgical patients: Antithrombotic therapy and prevention of thrombosis, 9th ed: American College of Chest Physicians evidence-based clinical practice guidelines. *Chest*, **2012**, *141*:e195S–e226S.

Kearon C, et al. Antithrombotic therapy for VTE disease: chest guideline and expert panel report. *Chest*, **2016**, *149*:315–352.

Keating G. Cangrelor: a review in percutaneous coronary intervention. *Drug*, **2015**, *75*:1425–1434.

Kelton JG, et al. Nonheparin anticoagulants for heparin-induced thrombocytopenia. *N Engl J Med*, **2013**, *368*:737–744.

Lhermusier T, Waksman R. Prasugrel hydrochloride for the treatment of acute coronary syndromes. *Expert Opin Pharmacother*, **2015**, *16*:585–596.

Limdi NA, et al. Race influences warfarin dose changes associated with genetic factors. *Blood*, **2015**, *126*:539–545.

McClain MR, et al. A rapid-ACCE review of CYP2C9 and VKORC1 alleles testing to inform warfarin dosing in adults at elevated risk for thrombotic events to avoid serious bleeding. *Genet Med*, **2008**, *10*:89–98.

Meyer G, et al. Fibrinolysis for patients with intermediate-risk pulmonary embolism. *N Engl J Med*, **2014**, *370*:1402–1411.

Moschonas IC, et al. Protease-activated receptor-1 antagonists in long-term antiplatelet therapy. Current state of evidence and future perspectives. *Int J Cardiol*, **2015**, *185*:9–18.

Park Y, et al. Update on oral antithrombotic therapy for secondary prevention following non-ST segment elevation myocardial infarction. *Trends Cardiovasc Med*, **2016**, *26*:321–334.

Patel MR, et al. Rivaroxaban versus warfarin in nonvalvular atrial fibrillation. *N Engl J Med*, **2011**, *365*:883–891.

Pollack CV, et al. Idarucizumab for dabigatran reversal. *N Engl J Med*, **2015**, *373*:511–520.

Roffi M, et al. 2015 ESC guidelines for the management of acute coronary syndromes in patients presenting without persistent ST-segment elevation. *Eur Heart J*, **2015**, doi:10.1093/eurheartj/ehv320.

Schulman S, et al. Dabigatran versus warfarin in the treatment of acute venous thromboembolism. *N Engl J Med*, **2009**, *361*:2342–2352.

Shi C, et al. Pharmacogenetics-based versus conventional dosing of warfarin: a meta-analysis of randomized controlled trials. *PLoS One*, **2015**, *10*:e0144511.

Siegal DM, et al. Andexanet alfa for the reversal of factor Xa inhibitor activity. *N Engl J Med*, **2015**, *373*:2413–2424.

Zhang Q, et al. Aspirin plus clopidogrel as secondary prevention after stroke or transient ischemic attack: a systematic review and meta-analysis. *Cerebrovasc Dis*, **2015**, *39*:13–22.

SECTION III MODULATION OF PULMONARY, RENAL, AND CARDIOVASCULAR FUNCTION

Chapter 33

Drug Therapy for Dyslipidemias

Holly E. Gurgle and Donald K. Blumenthal

Dyslipidemia is a major cause of ASCVDs, such as CHD, ischemic cerebrovascular disease, and peripheral vascular disease. Cardiovascular disease represents the number one cause of death among adults in many developed nations (Mozaffarian et al., 2015). Both genetic disorders and lifestyle contribute to the dyslipidemias, including hypercholesterolemia and low levels of HDL-C.

Classes of drugs that modify cholesterol levels include the following:

- Inhibitors of HMG-CoA reductase (*statins*)
- Bile acid–binding resins
- Nicotinic acid (*niacin*)
- Fibric acid derivatives (*fibrates*)
- Inhibitor of cholesterol absorption (*ezetimibe*)
- Omega-3 fatty acid ethyl esters (fish oil)
- PCSK9 inhibitors
- MTP inhibitor (*lomitapide*)
- Inhibitor of apolipoprotein B-100 synthesis (*mipomersen*)

The 2014 ACC/AHA Guideline on the Treatment of Blood Cholesterol to Reduce Atherosclerotic Cardiovascular Risk in Adults (Stone et al., 2014) recommends a substantial shift in approach to cholesterol management compared to the ATPIII (Grundy et al., 2004; NCEP, 2002). Whereas ATPIII advocated treating to specific lipoprotein targets, the 2014 ACC/AHA guideline focuses on offering fixed doses of statins to patients in four statin benefit groups to reduce morbidity and mortality. Since the 2014 release of the ACC/AHA guideline, several additional expert consensus recommendations have been published, providing alternative opinions on cholesterol management (Jacobson et al., 2015) and recommendations regarding the role of nonstatin cholesterol treatments (Lloyd-Jones et al., 2016) in reduction of ASCVD risk (see Table 33–1).

Plasma Lipoprotein Metabolism

Lipoproteins are macromolecular assemblies that contain lipids and proteins. The lipid constituents include free and esterified cholesterol, triglycerides, and phospholipids. The protein components, known as *apolipoproteins* or *apoproteins*, provide structural stability to the lipoproteins and also may function as ligands in lipoprotein-receptor interactions or as cofactors in enzymatic processes that regulate lipoprotein metabolism. The major classes of lipoproteins and their properties are summarized in Table 33–2. Apoproteins have well-defined roles in plasma lipoprotein metabolism (Table 33–3). Mutations in lipoproteins or their receptors can lead to familial dyslipidemias and premature death due to accelerated atherosclerosis.

In all spherical lipoproteins, the most water-insoluble lipids (cholesteryl esters and triglycerides) are core components, and the more polar, water-soluble components (apoproteins, phospholipids, and unesterified cholesterol) are located on the surface. Except for apo(a), the lipid-binding regions of all apoproteins contain amphipathic helices that interact with the polar, hydrophilic lipids (such as surface phospholipids) and with the aqueous plasma environment in which the lipoproteins circulate. Differences in the non–lipid-binding regions determine the functional specificities of the apolipoproteins.

Figure 33–1 summarizes the pathways involved in the uptake and transport of dietary fat and cholesterol, pathways that involve the lipoprotein structures described next.

Chylomicrons

Chylomicrons are synthesized from the fatty acids of dietary triglycerides and cholesterol absorbed by epithelial cells in the small intestine. Chylomicrons are the largest and lowest-density plasma lipoproteins. In normolipidemic individuals, chylomicrons are present in plasma for 3–6 h after a fat-containing meal has been ingested. Intestinal cholesterol absorption is mediated by *NPC1L1*, which appears to be the target of *ezetimibe*, a cholesterol absorption inhibitor.

After their synthesis in the endoplasmic reticulum, triglycerides are transferred by *MTP* to the site where newly synthesized apo B-48 is available to form chylomicrons. Apo B-48, synthesized only by intestinal epithelial cells, is unique to chylomicrons and functions primarily as a structural component of chylomicrons. Dietary cholesterol is esterified by the ACAT-2. ACAT-2 is found in the intestine and in the liver, where cellular free cholesterol is esterified before triglyceride-rich lipoproteins (chylomicrons and *VLDLs*) are assembled.

After entering the circulation via the thoracic duct, chylomicrons are metabolized initially at the capillary luminal surface of tissues that synthesize LPL (see Figure 33–1), including adipose tissue, skeletal and cardiac muscle, and breast tissue of lactating women. The resulting free fatty acids are taken up and used by the adjacent tissues. The interaction of chylomicrons and LPL requires apo C-II as a cofactor.

Abbreviations

ACAT-2: type 2 isozyme of acyl coenzyme A:cholesterol acyltransferase
ACC: American College of Cardiology
AHA: American Heart Association
ALT: alanine aminotransferase
apo(a): apolipoprotein (a)
ASCVD: atherosclerotic cardiovascular disease
AST: aspartate aminotransferase
ATPIII: 2002 Third Report of the Expert Panel on Detection, Evaluation, and Treatment of High Blood Cholesterol in Adults
CETP: cholesteryl ester transfer protein
CHD: coronary heart disease
DHA: docosahexaenoic acid
DM: diabetes mellitus
EPA: eicosapentaenoic acid
ER: extended release
FH: familial hypercholesterolemia
FRS: Hard CHD Framingham Risk Score
HDL: high-density lipoprotein
HDL-C: high-density lipoprotein cholesterol
heFH: heterozygous familial hypercholesterolemia
HL: hepatic lipase
HMG-CoA: 3-hydroxy-3-methylglutaryl coenzyme A
hoFH: homozygous familial hypercholesterolemia
HSL: hormone-sensitive lipase
IDL: intermediate-density lipoprotein
LCAT: lecithin:cholesterol acyltransferase
LDL: low-density lipoprotein
LDL-C: low-density lipoprotein cholesterol
LDLR: LDL receptor
LP(a): lipoprotein (a)
LPL: lipoprotein lipase
LRP: LDL receptor–related protein
MTP: microsomal triglyceride transfer protein
NCEP: National Cholesterol Education Program
NHLBI: National Heart, Lung, and Blood Institute
NLA: National Lipid Association
NPC1L1: Niemann-Pick C1–like 1 protein
OTC: over the counter
PCE: pooled cohort equation
PCSK9: proprotein convertase subtilisin/kexin type 9
PPAR: peroxisome proliferator–activated receptor
SR: scavenger receptor
SREBP: sterol regulatory element–binding protein
USPSTF: U.S. Preventive Services Task Force
VLDL: very low-density lipoprotein

Chylomicron Remnants

After LPL-mediated removal of much of the dietary triglycerides, the *chylomicron remnants*, with all of the dietary cholesterol, detach from the capillary surface and within minutes are removed from the circulation by the liver (see Figure 33–1). First, the remnants are sequestered by the interaction of apo E with heparan sulfate proteoglycans on the surface of hepatocytes and are processed by *HL*, further reducing the remnant triglyceride content. Next, apo E mediates remnant uptake by interacting with the hepatic *LDL* receptor or the *LRP*.

During the initial hydrolysis of chylomicron triglycerides by LPL, apo A-I and phospholipids are shed from the surface of chylomicrons and remain in the plasma. This is one mechanism by which nascent (precursor) HDL are generated. Chylomicron remnants are not precursors of LDL, but the dietary cholesterol delivered to the liver by remnants increases plasma LDL levels by reducing LDL receptor–mediated catabolism of LDL by the liver.

Very Low-Density Lipoproteins

The VLDLs are produced in the liver when triglyceride production is stimulated by an increased flux of free fatty acids or by increased *de novo* synthesis of fatty acids by the liver. Apo B-100, apo E, and apo C-I, C-II, and C-III are synthesized constitutively by the liver and incorporated into VLDLs (see Table 33–3). Triglycerides are synthesized in the endoplasmic reticulum, and along with other lipid constituents, are transferred by MTP to the site in the endoplasmic reticulum where newly synthesized apo B-100 is available to form nascent (precursor) VLDL. Small amounts of apo E and the C apoproteins are incorporated into nascent particles within the liver before secretion, but most of these apoproteins are acquired from plasma HDL after the VLDLs are secreted by the liver. Mutations of MTP that result in the inability of triglycerides to be transferred to either apo B-100 in the liver or apo B-48 in the intestine prevent VLDL and chylomicron production and cause the genetic disorder *abetalipoproteinemia*.

Plasma VLDL is catabolized by LPL in the capillary beds in a process similar to the lipolytic processing of chylomicrons (see Figure 33–1). When triglyceride hydrolysis is nearly complete, the VLDL remnants, usually termed *IDLs*, are released from the capillary endothelium and reenter the circulation. Apo B-100–containing small VLDLs and IDLs, which have a $t_{1/2}$ of less than 30 min, have two potential fates. About 40%–60% are cleared from the plasma by the liver via apo B-100– and apo E–mediated interaction with LDL receptors and LRP. LPL and HL convert the remainder of the IDLs to LDLs by removal of additional triglycerides. The C apoproteins, apo E, and apo A-V redistribute to HDL.

Apolipoprotein E plays a major role in the metabolism of triglyceride-rich lipoproteins (chylomicrons, chylomicron remnants, VLDLs, and IDLs). About half of the apo E in the plasma of fasting subjects is associated with triglyceride-rich lipoproteins, and the other half is a constituent of HDL.

Low-Density Lipoproteins

Virtually all of the LDL particles in the circulation are derived from VLDL. The LDL particles have a $t_{1/2}$ of 1.5–2 days. In subjects without

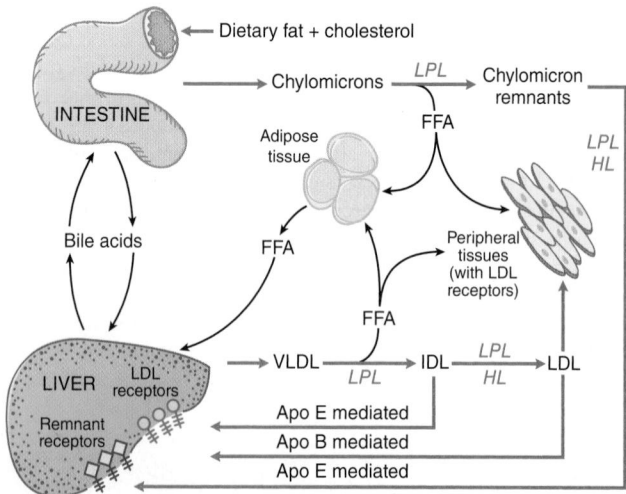

Figure 33–1 *The major pathways involved in the metabolism of chylomicrons synthesized by the intestine and VLDL synthesized by the liver.* Chylomicrons are converted to chylomicron remnants by the hydrolysis of their triglycerides by LPL. Chylomicron remnants are rapidly cleared from the plasma by the liver. "Remnant receptors" include the LRP, LDL receptors, and perhaps other receptors. FFA released by LPL is used by muscle tissue as an energy source or taken up and stored by adipose tissue.

TABLE 33–1 ■ COMPARISON OF KEY CLINICAL GUIDELINES FOR THE MANAGEMENT OF CHOLESTEROL IN ADULTS

	ATPIII 2004	ACC/AHA 2014	NLA 2015	USPSTF 2016
Risk assessment strategy	10-year FRS; CHD risk factors	10-year PCE	ASCVD risk factors used; FRS, PCE, or other	10-year PCE
Candidates for treatment	Patients above LDL goal	Patients in four statin benefit groups	Patients above LDL goal	Primary prevention in patients with risk
Recommended statin intensity	Titrated to achieve LDL goal	Moderate-to-high intensity	Titrated to achieve LDL goal	Low-to-moderate intensity
Recommendations	*Risk groups and LDL goals:* • High risk (LDL goal < 100, < 70 optional) if CHD, risk equivalent, or FRS ≥ 20% • Moderate-high risk (LDL goal < 130, < 100 optional) if ≥ 2 risk factors or FRS 10% to < 20% • Moderate risk (LDL goal <130, therapy started if LDL >160) if ≥2 risk factors or FRS <10% • Lower risk (LDL goal <160, therapy started if LDL >190) if 0 or 1 risk factor	*Four statin benefit groups:* • If ≥ 21 years old, clinical ASCVD, high-intensity statin (or moderate if > 75 years old) • If ≥ 21 years old and LDL ≥ 190, high-intensity statin • 40–75 years old with DM and LDL 70–189, moderate intensity (or high intensity if ASCVD ≥ 7.5%) • 40–75 years old with LDL 70–189, moderate-to-high intensity if ASCVD ≥ 7.5%	*Risk groups and LDL goals:* • Very high risk (LDL goal < 70) if ASCVD or DM + multiple risk factors or end-organ damage • High risk (LDL goal < 100) if 3 or more risk factors, DM + 0–1 risk factors, chronic kidney disease, LDL > 190, or high risk per calculator • Moderate risk (LDL goal < 100) if ≥ 2 risk factors or high risk per calculator • Low risk (LDL goal < 100) if 0–1 risk factors	• Statins recommended if 10-year risk ≥ 10% and 40 to 75 years old • Patient-specific approach if 10-year risk 7.5% to < 10% and with 1 or more cardiovascular risk factors • Statins not recommended if ≥ 75 years old

Refer to Table 33–4 for discussion of ASCVD risk factors.

Source: Data from ATPIII (Grundy et al., 2004; NCEP, 2002), ACC/AHA (Stone et al., 2014), NLA (Jacobson et al., 2015), USPSTF (2016).

hypertriglyceridemia, two-thirds of plasma cholesterol is found in the LDL. Plasma clearance of LDL is mediated primarily by LDL receptors (apo B-100 binds LDL to its receptor); a small component is mediated by non-receptor clearance mechanisms.

The most common cause of autosomal dominant hypercholesterolemia involves mutations of the LDL receptor gene. Defective or absent LDL receptors cause high levels of plasma LDL and *FH*. Treatment of hoFH, which is associated with accelerated ASCVD and premature death at the age of 30 or before, is treated by inhibiting apo B-100 synthesis with *mipomersen*, as well as by inhibiting cholesterol synthesis with statins. LDL becomes atherogenic when modified by oxidation, a required step for LDL uptake by the SRs of macrophages. This process leads to foam cell formation in arterial lesions. At least two SRs are involved (SR-AI/II and CD36). SR-AI/II appears to be expressed more in early atherogenesis, and CD36 expression is greater as foam cells form during lesion progression. The liver expresses a large complement of LDL receptors and removes about 75% of all LDL from the plasma. Consequently, manipulation of hepatic LDL receptor gene expression is a most effective way to modulate plasma LDL-C levels. *The most effective dietary alteration (decreased consumption of saturated fat and cholesterol) and pharmacological treatment (statins) for hypercholesterolemia act by enhancing hepatic LDL receptor expression.*

TABLE 33–2 ■ CHARACTERISTICS OF PLASMA LIPOPROTEINS

LIPOPROTEIN CLASS	DENSITY (g/mL)	MAJOR LIPID CONSTITUENT	TG:CHOL	SIGNIFICANT APOPROTEINS	SITE OF SYNTHESIS	CATABOLIC PATHWAY
Chylomicrons and remnants	<1.006	Dietary triglycerides and cholesterol	10:1	B-48, E, A-I, A-IV, C-I, C-II, C-III	Intestine	Triglyceride hydrolysis by LPL; apo E–mediated remnant uptake by liver
VLDL	<1.006	"Endogenous" or hepatic triglycerides	5:1	B-100, E, C-I, C-II, C-III	Liver	Triglyceride hydrolysis by LPL
IDL	1.006–1.019	Cholesteryl esters and "endogenous" triglycerides	1:1	B-100, E, C-II, C-III	Product of VLDL catabolism	50% converted to LDL mediated by HL; 50% apo E–mediated uptake by liver
LDL	1.019–1.063	Cholesteryl esters	NS	B-100	Product of VLDL catabolism	Apo B-100-mediated uptake by LDL receptor (~75% in liver)
HDL	1.063–1.21	Phospholipids, cholesteryl esters	NS	A-I, A-II, E, C-I, C-II, C-III	Intestine, liver, plasma	Complex: transfer of cholesteryl ester to VLDL and LDL; uptake of HDL cholesterol by hepatocytes
Lp(a)	1.05–1.09	Cholesteryl esters	NS	B-100, apo(a)	Liver	Unknown

CHOL, cholesterol; NS, not significant (triglyceride is < 5% of LDL and HDL); TG, triglyceride.

SECTION III MODULATION OF PULMONARY, RENAL, AND CARDIOVASCULAR FUNCTION

TABLE 33–3 ■ APOLIPOPROTEINS

APOLIPOPROTEIN (MW in kDa)	AVERAGE CONCENTRATION (mg/dL)	SITES OF SYNTHESIS	FUNCTIONS
apo A-I (~29)	130	Liver, intestine	Structural in HDL; LCAT cofactor; ligand of ABCA1 receptor; reverse cholesterol transport
apo A-II (~17)	40	Liver	Forms -S-S- complex with apo E-2 and E-3, which inhibits E-2 and E-3 binding to lipoprotein receptors
apo A-V (~40)	<1	Liver	Modulates triglyceride incorporation into hepatic VLDL; activates LPL
apo B-100 (~513)	85	Liver	Structural protein of VLDL, IDL, LDL; LDL receptor ligand
apo B-48 (~241)	Fluctuates according to dietary fat intake	Intestine	Structural protein of chylomicrons
apo C-I (~6.6)	6	Liver	LCAT activator; modulates receptor binding of remnants
apo C-II (8.9)	3	Liver	Lipoprotein lipase cofactor
apo C-III (8.8)	12	Liver	Modulates receptor binding of remnants
apo E (34)	5	Liver, brain, skin, gonads, spleen	Ligand for LDL receptor and receptors binding remnants; reverse cholesterol transport (HDL with apo E)
apo (a) (Variable)	Variable (under genetic control)	Liver	Modulator of fibrinolysis

High-Density Lipoproteins

The HDLs are protective lipoproteins that decrease the risk of CHD; thus, high levels of HDL are desirable. This protective effect may result from the participation of HDL in reverse cholesterol transport, the process by which excess cholesterol is acquired from cells and transferred to the liver for excretion. HDL effects also include putative anti-inflammatory, antioxidative, platelet antiaggregatory, anticoagulant, and profibrinolytic activities. Apo A-I is the major HDL apoprotein and its plasma concentration is a more powerful inverse predictor of CHD risk than is the HDL-C level. Apo A-I synthesis is required for normal production of HDL.

Mutations in the apo A-I gene that cause HDL deficiency often are associated with accelerated atherogenesis. In addition, two major subclasses of mature HDL particles in the plasma can be differentiated by their content of the major HDL apoproteins, apo A-I and apo A-II. Epidemiologic evidence in humans suggests that apo A-II may be atheroprotective.

The membrane transporter ABCA1 facilitates the transfer of free cholesterol from cells to HDL. After free cholesterol is acquired by the pre-β1 HDL, it is esterified by LCAT. The newly esterified and nonpolar cholesterol moves into the core of the particle, which becomes progressively more spherical, larger, and less dense with continued cholesterol acquisition and esterification. As the cholesteryl ester content of the particle (now called HDL$_2$) increases, the cholesteryl esters of these particles begin to be exchanged for triglycerides derived from any of the triglyceride-containing lipoproteins (chylomicrons, VLDLs, remnant lipoproteins, and LDLs). This exchange, mediated by the CETP, accounts for the removal of about two-thirds of the cholesterol associated with HDL in humans. The transferred cholesterol subsequently is metabolized as part of the lipoprotein into which it was transferred. Treatments that target CETP and the ABC transporters have yielded equivocal results in humans. While CETP inhibitors effectively reduce LDL, they also paradoxically increase the frequency of adverse cardiovascular events (angina, revascularization, myocardial infarction, heart failure, and death).

The triglyceride that is transferred into HDL$_2$ is hydrolyzed in the liver by HL, a process that regenerates smaller, spherical HDL$_3$ particles that recirculate and acquire additional free cholesterol from tissues containing excess free cholesterol. HL activity is regulated and modulates HDL-C levels. Androgens increase HL gene expression/activity, which accounts for the lower HDL-C values observed in men than in women. Estrogens reduce HL activity, but their impact on HDL-C levels in women is substantially less than that of androgens on HDL-C levels in men. HL appears to have a pivotal role in regulating HDL-C levels, as HL activity is increased in many patients with low HDL-C levels.

Lipoprotein (a)

Lipoprotein (a) [Lp(a)] is composed of an LDL particle that has a second apoprotein, apo(a), in addition to apo B-100. Apo(a) of Lp(a) is structurally related to plasminogen and appears to be atherogenic.

Atherosclerotic Cardiovascular Disease Risk Assessment

Therapy for dyslipidemias is based on reducing the risk of fatal and nonfatal atherosclerotic cardiovascular events, including myocardial infarction and stroke. A flowchart that illustrates the assessment and management of ASCVD risk is shown in Figure 33–2.

The major conventional risk factors for ASCVD are elevated LDL-C, reduced HDL-C, cigarette smoking, hypertension, type 2 diabetes mellitus, advancing age, and a family history of premature CHD events (men < 55 years; women < 65 years) in a first-degree relative (Table 33–4).

Primary prevention involves management of risk factors to prevent a first-ever ASCVD event. Secondary prevention is aimed at patients who have had a prior ASCVD event (myocardial infarction, stroke, or revascularization) and whose risk factors must be treated aggressively. In addition to cholesterol management, a comprehensive approach to ASCVD risk reduction includes smoking cessation, weight management, physical activity, healthy eating habits, antiplatelet use, and glucose and blood pressure management. All treatment plans to reduce ASCVD risk must include patient counseling to effect lifestyle changes. Secondary causes of dyslipidemias (Table 33–5), including medications that affect cholesterol, should also be considered prior to initiating treatment. Patients should also be evaluated for metabolic syndrome, which affects more than one in three adults and includes insulin resistance, obesity, hypertension, low HDL-C levels, a procoagulant state, vascular inflammation, and substantially increased risk of cardiovascular disease.

The PCE, published as part of the 2014 ACC/AHA guideline on the assessment of cardiovascular risk, was developed based on data from nine NHLBI-funded cohort studies and included data from geographically and racially diverse patient populations. The PCE estimates an individual patient's 10-year risk of ASCVD (defined as nonfatal myocardial infarction,

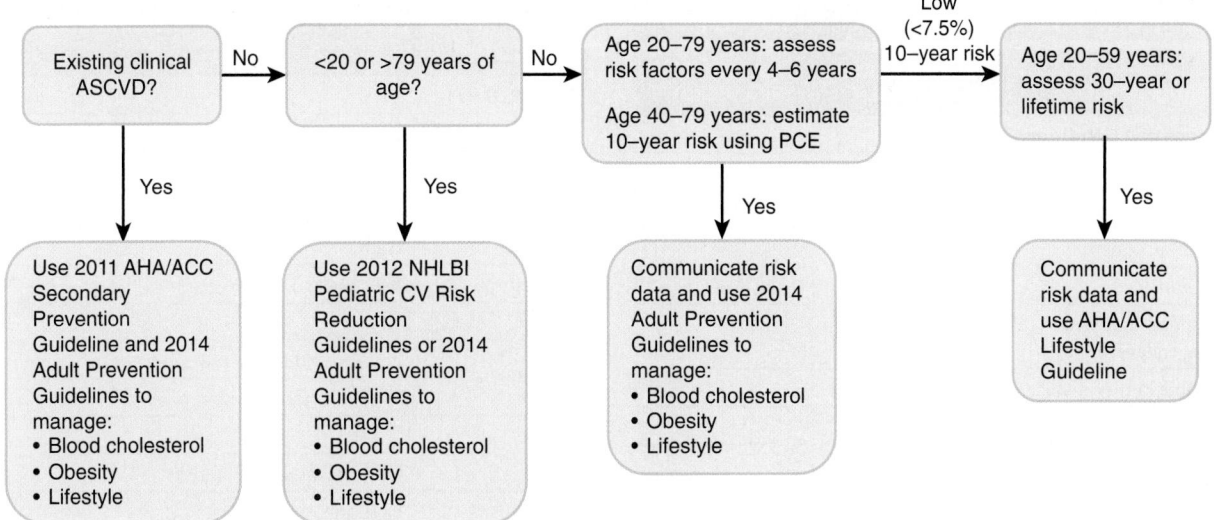

Figure 33–2 *Flowchart for assessing and managing ASCVD risk.* This chart is based on the 2014 ACC/AHA guideline on the assessment of cardiovascular risk. Refer to Table 33–1 and the ACC/AHA guidelines (Stone et al., 2014) for additional details.

CHD death, or fatal or nonfatal stroke) based on age, gender, total cholesterol, HDL-C, race, systolic blood pressure, smoking status, and history of diabetes, and hypertension. The ASCVD risk assessment calculator using the PCE is available online (https://tools.acc.org/ASCVD-Risk-Estimator/) and as a mobile app. Cardiovascular risk assessment calculators have also been developed for lifetime risk of cardiovascular disease.

Statin Drug Therapy

Although an understanding of optimal lipoprotein levels is helpful (see ranges in Table 33–6), the 2014 ACC/AHA guideline recommends the use of fixed statin doses for at-risk patients, instead of titration to specific lipoprotein goals. The ACC/AHA guidelines identify four statin benefit groups or patient populations most likely to benefit from statin therapy.

TABLE 33–4 ■ RISK FACTORS FOR ATHEROSCLEROTIC CARDIOVASCULAR DISEASE

Age

Male > 45 years of age or female > 55 years of age

Family history of premature CHD[a]

A first-degree relative (male < 55 years of age or female < 65 years of age when the first CHD clinical event occurs)

Current cigarette smoking

Defined as smoking within the preceding 30 days

Hypertension

Systolic blood pressure ≥ 140, diastolic pressure ≥ 90 or use of antihypertensive medication, irrespective of blood pressure

Low HDL-C

< 40 mg/dL (consider < 50 mg/dL as "low" for women)

Obesity

Body mass index > 25 kg/m² and waist circumference > 40 inches (men) or > 35 inches (women)

Type 2 diabetes mellitus[b]

[a]CHD defined as myocardial infarction, coronary death, or a coronary revascularization procedure.
[b]Diabetes mellitus is considered a high or very high risk condition for ASCVD.
Source: Data from 2015 NLA recommendations, part 1 (Jacobson et al, 2015).

Patients with known history of clinical ASCVD and those with elevated LDL-C greater than or equal to 190 mg/dL should be offered statins.

For primary prevention in patients 40 through 79 years of age with LDL 70 to 189 mg/dL, use of the PCE is recommended to identify patients more likely to benefit from treatment. Table 33–1 summarizes ACC/AHA recommendations for use of statins in adults. In November 2016, the USPSTF released recommendations for the use of statins in primary prevention populations (USPSTF, 2016). These recommendations build on those in the ACC/AHA guideline in helping to further identify higher-risk primary prevention patients. USPSTF also questions the use of higher-intensity statins in the 2014 ACC/AHA guideline and instead recommends low-to moderate-intensity statins for primary prevention patients.

Because the overwhelming body of evidence for ASCVD risk reduction with lipid-lowering therapies is from statin trials, evidence-based statin therapy of appropriate intensity is the hallmark of drug therapy of dyslipidemias. These drugs are competitive inhibitors of HMG-CoA reductase, which catalyzes an early, rate-limiting step in cholesterol biosynthesis. Higher doses of the more potent statins (e.g., atorvastatin, simvastatin, and rosuvastatin) also can reduce triglyceride levels caused by elevated VLDL levels. Figure 33–3 shows a representative statin structure and the reaction catalyzed by HMG-CoA reductase.

Mechanism of Action

Statins exert their major effect—reduction of LDL levels—through a mevalonic acid–like moiety that competitively inhibits HMG-CoA reductase. By reducing the conversion of HMG-CoA to mevalonate, statins inhibit an early and rate-limiting step in cholesterol biosynthesis. Statins affect blood cholesterol levels by inhibiting hepatic cholesterol synthesis, which results in increased expression of the LDL receptor gene. Some studies suggested that statins also can reduce LDL levels by enhancing the removal of LDL precursors (VLDL and IDL) and by decreasing hepatic VLDL production. The reduction in hepatic VLDL production induced by statins is thought to be mediated by reduced synthesis of cholesterol, a required component of VLDLs.

ADME

After oral administration, intestinal absorption of the statins is variable (30%–85%). All the statins, except simvastatin and lovastatin, are administered in the β-hydroxy acid form, which is the form that inhibits HMG-CoA reductase. Simvastatin and lovastatin are administered as inactive lactones that must be transformed in the liver to their respective β-hydroxy acids, simvastatin acid, and lovastatin acid. There is extensive first-pass hepatic uptake of all statins, mediated primarily by the organic

TABLE 33–5 ■ SECONDARY CAUSES OF DYSLIPIDEMIA

SECONDARY CAUSE	ELEVATED LDL-C	ELEVATED TRIGLYCERIDES
Disorders and Conditions		
Diabetes mellitus		+
Nephrotic syndrome	+	+
Excess alcohol use		+
Pregnancy	+	+
Menopause transition (declining estrogen levels)	+	+
Chronic kidney disease	+	+
Hypothyroidism	+	+
Obstructive liver disease	+	
Metabolic syndrome		+
HIV infection	+	+
Autoimmune disorders	+	+
Polycystic ovary syndrome	+	+
Drug Therapies		
Oral estrogens		+
Some progestins	+	
Glucocorticoids	+	+
Immunosuppressive drugs	+	+
Thiazide diuretics	+	+
Anabolic steroids	+	
Thiazolidinediones	+	
Rosiglitazone		+
β blockers (especially non-β_1 selective)		+
Fibric acids (in severe hypertriglyceridemia)	+	
Bile acid sequestrants		+
Amiodarone	+	
Danazol	+	
Isotretinoin	+	
Long chain ω-3 fatty acids (in severe hypertriglyceridemia) with docosahexanoate)	+	
Tamoxifen		+
Raloxifene		+
Interferon		+
Atypical antipsychotic drugs (clozapine, olanzapine)		+
Protease inhibitors		+
L-Asparaginase		+
Cyclophosphamide		+

Source: Data from 2015 NLA recommendations, part 1 (Jacobson et al, 2015).

TABLE 33–6 ■ CLASSIFICATION OF PLASMA LIPID LEVELS (mg/dL)

Non–HDL-C	
<130	Desirable
130–159	Above desirable
160–189	Borderline high
190–219	High
≥220	Very high
HDL-C	
<40	Low (consider < 50 mg/dL as low for women)
>60	High (desirable because of negative risk)
LDL-C	
<70	Optimal for very high risk[a]
<100	Desirable
100–129	Above desirable
130–159	Borderline high
160–189	High
≥190	Very high
Triglycerides	
<150	Normal
150–199	Borderline high
200–499	High
≥500	Very high

[a]Some consider LDL < 70 the optimal goal for patients with CHD or risk equivalents.

Source: Reproduced with permission from Jacobson TA, et al. National lipid association recommendations for patient-centered management of dyslipidemia: part 1—full report. *J Clin Lipidol*, **2015**, 9:129–169. Copyright © 2015 National Lipid Association. Published by Elsevier Inc. All rights reserved.

Due to extensive first-pass hepatic uptake, systemic bioavailability of the statins and their hepatic metabolites varies between 5% and 30% of administered doses. The metabolites of all statins, except fluvastatin and pravastatin, have some HMG-CoA reductase inhibitory activity. Under steady-state conditions, small amounts of the parent drug and its metabolites produced in the liver can be found in the systemic circulation. In the plasma, more than 95% of statins and their metabolites are protein bound, with the exception of pravastatin and its metabolites, which are only 50% bound. Peak plasma concentrations of statins are achieved in 1–4 h. The $t_{1/2}$ of the parent compounds are 1–4 h, except in the case of atorvastatin and rosuvastatin, which have half-lives of about 20 h, and simvastatin with a $t_{1/2}$ of about 12 h. The longer $t_{1/2}$ of atorvastatin and rosuvastatin may contribute to their greater cholesterol-lowering efficacy. The liver biotransforms all statins, and more than 70% of statin metabolites are excreted by the liver, with subsequent elimination in the feces.

Therapeutic Effects

Triglyceride Reduction by Statins

Triglyceride levels greater than 250 mg/dL are reduced substantially by statins, and the percentage reduction achieved is similar to the percentage reduction in LDL-C.

Effect of Statins on HDL-C Levels

Most studies of patients treated with statins have systematically excluded patients with low HDL-C levels. In studies of patients with elevated LDL-C levels and gender-appropriate HDL-C levels (40–50 mg/dL for men; 50–60 mg/dL for women), an increase in HDL-C of 5%–10% was observed, irrespective of the dose or statin employed. However, in patients with reduced HDL-C levels (<35 mg/dL), statins may differ in their effects on HDL-C levels. More studies are needed to ascertain

anion transporter OATP1B1 (see Chapter 5). *Hepatic cholesterol synthesis is maximal between midnight and 2:00 AM. Thus, statins with $t_{1/2}$ of 4 h or less (all but atorvastatin and rosuvastatin) should be taken in the evening.* Atorvastatin and rosuvastatin both have longer half-lives and may be taken at other times of day to optimize adherence.

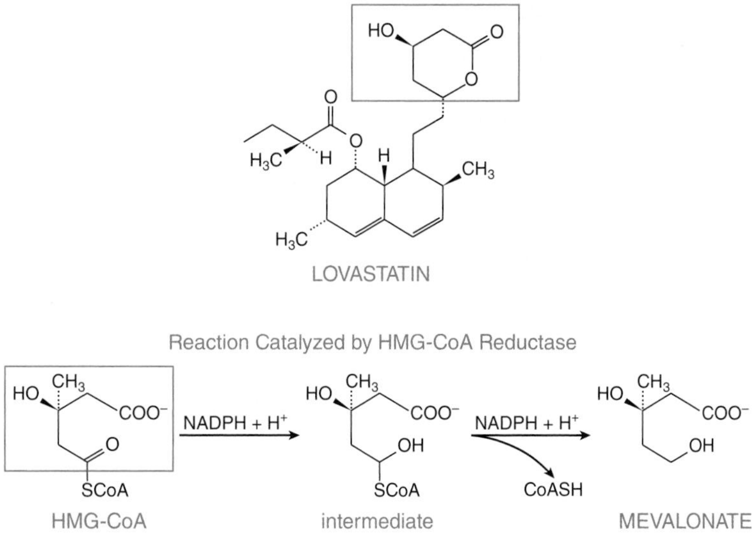

Figure 33–3 *Lovastatin and the HMG-CoA reductase reaction.*

whether the effects of statins on HDL-C in patients with low HDL-C levels are clinically significant.

Effects of Statins on LDL-C Levels

Dose-response relationships for all statins demonstrate that the efficacy of LDL-C lowering is log linear; LDL-C is reduced by about 6% (from baseline) with each doubling of the dose. Maximal effects on plasma cholesterol levels are achieved within 7–10 days. The statins are effective in almost all patients with high LDL-C levels. The exception is patients with *hoFH*, who have very attenuated responses to the usual doses of statins because both alleles of the LDL receptor gene code for dysfunctional LDL receptors.

Adverse Effects and Drug Interactions

Hepatotoxicity

Serious hepatotoxicity is rare and unpredictable, with a rate of about 1 case per million person-years of use. ACC/AHA guidelines recommend measuring ALT at baseline prior to initiation of statins. However since 2012, the FDA has no longer recommended routine monitoring of ALT or other liver enzymes following the initiation of statin therapy because routine periodic monitoring does not appear to be effective in detecting or preventing serious liver injury. Liver enzymes should be evaluated in patients with clinical symptoms suggestive of liver injury following initiation or changes in statin treatment (FDA, 2012).

Myopathy

The major adverse effect associated with statin use is myopathy. Myopathy refers to a broad spectrum of muscle complaints, ranging from mild muscle soreness or weakness (myalgia) to life-threatening rhabdomyolysis. The risk of muscle adverse effects increases in proportion to statin dose and plasma concentrations. Consequently, factors inhibiting statin catabolism are associated with increased myopathy risk, including advanced age (especially > 80 years of age), hepatic or renal dysfunction, perioperative periods, small body size, and untreated hypothyroidism. Measurements of creatinine kinase are not routinely necessary unless the patient also is taking a drug that enhances the risk of myopathy. Concomitant use of drugs that diminish statin catabolism or interfere with hepatic uptake is associated with increased risk of myopathy and rhabdomyolysis. The most common statin interactions occur with fibrates, especially *gemfibrozil* (38%), and with *cyclosporine* (4%), *digoxin* (5%), *warfarin* (4%), macrolide antibiotics (3%), and azole antifungals (1%). Other drugs that increase the risk of statin-induced myopathy include niacin (rare), HIV protease inhibitors, *amiodarone*, and *nefazodone*.

Gemfibrozil, the drug most commonly associated with statin-induced myopathy, both inhibits uptake of the active hydroxy acid forms of statins into hepatocytes by OATP1B1 and interferes with the transformation of most statins by glucuronidases. Coadministration of gemfibrozil nearly doubles the plasma concentration of the statin hydroxy acids. When statins are administered with niacin, the myopathy probably is caused by an enhanced inhibition of skeletal muscle cholesterol synthesis (a pharmacodynamic interaction). In 2016, the FDA withdrew approval for statin drug combinations containing fibrates or niacin (FDA, 2016).

Drugs that interfere with statin oxidation are those metabolized primarily by CYP3A4 and include certain macrolide antibiotics (e.g., *erythromycin*); azole antifungals (e.g., *itraconazole*); cyclosporine; *nefazodone*, a phenylpiperazine antidepressant; HIV protease inhibitors; and amiodarone. These pharmacokinetic interactions are associated with increased plasma concentrations of statins and their active metabolites. Atorvastatin, lovastatin, and simvastatin are primarily metabolized by CYPs 3A4 and 3A5. Fluvastatin is mostly (50%–80%) metabolized by CYP2C9 to inactive metabolites, but CYP3A4 and CYP2C8 also contribute to its metabolism. Pravastatin, however, is not metabolized to any appreciable extent by the CYP system and is excreted unchanged in the urine. Because pravastatin, fluvastatin, and rosuvastatin are not extensively metabolized by CYP3A4, these statins may be less likely to cause myopathy when used with one of the predisposing drugs. However, the benefits of combined therapy with any statin should be carefully weighed against the risk of myopathy.

Other Considerations

The choice of statins should be patient specific and based on factors such as cost, drug interactions, possible adverse effects, and desired intensity. Statin doses are characterized as low, moderate, or high intensity (Table 33–7), based on the degree of LDL-C lowering expected (range 30%–60%).

Rosuvastatin and pravastatin may be better tolerated than other statins and should be considered in patients with a history of myalgias with other statins. Lovastatin absorption is increased when taken with food, and patients should be encouraged to take with their evening meal. According to a 2012 FDA warning, simvastatin should not be used in combination with cyclosporine, HIV protease inhibitors, erythromycin, or gemfibrozil. In patients taking amlodipine or amiodarone, the daily dose of simvastatin should not exceed 20 mg. No more than 10 mg of simvastatin should be used in combination with diltiazem or verapamil. Concerns have been raised about possible cognitive impairment with statins, although review of the published data do not suggest that statins harm cognition. In contrast, other studies suggested statins may have a role in the prevention of dementias. Statins, especially at higher doses, likely confer a small increased risk of developing diabetes. However, the beneficial effects of

TABLE 33–7 ■ INTENSITY OF STATINS BY APPROXIMATE REDUCTIONS IN LDL-C WITH DAILY DOSING

HIGH-INTENSITY STATINS	MODERATE-INTENSITY STATINS	LOW-INTENSITY STATINS
LOWER LDL-C BY APPROXIMATELY 50% OR MORE	LOWER LDL-C BY APPROXIMATELY 30% TO LESS THAN 50%	LOWER LDL-C, ON AVERAGE, BY LESS THAN 30%
Atorvastatin 40–80 mg **Rosuvastatin 20–40 mg**	**Atorvastatin 10–20 mg** **Fluvastatin 40 mg twice daily** Fluvastatin XL 80 mg **Lovastatin 40 mg** Pitavastatin 2–4 mg **Pravastatin 40–80 mg** **Rosuvastatin 5–10 mg** **Simvastatin 20–40 mg**	Fluvastatin 20–40 mg Lovastatin 20 mg Pitavastatin 1 mg **Pravastatin 10–20 mg** Simvastatin 10 mg

Bold type signifies statins and doses used in randomized controlled trials demonstrating a reduction in major cardiovascular events or death.

Source: Data from Table 5 in 2014 ACC/AHA guidelines (Stone et al., 2014) and Table 2 in "2016 ACC Expert Consensus Decision Pathway on the Role of Non-Statin Therapies" (Lloyd-Jones et al., 2016).

statins on ASCVD events and mortality outweigh any increased risk conferred by promoting the development of diabetes. Atorvastatin is often the statin of choice for patients with severe renal dysfunction as it does not require dose adjustment.

Some statins have been approved for use in children with heFH. Atorvastatin, lovastatin, and simvastatin are indicated for children 11 years and older. Pravastatin is approved for children 8 years and older. *Statins are contraindicated during pregnancy and should be discontinued prior to conception if possible.* Data regarding statin use while breastfeeding are limited, and use should be discouraged.

Nonstatin Drug Therapies

The 2014 ACC/AHA guideline focuses on the use of statins to reduce ASCVD risk. However, several important clinical trials have evaluated whether fibrates, niacin, ezetimibe, and fish oil result in further reductions in ASCVD risk when used in addition to statins (ACCORD, 2010; AIM-HIGH, 2011; Cannon et al., 2015; HPS2-THRIVE, 2014; ORIGIN, 2012). The National Lipid Association released recommendations in 2015 that continued to emphasize specific LDL goals and encouraged the use of nonstatin therapies in addition to statins in high-risk individuals (Jacobson et al., 2015). In April 2016, the FDA withdrew approval for niacin ER or fenofibrate when used in addition to statins, citing studies that demonstrated no additional reduction in ASCVD events versus monotherapy with a statin (FDA, 2016). In July 2016, the ACC also released an expert consensus decision pathway to aid clinicians in the use of nonstatins (bile acid sequestrants, PCSK9 inhibitors, or ezetimibe) in addition to statins for the management of ASCVD risk (Lloyd-Jones et al., 2016). The use of nonstatins in high-risk patient populations requires careful shared decision-making.

Elevated triglycerides are an important risk factor for pancreatitis. Treatment with agents most effective at reducing levels of triglycerides (fibrate or fish oil) are recommended in patients with very elevated triglycerides (>1000 mg/dL) to reduce the risk of pancreatitis. These therapies may be used in addition to statin treatment if the patient otherwise has risk factors for ASCVD that make the patient an appropriate candidate for statin therapy.

Bile Acid Sequestrants

Cholestyramine, Colestipol, Colesevelam

The bile acid sequestrants cholestyramine and colestipol are among the oldest of the hypolipidemic drugs and are probably the safest because they are not absorbed from the intestine. These resins also are recommended for patients 11–20 years of age. Although statins are remarkably effective as monotherapy, the resins could be utilized as a second agent if statin therapy does not lower LDL-C levels sufficiently or in cases of statin intolerance.

Mechanism of Action. The bile acid sequestrants are highly positively charged and bind negatively charged bile acids. Because of their large size, the resins are not absorbed, and the bound bile acids are excreted in the stool. Because more than 95% of bile acids are normally reabsorbed, interruption of this process depletes the pool of bile acids, and hepatic bile acid synthesis increases. As a result, hepatic cholesterol content declines, stimulating the production of LDL receptors, an effect similar to that of statins. The increase in hepatic LDL receptors increases LDL clearance and lowers LDL-C levels, but this effect is partially offset by the enhanced cholesterol synthesis caused by upregulation of HMG-CoA reductase. Inhibition of reductase activity by a statin substantially increases the effectiveness of the resins. The resin-induced increase in bile acid production is accompanied by an increase in hepatic triglyceride synthesis, which is of consequence in patients with significant hypertriglyceridemia (baseline triglyceride level > 250 mg/dL). Use of colesevelam to lower LDL-C levels in hypertriglyceridemic patients should be accompanied by frequent (every 1–2 weeks) monitoring of fasting triglyceride levels.

Effects on Lipoprotein Levels. The reduction in LDL-C by resins is dose dependent. Doses of 8–12 g of cholestyramine or 10–15 g of colestipol are associated with 12%–18% reductions in LDL-C. Colesevelam lowers LDL-C by 18% at its maximum dose. Maximal doses (24 g of cholestyramine, 30 g of colestipol) may reduce LDL-C by as much as 25% but will cause GI side effects, which are often unacceptable. One to 2 weeks is sufficient to attain maximal LDL-C reduction by a given resin dose. In patients with normal triglyceride levels, triglycerides may increase transiently and then return to baseline. When used with a statin, resins are usually prescribed at submaximal doses due to poor tolerability.

Preparations and Use. The powdered forms of cholestyramine (4 g/dose) and colestipol (5 g/dose) are either mixed with a fluid (water or juice) and drunk as a slurry or mixed with crushed ice in a blender. Ideally, patients should take the resins before breakfast and before supper, starting with 1 scoop or packet twice daily and increasing the dosage after several weeks or longer as needed and as tolerated. Patients generally will not take more than 2 doses (scoops or packets) twice daily. Colesevelam hydrochloride is available as a solid tablet containing 0.625 g of colesevelam and as a powder in packets of 3.75 g or 1.875 g. The starting dose is either 3 tablets taken twice daily with meals or all 6 tablets taken with a meal. The tablets should be taken with a liquid. The maximum daily dose is 7 tablets (4.375 g).

Adverse Effects and Drug Interactions. The resins are generally safe, as they are not systemically absorbed. Because they are administered as chloride salts, rare instances of hyperchloremic acidosis have been reported. Severe hypertriglyceridemia is a contraindication to the use of cholestyramine and colestipol because these resins increase triglyceride levels. At present, there are insufficient data on the effect of colesevelam on triglyceride levels.

Drinking a slurry of powdered cholestyramine or colestipol produces a gritty sensation that is unpleasant but generally tolerated. Colestipol is available in a tablet form. Colesevelam is available as a hard capsule that absorbs water and creates a soft, gelatinous material that allegedly minimizes the potential for GI irritation. Patients taking cholestyramine and colestipol complain of bloating and dyspepsia. These symptoms can be substantially reduced if the drug is completely suspended in liquid several hours before ingestion. Constipation may occur but sometimes can be prevented by adequate daily water intake and psyllium. Colesevelam may be less likely than colestipol to cause the dyspepsia, bloating, and constipation.

The effect of cholestyramine and colestipol on the absorption of most drugs has not been studied. Cholestyramine and colestipol bind and interfere with the absorption of many drugs, including some thiazides, *furosemide*, *propranolol*, L-*thyroxine*, digoxin, warfarin, and some of the statins.

Colesevelam does not appear to interfere with the absorption of fat-soluble vitamins or of drugs such as digoxin, lovastatin, warfarin, *metoprolol*, *quinidine*, and *valproic acid*. Colesevelam reduces the maximum concentration and the area under the curve of sustained-release *verapamil* by 31% and 11%, respectively. In the absence of information to the contrary, prudence suggests that patients take other medications 1 h before or 3–4 h after a dose of colesevelam or colestipol. The safety and efficacy of colesevelam have not been studied in pediatric patients or pregnant women.

Niacin (Nicotinic Acid)

Niacin is a water-soluble B-complex vitamin that functions as a vitamin only after conversion to NAD or NADP, in which it occurs as an amide. Both niacin and its amide may be given orally as a source of niacin for its functions as a vitamin, but only niacin affects lipid levels. The hypolipidemic effects of niacin require larger doses than are required for its vitamin effects.

NICOTINIC ACID   NICOTINAMIDE

Mechanism of Action

In adipose tissue, niacin inhibits the lipolysis of triglycerides by HSL, thereby reducing transport of free fatty acids to the liver and decreasing hepatic triglyceride synthesis. Niacin may exert its effects on lipolysis by stimulating a G protein–coupled receptor (GPR109A) that couples to G_i and inhibits cyclic AMP production in adipocytes. In the liver, niacin reduces triglyceride synthesis by inhibiting both the synthesis and the esterification of fatty acids, effects that increase apo B degradation. Reduction of triglyceride synthesis reduces hepatic VLDL production, which accounts for the reduced LDL levels. Niacin also enhances LPL activity, an action that promotes the clearance of chylomicrons and VLDL triglycerides. Niacin raises HDL-C levels by decreasing the fractional clearance of apo A-I in HDL rather than by enhancing HDL synthesis.

ADME

The doses of regular (crystalline) niacin used to treat dyslipidemia are almost completely absorbed, and peak plasma concentrations (up to 0.24 mmol) are achieved within 30–60 min. The $t_{1/2}$ is about 60 min, which necessitates dosing two to three times daily. At lower doses, most niacin is taken up by the liver; only the major metabolite, nicotinuric acid, is found in the urine. At higher doses, a greater proportion of the drug is excreted in the urine as unchanged nicotinic acid.

Effects on Plasma Lipoprotein Levels

Regular or crystalline niacin in doses of 2–6 g/d reduces triglycerides by 35%–50% (as effectively as fibrates and statins); the maximal effect occurs within 4–7 days. Reductions of 25% in LDL-C levels are possible with doses of 4.5–6 g/d; 3–6 weeks are required for maximal effect. Niacin is the most effective agent available for increasing HDL-C (30%–40%), but the effect is less in patients with HDL-C levels less than 35 mg/dL. Niacin also is the only lipid-lowering drug that reduces Lp(a) levels significantly. Despite salutary effect on lipids, niacin's side effects limit its use (see Adverse Effects).

Therapeutic Use

Niacin is indicated for hypertriglyceridemia and elevated LDL-C. There are two commonly available forms of niacin. Crystalline niacin (immediate release or regular) refers to niacin tablets that dissolve quickly after ingestion. Sustained-release niacin refers to preparations that continuously release niacin for 6–8 h after ingestion. Niacin ER is the only preparation of niacin that is FDA-approved for treating dyslipidemia and that requires a prescription.

Crystalline niacin tablets are available OTC in a variety of strengths, from 50- to 500-mg tablets. The dose may be increased stepwise every 7 days

to a total daily dose of 1.5–2 g. After 2–4 weeks at this dose, transaminases, serum albumin, fasting glucose, and uric acid levels should be measured. After a stable dose is attained, blood should be drawn every 3–6 months to monitor for the various toxicities. OTC, sustained-release niacin preparations, and niacin ER are effective up to a total daily dose of 2 g. All doses of sustained-release niacin, but particularly doses above 2 g/d, have been reported to cause hepatotoxicity, which may occur soon after beginning therapy or after several years of use. The potential for severe liver damage should preclude use of OTC preparations in most patients. Niacin ER may be less likely to cause hepatotoxicity.

Concurrent use of niacin and a statin can cause myopathy. Two randomized trials evaluating niacin as add-on therapy to a statin versus statin monotherapy demonstrated no further reduction in ASCVD risk, despite improved lipoprotein parameters. Given this evidence, the FDA removed the indication for niacin use in addition to statin therapy and withdrew approval for statin combination formulations containing niacin (FDA, 2016). Niacin could still be considered as monotherapy in a statin-intolerant patient.

Adverse Effects

Two of niacin's side effects, flushing and dyspepsia, limit patient compliance. The cutaneous effects include flushing and pruritus of the face and upper trunk, skin rashes, and acanthosis nigricans. Flushing and associated pruritus are prostaglandin-mediated, thus taking an aspirin each day can alleviate the flushing in many patients. Flushing is worse when therapy is initiated or the dosage is increased but ceases in most patients after 1–2 weeks of a stable dose. Flushing is more likely to occur when niacin is consumed with hot beverages or with alcohol. Flushing is minimized if therapy is initiated with low doses (100–250 mg twice daily) and if the drug is taken after a meal. Dry skin, a frequent complaint, can be dealt with by using skin moisturizers, and acanthosis nigricans can be dealt with by using lotions containing *salicylic acid*. Dyspepsia and rarer episodes of nausea, vomiting, and diarrhea are less likely to occur if the drug is taken after a meal. Patients with any history of peptic ulcer disease should not take niacin.

The most common, medically serious side effects are hepatotoxicity, manifested as elevated serum transaminases, and hyperglycemia. Both regular (crystalline) niacin and sustained-release niacin, which was developed to reduce flushing and itching, have been reported to cause severe liver toxicity. Niacin ER appears to be less likely to cause severe hepatotoxicity, perhaps simply because it is administered once daily. The incidence of flushing and pruritus with this preparation is not substantially different from that with regular niacin. Severe hepatotoxicity is more likely to occur when patients take more than 2 g of sustained-release OTC preparations. Affected patients experience flu-like fatigue and weakness; usually, aspartate transaminase and ALT are elevated, serum albumin levels decline, and total cholesterol and LDL-C levels decline substantially.

In patients with diabetes mellitus, niacin should be used cautiously because niacin-induced insulin resistance can cause severe hyperglycemia. If niacin is prescribed for patients with known or suspected diabetes, blood glucose levels should be monitored at least weekly until proven to be stable. Niacin also elevates uric acid levels and may reactivate gout. A history of gout is a relative contraindication for niacin use. Rarer reversible side effects include toxic amblyopia and toxic maculopathy. Atrial tachyarrhythmias and atrial fibrillation have been reported, more commonly in elderly patients. *Niacin, at doses used in humans, has been associated with birth defects in experimental animals and should not be taken by pregnant women.*

Fibric Acid Derivatives

Clofibrate is a halogenated fibric acid derivative. Gemfibrozil is a nonhalogenated acid that is distinct from the halogenated fibrates. A number of fibric acid analogues (e.g., fenofibrate, *bezafibrate*, *ciprofibrate*) have been developed and are used in Europe and elsewhere.

Mechanism of Action

The mechanisms by which fibrates lower lipoprotein levels, or raise HDL levels, remain unclear. Many of the effects of these compounds on blood lipids are mediated by their interaction with PPARs, which regulate gene transcription. Fibrates bind to PPARα and reduce triglycerides through PPARα-mediated stimulation of fatty acid oxidation, increased LPL synthesis, and reduced expression of apo C-III. Increased LPL synthesis would enhance the clearance of triglyceride-rich lipoproteins. Reduced hepatic production of apo C-III, which serves as an inhibitor of lipolysis and receptor-mediated clearance, would enhance the clearance of VLDLs. Fibrate-mediated increases in HDL-C are due to PPARα stimulation of apo A-I and apo A-II expression, which increases HDL levels. Fenofibrate is more effective than gemfibrozil at increasing HDL levels. Most fibrates have potential antithrombotic effects, including inhibition of coagulation and enhancement of fibrinolysis.

ADME

Fibrates are absorbed rapidly and efficiently (>90%) when given with a meal but less efficiently when taken on an empty stomach. Peak plasma concentrations are attained within 1–4 h. More than 95% of these drugs in plasma are bound to protein, nearly exclusively to albumin. The $t_{1/2}$ of fibrates range from 1.1 (gemfibrozil) to 20 h (fenofibrate). The drugs are widely distributed throughout the body, and concentrations in liver, kidney, and intestine exceed the plasma level. Gemfibrozil is transferred across the placenta. The fibrate drugs are excreted predominantly as glucuronide conjugates (60%–90%) in the urine, with smaller amounts appearing in the feces. Excretion of these drugs is impaired in renal failure.

Effects on Lipoprotein Levels

Effects of fibric acid agents on lipoprotein levels differ widely, depending on the starting lipoprotein profile, the presence or absence of a genetic hyperlipoproteinemia, the associated environmental influences, and the specific fibrate used. Patients with type III hyperlipoproteinemia (*dysbetalipoproteinemia*) are among the most sensitive responders to fibrates. Elevated triglyceride and cholesterol levels are dramatically lowered, and tuberoeruptive and palmar xanthomas may regress completely. Angina and intermittent claudication also improve.

In patients with mild hypertriglyceridemia (e.g., triglycerides < 400 mg/dL), fibrate treatment decreases triglyceride levels by up to 50% and increases HDL-C concentrations by about 15%; LDL-C levels may be unchanged or increase. Normotriglyceridemic patients with heFH usually experience little change in LDL levels with gemfibrozil; with the other fibric acid agents, reductions as great as 20% may occur in some patients. Fibrates usually are the drugs of choice for treating severe hypertriglyceridemia and the chylomicronemia syndrome. While the primary therapy is to remove alcohol and lower dietary fat intake as much as possible, fibrates assist by increasing triglyceride clearance and decreasing hepatic triglyceride synthesis. In patients with chylomicronemia syndrome, fibrate maintenance therapy and a low-fat diet keep triglyceride levels well below 1000 mg/dL and thus prevent episodes of pancreatitis.

Therapeutic Use

Gemfibrozil usually is administered as a 600-mg dose taken twice daily, 30 min before the morning and evening meals. Fenofibrate is available in tablets of 48 and 145 mg or capsules containing 67, 134, and 200 mg. The choline salt of fenofibric acid is available in capsules of 135 and 45 mg. Equivalent doses of fenofibrate formulations are 135 mg of choline salt, 145-mg tablets, and 200-mg capsules. Fibrates are the drugs of choice for treating hyperlipidemic subjects with type III hyperlipoproteinemia, as well as subjects with severe hypertriglyceridemia (triglycerides > 1000 mg/dL) who are at risk for pancreatitis. A randomized clinical trial of fenofibrate added on to background statin therapy resulted in no further reduction of ASCVD risk (ACCORD, 2010). In 2016, the FDA withdrew approval for use of fenofibrate in addition to statin therapy for ASCVD risk reduction.

Adverse Effects and Drug Interactions

Fibric acid compounds usually are well tolerated. GI side effects occur in up to 5% of patients. Infrequent side effects include rash, urticaria, hair loss, myalgias, fatigue, headache, impotence, and anemia. Minor increases in liver transaminases and alkaline phosphatase have been reported. Clofibrate, bezafibrate, and fenofibrate reportedly potentiate the action of warfarin. Careful monitoring of the prothrombin time and reduction in dosage of warfarin may be appropriate.

A myopathy syndrome occasionally occurs in subjects taking clofibrate, gemfibrozil, or fenofibrate and may occur in up to 5% of patients treated with a combination of gemfibrozil and higher doses of statins. Gemfibrozil inhibits hepatic uptake of statins by OATP1B1 and competes for the same glucuronosyl transferases that metabolize most statins. Thus, levels of both drugs may be elevated when they are coadministered. Patients taking this combination should be followed at 3-month intervals with careful history and determination of creatine kinase values until a stable pattern is established. Patients taking fibrates with rosuvastatin should be followed especially closely even if low doses (5–10 mg) of rosuvastatin are employed. Fenofibrate is glucuronidated by enzymes that are not involved in statin glucuronidation; thus, fenofibrate-statin combinations are less likely to cause myopathy than combination therapy with gemfibrozil and statins.

All of the fibrates increase the lithogenicity of bile. Clofibrate use has been associated with increased risk of gallstone formation. Renal failure is a relative contraindication to the use of fibric acid agents, as is hepatic dysfunction. *Fibrates should not be used by children or pregnant women.*

Inhibitor of Cholesterol Absorption

Ezetimibe is the first compound approved for lowering total and LDL-C levels that inhibits cholesterol absorption by enterocytes in the small intestine. It lowers LDL-C levels by about 20% and may be used as adjunctive therapy with statins.

Mechanism of Action

Ezetimibe inhibits luminal cholesterol uptake by jejunal enterocytes, by inhibiting the transport protein NPC1L1. In human subjects, ezetimibe reduces cholesterol absorption by 54%, precipitating a compensatory increase in cholesterol synthesis that can be inhibited with a cholesterol synthesis inhibitor (e.g., a statin). The consequence of inhibiting intestinal cholesterol absorption is a reduction in the incorporation of cholesterol into chylomicrons; this diminishes the delivery of cholesterol to the liver by chylomicron remnants. The diminished remnant cholesterol content may decrease atherogenesis directly, as chylomicron remnants are very atherogenic lipoproteins. Reduced delivery of intestinal cholesterol to the liver by chylomicron remnants stimulates expression of the hepatic genes regulating LDL receptor expression and cholesterol biosynthesis. The greater expression of hepatic LDL receptors enhances LDL-C clearance from the plasma. Ezetimibe reduces LDL-C levels by 15%–20%.

ADME

Ezetimibe is highly water insoluble, precluding studies of its bioavailability. After ingestion, it is glucuronidated in the intestinal epithelium and absorbed and then enters an enterohepatic recirculation. Pharmacokinetic studies indicated that about 70% is excreted in the feces and about 10% in the urine (as a glucuronide conjugate). Bile acid sequestrants inhibit absorption of ezetimibe, and the two agents should not be administered together.

Therapeutic Use

Ezetimibe is available as a 10-mg tablet that may be taken at any time during the day, with or without food. Ezetimibe may be taken in combination with other dyslipidemia medications except bile acid sequestrants, which inhibit its absorption.

The role of ezetimibe as monotherapy of patients with elevated LDL-C levels is generally limited to the small group of statin-intolerant patients. The actions of ezetimibe are complementary to those of statins. Dual therapy with these two classes of drugs prevents both the enhanced cholesterol synthesis induced by ezetimibe and the increase in cholesterol absorption induced by statins, providing additive reductions in LDL-C levels. A combination tablet containing ezetimibe, 10 mg, and various doses of simvastatin (10, 20, 40, and 80 mg) has been approved. LDL reduction at the highest simvastatin dose plus ezetimibe is similar to that of high-intensity statins.

Adverse Effects and Drug Interactions

Other than rare allergic reactions, specific adverse effects have not been observed in patients taking ezetimibe. *Because all statins are contraindicated in pregnant and nursing women, combination products containing ezetimibe and a statin should not be used by women in childbearing years in the absence of contraception.*

Omega-3 Fatty Acid Ethyl Esters

Mechanism of Action

Omega-3 fatty acids, commonly EPA and DHA ethyl esters, reduce VLDL triglycerides and are used as an adjunct to diet for treatment of adult patients with severe hypertriglyceridemia. The recommended daily oral dose for patients with severe hypertriglyceridemia is 3–4 g/d administered with food.

ADME

The small intestine absorbs EPA and DHA, which are mainly oxidized in the liver, similar to fatty acids derived from dietary sources. The $t_{1/2}$ of elimination is approximately 50 to 80 h.

Therapeutic Use

Fish oil or other products containing omega-3 fatty acids are among the most common OTC herbal, vitamin, or nutritional supplements purchased by consumers each year. Doses and formulations of OTC items vary considerably. The AHA recommends that consumers eat a variety of fish at least twice a week and that fish oil supplements should only be considered for individuals with heart disease or high triglyceride levels in consultation with a medical professional. In addition to OTC fish oil products, several prescription-only products are available, generally at higher doses than those used OTC (1–1.2 g) and containing a combination of EPA and DHA. Icosapent ethyl, an ethyl ester derivative of EPA, does not contain DHA. Mixtures containing both EPA and DHA have increased LDL-C in patients with severe hypertriglyceridemia, whereas studies of EPA-only products suggest they may not significantly increase LDL-C while still reducing triglycerides. Controversy exists about when to treat hypertriglyceridemia. Modifiable secondary causes of high triglycerides such as uncontrolled diabetes and excessive alcohol intake should always be addressed prior to initiating therapy. While prescription omega-3 products generally have FDA indications for triglycerides 500 mg/dL or greater, many professional organizations advocate that such products be limited to patients with levels of 1000 mg/dL or greater who are at greatest risk for pancreatitis. The ORIGIN trial found no additional reduction in ASCVD risk associated with the use of omega-3 fatty acids versus background therapy with statins alone, calling into question the common use of fish oil supplements for "heart protection" by consumers.

Adverse Effects and Drug Interactions

Adverse effects may include arthralgia, nausea, fishy burps, dyspepsia, and increased LDL. Because omega-3 fatty acids may prolong bleeding time, patients taking anticoagulants should be monitored.

PCSK9 Inhibitors

Mechanism of Action

Proprotein convertase subtilisin/kexin type 9 is a protease that binds to the LDL receptor on the surface of hepatocytes and enhances lysosomal degradation of the LDL receptor, resulting in higher plasma LDL concentrations. Loss-of-function mutations of PCSK9 are associated with reduced LDL and lowered risk of ASCVD. Conversely, mutations leading to increased PCSK9 expression result in increased LDL levels and higher risk of ASCVD events. Two PCSK9 inhibitors, *alirocumab* and *evolocumab*, antibodies to PCSK9, are FDA-approved as adjunctive therapy to diet and maximally tolerated statin therapy in adult patients with hoFH and heFH or established ASCVD requiring additional LDL lowering. Evolocumab and alirocumab are fully humanized monoclonal antibodies that bind free PCSK9, thereby interfering with its binding to the LDL receptor, leading to increased liver clearance of LDL from the circulation and lower serum LDL levels (see Figure 33–4).

Although studies are ongoing, ORION-1 describes a novel RNA interference therapeutic, inclisiran, that targets PCSK9 mRNA and thus blocks PCSK9 protein synthesis (Ray et al., 2017). Early clinical trials showed promise for an RNA interference therapeutic (ALN-PCS) that targets PCSK9 mRNA and thus blocks PCSK9 protein synthesis. Low-volume subcutaneous injections of inclisiran resulted in persistent reductions in LDL-C and other atherogenic lipids for 180 days, suggesting that a biannual subcutaneous dosing regimen might be possible.

ADME

The PCSK9 inhibitors are administered as subcutaneous injections either every 2 weeks or once monthly, depending on the dose and indication. Evolocumab is administered as a 140-mg injection every 2 weeks or 420 mg once monthly. For hoFH, evolocumab 420 mg is administered once monthly or every 2 weeks, and alirocumab (75 mg or 150 mg) is administered once every 2 weeks. Administration requirements and storage of these medications are barriers when compared with the ease of oral dosage forms of other medications.

The LDL-C plasma levels may be measured 4 to 8 weeks after initiating therapy or changing doses. These medications inhibit PCSK9 availability for 2 to 3 weeks after administration (half-life of elimination is 11 to 20 days), after which LDL levels begin to rise. Limited data are available in individuals with renal or hepatic impairment, although dose adjustments are not expected to be necessary. *PCKS9 inhibitors should not be used in pregnancy because transmission across the placenta is expected. It is not known to what degree the medications will be present in breast milk, so use during lactation is not recommended.*

Therapeutic Use

The effects of PCSK9 inhibitors are complementary to those of statins. While statins interfere with cholesterol production and stimulate the production of LDL receptors, PCSK9 inhibitors enable more LDL receptors to be available on the surface of liver cells. PCSK9 inhibitors reduce LDL-C in a dose-dependent manner by as much as 70% when used as monotherapy or by as much as 60% in patients already on statin therapy. Indications and approvals of these agents vary between countries. Currently, PCSK9 inhibitors are not FDA-approved for treatment of dyslipidemias in statin-intolerant patients without known ASCVD, although they are being used in this population elsewhere. Among patients with known ASCVD and LDL >70 despite treatment with moderate-high intensity statins, the addition of evolucumab further reduced the risk of ASCVD events, but not death, in the FOURIER trial (Sabatine et al., 2017). Given the high cost of treatment with PCSK9 inhibitors versus relatively inexpensive statin treatment, cost-effectiveness studies will also need to be conducted in a variety of patient populations to provide further recommendations on the patients most likely to benefit from these therapies. Currently, and because of cost-effectiveness, treatment with maximally tolerated doses of statins and ezetimibe is recommended prior to initiation of PCKS9 inhibitors.

Adverse Effects and Drug Interactions

Several clinical trials have identified a small (<1%) risk of neurocognitive effects in patients treated with PCSK9 inhibitors compared to placebo. Additional studies are under way to better understand the long-term neurocognitive effects of these medications, if any. Unlike other medications used to treat dyslipidemias, PCSK9 inhibitors do not appear to substantially increase the risk of myopathies when used as monotherapy or in combination with statins. Similar to other monoclonal antibodies, risk of infections, including nasopharyngitis, urinary tract infections, or upper respiratory infections, is slightly increased. Injection site reactions are the most frequent adverse effect, although these occur in less than 10% of patients. There are no expected drug interactions with PCSK9 inhibitors.

Inhibitor of Microsomal Triglyceride Transfer

Lomitapide

Mechanism of Action. Lomitapide mesylate is the first drug that acts by inhibiting MTP, which is essential for the formation of VLDLs.

ADME. Lomitapide is administered with water and without food (or at least 2 h after the evening meal) because administration with food may

A. No PCSK9

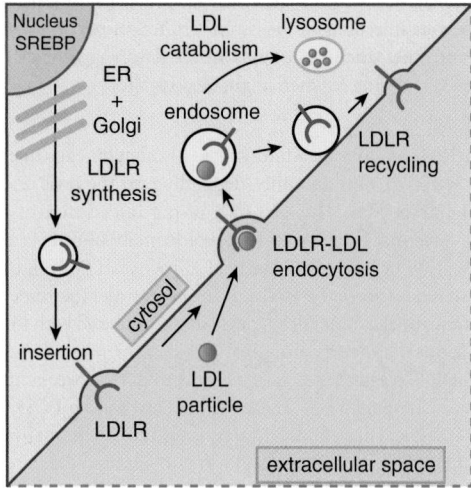

B. + PCSK9

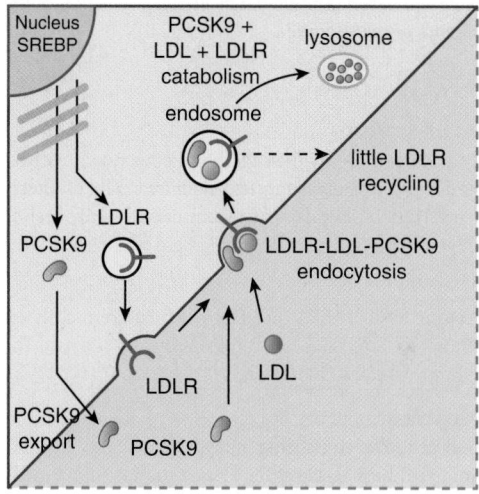

C. + PCSK9 + Ab^PCSK9

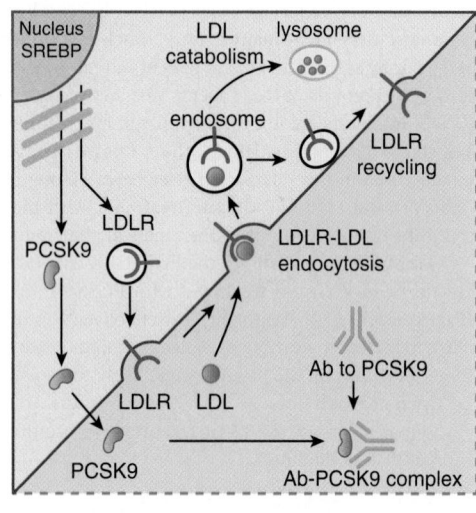

D. + PCSK9 + Ab^PCSK9 + statin

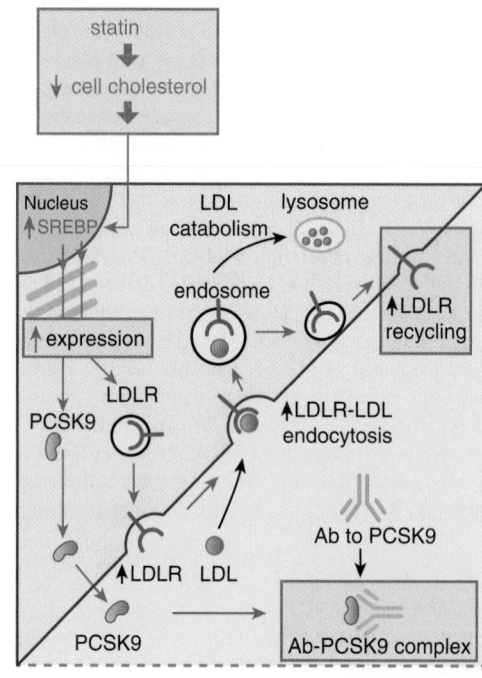

Figure 33–4 *LDL catabolism: effects of PCSK9, antibody to PCSK9, and statins.* Hepatic LDL uptake varies with the density of LDLRs in the hepatocyte membrane. The extent of LDLR synthesis and recycling affect the availability of LDLRs, variables that PCSK9, antibody to PCSK9, and statins can influence. **A.** *In the absence of PCSK9,* the LDLR is synthesized and inserted into the plasma membrane, where it binds LDL. The LDLR-LDL complex enters the hepatocyte by endocytosis. The complex dissociates within the endosome, the LDL entering the lysosomal pathway (degradation), and the LDLR being recycled to the membrane. **B.** *In the presence of PCSK9 biosynthesis,* however, PCSK9 is exported into the circulation. At the surface of the hepatocyte, PCSK9 interacts with the LDLR-LDL complex, entering the endosome and preventing the dissociation of LDLRs from LDL. As a consequence, the entire LDLR-LDL-PCSK9 complex enters the lysosomal pathway for degradation. Little or no LDLR is recycled, and future LDL uptake is reduced. There are gain-of-function mutations that enhance PCSK9 activity (see text). **C.** *In the presence of PCSK9 and antibody to PCSK9,* antibody to PCSK9 (Ab^PCSK9) prevents the binding of PCSK9 to the LDLR-LDL complex, returning the fate of the LDLR-LDL complex to that described in **A,** lysosomal degradation of LDL and recycling of LDLR to the membrane. **D.** *In the presence of PCSK9, antibody to PCSK9, and a statin,* levels of LDLR are increased by two different mechanisms. Statins, by inhibiting HMG-CoA reductase, reduce cell cholesterol, thereby activating SREBP and upregulating transcription of genes under its control; those include genes for LDLR and PCSK9. Expression of LDLR and PCSK9 increases. The newly synthesized LDLR molecules are inserted into the plasma membrane; the newly synthesized PCSK9 is exported. *In the absence of Ab^PCSK9,* the increased extracellular PCSK9 will bind to LDLR-LDL complexes, cause their lysosomal destruction, and thereby counteract some the statin's effect on circulating LDL and its uptake by hepatic LDLRs. *In the presence of antibody to PCSK9,* however, PCSK9 is complexed by Ab^PCSK9 and rendered inactive, permitting an increase in LDLR presence on the hepatocyte membrane and an increase in recycling of used LDLR to the membrane. Thus, by protecting LDLRs from degradation and enhancing synthesis of new LDLRs, the combination of a statin and Ab^PCSK9 can have a greater LDL-lowering effect than would the statin alone.

increase risk of GI adverse effects. The drug is metabolized by CYP3A4 and is contraindicated with inhibitors of CYP3A4.

Therapeutic Use. Lomitapide is FDA-approved as an adjunct to diet for lowering LDL-C, total cholesterol, apo B, and non–HDL-C lipoproteins in patients with hoFH. Lomitapide reduces LDL by up to 50% and should be used in combination with maximally tolerated statin therapy. The recommended starting oral dose (5 mg/d) is titrated upward at 4-week intervals to a maximum dose of 60 mg daily. The long-term cardiovascular effects of lomitapide are currently unknown.

Adverse Effects and Drug Interactions. Reported adverse effects commonly include significant diarrhea, vomiting, and abdominal pain in most patients. A strict low-fat diet may improve tolerability. Serious concerns also exist regarding hepatotoxicity and liver steatosis. In clinical trials, a third of patients experienced elevations in ALT or AST greater than three times the upper limit of normal. Lomitapide also increases hepatic fat, with or without concomitant increases in transaminases. The agent is used under an FDA risk evaluation and mitigation strategy due to its concerning side-effect profile. Lomitapide may be embryotoxic, and women of childbearing potential should have a negative pregnancy test before starting treatment and use effective contraception during treatment.

Inhibitor of Apolipoprotein B-100 Synthesis

Mipomersen

Mechanism of Action. Mipomersen is the first antisense oligonucleotide inhibitor of apo B-100 synthesis. Mipomersen binds to the mRNA of apo B-100 in a sequence-specific manner, which results in degradation or disruption of the apo B-100 mRNA, thereby reducing expression of apo B-100 protein.

ADME. The recommended dose is 1 mL of a 200-mg/mL solution, injected subcutaneously, once a week. It is metabolized in tissues by endonucleases to form shorter oligonucleotides available for further metabolism by exonucleases. The $t_{1/2}$ is 1 to 2 months. Maximal LDL reduction occurs after 6 months of treatment. Use is contraindicated in individuals with liver disease.

Therapeutic Use. In 2013, mipomersen was approved by the FDA as an addition to lipid-lowering medications and diet for patients with hoFH. However, given the side-effect profile of the medication, it was not approved elsewhere, including in Europe. LDL levels are reduced 30% to 50% with this treatment, although the discontinuation rates were high in clinical trials with this drug.

Adverse Effects and Drug Interactions. Injection site reactions are common (80%) and include erythema, pain, itching, and hematoma. Other common adverse effects include flu-like symptoms (30%), fatigue, and headache (15%). The agent is used under an FDA risk evaluation and mitigation strategy due to concerns about hepatotoxicity. Elevations in liver enzymes greater than three times the upper limit of normal occurred in approximately 10%–15% of patients in clinical trials.

Acknowledgement: *Thomas P. Bersot and Robert W. Mahley contributed to this chapter in recent editions of this book. We have retained some of their text in the current edition.*

Drug Facts for Your Personal Formulary: *Therapy for Dyslipidemias*

Drugs	Therapeutic Uses	Clinical Pharmacology and Tips
HMG-CoA Reductase Inhibitors (Statins)		
Atorvastatin Simvastatin Rosuvastatin Lovastatin Pravastatin Fluvastatin Pitavastatin	• The most effective and best-tolerated agents to treat dyslipidemias, especially elevated LDL-C	• *Safety of statins during pregnancy has not been established.* Women wishing to conceive and nursing mothers should not take statins. During their childbearing years, women taking statins should use highly effective contraception. • Hepatotoxicity (one case per million person-years of use); measure liver enzymes (ALT) at baseline and thereafter only when clinically indicated. • Myopathy and rhabdomyolysis (one death per million prescriptions (30-day supply); risk ↑ with dose and concomitant administration of drugs that interfere with statin catabolism or hepatic uptake.
Bile Acid–Binding Resins (Bile Acid Sequestrants)		
Cholestyramine Colestipol Colesevelam	• Probably safest lipid-lowering drugs (not absorbed systemically) • Recommended for patients 11–20 years of age	• Common GI side effects: bloating, dyspepsia, constipation. • Cholestyramine and colestipol bind and interfere with absorption of many drugs; administer all other drugs either 1 h before or 3–4 h after dose of a bile acid resin. • Severe hypertriglyceridemia is a contraindication to the use of cholestyramine and colestipol; they ↑ triglyceride levels.
Nicotinic Acid		
Niacin	• Favorably affects all lipid parameters; most effective agent for increasing HDL-C; also lowers triglycerides and reduces LDL-C	• *Should not be taken by pregnant women.* • Flushing, pruritus, and dyspepsia limit patient compliance. • Rarer episodes of nausea, vomiting, and diarrhea. • Hepatotoxicity, manifested as ↑ serum transaminases. • Hyperglycemia and niacin-induced insulin resistance; in patients with known or suspected diabetes, blood glucose levels should be monitored at least weekly until stable. • Concurrent use of niacin and a statin can cause myopathy and is contraindicated. • Contraindicated if any history of peptic ulcer disease. • Gout is a relative contraindication.
Fibric Acid (Fibrates)		
Gemfibrozil Fenofibrate *Not in the U.S.:* Ciprofibrate Bezafibrate	• Usual drugs of choice for treating chylomicronemia, hyperlipidemia with type III hyperlipoproteinemia, severe hypertriglyceridemia (triglycerides > 1000 mg/dL)	• GI side effects occur in up to 5% of patients. • *Fibrates should not be used by children or pregnant women.* • A myopathy syndrome may occur in subjects taking clofibrate, gemfibrozil, or fenofibrate. • The FDA has withdrawn approval for coadministration of fibrates with statins. • Renal failure and hepatic dysfunction are relative contraindications to the use of fibrates.

Drug Facts for Your Personal Formulary: *Therapy for Dyslipidemias (continued)*

Drugs	Therapeutic Uses	Clinical Pharmacology and Tips
Cholesterol Absorption Inhibitor		
Ezetimibe	• Monotherapy in patients with ↑ LDL-C who are statin intolerant • Combination with statin ⇒ additive reductions in LDL-C	• Bile-acid sequestrants inhibit absorption of ezetimibe; avoid concurrent use. • *Combination products containing ezetimibe and a statin should not be used by women in childbearing years in the absence of contraception.* • Generally well tolerated agent.
PCSK9 Inhibitors (Monoclonal Antibodies)		
Alirocumab Evolocumab	• Adjunct to diet and maximally tolerated statin therapy for adults with hoFH, heFH or clinical ASCVD who require additional lowering of LDL-C	• Hypersensitivity or injection site reactions are possible. • Most effective agents at reducing LDL-C. • Like other monoclonal antibodies, influenza-like symptoms, nasopharyngitis, upper respiratory infections may occur. • Used in addition to maximally tolerated statin doses (complementary mechanism; see Figure 33–4).
Omega-3 Fatty Acid Ethyl Esters		
Omega-3 fatty acids (EPA and DHA)	• Adjunct for treating severe hypertriglyceridemia (triglycerides > 1000 mg/dL)	• Adverse effects may include arthralgia, nausea, fishy burps, dyspepsia, and increased LDL. • Since omega-3-fatty acids may prolong bleeding time, patients taking anticoagulants should be monitored.
Inhibitor of Apo B-100 Synthesis (Antisense Oligonucleotide)		
Mipomersen	• Used as an adjunct to lipid-lowering agents and diet in patients with hoFH	• Common adverse effects include injection site reactions, flu-like symptoms, headache, and elevation of liver enzymes. • The agent is used under an FDA risk evaluation and mitigation strategy.
Inhibitor of Liver Microsomal Triglyceride Transfer Protein		
Lomitapide	• Used as an adjunct to diet for lowering LDL-C, total cholesterol, apo B, and non–HDL-C in patients with hoFH	• In patients with hoFH, treatment can reduce LDL-C by 40%–50%. • Adverse effects include GI symptoms, elevation of serum liver enzymes, and increased liver fat in most patients. • The agent is used under an FDA risk evaluation and mitigation strategy.

CHAPTER 33 DRUG THERAPY FOR DYSLIPIDEMIAS

Bibliography

ACCORD Study Group. Effects of combination lipid therapy in type 2 diabetes mellitus. *N Engl J Med*, **2010**, 362:1563–1574.

AIM-HIGH Investigators. Niacin in patients with low HDL cholesterol levels receiving intensive statin therapy. *N Engl J Med*, **2011**, 365: 2255–2267.

Cannon CP, et al. IMPROVE-IT Investigators. Ezetimibe added to statin therapy after acute coronary syndromes. *N Engl J Med*, **2015**, 372:2387–2397.

FDA. FDA drug safety communication: important safety label changes to cholesterol-lowering statin drugs. **January 2012**. Available at: https://www.fda.gov/drugs/drugsafety/ucm293101.htm. Accessed February 27, 2017.

FDA. Withdrawal of approval of indications related to the coadministration with statins in applications for niacin extended-release tablets and fenofibric acid delayed-release capsules. **April 2016**. Available at: https://www.federalregister.gov/documents/2016/04/18/2016-08887/abbvie-inc-et-al-withdrawal-of-approval-of-indications-related-to-the-coadministration-with-statins. Accessed February 27, 2017.

Grundy SM, et al. Implications of recent clinical trials for the National Cholesterol Education Program Adult Treatment Panel III Guidelines. *J Am Coll Cardiol*, **2004**, 44:720–732.

HPS2-THRIVE Collaborative Group. Effects of extended-release niacin with laropiprant in high-risk patients. *N Engl J Med*, **2014**, 371:203–212.

Jacobson TA, et al. National lipid association recommendations for patient-centered management of dyslipidemia—full report. *J Clin Lipidol*, **2015**, 9:129–169.

Lloyd-Jones DM, et al. 2016 ACC expert consensus decision pathway on the role of non-statin therapies for LDL-cholesterol lowering in the management of atherosclerotic cardiovascular disease risk. *J Am Coll Cardiol*, **2016**, 68:92–125.

Mozaffarian D, et al. Heart disease and stroke statistics—2015 update: a report from the American Heart Association. *Circulation*, **2015**, 131:e29–e322.

National Cholesterol Education Program (NCEP). Third report of the National Cholesterol Education Program (NCEP) Expert Panel on Detection, Evaluation, and Treatment of High Blood Cholesterol in Adults (Adult Treatment Panel III) final report. *Circulation*, **2002**, 106:3143–3421.

ORIGIN Trial Investigators. n–3 Fatty acids and cardiovascular outcomes in patients with dysglycemia. *N Engl J Med*, **2012**, 367:309–318.

Ray KK, et al. Inclisiran in patients at high cardiovascular risk with elevated LDL cholesterol. *N Engl J Med*, **2017**, 376:1430-1440.

Sabatine MS, et al. Evolocumab and clinical outcomes in patients with cardiovascular disease. *N Engl J Med*, **2017**, 376:1713-1722.

Stone NJ, et al. 2013 ACC/AHA guideline on the treatment of blood cholesterol to reduce atherosclerotic cardiovascular risk in adults: a report of the American College of Cardiology/American Heart Association Task Force on Practice Guidelines. *Circulation*, **2014**, 129(25)(suppl 2):S1–S45.

USPSTF. Statin use for the primary prevention of cardiovascular disease in adults US Preventive Services Task Force recommendation statement. *JAMA*, **2016**, 316:1997–2007.

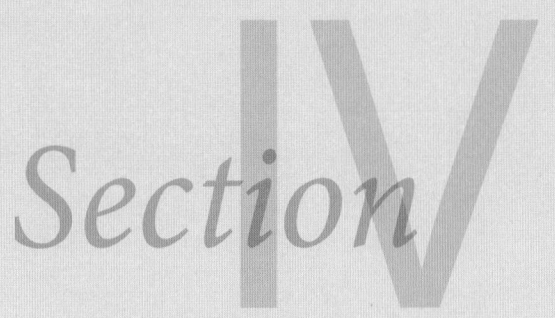

Section IV

Inflammation, Immunomodulation, and Hematopoiesis

Chapter 34

Introduction to Immunity and Inflammation

Nancy Fares-Frederickson and Michael David

The introduction of pathogens and foreign proteins into the human body can stimulate immune recognition, leading to inflammatory and allergic responses. Aspects of these responses are subject to pharmacological modulation. Before describing the actions of pharmacological agents affecting allergy and immunity, this chapter describes the cellular and molecular basis of immune and allergic responses and the points of pharmacological intervention. Subsequent chapters in this section cover in detail the classes of agents that can alter allergic and immune responses, as well as the biology and pharmacology of inflammation.

Cells and Organs of the Immune System

Hematopoiesis

All blood cells, including immune cells, originate from pluripotent hematapoietic stem cells (HSCs) of the bone marrow. HSCs are a population of undifferentiated progenitor cells that are capable of self-renewal. On exposure to cytokines and contact with the surrounding stromal cells, HSCs can differentiate into megakaryocytes (the source of platelets), erythrocytes (red blood cells), and leukocytes (white blood cells). This process is known as hematopoiesis (Figure 34–1).

The HSC pool can be divided in two populations: long-term (LT) and short-term (ST) HSCs. LT-HSCs are capable of lifelong self-renewal, allowing for continuous hematopoiesis throughout life. ST-HSCs have limited self-renewing capability, and differentiate into multipotent progenitors—the common myeloid progenitor (CMP) and the common lymphoid progenitor (CLP). The CMP gives rise to the myeloid lineage of cells that includes megakaryocytes; erythrocytes; granulocytes (neutrophils, eosinophils, basophils, mast cells); monocytes; macrophages; and dendritic cells (DCs).. In contrast, the CLP gives rise to the lymphoid lineage of cells that includes natural killer (NK) cells, B lymphocytes (B cells), and T lymphocytes (T cells) (Doulatov et al., 2012; Eaves, 2015).

Cells of the Innate Immune System

Innate immunity refers to the host defense mechanisms that are immediately available on exposure to pathogens.

Granulocytes

Granulocytes have characteristic cytoplasmic granules containing substances that, in addition to killing invading pathogens, enhance inflammation at the site of infection or injury. Neutrophils are the most abundant of the granulocytes and are generally the first cells to arrive at the site of injury. They are specialized at engulfing and killing pathogens—a process known as phagocytosis. Like neutrophils, eosinophils are also motile phagocytic cells. These cells defend against parasitic organisms such as helminths by releasing the contents of their granules, which are thought to damage the parasite membrane. Basophils and mast cells have granules that contain histamine and other pharmacologically active substances. In addition to their protective function, these cells can become dysregulated during the generation of allergic responses, in which they play an important role (see Hypersensitivity Reactions).

Mononuclear Phagocytes

Mononuclear phagocytes consist of monocytes and macrophages. Monocytes circulate in the blood and then migrate into tissues where they differentiate into macrophages, increase 5- to 10-fold in size, and acquire enhanced phagocytic and microbicidal activity. Macrophages engulf and eliminate pathogens, dead cells, and cellular debris. Macrophages can remain motile and travel throughout the tissues by amoeboid movements, and they can also take up residence in specific tissues, becoming tissue-resident macrophages. In addition to their role as phagocytes, macrophages release pro-inflammatory molecules, such as cytokines and eicosanoids, that recruit other immune cells to the site of infection (see Inflammation).

Natural Killer Cells

Natural killer cells are cytotoxic, granular lymphocytes that target tumor and virus-infected cells. NK cell receptors selectively target damaged or infected host cells by recognizing abnormal expression of surface molecules seen on damaged, but not healthy, cells.

Dendritic Cells

Dendritic cells are specialized cells that reside in tissues and stimulate adaptive immune responses. Immature DCs patrol peripheral tissues and sample their environment for infection by capturing pathogens through

Abbreviations

Ag: antigen
APC: antigen presenting cell
BCR: B-cell receptor
C#: complement component # (e.g. C3, C5)
CD: cluster of differentiation
CLL: chronic lymphocytic leukemia
CR#: complement receptor #
CTL: cytotoxic T lymphocyte
CTLA-4: cytotoxic T-lymphocyte–associated protein 4
DC: dendritic cell
HLA: human leukocyte antigen
HSC: hematopoietic stem cell
IFN: interferon
Ig: immunoglobulin
IL: interleukin
iNOS: inducible nitric oxide synthase: NOS2
IRF#: interferon regulatory factor #
ISG: interferon-stimulated gene
ISRE: interferon-stimulated response element
LTB$_4$: Leukotriene B$_4$
MADCAM-1: mucosal vascular addressin cell adhesion molecule 1
MALT: mucosa-associated lymphoid tissue
MHC: major histocompatibility complex
NK cell: natural killer cell
NO: nitric oxide
NSAID: nonsteroidal anti-inflammatory drug
PAMP: pathogen-associated molecular pattern
PD1: programmed cell death protein 1
PRR: pattern recognition receptor
Rh: rhesus
ROS: reactive oxygen species
ST: short term
TAP: transporter associated with antigen processing
T$_C$: cytotoxic T cell
TCR: T-cell receptor
T$_{FH}$: follicular helper T cells
T$_H$: helper T cell
TLR: toll-like receptor
TNF-α: tumor necrosis factor alpha
T$_{Reg}$: T-regulatory cells

phagocytosis, receptor-mediated endocytosis, and pinocytosis. After maturation, DCs shift from a phenotype that promotes antigen capture, to one that supports antigen presentation. Mature DCs migrate from the peripheral tissues to lymphoid organs and present antigens to activate helper and cytotoxic T cells (see Antigen Processing and Presentation).

Cells of the Adaptive Immune System

Adaptive immunity (also known as the acquired immune system) represents a branch of the immune system that is characterized by antigen specificity and immunological memory. It is mediated by B and T lymphocytes following exposure to specific antigens and is more complex than innate immunity in that it requires prior antigen processing and recognition to launch lymphocyte responses. Furthermore, in contrast to innate immune responses, which occur within hours after infection, B- and T-lymphocyte responses take days to develop.

B Cells

The B lymphocytes, also known as B cells, express cell surface pathogen receptors called immunoglobulins. When a naïve B cell (one that has not previously encountered antigen) detects a pathogen through binding of its immunoglobulin, it begins to proliferate. Its progeny can differentiate into plasma cells or memory B cells. Plasma cells are short-lived effector cells that specialize in secreting antibodies—the soluble form of immunoglobulins. Memory B cells are long-lived and persist for years following an infection. Because memory B cells express the same immunoglobulin as their parent B cell, they mount an enhanced secondary response to a pathogen on reinfection and are the basis for B cell–mediated immunity.

T Cells

The T lymphocytes, also known as T cells, express cell surface pathogen receptors called TCRs. Unlike immunoglobulins, which independently recognize antigens, TCRs only recognize antigens presented on MHC molecules on the surface of DCs or other APCs. T cells are divided into two subpopulations—T$_C$ cells and T$_H$ cells. T$_C$ cells or killer T cells destroy host cells that are infected with intracellular pathogens, whereas T$_H$ cells secrete cytokines that help enhance the function of other immune cells to mediate pathogen clearance. Activated T cells can differentiate into effector cells—cells that carry out immediate functions to help clear the infection—or memory cells. Memory T cells, like memory B cells, persist for years following an infection and mount an enhanced response on reexposure to the same pathogen (see Immunological Memory).

Organs of the Immune System

The organs of the immune system are divided into two categories based on their function: *primary lymphoid organs* and *secondary lymphoid organs*. Lymphocyte maturation and development take place in the primary lymphoid organs, whereas secondary lymphoid organs provide sites for mature lymphocytes to interact with APCs. These lymphoid organs are interconnected by blood and lymphatic vessels.

Primary Lymphoid Organs

The bone marrow and thymus make up the primary lymphoid organs. Both B-cell and T-cell precursors originate in the bone marrow from HSCs. B cells complete their maturation in the bone marrow, whereas T-cell precursors migrate to the thymus to complete their development.

The bone marrow tissue is composed of a meshwork of stromal cells (e.g., endothelial cells, adipocytes, fibroblasts, osteoclasts, osteoblasts, and macrophages). Immature B cells proliferate and differentiate within the bone marrow with direct (cell-cell contact) and indirect (cytokine release) help from stromal cells. IL-1, IL-6, and IL-7 are the most important cytokines guiding the B-cell differentiation process (Hoggatt et al., 2016).

The thymus is a bilobe organ that sits above the heart. Each lobe is divided into smaller lobules that consist of an outer compartment (cortex) and an inner compartment (medulla). Both the cortex and the medulla contain a stromal cell network comprising epithelial cells, DCs, and macrophages that present self-antigens to maturing T cells. This stromal cell network is responsible for the maturation process, and the cytokines IL-1, IL-2, IL-6, and IL-7 also play an important role in this process. The thymus begins to atrophy after puberty (as the thymic stroma is eventually replaced with adipose tissue), causing a decline in T-cell output. By age 35, T-cell production drops to 20% compared to that of newborn levels, and by age 65 this number further decreases to 2% (Palmer, 2013). Importantly, once the periphery is seeded with mature T cells, the host is equipped with a diversity of naïve T cells that will respond to any pathogen encounter, irrespective of diminished thymic output.

Secondary Lymphoid Organs

The secondary lymphoid organs, including the spleen, lymph nodes, and mucosa-associated lymphoid tissue MALT, are the sites where adaptive immune responses are initiated. The spleen is the largest lymphoid organ, consisting of red pulp and white pulp. The red pulp is a sponge-like tissue where old or damaged erythrocytes are recycled, whereas the white pulp region consists of lymphocytes. The spleen is the only lymphoid organ that is not connected to the lymphatic vessels. Instead, immune cells enter and exit the spleen through blood vessels.

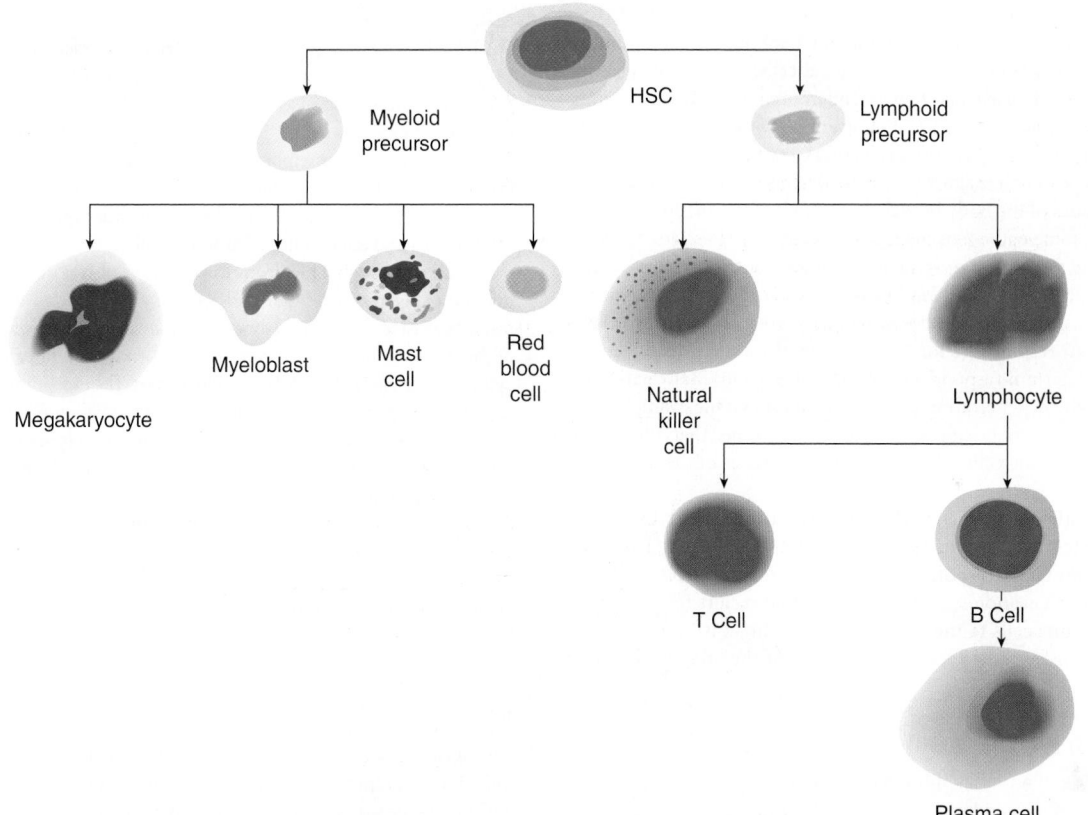

Figure 34–1 *Development of myeloid and lymphoid lineage cells from HSCs in the bone marrow.* HSCs give rise to lineage-specific precursors, which differentiate into all myeloid and lymphoid cells.

Lymph nodes are round, specialized structures that are positioned along the lymphatic vessels like beads on a chain. They collect the lymph (containing immune cells and antigens) that drains from the skin and internal organs and provide the physical location where antigen presentation and lymphocyte activation occur. The MALTs are loosely organized lymphoid tissues located in the submucosal surfaces of the gastrointestinal (GI) tract, respiratory system, and urinary tract (Neely and Flajnik, 2016).

The Lymphatic System

The "lymphatic system" or "lymphatics" represent a network of lymphatic vessels (similar to the circulatory system's veins and capillaries) that are connected to lymph nodes. Similar to their circulatory counterparts, small lymph capillaries are made up of single endothelial cell layers, whereas in larger lymph vessels the endothelial cells are surrounded by layers of smooth muscle cells. Additional parts of the lymphatic system are the tonsils, adenoids, spleen, and thymus. The lymphatics collect plasma continuously leaking out from blood vessels into the interstitial spaces and return this fluid, now called lymph, to the blood (after filtration in the lymph nodes) into the subclavian veins located on either side of the neck near the clavicles. Unlike blood movement, which is driven by a pump and flows throughout the body in a continuous loop, lymph flows in only one direction—upward toward the neck—and movement originates from rhythmic contractions of the smooth muscle cells, with directionality achieved via semilunar valves inside the vessels. The lymphatics therefore have an important function in regulating both immune and fluid homeostasis.

The B and T cells, unlike other blood cells, traffic through the body via both blood and lymph (hence the term *lymphocyte*). After completing their development in the primary lymphoid organs, B and T cells enter the bloodstream. When lymphocytes reach blood capillaries that empty into secondary lymphoid tissues, they enter these tissues. If a naïve lymphocyte encounters antigen, it will remain in the secondary lymphoid tissue and become activated. Otherwise, if no antigen is detected, the lymphocyte

then exits through the efferent lymph and reenters the bloodstream. This pattern of movement between the blood and lymph is referred to as lymphocyte recirculation, and it allows the lymphocyte population to continuously monitor the secondary lymphoid organs for signs of infection (Masopust and Schenkel, 2013; Thomas et al., 2016).

Innate Immunity

Innate immunity refers to the defense mechanisms that are immediately available on exposure to pathogens. These mechanisms consist of anatomical barriers, soluble mediators, and cellular responses. To establish an infection, a pathogen must first penetrate a host's anatomical barriers, including the skin and mucous membranes. If a pathogen manages to breach these anatomical barriers, the cellular innate immune response initiates rapidly, within a matter of minutes, to activate further mechanisms of the immune response.

Anatomical Barriers

The skin and mucosal surfaces form the first line of defense against pathogens. The skin is made up of a thin outer layer (epidermis) of tightly packed epithelial cells and an inner layer (dermis) of connective tissue containing blood vessels, sebaceous glands, and sweat glands. The respiratory, GI, and urogenital tracts are lined by mucous membranes. Like skin, mucous membranes consist of an outer layer of epithelial cells and an underlying layer of connective tissue. These anatomical surfaces act as more than just passive barriers against pathogens. All epithelial surfaces secrete antimicrobial peptides called host defense peptides (HDPs). HDPs kill bacteria, fungi, and viruses by disrupting their membranes (Hancock et al., 2016). The sebum secreted by the sebaceous glands contains fatty acids and lactic acids that inhibit bacterial growth on the skin. Mucosal surfaces are continuously covered in mucus (a viscous fluid secreted by epithelial cells of mucous membranes) containing antimicrobial substances that trap foreign microorganisms and help limit the spread of infection. In the respiratory tract, this mucous is continually removed by the action of cilia on epithelial cells. In addition, all these anatomical surfaces harbor commensal microorganisms. These commensals help protect against disease by preventing colonization by harmful microorganisms. These physical, mechanical, chemical, and microbiological barriers prevent a majority of pathogens from gaining access to the cells and tissues of the body (Belkaid and Tamoutounour, 2016).

However, some pathogens manage to breach these barriers. Microbes can enter the skin through scratches, wounds, or insect bites, such as those from mosquitoes (e.g., *Plasmodium falciparum,* the protozoan species predominantly responsible for malaria); ticks (e.g., *Borrelia burgdorferi,* the bacterium responsible for Lyme disease); and fleas (e.g., *Yersinia pestis,* the bacterium responsible for bubonic plague). Many pathogens enter the body by penetrating mucous membranes. One example is the influenza virus, which expresses a surface molecule that allows it to attach to and invade cells in the mucous membranes of the respiratory tract.

Once a pathogen breaches these anatomical barriers, the innate immune system first responds by detecting the pathogen. This initiates an inflammatory response—mediated by soluble effectors such as complement, eicosanoids, and cytokines—that results in the recruitment of immune cells to the site of infection, direct lysis or phagocytosis of pathogens, and eventual activation of the adaptive immune response.

Pathogen Recognition

The first phase of an innate immune response involves pathogen detection, which is mediated by secreted and cell surface pathogen receptors. Innate immune cells recognize broad structural patterns that are conserved within microbial species but are absent from host tissues. These broad structural patterns are referred to as *PAMPs* and the receptors that recognize them are called *PRRs*. PRRs can be broadly divided into three classes: secreted, endocytic, and signaling PRRs.

Secreted PRRs and the Complement System

Secreted PRRs are opsonins (molecules that enhance phagocytosis) that bind to microbial cell walls and tag them for destruction by the complement system or by phagocytes. C-reactive protein and mannose-binding lectin are two examples of secreted PRRs; both are components of the acute-phase response (see Inflammation).

The plasma proteins known as the complement system are some of the first to act following pathogen entry into host tissues. Over 30 proteins make up the complement system. These proteins circulate in blood and interstitial fluid in inactive forms that become activated in sequential cascades in response to interaction with molecular components of pathogens, leading to the activation of C3, which plays the most important role in pathogen detection and clearance. Complement activation leads to the cleavage of C3 into C3b and C3a fragments. The large C3b fragment (an opsonin) attaches to pathogen surfaces in a process called complement fixation and can activate C5 and a lytic pathway that can damage the plasma membrane of adjacent cells and microorganisms. The C5a fragment attracts macrophages and neutrophils and can activate mast cells. The small C3a fragment (anaphylatoxin) also promotes inflammation. Thus, complement fixation has two functions: the formation of protein complexes that damage the pathogen's membrane and marking the pathogen for destruction by phagocytes (Morgan and Harris, 2015).

Endocytic PRRs

Endocytic PRRs are expressed on the surface of phagocytic cells. These receptors mediate the uptake and transport of microbes into lysosomes, where they are degraded. The degraded microbial peptides are processed and presented to T cells by members of the MHC family of cell surface proteins. (In humans, the MHC is also called *human leukocyte antigen* or *HLA*). The mannose, glucan, and scavenger receptors are part of this class of receptors.

Signaling PRRs

On PAMP detection, signaling PRRs trigger intracellular signaling cascades that eventually result in the production of cytokines that orchestrate the early immune response. The most-studied group of signaling PRRs are the TLRs. TLRs are a family of PRRs that recognize a variety of microbial products. These transmembrane proteins are composed of an extracellular domain that detects pathogens and a cytoplasmic signaling domain that relays information to the nucleus. TLRs are expressed on the plasma membranes and endosomes of immune cells.

Signaling through TLRs leads to activation of two distinct signal transduction pathways (see PAMPs, PRRs, and the Induction of Interferons on next page). Most TLRs signal through a pathway that promotes the activation of the transcription factor NF-κB and the production of pro-inflammatory cytokines such as IL-1, IL-6, IL-12, and TNF-α. The exception is TLR3, which signals through a pathway that leads to the activation of the transcription factor IRF3, and the production of interferon (IFN) types I and III TLR4 is unique in that it signals through both pathways (Cao, 2016).

Type I (IFN-α and IFN-β) and type III (IFN-λ) IFNs promote the production of ISGs in infected and neighboring cells, the products of which induce an intracellular antimicrobial program that limits the spread of infectious pathogens, particularly viruses. Type I IFNs also augment antigen presentation and cytokine production by innate immune cells, leading to enhanced adaptive immune responses (Gonzalez-Navajas et al., 2012).

Pathogen Clearance

Pathogens vary in the manner by which they live and replicate within their hosts. Extracellular pathogens replicate on epithelial surfaces, or within the interstitial spaces, blood, and lymph of their host. Intracellular pathogens establish infections within host cells, either in the cytoplasm or in cellular vesicles. Depending on the nature of the infection, different immune cells and effector mechanisms are involved in the control and elimination of the pathogen.

Extracellular Pathogens

Unlike pathogens that replicate within host cells, extracellular pathogens are accessible to soluble effector proteins. Pathogens that replicate within interstitial spaces, blood, and lymph are detected by secreted PRRs and complement proteins. Complement fixation triggers direct lysis of the pathogen and enhances pathogen uptake by phagocytic cells. The phagocytic cells involved in the clearance of extracellular pathogens are macrophages and neutrophils. Tissue-resident macrophages are long-lived cells that are present from the start of an infection. They engulf pathogens and release inflammatory mediators to alert host cells of an attack. Neutrophils, in contrast, are short-lived, circulating phagocytes. Inflammatory cues, such as those released by macrophages, recruit neutrophils to the site of infection, where they soon become the dominant phagocyte.

On entry into host tissues, the first immune cells a pathogen encounters are the tissue-resident macrophages. Macrophages phagocytize microorganisms in a nonspecific fashion through their phagocytic receptors. Proteins of the complement system enhance this process by binding to receptors expressed by macrophages. One such receptor is complement receptor 1 (CR1). CR1 molecules interact with C3b fragments that have been deposited on the pathogen's surface, facilitating the engulfment and destruction of the pathogen.

In addition to engulfing invading pathogens, macrophages alert host cells of an infection. TLR4 engagement on macrophages leads to the production of pro-inflammatory cytokines such as IL-1, IL-6, IL-12, TNF-α, and CXCL8 (see Inflammation). These cytokines recruit immune cells, the most prominent of which are neutrophils, to the infected tissue (Lavin et al., 2015).

Circulating neutrophils have an average life span of less than 2 days. Mature neutrophils are kept in the bone marrow for up to 5 days before being released into circulation, ensuring a large reserve that can be summoned during an infection. When neutrophils sense inflammatory signals such as cytokines, chemokines, eicosanoids, ROS, or NO, they migrate to the site of infection, where they engulf and kill the invading pathogen.

PAMPs, PRRs, and the Induction of Interferons

Cells of the innate immune system—predominantly dendritic cells and macrophages—recognize broad structural patterns that are conserved within microbial species but are absent from host tissues. These patterns are called *pathogen-associated molecular patterns* (PAMPs); *Pattern recognition receptors* (PRRs) recognize PAMPS. There are three broad classes of PRRs: secreted, endocytic, and signaling PRRs.

Activation of signaling PRRs results in the production of cytokines that orchestrate the early immune response. The most well-studied group of signaling PRRs are the 11 Toll-like receptors (TLRs), each of which displays specificity for a distinct PAMP (e.g., TLR4 recognizes lipopolysaccharide (LPS); TLR3 binds double-stranded RNA [dsRNA]; TLR9 interacts with foreign DNA, etc.). Another receptor group, C-type lectin-like receptors, recognizes unique carbohydrate structures on invading microorganisms. Other signaling PRRs are cytosolic, such as retinoic acid–inducible gene (RIG)-I-like receptors (RLRs) that are activated by cytoplasmic double-stranded and 5′-triphosphorylated RNA species, and the nucleotide-binding oligomerization domain (NOD)-like receptor (NLRs) that detect cytosolic endotoxins. Signaling through most PRRs leads to broad cytokine responses, mediated by nuclear factor kappa B (NF-κB) and resulting in the production of pro-inflammatory cytokines such as interleukin (IL) 1, IL-6, IL-12, and tumor necrosis factor alpha (TNF-α).

In response to attack by viruses, bacteria, parasites, and tumor cells, membrane-bound and cytosolic (endosomal) signaling PRRs, including TLRs, work via several convergent pathways to stimulate the production of yet another class of cytokines, the interferons (IFNs). There are three types of IFNs: type I IFN (mainly IFN-α and IFN-β, plus other minor forms such as IFN-ε or IFN-ω); type II IFN (IFN-γ); and type III IFN (IFN-λ). IFNs are about 145 amino acid glycoproteins, with molecular masses of approximately 19–24 kDa, depending on the extent of glycosylation. Viral infections are the major inducers of the transcription of genes encoding type I IFNs. Pathways leading to IFN production are complex. The contemporary model now encompasses the concept that PRRs trigger intracellular signaling cascades that involve receptor-associated adapters (e.g., TRIM, TIRAP, MyD88, etc.) and the assembly of a signalosome containing various kinases (e.g., TBK1, IKKε, TAK, ASK1, etc.). Activation of these kinases in response to pathogen recognition leads to the phosphorylation and activation of the latent cytoplasmic transcription factors termed interferon regulatory factors (IRFs). Activation of IRF3 and IRF7, sometimes in combination with other transcription factors, activates transcription of the genes encoding type I IFNs.

Actions of IFNs

The IFNs are unique among the cytokine superfamily in that they produce an array of pleiotropic effects when they bind to their specific receptor. IFNs convey antiviral, antiproliferative, and immunomodulatory functions onto their target cells.

The IFNs are the most crucial cytokines in the defense against invading microorganisms, particularly viruses. IFN-α, IFN-β, and the more recently discovered IFN-λ, are vital elements in these defense mechanisms. Type I IFNs promote the production of interferon-stimulated genes (ISGs) in infected and neighboring cells, the products of which induce an intracellular antimicrobial program that limits the spread of infectious pathogens. Type I IFNs also augment antigen presentation, costimulation, and cytokine production by innate immune cells, leading to enhanced adaptive immune responses.

Produced by activated helper T (T_H) and natural killer (NK) cells, IFN-γ enhances the microbicidal activity of macrophages by inducing mammalian inducible nitric oxide synthase (iNOS, also called NOS2), thereby increasing their production of nitric oxide (NO) and their capacity to kill intracellular pathogens. Furthermore, CD8+ T cells utilize IFN-γ to directly kill infected cells and tumors. Indeed, IFN-γ contributes significantly to the adaptive immune system, where it also influences developmental processes such as immunoglobulin (Ig) isotype switching in B cells and T_H1 cell differentiation.

Cellular Signaling in Responses to IFNs

Interferon signaling is a complex mechanism that elicits the appropriate antimicrobial program in target cells. IFNs bind to distinct heteromeric membrane receptors. Binding of the type I IFNs to their specific cell surface receptors leads to cross tyrosine phosphorylation, recruitment and activation of the STAT (Janus kinase/signal transducer and activator of transcription) pathway. Several members of the STAT family of transcription factors and IRF9 cooperatively form the DNA binding protein complex ISGF3, which is required for expression of ISGs through activation of the interferon-stimulated response element (ISRE) in their promoters. Transcriptional induction of these immediate early response genes facilitates the establishment of an antiviral state, achieves antiproliferation in normal and tumor cells, and influences adaptive immune responses (e.g., via modulation of IL-2 production and expression of the α chain [CD25] of the IL-2R complex; see Figure 35–2).

Numerous genes contain an ISRE. Their gene products are components of the antiviral defense: 2′-5′ poly-A-synthase, dsRNA activated protein kinase (PKR), cell surface proteins such as ICAM and the major histocompatibility complex (MHC) I and II classes, chemokines (e.g., ISG15 and the IP10), and myriad genes of unknown function. More recently, numerous micro-RNAs have been added to the repertoire of IFN-induced response genes that contribute to control of pathogens.

In addition, neutrophils can release extracellular DNA nets that trap bacterial pathogens (von Kockritz-Blickwede and Nizet, 2009). Neutrophils die within 2 h of entry into infected tissues, forming the characteristic pus that develops at sites of infection (Kruger et al., 2015).

Intracellular Pathogens

The NK cells provide an early defense against intracellular pathogens. Like neutrophils, these circulating leukocytes migrate from the blood to the site of infection in response to inflammatory cues. Once at the site of infection, NK cells target and kill infected host cells.

The NK cells express receptors that deliver either activating or inhibitory signals. The ligands for the activating NK cell receptors are typically cell surface proteins whose expression is altered during infection or trauma. Healthy cells are protected from attack by NK cells because the signals generated from the inhibitory NK cell receptors dominate those generated from the activating receptors. In contrast, interaction between NK cells and infected or damaged cells shifts the balance of inhibitory and activating signals to favor an attack. This system allows NK cells to discriminate between healthy cells that should be protected and infected cells that should be destroyed.

The NK cells are stimulated by cytokines, including type I IFNs, IL-12, and TNF-α. IFN-α and IFN-β enhance NK cell cytotoxicity and induce NK cell proliferation, whereas IL-12 enhances cytokine production. The key cytokine produced by NK cells is IFN-γ, also called type II IFN. One function of IFN-γ is to activate macrophages. Activated macrophages exhibit enhanced microbicidal activity. One mechanism of their microbicidal activity is the induction of iNOS and the production of prodigious amounts of NO (Bjorkstrom et al., 2016).

Adaptive Immunity

Adaptive immunity refers to the arm of the immune response that changes (adapts) with each new infection. The cells responsible for adaptive immunity are B cells and T cells. The effector mechanisms used by B and T cells

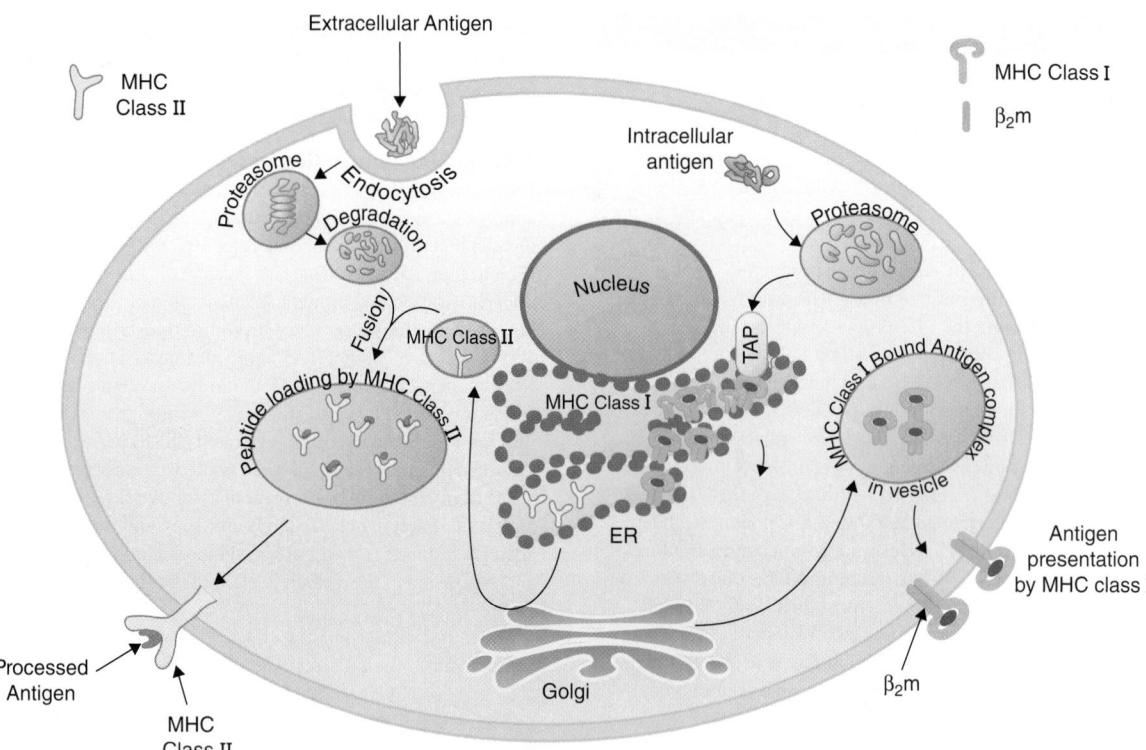

Figure 34–2 *Antigen processing and presentation via the MHC class I and II pathways.* Endogenous peptides from a variety of sources are processed by proteasomes; the resulting peptides are transported via the TAP complex into the ER, where they encounter MHC class I–β_2M (β_2-microglobulin) heterodimers. After the peptide loading of the MHC class I complex, the final peptide–MHC class I complexes migrate through the Golgi and are delivered to the cell surface to engage CD8$^+$ T cells. Exogenous antigens are endocytosed and processed by a lysosome/proteasome. The MHC class II complex is assembled in the ER, migrates through the Golgi, and subsequently fuses with the vesicle containing processed antigen fragments. These peptide cleavage products are loaded into the peptide-binding groove of the MHC class II, and the peptide–MHC class II complexes are transported to the cell surface and presented to CD4$^+$ T cells.

are similar to those used by innate immune cells; however, the important distinction between innate and adaptive immunity lies in their mode of pathogen recognition. Whereas the PRRs of the innate immune response recognize broad microbial patterns, B cells and T cells express receptors that recognize highly specific molecular structures. Following pathogen exposure, B and T cells with receptors that recognize the invading pathogen proliferate robustly and differentiate into effector lymphocytes. Soon after pathogen clearance, a large number of effector B and T cells die, but a small population of memory cells survives. Those cells have the ability to mount a rapid and specific response on reexposure to the same pathogen. This memory response, unique to adaptive immunity, is the basis for vaccination (see Chapter 36).

Initiation of the Adaptive Immune Response

The skin and mucosal surfaces prevent the majority of pathogens from entering host tissues and causing infections. Innate immune responses generally eliminate microorganisms that breach these barriers, typically within a few days. However, some pathogens establish an infection that cannot be controlled entirely by the innate immune response. In these cases, pathogen clearance requires the adaptive immune response.

Dendritic cells provide an essential link between innate and adaptive immunity. DCs engulf pathogens at the site of infection and travel to the lymphoid organs. Once there, they activate T cells by presenting them with fragments of the engulfed pathogen loaded on MHC molecules (see section on Antigen Processing and Presentation).

Pathogen Recognition

The innate immune system detects pathogens by a fixed repertoire of soluble and cell-surface receptors that recognize broad structures shared by different pathogens. The genes encoding these pathogen receptors are inherited from one generation to the next in a stable form.

The adaptive immune system uses a more focused strategy of pathogen recognition. B and T cells recognize pathogens by using cell surface receptors of one molecular type: BCRs and TCRs. In contrast to the stably inherited genes encoding innate immune pathogen receptors, the genes encoding BCRs and TCRs rearrange during the course of lymphocyte development. This gene rearrangement enables the development of millions of pathogen receptors with unique binding sites, each expressed by a small subset of lymphocytes. On pathogen exposure, only those lymphocytes with receptors that recognize specific components of the invading pathogen (referred to as the receptor's *cognate antigen*) are selected to proliferate and differentiate into effector cells.

Pathogen Receptors: BCRs and TCRs

The BCRs and TCRs are structurally related molecules. The BCR, also called immunoglobulin, is composed of two identical heavy chains and two identical light chains. Each polypeptide chain expresses an amino-terminal variable region, which contains the antigen-binding site, and a carboxy-terminal constant region. Immunoglobulins are anchored in the B-cell membrane by two transmembrane regions at the end of each heavy chain. Immunoglobulins are initially surface bound but become soluble when a B cell differentiates into a plasma cell. The soluble forms of immunoglobulins are called antibodies.

The TCR is composed of an α chain (TCRα) and a β chain (TCRβ), both anchored in the T-cell membrane by a transmembrane region. The α and β chains consist of a variable region that contains the antigen-binding site and a constant region. In contrast to immunoglobulins, TCRs remain membrane bound and are not secreted.

Both BCRs and TCRs develop through gene rearrangement. This genetic recombination process (which B cells complete in the bone marrow and T cells in the thymus) is a defining feature of the adaptive immune system. The human BCR and its soluble derivative, the antibody, are composed from genes of three loci, the *IG heavy chain*, the *IG κ light chain*, and the *IG λ light chain*, yielding a repertoire of more than 10^{11} possible combinations. In close resemblance, the TCR comprises either an α and a β chain (most common) or a γ and a δ chain. Two of the key enzymes involved are RAG1 and RAG2 (RAG, recombination-activating gene; deficiencies in these enzymes result in a complete absence of mature lymphocytes) and the terminal deoxynucleotidyl transferase, albeit the full complexity of the DNA repair machinery is required to accomplish a productive rearrangement. Failure to do so will lead to the elimination of the unsuccessful B or T cells by programmed cell death (Nemazee, 2006). These recombination and subsequent somatic hypermutation events are vital for an optimally performing adaptive immune system. They remain unutilized as pharmacological targets.

Antigen Processing and Presentation

Immunoglobulins are capable of recognizing antigens in their native form. TCRs, in contrast, only recognize processed antigen fragments presented by specialized molecules encoded by the MHC (Figure 34–2). The MHC was first identified as a genetic complex that determines an organism's ability to accept or reject transplanted tissue. Further studies highlighted the importance of MHC molecules in generating T_H- and T_C-cell responses.

There are two types of MHC molecules involved in antigen presentation: MHC class I and MHC class II. These structurally related molecules are expressed on different cell types but perform parallel functions in priming T-cell responses.

MHC Class I

MHC class I molecules consist of a transmembrane glycoprotein α chain noncovalently associated with a $β_2m$ molecule. MHC class I molecules are expressed on the surface of nearly all nucleated cells and present peptides from endogenous antigens to CD8 T_C cells.

MHC Class II

MHC class II molecules consist of two noncovalently associated transmembrane glycoproteins, an α chain and a β chain. MHC class II molecules are primarily expressed on the surface of professional APCs (DCs, macrophages, B cells) and present peptides from exogenous antigens to CD4 T_H cells.

Antigen Processing for Presentation by MHC

Unlike immunoglobulins, which recognize a wide range of molecular structures in their native form, TCRs can only recognize antigens in the form of a peptide bound to an MHC molecule. For a pathogen to be recognized by a T cell, pathogen-derived proteins need to be degraded into peptides—an event referred to as antigen processing (Figure 34-2). Endogenous antigens, those derived from intracellular pathogens, are processed by the cytosolic pathway for presentation by MHC class I molecules. Proteins in the cytosol are degraded into peptides by the proteosome. The resultant peptides are then transported out of the cytosol and into the ER by a protein called the *TAP*, which is embedded in the ER membrane. Once newly synthesized MHC class I α chains and $β_2m$ molecules are translocated into the ER membrane, the α chains and $β_2m$ molecules associate and bind peptide, forming a peptide-MHC complex. These peptide-MHC complexes make their way to the plasma membrane in membrane-enclosed vesicles of the Golgi apparatus.

Exogenous antigens, those derived from extracellular pathogens, are processed by the endocytic pathway for presentation by MHC class II molecules. In this pathway, extracellular pathogens are internalized by host cells through endocytosis or phagocytosis and are degraded by proteolytic enzymes within endocytic vesicles. Newly synthesized MHC class II α and β chains are translocated into the ER membrane, where they associate with a third chain, called the invariant chain. The invariant chain prevents MHC class II molecules from binding peptides in the ER and delivers MHC class II molecules to endocytic vesicles. Once in the endocytic vesicles, MHC class II molecules bind peptide and are carried to the cell surface by outgoing vesicles.

All T cells require peptide-MHC presentation by professional APCs for activation (see Primary Responses). If an intracellular pathogen does not infect a professional APC, CD8 T_C-cell responses can be generated through a third pathway of antigen presentation called *cross-presentation*. Cross-presentation involves the uptake of extracellular material by professional APCs and its delivery to the MHC class I presentation pathway instead of the MHC class II presentation pathway via a mechanism that remains incompletely understood (Blum et al., 2013).

Note that protein degradation occurs continuously, even in the absence of infection. In uninfected cells, MHC molecules carry self-peptides—derived from normal cellular protein turnover—to the cell surface. While these peptide-MHC complexes do not normally provoke an immune response, recognition of these self-peptides by autoreactive T cells can result in the development of *autoimmunity* (see *Autoimmunity: A Breach of Tolerance*).

Lymphocyte Development and Tolerance

Innate immune PRRs are fixed receptors that recognize broad microbial structures or structures associated with damaged host cells. These receptors rarely, if ever, recognize self-antigens expressed by healthy cells. In contrast, because BCRs and TCRs develop from gene rearrangement, receptors that recognize self-antigens expressed by healthy host cells can arise. The goal of lymphocyte development is to produce cells with functional pathogen receptors but eliminate cells whose receptors recognize self-antigens. Next, we describe the processes of B-cell and T-cell development and highlight the mechanisms that maintain self-tolerance.

B-Cell Development

B-cell development takes place in the bone marrow and is driven by interaction with bone marrow stromal cells and the local cytokine environment. B-cell development can be broadly divided into pro-B-, pre-B-, immature B-, and mature B-cell stages. BCR gene rearrangement starts at the early pro-B stage and continues throughout the pre-B stage. By the immature B-cell stage, B cells express fully rearranged IgM immunoglobulins on their cell surface. At this stage, immature B cells leave the bone marrow and complete their maturation in the periphery. Mature B cells express both IgM and IgD immunoglobulins on their cell surfaces (LeBien and Tedder, 2008).

Because B-cell activation depends on help from CD4 T_H cells, negative selection of T cells whose receptors recognize self-antigens also ensures that B cells whose receptors bind to the same self-antigen will not be activated. Consequently, B cells do not undergo as rigorous of a selection process as T cells. However, B cells whose receptors recognize components of the bone marrow are negatively selected and die by apoptosis.

T-Cell Development

Unlike B cells, which develop in the bone marrow, T-cell precursors complete their development in the thymus. T-cell precursors enter the thymus as $CD4^-$ $CD8^-$ DN (double negative) cells, not yet committed to the T-cell lineage.

The DN T cells can be divided into four subsets—DN1 to DN4—based on the expression of certain cell surface molecules. Gene rearrangement of the TCRB chain begins during the DN2 stage and continues through the DN3 stage. After β-chain rearrangement is complete, the newly synthesized β-chain combines with a protein known as the pre-Tα chain, forming the pre-TCR. DN3 cells then progress to the DN4 stage and express both the CD4 and CD8 coreceptors. These cells are now referred to as $CD4^+CD8^+$ DP (double positive) cells. DP T cells proliferate rapidly, generating clones of cells expressing the same β chain. After this period of rapid proliferation, T cells begin to rearrange their α-chain genes. Because cells within each clone can rearrange a different α chain, they generate a more diverse population than if the original cell had rearranged both the β chain and α chain before proliferating. Once a DP T cell expresses a fully rearranged TCR, it undergoes the processes of positive and negative selection.

The T cells migrate into the thymic cortex to undergo positive selection. The purpose of positive selection is to select for T cells whose TCRs can interact with an individual's own MHC molecules. In the cortex, T cells interact with cortical thymic epithelial cells, which express both MHC class I and MHC class II molecules. T cells with TCRs that do not recognize self-MHC molecules die by apoptosis. T cells with TCRs that can successfully bind to self-MHC molecules are signaled to survive and proceed to the thymic medulla. As a result of positive selection, DP thymocytes mature into single-positive T cells that express just one coreceptor (CD4 or CD8). T cells that successfully interact with MHC class I molecules develop into CD8 T cells, whereas T cells that interact with MHC class II molecules become CD4 cells.

After positive selection, T cells migrate to the thymic medulla to undergo negative selection. The purpose of negative selection is to eliminate T cells whose TCRs recognize self-antigens. This is accomplished by medullary thymic epithelial cells, which promiscuously express self-peptides on their MHC molecules. If T cells interact with self-peptides with high affinity, they are deleted by apoptosis (Shah and Zuniga-Pflucker, 2014).

The positive and negative selection processes responsible for generating self-MHC restricted and self-tolerant T cells are rigorous. It is estimated that over 98% of thymocytes die by apoptosis within the thymus, with the majority failing at the positive selection stage. The T cells that manage to successfully complete both positive and negative selection leave the thymus and take up residence in the secondary lymphoid structures.

Primary Responses

The processes of lymphocyte development and gene rearrangement generate millions of unique lymphocytes that each express pathogen receptors of a single specificity. During an infection, only a small portion of these B and T cells express receptors that can recognize the invading pathogen. To increase their numbers, each lymphocyte that recognizes the invading pathogen becomes activated and proliferates, giving rise to clones expressing identical immunoglobulins or TCRs. These processes, referred to as *clonal selection* and *clonal expansion*, are essential features of lymphocyte activation and differentiation, and facilitate the effector mechanisms that B and T cells use to combat infection.

B-Cell Activation and Antibody Production

In the majority of primary immune responses, B-cell activation and subsequent antibody production are dependent on help from CD4 T_H cells. When circulating B cells home to secondary lymphoid tissues, they first enter at the T-cell zone. If a B cell encounters its specific antigen, cross-linking of the BCR and coreceptor induces a signal transduction cascade that mediates changes in cell surface expression of adhesion molecules and chemokine receptors, preventing the B cells from leaving the T-cell zone.

After immunoglobulins bind their cognate antigen, they internalize the antigen by receptor-mediated endocytosis and process the antigen for display by MHC class II molecules. If a CD4 T_H cell recognizes its antigen, the B and T cell form a conjugate pair. This cognate interaction facilitates the delivery of T cell–derived cytokines to B cells. The most important of these cytokines is IL-4, which is essential for B-cell proliferation and differentiation into antibody-secreting plasma cells.

The initial antibodies produced by plasma cells are of generally low affinity. They help to keep the infection under control until a stronger antibody response is generated. Antibody quality improves over the course of the infection due to two processes: somatic hypermutation and isotype switching. Somatic hypermutation introduces random single-nucleotide substitutions throughout the immunoglobulin variable regions. These changes can result in immunoglobulin molecules with increased affinity for the pathogen. B cells producing these improved immunoglobulin molecules outcompete for binding to the invading pathogen and are preferentially selected to become plasma cells. As an infection proceeds, antibodies of higher affinity are produced—a process referred to as *affinity maturation* (Di Noia and Neuberger, 2007).

Isotype Switching.
Immunoglobulins can be divided into five classes (isotypes) called IgA, IgD, IgE, IgG, and IgM. These isotypes differ in their heavy-chain constant regions and have specialized effector functions. IgM is the first antibody secreted following B-cell activation and marks pathogens for destruction by the complement system. As an infection proceeds, antibodies with additional effector functions are generated by isotype switching. Isotype switching is a process by which proliferating B cells

rearrange their DNA to change their immunoglobulin constant regions. This process is strongly influenced by cytokines secreted by the B cell's cognate T cell (Xu et al., 2012).

Role of Antibodies in Pathogen Clearance.
Antibodies can aid in pathogen clearance in a number of ways. They can bind to a pathogen (or toxin) and prevent it from interacting with host cells. These antibodies are called neutralizing antibodies. Antibodies can also function as opsonins—coating of pathogens with antibodies can facilitate their engulfment by phagocytic cells, which often express receptors for the constant regions of antibodies. In addition, antibody deposition can activate the complement system, leading to the direct lysis of pathogens.

T-Cell Activation

Naïve T cells first encounter antigen presented by DCs in the secondary lymphoid tissues. For T cells to become fully activated, they need to receive two signals (Figure 34–3):

- a primary signal generated through ligation of the TCR
- a costimulatory signal generated through ligation of a T-cell surface protein called CD28

Both of these signals must be delivered by ligands on the same APC.

The primary signal is generated when the TCR engages a peptide-MHC complex. The TCR associates with an accessory molecule called CD3, forming the TCR-CD3 complex. CD3 does not influence the interaction of the TCR with its antigen but participates in the signal transduction that occurs after antigen engagement. The T-cell coreceptors CD4 and CD8 bind to the conserved regions of MHC molecules, strengthening and stabilizing the interaction between the TCR and the peptide-MHC complex. CD4 and CD8 also participate in signal transduction.

The costimulatory signal is generated when CD28 binds to its ligands, called B7-1 (CD80) and B7-2 (CD86). These costimulatory B7 molecules are only expressed on activated professional APCs, highlighting their importance in T-cell activation.

Engagement of the TCR complex activates signal transduction cascades that induce the expression of multiple genes, including NFAT, AP-1, and NF-κB. One of the most important downstream targets of these genes is IL-2, a cytokine that is essential for T-cell proliferation and survival. The IL-2 receptor, CD25, is expressed on activated T cells. When T cells become activated, they begin to express a cell surface protein called CTLA-4. This protein resembles CD28 and binds to the costimulatory B7 molecules with higher affinity than does CD28. Whereas CD28 ligation promotes T-cell activation, CTLA-4 ligation dampens T-cell activation. This inhibitory molecule serves to keep T-cell responses in check (Brownlie and Zamoyska, 2013). In addition to CTLA-4, T cells upregulate expression of other inhibitory coreceptors such as PD1 and PSGL-1 that help to fine-tune the ensuing T-cell response (Attanasio et al., 2016; Tinoco et al., 2016).

T-Cell Anergy.
For a naïve T cell to become fully activated, it must receive a signal through the TCR and CD28. If a T cell engages a peptide-MHC complex in the absence of a sufficient costimulatory signal, it enters a state of nonresponsiveness referred to as clonal anergy. Anergy is defined by the inability of T cells to proliferate after engaging a peptide-MHC complex due to a lack of IL-2 production and signaling (see Figure 35–2).

CD4 T_H-Cell Differentiation and Effector Functions.
Following activation, naïve CD4 T_H cells can differentiate into specialized T_H-cell subsets. These T_H-cell subsets display unique patterns of cytokine production and perform distinct effector functions. The initial studies on T_H-cell differentiation generated a biphasic model in which activated T_H cells differentiate into either T_H1 cells, which defend mainly against intracellular pathogens, or T_H2 cells, which aid in the clearance of extracellular pathogens. More recent models of T_H-cell differentiation have been expanded to include T_H9, T_H17, T_H22, T_{FH}, and T_{Reg} cells (DuPage and Bluestone, 2016).

As their name implies, CD4 T_H cells help activate other immune cells. T_H1 cells secrete IFN-γ and TNF-α, which activate macrophages to kill pathogens located within their phagosomes. These cytokines also activate CD8 T_C cells to kill infected host cells. T_H2 cells, which produce IL-4 and

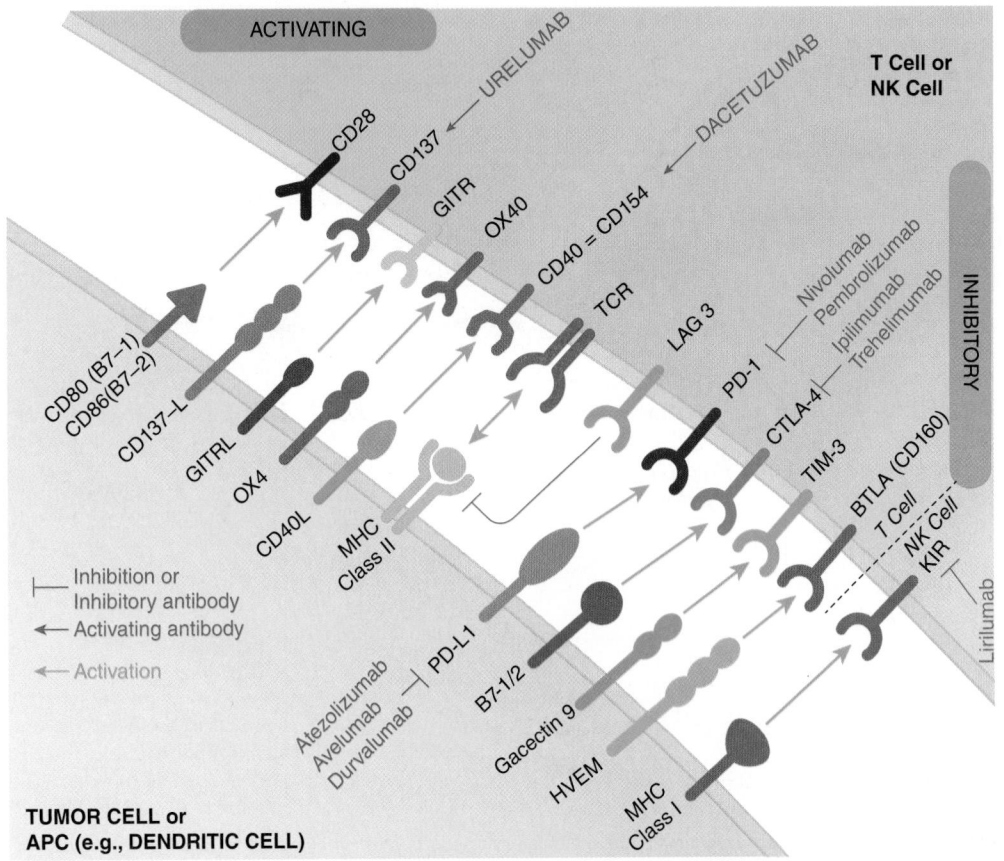

Figure 34–3 *T-cell receptor signaling.* TCR signaling on CD4⁺ cells after engagement with an MHC class II–peptide complex is enhanced by activating coreceptors (green-shaded area) or attenuated by inhibitory coreceptors (red-shaded area) after these bind their respective ligands on APCs or tumor cells. Numerous activating (→) or blocking (—⊣) monoclonal antibodies interfere with this fine-tuning of TCR signaling, thus allowing for the pharmacological modulation of the resulting immune response.

IL-5, defend against extracellular pathogens by enhancing humoral immunity. IL-4 activates B cells to differentiate into antibody-secreting plasma cells. T_H2-derived cytokines also induce class switching to IgA and IgE. Another subset of CD4 T_H cell, the T_{Reg} cell, is responsible for maintaining peripheral tolerance. Through various mechanisms, these cells suppress the proliferation of effector T cells, keeping the T-cell response under control.

CD8 T_C-Cell Effector Functions. The main role of CD8 T_C cells is to induce cytolysis of infected host cells expressing peptide-MHC class I complexes. Activated CD8 T_C cells kill their target cells by two distinct pathways: the granule exocytosis pathway and the Fas-FasL pathway. The granule exocytosis pathway involves the release of perforin and granule enzymes (granzymes A and B). Perforin molecules form pores in the target cell membrane, allowing the granzyme molecules to enter the cell. Upregulation of FasL (CD95L) on activated T_C cells induces the aggregation of Fas (CD95) on target cells. Both of these pathways activate the caspase cascade in the target cell, resulting in programmed cell death.

In addition to their cytolytic activity, activated CD8 T_C cells release pro-inflammatory cytokines, including IFN-γ and TNF-α. These cytokines further aid in pathogen clearance by enhancing the activity of macrophages and neutrophils (Harty et al., 2000).

Leukocyte Extravasation: Diapedesis

Leukocytes fulfill most of their immunological functions outside the bloodstream in the surrounding tissues. Consequently, traversing the blood endothelial cell layer barrier is a crucial step in this process. Extravasation (diapedesis) refers to the movement of leukocytes out of the blood into the site of infection or physical tissue damage (Figure 34–4). In the case of blood monocytes, extravasation also occurs in the absence of pathophysiological events and facilitates their conversion into tissue macrophages. On a molecular level, diapedesis can be dissected into four

mechanistic steps: *chemoattraction, rolling adhesion, tight adhesion,* and *transmigration* (Vestweber, 2015).

While initially believed to play its most important role in innate immunity, diapedesis has garnered more attention in recent years as a pharmacological target in the treatment of chronic (inflammatory) autoimmune diseases such as *multiple sclerosis* or *Crohn disease* (see Autoimmunity). The leukocyte cell surface adhesion molecule $α_4β_1$ integrin (VLA-4) that facilitates extravasation of CD4⁺ T cells interacts with VCAM-1 on vascular endothelial cells. Natalizumab is a humanized monoclonal antibody directed against $α_4$ integrin whose interference with the $α_4β_1$ integrin–VCAM-1 interaction leads to a blockade of autoreactive T-cell diapedesis into the brain and thus prevents attack on the myelin composing the nerve shielding. Similarly, natalizumab-mediated prevention of $α_4β_7$ integrin binding to the adhesion molecule MADCAM-1 found on endothelial cells of venules is responsible for the efficacy of the drug against Crohn disease. Another monoclonal antibody recently approved for the treatment of Crohn disease and ulcerative colitis is vedolizumab, which produces fewer side effects due to its $α_4β_7$-restricted binding specificity. Preventing entry of effector cells to inflammatory sites through the use of neutralizing antibodies has shown high therapeutic potential in multiple disease settings.

Immunological Memory

The B- and T-cell numbers decline after pathogen clearance, leaving behind a small population of memory cells. These memory cells have the ability to mount an enhanced secondary immune response on reexposure to the same pathogen.

Due to their expression of certain cell surface molecules, memory T cells are more sensitive to TCR-mediated activation by peptide-MHC complexes than naïve T cells. In addition, memory T cells have less-stringent requirements for costimulatory signals, allowing them to respond to

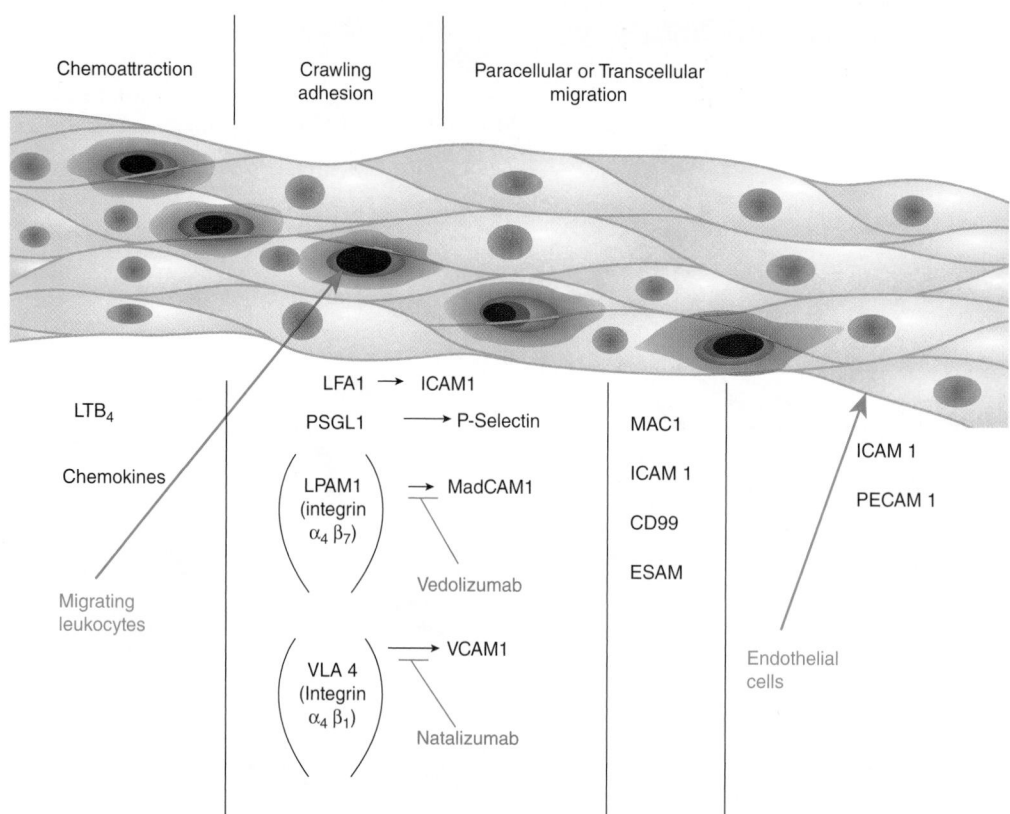

Figure 34–4 *Leukocyte diapedesis.* Leukocytes are recruited to the site of injury or infection by various chemoattractants. The expression of specific, complementary adhesion molecules on the surfaces of both the endothelial cells and the leukocytes facilitates the initial capture and subsequently the "rolling" binding of the leukocyte. After engagement of additional adhesion molecules, the leukocyte enters the subendothelial space, either by squeezing between endothelial cells (paracellular migration) or via movement through individual endothelial cells (transcellular migration). CAM, cellular adhesion molecule; ESAM, endothelial CAM; VCAM-1, vascular CAM 1; MADCAM-1, mucosal vascular addressin CAM 1; ICAM, inter-CAM; PSGL-1, P-selectin glycoprotein ligand 1; CD99, cluster of differentiation 99 antigen; MAC-1, macrophage-1 antigen.

peptide-MHC complexes displayed on cells that lack the costimulatory B7 molecules (Farber et al., 2014). Memory B cells produce better antibodies than naïve B cells because they express immunoglobulins that underwent somatic hypermutation and isotype switching during the first antigen encounter (Kurosaki et al., 2015). Combined, these properties allow for a faster and stronger secondary immune response, features that form the foundation of vaccination and subsequent "booster" or "refresher" inoculations (see Chapter 36).

Summary: Innate and Adaptive Immunity in Infectious Diseases

As described, the innate and adaptive immune systems work together to keep the host healthy. The innate immune response is the body's first line of defense and eliminates the majority of pathogens on its own. In the case that the innate immune system is insufficient to eliminate the pathogen, it keeps the infection in check until the adaptive immune system is able to mount a response. Pathogens will be cleared (acute infections), or they may evade the immune response and persist (chronic infections). Chronic infections such as HIV/AIDS and hepatitis B and C lead to immune system suppression that results in susceptibility to secondary infections or cancers associated with infection.

Inflammation

What Is Inflammation, and What Purpose Does It Serve?

The inflammatory response, or inflammation, is a physiologic response to tissue injury and infection, although it should be clear that *inflammation*

is not a synonym for *infection*. The Romans described the characteristics of this response almost 2000 years ago: pain (*dolor*), heat (*calor*), redness (*rubor*), and swelling (*tumor*). Within minutes of tissue injury and infection, plasma proteins mediate an increase in vascular diameter (vasodilation) and vascular permeability. Vasodilation increases blood flow to the area of injury, resulting in the heating and reddening of the tissue. Increased vascular permeability allows leakage of fluid into the blood vessels into the damaged tissue, resulting in swelling (edema). Within a few hours of these vascular changes, leukocytes arrive at the site of injury. They adhere to activated endothelial cells in the inflamed region and pass through the capillary walls into the tissue (extravasation). These leukocytes phagocytize the invading pathogens and release soluble mediators—cytokines, prostaglandins, leukotrienes—that further contribute to the inflammatory response and the recruitment and activation of effector cells.

Inflammation can be acute, as in response to tissue injury, or it may be chronic, leading to progressive tissue destruction, as seen in chronic infections, autoimmunity, and certain cancers. Next, we discuss both forms of inflammation, including their triggers, the soluble mediators and cell types involved, and the resulting tissue pathology.

Acute Inflammatory Response

The acute inflammatory response provides protection following tissue injury and infection by restricting damage to the localized site, recruiting immune cells to eliminate the invading pathogen, and initiating the process of wound repair.

Following tissue damage, a number of plasma proteins are activated, including those of the clotting and kinin systems. The enzymatic cascade of the clotting system produces fibrin strands that accumulate to form clots, limiting the spread of infection into the blood. The enzymatic cascade of the kinin system results in the production of bradykinin—a peptide that induces vasodilation and enhanced vascular permeability (see Chapter 39). In addition, the complement products C3a and C5a bind to receptors on local mast cells, facilitating their degranulation. The resulting release of histamine, prostaglandins, and leukotrienes contributes to vascular changes by inducing vasodilation and enhancing vascular permeability. Prostaglandins and leukotrienes also serve as chemoattractants for neutrophils (see Chapter 37).

Within a few hours of these vascular changes, neutrophils bind to the endothelial cells of the inflamed region and extravasate into the tissue (see previous section, Diapedesis). They phagocytize the invading pathogens and release soluble inflammatory mediators, including macrophage inflammatory proteins (MIPs) 1α and 1β, which are chemokines that attract macrophages to the site of inflammation. Macrophages arrive at the damaged tissue 5 to 6 h after the onset of the inflammatory response. Activated macrophages secrete three major pro-inflammatory cytokines: IL-1, IL-6, and TNF-α. These cytokines induce coagulation, increase vascular permeability, and promote the acute-phase response. IL-1 and TNF-α also induce increased expression of adhesion molecules on endothelial cells, allowing for circulating leukocytes (neutrophils, macrophages, granulocytes, and lymphocytes) to interact with the endothelium and extravasate into the inflamed tissues. Acute inflammation displays a rapid onset following tissue injury and resolves relatively quickly. The resulting tissue pathology is typically mild and localized.

Chronic Inflammation

Chronic inflammation results from continuous exposure to the offending element. This can be due to pathogen persistence, autoimmune diseases in which self-antigens continuously activate T cells, and cancers. The hallmark of chronic inflammation is the accumulation and activation of macrophages and lymphocytes, as well as fibroblasts that replace the original, damaged, or necrotic tissue. Soluble factors released by macrophages and lymphocytes play an important role in the development of chronic inflammation. While during acute inflammation non-protein–based soluble factors (e.g., eicosanoids, bioamines, etc.) dominate the landscape, chronic inflammation is largely caused not only by cytokines, chemokines, growth factors, and secreted/released enzymes, but also by ROS. For instance, cytotoxic T cells and Th1 cells release IFN-γ, which activates macrophages and DCs. These, in turn, release a variety of soluble factors, such as IL-6 and TNF-α, that ultimately result in tissue injury and cell death. Replacement of tissue lost this way by fibroblasts leads to fibrosis—an excessive deposition of fibrous tissue that can interfere with normal tissue function—due to excessive amounts of growth factors (platelet-derived growth factor, transforming growth factor-β), fibrogenic cytokines (IL-1 and TNF-α), and angiogenic factors (fibroblast growth factor, vascular endothelial growth factor). Chronic inflammation can also lead to the formation of granulomas—a mass of cells consisting of activated macrophages surrounded by activated lymphocytes.

Many mediators of acute and chronic inflammation have been identified, and there are myriad anti-inflammatory drugs available. The oldest class, NSAIDs, includes aspirin, which entered the market over a century ago, and the more recently introduced agents acetaminophen (1956) and ibuprofen (1969). NSAIDs target cyclooxygenase (COX), the rate-limiting enzyme in the production of prostaglandins, but can lead to an increase in leukotriene production. In contrast, glucocorticoids prevent the liberation of arachidonic acid from plasma-membrane phospholipids and thus reduce the synthesis of both classes of eicosanoids. The newest group of anti-inflammatory agents, whose use is limited to chronic inflammatory conditions, aims to eliminate pro-inflammatory cytokines through the use of monoclonal antibodies, or soluble receptors (typically a truncated receptor encompassing only the ligand-binding, extracellular domain). Infliximab, adalimumab, certolizumab, and golilumab are monoclonal antibodies that bind and neutralize TNF-α; etanercept is a TNF-α receptor fusion protein with the same goal.

Immune System–Related Conditions

There are pathologic conditions to which the immune system contributes, such as overreactions (allergy, autoimmunity, transplant rejection) or insufficient responses (immune deficiencies, cancer).

Hypersensitivity Reactions

The immune system mobilizes a number of effector mechanisms to eliminate pathogens from the body. These effector mechanisms typically generate a localized inflammatory response that effectively eliminates the pathogen, with minimal collateral damage to the surrounding tissue. Besides pathogens, humans come into contact with numerous foreign antigens, such as plant pollen and food. Contact with these environmental antigens does not elicit an immune response in the majority of individuals. However, in certain predisposed individuals, the immune system can mount a response to these generally innocuous antigens, resulting in tissue damage that ranges from mild irritation to life-threatening anaphylactic shock. These immune responses are referred to as allergic reactions or hypersensitivity reactions. Hypersensitivity reactions can be divided into four categories, type I to type IV, distinguished by the cell types and effector molecules involved (Burmester et al., 2003).

Type I Hypersensitivity: Immediate Hypersensitivity Reactions

Type I hypersensitivity reactions require that an individual first produces IgE antibodies on initial encounter with an antigen, also referred to as an allergen. After the antigen is cleared, the remaining antigen-specific IgE molecules will be bound by mast cells, basophils, and eosinophils that express receptors for the IgE constant region (FcεR1). This process is referred to as sensitization. On subsequent exposure to antigen, cross-linking of the IgE molecules on sensitized cells induces their immediate degranulation. The release of inflammatory mediators such as histamine, leukotrienes, and prostaglandins causes vasodilation, bronchial smooth muscle contraction, and mucus production similar to that seen during inflammatory responses to tissue injury and infection. Type I hypersensitivity reactions can be local or systemic. Systemic reactions against peanut or bee venom antigens can result in anaphylaxis, a potentially life-threatening condition.

Allergic asthma is an example of type I hypersensitivity. On exposure to certain allergens (typically inhaled), individuals with allergic asthma experience inflammation of the airways, characterized by tissue swelling and excessive mucus production. This narrowing of the airways makes it difficult to breathe (see Chapter 40).

Type II Hypersensitivity: Antibody-Mediated Cytotoxic Reactions

Type II hypersensitivities are antibody-mediated cytotoxic reactions. One example is the immunization to erythrocyte antigens during pregnancy. In an Rh-negative mother with an Rh-positive fetus (Rh inherited from the father), the mother forms antibodies against the Rh antigen when fetal blood cells come into contact with the maternal immune system, typically during delivery. If a subsequent pregnancy with an Rh-positive fetus occurs, maternal IgG antibodies can cross the placenta and cause hemolysis of fetal Rh-positive erythrocytes. Close monitoring and adequate symptomatic treatments (e.g., plasma exchange, intrauterine infusion, Rh immunoglobulin) are prescribed, as fetal symptoms can range from mild to potential fetal death from heart failure.

Type III Hypersensitivity: Immune Complex–Mediated Reactions

Type III hypersensitivity reactions are mediated by antibody-antigen complexes that form during an immune response (Figures 34–3 and 34–5). When not properly cleared, these immune complexes can settle into various tissues, where they induce complement activation. These immune complexes are of particular concern in the kidney, where they can lead to glomerulonephritis and kidney failure. While in the past

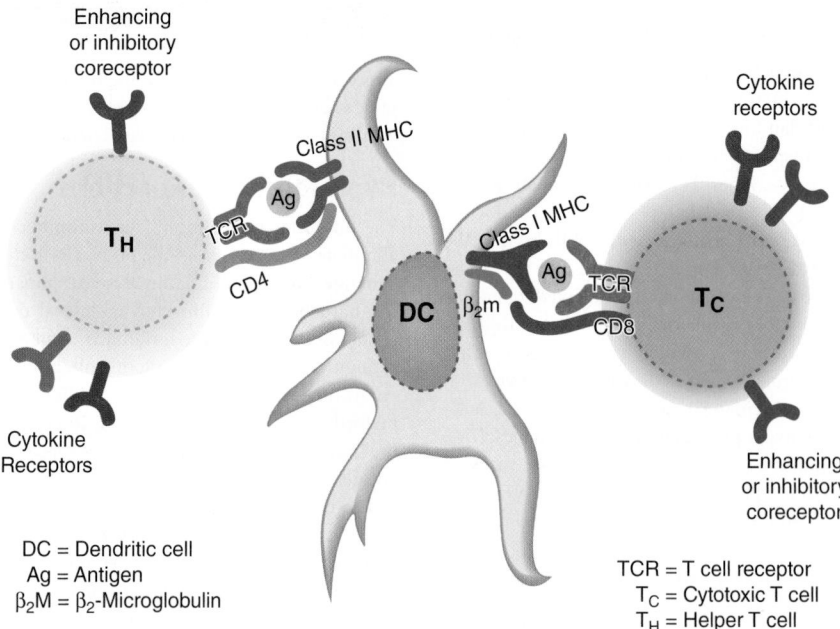

Figure 34–5 *Professional APCs.* APCs such as DCs display peptide-loaded MHC class I and class II complexes on their cell surface. CD8⁺ or CD4⁺ T cells, respectively, engage these MHC-antigen complexes, leading to signaling via the TCR. Simultaneous occupation of activating or inhibitory coreceptors, as well as various cytokine receptors, determines the ultimate T-cell response.

type III hypersensitivity reactions fell largely in the realm of autoimmune diseases (e.g., systemic lupus erythematosus), their incidence rate has significantly risen with the introduction of nonhuman or nonhumanized monoclonal antibodies as pharmacological agents (human antimouse antibodies). Murine or murine-human chimeric therapeutic monoclonal antibodies are "mistaken" by the patient's immune system as potentially dangerous, foreign antigens. The resulting immune response not only "defuses" the therapeutic antibody, but also promotes the formation of antibody(mu)-antibody(hu) or antibody(chim)-antibody(hu) complexes that trigger type III hypersensitivity reactions.

Type IV Hypersensitivity: Delayed Hypersensitivity Reactions

Unlike type I–III hypersensitivity reactions, which are antibody mediated, type IV reactions are mediated by T cells. However, all these hypersensitivity reactions are memory responses. Haptens are molecules that are too small to function as antigens on their own. These molecules penetrate the epidermis and bind to carrier proteins in the skin. Hapten-carrier complexes are detected by APCs in the skin (Langerhans cells), which then migrate to the lymph nodes and prime T-cell responses. When an individual is reexposed to the hapten, antigen-specific T cells migrate to the skin, causing local inflammation and edema. Nickel in clothing and jewelry is a common trigger of type IV hypersensitivity reactions.

Autoimmunity, Immune Deficiency, and Transplant Rejection

Just as for a regular and, appropriate immune response, autoimmunity is founded in either humoral (autoantibody) or cellular (T-cell) responses. As described in the section on lymphocyte development, the process of central tolerance limits the development of autoreactive B and T cells. This process is imperfect, and mechanisms of peripheral tolerance are in place to limit the activity of self-reactive lymphocytes that manage to escape thymic deletion. Peripheral tolerance is primarily mediated by two mechanisms: the action of T_Reg cells (see section on CD4 T_H-cell effector functions), and the induction of T-cell anergy. Naïve T cells require costimulatory signals to become activated. Consequently,

autoreactive T cells typically will not become activated if they interact with an MHC molecule expressing self-antigen because most tissues do not express costimulatory molecules. Induction of anergy leaves T cells unresponsive, even on subsequent exposure to antigen with sufficient costimulation.

Autoimmunity: A Breach of Tolerance

Several theories exist that aim to explain the origins of individual autoimmune disorders:

- *Molecular Mimicry.* The hypothesis of "molecular mimicry" reasons that unique pathogen-derived antigens resemble endogenous host antigens. If an infection occurs, the immune system's defensive arsenal (antibodies, CTLs, and NK cells) not only attack the pathogen-derived antigen but also assault the host's structurally similar antigen, thus causing autoimmunity in the form of "collateral damage."
- *Relationship Between Autoimmunity and the HLA System.* Individuals with specific HLA types are more likely to develop certain autoimmune diseases (e.g., type I diabetes, ankylosing spondylitis, celiac disease, systemic lupus erythematosus). A reasonable explanation for this observation might be found in the fact that particular HLA proteins are more "efficient" than others in presenting antigens and consequently might erroneously activate T cells.
- *Altered Thymic Function.* Thymic T-cell selection is crucial to central tolerance, and type I IFNs, which are highly induced during infectious events, also govern several steps in T-cell selection. Therefore, pathogen-induced disturbances to thymic events might negatively affect elimination of autoreactive T cells. Regardless of the mechanism, central tolerance has thus far not been exploited for pharmacological intervention.

Immune Deficiencies

Primary immunodeficiency encompasses genetic or developmental defects in the immune system that leave the individual susceptible to infections to various degrees. Severe forms (severe combined immunodeficiency) are typically diagnosed in early childhood and are associated with significantly reduced life expectancy. Presently, nine classes of primary immunodeficiency are recognized, totaling over 120 unique conditions. Unfortunately, current treatment options are limited to supportive therapy in the form of antiviral, antifungal, and antibacterial drugs.

	CURRENT MONOCLONAL ANTIBODY NOMENCLATURE			
UNIQUE PREFIX	**TARGET TISSUE**		**SOURCE ORGANISM**	**CONSERVED SUFFIX**
variable	*-o(s)-*	bone	*-u-*	human	-mab
	-vi(r)-	viral	*-o-*	mouse	
	-ba(c)-	bacterial	*-a-*	rat	
	-li(m)-	immune	*-e-*	hamster	
	-le(s)-	infectious lesions	*-i-*	primate	
	-ci(r)-	cardiovascular	*-xi-*	chimeric	
	-mu(l)-	musculoskeletal	*-zu-*	humanized	
	-ki(n)-	interleukin	*-axo-*	rat/murine hybrid	
	-co(l)-	colonic tumor			
	-me(l)-	melanoma			
	-ma(r)-	mammary tumor			
	-go(t)-	testicular tumor			
	-go(v)-	ovarian tumor			
	-pr(o)-	prostate tumor			
	-tu(m)-	miscellaneous tumor			
	-neu(r)-	nervous system			
	-tox(a)-	toxin as target			

Examples:				
Beva	ci		zu	mab
Ri	tu		xi	mab
Ala	ci		zu	mab
Glemba	tum		u	mab

Figure 34–6 *Current nomenclature for therapeutic monoclonal antibodies.* Current nomenclature incorporates information on the source of the antibody as well as the intended target tissue. An older nomenclature, still used by some workers, focused on the source of the antibody (Figure 34–7).

Acquired immunodeficiency refers to the loss of immune function due to environmental exposure. These conditions encompass patients receiving immune-suppressive therapy for autoimmune disorders or to prevent transplant rejections. Acquired immunodeficiency is also commonly observed in patients suffering from hematopoietic malignancies, as tumor cells outcompete functional leukocytes for space in the bone marrow or blood. Probably the most common use for the term, however, is in connection with HIV infection, the underlying cause for AIDS (see Chapter 64).

Transplant Rejection

"Host-versus-graft disease" or "graft-versus-host disease" results from the immunological rejection of a transplanted tissue by the recipient's immune system, or in cases where bone marrow is transplanted, the "new" immune system might attack the host's tissues. The intensity of rejection is minimized with increased compatibility between donor and recipient; however, a lifelong regimen of immunosuppressive drugs is unavoidable (see Chapter 35).

Classical immunosuppressive therapy employs glucocorticoids (e.g., prednisone), inhibitors of T-cell activation (e.g., cyclosporine), T-cell proliferation inhibitors (e.g., mycophenolic acid) or mTOR inhibitors (e.g., sirolimus) that inhibit production of IL-2, a cytokine essential for T-cell activation and proliferation. Treatment of transplant rejection also has benefitted from advances in monoclonal antibody therapy, and antibodies directed against the IL-2 receptor (e.g., daclizumab) or CD20 (e.g., rituximab) are now available to prevent transplant rejection (Figure 35–2).

Cancer Immunotherapy

As described previously, T-cell responses are modulated by a balance between costimulatory signals, exemplified by CD28 ligation, and coinhibitory signals, such as those provided by CTLA-4 or PD1 ligation. *Immune checkpoints* refer to inhibitory (often negative-feedback) pathways that limit the amplitude and duration of an immune response. Under normal physiological conditions, immune checkpoints protect tissues from damage during an immune response and contribute to the maintenance of self-tolerance. In conditions of chronic viral infections and cancers, chronic antigen persistence results in the development of dysfunctional "exhausted" T cells. Exhausted T cells are actively suppressed by inhibitory signals that limit their effector functions and turn off their target cell–killing capacity. These inhibitory pathways resulting in T-cell exhaustion have been documented in mice, monkeys, and humans, highlighting their importance in modulating T-cell function.

Cancer cells express a variety of genetic and epigenetic alterations that distinguish them from their normal counterparts. These tumor-associated antigens can be recognized by the host immune system; antitumor T cells are generated, which then eliminate these transformed cells. However, tumors frequently develop immune resistance mechanisms that evade the host's immune attack. One of these evasion strategies involves the manipulation of immune-inhibitory pathways or immune checkpoints. Tumors avoid being destroyed by actively stimulating these inhibitory receptors to turn off antitumor T cells. Figure 34–7 provides an overview of activating and inhibitory coreceptors and the drugs (monoclonal antibodies) that target them. In general, these antibodies work by releasing the brake on

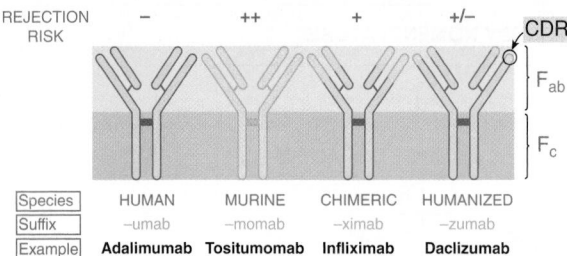

REJECTION RISK   −   ++   +   +/−   CDR

F_ab   F_c

Species	HUMAN	MURINE	CHIMERIC	HUMANIZED
Suffix	–umab	–momab	–ximab	–zumab
Example	**Adalimumab**	**Tositumomab**	**Infliximab**	**Daclizumab**

Figure 34–7 *Former nomenclature of therapeutic monoclonal antibodies.* This older nomenclature, still in use by some workers, focused primarily on the source of the antibody (murine, human, chimeric, or humanized). Current nomenclature (Figure 34–6) incorporates information on the target tissue as well. Fab, antigen-binding fragment; Fc, crystallizable fragment; CDR, complementarity-determining regions of the variable domains, also called hypervariable regions.

antitumor T cells and reinvigorating them to kill tumors. It is important to be aware that whereas some monoclonal antibodies block their respective target (PD1), others block the respective ligand (PD-L1). The therapeutic goal is to interfere with this inhibitory interaction that is actively suppressing T cells in the tumor microenvironment.

The two immune checkpoint receptors that have been the most extensively characterized in the context of cancer immunotherapy are CTLA-4 and PD1. These inhibitory molecules are highly expressed on antitumor T cells. When bound by their respective ligands (CD80/86 and PD-L1/PD-L2) on APCs or tumor cells, these inhibitory receptors dampen the T-cell response, albeit by different intracellular pathways. As antitumor T cells express PD1, tumor cells engage it through their expression of PD-L1. The tumor effectively inactivates the T cells and the tumor continues to grow (Pardoll, 2012; Tang et al., 2016). These pathways are further discussed in the cancer therapy chapters (Chapters 65–68).

Immunotherapy to cancers holds great promise for treating patients with advanced disease, as evidenced by the success of clinical trials using this technology. Biologics to stimulate antitumor T cells have been rapidly approved by the FDA and have become the first line of treatment of cancers such as metastatic melanoma, non–small cell lung cancer, and renal cell carcinoma. In addition, anti-PD1, anti–PD-L1, and anti–CTLA-4 therapies are currently in clinical trials to assess their efficacy in head and neck cancers, breast cancer, small cell lung cancer, Hodgkin lymphoma, gastric cancer, hepatocellular carcinoma, bladder cancer, ovarian cancer, colon cancer, and Merkel cell carcinoma. It is important to note that only a small fraction of patients respond to checkpoint monotherapy, and this frequency can increase when patients are given combination therapy, such as administering both anti-PD1 and anti–CTLA-4 antibodies. Furthermore, combination strategies that include checkpoint blockade paired with radiation or chemotherapy may further increase responsiveness in cancer patients.

One consequence of checkpoint blockade is that autoreactive T cells are also unleashed after therapy. Patients can develop toxicities that include hepatic, pneumonitis, colitis, rash, vitiligo, and endocrine pathology. Greater immunotherapy efficacy will likely be achieved when drugs are developed to target other inhibitory pathways and are used in combination, but caution must be evaluated to ensure patient safety (Callahan et al., 2016).

In addition to solid tumors, liquid tumors like CLL are also being targeted by immunotherapeutic approaches. Patient T cells are engineered to express chimeric antigen receptors (CARs) comprising antibody-binding domains connected to domains that activate T cells. In the case of CLL, CAR T cells recognize CD19 on B cells, and their chimeric receptor sustains T activation. CAR T cells are engineered from patient blood, expanded in vitro; then, millions are infused into the same patient. These cells then circulate in the patient and recognize all B cells expressing CD19 and destroy them. This cellular therapy has shown promise in patients with CLL with high durable objective responses (Kalos et al., 2011).

Bibliography

Attanasio J, Wherry EJ. Costimulatory and coinhibitory receptor pathways in infectious disease. *Immunity*, **2016**, *44*:1052–1068.

Belkaid Y, Tamoutounour S. The influence of skin microorganisms on cutaneous immunity. *Nat Rev Immunol*, **2016**, *16*(6):353–66.

Bjorkstrom NK, et al. Emerging insights into natural killer cells in human peripheral tissues. *Nat Rev Immunol*, **2016**, *16*(5):310–320.

Blum JS, et al. Pathways of antigen processing. *Annu Rev Immunol*, **2013**, *31*:443–473.

Brownlie RJ, Zamoyska R. T cell receptor signalling networks: branched, diversified and bounded. *Nat Rev Immunol*, **2013**, *13*(4):257–269.

Burmester G-Rd, et al. *Color Atlas of Immunology.* Thieme flexibook. Thieme, New York, **2003**, xiv, 322.

Callahan MK, et al. Targeting T cell co-receptors for cancer therapy. *Immunity*, **2016**, *44*:1069–1078.

Cao X. Self-regulation and cross-regulation of pattern-recognition receptor signalling in health and disease. *Nat Rev Immunol*, **2016**, *16*(1):35–50.

Di Noia JM, Neuberger MS. Molecular mechanisms of antibody somatic hypermutation. *Annu Rev Biochem*, **2007**, 76:1–22.

Doulatov S, et al. Hematopoiesis: a human perspective. *Cell Stem Cell*, **2012**, *10*(2):120–136.

DuPage M, Bluestone JA. Harnessing the plasticity of CD4(+) T cells to treat immune-mediated disease. *Nat Rev Immunol*, **2016**, *16*(3):149–163.

Eaves CJ. Hematopoietic stem cells: concepts, definitions, and the new reality. *Blood*, **2015**, *125*(17):2605–2613.

Farber DL, et al. Human memory T cells: generation, compartmentalization and homeostasis. *Nat Rev Immunol*, **2014**, *14*(1):24–35.

Gonzalez-Navajas JM, et al. Immunomodulatory functions of type I interferons. *Nat Rev Immunol*, **2012**, *12*(2):125–135.

Hancock RE, et al. The immunology of host defence peptides: beyond antimicrobial activity. *Nat Rev Immunol*, **2016**, *16*(5):321–334.

Harty JT, et al. CD8+ T cell effector mechanisms in resistance to infection. *Annu Rev Immunol*, **2000**, 18:275–308.

Hoggatt J, et al. Hematopoietic stem cell niche in health and disease. *Annu Rev Pathol*, **2016**, 11:555–581.

Kalos M, et al. T cells with chimeric antigen receptors have potent antitumor effects and can establish memory in patients with advanced leukemia. *Sci Transl Med*, **2011**, 3:95ra73.

Kruger P, et al. Neutrophils: between host defence, immune modulation, and tissue injury. *PLoS Pathog*, **2015**, *11*(3):e1004651.

Kurosaki T, et al. Memory B cells. *Nat Rev Immunol*, **2015**, *15*(3): 149–159.

Lavin Y, et al. Regulation of macrophage development and function in peripheral tissues. *Nat Rev Immunol*, **2015**, *15*(12):731–744.

LeBien TW, Tedder TF. B lymphocytes: how they develop and function. *Blood*, **2008**, *112*(5):1570–1580.

Masopust D, Schenkel JM. The integration of T cell migration, differentiation and function. *Nat Rev Immunol*, **2013**, *13*(5): 309–320.

Morgan BP, Harris CL. Complement, a target for therapy in inflammatory and degenerative diseases. *Nat Rev Drug Discov*, **2015**, *14*(12): 857–877.

Neely HR, Flajnik MF. Emergence and evolution of secondary lymphoid organs. *Annu Rev Cell Dev Biol*, **2016**, *32*:693–711.

Nemazee D. Receptor editing in lymphocyte development and central tolerance. *Nat Rev Immunol*, **2006**, *6*(10):728–740.

Palmer DB. The effect of age on thymic function. *Front Immunol*, **2013**. 4:316.

Pardoll DM. The blockade of immune checkpoints in cancer immunotherapy. *Nat Rev Cancer*, **2012**, *12*(4):252–264.

Shah DK, Zuniga-Pflucker JC. An overview of the intrathymic intricacies of T cell development. *J Immunol*, **2014**, *192*(9):4017–4023.

Tang H, et al. Immunotherapy and tumor microenvironment. *Cancer Lett*, **2016**, *370*(1):85–90.

Thomas SN, et al. Implications of lymphatic transport to lymph nodes in immunity and immunotherapy. *Annu Rev Biomed Eng*, **2016**, *18*:207–233.

Tinoco R, et al. PSGL-1 is an immune checkpoint regulator that promotes T cell exhaustion. *Immunity,* **2016**, *44*:1190–1203.

Vestweber D. How leukocytes cross the vascular endothelium. *Nat Rev Immunol*, **2015**, *15*(11):692–704.

von Köckritz-Blickwede M, Nizet V. Innate immunity turned inside-out: antimicrobial defense by phagocyte extracellular traps. *J Mol Med (Berl),* **2009**, *87*:775–783.

Xu Z, et al. Immunoglobulin class-switch DNA recombination: induction, targeting and beyond. *Nat Rev Immunol*, **2012**, *12*(7): 517–531.

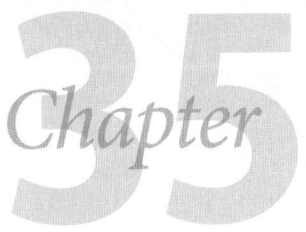

Chapter 35

Immunosuppressants and Tolerogens

Alan M. Krensky, Jamil R. Azzi, and David A. Hafler

This chapter reviews the components of the immune response and drugs that modulate immunity via immunosuppression or tolerance. Four major classes of immunosuppressive drugs are discussed: glucocorticoids (see Chapter 46), calcineurin inhibitors, antiproliferative and antimetabolic agents (see Chapter 66), and antibodies. While there are similarities, the approach to the use of immunosuppressant drugs in transplant rejection has evolved separately from the approaches used to treat autoimmune disease and thus is presented separately. Finally, the chapter ends with a brief case study of immunotherapy for the autoimmune disease MS.

The Immune Response

The immune system evolved to discriminate self from nonself. *Innate immunity* (natural immunity) is primitive, does not require priming, and is of relatively low affinity, but it is broadly reactive. *Adaptive immunity* (learned immunity) is antigen specific, depends on antigen exposure or priming, and can be of very high affinity. The two arms of immunity work closely together, with the innate immune system most active early in an immune response and adaptive immunity becoming progressively dominant over time.

The major effectors of *innate immunity* are complement, granulocytes, monocytes/macrophages, NK cells, mast cells, and basophils. The major effectors of *adaptive immunity* are B and T lymphocytes. B lymphocytes make antibodies; T lymphocytes function as helper, cytolytic, and regulatory (suppressor) cells. These cells not only are important in the normal immune response to infection and tumors but also mediate transplant rejection and autoimmunity.

Immunoglobulins (antibodies) on the B-lymphocyte surface are receptors for a large variety of specific structural conformations. In contrast, T lymphocytes recognize antigens as peptide fragments in the context of self MHC antigens (called HLAs in humans) on the surface of APCs, such as dendritic cells, macrophages, and other cell types expressing MHC class I and class II antigens. Once activated by specific antigen recognition, both B and T lymphocytes are triggered to differentiate and divide, leading to release of soluble mediators (cytokines, lymphokines) that perform as effectors and regulators of the immune response. Chapter 34 presents a more detailed view of the immune system at the levels of the molecules, cells, and organs involved in immunity.

Immunosuppression

Immunosuppressive drugs are used to dampen the immune response in organ transplantation and autoimmune disease. In transplantation, the major classes of immunosuppressive drugs used today are the following:

- Glucocorticoids
- Calcineurin inhibitors
- Antiproliferative/antimetabolic agents
- Biologicals (antibodies)

Table 35–1 summarizes the sites of action of representative immunosuppressants on T-cell activation. These drugs are successful in treating conditions such as acute immune rejection of organ transplants and autoimmune diseases. However, such therapies often require lifelong use and nonspecifically suppress the entire immune system, exposing patients in some instances to higher risks of infection and cancer. The calcineurin inhibitors and daily glucocorticoids, in particular, are nephrotoxic and diabetogenic, respectively, thus restricting their usefulness in a variety of clinical settings.

Monoclonal and polyclonal antibody preparations directed at both T cells and B cells or against cytokines such as TNF-α are important therapies providing an opportunity to more specifically target immune pathways. Finally, newer small molecules and antibodies have expanded the arsenal of immunosuppressives. In particular, mTOR inhibitors (*sirolimus, everolimus, temsirolimus*) (Budde et al., 2011; Euvrard et al., 2012), and anti-CD25 (IL-2R) antibodies (*basiliximab, daclizumab*) (Nashan, 2005) target growth factor pathways. *Belatacept* (Satyananda and Shapiro, 2014) inhibits T-cell costimulation. Thus, there are useful pharmacological tools that can substantially limit clonal expansion and potentially promote tolerance (Goldfarb-Rumyantzev et al., 2006; Krensky et al., 1990).

General Approach to Organ Transplantation Therapy

Organ transplantation therapy is organized around five general principles.

1. Carefully prepare the patient and select the best available ABO blood type–compatible HLA match for organ donation.
2. Employ multitier immunosuppressive therapy; simultaneously use several agents, each of which is directed at a different molecular target within the allograft response. Synergistic effects permit use of the

Abbreviations

ALG: antilymphocyte globulin
APC: antigen-presenting cell
ATG: antithymocyte globulin
AUC: area under the curve
CD: cluster of differentiation
CLL: chronic lymphocytic leukemia
CNS: central nervous system
CTL: cytotoxic T lymphocyte
CTLA4: cytotoxic T-lymphocyte–associated antigen 4
FKBP-12: FK506-binding protein 12
CYP: cytochrome P450
GVHD: graft-versus-host disease
HLA: human leukocyte antigen
HRPT: hypoxanthine–guanine phosphoribosyl transferase
IFN-β: interferon type I beta
Ig: immunoglobulin
IL: interleukin
IL-1RA: IL-1 receptor antagonist
IL-2R: interleukin 2 receptor
JCV: polyomavirus JC
LDL: low-density lipoprotein
LFA: lymphocyte function–associated antigen
mAb: monoclonal antibody
MHC: histocompatibility complex
MMF: mycophenolate mofetil
6-MP: 6-mercaptopurine
MPA: mycophenolic acid
MPAG: MPA glucuronide
MS: multiple sclerosis
mTOR: mammalian target of rapamycin
NFAT: nuclear factor of activated T lymphocytes
NHP: nonhuman primate
NK: natural killer
NSAID: nonsteroidal anti-inflammatory drug
PD1: programmed cell death protein 1
PD-L1: programmed death ligand 1
PML: progressive multifocal leukoencephalopathy
RA: rheumatoid arthritis
S1P-R: sphingosine-1-phosphate receptor
TCR: T-cell receptor
VZV: varicella zoster virus
WBC: white blood cell

TABLE 35–1 ■ SITES OF ACTION OF SELECTED IMMUNOSUPPRESSIVE AGENTS ON T-CELL ACTIVATION

DRUG	SITE (AND MECHANISM) OF ACTION
Glucocorticoids	Glucocorticoid response elements in DNA (regulate gene transcription)
Cyclosporine	Calcineurin (inhibits phosphatase activity)
Tacrolimus	Calcineurin (inhibits phosphatase activity)
Azathioprine	DNA (false nucleotide incorporation)
Mycophenolate mofetil	Inosine monophosphate dehydrogenase (inhibits activity)
Sirolimus	mTOR, protein kinase involved in cell-cycle progression (inhibits activity)
Everolimus	mTOR, protein kinase involved in cell-cycle progression (inhibits activity)
Belatacept	Costimulatory ligands (CD80 and CD86) present on antigen presenting cells (inhibits activity)
Alemtuzumab	CD52 protein, widely expressed on B cells, T cells, macrophages, NK cells (induces lysis)
Muromonab-CD3	T-cell receptor complex (blocks antigen recognition)
Daclizumab, basiliximab	IL-2R (block IL-2–mediated T-cell activation)

intensify the initial immunosuppressive therapy in patients at high risk of rejection (i.e., repeat transplants, broadly presensitized patients, African American patients, or pediatric patients). This strategy has been an important component of immunosuppression since the 1960s, when Starzl and colleagues demonstrated the beneficial effect of antilymphocyte globulin (ALC) in the prophylaxis of rejection. Two preparations are FDA-approved for use in transplantation: lymphocyte immune globulin (Atgam) and antithymocyte globulin (ATG; Thymoglobulin) (Brennan et al., 2006; Nashan, 2005). ATG is the most frequently used depleting agent. Alemtuzumab, a humanized anti-CD52 mAb that produces prolonged lymphocyte depletion, is approved for use in CLL and MS but is increasingly used off label as induction therapy in transplantation (Jones and Coles, 2014).

Most limitations of murine-based mAbs generally were overcome by the introduction of chimeric or humanized mAbs that lack antigenicity and have a prolonged serum $t_{1/2}$. Antibodies derived from transgenic mice carrying human antibody genes are labeled "humanized" (90%–95% human) or "fully human" (100% human); antibodies derived from human cells are labeled "human." However, all three types of antibodies are of equal efficacy and safety. Chimeric antibodies generally contain about 33% mouse protein and 67% human protein and can still produce an antibody response that results in reduced efficacy and shorter $t_{1/2}$ compared to humanized antibodies.

Biological agents for induction therapy in the prophylaxis of rejection currently are used in about 70% of de novo transplant patients. Biological agents for induction can be divided into two groups: the *depleting agents* and the *immune modulators*. The depleting agents consist of lymphocyte immune globulin, ATG, and muromonab-CD3 mAb; their efficacy derives from their ability to deplete the recipient's CD3-positive cells at the time of transplantation and antigen presentation. The second group of biological agents, the anti–IL-2R mAbs, do not deplete T lymphocytes, but rather block IL-2–mediated T-cell activation by binding to the α chain of IL-2R (CD25). For patients with high levels of anti-HLA antibodies and humoral rejection, more aggressive therapies include plasmapheresis, intravenous immunoglobulin, and rituximab, a chimeric anti-CD20 mAb (Brennan et al., 2006; Chan et al., 2011; Guerra et al., 2011; Nashan, 2005; Sureshkumar et al., 2012).

various agents at relatively low doses, thereby limiting specific toxicities while maximizing the immunosuppressive effect.

3. Employ intensive induction and lower-dose maintenance drug protocols; greater immunosuppression is required to gain early engraftment or to treat established rejection than to maintain long-term immunosuppression. The early high risk of acute rejection is replaced over time by the increased risk of the medications' side effects, necessitating a slow reduction of maintenance immunosuppressive drugs.

4. Investigation of each episode of transplant dysfunction is required, including evaluation for recurrence of the disease, rejection, drug toxicity, and infection (keeping in mind that these various problems can and often do coexist).

5. Reduce dosage or withdraw a drug if its toxicity exceeds its benefit (Danovitch et al., 2007).

Biological Induction Therapy

In many transplant centers, induction therapy with biological agents is used to delay the use of the nephrotoxic calcineurin inhibitors or to

Maintenance Immunotherapy

Basic immunosuppressive therapy uses multiple drugs simultaneously, typically a calcineurin inhibitor, glucocorticoids, and mycophenolate (a purine metabolism inhibitor), each directed at a discrete step in T-cell activation (Vincenti et al., 2008). Glucocorticoids, azathioprine, cyclosporine, tacrolimus, mycophenolate, sirolimus, belatacept, and various mAbs and polyclonal antibodies all are approved for use in transplantation.

Therapy for Established Rejection

Low doses of prednisone, calcineurin inhibitors, purine metabolism inhibitors, sirolimus, or belatacept are effective in preventing acute cellular rejection; they are less effective in blocking activated T lymphocytes and thus are not very effective against established, acute rejection or for the total prevention of chronic rejection. Therefore, treatment of established rejection requires the use of agents directed against activated T cells. These include glucocorticoids in high doses (pulse therapy), polyclonal antilymphocyte antibodies, or muromonab-CD3 (licensed by the FDA but not currently marketed in the U.S. due to decreased use).

Glucocorticoids

The introduction of glucocorticoids as immunosuppressive drugs in the 1960s played a key role in making organ transplantation possible. Prednisone, prednisolone, and other glucocorticoids are used alone and in combination with other immunosuppressive agents for treatment of transplant rejection and autoimmune disorders. The pharmacological properties of glucocorticoids are described in Chapter 46.

Mechanism of Action

Glucocorticoids have broad anti-inflammatory effects on multiple components of cellular immunity, but relatively little effect on humoral immunity. Glucocorticoids bind to receptors inside cells and regulate the transcription of numerous other genes (see Chapter 46). Glucocorticoids also curtail activation of NF-κB, suppress formation of pro-inflammatory cytokines such as IL-1 and IL-6, inhibit T cells from making IL-2 and proliferating, and inhibit the activation of CTLs. In addition, glucocorticoid-treated neutrophils and monocytes display poor chemotaxis and decreased lysosomal enzyme release.

Therapeutic Uses

There are numerous therapeutic indications for glucocorticoids. They commonly are combined with other immunosuppressive agents to prevent and treat transplant rejection. Glucocorticoids also are efficacious for treatment of GVHD in bone marrow transplantation. Glucocorticoids are routinely used to treat autoimmune disorders such as rheumatoid and other arthritides, systemic lupus erythematosus, systemic dermatomyositis, psoriasis and other skin conditions, asthma and other allergic disorders, inflammatory bowel disease, inflammatory ophthalmic diseases, autoimmune hematological disorders, and acute exacerbations of MS (see multiple sclerosis section). Lower-dose oral glucocorticoids, however, appear to have different biologic effects; low-dose oral prednisone made optic neuritis worse compared to high-dose intravenous solumedrol (Beck et al., 1992). In addition, glucocorticoids limit allergic reactions that occur with other immunosuppressive agents and are used in transplant recipients to block first-dose cytokine storm caused by treatment with muromonab-CD3 and to a lesser extent ATG (see Antithymocyte Globulin). Most transplant centers use an initial high dose of intravenous solumedrol with tapering to a maintenance dose of 5–10 mg/d in the long term. Currently, more than one-third of kidney transplant centers in the U.S. aim to withdraw steroids within the first 3 months after transplantation (Bergmann et al., 2012).

Toxicity

Extensive glucocorticoid use often results in disabling and life-threatening adverse effects. These effects include growth retardation in children, avascular necrosis of bone, osteopenia, increased risk of infection, poor wound healing, cataracts, hyperglycemia, and hypertension (see Chapter 46). The advent of combined glucocorticoid/calcineurin inhibitor regimens has allowed reduced doses or rapid withdrawal of steroids, resulting in lower steroid-induced morbidities (Vincenti et al., 2008).

Calcineurin Inhibitors

The most effective immunosuppressive drugs in routine use are the calcineurin inhibitors *cyclosporine* and *tacrolimus* (Figure 35–1), which target intracellular signaling pathways induced as a consequence of TCR activation (Figure 35–2). Cyclosporine and tacrolimus bind to an immunophilin (cyclophilin for cyclosporine or FKBP-12 for tacrolimus), resulting in subsequent interaction with calcineurin to block its phosphatase activity. Calcineurin-catalyzed dephosphorylation is required for movement of a component of the NFAT into the nucleus. NFAT, in turn, is required to induce a number of cytokine genes, including IL-2, a prototypic T-cell growth and differentiation factor (Verghese et al., 2014).

Tacrolimus

Tacrolimus is a macrolide antibiotic produced by *Streptomyces tsukubaensis*. Because of perceived slightly greater efficacy and ease of blood level monitoring, tacrolimus has become the preferred calcineurin inhibitor in most transplant centers (Ekberg et al., 2007).

Mechanism of Action. Like cyclosporine, tacrolimus inhibits T-cell activation by inhibiting calcineurin. Tacrolimus binds to an intracellular protein, FKBP-12, an immunophilin structurally related to cyclophilin. A complex of tacrolimus–FKBP-12, Ca^{2+}, calmodulin, and calcineurin then forms, and calcineurin phosphatase activity is inhibited (see Figure 35–2). Inhibition of phosphatase activity prevents dephosphorylation and nuclear translocation of NFAT and inhibits T-cell activation. Thus, although the intracellular receptors differ, cyclosporine and tacrolimus target the same pathway for immunosuppression.

ADME. *Tacrolimus* is available for oral administration as capsules and extended-release capsules (0.5, 1, and 5 mg); extended-release tablets (0.75, 1, and 4 mg); and a solution for injection (5 mg/mL). Sublingual tacrolimus has been used off label for the short term in patients who are unable to receive medications orally. Because of intersubject variability in pharmacokinetics, individualized dosing is required for optimal therapy. For tacrolimus, whole blood is the preferred sampling compartment; the trough drug level in whole blood seems to correlate better with clinical events for tacrolimus than for cyclosporine. Target concentrations are 10–15 ng/mL in the early preoperative period and 6–8 ng/mL at 3 months posttransplantation. Gastrointestinal absorption is incomplete and variable. Target concentrations are dependent on sampling technique and on product-release characteristics, immediate- versus extended-release forms. Food decreases the rate and extent of absorption. Plasma protein binding of tacrolimus is 75%–99%, involving primarily albumin and $α_1$-acid glycoprotein. The $t_{1/2}$ of tacrolimus is about 12 h. Tacrolimus is extensively metabolized in the liver by CYP3A; some of the metabolites are active. The bulk of excretion of the parent drug and metabolites is in the feces.

Therapeutic Uses. Tacrolimus is indicated for the prophylaxis of solid-organ allograft rejection in a manner similar to cyclosporine (see Cyclosporine) and is used off label as rescue therapy in patients with rejection episodes despite "therapeutic" levels of cyclosporine. Recommended initial oral doses are 0.2 mg/kg/d for adult kidney transplant patients, 0.1–0.15 mg/kg/d for adult liver transplant patients, 0.075 mg/kg/d for adult heart transplant patients, and 0.15–0.2 mg/kg/d for pediatric liver transplant patients in two divided doses 12 h apart. These dosages are intended to achieve typical blood trough levels in the 5- to 20-ng/mL range (Goring et al., 2014). Note that the oral dose of tacrolimus depends on product release characteristics (immediate- vs. extended-release formulation) and the specific cocktail of medications selected for prophylaxis.

Toxicity. Nephrotoxicity; neurotoxicity (e.g., tremor, headache, motor disturbances, seizures); GI complaints; hypertension; hyperkalemia; hyperglycemia; and diabetes all are associated with tacrolimus use. Tacrolimus has a negative effect on pancreatic islet β cells, and glucose intolerance and diabetes mellitus are well-recognized complications of

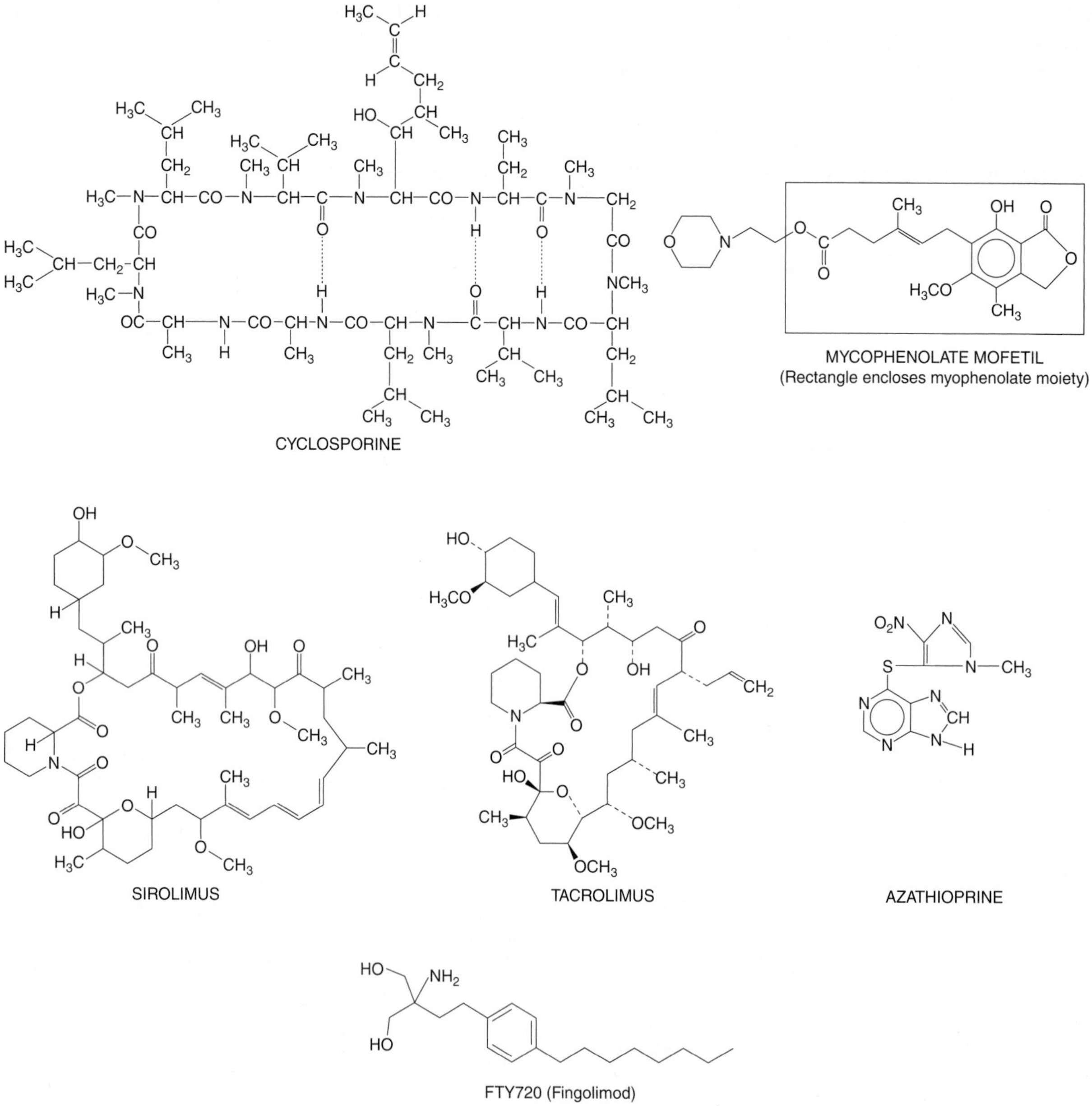

Figure 35–1 *Structures of selected immunosuppressive drugs.*

tacrolimus-based immunosuppression. While combined use of calcineurin inhibitors and glucocorticoids is particularly diabetogenic, new-onset diabetes after transplantation (NODAT) incidence was significantly higher with tacrolimus compared to cyclosporine, the other calcineurin inhibitor. Obese patients, African American or Hispanic transplant recipients, or those with a family history of type 2 diabetes or obesity are especially at risk. As with other immunosuppressive agents, there is an increased risk of secondary tumors and opportunistic infections. Notably, tacrolimus does not adversely affect uric acid or LDL cholesterol. Diarrhea and alopecia are common in patients on concomitant mycophenolate therapy.

Drug Interactions. Because of its potential for nephrotoxicity, tacrolimus blood levels and renal function should be monitored closely. Coadministration with cyclosporine results in additive or synergistic nephrotoxicity; therefore, a delay of at least 24 h is required when switching a patient from cyclosporine to tacrolimus. Because tacrolimus is metabolized mainly by CYP3A, the potential interactions described in the following section for cyclosporine also apply for tacrolimus. Per the label, concomitant use of tacrolimus with cyclosporine or sirolimus is not recommended for prophylaxis against renal transplant rejection.

Cyclosporine

Cyclosporine (cyclosporin A) is a cyclic polypeptide of 11 amino acids, produced by the fungus *Beauveria nivea,* that inhibits calcineurin activity (Azzi et al., 2013).

Mechanism of Action. Cyclosporine forms a complex with cyclophilin, a cytoplasmic-receptor protein present in target cells (Figure 35–2). This complex binds to calcineurin, inhibiting Ca^{2+}-stimulated dephosphorylation of the cytosolic component of NFAT. When cytoplasmic NFAT is dephosphorylated, it translocates to the nucleus and complexes with nuclear components required for complete T-cell activation, including transactivation of IL-2 and other lymphokine genes. Calcineurin phosphatase activity is inhibited after physical interaction with the cyclosporine/cyclophilin complex.

At the level of immune system function, cyclosporine suppresses some humoral immunity but is more effective against T-cell–dependent immune mechanisms such as those underlying transplant rejection and some forms of autoimmunity. It preferentially inhibits antigen-triggered signal transduction in T lymphocytes, blunting expression of many lymphokines, including IL-2, and the expression of antiapoptotic proteins.

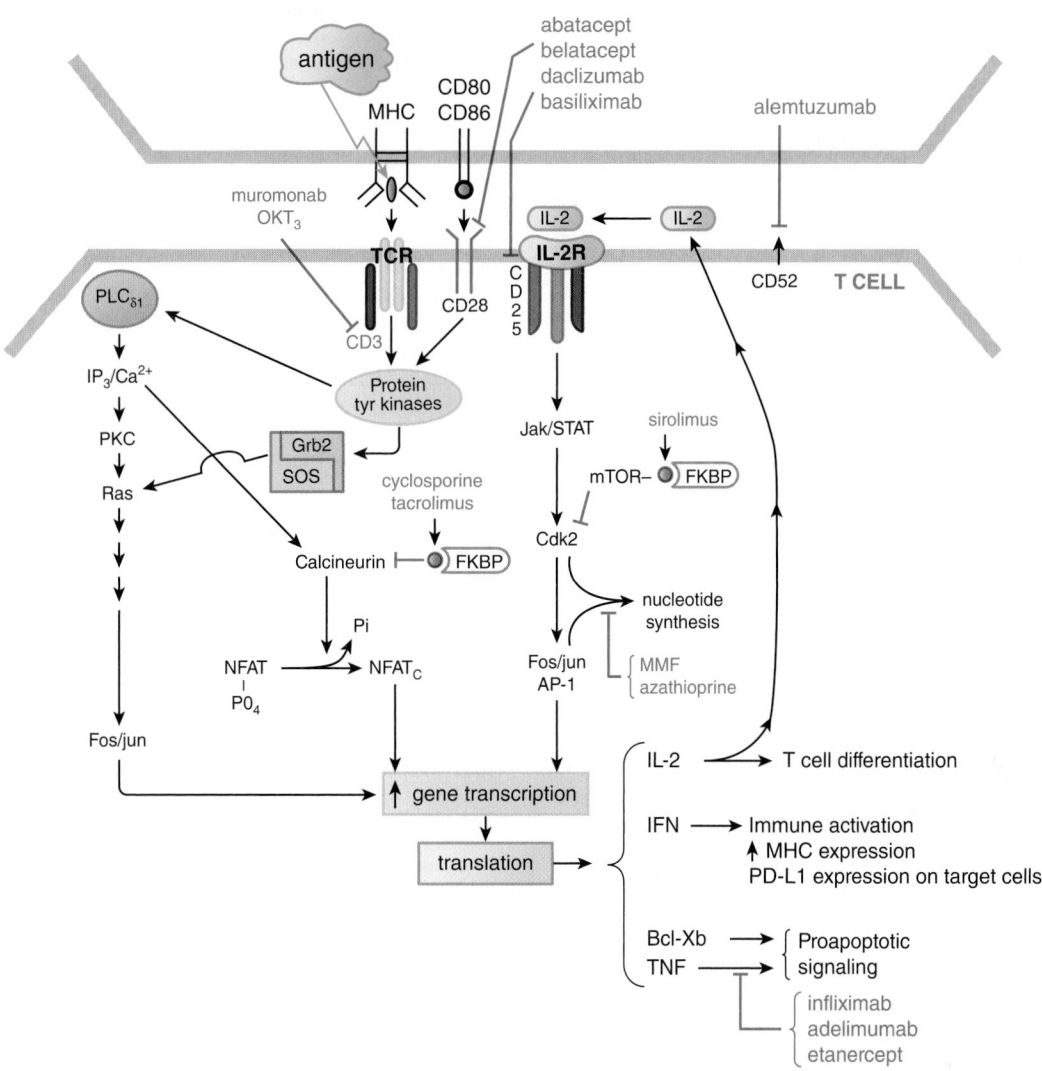

Figure 35–2 *T-cell activation and sites of action of immunosuppressive agents.* The TCR recognizes antigens bound to the MHC. A costimulatory signal is required for T-cell activation: The CD80/CD86-CD28 interaction from the APC to the T cell. Activation leads to IL-2 production (in a positive-feedback loop) and a host of other events, some of which are bracketed in the lower right-hand corner. Numerous agents are available to suppress T-cell activation. Cyclosporine and tacrolimus bind to immunophilins (cyclophilin and FKBP, respectively), forming a complex that inhibits the phosphatase calcineurin and the calcineurin-catalyzed dephosphorylation that permits translocation of NFAT into the nucleus. NFAT is required for transcription of IL-2 and other growth and differentiation–associated cytokines (lymphokines). Sirolimus (rapamycin) works downstream of the IL-2R, binding to FKBP; the FKBP-sirolimus complex binds to and inhibits the mTOR, a kinase involved in cell cycle progression (proliferation). MMF and azathioprine inhibit nucleic acid synthesis, thereby inhibiting T-cell proliferation. The antibody muromunab (OKT3) inhibits TCR function via interaction with its CD3 component. Daclizumab and basilixmab block IL-2 signaling by interacting with the alpha subunit of the IL-2R complex (CD25). Several antibodies can block the systemic effects of released TNF. Alemtuzumab, by binding to CD52, marks the cell for destruction, thereby depleting CD52+ cells.

Cyclosporine also increases expression of TGF-β, a potent inhibitor of IL-2–stimulated T-cell proliferation and generation of CTLs (Colombo and Ammirati, 2011; Molnar et al., 2015).

ADME. Because cyclosporine is lipophilic and highly hydrophobic, it is formulated for clinical administration using castor oil or other strategies to ensure solubilization. Cyclosporine can be administered intravenously or orally. The intravenous preparation is provided as a solution in an ethanol–polyoxyethylated castor oil vehicle that must be further diluted in 0.9% sodium chloride solution or 5% dextrose solution before injection. The oral dosage forms include soft gelatin capsules and oral solutions. Cyclosporine supplied in the original soft gelatin capsule is absorbed slowly, with 20%–50% bioavailability. A modified microemulsion formulation, NEORAL, has become the most widely used preparation. It has more uniform and slightly increased bioavailability compared to the original formulation. It is provided as 25- and 100-mg soft gelatin capsules and

a 100-mg/mL oral solution. The original and microemulsion formulations are *not bioequivalent* and cannot be used interchangeably without heightened monitoring of drug concentrations and assessment of graft function. A second modified formulation, GENGRAF, is also marketed, and like NEORAL, is *not interchangeable* with nonmodified cyclosporine formulations. Transplant units need to educate patients that the cyclosporine preparation know as SANDIMMUNE and its generics are not the same as NEORAL and its generics, such that one preparation cannot be substituted for another without risk of inadequate immunosuppression or increased toxicity. The danger of unauthorized, inadvertent, unmonitored, or inappropriate substitution of nonequivalent formulations can result in graft loss and other adverse patient outcomes.

Blood levels taken 2 h after a dose administration (so-called C_2 levels) may correlate better with the AUC than other single points, but no single time point can simulate the exposure better than more frequent drug sampling. In practice, if a patient has clinical signs or symptoms of toxicity or if there is unexplained rejection or renal dysfunction, a pharmacokinetic profile can be used to estimate that person's systemic exposure to the drug.

Cyclosporine absorption is incomplete following oral administration and varies with the individual patient and the formulation used. Cyclosporine is distributed extensively outside the vascular compartment. After intravenous dosing, the steady-state volume of distribution reportedly is as high as 3–5 L/kg in solid-organ transplant recipients. The elimination of cyclosporine from the blood generally is biphasic, with a terminal $t_{1/2}$ of 5–18 h. After intravenous infusion, clearance is about 5–7 mL/min/kg in adult recipients of renal transplants, but results differ by age and between different patient populations. For example, clearance is slower in cardiac transplant patients and more rapid in children. Thus, the intersubject variability is so large that individual monitoring is required.

After oral administration of cyclosporine (as NEORAL), the time to peak blood concentrations is 1.5–2 h. Administration with food delays and decreases absorption. High- and low-fat meals consumed within 30 min of administration decrease the AUC by about 13% and the maximum concentration by 33%. This makes it imperative to individualize dosage regimens for outpatients. Cyclosporine is extensively metabolized in the liver by hepatic CYP3A and to a lesser degree in the GI tract and kidneys. At least 25 metabolites have been identified in human bile, feces, blood, and urine. All of the metabolites have reduced biological activity and toxicity compared to the parent drug. Cyclosporine and its metabolites are excreted principally through the bile into the feces, with about 6% excreted in the urine. Cyclosporine also is excreted in human milk. In the presence of hepatic dysfunction, dosage adjustments are required. No adjustments generally are necessary for patients on dialysis or with renal failure.

Therapeutic Uses. Clinical indications for cyclosporine are kidney, liver, heart, and other organ transplantation; rheumatoid arthritis; psoriasis; and xerophthalmia. Its use in dermatology is discussed in Chapter 70. Cyclosporine usually is combined with other agents, especially glucocorticoids and either azathioprine or mycophenolate, and, most recently, sirolimus. The dose of cyclosporine varies, depending on the organ transplanted and the other drugs used in the specific treatment protocol(s). The initial dose generally is not given before the transplant because of the concern about nephrotoxicity. For renal transplant patients, therapeutic algorithms have been developed to delay cyclosporine or tacrolimus introduction until a threshold renal function has been attained. Dosing is guided by signs of rejection (too low a dose), renal or other toxicity (too high a dose), and close monitoring of blood levels. Great care must be taken to differentiate renal toxicity from rejection in kidney transplant patients. Ultrasound-guided allograft biopsy is the best way to assess the basis for renal dysfunction. Because adverse reactions have been ascribed more frequently to the intravenous formulation, this route of administration is discontinued as soon as the patient can take the drug orally.

In rheumatoid arthritis, cyclosporine is used in severe cases that have not responded to methotrexate. Cyclosporine can be combined with methotrexate, but the levels of both drugs must be monitored closely. In psoriasis, cyclosporine is indicated for treatment of adult immunocompetent patients with severe and disabling disease for whom other systemic therapies are contraindicated or have failed. Because of its mechanism of action, there is a theoretical basis for the use of cyclosporine in a variety of other T-cell–mediated diseases. Cyclosporine reportedly is effective in Behçet's, acute ocular syndrome, endogenous uveitis, atopic dermatitis, inflammatory bowel disease, and nephrotic syndrome, even when standard therapies have failed.

Toxicity. The principal adverse reactions to cyclosporine therapy are renal dysfunction and hypertension; tremor, hirsutism, hyperlipidemia, and gum hyperplasia also are frequently encountered. Hypertension occurs in about 50% of renal transplant and almost all cardiac transplant patients. Hyperuricemia may lead to worsening of gout, increased P-glycoprotein activity, and hypercholesterolemia (see Chapters 5, 33, and 38). Nephrotoxicity occurs in the majority of patients and is the

major reason for cessation or modification of therapy. Combined use of calcineurin inhibitors and glucocorticoids is particularly diabetogenic, although this seems more problematic in patients treated with tacrolimus (see previous Tacrolimus section). Cyclosporine, as opposed to tacrolimus, is more likely to produce elevations in LDL cholesterol.

Drug Interactions. Cyclosporine interacts with a wide variety of commonly used drugs, and close attention must be paid to drug interactions. Any drug that affects CYPs, especially CYP3A, may affect cyclosporine blood concentrations. Substances that inhibit this enzyme can decrease cyclosporine metabolism and increase blood concentrations. These include Ca^{2+} channel blockers (e.g., *verapamil, nicardipine*); antifungal agents (e.g., *fluconazole, ketoconazole*); antibiotics (e.g., *erythromycin*); glucocorticoids (e.g., *methylprednisolone*); HIV-protease inhibitors (e.g., *indinavir*); and other drugs (e.g., *allopurinol, metoclopramide*). Grapefruit juice inhibits CYP3A and the P-glycoprotein multidrug efflux pump and thereby can increase cyclosporine blood concentrations. In contrast, drugs that induce CYP3A activity can increase cyclosporine metabolism and decrease blood concentrations. Such drugs include antibiotics (e.g., *nafcillin, rifampin*); anticonvulsants (e.g., *phenobarbital, phenytoin*); and others (e.g., *octreotide, ticlopidine*).

Interactions between cyclosporine and sirolimus require that administration of the two drugs be separated by time. Sirolimus aggravates cyclosporine-induced renal dysfunction, while cyclosporine increases sirolimus-induced hyperlipidemia and myelosuppression. Additive nephrotoxicity may occur when cyclosporine is coadministered with *NSAIDs* and other drugs that cause renal dysfunction; elevation of methotrexate levels may occur when the two drugs are coadministered, as can reduced clearance of other drugs, including prednisolone, digoxin, and statins (Azzi et al., 2013; Ekberg et al., 2007).

Antiproliferative and Antimetabolic Drugs

Sirolimus

Sirolimus (rapamycin) is a macrocyclic lactone produced by *Streptomyces hygroscopicus.*

Mechanism of Action. Sirolimus inhibits T-lymphocyte activation and proliferation downstream of the IL-2 and other T-cell growth factor receptors (see Figure 35–2). Like cyclosporine and tacrolimus, therapeutic action of sirolimus requires formation of a complex with an immunophilin, in this case *FKBP-12*. The *sirolimus–FKBP-12 complex* does not affect calcineurin activity; rather, it binds to and inhibits the protein kinase *mTOR*, which is a key enzyme in cell cycle progression. Inhibition of mTOR blocks cell cycle progression at the $G_1 \rightarrow S$ phase transition.

In animal models, sirolimus not only inhibits transplant rejection, GVHD, and a variety of autoimmune diseases, but also has effects for several months after discontinuation, suggesting a tolerizing effect (see Tolerance). A newer indication for sirolimus is the avoidance of calcineurin inhibitors, even when patients are stable, to protect kidney function (Schena et al., 2009).

ADME. After oral administration, sirolimus is absorbed rapidly and reaches a peak blood concentration within about 1 h after a single dose in healthy subjects and within about 2 h after multiple oral doses in renal transplant patients. Systemic availability is about 15%, and blood concentrations are proportional to dose between 3 and 12 mg/m². A high-fat meal decreases peak blood concentration by 34%; sirolimus therefore should be taken consistently either with or without food, and blood levels should be monitored closely. About 40% of sirolimus in plasma is protein bound, especially to albumin. The drug partitions into formed elements of blood (blood-to-plasma ratio = 38 in renal transplant patients). Sirolimus is extensively metabolized by CYP3A4 and is transported by P-glycoprotein. The bulk of total excretion is via the feces. Although some of its metabolites are active, sirolimus itself is the major active component in whole blood and contributes more than 90% of the immunosuppressive effect. The blood $t_{1/2}$ after multiple doses in stable renal transplant patients is 62 h. A loading dose of three times the maintenance dose will provide nearly steady-state concentrations within 1 day in most patients.

Therapeutic Uses. Sirolimus is indicated for prophylaxis of organ transplant rejection, usually in combination with a reduced dose of calcineurin inhibitor and glucocorticoids. Sirolimus has been used with glucocorticoids and mycophenolate to avoid permanent renal damage. Sirolimus dosing regimens are relatively complex, with blood levels generally targeted between 5 and 15 ng/mL. It is recommended that the daily maintenance dose be reduced by approximately one-third in patients with hepatic impairment. Sirolimus also has been incorporated into stents to inhibit local cell proliferation and blood vessel occlusion (Moes et al., 2015).

Toxicity. The use of sirolimus in renal transplant patients is associated with a dose-dependent increase in serum cholesterol and triglycerides that may require treatment. Although immunotherapy with sirolimus per se is not considered nephrotoxic, patients treated with cyclosporine plus sirolimus have impaired renal function compared to patients treated with cyclosporine alone. Sirolimus can worsen proteinuria and should be used with caution in patients with GFR below 30% or proteinuria; these conditions can worsen renal failure. Renal function and proteinuria therefore must be monitored closely in such patients. Lymphocele, a known surgical complication associated with renal transplantation, is increased in a dose-dependent fashion by sirolimus, requiring close postoperative follow-up.

Other adverse effects include anemia, leukopenia, thrombocytopenia, mouth ulcer, hypokalemia, and GI effects. Delayed wound healing may occur with sirolimus use. This mTOR inhibitor has been shown to have anticancer effect, especially on skin cancer; it is considered the immunosuppressant of choice in patients with a history of malignancy. Temsirolimus is specifically approved for kidney (but not skin) cancer, while everolimus is approved for a variety of cancers (but not skin cancer). As with other immunosuppressive agents, there is an increased risk of infections.

Drug Interactions. Because sirolimus is a substrate for CYP3A4 and is transported by P-glycoprotein, close attention to interactions with other drugs that are metabolized or transported by these proteins is required (see Chapters 5 and 6). Dose adjustment may be required when sirolimus is coadministered with CYP3A4 and P-glycoprotein inhibitors (such as diltiazem) or strong inducers (such as rifampin) (Alberú et al., 2011; Euvrard et al., 2012).

Everolimus

Everolimus [40-O-(2-hydroxyethyl)-rapamycin] is FDA-approved for treatment of astrocytoma, breast cancer, kidney and liver transplant rejection prophylaxis, pancreatic neuroendocrine tumor, renal angiomyolipoma, and renal cell cancer. It is chemically closely related to sirolimus but has distinct pharmacokinetics. The main difference is a shorter $t_{1/2}$ and thus a shorter time to achieve steady-state concentrations of the drug. Dosage on a milligram per kilogram basis is similar to (but not the same as) that of sirolimus. In kidney transplant rejection prophylaxis, the initial dose of everolimus is 0.75 mg twice daily, with later adjustment based on serum concentrations. As with sirolimus, the combination of a calcineurin inhibitor and an mTOR inhibitor produces worse renal function at 1 year than does calcineurin inhibitor therapy alone, suggesting a drug interaction between the mTOR inhibitors and the calcineurin inhibitors that reduces rejection but enhances toxicity. The toxicity of everolimus and the potential for drug interactions seem to be the same as with sirolimus (Budde et al., 2011; Moes et al., 2015). Like sirolimus, individualization of drug dose through therapeutic drug monitoring is required.

Azathioprine

Azathioprine is a purine antimetabolite. It is an imidazolyl derivative of 6-mercaptopurine, metabolites of which can inhibit purine synthesis.

Mechanism of Action. Following exposure to nucleophiles such as glutathione, azathioprine is cleaved to 6-MP, which in turn is converted to additional metabolites that inhibit de novo purine synthesis (see Chapter 66). A fraudulent nucleotide, 6-thio-IMP, is converted to 6-thio-GMP and finally to 6-thio-GTP, which is incorporated into DNA. Cell proliferation thereby is inhibited, impairing a variety of lymphocyte functions. Azathioprine appears to be a more potent immunosuppressive agent than 6-MP (Hardinger et al., 2013).

ADME. Azathioprine is well absorbed orally and reaches maximum blood levels within 1–2 h after administration. The $t_{1/2}$ of azathioprine is about 10 min, and the $t_{1/2}$ of 6-MP is about 1 h. Other metabolites have a $t_{1/2}$ of up to 5 h. Blood levels have limited predictive value because of extensive metabolism, significant activity of many different metabolites, and high tissue levels attained. Azathioprine and mercaptopurine are moderately bound to plasma proteins and are partially dialyzable. Both are rapidly removed from the blood by oxidation or methylation in the liver or erythrocytes. Renal clearance has little impact on the biological effectiveness or toxicity.

Therapeutic Uses. Azathioprine is indicated as an adjunct for prevention of organ transplant rejection and in severe rheumatoid arthritis. The usual starting dose of azathioprine is 3–5 mg/kg/d. Lower initial doses (1 mg/kg/d) are used in treating rheumatoid arthritis. Complete blood count and liver function tests should be monitored.

Toxicity. The major side effect of azathioprine is bone marrow suppression, including leukopenia (common), thrombocytopenia (less common), or anemia (uncommon). Other important adverse effects include increased susceptibility to infections (especially varicella and herpes simplex viruses), hepatotoxicity, alopecia, GI toxicity, pancreatitis, and increased risk of neoplasia.

Drug Interactions. Xanthine oxidase, an enzyme of major importance in the catabolism of azathioprine metabolites, is blocked by allopurinol. Hence, the combination of azathioprine with allopurinol should be avoided. Adverse effects resulting from coadministration of azathioprine with other myelosuppressive agents or angiotensin-converting enzyme inhibitors include leukopenia, thrombocytopenia, and anemia as a result of myelosuppression.

Mycophenolate Mofetil

Mycophenolate mofetil is the 2-morpholinoethyl ester of MPA (Darji et al., 2008; Molnar et al., 2015).

Mechanism of Action. Mycophenolate mofetil is a prodrug that is rapidly hydrolyzed to the active drug MPA, a selective, noncompetitive, reversible inhibitor of inosine monophosphate dehydrogenase (IMPDH), an enzyme in the de novo pathway of guanine nucleotide synthesis. B and T lymphocytes are highly dependent on this pathway for cell proliferation; MPA thus selectively inhibits lymphocyte proliferation and functions, including antibody formation, cellular adhesion, and migration.

ADME. Mycophenolate mofetil undergoes rapid and complete metabolism to MPA after oral or intravenous administration. MPA is then metabolized to the inactive glucuronide MPAG. The parent drug is cleared from the blood within a few minutes. The $t_{1/2}$ of MPA is ~16 h. Most (87%) is excreted in the urine as MPAG. Plasma concentrations of MPA and MPAG are increased in patients with renal insufficiency.

Therapeutic Uses. Mycophenolate mofetil is indicated for prophylaxis of transplant rejection, and it typically is used in combination with glucocorticoids and a calcineurin inhibitor but not with azathioprine. Combined treatment with sirolimus is possible, although potential drug interactions necessitate careful monitoring of drug levels. The approved dose for liver transplantation rejection prophylaxis is 1 g twice daily. For renal transplants, 1 g is administered orally or intravenously (over 2 h) twice daily (2 g/d). A higher dose, 1.5 g twice daily (3 g/d), may be recommended for African American renal transplant patients and all liver and cardiac transplant patients. MMF is increasingly used off label in systemic lupus. MMF has been used to treat a number of different inflammatory disorders, including MS and sarcoidosis. A delayed-release formulation of MPA is available; it does not release MPA under acidic conditions (pH < 5), as in the stomach, but is soluble in neutral pH, as in the intestine. The enteric coating results in a delay in the time to reach maximum MPA concentrations (Darji et al., 2008).

Toxicity. The principal toxicities of MMF are GI and hematologic: leukopenia, pure red cell aplasia, diarrhea, and vomiting. The MPA formulation has been introduced to reduce the frequent GI upset and has had variable results. There also is an increased incidence of some infections, especially sepsis associated with cytomegalovirus. Tacrolimus in combination with

MMF has been associated with activation of polyoma viruses such as BK virus, which can cause interstitial nephritis. The use of mycophenolate in pregnancy is associated with congenital anomalies and increased risk of pregnancy loss.

Drug Interactions. Tacrolimus delays elimination of MMF by impairing the conversion of MPA to MPAG. This may enhance GI toxicity. Coadministration with antacids containing aluminum or magnesium hydroxide leads to decreased absorption of MMF; thus, these drugs should not be administered simultaneously. MMF should not be administered with cholestyramine or other drugs that affect enterohepatic circulation. Such agents decrease plasma MPA concentrations, probably by binding free MPA in the intestines. Acyclovir and ganciclovir may compete with MPAG for tubular secretion, possibly resulting in increased concentrations of both MPAG and the antiviral agents in the blood, an effect that may be compounded in patients with renal insufficiency. Mycophenolate serum level monitoring is not performed routinely (Darji et al., 2008; Goldfarb-Rumyantzev et al., 2006).

Other Antiproliferative and Cytotoxic Agents

Many of the cytotoxic and antimetabolic agents used in cancer chemotherapy (see Chapter 66) are immunosuppressive due to their action on lymphocytes and other cells of the immune system. Other cytotoxic drugs that have been used both on and off label as immunosuppressive agents include methotrexate, cyclophosphamide, thalidomide, and chlorambucil. *Methotrexate* is used for prophylaxis against GVHD and treatment of rheumatoid arthritis, psoriasis, bullous pemphigoid, and some cancers. *Cyclophosphamide* and *chlorambucil* are used in leukemia and lymphomas and a variety of other malignancies. Cyclophosphamide also is FDA-approved for childhood nephrotic syndrome and is used widely off label for treatment of severe systemic lupus erythematosus, MS, and vasculitides such as Wegener granulomatosis. *Leflunomide* is a pyrimidine synthesis inhibitor indicated for the treatment of adults with rheumatoid arthritis. This drug has found increasing empirical use in the treatment of polyomavirus nephropathy seen in immunosuppressed renal transplant recipients. There are no controlled studies showing efficacy compared with control patients treated with only withdrawal or reduction of immunosuppression alone in BK virus nephropathy. The drug inhibits dihydroorotate dehydrogenase in the de novo pathway of pyrimidine synthesis. It is hepatotoxic and can cause fetal injury when administered to pregnant women.

Fingolimod

Fingolimod is the first agent in a new class of small molecules, S1P-R agonists. This S1P-R prodrug reduces recirculation of lymphocytes from the lymphatic system to the blood and peripheral tissues, thereby shunting lymphocytes away from inflammatory lesions and organ grafts.

Mechanism of Action. *Fingolimod* specifically and reversibly causes sequestration of host lymphocytes into the lymph nodes and Peyer patches and thus away from the circulation, thereby protecting lesions and grafts from T-cell–mediated attack. Fingolimod does not impair T- and B-cell functions. Sphingosine kinase 2 phosphorylates fingolimod; the fingolimod-phosphate product is a potent agonist at S1P-Rs, producing the altered lymphocyte traffic.

Therapeutic Uses. Fingolimod is not useful for treatment of transplant rejection but is effective and FDA-approved as a first-line therapy in the MS (see section on MS; Pelletier and Hafler, 2012).

Toxicity. Lymphopenia, the predictable and most common side effect of fingolimod, reverses on discontinuation of the drug. Of greater concern is the negative chronotropic effect on the heart, which has been observed with the first dose in up to 30% of patients (Vincenti and Kirk, 2008). In most patients, the heart rate returns to baseline within 48 h, with the remainder returning to baseline thereafter.

Immunosuppression Antibodies and Fusion Receptor Protein

Polyclonal and mAbs against lymphocyte cell surface antigens are widely used for prevention and treatment of organ transplant rejection.

Polyclonal antisera are generated by repeated injections of human thymocytes (ATG) or lymphocytes (ALG) into animals and then purifying the serum immunoglobulin fraction. These preparations vary in efficacy and toxicity from batch to batch.

The capacity to produce mAbs (Figure 35–3) has overcome the problems of variability in efficacy and toxicity seen with the polyclonal products, but mAbs are more limited in their target specificity. The first-generation murine mAbs have been replaced by newer humanized or fully human mAbs that lack antigenicity, have a prolonged $t_{1/2}$, and can be mutagenized to alter their affinity to Fc receptors.

Another class of biological agents being developed for both autoimmunity and transplantation are fusion receptor proteins. These agents consist of the ligand-binding domains of receptors bound to the Fc region of an immunoglobulin (usually IgG1) to provide a longer $t_{1/2}$ (Baldo, 2015). Examples of such agents include *abatacept* (CTLA4-Ig) and *belatacept* (a second-generation CTLA4-Ig), discussed in the Costimulatory Blockade section.

Antithymocyte Globulin

Antithymocyte globulin is a purified gamma globulin from the serum of rabbits immunized with human thymocytes (Thiyagarajan et al., 2013). It is provided as a sterile, freeze-dried product for intravenous administration after reconstitution with sterile water. ATG is one of many immune globulin preparations used therapeutically, generally for passive immunization (see Table 35–2 and Chapter 36).

Mechanism of Action. Antithymocyte globulin contains cytotoxic antibodies that bind to CD2, CD3, CD4, CD8, CD11a, CD18, CD25, CD44, CD45, and HLA class I and II molecules on the surface of human T lymphocytes. The antibodies deplete circulating lymphocytes by direct cytotoxicity (both complement and cell mediated) and block lymphocyte function by binding to cell surface molecules involved in the regulation of cell function.

Therapeutic Uses. Antithymocyte globulin is used for induction immunosuppression, although the approved indications are for the treatment and prophylaxis of acute renal transplant rejection in combination with other immunosuppressive agents and for the treatment of aplastic anemia. Antilymphocyte-depleting agents (Thymoglobulin, Atgam, and OKT3) are not registered for use as induction immunosuppression. A course of antithymocyte-globulin often is given to renal transplant patients with delayed graft function to avoid early treatment with the nephrotoxic calcineurin inhibitors, thereby aiding in recovery from ischemic reperfusion injury. The recommended dose of Thymoglobulin for acute rejection of renal grafts is 1.5 mg/kg/d (over 4–6 h) for 7–14 days. Mean T-cell counts fall by day 2 of therapy. The recommended dose of Atgam for acute rejection of renal grafts is 10–15 mg/kg/d for 14 days. ATG also is used for acute rejection of other types of organ transplants and for prophylaxis of rejection.

Toxicity. Polyclonal antibodies are xenogeneic proteins that can elicit major side effects, including fever and chills with the potential for hypotension. Premedication with corticosteroids, acetaminophen, or an antihistamine and administration of the antiserum by slow infusion (over 4–6 h) into a large-diameter vessel minimize such reactions. Serum sickness and glomerulonephritis can occur; anaphylaxis is rare. Hematologic complications include leukopenia and thrombocytopenia. As with other immunosuppressive agents, there is an increased risk of infection and malignancy, especially when multiple immunosuppressive agents are combined. No drug interactions have been described; anti-ATG antibodies develop but do not limit repeated use.

Monoclonal Antibodies

Immunotherapy and the Nature of Costimulation and Inhibition

Multiple costimulatory and inhibitory molecules interact to regulate T-cell responses. Immune activation requires two signals that emanate from the interaction of membrane proteins on APCs and T cells

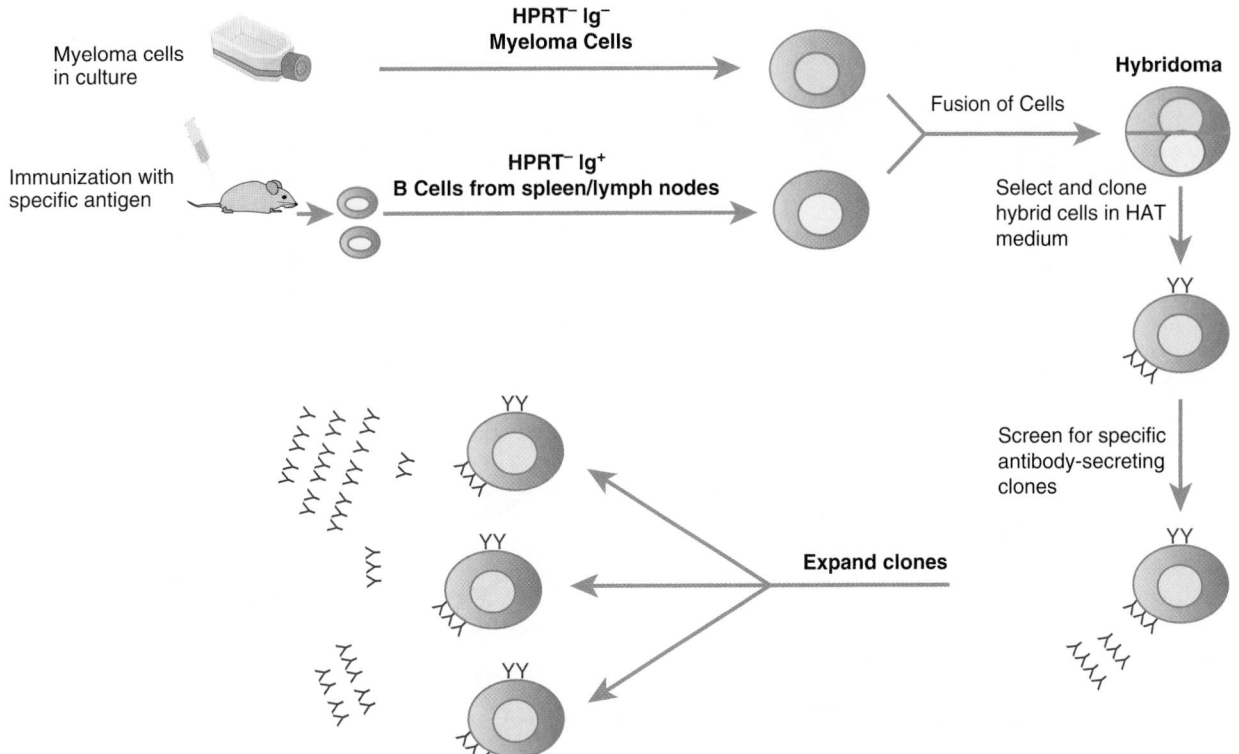

Figure 35–3 *Generation of mAbs.* Mice are immunized with the selected antigen, and the spleen or lymph node is harvested and B cells separated. These B cells are fused to a suitable B-cell myeloma selected for its ability to grow in medium supplemented with HAT (hypoxanthine, aminopterin, and thymidine). Only myeloma cells that fuse with B cells can survive in HAT-supplemented medium. The hybridomas expand in culture. Hybridomas of interest are selected based on a specific screening technique and then cloned by limiting dilution. The mAbs can be used directly as supernatants or ascites fluid for experimental use but are purified for clinical use.

TABLE 35–2 ■ SELECTED IMMUNE GLOBULIN PREPARATIONS

GENERIC NAME	COMMON SYNONYMS	ORIGIN
Antithymocyte globulin	ATG	Rabbit
Botulism immune globulin intravenous	BIG-IV	Human
Cytomegalovirus immune globulin intravenous	CMV-IGIV	Human
Hepatitis B immune globulin	HBIG	Human
Immune globulin intramuscular	Gamma globulin, IgG, IGIM	Human
Immune globulin intravenous	IVIG	Human
Immune globulin subcutaneous	IGSC	Human
Lymphocyte immune globulin	ALG, antithymocyte globulin (equine), ATG (equine)	Equine
Rabies immune globulin	RIG	Human
Rho(D) immune globulin intramuscular	Rho[D] IGIM	Human
Rho(D) immune globulin intravenous	Rho[D] IGIV	Human
Rho(D) immune globulin microdose	Rho[D] IG microdose	Human
Tetanus immune globulin	TIG	Human
Vaccinia immune globulin intravenous	VIGIV	Human

(Figures 34–5A and 34–5B). A growing number of antibodies directed at these interacting proteins permits interruption of immune activation to produce a state of immune suppression. Figures 35–2 and 35–4 point out some of these antibodies, which are especially useful in preventing rejection after organ transplantation, as summarized in the material that follows.

In what might be considered an antiparallel system to activation, inhibitory regulation of T-cell activity can also result from the interaction of paired membrane ligands of APCs and T cells (Figure 35–4C). These points of negative regulation are called *immune checkpoints*. By targeting and blocking these immune checkpoints, antibodies can permit T-cell activation to proceed, unfettered by downregulation (Figure 35–4C and 35–4D). Activating immune attacks of tumor cells by blockade of immune checkpoints is producing new therapeutic options for cancer therapy (Callahan et al., 2016; Topalian et al., 2015). Chapter 67 presents the use of immunotherapy in cancer treatment.

Anti-CD3 Monoclonal Antibodies

CD3 is a component of the TCR complex on the surface of human T lymphocytes (Figure 35–2). Antibodies directed at the ε chain of CD3 have been used with considerable efficacy in human transplantation. The anti-CD3 antibody is monoclonal and targets the CD3 chain of the TCR, inducing its endocytosis and T-cell inactivation and removal through phagocytosis. The original mouse IgG2a antihuman CD3 mAb, *muromonab-CD3* (OKT3), is no longer marketed due to its side effects: It frequently causes cytokine release syndrome and severe pulmonary edema. Nevertheless, muromonab remains FDA-registered and could be reintroduced to the market at any time.

Recently, genetically altered anti-CD3 mAbs have been developed that are "humanized" to minimize the occurrence of antiantibody responses and mutated to prevent binding to Fc receptors. In initial clinical trials, a humanized anti-CD3 mAb that does not bind to Fc receptors reversed acute renal allograft rejection without causing the first-dose

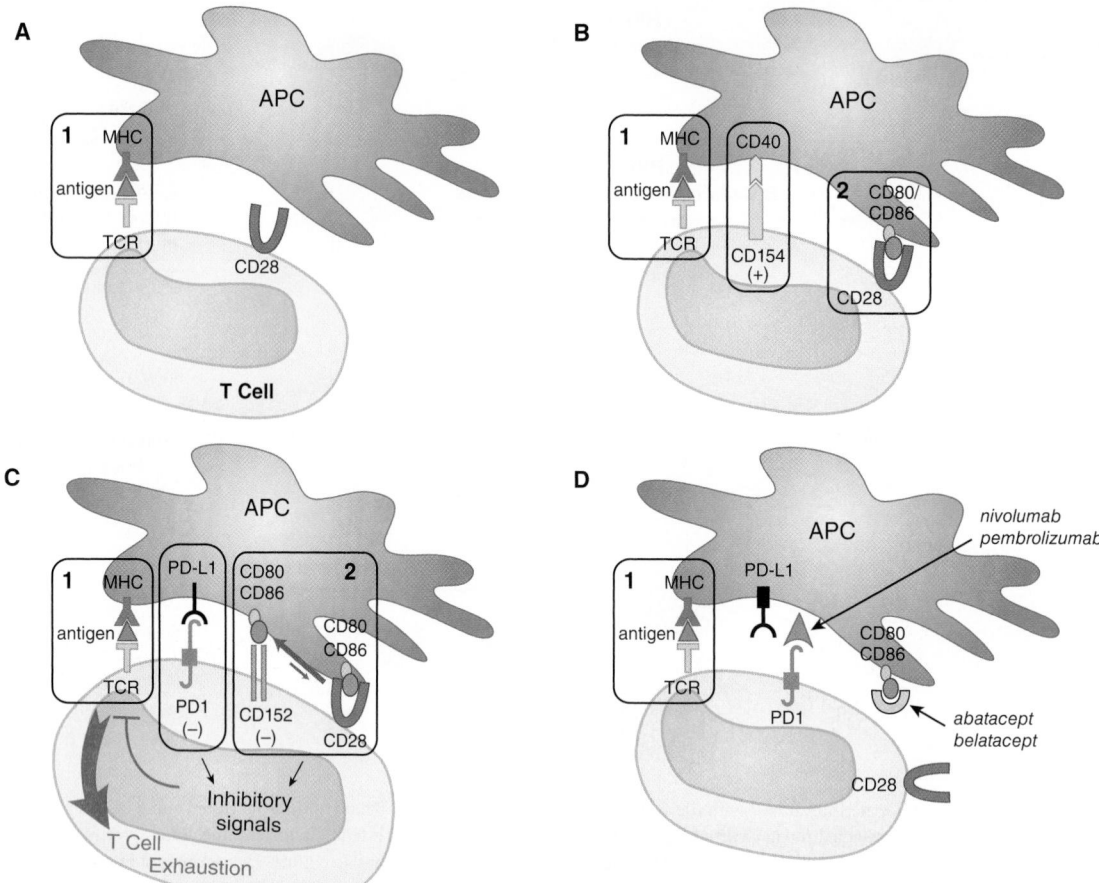

Figure 35–4   *T-cell activation: costimulation and coinhibitory checkpoints.* Numerous membrane CD proteins may be expressed on the APC and the T cell that lead to signaling interactions between ligands and receptors. These interactions can enhance or reduce the activation state of the T cell. Two signals are required for T-cell activation: presentation of an antigen ligand to the TCR and signaling by an additional "costimulatory" pair. **A.** The primary signal, *signal 1*, is the interaction of the TCR with the MHC-antigen complex on the APC. Activation requires a second, costimulatory interaction. **B**. *Signal 2*, the costimulatory interaction between CD28 on the T cell (the costimulatory receptor) and the costimulatory ligand on the APC, CD80/CD86, leads to T-cell activation. Additional costimulatory signals, such as the interaction of CD154 with CD40 on the APC, can further enhance T-cell activation (+). In the absence of costimulation, a T cell can become anergic or unresponsive. **C.** Additional APC–T-cell interactions can occur after T-cell activation, and some can be inhibitory, providing *immune checkpoints* that are important for reducing autoimmunity and for regulating the size and extent of immune responses. For example, the interaction of CD152 (CTLA4) with CD80/86 produces inhibitory signals that attenuate T-cell activation and proliferation (−). CD28 and CD152 compete for binding to CD80/CD86. As the figure suggests, the affinity of CD152 for CD80/CD86 exceeds that of CD28, and the equilibrium lies toward the formation of the inhibitory signaling complex, CD152-CD80/CD86. T cells may express varying amounts of another important modifier, PD1 (CD279). When liganded by PD-L1, PD1 produces inhibitory signals (↑ protein phosphatase activity, ↓ signaling by TCR, ↓ MAPK activity; see Figure 35–2) and reduces T-cell proliferation, leading to T-cell exhaustion, a state of hyporesponsiveness. When PD1 is highly expressed, as during conditions of chronic viral infection and cancer, suppression of T-cell activity via this pathway can be very effective; this pathway can facilitate continued viral replication and tumor progression. **D.** These immune checkpoints are useful sites for pharmacological regulation of T-cell activation. For instance, the agents abatacept and belatacept are fusion proteins that contain the CTLA4 domain of CD154 and act as decoys. These agents block costimulation of T cells by binding CD80/CD86 (see additional examples in Figure 35–2). Nivolumab and pembrolizumab are antibodies to PD1 and block interaction of PD1 with PD-L1, thereby blocking the immune suppression that would normally ensue and producing a state of immune hyperactivity. Checkpoint inhibitors that enhance immune responses are being used in cancer therapy (see Chapter 67). Antibodies can also be designed to be stimulatory ligands at checkpoints, to aid in generating a state of immune suppression that would be useful in treating autoimmune diseases.

cytokine release syndrome. Humanized anti-CD3 mAbs are also in phase 3 trials in patients with type 1 autoimmune diabetes.

Anti-CD52 Monoclonal Antibody (Alemtuzumab)

Alemtuzumab is a depleting humanized anti-CD52 mAb.

Mechanism of Action. Alemtuzumab binds the CD52 protein that is wildly expressed on B cells and T-cells, as well as macrophages, NK cells, and some granulocytes. Alemtuzumab binding to CD52 induces an antibody-dependent lysis of cells and a profound leukopenia that may last for more than a year (Jones and Coles, 2014).

Therapeutic Uses. *Alemtuzumab* is used mainly for induction of immunosuppressive therapy and allows the avoidance of the early high dose of steroids. For transplants, the most common regimen is a single

intraoperative dose of 30 mg. Alemtuzumab is also used for the treatment of refractory acute cellular- and antibody-mediated rejections with the same dose used during induction. The drug is licensed for the management of CLL and MS (CAMMS223 Investigators et al., 2008).

Toxicity. Neutropenia remains the most common adverse effect seen with *alemtuzumab*. Almost half of the patients will also experience thrombocytopenia and anemia. Another major side effect is autoimmune hemolytic anemia and other autoimmune diseases thought to be due to immune reconstitution after the profound lymphocyte depletion.

Anti-IL-2 Receptor (Anti-CD25) Antibodies

Daclizumab is a humanized murine complementarity-determining region/human IgG1 chimeric mAb. *Basiliximab* is a murine-human chimeric mAb. Both are licensed for use in conjunction with cyclosporine and corticosteroids for the prophylaxis of acute organ rejection in patients receiving renal transplants.

Mechanism of Action. The anti-CD25 mAbs bind with high affinity to the α subunit of the IL-2 receptor (Figure 35–2) and act as a receptor antagonist, inhibiting T-cell activation and proliferation without inducing cell lysis (Table 35–1). *Daclizumab* has a somewhat lower affinity but a longer $t_{1/2}$ (20 days) than *basiliximab* (Brennan et al., 2006). In addition, the induction of CD56[+] CD4[+] T cells is associated with response to therapy in patients with MS (D'Amico et al., 2015).

Therapeutic Uses. Anti-CD25 mAbs are used for induction therapy in solid-organ transplantation. They are also in phase 3 clinical trials in patients with MS. The long $t_{1/2}$ of daclizumab (20 days) results in saturation of the IL-2Rα on circulating lymphocytes for up to 120 days after transplantation. Daclizumab is administered in five doses (1 mg/kg given intravenously over 15 min in 50–100 mL of normal saline) starting immediately preoperatively and subsequently at biweekly intervals.

The $t_{1/2}$ of basiliximab is 7 days. In trials, basiliximab was administered in a fixed dose of 20 mg preoperatively and on days 0 and 4 after transplantation. This regimen of basiliximab saturated IL-2R on circulating lymphocytes for 25–35 days after transplantation. Basiliximab was used with a maintenance regimen consisting of cyclosporine and prednisone and was found to be safe and effective when used in a maintenance regimen consisting of cyclosporine, MMF, and prednisone.

While daclizumab and basiliximab are comparable in effectiveness, daclizumab has a more costly dosing regimen. The higher cost has reduced demand, and daclizumab is now produced only for use in treating MS.

Toxicity. *Basiliximab* and *daclizumab* seem to be relatively safe as induction agents, with most of the clinical trials reporting adverse reactions rates comparable to placebo. No cytokine-release syndrome has been noted, but anaphylactic reactions and rare lymphoproliferative disorders and opportunistic infections may occur. No drug interactions have been described.

Belatacept, a Fusion Protein

Belatacept is a fusion protein composed of a modified Fc fragment of a human immunoglobulin linked to the extracellular domain of the CTLA4 (CD152) that is present on T cells (Figure 35–5). This second-generation CTLA4-Ig has two amino acid substitutions, increasing its affinity for CD80 (2-fold) and CD86 (4-fold), yielding a 10-fold increase in potency in vitro compared to CTLA4-Ig (Chinen et al., 2015).

Mechanism of Action. Induction of specific immune responses by T lymphocytes requires two signals: an antigen-specific signal via the TCR and a costimulatory signal provided by the interaction of molecules such as CD28 on CD4 lymphocyte with CD80 and CD86 on APCs and CD2 engagement by LFA-3 (CD58) on CD8 cells (Figure 35–4) (Riella and Sayegh, 2013). *Belatacept* is a selective T-cell costimulation blocker that potently binds the cell surface costimulatory ligands (CD80 and CD86) present on APCs, interrupting their interaction with CD28 on T cells (signal 2). The inhibition of signal 2 inhibits T-cell activation, promoting anergy and apoptosis.

Disposition and Pharmacokinetics. *Belatacept* is the first intravenous maintenance therapy in solid-organ transplantation. Belatacept's pharmacokinetics were determined to be linear, with zero-order intravenous infusion and first-order elimination within the standard dose range of 5–10 mg/kg. The $t_{1/2}$ of *belatacept* is about 11 days.

Therapeutic Uses. Preclinical renal transplant studies showed that belatacept did not induce tolerance but did prolong graft survival. *Belatacept* is FDA approved as an alternative to calcineurin inhibitors as a strategy to prevent long-term calcineurin inhibitor toxicity (Satyananda and Shapiro, 2014; Talawila and Pengel, 2015). *Belatacept* has been approved specifically for prophylaxis of organ rejection in adult patients receiving a kidney transplant in combination with basiliximab induction, MMF, and corticosteroids.

The BENEFIT trial compared two *belatacept*-based regimens to cyclosporine and showed better kidney function and metabolic profile with

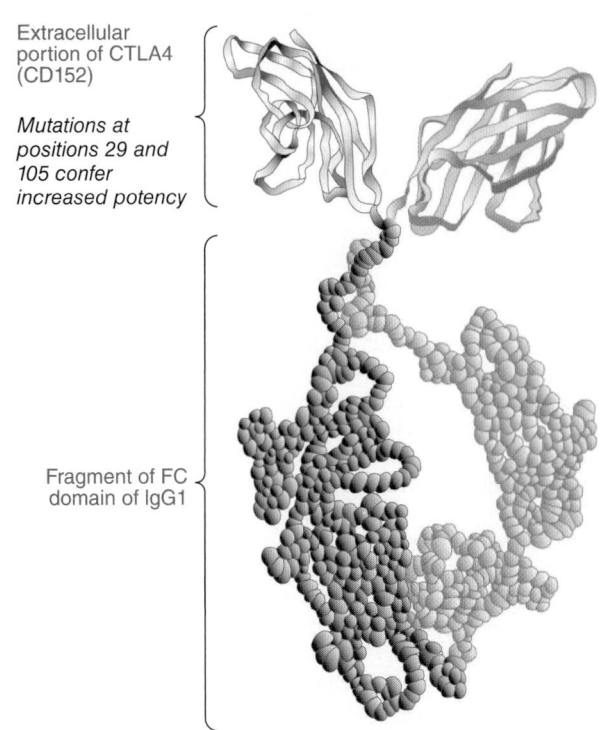

Extracellular portion of CTLA4 (CD152)

Mutations at positions 29 and 105 confer increased potency

Fragment of FC domain of IgG1

Figure 35–5 *Structure of belatacept, a CLTA4-Ig congener.* For details, see the text and Figure 35–4.

belatacept-treated patients compared to cyclosporine. Patients were induced with basiliximab and maintained on MMF and a prednisone taper. While infusions of belatacept are required relatively frequently early after transplantation, it becomes once/month by the end of the first or third month, depending on the dosage regimen chosen (Masson et al., 2014).

Toxicity. An increased risk of posttransplant lymphoproliferative disorder in Epstein-Barr virus seronegative patients has been observed with *belatacept* treatment. Hence, its use is restricted to Epstein-Barr virus seropositive patients. Infusion-related reactions occur infrequently, and the drug is generally well tolerated (Masson et al., 2014).

Drug Interactions. No specific pharmacokinetic drug-drug interactions have been reported with belatacept (Pestana et al., 2012).

General Approach to Treatment of Autoimmune Diseases

Genome-wide association scans have clearly clustered genetic variants around a group of diseases that appear to be mediated by autoimmune responses (Farh et al., 2015). Therapeutically, these diseases respond well to immunosuppression and the use of mAbs directed against cytokine pathways. However, these genetic investigations have revealed that a risk variant in one disease may be protective in another (Maier et al., 2009), consistent with the observation that inhibiting cytokine responses in one disease state, such as anti–TNF-α in rheumatoid arthritis, may lead to flare-ups in another disease (MS).

Anti–IL-2 Receptor (Anti-CD25) Antibodies

Anti–IL-2R mAbs discussed previously have been FDA-approved as a second line drug for patients with MS.

Anti-CD52

Mature lymphocytes express CD52 (CAMPATH-1 antigen), a negatively charged membrane dodecapeptide. *Alemtuzumab,* discussed previously, is a humanized mAb that binds to CD52 and targets the lymphocyte for destruction. In addition to the uses mentioned, alemtuzumab is approved for use in CLL and MS.

Anti-TNF Reagents

Tumor necrosis factor alpha is a pro-inflammatory cytokine that has been implicated in the pathogenesis of several immune-mediated intestinal, skin, and joint diseases. Several diseases (rheumatoid arthritis, Crohn disease) are associated with elevated levels of TNF-α. As a result, a number of anti-TNF agents have been developed as treatments.

Infliximab is a chimeric IgG1 mAb containing a human constant (Fc) region and a murine variable region. It binds with high affinity to TNF-α and prevents the cytokine from binding to its receptors. Infliximab is approved in the U.S. for treating the symptoms of rheumatoid arthritis and is typically used in combination with methotrexate in patients who do not respond to methotrexate alone. Infliximab also is approved for treatment of symptoms of moderate-to-severe Crohn disease in patients who have failed to respond to conventional therapy (see Chapter 51). Other FDA-approved indications include ankylosing spondylitis, plaque psoriasis, psoriatic arthritis, and ulcerative colitis. About 1 in 6 patients receiving infliximab experiences an infusion reaction characterized by fever, urticaria, hypotension, and dyspnea within 1–2 h after antibody administration. The development of antinuclear antibodies, and rarely a lupus-like syndrome, has been reported after treatment with infliximab (Meroni et al., 2015).

Etanercept is a fusion protein that targets TNF-α. Etanercept contains the ligand-binding portion of a human TNF-α receptor fused to the Fc portion of human IgG1 and binds to TNF-α and prevents it from interacting with its receptors. It is approved for treatment of the symptoms of rheumatoid arthritis, ankylosing spondylitis, plaque psoriasis, polyarticular juvenile idiopathic arthritis, and psoriatic arthritis. Etanercept can be used in combination with methotrexate in patients who have not responded adequately to methotrexate alone. Injection-site reactions (i.e., erythema, itching, pain, or swelling) have occurred in more than one-third of etanercept-treated patients.

Adalimumab is another anti-TNF product for intravenous use. This recombinant human IgG1 mAb is approved for use in rheumatoid arthritis, ankylosing spondylitis, Crohn disease, juvenile idiopathic arthritis, plaque psoriasis, psoriatic arthritis, and ulcerative colitis.

Golimumab is a human IgG1 (anti–TNF-α) monoclonal antibody. Golimumab alone or in combination with methotrexate is approved for treatment of moderately to severely active rheumatoid arthritis and active psoriatic arthritis. It is also approved for treatment of patients with ankylosing spondylitis and moderately to severely active ulcerative colitis. Golimumab is administered by subcutaneous injections and is available in 50- and 100-mg doses.

Certolizumab pegol is a humanized pegylated antibody specific to TNF-α. Pegylation of the Fab' fragment provides sustained activity. This agent is approved for the treatment of adults with Crohn disease and rheumatoid arthritis, active psoriatic arthritis, and active ankylosing spondylitis. It is available as 200 mg lyophilized powder or 200-mg/mL prefilled sterile injections for subcutaneous administration.

Toxicity. All anti-TNF agents (i.e., *infliximab, etanercept, adalimumab, golimumab, certolizumab*) increase the risk of serious infections, lymphomas, and other malignancies. For example, fatal hepatosplenic T-cell lymphomas have been reported in adolescent and young adult patients with Crohn disease treated with infliximab in conjunction with azathioprine or 6-MP.

IL-1 Inhibition

Plasma IL-1 levels are increased in patients with active inflammation (see Chapter 34). In addition to the naturally occurring IL-1RA, several IL-1RAs are in development, and a few have been approved for clinical use.

Anakinra is an FDA-approved recombinant, nonglycosylated form of human IL-1RA for the management of joint disease in rheumatoid arthritis. *Anakinra* is also approved for cryopyrin-associated periodic syndromes (CAPS), a group of rare inherited inflammatory diseases associated with overproduction of IL-1 that includes familial cold autoinflammatory and Muckle-Wells syndromes and for treatment of neonatal-onset multisystem inflammatory disease. It can be used alone or in combination with anti-TNF agents such as etanercept, infliximab, or adalimumab.

Canakinumab is an IL-1β mAb that is FDA approved for CAPS and active systemic juvenile idiopathic arthritis. *Canakinumab* is being evaluated for use in chronic obstructive pulmonary disease.

Rilonacept, a fusion protein that binds IL-1, is being evaluated for gout. IL-1 is an inflammatory mediator of joint pain associated with elevated uric acid crystals.

Other Interleukin Antagonists

Tocilizumab, an IL-6R, is FDA-approved for treatment of rheumatoid arthritis and systemic juvenile idiopathic arthritis; *siltuximab*, another IL-6 antagonist, is FDA approved for treatment of multicentric Castleman disease if the patient is HIV and human herpesvirus 8 negative. *Ustekinumab* is a human IL-12 and IL-23 antagonist indicated for the treatment of plaque psoriasis and psoriatic arthritis.

Secukinumab is a human anti-IL-17A antagonist indicated for treatment of plaque psoriasis.

Inhibition of Lymphocyte Function–Associated Antigen

Efalizumab is a humanized IgG1 mAb targeting the CD11a chain of LFA-1. Efalizumab binds to LFA-1 on lymphocytes and prevents LFA-1 interaction with intercellular adhesion molecule (ICAM), thereby inhibiting T-cell adhesion, trafficking, and activation. Efalizumab was approved for use in patients with psoriasis but has been withdrawn from the market because of excessive progressive multifocal leukoencephalopathy (Prater et al., 2014).

Alefacept is a human LFA-3–IgG1 fusion protein. The LFA-3 portion of alefacept binds to CD2 on T lymphocytes, blocking the interaction between LFA-3 and CD2 and interfering with T-cell activation. Alefacept is approved for use in psoriasis. Treatment with alefacept has been shown to produce a dose-dependent reduction in T-effector memory cells (CD45, RO⁺) but not in naïve cells (CD45, RA⁺) (Vincenti and Kirk, 2008). This effect has been related to its efficacy in psoriatic disease and is of significant interest in transplantation because T-effector memory cells are associated with costimulation blockade-resistant and depletional induction-resistant rejection. Alefacept delays rejection in NHP cardiac transplantation and has synergistic potential when used with costimulation blockade or sirolimus-based regimens in NHPs (Vincenti and Kirk, 2008). A phase II multicenter study to assess the safety and efficacy of maintenance therapy with alefacept in kidney transplant recipients showed no difference from placebo controls (Rostaing et al., 2013).

Cytokine Therapy: Interferon

For a description of IFN induction and signaling and the major actions of IFN, see Chapter 34. Interferon-β (IFN-β) was among the first cytokines used for the treatment of autoimmune diseases, particularly MS. IFNs are endogenous regulatory cytokines that increase or decrease transcriptional initiation of hundreds of genes in a cell-dependent fashion with multiple mechanisms of action, including induction of IL-10. The different IFN-β formulations have modest therapeutic efficacy, decreasing the exacerbation rate in MS by approximately 30%. They are relatively safe; fatigue is the major side effect. There are multiple preparations of IFN-β in the market that are administered either by the intramuscular or subcutaneous routes. IFN-β preparations are usually used for MS and IFN-α/γ preparations are used for infections. Three IFN-β preparations are currently on the market: AVONEX and REBIF are 1α formulations for MS; BETASERON, EXTAVIA (1β preparations) and *peginterferon* (1α) are indicated for relapsing MS. There are no significant differences between these IFN preparations, and as more efficacious drugs are now available, they should no longer be considered first-line drugs for the treatment of MS.

Targeting B Cells

Most of the advances in transplantation can be attributed to drugs designed to inhibit T-cell responses. As a result, T-cell–mediated acute rejection has been become much less of a problem, while B-cell–mediated responses such as antibody-mediated rejection and other effects of donor-specific antibodies have become more evident. Both biologicals and small molecules with B-cell–specific effects now are in development for transplantation, including humanized mAbs to CD20 and inhibitors of the two B-cell–activation factors, BLYS and APRIL, and their respective receptors. *Belimumab*, a mAb that targets BLYS, was recently approved for use in patients with systemic lupus erythromatosus.

The CD20 antibodies *rituximab* and *ocrelizumab* deplete circulating mature B lymphocytes (though they may remain to some degree in lymph nodes), and positive results from clinical trials in patients with rheumatoid arthritis and MS strongly suggest that B cells play a critical part in disease pathogenesis. Genetic fine mapping studies demonstrated a potentially pathogenic role of B cells in MS and rheumatoid arthritis that were not limited to antibody production. In particular, a definitive genetic modeling study pointed to the crucial role of B cells as APCs (Farh et al., 2015).

Tolerance

Immunosuppression has concomitant risks of opportunistic infections and secondary tumors. Therefore, the ultimate goal of research on organ transplantation and autoimmune diseases is to induce and maintain immunological tolerance, the active state of antigen-specific nonresponsiveness (Krensky and Clayberger, 1994). Tolerance, if attainable, would represent a true cure for conditions discussed previously in this section without the side effects of the various immunosuppressive therapies. The calcineurin inhibitors prevent tolerance induction in some, but not all, preclinical models. In these same model systems, *sirolimus* does not prevent tolerance and may even promote tolerance (Kawai et al., 2014; Krensky and Clayberger, 1994). In experimental animals, *sirolimus* promotes regulatory T cells, a subtype of T cells shown to suppress all immunity, and promotes tolerance. Studies in kidney transplant recipients showed that *sirolimus* spared regulatory T cells in the periphery, unlike calcineurin inhibitors, which reduced their percentage (Segundo et al., 2006).

Costimulatory Blockade

Inhibition of the costimulatory signal has been shown to induce tolerance (Figure 35–4).

Abatacept is a fusion protein (see previous discussion) that contains the binding region of CTLA4 (CD152), which is a CD28 homolog, and the Fc region of the human IgG1. CTLA4-Ig competitively inhibits CD28 binding to CD80 and CD86 and thus activation of T cells. CTLA4-Ig is effective in the treatment of rheumatoid arthritis in patients resistant to other drugs.

A second costimulatory pathway involves the interaction of CD40 on activated T cells with CD40 ligand (CD154) on B cells, endothelium, or APCs (see Figure 35–4). Among the purported activities of anti-CD154 antibody treatment is the blockade of B7 expression induced by immune activation. Two humanized anti-CD154 mAbs have been used in clinical trials in renal transplantation and autoimmune diseases. The development of these antibodies, however, is on hold because of associated thromboembolic events. An alternative approach to block the CD154-CD40 pathway is to target CD40 with mAbs. These antibodies are undergoing trials in non-Hodgkin lymphoma but are also likely to be developed for autoimmunity and transplantation.

Donor Cell Chimerism

A promising approach is induction of chimerism (coexistence of cells from two genetic lineages in a single individual) by first dampening or eliminating immune function in the recipient with ionizing radiation, drugs such as cyclophosphamide, or antibody treatment and then providing a new source of immune function by adoptive transfer (transfusion) of bone marrow or hematopoietic stem cells. On reconstitution of immune function, the recipient no longer recognizes new antigens provided during a critical period as "nonself." Such tolerance is long lived and less likely to be complicated by the use of calcineurin inhibitors.

Antigens

Specific antigens induce immunological tolerance in preclinical models of diabetes mellitus, arthritis, and MS. In vitro and preclinical in vivo studies demonstrated that one can selectively inhibit immune responses to specific antigens without the associated toxicity of immunosuppressive therapies. With these insights comes the promise of specific immune therapies to treat an array of immune disorders from autoimmunity to transplant rejection (Riedhammer and Weissert, 2015). To date, this approach has only worked in animal models of autoimmune disease.

Soluble HLA

In the precyclosporine era, blood transfusions were shown to be associated with improved outcomes in renal transplant patients. These findings gave rise to donor-specific transfusion protocols that improved outcomes. After the introduction of cyclosporine, however, these effects of blood transfusions disappeared, presumably due to the efficacy of this drug in blocking T-cell activation. Nevertheless, the existence of tolerance-promoting effects of transfusions is irrefutable. It is possible that this effect is due to HLA molecules on the surface of cells or in soluble forms. Soluble HLA and peptides corresponding to linear sequences of HLA molecules can induce immunological tolerance in animal models via a variety of mechanisms (Murphy and Krensky, 1999).

Immunotherapy for Multiple Sclerosis

Clinical Features and Pathology

Multiple sclerosis is a genetically mediated demyelinating inflammatory disease of the CNS white matter, characterized by mononuclear cell infiltration into the white matter with relative demyelination to axonal loss. Dense meningeal infiltrates are found in the subarachnoid spaces of patients, and these infiltrates are intimately associated with subpial demyelination, neuronal and neuritic damage, oligodendrocyte loss, cortical atrophy, and parenchymal microglial activation in the outer cortical layers. Inflammatory cortical demyelination occurs early in MS, preceding the appearance of classic white matter plaques with neurodegenerative changes, including oligodendrocyte loss, reactive astrocytosis, and axonal and neuronal injury within these cortical plaques on a background of inflammation. MS may be episodic or progressive and occurs with prevalence increasing from late adolescence to 35 years of age and then declining. MS is 3-fold more common in females than in males and occurs mainly in higher latitudes of the temperate climates. Epidemiologic studies suggest a role for environmental factors in the pathogenesis of MS, including low vitamin D, smoking, increases in body mass index, and high salt intake (Ransohoff et al., 2015).

Genome-wide association studies have identified genetic variants associated with MS susceptibility (International Multiple Sclerosis Genetics Consortium, et al., 2007), now with 200 variants identified. Although each of these contributes only a small increase in the complex phenotype of disease risk, the biological functions associated with individual allelic variants have been striking. Many of these variants fall within specific signaling cascades, which suggests that alterations in pathways—rather than individual genes—may be useful in predicting response to therapy. Over half of genetic variants associated with MS risk are also found in other putative autoimmune diseases, and risk alleles are primarily associated with genes that regulate immune function. Approximately 60% of probable causal variants mapped to enhancer-like elements, with preferential correspondence to stimulus-dependent CD4+ T-cell enhancers. By overlapping causal single-nucleotide variants with transcription factor–binding maps generated by ENCODE, single-nucleotide variants were strongly enriched within binding sites for immune-related transcription factors (Farh et al., 2015). In patients with MS, there are activated T cells that are reactive to different myelin antigens, including myelin basic protein, and these T cells secrete pro-inflammatory cytokines, whereas in healthy controls, T cells secrete the anti-inflammatory IL-10 cytokine (Cao et al., 2015). It is difficult to vigorously find autoantibodies to myelin antigens in patients with MS, distinguishing MS from other autoimmune diseases.

Attacks are classified by type and severity and likely correspond to specific degrees of CNS damage and pathological processes. Thus, physicians refer to relapsing-remitting MS (the form in 85% of younger patients), secondary progressive MS (progressive neurological deterioration following a long period of relapsing-remitting disease), and primary progressive MS (~15% of patients, wherein deterioration with relatively little inflammation is apparent at onset).

Pharmacotherapy

There have been major advances in the treatment of MS. Table 35-3 summarizes current immunomodulatory therapies for MS. Specific therapies are aimed at resolving acute attacks, reducing recurrences and exacerbations, and slowing the progression of disability. MS exacerbations are treated with 3 to 5 days of 1000 mg of intravenous methylprednisolone, as oral prednisone alone is an ineffective treatment that increases the risk of new attacks. The so-called first-generation (but not necessarily "first-line") drugs include a variety of *IFN-β* (discussed previously in Cytokine Therapy) and random polymers that contain amino acids commonly used as MHC anchors, and TCR contact residues have been proposed as possible "universal altered peptide ligands." Glatiramer acetate (GA), a random-sequence polypeptide consisting of four amino acids (alanine [A], lysine [K], glutamate [E], and tyrosine [Y]) with an average length of 40–100 amino acids, binds efficiently to MHC class II DR molecules in vitro. In clinical trials, GA, administered subcutaneously to patients with relapsing-remitting MS, decreased the rate of exacerbations by about 30%, similar to the efficacy of IFN-β. In vivo administration of GA induces highly cross-reactive CD4⁺ T cells that are immune deviated to secrete anti-inflammatory Th2 cytokines such as IL-4 and IL-13. Administration of GA also prevents the appearance of new lesions detectable by MRI (Duda et al., 2000). This represents one of the first successful uses of an agent that ameliorates autoimmune disease by altering signals through the TCR complex.

The long-term treatment of patients with MS is in transition, having moved from the use of first-era therapies of IFN-β and GA to more effective treatments. The anti-CD20 B cell depletion therapy with *ocrelizumab* is currently the most efficacious treatment (Hauser et al., 2017) and should in most instances be considered as a first line therapy. There is no rationale for the use of step therapy with IFN-β and GA before using the more effective drugs such as ocrelizumab and natalizumab.

The mAb *natalizumab*, directed against the adhesion molecule α_4 integrin, antagonizes interactions with integrin heterodimers containing α_4 integrin, such as $\alpha_4\beta_1$ integrin that is expressed on the surface of activated lymphocytes and monocytes. An interaction of $\alpha_4\beta_1$ integrin with vascular cell adhesion molecule 1 is critical for T-cell trafficking from the periphery into the CNS; blocking this interaction has been highly effective in inhibiting disease exacerbations.

Similarly, the S1P agonist *fingolimod* (mechanism discussed previously) is FDA-approved as a first-line therapy in MS, decreasing the exacerbation rate by about 50%. Use of natalizumab is associated with the development of progressive multifocal leukoencephalopathy, and availability is limited to a special distribution program (Touch) administered by the manufacturer that dictates measurement of JCV antibodies. Patients negative for JCV are often recommended to begin natalizumab, while JCV-positive persons are tested for VZV to evaluate fingolimod treatment. If the result is positive, indicating VZV immunity, fingolimod can be begun. If not, fingolimod treatment should follow VZV immunization. Regarding safety, natalizumab seems to be safe in patients negative for JCV antibody. In patients with cardiac issues—particularly with bundle branch blocks—fingolimod should be avoided.

Dimethyl fumarate appears to have multiple immunomodulatory effects and is an activator of *nrf2* that mediates antioxidative response. In two pivotal phase 3 trials, dimethyl fumarate reduced relapse rates by about 50% as compared with placebo, with a significant reduction of gadolinium-enhanced lesions as well as T2 lesions on MRI. The drug seems to be safe, although gastrointestinal side effects can occasionally cause difficulties.

Monoclonal antibodies directed against CD52 (*alemtuzumab*) were recently approved for relapsing-remitting MS (discussed previously). While it appears to be highly effective and long lived in terms of response, secondary autoimmune responses that emerge in patients with MS but

TABLE 35–3 ■ EFFICACY RANKING OF APPROVED THERAPIES FOR MULTIPLE SCLEROSIS[a]

DRUG	ERA OF DEVELOPMENT	MECHANISM OF ACTION	KEY CONSIDERATIONS
Most effective			
Natalizumab	Second	Monoclonal antibody against integrin α4	Risk of PML must be assessed via presence of JCV antibodies.
Ocrelizumab	Third	mAB against CD20 (B cells)	Low risk PML, slight increase in infections
Alemtuzumab	Third	mAB against CD52	High risk of 2° thyroiditis & other autoimmune disease
Highly effective			
Fingolimod	Second	Sphingosine S1P-R modulator	Cardiac complications preclude use in individuals over the age of 50 and those with history of cardiac disease. VZV antibody testing must be conducted to mitigate risk of disseminated herpes zoster.
Dimethyl fumarate	Third	Immunomodulator	Necessary to monitor lymphocyte count as risk mitigation against PML. GI complications may limit use.
Moderately effective			
IFN-β	First	Immunomodulator	Well-characterized long-term safety and efficacy profiles. Patients should not be required to "fail" before receiving alternative treatments.
Glatiramer acetate	First	Immunomodulator	Best safety profile for pregnant women with mild disease. Patients should not be required to "fail" before receiving alternative treatments.
Teriflunomide	Third	Pyrimidine-synthesis inhibitor	Risk of teratogenicity precludes use in women who are, or intend to become, pregnant.

[a]Rankings are estimated on the basis of clinical trials, postapproval studies, and few head-to-head comparisons. The factors that determine drug efficacy in any individual patient are largely undefined, and good clinical judgment is essential for treatment selection. For details, see Ransohoff et al., 2015.

not in those with CLL are thyroiditis and, more rarely, idiopathic thrombocytopenic purpura. The anti-CD20 antibody *ocrelizumab* has recently completed a phase 3 trial and has the most dramatic efficacy in treating MS, leading to FDA approval. It is now considered a first line drug in the treatment of relapsing remitting MS.

With all of these agents, the earlier in the course of MS that they are used, the more effective they are in preventing disease relapses. What is not clear is whether any of these agents will prevent or diminish the later onset of secondary progressive disease, which causes more severe disability.

Drug Facts for Your Personal Formulary: *Immunosuppressants and Tolerogens*

Drugs	Therapeutic Uses	Clinical Pharmacology and Tips
Glucocorticoids		
• Prednisone The liver converts prednisone to prednisolone.	Prevent and treat transplant rejection, treat GVHD in bone marrow transplant, autoimmune disease, rheumatoid arthritis, ulcerative colitis, multiple sclerosis, systemic lupus erythematosus	• Broad effects on cellular immunity • Affects transcription of many genes; ↓ NF-κB activation, ↓ pro-inflammatory cytokines IL-1 and IL-6 • ↓ T-cell proliferation, cytotoxic T-lymphocyte activation and neutrophil and monocyte function • Can cause ↑ blood glucose, hypertension, Cushingoid habitus, ↑ weight, ↑ risk of infection, osteoporosis, glaucoma, cataracts, depression, anxiety, psychosis • Long-term treatment ⇒ adrenal suppression; withdraw slowly on alternate days
• Prednisolone	Rheumatoid arthritis, uveitis, ulcerative colitis, multiple sclerosis, vasculitis, sarcoidosis, systemic lupus erythematosus	• As above
• Methylprednisolone	Systemic lupus erythematosus, multiple sclerosis	• As above
• Dexamethasone	Rheumatoid arthritis, idiopathic thrombocytopenic purpura	• As above
Calcineurin Inhibitors		
• Cyclosporine	Transplant rejection prophylaxis, transplant rejection rescue therapy, rheumatoid arthritis, psoriasis and other skin diseases, xerophthalmia	• Use algorithms to delay dosing until renal function OK in kidney transplant patients • Monitor C_p to avoid side effects • Side effects: tremor, hallucinations, drowsiness, coma, nephrotoxicity, hypertension, hirsutism, hyperlipidemia, gum hyperplasia • Metabolized by CYP3A ⇒ drug interactions • Severe interactions with antiarrhythmics
• Tacrolimus	Transplant rejection prophylaxis, transplant rejection rescue therapy	• GI absorption is incomplete and variable • Side effects include nephrotoxicity, neurotoxicity, GI complaints, and hypertension • Glucose intolerance and diabetes mellitus • Monitor blood levels to avoid nephrotoxicity
Antiproliferative and Antimetabolic Agents		
• Azathioprine	Purine metabolism inhibitor, adjunct for prevention of organ transplant rejection, rheumatoid arthritis	• Renal clearance has little effect on efficacy or toxicity • Side effects include bone marrow suppression (leukopenia > thrombocytopenia > anemia) • Susceptibility to infections, hepatotoxicity, alopecia, GI toxicity • Avoid allopurinol
• Mycophenolate mofetil	Purine metabolism inhibitor, prophylaxis of transplant rejection, used off label for systemic lupus erythematosus, multiple sclerosis, sarcoidosis	• Side effects include GI (diarrhea and vomiting) and hematologic (leukopenia, pure red cell aplasia) problems • Contraindicated in pregnancy
• Sirolimus	mTOR inhibitor, prophylaxis of organ transplant rejection, incorporated into stents to inhibit occlusion	• Monitor blood levels • Hyperlipidemia • Anemia, leukopenia, thrombocytopenia • GI effects, mouth ulcers, hyperkalemia • Anticancer effects • Metabolized by CYP3A; requires close attention to drug interactions
• Everolimus	mTOR inhibitor, astrocytoma, breast cancer, kidney and liver transplant reception prophylaxis, pancreatic neuroendocrine tumor, renal angiomyolipoma, renal cell cancer	• Pharmacokinetics distinct from sirolimus • Toxicity similar to sirolimus
• Temsirolimus	mTOR inhibitor	
T-cell costimulatory blocker		
• Belatacept	Prevention of renal transplant rejection	• Due to an increased risk of post-transplant lymphoproliferative disorder predominantly involving the CNS, progressive multifocal leukoencephalopathy, and serious CNS infections, administration of higher than the recommended doses or more frequent dosing is NOT recommended.

Drug Facts for Your Personal Formulary: *Immunosuppressants and Tolerogens* (*continued*)

Drugs	Therapeutic Uses	Clinical Pharmacology and Tips
Antibodies		
Antilymphocyte globulin • ATGAM • Thymoglobulin	Prevention and treatment of organ transplant rejection, aplastic anemia	• Contains antibodies against numerous T-cell surface molecules • Can elicit fever, chills, and potentially hypotension; use premedication: steroid/acetaminophen/antihistamine • Serum sickness, glomerulonephritis, anaphylaxis: rare • Watch for leukopenia, thrombocytopenia
Muromonab-CD3	In trials for autoimmune diseases	• Depletes CD3-positive cells
Anti-CD25 ***(anti–IL-2 receptor*** ***antibodies)*** • Basailixmab • Daclizumab	Prophylaxis of acute organ transplant rejection, multiple sclerosis (in clinical trial)	• β Adrenergic blocking effects (worsening of heart failure and bronchospasm) • Block T-cell activation • Do not deplete • Good safety profile
• Abetacept • Belatacept	Prophylaxis of organ transplant rejection, autoimmunity trials	• CTLA4-Ig fusion protein • Risk for posttransplant lymphoproliferative disorder
Anti-CD52 • Alemtuzumab	Chronic lymphocytic leukemia, multiple sclerosis, prevention and treatment of transplant rejection	• Prolonged lymphocyte depletion (neutropenia, thrombocytopenia as side effects) • Secondary autoimmunity
Anti-CD154 (CD40 ligand)	Renal transplantation, autoimmune diseases	• Blockade of B7 protein expression • On hold due to thromboembolic events
Anti-CD20 • Rituximab • Ocrelizumab	Rheumatoid arthritis, multiple sclerosis	• Deplete circulating mature B lymphocytes
Anti-TNF • Infliximab • Etanercept • Adalimumab • Golimumab • Certolizumab	Rheumatoid arthritis, Crohn disease, ankylosing spondylitis, plaque psoriasis, psoriatic arthritis, ulcerative colitis	• Infusion reaction with fever, urticaria, hypotension, and dyspnea can occur • Risk of serious infections, lymphoma, other malignancies
Anti–IL-1 • Anakinra • Canakininumab • Rilonacept	Rheumatoid arthritis, cryopyrin-associated syndromes, evaluated in gout	
Anti–LFA-1 • Efalizumab	Psoriasis	• Withdrawn: excessive progressive multifocal leukoencephalopathy
Anti-CD2 • Alefacept	Psoriasis	
• Belimumab (anti-BLYS)	Systemic lupus erythematosus	
Anti-VLA-4 • Natalizumab	Multiple sclerosis, Crohn disease	• Targets α-4 integrin blocking T-cell traffic to organ • Progressive multifocal leukoencephalopathy
Therapy for MS (Table 35–2 Summarizes More Detailed Therapies for MS.)		
• Ocrelizumab • Natalizumab • Alemtuzumab	Multiple sclerosis	• β cell depleting. First line drug. Highly efficacious. • Anti-VLA-4, blocks T cell traffic. Very efficacious. • Anti-CD52. Highly efficacious. Second line drug due to side effects.
• IFN-β	Multiple sclerosis	• Modest efficacy but safe • No longer first-line drug
• Fingolomod	Multiple sclerosis	• S1P-R agonist • Potential cardiac complications
• Tecfidera	Multiple sclerosis	• Monitor WBCs; slight risk of progressive multifocal leukoencephalopathy
• Glatiramer acetate	Multiple sclerosis	• Potentially safe in pregnancy but less efficacious
• Teriflunomide	Multiple sclerosis	• Pyrimidine-synthesis inhibitor; pregnancy risk

WBCs, white blood cells

Bibliography

Alberú J, et al. Lower malignancy rates in renal allograft recipients converted to sirolimus-based, calcineurin inhibitor-free immunotherapy: 24-month results from the CONVERT trial. *Transplantation,* **2011,** *92:*303–310.

Azzi JR, et al. Calcineurin inhibitors: 40 years later, can't live without. *J Immunol,* **2013,** *191:*5785–5791.

Baldo BA. Chimeric fusion proteins used for therapy: indications, mechanisms, and safety. *Drug Saf,* **2015,** *38:*455–479.

Beck RW, et al. A randomized controlled trial of corticosteroids in the treatment of acute optic neuritis. The Optic Neuritis Group. *N Engl J Med,* **1992,** *326:*581–588.

Bergmann TK, et al. Clinical pharmacokinetics and pharmacodynamics of prednisolone and prednisone in solid organ transplantation. *Clin Pharmacokinet,* **2012,** *51:*711–741.

Brennan DC, et al, and The Thymoglobulin Induction Study Group. Rabbit antithymocyte globulin versus basiliximab in renal transplantation. *N Engl J Med,* **2006,** *355:*1967–1977.

Budde K, et al. Everolimus-based, calcineurin-inhibitor-free regimen in recipients of de-novo kidney transplants: an open-label, randomised, controlled trial. *Lancet,* **2011,** *377:*837–847.

Callahan MK, et al. Targeting T cell co-receptors for cancer therapy. *Immunity,* **2016,** 44:1079–1078.

CAMMS223 Investigators, et al. Alemtuzumab vs. interferon beta-1a in early multiple sclerosis. *N Engl J Med,* **2008,** *359:*1786–1801.

Cao Y, et al. Functional inflammatory profiles distinguish myelin-reactive T cells from patients with multiple sclerosis. *Sci Transl Med,* **2015,** *7:*287ra274.

Chan K, et al. Kidney transplantation with minimized maintenance: alemtuzumab induction with tacrolimus monotherapy—an open label, randomized trial. *Transplantation,* **2011,** *92:*774–780.

Chinen J, et al. Advances in basic and clinical immunology in 2014. *J Allergy Clin Immunol,* **2015,** *135:*1132–1141.

Colombo D, Ammirati E. Cyclosporine in transplantation—a history of converging timelines. *J Biol Regul Homeost Agents,* **2011,** *25:* 493–504.

D'Amico E, et al. A critical appraisal of daclizumab use as emerging therapy in multiple sclerosis. *Expert Opin Drug Saf,* **2015,** *14:*1157–1168.

Danovitch GM, et al. Immunosuppression of the elderly kidney transplant recipient. *Transplantation,* **2007,** *84:*285–291.

Darji P, et al. Conversion from mycophenolate mofetil to enteric-coated mycophenolate sodium in renal transplant recipients with gastrointestinal tract disorders. *Transplant Proc,* **2008,** *40:*2262–2267.

Duda PW, et al. Glatiramer acetate (Copaxone) induces degenerate, Th2-polarized immune responses in patients with multiple sclerosis. *J Clin Invest,* **2000,** *105:*967–976.

Ekberg H, et al. Reduced exposure to calcineurin inhibitors in renal transplantation. *N Engl J Med,* **2007,** *357:*2562–2575.

Euvrard S, et al. Sirolimus and secondary skin-cancer prevention in kidney transplantation. *N Engl J Med,* **2012,** *367:*329–339.

Farh KK, et al. Genetic and epigenetic fine mapping of causal autoimmune disease variants. *Nature,* **2015,** *518:*337–343.

Goldfarb-Rumyantzev AS, et al. Role of maintenance immunosuppressive regimen in kidney transplant outcome. *Clin J Am Soc Nephrol,* **2006,** *1:*563–574.

Goring SM, et al. A network meta-analysis of the efficacy of belatacept, cyclosporine and tacrolimus for immunosuppression therapy in adult renal transplant recipients. *Curr Med Res Opin,* **2014,** *30:*1473–1487.

Guerra G, et al. Randomized trial of immunosuppressive regimens in renal transplantation. *J Am Soc Nephrol,* **2011,** *22:*1758–1768.

Hardinger KL, et al. Selection of induction therapy in kidney transplantation. *Transpl Int,* **2013,** *26:*662–672.

Hauser SL et al, and The OPERA I and OPERA II Clinical Investigators. Ocrelizumab versus Interferon Beta-1a in Relapsing Multiple Sclerosis. *N Engl J Med,* **2017,** *376:*221–234.

International Multiple Sclerosis Genetics Consortium, et al. Risk alleles for multiple sclerosis identified by a genomewide study. *N Engl J Med,* **2007,** *357:*851–862.

Jones JL, Coles AJ. Mode of action and clinical studies with alemtuzumab. *Exp Neurol,* **2014,** *262*(pt A):37–43.

Kappos KG, et al. Wide-QRS-complex tachycardia with a negative concordance pattern in the precordial leads: are the ECG criteria always reliable? *Pacing Clin Electrophysiol,* **2006,** *29:*63–66.

Kawai T, et al. Tolerance: one transplant for life. *Transplantation,* **2014,** *98:*117–121.

Krensky AM, Clayberger C. Prospects for induction of tolerance in renal transplantation. *Pediatr Nephrol,* **1994,** *8:*772–779.

Krensky AM, et al. T-lymphocyte-antigen interactions in transplant rejection. *N Engl J Med,* **1990,** *322:*510–517.

Maier LM, et al. IL2RA genetic heterogeneity in multiple sclerosis and type 1 diabetes susceptibility and soluble interleukin-2 receptor production. *PLoS Genet,* **2009,** *5:*e1000322.

Masson P, et al. Belatacept for kidney transplant recipients. *Cochrane Database Syst Rev,* **2014,** (11):CD010699.

Meroni PL, et al. New strategies to address the pharmacodynamics and pharmacokinetics of tumor necrosis factor (TNF) inhibitors: a systematic analysis. *Autoimmunol Rev,* **2015,** *14:*812–829.

Moes DJ, et al. Sirolimus and everolimus in kidney transplantation. *Drug Discov Today,* **2015,** *20:*1243–1249.

Molnar AO, et al. Generic immunosuppression in solid organ transplantation: systematic review and meta-analysis. *BMJ,* **2015,** *350:*h3163.

Murphy B, Krensky AM. HLA-derived peptides as novel immunomodulatory therapeutics. *J Am Soc Nephrol,* **1999,** *10:*1346–1355.

Nashan B. Antibody induction therapy in renal transplant patients receiving calcineurin-inhibitor immunosuppressive regimens: a comparative review. *BioDrugs,* **2005,** *19:*39–46.

Pelletier D, Hafler DA. Fingolimod for multiple sclerosis. *N Engl J Med,* **2012,** *366:*339–347.

Pestana JO, et al. Three-year outcomes from BENEFIT-EXT: a phase III study of belatacept versus cyclosporine in recipients of extended criteria donor kidneys. *Am J Transplant,* **2012,** *12:*630–639.

Polman CH, et al. A randomized, placebo-controlled trial of natalizumab for relapsing multiple sclerosis. *N Engl J Med,* **2006,** *354:*899–910.

Prater EF, et al. A retrospective analysis of 72 patients on prior efalizumab subsequent to the time of voluntary market withdrawal in 2009. *J Drugs Dermatol,* **2014,** *13:*712–718.

Ransohoff RM, et al. Multiple sclerosis-a quiet revolution. *Nat Rev Neurol,* **2015,** *11:*134–142.

Riedhammer C, Weissert R. Antigen presentation, autoantigens, and immune regulation in multiple sclerosis and other autoimmune diseases. *Front Immunol,* **2015,** *6:*322.

Riella LV, Sayegh MH. T-cell co-stimulatory blockade in transplantation: two steps forward one step back! *Expert Opin Biol Ther,* **2013,** *13:*1557–1568.

Rostaing L, et al. Alefacept combined with tacrolimus, mycophenolate mofetil and steroids in de novo kidney transplantation: a randomized controlled trial. *Am J Transplant,* **2013,** *13:*1724–1733.

Satyananda V, Shapiro R. Belatacept in kidney transplantation. *Curr Opin Organ Transplant,* **2014,** *19:*573–577.

Schena FP, et al, and The Sirolimus CONVERT Trial Study Group. Conversion from calcineurin inhibitors to sirolimus maintenance therapy in renal allograft recipients: 24-month efficacy and safety results from the CONVERT trial. *Transplantation,* **2009,** *87:*233–242.

Segundo DS, et al. Calcineurin inhibitors, but not rapamycin, reduce percentages of CD4$^+$CD25$^+$FOXP3$^+$ regulatory T cells in renal transplant recipients. *Transplantation,* **2006,** *82:*550–557.

Sureshkumar KK, et al. Influence of induction modality on the outcome of deceased donor kidney transplant recipients discharged on steroid-free maintenance immunosuppression. *Transplantation,* **2012,** *93:*799–805.

Talawila N, Pengel LH. Does belatacept improve outcomes for kidney transplant recipients? A systematic review. *Transpl Int,* **2015,** *28:*1251–1264.

Thiyagarajan UM, et al. Thymoglobulin and its use in renal transplantation: a review. *Am J Nephrol,* **2013,** *37:*586–601.

Topalian SL, et al. Immune checkpoint blockade: a common denominator approach to cancer therapy. *Cancer Cell,* **2015,** *4:*450–461.

Verghese PS, et al. Calcineurin inhibitors in HLA-identical living related donor kidney transplantation. *Nephrol Dial Transplant,* **2014,** *29:*209–218.

Vincenti F, Kirk AD. What's next in the pipeline. *Am J Transplant,* **2008,** *8:*1972–1981.

Vincenti F, et al. A randomized, multicenter study of steroid avoidance, early steroid withdrawal or standard steroid therapy in kidney transplant recipients. *Am J Transplant,* **2008,** *8:*307–316.

Immune Globulins and Vaccines

Roberto Tinoco and James E. Crowe, Jr.

Historical Perspective

The historical impact of infectious diseases is evident in the high mortality rates in young children and adults and the disruption that these diseases have caused in emerging societies. The rise of civilization in conjunction with the domestication of plants and animals permitted people to live in denser communities with each other and with their animals. Such proximity provided ideal breeding grounds for infectious pathogens, and their spread resulted in epidemics throughout the world. As people began to question the underlying causes of disease and the apparent protection to reinfection afforded to some survivors of a disease, ideas of immunity and disease prevention were born, apparently as early as the 5th century.

The concept of immunity goes back at least to the 17th century when emperor K'ang of China documented his practice of variolation, or inoculation, of his troops and his own children with smallpox to confer protection from the disease (Hopkins, 2002). Variolation involved taking liquid from a smallpox pustule of an infected patient, cutting the skin of an uninfected person, and then introducing the inoculum. Records from the 18th century note that Africans brought to the U.S. as slaves bore scars from smallpox variolation and were under the belief that they were immune to the disease. Variolation against smallpox was also reported by Lady Mary Montagu during her time in Constantinople (1716–1718). Lady Montagu, herself a survivor of smallpox, reported that certain Turkish women would open a wound in healthy individuals and introduce the contents of a smallpox vesicle with a large needle, thereby providing a level of protection against smallpox. About 2%–3% died after variolation, whereas 20%–30% died from natural infection. Lady Montagu had herself and a son variolated and later had a daughter successfully variolated in London under the auspices of physicians of the Royal Society. Positive outcomes notwithstanding, fear of the procedure persisted.

Around the same time, in Boston, Cotton Mather and Dr. Zabdiel Boylston began a program of variolation against smallpox. The program met with general success but was opposed by many physicians, fearful that inoculation spread the disease and worried by deaths after inoculation (~2% of those inoculated). One Puritan religious leader, Edmund Massey, preached against inoculation, quoting from the book of Job (Job 2:7: "So Satan went forth from the presence of the Lord and smote Job with sore boils.") and arguing that Satan was the prime practitioner of inoculation and that such diseases as smallpox were a necessary trial of faith or punishment for sins, the fear of which "is a happy restraint upon many people" (Gross and Sepkowitz, 1998). Medical practice in Boston has come a long way since that time.

In 1796, Edward Jenner, who coined the term *vaccination*, from *vacca*, Latin for "cow," helped to advance vaccine safety. He tested the hypothesis that smallpox protection could be achieved by using cowpox, a nonfatal, self-limited disease in humans caused by a virus of the Poxviridae family that includes monkeypox and smallpox and that can spread from cows to

Abbreviations

ACIP: Advisory Committee on Immunization Practices
ADCC: antibody-dependent cell-mediated cytotoxicity
AID: activation-induced cytidine deaminase
aP: acellular pertussis
APC: antigen-presenting cell
ASD: autism spectrum disorder
AVA: anthrax vaccine adsorbed
BCG: bacille Calmette-Guérin
BCR: B cell receptor
CDC: Centers for Disease Control and Prevention
CoP: correlate of protection
CRM: cross-reactive material
DTaP: diphtheria and tetanus toxoids and acellular pertussis
DTP: diphtheria and tetanus toxoids and pertussis
EMA: European Medicines Agency
Fab: fragment, antigen-binding
Fc: fragment crystallizable
GBS: Guillian-Barré syndrome
H1N1: hemagglutinin type 1 and neuraminidase type 1
H2N2: hemagglutinin type 2 and neuraminidase type 2
H3N2: hemagglutinin type 3 and neuraminidase type 2
HA: hemagglutinin
HbOC: *Haemophilus influenzae* type b oligosaccharide conjugate
Hib: *Haemophilus influenzae* type b
HIV: human immunodeficiency virus
HPV: human papillomavirus
IgG: immunoglobulin, class G
IIV: inactivated influenza vaccine
IOM: Institute of Medicine
IPV: inactivated poliovirus (vaccine)
JE: Japanese encephalitis
JE-MB: Japanese encephalitis mouse brain
JE-VC: Japanese encephalitis Vero cell
mCoP: mechanistic correlates of protection
MCV4: meningococcal vaccine 4
MeV: measles virus
MMR: measles-mumps-rubella
MMRV: measles-mumps-rubella-varicella
MVA: modified vaccinia Ankara
NA: neuraminidase
nCoP: nonmechanistic correlates of protection
PCV13: pneumococcal conjugate vaccine 13 valent
PRP: polyribosylribitol phosphate
PRP-OMPC: polyribosylribitol phosphate outer membrane protein conjugate
PRP-T: polyribosylribitol phosphate tetanus
RAG: recombination-activating gene
RSV: respiratory syncytial virus
SAE: serious adverse event
SAGE: Strategic Advisory Group of Experts
SIDS: sudden infant death syndrome
TB: *Mycobacterium tuberculosis*
Td: tetanus toxoid and reduced diphtheria toxoid
Tdap: tetanus toxoid, reduced diphtheria toxoid, acellular pertussis
VDJ: variable, diversity, joining
VLP: virus-like particle
VZV: varicella zoster virus
WHO: World Health Organization

humans. Jenner infected a boy with cowpox pus from an infected milkmaid; the boy got mildly ill from cowpox, recovered, and when challenged with smallpox collected from scabs of a smallpox patient, was unaffected, showed no symptoms, and was fully protected against the disease. Thus, it was possible to inoculate against a disease using material from a related but less-harmful disease.

By the early to mid-19th century, vaccination was accepted widely, and governments in the U.S. and Europe began to require vaccination of children. As in our own era, there was organized resistance from antivaccination groups. There was also a sense that immunity waned with time, and revaccinations were introduced, producing a sustained diminution of smallpox.

The work of Pasteur and Koch established a link between microorganisms and disease and provided the scientific understanding to develop more specific vaccines. Preservatives (glycerol was an early additive) and refrigeration increased shelf life of vaccines and permitted their wider distribution. The cells of the immune system began to be identified around 1890, followed by the discovery of antibodies and hyperimmune serum and demonstration of the efficacy of adjuvants (aluminum was the first) to increase immunogenicity (Marrack et al., 2009). In the 1950s, freeze-drying became standard, permitting worldwide distribution of purified vaccines. Through the coordinating efforts of the WHO, smallpox was declared "eliminated" in 1979.

Other scourges were attacked by vaccination in the mid-20th century. One was polio, an incurable neurological disease causing muscle wasting, paralysis, and death if the diaphragm is affected. In 1955, Jonas Salk released a vaccine against poliovirus. The Salk vaccine, an inactivated virus preparation administered by injection, was followed in 1961 by the Sabin oral vaccine, which employs an attenuated poliovirus that provides immunity to all three types of poliovirus. As a result of the polio vaccines, the annual number of cases in the U.S. fell to 161 in 1961 from 35,000 in 1955 (Hinman, 1984). Eradication of polio depends on interruption of person-to-person transmission, which requires that a high percentage of the susceptible population be inoculated. Most adults in developed countries are immune, but when a significant fraction of children is unvaccinated, there is the potential for an outbreak because wild polioviruses circulate.

These fundamental observations and experiments paved the way for the modern vaccines that have reduced mortality and morbidity rates from infectious pathogens across the globe. Modern laboratory technologies have rendered vaccines safe and highly effective against infectious pathogens and virus-transforming cancers and against neoantigens on cancerous cells. Vaccination strategies are a public health success, as shown by the complete worldwide eradication of smallpox and the elimination of polio in the Americas in 1994, Europe in 2002, and South-East Asia in 2014, with remaining endemic cases only in Pakistan, Afghanistan, and Nigeria in 2016 according to WHO. In 2016, WHO and the Pan American Health Organization declared the Americas free of endemic measles, credited to immunization campaigns. The current recommendations for childhood vaccinations are summarized in Table 36–1. The issue of nonvaccinators is presented further in the chapter.

Vaccination Induces Development of Immunological Memory

The hallmarks of an immune response to pathogens are the recognition and activation of the innate immune response that limits pathogen spread when microbes breach the host's natural protective barriers, such as the skin, the respiratory epithelium, or the GI epithelium. If the pathogen is not controlled, the innate immune system then recruits the humoral (antibody-secreting B cell) and cellular (T cell) arms of the adaptive immune response to specifically target and destroy the invading pathogen. Once the microbe is eliminated during this primary response, small numbers of pathogen-specific B and T cells survive long term, sometimes

TABLE 36–1 ■ RECOMMENDED IMMUNIZATION SCHEDULE FOR CHILDREN AND ADOLESCENTS AGED 18 YEARS OR YOUNGER, U.S., 2017.

Vaccine	Birth	1 mo	2 mos	4 mos	6 mos	9 mos	12 mos	15 mos	18 mos	19-23 mos	2-3 yrs	4-6 yrs	7-10 yrs	11-12 yrs	13-15 yrs	16 yrs	17-18 yrs
Hepatitis B (HepB)	1st dose	←----- 2nd dose ----→			←-------------------- 3rd dose --------------------→												
Rotavirus (RV) RV1 (2-dose series); RV5 (3-dose series)			1st dose	2nd dose	See footnote												
Diphtheria, tetanus, & acellular pertussis(DTaP: <7 yrs)			1st dose	2nd dose	3rd dose		←------- 4th dose -------→					5th dose					
Haemophilus influenzae type b (Hib)			1st dose	2nd dose	See footnote		←-- 3rd or 4th dose, See footnote --→										
Pneumococcal conjugate (PCV13)			1st dose	2nd dose	3rd dose		←------- 4th dose -------→										
Inactivated poliovirus (IPV: <18 yrs)			1st dose	2nd dose	←-------------------- 3rd dose --------------------→							4th dose					
Influenza (IIV)					←------------------ Annual vaccination (IIV) 1 or 2 doses ------------------→								Annual vaccination (IIV) 1 dose only				
Measles, mumps, rubella (MMR)							←------- 1st dose -------→					2nd dose					
Varicella(VAR)							←------- 1st dose -------→					2nd dose					
Hepatitis A (HepA)							←------- 2-dose series, See footnote -------→										
Meningococcal(Hib-MenCY ≥6 weeks; MenACWY-D≥9 mos; MenACWY-CRM ≥2 mos)							←---------------------------- See footnote ----------------------------→							1st dose		2nd dose	
Tetanus, diphtheria, & acellular pertussis(Tdap:≥7 yrs)														Tdap			
Human papillomavirus (HPV)													See footnote	See footnote			
Meningococcal B															See footnote		
Pneumococcal polysaccharide (PPSV23)											See footnote						

Legend:
- Range of recommended ages for all children
- Range of recommended ages for catch-up immunization
- Range of recommended ages for certain high-risk groups
- Range of recommended ages for non-high-risk groups that may receive vaccine, subject to individual clinical decision making
- No recommendation

These recommendations are reprinted from the website of the Centers for Disease Control and Prevention (CDC) and should be read with the footnotes provided on the CDC website: https://www.cdc.gov/vaccines/schedules/. For those who fall behind or start late, provide catch-up vaccination at the earliest opportunity as indicated by the green bars. To determine minimum intervals between doses, see the catch-up schedule on the CDC website. School entry and adolescent vaccine age groups are shaded in gray.

for the entire life of the host, as *memory B and T cells*. These memory cells confer host protection against reinfection with the same pathogen. During a second response, memory cells use their specific antigen receptors to recognize the invading pathogen. This results in their activation and expansion to directly kill infected cells (via T cells) or generate antibodies (via B cells) that will neutralize the pathogen.

Vaccination technology takes advantage of this paradigm. As a means of generating immunological memory, uninfected individuals are given a controlled infection or exposed to antigen that elicits an immune response. When these vaccinated individuals are subsequently infected with these pathogens in their environment, the responses of their memory T and B cells outpace the invading microbes to neutralize and prevent their spread in a much more rapid and greater magnitude secondary response.

B cell clonal expansion results in the differentiation of long-lived memory B cells and emergence of shorter-lived plasma cells that produce antibodies. During the primary response, following the vaccination, B cells will undergo this differentiation process and will initially secrete IgM antibodies. IgM antibodies are large and provide some protection. Days after the response is initiated, B cells will undergo clonal selection and will produce IgG, which is a higher-affinity antibody with enhanced pathogen neutralization capacity.

Differentiated plasma cells can also produce other antibody classes, such as IgA, IgD, and IgE, that have unique functions. IgD can be expressed on the surface of B cells; its function continues to be investigated. IgA antibodies are concentrated in mucous secretions, breast milk, and tears. IgE antibodies are important in the elimination of parasitic infections. *Because IgG antibodies have undergone a selection process that increases their affinity, these antibody types are the targets of vaccine design.* Secondary responses after vaccination therefore elicit a faster and larger B-cell response, and these B cells primarily make IgG antibodies (Clem, 2011).

Cellular immunity involving both CD4+ and CD8+ T cells is also a target of vaccine design. Unlike B cells, T cells target intracellular pathogens that have infected host cells. CD4+ T cells or helper T cells, stimulate B cells to produce antibody. CD8+ T cells kill infected cells. Like B cells, antigen-memory T cells survive long term and provide protection for future encounters with their specific antigen.

Immunization Strategies

Immunity can be achieved from either passive or active methods involving exposure to natural infection or through artificial human-made antigens. Individuals can develop antibodies from natural infection or after vaccination.

Passive

Passive immunity involves the transfer of preformed antibodies from an immune individual to a nonimmune individual to confer temporary immunity. An example of passive natural immunity is the transfer of antibodies from mother to fetus during pregnancy and through breast milk and colostrum consumed by an infant. These antibodies enter the body and provide a first line of defense to the fetus or infant, which otherwise has no immunity to any pathogen.

An example of *artificial passive immunization* is the injection of antivenom antibodies. Animals are immunized with venom antigen and their hyperimmunized serum is transfused into the patient. Antivenom can be monovalent, effective against one type of venom, or polyvalent and effective against venom from multiple species. An antivenom binds and neutralizes a toxin. Early administration after injury is critical because antivenom can halt but not reverse venom damage. Even though antivenom is purified, trace proteins remain, and these can trigger anaphylaxis or serum sickness in patients. Most antivenoms are administered intravenously but can also be injected intramuscularly against stonefish and redback spider venom. Antivenoms have been developed against venomous spiders, acarids, insects, scorpions, marine animals, and snakes. Passive immunization is used for a variety

TABLE 36–2 ■ AVAILABLE IMMUNE GLOBULINS
Human intravenous immune globulin
Human subcutaneous immune globulin
Human hyperimmune globulins
Anthrax immune globulin, intravenous
Botulism immune globulin, intravenous
Cytomegalovirus immune globulin, intravenous
Hepatitis B immune globulin, intravenous
Rho(D) immune globulin, intravenous
Vaccinia immune globulin, intravenous
Varicella zoster immune globulin
Animal-derived immune globulin products
Equine
Lymphocyte immune globulin, antithymocyte globulin
Centruroides (scorpion) immune F(ab')$_2$ injection
Crotalidae immune F(ab')$_2$
Black widow spider antivenin
Botulism antitoxin bivalent types A and B
Botulism antitoxin heptavalent (A, B, C, D, E, F, G)
Ovine
Crotalidae polyvalent immune Fab
Digoxin immune Fab
Rabbit
Antithymocyte globulin

of toxins and infections; a list of available immunoglobulins is shown in Table 36–2.

Active

A natural infection that stimulates the immune response in uninfected individuals may lead to development of immunological memory and protection from reinfection, as in the case of infection with the MeV. This only occurs if the individual survives the primary infection, which is not always the case for viruses like measles, influenza, or ebola. Active immunization through injection of artificial antigens elicits a controlled immune response leading to the generation of immunological memory. This type of immunization, compared to natural infection, does not cause infectious disease or compromise the life of the individual. Thus, vaccine technologies through active stimulation of the immune system ensure that the individual survives and has protection against the pathogen in the natural environment.

Vaccine Types

Advanced technologies are currently used to generate vaccines to prevent many infectious diseases and to deter infectious pathogens that cause cancer such as hepatitis viruses that can lead to hepatocellular carcinoma and HPVs, which can cause cervical, anal, vaginal, and penile cancers. Effective vaccines activate both the innate and the adaptive immune systems. There are many different types of vaccines, each with advantages and disadvantages. Vaccine design involves an understanding of the nature of the microbe, the tropism of the pathogen, and the practical need in certain regions of the world. The following section summarizes current methods used in vaccine design. For a list of vaccines approved by the U.S. Food and Drug Administration, see Table 36–3.

Live Attenuated

Live attenuated vaccines use a weakened form of a virus that contains antigens that appropriately stimulate an immune response. Such viruses have been passaged to reduce their virulence but retain immunogenic antigens that elicit strong humoral and cellular responses and the development of memory cells after one or two doses. A virus, for example, can be isolated

TABLE 36-3 ■ APPROVED VACCINES IN THE U.S.

Toxoids

Tetanus and diphtheria toxoids adsorbed for adult use

Tetanus toxoid adsorbed

Tetanus toxoid, reduced diphtheria toxoid and acellular pertussis vaccine, adsorbed

Bacterial polysaccharide

Meningococcal polysaccharide vaccine, groups A, C, Y, and W-135 combined

Pneumococcal vaccine, polyvalent

Typhoid Vi polysaccharide vaccine

Bacterial conjugate vaccines

Haemophilus b conjugate vaccine (meningococcal protein conjugate)

Haemophilus b conjugate vaccine (tetanus toxoid conjugate)

Pneumococcal 7-valent conjugate vaccine (diphtheria CRM_{197} protein)

Pneumococcal 13-valent conjugate vaccine (diphtheria CRM_{197} protein)

Meningococcal (groups A, C, Y, and W-135) oligosaccharide diphtheria CRM_{197} conjugate vaccine

Meningococcal groups C and Y and *Haemophilus* b tetanus toxoid conjugate vaccine

Meningococcal (groups A, C, Y, and W-135) polysaccharide diphtheria toxoid conjugate vaccine

Meningococcal group B vaccine

Live bacterial

BCG live

Typhoid vaccine live oral Ty21a

Cholera vaccine live oral

Inactivated bacterial

Plague vaccine

Live Viral

Measles and mumps virus vaccine, live

Measles, mumps, and rubella virus vaccine, live

Measles, mumps, rubella and varicella virus vaccine, live

Varicella virus vaccine, live

Zoster vaccine, live

Rotavirus vaccine, live, oral

Rotavirus vaccine, live, oral, pentavalent

Influenza vaccine, live, intranasal (quadrivalent, types A and types B)

Adenovirus type 4 and type 7 vaccine, live, oral

Yellow fever vaccine

Smallpox (vaccinia) vaccine, live

Inactivated or subunit viral

Poliovirus vaccine inactivated (human diploid cell)

Poliovirus vaccine inactivated (monkey kidney cell)

Hepatitis A vaccine, inactivated

Hepatitis B (recombinant) vaccine

Hepatitis A vaccine, inactivated, and Hepatitis B (recombinant) vaccine

Influenza A (H1N1) 2009 monovalent vaccine

Influenza virus vaccine, H5N1 (for national stockpile)

Influenza A (H5N1) virus monovalent vaccine, adjuvanted

Influenza virus vaccine (trivalent, types A and B)

Influenza virus vaccine (quadrivalent, types A and B)

Human papillomavirus bivalent (types 16, 18) vaccine, recombinant

Human papillomavirus quadrivalent (types 6, 11, 16, 18) vaccine, recombinant

Human papillomavirus 9-valent vaccine, recombinant

Japanese encephalitis virus vaccine, inactivated

Japanese encephalitis virus vaccine, inactivated, adsorbed

Rabies vaccine

Rabies vaccine adsorbed

from humans and then used to infect monkey cells. After several passages, the virus can no longer infect human cells but retains immunogenic capacity. These attenuated viruses can elicit a robust immune response because they are similar to the natural pathogen.

Several drawbacks exist with these vaccines. Because these are live viruses, they generally must be refrigerated to retain their activity. In remote areas of the world where refrigeration is not available, obtaining and storing this type of vaccine can be limiting. Because viruses can mutate and change in the host, it may be possible that viruses can become virulent again and cause disease, although the frequency of adverse reactions using these vaccines is very low. Furthermore, attenuated vaccines cannot be utilized in immune-compromised individuals (e.g., patients with HIV or cancer). In addition, these vaccines are usually not given during pregnancy. Measles, polio, rotavirus, yellow fever, and chickenpox viruses are examples of pathogens for which live attenuated vaccines have been generated. Attenuated vaccines for bacteria are more challenging to generate than for viruses because bacteria have more complex genomes; however, recombinant DNA technology can be utilized to remove virulence but retain immunogenicity. A vaccine against *Vibrio cholera* has been generated this way (currently not approved in the U.S.). A live attenuated vaccine for tuberculosis also has been developed.

Inactivated

Polio, influenza, and rabies viruses and typhoid and plague bacteria have been utilized to generate inactivated vaccines. Killing pathogens through the use of heat, radiation, or chemicals to inactivate them generates the antigenic starting materials. The dead pathogens can no longer replicate or mutate to their disease-causing state and thus are safe. These types of vaccines are useful because they can be freeze-dried and transported without refrigeration, an important consideration in reaching developing countries. A drawback with inactivated vaccines is that they induce an immune response that is much weaker than that induced by the natural infection; thus, patients require multiple doses to sustain immunity to the pathogen. In areas where people have limited access to healthcare, ensuring that these multiple doses are delivered on time can be problematic and may result in reduced immunity to the pathogen, as in the case of poliovirus endemic disease.

Subunit Vaccines

As with inactivated vaccines, subunit vaccines do not contain live pathogens; rather, subunit vaccines use a component of the microorganism as a vaccine antigen to mimic exposure to the organism itself. Subunit vaccines typically contain *polysaccharides* or proteins (*surface proteins* or *toxoids*). Compared to live attenuated vaccines, subunit vaccines induce a less-robust immune response. The selection of antigenic subunit and the design and development of the vaccine can be lengthy and costly because the pathogen's subunit antigens and their combination must be thoroughly tested to ensure they elicit an effective immune response. Scientists can identify the more immunogenic antigens in the laboratory and manufacture these antigen molecules via recombinant DNA technology, producing *recombinant subunit vaccines*. For example, the hepatitis B vaccine is generated by the insertion into baker's yeast of hepatitis B genes coding for selected antigens. The yeast cells express these antigens, which are then purified and used in making a vaccine. A drawback to these vaccines is that even though they elicit an immune response, immunity is not guaranteed. Subunit vaccines usually are considered safe because they have no live replicating pathogen present.

Polysaccharides. Polysaccharide subunit vaccines utilize polysaccharide (sugar) antigens to induce an immune response. Bacterial cell walls are composed of peptidoglycan polysaccharides that help pathogens evade the immune system. This evasion mechanism is highly effective in infants and young children, making them more susceptible to infection. Unfortunately, these polysaccharides are not very immunogenic. Furthermore, the vaccines produced to sugar antigens cause suboptimal immune responses that result in only short-term immunity. Meningococcal infection caused by *Neisseria meningitidis* (groups A, C, W-135, and Y) and *pneumococcal* disease are polysaccharide subunit vaccines against bacterial pathogens. Conjugate subunit vaccines use a technology to bind polysaccharide from the bacterial capsule to a carrier protein, often diphtheria or tetanus toxoid. This sort of antigen combination can induce long-term protection in infants and adults. These vaccines provide protection against pathogens where plain polysaccharide vaccines fail to work in infants and also provide more long-term protection in young children and adults. The *Haemophilus influenzae* type b (Hib) and *Pneumococcal* (PCV7 valent, PCV10 valent, PCV13 valent) are conjugate subunit vaccines recommended for children (see Table 36–1). The *meningococcal A* vaccine used in Africa is also an example of a conjugate subunit vaccine.

Surface Protein Subunit Vaccines. T protein–based subunit vaccines utilize purified proteins from the pathogen to induce an immune response. Because these proteins may not be presented in native form (i.e., as in the live pathogen), antibodies generated against these antigens may not bind efficiently to the live pathogen. Acellular pertussis (aP) and hepatitis B vaccines are examples of protein-based subunit vaccines. The hepatitis B vaccine contains the hepatitis B virus envelope protein made as an antigen produced in yeast cell culture.

Toxoids. Pathogenic bacteria such as *Clostridium tetani* and *Corynebacterium diphtheria* induce disease (tetanus or diphtheria, respectively) through production of their toxins. Vaccines against these toxins, known as toxoid vaccines, are effective because they elicit an immune response that results in the production of antibodies that can bind and neutralize these toxins, preventing cell damage in the patient. Inactivated or killed toxins are used as the immunogen; however, because they are not highly immunogenic, they must be adsorbed to adjuvants (aluminum or calcium salts) to increase their capacity to stimulate the immune response. Toxoid vaccines are safe because they do not contain live pathogens. In addition, they are stable over a wide range of temperatures and humidities (Baxter, 2007).

DNA Vaccines

Sequencing the genome of a pathogen provides information that enables the production of a DNA vaccine against selected genetic material. A microbe's antigenic genes are selected and incorporated in synthetic DNA. Intramuscular or intradermal injection delivers this engineered DNA to APCs, which uptake the DNA and transcribe and translate it to produce antigenic proteins. These APCs present these antigens to both humoral and cellular immune system components to generate immunity. This type of vaccine poses no risk of infection, can easily be developed and produced, is cost-effective, is stable, and provides long-term protection (Robinson et al., 2000). Disadvantages include its limit to protein antigens and the possibility of generating tolerance to that antigen because of low immunogenicity, thereby rendering ineffective immunity.

Many of these vaccines are currently in experimental phases, but none has been licensed in the U.S. DNA vaccines for influenza virus, herpesvirus, flaviviruses like Zika virus, and others are in the early stages of development. A DNA vaccine against West Nile virus has been approved for veterinary use. Delivery platforms for enhancing efficacy of DNA vaccines (such as electroporation) are being developed. There is also an emerging research field to use RNA as a vaccine delivery platform.

Recombinant Vectors

A vector is a virus or bacterium that is used to deliver heterologous microbial genes to cells for expression in the vaccinee to elicit an immune response. Once the vector infects or transduces host cells, the selected antigens will be presented during the immune response to generate immunity. Both viruses and bacteria are being investigated as recombinant vectors for candidate vaccines. Virus vectors that have been used in candidate vaccines include many poxviruses (vaccinia virus, modified vaccinia Ankara, avian poxviruses, and others), a large number of adenoviruses (of both human and primate origin), and other families of viruses.

Immunoglobulins

Structure

Vaccination results in the expansion and differentiation of B cells into long-lived memory cells that provide long-term protection to secondary challenge, and plasma cells, which are immunoglobulin (antibody)–generating cells that produce large quantities of these proteins. Antibodies in the body are found in two forms, either membrane bound on B cells as BCRs that can deliver signals to activate and induce B-cell differentiation after antigen ligation or as soluble effector molecules that neutralize antigens throughout the body. Antibodies are heterodimeric proteins composed of two chains, the light and heavy chains. Both light and heavy chains contain variable regions in the N-terminal region of the protein that engage antigens. Naïve B cells express BCRs with low affinity to antigen. These BCRs can be selected through VDJ recombination via the activity of RAG enzymes. Antibody diversity is achieved through antigen-binding site region variation, combinatorial diversity of gene segments, and combination of light and heavy regions, an overall diversity program that can result in an antibody repertoire of potentially 10^{16} to 10^{18} different molecules, ensuring that a unique B cell in the body will exist to recognize any foreign antigen. In addition to this diversity, antibodies also can undergo class-switch recombination in which the constant region of the heavy chain can be switched, based on cytokine signals by T cells, to tailor antibody specificity and function. It is this portion of the antibody that determines the five main isotypes: IgM, IgD, IgG, IgA, and IgE. These isotypes differ in size, Fc receptor binding, ability to fix complement, and appropriate isotypes for specific pathogens (Schroeder and Cavacini, 2010).

Antibody diversity can be further enhanced on antigen recognition by B cells and help from CD4$^+$ T cells. B cells can further strengthen their antibody affinity by mutating their variable regions, and with repetitive antigen stimulation, the affinity of binding to antigen can increase further. This mechanism explains why some vaccines, like the one for hepatitis B, are most immunogenic when delivered in three doses. This repeated antigen stimulation induces somatic hypermutation of antibody variable genes to increase antibody efficacy. AID is a key enzyme in mediating class-switch recombination and somatic hypermutation. Human patients with defective AID suffer from hyper-IgM syndrome and are unable to class switch their antibodies, which makes them more susceptible to certain infections.

Manufactured antibodies can be used for passive immunization; for a list of available antibodies, see Table 36–4. Such monoclonal antibodies are biologicals that have become some of the most important drugs of our era. To date, monoclonal antibodies have been implemented most effectively for use in cancer immunotherapy and management of autoimmune diseases. Palivizumab is a humanized murine monoclonal antibody that is licensed for use in high-risk infants to prevent hospitalization due to RSV. As the cost of production of monoclonal antibodies continues to fall, more of these biologicals will likely be used for prophylaxis or treatment of infectious diseases.

Antibody Classes and Functions

Immunoglobulin M

The first antibody class expressed by B cells is IgM. IgM molecules are membrane-bound monomers found on circulating mature B cells. When mature B cells are antigen stimulated, they generate IgM pentamers that are secreted. IgM antibodies, also called natural antibodies, have low affinity as monomers, but their avidity can increase in their pentameric structure, which improves epitope binding to repeating antigens on pathogens. These antibodies are found at mucosal surfaces and constitute 10% of the antibody content of serum. These antibodies are associated with a primary immune response. IgM molecules function by coating their specific antigen to target the pathogen for destruction via phagocytosis or to induce complement fixation to kill the pathogen (Schroeder and Cavacini, 2010).

TABLE 36–4 ■ THERAPEUTIC MONOCLONAL ANTIBODIES APPROVED IN THE E.U. AND THE U.S.

ANTIBODY	TARGET; *Ab Type*	THERAPEUTIC USE
Abciximab	GPIIb/IIIa; *chimeric IgG1 Fab*	Prevention of blood clots in angioplasty
Adalimumab	TNF; *human IgG1*	Rheumatoid arthritis
Ado-trastuzumab emtansine	HER2; *humanized IgG1; immunoconjugate*	Breast cancer
Alemtuzumab	CD52; *humanized IgG1*	Multiple sclerosis
Alirocumab	PCSK9; *human IgG1*	Lowering cholesterol
Atezolizumab[a]	PD-L1; *humanized IgG1*	Bladder cancer
Avelumab	PD-L1/*human IgG1*	Merkel cell carcinoma
Basiliximab	IL-2R; *chimeric IgG1*	Prevention of kidney transplant rejection
Belimumab	BLyS; *human IgG1*	Systemic lupus erythematosus
Bevacizumab	VEGF; *humanized IgG1*	Colorectal cancer
Bezlotoxumab	*Clostridium difficile* toxin B/*human IgG1*	*Clostridium difficile* infections
Blinatumomab	CD19, CD3; *murine bispecific tandem scFv*	Acute lymphoblastic leukemia
Brentuximab vedotin	CD30; *chimeric IgG1; immunoconjugate*	Hodgkin lymphoma, systemic anaplastic large cell lymphoma
Brodalumab	IL-17RA/*human IgG2*	Plaque psoriasis
Canakinumab	IL-1β; *human IgG1*	Muckle-Wells syndrome
Catumaxomab[b]	EPCAM/CD3; *rat/mouse bispecific mAb*	Malignant ascites
Certolizumab pegol	TNF; *humanized Fab, pegylated*	Crohn disease
Cetuximab	EGFR; *chimeric IgG1*	Colorectal cancer
Daclizumab	IL-2R; *humanized IgG1*	Multiple sclerosis
Daratumumab	CD38; *human IgG1*	Multiple myeloma
Denosumab	RANK-L; *human IgG2*	Bone loss
Dinutuximab	GD2; *chimeric IgG1*	Neuroblastoma
Dupilumab	IL-4Rα/*human IgG4*	Eczema
Durvalumab	PD-L1/*human IgG1*	Urothelial carcinoma
Eculizumab	C5; *humanized IgG2/4*	Paroxysmal nocturnal hemoglobinuria
Efalizumab	CD11a; *humanized IgG1*	Psoriasis
Elotuzumab	SLAMF7; *humanized IgG1*	Multiple myeloma
Evolocumab	PCSK9; *human IgG2*	Lowering cholesterol
Gemtuzumab ozogamicin[a]	CD33; *humanized IgG4*	Acute myeloid leukemia
Golimumab	TNF; *human IgG1*	Rheumatoid and psoriatic arthritis, ankylosing spondylitis
Ibritumomab tiuxetan	CD20; *murine IgG1*	Non-Hodgkin lymphoma
Idarucizumab	Dabigatran; *humanized Fab*	Dabigatran excess (reversing anticoagulation)
Infliximab	TNF; *chimeric IgG1*	Crohn disease
Ipilimumab	CTLA-4; *human IgG1*	Metastatic melanoma
Ixekizumab	IL-17a; *humanized IgG4*	Psoriasis
Mepolizumab	IL-5; *hIgG1*	Severe eosinophilic asthma
Muromonab-CD3	CD3; *murine IgG2a*	Reversal of kidney transplant rejection
Natalizumab	a4 integrin; *humanized IgG4*	Multiple sclerosis
Necitumumab	EGFR; *human IgG1*	Non–small cell lung cancer
Nivolumab	PD1; *human IgG4*	Melanoma, non–small cell lung cancer, renal cell carcinoma, non small cell carcinoma
Obiltoxaximab[a]	Protective antigen *of B. anthracis* exotoxin[c]; *chimeric IgG1*	Prevention of inhalational anthrax
Obinutuzumab	CD20; *humanized IgG1; glycoengineered*	Chronic lymphocytic leukemia
Ocrelizumab	CD20/*human IgG1*	Multiple Sclerosis
Ofatumumab	CD20; *human IgG1*	Chronic lymphocytic leukemia

(Continued)

SECTION IV

INFLAMMATION, IMMUNOMODULATION, AND HEMATOPOIESIS

TABLE 36–4 ■ THERAPEUTIC MONOCLONAL ANTIBODIES APPROVED IN THE E.U. AND THE U.S.(*CONTINUED*)

ANTIBODY	TARGET; *Ab Type*	THERAPEUTIC USE
Olaratumab	PDGFR/*human IgG1*	Soft tissue sarcoma
Omalizumab	IgE; *humanized IgG1*	Asthma
Palivizumab	RSV; *humanized IgG1*	Prevention of respiratory syncytial virus infection
Panitumumab	EGFR; *human IgG2*	Colorectal cancer
Pembrolizumab	PD1; *humanized IgG4*	Melanoma, non-small cell carcinoma
Pertuzumab	HER2; *humanized IgG1*	Breast cancer
Ramucirumab	VEGFR2; *human IgG1*	Gastric cancer
Ranibizumab	VEGF; *humanized IgG1 Fab*	Macular degeneration
Raxibacumab[a]	*B. anthrasis* protective antigen[c]; *human IgG1*	Prevention of inhalational anthrax
Reslizumab	IL-5; *humanized IgG4*	Asthma
Rituximab	CD20; *chimeric IgG1*	Non-Hodgkin lymphoma
Sarilumab	IL-6R/*human IgG1*	Rheumatoid arthritis
Secukinumab	IL-17a; *human IgG1*	Psoriasis
Siltuximab	IL-6; *chimeric IgG1*	Castleman disease
Tocilizumab	IL-6R; *humanized IgG1*	Rheumatoid arthritis
Tositumomab-I[131][a]	CD20; *murine IgG2a*	Non-Hodgkin lymphoma
Trastuzumab	HER2; *hIgG1*	Breast cancer
Ustekinumab	IL-12/23; *human IgG1*	Psoriasis
Vedolizumab	α4β7 integrin; *humanized IgG1*	Ulcerative colitis, Crohn disease

[a]Not approved in the E.U.
[b]Not approved in the U.S.
[c]Inhibits the binding of the protective antigen to its membrane receptors, thereby preventing the intracellular entry of the anthrax lethal factor and edema factor, the enzymatic toxin components responsible for the pathogenic effects of anthrax toxin.

Immunoglobulin D

Like IgM molecules, IgD molecules are also expressed on naïve B cells that have not been activated by their specific antigen and thus have not undergone somatic hypermutation. They are expressed as monomers on the surface of B cells and can also be secreted; they represent less than 0.5% of the antibody in the serum (Schroeder and Cavacini, 2010). The exact function of this antibody is not fully known, but it can bind bacterial proteins through the constant region (Riesbeck and Nordstrom, 2006).

Immunoglobulin G

The IgG antibodies exist as monomers, represent about 70% of the antibody in circulation, and have been the most studied. They have the longest $t_{1/2}$ in serum and are generated with high affinity after affinity maturation. The constant region of the heavy chain can further lead to diversity in the structure of these antibodies to generate four subclasses: IgG1, IgG2, IgG3, and IgG4. These subclasses are named based on their concentrations in serum, with IgG1 the most abundant and IgG4 the least. IgG1, IgG2, and IgG3 subclasses can activate complement to opsonize pathogens, but IgG4 cannot. These antibodies can also differ in their ability and affinity to engage Fc receptors, which further enhances their effector functions. All IgG subclasses cross the placenta to provide passive immunity to the fetus.

Vaccines predominantly induce these antibody types, which become important during the secondary immune response to inactivate pathogens. Different subclasses are selected during the secondary antibody response. In designing vaccines, scientists must determine which antibody subclass will provide the optimal response. In addition to complement and opsonization, IgG antibodies can directly neutralize toxins and viruses (Schroeder and Cavacini, 2010).

Immunoglobulin A

The IgA antibody class is expressed as monomers or dimers and represents about 15% of the antibodies in serum, slightly higher than IgM antibodies. At mucosal surfaces, saliva, and breast milk, however, IgA antibodies are found at the highest concentrations (Woof and Mestecky, 2005). In late pregnancy and the early post-natal period, female mammary glands produce colostrum; more than half of the protein content of colostrum that breast-feeding neonates consume is IgA antibodies. IgA is primarily a monomer in the serum but a dimer at mucosal sites.

IgA antibodies have two subclasses, IgA1 and IgA2, that differ only slightly in their structures. IgA1 antibodies are longer than IgA2 antibodies and are therefore more sensitive to degradation. IgA2 is more stable and is found primarily in mucosal secretions, in contrast to IgA1, which predominates in serum. IgA antibodies work via direct neutralization of viruses, bacteria, and toxins to protect mucosal tissues. They prevent antigen binding to host cells that damage or infect them. IgA antibodies within cells may also prevent pathogen tropism. Even though IgA antibodies do not lead to complement fixation, neutrophils can uptake them to mediate ADCC (Schroeder and Cavacini, 2010).

Immunoglobulin E

The IgE antibody class is present at the lowest serum concentration, less than 0.01% of circulating antibodies, and has the shortest $t_{1/2}$. IgE binds to Fcγ receptors with very high affinity. Langerhans and mast cells, basophils, and eosinophils express Fcγ receptors that bind IgE antibodies. Fc receptor engagement also results in FcγR upregulation on bound cells. These antibodies recognize antigens on parasitic worms when they are cross-linked on granulocytes; the cells degranulate to release inflammatory mediators to destroy the parasite. IgE antibodies are also relevant in mediating allergic reactions by recognizing innocuous antigens, such as bee venom and peanut antigen.

Patients who develop allergic reactions generate memory B cells that produce IgE antibodies to specific antigens. The granulocytes become coated with IgE antibodies and on antigen reexposure such as a bee's sting or peanuts, the antigen cross-links IgEs, leading to granulocyte degranulation, which can result in anaphylactic shock. Therapies are in development to generate and use antibodies against soluble IgE molecules to prevent their uptake by granulocytes. For a list of approved monoclonal antibodies, see Table 36–4.

Specific Conventional Vaccines Recommended in the U.S.

The CDC maintains tables listing currently recommended vaccinations for various susceptibilities throughout life. Next is a discussion of the properties and schedule of administration for the vaccinations recommended from birth to elder adulthood. The vaccines are grouped by the target type (bacterium, virus, etc.) and then by vaccine type, as discussed in the previous section. See Table 36–1 for infant and childhood vaccination schedules. For a complete list of the adult recommended immunization schedule, see Tables 36-5 and 36-6.

Vaccines for Bacteria

Bacterial Toxoid Vaccines: Diphtheria and Tetanus

Tetanus Toxoid Vaccine. Tetanus is a disease characterized by prolonged spasms and tetany caused by the toxin secreted by the bacterium *C. tetani*, which enters from environmental sources through wounds. Tetanus toxin enters the nervous system and by retrograde transport reaches the inhibitory interneurons of the spinal cord, where the active fragment cleaves synaptobrevin (see Figures 8–3 to 8–6), thereby inhibiting exocytosis of neurotransmitter from these nerve cells and resulting in uninhibited skeletal muscle contraction. The toxoid is produced by deactivating toxin isolated from the bacterium using formaldehyde. Immunization usually begins at about age 2 months, as a component of the combination vaccine DTaP that is given to infants. Tetanus toxoid is included in several combination vaccine formulations. DTaP is the vaccine used in children younger than age 7; Tdap and Td, given at later ages, are booster immunizations that offer continued protection from those diseases for adolescents and adults. In these designations, upper- and lowercase letters represent the comparative quantity of antigen present. Thus, the shared uppercase *T* indicates there is about the same amount of tetanus toxoid in DTaP, Tdap, and Td. The uppercase *D* and *P* in the childhood formulation indicate that there is more diphtheria and pertussis antigen in DTaP than in Tdap or Td.

Diphtheria Toxoid Vaccines. Diphtheria is a disease caused by a secreted toxin of the aerobic gram-positive bacterium *C. diphtheria*; toxin production is under control of the bacterial systems, but the structural gene for toxin production is contributed by a β phage that infects all pathogenic strains of *C. diphtheria*. The A subunit of the toxin is an ADP-ribosylase; following its entry into a cell, it ADP-ribosylates eukaryotic elongation factor 2 (eEF-2) and thereby inhibits protein translation in human cells (Gill et al., 1973). The throat of the victim becomes swollen and sore during infection, and the toxin causes damage to myelin sheaths in the nervous system, leading to loss of sensation or motor control. The vaccine, which has been used for nearly 80 years, is a toxoid that is produced by treating toxin with formalin. The toxoid is used to immunize infants beginning at about 2 months, typically as part of the combination DTaP vaccine. The diphtheria toxin also has been detoxified genetically by introduction of point mutations that abrogate enzymatic activity but allow retention of binding activity; for instance, the mutant diphtheria toxin protein CRM_{197} is the protein carrier for a licensed Hib vaccine.

Pertussis Vaccines. Pertussis, or whooping cough, is a respiratory tract disease characterized by prolonged paroxysmal coughing and sometimes respiratory failure; it is caused by the gram-negative coccobacillus *Bordetella pertussis*. The secreted pertussis toxin has an A subunit that, once in the cell cytosol, ADP-ribisylates the α subunit of the G_i protein that couples inhibitory GPCR signaling to adenylyl cyclase to reduce cyclic AMP production. After ADP-ribosylation, $G_{i\alpha}$ becomes inactive, and GPCR-mediated reduction of cyclic AMP production is abolished. The physiological sequelae of this action of pertussis toxin are thought to contribute

to the constellation of symptoms of whooping cough. Routine vaccination typically begins as part of the childhood combination DTaP vaccine series. It is also appropriate to immunize healthy adults, adolescents, and pregnant mothers as pertussis does occur throughout life due to waning immunity. There are two licensed pertussis vaccines, the historical inactivated organism "whole-cell" vaccine used in the past in the U.S. and still in many other countries and a second "acellular" formulation that incorporates antigen fragments derived from the organism. Both vaccines are immunogenic and protective. The whole-cell vaccine appears to induce more durable immunity, but the acellular vaccine causes about a 10-fold lower rate of side effects such as fever or injection site pain and erythema. Most developed countries now use acellular pertussis vaccine to reduce the reactivity profile, but many other countries continue to use the whole-cell vaccine successfully because the response is equally efficacious and more durable and the vaccine is economical.

Conjugated Bacterial Polysaccharide Vaccines

Haemophilus influenzae Type B Vaccine. *Haemophilus influenzae* is a major cause of life-threatening childhood bacterial diseases, including buccal, preseptal and orbital cellulitis, epiglottitis, bacteremia with sepsis, and meningitis. Universal vaccination with the Hib vaccine has nearly eliminated these diseases in the U.S. The Hib vaccine is a polysaccharide-protein conjugate that confers immunity to the disease by inducing antibodies to the capsular polysaccharide PRP. The Hib polysaccharide has been conjugated to diverse proteins, including the mutant diphtheria protein CRM_{197} (a vaccine termed HbOC); the meningococcal group B outer membrane protein C (a vaccine termed PRP-OMPC); and tetanospasmin, which is a toxoid of the *C. tetani* neurotoxin (a vaccine termed PRP-T). The vaccines all exhibit a high level of safety and immunogenicity. Interestingly, widespread immunization not only reduces disease in those vaccinated, but also reduces nasal carriage of the bacterium, resulting in reduced transmission to even those not vaccinated and providing evidence of herd immunity.

Streptococcus pneumoniae Vaccines. The gram-positive encapsulated bacterium *S. pneumoniae* causes invasive diseases in infants and young children, including meningitis, bacteremia and sepsis, and pneumonia. There are myriad *S. pneumoniae* types, based on the capsular polysaccharide; thus, polyvalent vaccines are needed. Vaccines confer immunity by inducing type-specific antipolysaccharide antibodies. Two types of vaccines are available, *polysaccharide* and *conjugate* vaccines. The 23-valent polysaccharide vaccine contains long chains of capsular polysaccharides that are collected from inactivated bacteria. Polysaccharide vaccine is used in children older than 2 years and in at-risk adults. PCVs have been developed, and increasing numbers of serotypes have been incorporated over time. The combined 13 serotypes in PCV13 protect against most invasive disease in the U.S. Infants are given a primary series of PCV13 at ages 2, 4, and 6 months, with a booster at 12 to 15 months.

Neisseria meningitidis Vaccines. *Neisseria meningitidis* is a significant cause of invasive bacterial disease in childhood, causing sepsis and meningitis. As with *S. pneumoniae*, there are diverse types of polysaccharide; thus, type-specific anticapsular polysaccharide antibodies mediate protection against invasive disease. Therefore, multivalent vaccines are required. A licensed quadrivalent polysaccharide vaccine protects against four subtypes of meningococcus—designated A, C, Y, and W-135. The polysaccharide vaccine works only in children older than 2 years. A tetravalent meningococcal conjugate vaccine, also containing the A, C, Y, and W-135 subtypes, is used in persons 9 months to 55 years of age. In 2013, the European Commission licensed a four-component, protein-based meningococcal B vaccine (incorporating fHbp, NadA, NHBA, and PorA P1.4 proteins) to prevent septicemia and meningitis.

Vaccines for Viruses

Poliovirus Vaccines

Polio is a characterized by acute flaccid paralysis, against which the WHO and others are conducting a worldwide eradication campaign. There are two types of poliovirus vaccines in use. The first is a *live attenuated oral*

TABLE 36–5 ■ RECOMMENDED IMMUNIZATION SCHEDULE FOR ADULTS AGED 19 YEARS OR OLDER BY AGE GROUP, U.S., 2017.

Vaccine	19–21 years	22–26 years	27–59 years	60–64 years	≥ 65 years
Influenza*	1 dose annually				
Td/Tdap*	Substitute Tdap for Td once, then Td booster every 10 yrs				
MMR*	1 or 2 doses depending on indication				
VAR*	2 doses				
HZV*				1 dose	
HPV–Female*	3 doses				
HPV–Male*	3 doses				
PCV13*				1 dose	
PPSV23*	1 or 2 doses depending on indication				1 dose
HepA*	2 or 3 doses depending on vaccine				
HepB*	3 doses				
MenACWY or MPSV*	1 or more doses depending on indication				
MenB*	2 or 3 doses depending on vaccine				
Hib*	1 or 3 doses depending on indication				

Recommended for adults who meet the age requirement, lack documentation of vaccination, or lack evidence of past infection

Recommended for adults with additional medical conditions or other indications

No recommendation

*NOTE: The above recommendations are reprinted from the website of the Centers for Disease Control and Prevention (CDC) and should be read along with the footnotes of this schedule available on the CDC website: https://www.cdc.gov/vaccines/schedules/.

TABLE 36–6 ■ RECOMMENDED IMMUNIZATION SCHEDULE FOR ADULTS AGED 19 YEARS OR OLDER BY MEDICAL CONDITION AND OTHER INDICATIONS, UNITED STATES, 2017.

Vaccine	Pregnancy	Immuno-compromised (excluding HIV infection)	HIV infection CD4+ count (cells/µL) <200	HIV infection CD4+ count (cells/µL) ≥200	Asplenia, persistent complement deficiencies	Kidney failure, end-stage renal disease, on hemodialysis	Heart or lung disease, chronic alcoholism	Chronic liver disease	Diabetes	Healthcare personnel	Men who have sex with men
Influenza				1 dose annually							
Td/Tdap	1 dose Tdap each pregnancy			Substitute Tdap for Td once, then Td booster every 10 yrs							
MMR	contraindicated	contraindicated	contraindicated		1 or 2 doses depending on indication						
VAR	contraindicated	contraindicated	contraindicated		2 doses						
HZV	contraindicated	contraindicated	contraindicated		1 dose						
HPV–Female		3 doses through age 26 yrs			3 doses through age 26 yrs						
HPV–Male		3 doses through age 26 yrs			3 doses through age 21 yrs						3 doses through age 26 yrs
PCV13				1 dose							
PPSV23				1, 2, or 3 doses depending on indication							
HepA				2 or 3 doses depending on vaccine							
HepB				3 doses							
MenACWY or MPSV4				1 or more doses depending on indication							
MenB				2 or 3 doses depending on vaccine							
Hib		3 doses post-HSCT recipients only		1 dose							

Recommended for adults who meet the age requirement, lack documentation of vaccination, or lack evidence of past infection

Recommended for adults with additional medical conditions or other indications

Contraindicated

No recommendation

*NOTE: The above recommendations are reprinted from the website of the Centers for Disease Control and Prevention (CDC) and should be read along with the footnotes of this schedule available on the CDC website: https://www.cdc.gov/vaccines/schedules/.

vaccine in use since the early 1960s (the "Sabin vaccine"), containing attenuated poliovirus types I, II, and III, produced in monkey kidney cell tissue culture. The vaccine replicates in the intestine and induces systemic and mucosal immunity, but also is shed in the stool, sometimes transmitting to close contacts. Infection of most close contacts contributes to herd immunity in the human population. Rarely (about one case per million doses), partial revertant viruses occur that cause vaccine-associated paralytic poliomyelitis in contacts. In many parts of the world, live poliovirus vaccine is still used. The last known case of naturally acquired poliovirus disease acquired in the U.S. occurred in 1979; the U.S. discontinued use of the live vaccine in 2000. Live poliovirus vaccine is contraindicated in subjects with primary immunodeficiency. Pregnant women and children with symptomatic HIV infection should receive IPV vaccine.

The second type of vaccine is a *killed virus* preparation called *IPV* (the "Salk vaccine"). Killed vaccine induces mainly humoral immunity but still exhibits excellent efficacy against disease. IPV does not transmit virus to contacts and does not cause vaccine-associated paralysis. An enhanced-potency IPV vaccine has been available since 1998, and this IPV preparation is now a component of some combination vaccines.

Measles Virus Vaccines

The current measles vaccine is a live attenuated strain given subcutaneously. A live, "more attenuated" preparation of the Enders-Edmonston virus strain (designated the "Moraten" strain) is the MeV vaccine currently used in the U.S. Vaccination is initiated at 12 to 15 months of age in the U.S. because transplacentally acquired maternal antibodies inhibit immunogenicity of vaccine in the first year of life.

Mumps Virus Vaccine

Mumps virus causes a febrile illness most commonly associated with inflammation of the parotids and sometimes with more severe conditions, including aseptic meningitis. A live attenuated virus vaccine has been used exclusively since the 1970s. The Jeryl-Lynn vaccine (from a mixture of two strains) was isolated from the throat of the daughter of Maurice Hilleman, a noted vaccine developer. The vaccine is typically given as a component of the combination MMR or MMRV vaccine at 12 to 15 months of age.

Rubella Virus Vaccine

Rubella virus, a member of the Togaviridae family, is spread by respiratory droplets and causes a mild infection with viremia. Rubella is harmful only to fetuses, and the effects can be devastating. A rubella infection during pregnancy can cause miscarriage, preterm birth, stillbirth, or various birth defects. The risks decrease as pregnancy progresses. The main goal of rubella immunization is to prevent congenital rubella syndrome. The live attenuated rubella virus vaccine is given subcutaneously, now usually as a component of MMR or MMRV vaccine, beginning between 12 and 15 months of age. The live rubella virus vaccine strain RA 27/3 is grown in human diploid cell culture. In the U.S., universal immunization (both boys and girls) is used to reduce infection of pregnant women. As a result, rubella and congenital rubella syndrome have been eliminated in the U.S. Rubella vaccine is part of MMR or MMRV combination vaccines for universal immunization starting at 12 to 15 months, followed by a booster dose at school entry (~5 to 6 years).

Varicella Zoster Virus Vaccine

Varicella zoster virus is one of the most infectious among agents that affect humans. It is spread by the respiratory route by small aerosol particles (cough, sneeze, etc.). Infection causes a febrile syndrome with vesicular rash, sometimes complicated by pneumonia or invasive bacterial skin disease. Congenital varicella syndrome can occur if varicella infection occurs during pregnancy. The vaccine used is the Oka strain of live attenuated VZV attenuated by sequential passage in cell monolayer cultures; it was licensed for universal immunization in the U.S. in 1995. The virus in the Oka/Merck vaccine in current use in the U.S. was further passaged in MRC-5 human diploid-cell cultures. The vaccine is often given as a part of the combination MMRV vaccine.

Hepatitis A Virus Vaccines

Hepatitis A virus infection causes acute liver disease after transmission by the fecal-oral route. An inactivated vaccine is recommended for all children, starting at 1 year of age. Two hepatitis A vaccines and one hepatitis A vaccine/hepatitis B combovaccine are licensed in the U.S. The vaccine is given as a two-dose series.

Hepatitis B Virus Vaccines

Hepatitis B virus is transmitted between people by contact with blood or other bodily fluids, including by sexual contact and maternal transfer to fetus or infant. Hepatitis B virus can cause a life-threatening and sometimes chronic liver disease. All infants receive the hepatitis B vaccine. When the mother has active infection, the neonate is treated with both the vaccine and hepatitis B immune globulin. The vaccine is a recombinant protein produced in yeast that is the protective antigen, hepatitis B surface antigen (see also Chapter 63).

Rotavirus Vaccines

Throughout the world, rotavirus is the most common cause of dehydrating diarrhea in infants. Four or five types (based on the surface proteins) cause severe disease. An early live attenuated vaccine (Rotashield) was withdrawn after association with intussusception (a segmental, telescoping collapse of the intestine). Two similar vaccines are now used that are safe and immunogenic. One is an oral pentavalent human-bovine reassortant rotavirus vaccine (containing five reassortant rotaviruses developed from human and the Wistar Calf 3 bovine parent rotaviral strains) first licensed in the U.S. in 2006 (RotaTeq). This vaccine is administered in a three-dose schedule, at 2, 4, and 6 months of age. Another oral live attenuated rotavirus vaccine licensed in the U.S. is based on a single attenuated human strain (Rotarix) using a two-dose schedule, beginning at 2 months of age. Rotavirus vaccines are used for universal immunization during infancy, with care to keep the initiation of the two- or three-dose series at a young age, as the rare rotavirus-associated intussusception risk with infection appears slightly higher at older ages.

Influenza Virus Vaccines

The orthomyxovirus influenza virus is a respiratory virus spread person-to-person by large-particle aerosols and fomites. The virus circulates in humans in two major serotypes (types A and B); two distinct A subtypes, designated H1N1 and H3N2, currently cause disease ("the flu") in humans. Current seasonal influenza vaccines are trivalent, including A/H1N1, A/H3N2, and B antigens, or quadrivalent with a second type B antigen. Experimental vaccines are being tested for some avian influenza viruses (such as A/H5N1 and A/H7N9) that have infected humans and have pandemic potential. During each annual seasonal epidemic, point mutations occur in genes encoding the hemagglutinin and neuraminidase proteins, which are the principal targets for protective antibodies. This antigenic drift in circulating influenza strains has led to a process in which regulatory officials and manufacturers adjust the virus antigens in influenza vaccines every year. Occasionally, the segmented virus genome reasserts during coinfection of an animal with a human and an avian virus, a new virus arises (antigenic shift), and a pandemic occurs. Major worldwide pandemics occurred in 1918 (H1N1), 1957 (H2N2), 1968 (H3N2), and 2009 (a novel H1N1). Major adjustments of vaccines must be made in such instances.

Two principal types of influenza vaccines are licensed at present, inactivated vaccine and live attenuated virus vaccine. The inactivated vaccine is prepared by treating wild-type viruses prepared in eggs or cell culture with an inactivating agent. Inactivated vaccine often prevents more than half of serious influenza-related disease when the viruses chosen for the seasonal vaccine antigenically match the eventual epidemic virus well. The vaccine is most effective at preventing severe respiratory disease and influenza-related hospitalizations.

All persons aged 6 months and above should be vaccinated. Those at most risk of severe disease and in most need of vaccine are infants, young children, people older than 65 years, pregnant women, and those with chronic health conditions or immunodeficiency. This vaccine is contraindicated in those who have had a life-threatening allergic reaction after a dose of influenza vaccine or have a severe allergy to any component of the vaccine, some of which contain a small amount of egg protein. Some people with a history of Guillain-Barré syndrome should not receive this vaccine. The vaccine is usually given as a single dose each year, although children 6 months through 8 years of age may need two doses during a single influenza season. Some IIVs contain a small amount of the preservative thimerosal (see Preservatives, Including Thimerosal). Although any association with developmental disorders has been disproven, public concern about this topic has led to the development of thimerosal-free IIVs.

The second principal type of influenza vaccine is a trivalent or quadrivalent live attenuated virus vaccine that is administered topically by nasal spray. New vaccines are prepared each year to address antigenic drift by reasserting genes encoding the current HA and NA antigens with a virus genetic background containing internal viral genes with well-defined attenuating mutations. The vaccine is licensed in the U.S. for persons 2 to 49 years of age. In some pediatric studies, the live attenuated vaccine appeared to provide a higher level of protection than inactivated vaccine; however, CDC vaccine effectiveness data from the influenza seasons in 2013–2016 in the U.S. indicated that the quadrivalent live attenuated vaccine did not demonstrate statistically significant effectiveness in children 2–17 years of age. Therefore, the CDC provided an interim recommendation that the vaccine should not be used in any setting in the U.S. for the 2016–2017 influenza season. Practitioners should check regularly for updated guidelines from the CDC on this point.

Human Papillomavirus Vaccines

Human papillomaviruses cause nearly all cases of cervical and anal cancer and a majority of oropharyngeal cancers. Most such cancers are caused by just two of the many HPV serotypes, types 16 and 18. Remarkably, even though the virus cannot be grown efficiently in culture, effective HPV vaccines were developed using VLPs that are formed by HPV surface components. All licensed HPV vaccines protect against at least these two types and some protect against four or nine types of HPV, with effectiveness against vaginal and vulvar cancers in women, as well as most cases of anal cancer and genital warts in both females and males. HPV vaccines are recommended for all 11- and 12-year-olds to protect against HPV infection and for women 13 to 26 years old and men 13 to 21 years old not previously vaccinated. HPV vaccination is also recommended for any man who has sex with a man. The vaccines are given in a three-dose regimen on a schedule of 0, 1-2, and 6 months.

Maternal Immunization

Maternal immunization during pregnancy can enhance newborn protection after birth by providing passive immunity to the neonate. Immunizing pregnant mothers is safe and protects the child from deadly infectious pathogens early in life when the immune system is not fully developed. One of the most successful maternal immunization protocols involves injection of tetanus toxoid to stimulate the production of IgG antibodies that have high neutralizing capacity and can cross the placenta. Vaccines for group B *Streptococcus*, Hib, RSV, *Streptococcus pneumoniae*, *Bordetella pertussis*, and trivalent *IIVs* have been tested in pregnant women. For a complete list of maternal vaccines, see Table 36–7.

Vaccines for Travel

International travelers should ensure that their vaccination status is current for conventional vaccines, including diphtheria, tetanus, pertussis, hepatitis A and B, and poliovirus; exposures to these agents may be more common in some international settings. There are additional vaccines that may be of benefit as preventive vaccines; these are listed next.

Japanese Encephalitis Virus Vaccine

Japanese encephalitis is a serious mosquito-borne flavivirus infection (not spread person to person) that can cause mild infections with fever and headache, serious neurological sequelae, and even death. Travelers who spend a month or longer in some rural parts of Korea, Japan, China, and eastern areas of Russia should consider vaccination. Two JE vaccines

TABLE 36-7 ■ VACCINES THAT MAY BE USED IN MOTHERS BEFORE, DURING, OR AFTER PREGNANCY[a]

VACCINE	BEFORE PREGNANCY	DURING PREGNANCY	AFTER PREGNANCY	TYPE OF VACCINE
Influenza	Yes	Yes, during season	Yes	Inactivated
Tdap	May be recommended; better to vaccinate during pregnancy when possible	Yes, during each pregnancy	Yes, immediately postpartum, if Tdap never received in lifetime; it is better to vaccinate during pregnancy	Toxoid/inactivated
Td	May be recommended	May be recommended, but Tdap is preferred	May be recommended	Toxoid
Hepatitis A	May be recommended	May be recommended	May be recommended	Inactivated
Hepatitis B	May be recommended	May be recommended	May be recommended	Inactivated
Meningococcal	May be recommended	Base decision on risk vs. benefit; inadequate data for specific recommendation	May be recommended	Inactivated
Pneumococcal	May be recommended	Base decision on risk vs. benefit; inadequate data for specific recommendation	May be recommended	Inactivated
HPV	May be recommended (through 26 years of age)	No	May be recommended (through 26 years of age)	Inactivated
MMR	May be recommended; once received, avoid conception for 4 weeks	No	May be recommended	Live
Varicella	May be recommended; once received, avoid conception for 4 weeks	No	May be recommended	Live

[a]Adapted from CDC guidance: http://www.cdc.gov/vaccines/pregnancy/downloads/immunizations-preg-chart.pdf.

are licensed in the U.S.: an inactivated mouse brain–derived JE vaccine (JE-MB) for use in travelers aged 1 year or older and an inactivated Vero cell culture–derived JE vaccine (JE-VC) for persons aged 17 years or older.

Yellow Fever Virus Vaccine

Yellow fever is a mosquito-borne flaviviral disease with a wide range of systemic symptoms. In severe cases, the disease causes hepatitis, hemorrhagic fever, and death. The CDC recommends this vaccine for children older than 9 months and adults who will be traveling to high-risk areas. There is generally a requirement for documentation of vaccination for travel to and from infected areas. The vaccine is a live attenuated virus vaccine that has been used successfully for many decades. For international travel, yellow fever virus vaccine must be approved by WHO and must be administered by an approved yellow fever vaccination center that can provide both vaccination and a validated International Certificate of Vaccination. The vaccine should be given at least 10 days before travel to an endemic area. Generally, a single dose suffices.

Typhoid Vaccine

Typhoid fever is an acute illness caused by the bacterium S. typhi, which is transmitted by ingestion of contaminated water or food. Typhoid vaccination is recommended for international travelers who will visit rural areas or villages that have inadequate sanitation. Symptoms include fever, headache, anorexia, and abdominal discomfort; the disease can be fatal. Treatment is challenging, and there has been an increase in the number of drug-resistant strains of S. typhi over the last several decades. There are two vaccines available to prevent infection: a single-dose, injectable, inactivated typhoid vaccine and an oral live typhoid vaccine that is taken in a four-dose course.

Rabies Virus Vaccine

Rabies is caused by a lyssavirus transmitted to humans from the bite of infected mammals; the untreated infection is nearly always fatal in humans. Rabies vaccination is used in two ways, first as a preventive vaccine prior to exposure and second as a postexposure intervention to prevent progression to fatal disease. Candidates for preexposure vaccination are people at high risk of exposure to natural rabies (veterinarians, animal handlers, spelunkers, et al.) or to laboratory strains or tissues (such as those involved in production of rabies biologicals). Preventive vaccination should be offered to international travelers who are likely to come in contact with animals in parts of the world where rabies is common (see CDC website). The vaccine is given in a three-dose series on days 0, 7, and 28. For those who may be repeatedly exposed to rabies virus, periodic testing for immunity is recommended, and booster doses can be administered as needed to maintain immunity. Postexposure vaccination is used in emergency settings following a bite or close exposure to an animal that may be rabid. In this setting, the vaccine is given in a four-dose series on days 0, 3, 7, and 14, concomitant with two injections of rabies immune globulin on day 0, one locally into the bite site and a second in an intramuscular injection for systemic administration of antibodies. A bite victim who has been previously vaccinated should receive two doses of rabies vaccine on days 0 and 3 but does not need rabies immune globulin.

Specialty Vaccines

There are limited-use vaccines that are offered in special circumstances to at-risk persons.

Anthrax Vaccine

Anthrax vaccine is offered to certain at-risk adults 18 to 65 years of age, including some members of the U.S. military, laboratory workers who work with anthrax, and some veterinarians or other individuals who handle animals or animal products. Anthrax is a serious disease in animals and human caused by Bacillus anthracis. People can contract anthrax from contact with infected animals or animal products. Usually, the cutaneous infection causes ulcers on the skin and systemic symptoms, including fever and malaise; up to 20% of untreated cases are fatal. Inhaled spores of B. anthracis usually cause fatal infection. AVA, given as multiple booster injections, protects against cutaneous and inhalation anthrax acquired by exposure on skin or by inhalation. The CDC recommends anthrax intramuscular booster shots 4 weeks, 6 months, 12 months, 18 months, and then annually.

Vaccinia Virus (Smallpox Vaccine)

Vaccinia vaccine is a live attenuated orthopoxvirus vaccine developed by multiple passages in cell culture to isolate viral variants that cause only limited infection in humans. The virus is produced as purified calf lymph and given percutaneously with a bifurcated needle. This vaccine was used in the first successful worldwide efforts to eradicate a human virus, variola or smallpox. Routine universal vaccinia immunization was discontinued around 1980, following the declaration by WHO that variola (smallpox) was eradicated, but the vaccine is still available. The nonemergency use of vaccinia vaccine includes vaccination of laboratory and healthcare workers exposed occupationally to vaccinia virus, to recombinant vaccinia viruses, or other orthopoxviruses that can infect humans, such as monkeypox virus and cowpox virus. Because there are still laboratory stocks of variola in research use in several countries, including the U.S., the U.S. ACIP has developed recommendations for the use of vaccinia vaccine if variola virus were used as an agent of biological terrorism or if a smallpox outbreak occurred accidentally. Large-scale use in the military and consideration of use in medical first responders in the U.S. has been implemented in recent decades. A derivative of conventional vaccinia virus vaccine has been developed that has desirable properties. MVA virus is a highly attenuated strain of vaccinia virus isolated after more than 500 passages in chicken embryo fibroblasts, during which the virus lost about 10% of the vaccinia genome and the ability to replicate productively in human and other primate cells.

Other Vaccines for Biodefense and Special Pathogens

There are a number of limited-use vaccines, such as those for workers in high-containment facilities conducting research on highly pathogenic agents that are emerging infectious diseases or potential agents for use in bioterrorism or biowarfare. Typically, these vaccines are used only under Investigational New Drug status. Examples include vaccines for Eastern equine encephalitis (EEE) virus, Venezuelan equine encephalitis (VEE) virus, Rift Valley fever virus, botulinum toxin, and others.

International Vaccines

There are additional vaccines pertinent to exposures in other countries that are licensed in some areas, but not yet in the U.S.

Dengue Virus Vaccine

Dengue fever is another mosquito-borne flaviviral disease caused by four different viral serotypes and annually affecting about 400 million people worldwide. The disease can be a mild systemic febrile illness during primary infection but can cause severe dengue disease and death during a second infection with virus of a different serotype. It is thought that cross-reactive nonneutralizing antibodies induced by one infection enhance the disease caused by subsequent infection with a heterologous serotype virus. This antibody-dependent enhancement concern has been a significant barrier to vaccine development efforts. Nevertheless, much progress has been made recently in dengue vaccine development.

There is currently no dengue vaccine approved for use in the U.S.; however, CYD-TDV developed by Sanofi Pasteur is a recombinant tetravalent (four-serotype) live attenuated virus vaccine that was first licensed in Mexico in December 2015 for use in individuals 9–45 years of age living in endemic areas. It is given as a three-dose series on a 0-, 6-, 12-month schedule. Additional dengue vaccine candidates are in clinical development.

Malaria Vaccine

The RTS,S vaccine is a recombinant protein-based malaria vaccine with AS01 adjuvant against *Plasmodium falciparum* that was developed by a large international public-private consortium and is the first malaria vaccine to complete efficacy trial testing with a positive review of the outcome. It is relevant for *P. falciparum*, which is common in sub-Saharan Africa, but does not protect against *Plasmodium vivax* malaria, which is more common in many countries outside Africa. The EMA issued a "European scientific opinion" on the vaccine, and WHO and its SAGE have advocated its use in large-scale implementation pilot tests in Africa.

BCG Vaccine

BCG vaccine is used to prevent severe disease due to *Mycobacterium tuberculosis* (TB). BCG vaccine is produced using a live attenuated bovine bacillus strain, *Mycobacterium bovis,* that has lost its ability to cause severe disease in humans. The vaccine typically is given as a single intradermal dose, often to infants near the time of birth. The efficacy of BCG vaccine against TB is uncertain in many settings, but the consensus is that the vaccine does protect against the most severe forms of disseminated TB, such as miliary disease and TB meningitis. The vaccine is a WHO essential medicine for endemic areas but is not used for universal vaccination in the U.S.

The Future of Vaccine Technology

Vaccination technology and improved methods to generate vaccines have led to the prevention of many infectious diseases. People no longer die at the high rates that prevailed before vaccines were developed. In the developing world, however, according to WHO reports, over 40% of deaths are due to infectious diseases, highlighting a continued need to improve existing vaccines, develop new vaccines, and improve delivery methods to increase efficacy. Viruses, bacteria, parasites, and antigens on cancerous cells are all future vaccine targets. New vaccines for pregnant mothers will be available to prevent diseases that can become chronic if the fetus becomes infected in utero, as is the case with malaria. Furthermore, an increasing elderly population will need access to better vaccines that can stimulate their aging immune systems, which are susceptible to infections like influenza and varicella viruses. Delivery methods are being explored to utilize nanoparticles and alternative adjuvants to improve vaccine immunogenicity so people will only need one vaccine dose rather than several. Needle-less delivery is already possible, as in the case of oral polio vaccine or via nasal sprays for influenza. Investigation continues on developing new edible vaccines using plants, microneedles, and needle-free dermal patches.

Most vaccines work through preventing disease due to acute infections; the challenge remains to develop vaccines against chronic viral infections where the host is immunosuppressed. These pathogens evade the immune system and persist in the host's own cells. To overcome these chronic pathogens, vaccines need to elicit both antibody and T cell responses, where B cells can neutralize the pathogen and T cells can actively kill and destroy infected cells. Vaccines against HPV and hepatitis B viruses protect not only from viral infection but also from developing infection-associated cancers.

New vaccines for other viral pathogens that can cause further complications are needed. For example, infection with group A streptococcus can lead to rheumatic fever, *Helicobacter pylori* may result in stomach cancer, and chlamydia infection can cause blindness and infertility. Vaccines provide effective prophylaxis; however, the frontier in vaccine technology will involve vaccines as therapies for already-established disease. Vaccines can be utilized against pathogens that become chronic, as in shingles, and also in conditions of autoimmunity and cancer, where the immune response is dysregulated. In the case of cancer, vaccines can be utilized to augment immunity to tumors to prevent their growth and metastasis. In the case of autoimmunity, the goal of this "negative vaccination" is to use vaccines to dampen immune function to prevent self-tissue destruction (Nossal, 2011).

Vaccine Safety: Myths, Truths, and Consequences

Vaccine Adjuvants and Safety

Adjuvants are substances added to vaccines to enhance the magnitude, quality, and duration of the protective immune response. Adjuvants are useful in vaccines because they stimulate the innate immune system that subsequently activates a strong adaptive immune response to ensure immune protection. Because many modern vaccines do not contain live pathogens, they must include adjuvants to ensure vaccine efficacy. Adjuvants are particularly useful in subunit protein vaccines, which often are inadequately immunogenic without enhancement.

There is extensive experience in human vaccines with two adjuvants, aluminum and monophosphoryl lipid A. Aluminum, in the form of alum, has been used for nearly 90 years in vaccines; aluminum hydroxide [$Al(OH)_3$] and aluminum phosphate ($AlPO_4$) are currently used. Aluminum is used in many childhood vaccines in the U.S. targeted to diphtheria-tetanus-pertussis, Hib and pneumococcus, hepatitis A and B, and HPV. Monophosphoryl lipid A (isolated from bacteria) has been used in the HPV vaccine Cervarix since 2009. A new influenza vaccine licensed for the 2016–2017 season included the adjuvant MF59, an oil-in-water emulsion of squalene oil. Another new influenza vaccine that is targeted to influenza H5N1 contains a new adjuvant termed AS03 (an "adjuvant system" containing α-tocopherol and squalene in an oil-in-water emulsion) and was licensed for inclusion in the U.S. pandemic influenza vaccine stockpile. Live attenuated virus vaccines do not contain adjuvants; thus, adjuvant-free vaccines include those directed against measles, mumps, rubella, chickenpox, rotavirus, polio, and live attenuated seasonal influenza virus.

Vaccines Do Not Cause Autism

Autism spectrum disorder rates have increased in the U.S. and other parts of the world in parallel with expansion in the diagnostic criteria of autism that that now include spectrum disorders with a broader array of symptoms (Hansen et al., 2015). The CDC found that 1 of 68 children in the U.S. has ASD. Patients with this disorder have development impairments that affect their communication, behavior, and social interactions. Even though some people have been concerned with a causal link between vaccines and autism, many large scientific studies have failed to detect any such link (Hviid et al., 2003; Madsen et al., 2002; Schechter and Grether, 2008; Taylor et al., 2014). The IOM (now termed the National Academy of Medicine) conducted thorough reviews and concluded that current childhood and adult vaccines are very safe. In 2014, a CDC study added to reports around the world that vaccines do not cause ASD. They concluded that the total amount of antigen received from vaccines did not differ between children with ASD and those without the disorder. Vaccination with the MMR vaccine also is not associated with development of ASD in children.

Preservatives, Including Thimerosal

Preservatives added to vaccine preparations are designed to kill or inhibit the growth of bacteria and fungi that could contaminate a vaccine vial. There are historical reports of severe adverse events or death due to bacterial contamination of multidose vials lacking preservative. The highest risk of contamination is probably due to repetitive puncture of a multidose vaccine vial that is stored over time. Therefore, The U.S. *Code of Federal Regulations* requires the addition of a preservative to multidose vials of vaccines. Preservatives eliminate or reduce contamination in this setting. Several preservatives have been incorporated into licensed vaccines, including 2-phenoxyethanol, benzethonium chloride, phenol, and thimerosal.

thimerosal-Na⁺

Thimerosal, known to many by the trade name Merthiolate, has been one of the most commonly used preservatives; it is an organomercurial, an organic compound containing mercury. Thimerosal has been used safely since the early 20th century as a preservative in biologics, including many vaccines, and has a long history of use. Over time, concerns were raised about its safety because some organomercurials were increasingly associated with neurotoxicity, and children began receiving increasing numbers of licensed vaccines. The FDA chose to work with manufacturers toward reduction or elimination of thimerosal from childhood vaccines because of these *theoretical concerns*. As a result, thiomersal has been eliminated or reduced to trace amounts in nearly all childhood vaccines except some IIVs.

In terms of toxicity from mercury, most of the data in the field pertains to methylmercury, whereas thimerosal is a derivative of ethylmercury, which is cleared more rapidly. Thimerosal does not have significant toxic effects at the concentrations used in vaccine formulations. However, questions were raised about the potential association of thimerosal-containing vaccines in children and the occurrence of neurodevelopmental disorders, especially autism. A rather sordid history of fraud, conflict of interest, and other irregularities has been revealed pertaining to the now-debunked association studies of thimerosal and autism; decades of studies have been conducted in safety reviews around this matter.

The National Vaccine Advisory Committee, ACIP of the CDC, and the IOM's Immunization Safety Review Committee have all conducted extensive reviews of association studies, and the conclusion is that autism is not associated with the amount of thimerosal in childhood vaccines. In any event, recognizing public concern, between 2001 and 2003, thimerosal was eliminated from or reduced in childhood vaccines (except for flu) for children under 6 years old in hopes of encouraging childhood vaccination. The CDC has compiled a thorough review and list of articles relating to this issue (CDC, 2015).

Adverse Events With Vaccines

For injectable vaccines, common adverse effects include minor *local reactions* to vaccines at the injection site (pain, swelling, and redness). More widespread effects, termed *systemic reactions*, may include fever, rash, irritability, drowsiness, and other symptoms, depending on the vaccine. The profile of reactions seen in large-scale trials is carefully documented in package inserts. During vaccine candidate testing, any occurrence of serious adverse events (SAEs) are examined carefully. SAEs are events following vaccination that involve hospitalization, life-threatening events, death, disability, permanent damage, congenital anomaly/birth defect, or other conditions requiring medical intervention. Vaccines with clear association with SAEs are typically not licensed. In some cases, to increase the likelihood of detecting of rare SAEs, the FDA requires phase 4 studies (postmarketing surveillance) to follow the performance of vaccines as use expands beyond the size of the trials leading to licensure. The government also collects data after licensure through the vaccine adverse event reporting system (VAERS). Vaccines can be withdrawn from market if concerns arise. For example, licensure for use of the live oral rotavirus vaccine Rotashield, which was recommended for routine immunization of the U.S. infants in 1998, was withdrawn in 1999 when reports in VAERS suggested an association between the vaccine and intussusception, a form of bowel obstruction.

Allergic Reactions

Allergy to components of vaccine formulations also can cause reactions. Trace amounts of antibiotics like neomycin, used to ensure sterility in some vaccines (e.g., MMR, trivalent IPV, and varicella vaccine), may cause adverse reactions. A history of anaphylactic reaction (but not local reaction) to neomycin is a contraindication to future immunization with those vaccines. Persons with a history of egg allergy should not be given an influenza vaccine prepared in eggs. Gelatin, which is used as a stabilizer in some virus vaccines like varicella and MMR vaccines, may cause allergic reaction in some.

Fainting

Fainting, or syncope, also has been reported in people after vaccination. Fainting is more common in adolescents than in children or adults and thus is more common after vaccination with HPV, MCV4, and Tdap. Immediate fainting episodes following vaccination procedures is triggered by pain or anxiety, rather than the contents of the vaccines. While fainting is not serious, falling while fainting can cause injury, with head injuries the most serious. Clinicians can give patients drinks and snacks to prevent some fainting and can prevent falls by having patients lie down or sit during the procedure. Patients who faint after vaccination will recover after a few minutes, and clinicians should observe patients for at least 15 min after vaccination (a recommendation of the CDC).

Febrile Seizure

Fevers of 102°F (38.9°C) or higher can cause children to experience febrile seizures, which are characterized by body spasms and jerky movements that may last for up to 2 min. About 5% of children will experience a febrile seizure in their lifetime, with most occurring at 14–18 months of age. Children experiencing simple febrile seizures recover quickly without long-term harm. These common seizures also are caused by febrile illnesses associated with viral infections, especially roseola, ear infections, and other common childhood illnesses. Current vaccines sometimes induce fevers, usually low grade in nature, but rarely result in febrile seizures. Although fever following vaccination with most vaccines rarely causes febrile seizure, there is a small increase in risk after MMR and MMRV vaccines. The CDC also has reported a small increase in febrile seizures after a child receives the IIV together with PCV13 vaccine or in combination with diphtheria, tetanus, or DTaP vaccines. The increase of febrile seizures when combining these vaccines is small, and the CDC does not recommend delivering them on separate days. Importantly, vaccine usage can help prevent febrile seizures by providing vaccinated children protection against measles, mumps, rubella, chickenpox, influenza, and pneumococcal infectious pathogens that may result in febrile seizures.

Guillain-Barré Syndrome

Guillian-Barré syndrome is a rare disease that affects the nervous system. Patients with GBS display muscle weakness and sometimes paralysis that results when their own immune system injures their neurons. GBS often occurs after an infection with bacteria or virus; most patients with GBS recover fully. However, some subjects can have permanent nerve damage. The incidence of GBS in the U.S. currently is about 3000–6000 cases per year; thus, it is rare in a population of about 350 million. GBS is more common in older adults, with people older than 50 years at greater risk. GBS may have several underlying causes, but scientists report that two-thirds of GBS cases occurred after patients were ill with gastroenteritis or respiratory tract infections. Infection with *Campylobacter jejuni* is the most common risk factor for the disease, but GBS also has been reported commonly after influenza virus, cytomegalovirus, or Epstein-Barr viral infection. GBS after vaccination is reported but rare.

An IOM study reported that widespread use of the 1976 swine influenza virus vaccine was associated with a small increase in risk for GBS, with an additional case of GBS per 100,000 people who were vaccinated, although later statistical review called this association into question. Current assessments are that the there is no significant risk of GBS after obtaining a seasonal influenza vaccine, or if there is an association, the risk is approximately one case per million vaccinated individuals, a low rate that is difficult to detect with certainty. Studies have shown that a person is more likely to get GBS after influenza infection than vaccination. Importantly, severe morbidity and mortality are a significant risk after influenza infection, and preventing complications and death can be achieved by getting vaccinated.

Sudden Infant Death Syndrome

Sudden infant death syndrome peaks when babies are between 2 and 4 months old, and infants are also given many vaccines during this period. The temporal overlap of peak SIDS incidence and the period of initiation of childhood vaccination series led to questions about any causal relationship between vaccines and SIDS. Numerous studies have failed to detect a causative association for vaccines and SIDS (Silvers et al., 2001). The IOM 2003 report reviewed the relationship of SIDS and vaccines and concluded that vaccines do not cause SIDS. Infant death by SIDS has decreased dramatically due to the 1992 American Academy of Pediatrics recommendations to place infants on their backs to sleep and the 1994 National Institute of Child Health and Human Development campaign efforts.

Safety of Multiple Vaccinations

Children are exposed to a large number of bacteria and viruses in their environment through food, teething of objects, and exposure to pets and to other humans. The typical viral infection results in exposure of the immune system to a dozen or more antigens; some bacteria express hundreds of antigens during infection. Each recommended childhood vaccine protects against 1 to 69 antigens. When a child is given the full recommended vaccines on the 2014 schedule, they are exposed to up to 315 antigens by age 2, which provides them critical protection against pathogens in the environment (CDC, 2016). Vaccinating patients against multiple antigens has been shown to be safe when they are delivered in combination at the same time. This strategy is advantageous for patients, especially children, because they lack immunity to most vaccine preventable diseases, so receiving this protection during the relatively vulnerable period of early development is important. The patient also has fewer doctor visits with combination or multiple vaccinations, reducing cost in terms of money and time for parents and disruption for children. Numerous studies have shown that giving various vaccine combinations does not cause chronic disease. Furthermore, each time a combination vaccine or multiple vaccination schedule is licensed, that intervention already has been tested for safety and efficacy in combination with the vaccines previously recommended for that age group. The ACIP and the Academy of Pediatrics recommend receiving multiple vaccines at the same time (CDC, 2016).

Vaccine Myths and Their Public Health Consequences

The public health success of vaccines is demonstrated by the decreased rates of mortality and morbidity due to infectious diseases contracted in childhood and adulthood. A dramatic example of success is the worldwide eradication of smallpox, a pathogen responsible for epidemics that killed 300–500 million people in the 20th century and disfigured many survivors. In the 20th century, poliovirus and MeV also incapacitated and killed infected individuals, especially young children. New generations have never seen the debilitating effects of these infectious diseases, thanks to decades of successful public health vaccination strategies. Infectious diseases, however, continue to affect the lives of many people in the developing world who have less access to healthcare or are affected by wars or famine. Recently, preventable diseases are arising again in the developed world because of vaccine myths that have reduced vaccination rates in these countries.

One of these myths concerns autism. A study that has been retracted and discredited claimed there was a link between vaccination in children and autism (Wakefield et al., 1998). Despite major shortcomings and incorrect interpretations, this study changed public perceptions regarding vaccine safety, and its influence persists. Experimental studies in different parts of the world with large cohorts, statistical power, and rigor have found no evidence that vaccines cause autism (American Academy of Pediatrics, 2017; Madsen et al., 2002). Researchers have found that autism occurs in families, may have a genetic component, and may be affected by environmental triggers such as insecticides, certain drugs, and rubella virus. The exact causes of ASDs are unknown and continue to be investigated (Landrigan, 2010).

Nonetheless, the antivaccination movement has gained momentum, with celebrities, politicians, and social media continuing to propagate erroneous vaccine information and conspiracy theories. According to the CDC, vaccination rates have fallen in many parts of the U.S. In nine U.S. states, fewer than two-thirds of children ages 19 to 35 months have been vaccinated with the recommended seven-vaccination regimen. This dismissal of scientific evidence on vaccines can have deadly consequences. Infectious epidemics due to preventable agents like poliovirus and MeV can reemerge. Unvaccinated children will be more susceptible to infection,

and many of them will not survive. Furthermore, unvaccinated subjects contribute to reducing the benefits of herd immunity that protects people who cannot be vaccinated for medical reasons, such as cancer, HIV infection, and other types of immunodeficiency.

Diseases due to pertussis, polio, measles, *H. influenzae*, and rubella virus once affected hundreds of thousands of people and killed thousands. Following the introduction of universal vaccinations, the rates of these diseases decreased to near-zero levels in the U.S. Some believe that because these diseases have been nearly eliminated in the U.S., vaccination is no longer needed. This thinking is incorrect. Vaccine-preventable diseases are communicable diseases, spreading from person to person, and the causative viruses and bacteria survive in nature. People, especially the unvaccinated, can be infected, and infected individuals will spread the disease to unvaccinated individuals. A greater fraction of vaccinated individuals in a population leads to fewer opportunities for the disease to spread (herd immunity).

Parental vaccine concerns should be taken seriously, and misconceptions should be thoroughly discussed by providers to ensure that patients have scientific information and are informed about the risks associated with failure to vaccinate. By providing parental education, pediatricians and other primary care medical providers can help reduce vaccine hesitancy.

Licensure and Monitoring of Vaccines

Immune Correlates and Mechanisms

During the process of vaccine development and testing, manufacturers seek to define laboratory tests and parameters that are associated with efficacy, which have been designated immune CoPs. First, it is important theoretically to understand some features of the biological mechanism of protection to optimize development and use of vaccines. At a practical level, identification of a correlate allows monitoring of the reproducibility of vaccines during repetitive manufacture, monitoring the expected impact of new combinations of vaccine antigens on immunogenicity of existing vaccines, and other critical issues.

Plotkin and others have developed terminology for principal types of correlates (Plotkin and Gilbert, 2012). A CoP is a marker of immune function that statistically correlates with protection. Such markers can be simply associated with protection (termed nCoP) or alternatively may be known to measure directly the immune effectors that mediate protection (mCoP). From a practical standpoint, either an nCoP or an mCoP can enable monitoring and prediction of effective vaccination.

The ideal CoP is one that is quantitative and derives from a reproducible laboratory test that has been validated under good laboratory practice conditions. The type of protection suggested for a particular correlate may vary because vaccines may be designed to prevent differing classes of infection, such as local versus systemic infection or severe disease versus any disease. Examples of quantitative CoPs in use include a threshold of 10 mIU/mL in serum of hepatitis B antibodies detected in a standardized ELISA (enzyme-linked immunosorbent assay), serum diphtheria toxin neutralization concentration of 0.01 to 0.1 IU/mL, a serum virus neutralization dilution titer of 1/5 for yellow fever virus, or a 1/40 dilution of serum in influenza hemagglutination inhibition titer.

Regulatory and Advisory Bodies

The Center for Biologics Evaluation and Research (CBER) of the FDA regulates vaccine products in the U.S., with recommendations from its Vaccines and Related Biological Products Advisory Committee. The EMA regulates in Europe. Manufacturers conduct phase 1 (safety and immunogenicity studies) in a small number of closely monitored subjects; phase 2 studies (dose-ranging studies) typically in several hundred subjects; and then phase 3 trials (efficacy studies) typically in thousands of subjects. If successful, the sponsor submits a Biologics License Application (BLA) to the FDA, which may lead to licensure. Licensure allows use, but decisions on whether vaccines are recommended for specific populations or for universal use are made by additional advisory bodies. The CDC hosts the ACIP, a committee of public health and medical experts, which makes recommendations for use of vaccines in the U.S. Various professional medical societies also publish recommendations, for instance, the American Academy of Pediatrics publishes the *AAP Red Book*, or "Report of the Committee on Infectious Diseases of the American Academy of Pediatrics," which contains vaccine recommendations. Finally, third-party payers, such as insurance companies, affect usage through reimbursement policies; thus, issues of cost, benefit, and profitability become considerations, as examined in Chapter 1.

Bibliography

American Academy of Pediatrics. Vaccine safety: examine the evidence. January 26, **2017**. Available at: https://www.healthychildren.org/English/safety-prevention/immunizations/Pages/Vaccine-Studies-Examine-the-Evidence.aspx. Accessed March 4, 2017.

Baxter D. Active and passive immunity, vaccine types, excipients and licensing. *Occup Med (Lond),* **2007**, *57*:552–556.

CDC. Vaccines do not cause autism. Update of November 23, **2015**. Available at: https://www.cdc.gov/vaccinesafety/concerns/autism.html. Accessed March 7, 2017.

CDC. Safety Information About Specific Vaccines. Update of January 21, **2016**. Available at: https://www.cdc.gov/vaccinesafety/vaccines/index.html. Accessed June 15, 2017.

Clem AS. Fundamentals of vaccine immunology. *J Glob Infect Dis,* **2011**, *3*:73–78.

Gill DM, et al. Diphtheria toxin, protein synthesis, and the cell. *Fed Proc,* **1973**, *32*:1508–1515.

Gross CP, Sepkowitz KA. The myth of the medical breakthrough: smallpox, vaccination, and Jenner reconsidered. *Int J Infect Dis,* **1998**, *3*:54–60.

Hansen SN, et al. Explaining the increase in the prevalence of autism spectrum disorders: the proportion attributable to changes in reporting practices. *JAMA Pediatr,* **2015**, *169*:56–62.

Hinman A. Landmark perspective: mass vaccination against polio. *JAMA,* **1984**, *251*:2994–2996.

Hopkins DR. *The Greatest Killer: Smallpox in History.* University of Chicago Press, Chicago, **2002**.

Hviid A, et al. Association between thimerosal-containing vaccine and autism. *JAMA,* **2003**, *290*:1763–1766.

Madsen KM, et al. A population-based study of measles, mumps, and rubella vaccination and autism. *N Engl J Med,* **2002**, *347*:1477–1482.

Marrack P, et al. Towards an understanding of the adjuvant action of aluminium. *Nat Rev Immunol,* **2009**, *9*:287–293.

Landrigan PJ. What causes autism? Exploring the environmental contribution. *Curr Opin Pediatr,* **2010**, *22*:219–225.

Nossal GJ. Vaccines of the future. *Vaccine,* **2011**, *29*(suppl 4):D111–D115.

Plotkin SA, Gilbert PB. Nomenclature for immune correlates of protection after vaccination. *Clin Infect Dis,* **2012**, *54*:1615–1617.

Riesbeck K, Nordstrom T. Structure and immunological action of the human pathogen *Moraxella catarrhalis* IgD-binding protein. *Crit Rev Immunol,* **2006**, *26*:353–376.

Robinson HL, et al. DNA vaccines for viral infections: basic studies and applications. *Adv Virus Res,* **2000**, *55*:1–74.

Schechter R, Grether JK. Continuing increases in autism reported to California's developmental services system: mercury in retrograde. *Arch Gen Psychiatry,* **2008**, *65*:19–24.

Schroeder HW Jr, Cavacini L. Structure and function of immunoglobulins. *J Allergy Clin Immunol,* **2010**, *125*:S41–S52.

Silvers LE, et al. The epidemiology of fatalities reported to the vaccine adverse event reporting system 1990–1997. *Pharmacoepidemiol Drug Saf,* **2001**, *10*:279–285.

Taylor LE, et al. Vaccines are not associated with autism: an evidence-based meta-analysis of case-control and cohort studies. *Vaccine,* **2014**, *32*:3623–3629.

Wakefield AJ, et al. Ileal-lymphoid-nodular hyperplasia, non-specific colitis, and pervasive developmental disorder in children. *Lancet,* **1998**, *351*: 637–641. Article retracted: *Lancet,* **2010**, *375*:445.

Woof JM, Mestecky J. Mucosal immunoglobulins. *Immunol Rev,* **2005**, *206*:64–82.

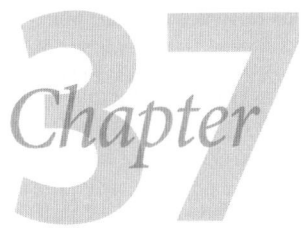

Chapter 37

Lipid-Derived Autacoids: Eicosanoids and Platelet-Activating Factor

Emer M. Smyth, Tilo Grosser, and Garret A. FitzGerald

Eicosanoids	Platelet-Activating Factor
▪ Biosynthesis	▪ Chemistry and Biosynthesis
▪ Inhibitors of Eicosanoid Biosynthesis	▪ Sites of PAF Synthesis
▪ Eicosanoid Degradation	▪ Mechanism of Action of PAF
▪ Pharmacological Properties	▪ Physiological and Pathological Functions of PAF
▪ Physiological Actions and Pharmacological Effects	▪ PAF Receptor Antagonists
▪ Therapeutic Uses	

Membrane lipids supply the substrate for the synthesis of *eicosanoids* and *platelet-activating factor* (PAF). Arachidonic acid (AA) metabolites, including *PGs, PGI₂, TxA₂, LTs*, and *epoxygenase products* of CYPs, collectively the eicosanoids, are not stored but are produced by most cells when a variety of physical, chemical, and hormonal stimuli activate acyl hydrolases that make arachidonate available. *Membrane glycerophosphocholine* derivatives can be modified enzymatically to produce PAF. PAF is formed by a smaller number of cell types, principally leukocytes, platelets, and endothelial cells. Eicosanoids and PAF lipids function as signaling molecules in many biological processes, including the regulation of vascular tone, renal function, hemostasis, parturition, GI mucosal integrity, and stem cell function. They are also important mediators of innate immunity and inflammation. Several classes of drugs, most notably NSAIDs (see Chapter 38), including aspirin, owe their principal therapeutic effects—relief of inflammatory pain and antipyresis—to blockade of PG formation.

Eicosanoids

Eicosanoids, from the Greek *eikosi* ("twenty") are formed from precursor essential fatty acids that contain 20 carbons and 3, 4, or 5 double bonds: 8,11,14-eicosatrienoic acid (dihomo-γ-linolenic acid), 5,8,11,14-eicosatetraenoic acid (AA; Figure 37–1), and EPA. AA is the most abundant precursor, derived from the dietary omega-6 fatty acid, linoleic acid (9,12-octadecadienoic acid), or ingested directly as a dietary constituent. EPA is a major constituent of oils from fatty fish such as salmon.

History

In 1930, American gynecologists Kurzrok and Lieb observed that strips of uterine myometrium relax or contract when exposed to semen. Subsequently, Goldblatt in England and von Euler in Sweden reported independently on smooth muscle contracting and vasodepressor activities in seminal fluid and accessory reproductive glands. In 1935, von Euler identified the active material as a lipid-soluble acid, which he named *prostaglandin*. Samuelsson, Bergström, and their colleagues elucidated the structures of PGE₁ and PGF₁α in 1962. In 1964, Bergström and coworkers and van Dorp and associates independently achieved biosynthesis of PGE₂ from AA. Discovery of TxA₂, PGI₂, and the LTs followed. Vane, Smith, and Willis in 1971 reported that aspirin and NSAIDs act by inhibiting PG biosynthesis. This remarkable period of discovery linked the Nobel Prize of von Euler in 1970 to that of Bergström, Samuelsson, and Vane in 1982.

Biosynthesis

Biosynthesis of eicosanoids is limited by the availability of AA and depends primarily on the release of esterified AA from membrane phospholipids or other complex lipids by acyl hydrolases, notably PLA₂. Once liberated, AA is metabolized rapidly to oxygenated products by *COXs, LOXs*, and CYPs (Figure 37–1).

Chemical and physical stimuli activate the Ca²⁺-dependent translocation of group IV_A cytosolic phospholipase A_2 (cPLA₂) to the membrane, where it hydrolyzes the *sn*-2 ester bond of membrane phosphatidylcholine and phosphatidylethanolamine, releasing AA. Multiple additional PLA₂ isoforms (secretory [s] and Ca²⁺-independent [i] forms) have been characterized. Under basal conditions, AA liberated by iPLA₂ is reincorporated into cell membranes. During stimulation, cPLA₂ dominates the acute release of AA, while an inducible sPLA₂ contributes to AA release under conditions of sustained or intense stimulation. sPLA₂ contributes to platelet microparticle generation of eicosanoids that then direct microparticle internalization by neutrophils driving inflammation (Duchez et al., 2015).

Products of Cyclooxygenases (Prostaglandin G/H Synthases)

Prostaglandin endoperoxide G/H synthase is called *cyclooxygenase* or *COX* colloquially. Products of this pathway are PGs, PGI₂, and TxA₂, collectively termed *prostanoids*. The pathway is described by Figure 37–1 and its legend.

Prostanoids are distinguished by substitutions on their cyclopentane rings the number of double bonds in their side chains, as indicated by numerical subscripts (dihomo-γ-linolenic acid is the precursor of *series₁*, AA for *series₂*, and EPA for *series₃*). Prostanoids derived from AA carry the subscript 2 and are the major series in mammals.

There are two distinct COX isoforms, COX-1 and COX-2 (Rouzer and Marnett, 2009; Smith et al., 2011). COX-1, expressed constitutively in most cells, is the dominant source of prostanoids for housekeeping functions, such as cytoprotection of the gastric epithelium (see Chapter 49). COX-2, in contrast, is upregulated by cytokines, shear stress, and growth factors and is the principal source of prostanoid formation in inflammation and cancer. However, this distinction is not absolute; both enzymes may contribute to the generation of autoregulatory and homeostatic prostanoids during physiologic and pathophysiologic processes.

With 61% amino acid identity, COX-1 and COX-2 have remarkably similar crystal structures. Both isoforms are expressed as dimers homotypically inserted into the endoplasmic reticular membrane. Through sequential COX and POX activity, both COXs convert AA to two unstable intermediates that are then converted to the prostanoids

Abbreviations

AA: arachidonic acid
ACTH: corticotropin (formerly adrenocorticotrophic hormone)
BLT1/2: LTB4 receptors
cAMP: cyclic adenosine monophosphate
COX: cyclooxygenase
CYP: cytochrome P450
CysLT: cysteinyl leukotriene
CysLT1/2: CysLT receptors
DP$_2$: a member of the fMLP-receptor superfamily, CRTH2
DP: PGD$_2$ receptor
EDHF: endothelium-derived hyperpolarizing factor
EET: epoxyeicosatrienoic acid
EP: PGE$_2$ receptor
EPA: 5,8,11,14,17-eicosapentaenoic acid
FLAP: 5-LOX–activating protein
FP: PGF$_2\alpha$ receptor
fMLP: formyl-methionyl-leucyl-phenylalanine
GPCR: G protein–coupled receptor
HETE: hydroxyeicosatetraenoic acid
HPETE: hydroxyperoxyeicosatetraenoic acid
IL: interleukin
IP$_3$: inositol 1,4,5-trisphosphate
IP: PGI$_2$ receptor
iPLA$_2$: independent PLA$_2$
IsoP: isoprostane
LOX: lipoxygenase
LT: leukotriene
LX*: lipoxin*, e.g., LXA, LXB
NSAID: nonsteroidal anti-inflammatory drug
PAF: platelet-activating factor
PAF-AH: PAF acetylhydrolyase
PG: prostaglandin
PGDH: PG 15-OH dehydrogenase
PGI$_2$: prostacyclin
PL*: phospholipase*, e.g., PLA, PLC
PMN: polymorphonuclear leukocyte
POX: peroxidase
TNF: tumor necrosis factor
TP: TxA$_2$ receptor
TxA: thromboxane A

by synthases, expressed in a relatively cell-specific fashion. For example, COX-1–derived TxA$_2$ is the dominant product in platelets, whereas COX-2–derived PGE$_2$ and TxA$_2$ dominate in activated macrophages. Prostanoids are released from cells by diffusion, although transport may be facilitated through the multidrug resistance-associated protein (MRP) transporter (Schuster, 2002).

Lipoxygenase Products

Major products of the LOX pathways are hydroxy fatty acid derivatives known as HETEs, LTs, and LXs (Figure 37–2) (Haeggström and Funk, 2011; Powell and Rokach, 2015). LTs play a major role in the development and persistence of the inflammatory response.

The LOXs are a family of enzymes containing nonheme iron; LOXs catalyze the oxygenation of polyenic fatty acids to corresponding lipid hydroperoxides. The enzymes require a fatty acid substrate with two cis double bonds separated by a methylene group. AA, which contains several double bonds in this configuration, is metabolized to HPETEs, which vary in the site of insertion of the hydroperoxy group. HPETEs are converted to their corresponding HETEs either nonenzymatically or by a POX.

There are five active human LOXs—5(S)-LOX, 12(S)-LOX, 12(R)-LOX, 15(S)-LOX-1, and 15(S)-LOX-2—classified according to the site of hydroperoxy group insertion. Their expression is frequently cell specific; platelets have only 12(S)-LOX, whereas leukocytes contain both 5(S)- and 12(S)-LOX (Figure 37–2). 12(R)-LOX is restricted in expression mostly to the skin. The epidermal LOXs, which constitute a distinct LOX subgroup, also include 15-LOX-2 and eLOX-3, the most recently identified family member. eLOX-3 has been reported to metabolize further 12(R)-HETE, the product of 12(R)-LOX, to a specific epoxyalcohol product.

The 5-LOX pathway leads to the synthesis of the LTs. When eosinophils, mast cells, PMNs, or monocytes are activated, 5-LOX translocates to the nuclear membrane and associates with FLAP, an integral membrane protein that facilitates AA to 5-LOX interaction (Evans et al., 2008). Drugs that inhibit FLAP block LT production. A two-step reaction is catalyzed by 5-LOX: oxygenation of AA to form 5-HPETE followed by dehydration to an unstable epoxide, LTA$_4$. LTA$_4$ is transformed by distinct enzymes to LTB$_4$ or LTC$_4$. Extracellular metabolism of the peptide moiety of LTC$_4$ generates LTD$_4$ and LTE$_4$ (Peters-Golden and Henderson, 2007). Collectively, LTC$_4$, LTD$_4$, and LTE$_4$ are the *CysLTs*. LTB$_4$ and LTC$_4$ are actively transported out of the cell. LTA$_4$, the primary product of the 5-LOX pathway, is metabolized by 12-LOX to form LXA$_4$ and LXB$_4$. These mediators also can arise through 5-LOX metabolism of 15-HETE.

Products of CYPs

The CYP epoxygenases, primarily CYP2C and CYP2J, metabolize AA to EETs (Fleming, 2014). In endothelial cells, EETs function as EDHFs, particularly in the coronary circulation. EET biosynthesis can be altered by pharmacological, nutritional, and genetic factors that affect CYP expression.

Other Pathways

The isoeicosanoids, a family of eicosanoid isomers, are generated by nonenzymatic free radical catalyzed oxidation of AA. Unlike PGs, these compounds are initially formed esterified in phospholipids and released by PLs; the isoeicosanoids then circulate and are metabolized and excreted into urine. Their production is not inhibited in vivo by inhibitors of COX-1 or COX-2, but their formation is suppressed by antioxidants. Isoprostanes correlate with cardiovascular risk factors, and increased levels are found in a large number of clinical conditions (Milne et al., 2015). Their relevance as biologically active mediators remains unclear. A series of compounds, *LXs, maresins, resolvins*, when synthesized and administered to certain models of inflammation, hasten its resolution. It remains to be established whether the endogenous compounds are formed in quantities sufficient to exert this effect in vivo (Skarke et al., 2015).

Inhibitors of Eicosanoid Biosynthesis

Inhibition of PLA$_2$ decreases the release of the precursor fatty acid and the synthesis of all its metabolites. PLA$_2$ may be inhibited by drugs that reduce the availability of Ca^{2+}. *Glucocorticoids* inhibit PLA$_2$ indirectly by inducing the synthesis of a group of proteins termed *annexins* that modulate PLA$_2$ activity. Glucocorticoids also downregulate induced expression of COX-2 but not of COX-1 (see Chapter 46). Aspirin and NSAIDs inhibit the COX, but not the POX, moiety of both COX enzymes and thus the formation of downstream prostanoids. These drugs do not inhibit LOXs and may cause increased formation of LTs by shunting of substrate to the LOX pathway. Dual inhibitors of COX and 5-LOX have proven effective in some models of inflammation and tissue injury (Minutoli et al., 2015; Oak et al., 2014). LTs may contribute to the GI side effects associated with NSAIDs (Janusz et al., 1998; Xu et al., 2009).

Differences in the sensitivity of COX-1 and COX-2 to inhibition by certain anti-inflammatory drugs led to the development of selective inhibitors of COX-2, including the coxibs (Grosser et al., 2010) (see Chapter 38). These drugs were hypothesized to offer therapeutic advantages over older NSAIDs (many of which are nonselective COX inhibitors) because COX-2 was thought to be the predominant source of PGs in inflammation, whereas COX-1 is the major source

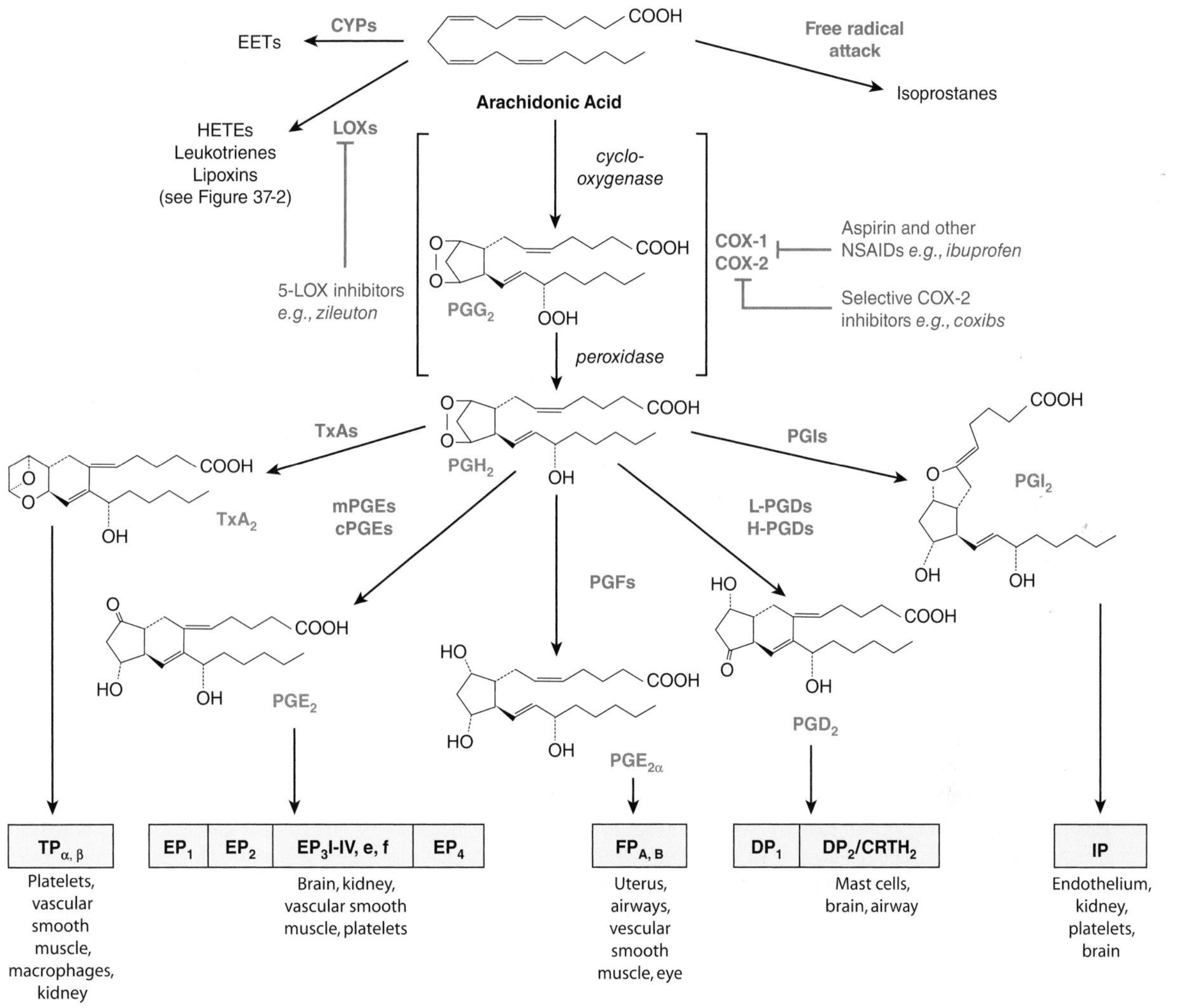

Figure 37–1 *Metabolism of AA.* Cyclic endoperoxides (PGG$_2$ and PGH$_2$) arise from the sequential COX and hydroperoxidase actions of COX-1 or COX-2 on AA released from membrane phospholipids. Subsequent products are generated by tissue-specific synthases and transduce their effects via membrane-bound receptors (blue boxes). EETs and isoprostanes are generated via CYP activity and nonenzymatic free radical attack, respectively. Aspirin and nonselective NSAIDs are nonselective inhibitors of COX-1 and COX-2 but do not affect LOX activity. See the text and the Abbreviations list for further definitions.

of cytoprotective PGs in the GI tract. Randomized trials of selective COX-2 inhibitors reported their superiority in GI safety over nonselective NSAID comparators.

However, there now is compelling evidence that COX-2 inhibitors confer a spectrum of cardiovascular hazards (myocardial infarction, stroke, systemic and pulmonary hypertension, congestive heart failure, and sudden cardiac death) (Grosser et al., 2010). The hazards can be explained sufficiently by suppression of cardioprotective COX-2–derived PGs, especially PGI$_2$, and the unrestrained effects of endogenous stimuli, such as platelet COX-1–derived TxA$_2$, on platelet activation, vascular proliferation and remodeling, hypertension, and atherogenesis.

Because LTs mediate inflammation, efforts have focused on development of LT receptor antagonists and selective inhibitors of the LOXs. *Zileuton*, an inhibitor of 5-LOX, and selective CysLT$_1$ receptor antagonists (*zafirlukast, pranlukast,* and *montelukast*) have established efficacy in the treatment of mild-to-moderate asthma (see Chapter 40). These treatments remain, however, less effective than inhaled corticosteroids. A common polymorphism in the gene for LTC$_4$ synthase that correlates with increased LTC$_4$ generation may be associated with higher asthma risk in some populations and with the efficacy of anti-LT therapy. Interestingly, although polymorphisms in the genes encoding 5-LOX or FLAP have yet to be linked to asthma, studies have demonstrated an association of these genes with myocardial infarction, stroke, and atherosclerosis (Peters-Golden and Henderson, 2007); thus, inhibition of LT biosynthesis may eventually prove to be useful in the prevention of cardiovascular disease.

Eicosanoid Degradation

Most eicosanoids are efficiently and rapidly inactivated (Figure 37–3). The enzymatic catabolic reactions are of two types:

- a rapid initial step, catalyzed by widely distributed PG-specific enzymes, wherein PGs lose most of their biological activity; and
- a second step in which these metabolites are oxidized, probably by enzymes identical to those responsible for the β and ω oxidation of fatty acids.

The lung, kidney, and liver play prominent roles in the enzymatically catalyzed reactions. Metabolic clearance requires an energy-dependent cellular uptake PG transporter and possibly other transporters (Schuster et al., 2002). The initial step is the oxidation of the 15-OH group to the corresponding ketone by PGDH. PGI$_2$ and TxA$_2$, however, undergo spontaneous hydrolysis as a first degradative step. LTC$_4$ degradation also occurs in the lungs, kidney, and liver but may also occur in LTC$_4$ via CYP4F enzymes. Inactivation of 15-hydroxyprostaglandin dehydrogenase, which elevates the capacity of tissues to form PGE$_2$, enhances tissue regeneration after hematopoietic stem cell transplantation and after hemihepatectomy (Zhang et al., 2015).

Pharmacological Properties

The eicosanoids function through activation of specific GPCRs (Table 37–1) that couple to intracellular second-messenger systems to modulate cellular activity (Figure 37–4).

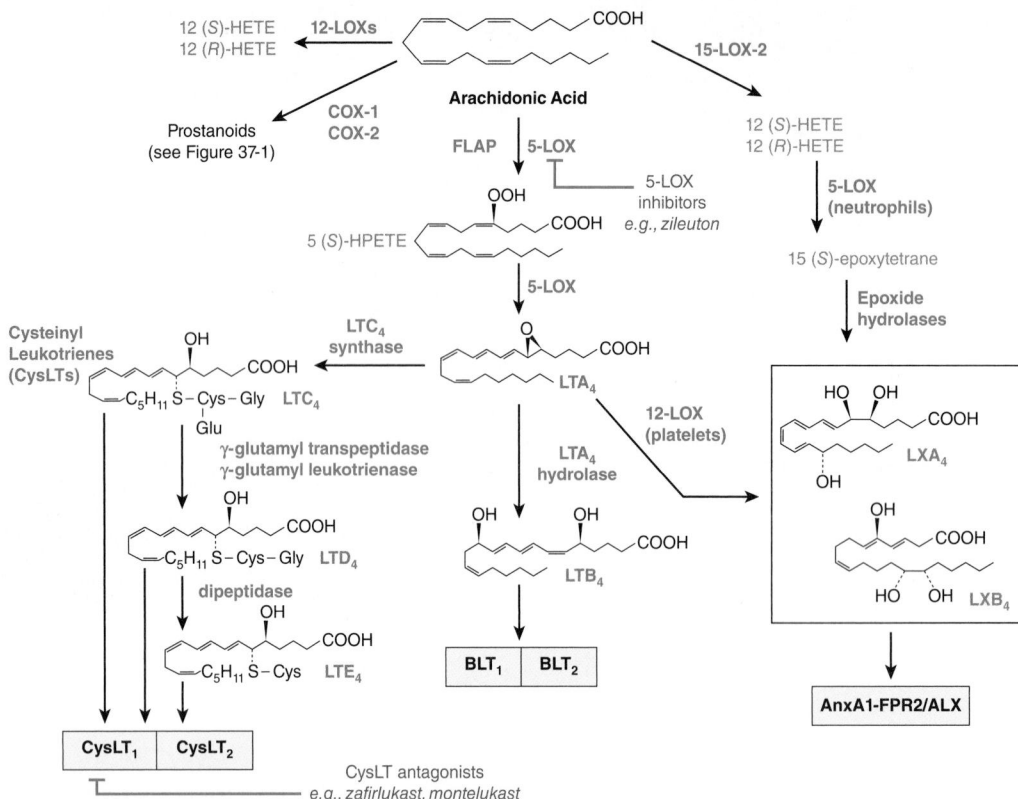

Figure 37–2 *Lipoxygenase pathways of AA metabolism.* FLAP presents AA to 5-LOX, leading to the generation of the LTs and CysLTs. LXs (boxed) are products of cellular interaction via a 5-LOX–12-LOX pathway or via a 15-LOX–5-LOX pathway. Biological effects are transduced via membrane-bound receptors (blue boxes). While its biological relevance remains controversial, LXA$_4$ can activate a GPCR also activated by Annexin A1 and by the formyl peptide. This GPCR is termed the AnxA1-Formyl peptide receptor 2/ALX receptor (AnxA1-FPR2/ALX) to reflect the range of its putative ligands. Zileuton inhibits 5-LOX but not the COX pathways (expanded in Figure 37–1). CysLT antagonists prevent activation of the CysLT$_1$ receptor. See the text and the Abbreviations list for further definitions.

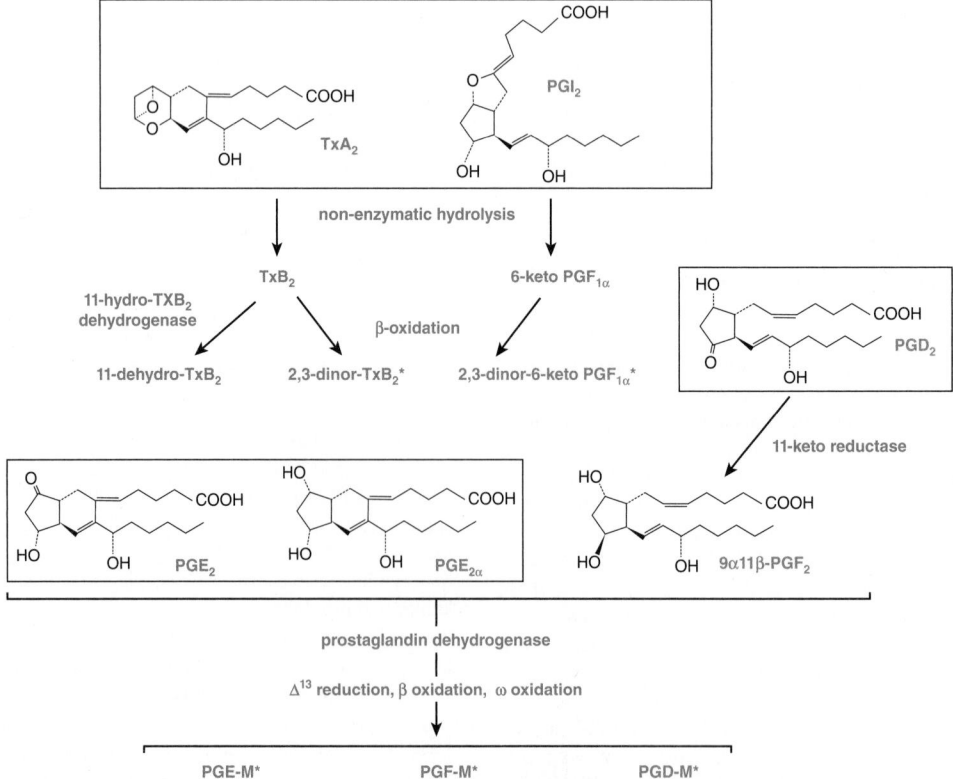

Figure 37–3 *Major pathways of prostanoid degradation.* Active metabolites are boxed. *Major urinary metabolites (M). See the text and the Abbreviations list for further definitions.

TABLE 37–1 ■ HUMAN EICOSANOID RECEPTORS

RECEPTOR	LIGANDS 1° (2°)	PRIMARY COUPLING	MAJOR PHENOTYPE IN KNOCKOUT MICE
DP_1	PGD_2	G_s	↓ Allergic asthma
$DP_2/CHRT_2$	PGD_2 (15d-PGJ_2)	G_i	↑ or ↓ Allergic airway inflammation
EP_1	PGE_2 (PGI_2)	G_q	↓ Response of colon to carcinogens
EP_2	PGE_2	G_s	Impaired ovulation and fertilization Salt-sensitive hypertension
EP_3 I–VI, e, f	PGE_2	G_i; G_s; G_q	Resistance to pyrogens ↓ Acute cutaneous inflammation
EP_4	PGE_2	G_s	Patent ductus arteriosus ↓ Bone mass/density in aged mice ↑ Bowel inflammatory response ↓ Colon carcinogenesis
$FP_{A,B}$	$PGF_{2\alpha}$ (IsoPs)	G_q	Failure of parturition
IP	PGI_2 (PGE_2)	G_s	↑ Thrombotic response ↓ Response to vascular injury ↑ Atherosclerosis ↑ Cardiac fibrosis Salt-sensitive hypertension ↓ Joint inflammation
$TP_{\alpha\beta}$	TxA_2 (IsoPs)	G_q, G_i, $G_{12/13}$, G_{16}	↑ Bleeding time ↓ Response to vascular injury ↓ Atherosclerosis ↑ Survival after cardiac allograft
BLT_1	LTB_4	G_{16}, G_i	Some suppression of inflammatory response
BLT_2	LTB_4 [12(S)-HETE, 12(R)-HETE]	G_q-like, G_i-like, G_z-like	? (Reports of altered inflammatory processes)
$CysLT_1$	LTD_4 (LTC_4/LTE_4)	G_q	↓ Innate and adaptive immune vascular permeability response ↑ Pulmonary inflammatory and fibrotic response
$CysLT_2$	LTC_4/LTD_4 (LTE_4)	G_q	↓ Pulmonary inflammatory and fibrotic response

This table lists the major classes of eicosanoid receptors and their signaling characteristics. Splice variants for EP_3, TP, and FP are indicated.

Prostaglandin Receptors

The PGs activate membrane receptors locally near their sites of formation. Eicosanoid receptors interact with G_s, G_i, and G_q to modulate the activities of adenylyl cyclase and PLC (see Chapter 3). Single-gene products have been identified for the receptors for PGI_2 (the IP), $PGF_{2\alpha}$ (the FP), and TxA_2 (the TP). Four distinct PGE_2 receptors (EP_{1-4}) and two PGD_2 receptors (DP_1 and DP_2—also known as $CRTH_2$) have been cloned. Additional isoforms of the TP (α and β), FP (A and B), and EP_3 (I-VI, e, f) receptors can arise through differential messenger RNA splicing (Smyth et al., 2009; Woodward et al., 2011). The prostanoid receptors appear to derive from an ancestral EP receptor and share high homology. Phylogenetic comparison of this receptor family reveals three subclusters (Figure 37–4):

- the relaxant receptors EP_2, EP_4, IP, and DP_1, which increase cellular cyclic AMP generation;
- the contractile receptors EP_1, FP, and TP, which increase cytosolic levels of Ca^{2+}; and
- EP_3, which can couple to both elevation of cytosolic [Ca^{2+}] and inhibition of adenylyl cyclase.

The DP_2 receptor is an exception and is unrelated to the other prostanoid receptors; rather, it is a member of the fMLP receptor superfamily.

Leukotriene Receptors

Two receptors exist for both LTB_4 (BLT_1 and BLT_2) and $CysLT_1$ and $CysLT_2$ (Bäck et al., 2011, 2014). The fMLP-2 receptor also binds LXA_4, but the functional importance of this ligand in vivo remains controversial. All

are GPCRs and couple with G_q and other G proteins, depending on the cellular context. BLT_1 is expressed predominantly in leukocytes, thymus, and spleen, whereas BLT_2, the low-affinity receptor for LTB_4, is found in spleen, leukocytes, ovary, liver, and intestine.

$CysLT_1$ binds LTD_4 with higher affinity than LTC_4, while $CysLT_2$ shows equal affinity for both LTs. Both receptors bind LTE_4 with low affinity. Activation of G_q, leading to mobilization of intracellular Ca^{2+}, is the primary signaling pathway reported. Studies also have placed G_i downstream of $CysLT_2$. $CysLT_1$ is expressed in lung and intestinal smooth muscle, spleen, and peripheral blood leukocytes, whereas $CysLT_2$ is found in heart, spleen, peripheral blood leukocytes, adrenal medulla, and brain.

Other Agents

Other AA-derived products (e.g., isoprostanes, EETs) have potent biological activities, and there is evidence for distinct receptors for some of these substances. An orphan receptor, GPR31, has been identified as a receptor for 12(S)-HETE (Powell and Rokach, 2015). Specific receptors for the HETEs and EETs have been proposed, and evidence that the orphan receptor GPR75 functions as a receptor for 20-HETE has recently been provided (Garcia et al 2017).

Physiological Actions and Pharmacological Effects

The widespread biosynthesis and myriad pharmacological actions of eicosanoids are reflected in their complex physiology and pathophysiology. Knowledge of the distribution of the major eicosanoid receptors helps to put the complexity into perspective (Figure 37–1). The development of mice with targeted disruptions of genes regulating eicosanoid biosynthesis

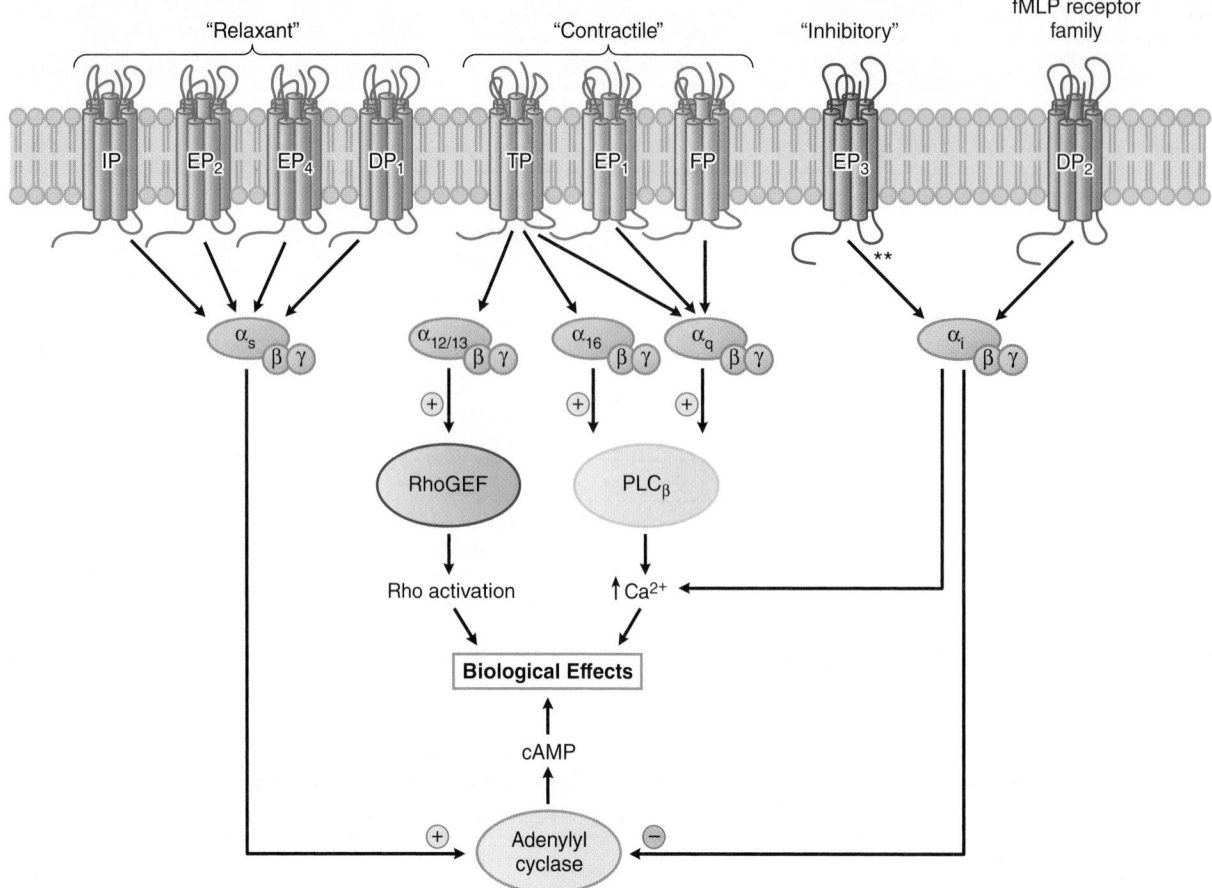

Figure 37–4 *Prostanoid receptors and their primary signaling pathways.* Prostanoid receptors are heptaspanning GPCRs. The terms *relaxant, contractile,* and *inhibitory* refer to the phylogenetic characterization of their primary effects. All EP_3 isoforms couple through G_i; some can also activate G_s or $G_{12/13}$ pathways. RhoGEF, Rho Guanine nucleotide Exchange Factor.

and eicosanoid receptors has revealed unexpected roles for these autacoids and has clarified hypotheses about their function (see Table 37–1). These topics, summarized here, were well reviewed by Smyth et al. (2011).

Cardiovascular System

Because of their short $t_{1/2}$, prostanoids act locally and generally are considered not to affect systemic vascular tone directly. They may modulate vascular tone locally at their sites of biosynthesis or through renal or other indirect effects. PGI_2, the major arachidonate metabolite released from the vascular endothelium, is derived primarily from COX-2 in humans. PGI_2 generation and release is regulated by shear stress and by both vasoconstrictor and vasodilator autacoids. In most vascular beds, PGE_2, PGI_2, and PGD_2 elicit vasodilation and a drop in blood pressure; physiologically, these responses are quite local because endogenous prostanoids are paracrine mediators that do not circulate (Smyth et al., 2009). Responses to $PGF_{2\alpha}$ is a potent constrictor of both pulmonary arteries and veins. TxA_2 is a potent vasoconstrictor and a mitogen in smooth muscle cells.

Prostaglandin E_2 can also cause vasoconstriction through activation of EP_1 and EP_3. Infusion of PGD_2 in humans results in flushing, nasal stuffiness, and hypotension. Local subcutaneous release of PGD_2 contributes to dilation of the vasculature in the skin, which causes facial flushing associated with niacin treatment in humans. Subsequent formation of F-ring metabolites from PGD_2 may result in hypertension. PGI_2, the major prostanoid released from the vascular endothelium, relaxes vascular smooth muscle, causing hypotension and reflex tachycardia on intravenous administration. PGI_2 limits pulmonary hypertension induced by hypoxia and systemic hypertension induced by AngII and lowers pulmonary resistance in patients with pulmonary hypertension.

Cyclooxygenase 2–derived PGE_2, acting via the EP_4 maintains the ductus arteriosus patent until birth, when reduced PGE_2 levels (a consequence

of increased PGE_2 metabolism) permit closure. The traditional NSAIDs induce closure of a patent ductus in neonates (see Chapter 38). Contrary to expectation, animals lacking the EP_4 die with a patent ductus during the perinatal period (Table 37–1) because the mechanism for control of the ductus in utero, and its remodeling at birth, is absent.

Infusion of PGs of the E and F series generally increases cardiac output. Weak, direct inotropic effects have been noted in various isolated preparations. In the intact animal, however, increased force of contraction and increased heart rate are, in large measure, a reflex consequence of a fall in total peripheral resistance. PGI_2 and PGE_2, acting on the IP or the EP_3, respectively, protect against oxidative injury in cardiac tissue.

Studies suggest a role for COX-2 in cardiac function. PGI_2 and PGE_2, acting on the IP or the EP_3, respectively, protect against oxidative injury in cardiac tissue. IP deletion augments myocardial ischemia/reperfusion injury, and both mPGE synthase-1 (mPGES-1) deletion and cardiomyocyte-specific deletion of the EP_4 exacerbate the decline in cardiac function after experimental myocardial infarction. COX-2–derived TxA_2 contributed to oxidant stress, isoprostane generation, and activation of the TP, and also possibly the FP, to increase cardiomyocyte apoptosis and fibrosis in a model of heart failure. Selective deletion of COX-2 in cardiomyocytes results in mild heart failure and a predisposition to arrhythmogenesis (Wang et al., 2009).

Leukotriene C_4 and LTD_4 can constrict or relax isolated vascular smooth muscle preparations, depending on the concentrations used and the vascular bed (Bäck et al., 2011). Although LTC_4 and LTD_4 have little effect on most large arteries or veins, nanomolar concentrations of these agents contract coronary arteries and distal segments of the pulmonary artery. The renal vasculature is resistant to this constrictor action, but the mesenteric vasculature is not. LTC_4 and LTD_4 act in the microvasculature to increase permeability of postcapillary venules; they are about 1000-fold more potent than histamine in this regard. At higher concentrations, LTC_4 and LTD_4 can constrict arterioles and reduce exudation of plasma. There is evidence for a role of the LTs in cardiovascular disease (Peters-Golden and Henderson, 2007). Human genetic studies have demonstrated a link between cardiovascular disease and polymorphisms in the LT biosynthetic enzymes and FLAP.

The EETs cause vasodilation in a number of vascular beds by activating the large conductance Ca^{2+}-activated K^+ channels of smooth muscle cells, thereby hyperpolarizing the smooth muscle and causing relaxation. EETs likely also function as EDHFs, particularly in the coronary circulation. Endogenous biosynthesis of EETs is increased in human syndromes of hypertension.

Platelets

Platelet aggregation leads to activation of membrane phospholipases, with the release of AA and consequent eicosanoid biosynthesis. In human platelets, TxA_2 and 12-HETE are the two major eicosanoids formed, although eicosanoids from other sources (e.g., PGI_2 derived from vascular endothelium) also affect platelet function. Mature platelets express only COX-1. TxA_2, the major product of COX-1 in platelets, induces platelet aggregation and amplifies the signal for other, more potent platelet agonists, such as thrombin and ADP. The importance of the TxA_2 pathway is evident from the efficacy of platelet COX-1 inhibition with low-dose aspirin in the secondary prevention of myocardial infarction and ischemic stroke. The total biosynthesis of TxA_2, as determined by excretion of its urinary metabolites, is augmented in clinical syndromes of platelet activation, including unstable angina, myocardial infarction, and stroke. Deletion of the TP in the mouse prolongs bleeding time, renders platelets unresponsive to TP agonists, and blunts the response to vasopressors and the proliferative response to vascular injury (Smyth et al., 2009). TxA_2 induces platelet shape change, through G_{12}/G_{13}-mediated Rho/Rho kinase–dependent regulation of myosin light-chain phosphorylation, and aggregation through G_q-dependent activation of PKC. The actions of TxA_2 on platelets are restrained by its short $t_{1/2}$ (~30 sec), by rapid TP desensitization, and by endogenous inhibitors of platelet function, including NO and PGI_2.

Low concentrations of PGE_2, via the EP_3, enhance platelet aggregation. In contrast, higher concentrations of PGE_2, acting via the IP or possibly EP_2 or EP_4 inhibit platelet aggregation. Both PGI_2 and PGD_2 inhibit the aggregation of platelets. PGI_2 limits platelet activation by TxA_2, and disaggregates preformed platelet clumps. The increased incidence of myocardial infarction and stroke in patients receiving selective inhibitors of COX-2, explained by inhibition of COX-2–dependent PGI_2 formation, supports this concept (Grosser et al., 2010).

Inflammation and Immunity

Eicosanoids play a major role in inflammatory and immune responses. LTs generally are pro-inflammatory and interact with PGs to promote and sustain inflammation (Ricciotti and FitzGerald, 2011), although there are some exceptions, such as the inhibitory actions of PGE_2 on mast cell activation. PGs and LXs and related compounds may also contribute to the resolution of inflammation (Buckley et al., 2014). COX-2 is the major source of prostanoids formed during and after an inflammatory response.

Prostaglandin E_2 and PGI_2 are the predominant pro-inflammatory prostanoids as a result of increased vascular permeability and blood flow in the inflamed region. TxA_2 can increase platelet-leukocyte interaction. PGD_2 may contribute to the resolution of inflammation. Lymphocytes have a minimal capacity to form PGs, yet they are a primary target of their action. PGs generally inhibit lymphocyte function and proliferation, suppressing the immune response. PGE_2 depresses the humoral antibody response by inhibiting the differentiation of B lymphocytes into antibody-secreting plasma cells. PGE_2 acts on T lymphocytes to inhibit mitogen-stimulated proliferation and lymphokine release by sensitized cells. PGE_2 and TxA_2 also may play a role in T-lymphocyte development by regulating apoptosis of immature thymocytes. PGE_2, acting via EP2 and EP4, has been shown to interact with the programmed cell death ligand to restrain cytotoxic T-cell function and survival during chronic infection

in mice (Chen et al., 2015). The COX-2/mPGES-1/PGE2 pathway can regulate PD-L1 expression in tumor infiltrating myeloid cells (Prima et al 2017). Given the efficacy of blockade of this pathway in a range of cancers, the possibility that blockade of PGE2 synthesis or action might augment this effect has been suggested. PGD_2 is a potent leukocyte chemoattractant, primarily through the DP_2.

The LTs are potent mediators of inflammation. Deletion of either 5-LOX or FLAP reduces inflammatory responses in model systems. LTB_4 is a potent chemotactic agent for neutrophils, T lymphocytes, eosinophils, monocytes, dendritic cells, and possibly also mast cells (Bäck et al., 2011). LTB_4 stimulates the aggregation of eosinophils and promotes degranulation and the generation of superoxide. LTB_4 promotes adhesion of neutrophils to vascular endothelial cells and their transendothelial migration and stimulates synthesis of pro-inflammatory cytokines from macrophages and lymphocytes.

The CysLTs are chemotaxins for eosinophils and monocytes. They also induce cytokine generation in eosinophils, mast cells, and dendritic cells. At higher concentrations, these LTs also promote eosinophil adherence, degranulation, cytokine or chemokine release, and oxygen radical formation. In addition, CysLTs contribute to inflammation by increasing endothelial permeability, thus promoting migration of inflammatory cells to the site of inflammation.

Bronchial and Tracheal Muscle

A complex mixture of autacoids is released when sensitized lung tissue is challenged by the appropriate antigen, including COX-derived bronchodilator and bronchoconstrictor substances. Amongst these, TxA_2, $PGF_{2\alpha}$, and PGD_2 contract, and PGE_2 and PGI_2 relax, bronchial and tracheal muscle. PGI_2 causes bronchodilation in most species; human bronchial tissue is particularly sensitive. PGI_2 antagonizes bronchoconstriction induced by other agents. PGD_2 appears to be the primary bronchoconstrictor prostanoid of relevance in humans. Polymorphisms in the genes for PGD_2 synthase and the TP have been associated with asthma in humans.

Roughly 10% of people given aspirin or NSAIDs develop bronchospasm. This appears attributable to a shift in AA metabolism to LT formation. This substrate diversion appears to involve COX-1, not COX-2. CysLTs are bronchoconstrictors that act principally on smooth muscle in the airways and are a thousand times more potent than histamine. They also stimulate bronchial mucus secretion and cause mucosal edema.

The CysLTs probably dominate during allergic constriction of the airway. Deficiency of 5-LOX leads to reduced influx of eosinophils in airways and attenuates bronchoconstriction. Furthermore, unlike COX inhibitors and histaminergic antagonists, CysLT receptor antagonists and 5-LOX inhibitors are effective in the treatment of human asthma (see Inhibitors of Eicosanoid Biosynthesis). The relatively slow LT metabolism in lung contributes to the long-lasting bronchoconstriction that follows challenge with antigen and may be a factor in the high bronchial tone that is observed in asthmatic patients in periods between acute attacks (see Chapter 40).

GI Smooth Muscle

Prostaglandin E_2 and PGF_2 stimulate contraction of the main longitudinal muscle from stomach to colon. PG endoperoxides, TxA_2, and PGI_2 also produce contraction but are less active. Circular muscle generally relaxes in response to PGE_2 and contracts in response to $PGF_{2\alpha}$. The LTs have potent contractile effects. PGs reduce transit time in the small intestine and colon. Diarrhea, cramps, and reflux of bile have been noted in response to oral PGE. PGEs and PGFs stimulate the movement of water and electrolytes into the intestinal lumen. Such effects may underlie the watery diarrhea that follows their oral or parenteral administration. PGE_2 appears to contribute to the water and electrolyte loss in cholera, a disease that is somewhat responsive to therapy with NSAIDs.

GI Secretion

In the stomach, PGE_2 and PGI_2 contribute to increased mucus secretion (*cytoprotection*), reduced acid secretion, and reduced pepsin content. PGE_2 and its analogues also inhibit gastric damage caused by a variety of ulcerogenic agents and promote healing of duodenal and gastric ulcers (see Chapter 49). Although COX-1 may be the dominant source of such cytoprotective PGs under physiological conditions, COX-2 predominates during ulcer healing. Selective inhibitors of COX-2 and deletion of the enzyme delay ulcer healing in rodents, but the impact of COX-2 inhibitors in humans is unclear. CysLTs, by constricting gastric blood vessels and enhancing production of pro-inflammatory cytokines, may contribute to the gastric damage.

Uterus

Strips of nonpregnant human uterus are contracted by $PGF_{2\alpha}$ and TxA_2 but are relaxed by PGEs. Sensitivity to the contractile response is most prominent before menstruation, whereas relaxation is greatest at midcycle. PGE_2, together with oxytocin, is essential for the onset of parturition. PGI_2 and high concentrations of PGE_2 produce relaxation. The intravenous infusion of low concentrations of PGE_2 or $PGF_{2\alpha}$ to pregnant women produces a dose-dependent increase in uterine tone and in the frequency and intensity of rhythmic uterine contractions. PGEs and PGFs are used to terminate pregnancy. Uterine responsiveness to PGs increases as pregnancy progresses but remains smaller than the response to oxytocin.

Kidney

Cyclooxygenase-2–derived PGE_2 and PGI_2 increase medullary blood flow, resulting in pressure diuresis, and inhibit tubular sodium reabsorption (Hao and Breyer, 2007). Expression of medullary COX-2 is increased during high salt intake. COX-1–derived products promote salt excretion in the collecting ducts. Cortical COX-2–derived PGE_2 and PGI_2 increase renal blood flow and glomerular filtration through their local vasodilating effects and as part of the tubuloglomerular feedback mechanism that controls renin release. Expression of COX-2 in macula densa cells increases in conditions of low distal tubular flow during low dietary salt intake or volume depletion. COX-2–derived PGE_2, and also possibly PGI_2, results in increased renin release, leading to sodium retention and elevated blood pressure.

TxA_2, generated at low levels in the normal kidney, has potent vasoconstrictor effects that reduce renal blood flow and glomerular filtration rate. Infusion of $PGF_{2\alpha}$ causes both natriuresis and diuresis. Conversely, $PGF_{2\alpha}$ may activate the renin-angiotensin system, contributing to elevated blood pressure. CYP epoxygenase products may regulate renal function. Both 20-HETE and the EETs are generated in renal tissue; 20-HETE constricts the renal arteries, while EETs mediate vasodilation and natriuresis.

Bartter syndrome is an autosomal recessive trait that manifests as hypokalemic metabolic alkalosis. The antenatal variant of Bartter syndrome is due to dysfunctional ROMK2 (Kir1.1), the K^+ channel that recycles K^+ into the tubular fluid. This syndrome also is known as *hyperPGE syndrome*. The relationship between dysfunctional ROMK2 and elevated PGE_2 synthesis is not clear; however, in patients with antenatal Bartter syndrome, inhibition of COX-2 ameliorates many of the clinical symptoms.

Eye

Prostaglandin $F_{2\alpha}$ induces constriction of the iris sphincter muscle, but its overall effect in the eye is to decrease intraocular pressure by increasing the aqueous humor outflow. A variety of FP agonists have proven effective in the treatment of open-angle glaucoma, a condition associated with the loss of COX-2 expression in the pigmented epithelium of the ciliary body (see Chapter 69).

Central Nervous System

Prostaglandin E_2 induces fever. The hypothalamus regulates the body temperature set point, which is elevated by endogenous pyrogens such as IL-1β, IL-6, TNF-α, and interferons (Morrison and Nakamura, 2011). The response is mediated by coordinate induction of COX-2 and mPGES-1 in the endothelium of blood vessels in the preoptic hypothalamic area to form PGE_2. PGE_2 can cross the blood-brain barrier and act on the EP_3 (and perhaps EP_1) on thermosensitive neurons, triggering the hypothalamus to elevate body temperature. Exogenous $PGF_{2\alpha}$ and PGI_2 induce fever but do not contribute to the endogenous pyretic response. PGD_2 appears to act on arachnoid trabecular cells in the basal forebrain to mediate an increase in extracellular adenosine that, in turn, facilitates induction of sleep. COX-2–derived prostanoids also have been implicated in the pathogenesis of several CNS degenerative disorders (e.g., Alzheimer disease, Parkinson disease; see Chapter 18).

Pain

Inflammatory mediators, including LTs and PGs, increase the sensitivity of nociceptors and potentiate pain perception. Centrally, both COX-1 and COX-2 are expressed in the spinal cord under basal conditions and release PGs in response to peripheral pain stimuli. Both PGE_2, through the EP_1 and EP_4 and PGI_2, via the IP, reduce the threshold to stimulation of nociceptors, causing "peripheral sensitization." PGE_2, and perhaps PGD_2, PGI_2, and $PGF_{2\alpha}$, can increase excitability in pain transmission neuronal pathways in the spinal cord, causing hyperalgesia and allodynia. LTB_4 also produces hyperalgesia. The release of these eicosanoids during the inflammatory process thus serves as an amplification system for the pain mechanism. The role of PGE_2 and PGI_2 in inflammatory pain is discussed in more detail in Chapter 38.

Endocrine System

The systemic administration of PGE_2 increases circulating concentrations of ACTH, growth hormone, prolactin, and gonadotropins. Other effects include stimulation of steroid production by the adrenals, stimulation of insulin release, and thyrotropin-like effects on the thyroid. PGE_2 works as part of a positive-feedback loop to induce oocyte maturation required for fertilization during and after ovulation. The critical role of $PGF_{2\alpha}$ in parturition relies on its ability to induce an oxytocin-dependent decline in progesterone levels. LOX metabolites also have endocrine effects. 12-HETE stimulates the release of aldosterone from the adrenal cortex and mediates a portion of the aldosterone release stimulated by AngII, but not that which occurs in response to ACTH.

Bone

Prostaglandins are strong modulators of bone metabolism. COX-1 is expressed in normal bone, while COX-2 is upregulated in settings such as inflammation and during mechanical stress. PGE_2 stimulates bone formation by increasing osteoblastogenesis and bone resorption via activation of osteoclasts.

Cancer

Pharmacological inhibition or genetic deletion of COX-2 restrains tumor formation in models of colon, breast, lung, and other cancers. Large human epidemiological studies reported that the incidental use of NSAIDs is associated with significant reductions in relative risk for developing these and other cancers. PGE_2 has been implicated as the primary pro-oncogenic prostanoid in multiple studies.

Therapeutic Uses

Inhibitors and Antagonists

The NSAIDs are used widely as anti-inflammatory drugs, whereas low-dose aspirin is employed frequently for cardioprotection (see Chapter 38). LT antagonists are useful clinically in the treatment of asthma, and FP agonists are used in the treatment of open-angle glaucoma (see Chapter 69). EP agonists are used to induce labor and to ameliorate gastric irritation owing to NSAIDs. DP_1 antagonists may be useful in offsetting the facial flushing associated with niacin. Orally active antagonists of LTC_4 and D_4, which block the $CysLT_1$ are used in the treatment of asthma that is mild to moderately severe (see Chapter 40). Their effectiveness in patients with aspirin-induced asthma also has been shown.

Prostanoids and Their Analogues

Prostanoids have a short $t_{1/2}$ in the circulation, and their systemic administration produces significant adverse effects. Nonetheless, several prostanoids are of clinical utility in the following situations.

Labor and Therapeutic Abortion. Prostaglandin E_2, $PGF_{2\alpha}$, and their analogues are used to induce labor at term and terminate pregnancy at any stage by promoting uterine contractions. These agents facilitate labor by promoting ripening and dilation of the cervix. Dinoprostone or misoprostol, synthetic analogues of PGE_2 and PGE_1, are used for cervical ripening and induction of labor and as abortifacients in the second trimester of pregnancy. Misoprostol, in combination with the antiprogesterone mifepristone (RU486), is highly effective in the termination of pregnancy.

An analogue of $PGF_{2\alpha}$, carboprost tromethamine, is used to induce second-trimester abortions and to control postpartum hemorrhage that does not respond to conventional methods.

Maintenance of Patent Ductus Arteriosus. The ductus arteriosus in neonates is highly sensitive to vasodilation by PGE_1. Maintenance of a patent ductus may be important hemodynamically in some neonates with congenital heart disease. PGE_1 (alprostadil) is highly effective for palliative therapy to maintain temporary patency until surgery can be performed. Apnea is observed in about 10% of neonates treated, particularly those who weigh less than 2 kg at birth.

Gastric Cytoprotection. Several PG analogues are used to suppress gastric ulceration. Misoprostol, a PGE_1 analogue, is approved for prevention of NSAID-induced gastric ulcers and is about as effective as the proton pump inhibitor omeprazole (Chapter 49).

Impotence. Prostaglandin E_1 (alprostadil), given as an intracavernous injection or urethral suppository, is a second-line treatment of erectile dysfunction. Phosphodiesterase 5 inhibitors (e.g., sildenafil, tadalafil, vardenafil, and avanafil; see Chapter 45) have superseded PGE_1 as the preferred treatment of this condition.

Pulmonary Hypertension. Long-term therapy with PGI_2 (epoprostenol), via continuous intravenous infusion, improves symptoms and can delay or preclude the need for lung or heart-lung transplantation in a number of patients. Several orally available PGI_2 analogues with longer $t_{1/2}$ have been used clinically. Iloprost can be inhaled or delivered by intravenous administration (injectable form is not available in the U.S.). Treprostinil ($t_{1/2} \sim 4$ h) may be delivered by continuous subcutaneous or intravenous infusion. Chapter 31 presents a comprehensive picture of the treatment of pulmonary artery hypertension.

Glaucoma. Latanoprost, a stable, long-acting $PGF_{2\alpha}$ derivative, was the first prostanoid used for glaucoma. Similar prostanoids with ocular hypotensive effects include bimatoprost, tafluprost, and travoprost. These drugs act as agonists at the FP and are administered as ophthalmic drops (see Chapter 69).

Platelet-Activating Factor

In 1971, Henson demonstrated that a soluble factor released from leukocytes caused platelets to aggregate. Benveniste and his coworkers characterized the factor as a polar lipid and named it *platelet-activating factor*. During this period, Muirhead described an antihypertensive polar renal lipid (APRL) produced by interstitial cells of the renal medulla that proved to be identical to PAF. Hanahan and coworkers then synthesized acetyl glyceryl ether phosphorylcholine (AGEPC) and determined that this phospholipid had chemical and biological properties identical to those of platelet activating factor (PAF). Independent determination of the structures of PAF and APRL showed them to be structurally identical to AGEPC. The commonly accepted name for this substance is PAF; however, its actions extend far beyond platelets.

Chemistry and Biosynthesis

Platelet-activating factor (1-*O*-alkyl-2-acetyl-*sn*-glycero-3-phosphocholine) represents a family of phospholipids because the alkyl group at position 1 can vary in length from 12 to 18 carbon atoms (Prescott et al., 2000). In human neutrophils, PAF consists predominantly of a mixture of the 16- and 18-carbon ethers, but its composition may change when cells are stimulated.

PLATELET-ACTIVATING FACTOR (n = 11 to 17)

Synthesis of eicosanoids and PAF depends on PLA_2 activity. The major biosynthetic pathway for PAF, the remodeling pathway, involves the precursor 1-*O*-alkyl-2-acyl-glycerophosphocholine, a membrane lipid; the 2-acyl substituents include AA. PAF is synthesized from this substrate in two steps (Figure 37–5). The rate-limiting step is the second one, acetyl-coenzyme-A-lyso-PAF acetyltransferase. The synthesis of PAF may be stimulated during antigen-antibody reactions or by a variety of agents, including chemotactic peptides, thrombin, collagen, and other autacoids; PAF also can stimulate its own formation. Both the PL and acetyltransferase are Ca^{2+}-dependent enzymes; thus, PAF synthesis is regulated by the availability of Ca^{2+}. The inactivation of PAF is catalyzed by PAF-AHs. PAF is inactivated by PAF-AH–catalyzed hydrolysis of the acetyl group, generating Lyso-PAF, which is then converted to a 1-*O*-alkyl-2-acyl-glycerophosphocholine by an acyltransferase (McIntyre et al., 2009; Stafforini et al., 2003).

Synthesis of PAF also can occur de novo by transfer of a phosphocholine substituent to alkyl acetyl glycerol by a lyso-glycerophosphate acetyl–coenzyme A transferase. This pathway may contribute to physiological levels of PAF for normal cellular functions. PAF-like molecules can be formed from oxidized phospholipids (oxPLs) (Stafforini et al., 2003). These compounds are increased in settings of oxidant stress, such as cigarette smoking, and differ structurally from PAF in that they contain a fatty acid at the *sn*-1 position of glycerol joined through an ester bond and various short-chain acyl groups at the *sn*-2 position. oxPLs mimic the structure of PAF, bind to its receptor, and elicit the same responses. Unlike the synthesis of PAF, which is highly controlled, oxPL production is unregulated. Degradation of oxPLs by PAF-AH is therefore necessary to suppress toxicity. Increased levels of plasma PAF-AH have been reported in colon cancer, cardiovascular disease, and stroke.

Sites of PAF Synthesis

Platelet-activating factor is not stored in cells but is synthesized in response to stimulation. PAF is synthesized by platelets, neutrophils, monocytes, mast cells, eosinophils, renal mesangial cells, renal medullary cells, and vascular endothelial cells. Depending on cell type, PAF can either remain cell associated or be secreted. For example, PAF is released from monocytes but retained by leukocytes and endothelial cells. In endothelial cells,

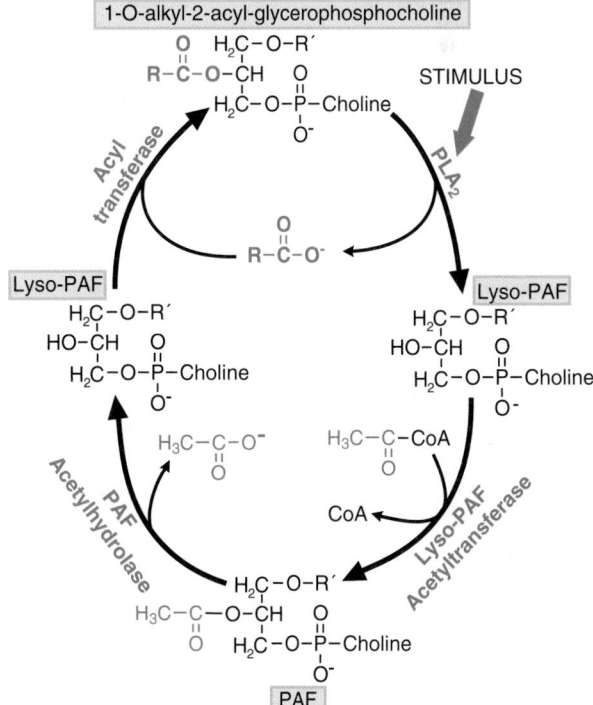

Figure 37–5 *Synthesis and degradation of PAF.* RCOO⁻ is a mixture of fatty acids but is enriched in AA that may be metabolized to eicosanoids.

PAF is displayed on the surface for juxtacrine signaling and stimulates adherent leukocytes.

Mechanism of Action of PAF

Extracellular PAF exerts its actions by stimulating a specific GPCR (Honda et al., 2002). The PAF receptor couples to Gq (to activate the PLC-IP$_3$–Ca^{2+} pathway) and to Gi (to inhibit adenylyl cyclase). Consequent activation of PLs A$_2$, C, and D gives rise to second messengers, including AA-derived PGs, TxA$_2$, or LTs, which may function as mediators of the effects of PAF.

In addition, p38 mitogen-activated protein kinase is activated downstream of the PAF-receptor–Gq interaction, while extracellular signal–regulated kinase activation can occur via interaction of activated PAF receptor with Gq, Go, or their βγ subunits, or via transactivation of the EGF receptor, leading to nuclear factor kappa B activation. PAF exerts many of its important pro-inflammatory actions without leaving its cell of origin. For example, PAF is synthesized in a regulated fashion by endothelial cells stimulated by inflammatory mediators. This PAF is presented on the surface of the endothelium, where it activates the PAF receptor on juxtaposed cells, including platelets, PMNs, and monocytes, and acts cooperatively with P selectin to promote adhesion. This function of PAF is important for orchestrating the interaction of platelets and circulating inflammatory cells with the inflamed endothelium.

Physiological and Pathological Functions of PAF

Platelet-activating factor generally is viewed as a mediator of pathological events and has been implicated in allergic asthma, endotoxic shock, acute pancreatitis, certain cancers, dermal inflammation, and inflammatory cardiovascular diseases such as atherosclerosis.

Inflammatory and Allergic Responses

Experimental administration of PAF reproduces many of the signs and symptoms in anaphylactic shock. However, the effects of PAF antagonists in the treatment of inflammatory and allergic disorders have been disappointing. In patients with asthma, PAF antagonists partially inhibit the bronchoconstriction induced by antigen challenge but not by challenges by methacholine, exercise, or inhalation of cold air. These results may reflect the complexity of these pathological conditions and the likelihood that other mediators contribute to the inflammation associated with these disorders.

Cardiovascular System

Platelet-activating factor is a potent vasodilator in most vascular beds; when administered intravenously, it causes hypotension. PAF-induced vasodilation is independent of effects on sympathetic innervation, the renin-angiotensin system, or AA metabolism and likely results from a combination of direct and indirect actions. PAF may, alternatively, induce vasoconstriction depending on the concentration, vascular bed, and involvement of platelets or leukocytes. For example, the intracoronary administration of very low concentrations of PAF increases coronary blood flow by a mechanism that involves the release of a platelet-derived vasodilator. Coronary blood flow is decreased at higher doses by the formation of intravascular aggregates of platelets or the formation of TxA$_2$. The pulmonary vasculature also is constricted by PAF, and a similar mechanism is thought to be involved.

Intradermal injection of PAF causes an initial vasoconstriction followed by a typical wheal and flare. PAF increases vascular permeability and edema in the same manner as histamine and bradykinin. The increase in permeability is due to contraction of venular endothelial cells, but PAF is more potent than histamine or bradykinin by three orders of magnitude.

Platelets

The PAF receptor is constitutively expressed on the surface of platelets. PAF potently stimulates platelet aggregation. The intravenous injection of PAF causes formation of intravascular platelet aggregates and thrombocytopenia. Although this is accompanied by the release of TxA$_2$ and the granular contents of the platelet, PAF does not require the presence of TxA$_2$ or other aggregating agents to produce this effect. PAF antagonists fail to block thrombin-induced aggregation, even though they prolong bleeding time and prevent thrombus formation in some experimental models. Thus, PAF may contribute to thrombus formation, but it does not function as an independent mediator of platelet aggregation.

Leukocytes

Platelet-activating factor is a potent and common activator of inflammatory cells. PAF stimulates a variety of responses in PMNs (eosinophils, neutrophils, and basophils). PAF stimulates PMNs to aggregate, degranulate, and generate free radicals and LTs. PAF is a potent chemotactic for eosinophils, neutrophils, and monocytes and promotes PMN-endothelial adhesion contributing, along with other adhesion molecular systems, to leukocyte rolling, tight adhesion, and migration through the endothelial monolayer. PAF also stimulates basophils to release histamine, activates mast cells, and induces cytokine release from monocytes. In addition, PAF promotes aggregation of monocytes and degranulation of eosinophils.

Smooth Muscle

Platelet-activating factor contracts GI, uterine, and pulmonary smooth muscle. PAF enhances the amplitude of spontaneous uterine contractions; these contractions are inhibited by inhibitors of PG synthesis. PAF does not affect tracheal smooth muscle but contracts airway smooth muscle. When given by aerosol, PAF increases airway resistance as well as the responsiveness to other bronchoconstrictors. PAF also increases mucus secretion and the permeability of pulmonary microvessels.

Stomach

In addition to contracting the fundus of the stomach, PAF is the most potent known ulcerogen. When given intravenously, it causes hemorrhagic erosions of the gastric mucosa that extend into the submucosa.

Kidney

Platelet-activating factor decreases renal blood flow, glomerular filtration rate, urine volume, and excretion of Na$^+$ without changes in systemic hemodynamics. PAF exerts a receptor-mediated biphasic effect on afferent arterioles, dilating them at low concentrations and constricting them at higher concentrations. The vasoconstrictor effect appears to be mediated, at least in part, by COX products, whereas vasodilation is a consequence of the stimulation of NO production by endothelium.

Other

Platelet-activating factor, a potent mediator of angiogenesis, has been implicated in breast and prostate cancer. PAF-AH deficiency has been associated with small increases in a range of cardiovascular and thrombotic diseases in some human populations.

PAF Receptor Antagonists

Several experimental PAF receptor antagonists exist that selectively inhibit the actions of PAF in vivo and in vitro. None has proven clinically useful. Thus, synthetic PAF, when administered in sufficient quantities, exerts a broad spectrum of effects. However, the evidence of its importance as an endogenous mediator remains to be established. Interestingly, inhibition of PAF-AH, which would be expected to elevate endogenous levels of PAF, was pursued as the protein also functions as a lipoprotein-associated PLA$_2$. Trials of an inhibitor, darapladib, failed to establish either clinical efficacy attributable to eicosanoid suppression or an adverse effect profile potentially attributable to increased levels of PAF (O'Donoghue et al., 2014).

Acknowledgment: *Jason D. Morrow, L. Jackson Roberts II, and Anne Burke contributed to this chapter in earlier editions of this book. We have retained some of their text in the current edition.*

Drug Facts for Your Personal Formulary: *Eicosanoids*

Drug	Therapeutic Uses	Clinical Pharmacology and Tips
Prostanoids and Prostanoid Analogues: PGE₁/PGE₂		
Alprostadil (PGE₁)	• Erectile dysfunction • Temporary maintenance of patent ductus arteriosus in neonates	• Rapidly metabolized • Prolonged erection (4–6 h) in 4% of patients • Apnea in 10%–12% of neonates with congenital heart defects; ventilator assistance should be available during treatment
Misoprostol (PGE₁ analogue)	• Protection from NSAID-induced gastric toxicity	• Contraindicated for use in pregnant women; women who may become pregnant must use birth control when taking misoprostol • Combined with mifepristone to terminate early pregnancy
Dinoprostone (PGE₂)	• Labor induction	• Rapidly metabolized
Prostanoids and Prostanoid Analogues: PGI₂ (Prostacyclin)		
Epoprostenol (PGI₂)	• Pulmonary arterial hypertension	• Rapidly metabolized • Administered by intravenous infusion • Most common dose-limiting adverse effects are nausea, vomiting, headache, hypotension, and flushing
Iloprost (PGI₂ analogue)	• Pulmonary arterial hypertension	• Administered by inhalation • Synthetic PGI₂ analogue with longer $t_{1/2}$ • May increase risk of bleeding when used with anticoagulants or platelet inhibitors
Treprostinil (PGI₂ analogue)	• Pulmonary arterial hypertension	• May be administered by subcutaneous/intravenous infusion or by inhalation • Adverse events similar to Iloprost
Prostanoids and Prostanoid Analogues: PGF₂ₐ		
Carboprost tromethamine	• Abortifacient (second trimester) • Postpartum hemorrhage	• Common adverse effects are vomiting, diarrhea, nausea, fever, flushing
Bimatoprost	• Ocular hypertension • Open-angle glaucoma • Hypotrichosis of the eyelashes	• Upper respiratory tract infections in about 10% of patients • May cause changes in pigmentation and hair growth
Latanoprost	• Ocular hypertension • Open-angle glaucoma	• Increased iris pigmentation with time
Tafluprost	• Ocular hypertension • Open-angle glaucoma	• Metabolized to active drug in the eye • May cause increased iris pigmentation
Travoprost	• Ocular hypertension • Open-angle glaucoma	• May cause increased iris pigmentation
Nonsteroidal Anti-Inflammatory Drugs		
Listed in Chapter 38		
Cysteinyl Leukotriene Receptor Antagonists/5-Lipoxygenase Inhibitors		
Listed in Chapter 40		

Bibliography

Bäck M, et al. International Union of Basic and Clinical Pharmacology. LXXXIV: leukotriene receptor nomenclature, distribution, and pathophysiological functions. *Pharmacol Rev,* **2011,** 63:539–584.

Bäck M, et al. Update on leukotriene, lipoxin and oxoeicosanoid receptors: IUPHAR Review 7. *Br J Pharmacol,* **2014,** 171:3551–3574.

Buckley CD, et al. Proresolving lipid mediators and mechanisms in the resolution of acute inflammation. *Immunity,* **2014,** 40:315–327.

Chen JH, et al. Prostaglandin E₂ and programmed cell death 1 signaling coordinately impair CTL function and survival during chronic viral infection. *Nat Med,* **2015,** 4:327–334.

Duchez AC, et al. Platelet microparticles are internalized in neutrophils via the concerted activity of 12-lipoxygenase and secreted phospholipase A2-IIA. *Proc Natl Acad Sci U S A,* **2015,** 112:E3564–E3573.

Evans JF, et al. What's all the FLAP about? 5-Lipoxygenase-activating protein inhibitors for inflammatory diseases. *Trends Pharmacol Sci,* **2008,** 29:72–78.

Fleming I. The pharmacology of the cytochrome P450 epoxygenase/soluble epoxide hydrolase axis in the vasculature and cardiovascular disease. *Pharmacol Rev,* **2014,** 66:1106–1140.

Garcia, V et al. 20-HETE signals through G-protein–coupled receptor GPR75 (Gq) to affect vascular function and trigger hypertension. *Circ Res,* **2017,** 120:1776–1788.

Grosser T, et al. Emotion recollected in tranquility: lessons learned from the COX-2 saga. *Annu Rev Med,* **2010,** 61:17–33.

Haeggström JZ, Funk CD. Lipoxygenase and leukotriene pathways: biochemistry, biology, and roles in disease. *Chem Rev,* **2011,** 111: 5866–5898.

Hao CM, Breyer MD. Physiologic and pathophysiologic roles of lipid mediators in the kidney. *Kidney Int,* **2007,** 71:1105–1115.

Honda Z, et al. Platelet-activating factor receptor. *J Biochem,* **2002,** 131:773–779.

Janusz JM, et al. New cyclooxygenase-2/5-lipoxygenase inhibitors. 1. 7-tert-buty1–2,3-dihydro-3-dimethylbenzofuran derivatives as gastrointestinal safe antiinflammatory and analgesic agents: discovery and variation of the 5-keto substituent. *J Med Chem,* **1998,** 41:1112–1123.

McIntyre TM, et al. The emerging roles of PAF acetylhydrolase. *J Lipid Res,* **2009,** 50(suppl):S255–S259.

Milne GL, et al. The isoprostanes-25 years later. *Biochim Biophys Acta,* **2015,** 1851:433–445.

Minutoli L, et al. A dual inhibitor of cyclooxygenase and 5-lipoxygenase protects against kainic acid-induced brain injury. *Neuromolecular Med,* **2015,** *17*:192–201.

Morrison SF, Nakamura K. Central neural pathways for thermoregulation. *Front Biosci,* **2011,** *16*:74–104.

Oak NR, et al. Inhibition of 5-LOX, COX-1, and COX-2 increases tendon healing and reduces muscle fibrosis and lipid accumulation after rotator cuff repair. *Am J Sports Med,* **2014,** *42*:2860–2868.

O'Donoghue ML, et al. Effect of darapladib on major coronary events after an acute coronary syndrome: the SOLID-TIMI 52 randomized clinical trial. *JAMA,* **2014,** *312*:1006–1015.

Peters-Golden M, Henderson WR Jr. Leukotrienes. *N Engl J Med,* **2007,** *357*:1841–1854.

Prima V, et al. COX2/mPGES1/PGE2 pathway regulates PD-L1 expression in tumor-associated macrophages and myeloid-derived suppressor cells. *Proc Natl Acad Sci USA,* **2017,** *114*:1117–1122.

Powell WS, Rokach J. Biosynthesis, biological effects, and receptors of hydroxyeicosatetraenoic acids (HETEs) and oxoeicosatetraenoic acids (oxo-ETEs) derived from arachidonic acid. *Biochim Biophys Acta,* **2015,** *1851*:340–355.

Prescott SM, et al. Platelet-activating factor and related lipid mediators. *Annu Rev Biochem,* **2000,** *69*:419–445.

Ricciotti EI, FitzGerald GA. Prostaglandins and inflammation. *Arterioscler Thromb Vasc Biol,* **2011,** *5*:986–1000.

Rouzer CA, Marnett LJ. Cyclooxygenases: structural and functional insights. *J Lipid Res,* **2009,** *50*(suppl):S29–S34.

Schuster VL. Prostaglandin transport. *Prostaglandins Other Lipid Mediat,* **2002,** *68*–*69*:633–647.

Skarke C, et al. Bioactive products formed in humans from fish oils. *J Lipid Res,* **2015,** *56*:1808–20.

Smith WL, et al. Enzymes of the cyclooxygenase pathways of prostanoid biosynthesis. *Chem Rev,* **2011,** *111*:5821–5865.

Smyth EM, et al. Lipid-derived autacoids. In: Brunton L, Chabner B, Knollmann B, eds. *The Pharmacological Basis of Therapeutics.* 12th ed. McGraw-Hill, New York, **2011,** 942–948.

Smyth EM, et al. Prostanoids in health and disease. *J Lipid Res,* **2009,** *50*(suppl):S423–S428.

Stafforini DM, et al. Platelet-activating factor, a pleiotrophic mediator of physiological and pathological processes. *Crit Rev Clin Lab Sci,* **2003,** *40*:643–672.

Wang D, et al. Cardiomyocyte cyclooxygenase-2 influences cardiac rhythm and function. *Proc Natl Acad Sci USA,* **2009,** *109*:7548–7552.

Woodward DF, et al. International Union of Basic and Clinical Pharmacology. LXXXIII: classification of prostanoid receptors, updating 15 years of progress. *Pharmacol Rev,* **2011,** *63*:471–538.

Xu GL, et al. Anti-inflammatory effects and gastrointestinal safety of NNU-hdpa, a novel dual COX/5-LOX inhibitor. *Eur J Pharmacol,* **2009,** *611*:100–106.

Zhang Y, et al. Tissue regeneration. Inhibition of the prostaglandin-degrading enzyme 15-PGDH potentiates tissue regeneration. *Science,* **2015,** *348*:aaa2340.

Chapter 38

Pharmacotherapy of Inflammation, Fever, Pain, and Gout

Tilo Grosser, Emer M. Smyth, and Garret A. FitzGerald

This chapter describes the non-steroidal anti-inflammatory drugs (NSAIDs) used to treat inflammation, pain, and fever and the drugs used for hyperuricemia and gout. The NSAIDs are first considered by class, then by groups of chemically similar agents described in more detail. Many of the basic properties of these drugs are summarized in Tables 38–1, 38–2, and 38–3.

The NSAIDs act by inhibiting the prostaglandin (PG) G/H synthase enzymes, colloquially known as the cyclooxygenases (COXs) (see Chapter 37). There are two forms, COX-1 and COX-2. The inhibition of COX-2 is thought to mediate, in large part, the antipyretic, analgesic, and anti-inflammatory actions of NSAIDs. Adverse reactions are largely caused by the inhibition of COX-1 and COX-2 in tissues in which they fulfill physiological functions, such as the GI tract, the kidney, and the cardiovascular system. Aspirin is the only irreversible inhibitor of the COX enzymes in clinical use. All other NSAIDs bind the COXs reversibly and act either by competing directly with arachidonic acid (AA) at the active site of COX-1 and COX-2 or by changing their steric confirmation in a way that alters their ability to bind arachidonic acid. Acetaminophen (paracetamol) is effective as an antipyretic and analgesic agent at typical doses that partly inhibit COXs and has only weak anti-inflammatory activity. Purposefully designed selective inhibitors of COX-2 (celecoxib, etoricoxib) are a subclass of NSAIDs; several of the older traditional NSAIDs, such as diclofenac and meloxicam (see Figure 38–1) also selectively inhibit COX-2 at therapeutic doses.

Inflammation, Pain, and Fever

Inflammation

The inflammatory process is the immune system's protective response to an injurious stimulus. It can be evoked by noxious agents, infections, and physical injuries, which release damage- and pathogen-associated molecules that are recognized by cells charged with immune surveillance (Tang et al., 2012). The ability to mount an inflammatory response is essential for survival in the face of environmental pathogens and injury. In some situations and diseases, inflammation may be exaggerated and sustained

HISTORICAL PERSPECTIVE

The history of aspirin provides an interesting example of the translation of a compound from the realm of herbal folklore to contemporary therapeutics. The use of willow bark and leaves to relieve fever has been attributed to Hippocrates but was most clearly documented by Edmund Stone in a 1763 letter to the president of the Royal Society. Similar properties were attributed to potions from meadowsweet (*Spiraea ulmaria*), from which the name aspirin is derived. Salicin was crystallized in 1829 by Leroux, and Pina isolated salicylic acid in 1836. In 1859, Kolbe synthesized salicylic acid, and by 1874, it was being produced industrially. It soon was being used for rheumatic fever and gout and as a general antipyretic. However, its unpleasant taste and adverse GI effects made it difficult to tolerate for more than short periods. In 1899, Hoffmann, a chemist at Bayer Laboratories, sought to improve the adverse effect profile of salicylic acid (which his father was taking with difficulty for arthritis). Hoffmann came across the earlier work of the French chemist Gerhardt, who had acetylated salicylic acid in 1853, apparently ameliorating its adverse effect profile, but without improving its efficacy, and therefore abandoned the project. Hoffmann resumed the quest, and Bayer began testing acetylsalicylic acid (ASA) in animals by 1899 and proceeded soon thereafter to human studies and the marketing of aspirin.

Acetaminophen was first used in medicine by von Mering in 1893. However, it gained popularity only after 1949, when it was recognized as the major active metabolite of both acetanilide and phenacetin. Acetanilide is the parent member of this group of drugs. It was introduced into medicine in 1886 under the name antifebrin by Cahn and Hepp, who had discovered its antipyretic action accidentally. However, acetanilide proved to be excessively toxic. A number of chemical derivatives were developed and tested. One of the more satisfactory of these was phenacetin. It was introduced into therapy in 1887 and was extensively employed in analgesic mixtures until it was implicated in analgesic abuse nephropathy, hemolytic anemia, and bladder cancer; it was withdrawn in the 1980s.

Abbreviations

AA: arachidonic acid
ACE: angiotensin-converting enzyme
ASA: acetylsalicylic acid/aspirin
AUC: area under the curve
COX: cyclooxygenase
CSF: cerebrospinal fluid
G6PD: glucose-6-phosphate dehydrogenase
GSH: glutathione
15(R)-HETE: 15(R)-hydroxyeicosatetraenoic acid
5-HIAA: 5-hydroxyindoleacetic acid
5HT: 5-hydroxytryptamine/serotonin
Ig: immunoglobulin
IL: interleukin
IM: intramuscular
IV: intravenous
LOX: lipooxygenase
LT: leukotriene
MI: myocardial infarction
NAC: N-acetylcysteine
NAPQI: N-acetyl-p-benzoquinone imine
NSAID: nonsteroidal anti-inflammatory drug
OAT: organic anion transporter
OTC: over the counter
PAF: platelet-activating factor
PG: prostaglandin
PGI$_2$: prostacyclin
PPI: proton pump inhibitor
TNF: tumor necrosis factor
Tx: thromboxane
UGT: uridine diphosphate glucuronosyltransferase
URAT: urate transporter
XO: xanthine oxidase

without apparent benefit and even with severe adverse consequences (e.g., hypersensitivity, autoimmune diseases, chronic inflammation). The inflammatory response is characterized mechanistically by

- transient local vasodilation and increased capillary permeability;
- infiltration of leukocytes and phagocytic cells; and
- resolution with or without tissue degeneration and fibrosis.

Many molecules are involved in the promotion and resolution of the inflammatory process. Histamine, bradykinin, 5HT, prostanoids, LTs, PAF, and an array of cytokines are important mediators (see Chapters 34, 37, and 39). Prostanoid biosynthesis is significantly increased in inflamed tissue. PGE$_2$ and prostacyclin (PGI$_2$) are the primary prostanoids that mediate inflammation. They increase local blood flow, vascular permeability, and leukocyte infiltration through activation of their respective receptors, EP$_2$ and IP. PGD$_2$, a major product of mast cells, contributes to inflammation in allergic responses, particularly in the lung.

Activation of endothelial cells plays a key role in recruiting circulating cells to inflammatory sites (Muller, 2011). Endothelial activation results in leukocyte rolling and adhesion as the leukocytes recognize newly expressed selectins, integrins, and adhesion molecules. PGE$_2$ and TxA$_2$ enhance leukocyte chemoattraction and endothelial adhesion.

The recruitment of inflammatory cells to sites of injury also involves the concerted interactions of the complement factors PAF, and eicosanoids such as LTB$_4$ (see Chapter 37). All can act as chemotactic agonists. Cytokines play essential roles in orchestrating the inflammatory process, especially TNF and IL-1. Several biological anti-inflammatory therapeutics target these cytokines or their signaling pathways (see Chapter 35). Other cytokines and growth factors (e.g., IL-2, IL-6, IL-8, granulocyte-macrophage colony-stimulating factor) contribute to manifestations of the inflammatory response. The concentrations of many of these factors are increased in the synovia of patients with inflammatory arthritis. Glucocorticoids interfere with the synthesis and actions of cytokines, such as IL-1 or TNF-α (see Chapter 35). Although some of the actions of these cytokines are accompanied by the release of PGs and TxA$_2$, COX inhibitors appear to block primarily their pyrogenic effects.

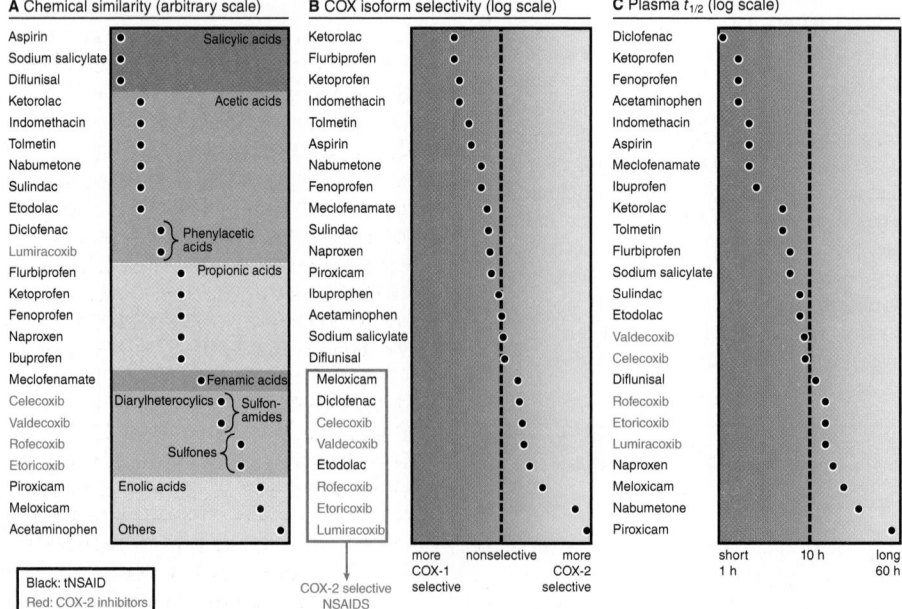

Figure 38–1 *Classification of NSAIDs by chemical similarity (**A**), COX isoform selectivity (**B**), and plasma t$_{1/2}$ (**C**).* The COX selectivity chart is plotted from data published in Warner T., et al. Nonsteroid drug selectivities for cyclooxygenase-1 rather than cyclooxygenase-2 are associated with human gastrointestinal toxicity: a full in vitro analysis. *Proc Natl Acad Sci U S A*, **1999**, *96*:7563–7568; and FitzGerald GA, Patrono C. The coxibs, selective inhibitors of cyclooxygenase-2. *N Engl J Med*, **2001**, *345*:433–442.

Pain

Nociceptors, peripheral terminals of primary afferent fibers that sense pain, can be activated by various stimuli, such as heat, acids, or pressure. Inflammatory mediators released from nonneuronal cells during tissue injury increase the sensitivity of nociceptors and potentiate pain perception. Among these mediators are bradykinin, H^+, 5HT, ATP, neurotrophins (nerve growth factor), LTs, and PGs. PGE_2 and PGI_2 reduce the threshold to stimulation of nociceptors, causing *peripheral sensitization*. Reversal of peripheral sensitization is thought to represent the mechanistic basis for the peripheral component of the analgesic activity of NSAIDs. NSAIDs may also have important central actions in the spinal cord and brain. Both COX-1 and COX-2 are expressed in the spinal cord under basal conditions and release PGs in response to peripheral pain stimuli.

Centrally active PGE_2 and perhaps also PGD_2, PGI_2, and $PGF_{2\alpha}$ contribute to *central sensitization*, an increase in excitability of spinal dorsal horn neurons that causes hyperalgesia and allodynia in part by disinhibition of glycinergic pathways (Chen et al., 2013). Central sensitization reflects the plasticity of the nociceptive system that is invoked by injury. This usually is reversible within hours to days following adequate responses of the nociceptive system (e.g., in postoperative pain). However, chronic inflammatory diseases may cause persistent modification of the architecture of the nociceptive system, which may lead to long-lasting changes in its responsiveness. These mechanisms contribute to chronic pain.

Fever

The hypothalamus regulates the set point at which body temperature is maintained. This set point is elevated in fever, reflecting an infection, or resulting from tissue damage, inflammation, graft rejection, or malignancy. These conditions all enhance formation of cytokines such as IL-1β, IL-6, TNF-α, and interferons, which act as endogenous pyrogens. The initial phase of the thermoregulatory response to such pyrogens may be mediated by ceramide release in neurons of the preoptic area in the anterior hypothalamus (Sanchez-Alavez et al., 2006). The second phase is mediated by coordinate induction of COX-2 and formation of PGE_2 (Engblom et al., 2003). PGE_2 can cross the blood-brain barrier and acts on EP_3 and perhaps EP_1 receptors on thermosensitive neurons. This triggers the hypothalamus to elevate body temperature by promoting an increase in heat generation and a decrease in heat loss. NSAIDs suppress this response by inhibiting COX-2–dependent PGE_2 synthesis.

Nonsteroidal Anti-inflammatory Drugs

The NSAIDs are mechanistically classified as *isoform nonselective NSAIDs*, which inhibit both COX-1 and COX-2, and *COX-2–selective NSAIDs* (FitzGerald and Patrono, 2001). Most NSAIDs are competitive, noncompetitive, or mixed reversible inhibitors of the COX enzymes. Aspirin (ASA) is a noncompetitive, irreversible inhibitor because it acetylates the isozymes in the AA-binding channel. Acetaminophen, which is antipyretic and analgesic but largely devoid of anti-inflammatory activity, acts as a noncompetitive reversible inhibitor by reducing the peroxide site of the enzymes.

The majority of NSAIDs are organic acids with relatively low pK_a values. As organic acids, the compounds generally are well absorbed orally, highly bound to plasma proteins, and excreted either by glomerular filtration or by tubular secretion. They also accumulate in sites of inflammation, where the pH is lower, potentially confounding the relationship between plasma concentrations and duration of drug effect. Most COX-2–selective NSAIDs have a relatively bulky side group, which aligns with a large side pocket in the AA-binding channel of COX-2 but hinders its optimal orientation in the smaller binding channel of COX-1 (Smith et al., 2011). Both isoform nonselective NSAIDs and the COX-2–selective NSAIDs generally are hydrophobic drugs, a feature that allows them to access the hydrophobic AA-binding channel and results in shared pharmacokinetic characteristics. Again, aspirin and acetaminophen are exceptions to this rule.

Cyclooxygenase Inhibition

The principal therapeutic effects of NSAIDs derive from their ability to inhibit PG production. The first enzyme in the PG synthetic pathway is COX, also known as PG G/H synthase. This enzyme converts AA to the unstable intermediates PGG_2 and PGH_2 and leads to the production of the prostanoids, TxA_2, and a variety of PGs (see Chapter 37). COX-1, expressed constitutively in most cells, is the dominant source of prostanoids for housekeeping functions, such as hemostasis. Conversely, COX-2, induced by cytokines, shear stress, and tumor promoters, is the more important source of prostanoid formation in inflammation and perhaps in cancer (see Chapter 37). However, both enzymes contribute to the generation of autoregulatory and homeostatic prostanoids with important functions in normal physiology (see Chapter 37). The indiscriminant inhibition of both inflammatory and homeostatic prostanoids by NSAIDs explains mechanistically most adverse reactions to this drug class. For example, inhibition of COX-1 accounts largely for the gastric adverse events and bleeding that complicate therapy because COX-1 is the dominant cytoprotective isoform in gastric epithelial cells and forms TxA_2 in platelets, which amplifies platelet activation and constricts blood vessels at the site of injury. Similarly, COX-2–derived products play important roles in blood pressure regulation and act as endogenous inhibitors of hemostasis. Inhibition of COX-2 can cause or exacerbate hypertension and increases the likelihood of thrombotic events.

While the functional COX enzymes are sequence homodimers, they are configured as conformational heterodimers in which one of the monomers functions as the catalytic subunit with heme bound and the other, without heme, serves as the allosteric subunit. Most NSAIDs inhibit the catalytic subunits of COX-1 and COX-2. However, COX-2 inhibition by naproxen, and flurbiprofen occurs primarily on the allosteric subunit (Dong et al., 2011; Zou et al., 2012).

Irreversible Cyclooxygenase Inhibition by Aspirin

Aspirin covalently acetylates the catalytic subunits of the COX-1 and COX-2 dimers, irreversibly inhibiting COX activity. This is an important distinction from all the other NSAIDs because the duration of aspirin's effects is related to the turnover rate of the COXs in different target tissues.

The importance of enzyme turnover in recovery from aspirin action is most notable in platelets, which, being anucleate, have a markedly limited capacity for protein synthesis. Thus, the consequences of inhibition of platelet COX-1 last for the lifetime of the platelet. Inhibition of platelet COX-1–dependent TxA_2 formation therefore is cumulative with repeated doses of aspirin (at least as low as 30 mg/d) and takes 8–12 days (the platelet turnover time) to recover fully once therapy has been stopped. Importantly, even a partially recovered platelet pool—just a few days after the last aspirin dose—may afford recovery of sufficient hemostatic integrity for some types of elective surgery to be performed. However, such a partial platelet function also may predispose noncompliant patients on low-dose aspirin for antiplatelet therapy to thrombotic events. The unique sensitivity of platelets to inhibition by low doses of aspirin is related to their presystemic inhibition in the portal circulation before aspirin is deacetylated to salicylate on first pass through the liver (Pedersen and FitzGerald, 1984). In contrast to aspirin, salicylic acid has no acetylating capacity. It is a relatively weak, reversible inhibitor of COX. Salicylic acid derivates, rather than the acid, are available for clinical use.

The COXs are configured such that the active site is accessed by the AA substrate via a hydrophobic channel. Aspirin acetylates serine 529 of COX-1, located high up in the hydrophobic channel. Interposition of the bulky acetyl residue prevents the binding of AA to the active site of the enzyme and thus impedes the ability of the enzyme to make PGs. Aspirin acetylates a homologous serine at position 516 in COX-2. Although covalent modification of COX-2 by aspirin also blocks the COX activity of this isoform, an interesting property not shared by COX-1 is that acetylated COX-2 synthesizes 15(R)-HETE. This may be metabolized, at least in vitro, by 5-LOX to yield 15-epi-lipoxin A_4, which has anti-inflammatory properties in model systems (see Chapter 37).

Selective Inhibition of Cyclooxygenase 2

The chronic use of the NSAIDs is limited by their poor GI tolerability. Selective inhibitors of COX-2 were developed to afford efficacy similar to traditional NSAIDs with better GI tolerability (FitzGerald and Patrono, 2001). Six such COX-2 inhibitors, the coxibs, were initially approved for clinical use: celecoxib, rofecoxib, valdecoxib (approved in the U.S.) and its prodrug parecoxib, etoricoxib, and lumiracoxib. Most coxibs have been either restricted in their use or withdrawn from the market in view of their adverse cardiovascular risk profile (Grosser et al., 2010). Celecoxib currently is the only COX-2 inhibitor licensed for use in the U.S. Some older NSAID compounds—diclofenac, etodolac, meloxicam, and nimesulide (the last not available in the U.S.)—exhibit selectivity for COX-2 that is close to that of celecoxib (Figure 38–1).

ADME

Absorption. The NSAIDs are rapidly absorbed following oral ingestion, and peak plasma concentrations are reached within 2–3 h. The poor aqueous solubility of most NSAIDs often is reflected by a less-than-proportional increase in the AUC of plasma concentration–time curves, due to incomplete dissolution, when the dose is increased. Food intake may delay absorption and systemic availability (i.e., fenoprofen, sulindac). Antacids, commonly prescribed to patients on NSAID therapy, variably delay absorption. Some compounds (e.g., diclofenac, nabumetone) undergo first-pass or presystemic elimination. Aspirin begins to acetylate platelets within minutes of reaching the presystemic circulation (Pedersen and FitzGerald, 1984).

Distribution. Most NSAIDs are extensively bound (95%–99%) to plasma proteins, usually albumin. Conditions that alter plasma protein concentration may result in an increased free drug fraction with potential toxic effects. Highly protein bound NSAIDs have the potential to displace other drugs if they compete for the same binding sites. Most NSAIDs are distributed widely throughout the body and readily penetrate arthritic joints, yielding synovial fluid concentrations in the range of half the plasma concentration (i.e., ibuprofen, naproxen, piroxicam) (Day et al., 1999). Most NSAIDs achieve sufficient concentrations in the CNS to have a central analgesic effect. Celecoxib is particularly lipophilic and moves readily into the CNS. Multiple NSAIDs are marketed in formulations for topical application on inflamed or injured joints. However, direct transport of topically applied NSAIDs into inflamed tissues and joints appears to be minimal, and detectable concentrations in synovial fluid of some agents (i.e., diclofenac) following topical use are primarily attained via dermal absorption and systemic circulation. Methods designed to enhance transdermal delivery, such as iontophoresis or chemical penetration enhancers, are under investigation. Topical application is also being explored as a delivery route for drug combinations containing narcotics and NSAIDs.

Metabolism and Excretion. Hepatic biotransformation and renal excretion are the principal routes of metabolism and elimination of the majority of NSAIDs. Plasma $t_{1/2}$ varies considerably among NSAIDs. Ibuprofen, diclofenac, and acetaminophen have a $t_{1/2}$ of 1–4 h, while piroxicam has a $t_{1/2}$ of about 50 h at steady state. Naproxen has a comparatively long but highly variable $t_{1/2}$ ranging from 9 to 25 h. Genetic variation in the major metabolizing enzymes and variation in the composition of intestinal microbiota may contribute to variability in metabolism and elimination. Elimination pathways frequently involve oxidation or hydroxylation. Acetaminophen, at therapeutic doses, is oxidized only to a small degree to form traces of the highly reactive metabolite NAPQI. Following overdose, however, the principal metabolic pathways are saturated, and hepatotoxic NAPQI concentrations can be formed (see Figure 4–5). Several NSAIDs or their metabolites are glucuronidated or otherwise conjugated. In some cases, such as the propionic acid derivatives naproxen and ketoprofen, the glucuronide metabolites can hydrolyze back to form the active parent drug when the metabolite is not removed efficiently due to renal insufficiency or competition for renal excretion with other drugs. This may prolong elimination of the NSAID significantly. In general, NSAIDs are not recommended in the setting of advanced hepatic or renal disease due to their adverse pharmacodynamic effects. NSAIDs usually are not removed by hemodialysis due to their extensive plasma protein binding; salicylic acid is an exception to this rule.

Therapeutic Uses

The NSAIDs are antipyretic, analgesic, and anti-inflammatory, with the exception of acetaminophen, which is antipyretic and analgesic but is largely devoid of anti-inflammatory activity.

Inflammation

The NSAIDs provide mostly symptomatic relief from pain and inflammation associated with musculoskeletal disorders, such as rheumatoid arthritis and osteoarthritis. Some NSAIDs are approved for the treatment of ankylosing spondylitis and gout. Patients with more debilitating disease may not respond adequately to full therapeutic doses of NSAIDs and may require aggressive therapy with second-line agents.

Pain

The NSAIDs are effective against inflammatory pain of low-to-moderate intensity. Although their maximal efficacy is generally less than the opioids, NSAIDs lack the unwanted adverse effects of opiates in the CNS, including respiratory depression and the potential for development of physical dependence. Coadministration of NSAIDs can reduce the opioid dose needed for sufficient pain control and reduce the likelihood of adverse opioid effects. For example, acetaminophen can be prescribed in combination with hydrocodone. NSAIDs do not change the perception of sensory modalities other than pain. NSAIDs are particularly effective when inflammation has caused sensitization of pain perception (see other discussion in this section on inflammation, pain, and fever). Thus, postoperative pain or pain arising from inflammation, such as arthritic pain, is controlled well by NSAIDs, whereas pain arising from the hollow viscera usually is not relieved. An exception to this is menstrual pain. Treatment of menstrual pain with NSAIDs has met with considerable success because cramps and other symptoms of primary dysmenorrhea are caused by the release of PGs by the endometrium during menstruation. NSAIDs are commonly used to treat migraine attacks and can be combined with drugs such as the triptans or with antiemetics to aid relief of the associated nausea. NSAIDs generally lack efficacy in neuropathic pain.

Fever

Antipyretic therapy is reserved for patients in whom fever in itself may be deleterious and for those who experience considerable relief when fever is lowered. NSAIDs reduce fever in most situations, but not the circadian variation in temperature or the rise in response to exercise or increased ambient temperature.

Fetal Circulatory System

The PGs are implicated in the maintenance of patency of the ductus arteriosus, and indomethacin, ibuprofen, and other NSAIDs have been used in neonates to close the inappropriately patent ductus. Conversely, infusion of prostandoid analogues maintains ductal patency after birth (see Chapter 37).

Cardioprotection

Ingestion of aspirin prolongs bleeding time. This effect is due to irreversible acetylation of platelet COX and the consequent inhibition of platelet function. It is the permanent suppression of platelet TxA_2 formation that is thought to underlie the cardioprotective effect of aspirin.

Aspirin reduces the risk of serious vascular events in high-risk patients (e.g., those with previous myocardial infarction) by 20%–25%. The reduction of subsequent thrombotic strokes is somewhat less, roughly 10%–15% (Antithrombotic Trialists' Collaboration et al., 2009). Low-dose aspirin (≤100 mg/d) is associated with a lower risk for GI adverse events than higher doses (e.g., 325 mg/d) and is often used following percutaneous coronary intervention (Xian et al., 2015). Low doses of aspirin are associated with a small (roughly 2-fold) but detectable increase in the incidence of serious GI bleeds and intracranial bleeds in placebo-controlled trials. The benefit from aspirin, however, outweighs these risks in the case of secondary prevention of cardiovascular disease. The issue is much more nuanced in patients who have never had a serious atherothrombotic event (primary prevention); here, prevention of myocardial infarction by aspirin is numerically balanced by the serious GI bleeds it precipitates (Patrono, 2015). Given their relatively short $t_{1/2}$ and reversible COX inhibition, most other NSAIDs are not thought to afford cardioprotection. Data suggest that cardioprotection is lost when combining low-dose aspirin with NSAIDs through a drug-drug interaction at the aspirin target site in platelet COX-1 (Catella-Lawson et al., 2001; Farkouh et al., 2004; Li et al., 2014). COX-2–selective NSAIDs are devoid of antiplatelet activity, as mature platelets do not express COX-2.

Other Clinical Uses

Systemic Mastocytosis. Systemic mastocytosis is a condition in which there are excessive mast cells in the bone marrow, reticuloendothelial system, GI system, bones, and skin (Theoharides et al., 2015). In patients with systemic mastocytosis, PGD_2, released from mast cells is the major mediator of severe episodes of flushing, vasodilation, and hypotension; this PGD_2 effect is resistant to antihistamines. The addition of aspirin or ketoprofen (off-label use) may be beneficial in patients with high levels of urinary PGD metabolites who have flushing and angioedema. However, NSAIDs can cause degranulation of mast cells, so blockade with histamine receptor antagonists should be established before NSAIDs are initiated.

Niacin Tolerability. Large doses of niacin (nicotinic acid) effectively lower serum cholesterol levels, reduce low-density lipoprotein, and raise high-density lipoprotein (see Chapter 33). However, niacin induces intense facial flushing mediated largely by release of PGD_2 from the skin, which can be inhibited by treatment with aspirin (Song et al., 2012).

Bartter Syndrome. Bartter syndrome includes a series of rare disorders (frequency ≤ 1/100,000 persons) characterized by hypokalemic, hypochloremic metabolic alkalosis with normal blood pressure and hyperplasia of the juxtaglomerular apparatus. Fatigue, muscle weakness, diarrhea, and dehydration are the main symptoms. Distinct variants are caused by mutations in a Na^+-K^+-$2Cl^-$ cotransporter, an apical ATP-regulated K^+ channel, a basolateral Cl^- channel, a protein (barttin) involved in cotransporter trafficking, and the extracellular Ca^{2+}-sensing receptor. Renal COX-2 is induced, and biosynthesis of PGE_2 is increased. Treatment with indomethacin, combined with potassium repletion and spironolactone, is associated with improvement in the biochemical derangements and symptoms. Selective COX-2 inhibitors also have been used (Nusing et al., 2001).

Cancer Chemoprevention. Epidemiological studies suggested that daily use of aspirin is associated with a 24% decrease in the incidence of colon cancer (Rothwell et al., 2010). Similar observations have been made with NSAID use in this and other cancers. NSAIDs have been used in patients with familial adenomatous polyposis, an inherited disorder characterized by multiple adenomatous colon polyps developing during adolescence and the inevitable occurrence of colon cancer by the sixth decade.

Adverse Effects of NSAID Therapy

Adverse events common to aspirin and NSAIDs are outlined in Table 38–1. To minimize potential adverse events of NSAIDs, the lowest effective dose should be used for the shortest feasible length of time. Age generally is correlated with an increased probability of developing serious adverse reactions to NSAIDs, and caution is warranted in choosing a lower starting dose for elderly patients. NSAIDs are labeled with a black-box warning related to cardiovascular risks and are specifically contraindicated following coronary artery bypass graft (CABG) surgery.

Gastrointestinal

The most common symptoms associated with these drugs are GI (~40% of patients), including dyspepsia, abdominal pain, anorexia, nausea, and diarrhea. However, these symptoms are not predictive of gastric or intestinal lesions such as subepithelial hemorrhages, erosions, and ulcers, which can be endoscopically detected in about 30%–50% of NSAID users, but are often asymptomatic and tend to heal spontaneously. Serious complications—bleeding, perforation, or obstruction—occur at an annual

TABLE 38–1 ■ SOME SHARED ADVERSE EFFECTS OF NSAIDs[a]

SYSTEM	MANIFESTATIONS
Gastrointestinal	Abdominal pain, bleeding, constipation, diarrhea, dyspepsia, dysphagia, eructation,[b] esophageal stricture/ulceration, esophagitis, flatulence, gastritis, hematemesis,[b] melena,[b] nausea, odynophagia, perforation, pyrosis, stomatitis, ulcers, vomiting, xerostomia[b]
Platelets	Inhibited platelet activation,[b] propensity for bruising,[b] increased risk of hemorrhage,[b] platelet dysfunction,[b] thrombocytopenia[b]
Renal	Azotemia,[b] cystitis,[b] dysuria,[b] hematuria, hyponatremia, interstitial nephritis, nephrotic syndrome,[b] oliguria,[b] polyuria,[b] renal failure, renal papillary necrosis, proteinuria, salt and water retention, hypertension, worsening of renal function in renal/cardiac/cirrhotic patients, ↓ effectiveness of antihypertensives and diuretics, hyperkalemia,[b] ↓ urate excretion (especially with aspirin)
Cardiovascular	Edema,[b] heart failure,[c] hypertension, MI,[c] palpitations,[b] premature closure of ductus arteriosus, sinus tachycardia,[b] stroke,[c] thrombosis,[c] vasculitis[b]
Neurologic	Anorexia,[b] anxiety,[b] aseptic meningitis, confusion,[b] depression, dizziness, drowsiness,[b] headache, insomnia,[b] malaise,[b] paresthesias, tinnitus, seizures,[b] syncope,[b] vertigo[b]
Reproductive	Prolongation of gestation, inhibition of labor, delayed ovulation
Hypersensitivity	Anaphylactoid reactions, angioedema, severe bronchospasm, urticaria, flushing, hypotension, shock
Hematologic	Anemia, agranulocytosis, aplastic anemia,[b] hemolytic anemia,[b] leukopenia[b]
Hepatic	Elevated enzymes, hepatitis, hepatic failure,[b] jaundice
Dermatologic	Diaphoresis,[b] exfoliative dermatitis, photosensitivity,[b] pruritus, purpura,[b] rash, Stevens-Johnson syndrome, toxic epidermal necrolysis, urticaria
Respiratory	Dyspnea,[b] hyperventilation (salicylates)
Other	Alopecia,[b] blurred vision,[b] conjunctivitis,[b] epistaxis,[b] fever,[b] hearing loss,[b] pancreatitis,[b] paresthesias, visual disturbance,[b] weight gain[b]

[a]Refer to product label for specific information.
[b]Reported for most, but not all, NSAIDs.
[c]With the exception of low-dose aspirin.

rate of 1%–2% in regular NSAID users. Many patients who develop a serious upper GI adverse event while receiving NSAID therapy are asymptomatic prior to diagnosis. The risk is particularly high in those with *Helicobacter pylori* infection, heavy alcohol consumption, or other risk factors for mucosal injury, including the concurrent use of glucocorticoids. All selective COX-2 inhibitors are less prone to induce gastric ulcers than equally efficacious doses of isoform nonselective NSAIDs (Sostres et al., 2013).

Several mechanisms contribute to NSAID-induced GI complications (see Chapter 37). Inhibition of COX-1 in gastric epithelial cells depresses mucosal cytoprotective PGs, especially PGI_2 and PGE_2. These eicosanoids inhibit acid secretion by the stomach, enhance mucosal blood flow, and promote the secretion of cytoprotective mucus in the intestine. COX-2 also contributes to constitutive formation of these PGs by human gastric epithelium, and products of COX-2 may contribute to ulcer healing. Another factor that may play a part in the formation of ulcers is the local irritation from contact of orally administered NSAIDs—most of which are organic acids—with the gastric mucosa. However, the incidence of serious GI adverse events is not significantly reduced by formulations devised to limit drug contact with the gastric mucosa, such as enteric coating or efferent solutions, suggesting that the contribution of direct irritation to the overall risk is minor. Platelet inhibition by NSAIDs increases the likelihood of bleeds when mucosal damage has occurred. Coadministration of proton pump inhibitors or H_2 antagonists in conjunction with NSAIDs reduces the rate of duodenal and gastric ulceration (see Chapter 49, Figure 49-1).

Cardiovascular

The COX-2–selective NSAIDs were developed to improve GI safety. However, COX-2 inhibitors depress formation of PGI_2 but do not inhibit the COX-1–catalyzed formation of platelet TxA_2. PGI_2 inhibits platelet aggregation and constrains the effect of prothrombotic and atherogenic stimuli by TxA_2 (Grosser et al., 2006, 2010, 2017), and renal PGI_2 and PGE_2 formed by COX-2 contribute to arterial pressure homeostasis (see Chapter 37). Genetic deletion of the PGI_2 receptor, IP, in mice augments the thrombotic response to endothelial injury, accelerates experimental atherogenesis, increases vascular proliferation, and adds to the effect of hypertensive stimuli (Cheng et al., 2002, 2006; Egan et al., 2004; Kobayashi et al., 2004). Tissue-specific genetic deletion of COX-2 in the vasculature accelerates the response to thrombotic stimuli and raises blood pressure (Yu et al., 2012). Together, these mechanisms would be expected to alter the cardiovascular risk of humans, as COX-2 inhibition in humans depresses PGI_2 synthesis (Catella-Lawson et al., 1999; McAdam et al., 1999). Indeed, a human mutation of the IP, which disrupts its signaling, is associated with increased cardiovascular risk (Arehart et al., 2008).

Clinical trials—with celecoxib, valdecoxib (withdrawn), and rofecoxib (withdrawn)—revealed an increase in the incidence of myocardial infarction, stroke, and vascular death by approximately 1.4-fold (Coxib and Traditional NSAID Trialists' Collaboration et al., 2013). The risk extends to diclofenac, which is almost as COX-2 selective as celecoxib, and to some of the other older NSAIDs. An exception in some individuals may be naproxen. There is considerable between-person variation in the $t_{1/2}$ of naproxen, and platelet inhibition might be anticipated throughout the dosing interval in some, but not all, individuals on naproxen (Capone et al., 2005). While this is supported by randomized controlled trials (Coxib and Traditional NSAID Trialists' Collaboration et al., 2013), identifying individuals who fall into the long-acting group is currently not practical in clinical routine. The FDA has determined that the data differentiating the risk between distinct NSAIDs is not sufficient to distinguish between drugs on the regulatory level; thus, a cardiovascular risk warning is included on the label of all NSAIDs (U.S. Food and Drug Administration, 2015). Similarly, all NSAIDs share a class black-box warning contraindicating their use for the treatment of perioperative pain in the setting of CABG surgery.

The NSAIDs with selectivity for COX-2 should be reserved for patients at high risk for GI complications. The cardiovascular risk appears to be conditioned by factors influencing drug exposure, such as dose, $t_{1/2}$, degree of COX-2 selectivity, potency, and treatment duration. Thus, the lowest possible dose should be prescribed for the shortest possible period.

Blood Pressure and Renal Adverse Events

All NSAIDs have been associated with renal and renovascular adverse events. Up to 5% of regular NSAID users can be expected to develop hypertension. Clinical studies suggest that hypertensive complications occur more commonly in patients treated with COX-2–selective than with nonselective NSAIDs. Heart failure risk is roughly doubled.

The NSAIDs have little effect on renal function or blood pressure in healthy human subjects because of the redundancy of systems that regulate renal function. In situations that challenge the regulatory systems, such as dehydration, hypovolemia, congestive heart failure, hepatic cirrhosis, chronic kidney disease, and other states of activation of the sympathoadrenal or renin-angiotensin systems, regulation of renal function by PG formation becomes crucial (see Chapter 37). NSAIDs impair the PG-induced inhibition of both the reabsorption of Cl^- and the action of antidiuretic hormone, which may result in the retention of salt and water. Inhibition of COX-2–derived PGs that contribute to the regulation of renal medullary blood flow may lead to a rise in blood pressure, increasing the risk of cardiovascular thrombotic events and heart failure. NSAIDs promote reabsorption of K^+ as a result of decreased availability of Na^+ at distal tubular sites and suppression of the PG-induced secretion of renin. The last effect may account in part for the usefulness of NSAIDs in the treatment of Bartter syndrome (see Bartter Syndrome section).

Analgesic Nephropathy. Analgesic nephropathy is a condition of slowly progressive renal failure, decreased concentrating capacity of the renal tubule, and sterile pyuria. Risk factors are the chronic use of high doses of combinations of NSAIDs and frequent urinary tract infections. If recognized early, discontinuation of NSAIDs may permit recovery of renal function.

Pregnancy

Myometrial COX-2 expression and levels of PGE_2 and $PGF_{2\alpha}$ increase markedly in the myometrium during labor. Prolongation of gestation by NSAIDs has been demonstrated in humans. Some NSAIDs, particularly indomethacin, have been used off label to stop preterm labor. However, this use is associated with closure of the ductus arteriosus and impaired fetal circulation in utero, particularly in fetuses older than 32 weeks of gestation. COX-2–selective inhibitors have been used off label as tocolytic agents; this use has been associated with stenosis of the ductus arteriosus and oligohydramnios. Low-dose aspirin (81 mg/d) reduces the risk of preeclampsia by 24% when used as (off-label) preventive medication after 12 weeks of gestation in women who are at high risk (LeFevre and Force, 2014).

Hypersensitivity

Hypersensitivity symptoms to aspirin and NSAIDs range from vasomotor rhinitis, generalized urticaria, and bronchial asthma to laryngeal edema, bronchoconstriction, flushing, hypotension, and shock. Aspirin intolerance (including aspirin-associated asthma) is a contraindication to therapy with any other NSAID because of cross sensitivity. Although less common in children, this cross sensitivity may occur in 10%–25% of patients with asthma, nasal polyps, or chronic urticaria and in 1% of apparently healthy individuals. It is provoked by even low doses (<80 mg) of aspirin and apparently involves COX inhibition. Treatment of aspirin hypersensitivity is similar to that of other severe hypersensitivity reactions, with support of vital organ function and administration of epinephrine.

Aspirin Resistance

All forms of treatment failure with aspirin have been collectively called *aspirin resistance*, but pharmacological resistance to aspirin is rare. Pseudoresistance, reflecting delayed and reduced drug absorption, complicates enteric-coated, but not immediate-release aspirin administration (Grosser et al., 2013).

Hepatotoxicity

Liver injury occurs in 17% of adults with unintentional acetaminophen overdose (Blieden et al., 2014). Liver toxicity from therapeutic doses of acetaminophen is extremely rare (see Acetaminophen section). By contrast, therapeutic dosing of diclofenac may be complicated by hepatotoxicity.

While the entire class of NSAIDs has a rate of less than 1 liver injury per 100,000 patients on average, chronic consumption of diclofenac is associated with a risk of 6–11 liver injuries per 100,000 users (Bjornsson et al., 2013; de Abajo et al., 2004) (see Diclofenac section). NSAIDs are not recommended in advanced hepatic or renal disease.

Reye Syndrome

Due to the possible association with Reye syndrome, aspirin and other salicylates are contraindicated in children and young adults less than 20 years of age with viral illness–associated fever (Schrör, 2007). Reye syndrome, a severe and often fatal disease, is characterized by the acute onset of encephalopathy, liver dysfunction, and fatty infiltration of the liver and other viscera. Although a mechanistic understanding is lacking, the epidemiologic association between aspirin use and Reye syndrome is sufficiently strong that aspirin and bismuth subsalicylate labels must indicate the risk. As the use of aspirin in children has declined dramatically, so has the incidence of Reye syndrome. Acetaminophen and ibuprofen have not been implicated in Reye syndrome and are the agents of choice for antipyresis in children and youths.

Drug Interactions

Refer to the individual product labels for a comprehensive listing of NSAID drug-drug interactions.

Concomitant NSAIDs and Low-Dose Aspirin

Many patients consume both an NSAID for chronic pain and low-dose aspirin for cardioprevention. Epidemiological studies suggest that this combination therapy increases significantly the likelihood of GI adverse events over either class of NSAID alone. In addition, prior occupancy of platelet COX-1 by the NSAID can impede access of aspirin to its acetylation target Ser 529 and prevents irreversible inhibition of platelet function (Catella-Lawson et al., 2001). This has been unequivocally shown to occur with ibuprofen and naproxen and may also affect other isoform nonselective NSAIDs (Li et al., 2014). This drug-drug interaction may undermine the cardioprotective effect of aspirin. Celecoxib is unlikely to cause this drug-drug interaction in vivo, but confers a direct cardiovascular hazard (Grosser et al., 2017). Thus, pain management in patients with preexisting cardiovascular disease remains a particular challenge because of the cardiovascular adverse effects of NSAIDs and the risk of drug-drug interactions that might undermine the antiplatelet effects of aspirin.

Other Drug-Drug Interactions

The ACE inhibitors act, at least partly, by preventing the breakdown of kinins that stimulate PG production (see Figure 39–4). Thus, NSAIDs may attenuate the effectiveness of ACE inhibitors by blocking the production of vasodilator and natriuretic PGs. The combination of NSAIDs and ACE inhibitors also can produce marked hyperkalemia, leading to cardiac arrhythmia, especially in the elderly and in patients with hypertension, diabetes mellitus, or ischemic heart disease. Corticosteroids and selective serotonin reuptake inhibitors may increase the frequency or severity of GI complications when combined with NSAIDs.

The NSAIDs may augment the risk of bleeding in patients receiving warfarin both because almost all NSAIDs suppress normal platelet function temporarily during the dosing interval and because some NSAIDs also increase warfarin levels by interfering with its metabolism. Thus, concurrent administration should be avoided.

Many NSAIDs are highly bound to plasma proteins, so they may displace other drugs from their binding sites. Such interactions can occur in patients given salicylates or other NSAIDs together with warfarin, sulfonylurea hypoglycemic agents, or methotrexate; the dosage of such agents may require adjustment to prevent toxicity. Patients taking lithium should be monitored because NSAIDs, including aspirin, reduce the renal excretion of this drug and can lead to toxicity.

Pediatric and Geriatric Use

Therapeutic Uses in Children

Therapeutic uses for NSAIDs in children include fever (acetaminophen, ibuprofen); pain (acetaminophen, ibuprofen); postoperative pain (ketorolac injection [single-dose only]); inflammatory disorders, such as juvenile arthritis (celecoxib, etodolac, meloxicam, naproxen, oxaprozin, tolmetin) and Kawasaki disease (off-label high-dose aspirin); and relief of ocular itching due to seasonal allergic rhinitis and postoperative inflammation after cataract extraction (ketorolac ophthalmic solution).

Kawasaki Disease. Aspirin generally is avoided in pediatric populations due to its potential association with Reye syndrome (see Reye Syndrome). However, high doses of aspirin (30–100 mg/kg/d) are used to treat children during the acute phase of Kawasaki disease, followed by low-dose antiplatelet therapy in the subacute phase.

Pharmacokinetics in Children

The NSAID dosing recommendations frequently are based on extrapolation of pharmacokinetic data from adults or children older than 2 years, and there are often insufficient data for dose selection in younger infants. For example, the pharmacokinetics of the most commonly used NSAID in children, acetaminophen, differ substantially between the neonatal period and older children or adults. The systemic bioavailability of rectal acetaminophen formulations in neonates and preterm babies is higher than in older patients. Acetaminophen clearance is reduced in preterm neonates, probably due to their immature glucuronide conjugation system (sulfation is the principal route of biotransformation at this age). Therefore, acetaminophen dosing intervals need to be extended (8–12 h) or daily doses reduced to avoid accumulation and liver toxicity.

Aspirin elimination also is delayed in neonates and young infants compared to adults, raising the risk of accumulation. Disease also may affect NSAID disposition in children. For example, ibuprofen plasma concentrations are reduced and clearance increased (~80%) in children with cystic fibrosis. This is probably related to the GI and hepatic pathologies associated with this disease. Aspirin's kinetics are markedly altered during the febrile phase of rheumatic fever or Kawasaki vasculitis. The reduction in serum albumin associated with these conditions causes an elevation of the free salicylate concentration, which may saturate renal excretion and result in salicylate accumulation to toxic levels. In addition to dose reduction, monitoring of the free drug may be warranted in these situations.

Pharmacokinetics in the Elderly

The clearance of many NSAIDs is reduced in the elderly due to changes in hepatic metabolism and creatine clearance. NSAIDs with a long $t_{1/2}$ and primarily oxidative metabolism (i.e., piroxicam, tenoxicam, celecoxib) have elevated plasma concentrations in elderly patients. For example, plasma concentrations after the same dose of celecoxib may rise up to 2-fold higher in patients older than 65 years than in patients younger than 50 years of age, warranting dose adjustment. The capacity of plasma albumin to bind drugs is diminished in older patients and may result in higher concentrations of unbound NSAIDs. For example, free naproxen concentrations are markedly increased in older patients, although total plasma concentrations essentially are unchanged, and the higher susceptibility of older patients to GI complications may be due in part to elevated total or free NSAID concentrations. Generally, it is advisable to start most NSAIDs at a low dosage in the elderly and increase the dosage only if the therapeutic efficacy is insufficient.

Specific Properties of Individual NSAIDs

General properties shared by NSAIDs were considered in the section, Nonsteroidal Anti-inflammatory Drugs. In this section, important characteristics of individual substances are discussed. NSAIDs are grouped by their chemical similarity, as in Figure 38–1.

Aspirin and Other Salicylates

The salicylates include aspirin, salicylic acid, methyl salicylate, diflunisal, salsalate (an unapproved marketed drug in the U.S.), olsalazine, sulfasalazine, balsalazide, choline magnesium trisalicylate (an unapproved marketed drug in the U.S.), magnesium salicylate, mesalamine, and salicylamide (a carboxamide derivative of salicylic acid contained as an ingredient in some OTC combination pain relievers). Salicylic acid is so irritating that it can only be used externally; therefore, the various derivatives of this acid have been synthesized for systemic use. For example, aspirin is the acetate ester of salicylic acid (ASA). Aspirin is a widely consumed analgesic, antipyretic, and anti-inflammatory agent. Because aspirin is so available, the possibility of misuse and serious toxicity is underappreciated, and it remains a cause of fatal poisoning in children.

SALICYLIC ACID   ASPIRIN

Table 38–2 summarizes the clinical pharmacokinetic properties of two salicylates, aspirin and diflunisal.

Mechanism of Action

The effects of aspirin are largely caused by its capacity to acetylate proteins, as described in Irreversible Cyclooxygenase Inhibition by Aspirin. Other salicylates generally act by virtue of their content of salicylic acid, which is a relatively weak inhibitor of the purified COX enzymes. Salicylic acid may also suppress inflammatory upregulation of COX-2 by interfering with transcription factor binding to the COX-2 promoter.

ADME

Absorption. Orally ingested salicylates are absorbed rapidly, partly from the stomach, but mostly from the upper small intestine. The peak plasma level is reached in about 1 h. The rate of absorption is determined by disintegration and dissolution rates of the tablets administered, the pH at the mucosal surface, and gastric emptying time. Even though salicylate is more ionized as the pH is increased, a rise in pH also increases the solubility of salicylate and thus dissolution of the tablets. The overall effect is to enhance absorption. The presence of food delays absorption of salicylates. Rectal absorption of salicylate usually is slower than oral absorption and is incomplete and inconsistent.

Salicylic acid is absorbed rapidly from the intact skin, especially when applied in oily liniments or ointments, and systemic poisoning has occurred from its application to large areas of skin. Methyl salicylate likewise is speedily absorbed when applied cutaneously; however, its GI absorption may be delayed many hours, making gastric lavage effective for removal even in poisonings that present late after oral ingestion.

Enteric coating delays and reduces the bioavailability of aspirin by roughly half and renders absorption more variable in the presence of food (Bogentoft et al., 1978), which is likely the cause of "pseudoresistance" to aspirin (see Aspirin Resistance).

Distribution. After absorption, salicylates are distributed throughout most body tissues and transcellular fluids, primarily by pH-dependent processes. Salicylates are transported actively out of the CSF across the choroid plexus. The drugs readily cross the placental barrier. Ingested aspirin mainly is absorbed as such, but some enters the systemic circulation as salicylic acid after hydrolysis by esterases in the GI mucosa and liver. Roughly 80%–90% of the salicylate in plasma is bound to proteins, especially albumin; the proportion of the total that is bound declines as plasma concentrations increase. Hypoalbuminemia, as may occur in rheumatoid arthritis, is associated with a proportionately higher level of free salicylate in the plasma. Salicylate competes with a variety of compounds for plasma protein-binding sites; these include thyroxine, triiodothyronine, penicillin, phenytoin, sulfinpyrazone, bilirubin, uric acid, and other NSAIDs, such as naproxen. Aspirin is bound to a more limited extent; however, it acetylates human plasma albumin in vivo by reaction with the ε-amino group of lysine and may change the binding of other drugs to albumin. Aspirin also acetylates other plasma and tissue proteins, but there is no evidence that this contributes to clinical efficacy or adverse events.

Metabolism and Excretion. Aspirin is rapidly deacetylated to form salicylic acid by spontaneous hydrolysis or esterases located in the intestinal wall, red blood cells, and the liver. The three chief metabolic products are salicyluric acid (the glycine conjugate), the ether or phenolic glucuronide, and the ester or acyl glucuronide. Salicylates and their metabolites are excreted in the urine. The excretion of free salicylates is variable and depends on the dose and the urinary pH. For example, the clearance of salicylate is about four times as great at pH 8 as at pH 6, and it is well above the glomerular filtration rate at pH 8. High rates of urine flow decrease tubular reabsorption, whereas the opposite is true in oliguria. The plasma $t_{1/2}$ for aspirin is about 20 min, and for salicylate is 2–3 h at antiplatelet doses, rising to 12 h at usual anti-inflammatory doses. The $t_{1/2}$ of salicylate may rise to 15–30 h at high therapeutic doses or when there is intoxication. This dose-dependent elimination is the result of the limited capacity of the liver to form salicyluric acid and the phenolic glucuronide, resulting in a larger proportion of unchanged drug being excreted in the urine at higher doses. Salicylate metabolism shows high intersubject variability due to the variable contribution of different metabolic pathways. Women frequently exhibit higher plasma concentrations, perhaps due to lower intrinsic esterase activity and gender differences in hepatic metabolism. Salicylate clearance is reduced and salicylate exposure is significantly increased in the elderly. The plasma concentration of salicylate is increased by conditions that decrease the glomerular filtration rate or reduce proximal tubule secretion, such as renal disease, or the presence of inhibitors that compete for the transport system (e.g., probenecid). In case of an overdose, hemodialysis and hemofiltration techniques remove salicylic acid effectively from the circulation.

Monitoring of Plasma Salicylate Concentrations. Aspirin is one of the NSAIDs for which plasma salicylate can provide a means to monitor therapy and toxicity. Intermittent analgesic-antipyretic doses of aspirin typically produce plasma aspirin levels of less than 20 μg/mL and plasma salicylate levels of less than 60 μg/mL. The daily ingestion of anti-inflammatory doses of 4–5 g of aspirin produces plasma salicylate levels in the range of 120–350 μg/mL. Optimal anti-inflammatory effects for patients with rheumatic diseases require plasma salicylate concentrations of 150–300 μg/mL. Significant adverse effects can be seen at levels greater than 300 μg/mL. At lower concentrations, the drug clearance is nearly constant (despite the fact that saturation of metabolic capacity is approached) because the fraction of drug that is free, and thus available for metabolism or excretion, increases as binding sites on plasma proteins are saturated. The total concentration of salicylate in plasma is therefore a relatively linear function of dose at lower concentrations. At higher concentrations, however, as metabolic pathways of disposition become saturated, small increments in dose can disproportionately increase plasma salicylate concentration. Failure to anticipate this phenomenon can lead to toxicity.

Therapeutic Uses

Systemic Uses. The *analgesic-antipyretic* dose of aspirin for adults is 325–1000 mg orally every 4–6 h. It is only rarely used for inflammatory diseases such as *arthritis, spondyloarthropathies,* and *systemic lupus erythematosus*; NSAIDs with a better GI safety profile are preferred. The anti-inflammatory doses of aspirin, as might be given in rheumatic fever, range from 4 to 8 g/d in divided doses. The maximum recommended daily dose of aspirin for adults and children 12 years or older is 4 g. The rectal administration of aspirin suppositories may be preferred in infants or when the oral route is unavailable. Aspirin suppresses clinical signs and improves tissue inflammation in acute rheumatic fever. Other salicylates available for systemic use include salsalate (salicylsalicylic acid), magnesium salicylate, diflunisal, and a combination of choline salicylate and magnesium salicylate (choline magnesium trisalicylate).

Diflunisal is a difluorophenyl derivative of salicylic acid that is not converted to salicylic acid in vivo. It is a competitive inhibitor of COX and a potent anti-inflammatory drug but is largely devoid of antipyretic effects, perhaps because of poor penetration into the CNS. The drug has been used primarily as an analgesic in the treatment of osteoarthritis and musculoskeletal strains or sprains; in these circumstances, it is about three to four times more potent than aspirin. For rheumatoid arthritis or osteoarthritis, 250–1000 mg/d is administered in two divided doses; maintenance dosage should not exceed 1.5 g/d. Diflunisal may produce

TABLE 38–2 ■ NSAIDS: SALICYLATES, ACETAMINOPHEN, AND ACETIC ACID DERIVATIVES

CLASS/DRUG	PHARMACOKINETICS	DOSING	COMMENTS	COMPARED TO ASPIRIN
Salicylates				
Aspirin	Peak C_p, 1 h Protein binding, 80–90% Metabolite, Salicyluric acid $t_{1/2}$, therapeutic, 2–3 h $t_{1/2}$, toxic dose, 15–30 h	Antiplatelet, 40–80 mg/day Pain/fever, 325–650 mg 4–6 h Rheumatic fever, Children 1 g/ 4–6 h or 10 mg/kg 4–6 h	Permanent platelet COX-1 inhibition Adverse effects: GL, ↑clotting time hypersensitivity Avoid in children with acute febrile illness (Reye syndrome)	
Diflunisal	Peak C_p, 2–3 h Protein binding, 99% Metabolite, Glucuronide $t_{1/2}$, 8–12 h	250–500 mg every 8–12 h (maximum = 1 g/dose and 4 g/d); children <12 y: 10–15 mg/kg every 4 h (maximum 5 doses/24 h) IV (>50 kg): 1000 mg every 6 h or 650 mg every 4 h; (<50 kg): 15 mg/kg every 6 h or 12.5 mg/kg 4h	Not metabolized to salicylic, competitive COX inhibitor, excreted into breast milk.	Analgesic and anti-inflammatory, 4–5× more potent Antipyretic, weaker Fewer platelet and GI side effects.
Para-aminophenol derivative				
Acetaminophen	Peak C_p, 30–60 min Protein binding, 20–50% Metabolites, Glucuronides (60%); sulfates (35%) $t_{1/2}$, 2 h	650 mg or less every 4 h (maximum of 4000 mg/24 h)	Weak nonspecific COX inhibitor at common doses Potency may be modulated by peroxidase Overdose ⇒ toxic metabolite, (NAPQI) liver necrosis	Analgesic/antipyretic, equivalent Anti-inflammatory, GI, and platelet effects < aspirin at 1000 mg/day
Acetic acid derivatives				
Indomethacin	Peak C_p, 1–2 h Protein binding, 99% Metabolites, O–demethyl (50%); unchanged (20%) $t_{1/2}$, 2 h	25 mg 2–3 times/day; 75–100 mg at night	Side effects (3–50%); frontal headache, neutropenia, thrombocytopenia; 20% discontinue	10–40× more potent; intolerance typically limits dose
Sulindac (sulfoxide prodrug)	Peak C_p 1–2 h; active metabolite 8 h, extensive enterohepatic circulation Metabolites, sulfone/conjugates (30%); sulindac/conjugate (25%) $t_{1/2}$, 7 h; 18 h for active sulfone metabolite	150–200 mg twice/day	20% GI side effects; 10% CNS side effects (headache, dizziness rash)	Efficacy comparable
Etodolac	Peak C_p, 1 h Protein binding, 99% Metabolism, Hepatic $t_{1/2}$, 7 h	200–400 mg 3–4 times/day, max: 1200 mg/d or 1000 mg/d (extended release) > 6 years (extended release): 400 mg/d (20–30 kg); add 200 mg/15 kg more wgt.	Some COX-2 selectivity in vitro Adverse effects similar to sulindac, but ~ half as frequent	100 mg etodolac efficacy ≈ 650 mg of aspirin, may be better tolerated
Tolmetin	Peak C_p, 20–60 min Protein binding, 99% Metabolites, Carboxylate conjugates $t_{1/2}$, 5 h	Adults: 400–600 mg 3 times/d Children > 2 y: 20 mg/kg/d in 3–4 divided doses	Food delays anti decreases peak absorption. May persist in synovial fluid ⇒ biological efficacy >plasma $t_{1/2}$	Efficacy similar; 25–40% develop side effects; 5–10% discontinue drug
Ketorolac	Peak C_p, 30–60 min Protein binding, 99% Metabolite, Glucuronide (90%) $t_{1/2}$, 4–6 h	See FDA Package insert	Parenterally (60 mg IM, then 30 mg every 6 h, or 30 mg IV every 6 h) Available as ocular prep	Potent analgesic, poor anti-inflammatory

SECTION IV
INFLAMMATION, IMMUNOMODULATION, AND HEMATOPOIESIS

(Continued)

TABLE 38–2 ■ NSAIDS: SALICYLATES, ACETAMINOPHEN, AND ACETIC ACID DERIVATIVES (*CONTINUED*)

CLASS/DRUG	PHARMACOKINETICS	DOSING	COMMENTS	COMPARED TO ASPIRIN
Diclofenac	Peak C_p, 1 h; extended release, 5 h Protein binding, 99% Metabolites, Glucuronide and sulfide (renal 65%, bile 35%) $t_{1/2}$ 1.2–2 h (immediate-release tabs); 12 h (topical epolamine patch)	50 mg 3 times/day or 75 mg twice/day	As topical gel, ocular solution, oral tablets combined with misoprostol First-pass effect; oral bioavailability, 50%	More potent; 20%, side effects; 2% discontinue; 15%, elevated liver enzymes Substrate for CYPs 2C9 are 3A4
Nabumetone (6-methoxy-2-napthylacetic acid prodrug)	Peak C_p, ~3 h Protein binding, 99% Metabolites, conjugates $t_{1/2}$, 19–26 h; 22–38 h (elderly)	500–1000 mg 1–2 times/d (maximum 2000 mg/d); Patients < 50 kg less likely to require more than 1000 mg/d	First-pass effects, 35% conversion of prodrug to active metabolite; preferential COX-2 inhibition at low doses; Adverse effects (13%): GI upset, abdominal pain	Less fecal blood loss during short-term therapy

Time to peak plasma drug concentration C_p is after a single dose. In general, food delays absorption but does not decrease peak concentration. The majority of NSAIDs undergo hepatic metabolism, and the metabolites are excreted in the urine. Major metabolites or disposal pathways are listed. Typical $t_{1/2}$ is listed for therapeutic doses; if $t_{1/2}$ is much different with the toxic dose, this is also given. Typical adult oral doses are listed unless otherwise noted. Refer to the current product labeling for complete prescribing information, including current labeled pediatric indications

fewer auditory side effects (see Ototoxic Effects) and appears to cause fewer and less-intense GI and antiplatelet effects than does aspirin.

Local Uses. Mesalamine (5-aminosalicylic acid) is a salicylate that is used for its local effects in the treatment of *inflammatory bowel disease* (see Figure 51–4). Oral formulations that deliver drug to the lower intestine are efficacious in the treatment of inflammatory bowel disease (in particular, ulcerative colitis). These preparations rely on pH-sensitive coatings and other delayed-release mechanisms such as linkage to another moiety to create a poorly absorbed parent compound that must be cleaved by bacteria in the colon to form the active drug. Mesalamine is available as a rectal enema for treatment of mild-to-moderate ulcerative colitis, proctitis, and proctosigmoiditis and as a rectal suppository for the treatment of active ulcerative proctitis. Mesalamine derivatives in clinical use include *balsalazide, sulfasalazine,* and *olsalazine.* Sulfasalazine (salicylazosulfapyridine) contains mesalamine linked covalently to sulfapyridine, and balsalazide contains mesalamine linked to the inert carrier molecule 4-aminobenzoyl-β-alanine. Sulfasalazine and olsalazine have been used in the treatment of rheumatoid arthritis and ankylosing spondylitis. Some OTC medications to relieve indigestion and diarrhea agents contain bismuth subsalicylate and have the potential to cause salicylate intoxication, particularly in children.

The keratolytic action of free salicylic acid is employed for the local treatment of warts, corns, fungal infections, and certain types of eczematous dermatitis. After treatment with salicylic acid, tissue cells swell, soften, and desquamate. Methyl salicylate (oil of wintergreen) is a common ingredient of ointments and deep-heating liniments used in the management of musculoskeletal pain; it also is available in herbal medicines and as a flavoring agent. The cutaneous application of methyl salicylate can result in pharmacologically active, and even toxic, systemic salicylate concentrations and has been reported to increase prothrombin time in patients receiving warfarin.

Adverse Effects and Toxicity

Respiration. Salicylates increase O_2 consumption and CO_2 production (especially in skeletal muscle) at anti-inflammatory doses, a result of uncoupling oxidative phosphorylation. The increased production of CO_2 stimulates respiration. Salicylates also stimulate the respiratory center directly in the medulla. Respiratory rate and depth increases, the P_{CO_2} falls, and respiratory alkalosis ensues.

Acid-Base and Electrolyte Balance and Renal Effects. Therapeutic doses of salicylate produce definite changes in the acid-base balance and electrolyte pattern. Compensation for the initial event, respiratory alkalosis, is achieved by increased renal excretion of bicarbonate, which is accompanied by increased Na^+ and K^+ excretion; plasma bicarbonate is thus lowered, and blood pH returns toward normal. This stage of compensatory renal acidosis was often seen in adults given intensive salicylate therapy before the development of safer alternatives. Today, it is an indicator of ensuing intoxication (see Salicylate Intoxication). Salicylates can cause retention of salt and water, as well as acute reduction of renal function in patients with congestive heart failure, renal disease, or hypovolemia. Although long-term use of salicylates alone rarely is associated with nephrotoxicity, the prolonged and excessive ingestion of analgesic mixtures containing salicylates in combination with other NSAIDs can produce papillary necrosis and interstitial nephritis (see Analgesic Nephropathy).

Cardiovascular Effects. Low-dose aspirin (≤100 mg daily) lowers cardiovascular risk and is recommended for the prevention of myocardial infarction and stroke in patients at elevated risk (see Cardioprotection section) (Patrono, 2015). At high therapeutic doses (≥3 g daily), salt and water retention can lead to an increase (≤20%) in circulating plasma volume and decreased hematocrit (via a dilutional effect). There is a tendency for the peripheral vessels to dilate because of a direct effect on vascular smooth muscle. Cardiac output and work are increased. Those with carditis or compromised cardiac function may not have sufficient cardiac reserve to meet the increased demands, and congestive cardiac failure and pulmonary edema can occur. High doses of salicylates can produce noncardiogenic pulmonary edema, particularly in older patients who ingest salicylates regularly over a prolonged period.

GI Effects. Ingestion of salicylates may result in epigastric distress, heartburn, dyspepsia, nausea, and vomiting. Salicylates also may cause erosive gastritis and GI ulceration and hemorrhage. These effects occur primarily with acetylated salicylates (i.e., aspirin). Because nonacetylated salicylates lack the ability to acetylate COX and thereby irreversibly inhibit its activity, they are weaker inhibitors than aspirin.

Aspirin-induced gastric bleeding sometimes is painless and, if unrecognized, may lead to iron-deficiency anemia. The daily ingestion of anti-inflammatory doses of aspirin (3–4 g) results in an average fecal blood loss of between 3 and 8 mL/d, as compared with about 0.6 mL/d in untreated subjects. Gastroscopic examination of aspirin-treated subjects often reveals discrete ulcerative and hemorrhagic lesions of the gastric mucosa; in many cases, multiple hemorrhagic lesions with sharply demarcated areas of focal necrosis are observed.

Hepatic Effects. Salicylates can cause hepatic injury, usually after high doses that result in plasma salicylate concentrations greater than 150 μg/mL. The injury is not an acute effect; rather, the onset characteristically occurs after several months of high-dose treatment. The majority of cases occur in patients with connective tissue disorders. There usually are no symptoms, simply an increase in serum levels of hepatic transaminases, but some patients note right upper quadrant abdominal discomfort and tenderness. Overt jaundice is uncommon. The injury usually is reversible on discontinuation of salicylates. However, the use of salicylates is contraindicated in patients with chronic liver disease. Considerable evidence implicates the use of salicylates as an important factor in the severe hepatic injury and encephalopathy observed in Reye syndrome. Large doses of salicylates may cause hyperglycemia and glycosuria and deplete liver and muscle glycogen.

Uricosuric Effects. The effects of salicylates on uric acid excretion are markedly dependent on dose. Low doses (1 or 2 g/d) may decrease urate excretion and elevate plasma urate concentrations; intermediate doses (2 or 3 g/d) usually do not alter urate excretion. Larger-than-recommended doses (>5 g/d) induce uricosuria and lower plasma urate levels; however, such large doses are tolerated poorly. Even small doses of salicylate can block the effects of probenecid and other uricosuric agents that decrease tubular reabsorption of uric acid.

Hematologic Effects. Irreversible inhibition of platelet function underlies the cardioprotective effect of aspirin. If possible, aspirin therapy should be stopped at least 1 week before surgery; however, preoperative aspirin often is recommended prior to cardiovascular surgery and percutaneous interventions. Patients with severe hepatic damage, hypoprothrombinemia, vitamin K deficiency, or hemophilia should avoid aspirin because the inhibition of platelet hemostasis can result in hemorrhage. Salicylates ordinarily do not alter the leukocyte or platelet count, the hematocrit, or the hemoglobin content. However, doses of 3–4 g/d markedly decrease plasma iron concentration and shorten erythrocyte survival time. Aspirin can cause a mild degree of hemolysis in individuals with a deficiency of G6PD.

Endocrine Effects. Long-term administration of salicylates decreases thyroidal uptake and clearance of iodine, but increases O_2 consumption and the rate of disappearance of thyroxine and triiodothyronine from the circulation. These effects probably are caused by the competitive displacement by salicylate of thyroxine and triiodothyronine from transthyretin and the thyroxine-binding globulin in plasma (see Chapter 43).

Ototoxic Effects. Hearing impairment, alterations of perceived sounds, and tinnitus commonly occur during high-dose salicylate therapy and are sometimes observed at low doses. Ototoxic symptoms are caused by increased labyrinthine pressure or an effect on the hair cells of the cochlea, perhaps secondary to vasoconstriction in the auditory microvasculature. Symptoms usually resolve within 2 or 3 days after withdrawal of the drug. As most competitive COX inhibitors are not associated with hearing loss or tinnitus, a direct effect of salicylic acid rather than suppression of PG synthesis is likely.

Salicylates and Pregnancy. Infants born to women who ingest salicylates for long periods may have significantly reduced birth weights. When administered during the third trimester, there also is an increase in perinatal mortality, anemia, antepartum and postpartum hemorrhage, prolonged gestation, and complicated deliveries; thus, its use during this period should be avoided. NSAIDs during the third trimester of pregnancy also can cause premature closure of the ductus arteriosus and should be avoided.

Local Irritant Effects. Salicylic acid is irritating to skin and mucosa and destroys epithelial cells.

Salicylate Intoxication. Salicylate poisoning or serious intoxication most often occurs in children and sometimes is fatal. CNS effects, intense hyperpnea, and hyperpyrexia are prominent symptoms. Death has followed use of 10–30 g of sodium salicylate or aspirin in adults, but much larger amounts (130 g of aspirin in one case) have been ingested without a fatal outcome. The lethal dose of methyl salicylate (also known as oil of wintergreen, sweet birch oil, gaultheria oil, betula oil) is considerably less than that of sodium salicylate. As little as a 4 mL (4.7 g) of methyl salicylate may cause severe systemic toxicity in children. Mild chronic salicylate intoxication is called *salicylism*. When fully developed, the syndrome includes headache, dizziness, tinnitus, difficulty hearing, dimness of vision, mental confusion, lassitude, drowsiness, sweating, thirst, hyperventilation, nausea, vomiting, and occasionally diarrhea.

Neurological Effects. In high doses, salicylates have toxic effects on the CNS, consisting of stimulation (including convulsions) followed by depression. Confusion, dizziness, tinnitus, high-tone deafness, delirium, psychosis, stupor, and coma may occur. Salicylates induce nausea and vomiting, which result from stimulation of sites that are accessible from the CSF, probably in the medullary chemoreceptor trigger zone.

Respiration. The respiratory effects of salicylates contribute to the serious acid-base balance disturbances that characterize poisoning by this class of compounds. Salicylates stimulate respiration indirectly by uncoupling of oxidative phosphorylation and directly by stimulation of the respiratory center in the medulla (described previously). Uncoupling of oxidative phosphorylation also leads to excessive heat production, and salicylate toxicity is associated with hyperthermia, particularly in children. Prolonged exposure to high doses of salicylates leads to depression of the medulla, with central respiratory depression and circulatory collapse, secondary to vasomotor depression. Because enhanced CO_2 production continues, respiratory acidosis ensues. Respiratory failure is the usual cause of death in fatal cases of salicylate poisoning. Elderly patients with chronic salicylate intoxication often develop noncardiogenic pulmonary edema, which is considered an indication for hemodialysis.

Acid-Base Balance and Electrolytes. High therapeutic doses of salicylate are associated with a primary respiratory alkalosis and compensatory metabolic acidosis. The phase of primary respiratory alkalosis rarely is recognized in children with salicylate toxicity. They usually present in a state of mixed respiratory and metabolic acidosis, characterized by a decrease in blood pH, a low plasma bicarbonate concentration, and normal or nearly normal plasma P_{CO_2}. Direct salicylate-induced depression of respiration prevents adequate respiratory hyperventilation to match the increased peripheral production of CO_2. Consequently, plasma P_{CO_2} increases and blood pH decreases. Because the concentration of bicarbonate in plasma already is low due to increased renal bicarbonate excretion, the acid-base status at this stage essentially is an uncompensated respiratory acidosis.

Superimposed, however, is a true metabolic acidosis caused by accumulation of acids as a result of three processes. First, toxic concentrations of salicylates displace plasma bicarbonate. Second, vasomotor depression caused by toxic doses of salicylates impairs renal function, with consequent accumulation of sulfuric and phosphoric acids; renal failure can ensue. Third, salicylates in toxic doses may decrease aerobic metabolism as a result of inhibition of various enzymes. This derangement of carbohydrate metabolism leads to the accumulation of organic acids, especially pyruvic, lactic, and acetoacetic acids.

The same series of events also causes alterations of water and electrolyte balance. The low plasma P_{CO_2} leads to decreased renal tubular reabsorption of bicarbonate and increased renal excretion of Na^+, K^+, and water. Water also is lost by salicylate-induced sweating (especially in the presence of hyperthermia) and hyperventilation. Dehydration, which can be profound, particularly in children, rapidly occurs. Because more water than electrolyte is lost through the lungs and by sweating, the dehydration is associated with hypernatremia.

Cardiovascular Effects. Toxic doses of salicylates lead to an exaggeration of the unfavorable cardiovascular responses seen at high therapeutic doses, and central vasomotor paralysis occurs. Petechiae may be seen due to defective platelet function.

Metabolic Effects. Large doses of salicylates may cause hyperglycemia and glycosuria and deplete liver and muscle glycogen; these effects are partly explained by the release of epinephrine. Such doses also reduce aerobic metabolism of glucose, increase glucose-6-phosphatase activity, and promote the secretion of glucocorticoids. There is a greater risk of hypoglycemia and subsequent permanent brain injury in children. Salicylates in toxic doses cause a significant negative nitrogen balance, characterized by an aminoaciduria. Adrenocortical activation may contribute to the negative nitrogen balance by enhancing protein catabolism. Salicylates reduce lipogenesis by partially blocking incorporation of acetate into fatty acids; they also inhibit epinephrine-stimulated lipolysis in fat cells and displace long-chain fatty acids from binding sites on human plasma proteins. The combination of these effects leads to increased entry and enhanced oxidation of fatty acids in muscle, liver, and other tissues and to decreased plasma concentrations of free fatty acids, phospholipid, and cholesterol; the oxidation of ketone bodies also is increased.

Management of Salicylate Overdose. Salicylate poisoning represents an acute medical emergency, and death may result despite maximal therapy. Monitoring of salicylate levels is a useful guide to therapy but must be used in conjunction with an assessment of the patient's overall clinical condition, acid-base balance, formulation of salicylate ingested, timing, and dose. There is no specific antidote for salicylate poisoning.

Drug Interactions

The plasma concentration of salicylates generally is little affected by other drugs, but concurrent administration of aspirin lowers the concentrations of indomethacin, naproxen, ketoprofen, and fenoprofen, at least in part by displacement from plasma proteins. Important adverse interactions of aspirin with warfarin, sulfonylureas, and methotrexate were mentioned previously (in Drug Interactions). Other interactions of aspirin include the antagonism of spironolactone-induced natriuresis and the blockade of the active transport of penicillin from CSF to blood. Magnesium-aluminum hydroxide antacids can alkalize the urine enough to increase salicylic acid clearance significantly and reduce steady-state concentrations. Conversely, discontinuation of antacid therapy can increase plasma concentrations to toxic levels.

Acetaminophen

Acetaminophen (paracetamol; *N*-acetyl-*p*-aminophenol) is the active metabolite of phenacetin.

ACETAMINOPHEN

Acetaminophen raises the threshold to painful stimuli, thus exerting an analgesic effect against pain due to a variety of etiologies. Acetaminophen is available without a prescription and is used as a common household analgesic by children and adults. It also is available in fixed-dose combinations containing narcotic and nonnarcotic analgesics (including aspirin and other salicylates), barbiturates, caffeine, vascular headache remedies, sleep aids, toothache remedies, antihistamines, antitussives, decongestants, expectorants, cold and flu preparations, and sore throat treatments. Acetaminophen is well tolerated; however, overdosage—two-thirds of which are intentionally induced—can cause severe hepatic damage (see Figure 4–4); it leads to nearly 80,000 emergency department visits and 30,000 hospitalizations annually in the U.S. (Blieden et al., 2014). The maximum FDA-recommended dose of acetaminophen is 4 g/d.

Mechanism of Action

Acetaminophen has analgesic and antipyretic effects similar to those of aspirin, but only weak anti-inflammatory effects. It is a nonselective COX inhibitor, which acts at the peroxide site of the enzyme and is thus distinct among NSAIDs. The presence of high concentrations of peroxides, as occur at sites of inflammation, reduces its COX-inhibitory activity.

ADME

Oral acetaminophen has excellent bioavailability. Peak plasma concentrations occur within 30–60 min, and the $t_{1/2}$ in plasma is about 2 h. Acetaminophen is relatively uniformly distributed throughout most body fluids. Binding of the drug to plasma proteins is variable, but less than with other NSAIDs. Some 90%–100% of drug may be recovered in the urine within the first day at therapeutic dosing, primarily after hepatic conjugation with glucuronic acid (~60%), sulfuric acid (~35%), or cysteine (~3%); small amounts of hydroxylated and deacetylated metabolites also have been detected (see Table 38–2). Children have less capacity for glucuronidation of the drug than do adults. A small proportion of acetaminophen

undergoes CYP-mediated *N*-hydroxylation to form NAPQI, a highly reactive intermediate. This metabolite normally reacts with sulfhydryl groups in GSH and thereby is rendered harmless. However, after ingestion of large doses of acetaminophen, the metabolite is formed in amounts sufficient to deplete hepatic GSH and contributes significantly to the toxic effects of overdose (see Acetaminophen Intoxication).

Therapeutic Uses

Acetaminophen is suitable for analgesic or antipyretic uses; it is particularly valuable for patients in whom aspirin is contraindicated (e.g., those with aspirin hypersensitivity, children with a febrile illness, patients with bleeding disorders). The conventional oral dose of acetaminophen is 325–650 mg every 4–6 h; total daily doses should not exceed 4 g (2 g/d for chronic alcoholics). Single doses for children 2–11 years old depend on age and weight (~10–15 mg/kg); no more than five doses should be administered in 24 h. An injectable preparation is available. Particular attention is warranted due to the availability of a wide variety of prescription and nonprescription multi-ingredient medications that represent potentially toxic overlapping sources of acetaminophen.

Adverse Effects and Toxicity

Acetaminophen usually is well tolerated. Therapeutic doses of acetaminophen have no clinically relevant effects on the cardiovascular and respiratory systems, platelets, or coagulation. The GI adverse effects are less common than with therapeutic doses of NSAIDs. Rash and other allergic reactions occur occasionally, but sometimes these are more serious and may be accompanied by drug fever and mucosal lesions. Patients who show hypersensitivity reactions to the salicylates only rarely exhibit sensitivity to acetaminophen. The most serious acute adverse effect of overdosage of acetaminophen is a potentially fatal hepatic necrosis (Graham et al., 2005). Hepatic injury with acetaminophen involves its conversion to the toxic metabolite NAPQI. The glucuronide and sulfate conjugation pathways become saturated, and increasing amounts undergo CYP-mediated *N*-hydroxylation to form NAPQI. This is eliminated rapidly by conjugation with GSH and then further metabolized to a mercapturic acid and excreted into the urine. In the setting of acetaminophen overdose, hepatocellular levels of GSH become depleted. The highly reactive NAPQI metabolite binds covalently to cell macromolecules, leading to dysfunction of enzymatic systems and structural and metabolic disarray. Furthermore, depletion of intracellular GSH renders the hepatocytes highly susceptible to oxidative stress and apoptosis. Renal tubular necrosis and hypoglycemic coma also may occur.

In adults, hepatotoxicity may occur after ingestion of a single dose of 10–15 g (150–250 mg/kg) of acetaminophen; doses of 20–25 g or more are potentially fatal. Conditions of CYP induction (e.g., heavy alcohol consumption) or GSH depletion (e.g., fasting or malnutrition) increase the susceptibility to hepatic injury, which has been documented, albeit uncommonly, with doses in the therapeutic range. Plasma transaminases become elevated, sometimes markedly so, beginning about 12–36 h after ingestion. Symptoms that occur during the first 2 days of acute poisoning by acetaminophen reflect gastric distress (e.g., nausea, abdominal pain, anorexia) and belie the potential seriousness of the intoxication. Clinical indications of hepatic damage manifest within 2–4 days of ingestion of toxic doses, with right subcostal pain, tender hepatomegaly, jaundice, and coagulopathy. Renal impairment or frank renal failure may occur. Liver enzyme abnormalities typically peak 72–96 h after ingestion. Biopsy of the liver reveals centrilobular necrosis with sparing of the periportal area. In nonfatal cases, the hepatic lesions are reversible over a period of weeks or months.

Management of Acetaminophen Intoxication. Severe liver damage occurs in 90% of patients with plasma concentrations of acetaminophen greater than 300 μg/mL at 4 h or 45 μg/mL at 15 h after the ingestion of the drug. Activated charcoal, if given within 4 h of ingestion, decreases acetaminophen absorption by 50%–90% and should be administered if the ingested dose is suspected to exceed 7.5 g. NAC is indicated for those at risk of hepatic injury. NAC functions by detoxifying NAPQI. It both repletes GSH stores and may conjugate directly with NAPQI by serving as a GSH substitute. In addition to NAC therapy, aggressive supportive care is warranted. This includes management of hepatic and renal failure, if they occur, and intubation if the patient becomes obtunded. Hypoglycemia can result from liver failure, and plasma glucose should be monitored closely. Fulminant hepatic failure is an indication for liver transplantation.

Acetic Acid Derivatives

Diclofenac

Diclofenac, a phenylacetic acid derivative, is among the most commonly used NSAIDs in Europe. Diclofenac has analgesic, antipyretic, and anti-inflammatory activities. Its potency is substantially greater than that of other NSAIDs. Although it was not developed to be a COX-2 selective drug, the selectivity of diclofenac for COX-2 resembles that of celecoxib (see Figure 38–1).

ADME. Diclofenac displays rapid absorption, extensive protein binding, and a $t_{1/2}$ of 1–2 h (see Table 38–2). The short $t_{1/2}$ makes it necessary to give doses of diclofenac considerably higher than would be required to inhibit COX-2 fully at peak plasma concentrations to afford sustained COX inhibition throughout the dosing interval. Thus, both COX isoforms are inhibited for the first phase of the dosing interval. However, as plasma levels decrease, diclofenac behaves like a COX-2 inhibitor in the later phase of the dosing interval. There is a substantial first-pass effect, such that only about 50% of diclofenac is available systemically. The drug accumulates in synovial fluid after oral administration, which may explain why its duration of therapeutic effect is considerably longer than its plasma $t_{1/2}$. Diclofenac is metabolized in the liver by a member of the CYP2C subfamily to 4-hydroxydiclofenac, the principal metabolite, and other hydroxylated forms; after glucuronidation and sulfation, the metabolites are excreted in the urine (65%) and bile (35%).

Therapeutic Uses. Diclofenac is approved in the U.S. for the long-term symptomatic treatment of rheumatoid arthritis, osteoarthritis, ankylosing spondylitis, pain, primary dysmenorrhea, and acute migraine. Multiple oral formulations are available, providing a range of release times; the usual daily oral dosage is 50–150 mg, given in several divided doses. For acute pain such as migraine, a powdered form for dissolution in water and a solution for intravenous injection are available. Diclofenac also is available in combination with misoprostol, a PGE_1 analogue; this combination retains the efficacy of diclofenac while reducing the frequency of GI ulcers and erosions. A 1% topical gel, a topical solution, and a transdermal patch are available for short-term treatment of pain due to minor strains, sprains, and bruises. A 3% gel formulation is indicated for topical treatment of actinic keratosis. In addition, an ophthalmic solution of diclofenac is available for treatment of postoperative inflammation following cataract extraction and for the temporary relief of pain and photophobia in patients undergoing corneal refractive surgery.

Adverse Effects. Diclofenac produces side effects (particularly GI) in about 20% of patients. The incidence of serious GI adverse effects, hypertension, and myocardial infarction are similar to the COX-2–selective inhibitors (Cannon et al., 2006). Hypersensitivity reactions have occurred following topical application and systemic administration. Severe liver injury occurs in 6–11 per 100,000 regular users annually (Bjornsson et al., 2013; de Abajo et al., 2004). Elevation of hepatic transaminases in plasma by more than three times the upper normal limit, indicating significant liver damage, occurs in about 4% of patients (Rostom et al., 2005). Transaminases should be monitored during the first 8 weeks of therapy with diclofenac. Other untoward responses to diclofenac include CNS effects, rashes, fluid retention, edema, and renal function impairment. The drug is not recommended for children, nursing mothers, or pregnant women.

Diclofenac is extensively metabolized. One metabolite, 4′-hydroxy diclofenac, can form reactive benzoquinone imines (similar to acetaminophen's metabolite NAPQI) that deplete hepatic GSH. Another highly reactive metabolite, diclofenac acyl glucuronide, is primarily catalyzed by UGT2B7 (King et al., 2001). Genetic variation that causes higher catalytic activity of UGT2B7 is associated with an increased risk of hepatotoxicity among patients taking diclofenac (Daly et al., 2007).

Indomethacin

Indomethacin is a methylated indole derivative indicated for the treatment of moderate-to-severe rheumatoid arthritis, osteoarthritis, and ankylosing spondylitis; acute gouty arthritis; and acute painful shoulder. Although indomethacin is still used clinically, mainly as a steroid-sparing agent, toxicity and the availability of safer alternatives have limited its use.

Indomethacin is a potent nonselective inhibitor of the COXs. It also inhibits the motility of polymorphonuclear leukocytes, depresses the biosynthesis of mucopolysaccharides, and may have a direct, COX-independent vasoconstrictor effect. Indomethacin has prominent anti-inflammatory and analgesic-antipyretic properties similar to those of the salicylates.

ADME. Oral indomethacin has excellent bioavailability. Peak concentrations occur 1–2 h after dosing (Table 38–2). The concentration of the drug in the CSF is low, but its concentration in synovial fluid is equal to that in plasma within 5 h of administration. There is enterohepatic cycling of the indomethacin metabolites and probably of indomethacin itself. The $t_{1/2}$ in plasma is variable, perhaps because of enterohepatic cycling, but averages about 2.5 h.

Therapeutic Uses. While indomethacin is estimated to be about 20 times more potent than aspirin, a high rate of intolerance limits its use. An intravenous formulation of indomethacin is approved for closure of persistent patent ductus arteriosus in premature infants. The regimen involves intravenous administration of 0.1–0.25 mg/kg every 12 h for three doses, with the course repeated one time if necessary. Successful closure can be expected in more than 70% of neonates treated. The principal limitation of treating neonates is renal toxicity, and therapy is interrupted if the output of urine falls significantly (<0.6 mL/kg/h). An injectable formulation of ibuprofen is an alternative for the treatment of patent ductus arteriosus.

Adverse Effects. A very high percentage (35%–50%) of patients receiving indomethacin experience adverse drug reactions. GI adverse events are common and can be fatal; elderly patients are at significantly greater risk. Diarrhea may occur and sometimes is associated with ulcerative lesions of the bowel. Acute pancreatitis has been reported, as have rare, but potentially fatal, cases of hepatitis. The most frequent CNS effect is severe frontal headache. Dizziness, vertigo, light-headedness, and mental confusion may occur. Seizures have been reported, as have severe depression, psychosis, hallucinations, and suicide. Caution is advised when administering indomethacin to elderly patients or to those with underlying epilepsy, psychiatric disorders, or Parkinson disease because they are at greater risk for the development of serious CNS adverse effects. Hematopoietic reactions include neutropenia, thrombocytopenia, and rarely aplastic anemia.

The total plasma concentration of indomethacin plus its inactive metabolites is increased by concurrent administration of probenecid. Indomethacin antagonizes the natriuretic and antihypertensive effects of furosemide and thiazide diuretics and blunts the antihypertensive effect of β receptor antagonists, AT_1-receptor antagonists, and ACE inhibitors.

Sulindac

Sulindac is a congener of indomethacin. Sulindac is a prodrug whose anti-inflammatory activity resides in its sulfide metabolite, which is more than 500 times more potent than sulindac as an inhibitor of COX but less than half as potent as indomethacin (see Figure 38–1). ADME data are summarized in Table 38–2. Sulindac is used for the treatment of rheumatoid arthritis, osteoarthritis, ankylosing spondylitis, painful shoulder, and gouty arthritis. Its analgesic and anti-inflammatory effects are comparable to those achieved with aspirin. The most common dosage for adults is 150–200 mg twice a day. Although the incidence of toxicity is lower than with indomethacin, adverse reactions to sulindac are common. The typical NSAID GI side effects are seen in nearly 20% of patients. CNS side effects as described for indomethacin are seen in 10% or fewer of patients. Rash occurs in (3%–9%) of patients, and pruritus occurs in 1%–3% of patients. Transient elevations of hepatic transaminases in plasma are less common. The same precautions that apply to other NSAIDs regarding patients at risk for GI toxicity, cardiovascular risk, and renal impairment also apply to sulindac.

Etodolac

Etodolac is an acetic acid derivative with some degree of COX-2 selectivity (see Table 38–2, Figure 38–1). A single oral dose (200–400 mg) of etodolac provides postoperative analgesia that lasts for 6–8 h. Etodolac also is effective in the treatment of osteoarthritis, rheumatoid arthritis, and mild-to-moderate pain, and the drug appears to be uricosuric. Sustained-release preparations are available. Etodolac is relatively well tolerated. About 5% of patients who have taken the drug for 1 year or less discontinue treatment because of GI side effects, rashes, and CNS effects.

Tolmetin

Tolmetin is approved for the treatment of osteoarthritis, rheumatoid arthritis, and juvenile rheumatoid arthritis and has been used in the treatment of ankylosing spondylitis. ADME and comparison to aspirin are in Table 38–2. Tolmetin recommended doses for adults (200–600 mg three times/d) are typically given with meals, milk, or antacids to lessen abdominal discomfort. However, peak plasma concentrations and bioavailability are reduced when the drug is taken with food. Side effects occur in 25%–40% of patients who take tolmetin. GI side effects are the most common (~15%), and gastric ulceration has been observed. CNS side effects similar to those seen with indomethacin and aspirin occur, but they are less common and less severe.

Ketorolac

Ketorolac is a potent analgesic but only a moderately effective anti-inflammatory drug. The use of ketorolac is limited to 5 days or less for acute pain and can be administered orally, intravenously, intramuscularly, or intranasally. Typical doses are 30–60 mg (intramuscular), 15–30 mg (intravenous), 10–20 mg (oral), and 31.5 mg (intranasal). Pediatric patients aged between 2 and 16 years may receive a single intramuscular (1 mg/kg up to 30 mg) or intravenous (0.5 mg/kg up to 15 mg) dose of ketorolac for severe acute pain. Ketorolac has a rapid onset of action and a short duration of action (see Table 38–2). It is widely used in postoperative patients, but it should not be used for routine obstetric analgesia. Topical (ophthalmic) ketorolac is approved for the treatment of seasonal allergic conjunctivitis and postoperative ocular inflammation. Ketorolac in a fixed-dose combination with phenylephrine is indicated as an irrigation during cataract or intraocular lens replacement surgery to maintain pupil size, prevent miosis, and reduce postoperative pain. Side effects of systemic ketorolac include somnolence (6%), dizziness (7%), headache (17%), GI pain (13%), dyspepsia (12%), nausea (12%), and pain at the site of injection (2%). Serious adverse GI, renal, bleeding, and hypersensitivity reactions to ketorolac may occur. Patients receiving greater than recommended doses or concomitant NSAID therapy, and the elderly, appear to be particularly at risk.

Nabumetone

Nabumetone is the prodrug of 6-methoxy-2-naphthylacetic acid. Nabumetone is approved for the treatment of rheumatoid arthritis and osteoarthritis. Its comparative pharmacokinetic properties are summarized in Table 38–2. Nabumetone is associated with crampy lower abdominal pain (12%) and diarrhea (14%). Other side effects include rash (3%–9%); headache (3%–9%); dizziness (3%–9%); heartburn, tinnitus, and pruritus (3%–9%).

Propionic Acid Derivatives

The propionic acid derivatives *ibuprofen, naproxen, flurbiprofen, fenoprofen, ketoprofen,* and *oxaprozin* are available in the U.S. (see Table 38–3). Ibuprofen is the most commonly used NSAID in the U.S. and is available with or without a prescription. Naproxen, also available with or without a prescription, has a longer but variable $t_{1/2}$. Oxaprozin also has a long $t_{1/2}$ and may be given once daily.

Mechanism of Action

Propionic acid derivatives are nonselective COX inhibitors with the effects and side effects common to other NSAIDs. Some of the propionic acid derivatives, particularly naproxen, have inhibitory effects on leukocyte function, and some evidence suggests that naproxen may have slightly better efficacy with regard to analgesia and relief of morning stiffness.

This suggestion of benefit accords with the longer $t_{1/2}$ of naproxen in comparison to other propionic acid derivatives.

Therapeutic Uses

Propionic acid derivatives are approved for use in the symptomatic treatment of rheumatoid arthritis, juvenile arthritis, and osteoarthritis. Some also are approved for pain, ankylosing spondylitis, acute gouty arthritis, tendinitis, bursitis, headache, postoperative dental pain and swelling, and primary dysmenorrhea. These agents may be comparable in efficacy to aspirin for the control of the signs and symptoms of rheumatoid arthritis and osteoarthritis.

Drug Interactions

Ibuprofen and naproxen have been shown to interfere with the antiplatelet effects of aspirin (Catella-Lawson et al., 2001; Li et al., 2014). Propionic acid derivatives have not been shown to alter the pharmacokinetics of the oral hypoglycemic drugs or warfarin. Refer to the full product labeling for a comprehensive listing of other drug interactions.

Ibuprofen

ADME. Table 38–3 summarizes the comparative pharmacokinetics of ibuprofen. Ibuprofen is absorbed rapidly, bound avidly to protein, and undergoes hepatic metabolism (90% is metabolized to hydroxylate or carboxylate derivatives) and renal excretion of metabolites. The $t_{1/2}$ is about 2 h. Slow equilibration with the synovial space means that its antiarthritic effects may persist after plasma levels decline. In experimental animals, ibuprofen and its metabolites readily cross the placenta.

Therapeutic Uses. Ibuprofen is supplied as tablets, chewable tablets, capsules, caplets, and gelcaps containing 50–600 mg; as oral drops; and as an oral suspension. An injectable formulation of ibuprofen is approved to close patent ductus arteriosus in premature infants. Solid oral dosage forms containing 200 mg or less are available without a prescription. Ibuprofen is licensed for marketing alone and in fixed-dose combinations with antihistamines, decongestants, famotidine, oxycodone, and hydrocodone. It is short acting, with a $t_{1/2}$ of about 2 h. The usual dose for mild-to-moderate pain is 400 mg every 4–6 h as needed.

Adverse Effects. Ibuprofen is better tolerated than aspirin and indomethacin and has been used in patients with a history of GI intolerance to other NSAIDs. Nevertheless, 5%–15% of patients experience GI side effects. Less-frequent adverse effects of ibuprofen include rashes (3%–9%), thrombocytopenia (<1%), headache (1%–3%), dizziness (3%–9%), blurred vision (<1%), and, in a few cases, toxic amblyopia (<1%), fluid retention (1%–3%), and edema (1%–3%). Patients who develop ocular disturbances should discontinue the use of ibuprofen and have an ophthalmic evaluation. Ibuprofen can be used occasionally by pregnant women; however, the concerns apply regarding third-trimester effects, including delay of parturition. Excretion into breast milk is thought to be minimal, so ibuprofen also can be used with caution by women who are breastfeeding.

Naproxen

Naproxen is supplied as tablets, delayed-release tablets, extended-release tablets, gelcaps, and caplets containing 200–500 mg of naproxen or naproxen sodium and as an oral suspension and suppositories. Solid oral dosage forms containing 200 mg or less are available without a prescription. Naproxen is licensed for marketing alone and in fixed-dose combinations with pseudoephedrine, diphenhydramine, esomeprazole, and sumatriptan; it is copackaged with lansoprazole. Naproxen is indicated for juvenile and rheumatoid arthritis, osteoarthritis, ankylosing spondylitis, pain, primary dysmenorrhea, tendonitis, bursitis, and acute gout.

ADME. Naproxen is absorbed fully after oral administration. Naproxen also is absorbed rectally but more slowly than after oral administration. Naproxen is almost completely (99%) bound to plasma proteins after normal therapeutic doses. The $t_{1/2}$ of naproxen in plasma is variable, 9 to 25 h. Age plays a role in the variability of the $t_{1/2}$ because of the age-related decline in renal function (and consequently longer $t_{1/2}$) (see Table 38–3). Low doses should be prescribed in the elderly. Naproxen is extensively metabolized in the liver. About 30% of the drug undergoes 6-desmethylation, and most of this metabolite, as well as naproxen

TABLE 38–3 ■ COMPARISON OF REPRESENTATIVE NSAIDS: FENAMATES AND PROPIONIC ACID DERIVATIVES

CLASS/DRUG	PHARMACOKINETICS	DOSING	COMMENTS	COMPARED TO ASPIRIN
Fenamates				
Mefenamic acid	Peak C_p, 2–4 h Protein binding, >90% Metabolism, CYP2C9 oxidation; glucuronidation of parent drug and metabolites $t_{1/2}$, 2–4 h	500 mg load, then 250 mg every 6 h	Therapy usually should not exceed 7 days or 2–3 days (dysmenorrhea); 15% elevated liver enzymes; excreted in breast milk	Efficacy similar
Meclofenamate	Peak C_p, 0.5–2 h; 3–4 h (with food) Protein binding, 99% Metabolism, Oxidation to 3–OH (~20% activity of parent) $t_{1/2}$, 0.8–2.1 h (parent); 0.5–4 h (active metabolite)	50–100 mg 4–6 times/d (maximum 400 mg/d)	Side effects: CNS, GI, and rash (all > 10%); administration with food ↓ rate/extent of absorption	Efficacy similar
Propionic acid derivatives				
Ibuprofen	Peak C_p, 2 h (tablets) , 1 h (chewable tablets), 0.75 h (liquid) Protein binding, 99% Metabolites, CYP2C9 oxidation to 2- and 3-hydroxylates; conjugation to acyl glucuronides $t_{1/2}$, 2–4 h (adults); 23–75 h (premature infants); 0.9–2.3 h (children)	200–800 mg 3–6 times/d with food (maximum 3.2 g/d); Canadian and U.S. pediatric max 2.4 g/d Children: 4–10 mg/kg/dose, 3–4 times/d	10%–15% discontinue; may increase risk of aseptic meningitis; excreted in breast milk Racemate: 60% of R-enantiomer converts to S-ibuprofen	Equipotent
Naproxen	Peak C_p, 2–4 h (base tabs); 1–4 h (liquid); 1–2 h (sodium salt); 4–12 h (delayed-release tabs) Protein binding, 99% (↑ free fraction in elderly) Metabolism, CYPs 2C9, 1A2, 2C8 oxidation to 6-O-desmethyl and other metabolites $t_{1/2}$, 9–25 h	250 mg 3–4 times/d; 250–550 mg 2 times/d; 750–1000 mg daily (extended release) Children: 5 mg/kg 2 times/d (max 15 mg/kg/d)	Peak anti-inflammatory effects after 2–4 weeks; ↑ free fraction and ↓ excretion ⇒ ↑ risk of toxicity in elderly; may increase risk of aseptic meningitis; excreted in breast milk; variably prolonged $t_{1/2}$ may afford cardioprotection in some individuals	Usually better tolerated
Fenoprofen	Peak C_p, 2 h Protein binding, 99% Metabolites, 4-OH metabolite; glucuronide conjugates $t_{1/2}$, 2.5–3 h	200 mg 4–6 times/d or 300–600 mg 3–4 times/d (max 3.2 g/d)	Peak anti-inflammatory effects after 2–3 weeks; 15% experience side effects; few discontinue use; excreted in breast milk	Generally better tolerated
Ketoprofen	Peak C_p, 1.2 h; 6.8 h (extended-release) Protein binding, 99% Metabolites, Glucuronide conjugates; enterohepatic recirculation? $t_{1/2}$, 0.9–3.3 h	25–50 mg 3–4 times/d; 75 mg 3 times/d; 200 mg daily (extended release); max 300 mg/d Anti–inflammatory, 50–75 mg, 3–4/d	30% develop side effects (usually GI, usually mild); ~13% liver function abnormalities; unbound fraction, systemic exposure, and $t_{1/2}$ ↑ with age in elderly; excreted in breast milk	Generally better tolerated; biological efficacy > plasma $t_{1/2}$
Flurbiprofen	Peak C_p, ~2 h Protein binding, 99% Metabolism, CYP2C9 oxidation, UGTB7 glucuronidation of parent and 4′-OH metabolite $t_{1/2}$, 7.5 h	200–300 mg/d in 2–4 divided doses (maximum 100 mg/dose)	Racemate; excreted in breast milk; available for ophthalmic use	Generally better tolerated

(Continued)

TABLE 38–3 ■ COMPARISON OF REPRESENTATIVE NSAIDS: FENAMATES AND PROPIONIC ACID DERIVATIVES (*CONTINUED*)

CLASS/DRUG	PHARMACOKINETICS	DOSING	COMMENTS	COMPARED TO ASPIRIN
Oxaprozin	Peak C_p, 2.4–3 h Protein binding, 99% Metabolism, 65% oxidates, 35% glucuronides $t_{1/2}$, 41–55 h	600–1200 mg daily (maximum 1800 mg); children > 21 kg: 600–1200 mg daily based on weight (maximum 1200 mg)	Slow onset, not indicated for fever or acute pain; dose in elderly adjusted on the basis of weight; expected to be excreted in breast milk	Generally better tolerated

Time to peak plasma drug concentration C_p is after a single dose. In general, food delays absorption but does not decrease peak concentration. The majority of NSAIDs undergo hepatic metabolism, and the metabolites are excreted in the urine. Major metabolites or disposal pathways are listed. Typical $t_{1/2}$ is listed for therapeutic doses; if $t_{1/2}$ is much different with the toxic dose, this is also given. Typical adult oral doses are listed unless otherwise noted. Refer to the current product labeling for complete prescribing information, including current labeled pediatric indications.

itself, is excreted as the glucuronide or other conjugates. Metabolites of naproxen are excreted almost entirely in the urine. Naproxen crosses the placenta and appears in the milk of lactating women at about 1% of the maternal plasma concentration.

Adverse Effects. Although the best available data were consistent with the suggestion that naproxen is an NSAID that is not associated with an increase in myocardial infarction rate (Coxib and Traditional NSAID Trialists' Collaboration et al., 2013), the FDA in 2015, based on the advisory committee recommendations, has issued a warning that NSAIDs can cause heart attacks and strokes, and that there is inconclusive evidence regarding whether the particular risk of any NSAID is definitively higher or lower than another NSAID (https://www.fda.gov/Drugs/DrugSafety/ucm451800.htm).

About 1%–10% of patients taking naproxen experience GI adverse effects that include heartburn, abdominal pain, constipation, diarrhea, nausea, dyspepsia, and stomatitis. Adverse effects with naproxen occur at approximately the same frequency as with indomethacin and other NSAIDs (see Table 38–1). CNS side effects include drowsiness (3%–9%), headache (3%–9%), dizziness (≤9%), vertigo (<3%), and depression (<1%). Other common reactions include pruritus (3%–9%) and diaphoresis (<3%). Rare instances of jaundice, impairment of renal function, angioedema, thrombocytopenia, and agranulocytosis have been reported.

Fenamates

The fenamates (anthranilic acids) include *mefenamic acid*, *meclofenamate*, and *flufenamic acid*. The pharmacological properties of the fenamates are those of typical NSAIDs, and therapeutically, they have no advantages over others in the class (see Table 38–3). Mefenamic acid and meclofenamate sodium are used in the short-term treatment of pain in soft-tissue injuries, dysmenorrhea, and rheumatoid and osteoarthritis. These drugs are not recommended for use in children or pregnant women. Roughly 5% of patients develop a reversible elevation of hepatic transaminases. Diarrhea, which may be severe and associated with steatorrhea and inflammation of the bowel, also is relatively common. Autoimmune hemolytic anemia is a potentially serious but rare side effect.

Enolic Acids (Oxicams)

The oxicam derivative *piroxicam* is the nonselective COX inhibitor with the longest $t_{1/2}$. *Meloxicam* shows modest COX-2 selectivity comparable to celecoxib (see Figure 38–1) and was approved as a COX-2–selective NSAID in some countries. These agents are similar in efficacy to aspirin, indomethacin, or naproxen for the long-term treatment of rheumatoid arthritis or osteoarthritis. The main advantage suggested for these compounds is their long $t_{1/2}$, which permits once-a-day dosing (see comparative pharmacokinetic and dosing data in Table 38–4).

Piroxicam

Piroxicam may inhibit activation of neutrophils, apparently independently of its ability to inhibit COX; hence, additional modes of anti-inflammatory action have been proposed, including inhibition of proteoglycanase and collagenase in cartilage.

Piroxicam is approved for the treatment of rheumatoid arthritis and osteoarthritis. Due to its slow onset of action and delayed attainment of steady state, it is less suited for acute analgesia but has been used to treat acute gout.

ADME. The pharmacokinetics of piroxicam are described in Table 38–4. The usual daily dose is 20 mg. Piroxicam is absorbed completely after oral administration and undergoes enterohepatic recirculation. Estimates of the $t_{1/2}$ in plasma have been variable; the average is about 50 h. Steady-state blood levels are reached in 7–12 days. Less than 5% of the drug is excreted into the urine unchanged. The major metabolic transformation in humans is hydroxylation of the pyridyl ring (predominantly by an isozyme of the CYP2C subfamily), and this inactive metabolite and its glucuronide conjugate account for about 60% of the drug excreted in the urine and feces.

Adverse Effects. Approximately 20% of patients experience side effects with piroxicam, and about 5% of patients discontinue use because of these effects. Piroxicam may be associated with more GI and serious skin reactions than other nonselective NSAIDs. In 2007, the European Medicines Agency reviewed the safety of orally administered piroxicam and concluded that its benefits outweigh its risks, but advised it should no longer considered a first-line agent or be used for the treatment of acute (short-term) pain and inflammation.

Meloxicam

Meloxicam is approved for use in osteoarthritis, rheumatoid arthritis, and juvenile rheumatoid arthritis. The recommended adult dose of meloxicam is 7.5–15 mg once daily. Meloxicam demonstrates some COX-2 selectivity (see Figure 38–1). There is significantly less gastric injury compared to piroxicam (20 mg/d) in subjects treated with 7.5 mg/d of meloxicam, but the advantage is lost with a dosage of 15 mg/d (Patoia et al., 1996).

Purpose-Developed COX-2 Selective NSAIDs

Selective inhibitors of COX-2 are molecules with side chains that fit within its hydrophobic pocket but are too large to block COX-1 with equally high affinity. Celecoxib is the only purposefully developed COX-2 inhibitor still approved in the U.S. (see its clinical pharmacokinetic properties and precautions in Table 38–4). As mentioned, other, older compounds (diclofenac, etodolac, meloxicam, nimesulide) have been retrospectively found to have a certain degree of selectivity for COX-2 (see Figure 38–1). Etoricoxib is approved in several countries, but restricted in its indications; rofecoxib, valdecoxib, and lumiracoxib were withdrawn worldwide because of the cardiovascular complications caused by suppression of cardioprotective COX-2–derived PGs, especially PGI_2, and the unrestrained effects of endogenous stimuli, such as platelet COX-1–derived TxA_2, on platelet activation, vascular proliferation and remodeling, hypertension, and atherogenesis. COX-2–selective NSAIDs should be avoided in patients prone to cardiovascular or cerebrovascular disease. While the purposefully developed COX-2 inhibitors have generally been shown to reduce severe GI complications when compared to isoform nonselective compounds, none of the COX-2–selective NSAIDs has established superior efficacy.

TABLE 38–4 ■ REPRESENTATIVE NSAIDS: ENOLIC ACID DERIVATIVES AND COXIBS

CLASS/DRUG	PHARMACOKINETICS	DOSING	COMMENTS	COMPARED TO ASPIRIN
Enolic acid derivatives				
Piroxicam	Peak C_p, 3–5 h Protein binding, 99% Metabolites, CYP2C9 hydroxylation, conjugation, *N*-demethylation $t_{1/2}$, ~50 h	20 mg daily	20% side effects; 5% discontinue; slow onset, not indicated for fever or acute pain; excreted in breast milk	Equipotent with lower incidence of minor GI effects
Meloxicam	Peak C_p, 4–5 h (and 12–14 h due to biliary recycling) Protein binding, 99% Metabolism, Hydroxylation $t_{1/2}$, 15–20 h	7.5 mg daily (maximum 15 mg/d); Children ≥ 2: lowest effective dose, 0.125 mg/kg daily (maximum 7.5 mg daily)	Some COX-2 selectivity, especially at lower doses; elderly females have higher systemic exposure and peak plasma concentrations than men and young women; excretion in breast milk unknown	—
Diaryl heterocyclic nsaids (*COX-2 selective*)				
			Evidence for cardiovascular adverse events	Decrease in GI side effects and in platelet effects
Celecoxib	Peak C_p, ~3 h Protein binding, 97% Metabolism, CYPs 2C9 (major) and 3A4 (minor), glucuronide $t_{1/2}$, 11.2 h	100–200 mg 1–2 times/d; 400 mg followed by 200 mg if needed on first day (acute pain); maximum, 800 mg/d. Children > 2 y: 50 mg (10–25 kg) or 100 mg (>25 kg) 2 times/d	CYP2D6 and CYP2D8 inhibitor; Adverse effects: GI complaints (5%); aseptic meningitis and methemoglobinemia have been reported; disseminated intravascular coagulation risk in pediatric patients; 40% higher systemic exposure in blacks and elderly females; excreted in breast milk	Usually better tolerated; does not usually prolong bleeding time

Time to peak plasma drug concentration C_p is after a single dose. In general, food delays absorption but does not decrease peak concentration. The majority of NSAIDs undergo hepatic metabolism, and the metabolites are excreted in the urine. Major metabolites or disposal pathways are listed. Typical $t_{1/2}$ is listed for therapeutic doses; if $t_{1/2}$ is much different with the toxic dose, this is also given. Typical adult oral doses are listed unless otherwise noted. Refer to the current product labeling for complete prescribing information, including current labeled pediatric indications.

Celecoxib

ADME. The bioavailability of oral celecoxib is not known; peak plasma levels occur at 2–4 h after administration. The elderly (≥65 years of age) may have up to 2-fold higher peak concentrations and AUC values than younger patients (≤55 years of age). Celecoxib is bound extensively to plasma proteins. Most is excreted as carboxylic acid and glucuronide metabolites in the urine and feces. The elimination $t_{1/2}$ is about 11 h. The drug commonly is given once or twice daily during chronic treatment. Plasma concentrations are increased in patients with mild and moderate hepatic impairment, requiring reduction in dose. Celecoxib is metabolized predominantly by CYP2C9 and inhibits CYP2D6. Clinical vigilance is necessary during coadministration of drugs that are known to inhibit CYP2C9 and drugs that are metabolized by CYP2D6.

Therapeutic Uses. Celecoxib is used for the management of acute pain for the treatment of osteoarthritis, rheumatoid arthritis, juvenile rheumatoid arthritis, ankylosing spondylitis, and primary dysmenorrhea. The recommended dose for treating osteoarthritis is 200 mg/d as a single dose or divided as two doses. In the treatment of rheumatoid arthritis, the recommended dose is 100–200 mg twice daily. Due to cardiovascular hazard, physicians are advised to use the lowest possible dose for the shortest possible duration.

Adverse Effects. Celecoxib confers a risk of myocardial infarction and stroke, and this appears to relate to dose and the underlying risk of cardiovascular disease. Effects attributed to inhibition of PG production in the kidney—hypertension and edema—occur with nonselective COX inhibitors and also with celecoxib. Selective COX-2 inhibitors lose their GI advantage over other NSAIDs alone when used in conjunction with aspirin. Chronic use of celecoxib may decrease bone mineral density, particularly in older male patients. There is some suggestion that celecoxib may slow fracture healing and tendon-to-bone healing.

Etoricoxib

Etoricoxib is a COX-2–selective inhibitor with selectivity second only to that of lumiracoxib (see Figure 38–1). Etoricoxib is incompletely (~80%) absorbed and has a long $t_{1/2}$ of 20–26 h. It is extensively metabolized before excretion. Patients with hepatic impairment are prone to drug accumulation. Renal insufficiency does not affect drug clearance. Etoricoxib is used for symptomatic relief in the treatment of osteoarthritis, rheumatoid arthritis, and acute gouty arthritis, as well as for the short-term treatment of musculoskeletal pain, postoperative pain, and primary dysmenorrhea. The drug is associated with the increased risk of heart attack and stroke. Etoricoxib is not available in the U.S.

Disease-Modifying Antirheumatic Drugs

Rheumatoid arthritis is an autoimmune disease that affects about 1% of the population. The pharmacological management of rheumatoid arthritis includes symptomatic relief through the use of NSAIDs. However, although they have anti-inflammatory effects, NSAIDs have minimal, if any, effect on progression of joint deformity. Disease-modifying antirheumatic drugs (DMARDs), on the other hand, reduce the disease activity of rheumatoid arthritis and retard the progression of arthritic tissue destruction. DMARDs include a diverse group of small-molecule nonbiological and biological agents (mainly antibodies or binding proteins), as summarized in Table 38–5.

Biological DMARDs remain reserved for patients with persistent moderate or high disease activity and indicators of poor prognosis. Therapy is tailored to the individual patient, and the use of these agents must be weighed against their potentially serious adverse effects. The combination of NSAIDs with these agents is common.

TABLE 38–5 ■ DISEASE-MODIFYING ANTIRHEUMATIC DRUGS

DRUG	CLASS OR ACTION	CHAPTER NUMBER
Small molecules		
Methotrexate	Antifolate	66
Leflunomide	Pyrimidine synthase inhibitor	66
Hydroxychloroquine	Antimalarial	53
Minocycline	5-Lipoxygenase inhibitor, tetracycline antibiotic	37, 59
Sulfasalazine	Salicylate	38, 51
Azathioprine	Purine synthase inhibitor	66
Cyclosporine	Calcineurin inhibitor	35
Cyclophosphamide	Alkylating agent	66
Penicillamine	Chelating agent	71
Auranofin	Gold compound	71
Biologicals		
Adalimumab	Ab, TNF-α antagonist	
Golimumab	Ab, TNF-α antagonist	
Etanercept	Ab, TNF-α antagonist	34, 35
Infliximab	IgG-TNF receptor fusion protein (anti-TNF)	
Certolizumab	Fab fragment toward TNF-α	
Abatacept	T-cell costimulation inhibitor (binds B7 protein on antigen-presenting cell)	34, 35
Rituximab	Ab toward CD20 (cytotoxic toward B cells)	67
Anakinra	IL-1 receptor antagonist	35, 67
Tocilizumab	IL-6 receptor antagonist	35, 67
Tofacitinib	Janus kinase inhibitor	67

Pharmacotherapy of Gout

Gout results from the precipitation of urate crystals in the tissues and the subsequent inflammatory response. Acute gout usually causes painful distal monoarthritis and can cause joint destruction, subcutaneous deposits (tophi), and renal calculi and damage. Gout affects 3% of the adult population of Western countries.

The pathophysiology of gout is incompletely understood. Hyperuricemia, while a prerequisite, does not inevitably lead to gout. Uric acid, the end product of purine metabolism, is relatively insoluble compared to its hypoxanthine and xanthine precursors, and normal serum urate levels (~5 mg/dL, or 0.3 mM) approach the limit of solubility. In most patients with gout, hyperuricemia arises from underexcretion rather than overproduction of urate. Mutations of one of the renal URATs, URAT-1, are associated with hypouricemia. Urate tends to crystallize as monosodium urate in colder or more acidic conditions. Monosodium urate crystals activate monocytes/macrophages via the toll-like receptor pathway mounting an innate immune response. This results in the activation of the cryopyrin inflammasome, the secretion of cytokines, including IL-1β and TNF-α, endothelial activation, and attraction of neutrophils to the site of inflammation. Neutrophils secrete inflammatory mediators that lower the local pH and lead to further urate precipitation. The aims of treatment are to:

- decrease the symptoms of an acute attack;
- decrease the risk of recurrent attacks; and
- lower serum urate levels.

The following substances are available for these purposes:

- Drugs that relieve inflammation and pain (NSAIDs, colchicine, glucocorticoids)
- Drugs that prevent inflammatory responses to crystals (colchicine and NSAIDs)
- Drugs that act by inhibition of urate formation (e.g., allopurinol, febuxostat) or to augment urate excretion (probenecid)

The NSAIDs have been discussed previously. Glucocorticoids are discussed in Chapter 46. This section focuses on *colchicine, allopurinol, febuxostat, pegloticase, rasuricase,* and the uricosuric agents *probenecid* and *benzbromarone*. Some other drugs used off label to reduce uric acid levels or treat gout include losartan, fenofibrate, and canakinumab; in 2011, the FDA denied a license application for canakinumab, citing an unfavorable risk-versus-benefit safety profile.

Colchicine

Colchicine is one of the oldest available therapies for acute gout. Plant extracts containing colchicine were used for joint pain in the 6th century. Colchicine is considered second-line therapy because it has a narrow therapeutic window and a high rate of side effects, particularly at higher doses.

Mechanism of Action

Colchicine exerts a variety of pharmacological effects, but how these relate to its activity in gout is partially understood (Leung et al., 2015). It has antimitotic effects, arresting cell division in G_1 by interfering with microtubule and spindle formation (an effect shared with vinca alkaloids). This effect is greatest on cells with rapid turnover (e.g., neutrophils, GI epithelium). Depolymerization of microtubules by colchicine reduces neutrophil recruitment to inflamed tissue and neutrophil adhesion. Colchicine may alter neutrophil motility and decreases the secretion of chemotactic factors and superoxide anions by activated neutrophils. Colchicine limits monosodium urate crystal–induced NALP3 inflammasome activation and subsequent formation of IL-1β and IL-18. This mechanism may explain its therapeutic activity in familial Mediterranean fever and other inflammatory diseases. Colchicine inhibits the release of histamine-containing granules from mast cells, the secretion of insulin from pancreatic β cells, and the movement of melanin granules in melanophores.

Colchicine also exhibits a variety of other pharmacological effects. It lowers body temperature, increases the sensitivity to central depressants, depresses the respiratory center, enhances the response to sympathomimetic agents, constricts blood vessels, and induces hypertension by central vasomotor stimulation. It enhances GI activity by neurogenic stimulation, but depresses it by a direct effect, and alters neuromuscular function.

ADME

Absorption of oral colchicine is rapid but variable. Peak plasma concentrations occur 0.5–2 h after dosing. Food does not affect the rate or extent of colchicine absorption. In plasma, 39% of colchicine is protein bound, primarily to albumin. The formation of colchicine-tubulin complexes in many tissues contributes to its large volume of distribution. There is significant enterohepatic circulation. The exact metabolism of colchicine in humans is unknown, but in vitro studies indicated that it may undergo oxidative demethylation by CYP3A4; glucuronidation may also be involved. In healthy volunteers, 40%–65% of the total absorbed oral dose of colchicine is recovered unchanged in the urine. The kidney, liver, and spleen also contain high concentrations of colchicine, but it apparently is largely excluded from heart, skeletal muscle, and brain. Colchicine is a substrate of P-glycoprotein efflux. The plasma $t_{1/2}$ of colchicine is about 31 h. The drug is contraindicated in patients with hepatic or renal impairment requiring concomitant therapy with CYP3A4 or P-glycoprotein inhibitors. Colchicine is not removed by hemodialysis.

Therapeutic Uses

The dosing regimen for colchicine must be individualized on the basis of age, renal and hepatic function, concomitant use of other medications, and disease severity. A minimum of 3 days, but preferably 7–14 days, should elapse between courses of gout treatment with colchicine to avoid cumulative toxicity. Patients with hepatic or renal disease and dialysis patients should receive reduced doses or less-frequent therapy. For elderly patients, adjust the dose for renal function. For those with cardiac, renal, hepatic, or GI disease, NSAIDs or glucocorticoids may be preferred.

Acute Gout. Colchicine dramatically relieves acute attacks of gout. It is effective in roughly two-thirds of patients if given within 24 h of attack onset. Pain, swelling, and redness abate within 12 h and are completely gone within 48–72 h. The regimen approved for adults recommends a total of two doses taken 1 h apart: 1.2 mg (2 tablets) at the first sign of a gout flare followed by 0.6 mg (1 tablet) 1 h later. Patients with severe renal or hepatic dysfunction and patients receiving dialysis should not receive repeat courses of therapy more frequently than every 2 weeks.

Prevention of Acute Gout. Colchicine is used in the prevention of recurrent gout, particularly in the early stages of antihyperuricemic therapy. The typical dose for prophylaxis in patients with normal renal and hepatic function is 0.6 mg taken orally 3 or 4 days/week for patients who have less than 1 attack per year, 0.6 mg daily for patients who have more than 1 attack per year, and 0.6 mg up to two times daily for patients who have severe attacks.

Adverse Effects

Exposure of the GI tract to large amounts of colchicine and its metabolites via enterohepatic circulation and the rapid rate of turnover of the GI mucosa may explain why the GI tract is particularly susceptible to colchicine toxicity. Nausea, vomiting, diarrhea, and abdominal pain are the most common untoward effects and the earliest signs of impending colchicine toxicity. Drug administration should be discontinued as soon as these symptoms occur. There is a latent period, which is not altered by dose, of several hours or more between the administration of the drug and the onset of symptoms. A dosing study demonstrated that one dose initially and a single additional dose after 1 h was much less toxic than the traditional hourly dosing regimen for acute gout flares. Acute intoxication causes hemorrhagic gastropathy.

Other serious side effects of colchicine therapy include myelosuppression, leukopenia, granulocytopenia, thrombopenia, aplastic anemia, and rhabdomyolysis. Life-threatening toxicities are associated with administration of concomitant therapy with P-glycoprotein or CYP3A4 inhibitors. The FDA suspended the U.S. marketing of all injectable dosage forms of colchicine in 2008. Colchicine is marketed in a fixed-dose combination with probenecid for the management of frequent recurrent gout attacks.

Allopurinol

History

Allopurinol initially was synthesized as a candidate antineoplastic agent but was found to lack antineoplastic activity. Subsequent testing showed it to be an inhibitor of XO that was useful clinically for the treatment of gout.

Allopurinol inhibits XO and prevents the synthesis of urate from hypoxanthine and xanthine. Allopurinol is used to treat hyperuricemia in patients with gout and to prevent it in those with hematological malignancies about to undergo chemotherapy (acute tumor lysis syndrome). Even though underexcretion rather than overproduction is the underlying defect in most gout patients, allopurinol remains effective therapy.

Allopurinol is an analogue of hypoxanthine. Its active metabolite, oxypurinol, is an analogue of xanthine.

ALLOPURINOL   XANTHINE   URIC ACID

Mechanism of Action

Both allopurinol and its primary metabolite, oxypurinol (alloxanthine), reduce urate production by inhibiting XO, which converts xanthine to uric acid. Allopurinol competitively inhibits XO at low concentrations and is a noncompetitive inhibitor at high concentrations. Allopurinol also is a substrate for XO; the product of this reaction, oxypurinol, also is a noncompetitive inhibitor of the enzyme. The formation of oxypurinol, together with its long persistence in tissues, is responsible for much of the pharmacological activity of allopurinol.

In the absence of allopurinol, the dominant urinary purine is uric acid. During allopurinol treatment, the urinary purines include hypoxanthine, xanthine, and uric acid. Because each has its independent solubility, the concentration of uric acid in plasma is reduced and purine excretion is increased, without exposing the urinary tract to an excessive load of uric acid. Despite their increased concentrations during allopurinol therapy, hypoxanthine and xanthine are efficiently excreted, and tissue deposition does not occur. There is a small risk of xanthine stones in patients with a very high urate load before allopurinol therapy, which can be minimized by liberal fluid intake and urinary alkalization.

Allopurinol facilitates the dissolution of tophi and prevents the development or progression of chronic gouty arthritis by lowering the uric acid concentration in plasma below the limit of its solubility. The formation of uric acid stones virtually disappears with therapy, which prevents the development of nephropathy. Once significant renal injury has occurred, allopurinol cannot restore renal function but may delay disease progression. The incidence of acute attacks of gouty arthritis may increase during the early months of allopurinol therapy as a consequence of mobilization of tissue stores of uric acid. Coadministration of colchicine helps suppress such acute attacks. In some patients, the allopurinol-induced increase in excretion of oxypurines is less than the reduction in uric acid excretion; this disparity primarily is a result of reutilization of oxypurines and feedback inhibition of de novo purine biosynthesis.

ADME

Allopurinol is absorbed relatively rapidly after oral ingestion, and peak plasma concentrations are reached within 60–90 min. About 20% is excreted in the feces in 48–72 h, presumably as unabsorbed drug, and 10%–30% is excreted unchanged in the urine. The remainder undergoes metabolism, mostly to oxypurinol. Oxypurinol is excreted slowly in the urine by glomerular filtration, counterbalanced by some tubular reabsorption. The plasma $t_{1/2}$ of allopurinol and oxypurinol is about 1–2 h and about 18–30 h (longer in those individuals with renal impairment), respectively. This allows for once-daily dosing and makes allopurinol the most commonly used antihyperuricemic agent. Allopurinol and its active metabolite oxypurinol are distributed in total tissue water, with the exception of brain, where their concentrations are about one-third of those in other tissues. Neither compound is bound to plasma proteins. The plasma concentrations of the two compounds do not correlate well with therapeutic or toxic effects.

Therapeutic Uses

Allopurinol is available for oral and intravenous use. Oral therapy provides effective therapy for primary and secondary gout, hyperuricemia secondary to malignancies, and calcium oxalate calculi. The goal of therapy is to reduce the plasma uric acid concentration to less than 6 mg/dL (<360 μmol/L) and typically less than 5 mg/dL (<297 μmol/L) in patients with tophi to accelerate the clearance of monosodium urate. In the management of gout, it is customary to antecede allopurinol therapy with colchicine and to avoid starting allopurinol during an acute attack. Fluid intake should be sufficient to maintain daily urinary volume greater than 2 L; slightly alkaline urine is preferred. An initial daily dose of 100 mg in patients with estimated glomerular filtration rates greater than 40 mg/min is increased by 100-mg increments at weekly intervals. Most patients can be maintained on 300 mg/d. Patients with reduced glomerular filtration require a lower dose to achieve the targeted uric acid concentration, and their clinical and pharmacological response needs be monitored frequently. Those with hematological malignancies may need up to 800 mg/d beginning 2–3 days before the start of chemotherapy. Daily doses greater than 300 mg should be divided.

The usual daily dose in children with secondary hyperuricemia associated with malignancies is 150–300 mg, depending on age. Allopurinol also is useful in lowering the high plasma concentrations of uric acid in patients with Lesch-Nyhan syndrome (orphan designation) and thereby prevents the complications resulting from hyperuricemia; there is no evidence that it alters the progressive neurological and behavioral abnormalities that are characteristic of the disease. Other orphan uses for allopurinol include Chagas disease and the ex vivo preservation of cadaveric kidneys prior to transplantation.

Adverse Effects

Allopurinol generally is well tolerated. The most common adverse effects are hypersensitivity reactions that may manifest after months or years of therapy. Serious hypersensitivity reactions preclude further use of the drug. The cutaneous reaction caused by allopurinol is predominantly a pruritic, erythematous, or maculopapular eruption, but occasionally the lesion is urticarial or purpuric.

Rarely, toxic epidermal necrolysis or Stevens-Johnson syndrome occurs, which can be fatal. The risk for Stevens-Johnson syndrome is limited primarily to the first 2 months of treatment. Because the rash may precede severe hypersensitivity reactions, patients who develop a rash should discontinue allopurinol. If indicated, desensitization to allopurinol can be carried out starting at 10–25 μg/d, with the drug diluted in oral suspension and doubled every 3–14 days until the desired dose is reached. This is successful in approximately half of patients.

Oxypurinol has orphan drug status and is available for compassionate use in the U.S. for patients intolerant of allopurinol. Fever, malaise, and myalgias also may occur in about 3% of patients, more frequently in those with renal impairment. Transient leukopenia or leukocytosis and eosinophilia are rare reactions that may require cessation of therapy. Hepatomegaly and elevated levels of transaminases in plasma and progressive renal insufficiency also may occur.

Allopurinol is contraindicated in patients who have exhibited serious adverse effects or hypersensitivity reactions to the medication and in nursing mothers and children, except those with malignancy or certain inborn errors of purine metabolism (e.g., Lesch-Nyhan syndrome). Allopurinol generally is used in patients with hyperuricemia posttransplantation. It can be used in conjunction with a uricosuric agent.

Drug Interactions

Allopurinol increases the $t_{1/2}$ of probenecid and enhances its uricosuric effect, while probenecid increases the clearance of oxypurinol, thereby increasing dose requirements of allopurinol. Allopurinol inhibits the enzymatic inactivation of mercaptopurine and its derivative azathioprine by XO. Thus, when allopurinol is used concomitantly with oral mercaptopurine or azathioprine, dosage of the antineoplastic agent must be reduced to 25%–33% of the usual dose (see Chapters 35 and 66). This is of importance when treating gout in the transplant recipient. The risk of bone marrow suppression also is increased when allopurinol is administered with cytotoxic agents that are not metabolized by XO, particularly cyclophosphamide. Allopurinol also may interfere with the hepatic inactivation of other drugs, including warfarin. Although the effect is variable, increased monitoring of prothrombin activity is recommended in patients receiving both medications.

It remains to be established whether the increased incidence of rash in patients receiving concurrent allopurinol and ampicillin should be ascribed to allopurinol or to hyperuricemia. Hypersensitivity reactions have been reported in patients with compromised renal function, especially those who are receiving a combination of allopurinol and a thiazide diuretic. The concomitant administration of allopurinol and theophylline leads to increased accumulation of an active metabolite of theophylline, 1-methylxanthine; the concentration of theophylline in plasma also may be increased (see Chapter 40).

Febuxostat

Febuxostat is an XO inhibitor approved for treatment of hyperuricemia in patients with gout.

Mechanism of Action

Febuxostat is a nonpurine inhibitor of XO. Unlike oxypurinol, the active metabolite of allopurinol, which inhibits the reduced form of XO, febuxostat forms a stable complex with both the reduced and oxidized enzymes and inhibits catalytic function in both states.

ADME

Febuxostat is rapidly absorbed with maximum plasma concentrations at 1–1.5 h postdose. The absolute bioavailability is unknown. Magnesium hydroxide and aluminum hydroxide delay absorption by about 1 h. Food reduces absorption slightly. Febuxostat, $t_{1/2}$ of 5–8 h, is extensively metabolized by both conjugation via UGT enzymes, including UGT1A1, UGT1A3, UGT1A9, and UGT2B7, and oxidation by CYPs 1A2, 2C8, and 2C9 and non-CYP enzymes and has elimination by both hepatic and renal pathways. Mild-to-moderate renal or hepatic impairment does not affect its elimination kinetics relevantly.

Therapeutic Use

Febuxostat is approved for hyperuric patients with gout attacks but is not recommended for treatment of asymptomatic hyperuricemia. It is available in 40- and 80-mg oral tablets. A dose of 40-mg/d febuxostat lowered serum uric acid to similar levels as 300-mg/d allopurinol. More patients reached the target concentration of 6.0 mg/dL (360 μmol/L) on 80-mg/d febuxostat than on 300-mg/d allopurinol. Thus, therapy should be initiated with 40 mg/d and the dose increased if the target serum uric acid concentration is not reached within 2 weeks.

Adverse Events

The most common adverse reactions in clinical studies were liver function abnormalities, nausea, joint pain, and rash. Liver function should be monitored periodically. An increase in gout flares was frequently observed after initiation of therapy, due to reduction in serum uric acid levels resulting in mobilization of urate from tissue deposits. Concurrent prophylactic treatment with an NSAID or colchicine is usually required. There was a higher rate of myocardial infarction and stroke in patients on febuxostat than on allopurinol. Whether there is a causal relationship between the cardiovascular events and febuxostat therapy or whether these were due to chance is not clear. Meanwhile patients should be monitored for cardiovascular complications.

Drug Interactions

Plasma levels of drugs metabolized by XO (e.g., theophylline, mercaptopurine, azathioprine) will increase when administered concurrently with febuxostat. Thus, febuxostat is contraindicated in patients on azathioprine or mercaptopurine; care should be exercised with concomitant administration of theophylline due to a 400-fold increase in the urinary excretion of the 1-methylxanthine metabolite.

Uricase

Pegloticase is a pegylated uricase (urate oxidase) that catalyzes the enzymatic oxidation of uric acid into allantoin, a more soluble and inactive metabolite. The recombinant enzyme, based on the porcine uricase, is administered by infusion. Pegloticase is used for the treatment of severe, treatment-refractory, chronic gout or when use of other urate-lowering therapies is contraindicated.

The drug's efficacy may be hampered by the production of antibodies against the drug. Pegloticase antibodies develop in nearly 90% of people, and high titers are associated with loss of the urate-lowering effect and with an elevated risk for infusion reactions. Anaphylactic reactions, and hemolysis in G6PD-deficient patients, have been associated with the use of pegloticase. Other frequently observed adverse reactions include vomiting, nausea, chest pain, constipation, diarrhea, and erythema, pruritus, and urticaria.

Rasburicase is a recombinant uricase that has been shown to lower urate levels more effectively than allopurinol. It is indicated for the initial management of elevated plasma uric acid levels in pediatric and adult patients with leukemia, lymphoma, and solid tumor malignancies who are receiving anticancer therapy expected to result in tumor lysis and significant hyperuricemia. The experience with rasburicase for treatment of gout is limited because of the formation of activity-limiting antibodies against the drug. Hemolysis in G6PD-deficient patients, methemoglobinemia, acute renal failure, and anaphylaxis have been associated with the use of rasburicase. Other frequently observed adverse reactions include vomiting, fever, nausea, headache, abdominal pain, constipation, diarrhea, and mucositis. Rasburicase causes enzymatic degradation of the uric acid in blood samples, and special handling is required to prevent spuriously low values for plasma uric acid in patients receiving the drug.

Uricosuric Agents

Uricosuric agents increase the excretion of uric acid. These agents are typically reserved for patients who underexcrete uric acid relative to their plasma levels. In humans, urate is filtered, secreted, and reabsorbed by the kidneys. Reabsorption is robust, such that the net amount excreted usually is about 10% of that filtered. Reabsorption is mediated by an OAT family member, URAT-1, which can be inhibited.

Urate is exchanged by URAT-1 for either an organic anion such as lactate or nicotinate or less potently for an inorganic anion such as chloride. Uricosuric drugs such as probenecid, benzbromarone (not available in the U.S.), and losartan compete with urate for the transporter, thereby inhibiting its reabsorption via the urate–anion exchanger system. However, transport is bidirectional, and depending on dosage, a drug may either decrease or increase the excretion of uric acid.

There are two mechanisms by which a drug may nullify the uricosuric action of another. First, the drug may inhibit the secretion of the uricosuric agent, thereby denying it access to its site of action, the luminal aspect of the brush border. Second, the inhibition of urate secretion by one drug may counterbalance the inhibition of urate reabsorption by the other.

Probenecid

Probenecid is a highly lipid-soluble benzoic acid derivative (pK_a 3.4).

PROBENECID

Mechanism of Action. Inhibition of Organic Acid Transport. The actions of probenecid are confined largely to inhibition of the transport of organic acids across epithelial barriers. Probenecid inhibits the reabsorption of uric acid by OATs, principally URAT-1. Uric acid is the only important endogenous compound whose excretion is known to be increased by probenecid. The uricosuric action of probenecid is blunted by the coadministration of salicylates.

Inhibition of Transport of Miscellaneous Substances. Probenecid inhibits the tubular secretion of a number of drugs, such as methotrexate and the active metabolite of clofibrate. It inhibits renal secretion of the inactive glucuronide metabolites of NSAIDs such as naproxen, ketoprofen, and indomethacin and thereby can increase their plasma concentrations. Probenecid inhibits the transport of 5-HIAA and other acidic metabolites of cerebral monoamines from the CSF to the plasma. The transport of drugs such as penicillin G also may be affected, and probenecid is used therapeutically to elevate and prolong plasma β-lactam levels. Probenecid depresses the biliary secretion of certain compounds, including the diagnostic agents indocyanine green and bromosulfophthalein. It also decreases the biliary secretion of rifampin, leading to higher plasma concentrations.

ADME. Probenecid is absorbed completely after oral administration. Peak plasma concentrations are reached in 2–4 h. The $t_{1/2}$ of the drug in plasma is dose dependent and varies from less than 5 to more than 8 h. Between 85% and 95% of the drug is bound to plasma albumin; the 5%–15% of unbound drug is cleared by glomerular filtration and active secretion by the proximal tubule. A small amount of probenecid glucuronide appears in the urine. It also is hydroxylated to metabolites that retain their carboxyl function and have uricosuric activity.

Therapeutic Uses. Probenecid is marketed for oral administration, alone and in combination with colchicine. The starting dose is 250 mg twice daily, increasing over 1–2 weeks to 500–1000 mg twice daily. Probenecid increases urinary urate levels. Liberal fluid intake therefore should be maintained throughout therapy to minimize the risk of renal stones. Probenecid should not be used in gouty patients with nephrolithiasis or with overproduction of uric acid. Concomitant colchicine or NSAIDs are indicated early in the course of therapy to avoid precipitating an attack of gout, which may occur in 20% or fewer of gouty patients treated with probenecid alone. After 6 months, if serum uric acid levels are within normal limits and there have been no gout attacks, the dose of probenecid may be tapered off by 500 mg every 6 months.

Combination With Penicillin. Higher doses of probenecid (1–2 g/d) are used as an adjuvant to prolong the dwell time of penicillin and other β-lactam antibiotics in the body (see Chapter 57).

Adverse Effects. Probenecid is well tolerated. Approximately 2% of patients develop mild GI irritation. The risk is increased at higher doses. It is ineffective in patients with renal insufficiency and should be avoided in those with creatinine clearance of less than 50 mL/min. Hypersensitivity reactions usually are mild and occur in 2%–4% of patients. Substantial overdosage with probenecid results in CNS stimulation, convulsions, and death from respiratory failure.

Benzbromarone

Benzbromarone is a potent uricosuric agent that has been marketed in several countries since 1970. It is a reversible inhibitor of the urate–anion exchanger in the proximal tubule. Hepatotoxicity reported in conjunction with its use has limited its availability. The drug is absorbed readily after oral ingestion; peak plasma levels are achieved in about 4 h. It is metabolized to monobrominated and dehalogenated derivatives, both of which have uricosuric activity, and is excreted primarily in the bile.

As the micronized powder, it is effective in a single daily dose ranging from 25 to 100 mg. It is effective in patients with renal insufficiency and may be prescribed to patients who are either allergic or refractory to other drugs used for the treatment of gout. Preparations that combine allopurinol and benzbromarone are more effective than either drug alone in lowering serum uric acid levels, in spite of the fact that benzbromarone lowers plasma levels of oxypurinol, the active metabolite of allopurinol. The uricosuric action is blunted by aspirin or sulfinpyrazone.

Lesinurad

Lesinurad is FDA approved for combination therapy with an XO inhibitor in treating hyperuricemia.

Mechanism of Action. Lesinurad inhibits the URAT-1 and OAT-4 transporters, thereby reducing renal uric acid reabsorption.

ADME. Lesinurad is rapidly absorbed after oral administration and has bioavailability of about 100%. Lesinurad is largely bound to plasma albumin and other plasma proteins (<98%). The elimination $t_{1/2}$ is about 5 h (clearance ~ 6 L/h). CYP2C9 is the major metabolizing enzyme. Lesinurad (30% unchanged) and its metabolites are excreted in the urine (>60% of dose) and feces. Renal impairment increases exposure, and lesinurid

should not be used when the renal function is severely reduced (estimated creatinine clearance < 45 mL/min).

Therapeutic Uses. Lesinurad (200 mg/d) is marketed for the treatment of gout in patients who have not achieved the target serum uric acid levels with an XO inhibitor alone. It should not be used for the treatment of asymptomatic hyperuricemia or as monotherapy.

Adverse Effects. Lesinurad has been labeled with a black-box warning because of a risk of acute renal failure that is more common when it is used without an XO inhibitor. Increases in blood creatinine levels (1.5- to 2-fold) were observed with a frequency of approximately 4% during combination therapy and 8% during monotherapy. Renal failure occurred in less than 1% of patients during combination therapy and approximately 9% during monotherapy. Similarly, the risk of nephrolithiasis is increased when lesinurad is given alone. Thus, if treatment with the XO inhibitor is interrupted, lesinurid dosing should also be interrupted. Other adverse reactions reported by patients during clinical trials include headache (~5%), influenza-like symptoms (~5%), and gastroesophageal reflux (~3%).

Acknowledgment: Jason D. Morrow, L. Jackson Roberts II, and Anne Burke contributed to this chapter in earlier editions of this book. We have retained some of their text in the current edition.

Drug Facts For Your Personal Formulary: *NSAIDs* (see also Tables 38–1, 38–2, and 38–3)

Drugs	Therapeutic Uses	Clinical Pharmacology and Tips
Salicylates • Used to treat pain, fever, inflammation • Adverse Effects: Primarily GI and CV, salicylate intoxication		
Aspirin	• Vascular indications • Pain/fever • Rheumatoid disease / Rheumatic fever	• Irreversible COX inhibitor ⇒ long-acting inhibition of platelet function at low doses • At higher concentrations, small increments in dose disproportionately ↑ C_p and toxicity • Use in children: limited due to Reye's syndrome association • Reduces the risk of recurrent adenomas in persons with a history of colorectal cancer or adenomas • Prolongs bleeding time for ~ 36 h after a dose
Salsalate	• Arthritis • Rheumatic disorders	• Prodrug of salicylic acid • Not approved in the US
Diflunisal	• Mild to moderate pain • Osteoarthritis/Rheumatoid arthritis	• Salicylic acid derivative • Largely devoid of antipyretic effects • $t_{1/2}$ prolonged with renal impairment
Mesalamine (5-aminosalicylic acid)	• Inflammatory bowel disease	• Oral formulation delivers 5-aminosalicylic acid to lower GI tract; relative bowel specificity reduces side effects • May cause an acute intolerance syndrome (difficult to discern from an exacerbation)
Sulfasalazine	• Rheumatoid arthritis • Inflammatory bowel disease	• Active metabolite 5-aminosalicylic acid (see mesalamine) released by colonic bacteria • With G6PD deficiency: susceptibility to hemolytic anemia
Olsalazine	• Inflammatory bowel disease	• Active metabolite 5-aminosalicylic acid (see mesalamine) is released by colonic bacteria.
Balsalazide	• Inflammatory bowel disease	• Active metabolite, 5-aminosalicylic acid (see mesalamine), is released by colonic bacteria.
Para-Aminophenol Derivative • Only acetaminophen remains on the market		
Acetaminophen	• Pain • Fever	• Weak nonspecific COX inhibitor at common doses • Low anti-inflammatory activity • Little effect on platelets • Overdose results in formation of hepatotoxic metabolite (NAPQI) • Toxicity risk ↑ with liver impairment, ethanol consumption ≥3 drinks/day, or malnutrition

Acetic Acid Derivatives

Indomethacin	• Acute pain • Arthritis, inflammatory conditions • Patent ductus arteriosus	• Potent anti-inflammatory with frequent adverse events (20% discontinue) • High-risk medication in patients ≥ 65 years
Sulindac	• Inflammatory diseases including osteoarthritis, rheumatoid arthritis, acute gouty arthritis, ankylosing spondylitis, acute painful shoulder	• Sulfoxide prodrug
Etodolac	• Pain, osteoarthritis, rheumatoid arthritis, juvenile arthritis	• Some COX-2 selectivity
Tolmetin	• Osteoarthritis, rheumatoid arthritis, juvenile arthritis	• ~33% of patients experience side effects
Ketorolac	• Moderate-to-severe acute pain • Off label: pericarditis, migraine • Ocular pain, seasonal allergic conjunctivitis	• Potent analgesic, poor anti-inflammatory • Max total systemic therapy: 5 days • Oral, IM, IV, nasal, and ophthalmic administration
Diclofenac	• Pain • Dysmenorrhea • Migraine (oral solution) • Osteoarthritis, rheumatoid arthritis • Ankylosing spondylitis	• Some COX-2 selectivity • Short $t_{1/2}$ requires relatively high doses to extend dosing interval • Rate of CV toxicity similar to that of COX-2 inhibitors • Liver toxicity (4%); severe liver injury in ~8 per 100,000 regular users annually
Nabumetone	• Osteoarthritis, rheumatoid arthritis	• Some COX-2 selectivity • 6-methoxy-2-napthylacetic acid prodrug

Fenamates • Anthranilic acids; Nonselective COX inhibitors with effects similar to other NSAIDs

Mefenamic acid	• Pain • Dysmenorrhea	• For patients ≥ 14 years and ≤ 7 days of treatment • ↑ hepatic enzymes in 5%
Meclofenamate	• Pain/fever, dysmenorrhea • Osteoarthritis, rheumatoid arthritis, juvenile arthritis • Ankylosing spondylitis, acute gouty arthritis, acute painful shoulder	• For patients ≥ 14 years • ↑ hepatic enzymes in 5%

Propionic Acid Derivatives • Nonselective COX inhibitors with the effects and side effects common to other NSAIDs

Ibuprofen	• Pain/fever, dysmenorrhea • Osteoarthritis, rheumatoid arthritis • Inflammatory diseases • Patent ductus arteriosus	• Over-the-counter NSAID • Injectable solution available • $t_{1/2}$: 2–4 h (adults); 23–75 h (premature infants); 0.9–2.3 h (children) • Interacts with aspirin's antiplatelet effect
Naproxen	• Pain, dysmenorrhea • Osteoarthritis, rheumatoid arthritis, ankylosing spondylitis; gout; juvenile arthritis, inflammatory diseases • Patent ductus arteriosus	• Over-the-counter NSAID • $t_{1/2}$ variable (9–25 h), age-related • FDA warning: naproxen may not have a lower risk of CV side effects compared to other NSAIDs • Interacts with aspirin's antiplatelet effect
Fenoprofen	• Pain • Osteoarthritis, rheumatoid arthritis	
Ketoprofen	• Pain, dysmenorrhea • Osteoarthritis, rheumatoid arthritis	• 30% develop side effects (usually GI, usually mild) • ↑ hepatic enzymes ~1%
Flurbiprofen	• Osteoarthritis, rheumatoid arthritis	• ↑ hepatic enzymes > 1%
Oxaprozin	• Osteoarthritis, rheumatoid arthritis, juvenile arthritis	• $t_{1/2}$: 41-55 h • Slow onset, not indicated for fever or acute pain

Enolic Acid Derivatives

Piroxicam	• Osteoarthritis, rheumatoid arthritis	• nonselective COX inhibitor with the longest $t_{1/2}$ ~50 h • Slow onset, not indicated for fever or acute pain • Adverse effects, 20%, 5% of patients discontinue; more GI and serious skin reactions than other NSAIDs
Meloxicam	• Osteoarthritis, rheumatoid arthritis, juvenile arthritis	• Some COX-2 selectivity • $t_{1/2}$: 15-20 h

Diaryl Heterocyclic NSAIDs

Celecoxib	• Pain • Dysmenorrhea • Osteoarthritis, rheumatoid arthritis, juvenile arthritis • ankylosing spondylitis • Off label use: gout	• COX-2 selective • Sulfonamide • Risk of myocardial infarction observed in randomized placebo controlled trials.

Drug Facts For Your Personal Formulary: *Gout*

Drugs	Therapeutic Uses	Clinical Pharmacology and Tips
Drugs that relieve inflammation and pain		
NSAIDs	• *See* NSAIDs, above	• *See* NSAIDs, above
Glucocorticoids	• *See* Chapter 46	• *See* Chapter 46
Colchicine	• Prophylaxis and the treatment of acute gout flares	• Depolymerizes microtubules $\Rightarrow$ ↓neutrophil migration into inflamed area • Narrow therapeutic index; toxic effects related to antimitotic activity • $t_{1/2}$: 31 h (21–50 h) • Individualize dose on the basis of age, hepatic and renal function • Contraindicated in patients with GI, renal, hepatic or cardiac disorders • Adverse effects: primarily GI • Drug interactions with P-gp and CYP3A4 inhibitors
Xanthine oxidase (XO) inhibitors • Inhibit urate synthesis		
Allopurinol	• Hyperuricemia in patients with gout gout • Calcium oxalate calculi • Hyperuricemia associated with cancer treatment	• active metabolite: oxypurinol • $t_{1/2}$: allopurinol 1–2 h, oxypurinol 18–30h; adjust dose in renal impairment • Rash, diarrhea, nausea frequent • Risk of gout attacks during the early months of therapy (tissue urate mobilization) • Serum [urate] usually ↓ in 24–48 h, normal 1–3 weeks
Febuxostat	• Hyperuricemia	• non-purine • more selective for XO than allopurinol • $t_{1/2}$: 5 to 8 h • Liver function abnormalities (5–7%)
Uricase • Oxidizes uric acid to allantoin (more soluble and inactive metabolite)		
Pegloticase	• Chronic gout refractory to conventional therapy	• $t_{1/2}$, 14 days • ↓Blood urate within hours of initial administration • Antibody development against drug may limit efficacy, cause hypersensitivity reactions • Adverse effects: bruising (11%), urticaria (11%), nausea (11%), gout flare during early therapy (74%), chest pain (6%)
Rasburicase	• Hyperuricemia associated with malignancy (pediatric and adult patients)	• $t_{1/2}$: 16 to 23 h • ↓Uric acid levels within hours of initial administration • Not suitable for chronic gout; activity-limiting antibodies form against the drug.
Uricosuric drugs–Inhibit of reabsorption of uric acid by organic anion transporters, thereby increasing excretion of uric acid		
Probenecid	• Hyperuricemia associated with gout (but not for acute attacks) • Prolongation and elevation of beta-lactam plasma levels	• Interferes with renal tubular handling of organic acids • $t_{1/2}$: 6-12 h (dose–dependent) • Risk of gout attacks during the early months of therapy (tissue urate mobilization) • ineffective in patients with renal insufficiency
Lesinurad	• Gout in patients who have not achieved the target serum uric acid levels with XO inhibitor alone	• $t_{1/2}$: 5 h • CYP2C9 substrate, so caution is recommended in patients who are CYP2C9 poor metabolizers • Must be used together with XO inhibitor due to renal failure risk

Bibliography

Antithrombotic Trialists' Collaboration, et al. Aspirin in the primary and secondary prevention of vascular disease: collaborative meta-analysis of individual participant data from randomised trials. *Lancet*, **2009**, *373*:1849–1860.

Arehart E, et al. Acceleration of cardiovascular disease by a dysfunctional prostacyclin receptor mutation: potential implications for cyclooxygenase-2 inhibition. *Circ Res*, **2008**, *102*:986–993.

Bjornsson ES, et al. Incidence, presentation, and outcomes in patients with drug-induced liver injury in the general population of Iceland. *Gastroenterology*, **2013**, *144*:1419–1425, 1425, e1411–e1413; quiz e1419–e1420.

Blieden M, et al. A perspective on the epidemiology of acetaminophen exposure and toxicity in the United States. *Expert Rev Clin Pharmacol*, **2014**, *7*:341–348.

Bogentoft C, et al. Influence of food on the absorption of acetylsalicylic acid from enteric-coated dosage forms. *Eur J Clin Pharmacol*, **1978**, *14*:351–355.

Cannon CP, et al. Cardiovascular outcomes with etoricoxib and diclofenac in patients with osteoarthritis and rheumatoid arthritis in the Multinational Etoricoxib and Diclofenac Arthritis Long-term (MEDAL) programme: a randomised comparison. *Lancet*, **2006**, *368*:1771–1781.

Capone ML, et al. Pharmacodynamic interaction of naproxen with low-dose aspirin in healthy subjects. *J Am Coll Cardiol*, **2005**, *45*:1295–1301.

Catella-Lawson F, et al. Cyclooxygenase inhibitors and the antiplatelet effects of aspirin. *N Engl J Med*, **2001**, *345*:1809–1817.

Catella-Lawson F, et al. Effects of specific inhibition of cyclooxygenase-2 on sodium balance, hemodynamics, and vasoactive eicosanoids. *J Pharmacol Exp Ther*, **1999**, *289*:735–741.

Chen L, et al. Prostanoids and inflammatory pain. *Prostaglandins Other Lipid Mediat*, **2013**, 104–105 58–66.

Cheng Y, et al. Role of prostacyclin in the cardiovascular response to thromboxane A$_2$. *Science*, **2002**, *296*:539–541.

Cheng Y, et al. Cyclooxygenases, microsomal prostaglandin E synthase-1, and cardiovascular function. *J Clin Invest*, **2006**, *116*:1391–1399.

Coxib and Traditional NSAID Trialists' Collaboration, et al. Vascular and upper gastrointestinal effects of non-steroidal anti-inflammatory drugs: meta-analyses of individual participant data from randomised trials. *Lancet*, **2013**, *382*:769–779.

Daly AK, et al. Genetic susceptibility to diclofenac-induced hepatotoxicity: contribution of UGT2B7, CYP2C8, and ABCC2 genotypes. *Gastroenterology*, **2007**, *132*:272–281.

Day RO, et al. Pharmacokinetics of nonsteroidal anti-inflammatory drugs in synovial fluid. *Clin Pharmacokinet*, **1999**, *36*:191–210.

de Abajo FJ, et al. Acute and clinically relevant drug-induced liver injury: a population based case-control study. *Br J Clin Pharmacol*, **2004**, *58*:71–80.

Dong L, et al. Human cyclooxygenase-2 is a sequence homodimer that functions as a conformational heterodimer. *J Biol Chem*, **2011**, *286*:19035–19046.

Egan KM, et al. COX-2-derived prostacyclin confers atheroprotection on female mice. *Science*, **2004**, *306*:1954–1957.

Engblom D, et al. Microsomal prostaglandin E synthase-1 is the central switch during immune-induced pyresis. *Nat Neurosci*, **2003**, *6*(11):1137–1138.

Farkouh ME, et al. Comparison of lumiracoxib with naproxen and ibuprofen in the Therapeutic Arthritis Research and Gastrointestinal Event Trial (TARGET), cardiovascular outcomes: randomised controlled trial. *Lancet*, **2004**, *364*:675–684.

FitzGerald GA, Patrono C. The coxibs, selective inhibitors of cyclooxygenase-2. *N Engl J Med*, **2001**, *345*:433–442.

Graham GG, et al. Tolerability of paracetamol. *Drug Saf*, **2005**, *28*:227–240.

Grosser T, et al. Drug resistance and pseudoresistance: an unintended consequence of enteric coating aspirin. *Circulation*, **2013**, *127*:377–85.

Grosser T, et al. Biological basis for the cardiovascular consequences of COX-2 inhibition: therapeutic challenges and opportunities. *J Clin Invest*, **2006**, *116*:4–15.

Grosser T, et al. The Cardiovascular Pharmacology of Nonsteroidal Anti-Inflammatory Drugs. *Trends Pharmacol Sci*, **2017**, *38*:733–748.

Grosser T, et al. Emotion recollected in tranquility: lessons learned from the COX-2 saga. *Annu Rev Med*, **2010**, *61*:17–33.

King C, et al. Characterization of rat and human UDP-glucuronosyltransferases responsible for the in vitro glucuronidation of diclofenac. *Toxicol Sci*, **2001**, *61*:49–53.

Kobayashi T, et al. Roles of thromboxane A_2 and prostacyclin in the development of atherosclerosis in apoE-deficient mice. *J Clin Invest*, **2004**, *114*:784–794.

LeFevre ML, Force U. Low-dose aspirin use for the prevention of morbidity and mortality from preeclampsia: U.S. Preventive Services Task Force recommendation statement. *Ann Intern Med*, **2014**, *161*:819–826.

Leung YY, et al. Colchicine—update on mechanisms of action and therapeutic uses. *Semin Arthritis Rheum*, **2015**, *45*:341–350.

Li X, et al. Differential impairment of aspirin-dependent platelet cyclooxygenase acetylation by nonsteroidal antiinflammatory drugs. *Proc Natl Acad Sci U S A*, **2014**, *111*:16830–16835.

McAdam BF, et al. Systemic biosynthesis of prostacyclin by cyclooxygenase (COX)-2: the human pharmacology of a selective inhibitor of COX-2. *Proc Natl Acad Sci U S A*, **1999**, *96*:272–277.

Muller WA. Mechanisms of leukocyte transendothelial migration. *Annu Rev Pathol*, **2011**, *6*:323–344.

Nusing RM, et al. Pathogenetic role of cyclooxygenase-2 in hyperprostaglandin E syndrome/antenatal Bartter syndrome: therapeutic use of the cyclooxygenase-2 inhibitor nimesulide. *Clin Pharmacol Ther*, **2001**, *70*:384–390.

Patoia L, et al. A 4-week, double-blind, parallel-group study to compare the gastrointestinal effects of meloxicam 7.5 mg, meloxicam 15 mg, piroxicam 20 mg and placebo by means of faecal blood loss, endoscopy and symptom evaluation in healthy volunteers. *Br J Rheumatol*. **1996**, *35*(suppl 1):61–67.

Patrono C. The multifaceted clinical readouts of platelet inhibition by low-dose aspirin. *J Am Coll Cardiol*, **2015**, *66*:74–85.

Pedersen AK, FitzGerald GA. Dose-related kinetics of aspirin. Presystemic acetylation of platelet cyclooxygenase. *N Engl J Med*, **1984**, *311*:1206–1211.

Rostom A, et al. Nonsteroidal anti-inflammatory drugs and hepatic toxicity: a systematic review of randomized controlled trials in arthritis patients. *Clin Gastroenterol Hepatol*, **2005**, *3*:489–498.

Rothwell PM, et al. Long-term effect of aspirin on colorectal cancer incidence and mortality: 20-year follow-up of five randomised trials. *Lancet*, **2010**, *376*(9754):1741–1750.

Sanchez-Alavez M, et al. Ceramide mediates the rapid phase of febrile response to IL-1beta. *Proc Natl Acad Sci U S A*, **2006**, *103*:2904–2908.

Schrör K. Aspirin and Reye syndrome: a review of the evidence. *Paediatr Drugs*, **2007**, *9*:195–204.

Smith WL, et al. Enzymes of the cyclooxygenase pathways of prostanoid biosynthesis. *Chem Rev*, **2011**, *111*: 5821–5865.

Song WL, et al. Niacin and biosynthesis of PGD(2)by platelet COX-1 in mice and humans. *J Clin Invest*, **2012**, *122*:1459–1468.

Sostres C, et al. Nonsteroidal anti-inflammatory drugs and upper and lower gastrointestinal mucosal damage. *Arthritis Res Ther*, **2013**, *15*(suppl 3):S3.

Tang D, et al. PAMPs and DAMPs: signal 0s that spur autophagy and immunity. *Immunol Rev*, **2012**, *249*:158–175.

Theoharides T, et al. Mast cells, mastocytosis, and related disorders. *N Engl J Med*, **2015**, *373*:163–172.

U.S. Food and Drug Administration. FDA Drug Safety Communication: FDA strengthens warning that non-aspirin nonsteroidal anti-inflammatory drugs (NSAIDs) can cause heart attacks or strokes. 2015. Available at: http://www.fda.gov/Drugs/DrugSafety/ucm451800.htm. Accessed June 1, 2016.

Warner T, et al. Nonsteroid drug selectivities for cyclo-oxygenase-1 rather than cyclo-oxygenase-2 are associated with human gastrointestinal toxicity: a full in vitro analysis. *Proc Natl Acad Sci U S A*, **1999**, *96*:7563–7568.

Xian Y, et al. Association of discharge aspirin dose with outcomes after acute myocardial infarction: insights from the Treatment With ADP Receptor Inhibitors: Longitudinal Assessment of Treatment Patterns and Events After Acute Coronary Syndrome (TRANSLATE-ACS) study. *Circulation*, **2015**, *132*:174–181.

Yu Y, et al. Vascular COX-2 modulates blood pressure and thrombosis in mice. *Sci Transl Med*, **2012**, *4*:132–154.

Zou H, et al. Human cyclooxygenase-1 activity and its responses to COX inhibitors are allosterically regulated by nonsubstrate fatty acids. *J Lipid Res*, **2012**, *53*:1336–1347.

Chapter 39

Histamine, Bradykinin, and Their Antagonists

Randal A. Skidgel

Endogenous histamine plays a role in the immediate allergic response and is an important regulator of gastric acid secretion. More recently, a role for histamine as a modulator of neurotransmitter release in the central and peripheral nervous systems has emerged. The cloning of four receptors for histamine and the development of subtype-specific receptor antagonists have enhanced our understanding of the physiological and pathophysiological roles of histamine. Competitive antagonists of H_1 receptors are used therapeutically in treating allergies, urticaria, anaphylactic reactions, nausea, motion sickness, and insomnia. Antagonists of the H_2 receptor are effective in reducing gastric acid secretion.

The peptides bradykinin and kallidin, released after activation of the kallikrein-kinin system, have cardiovascular effects similar to those of histamine and play prominent roles in inflammation and nociception. Icatibant, a competitive antagonist of the bradykinin B_2 receptor, and ecallantide, a specific plasma kallikrein inhibitor, are approved for the treatment of acute episodes of edema in patients with hereditary angioedema.

Histamine

Histamine is a hydrophilic molecule consisting of an imidazole ring and an amino group connected by an ethylene group; histamine is biosynthesized from histidine by decarboxylation (Figure 39–1). Histamine acts through four classes of receptors, designated H_1 through H_4. The four histamine receptors, all GPCRs, can be differentially activated by analogues of histamine (Figure 39–2) and inhibited by specific antagonists (Table 39–1).

Distribution and Biosynthesis

Distribution

Almost all mammalian tissues contain histamine in amounts ranging from less than 1 to more than 100 μg/g. Concentrations in plasma and other body fluids are generally very low, but they are significant in human CSF.

The concentration of histamine is particularly high in tissues that contain large numbers of mast cells, such as skin, bronchial mucosa, and intestinal mucosa.

Synthesis, Storage, and Metabolism

Histamine is formed by the decarboxylation of histidine by the enzyme *L-histidine decarboxylase* (Figure 39–1). Mast cells and basophils synthesize histamine and store it in secretory granules. At the secretory granule pH of about 5.5, histamine is positively charged and ionically complexed with negatively charged acidic groups on other granule constituents, primarily proteases and heparin or chondroitin sulfate proteoglycans. The turnover rate of histamine in secretory granules is slow (days to weeks). Non–mast cell sites of histamine formation include the epidermis, enterochromaffin-like cells of the gastric mucosa, neurons within the CNS, and cells in regenerating or rapidly growing tissues. Turnover is rapid at these non–mast cell sites because the histamine is released continuously rather than stored. Non–mast cell sites of histamine production contribute significantly to the daily excretion of histamine metabolites in the urine. Because L-histidine decarboxylase is an inducible enzyme, the histamine-forming capacity at such sites is subject to regulation. Histamine that is released or ingested is rapidly metabolized by either ring methylation catalyzed by *histamine-N-methyltransferase* or oxidative deamination catalyzed by *diamine oxidase* (Figure 39–1), and the metabolites are eliminated in the urine.

Release and Functions of Endogenous Histamine

Histamine is released from storage granules as a result of the interaction of antigen with IgE antibodies on the mast cell surface. Histamine plays a central role in immediate hypersensitivity and allergic responses. The actions of histamine on bronchial smooth muscle and blood vessels account for many of the symptoms of the allergic response. Histamine is a leukocyte chemoattractant, plays a major role in regulating gastric acid secretion, and modulates neurotransmitter release. In addition, some drugs act directly on mast cells to release histamine, causing untoward effects.

Role in Allergic Responses

The principal target cells of immediate hypersensitivity reactions are mast cells and basophils (Schwartz, 1994). As part of the allergic response to an antigen, IgE antibodies are generated and bind to the surfaces of mast cells and basophils via specific high-affinity F_c receptors. This receptor, FcεRI, consists of α, β, and two γ chains (see Chapter 34). Antigen bridges the IgE molecules and via FcεRI activates signaling pathways in mast cells or

Abbreviations

ACE: angiotensin I converting enzyme
ACh: acetylcholine
ADHD: attention-deficit/hyperactivity disorder
Ang: angiotensin
AT: angiotensin receptor
AV: atrioventricular
CNS: central nervous system
CPM/N: carboxypeptidase M/N
CSF: cerebrospinal fluid
EDHF: endothelial-derived hyperpolarizing factor
EET: epoxyeicosatrienoic acid
eNOS: endothelial nitric oxide synthase
GABA: gamma-aminobutyric acid
GPCR: G protein–coupled receptor
HMW: high molecular weight
5HT: serotonin
IgE: immunoglobulin E
IL-1: interleukin 1
iNOS: inducible nitric oxide synthase
IP$_3$: inositol triphosphate
JNK1/2: c-Jun N-terminal kinase1/2
LMW: low molecular weight
MAO: monoamine oxidase
PAF: platelet-activating factor
PG: prostaglandin
TNF-α: tumor necrosis factor alpha

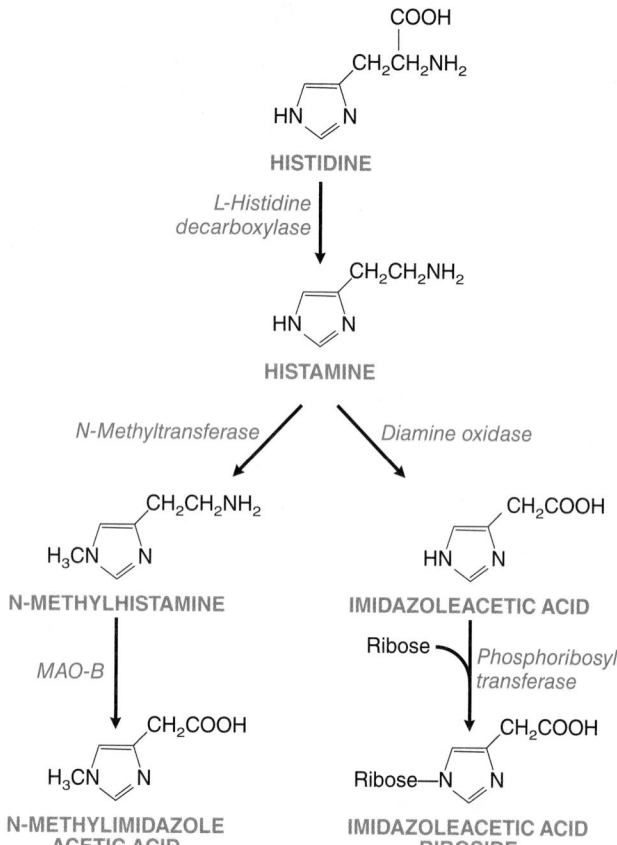

Figure 39–1 *Pathways of histamine synthesis and metabolism in humans.* Histamine is synthesized from histidine by decarboxylation. Histamine is metabolized via two pathways, predominantly by methylation of the ring followed by oxidative deamination (left side of figure) and secondarily by oxidative deamination and then conjugation with ribose.

basophils involving tyrosine kinases and subsequent phosphorylation of multiple protein substrates within 5–15 sec of contact with antigen. These events trigger the exocytosis of the contents of secretory granules that, in addition to histamine, includes serotonin, proteases, lysosomal enzymes, cytokines, and proteoglycans (Schwartz, 1994).

Release of Other Autacoids

Stimulation of IgE receptors also activates PLA$_2$, leading to the production of a host of mediators, including PAF and metabolites of arachidonic acid such as leukotrienes C$_4$ and D$_4$, which contract bronchial smooth muscle (Chapters 37 and 40). Kinins also are generated during some allergic responses. Thus, the mast cell secretes a variety of inflammatory mediators in addition to histamine, each contributing to aspects of the allergic response (see discussion that follows).

Histamine Release by Drugs, Peptides, Venoms, and Other Agents

Mechanical injury and many compounds, including a large number of therapeutic agents, stimulate the release of histamine from mast cells directly and without prior sensitization. Responses of this sort are most likely to occur following intravenous injections of certain categories of substances, particularly organic bases. Tubocurarine, succinylcholine, morphine, some antibiotics, radiocontrast media, and certain carbohydrate plasma expanders also may elicit the response. The phenomenon is one of clinical concern and may account for unexpected anaphylactoid reactions. Basic polypeptides often are effective histamine releasers, and over a limited range, their potency generally increases with the number of basic groups. For example, bradykinin is a poor histamine releaser, whereas kallidin (Lys-bradykinin) and substance P, with more positively charged amino acids, are more active (Johnson and Erdos, 1973). Some venoms, such as that of the wasp, contain potent histamine-releasing peptides. Basic polypeptides released on tissue injury constitute pathophysiological stimuli for secretion from mast cells and basophils.

Within seconds of the intravenous injection of a histamine liberator, human subjects experience a burning, itching sensation. This effect, most marked in the palms of the hand and in the face, scalp, and ears, is soon followed by a feeling of intense warmth. The skin reddens, and the color rapidly spreads over the trunk. Blood pressure falls, the heart rate accelerates, and the subject usually complains of headache. After a few minutes, blood pressure recovers, and crops of hives usually appear on the skin. Colic, nausea, hypersecretion of acid, and moderate bronchospasm also frequently occur. The effect becomes less intense with successive administration of the secretagogue as mast cell stores of histamine are depleted. Histamine liberators do not deplete histamine from non–mast cell sites. The mechanism by which basic secretagogues release histamine likely involves their direct interaction with G proteins or activation of a mast cell–specific cell surface GPCR named MRGRX2 (Seifert, 2015).

Increased Proliferation of Mast Cells and Basophils; Gastric Carcinoid Tumors

In urticaria pigmentosa (cutaneous mastocytosis), mast cells aggregate in the upper corium and give rise to pigmented cutaneous lesions that sting when stroked. In systemic mastocytosis, overproliferation of mast cells is also found in other organs. Patients with these syndromes suffer a constellation of signs and symptoms attributable to excessive histamine release, including urticaria, dermographism, pruritus, headache, weakness, hypotension, flushing of the face, and a variety of GI effects, such as diarrhea or peptic ulceration. A variety of stimuli, including exertion, insect stings, exposure to heat, allergens (including drugs to which a patient is allergic), can activate mast cells and cause histamine release, as can organic bases (many drugs) that cause histamine release directly. In

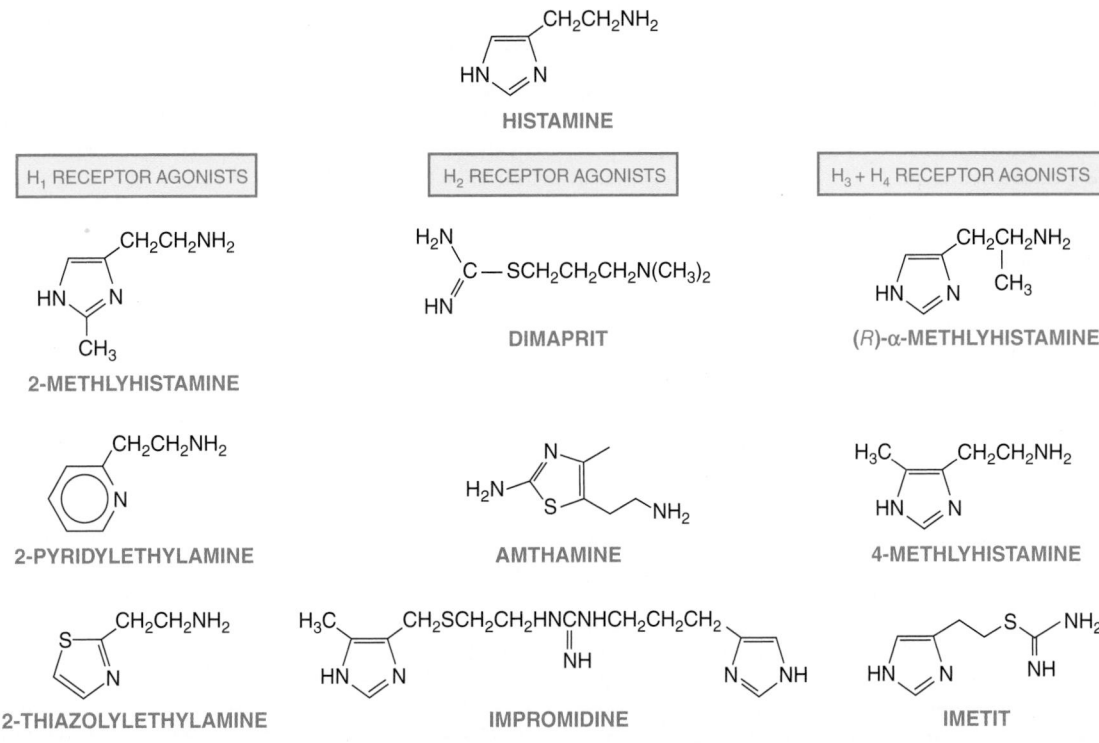

Figure 39–2 *Structure of histamine and some H_1, H_2, H_3, and H_4 agonists.* Dimaprit and 4-methylhistamine, originally identified as specific H_2 agonists, have a much higher affinity for the H_4 receptor; 4-methylhistamine is the most specific available H_4 agonist, with about 10-fold higher affinity than dimaprit, a partial H_4 agonist. Impromidine not only is among the most potent H_2 agonists but also is an antagonist at H_1 and H_3 receptors and a partial agonist at H_4 receptors. (R)-α-Methylhistamine and imetit are high-affinity agonists of H_3 receptors and lower-affinity full agonists at H_4 receptors.

myelogenous leukemia, elevation of blood basophils can result in histamine content high enough to cause flushing, pruritus, and hypotension. Management of these patients can be complicated by a large release of histamine after cytolysis, causing shock. Gastric carcinoid tumors secrete histamine, which is responsible for episodes of vasodilation as part of the patchy "geographical" flush.

Gastric Acid Secretion

Histamine acting at H_2 receptors is a powerful gastric secretagogue, evoking copious secretion of acid from parietal cells (see Figure 49–1); it also increases the output of pepsin and intrinsic factor. The secretion of gastric acid from parietal cells also is caused by stimulation of the vagus nerve and by the enteric hormone gastrin. However, histamine is the dominant physiological mediator of acid secretion; blockade of H_2 receptors not only antagonizes acid secretion in response to histamine but also inhibits responses to gastrin and vagal stimulation (see Chapter 49).

CNS

Histamine-containing neurons affect both homeostatic and higher brain functions, including regulation of the sleep-wake cycle, circadian and feeding rhythms, immunity, learning, memory, drinking, and body temperature. However, no human disease has yet been directly linked to dysfunction of the brain histamine system. Histamine, histidine decarboxylase, enzymes that metabolize histamine, and H_1, H_2, and H_3 receptors are distributed widely but nonuniformly in the CNS. H_1 receptors are associated with both neuronal and nonneuronal cells and are concentrated in regions that control neuroendocrine function, behavior, and nutritional state. Distribution of H_2 receptors is more consistent with histaminergic projections than that of H_1 receptors, suggesting that they mediate many of the postsynaptic actions of histamine. H_3 receptors are concentrated in areas known to receive histaminergic projections, consistent with their function as presynaptic autoreceptors. Histamine inhibits appetite and increases wakefulness via H_1 receptors.

TABLE 39–1 ■ CHARACTERISTICS OF HISTAMINE RECEPTORS

	H_1	H_2	H_3[a]	H_4
Size (amino acids)	487	359	329–445	390
G protein coupling (second messengers)	$G_{q/11}$ (↑ Ca^{2+}; ↑ NO and ↑ cGMP)	G_s (↑ cAMP)	$G_{i/o}$ (↓ cAMP; ↑ MAP kinase)	$G_{i/o}$ (↓ cAMP; ↑ Ca^{2+})
Distribution	Smooth muscle, endothelial cells, CNS	Gastric parietal cells, cardiac muscle, mast cells, CNS	CNS: pre- and post-synaptic	Cells of hematopoietic origin
Representative agonist	2-CH_3-histamine	Amthamine	(R)-α-CH_3-histamine	4-CH_3-histamine
Representative antagonist	Chlorpheniramine	Ranitidine	Tiprolisant	JNJ7777120

[a]At least 20 alternately spliced H_3 isoforms have been detected at the mRNA level. Eight of these isoforms, ranging in size from 329 to 445 residues, were found to be functionally competent by binding or signaling assays (see Esbenshade et al., 2008).

Physiological and Pharmacological Effects

Receptor-Effector Coupling and Mechanisms of Action

Histamine receptors are GPCRs, coupling to second-messenger systems and producing effects (Simons, 2004) as noted in Table 39–1. H_1 receptors couple to $G_{q/11}$ and activate the PLC-IP$_3$-Ca^{2+} pathway and its many possible sequelae, including activation of PKC, Ca^{2+}-calmodulin–dependent enzymes (eNOS and various protein kinases), and PLA$_2$. H_2 receptors link to G_s to activate the adenylyl cyclase–cyclic AMP–PKA pathway; H_3 and H_4 receptors couple to $G_{i/o}$ to inhibit adenylyl cyclase and decrease cellular cyclic AMP. Activation of H_3 receptors also can activate MAP kinase and inhibit the Na$^+$/H$^+$ exchanger; activation of H_4 receptors can mobilize stored Ca^{2+} (Simons and Simons, 2011). H_3 and H_4 receptors have about 1000-fold higher affinity for histamine (low nanomolar range) than do H_1 and H_2 receptors (low micromolar range). Activation of H_1 receptors on vascular endothelium stimulates eNOS to produce NO, which diffuses to nearby smooth muscle cells to increase cyclic GMP and cause relaxation. Stimulation of H_1 receptors on smooth muscle will mobilize Ca^{2+} and cause contraction, whereas activation of H_2 receptors on the same smooth muscle cell will link via G_s to enhanced cyclic AMP accumulation, activation of PKA, and then to relaxation.

Pharmacological definition of H_1, H_2, and H_3 receptors was possible through the use of relatively specific agonists and antagonists. Because the H_4 receptor exhibits 35%–40% homology to isoforms of the H_3 receptor, the two were initially harder to distinguish pharmacologically, but this has been resolved by the development of several H_3- and H_4-selective antagonists (Sander et al., 2008; Thurmond, 2015). 4-Methylhistamine and dimaprit, previously identified as specific H_2 agonists, are actually more potent H_4 agonists.

H_1 and H_2 Receptors

H_1 and H_2 receptors are distributed widely in the periphery and in the CNS and their activation by histamine can exert local or widespread effects (Simons and Simons, 2011). For example, histamine causes itching and stimulates secretion from nasal mucosa. It contracts many smooth muscles, such as those of the bronchi and gut, but markedly relaxes others, including those in small blood vessels. Histamine also is a potent stimulus of gastric acid secretion. Other, less-prominent effects include formation of edema and stimulation of sensory nerve endings. Bronchoconstriction and contraction of the gut are mediated by H_1 receptors. In the CNS, H_1 activation inhibits appetite and increases wakefulness. Gastric secretion results from the activation of H_2 receptors. Some responses, such as vascular dilation, are mediated by both H_1 and H_2 receptor stimulation.

H_3 and H_4 Receptors

The H_3 receptors are expressed mainly in the CNS, especially in the basal ganglia, hippocampus, and cortex (Haas et al., 2008). Presynaptic H_3 receptors function as autoreceptors on histaminergic neurons, inhibiting histamine release and modulating the release of other neurotransmitters. H_3 receptors are also found postsynaptically, especially in the basal ganglia, but their function is still being unraveled (Ellenbroek and Ghiabi, 2014). H_3 agonists promote sleep, and H_3 antagonists promote wakefulness.

The H_4 receptors primarily are found in eosinophils, dendritic cells, mast cells, monocytes, basophils, and T cells but have also been detected in the GI tract, dermal fibroblasts, CNS, and primary sensory afferent neurons (Thurmond, 2015). Activation of H_4 receptors has been associated with induction of cellular shape change, chemotaxis, secretion of cytokines, and upregulation of adhesion molecules, suggesting that H_4 antagonists may be useful inhibitors of allergic and inflammatory responses (Thurmond, 2015).

Although specific H_3 and H_4 receptor antagonists have been developed, none of these agents has yet been FDA-approved for clinical use. Based on the functions of H_3 receptors in the CNS, H_3 antagonists have potential in the treatment of sleeping disorders, ADHD, epilepsy, cognitive impairment, schizophrenia, obesity, neuropathic pain, and Alzheimer disease. Because of the unique localization and function of H_4 receptors, H_4 antagonists are promising candidates to treat inflammatory conditions such as allergic rhinitis, asthma, rheumatoid arthritis, and possibly pruritus and neuropathic pain.

Feedback Regulation of Release

Stimulation of H_2 receptor increases cyclic AMP and leads to feedback inhibition of histamine release from mast cells and basophils, whereas activation of H_3 and H_4 receptors has the opposite effect by decreasing cellular cyclic AMP. Activation of presynaptic H_3 receptors inhibits histamine release from histaminergic neurons. Because H_3 receptors have high constitutive activity, histamine release is tonically inhibited. H_3 inverse agonists thus reduce receptor activation and increase histamine release from histaminergic neurons.

Cardiovascular System

Histamine dilates resistance vessels, increases capillary permeability, and lowers systemic blood pressure. In some vascular beds, histamine constricts veins, contributing to the extravasation of fluid and edema formation upstream in capillaries and postcapillary venules.

Vasodilation. Vasodilation is the most important vascular effect of histamine in humans and can result from activation of either the H_1 or H_2 receptor. H_1 receptors have a higher affinity for histamine and cause Ca^{2+}-dependent activation of eNOS in endothelial cells; NO diffuses to vascular smooth muscle, increasing cyclic GMP (see Table 39–1) and causing rapid and short-lived vasodilation. By contrast, activation of H_2 receptors on vascular smooth muscle stimulates the cyclic AMP–PKA pathway, causing dilation that develops more slowly and is more sustained. As a result, H_1 antagonists effectively counter small dilator responses to low concentrations of histamine but blunt only the initial phase of larger responses to higher concentrations of the amine.

Increased Capillary Permeability. Histamine's effect on small vessels results in efflux of plasma protein and fluid into the extracellular spaces and an increase in lymph flow, causing edema. H_1 receptor activation on endothelial cells is the major mediator of this response, leading to G_q-mediated activation of RhoA and ROCK, which stimulates the contractile machinery of the cells and disrupts interendothelial junctions (Mikelis et al., 2015). The gaps between endothelial cells also may permit passage of circulating cells recruited to tissues during the mast cell response. Recruitment of circulating leukocytes is enhanced by H_1 receptor–mediated expression of adhesion molecules (e.g., P-selectin) on endothelial cells.

Triple Response of Lewis. If histamine is injected intradermally, it elicits a characteristic phenomenon known as the *triple response*. This consists of the following:

- a localized "reddening" around the injection site, appearing within a few seconds, and maximal at about 1 min;
- a "flare" or red flush extending about 1 cm beyond the original red spot and developing more slowly; and
- a "wheal" or swelling that is discernible in 1–2 min at the injection site.

The initial red spot (a few millimeters) results from the direct vasodilating effect of histamine (H_1 receptor–mediated NO production). The flare is due to histamine-induced stimulation of axon reflexes that cause vasodilation indirectly, and the wheal reflects histamine's capacity to increase capillary permeability (edema formation).

Heart. Histamine affects both cardiac contractility and electrical events directly. It increases the force of contraction of both atrial and ventricular muscle by promoting the influx of Ca^{2+}, and it speeds heart rate by hastening diastolic depolarization in the SA node. It also directly slows AV conduction to increase automaticity and, in high doses, can elicit arrhythmias. The slowed AV conduction involves mainly H_1 receptors, while the other effects are largely attributable to H_2 receptors and cyclic AMP accumulation. The direct cardiac effects of histamine given intravenously are overshadowed by baroreceptor reflexes stimulated by reduced blood pressure.

Extravascular Smooth Muscle

Histamine directly contracts or, more rarely, relaxes various extravascular smooth muscles. Contraction is due to activation of H_1 receptors on smooth muscle to increase intracellular Ca^{2+}, and relaxation is mainly due to activation of H_2 receptors. Although the spasmogenic influence of H_1 receptors is dominant in human bronchial muscle, H_2 receptors with dilator function also are present. Thus, histamine-induced bronchospasm in vitro is potentiated slightly by H_2 blockade. Patients with bronchial asthma and certain other pulmonary diseases are much more sensitive to the bronchoconstrictor effects of histamine.

Peripheral Nerve Endings

Histamine stimulates various nerve endings, causing sensory effects. In the epidermis, it causes itch; in the dermis, it evokes pain, sometimes accompanied by itching. Stimulant actions on nerve endings, including autonomic afferents and efferents, contribute to the "flare" component of the triple response and to indirect effects of histamine on the bronchi and other organs.

Histamine Shock

Histamine given in large doses or released during systemic anaphylaxis causes a profound and progressive fall in blood pressure. As the small blood vessels dilate, they trap large amounts of blood, their permeability increases, and plasma escapes from the circulation. These effects, resembling surgical or traumatic shock, diminish effective blood volume, reduce venous return, and greatly lower cardiac output.

Histamine Toxicity From Ingestion

Histamine is the toxin in food poisoning from spoiled scombroid fish such as tuna. Symptoms include severe nausea, vomiting, headache, flushing, and sweating. Histamine toxicity also can follow red wine consumption in persons with a diminished ability to degrade histamine. The symptoms of histamine poisoning can be suppressed by H_1 antagonists.

Histamine Receptor Antagonists

H_1 Receptor Antagonists

> **HISTORY**
>
> Antihistamine activity was first demonstrated by Bovet and Staub in 1937 with one of a series of amines with a phenolic ether moiety. The substance, 2-isopropyl-5-methylphenoxy-ethyldiethyl-amine, protected guinea pigs against several lethal doses of histamine but was too toxic for clinical use. By 1944, Bovet and his colleagues had described *pyrilamine maleate*, an effective histamine antagonist of this category. The discovery of highly effective *diphenhydramine* and *tripelennamine* soon followed. In the 1980s, nonsedating H_1 histamine receptor antagonists were developed for treatment of allergic diseases. Despite success in blocking allergic responses to histamine, the H_1 antihistamines failed to inhibit a number of other responses, notably gastric acid secretion. The discovery of H_2 receptors and H_2 antagonists by Black and colleagues provided a new class of agents that antagonized histamine-induced acid secretion (Black et al., 1972); the pharmacology of these drugs (e.g., *cimetidine, famotidine*) is described in Chapter 49.

Pharmacological Properties

All the available H_1 receptor "antagonists" are actually inverse agonists (see Chapter 3) that reduce constitutive activity of the receptor and compete with histamine binding to the receptor (Simons, 2004). The pharmacological actions and therapeutic applications of these antagonists can be largely predicted from knowledge of the location and mode of signaling of the histamine receptors.

Chemistry. Like histamine, many H_1 antagonists contain a substituted ethylamine moiety (the black portion on the figure that follows). Unlike histamine, which has a primary amino group and a single aromatic ring, most H_1 antagonists have a tertiary amino group linked by a two- or three-atom chain to two aromatic substituents (in red) and conform to the general formula:

$$\begin{array}{c} Ar_1 \\ \\ Ar_2 \end{array} X - \overset{|}{\underset{|}{C}} - \overset{|}{\underset{|}{C}} - N \begin{array}{c} \diagup \\ \diagdown \end{array}$$

where Ar is aryl and X is a nitrogen or carbon atom or a —C—O— ether linkage to the β-aminoethyl side chain. Sometimes, the two aromatic rings are bridged, as in the tricyclic derivatives, or the ethylamine may be part of a ring structure. Figure 39–3 shows the varied structures of representative H_1 antagonists built around this framework and constitute the several generations of compounds.

Effects on Physiological Systems

Smooth Muscle. The H_1 antagonists inhibit most of the effects of histamine on smooth muscles, especially the constriction of respiratory smooth muscle. H_1 antagonists inhibit the more rapid vasodilator effects mediated by activation of H_1 receptors on endothelial cells (synthesis/release of NO and other mediators) at lower doses of histamine. They also inhibit venous constriction seen in some vascular beds.

Capillary Permeability. H_1 antagonists strongly block the increased capillary permeability and formation of edema and wheal caused by histamine.

Flare and Itch. H_1 antagonists suppress the action of histamine on nerve endings, including the flare component of the triple response and the itching caused by intradermal injection.

Exocrine Glands. H_1 antagonists do not suppress gastric secretion. However, the antimuscarinic properties of many H_1 antagonists may contribute to lessened secretion in cholinergically innervated glands and reduce ongoing secretion in, for example, the respiratory tree.

Immediate Hypersensitivity Reactions: Anaphylaxis and Allergy. During hypersensitivity reactions, histamine is one of the many potent autacoids released, and its relative contribution to the ensuing symptoms varies widely with species and tissue. The protection afforded by H_1 antagonists varies accordingly. In humans, edema formation and itch are effectively suppressed. Other effects, such as hypotension, are less well antagonized. H_1 antagonists are ineffective in blocking bronchoconstriction due to asthma.

Mast Cell–Stabilizing and Anti-inflammatory Properties. Many second-generation H_1 antagonists (e.g., cetirizine, desloratadine, fexofenedine, olopatadine, ketotifen, alcaftadine, and others) exhibit mast cell–stabilizing effects, resulting in reduced release of mast cell mediators during an allergic response (Levi-Schaffer and Eliashar, 2009). These agents also have anti-inflammatory properties, which can include reduced cytokine secretion, decreased adhesion molecule expression, and inhibition of eosinophil infiltration. These effects can be both H_1 receptor dependent and independent, but precise mechanisms are still unclear, and it is unknown what role they play at normal therapeutic doses of these drugs. There is some evidence that H_1 antagonists with these additional properties may be more effective in the topical treatment of allergic conjunctivitis (Abelson et al., 2015).

CNS. The first-generation H_1 antagonists can both stimulate and depress the CNS (Simons and Simons, 2011). Stimulation occasionally is encountered in patients given conventional doses; the patients become restless, nervous, and unable to sleep. Central excitation also is a striking feature of overdose, which commonly results in convulsions, particularly in infants. Central depression, on the other hand, usually accompanies therapeutic doses of the older H_1 antagonists. Diminished alertness, slowed reaction times, and somnolence are common manifestations. Patients vary in their susceptibility and responses to individual drugs. The ethanolamines (e.g., diphenhydramine) are particularly prone to causing sedation. Because of

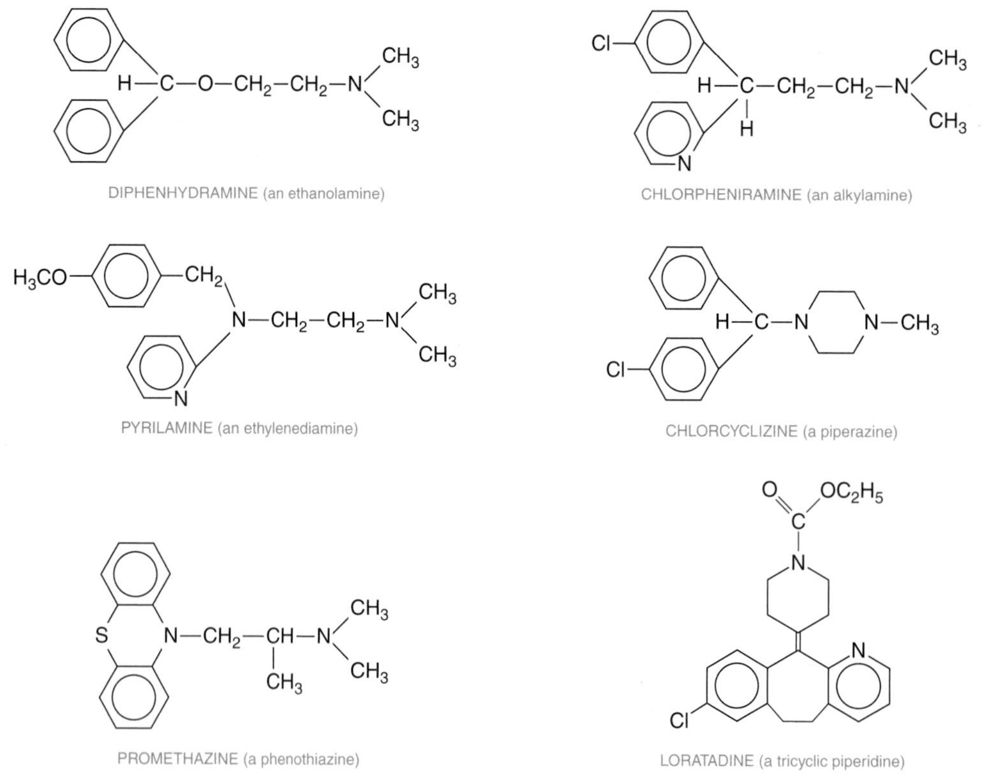

Figure 39–3 *Representative H₁ antagonists.*

the sedation that occurs with first-generation antihistamines, these drugs cannot be tolerated or used safely by many patients except at bedtime. Even then, patients may experience an antihistamine "hangover" in the morning, resulting in sedation with or without psychomotor impairment. Second-generation H₁ antagonists are termed *nonsedating* because they do not cross the blood-brain barrier appreciably. This is due to their decreased lipophilicity and because they are substrates of P-glycoprotein, which pumps them out of the blood-brain barrier capillary endothelial cells and back into the capillary lumen (see Chapter 5 and Simons and Simons, 2011).

Many antipsychotic agents are H₁ and H₂ receptor antagonists, but it is unclear whether this property plays a role in the antipsychotic effects of these agents. In test systems, the atypical antipsychotic agent *clozapine* is an effective H₁ antagonist, a weak H₃ antagonist, and an H₄ receptor agonist. The H₁ antagonist activity of typical and atypical antipsychotic drugs is responsible for the propensity of these agents to cause weight gain.

Anticholinergic Effects. Many of the first-generation H₁ antagonists tend to inhibit muscarinic cholinergic responses and may be manifest during clinical use (Simons and Simons, 2011). Some H₁ antagonists also can be used to treat motion sickness (see Chapters 9 and 50), probably as a result of their anticholinergic properties. Indeed, promethazine has perhaps the strongest muscarinic-blocking activity among these agents and is the most effective H₁ antagonist in combating motion sickness. The second-generation H₁ antagonists have no effect on muscarinic receptors (Simons and Simons, 2011).

Local Anesthetic Effect. Some H₁ antagonists have local anesthetic activity, and a few are more potent than procaine. Promethazine is especially active. However, the concentrations required for this effect are much higher than those that antagonize histamine's interactions with its receptors.

ADME. The H₁ antagonists are well absorbed from the GI tract. Following oral administration, peak plasma concentrations are achieved in 1–3 h, and effects usually last 4–6 h for first-generation agents; however, some of the drugs are much longer acting, as are most second-generation H₁

antagonists (del Cuvillo et al., 2006; Simons, 2004) (Table 39–2). These agents are distributed widely throughout the body, including the CNS for the first-generation agents. Peak concentrations of these drugs in the skin may persist long after plasma levels have declined. Thus, inhibition of "wheal-and-flare" responses to the intradermal injection of histamine or allergen can persist for 36 h or more after initial treatment and up to 7 days after discontinuation of treatment in patients who regularly use an H₁ antagonist for 1 week or more (del Cuvillo et al., 2006).

All first-generation and most second-generation H₁ antagonists are metabolized by CYPs and little, if any, is excreted unchanged in the urine; most appears there as metabolites (Bartra et al., 2006; Simons, 2004). Exceptions are cetirizine and acrivastine (<40% metabolized) and fexofenadine, levocetirizine, and epinastine (<10% metabolized). Cetirizine, levocetirizine, and acrivastine are excreted primarily into the urine; fexofenadine is mainly excreted in the feces, and epinastine is excreted in both urine (55%) and feces (30%).

The H₁ antagonists that are metabolized are eliminated more rapidly by children than by adults and more slowly in those with severe liver disease. These antagonists also have higher potential for drug interactions. For example, plasma levels of H₁ antagonists may be reduced when coadministered with drugs that induce CYP synthesis (e.g., benzodiazepines) or elevated when taken with drugs that compete with or inhibit the same CYP isoform (e.g., erythromycin, ketoconazole, antidepressants) (Bartra et al., 2006; Simons, 2004). Clinically relevant interactions are more likely with first-generation than second-generation drugs, which have a higher therapeutic index. However, two second-generation H₁ antagonists marketed previously, *terfenadine* and *astemizole*, were found in rare cases to prolong the QTc interval and induce a potentially fatal arrhythmia, torsade de pointes, due to their capacity to inhibit a cardiac K⁺ channel, I_{Kr}, when their metabolism was impaired and their plasma concentrations rose too high, due, for instance, to liver disease or to drugs that inhibited the CYP3A family (Bartra et al., 2006; Simons, 2004) (see Chapter 30). This led to the withdrawal of terfenadine and astemizole from the market. Astemizole and an active hydroxylated metabolite naturally have very long half-lives. Terfenadine is a prodrug,

TABLE 39–2 ■ PREPARATIONS AND DOSAGE OF REPRESENTATIVE H$_1$ RECEPTOR ANTAGONISTS[a]

CLASS *Generic name*	DURATION OF ACTION (h)[b]	PREPARATIONS[c]	SINGLE DOSE (adult)
First-generation agents			
Tricyclic dibenzoxepins			
Doxepin HCl	6–24	O, L, T	10–150 mg; insomnia: 6 mg (O)
			Pruritus: thin film 4 times/d (T)
Ethanolamines			
Carbinoxamine maleate	3–6	O, L	4–8 mg; 6–16 mg (SR)
Clemastine fumarate	12	O, L	1.34–2.68 mg
Diphenhydramine HCl	12	O, L, I, T	25–50 mg (O/L/I)
Dimenhydrinate[d]	4–6	O, I	50–100 mg
Ethylenediamines			
Pyrilamine maleate (only in combination products)	4–6	O, L	7.5–30 mg
Alkylamines			
Chlorpheniramine maleate	24	O, L, I, SR	4 mg, 12 mg (SR)
Brompheniramine maleate	4–6	O, L, I, SR	2 mg
Piperazines			
Hydroxyzine HCl	6–24	O, L, I	25–100 mg
Hydroxyzine pamoate	6–24	O, L (not in the U.S.)	25–100 mg
Cyclizine HCl	4–6	O	50 mg
Cyclizine lactate (not in the U.S.)	4–6	I	50 mg
Meclizine HCl	12–24	O	25–50 mg
Phenothiazines			
Promethazine HCl	4–6	O, L, I, S	12.5–50 mg
Piperidines			
Cyproheptadine HCl[e]	4–6	O, L	1–6.5 mg
Second-generation agents			
Tricyclic dibenzoxepins			
Olopatadine HCl	6–12	T	2 sprays/nostril; 1 drop/eye
Alkylamines			
Acrivastine[f]	6–8	O	8 mg
Piperazines			
Cetirizine HCl[f]	12–24	O, L	5–10 mg
Levocetirizine HCl	12–24	O, L	2.5–5 mg
Piperidines			
Alcaftadine	16–24	T	1 drop/eye
Bepotastine besilate	8	T	1 drop/eye
Desloratadine	24	O, L	5 mg
Fexofenadine HCl	12–24	O, L	60–180 mg
Ketotifen fumarate	8–12	T	1 drop/eye
Loratadine	24	O, L	10 mg
Other second-generation drugs			
Azelastine HCl[f]	12–24	T	2 sprays/nostril; 1 drop/eye
Emedastine	8–12	T	1 drop/eye
Epinastine	8–12	T	1 drop/eye

[a]For a discussion of phenothiazines, see Chapter 16.
[b]Duration of action of H$_1$ antihistamines by objective assessment of suppression of histamine- or allergen-induced symptoms is longer than expected from measurement of plasma concentrations or terminal elimination $t_{1/2}$ values.
[c]Preparations are designated as follows: O, oral solids; L, oral liquids; I, injection; S, suppository; SR, sustained release; T, topical. Many H$_1$ receptor antagonists also are available in preparations that contain multiple drugs. SR forms dissuade pseudoephedrine extraction for methamphetamine production.
[d]Dimenhydrinate is a combination of diphenhydramine and 8-chlorotheophylline in equal molecular proportions.
[e]Also has antiserotonin properties.
[f]Has mild sedating effects.

metabolized by hepatic CYP3A4 to fexofenadine, which is its replacement and lacks noticeable cardiotoxicity. In vitro testing for a new drug's capacity to inhibit I_{Kr} is now available.

Therapeutic Uses

The H_1 antagonists are used for treatment of various immediate hypersensitivity reactions. The central properties of some of the drugs also are of therapeutic value for suppressing motion sickness or for sedation.

Allergic Diseases. H_1 antagonists are useful in acute types of allergy that present with symptoms of rhinitis, urticaria, and conjunctivitis (Simons and Simons, 2011). Their effect is confined to the suppression of symptoms attributable to the histamine released by the antigen-antibody reaction. In bronchial asthma, histamine antagonists have limited efficacy and are not used as sole therapy (see Chapters 38 and 40). In the treatment of systemic anaphylaxis, where autacoids other than histamine are important, the mainstay of therapy is *epinephrine*; histamine antagonists have only a subordinate and adjuvant role. The same is true for severe angioedema, in which laryngeal swelling constitutes a threat to life (see Chapter 12).

Certain allergic dermatoses respond favorably to H_1 antagonists. The benefit is most striking in acute urticaria. H_1 antagonists are also first-line therapy for chronic urticaria but may require doses up to four times higher than that approved for treating rhinitis; patients refractory to high-dose H_1 antagonists should be switched to drugs targeting the immune response (Viegas et al., 2014). H_1 antagonists have a place in the treatment of pruritus. Some relief may be obtained in many patients with atopic and contact dermatitis (although topical corticosteroids are more effective) and in such diverse conditions as insect bites and poison ivy. The urticarial and edematous lesions of serum sickness respond to H_1 antagonists, but fever and arthralgia often do not.

Common Cold. H_1 antagonists are without value in combating the common cold. The weak anticholinergic effects of the older agents may tend to lessen rhinorrhea, but this drying effect may do more harm than good, as may their tendency to induce somnolence.

Motion Sickness, Vertigo, and Sedation. Scopolamine, the muscarinic antagonist, given orally, parenterally, or transdermally, is the most effective drug for the prophylaxis and treatment of motion sickness. Some H_1 antagonists are useful for milder cases and have fewer adverse effects. These drugs include dimenhydrinate and the piperazines (e.g., cyclizine, meclizine). Promethazine, a phenothiazine, is more potent and more effective, and its additional antiemetic properties may be of value in reducing vomiting; however, its pronounced sedative action usually is disadvantageous. Whenever possible, the various drugs should be administered about 1 h before the anticipated motion. Treatment after the onset of nausea and vomiting rarely is beneficial. Some H_1 antagonists, notably dimenhydrinate and meclizine, often are of benefit in vestibular disturbances such as Ménière disease and in other types of true vertigo. Only promethazine is useful in treating the nausea and vomiting subsequent to chemotherapy or radiation therapy for malignancies; however, other, more effective, antiemetic drugs (e.g., $5HT_3$ antagonists) are available (see Chapter 50). Diphenhydramine can reverse the extrapyramidal side effects caused by antipsychotics (see Chapter 16). The tendency of some H_1 receptor antagonists to produce somnolence has led to their use as hypnotics. H_1 antagonists, principally diphenhydramine, often are present in various proprietary over-the-counter remedies for insomnia. The sedative and mild antianxiety activities of hydroxyzine contribute to its use as an anxiolytic.

Adverse Effects

The most frequent side effect of first-generation H_1 antagonists is sedation. Concurrent ingestion of alcohol or other CNS depressants produces an additive effect that impairs motor skills. Other untoward central actions include dizziness, tinnitus, lassitude, incoordination, fatigue, blurred vision, diplopia, euphoria, nervousness, insomnia, and tremors. Other potential side effects, including loss of appetite, nausea, vomiting, epigastric distress, and constipation or diarrhea, may be reduced by taking the drug with meals. H_1 antagonists such as cyproheptadine may increase appetite and cause weight gain. Other side effects, owing to the antimuscarinic actions of some first-generation H_1 antagonists, include dryness of the mouth and respiratory passages (sometimes inducing cough), urinary retention or frequency, and dysuria. These effects are not observed with second-generation H_1 antagonists. Allergic dermatitis is not uncommon; other hypersensitivity reactions include drug fever and photosensitization. Hematological complications, such as leukopenia, agranulocytosis, and hemolytic anemia, are very rare.

Because H_1 antihistamines cross the placenta, caution is advised for women who are or may become pregnant (Simons and Simons, 2011). Several antihistamines (e.g., azelastine, hydroxyzine, fexofenadine) had teratogenic effects in animal studies, whereas others (e.g., chlorpheniramine, diphenhydramine, cetirizine, loratadine) did not. A recent systematic review concluded that antihistamines are unlikely to be strong risk factors for major birth defects (Gilboa et al., 2014). A combination drug consisting of the H_1 antagonist doxylamine and vitamin B_6 (pyridoxine) was approved in 1956 for treating the nausea and vomiting of pregnancy and then voluntarily removed in 1983 due to concerns over birth defects. Subsequent analyses showed the drug caused no increased risk of birth defects, and in 2013 it was reapproved for the same indication in a fixed-dose, delayed-release formulation. Antihistamines can be excreted in small amounts in breast milk, and first-generation antihistamines taken by lactating mothers may cause symptoms such as irritability, drowsiness, or respiratory depression in the nursing infant.

In acute poisoning with first-generation H_1 antagonists, their central excitatory effects constitute the greatest danger. The syndrome includes hallucinations, excitement, ataxia, incoordination, athetosis, and convulsions, fixed, dilated pupils with a flushed face, together with sinus tachycardia, urinary retention, dry mouth, and fever. The syndrome exhibits a remarkable similarity to that of atropine poisoning. Terminally, there is deepening coma with cardiorespiratory collapse and death usually within 2–18 h. Treatment is along general symptomatic and supportive lines. Overdoses of second-generation H_1 antagonists have not been associated with significant toxicity (Simons and Simons, 2011).

Pediatric and Geriatric Indications and Problems. Although little clinical testing has been done, second-generation antihistamines are preferred for elderly patients (>65 years of age), especially those with impaired cognitive function, because of the sedative and anticholinergic effects of first-generation drugs (Simons, 2004). In addition, a recent prospective study in participants 65 years old and older without dementia showed a significant 10-year cumulative dose-response relationship between use of anticholinergics (first-generation H_1 antagonists among the most common) and risk of dementia, primarily Alzheimer disease (Gray et al., 2015).

First-generation antihistamines are not recommended for use in children because their sedative effects can impair learning and school performance. The second-generation drugs have been approved by the FDA for use in children and are available in appropriate lower-dose formulations (e.g., chewable or rapidly dissolving tablets, syrup). Use of over-the-counter cough and cold medicines (containing mixtures of antihistamines, decongestants, antitussives, expectorants) in young children has been associated with serious side effects and deaths. In 2008, the FDA recommended that they should not be used in children less than 2 years of age, and drug manufacturers affiliated with the Consumer Healthcare Products Association voluntarily relabeled products "do not use" for children less than 4 years of age.

Available H₁ Antagonists

Summarized next are notable properties of a number of H_1 antagonists, grouped by their chemical structures. Representative preparations are listed in Table 39–2.

First-Generation Dibenzoxepin Tricyclic (Doxepin). Doxepin is marketed as a tricyclic antidepressant (see Chapter 15). It also is one of the most potent H_1 antagonists and has significant H_2 antagonist activity, but this does not translate into greater clinical effectiveness. It can cause drowsiness and is associated with anticholinergic effects. Doxepin is better tolerated by patients with depression than those who are not depressed, for whom even small doses may cause disorientation and confusion.

Second-Generation Dibenzoxepin Tricyclic (Olopatadine). Olopatadine is a topical H_1 antagonist with additional mast cell–stabilizing and anti-inflammatory properties. In drop form, it is an effective treatment of allergic conjunctivitis and as a spray helps reduce the nasal symptoms of allergic rhinitis.

Ethanolamines (Prototype: Diphenhydramine). The ethanolamines possess significant antimuscarinic activity and have a pronounced tendency to induce sedation. About half of those treated acutely with conventional doses experience somnolence. The incidence of GI side effects, however, is low with this group.

Ethylenediamine (Prototype: Pyrilamine). Pyrilamine is among the most specific H_1 antagonists. Although its central effects are relatively feeble, somnolence occurs in a fair proportion of patients. GI side effects are common.

First-Generation Alkylamines (Prototype: Chlorpheniramine). The first-generation alkylamines are among the most potent H_1 antagonists. The drugs are less prone to produce drowsiness and are more suitable for daytime use, but a significant proportion of patients still experience sedation. Side effects involving CNS stimulation are more common than with other groups.

Second-Generation Alkylamine (Acrivastine). The second-generation alkylamine is a derivative of the first-generation alkylamine triprolidine and may exhibit a somewhat higher incidence of mild sedation than other second-generation H_1 antagonists.

First-Generation Piperazines. Hydroxyzine is a long-acting compound that is used widely for skin allergies; its considerable CNS-depressant activity may contribute to its prominent antipruritic action, and it is also used as a sedative and antianxiety agent. Cyclizine and meclizine have been used primarily to counter motion sickness, although promethazine and diphenhydramine are more effective (as is the antimuscarinic scopolamine).

Second-Generation Piperazines (Cetirizine). Cetirizine has minimal anticholinergic effects. It also has negligible penetration into the brain but is associated with a somewhat higher incidence of drowsiness than most other second-generation H_1 antagonists. The active enantiomer levocetirizine has slightly greater potency and may be used at half the dose with less resultant sedation. Cetirizine and levocetirizine have additional mast cell–stabilizing and anti-inflammatory properties.

Phenothiazines (Prototype: Promethazine). Promethazine, which has prominent sedative and considerable anticholinergic effects, and its many congeners are used primarily for their antiemetic effects (see Chapter 50).

First-Generation Piperidine (Cyproheptadine). Cyproheptadine uniquely has both antihistamine and antiserotonin activity by antagonizing the $5HT_{2A}$ receptor. Cyproheptadine causes drowsiness; it also has significant anticholinergic effects and can increase appetite.

Second-Generation Piperidines (Prototype: Loratadine). Terfenadine and astemizole, early second-generation drugs, are no longer marketed because of their potential for causing a rare, but potentially fatal, arrhythmia, torsade de pointes (see previous discussion). Terfenadine was replaced by fexofenadine, an active metabolite that lacks the toxic side effects of terfenadine, is not sedating, and retains the antiallergic properties of the parent compound. Another antihistamine of this class developed using this strategy is *desloratadine*, an active metabolite of loratadine. These agents lack significant anticholinergic actions and penetrate poorly into the CNS. Taken together, these properties appear to account for the low incidence of side effects of piperidine antihistamines. All members of this class have mast cell–stabilizing and anti-inflammatory properties. Although the therapeutic significance of these additional effects are unclear for the drugs administered orally, they appear to provide additional benefit when used in topical formulations to treat allergic conjunctivitis. Alcaftadine has additional antagonist activity on H_4 receptors, which likely explains

its superiority to other topical H_1 antagonists in reducing the ocular itch of allergic conjunctivitis (Thurmond, 2015).

Other Second-Generation H_1 Antagonists. Drugs in this group (azelastine, emedastine, and epinastine) have divergent structures with therapeutic efficacy and side effects similar to other second-generation H_1 antagonists. They all are marketed as topical eye drops for the treatment of allergic conjunctivitis; azelastine is also available as a nasal spray for treating symptoms of allergic or vasomotor rhinitis. Epinastine has both H_1 and H_2 antagonist activity, which may help reduce eyelid edema. Epinastine and azelastine exhibit mast cell–stabilizing and anti-inflammatory properties. Emedastine is a highly selective H_1 antagonist without these additional actions.

H_2 Receptor Antagonists

The pharmacology and clinical utility of H_2 antagonists (e.g., cimetidine, ranitidine) for inhibiting gastric acid secretion in the treatment of GI disorders are described in Chapter 50.

H_3 Receptor Antagonists

The H_3 receptors are presynaptic autoreceptors on histaminergic neurons that originate in the tuberomammillary nucleus in the hypothalamus and project throughout the CNS, most prominently to the hippocampus, amygdala, nucleus accumbens, globus pallidus, striatum, hypothalamus, and cortex (Haas et al., 2008; Sander et al., 2008). The activated H_3 receptor depresses neuronal firing at the level of cell bodies/dendrites and decreases histamine release from depolarized terminals. Thus, H_3 agonists decrease histaminergic transmission, and antagonists increase it.

The H_3 receptors also are presynaptic heteroreceptors on a variety of neurons in brain and peripheral tissues, and their activation inhibits transmitter release from noradrenergic, serotoninergic, GABAergic, cholinergic, and glutamatergic neurons, as well as pain-sensitive C fibers. H_3 receptors in the brain have significant constitutive activity in the absence of agonist; consequently, inverse agonists reduce this constitutive activity, withdraw inhibition of transmitter release, and thereby promote transmitter release (activation of these neurons).

The H_3 antagonists/inverse agonists have a wide range of central effects; for example, they promote wakefulness, improve cognitive function (e.g., enhance memory, learning, and attention), and reduce food intake. As a result, there is considerable interest in developing H_3 antagonists for possible treatment of sleeping disorders, ADHD, epilepsy, cognitive impairment, schizophrenia, obesity, neuropathic pain, and Alzheimer disease (Haas et al., 2008; Sander et al., 2008). Thioperamide was the first "specific" H_3 antagonist/inverse agonist available experimentally, but it was equally effective at the H_4 receptor. A number of other imidazole derivatives have been developed as H_3 antagonists, including clobenpropit, ciproxifan, and proxyfan, but the imidazole ring enhances binding to the H_4 receptor and CYPs. Because of this, more selective nonimidazole H_3 antagonists/inverse agonists (e.g., tiprolisant) were developed (Haas et al., 2008; Sander et al., 2008), and some are now in phase 2 and 3 clinical trials.

H_4 Receptor Antagonists

The H_4 receptors are expressed on cells with inflammatory or immune functions and can mediate histamine-induced chemotaxis, induction of cell shape change, secretion of cytokines, and upregulation of adhesion molecules (Thurmond et al., 2008). The H_4 receptors also have a role in pruritus and neuropathic pain. Because of the unique localization and function of H_4 receptors, H_4 antagonists are promising candidates to treat inflammatory conditions and possibly pruritus and neuropathic pain (Thurmond, 2015). The H_4-specific antagonist JNJ-39758979 has been tested in phase 1 and 2 clinical trials for treatment of persistent asthma, pruritis, dermatitis, and rheumatoid arthritis.

The H_4 receptor has the highest homology with the H_3 receptor and binds many H_3 ligands, especially those with imidazole rings, although sometimes with different effects (Thurmond et al., 2008). For example, thioperamide is an effective inverse agonist at both H_3 and H_4 receptors, whereas H_3 inverse agonist clobenpropit is a partial agonist of the H_4

receptor; impentamine (an H_3 agonist) and iodophenpropit (an H_3 inverse agonist) are both neutral H_4 antagonists.

Bradykinin, Kallidin, and Their Antagonists

In the 1920s and 1930s, Frey, Kraut, and Werle characterized a hypotensive substance in urine, which was also found in other fluids and tissues, and named this material *kallikrein* after a Greek synonym for the pancreas, an especially rich source (Werle, 1970). It was established that kallikrein generates a pharmacologically active substance from an inactive precursor present in plasma; the active substance, *kallidin*, proved to be a polypeptide cleaved from a plasma globulin (Werle, 1970). Rocha e Silva, Beraldo, and associates later reported that trypsin and certain snake venoms acted on plasma globulin to produce a substance that lowered blood pressure and caused a slowly developing contraction of the gut (Rocha e Silva et al., 1949); they named it *bradykinin*, derived from the Greek words *bradys*, meaning "slow," and *kinein*, meaning "to move." In 1960, bradykinin, a nine amino acid peptide, was isolated and synthesized; shortly thereafter, kallidin was identified as bradykinin with an additional N-terminal Lys residue. The kinins have short half-lives because they are destroyed by plasma and tissue peptidases (Erdös and Skidgel, 1997). Two types of kinin receptors, B_1 and B_2, were identified based on the rank order of potency of kinin analogues and later validated by cloning (Leeb-Lundberg et al., 2005). The development of receptor-specific antagonists and receptor knockout mice have furthered our understanding of the role of kinins in the regulation of cardiovascular homeostasis and inflammatory processes (Leeb-Lundberg et al., 2005).

Tissue damage, allergic reactions, viral infections, and other inflammatory events activate a series of proteolytic reactions that generate bradykinin and kallidin in tissues. These peptides contribute to inflammatory responses as autacoids that act locally to produce pain, vasodilation, and increased vascular permeability but can also have beneficial effects, for example, in the heart, kidney, and circulation (Bhoola et al., 1992). Much of their activity is due to stimulation of the release of potent mediators such as prostaglandins, NO, or EDHF.

The Endogenous Kallikrein-Kininogen-Kinin System

The nonapeptide bradykinin and decapeptide kallidin (*lysyl-bradykinin*) (Table 39–3) are cleaved from α_2 globulins termed *kininogens* (Figure 39–4). There are two kininogens: HMW kininogen and LMW kininogen. A number of serine proteases will generate kinins, but the two highly specific proteases that release bradykinin and kallidin from the kininogens are termed *kallikreins*.

Kallikreins

Bradykinin and kallidin are cleaved from HMW or LMW kininogens by plasma or tissue kallikrein, respectively (see Figure 39–4). Plasma kallikrein and tissue kallikrein are distinct enzymes that are activated by different mechanisms (Bhoola et al., 1992). Plasma prekallikrein is an inactive protein of about 88 kDa that complexes with its substrate, HMW kininogen. The ensuing proteolytic cascade is normally restrained by the protease inhibitors present in plasma, most importantly the activated first component of complement (C1-INH) and α_2 macroglobulin. Under experimental conditions, the kallikrein-kinin system is activated by the binding of factor XII (*Hageman factor*) to negatively charged surfaces. Bound factor XII, a protease that is common to both the kinin and the intrinsic coagulation cascades (see Chapter 32), slowly undergoes autoactivation and, in turn, activates prekallikrein. Importantly, kallikrein rapidly further activates factor XII, thereby exerting a positive feedback on the system. In vivo, the order of this process can be reversed. The binding of the HMW kininogen–prekallikrein heterodimer to a multiprotein-receptor complex on endothelial cells leads to activation of the prekallikrein-HMW kininogen complex by either heat shock protein 90 (Hsp90) or prolylcarboxypeptidase to generate kallikrein, which can then activate factor XII to start the positive-feedback loop, and cleave HMW

TABLE 39–3 ■ STRUCTURE OF KININ AGONISTS AND ANTAGONISTS

NAME	STRUCTURE	FUNCTION
Bradykinin	Arg-Pro-Pro-Gly-Phe-Ser-Pro-Phe-Arg	Agonist, B_2
Kallidin	Lys-Arg-Pro-Pro-Gly-Phe-Ser-Pro-Phe-Arg	Agonist, B_2
[des-Arg^9]-Bradykinin	Arg-Pro-Pro-Gly-Phe-Ser-Pro-Phe	Agonist, B_1
[des-Arg^{10}]-Kallidin	Lys-Arg-Pro-Pro-Gly-Phe-Ser-Pro-Phe	Agonist, B_1
des-Arg^{10}-[Leu^9]-Kallidin	Lys-Arg-Pro-Pro-Gly-Phe-Ser-Pro-Leu	Antagonist, B_1
NPC-349	[D-Arg]-Arg-Pro-Hyp-Gly-Thi-Ser-D-Phe-Thi-Arg	Antagonist, B_2
HOE-140	[D-Arg]-Arg-Pro-Hyp-Gly-Thi-Ser-Tic-Oic-Arg	Antagonist, B_2
[des-Arg^{10}]-HOE-140	[D-Arg]-Arg-Pro-Hyp-Gly-Thi-Ser-Tic-Oic	Antagonist, B_1
FR173657	See Figure 32–3 of the 12th edition	Antagonist, B_2
FR190997		Agonist, B_2
SSR240612		Antagonist, B_1

Hyp, trans-4-hydroxy-Pro; Thi, β-(2-thienyl)-Ala; Tic, [D]-1,2,3,4-tetrahydroisoquinolin-3-yl-carbonyl; Oic, (3as,7as)-octahydroindol-2-yl-carbonyl.

kininogen to generate bradykinin (Kaplan and Joseph, 2014). This process may contribute to the symptoms of hereditary angioedema in patients that lack C1-INH.

Human tissue kallikrein is 1 of 15 gene family members with high sequence identity that are clustered at chromosome 19q13.4 (Prassas et al., 2015). However, the classical "tissue kallikrein," hK1, is the only family member to readily generate kallidin from LMW kininogen. Tissue kallikrein is synthesized as a 29-kDa preprotein in the epithelial cells or secretory cells in several tissues, including salivary glands, pancreas, prostate, and renal distal nephron (Bhoola et al., 1992). Tissue kallikrein also is expressed in human neutrophils; it acts locally near its sites of origin. The synthesis of tissue prokallikrein is controlled by a number of factors, including aldosterone in the kidney and salivary gland and androgens in certain other glands. The activation of tissue prokallikrein to kallikrein requires proteolytic cleavage to remove a seven–amino acid propeptide, which can be accomplished in vitro by plasma kallikrein and by some serine and metalloproteases. However, the activating enzyme(s) in vivo is unknown.

Kininogens

The two substrates for the kallikreins, HMW kininogen (120 kDa) and LMW kininogen (66 kDa), are derived from a single gene by alternative splicing. The first 401 amino acids are identical (through the bradykinin sequence and 12 additional residues) and then the sequences diverge, with HMW kininogen containing a 56-kDa C-terminal light chain and LMW kininogen a 4-kDa light chain (Bhoola et al., 1992). HMW kininogen is cleaved by both plasma and tissue kallikrein to yield bradykinin and kallidin, respectively, whereas LMW kininogen is cleaved only by tissue kallikrein to produce kallidin.

Metabolism of Kinins

The decapeptide kallidin is about as active as the nonapeptide bradykinin, even without conversion to bradykinin, which occurs when the N-terminal lysine residue is removed by an aminopeptidase (see Figure 39–4). The $t_{1/2}$ of kinins in plasma is only about 15 sec; 80%–90% of the kinins may

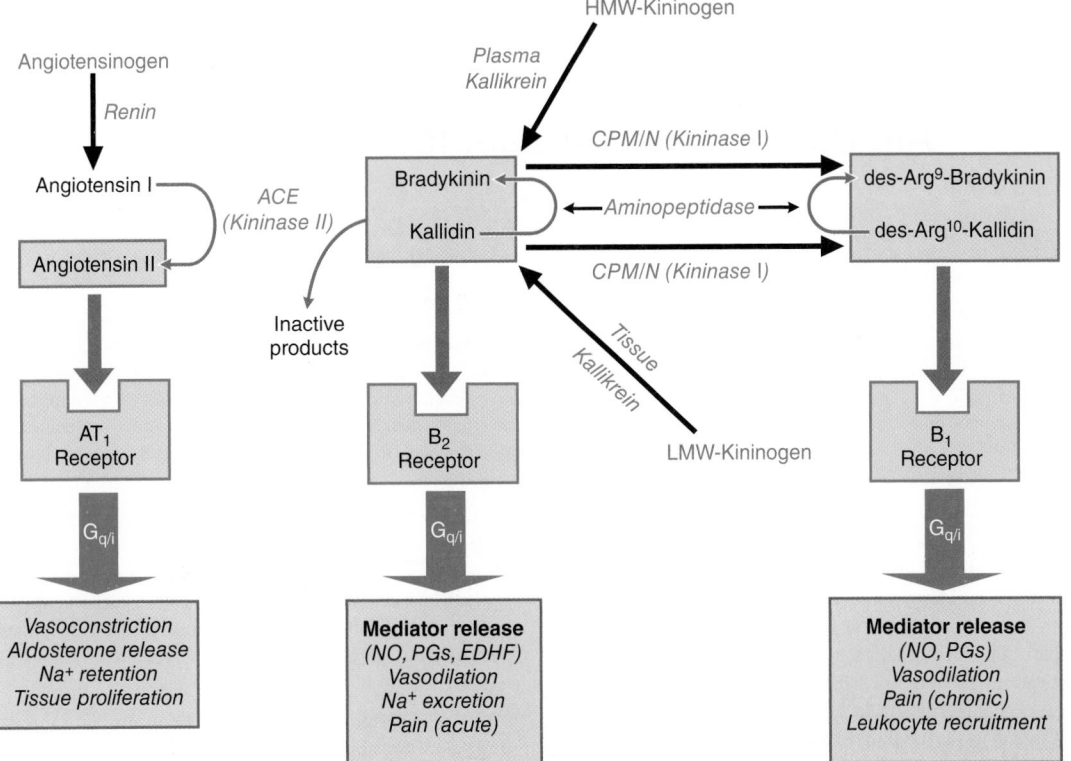

Figure 39–4 *Synthesis and receptor interactions of active peptides generated by the kallikrein-kinin and renin-angiotensin systems.* Bradykinin is generated by the action of plasma kallikrein on HMW kininogen, whereas kallidin (Lys1-bradykinin) is released by the hydrolysis of LMW kininogen by tissue kallikrein. Kallidin and bradykinin are the natural ligands of the B$_2$ receptor but can be converted to corresponding agonists of the B$_1$ receptor by removal of the C-terminal Arg by kininase I–type enzymes: the plasma membrane–bound CPM or soluble plasma CPN. Kallidin or [des-Arg^{10}]-kallidin can be converted to the active peptides bradykinin or to [des-Arg^9]-bradykinin by aminopeptidase cleavage of the N-terminal Lys residue. In a parallel fashion, the inactive decapeptide AngI is generated by the action of renin on the plasma substrate angiotensinogen. By removal of the C-terminal His-Leu dipeptide, ACE generates the active peptide AngII. These two systems have opposing effects. AngII is a potent vasoconstrictor that also causes aldosterone release and Na$^+$ retention via activation of the AT$_1$ receptor; bradykinin is a vasodilator that stimulates Na$^+$ excretion by activating the B$_2$ receptor. ACE generates active AngII and, at the same time, inactivates bradykinin and kallidin; thus, its effects are prohypertensive, and ACE inhibitors are effective antihypertensive agents. The B$_2$ receptor mediates most of bradykinin's effects under normal circumstances, whereas synthesis of the B$_1$ receptor is induced by inflammatory mediators in inflammatory conditions. Both B$_1$ and B$_2$ receptors couple through G$_q$ to activate PLC and increase intracellular Ca^{2+}; the physiological response depends on receptor distribution on particular cell types and occupancy by agonist peptides. For instance, on endothelial cells, activation of B$_2$ receptors results in Ca^{2+}-calmodulin–dependent activation of eNOS and generation of NO, which causes cyclic GMP accumulation and relaxation in neighboring smooth muscle cells. However, in endothelial cells under inflammatory conditions, B$_1$ receptor stimulation results in prolonged NO production via G$_i$ and an acute MAP kinase–dependent activation of iNOS. On smooth muscle cells, activation of kinin receptors coupling through G$_q$ results in an increased [Ca^{2+}]i and contraction. B$_1$ and B$_2$ receptors also can couple through G$_i$ to activate PLA$_2$, causing the release of arachidonic acid and the local generation of prostanoids (PGs) and other metabolites such as EDHF. Kallikrein also plays a role in the intrinsic blood coagulation pathway (see Chapter 32).

be destroyed in a single passage through the pulmonary vascular bed by enzymes present on the large endothelial surface area of the lung (Erdös and Skidgel, 1997). Plasma concentrations of bradykinin are difficult to measure because inadequate inhibition of kininogenases or kininases in the blood can lead to artifactual formation or degradation of bradykinin during blood collection. When care is taken to inhibit these processes, the reported physiological concentrations of bradykinin in blood are in the picomolar range.

The principal catabolizing enzyme in the lung and other vascular beds is kininase II, or ACE, a membrane-anchored peptidase on the surface of endothelial cells (see Chapter 26). Removal of the C-terminal dipeptide by ACE or neutral endopeptidase 24.11 (neprilysin) inactivates kinins (Figure 39–5) (Erdös and Skidgel, 1997). A slower-acting plasma enzyme, carboxypeptidase N (lysine carboxypeptidase, kininase I), releases the C-terminal arginine residue, producing [desArg^9]-bradykinin or [des-Arg^{10}]-kallidin (see Table 39–3 and Figures 39–4 and 39–5) (Skidgel and Erdös, 2007), either of which no longer activate B$_2$ receptors but are potent B$_1$ receptor agonists. Carboxypeptidase N is expressed in the liver and constitutively secreted into the blood. A rare familial

carboxypeptidase N deficiency was associated with angioedema or urticaria, possibly due to increased bradykinin (Skidgel and Erdös, 2007). Carboxypeptidase M, which cleaves the C-terminal Arg of bradykinin about 3-fold faster than carboxypeptidase N, is a widely distributed plasma membrane–bound enzyme that is also found on lung microvascular endothelial cells (Zhang et al., 2013a). Finally, aminopeptidase P is a membrane enzyme on epithelial and endothelial cells that can cleave the N-terminal arginine of bradykinin, rendering it inactive and susceptible to further cleavage by dipeptidyl peptidase IV (Erdös and Skidgel, 1997) (Figure 39–5).

Kinin Receptors and Their Signaling Pathways

The B$_1$ and B$_2$ kinin receptors are GPCRs whose signaling mediates most of the biological effects of the kallikrein-kinin system (Leeb-Lundberg et al., 2005). The B$_2$ receptor is expressed in most normal tissues, where it selectively binds intact bradykinin and kallidin (see Table 39–3 and Figure 39–4). The B$_2$ receptor mediates the effects of bradykinin and kallidin under normal circumstances, whereas synthesis of the B$_1$ receptor is induced by inflammatory conditions. The B$_1$ receptor is activated by the

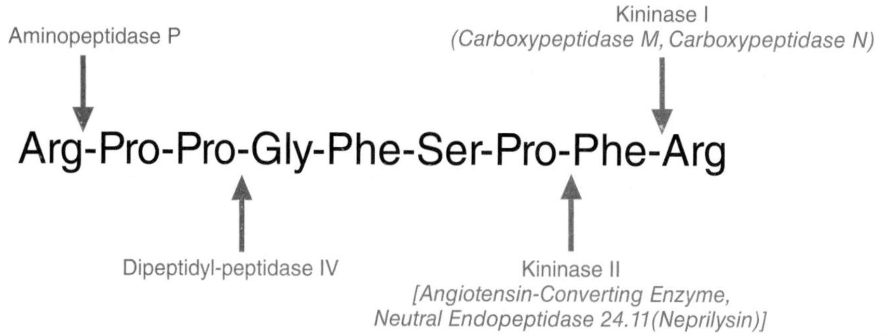

Aminopeptidase P

Kininase I
(Carboxypeptidase M, Carboxypeptidase N)

$$\text{Arg-Pro-Pro-Gly-Phe-Ser-Pro-Phe-Arg}$$

Dipeptidyl-peptidase IV

Kininase II
*[Angiotensin-Converting Enzyme,
Neutral Endopeptidase 24.11(Neprilysin)]*

Figure 39–5 *Schematic diagram of the degradation of bradykinin.* Arrows denote the primary cleavage sites in bradykinin. Bradykinin and kallidin are inactivated in vivo primarily by kininase II (ACE). Neutral endopeptidase 24.11 (neprilysin) cleaves bradykinin and kallidin at the same Pro-Phe bond as ACE and also is classified as a kininase II–type enzyme. In addition, aminopeptidase P can inactivate bradykinin by hydrolyzing the N-terminal Arg1-Pro2 bond, leaving bradykinin susceptible to further degradation by dipeptidyl peptidase IV. Bradykinin and kallidin are converted to their respective des-Arg^9 or des-Arg^{10} metabolites by kininase I–type carboxypeptidases M and N. Unlike the parent peptides, these kinin metabolites are potent ligands for B$_1$ kinin receptors but not B$_2$ kinin receptors.

C-terminal des-Arg metabolites of bradykinin and kallidin produced by the actions of carboxypeptidases N and M. Interestingly, carboxypeptidase M and the B$_1$ receptor interact on the cell surface to form an efficient signaling complex that enhances B$_1$ receptor agonist affinity and can lead to allosteric activation of B$_1$ receptor signaling by substrate binding to carboxypeptidase M (Zhang et al., 2013a, 2013b). B$_1$ receptors are normally absent or expressed at low levels in most tissues. B$_1$ receptor expression is upregulated by tissue injury and inflammation and by cytokines, endotoxins, and growth factors. Carboxypeptidase M expression also is increased by cytokines, to such a degree that B$_1$ receptor effects may predominate over B$_2$ effects (Zhang et al., 2013a).

Both B$_1$ and B$_2$ receptors couple through G$_q$ to activate PLC and increase intracellular Ca^{2+}; the physiological response depends on receptor distribution on particular cell types, the cell environment, and mediators generated (Leeb-Lundberg et al., 2005). For example, on normal endothelial cells, activation of B$_2$ receptors results in G$_q$ and Ca^{2+}-calmodulin-dependent activation of eNOS and short-term generation of NO, which causes cyclic GMP accumulation and relaxation in neighboring smooth muscle cells. However, direct activation of B$_1$ or B$_2$ receptors on smooth muscle cells leads to coupling through G$_q$ and increased [Ca^{2+}]$_i$, resulting in contraction.

Inflammatory conditions alter receptor signaling in endothelial cells, such that B$_2$ receptor stimulation leads to prolonged eNOS-derived NO that depends on G$_i$-mediated activation of MEK1/2 and JNK1/2, whereas B$_1$ receptor activation couples through G$_i$ and MAP kinase activation to cause ERK1/2-mediated phosphorylation and activation of iNOS, which generates prolonged, high-output NO (Kuhr et al., 2010; Lowry et al., 2013). Both B$_1$ and B$_2$ receptor stimulation activate the pro-inflammatory transcription factor NF-κB coupled through Gα$_q$ and βγ subunits and also activate the MAP kinase pathway (Leeb-Lundberg et al., 2005). B$_1$ and B$_2$ receptors also can couple through G$_i$ to activate PLA$_2$, causing the release of arachidonic acid and the local generation of metabolites such as prostaglandins and vasodilator EETs (Campbell and Falck, 2007).

The B$_1$ and B$_2$ receptors differ in their time courses of downregulation after agonist stimulation; the B$_2$ receptor response is rapidly desensitized, whereas the B$_1$ response is not (Leeb-Lundberg et al., 2005). This likely is due to modification at a Ser/Thr-rich cluster present in the C-terminal tail of the B$_2$ receptor that is not conserved in the B$_1$ receptor sequence. However, the B$_1$ receptor can heterodimerize with the B$_2$ receptor and in this form can be cross desensitized by activation of the B$_2$ receptor with agonist (Zhang et al., 2015).

Functions and Pharmacology of Kallikreins and Kinins

The utility of specific kinin receptor antagonists currently is being investigated in diverse areas such as pain, inflammation, chronic inflammatory diseases, and the cardiovascular system (Campos et al., 2006). The beneficial effects of ACE inhibitor therapy rest in part on enhancing bradykinin activity (e.g., on the heart, kidney, blood pressure; see Chapter 26); this has led to the suggestion that kinin agonists could be therapeutically beneficial (Heitsch, 2003).

Pain. The kinins are powerful algesic agents that cause an intense burning pain when applied to the exposed base of a blister. Bradykinin excites primary sensory neurons and provokes the release of neuropeptides such as substance P, neurokinin A, and calcitonin gene–related peptide. Although there is overlap, B$_2$ receptors generally mediate acute bradykinin algesia, whereas the pain of chronic inflammation appears to involve increased numbers and activation of B$_1$ receptors.

Inflammation. Kinins participate in a variety of inflammatory conditions (Bhoola et al., 1992; Leeb-Lundberg et al., 2005). Plasma kinins increase permeability in the microcirculation, acting on the small venules to cause disruption of the interendothelial junctions. This, together with an increased hydrostatic pressure gradient, causes edema. Edema, coupled with stimulation of nerve endings, results in a wheal-and-flare response to intradermal injection. In acute attacks of hereditary angioedema, excess bradykinin is formed, as reflected by depletion of the upstream components of the kinin cascade, and is a primary mediator of swelling, laryngeal edema, and abdominal pain (Walford and Zuraw, 2014).

The B$_1$ receptors on inflammatory cells (e.g., macrophages) can elicit production of the inflammatory mediators IL-1 and TNF-α. Kinin levels are increased in a number of chronic inflammatory diseases and may be significant in gout, disseminated intravascular coagulation, inflammatory bowel disease, rheumatoid arthritis, or asthma. In addition, kinins and their receptors are associated with a variety of neuroinflammatory disorders, including neuropathic pain in diabetes, autoimmune encephalomyelitis, and Alzheimer disease. Kinins may contribute to the skeletal changes seen in chronic inflammatory states; kinins stimulate bone resorption through B$_1$ and possibly B$_2$ receptors, perhaps by osteoblast-mediated osteoclast activation (see Chapter 44).

Respiratory Disease. The kinins have been implicated in allergic airway disorders such as asthma and rhinitis (Abraham et al., 2006). Inhalation of kinins causes bronchospasm mimicking an asthma attack in asthmatic patients but not in normal individuals. This bradykinin-induced bronchoconstriction is blocked by anticholinergic agents but not by antihistamines or cyclooxygenase inhibitors. Similarly, nasal challenge with bradykinin is followed by sneezing and glandular secretions in patients with allergic rhinitis, but not normal individuals or those with nonallergic, noninfectious perennial rhinitis.

Cardiovascular System. Infusion of bradykinin causes vasodilation and lowers blood pressure. Bradykinin causes vasodilation by activating its B$_2$ receptor on endothelial cells, resulting in the generation of NO, prostacyclin, and a hyperpolarizing EET that is a CYP-derived metabolite of arachidonate (Campbell and Falck, 2007). The endogenous kallikrein-kinin system plays a minor role in the regulation of normal blood pressure, but it may be important in hypertensive states. Urinary kallikrein concentrations are decreased in individuals with high blood pressure.

The kallikrein-kinin system is cardioprotective. Many of the beneficial effects of ACE inhibitors on heart function are attributable to enhancement of bradykinin effects, such as their antiproliferative activity or ability to increase tissue glucose uptake (Heitsch, 2003; Madeddu et al., 2007). Bradykinin contributes to the beneficial effect of preconditioning to protect the heart against ischemia and reperfusion injury. Bradykinin also stimulates tissue plasminogen activator release from the vascular endothelium and may contribute to the endogenous defense against some cardiovascular events, such as myocardial infarction and stroke (Heitsch, 2003; Madeddu et al., 2007).

Kidney. Renal kinins act in a paracrine manner to regulate urine volume and composition. Kallikrein is synthesized and secreted by the connecting cells of the distal nephron. Tissue kininogen and kinin receptors are present in the cells of the collecting duct. Like other vasodilators, kinins increase renal blood flow. Bradykinin also causes natriuresis by inhibiting Na^+ reabsorption at the cortical collecting duct. Treatment with mineralocorticoids, ACE inhibitors, and neutral endopeptidase (neprilysin) inhibitors increases renal kallikrein.

Other Effects. Kinins promote dilation of the fetal pulmonary artery, closure of the ductus arteriosus, and constriction of the umbilical vessels, all of which occur in the transition from fetal to neonatal circulation. Kinins also affect the CNS, disrupting the blood-brain barrier and allowing increased CNS penetration. Kinins and kinin receptor signaling have been associated with neuroinflammatory disorders, such as neuropathic pain in diabetes, autoimmune encephalomyelitis and Alzheimer disease.

Kallikrein Inhibitors

Aprotinin is a natural proteinase inhibitor that inhibits mediators of the inflammatory response, fibrinolysis, and thrombin generation following cardiopulmonary bypass surgery, including kallikrein and plasmin. Aprotinin was employed clinically to reduce blood loss in patients undergoing coronary artery bypass surgery, but unfavorable survival statistics in retrospective and prospective studies resulted in its discontinuation.

Ecallantide is a synthetic plasma kallikrein inhibitor approved for the treatment of acute attacks of hereditary angioedema in patients 12 years and older. It is administered by a healthcare professional (with appropriate medical support to manage possible anaphylaxis) subcutaneously at a total dose of 30 mg, divided into three 10-mg injections of 1 mL each. An additional dose of 30 mg may be administered within a 24-h period if the attack persists. The most common side effects (~3%–8% of patients) include headache, nausea, diarrhea, fever, injection site reactions, and nasopharyngitis. Safety has not been tested in pregnant or nursing women. Anaphylaxis has been reported in about 4% of treated patients, occurring within 1 h after dosing. Approximately 20% of patients treated with ecallantide develop antibodies to the drug and may be at a higher risk of hypersensitivity reactions on subsequent exposure. Ecallantide is currently being investigated as a potential treatment of other forms of angioedema (Zuraw et al., 2013).

Bradykinin and the Effects of ACE Inhibitors

The ACE inhibitors, widely used in the treatment of hypertension, congestive heart failure, and diabetic nephropathy, block the conversion of AngI to AngII and also block the degradation of bradykinin by ACE (see Figure 39–4 and Chapter 26). Numerous studies demonstrated that bradykinin contributes to many of the protective effects of ACE inhibitors (Heitsch, 2003; Madeddu et al., 2007). The search is on to find a suitable stable B_2 agonist for clinical evaluation that provides cardiovascular benefit without pro-inflammatory effects.

A rare side effect of ACE inhibitors is angioedema, which is likely due to the inhibition of kinin metabolism by ACE (Zuraw et al., 2013). A common side effect of ACE inhibitors that may be related to enhanced kinin levels is a chronic, nonproductive cough that dissipates when the drug is stopped. Bradykinin may also contribute to the therapeutic effects of the AT_1 receptor antagonists. During AT_1 receptor blockade, AngII signaling through the unopposed AT_2 subtype receptor is enhanced, causing an increase in bradykinin concentrations, which has beneficial effects on cardiovascular and renal function (Padia and Carey, 2013). However, the increase in bradykinin levels is likely more modest than that achieved by ACE inhibitors, as reflected by the lower incidence of angioedema in patients taking AT_1 receptor antagonists (Zuraw et al., 2013).

Kinin Receptor Antagonists

The selective B_2 receptor antagonist *icatibant* has been approved in the E.U. and recently in the U.S. for treatment of acute episodes of swelling in patients more than 18 years of age with hereditary angioedema. It is administered by a healthcare professional, or self-administered by the patient after training, at a dose of 30 mg in 3 mL of solution by subcutaneous injection in the abdomen. Additional doses may be administered at intervals of at least 6 h if the response is inadequate or symptoms recur, not to exceed three doses in any 24-h period. A common side effect experienced by most patients is a local reaction at the injection site (e.g., redness, bruising, swelling, burning, itching, etc.). A small percentage of patients experienced fever, elevated transaminase, dizziness, nausea, headache, or rash. Safety has not been tested in pregnant or nursing women. Although icatibant has the potential to attenuate the antihypertensive effects of ACE inhibitors, it is unclear if this is clinically significant, since patients taking ACE inhibitors were excluded from clinical trials with icatibant. Icatibant is currently being investigated as treatment of ACE inhibitor–induced angioedema, and initial results of small trials and individual case reports indicate that it is effective (Zuraw et al., 2013). Other forms of angioedema are under investigation for responsiveness to icatibant.

Acknowledgment: *Nancy J. Brown, L. Jackson Roberts II, Ervin G. Erdös, and Allen P. Kaplan contributed to this chapter in earlier editions of this book. We have retained some of their text in the current edition.*

Drug Facts for Your Personal Formulary: H_1 Antagonists

Drugs	Therapeutic Uses	Clinical Pharmacology and Tips
First-Generation Antihistamines: H_1 receptor inverse agonists • Most have central and anticholinergic effects • Use with caution in children and in adults > 65 years of age		
Doxepin	• Tricyclic antidepressant • Insomnia • Pruritis (topical cream) • Pruritis (atopic dermatitis, eczema, lichen simplex) (cream)	• Causes significant sedation/drowsiness • Anticholinergic effects • Increased risk of suicidal thoughts (children, adolescents, and young adults)
Carbinoxamine Clemastine Diphenhydramine Dimenhydrinate	• Symptoms of allergic response • Mild urticaria • Insomnia (diphenhydramine) • Motion sickness (dimenhydrinate, diphenhdramine)	• Pronounced tendency to cause sedation • Significant anticholinergic effects • GI side effects are low • Carbinoxamine and diphenhydramine: adjunct to epinephrine for anaphylaxis
Pyrilamine (only available as an ingredient in OTC combination preparations)	• Symptoms of allergic response	• Anticholinergic effects • Central effects < other first-generation drugs • GI side effects are quite common
Chlorpheniramine Dexchlorpheniramine Brompheniramine Dexbrompheniramine (component of cold medicine)	• Allergic conjunctivitis • Allergic rhinitis • Anaphylaxis (adjunct), histamine-mediated angioedema, dermatographism, pruritus, sneezing, urticaria (brompheniramine) • Symptoms of allergic response	Less drowsiness than other first-generation drugs; CNS stimulation side effects more common
Hydroxyzine	• Pruritis • Sedation • Antianxiety • Atopic dermatitis • Antiemetic • Urticaria	• CNS depressant action may contribute to antipruritic effects
Cyclizine (discontinued in the U.S.) Meclizine (not for use in children)	• Motion sickness • Nausea/vomiting • Vertigo	• Antinausea properties due to prominent anticholinergic effects • Less likely to cause drowsiness than other first-generation drugs • Meclizine, most used, long effect (≥8 h)
Promethazine	• Antiemetic • Motion sickness • Pruritus • Sedation • Symptoms of allergic response (off-label use)	• Risk of fatal respiratory depression in children, especially < 2 years • May lower seizure threshold • Has local anesthetic activity • Most potent antihistamine antiemetic
Cyproheptadine	• Allergic conjunctivitis • Allergic rhinitis • Anaphylaxis • Histamine-mediated angioedema • Pruritus, allergy • Vasomotor rhinitis • Urticaria • Dermatographism	• May increase appetite, cause weight gain • Has significant anticholinergic activity • Also blocks serotonin effects by antagonizing the $5HT_{2A}$ receptor
Second-Generation Antihistamines: H_1 receptor inverse agonists • Lack significant central and anticholinergic effects		
Olopatadine (nasal and ophthalmic only)	• Allergic conjunctivitis • Allergic rhinitis • Ocular pruritus • Rhinorrhea • Sneezing	• Approved for once-daily dosing • Eye drops may cause headaches in some • Nasal spray can cause epistaxis and nasal ulceration or septal perforation • Some increase in risk of somnolence with nasal spray • Nasal spray minor side effects include bitter taste and headache
Acrivastine (only marketed in combination with pseudoephedrine)	• Allergic rhinitis • Nasal congestion • Allergic symptoms	• ~40% metabolized by CYPs, reducing potential for drug interactions • Somewhat higher risk of mild sedation than other second-generation drugs
Cetirizine Levocetirizine	• Allergic rhinitis • Atopic dermatitis (cetirizine) • Urticaria (chronic idiopathic)	• Somewhat higher risk of mild sedation than other second-generation drugs; more potent levocetirizine can be used at lower dose with less risk of sedation • Only ~30% (cetirizine) or ~1% (levocetirizine) metabolized by CYPs, reducing potential for drug interactions

Second-Generation Antihistamines: H_1 receptor inverse agonists • Lack significant central and anticholinergic effects (continued)		
Loratadine Desloratadine	• Allergic rhinitis • Chronic idiopathic urticaria • Exercise-induced bronchospasm prophylaxis (loratadine) • Pruritus (desloratadine)	• Desloratadine is the active metabolite of loratadine • 24-h duration of activity so only once-a-day dosing is required
Fexofenadine	• Allergic rhinitis • Chronic idiopathic urticaria	• Is the active metabolite of terfenadine (withdrawn from the market due to risk of torsades de pointes) • Only ~8% metabolized by CYPs, reducing potential for drug interactions
Alcaftadine (ophthalmic only)	• Allergic conjunctivitis • Ocular pruritus	• In addition to mast cell–stabilizing and anti-inflammatory properties, its H_4 antagonist activity may give superior relief from ocular itching • Approved for once-daily dosing • Most common adverse reactions (<4%) are eye irritation, redness, and pruritis
Bepotastine (ophthalmic only)	• Allergic conjunctivitis • Ocular pruritus	• Has mast cell–stabilizing and anti-inflammatory properties • Most common (~25%) adverse reaction is mild taste • Other minor (2%–5%) reactions are eye irritation, headache, and nasopharyngitis
Ketotifen (ophthalmic only)	• Allergic conjunctivitis • Ocular pruritus	• Has mast cell–stabilizing and anti-inflammatory properties • Most common (~10%–25%) adverse reactions are red eyes and mild headache or rhinitis
Azelastine (nasal and ophthalmic only)	• Allergic conjunctivitis • Allergic rhinitis (alone and combined with fluticasone) • Ocular pruritus • Vasomotor rhinitis	• Has mast cell–stabilizing and anti-inflammatory properties • Eye drops may cause transient eye burning/stinging • Some increase in risk of somnolence with nasal spray • Minor side effects with eye drops and nasal spray include bitter taste and headache
Emedastine (ophthalmic only)	• Allergic conjunctivitis • Ocular pruritus	• Lacks mast cell–stabilizing and anti-inflammatory properties • Common side effect: headache (~11%) • Minor reactions (<5%): abnormal dreams, bad taste, eye irritation
Epinastine (ophthalmic only)	• Allergic conjunctivitis • Ocular pruritus	• In addition to mast cell–stabilizing and anti-inflammatory properties, its H_2 antagonist activity may reduce eyelid edema • Common side effect (~10%): symptoms of upper respiratory infection • Minor ocular reactions: burning sensation, folliculosis, hyperemia, and pruritis

Bibliography

Abelson MB, et al. Advances in pharmacotherapy for allergic conjunctivitis. *Expert Opin Pharmacother*, **2015**, *16*:1219–1231.

Abraham WM, et al. Peptide and non-peptide bradykinin receptor antagonists: role in allergic airway disease. *Eur J Pharmacol*, **2006**, *533*:215–221.

Bartra J, et al. Interactions of the H_1 antihistamines. *J Investig Allergol Clin Immunol*, **2006**, *16*(suppl 1):29–36.

Bhoola KD, et al. Bioregulation of kinins: kallikreins, kininogens, and kininases. *Pharmacol Rev*, **1992**, *44*:1–80.

Black JW, et al. Definition and antagonism of histamine H_2-receptors. *Nature*, **1972**, *236*:385–390.

Campbell WB, Falck JR. Arachidonic acid metabolites as endothelium-derived hyperpolarizing factors. *Hypertension*, **2007**, *49*:590–596.

Campos MM, et al. Non-peptide antagonists for kinin B_1 receptors: new insights into their therapeutic potential for the management of inflammation and pain. *Trends Pharmacol Sci*, **2006**, *27*:646–651.

del Cuvillo A, et al. Comparative pharmacology of the H_1 antihistamines. *J Investig Allergol Clin Immunol*, **2006**, *16*(suppl 1):3–12.

Ellenbroek BA, Ghiabi B. The other side of the histamine H_3 receptor. *Trends Neurosci*, **2014**, *37*:191–199.

Emanuel MB. Histamine and the antiallergic antihistamines: a history of their discoveries. *Clin Exp Allergy*, **1999**, *29*(suppl 3):1–11.

Erdös EG, Skidgel RA. Metabolism of bradykinin by peptidases in health and disease. In: Farmer SG, ed. *The Kinin System*. Academic Press, London, **1997**, 111–141.

Esbenshade TA, et al. The histamine H_3 receptor: an attractive target for the treatment of cognitive disorders. *Br J Pharmacol*, **2008**, *154*:1166–1181.

Gilboa SM, et al. Antihistamines and birth defects: a systematic review of the literature. *Expert Opin Drug Saf*, **2014**, *13*:1667–1698.

Gray SL, et al. Cumulative use of strong anticholinergics and incident dementia: a prospective cohort study. *JAMA Intern Med*, **2015**, *175*:401–407.

Haas HL, et al. Histamine in the nervous system. *Physiol Rev*, **2008**, *88*:1183–1241.

Heitsch H. The therapeutic potential of bradykinin B_2 receptor agonists in the treatment of cardiovascular disease. *Expert Opin Investig Drugs*, **2003**, *12*:759–770.

Johnson AR, Erdos EG. Release of histamine from mast cells by vasoactive peptides. *Proc Soc Exp Biol Med*, **1973**, *142*:1252–1256.

Kaplan AP, Joseph K. Pathogenic mechanisms of bradykinin mediated diseases: dysregulation of an innate inflammatory pathway. *Adv Immunol*, **2014**, *121*:41–89.

Kuhr F, et al. Differential regulation of inducible and endothelial nitric oxide synthase by kinin B_1 and B_2 receptors. *Neuropeptides*, **2010**, *44*:145–154.

Leeb-Lundberg LM, et al. International union of pharmacology. XLV. Classification of the kinin receptor family: from molecular mechanisms to pathophysiological consequences. *Pharmacol Rev*, **2005**, *57*:27–77.

Levi-Schaffer F, Eliashar R. Mast cell stabilizing properties of antihistamines. *J Invest Dermatol*, **2009**, *129*:2549–2551.

Lowry JL, et al. Endothelial nitric-oxide synthase activation generates an inducible nitric-oxide synthase-like output of nitric oxide in inflamed endothelium. *J Biol Chem*, **2013**, *288*:4174–4193.

Madeddu P, et al. Mechanisms of disease: the tissue kallikrein-kinin system in hypertension and vascular remodeling. *Nat Clin Pract Nephrol*, **2007**, *3*:208–221.

Mikelis CM, et al. RhoA and ROCK mediate histamine-induced vascular leakage and anaphylactic shock. *Nat Commun*, **2015**, *6*:6725.

Padia SH, Carey RM. AT$_2$ receptors: beneficial counter-regulatory role in cardiovascular and renal function. *Pflugers Arch*, **2013**, *465*: 99–110.

Prassas I, et al. Unleashing the therapeutic potential of human kallikrein-related serine proteases. *Nat Rev Drug Discov*, **2015**, *14*:183–202.

Rocha e Silva M, et al. Bradykinin, a hypotensive and smooth muscle stimulating factor released from plasma globulin by snake venoms and by trypsin. *Am J Physiol*, **1949**, *156*:261–273.

Sander K, et al. Histamine H$_3$ receptor antagonists go to clinics. *Biol Pharm Bull*, **2008**, *31*:2163–2181.

Schwartz LB. Mast cells: function and contents. *Curr Opin Immunol*, **1994**, *6*:91–97.

Seifert R. How do basic secretagogues activate mast cells? *Naunyn Schmiedebergs Arch Pharmacol*, **2015**, *388*:279–281.

Simons FE. Advances in H$_1$-antihistamines. *N Engl J Med*, **2004**, *351*: 2203–2217.

Simons FE, Simons KJ. Histamine and H1-antihistamines: celebrating a century of progress. *J Allergy Clin Immunol*, **2011**, *128*:1139–1150.

Skidgel RA, Erdös EG. Structure and function of human plasma carboxypeptidase N, the anaphylatoxin inactivator. *Int Immunopharmacol*, **2007**, *7*:1888–1899.

Thurmond RL. The histamine H$_4$ receptor: from orphan to the clinic. *Front Pharmacol*, **2015**, *6*:65.

Thurmond RL, et al. The role of histamine H$_1$ and H$_4$ receptors in allergic inflammation: the search for new antihistamines. *Nat Rev Drug Discov*, **2008**, *7*:41–53.

Viegas LP, et al. The maddening itch: an approach to chronic urticaria. *J Investig Allergol Clin Immunol*, **2014**, *24*:1–5.

Walford HH, Zuraw BL. Current update on cellular and molecular mechanisms of hereditary angioedema. *Ann Allergy Asthma Immunol*, **2014**, *112*:413–418.

Werle E. Discovery of the most important kallikreins and kallikrein inhibitors. In: Erdös EG, ed. *Handbook of Experimental Pharmacology*. *Vol. 25*. Springer-Verlag, Heidelberg, **1970**, 1–6.

Zhang X, et al. Carboxypeptidase M augments kinin B$_1$ receptor signaling by conformational crosstalk and enhances endothelial nitric oxide output. *Biol Chem*, **2013a**, *394*:335–345.

Zhang X, et al. Carboxypeptidase M is a positive allosteric modulator of the kinin B1 receptor. *J Biol Chem*, **2013b**, *288*:33226–33240.

Zhang X, et al. Downregulation of kinin B$_1$ receptor function by B$_2$ receptor heterodimerization and signaling. *Cell Signal*, **2015**, *27*:90–103.

Zuraw BL, et al. A focused parameter update: hereditary angioedema, acquired C1 inhibitor deficiency, and angiotensin-converting enzyme inhibitor-associated angioedema. *J Allergy Clin Immunol*, **2013**, *131*: 1491–1493.

Pulmonary Pharmacology

Peter J. Barnes

Pulmonary pharmacology concerns understanding how drugs act on the lung and the pharmacological therapy of pulmonary diseases. Much of pulmonary pharmacology is concerned with the effects of drugs on the airways and the therapy of airway obstruction, particularly asthma and COPD, which are among the most common chronic diseases in the world. Both asthma and COPD are characterized by chronic inflammation of the airways, although there are marked differences in inflammatory mechanisms and response to therapy between these diseases (Barnes, 2008b; Postma and Rabe, 2015). This chapter discusses the pharmacotherapy of obstructive airways disease, particularly therapy with bronchodilators, which act mainly by reversing airway smooth muscle contraction, and anti-inflammatory drugs, which suppress the inflammatory response in the airways. This chapter focuses on the pulmonary pharmacology of β_2 adrenergic agonists and corticosteroids; the basic pharmacology of these classes of agents is presented elsewhere (Chapters 12 and 46).

This chapter also discusses other drugs used to treat obstructive airway diseases, such as mucolytics and respiratory stimulants, and covers the drug therapy of cough, the most common respiratory symptom. Drugs used in the treatment of pulmonary hypertension (Chapter 31) or lung infections, including tuberculosis (Chapter 60), are covered elsewhere.

Mechanisms of Asthma

Asthma is a chronic inflammatory disease of the airways that is characterized by activation of *mast cells*, infiltration of *eosinophils, T helper 2 (T_H2) lymphocytes, and innate type 2 lymphocytes (ILC2)* (Figure 40–1)

(Barnes, 2011b; Lambrecht and Hammad, 2015). Mast cell activation by allergens and physical stimuli releases *bronchoconstrictor mediators*, such as *histamine, LTD_4, and prostaglandin D_2*, which cause bronchoconstriction, microvascular leakage, and plasma exudation. Increased numbers of mast cells in airway smooth muscle are a characteristic of asthma.

Many of the symptoms of asthma are due to airway smooth muscle contraction, and therefore bronchodilators are important as symptom relievers. Whether airway smooth muscle is intrinsically abnormal in asthma is not clear, but increased contractility of airway smooth muscle may contribute to airway hyperresponsiveness, the physiological hallmark of asthma.

The mechanism of chronic inflammation in asthma is still not well understood. It may initially be driven by allergen exposure, but it appears to become autonomous so that asthma is essentially incurable. The inflammation may be orchestrated by dendritic cells that regulate T_H2 cells that drive eosinophilic inflammation and also IgE formation by B lymphocytes.

Airway epithelium plays an important role through the release of multiple inflammatory mediators and through the release of growth factors in an attempt to repair the damage caused by inflammation. The inflammatory process in asthma is mediated through the release of more than 100 inflammatory mediators (Hall and Agrawal, 2014). Complex cytokine networks, including chemokines and growth factors, play important roles in orchestrating the inflammation process (Barnes, 2008a).

Chronic inflammation may lead to structural changes (remodeling) in the airways, including an increase in the number and size of airway smooth muscle cells, blood vessels, and mucus-secreting cells. A characteristic

Abbreviations

AC: adenylyl cyclase
ACh: acetylcholine
ALT: alanine aminotransferase
BDP: beclomethasone dipropionate
cAMP: cyclic adenosine monophosphate
CCR3: C-C chemokine receptor type 3
COMT: catechol-O-methyl transferase
COPD: chronic obstructive pulmonary disease
CRTh2: chemokine receptor homologous molecule expressed on Th2 lymphocytes
CXCR2: C-X-C motif chemokine receptor 2
cys-LT: cysteinyl-leukotriene
DPI: dry powder inhaler
FDA: Food and Drug Administration
FEV$_1$: forced expiratory volume in 1 second
FFA: free fatty acid
GABA: γ-aminobutyric acid
GR: glucocorticoid receptor
HDAC2: histone deacetylase 2
HFA: hydrofluoroalkane
ICS: inhaled corticosteroid
Ig: immunoglobulin
IL: interleukin
ILC2: innate type 2 lymphocyte
IM: intramuscular
IP$_3$: inositol 1,4,5-trisphosphate
IV: intravenous
LABA: long-acting inhaled β$_2$ agonist
LAMA: long-acting muscarinic antagonist
5-LO: 5′-lipoxygenase
LT: leukotriene
MAO: monoamine oxidase
MDI: metered-dose inhaler
MMAD: mass median aerodynamic diameter
MMP: matrix metalloproteinase
MOR: μ opioid receptor
NF-κB: nuclear factor kappa B
NMDA: N-methyl-D-aspartate
PAF: platelet-activating factor
PDE: phosphodiesterase
PG: prostaglandin
PKA: protein kinase A
PLC: phospholipase C
pMDI: pressurized metered-dose inhaler
SABA: short-acting β$_2$ agonists
SAMA: short-acting muscarinic antagonist
TAS2R: taste 2 receptor
Tc1 cell: cytotoxic T lymphocyte
Th17: T helper-17 cell
T$_H$2: T helper 2 lymphocyte
TNF: tumor necrosis factor
TRP: transient receptor potential
VIP: vasoactive intestinal polypeptide

histological feature of asthma is collagen deposition (fibrosis) below the basement membrane of the airway epithelium (Figure 49–1). This appears to be the result of eosinophilic inflammation and is found even at the onset of asthmatic symptoms. The complex inflammation of asthma is suppressed by corticosteroids in most patients, but even if asthma is well controlled, the inflammation and symptoms return if corticosteroids

are discontinued. Asthma usually starts in early childhood, then may disappear during adolescence and reappear in adulthood. It is characterized by variable airflow obstruction and typically shows a good therapeutic response to bronchodilators and corticosteroids. Asthma severity usually does not change, so that patients with mild asthma rarely progress to severe asthma and patients with severe asthma usually have this from the onset, although some patients, particularly with late-onset asthma, show a progressive loss of lung function like patients with COPD. Patients with severe asthma may have a pattern of inflammation more similar to COPD and are characterized by reduced responsiveness to corticosteroids (Trejo Bittar et al., 2015).

Mechanisms of COPD

Chronic obstructive pulmonary disease involves inflammation of the respiratory tract with a pattern that differs from that of asthma. In COPD, there is a *predominance of neutrophils, macrophages, cytotoxic T lymphocytes (Tc1 cells), and T helper-17 (Th17) cells*. The inflammation *predominantly affects small airways*, resulting in progressive small-airway narrowing and fibrosis (chronic obstructive bronchiolitis) and destruction of the lung parenchyma with destruction of the alveolar walls (emphysema) (Figure 40–2) (Barnes et al., 2015). These pathological changes result in airway closure on expiration, leading to air trapping and hyperinflation, particularly on exercise (dynamic hyperinflation). This accounts for shortness of breath on exertion and exercise limitation that are characteristic symptoms of COPD.

Bronchodilators reduce air trapping by dilating peripheral airways and are the mainstay of treatment in COPD. In contrast to asthma, the airflow obstruction of COPD tends to be progressive. The inflammation in the peripheral lung of patients with COPD is mediated by multiple inflammatory mediators and cytokines, although the pattern of mediators differs from that of asthma (Barnes, 2004). In contrast to asthma, the inflammation in patients with COPD is largely corticosteroid resistant, and there are currently no effective anti-inflammatory treatments. Many patients with COPD have comorbidities, including ischemic heart disease, hypertension, congestive heart failure, diabetes, osteoporosis, skeletal muscle wasting, depression, chronic renal disease, and anemia (Barnes and Celli, 2009). These diseases may occur together as part of multimorbidity, as diseases of accelerated aging with common pathogenetic mechanisms (Barnes, 2015).

Routes of Drug Delivery to the Lungs

Drugs may be delivered to the lungs by oral or parenteral routes and also by inhalation. The choice depends on the drug and on the respiratory disease.

Inhaled Route

Inhalation (Figure 40–3) is the preferred mode of delivery of many drugs with a direct effect on airways, particularly for asthma and COPD (Sanchis et al., 2013). It is the only way to deliver some drugs, such as cromolyn sodium and anticholinergic drugs, and is the preferred route of delivery for β$_2$ agonists and corticosteroids to reduce systemic side effects. Antibiotics may be delivered by inhalation in patients with chronic respiratory sepsis (e.g., in cystic fibrosis). The major advantage of inhalation is the delivery of drug to the airways in doses that are effective with a much lower risk of systemic side effects. This is particularly important with the use of ICS, which largely avoids systemic side effects. In addition, inhaled bronchodilators have a more rapid onset of action than when taken orally.

Particle Size

The size of particles for inhalation is of critical importance in determining the site of deposition in the respiratory tract. The optimum size for particles to settle in the airways is 2- to 5-μm MMAD. Larger particles settle out in the upper airways, whereas smaller particles remain suspended and are therefore exhaled. There is increasing interest in delivering drugs to small airways, particularly in COPD and severe asthma (Usmani and

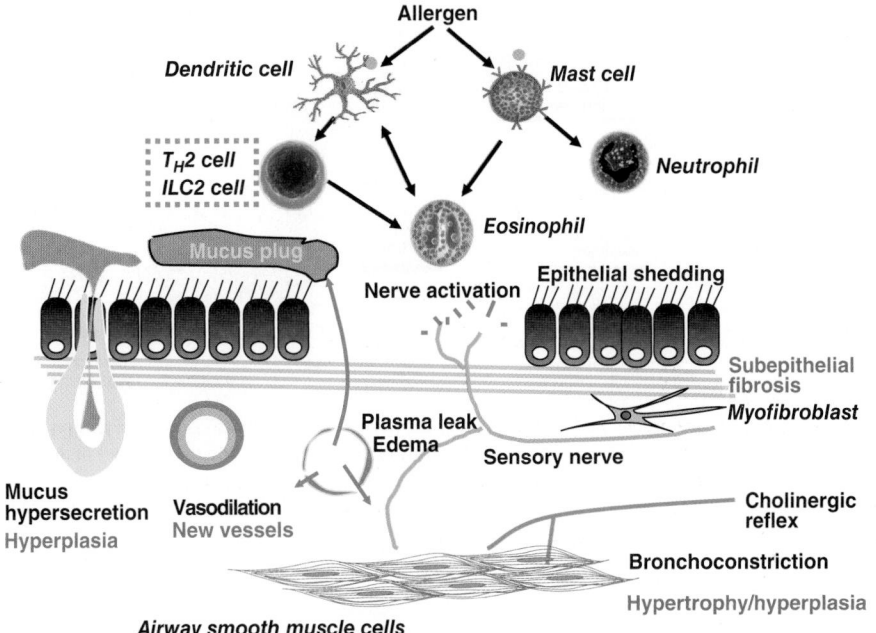

Figure 40–1 *Cellular mechanisms of asthma.* Myriad inflammatory cells are recruited and activated in the airways, where they release multiple inflammatory mediators, which can also arise from structural cells. These mediators lead to bronchoconstriction, plasma exudation and edema, vasodilation, mucus hypersecretion, and activation of sensory nerves. Chronic inflammation leads to structural changes, including subepithelial fibrosis (basement membrane thickening), airway smooth muscle hypertrophy and hyperplasia, angiogenesis, and hyperplasia of mucus-secreting cells.

Barnes, 2012). This involves delivering drug particles of about 1-µm MMAD, which is now possible using drugs formulated in HFA propellant.

Pharmacokinetics

Of the total drug delivered, only 10%–20% enters the lower airways with a conventional pMDI. Drugs are absorbed from the airway lumen and have direct effects on target cells of the airway. Drugs may also be absorbed into the bronchial circulation and then distributed to more peripheral airways. Drugs with higher molecular weights tend to be retained to a greater extent in the airways. Nevertheless, several drugs have greater therapeutic efficacy when given by the inhaled route. The ICS *ciclesonide* is a prodrug activated by esterases in the respiratory tract to the active principle des-ciclesonide. More extensive pulmonary distribution of a drug with a smaller MMAD increases alveolar deposition and thus is likely to increase absorption from the lungs into the general circulation, resulting in more systemic side effects. Thus, although HFA pMDIs deliver more ICS to smaller airways, there is also increased systemic absorption, so that the therapeutic ratio may not be changed.

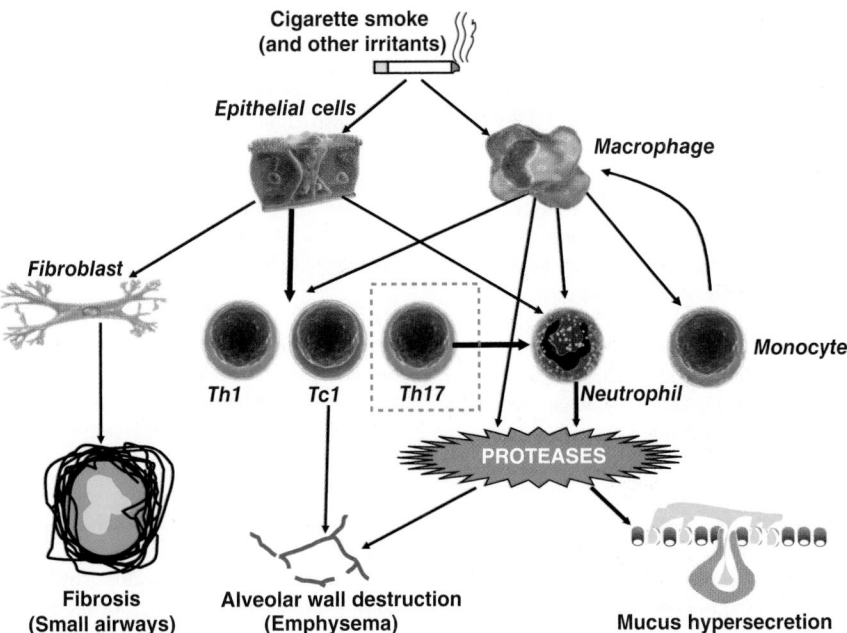

Figure 40–2 *Cellular mechanisms in COPD.* Cigarette smoke and other irritants activate epithelial cells and macrophages in the lung to release mediators that attract circulating inflammatory cells, including monocytes (which differentiate to macrophages within the lung), neutrophils, and T lymphocytes (T_H1, T_C1, and Th17 cells). Fibrogenic factors released from epithelial cells and macrophages lead to fibrosis of small airways. Release of proteases results in alveolar wall destruction (emphysema) and mucus hypersecretion (chronic bronchitis).

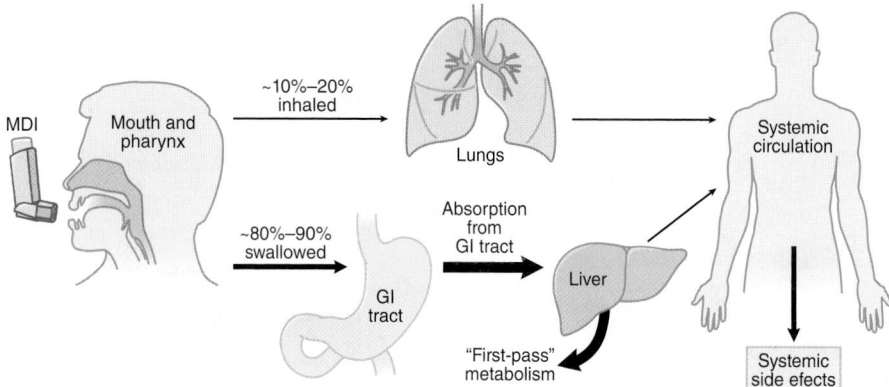

Figure 40–3 *Schematic representation of the deposition of inhaled drugs (e.g., corticosteroids, β₂ agonists).* Inhalation therapy deposits drugs directly, but not exclusively, in the lungs. Distribution between lungs and oropharynx depends mostly on the particle size and the efficiency of the delivery method. Most material will be swallowed and absorbed, entering systemic circulation after undergoing the first-pass effect in the liver. Some drug will also be absorbed into the systemic circulation from the lungs. Use of a large-volume spacer will reduce the amount of drug deposited on the oropharynx, thereby reducing the amount swallowed and absorbed from the GI tract, thus limiting systemic effects.

Delivery Devices

Pressurized Metered-Dose Inhalers. Drugs are propelled from a canister in the pMDI with the aid of a propellant, previously with a chlorofluorocarbon (Freon) but now replaced by an *HFA* that is "ozone friendly." These devices are convenient, portable, and typically deliver 50–200 doses of drug.

Spacer Chambers. Large-volume spacer devices between the pMDI and the patient reduce the velocity of particles entering the upper airways and the size of the particles by allowing evaporation of liquid propellant. This reduces the amount of drug that impinges on the oropharynx and increases the proportion of drug inhaled into the lower airways. Application of spacer chambers is useful in the reduction of the oropharyngeal deposition of ICS and the consequent reduction in the local side effects of these drugs. Spacer devices are also useful in delivering inhaled drugs to small children who are not able to use a pMDI. Children as young as 3 years of age are able to use a spacer device fitted with a face mask.

Dry Powder Inhalers. Drugs may also be delivered as a dry powder using devices that scatter a fine powder dispersed by air turbulence on inhalation. Children less than 7 years of age find it difficult to use a DPI. DPIs have been developed to deliver peptides and proteins, such as insulin, systemically but have proved to be problematic because of consistency of dosing.

Nebulizers. Two types of nebulizer are available. *Jet nebulizers* are driven by a stream of gas (air or oxygen), whereas *ultrasonic nebulizers* use a rapidly vibrating piezoelectric crystal and thus do not require a source of compressed gas. The nebulized drug may be inspired during tidal breathing, and it is possible to deliver much higher doses of drug compared with a pMDI. Nebulizers are therefore useful in treating acute exacerbations of asthma and COPD, for delivering drugs when airway obstruction is extreme (e.g., in severe COPD), for delivering inhaled drugs to infants and small children who cannot use the other inhalation devices, and for giving drugs such as antibiotics when relatively high doses must be delivered.

Oral Route

Drugs for treatment of pulmonary diseases may also be given orally. The oral dose is much higher than the inhaled dose required to achieve the same effect (typically by a ratio of about 20:1), so that systemic side effects are more common. *When there is a choice of inhaled or oral route for a drug (e.g., β₂ agonist or corticosteroid), the inhaled route is always preferable*, and the oral route should be reserved for the few patients unable to use inhalers (e.g., small children, patients with physical problems such as severe arthritis of the hands). Theophylline is ineffective by the inhaled route and therefore must be given systemically.

Corticosteroids may have to be given orally for parenchymal lung diseases (e.g., in interstitial lung diseases).

Parenteral Route

The intravenous route should be reserved for delivery of drugs in the severely ill patient who is unable to absorb drugs from the GI tract. Side effects are generally frequent due to the high plasma concentrations.

Bronchodilators

Bronchodilator drugs relax constricted airway smooth muscle in vitro and cause immediate reversal of airway obstruction in asthma in vivo (Cazzola et al., 2012). They also prevent bronchoconstriction (and thereby provide bronchoprotection). Three main classes of bronchodilator are in current clinical use:

- β₂ Adrenergic agonists (sympathomimetics)
- Theophylline (a methylxanthine)
- Anticholinergic agents (muscarinic receptor antagonists)

Drugs such as *cromolyn sodium*, which prevent bronchoconstriction, have no direct bronchodilator action and are ineffective once bronchoconstriction has occurred. *Anti-LTs* (LT receptor antagonists and 5'-lipoxygenase inhibitors) have a small bronchodilator effect in some asthmatic patients and appear to prevent bronchoconstriction. *Corticosteroids*, although gradually improving airway obstruction, have no direct effect on contraction of airway smooth muscle and are not therefore considered to be bronchodilators.

β₂ Adrenergic Agonists

Inhaled β₂ agonists are the bronchodilator treatment of choice in asthma because they are the most effective bronchodilators and have minimal side effects when used correctly. Systemic, short-acting, and nonselective β agonists, such as isoproterenol (isoprenaline) or metaproterenol, should only be used as a last resort.

Chemistry

The development of β₂ agonists is based on substitutions in the catecholamine structure of norepinephrine and epinephrine (see Chapters 8 and 12). The catechol ring consists of hydroxyl groups in the 3 and 4 positions of the benzene ring. Norepinephrine differs from epinephrine only in the terminal amine group; in general, further modification at this site confers β receptor selectivity. Many β₂-selective agonists have now been introduced, and although there may be differences in potency, there are no clinically significant differences in selectivity. Inhaled β₂-selective drugs in current clinical use have a similar duration of action (3–6 h).

The inhaled LABAs, salmeterol and formoterol, have a much longer duration of effect, providing bronchodilation and bronchoprotection for more than 12 h (Cazzola et al., 2013b). Formoterol has a bulky substitution in the aliphatic chain and has moderate lipophilicity, which appears to keep the drug in the membrane close to the receptor, so it behaves as a slow-release drug. Salmeterol has a long aliphatic chain, and its long duration may be due to binding within the receptor binding cleft ("exosite") that anchors the drug in the binding cleft. Once-daily β₂ agonists, such as indacaterol, vilanterol, and olodaterol, with a duration of action more than 24 h have now been developed.

Mode of Action

Occupation of β_2 receptors by agonists results in the activation of the G_s-adenylyl cyclase-cAMP-PKA pathway, resulting in phosphorylative events leading to bronchial smooth muscle relaxation (Figure 40–4). β_2 Receptors are localized to several different airway cells, where they may have additional effects. β_2 Agonists may cause bronchodilation also *indirectly* by inhibiting the release of bronchoconstrictor mediators from inflammatory cells and of bronchoconstrictor neurotransmitters from airway nerves. These mechanisms include the following:

- Prevention of mediator release from isolated human lung mast cells (via β_2 receptors)
- Prevention of microvascular leakage and thus the development of bronchial mucosal edema after exposure to mediators, such as histamine, LTD_4, and prostaglandin D_2
- Increase in *mucus secretion* from submucosal glands and *ion transport* across airway epithelium (may enhance mucociliary clearance, reversing defective clearance found in asthma)
- *Reduction in neurotransmission* in human airway *cholinergic nerves* by an action at presynaptic β_2 receptors to inhibit ACh release

Although these additional effects of β_2 agonists may be relevant to the prophylactic use of these drugs against various challenges, their rapid bronchodilator action is probably attributable to a direct effect on smooth muscle of all airways.

Anti-inflammatory Effects

Whether β_2 agonists have anti-inflammatory effects in asthma is controversial. The inhibitory effects of β_2 agonists on mast cell mediator release and microvascular leakage are clearly anti-inflammatory, suggesting that β_2 agonists may modify *acute* inflammation. However, β_2 agonists do not appear to have a significant inhibitory effect on the *chronic* inflammation of asthmatic airways, which is suppressed by corticosteroids. This has now been confirmed by several biopsy and bronchoalveolar lavage studies in patients with asthma who are taking regular β_2 agonists (including LABAs), that demonstrated no significant reduction in the number or activation in inflammatory cells in the airways, in contrast to resolution of the inflammation that occurs with ICS. This may be related to the fact that effects of β_2 agonists on macrophages, eosinophils, and lymphocytes are rapidly desensitized.

Clinical Use

Short-Acting β₂ Agonists.
Inhaled SABAs are the most widely used and effective bronchodilators in the treatment of asthma due to their functional antagonism of bronchoconstriction. When inhaled from pMDIs or DPIs, they are convenient, easy to use, rapid in onset, and without significant systemic side effects. These agents are effective in protecting against various asthma triggers, such as exercise, cold air, and allergens. SABAs are the bronchodilators of choice in treating acute severe asthma. The nebulized route of administration is easier and safer than intravenous administration and just as effective. Inhalation is preferable to oral administration because systemic side effects are less. *SABAs, such as albuterol, should be used "as required" by symptoms and not on a regular basis in the treatment of mild asthma; increased use indicates the need for more anti-inflammatory therapy.*

Oral β_2 agonists are occasionally indicated as an additional bronchodilator. Slow-release preparations (e.g., slow-release albuterol and bambuterol [not available in the U.S.]) may be indicated in nocturnal asthma; however, these agents have an increased risk of side effects. Several SABAs are available; they are resistant to uptake and enzymatic degradation by COMT and MAO; all are usable by inhalation and orally, have a similar duration of action (~3–4 h; less in severe asthma), and similar side effects. Differences in β_2 receptor selectivity have been claimed but are not clinically important. Drugs in clinical use include *albuterol (salbutamol), levalbuterol, metaproterenol, terbutaline, pirbuterol*, as well as several not available in the U.S. (*fenoterol, tulobuterol, and rimiterol*).

Long-Acting Inhaled β₂ Agonists.
The LABAs *salmeterol, formoterol, and arformoterol* have proved to be a significant advance in asthma and COPD therapy. These drugs have a bronchodilator action of more than 12 h and also protect against bronchoconstriction for a similar period

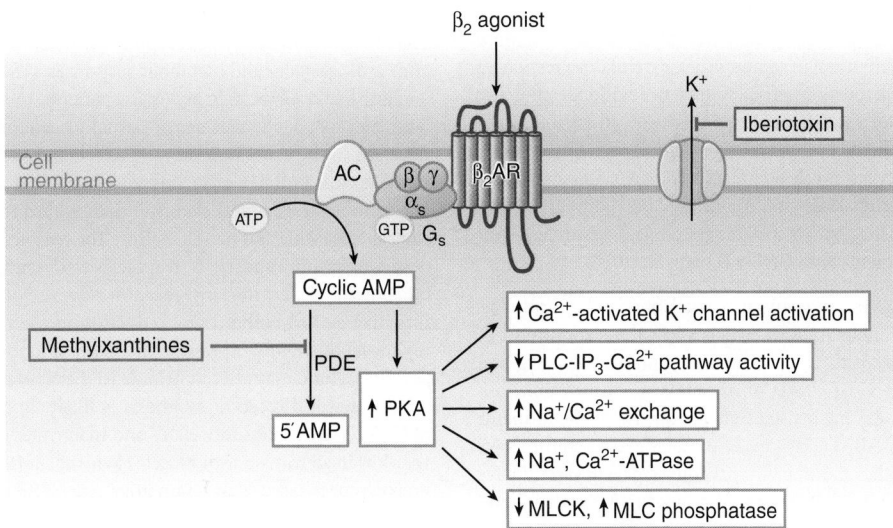

Figure 40–4 *Molecular actions of β₂ agonists to induce relaxation of airway smooth muscle cells.* Activation of β_2 receptors (β_2AR) results in activation of AC via G_s, leading to an increase in intracellular cAMP and activation of PKA. PKA phosphorylates a variety of target substrates, resulting in opening of Ca^{2+}-activated K^+ channels (K_{Ca}), thereby facilitating hyperpolarization, decreased PI hydrolysis, increased Na^+/Ca^{2+} exchange, increased Na^+, Ca^{2+}-ATPase activity, and decreased myosin light chain kinase (MLCK) activity and increased myosin light chain (MLC) phosphatase. β_2 Receptors may also couple to K_{Ca} via G_s. PDE, cyclic nucleotide phosphodiesterase.

(Cazzola et al., 2013b). They improve asthma control (when given twice daily) compared with regular treatment with SABAs (four to six times daily). Once-daily LABAs, such as *indacaterol, vilanterol,* and *olodaterol,* with a duration of over 24 h have now been developed and are more effective in patients with COPD than twice-daily LABAs and more frequent SABAs.

Tolerance to the bronchodilator effect of formoterol and the bronchoprotective effects of formoterol and salmeterol have been demonstrated but is of doubtful clinical significance. Although both formoterol and salmeterol have a similar duration of effect in clinical studies, there are differences. Formoterol has a more rapid onset of action and is an almost-full agonist, whereas salmeterol is a partial agonist with a slower onset of action. These differences might confer a theoretical advantage for formoterol in more severe asthma, whereas it may also make it more likely to induce tolerance. However, no significant clinical differences between salmeterol and formoterol have been found in the treatment of patients with severe asthma (Nightingale et al., 2002).

In COPD, LABAs are effective bronchodilators that may be used alone or in combination with anticholinergics or ICSs. LABAs improve symptoms and exercise tolerance by reducing both air trapping and exacerbations. *In patients with asthma, LABAs should never be used alone because they do not treat the underlying chronic inflammation, and this may increase the risk of life-threatening and fatal asthma exacerbations; rather, LABAs should always be used in combination with an ICS in a fixed-dose combination inhaler.* LABAs are an effective add-on therapy to ICSs and are more effective than increasing the dose of an ICS when asthma is not controlled at low doses.

Combination Inhalers. Combination inhalers that contain a LABA and a corticosteroid (e.g., *fluticasone/salmeterol, budesonide/formoterol*) are now widely used in the treatment of asthma and COPD. In asthma, combining a LABA with a corticosteroid offers complementary synergistic actions (Barnes, 2002). The combination inhaler is more convenient for patients, simplifies therapy, and improves adherence with the ICS. Also, delivering the two drugs in the same inhaler ensures they are delivered simultaneously to the same cells in the airways, allowing the beneficial molecular interactions between LABAs and corticosteroids to occur. Combination inhalers are now the preferred therapy for patients with persistent asthma. These combination inhalers are also more effective in patients with COPD than a LABA and an ICS alone, but the mechanisms accounting for this beneficial interaction are less well understood than in patients with asthma.

Stereoselective β₂ Agonists. Albuterol is a racemic mixture of active *R*- and inactive *S*-isomers. Although *R*-albuterol (levalbuterol) was more potent than racemic *R/S*-albuterol in some studies, careful dose responses showed no advantage in terms of efficacy and no evidence that the *S*-albuterol is detrimental in asthmatic patients (Lotvall et al., 2001). Because levalbuterol is usually more expensive than normally used racemic albuterol, this therapy has no clear clinical advantage. Stereoselective formoterol (*R,R*-formoterol, arformoterol) has now been developed as a nebulized solution but also appears to offer no clinical advantage over racemic formoterol in patients with COPD (Loh et al., 2015).

β₂ Receptor Polymorphisms. Several single-nucleotide polymorphisms and haplotypes of the human *ADRβ2*, which affect the structure of β₂ receptors, have been described. The common variants are $Gly^{16}Arg$ and $Gln^{27}Glu$, which have in vitro effects on receptor desensitization, but clinical studies have shown inconsistent effects on the bronchodilator responses to SABAs and LABAs (Hawkins et al., 2008). Some studies have shown that patients with the common homozygous $Arg^{16}Arg$ variant have more frequent adverse effects and a poorer response to SABAs than heterozygotes or $Gly^{16}Gly$ homozygotes, but overall these differences are small, and there appears to be no clinical value in measuring *ADRβ2* genotype. No differences have been found with responses to LABA between these genotypes (Bleecker et al., 2007).

Side Effects. Unwanted effects are dose related and due to stimulation of extrapulmonary β receptors (Table 40–1 and Chapter 12). Side effects

TABLE 40–1 ■ SIDE EFFECTS OF β₂ AGONISTS

- Muscle tremor (direct effect on skeletal muscle β₂ receptors)
- Tachycardia (direct effect on atrial β₂ receptors, reflex effect from increased peripheral vasodilation via β₂ receptors)
- Hypokalemia (direct β₂ effect on skeletal muscle uptake of K^+)
- Restlessness
- Hypoxemia ($\uparrow \dot{V}/\dot{Q}$ mismatch due to reversal of hypoxic pulmonary vasoconstriction)
- Metabolic effects ($\uparrow$ FFA, glucose, lactate, pyruvate, insulin)

are not common with inhaled therapy but quite common with oral or intravenous administration.

- *Muscle tremor* due to stimulation of β₂ receptors in skeletal muscle is the most common side effect. It may be more troublesome with elderly patients and so is a more frequent problem in patients with COPD.
- *Tachycardia* and *palpitations* are due to reflex cardiac stimulation secondary to peripheral vasodilation, from direct stimulation of atrial β₂ receptors (human heart has a relatively high proportion of β₂ receptors; see Chapter 12), and possibly also from stimulation of myocardial β₁ receptors as the doses of β₂ agonist are increased.
- *Hypokalemia* is a potentially serious side effect. This is due to β₂ receptor stimulation of potassium entry into skeletal muscle, which may be secondary to a rise in insulin secretion. Hypokalemia might be serious in the presence of hypoxia, as in acute asthma, when there may be a predisposition to cardiac arrhythmias (Chapter 30). In practice, however, significant arrhythmias after nebulized β₂ agonists are rarely observed in acute asthma or patients with COPD.
- *Ventilation-perfusion* V/Q *mismatch* due to pulmonary vasodilation in blood vessels previously constricted by hypoxia results in the shunting of blood to poorly ventilated areas and a fall in arterial oxygen tension. Although in practice the effect of β₂ agonists on Pao_2 is usually very small (<5 mm Hg fall), occasionally in severe COPD it can be large, although it may be prevented by giving additional inspired oxygen.
- *Metabolic* effects (increase in free fatty acid, insulin, glucose, pyruvate, and lactate) are usually seen only after large systemic doses.

Tolerance. Continuous treatment with an agonist often leads to tolerance, which may be due to downregulation of the receptor (Chapter 12). Tolerance of nonairway β₂ receptor–mediated responses, such as tremor and cardiovascular and metabolic responses, is readily induced in normal and asthmatic subjects. In asthmatic patients, tolerance to the bronchodilator effects of β₂ agonists has not usually been found. However, tolerance develops to the bronchoprotective effects of β₂ agonists, and this is more marked with indirect bronchoconstrictors that activate mast cells (e.g., adenosine, allergen, and exercise) than with direct bronchoconstrictors, such as histamine and methacholine. The reason for the relative resistance of airway smooth muscle β₂ responses to desensitization remains uncertain but may reflect the large receptor reserve: More than 90% of β₂ receptors may be lost without any reduction in the relaxation response. The high level of *ADRβ2 expression* in airway smooth muscle compared with peripheral lung may also contribute to the resistance to tolerance because a high rate of β receptor synthesis is likely. In addition, the expression of GRK2, which phosphorylates and inactivates occupied β₂ receptors, is very low in airway smooth muscle (Penn et al., 1998). By contrast, there is no receptor reserve in inflammatory cells, GRK2 expression is high, and tolerance to β₂ agonists rapidly develops at these sites.

Experimental studies have shown that corticosteroids prevent the development of tolerance in airway smooth muscle and prevent and reverse the fall in pulmonary β receptor density (Mak et al., 1995). However, ICSs fail to prevent the tolerance to the bronchoprotective effect of inhaled β₂ agonists, possibly because they do not reach airway smooth muscle in a high enough concentration.

Long-Term Safety. Because of a possible relationship between adrenergic drug therapy and the rise in asthma deaths in several countries during the early 1960s, doubts were cast on the long-term safety of β agonists. A particular $β_2$ agonist, fenoterol, was linked to the rise in asthma deaths in New Zealand in the early 1990s because significantly more of the fatal cases were prescribed fenoterol than the case-matched control patients (Beasley et al., 1999). An epidemiological study examining the links between drugs prescribed for asthma and death or near death from asthma attacks found a marked increase in the risk of death with high doses of all inhaled $β_2$ agonists. The risk was greater with fenoterol, but when the dose is adjusted to the equivalent dose for albuterol, there is no significant difference in the risk for these two drugs.

The link between high $β_2$ agonist usage and increased asthma mortality does not prove a causal association because patients with more severe and poorly controlled asthma, who are more likely to have an increased risk of fatal attacks, are more likely to be using higher doses of $β_2$ agonist inhalers and less likely to be using effective anti-inflammatory treatment. Indeed, in the patients who used regular inhaled steroids, there was a significant reduction in risk of death.

Regular use of inhaled $β_2$ agonists has also been linked to increased asthma morbidity. Regular use of fenoterol was associated with worse asthma control and a small increase in airway hyperresponsiveness compared with patients using fenoterol "on demand" for symptom control over a 6-month period (Sears, 2002). However, this was not found in a study with regular albuterol (Dennis et al., 2000). There is some evidence that regular inhaled $β_2$ agonists may increase allergen-induced asthma and sputum eosinophilia (Gauvreau et al., 1997).

SABAs should only be used on demand for symptom control, and if they are required frequently (more than three times weekly), an ICS is needed.

The safety of LABAs in asthma remains controversial. A large study of the safety of salmeterol showed an excess of respiratory deaths and near deaths in patients prescribed salmeterol, but these deaths occurred mainly in African Americans living in inner cities who were not taking ICSs (Nelson and Dorinsky, 2006). Similar data have also raised concerns about formoterol. However, concomitant treatment with an ICS appears to obviate such risk, so it is recommended that LABAs should only be used when ICSs are also prescribed (preferably in the form of a combination inhaler so that the LABAs can never be taken without the ICSs) (Cates et al., 2014). All LABAs approved in the U.S. carry a black-box warning cautioning against overuse. There are fewer safety concerns with LABA use in COPD. No major adverse effects were reported in several large and prolonged studies and no evidence of cardiovascular problems (Kew et al., 2013).

Future Developments

The β agonists will continue to be the bronchodilators of choice for asthma because they are effective in all patients and have few or no side effects when used in low doses. When used as required for symptom control, inhaled $β_2$ agonists appear safe. Use of large doses of inhaled $β_2$ agonists indicates poor asthma control; such patients should be assessed and appropriate controller medication used. LABAs are a useful option for long-term control in asthma and COPD. In patients with asthma, LABAs should probably only be used in a fixed combination with an ICS to prevent the potential danger associated with LABAs alone. There is little advantage to be gained by improving $β_2$ receptor selectivity because most of the side effects of these agents are due to $β_2$ receptor stimulation (muscle tremor, tachycardia, hypokalemia). Once-daily inhaled $β_2$ agonists are useful in patients with COPD and may have additive effects with LAMAs.

Methylxanthines

Methylxanthines, such as theophylline, which are related to caffeine, have been used in the treatment of asthma since 1930, and theophylline is still widely used in developing countries because it is inexpensive. Theophylline became more useful with the introduction of reliable slow-release preparations. However, inhaled $β_2$ agonists are far more effective as bronchodilators, and ICSs have a greater anti-inflammatory effect. In patients

with severe asthma and COPD, it still remains a useful drug as an add-on therapy (Barnes, 2013c).

THEOPHYLLINE   ADENOSINE   CYCLIC AMP

Chemistry

Theophylline is a methylxanthine similar in structure to the common dietary xanthines caffeine and theobromine. Several substituted derivatives have been synthesized, but only two appear to have any advantage over theophylline: *Enprofylline* is a more potent bronchodilator and may have fewer toxic effects because it does not antagonize adenosine receptors; *doxofylline*, a novel methylxanthine available in some countries, has an inhibitory effect on PDEs similar to that of theophylline but is less active as an adenosine antagonist and has a more favorable side-effect profile (Akram et al., 2012). Many salts of theophylline have also been marketed; the most common is aminophylline. Other salts do not have any advantage. Theophylline remains the major methylxanthine in clinical use.

Mechanism of Action

The mechanisms of action of theophylline are still uncertain. In addition to its bronchodilator action, theophylline has many nonbronchodilator effects that may be relevant to its effects in asthma and COPD (Figure 40–5). Several molecular mechanisms of action have been proposed:

- *Inhibition of PDEs.* Theophylline is a nonselective PDE inhibitor, but the degree of inhibition is relatively minimal at concentrations of theophylline that are within the therapeutic range. PDE inhibition and the concomitant elevation of cellular cAMP and cyclic GMP likely account for the bronchodilator action of theophylline. Several isoenzyme families of PDE have now been recognized, and those important in smooth muscle relaxation include PDE3, PDE4, and PDE5.

- *Adenosine receptor antagonism.* Theophylline antagonizes adenosine receptors at therapeutic concentrations. Adenosine causes bronchoconstriction in airways from asthmatic patients by releasing histamine and LTs. Antagonism of A_1 receptors may be responsible for serious side effects, including cardiac arrhythmias and seizures.

- *Interleukin 10 release.* IL-10 has a broad spectrum of anti-inflammatory effects, and there is evidence that its secretion is reduced in asthma. IL-10 release is increased by theophylline, and this effect may be mediated via inhibition of PDE activities, although this has not been seen at the low doses that are effective in asthma.

- *Effects on gene transcription.* Theophylline prevents the translocation of the pro-inflammatory transcription factor NF-κB into the nucleus, potentially reducing the expression of inflammatory genes in asthma and COPD (Ichiyama et al., 2001). However, these effects are seen at high concentrations and may be mediated by inhibition of PDE.

- *Effects on apoptosis.* Prolonged survival of granulocytes due to a reduction in apoptosis may be important in perpetuating chronic inflammation in asthma (eosinophils) and COPD (neutrophils). Theophylline promotes apoptosis in eosinophils and neutrophils in vitro. This is associated with a reduction in the antiapoptotic protein Bcl-2 (Chung et al., 2000). This effect is not mediated via PDE inhibition, but in neutrophils may be mediated by antagonism of adenosine A_{2A} receptors (Yasui et al., 2000). Theophylline also induces apoptosis in T lymphocytes via PDE inhibition.

- *Histone deacetylase activation.* Recruitment of HDAC2 by GRs switches off inflammatory genes. Therapeutic concentrations of theophylline activate HDAC, thereby enhancing the anti-inflammatory effects of corticosteroids (Cosio et al., 2004). This mechanism appears to be mediated by inhibition of PI_3-kinase-δ, which is activated by oxidative stress (To et al., 2010).

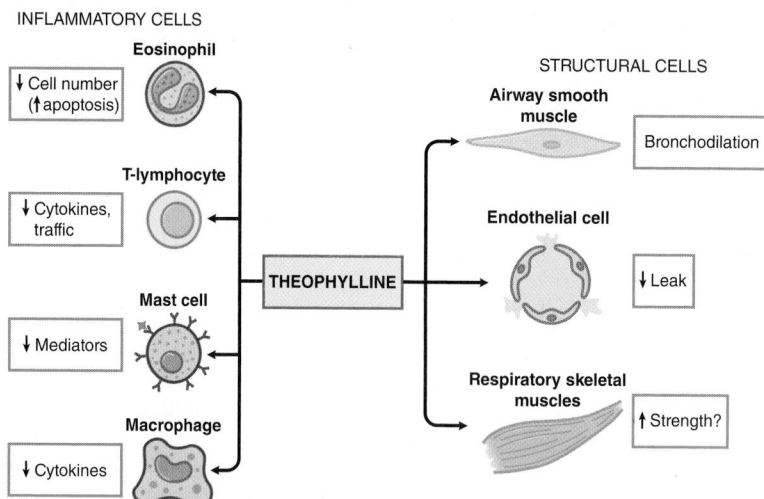

Figure 40–5 *Theophylline affects multiple cell types in the airway.*

Nonbronchodilator Effects

Theophylline has clinical benefit in asthma and COPD at plasma concentrations less than 10 mg/L, sufficiently low that such effects are unlikely to be explained by theophylline's bronchodilator action. There is increasing evidence that theophylline has anti-inflammatory effects in asthma (Barnes, 2013c). In patients with mild asthma, chronic oral treatment with theophylline inhibits the late response to inhaled allergen and reduces infiltration of eosinophils and CD4⁺ lymphocytes into the airways after allergen challenge (Lim et al., 2001). In patients with COPD, theophylline reduces the total number and proportion of neutrophils in induced sputum, the concentration of IL-8, and neutrophil chemotactic responses (Culpitt et al., 2002). Theophylline withdrawal in patients with COPD results in worsening of disease. In vitro theophylline is able to increase responsiveness to corticosteroids and to reverse corticosteroid resistance in cells from subjects with COPD (Cosio et al., 2004).

Pharmacokinetics and Metabolism

Theophylline has antiasthma effects other than bronchodilation below 10 mg/L, so the therapeutic range is now taken as 5–15 mg/L. The dose of theophylline required to give these therapeutic concentrations varies among subjects, largely because of differences in clearance of the drug. In addition, there may be differences in bronchodilator response to theophylline; furthermore, with acute bronchoconstriction, higher concentrations may be required to produce bronchodilation. Theophylline is rapidly and completely absorbed, but there are large interindividual variations in clearance due to differences in hepatic metabolism. Theophylline is metabolized in the liver, mainly by CYP1A2; myriad factors influence hepatic metabolism and clearance of of theophylline (see Table 40–2).

Because of these variations in clearance, individualization of theophylline dosage is required, and plasma concentrations should be measured 4 h after the last dose with slow-release preparations when steady state has been achieved. There is no significant circadian variation in theophylline metabolism, although there may be delayed absorption at night related to supine posture.

Preparations and Routes of Administration

Intravenous aminophylline, an ethylene diamine ester of theophylline that is water soluble, has been used for many years in the treatment of acute severe asthma. The recommended dose is 6 mg/kg given intravenously over 20–30 min, followed by a maintenance dose of 0.5 mg/kg per hour. If the patient is already taking theophylline, or there are any factors that decrease clearance, these doses should be halved and the plasma level checked more frequently. Nebulized β₂ agonists are now preferred over intravenous aminophylline for acute exacerbations of asthma and COPD.

Oral immediate-release theophylline tablets or elixirs, which are rapidly absorbed, give wide fluctuations in plasma levels and are not recommended. Several sustained-release preparations are now available that are absorbed at a constant rate and provide steady plasma concentrations over a 12- to 24-h period. Both slow-release aminophylline and theophylline are available and are equally effective (although the ethylene diamine component of aminophylline has been implicated in allergic reactions). For continuous treatment, twice-daily therapy (~8 mg/kg twice daily) is needed. For nocturnal asthma, a single dose of slow-release theophylline at night is often effective. Once optimal doses have been determined, routine monitoring of plasma concentrations is usually not necessary unless a change in clearance is suspected or evidence of toxicity emerges.

Clinical Use

In patients with acute asthma, intravenous aminophylline is less effective than nebulized β₂ agonists and should therefore be reserved for those patients who fail to respond to, or are intolerant of, β agonists. Theophylline should not be added routinely to nebulized β₂ agonists because it does not increase the bronchodilator response and may increase their side effects. Theophylline has been used as a controller in the management of mild persistent asthma, although it is usually found to be less effective than low doses of ICSs. Addition of low-dose theophylline to an ICS in patients who are not adequately controlled provides better symptom control and lung function than doubling the dose of inhaled steroid (Lim et al., 2001). LABAs are more effective as an add-on therapy, but theophylline is

TABLE 40–2 ■ FACTORS AFFECTING CLEARANCE OF THEOPHYLLINE

Increased clearance

- Enzyme induction (mainly CYP1A2) by coadministered drugs (e.g., rifampicin, barbiturates, ethanol)
- Smoking (tobacco, marijuana) via CYP1A2 induction
- High-protein, low-carbohydrate diet
- Barbecued meat
- Childhood

Decreased clearance

- CYP inhibition (cimetidine, erythromycin, ciprofloxacin, allopurinol, fluvoxamine, zileuton, zafirlukast)
- Congestive heart failure
- Liver disease
- Pneumonia
- Viral infection and vaccination
- High-carbohydrate diet
- Old age

TABLE 40–3 ■ SIDE EFFECTS OF THEOPHYLLINE AND MECHANISMS

SIDE EFFECT	PROPOSED MECHANISM
Nausea and vomiting	PDE4 inhibition
Headaches	PDE4 inhibition
Gastric discomfort	PDE4 inhibition
Diuresis	A_1 receptor antagonism
Behavioral disturbance (?)	?
Cardiac arrhythmias	PDE3 inhibition, A_1 receptor antagonism
Epileptic seizures	A_1 receptor antagonism

A, adenosine.

considerably less expensive and may be the only affordable add-on treatment when the costs of medication are limiting.

Theophylline is still used as a bronchodilator in COPD, but inhaled anticholinergics and β_2 agonists are preferred. Theophylline tends to be added to these inhaled bronchodilators in patients with more severe disease and has been shown to give additional clinical improvement when added to a LABA.

Side Effects

Unwanted effects of theophylline are usually related to plasma concentration and tend to occur at C_p greater than 15 mg/L. The most common side effects are headache, nausea, and vomiting (due to inhibition of PDE4), abdominal discomfort, and restlessness (Table 40–3). There may also be increased acid secretion (due to PDE inhibition) and diuresis (due to inhibition of adenosine A_1 receptors). Theophylline may lead to behavioral disturbance and learning difficulties in schoolchildren. At high concentrations, cardiac arrhythmias may occur as a consequence of inhibition of cardiac PDE3 and antagonism of cardiac A_1 receptors. At very high concentrations, seizures may occur due to central A_1 receptor antagonism. Use of low doses of theophylline, targeting plasma concentrations of 5–10 mg/L, largely avoids side effects and drug interactions.

Summary and Future Developments

Theophylline use has been declining, partly because of the problems with side effects, but mainly because more effective therapy with β_2 agonists and ICSs have been introduced. Oral theophylline remains a useful add-on treatment in some patients with difficult asthma and appears to have effects beyond those provided by steroids. Rapid-release theophylline preparations are the only affordable antiasthma medication in some developing countries. There is increasing evidence that theophylline has some antiasthma effect at doses that are lower than those needed for bronchodilation, and plasma levels of 5–15 mg/L are recommended.

Muscarinic Cholinergic Antagonists

The basic pharmacology of the antimuscarinic agents is presented in Chapter 9.

HISTORY

Datura stramonium (jimson weed) and related species of the nightshade family contain a mixture of muscarinic antagonists (atropine, hyoscyamine, scopolamine) and were smoked for relief of asthma two centuries ago. Subsequently, the purified plant alkaloid atropine was introduced for treating asthma. Due to the significant side effects of atropine, particularly drying of secretions, less-soluble quaternary compounds, such as atropine methylnitrate and ipratropium bromide, have been developed. These compounds are topically active and are not significantly absorbed from the respiratory or GI tracts.

Mode of Action

As competitive antagonists of endogenous ACh at muscarinic receptors, these agents inhibit the direct constrictor effect on bronchial smooth muscle mediated via the M_3-G_q-PLC-IP_3-Ca^{2+} pathway (see Chapters 3 and 9). The efficacy stems from the role played by the parasympathetic nervous system in regulating bronchomotor tone. The effects of ACh on the respiratory system include bronchoconstriction and tracheobronchial mucus secretion. Thus, antimuscarinic drugs antagonize these effects of ACh, resulting in bronchodilation and reduced mucus secretion.

Acetylcholine may also be released from other airway cells, including epithelial cells (Wessler and Kirkpatrick, 2008). The synthesis of ACh in epithelial cells is increased by inflammatory stimuli (such as TNF-α), which increase the expression of choline acetyltransferase, which could contribute to cholinergic effects in airway diseases. Muscarinic receptors are expressed in airway smooth muscle of small airways that do not appear to be significantly innervated by cholinergic nerves; these receptors may be a mechanism of cholinergic narrowing in peripheral airways that could be relevant in COPD, responding to locally synthesized, nonneuronal ACh.

Myriad mechanical, chemical, and immunological stimuli elicit reflex bronchoconstriction via vagal pathways, and cholinergic pathways may play an important role in regulating acute bronchomotor responses in animals. Anticholinergic drugs will only inhibit reflex ACh-mediated bronchoconstriction and have no blocking effect on the *direct* effects of inflammatory mediators, such as histamine and LTs, on bronchial smooth muscle. Furthermore, cholinergic antagonists probably have little or no effect on mast cells, microvascular leak, or the chronic inflammatory response.

Clinical Use

In asthmatic patients, anticholinergic drugs are less effective as bronchodilators than β_2 agonists and offer less-efficient protection against bronchial challenges. Anticholinergics are currently used as an additional bronchodilator in asthmatic patients not controlled on a LABA. Nebulized anticholinergic drugs are effective in acute severe asthma but less effective than β_2 agonists. In the acute and chronic treatment of asthma, anticholinergic drugs may have an additive effect with β_2 agonists and should therefore be considered when control of asthma is not adequate with nebulized β_2 agonists. A muscarinic antagonist should be considered when there are problems with theophylline or when inhaled β_2 agonists cause a troublesome tremor in elderly patients.

In COPD, anticholinergic drugs may be as effective as or even superior to β_2 agonists. Their relatively greater effect in COPD than in asthma may be explained by an inhibitory effect on vagal tone, which, although not necessarily increased in COPD, may be the only reversible element of airway obstruction and one that is exaggerated by geometric factors in the narrowed airways of patients with COPD (Figure 40–6). Anticholinergic drugs reduce air trapping and improve exercise tolerance in patients with COPD.

Therapeutic Choices

The *SAMA* ipratropium bromide is available as a pMDI and nebulized preparation. The onset of bronchodilation is relatively slow and is usually maximal 30–60 min after inhalation but may persist for 6–8 h. It is usually given by MDI three or four times daily on a regular basis, rather than intermittently for symptom relief, in view of its slow onset of action, but has now been replaced by *LAMAs*, such as tiotropium bromide.

Long-Acting Muscarinic Antagonists

Several LAMAs have now been developed from the treatment of COPD and, more recently, severe asthma. *Tiotropium bromide* is a long-acting anticholinergic drug that is suitable for once-daily dosing as a DPI (Spiriva) or via a soft mist mininebulizer device and was more effective than *ipratropium* four times daily in several studies; it also significantly reduces exacerbations (Cheyne et al., 2015). Tiotropium binds to all muscarinic receptor subtypes but dissociates slowly from M_3 and M_1 receptors, giving it a degree of kinetic receptor selectivity for these receptors compared with M_2 receptors, from which it dissociates more rapidly. Thus, compared with ipratropium, tiotropium is less likely to antagonize M_2-mediated inhibition of ACh release (the resulting increase in ACh could counteract the

$$\text{Resistance} \propto \frac{1}{r^4}$$

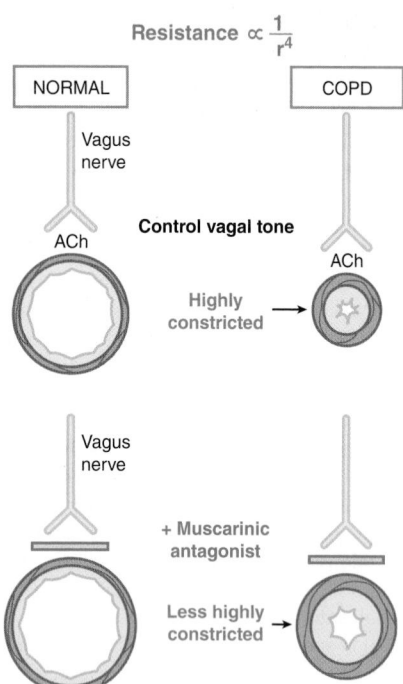

Figure 40–6 *Anticholinergic drugs inhibit vagally mediated airway tone, thereby producing bronchodilation.* This effect is small in normal airways but is greater in airways of patients with COPD, which are structurally narrowed and have higher resistance to airflow because airway resistance is inversely related to the fourth power of the radius r.

blockade of M_3 receptor–mediated bronchoconstriction) (Chapter 9). Over a 4-year period, tiotropium improved lung function and health status and reduced exacerbations and all-cause mortality, although there was no effect on disease progression (Tashkin et al., 2008).

Glycopyrronium bromide and *umeclidinium bromide* are also once-daily LAMAs with very similar clinical effects to tiotropium, whereas *aclidinium bromide* has to be given twice daily (Cazzola et al., 2013a). LAMAs are now becoming the bronchodilators of choice for patients with COPD. LAMAs are also effective as additional bronchodilators in patient with asthma not adequately controlled with maximal ICS/LABA therapy, although not all patients respond (Kerstjens et al., 2015).

Combination Inhalers

There are additive bronchodilator effects between anticholinergics and β_2 agonists in patients with COPD, which has led to the development of fixed-dose combinations. SABA/SAMA combinations, such as *albuterol/ipratropium*, are popular. Several studies have demonstrated additive effects of these two drugs, thus providing an advantage over increasing the dose of β_2 agonist in patients who have side effects.

LABA/LAMA dual combination inhalers have also been developed, including *indacaterol/glycopyrronium, vilanterol/umeclidinium bromide, olodaterol/tiotropium bromide* (all once daily), and *formoterol/glycopyrronium bromide, formoterol/aclidinium bromide* (twice daily), which all sow beneficial effects on lung function compared with either LABA or LAMA alone, although they may not be clearly beneficial in terms of reducing exacerbations (Calzetta et al., 2016).

Adverse Effects

Inhaled anticholinergic drugs are generally well tolerated. On stopping inhaled anticholinergics, a small rebound increase in airway responsiveness has been described. Systemic side effects after SAMA or LAMA are uncommon during normal clinical use because there is little systemic absorption. Because cholinergic agonists can stimulate *mucus secretion*, there has been concern that anticholinergics may reduce secretion and lead to more viscous mucus. However, ipratropium bromide and tiotropium bromide, even in high doses, have no detectable effect on mucociliary

clearance in either normal subjects or in patients with airway disease. A significant unwanted effect is the unpleasant *bitter taste* of inhaled ipratropium, which may contribute to poor compliance. Nebulized ipratropium bromide may precipitate *glaucoma* in elderly patients due to a direct effect of the nebulized drug on the eye. This may be prevented by nebulization with a mouthpiece rather than a face mask.

Reports of *paradoxical bronchoconstriction* with ipratropium bromide, particularly when given by nebulizer, were largely explained as effects of the hypotonic nebulizer solution and by antibacterial additives, such as benzalkonium chloride and EDTA. This problem has not been described with tiotropium bromide or other LAMAs. Occasionally, bronchoconstriction may occur with ipratropium bromide given by MDI. It is possible that this is due to blockade of prejunctional M_2 receptors on airway cholinergic nerves that normally inhibit ACh release.

LAMAs cause dryness of the mouth in 10%–15% of patients, but this usually disappears during continued therapy. Urinary retention is occasionally seen in elderly patients.

Future Developments

The LABA/LAMA fixed-combination inhalers are likely to become the bronchodilators of choice in patients with COPD, and LAMAs are added to ICS/LABA combinations in severe asthma. Some triple inhalers that have the ICS/LABA/LAMA combination, such as *budesonide/formoterol/glycopyrronium, mometasone/indacaterol/glycopyrronium*, and *fluticasone furoate/umeclidinium/vilanterol*, are in development for use in patients with severe asthma and asthma-COPD overlap. Dual-action drugs that are both muscarinic antagonists and β_2 agonist are also in clinical development, but it has proved difficult to balance the β agonist and anticholinergic activities (Ray and Alcaraz, 2009).

Novel Classes of Bronchodilator

Currently, the most effective bronchodilators are LABAs for asthma and a LAMA for COPD. Inventing new classes of bronchodilator has been difficult; several agents have had problems with vasodilator side effects because they relax vascular smooth muscle to a greater extent than airway smooth muscle. Nonetheless, there are several classes of bronchodilators under development, as described next.

Magnesium Sulfate

Magnesium sulfate ($MgSO_4$) is useful as an additional bronchodilator in children and adults with acute severe asthma. Intravenous or nebulized $MgSO_4$ benefits adults and children with severe exacerbations ($FEV_1 < 30\%$ of predicted value), giving improvement in lung function when added to nebulized β_2 agonist and a reduction in hospital admissions (Kew et al., 2014). The treatment is cheap and well tolerated, although the clinical benefit appears small. Side effects include flushing and nausea but are usually minor. Magnesium sulfate appears to act as a bronchodilator and may reduce cytosolic Ca^{2+} concentrations in airway smooth muscle cells. The concentration of magnesium is lower in serum and erythrocytes of asthmatic patients than in normal controls and correlates with airway hyperresponsiveness, although the improvement in acute severe asthma after magnesium does not correlate with plasma concentrations. The effects of intravenous $MgSO_4$ in COPD are minimal, and there are too few studies to make any firm recommendation (Shivanthan and Rajapakse, 2014).

Potassium Channel Openers

The K^+ channel openers such as *cromakalim* or *levcromakalim* (the *levo*-isomer of cromakalim) open ATP-dependent K^+ channels in smooth muscle, leading to membrane hyperpolarization and relaxation of airway smooth muscle. This suggests that K^+ channel activators may be useful as bronchodilators (Pelaia et al., 2002). Clinical studies in asthma, however, have been disappointing, with no bronchodilation or protection against bronchoconstrictor challenges. The cardiovascular side effects of these drugs (postural hypotension, flushing) limit the oral dose; furthermore, inhaled formulations are problematic. New developments include K^+ channel openers that open Ca^{2+}-activated large conductance K^+ channels (maxi-K channels) that are also opened by β_2 agonists; these drugs may be better tolerated. Maxi-K channel openers also inhibit mucus secretion and cough, and they may be of particular value in the treatment of COPD. So far, none of these drugs has been studied in patients with airway disease.

Vasoactive Intestinal Polypeptide Analogues

Vasoactive intestinal polypeptide is a peptide that has 28 amino acids; it binds to two GPCRs, VPAC$_1$ and VPAC$_2$, both of which couple primarily to G$_s$ to stimulate the adenylyl cyclase-cAMP-PKA pathway leading to relaxation of smooth muscle. VIP is a potent dilator of human airway smooth muscle in vitro but is not effective in patients because it is rapidly metabolized (plasma $t_{1/2} \sim 2$ min); in addition, VIP causes vasodilator side effects. More stable analogues of VIP, such as Ro 25-1533, which selectively stimulates VIP receptors in airway smooth muscle (via VPAC$_2$), have been synthesized. Inhaled Ro 25-1533 has a rapid bronchodilator effect in asthmatic patients, but it is not as prolonged as formoterol (Linden et al., 2003).

Bitter Taste Receptor Agonists

Bitter taste receptors (TAS2R) are GPCRs that are expressed in airway smooth muscle and mediate bronchodilation in response to agonists, such as *quinine* and *chloroquine*, even after β$_2$ receptor desensitization (An et al., 2012). However, these agonists are weak, so more potent drugs are needed.

Other Inhibitors of Smooth Muscle Contraction

Agents that inhibit the contractile machinery of airway smooth muscle, including rho kinase inhibitors, inhibitors of myosin light chain kinase, and myosin inhibitors, are also in development. Because these agents also cause vasodilation, it will be necessary to administer them by inhalation.

Corticosteroids

The introduction of *ICSs*, as a way of reducing the requirement and side effects of oral steroids, has revolutionized the treatment of chronic asthma (Barnes et al., 1998b). Because asthma is a chronic inflammatory disease, ICSs are considered first-line therapy in all but patients with the mildest disease. In marked contrast, ICSs are much less effective in COPD and should only be used in patients with severe disease who have frequent exacerbations. Oral corticosteroids remain the mainstay of treatment of several other pulmonary diseases, such as sarcoidosis, interstitial lung diseases, and pulmonary eosinophilic syndromes. The general pharmacology of corticosteroids is presented in Chapter 46.

Mechanism of Action

Corticosteroids enter target cells and bind to GRs in the cytoplasm (Chapter 46). There is only one type of GR that binds corticosteroids and no evidence for the existence of subtypes that might mediate different aspects of corticosteroid action (Barnes, 2011a). The steroid-GR complex moves into the nucleus, where it binds to specific sequences on the upstream regulatory elements of certain target genes, resulting in increased (or, rarely, decreased) transcription of the gene, with subsequent increased (or decreased) synthesis of the gene products.

The GRs may also interact with protein transcription factors and coactivator molecules in the nucleus and thereby influence the synthesis of certain proteins independently of any direct interaction with DNA. The repression of transcription factors, such as AP-1 and NF-κB, is likely to account for many of the anti-inflammatory effects of steroids in asthma. In particular, corticosteroids reverse the activating effect of these pro-inflammatory transcription factors on histone acetylation by recruiting HDAC2 to inflammatory genes that have been activated through acetylation of associated histones (Figure 40–7). GRs are acetylated when corticosteroids are bound and bind to DNA in this acetylated state as dimers, whereas the acetylated GR has to be deacetylated by HDAC2 to interact with inflammatory genes and NF-κB (Ito et al., 2006).

There may be additional mechanisms that are also important in the anti-inflammatory actions of corticosteroids. Corticosteroids have potent inhibitory effects on MAP kinase signaling pathways through the induction of MAP kinase phosphatase 1, which may inhibit the expression of multiple inflammatory genes (Clark, 2003)

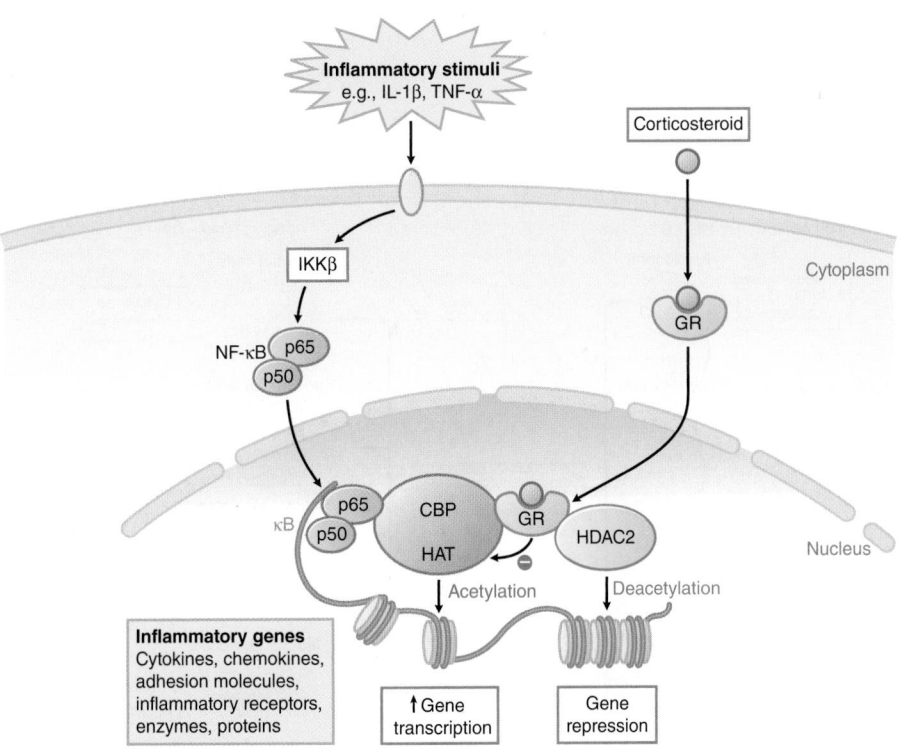

Figure 40–7 *Mechanism of anti-inflammatory action of corticosteroids in asthma.* Inflammatory stimuli (IL-1β, TNF-α, etc.) activate IKKβ, which activates the transcription factor NF-κB. A dimer of p50 and p65 NF-κB proteins translocates to the nucleus and binds to specific κB recognition sites and to coactivators, such as the CREB-binding protein (CBP), which have intrinsic histone acetyltransferase (HAT) activity. This results in acetylation of core histones and consequent increased expression of genes encoding multiple inflammatory proteins. Cytosolic GRs bind corticosteroids; the receptor-ligand complexes translocate to the nucleus and bind to coactivators to inhibit HAT activity in two ways: directly and, more importantly, by recruiting HDAC2, which reverses histone acetylation, leading to the suppression of activated inflammatory genes.

Anti-inflammatory Effects in Asthma

Corticosteroids have widespread effects on gene transcription, increasing the transcription of several anti-inflammatory genes and suppressing transcription of many inflammatory genes. Steroids have inhibitory effects on many inflammatory and structural cells that are activated in asthma and prevent the recruitment of inflammatory cells into the airways (Figure 40–8). In patients with mild asthma, the inflammation may be completely resolved after inhaled steroids.

Steroids potently inhibit the formation of multiple inflammatory cytokines, particularly cytokines released from T_H2 cells. Corticosteroids also decrease eosinophil survival by inducing apoptosis. Corticosteroids inhibit the expression of multiple inflammatory genes in airway epithelial cells, probably the most important action of ICSs in suppressing asthmatic inflammation. Corticosteroids also prevent and reverse the increase in vascular permeability due to inflammatory mediators and may therefore lead to resolution of airway edema. Steroids have a direct inhibitory effect on mucus glycoprotein secretion from airway submucosal glands, as well as indirect inhibitory effects by downregulation of inflammatory stimuli that stimulate mucus secretion.

Corticosteroids have no direct effect on contractile responses of airway smooth muscle; improvement in lung function after ICSs is presumably due to an effect on the chronic airway inflammation, edema, and airway hyperresponsiveness. A single dose of an ICS has no effect on the early response to allergen (reflecting the ICSs lack of effect on mast cell mediator release) but inhibits the late response (which may be due to an effect on macrophages, eosinophils, and airway wall edema) and also inhibits the increase in airway hyperresponsiveness.

The ICSs have rapid anti-inflammatory effects, reducing airway hyperresponsiveness and inflammatory mediator concentrations in sputum within a few hours (Erin et al., 2008). However, it may take several weeks or months to achieve maximal effects on airway hyperresponsiveness, presumably reflecting the slow healing of the damaged inflamed airway. It is important to recognize that corticosteroids *suppress* inflammation in the airways but do not cure the underlying disease. When steroids are withdrawn, there is a recurrence of the same degree of airway hyperresponsiveness, although in patients with mild asthma it may take several months to return.

Effect on β₂ Adrenergic Responsiveness

Steroids potentiate the effects of β agonists on bronchial smooth muscle and prevent and reverse β receptor desensitization in airways in vitro *and*

in vivo (Barnes, 2002; Black et al., 2009). At a molecular level, corticosteroids increase the transcription of the β_2 receptor gene in human lung in vitro and in the respiratory mucosa in vivo and also increase the stability of its messenger RNA. They also prevent or reverse uncoupling of β_2 receptors to G_s. In animal systems, corticosteroids prevent downregulation of β_2 receptors.

β_2 Agonists also enhance the action of GRs, resulting in increased nuclear translocation of liganded GR receptors and enhancing the binding of GRs to DNA. This effect has been demonstrated in sputum macrophages of asthmatic patients after an ICS and inhaled LABA (Barnes, 2011a). This suggests that β_2 agonists and corticosteroids enhance each other's beneficial effects in asthma therapy.

Pharmacokinetics

The pharmacokinetics of oral corticosteroids are described in Chapter 46. The pharmacokinetics of ICSs are important in relation to systemic effects (Barnes et al., 1998b). The fraction of steroid that is inhaled into the lungs acts locally on the airway mucosa but may be absorbed from the airway and alveolar surface. Thus, a portion of an inhaled dose reaches the systemic circulation. Furthermore, the fraction of inhaled steroid that is deposited in the oropharynx is swallowed and absorbed from the gut. The absorbed fraction may be metabolized in the liver (first-pass metabolism) before reaching the systemic circulation (Figure 40–3). The use of a spacer chamber reduces oropharyngeal deposition and therefore reduces systemic absorption of ICSs, although this effect is minimal in corticosteroids with a high first-pass metabolism. Mouth rinsing and discarding the rinse have a similar effect, and this procedure should be used with high-dose dry powder steroid inhalers when spacer chambers cannot be used.

Beclomethasone dipropionate and *ciclesonide* are prodrugs that release the active corticosteroid after the ester group is cleaved by esterases in the lung. Ciclesonide is available as an MDI for asthma and as a nasal spray for allergic rhinitis. *Budesonide* and *fluticasone propionate* have a greater first-pass metabolism than BDP and are therefore less likely to produce systemic effects at high inhaled doses.

Routes of Administration and Dosing

Inhaled Corticosteroids in Asthma

Inhaled corticosteroids are recommended as first-line therapy for patients with persistent asthma. They should be started in any patient who needs to use a β₂ agonist inhaler for symptom control more than twice weekly.

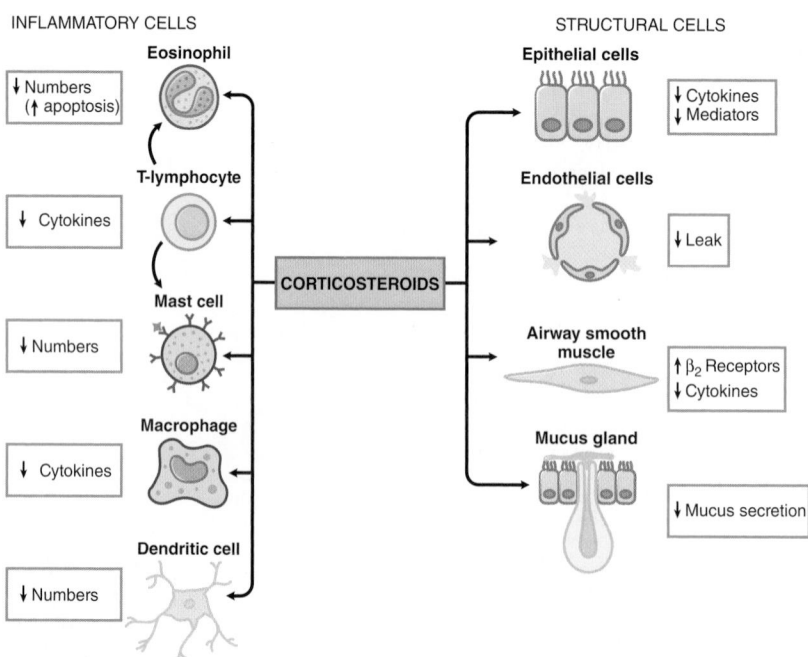

Figure 40–8 *Effect of corticosteroids on inflammatory and structural cells in the airways.*

They are effective in mild, moderate, and severe asthma and in children as well as adults (Barnes et al., 1998b).

Most of the benefit may be obtained from doses of less than 400 μg BDP or equivalent. However, some patients (with relative corticosteroid resistance) may benefit from higher doses (up to 2000 μg/d). For most patients, ICSs should be used twice daily, a regimen that improves adherence once control of asthma has been achieved (which may require four-time daily dosing initially or a course of oral steroids if symptoms are severe). Administration once daily of some steroids (e.g., budesonide, mometasone, and ciclesonide in mild asthma and fluticasone furoate in all patients) is effective when doses of 400 μg or less are needed. If a dose greater than 800 μg daily via pMDI is used, a spacer device should be employed to reduce the risk of oropharyngeal side effects. ICSs may be used in children in the same way as in adults; at doses of 400 μg/d or less, there is no evidence of significant growth suppression (Pedersen, 2001). The dose of ICS should be the minimal dose that controls asthma; once control is achieved, the dose should be slowly reduced (Hawkins et al., 2003). Nebulized corticosteroids (e.g., budesonide) are useful in the treatment of small children who are not able to use other inhaler devices.

Inhaled Corticosteroids in COPD

Patients with COPD occasionally respond to steroids, and these patients are likely to have concomitant asthma. Corticosteroids do not appear to have any significant anti-inflammatory effect in COPD; there appears to be an active resistance mechanism, which may be explained by impaired activity of HDAC2 as a result of oxidative stress (Barnes, 2013a). ICSs have no effect on the progression of COPD, even when given to patients with presymptomatic disease; in addition, ICSs have no effect on mortality (Yang et al., 2012). ICSs reduce the number of exacerbations in patients with severe COPD ($FEV_1 < 50\%$ predicted) who have frequent exacerbations and are recommended in these patients, although there is debate about whether these effects are due to inappropriate analysis of the data (Ernst et al., 2015). Oral corticosteroids are used to treat acute exacerbations of COPD, but the effect is very small (Niewoehner et al., 1999).

Patients with cystic fibrosis and bronchiectasis, which involve chronic neutrophilic inflammation of the airways, are also resistant to high doses of ICS.

Systemic Steroids

Intravenous steroids are indicated in acute asthma if lung function is less than 30% predicted and in patients who show no significant improvement with nebulized β_2 agonist. *Hydrocortisone* is the steroid of choice because it has the most rapid onset (5–6 h after administration), compared with 8 h with *prednisolone*. It is common to give hydrocortisone 4 mg/kg initially, followed by a maintenance dose of 3 mg/kg every 6 h. *Methylprednisolone* is also available for intravenous use. Intravenous therapy is usually given until a satisfactory response is obtained, and then oral prednisolone may be substituted. *Oral prednisone or prednisolone* (40–60 mg) has a similar effect to intravenous hydrocortisone and is easier to administer. A high dose of *inhaled fluticasone propionate* (2000 μg daily) is as effective as a course of oral prednisolone in controlling acute exacerbations of asthma in a family practice setting and in children in an emergency department setting, although this route of delivery is more expensive (Manjra et al., 2000).

Prednisone and *prednisolone* are the most commonly used oral steroids. Maximal beneficial effect is usually achieved with 30–40 mg prednisone daily, although a few patients may need 60–80 mg daily to achieve control of symptoms. The usual maintenance dose is about 10–15 mg/d. Short courses of oral steroids (30–40 mg prednisolone daily for 1–2 weeks) are indicated for exacerbations of asthma; the dose may be tapered over 1 week after the exacerbation is resolved (the taper is not strictly necessary after a short course of therapy, but patients find it reassuring). Oral steroids are usually given as a single dose in the morning because this coincides with the normal diurnal increase in plasma cortisol and produces less adrenal suppression than if given in divided doses or at night.

Adverse Effects

Corticosteroids inhibit corticotropin and cortisol secretion by a negative-feedback effect on the pituitary gland (see Chapter 46).

Hypothalamic-pituitary-adrenal (HPA) axis suppression depends on dose and usually only occurs with doses of prednisone greater than 7.5–10 mg/d. Significant suppression after short courses of corticosteroid therapy is not usually a problem, but prolonged suppression may occur after several months or years. *Steroid doses after prolonged oral therapy must be reduced slowly.* Symptoms of "steroid withdrawal syndrome" include lassitude, musculoskeletal pains, and, occasionally, fever. HPA suppression with inhaled steroids is usually seen only when the daily inhaled dose exceeds 2000 μg BDP or its equivalent daily.

Side effects of long-term oral corticosteroid therapy include fluid retention, increased appetite, weight gain, osteoporosis, capillary fragility, hypertension, peptic ulceration, diabetes, cataracts, and psychosis. Their frequency tends to increase with age. Very occasionally adverse reactions (such as anaphylaxis) to intravenous hydrocortisone have been described, particularly in aspirin-sensitive asthmatic patients.

The incidence of systemic side effects after ICSs is an important consideration, particularly in children (Lipworth, 1999) (Table 40–4). Initial studies suggested that adrenal suppression occurred only with inhaled doses greater than 1500–2000 μg/d. More sensitive measurements of systemic effects include indices of bone metabolism, such as serum osteocalcin and urinary pyridinium cross-links, and in children, knemometry, which may be increased with inhaled doses as low as 400 μg/d BDP in some patients. The clinical relevance of these measurements is not yet clear, however. Nevertheless, it is important to reduce the likelihood of systemic effects by using the lowest dose of inhaled steroid needed to control the asthma and by use of a large-volume spacer to reduce oropharyngeal deposition.

Several systemic effects of inhaled steroids have been described and include dermal thinning and skin capillary fragility (relatively common in elderly patients after high-dose inhaled steroids). Other side effects, such as cataract formation and osteoporosis, are reported but often in patients who are also receiving courses of oral steroids. There is some evidence that use of high-dose ICSs is associated with cataract and glaucoma, but it is difficult to dissociate the effects of ICS from the effects of courses of oral steroids that these patients usually require. There has been particular concern about the use of inhaled steroids in children because of growth suppression (Zhang et al., 2014).

The ICSs may have *local side effects* due to the deposition of inhaled steroid in the oropharynx. The most common problem is hoarseness and weakness of the voice (dysphonia) due to atrophy of the vocal cords following laryngeal deposition of steroid; it may occur in up to 40% of patients and is noticed particularly by patients who need to use their voices during their work (lecturers, teachers, and singers). Throat irritation and coughing after inhalation are common with MDIs and appear to be due to additives because these problems are not usually seen if the patient switches to a DPI. There is no evidence for atrophy of the lining of the airway. Oropharyngeal candidiasis occurs in about 5% of patients. There is no evidence for increased lung infections, including tuberculosis, in patients with asthma.

TABLE 40–4 ■ SIDE EFFECTS OF INHALED CORTICOSTEROIDS

Local side effects
  Dysphonia
  Oropharyngeal candidiasis
  Cough

Systemic side effects
  Adrenal suppression and insufficiency
  Growth suppression
  Bruising
  Osteoporosis
  Cataracts
  Glaucoma
  Metabolic abnormalities (glucose, insulin, triglycerides)
  Psychiatric disturbances (euphoria, depression)
  Pneumonia

Growing evidence suggests that high doses of ICSs increase the risk of pneumonia in patients with COPD (Finney et al., 2014); the risk appears to be higher with fluticasone propionate than budesonide.

Corticosteroid MDIs with HFA propellants produce smaller aerosol particles and may have a more peripheral deposition, making them useful in treating patients with more severe asthma.

Therapeutic Choices

Numerous ICSs are now available, including *BDP, triamcinolone, flunisolide, budesonide, hemihydrate, fluticasone propionate, mometasone furoate, ciclesonide,* and *fluticasone furoate.* All are equally effective as antiasthma drugs, but there are differences in their pharmacokinetics: Budesonide, fluticasone, mometasone, and ciclesonide have a lower oral bioavailability than BDP because they are subject to greater first-pass hepatic metabolism; this results in reduced systemic absorption from the fraction of the inhaled drug that is swallowed (Derendorf et al., 2006) and thus reduced adverse effects. At high doses (>1000 μg), budesonide and fluticasone propionate have fewer systemic effects than BDP and triamcinolone (not marketed in the U.S.), and they are preferred in patients who need high doses of ICSs and in children. Ciclesonide is another choice; it is a prodrug that is converted to the active metabolite by esterases in the lung, giving it low oral bioavailability and a high therapeutic index (Derendorf, 2007). Fluticasone furoate has the longest duration of action and is suitable for once-daily dosing (Woodcock et al., 2011).

When doses of inhaled steroid exceed 800 μg BDP or equivalent daily, a large-volume spacer is recommended to reduce oropharyngeal deposition and systemic absorption in the case of BDP. All currently available ICSs are absorbed from the lung into the systemic circulation, so that some systemic absorption is inevitable. However, the amount of drug absorbed does not appear to have clinical effects in doses of less than 800 μg BDP equivalent. Although there are potency differences among corticosteroids, there are relatively few comparative studies, partly because dose comparison of corticosteroids is difficult due to their long time course of action and the relative flatness of their dose-response curves.

Future Developments

Early treatment with ICSs in both adults and children may give a greater improvement in lung function than if treatment is delayed (Busse et al., 2008), likely reflecting the fact that corticosteroids are able to modify the underlying inflammatory process and prevent structural changes (fibrosis, smooth muscle hyperplasia, etc.). ICSs are currently recommended for patients with persistent asthmatic symptoms (e.g., need for an inhaled β_2 agonist more than twice a week).

Developing new corticosteroids with fewer systemic effects is desirable. It has been possible to develop corticosteroids that dissociate the DNA-binding effect of corticosteroids (which mediates most of the adverse effects) from the inhibitory effect on transcription factors such as NF-κB (which mediates much of the anti-inflammatory effect). Such "dissociated steroids" or selective GR agonists should, theoretically, retain anti-inflammatory activity but have a reduced risk of adverse effects; achieving this separation of desired and adverse effects is difficult in vivo (Belvisi et al., 2001). Nonsteroidal selective GR agonists are now in development.

Corticosteroid resistance is a major barrier to effective therapy in patients with severe asthma, in asthmatic patients who smoke, and in patients with COPD and cystic fibrosis (Barnes, 2013a; Barnes and Adcock, 2009). "Steroid-resistant" asthma is thought to be due to reduced anti-inflammatory actions of corticosteroids. In those with COPD and some patients with severe asthma, there is a reduction in HDAC2 expression that reduces corticosteroid responsiveness; this is potentially reversible by existing treatments, such as low-dose theophylline and nortriptyline.

Cromones

Cromolyn sodium (sodium cromoglycate) is a derivative of *khellin,* an Egyptian herbal remedy, and was found to protect against allergen challenge without any bronchodilator effect. A structurally related drug, *nedocromil sodium,* which has a similar pharmacological profile to cromolyn, was subsequently developed. Although cromolyn was popular in the past because of its good safety profile, its use has sharply declined with the more widespread use of the more effective ICSs, particularly in children.

Phosphodiesterase Inhibitors

The PDE inhibitors relax smooth muscle and inhibit inflammatory cells through an increase in cellular cAMP. PDE4 is the predominant PDE isoform in inflammatory cells, including mast cells, eosinophils, neutrophils, T lymphocytes, macrophages, and structural cells such as sensory nerves and epithelial cells (Hatzelmann et al., 2010), suggesting that PDE4 inhibitors could be useful as an anti-inflammatory treatment in both asthma and COPD.

In animal models of asthma, PDE4 inhibitors reduce eosinophil infiltration and responses to allergen, whereas in COPD they are effective against smoke-induced inflammation and emphysema. In COPD, an oral PDE4 inhibitor, *roflumilast,* has been approved for patients with COPD with severe disease (FEV_1 < 50% predicted, frequent exacerbations, and chronic bronchitis). Given once daily by mouth, it reduces exacerbations but has little effect on symptoms and lung function (Calverley et al., 2009), although it is effective on top of long-acting bronchodilators and ICSs (Martinez et al., 2015). The relatively weak efficacy is due to dose limitations as a result of side effects, particularly diarrhea, headaches, and nausea.

Of the four subfamilies of PDE4, PDE4D is the major form whose inhibition is associated with vomiting; inhibition of PDE4B is important for anti-inflammatory effects. Thus, selective PDE4B inhibitors may have a greater therapeutic index. Inhaled PDE4 inhibitors, to reduce systemic absorption and adverse responses, have proved to be ineffective. A dual PDE3/4 inhibitor gives bronchodilation in patients with COPD when given by nebulization, but it is uncertain whether there are significant anti-inflammatory effects (Franciosi et al., 2013).

Mediator Antagonists

Both H_1 antihistamines and anti-LTs have been applied to airway disease, but their added benefit over β_2 agonists and corticosteroids is slight (Barnes, 2004; Barnes et al., 1998a).

Antihistamines

Histamine mimics many of the features of asthma and is released from mast cells in acute asthmatic responses, suggesting that antihistamines may be useful in asthma therapy. There is little evidence that histamine H_1 receptor antagonists provide any useful clinical benefit, as demonstrated by a meta-analysis (van Ganse et al., 1997). Newer antihistamines, including *cetirizine* and *azelastine,* have some beneficial effects, but this may be unrelated to H_1 receptor antagonism. Antihistamines are not recommended in the routine management of asthma.

Antileukotrienes

There is considerable evidence that cys-LTs are produced in asthma and that they have potent effects on airway function, inducing bronchoconstriction, airway hyperresponsiveness, plasma exudation, mucus secretion, and eosinophilic inflammation (Figure 40–9; also see Chapter 37). These findings led to the development of 5′-lipoxygenase (5-LO) enzyme inhibitors (of which *zileuton* is the only drug marketed) and several antagonists of the cys-LT_1 receptor, including *montelukast* (s, *zafirlukast,* and *pranlukast* (not available in the U.S.).

Clinical Studies

In patients with mild-to-moderate asthma, anti-LTs cause a significant improvement in lung function and asthma symptoms, with a reduction in the use of rescue inhaled β_2 agonists. Several studies showed evidence for a bronchodilator effect, with an improvement in baseline lung function, suggesting that LTs are contributing to the baseline bronchoconstriction

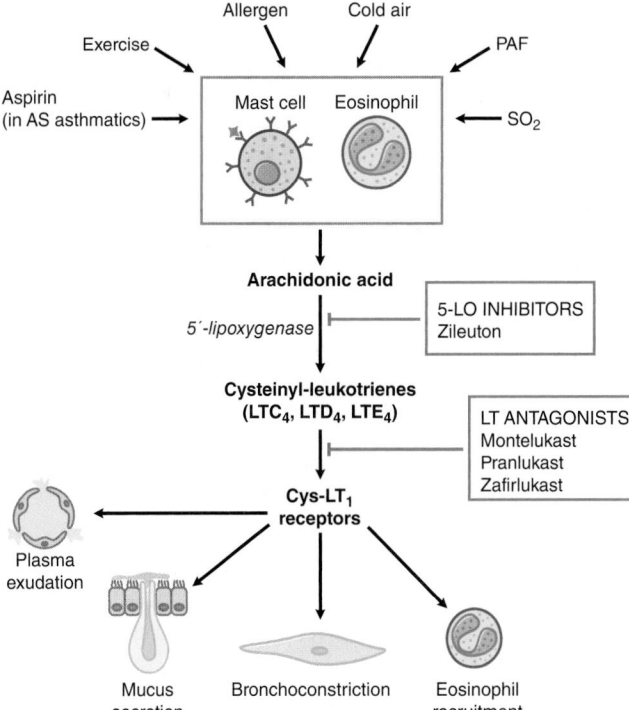

Figure 40–9 *Effects of cysteinyl-LTs on the airways and their inhibition by anti-LTs. AS, aspirin sensitive.*

in asthma, although this varies among patients. However, anti-LTs are considerably less effective than ICSs in the treatment of mild asthma and cannot be considered the treatment of first choice (Chauhan and Ducharme, 2012). Anti-LTs are indicated as an add-on therapy in patients who are not well controlled on ICSs. The added benefit is small, equivalent to doubling the dose of ICS, and less effective than adding a LABA. Anti-LTs have a beneficial effect in allergic rhinitis and have a similar efficacy to antihistamines (Grayson and Korenblat, 2007).

In patients with severe asthma who are not controlled on high doses of ICS and LABA, anti-LTs do not appear to provide any additional benefit (Robinson et al., 2001). Theoretically, anti-LTs should be of particular value in patients with aspirin-sensitive asthma because they block the airway response to aspirin challenge; however, their benefit is no greater here than in other types of asthma.

Anti-LTs are effective in preventing exercise-induced asthma, with efficacy similar to that of LABAs (Coreno et al., 2000). Anti-LTs appear to act mainly as antibronchoconstrictor drugs, and they are clearly less broadly effective than β_2 agonists because they antagonize only one of several bronchoconstrictor mediators.

The cys-LT_1 receptor antagonists have no role in the therapy of COPD. By contrast, LTB_4, a potent neutrophil chemoattractant, is elevated in COPD, indicating that 5-LO inhibitors that inhibit LTB_4 synthesis may have some potential benefit by reducing neutrophil inflammation. However, a pilot study failed to indicate any clear benefit of a 5-LO inhibitor in patients with COPD (Bernstein et al., 2011).

Adverse Effects

Zileuton, zafirlukast, and montelukast are all associated with rare cases of hepatic dysfunction; thus, liver-associated enzymes should be monitored. Several cases of Churg-Strauss syndrome have been associated with the use of zafirlukast and montelukast. Churg-Strauss syndrome is a rare vasculitis that may affect the heart, peripheral nerves, and kidney and is associated with increased circulating eosinophils and asthma. Cases of Churg-Strauss syndrome have been described in patients on anti-LTs who were not on concomitant corticosteroid therapy, suggesting there is a causal link (Nathani et al., 2008).

Future Developments

One of the major advantages of anti-LTs is their effectiveness in tablet form. This may increase compliance with chronic therapy and makes treatment of children easier. Montelukast is effective as a once-daily preparation (10 mg in adults, 5 mg in children). In addition, oral administration may treat concomitant allergic rhinitis. However, the clinical studies indicated a modest effect on lung function and symptom control. This is not surprising. There are many mediators besides cys-LTs involved in the pathophysiology of asthma, and anti-LTs are unlikely to be as effective as a β_2 agonist, which will counteract bronchoconstriction regardless of the spasmogen. It is likely that anti-LTs will be used less in the future because combination inhalers are the mainstay of asthma therapy.

Some patients appear to show better responses than others, suggesting that LTs may play a more important role in some patients. The variability in response to anti-LTs may reflect differences in production of or responses to LTs in different patients, and this in turn may be related to polymorphisms of 5-LO, LTC_4 synthase, or cys-LT_1 receptors that are involved in the synthesis of LTs (Tantisira and Drazen, 2009).

Immunomodulatory Therapies

Immunosuppressive Therapy

Immunosuppressive therapy (e.g., *methotrexate, cyclosporine A, gold, intravenous immunoglobulin*) has been considered in asthma when other treatments have been unsuccessful or to reduce the dose of oral steroids required. However, immunosuppressive treatments are less effective and have a greater propensity for side effects than oral corticosteroids and therefore cannot be routinely recommended.

Anti-IgE Receptor Therapy

Increased specific IgE is a fundamental feature of allergic asthma. *Omalizumab* is a humanized monoclonal antibody that blocks the binding of IgE to high-affinity IgE receptors (FcεR1) on mast cells and thus prevents their activation by allergens (Figure 40–10). It also blocks binding on IgE to low-affinity IgE receptors (FcεRII, CD23) on other inflammatory cells, including T and B lymphocytes, macrophages, and possibly eosinophils, to inhibit chronic inflammation. *Omalizumab* also reduces levels of circulating IgE.

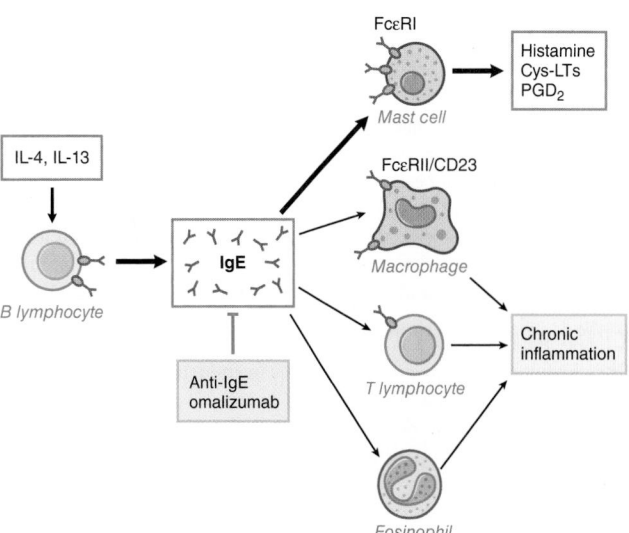

Figure 40–10 *Immunoglobulin E plays a central role in allergic diseases.* Blocking IgE using an antibody, such as omalizumab, is a rational therapeutic approach. IgE may activate high-affinity receptors (FcεRI) on mast cells as well as low-affinity receptors (FcεRII, CD23) on other inflammatory cells. Omalizumab prevents these interactions and the resulting inflammation..

Clinical Use

Omalizumab is used for the treatment of patients with severe asthma (Humbert et al., 2014). The antibody is administered by subcutaneous injection every 2–4 weeks, and the dose is determined by the titer of circulating total IgE. Omalizumab reduces the requirement for oral and ICSs and markedly reduces asthma exacerbations. Not all patients respond, and there are no clear clinical predictors of clinical response, necessitating a trial of therapy (usually over 4 months). Because of its high cost, this treatment is generally used only in patients with very severe asthma who are poorly controlled even on oral corticosteroids and in patients with very severe concomitant allergic rhinitis (Normansell et al., 2014). It may also be of value in protecting against anaphylaxis during specific immunotherapy. A recent study suggested that omalizumab may be effective in preventing asthma exacerbations if administered prior to the exacerbation season (Teach et al., 2015); this is linked to increased expression of type I interferons, which boost antiviral immunity. The major side effect of omalizumab is an anaphylactic response, which is uncommon (<0.1%).

Specific Immunotherapy

Although specific immunotherapy is effective in allergic rhinitis due to single allergens, there is little evidence that desensitizing injections to common allergens are effective in controlling chronic asthma (Rolland et al., 2009). Specific immunotherapy induces the secretion of the anti-inflammatory cytokine IL-10 from regulatory helper T lymphocytes, and this blocks costimulatory signal transduction in T cells (via CD28) so that they are unable to react to allergens presented by antigen-presenting cells (Ozdemir et al., 2016). Applying an understanding of the cellular processes involved might lead to safer and more effective approaches in the future. More specific immunotherapies may be developed with cloned allergen epitopes, T-cell peptide fragments of allergens, CpG oligonucleotides, and vaccines of conjugates of allergen and toll-like receptor 9 to stimulate T_H1 immunity and suppress T_H2 immunity (Broide, 2009).

New Drugs in Development for Airway Disease

Several new classes of drug are in development for asthma and COPD, but clinical development has been slow, and many treatments have either proved to be ineffective or are limited by toxicology and side-effect profiles (Barnes, 2012, 2013b)

Novel Mediator Antagonists

Blocking the receptors or synthesis of inflammatory mediators is a logical approach to the development of new treatments for asthma and COPD. However, in both diseases many different mediators are involved, and therefore blocking a single mediator is unlikely to be effective unless it plays a unique and key role in the disease process. Several specific mediator antagonists have been found to be ineffective in asthma, including antagonists/inhibitors of thromboxane, platelet-activating factor, bradykinin, and tachykinins. However, these blockers have often not been tested in COPD, in which different mediators are involved. A number of other approaches are under study, as noted next.

CRTh2 Antagonists

The chemotactic factor for T_H2 cells has been identified as prostaglandin D_2, which acts on a DP_2 receptor (Chapter 37). Several DP2/CRTh2 antagonists are now in development for asthma, with some promising initial results in patients with eosinophilic inflammation (Townley and Agrawal, 2012).

Antioxidants

Oxidative stress is important in severe asthma and COPD and may contribute to corticosteroid resistance. Existing antioxidants include vitamins C and E and *N*-acetyl-cysteine. These drugs have weak effects, but more potent antioxidants are in development, including activators of the transcription factor Nrf2 (Kirkham and Barnes, 2013).

Cytokine Modifiers

Cytokines play a critical role in perpetuating and amplifying the inflammation in asthma and COPD, suggesting that anticytokines may be beneficial as therapies (Barnes, 2008a). Although most attention has focused on inhibition of cytokines, some cytokines are anti-inflammatory and may have therapeutic potential. Several cytokine or cytokine receptor–blocking antibodies are in clinical development for asthma (Chung, 2015), but there has been less progress in COPD.

Interleukin 5 plays a pivotal role in eosinophilic inflammation and is also involved in eosinophil survival and priming. Anti-IL-5 and anti–IL-5 receptor (IL-5Rα) antibodies inhibit eosinophilic inflammation and airway hyperresponsiveness in patients with mild asthma but has no effect on allergen challenge (Leckie et al., 2000) or clinical benefits in unselected asthmatic patients (Flood-Page et al., 2007). In carefully selected patients with severe asthma and persistent eosinophilia despite high doses of corticosteroids, there is a significant reduction in exacerbations and sparing or oral steroids with an anti-IL-5 antibody, *mepolizumab* (Castro et al., 2014; Pavord et al., 2012). *Mepolizumab* has now been FDA approved for use in highly selected patients with severe asthma.

Blocking IL-4, which determines IgE synthesis and eosinophilic inflammation, has been ineffective in clinical studies. However, blocking IL-13 or its shared receptor with IL-4 (IL-4Rα) provides some clinic benefit and reduces exacerbations but is not yet approved (Hanania et al., 2015; Wenzel et al., 2013).

Production of TNF-α is increased in asthma and COPD and may play a key role in amplifying airway inflammation, through the activation of NF-κB, AP-1, and other transcription factors. However, in patients with COPD and in patients with severe asthma, anti–TNF-α blocking antibodies have been ineffective, at the expense of increasing infections and malignancies (Rennard et al., 2007; Wenzel et al., 2009).

Chemokine Receptor Antagonists

Many chemokines are involved in asthma and COPD and play a key role in recruitment of inflammatory cells, such as eosinophils, neutrophils, macrophages, and lymphocytes, into the lungs. Chemokine receptors are attractive targets because they are GPCRs; small-molecule inhibitors are now in development (Donnelly and Barnes, 2006). In asthma, *CCR3 antagonists*, which should block eosinophil recruitment into the airways, are the most favored target, but several small-molecule CCR3 antagonists have failed in development because of toxicity. In COPD, CXCR2 antagonists, which prevent neutrophil and monocyte chemotaxis due to CXC chemokines, such as CXCL1 and CXCL8, have been effective in animal models of COPD and in neutrophilic inflammation in normal subjects, but in clinical trials in patients with COPD, an oral CXCR2 antagonist provided little clinical benefit (Rennard et al., 2015).

Protease Inhibitors

Several proteolytic enzymes are involved in the chronic inflammation of airway diseases. Mast cell tryptase has several effects on airways, including increasing responsiveness of airway smooth muscle to constrictors, increasing plasma exudation, potentiating eosinophil recruitment, and stimulating fibroblast proliferation. Some of these effects are mediated by activation of protease-activated receptor, PAR2. Tryptase inhibitors have so far proved to be disappointing in clinical studies.

Proteases are involved in the degradation of connective tissue in COPD, particularly enzymes that break down elastin fibers, such as neutrophil elastase and MMPs, which are involved in emphysema. Neutrophil elastase inhibitors have been difficult to develop, and there are no positive clinical studies in patients with COPD. MMP9 appears to be the predominant elastolytic enzyme in emphysema, and several selective inhibitors are now in development.

New Anti-inflammatory Drugs

NF-κB Inhibitors

An important role is played by NF-κB in the orchestration of chronic inflammation (Figure 40–7); many of the inflammatory genes that are expressed in asthma and COPD are regulated by this transcription factor.

This has prompted a search for specific blockers of these transcription factors. NF-κB is naturally inhibited by IκB, which is degraded after activation by specific kinases. Small-molecule inhibitors of the IκB kinase IKK2 (or IKKβ) are in clinical development (Ziegelbauer et al., 2005). These drugs may be of particular value in COPD, for which corticosteroids are largely ineffective. However, there are concerns that inhibition of NF-κB may cause side effects such as increased susceptibility to infections, which has been observed in gene disruption studies when components of NF-κB are inhibited.

Mitogen-Activated Protein Kinase Inhibitors

The MAP kinase pathways are involved in chronic inflammation. There has been particular interest in the p38 MAP kinase pathway that is blocked by a novel class of drugs, such as *losmapimod* (Norman, 2015). These drugs inhibit the synthesis of many inflammatory cytokines, chemokines, and inflammatory enzymes. The p38 MAP kinase inhibitors are in development for the treatment of asthma (they inhibit T_H2 cytokine synthesis) and for COPD (they inhibit neutrophilic inflammation and signaling of inflammatory cytokines and chemokines). However, clinical studies have given disappointing results in patients with COPD, and the dose is limited by side effects (MacNee et al., 2013). Several inhaled p38 inhibitors are in development to reduce the risk of side effects (Millan, 2011).

Mucoregulators

Mucus hypersecretion occurs in chronic bronchitis, COPD, cystic fibrosis, and asthma (Fahy and Dickey, 2010). In chronic bronchitis, mucus hypersecretion is related to chronic irritation by cigarette smoke and may involve neural mechanisms and the activation of neutrophils to release enzymes such as neutrophil elastase and proteinase 3 that have powerful stimulatory effects on mucus secretion. Mast cell–derived chymase is also a potent mucus secretagogue. This suggests that several classes of drugs may be developed to control mucus hypersecretion. Mucus secretion is regulated by epidermal growth factor receptors, which lead to increased mucin gene *MUC5AC* expression, but a nebulized epidermal growth factor receptor inhibitor has been ineffective in COPD (Woodruff et al., 2010).

Systemic anticholinergic drugs appear to reduce mucociliary clearance, but this is not observed with either ipratropium bromide or tiotropium bromide, presumably reflecting their poor absorption from the respiratory tract. β_2 Agonists increase mucus production and mucociliary clearance and have been shown to increase ciliary beat frequency in vitro. Because inflammation leads to mucus hypersecretion, anti-inflammatory treatments should reduce mucus hypersecretion; ICSs are very effective in reducing increased mucus production in asthma.

Mucolytics

Several agents can reduce the viscosity of sputum in vitro. One group consists of derivatives of cysteine that reduce the disulfide bridges that bind glycoproteins to other proteins, such as albumin and secretory IgA. These drugs also act as antioxidants and may therefore reduce airway inflammation. Only *N-acetylcysteine* is available in the U.S.; *carbocysteine, methylcysteine, erdosteine,* and *bromhexine* are available elsewhere. Orally administered, these agents are relatively well tolerated, but clinical studies in chronic bronchitis, asthma, and bronchiectasis have been disappointing. A large controlled study of oral *N-acetylcysteine* in patients with COPD showed no effect in disease progression or in preventing exacerbations, although there was some benefit in the patients not treated with ICSs (Decramer et al., 2005), as confirmed in a subsequent studies of carbocysteine and *N-acetylcysteine* in patients with COPD not treated with other medications (Zheng et al., 2008, 2014). *N-Acetylcysteine* is not currently recommended for COPD management.

DNAse (dornase alfa) reduces mucus viscosity in sputum of patients with cystic fibrosis and is indicated if there is significant symptomatic and lung function improvement after a trial of therapy (Henke and Ratjen, 2007). There is no evidence that dornase alfa is effective in COPD or asthma, however.

Expectorants

Expectorants are oral drugs that are supposed to enhance the clearance of mucus. Although expectorants were once commonly prescribed, there is little or no objective evidence for their efficacy. Such drugs are often emetics that are given in subemetic doses on the basis that gastric irritation may stimulate an increase in mucus clearance via a reflex mechanism. Lacking evidence for their efficacy, the FDA has removed most expectorants from the market in a review of over-the-counter drugs. With the exception of *guaifenesin*, no agents are approved as expectorants in the U.S. In patients who find it difficult to clear mucus, adequate hydration and inhalation of steam may be of some benefit.

Antitussives

Despite the fact that cough is a common symptom of airway disease, its mechanisms are poorly understood, and current treatment is unsatisfactory (Pavord and Chung, 2008). Viral infections of the upper respiratory tract are the most common cause of cough; postviral cough is usually self-limiting and commonly patient medicated. Their wide use notwithstanding, over-the-counter cough medications are largely ineffective (Dicpinigaitis et al., 2014). Because cough is a defensive reflex, its suppression may be inappropriate in bacterial lung infection. Before treatment with antitussives, it is important to identify underlying causal mechanisms that may require therapy.

Whenever possible, treat the underlying cause, not the cough. Asthma commonly presents as cough, and the cough will usually respond to ICSs. A syndrome characterized by cough in association with sputum eosinophilia but no airway hyperresponsiveness, termed *eosinophilic bronchitis*, also responds to ICSs (Birring et al., 2003). Nonasthmatic cough does not respond to ICSs but sometimes responds to anticholinergic therapy. The cough associated with postnasal drip of sinusitis responds to antibiotics (if warranted), nasal decongestants, and intranasal steroids. The cough associated with ACE inhibitors (in ~ 15% of patients treated) responds to lowering the dose or withdrawal of the drug and substitution of an AT_1 receptor antagonist (see Chapter 26). Gastroesophageal reflux is a common cause of cough through a reflex mechanism and occasionally as a result of acid aspiration into the lungs. This cough may respond to suppression of gastric acid with an H_2 receptor antagonist or a proton pump inhibitor (see Chapter 49). Some patients have a chronic cough with no obvious cause, and this chronic idiopathic cough or cough hypersensitivity syndrome may be due to airway sensory neural hyperesthesia (Haque et al., 2005). There are several treatments that have been assessed in the treatment of refractory cough (Gibson et al., 2016).

Opiates

Opiates have a central mechanism of action on MORs in the medullary cough center, but there is some evidence that they may have additional peripheral action on cough receptors in the proximal airways. *Codeine* and *pholcodine* (not available in the U.S.) are commonly used, but there is little evidence that they are clinically effective, particularly on postviral cough; in addition, they are associated with sedation and constipation. *Morphine* and *methadone* are effective but indicated only for intractable cough associated with bronchial carcinoma.

Dextromethorphan

Dextromethorphan is a centrally active NMDA receptor antagonist. It may also antagonize opioid receptors. Despite the fact that it is in numerous over-the-counter cough suppressants and used commonly to treat cough, it is poorly effective. In children with acute nocturnal cough, it is not significantly different from placebo in reducing cough (Dicpinigaitis et al., 2014). It can cause hallucinations at higher doses and has significant abuse potential.

Local Anesthetics

Benzonatate, a local anesthetic, acts peripherally by anesthetizing the stretch receptors located in the respiratory passages, lungs, and pleura. By dampening the activity of these receptors, benzonatate may reduce the cough reflex. The recommended dose is 100 mg, three times per day, and up to 600 mg/d, if needed. Although clinical studies shortly after its approval showed some efficacy, benzonatate (200 mg) was not effective in suppressing experimentally induced cough (Dicpinigaitis et al., 2009). Side effects include dizziness and dysphagia. Seizures and cardiac arrest have occurred following an acute ingestion. Severe allergic reactions have been reported in patients allergic to *para-aminobenzoic acid*, a metabolite of benzonatate.

Neuromodulators

Gabapentin and *pregabalin* are GABA analogues that inhibit neurotransmission and have been used in neuropathic pain syndromes. They have been shown to benefit chronic idiopathic cough, which also involved neural hypersensitivity (Gibson and Vertigan, 2015). Side effects of somnolence and dizziness are common at higher doses, so it is usual to initiate therapy at lower doses.

Other Drugs

Several other drugs reportedly have small benefits in protecting against cough challenges or in reducing cough in pulmonary diseases. These drugs include *moguisteine* (not available in the U.S.), which acts peripherally and appears to open ATP-sensitive K^+ channels. *Theobromine*, a naturally occurring methylxanthine, reduces cough induced by tussive agents. Although the expectorant *guaifenesin* is not typically known as a cough suppressant, it is significantly better than placebo in reducing acute viral cough and inhibits cough-reflex sensitivity in patients with upper respiratory tract infections (Dicpinigaitis et al., 2009).

Novel Antitussives

There is clearly a need to develop new, more effective therapies for cough, particularly drugs that act peripherally to avoid sedation. There are close analogies between chronic cough and sensory hyperesthesia, so new therapies with novel antitussives are likely to arise from pain research.

Transient Receptor Potential Antagonists

Several types of TRP ion channels have been described on airway sensory nerves and may be activated by various mediators and physical factors, resulting in cough. TRPV1 (previously called the *vanilloid receptor*) is activated by capsaicin, H^+, and bradykinin, all of which are potent tussive agents. *TRPV1 inhibitors* block cough induced by capsaicin and bradykinin and are effective in some models of cough (McLeod et al., 2008). In a clinical study of an oral TRPV1 inhibitor, there was protection against capsaicin-induced cough but no clinical improvement in chronic idiopathic cough after long-term treatment (Khalid et al., 2014). A side effect of these drugs is loss of temperature regulation and hyperthermia, which has prevented clinical development.

Transient receptor potential A1 is emerging as a more promising novel target for antitussives (Grace and Belvisi, 2011). This channel is activated by oxidative stress and many irritants and may be sensitized by inflammatory cytokines (Bonvini et al., 2015). Several selective TRPA1 antagonists are now in development. TRPV4 may also activate cough and may be activated by ATP (Bonvini et al., 2016).

ATP Receptor Antagonists

Adenosine triphosphate is a potent tussive agent and stimulates cough in patients with asthma and COPD via activation of P2X3 receptors on afferent nerves (Basoglu et al., 2015). A *P2X3 antagonist* (AF-219) is effective in reducing chronic idiopathic cough, although abnormal taste (dysgeusia) is a frequent side effect (Abdulqawi et al., 2015).

Drugs for Dyspnea and Ventilatory Control

Drugs for Dyspnea

Bronchodilators should reduce breathlessness in patients with airway obstruction. Chronic oxygen use may have a beneficial effect, but in a few patients dyspnea may be extreme. Drugs that reduce breathlessness may also depress ventilation in parallel and may therefore be dangerous in severe asthma and COPD. Some patients show a beneficial response to dihydrocodeine and diazepam; however, these drugs must be used with great caution because of the risk of ventilatory depression (Currow et al., 2014). Slow-release morphine tablets may also be helpful in patients with COPD with extreme dyspnea (Currow and Abernethy, 2007). Nebulized morphine may also reduce breathlessness in COPD and could act in part on opioid receptors in the lung. Nebulized furosemide has some efficacy in treating dyspnea from a variety of causes, but the evidence is not yet sufficiently convincing to recommend this as routine therapy (Newton et al., 2008).

Ventilatory Stimulants

Selective respiratory stimulants are indicated if ventilation is impaired as a result of overdose with sedatives, in postanesthetic respiratory depression, and in idiopathic hypoventilation. Respiratory stimulants are rarely indicated in COPD because respiratory drive is already maximal, and further stimulation of ventilation may be counterproductive because of the increase in energy expenditure caused by the drugs.

Doxapram

At low doses (0.5 mg/kg IV), doxapram stimulates carotid chemoreceptors; at higher doses, it stimulates medullary respiratory centers. Its effect is transient; thus, intravenous infusion (0.3–3 mg/kg per min) is needed for sustained effect. Unwanted effects include nausea, sweating, anxiety, and hallucinations. At higher doses, increased pulmonary and systemic pressures may occur. Both the kidney and the liver participate in the clearance of doxapram, which should be used with caution if hepatic or renal function is impaired. In COPD, the infusion of doxapram is restricted to 2 h. The use of doxapram to treat ventilatory failure in COPD has now largely been replaced by noninvasive ventilation.

Almitrine

Almitrine bismesylate is a piperazine derivative that appears to selectively stimulate peripheral chemoreceptors and is without central actions. Almitrine stimulates ventilation only when there is hypoxia. Long-term use of almitrine is associated with peripheral neuropathy, limiting its availability in most countries, including the U.S.

Acetazolamide

The carbonic anhydrase inhibitor acetazolamide (see Chapter 25) induces metabolic acidosis and thereby stimulates ventilation, but it is not widely used because the metabolic imbalance it produces may be detrimental in the face of respiratory acidosis. It has a small beneficial effect in respiratory failure in patients with COPD. The drug has proved useful in prevention of high-altitude (mountain) sickness (Faisy et al., 2016).

Naloxone

Naloxone is a competitive opioid antagonist that is indicated only if ventilatory depression is due to overdose of opioids.

Flumazenil

Flumazenil is a benzodiazepine receptor antagonist that can reverse respiratory depression due to overdose of benzodiazepines (Veiraiah et al., 2012).

Acknowledgment: *Bradley J. Undem and Lawrence M. Lichtenstein contributed to this chapter in earlier editions of this book. We have retained some of their text in the current edition.*

Drug Facts for Your Personal Formulary: *Asthma and COPD Therapeutics*

Drug	Therapeutic Uses	Clinical Tips
Short-Acting β₂ Agonists: Inhaled bronchodilators for symptom relief and acute bronchodilation		
Albuterol (salbutamol)	• Asthma, COPD, and exercise-induced bronchospasm • Inhaled: 180 µg (2 puffs) every 4 to 6 h as needed • Nebulized: 2.5 mg via oral inhalation every 6–8 h as needed over 5 to 15 min • Oral: 2–4 mg by mouth every 6–8 h	• Also available nebulized and inhaled as levalbuterol (active isomer, so half the dose) • May need to be nebulized with oxygen in severe exacerbation • Adverse effects: tachycardia, palpitations, muscle tremors, and hyperkalemia
Levalbuterol (L-albuterol)	• Bronchodilator • Inhaled (MDI nebulizer)	• Half of doses of racemic albuterol • No advantage over racemic albuterol • Adverse effects: tachycardia, palpitations, muscle tremors, and hyperkalemia
Pirbuterol	• 400 µg (2 puffs) every 4–6 h as needed • Inhaled (MDI nebulizer)	• Similar to albuterol • Adverse effects: tachycardia, palpitations, muscle tremors, and hyperkalemia
Long-Acting β₂ Agonists: Add-on therapy to ICSs in asthma; can be used alone in COPD		
Formoterol	• Asthma as add-on to ICS • Maintenance and treatment of severe COPD • Inhaled: 12 µg (contents of 1 capsule) every 12 h • Nebulized 20 µg in 2 mL, twice per day	• Used as maintenance, usually in a combination with an ICS • Can also be used as a reliever of bronchospasm • Adverse effects: tachycardia, palpitations, muscle tremors, and hyperkalemia
Arformoterol Salmeterol Indacaterol Olodaterol	• Arformoterol for severe COPD • Maintenance treatment for COPD • Arformoterol, inhaled (nebulized), 15 µg in 2 mL twice daily • Salmeterol, inhaled 50 µg twice daily • Indacaterol, inhaled (DPI) 75 cetazolamide once daily • Olodaterol, inhaled 2.5 cetazolamide once daily	• Cannot be used as a reliever, only for maintenance treatment for COPD • Adverse effects: tachycardia, palpitations, muscle tremors, and hyperkalemia
Anticholinergics: Muscarinic receptor antagonists inhaled as bronchodilators		
Ipratropium bromide Albuterol/ipratropium combination	• Inhaled, 2 puffs (17 µg/puff) 3–4 times/d • Combination albuterol 103 µg/ipratropium 18 µg/puff; 2 puffs 4 times daily	• Largely replaced by LAMAs • Avoid spraying in eyes • Adverse effects include dry mouth, tachycardia, urinary retention, glaucoma • Combination with albuterol may be used as a reliever
Tiotropium Bromide	• 2.5 µg via oral inhalation (2 puffs of 1.25 µg/actuation) once daily	• Caution in patients with urinary retention or glaucoma history
Umeclidinium bromide	• Inhaled (DPI) 62.5 µg (1 puff) once daily	
Aclidinium bromide	• Inhaled (DPI) 400 µg (1 puff) twice daily	
Glycopyrrolate	• Inhaled (DPI) 1 capsule (15.6 µg) inhaled twice daily	
LAMA-LABA Combination Inhalers: Maintenance treatment for COPD		
Glycopyrrolate/indacaterol	• Inhaled (DPI) 1 inhalation (glycopyrrolate 15.6 µg/indacaterol 27.5 µg) twice daily	• Side effects of anticholinergics and β₂ agonists as above • Maintenance treatment for COPD
Umeclidinium/vilanterol	• Inhaled (DPI) 1 inhalation (umeclidinium 62.5 µg/25 µg vilanterol) once daily	
Tiotropium/olodaterol	• Inhaled (mist inhaler), 2 inhalations (containing 2.5 µg tiotropium/2.5 µg of olodaterol per inhalation) once daily	
Inhaled Corticosteroids: Maintenance treatment for asthma		
Beclomethasone dipropionate (BDP)	• Inhaled (MDI, DPI); 88 µg (1 spray = 44 µg) twice daily • Not to exceed 440 µg twice daily	• More systemic effects than other ICSs: orally bioavailable BDP is converted to an active metabolite, beclomethasone monopropionate, following absorption • Local effects: hoarse voice, candidiasis • Systemic effects: growth suppression, bruising, adrenal suppression
Fluticasone propionate	• Inhaled (MDI, DPI); 50, 100, 250 µg 2 puffs, twice daily • Do not exceed 1000 µg daily	• Fewer systemic effects than BDP • Local: hoarse voice, candidiasis
Budesonide	• Inhaled via jet nebulizer either once daily or divided into 2 doses (maximum daily dose 0.5 mg/d)	• Fewer systemic effects than BDP • Used in children less than 8 who cannot use PDI • Local: hoarse voice, candidiasis
Ciclesonide	• Inhaled (MDI) 80 µg twice daily	• Least-systemic effects of all ICSs; may be effective once daily • Local: hoarse voice, candidiasis

Drug Facts for Your Personal Formulary: *Asthma and COPD Therapeutics* (*continued*)

Drug	Therapeutic Uses	Clinical Tips
ICS/LABA Combination Inhalers: Maintenance treatment in asthma and COPD		
Fluticasone propionate/salmeterol	• Inhaled (DPI) • Starting dosage based on asthma severity	• Use lowest dose that maintains asthma control • Use only in severe COPD or asthma-COPD overlap • Adverse effects as for ICSs and LABAs
Budesonide/formoterol	• Inhaled (MDI) (80 µg budesonide and 4.5 µg formoterol per inhalation) twice daily	
Fluticasone furoate/vilanterol	• Inhaled (DPI) 1 inhalation (fluticasone furoate 100 µg/vilanterol 25 µg) once daily	
Systemic Corticosteroids: Short course or oral maintenance for asthma (and COPD)		
Prednisone Prednisolone	• Oral: 40–80 mg once daily or divided dose for 3–10 days for acute exacerbation • Minimal dose for maintenance	• Prednisone converted to prednisolone in the liver • Bruising, weight gain, edema, osteoporosis, diabetes, cataracts, adrenal suppression (see Chapter 46)
Hydrocortisone succinate	• IM/IV: 100–500 mg every 12 h for acute severe asthma	• Only if patient not able to take oral steroids
Methylprednisolone	• IV: 100–1000 mg for acute severe asthma	• Rarely indicated because of steroid side effects
Antileukotrienes (Leukotriene Modifiers) for Asthma Maintenance		
Montelukast (10 Zafirlukast) Zileuton	• Oral: montelukast (10 mg once/d); zafirlukast (20 mg twice/d); zileuton (600 mg four times/d or 1200 mg twice/d)	• Less effective than ICS in asthma • Headache, Churg-Strauss syndrome • Zileuton may cause hepatic dysfunction (do not use if ALT increased)
Methylxanthines: Add-on maintenance treatment of severe asthma and COPD		
Theophylline (oral) Aminophylline (IV)	• Aminophylline (IV) is indicated for severe exacerbation that does not respond to nebulized β agonists; shorter action than theophylline	• Interaction with drugs that affect CYP450 • Nausea, headaches, diuresis, arrhythmias, seizures
Phosphodiesterase 4 Inhibitor: Maintenance for severe COPD		
Roflumilast	• Severe COPD • Oral administration 500 µg once daily	• Add to maximal inhaled therapy if severe disease with acute exacerbations and chronic bronchitis
Anti-IgE: Maintenance Treatment for severe asthma		
Omalizumab	• Severe asthma • Subcutaneous administration • Dose depends on total IgE; given every 2–4 weeks	• Expensive, so mainly indicated in severe asthma that is difficult to control • Well tolerated; occasional headache • Occasional anaphylaxis

Bibliography

Abdulqawi R, et al. P2X3 receptor antagonist (AF-219) in refractory chronic cough: a randomised, double-blind, placebo-controlled phase 2 study. *Lancet*, **2015**, *385*:1198–1205.

Akram MF, et al. Doxofylline and theophylline: a comparative clinical study. *J Clin Diagnos Res*, **2012**, *6*:1681–1684.

An SS, et al. TAS2R activation promotes airway smooth muscle relaxation despite beta(2)-adrenergic receptor tachyphylaxis. *Am J Physiol*, **2012**, *303*:L304–L311.

Barnes PJ. Scientific rationale for combination inhalers with a long-acting β2-agonists and corticosteroids. *Eur Respir J*, **2002**, *19*:182–191.

Barnes PJ. Mediators of chronic obstructive pulmonary disease. *Pharm Rev*, **2004**, *56*:515–548.

Barnes PJ. Cytokine networks in asthma and chronic obstructive pulmonary disease. *J Clin Invest*, **2008a**, *118*:3546–3556.

Barnes PJ. Immunology of asthma and chronic obstructive pulmonary disease. *Nat Immunol Rev*, **2008b**, *8*:183–192.

Barnes PJ. Glucocorticosteroids: current and future directions. *Br J Pharmacol*, **2011a**, *163*:29–43.

Barnes PJ. Pathophysiology of allergic inflammation. *Immunol Rev*, **2011b**, *242*:31–50.

Barnes PJ. New drugs for asthma. *Semin Respir Crit Care Med*, **2012**, *33*:685–694.

Barnes PJ. Corticosteroid resistance in patients with asthma and chronic obstructive pulmonary disease. *J Allergy Clin Immunol*, **2013a**, *131*:636–645.

Barnes PJ. New anti-inflammatory treatments for chronic obstructive pulmonary disease. *Nat Rev Drug Discov*, **2013b**, *12*:543–559.

Barnes PJ. Theophylline. *Am J Respir Crit Care Med*, **2013c**, *188*:901–906.

Barnes PJ. Mechanisms of development of multimorbidity in the elderly. *Eur Respir J*, **2015**, *45*:790–806.

Barnes PJ, Adcock IM. Glucocorticoid resistance in inflammatory diseases. *Lancet*, **2009**, *342*:1905–1917.

Barnes PJ, et al. Chronic obstructive pulmonary disease. *Nat Rev Primers*, **2015**, *1*:1–21.

Barnes PJ, Celli BR. Systemic manifestations and comorbidities of COPD. *Eur Respir J*, **2009**, *33*:1165–1185.

Barnes PJ, et al. Inflammatory mediators of asthma: an update. *Pharmacol Rev*, **1998a**, *50*:515–596.

Barnes PJ, et al. Efficacy and safety of inhaled corticosteroids: an update. *Am J Respir Crit Care Med*, **1998b**, *157*: S1–S53.

Basoglu OK, et al. Effects of aerosolized adenosive 5′-triphosphate in smokers and patients with chronic obstructive pulmonary disease. *Chest*, **2015**, *148*:430–435.

Beasley R, et al. Beta-agonists: what is the evidence that their use increases the risk of asthma morbidity and mortality? *J Allergy Clin Immunol*, **1999**, *104*:S18–S30.

Belvisi MG, et al. Therapeutic benefit of a dissociated glucocorticoid and the relevance of in vitro separation of transrepression from transactivation activity. *J Immunol*, **2001**, *166*:1975–1982.

Bernstein JA, et al. MK-0633, a potent 5-lipoxygenase inhibitor, in chronic obstructive pulmonary disease. *Respir Med*, **2011**, *105*:392–401.

Birring SS, et al. Eosinophilic bronchitis: clinical features, management and pathogenesis. *Am J Respir Med*, **2003**, *2*:169–173.

Black JL, et al. Molecular mechanisms of combination therapy with inhaled corticosteroids and long-acting beta-agonists. *Chest*, **2009**, *136*:1095–1100.

Bleecker ER, et al. Effect of ADRB2 polymorphisms on response to long-acting beta2-agonist therapy: a pharmacogenetic analysis of two randomised studies. *Lancet*, **2007**, *370*:2118–2125.

Bonvini SJ, et al. Transient receptor potential cation channel, subfamily V, member 4 and airway sensory afferent activation: role of adenosine triphosphate. *J Allergy Clin Immunol*, **2016**, *138*:249–261.

Bonvini SJ, et al. Targeting TRP channels for chronic cough: from bench to bedside. *Naunyn Schmiedebergs Arch Pharmacol*, **2015**, *388*:401–420.

Broide DH. Immunomodulation of allergic disease. *Annu Rev Med*, **2009**, *60*:279–291.

Busse WW, et al. The Inhaled Steroid Treatment As Regular Therapy in Early Asthma (START) study 5-year follow-up: effectiveness of early intervention with budesonide in mild persistent asthma. *J Allergy Clin Immunol*, **2008**, *121*:1167–1174.

Calverley PM, et al. Roflumilast in symptomatic chronic obstructive pulmonary disease: two randomised clinical trials. *Lancet*, **2009**, *374*:685–694.

Calzetta L, et al. A systematic review with meta-analysis of dual bronchodilation with LAMA/LABA for the treatment of stable COPD. *Chest*, **2016**, *149*:1181–1196.

Castro M, et al. Benralizumab, an anti-interleukin 5 receptor alpha monoclonal antibody, versus placebo for uncontrolled eosinophilic asthma: a phase 2b randomised dose-ranging study. *Lancet Respir Med*, **2014**, *2*:879–890.

Cates CJ, et al. Safety of regular formoterol or salmeterol in adults with asthma: an overview of Cochrane reviews. *Cochrane Database Syst Rev*, **2014**, (2):CD010314.

Cazzola M, et al. Long-acting muscarinic receptor antagonists for the treatment of respiratory disease. *Pulm Pharmacol Ther*, **2013a**, *26*:307–317.

Cazzola M, et al. Pharmacology and therapeutics of bronchodilators. *Pharmacol Rev*, **2012**, *64*:450–504.

Cazzola M, et al. beta2-Agonist therapy in lung disease. *Am J Respir Crit Care Med*, **2013b**, *187*:690–696.

Chauhan BF, Ducharme FM. Anti-leukotriene agents compared to inhaled corticosteroids in the management of recurrent and/or chronic asthma in adults and children. *Cochrane Database Syst Rev*, **2012**, (5):CD002314.

Cheyne L, et al. Tiotropium versus ipratropium bromide for chronic obstructive pulmonary disease. *Cochrane Database Syst Rev*, **2015**, (9):CD009552.

Chung KF. Targeting the interleukin pathway in the treatment of asthma. *Lancet*, **2015**, *386*:1086–1096.

Chung IY, et al. The downregulation of bcl-2 expression is necessary for theophylline-induced apoptosis of eosinophil. *Cell Immunol*, **2000**, *203*:95–102.

Clark AR. MAP kinase phosphatase 1: a novel mediator of biological effects of glucocorticoids? *J Endocrinol*, **2003**, *178*:5–12.

Coreno A, et al. Comparative effects of long-acting beta2-agonists, leukotriene receptor antagonists, and a 5-lipoxygenase inhibitor on exercise-induced asthma. *J Allergy Clin Immunol*, **2000**, *106*:500–506.

Cosio BG, et al. Theophylline restores histone deacetylase activity and steroid responses in COPD macrophages. *J Exp Med*, **2004**, *200*:689–695.

Culpitt SV, et al. Effect of theophylline on induced sputum inflammatory indices and neutrophil chemotaxis in COPD. *Am J Respir Crit Care Med*, **2002**, *165*:1371–1376.

Currow DC, et al. Opioids for chronic refractory breathlessness: right patient, right route? *Drugs*, **2014**, *74*:1–6.

Currow DC, Abernethy AP. Pharmacological management of dyspnoea. *Curr Opin Support Palliat Care*, **2007**, *1*:96–101.

Decramer M, et al. Effects of N-acetylcysteine on outcomes in chronic obstructive pulmonary disease (Bronchitis Randomized on NAC Cost-Utility Study, BRONCUS): a randomised placebo-controlled trial. *Lancet*, **2005**, *365*:1552–1560.

Dennis SM, et al. Regular inhaled salbutamol and asthma control: the TRUST randomised trial. *Lancet*, **2000**, *355*: 1675–1679.

Derendorf H. Pharmacokinetic and pharmacodynamic properties of inhaled ciclesonide. *J Clin Pharmacol*, **2007**, *47*:782–789.

Derendorf H, et al. Relevance of pharmacokinetics and pharmacodynamics of inhaled corticosteroids to asthma. *Eur Respir J*, **2006**, *28*: 1042–1050.

Dicpinigaitis PV, et al. Inhibition of cough-reflex sensitivity by benzonatate and guaifenesin in acute viral cough. *Respir Med*, **2009**, *103*:902–906.

Dicpinigaitis PV, et al. Antitussive drugs—past, present, and future. *Pharmacol Rev*, **2014**, *66*:468–512.

Donnelly LE, Barnes PJ. Chemokine receptors as therapeutic targets in chronic obstructive pulmonary disease. *Trends Pharmacol Sci*, **2006**, *27*:546–553.

Erin EM, et al. Rapid anti-inflammatory effect of inhaled ciclesonide in asthma: a randomised, placebo-controlled study. *Chest*, **2008**, *134*:740–745.

Ernst P, et al. Inhaled corticosteroids in COPD: the clinical evidence. *Eur Respir J*, **2015**, *45*:525–537.

Fahy JV, Dickey BF. Airway mucus function and dysfunction. *N Engl J Med*, **2010**, *363*:2233–2247.

Faisy C, et al. Effect of acetazolamide vs placebo on duration of invasive mechanical ventilation among patients with chronic obstructive pulmonary disease: a randomized clinical trial. *JAMA*, **2016**, *315*:480–488.

Finney L, et al. Inhaled corticosteroids and pneumonia in chronic obstructive pulmonary disease. *Lancet Respir Medicine*, **2014**, *2*:919–932.

Flood-Page P, et al. A study to evaluate safety and efficacy of mepolizumab in patients with moderate persistent asthma. *Am J Respir Crit Care Med*, **2007**, *176*:1062–1071.

Franciosi LG, et al. Efficacy and safety of RPL554, a dual PDE3 and PDE4 inhibitor, in healthy volunteers and in patients with asthma or chronic obstructive pulmonary disease: findings from four clinical trials. *Lancet Respir Med*, **2013**, *1*:714–727.

Gauvreau GM, et al. Effect of regular inhaled albuterol on allergen-induced late responses and sputum eosinophils in asthmatic subjects. *Am J Respir Crit Care Med*, **1997**, *156*:1738–1745.

Gibson P, et al. Treatment of unexplained chronic cough: CHEST guideline and expert panel report. *Chest*, **2016**, *149*:27–44.

Gibson PG, Vertigan AE. Gabapentin in chronic cough. *Pulm Pharmacol Ther*, **2015**, *35*:145–148.

Grace MS, Belvisi MG. TRPA1 receptors in cough. *Pulm Pharmacol Ther*, **2011**, *24*:286–288.

Grayson MH, Korenblat PE. The role of antileukotriene drugs in management of rhinitis and rhinosinusitis. *Curr Allergy Asthma Rep*, **2007**, *7*:209–215.

Hall S, Agrawal DK. Key mediators in the immunopathogenesis of allergic asthma. *Int Immunopharmacol*, **2014**, *23*:316–329.

Hanania NA, et al. Lebrikizumab in moderate-to-severe asthma: pooled data from two randomised placebo-controlled studies. *Thorax*, **2015**, *70*:748–756.

Haque RA, et al. Chronic idiopathic cough: a discrete clinical entity? *Chest*, **2005**, *127*:1710–1713.

Hatzelmann A, et al. The preclinical pharmacology of roflumilast—a selective, oral phosphodiesterase 4 inhibitor in development for chronic obstructive pulmonary disease. *Pulm Pharmacol Ther*, **2010**, *23*:235–256.

Hawkins G, et al. Stepping down inhaled corticosteroids in asthma: randomised controlled trial. *BMJ*, **2003**, *326*:1115.

Hawkins GA, et al. Clinical consequences of ADRbeta2 polymorphisms. *Pharmacogenomics*, **2008**, *9*:349–358.

Henke MO, Ratjen F. Mucolytics in cystic fibrosis. *PaediatrRespir Rev*, **2007**, *8*:24–29.

Humbert M, et al. Omalizumab in asthma: an update on recent developments. *J Allergy Clin Immunol Pract*, **2014**, 2:525–536.e521.

Ichiyama T, et al. Theophylline inhibits NF-κB activation and IκBα degradation in human pulmonary epithelial cells. *Naunyn Schmied Arch Pharmacol*, **2001**, 364:558–561.

Ito K, et al. Histone deacetylase 2-mediated deacetylation of the glucocorticoid receptor enables NF-κB suppression. *J Exp Med*, **2006**, 203:7–13.

Kerstjens HA, et al. Tiotropium or salmeterol as add-on therapy to inhaled corticosteroids for patients with moderate symptomatic asthma: two replicate, double-blind, placebo-controlled, parallel-group, active-comparator, randomised trials. *Lancet Resp Med*, **2015**, 3:367–376.

Kew KM, et al. Intravenous magnesium sulfate for treating adults with acute asthma in the emergency department. *Cochrane Database Syst Rev*, **2014**, (5):CD010909.

Kew KM, et al. Long-acting beta2-agonists for chronic obstructive pulmonary disease. *Cochrane Database Syst Rev*, **2013**, (10):CD010177.

Khalid S, et al. Transient receptor potential vanilloid 1 (TRPV1) antagonism in patients with refractory chronic cough: a double-blind randomized controlled trial. *J Allergy Clin Immunol*, **2014**, 134:56–62.

Kirkham PA, Barnes PJ. Oxidative stress in COPD. *Chest*, **2013**, 144:266–273.

Lambrecht BN, Hammad H. The immunology of asthma. *Nature Immunol*, **2015**, 16:45–56.

Leckie MJ, et al. Effects of an interleukin-5 blocking monoclonal antibody on eosinophils, airway hyperresponsiveness and the late asthmatic response. *Lancet*, **2000**, 356:2144–2148.

Lim S, et al. Low-dose theophylline reduces eosinophilic inflammation but not exhaled nitric oxide in mild asthma. *Am J Respir Crit Care Med*, **2001**, 164:273–276.

Linden A, et al. Bronchodilation by an inhaled VPAC(2) receptor agonist in patients with stable asthma. *Thorax*, **2003**, 58:217–221.

Lipworth BJ. Systemic adverse effects of inhaled corticosteroid therapy: a systematic review and meta-analysis [see comments]. *Arch Intern Med*, **1999**, 159:941–955.

Loh CH, et al. Review of drug safety and efficacy of arformoterol in chronic obstructive pulmonary disease. *Exp Opinion Drug Safety*, **2015**, 14:463–472.

Lotvall J, et al. The therapeutic ratio of R-albuterol is comparable with that of RS-albuterol in asthmatic patients. *J Allergy Clin Immunol*, **2001**, 108:726–731.

MacNee W, et al. Efficacy and safety of the oral p38 inhibitor PH-797804 in chronic obstructive pulmonary disease: a randomised clinical trial. *Thorax*, **2013**, 68:738–745.

Mak JCW, et al. Protective effects of a glucocorticoid on down-regulation of pulmonary β_2 adrenergic receptors in vivo. *J Clin Invest*, **1995**, 96:99–106.

Manjra AI, et al. Efficacy of nebulized fluticasone propionate compared with oral prednisolone in children with an acute exacerbation of asthma. *Respir Med*, **2000**, 94:1206–1214.

Martinez FJ, et al. Effect of roflumilast on exacerbations in patients with severe chronic obstructive pulmonary disease uncontrolled by combination therapy (REACT): a multicentre randomised controlled trial. *Lancet*, **2015**, 385:857–866.

McLeod RL, et al. TRPV1 antagonists as potential antitussive agents. *Lung*, **2008**, 186 (Suppl 1):S59–S65.

Millan DS. What is the potential for inhaled p38 inhibitors in the treatment of chronic obstructive pulmonary disease? *Future Med Chem*, **2011**, 3:1635–1645.

Nathani N, et al. Churg-Strauss syndrome and leukotriene antagonist use: a respiratory perspective. *Thorax*, **2008**, 63:883–888.

Nelson HS, Dorinsky PM. Safety of long-acting beta-agonists. *Ann Intern Med*, **2006**, 145:706–710.

Newton PJ, et al. Nebulized furosemide for the management of dyspnea: does the evidence support its use? *J Pain Symptom Manage*, **2008**, 36:424–441.

Niewoehner DE, et al. Effect of systemic glucocorticoids on exacerbations of chronic obstructive pulmonary disease. *N Engl J Med*, **1999**, 340:1941–1947.

Nightingale JA, et al. Comparison of the effects of salmeterol and formoterol in patients with severe asthma. *Chest*, **2002**, 121:1401–1406.

Norman P. Investigational p38 inhibitors for the treatment of chronic obstructive pulmonary disease. *Expert Opin Investig Drugs*, **2015**, 24:383–392.

Normansell R, et al. Omalizumab for asthma in adults and children. *Cochrane Database Syst Rev*, **2014**, (1):CD003559.

Ozdemir C, et al. Mechanisms of aeroallergen immunotherapy: subcutaneous immunotherapy and sublingual immunotherapy. *Immunol Allergy Clin North Am*, **2016**, 36:71–86.

Pavord ID, Chung KF. Management of chronic cough. *Lancet*, **2008**, 371:1375–1384.

Pavord ID, et al. Mepolizumab for severe eosinophilic asthma (DREAM): a multicentre, double-blind, placebo-controlled trial. *Lancet*, **2012**, 380:651–659.

Pedersen S. Do inhaled corticosteroids inhibit growth in children? *Am J Respir Crit Care Med*, **2001**, 164:521–535.

Pelaia G, et al. Potential role of potassium channel openers in the treatment of asthma and chronic obstructive pulmonary disease. *Life Sci*, **2002**, 70:977–990.

Penn RB, et al. Mechanisms of acute desensitization of the beta2AR-adenylyl cyclase pathway in human airway smooth muscle. *Am J Respir Cell Mol Biol*, **1998**, 19:338–348.

Postma DS, Rabe KF. The asthma-COPD overlap syndrome. *N Engl J Med*, **2015**, 373:1241–1249.

Ray NC, Alcaraz L. Muscarinic antagonist-beta-adrenergic agonist dual pharmacology molecules as bronchodilators: a patent review. *Expert Opin Ther Pat*, **2009**, 19:1–12.

Rennard SI, et al. CXCR2 antagonist MK-7123—a phase 2 proof-of-concept trial for chronic obstructive pulmonary disease. *Am J Respir Crit Care Med*, **2015**, 191:1001–1011.

Rennard SI, et al. The safety and efficacy of infliximab in moderate-to-severe chronic obstructive pulmonary disease. *Am J Respir Crit Care Med*, **2007**, 175:926–934.

Robinson DS, et al. Addition of an anti-leukotriene to therapy in chronic severe asthma in a clinic setting: a double-blind, randomised, placebo-controlled study. *Lancet*, **2001**, 357:2007–2011.

Rolland JM, et al. Allergen-related approaches to immunotherapy. *Pharmacol Ther*, **2009**, 121:273–284.

Sanchis J, et al. Inhaler devices—from theory to practice. *Respir Med*, **2013**, 107:495–502.

Sears MR. Adverse effects of beta-agonists. *J Allergy Clin Immunol*, **2002**, 110:S322–S328.

Shivanthan MC, Rajapakse S. Magnesium for acute exacerbation of chronic obstructive pulmonary disease: a systematic review of randomised trials. *Ann Thorac Med*, **2014**, 9:77–80.

Tantisira KG, Drazen JM. Genetics and pharmacogenetics of the leukotriene pathway. *J Allergy Clin Immunol*, **2009**, 124:422–427.

Tashkin DP, et al. A 4-year trial of tiotropium in chronic obstructive pulmonary disease. *N Engl J Med*, **2008**, 359:1543–1554.

Teach SJ, et al. Preseasonal treatment with either omalizumab or an inhaled corticosteroid boost to prevent fall asthma exacerbations. *J Allergy Clin Immunol*, **2015**, 136:1476–1485.

To Y, et al. Targeting phosphoinositide-3-kinase-δ with theophylline reverses corticosteroid insensitivity in COPD. *Am J Respir Crit Care Med*, **2010**, 182:897–904.

Townley RG, Agrawal S. CRTH2 antagonists in the treatment of allergic responses involving TH2 cells, basophils, and eosinophils. *Ann Allergy Asthma Immunol*, **2012**, 109:365–374.

Trejo Bittar HE, et al. Pathobiology of severe asthma. *Annu Rev Pathol*, **2015**, 10:511–545.

Usmani OS, Barnes PJ. Assessing and treating small airways disease in asthma and chronic obstructive pulmonary disease. *Ann Med*, **2012**, 44:146–156.

van Ganse E, et al. Effects of antihistamines in adult asthma: a meta-analysis of clinical trials. *Eur Respir J*, **1997**, 10:2216–2224.

Veiraiah A, et al. Flumazenil use in benzodiazepine overdose in the UK: a retrospective survey of NPIS data. *Emerg Med J*, **2012**, 29:565–569.

Wenzel S, et al. Dupilumab in persistent asthma with elevated eosinophil levels. *N Engl J Med*, **2013**, 368:2455–2466.

Wenzel SE, et al. A randomized, double-blind, placebo-controlled study of TNF-α blockade in severe persistent asthma. *Am J Respir Crit Care Med*, **2009**, *179*:549–558.

Wessler I, Kirkpatrick CJ. Acetylcholine beyond neurons: the non-neuronal cholinergic system in humans. *BrJ Pharmacol*, **2008**, *154*: 1558–1571.

Woodcock A, et al. Efficacy in asthma of once-daily treatment with fluticasone furoate: a randomized, placebo-controlled trial. *Respir Res*, **2011**, *12*:132.

Woodruff PG, et al. Safety and efficacy of an inhaled epidermal growth factor receptor inhibitor (BIBW 2948 BS) in chronic obstructive pulmonary disease. *Am J Respir Crit Care Med*, **2010**, *181*:438–445.

Yang IA,et al. Inhaled corticosteroids for stable chronic obstructive pulmonary disease. *Cochrane Database Syst Rev*, **2012**, (7):CD002991.

Yasui K, et al. Theophylline induces neutrophil apoptosis through adenosine A_{2A} receptor antagonism. *J Leukoc Biol*, **2000**, *67*:529–535.

Zhang L, et al. Inhaled corticosteroids in children with persistent asthma: effects on growth. *Cochrane Database Syst Rev*, **2014**, (7):CD009471.

Zheng JP, et al. Effect of carbocisteine on acute exacerbation of chronic obstructive pulmonary disease (PEACE Study): a randomised placebo-controlled study. *Lancet*, **2008**, *371*:2013–2018.

Zheng JP, et al. Twice daily *N*-acetylcysteine 600 mg for exacerbations of chronic obstructive pulmonary disease (PANTHEON): a randomised, double-blind placebo-controlled trial. *Lancet Respir Med*, **2014**, *2*:187–194.

Ziegelbauer K, et al. A selective novel low-molecular-weight inhibitor of IkappaB kinase-beta (IKK-beta) prevents pulmonary inflammation and shows broad anti-inflammatory activity. *Br J Pharmacol*, **2005**, *145*:178–192.

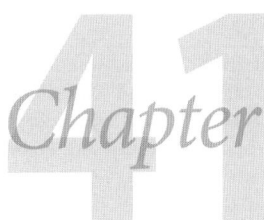

Chapter 41

Hematopoietic Agents: Growth Factors, Minerals, and Vitamins

Kenneth Kaushansky and Thomas J. Kipps

HEMATOPOIESIS

GROWTH FACTOR PHYSIOLOGY

ERYTHROPOIESIS-STIMULATING AGENTS
- Erythropoietin

MYELOID GROWTH FACTORS
- Granulocyte-Macrophage Colony-Stimulating Factor
- Granulocyte Colony-Stimulating Factor

THROMBOPOIETIC GROWTH FACTORS
- Interleukin 11
- Thrombopoietin Receptor Agonists

IRON DEFICIENCY AND OTHER HYPOCHROMIC ANEMIAS
- Bioavailability of Iron
- Metabolism of Iron
- Iron Requirements; Availability of Dietary Iron
- Treatment of Iron Deficiency
- Copper, Pyridoxine, and Riboflavin

VITAMIN B$_{12}$, FOLIC ACID, AND MEGALOBLASTIC ANEMIAS
- Cellular Roles of Vitamin B$_{12}$ and Folic Acid
- Vitamin B$_{12}$ and Human Health
- Folic Acid and Human Health

Hematopoiesis

The finite life span of most mature blood cells requires their continuous replacement, a process termed *hematopoiesis*. New cell production must respond to basal needs and states of increased demand. Erythrocyte production can increase more than 20-fold in response to anemia or hypoxemia, leukocyte production increases dramatically in response to systemic infections, and platelet production can increase 10- to 20-fold when platelet consumption results in thrombocytopenia.

The regulation of blood cell production is complex. Hematopoietic stem cells are rare marrow cells that manifest self-renewal and lineage commitment, resulting in cells destined to differentiate into the 10 or more distinct blood cell lineages. For the most part, this process occurs in the marrow cavities of the skull, vertebral bodies, pelvis, and proximal long bones; it involves interactions among hematopoietic stem and progenitor cells and the cells and complex macromolecules of the marrow stroma and is influenced by a number of soluble and membrane-bound hematopoietic growth factors. Several hormones and cytokines have been identified and cloned that affect hematopoiesis, permitting their production in quantities sufficient for research and, in some cases, therapeutic use. Clinical applications range from the treatment of primary hematologic diseases (e.g., aplastic anemia, congenital neutropenia) to use as adjuncts in the treatment of severe infections and in the management of patients with kidney failure or those undergoing cancer chemotherapy or marrow transplantation.

Hematopoiesis also requires an adequate supply of minerals (e.g., iron, cobalt, and copper) and vitamins (e.g., folic acid, vitamin B$_{12}$, pyridoxine, ascorbic acid, and riboflavin); deficiencies generally result in characteristic anemias or, less frequently, a general failure of hematopoiesis (Hoffbrand and Herbert, 1999). Therapeutic correction of a specific deficiency state depends on the accurate diagnosis of the anemic state and on knowledge about the correct dose, the use of these agents in appropriate combinations, and the expected response.

Growth Factor Physiology

Steady-state hematopoiesis encompasses the tightly regulated production of more than 400 billion blood cells each day. The hematopoietic organ also is unique in adult physiology in that several mature cell types are derived from a much smaller number of multipotent progenitors, which develop from a more limited number of pluripotent hematopoietic stem cells. Such cells are capable of maintaining their own number and differentiating under the influence of cellular and humoral factors to produce the large and diverse number of mature blood cells.

Our understanding of stem cell differentiation owes much to the in vitro culture of marrow cells. Using the results from clonal cultures in semisolid medium, stem cell differentiation can be described as a series of developmental steps that produce mixed blood cell lineage colonies, which give rise to large, immature and small, mature single-lineage burst-forming units (BFUs) and colony-forming units (CFUs), respectively, for each of the major blood cell types. These early progenitors (BFUs and CFUs) are capable of further proliferation and differentiation, increasing their number by some 30-fold. It is at this most mature stage of development that the lineage-committed growth factors (G-CSF, M-CSF, erythropoietin, and thrombopoietin) exert their primary proliferative and differentiative effects. Overall, proliferation and maturation of the CFU for each cell line can amplify the resulting mature cell product by another 30-fold or more, generating more than 1000 mature cells from each committed stem cell.

Hematopoietic and lymphopoietic growth factors are glycoproteins produced by a number of marrow cells and peripheral tissues. They are active at very low concentrations and typically affect more than one committed cell lineage. Most interact synergistically with other factors and stimulate production of additional growth factors, a process termed *networking*. Growth factors generally exert actions at several points in the processes of cell proliferation and differentiation and in mature cell function. However, the network of growth factors that contributes to any given cell lineage depends absolutely on a nonredundant, lineage-specific

Abbreviations

BFU: burst-forming units
BFU-E: BFU erythrocyte
CFU: colony-forming units
CFU-E: CFU erythrocyte
CFU-GEMM: CFU granulocyte, erythrocyte, monocyte and megakaryocyte
CFU-GM: CFU granulocyte and macrophage
CFU-Meg: CFU megakaryocyte
CH_3B_{12}: methylcobalamin
$CH_3H_4PteGlu_1$: methyltetrahydrofolate
CSF: colony stimulating factor
dTMP: thymidylate
dUMP: deoxyuridylate
EPO: erythropoietin
ESA: erythropoiesis-stimulating agent
FIGLU: formiminoglutamic acid
FL: FLT3 (FMS tyr kinase 3) ligand
FMS3: FMS tyr kinase 3
G-CSF: granulocyte colony-stimulating factor
GM-CSF: granulocyte-macrophage colony-stimulating factor
GVHD: graft-versus-host disease
HAART: highly active antiretroviral therapy
HFE: high Fe, hemochromatosis protein
HIF: hypoxia-inducible factor
HIV: human immunodeficiency virus
IFN: interferon
IL: interleukin
LAK: lymphokine-activated killer cell
M-CSF: monocyte-/macrophage-stimulating factor
NK: natural killer
PBSC: peripheral blood stem cell
PteGlu: pteroylglutamic acid, folic acid
SAM: S-adenosylmethionine
SCF: stem cell factor
TcII: transcobalamin II
TRA: thrombopoietin receptor agonist

factor, such that absence of factors that stimulate developmentally early progenitors is compensated for by redundant cytokines, but loss of the lineage-specific factor leads to a specific cytopenia.

Some of the overlapping and nonredundant effects of the more important hematopoietic growth factors are illustrated in Figure 41–1 *and* Table 41–1.

Erythropoiesis-Stimulating Agents

Erythropoiesis-stimulating agent (ESA) is the term given to a pharmacological substance that stimulates red blood cell production.

Erythropoietin

Erythropoietin is the most important regulator of the proliferation of committed erythroid progenitors (CFU-E) and their immediate progeny. In its absence, severe anemia is invariably present, commonly seen in patients with renal failure. Erythropoiesis is controlled by a feedback system in which a sensor in the kidney detects changes in oxygen delivery to modulate the erythropoietin secretion. The sensor mechanism is now understood at the molecular level (Haase, 2010).

Hypoxia-inducible factor, a heterodimeric (HIF-1α and HIF-1β) transcription factor, enhances expression of multiple hypoxia-inducible genes,

HISTORICAL PERSPECTIVE

Modern concepts of hematopoietic cell growth and differentiation derive from experiments done in the 1950s. Till and McCulloch demonstrated that individual hematopoietic cells could form macroscopic hematopoietic colonies in the spleens of irradiated mice, thereby establishing the concept of discrete hematopoietic stem cells (i.e., the presence of a multilineage clonal splenic colony appearing 11 days after transplantation implied that a single cell lodged and expanded into several cell lineages). This concept now has been expanded to include normal human marrow cells. Moreover, such cells now can be prospectively identified.

The basis for identifying soluble growth factors was provided by Sachs and independently by Metcalf, who developed clonal, in vitro assays for hematopoietic progenitor cells. Such hematopoietic colonies first developed only in the presence of conditioned culture medium from leukocytes or tumor cell lines. Individual growth factors then were isolated based on their activities in clonal in vitro assays, assays that were instrumental in purifying a hierarchy of progenitor cells committed to individual and combinations of mature blood cells (Kondo et al., 2003).

In 1906, Paul Carnot postulated the existence of a circulating growth factor that controls red blood cell development. He observed an increase in the red cell count in rabbits injected with serum obtained from anemic animals and postulated the existence of a factor that he called hemopoietin. Only in the 1950s did Reissmann, Erslev, and Jacobsen and coworkers define the origin and actions of the hormone, now called erythropoietin. Subsequently, extensive studies of erythropoietin were carried out in patients with anemia and polycythemia, leading to the purification of erythropoietin from urine and the subsequent cloning of the erythropoietin gene. The high-level expression of erythropoietin in cell lines has allowed for its purification and use in humans with anemia.

Similarly, the existence of specific leukocyte growth factors was suggested by the capacity of different conditioned culture media to induce the in vitro growth of colonies containing different combinations of granulocytes and monocytes. An activity that stimulated the production of both granulocytes and monocytes was purified from murine lung-conditioned medium, leading to cloning of GM-CSF, first from mice (Gough et al., 1984) and subsequently from humans (Wong et al., 1985). Finding an activity that stimulated the exclusive production of neutrophils permitted the cloning of G-CSF (Welte et al., 1985). Subsequently, a megakaryocyte colony-stimulating factor termed thrombopoietin was purified and cloned (Kaushansky, 1998).

Growth factors that support lymphocyte growth were identified using assays that measured the capacity of the cytokine to promote lymphocyte proliferation in vitro. This permitted the identification of the growth-promoting properties of IL-7, IL-4, or IL-15 for all lymphocytes, B cells, or NK cells, respectively (Goodwin et al., 1989; Grabstein et al., 1994). Recombinant expression of these complementary DNAs permitted production of sufficient quantities of biologically active growth factors for clinical investigations, allowing for the demonstration of the potential clinical utility of such factors.

such as vascular endothelial growth factor and erythropoietin. HIF-1α is labile due to its prolyl hydroxylation and subsequent polyubiquitination and degradation, aided by the von Hippel-Lindau (VHL) *protein.* During states of hypoxia, the prolyl hydroxylase is inactive, allowing the accumulation of HIF-1α and activating erythropoietin expression, which in turn stimulates rapid expansion of erythroid progenitors. Specific alteration of VHL leads to an oxygen-sensing defect, characterized by constitutively elevated levels of HIF-1α and erythropoietin, with resultant polycythemia (Gordeuk et al., 2004). A second isoform of HIF, HIF-2α, is an important

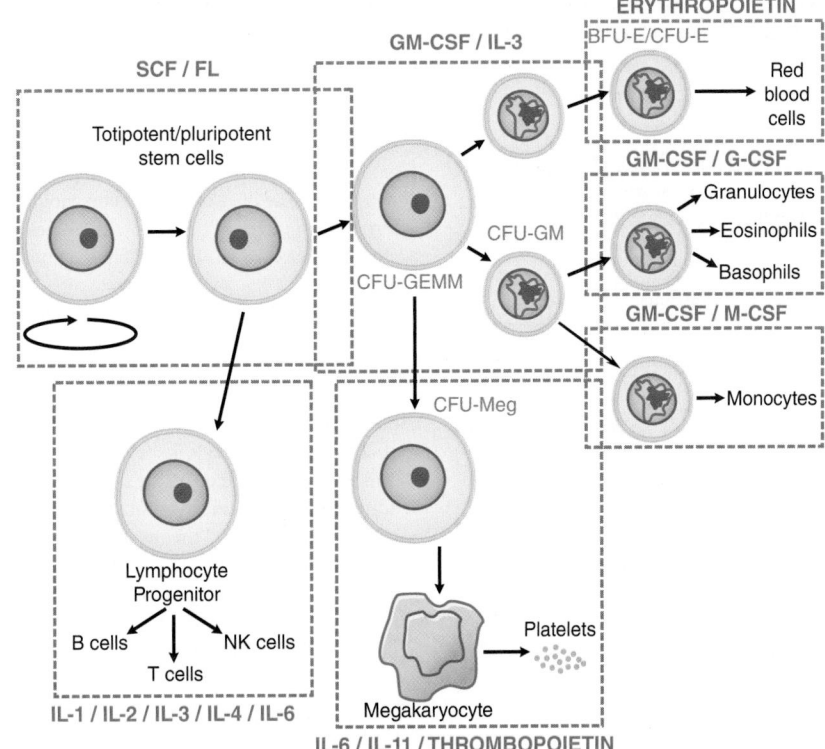

Figure 41–1 *Sites of action of hematopoietic growth factors in the differentiation and maturation of marrow cell lines.* A self-sustaining pool of marrow stem cells differentiates under the influence of specific hematopoietic growth factors to form a variety of hematopoietic and lymphopoietic cells. SCF, FL, IL-3, and GM-CSF, together with cell-cell interactions in the marrow, stimulate stem cells to form a series of BFUs and CFUs: CFU-GEMM, CFU-GM, CFU-Meg, BFU-E, and CFU-E. After considerable proliferation, further differentiation is stimulated by synergistic interactions with growth factors for each of the major cell lines—G-CSF, M-CSF, thrombopoietin, and erythropoietin. Each of these factors also influences the proliferation, maturation, and in some cases the function, of the derivative cell line (Table 41–1).

regulator of the expression of genes that contribute to iron absorption (Mastrogiannaki et al., 2013); a genetic gain-of-function mutation in HIF-2α also induces erythrocytosis in patients (Percy et al., 2008).

Erythropoietin is expressed primarily in peritubular interstitial cells of the kidney. Erythropoietin contains 193 amino acids, of which the first 27 are cleaved during secretion. The final hormone is heavily glycosylated and has a molecular mass of about 30 kDa. After secretion, erythropoietin binds to a receptor on the surface of committed erythroid progenitors in the marrow and is internalized. With anemia or hypoxemia, synthesis rapidly increases by 100-fold or more, serum erythropoietin levels rise, and marrow progenitor cell survival, proliferation, and maturation are dramatically stimulated. This finely tuned feedback loop can be disrupted by kidney disease, marrow damage, or a deficiency in iron or an essential vitamin. With an infection or an inflammatory state, erythropoietin secretion, iron delivery, and progenitor proliferation all are suppressed by inflammatory cytokines, but this accounts for only part of the resultant anemia; interference with iron metabolism also is an effect of inflammatory mediator effects on the hepatic protein *hepcidin* (Drakesmith and Prentice, 2012). Loss of hepcidin-producing liver mass or genetic or acquired conditions that repress hepcidin production by the liver may lead to iron overload (Pietrangelo, 2016).

Preparations

Preparations of recombinant human erythropoietin include *epoetin alfa, epoetin beta, epoetin omega,* and *epoetin zeta,* which differ almost exclusively in carbohydrate modifications due to manufacturing differences and are supplied in single-use vials or syringes containing 500–40,000 units for intravenous or subcutaneous administration. When injected intravenously, epoetin alfas are cleared from plasma with a $t_{1/2}$ of 4–8 h. However, the effect on marrow progenitors lasts much longer, and once-weekly dosing can be sufficient to achieve an adequate response. An engineered epoetin

alfa, darbepoetin, which displays a longer circulatory half-life, is also available for use in patients with indications similar to those for other epoetins. Based on phage display technology, small peptide agonists of the erythropoietin receptor were identified and developed into clinical agents by coupling to polyethylene glycol. One such erythropoiesis-stimulating peptide, peginesatide, was approved for the treatment of anemia due to chronic kidney disease; postmarketing reports of serious hypersensitivity reactions and anaphylaxis necessitated its removal from the market.

Recombinant human erythropoietin (*epoetin alfa*) is nearly identical to the endogenous hormone. The carbohydrate modification pattern of epoetin alfa differs slightly from the native protein, but this difference apparently does not alter kinetics, potency, or immunoreactivity of the drug. Modern assays can detect these differences and thereby identify athletes who use the recombinant product for "blood doping."

Therapeutic Uses, Monitoring, and Adverse Effects

Recombinant erythropoietin therapy, in conjunction with adequate iron intake, can be highly effective in a number of anemias, especially those associated with poor erythropoietic response. Epoetin alfa is effective in the treatment of anemias associated with surgery, AIDS, cancer chemotherapy, prematurity, and certain chronic inflammatory conditions. Darbepoetin alfa also has been approved for use in patients with anemia associated with chronic kidney disease. A Cochrane analysis could not demonstrate the superiority of one form of ESA over any another.

During erythropoietin therapy, absolute or functional iron deficiency may develop. Functional iron deficiency (i.e., normal ferritin levels but low transferrin saturation) presumably results from the inability to mobilize iron stores rapidly enough to support the increased erythropoiesis. Supplemental iron therapy is recommended for all patients whose serum ferritin is less than 100 μg/L or whose serum transferrin saturation is below 20%. During initial therapy and after any dosage adjustment, the

TABLE 41–1 ■ HEMATOPOIETIC GROWTH FACTORS

Erythropoietin (EPO)
- Stimulates proliferation and maturation of committed erythroid progenitors to increase red cell production

Stem cell factor (SCF, c-kit ligand, Steel factor) and FLT 3 ligand (FL)
- Act synergistically with a wide range of other colony-stimulating factors and interleukins to stimulate pluripotent and committed stem cells
- FL also stimulates both dendritic and NK cells (antitumor response)
- SCF also stimulates mast cells and melanocytes

Interleukins

IL-1, IL-3, IL-5, IL-6, IL-9, and IL-11
- Act synergistically with each other and SCF, GM-CSF, G-CSF, and EPO to stimulate BFU-E, CFU-GEMM, CFU-GM, CFU-E, and CFU-Meg growth
- Numerous immunologic roles, including stimulation of B-cell and T-cell growth

IL-5
- Controls eosinophil survival and differentiation

IL-6
- IL-6 stimulates human myeloma cells to proliferate
- IL-6 and IL-11 stimulate BFU-Meg to increase platelet production

IL-1, IL-2, IL-4, IL-7, and IL-12
- Stimulate growth and function of T cells, B cells, NK cells, and monocytes
- Costimulate B, T, and LAK cells

IL-8 and IL-10
- Numerous immunological activities involving B- and T-cell functions
- IL-8 acts as a chemotactic factor for basophils and neutrophils

Granulocyte-macrophage colony-stimulating factor (GM-CSF)
- Acts synergistically with SCF, IL-1, IL-3, and IL-6 to stimulate CFU-GM and CFU-Meg to increase neutrophil and monocyte production
- With EPO may promote BFU-E formation
- Enhances migration, phagocytosis, superoxide production, and antibody-dependent cell-mediated toxicity of neutrophils, monocytes, and eosinophils
- Prevents alveolar proteinosis

Granulocyte colony-stimulating factor (G-CSF)
- Stimulates CFU-G to increase neutrophil production
- Enhances phagocytic and cytotoxic activities of neutrophils

Monocyte/macrophage colony-stimulating factor (M-CSF, CSF-1)
- Stimulates CFU-M to increase monocyte precursors
- Activates and enhances function of monocyte/macrophages

Macrophage colony-stimulating factor (M-CSF)
- Stimulates CFU-M to increase monocyte/macrophage precursors
- Acts in concert with tissues and other growth factors to determine the proliferation, differentiation, and survival of a range of cells of the mononuclear phagocyte system

Thrombopoietin (TPO, *Mpl* ligand)
- Stimulates the self-renewal and expansion of hematopoietic stem cells
- Stimulates stem cell differentiation into megakaryocyte progenitors
- Selectively stimulates megakaryocytopoiesis to increase platelet production
- Acts synergistically with other growth factors, especially IL-6 and IL-11

hematocrit is determined once a week (patients infected with HIV and those with cancer) or twice a week (patients with renal failure) until it has stabilized in the target range and the maintenance dose has been established; the hematocrit then is monitored at regular intervals. If the hematocrit increases by more than 4 points in any 2-week period, the dose should be decreased. Due to the time required for erythropoiesis and the erythrocyte half-life, hematocrit changes lag behind dosage adjustments by 2–6 weeks. The dose of darbepoetin should be decreased if the hemoglobin increase exceeds 1 g/dL in any 2-week period because of the association of excessive rate of rise of hemoglobin with adverse cardiovascular events.

During hemodialysis, patients receiving epoetin alfa or darbepoetin may require increased anticoagulation. The risk of thrombotic events is higher in adults with ischemic heart disease or congestive heart failure receiving epoetin alfa therapy with the goal of reaching a normal hematocrit (42%) than in those with a lower target hematocrit of 30% (Bennett et al., 2008). ESA use is associated with increased rates of cancer recurrence and decreased on-study survival in patients in whom the drugs are administered for cancer-induced or for chemotherapy-induced anemia (Bohlius et al., 2009). The most common side effect of epoetin alfa therapy is aggravation of hypertension, which occurs in 20%–30% of patients and most often is associated with a rapid rise in hematocrit. ESAs should not be used in patients with preexisting uncontrolled hypertension. Patients may require initiation of, or increases in, antihypertensive therapy. Hypertensive encephalopathy and seizures have occurred in patients with chronic renal failure treated with epoetin alfa. Headache, tachycardia, edema, shortness of breath, nausea, vomiting, diarrhea, injection site stinging, and flu-like symptoms (e.g., arthralgias and myalgias) also have been reported in conjunction with epoetin alfa therapy.

Anemia of Chronic Renal Failure Patients with anemia secondary to chronic kidney disease are ideal candidates for epoetin alfa therapy as the disease represents a true hormone deficiency state. The response in predialysis, peritoneal dialysis, and hemodialysis patients depends on the severity of the renal failure, the erythropoietin dose and route of administration, and iron availability (Besarab et al., 1999; Kaufman et al., 1998). The subcutaneous route of administration is preferred over the intravenous route because absorption is slower and the amount of drug required is reduced by 20%–40%. The dose of epoetin alfa should be adjusted to obtain a gradual rise in the hematocrit over a 2- to 4-month period to a final hematocrit of 33%–36%. Treatment to hematocrit levels greater than 36% is not recommended.

Patients are started on doses of 80–120 units/kg of epoetin alfa, given subcutaneously, three times a week. The final maintenance dose of epoetin alfa can vary from 10 units/kg to more than 300 units/kg, with an average dose of 75 units/kg, three times a week. Children less than 5 years of age generally require a higher dose. Resistance to therapy is common in patients who develop an inflammatory illness or become iron deficient, so close monitoring of general health and iron status is essential. Less-common causes of resistance include occult blood loss, folic acid deficiency, carnitine deficiency, inadequate dialysis, aluminum toxicity, and osteitis fibrosa cystica secondary to hyperparathyroidism. Darbepoetin alfa is approved for use in patients who are anemic secondary to chronic kidney disease. The recommended starting dose is 0.45 μg/kg administered intravenously or subcutaneously once weekly or 0.75 μg/kg administered every 2 weeks, with dose adjustments depending on the response. Like epoetin alfa, side effects tend to occur when patients experience a rapid rise in hemoglobin concentration; a rise of less than 1 g/dL every 2 weeks generally is considered safe.

Anemia in Patients With AIDS Epoetin alfa therapy has been approved for the treatment of HIV-infected patients, especially those on zidovudine therapy (Fischl et al., 1990). Excellent responses to doses of 100–300 units/kg, given subcutaneously three times a week, generally are seen in patients with zidovudine-induced anemia. However, a more recent analysis of erythropoietin therapy in patients with HIV infection failed to support its routine use (Martí-Carvajal et al., 2011). The reason for the difference between 1990 and 2011 may lay in far more effective therapy for HIV in the HAART era, such that the origin of anemia in HIV-infected individuals today is different from what it was at the onset of the AIDS epidemic.

Cancer-Related Anemias Epoetin alfa therapy, 150 units/kg three times a week or 450–600 units/kg once a week, can reduce the transfusion requirement in patients with cancer undergoing chemotherapy as well as lead to reduced anemia-related symptoms. Previous therapeutic guidelines (Rizzo et al., 2002) recommended the use of epoetin alfa in patients with chemotherapy-associated anemia when hemoglobin levels fall below 10 g/dL, basing the decision to treat less-severe anemia (hemoglobin 10–12 g/dL) on clinical circumstances. For anemia associated with hematologic malignancies, the guidelines support the use of recombinant erythropoietin in patients with low-grade myelodysplastic syndrome. In this setting, neutropenia often dictates the use of G-CSF, which frequently augments the erythroid response to erythropoietin. In responding patients, the response duration is usually 2–3 years. A baseline serum erythropoietin level may help to predict the response; most patients with blood levels greater than 500 IU/L are unlikely to respond to any dose of the drug. Most patients treated with epoetin alfa experience an improvement in their anemia and their sense of well-being (Littlewood et al., 2001). Following these recommendations, case reports suggested a direct effect of both epoetin alfa and darbepoetin alfa in stimulation of tumor cells. A meta-analysis of a large number of patients and clinical trials estimated the risk at about 10% higher than for cancer patients not treated (Bohlius et al., 2009). Following on these results, new guidelines were issued (Rizzo et al., 2010). This finding is continuing to be evaluated by the FDA and warrants serious attention.

Use in Perioperative Patients Epoetin alfa has been used perioperatively to treat anemia (hematocrit 30%–36%) and reduce the need for allogeneic erythrocyte transfusion in nonanemic patients during and following surgery in patients with moderate or large anticipated blood loss. Patients undergoing elective orthopedic and cardiac procedures have been treated with 150–300 units/kg of epoetin alfa once daily for the 10 days preceding surgery, on the day of surgery, and for 4 days after surgery. As an alternative, 600 units/kg can be given on days 21, 14, and 7 before surgery, with an additional dose on the day of surgery. Using these dosing regimens, an average of four units of autologous blood can be obtained for postoperative use in a typical, nonanemic patient.

Other Uses Epoetin alfa has received orphan drug status from the FDA for the treatment of the anemia of prematurity, HIV infection, and myelodysplasia. In the last case, even very high doses (>1000 units/kg two to three times a week) sometimes have limited success. Highly competitive athletes have used epoetin alfa to increase their hemoglobin levels ("blood doping") and improve performance. Unfortunately, this misuse of the drug has been implicated in the deaths of several athletes and is strongly discouraged.

Myeloid Growth Factors

The myeloid growth factors are glycoproteins that stimulate the proliferation and differentiation of one or more myeloid cell types. Recombinant forms of several growth factors have been produced, including GM-CSF, G-CSF, IL-3, M-CSF or CSF-1, and stem cell factor (SCF) (see Table 41–1), although only G-CSF and GM-CSF have found meaningful clinical applications.

Myeloid growth factors are produced naturally by a number of different cells, including fibroblasts, endothelial cells, macrophages, and T cells (Figure 41–2). These factors are active at extremely low concentrations and act via membrane receptors of the cytokine receptor superfamily to activate the Jak/STAT signal transduction pathway. GM-CSF can stimulate proliferation, differentiation, and function of a number of the myeloid cell lineages (see Figure 41–1). It acts synergistically with other growth factors, including erythropoietin, at the level of the BFU. GM-CSF stimulates CFU-GM, CFU-M, CFU-E, and CFU-Meg to increase cell production. GM-CSF also enhances the migration, phagocytosis, superoxide production, and antibody-dependent cell-mediated toxicity of neutrophils, monocytes, and eosinophils (Weisbart et al., 1987).

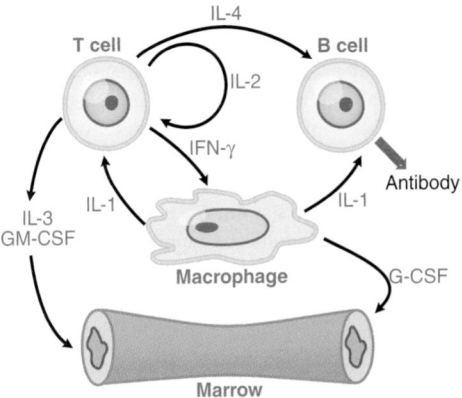

Figure 41–2 *Cytokine-cell interactions.* Macrophages, T cells, B cells, and marrow stem cells interact via several cytokines (IL-1, IL-2, IL-3, IL-4, IFN-γ, GM-CSF, and G-CSF) in response to a bacterial or a foreign antigen challenge. See Table 41–1 for the functional activities of these various cytokines.

The activity of G-CSF is restricted to neutrophils and their progenitors, stimulating their proliferation, differentiation, and function. It acts primarily on CFU-G, although it also can play a synergistic role with IL-3 and GM-CSF in stimulating other cell lines. G-CSF enhances phagocytic and cytotoxic activities of neutrophils. G-CSF reduces inflammation by inhibiting IL-1, tumor necrosis factor, and interferon gamma. G-CSF also mobilizes primitive hematopoietic cells, including hematopoietic stem cells, from the marrow into the peripheral blood (Sheridan et al., 1992). This observation has virtually transformed the practice of stem cell transplantation, such that more than 90% of all such procedures today use G-CSF–mobilized peripheral blood cells as the donor stem cell product.

Granulocyte-Macrophage Colony-Stimulating Factor

Recombinant human GM-CSF (*sargramostim*) is a glycoprotein with 127 amino acids. The primary therapeutic effect of sargramostim is to stimulate myelopoiesis.

The initial clinical application of sargramostim was in patients undergoing autologous marrow transplantation. By shortening the duration of neutropenia, transplant morbidity was significantly reduced without a change in long-term survival or risk of inducing an early relapse of the malignant process (Brandt et al., 1988).

The role of GM-CSF therapy in allogeneic transplantation is less clear. Its effect on neutrophil recovery is less pronounced in patients receiving prophylactic treatment of graft-versus-host disease (GVHD). However, it may improve survival in transplant patients who exhibit early graft failure (Nemunaitis et al., 1990).

It also has been used to mobilize CD34-positive progenitor cells for peripheral blood stem cell (PBSC) collection for transplantation after myeloablative chemotherapy (Haas et al., 1990). Sargramostim has been used to shorten the period of neutropenia and reduce morbidity in patients receiving intensive cancer chemotherapy (Gerhartz et al., 1993). It also stimulates myelopoiesis in some patients with cyclic neutropenia, myelodysplasia, aplastic anemia, or AIDS-associated neutropenia.

Sargramostim is administered by subcutaneous injection or slow intravenous infusion at doses of 125–500 μg/m²/d. Plasma levels of GM-CSF rise rapidly after subcutaneous injection and then decline with a $t_{1/2}$ of 2–3 h. When given intravenously, infusions should be maintained over 3–6 h. With the initiation of therapy, there is a transient decrease in the absolute leukocyte count secondary to cell margination and pulmonary vascular sequestration. This is followed by a dose-dependent, biphasic increase in leukocyte counts over the next 7–10 days. Once the drug is discontinued, the leukocyte count returns to baseline within 2–10 days. When GM-CSF is given in lower doses, the response is primarily neutrophilic, whereas monocytosis and eosinophilia are observed at larger doses. After hematopoietic stem cell transplantation or intensive chemotherapy, sargramostim is given daily during the period of maximum neutropenia until a sustained rise in the granulocyte count is observed. Frequent blood counts are essential to avoid an excessive rise in the granulocyte count. Higher doses are associated with more pronounced side effects, including bone pain, malaise, flu-like symptoms, fever, diarrhea, dyspnea, and rash. An acute reaction to the first dose, characterized by flushing, hypotension, nausea, vomiting, and dyspnea, with a fall in arterial oxygen saturation due to granulocyte sequestration in the pulmonary circulation, occurs in sensitive patients. With prolonged administration, a few patients may develop a capillary leak syndrome, with peripheral edema and pleural and pericardial effusions. Other serious side effects include transient supraventricular arrhythmia, dyspnea, and elevation of serum creatinine, bilirubin, and hepatic enzymes.

Granulocyte Colony-Stimulating Factor

Recombinant human G-CSF, *filgrastim*, is a glycoprotein with 175 amino acids. The principal action of filgrastim is the stimulation of CFU-G to increase neutrophil production (see Figure 41–1). Several forms of G-CSF are now available, including two longer-acting pegylated forms, pegfilgrastim and lipegfilgrastim.

Filgrastim is effective in the treatment of severe neutropenia after autologous hematopoietic stem cell transplantation and high-dose cancer chemotherapy (Lieschke and Burgess, 1992). Like GM-CSF, filgrastim shortens the period of severe neutropenia and reduces morbidity secondary to bacterial and fungal infections (Hammond et al., 1989). G-CSF also is effective in the treatment of severe congenital neutropenias. Filgrastim therapy can improve neutrophil counts in some patients with myelodysplasia or marrow damage (moderately SAA or tumor infiltration of the marrow). The neutropenia of patients with AIDS receiving zidovudine also can be partially or completely reversed.

Filgrastim is routinely used in patients undergoing PBSC collection for stem cell transplantation. It promotes the release of CD34$^+$ progenitor cells from the marrow, reducing the number of collections necessary for transplant. G-CSF–induced mobilization of stem cells into the circulation also has the potential to enhance repair of other damaged organs in which PBSCs might play a role. PBSC grafts have a higher cell dose and somewhat more committed progenitor cells than steady-state marrow grafts, resulting in faster engraftment and faster immunological reconstitution.

Filgrastim is administered by subcutaneous injection or intravenous infusion over at least 30 min at doses of 1–20 μg/kg/d. The usual starting dose in a patient receiving myelosuppressive chemotherapy is 5 μg/kg/d. The distribution and clearance rate from plasma ($t_{1/2}$ of 3.5 h) are similar for both routes of administration. The recommended dose for pegfilgrastim is fixed at 6 mg for patients weighing more than 20 kg, administered subcutaneously once per chemotherapy cycle. As with GM-CSF therapy, G-CSF administered after hematopoietic stem cell transplantation or intensive cancer chemotherapy will increase granulocyte production and shorten the period of severe neutropenia. Frequent blood cell counts should be obtained to determine the effectiveness of the treatment and guide dosage adjustment. In patients who received intensive myelosuppressive cancer chemotherapy, daily administration of G-CSF for 14–21 days or more may be necessary to correct the neutropenia.

Adverse Reactions

Adverse reactions to filgrastim include mild-to-moderate bone pain in patients receiving high doses over a protracted period, local skin reactions following subcutaneous injection, and rare cutaneous necrotizing vasculitis. Patients with a history of hypersensitivity to proteins produced by *Escherichia coli* should not receive the drug; the same holds for patients with sickle cell anemia, as it has been known to precipitate severe crises and even death. Mild-to-moderate splenomegaly has been observed in patients on long-term therapy.

Patients with sickle cell anemia should not be administered G-CSF as it is reported to trigger severe crises. In 2004 and 2006, two papers were published suggesting that previously healthy stem cell donors receiving human G-CSF for mobilization displayed marrow cell changes concerning for the development of future malignancy. Previous studies have shown an increase in

myeloid leukemia in patients with breast cancer receiving G-CSF for neutropenia. However, careful follow-up has failed to reveal any meaningful increase in myeloid leukemia in normal stem cell donors administered G-CSF.

Thrombopoietic Growth Factors

Interleukin 11

Interleukin 11 is a cytokine that stimulates hematopoiesis, intestinal epithelial cell growth, and osteoclastogenesis and inhibits adipogenesis. IL-11 also enhances megakaryocyte maturation in vitro. Recombinant human IL-11, *oprelvekin*, $t_{1/2}$ about 7 h, leads to a thrombopoietic response in 5–9 days when administered daily to normal subjects.

The drug is administered to patients at 25–50 μg/kg per day subcutaneously. Oprelvekin is approved for use in patients undergoing chemotherapy for nonmyeloid malignancies with severe thrombocytopenia (platelet count $< 20 \times 10^9$/L), and it is administered until the platelet count returns to more than 100×10^9/L. The major complications of therapy are fluid retention and associated cardiac symptoms, such as tachycardia, palpitation, edema, and shortness of breath; this is a significant concern in elderly patients and often requires concomitant therapy with diuretics. Also reported are blurred vision, injection site rash or erythema, and paresthesias.

Thrombopoietin Receptor Agonists

Thrombopoietin

Thrombopoietin, a glycoprotein produced by the liver, marrow stromal cells, and other organs, is the primary regulator of platelet production. Two forms of recombinant thrombopoietin have been tested for clinical use. One is a truncated version of the native protein, termed recombinant human megakaryocyte growth and development factor (rHuMGDF) that is covalently modified with polyethylene glycol to increase the circulatory $t_{1/2}$. The second is the full-length polypeptide termed recombinant human thrombopoietin (rHuTPO).

While use in thrombocytopenic clinical trial subjects was found to be safe, the use of rHuMGDF in a clinical trial of normal platelet donors, designed to boost the quantity of donated platelets, led to donor thrombocytopenia in several subjects due to the immunogenicity of this agent (Li et al., 2001). This experience led to both agents being abandoned for clinical use and to the development of small-molecular mimics of recombinant thrombopoietin, termed TRAs. Two of these agents are FDA approved for use in patients with immune thrombocytopenia (ITP), and one of the TRAs is also approved for use in patients with severe aplastic anemia (SAA) who have failed to respond to more conventional treatments. *Romiplostim* contains four copies of a small peptide that binds with high affinity to the thrombopoietin receptor, grafted onto an immunoglobulin scaffold. Romiplostim is safe and efficacious in patients with ITP (Kuter et al., 2008). The drug is administered weekly by subcutaneous injection, starting with a dose of 1 μg/kg, titrated to a maximum of 10 μg/kg, until the platelet count increases above 50×10^9/L. *Eltrombopag* is a small organic TRA that is administered orally; the recommended starting dose is 50 mg/d, titrated to 75 mg depending on platelet response. These and additional TRAs are undergoing clinical trials, in ITP and SAA, as well as in chemotherapy-induced thrombocytopenia and in several marrow disorders, including myelodysplastic syndromes.

Iron Deficiency and Other Hypochromic Anemias

The Bioavailability of Iron

Iron exists in the environment largely as ferric oxide, ferric hydroxide, and polymers. In this state, its biological availability is limited unless solubilized by acid or chelating agents. For example, bacteria and some plants produce high-affinity chelating agents that extract iron from the surrounding environment. Most mammals have little difficulty in acquiring iron; this is explained by ample iron intake and perhaps also by a greater efficiency in absorbing iron. Humans, however, appear to be an exception. Although total dietary intake of elemental iron in humans usually exceeds requirements, the bioavailability of the iron in the diet is limited.

HISTORICAL PERSPECTIVE

The modern understanding of iron metabolism began in 1937 with the work of McCance and Widdowson on iron absorption and excretion and Heilmeyer and Plotner's measurement of iron in plasma (Beutler, 2002). In 1947, Laurell described a plasma iron transport protein that he called *transferrin* (Laurell, 1951). Around the same time, Hahn and coworkers used radioisotopes to measure iron absorption and define the role of the intestinal mucosa to regulate this function (Hahn, 1948). In the next decade, Huff and associates initiated isotopic studies of internal iron metabolism. The subsequent development of practical clinical measurements of serum iron, transferrin saturation, plasma ferritin, and red cell protoporphyrin permitted the definition and detection of the body's iron store status and iron-deficient erythropoiesis. In 1994, Feder and colleagues identified the HFE gene, which is mutated in type 1 hemochromatosis (Feder et al., 1996). Subsequently, Ganz and colleagues discovered a peptide produced by the liver, which was termed *hepcidin* (Park et al., 2001), now known to be the master regulator of iron homeostasis and to play a role in anemia of chronic disease (Ganz and Nemeth, 2011).

Iron deficiency is the most common nutritional cause of anemia in humans. It can result from inadequate iron intake, malabsorption, blood loss, or an increased requirement, as with pregnancy. When severe, it results in a characteristic microcytic, hypochromic anemia. In addition to its role in hemoglobin, iron is an essential component of myoglobin, heme enzymes (e.g., cytochromes, catalase, and peroxidase), and the metalloflavoprotein enzymes (e.g., xanthine oxidase and α-glycerophosphate oxidase). Iron deficiency can affect metabolism in muscle independently of the effect of anemia on O_2 delivery. This may reflect a reduction in the activity of iron-dependent mitochondrial enzymes. Iron deficiency also has been associated with behavioral and learning problems in children, abnormalities in catecholamine metabolism, and possibly impaired heat production.

Metabolism of Iron

The body store of iron is divided between essential iron-containing compounds and excess iron, which is held in storage (Table 41–2). *Hemoglobin* dominates the essential fraction. Each hemoglobin molecule contains four atoms of iron, amounting to 1.1 mg (20 μmol) of iron/mL of red blood cells. Other forms of essential iron include *myoglobin* and a variety of heme and nonheme iron-dependent enzymes. *Ferritin* is a protein-iron storage complex that exists as individual molecules or as aggregates. *Apoferritin* (MW ~ 450 kDa) is composed of 24 polypeptide subunits that form an outer shell around a storage cavity for polynuclear hydrous ferric oxide phosphate. More than 30% of the weight of ferritin may be iron (4000 atoms of iron per ferritin molecule). Ferritin aggregates, referred to as *hemosiderin* and visible by light microscopy, constitute about one-third of normal stores. The two predominant sites of iron storage are the reticuloendothelial system and the hepatocytes.

Internal exchange of iron is accomplished by the plasma protein *transferrin*, a 76-kDa glycoprotein that has two binding sites for ferric iron. Iron is delivered from transferrin to intracellular sites by means of specific transferrin receptors in the plasma membrane. The iron-transferrin complex binds to the receptor, and the ternary complex is internalized through clathrin-coated pits by receptor-mediated endocytosis. A proton-pumping ATPase lowers the pH of the intracellular vesicular compartment (the endosomes) to about 5.5. Iron subsequently dissociates, and the receptor returns the apotransferrin to the cell surface, where it is released into the extracellular environment. Cells regulate their expression of transferrin receptors and intracellular ferritin in response to the iron supply (De Domenico et al., 2008). The synthesis of apoferritin and transferrin receptors is regulated posttranscriptionally by two iron-regulating proteins, IRP1 and IRP2. These IRPs are cytosolic RNA-binding proteins that bind to iron-regulating elements (IREs) present in the 5′ or 3′ untranslated regions of mRNA encoding apoferritin or the transferrin receptors, respectively. Binding of these IRPs to the 5′ IRE of apoferritin mRNA represses translation, whereas binding to the 3′ IRE of mRNA encoding the transferrin receptors enhances transcript stability, thereby increasing protein production.

The flow of iron through the plasma amounts to a total of 30–40 mg/d in the adult (~0.46 mg/kg of body weight). The major internal circulation of iron involves the erythron and reticuloendothelial cells (Figure 41–3). About 80% of the iron in plasma goes to the erythroid marrow to be packaged into new erythrocytes; these normally circulate for about 120 days before being catabolized by the reticuloendothelial system. At that time, a portion of the iron is immediately returned to the plasma bound to transferrin, while another portion is incorporated into the ferritin stores of reticuloendothelial cells and returned to the circulation more gradually. With abnormalities in erythrocyte maturation, the predominant portion of iron assimilated by the erythroid marrow may be rapidly localized in the reticuloendothelial cells as defective red cell precursors are broken down; this is termed *ineffective erythropoiesis*. The rate of iron turnover in plasma may be reduced by half or more with red cell aplasia, with all the iron directed to the hepatocytes for storage.

The human body conserves its iron stores to a remarkable degree. Only 10% of the total is lost per year by normal men (i.e., ~ 1 mg/d). Two-thirds of this iron is excreted from the GI tract as extravasated red cells, iron in bile, and iron in exfoliated mucosal cells. The other third is accounted for by small amounts of iron in desquamated skin and in the urine. Additional losses of iron occur in women due to menstruation. Although the average loss in menstruating women is about 0.5 mg per day, 10% of menstruating

TABLE 41–2 ■ THE BODY CONTENT OF IRON		
	BODY WEIGHT, mg/kg	
	MALE	**FEMALE**
Essential iron		
Hemoglobin	31	28
Myoglobin and enzymes	6	5
Storage iron	13	4
Total	50	37

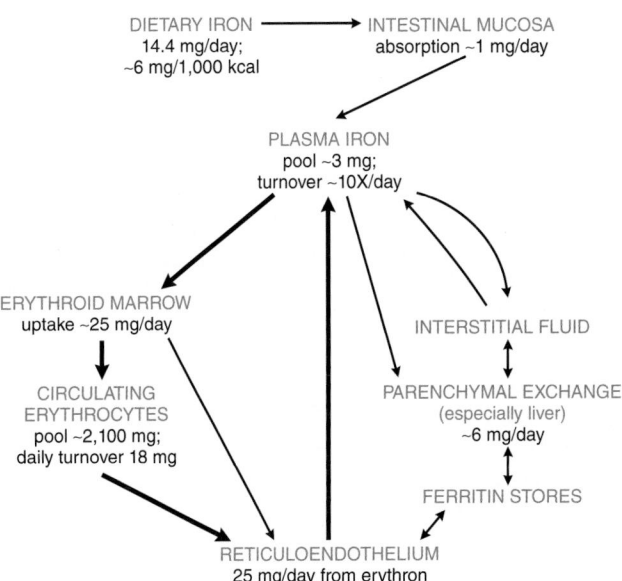

Figure 41–3 *Iron metabolism in humans (excretion omitted).*

TABLE 41–3 ■ IRON REQUIREMENTS FOR PREGNANCY

	AVERAGE (mg)	RANGE (mg)
External iron loss	170	150–200
Expansion of red cell mass	450	200–600
Fetal iron	270	200–370
Iron in placenta and cord	90	30–170
Blood loss at delivery	150	90–310
Total requirement[a]	980	580–1340
Cost of pregnancy[b]	680	440–1050

[a]Blood loss at delivery not included.

[b]Iron lost by the mother; expansion of red cell mass not included.

Source: Council on Foods and Nutrition. Iron deficiency in the United States. *JAMA*, **1968**, *203*:407–412. Used with permission. Copyright © 1968 American Medical Association. All rights reserved.

women lose more than 2 mg per day. Pregnancy and lactation impose an even greater requirement for iron (Table 41–3). Other causes of iron loss include blood donation, the use of anti-inflammatory drugs that cause bleeding from the gastric mucosa, and GI disease with associated bleeding.

The limited physiological losses of iron point to the primary importance of absorption in determining the body's iron content (Garrick and Garrick, 2009). After acidification and partial digestion of food in the stomach, iron is presented to the intestinal mucosa as either inorganic iron or heme iron. A ferrireductase, duodenal cytochrome B, located on the luminal surface of absorptive cells of the duodenum and upper small intestine, reduces the iron to the ferrous state, which is the substrate for divalent metal (ion) transporter 1 (DMT1, SLC11A2). DMT1 transports the iron to the basolateral membrane, where it is taken up by another transporter, *ferroportin* (Fpn; SLC40A1), and subsequently reoxidized to Fe^{3+}, primarily by *hephaestin* (Hp; *HEPH*), a transmembrane copper-dependent ferroxidase. Apotransferrin binds the resultant oxidized Fe^{3+}. The hepatic protein, hepcidin, binds to ferroportin, inducing its internalization and degradation, thus limiting the amount of iron released into the blood (Camaschella, 2013). Conditions that enhance the levels of hepcidin, such as inflammation, can result in decreased gut iron absorption, reduced serum iron, and inadequate iron available for developing red blood cells. Conversely, when hepcidin levels are low, such as in hemochromatosis, iron overload occurs due to excessive ferroportin-mediated iron influx.

Genetic polymorphism and consequent dysfunction in hepcidin or in proteins regulating its expression can result in inadequate levels of hepcidin and cause hereditary hemochromatosis (Pietrangelo, 2016). This can be due to polymorphism in *HFE*, resulting in a Cys→Tyr change at position 282 (C282Y) in the HFE protein, or pathogenic mutations in

hepcidin (*HAMP*), ferroportin (*FPN*), hemojuvelin (*HJV*), or transferrin receptor 2 (*TfR2*). The phenotype may vary, ranging from severe, as in *HJV–* or *HAMP*-juvenile-onset hemochromatosis, to relatively milder forms of adult-onset hemochromatosis, resulting from defects in *FPN* or *TfR2*. Acquired hemochromatosis can result from excessive amounts of parenteral iron, such as may occur in multiple transfusions for hereditary anemia or acquired aplastic anemia, from loss of hepcidin-producing liver mass, or with disease factors such as hepatitis C or chronic alcoholism that impair the production of hepcidin.

Iron Requirements; Availability of Dietary Iron

Adult men must absorb only 13 µg of iron/kg of body weight/d (~1 mg/d), whereas menstruating women require about 21 µg/kg (~1.4 mg) per day. In the last two trimesters of pregnancy, requirements increase to about 80 µg/kg (5–6 mg) per day; infants have similar requirements due to their rapid growth (Table 41–4).

The difference between dietary supply and requirements is reflected in the size of iron stores, which are low or absent when iron balance is precarious and high when iron balance is favorable. In infants after the third month of life and in pregnant women after the first trimester, stores of iron are negligible. Menstruating women have approximately one-third the stored iron found in adult men (see Table 41–2).

Although the iron content of the diet obviously is important, of greater nutritional significance is the bioavailability of iron in food. Heme iron, which constitutes only 6% of dietary iron, is far more available and is absorbed independent of the diet composition; it therefore represents 30% of iron absorbed (Conrad and Umbreit, 2000). The nonheme fraction represents the larger amount of dietary iron ingested by the economically underprivileged. In a vegetarian diet, nonheme iron is absorbed poorly because of the inhibitory action of a variety of dietary components, particularly phosphates. Ascorbic acid and meat facilitate the absorption of nonheme iron. In developed countries, the normal adult diet contains about 6 mg of iron per 1000 calories, providing an average daily intake for adult men of between 12 and 20 mg and for adult women of between 8 and 15 mg. Foods high in iron (>5 mg/100 g) include organ meats such as liver and heart, brewer's yeast, wheat germ, egg yolks, oysters, and certain dried beans and fruits; foods low in iron (<1 mg/100 g) include milk and milk products and most nongreen vegetables. Iron also may be added from cooking in iron pots. In assessing dietary iron intake, it is important to consider not only the amount of iron ingested but also its bioavailability.

Iron Deficiency

The prevalence of iron deficiency anemia in the U.S. is on the order of 1%–4% and depends on the economic status of the population (McLean et al., 2009). In developing countries, up to 20%–40% of infants and pregnant women may be affected. Better iron balance has resulted from the practice of fortifying flour, the use of iron-fortified formulas

TABLE 41–4 ■ DAILY IRON ABSORPTION REQUIREMENT

SUBJECT	IRON REQUIREMENT (µg/kg)	AVAILABLE IRON POOR DIET–GOOD DIET (µg/kg)	SAFETY FACTOR: AVAILABLE/REQUIREMENT
Infant	67	33–66	0.5–1
Child	22	48–96	2–4
Adolescent (male)	21	30–60	1.5–3
Adolescent (female)	20	30–60	1.5–3
Adult (male)	13	26–52	2–4
Adult (female)	21	18–36	1–2
Mid-to-late pregnancy	80	18–36	0.22–0.45

The numbers in columns 2 and 3 refer to iron absorption via the GI tract in micrograms per kilogram body weight. As noted in Figure 41–3, of 14.4 mg of dietary iron presented to the GI tract each day, only about 1 mg is absorbed. See text concerning factors influencing iron absorption and differential absorption of heme versus nonheme iron.

for infants, and the prescription of medicinal iron supplements during pregnancy.

Iron deficiency anemia results from dietary intake of iron that is inadequate to meet normal requirements (nutritional iron deficiency), blood loss, or interference with iron absorption (Camaschella, 2015). More severe iron deficiency is usually the result of blood loss, either from the GI tract or, in women, from the uterus. Finally, treatment of patients with erythropoietin can result in a functional iron deficiency. Iron deficiency in infants and young children can lead to behavioral disturbances and can impair development, which may not be fully reversible. Iron deficiency in children also can lead to an increased risk of lead toxicity secondary to pica and an increased absorption of heavy metals. Premature and low-birthweight infants are at greatest risk for developing iron deficiency, especially if they are not breast fed or do not receive iron-fortified formula (Finch, 2015). After the age of 2–3 years, the requirement for iron declines until adolescence, when rapid growth combined with irregular dietary habits again increase the risk of iron deficiency. Adolescent girls are at greatest risk; the dietary iron intake of most girls ages 11–18 is insufficient to meet their requirements.

Treatment of Iron Deficiency

General Therapeutic Principles

The response of iron deficiency anemia to iron therapy is influenced by several factors, including the severity of anemia, the ability of the patient to tolerate and absorb medicinal iron, and the presence of other complicating illnesses. Therapeutic effectiveness is best measured by the resulting increase in the rate of production of red cells. The magnitude of the marrow response to iron therapy is proportional to the severity of the anemia (level of erythropoietin stimulation) and the amount of iron delivered to marrow precursors.

The patient's ability to tolerate and absorb medicinal iron is a key factor in determining the rate of response to therapy. The small intestine regulates absorption and, with increasing doses of oral iron, limits the entry of iron into the bloodstream. This provides a natural ceiling on how much iron can be supplied by oral therapy. In the patient with moderately severe iron deficiency anemia, tolerable doses of oral iron will deliver, at most, 40–60 mg of iron per day to the erythroid marrow. This is an amount sufficient for production rates of two to three times normal.

Clinically, the effectiveness of iron therapy is best evaluated by tracking the reticulocyte response and the rise in the hemoglobin or the hematocrit. An increase in the reticulocyte count is not observed for at least 4–7 days after beginning therapy. A measurable increase in the hemoglobin level takes even longer. A decision regarding the effectiveness of treatment should not be made for 3–4 weeks after the start of treatment. An increase of 20 g/L or more in the concentration of hemoglobin by that time should be considered a positive response, assuming that no other change in the patient's clinical status can account for the improvement and that the patient has not been transfused.

If the response to oral iron is inadequate, the diagnosis must be reconsidered. A full laboratory evaluation should be conducted, and poor compliance by the patient or the presence of a concurrent inflammatory disease must be explored. A source of continued bleeding obviously should be sought. If no other explanation can be found, an evaluation of the patient's ability to absorb oral iron should be considered. There is no justification for merely continuing oral iron therapy beyond 3–4 weeks if a favorable response has not occurred.

Once a response to oral iron is demonstrated, therapy should be continued until the hemoglobin returns to normal. Treatment may be extended if it is desirable to replenish iron stores. This may require a considerable period of time because the rate of absorption of iron by the intestine will decrease markedly as iron stores are reconstituted. The prophylactic use of oral iron should be reserved for patients at high risk, including pregnant women, women with excessive menstrual blood loss, and infants. Iron supplements also may be of value for rapidly growing infants who are consuming substandard diets and for adults with a recognized cause of chronic blood loss. Except for infants, in whom the use of supplemented

formulas is routine, the use of over-the-counter mixtures of vitamins and minerals to prevent iron deficiency should be discouraged.

Therapy With Oral Iron

Orally administered ferrous sulfate is the treatment of choice for iron deficiency. Ferrous salts are absorbed about three times as well as ferric salts. Variations in the particular ferrous salt have relatively little effect on bioavailability; the sulfate, fumarate, succinate, gluconate, aspartate, other ferrous salts, and polysaccharide-ferrihydrite complex are absorbed to approximately the same extent. The effective dose of all of these preparations is based on iron content.

Other iron compounds have utility in fortification of foods. Reduced iron (metallic iron, elemental iron) is as effective as ferrous sulfate, provided that the material employed has a small particle size. Large-particle ferrum reductum and iron phosphate salts have much lower bioavailability. Ferric edetate has been shown to have good bioavailability and to have advantages for maintenance of the normal appearance and taste of food. The amount of iron in iron tablets is important. It also is essential that the coating of the tablet dissolve rapidly in the stomach. Delayed-release preparations are available, but absorption from such preparations varies. Ascorbic acid (≥200 mg) increases the absorption of medicinal iron by at least 30%. However, the increased uptake is associated with an increase in the incidence of side effects. Preparations that contain other compounds with therapeutic action, such as vitamin B_{12}, folate, or cobalt, are not recommended because the patient's response to the combination cannot easily be interpreted.

The average dose for the treatment of iron deficiency anemia is about 200 mg of iron per day (2–3 mg/kg), given in three equal doses of 65 mg. Children weighing 15–30 kg can take half the average adult dose; small children and infants can tolerate relatively large doses of iron (e.g., 5 mg/kg). When the object is the prevention of iron deficiency in pregnant women, for example, doses of 15 to 30 mg of iron per day are adequate. Bioavailability of iron is reduced with food and by concurrent antacids. For a rapid response or to counteract continued bleeding, as much as 120 mg of iron may be administered four times a day.

The duration of treatment is governed by the rate of recovery of hemoglobin (Table 41–5) and the desire to create iron stores. The former depends on the severity of the anemia. With a daily rate of repair of 2 g of hemoglobin per liter of whole blood, the red cell mass usually is reconstituted within 1–2 months. Thus, an individual with a hemoglobin of 50 g per liter may achieve a normal complement of 150 g/L in about 50 days, whereas an individual with a hemoglobin of 100 g/L may take only half that time. The creation of stores of iron requires many months of oral iron administration. The rate of absorption decreases rapidly after recovery from anemia, and after 3–4 months of treatment, stores may increase at a rate of not much more than 100 mg/month. Much of the strategy of continued therapy depends on the estimated future iron balance. Patients with an inadequate diet may require continued therapy with low doses of iron. If the bleeding has stopped, no further therapy is required after the hemoglobin has returned to normal. With continued bleeding, long-term, high-dose therapy clearly is indicated.

Untoward Effects of Oral Preparations of Iron. Side effects of oral iron preparations include heartburn, nausea, upper gastric discomfort, and diarrhea or constipation. A good policy is to initiate

TABLE 41–5 ■ AVERAGE RESPONSE TO ORAL IRON

TOTAL DOSE OF IRON (mg/d)	ESTIMATED ABSORPTION		INCREASE IN BLOOD HEMOGLOBIN (g/L/d)
	%	mg	
35	40	14	0.7
105	24	25	1.4
195	18	35	1.9
390	12	45	2.2

therapy at a small dosage and then gradually to increase the dosage to that desired. Only individuals with underlying disorders that augment the absorption of iron run the hazard of developing iron overload (hemochromatosis).

Iron Poisoning. Large amounts of ferrous salts are toxic, but fatalities are rare in adults. Most deaths occur in children, particularly between the ages of 12 and 24 months. As little as 1–2 g of iron may cause death, but 2–10 g usually is ingested in fatal cases. All iron preparations should be kept in childproof bottles. Signs and symptoms of severe poisoning may occur within 30 min after ingestion or may be delayed for several hours. They include abdominal pain, diarrhea, or vomiting of brown or bloody stomach contents containing pills. Of particular concern are pallor or cyanosis, lassitude, drowsiness, hyperventilation due to acidosis, and cardiovascular collapse. If death does not occur within 6 h, there may be a transient period of apparent recovery, followed by death in 12–24 h. The corrosive injury to the stomach may result in pyloric stenosis or gastric scarring.

In the evaluation of a child thought to have ingested iron, a color test for iron in the gastric contents and determination of the concentration of iron in plasma can be performed. If the latter is less than 63 μmol (3.5 mg/L), the child is not in immediate danger. However, vomiting should be induced when there is iron in the stomach, and an X-ray should be taken to evaluate the number of pills remaining in the small bowel (iron tablets are radiopaque). When the plasma concentration of iron is greater than the total iron-binding capacity (63 μmol; 3.5 mg/L), *deferoxamine* should be administered (see Chapter 71). The speed of diagnosis and therapy is important. With early treatment, the mortality from iron poisoning can be reduced from 45% to about 1%. *Deferiprone* and *deferasirox* are oral iron chelators approved by the FDA for treatment of patients with thalassemia who have iron overload.

Therapy With Parenteral Iron

When oral iron therapy fails, parenteral iron administration may be an effective alternative. Common indications are iron malabsorption (e.g., sprue, short-bowel syndrome), severe oral iron intolerance, as a routine supplement to total parenteral nutrition, and in patients who are receiving erythropoietin. Parenteral iron can be given to iron-deficient patients and pregnant women to create iron stores, something that would take months to achieve by the oral route. The indications for parenteral iron therapy include documented iron deficiency and intolerance or irresponsiveness to oral iron.

The rate of hemoglobin response is determined by the balance between the severity of the anemia (the level of erythropoietin stimulus) and the delivery of iron to the marrow from iron absorption and iron stores. When a large intravenous dose of iron dextran is given to a severely anemic patient, the hematologic response can exceed that seen with oral iron for 1–3 weeks. Subsequently, however, the response is no better than that seen with oral iron.

Parenteral iron therapy should be used only when clearly indicated because acute hypersensitivity, including anaphylactic and anaphylactoid reactions, can occur. Other reactions to intravenous iron include headache, malaise, fever, generalized lymphadenopathy, arthralgias, urticaria, and, in some patients with rheumatoid arthritis, exacerbation of the disease.

Several iron formulations are available in the U.S. (Larson and Coyne, 2014). These include iron dextran, sodium ferric gluconate, ferumoxytol, iron sucrose, and ferric carboxymaltose. Ferumoxytol is a semisynthetic carbohydrate-coated superparamagnetic iron oxide nanoparticle approved for treatment of iron deficiency anemia in patients with chronic kidney disease; the ferumoxytol has to be administered safely as a 1.02-g infusion over a relatively short infusion time of 15 min (Auerbach et al., 2013). Indications for ferric gluconate and iron sucrose are limited to patients with chronic kidney disease and documented iron deficiency, although broader applications are being advocated (Larson and Coyne, 2014).

Iron Dextran. Iron dextran injection is a colloidal solution of ferric oxyhydroxide complexed with polymerized dextran (molecular weight ~ 180,000 Da) that contains 50 mg/mL of elemental iron. The use of

low-molecular-weight iron dextran has reduced the incidence of toxicity relative to that observed with high-molecular-weight preparations. Iron dextran can be administered by intravenous (preferred) or intramuscular injection. Injection of a therapeutic dose should be initiated only after a test dose of 0.5 mL (25 mg of iron). Given intravenously in a dose less than 500 mg, the iron dextran complex is cleared with a plasma $t_{1/2}$ of 6 h. When 1 g or more is administered intravenously as total-dose therapy, reticuloendothelial cell clearance is constant at 10–20 mg/h.

Intramuscular injection of iron dextran should be initiated only after a test dose of 0.5 mL (25 mg of iron). If no adverse reactions are observed, the injections can proceed. The daily dose ordinarily should not exceed 0.5 mL (25 mg of iron) for infants weighing less than 4.5 kg, 1 mL (50 mg of iron) for children weighing less than 9 kg, and 2 mL (100 mg of iron) for other patients. However, local reactions and the concern about malignant change at the site of injection make intramuscular administration inappropriate except when the intravenous route is inaccessible. The patient should be observed for signs of immediate anaphylaxis and for an hour after injection for any signs of vascular instability or hypersensitivity, including respiratory distress, hypotension, tachycardia, or back or chest pain. Delayed hypersensitivity reactions also are observed, especially in patients with rheumatoid arthritis or a history of allergies. Fever, malaise, lymphadenopathy, arthralgias, and urticaria can develop days or weeks following injection and last for prolonged periods of time. Use iron dextran with extreme caution in patients with rheumatoid arthritis or other connective tissue diseases and during the acute phase of an inflammatory illness. Once hypersensitivity is documented, iron dextran therapy must be abandoned.

With multiple total-dose infusions such as those sometimes used in the treatment of chronic GI blood loss, accumulations of slowly metabolized iron dextran stores in reticuloendothelial cells can be impressive. The plasma ferritin level also can rise to levels associated with iron overload. It seems prudent, however, to withhold the drug whenever the plasma ferritin rises above 800 μg/L.

Sodium Ferric Gluconate. Sodium ferric gluconate is an intravenous iron preparation with a molecular size of about 295 kDa and an osmolality of 990 mOsm/kg^{-1}. Administration of ferric gluconate at doses ranging from 62.5 to 125 mg during hemodialysis is associated with transferrin saturation exceeding 100%. Unlike iron dextran, which requires processing by macrophages that may require several weeks, about 80% of sodium ferric gluconate is delivered to transferrin within 24 h. Sodium ferric gluconate also has a lower risk of inducing serious anaphylactic reactions than iron dextran (Sengolge et al., 2005).

Iron Sucrose. Iron sucrose is a complex of polynuclear iron (III)–hydroxide in sucrose (Beguin and Jaspers, 2014). Following intravenous injection, the complex is taken up by the reticuloendothelial system, where it dissociates into iron and sucrose. Iron sucrose is generally administered in daily amounts of 100–200 mg within a 14-day period to a total cumulative dose of 1000 mg. Like sodium ferric gluconate, iron sucrose appears to be better tolerated and to cause fewer adverse events than iron dextran (Hayat, 2008). This agent is FDA-approved for the treatment of iron deficiency in patients with chronic kidney disease. Chronic use has the potential to cause renal tubulointerstitial damage (Agarwal, 2006).

Ferric Carboxymaltose. Ferric carboxymaltose is an iron complex consisting of a ferric hydroxide core and a carbohydrate shell (Keating, 2015). With this preparation, a replenishment dose of up to 1000 mg of iron can be administered in 15 min. Intravenous administration results in transient elevations in serum iron, serum ferritin, and transferrin saturation, with subsequent correction in hemoglobin levels and replenishment of depleted iron stores. Ferric carboxymaltose is rapidly cleared from the circulation, becoming distributed (~80%) in the marrow, as well as the liver and spleen. Common reported drug-related adverse effects include headache, dizziness, nausea, abdominal pain, constipation, diarrhea, rash, and injection site reactions. However, the incidence of drug-related adverse events appears similar to those of patients treated with oral ferrous sulfate.

Ferric carboxymaltose is FDA-approved for therapy of iron deficiency anemia.

Copper , Pyridoxine, and Riboflavin

Copper

Copper has redox properties similar to those of iron, which simultaneously are essential and potentially toxic to the cell. Cells have virtually no free copper. Instead, copper is stored by metallothioneins and distributed by specialized chaperones to sites that make use of its redox properties. Transfer of copper to nascent cuproenzymes is performed by individual or collective activities of P-type ATPases, ATP7A and ATP7B, which are expressed in all tissues (Nevitt et al., 2012). In mammals, the liver is the organ most responsible for the storage, distribution, and excretion of copper. Mutations in ATP7A or ATP7B that interfere with this function have been found responsible for Wilson disease or Menkes syndrome (steely hair syndrome) (de Bie et al., 2007), respectively, which can result in life-threatening hepatic failure.

Copper deficiency is extremely rare; the amount present in food is more than adequate to provide the needed body complement of slightly more than 100 mg. Even in clinical states associated with hypocupremia (sprue, celiac disease, and nephrotic syndrome), effects of copper deficiency usually are not demonstrable. Anemia due to copper deficiency has been described in individuals who have undergone intestinal bypass surgery, in those who are receiving parenteral nutrition, in malnourished infants, and in patients ingesting excessive amounts of zinc (Willis et al., 2005). Copper deficiency interferes with the absorption of iron and its release from reticuloendothelial cells. In humans, the prominent findings have been leukopenia, particularly granulocytopenia, and anemia. Concentrations of iron in plasma are variable, and the anemia is not always microcytic. When a low plasma copper concentration is determined in the presence of leukopenia and anemia, a therapeutic trial with copper is appropriate. Daily doses up to 0.1 mg/kg of cupric sulfate have been given by mouth, or 1–2 mg per day may be added to the solution of nutrients for parenteral administration.

Pyridoxine

Patients with either hereditary or acquired sideroblastic anemia characteristically have impaired hemoglobin synthesis and accumulate iron in the perinuclear mitochondria of erythroid precursor cells, so-called ringed sideroblasts. Hereditary sideroblastic anemia is an X-linked recessive trait with variable penetrance and expression that results from mutations in the erythrocyte form of δ-aminolevulinate synthase.

Oral therapy with pyridoxine is of proven benefit in correcting the sideroblastic anemias associated with the antituberculosis drugs isoniazid and pyrazinamide, which act as vitamin B_6 antagonists. A daily dose of 50 mg of pyridoxine completely corrects the defect without interfering with treatment, and routine supplementation of pyridoxine often is recommended (see Chapter 56). In contrast, if pyridoxine is given to counteract the sideroblastic abnormality associated with administration of levodopa, the effectiveness of levodopa in controlling Parkinson disease is decreased. Pyridoxine therapy does not correct the sideroblastic abnormalities produced by chloramphenicol or lead. Patients with idiopathic acquired sideroblastic anemia generally fail to respond to oral pyridoxine, and those individuals who appear to have a pyridoxine-responsive anemia require prolonged therapy with large doses of the vitamin, 50–500 mg/d. The occasional patient who is refractory to oral pyridoxine may respond to parenteral administration of pyridoxal phosphate. However, oral pyridoxine in doses of 200–300 mg per day produces intracellular concentrations of pyridoxal phosphate equal to or greater than those generated by therapy with the phosphorylated vitamin.

Riboflavin

The spontaneous appearance in humans of red cell aplasia due to riboflavin deficiency undoubtedly is rare, if it occurs at all. Riboflavin deficiency has been described in combination with infection and protein deficiency, both of which are capable of producing hypoproliferative anemia. However, it seems reasonable to include riboflavin in the nutritional management of patients with gross, generalized malnutrition.

Vitamin B_{12}, Folic Acid, and the Treatment of Megaloblastic Anemias

Vitamin B_{12} and folic acid are dietary essentials. A deficiency of either vitamin impairs DNA synthesis in any cell in which chromosomal replication and division are taking place. Because tissues with the greatest rate of cell turnover show the most dramatic changes, the hematopoietic system is especially sensitive to deficiencies of these vitamins.

Cellular Roles of Vitamin B_{12} and Folic Acid

The major roles of vitamin B_{12} and folic acid in intracellular metabolism are summarized in Figure 41–4. Intracellular vitamin B_{12} is maintained as two active coenzymes: *methylcobalamin* and *deoxyadenosylcobalamin*.

Methylcobalamin (CH_3B_{12}) supports the *methionine synthetase* reaction, which is essential for normal metabolism of folate (Weissbach, 2008). Methyl groups contributed by methyltetrahydrofolate ($CH_3H_4PteGlu_1$) are used to form methylcobalamin, which then acts as a methyl group donor for the conversion of homocysteine to methionine. This folate-cobalamin interaction is pivotal for normal synthesis of purines and pyrimidines, and therefore of DNA. The methionine synthetase reaction is largely responsible for the control of the recycling of folate cofactors; the maintenance of intracellular concentrations of folylpolyglutamates; and, through the synthesis of methionine and its product *SAM*, the maintenance of a number of methylation reactions.

Deoxyadenosylcobalamin (deoxyadenosyl B_{12}) is a cofactor for the *mitochondrial mutase* enzyme that catalyzes the isomerization of l-methylmalonyl CoA to succinyl CoA, an important reaction in

HISTORY

The discovery of vitamin B_{12} and folic acid is a dramatic story that began almost 200 years ago and includes two Nobel Prize–winning discoveries. Beginning in 1824, Combe and Addison wrote a series of case reports describing what must have been megaloblastic anemias (still known as Addisonian pernicious anemia). Austin Flint in 1860 first described a severe gastric atrophy and called attention to its possible relationship to the anemia. After Whipple's observation in 1925 that liver is a source of a potent hematopoietic substance for iron-deficient dogs, Minot and Murphy carried out Nobel Prize–winning experiments that demonstrated the effectiveness of the feeding of liver to reverse pernicious anemia. Soon thereafter, Castle defined the need for both intrinsic factor, a substance secreted by the parietal cells of the gastric mucosa, and extrinsic factor, the vitamin-like material provided by crude liver extracts. Nearly 20 years passed before Rickes and coworkers and Smith and Parker isolated and crystallized vitamin B_{12}; Dorothy Hodgkin received the Nobel Prize for determining its X-ray crystal structure.

As attempts were being made to purify extrinsic factor, Wills and her associates described a macrocytic anemia in women in India that responded to a factor present in crude liver extracts but not in the purified fractions known to be effective in pernicious anemia. This factor, first called Wills' factor and later vitamin M, is now known to be folic acid. The term *folic acid* was coined by Mitchell and coworkers in 1941, after its isolation from leafy vegetables. From more recent work, we know that neither vitamin B_{12} nor folic acid as purified from foodstuffs is the active coenzyme in humans. During extraction, active labile forms are converted to stable congeners of vitamin B_{12} and folic acid, cyanocobalamin and PteGlu, respectively. These congeners must be modified in vivo to be effective. Despite our knowledge of the intracellular metabolic pathways in which these vitamins function as required cofactors, many questions remain, among them, What is the relationship of vitamin B_{12} deficiency to the neurological abnormalities that occur in megaloblastic anemia?

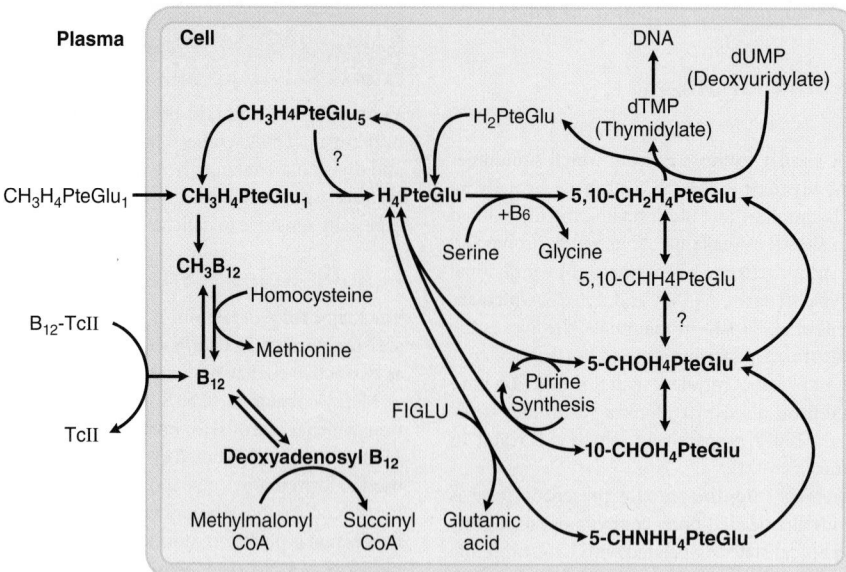

Figure 41–4 *Interrelationships and metabolic roles of vitamin B$_{12}$ and folic acid.* See text for explanation and Figure 41–5 for structures of the various folate coenzymes. FIGLU, formiminoglutamic acid, which arises from the catabolism of histidine; TcII, transcobalamin II.

carbohydrate and lipid metabolism. This reaction has no direct relationship to the metabolic pathways that involve folate.

Because methyltetrahydrofolate is the principal folate congener supplied to cells, the transfer of the methyl group to cobalamin is essential for the adequate supply of tetrahydrofolate (H$_4$PteGlu$_1$). Tetrahydrofolate is a precursor for the formation of intracellular folylpolyglutamates; it also acts as the acceptor of a one-carbon unit in the conversion of serine to glycine, with the resultant formation of 5,10-methylenetetrahydrofolate (5,10-CH$_2$H$_4$PteGlu). The last derivative donates the methylene group to dUMP for the synthesis of dTMP—an extremely important reaction in DNA synthesis. In the process, the 5,10-CH$_2$H$_4$PteGlu is converted to dihydrofolate (H$_2$PteGlu). The cycle then is completed by the reduction of the H$_2$PteGlu to H$_4$PteGlu by dihydrofolate reductase, the step that is blocked by folate antagonists such as methotrexate (see Chapter 66). As shown in Figure 41–4, other pathways also lead to the synthesis of 5,10-methylenetetrahydrofolate. These pathways are important in the metabolism of FIGLU and purines and pyrimidines.

Deficiency of either vitamin B$_{12}$ or folate decreases the synthesis of methionine and SAM and consequently interferes with protein biosynthesis, a number of methylation reactions, and the synthesis of polyamines. In addition, the cell responds to the deficiency by redirecting folate metabolic pathways to supply increasing amounts of methyltetrahydrofolate; this tends to preserve essential methylation reactions at the expense of nucleic acid synthesis. With vitamin B$_{12}$ deficiency, methylenetetrahydrofolate reductase activity increases, directing available intracellular folates into the methyltetrahydrofolate pool (not shown in Figure 41–4). The methyltetrahydrofolate then is trapped by the lack of sufficient vitamin B$_{12}$ to accept and transfer methyl groups, and subsequent steps in folate metabolism that require tetrahydrofolate are deprived of substrate. This process provides a common basis for the development of megaloblastic anemia with deficiency of either vitamin B$_{12}$ or folic acid.

The mechanisms responsible for the neurological lesions of vitamin B$_{12}$ deficiency are less well understood (Solomon, 2007). Damage to the myelin sheath is the most obvious lesion in this neuropathy. This observation led to the early suggestion that the deoxyadenosyl B$_{12}$–dependent methylmalonyl CoA mutase reaction, a step in propionate metabolism, is related to the abnormality. However, other evidence suggests that the deficiency of methionine synthetase and the block of the conversion of methionine to SAM are more likely to be responsible.

Vitamin B$_{12}$ and Human Health

Humans depend on exogenous sources of vitamin B$_{12}$ (see structure in Figure 41–5). In nature, the primary sources are certain microorganisms that grow in soil or the intestinal lumen of animals that synthesize the vitamin. The daily nutritional requirement of 3–5 μg must generally be obtained from animal by-products in the diet. However, some vitamin B$_{12}$ is available from legumes, which are contaminated with bacteria that can synthesize vitamin B$_{12}$, and vegetarians often fortify their diets with a wide range of vitamins and minerals; thus, strict vegetarians rarely develop vitamin B$_{12}$ deficiency. The terms *vitamin B$_{12}$* and *cyanocobalamin* are used interchangeably as generic terms for all of the cobamides active in humans. Preparations of vitamin B$_{12}$ for therapeutic use contain either cyanocobalamin or hydroxocobalamin because only these derivatives remain active after storage.

Metabolic Functions. The active coenzymes methylcobalamin and 5-deoxyadenosylcobalamin are essential for cell growth and replication. Methylcobalamin is required for the conversion of homocysteine to methionine and its derivative S-adenosylmethionine. In addition, when concentrations of vitamin B$_{12}$ are inadequate, folate becomes "trapped" as methyltetrahydrofolate to cause a functional deficiency of other required intracellular forms of folic acid. The hematologic abnormalities in vitamin B$_{12}$–deficient patients result from this process. Deoxyadenosylcobalamin is required for the rearrangement of methylmalonyl CoA to succinyl CoA.

ADME and Daily Requirements

In the presence of gastric acid and pancreatic proteases, dietary vitamin B$_{12}$ is released from food and salivary-binding protein and bound to gastric intrinsic factor. When the vitamin B$_{12}$–intrinsic factor complex reaches the ileum, it interacts with a receptor on the mucosal cell surface and is actively transported into circulation. Vitamin B$_{12}$ deficiency in adults is rarely the result of a deficient diet per se; rather, it usually reflects a defect in one or another aspect of this complex sequence of absorption (Figure 41–6). Antibodies to parietal cells or intrinsic factor complex also can play a prominent role in producing a deficiency. Several intestinal conditions can interfere with absorption, including pancreatic disorders (loss of pancreatic protease secretion), bacterial overgrowth, intestinal parasites, sprue, and localized damage to ileal mucosal cells by disease or as a result of surgery.

Absorbed vitamin B$_{12}$ binds to transcobalamin II, a plasma β globulin, for transport to tissues. The supply of vitamin B$_{12}$ available for tissues is

Figure 41–5 *The structures and nomenclature of vitamin B_{12} congeners.* The vitamin B_{12} molecule has three major portions: (1) a planar group porphyrin-like ring structure with four reduced pyrrole rings (A–D) linked to a central cobalt atom and extensively substituted with methyl, acetamide, and propionamide residues; (2) a 5,6-dimethylbenzimidazolyl nucleotide, which links almost at right angles to the planar nucleus with bonds to the cobalt atom and to the propionate side chain of the C pyrrole ring; and (3) a variable R group—the most important of which are found in the stable compounds cyanocobalamin and hydroxocobalamin and the active coenzymes methylcobalamin and 5-deoxyadenosylcobalamin.

Vitamin B_{12} Congeners	
Permissive Name	*R Group*
Cyanocobalamin (Vitamin B_{12})	–CN
Hydroxocobalamin	–OH
Methylcobalamin	–CH₃
5'-Deoxyadenosylcobalamin	–5'-Deoxyadenosyl

directly related to the size of the hepatic storage pool and the amount of vitamin B_{12} bound to transcobalamin II (see Figure 41–6). Vitamin B_{12} bound to transcobalamin II is rapidly cleared from plasma and preferentially distributed to hepatic parenchymal cells. As much as 90% of the body's stores of vitamin B_{12}, from 1 to 10 mg, is in the liver. Vitamin B_{12} is stored as the active coenzyme with a turnover rate of 0.5–8 µg per day. The recommended daily intake of the vitamin in adults is 2.4 µg. Approximately 3 µg of cobalamins are secreted into bile each day, 50%–60% of which is not destined for reabsorption. Interference with reabsorption by intestinal disease can progressively deplete hepatic stores of the vitamin.

Vitamin B_{12} Deficiency

The plasma concentration of vitamin B_{12} is the best routine measure of B_{12} deficiency and normally ranges from 150 to 660 pM (~200–900 pg/mL).

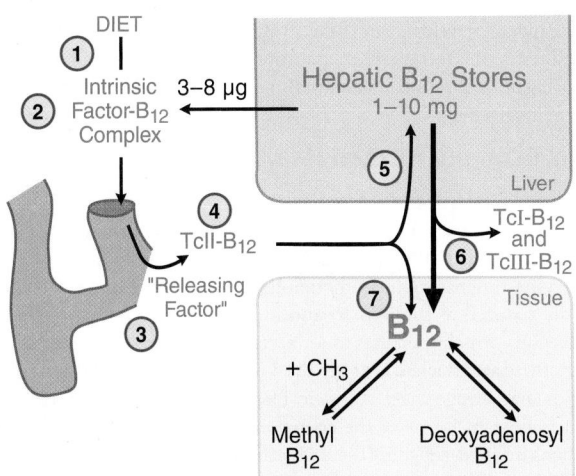

Figure 41–6 *Absorption and distribution of vitamin B_{12}.* Deficiency of vitamin B_{12} can result from a congenital or acquired defect in (1) inadequate dietary supply; (2) inadequate secretion of intrinsic factor (classical pernicious anemia); (3) ileal disease; (4) congenital absence of TcII; or (5) rapid depletion of hepatic stores by interference with reabsorption of vitamin B_{12} excreted in bile. The utility of measurements of the concentration of vitamin B_{12} in plasma to estimate supply available to tissues can be compromised by liver disease and (6) the appearance of abnormal amounts of TcI and TcIII in plasma. The formation of methylcobalamin requires (7) normal transport into cells and an adequate supply of folic acid as $CH_3H_4PteGlu_1$.

Deficiency should be suspected whenever the concentration falls below 150 pM. The correlation is excellent except when the plasma concentrations of transcobalamin I and III are increased, as occurs with hepatic disease or a myeloproliferative disorder. Inasmuch as the vitamin B_{12} bound to these transport proteins is relatively unavailable to cells, tissues can become deficient when the concentration of vitamin B_{12} in plasma is normal or even high. In subjects with congenital absence of transcobalamin II, megaloblastic anemia occurs despite relatively normal plasma concentrations of vitamin B_{12}; the anemia will respond to parenteral doses of vitamin B_{12} that exceed the renal clearance.

Vitamin B_{12} deficiency is recognized clinically by its impact on the hematopoietic and nervous systems. The sensitivity of the hematopoietic system relates to its high rate of cell turnover. Other tissues with high rates of cell turnover (e.g., mucosa and cervical epithelium) also have high requirements for the vitamin. As a result of an inadequate supply of vitamin B_{12}, DNA replication becomes highly abnormal. Once a hematopoietic stem cell is committed to enter a programmed series of cell divisions, the defect in chromosomal replication results in an inability of maturing cells to complete nuclear divisions while cytoplasmic maturation continues at a relatively normal rate. This results in the production of morphologically abnormal cells and death of cells during maturation, a phenomenon referred to as *ineffective hematopoiesis*. Severe deficiency affects all cell lines, and pronounced pancytopenia results.

The diagnosis of a vitamin B_{12} deficiency usually can be made using measurements of the serum vitamin B_{12} or serum methylmalonate (which is somewhat more sensitive and useful in identifying metabolic deficiency in patients with normal serum vitamin B_{12} levels). In managing a patient with severe megaloblastic anemia, a therapeutic trial using very small doses of the vitamin can be used to confirm the diagnosis. Serial measurements of the reticulocyte count, serum iron, and hematocrit are performed to define the characteristic recovery of normal red cell production. The *Schilling test* can be used to measure the absorption of the vitamin and delineate the mechanism of the disease. By performing the Schilling test with and without added intrinsic factor, it is possible to discriminate between intrinsic factor deficiency by itself and primary ileal cell disease. *Vitamin B_{12} deficiency can irreversibly damage the nervous system.* Because the neurological damage can be dissociated from the changes in the hematopoietic system, vitamin B_{12} deficiency must be considered in elderly patients with dementia or psychiatric disorders, even if they are not anemic (Spence, 2016).

Vitamin B_{12} Therapy

Vitamin B_{12} has an undeserved reputation as a health tonic and has been used for a number of disease states. A number of multivitamin preparations are marketed either as nutritional supplements or for the treatment of anemia; many are supplemented with intrinsic factor. Although the combination of oral vitamin B_{12} and intrinsic factor would appear to be ideal for patients with an intrinsic factor deficiency, such preparations are not reliable.

Vitamin B_{12} is available for injection or oral administration; combinations with other vitamins and minerals also can be given orally or parenterally. The choice of a preparation always depends on the cause of the deficiency. Oral administration cannot be relied on for effective therapy in the patient with a marked deficiency of vitamin B_{12} and abnormal hematopoiesis or neurological deficits. The treatment of choice for vitamin B_{12} deficiency is cyanocobalamin administered by intramuscular or subcutaneous injection, never intravenously. Cyanocobalamin is administered in doses of 1–1000 μg. Tissue uptake, storage, and utilization depend on the availability of transcobalamin II. Doses greater than 100 μg are cleared rapidly from plasma into the urine, and administration of larger amounts of vitamin B_{12} will not result in greater retention of the vitamin. Administration of 1000 μg is of value in the performance of the Schilling test. After isotopically labeled vitamin B_{12} is administered orally, the compound that is absorbed can be quantitatively recovered in the urine if 1000 μg of cyanocobalamin is administered intramuscularly. This unlabeled material saturates the transport system and tissue binding sites, so more than 90% of the labeled and unlabeled vitamin is excreted during the next 24 h.

Effective use of the vitamin B_{12} depends on accurate diagnosis and an understanding of the following general principles of therapy:

- Vitamin B_{12} should be given prophylactically only when there is a reasonable probability that a deficiency exists or will exist (i.e., dietary deficiency in the strict vegetarian, the predictable malabsorption of vitamin B_{12} in patients who have had a gastrectomy, and certain diseases of the small intestine) (Del Villar Madrigal et al., 2015). When GI function is normal, an oral prophylactic supplement of vitamins and minerals, including vitamin B_{12}, may be indicated. Otherwise, the patient should receive monthly injections of cyanocobalamin.
- The relative ease of treatment with vitamin B_{12} should not prevent a full investigation of the etiology of the deficiency. The initial diagnosis usually is suggested by macrocytic anemia or an unexplained neuropsychiatric disorder.
- Therapy always should be as specific as possible. Although a large number of multivitamin preparations are available, the use of shotgun vitamin therapy in the treatment of vitamin B_{12} deficiency can be dangerous: Sufficient folic acid may be given to result in a hematologic recovery that can mask continued vitamin B_{12} deficiency and permit neurological damage to develop or progress.
- Although a classical therapeutic trial with small amounts of vitamin B_{12} can help confirm the diagnosis, acutely ill elderly patients may not be able to tolerate the delay in the correction of a severe anemia. Such patients require supplemental blood transfusions and immediate therapy with folic acid and vitamin B_{12} to guarantee rapid recovery.
- Long-term therapy with vitamin B_{12} must be evaluated at intervals of 6–12 months in patients who are otherwise well. If there is an additional illness or a condition that may increase the requirement for the vitamin (e.g., pregnancy), reassessment should be performed more frequently.

Treatment of the Acutely Ill Patient. The therapeutic approach depends on the severity of the illness. In uncomplicated pernicious anemia, in which the abnormality is restricted to a mild or moderate anemia without leukopenia, thrombocytopenia, or neurological signs or symptoms, the administration of vitamin B_{12} alone will suffice. Moreover, therapy may be delayed until other causes of megaloblastic anemia have been excluded and sufficient studies of GI function have been performed to reveal the underlying cause of the disease. In this situation, a therapeutic trial with small amounts of parenteral vitamin B_{12} (1–10 μg per day) can confirm the presence of an uncomplicated vitamin B_{12} deficiency.

In contrast, patients with neurological changes or severe leukopenia or thrombocytopenia associated with infection or bleeding require emergency treatment. Effective therapy must not wait for detailed diagnostic tests. Once

the megaloblastic erythropoiesis has been confirmed and sufficient blood collected for later measurements of vitamin B_{12} and folic acid, the patient should receive intramuscular injections of 100 μg of cyanocobalamin and 1–5 mg of folic acid. For the next 1–2 weeks, the patient should receive daily intramuscular injections of 100 μg of cyanocobalamin, together with a daily oral supplement of 1 to 2 mg of folic acid. Because an effective increase in red cell mass will not occur for 10–20 days, the patient with a markedly depressed hematocrit and tissue hypoxia also should receive a transfusion of 2–3 units of packed red blood cells. If congestive heart failure is present, diuretics can be administered to prevent volume overload.

The first objective hematologic change is the disappearance of the megaloblastic morphology of the marrow. As the ineffective erythropoiesis is corrected, the concentration of iron in plasma falls dramatically as the metal is used in the formation of hemoglobin, usually within the first 48 h. Full correction of precursor maturation in marrow with production of an increased number of reticulocytes begins about the second or third day and peaks 3–5 days later. Patients with complicating iron deficiency, an infection or other inflammatory state, or renal disease may be unable to correct their anemia. Therefore, it is important to monitor the reticulocyte index over the first several weeks. If it does not continue at elevated levels while the hematocrit is below 35%, plasma concentrations of iron and folic acid should again be determined and the patient reevaluated for an illness that could inhibit the response of the marrow. The degree and rate of improvement of neurological signs and symptoms depend on the severity and the duration of the abnormalities. Those that have been present for only a few months usually disappear relatively rapidly. When a defect has been present for many months or years, full return to normal function may never occur.

Long-Term Therapy With Vitamin B_{12}. Once begun, vitamin B_{12} therapy must be maintained for life. This fact must be impressed on the patient and family, and a system must be established to guarantee continued monthly injections of cyanocobalamin.

Intramuscular injection of 100 μg of cyanocobalamin every 4 weeks is usually sufficient. Patients with severe neurological symptoms and signs may be treated with larger doses of vitamin B_{12} in the period immediately after the diagnosis. Doses of 100 μg per day or several times per week may be given for several months with the hope of encouraging faster and more complete recovery. It is important to monitor vitamin B_{12} concentrations in plasma and to obtain peripheral blood counts at intervals of 3–6 months to confirm the adequacy of therapy. Because refractoriness to therapy can develop at any time, evaluation must continue throughout the patient's life. Intranasal preparations are available for maintenance following normalization of vitamin B_{12}–deficient patients without nervous system involvement.

Folic Acid and Human Health

Biochemical Roles of Folate

Pteroylglutamic acid (Figure 41–7) is the common pharmaceutical form of folic acid. It is not the principal folate congener in food or the active coenzyme for intracellular metabolism. After absorption, PteGlu is rapidly reduced at the 5, 6, 7, and 8 positions to *tetrahydrofolic acid* (H_4PteGlu), which then acts as an acceptor of a number of one-carbon units. These are attached at either the 5 or the 10 position of the pteridine ring or may bridge these atoms to form a new five-member ring. The most important forms of the coenzyme that are synthesized by these reactions are listed in Figure 41–4, and each plays a specific role in intracellular metabolism:

- *Conversion of Homocysteine to Methionine.* This reaction requires CH_3H_4PteGlu as a methyl donor and uses vitamin B_{12} as a cofactor.
- *Conversion of Serine to Glycine.* This reaction requires tetrahydrofolate as an acceptor of a methylene group from serine and uses pyridoxal phosphate as a cofactor. It results in the formation of 5,10-CH_2H_4PteGlu, an essential coenzyme for the synthesis of dTMP.
- *Synthesis of Thymidylate.* 5,10-CH_2H_4PteGlu donates a methylene group and reducing equivalents to dUMP for the synthesis of dTMP—a rate-limiting step in DNA synthesis.

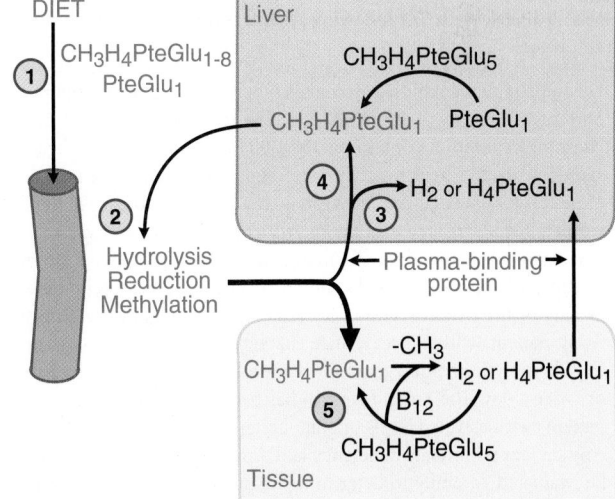

Position	Radical		Congener
N^5	—CH$_3$	CH$_3$H$_4$PteGlu	Methyltetrahydrofolate
N^5	—CHO	5-CHOH$_4$PteGlu	Folinic acid (citrovorum factor)
N^{10}	—CHO	10-CHOH$_4$PteGlu	10-Formyltetrahydrofolate
$N^{5,10}$	=CH—	5,10-CHH$_4$PteGlu	5,10-Methenyltetrahydrofolate
$N^{5,10}$	—CH$_2$—	5,10-CH$_2$H$_4$PteGlu	5,10-Methylenetetrahydrofolate
N^5	—CHNH	CHNHH$_4$PteGlu	Formiminotetrahydrofolate
N^{10}	—CH$_2$OH	CH$_2$OHH$_4$PteGlu	Hydroxymethyltetrahydrofolate

Figure 41–7 *The structures and nomenclature of PteGlu (folic acid) and its congeners.* X represents additional residues of glutamate; polyglutamates are the storage and active forms of the vitamin. The number of residues of glutamate is variable.

- *Histidine Metabolism.* H$_4$PteGlu also acts as an acceptor of a formimino group in the conversion of FIGLU to glutamic acid.
- *Synthesis of Purines.* Two steps in the synthesis of purine nucleotides require the participation of 10-CHOH$_4$PteGlu as a formyl donor in reactions catalyzed by ribotide transformylases: the formylation of glycinamide ribonucleotide and the formylation of 5-aminoimidazole-4-carboxamide ribonucleotide. By these reactions, carbon atoms at positions 8 and 2, respectively, are incorporated into the growing purine ring.
- *Utilization or Generation of Formate.* This reversible reaction uses H$_4$PteGlu and 10-CHOH$_4$PteGlu.

Daily Requirements. Many food sources are rich in folates, especially fresh green vegetables, liver, yeast, and some fruits. However, lengthy cooking can destroy up to 90% of the folate content of such food. Generally, a standard U.S. diet provides 50–500 μg of absorbable folate per day, although individuals with high intakes of fresh vegetables and meats will ingest as much as 2 mg per day. In the normal adult, the recommended daily intake is 400 μg; pregnant or lactating women and patients with high rates of cell turnover (such as patients with a hemolytic anemia) may require 500–600 μg or more per day. For the prevention of neural tube defects, a daily intake of at least 400 μg of folate in food or in supplements beginning a month before pregnancy and continued for at least the first trimester is recommended. Folate supplementation also is being considered in patients with elevated levels of plasma homocysteine.

ADME. As with vitamin B$_{12}$, the diagnosis and management of deficiencies of folic acid depend on an understanding of the transport pathways and intracellular metabolism of the vitamin (Figure 41–8). Folates present in food are largely in the form of reduced polyglutamates, and absorption requires transport and the action of a *pteroylglutamyl carboxypeptidase* associated with mucosal cell membranes. The mucosae of the duodenum and upper part of the jejunum are rich in *dihydrofolate reductase* and can methylate most or all of the reduced folate that is absorbed. Because most absorption occurs in the proximal portion of the small intestine, it is not unusual for folate deficiency to occur when the jejunum is diseased. Both nontropical and tropical sprues are common causes of folate deficiency and megaloblastic anemia.

Once absorbed, folate is transported rapidly to tissues as CH$_3$H$_4$PteGlu. Although certain plasma proteins do bind folate derivatives, they have a greater affinity for nonmethylated analogues. The role of such binding proteins in folate homeostasis is not well understood. An increase in binding capacity is detectable in folate deficiency and in certain disease states, such as uremia, cancer, and alcoholism. A constant supply of CH$_3$H$_4$PteGlu is maintained by food and by an enterohepatic cycle of the vitamin. The liver actively reduces and methylates PteGlu (and H$_2$ or H$_4$PteGlu) and then transports the CH$_3$H$_4$PteGlu into bile for reabsorption by the gut and subsequent delivery to tissues. This pathway may provide 200 μg or more of folate each day for recirculation to tissues. The importance of the enterohepatic cycle was suggested by animal studies that showed a rapid reduction of the plasma folate concentration after either drainage of bile or ingestion of alcohol, which apparently blocks the release of CH$_3$H$_4$PteGlu from hepatic parenchymal cells.

Folate Deficiency. Folate deficiency is a common complication of diseases of the small intestine that interferes with the absorption of folate

Figure 41–8 *Absorption and distribution of folate derivatives.* Dietary sources of folate polyglutamates are hydrolyzed to the monoglutamate, reduced, and methylated to CH$_3$H$_4$PteGlu$_1$ during GI transport. Folate deficiency commonly results from (1) inadequate dietary supply and (2) small intestinal disease. In patients with uremia, alcoholism, or hepatic disease, there may be defects in (3) the concentration of folate-binding proteins in plasma and (4) the flow of CH$_3$H$_4$PteGlu$_1$ into bile for reabsorption and transport to tissue (the folate enterohepatic cycle). Finally, vitamin B$_{12}$ deficiency will (5) "trap" folate as CH$_3$H$_4$PteGlu, thereby reducing the availability of H$_4$PteGlu$_1$ for its essential roles in purine and pyrimidine synthesis.

from food and the recirculation of folate through the enterohepatic cycle. The prevalence of folate deficiency in persons over age 65 is relatively high due to reduced dietary intake or intestinal malabsorption (Araujo et al., 2015). In acute or chronic alcoholism, daily intake of folate in food may be severely restricted, and the enterohepatic cycle of the vitamin may be impaired by toxic effects of alcohol on hepatic parenchymal cells; this is the most common cause of folate-deficient megaloblastic erythropoiesis and the most amenable to therapy, via reinstitution of a normal diet. Disease states characterized by a high rate of cell turnover, such as hemolytic anemias, also may be complicated by folate deficiency. In addition, drugs that inhibit dihydrofolate reductase (e.g., methotrexate and trimethoprim) or that interfere with the absorption and storage of folate in tissues (e.g., certain anticonvulsants and oral contraceptives) can lower the concentration of folate in plasma and may cause a megaloblastic anemia (Hesdorffer and Longo, 2015).

Folate deficiency is recognized by its impact on the hematopoietic system. As with vitamin B_{12}, this fact reflects the increased requirement associated with high rates of cell turnover. The megaloblastic anemia that results from folate deficiency cannot be distinguished from that caused by vitamin B_{12} deficiency. In contrast to vitamin B_{12} deficiency, folate deficiency is rarely, if ever, associated with neurological abnormalities. After deprivation of folate, megaloblastic anemia develops much more rapidly than it does following interruption of vitamin B_{12} absorption (e.g., gastric surgery). This observation reflects the fact that body stores of folate are limited. Although the rate of induction of megaloblastic erythropoiesis may vary, a folate-deficiency state may appear in 1–4 weeks, depending on the individual's dietary habits and stores of the vitamin.

Folate deficiency is implicated in the incidence of neural tube defects (Wallingford et al., 2013). An inadequate intake of folate also can result in elevations in plasma homocysteine. Because even moderate hyperhomocysteinemia is considered an independent risk factor for coronary artery and peripheral vascular disease and for venous thrombosis, the role of folate as a methyl donor in the homocysteine-to-methionine conversion is receiving increased attention (Stanger and Wonisch, 2012).

General Principles of Therapy.

The therapeutic use of folic acid is limited to the prevention and treatment of deficiencies of the vitamin. As with vitamin B_{12} therapy, effective use of the vitamin depends on accurate diagnosis and an understanding of the mechanisms that are operative in a specific disease state. The following general principles of therapy should be respected:

- Dietary supplementation is necessary when there is a requirement that may not be met by a "normal" diet. The daily ingestion of a multivitamin preparation containing 400–500 μg of folic acid has become standard practice before and during pregnancy to reduce the incidence of neural tube defects and for as long as a woman is breastfeeding. In women with a history of a pregnancy complicated by a neural tube defect, an even larger dose of 4 mg/d has been recommended. Patients on total parenteral nutrition should receive folic acid supplements as part of their fluid regimen because liver folate stores are limited. Adult patients with a disease state characterized by high cell turnover (e.g., hemolytic anemia) generally require 1 mg of folic acid given once or twice a day. The 1-mg dose also has been used in the treatment of patients with elevated levels of homocysteine.

- Any patient with folate deficiency and a megaloblastic anemia should be evaluated carefully to determine the underlying cause of the deficiency state. This should include evaluation of the effects of medications, the amount of alcohol intake, the patient's history of travel, and the function of the GI tract.

- Therapy always should be as specific as possible. Multivitamin preparations should be avoided unless there is good reason to suspect deficiency of several vitamins.

- The potential danger of mistreating a patient who has vitamin B_{12} deficiency with folic acid must be kept in mind. The administration of large doses of folic acid can result in an apparent improvement of the megaloblastic anemia, inasmuch as PteGlu is converted by dihydrofolate

reductase to $H_4PteGlu$; this circumvents the methylfolate "trap." However, folate therapy does not prevent or alleviate the neurological defects of vitamin B_{12} deficiency, and these may progress and become irreversible.

Therapeutic Use of Folate.

Folic acid is marketed as oral tablets containing PteGlu or l-methylfolate, as an aqueous solution for injection (5 mg/mL), and in combination with other vitamins and minerals. Folinic acid (leucovorin calcium, citrovorum factor) is the 5-formyl derivative of tetrahydrofolic acid. The principal therapeutic uses of folinic acid are to circumvent the inhibition of dihydrofolate reductase as a part of high-dose methotrexate therapy and to potentiate fluorouracil in the treatment of colorectal cancer (see Chapter 66). It also has been used as an antidote to counteract the toxicity of folate antagonists such as pyrimethamine or trimethoprim. Folinic acid provides no advantage over folic acid, is more expensive, and therefore is not recommended. A single exception is the megaloblastic anemia associated with congenital dihydrofolate reductase deficiency.

Evaluation of the serum folate level can help exclude folate deficiency, but only in patients whose serum folate levels exceed 5.0 ng/mL; 2%–5% of healthy adults can have serum folate levels that are below this level. Red cell folate levels (reference range > 140 ng/mL) reflect chronic folate levels, are less affected by acute ingestion of folate than are serum levels, but are more time consuming and costly to measure. Serum folate concentrations more frequently show a higher correlation with serum homocysteine, which is a sensitive marker of deficiency (Farrell et al., 2013). In any case, a patient with a low serum or red cell folate level should have follow-up tests that include serum homocysteine (reference range 5–16 mmol/L), which is elevated in B_{12} and folate deficiency, and serum methylmalonic acid (reference range 70–270 mmol/L), which is elevated only in B_{12} deficiency.

Untoward Effects.

There have been rare reports of reactions to parenteral injections of folic acid and leucovorin. Oral folic acid usually is not toxic. Folic acid in large amounts may counteract the antiepileptic effect of phenobarbital, phenytoin, and primidone and increase the frequency of seizures in susceptible children. The FDA recommends that oral tablets of folic acid be limited to strengths of 1 mg or less.

Acknowledgment: *Robert S. Hillman contributed to this chapter in a prior edition of this book. We have retained some of his text in the current edition.*

Bibliography

Agarwal R. Proinflammatory effects of iron sucrose in chronic kidney disease. *Kidney Int*, **2006**, 69:1259–1263.

Araujo JR, et al. Folates and aging: role in mild cognitive impairment, dementia and depression. *Ageing Res Rev*, **2015**, 22:9–19.

Auerbach M, et al. Safety and efficacy of total dose infusion of 1020 mg of ferumoxytol administered over 15 min. *Am J Hematol*, **2013**, 88: 944–947.

Beguin Y, Jaspers A. Iron sucrose—characteristics, efficacy and regulatory aspects of an established treatment of iron deficiency and iron-deficiency anemia in a broad range of therapeutic areas. *Expert Opin Pharmacother*, **2014**, 15:2087–2103.

Bennett CL, et al. Venous thromboembolism and mortality associated with recombinant erythropoietin and darbepoetin administration for the treatment of cancer-associated anemia. *JAMA*, **2008**, 299:914–924.

Besarab A, et al. A study of parental iron regimens in hemodialysis patients. *Am J Kidney Dis*, **1999**, 34:21–28.

Beutler E. History of iron in medicine. *Blood Cells Mol Dis*, **2002**, 29:297–308.

Bohlius J, et al. Erythropoietin or darbepoetin for patients with cancer: meta-analysis based on individual patient data. *Cochrane Database Syst Rev*, **2009**, 3: CD007303. doi:10.1002/14651858. CD007303.pub2. Accessed July 23, 2017.

Brandt SJ, et al. Effect of recombinant human granulocyte-macrophage colony-stimulating factor on hematopoietic reconstitution after high-dose chemotherapy and autologous bone marrow transplantation. *N Engl J Med*, **1988**, 318:869–876.

Camaschella C. Iron and hepcidin: a story of recycling and balance. *Hematology Am Soc Hematol Educ Program*, **2013**, *2013*:1–8.

Camaschella C. Iron-deficiency anemia. *N Engl J Med*, **2015**, *372*: 1832–1843.

Conrad ME, Umbreit JM. Iron absorption and transport - an update. *Am J Hematol*, **2000**, *64*:287–298

de Bie P, et al. Molecular pathogenesis of Wilson and Menkes disease: correlation of mutations with molecular defects and disease phenotypes. *J Med Genet*, **2007**, *44*:673–688.

De Domenico I, et al. The hepcidin-binding site on ferroportin is evolutionarily conserved. *Cell Metab*, **2008**, *8*:146–156.

Del Villar Madrigal E, et al. Anemia after Roux-en-Y gastric bypass. How feasible to eliminate the risk by proper supplementation? *Obes Surg*, **2015**, *25*:80–84.

Drakesmith H, Prentice AM. Hepcidin and the iron-infection axis. *Science*, **2012**, *338*:768–772.

Farrell CJ, et al. Red cell or serum folate: what to do in clinical practice? *Clin Chem Lab Med*, **2013**, *51*:555–569.

Feder JN, et al. A novel MHC class I-like gene is mutated in patients with hereditary haemochromatosis. *Nat Genet*, **1996**, *13*:399–408.

Finch CW. Review of trace mineral requirements for preterm infants: what are the current recommendations for clinical practice? *Nutr Clin Pract*, **2015**, *30*:44–58.

Fischl M, et al. Recombinant human erythropoietin for patients with AIDS treated with zidovudine. *N Engl J Med*, **1990**, *322*:1488–1493.

Ganz T, Nemeth E. Hepcidin and disorders of iron metabolism. *Annu Rev Med*, **2011**, *62*:347–360.

Garrick MD, Garrick LM. Cellular iron transport. *Biochim Biophys Acta*, **2009**, *1790*:309–325.

Gerhartz HH, et al. Randomized, double-blind, placebo-controlled, phase III study of recombinant human granulocyte-macrophage colony-stimulating factor as adjunct to induction treatment of high-grade malignant non-Hodgkin's lymphomas. *Blood*, **1993**, *82*:2329–2339.

Goodwin RG, et al. Human interleukin 7: molecular cloning and growth factor activity on human and murine B-lineage cells. *Proc Natl Acad Sci U S A*, **1989**, *86*:302–306.

Gordeuk VR, et al. Congenital disorder of oxygen sensing: association of the homozygous Chuvash polycythemia VHL mutation with thrombosis and vascular abnormalities but not tumors. *Blood*, **2004**, *103*:3924–3932.

Gough NM, et al. Molecular cloning of cDNA encoding a murine hematopoietic growth regulator, granulocyte-macrophage colony stimulating factor. *Nature*, **1984**, *309*:763–767.

Grabstein KH, et al. Cloning of a T cell growth factor that interacts with the β chain of the interleukin-2 receptor. *Science*, **1994**, *264*:965–968.

Haas R, et al. Successful autologous transplantation of blood stem cells mobilized with recombinant human granulocyte-macrophage colony-stimulating factor. *Exp Hematol*, **1990**, *18*:94–98.

Haase VH. Hypoxic regulation of erythropoiesis and iron metabolism. *Am J Physiol*, **2010**, *299*:F1–13.

Hahn PF. The use of radioactive isotopes in the study of iron and hemoglobin metabolism and the physiology of the erythrocyte. *Adv Biol Med Phys*, **1948**, *1*:287–319.

Hammond WPT, et al. Treatment of cyclic neutropenia with granulocyte colony-stimulating factor. *N Engl J Med*, **1989**, *320*:1306–1311.

Hayat A. Safety issues with intravenous iron products in the management of anemia in chronic kidney disease. *Clin Med Res*, **2008**, *6*:93–102.

Hesdorffer CS, Longo DL. Drug-induced megaloblastic anemia. *N Engl J Med*, **2015**, *373*:1649–1658.

Hoffbrand AV, Herbert V. Nutritional anemias. *Semin Hematol*, **1999**, *36*:13–23.

Kaufman JS, et al. Subcutaneous compared with intravenous epoetin in patients receiving hemodialysis. Department of Veterans Affairs Cooperative Study Group on Erythropoietin in Hemodialysis Patients. *N Engl J Med*, **1998**, *339*:578–583.

Kaushansky K. Thrombopoietin. *N Engl J Med*, **1998**, *339*:746–754.

Keating GM. Ferric carboxymaltose: a review of its use in iron deficiency. *Drugs*, **2015**, *75*:101–127.

Nevitt T, et al. Charting the travels of copper in eukaryotes from yeast to mammals. *Biochim Biophys Acta Mol Cell Res*, **2012**, *1823*:1580–1593.

Kondo M, et al. Biology of hematopoietic stem cells and progenitors: implications for clinical application. *Annu Rev Immunol*, **2003**, *21*:759–806.

Kuter DJ, et al. Efficacy of romiplostim in patients with chronic immune thrombocytopenic purpura: a double-blind randomised controlled trial. *Lancet*, **2008**, *371*:395–403.

Larson DS, Coyne DW. Update on intravenous iron choices. *Curr Opin Nephrol Hypertens*, **2014**, *23*:186–191.

Laurell CB. What is the function of transferrin in plasma? *Blood*, **1951**, *6*:183–187.

Li J, et al. Thrombocytopenia caused by the development of antibodies to thrombopoietin. *Blood*, **2001**, *98*:3241–3248.

Lieschke GJ, Burgess AW. Granulocyte colony-stimulating factor and granulocyte-macrophage colony-stimulating factor (2). *N Engl J Med*, **1992**, *327*:99–106.

Littlewood TJ, et al. Effects of epoetin alfa on hematologic parameters and quality of life in cancer patients receiving nonplatinum chemotherapy: results of a randomized, double-blind, placebo-controlled trial. *J Clin Oncol*, **2001**, *19*:2865–2874.

Martí-Carvajal AJ, et al. Treatment for anemia in people with AIDS. *Cochrane Database Syst Rev*, **2011**, (10):CD004776. doi:10.1002/14651858. Accessed March 28, 2016.

Mastrogiannaki M, et al. The gut in iron homeostasis: role of HIF-2 under normal and pathological conditions. *Blood*, **2013**, *122*:885–892.

McLean E, et al. Worldwide prevalence of anaemia, WHO Vitamin and Mineral Nutrition Information System, 1993–2005. *Public Health Nutr*, **2009**, *12*:444–454.

Nemunaitis J, et al. Use of recombinant human granulocyte-macrophage colony-stimulating factor in graft failure after bone marrow transplantation. *Blood*, **1990**, *76*:245–253.

Park CH, et al. Hepcidin, a urinary antimicrobial peptide synthesized in the liver. *J Biol Chem*, **2001**, *276*:7806–7810.

Percy MJ, et al. Novel exon 12 mutations in the HIF2A gene associated with erythrocytosis. *Blood*, **2008**, *111*:5400–5402.

Pietrangelo A. Iron and the liver. *Liver Int*, **2016**, *36*(suppl 1):116–123.

Rizzo JD, et al. Use of epoetin in patients with cancer: evidence-based clinical practice guidelines of the American Society of Clinical Oncology and the American Society of Hematology. *Blood*, **2002**, *100*:2303–2320.

Rizzo JD, et al. American Society of Hematology and the American Society of Clinical Oncology clinical practice guideline update on the use of epoetin and darbepoetin in adult patients with cancer. *Blood*, **2010**, *116*:4045–4059.

Sengolge G, et al. Intravenous iron therapy: well-tolerated, yet not harmless. *Eur J Clin Invest*, **2005**, *35*(suppl 3):46–51.

Sheridan WP, et al. Effect of peripheral-blood progenitor cells mobilised by filgrastim (G-CSF) on platelet recovery after high-dose chemotherapy. *Lancet*, **1992**, *339*:640–644.

Solomon LR. Disorders of cobalamin (vitamin B_{12}) metabolism: emerging concepts in pathophysiology, diagnosis and treatment. *Blood Rev*, **2007**, *21*:113–130.

Spence JD. Metabolic B_{12} deficiency: a missed opportunity to prevent dementia and stroke. *Nutr Res*, **2016**, *36*:109–116.

Stanger O, Wonisch W. Enzymatic and non-enzymatic antioxidative effects of folic acid and its reduced derivates. *Subcell Biochem*, **2012**, *56*:131–161.

Wallingford JB, et al. The continuing challenge of understanding, preventing, and treating neural tube defects. *Science*, **2013**, *339*:1222002.

Weisbart RH, et al. Human GM-CSF primes neutrophils for enhanced oxidative metabolism in response to the major physiological chemoattractants. *Blood*, **1987**, *69*:18–21.

Weissbach H. The isolation of the vitamin B_{12} coenzyme and the role of the vitamin in methionine synthesis. *J Biol Chem*, **2008**, *283*:23497–23504.

Welte K, et al. Purification and biochemical characterization of human pluripotent hematopoietic colony-stimulating factor. *Proc Natl Acad Sci U S A*, **1985**, *82*:1526–1530.

Willis MS, et al. Zinc-induced copper deficiency: a report of three cases initially recognized on bone marrow examination. *Am J Clin Pathol*, **2005**, *123*:125–131.

Wong GG, et al. Human GM-CSF: molecular cloning of the complementary DNA and purification of the natural and recombinant proteins. *Science*, **1985**, *228*:810–815.

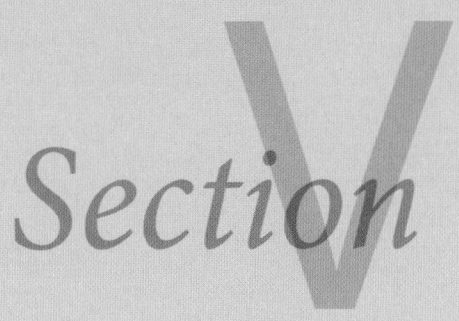

Section V

Hormones and Hormone Antagonists

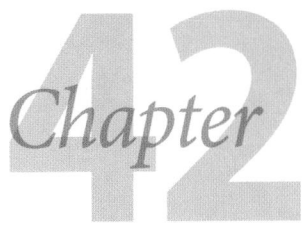

Chapter 42

Introduction to Endocrinology:
The Hypothalamic-Pituitary Axis

Mark E. Molitch and Bernard P. Schimmer

Endocrinology and Hormones: General Concepts

Endocrinology analyzes the biosynthesis of hormones, their sites of production, and the sites and mechanisms of their action and interaction. The term *hormone* is of Greek origin and classically refers to a chemical messenger that circulates in body fluids and produces specific effects on cells distant from the hormone's point of origin. The major functions of hormones include the regulation of energy storage, production, and utilization; the adaptation to new environments or conditions of stress; the facilitation of growth and development; and the maturation and function of the reproductive system. Although hormones were originally defined as products of ductless glands, we now appreciate that many organs not classically considered as "endocrine" (e.g., the heart, kidneys, GI tract, adipocytes, and brain) synthesize and secrete hormones that play key physiological roles. In addition, the field of endocrinology has expanded to include the actions of growth factors acting by means of autocrine and paracrine mechanisms, the influence of neurons—particularly those in the hypothalamus—that regulate endocrine function, and the reciprocal interactions of cytokines and other components of the immune system with the endocrine system.

Conceptually, hormones may be divided into two classes:

- Hormones that act predominantly via *nuclear receptors* to modulate transcription in target cells (e.g., steroid hormones, thyroid hormone, and vitamin D)
- Hormones that typically act via *membrane receptors* to exert rapid effects on signal transduction pathways (e.g., peptide and amino acid hormones)

The receptors for both classes of hormones provide tractable targets for a diverse group of compounds that are among the most widely used drugs in clinical medicine.

The Hypothalamic-Pituitary-Endocrine Axis

Many of the classic endocrine hormones (e.g., cortisol, thyroid hormone, sex steroids, GH) are regulated by complex reciprocal interactions among the hypothalamus, anterior pituitary, and endocrine glands (Table 42–1). The basic organization of the hypothalamic-pituitary-endocrine axis is summarized in Figure 42–1.

Discrete sets of hypothalamic neurons produce different releasing and inhibiting hormones, which are axonally transported to the median eminence. On stimulation, these neurons secrete their respective hypothalamic hormones into the hypothalamic-adenohypophyseal portal veins, which connect to the anterior pituitary gland. The *hypothalamic hormones* bind to membrane receptors on specific subsets of pituitary cells and regulate the secretion of the corresponding *pituitary hormones*. The pituitary hormones, which can be thought of as the *master signals*, circulate to the target endocrine glands or other tissues, where they activate specific receptors to stimulate the synthesis and secretion of the target *endocrine hormones or exert other tissue-specific effects*. These interactions are *feed-forward regulation* in which the master (signal) hormones stimulate the production of target hormones by the endocrine organs.

Superimposed on this positive feed-forward regulation is *negative-feedback* regulation, which permits precise control of hormone levels (see Figures 42–2 and 42–6). Typically, the endocrine target hormone circulates to both the hypothalamus and pituitary, where it acts via specific receptors to inhibit the production and secretion of both its hypothalamic-releasing hormone and the regulatory pituitary hormone. In addition, other brain regions have inputs to the hypothalamic hormone–producing neurons, further integrating the regulation of hormone levels in response to diverse stimuli.

Abbreviations

AC: adenylyl cyclase
ACTH: corticotropin, formerly adrenocorticotrophic hormone
CG: chorionic gonadotropin
CRH: corticotropin-releasing hormone
DA: dopamine
FSH: follicle-stimulating hormone, follitropin
GH: growth hormone
GHRH: growth hormone–releasing hormone
GnRH: gonadotropin-releasing hormone
GPCR: G protein –coupled receptor
hCG: human chorionic gonadotropin
5HT: 5-hydroxytryptamin serotonin
IGF-1: insulin-like growth factor 1
IGFBP: IGF-binding protein
IRS: insulin receptor substrate
LH: luteinizing hormone; lutropin
NPY: neuropeptide Y
OXTR: oxytocin receptor
POMC: pro-opiomelanocortin
PRL: prolactin
SC: subcutaneous
SHC: Src homology-containing protein
SHP2: Src-homology-2-domain-containing protein tyrosine phosphatase 2
SST: somatostatin
SSTR: SST receptor
TRH: thyrotropin-releasing hormone
TSH: thyroid-stimulating hormone, thyrotropin
VIP: vasoactive intestinal peptide

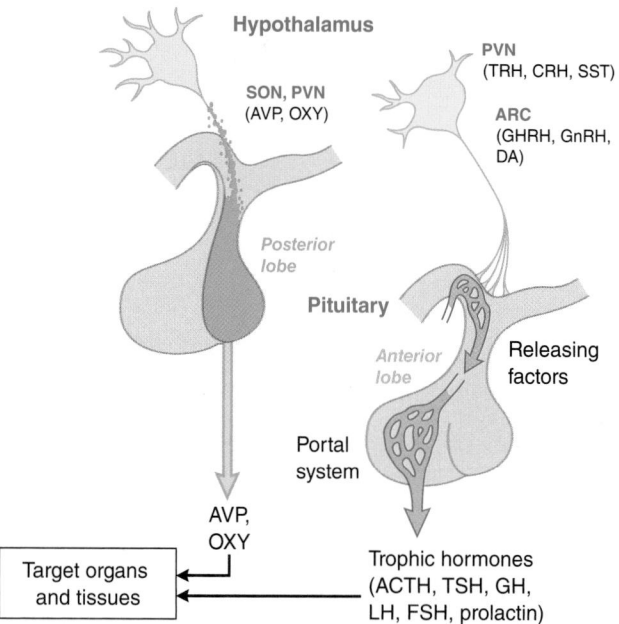

Figure 42–1 *Organization of the anterior and posterior pituitary gland.* Hypothalamic neurons in the supraoptic (SON) and paraventricular (PVN) nuclei synthesize arginine vasopressin (AVP) or oxytocin (OXY). Most of their axons project directly to the posterior pituitary, from which AVP and OXY are secreted into the systemic circulation to regulate their target tissues. Neurons that regulate the anterior lobe cluster in the mediobasal hypothalamus, including the PVH and the arcuate (ARC) nuclei. They secrete hypothalamic releasing hormones, which reach the anterior pituitary via the hypothalamic-adenohypophyseal portal system and stimulate distinct populations of pituitary cells. These cells, in turn, secrete the trophic (signal) hormones, which regulate endocrine organs and other tissues. ARC, arcuate; AVP, arginine vasopressin; OXY, oxytocin; PVN, paraventricular nuclei; SON, supraoptic nuclei; See Abbreviations list for other abbreviations.

Pituitary Hormones and Their Hypothalamic-Releasing Factors

The anterior pituitary hormones can be classified into three different groups based on their structural features (Table 42–2):

- POMC-derived hormones include *corticotropin* (ACTH) and α-MSH. These are derived from POMC by proteolytic processing (see Chapters 20 and 46).

- Somatotropic family of hormones *include GH and PRL*. In humans, the somatotropic family also includes placental lactogen.
- The glycoprotein hormones—*TSH* (also called thyrotropin), *LH* (also called lutropin), and *FSH* (also called follitropin). In humans, the glycoprotein hormone family also includes hCG.

The synthesis and release of *anterior pituitary hormones* are influenced by the CNS. Their secretion is positively regulated by a group of peptides referred to as *hypothalamic-releasing hormones* (see Figure 42–1).

TABLE 42–1 ■ HORMONES THAT INTEGRATE THE HYPOTHALAMIC-PITUITARY-ENDOCRINE AXIS

HYPOTHALAMIC HORMONE	EFFECT ON PITUITARY TROPHIC (SIGNAL) HORMONE	TARGET HORMONE(S)
Growth hormone-releasing hormone	↑↑ Growth hormone	IGF-1
Somatostatin	↓ Growth hormone	
	↓ Thyroid-stimulating hormone	
Dopamine	↓ Prolactin	—
Corticotropin-releasing hormone	↑ Corticotropin	Cortisol
Thyrotropin-releasing hormone	↑ Thyroid-stimulating hormone	Thyroid hormone
	↑ Prolactin	
Gonadotropin-releasing hormone	↑ Follicle-stimulating hormone	Estrogen (f)
	↑ Luteinizing hormone	Progesterone/estrogen (f)
		Testosterone (m)

f, female; m, male; ↑, increased production; ↓, decreased production.

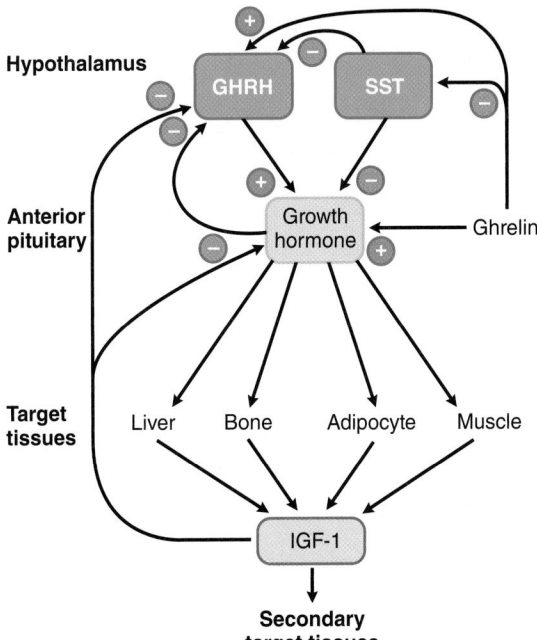

Growth Hormone and Prolactin

Growth hormone and PRL are structurally related members of the somatotropic hormone family and share many biological features. The somatotropes and lactotropes, the pituitary cells that produce and secrete GH and PRL, respectively, are subject to strong inhibitory input from hypothalamic neurons; for PRL, dopaminergic input is the dominant negative regulator of secretion. GH and PRL act via membrane receptors that belong to the cytokine receptor family and modulate target cell function via very similar signal transduction pathways (see Chapter 3).

Structures of GH and PRL

Table 42–2 presents some features of the somatotrophic family of hormones. GH is secreted by somatotropes as a heterogeneous mixture of peptides; the principal form is a single polypeptide chain of 22 kDa that has two disulfide bonds and is not glycosylated. Alternative splicing produces a smaller form (~20 kDa) with equal bioactivity that makes up 5%–10% of circulating GH. Recombinant human GH consists entirely of the 22-kDa form, which provides a way to detect GH abuse. In the circulation, a 55-kDa protein, which is derived from the extracellular domain of the proteolytically cleaved GHRH receptor, binds approximately 45% of the 22-kDa and 25% of the 20-kDa forms. A second protein unrelated to the GHR also binds approximately 5%–10% of circulating GH with lower affinity. Bound GH is cleared more slowly and has a biological $t_{1/2}$ about 10 times that of unbound GH, suggesting that the bound hormone may provide a GH reservoir that dampens acute fluctuations in GH levels associated with its pulsatile secretion.

Human PRL is synthesized by lactotropes; a portion of the secreted hormone is glycosylated at a single Asn residue. In the circulation, multimeric forms of PRL occur, as do degradation products of 16 kDa and 18 kDa. As with GH, the biological significance of these polymeric and degraded forms is not known.

Human placental lactogen, structurally similar to GH and PRL, occurs in pregnant females, with maximal levels near term. Human placental lactogen alters the mother's metabolism to favor fetal nutrition (mainly elevated blood glucose, secondary to reduced maternal insulin sensitivity).

Regulation of Secretion

GH Secretion

Daily GH secretion varies throughout life. GH secretion is high in children, peaks during puberty, and then decreases in an age-related manner in adulthood. GH is secreted in discrete but irregular pulses.

Figure 42–2 *Growth hormone secretion and actions.* Two hypothalamic factors, GHRH and SST, stimulate or inhibit the release of GH from the pituitary, respectively. IGF-1, a product of GH action on peripheral tissues, causes negative-feedback inhibition of GH release by acting at the hypothalamus and the pituitary. The actions of GH can be direct or indirect (mediated by IGF-1). See text for discussion of the other agents that modulate GH secretion and of the effects of locally produced IGF-1. Inhibition, –; stimulation, +.

These include *CRH, GHRH, GnRH,* and *TRH. SST,* another hypothalamic peptide, negatively regulates secretion of pituitary GH and TSH. The neurotransmitter DA inhibits the secretion of PRL by lactotropes.

The *posterior pituitary gland,* also known as the neurohypophysis, contains the endings of nerve axons arising from the hypothalamus that synthesize either *arginine vasopressin* or *oxytocin* (see Figure 42–1). Arginine vasopressin plays an important role in water homeostasis (see Chapter 25); oxytocin plays important roles in labor and parturition and in milk letdown, as discussed in the sections that follow.

TABLE 42–2 ■ PROPERTIES OF THE PROTEIN HORMONES OF THE HUMAN ADENOHYPOPHYSIS AND PLACENTA

CLASS Hormone	MASS (daltons)	PEPTIDE CHAINS	AMINO ACID RESIDUES	Comments
POMC-derived hormones[a]				These peptides are derived by proteolytic processing of the common precursor, POMC.
Corticotropin	4500	1	39	
α-Melanocyte–stimulating hormone	1650		13	
Somatotropic family of hormones				
Growth hormone	22,000		191	Receptors for these hormones belong to the cytokine superfamily.
Prolactin	23,000	1	199	
Placental lactogen	22,125		190	
Glycoprotein hormones				
Luteinizing hormone	29,400		β-121	These are heterodimeric glycoproteins with a common α subunit of 92 amino acids and unique β subunits that determine biological specificity and $t_{1/2}$.
Follicle-stimulating hormone	32,600	2	β-111	
Human chorionic gonadotropin	38,600		β-145	
Thyroid-stimulating hormone	28,000		β-118	

[a]See Chapter 46 for further discussion of POMC-derived peptides, including ACTH and α-MSH.

The amplitude of secretory pulses is greatest at night. GH secretion is stimulated by GHRH and ghrelin and subject to feedback inhibition by GH itself, SST, and IGF-1 (Figure 42–2).

Growth Hormone–Releasing Hormone. GHRH, a peptide with 44 amino acids produced by hypothalamic neurons, stimulates GH secretion (see Figure 42–2) by binding to a specific GPCR on somatotropes in the anterior pituitary. The stimulated GHRH receptor couples to G_s to raise intracellular levels of cAMP and Ca^{2+}, thereby stimulating GH synthesis and secretion. Loss-of-function mutations of the GHRH receptor cause a rare form of short stature in humans.

Ghrelin. Ghrelin, a 28-amino-acid peptide, stimulates GH secretion through actions on a GPCR called the GH secretagogue receptor. Ghrelin is synthesized predominantly in endocrine cells in the fundus of the stomach but also is produced at lower levels at a number of other sites, including the pituitary and hypothalamus. Hypothalamic ghrelin is thought to be a stimulus for GH release through actions on pituitary somatotrophs and hypothalamic GHRH-secreting neurons.

Both fasting and hypoglycemia increase circulating stomach-derived ghrelin levels, and this, in turn, stimulates appetite and increases food intake, apparently by central actions on NPY and agouti-related peptide neurons in the hypothalamus. The role of stomach-derived ghrelin in GH secretion is unclear because clinical studies attempting to correlate circulating levels of ghrelin with GH secretion have produced conflicting results (Nass et al., 2011).

Other Stimuli. Several neurotransmitters, drugs, metabolites, and other stimuli modulate the release of GHRH or SST and thereby affect GH secretion. DA, 5HT, and α_2 adrenergic receptor agonists stimulate GH release, as do hypoglycemia, exercise, stress, emotional excitement, and ingestion of protein-rich meals. In contrast, β adrenergic receptor agonists, free fatty acids, glucose, IGF-1, and GH itself inhibit release. Many of the physiological factors that influence PRL secretion also affect GH secretion. Thus, sleep, stress, hypoglycemia, exercise, and estrogen increase the secretion of both hormones.

Feedback Control of GH Secretion. Growth hormone and its major peripheral effector, *IGF-1*, act in negative-feedback loops to suppress GH secretion (Figure 42–2).

Insulin-like Growth Factor 1. The negative effect of IGF-1 is predominantly through direct effects on the anterior pituitary gland but also at the hypothalamus via stimulation of SST secretion. The negative-feedback action of GH is mediated in part by SST, synthesized in more widely distributed neurons (Ergun-Longmire and Wajnrajch, 2013).

After its synthesis and release, IGF-1 interacts with receptors on the cell surface that mediate its biological activities. The type 1 IGF receptor is closely related to the insulin receptor and consists of a heterotetramer with intrinsic tyrosine kinase activity. This receptor is present in essentially all tissues and binds IGF-1 and the related growth factor, IGF-2, with high affinity; insulin also can activate the type 1 IGF receptor but with an affinity approximately two orders of magnitude less than that of the IGFs. The signal transduction pathway for the insulin receptor is described in detail in Chapter 47.

Somatostatin. Somatostatin is synthesized as a 92-amino-acid precursor and processed by proteolytic cleavage to generate two peptides: SST-28 and SST-14 (Figure 42–3). SST exerts its effects by binding to and activating a family of five related GPCRs that signal through G_i to inhibit cAMP formation and to activate K^+ channels and protein phosphotyrosine phosphatases.

There are five SSTR subtypes. $SSTR_{1–4}$ bind the two forms of SST with approximately equal affinity; $SSTR_5$ has a 10- to 15-fold greater affinity for SST-28. $SSTR_2$ and $SSTR_5$ are the most important for regulation of GH secretion, and recent studies suggested that these two SSTRs form functional heterodimers with distinctive signaling behavior (Grant et al., 2008). SST exerts direct effects on somatotropes in the pituitary and indirect effects mediated via GHRH neurons in the arcuate nucleus.

PRL Secretion

Prolactin is unique among the anterior pituitary hormones in that hypothalamic regulation of its secretion is predominantly inhibitory. The major regulator of PRL secretion is DA, which interacts with the D_2 receptor, a

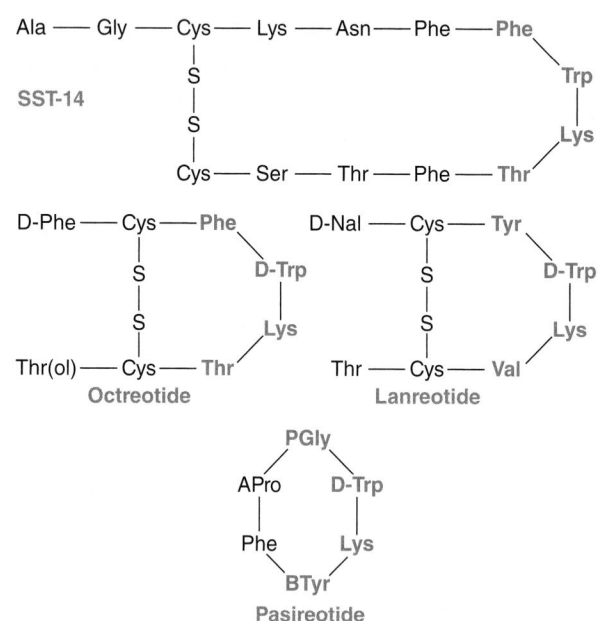

Figure 42–3 *Structures of SST-14 and selected synthetic analogues.* Residues that play key roles in binding to SST receptors are shown in red. Octreotide, lanreotide, and pasireotide are clinically available synthetic analogues of SST. APro, [(2-aminoethyl) aminocarboxyl oxy]-ʟ-proline; ᴅ-Nal, 3-(2-napthyl)-ᴅ-alanyl; PGly, phenylglycine; BTyr, benzyltyrosine.

GPCR on lactotropes, to inhibit PRL secretion (Figure 42–4). TRH and hypothalamic VIP have PRL-releasing properties, but their physiologic significance is uncertain. PRL acts predominantly in women, both during pregnancy and in the postpartum period in women who breastfeed. During pregnancy, the maternal serum PRL level starts to increase at 8 weeks of gestation, peaks to 150–250 ng/mL at term, and declines thereafter to prepregnancy levels unless the mother breastfeeds the infant. Suckling or breast manipulation in nursing mothers transmits signals from the breast to the hypothalamus via the spinal cord and the median forebrain bundle, causing elevation of circulating PRL levels. PRL levels can rise 10-fold within 30 min of stimulation. This response is distinct from milk letdown, which is mediated by oxytocin release from the posterior pituitary gland. The suckling response becomes less pronounced after several months of breastfeeding, and PRL concentrations eventually decline to prepregnancy levels. PRL also is synthesized by decidual cells early in pregnancy (accounting for the high levels of PRL in amniotic fluid during the first trimester of human pregnancy).

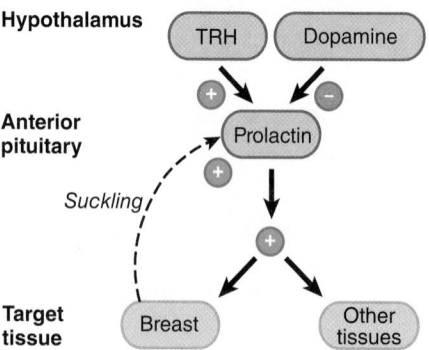

Figure 42–4 *Prolactin secretion and actions.* PRL is the only anterior pituitary hormone for which a unique stimulatory releasing factor has not been identified. TRH and VIP, however, can stimulate PRL release; DA inhibits it. Suckling induces PRL secretion, and PRL not only affects lactation and reproductive functions but also has effects on many other tissues. PRL is not under feedback control by peripheral hormones.

Molecular and Cellular Bases of GH and PRL Action

All of the effects of GH and PRL result from their interactions with specific membrane receptors on target tissues (Figure 42–5). Receptors for GH and PRL belong to the cytokine receptor superfamily and thus share structural similarity with the receptors for leptin, erythropoietin, granulocyte-macrophage colony-stimulating factor, and several of the interleukins. These receptors contain an extracellular hormone-binding domain, a single membrane-spanning region, and an intracellular domain that mediates signal transduction.

Growth hormone receptor activation results in the binding of a single GH to two receptor monomers to form a GH-[GHR]₂ ternary complex (initiated by high-affinity interaction of GH with one monomer of the GHR dimer [mediated by GH site 1], followed by a second, lower-affinity interaction of GH with the other GHR [mediated by GH site 2]). These interactions induce a conformational change that activates downstream signaling. The ligand-occupied GHR dimer lacks inherent tyrosine kinase activity but provides docking sites for two molecules of JAK2, a cytoplasmic tyrosine kinase of the Janus kinase family. The juxtaposition of the JAK2 molecules leads to *trans*-phosphorylation and autoactivation of JAK2, with consequent tyrosine phosphorylation of docking sites on the cytoplasmic segments of the GHR and of cytoplasmic proteins that mediate downstream signaling events (Figure 42–5; Chia, 2014). These include STAT proteins, SHC (an adapter protein that regulates the Ras/MAPK signaling pathway), and IRS-1 and IRS-2 (proteins that activate the PI3K pathway). One critical target of STAT5 is the gene encoding IGF-1, a mediator of many of the effects of GH (Figure 42–2). The fine control of GH action also involves feedback regulatory events that subsequently turn off the GH signal. As part of its action, GH induces the expression of a family of suppressor of cytokine signaling (SOC) proteins and a group of protein tyrosine phosphatases (including SHP2) that, by different mechanisms, disrupt the communication of the activated GHR with JAK2 (Flores-Morales et al., 2006).

Pegvisomant is a GH analogue with amino acid substitutions that disrupt the interaction at site 2; pegvisomant binds to the receptor and causes its internalization but cannot trigger the conformational change that stimulates downstream events in the signal transduction pathway.

The *effects of PRL* on target cells also result from interactions with a cytokine family receptor that is widely distributed and signals through many of the same pathways as the GHR (Bernard et al., 2015). Alternative splicing of the PRL receptor gene on chromosome 5 gives rise to multiple forms of the receptor that are identical in the extracellular domain but differ in their cytoplasmic domains. In addition, soluble forms that correspond to the extracellular domain of the receptor are found in circulation. Unlike human GH and placental lactogen, which also bind to the PRL receptor and thus are lactogenic, PRL binds specifically to the PRL receptor and has no somatotropic (GH-like) activity.

Physiological Effects of GH and PRL

The most striking physiological effect of GH is the stimulation of the longitudinal growth of bones. GH also increases bone mineral density after the epiphyses have closed. GH also increases muscle mass, increases the glomerular filtration rate, and stimulates preadipocyte differentiation into adipocytes. GH has potent anti-insulin actions in both the liver and peripheral tissues (e.g., adipocytes and muscle) that decrease glucose utilization and increase lipolysis, but most of its anabolic and growth-promoting effects are mediated indirectly through the induction of IGF-1. IGF-1 interacts with receptors on the cell surface that mediate its biological activities. Circulating IGF-1 is associated with a family of binding proteins (IGFBP) that serve as transport proteins and also may mediate certain aspects of IGF-1 signaling. Most IGF-1 in circulation is bound to IGFBP-3 and another protein called the acid-labile subunit.

The essential role of IGF-1 in growth is evidenced by patients with loss-of-function mutations in both alleles of the *IGF1* gene, whose severe intrauterine and postnatal growth retardation is unresponsive to GH but responsive to recombinant human IGF-1, and by the association of mutations in the IGF-1 receptor with intrauterine growth retardation (Walenkamp and Wit, 2008).

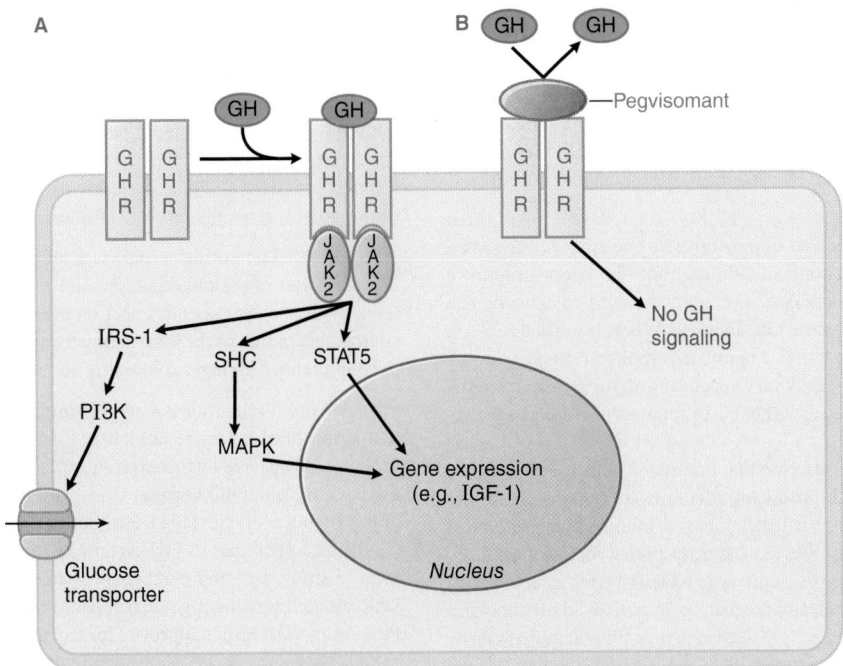

Figure 42–5 *Mechanisms of GH and PRL action and of GHR antagonism.* **A.** GH and two GHRs form a ternary complex that induces association and Tyr autophosphorylation of JAK2 and of docking sites on the cytoplasmic tail of GHRs. JAK2 phosphorylates cytoplasmic proteins that activate downstream signaling pathways, including STAT5 and mediators upstream of MAPK, which ultimately modulate gene expression. The structurally related PRL receptor also is a ligand-activated homodimer that recruits the JAK-STAT signaling pathway. GHR also activates IRS-1, which may mediate the increased expression of glucose transporters on the plasma membrane. **B.** Pegvisomant, a recombinant pegylated variant of human GH, is a high-affinity GH antagonist that interferes with GH binding.

The PRL effects are limited primarily to the mammary gland, where PRL plays an important role in inducing growth and differentiation of the ductal and lobuloalveolar epithelia and is essential for lactation. Target genes, by which PRL induces mammary development, include those encoding milk proteins (e.g., caseins and whey acidic protein), genes important for intracellular structure (e.g., keratins), and genes important for cell-cell communication (e.g., amphiregulin). PRL receptors are present in many other sites, including the hypothalamus, liver, adrenal, testes, ovaries, prostate, and immune system, suggesting that PRL may play multiple roles outside the breast. The physiological effects of PRL at these sites remain poorly characterized.

Pathophysiology of GH and PRL

Distinct endocrine disorders result from either excessive or deficient GH production. In contrast, PRL predominantly affects endocrine function when produced in excess.

Excess Production

Syndromes of excess secretion of GH and PRL typically are caused by somatotrope or lactotrope adenomas that oversecrete the respective hormones. These adenomas often retain some features of the normal regulation described previously, thus permitting pharmacological modulation of secretion—an important modality in therapy.

Clinical Manifestations of Excess GH. GH excess causes distinct clinical syndromes depending on the age of the patient. If the epiphyses are unfused, GH excess causes increased longitudinal growth, resulting in *gigantism*. In adults, GH excess causes *acromegaly*. The symptoms and signs of acromegaly (e.g., arthropathy, carpal tunnel syndrome, generalized visceromegaly, macroglossia, hypertension, glucose intolerance, headache, lethargy, excess perspiration, and sleep apnea) progress slowly, and diagnosis often is delayed. Mortality is increased at least 2-fold relative to age-matched controls, predominantly due to increased death from cardiovascular disease. Treatments that normalize GH and IGF-1 levels reverse this increased risk of mortality and ameliorate most of the other symptoms and signs.

Clinical Manifestations of Excess Prolactin. *Hyperprolactinemia* is a relatively common endocrine abnormality that can result from hypothalamic or pituitary diseases that interfere with the delivery of inhibitory dopaminergic signals, from renal failure, from primary hypothyroidism associated with increased TRH levels, or from treatment with DA receptor antagonists. Most often, hyperprolactinemia is caused by PRL-secreting pituitary adenomas. Manifestations of PRL excess in women include galactorrhea, amenorrhea, and infertility. In men, hyperprolactinemia causes loss of libido, erectile dysfunction, and infertility.

Diagnosis of Growth Hormone and Prolactin Excess. Although acromegaly should be suspected in patients with the appropriate symptoms and signs, diagnostic confirmation requires the demonstration of increased circulating GH or IGF-1. The "gold standard" diagnostic test for acromegaly is the oral glucose tolerance test. Whereas normal subjects suppress their GH level to less than 1 ng/mL in response to an oral glucose challenge (the absolute value may vary depending on the sensitivity of the assay), patients with acromegaly either fail to suppress or show a paradoxical increase in GH level.

In patients with hyperprolactinemia, the major question is whether conditions other than a PRL-producing adenoma are responsible for the elevated PRL level. A number of medications that inhibit DA signaling can cause moderate elevations in PRL (e.g., antipsychotics, metoclopramide), as can primary hypothyroidism, pituitary mass lesions that interfere with DA delivery to the lactotropes, and pregnancy. Thus, thyroid function and pregnancy tests are indicated, as is MRI to look for a pituitary adenoma or other defect that might elevate serum PRL.

Impaired Production

Clinical Manifestations of Growth Hormone Deficiency. Children with GH deficiency present with short stature, delayed bone age, and a low age-adjusted growth velocity. GH deficiency in adults is associated with decreased muscle mass and exercise capacity, decreased bone density, impaired psychosocial function, and increased mortality from cardiovascular causes. The diagnosis of GH deficiency should be entertained in children with height more than 2 to 2.5 standard deviations below normal, delayed bone age, a decreased growth velocity, and a predicted adult height substantially below the mean parental height. In adults, overt GH deficiency usually results from pituitary lesions caused by a functioning or nonfunctioning pituitary adenoma, secondary to trauma, or related to surgery or radiotherapy for a pituitary or suprasellar mass (Ergun-Longmire and Wajnrajch, 2013). Almost all patients with multiple deficits in other pituitary hormones also have deficient GH secretion.

Clinical Manifestations of Prolactin Deficiency. PRL deficiency may result from conditions that damage the pituitary gland. Inasmuch as the sole clinical manifestation of PRL deficiency is failure of postpartum lactation, PRL is not given as part of endocrine replacement therapy.

Pharmacotherapy of Disorders GH and PRL

Treatment of Growth Hormone Excess

The initial treatment modality in gigantism/acromegaly is selective removal of the adenoma by transsphenoidal surgery. Radiation and drugs that inhibit GH secretion or action are given if surgery does not result in cure (Katznelson et al., 2014). Pituitary irradiation may be associated with significant long-term complications, including visual deterioration and pituitary dysfunction. Thus, increased attention has been given to the pharmacological management of acromegaly.

Somatostatin Analogues

The development of synthetic analogues of SST has revolutionized the medical treatment of acromegaly. The goal of treatment is to decrease GH levels to less than 2.5 ng/mL after an oral glucose tolerance test and to bring IGF-1 levels to within the normal range for age and sex. The two SST analogues used widely are *octreotide* and *lanreotide*, synthetic derivatives that have longer half-lives than SST and bind preferentially to SST_2 and SST_5 receptors (see Figure 42–3).

Octreotide. Octreotide exerts pharmacologic actions similar to those of SST. Octreotide (100 µg) administered subcutaneously three times daily is 100% bioactive; peak effects are seen within 30 min, serum $t_{1/2}$ is about 90 min, and duration of action is about 12 h. An equally effective long-acting, slow-release form, *octreotide LAR*, is administered intramuscularly in a dose of 10, 20, or 30 mg once every 4 weeks. In addition to its effect on GH secretion, octreotide can decrease tumor size, although tumor growth generally resumes after octreotide treatment is stopped.

Lanreotide. Lanreotide autogel is a long-acting octapeptide SST analogue that causes prolonged suppression of GH secretion when administered by deep subcutaneous injection every 4 weeks. Its efficacy appears comparable to that of the long-acting formulation of octreotide. It is supplied in prefilled syringes containing 60, 90, or 120 mg.

Pasireotide. Pasireotide is a long-acting cyclohexapeptide SST analogue that is approved for the treatment of Cushing disease (excessive cortisol production triggered by increases in ACTH release due to a pituitary adenoma; see Chapter 46) in patients who are ineligible for pituitary surgery or in whom surgery has failed. Pasireotide binds to multiple SST receptors (1, 2, 3, and 5) but has its highest affinity for the SST_5 receptor. In a head-to-head study, a greater percentage of subjects administered pasireotide LAR reached treatment goals compared to those given octreotide LAR. Pasireotide LAR also is approved for treatment of acromegaly.

Adverse Effects. Gastrointestinal side effects—including diarrhea, nausea, and abdominal pain—occur in up to 50% of patients receiving all three SST analogues; the incidence and severity of these side effects are similar for the three analogues. The symptoms usually diminish over time and do not require cessation of therapy. Approximately 25% of patients receiving these drugs develop multiple tiny gallstones, presumably due to decreased gallbladder contraction and bile secretion. Bradycardia and QT prolongation may occur in patients with underlying cardiac disease. Inhibitory effects on TSH secretion rarely lead to hypothyroidism, but thyroid function should be evaluated periodically. Pasireotide suppresses ACTH secretion in Cushing disease and may lead to a decrease in cortisol secretion and to hypocortisolism. All SST analogues decrease insulin secretion, but the simultaneous reduction in GH levels results in a reduction in insulin resistance. For octreotide and lanreotide, most patients will experience no change in glucose tolerance; however, depending on the relative effects on insulin secretion versus resistance, some patients may experience a worsening and others an improvement in glucose tolerance. Pasireotide, in addition, decreases the secretion of glucagon-like peptide 1 and glucose insulinotropic peptide, two incretins that facilitate insulin secretion and inhibit glucagon secretion. As a result, glucose tolerance usually worsens significantly and antihyperglycemic therapy is often needed.

Other Therapeutic Uses. SST blocks not only GH secretion but also the secretion of other hormones, growth factors, and cytokines. Thus, the slow-release formulations of SST analogues have been used to treat symptoms associated with metastatic carcinoid tumors (e.g., flushing and diarrhea) and adenomas secreting VIP (e.g., watery diarrhea). Octreotide and lanreotide also can be used to treat patients who have failed surgery who have thyrotrope adenomas that oversecrete TSH. Octreotide is used for treatment of acute variceal bleeding and for perioperative prophylaxis in pancreatic surgery. Modified forms of octreotide labeled with indium or technetium have been used for diagnostic imaging of neuroendocrine tumors, such as pituitary adenomas and carcinoids; modified forms labeled with β emitters such as ^{90}Y have been used in selective destruction of SST_2 receptor-positive tumors.

Growth Hormone Antagonists

Pegvisomant. Pegvisomant is a GHR antagonist approved for the treatment of acromegaly. Pegvisomant binds to the GHR but does not activate JAK-STAT signaling or stimulate IGF-1 secretion (see Figure 42–5).

The drug is administered subcutaneously as a 40-mg loading dose, followed by administration of 10 mg/d. Based on serum IGF-1 levels, the dose is titrated at 4- to 6-week intervals to a maximum of 30 mg/d. Pegvisomant should not be used in patients with an unexplained elevation of hepatic transaminases, and liver function tests should be monitored in all patients. In addition, lipohypertrophy has occurred at injection sites, sometimes requiring cessation of therapy; this is believed to reflect the inhibition of direct actions of GH on adipocytes. Because of concerns that loss of negative feedback by GH and IGF-1 may increase the growth of GH-secreting adenomas, careful follow-up by pituitary MRI is strongly recommended.

Pegvisomant can also be given weekly, in addition to SST analogues, when IGF-1 levels are not fully controlled by the latter drugs (Lim and Fleseriu, 2017). Pegvisomant differs structurally from native GH and induces the formation of specific antibodies in about 15% of patients. Nevertheless, the development of tachyphylaxis due to these antibodies has not been reported.

Treatment of Prolactin Excess

The therapeutic options for patients with prolactinomas include transsphenoidal surgery, radiation, and treatment with DA receptor agonists that suppress PRL production via activation of D_2 receptors. Because of the very high efficacy of DA receptor agonists, they are generally regarded as the initial treatment of choice, with surgery and radiation reserved for patients who either do not respond or are intolerant of DA receptor agonists (Melmed et al., 2011).

Dopamine Receptor Agonists

Bromocriptine, cabergoline, and *quinagolide* effectively reduce PRL levels, thereby relieving the inhibitory effect of hyperprolactinemia on ovulation and permitting most patients with prolactinomas to become pregnant. Quinagolide should not be used when pregnancy is intended. These agents generally decrease both PRL secretion and the size of the adenoma. Over

time, especially with cabergoline, the prolactinoma may decrease in size to the extent that the drug can be discontinued without recurrence of the hyperprolactinemia.

Bromocriptine. Bromocriptine is the DA receptor agonist against which newer agents are compared. Bromocriptine is a semisynthetic ergot alkaloid (see Chapter 13) that interacts with D_2 receptors to inhibit release of PRL; to a lesser extent, it also activates D_1 dopamine receptors. The oral dose of bromocriptine is well absorbed; however, only 7% of the dose reaches the systemic circulation because of extensive first-pass metabolism in the liver. Bromocriptine has a short elimination $t_{1/2}$ (between 2 and 8 h) and thus is usually administered in divided doses. To avoid the need for frequent dosing, a slow-release oral form is available outside the U.S. Bromocriptine may be administered vaginally (2.5 mg once daily), with fewer GI side effects.

Bromocriptine normalizes serum PRL levels in 70%–80% and decreases tumor size in more than 50% of patients with prolactinomas. Hyperprolactinemia and tumor growth recur on cessation of therapy in most patients. At higher concentrations, bromocriptine is used in the management of Parkinson disease (see Chapter 18). Bromocriptine mesylate (1.6–4.8 mg/d) is approved as an adjunct to diet and exercise to improve glycemic control in adults with type 2 diabetes mellitus.

Adverse Effects. Frequent side effects include nausea and vomiting, headache, and postural hypotension, particularly on initial use. Less frequently, nasal congestion, digital vasospasm, and CNS effects such as psychosis, hallucinations, nightmares, or insomnia are observed. These adverse effects can be diminished by starting at a low dose (1.25 mg) administered at bedtime with a snack and then slowly increasing the dose as needed by monitoring PRL levels. Patients often develop tolerance to the adverse effects.

Cabergoline. Cabergoline is an ergot derivative with a longer $t_{1/2}$ (~65 h), higher affinity, and greater selectivity for the DA D_2 receptor compared to bromocriptine. Cabergoline undergoes significant first-pass metabolism in the liver.

Cabergoline is the preferred drug for the treatment of hyperprolactinemia because of greater efficacy and lower adverse effects. Therapy is initiated at a dose of 0.25 mg twice a week or 0.5 mg once a week. The dose can be increased to 1.5–2 mg two or three times a week as tolerated; the dose should be increased only once every 4 weeks. Doses of 2 mg/week or less normalize PRL levels in 80% of patients. Cabergoline induces remission in a significant number of patients with prolactinomas. At higher doses, cabergoline is used in some patients with acromegaly alone or in conjunction with SST analogues.

Adverse Effects. Compared to bromocriptine, cabergoline has a much lower tendency to induce nausea, although it still may cause hypotension and dizziness. Cabergoline has been linked to valvular heart disease, an effect proposed to reflect agonist activity at the serotonin $5HT_{2B}$ receptor; however, this is seen primarily at the high doses used in patients being treated for Parkinson disease and is not seen in the conventionally used doses (≤2 mg/week) for patients with prolactinomas.

Quinagolide. Quinagolide is a nonergot D_2 receptor agonist with a $t_{1/2}$ of about 22 h. Quinagolide is administered once daily at doses of 0.1–0.5 mg/d. It is not approved for use in the U.S. but has been used in the E.U. and Canada.

Treatment of Growth Hormone Deficiency

Somatropin

Replacement therapy is well established in GH-deficient children (Richmond and Rogol, 2010) and is gaining wider acceptance for GH-deficient adults (Molitch et al., 2011).

Humans do not respond to GH from nonprimate species. In the past, when GH for therapeutic use was purified from human cadaver pituitaries, GH was available in limited quantities and was ultimately linked to the transmission of Creutzfeldt-Jakob disease. Currently, human GH is produced by recombinant DNA technology. *Somatropin* refers to the many GH preparations whose sequences match that of native GH.

Pharmacokinetics. As a peptide hormone, GH is administered subcutaneously, with a bioavailability of 70%. Although the circulating $t_{1/2}$ of GH is only 20 min, its biological $t_{1/2}$ is considerably longer, and once-daily administration is sufficient.

Indications for Treatment. GH deficiency in children is a well-accepted cause of short stature. With the advent of essentially unlimited supplies of recombinant GH, therapy has been extended to children with other conditions associated with short stature despite adequate GH production, including Turner syndrome, Noonan syndrome, Prader-Willi syndrome, chronic renal insufficiency, children born small for gestational age, and children with idiopathic short stature (i.e., > 2.25 standard deviations below mean height for age and sex but with normal laboratory indices of GH levels). Severely affected GH-deficient adults may benefit from GH replacement therapy. The FDA also has approved GH therapy for AIDS-associated wasting and for malabsorption associated with the short-bowel syndrome (based on the finding that GH stimulates the adaptation of GI epithelial cells). Adults considered for GH treatment should have organic etiologies for the GH deficiency and must demonstrate low GH production in response to standardized stimulation tests or have at least three other pituitary hormone deficiencies.

Contraindications. GH should not be used in patients with acute critical illness due to complications after open heart or abdominal surgery, multiple accidental trauma, or acute respiratory failure. GH also should not be used in patients who have any evidence of active malignancy. GH replacement does not cause regrowth of pituitary tumor remnants when given to patients whose tumors have been resected. Other contraindications include proliferative retinopathy or severe nonproliferative diabetic retinopathy. In treating Prader-Willi syndrome, GH therapy must be carefully supervised. Sudden death has been observed when GH was given to children who were severely obese or who had severe respiratory impairment.

Therapeutic Uses. In GH-deficient children, somatropin typically is administered in a dose of 25–50 μg/kg/d subcutaneously in the evening; higher daily doses (e.g., 50–67 μg/kg) are employed for patients with Noonan syndrome or Turner syndrome, who have partial GH resistance. In children with overt GH deficiency, measurement of serum IGF-1 levels sometimes is used to monitor initial response and compliance; long-term response is monitored by close evaluation of height, sometimes in conjunction with measurements of serum IGF-1 levels. GH is continued until the epiphyses are fused and also may be extended into the transition period from childhood to adulthood. Children with idiopathic rather than organic GH deficiency need retesting after growth has ceased before continuing GH treatment as adults; many with this diagnosis will have normal GH levels on stimulation testing as adults.

Benefits of GH treatment in GH-deficient adults include increases in muscle mass, exercise capacity, energy, bone mineral density, and quality of life and a decrease in fat mass. For adults, a typical starting dose is 150–300 μg/d (these doses may vary depending on brand product), with higher doses used in younger patients transitioning from pediatric therapy. Either an elevated serum IGF-1 level or persistent side effects mandates a decrease in dose; conversely, the dose can be increased (typically by 100–200 μg/d) if serum IGF-1 has not reached the normal range after 2 months of GH therapy. Because estrogen inhibits GH action, women taking oral—but not transdermal—estrogen may require larger GH doses to achieve the target IGF-1 level.

Adverse Effects. In children, GH therapy is associated with remarkably few side effects. Rarely, patients develop intracranial hypertension, with papilledema, visual changes, headache, nausea, or vomiting. Because of this, funduscopic examination is recommended at the initiation of therapy and at periodic intervals thereafter. The consensus is that GH should not be administered in the first year after treatment of pediatric tumors, including leukemia, or during the first 2 years after therapy for medulloblastomas or ependymomas. Because an increased incidence of type 2 diabetes mellitus has been reported, fasting glucose levels should be

followed periodically during therapy. Finally, too-rapid growth may be associated with slipped epiphyses or scoliosis.

Side effects associated with the initiation of GH therapy in adults (peripheral edema, carpal tunnel syndrome, arthralgias, and myalgias) occur most frequently in older or obese patients and generally respond to a decrease in dose. Estrogens (e.g., birth control medications and estrogen supplements) inhibit GH action so that a larger dose is needed to maintain the same IGF-1 level. GH therapy can increase the metabolic inactivation of cortisol in the liver.

Drug Interactions. The effects of estrogen on GH therapy were noted above. This effect is much less marked with transdermal estrogen preparations. Recent studies suggested that GH therapy can increase the metabolic inactivation of glucocorticoids in the liver. Thus, GH may precipitate adrenal insufficiency in patients with occult secondary adrenal insufficiency or in patients receiving replacement doses of glucocorticoids. This has been attributed to the inhibition of the type 1 isozyme of steroid 11β-hydroxysteroid dehydrogenase, which normally converts inactive cortisone into the active 11-hydroxy derivative cortisol (see Chapter 46).

Insulin-like Growth Factor 1

Based on the hypothesis that GH predominantly acts via increases in IGF-1 (see Figure 42–2), IGF-1 has been developed for therapeutic use (Cohen et al., 2014). Recombinant human IGF-1 (*mecasermin*) and a combination of recombinant human IGF-1 with its binding protein, IGFBP-3 (*mecasermin rinfabate*), are FDA-approved. The latter formulation was subsequently discontinued for use in short stature due to patent issues, although it remains available for other conditions, such as severe insulin resistance, muscular dystrophy, and HIV-related adipose redistribution syndrome.

ADME. Mecasermin is administered by subcutaneous injection, and absorption is virtually complete. IGF-1 in circulation is bound by six proteins; a ternary complex that includes IGFBP-3 and the acid labile subunit accounts for more than 80% of the circulating IGF-1. This protein binding prolongs the $t_{1/2}$ of IGF-1 to about 6 h. Both the liver and kidney have been shown to metabolize IGF-1.

Therapeutic Uses. Mecasermin is FDA-approved for patients with impaired growth secondary to mutations in the GHR or postreceptor signaling pathway, patients who develop antibodies against GH that interfere with its action, and patients with IGF-1 gene defects that lead to primary IGF-1 deficiency. Typically, the starting dose is 40–80 μg/kg twice daily by subcutaneous injection, with a maximum of 120 μg/kg per dose twice daily. In patients with impaired growth secondary to GH deficiency or with idiopathic short stature, mecasermin stimulates linear growth but is less effective than conventional therapy using recombinant GH.

Adverse Effects. Side effects of mecasermin include hypoglycemia and lipohypertrophy. To diminish the frequency of hypoglycemia, mecasermin should be administered shortly before or after a meal or snack. Lymphoid tissue hypertrophy, including enlarged tonsils, also is seen and may require surgical intervention. Other adverse effects are similar to those associated with GH therapy.

Contraindications. Mecasermin should not be used for growth promotion in patients with closed epiphyses. It should not be given to patients with active or suspected neoplasia and should be stopped if evidence of neoplasia develops.

Growth Hormone–Releasing Hormone

Tesamorelin. Tesamorelin is a synthetic N-terminally modified form of human GHRH that is resistant to degradation by dipeptidyl peptidase 4 and therefore has a prolonged duration of action. Tesamorelin is able to increase the levels of GH and IGF-1, but its clinical effects are primarily to reduce visceral fat accumulation, with minimal effects on insulin resistance. Tesamorelin is FDA-approved for treatment of HIV-associated lipodystrophy but not for GH deficiency (Spooner and Olin, 2012).

The Glycoprotein Hormones: TSH and the Gonadotropins

The gonadotropins include *LH*, *FSH*, and *CG*. They are referred to as the gonadotropins because of their actions on the gonads. Together with TSH, they constitute the glycoprotein family of pituitary hormones (see Table 42–2). LH and FSH were named initially based on their actions on the ovary; appreciation of their roles in male reproductive function came later. LH and FSH are synthesized and secreted by gonadotropes, which make up about 10% of the hormone-secreting cells in the anterior pituitary. CG is produced by the placenta only in primates and horses. GnRH stimulates pituitary gonadotropin production, which is further regulated by feedback effects of the gonadal hormones (Figure 42–6; see Figure 44–2 and Chapters 44 and 45). TSH is measured in the diagnosis of thyroid disorders, and recombinant TSH (thyrotropin alfa) is used in the evaluation and treatment of well-differentiated thyroid cancer (see Chapter 43).

Structure-Function Aspects of the Gonadotropins

Each gonadotropic hormone is a glycosylated heterodimer containing a common α subunit and a distinct β subunit that confers specificity of action (see Table 42–2). The heterogeneity of glycosylation on the subunits produces myriad isoforms of these hormones and may affect receptor binding and signal transduction; terminal sialate residues seem to increase plasma half-lives of these gonadotropins (Mullen et al., 2013). Among the gonadotropin β subunits, that of CG is most divergent because it contains a carboxy-terminal extension of 30 amino acids and extra carbohydrate residues that prolong its $t_{1/2}$. The longer $t_{1/2}$ of hCG has some clinical relevance for its use in assisted reproduction technologies.

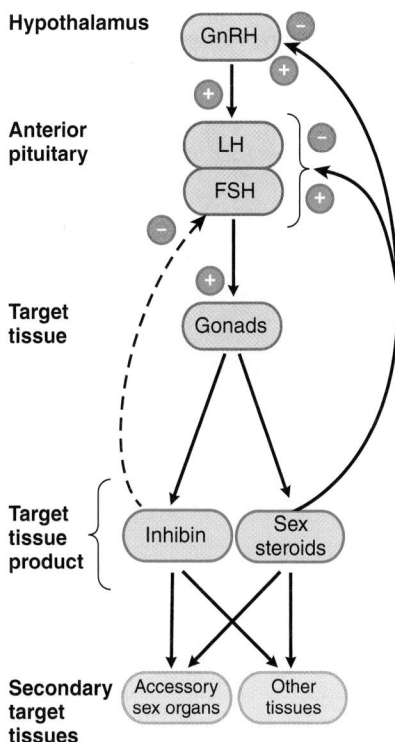

Figure 42–6 *The hypothalamic-pituitary-gonadal axis.* A single hypothalamic-releasing factor, GnRH, controls the synthesis and release of both gonadotropins (LH and FSH) in males and females. Gonadal steroid hormones (androgens, estrogens, and progesterone) exert feedback inhibition at the level of the pituitary and the hypothalamus. However, these feedback effects are dependent on sex, concentration, and time; the preovulatory surge of estrogen also can exert a stimulatory effect at the level of the pituitary and the hypothalamus. Inhibins, a family of polypeptide hormones produced by the gonads, specifically inhibit FSH secretion by the pituitary.

Physiology of the Gonadotropins

In men, LH acts on testicular Leydig cells to stimulate the de novo synthesis of androgens, primarily *testosterone*, from cholesterol. FSH acts on the Sertoli cells to stimulate the production of proteins and nutrients required for sperm maturation. In women, the actions of FSH and LH are more complex. FSH stimulates the growth of developing ovarian follicles and induces the expression of LH receptors on theca and granulosa cells. FSH also regulates the expression of aromatase in granulosa cells, thereby stimulating the production of *estradiol*. LH acts on the theca cells to stimulate the de novo synthesis of *androstenedione*, the major precursor of ovarian estrogens in premenopausal women (see Figure 44–1). LH also is required for the rupture of the dominant follicle during ovulation and for the synthesis of progesterone by the corpus luteum.

Regulation of Gonadotropin Synthesis and Secretion

The predominant regulator of gonadotropin synthesis and secretion is the hypothalamic peptide GnRH, a decapeptide with blocked amino and carboxyl termini derived by proteolytic cleavage of a precursor peptide with 92 amino acids.

Gonadotropin-releasing hormone release is pulsatile and is governed by a hypothalamic neural pulse generator (primarily in the arcuate nucleus) that controls the frequency and amplitude of GnRH release. Shortly before puberty, CNS inhibition decreases and the amplitude and frequency of GnRH pulses increase, particularly during sleep. As puberty progresses, the GnRH pulses increase further in amplitude and frequency until the normal adult pattern is established. The intermittent release of GnRH is crucial for the proper synthesis and release of the gonadotropins; the continuous administration of GnRH leads to desensitization and downregulation of GnRH receptors on pituitary gonadotropes.

Molecular and Cellular Bases of GnRH Action.
GnRH signals through a specific GPCR on gonadotropes that activates the $G_{q/11}$-PLC-IP$_3$-Ca^{2+} pathway (see Chapter 3), resulting in increased synthesis and secretion of LH and FSH. Although cAMP is not the major mediator of GnRH action, binding of GnRH to its receptor also increases adenylyl cyclase activity. GnRH receptors also are present in the ovary, testis, and other sites, where their physiological significance remains to be determined.

Other Regulators of Gonadotropin Production.
Gonadal steroids regulate gonadotropin production at the level of the pituitary and the hypothalamus, but effects on the hypothalamus predominate (see Figure 42–6). The feedback effects of gonadal steroids are dependent on sex, concentration, and time. In women, low levels of estradiol and progesterone inhibit gonadotropin production, largely through opioid action on the neural pulse generator. Higher and more sustained levels of estradiol have positive-feedback effects that ultimately result in the gonadotropin surge that triggers ovulation. In men, testosterone inhibits gonadotropin production, in part through direct actions and in part via its conversion by aromatase to estradiol. Gonadotropin production also is regulated by the *inhibins*, which are members of the bone morphogenetic protein family of secreted signaling proteins. *Inhibin A and B* are made by granulosa cells in the ovary and Sertoli cells in the testis in response to the gonadotropins and local growth factors. They act directly in the pituitary to inhibit FSH secretion without affecting that of LH. Inhibin A exhibits variation during the menstrual cycle, suggesting that it acts as a dynamic regulator of FSH secretion.

Molecular and Cellular Bases of Gonadotropin Action

The actions of LH and hCG on target tissues are mediated by the LH receptor; those of FSH are mediated by the FSH receptor. The FSH and LH receptors couple to G_s to activate the adenylyl cyclase–cAMP pathway. At higher ligand concentrations, the agonist-occupied gonadotropin receptors also activate PKC and Ca^{2+} signaling pathways via G_q-mediated effects on PLC$_\beta$. Most actions of the gonadotropins can be mimicked by cAMP analogues.

Clinical Disorders of the Hypothalamic-Pituitary-Gonadal Axis

Clinical disorders of the hypothalamic-pituitary-gonadal axis can manifest either as alterations in levels and effects of sex steroids (hyper- or hypogonadism) or as impaired reproduction. This section focuses on those conditions that specifically affect the hypothalamic-pituitary components of the axis and those for which gonadotropins are used diagnostically or therapeutically.

Deficient sex steroid production resulting from hypothalamic or pituitary defects is termed *hypogonadotropic hypogonadism* because circulating levels of gonadotropins are either low or undetectable. Hypogonadotropic hypogonadism in some patients results from GnRH receptor mutations; some of these mutations impair targeting of the GnRH receptor to the plasma membrane of gonadotropes, prompting efforts to develop pharmacological strategies to correct receptor trafficking and restore function (Conn et al., 2007). Many other disorders can impair gonadotropin secretion, including pituitary tumors, genetic disorders such as Kallmann syndrome, infiltrative processes such as sarcoidosis, and functional disorders such as exercise-induced amenorrhea.

In contrast, reproductive disorders caused by processes that directly impair gonadal function are termed *hypergonadotropic* because the impaired production of sex steroids leads to a loss of negative-feedback inhibition, thereby increasing the synthesis and secretion of gonadotropins.

- **Precocious Puberty.** Puberty normally is a sequential process requiring several years over which the GnRH neurons escape CNS inhibition and initiate pulsatile secretion of GnRH. This stimulates the secretion of gonadotropins and gonadal steroids, thus directing the development of secondary sexual characteristics appropriate for sex. Normally, the initial signs of puberty (breast development in girls and testes enlargement in boys) do not occur before age 8 in girls or age 9 in boys; the initiation of sexual maturation before this time is termed "precocious." GnRH-dependent excessive secretion of gonadotropins is rare and causes precocious puberty in children. This condition may be due to GnRH-producing hamartomas or other CNS abnormalities, but often no specific abnormality is found. This central precocious puberty must be

differentiated from that due to hormone-producing tumors of the gonads, in which case gonadotropin levels will be low. GnRH-independent precocious puberty results from peripheral production of sex steroids in a manner not driven by pituitary gonadotropins; etiologies include adrenal or gonadal tumors, activating mutations of the LH receptor in boys, and congenital adrenal hyperplasia. Synthetic GnRH analogues play important roles in the diagnosis and treatment of GnRH-dependent precocious puberty (see further discussion). In contrast, drugs that interfere with the production of sex steroids, including ketoconazole and aromatase inhibitors, are used in patients with GnRH-independent precocious puberty (Shulman et al., 2008), with varying success.

- **Sexual Infantilism.** The converse of precocious puberty is a failure to initiate the processes of pubertal development at the normal time. This can reflect defects in the GnRH neurons or gonadotropes (secondary hypogonadism) or primary dysfunction in the gonads. In either case, induction of sexual maturation using sex steroids (estrogen followed by estrogen/progesterone in females, testosterone in males) is standard therapy. This suffices to direct sex differentiation in the normal manner. If fertility is the goal, then therapy with either GnRH or gonadotropins is needed to stimulate appropriate germ cell maturation.

- **Infertility.** Infertility, or a failure to conceive after 12 months of unprotected intercourse, is seen in up to 10%–15% of couples and is increasing in frequency as women choose to delay childbearing. When the infertility is due to impaired synthesis or secretion of gonadotropins (hypogonadotropic hypogonadism), various pharmacological approaches are employed. In contrast, when infertility results from intrinsic processes affecting the gonads, pharmacotherapy generally is less effective. Therapeutic approaches to male infertility are described further in this chapter; strategies for female infertility are described in Chapter 44.

Treatment and Diagnosis of Gonadal Disorders

GnRH and Its Synthetic Agonist Analogues

A synthetic peptide comprising the native sequence of GnRH has been used both diagnostically and therapeutically in human reproductive disorders. In addition, a number of GnRH analogues with structural modifications have been synthesized and brought to market (Table 42–3).

TABLE 42–3 ■ STRUCTURES OF GONADOTROPIN-RELEASING HORMONE AND GNRH ANALOGUES

GNRH CONGENER	AMINO ACID RESIDUE										DOSAGE FORMS
	1	2	3	4	5	6	7	8	9	10	
Agonists											
GnRH	PyroGlu	His	Trp	Ser	Tyr	Gly	Leu	Arg	Pro	Gly-NH$_2$	IV, SC
Goserelin	—	—	—	—	—	D-Ser(tBu)	—	—	—	AzGly-NH$_2$	SC implant
Nafarelin	—	—	—	—	—	D-Nal	—	—	—	—	IN
Triptorelin	—	—	—	—	—	D-Trp	—	—	—	—	IM depot
Buserelin[a]	—	—	—	—	—	D-Ser(tBu)	—	—	Pro-NHEt		IN, SC
Deslorelin[a]	—	—	—	—	—	D-Trp	—	—	Pro-NHEt		IM, SC, depot
Histrelin	—	—	—	—	—	D-His(Bzl)	—	—	Pro-NHEt		SC implant
Leuprolide	—	—	—	—	—	D-Leu	—	—	Pro-NHEt		IM, SC, depot
Antagonists											
Cetrorelix	Ac-D-Nal	D-Cpa	D-Pal	—	—	D-Cit	—	—	—	D-Ala-NH$_2$	SC
Degarelix	AC-D-Nal	D-Cpa	D-Pal	—	D-Aph(L-Hor)	D-Aph(Cbm)	—	Lys(iPr)	—	D-Ala-NH$_2$	SC
Ganirelix	Ac-D-Nal	D-Cpa	D-Pal	—	—	D-hArg(Et)$_2$	—	D-hArg(Et)$_2$	—	D-Ala-NH$_2$	SC

Ac, acetyl; Aph, aminophenyl alanine; Bzl, benzyl; AzGly, azaglycyl; Cbm, carbamoyl; Cpa, chlorophenylalanyl; D-Nal, 3-(2-naphthyl)-D-alanyl; EtNH$_2$, *N*-ethylamide; hArg(Et)$_2$, ethyl homoarginine; Hor, hydroorotyl; Lys(iPr), isopropyl-lysyl; Pal, 3-pyridylalanyl; tBu, t butyl. A dash (—) denotes amino acid identity with GnRH. IM, intramuscular; IN, intranasal; IV, intravenous; SC, subcutaneous.

[a]Not available in the U.S.

GnRH Congeners

Synthetic agonist congeners of GnRH have longer half-lives than native GnRH. After a transient stimulation of gonadotropin secretion, they downregulate the GnRH receptor and inhibit gonadotropin secretion. The available GnRH agonists contain substitutions of the native sequence at position 6 that protect against proteolysis and substitutions at the carboxyl terminus that improve receptor-binding affinity. Compared to GnRH, these analogues exhibit enhanced potency and prolonged duration of action (Table 42–3).

Pharmacokinetics. The myriad formulations of GnRH agonists provide for diverse applications, including relatively short-term effects (e.g., assisted reproduction technology) and more prolonged action (e.g., depot forms that inhibit gonadotropin secretion in GnRH-dependent precocious puberty). The rates and extents of absorption thus vary considerably. The intranasal formulations have bioavailability (~4%) that is considerably lower than that of the parenteral formulations, which include products for implantation and injection (subcutaneous and intramuscular).

Clinical Uses. The depot form of the GnRH agonist leuprolide has been used diagnostically to differentiate between GnRH-dependent and GnRH-independent precocious puberty. Leuprolide depot (3.75 mg) is injected subcutaneously, and serum LH is measured 2 h later. A plasma LH level of more than 6.6 mIU/mL is diagnostic of GnRH-dependent (central) disease. Clinically, the various GnRH agonists are used to achieve pharmacological castration in disorders that respond to reduction in gonadal steroids (Fuqua, 2013). A clear indication is in children with GnRH-dependent precocious puberty, whose premature sexual maturation can be arrested with minimal side effects by chronic administration of a depot form of a GnRH agonist (Li et al., 2014).

Long-acting GnRH agonists are used for palliative therapy of hormone-responsive tumors (e.g., prostate or breast cancer), generally in conjunction with agents that block steroid biosynthesis or action to avoid transient increases in hormone levels (see Chapters 46 and 68). The GnRH agonists also are used to suppress steroid-responsive conditions such as endometriosis, uterine fibroids, acute intermittent porphyria, and priapism. They also have been evaluated off label for their potential to preserve follicles in women undergoing therapy with cytotoxic drugs for cancer treatment, although efficacy in this setting has not been established. Depot preparations can be administered subcutaneously or intramuscularly monthly or every 3 months. The long-lasting GnRH agonists have been used to avoid a premature LH surge, and thus ovulation, in various ovarian stimulation protocols for in vitro fertilization.

Adverse Effects. The long-acting agonists generally are well tolerated, and side effects are those that would be predicted to occur when gonadal steroidogenesis is inhibited (e.g., hot flashes and decreased bone density in both sexes, vaginal dryness and atrophy in women, and erectile dysfunction in men). Because of these effects, therapy in non–life-threatening diseases such as endometriosis or uterine fibroids generally is limited to 6 months. GnRH agonists are contraindicated in pregnant women.

Formulations and Indications. **Leuprolide.** Leuprolide is formulated in multiple doses for injection: subcutaneous (1 mg/d), subcutaneous depot (7.5 mg/month; 22.5 mg/3 months; 30 mg/4 months; 45 mg/6 months), and intramuscular depot (3.75 mg/month; 11.25 mg/3 months). It is approved for endometriosis, uterine fibroids, advanced prostate cancer, and precocious puberty. For endometriosis, leuprolide once-monthly injections (3.75 mg) or 3-month injections (11.25 mg) are also copackaged in combination with once-daily norethindrone (a steroidal progestin) 5-mg tablets for oral administration. Pediatric formulations of leuprolide also are approved for central precocious puberty.

Goserelin. Goserelin is formulated as a subcutaneous implant (3.6 mg/month; 10.8 mg/12 weeks). It is approved for endometriosis, for use as an endometrial-thinning agent prior to endometrial ablation for dysfunctional uterine bleeding, and for advanced prostate and breast cancer.

Histrelin. Histrelin is formulated as a subcutaneous implant (50 mg/12 months). It is approved for central precocious puberty and advanced prostate cancer.

Nafarelin. Nafarelin is formulated as a nasal spray (200 μg/spray). It is approved for endometriosis (400 μg/d) and central precocious puberty (1600 μg/d).

Triptorelin. Triptorelin is formulated for depot intramuscular injection (3.75 mg/month; 11.25 mg/12 weeks, 22.5 mg/24 weeks) and approved for advanced prostate cancer. *Buserelin* and *deslorelin* are not available in the U.S.

GnRH Antagonist Analogues

Ganirelix and Cetrorelix. Ganirelix acetate and cetrorelix acetate are FDA-approved to suppress the LH surge and thus prevent premature ovulation in ovarian-stimulation protocols as part of assisted reproduction technology (see Chapter 44).

Both GnRH antagonists are formulated for subcutaneous administration. Bioavailability exceeds 90% within 1–2 h, and the $t_{1/2}$ varies depending on the dose. Once-daily administration suffices for therapeutic effect. Hypersensitivity reactions, including anaphylaxis, have been noted in postmarketing surveillance, some with the initial dose. When used in conjunction with gonadotropin injections for assisted reproduction, the effects of estrogen withdrawal (e.g., hot flashes) are not seen. GnRH antagonists are contraindicated in pregnant women.

Cetrorelix is also used off label for endometriosis and uterine fibroids, both of which are estrogen dependent. As antagonists rather than agonists, these drugs do not transiently increase gonadotropin secretion and sex steroid biosynthesis.

Degarelix. Degarelix acetate is FDA-approved for treatment of advanced prostate cancer. Degarelix suppresses testosterone levels to 50 ng/dL or less (i.e., medical castration) and lowers prostate-specific antigen more rapidly than GnRH agonists without an initial testosterone surge (Shore, 2013).

ADME. Degarelix forms a depot gel at the site of injection and, as a consequence, is released in a biphasic pattern with a median plasma $t_{1/2}$ of 42 days for the starting dose and 28 days for the maintenance dose. Degarelix is distributed throughout total body water, is 90% protein bound, and is degraded by proteolysis via the hepatobiliary system; degraded protein fragments are eliminated in the feces, and unmetabolized drug is eliminated via the kidneys.

Adverse Effects. Adverse effects include injection site reactions, hot flashes, weight gain, increases in transaminase and γ-glutamyltransaminase levels, prolonged QT interval, and decreased bone mineral density.

Dosage and Route of Administration. Degarelix is administered subcutaneously in the abdomen, with the site of injection varied on a regular basis. The starting dose is 240 mg administered as two injections of 120 mg on each side of the abdomen, followed by a maintenance dose of 80 mg every 28 days.

Natural and Recombinant Gonadotropins

The gonadotropins are used for both diagnosis and therapy in reproductive endocrinology. For further discussion of the uses of gonadotropins in female reproduction, see Chapter 44.

The original gonadotropin preparations for clinical therapy were prepared from human urine and included *chorionic gonadotropin*, obtained from the urine of pregnant women, and *menotropins*, obtained from the urine of postmenopausal women. Because of their relatively low purity, these gonadotropins were administered intramuscularly to decrease the incidence of hypersensitivity reactions. Subsequently, urine-derived preparations were developed with sufficient purity to be administered subcutaneously. Highly purified preparations of human gonadotropins now are prepared using recombinant DNA technology and exhibit less batch-to-batch variation. This technology is being used to produce forms of gonadotropins with increased half-lives or higher clinical efficacy. One such "designer" gonadotropin, FSH-CTP, contains the β subunit of FSH fused to the carboxy-terminal extension of hCG, thereby increasing considerably the $t_{1/2}$ of the recombinant protein. In clinical trials, FSH-CTP has been shown to stimulate follicle maturation in vivo when injected weekly (Macklin et al., 2006).

Preparations

Follicle-Stimulating Hormone

Follicle-stimulating hormone has long been a mainstay of regimens for either ovarian stimulation or in vitro fertilization. The original *menotropins* formulations contained roughly equal amounts of FSH and LH, as well as a number of other urinary proteins, and were administered intramuscularly to diminish local reactions. *Urofollitropin*, prepared by immunoconcentration of FSH with monoclonal antibodies, is pure enough to be administered subcutaneously. The amount of LH contained in such preparations is diminished considerably.

Recombinant FSH is prepared by expressing cDNAs encoding the α and β subunits of human FSH in mammalian cell lines, yielding products whose glycosylation pattern mimics that of FSH produced by gonadotropes. The two available recombinant FSH preparations, *follitropin alfa* and *follitropin beta*, differ slightly in their carbohydrate structures: Both are more pure and exhibit less interbatch variability than do preparations purified from urine; thus, they can be administered subcutaneously. The relative advantages (i.e., efficacy, lower frequency of side effects such as ovarian hyperstimulation) of recombinant FSH versus urine-derived gonadotropins have not been definitively established (van Wely et al., 2011).

Human Chorionic Gonadotropin

The hCG used clinically originally came from the urine of pregnant women. Several urine-derived preparations are available; all of them are administered intramuscularly due to local reactions. Recombinant hCG (choriogonadotropin alfa) also is used clinically.

Recombinant Human LH

Menotropins contain considerable LH activity, thereby providing any LH activity that is needed to promote follicle maturation. Traditionally, LH was not used for ovulation induction because hCG produced identical effects via the LH receptor and had a longer $t_{1/2}$. Human LH produced using recombinant DNA technology and designated lutropin alfa has been discontinued from the U.S. market but is available elsewhere.

Diagnostic Uses

Pregnancy Testing

During pregnancy, the placenta produces significant amounts of hCG, which can be detected in maternal urine. Over-the-counter pregnancy kits containing antibodies specific for the unique β subunit of hCG qualitatively assay for the presence of hCG and can detect pregnancy within a few days after a woman's first missed menstrual period. Quantitative measurements of plasma hCG concentration by radioimmunoassay can indicate whether pregnancy is proceeding normally and can help to detect the presence of an ectopic pregnancy, hydatidiform mole, or choriocarcinoma. Such assays also are used to follow the therapeutic response of malignancies that secrete hCG, such as germ cell tumors.

Timing of Ovulation

Ovulation occurs about 36 h after the onset of the LH surge. Therefore, urinary concentrations of LH, as measured with an over-the-counter radioimmunoassay kit, can be used to predict the time of ovulation. Urine LH levels are measured every 12–24 h, beginning on day 10–12 of the menstrual cycle (assuming a 28-day cycle), to detect the rise in LH and estimate the time of ovulation. This estimate facilitates the timing of sexual intercourse to optimize the chance of achieving pregnancy.

Localization of Endocrine Disease

Measurements of plasma LH and FSH levels with β-subunit–specific radioimmunoassays are useful in the diagnosis of several reproductive disorders. Low or undetectable levels of LH and FSH are indicative of hypogonadotropic hypogonadism and suggest hypothalamic or pituitary disease, whereas high levels of gonadotropins suggest primary gonadal diseases. A plasma FSH level of 10–12 mIU/mL or greater on day 3 of the menstrual cycle is associated with reduced fertility. Elevated FSH levels also are diagnostic of menopause in women with amenorrhea in the appropriate age range.

Human CG can be used to stimulate testosterone production and thus to assess Leydig cell function in males suspected of having primary hypogonadism (e.g., in delayed puberty). A diminished response to multiple injections of hCG indicates Leydig cell failure; a normal response suggests a hypothalamic-pituitary disorder and normal Leydig cells.

Therapeutic Uses

Male Infertility

In men with impaired fertility secondary to gonadotropin deficiency (hypogonadotropic hypogonadism), gonadotropins can establish or restore fertility (Farhat et al., 2010). Treatment typically is initiated with hCG (1500–2000 IU intramuscularly or subcutaneously) three times per week until the plasma testosterone levels indicate full induction of steroidogenesis. Thereafter, the dose of hCG is reduced to 2000 IU twice a week or 1000 IU three times a week. If spermatogenesis does not occur with hCG alone, then recombinant FSH (typical dose of 150 IU) is added to fully induce spermatogenesis.

The most common side effect of gonadotropin therapy in males is gynecomastia, which occurs in up to a third of patients and presumably reflects increased production of estrogens due to the induction of aromatase. Maturation of the prepubertal testes typically requires treatment for more than 6 months, and optimal spermatogenesis in some patients may require treatment for up to 2 years. Once spermatogenesis has been initiated, ongoing treatment with hCG alone usually is sufficient to support sperm production.

Cryptorchidism

Cryptorchidism, the failure of one or both testes to descend into the scrotum, affects up to 3% of full-term male infants and becomes less prevalent with advancing postnatal age. Cryptorchid testes have defective spermatogenesis and are at increased risk for developing germ cell tumors. Hence, the current approach is to reposition the testes as early as possible, typically at 1 year of age but definitely before 2 years of age. The local actions of androgens stimulate descent of the testes; thus, hCG has been used by some to induce testicular descent if the cryptorchidism is not secondary to anatomical blockage. Therapy usually consists of injections of hCG (3000 IU/m² body surface area) intramuscularly every other day for six doses.

Posterior Pituitary Hormones: Oxytocin and Vasopressin

The neurohypophyseal hormones oxytocin and arginine vasopressin (also called antidiuretic hormone or ADH) are cyclic nonapeptides that differ by only two amino acids (Figure 42–7). The physiology and pharmacology of vasopressin are presented in Chapter 25.

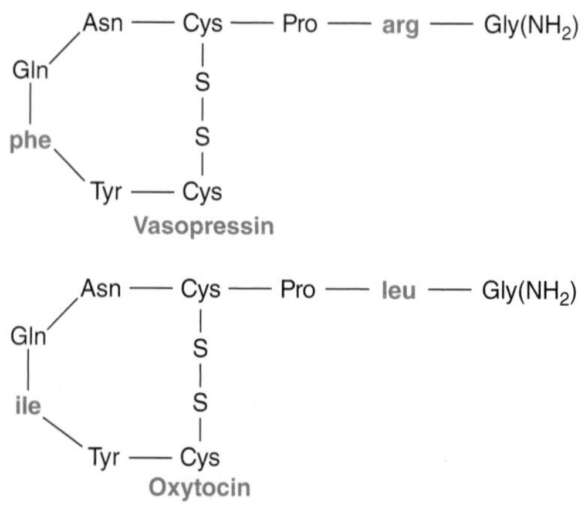

Figure 42–7 *The structures of vasopressin and oxytocin.* Vasopressin and oxytocin are cyclic nonapeptides that differ from each other by two amino acids (red).

Physiology of Oxytocin

Oxytocin is synthesized as a larger precursor in neurons whose cell bodies reside in the paraventricular nucleus and, to a lesser extent, the supraoptic nucleus in the hypothalamus. The precursor peptide is rapidly cleaved to the active hormone and its neurophysin, packaged into secretory granules as an oxytocin-neurophysin complex, and secreted from nerve endings that terminate primarily in the posterior pituitary gland (neurohypophysis). In addition, oxytocinergic neurons that regulate the autonomic nervous system project to regions of the hypothalamus, brainstem, and spinal cord. Other sites of oxytocin synthesis include the luteal cells of the ovary, the endometrium, and the placenta, but the physiologic significance of this is not known. Oxytocin acts via a specific GPCR (OXTR) closely related to the V_{1a} and V_2 vasopressin receptors. In the human myometrium, OXTR couples to G_q/G_{11}, activating the PLC_β-IP_3-Ca^{2+} pathway and enhancing activation of voltage-sensitive Ca^{2+} channels, stimulating muscle contraction (Figure 42–8). Oxytocin also increases local prostaglandin production, which further stimulates uterine contraction.

Stimuli for oxytocin secretion include sensory stimuli arising from dilation of the cervix and vagina and from suckling at the breast. Increases in circulating oxytocin in women in labor are difficult to detect, partly because of the pulsatile nature of oxytocin secretion and partly because of the activity of circulating oxytocinase. Nevertheless, increased oxytocin in maternal circulation is detected in the second stage of labor, likely triggered by sustained distension of the uterine cervix and vagina.

Estradiol stimulates oxytocin secretion, whereas the ovarian polypeptide *relaxin* inhibits its release. The inhibitory effect of relaxin appears to be the net result of a direct effect on oxytocin-producing cells and an inhibitory action mediated indirectly by endogenous opiates. Other factors that primarily affect vasopressin secretion also have some impact on oxytocin release: Ethanol inhibits release; pain, dehydration, hemorrhage, and hypovolemia stimulate release. Although peripheral actions of oxytocin appear to play no significant role in the response to dehydration,

hemorrhage, or hypovolemia, oxytocin may participate in the central regulation of blood pressure. Pharmacological doses of oxytocin can inhibit free water clearance by the kidney through arginine vasopressin-like activity at vasopressin V_2 receptors. As judged by the effects of intravenously administered oxytocin during labor induction, the plasma $t_{1/2}$ of oxytocin is about 13 min.

Sites of Oxytocin Action

Uterus

During the third trimester of pregnancy, spontaneous motor activity increases progressively until the sharp rise that constitutes the initiation of labor. Oxytocin stimulates the frequency and force of uterine contractions. Uterine responsiveness to oxytocin roughly parallels this increase in spontaneous activity and is highly dependent on estrogen, which increases the expression of the OXTRs.

Because of difficulties associated with the measurement of oxytocin levels and because loss of pituitary oxytocin apparently does not compromise labor and delivery, the physiological role of oxytocin in pregnancy is debated. Exogenous oxytocin can enhance rhythmic contractions at any time, but an 8-fold increase in uterine sensitivity to oxytocin occurs in the last half of pregnancy and is accompanied by a 30-fold increase in OXTR numbers. Progesterone antagonizes the stimulatory effect of oxytocin in vitro, and refractoriness to progesterone in late pregnancy may contribute to the normal initiation of human parturition.

Breast

Oxytocin plays an important physiological role in milk ejection. Stimulation of the breast through suckling or mechanical manipulation induces oxytocin secretion, causing contraction of the myoepithelium that surrounds alveolar channels in the mammary gland. This action forces milk from the alveolar channels into large collecting sinuses, where it is available to the suckling infant.

SECTION V HORMONES AND HORMONE ANTAGONISTS

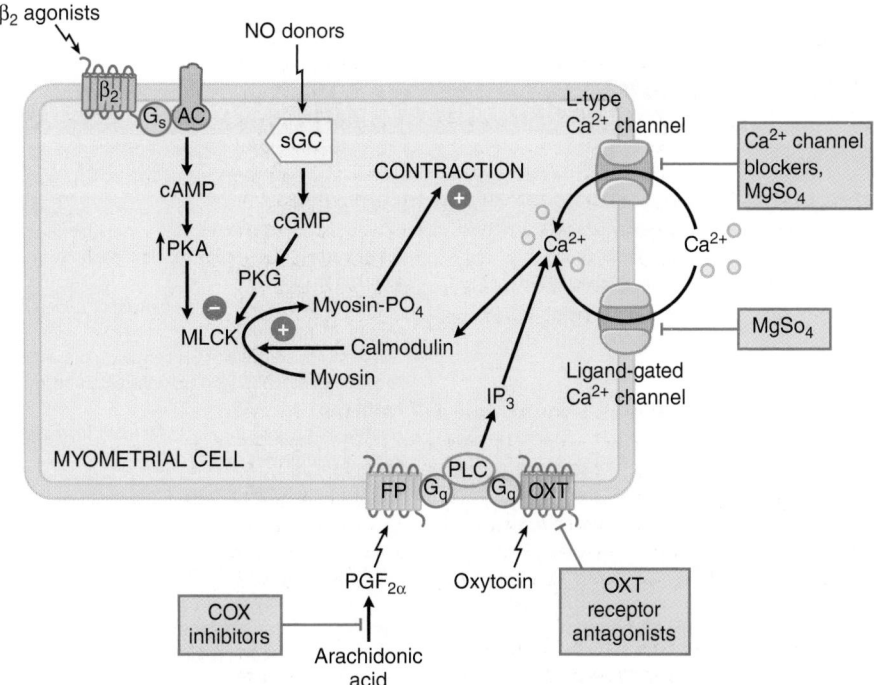

Figure 42–8 *Sites of action of oxytocin and tocolytic drugs in the uterine myometrium.* The elevation of cellular Ca^{2+} promotes contraction via the Ca^{2+}/calmodulin–dependent activation of myosin light chain kinase (MLCK). Relaxation is promoted by the elevation of cyclic nucleotides (cAMP and cGMP) and their activation of protein kinases, which cause phosphorylation/inactivation of MLCK. Pharmacological manipulations to reduce myometrial contraction include the following: (1) inhibiting Ca^{2+} entry (Ca^{2+} channel blockers, Mg_2SO_4); (2) reducing mobilization of intracellular Ca^{2+} by antagonizing GPCR-mediated activation of the G_q-PLC-IP_3-Ca^{2+}pathway (with antagonists of the FP and OXT receptors) or reducing production of the FP agonist $PGF_{2\alpha}$ (with COX inhibitors); and (3) enhancing relaxation by elevating cellular cAMP (with β_2 adrenergic agonists that activate G_s-AC) and cGMP (with NO donors that stimulate soluble guanylyl cyclase).

Brain

Studies in rodents have implicated oxytocin as an important CNS regulator of trust and of autonomic systems linked to anxiety and fear, but its importance in humans in this regard remains to be established.

Brain regions proposed to be critical in the response to fearful stimuli, including the amygdala, midbrain, and striatum, showed decreased activation in response to stressful stimuli following oxytocin treatment (Baumgartner et al., 2008; Huber et al., 2005). The role of perturbations of oxytocin signaling in mental conditions such as social phobia and autism and the possible therapeutic benefit of drugs that manipulate CNS oxytocin effects are exciting areas of ongoing investigation (Romano et al., 2016).

Clinical Use of Oxytocin

Oxytocin is used therapeutically only to induce or augment labor and to treat or prevent postpartum hemorrhage. Although widely used, oxytocin recently was added to a list of drugs "bearing a heightened risk of harm." In the U.S., the FDA-approved label contains this notice:

> Elective induction of labor is defined as the initiation of labor in a pregnant individual who has no medical indications for induction. Since the available data are inadequate to evaluate the benefits-to-risks considerations, Pitocin is not indicated for elective induction of labor.

Induction of Labor

Induction of labor is indicated when the perceived risk of continued pregnancy to the mother or fetus exceeds the risks of pharmacological induction. Oxytocin is the drug of choice for induction of labor for women with a suitably ripened cervix (see Chapter 37 for a discussion of prostaglandins in cervical ripening). It is administered by intravenous infusion of a diluted solution, has a $t_{1/2}$ of 12–15 min and achieves a steady-state uterine response after about 30 min. Both a high-dose protocol (starting with an infusion of 6 mU/min) and low-dose protocols (starting with an infusion dose of 0.5–2 mU/min) have been used

(American College of Obstetricians and Gynecologists, 2009). Uterine hyperstimulation is an adverse effect of oxytocin that should be avoided. Oxytocin at high doses activates the vasopressin V_2 receptor and has antidiuretic effects. Vasodilating actions of oxytocin also have been noted that may provoke hypotension and reflex tachycardia. Deep anesthesia may exaggerate the hypotensive effect of oxytocin by preventing the reflex tachycardia.

Augmentation of Dysfunctional Labor

Oxytocin also is used when spontaneous labor is not progressing at an acceptable rate. To augment hypotonic contractions, an infusion rate of 10 mU/min typically is sufficient. As with labor induction, potential complications of uterine overstimulation include trauma of the mother or fetus due to forced passage through an incompletely dilated cervix, uterine rupture, and compromised fetal oxygenation due to decreased uterine perfusion.

Prevention and Treatment of Postpartum Hemorrhage

Oxytocin (10 units IM) is given immediately after delivery to help maintain uterine contractions and tone. Alternatively, oxytocin (20 units) is diluted in 1 L of intravenous solution (yielding a concentration of 20 mU/mL) and infused at a rate of 10 mU/min until the uterus is contracted. The infusion rate then is reduced to 1–2 mU/min until the mother is ready for transfer to the postpartum unit.

Tocolytic Therapy for Established Preterm Labor

Inhibition of uterine contractions of preterm labor, or *tocolysis*, has been a focus of therapy (Figure 42–8). Although tocolytic agents delay delivery in ~80% of women, they neither prevent premature births nor improve adverse fetal outcomes, such as respiratory distress syndrome. Specific tocolytic agents include β adrenergic receptor agonists, $MgSO_4$, Ca^{2+} channel blockers, COX inhibitors, NO donors, and the oxytocin receptor antagonist *atosiban*. Atosiban is widely used in Europe but is not FDA-approved in the U.S. Chapter 44 presents additional information on tocolytic therapy.

Acknowledgment: Keith L. Parker contributed to this chapter in recent editions of this book. We have retained some of his text in the current edition.

Drug Facts for Your Personal Formulary: *Pituitary-Related Drugs*

Drugs	Therapeutic Uses	Clinical Pharmacology and Tips
Pituitary Hormones (Recombinant)		
Growth hormone (somatropin)	• Stimulating growth in childhood • In GH-deficient adults, replacing GH	• Given by daily SC injection to stimulate body growth, primarily through stimulation of IGF-1. As growth ceases, test for GH deficiency to determine if GH should be continued into adulthood. • Given only to adults with GH deficiency proven by GH stimulation tests or known organic childhood GH deficiency and low IGF-1 levels on testing off GH treatment. • Treatment in adults decreases fat mass, increases muscle mass, increases bone mass, and improves quality of life.
Oxytocin	• Augmentation of labor • Management of postpartum hemorrhage	• Administered by intravenous infusion. • Hyperstimulating the uterus should be avoided during augmentation of labor. • May provoke hypotension and reflex tachycardia.
Other Peptide Hormones		
Human chorionic gonadotropin	• Testing of Leydig cell function • Male infertility • Cryptorchidism in children	• Stimulates LH receptor, causing increased testicular testosterone production. • Induces testicular descent in children with cryptorchidism.
Tesamorelin	• Treatment of HIV-associated lipodystrophy	• N-Terminally modified version of human GHRH with primary effect of reducing visceral and other body fat in patients with HIV lipodystrophy.
Insulinlike growth factor 1 (mecasermin)	• Treatment of children with mutations in the GH receptor or transduction mechanisms mediating GH action or IGF-1 gene defects	• Adverse effects include hypoglycemia and lipohypertrophy.

Other Peptide Hormones (continued)

Gonadotropin-releasing hormone agonist analogues • Goserelin • Histrelin • Leuprolide • Nafarelin • Triptorelin	• Endometriosis • Diagnosis and treatment of precocious puberty • Palliative treatment of hormone-responsive tumors (prostate and breast cancer)	• Prolonged stimulation of the GnRH receptor by analogues results in downregulation of those receptors with decreased gonadotropin secretion.
Gonadotropin-releasing hormone antagonist analogues • Ganirelix • Cetrorelix • Degarelix	• Suppression of gonadotropin secretion and used in conjunction with exogenous gonadotropins for assisted reproduction • Palliative treatment of advanced prostate cancer (degarelix)	• Antagonism at the GnRH receptor results in decreased gonadotropin secretion without initial LH surge as seen with agonist analogues.

Somatostatin Analogues: Act on somatostatin receptors to reduce hormone secretion

Octreotide	• Acromegaly	• Long-acting release form is the standard type; given monthly.
Lanreotide	• Acromegaly	• Long-acting release form is the only available standard type; given monthly.
Pasireotide	• Acromegaly • Cushing disease	• Short-acting subcutaneous form is the only version FDA-approved for Cushing disease. • LAR form given monthly is the only version FDA-approved for acromegaly. • Additional adverse effects include significant hyperglycemia in many patients.

Dopamine Agonists: Act on dopamine receptors (D_2) to decrease prolactin secretion and prolactinoma size

Bromocriptine	• Treatment of hyperprolactinemia • Reduction in size of prolactinomas • Treatment of Parkinson disease	• An ergot derivative that has to be given one or more times daily. • Common adverse effects include nausea, vomiting, headache, and postural hypotension.
Cabergoline	• Treatment of hyperprolactinemia • Reduction in size of prolactinomas • Parkinson disease • Acromegaly	• A long-acting ergot derivative given once or twice weekly. • Has greater efficacy and tolerability than bromocriptine and may be active in patients who do not respond to bromocriptine. • At high doses used in patients with Parkinson disease; it cross reacts at the $5HT_{2B}$ receptor, causing cardiac valve abnormalities (not seen when used for patients with prolactinomas).
Quinagolide	• Treatment of hyperprolactinemia • Reduction in size of prolactinomas	• Not available in the U.S.

Hormone Receptor Blockers

Pegvisomant	• Treatment of acromegaly	• Blocks GH receptor and thus the activity of high GH levels and the generation of IGF-1 in acromegaly. Given by subcutaneous injections daily alone or weekly in combination with somatostatin analogues.

Bibliography

American College of Obstetricians and Gynecologists. ACOG Practice Bulletin No. 107: induction of labor. *Obstet Gynecol*, **2009**, *114*:386–397.

Baumgartner T, et al. Oxytocin shapes the neural circuitry of trust and trust adaptation in humans. *Neuron*, **2008**, *58*:639–650.

Bernard V, et al. New insights in prolactin: pathological implications. *Nat Rev Endocrinol*, **2015**, *11*:265–275.

Chia DJ. Minireview: mechanisms of growth hormone-mediated gene regulation. *Mol Endocrinol*, **2014**, *28*:1012–1025.

Cohen J, et al. Managing the child with severe primary insulin-like growth factor-1 deficiency (IGFD): IGFD diagnosis and management. *Drugs R D*, **2014**, *14*:25–29.

Conn PM, et al. G protein-coupled receptor trafficking in health and disease: lessons learned to prepare for therapeutic mutant rescue in vivo. *Pharmacol Rev*, **2007**, *59*:225–250.

Ergun-Longmire B, Wajnrajch M. Growth and growth disorders [updated 2013 May 22]. In: De Groot LJ, Beck-Peccoz P, Dungan K, et al., eds. *Endotext* [online]. MDText.com, South Dartmouth, MA, **2000**.

Farhat R, et al. Outcome of gonadotropin therapy for male infertility due to hypogonadotrophic hypogonadism. *Pituitary*, **2010**, *13*:105–110.

Flores-Morales A, et al. Negative regulation of growth hormone receptor signaling. *Mol Endocrinol*, **2006**, *20*:241–253.

Fuqua JS. Treatment and outcomes of precocious puberty: an update. *J Clin Endocrinol Metab*, **2013**, *98*:2198–2207.

Grant M, et al. Cell growth inhibition and functioning of human somatostatin receptor type 2 are modulated by receptor heterodimerization. *Mol Endocrinol*, **2008**, *22*:2278–2292.

Huber D, et al. Vasopressin and oxytocin excite distinct neuronal populations in the central amygdala. *Science*, **2005**, *308*:245–248.

Katznelson L, et al. Endocrine Society. Acromegaly: an Endocrine Society clinical practice guideline. *J Clin Endocrinol Metab*, **2014**, *99*:3933–3951.

Li P, et al. Gonadotropin releasing hormone agonist treatment to increase final stature in children with precocious puberty: a meta-analysis. *Medicine*, **2014**, *93*:e260.

Lim DS, Fleseriu M. The role of combination medical therapy in the treatment of acromegaly. *Pituitary*, **2017**, *20*:136–148.

Macklin NS, et al. The science behind 25 years of ovarian stimulation. *Endocr Rev*, **2006**, *27*:170–207.

Melmed S, et al. Endocrine Society. Diagnosis and treatment of hyperprolactinemia: an Endocrine Society clinical practice guideline. *J Clin Endocrinol Metab*, **2011**, *96*:273–288.

Molitch ME, et al. Endocrine Society. Evaluation and treatment of adult growth hormone deficiency: an Endocrine Society clinical practice guideline. *J Clin Endocrinol Metab*, **2011**, *96*:1587–1609.

Mullen MP, et al. Structural and functional roles of FSH and LH as glycoproteins regulating reproduction in mammalian species. In: Vizcarra J, ed. *Gonadotropin*. InTech, Rijeka, Croatia, **2013**, 155–180. doi:10.5772/2918. Accessed June 2, 2017.

SECTION V · HORMONES AND HORMONE ANTAGONISTS

786 Nass R, et al. The role of ghrelin in GH secretion and GH disorders. *Mol Cell Endocrinol*, **2011**, *340*:10–14.

Richmond E, Rogol AD. Current indications for growth hormone therapy for children and adolescents. *Endocr Dev*, **2010**, *18*:92–108.

Romano A, et al. From autism to eating disorders and more: the role of oxytocin in neuropsychiatric disorders. *Front Neurosci*, **2016**, *9*:497. doi:10.3389/fnins.2015.00497.

Shore ND. Experience with degarelix in the treatment of prostate cancer. *Ther Adv Urol*, **2013**, *5*:11–24.

Shulman DI et al. Use of aromatase inhibitors in children and adolescents with disorders of growth and adolescent development. *Pediatrics*, **2008**, *121*:e975–e983.

Spooner LM, Olin JL. Tesamorelin: a growth hormone-releasing factor analogue for HIV-associated lipodystrophy. *Ann Pharmacother*, **2012**, *46*:240–247.

Van Wely M, et al. Recombinant versus urinary gonadotrophin for ovarian stimulation in assisted reproductive technology cycles. *Cochrane Database Syst Rev*, **2011**, (2):CD005354. doi:10.1002/14651858. CD005354.pub2.

Walenkamp MJE, Wit JM. Single gene mutations causing SGA. *Best Pract Res Clin Endocrinol Metab*, **2008**, *22*:433–446.

Chapter 43

Thyroid and Antithyroid Drugs

Gregory A. Brent and Ronald J. Koenig

Thyroid hormone is essential for normal development, especially of the CNS. In the adult, thyroid hormone maintains metabolic homeostasis and influences the functions of virtually all organ systems. Thyroid hormone contains iodine, which must be supplied by nutritional intake. The thyroid gland contains large stores of thyroid hormone in the form of *thyroglobulin*. These stores maintain adequate systemic concentrations of thyroid hormone despite significant variations in iodine availability and nutritional intake. The thyroidal secretion is predominantly the prohormone T_4, which is converted in the liver and other tissues to supply the plasma with the active form, T_3. Local activation of T_4 also occurs in target tissues (e.g., brain and pituitary) and is increasingly recognized as an important regulatory step in thyroid hormone action. Similarly, local deactivation of T_3 is an important regulatory step. Serum concentrations of thyroid hormones are precisely regulated by the pituitary hormone *TSH* in a negative-feedback system. The predominant actions of thyroid hormone are mediated via nuclear TRs that modulate the transcription of specific genes.

Overt *hyperthyroidism* and *hypothyroidism*, thyroid hormone excess and deficiency, respectively, are associated with numerous clinical manifestations. Milder disease often has a subtler clinical presentation and may be identified based solely on abnormal biochemical tests of thyroid function. Maternal and neonatal hypothyroidism, due to iodine deficiency, remains a major preventable cause of mental retardation worldwide (Zimmermann, 2009). Treatment of the hypothyroid patient consists of thyroid hormone replacement (Biondi and Wartofsky, 2014). Treatments for hyperthyroidism include antithyroid drugs to decrease hormone synthesis and secretion, destruction of the gland by the administration of radioactive iodine, and surgical removal (Brent, 2008). In most patients, disorders of thyroid function can be either cured or controlled.

Likewise, thyroid malignancies are most often localized and resectable (Haugen and Sherman, 2013; Haugen et al., 2016). Metastatic disease often responds to radioiodine treatment but may become highly aggressive. Radioiodine-refractory, progressive thyroid cancers may respond to targeted chemotherapies such as tyrosine kinase inhibitors.

Thyroid Hormones

The thyroid gland produces two fundamentally different types of hormones. The thyroid follicle produces the iodothyronine hormones T_4 and T_3. The thyroid's parafollicular cells (C cells) produce *calcitonin*, a peptide with 32 amino acids that is not an important endogenous hormone but can be useful as a therapeutic agent in hypercalcemia and osteoporosis (see Chapter 48). Figures 43–1 and 43–2 show the structures of the thyroid hormones and their pathways of synthesis, storage, and release.

Chemistry of Thyroid Hormones

The principal hormones of the thyroid gland are the iodine-containing amino acid derivatives of thyronine (Figure 43–1). Following the isolation and the chemical identification of T_4, it was generally thought that all the hormonal activity of thyroid tissue could be accounted for by its content of T_4. However, careful studies revealed that crude thyroid preparations possessed greater calorigenic activity than could be accounted for by their T_4 content. The presence of a "second" thyroid hormone was debated, but T_3 was finally detected, isolated, and synthesized by Gross and Pitt-Rivers in 1952. T_3 has a much higher affinity for the nuclear TR compared with T_4 and is much more potent biologically on a molar basis. The subsequent demonstration of T_3 production from T_4 in athyreotic humans led to the practice of effective replacement in hypothyroidism with levothyroxine only.

Biosynthesis of Thyroid Hormones

The thyroid hormones are synthesized and stored as amino acid residues of *thyroglobulin*, a complex glycoprotein made up of two apparently identical subunits (330 kDa each) and constituting the vast majority of the thyroid follicular colloid. The thyroid gland is unique in storing great quantities of hormone precursor in this way, and extracellular thyroglobulin is proportional to the thyroid mass. The major steps in the synthesis,

Abbreviations

ADME: absorption, distribution, metabolism, excretion

Akt: protein kinase B

BAT: brown adipose tissue

CNS: central nervous system

CYP: cytochrome P450

D #: type # deiodinase, where # = 1, 2, or 3

DIT: diiodotyrosine

EOI: enzyme-linked species

ERK: extracellular signal-regulated kinase

FT$_4$: free thyroxine

HCN: hyperpolarization-activated, cyclic nucleotide–gated cation channel

HOI: hypoiodous acid

IP$_3$: inositol 1,4,5-trisphosphate

KISS: potassium iodide saturated solution

LDL: low-density lipoprotein

L-T$_3$: liothyronine

L-T$_4$: levothyroxine

MAP kinase: mitogen-activated protein kinase

MCT: monocarboxylic acid transporter

MHC: myosin heavy chain

MIT: monoiodotyrosine

MMI: methimazole

NIS: sodium iodide symporter

NO: nitric oxide

OATP1C1: solute carrier organic anion transporter family, member 1C1

PI3K: phosphoinositide 3-kinase

PKC: protein kinase C

PLC: phospholipase C

PTU: propylthiouracil

RAIU: radioactive iodine uptake

rT$_3$: 3,3′,5′-triiodothyronine, reverse T$_3$

SCN: thiocyanate

SECIS: selenocysteine insertion sequence

SST: somatostatin

T$_3$: 3,5,3′-triiodothyronine

T$_4$: thyroxine

TBG: thyroxine-binding globulin

Tetrac: tetraiodothyroacetic acid

Tg: thyroglobulin

T$_3$G: T$_3$ glucuronide

T$_4$G: T$_4$ glucuronide

T$_3$K: T$_3$ pyruvic acid

T$_4$K: T$_4$ pyruvic acid

TPO: thyroid peroxidase

TR: thyroid hormone receptor

TRH: thyrotropin-releasing hormone

Triac: triiodothyroacetic acid

T$_3$S: T$_3$ sulfate

T$_4$S: T$_4$ sulfate

TSH: thyroid-stimulating hormone, thyrotropin

---

storage, release, and interconversion of thyroid hormones are summarized in Figure 43–2 and described next.

Uptake of Iodide

Iodine ingested in the diet reaches the circulation in the form of iodide ion (I⁻). Normally, the I⁻ concentration in the blood is very low (0.2–0.4 μg/dL; ~ 15–30 nM). The thyroid actively transports the ion via

The thyroid is named for the Greek word for "shield shaped," from the shape of the nearby tracheal cartilage. The gland was first recognized as an organ of importance when thyroid enlargement was observed to be associated with changes in the eyes and heart in the condition we now call *hyperthyroidism*. Parry saw his first patient in 1786 but did not publish his findings until 1825. Graves reported the disorder in 1835, Basedow in 1840. Hypothyroidism was described later, in 1874, when Gull associated atrophy of the gland with the symptoms characteristic of *hypothyroidism*. The term *myxedema* was applied to the clinical syndrome in 1878 by Ord, in the belief that the characteristic thickening of the subcutaneous tissues was due to excessive formation of mucus. In 1891, Murray first treated a case of hypothyroidism by injecting an extract of sheep thyroid gland, later shown to be fully effective when given by mouth. The successful treatment of thyroid deficiency by administering thyroid extract was an important step toward modern endocrinology.

Extirpation experiments to elucidate the function of the thyroid were at first misinterpreted because of the simultaneous removal of the parathyroids. However, Gley's research on the parathyroid glands in the late 19th century allowed the functional differentiation of these two endocrine glands. The structure of parathyroid hormone, however, was not reported until the early 1970s. Calcitonin was discovered in 1961, demonstrating that the thyroid gland produced a second hormone.

---

a specific membrane-bound protein, termed the *NIS* (Kogai and Brent, 2012; Portulano et al., 2014). As a result, the ratio of [I⁻]$_{thyroid}$ to [I⁻]$_{plasma}$ is usually between 20 and 50 and can exceed 100 when the gland is stimulated. Iodide transport is inhibited by a number of ions, such as thiocyanate and perchlorate. TSH stimulates NIS gene expression and promotes insertion of NIS protein into the membrane in a functional configuration. Thus, decreased stores of thyroid iodine enhance iodide uptake, and the administration of iodide can reverse this situation by decreasing NIS protein expression. Iodine is accumulated by other tissues, including the salivary glands, gut, and lactating breast, and it is all mediated by a single NIS gene. Individuals with congenital NIS gene mutations have absent or defective iodine concentration in all tissues known to concentrate iodine.

Oxidation and Iodination

Transport of iodine from the thyroid follicular cell to the colloid is facilitated by the apical transporter *pendrin*. The oxidation of iodide to its active form is accomplished by *thyroid peroxidase*. The reaction results in the formation of MIT and DIT residues in thyroglobulin, a process referred to as *organification of iodine*, just prior to its extracellular storage in the lumen of the thyroid follicle.

Formation of Thyroxine and Triiodothyronine from Iodotyrosines

The remaining synthetic step is the coupling of two DIT residues to form T$_4$ or of an MIT and a DIT residue to form T$_3$. These oxidative reactions also are catalyzed by *thyroid peroxidase*. Intrathyroidal and secreted T$_3$ are also generated by the 5′-deiodination of T$_4$.

Synthesis and Secretion of Thyroid Hormones

Because T$_4$ and T$_3$ are synthesized and stored within thyroglobulin, proteolysis is an important part of the secretory process. This process is initiated by endocytosis of colloid from the follicular lumen at the apical surface of the cell, with the participation of a thyroglobulin receptor, *megalin*. This "ingested" thyroglobulin appears as intracellular colloid droplets, which apparently fuse with lysosomes containing the requisite proteolytic enzymes. TSH enhances the degradation of thyroglobulin by increasing the activity of lysisomal *thiol endopeptidases*, which selectively cleave thyroglobulin, yielding hormone-containing intermediates that subsequently are processed by exopeptidases. The liberated hormones then exit the cell

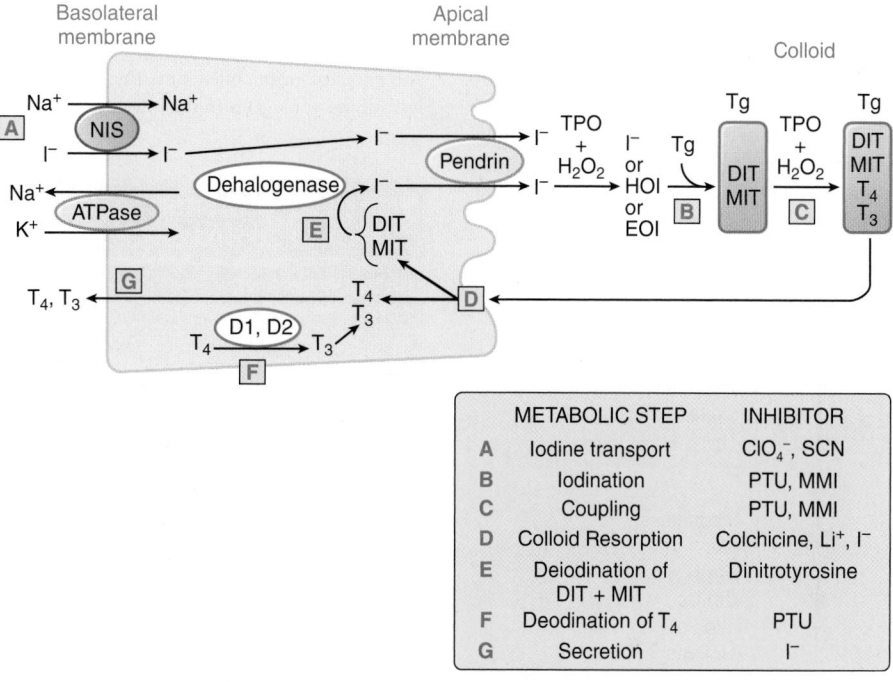

Figure 43–1 *Thyronine, thyroid hormones, and precursors.*

primarily as T_4 along with some T_3. The T_3 secreted by the thyroid derives partly from T_3 within mature thyroglobulin and partly from deiodination of T_4 (Figure 43–3), which also occurs peripherally (Figure 43–4).

Conversion of T_4 to T_3 in Peripheral Tissues

The normal daily production of T_4 is estimated to range between 80 and 100 µg; that of T_3 is between 30 and 40 µg. Although T_3 is secreted by the thyroid, metabolism of T_4 by 5′, or outer ring, deiodination in the peripheral tissues accounts for about 80% of circulating T_3 (Gereben et al., 2008). In contrast, removal of the iodine on position 5 of the inner ring produces the metabolically inactive 3,3′,5′-triiodothyronine (rT_3; Figure 43–3). Under normal conditions, about 40% of T_4 is converted to each of T_3 and rT_3, and about 20% is metabolized via other pathways, such as glucuronidation in the liver and excretion in the bile. Normal circulating concentrations of T_4 in plasma range from 4.5 to 11 µg/dL; those of T_3 are about 1/100 of that (60–180 ng/dL). T_3 has a much higher affinity for the nuclear TR compared with T_4 and is much more potent biologically on a molar basis.

There are three *iodothyronine deiodinases* (Marsili et al., 2011). Types 1 and 2 (D1, D2) convert T_4 to T_3. D1 is expressed primarily in the liver and kidney and also in the thyroid and pituitary (Figure 43–4). It is upregulated in hyperthyroidism, downregulated in hypothyroidism, and inhibited by the antithyroid drug *propylthiouracil*. D2 is expressed primarily in the CNS (including the pituitary and hypothalamus) and brown adipose tissue, also in the thyroid, and at low levels in skeletal muscle and other tissues. The activity of D2 is unaffected by propylthiouracil. D2 localizes to the endoplasmic reticulum, which facilitates access of D2-generated T_3 to the nucleus. Organs that express D2 use the locally generated T_3 in addition to plasma T_3 and therefore may have a relatively high fractional occupancy of TRs by T_3. T_4 induces ubiquitination and degradation of the D2 enzyme. This results in suppressed levels of D2 in hyperthyroidism and elevated levels in hypothyroidism, thus helping to maintain T_3 homeostasis. D3 catalyzes inner ring or 5-deiodination, the main inactivating pathway of T_3 metabolism; D1 performs this function to some extent. D3 is found at highest levels in the CNS and placenta and is also expressed in skin and uterus. D3 can be induced locally by inflammation and hypoxia and is highly expressed in certain tumors. Both D2 and D3 are expressed during development in time- and spatially-restricted patterns.

Figure 43–2 *Major pathways of thyroid hormone biosynthesis, storage as colloid, and release.*

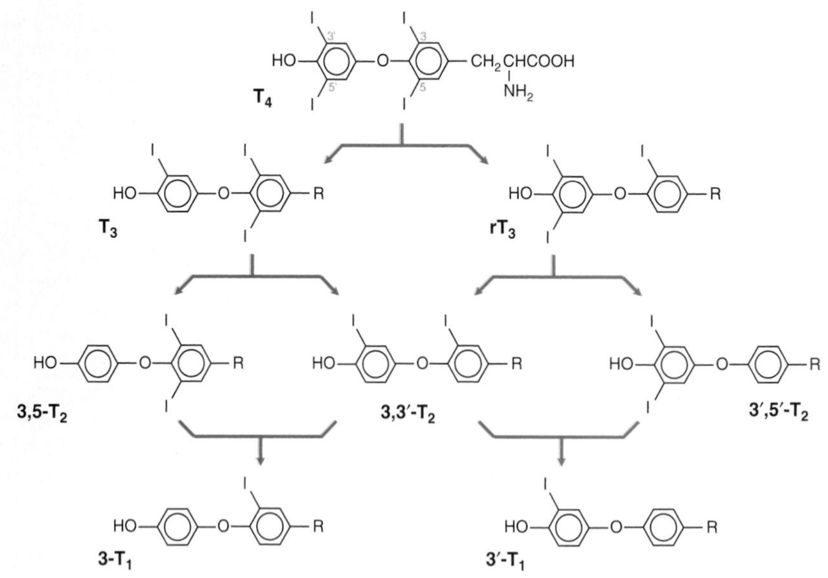

Figure 43–3 *Pathways of iodothyronine deiodination.*

The three deiodinases contain the rare amino acid *selenocysteine* in their active sites. Incorporation of selenocysteine into the growing peptide chain is a complex process involving multiple proteins. Mutations in one such protein, SECIS binding protein 2, are associated with abnormal circulating thyroid hormone levels (Dumitrescu et al., 2010).

Transport of Thyroid Hormones in the Blood

Iodine in the circulation is normally present in several forms, with 95% as organic iodine and about 5% as iodide. Most (90%–95%) organic iodine is T_4; T_3 represents a relatively minor fraction (~5%). The thyroid hormones are transported in the blood in strong but noncovalent association with several plasma proteins.

Thyroxine-binding globulin is the major carrier of thyroid hormones. It is a glycoprotein (mass of ~ 63,000 Da) that binds one molecule of T_4 per molecule of protein with a very high affinity (K_d, is ~ 10^{-10} M); T_3 is bound less avidly. T_4, but not T_3, also is bound by *transthyretin* (thyroxine-binding prealbumin), a retinol-binding protein. This protein is present in higher concentration than is TBG and binds T_4 with a K_d about 10^{-7} M. Albumin also can bind T_4 when the more avid carriers are saturated, but its physiological importance is unclear. Binding of thyroid hormones to plasma proteins protects the hormones from metabolism and excretion, resulting in their long half-lives in the circulation. The free (unbound) hormone is a small percentage (~0.03% of T_4 and ~ 0.3% of T_3) of the total hormone in plasma. The differential binding affinities for serum proteins also contribute to establishing the 10- to 100-fold differences in circulating hormone concentrations and half-lives of T_4 and T_3.

Essential to understanding the regulation of thyroid function is the "free hormone" concept: Only the unbound hormone has metabolic activity. Because of the high degree of binding of thyroid hormones to plasma proteins, changes in either the concentrations of these proteins or the affinities of the hormone-protein interactions have major effects on the total serum hormone levels. Certain drugs and a variety of pathological and physiological conditions can alter both the binding of thyroid hormones to plasma proteins and the amounts of these proteins (Table 43–1).

Degradation and Excretion of Thyroid Hormones

T_3 and T_4 not only can be deiodinated but also can be metabolized by ether cleavage, conjugation, and oxidative decarboxylation (Figure 43–5). T_4 is eliminated slowly from the body, with a $t_{1/2}$ of 6–8 days. In hyperthyroidism, the $t_{1/2}$ is shortened to 3–4 days, whereas in hypothyroidism it may be 9–10 days. In conditions associated with increased binding to TBG, such as pregnancy, clearance is retarded. The opposite effect is observed when binding to protein is inhibited by certain drugs (see Table 43–1). T_3, which is less avidly bound to protein, has a $t_{1/2}$ of about 1 day.

The liver is the major site of nondeiodinative degradation of thyroid hormones; T_4 and T_3 are conjugated with glucuronic and sulfuric acids and excreted in the bile. Some thyroid hormone is liberated by hydrolysis of the conjugates in the intestine and reabsorbed. A portion of the

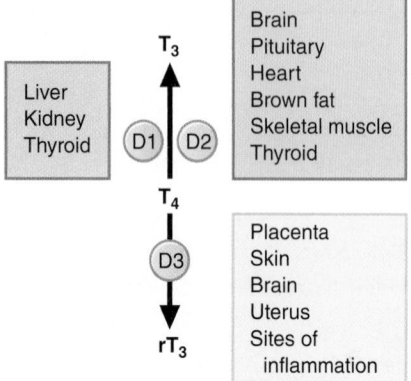

Figure 43–4 *Peripheral T4 → T3 conversion by deiodinase enzymes.*

TABLE 43–1 ■ FACTORS THAT ALTER BINDING OF THYROXINE TO THYROXINE-BINDING GLOBULIN	
INCREASE BINDING	**DECREASE BINDING**
Drugs	
Estrogens, tamoxifen	Corticosteroids, androgens
Selective estrogen receptor modulators	L-Asparaginase, furosemide
Methadone, heroin	Salicylates, mefenamic acid
Clofibrate, 5-fluorouracil	Antiseizure medications (phenytoin, carbamazepine)
Systemic factors	
Liver disease, porphyria	Acute and chronic illness
HIV infection	Inheritance
Inheritance	

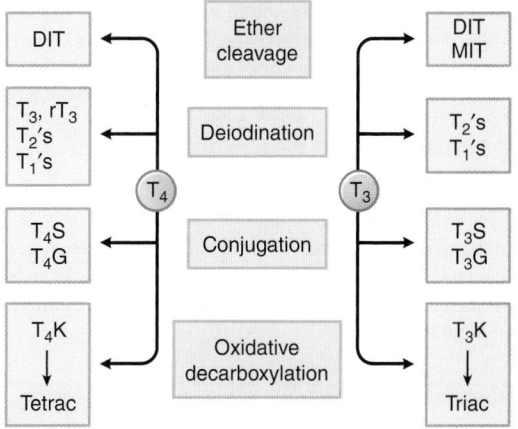

Figure 43–5 *Pathways of metabolism of T_4 and T_3.*

conjugated material reaches the colon unchanged, where it is hydrolyzed and eliminated in feces as the free compounds.

Factors Regulating Thyroid Hormone Secretion

Thyrotropin is a glycoprotein hormone that consists of an α subunit, common to pituitary glycoproteins such as gonadotropins, and a unique β subunit. TSH is secreted in a pulsatile manner and in a circadian pattern (levels are slightly higher during sleep at night) that is the inverse of the cortisol circadian pattern, reflecting the fact that cortisol reduces TSH secretion. TSH secretion is controlled by the hypothalamic peptide *TRH* and by the concentration of free thyroid hormones in the circulation. Increased thyroid hormone inhibits transcription of both the TRH gene and the genes encoding the α and β subunits of TSH, which suppresses the secretion of TSH and causes the thyroid to become inactive and regress. Any decrease in the normal rate of thyroid hormone secretion by the thyroid evokes an enhanced secretion of TSH. Additional mechanisms mediating the effect of thyroid hormone on TSH secretion appear to be a reduction in TRH secretion by the hypothalamus and a reduction in the number of TRH receptors on pituitary cells (Figure 43–6).

Thyrotropin-Releasing Hormone

Thyrotropin-releasing hormone stimulates the release of preformed TSH from secretory granules and also stimulates the subsequent synthesis of both α and β subunits of TSH. TRH is a tripeptide (L-pyroglutamyl-L-histidyl-L-proline amide) synthesized by the hypothalamus and released into the hypophyseal-portal circulation, where it interacts with TRH receptors on thyrotropes in the anterior pituitary. The binding of TRH to its receptor, a GPCR, stimulates the G_q-PLC-IP_3-Ca^{2+} pathway and activates PKC, ultimately stimulating the synthesis and release of TSH. Two TRH receptors have now been identified, TRH-R1 and TRH-R2, and there are receptor-selective TRH analogues. Somatostatin, dopamine, and glucocorticoids inhibit TRH-stimulated TSH secretion.

Actions of TSH on the Thyroid

Thyroid-stimulating hormone increases the synthesis and secretion of thyroid hormone. These effects follow the binding of TSH to its receptor (a GPCR) on the plasma membrane of thyroid cells. Binding of TSH to its receptor stimulates the G_s-adenylyl cyclase–cyclic AMP pathway. Higher concentrations of TSH activate the G_q-PLC pathway. Multiple mutations of the TSH receptor result in clinical thyroid dysfunction.

Iodine and Thyroid Function

Adequate iodine intake is essential for normal thyroid hormone production. When iodine intake is low, thyroid hormone production is reduced, TSH is secreted in excess, and the thyroid becomes hyperplastic and hypertrophic. The enlarged and stimulated thyroid becomes remarkably efficient at extracting the residual traces of iodide from the blood, developing an iodine gradient that may be 10 times normal; in mild-to-moderate iodine deficiency, the thyroid usually succeeds in producing sufficient hormone and preferentially secreting T_3. In more severe iodine deficiency,

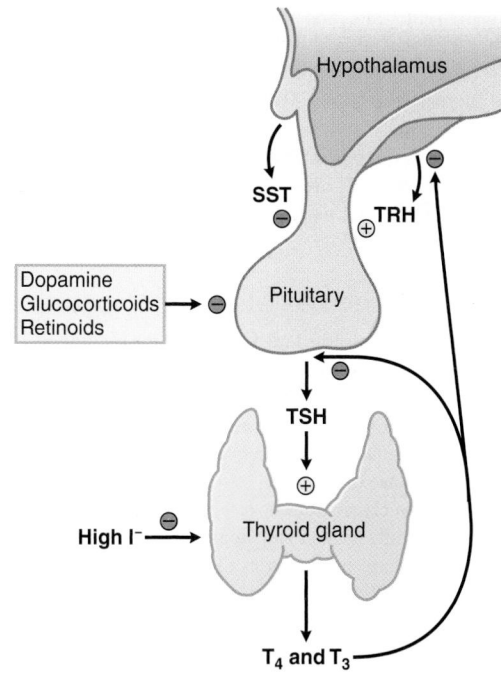

Figure 43–6 *Regulation of thyroid hormone secretion.* Myriad neural inputs influence hypothalamic secretion of TRH. TRH stimulates release of TSH from the anterior pituitary; TSH stimulates the synthesis and release of the thyroid hormones T_3 and T_4. T_3 and T_4 feed back to inhibit the synthesis and release of TRH and TSH. SST can inhibit TRH action, as can dopamine and high concentrations of glucocorticoids. Low levels of I^- are required for T_4 synthesis, but high levels inhibit T_4 synthesis and release.

adult hypothyroidism and cretinism may occur. High levels of iodine inhibit T_4 synthesis and release. In some areas of the world, simple or nontoxic goiter is prevalent because of insufficient dietary iodine. The addition of iodate to table salt (NaCl) provides a convenient iodine supplement. In the U.S., iodized salt provides 100 μg of iodine per gram. The recommended daily allowances for iodine range from 90 to 120 μg for children, 150 μg for adults, 220 μg for pregnancy, and 290 μg for lactation (Public Health Committee of the American Thyroid Association et al., 2006). Vegetables, meat, and poultry contain minimal amounts of iodine, whereas dairy products and fish are relatively high in iodine.

Iodized Salt

Iodine has been used empirically for the treatment of iodine-deficiency goiter for 150 years; however, its modern use evolved from extensive studies using iodine to prevent goiter in schoolchildren in Akron, Ohio, where endemic iodine-deficiency goiter was prevalent. The success of these experiments led to the adoption of iodine prophylaxis and therapy in many regions throughout the world where iodine-deficiency goiter was endemic. The most practical method for providing small supplements of iodine for large segments of the population is the addition of iodide or iodate to table salt; iodate is now preferred. The use of iodized salt is required by law in some countries, but in others, such as the U.S., the use is optional.

Transport of Thyroid Hormones Into and Out of Cells

The passage of thyroid hormones across the cell membrane is mediated by specific transporters, the most well-documented of which are two members of the SLC16A family of *MCTs*, MCTs 8 and 10 (Adijanto and Philip, 2012; van der Deure et al., 2010). MCT8 is widely expressed, including in liver, heart, and brain. MCT8 mutations cause Allan-Herndon-Dudley syndrome, characterized by neurodevelopmental defects that are likely due to impaired entry of T_4 and T_3 into the brain. MCT8 is also important for transport of T_4 out of the thyroid gland, which explains the finding of reduced serum T_4 concentration in patients with *Allan-Herndon-Dudley syndrome* (Bernal et al., 2015). MCT10 transports both T_4 and T_3 and is widely expressed, but its physiological importance for thyroid hormone transport in vivo is unknown. The organic anion transporter OATP1C1 preferentially transports T_4 over T_3 and is highly expressed in brain capillaries; in mice, OATP1C1 plays an important role in the transport of T_4 across the blood-brain barrier.

Mediation of Effects by Nuclear Receptors

Thyroid hormone action is mediated largely by the binding of T_3 to TRs, which are members of the nuclear receptor superfamily of transcription factors (Brent, 2012). This superfamily includes the receptors for steroid hormones, vitamin D, retinoic acid, a variety of small-molecule metabolites such as certain fatty acids and bile acids, and well as a number of "orphan receptors" (see Chapter 3).

The TRs have the classic nuclear receptor structure: an amino terminal domain, a centrally located zinc finger DNA-binding domain, and a ligand-binding domain that occupies the carboxyl terminal half of the protein. T_3 binds to TRs with about 10-fold greater affinity than does T_4, and T_4 is not thought to be biologically active in normal physiology. TRs bind to specific DNA sequences (thyroid hormone response elements) in the promoter/regulatory regions of target genes. The transcription of most target genes is repressed by unliganded TRs and induced in response to the binding of T_3. In the unliganded state, the TR ligand-binding domain interacts with a corepressor complex that includes *histone deacetylases* and other proteins. The binding of T_3 causes replacement of the corepressor complex by a coactivator complex that includes *histone acetyltransferases*, *methyltransferases*, and other proteins. Other thyroid hormone target genes, such as those encoding TRH and the TSH subunits, are negatively regulated by T_3. The mechanism is not well defined, but these genes tend to be induced by the unliganded TR in addition to being repressed by T_3.

Two genes encode TRs: *THRA* and *THRB*. *THRA* encodes the receptor TRα1. TRα1 is expressed in most cell types, but its major activities are in the regulation of heart rate, body temperature, skeletal muscle function, and the development of bone and small intestine. Patients with *THRA* mutations have been described with short stature, bony abnormalities, and chronic constipation, along with normal circulating TSH and low-normal T_4 levels, a syndrome termed *resistance to thyroid hormone alpha* (Refetoff et al., 2014; van Mullem et al., 2014).

The *THRB* gene has two promoters that lead to the production of TRβ1 and TRβ2. These receptors have unique amino terminal domains but otherwise are identical. TRβ1 is ubiquitous; TRβ2 has a highly restricted pattern of expression, including the pituitary and hypothalamus. TRβ1 mediates specific effects in liver metabolism (including the hypocholesterolemic effect of T_3); TRβ2 has roles in the negative feedback by T_3 on hypothalamic TRH and pituitary TSH and in the development of retinal cones and the inner ear. Mutations in *THRB* cause the syndrome of *resistance to thyroid hormone beta*. This syndrome is associated with goiter, tachycardia, impaired hearing, attention-deficit/hyperactivity disorder, and other abnormalities, and laboratory evaluation shows elevated levels of TSH, T_4, and T_3 (Refetoff, 1989).

Nongenomic Effects of Thyroid Hormone

Although nuclear receptors are generally thought of as DNA-binding transcription factors, nuclear receptors such as TRs also are found outside the nucleus where they can exert biological effects via rapid nongenomic mechanisms. A truncated form of TRα1 is palmitoylated and localizes to the plasma membrane, where it causes rapid T_3-dependent NO production as well as activation of ERK and Akt signaling (Kalyanaraman et al., 2014). Full-length TRα1 and TRβ1 reportedly associate in a T_3-dependent manner with the p85α subunit of PI3K, resulting in Akt activation (Hiroi et al., 2006). It is interesting to note that T_3 administration causes rapid vasodilation, which might be explained by the aforementioned generation of NO. There also is evidence for nongenomic actions of thyroid hormone

via a plasma membrane receptor within integrin αVβ3 (Lin et al., 2011). This putative receptor binds extracellular T_4 in preference to T_3, resulting in activation of MAP kinase. The importance of nongenomic actions in thyroid hormone physiology and pathophysiology remains uncertain.

Endogenous Thyroid Hormone–Related Compounds

3-Iodothyronamine and thyronamine are naturally occurring decarboxylated and deiodinated analogues of thyroid hormone that do not bind to TRs (Piehl et al., 2011). These compounds can serve as ligands for the GPCR trace amine–associated receptor 1, an interaction of unknown relevance in humans.

Major Clinical Effects of Thyroid Hormones

Growth and Development

Perhaps the most dramatic example of thyroid hormone action is amphibian metamorphosis, in which the tadpole is transmogrified into a frog by the actions of T_3. Not only does the animal grow limbs, lungs, and other terrestrial accoutrements, but also T_3 causes the tail to regress.

In humans, thyroid hormone plays a critical role in brain development by mechanisms that are incompletely understood (Abduljabbar and Afifi, 2012; Mayerl et al., 2014). The absence of thyroid hormone during the period of active neurogenesis (up to 6 months postpartum) leads to irreversible mental retardation (cretinism) and is accompanied by multiple morphological alterations in the brain. These severe morphological alterations result from disturbed neuronal migration, deranged axonal projections, and decreased synaptogenesis. Thyroid hormone supplementation begun during the first 2 weeks of postnatal life can prevent the development of these morphological changes. The actions of thyroid hormones are not limited to the brain; most tissues are affected by the administration of thyroid hormone or by its deficiency. The extensive defects in growth and development in cretins vividly illustrate the pervasive effects of thyroid hormones in normal individuals.

Cretinism is usually classified as *endemic* (caused by extreme iodine deficiency) or *sporadic* (a consequence of abnormal thyroid development or a defect in the synthesis of thyroid hormone). The affected child is dwarfed, with short extremities, mentally retardation, and listlessness. Other manifestations include puffy face, enlarged tongue, dry and doughy skin, slow heart rate, constipation, and decreased body temperature. For treatment to be fully effective, the diagnosis must be made shortly after birth and T_4 treatment initiated, long before these clinical manifestations are apparent. In regions of endemic iodine deficiency, iodine replacement is best instituted before pregnancy. Screening of newborn infants for deficient thyroid function is carried out in the U.S. and in most industrialized countries.

Thermogenic Effects

Thyroid hormone is necessary for both obligatory thermogenesis (the heat resulting from vital processes) and facultative or adaptive thermogenesis (Yehuda-Shnaidman et al., 2014). Only a few organs, including the brain, gonads, and spleen, are unresponsive to the thermogenic effects of T_3. Obligatory thermogenesis is the result of T_3 making most biological processes thermodynamically less efficient for the sake of producing heat. It is likely that multiple mechanisms contribute to this effect, such as the induction of futile cycling and changes in mitochondrial energetics, but the specific pathways involved and their quantitative contributions have yet to be fully defined. Although the induction by T_3 of uncoupling protein 1 is an important thermogenic mechanism in rodent brown adipose tissue, there is no convincing evidence that induction of uncoupling proteins plays a significant role in T_3-induced thermogenesis in other tissues (skeletal muscle, etc.). Regardless of the mechanism, thermogenesis is highly sensitive to thyroid hormone around the physiological range: Small changes in levothyroxine replacement doses may significantly alter resting energy expenditure in the hypothyroid patient. The capacity of

T_3 to stimulate thermogenesis has evolved along with ancillary effects to support this action, such as the stimulation of appetite and lipogenesis.

Cardiovascular Effects

Hyperthyroid patients have tachycardia, increased stroke volume, increased cardiac index, cardiac hypertrophy, decreased peripheral vascular resistance, and increased pulse pressure (Grais and Sowers, 2014). Hyperthyroidism is a relatively common cause of atrial fibrillation. Hypothyroid patients have bradycardia, decreased cardiac index, pericardial effusion, increased peripheral vascular resistance, decreased pulse pressure, and elevation of mean arterial pressure.

T_3 regulates myocardial gene expression primarily through TRα1, which is expressed at a higher level in cardiomyocytes than TRβ. T_3 shortens diastolic relaxation (lusitropic effect) by inducing expression of the sarcoplasmic reticulum ATPase SERCA2 and decreasing phospholamban, a SERCA2 inhibitor. T_3 increases the force of myocardial contraction (inotropic effect) in part by inducing expression of the ryanodine channel, the calcium channel of the sarcoplasmic reticulum (see Figure 29–6). T_3 induces the gene encoding the α isoform of MHC (MHCα) and decreases expression of the MHCβ gene. Because MHCα endows the myosin holoenzyme with greater ATPase activity, this is one mechanism by which T_3 enhances the velocity of contraction. The chronotropic effect of T_3 is mediated by increases in the pacemaker ion current I_f in the sinoatrial node (see Chapter 30). Several proteins that comprise the I_f channel are induced by T_3, including HCN2 and HCN4. T_3 also appears to have a direct nongenomic vasodilating effect on vascular smooth muscle, which may contribute to the decreased systemic vascular resistance and increased cardiac output of hyperthyroidism.

Metabolic Effects

Thyroid hormone stimulates the expression of hepatic LDL receptors and reduces apolipoprotein B levels through non-LDL receptor pathways (Goldberg et al., 2012; Mullur et al., 2014), such that hypercholesterolemia is a characteristic feature of hypothyroidism.

Thyroid hormone has complex effects on carbohydrate metabolism. Thyrotoxicosis is an insulin-resistant state. Postreceptor defects in the liver and peripheral tissues are manifested by depleted glycogen stores, enhanced gluconeogenesis, and an increase in the rate of glucose absorption from the gut. Compensatory increases in insulin secretion result in hyperinsulinemia. There may be impaired glucose tolerance or even diabetes, but the vast majority of hyperthyroid patients are euglycemic. Conversely, hypothyroidism results in decreased absorption of glucose from the gut, decreased insulin secretion, and a reduced rate of peripheral glucose uptake. Glucose metabolism generally is not affected in a clinically significant manner in nondiabetic hypothyroid patients, although insulin requirements may decrease in the hypothyroid patient with diabetes.

Disorders of Thyroid Function

Thyroid Hypofunction

Hypothyroidism, known as *myxedema* when severe, is the most common disorder of thyroid function. Worldwide, hypothyroidism resulting from iodine deficiency remains a common problem. In nonendemic areas where iodine is sufficient, chronic autoimmune thyroiditis (Hashimoto thyroiditis) accounts for most cases. This disorder is characterized by circulating antibodies directed against thyroid peroxidase and, sometimes, against thyroglobulin. These conditions are examples of *primary hypothyroidism,* failure of the thyroid gland itself. *Central hypothyroidism* occurs much less often and results from diminished stimulation of the thyroid by TSH because of pituitary failure (*secondary hypothyroidism*) or hypothalamic failure (*tertiary hypothyroidism*). Hypothyroidism present at birth (*congenital hypothyroidism*) is an important preventable cause of mental retardation in the world (Gruters and Krude, 2012).

Common symptoms of hypothyroidism include fatigue, lethargy, cold intolerance, mental slowness, depression, dry skin, constipation, mild

weight gain, fluid retention, muscle aches and stiffness, irregular menses, and infertility. Common signs include goiter (primary hypothyroidism only), bradycardia, delayed relaxation phase of the deep tendon reflexes, cool and dry skin, hypertension, nonpitting edema, and facial puffiness. Deficiency of thyroid hormone during the first few months of life causes feeding problems, failure to thrive, constipation, and sleepiness. Retardation of mental development is irreversible if not treated promptly. Childhood hypothyroidism impairs linear growth and bone maturation. Because the signs and symptoms of hypothyroidism are nonspecific, diagnosis requires the finding of an elevated serum TSH level and reduced or low-normal serum free T_4 or, in cases of central hypothyroidism, only a decreased serum free T_4.

Thyroid Hyperfunction

Thyrotoxicosis is a condition caused by elevated concentrations of circulating free thyroid hormones. Increased thyroid hormone production is the most common cause, with the common link of TSH receptor stimulation and increased iodine uptake by the thyroid gland, as established by the measurement of the percentage uptake of ^{123}I or ^{131}I in a 24-h RAIU test.

Thyroid-stimulating hormone receptor stimulation is either the result of TSH receptor stimulating antibodies in Graves disease or somatic activating TSH receptor mutations in autonomously functioning nodules or a toxic goiter. In contrast, thyroid inflammation or destruction resulting in excess "leak" of thyroid hormones or excess exogenous thyroid hormone intake results in a low 24-h RAIU test. The term *subclinical hyperthyroidism* is defined as those with a subnormal serum TSH and normal concentrations of free T_4 and T_3. Atrial arrhythmias, excess cardiac mortality, and excessive bone loss have been associated with this profile of thyroid function tests.

Graves disease is the most common cause of high RAIU thyrotoxicosis, accounting for 60%–90% of cases, depending on age and geographic region. Graves disease is an autoimmune disorder characterized by increased thyroid hormone production, diffuse goiter, and IgG antibodies that bind to and activate the TSH receptor. As with most types of thyroid dysfunction, women are affected more than men, with a ratio ranging from 5:1 to 7:1. Graves disease is more common between the ages of 20 and 50 but may occur at any age. Graves disease is commonly associated with other autoimmune diseases. The characteristic exophthalmos associated with Graves disease is an infiltrative ophthalmopathy and is considered an autoimmune-mediated inflammation of the periorbital connective tissue and extraocular muscles. Toxic uninodular/multinodular goiter accounts for 10%–40% of cases of hyperthyroidism and is more common in older patients. A low RAIU value is seen in the destructive thyroiditides and in thyrotoxicosis in patients taking excessive doses of thyroid hormone.

Most of the signs and symptoms of thyrotoxicosis stem from the excessive production of heat, increased motor activity, and increased sensitivity to catecholamines produced by the sympathetic nervous system. The skin is flushed, warm, and moist; the muscles are weak and tremulous; the heart rate is rapid, the heartbeat is forceful, and the arterial pulses are prominent and bounding. Increased expenditure of energy gives rise to increased appetite and, if intake is insufficient, to loss of weight. There also may be insomnia, difficulty in remaining still, anxiety and apprehension, intolerance to heat, and increased frequency of bowel movements. Angina, arrhythmias, and heart failure may be present in older patients. Older patients may experience less manifestations of sympathetic nervous system stimulation and reduced symptoms compared to younger individuals, sometimes referred to as "apathetic hyperthyroidism." Some individuals may show extensive muscular wasting as a result of thyroid myopathy. The most severe form of hyperthyroidism is thyroid storm (see section that follows on therapeutic uses of antithyroid drugs).

Thyroid Function Tests

Measurement of the total hormone concentration in plasma may not give an accurate picture of the activity of the thyroid gland; total hormone concentration changes with alterations in amount and affinity of TBG in plasma. Although equilibrium dialysis of undiluted serum and radioimmunoassay for FT_4 in the dialysate represent the gold standard for determining FT_4 concentrations, this assay is costly and typically unavailable in routine clinical laboratories. The most common assays used for estimating the free T_4 and free T_3 concentrations employ labeled analogues of these iodothyronines in chemiluminescence and enzyme-linked immunoassays. These assays are subject to influences of altered serum-binding proteins, nonthyroid disease states, acute illnesses, and other drugs. In individuals with normal pituitary function, serum measurement of TSH is the thyroid function test of choice because pituitary secretion of TSH is sensitively regulated in response to circulating concentrations of thyroid hormones. TSH is suppressed in patients with thyrotoxicosis and elevated in those with primary hypothyroidism, and these changes generally precede abnormalities in free T_4 and free T_3.

Therapeutic Uses of Thyroid Hormone

The major indications for the therapeutic use of thyroid hormone are for hormone replacement therapy in patients with hypothyroidism and for TSH suppression therapy in patients with thyroid cancer.

Thyroid Hormone Preparations

Synthetic preparations of the sodium salts of the natural isomers of the thyroid hormones are used for thyroid hormone therapy (Biondi and Wartofsky, 2014).

Levothyroxine

Levothyroxine sodium is available in tablets and liquid-filled capsules for oral administration and as a lyophilized powder for injection. Table 43–2 lists drugs and other factors that may influence levothyroxine dosage requirements. Absorption of levothyroxine occurs in the stomach and small intestine and is incomplete (~80% of the tablet dose is absorbed). Absorption

TABLE 43–2 ■ FACTORS INFLUENCING ORAL LEVOTHYROXINE THERAPY

Drugs and other factors that may increase levothyroxine dosage requirements

Impaired levothyroxine absorption

    Aluminum-containing antacids, proton pump inhibitors, sucralfate

    Bile acid sequestrants (cholestyramine, colestipol, colesevelam)

    Calcium carbonate (effect generally small), phosphate binders (lanthanum carbonate, sevelamer)

    Chromium picolinate, raloxifene, iron salts

    Food, soy products (effect generally very small), lactose intolerance (single case report)

Increased thyroxine metabolism, CYP3A4 induction

    Rifampin, carbamazepine, phenytoin, sertraline

Impaired $T_4 \rightarrow T_3$ conversion

    Amiodarone

Mechanisms uncertain or multifactorial

    Estrogen, pregnancy, lovastatin, simvastatin, ethionamide, Tyr kinase inhibitors

Drugs and other factors that may decrease levothyroxine dosage requirements

Advancing age (>65 years), androgen therapy in women

Drugs that may decrease TSH without changing free T_4 in levothyroxine-treated patients

Metformin

---

is slightly increased when the hormone is taken on an empty stomach, and it is associated with less variability in TSH levels when taken this way regularly (Bach-Huynh et al., 2009). Patients with gastrointestinal problems that result in poor absorption of tablet formulations may achieve better absorption with liquid-filled capsules (Vita et al., 2014). Serum T_4 peaks 2–4 h after oral ingestion, but changes are barely discernible with once-daily dosing due to the plasma $t_{1/2}$ of about 7 days. Given this long $t_{1/2}$, omission of one day's dose has only marginal effects on the serum TSH and free T_4, but to maintain consistent dosing, the patient should be instructed to take a double dose the next day. For any given serum TSH, the serum T_4/T_3 ratio is slightly higher in patients taking levothyroxine than in patients with endogenous thyroid function due to the fact that about 20% of circulating T_3 normally is supplied by direct thyroidal secretion (Gullo et al., 2011; Jonklaas et al., 2008). Follow-up blood tests typically are done about 6 weeks after any dosage change due to the 1-week plasma $t_{1/2}$ of T_4. If patients cannot take oral medications or intestinal absorption is in question, levothyroxine may be given intravenously once daily at a dose of about 80% of the patient's daily oral requirement.

Liothyronine

Liothyronine sodium is the salt of T_3 and is available in tablets and in an injectable form. Liothyronine absorption is nearly 100%, with peak serum levels 2–4 h following oral ingestion. Liothyronine may be used occasionally when a more rapid onset of action is desired, such as in the rare presentation of myxedema coma, or if rapid termination of action is desired, such as when preparing a patient with thyroid cancer for ^{131}I therapy. Liothyronine is less desirable for chronic replacement therapy due to the requirement for more-frequent dosing (plasma $t_{1/2}$ is 18–24 h), higher cost, and transient elevations of serum T_3 concentrations above the normal range. In addition, organs that express the D2 use the locally generated T_3 in addition to plasma T_3; hence, there is theoretical concern that these organs will not maintain physiological intracellular T_3 levels in the absence of plasma T_4. On a weight basis, the required daily dose of liothyronine (given three times a day to achieve steady serum T_3 levels) is about one-third that of L-T4 to achieve an equivalent TSH level in hypothyroid patients (Celi et al., 2011). However, normalization of circulating TSH results in an almost 2-fold higher serum T_3 compared with levothyroxine therapy because negative feedback on TSH normally relies in part on the local generation of T_3 from circulating T_4.

Other Preparations

A mixture of levothyroxine and T_3 around 4:1 by weight and desiccated thyroid preparations with a similar T_4:T_3 ratio also are available. A 60-mg (1-grain) desiccated thyroid tablet is approximately equivalent in activity to 80 μg of levothyroxine.

Thyroid Hormone Replacement Therapy in Hypothyroidism

Thyroxine is the hormone of choice for thyroid hormone replacement therapy due to its consistent potency and prolonged duration of action (Jonklaas et al., 2014). This therapy relies on D1 and D2 to convert T_4 to T_3 to maintain a steady serum level of free T_3.

The average daily adult full replacement dose of L-T_4 is 1.7 μg/kg body weight (0.8 μg/lb). Dosing should generally be based on lean body mass. The goal of therapy is to normalize the serum TSH (in primary hypothyroidism) or free T_4 (in secondary or tertiary hypothyroidism) and to relieve symptoms of hypothyroidism. In primary hypothyroidism, generally it is sufficient to follow TSH without free T_4. A patient with mild primary hypothyroidism will achieve a normal TSH with substantially less than a full replacement dose, but as the endogenous thyroid function declines, the dose will need to be increased. In individuals older than 60 years and those with known or suspected cardiac disease or with areas of autonomous thyroid function, institution of therapy at a subreplacement dose of L-T_4 (12.5–50 μg/d) is appropriate. The dose can be increased by 25 μg/d every 6 weeks until the TSH is normalized. The vast majority of controlled trials do not support the hypothesis that combination therapy with T_4 plus T_3 provides a better therapeutic response than does T_4 alone (Grozinsky-Glasberg et al., 2006), although for unclear reasons occasional patients say they feel better when taking combination therapies, such as desiccated thyroid. A double-blind crossover study of hypothyroid patients comparing levothyroxine and desiccated thyroid, maintaining the same reference range TSH, found that those who preferred desiccated thyroid had lost weight on this preparation (Hoang et al., 2013). Monotherapy with levothyroxine most closely mimics normal physiology and generally is preferred (Jonklaas et al., 2014).

Hypothyroidism During Pregnancy

Due to the increased serum concentration of TBG induced by estrogen, the expression of D3 by the placenta, and the small amount of transplacental passage of L-T_4 from mother to fetus, a higher dose of levothyroxine is usually required in pregnant patients. Overt hypothyroidism during pregnancy is associated with increased risk of miscarriage, fetal distress, preterm delivery, and impaired psychoneural and motor development in the progeny. Even mild maternal hypothyroidism may have subtle adverse effects. As part of prepregnancy planning, the dose of levothyroxine should be adjusted to maintain the TSH in the lower portion of the reference range. Women should increase their levothyroxine dose by about 30% as soon as pregnancy is confirmed, thus anticipating the increased need (Jonklaas et al., 2014). This can be achieved by taking two extra levothyroxine tablets per week. The serum TSH is measured in the first trimester, and the levothyroxine dose is further adjusted with the goal of maintaining the TSH in the lower portion of the reference range. Subsequent dosage adjustments are based on serum TSH, measured 4–6 weeks after each adjustment. TSH should be monitored periodically through to 20 weeks' gestation, when the dose adjustment is usually maximal, and then once between weeks 26 and 32 to confirm an adequate levothyroxine dose. The levothyroxine dose can be changed back to prepregnancy levels the day after delivery, with a follow-up TSH checked about 6 weeks later.

Isolated *hypothyroxinemia* during pregnancy, defined by a low serum free T4 concentration and normal serum TSH concentration, has been associated in a few studies with adverse neurocognitive development in the offspring. There are currently insufficient studies to recommend routine treatment of isolated hypothyroxinemia in pregnancy. Evaluation and treatment are further complicated by the influence of the elevated serum-binding proteins in pregnancy and lower values obtained for free T_4 by the analogue method, especially in the second and third trimesters. TSH remains the best test during pregnancy to evaluate thyroid status in pregnancy and response to treatment.

Myxedema Coma

Myxedema coma is a rare syndrome that represents the extreme expression of severe, long-standing hypothyroidism. Common precipitating factors include infection, congestive heart failure, and medical noncompliance. Myxedema coma occurs most often in elderly patients during the winter months. Cardinal features of myxedema coma are *hypothermia*, *respiratory depression*, and *decreased consciousness*.

Intravenous administration of thyroid hormone is advised (Jonklaas et al., 2014). Therapy with levothyroxine is begun with a loading dose of 200–400 μg followed by a daily full replacement dose. Some clinicians recommend adding liothyronine (10 μg intravenously followed by 2.5 to 10 μg every 8 h) until the patient is stable and conscious. Other important aspects of therapy include ventilatory support, passive warming with blankets, correction of hyponatremia, and treatment of the precipitating cause. Treatment with intravenous glucocorticoids is recommended until coexisting adrenal insufficiency is excluded.

Congenital Hypothyroidism

Success in the treatment of congenital hypothyroidism depends on the age at which therapy is started and the speed with which hypothyroidism is corrected. If therapy is instituted within the first 2 weeks of life, normal physical and mental development can be achieved (Gruters and Krude, 2012; Rose et al., 2006).

To rapidly normalize the serum T_4 concentration in the congenitally hypothyroid infant, an initial daily dose of levothyroxine of 10–15 μg/kg is recommended (Jonklaas et al., 2014; Leger et al., 2014). Because rapid normalization is even more important in infants with severe hypothyroidism,

doses on the higher side of the range mentioned are preferred in those infants. One published study found that brand-name and generic levothyroxine were not bioequivalent in infants with severe congenital hypothyroidism (Carswell et al., 2013), and this has led some experts to recommend against generic levothyroxine in this situation (Leger et al., 2014). The goal is to achieve a free T_4 in the upper half of the reference range and a TSH in the lower half, although some infants maintain a high TSH that seems to reflect mis-set feedback regulation. Laboratory evaluations of TSH and free T_4 are performed 2 and 4 weeks after treatment is initiated, every 1–2 months in the first 6 months, every 2–3 months between 6 months and 3 years of age, and every 6–12 months from age 3 years until the end of growth. Monitoring should be more frequent if the results are abnormal. Soy formula may impair levothyroxine absorption, necessitating a dosage increase.

Thyroid Hormone Replacement Therapy in Thyroid Cancer

The mainstays of therapy for well-differentiated thyroid cancer (papillary, follicular) are surgical thyroidectomy, radioiodine (discussed in material that follows), and levothyroxine to maintain a low TSH (Haugen et al, 2016). The rationale for TSH suppression is that TSH is a growth factor for thyroid cancer, but there are no randomized controlled trials that addressed the optimal TSH target range. A reasonable approach is to adjust the levothyroxine dose to maintain a low-normal TSH value in patients without persistent disease and at low risk for recurrence (Wang et al., 2015), a mildly subnormal TSH value (~0.1 mU/L) in patients at high risk for recurrence, and a more subnormal TSH level for patients with persistent disease. The benefits of TSH suppression need to be weighed against the risks, including osteoporosis and atrial fibrillation.

Thyroid Nodules

Nodular thyroid disease is the most common endocrinopathy. Thyroid nodules usually are asymptomatic, although they can cause neck discomfort, dysphagia, and a choking sensation. As with other forms of thyroid disease, nodules are more frequent in women. Exposure to ionizing radiation, especially in childhood, increases the rate of nodule development. Approximately 5% of thyroid nodules that come to medical attention are malignant. Most patients with thyroid nodules are euthyroid, which should be confirmed by TSH measurement. The most useful diagnostic procedures generally are ultrasound imaging and a fine-needle aspiration biopsy. The use of levothyroxine to suppress TSH in euthyroid individuals with thyroid nodules cannot be recommended as a general practice. However, if the TSH is elevated, it is appropriate to administer levothyroxine to bring the TSH into the lower portion of the reference range.

Adverse Effects of Thyroid Hormone

Adverse effects of thyroid hormone generally occur only on overtreatment and are similar to the consequences of hyperthyroidism. An excess of thyroid hormone can increase the risk of atrial fibrillation, especially in the elderly, and can increase the risk of osteoporosis, especially in postmenopausal women.

Antithyroid Drugs and Other Thyroid Inhibitors

Myriad compounds are capable of interfering, directly or indirectly, with the synthesis, release, or action of thyroid hormones (Tables 43–2 and 43–3). Several types are clinically useful:

- Antithyroid drugs, which interfere directly with the synthesis of thyroid hormones
- Ionic inhibitors, which block the iodide transport mechanism
- High concentrations of iodine, which decrease release of thyroid hormones from the gland and also may decrease hormone synthesis
- Radioactive iodine, which damages the thyroid gland with ionizing radiation

TABLE 43–3 ■ AGENTS THAT DISRUPT THYROID HORMONE SYNTHESIS, RELEASE, AND METABOLISM

MECHANISM	AGENT
Iodide uptake	Perchlorate, fluoroborate, thiocyanate, nitrate
Organification of iodine	Thionamides (propylthiouracil, methimazole, carbimazole), thiocyanate, sulfonamides
Coupling reaction	Sulfonamides, thionamides
Hormone release	Li$^+$ salts, iodide
Peripheral iodothyronine deiodination	Propylthiouracil, amiodarone, oral cholecystographic agents
Accelerated hepatic metabolism	Phenobarbital, rifampin, carbamazepine, phenytoin, sertraline, bexarotene

Adjuvant therapy with drugs that have no specific effects on thyroid hormone synthesis is useful in controlling the peripheral manifestations of thyrotoxicosis, including inhibitors of the peripheral deiodination of T$_4$ to T$_3$, β adrenergic receptor antagonists, and Ca^{2+} channel blockers.

Antithyroid Drugs

The antithyroid drugs with clinical utility are the *thioureylenes*, which belong to the family of thioamides. *Propylthiouracil* is the prototype (Figure 43–7).

HISTORICAL PERSPECTIVE

Studies on the mechanism of the development of goiter began with the observation that rabbits fed a diet composed largely of cabbage often developed goiters. This result was probably due to the presence of precursors of the thiocyanate ion in cabbage leaves. Later, two pure compounds were shown to produce goiter: sulfaguanidine, a sulfanilamide antimicrobial used to treat enteric infections, and phenylthiourea. Investigation of the effects of thiourea derivatives revealed that rats became hypothyroid despite hyperplastic changes in their thyroid glands that were characteristic of intense thyrotropic stimulation. After treatment was begun, no new hormone was made, and the goitrogen had no visible effect on the thyroid gland following hypophysectomy or the administration of thyroid hormone. This suggested that the goiter was a compensatory change resulting from the induced state of hypothyroidism and that the primary action of the compounds was to inhibit the formation of thyroid hormone. The therapeutic possibilities of such agents in hyperthyroidism were evident, and the substances so used became known as *antithyroid drugs*.

Mechanism of Action

Antithyroid drugs inhibit the formation of thyroid hormones by interfering with the incorporation of iodine into tyrosyl residues of thyroglobulin; they also inhibit the coupling of these iodotyrosyl residues to form iodothyronines (see Figure 43–2). These drugs are thought to inhibit the peroxidase enzyme. Inhibition of hormone synthesis results in the depletion of stores of iodinated thyroglobulin as the protein is hydrolyzed and the hormones are released into the circulation. In addition to blocking hormone synthesis, propylthiouracil partially inhibits the peripheral deiodination of T$_4$ to T$_3$. *Methimazole does not have this effect;* this provides a rationale for the choice of propylthiouracil over other antithyroid drugs in the treatment of severe hyperthyroid states or of thyroid storm (Angell et al., 2015).

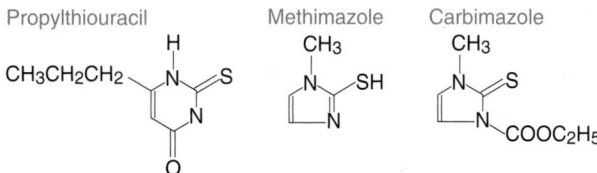

Figure 43–7 *Structures of antithyroid drugs of the thioamide type.*

ADME

The antithyroid compounds currently used in the U.S. are propylthiouracil (6-*n*-propylthiouracil) and methimazole (1-methyl-2-mercaptoimidazole). In Europe, carbimazole, a carbethoxy derivative of methimazole, is available, and its antithyroid action is due to its conversion to methimazole after absorption (Figure 43–7). Pharmacological properties of propylthiouracil and methimazole are shown in Table 43–4.

Absorption of effective amounts of propylthiouracil occurs within 20–30 min of an oral dose; the duration of action is brief. The effect of a dose of 100 mg of propylthiouracil begins to wane in 2–3 h; even a 500-mg dose is completely inhibitory for only 6–8 h. As little as 0.5 mg of methimazole similarly decreases the organification of radioactive iodine in the thyroid gland, but a single dose of 10–25 mg is needed to extend the inhibition to 24 h.

The $t_{1/2}$ of propylthiouracil in plasma is about 75 min; that of methimazole is 4–6 h. The drugs are concentrated in the thyroid, and methimazole, derived from the metabolism of carbimazole, accumulates after carbimazole is administered. Drugs and metabolites appear largely in the urine.

Therapeutic Uses

The antithyroid drugs are used in the treatment of hyperthyroidism in the following ways:

- As definitive treatment, to control the disorder in anticipation of a spontaneous remission in Graves disease
- In conjunction with radioactive iodine, to hasten recovery while awaiting the effects of radiation
- To control the disorder in preparation for surgical treatment

Methimazole is the drug of choice for Graves disease; it is effective when given as a single daily dose, has improved adherence, and is less toxic than propylthiouracil. Methimazole has a relatively long plasma and intrathyroidal $t_{1/2}$, as well as a long duration of action. The usual starting dose for methimazole is 15–40 mg per day. The usual starting dose of propylthiouracil is 100 mg every 8 h. When doses greater than 300 mg daily are

TABLE 43–4 ■ PHARMACOKINETIC FEATURES OF ANTITHYROID DRUGS

	PROPYLTHIOURACIL	METHIMAZOLE
Plasma protein binding	~75%	Nil
Plasma $t_{1/2}$	75 min	~4–6 h
Volume of distribution	~.0.4 L/kg	~0.7 L/kg
Concentrated in thyroid	Yes	Yes
Metabolism of drug during illness		
Severe liver disease	Normal	Decreased
Severe kidney disease	Normal	Normal
Dosing frequency	1–4 times daily	Once or twice daily
Transplacental passage	Low	Low
Levels in breast milk	Low	Low

needed, further subdivision of the time of administration to every 4–6 h is occasionally helpful. Once euthyroidism is achieved, usually within 12 weeks, the dose of antithyroid drug can be reduced, but not stopped, lest an exacerbation of Graves disease occur.

Response to Treatment

The thyrotoxic state usually improves within 3–6 weeks after the initiation of antithyroid drugs. The clinical response is related to the dose of antithyroid drug, the size of the goiter, and pretreatment serum T_3 concentration. The rate of response is determined by the quantity of stored hormone, the rate of turnover of hormone in the thyroid, the $t_{1/2}$ of the hormone in the periphery, and the completeness of the block in synthesis imposed by the dosage given. Hypothyroidism may develop as a result of overtreatment. After treatment is initiated, patients should be examined and thyroid function tests (serum FT_4 and total or free T_3 concentrations) measured every 2–4 months. Once euthyroidism is established, follow-up every 4–6 months is reasonable. Control of the hyperthyroidism is usually associated with a decrease in goiter size and normalization of serum TSH concentration. When this occurs, the dose of the antithyroid drug should be significantly decreased to avoid hypothyroidism.

Untoward Reactions

The incidence of side effects from propylthiouracil and methimazole as currently used is relatively low. Agranulocytosis is the most serious reaction, usually occurring in the first few weeks or months of therapy but sometimes later. Because agranulocytosis usually occurs rapidly and is not associated with a gradual reduction in granulocyte count, periodic prospective monitoring of granulocyte count is not generally helpful. Patients should be instructed to immediately report the development of sore throat or fever and should discontinue their antithyroid drug and obtain a granulocyte count. Agranulocytosis is reversible on discontinuation of the offending drug, and the administration of recombinant human granulocyte colony-stimulating factor may hasten recovery. Mild granulocytopenia, if noted, may be due to thyrotoxicosis or may be the first sign of this dangerous drug reaction; frequent leukocyte counts are then required.

The most common reaction is a mild urticarial papular rash that often subsides spontaneously without interrupting treatment but sometimes requires administration of an antihistamine and corticosteroids and changing to another antithyroid drug. Other less-frequent complications are pain and stiffness in the joints, paresthesias, headache, nausea, skin pigmentation, and loss of hair. Drug fever, hepatitis, and nephritis are rare, although abnormal liver function tests are not infrequent with higher doses of propylthiouracil. Although vasculitis was previously thought to be a rare complication, Antineutrophilic cytoplasmic antibodies (ANCAs) have been reported to occur in about 50% of patients receiving propylthiouracil and rarely with methimazole.

Thyrotoxicosis in Pregnancy

Thyrotoxicosis occurs in about 0.2% of pregnancies and is caused most frequently by Graves disease. Antithyroid drugs are the treatment of choice; radioactive iodine is clearly contraindicated. Both propylthiouracil and methimazole cross the placenta equally, and either may be used safely in the pregnant patient. Methimazole is usually avoided in the first trimester in favor of propylthiouracil due to methimazole-associated embryopathy, and then methimazole is used for the remainder of the pregnancy due to the concern for propylthiouracil-associated liver failure in pregnancy. Carbimazole is used in the E.U. during pregnancy and is rarely associated with congenital abnormalities. The antithyroid drug dosage should be minimized to keep the serum FT_4 index in the upper half of the normal range or slightly elevated. As pregnancy progresses, Graves disease often improves. Relapse or worsening of Graves disease is common after delivery, and patients should be monitored closely. Methimazole in nursing mothers, up to 20 mg daily, reportedly has no effect on thyroid function in the infant; propylthiouracil is thought to partition into breast milk even less than methimazole.

Adjuvant Therapy

Several drugs that have no intrinsic antithyroid activity are useful in the symptomatic treatment of thyrotoxicosis.

The *β Adrenergic receptor antagonists* (see Chapter 12) are effective in antagonizing the sympathetic/adrenergic effects of thyrotoxicosis—thereby reducing the tachycardia, tremor, and stare—and relieving palpitations, anxiety, and tension. Either propranolol, 20–40 mg four times daily, or atenolol, 50–100 mg daily, is usually given initially.

The *Ca^{2+} channel blockers* (diltiazem, 60–120 mg four times daily) can be used to control tachycardia and decrease the incidence of supraventricular tachyarrhythmias. Usually, only short-term treatment with β adrenergic receptor antagonists or Ca^{2+} channel blockers is required, 2–6 weeks, and it should be discontinued once the patient is euthyroid.

Immunotherapy has been used for Graves hyperthyroidism and ophthalmopathy. The B-lymphocyte–depleting agent rituximab, when used with methimazole, prolongs remission of Graves disease.

Thyroid Storm

Thyroid storm is an uncommon but life-threatening complication of thyrotoxicosis in which a severe form of the disease is usually precipitated by an intercurrent medical problem. It occurs in untreated or partially treated thyrotoxic patients. Precipitating factors associated with thyrotoxic crisis include infections, stress, trauma, thyroidal or nonthyroidal surgery, diabetic ketoacidosis, labor, heart disease, and, rarely, radioactive iodine treatment.

Clinical features are similar to those of thyrotoxicosis but more exaggerated. Cardinal features include fever (temperature usually >38.5°C) and tachycardia out of proportion to the fever. Nausea, vomiting, diarrhea, agitation, and confusion are frequent presentations. Coma and death may ensue in up to 20% of patients. Thyroid function abnormalities are similar to those found in uncomplicated hyperthyroidism. Therefore, thyroid storm is primarily a clinical diagnosis.

Treatment includes supportive measures such as intravenous fluids, antipyretics, cooling blankets, and sedation. Antithyroid drugs are given in large doses. Propylthiouracil is preferred over methimazole because it also impairs peripheral conversion of $T_4 \rightarrow T_3$. Oral iodides are used after the first dose of an antithyroid drug has been administered. Treatment of the underlying precipitating illness is essential.

Ionic Inhibitors

The *ionic inhibitors* are substances that interfere with the concentration of iodide by the thyroid gland. These agents are anions that resemble iodide: *thiocyanate*, *perchlorate*, and *fluoroborate*, all monovalent hydrated anions of a size similar to that of iodide.

Thiocyanate differs from the rest qualitatively; it is not concentrated by the thyroid gland but in large amounts may inhibit the organification of iodine. Perchlorate is 10 times as active as thiocyanate. Perchlorate (ClO_4^-) blocks the entrance of iodide into the thyroid by competitively inhibiting the NIS, and itself can be transported by NIS into the thyroid gland. The various NIS inhibitors (perchlorate, thiocyanate, and nitrate) are additive in inhibiting iodine uptake. Perchlorate can be used to control hyperthyroidism; however, when given in excessive amounts (2–3 g daily), it has caused fatal aplastic anemia. Perchlorate in doses of 750 mg daily has been used in the treatment of Graves disease, although it is not available in North America.

Perchlorate can be used to "discharge" inorganic iodide from the thyroid gland in a diagnostic test of iodide organification. Other ions, selected on the basis of their size, also have been found to be active; fluoroborate (BF_4^-) is as effective as perchlorate.

Lithium decreases secretion of T_4 and T_3, which can cause overt hypothyroidism in some patients taking Li^+ for the treatment of mania (see Chapter 16).

Iodine

Iodide is the oldest remedy for disorders of the thyroid gland. In high concentration, iodide can influence several of the important functions of the thyroid gland. Iodide limits its own transport and acutely and transiently inhibits the synthesis of iodotyrosines and iodothyronines (the *Wolff-Chaikoff effect*) (Pramyothin et al., 2011). An important clinical effect of high $[I^-]_{plasma}$ is inhibition of the release of thyroid hormone.

This action is rapid and efficacious in severe thyrotoxicosis. The effect is exerted directly on the thyroid gland and can be demonstrated in the euthyroid subject as well as in the hyperthyroid patient.

Response to Iodine in Hyperthyroidism

The response to iodine in patients with hyperthyroidism is often striking and rapid: Release of thyroid hormone into the circulation is rapidly blocked, and its synthesis is mildly decreased. In the thyroid gland, vascularity is reduced, the gland becomes much firmer, the cells become smaller, and colloid reaccumulates in the follicles as iodine concentration increases. The maximal effect occurs after 10–15 days of continuous therapy. Iodide therapy usually does not completely control the manifestations of hyperthyroidism, and the beneficial effect disappears. The uses of iodide in the treatment of hyperthyroidism are in the preoperative period in preparation for thyroidectomy and, in conjunction with antithyroid drugs and propranolol, in the treatment of thyrotoxic crisis.

Another use of iodide is to protect the thyroid from radioactive iodine fallout following a nuclear accident or military exposure. Because the uptake of radioactive iodine is inversely proportional to the serum concentration of stable iodine, the administration of 30–100 mg of iodine daily will markedly decrease the thyroid uptake of radioisotopes. Strong iodine solution (Lugol solution) consists of 5% iodine and 10% potassium iodide, yielding a dose of about 8 mg of iodine per drop. *KISS* also is available, containing 50 mg per drop. Typical doses include 16–36 mg (2–6 drops) of Lugol solution or 50–100 mg (1–2 drops) of KISS three times a day. A potassium iodide product (Thyroshield) is available over the counter to take in the event of a radiation emergency and block the uptake of radioiodine into the thyroid gland. The adult dose is 2 mL (130 mg) every 24 h, as directed by public health officials.

Euthyroid patients with a history of a wide variety of underlying thyroid disorders may develop iodine-induced hypothyroidism when exposed to large amounts of iodine present in many commonly prescribed drugs (Table 43–5), and these patients do not escape from the acute Wolff-Chaikoff effect (Pramyothin et al., 2011).

TABLE 43–5 ■ IODIDE CONTENT OF COMMONLY USED DRUGS AND COMPOUNDS

DRUGS	IODINE CONTENT
Oral or local	
Amiodarone	75 mg/200 mg tablet
Iodoquinol (diiodohydroxyquin)	134 mg/tablet
Echothiophate iodide ophthalmic solution	5–41 µg/drop
Iodoquinol	134 mg/tablet
Idoxuridine ophthalmic solution	18 µg/drop
Lugol solution	5–6 mg/drop
KI, saturated solution (KISS)	38 mg/drop
Topical antiseptics	
Clinoquinol cream	12 mg/g
Povidone-iodine	10 mg/mL
Radiographic contrast agents	
Diatrizoate meglumine sodium	370 mg/mL
Iothalamate	320 mg/mL
Ioxaglate	370 mg/ml
Iopamidol	370 mg/ml
Iohexol	350 mg/mL
Ioxilan	370 mg/mL

Untoward Reactions

Occasional individuals show a marked sensitivity to iodine. Angioedema is the prominent symptom, and laryngeal edema may lead to suffocation. Multiple cutaneous hemorrhages may be present; manifestations of the serum-sickness type of hypersensitivity (e.g., fever, arthralgia, lymph node enlargement, and eosinophilia) may appear. Thrombotic thrombocytopenic purpura and fatal periarteritis nodosa attributed to hypersensitivity to iodide also have been described.

The severity of symptoms of chronic intoxication with iodide (*iodism*) is related to the dose. The symptoms start with an unpleasant brassy taste and burning in the mouth and throat as well as soreness of the teeth and gums. Increased salivation, coryza, sneezing, and irritation of the eyes with swelling of the eyelids commonly occur. Mild iodism simulates a "head cold." Excess transudation into the bronchial tree may lead to pulmonary edema. In addition, the parotid and submaxillary glands may become enlarged and tender, and the syndrome may be mistaken for mumps parotitis. Skin lesions are common and vary in type and intensity. Rarely, severe and sometimes-fatal eruptions (ioderma) may occur after the prolonged use of iodides. The lesions are bizarre; they resemble those caused by bromism and generally involute quickly when iodide is withdrawn. Symptoms of gastric irritation are common, and diarrhea, which is sometimes bloody, may occur. Fever, anorexia, and depression may be present. The symptoms of iodism disappear within a few days after stopping the administration of iodide. Renal excretion of I⁻ can be increased by procedures that promote Cl⁻ excretion (e.g., osmotic diuresis, chloruretic diuretics, and salt loading). These procedures may be useful when the symptoms of iodism are severe.

Radioactive Iodine

The primary isotopes used for the diagnosis and treatment of thyroid disease are ^{123}I and ^{131}I. ^{123}I is primarily a short-lived γ-emitter with a $t_{1/2}$ of 13 h and is used in diagnostic studies. ^{124}I has been used successfully with positron emission tomographic/computed tomographic scanning for more precise dosimetry in high-risk thyroid cancer (Jentzen et al., 2014). ^{131}I has a $t_{1/2}$ of 8 days and emits both γ rays and β particles. More than 99% of its radiation is expended within 56 days. ^{131}I is used therapeutically for thyroid destruction of an overactive or enlarged thyroid and in thyroid cancer for thyroid ablation and treatment of metastatic disease.

The chemical behavior of the radioactive isotopes of iodine is identical to that of the stable isotope, ^{127}I. ^{131}I is rapidly and efficiently trapped by the thyroid, incorporated into the iodoamino acids, and deposited in the colloid of the follicles, from which it is slowly liberated. Thus, the destructive β particles originate within the follicle and act almost exclusively on the parenchymal cells of the thyroid, with little or no damage to surrounding tissue. The γ radiation passes through the tissue and can be quantified by external detection. The effects of the radiation depend on the dosage. With properly selected doses of ^{131}I, it is possible to destroy the thyroid gland completely without detectable injury to adjacent tissues.

Therapeutic Uses

Radioactive iodine finds its widest use in the treatment of hyperthyroidism and in the diagnosis of disorders of thyroid function. The clearest indication for radioactive iodine treatment is hyperthyroidism in older patients and in those with heart disease. Radioactive iodine also is an effective treatment when Graves disease has persisted or recurred after subtotal thyroidectomy and when prolonged treatment with antithyroid drugs has not led to remission. Finally, radioactive iodine is effective in patients with toxic nodular goiter. Sodium iodide ^{131}I is available as a solution or in capsules containing carrier-free ^{131}I suitable for oral administration. Sodium iodide ^{123}I is available for scanning procedures.

Hyperthyroidism

Radioactive iodine is a valuable alternative or adjunctive treatment of hyperthyroidism (Ross, 2011). Stable iodide (nonradioactive) may preclude treatment and imaging with radioactive iodine for weeks after the stable iodide has been discontinued. In those patients exposed to stable iodide, a 24-h radioiodine measurement of a tracer dose of ^{123}I should be performed before ^{131}I administration to ensure there is sufficient uptake to accomplish the desired ablation. The optimal dose of ^{131}I, expressed amount taken up, varies in different laboratories from 80 to 150 µCi per gram of thyroid tissue. The usual total dose is 4–15 mCi with a recommended target of delivering 8 mCi to the thyroid gland based on the 24-h radioiodine uptake (Alexander and Larsen, 2002; Brent, 2008).

Beginning a few weeks after treatment, the symptoms of hyperthyroidism gradually abate over a period of 2–3 months. If therapy has been inadequate, the necessity for further treatment is apparent within 6–12 months. It is not uncommon, however, for the serum TSH to remain low for several months after ^{131}I therapy. Thus, assessing radioactive iodine failure based on TSH concentrations alone may be misleading and should always be accompanied by determination of free T_4 and usually serum T_3 concentrations. Depending to some extent on the dosage schedule adopted, 80% of patients are cured by a single dose, about 20% require two doses, and a very small fraction require three or more doses before the disorder is controlled. β Adrenergic antagonists, antithyroid drugs, or both can be used to hasten the control of hyperthyroidism.

Advantages

With radioactive iodine treatment, the patient is spared the risks and discomfort of surgery. The cost is low, hospitalization is not required in the U.S., and patients can participate in their customary activities during the entire procedure, although there are recommendations to limit exposure in young children.

Disadvantages

The chief consequence of the use of radioactive iodine is the high incidence of delayed hypothyroidism. Although cancer death rate is not increased after radioiodine therapy, some studies suggest a small but significant increase in specific types of cancer, including stomach, kidney, and breast. This finding is especially significant because these tissues all express the iodine transporter NIS and may thus be especially susceptible to effects of radioactive iodine. Radioactive iodine treatment can induce a radiation thyroiditis, with release of preformed T_4 and T_3 into the circulation. In most patients, this is asymptomatic, but in some there can be worsening of symptoms of hyperthyroidism; rarely, cardiac manifestations (e.g., atrial fibrillation or ischemic heart disease); and very rarely thyroid storm. Pretreatment with antithyroid drugs should reduce or eliminate this complication.

The main contraindication for the use of ^{131}I therapy is pregnancy. After the first trimester, the fetal thyroid will concentrate the isotope and thus suffer damage; even during the first trimester, radioactive iodine is best avoided because there may be adverse effects of radiation on fetal tissues. In addition, the use of radioiodine to treat hyperthyroidism in children is controversial due to theoretical concern about causing neoplastic changes in the thyroid gland or other organs. Data are insufficient to resolve this issue, as the number of children who have been treated with radioiodine is relatively small. Many clinics decline to treat younger patients and reserve radioactive iodine for patients older than 25–30 years.

Thyroid Carcinoma

Because most well-differentiated thyroid carcinomas accumulate very little iodine, stimulation of iodine uptake with TSH is required to treat metastases effectively (Haugen and Sherman, 2013; Haugen et al., 2016). Endogenous TSH stimulation is promoted by withdrawal of thyroid hormone replacement therapy in patients previously treated with near-total or total thyroidectomy. An ablative dose of ^{131}I ranging from 30 to 150 mCi is administered, and a repeat total body scan is obtained several days to 1 week later.

Recombinant thyrotropin alpha (recombinant human TSH) can be used instead of thyroid hormone withdrawal to prepare a patient for radioiodine ablation of thyroid remnant tissue or to test the capacity of thyroid tissue, both normal and malignant, to take up radioactive iodine and to secrete thyroglobulin. Recombinant human TSH is not currently approved to prepare patients for radioiodine ablation of metastatic disease.

Papillary and Follicular Carcinomas

The majority of thyroid cancers derive from the thyroid follicular cells and are classified histologically as papillary or follicular carcinomas. Most of these carcinomas are adequately treated by surgery, radioiodine, and levothyroxine to suppress TSH. However, a small fraction progress despite these therapies, in which case they can be treated with the oral tyrosine kinase inhibitors *sorafenib* (Brose et al., 2014) or *lenvatinib* (Schlumberger et al., 2015) (see Chapter 67). The response to these drugs does not seem to be dependent on the presence or absence of specific oncogene mutations.

The recommended daily dose of sorafenib is 400 mg twice daily without food. Adverse reactions include palmar-plantar erythrodysesthesia, diarrhea, alopecia, fatigue, weight loss, hypertension, and others. The recommended daily dose of lenvatinib is 24 mg once daily with or without food, reduced to 14 mg in those with severe renal or hepatic impairment. Common adverse reactions include hypertension, diarrhea, fatigue, decreased appetite, decreased weight, nausea, stomatitis, and musculoskeletal pain, although there are multiple other toxicities, including treatment-related deaths.

Medullary Thyroid Carcinoma

A minor fraction of thyroid cancers originate from the parafollicular cells (C cells) that produce calcitonin and are denoted medullary thyroid carcinomas. Because they derive from the parafollicular cells, medullary carcinomas are not responsive to radioiodine or TSH suppression. Medullary carcinomas that progress despite surgery can be treated with either of the oral tyrosine kinase inhibitors *vandetanib* (Wells et al., 2012) and *cabozantinib* (Elisei et al., 2013) (see Chapter 67). These drugs can be prescribed for both the sporadic and inherited forms of medullary thyroid carcinoma without regard for *RET* gene mutational status because patients can respond even in the absence of *RET* mutations. However, the phase III vandetanib trial suggested a higher response rate in patients with tumors harboring the *RET* M918T mutation. The phase III cabozantinib trial demonstrated a longer progression-free survival in patients with *RET* M918T tumors and possibly also in patients with tumors harboring *RAS* mutations.

The dose of vandetanib is 300 mg once daily with or without food. The dose is reduced to 200 mg in moderate-to-severe renal impairment, and vandetanib is not recommended in moderate or severe hepatic impairment. Vandetanib has a black-box warning for QT prolongation. Additional adverse reactions include diarrhea, rash, nausea, hypertension, headache, and others.

The starting dose of cabozantinib is typically 60 to 100 mg on an empty stomach, which may be titrated to 140 mg as tolerated. It is not recommended in moderate or severe hepatic impairment. Cabozantinib has black-box warnings for GI perforations and fistulas (especially in patients receiving prior radiation therapy) and hemorrhage. Additional adverse reactions include diarrhea, palmar-plantar erythrodysesthesia, decreased weight and appetite, nausea, fatigue, and stomatitis.

General Comments

Treatment of thyroid cancer with tyrosine kinase inhibitors should continue until the patient is no longer clinically benefiting or until unacceptable toxicity occurs. Dosage reductions can mitigate toxicity. Resistance to one tyrosine kinase inhibitor does not necessarily imply resistance to another. *It is important to note that levothyroxine dosage requirements often increase in patients taking protein tyrosine kinase inhibitors; therefore, TSH levels should be monitored carefully* (Brose et al., 2014; Elisei et al., 2013; Schlumberger et al., 2015; Wells et al., 2012). The use of tyrosine kinase inhibitors is described in Chapter 67.

Acknowledgment: *Alan P. Farwell and Lewis E. Braverman contributed to this chapter in recent editions of this book. We have retained some of their text in the current edition.*

Drug Facts for Your Personal Formulary: *Thyroid and Antithyroid Drugs*

Drugs	Therapeutic Uses	Clinical Pharmacology and Tips
Thyroid Hormone Preparations: Replace T₄ or T₃ normally produced by the thyroid		
Levothyroxine (T_4)	• Hypothyroidism • TSH suppression in thyroid cancer	• Plasma $t_{1/2}$ ~ 1 week • Deiodinases convert circulating T_4 to the bioactive hormone T_3 • Dosage generally needs to increase during pregnancy • Congenital hypothyroidism requires rapid diagnosis and correction to allow normal physical and mental development • Overtreatment can lead to osteoporosis and atrial fibrillation
Liothyronine (T_3)	• When rapid onset of action is desired (sometimes for myxedema coma) • When rapid termination of action is desired (preparing patients with thyroid cancer for radioiodine therapy)	• Plasma $t_{1/2}$ ~ 18-24 h • Multiple daily doses needed to achieve needed C_{Pss} • Levothyroxine (T_4) generally preferred over liothyronine (T_3) for the long-term therapy of hypothyroidism
Desiccated thyroid and T_4-T_3 mixtures	• Generally not a preferred therapy, although occasional hypothyroid patients say they feel better than when taking levothyroxine	• Mixture of levothyroxine and liothyronine (2–5:1 by weight) • Supplies a relative excess of T_3 compared to normal thyroidal secretion, which is ~ 11:1 T_4 to T_3 by weight • No convincing evidence of greater efficacy than levothyroxine (T_4 alone)
Antithyroid Drugs: Thionamides: Interfere with incorporation of iodine into tyrosyl residues and inhibit iodotyrosyl-coupling reactions		
Methimazole	• Reduce thyroid hormone production	• Carbimazole (available in Europe) converted to methimazole after absorption • Long intrathyroidal $t_{1/2}$ allows once-daily dosing for most patients • Preferred antithyroid drug • Do not use in first trimester of pregnancy due to embryopathy
Propylthiouracil	• Reduce thyroid hormone production • May also reduce T_4 to T_3 conversion	• Major concern is liver toxicity; rare but more commonly seen in children and pregnancy • Only indications are for thyroid storm due to action on reducing T_4 to T_3 conversion and in the first trimester of pregnancy
Antithyroid Drugs: Ionic Inhibitors: Iodine uptake by antagonizing the sodium-iodide symporter		
Perchlorate	• Primarily used to enhance the response to thioamides in refractory Graves disease (e.g., that associated with amiodarone)	• Not available commercially; must be specialty compounded
Antithyroid Drugs: Iodide: Acute reduction in thyroid hormone		
Lugol solution	• Acutely reduce the secretion and synthesis of thyroid hormone	• "Escape" from thyroid inhibition after 7–10 days • Strictly contraindicated in pregnancy
KISS: potassium iodide saturated solution (or SSKI)	• Acutely reduce the secretion and synthesis of thyroid hormone	• "Escape" from thyroid inhibition after 7–10 days • Strictly contraindicated in pregnancy
Antithyroid Drugs: Radioactive Iodine: Used to destroy hyperfunctioning thyroid tissue		
¹³¹I	• Effective for permanent treatment of Graves disease and toxic nodule or toxic goiter • Destruction of iodide-avid thyroid cancer	• Highly effective for permanent cure to hyperthyroidism • Effective treatment of hyperthyroidism usually results in permanent hypothyroidism and lifelong requirement for levothyroxine replacement • Absolutely contraindicated in pregnancy • Treatment of thyroid cancer requires TSH stimulation (endogenous or exogenous)
Recombinant Human TSH Agonist for the TSH Receptor		
Thyrotropin alpha	• Stimulate radioiodine uptake and thyroglobulin release in patients with thyroid cancer after thyroidectomy • Prepare patients for radioiodine ablation of thyroid remnants after thyroidectomy for thyroid cancer	• Allows assessment of residual or recurrent thyroid cancer without stopping levothyroxine and becoming clinically hypothyroid • Allows radioiodine therapy of thyroid remnants without stopping levothyroxine and becoming clinically hypothyroid
Thyroid Cancer Chemotherapeutics: Tyrosine kinase inhibitors		
Sorafenib Lenvatinib	• Radioiodine-resistant, progressive papillary, or follicular thyroid cancer	• Response not predicted by presence or absence of specific oncogene mutations • Lack of response to one kinase inhibitor does not necessarily predict lack of response to others
Vandetanib Cabozantinib	• Progressive medullary thyroid cancer	• Can be used in hereditary or sporadic medullary thyroid cancer • Responses may be seen in patients with or without *RET* gene mutations

Bibliography

Abduljabbar MA, Afifi AM. Congenital hypothyroidism. *J Pediatr Endocrinol Metab*, **2012**, *25*:13–29.

Adijanto J, Philip NJ. The SLC16A family of monocarboxylate transporters (MCTs)—physiology and function in cellular metabolism, pH homeostasis, and fluid transport. *Curr Top Membr*, **2012**, *70*:275–311.

Alexander EK, Larsen PR. High dose of (131)I therapy for the treatment of hyperthyroidism caused by Graves' disease. *J Clin Endocrinol Metab*, **2002**, *87*:1073–1077.

Angell TE, et al. Clinical features and hospital outcomes in thyroid storm: a retrospective cohort study. *J Clin Endocrinol Metab*, **2015**, *100*:451–459.

Bach-Huynh TG, et al. Timing of levothyroxine administration affects serum thyrotropin concentration. *J Clin Endocrinol Metab*, **2009**, *94*:3905–3912.

Bernal J, et al. Thyroid hormone transporters—functions and clinical implications. *Nat Rev Endocrinol*, **2015**, *11*:406–417.

Biondi B, Wartofsky L. Treatment with thyroid hormone. *Endocr Rev*, **2014**, *35*:433–512.

Brent GA. Clinical practice. Graves' disease. *N Engl J Med*, **2008**, *358*:2594–2605.

Brent GA. Mechanisms of thyroid hormone action. *J Clin Invest*, **2012**, *122*:3035–3043.

Brose MS, et al. Sorafenib in radioactive iodine-refractory, locally advanced or metastatic differentiated thyroid cancer: a randomised, double-blind, phase 3 trial. *Lancet*, **2014**, *384*:319–328.

Carswell JM, et al. Generic and brand-name L-thyroxine are not bioequivalent for children with severe congenital hypothyroidism. *J Clin Endocrinol Metab*, **2013**, *98*:610–617.

Celi FS, et al. Metabolic effects of liothyronine therapy in hypothyroidism: a randomized, double-blind, crossover trial of liothyronine versus levothyroxine. *J Clin Endocrinol Metab*, **2011**, *96*:3466–3474.

Dumitrescu AM, et al. The syndrome of inherited partial SBP2 deficiency in humans. *Antioxid Redox Signal*, **2010**, *12*:905–920.

Elisei R, et al. Cabozantinib in progressive medullary thyroid cancer. *J Clin Oncol*, **2013**, *31*:3639–3646.

Gereben B, et al. Cellular and molecular basis of deiodinase-regulated thyroid hormone signaling. *Endocr Rev*, **2008**, *29*:898–938.

Goldberg IJ, et al. Thyroid hormone reduces cholesterol via a non-LDL receptor-mediated pathway. *Endocrinology*, **2012**, *153*:5143–5149.

Grais IM, Sowers JR. Thyroid and the heart. *Am J Med*, **2014**, *127*:691–698.

Grozinsky-Glasberg S, et al. Thyroxine-triiodothyronine combination therapy versus thyroxine monotherapy for clinical hypothyroidism: meta-analysis of randomized controlled trials. *J Clin Endocrinol Metab*, **2006**, *91*:2592–2599.

Gruters A, Krude H. Detection and treatment of congenital hypothyroidism. *Nat Rev Endocrinol*, **2012**, *8*:104–113.

Gullo D, et al. Levothyroxine monotherapy cannot guarantee euthyroidism in all athyreotic patients. *PLoS One*, **2011**, *6*:e22552.

Haugen BR, Sherman SI. Evolving approaches to patients with advanced differentiated thyroid cancer. *Endocr Rev*, **2013**, *34*:439–455.

Haugen BRM, et al. 2015 American Thyroid Association management guidelines for adult patients with thyroid nodules and differentiated thyroid cancer. *Thyroid*, **2016**, *26*:1–133.

Hiroi Y, et al. Rapid nongenomic actions of thyroid hormone. *Proc Natl Acad Sci U S A*, **2006**, *103*:14104–14109.

Hoang TD, et al. Desiccated thyroid extract compared with levothyroxine in the treatment of hypothyroidism: a randomized, double-blind, crossover study. *J Clin Endocrinol Metab*, **2013**, *98*:1982–1990.

Jentzen W, et al. Assessment of lesion response in the initial radioiodine treatment of differentiated thyroid cancer using 124I PET imaging. *J Nucl Med*, **2014**, *55*:1759-1765.

Jonklaas J, et al. Triiodothyronine levels in athyreotic individuals during levothyroxine therapy. *JAMA*, **2008**, *299*:769–777.

Jonklaas J, et al. Guidelines for the treatment of hypothyroidism: prepared by the American Thyroid Association Task Force on thyroid hormone replacement. *Thyroid*, **2014**, *24*:1670–1751.

Kalyanaraman H, et al. Nongenomic thyroid hormone signaling occurs through a plasma membrane-localized receptor. *Sci Signal*, **2014**, *7*:ra48.

Kogai T, Brent GA. The sodium iodide symporter (NIS): regulation and approaches to targeting for cancer therapeutics. *Pharmacol Ther*, **2012**, *135*:355–370.

Leger J, et al. European Society for Paediatric Endocrinology consensus guidelines on screening, diagnosis, and management of congenital hypothyroidism. *J Clin Endocrinol Metab*, **2014**, *99*:363–384.

Lin HY, et al. Identification and functions of the plasma membrane receptor for thyroid hormone analogues. *Discov Med*, **2011**, *11*:337–347.

Marsili A, et al. Physiological role and regulation of iodothyronine deiodinases: a 2011 update. *J Endocrinol Investig*, **2011**, *34*:395–407.

Mayerl S, et al. Transporters MCT8 and OATP1C1 maintain murine brain thyroid hormone homeostasis. *J Clin Invest*, **2014**, *124*:1987–1999.

Mullur R, et al. Thyroid hormone regulation of metabolism. *Physiol Rev*, **2014**, *94*:355–382.

Piehl S, et al. Thyronamines—past, present, and future. *Endocr Rev*, **2011**, *32*:64–80.

Portulano C, et al. The Na$^+$/I$^-$ symporter (NIS): mechanism and medical impact. *Endocr Rev*, **2014**, *35*:106–149.

Pramyothin P, et al. Clinical problem-solving. A hidden solution. *N Engl J Med*, **2011**, *365*:2123–2127.

Public Health Committee of the American Thyroid Association, et al. Iodine supplementation for pregnancy and lactation—United States and Canada: recommendations of the American Thyroid Association. *Thyroid*, **2006**, *16*:949–951.

Refetoff S. The syndrome of generalized resistance to thyroid hormone (GRTH). *Endocr Res*, **1989**, *15*:717–743.

Refetoff S, et al. Classification and proposed nomenclature for inherited defects of thyroid hormone action, cell transport, and metabolism. *J Clin Endocrinol Metab*, **2014**, *99*:768–770.

Rose SR, et al. Update of newborn screening and therapy for congenital hypothyroidism. *Pediatrics*, **2006**, *117*:2290–2303.

Ross DS. Radioiodine therapy for hyperthyroidism. *N Engl J Med*, **2011**, *364*:542–550.

Schlumberger M, et al. Lenvatinib versus placebo in radioiodine-refractory thyroid cancer. *N Engl J Med*, **2015**, *372*:621–630.

van der Deure WM, et al. Molecular aspects of thyroid hormone transporters, including MCT8, MCT10, and OATPs, and the effects of genetic variation in these transporters. *J Mol Endocrinol*, **2010**, *44*:1–11.

van Mullem AA, et al. Clinical consequences of mutations in thyroid hormone receptor-alpha1. *Eur Thyroid J*, **2014**, *3*:17–24.

Vita R, et al. The administration of l-thyroxine as soft gel capsule or liquid solution. *Expert Opin Drug Deliv*, **2014**, *11*:1103–1111.

Wang LY, et al. Thyrotropin suppression increases the risk of osteoporosis without decreasing recurrence in ATA low- and intermediate-risk patients with differentiated thyroid carcinoma. *Thyroid*, **2015**, *25*:300–307.

Wells SA Jr, et al. Vandetanib in patients with locally advanced or metastatic medullary thyroid cancer: a randomized, double-blind phase III trial. *J Clin Oncol*, **2012**, *30*:134–141.

Yehuda-Shnaidman E, et al. Thyroid hormone, thyromimetics, and metabolic efficiency. *Endocr Rev*, **2014**, *35*:35–58.

Zimmermann MB. Iodine deficiency. *Endocr Rev*, **2009**, *30*:376–408.

Chapter 44

Estrogens, Progestins, and the Female Reproductive Tract

Ellis R. Levin, Wendy S. Vitek, and Stephen R. Hammes

Estrogens and *progestins* are endogenous hormones that produce numerous physiological actions. In women, these include developmental effects, neuroendocrine actions involved in the control of ovulation, the cyclical preparation of the reproductive tract for fertilization and implantation, and major actions on mineral, carbohydrate, protein, and lipid metabolism. Estrogens also have important actions in males, including effects on bone, spermatogenesis, and behavior. Well-characterized receptors for each hormone mediate biological actions in both the unliganded and the liganded states.

The most common uses of estrogens and progestins are for contraception and menopausal hormone therapy (MHT) in women, but the specific compounds and dosages used in these two settings differ substantially. Antiestrogens are used in the treatment of hormone-responsive breast cancer and infertility. Selective estrogen receptor modulators (SERMs) that display tissue-selective agonist or antagonist activities are useful to prevent breast cancer and osteoporosis. The main use of antiprogestins has been for medical abortion.

A number of naturally occurring and synthetic environmental chemicals mimic, antagonize, or otherwise affect the actions of estrogens in experimental test systems. The precise effect of these agents on humans is unknown but is an area of active investigation.

Estrogens

Chemistry and Synthesis

Chemistry

Many steroidal and nonsteroidal compounds, some of which are shown in Table 44–1 and Figure 44–1, possess estrogenic activity. Estrogens interact with two receptors of the nuclear receptor superfamily, termed ERα and ERβ. The most potent naturally occurring estrogen in humans, for both ERα- and ERβ-mediated actions, is *17β-estradiol*, followed by *estrone* and *estriol*. Each contains a phenolic A ring with a hydroxyl group at carbon 3 and a β-OH or ketone in position 17 of ring D.

The phenolic A ring is the principal structural feature responsible for selective high-affinity binding to both receptors. Most alkyl substitutions on the A ring impair binding, but substitutions on ring C or D may be tolerated. Ethinyl substitutions at the C17 position greatly increase oral potency by inhibiting first-pass hepatic metabolism. Models for the ligand-binding sites of both ERs have been determined from structure-activity relationships and structural analysis (Pike et al., 2000). Selective ligands for ERα and ERβ are available for experimental studies but are not yet used therapeutically (Harrington et al., 2003).

Biosynthesis

Steroidal estrogens arise from androstenedione or testosterone (Figure 44–1) by aromatization of the A ring. The reaction is catalyzed by aromatase (CYP19), which uses NADPH and molecular oxygen as cosubstrates. A ubiquitous flavoprotein, NADPH–cytochrome P450 reductase, also is essential. Both proteins are localized in the endoplasmic reticulum of ovarian granulosa cells, testicular Sertoli and Leydig cells, adipose stroma, placental syncytiotrophoblasts, preimplantation blastocysts, bone, various brain regions, and many other tissues (Simpson et al., 2002).

The ovaries are the principal source of circulating estrogen in premenopausal women, with estradiol the main secretory product. Ovarian estradiol production is traditionally thought to require two cell types: theca cells and granulosa cells. The gonadotropin LH acts via receptors that couple to the G_s-adenylyl cyclase–cyclic AMP pathway to increase

Abbreviations

AF: activation function
CHD: coronary heart disease
COMT: catechol-*O*-methyl transferase
DES: diethylstilbestrol
ER: estrogen receptor
ERα: estrogen receptor α
ERβ: estrogen receptor β
ERE: estrogen response element
ERT: estrogen replacement therapy
FP: $PGF_{2α}$ receptor
FSH: follicle-stimulating hormone
GABA: γ-aminobutyric acid
GnRH: gonadotropin-releasing hormone
GPCR: G protein–coupled receptor
hCG: human chorionic gonadotropin
HDL: high-density lipoprotein
HERS: Heart and Estrogen/Progestin Replacement Study
HRT: hormone replacement therapy
HSP: heat shock protein
IGF: insulinlike growth factor
IU: intrauterine
IUD: intrauterine device
IUI: intrauterine insemination
IUS: intrauterine system
LDL: low-density lipoprotein
LH: luteinizing hormone
LNg: levonorgestrol, as in LNg-IUS
LNg14 or 20: LNg, 14 or 20 $μg/24h$
LPA: lipoprotein A
MHT: menopausal hormone therapy
MPA: medroxyprogesterone acetate
MWS: Million Women Study
NcoR: nuclear hormone receptor corepressor
NE: norepinephrine
OHSS: ovarian hyperstimulation syndrome
PAI-1: plasminogen activator inhibitor 1
PCOS: polycystic ovary syndrome
PG: prostaglandin
PID: pelvic inflammatory disease
PR: progesterone receptor
PRE: progesterone response element
PRM: progesterone receptor modulator
ROS: reactive oxygen species
SERM: selective estrogen receptor modulator
SHBG: sex hormone–binding globulin
SRC-1: steroid-receptor coactivator 1
WHI: Women's Health Initiative
WHIMS: Women's Health Initiative Memory Study

cholesterol (the precursors of all steroids) transport into the mitochondria of cells, where androgen precursors are produced. FSH then stimulates CYP19 production and activity in the granulosa cells, which converts the androgen precursors to estrogens. Notably, theca cells of the ovary contain a form of 17β-hydroxysteroid dehydrogenase (type I) that favors the production of testosterone and estradiol from androstenedione and estrone, respectively. However, in the liver, another form of this enzyme (type II) favors oxidation of circulating estradiol to estrone (Peltoketo et al., 1999), and both of these steroids are then converted to estriol (Figure 44–1). All three of these estrogens are excreted in the urine along with their glucuronide and sulfate conjugates.

HISTORY	Hormones in the Female Reproductive System

The hormonal nature of the ovarian control of the female reproductive system was firmly established in 1900 by Knauer when he found that ovarian transplants prevented the symptoms of gonadectomy, and by Halban, who showed that normal sexual development and function occurred when glands were transplanted. In 1923, Allen and Doisy devised a bioassay for ovarian extracts based on the vaginal smear of the rat. Frank and associates in 1925 detected an active sex principle in the blood of sows in estrus, and Loewe and Lange discovered in 1926 that a female sex hormone varied in the urine of women throughout the menstrual cycle. The excretion of estrogen in the urine during pregnancy also was reported by Zondek in 1928 and enabled Butenandt and Doisy in 1929 to crystallize an active substance.

Early investigations indicated that the ovary secretes two substances. Beard had postulated in 1897 that the corpus luteum serves a necessary function during pregnancy, and Fraenkel showed in 1903 that destruction of the corpora lutea in pregnant rabbits caused abortion. Several groups then isolated progesterone from mammalian corpora lutea in the 1930s.

In the early 1960s, pioneering studies by Jensen and colleagues suggested the presence of intracellular receptors for estrogens in target tissues. This was the first demonstration of receptors of the steroid/thyroid superfamily and provided techniques to identify receptors for the other steroid hormones. A second ER was identified in 1996 and was termed ERβ to distinguish it from the receptor identified by Jensen and others, termed ERα. Two protein isoforms, A and B, of the PR arise from a single gene by transcription initiation from different promoters.

In postmenopausal women, the principal source of circulating estrogen is adipose tissue stroma, where estrone is synthesized from dehydroepiandrosterone secreted by the adrenals. In men, estrogens are produced by the testes, but extragonadal production by aromatization of circulating C19 steroids (e.g., androstenedione and dehydroepiandrosterone) accounts for most circulating estrogens (Simpson, 2003).

Estrogens may be locally produced from androgens by the actions of aromatase or from estrogen conjugates by hydrolysis. Such local production of estrogens could play a causal or promotional role in the development of certain diseases, such as breast cancer, because mammary tumors contain both aromatase and hydrolytic enzymes. Estrogens also may be produced from androgens via aromatase in the CNS and other tissues and exert local effects near their production site (e.g., in bone, they affect bone mineral density).

The placenta uses fetal dehydroepiandrosterone and its 16α-hydroxyl derivative to produce large amounts of estrone and estriol. Human urine during pregnancy is thus an abundant source of natural estrogens. Pregnant mare's urine is the source of *conjugated equine estrogens*, which have been widely used therapeutically for many years.

Physiological Actions

Developmental Actions

Estrogens are largely responsible for pubertal changes in girls and secondary sexual characteristics. Estrogens cause growth and development of the vagina, uterus, and fallopian tubes and contribute to breast enlargement. They also contribute to molding the body contours, shaping the skeleton, and causing the pubertal growth spurt of the long bones and epiphyseal closure. Growth of axillary and pubic hair, pigmentation of the genital region, and the regional pigmentation of the nipples and areolae that occur after the first trimester of pregnancy are also estrogenic actions. Androgens may also play a secondary role in female sexual development (Chapter 45).

Estrogens appear to play important developmental roles in males. In boys, estrogen deficiency diminishes the pubertal growth spurt and delays

TABLE 44–1 ■ STRUCTURAL FORMULAS OF SELECTED ESTROGENS

STEROIDAL ESTROGENS

Derivative	R_1	R_2	R_3
Estradiol	—H	—H	—H
Estradiol valerate	—H	—H	$-\text{C(CH}_2)_3\text{CH}_3$ (O double bond)
Ethinyl estradiol	—H	—C≡CH	—H
Mestranol	—CH₃	—C≡CH	—H
Estrone sulfate	—SO₃H	—ᵃ	=Oᵃ
Equilinᵇ	—H	—ᵃ	=Oᵃ

ᵃDesignates C17 Ketone.
ᵇAlso contains 7, 8 double bond.

NONSTEROIDAL COMPOUNDS WITH ESTROGENIC ACTIVITY

Diethylstilbestrol

Bisphenol A

Genistein

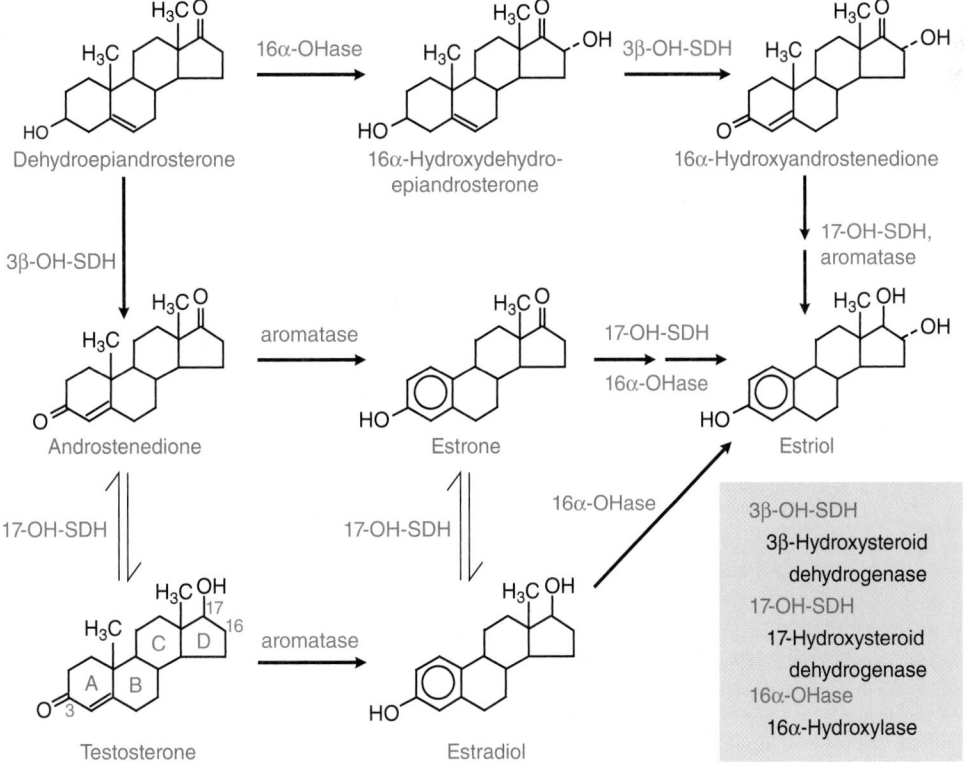

Figure 44–1 *The biosynthetic pathway for the estrogens.*

skeletal maturation and epiphyseal closure so that linear growth continues into adulthood. Estrogen deficiency in men leads to elevated gonadotropins, macroorchidism, and increased testosterone levels and also may affect carbohydrate and lipid metabolism and fertility in some individuals (Grumbach and Auchus, 1999).

Neuroendocrine Control of the Menstrual Cycle

A neuroendocrine cascade involving the hypothalamus, pituitary, and ovaries controls the menstrual cycle (Figure 44–2). A neuronal oscillator, or "clock," in the hypothalamus fires at intervals that coincide with bursts of GnRH release into the hypothalamic-pituitary portal vasculature (Chapter 42). GnRH interacts with its cognate receptor on pituitary gonadotropes to cause release of LH and FSH. The frequency of the GnRH pulses, which varies in the different phases of the menstrual cycle, controls the relative synthesis of the unique β subunits of FSH and LH.

The gonadotropins (LH and FSH) regulate the growth and maturation of the graafian follicle in the ovary and the ovarian production of estrogen and progesterone, which exert feedback regulation on the pituitary and hypothalamus. Because the release of GnRH is intermittent, LH and FSH secretion is pulsatile. The pulse *frequency* is determined by the neural clock (Figure 44–2), termed the *hypothalamic GnRH pulse generator* (Knobil, 1981), but the amount of gonadotropin released in each

pulse (i.e., the pulse *amplitude*) is largely controlled by the actions of estrogens and progesterone on the pituitary. The intermittent, *pulsatile* nature of hormone release is essential for the maintenance of normal ovulatory menstrual cycles because constant infusion of GnRH results in cessation of gonadotropin release and ovarian steroid production (Chapter 42). The neuropeptide kisspeptin 1, which is released from the hypothalamic anteroventral periventricular nucleus and the arcuate nucleus, may regulate GnRH pulsatility through its G protein–coupled receptor, GPR54, expressed in GnRH neurons. Inactivating mutations in GPR54 have been associated with hypogonadotropic hypogonadism (Seminara, 2006).

Although the precise mechanism that regulates the timing of GnRH release (i.e., pulse frequency) is unclear, hypothalamic cells appear to have an intrinsic ability to release GnRH episodically. The overall pattern of GnRH release likely is regulated by the interplay of intrinsic mechanism(s) and extrinsic synaptic inputs from opioid, catecholamine, and GABAergic neurons (Figure 44–2). Ovarian steroids, primarily progesterone, regulate the frequency of GnRH release, but the cellular and molecular mechanisms of this regulation are not well established.

At puberty the pulse generator is activated and establishes cyclic profiles of pituitary and ovarian hormones. Although the mechanism of activation is not entirely established, it may involve increases in circulating IGF-1

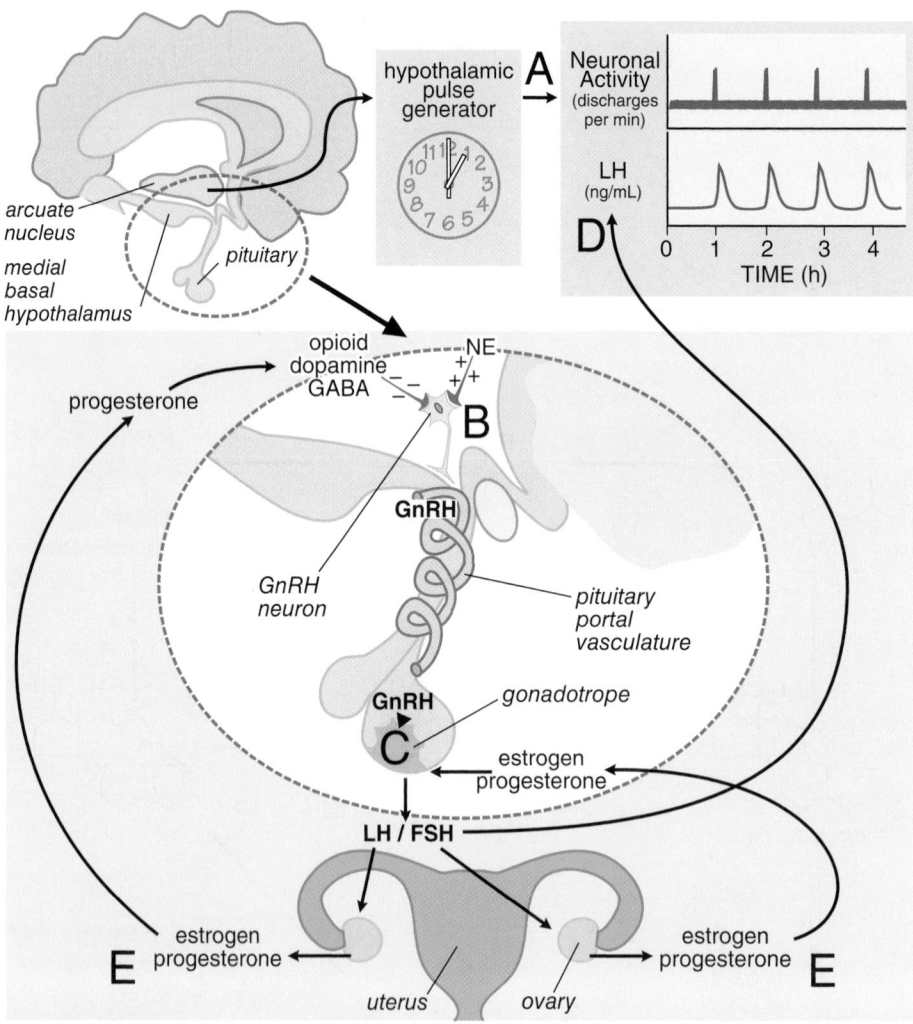

Figure 44–2 *Neuroendocrine control of gonadotropin secretion in females.* The hypothalamic pulse generator located in the arcuate nucleus of the hypothalamus functions as a neuronal "clock" that fires at regular hourly intervals (**A**). This results in the periodic release of GnRH from GnRH-containing neurons into the hypothalamic-pituitary portal vasculature (**B**). GnRH neurons (**B**) receive inhibitory input from opioid, dopamine, and GABA neurons and stimulatory input from noradrenergic neurons. The pulses of GnRH trigger the intermittent release of LH and FSH from pituitary gonadotropes (**C**), resulting in the pulsatile plasma profile (**D**). FSH and LH regulate ovarian production of estrogen and progesterone, which exert feedback controls (**E**). (See text and Figure 44–3 for additional details.)

and leptin levels, the latter acting to inhibit neuropeptide Y in the arcuate nucleus to relieve an inhibitory effect on GnRH neurons.

Figure 44–3 provides a schematic diagram of the profiles of gonadotropin and gonadal steroid levels in the menstrual cycle. The "average" plasma levels of LH throughout the cycle are shown in panel A of Figure 44–3; inserts illustrate the pulsatile patterns of LH during the proliferative and secretory phases in more detail. The average LH levels are similar throughout the early (follicular) and late (luteal) phases of the cycle, but the frequency and amplitude of the LH pulses are quite different in the two phases. This characteristic pattern of hormone secretions results from complex positive- and negative-feedback mechanisms (Hotchkiss and Knobil, 1994).

In the early follicular phase of the cycle, (1) the pulse generator produces bursts of neuronal activity with a frequency of about one per hour that correspond with pulses of GnRH secretion; (2) these cause a corresponding pulsatile release of LH and FSH from pituitary gonadotropes; and (3) FSH in particular causes the graafian follicle to mature and secrete estrogen. The effects of estrogens on the pituitary are inhibitory at this time and cause the amount of LH and FSH released from the pituitary to decline (i.e., the amplitude of the LH pulse decreases), so gonadotropin levels gradually fall (Figure 44–3). *Inhibin,* produced by the ovary, exerts negative feedback to selectively decrease serum FSH (Chapter 42). Activin and follistatin, two other peptides released from the ovary, may also regulate FSH production and secretion to a lesser extent, although their levels do not vary appreciably during the menstrual cycle.

At midcycle, serum estradiol rises above a threshold level of 150–200 pg/mL for about 36 h. This sustained elevation of estrogen no longer inhibits gonadotropin release but exerts a brief positive-feedback effect on the

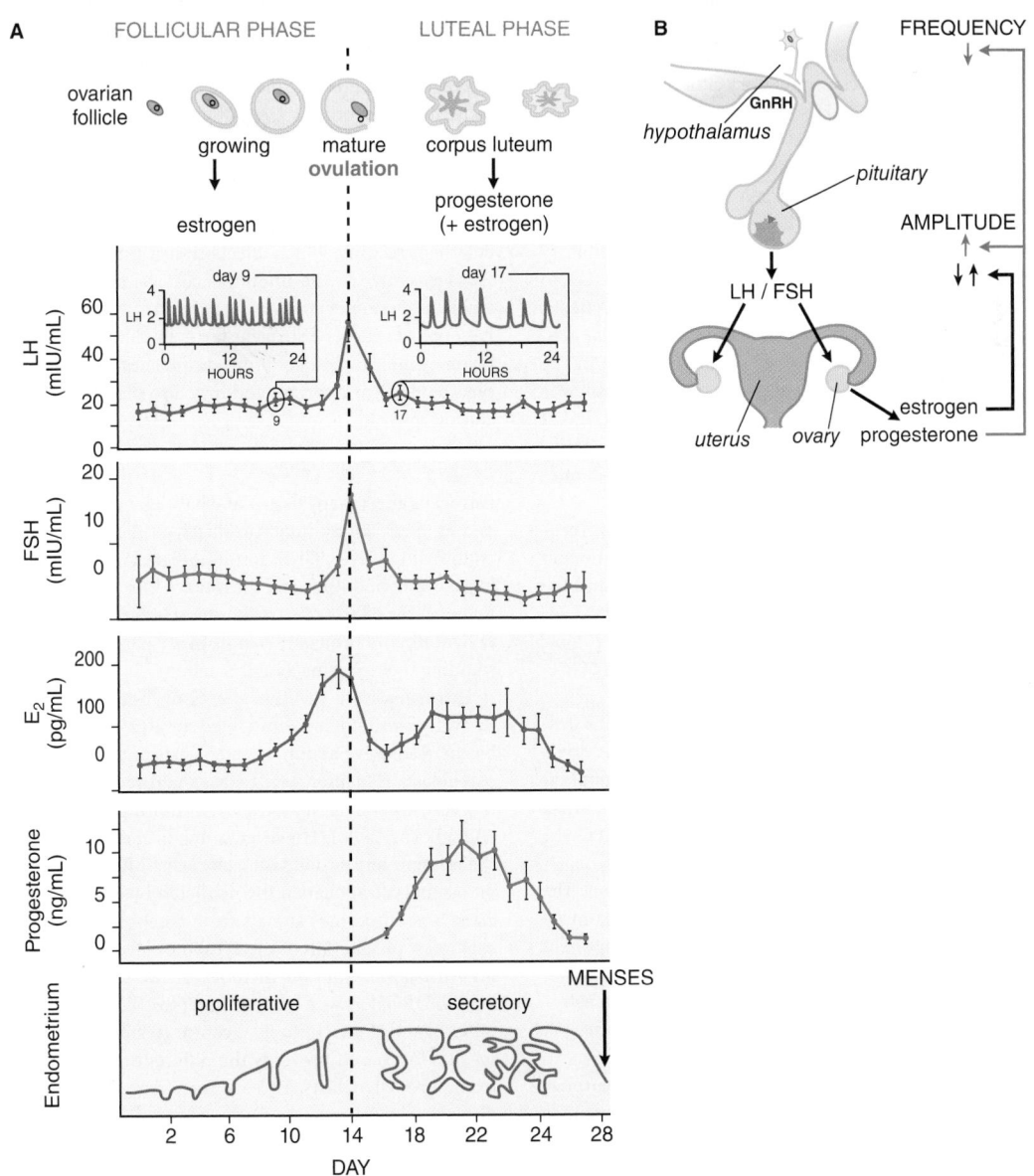

Figure 44–3 *Hormonal relationships of the human menstrual cycle.* **A.** Average daily values of LH, FSH, estradiol (E_2), and progesterone in plasma samples from women exhibiting normal 28-day menstrual cycles. Changes in the ovarian follicle (top) and endometrium (bottom) also are illustrated schematically. Frequent plasma sampling reveals pulsatile patterns of gonadotropin release. Characteristic profiles are illustrated schematically for the follicular phase (day 9, inset on left) and luteal phase (day 17, inset on right). Both the frequency (number of pulses per hour) and amplitude (extent of change of hormone release) of pulses vary throughout the cycle. (Modified from and reproduced with permission from Thorneycroft IH, et al. *Am J Obstet Gynecol,* **1971**, *111*:947–951. Copyright © Elsevier). **B.** Major regulatory effects of ovarian steroids on hypothalamic-pituitary function. Estrogen decreases the amount of FSH and LH released (i.e., gonadotropin pulse amplitude) during most of the cycle and triggers a surge of LH release only at midcycle. Progesterone decreases the frequency of GnRH release from the hypothalamus and thus decreases the frequency of plasma gonadotropin pulses. Progesterone also increases the amount of LH released (i.e., the pulse amplitude) during the luteal phase of the cycle.

pituitary to trigger the preovulatory surge of LH and FSH. This effect primarily involves a change in pituitary responsiveness to GnRH. Progesterone may contribute to the midcycle LH surge.

The midcycle surge in gonadotropins stimulates follicular rupture and ovulation within 1–2 days. The ruptured follicle then develops into the corpus luteum, which produces large amounts of progesterone and lesser amounts of estrogen under the influence of LH during the second half of the cycle. In the absence of pregnancy, the corpus luteum ceases to function, steroid levels drop, and menstruation occurs. When steroid levels drop, the pulse generator reverts to a firing pattern characteristic of the follicular phase, the entire system then resets, and a new ovarian cycle occurs.

Regulation of the frequency and amplitude of gonadotropin secretions by steroids may be summarized as follows: Estrogens act primarily on the pituitary to control the amplitude of gonadotropin pulses, and they may also contribute to the amplitude of GnRH pulses secreted by the hypothalamus.

In the follicular phase of the cycle, estrogens inhibit gonadotropin release but then have a brief midcycle stimulatory action that increases the amount released and causes the LH surge. Progesterone, acting on the hypothalamus, exerts the predominant control of the frequency of LH release. It decreases the firing rate of the hypothalamic pulse generator, an action thought to be mediated largely via inhibitory opioid neurons (containing PRs) that synapse with GnRH neurons. Progesterone also exerts a direct effect on the pituitary to oppose the inhibitory actions of estrogens and thus enhance the amount of LH released (i.e., to increase the amplitude of the LH pulses). These steroid feedback effects, coupled with the intrinsic activity of the hypothalamic GnRH pulse generator, lead to relatively frequent LH pulses of small amplitude in the follicular phase of the cycle and less-frequent pulses of larger amplitude in the luteal phase. Studies in knockout mice indicated that ERα (Hewitt and Korach, 2003) and PR-A (Conneely et al., 2002) mediate the major actions of estrogens and progestins, respectively, on the hypothalamic-pituitary axis.

When the ovaries are removed or cease to function, there is overproduction of FSH and LH, which are excreted in the urine. Measurement of urinary or plasma LH is valuable to assess pituitary function and the effectiveness of therapeutic doses of estrogen.

Effects of Cyclical Gonadal Steroids on the Reproductive Tract

The cyclical changes in estrogen and progesterone production by the ovaries regulate corresponding events in the fallopian tubes, uterus, cervix, and vagina. Physiologically, these changes prepare the uterus for implantation, and the proper timing of events in these tissues is essential for pregnancy. If pregnancy does not occur, the endometrium is shed as the menstrual discharge.

The uterus is composed of an *endometrium* and a *myometrium*. The endometrium contains an epithelium lining the uterine cavity and an underlying stroma; the myometrium is the smooth muscle component responsible for uterine contractions. These cell layers, the fallopian tubes, cervix, and vagina display a characteristic set of responses to both estrogens and progestins. The changes typically associated with menstruation occur largely in the endometrium (Figure 44–3).

The *luminal surface* of the endometrium is a layer of simple columnar epithelial secretory and ciliated cells that is continuous with the openings of numerous glands that extend through the underlying stroma to the myometrial border. Fertilization normally occurs in the fallopian tubes, so ovulation, transport of the fertilized ovum through the fallopian tube, and preparation of the endometrial surface must be temporally coordinated for successful implantation.

The *endometrial stroma* is a highly cellular connective tissue layer containing a variety of blood vessels that undergo cyclic changes associated with menstruation. The predominant cells are fibroblasts, but macrophages, lymphocytes, and other resident and migratory cell types also are present.

Menstruation marks the start of the menstrual cycle. During the follicular (or proliferative) phase of the cycle, estrogen begins the rebuilding

of the endometrium by stimulating proliferation and differentiation. An important response to estrogen in the endometrium and other tissues is induction of the PR, which enables cells to respond to this hormone during the second half of the cycle.

In the luteal (or secretory) phase of the cycle, elevated progesterone limits the proliferative effect of estrogens on the endometrium by stimulating differentiation. Major effects include stimulation of epithelial secretions important for implantation of the blastocyst and the characteristic growth of the endometrial blood vessels seen at this time. These effects are mediated by PR-A in animal models (Conneely et al., 2002). Progesterone is thus important in preparation for implantation and for the changes that take place in the uterus at the implantation site (i.e., the decidual response). There is a narrow "window of implantation," spanning days 19–24 of the endometrial cycle, when the epithelial cells of the endometrium are receptive to blastocyst implantation. If implantation occurs, hCG (Chapter 42), produced initially by the trophoblast and later by the placenta, interacts with the LH receptor of the corpus luteum to maintain steroid hormone synthesis during the early stages of pregnancy. Later, the placenta becomes the major site of estrogen and progesterone synthesis.

Estrogens and progesterone have important effects on the fallopian tube, myometrium, and cervix. In the fallopian tube, estrogens stimulate proliferation and differentiation, whereas progesterone inhibits these processes. Also, estrogens increase and progesterone decreases tubal muscular contractility, which affects transit time of the ovum to the uterus. Estrogens increase the amount of cervical mucus and its water content to facilitate sperm penetration of the cervix, whereas progesterone generally has opposite effects. Estrogens favor rhythmic contractions of the uterine myometrium, and progesterone diminishes contractions. These effects are physiologically important and may also play a role in the action of some contraceptives.

Metabolic Effects

Estrogens affect many tissues and have many metabolic actions in humans and animals. Many nonreproductive tissues, including bone, vascular endothelium, liver, CNS, immune system, GI tract, and heart, express low levels of both ERs, and the ratio of ERα to ERβ varies in a cell-specific manner. The effects of estrogens on selected aspects of mineral, lipid, carbohydrate, and protein metabolism are particularly important for understanding their pharmacological actions.

Estrogens have positive effects on bone mass (Riggs et al., 2002). Bone is continuously remodeled at sites called *bone-remodeling units* by the resorptive action of osteoclasts and the bone-forming action of osteoblasts (Chapter 48). Estrogens directly regulate osteoblasts and increase osteocyte survival by inhibiting apoptosis (Kousteni et al., 2002; Levin, 2008). However, a major effect of estrogens is to decrease the number and activity of osteoclasts. Much of the action of estrogens on osteoclasts appears to be mediated by altering cytokine (both paracrine and autocrine) signals from osteoblasts. Estrogens also increase osteoblast production of the cytokine osteoprotegerin (OPG), a soluble, non–membrane-bound member of the tumor necrosis factor superfamily. OPG acts as a "decoy" receptor that antagonizes the binding of OPG-ligand (OPG-L) to its receptor (termed *RANK*, or *receptor activator of NF-κB*) and prevents the differentiation of osteoclast precursors to mature osteoclasts. Estrogens increase osteoclast apoptosis, either directly or by increasing OPG. Estrogens affect bone growth and epiphyseal closure in both sexes. The importance of estrogen in the male skeleton is illustrated by a man with a completely defective ER who had osteoporosis, unfused epiphyses, increased bone turnover, and delayed bone age (Smith et al., 1994).

Estrogens slightly elevate serum triglycerides and slightly reduce total serum cholesterol levels. They increase HDL levels and decrease the levels of LDL and LPA (Chapter 33). This beneficial alteration of the ratio of HDL to LDL is an attractive but unproven effect of estrogen therapy in postmenopausal women. At relatively high concentrations, estrogens have antioxidant activity and may inhibit the oxidation of LDL by affecting superoxide dismutase. Estrogen actions on the vascular wall include increased production of NO, which occurs within minutes via a mechanism involving activation of Akt (protein kinase B) and induction of NO synthase (Simoncini et al., 2000). All of these changes promote vasodilation and retard atherogenesis. Estrogens also promote endothelial cell growth while inhibiting the proliferation of vascular smooth muscle cells.

The presence of ERs in the liver suggests that the beneficial effects of estrogen on lipoprotein metabolism are due partly to direct hepatic actions. Estrogens also alter bile composition by increasing cholesterol secretion and decreasing bile acid secretion. This leads to increased saturation of bile with cholesterol and appears to be the basis for increased gallstone formation in some women receiving estrogens. In general, estrogens increase plasma levels of cortisol-binding globulin, thyroxine-binding globulin, and SHBG, which binds both androgens and estrogens.

Estrogens alter a number of metabolic pathways that affect the clotting cascade (Mendelsohn and Karas, 1999). Systemic effects include changes in hepatic production of plasma proteins. Estrogens cause a small increase in coagulation factors II, VII, IX, X, and XII, and they decrease the anticoagulation factors protein C, protein S, and antithrombin III (Chapter 32). Fibrinolytic pathways also are affected, and several studies of women treated with estrogen alone or estrogen with a progestin have demonstrated decreased levels of PAI-1 protein with a concomitant increase in fibrinolysis (Koh et al., 1997). Thus, estrogens increase both coagulation and fibrinolytic pathways, and imbalance in these two opposing activities may cause adverse effects.

Estrogen Receptors

Estrogens exert their effects by interaction with receptors that are members of the superfamily of nuclear receptors. The two ER genes are located on separate chromosomes: ESR1 encodes ERα, and ESR2 encodes ERβ. Both ERs are estrogen-dependent nuclear transcription factors that have different tissue distributions and transcriptional regulatory effects on a wide number of target genes (Hanstein et al., 2004). Both ERα and ERβ exist as multiple mRNA isoforms due to differential promoter use and alternative splicing (reviewed by Kos et al., 2001; Lewandowski et al., 2002). The two human ERs are 44% identical in overall amino acid sequence and share the domain structure common to members of this family. There are significant differences between the two receptor isoforms in the ligand-binding domains and in both transactivation domains. Human ERβ does not appear to contain a functional AF-1 domain. The receptors appear to have different biological functions and respond differently to various estrogenic compounds (Kuiper et al., 1997). However, their high homology in the DNA-binding domains suggests that both receptors recognize similar DNA sequences and hence regulate many of the same target genes.

Estrogen receptor α is expressed most abundantly in the female reproductive tract—especially the uterus, vagina, and ovaries—as well as in the mammary gland, the hypothalamus, endothelial cells, and vascular smooth muscle. ERβ is expressed most highly in the prostate and ovaries, with lower expression in lung, brain, bone, and vasculature. Many cells express both ERα and ERβ, which can form either homo- or heterodimers. Both forms of ER are expressed on breast cancers, although ERα is believed to be the predominant form responsible for growth regulation (Chapter 67). When coexpressed with ERα, ERβ can inhibit ERα-mediated transcriptional activation in many cases (Hall and McDonnell, 1999). Polymorphic variants of ER have been identified, but attempts to correlate specific polymorphisms with the frequency of breast cancer (Han et al., 2003), bone mass (Kurabayashi et al., 2004), endometrial cancer (Weiderpass et al., 2000), or cardiovascular disease (Herrington and Howard, 2003) have led to contradictory results.

A cloned G protein–coupled receptor, GPR30, also appears to interact with estrogens in some cell systems, and its participation in the rapid effects of estrogen is an attractive idea. There may be interaction/cross-talk between membrane-associated ERα and membrane-localized GPR30 in some cancer cells, but in vivo confirmation is lacking (Levin, 2008; Olde and Leeb-Lundberg, 2009).

Mechanism of Action

Both ERs are ligand-activated transcription factors that increase or decrease the transcription of target genes (Figure 44–4). After entering the cell by passive diffusion through the plasma membrane, the hormone binds to an ER in the nucleus. In the nucleus, the ER is present as an inactive monomer bound to HSP90, and on binding estrogen, a change in ER conformation dissociates the HSPs and causes receptor dimerization, which increases the affinity and the rate of receptor binding to DNA (Cheskis et al., 1997). Homodimers of ERα or ERβ and ERα/ERβ heterodimers can be produced depending on the receptor complement in a given cell. The concept of ligand-mediated changes in ER conformation is central to understanding the mechanism of action of estrogen agonists and antagonists. The ER dimer binds to EREs, typically located in the promoter region of target genes. The ER/DNA complex recruits a cascade of coactivator and other proteins to the promoter region of target genes (Figure 44–4B) and allows the proteins that make up the general transcription apparatus to assemble and initiate transcription.

Besides coactivators and corepressors, both ERα and ERβ can interact physically with other transcription factors, such as Sp1 (Saville et al., 2000) or AP-1 (Paech et al., 1997), and these protein-protein interactions provide an alternate mechanism of action. In these circumstances, ER-ligand complexes interact with Sp1 or AP-1 that is already bound to its specific regulatory element, such that the ER complex does not interact directly with an ERE. This may explain how estrogens are able to regulate genes that lack a consensus ERE. Responses to agonists and antagonists mediated by these protein-protein interactions also are ER isoform and promoter specific. For example, 17β-estradiol induces transcription of a target gene controlled by an AP-1 site in the presence of an ERα/AP-1 complex but inhibits transcription in the presence of an ERβ/AP-1 complex. Conversely, antiestrogens are potent activators of ERβ/AP-1 but not of ERα/AP-1 complexes.

Other signaling systems may activate nuclear ER by ligand-independent mechanisms. Phosphorylation of ERα at serine 118 by MAPK activates the receptor (Kato et al., 1995). Similarly, PI3K-activated Akt directly phosphorylates ERα, causing ligand-independent activation of estrogen target genes (Simoncini et al., 2000). This provides a means of cross-talk between membrane-bound receptor pathways (i.e., EGF/IGF-1) that activate MAPK and the nuclear ER.

Some ERs are located on the plasma membrane of cells. These ERs are encoded by the same genes that encode ERα and ERβ but are transported to the plasma membrane and reside mainly in caveolae (Pedram et al., 2006). Translocation to the membrane by all sex steroid receptors is mediated by palmitoylation of a 9–amino acid motif in the respective E domains of the receptors (Levin, 2008). Membrane-localized ERs mediate the rapid activation of some proteins such as MAPK (phosphorylated in several cell types) and the rapid increase in cyclic AMP caused by the hormone. The finding that MAPK is activated by estradiol provides an additional level of cross-talk and complexity in estrogen signaling.

Pharmacology

ADME

Various estrogens are available for oral, parenteral, transdermal, or topical administration. Given the lipophilic nature of estrogens, absorption generally is good with the appropriate preparation. Aqueous or oil-based esters of estradiol are available for intramuscular injection, ranging in frequency from every week to once per month. Conjugated estrogens are available for intravenous or intramuscular administration. Transdermal patches that are changed once or twice weekly deliver estradiol continuously through the skin. Preparations are available for topical use in the vagina or for application to the skin. For many therapeutic uses, estrogen preparations are available in combination with a progestin. All estrogens are labeled with precautionary statements urging the prescribing of the lowest effective dose and for the shortest duration consistent with the treatment goals and risks for each individual patient.

Oral administration is common and may use estradiol, conjugated estrogens, esters of estrone and other estrogens, and *ethinyl estradiol*

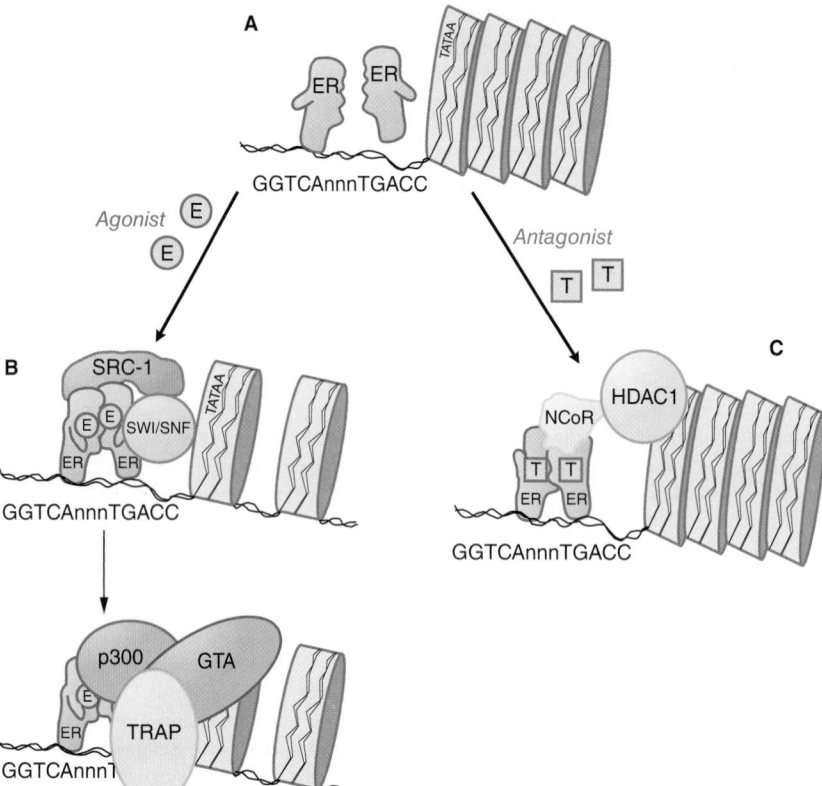

Figure 44–4 *Molecular mechanism of action of nuclear ER.* **A**. Unliganded ER exists as a monomer within the nucleus. **B**. Agonists such as 17β-estradiol (E) bind to the ER and cause a ligand-directed change in conformation that facilitates dimerization and interaction with specific ERE sequences in DNA. The ER-DNA complex recruits coactivators such as SWI/SNF that modify chromatin structure and coactivators such as SRC-1 that has histone acetyltransferase activity that further alters chromatin structure. This remodeling facilitates the exchange of the recruited proteins such that other coactivators (e.g., p300 and the TRAP complex) associate on the target gene promoter and proteins that comprise the general transcription apparatus (GTA) are recruited, with subsequent synthesis of mRNA. **C**. Antagonists such as tamoxifen (T) also bind to the ER but produce a different receptor conformation. The antagonist-induced conformation also facilitates dimerization and interaction with DNA, but a different set of proteins called corepressors, such as NcoR, are recruited to the complex. NcoR further recruits proteins such as histone deacetylase I (HDAC1) that act on histones to stabilize nucleosome structure and prevent interaction with the GTA.

(*in combination with a progestin*). Estradiol is available in nonmicronized and micronized preparations. The micronized formulations yield a large surface for rapid absorption to partially overcome low absolute oral bioavailability due to first-pass metabolism (Fotherby, 1996). Addition of the ethinyl substituent at C17 (ethinyl estradiol) inhibits first-pass hepatic metabolism. Other common oral preparations contain conjugated equine estrogens, which are primarily the sulfate esters of estrone, equilin, and other naturally occurring compounds; *esterified esters*; or mixtures of synthetic conjugated estrogens prepared from plant-derived sources. These are hydrolyzed by enzymes present in the lower gut that remove the charged sulfate groups and allow absorption of estrogen across the intestinal epithelium. In another oral preparation, *estropipate*, estrone is solubilized as the sulfate and stabilized with piperazine. Due largely to differences in metabolism, the potencies of various oral preparations differ widely; ethinyl estradiol, for example, is much more potent than conjugated estrogens.

A number of foodstuffs and plant-derived products, largely from soy, are available as nonprescription items and often are touted as providing benefits similar to those from compounds with established estrogenic activity. These products may contain flavonoids such as genistein (Table 44–1), which display estrogenic activity in laboratory tests, albeit generally much less than that of estradiol. In theory, these preparations could produce appreciable estrogenic effects, but their efficacy at relevant doses has not been established in human trials (Fitzpatrick, 2003).

Administration of estradiol via transdermal patches provides slow, sustained release of the hormone, systemic distribution, and more constant blood levels than oral dosing. Estradiol is also available as a topical emulsion applied to the upper thigh and calf or as a gel applied once daily to

the arm. The transdermal route does not lead to the high levels of the drug that occur in the portal circulation after oral administration, and it is thus expected to minimize hepatic effects of estrogens (e.g., effects on hepatic protein synthesis, lipoprotein profiles, and triglyceride levels).

When dissolved in oil and injected, esters of estradiol are well absorbed. Preparations available for intramuscular injection include compounds such as *estradiol valerate* or *estradiol cypionate* and may be absorbed over several weeks following a single intramuscular injection.

Preparations of estradiol and conjugated estrogen creams are available for topical administration to the vagina. These are effective locally, but systemic effects also are possible due to significant absorption. A 3-month vaginal ring may be used for slow release of estradiol, and tablets are also available for vaginal use (Vagifem).

Estradiol, ethinyl estradiol, and other estrogens are extensively bound to plasma proteins. Estradiol and other naturally occurring estrogens are bound mainly to SHBG and to a lesser degree to serum albumin. In contrast, ethinyl estradiol is bound extensively to serum albumin but not SHBG. Due to their size and lipophilic nature, unbound estrogens distribute rapidly and extensively.

Variations in estradiol metabolism occur and depend on the stage of the menstrual cycle, menopausal status, and several genetic polymorphisms (Herrington and Klein, 2001). In general, the hormone undergoes rapid hepatic biotransformation, with a plasma $t_{1/2}$ measured in minutes. Estradiol is converted primarily by 17β-hydroxysteroid dehydrogenase to estrone, which undergoes conversion by 16α-hydroxylation and 17-keto reduction to estriol, the major urinary metabolite. A variety of sulfate and glucuronide conjugates also are excreted in the urine. Lesser amounts of estrone or estradiol are oxidized to the 2-hydroxycatechols by CYP3A4 in the liver and by CYP1A in extrahepatic tissues or to 4-hydroxycatechols by CYP1B1 in extrahepatic sites, with the 2-hydroxycatechol formed to a greater extent. The 2- and 4-hydroxycatechols are largely inactivated by COMTs. However, smaller amounts may be converted by CYP- or peroxidase-catalyzed reactions to yield semiquinones or quinones that are capable of forming DNA adducts or of generating (via redox cycling) ROSs that could oxidize DNA bases (Yue et al., 2003).

Estrogens also undergo enterohepatic recirculation via (1) sulfate and glucuronide conjugation in the liver, (2) biliary secretion of the conjugates into the intestine, and (3) hydrolysis in the gut (largely by bacterial enzymes) followed by reabsorption.

Many other drugs and environmental agents (e.g., cigarette smoke) act as inducers or inhibitors of the various enzymes that metabolize estrogens and thus have the potential to alter their clearance. Consideration of the impact of these factors on efficacy and untoward effects is increasingly important with the decreased doses of estrogens currently employed for both MHT and contraception.

Ethinyl estradiol is cleared much more slowly than estradiol due to decreased hepatic metabolism, and the elimination-phase $t_{1/2}$ in various studies ranges from 13 to 27 h. Unlike estradiol, the primary route of biotransformation of ethinyl estradiol is via 2-hydroxylation and subsequent formation of the corresponding 2- and 3-methyl ethers. *Mestranol*, another semisynthetic estrogen and a component of some combination oral contraceptives, is the 3-methyl ether of ethinyl estradiol. In the body, it undergoes rapid hepatic demethylation to ethinyl estradiol, which is its active form (Fotherby, 1996).

Selective Estrogen Receptor Modulators and Antiestrogens

By altering the conformation of the two different ERs and thereby changing interactions with coactivators and corepressors in cell-specific and promoter-specific contexts, ligands may have a broad spectrum of activities from purely antiestrogenic in all tissues, to partially estrogenic in some tissues with antiestrogenic or no activities in others, to purely estrogenic activities in all tissues. The elucidation of these concepts has been a major breakthrough in estrogen pharmacology and should permit the rational design of drugs with selective patterns of estrogenic activity (Smith and O'Malley, 2004).

Selective Estrogen Receptor Modulators: Tamoxifen, Raloxifene, and Toremifene

Selective ER modulators, or SERMs, are compounds with tissue-selective actions. The pharmacological goal of these drugs is to produce beneficial estrogenic actions in certain tissues (e.g., bone, brain, and liver) during post-MHT but antagonist activity in tissues such as breast and endometrium, where estrogenic actions (e.g., carcinogenesis) might be deleterious. Currently approved drugs in the U.S. in this class are *tamoxifen citrate*, *raloxifene hydrochloride*, and *toremifene*, which is chemically related and has similar actions to tamoxifen. Tamoxifen and toremifene are used for the treatment of breast cancer, and raloxifene is used primarily for the prevention and treatment of osteoporosis and to reduce the risk of invasive breast cancer in high-risk postmenopausal women. They are considered in detail in Chapter 68.

Antiestrogens: Clomiphene and Fulvestrant

The antiestrogen compounds are distinguished from the SERMs in that they are pure antagonists in all tissues studied. Clomiphene is approved for the treatment of infertility in anovulatory women, and fulvestrant is used for the treatment of breast cancer in women with disease progression after tamoxifen.

Chemistry

The structures of the *trans*-isomer of tamoxifen, and of raloxifene, *trans*-clomiphene (enclomiphene), and fulvestrant are as follows:

ENCLOMIPHENE TAMOXIFEN

R_1: —CH_2CH_3 —CH_3
R_2: —Cl —CH_2CH_3

RALOXIFENE

FULVESTRANT (ICI 182, 780)

Tamoxifen is a triphenylethylene with the same stilbene nucleus as DES; compounds of this class display a variety of estrogenic and antiestrogenic activities. In general, the *trans* conformations have antiestrogenic activity, whereas the *cis* conformations display estrogenic activity. However, the pharmacological activity of the *trans* compound depends on the species, target tissue, and gene. Hepatic metabolism produces primarily *N*-desmethyltamoxifen, which has affinity for ER comparable to that of tamoxifen, and lesser amounts of the highly active 4-hydroxy metabolite, which has a 25–50 times higher affinity for both ERα and ERβ than does tamoxifen (Kuiper et al., 1997). Tamoxifen is marketed as the pure *trans*-isomer. Toremifene is a triphenylethylene with a chlorine substitution at the R2 position.

Raloxifene is a polyhydroxylated nonsteroidal compound with a benzothiophene core. Raloxifene binds with high affinity for both ERα and ERβ (Kuiper et al., 1997).

Clomiphene citrate is a triphenylethylene; its two isomers, zuclomiphene (*cis* clomiphene) and enclomiphene (*trans* clomiphene), are a weak estrogen agonist and a potent antagonist, respectively. Clomiphene binds to both ERα and ERβ, but the individual isomers have not been examined (Kuiper et al., 1997).

Fulvestrant is a 7α-alkylamide derivative of estradiol that interacts with both ERα and ERβ (Van Den Bemd et al., 1999).

Pharmacological Effects

All of these agents bind to the ligand-binding pocket of both ERα and ERβ and competitively block estradiol binding. However, the conformation of the ligand-bound ERs is different with different ligands (Smith and O'Malley, 2004), and this has two important mechanistic consequences. The distinct ER-ligand conformations recruit different coactivators and corepressors onto the promoter of a target gene by differential protein-protein interactions at the receptor surface. The tissue-specific actions of SERMs thus can be explained in part by the distinct conformation of the ER when occupied by different ligands, in combination with different coactivator and corepressor levels in different cell types that together affect the nature of ER complexes formed in a tissue-selective fashion.

Tamoxifen. Tamoxifen exhibits antiestrogenic, estrogenic, or mixed activity depending on the species and target gene measured. In clinical tests or laboratory studies with human cells, the drug's activity depends on the tissue and end point measured. For example, tamoxifen inhibits the proliferation of cultured human breast cancer cells and reduces tumor size and number in women (Jaiyesimi et al., 1995), and yet it stimulates proliferation of endometrial cells and causes endometrial thickening (Lahti et al., 1993). The drug has an antiresorptive effect on bone, and in humans it decreases total cholesterol, LDL, and LPA but does not increase HDL and triglycerides (Love et al., 1994). Tamoxifen treatment causes a 2- to 3-fold increase in the relative risk of deep vein thrombosis and pulmonary embolism and a roughly 2-fold increase in endometrial carcinoma (Smith, 2003). Tamoxifen produces hot flashes and other adverse effects, including cataracts and nausea. Due to its agonist activity in bone, it does not increase the incidence of fractures when used in this setting.

The conformation of ERs, especially in the AF-2 domain, determines whether a coactivator or a corepressor will be recruited to the ER-DNA complex (Smith and O'Malley, 2004). Tamoxifen induces a conformation that permits the recruitment of the corepressor to both ERα and ERβ, in contrast to 17α-estradiol, which induces a conformation that recruits coactivators to the receptor. The agonist activity of tamoxifen seen in tissues such as the endometrium is mediated by the ligand-independent AF-1 transactivation domain of ERα; because ERβ does not contain a functional AF-1 domain, tamoxifen does not activate ERβ (McInerney et al., 1998).

Raloxifene. Raloxifene is an estrogen agonist in bone, where it exerts an antiresorptive effect. The drug also acts as an estrogen agonist in reducing total cholesterol and LDL, but it does not increase HDL or normalize PAI-1 in postmenopausal women (Walsh et al., 1998). Studies indicated that raloxifene has an antiproliferative effect on ER-positive breast tumors and significantly reduces the risk of ER-positive but not ER-negative breast cancer (Cummings et al., 1999). Raloxifene does not alleviate the vasomotor symptoms associated with menopause. Adverse effects include hot flashes and leg cramps and a 3-fold increase in deep vein thrombosis and pulmonary embolism (Cummings et al., 1999).

Raloxifene acts as a partial agonist in bone but does not stimulate endometrial proliferation in postmenopausal women. Presumably this is due to some combination of differential expression of transcription factors in the two tissues and the effects of this SERM on ER conformation. Raloxifene induces a configuration in ERα that is distinct from that of tamoxifen-ERβ (Tamrazi et al., 2003), suggesting that a different set of coactivators/corepressors may interact with ER-raloxifene compared with ER-tamoxifen.

Fulvestrant. Fulvestrant is antiestrogenic. In clinical trials, it is efficacious in treating tamoxifen-resistant breast cancers (Robertson et al., 2003). Fulvestrant binds to ERα and ERβ with high affinity comparable to estradiol but represses transactivation. It also increases dramatically the intracellular proteolytic degradation of ERα while apparently protecting ERβ from degradation (Van Den Bemd et al., 1999). This effect on ERα protein levels may explain fulvestrant's efficacy in tamoxifen-resistant breast cancer.

Clomiphene. Clomiphene increases gonadotropin secretion and stimulates ovulation. It increases the amplitude of LH and FSH pulses without changing pulse frequency (Kettel et al., 1993). This suggests that the drug is acting largely at the pituitary level to block inhibitory actions of estrogen on gonadotropin release from the gland or is somehow causing the hypothalamus to release larger amounts of GnRH per pulse.

The most prominent effect of clomiphene in women was enlargement of the ovaries and the drug-induced ovulation in many patients with amenorrhea, polycystic ovarian syndrome, and dysfunctional bleeding with anovulatory cycles. Thus, clomiphene's major pharmacological use is to induce ovulation in women with a functional hypothalamic-hypophyseal-ovarian system and adequate endogenous estrogen production. In some cases, clomiphene is used in conjunction with human gonadotropins (Chapter 42) to induce ovulation.

ADME

Tamoxifen is given orally, and peak plasma levels are reached within 4–7 h. It has two elimination phases with half-lives of 7–14 h and 4–11 days. Due to the prolonged $t_{1/2}$, 3–4 weeks of treatment are required to reach steady-state plasma levels. Tamoxifen is metabolized in humans by multiple hepatic CYPs, some of which it also induces (Sridar et al., 2002). In humans and other species, 4-hydroxytamoxifen is produced via hepatic metabolism, and this compound is considerably more potent than the parent drug as an antiestrogen. The major route of elimination from the body involves N-demethylation and deamination. The drug undergoes enterohepatic circulation, and excretion is primarily in the feces as conjugates of the deaminated metabolite. Polymorphisms affect the rate of tamoxifen metabolism to its more potent 4-hydroxy metabolite and may affect its therapeutic activity in breast cancer (Chapter 67).

Raloxifene is absorbed rapidly after oral administration and has an absolute bioavailability of about 2%. The drug has a $t_{1/2}$ of about 28 h and is eliminated primarily in the feces after hepatic glucuronidation.

Clomiphene is well absorbed following oral administration, and the drug and its metabolites are eliminated primarily in the feces and to a lesser extent in the urine. The long plasma $t_{1/2}$ (5–7 days) is due largely to plasma-protein binding, enterohepatic circulation, and accumulation in fatty tissues.

Fulvestrant is administered monthly by intramuscular depot injections. Plasma concentrations reach maximal levels in 7 days and are maintained for a month. Numerous metabolites are formed in vivo, possibly by pathways similar to endogenous estrogen metabolism, but the drug is eliminated primarily (90%) via the feces in humans.

Therapeutic Uses

Breast Cancer. Tamoxifen is highly efficacious in the treatment of breast cancer. It is used alone for palliation of advanced breast cancer in women with ER-positive tumors, and it is now indicated as the hormonal treatment of choice for both early and advanced breast cancer in women of all ages (Jaiyesimi et al., 1995). Response rates are about 50% in women with ER-positive tumors. Tamoxifen increases disease-free survival and overall survival; treatment for 5 years reduces cancer recurrence by 50% and death by 27% and is more efficacious than shorter 1- to 2-year treatment periods. Tamoxifen reduces the risk of developing contralateral breast cancer and is approved for primary prevention of breast cancer in women at high risk, in whom it causes a 50% decrease in the development of new tumors. Prophylactic treatment should be limited to 5 years because effectiveness decreases thereafter. The most frequent side effect is hot flashes. Tamoxifen has estrogenic activity in the uterus, increases the risk of endometrial cancer by 2- to 3-fold, and also causes a comparable increase in the risk of thromboembolic disease that leads to serious risks for women receiving anticoagulant therapy (Smith, 2003) and women with a history of deep vein thrombosis or stroke.

Toremifene has therapeutic actions similar to tamoxifen, and fulvestrant may be efficacious in women who become resistant to tamoxifen. Untoward effects of fulvestrant include hot flashes, GI symptoms, headache, back pain, and pharyngitis.

Osteoporosis. Raloxifene reduces the rate of bone loss and may increase bone mass at certain sites. In a large clinical trial, raloxifene increased spinal bone mineral density by more than 2% and reduced the rate of vertebral fractures by 30%–50% but did not significantly reduce nonvertebral fractures (Delmas et al., 2002; Ettinger et al., 1999). Raloxifene does not appear to increase the risk of developing endometrial cancer. The drug has beneficial actions on lipoprotein metabolism, reducing both total cholesterol and LDL; however, HDL is not increased. Adverse effects include hot flashes, deep vein thrombosis, and leg cramps.

Infertility. Clomiphene citrate is a potent antiestrogen that primarily is used for treatment of anovulation in the setting of an intact hypothalamic-pituitary axis and adequate estrogen production (e.g., PCOS) or to induce superovulation in women with unexplained infertility. By inhibiting the negative-feedback effects of estrogen at hypothalamic and pituitary levels, clomiphene increases FSH levels and thereby enhances follicular maturation. The drug is relatively inexpensive, is orally active, and requires less-extensive monitoring than do other fertility protocols. However, the drug may exhibit untoward effects, including ovarian hyperstimulation, increased incidence of multiple births, ovarian cysts, hot flashes, and blurred vision. Prolonged use (e.g., ≥ 12 cycles) may increase the risk of ovarian cancer. The drug should not be administered to pregnant women due to reports of teratogenicity in animals, but there is no evidence of this when the drug has been used to induce ovulation.

Experimental SERM-Estrogen Combinations. There is considerable interest in MHT using combinations of a pure estrogen agonist (e.g., estradiol) with a SERM that has predominantly antagonist activity in the breast and endometrium but does not distribute to the CNS. The strategy is to obtain the beneficial actions of the agonist (e.g., prevention of hot flashes and bone loss) while the SERM blocks unwanted agonist action at peripheral sites (e.g., proliferative effects in breast and endometrium) but does not enter the brain to cause hot flashes. Animal studies have been encouraging (Labrie et al., 2003), but clinical efficacy and safety of this approach remain to be established.

Estrogen Synthesis Inhibitors

EXEMESTANE

ANASTROZOLE

Continual administration of GnRH agonists prevents ovarian synthesis of estrogens but not their peripheral synthesis from adrenal androgens (Chapter 42). *Aminoglutethimide* inhibits aromatase activity, but its use is limited by its lack of selectivity and its side effects (sedation). It was discontinued in the U.S. in 2008.

The recognition that locally produced as well as circulating estrogens may play a significant role in breast cancer has greatly stimulated interest in the use of aromatase inhibitors to selectively block production of estrogens (Chapter 68). Both steroidal (e.g., formestane and exemestane) and nonsteroidal (e.g., anastrozole, letrozole, and vorozole) agents are available. Steroidal, or type I, agents are substrate analogues that act as suicide inhibitors to irreversibly inactivate aromatase, whereas the nonsteroidal, or type II, agents interact reversibly with the heme groups of CYPs (Haynes et al., 2003). *Exemestane*, *letrozole*, and *anastrozole* are currently approved in the U.S. for the treatment of breast cancer.

As discussed in Chapter 68, these agents may be used as first-line treatment of breast cancer or as second-line drugs after tamoxifen. They are highly efficacious and actually superior to tamoxifen in adjuvant use for postmenopausal women (Coombes et al., 2004), and they are indicated either following tamoxifen for 2–5 years or as initial agents. They have the added advantage of not increasing the risk of uterine cancer or venous thromboembolism. Because they dramatically reduce circulating as well as local levels of estrogens, they produce hot flashes. They lack the beneficial effect of tamoxifen to maintain bone density and thus are usually administered with bisphosphonates. Their effects on plasma lipids remain to be established.

Progestins

HISTORY Progestins

Corner and Allen originally isolated a hormone in 1933 from the corpora lutea of sows and named it *progestin*. The next year, several European groups independently isolated the crystalline compound and called it *luteo-sterone*, unaware of the previous name. This difference in nomenclature was resolved in 1935 at a garden party in London given by Sir Henry Dale, who helped persuade all parties that the name *progesterone* was a suitable compromise.

Two major advances overcame the early difficulties and expense of obtaining progesterone from animal sources. The first was the synthesis of progesterone by Russel Marker from the plant product diosgenin in the 1940s, which provided a relatively inexpensive and highly pure product. The second was the synthesis of 19-nor compounds, the first orally active progestins, in the early 1950s by Carl Djerassi, who synthesized norethindrone at Syntex, and Frank Colton, who synthesized the isomer *norethynodrel* at Searle. These advances led to the development of effective oral contraceptives.

Chemistry

Compounds with biological activities similar to those of progesterone are referred to as progestins, progestational agents, progestagens, progestogens, gestagens, or gestogens. The progestins (Figure 44–5) include the naturally occurring hormone progesterone, 17α-acetoxyprogesterone derivatives in the pregnane series, 19-nortestosterone derivatives in the estrane series, and norgestrel and related compounds in the gonane series. MPA and megestrol acetate are C21 steroids in the pregnane family with selective activity very similar to that of progesterone itself. MPA and oral micronized progesterone are widely used with estrogens for MHT and other situations in which a selective progestational effect is desired. Furthermore, depot MPA is used as a long-acting injectable contraceptive. The 19-nortestosterone derivatives (estranes) were developed for use as progestins in oral contraceptives, and although their predominant activity is progestational, they exhibit androgenic and other activities. The gonanes are another family of "19-nor" compounds, containing an ethyl rather than a methyl substituent in the 13 position. They have diminished androgenic activity relative to the estranes. These two classes of 19-nortestosterone derivatives are the progestational components of most oral and some long-acting injectable contraceptives. The remaining oral contraceptives contain a class of progestins derived from spironolactone (e.g., drospirenone) that have antimineralocorticoid and antiandrogenic properties.

The structural features of several progestins are shown in Figure 44–5. Unlike the ER, which requires a phenolic A ring for high-affinity binding, the PR favors a Δ⁴-3-one A-ring structure in an inverted 1β,2α-conformation. Other steroid hormone receptors also bind this nonphenolic A-ring structure, although the optimal conformation differs from that for the PR. Thus, some synthetic progestins (especially the 19-nor compounds) display limited binding to glucocorticoid, androgen, and mineralocorticoid receptors, a property that probably accounts for some of their nonprogestational activities. The spectrum of activities of these compounds is highly dependent on specific substituent groups, especially the nature of the C17 substituent in the D ring, the presence of a C19 methyl group, and the presence of an ethyl group at position C13.

Biosynthesis and Secretion

Progesterone is secreted by the ovary, mainly from the corpus luteum, during the second half of the menstrual cycle (Figure 44–3). LH, acting via its G protein–coupled receptor, stimulates progesterone secretion during the normal cycle.

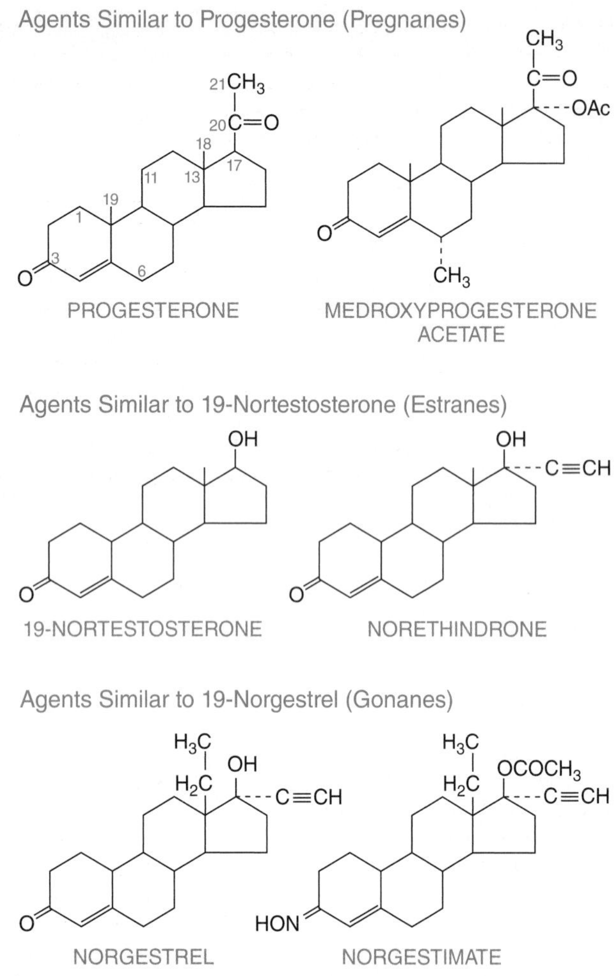

PROGESTERONE

MEDROXYPROGESTERONE ACETATE

Agents Similar to 19-Nortestosterone (Estranes)

19-NORTESTOSTERONE

NORETHINDRONE

Agents Similar to 19-Norgestrel (Gonanes)

NORGESTREL

NORGESTIMATE

Figure 44–5 *Structural features of various progestins.*

After fertilization, the trophoblast secretes hCG into the maternal circulation, which then stimulates the LH receptor to sustain the corpus luteum and maintain progesterone production. During the second or third month of pregnancy, the developing placenta begins to secrete estrogen and progesterone in collaboration with the fetal adrenal glands, and thereafter the corpus luteum is not essential to continued gestation. Estrogen and progesterone continue to be secreted in large amounts by the placenta up to the time of delivery.

Physiologic Actions

Neuroendocrine Actions

Progesterone produced in the luteal phase of the cycle has several physiological effects, including decreasing the frequency of GnRH pulses. This progesterone-mediated decrease in GnRH pulse frequency is critical for suppressing gonadotropin release and resetting the hypothalamic-pituitary-gonadal axis to transition from the luteal back to the follicular phase. Furthermore, GnRH suppression is the major mechanism of action of progestin-containing contraceptives.

Reproductive Tract. Progesterone decreases estrogen-driven endometrial proliferation and leads to the development of a secretory endometrium (Figure 44–3), and the abrupt decline in progesterone at the end of the cycle is the main determinant of the onset of menstruation. If the duration of the luteal phase is artificially lengthened, either by sustaining luteal function or by treatment with progesterone, decidual changes in the endometrial stroma similar to those seen in early pregnancy can be induced. Under normal circumstances, estrogen antecedes and accompanies progesterone in its action on the endometrium and is essential to the development of the normal menstrual pattern.

Progesterone also influences the endocervical glands, and the abundant watery secretion of the estrogen-stimulated structures is changed to a scant viscid material. As noted previously, these and other effects of progestins decrease penetration of the cervix by sperm.

The estrogen-induced maturation of the human vaginal epithelium is modified toward the condition of pregnancy by the action of progesterone, a change that can be detected in cytological alterations in the vaginal smear. If the quantity of estrogen concurrently acting is known to be adequate, or if it is ensured by giving estrogen, the cytological response to a progestin can be used to evaluate its progestational potency.

Progesterone is important for the maintenance of pregnancy. Progesterone suppresses menstruation and uterine contractility.

Mammary Gland. Development of the mammary gland requires both estrogen and progesterone. During pregnancy and to a minor degree during the luteal phase of the cycle, progesterone, acting with estrogen, brings about a proliferation of the acini of the mammary gland. Toward the end of pregnancy, the acini fill with secretions, and the vasculature of the gland notably increases; however, only after the levels of estrogen and progesterone decrease at parturition does lactation begin.

During the normal menstrual cycle, mitotic activity in the breast epithelium is very low in the follicular phase and then peaks in the luteal phase. This pattern is due to progesterone, which triggers a *single* round of mitotic activity in the mammary epithelium. This effect is transient because continued exposure to the hormone is rapidly followed by arrest of growth of the epithelial cells. Importantly, progesterone may be responsible for the increased risk of breast cancer associated with estrogen-progestin use in postmenopausal women, although controlled studies with only progestin have not been performed (Anderson et al., 2004; Rossouw et al., 2002).

CNS. During a normal menstrual cycle, an increase in basal body temperature of about 0.6°C (1°F) may be noted at midcycle; this correlates with ovulation. This increase is due to progesterone, but the exact mechanism of this effect is unknown. Progesterone also increases the ventilatory response of the respiratory centers to carbon dioxide and leads to reduced arterial and alveolar P_{CO_2} in the luteal phase of the menstrual cycle and during pregnancy. Progesterone also may have depressant and hypnotic actions in the CNS, possibly accounting for reports of drowsiness after hormone administration. This potential untoward effect may be abrogated by giving progesterone preparations at bedtime, which may even help some patients sleep.

Metabolic Effects. Progestins have numerous metabolic actions. Progesterone itself increases basal insulin levels and the rise in insulin after carbohydrate ingestion, but it does not normally alter glucose tolerance. However, long-term administration of more potent progestins, such as norgestrel, may decrease glucose tolerance. Progesterone stimulates lipoprotein lipase activity and seems to enhance fat deposition. Progesterone and analogues such as MPA have been reported to increase LDL and cause either no effects or modest reductions in serum HDL levels. The 19-norprogestins may have more pronounced effects on plasma lipids because of their androgenic activity.

Medroxyprogesterone acetate decreases the favorable HDL increase caused by conjugated estrogens during postmenopausal hormone replacement, but it does not significantly affect the beneficial effect of estrogens to lower LDL. In contrast, micronized progesterone does not significantly alter beneficial estrogen effects on either HDL or LDL profiles (Writing Group for the PEPI Trial, 1995); the spironolactone derivative drospirenone may actually have advantageous effects on the cardiovascular system due to its antiandrogenic and antimineralocorticoid activities. Progesterone also may diminish the effects of aldosterone in the renal tubule and cause a decrease in sodium reabsorption that may increase mineralocorticoid secretion from the adrenal cortex.

Pharmacology

Mechanism of Action

A single gene encodes two isoforms of the PR, PR-A and PR-B. The first 164 N-terminal amino acids of PR-B are missing from PR-A; this occurs by use of two distinct estrogen-dependent promoters in the PR gene (Giangrande and McDonnell, 1999). The ratios of the individual isoforms vary in reproductive tissues as a consequence of tissue type, developmental status, and hormone levels. Both PR-A and PR-B have AF-1 and AF-2 transactivation domains, but the longer PR-B also contains an additional AF-3 that contributes to its cell- and promoter-specific activity. Because the ligand-binding domains of the two PR isoforms are identical, there is no difference in ligand binding. In the absence of ligand, PR is present primarily in the nucleus in an inactive monomeric state bound to HSP90, HSP70, and p59. When receptors bind progesterone, the HSPs dissociate, and the receptors are phosphorylated and subsequently form dimers (homo- and heterodimers) that bind with high selectivity to PREs located on target genes (Giangrande and McDonnell, 1999). Transcriptional activation by PR occurs primarily via recruitment of coactivators such as SRC-1, NcoA-1, or NcoA-2 (Collingwood et al., 1999). The receptor-coactivator complex then favors further interactions with additional proteins, such as CBP and p300, which mediate other processes, including histone acetylase activity. Histone acetylation causes remodeling of chromatin that increases the accessibility of general transcriptional proteins, including RNA polymerase II, to the target promoter.

The biological activities of PR-A and PR-B are distinct and depend on the target gene. In most cells, PR-B mediates the stimulatory activities of progesterone; PR-A strongly inhibits this action of PR-B and is also a transcriptional inhibitor of other steroid receptors (McDonnell and Goldman, 1994). Current data suggest that coactivators and corepressors interact differentially with PR-A and PR-B (e.g., the corepressor SMRT binds much more tightly to PR-A than to PR-B) (Giangrande et al., 2000), and this may account, at least in part, for the differential activities of the two isoforms. Female PR-A knockout mice are infertile, with impaired ovulation and defective decidualization and implantation. Several uterine genes appear to be regulated exclusively by PR-A, including calcitonin and amphiregulin (Mulac-Jericevic et al., 2000), and the antiproliferative effect of progesterone on the estrogen-stimulated endometrium is lost in PR-A knockout mice. In contrast, knockout studies suggested that PR-B is largely responsible for mediating hormone effects in the mammary gland (Mulac-Jericevic et al., 2003).

Certain effects of progesterone, such as increased Ca^{2+} mobilization in sperm, can be seen in as little as 3 min (Blackmore, 1999) and are therefore considered transcription independent. Similarly, progesterone can promote oocyte maturation (meiotic resumption) independent of transcription (Hammes, 2004).

ADME

Progesterone undergoes rapid first-pass metabolism, but high-dose (e.g., 100–200 mg) preparations of micronized progesterone are available for oral use. Although the absolute bioavailability of these preparations is low (Fotherby, 1996), efficacious plasma levels nevertheless may be obtained. Progesterone also is available in oil solution for injection, as a vaginal gel, as a slow-release IUD for contraception, and as a vaginal insert for assisted reproductive technology.

Esters such as MPA are available for intramuscular administration, and MPA and megestrol acetate may be used orally. The 19-nor steroids have good oral activity because the ethinyl substituent at C17 significantly slows hepatic metabolism. Implants and depot preparations of synthetic progestins are available in many countries for release over very long periods of time (see section on contraceptives).

In the plasma, progesterone is bound by albumin and corticosteroid-binding globulin but is not appreciably bound to SHBG. 19-Nor compounds, such as norethindrone, norgestrel, and desogestrel, bind to SHBG and albumin, and esters such as MPA bind primarily to albumin. Total binding of all these synthetic compounds to plasma proteins is extensive, 90% or less, but the proteins involved are compound specific.

The elimination $t_{1/2}$ of progesterone is about 5 min, and the hormone is metabolized primarily in the liver to hydroxylated metabolites and their sulfate and glucuronide conjugates, which are eliminated in the urine. A major metabolite specific for progesterone is pregnane-3α,20α-diol; its measurement in urine and plasma is used as an index of endogenous

progesterone secretion. The synthetic progestins have much longer half-lives (e.g., ~ 7 h for norethindrone, 16 h for norgestrel, 12 h for gestodene, and 24 h for MPA). The metabolism of synthetic progestins is thought to be primarily hepatic, and elimination is generally via the urine as conjugates and various polar metabolites.

Antiprogestins and Progesterone Receptor Modulators

The first report of an antiprogestin, RU 38486 (often referred to as RU-486) or *mifepristone*, appeared in 1981; this drug is available for the termination of pregnancy (Christin-Maitre et al., 2000). In 2010, the FDA approved ulipristal acetate, a partial agonist at the progesterone receptor, for emergency contraception. Antiprogestins also have several other potential applications, including to prevent conception, to induce labor, and to treat uterine leiomyomas, endometriosis, meningiomas, and breast cancer (Spitz and Chwalisz, 2000).

Mifepristone

Chemistry

Mifepristone is a derivative of the 19-norprogestin norethindrone containing a dimethyl-aminophenol substituent at the 11β position. It effectively competes with both progesterone and glucocorticoids for binding to their respective receptors. Mifepristone is considered a PRM due to its context-dependent activity. Another widely studied antiprogestin is onapristone (or ZK 98299), which is similar in structure to mifepristone but contains a methyl substituent in the 13α rather than 13β orientation. More selective PRMs, such as asoprisnil, are being studied experimentally (DeManno et al., 2003).

MIFEPRISTONE

Pharmacological Effects

Mifepristone acts primarily as a competitive receptor antagonist for both PRs, although it may have some agonist activity in certain contexts. In contrast, onapristone appears to be a pure progesterone antagonist. PR complexes of both compounds antagonize the actions of progesterone-PR complexes and also appear to preferentially recruit corepressors (Leonhardt and Edwards, 2002).

When administered in the early stages of pregnancy, mifepristone causes decidual breakdown by blockade of uterine PRs. This leads to detachment of the blastocyst, which decreases hCG production. This in turn causes a decrease in progesterone secretion from the corpus luteum, which further accentuates decidual breakdown. Decreased endogenous progesterone coupled with blockade of PRs in the uterus increases uterine PG levels and sensitizes the myometrium to their contractile actions. Mifepristone also causes cervical softening, which facilitates expulsion of the detached blastocyst.

Mifepristone can delay or prevent ovulation depending on the timing and manner of administration. These effects are due largely to actions on the hypothalamus and pituitary rather than the ovary, although the mechanisms are unclear.

If administered for one or several days in the mid- to late luteal phase, mifepristone impairs the development of a secretory endometrium and produces menses. PR blockade at this time is the pharmacological equivalent of progesterone withdrawal, and bleeding normally ensues within several days and lasts for 1–2 weeks after antiprogestin treatment.

Mifepristone also binds to glucocorticoid and androgen receptors and exerts antiglucocorticoid and antiandrogenic actions. A predominant effect in humans is blockade of the feedback inhibition by cortisol of adenocorticotropic hormone secretion from the pituitary, thus increasing both corticotropin and adrenal steroid levels in the plasma.

ADME

Mifepristone is orally active with good bioavailability. Peak plasma levels occur within several hours, and the drug is slowly cleared, with a plasma $t_{1/2}$ of 20–40 h. In plasma, it is bound by α_1-acid glycoprotein, which contributes to the drug's long $t_{1/2}$. Metabolites are primarily the mono- and didemethylated products (thought to have pharmacological activity) formed via CYP3A4. The drug undergoes hepatic metabolism and enterohepatic circulation; metabolic products are found predominantly in the feces (Jang and Benet, 1997).

Therapeutic Uses

Mifepristone, in combination with misoprostol or other PGs, is available for the termination of early pregnancy. When mifepristone is used to produce a medical abortion, a PG is given 48 h after the antiprogestin to further increase myometrial contractions and ensure expulsion of the detached blastocyst. Intramuscular *sulprostone*, intravaginal *gemeprost*, and oral misoprostol have been used. The success rate with such regimens is greater than 90% among women with pregnancies of 49 days' duration or less. The most severe untoward effect is vaginal bleeding, which most often lasts 8–17 days but is only rarely (0.1% of patients) severe enough to require blood transfusions. High percentages of women also have experienced abdominal pain and uterine cramps, nausea, vomiting, and diarrhea due to the PG. Women receiving chronic glucocorticoid therapy should not be given mifepristone because of its antiglucocorticoid activity. In fact, due to its high affinity for the glucocorticoid receptor, high doses of mifepristone can result in adrenal insufficiency.

Perspective: Too Many People?

The incredible growth of the earth's human population stands out as one of the fundamental events of the last two centuries. The Old Testament dictum "be fruitful and multiply" (Genesis 9:1) has been followed too religiously by readers and nonreaders of the Bible alike. In 1798, Malthus started a great controversy by opposing the prevailing view of unlimited progress for humankind by making two postulates and a conclusion. Malthus postulated "that food is necessary for the existence of man" and that sexual attraction between female and male is necessary and likely to persist because "toward the extinction of the passion between the sexes, no progress whatever has hitherto been made," barring "individual exceptions." Malthus concluded that "the power of populations is infinitely greater than the power of the earth to produce subsistence for man," producing a "natural inequality" that would someday loom "insurmountable in the way to perfectibility of society."

Malthus was right: Passion between the sexes persists, and the power of populations is very great indeed, so much so that our sheer numbers have increased to the point that they are straining Earth's capacity to supply food, energy, and raw materials and to absorb the detritus of its human burden. Marine fisheries are being depleted, forests and aquifers are disappearing, and the atmosphere is accumulating greenhouse gases from combustion of the fossil fuels that provide the energy needs of 7 billion people, up from 1 billion in Malthus's day. Perhaps some of the blame can be laid at the feet of medical science: Advances in public health and medicine have led to a significant decline in mortality and an increased life expectancy. However, medical science has also begun to assume a portion of the responsibility for overpopulation and its adverse effects. To this end, drugs in the form of hormones and their analogues have been developed to control human fertility.

Ulipristal

Chemistry

Ulipristal, a derivative of 19-norprogesterone, functions as a selective progesterone receptor modulator, acting as a partial agonist at PRs. Unlike mifepristone, ulipristal appears to be a relatively weak glucocorticoid antagonist.

Pharmacological Effects

In high doses, ulipristal has antiproliferative effects in the uterus; however, its most relevant actions to date involve its capacity to inhibit ovulation. Ulipristal's antiovulatory actions likely occur due to progesterone regulation at many levels, including inhibition of LH release through the hypothalamus and pituitary and inhibition of LH-induced follicular rupture within the ovary.

A 30-mg dose of ulipristal can inhibit ovulation when taken up to 5 days after intercourse. Ulipristal can block ovarian rupture at or even just after the time of the LH surge, confirming that at least some of its effects are directly in the ovary. Ulipristal may also block endometrial implantation of the fertilized egg, although whether this contributes to its effects as an emergency contraceptive is not clear.

Therapeutic Uses

Ulipristal acetate is licensed in the E.U. and the U.S. as an emergency contraceptive. Studies comparing ulipristal to levonorgestrel (progesterone-only emergency contraception) demonstrate that ulipristal is at least as effective when taken up to 72 h after unprotected sexual intercourse. In addition, ulipristal remains effective up to 120 h (5 days) after intercourse, making ulipristal a more versatile emergency contraceptive than levonorgestrel, which does not work well beyond 72 h after unprotected intercourse. The most severe side effect in clinical trials using ulipristal has been a self-limited headache and some abdominal pain.

Therapeutic Uses of Estrogens and Progestins

Hormonal Contraception

Types of Hormonal Contraceptives

Combination Oral Contraceptives. The most frequently used agents in the U.S. are combination oral contraceptives containing both an estrogen and a progestin. These agents come in a variety of formulations and strengths (Table 44–2). Their theoretical efficacy generally is considered to be 99.9%. In practice, the 1-year failure rates of oral contraceptives are somewhat greater than 0.1% (Table 44–3). Combination oral contraceptives are available in many formulations. Almost all contain ethinyl estradiol as the estrogen and a 17α-alkyl-19-nortestosterone derivative as the progestin. Monophasic, biphasic, or triphasic pills are generally provided in 21-day packs. (Virtually all preparations come as 28-day packs, with the pills for the last 7 days containing only inert ingredients.) For the monophasic agents, fixed amounts of the estrogen and progestin are present in each pill, which is taken daily for 21 days, followed by a 7-day "pill-free" period. The biphasic and triphasic preparations provide two or three different pills containing varying amounts of active ingredients, to be taken at different times during the 21-day cycle. This reduces the total amount of steroids administered and more closely approximates the estrogen-to-progestin ratios that occur during the menstrual cycle. With these preparations, predictable menstrual bleeding generally occurs during the 7-day "off" period each month. However, several oral contraceptives are now available whereby progestin withdrawal is only induced every 3 months.

The estrogen content of current preparations ranges from 20 to 50 μg; most contain 30–35 μg. Preparations containing 35 μg or less of an estrogen are generally referred to as "low-dose" or "modern" pills. The dose of progestin is more variable because of differences in potency of the compounds used.

A transdermal preparation of norelgestromin and ethinyl estradiol is marketed for weekly application to the buttock, abdomen, upper arm, or torso for the first 3 consecutive weeks followed by a patch-free week for

Hormonal Contraception: A Brief History

Around the beginning of the 20th century, a number of European scientists, including Beard, Prenant, and Loeb, developed the concept that secretions of the corpus luteum suppressed ovulation during pregnancy. The Austrian physiologist Haberlandt then produced temporary sterility in rodents in 1927 by feeding them ovarian and placental extracts—a clear example of an oral contraceptive. In 1937, Makepeace and colleagues demonstrated that pure progesterone blocked ovulation in rabbits, and Astwood and Fevold found a similar effect in rats in 1939.

In the 1950s, Pincus, Garcia, and Rock found that progesterone and 19-norprogestins prevented ovulation in women. Ironically, this finding grew out of their attempts to treat infertility with estrogen-progestin combinations. The initial findings were that these treatments effectively blocked ovulation in most women. However, concern about cancer and other possible side effects of the estrogen they used (i.e., DES) led to the use of a progestin alone in their studies. One of the compounds used was norethynodrel, and early batches of this compound were contaminated with a small amount of mestranol. When mestranol was removed, it was noted that treatment with pure norethynodrel led to increased breakthrough bleeding and less-consistent inhibition of ovulation. Mestranol was thus reincorporated into the preparation, and this combination was employed in the first large-scale clinical trial of combination oral contraceptives.

Clinical studies in the 1950s in Puerto Rico and Haiti established the virtually complete contraceptive success of the norethynodrel/ mestranol combination. In early 1961, Enovid (norethynodrel plus mestranol; no longer marketed in the U.S.) was the first "Pill" approved by the FDA for use as a contraceptive agent in the U.S.; this was followed in 1962 by approval for Ortho-Novum (norethindrone plus mestranol). By 1966, numerous preparations using either mestranol or ethinyl estradiol with a 19-norprogestin were available. In the 1960s, the progestin-only minipill and long-acting injectable preparations were developed and introduced.

Millions of women began using oral contraceptives, and frequent reports of untoward effects began appearing in the 1970s. The recognition that these side effects were dose dependent and the realization that estrogens and progestins synergistically inhibited ovulation led to the reduction of doses and the development of so-called low-dose or second-generation contraceptives. The increasing use of biphasic and triphasic preparations throughout the 1980s further reduced steroid dosages; it may be that currently used doses are the lowest that will provide reliable contraception. In the 1990s, the "third-generation" oral contraceptives, containing progestins with reduced androgenic activity (e.g., norgestimate and desogestrel), became available in the U.S. after being used in Europe. A variety of contraceptive formulations are currently available, including pills, injections, skin patches, subdermal implants, vaginal rings, and IUDs that release hormones.

each 28-day cycle. A similar 3-week on/1-week off cycle is employed for the intravaginal ring containing ethinyl estradiol and etonogestrel.

Progestin-Only Contraceptives. Several agents are available for progestin-only contraception, with theoretical efficacies of 99%. Specific preparations include the "minipill"; low doses of progestins (e.g., 350 μg of norethindrone) taken daily without interruption; subdermal implants of 216 mg of norgestrel for long-term contraceptive action (e.g., up to 5 years) or 68 mg of etonogestrel for contraception lasting 3 years; and crystalline suspensions of MPA for intramuscular injection of 104 mg or 150 mg of drug. Each provides effective contraception for 3 months.

Intrauterine Devices. Two doses of levonorgestrel-releasing intrauterine systems (IUSs) are available in the U.S. The LNg20 contains 52 mg of levonorgesterel, which is initially released at a rate of 20 μg/d and declines

gradually to 10–14 μg/d after 5 years. A smaller LNg IUS is available for women with a small uterine cavity or cervical stenosis and may result in less pain with insertion. The LNg14 contains 13.5 mg of levonorgesterol, which is initially released at a rate of 14 μg/d and declines to 5 μg/d after 3 years. A copper IUD, TCu380A, is also available in the U.S. It contains 380 mm^2 of copper and is approved for 10 year' use. The TCu380A may be preferred over an LNg IUS in women who desire long-term contraception and wish to avoid exogenous hormones and hormonal side effects and can also be used as an emergency contraceptive.

Mechanism of Action

Combination Oral Contraceptives. Combination oral contraceptives act by preventing ovulation. Direct measurements of plasma hormone levels indicate that LH and FSH levels are suppressed, a midcycle surge of LH is absent, endogenous steroid levels are diminished, and ovulation does not occur. Although either component alone can be shown to exert these effects in certain situations, the combination synergistically decreases plasma gonadotropin levels and suppresses ovulation more consistently than either alone.

Given the multiple actions of estrogens and progestins on the hypothalamic-pituitary-ovarian axis during the menstrual cycle, several effects probably contribute to the blockade of ovulation.

Hypothalamic actions of steroids play a major role in the mechanism of oral contraceptive action. Progesterone diminishes the frequency of GnRH pulses. Because the proper frequency of LH pulses is essential for ovulation, this effect of progesterone likely plays a major role in the contraceptive action of these agents.

Multiple pituitary effects of both estrogen and progestin components are thus likely to contribute to oral contraceptive action. Oral contraceptives seem likely to decrease pituitary responsiveness to GnRH. Estrogens also suppress FSH release from the pituitary during the follicular phase of the menstrual cycle, and this effect seems likely to contribute to the lack of follicular development in oral contraceptive users. The progestin component may also inhibit the estrogen-induced LH surge at midcycle. Other effects may contribute to a minor extent to the extraordinary efficacy of oral contraceptives. Transit of sperm, the egg, and fertilized ovum are important to establish pregnancy, and steroids are likely to affect transport in the fallopian tube. In the cervix, progestin effects also are likely to produce a thick, viscous mucus to reduce sperm penetration and in the endometrium to produce a state that is not receptive to implantation. However, it is difficult to assess quantitatively the contributions of these effects because the drugs block ovulation so effectively.

Progestin-Only Contraceptives. Progestin-only pills and levonorgestrel implants are highly efficacious but block ovulation in only 60%–80% of cycles. Their effectiveness is thought to be due largely to a thickening of cervical mucus, which decreases sperm penetration, and to endometrial alterations that impair implantation; such local effects account for the efficacy of IUDs that release progestins. Depot injections of MPA are thought to exert similar effects, but they also yield plasma levels of drug high enough to prevent ovulation in virtually all patients, presumably by decreasing the frequency of GnRH pulses.

Intrauterine Devices. While the contraceptive benefit of the LNg IUS is attributed to the progestin-mediated effects of thickening of cervical mucous and endometrial alterations, the contraceptive mechanism of the copper IUD is related to an inflammatory reaction within the endometrium that impairs sperm viability, motility, and fertilization.

Untoward Effects

Combination Oral Contraceptives. Untoward effects of early hormonal contraceptives fell into several major categories: adverse cardiovascular effects, including hypertension, myocardial infarction, hemorrhagic or ischemic stroke, and venous thrombosis and embolism; breast, hepatocellular, and cervical cancers; and a number of endocrine and metabolic effects. The current consensus is that low-dose preparations pose minimal health risks in women who have no predisposing risk factors, and these drugs also provide many beneficial health effects (Burkman et al., 2004).

TABLE 44–2 ■ FORMULATIONS OF REPRESENTATIVE ORAL CONTRACEPTIVES

PRODUCT	FORMULATION	
COMBINATION[b] MONOPHASIC	**ESTROGEN (µg)**	**PROGESTIN (mg)**
Ethinyl estradiol/desogestrel	30	0.15
Ethinyl estradiol/drospirenone	30	3
Ethinyl estradiol/ethynodiol	35	1
	50	1
Ethinyl estradiol/levonorgestrel	20	0.1
Ethinyl estradiol/norgestrel	30	0.3
	50	0.5
Ethinyl estradiol/norethindrone	20	1
	30	1.5
	35	0.4
	50	1
Ethinyl estradiol/norgestimate	35	0.25
Mestranol/norethindrone	50	1
COMBINATION BIPHASIC	**ESTROGEN (µg)**	**PROGESTIN (mg)**
Ethinyl estradiol/desogestrel	20	0.15 (21 tabs)
Ethinyl estradiol/norethindrone	35	0.5 (10 tabs)
	35	1 (11 tabs)
COMBINATION TRIPHASIC	**ESTROGEN (µg)**	**PROGESTIN (mg)**
Ethinyl estradiol/desogestrel	25	0.1 (7 tabs)
	25	0.15 (7 tabs)
Ethinyl estradiol/levonorgestrel	30	0.05 (6 tabs)
	40	0.075 (5 tabs)
	30	0.125 (10 tabs)
Ethinyl estradiol/norethindrone	35	0.5 (7 tabs)
	35	1 (7 tabs)
Ethinyl estradiol/norgestimate	25 or 35	0.18 (7 tabs)
	25 or 35	0.215 (7 tabs)
	25 or 35	0.25 (7 tabs)
COMBINATION ESTROPHASIC	**ESTROGEN (µg)**	**PROGESTIN (mg)**
Ethinyl estradiol/norethindrone	20	1 (5 tabs)
	35	1 (9 tabs)
COMBINATION EXTENDED CYCLE	**ESTROGEN (µg)**	**PROGESTIN (mg)**
Ethinyl estradiol/drospirenone	20	3 (24 tabs)
Ethinyl estradiol/levonorgesterol	20	0.09 (28 tabs)
	30	0.15 (84 tabs)
Ethinyl estradiol/norethindrone	20	1 (24 tabs)
PROGESTIN ONLY	**ESTROGEN (µg)**	**PROGESTIN (mg)**
Norethindrone	—	0.35[c]
Norgestrel	—	0.075[c]

Unless otherwise indicated, the products are packaged with 21 active (hormone-containing) pills and 7 placebo tablets. For formulations that differ from this standard (e.g., multiphasic pills, extended-cycle formulations), the number of tablets of each pill strength are indicated.

[a]Some formulations also contain iron to diminish the risk of iron deficiency anemia; these are not listed separately here.

[b]Combination formulations contain both an estrogen and a progestin.

[c]Denotes continuous administration of active pills.

TABLE 44–3 ■ ONE-YEAR FAILURE RATE WITH VARIOUS FORMS OF CONTRACEPTION

BIRTH CONTROL METHOD	FAILURE (Perfect Use)	RATE (%) (Typical Use)
Combination oral contraceptive pills	0.3	8
Progestin-only minipill	0.5	8
Depo-Provera	0.3	3
Copper intrauterine device	0.6	0.8
Progestin intrauterine device	0.2	0.2
Implanon	0.05	0.05
Ortho Evra	0.3	8
NuvaRing	0.3	8
Condoms/diaphragms	2	15
Spermicides	18	9
Tubal ligation	0.5	0.5
Vasectomy	0.1	0.15
None	85	85

Cardiovascular Effects. The question of cardiovascular side effects has been reexamined for the newer low-dose oral contraceptives (Burkman et al., 2004). For nonsmokers without other risk factors such as hypertension or diabetes, there is no significant increase in the risk of myocardial infarction or stroke. There is a 28% increase in relative risk for venous thromboembolism, but the estimated absolute increase is very small because the incidence of these events in women without other predisposing factors is low (e.g., roughly half that associated with the risk of venous thromboembolism in pregnancy). The risk is significantly increased in women who smoke or have other factors that predispose to thrombosis or thromboembolism (Castelli, 1999). Postmarketing epidemiologic studies indicated that women using transdermal contraceptives have a higher-than-expected exposure to estrogen and are at increased risk for the development of venous thromboembolism. Early high-dose combination oral contraceptives caused hypertension in 4%–5% of normotensive women and increased blood pressure in 10%–15% of those with preexisting hypertension. This incidence is much lower with newer low-dose preparations, and most reported changes in blood pressure are not significant. Estrogens increase serum HDL and decrease LDL levels, and progestins tend to have the opposite effect. Recent studies of several low-dose preparations have not found significant changes in total serum cholesterol or lipoprotein profiles, although slight increases in triglycerides have been reported.

Cancer. Given the growth-promoting effects of estrogens, there has been a long-standing concern that oral contraceptives might increase the incidence of endometrial, cervical, ovarian, breast, and other cancers. These concerns were further heightened in the late 1960s by reports of endometrial changes caused by sequential oral contraceptives, which have since been removed from the market in the U.S. However, it is now clear that there is *not* a widespread association between oral contraceptive use and cancer (Burkman et al., 2004; Westhoff, 1999).

Epidemiological evidence suggests that combined oral contraceptive use may increase the risk of cervical cancer by about 2-fold but only in long-term (>5 years) users with persistent human papilloma virus infection (Moodley, 2004).

There have been reports of increases in the incidence of hepatic adenoma and hepatocellular carcinoma in oral contraceptive users. Current estimates indicate there is about a doubling in the risk of liver cancer after 4–8 years of use. However, these are rare cancers, and the absolute increases are small.

The major present concern about the carcinogenic effects of oral contraceptives is focused on breast cancer. The risk of breast cancer in women of childbearing age is very low, and current oral contraceptive users in this group have only a very small increase in relative risk of 1.1–1.2, depending on other variables. This small increase is not substantially affected by duration of use, dose or type of component, age at first use, or parity. Importantly, 10 years after discontinuation of oral contraceptive use, there is no difference in breast cancer incidence between past users and never users. In addition, breast cancers diagnosed in women who have ever used oral contraceptives are more likely to be localized to the breast and thus easier to treat (Westhoff, 1999).

Combination oral contraceptives decrease the incidence of endometrial cancer by 50%, an effect that lasts 15 years after the pills are stopped. This is thought to be due to the inclusion of a progestin, which opposes estrogen-induced proliferation, throughout the entire 21-day cycle of administration. These agents also decrease the incidence of ovarian cancer. There are accumulating data that oral contraceptive use decreases the risk of colorectal cancer (Fernandez et al., 2001).

Metabolic and Endocrine Effects. The effects of sex steroids on glucose metabolism and insulin sensitivity are complex (Godsland, 1996) and may differ among agents in the same class (e.g., the 19-norprogestins). Early studies with high-dose oral contraceptives generally reported impaired glucose tolerance; these effects have decreased as steroid dosages have been lowered, and current low-dose combination contraceptives may even improve insulin sensitivity. Similarly, the high-dose progestins in early oral contraceptives did raise LDL and reduce HDL levels, but modern low-dose preparations do not produce unfavorable lipid profiles (Sherif, 1999). There also have been periodic reports that oral contraceptives increase the incidence of gallbladder disease, but any such effect appears to be weak and limited to current or very long-term users (Burkman et al., 2004).

The estrogenic component of oral contraceptives may increase hepatic synthesis of a number of serum proteins, including those that bind thyroid hormones, glucocorticoids, and sex steroids. Although physiological feedback mechanisms generally adjust hormone synthesis to maintain normal "free" hormone levels, these changes can affect the interpretation of endocrine function tests that measure *total* plasma hormone levels and may necessitate dose adjustment in patients receiving thyroid hormone replacement.

The ethinyl estradiol present in oral contraceptives appears to cause a dose-dependent increase in several serum factors known to increase coagulation. However, in healthy women who do not smoke, there also is an increase in fibrinolytic activity, which exerts a countereffect so that overall there is a minimal effect on hemostatic balance. This compensatory effect is diminished in smokers (Fruzzetti, 1999).

Miscellaneous Effects. Nausea, edema, and mild headache occur in some individuals, and more severe migraine headaches may be precipitated by oral contraceptive use in a smaller fraction of women. Some patients may experience breakthrough bleeding during the 21-day cycle when the active pills are being taken. Withdrawal bleeding may fail to occur in a small fraction of women during the 7-day off period, thus causing confusion about a possible pregnancy. Acne and hirsutism are thought to be mediated by the androgenic activity of the 19-norprogestins.

Progestin-Only Contraceptives. Episodes of irregular, unpredictable spotting and breakthrough bleeding are the most frequently encountered untoward effect and the major reason women discontinue use of all three types of progestin-only contraceptives. With time, the incidence of these bleeding episodes decreases.

No evidence indicates that the progestin-only minipill preparations increase thromboembolic events, which are thought to be related to the estrogenic component of combination preparations. Acne may be a problem because of the androgenic activity of norethindrone-containing preparations. These preparations may be attractive for nursing mothers because they do not decrease lactation as do products containing estrogens.

Headache is the most commonly reported untoward effect of depot MPA. Mood changes and weight gain also have been reported, but controlled clinical studies of these effects are not available. Many studies have found decreases in HDL levels and increases in LDL levels, and there have been several reports of decreased bone density. These effects may be due to reduced endogenous estrogens because depot MPA is particularly effective in lowering gonadotropin levels. Because of the time required to completely eliminate the drug, the contraceptive effect of this agent may remain for 6–12 months after the last injection.

Progesterone-only medications have been associated with decreased bone mineral density, as noted by a black-box warning in the product label. Teenagers and younger women who have not achieved maximal bone density may be particularly at risk, although the data suggest that bone density returns to pretreatment levels fairly quickly after drug cessation.

Implants of norethindrone may be associated with infection, local irritation, pain at the insertion site, and, rarely, expulsion of the inserts. Headache, weight gain, and mood changes have been reported, and acne is seen in some patients. Ovulation occurs fairly soon after implant removal, reaching 50% in 3 months and almost 90% within 1 year.

Intrauterine Devices.

Intrauterine devices are generally well tolerated, although complications related to the device and side effects related to the progestin can occur. Expulsion of the device is greatest in the first year and has been reported in 3%–6% of women with an LNg20 and 3.2% in women with an LNg14. Malposition of the device, extending into the myometrium or the endocervical canal, occurs in 10% of women and is associated with difficult placement, uterine distortion, and obesity. Not all malpositioned devices need to removed, as this condition is often asymptomatic and does not compromise the contraceptive efficacy of the device.

Uterine perforation at the time of IUD insertion complicates approximately 1 in 1000 insertions. Symptoms of perforation may include pelvic pain and bleeding, although perforations are often asymptomatic. Surgical removal of the perforated IUD is preferred to minimize serious complications related to adhesions or perforation into the bowel, bladder, or blood vessels.

Pelvic inflammatory disease is infrequent at the time of insertion (1–10 per 1000 women undergoing insertion) and after insertion (1.4 women per 1000 women after insertion). Infections at the time of insertion or 1 month after insertion are generally related to new sexually transmitted infections. The LNg20 is associated with less risk of PID due to thickening of the cervical mucus. Oral antibiotic therapy may be attempted, and worsening infections should be treated with intravenous antibiotics and IUD removal.

Ectopic and intrauterine pregnancies rarely occur with an IUD in situ. Intrauterine pregnancies with an IUD in situ are at increased risk for adverse pregnancy outcomes if the IUD is left in place or removed. The decision to leave the IUD in place or remove it in pregnancy should be individualized based on the women's obstetrical history, the trimester when it is diagnosed, and the anticipated difficulty of removing the IUD.

While device-related complications are infrequent, side effects related to the progestin are common. Irregular bleeding in the first 3–6 months after insertion and amenorrhea at 1 year after insertion are common. Complaints of side effects such as hirsutism, acne, weight change, nausea, headache, mood change, and breast tenderness are related to systemic effects of levonorgestrel and are the most common reason for discontinuation (approximately 12% of women with the LNg20). The copper IUD may be an alternative for women who discontinue the LNg IUS due to hormonal side effects, but it is associated with intermenstrual bleeding and increased volume of bleeding.

Contraindications

Modern oral contraceptives are considered generally safe in most healthy women; *however, these agents can contribute to the incidence and severity of cardiovascular, thromboembolic, or malignant disease, particularly if other risk factors are present.* Contraindications for combination oral contraceptive use are the following: the presence or history of thromboembolic disease, cerebrovascular disease, myocardial infarction, coronary artery disease, or congenital hyperlipidemia; known or suspected carcinoma of the breast, carcinoma of the female reproductive tract; abnormal undiagnosed vaginal bleeding; known or suspected pregnancy; and past or present liver tumors or impaired liver function. *The risk of serious cardiovascular side effects is particularly marked in women more than 35 years of age who smoke heavily* (e.g., >15 cigarettes per day); even low-dose oral contraceptives are contraindicated in such patients.

Other relative contraindications include migraine headaches, hypertension, diabetes mellitus, obstructive jaundice of pregnancy or prior oral contraceptive use, and gallbladder disease. If elective surgery is planned, many physicians recommend discontinuation of oral contraceptives for several weeks to a month to minimize the possibility of thromboembolism after surgery. These agents should be used with care in women with prior gestational diabetes or uterine fibroids, and low-dose pills should generally be used in such cases.

Progestin-only contraceptives are contraindicated in the presence of undiagnosed vaginal bleeding, benign or malignant liver disease, and known or suspected breast cancer.

The Centers for Disease Control and Prevention U.S. medical eligibility criteria list all progestin-containing IUDs as category 2 for history of venous thromboembolism, which means a condition for which the advantages of using the method generally outweigh risks. The contraindications to IUDs are severe uterine distortion, active pelvic infection, and unexplained abnormal uterine bleeding. The copper IUD should be avoided in women with Wilson disease or a copper allergy.

Noncontraceptive Health Benefits

Oral contraceptives significantly reduce the incidence of ovarian and endometrial cancer within 6 months of use, and the incidence is decreased 50% after 2 years of use. Depot MPA injections also reduce very substantially the incidence of uterine cancer. This protective effect persists for up to 15 years after oral contraceptive use is discontinued. These agents also decrease the incidence of ovarian cysts and benign fibrocystic breast disease.

Oral contraceptives have major benefits related to menstruation in many women. These include more regular menstruation, reduced menstrual blood loss and less iron-deficiency anemia, and decreased frequency of dysmenorrhea. There also is a decreased incidence of PID and ectopic pregnancies, and endometriosis may be ameliorated. Some women also may obtain these benefits with progestin-only contraceptives. There are suggestions that MPA may improve hematological parameters in women with sickle cell disease (Cullins, 1996).

From a purely statistical perspective, fertility regulation by oral contraceptives is substantially safer than pregnancy or childbirth for most women, even without considering the additional health benefits of these agents.

In addition to effective pregnancy prevention, the LNg20 reduces dysmenorrhea and menstrual blood loss. One year after insertion, 30%–40% of women experience amenorrhea. The LNg20 can also be used to prevent and treat endometrial hyperplasia, although close monitoring is necessary, as endometrial adenocarcinoma has occurred in LNg20 users. While LNg14 is effective at preventing pregnancy, less is known regarding the noncontraceptive benefits of the LNg14.

Postcoital Contraception

Postcoital (or emergency) contraception is indicated for use in cases of mechanical failure of barrier devices or in circumstances of unprotected intercourse (Cheng et al., 2008). Because it is less effective than standard oral contraceptive regimens, it is not intended as a regular method of contraception. The mechanisms of action of the postcoital contraceptives are not fully understood, but their efficacy clearly cannot be accounted for solely by the inhibition of ovulation. Other potential mechanisms of action include effects on gamete function and survival and on implantation. These agents do not affect established pregnancies.

A copper iud is more effective than oral emergency contraceptive agents and can provide ongoing pregnancy prevention. The copper IUD can be inserted within 5–7 days after an unprotected act after a negative pregnancy test.

Selective progesterone-receptor modulators (PRMs) such as ulipristal are approved as an emergency contraceptive, effective up to 120 h after unprotected intercourse. Mifepristone in oral doses ranging from 10 to 50 mg when taken within 5 days after unprotected intercourse can also be used, but is not FDA approved.

Plan B, which contains two tablets of the progestin levonorgestrel (0.75 mg each), is marketed specifically for postcoital contraception and may be obtained in the U.S. without a prescription by women 18 years of age and older. Treatment is most effective if the first dose is taken within 72 h of intercourse, followed by a second dose 12 h later; a single dose of 1.5 mg within 72 h of intercourse appears to be equally effective.

Termination of Pregnancy

If contraception is not used or fails, either mifepristone (RU-486) or methotrexate (50 mg/m² intramuscularly or orally) can be used to terminate an unwanted pregnancy in settings outside surgical centers. A PG then is administered to stimulate uterine contractions and expel the detached conceptus; in the U.S., PGs used include dinoprostone (PGE_2) administered vaginally or the PGE_1 analogue misoprostol given orally or vaginally, both of which are used off label for this purpose. PGs used in other countries include the PGE_2 analogue sulprostone and the PGE_1 analogue gemeprost.

Mifepristone (600 mg) is FDA-approved for pregnancy termination within 49 days after the start of a woman's last menstrual period. The synthetic PGE_1 analogue misoprostol (400 μg) is administered orally 48 h later; vaginal administration is at least as effective but is not FDA approved. Complete abortion using this procedure exceeds 90%; when termination of pregnancy fails or is incomplete, surgical intervention is required. Other published regimens include lower doses of mifepristone (200 or 400 mg) and different time intervals between the mifepristone and misoprostol. Finally, repeated doses of misoprostol alone (e.g., 800 μg vaginally or sublingually every 3 h or every 12 h for three doses) also have been effective in settings where mifepristone is unavailable. Vaginal bleeding follows pregnancy termination and typically lasts from 1 to 2 weeks but rarely (in 0.1% of patients) is severe enough to require blood transfusion. A high percentage of women also experience abdominal pain and uterine cramps, nausea and vomiting, and diarrhea secondary to the PG. Myocardial ischemia and infarction have been reported in association with sulprostone and gemeprost.

Because mifepristone carries a risk of serious, and sometimes fatal, infections and bleeding following its use for medical abortion, a black-box warning has been added to the product labeling. Fulminant septic shock associated with *Clostridium sordellii* infections may result and is attributable to the combined effects of uterine infection and inhibition of glucocorticoid action by mifepristone (Cohen et al., 2007). Patients who develop symptoms and signs of infection, especially marked leukocytosis even without fever, should be treated aggressively with antibiotics effective against anaerobic organisms such as *C. sordellii* (e.g., penicillin, ampicillin, a macrolide, clindamycin, a tetracycline, or metronidazole).

Induction of Sexual Maturation

Estrogen Treatment in the Failure of Ovarian Development

In several conditions (e.g., Turner syndrome), the ovaries do not develop, and puberty does not occur. Therapy with estrogen at the appropriate time replicates the events of puberty, and androgens (Chapter 45) or growth hormone (Chapter 42) may be used concomitantly to promote normal growth. Although estrogens and androgens promote bone growth, they also accelerate epiphyseal fusion, and their premature use can thus result in shorter ultimate height.

Types of estrogens used and the treatment regimens may vary by country or individual preference. Examples include conjugated estrogens, 0.3–1.25 mg; micronized 17β-estradiol, 0.5–2.0 mg; ethinyl estradiol, 5–20 μg; and transdermal 17β-estradiol, 25–50 μg. To achieve optimal breast development, treatment typically is initiated with a low dose of estrogen (e.g., conjugated estrogens at a starting dosage of 0.3 mg/d or ethinyl estradiol at 5 μg/d) starting in patients between ages 10 and 12 years or immediately if the diagnosis is made after this age. After 3–6 months, the dosage is increased (e.g., 0.9–1.25 mg/d of conjugated estrogens or 20 μg/d of ethinyl estradiol). Once this is achieved, a progestin (e.g., medroxyprogesterone, 10 mg/d, or micronized progesterone,

200–400 μg/d) for 12 days each cycle is added to the regimen to optimize breast development and permit cyclical menses, thereby avoiding endometrial hyperplasia and its consequent risk of uterine cancer. Once menses are established, many clinicians will switch to a standard low-dose oral contraceptive pill or even may use an extended-cycle formulation.

Short stature, a universal feature of nonmosaic Turner syndrome, usually is treated with human growth hormone, often together with an androgen such as oxandrolone (see Chapter 45). Initiating treatment with human growth hormone and androgen and delaying the onset of estrogen therapy generally produces better growth response. Doses for growth hormone treatment in this context are higher than those in growth hormone–deficient children (e.g., 67 μg/kg/d; see Chapter 42 for further discussion of growth hormone replacement therapy).

Induction of Ovulation

Infertility (i.e., the failure to conceive after 1 year of unprotected sex) affects about 10%–15% of couples in developed nations and is increasing in incidence as more women choose to delay childbearing until later in life. The cause of infertility is attributed primarily to the woman in approximately one-third of cases, to the man in approximately one-third, and to both in approximately one-third.

Anovulation accounts for about 50% of female infertility and is a major focus of pharmacological interventions used to achieve conception. Although a history of regular cyclic bleeding is strong presumptive evidence for ovulation, assessment of urine LH levels with an ovulation predictor kit or measurement of the serum progesterone levels during the luteal phase provides more definitive information. Evaluation of anovulation may uncover PCOS, thyroid disorders, hyperprolactinemia, or hypogonadism, but the cause is often idiopathic.

A number of approaches have been used to stimulate ovulation in anovulatory women. Often, a stepwise approach is taken, initially using simpler and less-expensive treatments, followed by more complex and expensive regimens if initial therapy is unsuccessful.

Clomiphene

Clomiphene citrate was reviewed previously in this chapter. A typical regimen is 50 mg/d orally for 5 consecutive days starting between days 2 and 5 of the cycle in women who have spontaneous uterine bleeding or following a bleed induced by progesterone withdrawal in women who do not. If this regimen fails to induce ovulation, the dose of clomiphene is increased, first to the FDA-approved maximum of 100 mg/d and possibly to higher levels of 150 or 200 mg/d. Although clomiphene is effective in inducing ovulation in perhaps 75% of women, successful pregnancy ensues in only 40%–50% of those who ovulate. This has been attributed to clomiphene's inhibition of estrogen action on the endometrium, resulting in an environment that is not optimal for fertilization or implantation.

Aromatase Inhibitors

Aromatase inhibitors (e.g., letrozole, 2.5–7.5 mg/d for 5 days, typically starting on day 3 of the cycle) induce follicle development by inhibiting estrogen biosynthesis, thus decreasing estrogen negative feedback and increasing FSH levels and follicle development. In comparing letrozole and clomiphene for ovulation induction in women with PCOS and infertility, letrozole was associated with a higher pregnancy and live birth rate (Legro et al., 2014). Letrozole is associated with fewer estrogen deprivation side effects (hot flashes, mood change) and possibly fewer multifetal gestations than clomiphene.

Gonadotropins

The preparations of gonadotropins available for clinical use are detailed in Chapter 42. Gonadotropins are indicated for ovulation induction in anovulatory women with hypogonadotropic hypogonadism secondary to hypothalamic or pituitary dysfunction, gonadotropins also are used to induce ovulation in women with PCOS who do not respond to clomiphene.

Given the marked increases in maternal and fetal complications associated with multifetal gestation, the goal of ovulation induction in anovulatory women is to induce the formation and ovulation of a single dominant follicle. Generally, the increased risks of twin gestation will be accepted if two follicles are present.

As shown in Figure 44–6, a typical regimen for ovulation induction is to administer 75 iu of FSH daily in a "low-dose, step-up protocol." The dose is titrated based on the rise in estradiol and the growth rate of follicles as determined by estradiol levels and transvaginal ultrasonography. If three or more mature follicles are induced, gonadotropin therapy can be canceled, and barrier contraception can be used to prevent pregnancy, thereby avoiding multifetal pregnancy.

To complete follicular maturation and induce ovulation, hCG (5000–10,000 IU) is given 1 day after the last dose of gonadotropin. Fertilization of the oocyte(s) at 36 h after hCG administration then is attempted, by either intercourse or intrauterine insemination.

Gonadotropin induction also is used for ovarian stimulation in conjunction with IVF (Figure 44–6; Macklon et al., 2006). In this setting, larger doses of FSH (typically 225–300 IU/d) are administered to induce the maturation of multiple (ideally at least 5 and up to 20) oocytes that can be retrieved for IVF. To prevent the LH surge and subsequent premature luteinization of the ovarian follicles, gonadotropins typically are administered in conjunction with a GnRH agonist or a GnRH antagonist. The length of the IVF protocol is predicated by the initial flare of gonadotropin secretion that occurs in response to the GnRH agonists. In the long protocol, the agonist is started in the luteal phase of the previous cycle (generally on cycle day 21) and then maintained until the time of hCG injection to induce ovulation. Alternatively, in the "flare" protocol, the GnRH agonist is started on cycle day 2 (immediately after the start of menses), and gonadotropin injections are added 1 day later. In the GnRH antagonist "short protocol," the antagonist can be used to inhibit endogenous LH secretion and is typically started after follicular recruitment is initiated. Current regimens include daily injection in a dose of 0.25 mg (ganirelix or cetrorelix) starting on the fifth or sixth day of gonadotropin stimulation or a single dose of 3 mg of cetrorelix administered on day 8 or 9 of the late follicular phase. Adequate follicle maturation typically takes 8–12 days after gonadotropin therapy is initiated.

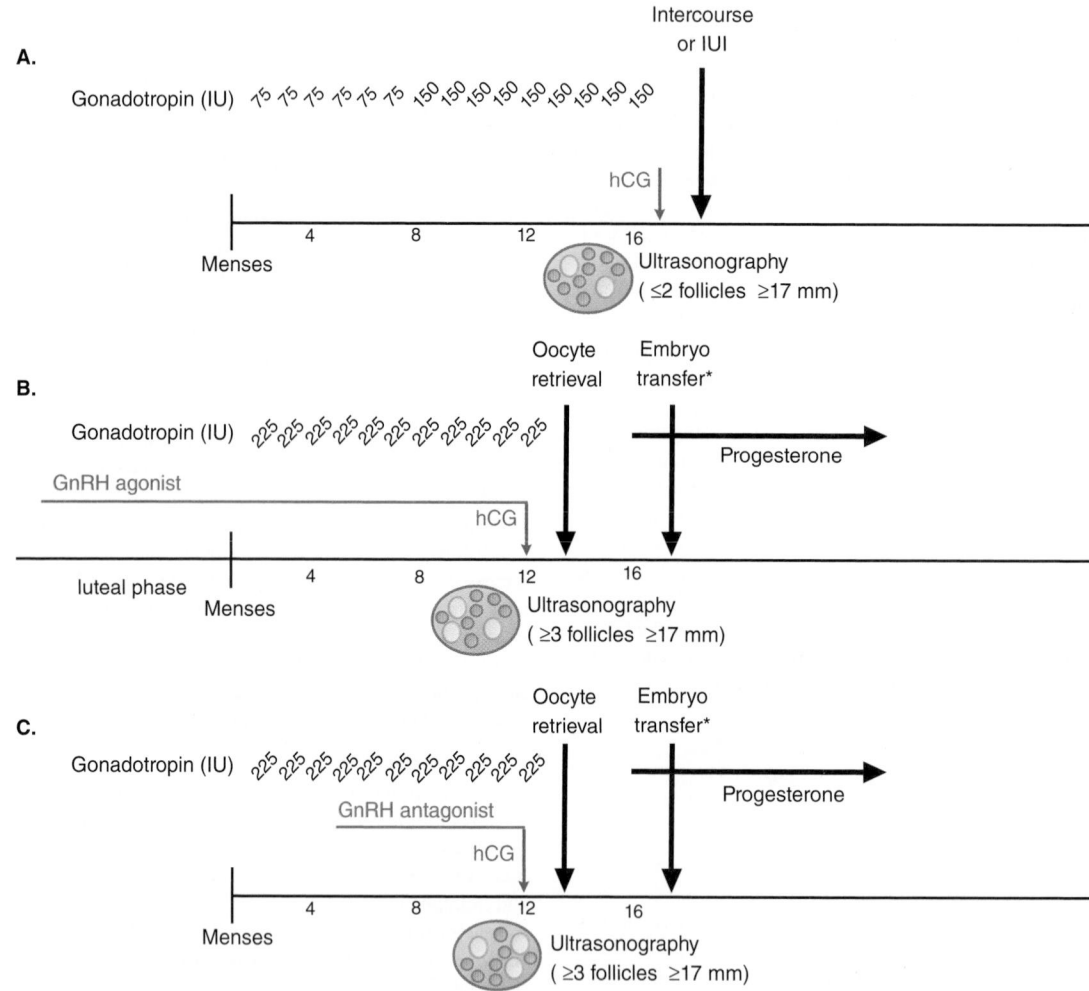

Figure 44–6 *Idealized regimens using exogenous gonadotropins for induction of fertility.* **A.** Step-up regimen for ovulation induction. After menses, daily injections of gonadotropin (75 IU) are started. Follicle maturation is assessed by serial measurement of plasma estradiol and follicle size, as discussed in the text. If an inadequate response is seen, the dose of gonadotropin is increased to 112 or 150 IU/d. When one or two follicles have achieved a diameter of 17 mm or greater, final follicle maturation and ovulation are induced by injection of hCG. Fertilization then is achieved at 36 h after hCG injection by intercourse or intrauterine insemination (IUI). If more than two mature follicles are seen, the cycle is terminated, and barrier contraception is used to avoid triplets or higher degrees of multifetal gestation. **B.** Long protocol for ovarian hyperstimulation using a gonadotropin-releasing hormone (GnRH) agonist to inhibit premature ovulation, followed by in vitro fertiliztion (IVF). After the GnRH agonist has inhibited endogenous secretion of gonadotropins, therapy with exogenous gonadotropins is initiated. Follicle maturation is assessed by serial measurements of plasma estradiol and follicle size by ultrasonography. When three or more follicles are 17 mm or larger in diameter, then ovulation is induced by injection of hCG. At 32–36 h after the hCG injection, the eggs are retrieved and used for IVF. Exogenous progesterone is provided to promote a receptive endometrium, followed by embryo transfer at 3–5 days after fertilization. **C.** Protocol for ovarian hyperstimulation in an IVF protocol using a GnRH antagonist. The cycle duration is shorter because the GnRH antagonist does not induce a transient flare of gonadotropin secretion that might disrupt the timing of the cycle, but many other elements of the cycle are analogous to those in **B.**

Using either the long or short protocols, hCG (at typical doses of 5000–10,000 IU of urine-derived product or 250 μg of recombinant hCG) is given to induce final oocyte development, and the mature eggs are retrieved from the preovulatory follicles at 36 h thereafter. The ova are retrieved by transvaginal ultrasound-guided aspiration and fertilized in vitro with sperm (IVF) or by intracytoplasmic sperm injection; one or two embryos then are transferred to the uterus 3–5 days after fertilization.

Because of the inhibitory effects of GnRH agonists or antagonists on pituitary gonadotropes, the secretion of LH that normally sustains the corpus luteum after ovulation does not occur. Repeated injections of hCG, while sustaining the corpus luteum, may increase the risk of OHSS. Thus, standard IVF regimens typically provide exogenous progesterone replacement to support the fetus until the placenta acquires the biosynthetic capacity to take over this function; regimens include progesterone in oil (50–100 mg/d intramuscularly) or micronized progesterone (180–300 mg twice daily vaginally). Vaginal preparations containing 100 or 90 mg of micronized progesterone are approved for administration two or three times daily as part of IVF.

Aside from the attendant complications of multifetal gestation, the major side effect of gonadotropin treatment is OHSS. This potentially life-threatening event is believed to result from increased ovarian secretion of substances that increase vascular permeability and is characterized by rapid accumulation of fluid in the peritoneal cavity, thorax, and even the pericardium. Symptoms and signs include abdominal pain or distention, nausea and vomiting, diarrhea, dyspnea, oliguria, and marked ovarian enlargement on ultrasonography. OHSS can lead to hypovolemia, electrolyte abnormalities, acute respiratory distress syndrome, thromboembolic events, and hepatic dysfunction.

In an effort to minimize OHSS in at-risk patients, the FSH can be withheld for a day or two ("coasting"). The rationale for this approach is that larger follicles become relatively gonadotropin independent and thus will continue to mature, while the smaller follicles undergo atresia in response to gonadotropin deprivation. Alternatively, an endogenous LH surge can be induced with a GnRH agonist during a GnRH antagonist short protocol, which nearly eliminates the incidence of OHSS by avoiding the use of HCG to trigger oocyte maturation.

The potential deleterious effects of gonadotropins are debated. Some studies have suggested that gonadotropins are associated with an increased risk of ovarian cancer, but this conclusion is controversial (Brinton et al., 2005).

Insulin Sensitizers

Polycystic ovary syndrome affects 4%–7% of women of reproductive age and is the most frequent cause of anovulatory infertility. Inasmuch as patients with PCOS often exhibit hyperinsulinemia and insulin resistance, insulin sensitizers such as metformin have been evaluated for their effects on ovulation and fertility (see Chapter 47). Although several small trials suggested that metformin increased ovulation relative to placebo in patients with PCOS, a trial failed to demonstrate a significant effect of metformin on fertility (Legro et al., 2007); metformin was less effective than clomiphene in inducing ovulation, promoting conception, or improving live birth rates, and there was no benefit of combining metformin with clomiphene on live births, except possibly in women resistant to clomiphene. Thus, except in women who exhibit glucose intolerance, the consensus is that metformin generally should not be used for fertility induction in women with PCOS (Thessaloniki ESHRE/ASRM-Sponsored PCOS Consensus Workshop Group, 2008).

Thiazolidinediones also have been evaluated for their ability to induce ovulation in patients with PCOS but are not used for this indication given an increased risk of congestive heart failure and myocardial ischemia.

Drug Therapy in Obstetrics

Pregnancy-Induced Hypertension/Preeclampsia

Hypertension affects up to 10% of pregnant women in the U.S.

Hypertension that precedes pregnancy or manifests before 20 weeks of gestation is believed to overlap considerably in pathogenesis with essential hypertension. These patients appear to be at increased risk for gestational diabetes and need careful monitoring. In contrast, pregnancy-induced hypertension, or preeclampsia, generally presents after 20 weeks of gestation as a new-onset hypertension with proteinuria (> 300 mg of urinary protein/24 h); preeclampsia is thought to involve placenta-derived factors that affect vascular integrity and endothelial function in the mother, thus causing peripheral edema, renal and hepatic dysfunction, and in severe cases, seizures. Chronic hypertension is an established risk factor for preeclampsia. The consensus panel recommended initiation of drug therapy in women with a diastolic blood pressure > 105 mm Hg or a systolic blood pressure > 160 mm Hg. If severe preeclampsia ensues, with marked hypertension and evidence of end-organ damage, then termination of the pregnancy by delivery of the baby is the treatment of choice, provided that the fetus is sufficiently mature to survive outside the uterus. If the baby is very preterm, then hospitalization and pharmacotherapy may be employed in an effort to permit further fetal maturation in utero.

Several drugs commonly used for hypertension in non-pregnant patients (e.g., angiotensin-converting enzyme inhibitors, angiotensin-receptor antagonists) should not be used in pregnant women due to unequivocal evidence of adverse fetal effects. Many experts will convert the patient to the centrally acting α adrenergic agonist α-methyldopa (250 mg twice daily) (FDA Category B), which rarely is used for hypertension in non-pregnant patients. Other drugs with reasonable evidence of safety (Category C) also may be used, including the combination α_1-selective, β-nonselective adrenergic antagonist labetalol (100 mg twice daily) and the Ca^{2+} channel blocker nifedipine (30 mg once daily).

If severe preeclampsia or impending labor requires hospitalization, blood pressure can be controlled acutely with hydralazine (5 or 10 mg IV or IM, with repeated dosing at 20-min intervals depending on blood pressure response) or labetalol (20 mg IV, with dose escalation to 40 mg at 10 min if blood pressure control is inadequate). In addition to receiving drugs for blood pressure control, women with severe preeclampsia or who have CNS manifestations (e.g., headache, visual disturbance, or altered mental status) are treated as inpatients with magnesium sulfate, based on its documented efficacy in seizure prevention and lack of adverse effects on the mother or baby. Such treatment also should be considered for postpartum women with CNS manifestations: ~20% of episodes of eclampsia occur in women more than 48 h post-delivery.

Prevention or Arrest of Preterm Labor

Scope of the Problem and Etiology

Preterm birth, defined as delivery before 37 weeks of gestation, occurs in more than 10% of pregnancies in the U.S. and is increasing in frequency; it is associated with significant complications, such as neonatal respiratory distress syndrome, pulmonary hypertension, and intracranial hemorrhage.

Although incompletely understood, risk factors for preterm labor include multifetal gestation, premature rupture of the membranes, intrauterine infection, and placental insufficiency. The more premature the baby, the greater the risk of complications, prompting efforts to prevent or interrupt preterm labor.

The therapeutic objective in preterm labor is to delay delivery so that the mother can be transported to a regional facility specializing in the care of premature babies and supportive agents can be administered; such supportive treatments include glucocorticoids to stimulate fetal lung maturation (see Chapter 46) and antibiotics (e.g., erythromycin, ampicillin) to diminish the frequency of neonatal infection with group B β-hemolytic *Streptococcus*. Based on concerns over deleterious effects of antibiotic therapy, it is essential that antibiotics not be administered indiscriminately to all women thought to have preterm labor, but rather be reserved for those with premature rupture of the membranes and evidence of infection.

Prevention of Preterm Labor: Progesterone Therapy

Progesterone levels in some species diminish considerably in association with labor, whereas administration of progesterone inhibits the secretion of pro-inflammatory cytokines and delays cervical ripening. Thus, progesterone and its derivatives have long been advocated to diminish the onset of preterm labor in women at increased risk due to previous preterm delivery. Despite considerable controversy, recent randomized trials have revived interest in this approach. Hydroxyprogesterone caproate at a dose of 250 mg administered weekly by intramuscular injection has been shown to reduce preterm birth by about one-third in women with a prior preterm birth of a singleton. Vaginal administration of progesterone (200 mg each night) has been shown to reduce preterm birth in women with midtrimester cervical shortening by ultrasound examination. The role of progesterone for prevention of preterm birth in multiple gestations is controversial.

Tocolytic Therapy for Established Preterm Labor

Inhibition of uterine contractions of preterm labor, or *tocolysis*, has been a focus of therapy (Simhan and Caritis, 2007). Although tocolytic agents delay delivery in about 80% of women, they neither prevent premature births nor improve adverse fetal outcomes such as respiratory distress syndrome.

Specific tocolytic agents include β adrenergic receptor agonists, MgSO$_4$, Ca^{2+} channel blockers, COX inhibitors, oxytocin receptor antagonists, and NO donors. The mechanisms of action of these agents are illustrated in Figure 44–7.

The β adrenergic receptor agonists relax the myometrium by activating the cyclic AMP-PKA signaling cascade that phosphorylates and inactivates MLCK, a key enzyme in uterine contraction. *Ritodrine*, a selective β$_2$ agonist, was specifically developed as a uterine relaxant and remains the only tocolytic drug to have gained FDA approval; it was voluntarily withdrawn from the U.S. market. *Terbutaline*, which is FDA-approved for asthma, has been used off label for this purpose and can be administered orally, subcutaneously, or intravenously. Terbutaline may delay births, but only during the first 48 h of treatment, and is associated with a number of adverse maternal effects, including tachycardia, hypotension, and pulmonary edema.

Similarly, Ca^{2+} channel blockers inhibit the influx of Ca^{2+} through depolarization-activated, voltage-sensitive Ca^{2+} channels in the plasma membrane, thereby preventing the activation of MLCK and the stimulation of uterine contraction. *Nifedipine*, the Ca^{2+} channel blocker used most commonly for this purpose, can be administered parenterally or orally. Relative to β$_2$ adrenergic agonists, nifedipine is more likely to improve fetal outcomes and less likely to cause maternal side effects.

Based on the role of PGs in uterine contraction, COX inhibitors (e.g., indomethacin) have been used to inhibit preterm labor, and some data suggest that they may reduce the number of preterm births. Because they also can inhibit platelet function and induce closure in utero of the ductus arteriosus, these inhibitors should not be employed in term pregnancies (or in pregnancies beyond 32 weeks of gestation, when the risk of severe complications of prematurity is relatively lower). Short courses of treatment (<72 h) pose less risk for impaired circulation in the fetus.

Despite numerous clinical trials, the superiority of any one therapy has not been established, and none of the drugs has been shown definitively to improve fetal outcome.

Initiation of Labor

Labor induction is indicated when the perceived risk of continued pregnancy to the mother or fetus exceeds the risks of delivery or pharmacological induction.

Prostaglandins and Cervical Ripening

Prostaglandins play key roles in parturition (see Chapter 37). Thus, PGE$_1$, PGE$_2$, and PGF$_{2\alpha}$ are used to facilitate labor by promoting ripening and dilation of the cervix. They can be administered either orally or via local administration (either vaginally or intracervically). The ability of certain

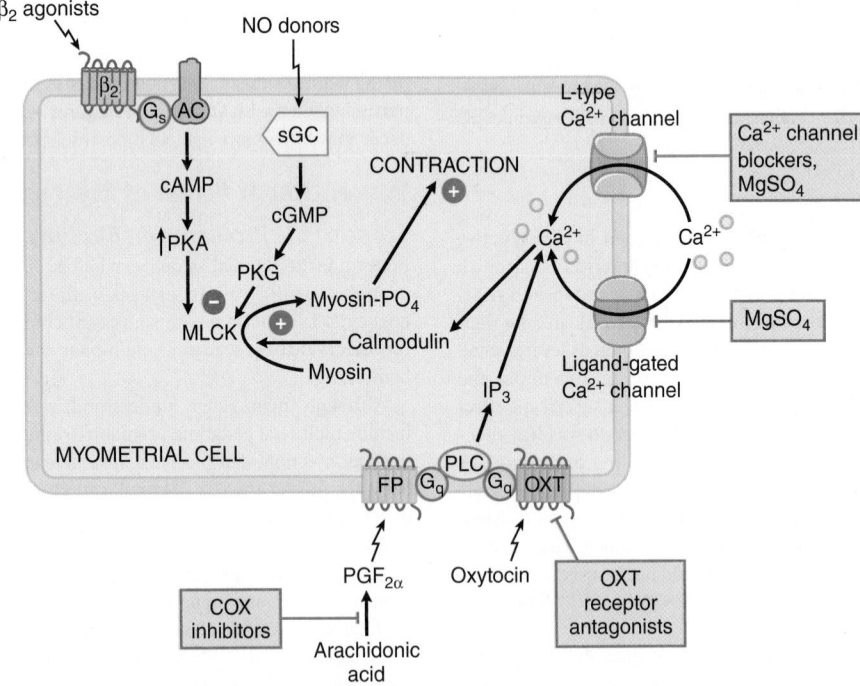

Figure 44–7 *Sites of action of tocolytic drugs in the uterine myometrium.* The elevation of cellular Ca^{2+} promotes contraction via the Ca^{2+}/calmodulin-dependent activation of MLCK. Relaxation is promoted by the elevation of cyclic nucleotides (cAMP and cGMP) and their activation of protein kinases, which cause phosphorylation/inactivation of MLCK. Pharmacological manipulations to reduce myometrial contraction include the following: (1) inhibiting Ca^{2+} entry (Ca^{2+} channel blockers, Mg$_2$SO$_4$); (2) reducing mobilization of intracellular Ca^{2+} by antagonizing GPCR-mediated activation of the G$_q$-PLC-IP$_3$-Ca^{2+} pathway (with antagonists of the FP and OXT receptors) or reducing production of the FP agonist, PGF$_2\alpha$ (with COX inhibitors); (3) enhancing relaxation by elevating cellular cAMP (with β$_2$ adrenergic agonists that activate G$_s$-AC) and cellular cGMP (with NO donors that stimulate sGC). Note that pharmacological activators of sGC (e.g., riociguat) are contraindicated in pregnancy (see Chapter 31). AC, adenylyl cyclase; COX, cyclooxygenase; FP, the PGF$_2$ receptor; OXT, the oxytocin receptor; PLC, phospholipase C; sGC, soluble guanylyl cyclase.

PGs to stimulate uterine contractions also makes them valuable agents in the therapy of postpartum hemorrhage.

Available preparations include dinoprostone (PGE_2), which is FDA approved to facilitate cervical ripening. Dinoprostone is formulated as a gel for intracervical administration via syringe in a dose of 0.5 mg or as a vaginal insert (pessary) in a dose of 10 mg; the latter is designed to release active PGE_2 at a rate of 0.3 mg/h for up to 12 h and should be removed at the onset of labor or 12 h after insertion. No more than three doses should be used in a 24-h period. Dinoprostone should not be used in women with a history of asthma, glaucoma, or myocardial infarction. The major adverse effect is uterine hyperstimulation, which may be reversed more rapidly using the vaginal insert by removing it with the attached tape.

Misoprostol, a synthetic derivative of PGE_1 (see Chapter 38) is used off label either orally or vaginally to induce cervical ripening; typical doses are 100 μg (orally) or 25 μg (vaginally). An advantage of misoprostol in this setting is its considerably lower cost. Adverse effects include uterine hyperstimulation and, rarely, uterine rupture. Misoprostol should be discontinued for at least 3 h before initiating oxytocin therapy.

Oxytocin

The structure and physiology of oxytocin are discussed in Chapter 42. This section presents therapeutic uses of oxytocin in obstetrics, which include the induction of labor, the augmentation of labor that is not progressing, and the prophylaxis or treatment of postpartum hemorrhage. Although widely used, oxytocin recently was added to a list of drugs "bearing a heightened risk of harm" (Clark et al., 2009), and its role and specific application to most deliveries in the U.S. remain open to debate. Thus, careful review of the appropriate indications for oxytocin administration and attention to the dose and progress of labor during induction are essential.

Labor Induction. Oxytocin is the drug of choice for labor induction; for this purpose, it is administered by intravenous infusion of a diluted solution, preferably via an infusion pump. Current protocols start with an oxytocin dose of 6 mIU/min, followed by advancement of dose as needed, up to 40 mIU/min. Uterine hyperstimulation should be avoided; however, if it occurs, as evidenced by too-frequent contractions (more than five contractions in a 10-min interval) or the development of uterine tetany, the oxytocin infusion should be discontinued immediately. Because the $t_{1/2}$ of intravenous oxytocin is relatively short (12–15 min), the hyperstimulatory effects of oxytocin will dissipate fairly rapidly after the infusion is discontinued. Thereafter, the infusion can be reinitiated at a dose of half that at which hyperstimulation occurred and increased cautiously as tolerated.

Because of its structural similarity to vasopressin, oxytocin at higher doses activates the vasopressin V_2 receptor and has antidiuretic effects. Particularly if hypotonic fluids (e.g., dextrose in water) are infused too liberally, water intoxication may result in convulsions, coma, and even death. Vasodilating actions of oxytocin also have been noted, particularly at high doses, which may provoke hypotension and reflex tachycardia. Deep anesthesia may exaggerate the hypotensive effect of oxytocin by preventing the reflex tachycardia.

Augmentation of Dysfunctional Labor. Oxytocin also is used when spontaneous labor is not progressing at an acceptable rate. To augment hypotonic contractions in dysfunctional labor, an infusion rate of 10 mIU/min typically is sufficient; doses in excess of 40 mIU/min rarely are effective when lower concentrations fail. As with labor induction, potential complications of uterine overstimulation include trauma of the mother or fetus due to forced passage through an incompletely dilated cervix, uterine rupture, and compromised fetal oxygenation due to decreased uterine perfusion.

Menopause and Hormone Therapy

Menopause refers to the permanent cessation of menstrual periods (i.e., for > 12 months) resulting from the loss of ovarian follicular activity; it usually occurs when women are between 45 and 60 years of age. The decline in estradiol levels produces a variety of symptoms and signs, including vasomotor disturbances (hot flashes or flushes), sweating,

irritability, sleep disturbances, and atrophy of estrogen-dependent tissue. In addition, postmenopausal women are at increased risk for osteoporosis, bone fractures, and CHD and experience increased memory loss and other cognitive difficulties.

Estrogens

Estrogens are most commonly used to treat vasomotor disturbances ("hot flashes") in postmenopausal women. Other important benefits are amelioration of the effects of urogenital atrophy, a decreased incidence of colon cancer, and prevention of bone loss. A variety of preparations, including oral, transdermal, and vaginal, are available. *Regardless of the specific drug(s) selected, treatment should use the minimum dose and duration for the desired therapeutic end point.*

In postmenopausal women with an *intact uterus*, a progestin is included to prevent endometrial cancer. *MPA* is used in the U.S., but micronized progesterone is preferred; *norethindrone* and *norgestrel/levonorgestrel* are also commonly used. Women *without a uterus* are administered estrogen alone. Postmenopausal hormone therapy and contraception are the most frequent uses of progestins.

The two major uses of estrogens are for *MHT* and as components of *combination oral contraceptives*, and the pharmacological considerations for their use and the specific drugs and doses used differ in these settings. Historically, conjugated equine estrogens have been the most common agents for postmenopausal use (0.625 mg/d). In contrast, most combination oral contraceptives in current use employ 20–35 μg/d of ethinyl estradiol. These preparations differ widely in their oral potencies (e.g., a dose of 0.625 mg of conjugated estrogens generally is considered equivalent to 5–10 μg of ethinyl estradiol). Thus, the "effective" dose of estrogen used for MHT is less than that in oral contraceptives when one considers potency. Furthermore, in the last two decades, the doses of estrogens employed in both settings have decreased substantially. The untoward effects of the 20- to 35-μg doses now commonly used thus have a lower incidence and severity than those reported in older studies (e.g., with oral contraceptives that contained 50–150 μg of ethinyl estradiol or mestranol).

Menopausal Hormone Therapy

The established benefits of estrogen therapy in postmenopausal women include amelioration of vasomotor symptoms and the prevention of bone fractures and urogenital atrophy.

Vasomotor Symptoms

The decline in ovarian function at menopause is associated with vasomotor symptoms in most women. The characteristic hot flashes may alternate with chilly sensations, inappropriate sweating, and (less commonly) paresthesias. Treatment with estrogen is specific and is the most efficacious pharmacotherapy for these symptoms (Belchetz, 1994). If estrogen is contraindicated or otherwise undesirable, other options may be considered. MPA may provide some relief of vasomotor symptoms for certain patients, and the α_2 adrenergic agonist clonidine diminishes vasomotor symptoms in some women, presumably by blocking the CNS outflow that regulates blood flow to cutaneous vessels. In many women, hot flashes diminish within several years; when prescribed for this purpose, the dose and duration of estrogen use should thus be the minimum necessary to provide relief.

Osteoporosis

Osteoporosis is a disorder of the skeleton associated with the loss of bone mass (Chapter 48). The result is thinning and weakening of the bones and an increased incidence of fractures, particularly compression fractures of the vertebrae and minimal-trauma fractures of the hip and wrist. The frequency and severity of these fractures and their associated complications (e.g., death and permanent disability) are a major public health problem, especially as the population continues to age. Osteoporosis is an indication for estrogen therapy, which clearly is efficacious in decreasing the incidence of fractures. However, because of the risks associated with estrogen use, first-line use of other drugs, such as bisphosphonates, should be considered (Chapter 48). Most fractures in the postmenopausal period occur in women without a prior history of osteoporosis, and estrogens are the most efficacious agents available for prevention of fractures at all sites in such women (Anderson et al., 2004; Rossouw et al., 2002).

Estrogens act primarily to decrease bone resorption; consequently, estrogens are more effective at preventing rather than restoring bone loss (Belchetz, 1994; Prince et al., 1991). Estrogens are most effective if treatment is initiated before significant bone loss occurs, and their maximal beneficial effects require continuous use; bone loss resumes when treatment is discontinued. An appropriate diet with adequate intake of Ca^{2+} and vitamin D and weight-bearing exercise enhance the effects of estrogen treatment.

Vaginal Dryness and Urogenital Atrophy

Loss of tissue lining the vagina or bladder leads to a variety of symptoms in many postmenopausal women (Robinson and Cardozo, 2003). These include dryness and itching of the vagina, dyspareunia, swelling of tissues in the genital region, pain during urination, a need to urinate urgently or often, and sudden or unexpected urinary incontinence. When estrogens are being used solely for relief of vulvar and vaginal atrophy, local administration as a vaginal cream, ring device, or tablets may be considered.

Cardiovascular Disease

The incidence of cardiovascular disease is low in premenopausal women, rising rapidly after menopause, and epidemiological studies consistently showed an association between estrogen use and reduced cardiovascular disease in postmenopausal women. Estrogens produce a favorable lipoprotein profile, promote vasodilation, inhibit the response to vascular injury, and reduce atherosclerosis. However, estrogens promote coagulation and thromboembolic events. Randomized prospective studies unexpectedly have indicated that the incidence of heart disease and stroke in older postmenopausal women treated with conjugated estrogens and a progestin was initially increased, although the trend reversed with time (Grady et al., 2002; Rossouw et al., 2002). Combined estrogen-progestin therapy is associated with a decrease in heart attacks in younger women.

Other Therapeutic Effects

Many other changes occur in postmenopausal women, including a general thinning of the skin; changes in the urethra, vulva, and external genitalia; and a variety of changes, including headache, fatigue, and difficulty concentrating. Chronic lack of sleep created by hot flashes and other vasomotor symptoms may be contributing factors. Estrogen replacement may help alleviate or lessen some of these via direct actions (e.g., improvement of vasomotor symptoms) or secondary effects resulting in an improved feeling of well-being (Belchetz, 1994). The WHI demonstrated that a conjugated estrogen in combination with a progestin reduces the risk of colon cancer by roughly one-half in postmenopausal women (Rossouw et al., 2002).

Menopausal Hormone Regimens

In the 1960s and 1970s, there was an increase in *estrogen-replacement therapy,* or ERT (i.e., estrogens alone) in postmenopausal women, primarily to reduce vasomotor symptoms, vaginitis, and osteoporosis. About 1980, epidemiological studies indicated that this treatment increased the incidence of endometrial carcinoma. This led to the use of *hormone-replacement therapy* (HRT), which includes a progestin to limit estrogen-related endometrial hyperplasia. Postmenopausal HRT, when indicated, should include both an estrogen and progestin for women with a uterus (Belchetz, 1994). For women who have undergone a hysterectomy, endometrial carcinoma is not a concern, and estrogen alone avoids the possible deleterious effects of progestins.

Conjugated estrogens and MPA historically have been used most commonly in menopausal hormone regimens, although estradiol, estrone, and estriol have been used as estrogens, and norethindrone, norgestimate, levonorgestrel, norethisterone, and progesterone also have been widely used (especially in Europe). Various "continuous" or "cyclic" regimens have been used; the latter regimens include drug-free days. An example of a cyclic regimen is as follows: (1) administration of an estrogen for 25 days; (2) the addition of MPA for the last 12–14 days of estrogen treatment; and (3) 5–6 days with no hormone treatment, during which withdrawal bleeding normally occurs due to breakdown and shedding of the endometrium. Continuous administration of combined estrogen plus progestin does not lead to regular, recurrent endometrial shedding but may cause intermittent spotting or bleeding, especially in the first year of use. Other regimens include a progestin intermittently (e.g., every third month), but the long-term endometrial safety of these regimens remains to be firmly established. Conjugated estrogens plus MPA given as a fixed dose daily and conjugated estrogens given for 28 days plus MPA given for 14 of 28 days are widely used combination formulations. Other combination products available in the U.S. are ethinyl estradiol plus norethindrone acetate, estradiol plus norethindrone, estradiol and norgestimate, and estradiol and drospirenone. Doses and regimens are usually adjusted empirically based on control of symptoms, patient acceptance of bleeding patterns, or other untoward effects.

Another pharmacological consideration is the route of estrogen administration. Oral administration exposes the liver to higher concentrations of estrogens than does transdermal administration and may increase SHBG, other binding globulins, and angiotensinogen and possibly the cholesterol content of the bile. Transdermal estrogen appears to cause smaller beneficial changes in LDL and HDL profiles (~50% of those seen with the oral route) (Walsh et al., 1994).

Tibolone is widely used in the E.U. for treatment of vasomotor symptoms and prevention of osteoporosis but is not currently approved in the U.S. The parent compound itself is devoid of activity, but it is metabolized in a tissue-selective manner to three metabolites that have predominantly estrogenic, progestogenic, and androgenic activities. The effects of this drug on fractures, breast cancer, and long-term outcomes remain to be established (Modelska and Cummings, 2002).

Regardless of the specific agent or regimen, MHT with estrogens should use the lowest dose and shortest duration necessary to achieve an appropriate therapeutic goal.

Untoward Responses

The use of unopposed estrogen for hormone treatment in postmenopausal women increases the risk of endometrial carcinoma by 5- to 15-fold (Shapiro et al., 1985). This increased risk can be prevented if a progestin is coadministered with the estrogen (Pike et al., 1997), and this is now standard practice.

The association between estrogen or estrogen-progestin use and breast cancer is of great concern. The results of two large randomized clinical trials of estrogen/progestin and estrogen only (i.e., the two arms of WHI) in postmenopausal women clearly established a small but significant increase in the risk of breast cancer in the CEE+MPA studies (CEE, conjugated equine estrogens) (Anderson et al., 2004; Rossouw et al., 2002). In the WHI study, CEE+MPA was associated with an increased relative risk of breast cancer by 25%; the absolute increase in attributable cases of disease was 6 per 1000 women and required 3 or more years of treatment. In women without a uterus who received CEE alone, the relative risk of breast cancer was actually decreased by 23%, and the decrease only narrowly missed reaching statistical significance. Interestingly, the incidence of colon cancer was reduced by 26% in the WHI trial.

The Million Women Study (MWS) in the U.K. was a cohort study rather than a clinical trial (Beral et al., 2003). It surveyed more than 1 million women; about half had received some type of hormone treatment, and half had never used this type of treatment. Those receiving an estrogen-progestin combination had an increased relative risk of invasive breast cancer of 2, and those receiving estrogen alone had an increased relative risk of 1.3, but the increase in actual attributable cases of the disease was again small.

Both the WHI and MWS data are thus consistent with earlier studies indicating that the progestin component (e.g., medroxyprogesterone) in combined HRT plays a major role in this increased risk of breast cancer (Ross et al., 2000; Schairer et al., 2000). Importantly, although long-term data have not accumulated for the WHI trials, the available data suggest that the excess risk of breast cancer associated with menopausal hormone use appears to abate 5 years after discontinuing therapy. Thus, HRT for 5 years or less is often prescribed to mitigate hot flashes and likely has a minimal effect on the risk of breast cancer.

Historically, the carcinogenic actions of estrogens were thought to be related to their trophic effects. However, if catechol estrogens, especially the 4-hydroxycatechols, are converted to semiquinones or quinones prior to "inactivation" by COMT, the generation of ROSs may cause direct chemical damage to DNA bases (Yue et al., 2003). In this regard, CYP1B1, which has specific estrogen-4-hydroxylase activity, is present in tissues such as uterus, breast, ovary, and prostate, which often give rise to hormone-responsive cancers.

Metabolic and Cardiovascular Effects

Although they may slightly elevate plasma triglycerides, estrogens themselves generally have favorable overall effects on plasma lipoprotein profiles. However, addition of progestins may reduce the favorable actions of estrogens. Estrogens do increase cholesterol levels in bile and cause a relative 2- to 3-fold increase in gallbladder disease. Currently prescribed doses of estrogens generally do not increase the risk of hypertension, and estrogen engaging the ERβ receptor typically reduces blood pressure.

Many studies and clinical trials suggested that estrogen therapy in postmenopausal women would reduce the risk of cardiovascular disease by 35%–50% (Manson and Martin, 2001). However, two recent randomized clinical trials have not found such protection. The HERS study followed women with established CHD and found that estrogen plus a progestin increased the relative risk of nonfatal myocardial infarction or CHD death within 1 year of treatment, but there was no overall change in 5 years (Hulley et al., 1998). The HERS II follow-up found no overall change in the incidence of CHD after 6.8 years of the treatment (Grady et al., 2002). In women *without* existing CHD (WHI trials), treated with an estrogen plus progestin, protective effects were seen but only when hormone replacement was initiated within 10 years of menopause (Rossouw et al., 2002).

It is clear, however, that oral estrogens increase the risk of thromboembolic disease in healthy women and in women with preexisting cardiovascular disease (Grady et al., 2000). The increase in absolute risk is small but significant. In the WHI, for example, an estrogen-progestin combination led to an increase in eight attributable cases of stroke per 10,000 older women and a similar increase in pulmonary embolism (Rossouw et al., 2002). The latter was seen mainly in women who concomitantly smoked cigarettes.

Effects on Cognition

Several retrospective studies had suggested that estrogens had beneficial effects on cognition and delayed the onset of Alzheimer disease (Green and Simpkins, 2000). However, the Women's Health Initiative Memory Study (WHIMS) of a group of women 65 years of age or older found that estrogen-progestin therapy was associated with doubling in the number of women diagnosed with probable dementia, and no benefit of hormone treatment on global cognitive function was observed (Rapp et al., 2003; Shumaker et al., 2003).

Other Potential Untoward Effects

Nausea and vomiting are an initial reaction to estrogen therapy in some women, but these effects may disappear with time and may be minimized by taking estrogens with food or just before sleep. Fullness and tenderness of the breasts and edema may occur, but sometimes can be diminished by lowering the dose.

Drug Therapy in Endometriosis, Hirsutism, and Gender Transition

Endometriosis

Endometriosis is an estrogen-dependent disorder that results from endometrial tissue ectopically located outside the uterine cavity (Farquhar, 2007). It predominantly affects women during their reproductive years, with a prevalence of 0.5%–5% in fertile women and 25%–40% in infertile women. Diagnosis typically is made at laparoscopy, either prompted by unexplained pelvic pain (dysmenorrhea or dyspareunia) or infertility. Although poorly understood, the infertility is thought to reflect involvement of the fallopian tubes with the underlying process and, possibly, impaired oocyte maturation.

Because the proliferation of ectopic endometrial tissue is responsive to ovarian steroid hormones, many symptomatic approaches to therapy aim to produce a relatively hypoestrogenic state. Combination oral contraceptives have been standard first-line treatment of symptoms of endometriosis, and ample evidence from observational trials supports their benefit. The predominant mechanism of action is believed to be suppression of gonadotropin secretion, with subsequent inhibition of estrogen biosynthesis. Progestins (e.g., medroxyprogesterone, dienogest) also have been used to promote decidualization of the ectopic endometrial tissue. The levonorgestrel IUS, which is approved for contraception, also has been used off label for this indication, as well as for menorrhagia.

Stable GnRH agonists can suppress gonadotropin secretion and thus effect medical castration. Drugs that carry an indication for endometriosis include leuprolide, goserelin, and nafarelin; other GnRH agonists also may be used off label for this purpose (see Chapter 42). Due to significant decreases in bone density and symptoms of estrogen withdrawal, "add-back" therapy with either a low-dose synthetic estrogen (e.g., conjugated equine estrogens, 0.625–1.25 mg) or a high-dose progestin (e.g., norethindrone, 5 mg) has been used when the duration of therapy has exceeded 6 months (Olive, 2008). Danazol, a synthetic androgen that inhibits gonadotropin production via feedback inhibition of the pituitary-ovarian axis, also is FDA approved for endometriosis therapy; it rarely is used now because of its significant adverse effects, including hirsutism and elevation of hepatic transaminases. In Europe and elsewhere, the antiprogestin gestrinone has been employed. By virtue of their ability to block the terminal step in estrogen biosynthesis, inhibitors of aromatase are under investigation for endometriosis (reviewed by Barbieri, 2008).

Hirsutism

Hirsutism, or increased hair growth in the male distribution, affects about 10% of women of reproductive age. It can be a relatively benign, idiopathic process or part of a more severe disorder of androgen excess that includes overt virilization (voice deepening, increased muscle mass, male pattern balding, clitoromegaly) and often results from ovarian or adrenal tumors. Specific etiologies associated with hirsutism include congenital adrenal hyperplasia, PCOS, and Cushing syndrome. After excluding serious pathology such as a steroid-producing malignancy, the treatment largely becomes empirical (Martin et al., 2008).

Pharmacotherapy is directed at decreasing androgen production and action. Initial therapy often involves treatment with combination oral contraceptive pills, which suppress gonadotropin secretion and thus the production of ovarian androgens. The estrogen also increases the concentration of SHBG, thereby diminishing the free concentration of testosterone. The full effect of this suppression may take up to 6–9 months. GnRH agonists downregulate gonadotropin secretion and also may be used to suppress ovarian steroid production.

In patients who fail to respond to ovarian suppression, efforts to block androgen action may be effective. Spironolactone, a mineralocorticoid receptor antagonist, and flutamide (see Chapter 45) inhibit the androgen receptor. In Europe and elsewhere, cyproterone (50–100 mg/d) is used as an androgen receptor blocker, often in conjunction with a combination oral contraceptive. Finasteride, an inhibitor of the type 2 isozyme of 5α-reductase that blocks the conversion of testosterone to dihydrotestosterone also is effective. Male offspring of women who become pregnant while taking any of these androgen inhibitors are at risk of impaired virilization secondary to impaired synthesis or action of dihydrotestosterone (pregnancy risk FDA category X; see Appendix I). The antifungal ketoconazole, which inhibits CYP steroid hydroxylases (see Chapters 46 and 61), also can block androgen biosynthesis but may cause liver toxicity. Topical eflornithine, an ornithine decarboxylase inhibitor, has been used with some success to decrease the rate of facial hair growth.

Nonpharmacological approaches include bleaching, depilatory treatments (e.g., shaving, treatment with hair-removing chemicals), or methods that remove the entire hair follicle (e.g., plucking, electrolysis, laser ablation).

Gender Transition

In the past 10–20 years, sex steroids have been used more frequently in transgender patients. Because no significant clinical trials have been performed, a great deal of variability exists in the approaches taken in both male-to-female and female-to-male transgender patients. In general, younger patients in their early teens are often held from natural puberty through the use of GnRH agonists until the individuals are old and mature enough to be certain of their decision. Once the decision is made, whether the patients are younger or older, the approaches can be myriad, although they follow the same principals: (1) suppress endogenous sex steroid production and (2) promote physical and mental features of the desired gender.

Male-to-Female Transitions

The primary medication used for male-to-female transition is some form of estrogen, whether it be oral estradiol (2–6 mg per day), transdermal estradiol (0.1–0.4 mg every 24 h), or injectable estrogens such as estradiol valerate or estradiol cypionate (5–10 mg IM every 2 weeks). Side effects with estrogens, including thrombosis and breast cancer (not really established in male-to-female transgender patients) must be discussed with patients. Target serum estradiol levels are usually in the range of 100–200 pg/mL. In many patients, estrogen treatment alone will be sufficient to suppress endogenous androgen production and therefore androgen-mediated effects; however, in patients where this is not possible, antiandrogens such as spironolactone (100–400 mg per day) can be used. Alternatively, endogenous androgen production can be suppressed with GnRH agonists. The advantage of using antiandrogens or GnRH agonists is that the dosages of estradiol can often be significantly lower.

Female-to-Male Transitions

The primary medication used in female-to-male transitions is some form of androgen, whether it be injectable, such as testosterone enanthate or cypionate (50–100 mg IM per week), or androgen gels (25–100 mg per day of testosterone). Target plasma androgen levels should be in the normal male range (300–500 mg per day). Side effects of excess androgens, including polycythemia and lipid abnormalities, should be discussed and monitored with all patients. In general, these doses of androgens are sufficient to suppress endogenous ovarian steroid hormone production; however, if breakthrough uterine bleeding still occurs, patients can be treated with depot medroxyprogesterone (150 mg every 3 months) until bleeding no longer occurs.

Acknowledgment: *David S. Loose and George M. Stancel contributed to this chapter in recent editions of this book. We have retained some of their text in the current edition.*

Drug Facts for Your Personal Formulary: *Estrogens, Progestins, GnRH, Gonadotropins*

Drug	Therapeutic Uses	Major Toxicity and Clinical Pearls
Estrogens		
Steroidal Estrogen and Derivatives Estradiol Estradiol valerate Estradiol cypionate Ethinyl estradiol Mestranol, equilin Estrone sulfate **Nonsteroidal Compounds** Diethylstilbestrol Bisphenol A, genistein	• Menopause hormone therapy • Components of oral contraceptives • Treatment of transgender individuals • Depending on the preparation, may be available for oral, parenteral, transdermal, or topical administration	• Act via ERα and ERβ • Precaution: prescribe the lowest effective dose for the shortest duration consistent with treatment goals and risks for each individual patient • Increased risk of thromboembolism • Potencies of various oral preparations differ due to differences in first-pass metabolism
Selective Estrogen Receptor Modulators		
Tamoxifen	• Treatment of breast cancer • Antiestrogenic, estrogenic, or mixed activity depending on tissue	• Tissue-selective actions on ERs • Beneficial estrogenic actions in bone, brain, and liver during postmenopausal hormone therapy • Antagonist activity in breast and endometrium • Increased risk of thromboembolism
Raloxifene	• Treatment of osteoporosis (estrogen agonist in bone) • Reduces total cholesterol and LDL but does not increase HDL • To reduce risk of breast cancer in high-risk postmenopausal women	
Toremifene	• Treatment of breast cancer	
Antiestrogens		
Clomiphene	• Treatment of infertility in anovulatory women	• Primarily a receptor antagonist but also has weak agonist activity
Fulvestrant	• Treatment of breast cancer in women with disease progression after tamoxifen • Used in women with resistance to aromatase inhibitors	• Receptor antagonist in all tissues

Estrogen Synthesis Inhibitors

Aromatase Inhibitors *Steroidal inhibitors* Formestane Exemestane *Nonsteroidal inhibitors* Anastrozole Letrozole, vorozole	• Treatment of breast cancer (exemestane, letrozole, and anastrozole approved in the U.S.)	• *Steroidal inhibitors:* substrate analogues that irreversibly inactivate aromatase • *Nonsteroidal inhibitors:* interact reversibly with the heme groups of CYPs • Risk of osteoporosis with long-term use

Progestins

Pregnanes Progesterone Medroxyprogesterone acetate Megestrol acetate	• Menopause hormone therapy • Contraception • Assisted reproductive technology • Depot MPA used as a long-acting injectable contraceptive	• Formulations: oral, injection, vaginal gel, slow-release intrauterine device, vaginal insert • Progesterone: rapid first-pass metabolism • MPA and high-dose micronized progesterone are available for oral use
Estranes Norethindrone 19-Norethindrone	• Used in oral and injectable contraceptives	• 19-Nortestosterone derivatives • Progestational activity but also some androgenic and other activities
Gonanes Norgestrel Norgestimate	• Used in oral and injectable contraceptives	• 19-Nortestosterone derivatives, ethyl rather than methyl group at position 13 • Progestational components of contraceptives

Antiprogestins and Progesterone Receptor Modulators

Mifepristone (RU 38486)	• Termination of early pregnancy	• Competitive receptor antagonist of both progesterone receptors • May have some agonist activity
Ulipristal acetate	• Emergency contraception	• Partial progesterone receptor agonist

GnRH Agonist and Antagonists

GnRH agonist Leuprolide	• Controlled ovarian hyperstimulation • Endometriosis • Uterine leiomyomas • Precocious puberty • Menstrual suppression in special circumstance (e.g., thrombocytopenia)	• Initial agonist action ("flare effect") results in increase in FSH and LH • After 1–3 weeks, desensitization and pituitary downregulation result in a hypogonadotropic, hypogonadal state • Risk of osteoporosis with long-term use
GnRH antagonist Cetrorelix, ganirelix Goserelin, buserelin Triptorelin, nafarelin	• Controlled ovarian hyperstimulation	• Competitive GnRH receptor antagonist • Immediate decline in LH and FSH levels • Risk of osteoporosis with long-term use

Gonadotropins

FSH *Recombinant FSH* Follitropin-alpha Follitropin-beta *Human menopausal menotropins* Menotropins Urofollitropins Highly purified urinary FSH	• Ovulation induction • Controlled ovarian hyperstimulation	• hMG may contain FSH, LH, and hCG and purification results in standardization of the FSH and LH activity • Injectable or intravenous
LH Recombinant LH	• Controlled ovarian hyperstimulation in women with LH deficiency due to hypogonadotropic hypogonadism	• Injectable or intravenous
hCG Recombinant hCG Urinary hCG Highly purified urinary hCG	• Promotes meiotic maturation from prophase I to metaphase II in oocytes	• Injectable or intravenous • Also used to stimulate testosterone and sperm production in men

SECTION V HORMONES AND HORMONE ANTAGONISTS

Bibliography

Anderson GL, et al. for The Women's Health Initiative Steering Committee. Effects of conjugated equine estrogen in postmenopausal women with hysterectomy: the Women's Health Initiative randomized controlled trial. *JAMA*, **2004**, *291*:1701–1712.

Barbieri RL. Update in female reproduction: A life-cycle approach. *J Clin Endocrinol Metab*, **2008**, *93*:2439–2446.

Belchetz PE. Hormonal treatment of postmenopausal women. *N Engl J Med*, **1994**, *330*:1062–1071.

Beral V, for the Million Women Study Collaborators. Breast cancer and hormone-replacement therapy in the Million Women Study. *Lancet*, **2003**, *362*:419–427.

Blackmore PF. Extragenomic actions of progesterone in human sperm and progesterone metabolites in human platelets. *Steroids*, **1999**, *64*:149–156.

Brinton LA, et al. Ovulation induction and cancer risk. *Fertil Steril*, **2005**, *83*:261–274.

Burkman R, et al. Safety concerns and health benefits associated with oral contraception. *Am J Obstet Gynecol*, **2004**, *190*(suppl 4):S5–S22.

Castelli WP. Cardiovascular disease: pathogenesis, epidemiology, and risk among users of oral contraceptives who smoke. *Am J Obstet Gynecol*, **1999**, *180*:349S–356S.

Cheng L, et al. Interventions for emergency contraception. *Cochrane Database Syst Rev*, **2008**, *16*:CD001324.

Cheskis BJ, et al. Estrogen receptor ligands modulate its interaction with DNA. *J Biol Chem*, **1997**, *272*:11384–11391.

Christin-Maitre S, et al. Medical termination of pregnancy. *N Engl J Med*, **2000**, *342*:946–956.

Clark SL, et al. Oxytocin: New perspectives on an old drug. *Am J Obstet Gynecol*, **2009**, *200*:35.e1–35.e6.

Cohen AL, et al. Toxic shock associated with Clostridium sordellii and Clostridium perfringens after medical and spontaneous abortion. *Obstet Gynecol*, **2007**, *110*:1027–1033.

Collingwood TN, et al Nuclear receptors: co-activators, co-repressors and chromatin remodeling in the control of transcription. *J Mol Endocrinol*, **1999**, *23*:255–275.

Conneely OM, et al. Reproductive functions of progesterone receptors. *Recent Prog Horm Res*, **2002**, *57*:339–355.

Coombes RC, et al., for the Intergroup Exemestane Study. A randomized trial of exemestane after two to three years of tamoxifen therapy in postmenopausal women with primary breast cancer. *N Engl J Med*, **2004**, *350*:1081–1092.

Cullins VE. Noncontraceptive benefits and therapeutic uses of depot medroxyprogesterone acetate. *J Reprod Med*, **1996**, *41*(suppl 5): 428–433.

Cummings SR, et al. The effect of raloxifene on risk of breast cancer in postmenopausal women: results from the MORE randomized trial. Multiple Outcomes of Raloxifene Evaluation. *JAMA*, **1999**, *281*:2189–2197.

Delmas PD, et al. Multiple Outcomes of Raloxifene Evaluation (MORE) Investigators. Efficacy of raloxifene on vertebral fracture risk reduction in postmenopausal women with osteoporosis: four-year results from a randomized clinical trial. *J Clin Endocrinol Metab*, **2002**, *87*:3609–3617.

DeManno D, et al. Asoprisnil (J867): A selective progesterone receptor modulator for gynecological therapy. *Steroids*, **2003**, *68*:1019–1032.

Ettinger B, et al. Reduction of vertebral fracture risk in postmenopausal women with osteoporosis treated with raloxifene: results from a 3-year randomized clinical trial. Multiple Outcomes of Raloxifene Evaluation (MORE) Investigators. *JAMA*, **1999**, *282*:637–645.

Farquhar C. Endometriosis. *BMJ*, **2007**, *334*:249–253.

Fernandez E, et al. Oral contraceptives and colorectal cancer risk: a meta-analysis. *Br J Cancer*, **2001**, *84*:722–727.

Fitzpatrick LA. Soy isoflavones: hope or hype? *Maturitas*, **2003**, *44* (suppl 1):S21–S29.

Fotherby K. Bioavailability of orally administered sex steroids used in oral contraception and hormone replacement therapy. *Contraception*, **1996**, *54*:59–69.

Fruzzetti F. Hemostatic effects of smoking and oral contraceptive use. *Am J Obstet Gynecol*, **1999**, *180*:S369–S374.

Giangrande PH, et al. The opposing transcriptional activities of the two isoforms of the human progesterone receptor are due to differential cofactor binding. *Mol Cell Biol*, **2000**, *20*:3102–3115.

Giangrande PH, McDonnell DP. The A and B isoforms of the human progesterone receptor: two functionally different transcription factors encoded by a single gene. *Recent Prog Horm Res*, **1999**, *54*:291–313.

Godsland IF. The influence of female sex steroids on glucose metabolism and insulin action. *J Intern Med Suppl*, **1996**, *738*:1–60.

Grady D, et al., for the HERS Research Group. Cardiovascular disease outcomes during 6.8 years of hormone therapy: Heart and Estrogen/progestin Replacement Study follow-up (HERS II). *JAMA*, **2002**, *288*: 49–57.

Grady D, et al. Postmenopausal hormone therapy increases risk for venous thromboembolic disease. Heart and Estrogen/progestin Replacement Study. *Ann Intern Med*, **2000**, *132*:689–696.

Green PS, Simpkins JW. Neuroprotective effects of estrogens: potential mechanisms of action. *Int J Dev Neurosci*, **2000**, *18*:347–358.

Grumbach MM, Auchus RJ. Estrogen: consequences and implications of human mutations in synthesis and action. *J Clin Endocrinol Metab*, **1999**, *84*:4677–4694.

Hall JM, McDonnell DP. The estrogen receptor β-isoform (ER β) of the human estrogen receptor modulates ER β transcriptional activity and is a key regulator of the cellular response to estrogens and antiestrogens. *Endocrinology*, **1999**, *140*:5566–5578.

Hammes SR. Steroids and oocyte maturation—a new look at an old story. *Mol Endocrinol*, **2004**, *18*:769–775.

Han W, et al. Full sequencing analysis of estrogen receptor-α gene polymorphism and its association with breast cancer risk. *Anticancer Res*, **2003**, *23*:4703–4707.

Hanstein B, et al. Insights into the molecular biology of the estrogen receptor define novel therapeutic targets for breast cancer. *Eur J Endocrinol*, **2004**, *150*:243–255.

Harrington WR, et al. Activities of estrogen receptor α- and β-selective ligands at diverse estrogen responsive gene sites mediating transactivation or transrepression. *Mol Cell Endocrinol*, **2003**, *206*: 13–22.

Haynes BP, et al. The pharmacology of letrozole. *J Steroid Biochem Mol Biol*, **2003**, *87*:35–45.

Herrington DM, Howard TD. ER-α variants and the cardiovascular effects of hormone replacement therapy. *Pharmacogenomics*, **2003**, *4*: 269–277.

Herrington DM, Klein KP. Pharmacogenetics of estrogen replacement therapy. *J Appl Physiol*, **2001**, *91*:2776–2784.

Hewitt SC, Korach KS. Oestrogen receptor knockout mice: roles for oestrogen receptors α and β in reproductive tissues. *Reproduction*, **2003**, *125*:143–149.

Hotchkiss J, Knobil E. The menstrual cycle and its neuroendocrine control. In: Knobil E, Neill JD, eds. *The Physiology of Reproduction*. 2nd ed. Raven Press, New York, **1994**, 711–749.

Hulley S, et al. Randomized trial of estrogen plus progestin for secondary prevention of coronary heart disease in postmenopausal women. Heart and Estrogen/progestin Replacement Study (HERS) Research Group. *JAMA*, **1998**, *280*:605–613.

Jaiyesimi IA, et al. Use of tamoxifen for breast cancer: twenty-eight years later. *J Clin Oncol*, **1995**, *13*:513–529.

Jang GR, Benet LZ. Antiprogestin pharmacodynamics, pharmacokinetics, and metabolism: implications for their long-term use. *J Pharmacokinet Biopharm*, **1997**, *25*:647–672.

Kato S, et al. Activation of the estrogen receptor through phosphorylation by mitogen-activated protein kinase. *Science*, **1995**, *270*:1491–1494.

Kettel LM, et al. Hypothalamic-pituitary-ovarian response to clomiphene citrate in women with polycystic ovary syndrome. *Fertil Steril*, **1993**, *59*:532–538.

Knobil E. Patterns of hypophysiotropic signals and gonadotropin secretion in the rhesus monkey. *Biol Reprod*, **1981**, *24*:44–49.

Koh KK, et al. Effects of hormone-replacement therapy on fibrinolysis in postmenopausal women. *N Engl J Med*, **1997**, *336*:683–690.

Kos M, et al. Minireview: genomic organization of the human ERalpha gene promoter region. *Mol Endocrinol*, **2001**, *15*:2057–2063.

Kousteni S, et al. Reversal of bone loss in mice by nongenotropic signaling of sex steroids. *Science*, **2002**, *298*:843–846.

Kuiper GG, et al. Comparison of the ligand binding specificity and transcript tissue distribution of estrogen receptors ER α and β. *Endocrinology*, **1997**, *138*:863–870.

Kurabayashi T, et al. Association of vitamin D and estrogen receptor gene polymorphism with the effects of long term hormone replacement therapy on bone mineral density. *J Bone Miner Metab*, **2004**, *22*:241–247.

Labrie F, et al. The combination of a novel selective estrogen receptor modulator with an estrogen protects the mammary gland and uterus in a rodent model: the future of postmenopausal women's health? *Endocrinology*, **2003**, *144*:4700–4706.

Lahti E, et al. Endometrial changes in postmenopausal breast cancer patients receiving tamoxifen. *Obstet Gynecol*, **1993**, *81*:660–664.

Legro RS, et al. Cooperative multicenter reproductive medicine network. *N Engl J Med*, **2007**, *356*(6):551–566.

Legro RS, et al. Letrozole versus clomiphene for infertility in the polycystic ovary syndrome. *N Engl J Med*, **2014**, *371*:119–129.

Leonhardt SA, Edwards DP. Mechanism of action of progesterone antagonists. *Exp Biol Med*, **2002**, *227*:969–980.

Levin ER. Rapid signaling by steroid receptors. *Am J Physiol*, **2008**, *295*:R1425–R1430.

Lewandowski S, et al. Estrogen receptor β. Potential functional significance of a variety of mRNA isoforms. *FEBS Lett*, **2002**, *524*:1–5.

Love RR, et al. Effects of tamoxifen on cardiovascular risk factors in postmenopausal women after 5 years of treatment. *J Natl Cancer Inst*, **1994**, *86*:1534–1539.

Manson JE, Martin KA. Clinical practice. Postmenopausal hormone-replacement therapy. *N Engl J Med*, **2001**, *345*:34–40.

Martin KA, et al. Evaluation and treatment of hirsutism in premenopausal women: An endocrine society clinical practice guideline. *J Clin Endocrinol Metab*, **2008**, *93*:1105–1120.

McDonnell DP, Goldman ME. RU486 exerts antiestrogenic activities through a novel progesterone receptor A form-mediated mechanism. *J Biol Chem*, **1994**, *269*:11945–11949.

McInerney EM, et al. Transcription activation by the human estrogen receptor subtype beta (ER beta) studied with ER beta and ER alpha receptor chimeras. *Endocrinology*, **1998**, *139*:4513–4522.

Mendelsohn ME, Karas RH. The protective effects of estrogen on the cardiovascular system. *N Engl J Med*, **1999**, *340*:1801–1811.

Modelska K, Cummings S. Tibolone for postmenopausal women: systematic review of randomized trials. *J Clin Endocrinol Metab*, **2002**, *87*:16–23.

Moodley J. Combined oral contraceptives and cervical cancer. *Curr Opin Obstet Gynecol*, **2004**, *16*:27–29.

Mulac-Jericevic B, et al. Defective mammary gland morphogenesis in mice lacking the progesterone receptor B isoform. *Proc Natl Acad Sci U S A*, **2003**, *100*:9744–9749.

Mulac-Jericevic B, et al. Subgroup of reproductive functions of progesterone mediated by progesterone receptor-B isoform. *Science*, **2000**, *289*:1751–1754.

Olde B, Leeb-Lundberg LM. GPR30/GPER1: searching for a role in estrogen physiology. *Trends Endocrinol Metab*, **2009**, *20*:409–416.

Olive DL. Gonadotropin-releasing hormone agonists for endometriosis. *N Engl J Med*, **2008**, *359*:1136–1142.

Paech K, et al. Differential ligand activation of estrogen receptors ERα and ERβ at AP1 sites. *Science*, **1997**, *277*:1508–1510.

Pedram A, et al. Nature of functional estrogen receptors at the plasma membrane. *Mol Endocrinol*, **2006**, *20*:1996–2009.

Peltoketo H, et al. Regulation of estrogen action: role of 17 β-hydroxysteroid dehydrogenases. *Vitam Horm*, **1999**, *55*:353–398.

Pike AC, et al. A structural biologist's view of the oestrogen receptor. *J Steroid Biochem Mol Biol*, **2000**, *74*:261–268.

Pike MC, et al. Estrogen-progestin replacement therapy and endometrial cancer. *J Natl Cancer Inst*, **1997**, *89*:1110–1116.

Prince RL, et al. Prevention of postmenopausal osteoporosis. A comparative study of exercise, calcium supplementation, and hormone-replacement therapy. *N Engl J Med*, **1991**, *325*:1189–1195.

Rapp SR, et al., for the WHIMS Investigators. Effect of estrogen plus progestin on global cognitive function in postmenopausal women: the Women's Health Initiative Memory Study: randomized controlled trial. *JAMA*, **2003**, *289*:2663–2672.

Riggs BL, et al. Sex steroids and the construction and conservation of the adult skeleton. *Endocr Rev*, **2002**, *23*:279–302.

Robertson JF, et al. Fulvestrant versus anastrozole for the treatment of advanced breast carcinoma in postmenopausal women: a prospective combined analysis of two multi-center trials. *Cancer*, **2003**, *98*:229–238.

Robinson D, Cardozo LD. The role of estrogens in female lower urinary tract dysfunction. *Urology*, **2003**, *62*(suppl 4A):45–51.

Ross RK, et al. Effect of hormone replacement therapy on breast cancer risk: estrogen versus estrogen plus progestin. *J Natl Cancer Inst*, **2000**, *92*(4):328–332.

Rossouw JE, et al., for the Writing Group for the Women's Health Initiative Investigators. Risks and benefits of estrogen plus progestin in healthy postmenopausal women: principal results from the Women's Health Initiative randomized controlled trial. *JAMA*, **2002**, *288*:321–333.

Saville B, et al. Ligand-, cell-, and estrogen receptor subtype (α/β)-dependent activation at GC-rich (Sp1) promoter elements. *J Biol Chem*, **2000**, *275*:5379–5387.

Schairer C, et al. Menopausal estrogen and estrogen-progestin replacement therapy and breast cancer risk. *JAMA*, **2000**, *283*:485–491.

Seminara SB. Mechanisms of disease: the first kiss—a crucial role for kisspeptin-1 and its receptor G-protein-coupled receptor 54, in puberty and reproduction. *Nat Clin Pract Endocrinol Metab*, **2006**, *2*:328–334.

Shapiro S, et al. Risk of localized and widespread endometrial cancer in relation to recent and discontinued use of conjugated estrogens. *N Engl J Med*, **1985**, *313*:969–972.

Sherif K. Benefits and risks of oral contraceptives. *Am J Obstet Gynecol*, **1999**, *180*:S343–S348.

Shumaker SA, et al., for the WHIMS Investigators. Estrogen plus progestin and the incidence of dementia and mild cognitive impairment in postmenopausal women: the Women's Health Initiative Memory Study: a randomized controlled trial. *JAMA*, **2003**, *289*:2651–2662.

Simhan HN, Caritis SN. Prevention of preterm delivery. *N Engl J Med*, **2007**, *357*:477–487.

Simoncini T, et al. Interaction of oestrogen receptor with the regulatory subunit of phosphatidylinositol-3-OH kinase. *Nature*, **2000**, *407*: 538–541.

Simpson ER. Sources of estrogen and their importance. *J Steroid Biochem Mol Biol*, **2003**, *86*:225–230.

Simpson ER, et al. Aromatase—a brief overview. *Annu Rev Physiol*, **2002**, *64*:93–127.

Smith CL, O'Malley BW. Coregulator function: a key to understanding tissue specificity of selective receptor modulators. *Endocr Rev*, **2004**, *25*:45–71.

Smith EP, et al. Estrogen resistance caused by a mutation in the estrogen-receptor gene in a man. *N Engl J Med*, **1994**, *331*:1056–1061.

Smith RE. A review of selective estrogen receptor modulators and national surgical adjuvant breast and bowel project clinical trials. *Semin Oncol* **2003**, *30*(suppl 16):4–13.

Spitz IM, Chwalisz K. Progesterone receptor modulators and progesterone antagonists in women's health. *Steroids*, **2000**, *65*:807–815.

Sridar C, et al. Effect of tamoxifen on the enzymatic activity of human cytochrome CYP2B6. *J Pharmacol Exp Ther*, **2002**, *301*:945–952.

Tamrazi A, et al. Molecular sensors of estrogen receptor conformations and dynamics. *Mol Endocrinol*, **2003**, *17*:2593–2602.

Thessaloniki ESHRE/ASRM-Sponsored PCOS Consensus. Workshop Group. Consensus on infertility treatment related to polycystic ovary syndrome. *Fertil Steril*, **2008**, *89*:505–522.

Thorneycroft IH, et al. The relation of serum 17-hydroxyprogesterone and estradiol-17β levels during the human menstrual cycle. *Am J Obstet Gynecol*, **1971**, *111*:947–951.

Van Den Bemd GJ, et al. Distinct effects on the conformation of estrogen receptor α and β by both the antiestrogens ICI 164,384 and ICI 182,780 leading to opposite effects on receptor stability. *Biochem Biophys Res Commun*, **1999**, *261*:1–5.

Walsh BW, et al. Effects of raloxifene on serum lipids and coagulation factors in healthy postmenopausal women. *JAMA*, **1998**, *279*:1445–1451.

Walsh BW, et al. Effects of postmenopausal hormone replacement with oral and transdermal estrogen on high density lipoprotein metabolism. *J Lipid Res*, **1994**, *35*:2083–2093.

Weiderpass E, et al. Estrogen receptor α gene polymorphisms and endometrial cancer risk. *Carcinogenesis*, **2000**, *21*:623–627.

Westhoff CL. Breast cancer risk: perception versus reality. *Contraception*, **1999**, *59*(suppl):25S–28S.

Writing Group for the PEPI Trial. Effects of estrogen or estrogen/progestin regimens on heart disease risk factors in postmenopausal women. The Postmenopausal Estrogen/Progestin Interventions (PEPI) Trial. *JAMA*, **1995**, *273*:199–208.

Yue W, et al. Genotoxic metabolites of estradiol in breast: potential mechanism of estradiol induced carcinogenesis. *J Steroid Biochem Mol Biol*, **2003**, *86*:477–486.

Chapter 45

Androgens and the Male Reproductive Tract

Peter J. Snyder

Testosterone and Other Androgens

In men, *testosterone* is the principal secreted androgen. *Leydig cells* synthesize the majority of testosterone by the pathways shown in Figure 45–1. In women, testosterone also is the principal androgen and is synthesized in the corpus luteum and the adrenal cortex by similar pathways. The testosterone precursors *androstenedione* and *DHEA* are weak androgens that can be converted peripherally to testosterone.

Secretion and Transport of Testosterone

Testosterone secretion is greater in men than in women at almost all stages of life, a difference that explains many of the other differences between men and women. In the first trimester in utero, the fetal testes begin to secrete testosterone, the principal factor in male sexual differentiation, probably stimulated by hCG from the placenta. By the beginning of the second trimester, the serum testosterone concentration is close to that of midpuberty, about 250 ng/dL (Figure 45–2). Testosterone production then falls by the end of the second trimester, but by birth the value is again about 250 ng/dL, possibly due to stimulation of the fetal Leydig cells by *LH* from the fetal pituitary gland. The testosterone value falls again in the first few days after birth, but it rises and peaks again at about 250 ng/dL at 2–3 months after birth and falls to less than 50 ng/dL by 6 months, where it remains until puberty. During puberty, from about 12 to 17 years of age, the serum testosterone concentration in males increases so that by early adulthood the serum testosterone concentration is 300 ng/dL to 800 ng/dL in men, compared to 30 ng/dL to 50 ng/dL in women. The magnitude of the testosterone concentration in the male is responsible for the pubertal changes that further differentiate men from women. As men age, their serum testosterone concentrations gradually decrease, which may contribute to other effects of aging in men.

Luteinizing hormone, secreted by the pituitary gonadotropes (see Chapter 42), is the principal stimulus of testosterone secretion in men, perhaps potentiated by *FSH*, also secreted by gonadotropes. The secretion of LH by gonadotropes is positively regulated by hypothalamic *GnRH*; testosterone directly inhibits LH secretion in a negative-feedback loop. LH is secreted in pulses, which occur approximately every 2 h and are greater in magnitude in the morning (Crowley et al., 1985). The pulsatility appears to result from pulsatile secretion of GnRH from the hypothalamus. Testosterone secretion is likewise pulsatile and diurnal, the highest plasma concentrations occurring at about 8 AM and the lowest at about 8 PM. The morning peaks diminish as men age. SHBG binds about 40% of circulating testosterone with high affinity, rendering the bound hormone unavailable for biological effects. Albumin binds almost 60% of circulating testosterone with low affinity, leaving about 2% unbound or free. In women, LH stimulates the *corpus luteum* (formed from the follicle after release of the ovum) to secrete testosterone. Under normal circumstances, however, *estradiol* and *progesterone*, not testosterone, are the principal inhibitors of LH secretion in women.

Metabolism of Testosterone to Active and Inactive Compounds

Testosterone has many different effects in tissues, both directly and through its metabolism to *dihydrotestosterone* and *estradiol* (Figure 45–3). The enzyme 5α-reductase catalyzes the conversion of

Abbreviations

AR: androgen receptor
AUC: area under the curve
cGMP: cyclic guanosine monophosphate
CYP: cytochrome P450
DHEA: dehydroepiandrosterone
eNOS: endothelial nitric oxide synthase, NOS3
FSH: follicle-stimulating hormone
GnRH: gonadotropin-releasing hormone
hCG: human chorionic gonadotropin
HDL: high-density lipoprotein
LDL: low-density lipoprotein
LH: luteinizing hormone
NANC: nonadrenergic/noncholinergic
NO: nitric oxide
PDE5: phosphodiesterase 5
PKG: protein kinase G
sGC: soluble guanylate cyclase
SHBG: sex hormone–binding globulin
THG: tetrahydrogestrinone

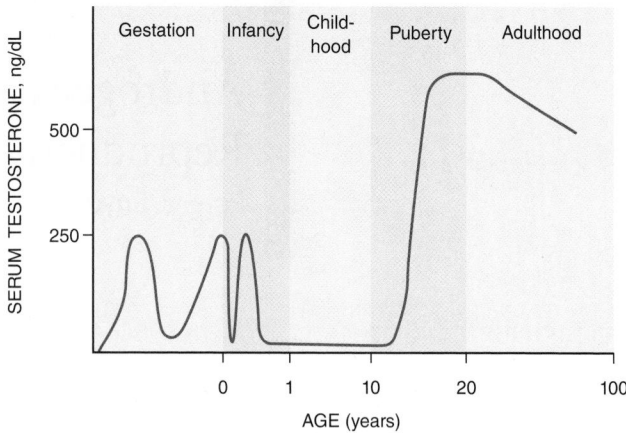

Figure 45–2 *Schematic representation of the serum testosterone concentration from early gestation to old age.*

Physiological and Pharmacological Effects of Androgens

Testosterone is the principal circulating androgen in men. At least three mechanisms contribute to the varied effects of testosterone:

- direct binding to the AR;
- conversion in certain tissues to dihydrotestosterone, which also binds to the AR; and
- conversion to estradiol, which binds to the estrogen receptor (Figure 45–4).

Effects That Occur Via the Androgen Receptor

Testosterone and dihydrotestosterone act as androgens via a single AR, a member of the nuclear receptor superfamily designated as NR3A. The AR has an amino-terminal domain that contains a polyglutamine repeat of variable length, a DNA-binding domain consisting of two Zn finger motifs, and a carboxyterminal ligand-binding domain. The polyglutamine

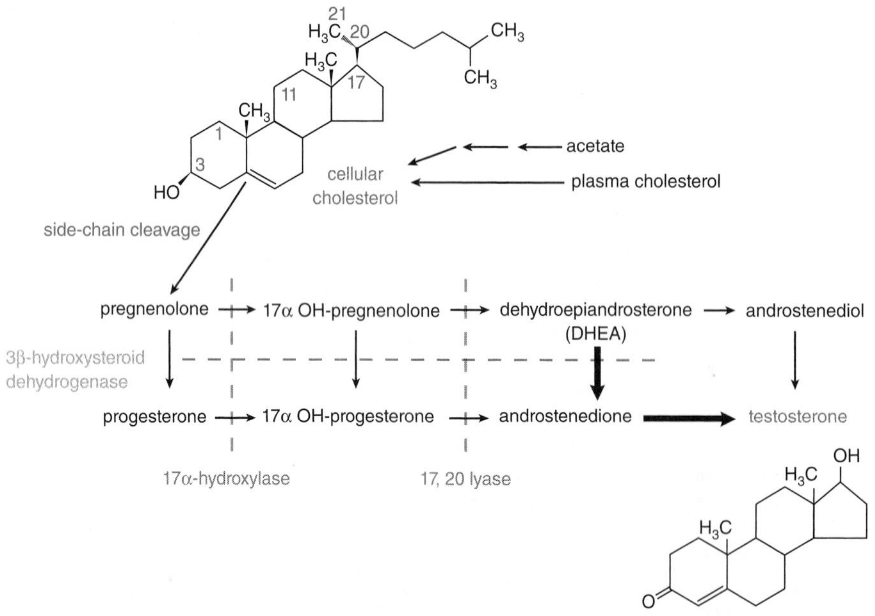

testosterone to dihydrotestosterone. Dihydrotestosterone binds to the *AR* with higher affinity than testosterone and activates gene expression more efficiently. Two forms of 5α-reductase have been identified: *type I*, which is found predominantly in nongenital skin, liver, and bone; and *type II*, which is found predominantly in urogenital tissue in men and genital skin in men and women. The enzyme complex aromatase, present in many tissues, catalyzes the conversion of testosterone to estradiol. This conversion accounts for about 85% of circulating estradiol in men; the remainder is secreted directly by the testes (MacDonald et al., 1979). Hepatic metabolism converts testosterone to the biologically inactive compounds androsterone and etiocholanolone (see Figure 45–3). Dihydrotestosterone is metabolized to androsterone, androstanedione, and androstanediol.

Figure 45–1 *Pathway of synthesis of testosterone in the Leydig cells of the testes.* In Leydig cells, the 11 and 21 hydroxylases (present in adrenal cortex) are absent, but CYP17 (17α-hydroxylase) is present. Thus, androgens and estrogens are synthesized; corticosterone and cortisol are not formed. Bold arrows indicate favored pathways.

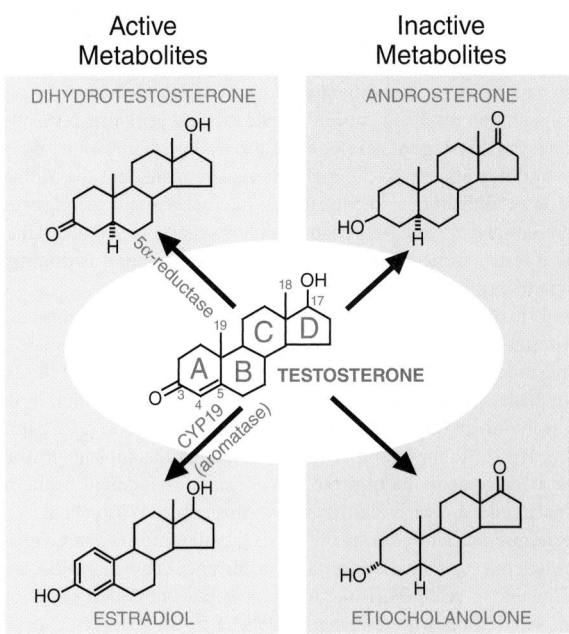

at the amino terminus of the molecule (Walcott and Merry, 2002). The result is very mild androgen resistance, manifest principally by gynecomastia, and progressively severe motor neuron atrophy (Dejager et al., 2002). The mechanism by which the neuronal atrophy occurs is unknown. Other mutations in AR may explain why metastatic prostate cancer often regresses initially in response to androgen deprivation treatment, but then becomes unresponsive to continued deprivation. AR continues to be expressed in androgen-independent prostate cancer, and its signaling remains active. The ligand-independent signaling may result from mutations in the AR gene or changes in AR coregulatory proteins. In some patients resistant to standard androgen deprivation therapy, the tumor responds to further depletion of androgens by inhibitors of adrenal androgen synthesis, such as *abiraterone*.

Effects That Occur Via the Estrogen Receptor

Certain effects of testosterone are mediated by its conversion to estradiol, catalyzed by CYP19 (aromatase). In rare cases in males deficient in CYP19 or the estrogen receptor, the epiphyses do not fuse, and long-bone growth continues indefinitely; moreover, such patients are osteoporotic. Administration of estradiol corrects the bone abnormalities in patients with aromatase deficiency but not in those with an estrogen-receptor defect. Because men have larger bones than women, and bone expresses the AR (Colvard et al., 1989), testosterone also may have an effect on bone via the AR. Administration of estradiol to a male with CYP19 deficiency can increase libido, suggesting that the effect of testosterone on male libido may be mediated by conversion to estradiol (Smith et al., 1994).

Suppression of testosterone production with a GnRH analogue and then replacing testosterone with or without *anastrozole*, an inhibitor of CYP19, also illustrates effects of testosterone that require conversion to estradiol. This paradigm demonstrated that the increase in sexual desire and erectile function and decrease in subcutaneous and abdominal fat require conversion of testosterone to estradiol but that the increase in lean mass and muscle strength do not (Finkelstein et al., 2013).

Effects of Androgens at Different Stages of Life

In Utero

When the fetal testes, stimulated by hCG, begin to secrete testosterone at about the eighth week of gestation, the high local concentration of testosterone around the testes stimulates the nearby Wolffian ducts to differentiate into the male internal genitalia: the epididymis, vas deferens,

Figure 45–3 *Metabolism of testosterone to its major active and inactive metabolites.*

repeat of variable length is unique to the AR; a shorter length appears to increase the receptor's activity.

In the absence of a ligand, the AR is located in the cytoplasm associated with a heat shock protein complex. When testosterone or dihydrotestosterone binds to the ligand-binding domain, the AR dissociates from the heat shock protein complex, dimerizes, and translocates to the nucleus. The dimer then binds via the DNA-binding domains to androgen response elements on certain responsive genes. The ligand-receptor complex recruits coactivators and acts as a transcription factor complex, stimulating or repressing expression of those genes (Agoulnik and Weigel, 2008).

Mutations in the hormone or DNA-binding regions of the AR result in resistance to the action of testosterone, beginning in utero (McPhaul and Griffin, 1999); as a consequence, male sexual differentiation and pubertal development are incomplete. Other AR mutations occur in patients with spinal and bulbar muscular atrophy, known as Kennedy disease. These patients have an expansion of the CAG repeat, which codes for glutamine,

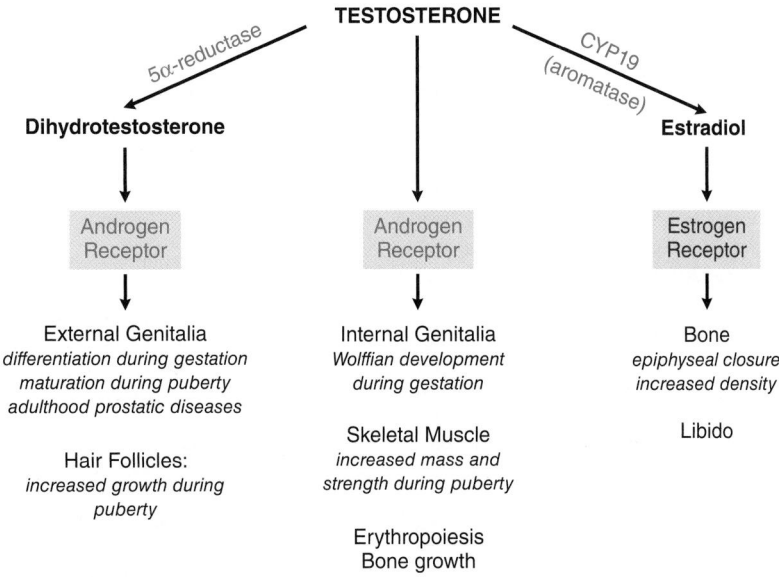

Figure 45–4 *Direct effects of testosterone and effects mediated indirectly via dihydrotestosterone or estradiol.*

and seminal vesicles. In the anlage of the external genitalia, testosterone is converted to dihydrotestosterone, which causes the development of the male external genitalia. The increase in testosterone at the end of gestation may result in further phallic growth.

Infancy

The consequences of the increase in testosterone secretion by the testes during the first few months of life are not yet known.

Puberty

Puberty in the male begins at a mean age of 12 years with an increase in the secretion of FSH and LH from the gonadotropes, stimulated by increased secretion of GnRH from the hypothalamus. The increased secretion of FSH and LH stimulates the testes. The increase in testosterone production by Leydig cells and the effect of FSH on the Sertoli cells stimulate the development of the seminiferous tubules, which eventually produce mature sperm. Increased secretion of testosterone into the systemic circulation affects many tissues simultaneously, and the changes in most of them occur gradually during the course of several years. The phallus enlarges in length and width, the scrotum becomes rugated, and the prostate begins secreting the fluid it contributes to the semen. The skin becomes coarser and oilier due to increased sebum production, which contributes to the development of acne. Sexual hair begins to grow, initially pubic and axillary hair, then hair on the lower legs, and finally other body hair and facial hair. Muscle mass and strength, especially of the shoulder girdle, increase, and subcutaneous fat decreases. Epiphyseal bone growth accelerates, resulting in the pubertal growth spurt, but epiphyseal maturation leads eventually to slowing and then cessation of growth. Bone also becomes thicker. Erythropoiesis increases, resulting in higher hematocrit and hemoglobin concentrations in men than boys or women. The larynx thickens, resulting in a lower voice. Libido develops. Other changes may result from the increase in testosterone during puberty; men tend to have a better sense of spatial relations than do women and to exhibit behavior that differs in some ways from that of women, including being more aggressive.

Adulthood

The serum testosterone concentration and the characteristics of the adult man are maintained largely during early adulthood and midlife. One change during this time is the gradual development of male pattern baldness, beginning with recession of hair at the temples or at the vertex.

Two other conditions are of great medical significance. One is benign *prostatic hyperplasia*, which occurs to a variable degree in almost all men, sometimes obstructing urine outflow by compressing the urethra as it passes through the prostate. This development is mediated by the conversion of testosterone to dihydrotestosterone by 5α-reductase II within prostatic cells (Wilson, 1980). The other change is the development of *prostate cancer*. Although no direct evidence suggests that testosterone causes the disease, prostate cancer depends on androgen stimulation. This dependency is the basis of treating metastatic prostate cancer by lowering the serum testosterone concentration or by blocking its action at the receptor.

Senescence

As men age, the serum testosterone concentration gradually declines (see Figure 43–2), and the SHBG concentration gradually increases, so that by age 80, the total testosterone concentration is about 80% and the free testosterone is about 40% of those at age 20 (Harman et al., 2001). This fall in serum testosterone could contribute to several other changes that occur with increasing age in men, including decreases in energy, libido, muscle mass and strength, and bone mineral density, as well as increased fat mass and fractures. Androgen deprivation also leads to insulin resistance, truncal obesity, and abnormal serum lipids, as observed in patients with metastatic prostate cancer receiving this treatment (see also Chapter 68).

Consequences of Androgen Deficiency

The consequences of androgen deficiency depend on the stage of life during which the deficiency first occurs and on the degree of the deficiency.

During Fetal Development

Testosterone deficiency in a male fetus during the first trimester in utero causes incomplete sexual differentiation. Complete deficiency of testosterone secretion results in entirely female external genitalia. Testosterone deficiency at this stage of development also leads to failure of the Wolffian ducts to differentiate into the male internal genitalia, but the Müllerian ducts do not differentiate into the female internal genitalia as long as testes are present and secrete Müllerian inhibitory substance. Similar changes occur if testosterone is secreted normally, but its action is diminished because of an abnormality of the AR or of the 5α-reductase.

Abnormalities of the AR can have quite varied effects. The most severe form results in complete absence of androgen action and a female phenotype; moderately severe forms result in partial virilization of the external genitalia; and the mildest forms permit normal virilization in utero and result only in impaired spermatogenesis in adulthood (McPhaul and Griffin, 1999). Abnormal 5α-reductase results in incomplete virilization of the external genitalia in utero but normal development of the male internal genitalia, which requires only testosterone (Wilson et al., 1993). Testosterone deficiency during the third trimester impairs phallus growth. The result, microphallus, is a common occurrence in boys later discovered to be unable to secrete LH due to abnormalities of GnRH secretion or action. In addition, with testosterone deficiency, the testes fail to descend into the scrotum; this condition, cryptorchidism, occurs commonly in boys whose LH secretion is subnormal (see Chapter 42).

Before Completion of Puberty

When a boy can secrete testosterone normally in utero but loses the capacity to do so before the anticipated age of puberty, the result is failure to complete puberty. All of the pubertal changes previously described, including those of the external genitalia, sexual hair, muscle mass, voice, and behavior, are impaired to a degree proportionate to the abnormality of testosterone secretion. In addition, if growth hormone secretion is normal when testosterone secretion is subnormal during the years of expected puberty, the long bones continue to lengthen because the epiphyses do not close. The result is longer arms and legs relative to the trunk. Another consequence of subnormal testosterone secretion during the age of expected puberty is enlargement of glandular breast tissue, called *gynecomastia*.

After Completion of Puberty

When testosterone secretion becomes impaired after puberty (e.g., castration or antiandrogen treatment), regression of the pubertal effects of testosterone depends on both the degree and the duration of testosterone deficiency. When the degree of testosterone deficiency is substantial, libido and energy decrease within a week or two, but other testosterone-dependent characteristics decline more slowly. A clinically detectable decrease in muscle mass in an individual does not occur for several years. A pronounced decrease in hematocrit and hemoglobin will occur within several months. A decrease in bone mineral density probably can be detected by dual-energy absorptiometry within 2 years, but an increase in fracture incidence would not be likely to occur for many years. A loss of sexual hair takes many years.

In Women

Loss of androgen secretion in women results in a decrease in sexual hair, but not for many years. Androgens may have other important effects in women, and the loss of androgens (especially with the severe loss of ovarian and adrenal androgens that occurs in panhypopituitarism) may result in the loss of effects associated with libido, energy, muscle mass and strength, and bone mineral density.

Therapeutic Androgen Preparations

Ingestion of testosterone is not an effective means of replacing testosterone deficiency due to the rapid hepatic catabolism. Most pharmaceutical preparations of androgens, therefore, are designed to bypass hepatic catabolism of testosterone.

TABLE 45–1 ■ ANDROGENS AVAILABLE FOR THERAPEUTIC USE

Testosterone
Testosterone Esters
Testosterone enanthate/undecanoate/cypionate
17α-Alkylated Androgens
Methyltestosterone, oxandrolone, stanozolol
Fluoxymesterone, danazol
Other
7α-Methyl-19-nortestosterone, tetrahydrogestrinone

Testosterone Esters

Esterifying a fatty acid to the 17α-hydroxyl group of testosterone creates a compound that is even more lipophilic than testosterone itself. When an ester, such as testosterone enanthate (heptanoate) or cypionate (cyclopentylpropionate) (Table 45–1), is dissolved in oil and administered intramuscularly every 1–2 weeks to hypogonadal men, the ester hydrolyzes in vivo and results in serum testosterone concentrations that range from higher than normal in the first few days after the injection to low normal just before the next injection (Figure 45–5). Attempts to decrease the frequency of injections by increasing the amount of each injection result in wider fluctuations and poorer therapeutic outcomes. The undecanoate ester of testosterone, when dissolved in oil and ingested orally, is absorbed into the lymphatic circulation, thus bypassing initial hepatic catabolism. *Testosterone undecanoate* in oil also can be injected and produces stable serum testosterone concentrations for 2 months.

Alkylated Androgens

Several decades ago, chemists found that adding an alkyl group to the 17α position of testosterone retards its hepatic catabolism. Consequently, 17α-alkylated androgens are androgenic when administered orally; however, they are less androgenic than testosterone and cause hepatotoxicity, whereas native testosterone does not. Some 17α-alkylated androgens show greater anabolic effects than androgenic effects compared to native testosterone in laboratory tests in rats; however, these "anabolic" steroids, so favored by athletes to illicitly improve performance, have not been convincingly demonstrated to have such a differential effect in human beings. Citing potentially serious health risks, the FDA has recommended against the use of body-building products that are marketed as containing steroids or steroid-like substances (FDA, 2009; FDA, 2016).

Transdermal Delivery Systems

To avoid the "first-pass" inactivation of testosterone by the liver, chemicals called excipients are used to facilitate the absorption of native testosterone across the skin in a controlled fashion. These transdermal preparations provide more stable serum testosterone concentrations than do injections of testosterone esters. Available preparations include gels applied to the skin or nasal mucosa, a transdermal patch, and a buccal tablet (see Figure 45–5).

Selective Androgen Receptor Modulators

Selective estrogen receptor modulators have been developed (see Chapter 44). Are selective AR modulators possible that exhibit desirable effects of testosterone in some tissues (such as muscle and bone) without the undesirable effects in other tissues, such as prostate? Nonsteroidal

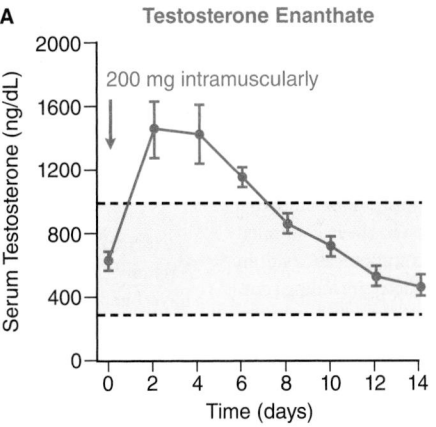
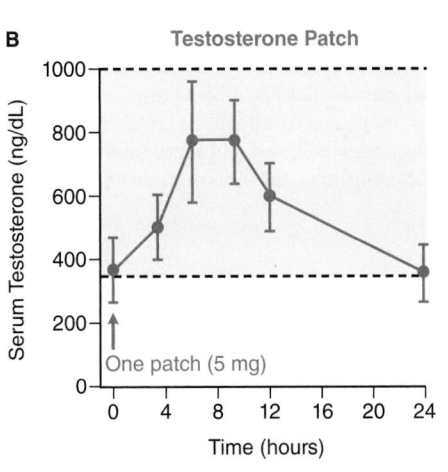
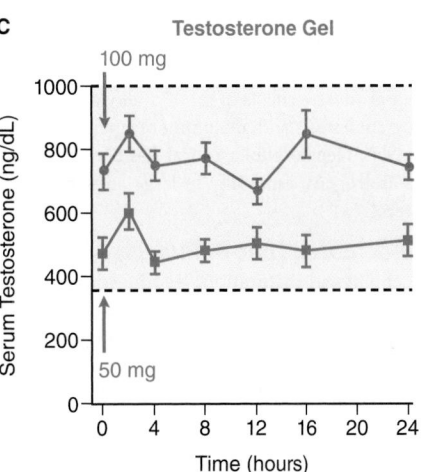

Figure 45–5 *Pharmacokinetic profiles of testosterone preparations during chronic administration to hypogonadal men.* Doses of each were given at time 0. Shaded areas indicate range of normal levels. (**A.** Data adapted from Snyder et al. 1980. **B.** Data adapted from Dobs et al. 1999. **C.** Data adapted from Swerdloff et al. 2000.)

molecules with these properties have been developed and have been tested in humans, but none has yet been effective.

Therapeutic Uses of Androgens

Male Hypogonadism

The best established indication for administration of androgens is testosterone deficiency in men. Any of the testosterone preparations or testosterone esters described can be used to treat testosterone deficiency.

Monitoring for Efficacy

The goal of administering testosterone to a hypogonadal man is to mimic as closely as possible the normal serum concentration (see Figure 45–5). Therefore, measuring the serum testosterone concentration during treatment is the most important aspect of monitoring testosterone treatment for efficacy. With testosterone gels, the serum testosterone concentration is relatively constant from one application to the next (Swerdloff et al., 2000). When the enanthate or cypionate ester of testosterone is administered once every 2 weeks, the serum testosterone concentration measured midway between doses should be normal; if not, the dosage schedule should be adjusted accordingly. If testosterone deficiency results from testicular disease, as indicated by an elevated serum LH concentration, adequacy of testosterone treatment also can be judged indirectly by the normalization of LH within 2 months of treatment initiation (Snyder and Lawrence, 1980).

Normalization of the serum testosterone concentration induces normal virilization in prepubertal boys and restores virilization in adult men who became hypogonadal as adults. Within a few months, and often sooner, libido, energy, and hematocrit return to normal. Within 6 months, muscle mass increases and fat mass decreases. Bone density, however, continues to increase for 2 years (Snyder et al., 2000).

Monitoring for Deleterious Effects

Testosterone administered by itself as a transdermal preparation has no "side effects" (i.e., no effects that endogenously secreted testosterone does not have), as long as the dose is not excessive. Modified testosterone compounds, such as the 17α-alkylated androgens, do have undesirable effects even when dosages are targeted at physiological replacement. Some of these undesirable effects occur shortly after testosterone administration is initiated, whereas others usually do not occur until administration has been continued for many years. Raising the serum testosterone concentration can result in undesirable effects similar to those that occur during puberty, including acne, gynecomastia, and more aggressive sexual behavior. Physiological amounts of testosterone do not appear to affect serum lipids or apolipoproteins.

Replacement of physiological levels of testosterone occasionally may have undesirable effects in the presence of concomitant illnesses. If the testosterone dose is excessive, erythrocytosis and, uncommonly, salt and water retention and peripheral edema occur even in men who have no predisposition to these conditions.

When a man is more than 40 years of age, he is subject to certain testosterone-dependent diseases, including benign prostatic hyperplasia and prostate cancer. The principal adverse effects of the 17α-alkylated androgens are hepatic, including cholestasis and, uncommonly, peliosis hepatitis, blood-filled hepatic cysts. Hepatocellular cancer has been reported rarely. The 17α-alkylated androgens, especially in large amounts, may lower serum HDL cholesterol.

Monitoring at the Anticipated Time of Puberty

Testosterone accelerates epiphyseal maturation, leading initially to a growth spurt but then to epiphyseal closure and permanent cessation of linear growth. Consequently, the height and growth hormone status of the boy being treated must be considered. Boys who are short because of growth hormone deficiency should be treated with growth hormone before their hypogonadism is treated with testosterone.

Male Senescence

Serum testosterone levels decrease as men age, and the parallels between the consequences of aging and those of hypogonadism due to pituitary or testicular disease, such as decreases in muscle mass and strength, sexual function, bone density, and hemoglobin, suggest the possibility that the decrease in testosterone with aging may contribute to these changes of aging. Several studies demonstrated that testosterone treatment of older men with low testosterone increased their muscle mass and decreased their fat mass. A new study of 788 men 65 years or older with low testosterone concentrations demonstrated that testosterone treatment, compared to placebo, for 1 year improved sexual function, mood, and depressive symptoms (Snyder et al., 2016).

No studies to date have been large enough to determine if testosterone treatment of older men will increase the risk of prostate cancer, urinary tract symptoms, or heart disease. The FDA, however, has become sufficiently concerned about the possible risk of cardiovascular disease, based on epidemiologic studies and small clinical trials, that it has required a label change for testosterone preparations to indicate that they are approved only for men with "classical hypogonadism," meaning hypogonadism due to discernible pituitary or testicular disease (Ngyuen et al., 2015).

Female Hypogonadism

Few data exist regarding whether increasing the serum testosterone concentrations of women whose serum testosterone concentrations are below normal will improve their libido, energy, muscle mass and strength, or bone mineral density. In a study of women with low serum testosterone concentrations due to panhypopituitarism, increasing the testosterone concentration to normal was associated with small increases in bone mineral density, fat-free mass, and sexual function compared to placebo (Miller et al., 2006).

Enhancement of Athletic Performance

Some athletes take drugs, including androgens, in an attempt to improve their performance. Because androgens for this purpose usually are taken surreptitiously, information about their possible effects is not as complete as that for androgens taken for treatment of male hypogonadism. Citing potentially serious health risks, the FDA has recommended against the use of body-building products that are marketed as containing steroids or steroid-like substances (FDA, 2009 and 2016).

Kinds of Androgens Used

Virtually all androgens produced for human or veterinary purposes have been taken by athletes. When such use by athletes began more than 30 years ago, 17α-alkylated androgens and other compounds (the so-called anabolic steroids) that were thought to have greater anabolic effects than androgen effects relative to testosterone were used most commonly. Because these compounds can be detected readily by organizations that govern athletic competitions, other agents that increase the serum concentration of testosterone itself, such as the testosterone esters or hCG, have increased in popularity. Testosterone precursors, such as *androstenedione* and DHEA, also have increased in popularity recently because they are treated as nutritional supplements and thus are not regulated by athletic organizations. A new development in use of androgens by athletes is *THG*, a potent androgen that appears to have been designed and synthesized to avoid detection by antidoping laboratories on the basis of its novel structure and rapid catabolism.

Tetrahydrogestrinone (THG)

Efficacy

The few controlled studies of the effects of pharmacological doses of androgens do suggest a dose-dependent effect of testosterone on muscle strength that acts synergistically with exercise (Bhasin et al., 1996). In one controlled study, 43 normal young men were randomized to one of four groups: strength training with or without 600 mg of testosterone enanthate once a week (more than six times the replacement dose) or no exercise with or without testosterone. The men who received testosterone experienced an increase in muscle strength compared to those who received placebo, and the men who exercised simultaneously experienced even greater increases (Bhasin et al., 1996). In another study, normal young men were treated with a GnRH analogue to reduce endogenous testosterone secretion severely and, in a random blinded fashion, weekly doses of testosterone enanthate from 25 to 600 mg. There was a dose-dependent effect of testosterone on muscle strength (Bhasin et al., 2001). In contrast, in a double-blind study of androstenedione, men who took 100 mg three times a day for 8 weeks did not experience an increase in muscle strength compared to men who took placebo. The treatment also did not increase the mean serum testosterone concentration (King et al., 1999).

Side Effects

All androgens suppress gonadotropin secretion when taken in high doses and thereby suppress endogenous testicular function. This decreases endogenous testosterone and sperm production, resulting in diminished fertility. If administration continues for many years, testicular size may diminish. Testosterone and sperm production usually return to normal within a few months of discontinuation but may take longer. High doses of androgens also cause erythrocytosis.

When administered in high doses, androgens that can be converted to estrogens, such as testosterone itself, cause gynecomastia. Androgens whose A ring has been modified so that it cannot be aromatized, such as dihydrotestosterone, do not cause gynecomastia even in high doses.

The 17α-alkylated androgens are the only androgens that cause hepatotoxicity. These androgens, when administered in high doses, affect serum lipid concentrations, specifically to decrease HDL cholesterol and increase LDL cholesterol. Women and children experience virilization, including facial and body hirsutism, temporal hair recession in a male pattern, and acne. Boys experience phallic enlargement, and women experience clitoral enlargement. Boys and girls whose epiphyses have not yet closed experience premature closure and stunting of linear growth.

Detection

An androgen other than testosterone can be detected by gas chromatography and mass spectroscopy if the athlete is still taking it when tested. Exogenous testosterone itself can be detected by one of two methods. One is the T/E ratio, the ratio of testosterone glucuronide to its endogenous epimer, epitestosterone glucuronide, in urine. Administration of exogenous testosterone suppresses secretion of both testosterone and epitestosterone and replaces them with only testosterone, so the T/E ratio is higher than normal. This technique is limited, however, by heterozygosity in the UDP-glucuronosyl transferase that converts testosterone to testosterone glucuronide. An athlete who has a deletion of one or both copies of the gene coding for this enzyme and who takes exogenous testosterone will have a much lower T/E ratio than one who has both copies (Schulze et al., 2008).

A second technique for detecting administration of exogenous testosterone employs gas chromatography-combustion-isotope ratio mass spectrometry to detect the presence of ^{13}C and ^{12}C compounds. Urinary steroids with a low $^{13}C/^{12}C$ ratio are likely to have originated from pharmaceutical sources as opposed to endogenous physiological sources (Aguilera et al., 2001).

Catabolic and Wasting States

Testosterone, because of its anabolic effects, has been used in attempts to ameliorate catabolic and muscle-wasting states, but this has not been generally effective. One exception is in the treatment of muscle wasting associated with AIDS, which often is accompanied by hypogonadism.

Treatment of men with AIDS-related muscle wasting and subnormal serum testosterone concentrations increases their muscle mass and strength (Bhasin et al., 2000).

Angioedema

Chronic androgen treatment of patients with angioedema effectively prevents attacks. The disease is caused by hereditary impairment of C1-esterase inhibitor or acquired development of antibodies against it. The 17α-alkylated androgens (e.g., stanozolol, danazol) stimulate hepatic synthesis of the esterase inhibitor. In women, virilization is a potential side effect. In children, virilization and premature epiphyseal closure prevent chronic use of androgens for prophylaxis, although they are used occasionally to treat acute episodes. Alternatively, concentrated C1-esterase inhibitor derived from human plasma may be used for protection in patients with hereditary angioedema.

Blood Dyscrasias

Androgens once were employed to attempt to stimulate erythropoiesis in patients with anemias of various etiologies, but the availability of erythropoietin has supplanted that use. Androgens, such as danazol, still are used occasionally as adjunctive treatment of hemolytic anemia and idiopathic thrombocytopenic purpura that are refractory to first-line agents.

Antiandrogens

Because some effects of androgens are undesirable, at least under certain circumstances, agents have been developed specifically to inhibit androgen synthesis or effects. Other drugs, originally developed for different purposes, have been accidentally found to be antiandrogens and now are used intentionally for this indication. See Chapter 68 for a more detailed discussion of androgen deprivation therapy for prostate cancer.

Inhibitors of Testosterone Secretion

Analogues of GnRH effectively inhibit testosterone secretion by inhibiting LH secretion. GnRH analogues, given repeatedly, downregulate the GnRH receptor and are available for treatment of prostate cancer.

Some antifungal drugs of the imidazole family, such as *ketoconazole* (see Chapter 61), inhibit CYPs and thereby block the synthesis of steroid hormones, including testosterone and cortisol. Because they may induce adrenal insufficiency and are associated with hepatotoxicity, these drugs generally are not used to inhibit androgen synthesis, but sometimes are employed in cases of glucocorticoid excess (see Chapter 46).

Inhibitors of Androgen Action

These drugs inhibit the binding of androgens to the AR or inhibit 5α-reductase.

Androgen Receptor Antagonists

Flutamide, Bicalutamide, Nilutamide, and Enzalutamide. The relatively potent AR antagonists flutamide, bicalutamide, nilutamide, and enzalutamide have limited efficacy when used alone because the increased LH secretion stimulates higher serum testosterone concentrations. They are used primarily in conjunction with a GnRH analogue in the treatment of metastatic prostate cancer (see Chapter 68). In this situation, they block the action of adrenal androgens, which are not inhibited by GnRH analogues. Flutamide also has been used to treat hirsutism in women; however, its association with hepatotoxicity warrants caution against its use for this cosmetic purpose.

Spironolactone. Spironolactone (see Chapter 25) is an inhibitor of aldosterone that also is a weak inhibitor of the AR and a weak inhibitor of testosterone synthesis. When the agent is used to treat fluid retention or hypertension in men, gynecomastia is a common side effect. In part because of this adverse effect, the selective mineralocorticoid receptor antagonist *eplerenone* was developed. Spironolactone can be used in women to treat hirsutism.

Cyproterone Acetate. Cyproterone acetate is a progestin and a weak antiandrogen by virtue of binding to the AR. It is moderately effective in reducing hirsutism alone or in combination with an oral contraceptive but is not approved for use in the U.S.

5α-Reductase Inhibitors

Finasteride and dutasteride are antagonists of 5α-reductase. They block the conversion of testosterone to dihydrotestosterone, especially in the male external genitalia. These drugs were developed to treat benign prostatic hyperplasia, and they are approved in the U.S. and many other countries for this purpose. When they are administered to men with moderately severe symptoms due to obstruction of urinary tract outflow, serum and prostatic concentrations of dihydrotestosterone decrease, prostatic volume decreases, and urine flow rate increases (McConnell et al., 1998). Impotence is a documented, albeit infrequent, side effect of this use. Gynecomastia is a rare side effect.

Finasteride also is approved for use in the treatment of male pattern baldness and is effective in the treatment of hirsutism.

Pharmacologic Treatment of Erectile Dysfunction

Normal erectile function depends on a combination of many factors, including visual, psychologic, hormonal, and neurologic factors, that act via the common mechanism of increasing the synthesis of NO by vascular endothelium in the arterioles supplying the corpora cavernosa and in the corpora cavernosa. NO diffuses to adjacent smooth muscle cells and causes vasodilation of arterioles and increased compliance of the cavernosal space, permitting its engorgement with blood. This accumulation of blood also restricts the outflow by compressing the veins against the surrounding sheath (*tunica albuginea*). The overall result is penile erection.

Erectile dysfunction can result from psychologic, hormonal, and vascular causes, including damage to endothelium and from side effects of various drugs, including some that are used in the therapy of hypertension; it is associated with a variety of disease states, including diabetes (Dean and Lue, 2005).

Erectile Signaling and Erectile Dysfunction

Nitric oxide acts by binding and activating sGC, which catalyzes the production of cyclic GMP from cellular GTP. Cyclic GMP is a second messenger that activates PKG, leading to phosphorylation of contractile proteins and ion channels to decrease the concentration of intracellular Ca^{++}, resulting in smooth muscle relaxation and increased blood flow to corpora cavernosa. PDE5 degrades cyclic GMP; thus, erectile dysfunction can be improved by drugs that retard the degradation of cyclic GMP by inhibiting PDE5 (Goldstein et al., 1998) (Figure 45–6).

PDE5 Inhibitors

Available inhibitors of PDE5 include sildenafil, vardenafil, tadalafil, and avanafil. All of these agents compete for cyclic GMP binding at the site of cyclic GMP hydrolysis on PDE5. PDE5 inhibitors are also used in treating pulmonary arterial hypertension (Chapter 31).

ADME

Table 45–2 summarizes a number of pharmacokinetic properties of the available PDE5 inhibitors. These agents are adequately absorbed orally, widely distributed, and act fairly quickly (within ~ 30 min). Their affinities, time to onset, and half-lives differ somewhat, giving patients options for onset and duration of effect. The drugs are cleared by hepatic CYP3A4, with minor contributions by CYP2C9 (20% for sildenafil). Excretion of metabolites is largely via the feces, with urinary excretion playing a secondary role in excretion of tadalafil (36%) (Mehrotra et al., 2007).

Clinical Use

All of these agents produce satisfactory results in most patients. The starting dose recommendations vary, and patients should start at the lowest recommended dose. This is especially important in patients over 65 years.

Adverse Effects, Precautions

Adverse effects are similar but not identical across this drug class owing to their similar mechanism of action but their differing specificities toward PDE5 compared to other PDE isoforms. Common complaints are headache, flushing, dyspepsia, nasal congestion, dizziness, and back pain. Some patients using sildenafil or vardenafil may notice blurred vision and a

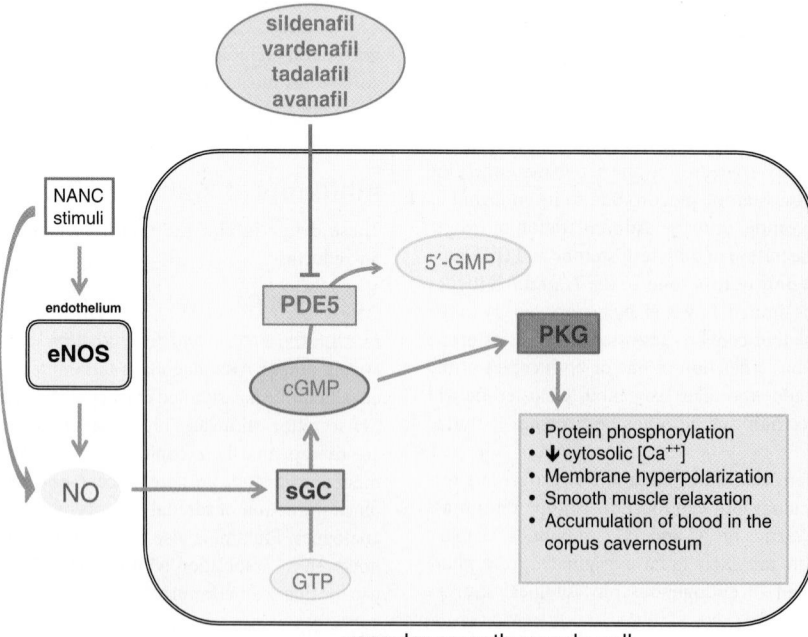

vascular smooth muscle cell

Figure 45–6 *Mechanism of action of PDE5 inhibitors in the corpus cavernosum.* Physiologically, penile erection is initiated by NANC neural stimulation that results in NO release from neurons and endothelial cells. PDE5 inhibitors enhance signaling through the NO-guanylyl cyclase-cGMP-PKG pathway by inhibiting the degradation of cGMP, thereby enhancing the activation of PKG. PKG activation leads to relaxation of cavernosal smooth muscle, which permits engorgement of the corpus cavernosum with blood, resulting in penile erection.

TABLE 45–2 ■ PHARMACOKINETIC PROPERTIES OF PDE5 INHIBITORS

	SILDENAFIL	VARDENAFIL	TADALAFIL	AVANAFIL
K_i (nM)	4	0.1	2	4
Plasma $t_{1/2}$ (h)	4	4	17.5	1.3–2
Oral bioavailability (%)	40	15	40	70
Onset of action (min)	30–60	30–60	30–120	15–30
Time to C_{Pmax} (min)	60	60	120	30
Maximum duration of action (h)[b]	12	10	36	6
Optic effects/PDE6	+	+	−	−
Food[a] alters AUC, C_{pmax}?	+	+	−	±

[a]High-fat meal; generally reduces AUC and C_{Pmax} but for avanafil, prolongs absorption period and time to C_{Pmax} (by 1 h), decreases C_{Pmax} (−24%) and increases AUC (+14%).
[b]Duration will vary with dose and rate of clearance.

For PK data on PDE5 inhibitors, see FDA, 2012, and Mehrotra et al., 2007.

blue-green tinting of vision, referable to inhibition of retinal PDE6, which is involved in phototransduction (see Figure 69-9).

Concomitant administration of potent CYP3A inducers (e.g., bosentan) will generally cause substantial decreases in plasma levels of drugs in this class. CYP3A inhibitors (e.g., protease inhibitors used in human immunodeficiency virus therapy, erythromycin, and cimetidine) inhibit metabolism of PDE5 inhibitors, thereby prolonging the half-lives and elevating blood levels of these agents. Consistent with their mechanism of action, potentiation of cyclic GMP signaling, PDE5 inhibitors potentiate the hypotensive effects of nitrate vasodilators, producing dangerously low blood pressures. Thus, the administration of PDE5 inhibitors to patients receiving organic nitrates is contraindicated. The patient's underlying cardiovascular status and concurrent use of hypotensive agents (e.g., nitrates, α adrenergic antagonists) must be considered prior to use of this class of drugs. Priapism (erection lasting longer than 4 h) induced by PDE5 inhibitors runs the risk of ischemic damage to the cavernosal smooth muscle and sinusoidal epithelium and requires medical attention.

Developing Therapies for Erectile Dysfunction

In addition to use of PDE5 inhibitors, alternative routes for regulating smooth muscle tone in the corpus cavernosum are being actively explored. For example, direct activators of guanylyl cyclase are now available (e.g., riociquat). Local inhibition of arginase may enhance NO production in cases where arginine, the substrate for NO synthase, limits NO production (Caldwell et al., 2015). Rho A and Rho kinase are highly expressed in penile smooth muscle, where Rho kinase phosphorylates and inhibits the regulatory subunit of myosin light chain phosphatase and helps to maintain a tonic contracted state of the cavernosal smooth muscle (an antierectile state), thereby promoting maintenance of the flaccid state. In experimental preparations, inhibitors of Rho kinase (e.g., fasudil) will elicit penile erection (Sopko et al., 2014). Mirabegron, a β_3 adrenergic agonist used in treatment of overactive bladder, relaxes isolated muscle strips from human and rodent corpus cavernosum (Gur et al., 2016), and H_2S has proerectile activity mediated by its effect on a large-conductance Ca^{++}-activated K^+ in cavernosal smooth muscle (Jupiter et al., 2015).

Drug Facts for Your Personal Formulary: *Androgens; PDE5 Inhibitors*

Drugs	Therapeutic Uses	Clinical Pharmacology and Tips
Testosterone Esters • Effective for weeks to months. Wide fluctuations in serum concentrations		
Testosterone enanthate testosterone cypionate	• Treatment of male hypogonadism	• Formulated as oils for injection • Administer as a deep I.M. injection every 1-2 weeks. • Generally effective in causing and maintaining virilization. • Fluctuations in serum concentrations result in fluctuations in energy, mood, and libido. • Available as gels, implants, buccal tabs
Testosterone undecanoate	• Treatment of male hypogonadism	• Formulated as oil for injection • Administer as a deep I.M. gluteal injection. Observe for 30 min after injection for anaphylaxis or pulmonary microembolism. • Administer every 10 weeks.
Testosterone undecanoate for oral administration (not available in the U.S.)	• Treatment of male hypogonadism	• Taken 2-3 times a day with food • Absorbed into lymphatics
Testosterone Transdermal Patch		
Several FDA-approved products	• Treatment of male hypogonadism	• Worn without interruption and changed once a day • High rate of skin rash
Transdermal Testosterone Gels		
Several FDA-approved products	• Treatment of male hypogonadism	• Applied once a day • Relatively steady serum testosterone concentration

Drug Facts for Your Personal Formulary: *Androgens; PDE5 Inhibitors* (*continued*)

Drugs	Therapeutic Uses	Clinical Pharmacology and Tips
17α- alkylated Androgens		
Danazol Stanozolol (not marketed in the U.S.)	• Treatment of angioedema • Treatment of hemolytic anemia • Angioedema prophylaxis • Endometriosis • Fibrocystic breast disease	• Risk of hepatoxicity
GnRH Analogs		
Leuprolide Goserelin Triptorelin Histrelin Buserelin (not available in the U.S.)	• Treatment of metastatic prostate cancer • Leuprolide also approved for endometriosis, precocious puberty, prostate cancer and uterine leiomyomata • Goserelin also approved for breast cancer, dysfunctional uterine bleeding, and endometriosis • Histrelin also approved for precocious puberty and prostate cancer	• Parenteral administration • Suppresses LH secretion and thereby causes profound hypogonadism
Androgen Receptor Antagonists		
Flutamide Bicalutamide Nilutamide Enzalutamide	• Adjuvant treatment of metastatic prostate cancer	• Used in conjunction with GnRH agonists
5α-reductase inhibitors		
Finasteride Dutasteride	• Treatment of lower urinary tract symptoms due to benign prostatic hyperplasia • Finasteride also approved for alopecia	• Shrinks the size of the prostate by decreasing the production of dihydrotestosterone in the prostate • Dutasteride also marketed as fixed-dose combination with tamsulosin
PDE5 Inhibitors		
Sildenafil, vardenafil, tadalafil, avanafil	• Male erectile dysfunction • Pulmonary arterial hypertension (sildenafil, tadalafil)	• Contraindicated in patients using nitrate vasodilators (can cause dangerously low blood pressure) • Side effects: headache, flushing, blue-green tinted vision • Erection lasting > 4h requires medical attention

Bibliography

Agoulnik IU, Weigel NL. Androgen receptor coactivators and prostate cancer. *Adv Exp Med Biol*, **2008**, *617*:245–255.

Aguilera R, et al. Performance characteristics of a carbon isotope ratio method for detecting doping with testosterone based on urine diols: controls and athletes with elevated testosterone/epitestosterone ratios. *Clin Chem*, **2001**, *47*:292–300.

Bhasin S, et al. The effects of supraphysiologic doses of testosterone on muscle size and strength in normal men. *N Engl J Med*, **1996**, *335*:1–7.

Bhasin S, et al. Testosterone replacement and resistance exercise in HIV-infected men with weight loss and low testosterone levels. *JAMA*, **2000**, *283*:763–770.

Bhasin S, et al. Testosterone dose response relationships in healthy young men. *Am J Physiol*, **2001**, *281*:E1172–1181.

Caldwell RB, et al. Arginase: an old enzyme with new tricks. *Trends Pharm Sci*, **2015**, *36*:395–405.

Colvard DS, et al. Identification of androgen receptors in normal osteoblast-like cells. *Proc Natl Acad Sci USA*, **1989**, *86*:854–857.

Crowley WF Jr, et al. The physiology of gonadotropin-releasing hormone (GnRH) secretion in men and women. *Recent Prog Horm Res*, **1985**, *41*:473–531.

Dean RC, Lue TF. Physiology of penile erection and pathophysiology of erectile dysfunction. *Urol Clin North Am*, **2005**, *32*:379–395.

Dejager S, et al. A comprehensive endocrine description of Kennedy's disease revealing androgen insensitivity linked to CAG repeat length. *J Clin Endocrinol Metab*, **2002**, *87*:3893–3901.

Dobs AS, et al. Pharmacokinetics, efficacy, and safety of a permeation-enhanced testosterone transdermal system in comparison with bi-weekly injections of testosterone enanthate for the treatment of hypogonadal men. *J Clin Endocrinol Metab*, **1999**, *84*:3469–3478.

FDA. Public health advisory: the FDA recommends that consumers should not use body building products marketed as containing steroids or steroid-like substances. **2016**. Available at: http://www.fda.gov/NewsEvents/Newsroom/PressAnnouncements/ucm174060.htm. Accessed April 19, 2016.

FDA. Clinical pharmacology and biopharmaceutics review (avanafil). **2012**. http://www.accessdata.fda.gov/drugsatfda_docs/nda/2012/202276Orig1s000ClinPharmR.pdf. Accessed June 24, 2016.

FDA. Warning on Body Building Products Marketed as Containing Steroids or Steroid-Like Substances. **2009**. Available at: https://www.fda.gov/For Consumers/ConsumerUpdates/ucm173739.htm. Accessed June 9, 2017.

Finkelstein JS, et al. Gonadal steroids and body composition, strength, and sexual function in man. *N Engl J Med*, **2013**, *369*:2457.

Goldstein I, et al. Oral sildenafil in the treatment of erectile dysfunction. *N Engl J Med*, **1998**, *338*:1397–1404.

Gur S, et al. Mirabegron causes relaxation of human and rat corpus cavernosum: could it be a potential therapy for erectile dysfunction? *BJU Int*, **2016**, *118*:464–474. doi:10.1111/bju.13515.

Harman SM, et al. Longitudinal effects of aging on serum total and free testosterone levels in healthy men. Baltimore Longitudinal Study of Aging. *J Clin Endocrinol Metab*, **2001**, *86*:724–731.

Jupiter RC, et al. Analysis of erectile responses to H_2S donors in the anesthetized rat. *Am J Physiol*, **2015**, *309*:H835–H843.

King DS, et al. Effect of oral androstenedione on serum testosterone and adaptation to resistance training in young men: a randomized controlled trial. *JAMA*, **1999**, *28*:2020–2028.

MacDonald PC, et al. Origin of estrogen in normal men and in women with testicular feminization. *J Clin Endocrinol Metab*, **1979**, *49*: 905–917.

McConnell JD, et al. The effect of finasteride on the risk of acute urinary retention and the need for surgical treatment among men with benign prostatic hyperplasia. Finasteride Long-Term Efficacy and Safety Study Group. *N Engl J Med*, **1998**, *338*:557–563.

McPhaul MJ, Griffin JE. Male pseudohermaphroditism caused by mutations of the human androgen receptor. *J Clin Endocrinol Metab*, **1999**, *84*:3435–3441.

Miller KK, et al. Effects of testosterone replacement in androgen-deficient women with hypopituitarism: a randomized, double-blind, placebo-controlled study. *J Clin Endocrinol Metab*, **2006**, *91*:1683–1690.

Nguyen CP, et al. Testosterone and "Age-related Hypogonadism"—FDA Concerns. *N Engl J Med*, **2015**, *373*:689–691.

Schulze JJ, et al. Genetic aspects of epitestosterone formation and androgen disposition: influence of polymorphisms in CYP17 and UGT2B enzymes. *Pharmacogenet Genomics*, **2008**, *18*:477–485.

Smith EP, et al. Estrogen resistance caused by a mutation in the estrogen-receptor gene in a man. *N Engl J Med*, **1994**, *331*:1056–1061.

Snyder PJ, et al. Effects of testosterone treatment in older men. *N Engl J Med*, **2016**, *374*:611–624.

Snyder PJ, Lawrence DA. Treatment of male hypogonadism with testosterone enanthate. *J Clin Endocrinol Metab*, **1980**, *51*:1535–1539.

Snyder PJ, et al. Effects of testosterone replacement in hypogonadal men. *J Clin Endocrinol Metab*, **2000**, *85*:2670–2677.

Sopko NA, et al. Understanding and targeting the Rho kinase pathway in erectile dysfunction. *Nat Rev Urol*, **2014**, *11*:622–628.

Swerdloff RS, et al. Long-term pharmacokinetics of transdermal testosterone gel in hypogonadal men. *J Clin Endocrinol Metab*, **2000**, *85*:4500–4510.

Walcott J, Merry D. Trinucleotide repeat disease. The androgen receptor in spinal and bulbar muscular atrophy. *Vitam Horm*, **2002**, *65*:127–147.

Wilson JD. The pathogenesis of benign prostatic hyperplasia. *Am J Med*, **1980**, *68*:745–756.

Wilson JD, et al. Steroid 5 alpha-reductase 2 deficiency. *Endocr Rev*, **1993**, *14*:577–593.

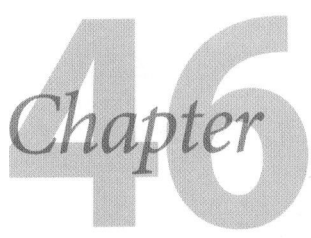

Chapter 46

Adrenocorticotropic Hormone, Adrenal Steroids, and the Adrenal Cortex

Bernard P. Schimmer and John W. Funder

The major physiological and pharmacological effects of *ACTH* result from the increase in circulating levels of *adrenocortical steroids* that ACTH causes. Synthetic derivatives of ACTH are used principally in the diagnostic assessment of adrenocortical function. Because corticosteroids mimic the therapeutic effects of ACTH, synthetic steroids generally are used therapeutically instead of ACTH.

Corticosteroids and their biologically active synthetic derivatives differ in their metabolic (glucocorticoid) and electrolyte-regulating (mineralocorticoid) activities. These agents are used at physiological doses as replacement therapy when endogenous production is impaired. Glucocorticoids potently suppress inflammation, and their use in inflammatory and autoimmune diseases makes them among the most frequently prescribed classes of drugs. Because glucocorticoids exert effects on almost every organ system, their administration and withdrawal may be complicated by serious side effects. Therefore, the decision to institute therapy with systemic glucocorticoids always requires careful consideration of the relative risks and benefits in each patient.

Corticotropin

Human ACTH, a peptide of 39 amino acids, is synthesized as part of a larger precursor protein, POMC, and is derived from the precursor by proteolytic cleavage at dibasic residues by the *serine endoprotease, prohormone convertase 1* (also known as prohormone convertase 3) (Figure 46–1). Other biologically important peptides, including *endorphins, lipotropins, and the MSHs,* also are produced by proteolytic processing of the same POMC precursor (see Chapter 20 and Takahashi and Mizusawa, 2013).

The actions of ACTH and the other melanocortins derived from POMC are mediated by their specific interactions with five MCR subtypes (MC_1R–MC_5R) comprising a subfamily of GPCRs (Cone, 2006; Montero-Melendez, 2015). The well-known effects of MSH on pigmentation result from interactions with MC_1R on melanocytes. ACTH, which is identical to α-MSH in its first 13 amino acids, exerts its effects on the adrenal cortex through MC_2R. The affinity of ACTH for MC_1R is much lower than for MC_2R; however, under pathological conditions in which ACTH levels are persistently elevated, such as primary adrenal insufficiency, ACTH also can signal through MC_1R and cause hyperpigmentation. β-MSH and possibly other melanocortins, acting via MC_4R and MC_3R in the hypothalamus, play a role in regulating appetite and body weight. The role of MC_5R is less well defined, but studies in rodents suggest

HISTORICAL PERSPECTIVE

Addison described fatal outcomes in patients with adrenal destruction in a presentation to the South London Medical Society in 1849. These studies were soon extended when Brown-Séquard demonstrated that bilateral adrenalectomy was fatal in laboratory animals. It later was shown that the adrenal cortex, rather than the medulla, was essential for survival in these ablation experiments, and that the adrenal cortex regulated both carbohydrate metabolism and fluid and electrolyte balance. The isolation and identification of the adrenal steroids by Reichstein and Kendall and the effects of these compounds on carbohydrate metabolism (hence the term *glucocorticoids*) culminated with the synthesis of *cortisone*, the first pharmacologically effective glucocorticoid to become readily available. Subsequently, Tait and colleagues isolated and characterized a distinct corticosteroid, *aldosterone*, which potently affected fluid and electrolyte balance and therefore was termed a *mineralocorticoid*. The isolation of distinct corticosteroids that regulated carbohydrate metabolism or fluid and electrolyte balance led to the concept that the adrenal cortex comprises two largely independent units: an outer zone that produces mineralocorticoids and an inner region that synthesizes glucocorticoids and androgen precursors (reviewed by Miller, 2013).

Studies of adrenocortical steroids also played a key part in delineating the role of the anterior pituitary in endocrine function. As early as 1912, Cushing described patients with hypercorticism, and he later recognized that pituitary basophilism caused the adrenal overactivity, thus establishing the link between the anterior pituitary and adrenal function. These studies led to the purification of ACTH and the determination of its chemical structure. ACTH was further shown to be essential for maintaining the structural integrity and steroidogenic capacity of the inner cortical zones. Harris established the role of the hypothalamus in pituitary control and postulated that a soluble factor produced by the hypothalamus activated ACTH release. These investigations culminated with the determination of the structure of CRH, a hypothalamic peptide that, together with AVP, regulates secretion of ACTH from the pituitary (Miller, 2013).

Shortly after synthetic cortisone became available, Hench and colleagues demonstrated its dramatic effect in the treatment of rheumatoid arthritis, setting the stage for the clinical use of corticosteroids in a wide variety of diseases, as discussed in this chapter.

Abbreviations

ACh: acetylcholine
ACTH: corticotropin (formerly adrenocorticotropic hormone)
AngII: angiotensin II
AP-1: activator protein 1
ATPase: adenosine triphosphatase
AVP: arginine vasopressin
CAH: congenital adrenal hyperplasia
CBG: corticosteroid-binding globulin
CIRCI: critical illness–related cortisol insufficiency
CNS: central nervous system
COX: cyclooxygenase
CRF: corticotropin-releasing factor (CRF$_1$, CRF$_2$)
CRH: corticotropin-releasing hormone
CYP: cytochrome P450
CYP11A1: cholesterol side-chain cleavage enzyme
CYP11B1: 11ß-hydroxylase
CYP11B2: aldosterone synthase
CYP17: 17α-hydroxylase
CYP19: aromatase
CYP21: steroid 21-hydroxylase
DHEA: dehydroepiandrosterone
ELAM-1: endothelial-leukocyte adhesion molecule 1
FDA: Food and Drug Administration
GM-CSF: granulocyte-macrophage colony-stimulating factor
GR: glucocorticoid receptor
GRE: glucocorticoid-response element
HPA: hypothalamic-pituitary-adrenal
3β-HSD: 3β-hydroxysteroid dehydrogenase
11β-HSD1: 11β-hydroxysteroid dehydrogenase (type 1)
11β-HSD2: 11β-hydroxysteroid dehydrogenase (type 2)
HSP70: 70-kDa heat shock protein
HSP90: 90-kDa heat shock protein
ICAM-1: intercellular adhesion molecule 1
Ig: immunoglobulin
IL: interleukin
IP: 56-kDa immunophilin
IP$_3$: inositol trisphosphate
LPH: lipotropin
LT: leukotriene
MCR: melanocortin receptor
MR: mineralocorticoid receptor
mRNA: messenger RNA
MSH: melanocyte-stimulating hormone
NE: norepinephrine
NF-κB: nuclear factor kappa B
NOS: nitric oxide synthase
PG: prostaglandin
PK: protein kinase
PLC: phospholipase C
POMC: pro-opiomelanocortin
RANK: receptor for activating NF-κB
SSTR: somatostatin receptor
TNF: tumor necrosis factor

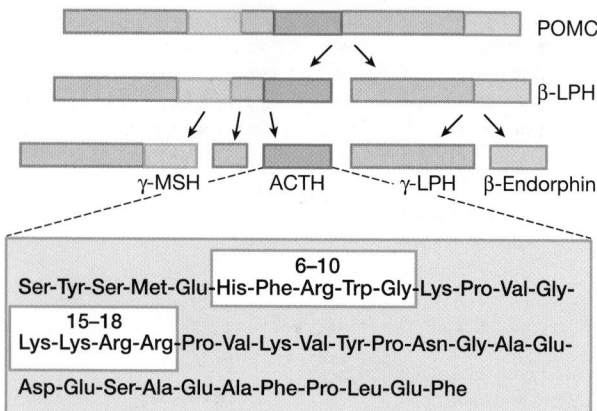

Figure 46–1 *Processing of POMC to ACTH.* POMC is converted to ACTH and other peptides in the anterior pituitary. The boxes within the ACTH structure indicate regions important for steroidogenic activity (residues 6–10) and binding to the ACTH receptor (15–18). α-MSH also derives from the POMC precursor and contains the first 13 residues of ACTH.

adrenal cortex histologically and functionally can be separated into three zones (Figure 46–2) that produce different steroid products under different regulatory influences:

- The *outer zona glomerulosa* secretes the mineralocorticoid aldosterone.
- The *middle zona fasciculata* secretes the glucocorticoid cortisol.
- The *inner zona reticularis* secretes DHEA and its sulfated derivative DHEA-S (plasma concentration 1000 times that of DHEA). DHEA sulfatase converts DHEA-S to DHEA in the periphery.

Cells of the outer zone have receptors for both ACTH and AngII and express *aldosterone synthase* (CYP11B2), the enzyme that catalyzes the terminal reactions in mineralocorticoid biosynthesis. Although ACTH acutely stimulates mineralocorticoid production by the zona glomerulosa, this zone is regulated predominantly by AngII and *extracellular K*$^+$ (see Chapter 25) and does not undergo atrophy in the absence of ongoing stimulation by the pituitary gland. With persistently elevated ACTH, mineralocorticoid levels initially increase and then return to normal (a phenomenon termed *ACTH escape*).

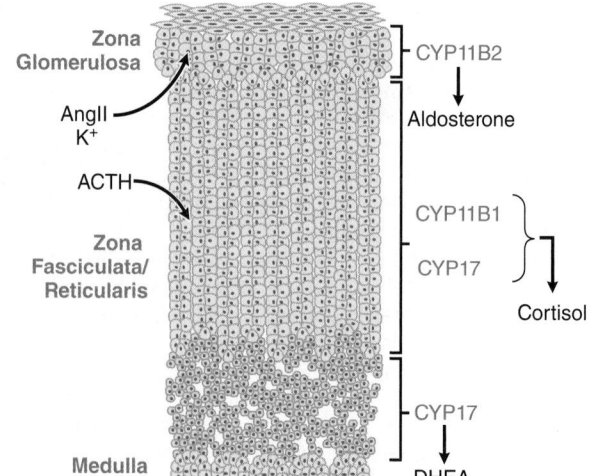

Figure 46–2 *The three anatomically and functionally distinct compartments of the adrenal cortex.* The major functional compartments of the adrenal cortex are shown, along with the steroidogenic enzymes that determine the unique profiles of corticosteroid products. Also shown are the predominant physiological regulators of steroid production: AngII and K$^+$ for the zona glomerulosa and ACTH for the zona fasciculata. The physiological regulator(s) of DHEA production by the zona reticularis are not known, although ACTH acutely increases DHEA biosynthesis.

roles in exocrine secretion and pheromone-related aggressive behavior (Morgan and Cone, 2006).

Actions on the Adrenal Cortex

Acting via MC$_2$R, ACTH stimulates the adrenal cortex to secrete *glucocorticoids*, *mineralocorticoids*, and the androgen precursor DHEA. The

Cells of the zona fasciculata have fewer receptors for AngII and express *steroid 17α-hydroxylase* (CYP17) and *11β-hydroxylase* (CYP11B1), enzymes that catalyze the production of glucocorticoids. In the zona reticularis, CYP17 carries out an additional C17–20 lyase reaction that converts C21 corticosteroids to C19 androgen precursors.

In the absence of the anterior pituitary and ACTH stimulation, the inner zones of the cortex atrophy, and the production of glucocorticoids and adrenal androgens is markedly impaired. Persistently elevated levels of ACTH, due either to repeated administration of large doses of ACTH or to excessive endogenous production, induce hypertrophy and hyperplasia of the inner zones of the adrenal cortex, with overproduction of cortisol and adrenal androgens. Adrenal hyperplasia is most marked in congenital disorders of steroidogenesis, in which ACTH levels are continuously elevated as a secondary response to impaired cortisol biosynthesis.

Mechanism of Action

Corticotropin stimulates the synthesis and release of adrenocortical hormones by increasing de novo biosynthesis. ACTH, binding to MC_2R, activates the G_s-adenylyl cyclase–cyclic AMP–PKA pathway. Cyclic AMP is the second messenger for most effects of ACTH on steroidogenesis.

Temporally, the response of adrenocortical cells to ACTH has two phases. The *acute phase*, which occurs within seconds to minutes, largely reflects an increased supply of cholesterol substrate to the steroidogenic enzymes. The *chronic phase*, which occurs over hours to days, results largely from increased transcription of the steroidogenic enzymes.

A number of transcriptional regulators participate in the induction of the steroidogenic enzymes by ACTH. Among these is the nuclear receptor NR5A1 (steroidogenic factor 1), a transcription factor required for the development of the adrenal cortex and for the expression of most of the steroidogenic enzymes (Schimmer and White, 2010). Pathways of adrenal steroid biosynthesis and the structures of the major steroid intermediates and products of the human adrenal cortex are shown in Figure 46–3. The rate-limiting step in steroid hormone production is the translocation of *cholesterol* across mitochondrial membranes by the *steroid acute regulatory protein*. Cholesterol is then converted to *pregnenolone* by the side-chain cleavage enzyme, CYP11A1, which represents the first enzymatic step in steroid hormone biosynthesis (Miller and Auchus, 2011). Most of the enzymes required for steroid hormone biosynthesis, including CYP11A1, are members of the cytochrome P450 superfamily (see Chapter 6). To ensure an adequate supply of substrate for steroidogenesis, the adrenal cortex uses multiple sources of cholesterol, including circulating cholesterol and cholesterol esters taken up via the low-density lipoprotein and high-density lipoprotein receptor pathways; endogenous cholesterol liberated from cholesterol ester stores via activation of cholesterol esterase; and endogenous cholesterol from de novo biosynthesis.

Extra-adrenal Effects of ACTH

In large doses, ACTH causes a number of metabolic changes in adrenalectomized animals, including ketosis, lipolysis, hypoglycemia (immediately after treatment), and resistance to insulin (later after treatment). Given the large doses of ACTH required, the physiological significance of these extra-adrenal effects is questionable.

Regulation of ACTH Secretion

Hypothalamic-Pituitary-Adrenal Axis

The rate of glucocorticoid secretion is determined by fluctuations in the release of ACTH by the pituitary corticotropes. These corticotropes are regulated by *CRH* and *AVP*, peptide hormones released by specialized neurons of the endocrine hypothalamus into the network of portal veins bathing the anterior pituitary (Papadimitriou and Priftis, 2009). This HPA axis forms an integrated system that maintains appropriate levels of glucocorticoids (Figure 46–4). The three characteristic modes of physiologic regulation of the HPA axis are

- *diurnal rhythm* in basal steroidogenesis
- *negative-feedback regulation* by adrenal corticosteroids
- marked *increases in steroidogenesis in response to stress.*

Pathologic elevation of steroidogenesis is seen in Cushing disease, the ectopic ACTH syndrome, and conditions where GRs or MRs are defective.

The *diurnal rhythm* is determined by circadian clocks in the hypothalamus, suprachiasmatic nucleus, and adrenal gland itself and is entrained by higher neuronal centers in response to sleep-wake cycles, such that levels of ACTH peak in the early morning hours, causing the circulating glucocorticoid levels to peak at about 8 AM. (Leliavski et al., 2015). *Negative-feedback regulation* occurs at multiple levels of the HPA axis and is the major mechanism that maintains circulating glucocorticoid levels in the appropriate range. *Stress* can override the normal negative-feedback control mechanisms, leading to marked increases in plasma concentrations of glucocorticoids.

Following release into the hypophyseal plexus, CRH is transported via this portal system to the anterior pituitary, where it binds to specific membrane receptors on corticotropes. On CRH binding, the CRH receptor activates the G_s-adenylyl cyclase–cyclic AMP pathway within corticotropes, ultimately stimulating both ACTH biosynthesis and secretion. CRH and CRH-related peptides called *urocortins* also are produced at other sites, including the amygdala and hindbrain, gut, skin, adrenal gland, adipose tissue, placenta, and additional sites in the periphery. The classical CRH receptor, now designated CRF_1 receptor, belongs to the class II family of GPCRs that includes receptors for calcitonin, parathyroid hormone, growth hormone–releasing hormone, secretin, glucagon, and glucagon-like peptide. A second CRH receptor, the CRF_2 receptor, is distinguished from the CRF_1 receptor in its binding specificities for CRH and the urocortins. The finding that the HPA axis often is altered in patients suffering from major depressive disorders illustrates the complex relationships between stress and mood and has stimulated considerable interest in the possible use of CRH antagonists in disorders such as anxiety and depression (Holsboer and Ising, 2008).

Arginine Vasopressin

Arginine vasopressin also acts as a secretagogue for corticotropes, significantly potentiating the effects of CRH. AVP is produced in the paraventricular nucleus and secreted into the pituitary portal veins from the median eminence. AVP binds to V_{1b} receptors and activates the G_q-PLC-IP_3-Ca^{2+} pathway to enhance the release of ACTH. In contrast with CRH, AVP does not increase ACTH synthesis.

Negative Feedback of Glucocorticoids

Glucocorticoids inhibit ACTH secretion via direct and indirect actions on CRH neurons to decrease CRH mRNA levels and CRH release and via direct effects on corticotropes. The indirect inhibitory effects on CRH neurons appear to be mediated by both corticosteroid receptors in the hippocampus. At lower cortisol levels, MRs, which have higher affinity for glucocorticoids than GRs, are the major receptor species occupied. As glucocorticoid concentrations rise and saturate MRs, the GRs become increasingly occupied. Both MRs and GRs apparently control the basal activity of the HPA axis, whereas feedback inhibition by glucocorticoids predominantly involves GRs. In the pituitary, glucocorticoids act through GRs to inhibit the release of ACTH from corticotropes and the expression of POMC. These effects are both rapid (occurring within seconds to minutes) and delayed (requiring hours and involving changes in gene transcription mediated through GRs).

The Stress Response

Stress overcomes negative-feedback regulation of the HPA axis, leading to a marked rise in corticosteroid production. Examples of stress signals include injury, hemorrhage, severe infection, major surgery, hypoglycemia, cold, pain, and fear. Although the precise mechanisms that underlie this stress response and the essential actions played by corticosteroids are not fully defined, increased corticosteroid secretion is vital to maintain homeostasis in these settings. As discussed further in the chapter, complex interactions between the HPA axis and the immune system may be a fundamental physiological component of this stress response.

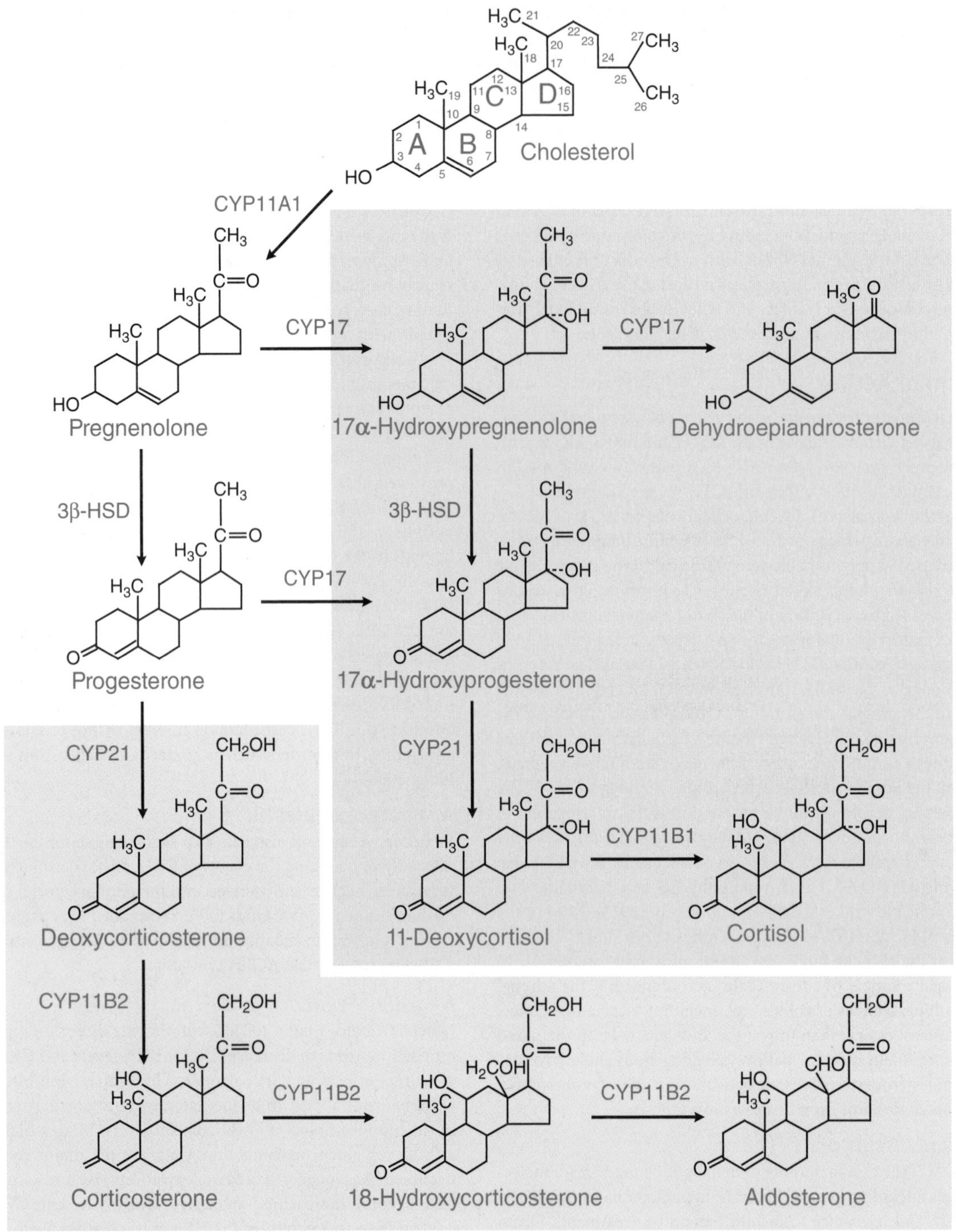

Figure 46–3 *Pathways of corticosteroid biosynthesis.* The steroidogenic pathways used in the biosynthesis of the corticosteroids are shown, along with the structures of the intermediates and products. The pathways unique to the zona glomerulosa are shown in the orange box; those that occur in the inner zona fasciculata and zona reticularis are shown in the gray box. The zona reticularis does not express 3β-HSD and thus preferentially synthesizes DHEA.

Therapeutic Uses and Diagnostic Applications of ACTH

Corticotropin has limited utility therapeutically. All proven therapeutic effects of ACTH can be achieved with appropriate doses of corticosteroids with a lower risk of side effects. Moreover, therapy with ACTH is less predictable and less convenient than therapy with corticosteroids. ACTH stimulates mineralocorticoid and adrenal androgen secretion and may therefore cause acute retention of salt and water, as well as virilization. Cosyntropin, a synthetic peptide that corresponds to residues 1–24 of human ACTH, is used in testing the integrity of the HPA axis. At the considerably supraphysiological dose of 250 μg, cosyntropin maximally stimulates adrenocortical steroidogenesis. An increase in the circulating

cortisol to a level greater than 18–20 μg/dL indicates a normal response. Cosyntropin may be used diagnostically in adrenal venous sampling to distinguish between unilateral and bilateral aldosterone oversecretion in primary aldosteronism.

CRH Stimulation Test

Ovine CRH (corticorelin) and human CRH (not available in the U.S.) are used for diagnostic testing of the HPA axis. In patients with documented ACTH-dependent hypercortisolism, CRH testing may help differentiate pituitary (i.e., Cushing disease) from ectopic sources of ACTH.

Assays for ACTH

Immunochemiluminescent assays that use two separate antibodies directed at distinct epitopes on the ACTH molecule now are widely

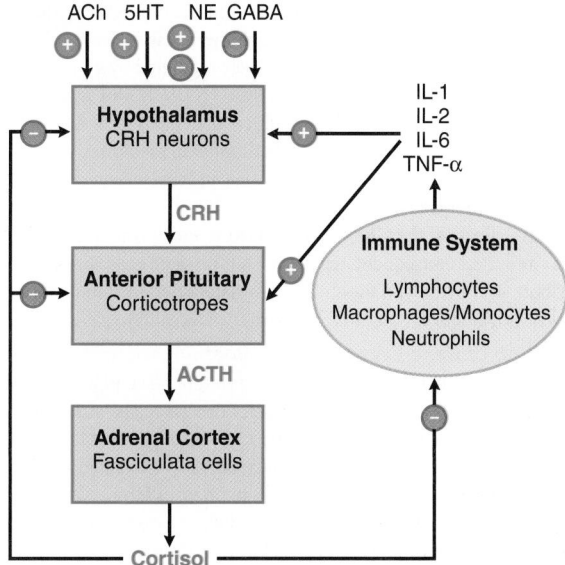

ACh 5HT NE GABA

Figure 46–4 *The HPA axis and the immune inflammatory network.* Inputs from higher neuronal centers regulate CRH secretion. + indicates a positive regulator, − indicates a negative regulator, + and − together indicate a mixed effect, as for NE. In addition, AVP stimulates release of ACTH from corticotropes.

available. These assays increase the ability to differentiate patients with primary hypoadrenalism due to intrinsic adrenal disease, who have high ACTH levels due to the loss of normal glucocorticoid feedback inhibition, from those with secondary forms of hypoadrenalism due to low ACTH levels resulting from hypothalamic or pituitary disorders. The immunochemiluminescent ACTH assays also are useful in differentiating ACTH-dependent from ACTH-independent forms of hypercortisolism: High ACTH levels are seen when the hypercortisolism results from pituitary adenomas (e.g., Cushing disease) or nonpituitary tumors that secrete ACTH (e.g., the syndrome of ectopic ACTH), whereas low ACTH levels are seen in patients with excessive glucocorticoid production due to primary adrenal disorders. One problem with the immunoassays for ACTH is that their specificity for intact ACTH can lead to falsely low values in patients with ectopic ACTH secretion; these tumors can secrete aberrantly processed forms of ACTH that have biological activity but do not react in the antibody assays.

Absorption, Fate, and Toxicity

Corticotropin is readily absorbed from parenteral sites. The hormone rapidly disappears from the circulation after intravenous administration; in humans, the $t_{1/2}$ in plasma is about 15 min, primarily due to rapid enzymatic hydrolysis. Aside from rare hypersensitivity reactions, the toxicity of ACTH is primarily attributable to the increased secretion of corticosteroids. Cosyntropin generally is less antigenic than native ACTH.

Adrenocortical Steroids

The adrenal cortex synthesizes two classes of steroids: the *corticosteroids* (glucocorticoids and mineralocorticoids; see Figure 46–3), which have 21 carbon atoms, and the *androgens*, which have 19 carbons (see Figure 45–3). The actions of corticosteroids historically were described as *glucocorticoid* (reflecting their carbohydrate metabolism–regulating activity) and *mineralocorticoid* (reflecting their electrolyte balance–regulating activity). In humans, *cortisol* is the main glucocorticoid, and aldosterone is the physiologic mineralocorticoid. Table 46–1 shows typical rates of secretion of cortisol and aldosterone, as well as their normal circulating concentrations.

Although the adrenal cortex is an important source of androgen precursors in women, patients with adrenal insufficiency can be restored to

TABLE 46–1 ■ NORMAL DAILY PRODUCTION RATES AND CIRCULATING LEVELS OF THE PREDOMINANT CORTICOSTEROIDS

	CORTISOL	ALDOSTERONE
Rate of secretion under optimal conditions	10 mg/d	0.125 mg/d
Concentration in peripheral plasma:		
8 AM	16 µg/100 mL	0.01 µg /100 mL
4 AM	4 µg/100 mL	0.01 µg /100 mL

normal life expectancy by replacement therapy with glucocorticoids and mineralocorticoids. Adrenal androgens are not essential for survival. The sulfated derivative DHEA-S is the most highly secreted adrenal steroid; levels of DHEA and DHEA-S peak in the third decade of life and decline progressively thereafter. Moreover, patients with a number of chronic diseases have very low DHEA levels, leading some to propose that DHEA treatment might at least partly alleviate the loss of libido, the decline in cognitive function, the decreased sense of well-being, and other adverse physiological consequences of aging. However, studies on the benefits of addition of DHEA to the standard replacement regimen in women with adrenal insufficiency have been inconclusive. Despite the absence of definitive data, DHEA is widely used as an over-the-counter nutritional supplement for its alleged health benefits.

Physiological Functions and Pharmacological Effects

Corticosteroids have numerous effects, which include alterations in carbohydrate, protein, and lipid metabolism; maintenance of fluid and electrolyte balance; and preservation of normal function of the cardiovascular system, the immune system, the kidney, skeletal muscle, the endocrine system, and the nervous system. In addition, corticosteroids endow the organism with the capacity to resist stressful and noxious stimuli and environmental changes. In the absence of adequate secretion of corticosteroids from the adrenal cortex, stresses such as infection, trauma, and extremes in temperature can be fatal.

The actions of corticosteroids are related to those of other hormones. For example, in the absence of lipolytic hormones, cortisol has virtually no effect on the rate of lipolysis by adipocytes. Conversely, in the absence of glucocorticoids, epinephrine and NE have only minor effects on lipolysis. Administration of a small dose of glucocorticoid, however, markedly potentiates the lipolytic action of these catecholamines. Those effects of corticosteroids that involve concerted actions with other hormonal regulators are termed *permissive* and most likely reflect steroid-induced changes in protein synthesis, which, in turn, modify tissue responsiveness to other hormones.

Corticosteroids are termed either *mineralocorticoids* or *glucocorticoids*, according to their relative potencies in Na⁺ retention and effects on carbohydrate metabolism (i.e., hepatic deposition of glycogen and gluconeogenesis). In general, the potencies of steroids on glucose metabolism closely parallel their potencies as anti-inflammatory agents. The effects on Na⁺ retention and the carbohydrate/anti-inflammatory actions are not closely related and reflect selective actions at distinct receptors. As noted in further discussion (see structure-activity relationships and Table 46–3), some steroid derivatives provide relative selectivity as stimulants of Na⁺ retention or anti-inflammatory effects.

General Mechanisms for Corticosteroid Effects

Corticosteroids bind to specific receptor proteins in target tissues to regulate the expression of corticosteroid-responsive genes, thereby changing the levels and array of proteins synthesized by the various target tissues (Figure 46–5). Many effects of corticosteroids are not immediate but become apparent after several hours; clinically, one often but not invariably sees a delay before beneficial effects of corticosteroid therapy become

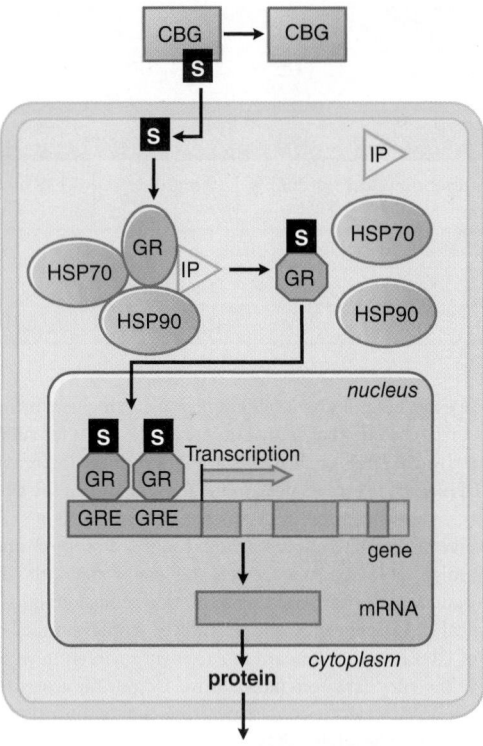

Altered cellular function

Figure 46–5 *Intracellular mechanism of action of the GR.* The figure shows the molecular pathway by which cortisol (labeled S) enters cells and interacts with the GR to change GR conformation (indicated by the change in shape of the GR), induce GR nuclear translocation, and activate transcription of target genes. Glucocorticoids also inhibit the expression of certain genes, including POMC expression by corticotropes. Here, GRE indicates the GREs in the DNA that are bound by GR, thus providing specificity to induction of gene transcription by glucocorticoids. Within the gene are introns (gray) and exons (red); transcription and mRNA processing leads to splicing and removal of introns and assembly of exons into mRNA.

manifest. Although corticosteroids predominantly act by increasing gene transcription, there are examples in which glucocorticoids decrease gene transcription. In addition, corticosteroids exert their immediate effects by nongenomic mechanisms, usually via classical GRs or MRs (Prigent et al., 2004).

Glucocorticoid Receptors. The receptors for corticosteroids are members of the nuclear receptor family of transcription factors. GRs (also called NR3C1, nuclear receptor subfamily 3, group C, member 1) reside predominantly in the cytoplasm in an inactive form complexed with other proteins. Steroid binding results in receptor activation and translocation to the nucleus (see Figure 46–5). Several GR isoforms result from alternative RNA splicing and from translation initiation at alternative sites. Of these, GRα is the prototypical glucocorticoid-responsive isoform. A second major GR isoform, GRβ, is a truncated, dominant, negative variant that lacks 35 amino acids at the C terminus and is unable to bind glucocorticoids or activate gene expression. Multiple polymorphisms in the human GR are associated with differences in GR function and have been linked to glucocorticoid insensitivity (Vandevyver et al., 2014).

Regulation of Gene Expression by Glucocorticoids. After ligand binding, GRs dissociate from their associated proteins and translocate to the nucleus. There, they interact with specific DNA sequences called GREs, which provide specificity in terms of induction of gene transcription by glucocorticoids. Genes can be activated or inhibited by GR-GRE interactions. The mechanisms whereby GR activate transcription are complex and not completely understood, but they involve interaction with transcriptional coactivators and with proteins that make up the basal transcription apparatus. In an example of transcriptional inhibition GRs

inhibit transcription of POMC by a direct interaction with a GRE in the *POMC* promoter, thereby contributing to the negative-feedback regulation of the HPA axis. Other genes negatively regulated by glucocorticoids include genes for COX-2, inducible NOS (NOS2), and inflammatory cytokines. Some inhibitory effects of glucocorticoids, such as downregulation of expression of genes encoding a number of cytokines, collagenase, and stromelysin, have been linked to protein-protein interactions between the GRs and other transcription factors (e.g., NF-κB and AP-1) rather than to negative effects of the GRs at specific GREs. Such protein-protein interactions and their consequent negative effects on gene expression appear to contribute significantly to the anti-inflammatory and immunosuppressive effects of the glucocorticoids (De Bosscher et al., 2003).

Regulation of Gene Expression by Mineralocorticoids. Like GRs, the MR also is a ligand-activated transcription factor and binds to a very similar hormone-responsive element. MRs also associate with HSP90 and GREs to activate the transcription of discrete sets of genes in target tissues. GRs and MRs differ in their ability to inhibit AP-1–mediated gene activation and, in terms of gene transcription, by their differential recruitment of other transcription factors. In addition, GRs are essentially ubiquitous, whereas MRs are expressed in epithelial tissues involved in electrolyte transport (i.e., the kidney, colon, salivary glands, and sweat glands) and in some nonepithelial tissues (e.g., hippocampus, heart, vasculature, and adipose tissue).

Aldosterone exerts its effects on Na⁺ and K⁺ homeostasis primarily via its actions on the principal cells of the distal renal tubules and collecting ducts, whereas effects on H⁺ secretion largely are exerted in the intercalated cells. The binding of aldosterone to the MRs in the kidney initiates a sequence of events that includes the rapid induction of *serum-* and *glucocorticoid-regulated kinase*, which in turn phosphorylates and activates amiloride-sensitive epithelial Na⁺ channels in the apical membrane. Thereafter, increased Na⁺ influx stimulates the Na⁺, K⁺-ATPase in the basolateral membrane. In addition to these rapid genomic actions, aldosterone increases the synthesis of the individual components of these membrane proteins as part of a more delayed effect.

Receptor-Independent Mechanism for Corticosteroid Specificity. Aldosterone (a classic mineralocorticoid) and cortisol (generally viewed as predominantly glucocorticoid) bind the MRs with equal affinity. In epithelial cells of the kidney, colon, and salivary glands, aldosterone specifically activates MRs in the face of much higher circulating levels of glucocorticoids due to the coexpression of the type 2 isozyme of *11β-HSD2*. This enzyme metabolizes glucocorticoids such as cortisol to inactive 11-keto derivatives such as cortisone (Figure 46–6). Aldosterone escapes this inactivation and maintains mineralocorticoid activity because its predominant physiological form is the hemiacetal derivative that is resistant to 11β-HSD action (Figure 46–7). In the absence of 11β-HSD2, as occurs in the inherited disease *syndrome of apparent mineralocorticoid excess*, the MR is activated by cortisol, leading to severe

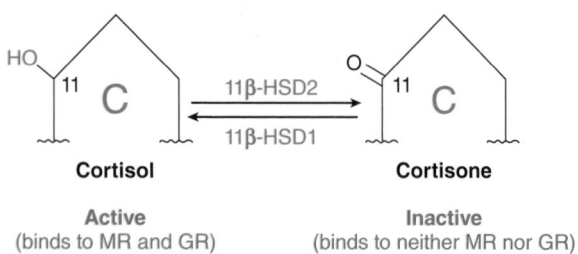

Cortisol
Active
(binds to MR and GR)

Cortisone
Inactive
(binds to neither MR nor GR)

Figure 46–6 *The 11β-HSD confers specificity of corticosteroid action.* 11β-HSD2 converts cortisol, which binds to both the MR and the GR, to cortisone, which binds to neither MR nor GR, thereby protecting the MR from the high circulating concentrations of cortisol. This inactivation allows specific responses to aldosterone in sites such as the distal nephron. 11β-HSD1 catalyzes the reverse reaction, which converts inactive cortisone to active cortisol in such tissues as liver and fat. Only ring C of the corticosteroid is depicted. Aldosterone is resistant to 11β-HSD2 by virtue of the condensation of its 11β-hydroxyl group with its 18-aldehyde to form a hemiacetal structure.

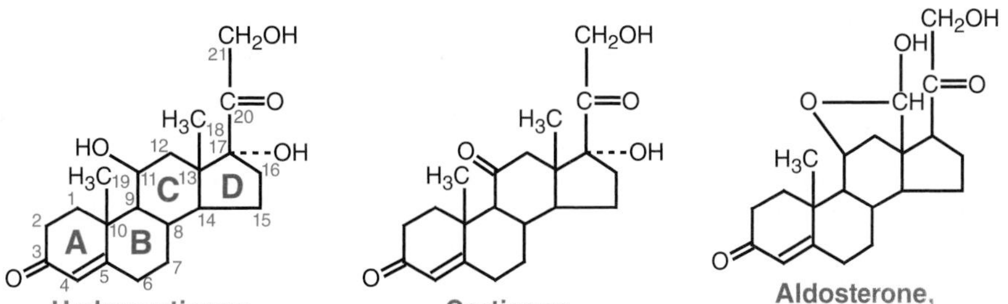

Figure 46–7 *Structure and nomenclature of GR and MR agonists.*

hypokalemia and mineralocorticoid-related hypertension. A state of mineralocorticoid excess also can be induced by inhibiting 11β-HSD with *glycyrrhizic acid*, a component of licorice implicated in licorice-induced hypertension.

Carbohydrate and Protein Metabolism

Glucocorticoids markedly affect carbohydrate and protein metabolism, which can be viewed as protecting glucose-dependent tissues (e.g., the brain and heart) from starvation. Glucocorticoids stimulate the liver to form glucose from amino acids and glycerol and to store glucose as glycogen. In the periphery, glucocorticoids diminish glucose utilization, increase protein breakdown and the synthesis of glutamine, and activate lipolysis, thereby providing amino acids and glycerol for gluconeogenesis. The net result is to increase blood glucose levels. Through their effects on glucose metabolism, glucocorticoids can worsen glycemic control in patients with overt diabetes and can precipitate the onset of hyperglycemia in susceptible patients.

Lipid Metabolism

Two effects of glucocorticoids on lipid metabolism are firmly established. The first is the dramatic redistribution of body fat that occurs in hypercortisolism, such as Cushing syndrome. In this setting, there is increased fat in the back of the neck ("buffalo hump"), face ("moon facies"), and supraclavicular area, coupled with a loss of fat in the extremities. The other is the permissive facilitation of the lipolytic effect of other agents, such as growth hormone and β adrenergic receptor agonists, resulting in an increase in free fatty acids after glucocorticoid administration.

Electrolyte and Water Balance

Aldosterone is by far the most potent endogenous corticosteroid with respect to fluid and electrolyte balance. Mineralocorticoids act on the distal tubules and collecting ducts of the kidney to enhance reabsorption of Na^+ from the tubular fluid; they also increase the urinary excretion of K^+ and H^+. These actions on electrolyte transport, in the kidney and in other tissues (e.g., colon, salivary glands, and sweat glands), appear to account for the physiological and pharmacological activities that are characteristic of mineralocorticoids. Thus, the primary features of hyperaldosteronism are positive Na^+ balance with consequent expansion of extracellular fluid volume, normal or slight increases in plasma Na^+ concentration, normal or low plasma K^+, and alkalosis. Mineralocorticoid deficiency, in contrast, leads to Na^+ wasting and contraction of the extracellular fluid volume, hyponatremia, hyperkalemia, and acidosis. Chronically, hyperaldosteronism causes hypertension, whereas aldosterone deficiency can lead to hypotension and vascular collapse.

Glucocorticoids also exert effects on fluid and electrolyte balance, largely due to permissive effects on tubular function and actions that maintain the glomerular filtration rate. Glucocorticoids play a permissive role in the renal excretion of free water. In part, the inability of patients with glucocorticoid deficiency to excrete free water results from the increased secretion of AVP, which stimulates water reabsorption in the kidney. In addition to their effects on monovalent cations and water, glucocorticoids exert multiple effects on Ca^{2+} metabolism, lowering Ca^{2+} uptake from the gut and increasing Ca^{2+} excretion by the kidney, collectively leading to decreased total body Ca^{2+} stores.

Cardiovascular System

The most striking effects of corticosteroids on the cardiovascular system result from mineralocorticoid-induced changes in renal Na^+ retention, as is evident in primary aldosteronism. MR activation has direct effects on the heart and vessel walls; aldosterone induces hypertension and interstitial cardiac fibrosis in animal models. The increased cardiac fibrosis appears to result from direct mineralocorticoid actions in the heart (Zannad and Radauceanu, 2005). The second major action of corticosteroids on the cardiovascular system is to enhance vascular reactivity to other vasoactive substances. Hypoadrenalism is associated with reduced responsiveness to vasoconstrictors such as NE and AngII, perhaps due to decreased expression of adrenergic receptors in the vascular wall. Conversely, hypertension is seen in patients with excessive glucocorticoid secretion, occurring in most patients with Cushing syndrome and in a subset of patients treated with synthetic glucocorticoids (even those lacking any significant mineralocorticoid action).

Skeletal Muscle

Permissive concentrations of corticosteroids are required for the normal function of skeletal muscle, and diminished work capacity is a prominent sign of adrenocortical insufficiency. In patients with Addison disease, weakness and fatigue are frequent symptoms. Excessive amounts of either glucocorticoids or mineralocorticoids also impair muscle function. In primary aldosteronism, muscle weakness results primarily from hypokalemia rather than from direct effects of mineralocorticoids on skeletal muscle. In contrast, glucocorticoid excess over prolonged periods, secondary to either glucocorticoid therapy or endogenous hypercortisolism, causes skeletal muscle wasting. This effect, *steroid myopathy*, accounts in part for weakness and fatigue in patients with glucocorticoid excess.

CNS

Corticosteroids exert a number of indirect effects on the CNS, through maintenance of blood pressure, plasma glucose concentrations, and electrolyte concentrations. Increasingly, direct effects of corticosteroids on the CNS have been recognized, including effects on mood, behavior, and brain excitability. Patients with adrenal insufficiency exhibit a diverse array of neurological manifestations, including apathy, depression, irritability, and even psychosis. Appropriate replacement therapy corrects these abnormalities. Conversely, glucocorticoid administration can induce multiple CNS reactions. Most patients respond with mood elevation, which may impart a sense of well-being despite the persistence of underlying disease. Some patients exhibit more pronounced behavioral changes, such as mania, insomnia, restlessness, and increased motor activity. A smaller but significant percentage of patients treated with glucocorticoids become anxious, depressed, or overtly psychotic. A high incidence of neuroses and psychoses is seen in patients with Cushing syndrome. These abnormalities usually disappear after cessation of glucocorticoid therapy or treatment of the Cushing syndrome.

Formed Elements of Blood

Glucocorticoids exert minor effects on hemoglobin and the erythrocyte content of blood, as evidenced by the frequent occurrence of polycythemia in Cushing syndrome and of normochromic, normocytic anemia in adrenal insufficiency. More profound effects are seen in the setting of autoimmune hemolytic anemia, in which the immunosuppressive effects of glucocorticoids can diminish erythrocyte destruction.

Corticosteroids also affect circulating white blood cells. Addison disease is associated with an increased mass of lymphoid tissue and lymphocytosis; in contrast, Cushing syndrome is characterized by lymphocytopenia and a decreased mass of lymphoid tissue. The administration of glucocorticoids leads to a decreased number of circulating lymphocytes, eosinophils, monocytes, and basophils. A single dose of hydrocortisone leads to a decline of these circulating cells within 4–6 h; this effect persists for 24 h and results from the redistribution of cells away from the periphery rather than from increased destruction. In contrast, glucocorticoids increase circulating polymorphonuclear leukocytes as a result of increased release from the marrow, diminished rate of removal from the circulation, and decreased adherence to vascular walls. Finally, glucocorticoids are effective in the treatment of certain lymphoid malignancies, possibly related to the capacity of glucocorticoids to activate apoptosis.

Anti-inflammatory and Immunosuppressive Actions

In addition to their effects on lymphocyte number, glucocorticoids profoundly alter the immune responses of lymphocytes. These effects are important facets of the anti-inflammatory and immunosuppressive actions of the glucocorticoids. Although the use of glucocorticoids as anti-inflammatory agents does not address the underlying cause of the disease, the suppression of inflammation is of enormous clinical utility and has made these drugs among the most frequently prescribed agents. Similarly, glucocorticoids are of immense value in treating diseases that result from undesirable immune reactions. These diseases range from conditions that predominantly result from humoral immunity, such as urticaria (see Chapter 70), to those that are mediated by cellular immune mechanisms, such as transplantation rejection (see Chapter 35). The immunosuppressive and anti-inflammatory actions of glucocorticoids are inextricably linked, perhaps because they both involve inhibition of leukocyte functions.

Multiple mechanisms are involved in the suppression of inflammation by glucocorticoids. Glucocorticoids inhibit the production by multiple cells of factors that are critical in generating the inflammatory response. As a result, there is decreased release of vasoactive and chemoattractive factors, diminished secretion of lipolytic and proteolytic enzymes, decreased extravasation of leukocytes to areas of injury, and ultimately, decreased fibrosis. Glucocorticoids can also reduce expression of pro-inflammatory cytokines, as well as COX-2 and NOS2. Some of the cell types and mediators that are inhibited by glucocorticoids are summarized in Table 46–2.

Among the pro-inflammatory cytokines, IL-1, IL-6, and TNF-α stimulate the HPA axis, with IL-1 having the broadest range of actions. IL-1 stimulates the release of CRH by hypothalamic neurons, interacts directly with the pituitary to increase the release of ACTH, and may directly stimulate the adrenal gland to produce glucocorticoids. The increased production of glucocorticoids, in turn, profoundly inhibits the immune system at multiple sites as discussed previously. Thus, the HPA axis and the immune system are capable of bidirectional interactions in response to stress, and these interactions appear to be important for homeostasis (Turnbull and Rivier, 1999).

ADME

Absorption

Hydrocortisone and numerous congeners, including the synthetic analogues, are orally effective. Certain water-soluble esters of hydrocortisone and its synthetic congeners are administered intravenously to achieve high concentrations of drug rapidly in systemic or targeted body fluids. More prolonged effects are obtained by intramuscular injection of suspensions of hydrocortisone, its esters, and congeners. Minor changes in chemical structure may markedly alter the rate of absorption, time of onset of effect, and duration of action. Glucocorticoids also are absorbed systemically from sites of local administration, such as synovial spaces, the conjunctival sac, skin, and respiratory tract. When administration is prolonged, when the site of application is covered with an occlusive dressing, or when large areas of skin are involved, absorption may be sufficient to cause systemic effects, including suppression of the HPA axis.

Distribution, Metabolism, and Excretion

After absorption, 90% or more of cortisol in plasma is reversibly bound to protein under normal circumstances. In most tissues, only the fraction of corticosteroid that is unbound is active and can enter cells. Two plasma proteins account for almost all of the steroid-binding capacity: *CBG* (also called *transcortin*) and *albumin*. CBG is an α globulin secreted by the liver that has high affinity for steroids (dissociation constant of ~1 nM) but relatively low total binding capacity, whereas albumin, also produced by the liver, has a relatively large binding capacity but low affinity (estimated dissociation constant of 1 mM). In tissues with prolonged capillary transit time (e.g., liver, spleen), steroid dissociates from albumin. At high steroid concentrations, the capacity of CBG binding is exceeded, and a slightly greater fraction of the steroid exists in the free state. CBG has relatively high affinity for cortisol and some of its synthetic congeners and low affinity for aldosterone and glucuronide-conjugated steroid metabolites; thus, greater percentages of these last steroids are found in the free form. A special state of physiological hypercortisolism occurs during pregnancy. The elevated circulating estrogen levels induce CBG production, and CBG and total plasma cortisol increase several-fold; the physiological significance of these changes remains to be established.

TABLE 46–2 ■ INHIBITORY EFFECTS OF GLUCOCORTICOIDS ON INFLAMMATORY/IMMUNE RESPONSES

CELL TYPE	FACTOR INHIBITED	COMMENTS
Macrophages and monocytes	Arachidonic acid, PGs, and LTs	Mediated by glucocorticoid inhibition of COX-2 and PLA$_2$.
	Cytokines: IL-l, IL-6, and TNF-α	Production and release are blocked; cytokines exert multiple effects on inflammation (e.g., ↑ T cells, ↑ fibroblast proliferation).
	Acute phase reactants	Including the third component of complement.
Endothelial cells	ELAM-1 and ICAM-1	ELAM-1 and ICAM-1 are critical for leukocyte localization.
	Acute-phase reactants Cytokines (e.g., IL-1) Arachidonic acid derivatives	Same as above for macrophages and monocytes.
Basophils	Histamine, LTC$_4$	IgE-dependent release ↓ by glucocorticoids.
Fibroblasts	Arachidonic acid metabolites	Same as above for macrophages and monocytes. Glucocorticoids ↓ growth factor–induced DNA synthesis and fibroblast proliferation.
Lymphocytes	Cytokines (IL-1, IL-2, IL-3, IL-6, TNF-α, GM-CSF, interferon γ)	Same as above for macrophages and monocytes.

The aldosterone levels also rise 3- to 10-fold in pregnancy, reflecting the activity of the elevated progesterone plasma levels as an MR antagonist. Because progesterone is also a GR antagonist, it may contribute to the elevated levels of cortisol.

As a general rule, the metabolism of steroid hormones involves sequential additions of O or H atoms, followed by conjugation to form water-soluble derivatives. Reduction of the 4,5 double bond (Figure 46–3) occurs at both hepatic and extrahepatic sites, yielding inactive compounds. Subsequent reduction of the 3-ketone substituent to the 3-hydroxyl derivative, forming tetrahydrocortisol, occurs only in the liver. Most of these A ring–reduced steroids are conjugated through the 3-hydroxyl group with sulfate or glucuronide by enzymatic reactions that take place in the liver and, to a lesser extent, in the kidney. The resultant sulfate esters and glucuronides are water soluble and are excreted in urine. Neither biliary nor fecal excretion is of quantitative importance in humans.

Synthetic steroids with an 11-keto group, such as cortisone and prednisone, must be enzymatically reduced to the corresponding 11β-hydroxy derivative before they are biologically active (Figure 46–6). The type 1 isozyme of 11β-HSD (11β-HSD1) catalyzes this reduction, predominantly in the liver, but also in specialized sites such as adipocytes, bone, eye, and skin. In settings in which this enzymatic activity is impaired, it is prudent to use steroids that do not require enzymatic activation (e.g., hydrocortisone or prednisolone rather than cortisone or prednisone). Such settings include individuals with severe hepatic failure and patients with the very rare condition of cortisone reductase deficiency.

Structure-Activity Relationships

Chemical modifications of the cortisol molecule have generated derivatives with greater separation of glucocorticoid and mineralocorticoid activity (Table 46–3); for a number of synthetic glucocorticoids, the effects on electrolytes are minimal even at the highest doses used. In addition, these modifications have led to derivatives with greater potencies and with longer durations of action. A vast array of steroid preparations is available for oral, parenteral, and topical use. Some of these are summarized in Table 46–4. None of these currently available derivatives effectively separates anti-inflammatory effects from effects on carbohydrate, protein, and fat metabolism or from suppressive effects on the HPA axis.

Estimates of Na+-retaining and anti-inflammatory potencies of representative steroids are listed in Table 46–3. Some steroids that are classified predominantly as glucocorticoids (e.g., cortisol) also possess modest but significant mineralocorticoid activity and thus may affect fluid and electrolyte handling in the clinical setting. At doses used for replacement therapy in patients with primary adrenal insufficiency, the mineralocorticoid effects of these "glucocorticoids" are insufficient to replace that of

aldosterone, and concurrent therapy with a more potent mineralocorticoid generally is needed. In contrast, aldosterone is exceedingly potent with respect to Na+ retention but has only minimal effects on carbohydrate metabolism. Even at levels that maximally affect electrolyte balance, aldosterone has no significant glucocorticoid activity and thus acts as a pure mineralocorticoid.

Toxicity of Adrenocortical Steroids

Two categories of toxic effects result from the therapeutic use of glucocorticoids: those resulting from withdrawal of steroid therapy and those resulting from continued use at supraphysiological doses. The side effects from both categories are potentially life threatening and require a careful assessment of the risks and benefits in each patient.

Withdrawal Therapy

The most frequent problem in steroid withdrawal is flare-up of the underlying disease for which steroids were prescribed. Several other complications are associated with steroid withdrawal. The most severe, acute adrenal insufficiency, results from overly rapid withdrawal of corticosteroids after prolonged therapy has suppressed the HPA axis. Many patients recover from glucocorticoid-induced HPA suppression within several weeks to months; however, in some individuals the time to full recovery can be a year or longer.

Protocols for discontinuing corticosteroid therapy in patients receiving long-term treatment have been proposed. Patients who have received supraphysiological doses of glucocorticoids for a period of 2–4 weeks within the preceding year should be considered to have some degree of HPA impairment. A characteristic glucocorticoid withdrawal syndrome consists of fever, myalgia, arthralgia, and malaise, which may be difficult to differentiate from some of the underlying diseases for which steroid therapy was instituted. Finally, *pseudotumor cerebri*, a clinical syndrome that includes increased intracranial pressure with papilledema, is a rare condition that sometimes is associated with reduction or withdrawal of corticosteroid therapy.

Continued Use of Supraphysiological Glucocorticoid Doses

Besides the consequences that result from the suppression of the HPA axis, a number of other complications result from prolonged therapy with glucocorticoids. These include fluid and electrolyte abnormalities, hypertension, hyperglycemia, increased susceptibility to infection, peptic ulcers, osteoporosis, myopathy, behavioral disturbances, cataracts, growth arrest, and the characteristic habitus of steroid overdose, including fat redistribution, striae, and ecchymoses.

Fluid and Electrolyte Handling. Alterations in fluid and electrolyte handling can cause hypokalemic alkalosis and hypertension, particularly

TABLE 46–3 ■ RELATIVE POTENCIES AND EQUIVALENT DOSES OF REPRESENTATIVE CORTICOSTEROIDS

COMPOUND	ANTI-INFLAMMATORY POTENCY	NA+-RETAINING POTENCY	DURATION OF ACTION[a]	EQUIVALENT DOSE (MG)[b]
Hydrocortisone[c]	1	1	S	20
Cortisone	0.8	0.8	S	25
Fludrocortisone	10	125	I	—[d]
Prednisone	4	0.8	I	5
Prednisolone	4	0.8	I	5
Methylprednisolone	5	0.5	I	4
Triamcinolone	5	0	I	4
Betamethasone	25	0	L	0.75
Dexamethasone	25	0	L	0.75

[a]Biological $t_{1/2}$: S, short (8–12 h); I, intermediate (12–36 h); L, long (36–72 h).
[b]Dose relationships apply only to oral or intravenous administration; potencies may differ greatly following intramuscular or intra-articular administration.
[c]The name for cortisol when used as a drug.
[d]This agent is used for its mineralocorticoid effects, not for glucocorticoid effects.

TABLE 46–4 ■ AVAILABLE PREPARATIONS OF ADRENOCORTICAL STEROIDS AND THEIR SYNTHETIC ANALOGUES

NONPROPRIETARY NAME	TYPE OF PREPARATION
Alclometasone dipropionate	Topical
Amcinonide	Topical
Beclomethasone dipropionate	Inhaled, Nasal
Betamethasone acetate	Injectable
Betamethasone sodium phosphate	Oral, injectable
Betamethasone valerate	Topical
Budesonide	Oral, inhaled, nasal, rectal
Ciclesonide	Inhaled, nasal
Clobetasol propionate	Topical, shampoo
Clocortolone pivalate	Topical
Desonide	Topical
Desoximetasone	Topical
Dexamethasone	Oralophthalmic, ocular implant
Dexamethasone sodium phosphate	Ophthalmic, injectable
Diflorasone diacetate	Topical
Fludrocortisone acetate[a]	Oral
Flunisolide	Inhaled Nasal
Fluocinolone acetonide	Topical, shampoo, otic, intravitreal implant
Fluocinonide	Topical
Fluorometholone	Ophthalmic
Fluorometholone acetate	Ophthalmic
Flurandrenolide	Impregnated dressing, topical
Halcinonide	Topical
Hydrocortisone	Topical, oral, rectal
Hydroxycortisone acetate	Topical, rectal
Hydroxycortisone butyrate	Topical
Hydrocortisone probutate	Topical
Hydrocortisone sodium succinate	Injectable
Hydrocortisone valerate	Topical
Methylprednisolone	Oral
Methylprednisolone acetate	Injectable
Methylprednisolone sodium succinate	Injectable
Mometasone furoate	Inhaled, nasal, topical
Prednisolone	Oral
Prednisolone acetate	Oral, ophthalmic
Prednisolone sodium phosphate	Oral, ophthalmic
Prednisone	Oral
Triamcinolone acetonide	Nasal, topical, injectable, dental
Triamcinolone hexacetonide	Injectable

Note: Topical preparations include agents for application to skin or mucous membranes in creams, solutions, ointments, gels, pastes (for oral lesions), and aerosols; *ophthalmic* preparations include solutions, suspensions, and ointments; *inhalation* preparations include agents for nasal or oral inhalation.

[a]Fludrocortisone acetate is intended for use as a mineralocorticoid.

in patients with primary hyperaldosteronism secondary to an adrenal adenoma or in patients treated with potent mineralocorticoids. Similarly, hypertension is a relatively common manifestation of exogenous glucocorticoid administration, even in patients treated with glucocorticoids lacking appreciable mineralocorticoid activity.

Metabolic Changes. The effects of glucocorticoids on intermediary metabolism were described previously. Hyperglycemia with glycosuria usually can be managed with diet or insulin, and its occurrence should not be a major factor in the decision to continue corticosteroid therapy or to initiate therapy in diabetic patients.

Immune Responses. Because of their multiple effects to inhibit the immune system and the inflammatory response, glucocorticoid use is associated with an increased susceptibility to infection and a risk for reactivation of latent tuberculosis. In the presence of known infections of some consequence, glucocorticoids should be administered only if absolutely necessary and concomitantly with appropriate and effective antimicrobial or antifungal therapy.

Possible Risk of Peptic Ulcers. There is considerable debate about the association between peptic ulcers and glucocorticoid therapy. The possible onset of hemorrhage and perforation in these ulcers and their insidious onset make peptic ulcers a serious therapeutic problem (Chapter 49). Prudence suggests vigilance for peptic ulcer formation in patients receiving therapy with corticosteroids, especially if administered concomitantly with aspirin or coxibs.

Myopathy. Myopathy, characterized by weakness of proximal limb muscles, can occur in patients taking large doses of corticosteroids and also is part of the clinical picture in patients with endogenous Cushing syndrome. It can be of sufficient severity to impair ambulation and is an indication for withdrawal of therapy. Attention also has focused on steroid myopathy of the respiratory muscles in patients with asthma or chronic obstructive pulmonary disease (Chapter 40); this complication can diminish respiratory function. Recovery from the steroid myopathies may be slow and incomplete.

Behavioral Changes. Behavioral disturbances are common after administration of corticosteroids and in patients who have Cushing syndrome secondary to endogenous hypercortism; these disturbances may take many forms, including nervousness, insomnia, changes in mood or psyche, and overt psychosis.

Cataracts. Cataracts are a well-established complication of glucocorticoid therapy and are related to dosage and duration of therapy. Children appear to be particularly at risk. Cessation of therapy may not lead to complete resolution of opacities, and the cataracts may progress despite reduction or cessation of therapy. Patients on long-term glucocorticoid therapy at prednisone doses of 10–15 mg/d or greater should receive periodic slit-lamp examinations to detect glucocorticoid-induced posterior subcapsular cataracts.

Osteoporosis. Osteoporosis, a frequent serious complication of glucocorticoid therapy, occurs in patients of both genders and all ages and is related to dosage and duration of therapy. About 30%–50% of all patients who receive chronic glucocorticoid therapy ultimately will develop osteoporotic fractures. Glucocorticoids preferentially affect trabecular bone and the cortical rim of the vertebral bodies; the ribs and vertebrae are the most frequent sites of fracture. Glucocorticoids decrease bone density by multiple mechanisms, including inhibition of gonadal steroid hormones, diminished GI absorption of Ca^{2+}, and inhibition of bone formation due to suppressive effects on osteoblasts and stimulation of resorption by osteoclasts via changes in the production of osteoprotegerin and RANK ligand (see Chapter 48). In addition, glucocorticoid inhibition of intestinal Ca^{2+} uptake may lead to secondary increases in parathyroid hormone, thereby increasing bone resorption.

The initiation of glucocorticoid therapy at 5 mg/d or more of prednisone (or its equivalent) for 3 months or longer is an indication for bone densitometry to detect abnormalities in trabecular bone. Because bone loss associated with glucocorticoids predominantly occurs within the first

6 months of therapy, densitometric evaluation of the lumbar spine and hip, along with prophylactic measures, should be initiated. Most authorities advocate maintaining a Ca^{2+} intake of 1500 mg/d by diet plus Ca^{2+} supplementation and vitamin D intake of 800 IU/d, assuming that these measures do not increase urinary calcium excretion above the normal range. An important advance in the prevention of glucocorticoid-related osteoporosis is the successful use of bisphosphonates (e.g., risedronate and zoledronic acid), which have been shown to decrease the decline in bone density and the incidence of fractures in patients receiving glucocorticoid therapy. Additional discussion of these issues is found in Chapters 44 and 48.

Osteonecrosis. Osteonecrosis (also known as avascular or aseptic necrosis) is a relatively common complication of glucocorticoid therapy. The femoral head is affected most frequently, but this process also may affect the humeral head and distal femur. Joint pain and stiffness usually are the earliest symptoms, and this diagnosis should be considered in patients receiving glucocorticoids who abruptly develop hip, shoulder, or knee pain. Although the risk increases with the duration and dose of glucocorticoid therapy, osteonecrosis also can occur when high doses of glucocorticoids are given for short periods of time. Osteonecrosis generally progresses, and most affected patients ultimately require joint replacement.

Regulation of Growth and Development. Growth retardation in children can result from administration of relatively small doses of glucocorticoids. Although the precise mechanism is unknown, there are reports that collagen synthesis and linear growth in these children can be restored by (off-label) treatment with growth hormone; further studies are needed to define the role of concurrent treatment with growth hormone in this setting. In experimental animals, antenatal exposure to glucocorticoids is clearly linked to cleft palate and altered neuronal development, ultimately resulting in complex behavioral abnormalities. The actions of glucocorticoids to promote cellular differentiation play important physiological roles in human development in late gestation and in the neonatal period (e.g., production of pulmonary surfactant and induction of hepatic gluconeogenic enzymes); those actions notwithstanding, antenatal steroids may lead to subtle abnormalities in fetal development. Babies born to women receiving large doses of corticosteroids during pregnancy should be monitored for signs of adrenal insufficiency and appropriate therapy initiated, if necessary.

Therapeutic Uses and Diagnostic Applications in Endocrine Diseases

With the exception of replacement therapy in deficiency states, the use of glucocorticoids largely is empirical. Given the number and severity of potential side effects, the decision to institute therapy with glucocorticoids always requires careful consideration of the relative risks and benefits in each patient. For any disease and in any patient, the optimal dose to achieve a given therapeutic effect must be determined by trial and error and periodic reevaluation as the activity of the underlying disease changes or as complications of therapy arise. *A single dose of glucocorticoid, even a large one, is virtually without harmful effects, and a short course of therapy (up to 1 week), in the absence of specific contraindications, is unlikely to be harmful. As the duration of glucocorticoid therapy is increased beyond 1 week, there are time- and dose-related increases in the incidence of disabling and potentially lethal effects.* Except in patients receiving replacement therapy, glucocorticoids are neither specific nor curative; rather, they are palliative by virtue of their anti-inflammatory and immunosuppressive actions. Finally, *abrupt cessation of glucocorticoids after prolonged therapy is associated with the risk of adrenal insufficiency, which may be fatal.*

When glucocorticoids are to be given over long periods, the dose, determined empirically, must be the lowest that will achieve the desired effect. When the therapeutic goal is relief of painful or distressing symptoms not associated with an immediately life-threatening disease, complete relief is not sought, and the steroid dose is reduced gradually until worsening symptoms indicate that the minimal acceptable dose has been found. Where possible, the substitution of other medications, such as nonsteroidal anti-inflammatory drugs, may facilitate tapering the glucocorticoid

dose once the initial benefit of therapy has been achieved. When therapy is directed at a life-threatening disease (e.g., pemphigus or lupus cerebritis), the initial dose should be a large one aimed at achieving rapid control of the crisis. If some benefit is not observed quickly, then the dose should be doubled or tripled. After initial control in a potentially lethal disease, dose reduction should be carried out under conditions that permit frequent accurate observations of the patient.

The lack of demonstrated deleterious effects of a single dose of glucocorticoids within the conventional therapeutic range justifies their administration to critically ill patients who may have adrenal insufficiency. If the underlying condition does result from deficiency of glucocorticoids, then a single intravenous injection of a soluble glucocorticoid may prevent immediate death and allow time for a definitive diagnosis. If the underlying disease is not adrenal insufficiency, the single dose will not harm the patient. Long courses of therapy at high doses should be reserved for life-threatening disease.

To diminish HPA axis suppression, the intermediate-acting steroid preparations (e.g., prednisone or prednisolone) should be given in the morning as a single dose. Alternate-day therapy with the same glucocorticoids is employed for patients who obtain adequate therapeutic responses on this regimen. Alternatively, pulse therapy with higher glucocorticoid doses (e.g., doses as high as 1–1.5 g/d IV of methylprednisolone for 3 days) frequently is used to initiate therapy in patients with fulminant, immunologically related disorders, such as acute exacerbations of multiple sclerosis, acute transplantation rejection, necrotizing glomerulonephritis, and lupus nephritis.

Replacement Therapy for Adrenal Insufficiency

Adrenal insufficiency can result from structural or functional lesions of the adrenal cortex (primary adrenal insufficiency or Addison disease) or from structural or functional lesions of the anterior pituitary or hypothalamus (secondary adrenal insufficiency). In developed countries, primary adrenal insufficiency most frequently is secondary to autoimmune adrenal disease, whereas tuberculous adrenalitis is the most frequent etiology in developing countries. Other causes include adrenalectomy, bilateral adrenal hemorrhage, neoplastic infiltration of the adrenal glands, AIDS, inherited disorders of the steroidogenic enzymes, and X-linked adrenoleukodystrophy. Secondary adrenal insufficiency resulting from pituitary or hypothalamic dysfunction generally presents in a more insidious manner than does the primary disorder, probably because mineralocorticoid biosynthesis is preserved.

Acute Adrenal Insufficiency. The life-threatening disease of acute adrenal insufficiency is characterized by GI symptoms (nausea, vomiting, and abdominal pain), dehydration, hyponatremia, hyperkalemia, weakness, lethargy, and hypotension. It usually is associated with disorders of the adrenal rather than the pituitary or hypothalamus and sometimes follows abrupt withdrawal of glucocorticoids used at high doses or for prolonged periods.

The immediate management of patients with acute adrenal insufficiency includes intravenous therapy with isotonic NaCl solution supplemented with 5% glucose and corticosteroids and appropriate therapy for precipitating causes such as infection, trauma, or hemorrhage. Because cardiac function often is reduced in the setting of adrenocortical insufficiency, the patient should be monitored for evidence of volume overload, such as rising central venous pressure or pulmonary edema. After an initial intravenous bolus of 100 mg, hydrocortisone should be given by continuous infusion at a rate of 50–100 mg every 8 h, a dose that confers sufficient mineralocorticoid activity to meet all requirements. As the patient stabilizes, the hydrocortisone dose may be decreased to 25 mg every 6–8 h. Thereafter, patients are treated in the same fashion as those with chronic adrenal insufficiency. For the initial management of unconfirmed acute adrenal insufficiency, 4 mg of dexamethasone sodium phosphate can be substituted for hydrocortisone; dexamethasone does not cross-react in the cortisol assay and will not interfere with the measurement of cortisol (either basally or in response to the cosyntropin [ACTH] stimulation test). Failure to respond to cosyntropin in this setting is diagnostic of adrenal insufficiency.

Chronic Adrenal Insufficiency. Patients with chronic adrenal insufficiency present with many of the same manifestations seen in adrenal crisis but with lesser severity. These patients require daily treatment with corticosteroids. The adequacy of corticosteroid replacement therapy is judged by clinical criteria and biochemical measurements. The subjective well-being of the patient is an important clinical parameter in primary and secondary disease. In primary adrenal insufficiency, the disappearance of hyperpigmentation and the resolution of electrolyte abnormalities are valuable indicators of adequate replacement. Overtreatment may cause manifestations of Cushing syndrome in adults and decreased linear growth in children. Plasma ACTH levels may be used to monitor therapy in patients with primary adrenal insufficiency; the early-morning ACTH level should not be suppressed but should be less than 100 pg/mL (22 pmol/L).

Traditional replacement regimens have used hydrocortisone in doses of 20–30 mg/d; however, some authorities use lower doses of 15–20 mg/d based on estimates of daily rates of cortisol production (Table 46–1). *Cortisone acetate*, which is inactive until converted to cortisol by 11β-HSD1, also has been used in doses ranging from 25 to 37.5 mg/d. In an effort to mimic the normal diurnal rhythm of cortisol secretion, these glucocorticoids generally have been given in divided doses, with two-thirds of the dose given in the morning and one-third given in the afternoon. Although some patients with primary adrenal insufficiency can be maintained on hydrocortisone and liberal salt intake, most of these patients also require mineralocorticoid replacement; fludrocortisone acetate generally is used in doses of 0.05–0.2 mg/d. In secondary adrenal insufficiency, the administration of a glucocorticoid alone is generally adequate because the zona glomerulosa, which makes mineralocorticoids, is usually intact.

When initiating treatment in patients with panhypopituitarism, administer glucocorticoids before initiating treatment with thyroid hormone because the administration of thyroid hormone may precipitate acute adrenal insufficiency by increasing the metabolism of cortisol. Dexamethasone and prednisone also have been used as chronic replacement therapy; however, careful monitoring for hypercorticoidism is required due to their increased potency and longer durations of action.

Standard doses of glucocorticoids often must be adjusted upward in patients who also are taking drugs that increase their metabolic clearance (e.g., phenytoin, barbiturates, or rifampin) or who suffer the stress of intercurrent illness. *All patients with adrenal insufficiency should wear a medical alert bracelet or tag that lists their diagnosis and carries information about their steroid regimen.* During minor illness, the glucocorticoid dose should be doubled. The patient and family members should also be trained to administer parenteral dexamethasone (4 mg intramuscularly) in the event that severe nausea or vomiting precludes the oral administration of medications; they then should seek medical attention immediately. Glucocorticoid doses also are adjusted when patients with adrenal insufficiency undergo surgery. In this setting, the doses are designed to approximate or exceed the maximal cortisol secretory rate of 200 mg/d; a standard regimen is hydrocortisone 100 mg parenterally every 8 h. Following surgery, the dose is halved each day until it is reduced to routine maintenance levels.

Congenital Adrenal Hyperplasia. CAH is a group of genetic disorders in which there is a deficiency in the activity of one of several enzymes required for the biosynthesis of glucocorticoids. The impaired production of cortisol and the consequent lack of negative-feedback inhibition lead to increased release of ACTH. As a result, other hormonally active steroids that are proximal to the enzymatic block in the steroidogenic pathway are produced in excess. CAH includes a spectrum of disorders for which precise clinical presentation, laboratory findings, and treatment depend on which of the steroidogenic enzymes is deficient. In about 90% of patients, CAH results from mutations in CYP21, the enzyme that carries out the 21-hydroxylation reaction (see Figure 46–3).

Clinically, patients are divided into those with classic CAH, who have severe defects in enzymatic activity and first present during childhood, and those with nonclassic CAH, who present after puberty with signs and symptoms of mild androgen excess, such as hirsutism, amenorrhea, infertility, and acne. Female patients with classic CAH frequently are born with virilized external genitalia (female pseudohermaphroditism) that result

from elevated production of adrenal androgen precursors at critical stages of sexual differentiation in utero and often require reconstructive genital surgery. Some medical centers have experimented with dexamethasone administration in utero with success; however, this approach is highly controversial because of concerns regarding abnormal behavioral development after prenatal exposure to glucocorticoids (Miller and Witchel, 2013). Males appear normal at birth and later may have precocious development of secondary sexual characteristics (isosexual precocious puberty). In both sexes, linear growth is accelerated in childhood, but the adult height is reduced by premature closure of the epiphyses. Some patients with classical CAH are unable to conserve Na$^+$ normally and thus are called "salt wasters."

All patients with classical CAH require replacement therapy with hydrocortisone or a suitable congener, and those with salt wasting also require mineralocorticoid replacement. The goals of therapy are to restore levels of physiological steroid hormones to the normal range and to suppress ACTH and thereby abrogate the effects of overproduction of adrenal androgens. The typical oral dose of hydrocortisone is about 0.6 mg/kg daily in two or three divided doses. The mineralocorticoid used is fludrocortisone acetate (0.05–0.2 mg/d). Many experts also administer table salt to infants (one-fifth of a teaspoon dissolved in formula daily) until the child is eating solid food. Therapy is guided by gain in weight and height, by plasma levels of 17-hydroxyprogesterone, and by blood pressure. Elevated plasma renin activity suggests that the patient is receiving an inadequate dose of mineralocorticoid. Sudden spurts in linear growth often indicate inadequate pituitary suppression and excessive androgen secretion, whereas growth failure suggests overtreatment with glucocorticoid.

Diagnostic Applications of Dexamethasone

In addition to its therapeutic uses, dexamethasone is used as a first-line agent to diagnose hypercortisolism and to differentiate among the different causes of Cushing syndrome (Arnaldi et al., 2003). To determine if patients with clinical manifestations suggestive of hypercortisolism have biochemical evidence of increased cortisol biosynthesis, an overnight dexamethasone suppression test has been devised. Patients are given 1 mg of dexamethasone orally at 11 PM, and cortisol is measured at 8 AM the following morning. Suppression of plasma cortisol to less than 1.8 µg/dL suggests strongly that the patient does not have Cushing syndrome. Drugs such as barbiturates that enhance dexamethasone metabolism or drugs (estrogens) or conditions (pregnancy) that increase the concentrations of CBG can interfere with suppression and compromise the test.

The formal dexamethasone suppression test is used in the differential diagnosis of biochemically documented Cushing syndrome. Following determination of baseline cortisol levels for 48 h, dexamethasone (0.5 mg every 6 h) is administered orally for 48 h. This dose markedly suppresses cortisol levels in normal subjects, including those who have nonspecific elevations of cortisol due to obesity or stress, but it does not suppress levels in patients with Cushing syndrome. In the high-dose phase of the test, dexamethasone is administered orally at 2 mg every 6 h for 48 h. Patients with pituitary-dependent Cushing syndrome (i.e., Cushing disease) generally respond with decreased cortisol levels. In contrast, patients with ectopic production of ACTH or with adrenocortical tumors generally do not exhibit decreased cortisol levels. Despite these generalities, dexamethasone may suppress cortisol levels in some patients with ectopic ACTH production, particularly with tumors such as bronchial carcinoids, and many experts prefer to use inferior petrosal sinus sampling after CRH administration to make this distinction.

Therapeutic Uses in Nonendocrine Diseases

There are important uses of glucocorticoids in diseases that do not directly involve the HPA axis. The disorders discussed next illustrate the principles governing glucocorticoid use in selected diseases. The dosage of glucocorticoids varies considerably depending on the nature and severity of the underlying disorder. Approximate doses of a representative glucocorticoid (e.g., prednisone) are provided.

Rheumatic Disorders

Glucocorticoids are used widely in the treatment of rheumatic disorders and are a mainstay in the treatment of the more serious inflammatory rheumatic diseases, such as systemic lupus erythematosus, and a variety of vasculitic disorders, such as polyarteritis nodosa, Wegener granulomatosis, Churg-Strauss syndrome, and giant cell arteritis. For these more serious disorders, the starting dose of glucocorticoids should be sufficient to suppress the disease rapidly and minimize resultant tissue damage. Initially, prednisone (1 mg/kg/d in divided doses) often is used, generally followed by consolidation to a single daily dose, with subsequent tapering to a minimal effective dose as determined by the clinical picture.

Glucocorticoids are often used in conjunction with other immunosuppressive agents such as cyclophosphamide and methotrexate, which offer better long-term control than steroids alone. The exception is giant cell arteritis, for which glucocorticoids remain superior to other agents. Caution should be exercised in the use of glucocorticoids in some forms of vasculitis (e.g., polyarteritis nodosa), for which underlying infections with hepatitis viruses may play a pathogenetic role. Intermediate-acting glucocorticoids, such as prednisone and prednisolone, are generally preferred over longer-acting steroids such as dexamethasone.

In rheumatoid arthritis, because of the serious and debilitating side effects associated with their chronic use, glucocorticoids are used as stabilizing agents for progressive disease that fails to respond to first-line treatments such as physiotherapy and nonsteroidal anti-inflammatory drugs. In this case, glucocorticoids provide relief until other, slower-acting antirheumatic drugs (e.g., methotrexate or agents targeted at TNF) take effect. A typical starting dose is 5–10 mg of prednisone per day. In the setting of an acute exacerbation, higher doses of glucocorticoids may be employed (typically 20–40 mg/d of prednisone or equivalent), with rapid taper thereafter. Alternatively, patients with major symptomatology confined to one or a few joints may be treated with intra-articular steroid injections. Depending on joint size, typical doses are 5–20 mg of the very long-lasting triamcinolone acetonide or its equivalent.

In noninflammatory degenerative joint diseases (e.g., osteoarthritis) or in a variety of regional pain syndromes (e.g., tendinitis or bursitis), glucocorticoids may be administered by local injection for the treatment of episodic disease flare-up. It is important to use a glucocorticoid that does not require bioactivation (e.g., prednisolone rather than prednisone) and to minimize the frequency of local steroid administration whenever possible. In the case of repeated intra-articular injection of steroids, there is a significant incidence of painless joint destruction, resembling Charcot arthropathy. It is recommended that intra-articular injections be performed with intervals of at least 3 months to minimize complications.

Renal Diseases

Patients with nephrotic syndrome secondary to minimal change disease generally respond well to steroid therapy, and glucocorticoids are the first-line treatment in both adults and children. Initial daily doses of prednisone are 1–2 mg/kg for 6 weeks, followed by a gradual tapering of the dose over 6–8 weeks, although some nephrologists advocate alternate-day therapy. Objective evidence of response, such as diminished proteinuria, is seen within 2–3 weeks in 85% of patients, and more than 95% of patients enter remission within 3 months. Patients with renal disease secondary to systemic lupus erythematosus also are generally given a therapeutic trial of glucocorticoids. In the case of membranous glomerulonephritis, many nephrologists recommend a trial of alternate-day glucocorticoids for 8–10 weeks (e.g., prednisone 120 mg every other day), followed by a 1- to 2-month period of tapering.

Allergic Diseases

The onset of action of glucocorticoids in allergic diseases is delayed, and patients with severe allergic reactions such as anaphylaxis require immediate therapy with epinephrine. The manifestations of allergic diseases of limited duration—such as hay fever, serum sickness, urticaria, contact dermatitis, drug reactions, bee stings, and angioneurotic edema—can be suppressed by adequate doses of glucocorticoids given as supplements to the primary therapy. In severe disease, intravenous glucocorticoids (methylprednisolone 125 mg IV every 6 h or equivalent) are appropriate. For allergic rhinitis, many experts recommend intranasal steroids.

Pulmonary Diseases

The use of glucocorticoids in bronchial asthma and other pulmonary diseases is discussed in Chapter 40. Antenatal glucocorticoids are used

frequently in the setting of premature labor, decreasing the incidence of respiratory distress syndrome, intraventricular hemorrhage, and death in infants delivered prematurely. Betamethasone (12 mg IM every 24 h for two doses) or dexamethasone (6 mg IM every 12 h for four doses) is administered to women with definitive signs of premature labor between 26 and 34 weeks of gestation. For women still at risk of preterm birth 7 or more days after receiving the initial glucocorticoid dose, a meta-analysis of 10 randomized clinical trials involving over 4730 women and 5700 infants showed that a second course of treatment reduced the risk of respiratory distress syndrome and serious neonatal morbidity without adverse effects in infants followed for 2 to 3 years after (McKinlay et al., 2012).

Infectious Diseases

Although the use of immunosuppressive glucocorticoids in infectious diseases may seem paradoxical, there are a limited number of settings in which they are indicated in the therapy of specific infectious pathogens. One example is in patients with AIDS with *Pneumocystis carinii* pneumonia and moderate-to-severe hypoxia; addition of glucocorticoids to the antibiotic regimen increases oxygenation and lowers the incidence of respiratory failure and mortality. Similarly, glucocorticoids clearly decrease the incidence of long-term neurological impairment associated with *Haemophilus influenzae* type b meningitis in infants and children 2 months of age or older.

Ocular Diseases

Glucocorticoids frequently are used to suppress inflammation in the eye and can preserve sight when used properly. They are administered topically for diseases of the outer eye and anterior segment and attain therapeutic concentrations in the aqueous humor after instillation into the conjunctival sac. For diseases of the posterior segment, intraocular injection or systemic administration is required. These uses of glucocorticoids are discussed in Chapter 69.

Skin Diseases

Glucocorticoids are remarkably efficacious in the treatment of a wide variety of inflammatory dermatoses. A typical regimen for an eczematous eruption is 1% hydrocortisone ointment applied locally twice daily. Effectiveness is enhanced by application of the topical steroid under an occlusive film, such as plastic wrap; unfortunately, the risk of systemic absorption also is increased by occlusive dressings, and this can be a significant problem when the more potent glucocorticoids are applied to inflamed skin. Glucocorticoids are administered systemically for severe episodes of acute dermatological disorders and for exacerbations of chronic disorders. The dose in these settings is usually 40 mg/d of prednisone. Systemic steroid administration can be lifesaving in pemphigus, which may require daily doses of up to 120 mg of prednisone. Chapter 70 presents the dermatologic uses of glucocorticoids.

Gastrointestinal Diseases

Patients with inflammatory bowel disease (chronic ulcerative colitis and Crohn disease) who fail to respond to more conservative management (i.e., rest, diet, and sulfasalazine) may benefit from glucocorticoids; steroids are most useful for acute exacerbations (see Chapter 51).

Hepatic Diseases

The use of corticosteroids in hepatic disease has been controversial. Glucocorticoids clearly are of benefit in autoimmune hepatitis; as many as 80% of patients show histological remission when treated with prednisone (40–60 mg daily initially, with tapering to a maintenance dose of 7.5–10 mg daily after serum transaminase levels fall). The role of corticosteroids in alcoholic liver disease is not fully defined; the most recent meta-analyses did not support a beneficial role of corticosteroids. In the setting of severe hepatic disease, prednisolone should be used instead of prednisone, which requires hepatic conversion to be active.

Malignancies

Glucocorticoids are used in the chemotherapy of acute lymphocytic leukemia and lymphomas because of their antilymphocytic effects, most commonly as a component of combination therapy (see Chapters 67 and 68). They also are used to manage chemotherapy-induced nausea and vomiting (Table 50–5) and to reduce hypersensitivity reactions and fluid retention associated with taxane chemotherapy (Chapter 66).

Cerebral Edema

Corticosteroids at very high doses (e.g., dexamethasone 4–16 mg every 6 h) are commonly used in the reduction or prevention of cerebral edema associated with parasites and neoplasms, especially those that are metastatic.

Miscellaneous Uses

Sarcoidosis. Corticosteroids are indicated therapy for patients with debilitating symptoms or life-threatening forms of sarcoidosis. Patients with severe pulmonary involvement are treated with 20–40 mg/d of prednisone, or an equivalent dose of alternative steroids, to induce remission. Higher doses may be required for other forms of this disease. Maintenance doses may be as low as 5 mg/d of prednisone. All patients who require chronic glucocorticoid therapy at doses exceeding the normal daily production rate are at increased risk of secondary tuberculosis; therefore, patients with a positive tuberculin reaction or other evidence of tuberculosis should be considered for prophylactic antituberculosis therapy.

Thrombocytopenia. In thrombocytopenia, prednisone (0.5 mg/kg) is used to decrease the bleeding tendency. In more severe cases, and for initiation of treatment of idiopathic thrombocytopenia, daily doses of prednisone (1–1.5 mg/kg) are employed. Patients with refractory idiopathic thrombocytopenia may respond to pulsed high-dose glucocorticoid therapy.

Autoimmune Destruction of Erythrocytes. Patients with autoimmune destruction of erythrocytes (i.e., hemolytic anemia with a positive Coombs test) are treated with prednisone (1 mg/kg/d). In the setting of severe hemolysis, higher doses may be used, with tapering as the anemia improves. Small maintenance doses may be required for several months in patients who respond.

Organ Transplantation. In organ transplantation, high doses of prednisone (50–100 mg) are given at the time of transplant surgery, in conjunction with other immunosuppressive agents, and most patients are kept on a maintenance regimen that includes lower doses of glucocorticoids (see Chapter 35). For some solid-organ transplants (e.g., pancreas), protocols that either withdraw corticosteroids early after transplantation or that avoid them completely have become more common (Niederhaus et al., 2013).

Spinal Cord Injury. Large doses of methylprednisolone sodium succinate (30 mg/kg initially followed by an infusion of 5.4 mg/kg/h for 23 h) are a treatment option for patients with acute spinal cord injury. Although, multicenter controlled trials have demonstrated decreases in neurological defects in patients with acute spinal cord injury treated within 8 h of injury (Bracken, 2012), concerns regarding statistical analysis, reproducibility of data, and potential side effects of treatment have caused some experts to advocate against use of methylprednisolone in this setting (Hurlbert et al., 2013).

Inhibitors of ACTH Secretion and the Biosynthesis and Actions of Adrenocortical Steroids

Hypercortisolism with its attendant morbidity and mortality is most frequently caused by corticotroph adenomas that overproduce ACTH (Cushing disease) or by adrenocortical tumors or bilateral hyperplasias that overproduce cortisol (Cushing syndrome). Less frequently, hypercortisolism may result from adrenocortical carcinomas or ectopic ACTH- or CRH-producing tumors. Although surgery is the treatment of choice, it is not always effective, and adjuvant therapy with pharmacological inhibitors becomes necessary. In these settings, inhibitors of ACTH secretion and of adrenal steroidogenesis are clinically useful. All of these agents pose the common risk of precipitating acute adrenal insufficiency; thus, they must be used in appropriate doses, and the status of the patient's HPA axis

must be carefully monitored. Most of the inhibitors discussed here are considered in detail in other chapters; mineralocorticoid antagonists are not considered here but are discussed in Chapter 25.

Inhibitors of ACTH Secretion

Pasireotide

Pasireotide is a somatostatin analogue that is an agonist at four of the five subtypes of SSTR, with especially high affinity for SSTR5. Through these interactions, pasireotide effectively inhibits growth hormone secretion and is used in the treatment of acromegaly (Chapter 42). Pasireotide also inhibits ACTH secretion and reduces the circulating levels of cortisol in patients with ACTH-producing pituitary tumors; the agent is FDA-approved for use in those patients with Cushing disease who are not candidates for surgery or who have recurrent disease. At subcutaneous doses of 0.6 or 0.9 mg twice daily, pasireotide reduces urinary free cortisol levels by at least 50% in approximately half the treated patients; depending on the dose, cortisol levels reach the normal range in 15%–26% of patients. Treatment improves signs and symptoms of hypercortisolism, including blood pressure, low-density lipoprotein cholesterol, and body mass index. Common adverse effects include hyperglycemia, gallstones, and transient GI discomfort (Colao et al., 2012).

Cabergoline

Cabergoline is a potent long-acting dopamine D_2 receptor agonist used primarily to treat hyperprolactinemia (Chapter 42). Cabergoline also inhibits ACTH secretion from corticotroph tumors, which are often D_2 receptor positive. Several small studies have shown that 37% of patients with recurrent Cushing disease achieve normal levels of free urinary cortisol when treated with cabergoline. The FDA has not yet approved cabergoline for this use.

Inhibitors of Steroidogenesis

Ketoconazole

Ketoconazole is an antifungal agent (see Chapter 61). In doses higher than those employed in antifungal therapy, it is an effective inhibitor of adrenal and gonadal steroidogenesis, primarily because it inhibits the activity of CYP17 (17α-hydroxylase). At even higher doses, ketoconazole also inhibits CYP11A1, effectively blocking steroidogenesis in all primary steroidogenic tissues. Ketoconazole is an effective inhibitor of steroid hormone biosynthesis in patients with hypercortisolism (although the FDA has not approved use for this indication). In most cases, a dosage regimen of 600–800 mg/d (in two divided doses) is required, and some patients may require up to 1200 mg/d (in two or three doses). Side effects include hepatic dysfunction with the possibility of severe hepatic injury. The potential of ketoconazole to alter drug transport and metabolism by inhibiting P-glycoprotein and CYP3A4 can lead to serious drug interactions (see Chapters 5 and 6).

Metyrapone

Metyrapone is a relatively selective inhibitor of CYP11B1 and thus inhibits the conversion of 11-deoxycortisol to cortisol, thereby reducing cortisol production and elevating precursor levels (e.g., 11-deoxycortisol and its precursor 11-deoxycorticosterone). Although the biosynthesis of aldosterone also is impaired, the elevated levels of 11-deoxycorticosterone and 11-deoxycortisol sustain mineralocorticoid-dependent functions. In a diagnostic test of the entire HPA axis, metyrapone (30 mg/kg, maximum dose of 3 g) is administered orally with a snack at midnight, and plasma cortisol and 11-deoxycortisol are measured at 8 AM the next morning. A plasma cortisol less than 8 μg/dL validates adequate inhibition of CYP11B1; in this setting, an 11-deoxycortisol level less than 7 μg/dL is highly suggestive of impaired HPA function.

Metyrapone has been used off label to treat the hypercortisolism resulting from either adrenal neoplasms or tumors ectopically producing ACTH. Maximal suppression of steroidogenesis requires doses of 4 g/d. More frequently, metyrapone is used as adjunctive therapy in patients who have received pituitary irradiation or in combination with other agents that inhibit steroidogenesis. In this setting, a dose of 500–750 mg three or four times daily is employed. The use of metyrapone in the treatment of Cushing syndrome secondary to pituitary hypersecretion of ACTH is more controversial. Chronic administration of metyrapone can cause hirsutism, which results from increased synthesis of adrenal androgens upstream from the enzymatic block, and hypertension, which results from elevated levels of 11-deoxycortisol/11-deoxycorticosterone. Other side effects include nausea, headache, sedation, and rash.

Etomidate

Etomidate, a substituted imidazole used primarily as an anesthetic agent and sedative, inhibits cortisol secretion at subhypnotic doses primarily by inhibiting CYP11B1 activity. Etomidate has been used off label to treat hypercortisolism when rapid control is required in a patient who cannot take medication by the oral route. Etomidate is administered as a bolus of 0.03 mg/kg intravenously, followed by an infusion of 0.1 mg/kg/h to a maximum of 0.3 mg/kg/h (Biller et al., 2008).

Mitotane

MITOTANE (o,p′ DDD)

Mitotane is an adrenocorticolytic agent used to treat inoperable adrenocortical carcinoma. Its cytolytic action is due to its metabolic conversion to a reactive acyl chloride by adrenal mitochondrial CYPs and subsequent reactivity with cellular proteins. It also inhibits CYP11A1 (cholesterol side-chain cleavage enzyme), thereby reducing steroid synthesis. Initial doses range from 2 to 6 g/d administered orally in three or four divided doses. The maintenance dose is 9–10 g/d in three or four divided doses. The maximal dose can be as high as 16 g/d, if tolerated. Its onset of action takes weeks to months, and GI disturbances and ataxia are its major toxicities. See Chapter 66 for the structure of mitotane and additional details on its use.

Glucocorticoid Antagonist

Mifepristone

Mifepristone (RU-486), is a progesterone receptor antagonist used to terminate early pregnancy (see Chapter 44). At higher doses, mifepristone also inhibits the GRs, blocking feedback regulation of the HPA axis and secondarily increasing endogenous ACTH and cortisol levels. Because of its capacity to inhibit glucocorticoid action, mifepristone also has been studied as a potential therapeutic agent in a small number of patients with hypercortisolism. Mifepristone has been granted orphan drug status in the U.S. for the treatment of hyperglycemia secondary to endogenous Cushing syndrome in patients who have type 2 diabetes mellitus or glucose intolerance and have failed surgery or are not candidates for surgery.

Drug Facts for Your Personal Formulary: *Adrenal Related*

Drugs	Therapeutic Uses	Clinical Pharmacology and Tips
Replacement Therapy		
Hydrocortisone/cortisone	Primary and secondary chronic adrenal insufficiency	• Hydrocortisone is the synthetic equivalent of cortisol. • Daily oral dose of hydrocortisone is 20–30 mg, preferably as divided doses. • Although nonphysiologic glucocorticoids are sometimes used, hydrocortisone or cortisone is preferred for replacement therapy. • Tip: Two-thirds of dose in the morning, one-third of dose in the evening.
Hydrocortisone, other glucocorticoids	Acute adrenal insufficiency Critical illness-related cortisol insufficiency (CIRCI)	• CIRCI reflects inadequate cortisol production or may occur with abrupt cessation of administered glucocorticoids. • High-dose intravenous hydrocortisone (50–100 mg/6 h) or a constant infusion of 10 mg/h is needed. • An alternative is prednisone at 1 mg/kg/d.
Fludrocortisone (9α-fluorocortisol)	Mineralocorticoid replacement	• Doses of 0.05–0.2 mg/d. • Lower dose is used initially and is titrated upward as required by blood pressure, plasma renin levels, and response to upright posture. • Fludrocortisone has a $t_{1/2} \geq 24$ h so divided doses are not necessary.
Anti-inflammatory Agents: Systemic		
Prednisolone, methylprednisolone Dexamethasone, budesonide Others	Across the spectrum of inflammatory disease Preterm (24–34 weeks) delivery	• Initial high-dose tapering to low dose in short-course therapy. • In early therapy—insomnia, weight gain, emotional lability • With high-dose/long-term therapy: psychosis, increased susceptibility to infection, osteoporosis, osteonecrosis, myopathy, HPA axis suppression. • On cessation of therapy: acute hypocortisolism. • Tip: Constant vigilance.
Anti-inflammatory Agents: Topical		
Betamethasone Hydrocortisone Beclomethasone Dexamethasone Triamcinolone acetonide	Dermatitis, pemphigus, atopic dermatitis, vitiligo, psoriasis, etc.	• Fluorinated steroids have better skin penetration than hydrocortisone. • Effects are magnified by occlusive dressings. • Local adverse events: atrophy, striae, and exacerbation of skin infection. • Tip: Skin-lightening cosmetics include corticosteroids and may produce serious systemic adverse events.

Drug Facts for Your Personal Formulary: *Adrenal Related* (*continued*)

Drugs	Therapeutic Uses	Clinical Pharmacology and Tips
Anti-inflammatory Agents: Ophthalmic		
Dexamethasone Triamcinolone acetonide Fluocinolone acetate (implant)	Macular disease (degeneration, edema, retinal vein occlusion) Postoperative inflammation Corneal injury Uveitis	• Commonly repeated at 3-month intervals • Adverse effects: glaucoma, cataract formation • Contraindications: glaucoma, eye infections
Anti-inflammatory Agents: Inhaled		
Beclomethasone, budesonide, ciclesonide, flunisolide, fluticasone, mometasone, triamcinolone acetonide	Asthma, chronic obstructive pulmonary disease	• Rapid metabolism postabsorption into blood is the key for lung selectivity and lower incidence of adverse events. • Chronic use in children may slow growth velocity without compromising final height. • Tip: Ciclesonide, a pro-drug converted to active des-ciclesonide in the lung, has low oral bioavailability and less HPA suppression.
Anti-inflammatory Agents: Intranasal		
Mometasone furoate Fluticasone furoate Fluticasone propionate	Allergic rhinitis, rhinosinusitis, rhinoconjunctivitis, nasal polyposis, postoperatively for sinus ostia stenosis surgery	• Potent localized activity, minimal systemic risk. • Tip: Avoid frequent use.
Anti-inflammatory Steroids: Intra-articular		
Hydrocortisone	Relief of joint pain	• Local and systemic adverse events rare. • Success varies with difficulty (e.g., vertebral facet joints versus knees).
Chemotherapy		
Dexamethasone Prednisolone Methylprednisolone Prednisone	Acute lymphatic leukemia Chronic lymphatic leukemia Thymoma Non-Hodgkin lymphoma Multiple myeloma, breast cancer	• Used in combination with a variety of chemotherapeutic agents. • Used for primary cytotoxic effects, plus relief of pain and nausea and appetite stimulation. • Tip: No place in acute or chronic myelogenous leukemia.
Diagnostics		
Dexamethasone	Cushing disease	• ↓ ACTH secretion from pituitary corticotrophs but not from ectopic sources.
Metyrapone	Integrity of entire HPA axis	• Inhibits CYP11B1, thereby reducing cortisol and ↑ levels of precursor steroids. • Failure to adequately ↑ precursor levels indicates impaired HPA function.
Cosyntropin (synthetic ACTH)	Ectopic ACTH secretion Adrenal insufficiency Lateralization of aldosterone overproduction	• Cosyntropin is a truncated synthetic form of ACTH used to test adrenal reserve. • Tip: Cosyntropin is commonly used as either a bolus before or a continuous infusion during adrenal venous sampling to distinguish between unilateral and bilateral aldosterone oversecretion in primary aldosteronism.
Stimulant of ACTH Secretion		
Corticorelin	Peritumoral brain edema postsurgery (off-label use); diagnostic testing	• A synthetic CRH, preferred to high-dose dexamethasone in relieving peritumoral brain edema. • Used diagnostically to distinguish Cushing disease from ectopic ACTH syndrome.
Inhibitors of ACTH Secretion		
Pasireotide	ACTH oversecretion (Cushing disease)	• Targets $SSTR_5$ (abundant on corticotrophs), ↓ ACTH secretion; used for recurrent or non-resectable ACTH-secreting adenomas
Cabergoline	ACTH oversecretion and hyperprolactinemia	• D_2 receptor agonist; ↓ ACTH secretion, ↓ prolactin secretion; useful but not FDA-approved for Cushing disease
Inhibitors of Corticosteroid Production		
Ketoconazole	Hypercortisolism (off-label use) (Used at lower doses as antifungal agent; see Chapter 61)	• ↓ CYP17 (17α-hydroxylase) and CYP11A1 (cholesterol side chain cleavage), ↓ adrenal and gonadal steroidogenesis • Adverse effects: hepatic toxicity; drug interactions due to inhibition of CYP3A4 and P-glycoprotein
Metyrapone	Hypercortisolism; adjunctive therapy after pituitary irradiation	• Inhibits CYP11B1 (11-deoxy cortisol → cortisol), • ↓ cortisol; 4 g/d to maximally ↓ steroidogenesis • chronic use may cause hirsutism & hypertension
Etomidate	Rapid control of hypercorticolism (off label use) (Also a short-acting anesthetic; see Chapter 21)	• Inhibits CYP11B1 (11-deoxy cortisol → cortisol), • ↓ cortisol production at sub-anesthetic doses • Administer as IV bolus, 0.03 mg/kg

Inhibitors of Corticosteroid Production (continued)		
Mitotane	Treating inoperable adrenocortical carcinoma (See also Chapter 66)	• Activated by adrenal cortical CYPs to an acyl chloride with cytolytic effects • Inhibits CYP11A1 (cholesterol side chain cleavage), ↓ steroidogenesis
Glucocorticoid Antagonist		
Mifepristone (RU486)	Hypercortisolism (Used at lower doses as anti-progesterone for termination of early pregnancy; see Chapter 44)	• GR antagonist, IC_{50}~2.2 nM (IC_{50} for anti-progesterone effect, ~0.025 nM) • Used at 300-1200 mg/d to treat inoperable hypercortisolism that is resistant to other agents

Bibliography

Arnaldi G, et al. Diagnosis and complications of Cushing's syndrome: a consensus statement. *J Clin Endocrinol Metab*, **2003**, *88*:5593–5602.

Biller BM, et al. Treatment of adrenocorticotropin-dependent Cushing's syndrome: a consensus statement. *J Clin Endocrinol Metab*, **2008**, *93*:2454–2462.

Bracken MB. Steroids for acute spinal cord injury. *Cochrane Database Syst Rev 1*, **2012**, (1):CD001046. doi:10.1002/14651858.CD001046.pub2. Accessed March, 2016.

Colao A, et al. Pasireotide B2305 Study Group. A 12-month phase 3 study of pasireotide in Cushing's disease. *N Engl J Med*, **2012**, *366*: 914–924.

Cone RD. Studies on the physiological functions of the melanocortin system. *Endocr Rev*, **2006**, *27*:736–749.

De Bosscher K, et al. The interplay between the glucocorticoid receptor and nuclear factor-kappaB or activator protein-1: molecular mechanisms for gene repression. *Endocr Rev*, **2003**, *24*:488–522.

Holsboer F, Ising M. Central CRH system in depression and anxiety—evidence from clinical studies with CRH1 receptor antagonists. *Eur J Pharmacol*, **2008**, *583*:350–357.

Hurlbert RJ, et al. Pharmacological therapy for acute spinal cord injury. *Neurosurgery*, **2013**, *72*(suppl 2):93–105.

Leliavski A, et al. Adrenal clocks and the role of adrenal hormones in the regulation of circadian physiology. *J Biol Rhythms*, **2015**, *30*:20–34.

McKinlay CJ, et al. Repeat antenatal glucocorticoids for women at risk of preterm birth: a Cochrane Systematic Review. *Am J Obstet Gynecol*, **2012**, *206*:187–194.

Miller WL. A brief history of adrenal research: steroidogenesis—the soul of the adrenal. *Mol Cell Endocrinol*, **2013**, *371*:5–14.

Miller WL, Auchus RJ. The molecular biology, biochemistry, and physiology of human steroidogenesis and its disorders. *Endocr Rev*, **2011**, *32*:81–151.

Miller WL, Witchel SF. Prenatal treatment of congenital adrenal hyperplasia: risks outweigh benefits. *Am J Obstet Gynecol*, **2013**, *208*:354–359.

Montero-Melendez T. ACTH: The forgotten therapy. *Semin Immunol*, **2015**, *27*:216–226.

Morgan C, Cone RD. Melanocortin-5 receptor deficiency in mice blocks a novel pathway influencing pheromone-induced aggression. *Behav Genet*, **2006**, *36*:291–300.

Niederhaus SV, et al. Induction therapy in pancreas transplantation. *Transpl Int*, **2013**, *26*:704–714.

Papadimitriou A, Priftis KN. Regulation of the hypothalamic-pituitary-adrenal axis. *Neuroimmunomodulation*, **2009**, *16*:265–271.

Prigent H, et al. Science review: mechanisms of impaired adrenal function in sepsis and molecular actions of glucocorticoids. *Crit Care*, **2004**, *8*:243–252.

Schimmer BP, White PC. Minireview: steroidogenic factor 1: its roles in differentiation, development, and disease. *Mol Endocrinol*, **2010**, *24*:1322–1337.

Takahashi A, Mizusawa K. Posttranslational modifications of proopiomelanocortin in vertebrates and their biological significance. *Front Endocrinol (Lausanne)*, **2013**, *4*:143.

Turnbull AV, Rivier CL. Regulation of the hypothalamic-pituitary-adrenal axis by cytokines: actions and mechanisms of action. *Physiol Rev*, **1999**, *79*:1–71.

Vandevyver S, et al. Comprehensive overview of the structure and regulation of the glucocorticoid receptor. *Endocr Rev*, **2014**, *35*:671–693.

Zannad F, Radauceanu A. Effect of MR blockade on collagen formation and cardiovascular disease with a specific emphasis on heart failure. *Heart Fail Rev*, **2005**, *10*:71–80.

SECTION V

HORMONES AND HORMONE ANTAGONISTS

Chapter 47

Endocrine Pancreas and Pharmacotherapy of Diabetes Mellitus and Hypoglycemia

Alvin C. Powers and David D'Alessio

Diabetes mellitus is a spectrum of metabolic disorders arising from myriad pathogenic mechanisms, all resulting in hyperglycemia. Both genetic and environmental factors contribute to its pathogenesis, which involves insufficient insulin secretion, reduced responsiveness to endogenous or exogenous insulin, increased glucose production, or abnormalities in fat and protein metabolism. The resulting hyperglycemia may lead to both acute symptoms and metabolic abnormalities. Major sources of the morbidity of diabetes are the chronic complications that arise from prolonged hyperglycemia, including retinopathy, neuropathy, nephropathy, and cardiovascular disease. These chronic complications can be mitigated in many patients by sustained control of the blood glucose and treatment of comorbidities such as hypertension and dyslipidemia (Nathan, 2014; Orchard et al., 2015). There are now a wide variety of treatment options for hyperglycemia that target different processes involved in glucose regulation or dysregulation (Nathan, 2015).

Physiology of Glucose Homeostasis

Regulation of Blood Glucose

The maintenance of glucose homeostasis, termed *glucose tolerance*, is a highly developed systemic process involving the integration of several major organs (Figure 47–1). Although the actions of insulin are of central importance, webs of interorgan communication via other hormones, nerves, local factors, and substrates also play vital roles. The pancreatic β cell is central in this homeostatic process, adjusting the amount of insulin secreted very precisely to promote glucose uptake after meals and to regulate glucose output from the liver during fasting.

In the *fasting state* (Figure 47–1A), the fuel demands of the body are met by the oxidation of fatty acids. The brain does not effectively use fatty acids to meet energy needs and in the fasting state requires glucose for normal function; glucose requirements are about 2 mg/kg/min in adult humans, largely to supply the CNS with an energy source. *Fasting glucose*

requirements are primarily provided by the liver. Liver glycogen stores provide some of this glucose; conversion of lactate, alanine, and glycerol into glucose accounts for the remainder. The dominant regulation of hepatic *glycogenolysis* and *gluconeogenesis* is controlled by the pancreatic islet hormones *insulin* and *glucagon*. Insulin inhibits hepatic glucose production, and the decline of circulating insulin concentrations in the postabsorptive state (fasting) is permissive for higher rates of glucose output. Glucagon maintains blood glucose concentrations at physiological levels in the absence of exogenous carbohydrate (overnight and in between meals) by stimulating gluconeogenesis and glycogenolysis by the liver. Insulin secretion is stimulated by *food ingestion*, nutrient absorption, and elevated blood glucose, and insulin promotes glucose, lipid, and protein anabolism (Figure 47–1B). The centrality of insulin in glucose metabolism is emphasized by the fact that all the forms of human diabetes have as a root cause some abnormality of insulin secretion or action.

Pancreatic *β cell* function is primarily controlled by plasma glucose concentrations. Elevations of blood glucose are necessary for insulin release above basal levels, and other stimuli are relatively ineffective when plasma glucose is in the fasting range (4.4–5.5 mM or 80–100 mg%). These other stimuli include nutrient substrates, *insulinotropic hormones* released from the GI tract, and autonomic neural pathways. Neural stimuli cause some increase of insulin secretion prior to food consumption. Neural stimulation of insulin secretion occurs throughout the meal and contributes significantly to glucose tolerance. Arrival of nutrient chyme to the intestine leads to the release of insulinotropic peptides from specialized endocrine cells in the intestinal mucosa. *GIP and GLP-1*, together termed *incretins*, are the essential gut hormones contributing to *glucose tolerance*. They are secreted in proportion to the nutrient load ingested and relay this information to the islet as part of a feed-forward mechanism that allows an insulin response appropriate to meal size. Insulin secretion rates in healthy humans are highest in the early digestive phase of meals, preceding and limiting the peak in blood glucose. This pattern of premonitory insulin secretion is an essential feature of normal glucose tolerance. Mimicking this pattern is one of the key challenges for successful insulin therapy in diabetic patients.

Abbreviations

AC: adenylyl cyclase
A1c: hemoglobin A_{1c}
ADA: American Diabetes Association
BP: blood pressure
CHF: congestive heart failure
CNS: central nervous system
CSII: continuous subcutaneous insulin infusion
CV: cardiovascular
CVD: cardiovascular disease
DPP-4: dipeptidyl peptidase IV
EPI: epinephrine
GDM: gestational diabetes mellitus
GEF: guanine nucleotide exchange factor
GFR: glomerular filtration rate
GIP: glucose-dependent insulinotropic polypeptide
GIRK: G protein–coupled inwardly rectifying K^+ channel
GK: glucokinase (hexokinase IV)
GLP: glucagon-like peptide
GLP-1RA: GLP-1 receptor agonist
GLUT: glucose transporter
G6P: glucose-6-phosphate
GPCR: G protein–coupled receptor
GRPP: glicentin-related pancreatic polypeptide
Hb: hemoglobin
HbA$_{1c}$: hemoglobin A_{1c}
HDL: high-density lipoprotein
HGP: hepatic glucose production
HNF: hepatocyte nuclear transcription factor
IAPP: islet amyloid polypeptide
ICU: intensive care unit
IFG: impaired fasting glucose
IFN: interferon
IGF-1: insulinlike growth factor 1
IGT: impaired glucose tolerance
IL: interleukin
IRS: insulin receptor substrate
K$_{ir}$: inward rectifying K^+ channel
LDL: low-density lipoprotein
MAOI: monoamine oxidase inhibitor
MODY: maturity onset diabetes of the young
mTOR: mammalian target of rapamycin
NE: norepinephrine
NPH: neutral protamine Hagedorn
NSAID: nonsteroidal anti-inflammatory drug
OCT: organic cation transporter
PC: prohormone convertase
PI3K: phosphatidylinositol-3-kinase
PIP3: phosphatidylinositol 3,4,5-trisphosphate
PLC: phospholipase
PPAR: peroxisome proliferator-activated receptor
SGLT2: sodium-glucose cotransporter 2
Shc: Src-homology-2-containing (protein)
SST: somatostatin
SUR: sulfonylurea receptor
TGF: transforming growth factor
TNF: tumor necrosis factor

Elevated circulating insulin concentrations lower glucose in blood by inhibiting hepatic glucose production (HGP) and stimulating the uptake and metabolism of glucose by muscle and adipose tissue. Production of glucose is inhibited half-maximally by an insulin concentration of about 120 pmol/L, whereas glucose utilization is stimulated half-maximally at about 300 pmol/L. Some of the effects of insulin on the liver occur rapidly, within the first 20 min of meal ingestion, whereas stimulation of peripheral glucose uptake may require up to an hour to reach significant rates. Insulin has potent effects to reduce lipolysis from adipocytes, primarily through the inhibition of hormone-sensitive lipase; insulin also increases lipid storage by promoting lipoprotein-lipase synthesis and adipocyte glucose uptake. In muscle and other tissues, insulin stimulates amino acid uptake and protein synthesis and inhibits protein degradation.

The limited glycogen stores in skeletal muscle are mobilized at the onset of physical activity, but most of the glucose support for exercise comes from hepatic gluconeogenesis. The dominant regulation of hepatic glucose production during exercise comes from EPI and NE. The catecholamines stimulate glycogenolysis and gluconeogenesis, inhibit insulin secretion, and enhance release of glucagon, all contributing to increased hepatic glucose output. In addition, catecholamines promote lipolysis, freeing fatty acids for oxidation in exercising muscle and glycerol for hepatic gluconeogenesis.

Pancreatic Islet Physiology and Insulin Secretion

The pancreatic islets comprise 1%–2% of the pancreatic volume. The pancreatic islet is a highly vascularized, highly innervated miniorgan containing five endocrine cell types: *α cells* that secrete *glucagon,* *β cells* that secrete *insulin,* *δ cells* that secrete *SST,* *PP cells* that secrete *pancreatic polypeptide,* and *ε cells* that secrete *ghrelin.*

Insulin is initially synthesized as a single polypeptide chain, *preproinsulin* (110 amino acids), which is processed first to *proinsulin* and then to *insulin* and *C-peptide* (Figure 47–2). This complex and highly regulated process involves the Golgi complex, the endoplasmic reticulum, and the secretory granules of the β cell. Secretory granules are critical in the cleavage and processing of the prohormone to the final secretion products, insulin and C-peptide, and in bringing insulin to the cell membrane for exocytosis. Equimolar quantities of insulin and C-peptide (31 amino acids) are cosecreted. Insulin has a $t_{1/2}$ of 5–6 min due to extensive hepatic clearance. C-peptide, in contrast, with no known physiological function or receptor, has a $t_{1/2}$ of about 30 min. The C-peptide is useful in assessment of β cell secretion and to distinguish endogenous and exogenous hyperinsulinemia (e.g., in the evaluation of insulin-induced hypoglycemia). The β cell also synthesizes and secretes IAPP or *amylin,* a 37–amino acid peptide. IAPP influences GI motility and the speed of glucose absorption. *Pramlintide* is an agent used in the treatment of diabetes that mimics the action of IAPP.

Insulin secretion is tightly regulated to provide stable concentrations of glucose in blood during both fasting and feeding. This regulation is achieved by the coordinated interplay of various nutrients, GI hormones, pancreatic hormones, and autonomic neurotransmitters. Glucose, amino acids, fatty acids, and ketone bodies promote the secretion of insulin. Glucose is the primary insulin secretagogue, and insulin secretion is tightly coupled to the extracellular glucose concentration. Insulin secretion is much greater when the same amount of glucose is delivered orally compared to intravenously, a response termed the *incretin effect* and attributed to insulinotropic GI peptides. Islets are richly innervated by both adrenergic and cholinergic nerves. Stimulation of α_2 adrenergic receptors inhibits insulin secretion, whereas β_2 adrenergic receptor agonists and vagal nerve stimulation enhance release. In general, any condition that activates the sympathetic branch of the autonomic nervous system (such as hypoxia, hypoglycemia, exercise, hypothermia, surgery, or severe burns) suppresses the secretion of insulin by stimulation of α_2 adrenergic receptors.

The molecular events controlling glucose-stimulated insulin secretion begin with the transport of glucose into the β cell via GLUT, a facilitative glucose transporter, primarily GLUT1 in human β cells (Figure 47–3). On entry into the β cell, glucose is quickly phosphorylated by GK (hexokinase

A Fasting state

Brain

Glucose
<100 mg/dL
(5.6 mM)

Fatty Acids
400 μM

Liver

Skeletal
muscle

Glucagon

Insulin

Insulin

Pancreatic
islet

Insulin

Adipose
tissue

B Prandial state

Brain

Glucose
120–140 mg/dL
(6.7–7.8 mM)

Fatty Acids
<400 **m**M

Liver

Skeletal
muscle

Dietary carbohydrate

Glucagon

Insulin

Insulin

GI tract

Incretins

Pancreatic
islet

Insulin

Adipose
tissue

Dietary lipids

Figure 47–1 *Insulin, glucagon, and glucose homeostasis.* **A.** *Fasting State*–In healthy humans, plasma glucose is maintained in a range from 4.4 to 5 mM and fatty acids near 400 μM. In the absence of nutrient absorption from the GI tract, glucose is supplied primarily from the liver and fatty acids from adipose tissue. With fasting, plasma insulin levels are low, and plasma glucagon is elevated, contributing to increased hepatic glycogenolysis and gluconeogenesis; low insulin also releases adipocytes from inhibition, permitting increased lipogenesis. Most tissues oxidize primarily fatty acids during fasting, sparing glucose for use by the CNS. **B.** *Prandial State*–During feeding, nutrient absorption causes an increases in plasma glucose, resulting in release of incretins from the gut and neural stimuli that promote insulin secretion. Under the control of insulin, the liver, skeletal muscle, and adipose tissue actively take up glucose. Hepatic glucose production and lipolysis are inhibited, and total body glucose oxidation increases. The brain senses plasma glucose concentrations and provides regulatory inputs contributing to fuel homeostasis. The boldness of the arrows reflects relative intensity of action; a dashed line indicates little or no activity.

IV); *this phosphorylation is the rate-limiting step in glucose metabolism in the β cell.* GK's distinctive affinity for glucose leads to a marked increase in glucose metabolism over the range of 5–10 mM glucose, where glucose-stimulated insulin secretion is most pronounced. The G6P produced by GK activity enters the glycolytic pathway, producing changes in NADPH

and the ratio of ADP/ATP. Elevated ATP inhibits an ATP-sensitive K^+ channel (K_{ATP} channel), leading to cell membrane depolarization. This heteromeric K_{ATP} channel consists of an inward rectifying K^+ channel (Kir6.2) and a closely associated protein known as the SUR. Mutations in the K_{ATP} channel are responsible for specific types of neonatal diabetes and hyperinsulinemic hypoglycemia. Membrane depolarization following K_{ATP} closure leads to opening of a voltage-dependent Ca^{2+} channel and increased intracellular Ca^{2+}, resulting in exocytotic release of insulin from storage vesicles. These intracellular events are modulated by changes in cAMP production, amino acid metabolism, and the level of transcription factors. GPCRs for glucagon, GIP, and GLP-1 and other regulatory peptides couple to G_s to stimulate adenylyl cyclase and insulin secretion; receptors for SST and α_2 adrenergic agonists couple to G_i to reduce cellular cAMP production and secretion.

The pancreatic α cell secretes *glucagon*, primarily in response to hypoglycemia. Glucagon biosynthesis begins with *preproglucagon*, which is processed in a cell-specific fashion to several biologically active peptides, such as glucagon, GLP-1, and GLP-2 (see Figure 47–9). *In general, glucagon and insulin secretion are regulated in a reciprocal fashion; that is, the agents or processes that stimulate insulin secretion inhibit glucagon secretion. Notable exceptions are arginine and SST: Arginine stimulates and SST inhibits the secretion of both hormones.*

Insulin Action

The insulin receptor is expressed on virtually all mammalian cell types. Tissues that are critical for regulation of blood glucose are liver, skeletal muscle, fat (Figure 47–1), and specific regions of the brain and the pancreatic islet. The actions of insulin are anabolic, and insulin signaling is critical for promoting the uptake, use, and storage of the major nutrients: glucose, lipids, and amino acids. Insulin stimulates glycogenesis, lipogenesis, and protein synthesis; it also inhibits the catabolism of these compounds. On a

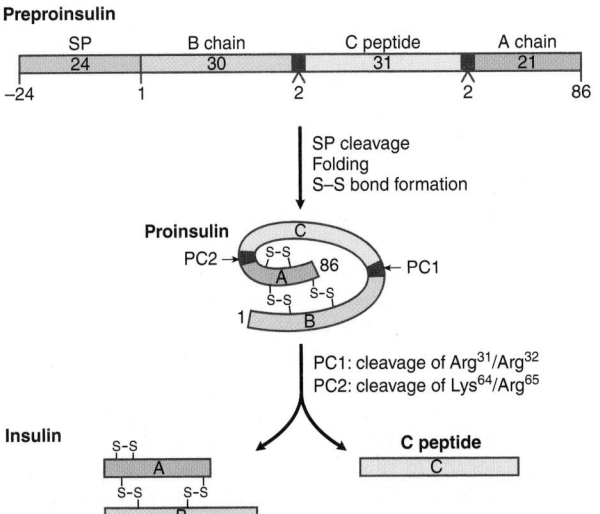

Figure 47–2 *Synthesis and processing of insulin.* The initial peptide, proinsulin (110 amino acids) consists of a signal peptide (SP), B chain, C-peptide, and A chain. The SP is cleaved and S-S bonds form as the proinsulin folds. Two prohormone convertases, PC1 and PC2, cleave proinsulin into insulin, C-peptide, and two dipeptides. Insulin and C-peptide are stored in granules and cosecreted in equimolar quantities.

Preproinsulin

SP	B chain	C peptide	A chain
24	30	31	21

−24 1   2   2   86

SP cleavage
Folding
S–S bond formation

Proinsulin

PC2   C   PC1
S-S   86
A
S-S   1   B

PC1: cleavage of Arg^{31}/Arg^{32}
PC2: cleavage of Lys^{64}/Arg^{65}

Insulin

S-S
A
S-S   S-S
B

C peptide

C

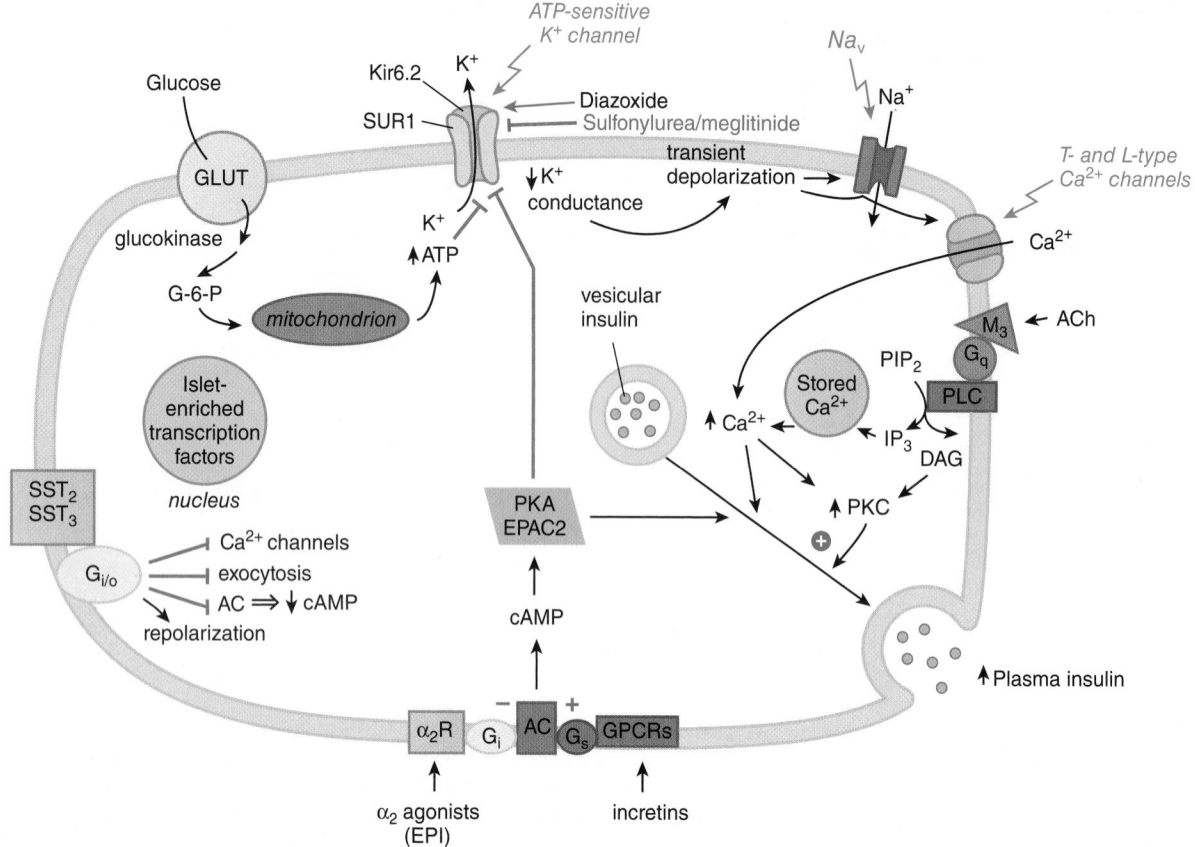

Figure 47–3 *Regulation of insulin secretion from a pancreatic β cell.* The pancreatic β cell in a resting state (fasting blood glucose) is hyperpolarized. Elevated plasma glucose enters the cell via GLUTs (primarily GLUT1 in humans). The resulting enhanced glucose metabolism elevates cellular ATP, which reduces K^+ conductance through the K_{ATP} channel; the decreased K^+ conductance results in local membrane depolarization and activation of Ca^{2+} and Na^+ channels; the increased $[Ca^{2+}]_{in}$ stimulates exocytosis of stored insulin, using the basic mechanisms described for exocytosis of neurotransmitters (Figures 8–4 to 8–6). ACh, acting via M_3 receptors, can activate the G_q-PLC-IP_3-Ca^{2+}-PKC pathway; incretins, also acting via GPCRs, can activate the G_s-AC-cAMP-PKA/EPAC2 pathway; both of these GPCR-activated pathways enhance exocytosis. Elevated cAMP also leads to inhibition of the K_{ATP} channel, enhancing depolarization and furthering exocytosis. The depolarization/exocytosis period is limited by closure of voltage-sensitive ion channels, by export of Ca^{2+} and Na^+, and by sequestration of Ca^{2+} within the SR by the SERCA transporter. SST, acting via SST2 and SST3 that couple to $G_{i/o}$, can aid in restoring the hyperpolarized state of the cell, as can α_2 agonists. The K_{ATP} channel has SUR1 and Kir 6.2 subunits; ATP binds to and inhibits Kir 6.2; sulfonylureas and meglitinides bind to and inhibit SUR1; all three agents thereby promote insulin secretion. Diazoxide and ADP-Mg^{2+} (low ATP) bind to and activate SUR1, thereby inhibiting insulin secretion. Mitochondrial mutations and isletenriched transcription factors can contribute to the development of diabetes. This schematic is a simplification; Rorsman and Braun (2013) have reviewed the subject in greater detail. G, G protein, with subtype indicated by subscript; AC, adenylyl cyclase; EPAC, exchange protein activated by cAMP; GLUT, GLUT1 glucose transporter; GPCR, G-protein coupled receptor; PKA, protein kinase A; PKC, protein kinase C; PLC, phospholipase C; SST2/3, somatostatin receptors.

cellular level, insulin stimulates transport of substrates and ions into cells, promotes translocation of proteins between cellular compartments, regulates the action of specific enzymes, and controls gene transcription and mRNA translation. Some effects of insulin (e.g., activation of glucose and ion transport systems, phosphorylation or dephosphorylation of specific enzymes) occur within seconds or minutes; other effects (e.g., those promoting protein synthesis and regulating gene transcription and cell proliferation) manifest over minutes to hours to days. The effects of insulin on cell proliferation and differentiation occur over a longer period of time.

The Insulin Receptor

Insulin action is transmitted through a receptor tyrosine kinase that bears functional similarity to the *IGF-1 receptor* (Samuel and Shulman, 2016). The insulin receptor is composed of linked α/β subunit dimers that are products of a single gene; dimers linked by disulfide bonds form a transmembrane heterotetramer glycoprotein composed of two extracellular α subunits and two membrane-spanning β subunits (Figure 47–4). The number of receptors varies from 40/cell on erythrocytes to 300,000/cell on adipocytes and hepatocytes.

The α subunits inhibit the inherent tyrosine kinase activity of the β subunits. Insulin binding to the α subunits releases this inhibition and allows transphosphorylation of one β subunit by the other and autophosphorylation at specific sites from the juxtamembrane region to the intracellular tail of the receptor. Activation of the insulin receptor initiates signaling by phosphorylating a set of intracellular proteins, including the IRSs and Shc protein. These proteins interact with effectors that amplify and extend the signaling cascade.

Insulin action on glucose transport depends on the activation of PI3K. PI3K is activated by interaction with IRS proteins and generates PIP3, which regulates the localization and activity of several downstream kinases, including PKB (Akt), atypical isoforms of PKC (ς and λ/τ), and mTOR. The isoform Akt2 appears to control the downstream steps that are important for glucose uptake in skeletal muscle and adipose tissue and to regulate glucose production in the liver. Substrates of Akt2 coordinate the translocation of GLUT4 to the plasma membrane through processes involving actin remodeling and other membrane trafficking systems. Actions of small G proteins, such as Rac and TC10, have also been implicated in the actin remodeling necessary for GLUT4 translocation.

867

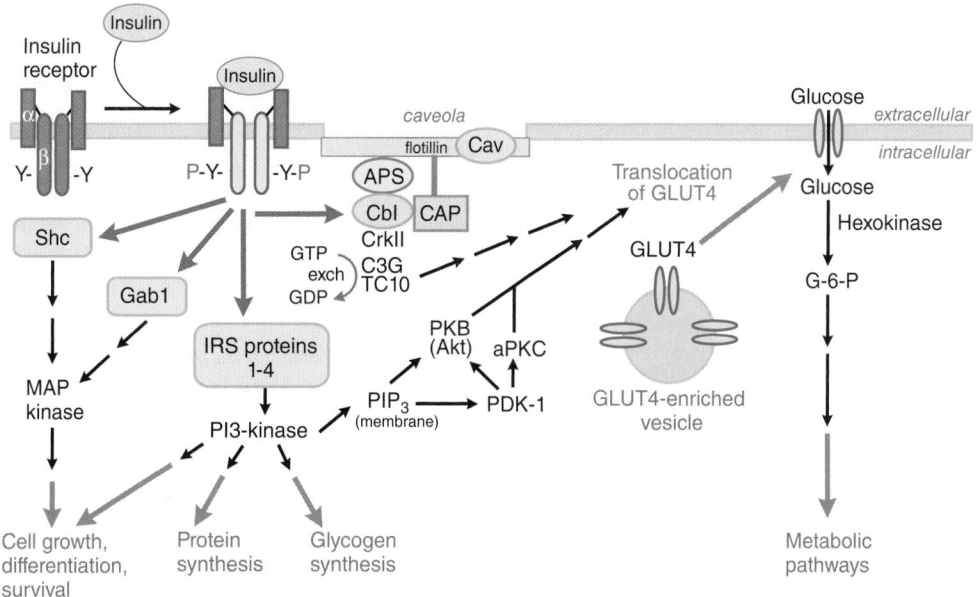

Figure 47–4 *Pathways of insulin signaling.* The binding of insulin to its plasma membrane receptor activates a cascade of downstream signaling events. Insulin binding activates the intrinsic tyrosine kinase activity of the receptor dimer, resulting in the tyrosine phosphorylation (Y-P indicates the phosphorylated tyrosine residue, Y) of the receptor's β subunits and a small number of specific substrates (yellow shapes): the IRS proteins Gab-1 and Shc; within the membrane, a caveolar pool of insulin receptor phosphorylates Cav, APS, and Cbl. These tyrosine-phosphorylated proteins interact with signaling cascades via SH2 and SH3 domains to mediate the effects of insulin, with specific effects resulting from each pathway. In the target tissues such as skeletal muscle and adipocytes, a key event is the translocation of GLUT4 from intracellular vesicles to the plasma membrane; this translocation is stimulated by both the caveolar and noncaveolar pathways. In the noncaveolar pathway, the activation of PI3K is crucial, and PKB/Akt (anchored at the membrane by PIP3) or an atypical form of PKC is involved. In the caveolar pathway, caveolar protein flotillin localizes the signaling complex to the caveola; the signaling pathway involves a series of SH2 domain interactions that add the adaptor protein CrkII, the guanine nucleotide exchange protein C3G, and small GTP-binding protein TC10. The pathways are inactivated by specific phosphoprotein phosphatases (e.g., PTB1B). In addition to the actions shown, insulin stimulates the plasma membrane Na^+, K^+-ATPase by a mechanism that is still being elucidated; the result is an increase in pump activity and a net accumulation of K^+ in the cell. APS, adaptor protein with PH and SH2 domains; CAP, Cbl associated protein; CAV, caveolin; CrkII, chicken tumor virus regulator of kinase II; Gab-1, Grb-2 associated binder; GLUT4, glucose transporter 4; PDK, phosphoinositide-dependent kinase; Y-P, phosphorylated tyrosine residue.

GLUT4

GLUT4 is expressed in insulin-responsive tissues such as skeletal muscle and adipose tissue. In the basal state, most GLUT4 resides in the intracellular space; following activation of insulin receptors, GLUT4 is shifted rapidly and in abundance to the plasma membrane (Saltiel, 2016), where it facilitates inward transport of glucose from the circulation. Insulin signaling also reduces GLUT4 endocytosis, increasing the residence time of the protein in the plasma membrane (Saltiel, 2016). Following the facilitated diffusion into cells along a concentration gradient, glucose is phosphorylated to G6P by hexokinases. Hexokinase II is found in association with GLUT4 in skeletal and cardiac muscle and in adipose tissue. Like GLUT4, hexokinase II is regulated transcriptionally by insulin. G6P can be isomerized to G1P and stored as glycogen (insulin enhances the activity of glycogen synthase); G6P can enter the glycolytic pathway (for ATP production) and the pentose phosphate pathway.

Pathophysiology and Diagnosis of Diabetes Mellitus

Glucose Homeostasis and the Diagnosis of Diabetes

Broad categories of glucose homeostasis are defined by the fasting blood glucose or the glucose level following an oral glucose challenge. These include the following:

- Normal glucose homeostasis: fasting plasma glucose < 5.6 mmol/L (100 mg/dL)
- Impaired fasting glucose (IFG) : 5.6–6.9 mmol/L (100–125 mg/dL)

- Impaired glucose tolerance (IGT): glucose level between 7.8 and 11.1 mmol/L (140 and 199 mg/dL) 120 min after ingestion of 75 g liquid glucose solution
- Diabetes mellitus (see Table 47–1)

The American Diabetes Association (ADA) and the World Health Organization (WHO) have adopted criteria for the diagnosis of diabetes based on the fasting blood glucose, the glucose value following an oral glucose challenge, or the level of HbA_{1c} (or more simply, A1c; exposure of

TABLE 47–1 ■ CRITERIA FOR THE DIAGNOSIS OF DIABETES

- Symptoms of diabetes plus random blood glucose concentration ≥ 11.1 mM (200 mg/dL)[a] or
- Fasting plasma glucose ≥ 7.0 mM (126 mg/dL)[b] or
- Two-hour plasma glucose ≥ 11.1 mM (200 mg/dL) during an oral glucose tolerance test[c]
- HbA_{1c} ≥ 6.5%

Note: In the absence of unequivocal hyperglycemia and acute metabolic decompensation, these criteria should be confirmed by repeat testing on a different day.
[a]*Random* is defined as without regard to time since the last meal.
[b]*Fasting* is defined as no caloric intake for at least 8 h.
[c]The test should be performed using a glucose load containing the equivalent of 75 g anhydrous glucose dissolved in water; this test is not recommended for routine clinical use.
Criteria compiled from *Diabetes Care*, **2017**, *40*:S11–524.

proteins to elevated glucose produces nonenzymatic glycation of proteins, including Hb, so the level of A1c represents a measure of the average glucose concentration to which the Hb has been exposed) (see Table 47–1). IFG and IGT portend a markedly increased risk of progressing to type 2 diabetes and are associated with increased risk of cardiovascular disease.

The four categories of diabetes include type 1 diabetes, type 2 diabetes, other forms of diabetes, and GDM (Table 47–2). Although hyperglycemia is common to all forms of diabetes, the pathogenic mechanisms leading to diabetes are quite distinct.

Screening for Diabetes and Categories of Increased Risk of Diabetes

Many individuals with type 2 diabetes are asymptomatic at the time of diagnosis, and diabetes is often found on routine blood testing for non–glucose-related reasons. The ADA recommends widespread screening for type 2 diabetes of adults with the following features:

- Age more than 45 years, or
- Body mass index greater than 25 kg/m^2 (or greater than 23 kg/m^2 in persons of Asian descent) with one of these additional risk factors: physical inactivity; hypertension; low HDL value; family history of type 2 diabetes; high-risk ethnic group (African American, Latino, Native American, Asian American, and Pacific Islander); abnormal glucose testing (IFG, IGT, A1c of 5.7%–6.4%); cardiovascular disease; features

TABLE 47–2 ■ DIFFERENT FORMS OF DIABETES MELLITUS

I. **Type 1 diabetes β-cell destruction,** usually leading to absolute insulin deficiency
   A. Immune mediated
   B. Idiopathic

II. **Type 2 diabetes** (may range from predominantly insulin resistance with relative insulin deficiency to a predominantly insulin secretory defect with insulin resistance)

III. **Other specific types of diabetes**
   A. Monogenic disorders of β-cell function
      1. HNF-4α (MODY 1)
      2. Glucokinase (MODY 2)
      3. HNF-1α (MODY 3)
      4. Other forms of MODY: insulin promoter factor 1, HNF-1β, NeuroD1, and others
      5. Permanent neonatal diabetes KCNJ11 gene encoding Kir6.2 subunit of β-cell K$_{ATP}$ channel, insulin gene
      6. Mitochondrial DNA
   B. Genetic defects in insulin action, including type A insulin resistance, leprechaunism, Rabson-Mendenhall syndrome, lipodystrophy syndromes
   C. Diseases of the exocrine pancreas—pancreatitis, pancreatectomy, neoplasia, cystic fibrosis, hemochromatosis, fibrocalculous pancreatopathy, mutations in carboxyl ester lipase
   D. Endocrinopathies—acromegaly, Cushing syndrome, glucagonoma, pheochromocytoma, hyperthyroidism, somatostatinoma, aldosteronoma
   E. Drug or chemical induced—pyrinuron (a rodenticide no longer sold in the U.S.); see drugs listed in Table 47–3
   F. Infections—congenital rubella, cytomegalovirus
   G. Uncommon forms of immune-mediated diabetes—"stiff-person" syndrome, anti-insulin receptor antibodies
   H. Other genetic syndromes sometimes associated with diabetes—Wolfram, Down, Klinefelter, Laurence-Moon-Biedl, Prader-Willi, and Turner syndromes; Friedreich ataxia; Huntington disease; myotonic dystrophy; porphyria

IV. **Gestational diabetes mellitus**

of insulin resistance; or women with polycystic ovary syndrome or who have previously delivered a large infant or had GDM

In screening for diabetes, fasting plasma glucose, A1c, and plasma glucose after an oral glucose tolerance test are equally valid, but the fasting glucose and A1c are used most commonly. Early diagnosis and treatment of type 2 diabetes should delay diabetes-related complications and reduce the burden of the disease. A number of interventions, including pharmacological agents and lifestyle modification, are effective. Screening for type 1 diabetes is not currently recommended.

Pathogenesis of Type 1 Diabetes

Type 1 diabetes accounts for 5%–10% of diabetes and results from autoimmune-mediated destruction of the β cells of the islet, leading to total or near-total insulin deficiency (Atkinson et al., 2014). Prior terminology included juvenile-onset diabetes mellitus or insulin-dependent diabetes mellitus. Type 1 diabetes can occur at any age. Individuals with type 1 diabetes and their families have an increased prevalence of autoimmune diseases such as Addison, Graves, and Hashimoto diseases; pernicious anemia; vitiligo; and celiac sprue. The concordance of type 1 diabetes in genetically identical twins is 40%–60%, indicating a significant genetic component. The major genetic risk (40%–50%) is conferred by HLA class II genes encoding HLA-DR and HLA-DQ. However, there likely is a critical interaction of genetics and an environmental or infectious agent. Most individuals with type 1 diabetes (about 75%) do not have a family member with type 1 diabetes, and the genes conferring genetic susceptibility are found in a significant fraction of the nondiabetic population.

Genetically susceptible individuals are thought to have a normal β cell number or mass until β cell–directed autoimmunity develops and β cell loss begins. The initiating or triggering stimulus for the autoimmune process is not known, but most favor exposure to viruses (enterovirus, etc.) or other ubiquitous environmental agents. The β cell destruction is likely cell mediated, and there is also evidence that infiltrating cells produce local inflammatory agents such as TNF-α, IFN-γ, and IL-1, all of which can lead to β cell death. The β cell destruction occurs over a period of months to years and when more than 80% of the β cells are destroyed, hyperglycemia ensues and the clinical diagnosis of type 1 diabetes is made. The ADA and others now recognize three stages of type 1 diabetes: 1) autoimmunity plus normal insulin secretion; 2) autoimmunity with dysglycemia; 3) autoimmunity with hyperglycemia (diabetes). Most patients report several weeks of polyuria and polydipsia, fatigue, and often abrupt and significant weight loss. Some adults with the phenotypic appearance of type 2 diabetes (obese, not insulin-requiring initially) have islet cell autoantibodies suggesting autoimmune-mediated β cell destruction and are diagnosed as having latent-autoimmune diabetes of adults (LADA).

Pathogenesis of Type 2 Diabetes

The type 2 diabetes condition is best thought of as a heterogeneous syndrome of dysregulated glucose homeostasis associated with impaired insulin secretion and action. Overweight or obesity is a common correlate of type 2 diabetes that occurs in about 80% of affected individuals. For the vast majority of persons developing type 2 diabetes, there is no clear inciting incident; rather, the condition is thought to develop gradually over years, with progression through an identifiable prediabetic stage. Type 2 diabetes results when there is insufficient insulin action to maintain plasma glucose levels in the normal range. Insulin action is the composite effect of plasma insulin concentrations (determined by islet β cell function) and insulin sensitivity of key target tissues (liver, skeletal muscle, and adipose tissue). These sites of regulation are all impaired to variable extents in patients with type 2 diabetes (Figure 47–5). The etiology of type 2 diabetes has a strong genetic component. It is a heritable condition with a relative 4-fold increased risk of disease for persons having a diabetic parent or sibling, increasing to 6-fold if both parents have type 2 diabetes. Although more than 80 genetic loci with clear associations to type 2 diabetes have been identified through recent genome-wide association studies, the contribution of each is relatively small (Fuchsberger et al., 2016).

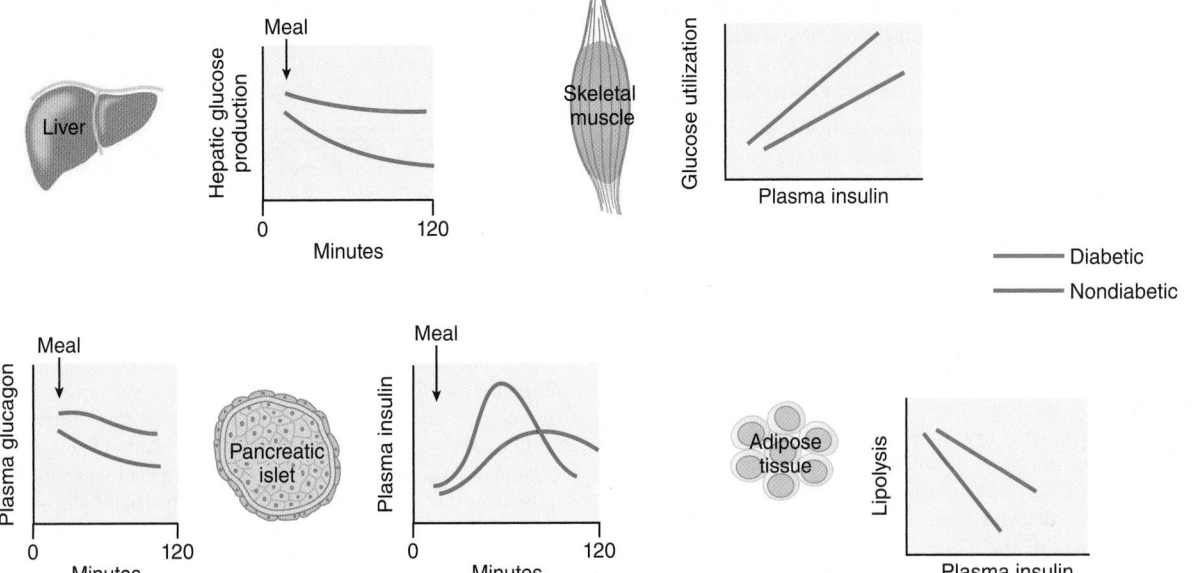

Figure 47–5 *Pathophysiology of type 2 diabetes mellitus.* Graphs show data from nondiabetic individuals (blue lines) and from individuals with diabetes (red lines), comparing postprandial insulin and glucagon secretion and hepatic glucose production, and comparing the sensitivities of muscle glucose use and adipocyte lipolysis to insulin.

Impaired β Cell Function

In type 2 diabetes, the sensitivity of the β cell to glucose is impaired, and there is also a loss of responsiveness to other stimuli, such as insulinotropic GI hormones and neural signaling. This results in delayed secretion of insufficient amounts of insulin, allowing the blood glucose to rise dramatically after meals, and failure to restrain liver glucose release during fasting. The absolute mass of β cells also is reduced in patients with type 2 diabetes. Progressive reduction of β cell mass and function explains the natural history of type 2 diabetes in most patients who require steadily increasing therapy to maintain glucose control.

Type 2 diabetic patients sometimes have elevated levels of fasting insulin, a result of their higher fasting glucose levels and insulin resistance. Another factor contributing to apparently high insulin levels early in the course of the disease is the presence of increased amounts of proinsulin. Proinsulin, the precursor to insulin, is inefficiently processed in the diabetic islet. Whereas healthy subjects have only 2%–4% of total circulating insulin as proinsulin, patients with type 2 diabetes can have 10%–20% of the measurable plasma insulin in this form. Proinsulin has a considerably attenuated effect for lowering blood glucose compared to insulin. Excessive and dysregulated glucagon secretion is another prominent feature of type 2 diabetes (D'Alessio, 2011).

Insulin Resistance

Insulin sensitivity is measured as the amount of glucose cleared from the blood in response to a fixed dose of insulin. The failure of normal amounts of insulin to elicit the expected response is referred to as *insulin resistance*. There is inherent variability of insulin sensitivity amongst cells, tissues, and individuals. Insulin sensitivity is affected by many factors, including age, body weight, physical activity levels, illness, and medications. Nonetheless, persons with type 2 diabetes or glucose intolerance have reduced responses to insulin and can be distinguished from groups with normal glucose tolerance (Samuel and Shulman, 2016).

The major insulin-responsive tissues are skeletal muscle, adipose tissue, and liver. Insulin resistance in muscle and fat is generally marked by a decrease in transport of glucose from the circulation. Hepatic insulin resistance generally refers to a blunted ability of insulin to suppress glucose production. Insulin resistance in adipocytes causes increased rates of lipolysis and release of fatty acids into the circulation, which can contribute to insulin resistance in liver and muscle, hepatic steatosis, and dyslipidemia. The sensitivity of humans to the effects of insulin administration is inversely related to the amount of fat stored in the abdominal cavity; more visceral adiposity leads to more insulin resistance. Intracellular lipid or its by-products may have direct effects to impede insulin signaling. Enlarged collections of adipose tissue, visceral or otherwise, are often infiltrated with macrophages and can become sites of chronic inflammation. Adipocytokines, secreted from adipocytes and immune cells, including TNF-α, IL-6, resistin, and retinol-binding protein 4, can also cause systemic insulin resistance.

Sedentary persons are more insulin resistant than active ones, and physical training can improve insulin sensitivity. Physical activity can decrease the risk of developing diabetes and improve glycemic control in persons who have diabetes. Insulin resistance is more common in the elderly, and within populations, insulin sensitivity decreases linearly with age. At the cellular level, insulin resistance involves blunted steps in the cascade from the insulin receptor tyrosine kinase to translocation of GLUT4 transporters, but the molecular mechanisms are incompletely defined. There have been more than 75 different mutations in the insulin receptor discovered, most of which cause significant impairment of insulin action. These mutations affect insulin receptor number, ligand binding, receptor phosphorylation, and trafficking. Mutations involving the insulin binding domains of the extracellular α-chain cause the most severe syndromes. Insulin sensitivity is under genetic control, but it is unclear whether insulin-resistant individuals have mutations in specific components of the insulin signaling cascade or whether they have a complement of signaling effectors that operate at the lower range of normal. Regardless, it is apparent that insulin resistance clusters in families and is a major risk factor for the development of diabetes.

Dysregulated Hepatic Glucose Metabolism

In type 2 diabetes, hepatic glucose output is excessive in the fasting state and inadequately suppressed after meals. Abnormal secretion of the islet hormones—insufficient insulin and excessive glucagon—accounts for a significant portion of dysregulated hepatic metabolism in type 2 diabetes. Increased concentrations of glucagon, especially in conjunction with hepatic insulin resistance, can lead to excessive hepatic gluconeogenesis and glycogenolysis and abnormally high fasting glucose concentrations. The liver is resistant to insulin action in type 2 diabetes, and the capacity of insulin to suppress HGP and promote hepatic glucose uptake and glycogen synthesis after meals is reduced. Despite ineffective insulin effects on hepatic glucose metabolism, the lipogenic effects of insulin in the liver are maintained and even accentuated by fasting hyperinsulinemia. This contributes to hepatic steatosis and further worsening of insulin resistance.

Pathogenesis of Other Forms of Diabetes

Mutations in key genes involved in glucose homeostasis cause monogenic diabetes, which is inherited in an autosomal dominant fashion (Hattersley and Patel, 2017). These fall in two broad categories: diabetes onset in the immediate neonatal period (<6 months of age) and diabetes in children or adults. Some forms of neonatal diabetes are caused by mutations in SUR or its accompanying inward rectifying K^+ channel or mutations in the insulin gene. Monogenic diabetes beyond the first year of life may appear clinically similar to type 1 or type 2 diabetes. In other instances, children, adolescents, and young adults may present with monogenic forms of diabetes known as MODY (maturity onset diabetes of the young). Phenotypically, these individuals are not obese or insulin resistant and may initially have only modest hyperglycemia. The most common causes are mutations in key islet-enriched transcription factors or GK (Table 47-2). Most individuals with MODY are treated similarly to those with type 2 diabetes; some may respond to a sulfonylurea.

Chronic diseases of the pancreas, such as pancreatitis or cystic fibrosis, or endocrinopathies such as acromegaly and Cushing disease (see Table 47–2) can cause diabetes. A number of medications promote hyperglycemia or lead to diabetes by impairing either insulin secretion or insulin action (Table 47–3).

Diabetes-Related Complications

Untreated diabetes can lead to severe metabolic disturbances that can be acutely life threatening, such as diabetic ketoacidosis and a hyperglycemic hyperosmolar state. These require hospitalization for insulin administration, rehydration with intravenous fluids, and careful monitoring of electrolytes and metabolic parameters. Chronic end-organ effects of diabetes are commonly divided into microvascular and macrovascular complications. Microvascular complications occur only in individuals with diabetes and include retinopathy, nephropathy, and neuropathy, which are specific to diabetes. Macrovascular complications related to atherosclerosis, such as myocardial infarction and stroke, occur more frequently in individuals with diabetes but are not diabetes specific. In the U.S., diabetes is the leading cause of blindness in adults, the leading reason for renal failure requiring dialysis or renal transplantation, and the leading cause of nontraumatic lower extremity amputations. Evidence from clinical trials indicated that most of these diabetes-related complications can be prevented, delayed, or reduced by chronic, effective glucose lowering.

The mechanisms by which long-standing hyperglycemia causes end-organ complications are unclear. There is experimental evidence to suggest roles for AGEs (advanced glycosylation end products), increased glucose metabolism via the sorbitol pathway, increased formation of diacylglycerol leading to PKC activation, and increased flux through the hexosamine pathway. Growth factors such as VEGF-A (vascular endothelial growth factor-A) may be involved in diabetic retinopathy and TGF-β in diabetic nephropathy.

Therapy of Diabetes

Goals of Therapy

The goals of therapy for diabetes are to alleviate the symptoms related to hyperglycemia (fatigue, polyuria, weight loss) and to prevent or reduce the acute metabolic decompensation and chronic end-organ complications.

Glycemic control is assessed using both short-term (blood glucose self-monitoring; continuous glucose monitoring) and long-term (A1c, fructosamine) metrics. Using capillary blood glucose measurements, patients can measure capillary blood glucose throughout their usual fasting and feeding periods and report these values to the diabetes management team. Continuous glucose monitoring of interstitial glucose is a rapidly evolving technology that allows near real-time tracking of blood glucose levels and is being used more frequently in the management of type 1 diabetes. A1c reflects glycemic control over the prior 3 months, whereas measures of glycosylated serum proteins or albumin (fructosamine) reflect glycemic control over the preceding 2 weeks.

The term *comprehensive diabetes care* describes optimal therapy, which involves more than glucose management and includes treatment of abnormalities in blood pressure and lipids and detection and management of diabetes-related complications (Figure 47-6). Table 47-4 shows the ADA-recommended treatment goals for comprehensive diabetes care for glucose, blood pressure, and lipids (see Chapters 28 and 33). The treatment goals should be individualized to the patient and take into account factors such as risk of hypoglycemia, life expectancy, age, other medical conditions, duration of diabetes, and advanced macrovascular/microvascular complications of diabetes (Cahn et al., 2015). (see Table 47–4). Also, the patient's attitude toward diabetes, expectations, resources, and support systems should be considered. Costs of the various agents are compared in Table 47–8.

Nonpharmacologic Aspects of Diabetes Therapy

The patient with diabetes should be educated about nutrition, exercise, and medications aimed at lowering the plasma glucose (American Diabetes Association, 2017). In type 1 diabetes, matching caloric intake and insulin dosing is important. In type 2 diabetes, the diet is directed at weight loss and reduction of blood pressure and atherosclerotic risk. There is now compelling evidence that metabolic surgery can prevent or even reverse type 2 diabetes, with clinical trials showing greater efficacy than medical management (Rubino et al., 2016).

Insulin Therapy

Insulin is the mainstay for treatment of virtually all patients with type 1 and many with type 2 diabetes (Cefalu et al., 2015). Although there are specific preparations of insulin that may be administered intramuscularly,

TABLE 47–3 ■ SOME DRUGS THAT MAY PROMOTE HYPERGLYCEMIA OR HYPOGLYCEMIA

HYPERGLYCEMIA	HYPOGLYCEMIA
Glucocorticoids; thyroid hormone	β Adrenergic antagonists
Antipsychotics (atypical, others)	Theophylline
Protease inhibitors	ACE inhibitors
β Adrenergic agonists; epinephrine	Salicylates, NSAIDs
Thiazide diuretics	LiCl
Hydantoins (phenytoin, others)	Ethanol
Opioids (fentanyl, morphine, others)	Pentamidine
Diazoxide; nicotinic acid	Bromocriptine
Interferons; amphotericin B	
Acamprosate; basiliximab; asparaginase	

For details and discussion of these issues, see Murad et al., 2009.

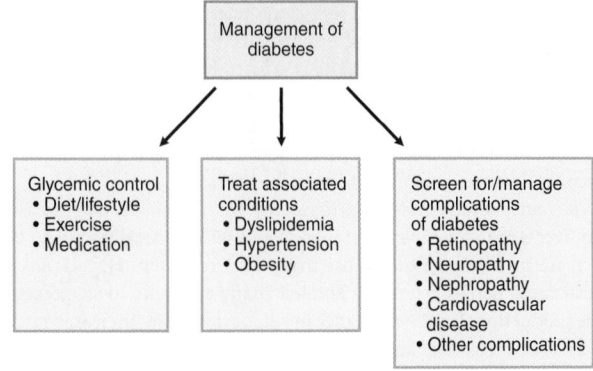

Figure 47–6 *Components of comprehensive diabetes care.*

TABLE 47–4 ■ GOALS OF THERAPY FOR DIABETES IN NONPREGNANT ADULTS

INDEX	GOAL[a]
Glycemic control[b]	
A_{1C}	<7.0%
Preprandial capillary plasma glucose	4.4–7.2 mmol/L (80–130 mg/dL)
Peak postprandial capillary plasma glucose	<10.0 mmol/L (<180 mg/dL)[c]
Blood pressure	<140/90[d]
Intensity of statin therapy for lipids[e]	
Age < 40 years	
-No ASCVD risk factors	None
-ASCVD risk factors	Moderate or high
-ASCVD	High
Age 40–75 years	
-No ASCVD risk factors	Moderate
-ASCVD risk factors	High
-ASCVD	High
Age > 75 years	
-No ASCVD risk factors	Moderate
-ASCVD risk factors	Moderate or high
-ASCVD	High

[a]Goals should be individualized for each patient and may be different for certain patient populations (lower or higher). According to the ADA, "Goals should be individualized based on duration of diabetes, age/life expectancy, comorbid conditions, known CVD or advanced microvascular complications, hypoglycemia unawareness, and individual patient considerations."
[b]Achieving A_{1C} value is primary goal.
[c]At 1–2 h after beginning of a meal.
[d]Lower BP targets (<130/80) may be appropriate for certain individuals with diabetes.
[e]For individuals with acute coronary syndrome and LDL > 50 mg/dL (1.3 mmol/L) or who cannot tolerate high-dose statins, see Chapter 33. More detailed recommendations can be found in American Diabetes Association, 2017. ASCVD, arteriosclerotic cardiovascular disease.

intravenously, or nasally, long-term treatment relies predominantly on subcutaneous injection. Subcutaneous administration of insulin delivered into the peripheral circulation can lead to near-normal glycemia but differs from physiological secretion of insulin in two major ways:

- The absorption kinetics do not reproduce the rapid rise and decline of endogenous insulin in response to changes in blood glucose.
- Injected insulin is delivered into the peripheral circulation instead of being released into the portal circulation. Thus, the portal/peripheral insulin concentration is not physiological, and this may alter the influence of insulin on hepatic metabolism.

Insulin Preparation and Chemistry

Human insulin, produced by recombinant DNA technology, is soluble in aqueous solution. Doses and concentrations of clinically used insulin preparations are expressed in international units. One international unit of insulin is defined as the bioequivalent of 34.7 μg of crystalline insulin; this is equivalent to the older working definition of a U.S. Pharmacopeia unit as the amount required to reduce the blood glucose concentration to 45 mg/dL (2.5 mM) in 2.2-kg rabbit fasted for 24 h. Most preparations of insulin are supplied in solution or suspension at a concentration of 100 units/mL, which is about 3.6 mg insulin per milliliter (0.6 mM) and termed U-100. Insulin also is available in more concentrated preparations (200 [degludec and lispro insulins], 300 [glargine insulin], or 500 [regular insulin] units/mL) for patients who are resistant to the hormone and require higher doses.

Insulin Formulations

Preparations of insulin are classified according to their duration of action into *short acting* and *long acting* (Table 47–5). Within the short-acting acting category, it is common to distinguish the *very rapid-acting insulins* (aspart, glulisine, lispro) from regular insulin. Likewise, some distinguish formulations with a *longer duration of action* (degludec, detemir, glargine) from NPH insulin. Two approaches are used to modify the absorption and pharmacokinetic profile of insulin. The first approach is based on formulations that slow the absorption following subcutaneous injection. The other approach is to alter the amino acid sequence or protein structure of human insulin so that it retains its ability to bind to the insulin receptor, but its behavior in solution or following injection is either accelerated or prolonged in comparison to native or regular insulin (Figure 47–7). There is wide variability in the kinetics of insulin action amongst individuals and even with repeated doses in the same individual. The time to peak hypoglycemic effect and insulin levels can vary by 50%, due in part by large variations in the rate of subcutaneous absorption.

Short-Acting Regular Insulin. Native or regular insulin molecules associate as hexamers in aqueous solution at a neutral pH, and this aggregation slows absorption following subcutaneous injection. Regular insulin should be injected 30–45 min before a meal. Regular, unbuffered, *100-units/mL* insulin also may be given intravenously or intramuscularly. However, unbuffered, regular insulin (*500 units/mL*) is for subcutaneous injection only and should not be given by intravenous or intramuscular injection.

Short-Acting Insulin Analogues. The short-acting insulin analogues are absorbed more rapidly from subcutaneous sites than regular insulin (see Figures 47–7 and 47–8; see Table 47–5) (Kerr et al., 2013). Insulin analogues should be injected 15 min or less before a meal. The time-action profile of these insulin analogues is similar. When used to treat glycemia after meals, the short-acting analogues have lower rates of hypoglycemia and modestly improved A1c levels compared to regular insulin.

Insulin lispro is identical to human insulin except at positions B28 and B29. Unlike regular insulin, lispro dissociates into monomers almost instantaneously following injection. This property results in the characteristic rapid absorption and shorter duration of action compared with regular insulin.

Insulin aspart is formed by the replacement of proline at B28 with aspartic acid, reducing self-association. Like lispro, insulin aspart dissociates rapidly into monomers following injection.

Insulin glulisine is formed when glutamic acid replaces lysine at B29 and lysine replaces asparagine at B3; these substitutions result in a reduction in self-association and rapid dissociation into active monomers.

Long-Acting Insulins. NPH insulin (insulin isophane) is a suspension of native insulin complexed with zinc and protamine in a phosphate buffer. This produces a cloudy or whitish solution in contrast to the clear appearance of other insulin solutions. NPH insulin dissolves more gradually when injected subcutaneously; thus, its duration of action is prolonged. NPH insulin is usually given either once a day (at bedtime) or twice a day in combination with short-acting insulin.

Insulin glargine is a long-acting analogue of human insulin. Two arginine residues are added to the C terminus of the B chain, and an asparagine molecule in position 21 on the A chain is replaced with glycine. Insulin glargine is a clear solution with a pH of 4.0, which stabilizes the insulin hexamer. When injected into the neutral pH of the subcutaneous space, aggregation occurs, resulting in prolonged, predictable, absorption from the injection site. Owing to insulin glargine's acidic pH, it cannot be mixed with short-acting insulin preparations that are formulated at a neutral pH. Glargine has a sustained peakless absorption profile and provides more predictable 24-h insulin coverage than NPH insulin when injected once daily. Clinical trial data suggest that glargine has a lower risk of hypoglycemia, particularly overnight compared to NPH insulin. Glargine may be administered at any time during the day with equivalent efficacy and does not accumulate after several injections. Different preparations are

TABLE 47–5 ■ TIME-ACTION PROFILES OF INSULIN PREPARATIONS

TYPE	PREPARATION	TIMES		
		ONSET (h)	PEAK (h)	EFFECTIVE DURATION (h)
Short acting				
	Aspart			
	Glulisine	<0.25	0.5–1.5	3–4
	Lispro			
	Regular	0.5–1.0	2–3	4–6
Long acting				
	Detemir	1–4	0	12–20
	Glargine[b]	1–4	0[a]	12–24
	Degludec	1–4	0	24–42
	NPH	1–2	6–10	10–16
Insulin combinations				
	Mixture: short acting (25%–50%) and long acting (50%–76%)	<0.25–1.0	1.5[c]	Up to 10–16
Inhaled insulin				
	Afrezza	<0.25	0.5–1.5	2–3

[a]Glargine, degludec, and detemir have minimal peak activity at steady-state.
[b]Available as a U-100 and U-300 preparation.
[c]Some mixtures will have dual peaks, one at 2-3 h, the second one several hours later.
[d]Discontinued by manufacturer in the US.

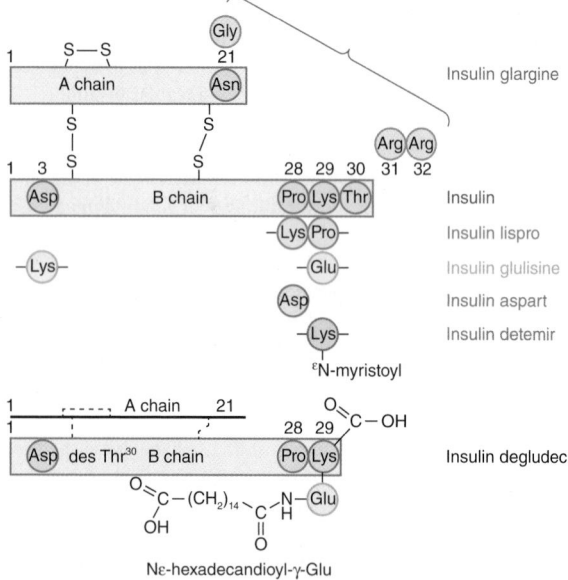

Figure 47–7 *Insulin analogues.* Modifications of native insulin can alter its pharmacokinetic profile. Reversing amino acids 28 and 29 in the B chain (lispro) or substituting Asp for Pro^{28B} (aspart) gives analogues with reduced tendencies for molecular self-association that are faster acting. Altering Asp^{3B} to Lys and Lys^{29B} to Glu produces an insulin (glulisine) with a more rapid onset and a shorter duration of action. Substituting Gly for Asn^{21A} and lengthening the B chain by adding Arg^{31} and Arg^{32} produces a derivative (glargine) with reduced solubility at pH 7.4 that is, consequently, absorbed more slowly and acts over a longer period of time. Deleting Thr^{30B} and adding a myristoyl group to the ε-amino group of Lys^{29B} (detemir) enhances reversible binding to albumin, thereby slowing transport across vascular endothelium to tissues and providing prolonged action. *Insulin degludec* is LysB29(Nε-hexadecandioyl-γ-Glu) des(B30) human insulin. When degludec is injected subcutaneously, it forms multihexameric complexes that slow absorption; degludec also binds well to albumin; these two characteristics contribute to the prolonged effect of degludec (>24 h at steady state).

formulated at different concentrations: *Lantus* is formulated at 100 units/mL and a new formulation, *Toujeo*, at 300 units/mL. Toujeo may have a longer duration of action than Lantus. Basiglar is a glargine biosimilar formulation.

Insulin detemir is an insulin analogue modified by the addition of a saturated fatty acid to the ε amino group of LysB29, yielding a myristoylated insulin. When insulin detemir is injected subcutaneously, it binds to albumin via its fatty acid chain. In patients with type 1 diabetes, insulin detemir, administered twice a day, has a smoother time-action profile and produces a reduced prevalence of hypoglycemia than NPH insulin. The absorption profiles of glargine and detemir insulin are similar, but detemir often requires twice-daily administration.

Insulin degludec is a modified insulin with one amino acid deleted (threonine at position B30) and is conjugated to hexadecanedioic acid via γ-L-glutamyl spacer at the amino acid lysine at position B29. Degludec, which is active at a physiologic pH, forms multihexamers after injection subcutaneously. It has less severe hypoglycemia than glargine.

Other Insulin Formulations. Stable combinations of short-acting and long-acting insulins provide convenience by reducing the number of daily injections.

Inhaled insulin (Afrezza) is formulated for inhalation using a manufacturer-specific device (Leahy, 2015). This formulation should be used in combination with a long-acting insulin and has a more rapid onset and shorter duration than injected insulin analogues. It is not widely used. Adverse events include cough and throat irritation. It should not be used in individuals who smoke.

Insulin Delivery

Most insulin is injected subcutaneously. Pen devices containing prefilled insulin have proven to be popular. Jet injector systems that enable patients to receive subcutaneous insulin injections without a needle are available. Intravenous infusions of insulin are useful in patients with ketoacidosis or when requirements for insulin may change rapidly, such as during the perioperative period, during labor and delivery, and in intensive care situations. Long-acting insulin should not be given intravenously or intramuscularly or in an infusion device.

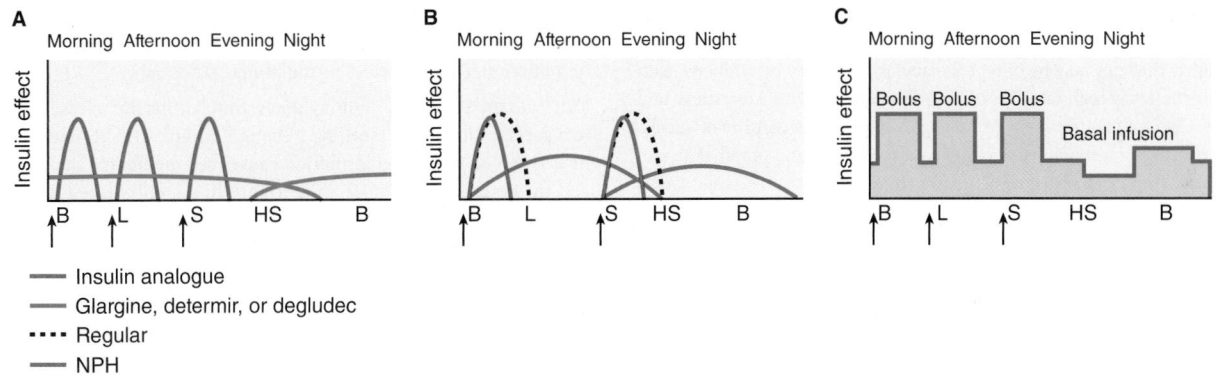

Figure 47–8 *Commonly used insulin regimens.* Panel **A** shows administration of a long-acting insulin like glargine (detemir or *degludec* could also be used; detemir may require twice-daily administration; degludec is used once daily; see text for details) to provide basal insulin and a premeal short-acting insulin analogue (see Table 47–5). Panel **B** shows a less-intensive insulin regimen with twice-daily injection of NPH insulin providing basal insulin and regular insulin or an insulin analogue providing mealtime insulin coverage. Only one type of short-acting insulin would be used. Panel **C** shows the insulin level attained following subcutaneous insulin (short-acting insulin analogue) by an insulin pump programmed to deliver different basal rates. At each meal, an insulin bolus is delivered. Here, B indicates breakfast, L lunch, S supper, and HS bedtime. An upward arrow shows insulin administration at mealtime. (Reprinted with permission from Kaufman FR, ed. *Medical Management of Type 1 Diabetes*, 6th ed. American Diabetes Association, Alexandria, VA, **2012**. Copyright © 2012 by the American Diabetes Association.)

Continuous Subcutaneous Insulin Infusion. Short-acting insulins are the only form of the hormone used in subcutaneous insulin infusion devices. A number of pumps are available for CSII therapy; this technology is rapidly evolving with improvements in hardware and software (McAdams and Rizvi, 2016). Insulin infusion devices provide a constant basal infusion of insulin and have the option of different infusion rates during the day and night to help avoid the rise in blood glucose that occurs just prior to awakening from sleep (the dawn phenomenon) and bolus injections that are programmed according to the size and nature of a meal. Selection of the most appropriate patients is extremely important for success with CSII. Pump insulin infusion devices can produce a more physiological profile of insulin replacement during exercise (where insulin production is decreased) and thus less hypoglycemia than traditional subcutaneous insulin injections provide. The technology for combining an insulin infusion device and continuous glucose monitoring is rapidly evolving with algorithms that alter the infusion rate (Thabit and Hovorka, 2016).

Factors That Affect Insulin Absorption

Factors that determine the rate of absorption of insulin after subcutaneous administration include the site of injection, the type of insulin, subcutaneous blood flow, smoking, regional muscular activity at the site of the injection, the volume and concentration of the injected insulin, and depth of injection (insulin has a more rapid onset of action if delivered intramuscularly rather than subcutaneously). Increased subcutaneous blood flow (brought about by massage, hot baths, or exercise) increases the rate of absorption. The abdomen currently is the preferred site of injection in the morning because insulin is absorbed 20%–30% faster from that site than from the arm. Rotation of insulin injection sites is recommended to avoid or limit subcutaneous scarring, lipohypertrophy, or lipoatrophy.

Insulin Dosing and Regimens

A number of commonly used dosage regimens that include mixtures of insulin given in two or more daily injections are depicted in Figure 47–8. For most patients, insulin-replacement therapy includes long-acting insulin (basal) and a short-acting insulin to provide postprandial needs. In a mixed population of patients with type 1 diabetes, the average dose of insulin is usually 0.6–0.7 units/kg body weight per day, with a range of 0.4–1 units/kg/d. Obese patients generally and pubertal adolescents may require more (about 1–2 units/kg/d) because of resistance of peripheral tissues to insulin. Patients who require less insulin than 0.5 units/kg/d may have some endogenous production of insulin or may be more sensitive to the hormone because of good physical conditioning. The basal dose is usually 40%–50% of the total daily dose, with the remainder as prandial or premeal insulin. The insulin dose at mealtime should reflect the anticipated carbohydrate intake. A supplemental scale of short-acting

insulin is added to the prandial insulin dose to allow correction of the blood glucose. *Insulin administered as a single daily dose of long-acting insulin, alone or in combination with short-acting insulin, is rarely sufficient to achieve euglycemia. More complex regimens that include multiple injections of long-acting or short-acting insulin are needed to reach this goal. In all patients, careful monitoring of therapeutic end points directs the insulin dose used. This approach is facilitated by self-monitoring of glucose, measurements of A1c, and individualization of the patient's therapeutic regimen (Table 47–4).* In patients who have gastroparesis or loss of appetite, injection of a short-acting analogue postprandially, based on the amount of food actually consumed, may provide smoother glycemic control.

Adverse Events

Hypoglycemia is the major risk that must be weighed against benefits of efforts to normalize glucose control. Insulin treatment of both type 1 and type 2 diabetes is associated with modest weight gain. Although uncommon, allergic reactions to recombinant human insulin may still occur as a result of reaction to the small amounts of aggregated or denatured insulin in preparations, to minor contaminants, or because of sensitivity to a component added to insulin in its formulation (protamine, Zn^{2+}, etc.). Atrophy of subcutaneous fat at the site of insulin injection (lipoatrophy) was a rare side effect of older insulin preparations. Lipohypertrophy (enlargement of subcutaneous fat depots) has been ascribed to the lipogenic action of high local concentrations of insulin.

Insulin Treatment of Ketoacidosis and Other Special Situations

Intravenous administration of insulin is most appropriate in patients with ketoacidosis or severe hyperglycemia with a hyperosmolar state (Umpierrez and Korytkowski, 2016). Insulin infusion inhibits lipolysis and gluconeogenesis completely and produces near-maximal stimulation of glucose uptake. In most patients with diabetic ketoacidosis, blood glucose concentrations will fall by about 10% per hour; the acidosis is corrected more slowly. As treatment proceeds, it often is necessary to administer glucose along with the insulin not only to prevent hypoglycemia but also to allow clearance of all ketones. Patients with a nonketotic hyperglycemic hyperosmolar state may be more sensitive to insulin than are those with ketoacidosis. Appropriate replacement of fluid and electrolytes, particularly K^+, is an integral part of the therapy in both situations because there is always a major K^+ deficit. A long-acting insulin should be administered subcutaneously before the insulin infusion is discontinued.

Treatment of Diabetes in Children or Adolescents

Diabetes is one of the most common chronic diseases of childhood, and rates of type 1 diabetes in American youth are estimated at 1 in 300. An unfortunate corollary of the growing rates of obesity over the past three decades is an increase in the numbers of children and adolescents with non-autoimmune, or type 2, diabetes. Current estimates are that 15%–20% of new cases of pediatric diabetes may be of type 2 diabetes; rates vary by ethnicity, with disproportionately high rates in Native Americans, African Americans, and Latinos. Current practice for type 1 diabetes is for intensive, physiologically based insulin replacement using combinations of basal and prandial insulin replacement or CSII with a goal of near-normal glucose control while avoiding hypoglycemia (Figure 47–7). The primary limiting factor of aggressive insulin therapy is hypoglycemia. In children and adolescents with type 1 diabetes, the recommended A1c goal is less than 7.5%, with a lower goal as appropriate. Insulin infusion devices and continuous glucose monitoring are being used with increasing frequency in the pediatric diabetic population and in older children and adolescents.

Because of the association of type 2 diabetes with obesity in the pediatric age group, lifestyle management is the recommended first step in therapy. Goals of reducing body weight and increasing physical activity are broadly recommended. The only medication currently approved by the FDA specifically for medical treatment of type 2 diabetes is *metformin*. Metformin is approved for children as young as 10 years of age and is available in a liquid formulation (100 mg/mL). Insulin is the typical second line of therapy after metformin; basal insulin can be added to oral agent therapy or multiple daily injections can be used when simpler regimens are not successful. Weight gain is a more significant problem than hypoglycemia with insulin treatment in pediatric type 2 diabetes.

Management of Diabetes in Hospitalized Patients

Hyperglycemia is common in hospitalized patients. Prevalence estimates of elevated blood glucose amongst inpatients with and without a prior diagnosis of diabetes range between 20% and 100% for patients treated in ICUs and 30% and 83% outside the ICU. Stress of illness has been associated with insulin resistance, possibly the result of counterregulatory hormone secretion, cytokines, and other inflammatory mediators. Food intake is often variable due to concurrent illness or preparation for diagnostic testing. Medications used in the hospital, such as glucocorticoids or dextrose-containing intravenous solutions, can exacerbate tendencies toward hyperglycemia. Finally, fluid balance and tissue perfusion can affect the absorbance of subcutaneous insulin and the clearance of glucose. Therapy of hyperglycemia in hospitalized patients needs to be adjusted for these variables. Emerging data indicate that hyperglycemia portends poor outcomes in hospitalized patients.

Insulin is the cornerstone of treatment of hyperglycemia in hospitalized patients. Oral agents have a limited place in treatment of hyperglycemic patients in the hospital because of slow onset of action, insufficient potency, need for intact GI function, and side effects. In noncritically ill hospitalized patients, a basal plus bolus correction insulin regimen, adjusted for oral intake, is optimal (Jacobi et al., 2012; McDonnell and Umpierrez, 2012). Using only short-acting insulins administered in response to hyperglycemia (i.e., sliding-scale regimens) to treat diabetes in the inpatient hospital setting is not appropriate therapy. For critically ill patients and those with variable blood pressure, edema, and tissue perfusion, intravenous insulin is the treatment of choice. Intravenous administration of insulin also is well suited to the treatment of diabetic patients during the perioperative period and during childbirth. The ADA suggests blood glucose targets of 140–180 m/dL (7.8–10.0 mM) in most hospitalized patients with more stringent goals, such as 110–140 mg/dL (6.1–7.8 mmol/L) in some critically ill patients (if achievable without significant hypoglycemia).

Insulin Secretagogues and Glucose-Lowering Agents

A variety of *sulfonylureas, meglitinides, GLP-1 agonists,* and *inhibitors of DPP-4* are used as secretagogues to stimulate insulin release (Table 47–6).

K_{ATP} Channel Modulators: Sulfonylureas

First-generation sulfonylureas (*tolbutamide, tolazamide,* and *chlorpropamide*) are rarely used now in the treatment of type 2 diabetes. The second, more potent, generation of hypoglycemic sulfonylureas includes *glyburide*

(glibenclamide), *glipizide*, and *glimepiride* (Kalra et al., 2015; Thule and Umpierrez, 2014). Some are available in an extended-release (glipizide) or a micronized (glyburide) formulation.

Mechanism of Action. Sulfonylureas stimulate insulin release by binding to a specific site on the β cell K_{ATP} channel complex (SUR) and inhibiting its activity. K_{ATP} channel inhibition causes cell membrane depolarization and the cascade of events leading to insulin secretion (see Figure 47–3). The acute administration of sulfonylureas to patients with type 2 diabetes increases insulin release from the pancreas. With chronic administration, circulating insulin levels decline to those that existed before treatment, but despite this reduction in insulin levels, reduced plasma glucose levels are maintained. The absence of acute stimulatory effects of sulfonylureas on insulin secretion during chronic treatment is attributed to downregulation of cell surface receptors for sulfonylureas on the pancreatic β cell.

ADME. Sulfonylureas are effectively absorbed from the GI tract. Food and hyperglycemia can reduce absorption. Sulfonylureas in plasma are largely (90%–99%) bound to protein, especially albumin. The volumes of distribution of most of the sulfonylureas are about 0.2 L/kg. Although their half-lives are short (3–5 h), their hypoglycemic effects are evident for 12–24 h, and they often can be administered once daily. The liver metabolizes all sulfonylureas, and the metabolites are excreted in the urine. Thus, sulfonylureas should be administered with caution to patients with either renal or hepatic insufficiency.

Therapeutic Uses. Sulfonylureas are used to treat hyperglycemia in type 2 diabetes. Of properly selected patients, 50%–80% respond to this class of agents. All members of the class appear to be equally efficacious. A significant number of patients who respond initially later cease to respond

TABLE 47–6 ■ PROPERTIES OF INSULIN SECRETAGOGUES

CLASS Generic name	DAILY DOSAGE[a](mg)	DURATION OF ACTION (hours or dosing frequency)
Sulfonylureas[b]		
Glimepiride	1–8	24
Glipizide	5–40	12–18
Glipizide (extended release)	5–20	24
Glyburide	1.25–20	12–24
Glyburide (micronized)	0.75–12	12–24
Nonsulfonylureas (Meglitinides)[c]		
Nateglinide	180–360	2–4
Repaglinide	0.5–16	2–6
GLP-1 Agonists		
Albiglutide	30–50	Weekly
Dulaglutide	0.75–1.5	Weekly
Exenatide[b]	2	Weekly
Liraglutide	0.6–1.8	Daily
Lixisenatide	0.010–0.020	Daily
Dipeptidyl Peptidase-4 Inhibitors		
Alogliptin	25	Daily
Linagliptin	5	Daily
Saxagliptin	2.5–5	Daily
Sitagliptin	25–100	12–16
Vildagliptin	50–100	Twice daily

[a]Dose should be lower in some patients.
[b]Older sulfonylureas are available, but rarely used (see text). Doses > 30 mg/d usually are divided into two doses.
[c]Labeled for administration 3–4 times daily.

to the sulfonylurea and develop unacceptable hyperglycemia (so-called secondary failure). This may occur as a result of a change in drug metabolism or more likely from a progression of β cell failure. Some individuals with neonatal diabetes or MODY- 3 respond to these agents. Contraindications to the use of these drugs include type 1 diabetes, pregnancy, lactation, and, for the older forms, significant hepatic or renal insufficiency.

Adverse Effects; Drug Interactions. Sulfonylureas may cause hypoglycemic reactions, including coma. Weight gain of 1–3 kg is a common side effect of improving glycemic control with sulfonylurea treatment. Less-frequent side effects include nausea and vomiting, cholestatic jaundice, agranulocytosis, aplastic and hemolytic anemias, generalized hypersensitivity reactions, and dermatological reactions. Rarely, patients treated with these drugs develop an alcohol-induced flush similar to that caused by disulfiram or hyponatremia. Whether this class of drugs is associated with an increase in cardiovascular mortality remains controversial.

The hypoglycemic effect of sulfonylureas may be enhanced by various mechanisms (decreased hepatic metabolism or renal excretion, displacement from protein-binding sites). Some drugs (sulfonamides, clofibrate, and salicylates) displace the sulfonylureas from binding proteins, thereby transiently increasing the concentration of free drug. Ethanol may enhance the action of sulfonylureas and cause hypoglycemia. Hypoglycemia may be more frequent in patients taking a sulfonylurea in combination with one or more of these agents: androgens, anticoagulants, azole antifungals, chloramphenicol, fenfluramine, fluconazole, gemfibrozil, H_2 antagonists, magnesium salts, methyldopa, MAOIs, probenecid, sulfinpyrazone, sulfonamides, tricyclic antidepressants, and urinary acidifiers. Other drugs may decrease the glucose-lowering effect of sulfonylureas by increasing hepatic metabolism, increasing renal excretion, or inhibiting insulin secretion (β blockers, Ca^{2+} channel blockers, cholestyramine, diazoxide, estrogens, hydantoins, isoniazid, nicotinic acid, phenothiazines, rifampin, sympathomimetics, thiazide diuretics, and urinary alkalinizers).

Dosage Forms Available. Treatment is initiated at the lower end of the dose range and titrated upward based on the patient's glycemic response. Some have a longer duration of action and can be prescribed in a single daily dose (glimepiride), whereas others are formulated as extended-release or micronized formulations to extend their duration of action (see Table 47–6). Sulfonylureas such as glipizide or glimepiride appear safer than longer-acting sulfonylureas in elderly individuals with type 2 diabetes, but even the short-duration agents should be used with caution in elderly patients.

K_{ATP} Channel Modulators: Nonsulfonylureas

Repaglinide. Repaglinide is an oral insulin secretagogue of the meglitinide class (see Table 47–6). Like sulfonylureas, it stimulates insulin release by closing K_{ATP} channels in pancreatic β cells (Chen et al., 2015).

The drug is absorbed rapidly from the GI tract, and peak blood levels are obtained within 1 h. The $t_{1/2}$ is about 1 h. These features allow for multiple preprandial use. Repaglinide is metabolized primarily by the liver (CYP3A4) to inactive derivatives. Because a small proportion (~10%) is metabolized by the kidney, dosing of the drug in patients with renal insufficiency also should be performed cautiously.

The major side effect of repaglinide is hypoglycemia. Repaglinide also is associated with a decline in efficacy (secondary failure) after initially improving glycemic control. Certain drugs may potentiate the action of repaglinide by displacing it from plasma protein-binding sites (β blockers, chloramphenicol, coumarin, MAOIs, NSAIDs, probenecid, salicylates, and sulfonamide) or altering its metabolism (gemfibrozil, itraconazole, trimethoprim, cyclosporine, simvastatin, clarithromycin).

Nateglinide. Nateglinide is an orally effective insulin secretagogue. Nateglinide stimulates insulin secretion by blocking K_{ATP} channels in pancreatic β cells (Chen et al., 2015). Nateglinide promotes a more rapid but less-sustained secretion of insulin than other available oral antidiabetic agents. The drug's major therapeutic effect is reducing postprandial glycemic elevations in patients with type 2 diabetes.

Nateglinide is most effective when administered at a dose of 120 mg, three times daily, 1–10 min before a meal. It is metabolized primarily by hepatic CYPs (2C9, 70%; 3A4, 30%) and should be used cautiously in patients with hepatic insufficiency. About 16% of an administered dose is excreted by the kidney as unchanged drug. Some drugs reduce the glucose-lowering effect of nateglinide (corticosteroids, rifamycins, sympathomimetics, thiazide diuretics, thyroid products); others (alcohol, NSAIDs, salicylates, MAOIs, and nonselective β blockers) may increase the risk of hypoglycemia with nateglinide. Nateglinide therapy may produce fewer episodes of hypoglycemia than other currently available oral insulin secretagogues, including repaglinide. As with sulfonylureas and repaglinide, secondary failure occurs.

Biguanides

Metformin is the only member of the biguanide class of oral hypoglycemic drugs available for use today. Previously available biguanides, phenformin and buformin, were removed from the market in the 1970s due to unacceptable rates of associated lactic acidosis.

Mechanism of Action. Several mechanisms have been proposed to explain the central pharmacologic action of metformin, the reduction of HGP primarily by limiting gluconeogenesis. Metformin has specific actions on mitochondrial respiration that reduce intracellular ATP and increase AMP. Experimental evidence supports activation of AMP-dependent protein kinase (AMPK) by metformin, leading to stimulation of hepatic fatty acid oxidation, glucose uptake, and nonoxidative glucose metabolism and reduction of lipogenesis and gluconeogenesis. Metformin also inhibits the mitochondrial glycerol phosphate dehydrogenase, thereby changing the redox state of the cell. More recent evidence implicates other mechanisms, including blunting the effects of glucagon, inhibiting conversion of lactate and glycerol to glucose, and shifting the liver toward negative lipid balance.

Most of the pharmacologic effects of metformin are mediated in the liver with little effect on glucose metabolism or insulin sensitivity in skeletal muscle. Metformin has little effect on blood glucose in normoglycemic states, does not stimulate the release of insulin or other islet hormones, and rarely causes hypoglycemia. However, even in persons with only mild hyperglycemia, metformin lowers blood glucose by reducing HGP and increasing glucose clearance. This last effect is not well understood because of the modest action of metformin to promote glucose uptake in peripheral tissues (e.g., skeletal muscle and adipose tissue). There is little information to support a direct effect of metformin on hepatic insulin signaling, but there are at least complementary effects of the drug to improve the dose-response relationship between insulin and hepatic glucose production.

ADME. Fixed-dose combinations of metformin in conjunction with glipizide, glyburide, pioglitazone, repaglinide, rosiglitazone, linagliptin, saxagliptin, sitagliptin, alogliptin, canagliflozin, dapagliflozin, and empagliflozin are available. Based on the pharmacokinetics of the common immediate-release form of metformin, it is now recommended for twice-daily administration at doses of 0.5–1.0 g. The maximum dose is 2550 mg, but therapeutic benefit starts to plateau at 2000 mg. A sustained-release preparation is available for once-daily dosing starting at 500 mg daily, with titration up to 2000 mg as necessary.

Metformin is absorbed primarily from the small intestine with a bioavailability of 70%–80%. Peak concentrations after an oral dose occur at about 2 h; the drug's plasma $t_{1/2}$ is 4–5 h. The drug does not bind to plasma proteins and is excreted unchanged in the urine. The transport of metformin into hepatocytes is mediated primarily by OCT 1; renal uptake is mediated by OCT 2. Export into the urine is by MATE1/2 (multidrug and toxin extrusion proteins).

Therapeutic Uses. Metformin is generally accepted as the first-line treatment of type 2 diabetes and is currently the most commonly used oral agent for this condition. Metformin is effective as monotherapy and in combination with other glucose lowering medications (Mearns et al., 2015). African Americans may have a better response to metformin than Caucasians.

Metformin has superior or equivalent efficacy of glucose lowering compared to other oral agents used to treat diabetes and reduces microvascular complications in patients with type 2 diabetes; more limited data support a beneficial effect to reduce macrovascular disease as well. Metformin does not typically cause weight gain and in some cases causes mild weight reduction. In persons with IGT, treatment with metformin delays the progression to diabetes. Metformin has been used as a treatment of infertility in women with polycystic ovarian syndrome. Although not formally approved for this purpose, metformin demonstrably improves ovulation and menstrual cyclicity and reduces circulating androgens and hirsutism.

Adverse Effects; Drug Interactions. The most common side effects (10%–25%) of metformin are GI: nausea, indigestion, abdominal cramps or bloating, diarrhea, or some combination of these. Metformin has direct effects on GI function, including interference with the absorption of glucose and bile salts. Use of metformin is also associated with 20%–30% lower blood levels of vitamin B_{12} and these levels should be monitored. Most adverse GI effects of metformin abate over time with continued use and can be minimized by starting at low doses and gradually titrating to a target dose over several weeks, as well as by having patients take the drug with meals. Most studies indicated that extended-release metformin has decreased GI side effects and can be substituted for immediate-release metformin in patients who are having difficulty tolerating the drug.

Because the previously available biguanides phenformin and buformin caused lactic acidosis, metformin has been carefully scrutinized for this side effect. Lactic acidosis associated with metformin has been rarely reported in patients with the setting of concurrent conditions that can cause poor tissue perfusion (e.g., sepsis, myocardial infarction, and congestive heart failure). However, recent analyses have raised doubts regarding whether the association of metformin with lactic acidosis is causal. Renal failure is a common comorbidity in patients with lactic acidosis associated with metformin use, and plasma metformin levels are inversely related to GFR due to reduced clearance of drug from the circulation (e.g., levels rise above the usual therapeutic range when creatinine clearance drops below 40–50 mL/min). However, in recent studies of patients with severe renal failure, including some requiring dialysis, rates of lactic acidosis were not increased in those taking metformin. The ADA suggests that metformin may be used safely when the GFR is greater than 45 mL/min/1.73 m^2, and that the dose should be reduced by 50%–75% when GFR is 30–45 mL/min/1.73 m^2.

It is important to assess renal function before starting metformin and to monitor function at least annually. Metformin should be discontinued preemptively if renal function could decline precipitously, such as before radiographic procedures that use contrast dyes and during admission to the hospital for severe illness. Metformin should not be used in patients with severe pulmonary disease, decompensated heart failure, severe liver disease, or chronic alcohol abuse. Cationic drugs that are eliminated by renal tubular secretion have the potential for interaction with metformin by competing for common renal tubular transport systems. Adjustment of metformin is recommended in patients who are taking cationic medications such as cimetidine, furosemide, and nifedipine.

Thiazolidinediones

Thiazolidinediones are ligands for the PPARγ receptor, a nuclear hormone receptor that has two isoforms and is involved in the regulation of genes related to glucose and lipid metabolism. Two thiazolidinediones are currently available to treat patients with type 2 diabetes, *rosiglitazone* and *pioglitazone*; a third, *troglitazone*, was removed from the market in 2000 due to hepatotoxicity.

Mechanism of Action; Pharmacological Effects. Thiazolidinediones activate PPARγ receptors, which are expressed primarily in adipose tissue with lesser expression in cardiac, skeletal, and smooth muscle cells; islet β cells; macrophages; and vascular endothelial cells. The endogenous ligands for PPARγ include small lipophilic molecules such as oxidized linoleic acid, arachidonic acid, and the prostaglandin metabolite 15d-PGJ2. Ligand binding to PPARγ causes heterodimer formation with the retinoid X receptor and interaction with PPAR response elements on specific genes (see Chapter 3). The principal response to PPARγ activation is

adipocyte differentiation. PPARγ activity also promotes uptake of circulating fatty acids into fat cells and shifts of lipid stores from extra-adipose sites to adipose tissue.

One consequence of the cellular responses to PPARγ activation is increased tissue sensitivity to insulin. Pioglitazone and rosiglitazone are insulin sensitizers and increase insulin-mediated glucose uptake by 30%–50% in patients with type 2 diabetes. Although adipose tissue seems to be the primary target for PPARγ agonists, both clinical and preclinical models support a role for skeletal muscle, the major site for insulin-mediated glucose disposal, in the response to thiazolidinediones. In addition to promoting glucose uptake into muscle and adipose tissue, the thiazolidinediones reduce HGP and increase hepatic glucose uptake. It is not clear whether thiazolidinedione-induced improvement of insulin resistance is due to direct effects on key target tissues (skeletal muscle and liver), indirect effects mediated by secreted products of adipocytes (e.g., adiponectin), or some combination of these.

Thiazolidinediones also affect lipid metabolism. Treatment with rosiglitazone or pioglitazone reduces plasma levels of fatty acids by increasing clearance and reducing lipolysis. These drugs also cause a shift of triglyceride stores from nonadipose to adipose tissues and from visceral to subcutaneous fat depots. Pioglitazone reduces plasma triglycerides by 10%–15%, raises HDL cholesterol levels, and increases LDL cholesterol. In contrast, rosiglitazone has minimal effects on plasma triglycerides, and the only consistent effect on circulating lipids is an increase of LDL cholesterol.

ADME. Rosiglitazone and pioglitazone are dosed once daily. The starting dose of rosiglitazone is 4 mg, and the maximum dose should not exceed 8 mg daily. The starting dose of pioglitazone is 15–30 mg, increased up to a maximum of 45 mg daily. Both agents are absorbed within 2–3 h, and bioavailability is unaffected by food. The thiazolidinediones are metabolized by the liver and may be administered to patients with renal insufficiency, but should not be used if there is active hepatic disease. Rifampin induces hepatic CYPs and causes a significant decrease in plasma concentrations of rosiglitazone and pioglitazone; gemfibrozil impedes metabolism of the thiazolidinediones and can increase plasma levels by about 2-fold; a dose reduction is suggested with this combination. The onset of action of thiazolidinediones is relatively slow; maximal effects on glucose homeostasis develop gradually over the course of 1–3 months.

Therapeutic Uses. Thiazolidinediones enhance insulin action on liver, adipose tissue, and skeletal muscle; confer improvements in glycemic control in persons with type 2 diabetes; and cause average reductions in A1c of 0.5%–1.4%. Thiazolidinediones require the presence of insulin for pharmacological activity and are not used to treat type 1 diabetes. Both pioglitazone and rosiglitazone are effective as monotherapy and as additive therapy to metformin, sulfonylureas, or insulin. In addition, pioglitazone is marketed in a fixed-dose combination with alogliptin.

Adverse Effects; Drug Interactions. The most common adverse effects of the thiazolidinediones are weight gain and edema. Thiazolidinediones cause an increase in body adiposity and an average weight gain of 2–4 kg over the first year of treatment. The use of insulin with thiazolidinedione treatment roughly doubles the incidence of edema and amount of weight gain compared with either drug alone. Macular edema has been reported in patients using both rosiglitazone and pioglitazone, but this was not a consistent finding in recent clinical trials (Ambrosius et al., 2010).

As with other side effects of thiazolidinediones, fluid retention is dose related. Use of thiazolidinediones is associated with a mild reduction of hematocrit, which may be an effect of fluid retention, although a primary effect on hematopoiesis has not been excluded.

Exposure to these drugs over several years in clinical trials has been associated with an increased incidence of heart failure of up to 2-fold (Home, 2012; Horita et al., 2015). This has generally been attributed to the effect of the drugs to cause plasma volume expansion in patients with type 2 diabetes who have an increased risk for heart failure. There does not appear to be an acute effect of pioglitazone or rosiglitazone to reduce myocardial contractility or ejection fraction.

The use of thiazolidinediones in diabetic patients without a history of heart failure, or with compensated heart failure, can be initiated, but monitoring for signs and symptoms of congestive heart failure is important, especially when insulin is also used. Thiazolidinediones should not be used in patients with moderate-to-severe heart failure. In the past, evidence suggested that rosiglitazone increased the risk of cardiovascular events (myocardial infarction, stroke). For this reason, the FDA restricted its use for several years, but this regulation has now been lifted. The connection of the drug to cardiovascular disease remains controversial; most evidence supports either mild beneficial effects of pioglitazone on overall cardiovascular events or a neutral impact. In a trial of nondiabetic individuals who had insulin resistance and a recent history of ischemic stroke or TIA, pioglitazone reduced the risk of subsequent stroke or myocardial infarction and diabetes (Kernan et al., 2016).

Treatment with thiazolidinediones has been associated with a consistent increased risk of bone fracture in women, with some studies also showing effects in men (Gilbert and Pratley, 2015). Therefore, the presence of osteoporosis and other risks for fracture should be considered before starting thiazolidinediones.

Pioglitazone and rosiglitazone are associated with a lowering of transaminases, probably reflective of reductions in hepatic steatosis (Singh et al., 2015); thus, thiazolidinediones should be withheld from patients with clinically apparent liver disease, and liver function should be monitored intermittently during treatment.

GLP-1–Based Agents

Incretins are GI hormones that are released after meals and stimulate insulin secretion. The best-known incretins are GLP-1 and GIP. GIP has reduced efficacy to stimulate insulin release and lower blood glucose in persons with type 2 diabetes, whereas GLP-1 is effective, and the GLP-1 signaling system has been a successful drug target.

Both GLP-1 and glucagon are derived from preproglucagon, a 180–amino acid precursor with five separately processed domains (Figure 47–9). An amino-terminal signal peptide is followed by glicentin-related pancreatic peptide, glucagon, GLP-1, and GLP-2. Processing of the protein is sequential and occurs in a tissue-specific fashion. Pancreatic α cells cleave proglucagon into glucagon and a large C-terminal peptide that includes both of the GLPs. Intestinal L cells and specific hindbrain neurons process proglucagon into a large N-terminal peptide that includes glucagon or GLP-1 and GLP-2. GLP-2 affects the proliferation of epithelial cells lining the GI tract. Teduglutide, a GLP-2 analogue, is approved for treatment of short-bowel syndrome (see Chapter 50).

Given intravenously to diabetic subjects in supraphysiologic amounts, GLP-1 stimulates insulin secretion, inhibits glucagon release, delays gastric emptying, reduces food intake, and normalizes fasting and postprandial insulin secretion. The insulinotropic effect of GLP-1 is glucose dependent in that insulin secretion at fasting glucose concentrations, even with high levels of circulating GLP-1, is minimal. GLP-1 is rapidly inactivated by the enzyme DPP-4, yielding a plasma $t_{1/2}$ of 1–2 min; thus, the natural peptide, itself, is not a useful therapeutic agent. Two broad strategies have been taken to applying GLP-1 to therapeutics: the development of injectable, DPP-4-resistant peptide agonists of the GLP-1 receptor and the creation of small-molecule inhibitors of DPP-4 (Figure 47–10; see Table 47–6).

GLP-1 Receptor Agonists

Five GLP-1RAs have been approved for treatment of diabetic patients in the U.S (Table 47–6); a fifth, lixisenatide, is available in Europe (Madsbad, 2016; Trujillo and Nuffer, 2014).

Exenatide. Exendin-4, is a naturally occurring 39–amino acid reptilian peptide with 53% sequence homology to GLP-1. This peptide is a potent GLP-1RA that shares many of the physiological and pharmacological effects of GLP-1. It is not metabolized by DPP-4 and so has extended activity following injection. Synthetic exendin-4, exenatide, is approved for use as monotherapy and as adjunctive therapy for patients with type 2 diabetes not achieving glycemic targets with other drugs.

In clinical trials, exenatide, alone or in combination with metformin, sulfonylurea, or thiazolidinedione, was associated with improved glycemic control, as reflected in an about 1% decrease in A1c and weight loss that averaged 2.5–4 kg. Evidence from clinical trials indicated that exenatide can also be used in conjunction with basal insulin. An extended-release form of exenatide is administered by subcutaneous injection once a week with greater effectiveness than twice-daily treatment.

Liraglutide. The liraglutide peptide is a long-acting, DPP-4-resistant form of GLP-1, but with a Lys34Arg substitution and addition of an α-glutamic acid spacer coupled to a C16 fatty acyl group at Lys[26]. The fatty acid side chain permits binding to albumin and other plasma proteins and accounts for an extended $t_{1/2}$ that permits once-daily administration; the fatty acid also seems to offer some protection from cleavage of the N-terminus by DPP-4. The pharmacodynamic profile of liraglutide mimics GLP-1 and exenatide. In clinical trials, liraglutide caused both improvement in glycemic control and weight loss. In a single comparative trial, liraglutide reduced A1c about 30% more than exenatide (Buse et al., 2009). Liraglutide is indicated for adjunctive therapy in patients not achieving glycemic control with oral agents. Liraglutide can be added to oral agents or basal insulin. In a recent report, liraglutide reduced the risk of cardiovascular death, nonfatal myocardial infarction, or nonfatal stroke in patients with type 2 diabetes and established cardiovascular disease. Similar positive effects on cardiovascular risk have also been demonstrated in a trial of semaglutide, a compound in development with similarities to liraglutide. Other GLP-1 receptor agonists (exenatide and lixisenatide) are neutral with regards to cardiovascular risk in the trials completed to date.

Albiglutide. Albiglutide is a fusion protein that includes two sequential GLP-1 moieties linked to human albumin; the GLP-1 sequences are modified to prevent DPP-4 cleavage. Albiglutide is also indicated for patients

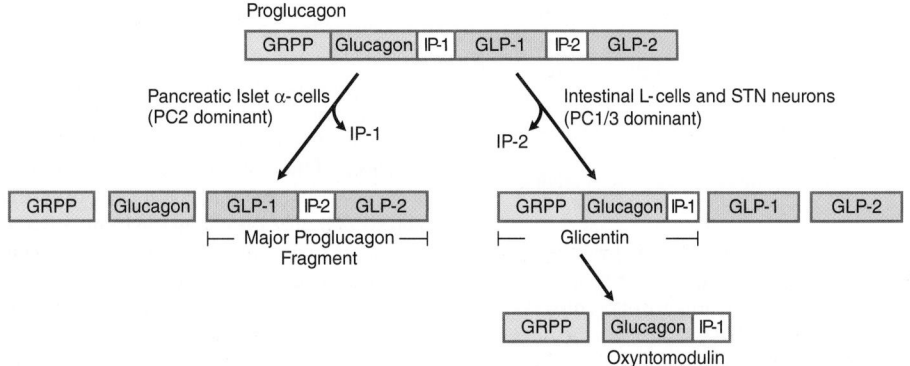

Figure 47–9 *Processing of proglucagon to glucagon, GLP-1, GLP-2, and GRPP.* Proglucagon is synthesized in islet α cells, intestinal enteroendocrine cells (L cells), and a subset of neurons in the hindbrain. In α cells, prohormone processing is primarily by proconvertase 2, releasing glucagon, GRPP, and a major proglucagon fragment containing the two GLPs. In L cells and neurons, proglucagon cleavage is mostly through proconvertase 1/3, giving glicentin, oxyntomodulin, GLP-1, and GLP-2. IP-1, intervening peptide—1; STN, solitary tract nucleus.

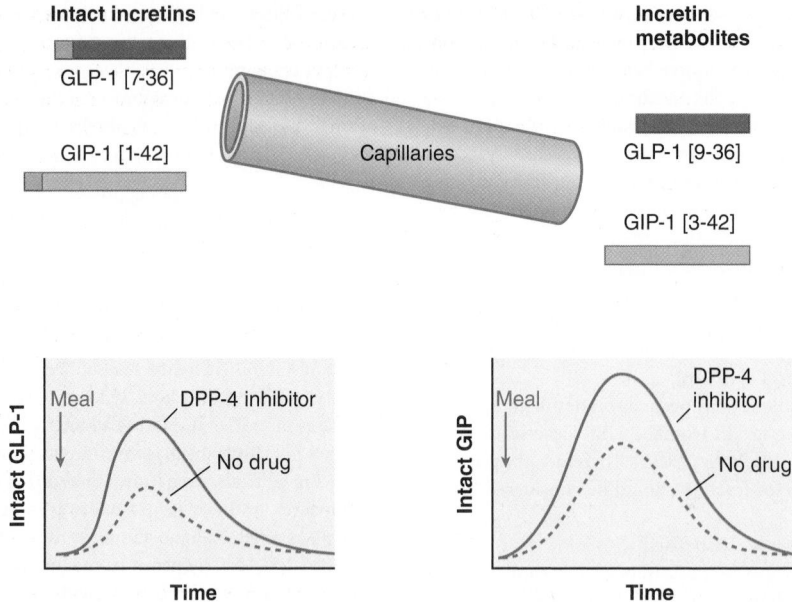

Figure 47–10 *Pharmacological effects of DDP-4 inhibition.* DPP-4, an ectoenzyme located on the luminal side of capillary endothelial cells metabolizes the incretins, GLP-1, and GIP, by removing the two N-terminal amino acids. The target for DPP-4 cleavage is a proline or alanine residue in the second position of the primary peptide sequence. The truncated metabolites GLP-1[9–36] and GIP[3–42] are the major forms of the incretins in plasma and are inactive as insulin secretagogues. Treatment with a DPP-4 inhibitor increases the concentrations of intact GLP-1 and GIP.

with type 2 diabetes with suboptimal glucose control and can be used in conjunction with oral agents and basal insulin.

Dulaglutide. Dulaglutide is a fusion protein consisting of two linked molecules that have a modified version of GLP-1 linked to the Fc portion of a human immunoglobulin; the GLP-1 sequences are modified to protect against the action of DPP-4. Pharmacodynamics are comparable to other GLP-1RAs, and the drug can be used with other antidiabetic agents.

Lixisenatide. Lixisenatide is a slightly longer form of exendin-4 that has comparable pharmacodynamics. Data from a recent clinical trial of diabetic subjects with a prior history of cardiovascular disease indicated no impact of lixisenatide on recurrent events.

While all of the GLP-1RAs have demonstrated efficacy as monotherapy, none is considered as a first-line agent. While there are several clinical trials available that directly compared different GLP-1RAs, in general the differences in efficacy are small relative to the overall effect of the drugs, and definitive differences await more comprehensive studies.

Mechanism of Action. All GLP-1RAs share a common mechanism, activation of the GLP-1 receptor, a member of glucagon receptor family of GPCRs (class B GPCRs). GLP-1 receptors are expressed by β cells, cells in the peripheral and central nervous systems, the heart and vasculature, kidney, lung, and GI mucosa. Binding of agonists to the GLP-1 receptor activates the cAMP-PKA pathway and several GEFs. GLP-1 receptor activation also initiates signaling via PKC and PI3K and alters the activity of several ion channels. In β cells, the end result of these actions is increased insulin biosynthesis and exocytosis in a glucose-dependent manner (see Figure 47–3). Activation of GLP-1 receptors in the CNS accounts for the effects of receptor agonists on food intake and gastric emptying and for side effects such as nausea.

ADME. *Exenatide* is given as a subcutaneous injection twice daily, typically before meals. It is rapidly absorbed, reaches peak concentrations in about 2 h, and has a plasma $t_{1/2}$ of 2–3 h. Clearance of the drug occurs primarily by glomerular filtration, with tubular proteolysis and minimal reabsorption. Exenatide is marketed as a pen that delivers 5 or 10 μg; dosing is typically started at the lower amount and increased as needed. There is a weekly preparation based on the embedding of exenatide in a polymeric microsphere that releases drug slowly after injection. Weekly exenatide is given as a suspension of 2 mg that is prepared from lyophilized

material and diluent immediately prior to injection. Once in the circulation, the drug is metabolized similarly to short-acting exenatide; however, based on the extended rate of delivery, 5–6 weekly doses are required to reach therapeutic steady state.

Liraglutide is given as a subcutaneous injection once daily. Peak levels occur in 8–12 h; the elimination $t_{1/2}$ is 12–14 h. There is little renal or intestinal excretion of liraglutide; clearance is primarily through the metabolic pathways of large plasma proteins. Liraglutide is supplied in a pen injector that delivers 0.6, 1.2, or 1.8 mg of drug; the lowest dose is for treatment initiation, with elevation to the higher doses based on clinical response.

Albiglutide has a $t_{1/2}$ of 5–7 days and can be dosed weekly. It is delivered through a pen device at doses of 30 or 50 mg following reconstitution. Clearance of the drug is primarily through enzymatic degradation, although renal clearance can be inferred from the increasing plasma levels in some patients with renal impairment.

Dulaglutide has similar pharmacokinetic properties to albiglutide; no effects of hepatic or renal impairment on these has been demonstrated.

Lixisenatide has an elimination $t_{1/2}$ of 3–4 h that involves a significant degree of renal clearance.

Adverse Effects; Drug Interactions. Intravenous or subcutaneous administration of GLP-1 causes nausea and vomiting; this is thought to be mediated through neural activation of specific CNS neurons that are activated following peripheral dosing of peptide. The doses above which GLP-1 causes GI side effects are higher than those needed to regulate blood glucose. Nonetheless, up to 30%–50% of subjects report nausea at the initiation of therapy with any of the GLP-1RAs, although the GI side effects of these drugs wane over time. Activation of GLP-1 receptors in the CNS mediates the typical delay of gastric emptying, and GLP-1 agonists may alter the pharmacokinetics of drugs that require rapid GI absorption, such as oral contraceptives and antibiotics. In the absence of other diabetes drugs that cause low blood glucose, hypoglycemia associated with GLP-1 agonist treatment is rare, but the combination of GLP-1 agonist with sulfonylurea drugs causes an increased rate of hypoglycemia compared to sulfonylurea treatment alone. Because of the reliance on renal clearance, exenatide, and probably lixisenatide, should not be given to persons with moderate-to-severe renal failure (creatinine clearance < 30 mL/min). Based on surveillance data, there is a possible association of exenatide treatment with pancreatitis; therefore, these drugs should not be used in persons with a history or predisposition to pancreatitis. The GLP-1 receptor is expressed by thyroid C cells. Although there is not an established clinical association with medullary carcinoma of the thyroid, GLP-1 agonists should not be given to these patients.

DPP-4 Inhibitors

Dipeptidyl peptidase IV is a serine protease that is widely distributed throughout the body, expressed as an ectoenzyme on vascular endothelial cells, on the surface of T lymphocytes, and in a circulating form. DPP-4 cleaves the two N-terminal amino acids from peptides with a proline or alanine in the second position (Deacon and Lebovitz, 2016) and seems to be especially critical for the inactivation of GLP-1 and GIP. DPP-4 inhibitors increase the AUC of GLP-1 and GIP as stimulated by ingestion of food (see Figure 47–10). Several agents provide nearly complete and long-lasting inhibition of DPP-4, thereby increasing the proportion of active GLP-1 from 10% to 20% of total circulating GLP-1 immunoreactivity to nearly 100%. *Sitagliptin, saxagliptin, linagliptin*, and *alogliptin* are available in the U.S.; *vildagliptin*, is available in the E.U.

Mechanism of Action; Pharmacological Effects. Alogliptin, linagliptin, and sitagliptin are competitive inhibitors of DPP-4; vildagliptin and saxagliptin bind the enzyme covalently. All five drugs can be given in doses that lower measurable activity of DPP-4 by more than 95% for 12 h. This causes a greater than 2-fold elevation of plasma concentrations of active GIP and GLP-1 and is associated with increased insulin secretion, reduced glucagon levels, and improvements in both fasting and postprandial hyperglycemia. Inhibition of DPP-4 does not appear to have direct effects on insulin sensitivity, gastric motility, or satiety; chronic treatment with a DPP-4 inhibitor also does not affect body weight. DPP-4 inhibitors, used as monotherapy in type 2 diabetic patients, reduce A1c levels by an average of about 0.8%. These compounds are also effective for chronic glucose control when added to the treatment of diabetic patients receiving metformin, thiazolidinediones, sulfonylureas, and insulin, with a further reduction of A1c by about 0.5%. The effects of DPP-4 inhibitors in combination regimens appear to be additive.

ADME. The recommended doses of the DPP4 inhibitors are alogliptin, 25 mg daily; linagliptin, 5 mg daily; saxagliptin, 5 mg daily; sitagliptin, 100 mg daily; and vildagliptin, 50 mg one or two times daily. DPP-4 inhibitors are absorbed effectively from the small intestine. Alogliptin, saxagliptin, sitagliptin, and vildagliptin circulate primarily in unbound form and are excreted largely unchanged in the urine; lower doses should be given to patients with reduced renal function. Linagliptin binds extensively to plasma proteins and is cleared primarily by the hepatobiliary system, with little renal clearance. Only saxagliptin is metabolized by hepatic microsomal enzymes, and its dose should be lowered to 2.5 mg daily when coadministered with strong CYP3A4 inhibitors (e.g., ketoconazole, atazanavir, clarithromycin, indinavir, itraconazole, nefazodone, nelfinavir, ritonavir, saquinavir, and telithromycin).

Adverse Effects. There are no consistent adverse effects that have been noted in clinical trials with any of the DPP-4 inhibitors. Large cardiovascular safety studies have been completed for alogliptin, saxagliptin, and sitagliptin. There was no impact of these drugs on the incidence of cardiovascular events in diabetic patients, although patients treated with saxagliptin had an increase in hospitalization for heart failure. The FDA has issued a warning that this class of drugs is rarely associated with severe joint pain. DPP-4 is expressed on lymphocytes; in the immunology literature, the enzyme is referred to as CD26. Effects on immune function bear scrutiny as more patients are treated with these compounds.

Alpha Glucosidase Inhibitors

α-Glucosidase inhibitors reduce intestinal absorption of starch, dextrin, and disaccharides by inhibiting the action of α-glucosidase in the intestinal brush border (Standl and Schnell, 2012). These drugs also increase the release of the glucoregulatory hormone GLP-1 into the circulation, which may contribute to their glucose-lowering effects. The drugs in this class are *acarbose, miglitol*, and *voglibose* (not available in the U.S.).

ADME. Dosing of acarbose and miglitol are similar. Both are provided as 25-, 50-, or 100-mg tablets that are taken before meals. Treatment should

start with lower doses and be titrated as indicated by balancing postprandial glucose, A1c, and GI symptoms. Acarbose is minimally absorbed; the small amount of drug reaching the systemic circulation is cleared by the kidney. Miglitol absorption is saturable, with 50%–100% of any dose entering the circulation. Miglitol is cleared almost entirely by the kidney, and dose reductions are recommended for patients with creatinine clearance less than 30 mL/min.

Adverse Effects; Drug Interactions. The most prominent adverse effects are malabsorption, flatulence, diarrhea, and abdominal bloating. Mild-to-moderate elevations of hepatic transaminases are reported with acarbose, but symptomatic liver disease is very rare. Cutaneous hypersensitivity has been described but is also rare. Hypoglycemia has been described when α-glucosidase inhibitors are added to insulin or an insulin secretagogue. Acarbose can decrease the absorption of digoxin; miglitol can decrease the absorption of propranolol and ranitidine. The α-glucosidase inhibitors are contraindicated in patients with stage 4 renal failure.

Therapeutic Use. α-Glucosidase inhibitors are indicated as adjuncts to diet and exercise in type 2 diabetic patients not reaching glycemic targets. They can also be used in combination with other oral antidiabetic agents or insulin. In clinical studies, α-glucosidase inhibitors reduced A1c by 0.5%–0.8%, fasting glucose by about 1 mM, and postprandial glucose by 2.0–2.5 mM. These agents do not cause weight gain or have significant effects on plasma lipids.

Na⁺-Glucose Transporter 2 Inhibitors

SGLT2 is a Na⁺-glucose cotransporter located almost exclusively in the proximal portion of the renal tubule. SGLT2 is a high-affinity, low-capacity transporter that moves glucose against a concentration gradient from the tubular lumen using energy generated from Na⁺ flux through the epithelial cells. Renal retention of glucose is nearly complete in nondiabetic persons, and SGLT2 accounts for 80%–90% of this reclamation; the remainder is recovered by SGLT1 more distally in the tubule. Early studies in diabetic animals demonstrated that hyperglycemia could be nearly ameliorated by the naturally occurring compound *phlorizin*, an SGLT inhibitor. Based on this proof of principle, drugs that are specific inhibitors of SGLT2 have been developed to treat diabetes (Mudaliar et al., 2015; White, 2015). These agents block glucose transport in the proximal tubule and lower blood glucose by promoting urinary loss.

Mechanism of Action; Pharmacological Effects. SGLT2 inhibitors reduce the rate of glucose reclamation in the proximal tubule and shift the renal threshold for glucose excretion from about 180 to 50 mg/dL (10 to 2.8 mM). In monotherapy, they reduce A1c by 0.7%–1.0%, cause weight loss of 2–4 kg, and decrease blood pressure by 2–4 mm Hg. There are currently three SGLP2 inhibitors available for clinical use—*canagliflozin, dapagliflozin* and *empagliflozin*—with several other members of this class still in development. These agents are indicated for use in combination with other oral agents and insulin; such use leads to an additional decrease of A1c of 0.5%–0.7%. SGLT2 inhibitors are available in combination with metformin and DPP-4 inhibitors; a combined SGLT1/SGLT2 inhibitor is under investigation.

ADME. Available SGLT2 inhibitors share favorable pharmacokinetic properties. They have good oral bioavailability (60%–80%) that is not affected by food and reach peak levels 1–2 h after ingestion. They are about 90% bound to circulating proteins with half-lives of about 12 h, making them suitable for once-daily dosing. The compounds are metabolized by glucuronidation and the inactive metabolites renally excreted; there is virtually no renal excretion of the parent drugs. All three drugs are available in two doses, dapagliflozin 5 and 10 mg, canagliflozin 100 and 300 mg, and empagliflozin 10 and 25 mg.

Adverse Effects; Drug Interactions. The side effects of SGLT2 inhibitors are predictable from their mechanism of action. There is a small (1%–2%) increase in lower urinary tract infections and a 3%–5% increase in genital mycotic infections. Urine glucose losses cause mild diuresis, which can lead to hypotension and associated symptoms in a small percentage of, usually older, patients. Importantly, because SGLT2 inhibitors ultimately depend on the rate of glucose filtration to be effective, potency decreases by 40%–80% across the spectrum of stage 3 kidney disease (GFR 60–30 mL/min). SGLT2 inhibitors do not cause hypoglycemia but can increase that likelihood when combined with drugs that do.

Recent analyses of clinical trials with SGLT inhibitors suggested that they may increase the risk of fractures (FDA warning), and there is preliminary evidence that these drugs affect mineral balance and circulating levels of parathyroid hormone and 1,25-hydroxy vitamin D. Studies are ongoing to see if this is a significant problem. There have been rare cases of diabetic ketoacidosis reported in patients treated with SGLT2 inhibitors. In phase 3 clinical trials, there was no evidence that SGLT2 inhibitors had adverse effects on cardiovascular disease. Data from controlled trials indicate that empagliflozin and canagliflozin reduce the risk for major cardiovascular events. (Zinman et al., 2015; Neal et al., 2017). Canagliflozin is associated with an increased risk of lower extremity amputation.

Other Glucose-Lowering Agents

Pramlintide. Islet amyloid polypeptide (amylin), is a 37–amino acid peptide produced in the pancreatic β cell and secreted with insulin. A synthetic form of amylin with several amino acid modifications to improve bioavailability, *pramlintide,* has been developed as a drug for the treatment of diabetes (Bower and Hay, 2016). Pramlintide likely acts through the amylin receptor in specific regions of the hindbrain. Activation of the amylin receptor reduces glucagon secretion, delays gastric emptying, and fosters a feeling of satiety.

ADME. Pramlintide is administered as a subcutaneous injection prior to meals. The drug is not extensively bound by plasma proteins and has a $t_{1/2}$ of 50 min. Metabolism and clearance are primarily renal. The doses in patients with type 1 diabetes start at 15 μg and are titrated upward to a maximum of 60 μg; in type 2 diabetes, the starting dose is 60 μg, and the maximum is 120 μg. Because of differences in the pH of the solutions, pramlintide should not be administered in the same syringe as insulin.

Adverse Effects; Drug Interactions. The most common adverse effects are nausea and hypoglycemia. Although pramlintide alone does not lower blood glucose, addition to insulin at mealtimes can cause increased rates of hypoglycemia, occasionally severe. It is currently recommended that prandial insulin doses be reduced 30%–50% at the time of pramlintide initiation and then retitrated. Because of its effects on GI motility, pramlintide is contraindicated in patients with gastroparesis or other disorders of motility. Pramlintide is a pregnancy category C drug. Pramlintide can be used in persons with moderate renal disease (creatinine clearance > 20 mL/min).

Therapeutic Uses. Pramlintide is approved for treatment of types 1 and 2 diabetes as an adjunct in patients who take insulin with meals. Pramlintide is now being evaluated as a drug for weight loss in nondiabetic persons.

Bile Acid–Binding Resins.
The only bile acid sequestrant specifically approved for the treatment of type 2 diabetes is *colesevelam.*

Mechanism of Action. Bile acid metabolism is abnormal in patients with type 2 diabetes, and there have been intermittent reports that bile acid–binding resins lower plasma glucose in diabetic patients. The mechanism by which bile acid binding and removal from enterohepatic circulation lowers blood glucose has not been established. Bile acid sequestrants could reduce intestinal glucose absorption, although there is no direct evidence of this. Bile acids also act as signaling molecules through nuclear receptors, some of which may act as glucose sensors.

ADME. Colesevelam is provided as a powder for oral solution and as 625-mg tablets; typical usage is 3 tablets twice daily before lunch and dinner or 6 tablets prior to the patient's largest meal. The drug is absorbed from the intestinal tract only in trace amounts, so its distribution is limited to the GI tract.

Adverse Effects; Drug Interactions. Common side effects of colesevelam are GI, with constipation, dyspepsia, abdominal pain, and nausea affecting up to 10% of treated patients. Like other bile acid–binding resins, colesevelam can increase plasma triglycerides in persons with an inherent tendency to hypertriglyceridemia and should be used cautiously in patients with plasma triglycerides greater than 200 mg/dL. Colesevelam can interfere with the absorption of commonly used agents (e.g., phenytoin, warfarin, verapamil, glyburide, L-thyroxine, and ethinyl estradiol

and fat-soluble vitamins). Colesevelam is a pregnancy category B drug that has no contraindications in patients with renal or liver disease.

Therapeutic Uses. Colesevelam is approved for treatment of hypercholesterolemia and may be used for treatment of type 2 diabetes as an adjunct to diet and exercise. In clinical trials, colesevelam reduced A1c by 0.5% when added to metformin, sulfonylurea, or insulin treatment in type 2 diabetic patients.

Bromocriptine. A formulation of bromocriptine, a dopamine receptor agonist, is approved for the treatment of type 2 diabetes. Bromocriptine is an established treatment of Parkinson disease and hyperprolactinemia (see Chapters 13, 18, and 42). Effects of bromocriptine on blood glucose are modest and may reflect an action in the CNS. The dose range for bromocriptine is 1.6 to 4.8 mg, taken with food in the morning within 3 h of awakening. Side effects include nausea, fatigue, dizziness, orthostatic hypotension, vomiting, and headache.

Combined Pharmacological Approaches to Type 2 Diabetes

Managing the Progression of Type 2 Diabetes.

For most patients, the pathologic changes causing hyperglycemia in type 2 diabetes progress over time. Thus, most patients require step-wise intensification of therapy to maintain glycemic goals. Several academic societies and health organizations have issued guidelines, approaches, algorithms, or flowcharts for the treatment of type 2 diabetes (Chamberlain et al., 2016; Garber et al., 2016). Figure 47–11 presents a simplified version; more details can be found in guidelines from the ADA, European Society for Study of Diabetes, American Association of Clinical Endocrinology, and National Institute for Health and Care Excellence (United Kingdom). Table 47–7 summarizes available pharmacological agents for the treatment of diabetes. While there is no consensus as to preferred combinations or the order in which they are used, in general selection involves consideration of side effect profile, cost and A1C goal. Recent results suggest that individuals with type 2 diabetes who are at high risk for cardiovascular disease benefit from SGLT2 inhibitors and GLP-1 agonists.

There is consensus that metformin and lifestyle changes should be the first interventions. After that, a number of pathways or combination of drugs can be used for treatment of type 2 diabetes if the glucose control does not reach the therapeutic target (Brietzke, 2015; Ismail-Beigi, 2012). For example, the addition of a second oral agent may provide good therapeutic results. Combinations of fixed doses of most of the oral agents are now available; while most oral agents have additive effects, no specific combinations have been demonstrated to have particular efficacy that can be predicted for most patients. Another approach is to introduce basal long-acting insulin (at bedtime) in combination with an oral glucose-lowering agent. This combination allows the oral agent to provide postprandial glycemic control, while the basal insulin provides the foundation for normalizing fasting or basal glucose levels. Long-acting insulin can be combined with almost all of the oral antihyperglycemic agents in Table 47–7. The exact combination of therapies can be guided by an estimation of the β cell secretory reserve in the patient (i.e., a measurement of C-peptide level) and individualized patient glycemic goals (Lathief and Inzucchi, 2016). The progressive insulin deficiency in type 2 diabetes often makes it increasingly difficult to achieve the glycemic goal solely with oral antihyperglycemic agents; thus, often insulin is required.

Costs of Diabetes Drugs.
Treatment of diabetes can be very expensive, especially because most patients use multiple agents, as well as drugs for associated conditions such as hypertension, dyslipidemia, and cardiovascular disease. Thus, cost has become a key issue in the management of diabetic patients, an issue that can affect adherence to and choice of treatment plans (Table 47–8). Newer agents are more costly, while older drug classes like sulfonylurea and biguanides are inexpensive and available in generic formulations. In recent years, the price of insulins has increased steadily despite the addition of numerous new products to the market. The balance of cost-benefit ratio and adverse

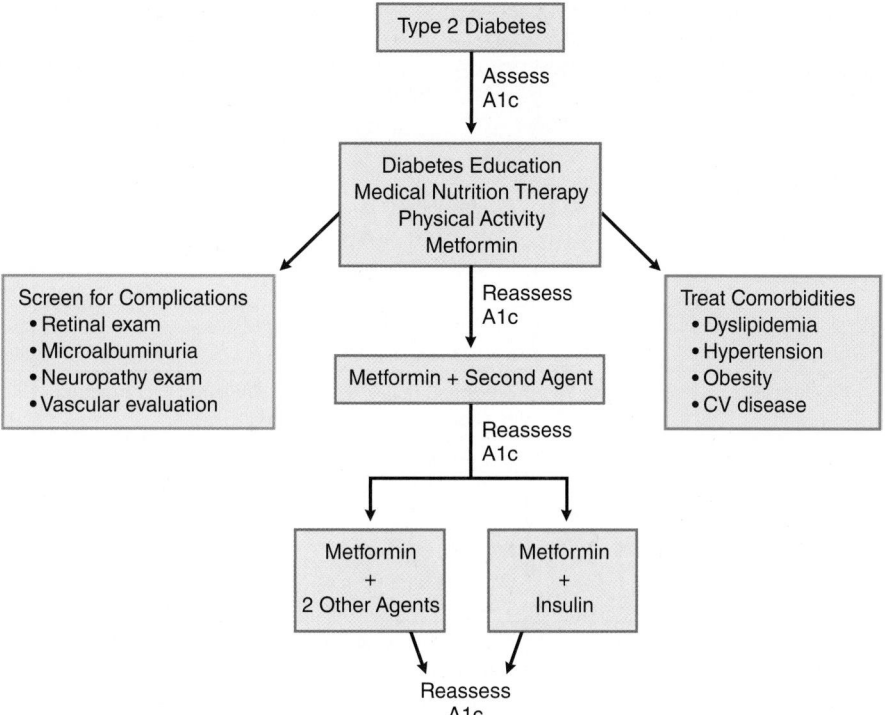

Figure 47–11 *Treatment algorithm for management of type 2 diabetes mellitus.* Patients diagnosed with type 2 diabetes, by fasting glucose, oral glucose tolerance testing, or A1c measurement, should have diabetes education that includes instruction on medical nutrition therapy and physical activity. Metformin is the consensus first line of therapy and should be started at the time of diagnosis. Failure to reach the glycemic target, generally A1c 7% or less within 2–3 months, should prompt the addition of a second agent (insulin, sulfonylurea, thiazolidinedione, DPP-IV inhibitor, GLP-1 agonist, or SGLT-2 inhibitor). Reinforce lifestyle interventions at every visit and check A1c every 3 months. Treatment may escalate to metformin plus insulin or metformin plus two other agents from the list given. See text for recommendations concerning individuals with, or at high risk for, cardiovascular disease.

profile of the new agents compared to older drugs remains controversial and incompletely defined.

Emerging Therapies for Diabetes

A number of immunomodulatory approaches are being investigated to prevent or block the autoimmune process central to type 1 diabetes, but none has yet shown efficacy outweighing adverse events. Activators of GK, glucagon antagonists, and inhibitors of 11β-hydroxysteroid dehydrogenase are being investigated as novel therapies for type 2 diabetes (Bailey et al., 2016). Advances in protein chemistry have allowed the development of peptides that activate more than one receptor to improve glucose regulation. Most of these incorporate GLP-1 receptor agonism with the capacity to activate receptors for glucagon, GIP, or gastrin. These compounds have been potent in pre-clinical models and are now in human trials. Some drugs developed for type 2 diabetes are being tested as adjunctive therapy for type 1 diabetes (Frandsen et al., 2016).

Hypoglycemia

In the absence of prolonged fasting, healthy humans almost never have blood glucose levels below 3.5 mM. This is due to a highly adapted neuroendocrine counterregulatory system that prevents acute hypoglycemia, a hazardous and potentially lethal situation. The three major clinical scenarios for hypoglycemia are as follows:

- Treatment of diabetes
- Inappropriate production of endogenous insulin or an insulinlike substance by a pancreatic islet tumor (insulinoma) or a nonislet tumor
- Treatment (purposeful or inadvertent) with a glucose-lowering agent in an individual without diabetes

Hypoglycemia in the first and third scenarios can occur in either the fasting or the fed state, whereas hypoglycemia secondary to neoplasms occurs almost exclusively in the fasting or postabsorptive state. Some drugs not used for the treatment of diabetes promote hypoglycemia (see Table 47–7).

Hypoglycemia is an adverse reaction to a number of oral therapies and is most pronounced and serious with insulin therapy. Hypoglycemia may result from an inappropriately large dose of insulin, from a mismatch between the time of peak delivery of insulin and food intake, or from superposition of additional factors that increase sensitivity to insulin (e.g., adrenal or pituitary insufficiency) or that increase insulin-independent glucose uptake (e.g., exercise). Hypoglycemia is the major risk that always must be weighed against benefits of efforts to normalize glucose control. Hypoglycemia is especially problematic in the elderly and should be given strong consideration when individualizing glycemic goals.

The first physiological response to hypoglycemia is a reduction of endogenous insulin secretion, which occurs at a plasma glucose level of about 70 mg/dL (3.9 mM); thereafter, the counterregulatory hormones (EPI, NE, glucagon, growth hormone, and cortisol) are released. Symptoms of hypoglycemia are first discerned at a plasma glucose level of 60–70 mg/dL (3.3–3.9 mM). Sweating, hunger, paresthesias, palpitations, tremor, and anxiety, principally of autonomic origin, usually are seen first. Difficulty in concentrating, confusion, weakness, drowsiness, a feeling of warmth, dizziness, blurred vision, and loss of consciousness (i.e., most important neuroglycopenic symptoms) usually occur at lower plasma glucose levels than do autonomic symptoms. Severe hypoglycemia can lead to seizure and coma.

In patients with type 1 and type 2 diabetes of longer duration, the glucagon secretory response to hypoglycemia becomes deficient. Diabetic patients thus become dependent on EPI for counterregulation, and if this mechanism becomes deficient, the incidence of severe hypoglycemia increases, especially in individuals with hypoglycemia unawareness and autonomic neuropathy. With the ready availability of home glucose

TABLE 47–7 ■ COMPARISON OF AGENTS USED FOR TREATMENT OF DIABETES

TYPE Agent	MECHANISM OF ACTION	HbA$_{1C}$ REDUCTION (%)[a]	AGENT-SPECIFIC ADVANTAGES	AGENT-SPECIFIC DISADVANTAGES	CONTRAINDICATIONS AND PRECAUTIONS
Oral					
Biguanides[c]	↓ Hepatic glucose production	1–2	Weight neutral, do not cause hypoglycemia, inexpensive	Diarrhea, nausea, lactic acidosis	GFR < 50 mL/min, CHF, radiographic contrast studies, seriously ill patients, acidosis
Dipeptidyl peptidase 4 inhibitors[c]	Prolong endogenous GLP-1 action	0.5–0.8	Do not cause hypoglycemia	Expensive	↓ Dose with renal disease
α-Glucosidase inhibitors[c]	↓ GI glucose absorption	0.5–0.8	↓ Postprandial glycemia	GI flatulence, liver function tests	Renal/liver disease
Insulin secretagogues— sulfonylureas[c]	↑ Insulin secretion	1–2	Inexpensive	Hypoglycemia, weight gain	Renal/liver disease
Insulin secretagogues— nonsulfonylureas[c]	↑ Insulin secretion	1–2	Rapid onset of action, lower postprandial glucose	Hypoglycemia, precautions for elderly and renal impairment	Renal/liver disease
SGLT2 inhibitors[c] (*the gliflozins*)	↑ Renal glucose excretion	0.9–1.2	Mild weight loss and BP reduction; do not cause hypoglycemia; CV benefit (empagliflozin, canagliflozin)	↑ Rate of lower urinary tract and genital mycotic infections; hypotension; rarely DKA; see text for canagliflozin	Renal disease
Thiazolidinediones[c] (*the glitazones*)	↓ Insulin resistance, ↑ glucose utilization	0.5–1.4	Lower insulin requirements	Peripheral edema, CHF, weight gain, fractures in females, macular edema	CHF, liver disease
Parenteral					
Insulin	↑ Glucose utilization, ↓ hepatic glucose production, and other anabolic actions	Not limited	Well-known safety/ adverse effect profile from much clinical experience	Injection, weight gain, hypoglycemia	Hypoglycemia
GLP-1R agonists[c]	↑ Insulin, ↓ glucagon, slow gastric emptying, satiety	0.5–1.5	Weight loss, CV benefit (liraglutide)	Injection, nausea, ↑ risk of hypoglycemia with insulin secretagogues	Renal disease, agents that also slow GI motility, pancreatitis, medullary carcinoma of thyroid
Amylin agonists[b,c]	Slow gastric emptying, ↓ glucagon	0.25–0.5	Reduce postprandial glycemia; weight loss	Injection, nausea, ↑ risk of hypoglycemia with insulin	Agents that also slow GI motility
Other					
Medical nutrition therapy and physical activity[c]	↓ Insulin resistance, ↑ insulin secretion	1–3	Weight loss, improved CV health	Compliance difficult, long-term success low	
Inhaled insulin[c,d]	↑ Glucose utilization, ↓ hepatic glucose production, other anabolic actions	0.25–0.5	Rapid onset of action	Limited clinical experience	Pulmonary disease, smoking

[a]A$_{1C}$ reduction (absolute) depends partly on starting A$_{1C}$ value.
[b]Used in conjunction with insulin for treatment of type 1 diabetes.
[c]Used for treatment of type 2 diabetes.
[d]Marketing discontinued in the U.S.
DKA, Diabetic ketoacidosis

monitoring, hypoglycemia can be documented in most patients who experience suggestive symptoms. Hypoglycemia that occurs during sleep may be difficult to detect but should be suspected from a history of morning headaches, night sweats, or symptoms of hypothermia. Mild-to-moderate hypoglycemia may be treated simply by ingestion of oral glucose (15–20 g of carbohydrate). When hypoglycemia is severe, it should be treated with intravenous glucose or an injection of glucagon.

Agents Used to Treat Hypoglycemia

Glucagon, a single-chain polypeptide of 29 amino acids now produced by recombinant DNA technology, interacts with the glucagon GPCR on the plasma membrane of target cells, most importantly the hepatocyte, activating the G$_s$-cAMP-PKA pathway. Glucagon should be prescribed for individuals at risk for severe hypoglycemia, and the patient's family or friends should be trained to inject this in an emergency. Glucagon is

TABLE 47–8 ■ RELATIVE COSTS OF THERAPEUTIC AGENTS FOR DIABETES

DRUG CLASS	AGENT	RELATIVE COST
α-Glucosidase inhibitors	Acarbose	+
	Miglitol	+++
Amylin analogue	Pramlintide	++++
Biguanides	Metformin, metformin ER	+
Dipeptidyl peptidase 4 inhibitors	Alogliptin, linagliptin, lixisenatide saxagliptin, sitagliptin, vildagliptin	++++
GLP-1 receptor agonists	Albiglutide, dulaglutide, exenatide, liraglutide	++++
Meglitinides	Nateglinide, repaglinide	++
SGLT2 inhibitors	Canagliflozin, dapagliflozine, empagliflozin	++++
Sulfonylureas, second generation	Glimepiride, glipizide, glyburide	+
Thiazolidinediones	Pioglitazone	+
	Rosiglitazone	+++
Recombinant human insulin	Humulin regular, NPH and U-500, Novolin regular and NPH	+++
Basal insulin analogues	Degludec, detemir, glargine	++++
Prandial insulin analogues	Aspart, glulisine, lispro	++++
Inhaled insulin[a]	Afrezza	+++

Cost scale is based on average 2016 retail prices in the U.S. +, < $10/month; ++, < $100/month; +++, $100–300/month; ++++, > $300/month
[a]Marketing discontinued in the U.S.

used to treat severe hypoglycemia when the diabetic patient cannot safely consume oral glucose and intravenous glucose is not available.

For hypoglycemic reactions, 1 mg is administered intravenously, intramuscularly, or subcutaneously. The intramuscular route is preferred in such an emergency. The hyperglycemic action of glucagon is transient and may be inadequate if hepatic stores of glycogen are depleted. After the initial response to glucagon, patients should be given oral glucose or urged to eat to prevent recurrent hypoglycemia. Nausea and vomiting are the most frequent adverse effects. Formulations of glucagon that can be administered as an intranasal powder have shown promising results in early phase trials.

Other Pancreatic Islet–Related Hormones or Drugs

Diazoxide

Diazoxide is an antihypertensive, antidiuretic benzothiadiazine derivative with potent hyperglycemic actions when given orally. Diazoxide interacts with the K_{ATP} channel on the β cell membrane and either prevents its closing or prolongs the open time. This effect, opposite to that of the sulfonylureas (see Figure 47–3), inhibits insulin secretion.

The usual oral dose is 3–8 mg/kg per day in adults and children and 8 to 15 mg/kg per day in infants and neonates. The drug can cause nausea and vomiting and thus usually is given in divided doses with meals. Diazoxide circulates largely bound to plasma proteins and has a $t_{1/2}$ of about 48 h.

Diazoxide has a number of adverse effects, including retention of Na^+ and fluid, hyperuricemia, hypertrichosis, thrombocytopenia, and leukopenia, which sometimes limit its use. Despite these side effects, the drug may be useful in patients with inoperable insulinomas and in children with neonatal hyperinsulinism.

Somatostatin

Somatostatin is produced by δ cells of the pancreatic islet, by cells of the GI tract, and in the CNS. SST, which circulates primarily as 14– or a 28–amino acid forms, acts through a family of five GPCRs, $SSTR_{1-5}$. SST inhibits a wide variety of endocrine and exocrine secretions, including TSH (thyroid stimulating hormone) and GH (growth hormone) from the pituitary, and gastrin, motilin, VIP, (vasoactive intestinal peptide) glicentin, insulin, glucagon, and pancreatic polypeptide from the GI tract/pancreatic islet. The physiological role of SST has not been defined precisely, but its short $t_{1/2}$ (3–6 min) prevents its use therapeutically. Longer-acting analogues such as octreotide and lanreotide are useful for treatment of severe secretory diarrhea (Chapter 50) and carcinoid tumors, glucagonomas, VIPomas, acromegaly, and Cushing disease (Chapter 42) (Baldelli et al., 2014). Gallbladder abnormalities (stones and biliary sludge) occur frequently with chronic use of the SST analogues, as do GI symptoms.

Acknowledgment: *Stephen N. Davis and Daryl K. Granner contributed to this chapter in earlier editions of this book. We have retained some of their text in the current edition.*

Drug Facts for Your Personal Formulary: *Agents for Diabetes and Hypoglycemia*

Drugs	Therapeutic Uses	Clinical Pharmacology and Tips
Insulin Formulations		
Insulin—short acting (regular)	• Type 1 and type 2 diabetes • Control prandial rise in blood glucose • Acute correction of hyperglycemia • Intravenous infusion for DKA and hyperglycemia in hospitalized setting	• Injected SC, IM, or IV • Onset of action 30–45 min after subcutaneous injection • Duration of action of 4–6 h after subcutaneous injection • Major adverse event: hypoglycemia
Insulin analogues—short acting (lispro, aspart, glulisine)	• Type 1 and type 2 diabetes • Control prandial rise in blood glucose • Used in insulin pump for treatment of diabetes	• Genetically modified to accelerate insulin absorption profile • Injected SC or IM • Onset of action 5–15 min after SC injection • Duration of action of 3–4 h after SC injection • Major adverse event: hypoglycemia
Insulin—long acting (NPH)	• Provide basal insulin in type 1 and type 2 diabetes • Reduce fasting hyperglycemia in type 2 diabetes	• Formulated to prolong insulin absorption • Usually requires twice-daily subcutaneous injection to provide 24-h basal insulin coverage • Combined with short-acting insulin in basal/bolus regimen • Given at bedtime in type 2 diabetes to reduce hepatic glucose production • Duration of action of 8–12 h • Major adverse event: hypoglycemia
Insulin analogues—long acting (glargine, detemir, degludec)	• Provide basal insulin in type 1 and type 2 diabetes	• Genetically modified to prolong absorption • Once-a-day subcutaneous injection ⇒ 24-h basal insulin coverage • Combined with shorting action insulin in basal/bolus regimen • Duration of action of 18–42 h • Major adverse event: hypoglycemia
Oral Glucose-Lowering Agents		
Biguanides (metformin)	• Therapy of type 2 diabetes • Usually initial agent in type 2 diabetes	• Reduce hepatic glucose production • Weight neutral • Do not cause hypoglycemia • Adverse events include diarrhea, nausea, lactic acidosis (black-box warning) • Use cautiously in renal insufficiency, hospitalized patients; temporarily discontinue therapy prior to potential renal insults (e.g., radiocontrast media) • Avoid use in patients with hepatic dysfunction • Can be combined with other agents • Inexpensive
α-Glucosidase inhibitors Acarbose, miglitol, voglibose	• Therapy of type 2 diabetes	• Reduce carbohydrate breakdown in GI tract • Adverse effects: GI flatulence, elevated liver function tests • Can be combined with other agents • Relatively modest glucose lowering
Dipeptidyl peptidase 4 inhibitors Sitagliptin, saxagliptin, linagliptin, alogliptin, vildagliptin	• Therapy of type 2 diabetes	• Prolong action of GLP-1; promotes insulin secretion • Can be combined with other agents • Relatively modest glucose lowering
Insulin secretagogues—sulfonylureas Second generation: glyburide, glibenclamide, glipizide, and others	• Therapy of type 2 diabetes	• Stimulate insulin secretion • Major adverse event is hypoglycemia • Adjustments needed in renal/liver disease • Newer agents more potent, may have better safety profile than first-generation agents. • Can be combined with other agents • Modest weight gain • Inexpensive
Insulin secretagogues—nonsulfonylureas Repaglinide, nateglinide	• Therapy of type 2 diabetes	• ↑ Insulin secretion; quicker onset and shorter duration than sulfonylureas • Major adverse event: hypoglycemia • Adjustments needed in renal/liver disease • Can be combined with other agents
SLGT2 inhibitors Canagliflozin, dapagliflozin, empagliflozin	• Therapy of type 2 diabetes	• Prevent glucose reabsorption and promote renal glucose excretion • Mild weight loss and BP reduction
		• Do not cause hypoglycemia • May ↑ rate of lower urinary tract and genital mycotic infections, hypotension, and DKA • Can be combined with other agents

Other Glucose-Lowering Agents (continued)

Thiazolidinediones Rosiglitazone, pioglitazone	• Therapy of type 2 diabetes	• Increase insulin sensitivity • Adverse effects: peripheral edema, CHF, weight gain, fractures, macular edema • Use with caution in CHF, liver disease • Can be combined with other agents

Other Glucose-Lowering Agents

GLP-1 agonists Albiglutide, dulaglutide, exenatide, liraglutide	• Therapy of type 2 diabetes	• ↑ Insulin secretion, ↓ gastric emptying, ↓ glucagon • Injected subcutaneously • Often associated with weight loss • Adverse events include nausea • Do not use with agents that ↓ GI motility • Risk of hypoglycemia with insulin
Amylin analogue Pramlintide	• Adjunctive therapy with insulin in type 1 and type 2 diabetes	• Slows gastric emptying, decreases glucagon • Injected subcutaneously • ↓ Postprandial glycemia • Often associated with weight loss • Adverse events include nausea • Do not use with agents that ↓ GI motility • Risk of hypoglycemia with insulin

Drugs to Reverse Hypoglycemia

Glucagon	• Emergency treatment of severe hypoglycemia • Diagnostic aid for GI radiographic examination	• Injected SC, IM, or IV • Quickly raises blood glucose • Relaxes smooth muscles of the GI tract • + Inotropism and chronotropism on heart

Other Pancreatic Islet-Related Hormones or Drugs

Diazoxide	• Treatment of hypertensive crisis • Treatment of pathologic hyperinsulinemia	• Inhibits insulin secretion • Adverse events include nausea, vomiting, fluid retention, hyperuricemia, hypertrichosis, thrombocytopenia, and leukopenia
Somatostatin analogues Octreotide, lanreotide	• Treatment of carcinoid tumors, glucagonomas, VIPomas, acromegaly, and Cushing disease	• Injected intramuscularly • Inhibits hormone release • Adverse events include gallbladder abnormalities

Bibliography

Ambrosius WT, et al. Lack of association between thiazolidinediones and macular edema in type 2 diabetes: the ACCORD eye substudy. *Arch Ophthalmol*, **2010**, *128*:312–318.

American Diabetes Association. Standards of Medical Care in Diabetes-2017. *Diabetes Care*, **2017**, *40*(Suppl. 1):S1–S135.

Atkinson MA, et al. Type 1 diabetes. *Lancet*, **2014**, *383*:69–82.

Bailey CJ, et al. Future glucose-lowering drugs for type 2 diabetes. *Lancet Diabetes Endocrinol*, **2016**, *4*:350–359.

Baldelli R, et al. Somatostatin analogs therapy in gastroenteropancreatic neuroendocrine tumors: current aspects and new perspectives. *Front Endocrinol*, **2014**, *5*:7. doi:10.3389/fendo.2014.00007.

Brietzke SA. Oral antihyperglycemic treatment options for type 2 diabetes mellitus. *Med Clin N Am*, **2015**, *99*:87–106.

Bower RL, Hay DL. Amylin structure-function relationships and receptor pharmacology: implications for amylin mimetic drug development. *Br J Pharmacol*, **2016**, *173*:1883–1898.

Buse JB et al. Liraglutide once a day versus exenatide twice a day for type 2 diabetes: a 26-week randomised, parallel-group, multinational, open-label trial (LEAD-6). *Lancet*, **2009**, *374*:39–47.

Cahn A, et al. Clinical assessment of individualized glycemic goals in patients with type 2 diabetes: formulation of an algorithm based on a survey among leading worldwide diabetologists. *Diabetes Care*, **2015**, *38*:2293–2300.

Cefalu WT, et al. Insulin's role in diabetes management: after 90 years, still considered the essential black dress. *Diabetes Care*, **2015**, *38*: 2200–2203.

Chamberlain JJ, et al. Diagnosis and management of diabetes: synopsis of the 2016 American Diabetes Association standards of medical care in diabetes. *Ann Intern Med*, **2016**, *164*:542–552.

Chen M, et al. Pharmacogenomics of glinides. *Pharmacogenomics*, **2015**,

D'Alessio D. The role of dysregulated glucagon secretion in type 2 diabetes. *Diabetes Obes Metab*, **2011**, *13*(suppl 1):126–132.

CF, Lebovitz HE. Comparative review of dipeptidyl peptidase-4 inhibitors and sulphonylureas. *Diabetes Obes Metab*, **2016**, *18*:333–347. doi:10.1111/dom.12610.

Frandsen CS, et al. Non-insulin drugs to treat hyperglycaemia in type 1 diabetes mellitus. *Lancet Diabetes Endocrinol*, **2016**, *4*:766–780.

Fuchsberger C, et al. The genetic architecture of type 2 diabetes. Nature, **2016**, *536*:41-47.

Garber AJ, et al. Consensus statement by the American Association of Clinical Endocrinologists and American College of Endocrinology on the comprehensive type 2 diabetes management algorithm–2016 executive summary. *Endocr Pract*, **2016**, *22*:84–113.

Gilbert MP, Pratley RE. The impact of diabetes and diabetes medications on bone health. *Endocr Rev*, **2015**, *36*:194–213.

Hattersley AT, Patel KA. Precision diabetes: learning from monogenic diabetes. Diabetologia, **2017**, *60*:769-777.

Home P. Cardiovascular disease and oral agent glucose-lowering therapies in the management of type 2 diabetes. *Diabetes Technol Ther*, **2012**, *14*(suppl 1):S33–S42.

Horita S, et al. Thiazolidinediones and edema: recent advances in the pathogenesis of thiazolidinediones-induced renal sodium retention. *PPAR Res*, **2015**, *2015*:646423.

Ismail-Beigi F. Clinical practice. Glycemic management of type 2 diabetes mellitus. *N Engl J Med*, **2012**, *366*:1319–1327. doi:10.1056/NEJMcp1013127.

Jacobi J, et al. Guidelines for the use of an insulin infusion for the management of hyperglycemia in critically ill patients. *Crit Care Med*, **2012**, *40*:3251–3276.

Kalra S, et al. Place of sulfonylureas in the management of type 2 diabetes mellitus in South Asia: a consensus statement. *Indian J Endocrinol Metab*, **2015**, *19*(5):577–596.

Kernan WN, et al. Pioglitazone after Ischemic Stroke or Transient Ischemic Attack. *N Engl J Med*, **2016**, *374*:1321-1331

Kerr D, et al. Stability and performance of rapid-acting insulin analogs used for continuous subcutaneous insulin infusion: a systematic review. *J Diabetes Sci Technol*, **2013**, *7*:1595–1606.

Lathief S, Inzucchi SE. Approach to diabetes management in patients with CVD. *Trends Cardiovasc Med*, **2016**, *26*:165–179.

Leahy JL. Technosphere inhaled insulin: is faster better? *Diabetes Care*, **2015**, *38*:2282–2284.

Madsbad S. Review of head-to-head comparisons of glucagon-like peptide-1 receptor agonists. *Diabetes Obes Metab*, **2016**, *18*(4):317–332.

McAdams BH, Rizvi AA. An overview of insulin pumps and glucose sensors for the generalist. *J Clin Med*, **2016**, *5*:5.

McDonnell ME, Umpierrez GE. Insulin therapy for the management of hyperglycemia in hospitalized patients. *Endocrinol Metab Clin North Am*, **2012**, *41*:175–201.

Mearns ES, et al. Efficacy and safety of antihyperglycaemic drug regimens added to metformin and sulphonylurea therapy in type 2 diabetes: a network meta-analysis. *Diabetic Med*, **2015**, *32*:1530–1540.

Mudaliar S, et al. Sodium-glucose cotransporter inhibitors: effects on renal and intestinal glucose transport: from bench to bedside. *Diabetes Care*, **2015**, *38*:2344–2353.

Nathan DM. The Diabetes Control and Complications Trial/Epidemiology of Diabetes Interventions and Complications Study at 30 years: overview. *Diabetes Care*, **2014**, *37*:9–16.

Nathan DM. Diabetes: advances in diagnosis and treatment. *JAMA*, **2015**, *314*:1052–1062.

Neal B, et al. Canagliflozin and cardiovascular and renal events in type 2 diabetes. *N Engl J Med*, **2017**. DOI: 10.1056/NEJMoa1611925. Accessed July 31, 2017.

Orchard TJ, et al. Association between 7 years of intensive treatment of type 1 diabetes and long-term mortality. *JAMA*, **2015**, *313*:45–53.

Rorsman P, Braun M. Regulation of insulin secretion in human pancreatic islets. *Annu Rev Physiol*, **2013**, *75*:155-179.

Rubino F, et al. Metabolic surgery in the treatment algorithm for type 2 diabetes: A joint statement by international diabetes organizations. *Diabetes Care*, **2016**, *39*:861-877.

Saltiel AR. Insulin signaling in the control of glucose and lipid homeostasis. *Handb Exp Pharmacol*, **2016**, *233*:51-71.

Samuel VT, Shulman GI. The pathogenesis of insulin resistance: integrating signaling pathways and substrate flux. *J Clin Investig*, **2016**, *126*:12–22.

Singh S, et al. Comparative effectiveness of pharmacological interventions for nonalcoholic steatohepatitis: a systematic review and network meta-analysis. *Hepatology*, **2015**, *62*:1417–1432.

Standl E, Schnell O. Alpha-glucosidase inhibitors 2012—cardiovascular considerations and trial evaluation. *Diabetes Vasc Dis Res*, **2012**, *9*:163–169.

Thabit H, Hovorka R. Coming of age: the artificial pancreas for type 1 diabetes. *Diabetologia*, **2016**, *59*:1795-1805.

Thule PM, Umpierrez G. Sulfonylureas: a new look at old therapy. *Curr Diab Rep*, **2014**, *14*:473.

Trujillo JM, Nuffer W. GLP-1 receptor agonists for type 2 diabetes mellitus: recent developments and emerging agents. *Pharmacotherapy*, **2014**, *34*:1174–1186.

Umpierrez G, Korytkowski M. Diabetic emergencies—ketoacidosis, hyperglycaemic hyperosmolar state and hypoglycaemia. **2016**, *12*(4):222–232.

White JR. Sodium glucose cotransporter 2 inhibitors. *Med Clin North Am*, **2015**, *99*:131–143.

Zinman B et al. Empagliflozin, cardiovascular outcomes, and mortality in type 2 diabetes. *N Engl J Med*, **2015**, *373*:2117-2128.

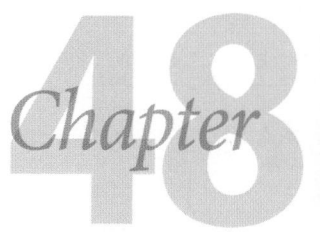

Chapter 48

Agents Affecting Mineral Ion Homeostasis and Bone Turnover

Thomas D. Nolin and Peter A. Friedman

This chapter presents a primer on mineral ion homeostasis and the endocrinology of Ca^{2+} and phosphate metabolism, then some relevant pathophysiology, and finally pharmacotherapeutic options in treating disorders of mineral ion homeostasis.

Physiology of Mineral Ion Homeostasis

Calcium

Elemental calcium is essential for many biological functions, ranging from muscle contraction and intracellular signaling (see Chapter 3) to blood coagulation and supporting the formation and continuous remodeling of the skeleton.

Extracellular Ca^{2+} is in the millimolar range, whereas intracellular free Ca^{2+} is maintained at submicromolar levels. Different mechanisms evolved that regulate Ca^{2+} over this 10,000-fold concentration span. Changes in cytosolic Ca^{2+} (whether released from intracellular stores or entering via membrane Ca^{2+} channels) can modulate effector targets, often by interacting with the ubiquitous Ca^{2+}-binding protein *calmodulin*. The rapid association-dissociation kinetics of Ca^{2+} permit effective regulation of cytosolic Ca^{2+} over the range of 100 nM to 1 μM.

The body content of calcium in healthy adult men and women, respectively, is about 1300 and 1000 g, of which more than 99% is in bone and teeth. Ca^{2+} in extracellular fluids is stringently regulated within narrow limits. In adult humans, the normal serum Ca^{2+} concentration ranges from 8.5 to 10.4 mg/dL (4.25–5.2 mEq/L, 2.1–2.6 mM) and includes three distinct chemical forms: *ionized* (50%), *protein bound* (40%), and *complexed* (10%). Thus, whereas total plasma Ca^{2+} concentration is about 2.5 mM, the concentration of ionized Ca^{2+} in plasma is about 1.2 mM. The various pools of Ca^{2+} are illustrated schematically in Figure 48–1.

Albumin accounts for some 90% of the serum Ca^{2+} bound to plasma proteins; a change of plasma albumin concentration of 1.0 g/dL from the normal value of 4.0 g/dL can be expected to alter total Ca^{2+} concentration by about 0.8 mg/dL. The remaining 10% of the serum Ca^{2+} is complexed with small polyvalent anions, primarily phosphate and citrate. Only diffusible Ca^{2+} (i.e., ionized plus complexed) crosses cell membranes. The degree of complex formation depends on the ambient pH and the concentrations of ionized Ca^{2+} and complexing anions. Ionized Ca^{2+} is the physiologically relevant component, mediating calcium's biological effects, and, when perturbed, produces the characteristic signs and symptoms of hypo- or hypercalcemia. Hormones that affect intestinal calcium absorption and renal calcium excretion tightly control the extracellular Ca^{2+} concentration; when needed, these same hormones regulate withdrawal from the large skeletal reservoir.

Calcium Stores

The skeleton contains 99% of total body calcium in a crystalline form resembling the mineral hydroxyapatite; other ions, including Na^+, K^+, Mg^{2+}, and F^-, also are present in the crystal lattice. The steady-state content of Ca^{2+} in bone reflects the net effect of bone resorption and bone formation. Although the bulk of skeletal calcium is not readily available for meeting short-term needs, a rapidly exchangeable calcium pool at the endosteal surface can be both mobilized and serve to sequester acute increases of extracellular calcium.

Calcium Absorption and Excretion

In the U.S., about 75% of dietary Ca^{2+} is obtained from milk and dairy products. Guidelines for daily vitamin D and calcium supplementation (Institute of Medicine, 2011) are shown in Table 48–1. Figure 48–2 illustrates the components of whole-body daily Ca^{2+} turnover. Ca^{2+} enters the body only through the intestine. *Vitamin D–dependent Ca^{2+} transport* occurs in the proximal duodenum, whereas most Ca^{2+} uptake is mediated by *passive absorption* throughout the small intestine. When calcium intake is adequate or high, passive calcium absorption in the jejunum and ileum

Abbreviations

BMD: bone mineral density
CaSR: calcium-sensing receptor
CGRP: calcitonin gene–related peptide
CKD-MBD: chronic kidney disease–mineral bone disease
CTR: calcitonin receptor
CYP: cytochrome P450
DHT: dihydrotachysterol
ERK: extracellular signal–regulated kinase
FGF: fibroblast growth factor
FGF23: fibroblast growth factor 23
FGFR: FGF receptor
FGFR/KL: FGF receptor/Klotho
FRS2α: FGFR substrate 2α
HRT: hormone replacement therapy
HVDDR: hereditary 1,25-dihydroxyvitamin D resistance
Ig: immunoglobulin
IL-1: interleukin 1
IP$_3$: inositol triphosphate
KL: klotho
MTC: medullary thyroid carcinoma
NF-κB: nuclear factor kappa B
25-OHD$_3$: 25-OH-cholecalciferol
OPG: osteoprotegerin
NPT2: Sodium-dependent phosphate transport protein 2
PDDR: pseudovitamin D–deficiency rickets
P$_i$: inorganic phosphate
PKC: protein kinase C
PLC: phospholipase C
PTH: parathyroid hormone
PTHR: PTH receptor
PTHrP: PTH-related protein
RANK: receptor for activating NF-κB
RANKL: RANK ligand
RDA: recommended daily allowance
REMS: Risk Evaluation and Mitigation Strategy
SERM: selective estrogen receptor modulator
SGK1: serum and glucocorticoid–regulated kinase 1
TK: tyrosine kinase
TRPV6: Transient receptor potential cation channel V6
VDDR-1: vitamin D–dependent rickets type I
VDR: vitamin D receptor
XLH: X-linked hypophosphatemia

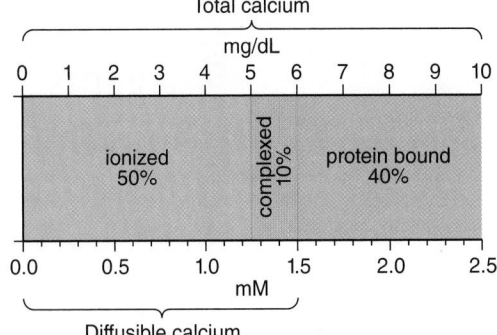

Figure 48–1 *Pools of calcium in serum.* Concentrations are expressed as milligrams per deciliter (top axis) and as millimoles per liter (bottom axis). The total serum calcium concentration is 10 mg/dL or 2.5 mM, divided into three pools: protein bound (40%), complexed with small anions (10%), and ionized calcium (50%). The complexed and ionized pools represent the diffusable forms of calcium that can enter cells.

filtered Na$^+$, the presence of nonreabsorbed anions, and diuretic agents (see Chapter 25). Sodium intake, and therefore Na$^+$ excretion, is directly related to urinary Ca^{2+} excretion. Diuretics that act on the ascending limb of the loop of Henle (e.g., furosemide) increase Ca^{2+} excretion. By contrast, thiazide diuretics uncouple the relationship between Na$^+$ and Ca^{2+} excretion, increasing sodium excretion but diminishing calcium excretion. Urinary Ca^{2+} excretion is a direct function of dietary protein intake, presumably owing to the effect of sulfur-containing amino acids on renal tubular function.

Phosphate

Phosphate is present in plasma, extracellular fluid, cell membrane phospholipids, intracellular fluid, collagen, and bone tissue. More than 80% of total body phosphorus is found in bone; about 15% is in soft tissue. In addition, phosphate is a dynamic constituent of intermediary and energy

TABLE 48–1 ■ RECOMMENDED DAILY ALLOWANCE OF CALCIUM AND VITAMIN D

LIFE STAGE GROUP	CALCIUM (mg/d)[a]	VITAMIN D (IU/d)[a,b]
Infants 0 to 6 months	200[c]	400[d]
Infants 6 to 12 months	260[c]	400[d]
1–3 years old	700	600
4–8 years old	1000	600
9–13 years old	1300	600
14–18 years old	1300	600
19–30 years old	1000	600
31–50 years old	1000	600
51–70 years old	1000	600
51- to 70-year-old females	1200	600
>70 years old	1200	600
14–18 years old, pregnant/lactating	1300	600
19–50 years old, pregnant/lactating	1000	600

[a]Intake covering needs of ≥ 97.5% of population.
[b]Covers all forms of vitamin D. For details, see Institute of Medicine, 2011.
[c]For infants 0 to 6 months of age, adequate intake is 200 mg/d; it is 260 mg/d for infants 6 to 12 months of age. RDAs have not been established for infants.
[d]For infants 0 to 6 months of age, adequate intake is 400 IU/d; it is 400 IU/d for infants 6 to 12 months of age. RDAs have not been established for infants.

is the major absorptive process. Conversely, when intake is low, vitamin D–dependent active calcium absorption is upregulated in the duodenum and accounts for the larger proportion of calcium that is absorbed.

This uptake, whether active or passive, is counterbalanced by an obligatory daily intestinal Ca^{2+} loss of about 150 mg/d that reflects the Ca^{2+} content of mucosal and biliary secretions and in sloughed intestinal cells. The efficiency of intestinal Ca^{2+} absorption is inversely related to calcium intake. Thus, a diet low in calcium leads to a compensatory increase in fractional absorption owing partly to activation of vitamin D. In older persons, this response is considerably less robust. Disease states associated with steatorrhea, chronic diarrhea, or malabsorption promote fecal loss of Ca^{2+}. Drugs such as glucocorticoids and phenytoin depress intestinal Ca^{2+} transport.

Urinary Ca^{2+} excretion is the difference between the amount filtered at the glomerulus and the quantity reabsorbed. About 9 g of calcium are filtered each day, of which more than 98% is reabsorbed by the tubules. The efficiency of reabsorption is highly regulated by PTH and is influenced by

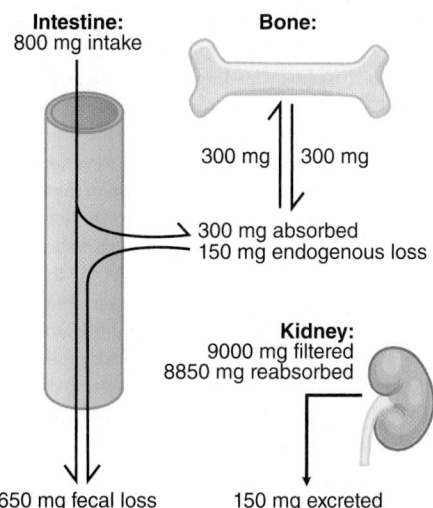

Figure 48–2 *Whole-body daily turnover of calcium.* In healthy adults, calcium intake is equal to calcium excretion, and no net gain or loss of skeletal calcium occurs. Daily dietary calcium intake averages 800 mg. Net intestinal absorption amounts to 150 mg and is balanced by an equivalent amount of calcium excretion by the kidneys. Fecal calcium excretion amounts to 650 mg. In the absence of a challenge to calcium homeostasis such as lactation, the kidneys are the primary site of calcium metabolism. (Adapted with permission from Yanagawa N, Lee DBN. Renal handling of calcium and phosphorus. In: Coe FL, Favus MJ, eds. *Disorders of Bone and Mineral Metabolism.* Raven Press, New York, **1992**, 3–40.)

metabolism and acts as a key regulator of enzyme activity when transferred by protein kinases from ATP to phosphorylatable serine, threonine, and tyrosine residues.

Biologically, phosphorus exists in both organic and inorganic (P_i) forms. Organic forms include phospholipids and various organic esters. In extracellular fluid, the bulk of phosphorus is present as inorganic phosphate in the form of NaH_2PO_4 and Na_2HPO_4. At pH 7.4, the ratio of disodium to monosodium phosphate is 4:1, so plasma phosphate has an intermediate valence of 1.8. Owing to its relatively low concentration in extracellular fluid, phosphate contributes little to buffering capacity. The aggregate level of P_i modifies tissue concentrations of Ca^{2+} and plays a major role in renal H^+ excretion. Within bone, phosphate is complexed with Ca^{2+} as hydroxyapatites and as calcium phosphate.

Absorption, Distribution, and Excretion

Phosphate is an abundant dietary component; even an inadequate diet rarely causes phosphate depletion. Phosphate is extensively absorbed from the GI tract primarily by passive movement (proportional to the concentration in the intestinal lumen), with a smaller fraction mediated by active vitamin D–dependent transport. The fact that most intestinal phosphate absorption is passive may explain why it continues in the presence of hyperphosphatemia, whereas renal phosphate transport is downregulated by elevated phosphate concentrations. The NPT2B Na-phosphate cotransporter mediates active GI phosphate transport, which proceeds through a classic feedback mechanism: Decreases of serum phosphate enhance the biogenesis of vitamin D, which in turn upregulates NPT2B expression.

In adults, about two-thirds of ingested phosphate is absorbed and is excreted almost entirely into the urine. Small amounts of phosphate are secreted into the intestine. In growing children, phosphate balance is positive, and plasma concentrations of phosphate are higher than in adults.

Renal phosphate excretion is the difference between the amount filtered and that reabsorbed. More than 90% of plasma phosphate is freely filtered at the glomerulus, and 80% is reabsorbed, predominantly by proximal tubules. Renal phosphate absorption is regulated by PTH and FGF23 and by other factors, primarily dietary phosphate. Additional

hormonal regulators of intestinal phosphate absorption include glucocorticoids, estradiol, and epidermal growth factor. Nonhormonal factors contributing to phosphate homeostasis include extracellular volume and acid-base status.

Dietary phosphate deficiency upregulates renal phosphate transporters and decreases excretion, whereas a high-phosphate diet increases phosphate excretion; these changes are independent of effects on plasma P_i, Ca^{2+}, PTH, or FGF23 (Bourgeois et al., 2013). PTH and FGF23 increase urinary phosphate excretion by blocking phosphate reabsorption. Expansion of plasma volume increases urinary phosphate excretion.

Role of Phosphate in Urine Acidification

Phosphate is concentrated progressively as it traverses the renal tubule and becomes the most abundant buffer system in the distal tubule and terminal nephron. The exchange of H^+ and Na^+ in the tubular urine converts Na_2HPO_4 to NaH_2PO_4, permitting the excretion of large amounts of acid without lowering the urine pH to a degree that would block H^+ transport.

Pharmacological Actions of Phosphate

Phosphate salts are employed as mild laxatives (see Chapter 50) and to acidify the urine and treat hypophosphatemia.

Hormonal Regulation of Calcium and Phosphate Homeostasis

A number of hormones interact to regulate extracellular Ca^{2+} and phosphate balance. The most important are PTH, FGF23, and *1,25-dihydroxyvitamin D₃ (calcitriol)*, which regulate mineral homeostasis by effects on the kidney, intestine, and bone (Figure 48–3).

Parathyroid Hormone

Parathyroid hormone is a polypeptide that helps to regulate plasma Ca^{2+} by affecting bone resorption/formation, renal Ca^{2+} excretion/reabsorption, and calcitriol synthesis (thus, GI Ca^{2+} absorption).

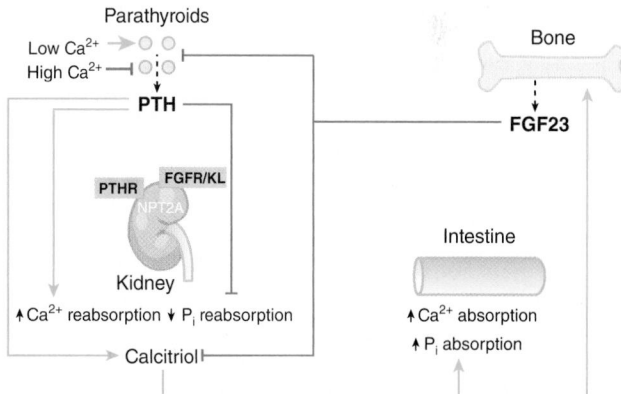

Figure 48–3 *Calcium homeostasis and its regulation by PTH, FGF23, and 1,25-dihydroxyvitamin D.* PTH, released from parathyroids (dotted line), has stimulatory effects on bone and kidney, increasing calcium mobilization and reabsorption, decreasing phosphate reabsorption, and stimulating 1α-hydroxylase activity in kidney mitochondria, leading to the production of 1,25-dihydroxyvitamin D (calcitriol) from 25-hydroxycholecalciferol (Figure 48–6). FGF23, released from bone (dotted line), likewise dampens renal phosphate reabsorption and augments calcium recovery but decreases the production of 1,25-dihydroxyvitamin D by inhibiting 25(OH)1-α-hydroxylase (*CYP27B1*) and increasing metabolism by inducing 1,25(OH)₂vitamin D 24-hydroxylase (*CYP24A1*). FGF23 also suppresses PTH release by the parathyroid glands. Calcitriol, the biologically active metabolite of vitamin D, increases intestinal calcium and phosphate absorption, and regulates FGF23 synthesis and release and calcium mobilization in bone.

HISTORY

Sir Richard Owen, the curator of the British Museum of Natural History, discovered the parathyroid glands in 1852 while dissecting a rhinoceros that had died in the London Zoo. Credit for discovery of the human parathyroid glands usually is given to Sandstrom, a Swedish medical student who published an anatomical report in 1890. In 1891, von Recklinghausen reported a new bone disease, which he termed *osteitis fibrosa cystica*, which Askanazy subsequently described in a patient with a parathyroid tumor in 1904. The glands were rediscovered a decade later by Gley, who determined the effects of their extirpation with the thyroid. Vassale and Generali then successfully removed only the parathyroids and noted that tetany, convulsions, and death quickly followed unless calcium was given postoperatively. MacCallum and Voegtlin first noted the effect of parathyroidectomy on plasma Ca^{2+}. The relation of low plasma Ca^{2+} concentration to symptoms was quickly appreciated, and a comprehensive picture of parathyroid function began to form. Active glandular extracts alleviated hypocalcemic tetany in parathyroidectomized animals and raised the level of plasma Ca^{2+} in normal animals. For the first time, the relation of clinical abnormalities to parathyroid hyperfunction was appreciated.

Chemistry

Parathyroid hormone is a single polypeptide chain of 84 amino acids with a molecular mass of about 9500 Da. Biological activity is associated with the N-terminal portion of the peptide; residues 1–27 are required for optimal binding to the PTHR and hormone activity. Derivatives lacking the first and second residue bind to PTHRs but do not activate the cyclic AMP or IP_3–Ca^{2+} signaling pathways. The PTH fragment lacking the first six amino acids inhibits PTH action.

Synthesis and Secretion

Parathyroid hormone is synthesized as a 115–amino acid peptide called *preproparathyroid hormone*, which is converted to *proparathyroid hormone* by cleavage of 25 amino-terminal residues in the endoplasmic reticulum. Proparathyroid hormone is converted in the Golgi complex to PTH by cleavage of six amino acids. PTH(1–84) resides within secretory granules until it is discharged into the circulation. PTH(1–84) has a $t_{1/2}$ in plasma of about 4 min; removal by the liver and kidney accounts for about 90% of its clearance. Proteolysis of PTH generates smaller fragments [e.g., a 33- to 36–amino acid N-terminal fragment that is fully active, a larger C-terminal peptide, and PTH(7–84)]. PTH(7–84) and other amino-truncated PTH fragments are normally cleared from the circulation predominantly by the kidneys, whereas intact PTH is also removed by extrarenal mechanisms.

Physiological Functions and Mechanism of Action

The primary function of PTH is to maintain a constant concentration of Ca^{2+} and P_i in the extracellular fluid. The principal processes regulated are renal Ca^{2+} and P_i absorption and mobilization of bone Ca^{2+} (see Figure 48–3). The actions of PTH on its target tissues are mediated by at least two GPCRs that can couple with G_s, G_q, and $G_{12/13}$ in cell type-specific manners (Garrido et al., 2009). The type I PTHR, which also binds PTHrP, mediates mineral-ion homeostasis and the skeletal actions of PTH. A second PTHR expressed in arterial and cardiac endothelium, brain, pancreas, placenta, and elsewhere binds PTH but not PTHrP. A third putative PTHR, designated the CPTH receptor, interacts with carboxy-terminal PTH fragments that are truncated in the amino-terminal region, contain most of the carboxy terminus, and are inactive at the PTH_1 receptor; CPTH receptors are expressed on osteocytes (Scillitani et al., 2011).

Regulation of Secretion. *Plasma Ca^{2+} is the major factor regulating PTH secretion.* As the concentration of Ca^{2+} diminishes, PTH secretion increases; hypocalcemia induces parathyroid hypertrophy and hyperplasia. Conversely, if the concentration of Ca^{2+} is high, PTH secretion decreases. Changes in plasma Ca^{2+} regulate PTH secretion by the plasma membrane–associated CaSR on parathyroid cells. The CaSR is a GPCR that couples with G_q and G_i. Occupancy of the CaSR by Ca^{2+} stimulates the G_q-PLC-IP_3-Ca^{2+} pathway leading to activation of PKC; this results in inhibition of PTH secretion, an unusual case in which elevation of cellular Ca^{2+} inhibits secretion (another being the granular cells in the juxtaglomerular complex of the kidney, where elevation of cellular Ca^{2+} inhibits renin secretion). Simultaneous activation of the CaSR-G_i pathway by Ca^{2+} reduces cyclic AMP synthesis and lowers the activity of PKA, also a negative signal for PTH secretion. Conversely, reduced occupancy of CaSR by Ca^{2+} reduces signaling through G_i and G_q, thereby promoting PTH secretion. Other agents that increase parathyroid cell cyclic AMP levels, such as β adrenergic receptor agonists and dopamine, also increase PTH secretion, but much less than does hypocalcemia. The active vitamin D metabolite 1,25-dihydroxyvitamin D (*calcitriol*) directly suppresses PTH gene expression. Severe hypermagnesemia or hypomagnesemia can inhibit PTH secretion.

Effects on Bone. Parathyroid hormone exerts both catabolic and anabolic effects on bone. Chronically elevated PTH enhances bone resorption and thereby increases Ca^{2+} delivery to the extracellular fluid, whereas intermittent exposure to PTH promotes anabolic actions. The primary skeletal target cell for PTH is the osteoblast.

Effects on Kidney. In the kidney, PTH enhances the efficiency of Ca^{2+} reabsorption, inhibits tubular reabsorption of phosphate, and stimulates conversion of vitamin D to its biologically active form, 1,25-dihydroxy vitamin D_3 (calcitriol; see Figure 48–3). As a result, filtered Ca^{2+} is avidly retained, and its concentration increases in plasma, whereas phosphate is excreted, and its plasma concentration falls. Newly synthesized 1,25-dihydroxy vitamin D_3 interacts with specific high-affinity receptors in the intestine to increase the efficiency of intestinal Ca^{2+} absorption, thereby contributing to the increase in plasma Ca^{2+}.

Calcitriol Synthesis. The final step in the activation of vitamin D to calcitriol occurs in kidney proximal tubule cells. Three primary regulators govern the enzymatic activity of the 25-hydroxyvitamin D_3-1α-hydroxylase that catalyzes this step: P_i, PTH, and Ca^{2+} (see discussion later in this chapter). Reduced circulating or tissue phosphate content rapidly increases calcitriol production, whereas hyperphosphatemia or hypercalcemia suppresses it. PTH powerfully stimulates calcitriol synthesis. Thus, when hypocalcemia causes a rise in PTH concentration, both the PTH-dependent lowering of circulating P_i and a more direct effect of the hormone on the 1α-hydroxylase lead to increased circulating concentrations of calcitriol.

Integrated Regulation of Extracellular Ca^{2+} and Phosphate by PTH. Even modest reductions of serum Ca^{2+} stimulate PTH secretion. For minute-to-minute regulation of Ca^{2+}, adjustments in renal Ca^{2+} handling suffice to maintain plasma calcium homeostasis. With prolonged hypocalcemia, the renal 1α-hydroxylase is induced, enhancing the synthesis and release of calcitriol that directly stimulates intestinal Ca^{2+} absorption (see Figure 48–3), and delivery of Ca^{2+} from bone into the extracellular fluid is augmented. With prolonged and severe hypocalcemia, new bone-remodeling units are activated to restore circulating Ca^{2+} concentrations, albeit at the expense of skeletal integrity.

When plasma Ca^{2+} activity rises, PTH secretion is suppressed, and tubular Ca^{2+} reabsorption decreases. The reduction in circulating PTH promotes renal phosphate conservation, and both the decreased PTH and the increased phosphate depress calcitriol production and thereby decrease intestinal Ca^{2+} absorption. Finally, bone remodeling is suppressed. These integrated physiological events ensure a coherent response to positive or negative excursions of plasma Ca^{2+} concentrations.

Fibroblast Growth Factor 23

Fibroblast growth factor 23 is a member of the FGF19 family of endocrine FGFs. Osteocytes and other bone cells, including osteoblasts, and lining cells are the primary source of FGF23. FGF23 is secreted in response to dietary phosphorus load and to changes in serum phosphate and 1,25-dihydroxyvitamin D. *Its main function is the promotion of urinary phosphate excretion and the suppression of active vitamin D production by the kidney.* FGF23, unlike PTH, also suppresses intestinal phosphate absorption.

Synthesis and Secretion

Fibroblast growth factor 23 is synthesized as a 251–amino acid peptide. Cleavage of the amino-terminal signal sequence and glycosylation produce the active protein consisting of an amino-terminal core sequence and a shorter carboxy-terminal fragment (Figure 48–4). FGF23 is extensively O-glycosylated, which shields it from proteolysis and enhances secretion. FGF23 possesses a furin cleavage site, ^{176}RXXR^{179}. Hydrolysis produces FGF23 fragments that are biologically inactive or act as antagonists. Phosphorylation at Ser^{180} inhibits O-glycosylation, thereby making FGF23 more susceptible to protease degradation.

Regulated FGF23 proteolysis may contribute to maintaining serum phosphate levels by generating more of a carboxy terminal cFGF23 peptide (cFGF23) relative to the amount of iFGF23 (intact FGF23). cFGF23 is now thought to inhibit FGF23 action by competitively blocking binding to FGFRs and klotho.

Unlike paracrine FGFs that require heparan sulfate for FGFR activation, FGF23 (and FGF19) bind heparan sulfate with very low affinity, and it is not necessary for signal transduction. FGF23 inhibits renal phosphate transport by activating FGFRs through a mechanism that entails the transmembrane form of α-klotho. *Klotho serves as an essential coreceptor for FGFR activation and transduction of FGF23 signaling.* Cleaved klotho increases FGF23 formation, while FGF23 decreases expression of transmembrane klotho (Smith et al., 2012). FGFRs are receptor TKs consisting of an extracellular domain with immunoglobulin-like loops and an intracellular region that harbors TK domains (Figure 48–4). The amino-terminal portion of FGF23 binds the FGFR, while the carboxy-terminal segment binds to klotho. This ternary complex (FGFR, klotho, and FGF23) then dimerizes, thereby enabling intracellular TK autophosphorylation of FGFR. Intracellular signaling is achieved primarily through ERKs and PLC.

Regulation of Secretion. Fibroblast growth factor 23 is released from bone into the circulation in response to elevations of serum phosphate, PTH, and 1,25 vitamin D. The sensing mechanism responding to these changes and its control over FGF23 secretion is unknown. Iron deficiency also influences FGF23 levels. FGF23 is normally released by both as iFGF23 and inactive cFGF23 fragments. In healthy individuals, low serum iron is associated with elevated cFGF23 levels, but not with iFGF23. The ratio of iFGF23:cFGF23 varies appreciably in disease states and in inherited disorders of FGF23 metabolism (Wolf and White, 2014).

Physiological Functions and Mechanism of Action

Effects on Kidney. Fibroblast growth factor 23 increases phosphate excretion and lowers vitamin D formation. The phosphaturic action of FGF23 is mediated by FGFR1c and to a lesser degree by FGFR4 (Gattineni et al., 2014). FGF23 and PTH reduce phosphate by mechanisms that involve endocytosis and downregulation of NPT2A and NPT2C, the principal Na-phosphate cotransporters that mediate phosphate retrieval from the tubular fluid. *Notably, although FGF23 and PTH exert parallel inhibitory actions on phosphate excretion, they have opposite effects on vitamin D metabolism. PTH stimulates the formation of the active form of vitamin D, whereas FGF23 reduces vitamin D levels by augmenting its metabolism to inactive forms.*

Exogenous FGF23 administration reduces serum P$_i$ and calcitriol synthesis. Although no clinical agents based on FGF23 have yet been developed, bioactive fragments or FGF23 inhibitors might become useful in counterbalancing the hyperphosphatemic actions of vitamin D therapy. The novel recombinant human IgG monoclonal antibody KRN23, which binds FGF23 and inhibits its activity, can increase P$_i$ reabsorption and serum concentrations of P$_i$ and calcitriol in patients with XLH (Carpenter et al., 2014; Imel et al., 2015).

Soluble klotho, a circulating cleavage product of membrane-associated klotho, when administered to mice increased serum levels of FGF23 and reduced bone mineral content with a concomitant increase in fracture incidence (Smith et al., 2012). These findings suggest that a scavenging antibody directed to the soluble klotho fragment might provide an additional means to reduce FGF23 levels in patients with secondary hyperparathyroidism or CKD-MBD.

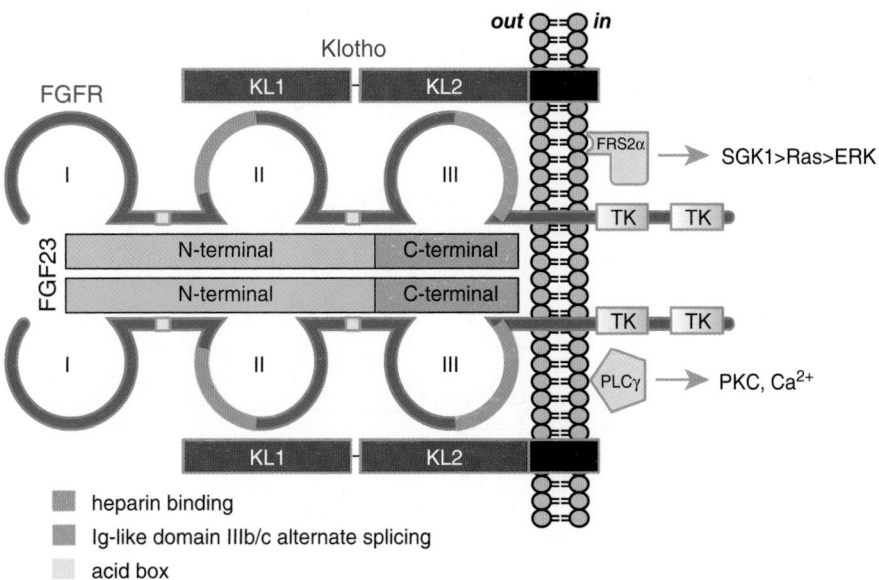

Figure 48–4 *FGF23-FGFR-Klotho complex.* FGF23 binding to the FGFR + klotho complex promotes dimerization of the ternary complex. FGFRs possess three Ig-like domains (I, II, III). Alternative splicing in domain III gives rise to FGFR1/2/3 isoforms. FGFR1c is believed to be the FGF23 receptor. FGF23 requires α-klotho to bind and activate FGFR1. FGF23 consists of a larger N-terminal region and shorter C-terminal segment. Intracellular proteolysis and inactivation of FGF23 occurs at a site separating the two domains. Klotho is a transmembrane protein with two large extracellular KL1 and KL2 domains that can be cleaved by a disintegrin and metalloproteinase 10 and 17 (ADAM10/17). Full-length klotho and the shed extracellular domain of KL have distinct functions. Notably, full-length klotho is coreceptor for FGFR1. Intracellular TK domains on FGFRs mediate downstream signaling, primarily through parallel pathways involving FRS2α, SGK1, ERK1/2 for FGF23 (Andrukhova et al., 2012), and PLCγ (which activates signaling by Ca²⁺-activating PKC) (Ornitz and Itoh, 2015).

HISTORY

Prior to the discovery of vitamin D, a high percentage of urban children living in temperate zones developed rickets. Some researchers believed that the disease was due to lack of fresh air and sunshine; others claimed a dietary factor was responsible. Mellanby and Huldschinsky showed both notions to be correct; addition of cod liver oil to the diet or exposure to sunlight prevented or cured the disease. In 1924, it was found that ultraviolet irradiation of animal rations was as efficacious at curing rickets as was irradiation of the animal itself. These observations led to the elucidation of the structures of chole- and ergocalciferol and eventually to the discovery that these compounds require further processing in the body to become active. The discovery of metabolic activation is attributable primarily to studies conducted in the laboratories of DeLuca and Kodicek (DeLuca, 1988).

Chemistry and Occurrence

Vitamin D is a hormone rather than a vitamin, and it plays an active role in Ca^{2+} homeostasis. The biological actions of vitamin D are mediated by the VDR, a nuclear receptor. Vitamin D is the name applied to two related fat-soluble substances, vitamin D_3 (cholecalciferol) and vitamin D_2 (ergocalciferol). Recent studies showed clearly that vitamin D_3 has a potency about 10-fold greater than that of vitamin D_2. This difference is likely attributable to the longer $t_{1/2}$ of vitamin D_3 and lower affinity of vitamin D_2 metabolites for the vitamin D–binding protein (Jones et al., 2014), dispelling the long-held notion that there is no practical difference between vitamin D_2 and vitamin D_3. The total concentration of serum 25-hydroxyvitamin D ($D_2 + D_3$) is now accepted as the clinical parameter for assessing vitamin D status and functional adequacy of vitamin D treatments.

The principal provitamin found in animal tissues is *7-dehydrocholesterol*, which is synthesized in the skin. Exposure of the skin to sunlight converts 7-dehydrocholesterol to *cholecalciferol* (vitamin D_3). *Ergosterol*, present only in plants and fungi, is the provitamin for *ergocalciferol* (vitamin D_2). Vitamin D_2 is the active constituent of a number of commercial vitamin preparations and is in irradiated bread and irradiated milk.

Human Requirements and Units

Although sunlight provides adequate vitamin D supplies in the equatorial belt, in temperate climates insufficient cutaneous solar radiation, especially in winter, may necessitate dietary vitamin D supplementation (Faurschou et al., 2012). Serum levels of vitamin D vary widely, likely reflecting genetic background, diet, latitude, time spent out of doors, body size, developmental stage, and state of health, as well as plasma levels of *vitamin D–binding protein*, a specific α globulin. The actions of vitamin D may differ with the expression of components of the synthetic and action pathways of vitamin D. Other factors contributing to the rise of vitamin D deficiency may include diminished consumption of vitamin D–fortified foods owing to concerns about fat intake; reduced intake of dairy products; an increased prevalence and duration of exclusive breastfeeding (human milk is a poor source of vitamin D); and increased use of sunscreens and decreased exposure to sunlight to reduce the risk of skin cancer and prevent premature aging from exposure to ultraviolet radiation. The recommended amount of sunscreen and SPF advised by the World Health Organization may abolish endogenous vitamin D production (Faurschou et al., 2012). The U.S. Institute of Medicine suggests achieving a serum level for 25-OH vitamin D of 50 nmol/L (20 ng/mL). The most recent recommended daily intakes of vitamin D and calcium are shown in Table 48–1.

Metabolic Activation

Vitamin D requires modification to become biologically active. The primary active metabolite, 1α,25-dihydroxy vitamin D (*calcitriol*), is the product of successive hydroxylations (see Figure 48–5).

25-Hydroxylation of Vitamin D. The initial hydroxylation occurs in the *liver* to generate 25-OH-cholecalciferol (25-OHD$_3$, or *calcifediol*) and 25-OHD$_2$ (ergocalciferol), respectively. 25-OHD$_3$ is the major circulating form of vitamin D$_3$; it has a biological $t_{1/2}$ of 19 days, and normal steady-state concentrations are 15–50 ng/mL, whereas 25-OHD$_2$ has a $t_{1/2}$ of 13 days.

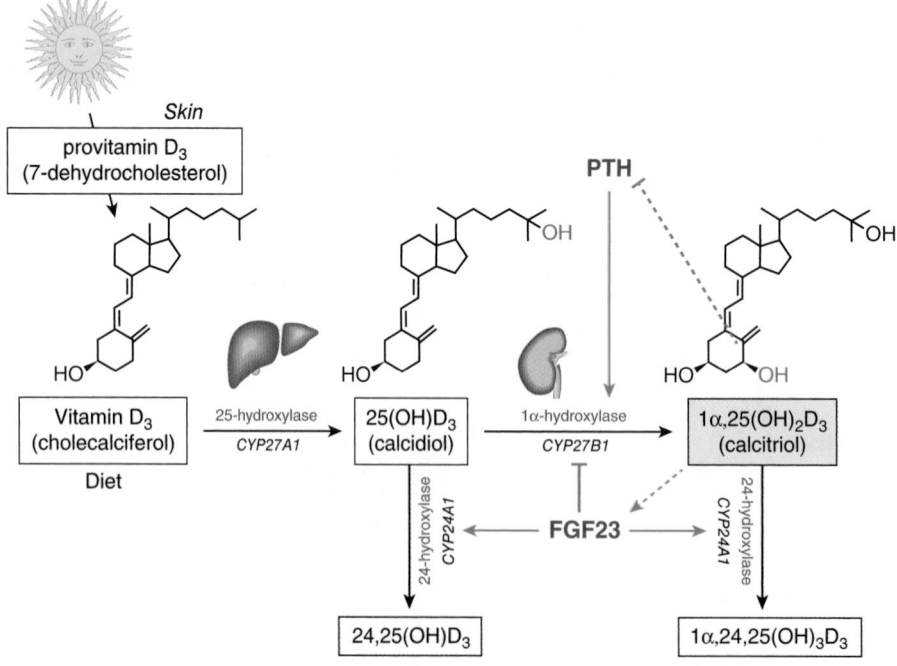

Figure 48–5 *Vitamin D metabolism.* Vitamin D (cholecalciferol) is formed in the skin by solar ultraviolet irradiation of 7-dehydrocholesterol or provided in the diet or by supplements. Sequential hydroxylation at position 25 (red) in the liver to 25(OH)D$_3$ (calcidiol) and at position 1 (red) in the kidneys produces biologically active 1α,25(OH)$_2$D$_3$ (calcitriol). Metabolism of calcidiol and calcitriol by 24-hydroxylase reduces serum levels of 1α,25(OH)$_2$D$_3$. PTH promotes the formation of 1α,25(OH)$_2$D$_3$, while FGF23 reduces 1α,25(OH)$_2$D$_3$ levels by stimulating 24-hydroxylation by *CYP24A1* and inhibiting 1α-hydroxylase (*CYP27B1*). Elevated calcitriol levels decrease PTH synthesis by parathyroid glands and stimulate FGF23 release from osteocytes.

1α-Hydroxylation of 25-OHD. After production in the liver, 25-OHD enters the circulation and is carried by vitamin D–binding globulin. Final activation occurs primarily in the *kidney*, where the enzyme 25-hydroxyvitamin D-1α-hydroxylase (*CYP27B1*) in the proximal tubules converts 25-OHD$_3$ to *calcitriol*. This process is highly regulated (Figures 48-3 and 48-5). Dietary deficiency of vitamin D, calcium, or phosphate stimulates 1α-hydroxylation of 25-OHD$_3$, increasing the formation of biologically active 1,25(OH)$_2$D$_3$. In contrast, when Ca^{2+} concentrations are elevated, 25-OHD$_3$ is inactivated by 24-hydroxylation. Similar reactions occur with 25-OHD$_2$ (ergocalciferol). Calcitriol controls 1α-hydroxylase activity by a negative-feedback mechanism that involves a direct action on the kidney, as well as inhibition of PTH secretion. The plasma $t_{1/2}$ of calcitriol is estimated at 3–5 days in humans.

24-Hydroxylation of Calcitriol. The 25(OH) vitamin D–24-hydroxylase enzyme *CYP24A1* catalyzes several steps of 1,25(OH)$_2$D$_3$ degradation. *CYP24A1* is upregulated by FGF23 and calcitriol and downregulated by PTH.

Physiological Functions and Mechanism of Action

Calcitriol augments absorption and retention of Ca^{2+} and phosphate and thereby helps to maintain normal concentrations of Ca^{2+} and phosphate in plasma. Calcitriol facilitates absorption of Ca^{2+} and phosphate in the small intestine, interacts with PTH to enhance their mobilization from bone, and decreases their renal excretion. The actions of calcitriol are mediated by the nuclear receptor VDR, a member of the steroid and thyroid hormone nuclear receptor superfamily. Calcitriol binds to cytosolic VDRs within target cells; the VDR-hormone complex translocates to the nucleus and interacts with DNA to modify gene transcription. Calcitriol also exerts rapid, nongenomic effects. These actions also involve the VDR but at an alternative site where calcitriol binds in a planar configuration.

Calcium is absorbed predominantly from the duodenum. In the absence of calcitriol, GI calcium absorption is inefficient and involves passive diffusion via a paracellular pathway. Ca^{2+} absorption is potently augmented by calcitriol. It is likely that calcitriol enhances all three steps involved in intestinal Ca^{2+} absorption (Kellett, 2011):

- entry across mucosal membranes mediated by TRPV6 and Ca(v)1.3 Ca^{2+} channels
- diffusion through the enterocytes
- active extrusion across serosal plasma membranes

Calcitriol upregulates the synthesis of FGF23, calbindin-D$_{9K}$, calbindin-D$_{28K}$, and the serosal plasma membrane Ca^{2+}-ATPase. Calbindin-D$_{9K}$ enhances the extrusion of Ca^{2+} by the Ca^{2+}-ATPase; the precise function of calbindin-D$_{28K}$ is unsettled.

The primary role of calcitriol is to stimulate intestinal absorption of Ca^{2+}, which in turn indirectly promotes bone mineralization. Hence, PTH and calcitriol act independently to enhance bone resorption. Osteoblasts, the cells responsible for bone formation, express VDR, and calcitriol induces production of several osteoblast proteins, including osteocalcin, a vitamin K–dependent protein that contains γ-carboxyglutamic acid residues, and IL-1, a lymphokine that promotes bone resorption. Thus, the current view is that calcitriol is a bone-mobilizing hormone but not a bone-forming hormone. In a healthy scenario, osteoblast and osteoclast activities are coupled. Osteoporosis is a disease in which that coupling is disturbed; osteoblast responsiveness to calcitriol is profoundly impaired, osteoclast activity predominates, and bone resorption exceeds formation.

Other Effects of Calcitriol. Effects of calcitriol extend well beyond calcium homeostasis. Receptors for calcitriol are distributed widely throughout the body. Calcitriol affects maturation and differentiation of mononuclear cells and influences cytokine production and immune function. Calcitriol inhibits epidermal proliferation, promotes epidermal differentiation, and is used as a treatment of plaque psoriasis (see Chapter 70).

Calcitonin

Calcitonin is a hypocalcemic hormone whose actions generally oppose those of PTH. The thyroid parafollicular C cells produce and secrete calcitonin.

Calcitonin is the most potent peptide inhibitor of osteoclast-mediated bone resorption and helps to protect the skeleton during periods of "calcium stress," such as growth, pregnancy, and lactation. Calcitonin acts through the CTR, a GPCR that links to G$_s$ and G$_q$.

HISTORY

Copp observed in 1962 that perfusion of canine parathyroid and thyroid glands with hypercalcemic blood caused transient hypocalcemia that occurred significantly earlier than that caused by total parathyroidectomy. He concluded that the parathyroid glands secreted a calcium-lowering hormone (calcitonin) in response to hypercalcemia and in this way normalized plasma Ca^{2+} concentrations. The physiological relevance of calcitonin has been challenged vigorously: Calcitonin normally circulates at remarkably low levels; surgical removal of the thyroids has no appreciable effect on calcium metabolism; and conditions associated with profound elevations of serum calcitonin concentration are not accompanied by hypocalcemia (Hirsch and Baruch, 2003). The primary interest in calcitonin arises from its pharmacological use in treating Paget disease and hypercalcemia and in its diagnostic use as a tumor marker for medullary carcinoma of the thyroid.

Regulation of Secretion

Calcitonin is a single-chain peptide of 32 amino acids with a disulfide bridge linking cys1 and cys7. Serum [Ca^{2+}] concentrations regulate the biosynthesis and secretion of calcitonin. Calcitonin secretion increases when serum Ca^{2+} is high and decreases when plasma Ca^{2+} is low. Thus, PTH secretion decreases and calcitonin release increases as serum calcium concentrations rise (Figure 48-6). The circulating concentrations of calcitonin are low, normally less than 15 and 10 pg/mL for males and females, respectively. The circulating $t_{1/2}$ of calcitonin is about 10 min. Abnormally elevated levels of calcitonin are characteristic of thyroid C cell hyperplasia and MTC. The calcitonin gene is localized on human chromosome 11p and contains six exons; differential splicing of the exons leads to tissue-specific production of calcitonin, katacalcin, and CGRP.

Bone Physiology

The skeleton is the primary structural support for the body and also provides a protected environment for hematopoiesis. It contains both a large mineralized matrix and a highly active cellular compartment.

Bone Mass

Bone mineral density and fracture risk in later years reflect the maximal bone mineral content at skeletal maturity (peak bone mass) and the subsequent rate of bone loss. Major increases in bone mass, accounting for about 60% of final adult levels, occur during adolescence, mainly during years of highest growth velocity. Inheritance accounts for much of the variance in bone acquisition; other factors include circulating estrogen and androgens, physical activity, and dietary calcium. Bone mass peaks during the third decade, remains stable until age 50, and then declines progressively. In women, loss of estrogen at menopause accelerates the rate of bone loss. *Primary regulators of adult bone mass include physical activity, reproductive endocrine status, and calcium intake. Optimal maintenance of BMD requires sufficiency in all three areas, and deficiency of one is not compensated by excessive attention to another.*

Bone Remodeling

Once new bone is laid down, it is subject to a continuous process of breakdown and renewal called *remodeling*, by which bone mass is adjusted throughout adult life. Remodeling is carried out by myriad independent "bone-remodeling units" throughout the skeleton. In response to physical or biochemical signals, recruitment of marrow precursor cells to the bone surface results in their fusion into the characteristic multinucleated

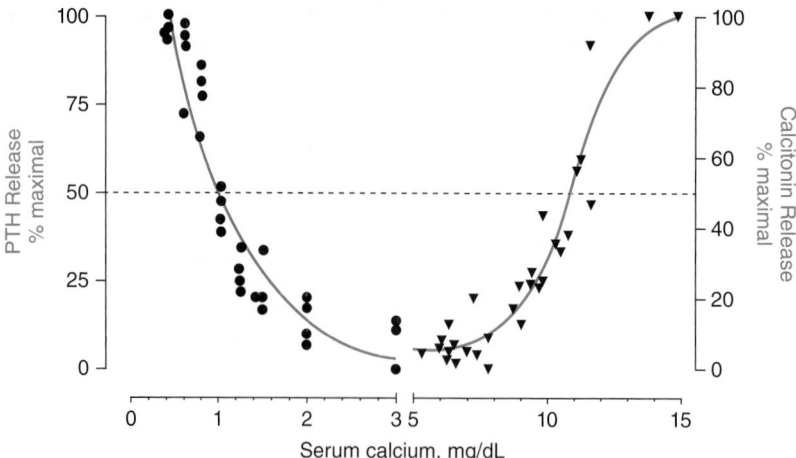

Figure 48–6 *Inverse relations between PTH and calcitonin release.* As serum calcium falls below its set point of about 1.2 mM, PTH secretion increases as a means to defend calcium homeostasis. Conversely, as calcium levels rise, PTH secretion is inhibited, while release of calcitonin increases. (Replotted from original observations; Imanishi et al., 2002; Torres et al., 1991).

osteoclasts that resorb, or excavate, a cavity into the bone. Osteoclast production is regulated by osteoblast-derived cytokines (e.g., IL-1 and IL-6). One important mechanism is RANK and its natural ligand, RANKL (previously called *osteoclast differentiation factor*). On binding to RANK, RANKL induces osteoclast formation (Figure 48–7). RANKL initiates the activation of mature osteoclasts, as well as the differentiation of osteoclast precursors. Osteoblasts produce OPG, which acts as a decoy ligand that inhibits osteoclast production by competing effectively with RANKL for binding to RANK. Under conditions favoring increased bone resorption, such as estrogen deprivation, OPG is suppressed, RANKL binds to RANK, and osteoclast production increases. When estrogen sufficiency is reestablished, OPG increases and competes effectively with RANKL for binding to RANK.

The resorption phase is followed by invasion of preosteoblasts into the base of the resorption cavity. These cells become osteoblasts and elaborate new bone matrix constituents that help form *osteoid*. Once the newly formed osteoid reaches a thickness of about 20 μM, mineralization begins. A complete remodeling cycle normally requires about 6 months. Small bone deficits persist on completion of each cycle, reflecting inefficient remodeling dynamics. Consequently, lifelong accumulation of remodeling

deficits underlies the well-documented phenomenon of age-related bone loss, a process that begins shortly after growth stops. *Alterations in remodeling activity represent the final pathway through which diverse stimuli, such as dietary sufficiency, exercise, hormones, and drugs, affect bone balance.*

Disorders of Mineral Homeostasis and Bone

Abnormal Calcium Metabolism

Hypercalcemia

In an outpatient setting, the most common cause of hypercalcemia is primary hyperparathyroidism, which results from hypersecretion of PTH by one or more parathyroid glands. Symptoms and signs of primary hyperparathyroidism include fatigue, exhaustion, weakness, polydipsia, polyuria, joint pain, bone pain, constipation, depression, anorexia, nausea, heartburn, nephrolithiasis, and hematuria. This condition frequently is accompanied by significant hypophosphatemia owing to the effects of PTH in diminishing renal tubular phosphate reabsorption.

Hypercalcemia in hospitalized patients is caused most often by a systemic malignancy, either with or without bony metastasis. PTHrP is a primitive, highly conserved protein that may be abnormally expressed in malignant tissue. PTHrP interacts with the PTHR in target tissues, thereby causing the hypercalcemia and hypophosphatemia seen in humoral hypercalcemia of malignancy (Grill et al., 1998). In some patients with lymphomas, hypercalcemia results from overproduction of 1,25-dihydroxyvitamin D by the tumor cells owing to stimulation of 25(OH) vitamin D–1α-hydroxylase.

Vitamin D excess may cause hypercalcemia if sufficient 25-OHD is present to stimulate intestinal Ca^{2+} hyperabsorption, leading to hypercalcemia and suppressing PTH and 1,25-dihydroxyvitamin D levels. Measurement of 25-OHD is diagnostic. Occasionally, patients with *hyperthyroidism* show mild hypercalcemia, presumably owing to increased bone turnover. *Immobilization* may lead to hypercalcemia in growing children and young adults but rarely causes hypercalcemia in older individuals unless bone turnover is already increased, as in Paget disease or hyperthyroidism. Hypercalcemia sometimes is noted in adrenocortical deficiency, as in Addison disease, or following removal of a hyperfunctional adrenocortical tumor. Hypercalcemia occurs following renal transplantation owing to persistent hyperfunctioning parathyroid tissue that resulted from the previous renal failure. Serum assays for PTH, PTHrP, and 25-OH- and 1,25-$(OH)_2$D permit accurate diagnosis in the great majority of cases.

Hypocalcemia

Combined deprivation of Ca^{2+} and vitamin D, as observed with malabsorption states, readily promotes hypocalcemia. When caused by

Figure 48–7 *Osteoclast formation.* Receptor for activating RANKL, acting on RANK, promotes osteoclast formation and subsequent resorption of bone matrix. OPG, a decoy receptor, binds to RANKL, reducing its interaction with RANK and thereby inhibiting osteoclast differentiation.

malabsorption, hypocalcemia is accompanied by low concentrations of phosphate, total plasma proteins, and magnesium. Mild hypocalcemia (i.e., serum Ca^{2+} in the range of 8–8.5 mg/dL [2–2.1 mM]), is usually asymptomatic. Patients exhibit greater symptoms if the hypocalcemia develops acutely.

Symptoms of hypocalcemia include tetany and related phenomena, such as paresthesias, increased neuromuscular excitability, laryngospasm, muscle cramps, and tonic-clonic convulsions. In chronic *hypoparathyroidism*, ectodermal changes (e.g., consisting of loss of hair, grooved and brittle fingernails, defects of dental enamel, and cataracts) occur. Psychiatric symptoms such as emotional lability, anxiety, depression, and delusions often are present. Hypoparathyroidism is most often a consequence of thyroid or neck surgery but also may be due to genetic or autoimmune disorders. *Pseudohypoparathyroidism* is a family of various hypocalcemic and hyperphosphatemic disorders. Pseudohypoparathyroidism results from resistance to PTH; this resistance is due to mutations in $G_s\alpha$ (*GNAS1*), which normally mediates hormone-induced adenylyl cyclase activation (Bastepe, 2008). Multiple hormonal abnormalities have been associated with the *GNAS1* mutation, but none is as severe as the deficient response to PTH.

Disturbed Phosphate Metabolism

Dietary inadequacy rarely causes phosphate depletion. Sustained use of antacids, however, can severely limit phosphate absorption and result in clinical phosphate depletion, manifest as malaise, muscle weakness, and osteomalacia (see Chapter 49). *Osteomalacia* is characterized by undermineralized bone matrix and may occur when sustained phosphate depletion is caused by inhibiting its absorption in the GI tract (as with aluminum-containing antacids) or by excess renal excretion owing to PTH action. *Hyperphosphatemia* occurs commonly in CKD. The increased phosphate level reduces the serum Ca^{2+} concentration, which in turn activates the parathyroid gland CaSR, stimulates PTH secretion, and exacerbates the hyperphosphatemia. The CaSR agonist *cinacalcet* suppresses PTH secretion and has been approved as treatment of secondary hyperparathyroidism in adult patients with CKD receiving chronic dialysis therapy, for hypercalcemia secondary to parathyroid cancer, and for primary hyperparathyroidism in patients unable to be managed surgically.

The investigational recombinant human monoclonal antibody KRN23 against FGF23 is extremely effective in correcting the hypophosphatemia associated with XLH, the most common form of hereditary rickets and osteomalacia. Monthly administration provides prolonged restoration of serum phosphate by reducing urinary phosphate excretion without adversely altering serum PTH or calcium levels (Carpenter et al., 2014; Imel et al., 2015). KRN23 was granted orphan drug status for treating XLH or other hypophosphatemic conditions in the E.U. in 2014, but it is not yet approved for use in the U.S.

Disorders of Vitamin D

Hypervitaminosis D

The acute or long-term administration of excessive amounts of vitamin D or enhanced responsiveness to normal amounts of the vitamin leads to derangements in calcium metabolism. In adults, hypervitaminosis D results from overtreatment of hypoparathyroidism and from faddist use of excessive doses. The amount of vitamin D necessary to cause hypervitaminosis varies widely. As a rough approximation, continued daily ingestion of 50,000 units or more may result in poisoning. The initial signs and symptoms of vitamin D toxicity are those associated with hypercalcemia.

Vitamin D Deficiency

Vitamin D deficiency results in inadequate absorption of Ca^{2+} and phosphate. The consequent decrease of plasma Ca^{2+} concentration stimulates PTH secretion, which acts to restore plasma Ca^{2+} at the expense of bone. FGF23 increases as well. Plasma concentrations of phosphate remain subnormal because of the phosphaturic effect of increased circulating PTH and FGF23. In children, the result is failure to mineralize newly formed bone and cartilage matrix, causing the defect in growth known as *rickets*.

In adults, vitamin D deficiency results in osteomalacia, a disease characterized by generalized accumulation of undermineralized bone matrix. Muscle weakness, particularly of large proximal muscles, is typical and may reflect both hypophosphatemia and inadequate vitamin D action on muscle. Gross deformity of bone occurs only in advanced stages of the disease. Circulating 25-OHD concentrations less than 8 ng/mL are highly predictive of osteomalacia.

Metabolic Rickets and Osteomalacia

The disorders of metabolic rickets and osteomalacia are characterized by abnormalities in calcitriol synthesis or response. Variants include the following:

- *Hypophosphatemic vitamin D–resistant rickets*: Usually, this is an X-linked disorder (XLH) of calcium and phosphate metabolism. Patients experience clinical improvement when treated with large doses of vitamin D, usually in combination with inorganic phosphate.
- *Vitamin D–dependent rickets*, also called *VDDR-1* or *PDDR*: This is an autosomal recessive disease caused by an inborn error of vitamin D metabolism involving defective conversion of 25-OHD to calcitriol due to mutations in CYP1α (1α-hydroxylase).
- *HVDDR*, also called *vitamin D–dependent rickets type II*: This is an autosomal recessive disorder that is characterized by hypocalcemia, osteomalacia, rickets, and total alopecia. Multiple heterogeneous mutations of the VDR cause this variant.
- *CKD-MBD (renal rickets)*: Refers to the disordered bone morphology that attends CKD. The variant is characterized by abnormalities of bone turnover, mineralization, volume, linear growth, or strength, as well as underlying defects in mineral ion, PTH, or vitamin D metabolism.

Osteoporosis

Osteoporosis is a condition of low bone mass and microarchitectural disruption that results in fractures with minimal trauma. Many women (30%–50%) and men (15%–30%) suffer a fracture related to osteoporosis. Characteristic sites of fracture include vertebral bodies, the distal radius, and the proximal femur, but osteoporotic individuals have generalized skeletal fragility, and fractures at sites such as ribs and long bones also are common. Fracture risk increases exponentially with age, and spine and hip fractures are associated with reduced survival.

Osteoporosis can be categorized as *primary* or *secondary*. *Primary osteoporosis* represents two different conditions: *type I osteoporosis*, characterized by loss of trabecular bone owing to estrogen lack at menopause, and *type II osteoporosis*, characterized by loss of cortical and trabecular bone in men and women due to long-term remodeling inefficiency, dietary inadequacy, and activation of the parathyroid axis with age. *Secondary osteoporosis* is due to systemic illness or chronic use of medications such as glucocorticoids or phenytoin. The most successful approaches to secondary osteoporosis are prompt resolution of the underlying cause and drug discontinuation. Whether primary or secondary, osteoporosis is associated with characteristic disordered bone remodeling, so the same therapies can be used in both conditions.

Paget Disease

Single or multiple sites of disordered bone remodeling characterize Paget disease. It affects up to 2%–3% of the population more than 60 years of age. The primary pathologic abnormality is increased bone resorption followed by exuberant bone formation. However, the newly formed bone is disorganized and of poor quality, resulting in characteristic bowing, stress fractures, and arthritis of joints adjoining the involved bone. The altered bone structure can produce secondary problems, such as deafness, spinal cord compression, high-output cardiac failure, and pain. Malignant degeneration to osteogenic sarcoma is a rare but lethal complication of Paget disease.

Chronic Kidney Disease–Mineral Bone Disease

Bone disease is a frequent consequence of CKD and dialysis treatment. Pathologically, lesions are typical of hyperparathyroidism (osteitis fibrosa), vitamin D deficiency (osteomalacia), or a mixture of both. The underlying pathophysiology reflects increased serum phosphate and decreased calcium, leading to the loss of bone.

Pharmacological Treatment of Disorders of Mineral Ion Homeostasis and Bone Metabolism

Hypercalcemia

Hypercalcemia can be life threatening. Such patients frequently are severely dehydrated because hypercalcemia compromises renal concentrating mechanisms. Thus, fluid resuscitation with large volumes of isotonic saline must be early and aggressive (6–8 L/d). Agents that augment Ca^{2+} excretion, such as loop diuretics (see Chapter 25), may help to counteract the effect of plasma volume expansion by saline but are contraindicated until volume is repleted.

Corticosteroids administered at high doses (e.g., 40–80 mg/d of prednisone) may be useful when hypercalcemia results from sarcoidosis, lymphoma, or hypervitaminosis D (see Chapter 46). The response to steroid therapy is slow; from 1 to 2 weeks may be required before plasma Ca^{2+} concentration falls. Calcitonin may be useful in managing hypercalcemia. Reduction in Ca^{2+} can be rapid, although "escape" from the hormone commonly occurs within several days. The recommended starting dose is 4 units/kg of body weight administered subcutaneously every 12 h; if there is no response within 1–2 days, the dose may be increased to a maximum of 8 units/kg every 12 h. If the response after 2 more days still is unsatisfactory, the dose may be increased to a maximum of 8 units/kg every 6 h. Calcitonin can lower serum calcium by 1–2 mg/dL.

Intravenous *bisphosphonates* (*pamidronate, zoledronate*) have proven very effective in the management of hypercalcemia (see further material for discussion of bisphosphonates). These agents potently inhibit osteoclastic bone resorption. Pamidronate is given as an intravenous infusion of 60–90 mg over 4–24 h. With pamidronate, resolution of hypercalcemia occurs over several days, and the effect usually persists for several weeks. Zoledronate has largely superseded pamidronate because of its more rapid normalization of serum Ca^{2+} and longer duration of action.

Plicamycin (mithramycin; discontinued in the U.S.) is a cytotoxic antibiotic that also decreases plasma Ca^{2+} concentrations by inhibiting bone resorption. Reduction in plasma Ca^{2+} concentrations occurs within 24–48 h when a relatively low dose of this agent is given (15–25 µg/kg of body weight) to minimize the high systemic toxicity of the drug; indeed, its toxicity generally precludes its use.

Once the hypercalcemic crisis has resolved, or in patients with milder calcium elevations, long-term therapy is initiated. Parathyroidectomy remains the only definitive treatment of primary hyperparathyroidism. As described further in this chapter, a calcium mimetic that stimulates the CaSR is an effective therapeutic option for hyperparathyroidism. Therapy of hypercalcemia of malignancy ideally is directed at the underlying cancer. When this is not possible, parenteral bisphosphonates often will maintain Ca^{2+} levels within an acceptable range.

Hypocalcemia and Other Therapeutic Uses of Calcium

Calcium is used in the treatment of calcium deficiency states and as a dietary supplement. Hypoparathyroidism is treated primarily with vitamin D and various calcium salts. *Calcium chloride* ($CaCl_2 \cdot 2H_2O$) contains 27% Ca^{2+}; it is valuable in the treatment of hypocalcemic tetany and laryngospasm. The salt is given intravenously and *must never be injected into tissues*. Injections of calcium chloride are accompanied by peripheral vasodilation and a cutaneous burning sensation. The usual intravenous preparation is a 10% solution (equivalent to 1.36 mEq Ca^{2+}/mL). The rate of injection should be slow (not more than 1 mL/min) to prevent cardiac arrhythmias from a high concentration of Ca^{2+}. The injection may induce a moderate fall in blood pressure owing to vasodilation.

Calcium gluceptate injection (a 22% solution; 18 mg or 0.9 mEq of Ca^{2+}/mL; not available in the U.S.) is administered intravenously at a dose of 5–20 mL for the treatment of severe hypocalcemic tetany. *Calcium gluconate* injection (a 10% solution; 9.3 mg of Ca^{2+}/mL) given intravenously is the treatment of choice for severe hypocalcemic tetany. Patients with moderate-to-severe hypocalcemia are typically treated by intravenous infusion of calcium gluconate at a dose of 10–15 mg of Ca^{2+}/kg of body weight over 4–6 h. Because the usual 10-mL vial of a 10% solution contains only 93 mg Ca^{2+}, many vials are needed. Treatment with intravenous Ca^{2+}, administered as calcium gluconate (10–30 mL of a 10% solution), also may be lifesaving in patients with extreme hyperkalemia (serum $K^+ > 7$ mEq/L).

Additional FDA-approved uses of intravenous Ca^{2+} include treatment of black widow spider envenomation and management of magnesium toxicity. The intramuscular route should not be employed because abscess formation at the injection site may result.

For control of milder hypocalcemic symptoms, oral medication suffices, frequently in combination with vitamin D or one of its active metabolites. Calcium carbonate is relatively inexpensive and well tolerated, so it is prescribed most frequently. *Calcium carbonate* and *calcium acetate* are used to restrict phosphate absorption in patients with CKD and oxalate absorption in patients with inflammatory bowel disease.

Vitamin D

The physiology and corresponding mechanism of action of vitamin D was described previously in this chapter.

ADME

Vitamin D is absorbed from the small intestine. Bile is essential for adequate absorption of vitamin D and is also the primary route of vitamin D excretion. Patients who have intestinal bypass surgery or inflammation of the small intestine may fail to absorb vitamin D sufficiently to maintain normal levels; hepatic or biliary dysfunction also may seriously impair vitamin D absorption. Absorbed vitamin D circulates in the blood in association with vitamin D–binding protein. The vitamin disappears from plasma with a $t_{1/2}$ of 20–30 h but is stored in fat depots for prolonged periods.

Therapeutic Uses for Vitamin D

The major therapeutic uses of vitamin D are the following:

- prophylaxis and cure of nutritional rickets
- treatment of metabolic rickets and osteomalacia, particularly in the setting of CKD
- treatment of hypoparathyroidism
- prevention and treatment of osteoporosis
- dietary supplementation

Nutritional Rickets. Nutritional rickets results from inadequate exposure to sunlight or deficiency of dietary vitamin D. The incidence of this condition in the U.S. is now increasing. Infants and children receiving adequate amounts of vitamin D–fortified food do not require additional vitamin D; however, breastfed infants or those fed unfortified formula should receive 400 units of vitamin D daily as a supplement (see Table 48–1) (Wagner et al., 2008), usually administered with vitamin A, for which purpose a number of balanced vitamin A and D preparations are available. *Because the fetus acquires* more than *85% of its calcium stores during the third trimester, premature infants are especially susceptible to rickets and may require supplemental vitamin D.* Treatment of fully developed rickets requires a larger dose of vitamin D than that used prophylactically. One thousand units daily will normalize plasma Ca^{2+} and phosphate concentrations in about 10 days, with radiographic evidence of healing in about 3 weeks. However, a larger dose of 3000–4000 units daily often is prescribed for more rapid healing, particularly when severe thoracic rickets compromises respiration.

Treatment of Osteomalacia and CKD-MBD. Osteomalacia, distinguished by undermineralization of bone matrix, occurs commonly during sustained phosphate depletion. Patients with CKD are at risk for developing osteomalacia but also may develop a complex bone disease called CKD-MBD, formerly known as *renal osteodystrophy*. In this setting, bone metabolism is stimulated by an increase in PTH and by a delay in bone mineralization that is due to decreased renal synthesis of calcitriol. In CKD-MBD, low BMD may be accompanied by high-turnover bone lesions, typically seen in patients with uncontrolled hyperparathyroidism or by low bone remodeling activity seen in patients with adynamic bone disease.

The therapeutic approach to the patient with CKD-MBD depends on its skeletal manifestation. In high-turnover (hyperparathyroid) or mixed high-turnover disease with deficient mineralization, dietary phosphate restriction, generally in combination with a phosphate binder, is recommended. Administration of calcium-containing phosphate binders along with calcitriol may contribute to oversuppression of PTH secretion and likewise result in adynamic bone disease. The increased calcium burden associated with calcium-based phosphate binders likely contributes to the increased incidence of vascular calcification in patients with CKD.

Non–calcium-containing phosphate binders are highly effective alternatives to traditional calcium-based agents. *Sevelamer hydrochloride* is a nonabsorbable polymer that acts as a nonselective anion exchanger. The drug is modestly water soluble, and only trace amounts are absorbed from the GI tract. Sevelamer not only effectively lowers serum phosphate concentration in hemodialysis patients but also binds bile acids, and to a lesser extent low-density lipoprotein cholesterol and fat-soluble vitamins. Side effects of sevelamer hydrochloride include vomiting, nausea, diarrhea, dyspepsia, and metabolic acidosis.

Sevelamer carbonate is equivalent to sevelamer hydrochloride in terms of safety and tolerability, with a lower likelihood of inducing metabolic acidosis. *Lanthanum carbonate* is a poorly permeable trivalent cation that is highly effective in treating the hyperphosphatemia associated with CKD-MBD but is associated with GI side effects.

Most recently, the FDA approved two novel iron-based phosphate binders. *Sucroferric oxyhydroxide* is a polynuclear iron(III)–oxyhydroxide compound that binds phosphate by ligand exchange. The drug exhibits similar phosphate control efficacy as sevelamer with a lower daily pill burden. *Ferric citrate* also exhibits comparable phosphate control efficacy to sevelamer and to calcium acetate. In addition, ferric citrate delivers a significant amount of iron, resulting in increased erythropoietic parameters and the possibility of iron overload with chronic dosing. Diarrhea is a common side effect of both iron-based phosphate binders (Shah et al., 2015).

Niacin and nicotinic acid lower serum phosphate and have been proposed as alternatives to the use of sevelamer. Recent studies suggested that extended-release niacin does not improve cardiovascular outcomes and is associated with greater all-cause mortality. Direct comparison of nicotinic acid and sevelamer in patients with CKD showed that although nicotinic acid reduced hyperphosphatemia, sevelamer exhibited greater efficacy in controlling hyperphosphatemia as well as the Ca•P product (Ahmadi et al., 2012; Kalil et al., 2015).

Hypoparathyroidism. Vitamin D and its analogues are the mainstay of the therapy of hypoparathyroidism. DHT, a reduced form of vitamin D_2, has a faster onset, shorter duration of action, and greater effect on bone mobilization than does vitamin D and traditionally has been a preferred agent; however, it is no longer available in the U.S. Although most hypoparathyroid patients respond to any form of vitamin D, calcitriol may be preferred for temporary treatment of hypocalcemia while awaiting effects of a slower-acting form of vitamin D.

Prevention and Treatment of Osteoporosis. This is described separately further in the chapter.

Dietary Supplementation. See Table 48–1.

Adverse Effects of Vitamin D Therapy

The primary toxicity associated with calcitriol reflects its potent effect to increase intestinal absorption of Ca^{2+} and phosphate, along with the potential to mobilize osseous Ca^{2+} and phosphate. Hypercalcemia, with or without hyperphosphatemia, commonly complicates calcitriol therapy and may limit its use at doses that effectively suppress PTH secretion. Noncalcemic vitamin D analogues provide alternative interventions, although they do not obviate the need to monitor serum Ca^{2+} and phosphorus

concentrations. Hypervitaminosis D is treated by immediate withdrawal of the vitamin, a low-calcium diet, administration of glucocorticoids, and vigorous fluid support; forced saline diuresis with loop diuretics is also useful. With this regimen, the plasma Ca^{2+} concentration falls to normal, and Ca^{2+} in soft tissue tends to be mobilized. Conspicuous improvement in renal function occurs unless kidney damage has been severe.

Available Vitamin D Analogues

Cholecalciferol (vitamin D_3) and *calcitriol* (1,25-dihydroxycholecalciferol) are available for oral administration or injection. Several derivatives of vitamin D are also used therapeutically.

Doxercalciferol (1α-hydroxyvitamin D_2), a prodrug that first must be activated by hepatic 25-hydroxylation, is approved for use in treating secondary hyperparathyroidism. *DHT* is a reduced form of vitamin D_2. In the liver, DHT is converted to its active form, 25-OH dihydrotachysterol. DHT is effective in mobilizing bone mineral at high doses; it therefore can be used to maintain plasma Ca^{2+} in hypoparathyroidism. DHT is well absorbed from the GI tract and maximally increases serum Ca^{2+} concentration after 2 weeks of daily administration. The hypercalcemic effects typically persist for 2 weeks but can last twice that long. DHT (not marketed in the U.S.) is available for oral administration in doses ranging from 0.2 to 1 mg/d (average 0.6 mg/d).

Ergocalciferol (calciferol) is vitamin D_2. It is available for oral administration. Ergocalciferol is indicated for the prevention of vitamin D deficiency and the treatment of familial hypophosphatemia, hypoparathyroidism, and vitamin D–resistant rickets type II, typically in doses of 50,000–200,000 units/d in conjunction with calcium supplements. *1α-Hydroxycholecalciferol* (1-OHD$_3$, alfacalcidol) is a synthetic vitamin D_3 derivative that is already hydroxylated in the 1α position and is rapidly hydroxylated by 25-hydroxylase to form 1,25-(OH)$_2$D$_3$. It is equivalent to calcitriol in assays for stimulation of intestinal absorption of Ca^{2+} and bone mineralization; it does not require renal activation. It is available in the U.S. for experimental purposes.

Analogues of Calcitriol. Several vitamin D analogues suppress PTH secretion by the parathyroid glands but have less or negligible hypercalcemic activity. They therefore offer a safer and more effective means of controlling secondary hyperparathyroidism.

Calcipotriene (Calcipotriol). Calcipotriol is a synthetic derivative of calcitriol with a modified side chain. Calcipotriol is less than 1% as active as calcitriol in regulating Ca^{2+} metabolism. Calcipotriol has been studied extensively as a treatment of psoriasis and is available for topical use (see Chapter 70).

Paricalcitol. Paricalcitol (1,25-dihydroxy-19-norvitamin D_2) is a synthetic calcitriol derivative that lacks the exocyclic C19 and has a vitamin D_2 rather than vitamin D_3 side chain. It reduces serum PTH levels without producing hypercalcemia or altering serum phosphorus (Mazzaferro et al., 2014). Paricalcitol administered orally or intravenously is FDA-approved for treating secondary hyperparathyroidism in patients with CKD.

Maxacalcitol. Known variously as 1,25-dihydroxy-22-oxavitamin D_3, OCT, and 22-oxacalcitriol, maxacalcitol differs from calcitriol only in the substitution of C-22 with an O atom. Oxacalcitriol has a low affinity for vitamin D–binding protein; thus, more of the drug circulates in the free (unbound) form and is metabolized more rapidly than calcitriol, with a consequent shorter $t_{1/2}$. Oxacalcitriol is a potent suppressor of PTH gene expression and shows very limited activity on intestine and bone. It is a useful compound in patients with overproduction of PTH in CKD. Oxacalcitriol is not available in the U.S.

Calcitonin

Mechanism of Action

The CTR, a GPCR that couples to multiple G proteins, mediates calcitonin's actions. The hypocalcemic and hypophosphatemic effects of calcitonin are caused predominantly by direct inhibition of osteoclastic bone resorption (Henriksen et al., 2010). The calcitonin peptide family also includes CGRP, the closely related peptide *adrenomedullin, intermedin,* and *amylin.* CGRP and adrenomedullin are potent endogenous vasodilators.

Diagnostic Use

Calcitonin is a sensitive and specific marker for the presence of MTC, a neuroendocrine malignancy originating in thyroid parafollicular C cells.

Therapeutic Use

Calcitonin lowers plasma Ca^{2+} and phosphate concentrations in patients with hypercalcemia. Calcitonin is administered through injection or nasal spray. Although calcitonin is effective for up to 6 h in the initial treatment of hypercalcemia, patients become refractory after a few days. This is likely due to receptor downregulation (Henriksen et al., 2010). Use of calcitonin does not substitute for aggressive fluid resuscitation, and the bisphosphonates are the preferred agents. Calcitonin is effective in disorders of increased skeletal remodeling, such as Paget disease, and in some patients with osteoporosis. For Paget disease, calcitonin generally is administered by subcutaneous injection because intranasal delivery is relatively ineffective owing to limited bioavailability. After initial therapy at 100 units/d, the dose typically is reduced to 50 units three times a week. Side effects of calcitonin include nausea, hand swelling, urticaria, and, rarely, intestinal cramping. Hypersensitivity reactions, including anaphylaxis, have also been reported.

Bisphosphonates

Chemistry

Bisphosphonates are analogues of pyrophosphate that contain two phosphonate groups attached to a geminal (central) carbon that replaces the oxygen in pyrophosphate (Figure 48–8). These agents form a three-dimensional structure capable of chelating divalent cations such as Ca^{2+} and have a strong affinity for bone, targeting especially bone surfaces undergoing remodeling. *First-generation bisphosphonates* (medronate, clodronate, and etidronate) contain minimally modified side chains or possess a chlorophenol group (tiludronate) and are the least-potent agents. *Second-generation aminobisphosphonates* (e.g., alendronate and pamidronate) contain a nitrogen group in the side chain and are 10–100 times more potent than first-generation compounds. *Third-generation bisphosphonates* (e.g., risedronate and zoledronate) contain a nitrogen atom within a heterocyclic ring and are up to 10,000 times more potent than first-generation agents (Ebetino et al., 2011).

Mechanism of Action

Bisphosphonates act by direct inhibition of bone resorption. Bisphosphonates concentrate at sites of active remodeling, remain in the matrix until the bone is remodeled, and then are released in the acid environment of the resorption lacunae and induce apoptosis in osteoclasts. Although bisphosphonates prevent hydroxyapatite dissolution, their antiresorptive action is due to direct inhibitory effects on osteoclasts rather than strictly physiochemical effects (Cremers and Papapoulos, 2011). The antiresorptive activity apparently involves two primary mechanisms: osteoclast apoptosis and inhibition of components of the cholesterol biosynthetic pathway.

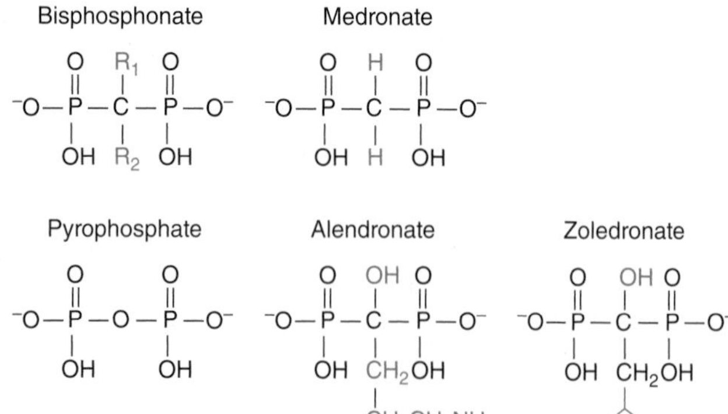

ADME

All oral bisphosphonates are poorly absorbed from the intestine. They have remarkably limited bioavailability (<1% [alendronate, risedronate] to 6% [etidronate, tiludronate]), which is further reduced by food and medications containing divalent cations such as calcium supplements, antacids, and iron. Hence, these drugs should be administered with a full glass of water following an overnight fast and at least 30 min before breakfast. Bisphosphonates distribute extensively into bone, undergo negligible hepatic clearance, and are excreted unchanged by the kidneys. Renal excretion of bisphosphonates declines proportionally with kidney function, and they are not recommended for patients with a creatinine clearance of less than 30 mL/min (Cremers and Papapoulos, 2011; Ott, 2015).

Therapeutic Uses

Bisphosphonates are used extensively in conditions characterized by osteoclast-mediated bone resorption, including Paget disease, tumor-associated osteolysis, and hypercalcemia. In particular, much interest is focused on the role of bisphosphonates in the treatment of osteoporosis, including postmenopausal osteoporosis and steroid-induced osteoporosis. Clinical trials showed that treatment is associated with increased BMD and protection against fracture. Bisphosphonates may also have direct antitumor action by inhibiting oncogene activation through their antiangiogenic effects. Randomized clinical trials of bisphosphonates in patients with breast cancer suggested that these agents delay or prevent development of metastases as a component of endocrine adjuvant therapy (Early Breast Cancer Trialists' Collaborative, 2015). Oral bisphosphonates have not been used widely in children or adolescents because of uncertainty of long-term effects of bisphosphonates on the growing skeleton.

Adverse Effects

Oral bisphosphonates can cause heartburn, esophageal irritation, or esophagitis. Other GI side effects include abdominal pain and diarrhea. Symptoms often abate when patients take the medication after an overnight fast, with tap or filtered water (not mineral water), and remain upright. Patients with active upper GI disease should not be given oral bisphosphonates. Initial parenteral infusion of pamidronate may cause skin flushing, flu-like symptoms, muscle and joint aches and pains, nausea and vomiting, abdominal discomfort, and diarrhea (or constipation) but mainly when given in higher concentrations or at faster rates than those recommended. These symptoms are short lived and generally do not recur with subsequent administration.

Zoledronate can cause severe hypocalcemia and has been associated with renal toxicity, deterioration of kidney function, and potential kidney disease. Infusion of zoledronate, 4 mg, should be performed over at least 15 min; patients should have standard laboratory and clinical parameters of kidney function assessed prior to treatment and periodically thereafter to monitor for deterioration in kidney function. Bisphosphonate use also is associated with osteonecrosis of the jaw (a rare event, with an incidence of ~ 2 in 100,000 patient-years in which the precise causal role of bisphosphonates has not been elucidated) as well as stress fractures in the lateral cortex of the femoral shaft (most commonly associated with alendronate and rarely with zoledronate; Reid, 2015).

Available Bisphosphonates

Etidronate sodium is used for treatment of Paget disease and may be used parenterally to treat hypercalcemia (although largely supplanted for this use by amidronate and zoledronate). *Pamidronate* (available in the U.S. only for parenteral administration) is approved for management of hypercalcemia associated with malignancy and Paget disease and for prevention of bone loss in breast cancer and multiple myeloma; it also is effective in other skeletal disorders. For treatment of hypercalcemia, pamidronate may be given as an intravenous infusion of 60–90 mg over 2–24 h.

Several newer bisphosphonates have been approved for treatment of Paget disease. These include *tiludronate*, *alendronate*, and *risedronate*.

Figure 48–8 *Pyrophosphate and bisphosphonates.* The substituents (R_1 and R_2) on the central carbon of the bisphosphonate parent structure are shown in blue. Examples of a first-generation bisphosphonate (medronate), a second-generation aminobisphosphonate (alendronate), and a third-generation bisphosphonate (zoledronate) are shown.

Tiludronate standard dosing is 400 mg/d orally for 3 months. Tiludronate in recommended doses does not interfere with bone mineralization, unlike etidronate. Zoledronate is approved for treating Paget disease; administered as a single 5-mg infusion, zoledronate decreases bone turnover markers for 6 months with no loss of therapeutic effect. Zoledronate is widely used for prevention of osteoporosis in patients with prostate and breast cancer receiving hormonal therapy. It reduces both vertebral and nonvertebral fractures. A 4-mg formulation is available for intravenous treatment of hypercalcemia of malignancy, multiple myeloma, or bone metastasis resulting from solid tumors. The potent bisphosphonate *ibandronate* is approved for the prevention and treatment of postmenopausal osteoporosis. The recommended oral dose is 2.5 mg daily or 150 mg once monthly.

For patients in whom oral bisphosphonates cause severe esophageal distress, *intravenous* zoledronate and ibandronate offer skeletal protection without causing adverse GI effects. For treatment of osteoporosis, ibandronate (3 mg) is given intravenously every 3 months. Zoledronate is the first bisphosphonate to be approved for once-yearly intravenous treatment of osteoporosis (5 mg annually).

Parathyroid Hormone

Continuous administration of PTH or high-circulating PTH levels achieved in primary hyperparathyroidism causes bone demineralization and osteopenia. However, *intermittent* PTH administration promotes bone growth. Although hypoparathyroidism was the last classic endocrine-deficiency disease to have the missing hormone as an available treatment option, PTH analogues are now available to these patients.

Chemistry

As described previously, PTH is a single-polypeptide chain of 84 amino acids with a molecular mass of about 9500 Da. The classic biological activity of PTH is associated with the N-terminal portion of the peptide; residues 1–27 are required for optimal binding to the PTHR and hormone activity. Currently available PTH analogues include teriparatide, a synthetic human 34–amino acid amino-terminal PTH fragment [hPTH(1–34)]; a full-length replica of endogenous PTH, recombinant human PTH consisting of 84 amino acids [rhPTH(1–84)] (Kim and Keating, 2015); and abaloparatide, a recently approved synthetic 34-amino acid analogue of human PTHrP, hPTHrP(1–34).

Mechanism of Action

The physiological functions and mechanism of action of PTH were described previously in the chapter.

ADME

These agents are peptides and are administered by subcutaneous injection (*see Drugs Available*). Pharmacokinetics and systemic actions of *teriparatide* on mineral metabolism are the same as for PTH. Serum PTH concentrations peak at 30 min after the injection and are undetectable within 3 h, whereas the serum Ca^{2+} concentration peaks at 4–6 h after administration. Teriparatide bioavailability averages 95%. The drug's volume of distribution is approximately 0.1 L/kg. The elimination of teriparatide proceeds by nonspecific enzymatic mechanisms in the liver, followed by renal excretion. Teriparatide systemic clearance averages 62 L/h in women and 94 L/h in men. The elimination $t_{1/2}$ of serum teriparatide is about 1 h when administered subcutaneously versus 5 min when administered intravenously.

Abaloparatide is supplied in an injector pen with 30 daily doses. The peptide is rapidly absorbed (bioavailabilty = 36%), achieving peak concentrations ~30 min following subcutaneous injection. Elimination half-life is ~1.7 h; clearance is presumed to be by proteolytic hydrolysis, with renal elimination of peptide fragments.

For *rhPTH(1–84)*, dose-proportional increases in serum Ca^{2+} concentration, which peaks at 10–12 h after subcutaneous administration, are exhibited. Bioavailability of rhPTH(1–84) is 53%, and its volume of distribution is 5.3 L. The liver and the kidneys are the major route of rhPTH(1–84) elimination, as for teriparatide. The elimination $t_{1/2}$ of rhPTH(1–84) is ~3 h (Clarke et al., 2014; Kim and Keating, 2015). Overall, the prolonged peak

effects and slower elimination of rhPTH(1–84) compared to teriparatide may explain why teriparatide typically requires multiple injections per day while rhPTH(1–84) requires only single-daily or alternate-day dosing.

Therapeutic Uses

Teriparatide (PTH1-34) and abaloparatide (PTHrP(1-34)) are the only anabolic agents currently available that increase new bone formation. They are approved for use in treating severe osteoporosis in patients at a high risk for fracture. In postmenopausal women with osteoporosis, teriparatide increases BMD and reduces the risk of vertebral and nonvertebral fractures. Candidates for treatment with teriparatide and abaloparatide include women who have a history of osteoporotic fracture, who have multiple risk factors for fracture, or who failed or are intolerant of previous osteoporosis therapy. Men with primary or hypogonadal osteoporosis are also candidates for treatment with these agents.

The *rhPTH(1–84)* is approved for treating hypocalcemia in patients with hypoparathyroidism whose serum Ca^{2+} concentrations cannot be controlled solely by calcium supplementation and active vitamin D treatment. Intermittent rhPTH(1–84) may soon be approved for use in osteoporosis, but its benefits over teriparatide remain to be established.

Adverse Effects

Adverse effects include hypercalcemia; the incidence with abaloparatide is lower than observed with teriparatide (Miller *et al.*, 2016). exacerbation of nephrolithiasis and elevation of serum uric acid levels. Development of osteosarcoma has been a serious concern in patients treated with teriparatide; however, postmarketing surveillance data suggest there is no causal association between teriparatide use and osteosarcoma (Andrews et al., 2012). Nevertheless, teriparatide and abaloparatide carry block box warnings and use should be limited to no more than 2 years and avoided in patients who are at increased baseline risk for osteosarcoma (including those with Paget disease of bone, unexplained elevations of alkaline phosphatase, open epiphyses, or prior radiation therapy involving the skeleton). Orthostatic hypotension may occur shortly after injection of abaloparatide.

Although clinical experience with rhPTH(1–84) is relatively limited to date, the most commonly reported adverse effects in clinical trials included paresthesia, hypo- and hypercalcemia, headache, and nausea. A potential risk of osteosarcoma is based on preclinical data, and the drug should not be used in patients who are at increased baseline risk for osteosarcoma (Kim and Keating, 2015).

Drugs Available

Teriparatide is administered by once-daily subcutaneous injection of 20 mcg into the thigh or abdomen. Abaloparatide is administered at a starting dose of 80 mcg by subcutaneous injection into the periumbilical region of the abdomen. The site of administration should be rotated, but the time at which the injection is made should be the same each day. The starting dose of rhPTH(1–84) is 50 mcg once daily, also administered subcutaneously into the thigh. Serum Ca^{2+} concentrations should be monitored every 3–7 days after initiating treatment or adjusting the dose. Subcutaneous administration of abaloparatide reduced the risk of new vertebral and nonvertebral fractures over a period of 18 months (Miller *et al.*, 2016). Shorter studies demonstrated increased lumbar spine and hip density that were greater than those achieved with teriparatide (Leder *et al.*, 2015). The dose of rhPTH(1–84) may be adjusted to maintain normal serum Ca^{2+} concentrations. The minimum recommended dose of rhPTH(1–84) is 25 µg daily; the dose should not exceed 100 µg daily.

Long-acting formulations of PTH (LA-PTH) currently are in development (Maeda et al., 2013). Such formulations may offer an advantage over teriparatide, which is limited by its short (4- to 6-h) duration of effect on serum Ca^{2+} concentrations. Another agent that consists of the N-terminal biologically active region of PTH linked to a collagen-binding domain exhibits sustained increases in BMD by more than 10% for 1 year in rodents after single-dose administration (Ponnapakkam et al., 2012). The advantages of these LA-PTH formulations over rhPTH(1–84) are not clear at this time.

A novel class of drugs that inhibit the CaSR (*calcilytics*) stimulate the secretion of PTH and decrease renal excretion of Ca^{2+}. The calcilytic *ronacaleret*, investigated for potential treatment of postmenopausal osteoporosis, was less effective than teriparatide, and its development was subsequently halted (Fitzpatrick et al., 2012). The role of calcilytics in the treatment of diseases involving hypocalcemia or hypercalciuria continues to be explored (Nemeth and Shoback, 2013).

Calcium-Sensing Receptor Mimetics

Calcimimetics are drugs that mimic the stimulatory effect of Ca^{2+} on the CaSR to inhibit PTH secretion by the parathyroid glands. *Cinacalcet*, the first and only approved drug in the class currently, offers a pharmacotherapeutic alternative to surgery for the treatment of PTH hypersecretion diseases.

Chemistry

Cinacalcet is available as a hydrochloride (Figure 48–9) and is formulated with one chiral center having an R-absolute configuration; the *R*-enantiomer is the more potent enantiomer and is primarily responsible for cinacalcet's pharmacodynamic activity.

Mechanism of Action

By enhancing the sensitivity of the CaSR to extracellular Ca^{2+}, calcimimetics lower the concentration of Ca^{2+} at which PTH secretion is suppressed. Inorganic di- and trivalent cations, along with polycations such as aminoglycosides (e.g., streptomycin, gentamicin, and neomycin) and polybasic amino acids (e.g., polylysine) are full agonists and are referred to as *type I calcimimetics*. They are able to activate the CaSR directly with no other cofactors. On the other hand, phenylalkylamine derivatives, including cinacalcet, that are allosteric CaSR modulators require the presence of Ca^{2+} or other full agonists to enhance the sensitivity of activation without altering the maximal response and are designated *type II calcimimetics* (Cianferotti et al., 2015; Filopanti et al., 2013).

ADME

Cinacalcet exhibits first-order absorption, with peak serum concentrations achieved 2–6 h after oral administration. Maximal effects on serum PTH occur 2–4 h after administration. It has an extraordinarily large volume of distribution of 1000 L and is metabolized by multiple hepatic CYPs, including CYPs 3A4, 2D6, and 1A2. Metabolites are eliminated by biliary (15%) and renal excretion (85%). Cinacalcet has an elimination $t_{1/2}$ of 30–40 h.

Therapeutic Uses

Cinacalcet is approved for the treatment of (1) secondary hyperparathyroidism in adults with CKD on dialysis; (2) hypercalcemia in adults with parathyroid carcinoma; and (3) hypercalcemia in adult patients with primary hyperparathyroidism who are not candidates for surgical parathyroidectomy. Treatment with cinacalcet lowers serum PTH levels in patients with normal or reduced kidney function (Nemeth and Shoback, 2013). In patients with secondary hyperparathyroidism on dialysis, treatment with cinacalcet significantly decreases bone turnover and improves bone histology (Behets et al., 2015). Moreover, by lowering serum FGF23 concentrations, cinacalcet treatment decreases the rate of cardiovascular death and major cardiovascular events (Moe et al., 2015).

Adverse Effects

The principal adverse event with cinacalcet is hypocalcemia. Thus, the drug should not be used if the initial serum $[Ca^{2+}]$ is less than 8.4 mg/dL;

serum Ca^{2+} and phosphorus concentrations should be measured within 1 week, and PTH should be measured within 4 weeks after initiating therapy and after changing dosage. Seizure threshold is lowered by significant reductions in serum Ca^{2+}, so patients with a history of seizure disorders should be monitored especially closely. Finally, adynamic bone disease may develop if the PTH level is less than 100 pg/mL, and the drug should be discontinued or the dose decreased if the PTH level falls below 150 pg/mL.

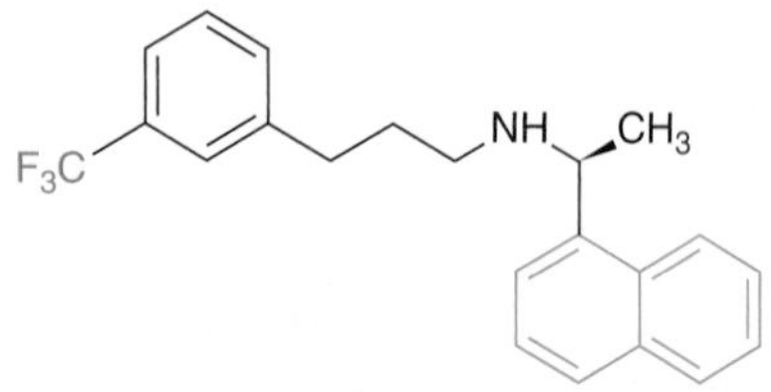

Drug Interactions

Drug interactions can be anticipated with drugs that interfere with Ca^{2+} homeostasis or that hinder cinacalcet absorption. Potentially interfering drugs include vitamin D analogues, phosphate binders, bisphosphonates, calcitonin, glucocorticoids, gallium, and cisplatin. Caution is recommended when cinacalcet is coadministered with strong inhibitors of CYP3A4 (e.g., ketoconazole, erythromycin, or itraconazole). Because cinacalcet is a strong inhibitor of CYP2D6, dose adjustment may be required for concomitant medications that are CYP2D6 substrates (e.g., many β adrenergic receptor blockers, flecainide, vinblastine, and most tricyclic antidepressants).

Drugs Available

Cinacalcet is available in 30-, 60-, and 90-mg tablets. The recommended starting dose for treatment of secondary hyperparathyroidism in patients with CKD on dialysis is 30 mg once daily, with a maximum of 180 mg/d. For treatment of parathyroid carcinoma, a starting dose of 30 mg twice daily is recommended, with a maximum of 90 mg four times daily. The starting dose is titrated upward every 2–4 weeks to maintain the PTH level between 150 and 300 pg/mL (secondary hyperparathyroidism) or to normalize serum calcium (parathyroid carcinoma).

Fluoride

Fluoride is discussed because of its effects on dentition and bone and its toxic properties.

Mechanism of Action

Sodium fluoride enhances osteoblast activity and increases bone volume. These effects may be bimodal, with low doses stimulating and higher doses suppressing osteoblasts. However, the apparent effects of fluoride in osteoporosis are slight compared with those achieved with PTH or others. Fluoride can inhibit several enzyme systems and diminish tissue respiration and anaerobic glycolysis.

ADME

Fluoride is obtained from the ingestion of plants and water, with absorption taking place largely in the intestine. A second route of absorption is through the lungs, and inhalation of fluoride present in dusts and gases constitutes the major route of industrial exposure. Fluoride is distributed widely in organs and tissues but is concentrated in bone and teeth, and the skeletal burden is related to intake and age. Bone deposition reflects skeletal turnover; growing bone shows greater deposition than mature bone. The kidneys are the major sites of fluoride excretion. Small amounts of fluoride also appear in sweat, milk, and intestinal secretions.

Therapeutic Use

Because it is concentrated in the bone, the radionuclide ^{18}F has been used in skeletal imaging. Sodium fluoride is a mainstay of therapy for the prevention of dental carries.

Fluoride and Dental Caries. Supplementation of water fluoride content to 1.0 ppm is a safe and practical intervention that substantially reduces the incidence of caries in permanent teeth. There are partial benefits for children who begin drinking fluoridated water at any age; however, optimal benefits are obtained at ages before permanent teeth erupt. Topical application of fluoride solutions by dental personnel appears to be effective on newly erupted teeth and can reduce the incidence of caries by 30%–40%. Dietary fluoride supplements should be considered for children less than 12 years of age whose drinking water contains less than 0.7 ppm fluoride. Adequate incorporation of fluoride into teeth hardens the outer layers of enamel and increases resistance to demineralization. The fluoride salts usually employed in dentifrices are sodium fluoride and

Figure 48–9 *Structure of cinacalcet* (depicted as free base). The compound is a phenyl-propylamine derivative with a 3-trifluoromethyl group (red) and naphthalene moiety (blue).

stannous fluoride. Sodium fluoride also is available in a variety of preparations for oral and topical use.

Regulation of the fluoride concentration of community water supplies periodically encounters vocal opposition, including allegations of putative adverse health consequences of fluoridated water. Careful examination of these issues indicates that cancer and all-cause mortalities do not differ significantly between communities with fluoridated and nonfluoridated water.

Acute Poisoning

Acute fluoride poisoning usually results from accidental ingestion of fluoride-containing insecticides or rodenticides. Initial symptoms (salivation, nausea, abdominal pain, vomiting, and diarrhea) are secondary to the local action of fluoride on the intestinal mucosa. Systemic symptoms are varied and severe: increased irritability of the CNS consistent with the Ca^{2+}-binding effect of fluoride and the resulting hypocalcemia; hypotension, presumably owing to central vasomotor depression as well as direct cardiotoxicity; and stimulation and then depression of respiration. Death can result from respiratory paralysis or cardiac failure. The lethal dose of sodium fluoride for humans is about 5 g, although there is considerable variation. Treatment includes the intravenous administration of glucose in saline and gastric lavage with limewater (0.15% calcium hydroxide solution) or other Ca^{2+} salts to precipitate the fluoride. Calcium gluconate is given intravenously for tetany; urine volume is kept high with vigorous fluid resuscitation.

Chronic Poisoning

In humans, the major manifestations of chronic ingestion of excessive fluoride are osteosclerosis and mottled enamel. Osteosclerosis is characterized by increased bone density secondary both to elevated osteoblastic activity and to the replacement of hydroxyapatite by the denser fluoroapatite. The degree of skeletal involvement varies from changes that are barely detectable radiologically to marked cortical thickening of long bones, numerous exostoses scattered throughout the skeleton, and calcification of ligaments, tendons, and muscle attachments. In its severest form, it is a disabling and crippling disease.

Mottled enamel, or dental fluorosis, was first described more than 60 years ago. In very mild mottling, small, opaque, paper-white areas are scattered irregularly over the tooth surface. In severe cases, discrete or confluent, deep brown– to black-stained pits give the tooth a corroded appearance. Mottled enamel results from a partial failure of the enamel-forming ameloblasts to elaborate and lay down enamel. Mottling is one of the first visible signs of excess fluoride intake during childhood. Continuous use of water containing about 1 ppm of fluoride may result in very mild mottling in 10% of children; at 4–6 ppm, the incidence approaches 100%, with a marked increase in severity. Severe dental fluorosis formerly occurred in regions where local water supplies had a very high fluoride content (e.g., Pompeii, Italy, and Pike's Peak, CO). Current regulations in the U.S. require lowering the fluoride content of the water supply or providing an alternative source of acceptable drinking water for affected communities. Sustained consumption of water with a fluoride content of 4 mg/L (4 ppm) is associated with deficits in cortical bone mass and increased rates of bone loss over time.

Integrated Approach to Prevention and Treatment of Osteoporosis

Osteoporosis is a major and growing public health problem in developed nations. Approximately 50% of women and 25% of men more than 50 years of age will experience an osteoporosis-related fracture. Important reductions in fracture risk can be achieved with attention to health (muscle-strengthening exercise; avoiding smoking and excessive alcohol use) and nutrition (i.e., increased dietary calcium or calcium or vitamin D supplements). Pharmacological agents used to manage osteoporosis act by decreasing the rate of bone resorption and thereby slowing the rate of bone loss (antiresorptive therapy) or by promoting bone formation (anabolic therapy). Because bone remodeling is a coupled process, antiresorptive

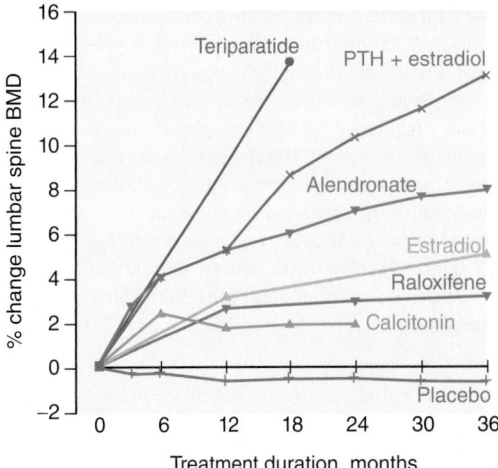

Figure 48–10 *Relative efficacy of different therapeutic interventions on BMD of the lumbar spine.* Teriparatide (40 μg) (Neer et al., 2001), PTH (25 μg) + estradiol, alendronate (10 mg), estradiol (0.625 mg/d), raloxifene (120 mg), calcitonin (200 IU). Typical results with placebo treatment underscore the inexorable bone loss without intervention. Some of the indicated treatment interventions involved combination therapy, and absolute comparisons should not be made.

drugs ultimately decrease the rate of bone formation and therefore do not promote substantial gains in BMD. Increases in BMD during the first years of antiresorptive therapy represent a constriction of the remodeling space to a steady-state level, after which BMD reaches a new plateau (Figure 48–10).

Pharmacological treatment of osteoporosis is aimed at restoring bone strength and preventing fractures. Antiresorptive drugs (such as the bisphosphonates, estrogen, the SERM raloxifene, and, to some extent, calcitonin) inhibit osteoclast-mediated bone loss, thereby reducing bone turnover. Although the administration of estrogen to women at menopause is a powerful intervention to preserve bone and protect against fracture, the detrimental effects of HRT have mandated a major reexamination of treatment options (see further and Chapter 44). In addition to antiresorptive agents, the FDA has approved the hPTH(1-34) fragment (*teriparatide*) and the hPTHrP(1-34) fragment (*abaloparatide*) for use in treating postmenopausal women with osteoporosis. Teriparatide is also approved for use in increasing bone mass in men with primary or hypogonadal osteoporosis.

Antiresorptive Agents

Bisphosphonates

Bisphosphonates are the most frequently used drugs for the prevention and treatment of osteoporosis. Second- and third-generation oral bisphosphonates, alendronate and risedronate, have sufficient potency to suppress bone resorption at doses that do not inhibit mineralization. Alendronate, risedronate, and ibandronate are used for prevention and treatment of osteoporosis and for the treatment of glucocorticoid-associated osteoporosis.

Denosumab

The ligand of RANK binds to its cognate receptor RANK on the surface of precursor and mature osteoclasts and stimulates these cells to mature and resorb bone. OPG, which competes with RANK for binding to RANKL, is the physiological inhibitor of RANKL. Denosumab is a human monoclonal antibody that binds with high affinity to RANKL, mimicking the effect of OPG and thereby reducing the binding of RANKL to RANK. Denosumab blocks osteoclast formation and activation. It increases BMD and decreases bone turnover markers when given subcutaneously, 60 mg once every 6 months. Osteonecrosis of the jaw and fractures of the femoral shaft have been reported with denosumab use. It is contraindicated in the setting of preexisting hypocalcemia.

Selective Estradiol Receptor Modulators

Considerable work has been undertaken to develop estrogenic compounds with tissue-selective activities. Raloxifene acts as an estrogen agonist on bone and liver, is inactive on the uterus, and acts as an antiestrogen on the breast (see Chapter 44). In postmenopausal women, raloxifene stabilizes and modestly increases BMD and reduces the risk of vertebral compression fracture (Komm and Mirkin, 2014). Raloxifene is approved for both the prevention and the treatment of osteoporosis. Adverse effects of raloxifene include worsening of vasomotor symptoms. The drug is also associated with an increased risk of deep vein thrombosis and pulmonary embolism, so it is contraindicated in adults with a history of venous thromboembolism.

Estrogen

Postmenopausal status or estrogen deficiency at any age significantly increases a patient's risk for osteoporosis and fractures. Likewise, overwhelming evidence supports the positive impact of estrogen replacement on the conservation of bone and protection against osteoporotic fracture after menopause (see Chapter 44). However, the Women's Health Initiative studies indicated that HRT significantly increases risks of heart disease and breast cancer; consequently, HRT is now reserved only for the short-term relief of vasomotor symptoms associated with menopause.

Calcium

The rationale for using supplemental calcium to protect bone varies with time of life. For preteens and adolescents, adequate substrate calcium is required for bone accretion. Higher Ca^{2+} intake during the third decade of life is positively related to the final phase of bone acquisition. There is controversy about the role of calcium during the early years after menopause, when the primary basis for bone loss is estrogen withdrawal. In elderly subjects, supplemental calcium suppresses bone turnover and improves BMD. Patients may increase calcium by dietary means and may choose from many palatable, low-cost calcium preparations. The most frequently prescribed is carbonate, which should be taken with meals to facilitate dissolution and absorption. Traditional dosing of calcium is about 1000 mg/d, nearly the amount present in a quart of milk. Adults more than 50 years of age need 1200 mg of calcium daily. More may be necessary to overcome endogenous intestinal calcium losses, but daily intakes of 2000 mg or more frequently are reported to be constipating.

Vitamin D and Its Analogues

Modest supplementation with vitamin D (400–800 IU/d) may improve intestinal Ca^{2+} absorption, suppress bone remodeling, and improve BMD in individuals with marginal or deficient vitamin D status. Supplemental vitamin D in combination with calcium reduces fracture incidence.

The use of calcitriol to treat osteoporosis is distinct from ensuring vitamin D nutritional adequacy. Here, the rationale is to suppress parathyroid function directly and reduce bone turnover. Higher doses of calcitriol appear to be more likely to improve BMD, but at the risk of developing hypercalciuria and hypercalcemia; therefore, close scrutiny of patients and dose are required. Restriction of dietary calcium may reduce toxicity during calcitriol therapy.

Calcitonin

Calcitonin inhibits osteoclastic bone resorption and modestly increases bone mass in patients with osteoporosis, most prominently in patients with high intrinsic rates of bone turnover. Calcitonin nasal spray (200 units/d) reduces the incidence of vertebral compression fractures by about 40% in osteoporotic women (Chesnut et al., 2000).

Thiazide Diuretics

Although not strictly antiresorptive, thiazides reduce urinary Ca^{2+} excretion and constrain bone loss in patients with hypercalciuria. Hydrochlorothiazide, 25 mg once or twice daily, may reduce urinary Ca^{2+} excretion substantially. Effective doses of thiazides for reducing urinary Ca^{2+} excretion generally are lower than those necessary for blood pressure control (see Chapters 25 and 28).

Anabolic Agents

Teriparatide

Teriparatide is the only anabolic agent currently available that increases new bone formation. It is FDA-approved for treatment of osteoporosis for up to 2 years in both men and postmenopausal women at high risk for fractures. Teriparatide increases predominantly trabecular bone at the lumbar spine and femoral neck; it has less-significant effects at cortical sites. Teriparatide is approved at the 20-mcg dose, administered once daily by subcutaneous injection in the thigh or abdominal wall. The most common adverse effects associated with teriparatide include injection-site pain, nausea, headaches, leg cramps, and dizziness.

Combination Therapies

Osteoporosis

Because teriparatide stimulates bone formation, whereas bisphosphonates reduce bone resorption, it was predicted that therapy combining the two would enhance the effect on BMD more than treatment with either one alone. However, addition of alendronate to PTH treatment provided no additional benefit for BMD and reduced the anabolic effect of PTH in both women and men. Sequential treatment with PTH(1–84) followed by alendronate increases vertebral BMD to a greater degree than alendronate or estrogen alone.

Paget Disease

Although most patients with Paget disease require no treatment, factors such as severe pain, neural compression, progressive deformity, hypercalcemia, high-output congestive heart failure, and repeated fracture risk are considered indications for treatment. Bisphosphonates and calcitonin decrease the elevated biochemical markers of bone turnover, such as plasma alkaline phosphatase activity and urinary excretion of hydroxyproline. An initial course of bisphosphonate typically is given once daily or once weekly for 6 months. With treatment, most patients experience a decrease in bone pain over several weeks. Such treatment may induce long-lasting remission. If symptoms recur, additional courses of therapy can be effective.

Optimal therapy for Paget disease varies among patients. Bisphosphonates are the standard therapy. Intravenous pamidronate induces long-term remission following a single infusion. Zoledronate exhibits greater response rates and a longer median duration of complete response. Compared with calcitonin, bisphosphonates have the advantage of oral administration, lower cost, lack of antigenicity, and generally fewer side effects.

Drug Facts for Your Personal Formulary: *Agents Affecting Mineral Ion Homeostasis and Bone Turnover*

Drugs	Therapeutic Uses	Clinical Pharmacology and Tips
Vitamin D Analogues		
Ergocalciferol	• Vitamin D deficiency • Nutritional rickets • Vitamin D–resistant rickets • Familial hypophosphatemia • Hypoparathyroidism • Osteomalacia/osteoporosis	• Vitamin D_2 • May cause hypercalcemia
Cholecalciferol		• Vitamin D_3 • May cause hypercalcemia
Doxercalciferol	• Secondary hyperparathyroidism in patients with CKD	• 1-Hydroxylated ergocalciferol (1-OH-D_2) • "Activated" in the liver by 25-hydroxylation • May cause hypercalcemia, hypercalciuria, or hyperphosphatemia
Alfacalcidol	• Secondary hyperparathyroidism in patients with CKD	• 1-Hydroxylated cholecalciferol (1-OH-D_3) • "Activated" in the liver by 25-hydroxylation • May cause hypercalcemia, hypercalciuria, or hyperphosphatemia
Dihydrotachysterol	• Familial hypophosphatemia • Hypoparathyroidism • Osteoporosis • Secondary hyperparathyroidism in patients with CKD	• Reduced form of ergocalciferol • "Activated" in the liver by 25-hydroxylation • May cause hypercalcemia, hypercalciuria, or hyperphosphatemia • Not available in the U.S.
Calcifediol	• Hypocalcemia • Secondary hyperparathyroidism in patients with CKD	• 25-Hydroxylated form of cholecalciferol • "Activated" in the kidney by 1-hydroxylation • Not available in the U.S.
Calcitriol	• Hypocalcemia • Secondary hyperparathyroidism in patients with CKD • Hypoparathyroidism	• 1,25-Dihydroxylated form of cholecalciferol • Activated form of vitamin D • May cause hypercalcemia, hypercalciuria, or hyperphosphatemia
Paricalcitol	• Secondary hyperparathyroidism in patients with CKD	• 1,25-Dihydroxy-19-norvitamin D_2 • Minimal effects on serum calcium and phosphorus
Maxacalcitol	• Secondary hyperparathyroidism in patients with CKD	• 1,25-Dihydroxy-22-oxavitamin D_3 • Shorter $t_{1/2}$ than calcitriol • Potent suppressor of PTH gene expression • Not marketed in the U.S.
Calcipotriol	• Psoriasis	• Negligible effects on serum calcium • For topical application only
Phosphate-Binding Agents • Taken with meals to reduce the amount of dietary phosphate absorbed		
Calcium carbonate	• Treatment and prevention of CKD-MBD	• Inexpensive, well tolerated, commonly used • 40% elemental calcium
Calcium acetate	• Treatment and prevention of CKD-MBD	• Well tolerated, commonly used • 25% elemental calcium
Sevelamer hydrochloride	• Treatment and prevention of CKD-MBD	• Nonabsorbable polymer that acts as a nonselective anion exchanger • Risk of metabolic acidosis
Sevelamer carbonate	• Treatment and prevention of CKD-MBD	• Same polymeric structure as sevelamer hydrochloride, with chloride replaced by carbonate • Decreased risk of metabolic acidosis
Lanthanum carbonate	• Treatment and prevention of CKD-MBD	• Risk of gastrointestinal obstruction and ileus • Contraindicated in bowel obstruction
Sucroferric oxyhydroxide (oral formulation)	• Treatment and prevention of CKD-MBD	• Polynuclear iron(III)–oxyhydroxide compound that binds phosphate by ligand exchange • Negligible absorption of iron • Injectable formulation is used for iron replacement therapy
Ferric citrate	• Treatment and prevention of CKD-MBD	• Iron absorption may lead to increased systemic iron parameters and toxicity

Drug Facts for Your Personal Formulary: *Agents Affecting Mineral Ion Homeostasis and Bone Turnover (continued)*

Drugs	Therapeutic Uses	Clinical Pharmacology and Tips
Bisphosphonates • Inhibit osteoclast-mediated bone resorption		
Etidronate	• Paget disease • Heterotopic ossification • Hypercalcemia	• Esophagitis, esophageal ulcers or erosions reported with oral administration • Contraindicated in those with abnormalities that delay esophageal emptying • Risk of nephrotoxicity • Osteonecrosis of the jaw reported
Clodronate	• Paget disease • Treatment and prevention of osteoporosis • Hypercalcemia of malignancy • Prevention of bone loss in breast cancer and multiple myeloma	• Risk of nephrotoxicity • Osteonecrosis of the jaw reported • Not commercially available in the U.S.
Tiludronate	• Paget disease	• Esophagitis, esophageal ulcers or erosions reported with oral administration • Caution in creatinine clearance < 35 mL/min • Osteonecrosis of the jaw reported
Pamidronate	• Paget disease • Hypercalcemia of malignancy • Prevention of bone loss in breast cancer and multiple myeloma	• 10–100 times more potent than etidronate • Risk of nephrotoxicity • Osteonecrosis of the jaw reported • Fractures of the femoral shaft reported • Available in the U.S. only for parenteral administration
Alendronate	• Paget disease • Treatment and prevention of osteoporosis	• 10–100 times more potent than etidronate • Esophagitis, esophageal ulcers or erosions reported with oral administration • Contraindicated in those with abnormalities that delay esophageal emptying • Osteonecrosis of jaw, fractures of femoral shaft reported
Ibandronate	• Treatment and prevention of osteoporosis	• Esophagitis, esophageal ulcers or erosions reported with oral administration • Contraindicated in those with abnormalities that delay esophageal emptying • Risk of nephrotoxicity • Osteonecrosis of jaw, fractures of the femoral shaft, anaphylaxis reported
Risedronate	• Paget disease • Treatment and prevention of osteoporosis	• Third-generation agent • 10,000 times more potent than etidronate • Esophagitis, esophageal ulcers or erosions reported with oral administration • Contraindicated in those with abnormalities that delay esophageal emptying • Osteonecrosis of jaw, fractures of the femoral shaft reported • Many dosing regimens (daily to 2 months)
Zoledronate	• Paget disease • Treatment and prevention of osteoporosis • Hypercalcemia of malignancy • Adjunctive treatment of bone metastases from solid tumors and osteolytic lesions of multiple myeloma	• Third-generation agent • 10,000 times more potent than etidronate • Contraindicated in hypocalcemia and creatinine clearance < 35 mL/min • May cause severe hypocalcemia • Risk of nephrotoxicity • Osteonecrosis of jaw, fractures of femoral shaft, anaphylaxis reported • Annual dosing for postmenopausal use
Parathyroid Hormone Analogues		
Teriparatide *[hPTH(1-34)]* Abaloparatide *[hPTHrP(1-34)]*	• Treatment of osteoporosis	• Anabolic agents • Increase new bone formation • Use should be limited to ≤ 2 years • Should not be used in patients who are at increased baseline risk for osteosarcoma
rhPTH	• Adjunctive treatment of hypocalcemia in patients with hypoparathyroidism	• Recombinant human parathyroid hormone [rhPTH(1-84)] • Severe hypercalcemia reported • Should not be used in patients who are at increased baseline risk for osteosarcoma • Only available under an REMS program
Long acting PTH	• Treatment of osteoporosis	• Increases serum calcium concentrations in rodents for almost 24 h • Investigational use only
Calcium-Sensing Receptor Mimetics • Cinacalcet		
Cinacalcet	• Secondary hyperparathyroidism in adults with CKD on dialysis • Hypercalcemia in adults with parathyroid carcinoma • Hypercalcemia in adults with primary hyperparathyroidism who are not candidates for surgical parathyroidectomy	• May cause severe hypocalcemia • Concomitant use of strong inhibitors of CYP3A4 should be avoided • Dose adjustment may be required for concomitant medications that are CYP2D6 substrates

Miscellaneous Antiresorptive Agents

Calcitonin	• Paget disease • Hypercalcemia • Postmenopausal osteoporosis	• Direct inhibitor of osteoclastic bone resorption • Anaphylaxis/hypersensitivity reported
Denosumab	• Treatment and prevention of osteoporosis • Treatment to increase bone mass in adults at high risk for fracture receiving cancer therapy	• Human monoclonal antibody that binds with high affinity to RANKL • Contraindicated in setting of preexisting hypocalcemia • Osteonecrosis of the jaw reported • Fractures of the femoral shaft reported
Raloxifene	• Treatment and prevention of osteoporosis	• Selective estrogen receptor modulator • Contraindicated in adults with history of venous thromboembolism; increased risk of deep vein thrombosis and pulmonary embolism
Hydrochlorothiazide	• Osteoporosis • Hypercalciuria	• Reduce urinary calcium excretion • Constrain bone loss in patients with hypercalciuria

Fluoride

Sodium fluoride	• Prophylaxis of dental caries	• Childhood consumption of fluoridated drinking water reduces incidence of caries in permanent teeth • Topical application can reduce the incidence of caries by 30%–40%

Bibliography

Ahmadi F, et al. Comparison of efficacy of the phosphate binders nicotinic acid and sevelamer hydrochloride in hemodialysis patients. *Saudi J Kidney Dis Transpl,* 2012, 23:934–938.

Andrews EB, et al. The U.S. postmarketing surveillance study of adult osteosarcoma and teriparatide: study design and findings from the first 7 years. *J Bone Miner Res,* 2012, 27:2429–2437.

Andrukhova O, et al. FGF23 acts directly on renal proximal tubules to induce phosphaturia through activation of the ERK1/2-SGK1 signaling pathway. *Bone,* 2012, 51:621–628.

Bastepe M. The GNAS locus and pseudohypoparathyroidism. *Adv Exp Med Biol,* 2008, 626:27–40.

Behets GJ, et al. Bone histomorphometry before and after long-term treatment with cinacalcet in dialysis patients with secondary hyperparathyroidism. *Kidney Int,* 2015, 87:846–856.

Bourgeois S, et al. The phosphate transporter NaPi-IIa determines the rapid renal adaptation to dietary phosphate intake in mouse irrespective of persistently high FGF23 levels. *Pflugers Arch,* 2013, 465:1557–1572.

Carpenter TO, et al. Randomized trial of the anti-FGF23 antibody KRN23 in X-linked hypophosphatemia. *J Clin Invest,* 2014, 124:1587–1597.

Chesnut CH, 3rd, et al. A randomized trial of nasal spray salmon calcitonin in postmenopausal women with established osteoporosis: the prevent recurrence of osteoporotic fractures study. PROOF Study Group. *Am J Med,* 2000, 109:267–276.

Cianferotti L, et al. The calcium-sensing receptor in bone metabolism: from bench to bedside and back. *Osteoporos Int,* 2015, 26:2055–2071.

Clarke BL, et al. Pharmacokinetics and pharmacodynamics of subcutaneous recombinant parathyroid hormone (1–84) in patients with hypoparathyroidism: an open-label, single-dose, phase I study. *Clin Ther,* 2014, 36:722–736.

Cremers S, Papapoulos S. Pharmacology of bisphosphonates. *Bone,* 2011, 49:42–49.

DeLuca HF. The vitamin D story: a collaborative effort of basic science and clinical medicine. *FASEB J,* 1988, 3:224–236.

Early Breast Cancer Trialists' Collaborative Group. Adjuvant bisphosphonate treatment in early breast cancer: meta-analyses of individual patient data from randomised trials. *Lancet,* 2015, 386:1353–1361.

Ebetino FH, et al. The relationship between the chemistry and biological activity of the bisphosphonates. *Bone,* 2011, 49:20–33.

Faurschou A, et al. The relation between sunscreen layer thickness and vitamin D production after ultraviolet B exposure: a randomized clinical trial. *Br J Dermatol,* 2012, 167:391–395.

Filopanti M, et al. Pharmacology of the calcium sensing receptor. *Clin Cases Miner Bone Metab,* 2013, 10:162–165.

Fitzpatrick LA, et al. Ronacaleret, a calcium-sensing receptor antagonist, increases trabecular but not cortical bone in postmenopausal women. *J Bone Miner Res,* 2012, 27:255–262.

Garrido JL, et al. Role of phospholipase D in parathyroid hormone receptor type 1 signaling and trafficking. *Mol Endocrinol,* 2009, 23:2048–2059.

Gattineni J, et al. Regulation of renal phosphate transport by FGF23 is mediated by FGFR1 and FGFR4. *Am J Physiol Renal Physiol,* 2014, 306:F351–F358.

Grill V, et al. Parathyroid hormone related protein (PTHrP) and hypercalcaemia. *Eur J Cancer,* 1998, 34:222–229.

Henriksen K, et al. Oral salmon calcitonin—pharmacology in osteoporosis. *Expert Opin Biol Ther,* 2010, 10:1617–1629.

Hirsch PF, Baruch H. Is calcitonin an important physiological substance? *Endocrine,* 2003, 21:201–228.

Imanishi Y, et al. A new method for in vivo analysis of parathyroid hormone-calcium set point in mice. *J Bone Miner Res,* 2002, 17:1656–1661.

Imel EA, et al. Prolonged correction of serum phosphorus in adults with X-linked hypophosphatemia using monthly doses of KRN23. *J Clin Endocrinol Metab,* 2015, 100:2565–2573.

Institute of Medicine. *Dietary Reference Intakes for Calcium and Vitamin D.* National Academies Press, Washington, DC, 2011, 1015.

Jones KS, et al. 25(OH)D$_2$ half-life is shorter than 25(OH)D$_3$ half-life and is influenced by DBP concentration and genotype. *J Clin Endocrinol Metab,* 2014, 99:3373–3381.

Kalil RS, et al. Effect of extended-release niacin on cardiovascular events and kidney function in chronic kidney disease: a post hoc analysis of the AIM-HIGH trial. *Kidney Int,* 2015, 87:1250–1257.

Kellett GL. Alternative perspective on intestinal calcium absorption: proposed complementary actions of Ca(v)1.3 and TRPV6. *Nutr Rev,* 2011, 69:347–370.

Kim ES, Keating GM. Recombinant human parathyroid hormone (1–84): a review in hypoparathyroidism. *Drugs,* 2015, 75:1293–1303.

Komm BS, Mirkin S. An overview of current and emerging SERMs. *J Steroid Biochem Mol Biol,* 2014, 143:207–222.

Leder, B.Z., et al. Effects of abaloparatide, a human parathyroid hormone-related peptide analog, on bone mineral density in postmenopausal women with osteoporosis. *J Clin Endocrinol Metab,* 2015, 100:697–706.

Maeda A, et al. Critical role of parathyroid hormone (PTH) receptor-1 phosphorylation in regulating acute responses to PTH. *Proc Natl Acad Sci U S A,* 2013, 110:5864–5869.

Mazzaferro S, et al. Vitamin D metabolites and/or analogs: which D for which patient? *Curr Vasc Pharmacol,* 2014, 12:339–349.

Miller PD, et al. Effect of abaloparatide vs placebo on new vertebral fractures in postmenopausal women with osteoporosis: a randomized clinical trial. *JAMA,* 2016, 316:722–733.

906 Moe SM, et al. Cinacalcet, fibroblast growth factor-23, and cardiovascular disease in hemodialysis: the Evaluation of Cinacalcet HCl Therapy to Lower Cardiovascular Events (EVOLVE) trial. *Circulation*, **2015**, *132*:27–39.

Neer RM, et al. Effect of parathyroid hormone (1–34) on fractures and bone mineral density in postmenopausal women with osteoporosis. *N Engl J Med*, **2001**, *344*:1434–1441.

Nemeth EF, Shoback D. Calcimimetic and calcilytic drugs for treating bone and mineral-related disorders. *Best Pract Res Clin Endocrinol Metab*, **2013**, *27*:373–384.

Ornitz DM, Itoh N. The fibroblast growth factor signaling pathway. *Wiley Interdiscip Rev Dev Biol*, **2015**, *4*:215–266.

Ott SM. Pharmacology of bisphosphonates in patients with chronic kidney disease. *Semin Dial*, **2015**, *28*:363–369.

Ponnapakkam T, et al. A single injection of the anabolic bone agent, parathyroid hormone-collagen binding domain (PTH-CBD), results in sustained increases in bone mineral density for up to 12 months in normal female mice. *Calcif Tissue Int*, **2012**, *91*:196–203.

Reid IR. Short-term and long-term effects of osteoporosis therapies. *Nat Rev Endocrinol*, **2015**, *11*:418–428.

Scillitani A, et al. Carboxyl-terminal parathyroid hormone fragments: biologic effects. *J Endocrinol Invest*, **2011**, *34*:23–26.

Shah HH, et al. Novel iron-based phosphate binders in patients with chronic kidney disease. *Curr Opin Nephrol Hypertens*, **2015**, *24*:330–335.

Smith RC, et al. Circulating αKlotho influences phosphate handling by controlling FGF23 production. *J Clin Invest*, **2012**, *122*:4710–4715.

Torres A, et al. Sigmoidal relationship between calcitonin and calcium: studies in normal, parathyroidectomized, and azotemic rats. *Kidney Int*, **1991**, *40*:700–704.

Wagner CL, Greer FR, American Academy of Pediatrics Section on Breastfeeding and Committee on Nutrition. Prevention of rickets and vitamin D deficiency in infants, children, and adolescents. *Pediatrics*, **2008**, *122*:1142–1152.

Wolf M, White KE. Coupling fibroblast growth factor 23 production and cleavage: iron deficiency, rickets, and kidney disease. *Curr Opin Nephrol Hypertens*, **2014**, *23*:411–419.

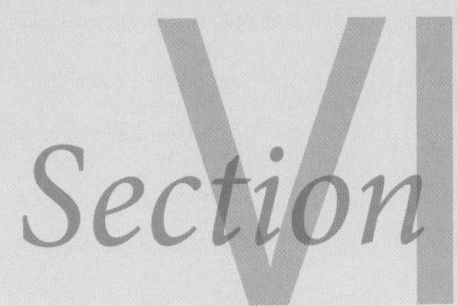

Section VI

Gastrointestinal Pharmacology

Pharmacotherapy for Gastric Acidity, Peptic Ulcers, and Gastroesophageal Reflux Disease

Keith A. Sharkey and Wallace K. MacNaughton

Gastric acid and pepsin in the stomach normally do not produce damage or symptoms of acid-peptic diseases because of intrinsic defense mechanisms. The stomach is protected by a number of factors, collectively referred to as "mucosal defense," many of which are stimulated by the local generation of PGs and NO. If these defenses are disrupted, a gastric or duodenal ulcer may form. The treatment and prevention of acid-related disorders are accomplished by decreasing gastric acidity and enhancing mucosal defense. The appreciation that an infectious agent, *Helicobacter pylori*, plays a key role in the pathogenesis of acid-peptic diseases revolutionized approaches to prevention and therapy of these common disorders.

Barriers to the reflux of gastric contents into the esophagus comprise the primary esophageal defense. If these protective barriers fail and reflux occurs, dyspepsia or erosive esophagitis may result. Therapies are directed at decreasing gastric acidity, enhancing the tone of the lower esophageal sphincter, and stimulating esophageal motility (see Chapter 50).

Physiology of Gastric Secretion

Gastric acid secretion is a complex and continuous process: Neuronal (ACh, GRP); paracrine (histamine); and endocrine (gastrin) factors regulate the secretion of H⁺ by parietal cells (acid-secreting cells) (Figure 49–1). Their specific receptors (M₃, BB₂, H₂, and CCK₂, respectively) are on the basolateral membrane of parietal cells in the body and fundus of the stomach. Some of these receptors are also present on ECL cells, where they regulate the release of histamine. The H₂ receptor is a GPCR that activates the Gₛ–adenylyl cyclase–cyclic AMP–PKA pathway (see Chapters 3 and 39). ACh and gastrin signal through GPCRs that couple to the Gₑ-PLC-IP₃-Ca²⁺ pathway in parietal cells; GRP uses the same signaling pathway to activate gastrin secretion from G cells. In parietal cells, the cyclic AMP and the Ca²⁺-dependent pathways activate H⁺,K⁺-ATPase (the proton pump), which exchanges H⁺ and K⁺ across the parietal cell membrane. This pump generates the largest ion gradient known in vertebrates, with an intracellular pH of about 7.3 and an intracanalicular pH of about 0.8.

The important structures for CNS stimulation of gastric acid secretion are the dorsal motor nucleus of the vagal nerve, the hypothalamus, and the solitary tract nucleus. Efferent fibers originating in the dorsal motor nuclei descend to the stomach via the vagus nerve and synapse with ganglion cells of the enteric nervous system. ACh release from postganglionic vagal fibers directly stimulates gastric acid secretion through muscarinic M₃ receptors on the basolateral membrane of parietal cells. The CNS predominantly modulates the activity of the enteric nervous system via ACh, stimulating gastric acid secretion in response to the sight, smell, taste, or anticipation of food (the "cephalic" phase of acid secretion). ACh also indirectly affects parietal cells by increasing the release of histamine from the ECL cells in the fundus of the stomach and of gastrin from G cells in the gastric antrum.

The ECL cells, the source of gastric histamine, are usually in close proximity to parietal cells. Histamine acts as a paracrine mediator, diffusing from its site of release to nearby parietal cells, where it activates H₂ receptors to stimulate gastric acid secretion.

Gastrin, produced by antral G cells, is the most potent inducer of acid secretion. Multiple pathways stimulate gastrin release, including CNS activation, local distention, and chemical components of the gastric contents. In addition to releasing ACh, some vagal fibers to the stomach also release GRP (a peptide of 27 amino acids); GRP activates the BB₂ bombesin receptor on G cells, activating the Gₑ-PLC-IP₃-Ca²⁺ pathway and causing secretion of gastrin. Gastrin stimulates acid secretion indirectly by inducing the release of histamine by ECL cells; a direct effect on parietal cells also plays a lesser role.

Somatostatin, produced by antral D cells, inhibits gastric acid secretion. Acidification of the gastric luminal pH to less than 3 stimulates somatostatin release, which in turn suppresses gastrin release in a negative-feedback loop. Somatostatin-producing cells are decreased in patients with *H. pylori* infection, and the consequent reduction of somatostatin's inhibitory effect may contribute to excess gastrin production.

Abbreviations

ACh: acetylcholine
cAMP: cyclic adenosine monophosphate
CCK: cholecystokinin
CNS: central nervous system
CYP: cytochrome P450
DU: duodenal ulcer
ECG: electrocardiogram
ECL: enterochromaffin-like cell
ENS: enteric nervous system
GERD: gastroesophageal reflux disease
GI: gastrointestinal
GPCR: G protein–coupled receptor
GRP: gastrin-releasing peptide
GU: gastric ulcer
HIST: histamine
IP$_3$: inositol 1,4,5-trisphosphate
NO: nitric oxide
NSAID: nonsteroidal anti-inflammatory drug
OTC: over the counter
PG: prostaglandin
PK: protein kinase
PLC: phospholipase C
PPI: proton pump inhibitor
SST: somatostatin

Parietal Cell H⁺,K⁺-ATPase

H$^+$,K$^+$-ATPase is the enzyme responsible for secreting protons into the lumen of the gastric gland (Shin et al., 2009). It is a heterodimeric protein composed of two subunits that are the products of two genes. The *ATP4A* gene encodes the α subunit that contains the catalytic sites of the enzyme and forms the membrane pore, and the *ATP4B* encodes the β subunit of the H$^+$,K$^+$-ATPase, which contains an N-terminal cytoplasmic domain, a transmembrane domain, and a highly glycosylated extracellular domain. Hydronium ions bind to three active sites present in the α subunit, and secretion involves conformational change that allows the movement of protons. This movement is balanced by the transport of K$^+$. The stoichiometry of transport is pH dependent, varying between two H$^+$ and two K$^+$ per molecule of ATP to one of each under more acidic conditions. Inhibiting the H$^+$,K$^+$-ATPase (or proton pump) is the mainstay of modern pharmacotherapy for acid-related disorders.

Gastric Defenses Against Acid

The extremely high concentration of H$^+$ in the gastric lumen requires robust defense mechanisms to protect the esophagus, stomach, and proximal small intestine (Wallace, 2008). The primary esophageal defense is the gastroesophageal junction—the lower esophageal sphincter in association with the diaphragm and angle of His—which prevents reflux of acidic gastric contents into the esophagus. The stomach protects itself from acid damage by a number of mechanisms that require adequate mucosal blood flow. One key defense is the secretion of a mucous layer that helps to protect gastric epithelial cells by trapping secreted bicarbonate at the cell surface. Gastric mucus is soluble when secreted but quickly forms an insoluble gel that coats the mucosal surface of the stomach, slows ion diffusion, and prevents mucosal damage by macromolecules such as pepsin. Mucus production is stimulated by PGs E$_2$ and I$_2$, which also directly inhibit gastric acid secretion by parietal cells. Thus, drugs that inhibit PG formation (e.g., NSAIDs, ethanol) decrease mucus secretion and predispose to the development of acid-peptic disease. The proximal part of the duodenum is protected from gastric acid through the production of bicarbonate, primarily from mucosal Brunner glands.

Figure 49–1 outlines the rationale and pharmacological basis for the therapy of acid-peptic disease. The PPIs are used most commonly, followed by the histamine H$_2$ receptor antagonists.

Proton Pump Inhibitors

The most potent suppressors of gastric acid secretion are inhibitors of the gastric H$^+$,K$^+$-ATPase or proton pump (Figure 49–2). These drugs diminish the daily production of acid (basal and stimulated) by 80%–95% (Shin and Sachs, 2008).

Mechanism of Action and Pharmacology

Six PPIs are available for clinical use: *omeprazole* and its S-isomer, *esomeprazole, lansoprazole* and its R-enantiomer, *dexlansoprazole, rabeprazole,* and *pantoprazole.* All PPIs have equivalent efficacy at comparable doses.

Proton pump inhibitors are prodrugs that require activation in an acid environment. After absorption into the systemic circulation, the prodrug diffuses into the parietal cells of the stomach and accumulates in the acidic secretory canaliculi. Here, it is activated by proton-catalyzed formation of a tetracyclic sulfenamide (see Figure 49–2), trapping the drug so that it cannot diffuse back across the canalicular membrane. The activated form then binds covalently with sulfhydryl groups of cysteines in the H$^+$,K$^+$-ATPase, irreversibly inactivating the pump molecule. Acid secretion resumes only after new pump molecules are synthesized and inserted into the luminal membrane, providing a prolonged (up to 24- to 48-h) suppression of acid secretion, despite the much shorter plasma $t_{1/2}$ of about 0.5–3 h of the parent compounds. Because they block the final step in acid production, the PPIs effectively suppress stimulated acid production, regardless of the physiological stimulus, as well as basal acid production.

The amount of H$^+$,K$^+$-ATPase increases after fasting; therefore, PPIs should be given before the first meal of the day. In most individuals, once-daily dosing is sufficient to achieve an effective level of acid inhibition, and a second dose, which is occasionally necessary, can be administered before an evening meal. Rebound acid hypersecretion occurs following prolonged treatment with PPIs, and clinical studies suggest that rebound after ceasing treatment can provoke symptoms such as dyspepsia.

To prevent degradation of PPIs by acid in the gastric lumen and improve oral bioavailability, oral dosage forms are supplied in different formulations:

- Enteric-coated pellets within gelatin capsules (*omeprazole, dexlansoprazole, esomeprazole, lansoprazole, rabeprazole*)
- Delayed-release tablets (omeprazole formulations)
- Delayed-release capsules (dexlansoprazole, esomeprazole formulations)
- Delayed-release oral suspension packets (esomeprazole, omeprazole, pantoprazole)
- Enteric-coated microgranules in orally disintegrating tablets (*lansoprazole*)
- Enteric-coated tablets (*pantoprazole, rabeprazole,* and *omeprazole*)
- Powdered omeprazole combined with sodium bicarbonate (capsules and oral suspension)

The delayed-release and enteric-coated tablets dissolve only at alkaline pH, whereas admixture of *omeprazole* with sodium bicarbonate simply neutralizes stomach acid; both strategies substantially improve the oral bioavailability of these acid-labile drugs. Patients for whom the oral route of administration is not available can be treated parenterally with *esomeprazole sodium* or *pantoprazole.*

ADME

Because an acidic pH in the parietal cell acid canaliculi is required for drug activation and food stimulates acid production, these drugs ideally should be given about 30 min before meals. Concurrent administration of food may reduce somewhat the rate of absorption of PPIs, but this effect is not thought to be clinically significant. Once in the small bowel, PPIs are rapidly absorbed, highly protein bound, and extensively metabolized by hepatic CYPs, particularly CYP2C19 and CYP3A4. Asians are more likely

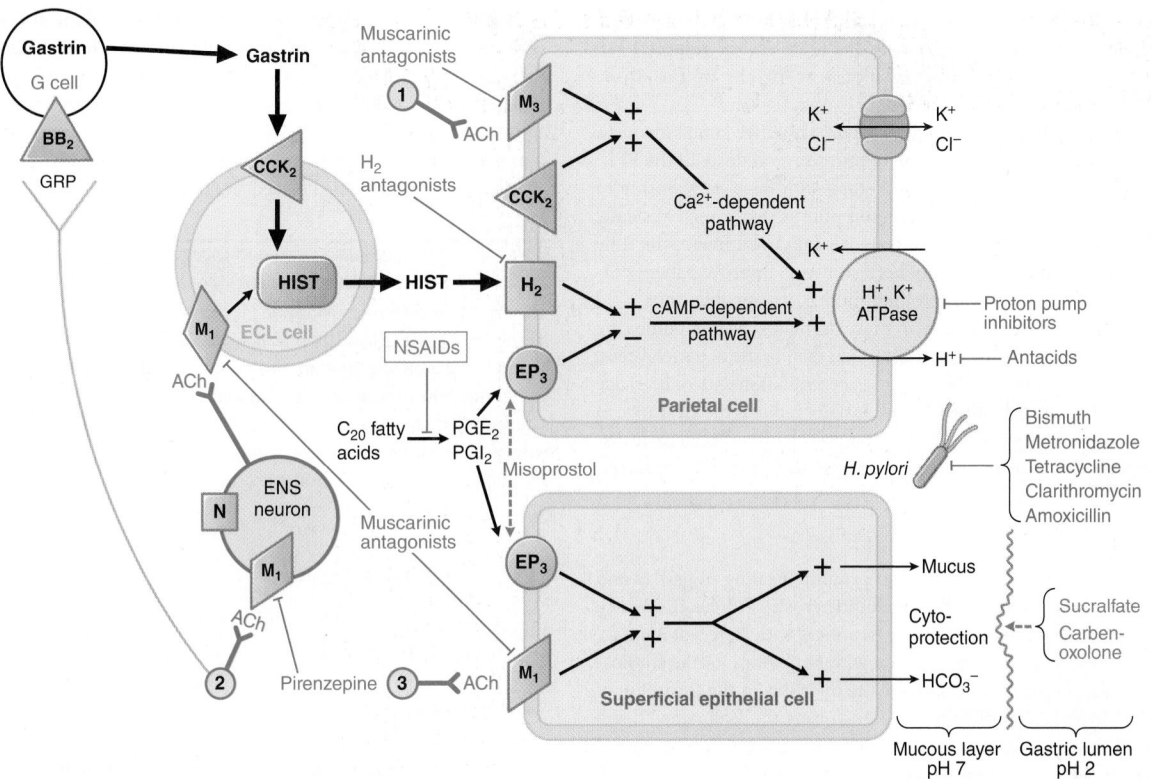

Figure 49–1 *Pharmacologist's view of gastric secretion and its regulation: the basis for therapy of acid-peptic disorders.* Shown are the interactions among neural input and a variety of enteroendocrine cells: an ECL cell that secretes histamine, a ganglion cell of the ENS, a G cell that secretes gastrin, a parietal cell that secretes acid, and a superficial epithelial cell that secretes mucus and bicarbonate. Physiological pathways, shown in solid black, may be stimulatory (+) or inhibitory (−). 1 and 3 indicate possible inputs from postganglionic cholinergic fibers; 2 shows neural input from the vagus nerve. Physiological agonists and their respective membrane receptors include ACh and its muscarinic (M) and nicotinic (N) receptors; GRP and its receptor, the BB_2 bombesin receptor; gastrin and its receptor, the CCK_2; HIST and the H_2 receptor; and PGE_2 and the EP_3 receptor. A red line with a T bar indicates sites of pharmacological antagonism. A light blue dashed arrow indicates a drug action that mimics or enhances a physiological pathway. Shown in red are drugs used to treat acid-peptic disorders. NSAIDs can induce ulcers via inhibition of cyclooxygenase. Not shown is a physiological pathway that reduces acid secretion: a D cell that secretes SST, which inhibits G-cell release of gastrin.

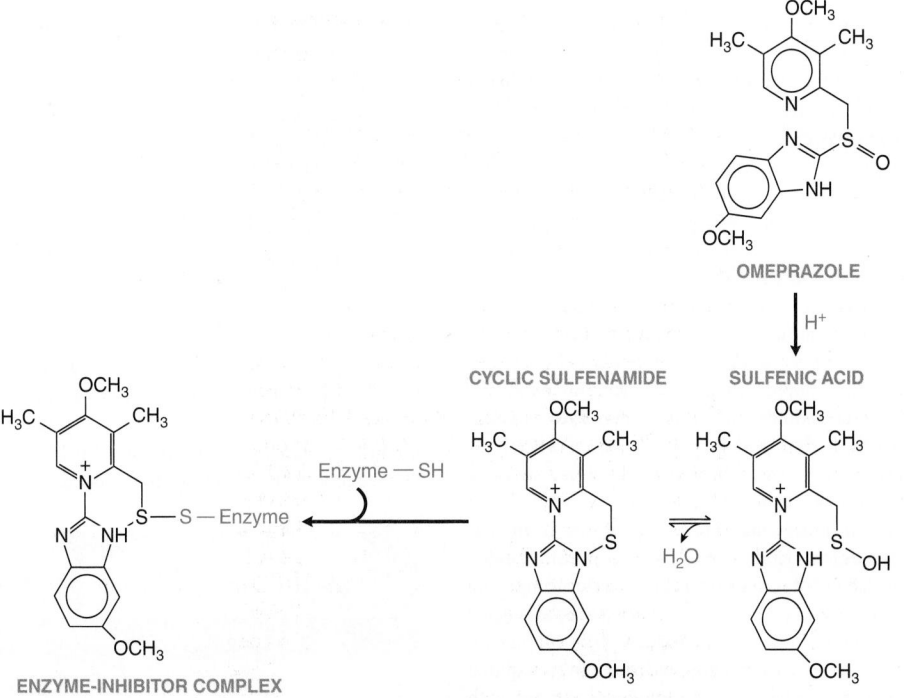

Figure 49–2 *Activation of a PPI from its prodrug form.* Omeprazole is converted to a sulfenamide in the acidic secretory canaliculi of the parietal cell. The sulfenamide interacts covalently with sulfhydryl groups in the proton pump, thereby irreversibly inhibiting its activity. Lansoprazole, rabeprazole, and pantoprazole undergo analogous conversions.

than Caucasians or African Americans to have the CYP2C19 genotype that correlates with slow metabolism of PPIs (23% vs. 3%, respectively), which may contribute to heightened efficacy or toxicity in this ethnic group (Camilleri, 2012).

Because not all pumps and all parietal cells are active simultaneously, maximal suppression of acid secretion requires several doses of the PPIs. For example, it may take 2–5 days of therapy with once-daily dosing to achieve the about 70% inhibition of proton pumps that is seen at steady state. More frequent initial dosing (e.g., twice daily) will reduce the time to achieve full inhibition but has not been shown to improve patient outcome. The resulting proton pump inhibition is irreversible; thus, acid secretion is suppressed for 24–48 h, or more, until new proton pumps are synthesized and incorporated into the luminal membrane of parietal cells. Chronic renal failure does not lead to drug accumulation with once-a-day dosing of the PPIs. Hepatic disease substantially reduces the clearance of esomeprazole and lansoprazole. Thus, in patients with severe hepatic disease, dose reduction is recommended for esomeprazole and lansoprazole.

Therapeutic Uses and Adverse Effects

Prescription PPIs are primarily used to promote healing of gastric and duodenal ulcers and to treat GERD, including erosive esophagitis, which is either complicated or unresponsive to treatment with H_2 receptor antagonists. They are also used in conjunction with antibiotics for the eradication of *Helicobacter pylori*. PPIs also are the mainstay in the treatment of pathological hypersecretory conditions, including the Zollinger-Ellison syndrome. *Lansoprazole, pantoprazole*, and *esomeprazole* are approved for treatment and prevention of recurrence of NSAID-associated gastric ulcers in patients who continue NSAID use. It is not clear if PPIs affect the susceptibility to NSAID-induced damage and bleeding in the small and large intestine. All PPIs are approved for reducing the risk of duodenal ulcer recurrence associated with *H. pylori* infections. Over-the-counter *omeprazole, esomeprazole*, and *lansoprazole* are approved for the self-treatment of acid reflux. Therapeutic applications of the PPIs are discussed further in the section Therapeutic Strategies for Specific Acid-Peptic Disorders.

The PPIs generally cause remarkably few adverse effects and have an excellent safety record (Chen et al., 2012; Reimer, 2013). The most common side effects are nausea, abdominal pain, constipation, flatulence, and diarrhea. Subacute myopathy, arthralgias, headaches, interstitial nephritis, and skin rashes also have been reported. PPIs are metabolized by hepatic CYPs and therefore may interfere with the elimination of other drugs cleared by this route. PPIs have been observed to interact with warfarin (*esomeprazole, lansoprazole, omeprazole*, and *rabeprazole*); diazepam (*esomeprazole* and *omeprazole*); and cyclosporine (*omeprazole* and *rabeprazole*). Among the PPIs, only omeprazole inhibits CYP2C19 (thereby decreasing the clearance of disulfiram, phenytoin, and other drugs) and induces the expression of CYP1A2 (thereby increasing the clearance of imipramine, several antipsychotic drugs, tacrine, and theophylline). There is some evidence that PPIs can inhibit conversion of clopidogrel (at the level of CYP2C19) to the active anticoagulating form, but this is controversial (Huang et al., 2012). *Pantoprazole* is less likely to result in this interaction; concurrent use of clopidogrel and PPIs (mainly *pantoprazole*) significantly reduces GI bleeding without increasing adverse cardiac events (see Chapter 32). Another drug interaction is between methotrexate and PPI therapy because PPIs can competitively inhibit methotrexate elimination and thereby increase methotrexate levels.

Chronic treatment with *omeprazole* decreases the absorption of vitamin B_{12}, but the clinical relevance of this effect is not clear. Loss of gastric acidity also may affect the bioavailability of such drugs as ketoconazole, ampicillin esters, and iron salts. Chronic use of PPIs has been reported to be associated with an increased risk of bone fracture and with increased susceptibility to certain infections (e.g., hospital-acquired pneumonia, community-acquired *Clostridium difficile*, spontaneous bacterial peritonitis in patients with ascites). Hypergastrinemia is more frequent and more severe with PPIs than with H_2 receptor antagonists and associated with this is ECL hyperplasia, fundic gland polyposis, and atrophic gastritis. This hypergastrinemia may

predispose to rebound hypersecretion of gastric acid on discontinuation of therapy and also may promote the growth of GI tumors, although the risk appears very low (Song et al., 2014). Recently, there have been associations made between long-term PPI use and increased risk of chronic kidney disease and dementia. These studies are not yet supported by well-controlled prospective trials and the evidence for these significant adverse effects remains very limited (Freedberg et al, 2017).

H_2 Receptor Antagonists

The arrival of selective histamine H_2 receptor antagonists was a landmark in the treatment of acid-peptic disease. Before the availability of the H_2 receptor antagonists, the standard of care was simply acid neutralization in the stomach lumen, generally with inadequate results. The long history of safety and efficacy with the H_2 receptor antagonists led to their availability without a prescription. Increasingly, however, PPIs are replacing the H_2 receptor antagonists in clinical practice.

Mechanism of Action and Pharmacology

The H_2 receptor antagonists inhibit acid production by reversibly competing with histamine for binding to H_2 receptors on the basolateral membrane of parietal cells (Black, 1993). Four different H_2 receptor antagonists, which differ mainly in their pharmacokinetics and propensity to cause drug interactions, are available in the U.S.: *cimetidine, ranitidine, famotidine*, and *nizatidine*. These drugs are less potent than PPIs but still suppress 24-hour gastric acid secretion by about 70%. Suppression of basal and nocturnal acid secretion is about 70%; because suppression of nocturnal acid secretion is important in the healing of duodenal ulcers, evening dosing of an H_2 receptor antagonist is adequate therapy in most cases. There is little evidence for the use of H_2 receptor antagonists for the treatment of bleeding ulcers, and they are no longer recommended for this purpose. All four H_2 receptor antagonists are available as prescription and over-the-counter formulations for oral administration. Intravenous and intramuscular preparations of cimetidine, ranitidine, and famotidine also are available for use in critically ill patients (Table 49–1)

ADME

The H_2 receptor antagonists are rapidly absorbed after oral administration, with peak serum concentrations within 1–3 h. Absorption may be enhanced by food or decreased by antacids, but these effects probably are unimportant clinically. Therapeutic levels are achieved rapidly after intravenous dosing and are maintained for 4–5 h (*cimetidine*), 6–8 h

TABLE 49–1 ■ INTRAVENOUS DOSES OF H_2 RECEPTOR ANTAGONISTS

	CIMETIDINE	RANITIDINE	FAMOTIDINE
Intermittent bolus	300 mg every 6–8 h	50 mg every 6–8 h	20 mg every 12 h
Continuous infusion	37.5–100 mg/h	6.25–12.5 mg/h	1.7–2.1 mg/h

(ranitidine), or 10–12 h (famotidine). The $t_{1/2}$ values of these agents after oral administration in adults range from 1 to 3.5 h; cimetidine clearance is faster in children, reducing its $t_{1/2}$ by about 30%. Only a small fraction of these drugs is protein bound. The kidneys excrete these drugs and their metabolites by filtration and renal tubular secretion, and it is important to reduce drug doses in patients with decreased creatinine clearance. Neither hemodialysis nor peritoneal dialysis clears significant amounts of these drugs. Hepatic metabolism accounts for a small fraction of clearance (from < 10% to about 35%), but liver disease per se is generally not an indication for dose adjustment.

Therapeutic Uses and Adverse Effects

The major therapeutic indications for H_2 receptor antagonists are to promote healing of gastric and duodenal ulcers, to treat uncomplicated GERD, and to prevent the occurrence of stress ulcers. For more information about the therapeutic applications of H_2 receptor antagonists, see Therapeutic Strategies for Specific Acid-Peptic Disorders.

The H_2 receptor antagonists generally are well tolerated, with a low (<3%) incidence of adverse effects (Sabesin, 1993). Side effects are minor and include diarrhea, headache, drowsiness, fatigue, muscular pain, and constipation. Less-common side effects include those affecting the CNS (confusion, delirium, hallucinations, slurred speech, and headaches), which occur primarily with intravenous administration of the drugs or in elderly subjects. Several reports have associated H_2 receptor antagonists with various blood disorders, including thrombocytopenia. H_2 receptor antagonists cross the placenta and are excreted in breast milk. Although no major teratogenic risk has been associated with these agents, caution is warranted when they are used in pregnancy.

All agents that inhibit gastric acid secretion may alter the rate of absorption and subsequent bioavailability of the H_2 receptor antagonists (see Antacids section). Drug interactions with H_2 receptor antagonists occur mainly with cimetidine, and its use has decreased markedly. Cimetidine inhibits CYPs (e.g., CYP1A2, CYP2C9, and CYP2D6) and thereby can increase the levels of a variety of drugs that are substrates for these enzymes. Ranitidine also interacts with hepatic CYPs, but with an affinity of only 10% of that of cimetidine. Famotidine and nizatidine are even safer in this regard. Slight increases in blood alcohol concentration may result from concomitant use of H_2 receptor antagonists and alcohol.

Tolerance and Rebound With Acid-Suppressing Medications

Tolerance to the acid-suppressing effects of H_2 receptor antagonists may develop within 3 days of starting treatment and may be resistant to increased doses of the medications (Sandevik et al., 1997). Diminished sensitivity to these drugs may result from the effect of the secondary hypergastrinemia to stimulate histamine release from ECL cells.

Agents That Enhance Mucosal Defense

Misoprostol

Misoprostol (15-deoxy-16-hydroxy-16-methyl-PGE_1) is a synthetic analogue of PGE_1 that is FDA approved to prevent NSAID-induced mucosal injury.

Mechanism of Action and Pharmacology

Prostaglandin E_2 and prostacyclin (PGI_2) are the major PGs synthesized by the gastric mucosa. Contrary to their cyclic AMP–elevating effects on many cells via EP_2 and EP_4 receptors, these prostanoids bind to the EP_3 receptor on parietal cells and stimulate the G_i pathway, thereby decreasing intracellular cyclic AMP and gastric acid secretion. PGE_2 also can prevent gastric injury by cytoprotective effects that include stimulation of mucin and bicarbonate secretion and increased mucosal blood flow. Acid suppression appears to be the most important effect clinically (Wolfe and Sachs, 2000).

Because NSAIDs diminish PG formation by inhibiting cyclooxygenase, synthetic PG analogues offer a logical approach to counteract NSAID-induced damage.

ADME

Misoprostol is rapidly absorbed after oral administration and is rapidly and extensively deesterified to form misoprostol acid, the principal and active metabolite of the drug. A single dose inhibits acid production within 30 min; the therapeutic effect peaks at 60–90 min and lasts for up to 3 h. Food and antacids decrease the rate of misoprostol absorption. The free acid is excreted mainly in the urine, with an elimination $t_{1/2}$ of 20–40 min.

Therapeutic Uses and Adverse Effects

Misoprostol is rarely used because of its side effects (Rostom et al., 2009). The degree of inhibition of gastric acid secretion by misoprostol is directly related to dose; oral doses of 100–200 μg significantly inhibit basal acid secretion (up to 85%–95% inhibition) or food-stimulated acid secretion (up to 75%–85% inhibition). The usual recommended dose for ulcer prophylaxis is 200 μg four times a day.

Diarrhea, with or without abdominal pain and cramps, occurs in up to 30% of patients who take *misoprostol*. Apparently dose related, it typically begins within the first 2 weeks after therapy is initiated and often resolves spontaneously within a week; more severe cases may necessitate drug discontinuation. *Misoprostol can cause clinical exacerbations of inflammatory bowel disease* (see Chapter 51). *Misoprostol is contraindicated for reducing the risk of NSAID-induced ulcer in women of childbearing potential unless the patient is at high risk of complications from gastric ulcers associated with use of the NSAID. It is also completely contraindicated during pregnancy* because it can increase uterine contractility.

Sucralfate

Mechanism of Action and Pharmacology

In the presence of acid-induced damage, pepsin-mediated hydrolysis of mucosal proteins contributes to mucosal erosion and ulcerations. This process can be inhibited by sulfated polysaccharides. *Sucralfate* consists of the octasulfate of sucrose to which $Al(OH)_3$ has been added. In an acid environment (pH < 4), sucralfate undergoes extensive cross-linking to produce a viscous, sticky polymer that adheres to epithelial cells and ulcer craters for up to 6 h after a single dose. In addition to inhibiting hydrolysis of mucosal proteins by pepsin, *sucralfate* may have other cytoprotective effects, including stimulation of local production of PGs and epidermal growth factor (Szabo, 2014). *Sucralfate* also binds bile salts; thus, some clinicians use *sucralfate* to treat individuals with the syndromes of biliary esophagitis or gastritis (the existence of which is controversial).

Therapeutic Uses and Adverse Effects

The use of *sucralfate* to treat peptic acid disease has diminished in recent years. Nevertheless, because increased gastric pH may be a factor in the development of nosocomial pneumonia in critically ill patients, sucralfate may offer an advantage over PPIs and H_2 receptor antagonists for the prophylaxis of stress ulcers. *Sucralfate* also has been used in conditions associated with mucosal inflammation/ulceration that may not respond to acid suppression, including oral mucositis (radiation and aphthous ulcers) and bile reflux gastropathy. Administered by rectal enema, sucralfate also has been used for radiation proctitis and solitary rectal ulcers. Because it is activated by acid, *sucralfate* should be taken on an empty stomach 1 h before meals. Use of antacids within 30 min of a dose of *sucralfate* should be avoided. The dose of sucralfate is 1 g four times daily (for active duodenal ulcer) or 1 g twice daily (for maintenance therapy). For children, it is given 40–80 mg/kg/d in divided doses every 6 h.

The most common side effect of *sucralfate* is constipation (about 2%). *Sucralfate* should be avoided in patients with renal failure who are at risk for aluminum overload (Marks, 1991). Likewise, aluminum-containing antacids should not be combined with *sucralfate* in these patients. *Sucralfate* forms a viscous layer in the stomach that may inhibit absorption of other drugs, including phenytoin, digoxin, cimetidine, ketoconazole, and fluoroquinolone antibiotics. *Sucralfate* therefore should be taken at least 2 h after the administration of other drugs. The "sticky" nature of the viscous gel produced by *sucralfate* in the stomach also may be responsible for the development of bezoars in some patients.

Antacids

Mechanism of Action and Pharmacology

There are far more effective and persistent agents than antacids, but their price, accessibility, and rapid action make them popular with consumers as OTC medications, and they can be used for the acute treatment of acid reflux ("heartburn") and esophagitis (see discussion that follows). Many factors, including palatability, determine the effectiveness and choice of antacid. Although sodium bicarbonate effectively neutralizes acid, it is very water soluble and rapidly absorbed from the stomach, and the alkali and sodium loads may pose a risk for patients with cardiac or renal failure. $CaCO_3$ rapidly and effectively neutralizes gastric H^+, but the release of CO_2 from bicarbonate- and carbonate-containing antacids can cause belching, nausea, abdominal distention, and flatulence. Calcium also may induce rebound acid secretion, necessitating more frequent administration. Combinations of Mg^{2+} (rapidly reacting) and Al^{3+} (slowly reacting) hydroxides provide a relatively balanced and sustained neutralizing capacity and are preferred by most experts. Magaldrate, a hydroxymagnesium aluminate complex, is converted rapidly in gastric acid to $Mg(OH)_2$ and $Al(OH)_3$, which are absorbed poorly and thus provide a sustained antacid effect. Although fixed combinations of Mg^{2+} and Al^{3+} theoretically counteract the adverse effects of each other on the bowel (Al^{3+} can relax gastric smooth muscle, producing delayed gastric emptying and constipation; Mg^{2+} exerts the opposite effects), such balance is not always achieved in practice. Simethicone, a surfactant that may decrease foaming and hence esophageal reflux, is included in many antacid preparations. However, other fixed combinations, particularly those with aspirin, that are marketed for "acid indigestion" are potentially unsafe in patients predisposed to gastroduodenal ulcers and should not be used.

Therapeutic Uses and Adverse Effects

Antacids are given orally 1 and 3 h after meals and at bedtime. For severe symptoms or uncontrolled reflux, antacids can be given as often as every 30–60 min. In general, antacids should be administered in suspension form because this probably has greater neutralizing capacity than powder or tablet dosage forms. Antacids are cleared from the empty stomach in about 30 min. However, the presence of food is sufficient to elevate gastric pH to about 5 for about 1 h and to prolong the neutralizing effects of antacids for about 2–3 h.

Antacids vary in the extent to which they are absorbed and hence in their systemic effects. In general, most antacids can elevate urinary pH by about 1 pH unit. Antacids that contain Al^{3+}, Ca^{2+}, or Mg^{2+} are absorbed less completely than are those that contain $NaHCO_3$. With renal insufficiency, absorbed Al^{3+} can contribute to osteoporosis, encephalopathy, and proximal myopathy. About 15% of orally administered Ca^{2+} is absorbed, causing transient hypercalcemia. The hypercalcemia from as little as 3–4 g of $CaCO_3$ per day can be problematic in patients with uremia. In the past, when large doses of $NaHCO_3$ and $CaCO_3$ were administered commonly with milk or cream for the management of peptic ulcer, the *milk-alkali syndrome* (alkalosis, hypercalcemia, and renal insufficiency) occurred frequently. Today, this syndrome is rare and generally results from the chronic ingestion of large quantities of Ca^{2+} (five to forty 500-mg tablets per day of calcium carbonate) taken with milk.

By altering gastric and urinary pH, antacids may affect a number of drugs (e.g., thyroid hormones, allopurinol, and imidazole antifungals), by altering rates of dissolution and absorption, bioavailability, and renal elimination). Al^{3+} and Mg^{2+} antacids also are notable for their propensity to chelate other drugs present in the GI tract and thereby decrease their absorption. Most interactions can be avoided by taking antacids 2 h before or after ingestion of other drugs.

Other Acid Suppressants and Cytoprotectants

The M_1 muscarinic receptor antagonists *pirenzepine* and *telenzepine* (see Chapter 9) can reduce basal acid production by 40%–50%. The ACh receptor on the parietal cell itself is of the M_3 subtype, and these drugs are

believed to suppress neural stimulation of acid production via actions on M_1 receptors of intramural ganglia (see Figure 49–1). Because of their relatively poor efficacy, significant and undesirable anticholinergic side effects, and risk of blood disorders (pirenzepine), they rarely are used today.

Rebamipide is used for ulcer therapy in parts of India and Asia. Its cytoprotective effects are exerted by increasing PG generation in gastric mucosa and by scavenging reactive oxygen species. Ecabet, which appears to increase the formation of PGE_2 and PGI_2, also is used for ulcer therapy, mostly in Japan. Carbenoxolone, a derivative of glycyrrhizic acid found in licorice root, has been used with modest success for ulcer therapy in Europe. Unfortunately, carbenoxolone inhibits the type I isozyme of 11β-hydroxysteroid dehydrogenase, which protects the mineralocorticoid receptor from activation by cortisol in the distal nephron; it therefore causes hypokalemia and hypertension due to excessive mineralocorticoid receptor activation (see Chapter 46). Bismuth compounds (see Chapter 50) are frequently prescribed in combination with antibiotics to eradicate *H. pylori* and prevent ulcer recurrence. Bismuth compounds bind to the base of the ulcer, promote mucin and bicarbonate production, and have significant antibacterial effects.

Therapeutic Strategies for Specific Acid-Peptic Disorders

Gastroesophageal Reflux Disease

Although most cases of acid reflux or gastroesophageal regurgitation follow a relatively benign course, these symptoms, often referred to as nonerosive reflux disease, can still be troubling (Boeckxstaens et al., 2014). More severe GERD is erosive esophagitis, characterized by endoscopically visible mucosal damage. This can lead to stricture formation and Barrett metaplasia (replacement of squamous by intestinal columnar epithelium), which is associated with a small but significant risk of adenocarcinoma. The goals of GERD therapy are complete resolution of symptoms and healing of esophagitis (Altan et al., 2012). PPIs clearly are more effective than H_2 receptor antagonists in achieving these goals (see Figure 49–3).

In general, the optimal dose for each patient is determined based on symptom control. Strictures associated with GERD also respond better to PPIs than to H_2 receptor antagonists. One of the complications of GERD, Barrett esophagus, appears to be more refractory to therapy because neither acid suppression nor antireflux surgery has been shown convincingly to produce regression of metaplasia.

Regimens for the treatment of GERD with PPIs and histamine H_2 receptor antagonists are listed in Table 49–2. Although some patients with

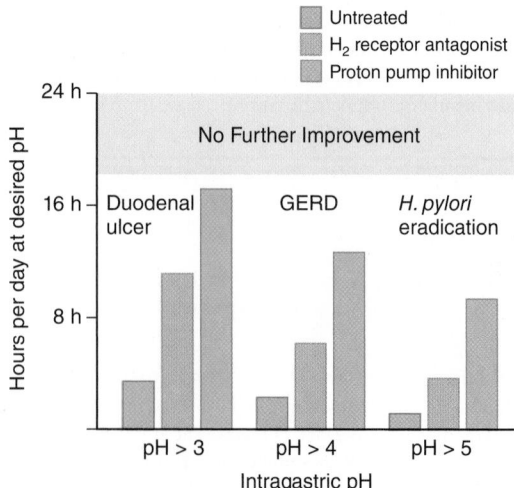

Figure 49–3 *Comparative success of therapy with PPIs and H_2 antagonists.* Data show the effects of a PPI (given once daily) and an H_2 receptor antagonist (given twice daily) in elevating gastric pH to the target ranges (i.e., pH 3 for duodenal ulcer, pH 4 for GERD, and pH 5 for antibiotic eradication of *H. pylori*).

TABLE 49–2 ■ ANTISECRETORY DRUG REGIMENS FOR TREATMENT OF GERD

DRUG	ADULT DOSAGE	PEDIATRIC DOSAGE
H$_2$ receptor antagonists[a]		
Cimetidine	400 mg 4 times daily or 800 mg twice daily for 12 weeks	20–40 mg/kg/d divided every 6 h for 8–12 weeks
Famotidine	20 mg twice daily for up to 12 weeks	0.5 mg/kg/d at bedtime or divided every 12 h (infants < 3 months)[b]
Nizatidine	150 mg twice daily	<12 years: 10 mg/kg/d[c] divided every 12 h >12 years: 150 mg twice daily
Ranitidine	150 mg twice daily	5–10 mg/kg/d divided, every 8–12 h
Proton pump inhibitors		
Esomeprazole magnesium	20–40 mg daily for 4–8 weeks	2.5 – 20 mg daily[d] up to 8 weeks
Esomeprazole sodium	20–40 mg daily (IV)[e]	IV[d,e]: 0.5 mg/kg daily (infants > 1 month). Children: 10 mg daily (<55 kg); 20 mg daily (>55 kg)
Esomeprazole strontium	24.65 or 49.3 mg daily for 4–8 weeks	
Dexlansoprazole	30 mg daily for 4 weeks (nonerosive GERD); erosive GERD: 60 mg daily up to 6 months, then 30 mg daily up to 6 months (maintenance therapy)	Safety/efficacy not established
Lansoprazole	15 mg (nonerosive GERD) or 30 mg (erosive GERD) daily up to 8 weeks	15–30 mg daily[d] for up to 12 weeks
Omeprazole	20 mg daily	5–20 mg daily[d]
Pantoprazole	40 mg daily (erosive GERD)	20–40 mg daily[d] for up to 8 weeks
Rabeprazole	20 mg daily (erosive GERD)	Children 1–11 years old: 5–10 mg daily up to 12 weeks Adolescents: 20 mg daily up to 8 weeks

[a]Not for erosive disease.

[b]For children and adolescents, individualize treatment duration and dose based on clinical response or pH determination (gastric or esophageal) and endoscopy. For infants, employ conservative measures (e.g., thickened feedings) and limit therapy to 8 weeks.

[c]Indicates off-label use.

[d]Varies by weight.

[e]Used when oral PPI cannot be given; short-term use only.

mild GERD symptoms may be managed by nocturnal doses of H$_2$ receptor antagonists, twice-daily dosing usually is required. Antacids are insufficient and are recommended only for the patient with mild, infrequent episodes of acute acid reflux. In general, prokinetic agents (see Chapter 50) are not particularly useful for GERD, either alone or in combination with acid-suppressant medications. There is reasonable evidence that PPIs, and, to a lesser extent, H$_2$ receptor antagonists, are safe and effective for the treatment of GERD in children (Tighe et al., 2014).

Severe Symptoms and Nocturnal Acid Breakthrough

In patients with severe symptoms or extraintestinal manifestations of GERD, twice-daily dosing with a PPI may be needed. However, it is difficult, if not impossible, to render patients achlorhydric, and two-thirds or more of subjects will continue to make acid, particularly at night. This phenomenon, called *nocturnal acid breakthrough*, has been invoked as a cause of refractory symptoms in some patients with GERD. However, decreases in gastric pH at night while on therapy generally are not associated with acid reflux into the esophagus, and the rationale for suppressing nocturnal acid secretion remains to be established. Patients with continuing symptoms on twice-daily PPIs are often treated by adding an H$_2$ receptor antagonist at night. Although this can further suppress acid production, the effect is short lived, probably due to the development of tolerance (Fackler et al., 2002).

Therapy for Extraintestinal Manifestations of GERD

Acid reflux has been implicated in a variety of atypical symptoms, including noncardiac chest pain, asthma, laryngitis, chronic cough, and other ear, nose, and throat conditions. PPIs (at higher doses) have been used with some success in certain patients with these disorders.

GERD and Pregnancy

Acid reflux is estimated to occur in 30%–50% of pregnancies, with an incidence approaching 80% in some populations (Richter, 2003). In the vast majority of cases, GERD ends soon after delivery and thus does not represent an exacerbation of a preexisting condition. Because of its high prevalence and the fact that it can contribute to the nausea of pregnancy, treatment often is required. Treatment choice in this setting is complicated by the paucity of safety data about use during pregnancy for the most commonly used drugs. In general, most drugs used to treat GERD fall in FDA category B, with the exception of *omeprazole* (FDA category C; see Appendix I for information on these categories). Mild cases of GERD during pregnancy should be treated conservatively; antacids or sucralfate are considered the first-line drugs. If symptoms persist, H$_2$ receptor antagonists can be used, with ranitidine having the most established track record in this setting. PPIs are reserved for women with intractable symptoms or complicated reflux disease. In these situations, omeprazole, lansoprazole, and pantoprazole are considered the safest choices (Ali and Egan, 2007).

Pediatric GERD

Reflux disease in infants and children is increasing at an alarming rate (Vandenplas, 2014). Children over 10 years can be diagnosed and treated similarly to adults, but infants and very young children require careful diagnosis to rule out cow's milk allergy or eosinophilic esophagitis. Many nonpharmacologic approaches can be used to alleviate some of the very troubling symptoms of this condition, which may not be due to acid reflux. If acid reduction is indicated, PPIs are more effective than H$_2$ receptor antagonists; however, the therapeutic efficacy of PPIs in newborns and infants is low, and there is an increased risk of adverse effects, including respiratory tract infections and gastroenteritis, which should be carefully considered. It is likely PPIs are overused in the treatment of pediatric GERD.

Peptic Ulcer Disease

Peptic ulcer disease is best viewed as an imbalance between mucosal defense factors (bicarbonate, mucin, PG, NO, and other peptides and growth factors) and injurious factors (acid and pepsin) (Hunt et al., 2015; Wallace, 2008). On average, patients with *duodenal ulcers* produce more acid than do control subjects, particularly at night (basal secretion). Although patients with *gastric ulcers* have normal or even diminished acid production, ulcers rarely, if ever, occur in the complete absence of acid. Presumably, weakened mucosal defense and reduced bicarbonate production contribute to the injury from the relatively lower levels of acid in these patients. *Helicobacter pylori* and exogenous agents such as NSAIDs interact in complex ways to cause an ulcer. Up to 60% of peptic ulcers are associated with *H. pylori* infection of the stomach. This infection may lead to impaired production of somatostatin by D cells and, in time, cause decreased inhibition of gastrin production, resulting in increased acid production and reduced duodenal bicarbonate production. Table 49–3 summarizes current recommendations for drug therapy of gastroduodenal ulcers.

The PPIs relieve symptoms of duodenal ulcers and promote healing more rapidly than do H_2 receptor antagonists, although both classes of drugs are effective in this setting (see Figure 49–3). A peptic ulcer represents a chronic disease, and recurrence within 1 year is expected in the majority of patients who do not receive prophylactic acid suppression. With the appreciation that *H. pylori* plays a major etiopathogenic role in the majority of peptic ulcers, prevention of relapse is focused on eliminating this organism from the stomach. Intravenous *esomeprazole* (80 mg IV over 30 min, followed by 8 mg/h continuous infusion for a total of 72 h, then 40 mg orally or another single daily dose oral PPI, for an appropriate duration; off-label use) and *pantoprazole* (off-label use) are the preferred therapy in patients with acute bleeding ulcers (Laine and Jensen, 2012; Wong and Sung, 2013). The theoretical benefit of maximal acid suppression in this setting is to accelerate healing of the underlying ulcer. In addition, a higher gastric pH enhances clot formation and retards clot dissolution.

The NSAIDs also are frequently associated with peptic ulcers and bleeding. The effects of these drugs are mediated systemically; in the stomach, NSAIDS suppress mucosal PG synthesis (particularly PGE_2 and PGI_2) and thereby reduce mucus production and cytoprotection (see Figure 49–1). Thus, minimizing NSAID use is an important adjunct to gastroduodenal ulcer therapy.

Treatment of *Helicobacter pylori* Infection

Helicobacter pylori, a gram-negative rod, has been associated with gastritis and the subsequent development of gastric and duodenal ulcers, gastric adenocarcinoma, and gastric B-cell lymphoma (Suerbaum and Michetti, 2002). Because of the critical role of *H. pylori* in the pathogenesis of peptic ulcers, eradicating this infection is standard care in patients with gastric or duodenal ulcers (Malfertheiner et al., 2013). Provided that patients are not taking NSAIDs, this strategy almost completely eliminates the risk of ulcer recurrence. Eradication of *H. pylori* also is indicated in the treatment of mucosa-associated lymphoid tissue lymphomas of the stomach, which can regress significantly after such treatment. *Helicobacter pylori* eradication is also indicated for treatment of chronic atrophic gastritis and presence of intestinal metaplasia/dysplasia (with positive *H. pylori* biopsies).

Five important considerations influence the selection of an eradication regimen (Table 49–4) (Chey and Wong, 2007; Malfertheiner et al., 2012):

- Single-antibiotic regimens are ineffective in eradicating *H. pylori* infection and lead to microbial resistance. Combination therapy with two or three antibiotics (plus acid-suppressive therapy) is associated with the highest rate of *H. pylori* eradication.
- A PPI significantly enhances the effectiveness of *H. pylori* antibiotic regimens containing amoxicillin and clarithromycin (see Figure 49–3).
- A regimen of 10–14 days of treatment appears to be better than shorter treatment regimens.
- Poor patient compliance is linked to the medication-related side effects experienced by as many as half of patients taking triple-agent regimens and to the inconvenience of three- or four-drug regimens administered several times per day. Packaging that combines the daily doses into one convenient unit is available and may improve patient compliance.

TABLE 49–3 ■ REGIMENS FOR TREATING GASTRODUODENAL ULCERS IN ADULTS[a]

DRUG	ACTIVE ULCER	MAINTENANCE THERAPY
Proton pump inhibitors[b]		
Esomeprazole magnesium	NSAID risk reduction: 20 or 40 mg daily for up to 6 months	
Esomeprazole strontium	NSAID risk reduction: 24.65 or 49.3 mg daily for up to 6 months	
Lansoprazole	15 mg (DU) daily for 4 weeks	15 mg daily
	15 mg (NSAID risk reduction) daily for up to 12 weeks	
	30 mg (GU including NSAID associated) daily for up to 8 weeks	30 mg daily[c]
Omeprazole	20 mg (DU) daily for 4–8 weeks	20 mg daily[c]
	40 mg (GU) daily for 4–8 weeks	
Pantoprazole	20 mg (NSAID risk reduction) daily[c]	20 mg daily[c]
	40 mg (GU) daily[c]	
Rabeprazole	20 mg (DU for up to 4 weeks; GU[c]) daily	
Prostaglandin analogue		
Misoprostol	200 µg four times daily (NSAID-associated ulcer prevention)[d]	

[a]There is little evidence for the use of H_2 receptor antagonists for the treatment of bleeding ulcers.
[b]Deslansoprazole is not labeled for the treatment of active ulcers.
[c]Off-label use.
[d]Only misoprostol 800 µg/d has been directly shown to reduce the risk of ulcer complications such as perforation, hemorrhage, or obstruction. (Rostom A, Moayyedi P, Hunt R. Canadian Association of Gastroenterology Consensus Group. Canadian consensus guidelines on long-term nonsteroidal anti-inflammatory drug therapy and the need for gastroprotection: benefits versus risks. *Aliment Pharmacol Ther,* **2009**, *29*:481–496.)

TABLE 49–4 ■ THERAPY OF *HELICOBACTER PYLORI* INFECTION

Triple therapy × 10–14 days: PPI + clarithromycin 500 mg + amoxicillin 1 g twice a day (metronidazole 500 mg twice a day can be substituted for amoxicillin)

Quadruple therapy × 10–14 days: PPI + metronidazole 250 mg + bismuth subsalicylate 525 mg + tetracycline 500 mg four times daily

or

Sequential therapy: PPI + amoxicillin 1 g twice a day for 5 days followed by PPI + clarithromycin 500 mg and tinidazole/metronidazole 500 mg twice a day for 5 days;

or

PPI + amoxicillin 1 g twice a day + levofloxacin 250 or 500 mg twice a day for 10 days

PPI *daily dosages*:

Omeprazole: 20 mg twice a day (triple therapy); 40 mg daily (dual therapy)

Lansoprazole: 30 mg twice a day (triple therapy); 30 mg three times daily for 14 days (dual therapy with amoxicillin)

Rabeprazole: 20 mg twice a day for 7 days

Pantoprazole: 40 mg twice a day[a]

Esomeprazole magnesium: 40 mg daily (triple therapy)

Esomeprazole strontium: 49.3 mg daily (triple therapy)

[a]Off-label use.
Data from Chey and Wong, 2007.

- The emergence of resistance to clarithromycin and metronidazole increasingly is recognized as an important factor in the failure to eradicate *H. pylori*. In the presence of in vitro evidence of resistance to metronidazole, amoxicillin should be used instead. In areas with a high frequency of resistance to clarithromycin and metronidazole, a 14-day quadruple-drug regimen (three antibiotics combined with a PPI) generally is effective therapy.

NSAID-Related Ulcers

Chronic NSAID users have a 2%–4% risk of developing a symptomatic ulcer, GI bleeding, or perforation. Ideally, NSAIDs should be discontinued in patients with an ulcer if at all possible. Healing of ulcers despite continued NSAID use is possible with the use of acid-suppressant agents, usually at higher doses and for a considerably longer duration than standard regimens (e.g., ≥ 8 weeks). PPIs are superior to H_2 receptor antagonists and misoprostol in promoting the healing of active ulcers and in preventing recurrence of gastric and duodenal ulcers in the setting of continued NSAID administration (Lanas and Hunt, 2006; Rostom et al., 2009). The FDA has approved fixed-dose combinations of NSAIDS with a PPI or H_2 antagonist; these combinations are intended to lower the risk of ulcers in patients who regularly use NSAIDs for arthritic pain.

Stress-Related Ulcers

Stress ulcers are ulcers of the stomach or duodenum that occur in the context of a profound illness or trauma requiring intensive care (Bardou et al., 2015). The etiology of stress-related ulcers differs somewhat from that of other peptic ulcers, involving acid and mucosal ischemia. Because of limitations on the oral administration of drugs in many patients with stress-related ulcers, intravenous H_2 receptor antagonists have been used extensively to reduce the incidence of GI hemorrhage due to stress ulcers. Now that intravenous preparations of PPIs are available, they are appropriate to consider. *However, there is some concern over the risk of pneumonia secondary to gastric colonization by bacteria in an alkaline milieu.* In this setting, sucralfate appears to provide reasonable prophylaxis against bleeding without increasing the risk of aspiration pneumonia.

Zollinger-Ellison Syndrome

Patients with Zollinger-Ellison syndrome develop pancreatic or duodenal gastrinomas that stimulate the secretion of very large amounts of acid, sometimes in the setting of multiple endocrine neoplasia, type I (Krampitz and Norton, 2013). This can lead to severe gastroduodenal ulceration and other consequences of uncontrolled hyperchlorhydria. PPIs are the drugs of choice, usually given at about twice the routine dosage for peptic ulcers (omeprazole 60 mg daily, esomeprazole 80 mg daily, lansoprazole 60 mg daily, rabeprazole 60 mg daily, or pantoprazole 120 mg daily); some patients need two to three times these doses to control acid secretion. However, once control of acid secretion has been achieved, dose reduction is usually possible. PPIs are well tolerated and safe even at very high doses. If PPIs are unable to control gastric acid secretion, the long-acting somatostatin analogue *octreotide* (off-label indication) can be given to inhibit secretion of gastrin. This is not a first-line agent due to unpredictable response rates and the side effects of the treatment.

Functional Dyspepsia

The term *functional dyspepsia* refers to ulcer-like symptoms in patients who lack overt gastroduodenal ulceration (Tack and Talley, 2013). Functional dyspepsia can be subdivided into postprandial distress syndrome and epigastric pain syndrome, based on the presence of symptoms related to meals. It is defined as the presence of one or more of the following: postprandial fullness, early satiation, epigastric pain or burning, and no evidence of structural disease. It may be associated with gastritis (with or without *H. pylori*) or with NSAID use, but the pathogenesis of this syndrome remains controversial.

The PPIs appear to be moderately effective in the treatment of patients with functional dyspepsia (Vanheel and Tack, 2014). In general, twice-daily PPIs are no better than once-daily PPIs. The dosing is as for GERD (Table 49–2). H_2 receptor antagonists are only marginally effective for the treatment of functional dyspepsia. Because central mechanisms may contribute to functional dyspepsia either through visceral hypersensitivity or other mechanisms, tricyclic antidepressants such as amitriptyline or desipramine (10 to 25 mg at night) (see Chapter 15) can be considered in patients with functional dyspepsia whose symptoms persist despite PPI therapy for 8 weeks. Prokinetic agents such as metoclopramide (see Chapter 50) are not considered for functional dyspepsia because of their side-effect profile. The novel gastroprokinetic agent *acotiamide* is being investigated for use in postprandial distress syndrome, and $5HT_{1A}$ serotonin receptor agonists that relax the fundus (see Chapter 13) are being tested in patients with postprandial distress syndrome with early satiation. Antacids are not generally helpful for the treatment of functional dyspepsia.

Functional Esophageal Disorders

Functional esophageal disorders are disorders that cause esophageal symptoms and that are diagnosed on the basis of negative results on standard esophageal tests, thereby excluding structural disorders, motility disorders like achalasia, and GERD (Amarasinghe and Sifrim, 2014). There are four of these fairly common disorders: (1) functional heartburn, (2) functional chest pain, (3) functional dysphagia, and (4) globus. PPI therapy (off-label use) as outlined previously is routinely used for the initial treatment of functional heartburn, functional chest pain, and globus. As in functional dyspepsia, central mechanisms contribute to these disorders and similar approaches follow for the treatment of functional heartburn and functional chest pain if PPI therapy is ineffective, including the use of tricyclic antidepressants or selective serotonin reuptake inhibitors. For the treatment of globus, gabapentin or pregabalin is used.

Acknowledgment: *Laurence L. Brunton, Willemijntje A. Hoogerwerf, Pankaj Jay Pasricha, and John L. Wallace contributed to this chapter in earlier editions of this book. We have retained some of their text in the current edition.*

Drug Facts for Your Personal Formulary: *Antisecretory Agents and Gastroprotectives*

Drugs	Therapeutic Uses	Clinical Pharmacology and Tips
Proton Pump Inhibitors		
Dexlansoprazole	• Gastroesophageal reflux disease • Erosive esophagitis	• Generally well tolerated • Possible interaction with clopidogrel (controversial) • Increased incidence of osteoporosis-related fractures of hip, wrist, or spine • Diarrhea • Interstitial nephritis • May cause cyanocobalamin (vitamin B_{12}) deficiency with daily long-term use (>3 years)
Esomeprazole Lansoprazole Omeprazole Pantoprazole	• Gastric ulcers • Duodenal ulcers • Erosive esophagitis • Gastroesophageal reflux disease • *Helicobacter pylori* eradication • Zollinger-Ellison syndrome	• OTC forms for acid reflux • Generally well tolerated • Possible interaction with clopidogrel (controversial) • Increased incidence of osteoporosis-associated fractures of hip, wrist, or spine • Diarrhea • Interstitial nephritis • May cause cyanocobalamin (vitamin B_{12}) deficiency with daily long-term use (>3 years) • Interactions with diagnostic investigations for neuroendocrine tumors
Rabeprazole	• Gastroesophageal reflux disease • *Helicobacter pylori* eradication • Zollinger-Ellison syndrome	• Generally well tolerated • Possible interaction with clopidogrel (controversial) • Increased incidence of osteoporosis-associated bone fractures of hip, wrist, or spine • Diarrhea • Interstitial nephritis
Histamine 2 Receptor Antagonists		
Cimetidine Famotidine Nizatidine Ranitidine	• Gastric ulcer (to promote healing) • Duodenal ulcer (to promote healing) • Gastroesophageal reflux disease	• No longer recommend for treating active ulcers • Generally well tolerated
Mucosal Defensive Agents		
Misoprostol	• Ulcer prophylaxis	• Rarely used because of side effects • Cannot be used in women of childbearing potential • Diarrhea • Marketed in combination with diclofenac
Sucralfate	• Ulcer prophylaxis	• Generally well tolerated • Constipation
Antacids	• Acid reflux • Esophagitis	• OTC; generally well tolerated • Na^+ and AL^{+3} loads: potential problems in CV and renal disease

Bibliography

Ali RA, Egan LJ. Gastroesophageal reflux disease in pregnancy. *Best Prac Res Clin Gastroenterol*, 2007, 21:793–806.

Altan E, Blondeau K, Pauwels A, Farré R, Tack J. Evolving pharmacological approaches in gastroesophageal reflux disease. *Expert Opin Emerg Drugs*, 2012, 17:347–359.

Amarasinghe G, Sifrim D. Functional esophageal disorders: pharmacological options. *Drugs*, 2014, 74:1335–1344.

Bardou M, Quenot JP, Barkun A. Stress-related mucosal disease in the critically ill patient. *Nat Rev Gastroenterol Hepatol*, 2015, 12:98–107.

Black J. Reflections on the analytical pharmacology of histamine H_2-receptor antagonists. *Gastroenterology*, 1993, 105:963–968.

Boeckxstaens G, El-Serag HB, Smout AJ, Kahrilas PJ. Symptomatic reflux disease: the present, the past and the future. *Gut*, 2014, 63:185–1193.

Camilleri M. The role of pharmacogenetics in nonmalignant gastrointestinal diseases. *Nat Rev Gastroenterol Hepatol*, 2012, 9:173–184.

Chen J, Yuan YC, Leontiadis GI, Howden CW. Recent safety concerns with proton pump inhibitors. *J Clin Gastroenterol*, 2012, 46:93–114.

Chey WD, Wong BCY. American College of Gastroenterology guideline on the management of *Helicobacter pylori* infection. *Am J Gastroenterol*, 2007, 102:1808–1825.

Fackler WK, Ours TM, Vaezi MF, Richter JE. Long-term effect of H2RA therapy on nocturnal gastric acid breakthrough. *Gastroenterology*, 2002, 122:625–632.

Freedberg DE, et al. The risks and benefits of long-term use of proton pump inhibitors: expert review and best practice advice from the American Gastroenterological Association. *Gastroenterology*, 2017, 152:706–715.

Huang B, Huang Y, Li Y, et al. Adverse cardiovascular effects of concomitant use of proton pump inhibitors and clopidogrel in patients with coronary artery disease: a systematic review and meta-analysis. *Arch Med Res*, 2012, 43:212–224.

Hunt RH, Camilleri M, Crowe SE, et al. The stomach in health and disease. *Gut*, 2015, 64:1650–1668. doi:10.1136/gutjnl-2014-307595.

Krampitz GW, Norton JA. Current management of the Zollinger-Ellison syndrome. *Adv Surg*, 2013, 47:59–79.

Laine L, Jensen DM. Management of patients with ulcer bleeding. *Am J Gastroenterol*, 2012, 107:345–360.

Lanas A, Hunt RH. Prevention of anti-inflammatory drug-induced gastrointestinal damage: benefits and risks of therapeutic strategies. *Ann Med*, 2006, 38:415–428.

Malfertheiner P, Megraud F, O'Morain CA, et al., European *Helicobacter* study group. Management of *Helicobacter pylori* infection—the Maastricht IV/Florence consensus report. *Gut*, 2012, 61:646–664.

CHAPTER 49 — PHARMACOTHERAPY FOR GASTRIC ACIDITY, PEPTIC ULCERS, AND GERD

Malfertheiner P, Venerito M, Selgrad M. *Helicobacter pylori* infection: selected aspects in clinical management. *Curr Opin Gastroenterol*, **2013**, 29:669–675.

Marks IN. Sucralfate-safety and side effects. *Scand J Gastroenterol Suppl*, **1991**, 185:36–42.

Reimer C. Safety of long-term PPI therapy. *Best Prac Res Clin Gastroenterol*, **2013**, 27:443–454.

Richter JE. Gastroesophageal reflux disease during pregnancy. *Gastroenterol Clin North Am*, **2003**, 32:235–261.

Rostom A, Moayyedi P, Hunt R. Canadian Association of Gastroenterology Consensus Group. Canadian consensus guidelines on long-term nonsteroidal anti-inflammatory drug therapy and the need for gastroprotection: benefits versus risks. *Aliment Pharmacol Ther*, **2009**, 29:481–496.

Sabesin SM. Safety issues relating to long-term treatment with histamine H_2-receptor antagonists. *Aliment Pharmacol Ther*, **1993**, 7(suppl 2): 35–40.

Sandevik AK, Brenna E, Waldum HL. Review article: the pharmacological inhibition of gastric acid secretion-tolerance and rebound. *Aliment Pharmacol Ther*, **1997**, 11:1013–1018.

Shin JM, Munson K, Vagin O, Sachs G. The gastric HK-ATPase: structure, function, and inhibition. *Pflugers Arch Eur J Physiol*, **2009**, 457:609–622.

Shin JM, Sachs G. Pharmacology of proton pump inhibitors. *Curr Gastroenterol Rep*, **2008**, 10:528–534.

Song H, Zhu J, Lu D. Long-term proton pump inhibitor (PPI) use and the development of gastric pre-malignant lesions. *Cochrane Database Syst Rev*, **2014**, (12):CD010623. doi:10.1002/14651858.CD010623.pub2.

Suerbaum S, Michetti P. *Helicobacter pylori* infection. *N Engl J Med*, **2002**, 347:1175–1186.

Szabo S. "Gastric cytoprotection" is still relevant. *J Gastroenterol Hepatol*, **2014**, 29(suppl 4):124–132.

Tack J, Talley NJ. Functional dyspepsia—symptoms, definitions and validity of the Rome III criteria. *Nat Rev Gastroenterol Hepatol*, **2013**, 10:134–141.

Tighe M, Afzal NA, Bevan A, Hayen A, Munro A, Beattie RM. Pharmacological treatment of children with gastro-oesophageal reflux. *Cochrane Database Syst Rev*, **2014**, (11):CD008550. doi:10.1002/14651858.CD008550.pub2.

Vandenplas Y. Management of pediatric GERD. *Nat Rev Gastroenterol Hepatol*, **2014**, 11:147–157.

Vanheel H, Tack, J. Therapeutic options for functional dyspepsia. *Dig Dis*, **2014**, 32:230–234.

Wallace JL. Prostaglandins, NSAIDs and mucosal defence. Why doesn't the stomach digest itself? *Physiol Rev*, **2008**, 88:1547–1565.

Wolfe MM, Sachs G. Acid suppression: optimizing therapy for gastroduodenal ulcer healing, gastroesophageal reflux disease, and stress-related erosive syndrome. *Gastroenterology*, **2000**, 118:S9–S31.

Wong SH, Sung JJY. Management of GI emergencies: peptic ulcer acute bleeding. *Best Prac Res Clin Gastroenterol*, **2013**, 27:639–647.

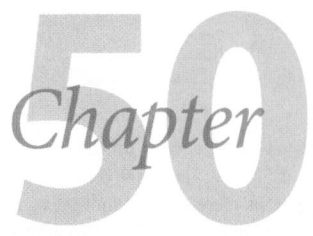

Chapter 50

Gastrointestinal Motility and Water Flux, Emesis, and Biliary and Pancreatic Disease

Keith A. Sharkey and Wallace K. MacNaughton

Gastrointestinal Motility

The GI tract is in a continuous contractile, absorptive, and secretory state. The control of this state is complex, with contributions by the muscle and epithelium, the enteric nervous system (ENS), the autonomic nervous system (ANS), and local and circulating hormones. Of these, perhaps the most important regulator of physiological gut function is the ENS (Figure 50–1) (Furness, 2006; Furness, 2012; Grundy et al., 2006).

The ENS is an extensive collection of nerves and glial cells that constitutes the third division of the ANS. It is the only part of the ANS truly capable of autonomous function if separated from the CNS. The ENS lies within the wall of the GI tract and is organized into two connected networks of neurons, nerve fibers, and glial cells: the *myenteric (Auerbach) plexus*, found between the circular and longitudinal muscle layers, and the *submucosal (Meissner) plexus*, located in the submucosa (Furness, 2012; Sharkey, 2015). The former is largely responsible for motor control, whereas the latter regulates secretion, fluid transport, and blood flow.

To prevent the unwanted translocation of toxins, antigen commensal bacteria, and other potentially pathogenic components of the luminal contents, an elaborate "intestinal barrier" has developed. This consists of a physical barrier, an immune barrier, and a secretory barrier, which includes the secretion of antimicrobial peptides, mucus, and fluid. The secretory and immune components of the intestinal barrier are regulated by ENS and ANS neural mechanisms that integrate the control of these components of barrier function with digestive processes in the gut (Mayer et al., 2014; Sharkey and Savidge, 2014).

Generation and Regulation of GI Motor Activity

The ENS is responsible for the largely autonomous nature of most GI activity. This activity is organized into relatively distinct programs that respond to input from the local environment of the gut, as well as the ANS-CNS. Each program consists of a series of complex, but coordinated, patterns of secretion and movement that show regional and temporal variation (Deloose et al., 2012). The *fasting program* of motor activity in the gut is called the MMC (*migrating myoelectric complex* when referring to electrical activity and *migrating motor complex* when referring to the accompanying contractions) and consists of a series of four phasic activities: I, quiescence; II, increasing frequencies of action potentials and smooth muscle contractions; III, peak contractile activity; and IV, declining activity toward a renewal of phase I. Phase II of the MMC is associated with the release of the peptide hormone *motilin*. Motilin agonists stimulate motility in the proximal gut. The most characteristic, phase III, consists of clusters of rhythmic contractions that occupy short segments of the intestine for a period of 6–10 min before proceeding caudally (toward the anus). One MMC cycle (i.e., all four phases) takes about 80–110 min. The MMC occurs in the fasting state, helping to sweep debris caudad in the gut and limiting the overgrowth of commensal luminal bacteria. The MMC is interrupted by the fed program in intermittently feeding animals such as humans. The *fed program* consists of high-frequency (12–15/min) contractions that either are propagated for short segments (*propulsive*) or are irregular and not propagated (*mixing*).

Peristalsis is a series of reflex responses to a bolus in the lumen of a given segment of the intestine; the *ascending excitatory reflex* results in contraction of the circular muscle on the oral side of the bolus, whereas the *descending inhibitory reflex* results in relaxation on the anal side. The net pressure gradient moves the bolus caudad. Motor neurons receive input from ascending and descending interneurons (which constitute the relay and programming systems), which are of two broad types, *excitatory* and *inhibitory*. The primary neurotransmitter of the *excitatory motor neurons* is ACh. The principal neurotransmitter in the *inhibitory motor neurons* is NO, although important contributions may also be made by ATP, VIP, and PACAP. Enterochromaffin cells, the major population of enteroendocrine cells, scattered throughout the epithelium of the intestine, release serotonin (5HT) to initiate many gut reflexes by acting locally on enteric neurons (Gershon and Tack, 2007). Excessive release of 5HT in the gut

Abbreviations

ACh: acetylcholine
ANS: autonomic nervous system
AQP: aquaporin
CA: carbonic anhydrase
CCK: cholecystokinin
CFTR: cystic fibrosis transmembrane conductance regulator
CTZ: chemoreceptor trigger zone
CYP: cytochrome P450
DOR: delta opioid receptor
DRA: downregulated in adenoma
ECG: electrocardiogram
ENaC: epithelial sodium channel
ENS: enteric nervous system
FDA: U.S. Food and Drug Administration
GC: guanyl cyclase
GERD: gastroesophageal reflux disease
GI: gastrointestinal
GLP: glucagon-like peptide
GPCR: G protein–coupled receptor
HERG: human ether-a-go-go related gene
HIV: human immunodeficiency virus
5HT: serotonin, 5-hydroxytryptamine
IBS: irritable bowel syndrome
KOR: kappa opioid receptor
MOR: mu opioid receptor
NEP: neutral endopeptidase
NHE: Na^+-H^+ exchanger
NK: neurokinin
NO: nitric oxide
NSAID: nonsteroidal anti-inflammatory drug
OTC: over the counter
PACAP: pituitary adenylyl cyclase–activating peptide
PAF: platelet-activating factor
PEG: polyethylene glycol
QT: ECG interval
SERT: serotonin transporter
SGLT: sodium-glucose cotransporter
SLC: solute carrier transporter
SSRI: selective serotonin reuptake inhibitor
SST: somatostatin
STN: solitary tract nucleus
TJ: tight junction
TMEM: transmembrane protein
USP: U.S. Pharmacopeia
VIP: vasoactive intestinal peptide

wall (e.g., by chemotherapeutic agents) leads to vomiting by actions of 5HT on vagal nerve endings in the proximal small intestine. Compounds targeting the 5HT system are important modulators of motility, secretion, and emesis.

Other cell types are also important in the regulation of GI motility, including interstitial cells of Cajal and various enteroendocrine cell populations. Interstitial cells of Cajal, which are distributed in networks within the gut wall, are responsible for setting the electrical rhythm and the pace of contractions in various regions of the gut (Huizinga and Chen, 2014). These cells also modulate excitatory and inhibitory neuronal communication to the smooth muscle. Enteroendocrine cell populations release locally acting hormones, such as *ghrelin*, *CCK*, *motilin*, and *GLP-1*, all of which can influence GI motility, before (e.g., ghrelin) or after meals (e.g., CCK and GLP-1) (Psichas et al., 2015).

Excitation Contraction Coupling in GI Smooth Muscle

Control of tension in GI smooth muscle is dependent on the intracellular Ca^{2+} concentration (Sanders et al., 2012). There are basically two types of excitation-contraction coupling in these cells. *Ionotropic receptors* can mediate changes in membrane potential, which in turn activate voltage-gated Ca^{2+} channels to trigger an influx of Ca^{2+} (electromechanical coupling); *metabotropic receptors* activate various signal transduction pathways to release Ca^{2+} from intracellular stores (pharmacomechanical coupling). Inhibitory receptors act via PKA and PKG and lead to hyperpolarization, decreased cytosolic $[Ca^{2+}]$, and reduced interaction of actin and myosin. As an example, NO may induce relaxation via activation of the guanylyl cyclase–cyclic GMP pathway and cause the opening of several types of K^+ channels.

Functional and Motility Disorders of the Bowel

Gastrointestinal motility disorders are a heterogeneous group of conditions (Drossman, 2006; Faure et al., 2012). Common motility disorders include achalasia of the esophagus (impaired relaxation of the lower esophageal sphincter associated with defective esophageal peristalsis that results in dysphagia and regurgitation), gastroparesis (delayed gastric emptying), GERD (chronic reflux of gastric contents into the esophagus due to an increased frequency of transient lower esophageal sphincter relaxations, ineffective esophageal peristalsis, or gastric dysmotility); intestinal pseudoobstruction (myopathic and neuropathic forms of intestinal dysmotility); constipation; Hirschsprung disease; anorectal dysfunction; and others. These disorders can be congenital, idiopathic, or secondary to systemic diseases (e.g., diabetes mellitus or scleroderma). Motility disorders also traditionally include the functional GI conditions, such as IBS, functional dyspepsia, and noncardiac chest pain. These are brain-gut disorders that are characterized by the presence of increased pain from the gut associated with GI motor abnormalities and other symptoms. For most of these disorders, treatment remains empirical and symptom based, reflecting limited understanding of the pathophysiology involved in most cases.

Prokinetic Agents and Other Stimulants of GI Motility

Prokinetic agents are medications that enhance coordinated GI motility and transit of material in the GI tract (Acosta and Camilleri, 2015; Altan et al., 2012; Corsetti and Tack, 2014; Tack and Zaninotto, 2015). These agents appear to enhance the release of excitatory neurotransmitter at the nerve-muscle junction without interfering with the normal physiological pattern and rhythm of motility. By contrast, activation of muscarinic receptors with the older cholinomimetic agents (see Chapter 9) or acetylcholinesterase inhibitors (see Chapter 10) enhances contractions in a relatively uncoordinated fashion that produces little or no net propulsive motor activity.

Dopamine Receptor Antagonists

Dopamine is present in significant amounts in the GI tract and has several inhibitory effects on motility, including reduction of lower esophageal sphincter and intragastric pressures. These effects, which result from suppression of ACh release from myenteric motor neurons, are mediated by D_2 dopaminergic receptors. Dopamine receptor antagonists are effective as prokinetic agents; they have the additional advantage of relieving nausea and vomiting by antagonism of dopamine receptors in the CTZ of the brainstem. Examples are *metoclopramide* and *domperidone* (Acosta and Camilleri, 2015; Reddymasu et al., 2007).

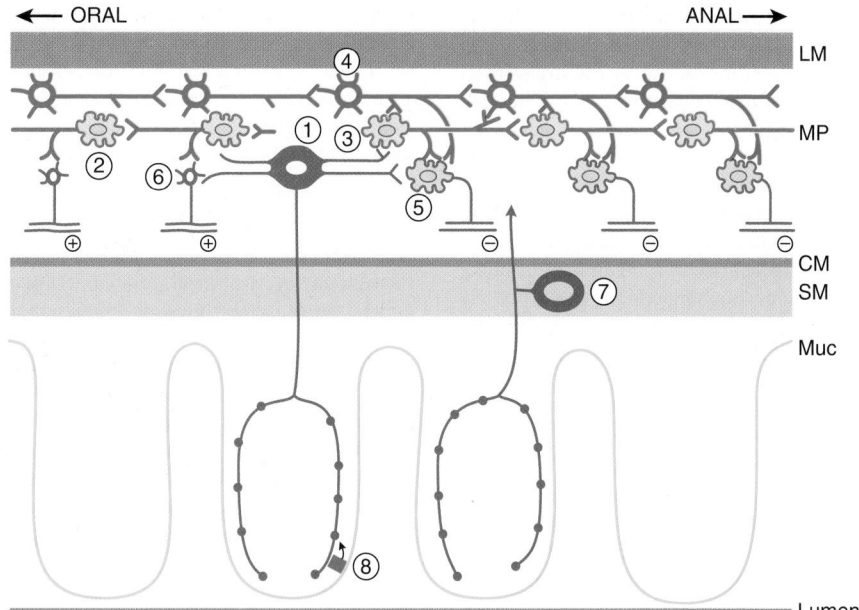

Figure 50–1 *The neuronal network that initiates and generates the peristaltic response.* Mucosal stimulation leads to release of serotonin by enterochromaffin cells (8), which excites the intrinsic primary afferent neurons (1), which then communicate with ascending (2) and descending (3) interneurons in the local reflex pathways. The reflex results in contraction at the oral end via the excitatory motor neuron (6) and aboral relaxation via the inhibitory motor neuron (5). The migratory myoelectric complex (see text) is shown here as being conducted by a different chain of interneurons (4). Another intrinsic primary afferent neuron with its cell body in the submucosa also is shown (7). MP, myenteric plexus; CM, circular muscle; LM, longitudinal muscle; SM, submucosa; Muc, mucosa. (Adapted with permission from Kunze WA, Furness JB. The enteric nervous system and regulation of intestinal motility. *Annu Rev Physiol*, **1999**, *61*:117–142. Permission conveyed via Copyright Clearance Center, Inc.)

Metoclopramide

METOCLOPRAMIDE

Mechanism of Action and Pharmacology. *Metoclopramide* and other substituted benzamides are derivatives of *para*-aminobenzoic acid and are structurally related to procainamide. The mechanisms of action of *metoclopramide* are complex and involve $5HT_4$ receptor agonism, vagal and central $5HT_3$ antagonism, and possible sensitization of muscarinic receptors on smooth muscle, in addition to dopamine receptor antagonism. Administration of *metoclopramide* results in coordinated contractions that enhance transit. Its effects are confined largely to the upper digestive tract, where it increases lower esophageal sphincter tone and stimulates antral and small intestinal contractions. *Metoclopramide* has no clinically significant effects on large-bowel motility (Acosta and Camilleri, 2015).

ADME. *Metoclopramide* is absorbed rapidly after oral ingestion, undergoes sulfation and glucuronide conjugation by the liver, and is excreted principally in the urine, with a $t_{1/2}$ of 4–6 h. Peak concentrations occur within 1 h after a single oral dose; the duration of action is 1–2 h.

Therapeutic Uses and Adverse Effects. *Metoclopramide* is indicated in patients with gastroparesis, in whom the drug may cause moderate improvements of gastric emptying. *Metoclopramide* injection is used as an adjunctive measure in medical or diagnostic procedures such as upper endoscopy or contrast radiography of the GI tract (single IV dose of 10 mg). Its greatest utility lies in its ability to ameliorate the nausea and vomiting that often accompany GI dysmotility syndromes. *Metoclopramide* is available in oral dosage forms (tablets and solution) and as a parenteral preparation for intravenous or intramuscular administration. The initial regimen is 10 mg orally, 30 min before each meal and at bedtime. The onset of action is within 30–60 min. In patients with severe nausea, an initial dose of 10 mg can be given intramuscularly (onset of action 10–15 min) or intravenously (onset of action 1–3 min). For prevention of chemotherapy-induced emesis, *metoclopramide* can be given as an infusion of 1–2 mg/kg administered over at least 15 min, beginning 30 min before the chemotherapy is begun and repeated as needed every 2 h for two doses, then every 3 h for three doses. Because of adverse effects related to drug exposure, the recommended duration of use is less than 12 weeks. *Metoclopramide* has a very limited use for the treatment of GERD in children because of significant safety concerns (see discussion that follows) and limited efficacy.

The major side effects of *metoclopramide* include extrapyramidal effects. Dystonias, usually occurring acutely after intravenous administration, and Parkinsonian-like symptoms that may occur several weeks after initiation of therapy generally respond to treatment with anticholinergic or antihistaminic drugs and reverse on discontinuation of *metoclopramide*. Tardive dyskinesia also can occur with chronic treatment and may be irreversible. Extrapyramidal effects appear to occur more commonly in children and young adults and at higher doses. *Metoclopramide* also can cause galactorrhea by blocking the inhibitory effect of dopamine on prolactin release (seen infrequently in clinical practice). Methemoglobinemia has been reported occasionally in premature and full-term neonates receiving metoclopramide.

Domperidone

Mechanism of Action and Pharmacology. In contrast to *metoclopramide*, *domperidone* predominantly antagonizes the D_2 receptor without major involvement of other receptors, but otherwise its mechanism of action is similar (Reddymasu et al., 2007).

ADME. *Domperidone* is rapidly absorbed, yielding peak concentrations in 30 min. The drug undergoes metabolism via hepatic CYP3A4, N-dealkylation, and hydroxylation; it has a $t_{1/2}$ of 7 h. It is excreted in the feces (~two-thirds) and urine (~one-third).

Therapeutic Uses and Adverse Effects. *Domperidone* is available for use in the U.S. only through an expanded access to investigational drugs with the FDA, but it is readily available in many other countries. It has modest prokinetic activity in doses of 10 mg three times a day. Although it does not readily cross the blood-brain barrier to cause extrapyramidal side effects, *domperidone* exerts effects in the parts of the CNS that lack this barrier, such as those regulating emesis, temperature, and prolactin release. *Domperidone* does not appear to have any significant effects on lower GI motility. Like metoclopramide, it has limited efficacy in children. There is an increased risk of serious ventricular arrhythmias, including sudden cardiac death, in association with domperidone use, especially in older persons (>60 years) and at doses above 30 mg/d. Like metoclopramide, it can also elevate prolactin levels, presenting as galactorrhea, gynecomastia, amenorrhea, or impotence.

Serotonin Receptor Agonists

Serotonin (5HT) plays an important role in the normal motor and secretory function of the gut (see Chapter 13) (Gershon and Tack, 2007). Indeed, more than 90% of the total 5HT in the body exists in the GI tract. The enterochromaffin cell produces most of this 5HT and rapidly releases it in response to chemical and mechanical stimulation (e.g., food boluses; chemotherapeutic agents such as cisplatin; certain microbial toxins; adrenergic, cholinergic, and purinergic receptor agonists). 5HT triggers the *peristaltic reflex* (see Figure 50–1) by stimulating intrinsic sensory neurons in the myenteric plexus (via $5HT_{1p}$ and $5HT_4$ receptors), as well as extrinsic vagal and spinal sensory neurons (via $5HT_3$ receptors). In addition, stimulation of submucosal intrinsic afferent neurons activates secretomotor reflexes, resulting in epithelial secretion.

The 5HT receptors occur on other neurons in the ENS, where they can be either stimulatory ($5HT_3$ and $5HT_4$) or inhibitory ($5HT_{1A}$). In addition, serotonin stimulates the release of other neurotransmitters. Thus, $5HT_1$ stimulation of the gastric fundus results in release of NO and reduction in smooth muscle tone. $5HT_4$ stimulation of excitatory motor neurons enhances ACh release at the neuromuscular junction, and both $5HT_3$ and $5HT_4$ receptors facilitate interneuronal signaling. Developmentally, 5HT acts as a *neurotrophic factor* for enteric neurons via the $5HT_{2B}$ and $5HT_4$ receptors. Reuptake of serotonin by enteric neurons and epithelium is mediated by the same transporter (SERT) as 5HT reuptake by serotonergic neurons in the CNS. This reuptake also is blocked by SSRIs (see Figure 15–1), which explains the common side effect of diarrhea that accompanies the use of these agents (Gershon, 2013).

Modulation of the multiple, complex, and sometimes-opposing effects of 5HT on gut motor function has become a major target for drug development. The availability of serotonergic prokinetic drugs has in recent years been restricted because of serious adverse cardiac events (Tack et al., 2012). In the U.S., *tegaserod* is only available as an emergency investigational new drug, and *cisapride* is available only via a limited-access protocol. A novel $5HT_4$ agonist, *prucalopride*, is approved in Europe and Canada for symptomatic treatment of chronic constipation in women in whom laxatives fail to provide adequate relief.

Cisapride

Mechanism of Action and Pharmacology. *Cisapride* is a $5HT_4$ agonist that stimulates adenylyl cyclase activity in neurons. It also has weak $5HT_3$ antagonistic properties and may directly stimulate smooth muscle.

Cisapride was a commonly used prokinetic agent; however, it no longer is generally available in the U.S. because of its potential to induce serious and occasionally fatal cardiac arrhythmias, including ventricular tachycardia, ventricular fibrillation, and torsades de pointes. These arrhythmias result from a prolonged QT interval through an interaction with pore-forming subunits of the *HERG* K^+ channel (see Chapter 30).

ADME. *Cisapride* is metabolized in the liver by CYP3A4 (see Chapter 6). It has an onset of action of 30–60 min and a $t_{1/2}$ of 6–12 h.

Therapeutic Uses and Adverse Effects. *Cisapride* is available only through an investigational, limited-access program for patients with GERD, gastroparesis, intestinal pseudoobstruction, refractory severe chronic constipation, and neonatal enteral feeding intolerance who have failed all standard therapeutic modalities and who have undergone a thorough diagnostic evaluation, including an ECG. It has modest prokinetic activity in doses of 5–10 mg four times a day before meals. *Cisapride* is contraindicated in patients with a history of prolonged QT interval, renal failure, ventricular arrhythmias, ischemic heart disease, congestive heart failure, respiratory failure, uncorrected electrolyte abnormalities, or concomitant medications known to prolong the QT interval.

Prucalopride

Mechanism of Action and Pharmacology. *Prucalopride* is a specific $5HT_4$ receptor agonist (Figure 50–2) that facilitates cholinergic neurotransmission. It acts throughout the length of the intestine, increasing oral-cecal transit and colonic transit without affecting gastric emptying in healthy volunteers.

ADME. *Prucalopride* has a time to peak action of 2–3 h and a $t_{1/2}$ of 24 h. It is primarily excreted in the urine as the unchanged drug.

Therapeutic Uses and Adverse Effects. Given in doses of 1–4 mg orally, once daily, the drug improved bowel habits; significantly increased the number of spontaneous, complete bowel movements; reduced the severity of symptoms; and improved quality of life in patients with severe chronic constipation. *Prucalopride* is approved or use in women with chronic constipation in whom laxatives fail to provide adequate relief. Nausea, diarrhea, abdominal pain, and headaches are common adverse effects. Cardiovascular risks do not seem to be elevated, but patients should be monitored (Diederen et al., 2015).

Motilin and Macrolide Antibiotics

Mechanism of Action and Pharmacology

Motilin, a 22–amino acid peptide hormone secreted by enteroendocrine M cells and by some enterochromaffin cells of the upper small bowel, is a potent contractile agent of the upper GI tract. Motilin levels fluctuate in association with the MMC and appear to be responsible for the amplification, if not the actual induction, of phase III activity. In addition, motilin receptors are GPCRs found on smooth muscle cells and enteric neurons.

The effects of motilin can be mimicked by *erythromycin*, a property shared to varying extents by other macrolide antibiotics (e.g., *azithromycin*, *clarithromycin*, etc.; see Chapter 59). In addition to its motilin-like effects, which are most pronounced at higher doses (250–500 mg), erythromycin at lower doses (e.g., 40–80 mg) also may act by other poorly defined mechanisms that may involve cholinergic facilitation. Erythromycin has multiple effects on upper GI motility, increasing lower esophageal pressure

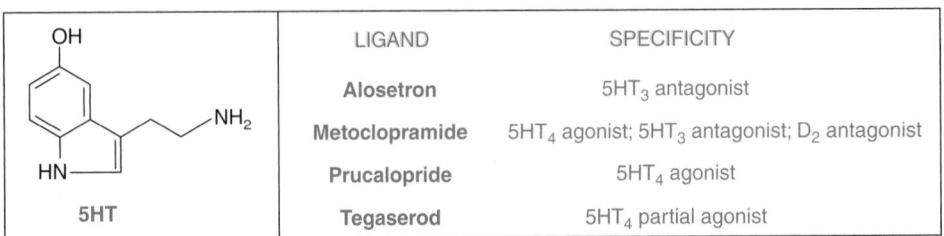

LIGAND	SPECIFICITY
Alosetron	$5HT_3$ antagonist
Metoclopramide	$5HT_4$ agonist; $5HT_3$ antagonist; D_2 antagonist
Prucalopride	$5HT_4$ agonist
Tegaserod	$5HT_4$ partial agonist

Figure 50–2 *Serotonergic agents modulating GI motility.*

and stimulating gastric and small-bowel contractility. By contrast, it has little or no effect on colonic motility. At doses higher than 3 mg/kg, it can produce a spastic type of contraction in the small bowel, resulting in cramps, impairment of transit, and vomiting.

ADME

Erythromycin is metabolized by demethylation in the liver by CYP3A4. The time to peak action is about 0.5–2.5 h (ethylsuccinate), and it has a $t_{1/2}$ of 2 h. It is primarily excreted in the feces.

Therapeutic Uses and Adverse Effects

Erythromycin is used as a prokinetic agent in patients with diabetic gastroparesis, where it can improve gastric emptying in the short term. *Erythromycin*-stimulated gastric contractions can be intense and result in "dumping" of relatively undigested food into the small bowel. This potential disadvantage can be exploited clinically to clear the stomach of undigestible residue such as bezoars. Rapid development of tolerance (~28 days) to *erythromycin*, possibly by downregulation of the motilin receptor, and antibiotic effects (undesirable in this context) limit the use of this drug as a prokinetic agent. A standard dose of *erythromycin* for gastric stimulation is 1.5–3 mg/kg intravenous infusion every 6 h in a hospital setting or 125 mg orally every 12 h (Acosta and Camilleri, 2015). For small-bowel stimulation, a smaller dose (e.g., 3 mg/kg IV every 8 h) may be more useful; higher doses may actually retard the motility. Tachyphylaxis to erythromycin and potential side effects limit its use in the management of gastroparesis. Concerns about GI toxicity, ototoxicity, pseudomembranous colitis, and the induction of resistant strains of bacteria, QT prolongation, and sudden death, particularly when used in patients taking medications that inhibit CYP3A4, limit the use of *erythromycin* to acute situations or in circumstances where patients are resistant to other medications.

Other macrolides (e.g., *azithromycin* and *clarithromycin*) accelerate gastric emptying, but because there are no clinical trials compared to other medications or placebo indicating any benefit, their additional cost, potential for risk, and antibiotic resistance would preclude consideration for their use in motility disorders.

Miscellaneous Agents for Stimulating Motility

The hormone CCK is released from the intestine in response to meals and delays gastric emptying, causes contraction of the gallbladder, stimulates pancreatic enzyme secretion, increases intestinal motility, and promotes satiety. The C-terminal octapeptide of CCK, *sincalide*, is useful for stimulating the gallbladder or pancreas and for accelerating barium transit through the small bowel for diagnostic testing of these organs. It is given by intravenous injection or infusion and has an onset of action of 5–15 min.

Currently, there are a number of agents under evaluation that stimulate motility whose mechanisms of action are based on well-established neurohumoral mechanisms (Camilleri, 2014). These include a novel *motilin receptor agonist* (camicinal), a *ghrelin receptor agonist* (relamorelin), and novel $5HT_4$ *agonists* (velusetrag and naronapride).

Agents That Suppress Motility

Smooth muscle relaxants such as organic nitrates, type 5 phosphodiesterase inhibitors, and Ca^{2+} channel antagonists produce temporary, if partial, relief of symptoms in motility disorders such as achalasia, in which the lower esophageal sphincter fails to relax, resulting in severe difficulty in swallowing (Pandolfino and Gawron, 2015). Preparations of botulinum toxin (onabotulinumtoxinA), injected directly into the lower esophageal sphincter via an endoscope, in doses of 80–100 units, inhibit ACh release from nerve endings and can produce partial paralysis of the sphincter muscle, with significant improvements in symptoms and esophageal clearance (Zhao and Pasricha, 2003). Other GI conditions in which botulinum toxin A has been used include gastroparesis, sphincter of Oddi dysfunction, and anal fissures, although currently there are no strong trial data to support its efficacy.

Laxatives, Cathartics, and Therapy for Constipation

Overview of GI Water and Electrolyte Flux

Water normally accounts for 70%–85% of total stool weight. Net stool fluid content reflects a balance between luminal input (ingestion of fluids and luminally directed secretion of water and electrolytes) and output (absorption) along the length of the GI tract. The daily challenge for the gut is to extract water, minerals, and nutrients from the luminal contents, leaving behind a manageable pool of fluid for proper expulsion of waste material via the process of defecation.

Normally, about 8–9 L of fluid enter the small intestine daily from exogenous and endogenous sources (Figure 50–3). Net absorption of the water occurs in the small intestine in response to osmotic gradients that result from the uptake and secretion of ions and the absorption of nutrients (mainly sugars and amino acids), with only about 1–1.5 L crossing the ileocecal valve. The colon then extracts most of the remaining fluid, leaving about 100 mL of fecal water daily. Under normal circumstances, these quantities are within the range of the total absorptive capacity of the small bowel (~16 L) and colon (4–5 L). Neurohumoral mechanisms, pathogens, and drugs can alter secretion and absorption of fluid by the intestinal epithelium (Figure 50–4). Altered motility also contributes in a general way to this process. With decreased motility and excess fluid removal, feces can become inspissated and impacted, leading to constipation. When the capacity of the colon to absorb fluid is exceeded, diarrhea occurs.

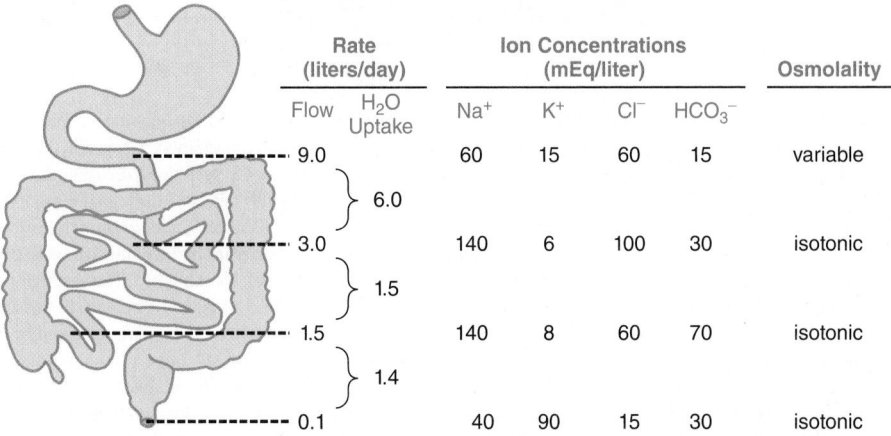

Figure 50–3 *Typical volume and composition of fluid that traverses the small and large intestines daily.* Of the 9 L of fluid typically presented to the small intestine each day, 2 L are from the diet and 7 L are from secretions (salivary, gastric, pancreatic, and biliary). The absorptive capacity of the colon is 4–5 L per day.

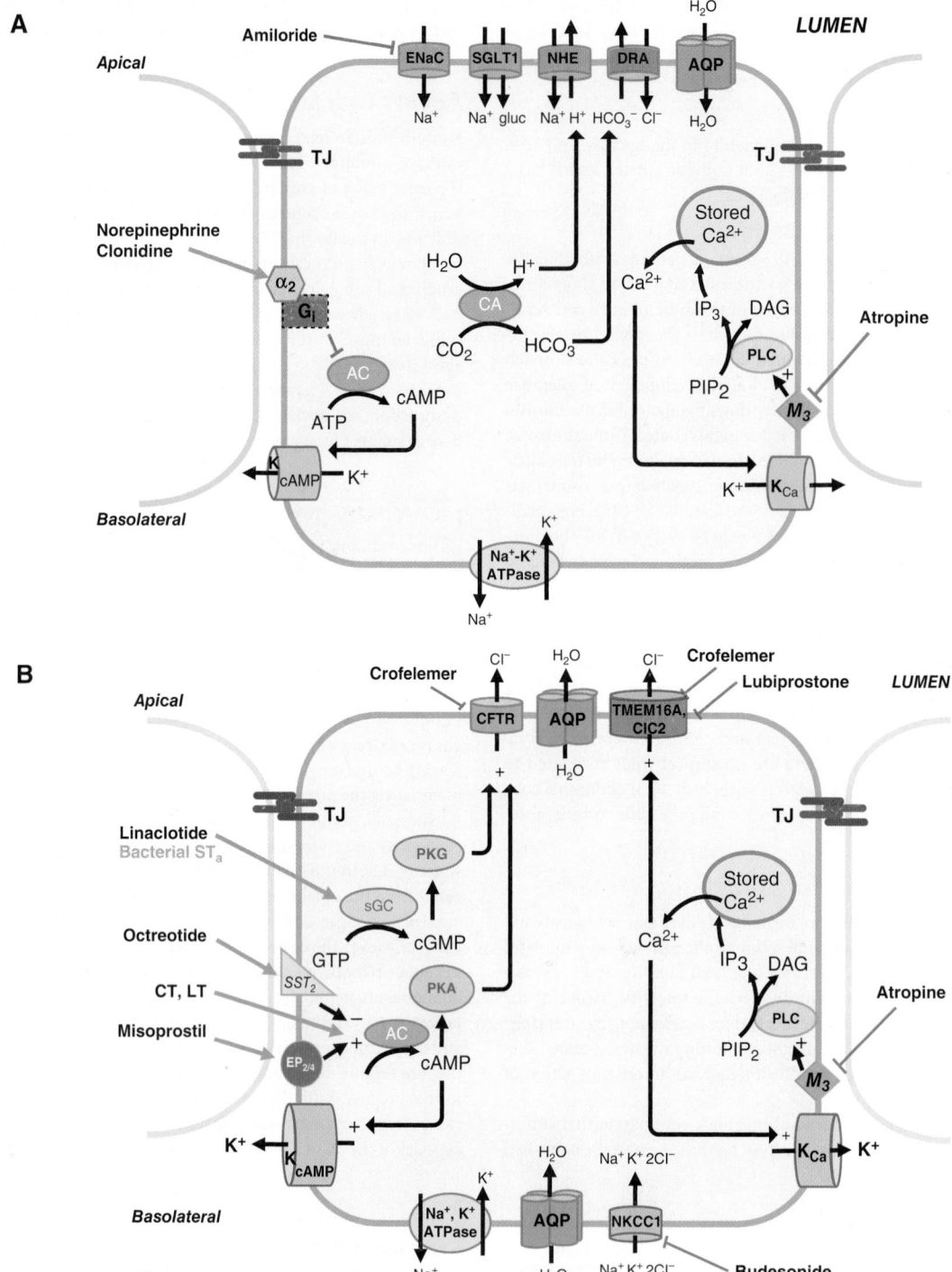

Figure 50–4 *Mechanism of action of drugs that alter intestinal epithelial secretion and absorption.* **A.** *Agents affecting intestinal epithelial secretion.* Secretion is driven in secretory enterocytes by the Na⁺ gradient established by the Na⁺,K⁺-ATPase. This Na⁺ gradient drives the symporter NKCC1 (SLC12A2), which allows for the accumulation of Cl⁻ in the cell. Regulation of chloride channels in the apical (luminal) membrane drives Cl⁻ secretion. Vectorial movement of chloride drives the secretion of water through the paracellular route and through AQP water channels. Chloride secretion is rapidly regulated through phosphorylation of CFTR by the cyclic nucleotide-dependent protein kinases, PKA and PKG. Thus, drugs that stimulate adenylyl cyclase (i.e., misoprostil, acting through prostanoid EP₂ or EP₄ receptors) or GC (linaclotide) will stimulate Cl⁻ and water secretion. Several bacterial toxins cause water efflux and diarrhea by these mechanisms: cholera toxin (CT) and heat-labile *Escherichia coli* toxin (LT) stimulate cyclic AMP synthesis in the enterocyte by ADP-ribosylating Gα$_s$, blocking its GTPase activity and leading to constitutive activation of adenylyl cyclase; the heat-stable enterotoxins (e.g., ST$_a$) stimulate the membrane-bound form of guanylyl cyclase. Drugs that inhibit adenylyl cyclase (e.g., octreotide, acting at SST2 receptors) inhibit secretion. Calcium-dependent chloride channels (TMEM 16A, ClC₂) are regulated by increases in cytosolic Ca²⁺, such as that induced by activation of muscarinic M₃ receptors that atropine blocks. Increases in cytosolic cyclic AMP and Ca²⁺ also regulate cyclic AMP–dependent and Ca²⁺-dependent K⁺ channels; this regulation is essential in maintaining the Na⁺ gradient necessary to facilitate secretion. Apical chloride channels (CFTR, TMEM 16A) can also be inhibited by drugs such as lubiprostone and crofelemer. Drugs such as budesonide inhibit NKCC1 function and thereby reduce secretion. **B.** *Agents affecting intestinal epithelial absorption.* Absorption is also driven by Na⁺,K⁺-ATPase in absorptive enterocytes, which creates the Na⁺ gradient that facilitates Na⁺ absorption through ENaC or through coupled transporters such as the Na⁺-glucose cotransporter SGLT1 (SLC5A1) and members of the NHE family. ENaC is blocked by amiloride and similar compounds. NHE and the bicarbonate-Cl⁻ exchanger, DRA, depend on the action of carbonic anhydrase (CA), which generates H⁺ and HCO₃⁻ from water and CO₂ in the cytosol. Water enters the cell through apical AQPs. As in secretion, regulation of K⁺ channels by cyclic AMP and Ca²⁺ is essential. Thus, drugs that act on α₂ adrenergic receptors (e.g., clonidine) will reduce adenylyl cyclase activity and lower enterocyte cyclic AMP levels, thereby reducing absorption.

Constipation: General Principles of Pathophysiology and Treatment

Patients use the term *constipation* not only for decreased frequency, but also for difficulty in initiation or passage of firm or small-volume feces or a feeling of incomplete evacuation.

Constipation has many reversible or secondary causes, including lack of dietary fiber, drugs, hormonal disturbances, neurogenic disorders, and systemic illnesses. In most cases of chronic constipation, no specific cause is found. Up to 60% of patients presenting with constipation have normal colonic transit. These patients either have IBS or define constipation in terms other than stool frequency. In the rest, attempts usually are made to categorize the underlying pathophysiology either as a disorder of delayed colonic transit because of an underlying defect in colonic motility or, less commonly, as an isolated disorder of defecation or evacuation (outlet disorder) due to dysfunction of the neuromuscular apparatus of the rectoanal region.

Colonic motility is responsible for mixing luminal contents to promote absorption of water and moving them from proximal to distal segments by means of propulsive contractions (Dinning et al., 2009). Mixing in the colon is accomplished in a way similar to that in the small bowel: by short- or long-duration, stationary (nonpropulsive) contractions. In any given patient, the predominant factor often is not obvious. Consequently, the pharmacological approach to constipation remains empirical and is usually based on nonspecific principles.

Constipation generally may be corrected by adherence to a fiber-rich (20–35 g daily) diet, adequate fluid intake, appropriate bowel habits and training, and avoidance of constipating drugs (Emmanuel et al., 2009; Lacy et al., 2014; Menees et al., 2012). Constipation related to medications can be corrected by use of alternative drugs where possible or adjustment of dosage. If nonpharmacological measures alone are inadequate, they may be supplemented with bulk-forming agents or osmotic laxatives.

When stimulant laxatives are used, they should be administered at the lowest effective dosage and for the shortest period of time to avoid abuse. In addition to perpetuating dependence on drugs, the laxative habit may lead to excessive loss of water and electrolytes; secondary aldosteronism may occur if volume depletion is prominent. Steatorrhea, protein-losing enteropathy with hypoalbuminemia, and osteomalacia due to excessive loss of calcium in the stool have been reported. Laxatives frequently are employed before surgical, radiological, and endoscopic procedures where an empty colon is desirable. The terms *laxatives*, *cathartics*, *purgatives*, *aperients*, and *evacuants* often are used interchangeably. There is a distinction, however, between *laxation* (the evacuation of formed fecal material from the rectum) and *catharsis* (the evacuation of unformed, usually watery, fecal material from the entire colon). Most of the commonly used agents promote laxation, but some are actually cathartics that act as laxatives at low doses.

Laxatives relieve constipation and promote evacuation of the bowel via the following:

- enhancing retention of intraluminal fluid by hydrophilic or osmotic mechanisms;
- decreasing net absorption of fluid by effects on small- and large-bowel fluid and electrolyte transport; and
- altering motility by inhibiting segmenting (nonpropulsive) contractions or stimulating propulsive contractions.

Laxatives can be classified based on their actions (Table 50–1) or by the pattern of effects produced by the usual clinical dosage (Table 50–2), with some overlap between classifications.

A variety of laxatives, both osmotic agents and stimulants, increases the activity of NO synthase and the biosynthesis of PAF (see Chapter 37) in the gut. PAF is a phospholipid pro-inflammatory mediator that stimulates colonic secretion and GI motility (Izzo et al., 1998). NO also may stimulate intestinal secretion and inhibit segmenting contractions in the colon, thereby promoting laxation. Agents that reduce the expression of NO synthase or its activity can prevent the laxative effects of castor oil, cascara, magnesium sulfate, and bisacodyl (but not senna).

TABLE 50–1 ■ CLASSIFICATION OF LAXATIVES

1. **Luminally active agents**
   Hydrophilic colloids; bulk-forming agents (bran, psyllium, etc.)
   Osmotic agents (nonabsorbable inorganic salts or sugars)
   Stool-wetting agents (surfactants) and emollients (docusate, mineral oil)

2. **Nonspecific stimulants or irritants (with effects on fluid secretion and motility)**
   Diphenylmethanes (bisacodyl)
   Anthraquinones (senna and cascara)
   Castor oil

3. **Prokinetic agents (acting primarily on motility)**
   $5HT_4$ receptor agonists
   Dopamine receptor antagonists
   Motilides (erythromycin)

Dietary Fiber and Supplements

Bulk, softness, and hydration of feces depend on the fiber content of the diet. Fiber is that part of food that resists enzymatic digestion and reaches the colon largely unchanged. Colonic bacteria ferment fiber to varying degrees, depending on its chemical nature and water solubility. Fermentation of fiber has two important effects: (1) It produces short-chain fatty acids that are trophic for colonic epithelium; (2) it increases bacterial mass. Although fermentation of fiber generally decreases stool water, short-chain fatty acids may have a prokinetic effect, and increased bacterial mass may contribute to increased stool volume. However, fiber that is not fermented can attract water and increase stool bulk. The net effect on bowel movement therefore varies with different compositions of dietary fiber (Table 50–3). In general, insoluble, poorly fermentable fibers, such as lignin, are most effective in increasing stool bulk and transit.

Bran, the residue left when flour is made from cereal grains, contains more than 40% dietary fiber. Wheat bran, with its high lignin content, is most effective at increasing stool weight (a dose of 1–3 g up to three times a day). Fruits and vegetables contain more *pectins* and *hemicelluloses*, which are more readily fermentable and produce less effect on stool transit. *Psyllium husk*, derived from the seed of the plantago herb (*Plantago ovata*; known as ispaghula or isbgol in many parts of the world), is a component of many commercial products for constipation. Psyllium husk contains

TABLE 50–2 ■ CLASSIFICATION AND COMPARISON OF REPRESENTATIVE LAXATIVES

LAXATIVE EFFECT AND LATENCY IN USUAL CLINICAL DOSAGE		
SOFTENING OF FECES, 1–3 DAYS	**SOFT OR SEMIFLUID STOOL, 6–8 H**	**WATERY EVACUATION, 1–3 H**
Bulk-forming laxatives	*Stimulant laxatives*	*Osmotic laxatives*[a]
Bran	Diphenylmethane derivatives	Magnesium sulfate
Psyllium preparations	Bisacodyl	Milk of magnesia
Methylcellulose		Magnesium citrate
Calcium polycarbophil		
Surfactant/osmotic laxatives	*Anthraquinone derivatives*	*Castor oil*
Docusates	Senna	
Poloxamers	Cascara sagrada	
Lactulose		

[a]Employed in high dosage for rapid cathartic effect and in lower dosage for laxative effect.

SECTION VI GASTROINTESTINAL PHARMACOLOGY

TABLE 50–3 ■ PROPERTIES OF DIFFERENT DIETARY FIBERS

TYPE OF FIBER	WATER SOLUBILITY	% FERMENTED
Nonpolysaccharides		
Lignin	Poor	0
Cellulose	Poor	15
Noncellulose polysaccharides		
Hemicellulose	Good	56–87
Mucilages and gums	Good	85–95
Pectins	Good	90–95

In general, insoluble, poorly fermentable fibers, such as lignin, are most effective in increasing stool bulk and transit.

a hydrophilic mucilloid that undergoes significant fermentation in the colon, leading to an increase in colonic bacterial mass; the usual dose is 2.5–4 g (1–3 teaspoons full in 250 mL of fruit juice), titrated upward until the desired goal is reached. A variety of semisynthetic celluloses—such as methylcellulose (~2 g three times a day) and the hydrophilic resin calcium polycarbophil (1–2 g/d), a polymer of acrylic acid resin—also are available. These poorly fermentable compounds absorb water and increase fecal bulk. Malt soup extract, an extract of malt from barley grains that contains small amounts of polymeric carbohydrates, proteins, electrolytes, and vitamins, is another orally administered bulk-forming agent. The onset of action of these bulk-forming laxatives is generally between 12 and 72 h. Bloating is the most common side effect of soluble fiber products (perhaps due to colonic fermentation), but it usually decreases with time (Lacy et al., 2014).

Osmotically Active Agents

Polyethylene Glycol–Electrolyte Solutions. Long-chain PEGs (MW ~ 3350 Da) are poorly absorbed and retain water via their high osmotic nature (Paré and Fedorak, 2014). When used in high volume, aqueous solutions of PEGs with electrolytes produce an effective catharsis and have replaced oral sodium phosphates as the most widely used preparations for colonic cleansing prior to radiological, surgical, and endoscopic procedures.

Usually, 240 mL of this solution is taken every 10 min until 4 L is consumed or the rectal effluent is clear. To avoid net transfer of ions across the intestinal wall, these preparations contain an isotonic mixture of sodium sulfate, sodium bicarbonate, sodium chloride, and potassium chloride. The osmotic activity of the PEG molecules retains the added water, and the electrolyte concentration ensures little or no net ionic shifts. A powder form of PEG 3350 is now available as an OTC product for the treatment of occasional constipation and for the treatment of more chronic constipation; the PEG preparation is suitable because it has such a benign side-effect profile. The usual dose is 8.5–34 g of powder per day in 8 oz of water, with an expected onset of action of 1–4 days. These laxatives may cause nausea, cramping, and bloating.

Saline Laxatives. Laxatives containing magnesium cations or phosphate anions commonly are called *saline laxatives*: magnesium sulfate, magnesium hydroxide, magnesium citrate, and sodium phosphate. Their cathartic action is believed to result from osmotic water retention, which then stimulates peristalsis. Other mechanisms may contribute, including the production of inflammatory mediators.

Magnesium-containing laxatives may stimulate the release of CCK, which leads to intraluminal fluid and electrolyte accumulation and to increased intestinal motility. For every additional milliequivalent of Mg^{2+} in the intestinal lumen, fecal weight increases by about 7 g. The usual dose of Mg^{2+} salts contains 40–120 mEq of Mg^{2+} and produces 300–600 mL of stool within 0.5–6 h. The most common side effects of these laxatives is urgency to defecate and watery stools.

Phosphate salts are better absorbed than Mg^{2+}-based agents and therefore need to be given in larger doses to induce catharsis. However, because of the risks of acute phosphate nephropathy, oral phosphates are not recommended for the treatment of constipation and should be completely avoided in patients at risk (the elderly, patients with known bowel pathology or renal dysfunction, and patients on angiotensin-converting enzyme inhibitors, angiotensin receptor blockers, and NSAIDs).

The Mg^{2+}-containing preparations must be used with caution or avoided in patients with renal insufficiency, cardiac disease, or preexisting electrolyte abnormalities and in patients on diuretic therapy.

Nondigestible Sugars and Alcohols. *Lactulose* is a synthetic disaccharide of galactose and fructose that resists intestinal disaccharidase activity. This and other nonabsorbable sugars such as *sorbitol* and *mannitol* are hydrolyzed in the colon to short-chain fatty acids, which stimulate colonic propulsive motility by osmotically drawing water into the lumen. Sorbitol and lactulose are equally efficacious in the treatment of constipation caused by opioids and vincristine, of constipation in the elderly, and of idiopathic chronic constipation. They are available as 70% solutions, which are given in doses of 15–30 mL at night, with increases as needed up to 60 mL/d in divided doses. Effects may not be seen for 24 to 48 h after dosing begins. Abdominal discomfort or distention and flatulence are relatively common but usually subside with continued administration.

Lactulose also is used to treat hepatic encephalopathy. Patients with severe liver disease have an impaired capacity to detoxify ammonia coming from the colon, where it is produced by bacterial metabolism of fecal urea. The drop in luminal pH that accompanies hydrolysis to short-chain fatty acids in the colon results in "trapping" of the ammonia by its conversion to the polar ammonium ion. Combined with the increases in colonic transit, this therapy significantly lowers circulating ammonia levels. The therapeutic goal in this condition is to give sufficient amounts of lactulose (usually 20–30 g three to four times per day) to produce two to three soft stools a day with a pH of 5–5.5.

Stool-Wetting Agents and Emollients

Docusate. Docusate salts are anionic surfactants that lower the surface tension of the stool to allow mixing of aqueous and fatty substances, softening the stool, and permitting easier defecation. These agents also stimulate intestinal fluid and electrolyte secretion (possibly by increasing mucosal cyclic AMP) and alter intestinal mucosal permeability. Docusate sodium (dioctyl sodium sulfosuccinate, 100 mg twice per day) and docusate calcium (dioctyl calcium sulfosuccinate, 240 mg per day) are well tolerated but have marginal efficacy in most cases of constipation.

Mineral Oil. Mineral oil is a mixture of aliphatic hydrocarbons obtained from petrolatum. The oil is indigestible and absorbed only to a limited extent. When mineral oil is taken orally for 2–3 days, it penetrates and softens the stool and may interfere with resorption of water. The side effects of mineral oil preclude its regular use and include interference with absorption of fat-soluble substances (such as vitamins), elicitation of foreign-body reactions in the intestinal mucosa and other tissues, and leakage of oil past the anal sphincter. Rare complications such as lipid pneumonitis due to aspiration also can occur, so "heavy" mineral oil should not be taken at bedtime and "light" (topical) mineral oil should never be administered orally.

Stimulant (Irritant) Laxatives

Stimulant laxatives have direct effects on enterocytes, enteric neurons, and GI smooth muscle and probably induce limited low-grade inflammation in the small and large bowel to promote accumulation of water and electrolytes and stimulate intestinal motility (Lacy et al., 2014; Paré and Fedorak, 2014). This group includes *diphenylmethane derivatives*, *anthraquinones*, and *ricinoleic acid*.

Diphenylmethane Derivatives. **Bisacodyl.** Bisacodyl is marketed as enteric-coated and regular tablets and as a suppository for rectal administration. The usual oral daily dose of bisacodyl is 10–30 mg for adults and 5–10 mg for children ages 6–12 years old. The drug requires hydrolysis by endogenous esterases in the bowel for activation, so the laxative effects after an oral dose usually are produced in 6–10 h. Suppositories (10 mg) work within 15–60 min. Due to the possibility of developing an atonic nonfunctioning colon, bisacodyl should not be used for more than

10 consecutive days. Bisacodyl is mainly excreted in the stool; about 5% is absorbed and excreted in the urine as a glucuronide. Overdosage can lead to catharsis and fluid and electrolyte deficits. The diphenylmethanes can damage the mucosa and initiate an inflammatory response in the small bowel and colon, and they can also cause colonic ischemia.

Sodium Picosulfate. Sodium picosulfate is a diphenylmethane derivative that is hydrolyzed by colonic bacteria to its active form and acts locally only in the colon. Effective doses of the diphenylmethane derivatives vary as much as 4- to 8-fold in individual patients. This agent is only used for bowel cleansing prior to colonoscopy. Significant adverse reactions include hypermagnesemia and reduced glomerular filtration rate. Caution should be exercised in patients with cardiac arrhythmias and those with renal impairment. *Phenolphthalein*, once among the most popular components of laxatives, has been withdrawn from the market in the U.S. because of potential carcinogenicity. *Oxyphenisatin* was withdrawn due to hepatotoxicity.

Anthraquinone Laxatives. These derivatives of plants such as aloe, cascara, and senna share a tricyclic anthracene nucleus modified with hydroxyl, methyl, or carboxyl groups to form monoanthrones, such as rhein and frangula. For medicinal use, monoanthrones (oral mucosal irritants) are converted to more innocuous dimeric (dianthrones) or glycoside forms. This process is reversed by bacterial action in the colon to generate the active forms.

Senna. Senna is obtained from the dried leaflets on pods of *Cassia acutifolia* or *Cassia angustifolia* and contains the rhein dianthrone glycosides sennoside A and B. The 15–30 mg is given as a single dose or a divided dose twice daily; it has an onset of action of 6–12 h. Chronic use of senna may lead to melanosis coli, and adverse effects include nausea and vomiting and abdominal cramping.

Cascara sagrada. Cascara sagrada is obtained from the bark of the buckthorn tree and contains the glycosides barbaloin and chrysaloin. The synthetic monoanthrone danthron was withdrawn from the U.S. market because of concerns over possible carcinogenicity.

The FDA has categorized aloe and cascara sagrada products sold as laxatives as not generally recognized as safe and effective for OTC use because of a lack of scientific information about potential carcinogenicity. These ingredients may still be sold OTC in the U.S., but legally they cannot be labeled for use as laxatives. This judgment is medically prudent but may provoke a wistfulness among Joyceans, who recall that cascara sagrada, the *sacred bark*, worked well for Leopold Bloom, in Dublin, on the morning of June 16, 1904:

Midway, his last resistance yielding, he allowed his bowels to ease themselves quietly as he read, reading still patiently that slight constipation of yesterday quite gone. Hope its not too big to bring on piles again. No, just right. So. Ah! Costive one tabloid of cascara sagrada. Life might be so. (*Ulysses*, James Joyce, 1922)

Castor Oil. A bane of childhood since the time of the ancient Egyptians, castor oil is derived from the bean of the castor plant, *Ricinus communis*. The castor bean is the source of an extremely toxic protein, ricin, as well as the oil (chiefly of the triglyceride of ricinoleic acid). The triglyceride is hydrolyzed in the small bowel by the action of lipases into glycerol and the active agent, *ricinoleic acid*, which acts primarily in the small intestine to stimulate secretion of fluid and electrolytes and speed intestinal transit. When taken on an empty stomach, as little as 4 mL of castor oil may produce a laxative effect within 1–3 h; however, the usual dose for a cathartic effect is 15–60 mL for adults. Because of its unpleasant taste and its potential toxic effects on intestinal epithelium and enteric neurons, castor oil is not recommended now.

Enemas and Suppositories. Enemas are employed either by themselves or as adjuncts to bowel preparation regimens to empty the distal colon or rectum of retained solid material. Bowel distention by any means will produce an evacuation reflex in most people, and almost any form of enema, including normal saline solution, can achieve this. Specialized enemas contain additional substances that are either osmotically active or irritant;

however, their safety and efficacy have not been studied. Repeated enemas with hypotonic solutions can cause hyponatremia; repeated enemas with sodium phosphate–containing solution can cause hypocalcemia.

Glycerin. Glycerin is absorbed when given orally but acts as a hygroscopic agent and lubricant when given rectally. The resultant water retention stimulates peristalsis and usually produces a bowel movement in less than an hour. Glycerin is for rectal use only and is given in a single daily dose as a 2- or 3-g rectal suppository or as 5–15 mL of an 80% solution in enema form. Rectal glycerin may cause local discomfort, burning, or hyperemia and (minimal) bleeding. *CEO-TWO* suppositories contain sodium bicarbonate and potassium bitartrate and make use of rectal distension to initiate laxation. When administered rectally, the suppository produces CO_2, which initiates a bowel movement in 5–30 min.

Prokinetic and Secretory Agents for Constipation

The term *prokinetic* is reserved for agents that enhance GI transit via interaction with specific receptors involved in the regulation of motility (Acosta and Camilleri, 2015; Altan et al., 2012; Corsetti and Tack, 2014; Tack and Zaninotto, 2015).

The potent $5HT_4$ receptor agonist *prucalopride* (1–4 mg per day) may be useful for the treatment of chronic constipation. *Misoprostol*, a synthetic prostaglandin analogue, is primarily used for protection against gastric ulcers resulting from the use of NSAIDs and for the medical termination of pregnancy (see Chapters 37, 44, and 49). Prostaglandins can stimulate colonic contractions, particularly in the descending colon; this may account not only for the diarrhea that limits the usefulness of misoprostol as a gastroprotectant, but also for misoprostol's utility in patients with intractable constipation. Doses of 200 µg daily or every other day can be effective when used with PEG. Misoprostol should not be used in women who could become pregnant because it induces labor. It can also increase menstrual bleeding. *Colchicine*, a microtubule formation inhibitor used for gout (see Chapter 38), also has been shown to be effective in constipation (1 mg per day), but its toxicity limits widespread use.

Three recently introduced secretory agents, *lubiprostone, linaclotide*, and plecanatide, with novel mechanisms of action restricted to the gut lumen, have demonstrated effectiveness in the treatment of chronic constipation in adults.

Lubiprostone. **Mechanism of Action and Pharmacology.** Lubiprostone is a prostanoid activator of Cl^- channels. The drug appears to bind to the EP_4 receptor for PGE_2, a GPCR that couples to G_s, activating adenylyl cyclase and leading to enhanced apical Cl^- conductance. The drug promotes the secretion of a chloride-rich fluid, thereby improving stool consistency and promoting increased frequency by reflexly activating motility (Wilson and Schey, 2015).

Therapeutic Uses and Adverse Effects. A dose of 8 µg twice daily was found to be effective in constipation-predominant IBS, although higher doses (24 µg twice daily) are given for chronic constipation and opioid-induced constipation (see discussion that follows). The drug is poorly bioavailable, acting only in the lumen of the bowel. Side effects of lubiprostone include nausea (in up to 30% of patients), headache, diarrhea, allergic reactions, and dyspnea.

Linaclotide. **Mechanism of Action and Pharmacology.** Another class of secretory agent is linaclotide, a 14–amino acid peptide agonist of the membrane-spanning GC-C. In the intestinal epithelium, GC-C is activated physiologically by guanylin and uroguanylin, pathologically by heat-stable bacterial toxins that cause diarrhea, and pharmacologically by linaclotide. Activation of GC-C results in increased synthesis of cyclic GMP, resulting in enhanced chloride and bicarbonate secretion into the intestinal lumen, leading in turn to water secretion and enhanced motility. Some cellular cyclic GMP may be exported and may reduce visceral pain by an action on primary afferent nerves innervating the GI tract (Yu and Rao, 2014).

Therapeutic Uses and Adverse Effects. This compound is approved in the treatment of constipation-predominant IBS and chronic constipation in adults at doses of 290 and 145 µg daily, respectively. Common side effects include diarrhea (which can be serious), gas, abdominal pain, and headaches. Linaclotide is contraindicated in children under 6 years old and is not recommended for older children.

Plecanatide. *Mechanism of Action and Pharmacology.* Plecanatide is a 16-amino acid peptide related to uroguanylin; it has essentially the same mechanism of action as linaclotide.

Therapeutic Uses and Adverse Effects. This agent is approved for the treatment of chronic idiopathic constipation in adults at a dose of 3 mg daily, with or without food. The most common adverse reaction is diarrhea (5%; severe in 0.6%). Plecanatide is contraindicated in children less than 6 years old and not advised in older children up to 18 years of age.

Opioid-Induced Constipation

Opioid analgesics can cause severe constipation. Laxatives and dietary strategies are frequently ineffective in the management of opioid-induced constipation. In addition to *lubiprostone*, a promising alternative strategy is the prevention of opioid-induced constipation with peripherally acting MOR antagonists that specifically target the underlying reason for this condition, without limiting centrally produced analgesia and limiting the symptoms of opioid withdrawal (Nelson and Camilleri, 2016).

Methylnaltrexone

Mechanism of Action and Pharmacology. The peripherally restricted MOR antagonist methylnaltrexone is approved for the treatment of opioid-induced constipation. The efficacy of this compound has been shown in randomized placebo-controlled trials (Nelson and Camilleri, 2016).

ADME. In patients who respond to the drug, its onset of action is 30–60 min. It is excreted largely unchanged in the urine and feces, but does undergo some hepatic metabolism including sulfation. The time to peak plasma concentration is 30 min and the $t_{1/2}$ is about 8 h.

Therapeutic Uses and Adverse Effects. *Methylnaltrexone* is given as a subcutaneous injection (12 mg per day) in adults with chronic noncancer pain after discontinuing other laxatives. In advanced illness (palliative care), dosing varies according to body weight (0.15 mg/kg), with dosing every other day to a maximum of daily injection if required. When administered repeatedly every other day for 2 weeks, bowel movements occurred in about 50% of patients, compared with 8%–15% of patients receiving placebo. Abdominal pain, flatulence, and nausea frequently accompany this treatment. Serious diarrhea sometimes occurs that requires discontinuing therapy. Patients with known or suspected GI obstruction are at increased risk of perforation. Opioid withdrawal may be precipitated in patients with a compromised blood-brain barrier.

Naldemedine

Mechanism of Action and Pharmacology. Naldemedine is a peripherally-restricted opioid antagonist. It is a derivative of naltrexone made more polar and larger in mass with the addition of a side-chain. It is also a substrate for the Pgp efflux transporter. These two properties limit its access to the CNS.

ADME. Following oral administration in the fasted state, naldemedine is rapidly absorbed, reaching peak concentrations in ~45 min. Food prolongs the time to peak (to ~2.5 h) but does not reduce the overall extent of absorption. Naldemedine is metabolized by hepatic CYP3A and is excreted in both the urine (57%) and feces (35%); its t1/2 is 11 h.

Therapeutic Uses and Adverse Effects. Naldemedine is approved for the treatment of opioid-induced constipation in adult patients with chronic noncancer pain; dose, 0.2 mg/d, orally. Common adverse reactions are abdominal pain, diarrhea, nausea, vomiting, and gastroenteritis. Naldemedine is contraindicated in patients with known or suspected obstruction of the GI tract. Opioid withdrawal may be precipitated with the use of this compound.

Naloxegol

Mechanism of Action and Pharmacology. Naloxegol is composed of the MOR antagonist naloxone conjugated to a PEG polymer. This limits blood-brain barrier permeability because it is a substrate for the P-glycoprotein efflux transporter, so it behaves as a peripherally restricted MOR antagonist. It is approved for the treatment of opioid-induced constipation. Randomized placebo-controlled trials have demonstrated the efficacy of this compound (Nelson and Camilleri, 2016).

ADME. The drug is given orally on an empty stomach and is rapidly absorbed. The time to peak plasma concentration is about 2 h with a secondary peak occurring 0.4–3 h after the first. Naloxegol is metabolized primarily by hepatic CYP3A; metabolites are excreted in the feces (68%) and urine (16%). The plasma $t_{1/2}$ is variable, 6–11 h.

Therapeutic Uses and Adverse Effects. *Naloxegol* is approved for opioid-induced constipation in adults, given orally 12.5 or 25 mg once per day after discontinuing other laxatives. Diarrhea, abdominal pain, flatulence, and nausea and vomiting are the major adverse reactions. Precautions are the same as for *methylnaltrexone*: Patients with known or suspected GI obstruction are at increased risk of perforation, and opioid withdrawal may be precipitated in patients with a compromised blood-brain barrier.

Naloxone and Oxycodone

Mechanism of Action and Pharmacology. A fixed-ratio (2:1 of oxycodone:naloxone) combination drug is given orally to relieve opioid-induced constipation when opioid pain relief is still required. The *naloxone* displaces oxycodone from the MOR in the GI tract without limiting the degree of central analgesia (Nelson and Camilleri, 2016). This combination drug carries with it the risks inherent with all opioids, including addiction and respiratory depression. Full details of this agent are given in Chapter 20.

Therapeutic Uses and Adverse Effects. Naloxone-oxycodone is approved in Canada and other countries for opioid-induced constipation in adults, but currently not for this purpose in the U.S. This oral medication dosing is for pain control and is individualized. A single dose of 40 mg oxycodone/20 mg naloxone every 12 h should not be exceeded. Adverse GI reactions include nausea and vomiting, constipation, and diarrhea.

Other Agents for Opioid-induced Constipation. In clinical trials, the MOR antagonist *alvimopan* (see separate discussion in the following material) increased spontaneous bowel movements and improved other symptoms of opioid-induced constipation without compromising analgesia. Alvimopan is approved for use in the U.S. for postoperative bowel recovery. However, due to significant cardiovascular adverse events, this drug is not FDA-approved for opioid-induced constipation, and further phase III trials are under way. In addition, the 5HT$_4$ agonist *prucalopride* and the GC-C agonist *linaclotide* (see previous discussion) are in clinical trials for this condition, as are other novel peripherally active MOR antagonists.

Postoperative Ileus

Postoperative ileus refers to the intolerance to oral intake and nonmechanical obstruction of the bowel that occurs after abdominal and nonabdominal surgery. The pathogenesis is complex and is a combination of activation of neural inhibitory reflexes involving sympathetic nerves, enteric MOR, and the activation of local inflammatory mechanisms that reduce smooth muscle contractility (Bragg et al., 2015). The condition is exacerbated by opioids, which are the mainstay of postoperative analgesia. Prokinetic agents typically do not have much effect in this condition, but a new therapeutic agent has been introduced to reduce GI recovery time after surgery.

Alvimopan

Mechanism of Action and Pharmacology. Alvimopan is an orally active, peripherally restricted MOR antagonist that is approved to accelerate the time to upper and lower GI recovery following partial large- or small-bowel resection surgery with primary anastomosis (Curran et al., 2008).

ADME. The drug is hydrolyzed by the gut flora to the active amide. The active metabolite is further metabolized by hepatic glucuronidases. The peak plasma concentration of the active metabolite occurs in about 36 h. The drug's $t_{1/2}$ is 10–18 h; the drug is excreted in the urine and feces.

Therapeutic Uses and Adverse Effects. The drug is given 30 min to 5 h prior to surgery (12 mg) and then twice daily for up to a maximum of 7 days or until discharge, not to exceed 15 doses total. Adverse effects include hypokalemia, dyspepsia, and anemia. Because of the risk of myocardial infarctions, this drug is only available through a restricted-access program in the U.S.

Antidiarrheal Agents

Diarrhea: General Principles and Approach to Treatment

Diarrhea (Greek and Latin: *dia*, "through," and *rheein*, "to flow or run") does not require any definition to people who suffer from "the too rapid evacuation of too fluid stools." Scientists usually define diarrhea as excessive fluid weight, with 200 g per day representing the upper limit of normal stool water weight for healthy adults in the Western world. Because stool weight is largely determined by stool water, most cases of diarrhea result from disorders of intestinal water and electrolyte transport.

An appreciation and knowledge of the underlying causative processes in diarrhea facilitates effective treatment (Thiagarajah et al., 2015). From a mechanistic perspective, diarrhea can be caused by an increased osmotic load within the intestine (resulting in retention of water within the lumen); excessive secretion of electrolytes and water into the intestinal lumen; exudation of protein and fluid from the mucosa; and altered intestinal motility resulting in rapid transit (and decreased fluid absorption). In most instances, multiple processes are affected simultaneously, leading to a net increase in stool volume and weight accompanied by increases in fractional water content.

Many patients with sudden onset of diarrhea have a *benign*, self-limited illness requiring no treatment or evaluation. *Acute diarrhea* is frequently due to infection with bacteria, viruses, or protozoa. In more severe cases of diarrhea and in infants and small children, dehydration and electrolyte imbalances are the principal risk. *Oral rehydration therapy* therefore is a cornerstone for patients with acute illnesses resulting in significant diarrhea. This therapy exploits the fact that nutrient-linked cotransport of water and electrolytes remains intact in the small bowel in most cases of acute diarrhea. Na^+ absorption links to glucose uptake by the enterocyte; this is followed by movement of water in the same direction. A balanced mixture of glucose and electrolytes in volumes matched to losses therefore can prevent dehydration. This can be provided by many commercial premixed formulas using glucose-electrolyte or rice-based physiological solutions.

Pharmacotherapy of diarrhea in adults should be reserved for patients with significant or persistent symptoms (Menees et al., 2012). Nonspecific antidiarrheal agents typically do not address the underlying pathophysiology responsible for the diarrhea. Many of these agents act by decreasing intestinal motility and should be avoided in acute diarrheal illnesses caused by invasive organisms. In such cases, these agents may mask the clinical picture, delay clearance of organisms, and increase the risk of systemic invasion by the infectious organisms.

Empiric Antibiotic Therapy

The use of empiric antibiotic therapy for acute diarrhea (therapy given in the absence of diagnostic evaluation) must be carefully balanced with the risks. In patients with suspected or proven enterohemorrhagic *Escherichia coli*, antibiotics should be avoided because of the risk of hemolytic uremic syndrome. Similarly, in patients with suspected *Clostridium difficile*, other antibiotics should be discontinued if possible. Treatment of traveler's diarrhea, bacterial diarrhea, and those with more severe conditions is appropriate under some conditions, based on the severity of diarrhea and the duration of the symptoms (Steffen et al., 2015). The first-line therapy for acute (most commonly, traveler's) diarrhea in adults is oral *fluoroquinolone* antibiotics (see Chapter 56 for specific drug details): *ciprofloxacin* (500 mg twice daily for up to 3 days), *norfloxacin* (400 mg twice daily for up to 3 days), *ofloxacin* (200 mg twice daily for up to 3 days), or *levofloxacin* (500 mg daily for up to 3 days). *Azithromycin* (500 mg per day for 1–3 days, or a maximum of 1000-mg single dose) and *rifaximin* (200 mg three times per day for up to 3 days) are alternative therapeutic agents. Trimethoprim/sulfamethoxazole is also FDA-approved for this use (1 double-strength tab [160/8000 mg] twice daily for 5 days). In children, the treatment of traveler's diarrhea remains controversial. *Azithromycin* (10 mg/kg to a maximum of 500-mg single dose) is the preferred treatment of children with traveler's diarrhea.

Bismuth Subsalicylate

Mechanism of Action and Pharmacology. Bismuth compounds are used to treat a variety of GI disorders, although their mechanism of action remains poorly understood (Menees et al., 2012). Bismuth subsalicylate is a popular OTC preparation that consists of trivalent bismuth and salicylate suspended in a mixture of magnesium aluminum silicate clay. In the low pH of the stomach, the bismuth subsalicylate reacts with hydrochloric acid to form bismuth oxychloride and salicylic acid.

Bismuth is thought to have antisecretory, anti-inflammatory, and antimicrobial effects. Bismuth also relieves nausea and abdominal cramps. The clay in bismuth subsalicylate and generic formulations may have some additional benefits in diarrhea, but this is not clear. Bismuth subsalicylate is used for the prevention and treatment of traveler's diarrhea, but it also is effective in other forms of episodic diarrhea and in acute gastroenteritis.

Therapeutic Uses and Adverse Effects. A recommended dose of the bismuth subsalicylate (30 mL of regular-strength liquid or 2 tablets) contains approximately equal amounts of bismuth and salicylate (262 mg each). For control of indigestion, nausea, or diarrhea, the dose is repeated every 30–60 min, as needed, up to eight times a day. Dark stools (sometimes mistaken for melena) and black staining of the tongue in association with bismuth compounds are caused by bismuth sulfide formed in a reaction between the drug and bacterial sulfides in the GI tract. Although 99% of the bismuth passes unaltered and unabsorbed into the feces, the salicylate is absorbed in the stomach and small intestine. Thus, the product carries the same warning regarding Reye syndrome as other salicylates and may also cause CNS side effects, hearing loss, and tinnitus.

Probiotics

The GI tract contains a vast and complex commensal microflora necessary for health. Alterations in the balance or composition of the microflora are responsible for antibiotic-associated diarrhea and possibly other disease conditions (see Chapter 51). Probiotic preparations containing a variety of bacterial strains have shown some degree of benefit in acute diarrheal conditions, antibiotic-associated diarrhea, and infectious diarrhea (Menees et al., 2012). In clinical trials, preparations containing *Lactobacillus* GG and *Saccharomyces boulardii* have been found to be effective for these conditions.

Antimotility and Antisecretory Agents

Opioids. Opioids continue to be widely used in the treatment of diarrhea. They act by several different mechanisms, mediated principally through either MORs or DORs on enteric nerves, epithelial cells, and muscle (see Chapter 20). These mechanisms include effects on intestinal motility (MOR), intestinal secretion (DOR), or absorption (MOR and DOR). Commonly used antidiarrheals such as *diphenoxylate*, *difenoxin*, and *loperamide* act principally via peripheral MOR and are preferred over opioids that penetrate the CNS.

Loperamide. ***Mechanism of Action and Pharmacology.*** *Loperamide*, a compound with MOR activity, is an orally active antidiarrheal agent (Hanauer, 2008; Menees et al., 2012). The drug is 40–50 times more potent than morphine as an antidiarrheal agent and penetrates the CNS poorly. It increases small intestinal and mouth-to-cecum transit times. *Loperamide* also increases anal sphincter tone. In addition, *loperamide* has antisecretory activity against cholera toxin and some forms of *E. coli* toxin, presumably by acting on G_i-linked receptors to counter the stimulation of adenylyl cyclase activity by the toxins.

ADME. *Loperamide* is available OTC in capsule, solution, and chewable tablet forms. It acts quickly after an oral dose, with peak plasma levels achieved within 3–5 h. It has a $t_{1/2}$ of about 11 h and undergoes extensive hepatic metabolism.

Therapeutic Uses and Adverse Effects. The usual adult dose is 4 mg initially followed by 2 mg after each subsequent loose stool, up to 16 mg per day. If clinical improvement in acute diarrhea does not occur within 48 h, loperamide should be discontinued. Recommended maximum daily doses for children are 3 mg for ages 2–5 years, 4 mg for ages 6–8 years, and 6 mg for ages 8–12 years. *Loperamide* is not recommended for use in children younger than 2 years. *Loperamide* is effective against traveler's diarrhea, used alone or in combination with antibiotics. It is used as adjunct treatment in many forms of chronic diarrheal disease (initially as for acute diarrhea, but with typical divided daily doses of 4–8 mg per day), with few adverse effects. *Loperamide* lacks significant abuse potential and is more effective in treating diarrhea than diphenoxylate. Overdosage, however, can result in constipation, CNS depression (especially in children), and paralytic ileus. In patients with active inflammatory bowel disease involving the colon (see Chapter 51), *loperamide* should be used with great caution, if at all, to avoid development of toxic megacolon.

Diphenoxylate and Difenoxin. **Mechanism of Action and Pharmacology.** *Diphenoxylate* and its active metabolite *difenoxin* (diphenoxylic acid) are related structurally to meperidine. As antidiarrheal agents, *diphenoxylate* and *difenoxin* are somewhat more potent than morphine (Menees et al., 2012). Both drugs are listed as schedule V controlled substances by the Drug Enforcement Agency, and both are coformulated with atropine to discourage habituation.

ADME. Both compounds are extensively absorbed after oral administration, with peak levels achieved within 1–2 h. *Diphenoxylate* is rapidly deesterified to *difenoxin*, which is eliminated with a $t_{1/2}$ of about 12 h.

Therapeutic Uses and Adverse Effects. Both drugs are indicated for the treatment of diarrhea. The usual dosage for adults is 2 tablets initially (*diphenoxylate* or *difenoxin*), then 1 tablet every 3–4 h, not to exceed 20 mg/d (diphenoxylate) or 8 mg/d (difenoxin). Acute diarrhea usually improves in 48 h if the medication is effective. If chronic diarrhea does not improve within 10 days at the maximum daily dose, then these agents are not likely to be effective. *Diphenoxylate* is also sold as an oral solution (2.5 mg per 5 mL), which is recommended if used cautiously in children. For children, the initial dose is 0.3–0.4 mg/kg/d in four divided doses to a maximum of 10 mg per day. Once symptoms are controlled, dosing should be reduced; if no effect is seen in 48 h, the drug is unlikely to be effective. Both drugs can produce CNS effects when used in higher doses (40–60 mg per day) and thus have a potential for abuse or addiction. They are available in preparations containing small doses of atropine (considered subtherapeutic) to discourage abuse and deliberate overdosage: 25 μg of atropine sulfate per tablet with either 2.5 mg *diphenoxylate* hydrochloride or 1 mg of *difenoxin* hydrochloride. With excessive use or overdose, constipation and (in inflammatory conditions of the colon) toxic megacolon may develop. In high doses, these drugs cause CNS effects as well as anticholinergic effects from the atropine (nausea, dry mouth, blurred vision, etc.) (see Chapter 9).

Other Opioids. Opioids used for diarrhea include codeine (in doses of 30 mg given three or four times daily) and opium-containing compounds. *Paregoric* (camphorated opium tincture) contains the equivalent of 2 mg of morphine per 5 mL (0.4 mg/mL); *deodorized tincture of opium*, which is 25 times stronger, contains the equivalent of 50 mg of morphine per 5 mL (10 mg/mL). The two tinctures sometimes are confused in prescribing and dispensing, resulting in dangerous overdoses. The antidiarrheal dose of opium tincture for adults is 0.6 mL (equivalent to 6 mg morphine) four times daily; the adult dose of paregoric is 5–10 mL (equivalent to 2–4 mg morphine) one to four times daily. *Paregoric* is used in children at a dose of 0.25–0.5 mL/kg (equivalent to 0.1–0.2 mg morphine/kg) one to four times daily.

Enkephalins. Enkephalins are endogenous opioids that are important enteric neurotransmitters; they can inhibit intestinal secretion without affecting motility. *Racecadotril* is an example.

Mechanism of Action and Pharmacology. *Racecadotril* (acetorphan), a prodrug, is rapidly converted in the body to thiorphan, a dipeptide inhibitor of enkephalinase (an NEP; EC 3.4.24.11) that does not penetrate into the CNS. By inhibiting peripheral enkephalin degradation, thiorphan potentiates the effects of endogenous enkephalins on the MOR in the GI tract to produce an antidiarrheal effect predominantly as an antisecretory agent (Thiagarajah et al., 2015). In addition to enkephalins, substrates of NEP include neuropeptide Y, atrial and brain natriuretic peptides, substance P, and neurotensins, among others (Erdös and Skidgel, 1989). Thus, inhibition of enkephalinase activity could elevate the levels of these messengers as well, complicating interpretation of racecadotril's effects on physiological systems.

Therapeutic Uses and Adverse Effects. *Racecadotril* is indicated for acute diarrhea. It is given orally as a 100 mg initial dose, which is repeated every 8 h as needed until diarrhea stops, for up to 7 days maximum. In children, it is given with oral rehydration solution according to body weight (1.5 mg/kg every 8 h), until symptoms improve or for a maximum of 7 days. This drug is available in many countries, but not the U.S., and is efficacious and safe in children with acute diarrhea. It produces less constipation than *loperamide* and has minimal other adverse effects (headache, itching).

α₂ Adrenergic Receptor Agonists

Mechanism of Action and Pharmacology. The α₂ adrenergic receptor agonists such as *clonidine* can interact with specific receptors on enteric neurons and enterocytes, thereby stimulating absorption and inhibiting secretion of fluid and electrolytes and increasing intestinal transit time. These agents may have a role for use by diabetics with chronic diarrhea.

Therapeutic Uses and Adverse Effects. Oral *clonidine* (beginning at 0.6 mg three times daily) has been used used in diabetic patients with chronic diarrhea; the use of a topical preparation may result in plasma levels of the drug that are more steady. *Clonidine* also may be useful in patients with diarrhea caused by opiate withdrawal. Side effects such as hypotension, depression, and perceived fatigue may be dose limiting in susceptible patients (see Chapter 12 for details of the pharmacology of clonidine).

Octreotide and Somatostatin

Mechanism of Action and Pharmacology. Octreotide (see Chapter 43) is an octapeptide analogue of SST that is effective in inhibiting the severe secretory diarrhea brought about by hormone-secreting tumors of the pancreas and the GI tract. *Octreotide* inhibits secretion of 5HT and various GI peptides. Its greatest utility may be in the "dumping syndrome" seen in some patients after gastric surgery and pyloroplasty, in whom octreotide inhibits the release of hormones (triggered by rapid passage of food into the small intestine) that are responsible for distressing local and systemic effects. *Octreotide* is widely available; SST is available in some countries, but not the U.S.

ADME. *Octreotide* has a $t_{1/2}$ of 1–2 h and is administered either subcutaneously or intravenously as a bolus dose. The time to peak is 0.4 h after subcutaneous injection and 1 h after intramuscular injection. It is metabolized in the liver and excreted in the urine. SST has a plasma $t_{1/2}$ of 1–2 min.

Therapeutic Uses and Adverse Effects. Standard initial therapy with *octreotide* is 50–100 μg, given subcutaneously two or three times a day, with titration to a maximum dose of 500 μg three times daily, based on clinical and biochemical responses. A long-acting preparation of *octreotide* acetate enclosed in biodegradable microspheres is available for use in the treatment of diarrhea associated with carcinoid tumors and VIP-secreting tumors, as well as in the treatment of acromegaly (see Chapter 42). This preparation is injected intramuscularly once per month in a dose of 20 mg. Side effects of octreotide depend on the duration of therapy: Transient nausea, bloating, or pain at sites of injection may occur in the short term, and gallstone formation and hypo- or hyperglycemia may happen in the long term. However, there are also numerous other side effects, including cardiovascular, endocrine, and CNS.

Variceal Bleeding. SST and octreotide are effective in reducing hepatic blood flow, hepatic venous wedge pressure, and azygos blood flow. These agents constrict the splanchnic arterioles by a direct action on vascular smooth muscle and by inhibiting the release of peptides contributing to the hyperdynamic circulatory syndrome of portal hypertension. *Octreotide* also may act through the ANS. For patients with variceal bleeding, therapy with *octreotide* usually is initiated while the patient is waiting for endoscopy (a 50-μg bolus dose followed by 50 μg hourly for 2–5 days) (Bhutta and Garcia-Tsao, 2015). Because of its short $t_{1/2}$ (1–2 min), SST can be given only by intravenous infusion (a 250-μg bolus dose followed by 250 μg hourly for 2–5 days). Higher doses (up to 500 μg/h) are more efficacious and can be used for patients who continue to bleed on the lower dose.

Intestinal Dysmotility. Octreotide has complex and apparently conflicting effects on GI motility, including inhibition of antral motor activity and colonic tone. However, *octreotide* also can rapidly induce phase III activity of the migrating motor complex in the small bowel to produce longer and faster contractions than those occurring spontaneously. Its use has been shown to result in improvement in selected patients with scleroderma and small-bowel dysfunction.

Pancreatitis. Both SST and *octreotide* inhibit pancreatic secretion and have been used for the prophylaxis and treatment of acute pancreatitis (Li et al., 2011). The rationale for their use is to rest the pancreas so inflammation by the continuing production of proteolytic enzymes is not aggravated, to reduce intraductal pressures, and to ameliorate pain. However, clinical trials have demonstrated that neither agent is effective in the treatment of acute pancreatitis, although octreotide confers some benefit when given prophylactically to prevent postendoscopic retrograde cholangiopancreatography pancreatitis.

Telotristat Ethyl

Mechanism of Action and Pharmacology. This drug reduces diarrhea associated with carcinoid tumors by inhibiting tryptophan hydroxylase, the rate-limiting enzyme of 5HT biosynthesis. 5HT secretion stimulates fluid secretion and motility in the GI tract.

ADME. Telotristat ethyl is absorbed after oral administration and converted to the active agent Teloristat by the action of carboxylesterases. Peak plasma levels of Teloristat occur 1-3 h after ingestion. Clearance occurs with a $t_{1/2}$ of 5 h; elimination is via the feces.

Therapeutic Uses and Adverse Effects. Telotristat is given in combination with somatostatin analog therapy for the treatment of diarrhea in carcinoid syndrome. A dose of 250 mg three times/d may be given to adult patients who are not adequately controlled by somatostatin analog therapy alone. The main adverse effects are constipation, nausea, headache, increased gamma glutamyl transferase levels, depression, peripheral edema, flatulence, reduced appetite and, pyrexia.

Berberine

Berberine is a plant alkaloid that has complex pharmacological actions that include antimicrobial effects, stimulation of bile flow, inhibition of ventricular tachyarrhythmias, and possible antineoplastic activity. It is used most commonly to treat bacterial diarrhea and cholera but is also apparently effective against intestinal parasites (Menees et al., 2012). The antidiarrheal effects in part may be related to its antimicrobial activity, as well as its ability to inhibit smooth muscle contraction and delay intestinal transit by antagonizing the effects of ACh (by competitive and noncompetitive mechanisms) and blocking the entry of Ca^{2+} into cells. In addition, it inhibits intestinal secretion. Berberine is not FDA-approved for use in the U.S.

Bulk-Forming and Hydroscopic Agents

Hydrophilic and poorly fermentable colloids or polymers such as *carboxymethylcellulose* and calcium polycarbophil absorb water and increase stool bulk (calcium polycarbophil absorbs 60 times its weight in water). They usually are used for constipation but are sometimes useful in acute episodic diarrhea and in mild chronic diarrhea in patients with IBS. Some of these agents also may bind bacterial toxins and bile salts.

Another bulk-forming agent is *dextranomer and hyaluronic acid*. Dextranomer microspheres are a network of dextran-sucrose beads with exposed hydroxy groups. When this complex is applied to an exudative wound surface, the exudate is drawn by capillary forces generated by the swelling of the beads. The sodium hyaluronate provides viscosity and facilitates injection of the dextranomer. This agent is licensed (as a device) for the treatment of fecal incontinence in adults. It is given as four time 1-mL submucosal injection in the anal canal, which can be repeated after at least 4 weeks if the first treatment is inadequate. The major adverse effects include injection area pain and bleeding.

Bile Acid Sequestrants

Cholestyramine, colestipol, and *colesevelam* effectively bind bile acids and some bacterial toxins (Menees et al., 2012). *Cholestyramine* is useful in the treatment of bile salt–induced diarrhea, as in patients with resection of the distal ileum or after cholecystectomy. In these patients, excessive concentrations of bile salts reach the colon and stimulate water and electrolyte secretion. Patients with extensive ileal resection (usually > 100 cm) eventually develop net bile salt depletion, which can produce steatorrhea because of inadequate micellar formation required for fat absorption. In such patients, the use of *cholestyramine* aggravates the diarrhea. In patients having bile salt–induced diarrhea, *cholestyramine* and *colesevelam* can be given as an off-label use at a dose of 4–12 g of the dried resin per day. If successful, the dose may be titrated down to achieve the desired stool frequency. The use of these agents is limited by GI side effects, including bloating, flatulence, abdominal discomfort, and constipation.

Crofelemer

Mechanism of Action and Pharmacology. Crofelemer is a purified oligomeric proanthocyanidin from "dragon's blood," the reddish latex-like sap of a South American euphorbia. This botanic extract is used for the treatment of diarrhea associated with antiretroviral therapy for HIV/AIDS (Crutchley et al., 2010). It is not approved for infectious or other diarrheas. This drug has minimal systemic absorption and works by inhibiting the cyclic AMP–stimulated CFTR Cl^- channel and Ca^{2+}-activated chloride ion channels on the luminal aspect of the enterocyte, thereby reducing the water loss associated with chloride secretion into the lumen.

Therapeutic Uses and Adverse Effects. This drug is given orally (125 mg twice daily) to adults. Infectious diarrhea must be ruled out before treatment. The main adverse effects include upper respiratory tract infections, cough, flatulence, nausea, joint and back pain, and some other GI conditions.

Irritable Bowel Syndrome

Irritable bowel syndrome affects up to 15% of the population in the U.S. and most other Western countries. Patients may complain of a variety of symptoms, the most characteristic of which is recurrent abdominal pain associated with altered bowel movements. IBS appears to result from a varying combination of disturbances in visceral motor and sensory function, often associated with significant affective disorders (Khan and Chang, 2010; Mayer et al., 2014). The disturbances in bowel function can be either constipation or diarrhea or both at different times. Considerable evidence suggests a specific enhancement of visceral (as opposed to somatic) sensitivity to noxious, as well as physiological, stimuli in this syndrome (Dekel et al., 2013; Mayer et al., 2014).

Many patients can be managed with dietary restrictions, notably by avoiding fermentable oligo-di-monosaccharides and polyols, lactose, or gluten, and fiber supplementation; many cannot. Treatment of bowel symptoms (either diarrhea or constipation) is predominantly symptomatic and nonspecific, using the agents discussed previously. An important role for serotonin in IBS has been suggested based on its involvement in sensitization of nociceptor neurons in inflammatory conditions and its role in the control of motility and secretion (Dekel et al., 2013). This has led to the development of specific receptor modulators for the treatment of IBS, such as the $5HT_3$ antagonist *alosetron* and the $5HT_4$ agonist *prucalopride* (see Figure 50–2).

An effective class of agents for IBS has been the tricyclic antidepressants (see Chapter 15), which can have neuromodulatory and analgesic properties independent of their antidepressant effect (Dekel et al., 2013). Tricyclic antidepressants have a proven track record in the management of chronic "functional" visceral pain in adults (off-label use). *Amitriptyline, nortriptyline, imipramine,* or *desimipramine* can be used at lower doses than those used to treat depression. Starting doses of 10–25 mg *amitriptyline, nortriptyline,* or *imipramine* or 12.5–25 mg *desimipramine* at bedtime, should be given for 3–4 weeks because of their delayed onset of action; doses can increased if tolerated and the patient is responsive to treatment. Although changes in mood usually do not occur at these doses, there may be some diminution of anxiety and restoration of sleep patterns. SSRIs (see Chapters 13 and 15) have fewer side effects and have been advocated particularly for patients with functional constipation because SSRIs can increase bowel movements and even cause diarrhea. However, they probably are not as effective as tricyclic antidepressants in the management of visceral pain. Antidepressant use in children is not strongly supported by clinical trials. α_2 Adrenergic agonists, such as clonidine (see Chapter 12), also can increase visceral compliance and reduce distention-induced pain.

Alosetron

Mechanism of Action and Pharmacology

The 5HT$_3$ receptor participates in sensitization of spinal sensory neurons, vagal signaling of nausea, and peristaltic reflexes. The clinical effect of 5HT$_3$ antagonism is a general reduction in GI contractility with decreased colonic transit, along with an increase in fluid absorption. *Alosetron*, a potent antagonist of the 5HT$_3$ receptor, was initially withdrawn from the U.S. market because of an unusually high incidence of ischemic colitis (up to 3 per 1000 patients), leading to surgery and even death in a small number of cases. Nevertheless, the FDA has reapproved this drug under a limited distribution system for women with severe diarrhea-predominant IBS (Camilleri, 2013). The manufacturer requires a prescription program that includes physician certification and an elaborate patient education and consent protocol before dispensing.

ADME

Alosetron is rapidly absorbed from the GI tract; its duration of action (~10 h) is longer than expected from its $t_{1/2}$ of 1.5 h. It is metabolized by hepatic CYPs and is excreted in the urine and feces.

Therapeutic Uses and Adverse Effects

The drug should be started at 1 mg/d divided into two doses for the first 4 weeks and, if tolerated, advanced to a maximum of 1 mg twice daily if necessary. If the response is inadequate after 4 weeks of 1 mg twice-daily dosing, treatment should be discontinued. The most serious adverse reactions are constipation and ischemic colitis, and therapy must be discontinued immediately in patients who develop those symptoms. Other adverse reactions include nausea and vomiting, GI discomfort and pain, diarrhea, flatulence, hemorrhoids, and others.

Additional 5HT$_3$ antagonists currently available in the U.S. are approved for nausea and vomiting (see further in this chapter and Chapter 13).

Eluxadoline

Mechanism of Action and Pharmacology

Eluxadoline is a mixed MOR agonist, DOR antagonist, and κ-opioid receptor agonist. It acts locally to reduce abdominal pain and diarrhea without producing constipation in patients with IBS. This opioid drug is FDA approved for the treatment of diarrhea-predominant IBS in adults (Hornby, 2015).

ADME

Eluxadoline's time to peak C_p is 1.5–2 h; its $t_{1/2}$ is 3.7–6 h. The route of eluxadoline's metabolism is not well established; the drug and its metabolic products are excreted in the feces.

Therapeutic Uses and Adverse Effects

In patients with diarrhea-predominant IBS with a gallbladder, the therapeutic dose is 100 mg twice daily with food; the dose may be decreased to 75 mg twice daily in patients unable to tolerate the 100-mg dose. In patients without a gallbladder, eluxadoline is dosed at 75 mg twice daily to reduce the risk of sphincter of Oddi spasm and the potential complication of pancreatitis. Patients with known or suspected biliary duct obstruction, sphincter of Oddi disease or dysfunction, or a history of pancreatitis or structural diseases of the pancreas, should not be given *eluxadoline*. There are also risks from constipation, and the drug should be discontinued if severe constipation occurs. There is some potential for addiction. The major adverse reactions to the drug are constipation, nausea, and abdominal pain.

Rifaximin

Mechanism of Action and Pharmacology

Antibiotics should not be used routinely in patients with IBS, but the FDA has approved the bacterial RNA synthesis inhibitor *rifaximin* for diarrhea-predominant IBS (Saadi and McCallum, 2013).

ADME

Rifaximin is well absorbed, with a time to peak less than 1 h. Its $t_{1/2}$ is 6 h; it is cleared by the action of hepatic CYP3A; metabolites are excreted in the feces.

Therapeutic Uses and Adverse Effects

In patients with diarrhea-predominant IBS, the therapeutic dose is 550 mg three times daily for 2 weeks. This regimen may be re-treated twice if symptoms recur. Adverse reactions include nausea, peripheral edema, dizziness, fatigue, and the development of ascites and elevation in serum alanine aminotransferase. If diarrhea worsens after treatment with rifaximin, then an evaluation for development of a severe infectious diarrhea, *C. difficile* enterocolitis, should be performed.

Antispasmodics

Anticholinergic agents ("spasmolytics" or "antispasmodics") often are used in patients with IBS. The most common agents of this class available in the U.S. are nonspecific antagonists of the muscarinic receptor (see Chapter 9) and include the tertiary amines *dicyclomine* and *hyoscyamine* and the quaternary ammonium compounds *glycopyrrolate* and *methscopolamine* (off-label use). The advantage of the last two compounds is that they have a limited propensity to cross the blood-brain barrier and hence a lower risk for neurological side effects such as light-headedness, drowsiness, or nervousness. These agents typically are given on either an as-needed basis or before meals to prevent the pain and fecal urgency that occur in some patients with IBS.

Dicyclomine is given in 20-mg doses orally every 6 h, increasing to 40 mg every 6 h unless limited by side effects. *Hyoscyamine* is available as sublingual tablets, orally disintegrating tablets, immediate-release oral capsules, tablets, elixir, and drops (all administered as 0.125–0.25 mg every 4 h as needed) and extended-release forms for oral use (0.25–0.375 mg every 12 h, or 0.375 mg every 8 h, as needed), and as an injection for intramuscular, intravenous, or subcutaneous use (0.25–0.5 mg every 4 h as needed). *Glycopyrrolate* is rarely used but is available as immediate-release tablets, as an oral solution, and as an injectable; the oral dose is 1–2 mg two or three times daily, not to exceed 6 mg/d. *Methscopolamine* is provided as 2.5-mg and 5-mg tablets; the dose is 2.5 mg a half hour before meals and 2.5–5 mg at bedtime.

Other Drugs

Cimetropium and acotiamide are muscarinic antagonists that are effective in patients with IBS but are not available in the U.S. *Acotiamide* appears to be a promising agent for the treatment of postprandial distress syndrome, one of two major forms of functional dyspepsia (Zala et al., 2015). *Otilonium* bromide is a quaternary ammonium salt with antimuscarinic effects that also appears to block Ca^{2+} channels and neurokinin NK$_2$ receptors; it is not available in the U.S. *Mebeverine* hydrochloride, a derivative of hydroxybenzamide, appears to have a direct effect on the smooth muscle cell, blocking K$^+$, Na$^+$, and Ca^{2+} channels. *Mebeverine* is used outside the U.S. as an antispasmodic agent. It is given orally, 100–135 mg three times daily or 200 mg twice daily, before meals.

Antinauseants and Antiemetics

Nausea and Vomiting

Emesis and the sensation of *nausea* that frequently accompanies it are generally viewed as components of a protective reflex that serve to rid the stomach and intestine of toxic substances (*emesis*) and prevent their further ingestion (*nausea* serves as an unconditioned aversive stimulus for learning and memory) (Horn, 2008; Hornby, 2001). *Vomiting* is a complex process that appears to be coordinated by a central emesis center in the lateral reticular formation of the midbrainstem adjacent to both the CTZ in the area postrema on the floor of the fourth ventricle and the STN. The lack of a blood-brain barrier at the CTZ permits monitoring of blood and cerebrospinal fluid constantly for toxic substances and

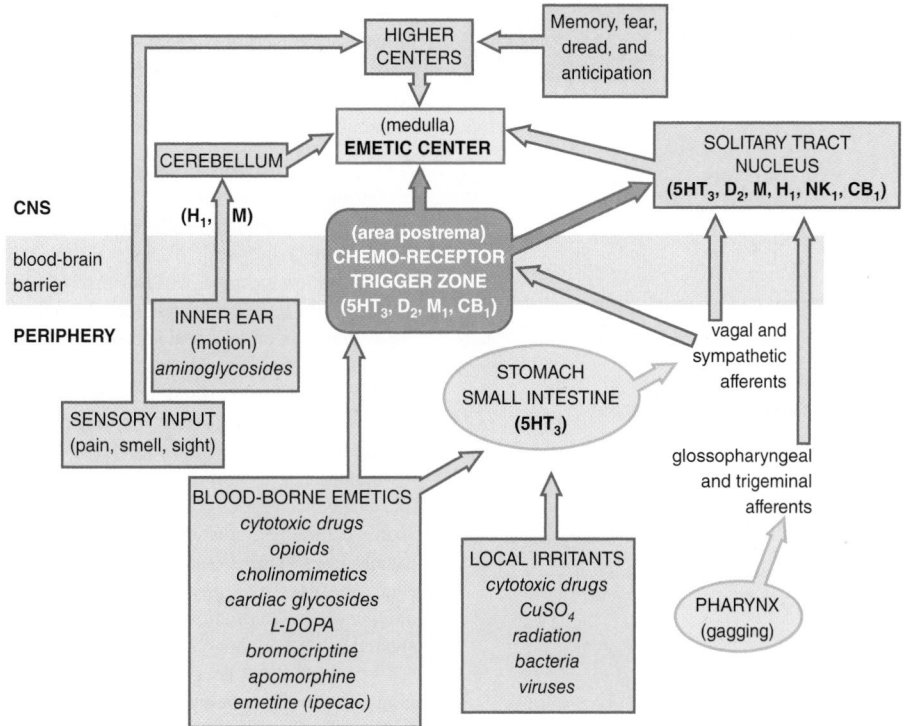

Figure 50–5 *Pharmacologist's view of emetic stimuli.* Many signaling pathways lead from the periphery to the emetic center. Stimulants of these pathways are noted in *italics*. These pathways involve specific neurotransmitters and their receptors (**bold** type). Receptors are shown for dopamine (D_2), ACh (muscarinic, M), histamine (H_1), cannabinoids (CB_1), substance P (NK_1), and $5HT_3$. Some of these receptors also may mediate signaling in the emetic center.

relaying information to the emesis center to trigger nausea and vomiting. The emesis center also receives information from the gut, principally by the vagus nerve (via the STN) and also by splanchnic afferents via the spinal cord. Two other important inputs to the emesis center come from the cerebral cortex (particularly in anticipatory nausea or vomiting) and the vestibular apparatus (in motion sickness). The CTZ has high concentrations of receptors for serotonin ($5HT_3$), dopamine (D_2), ACh (muscarinic M_1), neurokinin (NK_1), cannabinoid (CB_1), and opioids. The STN is rich in receptors for enkephalin, histamine, and ACh and also expresses $5HT_3$ receptors. Myriad neurotransmitter agonists for these receptors are involved in nausea and vomiting (Figure 50–5). Antiemetics generally are classified according to the predominant receptor on which they are proposed to act (Table 50–4). For treatment and prevention of the nausea and emesis associated with cancer chemotherapy, several antiemetic agents from different pharmacological classes may be used in combination (Table 50–5).

Nausea is distinct from emesis and is a frequent side effect of medications as well as a common feature of diseases that range from CNS disorders to GI disorders and infection. The brain centers involved in the sensation of nausea are located in higher brain regions than the emetic centers and include the insular, anterior cingulate, orbitofrontal, somatosensory, and prefrontal cortices. Most drugs used to treat emesis are relatively poor at preventing nausea (Andrews and Sanger, 2014).

5HT₃ Receptor Antagonists

Mechanism of Action and Pharmacology.
The $5HT_3$ antagonists are the most effective drugs for the treatment of chemotherapy-induced and postoperative nausea and vomiting in adults and children (Andrews and Sanger, 2014; Kovac, 2013; Navari, 2013). However, they are less effective at suppressing acute nausea than they are at suppressing acute vomiting, and they are ineffective at reducing instances of delayed (24 h later) nausea and vomiting and anticipatory nausea and vomiting.

Ondansetron is the prototypical drug in this class. Other agents in this class include the first-generation antagonists *granisetron*, *dolasetron* (not available in Canada), and *tropisetron* (not available in the U.S.) and the second-generation antagonist *palonosetron*. *Palonosetron* has higher

TABLE 50–4 ■ GENERAL CLASSIFICATION OF ANTIEMETIC AGENTS

ANTIEMETIC CLASS	EXAMPLES	MOST EFFECTIVE AGAINST
$5HT_3$ receptor antagonists[a]	Ondansetron	Cytotoxic drug-induced emesis
Centrally acting dopamine receptor antagonists	Metoclopramide[b] Promethazine[c]	Cytotoxic drug-induced emesis
Cannabinoid receptor agonists	Dronabinol nabilone	
Neurokinin receptor antagonists	Aprepitant	Cytotoxic drug-induced emesis (delayed vomiting)
Histamine H₁ antagonists	Cyclizine	Vestibular emesis (motion sickness)
Muscarinic receptor antagonists	Hyoscine (scopolamine)	

[a]The most effective agents for chemotherapy-induced nausea and vomiting are the $5HT_3$ antagonists and metoclopramide. In addition to their use as single agents, they are often combined with other drugs to improve efficacy and reduce incidence of side effects. See Table 50–5.

[b]Also has some peripheral activity at $5HT_3$ receptors.

[c]Also has some antihistaminic and anticholinergic activity.

receptor affinity, a longer $t_{1/2}$, and demonstrated superiority over first-generation antagonists (Navari, 2014).

The $5HT_3$ receptors are present in several critical sites involved in emesis, including vagal afferents, the STN (which receives signals from vagal afferents), and the area postrema itself (see Figure 50–5). Serotonin is released by the enterochromaffin cells of the small intestine in response to chemotherapeutic agents and stimulates vagal afferents (via $5HT_3$ receptors) to initiate the vomiting reflex. The highest concentrations of $5HT_3$ receptors in the

TABLE 50–5 ■ ANTIEMETIC AGENTS IN CANCER CHEMOTHERAPY[a]

Low risk of emesis:

Prechemotherapy
- Dexamethasone
- Metoclopramide ± diphenhydramine
- Prochlorperazine ± lorazepam

Postchemotherapy (delayed emesis)
- None

Moderate risk of emesis:

Prechemotherapy
- $5HT_3$ antagonist + dexamethasone
- $5HT_3$ antagonist + dexamethasone + NK_1 antagonist

Postchemotherapy (delayed emesis)
- Aprepitant (days 2 and 3)
- Dexamethasone or $5HT_3$ antagonist (days 2–3 or 4)
- Aprepitant (days 2–3, if used prechemo) ± dexamethasone (days 2–4) ± lorazepam (days 2–4)

High risk of emesis:

Prechemotherapy
- $5HT_3$ antagonist + dexamethasone + NK_1 antagonist ± lorazepam
- $5HT_3$ antagonist/NK_1 antagonist + dexamethasone

Postchemotherapy (delayed emesis)
- Dexamethasone + aprepitant
- Dexamethasone (days 2–4) + aprepitant (days 2 and 3) ± lorazepam (days 2–4)

[a]*Specific recommendations and doses are tailored to the patient and the chemotherapeutic regimen. For updated information, see the National Cancer Institute website (see Cancer Topics: Nausea and Vomiting). Some patients profit from cannabinoids (dronabinol, nabilone) with or without a phenothiazine or dexamethasone.*

CNS are found in the STN and CTZ, and antagonists of $5HT_3$ receptors also may suppress nausea and vomiting by acting at these sites.

ADME. These agents are absorbed well from the GI tract and have a rapid onset of action. *Ondansetron* is extensively metabolized in the liver by CYP1A2, CYP2D6, and CYP3A4, followed by glucuronide or sulfate conjugation. The $t_{1/2}$ is 3–6 h. Patients with hepatic dysfunction have reduced plasma clearance, and some adjustment in the dosage is advisable. *Granisetron* also is metabolized predominantly by the liver by the CYP3A family and has a $t_{1/2}$ of 6–9 h, depending on the route of administration. *Dolasetron* is converted rapidly by plasma carbonyl reductase to its active metabolite, hydrodolasetron. A portion of this compound then undergoes subsequent biotransformation by CYP2D6 and CYP3A4 in the liver, while about one-third of it is excreted unchanged in the urine. The $t_{1/2}$ of the active metabolite hydrodolasetron is 6–8 h. *Palonosetron* is metabolized principally by CYP2D6; the metabolized and the unchanged

forms are excreted in the urine in roughly equal proportions. The $t_{1/2}$ after intravenous injection is about 40 h in adults. The antiemetic effects of these drugs persist long after they disappear from the circulation, suggesting their continuing interaction at the receptor level; these drugs can be administered effectively just once a day.

Therapeutic Uses and Adverse Effects. These agents are most effective in treating chemotherapy-induced nausea and in treating nausea secondary to upper abdominal irradiation. They also are effective against hyperemesis of pregnancy and, to a lesser degree, postoperative nausea, but not against motion sickness. Unlike other agents in this class, *palonosetron* may be helpful in delayed emesis, perhaps reflecting its long $t_{1/2}$. These agents are available as tablets, oral solution, and intravenous preparations for injection. *Palonosetron*, in combination with the NK_1 receptor antagonist *netupitant* (see further discussion), is FDA approved for the treatment of acute and delayed nausea and vomiting. This combination is highly effective when combined with the corticosteroid *dexamethasone* (see further discussion). For patients on cancer chemotherapy, these drugs can be given in a single intravenous dose (Table 50–6) infused over 15 min, beginning 30 min before chemotherapy, or in two or three divided doses, with the first usually given 30 min before and subsequent doses at various intervals after chemotherapy. The drugs also can be used intramuscularly (*ondansetron* only) or orally. *Granisetron* is available as a transdermal formulation that is applied 24–48 h before chemotherapy and worn for up to 7 days.

In general, these drugs are very well tolerated, with the most common adverse effects being constipation or diarrhea, headache, and lightheadedness. Electrocardiogram interval changes (QT prolongation) are a feature of the first-generation antagonists; the injectable form of *dolasetron* is contraindicated for prophylactic therapy for chemotherapy-induced nausea and vomiting. The oral form is associated with a lower risk, but risk is still present. *Palonosetron* does not appear to increase QT intervals (Gonullu et al., 2012). These drugs have also been associated with serotonin syndrome and should be used cautiously if patients are taking other medications, such as SSRIs, that could increase 5HT levels.

Dopamine Receptor Antagonists

Mechanism of Action and Pharmacology. The principal mechanism of action of dopamine receptor antagonists is D_2 receptor antagonism at the CTZ, reducing excitatory neurotransmitter release (Andrews and Sanger, 2014; Kovac, 2013).

Phenothiazines. *Prochlorperazine*, and to a lesser extent *chlorpromazine* (see Chapter 16), are among the most commonly used "general-purpose" antinauseants and antiemetics in adults and children. These drugs are not uniformly effective in cancer chemotherapy-induced emesis, but they possess antihistaminic and anticholinergic activities that are of value in other forms of nausea and vomiting, such as motion sickness and that of GI origin. These drugs are available as tablets, injectables, or suppositories. Typical dosing of *prochlorperazine* is 5–10 mg orally every 6–8 h, 5–10 mg intramuscularly, or 2.5 mg to 10 mg intravenously every 3–4 h (maximum 40 mg/d), or 25 mg rectally every 12 h. The main adverse effects are extrapyramidal reactions, including dystonia, cardiac effects, and hypotension. These drugs are contraindicated due to increased mortality in elderly patients with dementia-related psychosis.

TABLE 50–6 ■ $5HT_3$ ANTAGONISTS IN CHEMOTHERAPY-INDUCED NAUSEA/EMESIS

DRUG	CHEMICAL NATURE	RECEPTOR INTERACTIONS	$t_{1/2}$	ADULT DOSE (IV)
Ondansetron	Carbazole derivative	$5HT_3$ antagonist, weak $5HT_4$ antagonist	3.9 h	0.15 mg/kg
Granisetron	Indazole	$5HT_3$ antagonist	9–11.6 h	10 μg/kg
Dolasetron (not approved in the U.S.)	Indole moiety	$5HT_3$ antagonist	7–9 h	1.8 mg/kg
Palonosetron	Isoquinoline	$5HT_3$ antagonist; highest affinity for $5HT_3$ receptor in class	40 h	0.25 mg

Benzamides. The prokinetic benzamide agents (see previous discussion) are moderately useful antiemetics, but are no longer the drugs of choice for acute chemotherapy-induced nausea and vomiting due to their lack of efficacy and side-effect profile. However, the antiemetic actions add to their value in the treatment of GI motor disturbances, and metoclopramide is a useful treatment of delayed emesis.

Trimethobenzamide is given for gastroenteritis and postoperative nausea and vomiting (orally at doses of 300 mg every 6 h or 200 mg IM).

Olanzapine. Olanzapine is an atypical (second-generation) antipsychotic that is a dopamine (D_{1-4}) and $5HT_2$ receptor antagonist (see Chapter 16). It is an effective agent for the prevention of chemotherapy-associated delayed nausea or vomiting (off-label use; used in combination with a corticosteroid and $5HT_3$ antagonist) (Fonte et al., 2015). It is also gaining attention for the treatment of refractory non–chemotherapy-induced nausea and vomiting. It is given orally, 10 mg once daily for 3 to 5 days, beginning on day 1 of chemotherapy or 5 mg once daily for 2 days before chemotherapy, followed by 10 mg once daily (beginning on the day of chemotherapy) for 3 to 8 days. The adverse reactions are extensive and include many CNS, cardiovascular, and metabolic side effects that are described in Chapter 16.

Antihistamines

Histamine H_1 antagonists are primarily useful for motion sickness and postoperative emesis. They act on vestibular afferents and within the brainstem. *Cyclizine*, *meclizine*, *promethazine*, and *diphenhydramine* are examples of this class of agents. *Cyclizine* has additional anticholinergic effects that may be useful for patients with abdominal cancer. Sedation is always a common side effect of these drugs. For a detailed discussion of these drugs, see Chapter 39.

Anticholinergic Agents

The most commonly used muscarinic receptor antagonist for motion sickness is *scopolamine* (hyoscine), which can be injected as the hydrobromide, but usually is administered as the free base in the form of a transdermal patch (1.5 mg every 3 days). Its principal utility is in the prevention and treatment of motion sickness, with some activity in postoperative nausea and vomiting. In general, however, anticholinergic agents have no role in chemotherapy-induced nausea. The principle side effects are dry mouth, visual disturbances, and drowsiness.

Neurokinin Receptor Antagonists

Mechanism of Action and Pharmacology. The nausea and vomiting associated with emetogenic chemotherapy (see Chapter 65) has two components: an acute phase that universally is experienced (within 24 h after chemotherapy) and a delayed phase that affects only some patients (on days 2–5). $5HT_3$ receptor antagonists are not very effective against delayed emesis. However, antagonists of the NK_1 receptors, the receptors for the neuropeptide substance P, such as *aprepitant* (and its parenteral formulation *fosaprepitant*), have antiemetic effects in delayed nausea and improve the efficacy of standard antiemetic regimens in patients receiving multiple cycles of chemotherapy (Aapro et al., 2015). A new, highly selective NK_1 antagonist, *rolapitant*, with an exceptionally long plasma $t_{1/2}$ (180 h) was FDA approved in September 2015 for prevention of chemotherapy-induced delayed emesis.

Aprepitant. The NK_1 antagonist aprepitant is typically given with a $5HT_3$ antagonist and dexamethasone.

> **ADME.** After absorption, *aprepitant* is bound extensively to plasma proteins (>95%); it is metabolized primarily by hepatic CYP3A4 and is excreted in the stools; its $t_{1/2}$ is 9–13 h. *Aprepitant* has the potential to interact with other substrates of CYP3A4, requiring adjustment of other drugs, including dexamethasone, methylprednisolone (whose dose may need to be reduced by 50%), and warfarin.
>
> **Therapeutic Uses and Adverse Effects.** *Aprepitant* is contraindicated in patients on cisapride or pimozide, in whom life-threatening QT prolongation has been reported. *Aprepitant* is supplied in 40-, 80-, and 125-mg capsules and is administered for 3 days in conjunction with highly emetogenic chemotherapy, along with a $5HT_3$ antagonist and

a corticosteroid. The injectable form, fosaprepitant, in a dose of 115 mg, may be substituted for the first dose of aprepitant at the start of the 3-day regimen. The recommended adult dosage of aprepitant is 125 mg administered 1 h before chemotherapy on day 1, followed by 80 mg once daily in the morning on days 2 and 3 of the treatment regimen.

Rolapitant. Rolapitant is a potent NK_1 receptor antagonist that is administered with a $5HT_3$ antagonist and dexamethasone to help prevent delayed phase chemotherapy-induced nausea and vomiting.

> **ADME.** After a single oral dose of 180 mg, rolapitant is well absorbed with peak C_p at 4 h and $t_{1/2}$ at about 180 h. *Rolapitant* is metabolized primarily by CYP3A4 to form an active metabolite, M19 (C4-pyrrolidine-hydroxylated rolapitant). M19 has a $t_{1/2}$ of about 158 h. Rolapitant is eliminated mainly via the hepatic/biliary route.
>
> **Therapeutic Uses and Adverse Effects.** A single 180-mg dose is administered orally 1–2 h prior to chemotherapy (together with $5HT_3$ antagonist and dexamethasone). The adverse effects include neutropenia, hiccups, decreased appetite, and dizziness. *Rolapitant* is a moderate inhibitor of CYP2D6 and of the Pgp and BCRP transporters. *Rolapitant* is contraindicated in patients receiving drugs that are CYP2D6 substrates, such as thioridazine or pimozide. A significant increase in plasma concentrations of thioridazine may result in QT prolongation and torsades de pointes.

Netupitant and Palonesetron Combination. A combination NK_1 *receptor antagonist* plus $5HT_3$ *receptor antagonist* (netupitant and palonesetron) was recently approved (Abramovitz and Gaertner, 2016).

> **ADME.** This combination is well absorbed; the drugs have a similar time to peak C_p (5 h) and very long half-lives (*netupitant*, ~ 80 h; *palonesetron*, ~ 48 h). They are excreted in the feces and urine. *Netupitant* is extensively metabolized by CYP3A4 (major) and CYP2C9 and CYP2D6 (minor) to active metabolites. *Palonesetron* is about 50% metabolized in the liver to inactive metabolites.
>
> **Therapeutic Uses and Adverse Effects.** A single capsule is administered orally about 1 h prior to chemotherapy (together with dexamethasone, at doses varying according to the type of chemotherapy). The adverse effects are the same as for the $5HT_3$ antagonists (see previous discussion).

Cannabinoids

Dronabinol. **Mechanism of Action and Pharmacology.** Dronabinol (Δ-9-tetrahydrocannabinol) is a naturally occurring cannabinoid that can be synthesized chemically or extracted from the marijuana plant, *Cannabis sativa*. The mechanism of the antiemetic action of dronabinol is related to stimulation of the CB_1 subtype of cannabinoid receptors on neurons in and around the CTZ and emetic center (see Figure 50–5) (Sharkey et al., 2014).

> **ADME.** Dronabinol is a highly lipid-soluble compound that is absorbed readily after oral administration; its onset of action occurs within an hour, and peak levels are achieved within 2–4 h. It undergoes extensive first-pass metabolism with limited systemic bioavailability after single doses (only 10%–20%). The principal active metabolite is 11-OH-delta-9-tetrahydrocannabinol. These metabolites are excreted primarily via the biliary-fecal route, with only 10%–15% excreted in the urine. Both dronabinol and its metabolites are highly bound (>95%) to plasma proteins. Because of its large volume of distribution, a single dose of dronabinol can result in detectable levels of metabolites for several weeks.
>
> **Therapeutic Uses and Adverse Effects.** Dronabinol is a useful prophylactic agent in patients receiving cancer chemotherapy when other antiemetic medications are not effective. It also can stimulate appetite and has been used in patients with AIDS and anorexia. As an antiemetic agent, it is administered at an initial dose of 5 mg/m² given 1–3 h before chemotherapy and then every 2–4 h afterward for a total of four to six doses. If this is inadequate, incremental increases can be made up to a maximum of 15 mg/m² per dose. For other indications, the usual starting dose is 2.5 mg twice a day; this can be titrated up to a maximum of 20 mg per day.

Dronabinol has complex effects on the CNS, including a prominent central sympathomimetic activity. This can lead to palpitations, tachycardia, vasodilation, hypotension, and conjunctival injection (bloodshot eyes). Patient supervision is necessary because marijuana-like "highs" (e.g., euphoria, somnolence, detachment, dizziness, anxiety, nervousness, panic, etc.) can occur, as can more disturbing effects such as paranoid reactions and abnormalities of thinking. After abrupt withdrawal of dronabinol, an abstinence syndrome (irritability, insomnia, and restlessness) can occur. Because of its high affinity for plasma proteins, dronabinol can displace other plasma protein-bound drugs, whose doses may have to be adjusted as a consequence. Dronabinol should be prescribed with great caution to persons with a history of substance abuse (alcohol, drugs) because it also may be abused by these patients.

Nabilone. **Mechanism of Action and Pharmacology.** Nabilone is a synthetic cannabinoid with a mode of action similar to that of dronabinol.

ADME. Nabilone is a highly lipid-soluble compound that is rapidly absorbed after oral administration; its onset of action occurs within an hour, and peak levels are achieved within 2 h. The $t_{1/2}$ is about 2 h for the parent compound and 35 h for metabolites. The metabolites are excreted primarily via the biliary-fecal route (60%), with only about 25% excreted in the urine.

Therapeutic Uses and Adverse Effects. Nabilone is a useful prophylactic agent in patients receiving cancer chemotherapy when other antiemetic medications are not effective. A dose (1–2 mg) can be given the night before chemotherapy; usual dosing starts 1–3 h before treatment and then every 8–12 h during the course of chemotherapy and for 2 days following its cessation. The adverse effects are largely the same as for dronabinol, with significant CNS actions in more than 10% of patients. Cardiovascular, GI, and other side effects are also common and, together with the CNS actions, limit the usefulness of this agent.

Glucocorticoids and Anti-inflammatory Agents

Glucocorticoids such as dexamethasone can be useful adjuncts (see Table 50–5) in the treatment of nausea in patients with widespread cancer, possibly by suppressing peritumoral inflammation and prostaglandin production. A similar mechanism has been invoked to explain beneficial effects of NSAIDs in the nausea and vomiting induced by systemic irradiation (Chu et al., 2014). For a detailed discussion of these drugs, see Chapters 38 and 46.

Benzodiazepines

Benzodiazepines, such as *lorazepam* and *alprazolam*, by themselves are not very effective antiemetics, but their sedative, amnesic, and antianxiety effects can be helpful in reducing the anticipatory component of nausea and vomiting in patients. For a detailed discussion of these drugs, see Chapter 19.

Phosphorated Carbohydrate Solutions

Aqueous OTC solutions of *glucose, fructose,* and *orthophosphoric* are available to relieve nausea. These solutions are given orally (15–30 mL, adults; 5–10 mL, children; repeated every 15 min until the symptoms alleviate. No more than five doses may be taken). Their mechanisms of action are unclear.

Doxylamine Succinate and Pyridoxine

Mechanism of Action and Pharmacology. Nausea commonly occurs in the early stages of pregnancy. This may or may not be accompanied by vomiting. The management of this condition depends of the severity of symptoms, which usually resolve by midpregnancy regardless of their severity. *Pyridoxine* (vitamin B_6) improves mild-to-moderate nausea and its efficacy is improved when it is combined with the histamine H_1 antagonist *doxylamine* (Fantasia, 2014). Considering the caveats associated with the use of antinausea medications during early pregnancy, readers may wish to review the history of this drug combination; see the work of Slaughter et al., 2014.

ADME. *Doxylamine* is metabolized in the liver by N-dealkylation. It has a $t_{1/2}$ of 10–12 h and is excreted in the urine. *Pyridoxine* is well absorbed and has a $t_{1/2}$ of 2–3 weeks.

Therapeutic Uses and Adverse Effects. This drug-vitamin combination is given for the treatment of nausea and vomiting of pregnancy. Initially, 2 delayed-release tablets (a total of *doxylamine* 20 mg and pyridoxine 20 mg) are taken at bedtime. The dose may be increased to 4 tablets per day as needed for more severe nausea (1 tablet in the morning, 1 tablet in the afternoon, 2 tablets at bedtime). The major side effects of this drug include drowsiness, dry mouth, light-headedness, and constipation.

Miscellaneous GI Disorders

Cystic Fibrosis, Chronic Pancreatitis, and Steatorrhea

Pancreatic Enzymes

Chronic pancreatitis is a debilitating syndrome that results in symptoms from loss of glandular function (exocrine and endocrine) and inflammation (pain). The goals of pharmacological therapy are prevention of malabsorption and palliation of pain (Trang et al., 2014). *Cystic fibrosis* is a genetic disorder that affects exocrine secretion. Exocrine pancreatic insufficiency occurs in the majority of patients with more severe forms of cystic fibrosis. Pharmacological therapy is used to treat these patients (Somaraju and Solis-Moya, 2014).

Enzyme Formulations. Pancreatic enzymes (lipase, amylase, and proteases) are secreted together; hence, lipase can be used to titrate the doses of pancreatic enzyme supplements, which are typically prescribed on the basis of the lipase content. Only *pancrelipase* is licensed for sale in the U.S. Pancrelipase products, of which there are six on the market, differ in their content of lipase, protease, and amylase and thus may not be interchangeable.

Replacement Therapy for Malabsorption. Fat malabsorption (*steatorrhea*) and protein maldigestion occur when the pancreas loses more than 90% of its ability to produce digestive enzymes. This occurs in chronic pancreatitis, following pancreatectomy, or in cystic fibrosis. The resultant diarrhea and malabsorption can be managed well if 90,000 USP units of pancreatic lipase are delivered to the duodenum during a 4-h period with and after meals. Alternatively, one can titrate the dosage to the fat content of the diet, with about 8000 USP units of lipase activity required for each 17 g of dietary fat. Available preparations of pancreatic enzymes contain 3000–40,000 USP units of lipase, 10,000–136,000 USP units of protease, and 15,000–218,000 USP units of amylase. In adults and children over 4 years, the initial dose of lipase is 500 USP units/kg/meal, increasing up to 2500 USP units/kg/meal. Children younger than 4 have increased needs for lipase, and initial doses are higher. There are also special dosing regimens for breastfeeding infants. In all cases, lipase dosing should not exceed maximum recommendations and generally should not exceed 2500 USP units/kg/meal or 10,000 USP unit/kg/d.

Enzymes for Pain. Pain is the other cardinal symptom of chronic pancreatitis. The rationale for its treatment with pancreatic enzymes is based on the principle of negative-feedback inhibition of the pancreas by the presence of duodenal proteases. The release of CCK, the principal secretagogue for pancreatic enzymes, is triggered by CCK-releasing monitor peptide in the duodenum, which normally is denatured by pancreatic trypsin. In chronic pancreatitis, trypsin insufficiency leads to persistent activation of this peptide and an increased release of CCK, which is thought to cause pancreatic pain because of continuous stimulation of pancreatic enzyme output and increased intraductal pressure. Delivery of active proteases to the duodenum (which can be done reliably only with uncoated preparations) therefore is important for the interruption of this loop. Although enzymatic therapy has become firmly entrenched for the treatment of painful pancreatitis, the evidence supporting this practice is equivocal at best.

Adverse Effects. Despite the fact that the enzymes are not absorbed and are excreted in feces, there are adverse effects, which include headache and abdominal pain; however, pancreatic enzyme preparations are tolerated extremely well by patients. Hyperuricosuria in patients with cystic fibrosis can occur, and malabsorption of folate and iron has been reported.

Gallstones and Primary Biliary Cirrhosis

Bile Acids

Bile acids and their conjugates are synthesized from cholesterol in the liver. Bile acids induce bile flow, feedback-inhibit cholesterol synthesis, promote intestinal excretion of cholesterol, and facilitate the emulsification and absorption of lipids and fat-soluble vitamins. After secretion into the biliary tract, bile acids are largely (95%) reabsorbed in the intestine, returned to the liver, and then again secreted in bile (enterohepatic circulation). Cholic acid, chenodeoxycholic acid, and deoxycholic acid constitute 95% of bile acids; lithocholic acid and ursodeoxycholic acid are minor constituents. The bile acids exist largely as glycine and taurine conjugates, the salts of which are called bile salts.

Traditional therapy for gallstones involves oral litholysis with *ursodeoxycholic acid* (ursodiol), but there is now evidence that inhibiting cholesterol synthesis (with statins) or intestinal cholesterol absorption (with ezetimibe) may have some beneficial effects to reduce gallstone formation (Portincasa et al., 2012). As for the treatment of gallstones, treatments for primary biliary cirrhosis also involve the use of *ursodeoxycholic acid*. New therapies are being developed that include *obeticholic acid*, a semisynthetic analogue of *chenodeoxycholic acid*, an endogenous ligand of the farnesoid X receptor (a nuclear receptor important for regulating bile acid and cholesterol metabolism), and treatment with fibrates, peroxisome proliferator-activated receptor alpha agonists. Another promising therapy includes combining *ursodeoxycholic acid* with the steroid budesonide (see Chapter 46) for the treatment of early-stage primary biliary cirrhosis (Tabibian and Lindor, 2015).

Ursodeoxycholic acid (ursodiol) (Figure 50–6) is a hydrophilic, dehydroxylated bile acid that is formed by epimerization of the bile acid chenodeoxycholic acid (chenodiol) in the gut by intestinal bacteria. Ursodiol is given for the prevention and treatment of gallstones and for the treatment of primary biliary cirrhosis (Portincasa et al., 2012; Tabibian and Lindor, 2015). When administered orally, litholytic bile acids such as chenodiol and ursodiol alter relative concentrations of bile acids, decrease biliary lipid secretion, and reduce the cholesterol content of the bile so that it is less lithogenic. *Ursodiol* also may have cytoprotective effects on hepatocytes and effects on the immune system that account for some of its beneficial effects in cholestatic liver diseases. For gallstone treatment, it is given orally 8–10 mg/kg/d in divided doses, for gallstone prevention 300 mg twice daily, and for primary biliary cirrhosis 13–15 mg/kg/d in two to four divided doses with food. Adverse effects at these doses are generally uncommon, but include headache, GI disturbances, and nausea. At higher-than-recommended doses, there may be serious adverse effects of *ursodiol*. Dissolution of gallstones by chenodiol is reserved for patients who are at increased surgical risk and have radiolucent stones.

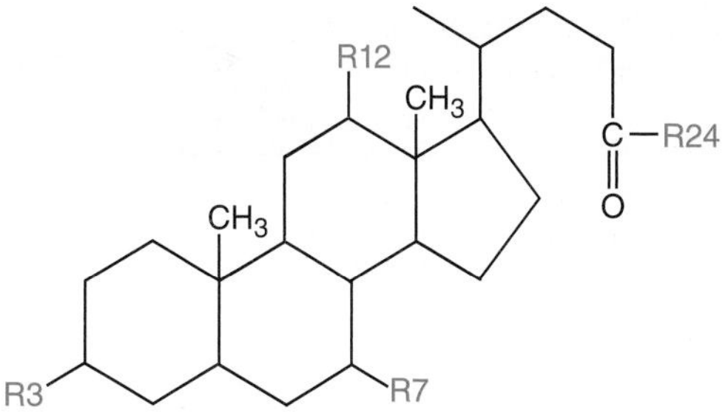

Flatulence

"Gas" is a common but relatively vague GI complaint, used in reference not only to flatulence and eructation but also bloating or fullness. OTC and herbal preparations are popular. *Simethicone*, a mixture of siloxane polymers stabilized with silicon dioxide, is an inert nontoxic, insoluble liquid. Because of its capacity to collapse bubbles by forming a thin layer on their surface, it is an effective antifoaming agent; whether this accomplishes a therapeutic effect in the GI tract is not clear. Simethicone is available in chewable tablets, liquid-filled capsules, suspensions, and orally disintegrating strips, either by itself or in combination with other OTC medications, including antacids and other digestants. The usual dosage in adults is 40–125 mg four times daily after meals; the pediatric

Figure 50–6 *Major bile acids in adults.*

Bile Acid	R3	R7	R12	R24
Cholic acid	–OH	–OH	–OH	
Chenodeoxycholic acid	–OH	–OH	–H	glycine (75%)
Deoxycholic acid	–OH	–H	–OH	taurine (24%)
Lithocholic acid	–SO₂⁻ / –OH	–H	–H	–OH (<1%)
Ursodeoxycholic acid	–OH	◄OH	–H	

dose is 20–50 mg four times daily after meals and at bedtime, depending on the age of the child. Activated charcoal may be used alone or in combination with simethicone but has not been shown conclusively to have much benefit. An α-galactosidase OTC preparation is available to reduce gas from baked beans.

Short-Bowel Syndrome

Short-bowel syndrome is a malabsorption disorder caused by removal of the small intestine or rarely because of a congenital bowel abnormality. Short-bowel syndrome requires total *parenteral nutrition*, and treatments are aimed at reducing the need for this, including supplemented specialized diets and implementing a therapy based on physiologic principles of the actions of gut hormones.

Teduglutide

Mechanism of Action and Pharmacology. The gut hormone GLP-2 is secreted by L cells of the ileum and colon and is the only intestinotrophic gut peptide. Among other actions, it enhances growth of the intestinal mucosa through the release of mediators, including insulin-like growth factor 1. *Teduglutide* is a 33–amino acid GLP-2 analogue recently approved for the treatment of short-bowel syndrome (Jeppesen, 2015).

ADME. The drug has a $t_{1/2}$ of 1–2 h and is excreted in the urine. It is catabolized by dipeptidyl peptidase 4, but more slowly than the native peptide because of the substituted amino acid structure.

Therapeutic Uses and Adverse Effects. *Teduglutide* is administered subcutaneously once daily (0.05 mg/kg) to help improve intestinal absorption of nutrients and thereby reduce the need for parenteral support. Common side effects include abdominal pain, nausea, headache, and flu-like symptoms. There is also the potential for *teduglutide* to cause cancer of the bowel; therefore, it is not recommended for patients with active malignancies.

Acknowledgment: *Laurence L. Brunton, Pankaj Jay Pasricha, and John L. Wallace contributed to this chapter in earlier editions of this book. We have retained some of their text in the current edition.*

Drug Facts for Your Personal Formulary: *Antisecretory Agents and Gastroprotectives*

Drugs	Therapeutic Uses	Clinical Pharmacology and Tips
Prokinetic Agents (agents acting through specific receptors to regulate GI motility)		
MOR antagonist Alvimopan	• Postoperative ileus	• Myocardial infarction • Hypokalemia • Dyspepsia

5HT$_4$ receptor agonists
  Cisapride
  Prucalopride
	• Gastroesophageal reflux disease
	• Gastroparesis
	• Intestinal pseudoobstruction
	• Severe constipation
	• Neonatal feeding intolerance
		• Serious cardiac risks
		• Headache
		• Diarrhea

D$_2$ receptor antagonist
  Domperidone
  Metoclopramide (also 5HT$_3$ receptor antagonist, 5HT$_4$ receptor agonist)
	• Gastroparesis
	• Prevention of nausea and vomiting
		• Serious cardiac risks, especially in older persons
		• Limited pediatric use
		• Tardive dyskinesia
		• Limited pediatric use
		• Short-term use only

Motilin receptors Erythromycin (stimulate motilin receptors on GI smooth muscle cells)	• Gastroparesis	• Short-term use only • Ototoxicity • Pseudomembranous colitis • Cardiac risks

CCK peptide analogue
  Sincalide
  (C-terminal octapeptide of CCK)
	• Intravenous injection
	• Gallbladder contraction
	• Pancreatic secretion
	• Intestinal motility
	• Accelerates barium transit through small bowel for diagnostic testing
		• Nausea, vomiting, diarrhea
		• Sweating
		• Light-headed
		• Headache
		• May cause serious allergic reactions

Laxatives		
Dietary Fiber		
Psyllium Methylcellulose	• Increase fecal bulk	• Bloating
Stool-Softening Agents		
Docusate	• Constipation	• Marginal efficacy
Mineral oil	• Constipation	• Side effects preclude regular use • Interferes with absorption of fat-soluble vitamins • Oil leakage
Osmotically Active Agents		
Polyethylene glycol–electrolyte solutions	• Colonic cleansing prior to examination • Constipation (powder form)	• Nausea • Cramping and bloating
Saline laxatives–Mg^{2+}	• Constipation	• Urgency • Watery stools • Renal insufficiency • Heart disease • Diuretic therapy

Nondigestible sugars and alcohols
  Lactulose
  Sorbitol
	• Constipation caused by opioids
	• Idiopathic chronic constipation
	• Lactulose also used to treat hepatic encephalopathy
		• Abdominal discomfort
		• Flatulence

Stimulant Laxatives		

Diphenylmethane derivatives
  Bisacodyl
  Sodium picosulfate
	• Constipation
	• Bowel cleansing prior to colonoscopy
		• Can damage mucosa
		• Inflammatory response
		• May cause hypermagnesemia
		• May decrease glomerular filtration rate

Anthraquinone laxatives Senna	• Constipation	• Plant derivatives • Melanosis coli • Nausea and vomiting • Cramping

Laxatives (continued)

Ricinoleic acid Castor oil	• Act on small intestine • Stimulate secretion • Increase intestinal transit	• Potential toxic effect from ricin • Not clinically recommended
Enemas and suppositories Glycerin	• Bowel distension • Glycerin for rectal use	• Discomfort

Pro-Secretory Agents

Guanylate cyclase-C agonist
    Linaclotide
    Plecanatide
	• Opioid-induced constipation	• Contraindicated in children up to 6 years
		• Diarrhea

Cl⁻ channel activator Lubiprostone	• Chronic idiopathic constipation • Opioid-induced constipation • IBS with constipation	• Nausea • Diarrhea

Drugs for Opioid-Induced Constipation

MOR antagonists
    Methylnaltrexone
    Naloxegol
    Naldemedine
	• Opioid-induced constipation	• Peripheral MOR antagonist
		• Diarrhea
		• Abdominal pain
		• Nausea and vomiting
		• Flatulence

Opioid receptor agonist/antagonist Oxycodone:naloxone (2:1 ratio)	• Opioid-induced constipation	• Respiratory depression • Addiction • Nausea and vomiting • Constipation • Diarrhea

Antidiarrheal Agents

5HT$_3$ receptor antagonist Alosetron	• Diarrhea-predominant IBS in women	• Ischemic colitis • Constipation

Antibiotics—empiric therapy
Fluoroquinolone
    Ciprofloxacin
    Levofloxacin
    Norfloxacin
    Ofloxacin
Alternative antibiotics
    Azithromycin
    Rifaxamin
	• Acute diarrhea
	• Traveler's diarrhea
	
	• Azithromycin: preferred treatment for children with traveler's diarrhea
	• Rifaxamin: preferred for diarrhea-predominant IBS
		• Avoid if *Escherichia coli* suspected
		• Avoid if *Clostridium difficile* suspected
		• Controversial in children (azithromycin is preferred for children)
		• Nausea
		• Peripheral edema
		• Dizziness

Bile acid sequestrants
    Cholestyramine
    Colesevelam
    Colestipol
	• Bile salt–induced diarrhea	• Bloating
		• Flatulence
		• Abdominal discomfort
		• Constipation

Bismuth subsalicylate	• Acute diarrhea • Nausea and abdominal cramping	• Dark stools
α$_2$ adrenergic receptor agonist Clonidine	• Diabetic diarrhea	• Hypotension • Depression • Drowsiness • Fatigue
Crofelemer (plant derived)	• HIV/AIDS diarrhea	• Infectious diarrhea must not be suspected • Inhibits CFTR and reduces Cl⁻secretion

MOR agonists
    Diphenoxylate
    Difenoxin
    Loperamide
	• Acute diarrhea
	• Chronic diarrhea
	• Traveler's diarrhea
		• Limit use to 10 days
		• Use with caution in children
		• Constipation
		• Toxic megacolon
		• CNS depression in children
		• Paralytic ileus

MOR/KOR agonist DOR antagonist Eluxadoline	• Diarrhea-predominant IBS	• Pancreatitis • Sphincter of Oddi spasm • Constipation
SST receptor agonist Octreotide	• Severe secretory diarrhea due to GI tumors • Postgastrectomy dumping syndrome	• Sinus bradycardia • Chest pain • Headache • Abdominal pain • Nausea • Diarrhea

SECTION VI GASTROINTESTINAL PHARMACOLOGY

Drug Facts for Your Personal Formulary: *Antisecretory Agents and Gastroprotectives (continued)*

Drugs	Therapeutic Uses	Clinical Pharmacology and Tips
Antidiarrheal Agents (continued)		
Enkephalinase inhibitor Racecadotril	• Acute diarrhea	• Proven safety in children

Tryptophan hydroxylase inhibitor
  Telotristat ethyl
	• Severe diarrhea due to carcinoid tumors	• Adverse Effects: Constipation, Nausea, Headache,
		  Depression

Antispasmodic Agents (Anticholinergics)		
Dicyclomine Glycopyrrolate Hyoscyamine Methscopolamine	• Abdominal and urgency in IBS	• Contraindicated in colitis, reflux esophagitis, and bowel obstruction • Dizziness • Dry mouth • Nausea • Blurred vision
Antiemetic Agents		

Antihistamines
  Cyclizine, diphenhydramine, meclizine,
  promethazine
	• Motion sickness
	• Nausea and vomiting
		• Sedation
		• Dry mouth
		• Promethazine is contraindicated in children < 2 years old

Doxylamine succinate and pyridoxine (H_1 receptor antagonist and vitamin B_6)	• Nausea and vomiting of pregnancy	• Drowsiness • Dry mouth • Light-headedness • Constipation

NK_1 *antagonists*
  Aprepitant
  Rolapitant
	• Chemotherapy-induced nausea and
	  vomiting
	• Postoperative nausea and vomiting
		• Given with dexamethasone and a $5HT_3$ antagonist
		• Contraindicated in patients on cisapride, pimozide, or thioridazine
		• Fatigue, constipation, hiccups

$5HT_3$ *antagonists*
  Dolasetron
  Granisetron
  Ondansetron
  Palonesetron
  Tropisetron
	• Chemotherapy-induced nausea and
	  vomiting
	• Radiation-induced nausea and vomiting
	• Postoperative nausea and vomiting
		• ECG effects
		• Serotonin syndrome
		• Headache
		• Constipation
		• Fatigue
		• Malaise

$NK_1/5HT_3$ *antagonists*
  Netupitant
  Palonesetron
	• Chemotherapy-induced nausea and
	  vomiting
		• Serotonin syndrome
		• Headache
		• Constipation
		• Fatigue

Cannabinoid receptor agonists
  Dronabinol
  Nabilone
	• Chemotherapy-induced nausea and
	  vomiting
		• Psychoactive
		• Many CNS side effects

Dopamine receptor antagonists
  Olanzapine ($5HT_{2A}$ and $5HT_{2C}$, D_{1-4}, H_1,
  α_1 adrenergic, and M receptor
  antagonists)
  Phenothiazines (D_2, H_1, $5HT_{2A}$, M, and
  α_1 receptor antagonists)
  Chlorpromazine
  Prochlorperazine
	• Chemotherapy-induced nausea and
	  vomiting
	• Refractory nausea and vomiting
		• D_2 antagonism at CTZ
		• Somnolence
		• Hypotension
		• Increased mortality in elderly patients with dementia-related
		  psychosis
		• Cardiac effects
		• Extrapyramidal reactions

Muscarinic receptor antagonist Scopolamine	• Motion sickness • Nausea and vomiting	• Cardiovascular actions • Constipation, drowsiness, dry mouth, blurred vision • Many other side effects
Miscellaneous Agents		
Pancreatic enzymes	• Malabsorption (postpancreatectomy; cystic fibrosis) • Pancreatitis pain	• Headache • Abdominal pain
Simethicone	• Flatulence, bloating	
Teduglutide (GLP-2 receptor analogue)	• Short-bowel syndrome	• Colonic polyps/malignancy • Pancreatitis • Abdominal pain and distention • Nausea, headache
Ursodeoxycholic acid (bile acid)	• Dissolution of gallstones	• Nausea, headache • GI disturbances

Aapro M, et al. Aprepitant and fosaprepitant: a 10-year review of efficacy and safety. *Oncologist*, **2015**, *20*:450–458.

Abramovitz RB, Gaertner KM. The role of netupitant and palonesetron in chemotherapy-induced nausea and vomiting. *J Oncol Pharm Pract*, **2016**, *22*:477–484.

Acosta A, Camilleri M. Prokinetics in gastroparesis. *Gastroenterol Clin N Am*, **2015**, *44*:97–111.

Altan E, et al. Evolving pharmacological approaches in gastroesophageal reflux disease. *Expert Opin Emerg Drugs*, **2012**, *17*:347–359.

Andrews PLR, Sanger GJ. Nausea and the quest for the perfect anti-emetic. *Eur J Pharmacol*, **2014**, *722*:108–121.

Bhutta AQ, Garcia-Tsao G. The role of medical therapy for variceal bleeding. *Gastrointest Endoscopy Clin N Am*, **2015**, *25*:479–490.

Bragg D, et al. Postoperative ileus: recent developments in pathophysiology and management. *Clin Nutr*, **2015**, *34*:367–376.

Camilleri M. Current and future pharmacological treatments for diarrhea-predominant irritable bowel syndrome. *Expert Opin Pharmacother*, **2013**, *14*:1151–1160.

Camilleri M. Novel therapeutic agents in neurogastroenterology: advances in the past year. *Neurogastroenterol Motil*, **2014**, *26*:1070–1078.

Chu CC, et al. The cellular mechanisms of the antiemetic action of dexamethasone and related glucocorticoids against vomiting. *Eur J Pharmacol*, **2014**, *722*:48–54.

Corsetti M, Tack J. New pharmacological treatment options for chronic constipation. *Expert Opin Pharmacother*, **2014**, *15*:927–941.

Crutchley RD, et al. Crofelemer, a novel agent for treatment of secretory diarrhea. *Ann Pharmacother*, **2010**, *44*:878–884.

Curran MP, et al. Alvimopan. *Drugs*, **2008**, *68*:2011–2019.

Dekel R, et al. The use of psychotropic drugs in irritable bowel syndrome. *Expert Opin Invest Drugs*, **2013**, *22*:329–339.

Deloose E, et al. The migrating motor complex: control mechanisms and its role in health and disease. *Nat Rev Gastroenterol Hepatol*, **2012**, *9*:271–285.

Diederen K, et al. Efficacy and safety of prucalopride in adults and children with chronic constipation. *Expert Opin Pharmacother*, **2015**, *16*:407–416.

Dinning PG, et al. Pathophysiology of colonic causes of chronic constipation. *Neurogastroenterol Motil*, **2009**, *21*(suppl 2): 20–30.

Drossman DA. The functional gastrointestinal disorders and the Rome III process. *Gastroenterology*, **2006**, *130*:1377–1390.

Emmanuel AV, et al. Pharmacological management of constipation. *Neurogastroenterol Motil*, **2009**, *21* (suppl 2):41–54.

Erdös EG, Skidgel RA. Neutral endopeptidase 24.11 (enkephalinase) and related regulators of peptide hormones. *FASEB J*, **1989**, *3*:145–151.

Fantasia HC. A new pharmacologic therapy for nausea and vomiting of pregnancy. *Nurs Womens Health*, **2014**, *18*:73–77.

Faure C, et al. (eds.) *Pediatric Neurogastroenterology*. Humana Press, Springer, New York, **2012**.

Fonte C, et al. A review of olanzapine as an antiemetic chemotherapy-induced nausea and vomiting and in palliative care patients. *Crit Rev Oncol Hematol*, **2015**, *95*:214–221.

Furness JB. *The Enteric Nervous System*. Wiley-Blackwell, Oxford, UK, **2006**, 286.

Furness JB. The enteric nervous system and neurogastroenterology. *Nat Rev Gastroenterol Hepatol*, **2012**, *9*:286–294.

Gershon MD. 5-Hydroxytryptamine (serotonin) in the gastrointestinal tract. *Curr Opin Endocrinol Diabetes Obes*, **2013**, *20*:14–21.

Gershon MD, Tack J. The serotonin signalling system: From basic understanding to drug development for functional GI disorders. *Gastroenterology*, **2007**, *132*:397–414.

Gonullu G, et al. Electrocardiographic findings of palonosetron in cancer patients. *Support Care Cancer*, **2012**, *20*:1435–1439.

Grundy D, et al. Fundamentals of neurogastroenterology: basic science. *Gastroenterology*, **2006**, *130*: 1391–1411.

Hanauer SB. The role of loperamide in gastrointestinal disorders. *Rev Gastroenterol Disord*, **2008**, *8*:15–20.

Horn CC. Why is the neurobiology of nausea and vomiting so important? *Appetite*, **2008**, *50*:430–434.

Hornby PJ. Central neurocircuitry associated with emesis. *Am J Med*, **2001**, *111*(suppl 8A):106S–112S.

Hornby PJ. Drug discovery approaches to irritable bowel syndrome. *Expert Opin Drug Saf*, **2015**, *10*:809–824.

Huizinga JD, Chen JH. Interstitial cells of Cajal: update on basic and clinical science. *Curr Gastroenterol Rep*, **2014**, *16*:363.

Izzo AA, et al. Recent findings on the mode of action of laxatives: the role of platelet activating factor and nitric oxide. *Trends Pharmacol Sci*, **1998**, *19*:403–405.

Jeppesen PB. Gut hormones in the treatment of short-bowel syndrome and intestinal failure. *Curr Opin Endocrinol Diabetes Obes*, **2015**, *22*:14–20.

Khan S, Chang L. Diagnosis and management of IBS. *Nat Rev Gastroenterol Hepatol*, **2010**, *10*:565–581.

Kovac AL. Update on the management of postoperative nausea and vomiting. *Drugs*, **2013**, *73*:1525–1547.

Lacy BE, et al. Treatment for constipation: new and old pharmacological strategies. *Neurogastroenterol Motil*, **2014**, *26*:749–763.

Li J, et al. Somatostatin and octreotide on the treatment of acute pancreatitis—basic and clinical studies for three decades. *Curr Pharm Des*, **2011**, *17*:1594–1601.

Mayer EA, et a. Brain-gut microbiome interactions and functional bowel disorders. *Gastroenterology*, **2014**, *146*:1500–1512.

Menees S, et al. Agents that act luminally to treat diarrhoea and constipation. *Nat Rev Gastroenterol Hepatol*, **2012**, *9*:881–674.

Navari RM. Management of chemotherapy-induced nausea and vomiting. *Drugs*, **2013**, *73*:249–262.

Navari RM. Palonosetron for the treatment of chemotherapy-induced nausea and vomiting. *Expert Opin Pharmacother*, **2014**, *15*:2599–2608.

Nelson AD, Camilleri M. Opioid-induced constipation: advances and clinical guidance. *Ther Adv Chronic Dis*, **2016**, *7*:121–134.

Pandolfino JE, Gawron AJ. Achalasia: a systematic review. *JAMA*, **2015**, *313*:1841–1852.

Paré P, Fedorak RN. Systematic review of stimulant and nonstimulant laxatives for the treatment of functional constipation. *Can J Gastroenterol Hepatol*, **2014**, *28*:549–557.

Portincasa P, et al. Therapy of gallstone disease: what it was, what it is and what it will be. *World J Gastrointest Pharmacol Ther*, **2012**, *3*:7–20.

Psichas A, et al. Gut chemosensing mechanisms. *J Clin Invest*, **2015**, *125*:908–917.

Reddymasu SC, et al. Domperidone: review of pharmacology and clinical applications in gastroenterology. *Am J Gastroenterol*, **2007**, *102*:2036–2045.

Saadi M, McCallum RW. Rifaximin in irritable bowel syndrome: rationale, evidence and clinical use. *Ther Adv Chronic Dis*, **2013**, *4*:71–75.

Sanders KM, et al. Regulation of gastrointestinal motility—insights from smooth muscle biology. *Nat Rev Gastroenterol Hepatol*, **2012**, *9*:633–645.

Sharkey KA. Emerging roles for enteric glia in gastrointestinal disorders. *J Clin Invest*, **2015**, *125*:918–925.

Sharkey KA, et al. Regulation of nausea and vomiting by cannabinoids and the endocannabinoid system. *Eur J Pharmacol*, **2014**, *722*:134–146.

Sharkey KA, et al. Savidge T. Role of enteric neurotransmission in host defense and protection of the gastrointestinal tract. *Auton Neurosci*, **2014**, *181*:94–106.

Slaughter SR, et al. FDA approval of doxylamine–pyridoxine therapy for use in pregnancy. *N Engl J Med*, **2014**, *370*:1081–1083.

Somaraju UR, Solis-Moya A. Pancreatic enzyme replacement therapy for people with cystic fibrosis. *Cochrane Database Syst Rev*, **2014**, (10):CD008227.

Steffen R, et al. Traveler's diarrhea: a clinical review. *JAMA*, **2015**, *313*:71–80.

Tabibian JH, Lindor KD. Primary biliary cirrhosis: safety and benefits of established and emerging therapies. *Expert Opin Drug Saf*, **2015**, *14*:1435–1444.

Thiagarajah JR, et al. Secretory diarrhoea: mechanisms and emerging therapies. *Nat Rev Gastroenterol Hepatol*, **2015**, *12*:446–457.

SECTION VI GASTROINTESTINAL PHARMACOLOGY

944 Tack J, et al. Systematic review: cardiovascular safety profile of 5HT(4) agonists developed for gastrointestinal disorders. *Aliment Pharmacol Ther*, **2012**, 35:745–767.

Tack J, Zaninotto G. Therapeutic options in esophageal dysphagia. *Nat Rev Gastroenterol Hepatol*, **2015**, 12:332–341.

Trang T, et al. Pancreatic enzyme replacement therapy for pancreatic exocrine insufficiency in the 21st century. *World J Gastrointest Pharmacol Ther*, **2014**, 20:11467–11485.

Wilson N, Schey R. Lubiprostone in constipation: clinical evidence and place in therapy. *Ther Adv Chronic Dis*, **2015**, 6:40–50.

Yu SW, Rao SS. Advances in the management of constipation-predominant irritable syndrome: the role of linaclotide. *Therap Adv Gastroenterol*, **2014**, 7:193–205.

Zala AV, et al. Emerging drugs for functional dyspepsia. *Expert Opin Emerg Drug*, **2015**, 20:221–233.

Zhao X, Pasricha PJ. Botulinum toxin for spastic GI disorders: a systematic review. *Gastrointest Endosc*, **2003**, 57:219–235.

Chapter 51

Pharmacotherapy of Inflammatory Bowel Disease

Wallace K. MacNaughton and Keith A. Sharkey

Inflammatory Bowel Disease

Inflammatory bowel disease is a spectrum of remitting and relapsing, chronic, inflammatory intestinal conditions. IBD causes significant GI symptoms that include diarrhea, abdominal pain, bleeding, anemia, and weight loss. IBD conventionally is divided into two major subtypes: *ulcerative colitis* and *Crohn disease*.

Ulcerative colitis is characterized by confluent mucosal inflammation of the colon starting at the anal verge and extending proximally for a variable extent (e.g., proctitis, left-sided colitis, or pancolitis) (Ordas et al., 2012). *Crohn disease*, by contrast, is characterized by transmural inflammation of any part of the GI tract but most commonly the area adjacent to the ileocecal valve (Sartor, 2006). The inflammation in Crohn disease is not necessarily confluent, frequently leaving "skip areas" of relatively normal mucosa. The transmural nature of the inflammation may lead to fibrosis and strictures or fistula formation. IBD is often associated with extraintestinal manifestations involving the joints, skin, or eyes (Ott and Scholmerich, 2013). Primary sclerosing cholangitis is a serious but infrequent complication of ulcerative colitis in which inflammation and fibrostenosis occurs in the intra- and extrahepatic biliary tree (Williamson and Chapman, 2014). Chronic, severe IBD is associated with an increased risk for the development of colorectal cancer (Beaugerie and Itzkowitz, 2015).

Pathogenesis of IBD

A summary of proposed pathogenic events and potential sites of therapeutic intervention is shown in Figure 51–1. Both diseases are associated with an aberrant immune response to the commensal microbiota of the gut in genetically susceptible individuals (Sartor, 2006). Recent evidence of dysbiosis of the microbiome in IBD supports this theory (Bellaguarda and Chang, 2015). Nevertheless, Crohn disease and ulcerative colitis result from distinct pathogenic mechanisms at the level of mucosal immune activation (Xavier and Podolsky, 2007). Histologically, the transmural lesions in *Crohn disease* exhibit marked infiltration of lymphocytes and macrophages, granuloma formation, and submucosal fibrosis, whereas the superficial lesions in *ulcerative colitis* have lymphocytic and neutrophilic infiltrates.

Our understanding of the pathogenesis of both Crohn disease and ulcerative colitis has increased dramatically in recent years (Kaser et al., 2010). Within the diseased bowel in *Crohn disease*, the cytokine profile includes increased levels of IL-12, IL-23, IFN-γ, and TNF-α, findings characteristic of T_H1-mediated inflammatory processes. In contrast, the inflammatory response in *ulcerative colitis* resembles aspects of that mediated by the T_H2 pathway. Understanding of the inflammatory processes has evolved with the description of regulatory T cells and pro-inflammatory T_H17 cells, a novel T-cell population that expresses IL-23 receptor as a surface marker and produces, among others, the pro-inflammatory cytokines IL-17, IL-21, IL-22, and IL-26. T_H17 cells seem to play a prominent role in intestinal inflammation, particularly in *Crohn disease*.

Medical therapy for IBD is problematic. Because of the multifactorial nature of disease etiology, current therapy for IBD seeks to dampen the generalized inflammatory response. Regrettably, no agent can reliably accomplish this, and the response of an individual patient to a given drug may be limited and unpredictable. Recently, mucosal healing has become an important therapeutic aim, as opposed to simply the relief of symptoms (Florholmen, 2015). Specific goals of pharmacotherapy in IBD include controlling acute exacerbations of the disease, maintaining remission, and treating specific complications, such as fistulas (D'Haens et al., 2014). The major therapeutic options are considered in the following material.

Classifications of Drugs to Treat IBD

Mesalamine-Based Therapy

First-line therapy for mild-to-moderate ulcerative colitis generally involves 5-ASA (Bressler et al., 2015). 5-ASA–based treatments have largely been abandoned in maintenance of remission Crohn disease (Sandborn et al., 2007) due to the fact that their anti-inflammatory effects are targeted topically to the mucosa, with limited effects on deeper inflammation, which has implications for long-term outcomes. The archetype for this class of medications is *sulfasalazine*, which consists of *5-ASA* linked to *sulfapyridine* by an *azo* bond (Figure 51–2).

Mechanism of Action, Pharmacological Properties, and Therapeutic Uses

Sulfasalazine is an oral prodrug that effectively delivers 5-ASA to the distal GI tract (Figure 51–3). The *azo* linkage in *sulfasalazine* prevents absorption in the stomach and small intestine, and the individual components are not liberated until colonic bacterial *azoreductases* cleave the bond for local effect (Peppercorn and Goldman, 1972). 5-ASA is the therapeutic moiety, with little, if any, contribution by *sulfapyridine*, a *sulfonamide antibiotic*. Although 5-ASA is a salicylate and can block COX, its mode of action does not appear to involve this activity; indeed, traditional NSAIDs

Abbreviations

APC: antigen-presenting cell
5-ASA: 5-aminosalicylic acid, mesalamine
COX: cyclooxygenase
FDA: Food and Drug Administration
GI: gastrointestinal
HGPRT: hypoxanthine-guanine phosphoribosyl transferase
HPA: hypothalamic-pituitary-adrenal (axis)
IBD: inflammatory bowel disease
IFN: interferon
IL: interleukin
6-MMP: 6-methyl-mercaptopurine
NSAID: nonsteroidal anti-inflammatory drug
PPAR-γ: peroxisome proliferator-activated receptor gamma
TGF: transforming growth factor
T$_H$: T helper (lymphocyte)
TNF-α: tumor necrosis factor alpha
TPMT: thiopurine methyltransferase
XO: xanthine oxidase

may exacerbate IBD and are strongly contraindicated. Many potential sites of action (effects on immune function and inflammation) have been demonstrated in vitro for *sulfasalazine* and *mesalamine* (Perrotta et al., 2015), including inhibition of the production of IL-1 and TNF-α, inhibition of the lipoxygenase pathway, scavenging of free radicals and oxidants, the inhibition of PPAR-γ, and inhibition of NF-κB, a transcription factor pivotal to production of inflammatory mediators. However, specific mechanisms of action underlying the efficacy of sulfasalazine/5-ASA in IBD have not been identified.

To preserve the therapeutic effect of 5-ASA without the adverse effects of sulfapyridine, several second-generation 5-ASA compounds have been developed. They are divided into two groups: *prodrugs* and *coated drugs*. Prodrugs contain the same azo bond as *sulfasalazine* but replace the linked *sulfapyridine* with either another 5-ASA (*olsalazine*) or an inert compound (*balsalazide*) (Jain et al., 2006). The alternative approaches employ mesalamine directly, using either a delayed-release formulation or a pH-sensitive coating. *Delayed-release mesalamine* releases drug throughout the GI tract, whereas *pH-sensitive mesalamine* is released in the small intestine and colon. These different distributions of drug delivery have potential therapeutic implications (Figure 51–4).

Oral *sulfasalazine* is effective in patients with mild or moderately active ulcerative colitis, with response rates of 60%–80%. The usual dose is 4 g/d in four divided doses with food; to avoid adverse effects, the dose is increased gradually from an initial dose of 500 mg twice a day. Doses as high as 6 g/d can be used but cause an increased incidence of side effects. For patients with severe colitis, *sulfasalazine* is of less-certain value, even though it is often added as an adjunct to systemic glucocorticoids. The drug plays a useful role in preventing relapses once remission has been achieved. Because they lack the dose-related side effects of sulfapyridine, the delayed- and pH-dependent formulations can be used to deliver *mesalamine* with improved safety and tolerability. The doses of *mesalamine* used to treat active disease are 2.4–4.8 g/d for up to 8 weeks, and current practice is to administer 5-ASA as a once-daily dose, which is as effective as a multiple daily dosing regimen (Feagan and Macdonald, 2012).

Topical preparations of *mesalamine* suspended in a wax matrix suppository or in a suspension enema are effective in active proctitis and distal ulcerative colitis, respectively. They appear to be superior to topical hydrocortisone in this setting, with response rates of 75%–90%. *Mesalamine* enemas (4 g/60 mL) should be used at bedtime and retained for at least 8 h; the suppository (500 and 1000 mg) should be used two to three times a day with the objective of retaining it for at least 3 h. Response to

local therapy with mesalamine may occur within 7–14 days; however, the usual course of therapy is from 8 to 16 weeks for induction of remission. Once remission has occurred, lower doses can be considered for maintenance, although increasingly the dose used for induction is continued for maintenance.

ADME

The pharmacokinetics of 5-ASA–based drugs are well described (Sandborn and Hanauer, 2003). About 20%–30% of orally administered *sulfasalazine* (mesalamine prodrug) is absorbed in the small intestine. Much of this is taken up by the liver and excreted unmetabolized in the bile; the rest (~10%) is excreted unchanged in the urine. The remaining 70% reaches the colon, where, if cleaved completely by bacterial enzymes, it generates 400 mg *mesalamine* for every gram of the parent compound. Thereafter, the individual components of *sulfasalazine* follow different metabolic pathways. *Sulfapyridine* is absorbed rapidly from the colon and undergoes extensive hepatic metabolism, including acetylation and hydroxylation, and conjugation with glucuronic acid, prior to excretion in the urine. The acetylation phenotype of the patient determines plasma levels of *sulfapyridine* and the probability of side effects; rapid acetylators have lower systemic levels of the drug and fewer adverse effects. Only 25% of *mesalamine* is absorbed from the colon, and most of the drug is excreted in the stool. The small amount that is absorbed is acetylated in the intestinal mucosal wall and liver and then excreted in the urine. Intraluminal concentrations of *mesalamine* therefore are very high (~1500 μg/mL).

The pH-sensitive coatings limit gastric and small intestinal absorption of mesalamine. The pharmacokinetics of delayed-release formulations differ somewhat. The ethylcellulose-coated microgranules are released in the upper GI tract as discrete prolonged-release units of *mesalamine*. Acetylated *mesalamine* can be detected in the circulation within an hour after ingestion, indicating some rapid absorption, although some intact microgranules can later be detected in the colon. Because the delayed-release drug is released in the small bowel, a greater fraction of the 5-ASA in the delayed-release formulations is absorbed systemically compared with the other 5-ASA preparations.

Adverse Effects

Side effects of *sulfasalazine* occur in 10%–45% of patients with ulcerative colitis and are related primarily to the sulfa moiety. Some are dose related, including headache, nausea, and fatigue; these can be minimized by giving the medication with meals or by decreasing the dose. Allergic reactions include rash, fever, Stevens-Johnson syndrome, hepatitis, pneumonitis, hemolytic anemia, and bone marrow suppression. *Sulfasalazine* reversibly decreases the number and motility of sperm but does not impair female fertility. *Sulfasalazine* inhibits intestinal folate absorption and is usually administered with folate. *Mesalamine* formulations generally are well tolerated. Headache, dyspepsia, and skin rash are the most common side effects. Diarrhea appears to be particularly common with *olsalazine* (occurring in 10%–20% of patients). Nephrotoxicity, although rare, is a more serious concern. *Mesalamine* has been associated with interstitial nephritis; renal function should be monitored in all patients receiving these drugs.

Both *sulfasalazine* and its metabolites cross the placenta but have not been shown to harm the fetus. The newer formulations also appear to be safe in pregnancy, but there have been some safety concerns about dibutyl phthalate, an inactive ingredient in the coating of some formulations, in the context of pregnancy.

Glucocorticoids

The glucocorticoids cortisone, dexamethasone, prednisolone, and triamcinolone are all FDA approved for the treatment of IBD.

Mechanism of Action, Pharmacological Properties, and Therapeutic Uses

The effects of glucocorticoids on the inflammatory response are numerous (see Chapters 42 and 46). Glucocorticoids are indicated for

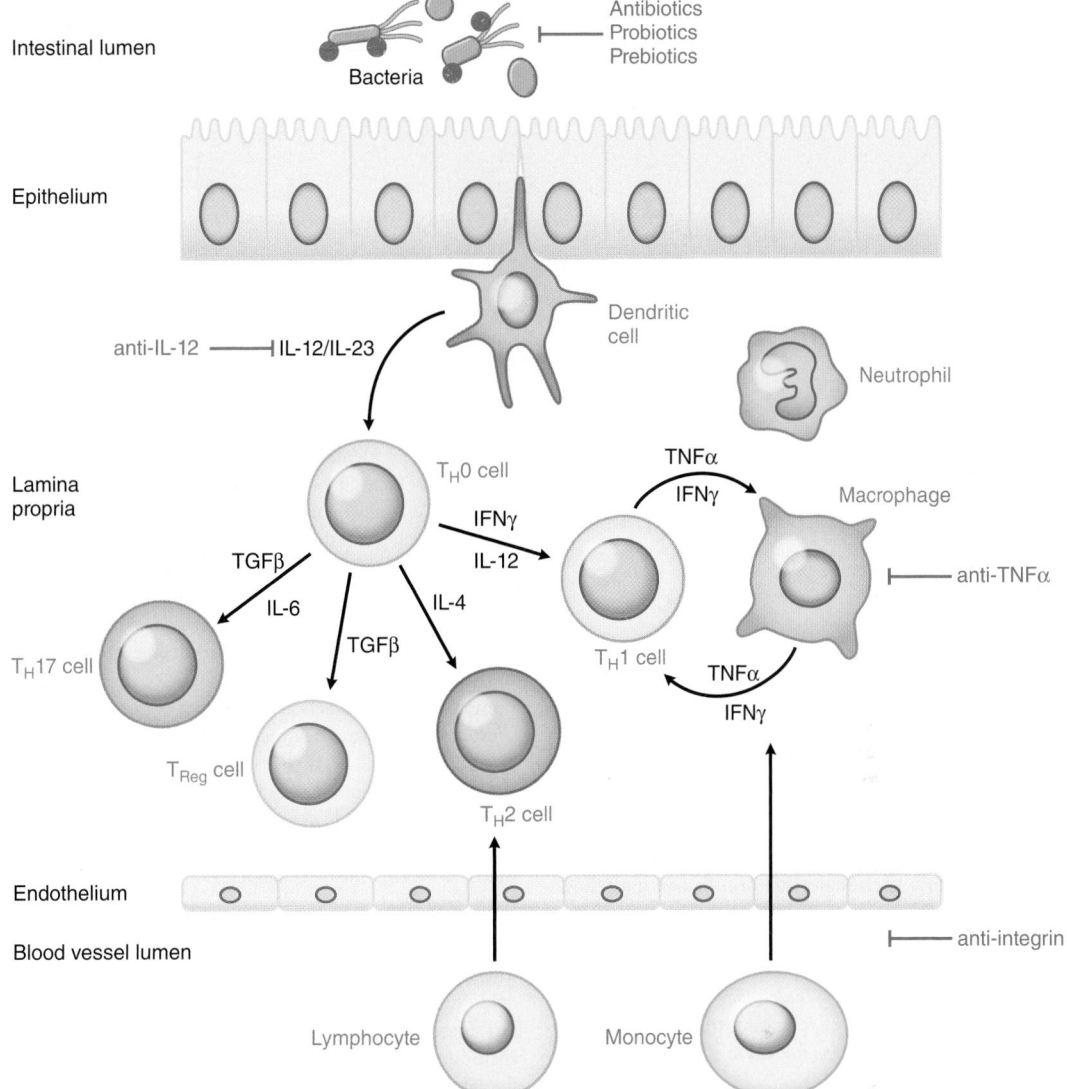

Figure 51–1 *Proposed pathogenesis of IBD and target sites for pharmacological intervention.* Shown are the interactions among bacterial antigens in the intestinal lumen and immune cells in the intestinal wall. If the epithelial barrier is impaired, bacterial antigens can gain access to APCs such as dendritic cells in the lamina propria. These cells then present the antigen(s) to CD4$^+$ lymphocytes and also secrete cytokines such as IL-12 and IL-18, thereby inducing the differentiation of T_H1 cells in Crohn disease (or, under the control of IL-4, T_H2 cells in ulcerative colitis). The balance of pro-inflammatory and anti-inflammatory events is also governed by regulatory T_H17 and T_{Reg} cells, both of which serve to limit immune and inflammatory responses in the GI tract. TGF-β and IL-6 are important cytokines that drive the expansion of the regulatory T-cell subsets. The T_H1 cells produce a characteristic array of cytokines, including IFN-γ and TNF-α, which in turn activate macrophages. Macrophages positively regulate T_H1 cells by secreting additional cytokines, including IFN-γ and TNF-α. Recruitment of a variety of leukocytes is mediated by activation of resident immune cells, including neutrophils. Cell adhesion molecules such as integrins are important in the infiltration of leukocytes, and novel biological therapeutic strategies aimed at blocking leukocyte recruitment are effective at reducing inflammation. General immunosuppressants (e.g., glucocorticoids, thioguanine derivatives, methotrexate, and cyclosporine) affect multiple sites of inflammation. More site-specific interventions involve intestinal bacteria (antibiotics, prebiotics, and probiotics) and therapy directed at TNF-α, IL-12/23, or integrins.

moderate-to-severe IBD. Patients with IBD segregate into three general groups with respect to their response to glucocorticoids:

- *Glucocorticoid-responsive patients* improve clinically within 1–2 weeks and remain in remission as the steroids are tapered and then discontinued.
- *Glucocorticoid-dependent patients* respond to glucocorticoids but then experience a relapse of symptoms as the steroid dose is tapered or discontinued.
- *Glucocorticoid-unresponsive* or *"steroid-resistant" patients* do not improve even with prolonged high-dose steroids.

Glucocorticoids induce a reduction in the inflammatory response and symptomatic remission in most patients with Crohn disease, with improvement generally occurring within 5 days of initiating treatment; however, some patients require treatment for several weeks before remission occurs. Glucocorticoids sometimes are used for prolonged periods to control symptoms in corticosteroid-dependent patients, as these patients will often experience a recurrence of their disease as the glucocorticoid is withdrawn. A proportion of patients with IBD are steroid resistant, and the failure to respond to steroids with prolonged remission (i.e., a disease relapse) should prompt consideration of adjunctive and alternative therapies, including immunosuppressive agents and biological therapies (Manz et al., 2012). Glucocorticoids are not a safe or practical means to maintain remission in either ulcerative colitis or Crohn disease due to the high rate of adverse events associated with their prolonged use. The most commonly used glucocorticoid in Crohn disease is *prednisone,* given orally or intravenously. For more severe cases, glucocorticoids such as *methylprednisolone* or *hydrocortisone* are given intravenously.

948

Sulfasalazine

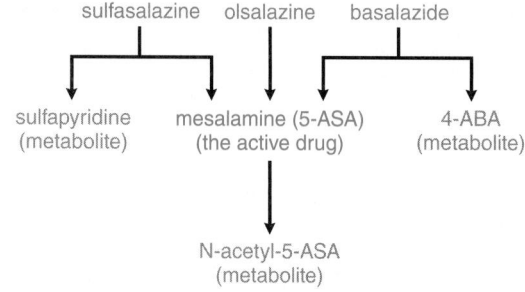

Figure 51–2 *Sulfasalazine and related agents.* The red N atoms indicate the diazo linkage that is cleaved to generate the active moiety.

The enteric-release form of the synthetic steroid, *budesonide,* is used for ileocecal Crohn disease. Its putative action is the delivery of therapeutic quantities of steroid to a specific portion of inflamed gut while minimizing systemic side effects, owing to its local release and extensive first-pass hepatic metabolism to inactive derivatives such that systemic levels remain low. Generally, however, oral *budesonide* is considered less effective than conventional glucocorticoids. *Budesonide* is FDA-approved for use in the short-term maintenance of remission (up to 3 months), although recent studies have suggested it is not more effective than placebo for this indication (Kuenzig et al., 2014).

Glucocorticoid enemas are useful mainly in patients whose disease is limited to the rectum and left colon. *Betamethasone* and *budesonide* are available as retention enemas. Patients with distal disease usually respond within 3–7 days. Absorption, although less than with oral preparations, is still substantial (up to 50%–75%). *Hydrocortisone* also can be given once or twice daily as a 10% foam suspension that delivers 80 mg *hydrocortisone* per application; this formulation can be useful in patients with very short areas of distal proctitis and difficulty retaining enemas.

ADME

Prednisone is the most commonly administered glucocorticoid and is used for the induction of remission of moderate-to-severe Crohn disease in patients who do not respond to 5-ASA drugs (Benchimol et al., 2008).

Figure 51–3 *Metabolic fates of the different oral formulations of 5-ASA.* Chemical structures are in Figure 51–2. 4-ABA, 4-aminobenzoyl-β-alanine.

It is sometimes given as a first-line therapeutic to induce remission. *Prednisone* is most often administered orally but can be administered intravenously when patients present with severe, acute flares of disease. Initial doses in IBD are 40–60 mg of *prednisone* or equivalent per day; higher doses are generally no more effective. Most patients respond within 10–14 days, at which point the dose is reduced by 5 mg per week (tapered) over several weeks to months. *Prednisone* is absorbed at a rate of 50%–90%; 65%–90% of the absorbed drug is protein bound in the serum. It is metabolized to the active compound, *prednisolone,* in the liver. The $t_{1/2}$ for *prednisone* about 3.5 h, with metabolized drug excreted in the urine. Because of the complex nature of the mechanism of action of glucocorticoids, numerous drug interactions have been reported.

Budesonide for the treatment of IBD is administered orally at a dose of 9 mg/d for up to 8 weeks (Kane et al., 2002). There is usually no therapeutic benefit of continuing treatment beyond 3 months. The bioavailability of orally administered *budesonide* is limited (9%–21%) by its high first-pass metabolism. The time to peak serum concentration is 7–19 h when given in capsule form. The $t_{1/2}$ is about 2–3.6 h. Excretion of metabolites is renal (60%) and fecal.

Adverse Effects

The significant adverse events associated with conventional glucocorticoids such as *prednisone* limit their long-term use. These are numerous, but among the more common are skin and soft tissue manifestations, including skin thinning and the development of Cushingoid features (weight redistribution and weight gain). Other side effects include cardiovascular events and psychiatric and cognitive effects. Conventional glucocorticoids can suppress the HPA axis, which can result in adrenal insufficiency when the drug is withdrawn abruptly. This effect necessitates the tapering of dose rather than quick withdrawal of the drug. The mechanisms underlying these and other adverse effects of conventional glucocorticoids are detailed in Chapter 46. *Budesonide* has a similar profile of adverse events, but with lower incidence due its extensive first-pass hepatic metabolism.

Immunomodulatory Agents

Several drugs developed for cancer chemotherapy or as immunosuppressive agents in organ transplants are also used for treatment of IBD.

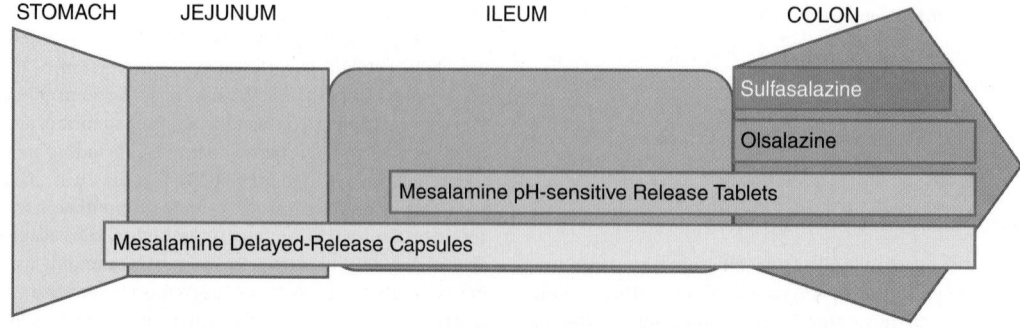

Figure 51–4 *Sites of release of mesalamine (5-ASA) in the GI tract from different oral formulations.*

Clinical experience has defined specific roles for each of these agents as mainstays in the pharmacotherapy of IBD. However, their potential for serious adverse effects mandates a careful assessment of risks and benefits in each patient.

Thiopurine Derivatives

The cytotoxic thiopurine derivatives *mercaptopurine* and *azathioprine* (see Chapters 35 and 66) are used off label to treat patients with severe IBD or those who are steroid resistant or steroid dependent (Coskun et al., 2016). These thiopurines impair purine biosynthesis and inhibit cell proliferation. Both are prodrugs: Azathioprine is converted to 6-mercaptopurine, which is subsequently metabolized to 6-thioguanine nucleotides, the putative active moieties (Figure 51–5).

Therapeutic Uses. These drugs are generally used interchangeably with appropriate dose adjustments, typically *azathioprine* (1.5–2.5 mg/kg) or *mercaptopurine* (1.5–2.0 mg/kg) in both Crohn disease and ulcerative colitis as an adjunct to glucocorticoids and biologics (Nielsen et al., 2001). They help maintain remission in both diseases; they also may prevent or delay recurrence of Crohn disease after surgical resection. Finally, they are used to treat fistulas in Crohn disease. The clinical response to *azathioprine* or *mercaptopurine* may take weeks to months, such that other drugs with a more rapid onset of action (e.g., *mesalamine*, glucocorticoids, or biologics) are preferred in the acute setting.

In general, physicians who treat IBD believe that the long-term risks of *azathioprine-mercaptopurine* are lower than those of steroids. Thus, these purines are used in glucocorticoid-unresponsive or glucocorticoid-dependent disease and in patients who have had recurrent flares of disease requiring repeated courses of steroids. In addition, patients who have not responded adequately to *mesalamine* but are not acutely ill may benefit by conversion from glucocorticoids to immunomodulatory drugs. Immunomodulators therefore may be viewed as steroid-sparing agents.

ADME. Favorable responses to *azathioprine-mercaptopurine* are seen in up to two-thirds of patients. *Mercaptopurine* has three metabolic fates (Figure 51–5):

- conversion by XO to 6-thiouric acid;
- metabolism by TPMT to 6-MMP; and
- conversion by HGPRT to 6-thioguanine nucleotides and other metabolites.

The relative activities of these different pathways may explain, in part, individual variations in efficacy and adverse effects.

The plasma $t_{1/2}$ of *mercaptopurine* is limited by its relatively rapid (i.e., within 1–2 h) uptake into erythrocytes and other tissues. Following this uptake, differences in TPMT activity determine the drug's fate. Approximately 80% of the U.S. population has what is considered "normal" metabolism, whereas 1 in 300 individuals have minimal TPMT activity. In the latter setting, *mercaptopurine* metabolism is shifted away from 6-MMP and driven toward 6-thioguanine nucleotides, which can severely suppress the bone marrow. About 10% of people have intermediate TPMT activity;

given a similar dose, these individuals will tend to have higher 6-thioguanine levels than the normal metabolizers. Finally, about 10% of the population are rapid metabolizers. In these individuals, *mercaptopurine* is shunted away from 6-thioguanine nucleotides toward 6-MMP, which has been associated with abnormal liver function tests. In addition, relative to normal metabolizers, the 6-thioguanine levels of these rapid metabolizers are lower for an equivalent oral dose, possibly reducing therapeutic response. Pharmacogenetic typing can guide therapy (see Chapter 7).

Xanthine oxidase in the small intestine and liver converts *mercaptopurine* to thiouric acid, which has no therapeutic activity. Inhibition of XO by allopurinol diverts *mercaptopurine* to more active metabolites, such as 6-thioguanine, increasing both immunomodulatory and potential toxic effects. Thus, patients on *mercaptopurine* should be warned about potentially serious interactions with medications used to treat gout or hyperuricemia, and the dose should be decreased to 25% of the standard dose in subjects who are already taking allopurinol.

Adverse Effects. Adverse effects of *azathioprine-mercaptopurine* can be either *idiosyncratic* or *dose related*. Adverse effects occur at any time after initiation of treatment and can affect up to 10% of patients. One of the most serious idiosyncratic reactions is pancreatitis, which affects about 5% of patients treated with these drugs. Fever, rash, and arthralgias are seen occasionally; nausea and vomiting are somewhat more frequent. The major dose-related adverse effect is bone marrow suppression, and blood counts should be monitored closely when therapy is initiated and at less-frequent intervals during maintenance therapy. Elevations in liver function tests also may be dose related. The serious adverse effect of cholestatic hepatitis is relatively rare. Thiopurines given in the setting of cancer chemotherapy or organ transplants have been associated with an increased incidence of malignancy, particularly non-Hodgkin lymphoma.

Methotrexate

Methotrexate is a folic acid analogue that inhibits *dihydrofolate reductase*, thereby blocking DNA synthesis and causing cell death (Coskun et al., 2016). The anti-inflammatory effects of *methotrexate* may involve mechanisms in addition to inhibition of dihydrofolate reductase. These include inhibition of purine metabolism, inhibition of T-cell activation and production of cytokines and intercellular adhesion molecules, and inhibition of IL-1β receptor binding.

Therapeutic Uses. *Methotrexate* is reserved for patients whose IBD is either steroid resistant or steroid dependent. In Crohn disease, it is used for maintenance of remission and as an adjunct to biologics to boost efficacy and reduce formation of antidrug antibodies (Patel et al., 2014). *Methotrexate* (15–25 mg/week) is generally administered parenterally. The choice of parenteral administration reflects the unpredictable intestinal absorption at higher doses of methotrexate and in the presence of intestinal disease. A dose of 25 mg weekly is often used for induction of the remission of the inflammatory response, with 15 mg given once weekly for maintenance of remission. *Methotrexate* is sometimes used in combination with anti–TNF-α antibody therapy (see discussion that follows).

ADME. *Methotrexate* is administered intramuscularly or subcutaneously for induction and maintenance of remission of Crohn disease. After administration, approximately 50% is bound to serum proteins. Methotrexate can cross the blood-brain barrier but occurs at much lower levels in cerebrospinal fluid than in serum. It has a $t_{1/2}$ of about 3–10 h at doses used for the treatment of Crohn disease (see Appendix II). Approximately 90% of administered *methotrexate* appears unaltered in the urine, likely as a result of active tubular secretion.

Adverse Effects. Drugs that inhibit renal excretion of MTX may increase treatment-related toxicity. These include NSAIDs, phenytoin, ciprofloxacin, penicillin-type drugs, probenecid, amiodarone, and proton pump inhibitors. *Methotrexate*, at the doses used for the treatment of Crohn disease, is generally well tolerated. When toxicity occurs, it manifests as nausea, loose stool, stomatitis, punctate cutaneous eruption, CNS symptoms (including headache, fatigue, and impaired ability to concentrate),

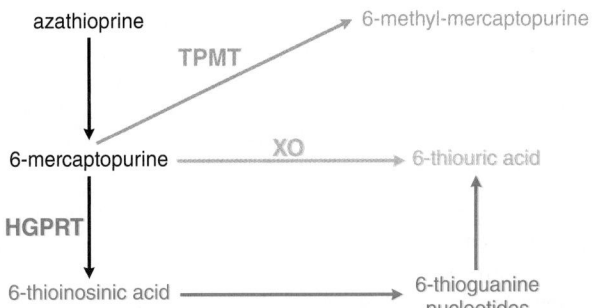

Figure 51–5 *Metabolism of azathioprine and 6-mercaptopurine.* The activities of these enzymes vary among humans because genetic polymorphisms are expressed differentially, explaining responses and side effects when azathioprine-mercaptopurine therapy is employed.

alopecia, fever (drug related or due to infection), and hematologic abnormalities, particularly macrocytosis.

Cyclosporine

Cyclosporine is an inhibitor of calcineurin and a potent immunomodulator used most frequently after organ transplantation (see Chapter 35). It is effective in specific clinical settings in IBD, but the high frequency of significant adverse effects limits its use as a first-line medication.

Therapeutic Uses. Between 50% and 80% of these severely ill patients with IBD improve significantly (generally within 7 days) in response to intravenous *cyclosporine* (2–4 mg/kg per day), sometimes avoiding emergent colectomy. Careful monitoring of *cyclosporine* levels is necessary to maintain a therapeutic level between 300 and 400 ng/mL of whole blood. Oral *cyclosporine* is less effective as maintenance therapy in Crohn disease, perhaps because of its limited intestinal absorption. In this setting, long-term therapy with formulations of *cyclosporine* that have increased oral bioavailability may be more effective. *Cyclosporine* can be used to treat fistulous complications of Crohn disease. A significant rapid response to intravenous *cyclosporine* has been observed; however, frequent relapses accompany oral *cyclosporine* therapy, and other medical strategies are required to maintain fistula closure. Thus, calcineurin inhibitors generally are used to treat specific problems over the short-term while providing a bridge to longer-term therapy.

ADME. *Cyclosporine* given orally is erratically and incompletely absorbed by the intestine. Following absorption, 90%–98% is bound to serum lipoproteins. Depending on the formulation, the $t_{1/2}$ is biphasic, with the terminal phase being about 9–18 h.

Adverse Effects. The significant adverse effects associated with the use of *cyclosporine* limit its use to specific types of severe IBD. These side effects most often include increased susceptibility to infections, renal insufficiency, hypertension, seizures, and peripheral neuropathy. Significant drug interactions have been reported.

Other immunosuppressants that are being evaluated in IBD include the calcineurin inhibitor *tacrolimus* (FK506) and the inhibitors of inosine monophosphate dehydrogenase, *mycophenolate mofetil* and *mycophenolate*, to which lymphocytes are especially susceptible (see Chapter 35).

Biological Therapies for IBD

Anti–TNF-α Monoclonal Antibodies

Infliximab, adalimumab, and *certolizumab pegol* are monoclonal immunoglobulins that have been developed for the treatment of chronic inflammatory diseases. *Infliximab* is a chimeric antibody (25% mouse, 75% human), whereas *adalimumab* is a fully humanized antibody. *Certolizumab pegol* is a humanized fragment antigen binding that is "pegylated" (i.e., bound to a polyethylene glycol polymer to increase serum half-life of the parent compound). These drugs bind to and neutralize both soluble and membrane-bound TNF-α, one of the principal cytokines mediating the T_H1 immune response characteristic of Crohn disease (see Figure 51–1), thereby preventing its binding to p55 and p75 receptors. Chapters 34 and 35 present more detailed and mechanistic view of Ab production and the use of Abs to regulate immune function.

Therapeutic Uses and ADME—Crohn Disease. Monoclonal anti–TNF-α antibodies are used for moderate-to-severe Crohn disease, including fistulizing disease that is resistant to other therapies (Peyrin-Biroulet et al., 2008). The antibody preparations are used for both the induction and the maintenance of remission in adults and children. Anti–TNF-α antibodies used in the treatment of Crohn disease are administered parenterally. *Infliximab* is given intravenously at an initial dose of 5 mg/kg, with subsequent doses of 5 mg/kg at weeks 2 and 6, followed by maintenance doses of 5 mg/kg every 8 weeks. The $t_{1/2}$ is about 8–10 days, although the clearance rate increases in patients who develop anti-infliximab antibodies. *Adalimumab* is given subcutaneously at an initial dose of 160 mg, with subsequent doses of 80 mg at week 2 and maintenance doses of 40 mg every second week starting on week 4. Bioavailability following a 40-mg

dose is about 64%; the $t_{1/2}$ is about 2 weeks. *Certolizumab pegol* is given at an induction dose of 400 mg subcutaneously at weeks 0, 2, and 4, and then every 4 weeks for maintenance of response. Bioavailability when given subcutaneously is about 80%; the $t_{1/2}$ is about 2 weeks. The clearance of monoclonal anti–TNF-α antibodies is not well understood but is likely due to proteolytic degradation. The polyethylene glycol moiety of *certolizumab pegol* is cleared by urinary excretion.

Adverse Effects. Both acute (fever, chills, urticaria, or even anaphylaxis) and subacute (serum sickness–like) reactions may develop after infliximab infusion. Antibodies to infliximab can decrease its clinical efficacy (Lichtenstein, 2013). Strategies to minimize the development of these antibodies (e.g., treatment with glucocorticoids or other immunosuppressives) may be critical to preserving infliximab efficacy but may increase the chance of infection. Because *adalimumab* and *certolizumab* are humanized antibodies, there is less chance for the development of an immune response against them. *Infliximab* therapy is associated with increased incidence of respiratory infections; of particular concern is potential reactivation of tuberculosis or development of opportunistic infections with subsequent dissemination. The FDA recommends that candidates for *infliximab* therapy be tested for latent tuberculosis with purified protein derivative; patients testing positive should be treated prophylactically with isoniazid. *Infliximab* is contraindicated in patients with severe congestive heart failure. There is concern about a possible increased incidence of non-Hodgkin lymphoma, but a causal role has not been established.

Although *infliximab* was designed specifically to target TNF-α, it may have more complex actions. *Infliximab* binds membrane-bound TNF-α and may cause lysis of these cells by antibody-dependent or cell-mediated cytotoxicity. Thus, *infliximab* may deplete specific populations of subepithelial inflammatory cells. These effects, together with its mean terminal plasma $t_{1/2}$ of 8–10 days, may explain the prolonged clinical effects of *infliximab*. *Infliximab* (5 mg/kg infused IV at intervals of every 6–8 weeks) decreases the frequency of acute flares in approximately two-thirds of patients with moderate-to-severe Crohn disease and also facilitates the closing of enterocutaneous fistulas associated with Crohn disease. Emerging evidence also supports its efficacy in maintaining remission and in preventing recurrence of fistulas. The combination of *infliximab* and *azathioprine* is more effective than infliximab alone in induction of remission and mucosal healing in steroid-resistant patients.

Other Monoclonal Antibodies for the Treatment of Crohn Disease

Vedolizumab is a humanized, monoclonal antibody that binds to and inhibits the $α_4$-integrin subunit and therefore blocks binding of $α_4β_1$ and $α_4β_7$ on lymphocytes to *addressin* (also known as mucosal vascular addressin cell adhesion molecule, MADCAM 1) on venular endothelial cells, thus preventing lymphocyte recruitment to the intestinal mucosa (Jovani and Danese, 2013). It is approved for use in the treatment of moderate-to-severe Crohn disease and ulcerative colitis. *Vedolizumab* is generally given at a dose of 300 mg at 0, 2, and 6 weeks, with maintenance doses given every 8 weeks thereafter. The main side effects are headache, hypersensitivity reactions, arthralgia, nasopharyngitis, and fatigue. Anti–TNF-α drugs may enhance the adverse effects of *vedolizumab*.

Ustekinumab is a monoclonal antibody that targets the p40 subunit common to the pro-inflammatory cytokines IL-12 and IL-23, thus preventing activation of IL-12β1 and IL-23 receptors on lymphocytes (Teng et al., 2015). Originally developed for the treatment of psoriasis, it shows efficacy in the induction and maintenance of remission in Crohn disease. Trials indicate effective induction and maintenance of remission at a dose of 6 mg/kg (Khanna et al., 2015). During the initial trials of *ustekinumab* for Crohn disease, side effects included headache, arthralgia, infection, nausea, and nasopharyngitis.

Therapeutic Uses and ADME—Ulcerative Colitis. Unlike Crohn disease, ulcerative colitis can be cured with surgery (colectomy). Thus, the cost and potential adverse events associated with monoclonal antibody therapy need to be balanced with the effectiveness of the drug at preventing the need for colonic resection. Biologics are well established in their use in ulcerative colitis, particularly in those patients for whom primary therapy with glucocorticoids, 5-ASA, or immunomodulators has failed. *Infliximab, adalimumab,* and *golimumab* have become mainstays in the treatment of ulcerative colitis, and *vedolizumab* is also now available. Large controlled clinical trials have demonstrated that anti–TNF-α agents significantly reduce the severity of the inflammation that characterizes ulcerative colitis. Similarly, *vedolizumab* is now indicated and approved for the treatment of moderate-to-severe ulcerative colitis. The administration, dosing, metabolism, and adverse events are similar for the use of these drugs in ulcerative colitis and Crohn disease.

Manipulating the Intestinal Microbiome to Treat IBD

Antibiotics and Probiotics

A balance normally exists in the GI tract among the mucosal epithelium, the normal gut flora, and the immune response (Biteen et al., 2016; Schreiner et al., 2015). Dysbiosis of the intestinal microbiome is now considered a key factor in the development of IBD (Dalal and Chang, 2014). Thus, certain bacterial strains may be either pro- (e.g., *Bacteroides*) or anti-inflammatory (e.g., *Lactobacillus*), prompting attempts to manipulate the colonic flora in patients with IBD. Traditionally, antibiotics have been used most prominently in Crohn disease.

Antibiotics can be used as:

- adjunctive treatment along with other medications for active IBD in severe cases where there is concern about coexisting sepsis
- treatment of perforating or fistulizing complications of Crohn disease
- prophylaxis for recurrence in postoperative Crohn disease

Metronidazole, ciprofloxacin, amoxicillin-clavulanate, and *piperacillin-tazobactam* are the antibiotics used most frequently. Crohn disease–related complications that may benefit from antibiotic therapy include intra-abdominal abscess and inflammatory masses, perianal disease (including fistulas and perirectal abscesses), small-bowel bacterial overgrowth secondary to partial small-bowel obstruction, secondary infections with organisms such as *Clostridium difficile,* and postoperative complications.

More recently, *probiotics* have been used to treat specific clinical situations in IBD. Probiotics are mixtures of putatively beneficial lyophilized bacteria given orally. Several studies have provided evidence for beneficial effects of probiotics in ulcerative colitis and pouchitis (Sokol, 2014). However, the utility of probiotics as a primary therapy for IBD remains unclear.

Fecal Transplant as Therapy in IBD

The recognition that the etiology of IBD involves dysbiosis of the intestinal microbiome has raised interest in methods to reestablish normal microflora in patients. Fecal transplant involves the instillation of a preparation of feces from a healthy donor into the colon, either by enema or during colonoscopy. This has proven to be an effective therapy for antibiotic-resistant *C. difficile* infection. Several clinical trials have assessed the efficacy of fecal transplant in Crohn disease and ulcerative colitis, with varying results (Hansen and Sartor, 2015).

Supportive Therapy in IBD

Analgesic, anticholinergic, and antidiarrheal agents play supportive roles in reducing symptoms and improving quality of life. Oral iron, folate, and

vitamin B$_{12}$ should be administered as indicated. *Loperamide* or *diphenoxylate* (see Chapter 50) can be used to reduce the frequency of bowel movements and relieve rectal urgency in patients with mild disease in selected circumstances; these agents are contraindicated in patients with severe disease because they may predispose to the development of toxic megacolon. *Cholestyramine* can be used to treat bile salt–induced colonic secretion in patients who have undergone limited ileocolic resections. Anticholinergic agents (dicyclomine hydrochloride, etc.; Chapter 10) are used to reduce abdominal cramps, pain, and rectal urgency. As with the antidiarrheal agents, they are contraindicated in severe disease or when obstruction is suspected.

Pediatric IBD

Children and adolescents remain the fastest-growing group of patients with IBD. On average, children present with more severe disease than do adults. In addition, while many children present with the classical symptoms of IBD, approximately 22% of children present with additional symptoms, such as growth failure, perianal disease, or other extraintestinal manifestations as the primary symptom, thus complicating diagnosis.

The drugs used for treating pediatric IBD are the same as those used for the treatment of these diseases in adults. Exclusive enteral nutrition is an effective alternative to 5-ASA compounds, glucocorticoids, immunosuppressants, and biologics. Indeed, 8–12 weeks of liquid formula as the sole source of calories is as effective as glucocorticoids in relieving symptoms and has the advantage of supporting growth (Rosen et al., 2015). In terms of drug therapy, a child's immunization status should be considered before commencing immunosuppressive therapy (glucocorticoids, *azathioprine-methotrexate,* anti–TNF-α drugs). Children should be tested for latent tuberculosis, particularly prior to treatment with anti–TNF-α drugs. During treatment, children may receive inactivated vaccines, but it is not recommended that they be given live vaccines.

Antibiotics have recently been shown to have some utility in treating mild-to-moderate pediatric Crohn disease. In particular, *ciprofloxacin, metronidazole,* and *rifaximin* were demonstrably effective in small clinical trials (Serban, 2015). Their role in the treatment of ulcerative colitis has yet to be established.

Therapy of IBD During Pregnancy

Inflammatory bowel disease is a chronic disease that affects women in their reproductive years. In general, decreased disease activity increases fertility and improves pregnancy outcomes. At the same time, limiting medication during pregnancy is always desired but sometimes conflicts with the goal of controlling the disease. The use of medical therapies to treat IBD during pregnancy and lactation has been reviewed (Nielsen et al., 2014), although studies that thoroughly investigated the use of medications to treat IBD in pregnancy are limited (Damas et al., 2015). *Mesalamine* and *glucocorticoids* are FDA category B drugs (see Appendix I) that are used frequently in pregnancy and generally are considered safe, whereas *methotrexate* is absolutely contraindicated in pregnant patients. There does not appear to be an increase in adverse outcomes in pregnant patients maintained on thiopurine-based immunosuppressives. Anti–TNF-α drugs, particularly *infliximab* and *adalimumab,* have been assessed for their safety for use during pregnancy and have been found to have low risk for adverse events (Khan et al., 2014).

Acknowledgment: Laurence L. Brunton, Syed Jafri, Joseph H. Sellin, Pankaj Jay Pasricha, and *John L. Wallace contributed to this chapter in earlier editions of this book. We have retained some of their text in the current edition.*

Drug Facts for Your Personal Formulary: *Drugs for the Treatment of Inflammatory Bowel Diseases*

Drugs	Therapeutic Uses	Clinical Pharmacology and Tips
Mesalamine-Based Drugs		
Mesalamine (5-ASA)	• Induction and maintenance of remission in mild-to-moderate ulcerative colitis • Used in combination with glucocorticoids for severe ulcerative colitis	• Effects are primarily topical with limited effects on deeper tissue inflammation • Following oral administration, jejunum is primary site of absorption, so utility in more distal disease is limited • Can be delivered as a suppository for rectal disease
Sulfasalazine	• Induction and maintenance of remission in mild-to-moderate ulcerative colitis • Used in combination with glucocorticoids for severe ulcerative colitis	• Prodrug, delivers 5-ASA to more distal GI regions following metabolism by colonic bacteria • Sulfapyridine is also released; may cause adverse effects in patients sensitive to sulfa drugs
Olsalazine	• Induction and maintenance of remission in mild-to-moderate ulcerative colitis • Used in combination with glucocorticoids for severe ulcerative colitis	• Prodrug with two azo-linked 5-ASA molecules • Eliminates the side effects associated with the sulfapyridine moiety of sulfasalazine
Balsalazide	• Induction and maintenance of remission in mild-to-moderate ulcerative colitis • Used in combination with glucocorticoids for severe ulcerative colitis	• Prodrug with a 5-ASA molecule linked to an inert, unabsorbable second moiety • Eliminates the side effects associated with the sulfapyridine moiety of sulfasalazine
Glucocorticoids: Minimize duration of use. Taper dose prior to stopping to minimize disease relapse and avoid adrenal insufficiency that follows rapid glucocorticoid withdrawal after prolonged therapy has suppressed the HPA axis.		
Prednisone	• Induction of remission in moderate-to-severe Crohn disease and ulcerative colitis	• Hepatic metabolism to active moiety, prednisolone • Not used for maintenance therapy due to serious adverse effects
Methylprednisolone	• Induction of remission in moderate-to-severe Crohn disease and ulcerative colitis	• Can be administered orally, intravenously, or intramuscularly to patients who respond poorly to oral prednisone • Preferred over hydrocortisone, which has higher incidence of Na$^+$ retention and K$^+$ wasting
Hydrocortisone	• Induction of remission in moderate-to-severe Crohn disease and ulcerative colitis	• Administered intravenously to patients who respond poorly to oral prednisone
Budesonide	• Induction of remission in mild-to-moderate Crohn disease and ulcerative colitis, particularly in distal disease • Not effective for long-term maintenance of clinical remission	• Prominent first-pass metabolism reduces side effects that can result from maintenance of higher systemic levels
Immunomodulatory Agents		
6-Mercaptopurine	• Used as an adjunct to glucocorticoids and biologics in the treatment of moderate-to-severe Crohn disease and ulcerative colitis • Effective in maintenance of remission	• Slow-acting drug; maximum therapeutic benefit may take months to achieve • Other metabolites also have anti-inflammatory activity • Fourfold increased risk of lymphoma in patients with IBD treated with thiopurines
Azathioprine	• Used as an adjunct to glucocorticoids and biologics in the treatment of moderate-to-severe Crohn disease and ulcerative colitis • Effective in maintenance of remission	• Prodrug metabolized nonenzymatically in blood to active form, 6-mercaptopurine • Other metabolites also have anti-inflammatory activity • Fourfold increased risk of lymphoma in patients with IBD treated with thiopurines
Methotrexate	• Maintenance of remission in Crohn disease, particularly steroid-resistant or steroid-dependent disease • Often used in combination with biologic agents	• Folic acid analogue that has anti-inflammatory activity of unclear mechanism • Administered parenterally • Cleared unaltered by the kidney, so inhibition of renal excretion mechanisms may lead to drug toxicity
Cyclosporine	• Used to treat specific cases of severe Crohn disease, including fistulizing disease • Not useful for maintenance of remission	• Erratic and incomplete absorption means blood levels must be monitored • Significant adverse events profile
Tacrolimus (FK506)	• Useful for the treatment of refractory Crohn disease	• Immunomodulator with similar mechanism as cyclosporine but with better oral absorption

Biologics: Anti–TNF-α		
Infliximab	• Induction or maintenance of remission in moderate-to-severe Crohn disease or ulcerative colitis in patients who have not responded well to other therapies	• Partly humanized, chimeric anti–TNF-α monoclonal antibody • Usually administered by intravenous infusion • Patients may develop antibodies against the drug
Adalimumab	• Induction or maintenance of remission in moderate-to-severe Crohn disease or ulcerative colitis in patients who have not responded well to other therapies	• Fully humanized anti–TNF-α monoclonal antibody; reduced incidence of antidrug antibodies • Administered subcutaneously • Useful for patients for whom infliximab has lost efficacy or has caused adverse reactions
Certolizumab pegol	• Induction or maintenance of remission in moderate-to-severe Crohn disease in patients who have not responded well to other therapies	• Humanized anti–TNF-α monoclonal antibody bound to PEG to increase plasma $t_{1/2}$ • Administered subcutaneously • Useful for patients for whom infliximab has lost efficacy or caused adverse reactions • May be a better option in pregnant women due to less drug crossing placental barrier
Biologics: Other		
Vedolizumab	• Induction or maintenance of remission in moderate-to-severe Crohn disease or ulcerative colitis in patients who have not responded to other therapies	• Humanized anti-$\alpha_4\beta_7$ monoclonal antibody • Given by intravenous infusion • May cause hypersensitivity reactions
Ustekinumab	• Induction or maintenance of remission in moderate-to-severe Crohn disease in patients who have not responded to other therapies	• Humanized monoclonal antibody against p40 subunit of IL-12 and IL-23 • Administered subcutaneously • Long-term safety profile has not yet been established
Antibiotics		
Metronidazole	• Used as adjunctive therapy in mild-to-moderate Crohn disease • Sometimes used in conjunction with ciprofloxacin • Used in pediatric IBD	• Modest therapeutic benefit in Crohn disease • Little to no benefit in ulcerative colitis
Ciprofloxacin	• Used as adjunctive therapy in mild-to-moderate Crohn disease • Sometimes used in conjunction with metronidazole • Used in pediatric IBD	• Modest therapeutic benefit in Crohn disease • Little to no benefit in ulcerative colitis
Rifaximin	• Used as adjunctive therapy in mild-to-moderate Crohn disease • Used in pediatric Crohn disease	• Less experience with this drug compared to metronidazole or ciprofloxacin
Probiotics		
Various types and formulations	• Some utility in ulcerative colitis and pouchitis, but few clinical trials	• Effects are transient; long-term colonic colonization rarely occurs • Watch for progress on fecal transplant therapy

Bibliography

Beaugerie L, Itzkowitz SH. Cancers complicating inflammatory bowel disease. *N Engl J Med*, **2015**, *372*:1441–1452.

Bellaguarda E, Chang EB. IBD and the gut microbiota: from bench to personalized medicine. *Curr Gastroenterol Rep*, **2015**, *17*:15. doi:10.1007/s11894-015-0439-z.

Benchimol EI, et al. Traditional corticosteroids for induction of remission in Crohn's disease. *Cochrane Database Syst Rev*, **2008**, (2):CD006792.

Biteen JS, et al. Tools for the microbiome: nano and beyond. *ACS Nano*, **2016**, *10*:6–37.

Bressler B, et al. Clinical practice guidelines for the medical management of nonhospitalized ulcerative colitis: the Toronto consensus. *Gastroenterology*, **2015**, *148*:1035–1058.

Coskun M, et al. Pharmacology and optimization of thiopurines and methotrexate in inflammatory bowel disease. *Clin Pharmacokinet*, **2016**, *55*:257–274.

Dalal SR, Chang EB. The microbial basis of inflammatory bowel diseases. *J Clin Invest*, **2014**, *124*:4190–4196.

Damas OM, et al. Treating inflammatory bowel disease in pregnancy: the issues we face today. *J Crohn's Colitis*, **2015**, *9*:928–936.

D'Haens GR, et al. Future directions in inflammatory bowel disease management. *J Crohn's Colitis*, **2014**, *8*:726–734.

Feagan BG, Macdonald JK. Oral 5-aminosalicylic acid for maintenance of remission in ulcerative colitis. *Cochrane Database Syst Rev*, **2012**,(10):CD000544.

Florholmen J. Mucosal healing in the era of biologic agents in treatment of inflammatory bowel disease. *Scand J Gastroenterol*, **2015**, *50*:43–52.

Hansen JJ, Sartor RB. Therapeutic manipulation of the microbiome in IBD: current results and future approaches. *Curr Treat Options Gastroenterol*, **2015**, *13*:105–120.

Jain A, et al. Azo chemistry and its potential for colonic delivery. *Crit Rev Ther Drug Carrier Syst*, **2006**, *23*:349–400.

Jovani M, Danese S. Vedolizumab for the treatment of IBD: a selective therapeutic approach targeting pathogenic α4β7 cells. *Curr Drug Targets*, **2013**, *14*:1433–1443.

Kane SV, et al. The effectiveness of budesonide therapy for Crohn's disease. *Aliment Pharmacol Ther*, **2002**, *16*:1509–1517.

Kaser A, et al. Inflammatory bowel disease. *Annu Rev Immunol*, **2010**, *28*:573–621.

Khan N, et al. Safety of anti-TNF therapy in inflammatory bowel disease during pregnancy. *Expert Opin Drug Saf*, **2014**, *13*:1699–1708.

954 Khanna R, et al. Anti-IL-12/23p40 antibodies for induction of remission in Crohn's disease. *Cochrane Database Syst Rev*, **2015**,(5):CD007572.

Kuenzig ME, et al. Budesonide for maintenance of remission in Crohn's disease. *Cochrane Database Syst Rev*. 2014 Aug 21;(8):CD002913. doi: 10.1002/14651858.CD002913.pub3.

Lichtenstein GR. Comprehensive review: antitumor necrosis factor agents in inflammatory bowel disease and factors implicated in treatment response. *Ther Adv Gastroenterol*, **2013**, 6:269–293.

Manz M, et al. Therapy of steroid-resistant inflammatory bowel disease. *Digestion*, **2012**, *86*(suppl 1):11–15.

Nielsen OH, et al. IBD medications during pregnancy and lactation. *Nat Rev Gastroenterol Hepatol*, **2014**, 11:116–127.

Nielsen OH, et al. Review article: the treatment of inflammatory bowel disease with 6-mercaptopurine or azathioprine. *Aliment Pharmacol Ther*, **2001**, 15:1699–1708.

Ordas I, et al. Ulcerative colitis. *Lancet*, **2012**, *380*:1606–1619.

Ott C, Scholmerich J. Extraintestinal manifestations and complications in IBD. *Nat Rev Gastroenterol Hepatol*, **2013**, 10:585–595.

Patel V, et al. Methotrexate for maintenance of remission in Crohn's disease. *Cochrane Database Syst Rev*, **2014**, 8:CD006884.

Peppercorn MA, Goldman P. The role of intestinal bacteria in the metabolism of salicylazosulfapyridine. *J Pharmacol Exp Ther*, **1972**, *181*:555–562.

Perrotta C, et al. Five-aminosalicylic acid: an update for the reappraisal of an old drug. *Gastroenterol Res Pract*, **2015**, *2015*:456895. doi:10.1155/2015/456895.

Peyrin-Biroulet L, et al. Efficacy and safety of tumor necrosis factor antagonists in Crohn's disease: meta-analysis of placebo-controlled trials. *Clin Gastroenterol Hepatol*, **2008**, 6:644–653.

Rosen MJ, et al. Inflammatory bowel disease in children and adolescents. *JAMA Pediatr*, **2015**, *169*:1053–1060. doi:10.1001/jamapediatrics.2015.1982.

Sandborn WJ, et al. Medical management of mild to moderate Crohn's disease: evidence-based treatment algorithms for induction and maintenance of remission. *Aliment Pharmacol Ther*, **2007**, *26*:987–1003.

Sandborn WJ, Hanauer SB. Systematic review: the pharmacokinetic profiles of oral mesalazine formulations and mesalazine pro-drugs used in the management of ulcerative colitis. *Aliment Pharmacol Ther*, **2003**, *17*:29–42.

Sartor RB. Mechanisms of disease: pathogenesis of Crohn's disease and ulcerative colitis. *Nat Clin Prac Gastroenterol Hepatol*, **2006**, 3:390–407.

Schreiner AB, et al. The gut microbiome in health and in disease. *Curr Opin Gastroenterol,* **2015**, *31*:69–75.

Serban DE. Microbiota in inflammatory bowel disease pathogenesis and therapy: is it all about diet? *Nutr Clin Pract*, **2015**, *pii*:0884533615606898.

Sokol H. Probiotics and antibiotics in IBD. *Dig Dis*, **2014**, *32*(suppl 1):10–17.

Teng MW, et al. IL-12 and IL-23 cytokines: from discovery to targeted therapies for immune-mediated inflammatory diseases. *Nat Med*, **2015**, *21*:719–729.

Williamson, KD, Chapman RW. Primary sclerosing cholangitis. *Dig Dis*, **2014**, *32*:438–445.

Xavier RJ, Podolsky DK. Unravelling the pathogenesis of inflammatory bowel disease. *Nature*, **2007**, *448*:427–434.

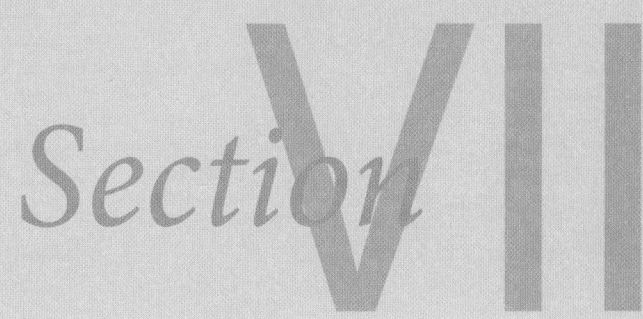

Section VII

Chemotherapy of Infectious Diseases

Chapter 52

General Principles of Antimicrobial Therapy

Tawanda Gumbo

Antimicrobial Chemotherapy: Classes and Actions

The *germ theory* of disease, based on the work of Louis Pasteur and Robert Koch, was a revolution in the human understanding of nature that linked specific microorganisms to specific diseases. The germ theory developed considerably in the 20th century, with identification and characterization of many microbial pathogens and their pathogenic mechanisms and the introduction of antimicrobial drugs. With the use of these drugs came issues of appropriate regimens, drug resistance, drug interactions, and toxicity.

This chapter reviews the general classes of antimicrobial drugs, their mechanisms of action, mechanisms of resistance, and patterns of kill by different classes of the drugs. Chapters 53 through 64 present the pharmacological properties and uses of individual classes of antimicrobials.

Microorganisms of medical importance fall into four categories: *bacteria, viruses, fungi,* and *parasites.* The first broad classification of antibiotics follows this classification closely, so that we have antibacterial, antiviral, antifungal, and antiparasitic agents. However, there are many antibiotics that work against more than one category of microbes, especially those that target evolutionarily conserved pathways. Within each of these major categories, drugs are further categorized by their biochemical properties.

Antimicrobial molecules should be viewed as ligands whose receptors are microbial proteins. The term *pharmacophore,* introduced by Ehrlich, defines that active chemical moiety of the drug that binds to the microbial receptor. The microbial proteins targeted by the antibiotic are essential components of biochemical reactions in the microbes, and interference with these physiological pathways kills the microorganisms. The biochemical processes commonly inhibited include cell wall synthesis in bacteria and fungi, cell membrane synthesis, synthesis of 30S and 50S ribosomal subunits, nucleic acid metabolism, function of topoisomerases, viral proteases, viral integrases, viral envelope entry/fusion proteins, folate synthesis in parasites, and parasitic chemical detoxification processes. Recently, *antisense antibiotics* have been developed; these work by inhibiting gene expression in bacteria in a sequence-specific manner. Furthermore, *interferon*-based products work by inducing specific antiviral activities of the infected human cells.

Classification of an antibiotic is based on the following:

- class and spectrum of microorganisms it kills
- biochemical pathway it interferes with
- chemical structure of its pharmacophore

Because antimicrobial agents are ligands that bind to their targets to produce effects, the relationship between drug concentration and effect on a population of organisms is modeled using the standard Hill-type curve for receptor and agonist (Chapters 2 and 3), characterized by three parameters:

- IC_{50} (also termed EC_{50}), the inhibitory concentration that is 50% effective, a measure of the antimicrobial agent's potency
- E_{max}, a measure of the maximal effect
- H, the slope of the curve, or Hill factor

In antimicrobial therapy, the relationship is often expressed as an inhibitory sigmoid E_{max} model (Figure 52–1), to take into account the *control bacterial population without treatment (E_{con})* as a fourth parameter (Equation 52–1 and Figure 52–1), where *E is effect as measured by microbial burden.*

$$E = E_{con} - E_{max} \times [IC]^H/([IC]^H + [IC_{50}]^H) \qquad \text{(Equation 52–1)}$$

Abbreviations

ABC: ATP binding cassette
AUC: area under the C_p-time curve
CCR5: chemokine receptor type 5
CD4: T-helper cells
CFU: colony-forming unit
CMV: cytomegalovirus
CNS: central nervous system
C_p: plasma concentration
C_{Pmax}: peak concentration
CSF: cerebrospinal fluid
DHFR: dihydrofolate reductase
DHPS: dihydropteroate synthase
E: effect
EC: effective concentration
ELF: epithelial lining fluid
E_{max}: maximal effect
H: the slope of the curve or Hill factor
HIV: human immunodeficiency virus
IC: inhibitory concentration
MALDI-TOF MS: matrix-assisted laser desorption/ionization time-of-flight mass spectrometry
mdr1: multidrug resistance gene
MEC: minimum effective concentration
MIC: minimum inhibitory concentration
PAE: post antibiotic effect
PCR: polymerase chain reaction
PK/PD: pharmacokinetics-pharmacodynamics
rpoB: RNA polymerase

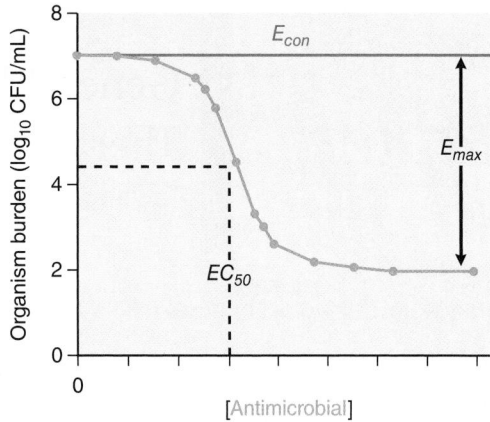

Figure 52–1 *Inhibitory sigmoid E_{max} curve.*

The Pharmacokinetic Basis of Antimicrobial Therapy

Penetration of Antimicrobial Agents Into Anatomic Compartments

In many infections, the pathogen causes disease not in the whole body, but in specific organs. Within an infected organ only specific pathological compartments may be infected. Antibiotics are often administered orally or parenterally, far away from these sites of infection. Therefore, in choosing an antimicrobial agent for therapy, a crucial consideration is whether the drug can penetrate to the site of infection.

For example, the antibiotic levofloxacin achieves a skin tissue/peak plasma concentration C_{Pmax} ratio of 1.4, ELF/(C_p)ratio of 2.8, and urine/(C_p) ratio of 67 (Chow et al., 2002; Conte et al., 2006; Wagenlehner et al., 2006). The two most important factors in predicting successful clinical and microbiological outcomes using levofloxacin in the patients are the site of infection and achieving a C_{Pmax} level of 12 times the MIC (C_{Pmax}/MIC ≥12). The failure rate of therapy is 0% in patients with urinary tract infections, 3% in patients with pulmonary infections, and 16% in patients with skin and soft tissue infections (Preston et al., 1998). Clearly, the poorer the penetration into the anatomical compartment, the higher the likelihood of failure.

The penetration of a drug into an anatomical compartment depends on the *physical barriers* that the molecule must traverse, the *chemical properties of the drug*, and the *presence of multidrug transporters*. The physical barriers are usually due to layers of epithelial and endothelial cells and the type of junctions formed between these cells. As discussed in Chapters 2 and 5, penetration across this physical barrier generally correlates the hydrophilicity or hydrophobicity of the drug. Hydrophobic molecules concentrate in the bilipid cell membrane bilayer, whereas hydrophilic molecules tend to concentrate in the blood, the cytosol, and other aqueous compartments. Thus, the greater its lipophilicity, the greater the likelihood that an antimicrobial agent will cross physical barriers erected by layers of cells. Conversely, *the more charged a molecule is, and the larger it is, the poorer its penetration across membranes and other physical barriers* (see Figure 2–3).

Another barrier is due to *membrane transporters*, which actively export drugs from the cellular or tissue compartment back into the blood (Figure 5–4). A well-known example is the *P-glycoprotein*. *P-glycoprotein exports structurally unrelated amphiphilic and lipophilic molecules of 3–4 kDa, reducing their effective penetration*. Examples of antimicrobial agents that are P-glycoprotein substrates include HIV protease inhibitors, the antiparasitic agent ivermectin, the antibacterial agent telithromycin, and the antifungal agent itraconazole.

CNS

The CNS is guarded by the blood-brain barrier. The movement of antibiotics across the blood-brain barrier is restricted by tight junctions that connect endothelial cells of cerebral microvessels to one another in the brain parenchyma, as well as by protein transporters (Daneman and Prat, 2015). Antimicrobial agents that are polar at physiological pH generally penetrate poorly; some, such as *penicillin G*, are actively transported out of the CSF and achieve CSF concentrations of only 0.5%–5% of the C_p. However, the integrity of the blood-brain barrier is diminished during active bacterial infection; tight junctions in cerebral capillaries open, leading to a marked increase in the penetration of even polar drugs. As the infection is eradicated and the inflammatory reaction subsides, penetration diminishes to normal. Because this may occur while viable microorganisms persist in the CSF, drug dosage should not be reduced as the patient improves.

Eye

Drug penetration into the eye is especially pertinent in the treatment of endophthalmitis and infections of the retina. There is generally poor penetration of drug from plasma to this compartment, so that the standard therapy is direct instillation of antibiotics into the ocular cavity (see Chapter 69). In patients with pulmonary infections such as pneumonia, drugs must penetrate into the ELF, where the pathogens are found (Kiem and Schentag, 2008).

Pericardium

Drug penetration into the pericardium is governed by physical barriers and also likely by some form of active transport. In patients treated for tuberculous pericarditis with the regimen of isoniazid, rifampin, pyrazinamide, and ethambutol, simultaneous blood and pericardial fluid concentrations were measured over 24 h (Shenje et al., 2015). Rifampin concentrations in pericardial fluid were only 20% those in plasma due to poor penetration as well as active clearance, while ethambutol C_{Pmax} was 55% due to poor penetration. On the other hand, isoniazid and pyrazinamide concentrations in pericardial fluid and blood were equivalent. Do not assume that different drugs penetrate equally to the compartment of concern.

Biofilms

Compartments requiring special drug penetration are endocardial vegetations and the biofilm formed by bacteria and fungi on prosthetic devices such as artificial heart valves, long-dwelling intravascular catheters, artificial hips, and devices for internal fixation of bone fractures. Bacterial and fungal biofilms are colonies of slowly growing cells enclosed within an exopolymer matrix. The exopolysaccharide is negatively charged and can bind positively charged antibiotics and restrict their access to the intended target. To be effective against infections in these compartments, antibiotics have to be able to penetrate the biofilm and endothelial barriers (Sun et al., 2013).

Pharmacokinetic Compartments

Once an antibiotic has penetrated to the site of infection, it may be subjected to processes of elimination and distribution that differ from those in the blood. Sites where the concentration-time profiles differ from each other are considered separate pharmacokinetic compartments; thus, the human body is viewed as *multicompartmental*. The concentration of antibiotic within each compartment is assumed to be homogeneous. If two compartments have similar concentration profiles, then they may be considered a single compartment. Antibiotic concentrations can be analyzed using any number of such compartments, with the best number of compartments chosen based on the least number of compartments that can adequately explain the findings. The model is also defined as *open* or *not open*; an open model is one in which the drug is eliminated out of the body from the compartment (e.g., kidneys). The kinetic order of the process must also be specified (Chapter 2): A *first-order process* is directly correlated to concentration of drug D, or $[D]^1$, as opposed to *zero order*, which is independent of [D] and reflects a process that is saturated at ambient levels of D (such as the elimination of ethanol; Chapter 23).

Consider a patient with pneumonia, with the pathogen in the lung ELF. The patient ingests an antibiotic that is absorbed via the GI tract (*g*) into blood or the central compartment (*compartment 1*) as a first-order input. In this process, the transfer constant from the GI tract to central compartment is termed the *absorption constant* and is designated k_a. The antibiotic in the central compartment is then delivered to the lungs, where it penetrates into the ELF (*compartment 2*). However, it also penetrates into other tissues of the body peripheral to the site of infection, termed the *peripheral compartment* (*compartment 3*). Thus, we have four compartments (including *g*, a specific compartment, the GI tract, from the set of initial absorption compartments in Figure 52–2), each with its own concentration-time profile. The penetration of drug from compartment 1 to 2 is based on the penetration factors discussed previously and is defined by the transfer constant k_{12}. However, the drug also redistributes from

compartment 2 back to 1, defined by transfer constant k_{21}. A similar process between the blood and peripheral tissues leads to transfer constants k_{13} and k_{31}. The drug may also be lost from the body (i.e., open system) via the lungs and other peripheral tissues (e.g., kidneys or liver) at a rate proportional to the concentration.

Antibiotic concentrations within each compartment change with time (the changes are described using standard differential equations). If *X* is the amount of antibiotic in a compartment, *SCL* the drug clearance, and V_c the volume of the central compartment, then equations for *absorption compartment* (Equation 52–2), *central compartment* (Equation 52–3), *site of infection* or compartment 2 (Equation 52–4), and *peripheral compartment* (Equation 52–5) are as follows:

$$dX_g/dt = -K_a \cdot X_g \qquad \text{(Equation 52–2)}$$

$$dX_1/dt = K_a \cdot X_g - [(SCL/V_c) + K_{12} + K_{13}] \cdot X_1 + K_{21} \cdot X_2 + K_{31} \cdot X_3$$
$$\text{(Equation 52–3)}$$

$$dX_2/dt = K_{12} \cdot X_1 - K_{21} \cdot X_2 \qquad \text{(Equation 52–4)}$$

$$dX_3/dt = K_{13} \cdot X_3 - K_{31} \cdot X_3 \qquad \text{(Equation 52–5)}$$

Such models have been used in conjunction with population pharmacokinetics to describe and model a plethora of antimicrobials used to treat bacteria, fungi, viruses, and parasites (Hope et al., 2007; Tarning et al., 2008; Wilkins et al., 2008). Semimechanistic models have been applied to relate pathogen response to drug concentrations within these pharmacokinetic compartments in preclinical disease models and in patients (Gumbo et al., 2006; Jumbe et al., 2003; Talal et al., 2006). These models can be made more complex and more predictive by adding parameters describing the effect of inoculum, delay in microbial effect, or splitting the drug-resistant population to smaller subpopulations based on a molecular mechanism of resistance (Bulitta et al., 2009).

Population Pharmacokinetics and Variability in Drug Response

When multiple patients are treated with the same dose of a drug, each patient will achieve unique pharmacokinetic parameters. This is termed *between-patient variability*. Even when the same dose is administered to the same patient on two separate occasions, the patient may achieve a different concentration-time profile of the drug between the two occasions.

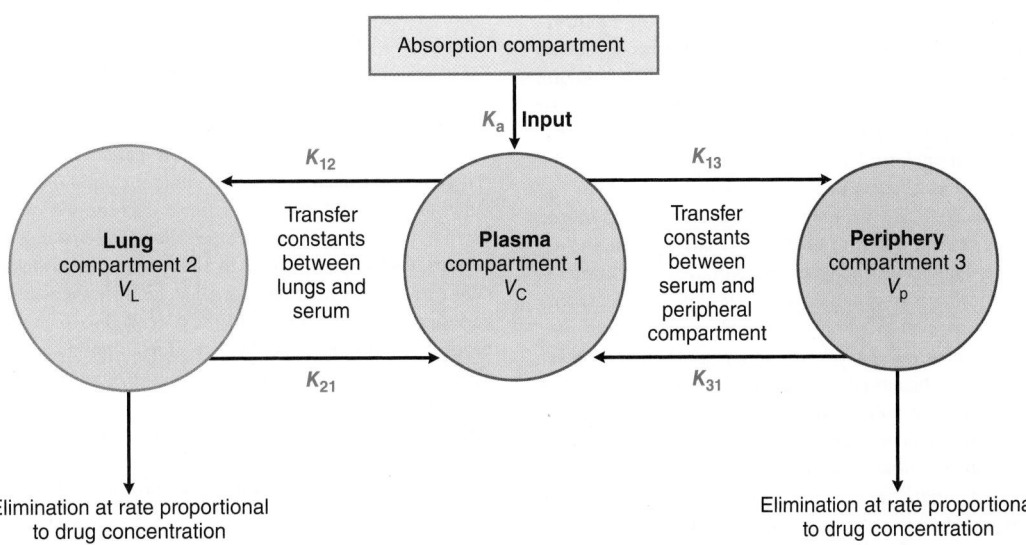

Figure 52–2 *Diagrammatic depiction of a multicompartment model.* K_a, absorption constant; V_c, central compartment volume; V_L, volume of lung compartment; V_p, peripheral compartment volume.

This is termed *interoccasion or within-patient variability*. The variability is reflected at the level of the compartmental pharmacokinetic parameters in Equations 52-2 to 52-5, such as k_a, k_{12}, k_{21}, SCL, V_c, and so on. Even when a recommended dose is administered, the drug may fail to reach a therapeutic concentration in some patients, purely because of the between-patient variability.

An important example of the consequences of between-patient variability involves antituberculosis drugs: In patients who are adherent to therapy, subtherapeutic concentrations of isoniazid, rifampin, pyrazinamide, and ethambutol account for more than 90% of therapy failure, slower sterilizing effect, and acquired drug resistance (Chigutsa et al., 2015; Pasipanodya et al., 2013). The same has been seen with antileishmania drugs and antifungal agents (Andes et al., 2011; Dorlo et al., 2014). In other patients, the drug may reach high and toxic concentrations because of the between-patient variability. Such variability could be due to genetic variability, weight, height, age, and comorbid conditions such as renal and liver dysfunction. An important driver of variability is the widespread problem of overweight and obesity, which increases the clearance and can alter the volume of distribution of many antibiotics. This emerging problem is prompting changes in dosing strategies.

Drug interactions are another important source of variability with potentially dangerous consequences. These interactions usually occur when one drug inhibits or induces uptake or clearance mechanisms affecting another drug (see Chapters 5 and 6).

The common practice of using an "average" value of data, or "naive pooling," has implications of smoothing out data and failing to recognize subgroups of patients at risk for therapeutic failure or increased toxicity of antibiotic. Knowledge of covariates associated with pharmacokinetic variability leads to better dose adjustments, switching therapy from one antibiotic to another, or changing concomitant medications.

Impact of Susceptibility Testing on Success of Antimicrobial Agents

The microbiology laboratory plays a central role in the decision to choose a particular antimicrobial agent over others. First, identification and isolation of the culprit organism takes place when the patients' specimens are sent to the microbiology laboratory. Once the microbial species causing the disease has been identified, a rational choice of the class of antibiotics likely to work in the patient can be made. The microbiology laboratory then plays a second role, which is to perform susceptibility testing.

Millions of individuals across the globe become infected by many different isolates of the same species of pathogen. Evolutionary processes cause each isolate to be slightly different from the next, so that each may have a unique susceptibility to antimicrobial agents. As the microorganisms divide within the patient, they may undergo further evolution between the time of infection and the time of diagnosis. Therefore, one observes a distribution of concentrations of antimicrobial agents that can kill the pathogens. Often, this distribution is Gaussian, with a skew that depends on where the patient lives. Such factors will affect the shape of the inhibitory sigmoid E_{max} model curve described by Equation 52-1.

With changes in susceptibility, the sigmoid E_{max} curve shifts in one of two basic ways. The first is a shift to the right, an increase in IC_{50} (Figure 52-3A), meaning that much higher concentrations of antimicrobials than before are now needed to show specific effect. *Susceptibility tests for bacteria, fungi, parasites, and viruses have been developed to determine whether these shifts have occurred at a sufficient magnitude to warrant higher doses of drug to achieve particular effect.* The change in IC_{50} may become so large that it is not possible to overcome the concentration deficit by increasing the antimicrobial dose without causing toxicity to the patient. At that stage, the organism is now "resistant" to the particular antibiotic.

A second possible change in the curve is decrease in E_{max} (Figure 52-3B), such that increasing the dose of the antimicrobial agent beyond a certain point will achieve no further effect; that is, changes in the microbe are such that eradication of the microbe by the particular drug can never be achieved. This occurs because the available target proteins have been reduced or the

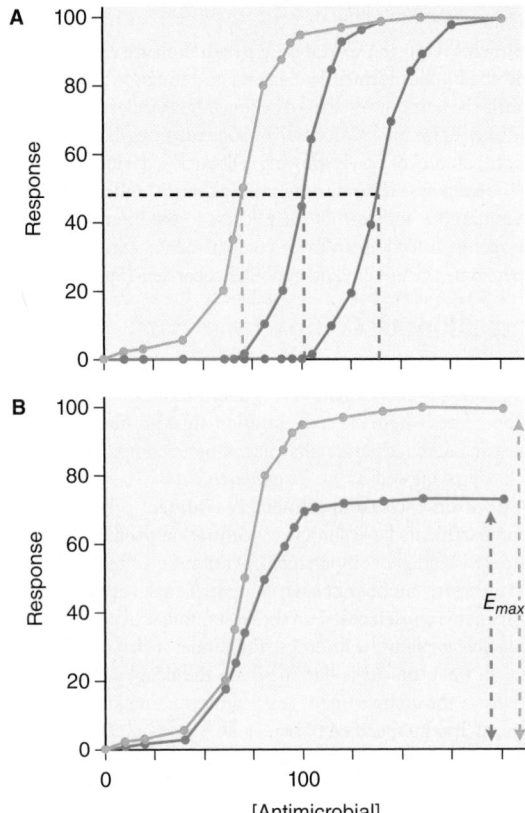

Figure 52–3 *Changes in sigmoid E_{max} model with increases in drug resistance.* An increase in resistance may show changes in IC_{50}: In **A**, the IC_{50} increases from 70 (orange line) to 100 (green line) to 140 (blue line). An increase in resistance may also show a decrease in E_{max}: In **B**, efficacy decreases from full response (orange line) to 70% (green line).

microbe has developed an alternative pathway to overcome the biochemical inhibition. For example, maraviroc is an allosteric, noncompetitive antagonist that binds to the CCR5 receptor of patient's CD4 cells to deny HIV entry into the cell. Viral resistance occurs by a mechanism that involves HIV adapting to use of the maraviroc-bound CCR5, which results in decrease of E_{max} in phenotypic susceptibility assays (Hirsch et al., 2008).

Bacteria

For bacteria, dilution tests employ antibiotics in serially diluted concentrations on solid agar or in broth medium that contains a culture of the test microorganism. The lowest concentration of the agent that prevents visible growth after 18–24 h of incubation is known as the *minimum inhibitory concentration* (MIC).

Recently, nucleic acid amplification–based reactions of specific bacterial genes have been used in the clinic for rapid diagnosis of drug resistance. The genes targeted are those encoding known drug resistance proteins or processes. For example, rifampin resistance in *Mycobacterium tuberculosis* has been difficult to ascertain in a timely fashion: The bacteria take 2 to 3 weeks to grow in order to identify them as a cause of disease, and then a similar amount of time is needed to form some version of the broth dilution tests. Small PCR reactors at points of care can purify and concentrate a patient's fluid sample, perform nucleic acid amplification of a target gene, identify mutations, and provide a result in less than 2 h. In other bacteria, MALDI-TOF MS is being used for identification of resistance to drugs such as vancomycin in *Staphylococcus aureus* and is being extended to many other compounds and bacterial species.

Fungi

For fungi that are yeasts (i.e., *Candida*), susceptibility testing methods are similar to those used for bacteria. However, the definitions of MIC differ based on drug and the type of yeast, so there are cutoff points of 50% decrease in turbidity compared to controls at 24 h, 80% at 48 h, or total clearance of the turbidity. Susceptibility tests and MICs for triazoles have been extensively shown to correlate with clinical outcomes.

Standardized tests for echinocandin antifungals and amphotericin B–based compounds are available. Susceptibility tests for molds have also been developed, especially for *Aspergillus species*. Different terminology from MICs is required when evaluating echinocandins against molds because the fungal burden cannot be readily measured, given that hyphae will break up into unpredictable numbers of discrete fungi when under antifungal pressure. Furthermore, echinocandins often do not completely inhibit mold growth, but instead cause damage reflected by morphological changes in hyphae. Thus, the *minimum effective concentration* (MEC) for echinocandins is the lowest drug concentration at which short, stubby, and highly branched hyphae are observed on microscopic examination.

Viruses

In HIV phenotypic assays, the patient's HIV-RNA is extracted from plasma, and genes for targets of antiretroviral drugs such as reverse transcriptase and protease are amplified. The genes are then inserted into a standard HIV vector that lacks an alogous gene sequences to produce a recombinant virus, which is coincubated with a drug of interest in a mammalian cell viability assay (Hanna and D'Aquila, 2001; Petropoulos et al., 2000). Growth is compared to a standardized wild-type control virus.

Genotypic tests are now a standard part of HIV care in many parts of the world. The simplest tests measure presence of mutations associated with loss of susceptibility to a drug, that is, that the organism is "resistant" to the drug and the drug should not be used to treat that patient.

Parasites

Susceptibility testing for parasites, especially those that cause malaria, has been performed in the laboratory. The tests are similar to the broth tests for bacteria, fungi, and viruses. *Plasmodium* species in the patient's blood are cultured ex vivo in the presence of different dilutions of antimalarial drug. A sigmoid E_{max} curve for effect versus drug concentration is used to identify IC_{50} and E_{max}. These susceptibility tests are usually field tests at sentinel sites that are used to determine if there is drug resistance in a particular area. In general, susceptibility tests for parasitic infections are not standardized. These tests are primarily used in the research setting and not for individualization of therapy.

Basis for Selection of Dose and Dosing Schedule

Although susceptibility testing in the laboratory is central to decision making, it does not completely predict patient response. In susceptibility tests, the drug concentration is constant; by contrast, in patients the drug concentration is dynamic and ever changing. Antibiotics are prescribed at a certain schedule (e.g., three times a day) so that there is a periodicity in the fluctuations of drug at the site of infection, and the microbe is exposed to a particular shape of the concentration-time curve. Harry Eagle performed studies on penicillin and discovered that the shape of the concentration-time profile was an important determinant of the efficacy of the antibiotic. This important observation was forgotten until William Craig and colleagues rediscovered it and performed systematic studies on several classes of antibiotics, initiating the era of antimicrobial PK/PD (Ambrose et al., 2007; Craig, 2007). These findings have now been extended to combination therapy and to microbes that require long treatment durations, such as *Mycobacterium tuberculosis* and HIV.

There are three precepts to follow in antimicrobial therapy:

First, apply knowledge of the susceptibility (either MIC or IC_{90}) of the organism to the antimicrobial agent and index drug exposure to MIC.

As an example, the pyrazinamide MIC is an important determinant of *M. tuberculosis* response and microbial measures of cure (Chigutsa et al., 2015). In fact, microbial response is driven by the ratio of the AUC to the MIC.

Similarly, in the treatment of candidemia, the rate of response is driven by the ratio dose/MIC (Rodríquez-Tudela et al., 2007). This is not a surprise because the IC_{50} shifts to the right with decrease in susceptibility (Figure 52–3A).

Second, use the optimal dose of the antibiotic for the patient, that is, the dose that achieves IC_{80} to IC_{90} exposures at the site of infection.

Dose by itself is a poor measure of drug exposure. Rather, actual drug concentration achieved at the site of infection is the important measure. The shape of the relationship between non–protein-bound antibiotic concentration (exposure) versus microbial kill is the inhibitory sigmoid E_{max} curve of Figure 52–1. Maximal kill is actually on an asymptote, so that non–protein-bound antimicrobial exposures associated with 80%–90% of E_{max} are termed *optimal* concentrations. This exposure can often be easily identified in preclinical models and directly applied to patient populations, provided interspecies differences in protein binding and pharmacokinetic variability are taken into account.

Third, use a dosing schedule that maximizes the antimicrobial effect; recognize that optimal microbial kill by the antibiotic may be best achieved by maximizing certain shapes of the concentration-time curve.

As an example, consider an antibiotic with a serum $t_{1/2}$ of 3 h that is being used to treat a bloodstream infection by a pathogen with an MIC of 0.5 mg/L; the antibiotic is administered with a dosing interval of 24 h (that is, a once-daily schedule). Figure 52–4A depicts the concentration-time curve of the antibiotic, with definitions of C_{Pmax}, AUC, and the fraction of the dosing interval for which the drug concentration remains above the

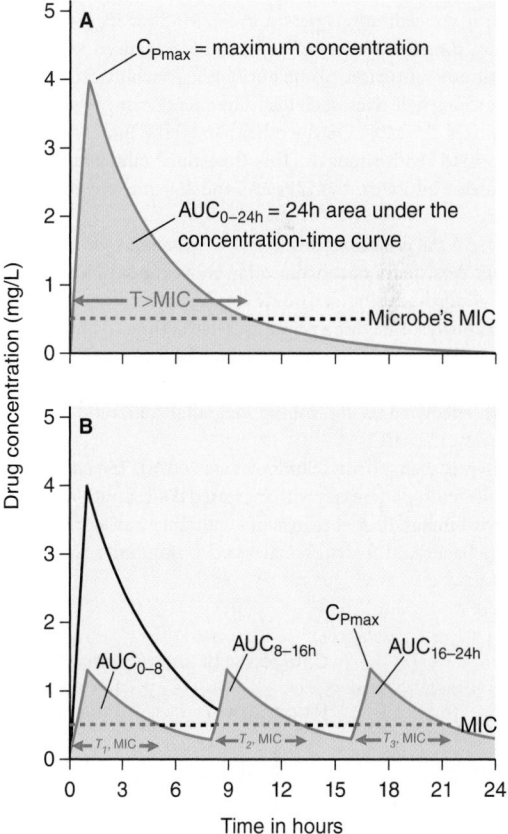

Figure 52–4 *Effect of different dose schedules on shape of the concentration-time curve.* The same total dose of a drug was administered as a single dose (panel **A**) and in three equal portions every 8 h (panel **B**). The total AUC for the fractionated dose in **B** is determined by adding AUC_{0-8h}, AUC_{8-16h}, and AUC_{16-24h}, which totals to the same AUC_{0-24h} in **A**. The time that the drug concentration exceeds MIC in **B** is also determined by adding $T_1 > MIC$, $T_2 > MIC$, and $T_3 > MIC$, which results in a fraction greater than that for **A**.

MIC (T > MIC), as shown. The AUC is a measure of the total concentration of drug and is calculated by taking an integral between two time points, 0–24 h (AUC_{0-24}) in this case.

Now, if one were to change the dosing schedule of the same antibiotic amount by splitting it into three equal doses administered at 0, 8, and 16 h, the shape of the concentration-time curve changes to that shown in Figure 52–4B. Because the same cumulative dose has been given for the dosing interval of 24 h, the AUC_{0-24} will be similar whether it was given once a day or three times a day. For the same pathogen, therefore, the change in dose schedule does not change the AUC_{0-24}/MIC. However, the C_{Pmax} will decrease by a third when the total dose is split into thirds and administered more frequently (Figure 52–4B). Thus, when a dose is fractionated and administered more frequently, the C_{Pmax}/MIC ratio *decreases*. In contrast, the time that the drug concentration persists above MIC (T > MIC) will *increase* with the more frequent dosing schedule, despite the same cumulative dose being administered. Which of the three indices (AUC/MIC, C_{Pmax}/MIC, or T > MIC) is the most important to the outcome being assessed (i.e., microbial kill)? A common approach to the answer is to determine which of these patterns best approximates a perfect inhibitory sigmoid E_{max} curve (based on various statistical assessments of goodness of fit) in Equation 52–1.

Some classes of antimicrobial agents kill best when concentration persists above MIC for longer durations of the dosing interval. Indeed, increasing the drug concentration beyond four to six times the MIC does not increase microbial kill for such antibiotics. Two good examples are β-lactam antibacterials (e.g., penicillin) and the antifungal agent 5-flourocytosine (Ambrose et al., 2007; Andes and van Ogtrop, 2000). There are usually good biochemical explanations for this pattern; the clinical implication, however, is that a drug optimized by T > MIC should be dosed more frequently, or if possible should have its $t_{1/2}$ prolonged by other drugs, so that drug concentrations persist above MIC (or EC_{95}) as long as possible. Thus, the effectiveness of penicillin is enhanced when it is given as a continuous infusion. Some antibiotics, such as ceftriaxone ($t_{1/2}$ = 8 h), have a long half-lives, such that infrequent dosing several times a day still optimizes T > MIC. On the other hand, HIV protease inhibitors are often "boosted" with ritonavir. This "boosting" inhibits the metabolism of the protease inhibitors by CYPs 3A4 and 2D6, thereby prolonging time above EC_{95}.

Conversely, the peak concentration is what matters for other antimicrobial agents. Persistence of concentration above the MIC has less relevance for these drugs, meaning that these drugs can be dosed more intermittently. Aminoglycosides are a prime example of this class; aminoglycosides are highly effective when given once a day. These C_{Pmax}/MIC–linked drugs can often be administered less frequently due to their long duration of PAE, with effectiveness continuing long after antibiotic concentrations decline below the MIC.

Rifampin is such a drug (Gumbo et al., 2007a). The entry of rifampin into *M. tuberculosis* increases with increased concentration in the bacillus microenvironment, likely because of a saturable transport process. Once inside the bacteria, the drug's macrocyclic ring binds the β subunit of DNA-dependent RNA polymerase (*rpoB*) to form a stable drug-enzyme complex within 10 min, a process not enhanced by longer incubation of drug and enzyme and only slowly reversed. The PAE of the rifampin is long and concentration dependent (Gumbo et al., 2007a).

There is a third group of drugs for which it is the cumulative dose that matters, and for which the daily dosing schedule has no effect on efficacy. Thus, it is more ratio of the total concentration (AUC) to MIC that matters and not the time that concentration persists above a certain threshold. Antibacterial agents such as daptomycin fall into this class (Louie et al., 2001). These agents also have a good PAE. The AUC/IC_{50} explains why tenofovir and emtricitabine (nucleoside analogue reverse transcriptase inhibitors) have been combined into one pill, administered once a day for the treatment of AIDS.

The shape of the concentration-time curve that optimizes resistance suppression is often different from that which optimizes microbial kill. In many instances, the drug exposure associated with resistance suppression is much higher than that for optimal kill. Ideally, this higher exposure should be achieved by each dose in patients for optimal effect, rather than the EC_{80} as discussed previously. However, this is often precluded by drug toxicity at higher dosages. Second, although the relationship between kill and exposure is based on the inhibitory sigmoid E_{max} model, experimental work with preclinical models demonstrated that this model does not apply to resistance suppression (Gumbo et al., 2007b; Tam et al., 2007).

To summarize:

- The optimal dose should be designed to achieve a high probability of exceeding the EC_{80} microbial PK/PD index, or an index associated with suppression of resistance, given the population pharmacokinetic variability and the MIC distribution of clinical microbe isolates.
- The dose schedule is chosen according to whether efficacy is driven by AUC/MIC (or AUC/EC_{95}), C_{Pmax}/MIC, or T > MIC. Duration of therapy is then chosen based on best-available evidence.

Types and Goals of Antimicrobial Therapy

A useful way to organize the types and goals of antimicrobial therapy is to consider where along the disease progression timetable therapy is initiated (Figure 52–5); therapy can be *prophylactic, preemptive, empirical, definitive,* or *suppressive.*

Prophylactic Therapy

Prophylaxis involves treating patients who are not yet infected or have not yet developed disease. The goal of prophylaxis is to prevent infection in some patients or to prevent development of a potentially dangerous disease in those who already have evidence of infection. *The main principle behind prophylaxis is targeted therapy.*

An important recent advance has been the understanding of the roles of the human microbiome in health. The biome is a critical defense against dangerous infections and important in uptake of vaccines. So extensive is

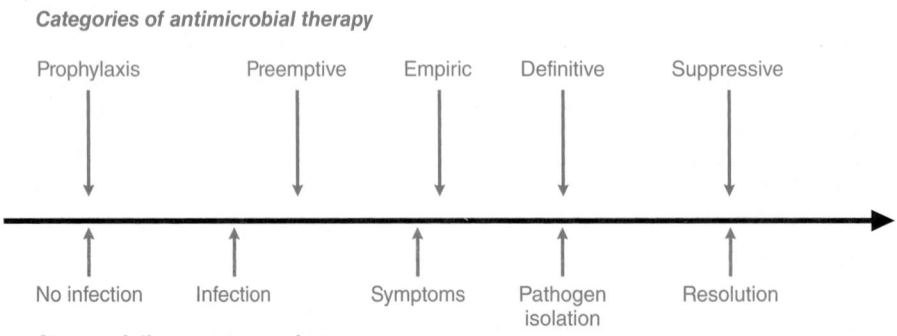

Categories of antimicrobial therapy

Prophylaxis   Preemptive   Empiric   Definitive   Suppressive

No infection   Infection   Symptoms   Pathogen isolation   Resolution

Stages of disease progression

Figure 52–5 *Antimicrobial therapy-disease progression timeline.*

the putative preventive role of the microbiome that the list of conditions when it is disrupted is long, but includes common conditions such as allergies, autism, cancer, antibiotic-associated colitis, diabetes, and obesity. Thus, in routine prophylaxis there is need to preserve the native biome as much as possible. Thus, consider the following:

- Consider narrow-spectrum antibiotics targeted at the most important (potential surgical site) infectious organisms and do not target all possible bacteria.
- Limit the duration of prophylaxis to be as short as the time in which maximum contamination is expected (e.g., during incisions and the surgical procedure) and do not prolong beyond this time.
- Apply PK/PD thinking, as described previously.

Prophylaxis in Immunosuppressed Patients

Prophylaxis is used in immunosuppressed patients such as those with HIV-AIDS or are posttransplantation and on antirejection medications. The efficacy of prophylaxis in these patients is based on excellent evidence (Centers for Disease Control and Prevention et al., 2000; DHHS Panel, 2015). In these groups of patients, specific antiparasitic, antibacterial, antiviral, and antifungal therapy is administered based on the well-defined pattern of pathogens that are major causes of morbidity during immunosuppression. A risk-benefit analysis determines choice and duration of prophylaxis. Prophylaxis of opportunistic infections in patients with AIDS is started when the CD4 count falls below 200 cells/mm³, and is discontinued when the CD4 count climbs above 200 cells/mm³. In posttransplant patients, prophylaxis depends on time since the transplant procedure, which is related to intensity of use and type of immunosuppressive therapy. Prophylaxis should be discontinued in patients who are doing well at certain benchmarks, such as 1 year posttransplant. Infections for which prophylaxis is given include *Pneumocystis jiroveci, Mycobacterium avium-intracellulare, Toxoplasma gondii, Candida* species, *Aspergillus* species, *Cytomegalovirus,* and other Herpesviridae. In general, the prophylactic dose is lower than when the same drug is used for acute treatment.

Chemoprophylaxis for Surgical Procedures

Wound infection results when a critical number of bacteria are present in the wound at the time of closure, and chemoprophylaxis can be used to prevent wound infections after surgical procedures. Antimicrobial agents directed against the invading microorganisms may reduce the number of viable bacteria below the critical level and thus prevent infection. Because *S. aureus* is consistently the most common organism causing surgical site infections, programs have been developed to decolonize the patient of this organism *prior to* cardiac and orthopedic surgery. Approaches to decrease surgical site infections involve screening by culturing the patient's nares and other colonization sites before surgery and decolonizing any *S. aureus* with intranasal mupirocin twice daily and chlorhexidine-gluconate baths daily for up to 5 days before the surgery, followed by the usual perioperative systemic antibiotics (Schweizer et al., 2015).

The systemic antibiotic used is chosen based on the pathogen most likely to contaminate the incision, which in turn depends on the site where surgery is being performed (Bratzler et al., 2013). The most common pathogens infecting incision sites after clean surgery are staphylococci, specifically *S. aureus* and coagulase-negative staphylococci. In clean contaminated surgery over the abdomen and pelvis, the same organisms remain important, but *Enterococcus* species and gram-negative rods are also common. The perioperative antimicrobial dose should be administered intravenously within 60 min prior to the surgical incision, so that concentrations are above the MIC of the organism at time of incision. The frequency of redosing during the procedure is based on the half-life of the drug in order to have adequate antibiotic concentrations above the MIC until closure of the surgical incision. This is especially important for those β-lactam antibiotics that have short half-lives; these should be redosed at intervals of two times the half-life. It is recommended that the duration of prophylaxis be shorter than 24 h postoperation and in many instances be just a single dose.

The types of surgical procedures for which systemic antibiotic prophylaxis is required has recently been expanded (Table 52–1) (Bratzler et al., 2013). The guidelines, based on consensus of opinion leaders, also suggest that the same principles for adults apply to children. However, note that the pharmacokinetics of the antibiotics may differ in children.

Prophylaxis in Patients at Risk of Infective Endocarditis

Patients at the highest risk for infective endocarditis for which prophylaxis is recommended fall into four groups (Wilson et al., 2007):

- those with a prosthetic material used for heart valve repair or replacement;
- patients having had previous infective endocarditis;
- patients with congenital heart disease such as unrepaired cyanotic heart disease, or within 6 months of repair of the heart disease with prosthetic material, or those with residual defects adjacent to prosthetic material; and
- postcardiac transplant patients with heart valve defects.

Chemoprophylaxis is reasonable when these patients undergo dental procedures if there is manipulation of gingival tissue or the periapical region of teeth or perforation of oral mucosa, but not for other dental procedures. Recommended therapy is a single dose of oral amoxicillin 30 min to 1 h before the procedure; intravenous ampicillin or ceftriaxone in those unable to take oral medication; or macrolide or clindamycin for patients allergic to β-lactam agents. Therapy may be administered no more than 2 h after the procedure for patients who failed to receive the prophylaxis prior to the procedure (Wilson et al., 2007).

Prophylaxis for Procedures on Infected Tissues

Prophylaxis is also reasonable for procedures that will involve infected skin and soft tissues as well as infected respiratory tract, but not in routine genitourinary and GI tract procedures. If the organism causing the infection is known, then the prophylactic antibiotic for patients undergoing these procedures should be tailored toward that organism.

Postexposure Prophylaxis

Postexposure prophylaxis may be used to protect healthy persons from acquisition of or invasion by specific microorganisms to which they are exposed. Successful examples of this practice include rifampin administration to prevent meningococcal meningitis in people who are in close contact with a case, prevention of gonorrhea or syphilis after contact with an infected person, and macrolides after contact with confirmed cases of pertussis.

For HIV, there is now clear evidence to use antiretroviral therapy as part of prophylaxis in four situations: (1) immediate antiretroviral therapy for the partner in a serodiscordant couple; (2) preexposure prophylaxis for all population groups at substantial risk of HIV infection; (3) prevention of mother-to-child transmission; and (4) postexposure prophylaxis, which is after accidental exposure to HIV in body fluids. It is recommended that at least three drugs be administered for at least 28 days.

For influenza, the neuraminidase inhibitor oseltamivir is recommended for prevention of influenza A and B in healthy adults and children with close contact of laboratory-confirmed cases (Hayden and Pavia, 2006). Finally, mother-to-child transmission of syphilis is also an important public health problem for which specific chemotherapeutic regimens have been devised, based on locality. Prophylactic therapy for syphilis during pregnancy is effective in reducing neonatal death and infant neurological, auditory, and bone malformations.

Preemptive Therapy

Preemptive therapy is used as a substitute for universal prophylaxis and as early targeted therapy in high-risk patients who already have a laboratory or other test indicating that an asymptomatic patient is infected. The principle is that delivery of therapy prior to development of symptoms aborts impending disease, and the therapy is for a short and defined duration. This has been applied in the clinic to therapy for CMV after both hematopoietic stem cell transplants and after solid-organ transplantation (Gerna et al., 2008). When rapid turnaround tests (e.g., PCR based) are available, the preemptive strategy is now more preferable than universal prophylaxis for CMV.

Empirical Therapy in the Symptomatic Patient

Should a symptomatic patient be treated immediately? *The reflex action to associate fever with treatable infections and prescribe antimicrobial therapy without further evaluation is irrational and potentially dangerous.*

TABLE 52–1 ■ PROPHYLACTIC ANTIMICROBIALS FOR SURGERY

ANATOMICAL REGION	TYPE OF PROCEDURE	RECOMMENDED ANTIBIOTICS
Head and neck	Neurosurgery: craniotomy and cerebrospinal fluid shunting	Cefazolin
	Clean contaminated cancer surgery	Cefazolin + metronidazole
		Cefuroxime + metronidazole
		Ampicillin-sulbactam
Thoracic/cardiac	Coronary artery bypass, cardiac device insertion	Cefazolin, cefuroxime
	Lobectomy, pneumonectomy, lung resection, thoracotomy	Cefazolin, ampicillin-sulbactam
	Transplantation of heart and lung	Cefazolin
Abdomen		
Gastroduodenal	Procedures that enter GI lumen or no GI entry but high-risk patients	Cefazolin
Biliary tract	Open procedure	Cefazolin, ampicillin-sulbactam, cefoxitin, ceftriaxone, cefotetan
Laparoscopy	High-risk procedures	Cefazolin, ampicillin-sulbactam, cefoxitin, ceftriaxone, cefotetan
Appendix	Appendectomy for appendicitis	Cefazolin + metronidazole, cefoxitin, cefotetan
Hernia	Hernia repair	Cefazolin
Colorectal	All	Cefazolin + metronidazole, ampicillin-sulbactam, cefoxitin, ceftriaxone, cefotetan, ceftriaxone + metronidazole ertapenem
Pancreas	Pancreas and pancreas-kidney transplantation	Cefazolin + fluconazole
Pelvis/gynecological		
Uterus	Hysterectomy	Cefazolin, ampicillin-sulbactam, cefoxitin, cefotetan
	Cesarean section	Cefazolin
Urologic	Lower tract instrumentation with risk factors for infection	Fluoroquinolone, trimethoprim-sulfamethoxazole, cefazolin
	Clean: with or without entry into urinary tract	Cefazolin
	Involving implanted prosthesis	Cefazolin + aminoglycoside, cefazolin, ampicillin-sulbactam
	Clean contaminated	Cefazolin + metronidazole, cefoxitin
Orthopedic	Spinal procedures, hip fracture repair, joint replacement	Cefazolin

The first consideration in selecting an antimicrobial is to determine if the drug is indicated. The diagnosis may be masked if therapy is started and appropriate cultures are not obtained. Antimicrobial agents are potentially toxic and may promote selection of resistant microorganisms. For some diseases, the risk in waiting a few days is low, and these patients can wait for microbiological evidence of infection without empirical treatment. If the risks of waiting are high, based either on the patient's immune status or other known risk factors, then initiation of optimal empirical antimicrobial therapy should rely on the clinical presentation and clinical experience. In addition, simple and rapid laboratory techniques are available for the examination of infected tissues.

The most valuable and time-tested method for immediate identification of bacteria is examination of the infected secretion or body fluid with Gram stain. In malaria-endemic areas, or in travelers returning from such an area, a simple thick-and-thin blood smear may mean the difference between a patient's survival on appropriate therapy or death while on the wrong therapy for a presumed bacterial infection. On the other hand, neutropenic patients with fever have high risks of mortality, and when febrile, they are presumed to have either a bacterial or a fungal infection. Thus, a broad-spectrum combination of antibacterial and antifungal agents that cover common infections encountered in granulocytopenic

patients is given. Performance of cultures is still mandatory with a view to modify antimicrobial therapy with culture results.

Definitive Therapy With Known Pathogen

Once a pathogen has been identified and susceptibility results are available, therapy should be streamlined to a narrow targeted antibiotic. *Monotherapy is preferred* to decrease the risk of antimicrobial toxicity and selection of antimicrobial-resistant pathogens. Proper antimicrobial doses and dose schedules are crucial to maximizing efficacy and minimizing toxicity. In addition, the duration of therapy should be as short as is necessary. Unnecessarily prolonged therapies lead to the emergence of resistance.

Combination therapy is an exception, rather than a rule. Once a pathogen has been isolated, there should be no reason to use multiple antibiotics, except when evidence overwhelmingly suggests otherwise. Using two antimicrobial agents where one suffices leads to increased toxicity and unnecessary damage to the patient's protective fungal and bacterial flora. There are special circumstances where evidence favors combination therapy:

- preventing resistance to monotherapy;
- accelerating the rapidity of microbial kill;

- enhancing therapeutic efficacy by use of synergistic interactions or enhancing kill by a drug based on a mutation generated by resistance to another drug;
- reducing toxicity (i.e., when sufficient efficacy of a single antibacterial agent can be achieved only at doses that are toxic to the patient and a second drug is coadministered to permit lowering the dose of the first drug)

Clinical situations for which combination therapy is advised include antiretroviral therapy for AIDS; antiviral therapy for hepatitis B and C; the treatment of tuberculosis, *M. avium-intracellulare,* and leprosy; fixed-dose combinations of antimalarial drugs; the treatment of *Cryptococcus neoformans* with flucytosine and amphotericin B; during empirical therapy for patients with febrile neutropenia; and for advanced AIDS with fever. The combination of a sulfonamide and an inhibitor of DHFR, such as trimethoprim, is synergistic owing to the inhibition of sequential steps in microbial folate synthesis; a fixed combination of sulfamethoxazole and trimethoprim is active against organisms that may be resistant to sulfonamides alone.

Posttreatment Suppressive Therapy

In some patients, the infection is controlled but not completely eradicated by the initial round of antimicrobial treatment, and the immunological or anatomical defect that led to the original infection is still present. In such patients, therapy is continued at a lower dose. This is common in patients with AIDS and patients posttransplant. The goal is more as secondary prophylaxis. Nevertheless, risks of toxicity from the long durations of therapy are still real. In this group of patients, the suppressive therapy is eventually discontinued if the patient's immune system improves.

Mechanisms of Resistance to Antimicrobial Agents

Antimicrobial agents were viewed as miracle cures when first introduced into clinical practice. However, as became evident soon after the discovery of penicillin, resistance develops and dims the luster of the miracle. This serious development is ever present with each new antimicrobial agent and threatens the end of the antimicrobial era. Today, every major class of antibiotic is associated with the emergence of significant resistance. *Two major factors are associated with emergence of antibiotic resistance: evolution and clinical/environmental practices.* When a microbial species is subjected to an existential threat, chemical or otherwise, that pressure will select for random mutations in the species' genome that permit survival. Pathogens will evolve to develop resistance to the chemical warfare to which we subject them. This evolution is greatly assisted by poor therapeutic practices by healthcare workers and the indiscriminant use of antibiotics in agriculture and animal husbandry.

Antimicrobial resistance can develop at any one or more of steps in the processes by which a drug reaches and combines with its target. Thus, resistance development may develop due to

- reduced entry of antibiotic into pathogen
- enhanced export of antibiotic by efflux pumps
- release of microbial enzymes that alter or destroy the antibiotic
- alteration of target proteins
- development of alternative pathways to those inhibited by the antibiotic

Mechanisms by which such resistance develops can include acquisition of genetic elements that code for the resistant mechanism, mutations that develop under antibiotic pressure, or constitutive induction.

Resistance Due to Reduced Entry of Drug Into Pathogen

The outer membrane of gram-negative bacteria is a semipermeable barrier that excludes large polar molecules from entering the cell. Small polar molecules, including many antibiotics, enter the cell through protein channels called *porins*. Absence of, mutation in, or loss of a favored porin channel can slow the rate of drug entry into a cell or prevent entry altogether, effectively reducing drug concentration at the target site. If the target is intracellular and the drug requires active transport across the cell membrane, a mutation or phenotypic change that slows or abolishes this transport mechanism can confer resistance. For example, *Trypanosoma brucei* is treated with suramin and pentamidine during early stages, but with melarsoprol and eflornithine when CNS disease (sleeping sickness) is present. Melarsoprol is actively taken up by the trypanosome P2 transporter. When the parasite lacks the P2 transporter or has a mutant form, resistance to melarsoprol and cross resistance to pentamidine occur due to reduced drug uptake (Ouellette, 2001).

Resistance Due to Drug Efflux

Microorganisms can overexpress efflux pumps and then expel antibiotics to which the microbes would otherwise be susceptible. There are five major systems of efflux pumps that are relevant to antimicrobial agents:

- The multidrug and toxin extruder
- The major facilitator superfamily transporters
- The small multidrug resistance system
- The resistance nodulation division exporters
- ABC transporters

Efflux pumps are a prominent mechanism of resistance for parasites, bacteria, and fungi. One of the tragic consequences of resistance emergence has been the development of drug resistance by *Plasmodium falciparum.* Drug resistance to most antimalarial drugs, specifically chloroquine, quinine, mefloquine, halofantrine, lumefantrine, and the artemether-lumefantrine combination is mediated by an ABC transporter encoded by *P. falciparum* multidrug resistance gene 1 (Pf*mdr1*) (Happi et al., 2009). Point mutations in the Pf*mdr1* gene lead to drug resistance and failure of chemotherapy.

Drug efflux sometimes works in tandem with chromosomal resistance, as is seen in *Streptococcus pneumoniae* and *M. tuberculosis.* In these situations, induction of efflux pumps occurs early, which increases the MIC only modestly. However, this MIC increase may suffice to allow further microbial replication, a continuation of mutation, and the development of resistance via more robust chromosomal mutations (Gumbo et al., 2007b; Jumbe et al., 2006; Schmalstieg et al., 2012).

Resistance Due to Destruction of Antibiotic

Drug inactivation is a common mechanism of drug resistance. Bacterial resistance to aminoglycosides and to β-lactam antibiotics usually is due to production of an aminoglycoside-modifying enzyme or β-lactamase.

Resistance Due to Altered Target Structure

A common consequence of either single- or multiple-point mutations is a change in amino acid composition and conformation of an antimicrobial's target protein. This change can lead to reduced affinity of drug for its target or of a prodrug for the enzyme that activates the prodrug. Such alterations may be due to mutation of the natural target (e.g., fluoroquinolone resistance), target modification (e.g., ribosomal protection type of resistance to macrolides and tetracyclines), or acquisition of a resistant form of the native, susceptible target (e.g., staphylococcal methicillin resistance caused by production of a low-affinity penicillin-binding protein) (Hooper, 2002; Lim and Strynadka, 2002; Nakajima, 1999). In HIV resistance, mutations associated with reduced affinity are encountered for protease inhibitors, integrase inhibitors, fusion inhibitors, and nonnucleoside reverse transcriptase inhibitors (Nijhuis et al., 2009). Similarly, benzimidazoles are used against myriad worms and protozoa and work by binding to the parasite's tubulin; point mutations in the β-tubulin gene lead to modification of the tubulin and drug resistance (Ouellette, 2001).

Incorporation of Drug

An uncommon situation occurs when an organism not only becomes resistant to an antimicrobial agent but also subsequently starts requiring it for growth. Enterococcus, which easily develops vancomycin resistance, can, after prolonged exposure to the antibiotic, develop vancomycin-requiring strains. In 1955, shortly after introduction of streptomycin for tuberculosis, Hashimoto isolated a streptomycin-dependent mutant of *M. tuberculosis*; it grows in the presence of the antibiotic but goes into dormancy in the absence of the streptomycin.

Resistance Due to Enhanced Excision of Incorporated Drug

Nucleoside reverse transcriptase inhibitors such as zidovudine are 2′-deoxyribonucleoside analogues that are converted to their 5′-triphosphate form and compete with natural nucleotides. These drugs are incorporated into the viral DNA chain and cause chain termination. When resistance emerges via mutations in the reverse transcriptase gene, phosphorolytic excision of the incorporated chain-terminating nucleoside analogue is enhanced (Arion et al., 1998).

Heteroresistance and Viral Quasi-Species

Heteroresistance occurs when a subset of the total microbial population is resistant, despite the total population being considered susceptible on testing (Falagas et al., 2008; Rinder, 2001). A subclone that has alterations in genes associated with drug resistance is expected to reflect the normal mutation rates (occurrence in 1 in 10^6 to 10^5 colonies). In bacteria, heteroresistance has been described especially for vancomycin in *S. aureus* and *Enterococcus faecium*; colistin in *Acinetobacter baumannii-calcoaceticus*; rifampin, isoniazid, and streptomycin in *M. tuberculosis*; and penicillin in *S. pneumoniae* (Falagas et al., 2008; Rinder, 2001). Increased therapeutic failures and mortality have been reported in patients with heteroresistant staphylococci and *M. tuberculosis* (Falagas et al., 2008; Hofmann-Thiel et al., 2009). For fungi, heteroresistance leading to clinical failure has been described for fluconazole in *C. neoformans* and *Candida albicans* (Marr et al., 2001; Mondon et al., 1999).

Viral replication is more error prone than replication in bacteria and fungi. Viral evolution under drug and immune pressure occurs relatively easily, commonly resulting in variants or quasi-species that may contain drug-resistant subpopulations. This is not often termed heteroresistance, but the principle is the same: A virus may be considered susceptible to a drug because either phenotypic or genotypic tests reveal "lack" of resistance, even though there is a resistant subpopulation just below the limit of assay detection. These minority quasi-species that are resistant to antiretroviral agents have been associated with failure of antiretroviral therapy (Metzner et al., 2009).

Evolutionary Basis of Resistance Emergence

Development of Resistance via Mutation Selection

Mutations are random events that confer a survival advantage when drug is present. Mutation and antibiotic selection of resistant mutants are the molecular basis for resistance for many bacteria, viruses, and fungi. Mutations may occur in the gene encoding the following:

- the target protein, altering its structure so that it no longer binds the drug
- a protein involved in drug transport
- a protein important for drug activation or inactivation
- in a regulatory gene or promoter affecting expression of the target, a transport protein, or an inactivating enzyme

In some instances, a single-step mutation results in a high degree of resistance. In *M. tuberculosis katG,* Ser315 mutations cause resistance to isoniazid; the M814V mutation in the reverse transcriptase gene of HIV-1 causes resistance to lamivudine; and *C. albicans fks1* Ser645 mutations cause resistance to echinocandins.

In other circumstances, however, it is the sequential acquisition of multiple mutations that leads to clinically significant resistance. For example, the combination of pyrimethamine (an inhibitor of DHFR) and sulfadoxine (an inhibitor of DHPS) blocks the folate biosynthetic pathway in *P. falciparum*. Clinically meaningful resistance occurs only when there is a single-point mutation in the *DHPS* gene accompanied by at least a double mutation in the *DHFR* gene.

Hypermutable Phenotypes

Genetic continuity is accomplished principally by the replicative and repair activities of DNA polymerases and postreplicative repair systems. The development of a defect in one of these repair mechanisms leads to a high degree of mutations in many genes; such isolates are termed *mutator (Mut) phenotypes* and may include mutations in genes causing antibiotic resistance (Giraud et al., 2002). This second-order selection of hypermutable (mutator) alleles based on alterations in DNA repair genes has been implicated in the emergence of multidrug-resistant strains of *M. tuberculosis* Beijing genotype (Rad et al., 2003).

Resistance by External Acquisition of Genetic Elements

As described, drug resistance may be acquired by mutation and selection, with passage of the trait *vertically* to daughter cells, provided the mutation is not lethal, does not appreciably alter virulence, and does not affect replication by the progeny. Drug resistance more commonly is acquired by *horizontal transfer* of resistance determinants from a donor cell, often of another bacterial species, by *transduction, transformation,* or *conjugation*. Resistance acquired by horizontal transfer can disseminate rapidly and widely either by clonal spread of the resistant strain or by subsequent transfers to other susceptible recipient strains. Horizontal transfer of resistance offers several advantages over mutation selection. Lethal mutation of an essential gene is avoided; the level of resistance often is higher than that produced by mutation, which tends to yield incremental changes. The gene, which still can be transmitted vertically, can be mobilized and rapidly amplified within a population by transfer to susceptible cells, and the resistance gene can be eliminated when it no longer offers a selective advantage.

Horizontal Gene Transfer

Horizontal transfer of resistance genes is greatly facilitated by mobile genetic elements. Mobile genetic elements include plasmids and transducing phages. Other mobile elements—*transposable elements, integrons,* and *gene cassettes*—also participate. *Transposable elements* are of three general types: *insertion sequences, transposons,* and *transposable phages.* Only insertion sequences and transposons are important for resistance. There are numerous modes of horizontal resistance transfer:

- *Insertion sequences* are short segments of DNA encoding enzymatic functions (e.g., transposase and resolvase) for site-specific recombination with inverted repeat sequences at either end. They can copy themselves and insert themselves into a chromosome or a plasmid. Insertion sequences do not encode resistance, but they function as sites for integration of other resistance-encoding elements (e.g., plasmids or transposons).
- *Transposons* are insertion sequences, mobile elements that excise and integrate in the bacterial genomic or plasmid DNA (i.e., from plasmid to plasmid, from plasmid to chromosome, or from chromosome to plasmid). Basically, a resistance gene can "hitchhike" with a transferable element out of the host and into a recipient.
- *Integrons* are not formally mobile and do not copy themselves, but they encode an integrase and provide a specific site into which mobile gene cassettes integrate.
- *Gene cassettes* encode resistance determinants, usually lacking a promoter, with a downstream repeat sequence. The integrase recognizes this repeat sequence and directs insertion of the cassette into position behind a strong promoter that is present on the integron. Integrons may be located within transposons or in plasmids and therefore may be mobilizable or located on the chromosome.
- *Transduction* is the acquisition of bacterial DNA from a phage (a virus that propagates in bacteria) that has incorporated DNA from a previous host bacterium within its outer protein coat. If the DNA includes a

Resistance Transfer in Action

A startling example of how the transfer mechanisms spread resistance is the recent description of the plasmid-mediated colistin resistance gene (*mcr*-1), which confers resistance to one of the last-resort antibiotics for multidrug-resistant gram-negative bacteria (Liu et al., 2016). Colistin is used in agriculture and animal husbandry. *Escherichia coli* strains carrying this gene were found in pigs, then in pork, and then in patients. The plasmid carrying *mcr-1* was mobilized by conjugation to *E. coli* at a frequency of 10^{-1} to 10^{-3} cells per recipient and could be spread and maintained in other gram-negative rods of clinical significance. The resistant bacteria were initially identified in China, but within months isolates were also identified in North America, South America, Europe, East Asia, and Africa and in other organisms, such as *Salmonella typhimurium*. The gene has now been demonstrated in gut microbiota of healthy individuals, suggesting integration in the human gut and the capacity to spread to organisms in the human microbiome.

gene for drug resistance, the newly infected bacterial cell may acquire resistance. Transduction is particularly important in the transfer of antibiotic resistance among strains of *S. aureus*.

- *Transformation* is the uptake and incorporation into the host genome by homologous recombination of free DNA released into the environment by other bacterial cells. Transformation is the molecular basis of penicillin resistance in pneumococci and *Neisseria*.

- *Conjugation* is gene transfer by direct cell-to-cell contact through a sex pilus or bridge, allowing the transfer of multiple resistance genes in a single event. The transferable genetic material consists of two different sets of plasmid-encoded genes on the same or different plasmids: one encoding the actual resistance, and another encoding genes necessary for bacterial conjugation. Conjugation with genetic exchange between nonpathogenic and pathogenic microorganisms probably occurs in the GI tract. The efficiency of transfer is low; however, antibiotics can exert a powerful selective pressure to allow emergence of the resistant strain. Genetic transfer by conjugation is common among gram-negative bacilli, and resistance is conferred on a susceptible cell as a single event. Enterococci also contain a broad range of host-range conjugative plasmids that are involved in the transfer and spread of resistance genes among gram-positive organisms.

Bibliography

Ambrose PG, et al. Pharmacokinetics-pharmacodynamics of antimicrobial therapy: It's not just for mice anymore. *Clin Infect Dis,* **2007**, *44*:79–86.

Andes D, et al. Use of pharmacokinetic-pharmacodynamic analyses to optimize therapy with the systemic antifungal micafungin for invasive candidiasis or candidemia. *Antimicrob Agents Chemother,* **2011**, *55*: 2113–2121.

Andes D, van Ogtrop M. In vivo characterization of the pharmacodynamics of flucytosine in a neutropenic murine disseminated candidiasis model. *Antimicrob Agents Chemother,* **2000**, *44*:938–942.

Arion D, et al. Phenotypic mechanism of HIV-1 resistance to 3′-azido-3′-deoxythymidine (AZT): increased polymerization processivity and enhanced sensitivity to pyrophosphate of the mutant viral reverse transcriptase. *Biochemistry,* **1998**, *37*: 15908–15917.

Bratzler DW, et al. Clinical practice guidelines for antimicrobial prophylaxis in surgery. *Am J Health Syst Pharm,* **2013**, *70*:195–283.

Bulitta JB, et al. Development and qualification of a pharmacodynamic model for the pronounced inoculum effect of ceftazidime against *Pseudomonas aeruginosa*. *Antimicrob Agents Chemother,* **2009**, *53*: 46–56.

Centers for Disease Control and Prevention, Infectious Disease Society of America, American Society of Blood and Marrow Transplantation. Guidelines for preventing opportunistic infections among hematopoietic stem cell transplant recipients. *MMWR Recomm Rep,* **2000**, *49*:1–7.

Chigutsa E, et al. Impact of nonlinear interactions of pharmacokinetics and MICs on sputum bacillary kill rates as a marker of sterilizing effect in tuberculosis. *Antimicrob Agents Chemother,* **2015**, *59*:38–45.

Chow AT, et al. Penetration of levofloxacin into skin tissue after oral administration of multiple 750 mg once-daily doses. *J Clin Pharm Ther,* **2002**, *27*:143–150.

Conte JE Jr, et al. Intrapulmonary pharmacokinetics and pharmacodynamics of high-dose levofloxacin in healthy volunteer subjects. *Int J Antimicrob Agents,* **2006**, *28*: 114–121.

Craig WA. Pharmacodynamics of antimicrobials: general concepts and applications. In: Nightangle CH, Ambrose PG, Drusano GL, Murakawa T, eds. *Antimicrobial Pharmacodynamics in Theory and Practice.* 2nd ed. Informa Healthcare USA, New York, **2007**, 1–19.

Daneman R, Prat A. The blood-brain barrier. *Cold Spring Harb Perspect Biol,* **2015**, *7*:1–23.

DHHS Panel. Guidelines for prevention and treatment of opportunistic infections in HIV-infected adults and adolescents. **2015**. Available at: https://aidsinfo.nih.gov/contentfiles/lvguidelines/Adult_OI.pdf.Accessed February 23, 2016.

Dorlo TP, et al. Failure of miltefosine in visceral leishmaniasis is associated with low drug exposure. *J Infect Dis,* **2014**, *210*:146–153.

Falagas ME, et al. Heteroresistance: a concern of increasing clinical significance? *Clin Microbiol Infect,* **2008**, *14*:101–104.

Gerna G, et al. Prophylaxis followed by preemptive therapy versus preemptive therapy for prevention of human cytomegalovirus disease in pediatric patients undergoing liver transplantation. *Transplantation,* **2008**, *86*:163–166.

Giraud A, et al. Mutator bacteria as a risk factor in treatment of infectious diseases. *Antimicrob Agents Chemother,* **2002**, *46*:863–865.

Gumbo T, et al. Anidulafungin pharmacokinetics and microbial response in neutropenic mice with disseminated candidiasis. *Antimicrob Agents Chemother,* **2006**, *50*:3695–3700.

Gumbo T, et al. Concentration-dependent *Mycobacterium tuberculosis* killing and prevention of resistance by rifampin. *Antimicrob Agents Chemother,* **2007a**, *51*:3781–3788.

Gumbo T, et al. Isoniazid bactericidal activity and resistance emergence: Integrating pharmacodynamics and pharmacogenomics to predict efficacy in different ethnic populations. *Antimicrob Agents Chemother,* **2007b**, *51*:2329–2336.

Hanna GJ, D'Aquila RT. Clinical use of genotypic and phenotypic drug resistance testing to monitor antiretroviral chemotherapy. *Clin Infect Dis,* **2001**, *32*:774–782.

Happi CT, et al. Selection of *Plasmodium falciparum* multidrug resistance gene 1 alleles in asexual stages and gametocytes by artemether-lumefantrine in Nigerian children with uncomplicated falciparum malaria. *Antimicrob Agents Chemother,* **2009**, *53*:888–895.

Hayden FG, Pavia AT. Antiviral management of seasonal and pandemic influenza. *J Infect Dis,* **2006**, *194*(suppl2):S119–S126.

Hirsch MS, et al. Antiretroviral drug resistance testing in adult HIV-1 infection: 2008 recommendations of an International AIDS Society-USA panel. *Clin Infect Dis,* **2008**, *47*: 266–285.

Hofmann-Thiel S, et al. Mechanisms of heteroresistance to isoniazid and rifampin of *Mycobacterium tuberculosis* in Tashkent, Uzbekistan. *Eur Respir J,* **2009**, *33*:368–374.

Hooper DC. Fluoroquinolone resistance among gram-positive cocci. *Lancet Infect Dis,* **2002**, *2*:530–538.

Hope WW, et al. Population pharmacokinetics of micafungin in pediatric patients and implications for antifungal dosing. *Antimicrob Agents Chemother,* **2007**, *51*:3714–3719.

Jumbe N, et al. Application of a mathematical model to prevent in vivo amplification of antibiotic-resistant bacterial populations during therapy. *J Clin Invest,* **2003**, *112*:275–285.

Jumbe NL, et al. Quinolone efflux pumps play a central role in emergence of fluoroquinolone resistance in *Streptococcus pneumoniae*. *Antimicrob Agents Chemother,* **2006**, *50*:310–317.

Kiem S, Schentag JJ. Interpretation of antibiotic concentration ratios measured in epithelial lining fluid. *Antimicrob Agents Chemother,* **2008**, *52*:24–36.

Lim D, Strynadka NC. Structural basis for the beta lactam resistance of PBP2a from methicillin-resistant *Staphylococcus aureus*. *Nat Struct Biol,* **2002**, *9*:870–876.

Liu YY, et al. Emergence of plasmid-mediated colistin resistance mechanism MCR-1 in animals and human beings in China: a microbiological and molecular biological study. *Lancet Infect Dis*, **2016**, *16*:161–168.

Louie A, et al. Pharmacodynamics of daptomycin in a murine thigh model of *Staphylococcus aureus* infection. *Antimicrob Agents Chemother*, **2001**, *45*:845–851.

Marr KA, et al. Inducible azole resistance associated with a heterogeneous phenotype in *Candida albicans*. *Antimicrob Agents Chemother*, **2001**, *45*:52–59.

Metzner KJ, et al. Minority quasi-species of drug-resistant HIV-1 that lead to early therapy failure in treatment-naive and -adherent patients. *Clin Infect Dis*, **2009**, *48*:239–247.

Mondon P, et al. Heteroresistance to fluconazole and voriconazole in *Cryptococcus neoformans*. *Antimicrob Agents Chemother*, **1999**, *43*:1856–1861.

Nakajima Y. Mechanisms of bacterial resistance to macrolide antibiotics. *J Infect Chemother*, **1999**, *5*:61–74.

Nijhuis M, et al. Antiviral resistance and impact on viral replication capacity: evolution of viruses under antiviral pressure occurs in three phases. *Handb Exp Pharmacol*, **2009**, *189*:299–320.

Ouellette M. Biochemical and molecular mechanisms of drug resistance in parasites. *Trop Med Int Health*, **2001**, *6*:874–882.

Pasipanodya JG, et al. Serum drug concentrations predictive of pulmonary tuberculosis outcomes. *J Infect Dis*, **2013**, *208*:1464–7143.

Petropoulos CJ, et al. A novel phenotypic drug susceptibility assay for human immunodeficiency virus type1. *Antimicrob Agents Chemother*, **2000**, *44*:920–928.

Preston SL, et al. Pharmacodynamics of levofloxacin: a new paradigm for early clinical trials. *JAMA*, **1998**, *279*:125–129.

Rad ME, et al. Mutations in putative mutator genes of *Mycobacterium tuberculosis* strains of the W-Beijing family. *Emerg Infect Dis*, **2003**, *9*:838–845.

Rinder H. Hetero-resistance: an under-recognised confounder in diagnosis and therapy? *J Med Microbiol*, **2001**, *50*:1018–1020.

Rodríguez-Tudela JL, et al. Correlation of the MIC and dose/MIC ratio of fluconazole to the therapeutic response of patients with mucosal candidiasis and candidemia. *Antimicrob Agents Chemother*, **2007**, *51*:3599–3604.

Schmalstieg AM, et al. The antibiotic resistance arrow of time: efflux pump induction is a general first step in the evolution of mycobacterial drug resistance. *Antimicrob Agents Chemother*, **2012**, *56*:4806–4815.

Schweizer ML, et al. Association of a bundled intervention with surgical site infections among patients undergoing cardiac, hip, or knee surgery. *JAMA*, **2015**, *313*:2162–2171.

Shenje J, et al. Poor penetration of antibiotics into pericardium in pericardial tuberculosis. *EBioMedicine*, **2015**, *2*:1640–1649.

Sun F, et al. Biofilm-associated infections: antibiotic resistance and novel therapeutic strategies. *Future Microbiol*, **2013**, *8*:877–886. doi:10.2217/fmb.13.58.

Talal AH, et al. Pharmacodynamics of PEG-IFN alpha differentiate HIV/HCV coinfected sustained virological responders from nonresponders. *Hepatology*, **2006**, *43*:943–953.

Tam VH, et al. The relationship between quinolone exposures and resistance amplification is characterized by an inverted U: a new paradigm for optimizing pharmacodynamics to counterselect resistance. *Antimicrob Agents Chemother*, **2007**, *51*:744–747.

Tarning J, et al. Population pharmacokinetics of piperaquine after two different treatment regimens with dihydroartemisinin-piperaquine in patients with *Plasmodium falciparum* malariain Thailand. *Antimicrob Agents Chemother*, **2008**, *52*:1052–1061.

Wagenlehner FM, et al. Concentrations in plasma, urinary excretion and bactericidal activity of levofloxacin (500 mg) versus ciprofloxacin (500 mg) in healthy volunteers receiving a single oral dose. *Int J Antimicrob Agents*, **2006**, *28*:551–519.

Wilkins JJ, et al. Population pharmacokinetics of rifampin in pulmonary tuberculosis patients, including a semimechanistic model to describe variable absorption. *Antimicrob Agents Chemother*, **2008**, *52*:2138–2148.

Wilson W, et al. Prevention of infective endocarditis: guidelines from the American Heart Association. *Circulation*, **2007**, *116*:1736–1754.

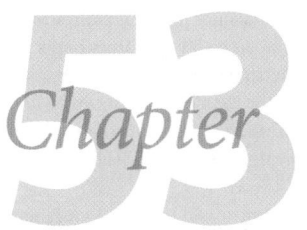

Chapter 53

Chemotherapy of Malaria

Joseph M. Vinetz

Global Impact of Malaria

Malaria remains among the top five causes of death among children younger than 5 years, affects about a quarter of a billion people, and causes almost 900,000 deaths annually (GBD_2013_Collaborators, 2015). Malarial transmission occurs in regions of Africa, Latin and South America, Asia, the Middle East, the South Pacific, and the Caribbean (Figure 53–1). This disease is caused by infection with protozoan parasites of the genus *Plasmodium*. Five *Plasmodium* spp. are known to infect humans: *P. falciparum*, *P. vivax*, *P. ovale*, *P. malariae*, and *P. knowlesi*. *Plasmodium falciparum* and *P. vivax* cause most malarial infections worldwide. *Plasmodium falciparum* accounts for the majority of the burden of malaria in sub-Saharan Africa and is associated with the most severe disease. *Plasmodium vivax* accounts for half of the malaria burden in South and East Asia and more than 80% of the malarial infections in the Americas and has been underappreciated as a cause of severe malaria (Baird, 2013).

Over the past half-century, malaria parasites worldwide—primarily *P. falciparum* and *P. vivax*—have become increasingly resistant to antimalarial drugs, including chloroquine (Djimde et al., 2001; Warhurst, 2001); mefloquine (White et al., 2014); quinine (White et al., 2014); sulfadoxine/pyrimethamine (Artimovich et al., 2015; Plowe et al., 1995, Sibley et al., 2001); and atovaquone (Garcia-Bustos et al., 2013; Kessl et al., 2007). In response, new, multiprong international public-private partnerships as well as other funding agencies and sources have emerged to create new pipelines that advance drug candidates from discovery to clinical development (Hemingway et al., 2016; Wells et al., 2010, 2015).

Biology of Malarial Infection

Malarial infection is initiated when a female anopheline mosquito injects *Plasmodium* sporozoites during a blood meal (Miller et al., 1998). After entering the dermis, sporozoites enter the bloodstream and, within minutes, arrive at the liver, where they infect individual hepatocytes via cell surface receptor-mediated events (Sinnis et al., 2013). This process initiates the *asymptomatic prepatent period*, or *exoerythrocytic stage* of infection, which typically lasts about 1 week.

During this period, the parasite undergoes asexual replication within hepatocytes, resulting in production of liver-stage *schizonts*. When an infected hepatocyte ruptures, tens of thousands of *merozoites* are released into the bloodstream and infect red blood cells. After the initial exoerythrocytic stage, *P. falciparum* and *P. malariae* are no longer found in the liver. *Plasmodium vivax* and *P. ovale*, however, can maintain a quiescent hepatocyte infection as a dormant form of the parasite known as the *hypnozoite* and can reinitiate symptomatic disease long after the initial symptoms of malaria are recognized and treated. Erythrocytic forms cannot reestablish infection of hepatocytes. Transmission of human-infecting malarial parasites is maintained in human populations by the persistence of hypnozoites (several months to a few years for *P. vivax* and *P. ovale*), by antigenic variation in *P. falciparum* (probably months), and by the putative antigen variation in *P. malariae* (for as long as several decades).

The *asexual erythrocytic stages* of malarial parasites are responsible for the clinical manifestations of malaria. This part of the *Plasmodium* life cycle is initiated by merozoite recognition of red blood cells and mediated by cell surface receptors that facilitate invasion of red blood cells.

Once inside a red blood cell, the merozoite develops into a ring form, which becomes a hemoglobin-metabolizing trophozoite (feeding stage) that matures into an asexually dividing blood-stage *schizont*. Schizont rupture at the end of the growth-and-division cycle releases 8–32 merozoites that invade new red blood cells. The erythrocytic replication cycle lasts for 24 h (for *P. knowlesi*), 48 h (for *P. falciparum*, *P. vivax*, and *P. ovale*), and 72 h (for *P. malariae*). Although most invading merozoites develop into schizonts, a small proportion becomes *gametocytes*, the form of the parasite infective to mosquitoes. Gametocytes are ingested by the mosquito during an infectious blood meal; on reaching the midgut of the mosquito, the gametocytes transform into gametes that fertilize to become zygotes. Zygotes mature into ookinetes that invade the mosquito midgut wall and transform into oocysts. Numerous rounds of asexual replication occur in the oocyst to generate sporozoites over 10–14 days. Fully developed sporozoites rupture from oocysts and invade the mosquito salivary glands, from which they can initiate a new infection during subsequent mosquito blood meals (Figure 53–2). Thus, the infection cycles from mosquito to human to mosquito.

Plasmodium falciparum has a family of binding proteins that recognize a variety of host cell molecules that this parasite species uses to invade all stages of erythrocytes (Lim et al., 2015; Weiss et al., 2016); high parasitemia may result from this mechanism. In contrast, *P. vivax* selectively binds to the Duffy chemokine receptor protein as well as reticulocyte-specific proteins (Chitnis et al., 2008; Paul et al., 2015). *Plasmodium falciparum* assembles cytoadherence proteins (e.g., PfEMP1) (Weiss et al., 2016), encoded by a highly variable family of *var* genes into structures called

Abbreviations

ACT: artemisinin-based combination therapy
AV: atrioventricular
CDC: Centers for Disease Control and Prevention
CNS: central nervous system
CSA: chondroitin sulfate A
CSF: cerebrospinal fluid
cytbc₁: cytochrome bc_1
DEET: N, N'-diethylmetatoluamide
ECG: electrocardiogram
FDA: Food and Drug Administration
GI: gastrointestinal
G6PD: glucose-6-phosphate dehydrogenase
5HT: serotonin
IND: investigational new drug (application)
pfCRT: *Plasmodium falciparum* chloroquine resistance transporter
pfMRP: Plasmodium facliparum multidrug resistance-associated protein

knobs that are presented on the erythrocyte surface (Hviid et al., 2015; Ukaegbu et al., 2015). Knobs allow the *P. falciparum*–parasitized erythrocyte to bind to postcapillary vascular endothelium to avoid spleen-mediated clearance and allow the parasite to grow in a low-O_2, high-CO_2 microenvironment.

Clinical Manifestations of Malaria

The cardinal signs and symptoms of malaria are high, spiking fevers (with or without periodicity), chills, headaches, myalgias, malaise, and GI symptoms (White et al., 2014). Severe headache, a characteristic early symptom in malaria caused by all *Plasmodium* spp., often heralds the onset of disease, even before fever and chills. *Plasmodium falciparum* causes the most severe disease and may lead to organ failure and death. Placental malaria, of particular danger for primigravidae, is due to *P. falciparum* adherence to CSA in the placenta. This often leads to severe complications, including miscarriage. When treated early, symptoms of malarial infection usually improve within 24–48 h. New insights into malaria clinical presentations indicate that—in the endemic setting where nonsterilizing clinical immunity is the rule, not the exception—the cardinal symptoms of malaria may be atypical or absent (Chen et al., 2016).

Acute illness due to *P. vivax* infection may appear severe due to high fever and prostration. Indeed, the pyrogenic threshold of this parasite (i.e., "blood stage" parasite burden associated with fever) is lower than that of *P. falciparum*. Nonetheless, *P. vivax* malaria generally has a low mortality rate. *Plasmodium vivax* malaria is characterized by relapses caused by the reactivation of latent tissue forms. Clinical manifestations of relapse are the same as those of primary infection. In recent years, severe *P. vivax* malaria from Oceania (Papua New Guinea, Indonesia) and India possess important similarities to severe malaria caused by *P. falciparum*. These include neurological symptoms (diminished consciousness, seizure) and pulmonary edema. Rare but life-threatening complications can occur, including splenic rupture, acute lung injury, and profound anemia.

Plasmodium ovale causes a clinical syndrome similar to that of *P. vivax* but may be milder with lower levels of parasitemia. It shares with *P. vivax* the ability to form the hypnozoite (dormant liver stage) that may relapse after months to 2 years later. *Plasmodium ovale* is more common in sub-Saharan Africa and some islands in Oceania.

Plasmodium malariae generally causes an indolent infection with very low levels of parasitemia and often does not produce clinical symptoms. This parasite can be found in all malaria-endemic areas but is most common in sub-Saharan Africa and the southwest Pacific. Interestingly, *P. malariae* prevalence increases during the dry season and can be found as a coinfection with *P. falciparum*. An uncommon but potentially fatal complication of *P. malariae* is a glomerulonephritis syndrome that does not respond to antimalarial treatment.

Plasmodium knowlesi infection is often misdiagnosed as *P. malariae* by light microscopy. This infection is distinguished by a shorter erythrocytic cycle (24 h compared with 72 h for *P. malariae*) and higher levels of parasitemia. Like *P. malariae*, *P. knowlesi* is generally sensitive to chloroquine, but patients presenting with advanced disease nonetheless may progress to death despite adequate drug dosing.

Asymptomatic *P. falciparum* and *P. vivax* infections are common in endemic regions and represent important potential reservoirs for malaria transmission. Although different studies are not entirely consistent in the definition of *asymptomatic*, generally this state implies a lack of fever, headache, and other systemic complaints, within a defined time period prior to a positive test for malaria parasitemia. Migration of asymptomatic individuals to areas where malaria is not present but vector mosquitoes are (i.e., anophelism without malaria) is an important mechanism for the introduction or reintroduction of malaria, in addition to facilitating the spread of drug-resistant isolates. Novel approaches to preventing transmission from asymptomatic reservoirs—whether through new drugs or vaccines—will be essential for future malaria control, elimination, and eradication strategies.

Classification of Antimalarial Agents

The various stages of the malarial parasite life cycle in humans differ in their drug sensitivity. Thus, antimalarial drugs can be classified based on their activities during this life cycle as well as by their intended use for either chemoprophylaxis or treatment. The spectrum of antimalarial drug activity leads to several generalizations.

The first relates to chemoprophylaxis: *Because no antimalarial drug kills sporozoites, it is not truly possible to prevent infection; drugs can only prevent the development of symptomatic malaria caused by the asexual erythrocytic forms, either in the bloodstream or as produced within and released by hepatocytes prior to erythrocyte invasion.*

The second relates to the treatment of an established infection: *No single antimalarial is effective against all hepatic and intraerythrocytic stages of the life cycle that may coexist in the same patient. Complete elimination of the parasite infection, therefore, may require more than one drug.*

The patterns of clinically useful antimalarial agents fall into three general categories (Table 53–1):

1. Agents (*artemisinins, chloroquine, mefloquine, quinine* and *quinidine, pyrimethamine, sulfadoxine,* and *tetracycline*) that are not reliably effective against primary or latent liver stages. Instead, their action is directed against the asexual blood stages responsible for disease. These drugs will treat, or prevent, clinically symptomatic malaria.
2. Drugs (typified by *atovaquone* and *proguanil*) that target not only the asexual erythrocytic forms but also the primary liver stages of *P. falciparum*. This additional activity shortens to several days the required period for postexposure chemoprophylaxis.
3. *Primaquine,* an eight-amino quinoline that is effective against primary and latent liver stages as well as gametocytes. Primaquine is used most commonly to eradicate the intrahepatic hypnozoites of *P. vivax* and *P. ovale* that are responsible for relapsing infections. *Tafenoquine,* an eight-amino quinolone, is a long half-life analogue of *primaquine*, has a similar spectrum of action as *primaquine*, and is in advanced clinical trials (Llanos-Cuentas et al., 2014).

Aside from their antiparasitic activity, the utility of antimalarials for chemoprophylaxis or therapy depends on their pharmacokinetics and

A. Eastern Hemisphere

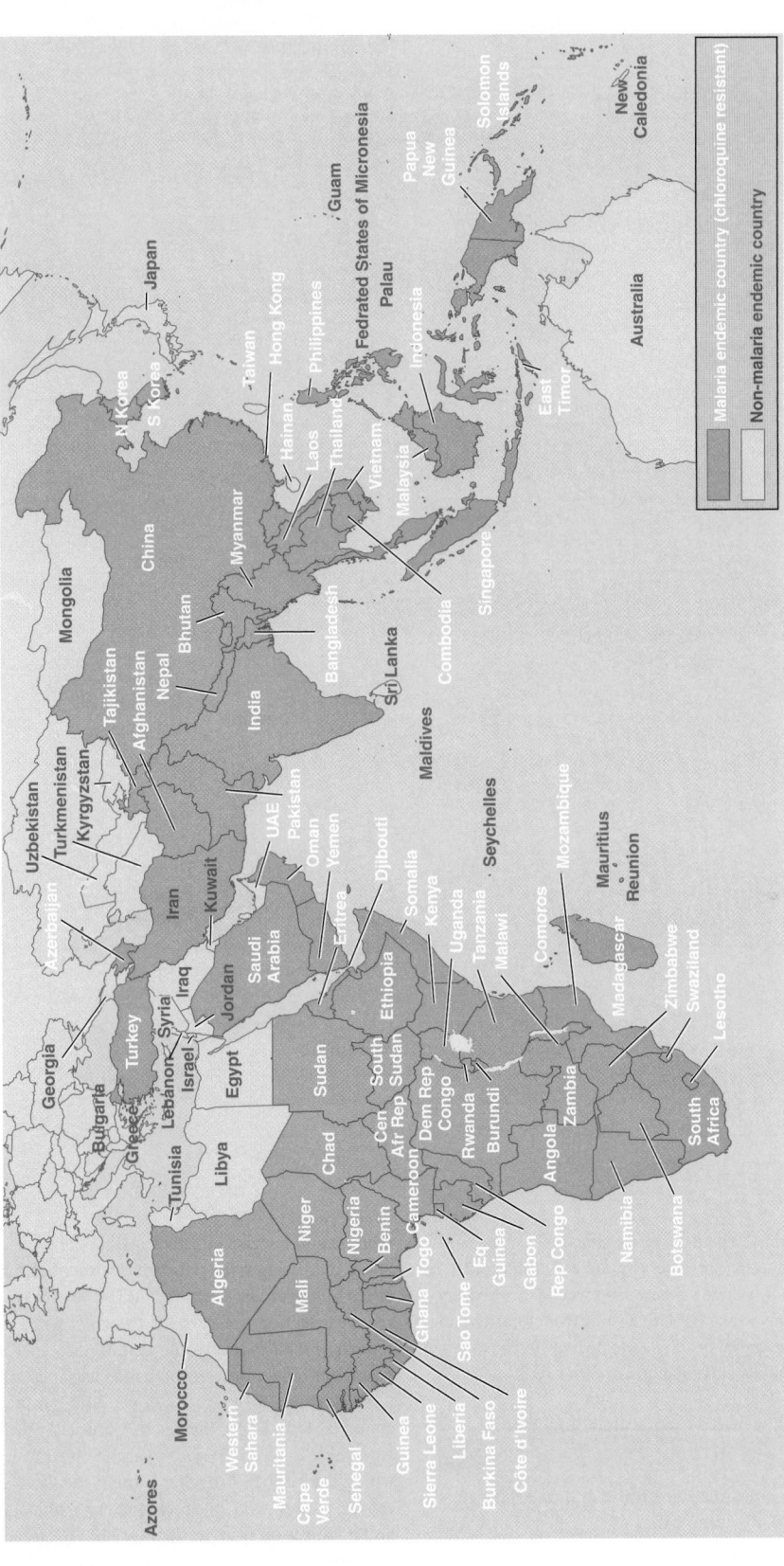

Figure 53–1 *Malaria-endemic countries.* **A.** Eastern Hemisphere; **B.** Western Hemisphere. A country is shaded orange even if malaria is endemic in just a portion of that country. Large regions not shown on the maps (e.g., Scandinavia, Russia, Canada, U.S.A., Tasmania, New Zealand) are non-endemic for malaria. (Reproduced from Centers for Disease Control and Prevention. https://wwwnc.cdc.gov/travel/yellowbook/2018/infectious-diseases-related-to-travel/malaria; accessed July 29, 2017). In areas of endemic malaria, the disease is largely chloroquine-resistant. For up-to-date information, consult the online CDC Malaria Map (https://www.cdc.gov/malaria/travelers/about_maps.html) and the CDC's Malaria Information and Prophylaxis, by Country (http://www.cdc.gov/malaria/travelers/country_table/a.html).

B. Western Hemisphere

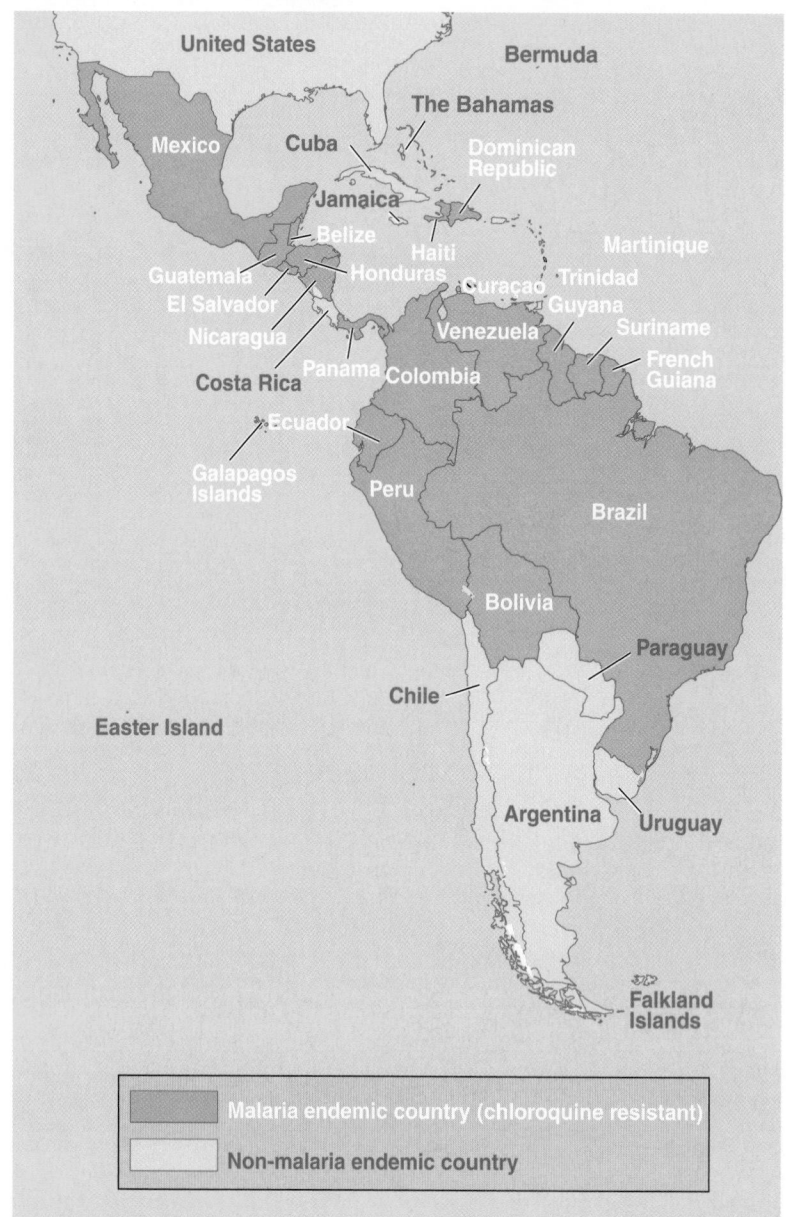

Figure 53–1 *(Continued)*

safety. Quinine and primaquine, which have significant toxicity and relatively short half-lives, generally are reserved for the treatment of established infection and are not used for chemoprophylaxis in a healthy traveler. By contrast, chloroquine, which is relatively free from toxicity and has a long $t_{1/2}$, is convenient for chemoprophylactic dosing (in those few areas still reporting chloroquine-sensitive malaria).

Specific Antimalarial Agents

For ease of reference, detailed information on the antimalarial drugs appears next in alphabetical order by drug name.

Artemisinin and Its Derivatives

Artemisinin and its three major semisynthetic derivatives in clinical use, dihydroartemisinin, artemether, and artesunate, are potent and fast-acting antimalarials. They are optimized for the treatment of severe *P. falciparum*

malaria and are also effective against the asexual erythrocytic stages of *P. vivax*. Increasingly, the standard treatment of malaria employs *artemisinin-based combination therapies* (ACTs) to increase treatment efficacy and reduce selection pressure for the emergence of drug resistance. Recent reports of *P. falciparum* artemisinin "resistance" do not indicate true resistance but reflect delayed parasite clearance time on the order of hours (Ashley et al., 2014; Huang et al., 2015); mutations in the *P. falciparum* gene *Pfk13* encoding the kelch13 propeller protein have been associated with these delayed parasite clearance times, although the mechanism by which the kelch13 propeller protein mediates delayed parasite clearance remains unknown. True resistance to artemisinin has not been reported, and no infection from this parasite has been reported to survive ACT due to delayed clearance times (van Schalkwyk et al., 2015). The clinical significance of *P. falciparum* artemisinin "resistance/delayed clearance" remains unclear (Fairhurst, 2015), but this mutation potential could threaten the future utility of this drug class. Moreover, in the presence of mutations that confer resistance to partner drugs (e.g., the ACT partner

ADME

The semisynthetic artemisinins have been formulated for oral (dihydroartemisinin, artesunate, and artemether); intramuscular (artesunate and artemether); intravenous (artesunate); and rectal (artesunate) routes. Bioavailability after oral dosing typically is 30% or less. Peak serum levels occur rapidly with artemisinins and in 2–6 h with intramuscular artemether. Both artesunate and artemether have modest levels of plasma protein binding, ranging from 43% to 82%. These derivatives are extensively metabolized and converted to dihydroartemisinin, which has a plasma $t_{1/2}$ of 1–2 h. Drug bioavailability via rectal administration is highly variable among individual patients. With repeated dosing, artemisinin and artesunate induce their own CYP-mediated metabolism, primarily via CYPs 2B6 and 3A4, which may enhance clearance by as much as 5-fold.

Therapeutic Uses

Given their rapid and potent activity against even multidrug-resistant parasites, the artemisinins are valuable for the treatment of severe *P. falciparum* malaria. The artemisinins generally are not used alone because of their limited ability to eradicate infection completely. Artemisinins are highly effective for the first-line treatment of malaria when combined with other antimalarials. Artemisinins should not be used for chemoprophylaxis because of their short $t_{1/2}$ values.

Toxicity and Contraindications

In pregnant rats and rabbits, artemisinins can cause increased embryo lethality or malformations early postconception. Preclinical toxicity studies have identified the brain (and brainstem), liver, and bone marrow as the principal target organs. However, no systematic neurological changes have been attributed to treatment in patients 5 years of age or older. Patients may develop dose-related and reversible decreases in reticulocyte and neutrophil counts and increases in transaminase levels. About 1 in 3000 patients develops an allergic reaction. Although studies of artemisinin treatment during the first trimester have found no evidence of adverse effects on fetal development, it is recommended that ACTs not be used during the first trimester of pregnancy or for the treatment of children 5 kg or less.

ACT Partner Drugs

Partner drugs for ACT are chosen for potency and $t_{1/2}$ that substantially exceeds that of the artemisinin partner. The primary ACT regimens that are well tolerated in adults and children 5 kg or more are artemether-lumefantrine, artesunate-amodiaquine, and dihydroartemisinin-piperaquine. In the U.S., artemether-lumefantrine is probably the drug of choice for all malaria cases if oral drug treatment is appropriate. Pyronaridine remains in clinical trials and is not licensed.

- **Lumefantrine** shares structural similarities with the arylamino alcohol drugs mefloquine and halofantrine and is formulated with artemether. This combination is highly effective for the treatment of uncomplicated malaria and is the most widely used first-line antimalarial across Africa. The pharmacokinetic properties of lumefantrine include a large apparent volume of distribution and a terminal elimination $t_{1/2}$ of 4–5 days. Administration with a high-fat meal is recommended because it significantly increases absorption. A sweetened dispersible formulation of artemether-lumefantrine has been approved for treatment of children.
- **Amodiaquine** is a congener of chloroquine that is no longer recommended in the U.S. for chemoprophylaxis of *P. falciparum* malaria because of toxicities (hepatic and agranulocytosis) generally associated with its prophylactic use. Amodiaquine is rapidly converted by hepatic CYPs into monodesethyl-amodiaquine. This metabolite, which retains substantial antimalarial activity, has a plasma $t_{1/2}$ of 9–18 days and reaches a peak concentration of about 500 nM 2 h after oral administration of the recommended dose. By contrast, amodiaquine has a $t_{1/2}$ of about 3 h, attaining a peak concentration of about 25 nM within 30 min of oral administration. Clearance rates of amodiaquine vary widely among individuals (78–943 mL/min/kg).
- **Piperaquine** is a potent and well-tolerated bisquinoline compound structurally related to chloroquine. Piperaquine has a large volume of

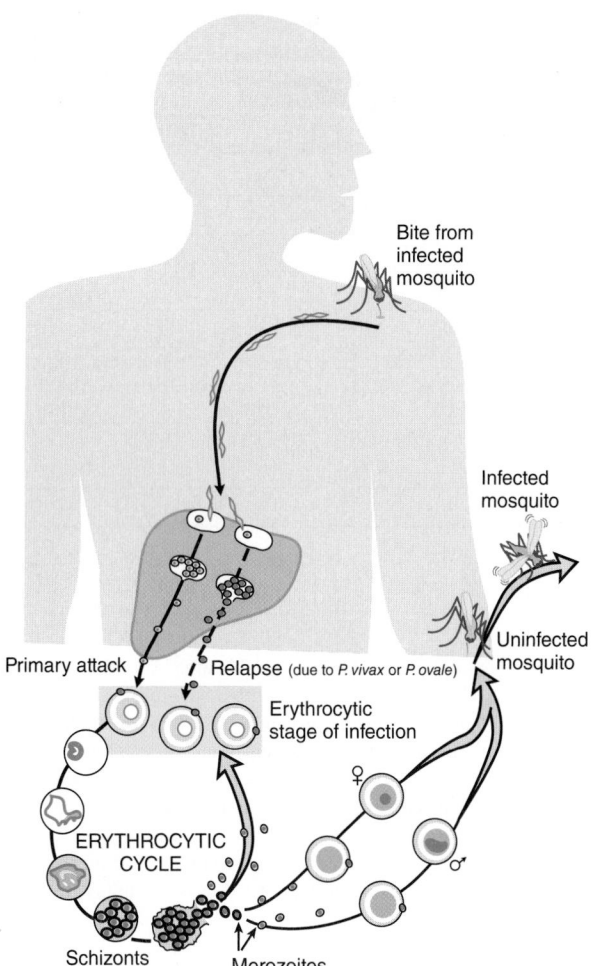

Figure 53–2 *Life cycle of malaria parasites.*

Bite from infected mosquito

Infected mosquito

Uninfected mosquito

Primary attack

Relapse (due to *P. vivax* or *P. ovale*)

Erythrocytic stage of infection

ERYTHROCYTIC CYCLE

Schizonts

Merozoites

drug piperaquine), clinically significant ACT failure is substantial, with recrudescence rates reported to exceed 50% (Amaratunga et al., 2016; Spring et al., 2015). Resistance of non–*P. falciparum* malaria parasites to artemisinin class drugs has not been reported.

H₃C, CH₃, H, O, O, H, O, O, CH₃

ARTEMISININ

Artemisinins cause a significant reduction of the parasite burden, with a 4-log$_{10}$ reduction in the parasite population for each 48-h cycle of intra-erythrocytic invasion, replication, and egress. Only three to four cycles (6–8 days) of treatment are required to remove all the parasites from the blood. In addition, artemisinins possess some gametocytocidal activity, leading to a decrease in malarial parasite transmission.

Mechanism of Action

The activity of artemisinin and derivatives seems to result from cleavage of the drug's peroxide bridge by reduced heme-iron, produced inside the highly acidic digestive vacuole of the parasite as it digests hemoglobin. The site of action of the putatively toxic heme-adducts is unclear. In addition, activated artemisinin might in turn generate free radicals that alkylate and oxidize macromolecules in the parasite.

TABLE 53–1 ■ SUSCEPTIBILTY TO DRUGS OF MALARIAL PARASITES AT VARIOUS DEVELOPMENTAL STAGES

GROUP	DRUGS	SPOROZOITE	LIVER STAGES		BLOOD STAGES	
			PRIMARY	HYPNOZOITE	ASEXUAL	GAMETOCYTE
1	Artemisinins	–	–	–	+	+
	Chloroquine	–	–	–	+	+/–
	Mefloquine	–	–	–	+	–
	Quinine/quinidine	–	–	–	+	+/–
	Pyrimethamine	–	–	–	+	–
	Sulfadoxine	–	–	–	+	–
	Tetracycline	–	–	–	+	–
2	Atovaquone/proguanil	–	+	–	+	+/–
3	Primaquine	–	+	+	–	+

–, no activity; +/–, low to moderate activity; **+, clinically important activity**.

distribution and reduced rates of excretion after multiple doses. It is rapidly absorbed, with a T_{max} (time to reach the highest concentration) of 2 h after a single dose. Piperaquine has the longest plasma $t_{1/2}$ (5 weeks) of all ACT partner drugs, a factor that could contribute to reducing rates of reinfection following treatment. Reduced efficacy of piperaquine in combination with dihydroartemisinin in Cambodia has been reported, primarily associated with mutations that led to piperaquine resistance but also in the *Pfk13* gene associated with delayed parasite clearance time (Amaratunga et al., 2016; Spring et al., 2015).

- **Pyronaridine**, an antimalarial structurally related to amodiaquine, is well tolerated and potent against both *P. falciparum* and *P. vivax*. Pyronaridine leads to fever resolution in 1–2 days and parasite clearance in 2–3 days. This drug, tested in clinical trials as a partner with artemisinin class drugs, has not yet been licensed.

Atovaquone

A fixed combination of *atovaquone* with *proguanil hydrochloride* is available in the U.S. for malaria chemoprophylaxis and for the treatment of uncomplicated *P. falciparum* malaria in adults and children.

Mechanism of Action, Selective Toxicity, Antimalarial Action, and Resistance

Atovaquone is a lipophilic analogue of ubiquinone (coenzyme Q), the electron acceptor for the parasite's cytbc$_1$ complex. Cytbc$_1$, situated on the inner mitochondrial membrane, supplies oxidized ubiquinone for dihydroorotate dehydrogenase, an essential enzyme in pyrimidine biosynthesis in the parasite. In addition, cytbc$_1$ is part of the respiratory chain and transports H$^+$ into the intramembranous space of mitochondria. By binding at the Q$_o$ site of cytbc1, atovaquone inhibits electron transport, collapses the mitochondrial membrane potential, and inhibits regeneration of ubiquinone. The selective toxicity of atovaquone for the *Plasmodium* genus and not the human host may stem from structural differences in the amino terminal regions of plasmodial and human cytochrome b (Capper et al., 2015).

The drug is highly active against *P. falciparum* asexual blood-stage parasites and the liver stages of *P. falciparum*, but not against *P. vivax* liver-stage hypnozoites. Synergy between proguanil and atovaquone results from the ability of nonmetabolized proguanil to enhance the mitochondrial toxicity of atovaquone. Resistance to atovaquone alone in *P. falciparum* develops easily and is conferred by single, nonsynonymous nucleotide polymorphisms in the cytochrome b gene located in the mitochondrial genome. Addition of proguanil markedly reduces the frequency of appearance of atovaquone resistance. However, once atovaquone resistance is present, the synergy of the partner drug proguanil diminishes.

ADME

Atovaquone absorption is slow and variable after an oral dose; absorption improves when the drug is taken with a fatty meal. More than 99% of the drug is bound to plasma protein; CSF levels are less than 1% of those in plasma. Profiles of drug concentration versus time often show a double peak, the first at 1–8 h, the second 1–4 days after a single dose; this pattern suggests enterohepatic circulation. Humans do not metabolize atovaquone significantly. The drug is excreted in bile, and more than 94% of the drug is recovered unchanged in feces. Atovaquone has a reported elimination $t_{1/2}$ from plasma of 2–3 days in adults and 1–2 days in children.

Therapeutic Uses

A tablet containing a fixed dose of 250 mg atovaquone and 100 mg proguanil hydrochloride, taken orally, is highly effective and safe in a 3-day regimen for treating mild-to-moderate attacks of chloroquine- or sulfadoxine-pyrimethamine–resistant *P. falciparum* malaria. The same regimen followed by a primaquine course is effective in treatment of *P. vivax* malaria. Atovaquone-proguanil is a standard agent for malaria chemoprophylaxis. Experience in prevention of non–*P. falciparum* malaria is limited. *Plasmodium vivax* infection may occur after drug discontinuation, indicating imperfect activity against exoerythrocytic stages of this parasite.

Toxicity

Atovaquone may cause side effects (abdominal pain, nausea, vomiting, diarrhea, headache, rash) that require cessation of therapy. Vomiting and diarrhea may decrease drug absorption, resulting in therapeutic failure. However, readministration of this drug within an hour of vomiting may still be effective in patients with *P. falciparum* malaria. Atovaquone occasionally causes transient elevations of serum transaminase or amylase.

Precautions and Contraindications

Although atovaquone is generally considered to be safe, it needs further evaluation in children weighing less than 11 kg, pregnant women, and lactating mothers. Atovaquone may compete with certain drugs for binding to plasma proteins. Therapy with rifampin reduces plasma levels of atovaquone substantially; the mechanism of this effect is not clear. Coadministration with tetracycline is associated with a 40% reduction in plasma concentration of atovaquone.

Diaminopyrimidines

Sulfadoxine-pyrimethamine was a primary treatment of uncomplicated *P. falciparum* malaria, especially against chloroquine-resistant strains. Due to widespread resistance, it is no longer recommended for the treatment of uncomplicated malaria.

Antimalarial Action and Resistance

Pyrimethamine is a slow-acting blood *schizontocide* with antimalarial effects in vivo resulting from inhibition of *folate biosynthesis* in *Plasmodium,* similar to proguanil. The efficacy of pyrimethamine against hepatic forms of *P. falciparum* is less than that of proguanil. At therapeutic doses, pyrimethamine fails to eradicate *P. vivax* hypnozoites or gametocytes of any *Plasmodium* species. The drug increases the number of circulating *P. falciparum* mature infecting gametocytes, likely leading to increased transmission to mosquitoes during the period of treatment.

Synergy of pyrimethamine and the sulfonamides or sulfones results from inhibition of two metabolic steps in folate biosynthesis in the parasite:

- the utilization of *p*-aminobenzoic acid for the synthesis of dihydropteroic acid, which is catalyzed by dihydropteroate synthase and inhibited by sulfonamides; and
- the reduction of dihydrofolate to tetrahydrofolate, which is catalyzed by dihydrofolate reductase and inhibited by pyrimethamine (see Figure 56–2).

Dietary *p*-aminobenzoic acid or folate may affect the therapeutic response to antifolates. Resistance to pyrimethamine has developed in regions of prolonged or extensive drug use and can be attributed to mutations in dihydrofolate reductase that decrease the binding affinity of pyrimethamine.

ADME

Oral pyrimethamine is slowly but completely absorbed, reaching peak plasma levels in 2–6 h. The compound is significantly distributed in the tissues and is about 90% bound to plasma proteins. Pyrimethamine is slowly eliminated from plasma, with a $t_{1/2}$ of 85–100 h. Concentrations that are suppressive for responsive *Plasmodium* strains remain in the blood for about 2 weeks. Pyrimethamine also enters the milk of nursing mothers.

Therapeutic Uses

Due to increasing drug resistance, pyrimethamine-sulfadoxine is no longer recommended for the treatment of uncomplicated malaria or for chemoprophylaxis. However, for those living in malaria-endemic areas, some still recommend it for the intermittent preventive treatment of malaria in pregnancy.

Toxicity, Precautions, and Contraindications

Antimalarial doses of pyrimethamine alone cause minimal toxicity except for occasional skin rashes and reduced hematopoiesis. Excessive doses can produce a megaloblastic anemia, resembling that of folate deficiency, which responds readily to drug withdrawal or treatment with folinic acid. At high doses, pyrimethamine is teratogenic in animals, and in humans the related combination, trimethoprim-sulfamethoxazole, may cause birth defects.

Sulfonamides or sulfones, rather than pyrimethamine, usually account for the toxicity associated with coadministration of these antifolate drugs. The combination of pyrimethamine and sulfadoxine causes severe and even fatal cutaneous reactions, such as erythema multiforme, Stevens-Johnson syndrome, or toxic epidermal necrolysis. It has also been associated with serum sickness–type reactions, urticaria, exfoliative dermatitis, and hepatitis. Pyrimethamine-sulfadoxine is contraindicated for individuals with previous reactions to sulfonamides, for lactating mothers, and for infants less than 2 months of age. Administration of pyrimethamine with dapsone, a drug combination unavailable in the U.S., has occasionally been associated with agranulocytosis.

Proguanil

The antimalarial activity of proguanil (chloroguanide) is ascribed to cycloguanil, a cyclic triazine metabolite (structurally related to pyrimethamine) and selective inhibitor of the bifunctional plasmodial dihydrofolate reductase-thymidylate synthetase that is crucial for parasite de novo purine and pyrimidine synthesis.

Antimalarial Action and Resistance

In drug-sensitive *P. falciparum* malaria, proguanil exerts activity against both the primary liver stages and the asexual red blood cell stages, thus adequately controlling the acute attack and usually eradicating the infection. Proguanil is also active against acute *P. vivax* malaria, but because the latent tissue stages of *P. vivax* are unaffected, relapses may occur after the drug is withdrawn. Proguanil treatment does not destroy gametocytes, but oocytes in the gut of the mosquito can fail to develop normally.

Cycloguanil selectively inhibits the bifunctional dihydrofolate reductase–thymidylate synthetase of sensitive plasmodia, causing inhibition of DNA synthesis and depletion of folate cofactors. A series of amino acid changes near the dihydrofolate reductase–binding site have been identified that cause resistance to cycloguanil, pyrimethamine, or both. The presence of *Plasmodium* dihydrofolate reductase is not required for the intrinsic antimalarial activity of proguanil or chlorproguanil; however, the molecular basis for this alternative activity is unknown. Proguanil accentuates the mitochondrial membrane-potential–collapsing action of atovaquone against *P. falciparum* but displays no such activity by itself. In contrast to cycloguanil, resistance to the parent drug, proguanil, either alone or in combination with atovaquone, is not well documented.

ADME

Proguanil is slowly but adequately absorbed from the GI tract. After a single oral dose, peak plasma concentrations are attained within 5 h. The mean plasma elimination $t_{1/2}$ is about 180–200 h or longer. The drug's activation and metabolism involve the CYP2C subfamily; about 3% of whites are deficient in this oxidation phenotype, contrasted with about 20% of Asians and Kenyans. Proguanil is oxidized to two major metabolites, the active cycloguanil and an inactive 4-chlorophenyl biguanide. On a daily dosage regimen of 200 mg-daily, plasma levels of cycloguanil in extensive metabolizers exceed the therapeutic range, whereas cycloguanil levels in poor metabolizers do not. Proguanil itself does not accumulate appreciably in tissues during long-term administration, except in red blood cells, where its concentration is about three times that in plasma. In humans, 40%–60% of the absorbed proguanil is excreted in urine, either as the parent drug or as the active metabolite.

Therapeutic Uses

Proguanil as a single agent is not available in the U.S. but has been prescribed as chemoprophylaxis in England and Europe for individuals traveling to malarious areas in Africa. Strains of *P. falciparum* resistant to proguanil emerge rapidly in areas where the drug is used exclusively, but breakthrough infections may also result from deficient conversion of proguanil to its active antimalarial metabolite. Proguanil is effective and tolerated well in combination with atovaquone, once daily for 3 days, to treat drug-resistant strains of *P. falciparum* or *P. vivax* (see section on atovaquone). *P. falciparum* readily develops clinical resistance to monotherapy with either proguanil or atovaquone; however, resistance to the combination is uncommon unless the strain is initially resistant to atovaquone.

Toxicity and Side Effects

In chemoprophylactic doses of 200–300 mg daily, proguanil causes relatively few adverse effects, except occasional nausea and diarrhea. Large doses (≥1 g daily) may cause vomiting, abdominal pain, diarrhea, hematuria, and the transient appearance of epithelial cells and casts in the urine. Doses as high as 700 mg twice daily have been taken for more than 2 weeks without serious toxicity. Proguanil is safe for use during pregnancy. It is remarkably safe when used in conjunction with other antimalarial drugs.

Quinolines and Related Compounds

Quinine is the chief alkaloid of cinchona, the powdered bark of the South American cinchona tree. Quinine and its many derivatives have been the mainstay of malarial treatment for four centuries. Structure-activity analysis of the cinchona alkaloids provided the basis for the discovery of more recent antimalarials, such as mefloquine.

QUININE

CHLOROQUINE

Antimalarial Action

Asexual malarial parasites flourish in host erythrocytes by digesting hemoglobin; this generates free radicals and iron-bound heme as highly reactive by-products. Heme is sequestered as an insoluble, chemically inert malarial pigment termed *hemozoin*. Quinolines interfere with heme sequestration. Failure to inactivate heme and drug-heme complexes is thought to kill the parasites via oxidative damage to membranes or other critical biomolecules.

Chloroquine and Hydroxychloroquine

Chloroquine, a weak base, concentrates in the highly acidic digestive vacuoles of susceptible *Plasmodium*, where it binds to heme and disrupts its sequestration. Hydroxychloroquine, in which one of the *N*-ethyl substituents of chloroquine is β-hydroxylated, is essentially equivalent to chloroquine against *P. falciparum* malaria.

Resistance. Resistance of erythrocytic asexual forms of *P. falciparum* to antimalarial quinolines, especially chloroquine, now is widespread (Figure 53–1). Chloroquine resistance results from mutations in the polymorphic gene *pfcrt* gene that encodes a putative transporter that resides in the membrane of the acidic digestive vacuole, the site of hemoglobin degradation and chloroquine action. In addition to PfCRT, the P-glycoprotein transporter encoded by *pfmdr1*, and other transporters, including *P. facliparum* multidrug resistance-associated protein (PfMRP), may play a modulatory role in chloroquine resistance.

ADME. Chloroquine is well absorbed from the GI tract and rapidly from intramuscular and subcutaneous sites. This drug extensively sequesters in tissues, particularly liver, spleen, kidney, lung, and, to a lesser extent, brain and spinal cord. Chloroquine binds moderately (60%) to plasma proteins. The actions of hepatic CYPs produce two active metabolites, desethylchloroquine and bisdesethylchloroquine. Renal clearance of chloroquine is about half of its total systemic clearance. Unchanged chloroquine and desethylchloroquine account for more than 50% and 25% of the urinary drug products, respectively, and their renal excretion is increased by urine acidification. To avoid potentially lethal toxicity, parenteral chloroquine is given either slowly by constant intravenous infusion or in small divided doses by the subcutaneous or intramuscular route. Chloroquine is safer when given orally because the rates of absorption and distribution are more closely matched. Peak plasma levels are achieved in about 3–5 h. The $t_{1/2}$ of chloroquine increases from a few days to weeks as plasma levels decline. The terminal $t_{1/2}$ ranges from 30 to 60 days, and traces of the drug can be found in the urine for years after a therapeutic regimen.

Therapeutic Uses. Chloroquine is highly effective against the erythrocytic forms of *P. vivax, P. ovale, P. malariae, P. knowlesi,* and chloroquine-sensitive strains of *P. falciparum.* For infections caused by *P. ovale* and *P. malariae,* it remains the agent of choice for chemoprophylaxis and treatment. For *P. falciparum,* ACTs have largely replaced chloroquine.

The utility of chloroquine has declined across most malaria-endemic regions of the world because of the spread of chloroquine-resistant *P. falciparum.* Except in areas where resistant strains of *P. vivax*

are reported, chloroquine is effective in chemoprophylaxis or treatment of acute attacks of malaria caused by *P. vivax, P. ovale,* and *P. malariae.* Chloroquine has no activity against primary or latent liver stages of the parasite. To prevent relapses in *P. vivax* and *P. ovale* infections, primaquine can be given either with chloroquine or used after a patient leaves an endemic area. Chloroquine rapidly controls the clinical symptoms and parasitemia of acute malarial attacks. Most patients become completely afebrile within 24–48 h after receiving therapeutic doses. If patients fail to respond during the second day of chloroquine therapy, resistant strains should be suspected and therapy instituted with quinine plus tetracycline or doxycycline or with atovaquone-proguanil, artemether-lumefantrine, or mefloquine if the others are not available. In comatose children, chloroquine is well absorbed and effective when given through a nasogastric tube. Tables 53–2 and 53–3 provide information about recommended chemoprophylactic and therapeutic dosage regimens involving chloroquine. Chloroquine and its analogues are also used to treat certain nonmalarial conditions, including hepatic amebiasis.

Toxicity and Side Effects. Taken in proper doses and for recommended total durations, chloroquine is safe, but its safety margin is narrow; a single dose of 30 mg/kg may be fatal. Acute chloroquine toxicity is encountered most frequently when therapeutic or high doses are administered too rapidly by parenteral routes. Cardiovascular effects include hypotension, vasodilation, suppressed myocardial function, cardiac arrhythmias, and eventual cardiac arrest. Confusion, convulsions, and coma may also result from overdose. Chloroquine doses of more than 5 g given parenterally usually are fatal. Prompt treatment with mechanical ventilation, epinephrine, and diazepam may be lifesaving.

Doses of chloroquine used for oral therapy of the acute malarial attack may cause GI upset, headache, visual disturbances, and urticaria. Pruritus also occurs most commonly among dark-skinned persons. Prolonged treatment with suppressive doses occasionally causes side effects such as headache, blurring of vision, diplopia, confusion, convulsions, lichenoid skin eruptions, bleaching of hair, widening of the QRS interval, and T-wave abnormalities. These complications usually disappear soon after the drug is withheld. Rare instances of hemolysis and blood dyscrasias have been reported. Chloroquine may cause discoloration of nail beds and mucous membranes. This drug has also been reported to interfere with the immunogenicity of certain vaccines. Irreversible retinopathy and ototoxicity can result from high daily doses (>250 mg) of chloroquine or hydroxychloroquine leading to cumulative total doses of more than 1 g/kg. Retinopathy presumably is related to drug accumulation in melanin-containing tissues and can be avoided if the daily dose is 250 mg or less. Prolonged therapy with high doses of chloroquine or hydroxychloroquine also can cause toxic myopathy, cardiopathy, and peripheral neuropathy. These reactions improve if the drug is withdrawn promptly. Rarely, neuropsychiatric disturbances, including suicide, may be related to overdose.

Precautions and Contraindications. Chloroquine is not recommended for treating individuals with epilepsy or myasthenia gravis and should be used cautiously, if at all, in the presence of advanced liver disease or severe GI, neurological, or blood disorders. The dose should be reduced in renal failure. In rare cases, chloroquine can cause hemolysis in patients with G6PD deficiency. Chloroquine should not be prescribed for patients with psoriasis or other exfoliative skin conditions. It should not be used to treat malaria in patients with porphyria cutanea tarda; however, it can be used in lower doses for treatment of manifestations of this form of porphyria.

Chloroquine inhibits CYP2D6 and thus can interact with a variety of different drugs. It attenuates the efficacy of the yellow fever vaccine when administered at the same time. It should not be given with mefloquine because of increased risk of seizures. Chloroquine opposes the action of anticonvulsants and increases the risk of ventricular arrhythmias when coadministered with amiodarone or halofantrine. By increasing plasma levels of digoxin and cyclosporine, chloroquine can increase the risk of toxicity from these agents. Patients receiving long-term, high-dose

TABLE 53–2 ■ CHEMOPROPHYLAXIS FOR PREVENTION OF MALARIA IN NONIMMUNE INDIVIDUALS

DRUG (USAGE)	ADULT DOSE	PEDIATRIC DOSE	COMMENTS
Atovaquone/proguanil (Prophylaxis in all areas)	Adult tablets contain 250 mg atovaquone and 100 mg proguanil hydrochloride; 1 adult tablet orally, daily	Pediatric tablets (62.5 mg atovaquone/25 mg proguanil HCl) 5–8 kg: 1/2 ped tab/day >8–10 kg: 3/4 ped tab/day >10–20 kg: 1 ped tab/day >20–30 kg: 2 ped tab/day >30–40 kg: 3 ped tab/day >40 kg: 1 adult tab daily	Begin 1–2 days before travel to malarious areas. Take daily at the same time each day while in the malarious area and for 7 days after leaving such areas. Contraindicated in persons with severe renal impairment (creatinine clearance < 30 mL/min). Take with food or a milky drink. Not recommended for prophylaxis for children weighing less than 5 kg, pregnant women, and women breastfeeding infants weighing less than 5 kg.
Chloroquine phosphate (Prophylaxis in areas with chloroquine-sensitive malaria)	300 mg base (500 mg salt) orally, once/week	5 mg/kg base (8.3 mg/kg salt) orally, once/week, up to maximum adult dose (300 mg base)	Begin 1–2 weeks before travel to malarious areas. Take weekly on the same day of the week while in the malarious area and for 4 weeks after leaving such areas. May exacerbate psoriasis.
Doxycycline (Prophylaxis in all areas)	100 mg orally, daily	≥8 years of age: 2 mg/kg up to adult dose of 100 mg/d	Begin 1–2 days before travel to malarious areas. Take daily at the same time each day while in the malarious area and for 4 weeks after leaving such areas. Contraindicated in children less than 8 years of age and pregnant women.
Hydroxychloroquine sulfate (Alternative to chloroquine for prophylaxis in areas with chloroquine-sensitive malaria)	310 mg base (400 mg salt) orally, once/week	5 mg/kg base (6.5 mg/kg salt) orally, once/week, up to maximum adult dose (310 mg base)	Begin 1–2 weeks before travel to malarious areas. Take weekly on the same day of the week while in the malarious area and for 4 weeks after leaving such areas.
Mefloquine (Prophylaxis in areas with mefloquine-sensitive malaria)	228 mg base (250 mg salt) orally, once/week	≤9 kg: 4.6 mg/kg base (5 mg/kg salt) orally, once/week >9–19 kg: 1/4 tab weekly >19–30 kg: 1/2 tab weekly >31–45 kg: 3/4 tab weekly ≥45 kg: 1 tablet weekly	Begin 1–2 weeks before travel to malarious areas. Take weekly on same day of the week while in malarious area and for 4 weeks after leaving such areas. Contraindicated in persons allergic to mefloquine or related compounds (e.g., quinine, quinidine) and in persons with active depression, recent history of depression, generalized anxiety disorder, psychosis, schizophrenia, other major psychiatric disorders, or seizures. Use with caution in persons with psychiatric disturbances or a previous history of depression. Not recommended for persons with cardiac conduction abnormalities.
Primaquine (Prophylaxis for short-duration travel to areas with principally *P. vivax*)	30 mg base (52.6 mg salt) orally, daily	0.5 mg/kg base (0.8 mg/kg salt) up to adult dose orally, daily	Begin 1–2 days before travel to malarious areas. Take daily at same time each day while in malarious area and for 7 days after leaving such areas. Contraindicated in persons with G6PD[a] deficiency and during pregnancy and lactation (unless the infant being breastfed has documented normal G6PD level).
Primaquine (For presumptive antirelapse therapy [terminal prophylaxis] to decrease the risk of relapses (*P. vivax*, *P. ovale*))	30 mg base (52.6 mg salt) orally, once/day for 14 days after departure from the malarious area.	0.5 mg/kg base (0.8 mg/kg salt) up to adult dose orally, once/day for 14 days after departure from the malarious area	Indicated for persons who have had prolonged exposure to *P. vivax* and *P. ovale* or both. Contraindicated in persons with G6PD[a] deficiency and during pregnancy and lactation (unless the infant being breastfed has documented normal G6PD level).

ped, pediatric; tab, tablet.

These regimens are based on published recommendations of the U.S. CDC. These recommendations may change over time. Up-to-date information should be obtained from https://wwwnc.cdc.gov/travel. Recommendations and available treatment differ among countries in the industrialized world, developing world, and malaria-endemic regions; in the last, some antimalarial treatments may be available without prescription, but the most effective drugs usually are controlled by governmental agencies.

[a]All persons who take primaquine should have a documented normal G6PD level before starting the medication.

Source: Arguin PM, Tan KR. Infectious diseases related to travel. http://wwwnc.cdc.gov/travel/yellowbook/2016/infectious-diseases-related-to-travel/malaria. Page last updated July 10, 2015. Accessed May 24, 2016.

therapy should undergo ophthalmological and neurological evaluations every 3–6 months.

Quinine and Quinidine

Oral quinine is FDA-approved for the treatment of uncomplicated *P. falciparum* malaria. Quinidine, a stereoisomer of quinine, is more potent as an antimalarial and more toxic than quinine.

Antimalarial Action and Resistance. Quinine acts against asexual erythrocytic forms and has no significant effect on hepatic forms of malarial parasites. This drug is more toxic and less effective than chloroquine against malarial parasites susceptible to both drugs. Compared to artemisinin class therapy, quinine produces poorer clinical outcomes. However, quinine, along with its stereoisomer quinidine, is especially

TABLE 53–3 ■ AGENTS FOR PRESUMPTIVE SELF-TREATMENT OF MALARIA[a]

DRUG	ADULT DOSE	PEDIATRIC DOSE	COMMENTS
Atovaquone-Proguanil			
Adult tablet: 250 mg atovaquone and 100 mg proguanil. *Pediatric tablet*: 62.5 mg atovaquone and 25 mg proguanil.	4 adult tablets, orally as a single daily dose for 3 consecutive days	Daily dose to be taken for 3 consecutive days: 5–8 kg: 2 pediatric tabs 9–10 kg: 3 pediatric tablets 11–20 kg: 1 adult tablet 21–30 kg: 2 adult tablets 31–40 kg: 3 adult tablets >41 kg: 4 adult tablets	Contraindicated in people with severe renal impairment (creatinine clearance < 30 mL/min). Not recommended for people on atovaquone-proguanil prophylaxis. Not recommended for children weighing <5 kg, pregnant women, and women breastfeeding infants weighing < 5 kg.

DRUG	DOSE		COMMENTS
Artemether-Lumefantrine			
A tablet contains 20 mg artemether and 120 mg lumefantrine.	A 3-day treatment schedule with a total of 6 oral doses is recommended for both adult and pediatric patients *based on weight*. The patient should receive the initial dose, followed by the second dose 8 h later, then 1 dose twice daily for the following 2 days. 5 to < 15 kg: 1 tablet per dose 15 to < 25 kg: 2 tablets per dose 25 to < 35 kg: 3 tablets per dose ≥35 kg: 4 tablets per dose		Not for people on mefloquine prophylaxis. Not recommended for children weighing < 5 kg, pregnant women, and women breastfeeding infants weighing < 5 kg.

[a]If used for presumptive self-treatment, medical care should be sought as soon as possible.

Source: Modified from www.cdc.gov/travel; accessed May 26, 2016.

valuable for the parenteral treatment of severe illness owing to drug-resistant strains of *P. falciparum*. Because of its toxicity and short $t_{1/2}$, quinine is generally not used for chemoprophylaxis. The antimalarial mechanism of quinine is presumably similar to that of chloroquine. The basis of *P. falciparum* resistance to quinine is complex. Patterns of *P. falciparum* resistance to quinine correlate in some strains with resistance to chloroquine yet in others correlate more closely with resistance to mefloquine and halofantrine. A number of transporter genes may confer resistance to quinine.

Action on Skeletal Muscle. Quinine not only increases the tension response to a single maximal stimulus delivered to muscle directly or through nerves, but also increases the refractory period of muscle so that the response to tetanic stimulation is diminished. The excitability of the motor end-plate region decreases so that responses to repetitive nerve stimulation and to acetylcholine are reduced. Quinine can antagonize the actions of physostigmine on skeletal muscle. Quinine may also produce alarming respiratory distress and dysphagia in patients with myasthenia gravis.

ADME. Quinine is readily absorbed when given orally or intramuscularly. Oral absorption occurs mainly from the upper small intestine and is more than 80% complete, even in patients with marked diarrhea. After an oral dose, plasma levels reach a maximum in 3–8 h and, after distributing into an apparent volume of about 1.5 L/kg, decline with a $t_{1/2}$ of about 11 h. The pharmacokinetics of quinine may change with severe malarial infection: The apparent volume of distribution and the systemic clearance of quinine decrease, such that the average elimination $t_{1/2}$ increases to 18 h. The high levels of plasma α_1-acid glycoprotein produced in severe malaria may prevent toxicity by binding quinine and thereby reducing the free fraction of drug. Concentrations of quinine are lower in erythrocytes (33%–40%) and CSF (2%–5%) than in plasma, and the drug readily reaches fetal tissues. The cinchona alkaloids are metabolized extensively, especially by hepatic CYP3A4; thus, only about

20% of an administered dose is excreted in an unaltered form in the urine. The major metabolite of quinine, 3-hydroxyquinine, retains some antimalarial activity and can accumulate and possibly cause toxicity in patients with renal failure. Renal excretion of quinine itself is more rapid when the urine is acidic.

Therapeutic Uses. Quinine and quinidine have long been treatments of choice for drug-resistant and severe *P. falciparum* malaria. However, the advent of oral and intravenous artemisinin therapy has changed this situation. Standard of care for severe illness, and only until artemisinin therapy can be started, is the prompt use of loading doses of intravenous quinine (or quinidine, where intravenous quinine is not available) can be lifesaving. Oral medication to maintain therapeutic concentrations is then given as soon as tolerated and is continued for 5–7 days. Especially for treatment of infections with multidrug-resistant strains of *P. falciparum*, slower-acting blood schizonticides such as tetracyclines or clindamycin are given concurrently to enhance quinine efficacy. Formulations of quinine and quinidine and specific regimens for their use in the treatment of *P. falciparum* malaria are shown in the Drug Facts table.

The therapeutic range for "free" quinine is 0.2 and 2.0 mg/L. Regimens needed to achieve this target vary based on patient age, severity of illness, and the responsiveness of *P. falciparum* to the drug. Dosage regimens for quinidine are similar to those for quinine, although quinidine binds less to plasma proteins and has a larger apparent volume of distribution, greater systemic clearance, and shorter terminal elimination $t_{1/2}$ than quinine. The CDC recommends a dose of quinidine of 10 mg salt/kg initially, followed by 0.02 mg salt/kg/min.

Nocturnal Leg Cramps. It is commonly believed that night cramps are relieved by quinine (200–300 mg) taken at bedtime. The FDA has required drug manufacturers to stop marketing over-the-counter quinine products for nocturnal leg cramps, stating that data supporting safety and efficacy of quinine for this indication were inadequate and that risks outweighed the potential benefits.

Toxicity and Side Effects. The fatal oral dose of quinine for adults is about 2–8 g. Quinine is associated with a triad of dose-related toxicities when given at full therapeutic or excessive doses: cinchonism, hypoglycemia, and hypotension. Mild forms of cinchonism (consisting of tinnitus, high-tone deafness, visual disturbances, headache, dysphoria, nausea, vomiting, and postural hypotension) occur frequently and disappear soon after the drug is withdrawn. Hypoglycemia is also common and can be life threatening if not treated promptly with intravenous glucose. Hypotension is rare and most often is associated with excessively rapid intravenous infusions of quinine or quinidine. Prolonged medication or high single doses also may produce GI, cardiovascular, and skin manifestations. GI symptoms (nausea, vomiting, abdominal pain, and diarrhea) result from the local irritant action of quinine, but the nausea and emesis also have a central basis. Cutaneous manifestations may include flushing, sweating, rash, and angioedema, especially of the face. Quinine and quinidine, even at therapeutic doses, may cause hyperinsulinemia and severe hypoglycemia through their powerful stimulatory effect on pancreatic beta cells.

Quinine rarely causes cardiac complications unless therapeutic plasma concentrations are exceeded. QTc prolongation is mild and does not appear to be affected by concurrent mefloquine treatment. Acute overdosage also may cause serious and even fatal cardiac dysrhythmias, such as sinus arrest, junctional rhythms, atrioventricular block, and ventricular tachycardia and fibrillation. Quinidine is even more cardiotoxic than quinine. Cardiac monitoring of patients on intravenous quinidine is advisable where possible.

Severe hemolysis can result from hypersensitivity to these cinchona alkaloids. Hemoglobinuria and asthma from quinine may occur more rarely. "Blackwater fever"—the triad of massive hemolysis, hemoglobinemia, and hemoglobinuria leading to anuria, renal failure, and in some instances death—is a rare hypersensitivity reaction to quinine therapy that can occur during treatment of malaria. Quinine occasionally may cause milder hemolysis, especially in people with G6PD deficiency. Thrombotic thrombocytopenic purpura also is rare but can occur even in response to ingestion of tonic water, which has about 4% the therapeutic oral dose per 12 oz ("cocktail purpura"). Other rare adverse effects include hypoprothrombinemia, leukopenia, and agranulocytosis.

Research in model systems indicated that quinine can inhibit a number of transport proteins, including Tat2p, which transports tryptophan, the precursor of 5HT. Quinine also competitively inhibits the rate-limiting step in 5HT biosynthesis, tryptophan hydroxylase (Islahudin et al., 2014; Khozoie et al., 2009). Whether these data relate to adverse effects of quinine in humans remains to be determined.

Precautions, Contraindications, and Drug Interactions. Quinine must be used with considerable caution, if at all, in patients who manifest hypersensitivity. Quinine should be discontinued immediately if evidence of hemolysis appears. This drug should be avoided in patients with tinnitus or optic neuritis. In patients with cardiac dysrhythmias, the administration of quinine requires the same precautions as for quinidine. Quinine appears to be safe in pregnancy and is used commonly for the treatment of pregnancy-associated malaria. However, glucose levels must be monitored because of the increased risk of hypoglycemia.

Quinine and quinidine are highly irritating and should not be given subcutaneously. Concentrated solutions may cause abscesses when injected intramuscularly or thrombophlebitis when infused intravenously. Antacids that contain aluminum can delay absorption of quinine from the GI tract. Quinine and quinidine can delay the absorption and elevate plasma levels of cardiac glycosides and warfarin and related anticoagulants. The action of quinine at neuromuscular junctions enhances the effect of neuromuscular blocking agents and opposes the action of acetylcholinesterase inhibitors. Prochlorperazine can amplify quinine's cardiotoxicity, as can halofantrine. The renal clearance of quinine can be decreased by cimetidine and increased by urine acidification and by rifampin.

Mefloquine

Mefloquine emerged from the Walter Reed Malaria Research Program as safe and effective against drug-resistant strains of *P. falciparum*.

Mechanisms of Action and Resistance. Mefloquine is a highly effective blood schizonticide. Mefloquine associates with intraerythrocytic hemozoin, suggesting similarities to the mode of action of chloroquine. However, increased *pfmdr1* copy numbers are associated with both reduced parasite susceptibility to mefloquine and increased PfMDR1-mediated solute import into the digestive vacuole of intraerythrocytic parasites, suggesting that the drug's target resides outside this vacuolar compartment. The (−)-enantiomer is associated with adverse CNS effects; the (+)-enantiomer retains antimalarial activity with fewer side effects. Mefloquine can be paired with artesunate to reduce the selection pressure for resistance. This combination has proved efficacious for the treatment of *P. falciparum* malaria, even in regions with high prevalence of mefloquine-resistant parasites.

ADME. Mefloquine is taken orally because parenteral preparations cause severe local reactions. The drug is absorbed rapidly but with marked variability. Probably owing to extensive enterogastric and enterohepatic circulation, plasma levels of mefloquine rise in a biphasic manner to their peak in about 17 h. Mefloquine has a variable and long $t_{1/2}$, 13–24 days, reflecting its high lipophilicity, extensive tissue distribution, and extensive binding (about 98%) to plasma proteins. The slow elimination of mefloquine fosters the emergence of drug-resistant parasites. Mefloquine is extensively metabolized in the liver by CYP3A4; this CYP can be inhibited by ketoconazole and induced by rifampicin. Excretion of mefloquine is mainly by the fecal route; about 10% of mefloquine appears unchanged in the urine.

Therapeutic Uses. Mefloquine should be reserved for the prevention and treatment of malaria caused by drug-resistant *P. falciparum* and *P. vivax*; it is no longer considered first-line treatment of malaria. The drug is especially useful as a chemoprophylactic agent for travelers spending weeks to years in areas where these infections are endemic (see Table 53–2). In areas where malaria is due to multiply drug-resistant strains of *P. falciparum*, mefloquine is more effective when used in combination with an artemisinin compound.

Toxicity and Side Effects. At chemoprophylactic dosages, while oral mefloquine is generally well tolerated, the U.S. FDA has added a "black box" warning to mefloquine labeling, noting the drug's potential to cause severe, possibly permanent, neurological and psychiatric adverse effects. Vivid dreams are common; significant neuropsychiatric signs and symptoms can occur in 10% or more of people receiving treatment doses; serious adverse events (psychosis, seizures) are rare. Short-term adverse effects of treatment include nausea, vomiting, and dizziness. Dividing the dose improves tolerance. The full dose should be repeated if vomiting occurs within the first hour. After treatment of malaria with mefloquine, CNS toxicity can be as high as 0.5%; symptoms include seizures, confusion or decreased sensorium, acute psychosis, and disabling vertigo. Such symptoms are reversible on drug discontinuation. Mild-to-moderate toxicities (e.g., disturbed sleep, dysphoria, headache, GI disturbances, and dizziness) occur even at prophylactic dosages. Adverse effects usually manifest after the first to third doses and often abate even with continued treatment. Cardiac abnormalities, hemolysis, and agranulocytosis are rare.

Contraindications and Drug Interactions. At very high doses, mefloquine is teratogenic in rodents. Studies have suggested an increased rate of stillbirths with mefloquine use, especially during the first trimester. Pregnancy should be avoided for 3 months after mefloquine use because of the prolonged $t_{1/2}$ of this agent. This drug is contraindicated for patients with a history of seizures, depression, bipolar disorder and other severe neuropsychiatric conditions, or adverse reactions to quinoline antimalarials. Although this drug can be taken safely 12 h after a last dose of quinine, taking quinine shortly after mefloquine can be hazardous because the latter is eliminated so slowly. Treatment with or after halofantrine or within 2 months of prior mefloquine administration is contraindicated. Controlled studies suggest that mefloquine does not impair performance in persons who tolerate the drug; nonetheless, some advise against the use of mefloquine for patients in occupations that require focused concentration, dexterity, and cognitive function.

Primaquine

Primaquine, in contrast to other antimalarials, acts on exoerythrocytic tissue stages of *Plasmodium* spp. in the liver to prevent and cure relapsing malaria. Patients should be screened for G6PD deficiency prior to therapy with this drug.

PRIMAQUINE

Antimalarial Action and Parasite Resistance. The mechanism of action of the 8-aminoquinolines has not been elucidated. Primaquine acts against primary and latent hepatic stages of *Plasmodium* spp. and prevents relapses in *P. vivax* and *P. ovale* infections. This drug and other 8-aminoquinolines also display gametocytocidal activity against *P. falciparum* and other *Plasmodium* species. However, primaquine is inactive against asexual blood-stage parasites.

ADME. Absorption of primaquine from the GI tract approaches 100%. Peak plasma concentration occurs within 3 h and then falls with a variable $t_{1/2}$ averaging 7 h. Primaquine is metabolized rapidly; only a small fraction of a dose is excreted as the parent drug. Importantly, primaquine induces CYP1A2. The major metabolite, carboxyprimaquine, is inactive.

Therapeutic Uses. Primaquine is used primarily for terminal chemoprophylaxis and radical cure of *P. vivax* and *P. ovale* (relapsing) infections because of its high activity against the latent tissue forms (hypnozoites) of these *Plasmodium* species. The compound is given together with a blood schizonticide, usually chloroquine, to eradicate erythrocytic stages of these plasmodia and reduce the possibility of emerging drug resistance. For terminal chemoprophylaxis, primaquine regimens should be initiated shortly before or immediately after a subject leaves an endemic area (see Table 53–2). Radical cure of *P. vivax* or *P. ovale* malaria can be achieved if the drug is given either during an asymptomatic latent period of presumed infection or during an acute attack. Simultaneous administration of a schizonticidal drug plus primaquine is more effective than sequential treatment in promoting a radical cure. Limited studies demonstrated efficacy in prevention of *P. falciparum* and *P. vivax* malaria when primaquine was taken as chemoprophylaxis. Primaquine is generally well tolerated when taken for up to 1 year.

Toxicity and Side Effects. Primaquine has few side effects when given in the usual therapeutic doses. Primaquine can cause mild-to-moderate abdominal distress in some individuals. Taking the drug at mealtime often alleviates these symptoms. Mild anemia, cyanosis (methemoglobinemia), and leukocytosis are less common. High doses (60–240 mg daily) worsen the abdominal symptoms. Methemoglobinemia can occur even with usual doses of primaquine and can be severe in individuals with congenital deficiency of NADH methemoglobin reductase (NADH-cytochrome b5 reductase [diaphorase 1]). Chloroquine and dapsone may synergize with primaquine to produce methemoglobinemia in these patients. Granulocytopenia and agranulocytosis are rare complications of therapy and usually are associated with overdosage. Other rare adverse reactions are hypertension, arrhythmias, and symptoms referable to the CNS.

Therapeutic or higher doses of primaquine may cause acute hemolysis and hemolytic anemia in humans with G6PD deficiency. Primaquine is the prototype of more than 50 drugs, including antimalarial tafenoquine and sulfonamides, that causes hemolysis in G6PD-deficient individuals.

Precautions and Contraindications. G6PD deficiency should be ruled out prior to administration of primaquine. Primaquine has been used cautiously in subjects with the A form of G6PD deficiency, although benefits of treatment may not necessarily outweigh the risks but should not be used in patients with more severe deficiency. If a daily dose of more than 30 mg primaquine base (>15 mg in potentially sensitive patients) is given, then

blood counts should be followed carefully. Patients should be counseled to look for dark or blood-colored urine, which would indicate hemolysis. Primaquine should not be given to pregnant women; in treating lactating mothers, primaquine should be prescribed only after ascertaining that the breastfeeding infant has a normal G6PD level. Primaquine is contraindicated for acutely ill patients suffering from systemic disease characterized by a tendency to granulocytopenia (e.g., active forms of rheumatoid arthritis and lupus erythematosus). Primaquine should not be given to patients receiving drugs capable of causing hemolysis or depressing the myeloid elements of the bone marrow.

Tafenoquine

As a derivative of primaquine, tafenoquine presumably has the same mechanism of action as primaquine; its reported toxicities and side effects are the same, particularly with relation to G6PD deficiency. Absorption after dosing is nearly complete but delayed over about 12 h in healthy volunteers (Charles et al., 2007). The main differences between primaquine and tafenoquine relate to ADME. There are no reported detectable QTc effects with tafenoquine. This agent has not been tested in pregnant women or children.

ADME. After oral administration (no parenteral formulation is available) tafenoquine is slowly absorbed, with maximum plasma concentrations occurring about 12 h after dosing in fasting healthy subjects; absorption and elimination are first order (Brueckner et al., 1998). The elimination $t_{1/2}$ of tafenoquine is about 14 days (Brueckner et al., 1998; Charles et al., 2007). The drug has a large volume of distribution and low clearance. In vivo metabolism of the parent drug and resultant metabolites is not well understood. Mild GI side effects include heartburn, gas, vomiting, and diarrhea. Methemoglobinemia, hemolytic anemia, thrombocytopenia, or changes in white blood cell counts or electrocardiograms are not observed in healthy fasting subjects without G6PD deficiency (Brueckner et al., 1998; Charles et al., 2007).

Therapeutic Uses, Toxicity, Side Effects, Precautions, and Contraindications. These are largely considered to be those of primaquine, but potentially exacerbated because of the long elimination half-life.

Sulfonamides and Sulfones

The sulfonamides and sulfones are slow-acting blood schizonticides and are more active against *P. falciparum* than *P. vivax*.

Mechanism of Action

Sulfonamides are *p*-aminobenzoic acid analogues that competitively inhibit *Plasmodium* dihydropteroate synthase. These agents are combined with an inhibitor of parasite dihydrofolate reductase to enhance their antimalarial action. See Figure 56–2 and neighboring text for details of these agents.

Drug Resistance

Sulfadoxine resistance is conferred by several point mutations in the dihydropteroate synthase gene. These sulfadoxine resistance mutations, when combined with mutations of dihydrofolate reductase and conferring pyrimethamine resistance, greatly increase the likelihood of sulfadoxine-pyrimethamine treatment failure. Sulfadoxine-pyrimethamine, given intermittently during the second and third trimesters of pregnancy, is a routine component of antenatal care throughout Africa. Intermittent preventive treatment strategies may also benefit infants. Generally, one can anticipate that, in the absence of novel antifolates effective against existing drug-resistant strains, the use of these antimalarials for either prevention or treatment will continue to decline.

Tetracyclines and Clindamycin

Tetracycline and doxycycline are useful in malaria treatment, as is clindamycin. These agents are slow-acting blood schizonticides that can be used alone for short-term chemoprophylaxis in areas with chloroquine- and mefloquine-resistant malaria (only doxycycline is recommended for malaria chemoprophylaxis).

These antibiotics act via a delayed-death mechanism resulting from their inhibition of protein translation in the parasite apicoplast (an organelle evolutionarily derived from plant chloroplasts). This effect on malarial parasites manifests as death of the progeny of drug-treated parasites, resulting in slow onset of antimalarial activity. Their relatively slow mode of action makes these drugs ineffective as single agents for malaria treatment. Dosage regimens for tetracyclines and clindamycin are listed in the Drug Facts table. Because of their adverse effects on bones and teeth, tetracyclines should not be given to pregnant women or to children younger than 8 years. For details of these agents, see Chapter 59.

Principles and Guidelines for Chemoprophylaxis and Chemotherapy of Malaria

Pharmacological prevention of malaria poses a difficult challenge because *P. falciparum*, which causes nearly all the deaths from human malaria, has become progressively more resistant to available antimalarial drugs. Oral artemether-lumefantrine is likely appropriate as first-line antimalarial treatment of uncomplicated malaria. Chloroquine remains effective against malaria caused by *P. ovale*, *P. malariae*, *P. knowlesi*, most strains of *P. vivax*, and chloroquine-sensitive strains of *P. falciparum* found in some geographic areas. However, chloroquine-resistant strains of *P. falciparum* are now the rule, not the exception, in most malaria-endemic regions (see Figure 53–1). Extensive geographic overlap also exists between chloroquine resistance and resistance to pyrimethamine-sulfadoxine. Multidrug-resistant *P. falciparum* malaria is especially prevalent and severe in Southeast Asia and Oceania. These infections may not respond adequately even to mefloquine or quinine. The following section presents an overview of the chemoprophylaxis and chemotherapy of malaria. Current CDC recommendations for drugs and dosing regimens for the chemoprophylaxis and treatment of malaria in nonimmune individuals are shown in Tables 53–2 and 53–3.

Drugs should not replace simple, inexpensive measures for malaria prevention. Individuals visiting malarious areas should take appropriate steps to prevent mosquito bites. One such measure is to avoid exposure to mosquitoes at dusk and dawn, usually the times of maximal feeding. Others include using insect repellents containing at least 30% DEET and sleeping in well-screened rooms or under bed nets impregnated with a pyrethrin insecticide such as permethrin.

Malaria Chemoprophylaxis

Regimens for malaria chemoprophylaxis include primarily three drugs: *atovaquone-proguanil* and *doxycycline*, which can both be used in all areas; and *mefloquine*, which can be used in areas with mefloquine-sensitive malaria. Other available options are chloroquine or hydroxychloroquine (but their use is restricted to the few areas with chloroquine-sensitive malaria) and primaquine (for short-duration travel to areas with principally *P. vivax*). In general, dosing should be started before exposure, ideally before the traveler leaves home (see Table 53–2).

In those few areas where chloroquine-sensitive strains of *P. falciparum* are found, chloroquine is still suitable for chemoprophylaxis. In areas where chloroquine-resistant malaria is endemic, mefloquine and atovaquone-proguanil are the regimens of choice for chemoprophylaxis. For chemoprophylaxis in long-term travelers, chloroquine is safe at the doses used, but some recommend yearly retinal examinations, and there is a finite dose limit for which chemoprophylaxis with chloroquine is recommended because of ocular toxicity. Mefloquine and doxycycline are well tolerated. Mefloquine is the best-documented drug for malaria prophylaxis in long-term travelers and, if well tolerated, can be used for prolonged periods. Atovaquone-proguanil has been studied for prophylactic use up to 20 weeks but probably is acceptable for years based on experience with the individual components.

Self-Treatment of Presumptive Malaria for Travelers

The CDC provides travelers' guidelines for self-treatment of presumptive malaria with appropriate drugs (atovaquone-proguanil, artemether-lumefantrine; as described in Table 53–3) when professional care is not available within 24 h. In such cases, medical care should be sought immediately after treatment. These recommendations may change over time and with specific locations. Consult the CDC Yellow Book (https://wwwnc.cdc.gov/travel/page/yellowbook-home-2014).

Diagnosis and Treatment of Malaria

The diagnosis of malaria must be considered for patients presenting with acute febrile illness after returning from a malaria-endemic region. An organized, rational approach to diagnosis, parasite identification, and appropriate treatment is crucial. Guidelines for treatment of malaria in the U.S. are provided by the CDC and are shown Figure 53–3, with details of the available agents summarized in Table 53–3. More information is available online (http://www.cdc.gov/malaria/resources/pdf/treatmenttable.pdf) and from the CDC Malaria Hotline (770-488-7788 and 770-488-7100).

Children and pregnant women are the most susceptible to severe malaria. The treatment of children generally is the same as for adults (pediatric dose should never exceed adult dose) (see the Drug Facts table). However, tetracyclines should not be given to children less than 8 years of age except in an emergency, and atovaquone-proguanil as treatment has been approved only for children weighing more than 5 kg.

Chemoprophylaxis and Treatment During Pregnancy

Chemoprophylaxis during pregnancy is complex, and women should evaluate with expert medical staff the benefits and risks of different strategies with regard to their particular situations. Severe malaria during pregnancy should be treated with intravenous antimalarial treatment according to the general guidelines for severe malaria, taking into account the drugs that should be avoided during pregnancy. In lactating mothers, treatment with most compounds is acceptable, although chloroquine and hydroxychloroquine are the preferred agents. The use of atovaquone-proguanil is not recommended unless breastfeeding infants weigh more than 5 kg. Also, the breastfeeding infant should be shown to have a normal G6PD level before receiving primaquine.

Treating the Mosquito Rather Than the Human

Recent technological developments seem likely to revolutionize mosquito control and mosquito susceptibility to malarial parasites. Isaacs et al. (2011) engineered resistance to infection by *P. falciparum* in mosquitoes by having the mosquitoes express single-chain antibodies that targeted antigens on the parasite's surface and inhibited the parasite's capacity to invade the midgut and salivary glands of the mosquito, effects that would reduce or eliminate the capacity of the mosquito to infect humans in the course of a blood meal.

The development of gene editing using CRISPR/cas9 (see Chapter 3) has opened up a new avenue for high-efficiency expression of resistance genes for treating the spread and prevalence of malaria. Gantz and Bier (2015) have described a "mutagenic chain reaction" based on CRISPR/cas9 that can spread a mutation from one chromosome to its homologous chromosome, converting heterozygous mutations to homozygosity in most germline and somatic cells in *Drosophila*. This gene drive system works in mosquitoes as well (Gantz et al., 2015), introducing antiplasmodium effector genes into the germline and thence into the progeny with very high frequency. Other CRISPR/cas9 endonuclease constructs have driven genes in the malarial vector *Anopheles gambiae,* targeting female reproduction and holding the promise of reducing the mosquito population in malarious areas to levels that will not support transmission of the disease (Hammond et al., 2016).

It seems likely that this gene editing–gene drive technology will be applicable to other vector-borne diseases. As Hammond et al. (2016) noted, "The success of gene drive technology for vector control will depend on the choice of suitable promoters to effectively drive homing during … gametogenesis, the phenotype of the disrupted genes, the robustness of the nuclease during homing and the ability of the target population to generate compensatory mutations". CRISPR/cas9 gene drives have not yet been released into the wild. Indeed, the use of these techniques in the field must be approached with caution and must await a full understanding of the ecological consequences and the ethical and regulatory issues.

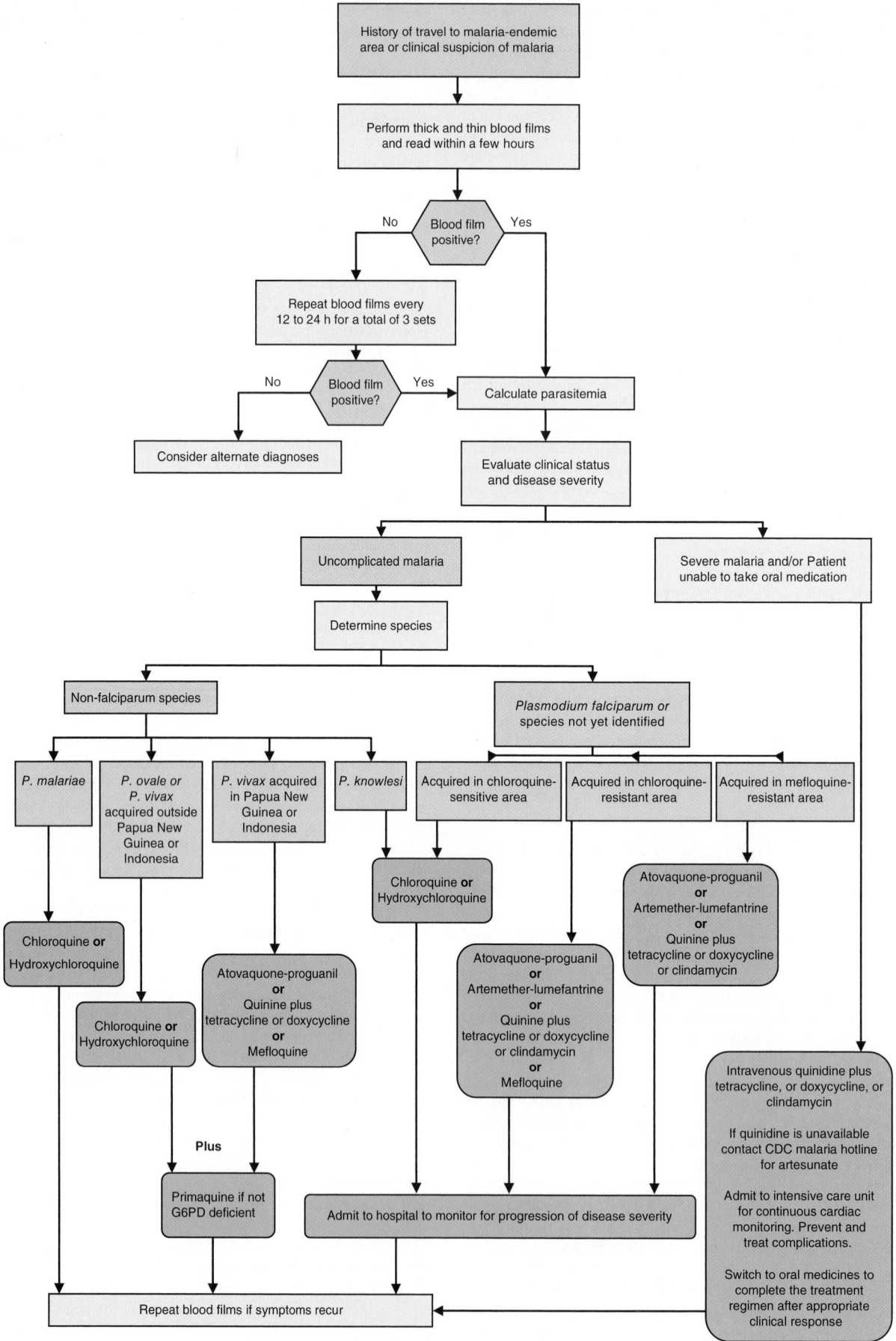

Figure 53–3 *Decision algorithm for the treatment of malaria.* Atovaquone-proguanil, mefloquine, artemether-lumefantrine, tetracycline, and doxycycline are not indicated during pregnancy (pregnancy category C). Tetracycline and doxycycline are not indicated in children younger than 8 years. (Modified from Centers for Disease Control and Prevention. Malaria. **n.d.** http://www.cdc.gov/malaria/resources/pdf/algorithm.pdf. Accessed May 24, 2016.)

Drug Facts for Your Personal Formulary: *Regimens for Malaria Treatment*

Drug Indication	Adult Dosage	Pediatric Dosage[a]	Potential Adverse Effects	Comments
Artemether-lumefantrine *P. falciparum* from chloroquine-resistant or unknown areas	Tablet: 20 mg artemether, lumefantrine. Dose: 4 tablets. Day 1: 2 doses separated by 8 h; thereafter twice daily × 2 days	Wgt (kg) Tablets/dose 5–15 1 15–25 2 25–<35 3 >35 4 Use same 3-day schedule as adults	Adults; headache anorexia, dizziness, asthenia, arthralgia myalgia Children: fever, cough, vomiting, loss of appetite, headache	Take with food or whole milk. If patient vomits within 30 min, repeat dose. Contraindicated in pregnancy.
Artesunate (IV; available from CDC) Severe malaria; see CDC guidelines.	U.S. treatment IND (CDC): 4 equal doses of artesunate (2.4 mg/kg each) over a 3-day period followed by oral treatment with atovaquone-proguanil, doxycycline, clindamycin, or mefloquine (to avoid emergence of resistance)		See Artemether	See Artemether CDC guidelines
Atovaquone-proguanil *P. falciparum* from chloroquine-resistant areas *P. vivax*	Adult tablet 250 mg atovaquone/100 mg proguanil 4 Adult tablets orally per day × 3 days	Pediatric tablet = 62.5 mg atovaquone/25 mg proguanil 5–8 kg: 2 ped tab orally/d × 3 d >8–10 kg: 3 ped tab daily × 3 d >10–20 kg: 1 adult tab daily × 3 d >20–30 kg: 2 adult tab daily × 3 d >30–40 kg: 3 adult tab daily × 3 d >40 kg: 4 adult tab daily × 3 d	Abdominal pain, nausea, vomiting, diarrhea, headache, rash, mild reversible elevations in liver aminotransferase levels	Not indicated for use in pregnant women due to limited data. Contraindicated if hypersensitivity to atovaquone or proguanil; severe renal impairment (creatinine clearance < 30 mL/min). Should be taken with food to increase absorption of atovaquone.
Chloroquine phosphate *P. falciparum* from chloroquine-sensitive areas *P. vivax* from chloroquine-sensitive areas All *P. ovale* All *P malariae* All *P. knowlesi*	600 mg base (1000 mg salt) orally immediately, followed by 300 mg base (500 mg salt) orally at 6, 24, and 48 h Total dose: 1500 mg base (2500 mg salt)	10 mg base/kg orally immediately, followed by 5 mg base/kg orally at 6, 24, and 48 h Total dose: 25 mg base/kg	Nausea, vomiting, rash, headache, dizziness, urticaria, abdominal pain, pruritus	Safe in children and pregnant women. Give for chemoprophylaxis (500 mg salt orally every week) in pregnant women with chloroquine-sensitive *P. vivax*. Contraindicated if retinal or visual field change; hypersensitivity to 4-aminoquinolines. Use with caution in those with impaired liver function since the drug is concentrated in the liver.
Clindamycin (oral or IV) *P. falciparum* from chloroquine-resistant areas *P. vivax* from chloroquine-resistant areas	Oral: 20 mg base/kg/d orally divided 3 times daily × 7 d IV: 10 mg base/kg loading dose IV followed by 5 mg base/kg IV every 8 h; switch to oral clindamycin (as above) as soon as patient can take oral meds; duration = 7 d	Oral: 20 mg base/kg/d orally divided 3 times daily × 7 d IV: 10 mg base/kg loading dose IV followed by 5 mg base/kg IV every 8 h; switch to oral clindamycin (oral dose as above) as soon as patient can take oral medication; treatment course = 7 d	Diarrhea, nausea, rash	Always use in combination with quinine-quinidine. Safe in children and pregnant women.
Doxycycline (oral or IV) *P. falciparum* and *P. vivax* from chloroquine-resistant areas	Oral: 100 mg orally twice daily × 7 d. IV: 100 mg IV every 12 h and then switch to oral doxycycline (as above) as soon as patient can take oral medication; treatment course = 7 d.	Oral: 2.2 mg/kg orally every 12 h × 7 d. IV: Only if patient is not able to take oral medication; for children < 45 kg, give 2.2 mg/kg IV every 12 h and then switch to oral doxycycline (dose as above) as soon as patient can take oral medication; for children > 45 kg, use same dosing as for adults; duration = 7 d.	Nausea, vomiting, diarrhea, abdominal pain, dizziness, photosensitivity, headache, esophagitis, odynophagia. Rarely hepatotoxicity, pancreatitis, and benign intracranial hypertension seen with tetracycline class of drugs.	Always use in combination with quinine or quinidine. Contraindicated in children < 8 y, pregnant women, and persons with known hypersensitivity to tetracyclines. Food, milk, and Ca^{2+} antacids decrease absorption and decrease GI disturbances. To prevent esophagitis, take tetracyclines with large amounts of fluids (patients should not lie down for 1 h after taking the drugs). Barbiturates, carbamazepine, or phenytoin may cause reduction in C_p of doxycycline.

Drug Facts for Your Personal Formulary: *Regimens for Malaria Treatment* (*continued*)

Drug Indication	Adult Dosage	Pediatric Dosage[a]	Potential Adverse Effects	Comments
Hydroxychloroquine (oral) Secondary alternative for treatment of *P. falciparum* and *P. vivax* from chloroquine-sensitive areas All *P. ovale* All *P. malariae*	620 mg base (= 800 mg salt) orally immediately, followed by 310 mg base (= 400 mg salt) orally at 6, 24, and 48 h Total dose: 1550 mg base (= 2000 mg salt)	10 mg base/kg orally immediately, followed by 5 mg base/kg orally at 6, 24, and 48 h Total dose: 25 mg base/kg	Nausea, vomiting, rash, headache, dizziness, urticaria, abdominal pain, pruritus[b]	Safe in children and pregnant women. Contraindicated if retinal or visual field change; hypersensitivity to 4-aminoquinolines. Use with caution in those with impaired liver function.
Mefloquine[c] *P. falciparum* from chloroquine-resistant areas, except Thailand-Burmese and Thailand-Cambodian border regions *P. vivax* from chloroquine-resistant areas	684 mg base (= 750 mg salt) orally as initial dose, followed by 456 mg base (= 500 mg salt) orally given 6–12 h after initial dose Total dose = 1250 mg salt	13.7 mg base/kg (= 15 mg salt/kg) orally as initial dose, followed by 9.1 mg base/kg (= 10 mg salt/kg) orally given 6–12 h after initial dose Total dose = 25 mg salt/kg	Nausea, vomiting, diarrhea, abdominal pain; dizziness, headache, somnolence, sleep disorders; myalgia, mild skin rash, and fatigue; moderate-to-severe neuropsychiatric reactions; ECG changes (sinus arrhythmia, sinus bradycardia, 1° AV block, QTc prolongation, and abnormal T waves.	Contraindicated if hypersensitive to the drug or to related compounds; cardiac conduction abnormalities; psychiatric disorders; and seizure disorders. Do not administer if patient has received related drugs (chloroquine, quinine, quinidine) less than 12 h ago
Primaquine phosphate Radical cure of *P. vivax* and *P. ovale* (to eliminate hypnozoites)	30 mg base orally per day × 14 d	0.5 mg base/kg orally per day × 14 d	GI disturbances, methemoglobinemia (self-limited), hemolysis in persons with G6PD deficiency	Must screen for G6PD deficiency prior to use. Contraindicated in persons with G6PD deficiency; pregnant women. Should be taken with food to minimize GI adverse effects.
Quinine sulfate (oral) *P. falciparum* from chloroquine-resistant areas *P. vivax* from chloroquine-resistant areas	542 mg base (650 mg salt)[d] orally 3 times daily × 3 d (infections acquired outside Southeast Asia) to 7 d (infections acquired in Southeast Asia)	8.3 mg base/kg (10 mg salt/kg) orally 3 times daily × 3 d (infections acquired outside Southeast Asia) to 7 d (infections acquired in Southeast Asia)	Cinchonism,[e] sinus arrhythmia, junctional rhythms, atrioventricular block, prolonged QT interval, ventricular tachycardia, ventricular fibrillation (these are rare and more commonly seen with quinidine), hypoglycemia	Combine with tetracycline, doxycycline, or clindamycin, except for *P. vivax* infections in children < 8 y or pregnant women. Contraindicated in hypersensitivity, including history of blackwater fever, thrombocytopenic purpura, or thrombocytopenia associated with quinine or quinidine use; many cardiac conduction defects and arrhythmias[f]; myasthenia gravis; optic neuritis.
Quinidine gluconate (intravenous) Severe malaria (all species, independently of chloroquine resistance) Patient unable to take oral medication Parasitemia > 10%	6.25 mg base/kg (= 10 mg salt/kg) loading dose IV over 1–2 h, then 0.0125 mg base/kg/min (0.02 mg salt/kg/min) continuous infusion for at least 24 h Note alternative regimen[g]	Same as adult	Cinchonism, tachycardia, prolongation of QRS and QTc intervals, flattening of T wave (effects are often transient). Ventricular arrhythmias, hypotension, hypoglycemia	Combine with tetracycline, doxycycline, or clindamycin. Contraindicated in hypersensitivity; history of blackwater fever including history of blackwater fever, thrombocytopenic purpura or thrombocytopenia associated with quinine or quinidine use; many cardiac conduction defects and arrhythmias[h;] myasthenia gravis; optic neuritis.

Drug Facts for Your Personal Formulary: *Regimens for Malaria Treatment* (*continued*)

Drug Indication	Adult Dosage	Pediatric Dosage[a]	Potential Adverse Effects	Comments
Tetracycline (oral or IV) *P. falciparum* and *P. vivax* from chloroquine-resistant areas (with quinine/quinidine)	Oral: 250 mg 4 times daily × 7 d IV: dosage same as for oral	25 mg/kg/d orally, divided, 4x daily × 7 d IV: dosage same as for oral	See doxycycline	See doxycycline.

These regimens are based on published recommendations of the U.S. CDC. Although current at the time of writing, these recommendations may change over time. Up-to-date information should be obtained from the CDC website at https://wwwnc.cdc.gov/travel. Recommendations and available treatment differ among countries in the industrialized world, developing world, and malaria-endemic regions; in the last, some antimalarial treatments may be available without prescription, but the most effective drugs usually are controlled by governmental agencies.

[a]Pediatric dosage should never exceed adult dosage.

[b]Extrapolated from chloroquine literature.

[c]Mefloquine should not be used to treat *P. falciparum* infections acquired in the following areas: borders of Thailand with Burma (Myanmar) and Cambodia, western provinces of Cambodia, eastern states of Burma (Myanmar), border between Burma and China, Laos along borders of Laos and Burma (and adjacent parts of Thailand-Cambodia border), and southern Vietnam due to resistant strains.

[d]Quinine sulfate capsule manufactured in the U.S. is in a 324-mg dose; therefore, 2 capsules should be sufficient for adult dosing.

[e]Nausea, vomiting, headache, tinnitus, deafness, dizziness, and visual disturbances.

[f]Refer to quinine sulfate, package insert (Mutual Pharmaceutical Inc., Philadelphia, PA, Rev. 08, November 2009).

[g]Alternative dosing hypoglycemia optic neuritis regimen for quinidine gluconate (IV): 15 mg base/kg (24 mg salt/kg) loading dose IV infused over 4 h, followed by 7.5 mg base/kg (= 12 mg salt/kg) infused over 4 h every 8 h, starting 8 h after the loading dose (see package insert); once parasite density < 1% and patient can take oral medication, complete treatment with oral quinine, dose as above. Quinidine or quinine course = 7 d in Southeast Asia (3 d in Africa or South America).

[h]Refer to quinidine gluconate, package insert (Eli Lilly Co., Indianapolis, IN, February 2002).

Sources: http://wwwnc.cdc.gov/travel/content/yellowbook/home-2010.aspx, and http://www.cdc.gov/malaria/diagnosis_treatment/clinicians2.html, accessed May 24, 2016.

Bibliography

Amaratunga C, et al. Dihydroartemisinin-piperaquine resistance in *Plasmodium falciparum* malaria in Cambodia: a multisite prospective cohort study. *Lancet Infect Dis*, **2016**, 16:357–365.

Artimovich E, et al. Persistence of sulfadoxine-pyrimethamine resistance despite reduction of drug pressure in Malawi. *J Infect Dis*, **2015**, 212:694–701.

Ashley EA, et al. Spread of artemisinin resistance in *Plasmodium falciparum* malaria. *N Engl J Med*, **2014**, 371:411–423.

Baird JK. Evidence and implications of mortality associated with acute *Plasmodium vivax* malaria. *Clin Microbiol Rev*, **2013**, 26:36–57.

Brueckner RP, et al. First-time-in-humans safety and pharmacokinetics of WR 238605, a new antimalarial. *Am J Trop Med Hyg*, **1998**, 58:645–649.

Capper MJ, et al. Antimalarial 4(1H)-pyridones bind to the Q_i site of cytochrome bc1. *Proc Natl Acad Sci U S A*, **2015**, 112:755–760.

Charles BG, et al. Population pharmacokinetics of tafenoquine during malaria prophylaxis in healthy subjects. *Antimicrob Agents Chemother*, **2007**, 51:2709–2715.

Chen I, et al. "Asymptomatic" malaria: a chronic and debilitating infection that should be treated. *PLoS Med*, **2016**, 13:e1001942.

Chitnis CE, et al. Targeting the *Plasmodium vivax* Duffy-binding protein. *Trends Parasitol*, **2008**, 24:29–34.

Djimde A, et al. Application of a molecular marker for surveillance of chloroquine-resistant falciparum malaria. *Lancet*, **2001**, 358:890–891.

Fairhurst RM. Understanding artemisinin-resistant malaria: what a difference a year makes. *Curr Opin Infect Dis*, **2015**, 28:417–425.

Garcia-Bustos JF, et al. Antimalarial drug resistance and early drug discovery. *Curr Pharm Des*, **2013**, 19:270–281.

Gantz VM, Bier E. Genome editing. The mutagenic chain reaction: a method for converting heterozygous to homozygous mutations. *Science,* **2015**, 348:442–444.

Gantz VM, et al. Highly efficient Cas9-mediated gene drive for population modification of the malaria vector mosquito *Anopheles stephensi*. *Proc Natl Acad Sci U S A*, **2015**, 112:E6736–E6743.

GBD_2013_Collaborators. Global, regional, and national age-sex specific all-cause and cause-specific mortality for 240 causes of death, 1990–2013: a systematic analysis for the Global Burden of Disease Study 2013. *Lancet*, **2015**, 385:117–171.

Hammond A, et al. A CRISPR-Cas9 gene drive system targeting female reproduction in the malaria mosquito vector *Anopheles gambiae*. *Nat Biotechnol*, **2016**, 34:78–83.

Hemingway J, et al. Tools and strategies for malaria control and elimination: what do we need to achieve a grand convergence in Malaria? *PLoS Biol*, **2016**, 14:e1002380.

Huang F, et al. A single mutation in K13 predominates in southern China and is associated with delayed clearance of *Plasmodium falciparum* following artemisinin treatment. *J Infect Dis*, **2015**, 212:1629–1635.

Hviid L, et al. PfEMP1—a parasite protein family of key importance in *Plasmodium falciparum* Malaria immunity and pathogenesis. *Adv Parasitol*, **2015**, 88:51–84.

Isaacs AT, et al. Engineered resistance to *Plasmodium falciparum* development in transgenic *Anopheles* stephensi. *PLoS Pathog*, **2011**, 7:e1002017.

Islahudin F, et al. The antimalarial drug quinine interferes with serotonin biosynthesis and action. *Sci Rep*, **2014**, 4:3618.

Kessl JJ, et al. Modeling the molecular basis of atovaquone resistance in parasites and pathogenic fungi. *Trends Parasitol*, **2007**, 23:494–501.

Khozoie C, et al. The antimalarial drug quinine disrupts Tat2p-mediated tryptophan transport and causes tryptophan starvation. *J Biol Chem*, **2009**, 284:17968–17974.

Lim NT, et al. Characterization of inhibitors and monoclonal antibodies that modulate the interaction between *Plasmodium falciparum* adhesin PfRh4 with its erythrocyte receptor complement receptor 1. *J Biol Chem*, **2015**, 290:25307–25321.

Llanos-Cuentas A, et al. Tafenoquine plus chloroquine for the treatment and relapse prevention of *Plasmodium vivax* malaria (DETECTIVE): a multicentre, double-blind, randomised, phase 2b dose-selection study. *Lancet*, **2014**, 383:1049–1058.

Miller LH, et al. Research toward vaccines against malaria. *Nat Med*, **1998**, 4:520–524.

Paul AS, et al. Host-parasite interactions that guide red blood cell invasion by malaria parasites. *Curr Opin Hematol*, **2015**, *22*:220–226.

Plowe C V, et al. Pyrimethamine and proguanil resistance-conferring mutations in *Plasmodium falciparum* dihydrofolate reductase: polymerase chain reaction methods for surveillance in Africa. *Am J Trop Med Hyg*, **1995**, *52*:565–568.

Sibley CH, et al. Pyrimethamine-sulfadoxine resistance in *Plasmodium falciparum*: what next? *Trends Parasitol*, **2001**, *17*:582–588.

Sinnis P, et al. Quantification of sporozoite invasion, migration, and development by microscopy and flow cytometry. *Methods Mol Biol*, **2013**, *923*:385–400.

Spring MD, et al. Dihydroartemisinin-piperaquine failure associated with a triple mutant including kelch13 C580Y in Cambodia: an observational cohort study. *Lancet Infect Dis*, **2015**, *15*:683–691.

Ukaegbu UE, et al. A unique virulence gene occupies a principal position in immune evasion by the malaria parasite *Plasmodium falciparum*. *PLoS Genet*, **2015**, *11*:e1005234.

van Schalkwyk DA, et al. Malaria resistance to non-artemisinin partner drugs: how to reACT. *Lancet Infect Dis*, **2015**, *15*:621–623.

Warhurst DC. A molecular marker for chloroquine-resistant falciparum malaria. *N Engl J Med*, **2001**, *344*:257–263.

Weiss GE, et al. Overlaying molecular and temporal aspects of malaria parasite invasion. *Trends Parasitol*, **2016**, *32*:284–295.

Wells TN, et al. Malaria medicines: a glass half full? *Nat Rev Drug Discov*, **2015**, *14*:424–442.

Wells TN, et al. When is enough enough? The need for a robust pipeline of high-quality antimalarials. *Discov Med*, **2010**, *9*:389–398.

White NJ, et al. Malaria. *Lancet*, **2014**, *383*:723–735.

Chapter 54

Chemotherapy of Protozoal Infections: Amebiasis, Giardiasis, Trichomoniasis, Trypanosomiasis, Leishmaniasis, and Other Protozoal Infections

Dawn M. Wetzel and Margaret A. Phillips

PROTOZOAL INFECTIONS OF HUMANS

- Amebiasis
- Giardiasis
- Trichomoniasis
- Toxoplasmosis
- Cryptosporidiosis
- Trypanosomiasis
- Leishmaniasis
- Other Protozoal Infections

ANTIPROTOZOAL DRUGS

- Amphotericin B
- Eflornithine
- 8-Hydroxyquinolines
- Melarsoprol
- Metronidazole and Tinidazole
- Miltefosine
- Nifurtimox and Benznidazole
- Nitazoxanide
- Paromomycin
- Pentamidine
- Sodium Stibogluconate
- Suramin

Humans host a wide variety of protozoal parasites that can be transmitted by insect vectors, directly from other mammalian reservoirs, or from one person to another. The immune system plays a crucial role in protecting against the pathological consequences of many protozoal infections. Thus, opportunistic infections with protozoa are prominent in infants, individuals with cancer, transplant recipients, those receiving immunosuppressive drugs or extensive antibiotic therapy, and persons with advanced HIV infection. Because effective vaccines are unavailable, chemotherapy has been the only practical way to both treat infected individuals and reduce transmission. Satisfactory agents for treating important protozoal infections such as African trypanosomiasis (sleeping sickness) and chronic Chagas disease still are lacking. Many effective antiprotozoal drugs are toxic at therapeutic doses; this problem is exacerbated by increasing drug resistance. For a list of drugs and doses used to treat these diseases see Drugs for Parasitic Infections (2013).

Protozoal Infections of Humans

Amebiasis

Amebiasis affects about 10% of the world's population, causing invasive disease in about 50 million people and death in about 100,000 of these annually (Stanley, 2003). Amebiasis is seen most commonly among individuals living in poverty, crowded conditions, and areas with poor sanitation (Petri 2014). Three morphologically identical but genetically distinct species of *Entamoeba—E. histolytica, E. dispar,* and *E. moshkovskii*—exist (Petri, 2014). In addition, *Entamoeba bangladeshi* was recently discovered in diarrheal samples and may be pathogenic (Royer et al., 2012). However, the major species that definitely requires treatment is *E. histolytica*, the third-leading cause of mortality by parasitic infection.

Humans are the only known hosts for these protozoa, which are transmitted by the fecal-oral route. Ingested *E. histolytica* cysts survive acid gastric contents and transform into *trophozoites* that reside in the large intestine (Petri, 2014). The outcome of *E. histolytica* infection is variable. Many individuals remain asymptomatic but excrete the infectious cyst form, making them a source for further infections. In other individuals,

E. histolytica trophozoites invade into the colonic mucosa with resulting colitis and bloody diarrhea (amebic dysentery). In a small proportion of patients, *E. histolytica* trophozoites invade through the colonic mucosa, reach the portal circulation, and travel to the liver, where they establish an amebic liver abscess (Haque et al., 2003). Both host and parasite factors influence the course and severity of the disease (Marie and Petri, 2014).

The cornerstone of therapy for amebiasis is metronidazole or its analogue tinidazole (Haque et al., 2003; Petri, 2014; Stanley, 2003). Because metronidazole is so well absorbed in the gut, levels may not be therapeutic in the colonic lumen. The drug is also less effective against cysts. Therefore, patients with amebic colitis or amebic liver abscess should receive a luminal agent in addition to metronidazole to eradicate any *E. histolytica* trophozoites residing within the gut lumen. Luminal agents are also used to treat asymptomatic individuals found to be infected with *E. histolytica*. The nonabsorbed aminoglycoside *paromomycin* and the 8-hydroxyquinoline compound *iodoquinol* are effective luminal agents (Haque et al., 2003). In addition, *nitazoxanide*, which is approved in the U.S. for treatment of cryptosporidiosis and giardiasis, has activity against *E. histolytica* (Adagu et al., 2002).

Giardiasis

Giardiasis, caused by the flagellated protozoan *Giardia intestinalis*, is prevalent worldwide and is the most commonly reported intestinal protozoal infection in the U.S. Infection results from ingestion of the cyst form of the parasite, which is found in fecally contaminated water or food. Cysts shed from animals or infected humans can contaminate recreational and drinking water supplies (Fletcher et al., 2012). Human-to-human transmission is common among children in day-care centers, institutionalized individuals, and male homosexuals (Escobedo, Almirall, et al., 2014). Infection with *Giardia* results in one of three syndromes:

- an asymptomatic carrier state
- acute self-limited diarrhea
- chronic diarrhea, characterized by signs of malabsorption (steatorrhea) and weight loss

Abbreviations

ADME: absorption, distribution, metabolism, excretion
CDC: Centers for Disease Control and Prevention
CNS: central nervous system
CSF: cerebrospinal fluid
DFMO: α-D,L-difluoromethylornithine
FDA: Food and Drug Administration
GI: gastrointestinal
HAART: highly active antiretroviral therapy
HIV: human immunodeficiency virus
IND: investigational new drug
NADH: reduced (hydrogenated) nicotinamide adenine dinucleotide
NECT: nifurtimox-eflornithine combination therapy
PCP: *Pneumocystis carini*
PCR: polymerase chain reaction
PFOR: pyruvate-ferredoxin oxidoreductase
PJP: *Pneumocystis jiroveci*
WHO: World Health Organization

Chemotherapy with a 5- to 7-day course of *metronidazole* usually is successful, although sometimes therapy may have to be repeated or prolonged (Escobedo, Hanevik, et al., 2014). A single dose of *tinidazole* may be superior to metronidazole. *Paromomycin* can be used to treat pregnant women to avoid any possible mutagenic effects of the other drugs (Hill and Nash, 2014). *Nitazoxanide* is also approved for the treatment of giardiasis in adults and immune-competent children less than 12 years of age (Drugs for Parasitic Infections, 2013).

Trichomoniasis

Trichomoniasis is caused by the flagellated protozoan *Trichomonas vaginalis* (Meites, 2013). This organism inhabits the human genitourinary tract, where it causes vaginitis in women and, uncommonly, urethritis in men. Trichomoniasis is the most common nonviral sexually transmitted disease. Infection with this organism is associated with an increased risk of acquiring HIV (Kissinger, 2015). Only *trophozoite* forms of *T. vaginalis* have been identified in infected secretions. Metronidazole remains the drug of choice for treating trichomoniasis (Secor et al., 2014). Tinidazole, another nitroimidazole, appears to be better tolerated than metronidazole and has been used successfully to treat metronidazole-resistant *T. vaginalis* (Schwebke, 2014).

Toxoplasmosis

Toxoplasmosis is a zoonotic infection caused by the obligate intracellular protozoan *Toxoplasma gondii*. Although cats and other feline species are the natural hosts, tissue cysts (*bradyzoites*) have been recovered from all mammalian species examined. Common routes of infection in humans are as follows:

* ingestion of undercooked meat containing tissue cysts;
* ingestion of contaminated vegetable matter containing infective *oocysts*;
* direct oral contact with feces of cats shedding oocysts; or
* transplacental fetal infection with *tachyzoites* from acutely infected mothers (Woodhall et al., 2014).

The acute illness is usually self-limiting, and treatment rarely is required. However, individuals who are immunocompromised, such as patients with AIDS, are at risk of developing toxoplasmic encephalitis from reactivation of tissue cysts deposited in the brain (Jones et al., 2014). Clinical manifestations of congenital toxoplasmosis vary, but chorioretinitis,

which may present decades after exposure, is the most common finding (Kieffer and Wallon, 2013).

The primary treatment of toxoplasmic encephalitis consists of the antifolates *pyrimethamine* and *sulfadiazine* along with *folinic acid* (*leucovorin*) (Woodhall et al., 2014). Therapy must be discontinued in about 40% of cases because of toxicity, primarily due to the sulfa compound (Yan et al., 2013). Pyrimethamine-clindamycin appears to have comparable efficacy to pyrimethamine-sulfadiazine for treating toxoplasmosis in immunocompromised patients, but this combination also causes substantial toxicity (Rajapakse et al., 2013). Alternative regimens combining azithromycin, clarithromycin, atovaquone, or dapsone with either trimethoprim-sulfamethoxazole or pyrimethamine are not only less toxic but also less effective (Rajapakse et al., 2013). *Spiramycin*, which concentrates in placental tissue, is used for the treatment of acute acquired toxoplasmosis in early pregnancy to prevent transmission to the fetus (Kieffer and Wallon, 2013). Spiramycin is available through the investigational new drug process at the U.S. FDA. If fetal infection occurs, the combination of pyrimethamine, sulfadiazine, and folinic acid is administered to the mother (only after the first 12–14 weeks of pregnancy) and to the newborn postnatally for 1 year (Contopoulos-Ioannidis and Montoya, 2012; Kieffer and Wallon, 2013).

Cryptosporidiosis

Cryptosporidia are coccidian protozoan parasites that cause diarrhea. *Cryptosporidium parvum* and the newly named *Cryptosporidium hominis* appear to account for almost all infections in humans (Checkley et al., 2015). Infectious *oocysts* in feces may be spread either by direct human-to-human contact or by contaminated water supplies. Groups at risk include travelers, children in day care, male homosexuals, animal handlers, and veterinary or healthcare personnel. After ingestion, the mature oocyte is digested, releasing *sporozoites* that invade host epithelial cells (Wilhelm and Yarovinsky, 2014). In most individuals, infection is self-limited. However, in patients with AIDS and other immunocompromised individuals, the severity of diarrhea may require hospitalization (Marcos and Gotuzzo, 2013).

Nitazoxanide has shown activity in treating cryptosporidiosis in immunocompetent children and adults (Wright, 2012). Its efficacy in children and adults with HIV/AIDS or other immunocompromising conditions is not clearly established (Cabada and White, 2010). The most effective therapy for cryptosporidiosis in immunocompromised patients is restoration of immune function (e.g., through HAART in patients with AIDS) (White, 2014).

Trypanosomiasis

African trypanosomiasis, or "sleeping sickness," is caused by subspecies of the hemoflagellate *Trypanosoma brucei* that are transmitted by bloodsucking tsetse flies of the genus *Glossina* (Kennedy, 2013). Largely restricted to sub-Saharan Africa, the infection causes serious human illness and also threatens livestock (*nagana*), leading to protein malnutrition. In humans, the infection is fatal unless treated. Sleeping sickness is found in 36 countries in Africa, but the caseload has dropped significantly due to renewed control efforts, and fewer than 10,000 cases were reported in 2013 (WHO, 2015a).

The parasite is entirely extracellular, and early human infection is characterized by the finding of replicating parasites in the bloodstream or lymph without CNS involvement (stage 1); stage 2 disease is characterized by CNS involvement (Kennedy, 2013). Symptoms of early-stage disease include febrile illness, lymphadenopathy, splenomegaly, and occasional myocarditis that result from systemic dissemination of the parasites. There are two types of African trypanosomiasis: The East African (Rhodesian; *T. brucei rhodesiense*) variety produces a progressive and rapidly fatal form of disease marked by early involvement of the CNS and frequent terminal cardiac failure; the West African type (Gambian; *T. brucei gambiense*) causes illness characterized by later involvement of the CNS and a more long-term course that progresses to the classical symptoms of sleeping sickness over months to years. Neurological symptoms include confusion, sensory deficits, psychiatric signs, disruption of the sleep cycle, and eventual progression into coma and death.

Standard therapy for early-stage disease is *pentamidine* for *T. brucei gambiense* and *suramin* for *T. brucei rhodesiense* (Barrett et al., 2007; Kennedy, 2013). Both compounds are given parenterally over long periods and are not effective against late-stage disease. The CNS phase was traditionally treated with melarsoprol (available from the CDC), a highly toxic agent that causes a fatal reactive encephalopathy in 2%–10% of treated patients.

Eflornithine (available from the CDC), an inhibitor of ornithine decarboxylase, a key enzyme in polyamine metabolism, is the only agent for the treatment of late-stage disease. It has efficacy against both early and late stages of human *T. brucei gambiense* infection; however, it is thought to be ineffective as monotherapy for infections of *T. brucei rhodesiense*. Notably, eflornithine has significantly fewer side effects than melarsoprol and is more effective than melarsoprol for treatment of late-stage Gambian trypanosomiasis. *NECT* (nifurtimox-eflornithine combination) allows shorter exposure to eflornithine with good efficacy and a reduction in adverse events; it has become the treatment of choice for late-stage *T. brucei gambiense* (Lutje et al., 2013; Yun et al., 2010). However, NECT is difficult to administer in a rural setting, and the lack of an alternative to melarsoprol to treat *T. brucei rhodesiense* is concerning. Two new orally available agents are currently in clinical trials, fexinidazole and SCYX-7158, which offer the potential for improved treatment of the disease if they successfully make it to registration (Eperon et al., 2014).

American trypanosomiasis, or *Chagas disease*, is a zoonotic infection caused by *Trypanosoma cruzi* (Bern et al., 2011; Chatelain, 2015; Messenger et al., 2015). The World Health Organization estimates that Chagas affects about 6–7 million worldwide. The spread of Chagas disease is primarily confined to Latin America, but due to immigration, a number of cases are now seen outside that region. Bloodsucking triatomid bugs infesting poor rural dwellings most commonly transmit this infection to young children; transplacental transmission may also occur. Within the Western Hemisphere, the United States has the seventh-highest caseload (300,000 identified cases), representing a significant public health concern because the parasite can also be transmitted by blood transfusion and organ transplantation (Bern et al., 2011; Hotez et al., 2013; Malik et al., 2015). Most cases in the U.S. arise through immigration, but the parasite and its vector are endemic in the southern half of the U.S. (Bern et al., 2011), and transmission within the U.S. can occur, as highlighted by five recent case reports from Texas (Garcia et al., 2015).

While the blood supply is now being monitored, lack of awareness of the disease can lead to nonoptimal care of those infected (Hotez et al., 2013). The clinical outcome of an infected patient can vary widely from asymptomatic to severe disease; whether genetic differences in *T. cruzi* isolates contribute to outcome is not firmly established (Kaplinski et al., 2015). The chronic form of the disease in adults is a major cause of cardiomyopathy, megaesophagus, megacolon, and death. Chagas heart disease is typically managed in accordance with American College of Cardiology/American Heart Association guidelines for treatment of heart failure, although whether doses of angiotensin-converting enzyme inhibitors and β adrenergic blockers should be adjusted downward is debated (Botoni et al., 2013; Malik et al., 2015; Ribeiro et al., 2012). Atypical clinical presentations and higher morbidity have been observed in immunosuppressed or compromised patients.

Two nitroheterocyclic drugs, *nifurtimox* and *benznidazole* (both available from the CDC), are used to treat this infection, although neither is approved by the U.S. FDA. Both agents suppress parasitemia and can cure the acute phase of Chagas disease. Treatment of intermediate- and late-stage disease is likely also beneficial, although the usefulness of treating at these stages is still debated. Both nifurtimox and benznidazole are toxic and must be taken for long periods. Increased awareness among physicians, better drugs, and better diagnostic methods are badly needed to help combat this disease.

Leishmaniasis

Leishmaniasis is a complex vector-borne zoonosis caused by about 20 different species of intramacrophage protozoa of the genus *Leishmania*. Small mammals and canines generally serve as reservoirs for these pathogens, which can be transmitted to humans by the bites of female phlebotomine sandflies (WHO, 2015b).

Various forms of leishmaniasis affect people in southern Europe and many tropical and subtropical regions throughout the world. Flagellated extracellular free *promastigotes*, regurgitated by feeding flies, enter the host, where they attach to and become phagocytized by tissue macrophages. These transform into *amastigotes*, which reside and multiply within phagolysosomes until the cell bursts. Released amastigotes then propagate the infection by invading more macrophages. Amastigotes taken up by feeding sandflies transform back into promastigotes, thereby completing the transformation cycle. The particular localized or systemic disease syndrome caused by *Leishmania* depends on the species or subspecies of infecting parasite, the distribution of infected macrophages, and especially the host's immune response.

In increasing order of systemic involvement and clinical severity, major syndromes of human leishmaniasis are classified into *cutaneous, mucocutaneous, diffuse cutaneous*, and *visceral (kala azar)* forms (WHO, 2015b). The disease syndrome manifested depends on the species of infecting parasite, the distribution of infected macrophages, and the host immune response (Podinovskaia and Descoteaux, 2015). As such, leishmaniasis is increasingly recognized as an AIDS-associated opportunistic infection (van Griensven et al., 2014). Cutaneous forms of leishmaniasis generally are self-limiting, with cures occurring 3–18 months after infection, but can leave disfiguring scars (Monge-Maillo and Lopez-Velez, 2013). Mucocutaneous, diffuse cutaneous, and visceral leishmaniasis do not resolve without therapy. Visceral disease caused by *Leishmania donovani* is fatal unless treated (Sundar and Chakravarty, 2015).

The classic therapy for all species of *Leishmania* is with *pentavalent antimony compounds* such as sodium stibogluconate (sodium antimony gluconate); resistance is widespread, particularly in India (Sundar and Chakravarty, 2015). Recently, treatment of leishmaniasis has undergone major changes owing to the success of the first orally active agent, *miltefosine, which has been FDA-approved for cutaneous, mucocutaneous, and visceral disease* (Miltefosine (Impavido) for Leishmaniasis, 2014). Miltefosine also appears to have promise for treating dogs, an important animal reservoir of the disease (Alvar et al., 2006). However, its teratogenic effects limit its utility in women of childbearing age (Sindermann and Engel, 2006). As an alternative, *liposomal amphotericin B* is a highly effective agent for visceral leishmaniasis (Magill, 2014) and is now recommended therapy in the U.S. in a recently released treatment guideline (Aronson et al., 2016). In addition, paromomycin has been used with some success as a parenteral agent for visceral disease, and topical formulations of paromomycin have also been used for cutaneous disease (Monge-Maillo and Lopez-Velez, 2013).

Other Protozoal Infections

Just a few of the many less-common protozoal infections of humans are highlighted in this section.

Babesiosis

Babesiosis, caused by either *Babesia microti* or *B. divergens*, is a tick-borne zoonosis that superficially resembles malaria in that the parasites invade erythrocytes and produce a febrile illness, hemolysis, and hemoglobinuria. Although this infection usually is mild and self-limiting, it can be severe or even fatal in asplenic or severely immunocompromised individuals. Therapy is with a combination of *clindamycin* and *quinine* for severe disease or the combination of *azithromycin* and *atovaquone* for mild or moderate infections (Gelfand and Vannier, 2014; Vannier et al., 2015).

Balantidiasis

Balantidiasis, caused by the ciliated protozoan *Balantidium coli*, is an infection of the large intestine that may be confused with amebiasis. However, unlike amebiasis, this infection usually responds to *tetracycline* therapy (Schuster and Ramirez-Avila, 2008; Suh et al., 2014).

Other Coccidia

Cyclospora cayetanensis (Szumowski and Troemel, 2015) causes self-limited diarrhea in normal hosts and can cause prolonged diarrhea in immunocompromised individuals. *Cystoisospora belli*, formerly known as *Isospora belli,* causes diarrhea in patients with AIDS. Both *Cyclospora* and *Cystoisospora* respond to *trimethoprim-sulfamethoxazole* (Legua and Seas, 2013; Suh et al., 2014).

Microsporidia

Microsporidia are spore-forming, unicellular, eukaryotic organisms that were once thought to be parasites but are now classified as fungi (Field and Milner, 2015). As such, they are discussed in Chapter 61 (on antifungal agents).

Antiprotozoal Drugs

For ease of reference, the myriad agents used to treat nonmalarial protozoal diseases are presented alphabetically.

Amphotericin B

The pharmacology, formulation, and toxicology of amphotericin B are presented in Chapter 61.

Antiprotozoal Effects

Amphotericin B is a highly effective antileishmanial agent that cures more than 90% of the cases of visceral leishmaniasis and is the drug of choice for antimonial-resistant cases (Mohamed-Ahmed et al., 2012). It is the recommended agent for visceral leishmaniasis in the U.S. (Aronson et al., 2016). Amphotericin B is also therapy for cutaneous or mucosal leishmaniasis and is effective for treating immunocompromised patients (van Griensven et al., 2014). Lipid preparations of the drug have reduced toxicity, but the cost of the drug and the difficulty of administration remain a problem in endemic regions (Bern et al., 2006).

Mechanism of Action

Amphotericin's activity against *Leishmania* is similar to its antifungal effects (see Chapter 61). Amphotericin complexes with ergosterol precursors in the cell membrane, forming pores that allow ions to enter the cell. *Leishmania* has similar sterol composition to fungi, and amphotericin binds fungal sterols preferentially over host cholesterol (Moen et al., 2009).

Therapeutic Uses

Typical regimens of 10–20 mg/kg total dose given in divided doses over 10–20 days by intravenous infusion have yielded cure rates of more than 95%. In the U.S., the FDA recommends 3 mg/kg intravenously on days 1–5, 14, and 21 for a total dose of 21 mg/kg to treat visceral leishmaniasis or 3 mg/kg/d for 7–10 days to treat cutaneous disease. Shorter courses of the drug for treatment of visceral leishmaniasis have demonstrated good efficacy and provide a potential cost-saving alternative, although only a limited number of patients have been tested (Monge-Maillo and Lopez-Velez, 2013). In addition, combining antileishmanial drugs may be effective; further studies are needed for such regimens (Sundar and Chakravarty, 2013).

Eflornithine

Eflornithine (DFMO) is an irreversible catalytic (suicide) inhibitor of ornithine decarboxylase, the enzyme that catalyzes the first and rate-limiting step in the biosynthesis of polyamines (putrescine, spermidine, and spermine) that are required for cell division and for normal cell differentiation (Jacobs et al., 2011). In trypanosomes, spermidine is required for the synthesis of trypanothione, a conjugate of spermidine and glutathione that replaces many of the functions of glutathione in the parasite. Eflornithine is transported into the cell via an amino acid transporter (*Tb* AAT6) (Vincent et al., 2010).

EFLORNITHINE   ORNITHINE

Eflornithine in combination with nifurtimox (NECT) is currently the drug of choice for treatment of late-stage West African (Gambian) trypanosomiasis caused by *T. brucei gambiense* (Jacobs et al., 2011). It is thought to be less effective against East African trypanosomiasis and thus is not recommended for this application. Eflornithine is no longer available for systemic use in the U.S. but is available for treatment of Gambian trypanosomiasis by special request from the CDC. NECT is safer and more efficacious than melarsoprol for late-stage gambiense sleeping sickness.

Antitrypanosomal Effects

Eflornithine is a cytostatic agent that has multiple biochemical effects on trypanosomes, all of which are a consequence of polyamine depletion (Jacobs et al., 2011). The parasite and human enzymes are equally susceptible to inhibition by eflornithine; however, the mammalian enzyme is turned over rapidly, whereas the parasite enzyme is stable, and this difference likely plays a role in the selective toxicity.

ADME

Eflornithine is given by intravenous infusion. The drug does not bind to plasma proteins but is well distributed and penetrates into the CSF, where estimated concentrations of at least 50 μM must be reached for parasite clearance (Burri and Brun, 2003). The mean $t_{1/2}$ is 3–4 h, and renal clearance after intravenous administration is rapid (2 mL/min/kg), with more than 80% of the drug cleared by the kidney largely in unchanged form (Sanderson et al., 2008).

Therapeutic Uses

Eflornithine in combination with nifurtimox (NECT) is used for the treatment of late-stage West African trypanosomiasis caused by *T. brucei gambiense*. The combination is logistically easier to administer and better tolerated than eflornithine alone. Importantly, compared to eflornithine alone, NECT achieves a higher cure rate (96.5% vs. 91.5%). Dosing is as follows: 200 mg/kg IV every 12 h by 2-h infusion for 7 days plus nifurtimox (orally at 15 mg/kg/d in three divided doses [every 8 h]) for 10 days (Priotto et al., 2009).

Toxicity and Side Effects

Eflornithine causes adverse reactions that are generally reversible on withdrawal of the drug. Abdominal pain and headache are the predominant complaints, followed by reactions at the injection sites. Tissue infections and pneumonia are also observed. The most severe reactions for eflornithine alone were reported to include fever peaks (6%), seizures (4%), and diarrhea (2%) (Balasegaram et al., 2009; Priotto et al., 2008). For NECT, severe adverse events were reduced compared to eflornithine alone (14% vs. 29%), and treatment-related deaths were also fewer (0.7% vs. 2%) (Priotto et al., 2009). The case fatality rate for eflornithine (0.7%–1.2%) and for NECT (0.2%) is significantly lower than for melarsoprol (4.9%), and overall either eflornithine alone or NECT is superior to melarsoprol with respect to both safety and efficacy. Reversible hearing loss can occur after prolonged therapy with oral doses. Therapeutic doses of eflornithine are large and require coadministration of substantial volumes of intravenous fluid. This poses significant practical limitations in remote settings and can cause fluid overload in susceptible patients.

8-Hydroxyquinolines

The halogenated 8-hydroxyquinolines iodoquinol (diiodohydroxyquin) and clioquinol (iodochlorhydroxyquin) can be used as luminal agents to eliminate intestinal colonization with *E. histolytica* and combined with metronidazole to treat amebic colitis or amebic liver abscess. Because of its superior adverse-event profile, paromomycin is preferred as the luminal agent for amebiasis. However, iodoquinol, the safer of the two 8-hydroxyquinolones, is available for use in the U.S. and is a reasonable alternative. When used at appropriate doses (never to exceed 2 g/d) for short periods of time (not greater than 20 days in adults), adverse effects are unusual (Haque et al., 2003). However, using these drugs at high doses for long periods carries significant risk. The most important toxic reaction, ascribed primarily to clioquinol, is subacute myelo-optic neuropathy (Meade, 1975). Administering iodoquinol in high doses to children with chronic diarrhea is associated with optic atrophy and permanent vision loss (Escobedo et al., 2009). Peripheral neuropathy is a less-severe manifestation of neurotoxicity from these drugs (Haque et al., 2003). For adults, the recommended dose of iodoquinol is 650 mg orally three times daily for 20 days, whereas children receive 30–40 mg/kg body weight orally, divided three times a day (not to exceed 1.95 g/d) for 20 days (Drugs for Parasitic Infections, 2013).

Melarsoprol

Despite the fact that it causes an often-fatal encephalopathy in 2%–10% of the patients treated with it, melarsoprol is the only drug for the treatment of late (CNS) stages of East African trypanosomiasis caused by *T. brucei rhodesiense* (Kennedy, 2013). Although melarsoprol is also effective against late-stage West African trypanosomiasis caused by *T. brucei gambiense*, NECT has become the first-line treatment of this disease.

MELARSOPROL

Melarsoprol is supplied as a 3.6% (w/v) solution in propylene glycol for intravenous administration. It is available in the U.S. only from the CDC.

Mechanism of Action; Antiprotozoal Effects

Melarsoprol is metabolized to melarsen oxide, the active drug (Barrett et al., 2007). Arsenoxides react avidly and reversibly with vicinal sulfhydryl groups and thereby inactivate many enzymes. Melarsoprol reacts with trypanothione, the spermidine-glutathione adduct that substitutes for glutathione in these parasites. Binding of melarsoprol to trypanothione results in a melarsen oxide–trypanothione adduct that inhibits trypanothione reductase. Treatment failure owing to resistance of trypanosomes to melarsoprol has risen sharply, and some of the resistant strains are an order of magnitude less sensitive to the drug. Resistance to melarsoprol arises due to transport defects linked to the aquaglyceroporin pore-forming protein (Munday et al., 2015).

ADME

Melarsoprol is always administered by slow intravenous injection, with care to avoid leakage into the surrounding tissues because the drug is intensely irritating. Melarsoprol is a prodrug and is metabolized rapidly (<30 min) to melarsen oxide, the active form of the drug (Barrett et al., 2007). Bioassays show that the active metabolite has a terminal $t_{1/2}$ of 43 h. A small but therapeutically significant amount of the drug enters the CSF and clears trypanosomes infecting the CNS.

Therapeutic Uses

Melarsoprol is the only effective drug available for treatment of the late meningoencephalitic stage of East African (Rhodesian) trypanosomiasis, which is nearly 100% fatal if untreated (Kennedy, 2013). The drug is also effective in the early hemolymphatic stage of these infections, but because of its toxicity, it is reserved for therapy of late-stage infections. Patients infected with *T. brucei rhodesiense* who relapse after a course of melarsoprol usually respond to a second course of the drug. In contrast, patients infected with *T. brucei gambiense* who are not cured with melarsoprol rarely benefit from repeated treatment with this drug. Such patients often respond well to eflornithine.

Dosing is 2.2 mg/kg/d IV for 10 days for both *T. brucei gambiense* (Pepin and Mpia, 2006) and *T. brucei rhodesiense* (Kuepfer et al., 2012).

Encephalopathy develops more frequently in patients with *T. brucei rhodesiense* compared to *T. brucei gambiense*. Concurrent administration of prednisolone is frequently employed throughout the treatment course to reduce the prevalence of encephalopathy.

Toxicity and Side Effects

Treatment with melarsoprol is associated with significant toxicity and morbidity (Barrett et al., 2007; Kennedy, 2013). A febrile reaction often occurs soon after drug injection, especially if parasitemia is high. The most serious complications involve the nervous system. A reactive encephalopathy occurs 9–11 days after treatment starts in about 5%–10% of patients, leading to death in about half of these. Peripheral neuropathy occurs in about 10% of patients receiving melarsoprol. Hypertension and myocardial damage are not uncommon, although shock is rare. Albuminuria occurs frequently, and evidence of renal or hepatic damage may necessitate modification of treatment. Vomiting and abdominal colic also are common, but their incidence can be reduced by injecting melarsoprol slowly into the supine, fasting patient.

Precautions and Contraindications

Melarsoprol should be given only to patients under hospital supervision. Initiation of therapy during a febrile episode has been associated with an increased incidence of reactive encephalopathy. Administration of melarsoprol to leprous patients may precipitate erythema nodosum. Use of the drug is contraindicated during epidemics of influenza. Severe hemolytic reactions have been reported in patients with deficiency of glucose-6-phosphate dehydrogenase. The drug may be used in pregnancy.

Metronidazole and Tinidazole

Metronidazole is active in vitro against a wide variety of anaerobic protozoal parasites and anaerobic bacteria. Other clinically effective 5-nitroimidazoles closely related in structure and activity to metronidazole include tinidazole, secnidazole, and ornidazole. Among these, only tinidazole is available in the U.S. Metronidazole is clinically effective in trichomoniasis, amebiasis, and giardiasis. Metronidazole manifests antibacterial activity against all anaerobic cocci; anaerobic gram-negative bacilli, including *Bacteroides* spp.; anaerobic spore-forming, gram-positive bacilli such as *Clostridium*; and microaerophilic bacteria such as *Helicobacter* and *Campylobacter* spp. Nonsporulating gram-positive bacilli often are resistant, as are aerobic and facultatively anaerobic bacteria (Lofmark et al., 2010). Please refer to Chapter 59 on protein synthesis inhibitors for additional details about the use of metronidazole in bacterial infections.

METRONIDAZOLE

Mechanism of Action

Metronidazole is a prodrug requiring reductive activation of the nitro group by susceptible organisms. Unlike their aerobic counterparts, anaerobic and microaerophilic pathogens (e.g., the amitochondriate protozoa *T. vaginalis*, *E. histolytica*, and *G. lamblia* and various anaerobic bacteria) contain electron transport components that have a sufficiently negative redox potential to donate electrons to metronidazole. The single-electron transfer forms a highly reactive nitro radical anion that kills susceptible organisms by radical-mediated mechanisms that target DNA. Metronidazole is catalytically recycled; loss of the active metabolite's electron regenerates the parent compound. Increasing levels of O_2 inhibit metronidazole-induced cytotoxicity because O_2 competes with metronidazole for electrons. Thus, O_2 can both decrease reductive activation of metronidazole and increase recycling of the activated drug. Anaerobic or microaerophilic organisms susceptible to metronidazole derive energy from the oxidative fermentation of ketoacids such as pyruvate. Pyruvate decarboxylation, catalyzed by PFOR, produces electrons that reduce ferredoxin, which in turn catalytically donates its electrons to biological electron acceptors or to metronidazole (Lamp et al., 1999).

Resistance

Clinical resistance to metronidazole is well documented for *T. vaginalis*, *G. lamblia*, and a variety of anaerobic and microaerophilic bacteria.

Resistance correlates with impaired oxygen-scavenging capabilities, leading to higher local O_2 concentrations, decreased activation of metronidazole, and futile recycling of the activated drug. Other resistant strains have lowered levels of PFOR and ferredoxin, perhaps explaining why they may still respond to higher doses of metronidazole (Townson et al., 1994).

ADME

Preparations of metronidazole are available for oral, intravenous, intravaginal, and topical administration. The drug usually is absorbed completely and promptly after oral intake and distributed to a volume approximating total body water; less than 20% of the drug is bound to plasma proteins. A linear relationship between dose and plasma concentration pertains for doses of 200–2000 mg. Repeated doses every 6–8 h result in some drug accumulation. The $t_{1/2}$ of metronidazole in plasma is about 8 h. With the exception of the placenta, metronidazole penetrates well into body tissues and fluids, including vaginal secretions, seminal fluid, saliva, breast milk, and CSF. After an oral dose, more than 75% of labeled metronidazole is eliminated in the urine, largely as metabolites formed by the liver from oxidation of the drug's side chains, a hydroxy derivative and an acid; about 10% is recovered as unchanged drug.

Two principal metabolites result. The hydroxy metabolite has a longer $t_{1/2}$ (~12 h) and has about 50% of the antitrichomonal activity of metronidazole. Formation of glucuronides also is observed. Small quantities of reduced metabolites are formed by the gut flora. The urine of some patients may be reddish brown owing to the presence of unidentified pigments derived from the drug. Oxidative metabolism of metronidazole is induced by phenobarbital, prednisone, rifampin, and possibly ethanol and is inhibited by cimetidine (Lamp et al., 1999; Martinez and Caumes, 2001).

Therapeutic Uses

Trichomoniasis. Metronidazole cures genital infections with *T. vaginalis* in more than 90% of cases. The preferred treatment regimen is 2 g metronidazole as a single oral dose for both males and females. Tinidazole, which has a longer $t_{1/2}$ than metronidazole, is also used at a 2-g single dose and appears to provide equivalent or better responses (Drugs for Parasitic Infections, 2013). When repeated courses or higher doses of the drug are required, it is recommended that intervals of 4–6 weeks elapse between courses. Leukocyte counts should occur before, during, and after each course. Treatment failures owing to the presence of metronidazole-resistant strains of *T. vaginalis* are becoming increasingly common. Most of these cases can be treated successfully by giving a second 2-g dose to both patient and sexual partner. In addition to oral therapy, the use of a 500- to 1000-mg vaginal suppository may be beneficial in refractory cases (Muzny and Schwebke, 2013).

Amebiasis. Metronidazole is the agent of choice for the treatment of all symptomatic forms of amebiasis, including amebic colitis and amebic liver abscess. The recommended dose is 500–750 mg metronidazole taken orally three times daily for 7–10 days (McCarthy et al., 2014) or, for children, 35–50 mg/kg/d given in three divided doses for 7–10 days (Drugs for Parasitic Infections, 2013). Amebic liver abscess has been treated successfully by short courses of metronidazole or tinidazole. *Entamoeba histolytica* persists in most patients who recover from acute amebiasis after metronidazole therapy, so it is recommended that all such individuals also be treated with a luminal amebicide.

Giardiasis. Tinidazole is approved for the treatment of giardiasis as a single 2-g dose and is appropriate first-line therapy (Hill and Nash, 2014). Although metronidazole has never been FDA-approved for treatment of giardiasis in the U.S., there are many years of experience with its use (Drugs for Parasitic Infections, 2013; Pasupuleti et al., 2014).

Toxicities and Contraindications

Common side effects are headache, nausea, dry mouth, and a metallic taste. Vomiting, diarrhea, and abdominal distress are experienced occasionally. Dysuria, cystitis, and a sense of pelvic pressure have been reported. Dizziness, vertigo, and, very rarely, encephalopathy, convulsions, incoordination, and ataxia are neurotoxic effects that warrant drug discontinuation.

Metronidazole also should be withdrawn if numbness or paresthesias of the extremities occur. Reversal of serious sensory neuropathies may be slow or incomplete.

Urticaria, flushing, and pruritus indicate drug sensitivity and can require withdrawal of metronidazole (Lofmark et al., 2010). Metronidazole is a rare cause of Stevens-Johnson syndrome, which may be more common among individuals receiving high doses of metronidazole and concurrent therapy with the antihelminthic mebendazole (Chen et al., 2003).

Drug Interactions

Metronidazole has a disulfiram-like effect, and some patients experience abdominal distress, vomiting, flushing, or headache if they drink alcoholic beverages during or within 3 days of therapy (Jang and Harris, 2007). Metronidazole and disulfiram or any disulfiram-like drug should not be taken together because confusional and psychotic states may occur. Metronidazole should be used cautiously in patients with active disease of the CNS because of potential neurotoxicity. The drug also may precipitate CNS signs of lithium toxicity in patients receiving high doses of lithium. Metronidazole can prolong the prothrombin time of patients receiving therapy with warfarin anticoagulants. The dosage of metronidazole should be reduced in patients with severe hepatic disease. Metronidazole use during the first trimester of pregnancy generally is not advised (Drugs for Parasitic Infections, 2013; Lofmark et al., 2010).

Miltefosine

Miltefosine is an alkylphosphocholine analogue developed originally as an anticancer agent. Its antiprotozoal activity was discovered in the 1980s as it was being evaluated for cancer chemotherapy. In 2002, it was approved in India as the first orally active treatment available for visceral leishmaniasis. It is highly curative against visceral leishmaniasis and also is effective against the cutaneous forms of the disease (Magill, 2014). Its main drawback is its teratogenicity; consequently, it must not be used in pregnant women (Miltefosine (Impavido) for Leishmaniasis, 2014).

MILTEFOSINE

Antiprotozoal Effects

Miltefosine is the first orally available therapy for leishmaniasis. It is a safe and effective treatment of visceral leishmaniasis and has shown greater than 90% efficacy against some species of cutaneous leishmaniasis, although significant strain variation has been noted in clinical trials (Sundar and Chakravarty, 2015). The mechanism of action of miltefosine is not understood. Studies suggest that the drug may alter ether-lipid metabolism, cell signaling, or glycosylphosphatidylinositol anchor biosynthesis (Dorlo et al., 2012). A transporter for miltefosine has been cloned by functional rescue of a laboratory-generated resistant strain of *L. donovani*. The transporter is a P-type ATPase that belongs to the aminophospholipid translocase subfamily. The basis for the drug resistance appears to be a point mutation in this transporter that leads to decreased drug uptake and thereby confers drug resistance (Perez-Victoria et al., 2003; Sundar and Chakravarty, 2015).

ADME

Miltefosine is well absorbed orally and distributed throughout the human body. Detailed pharmacokinetic data are lacking, with the exception that miltefosine has a long $t_{1/2}$ (1–4 weeks). Plasma concentrations are proportional to the dose (Miltefosine (Impavido) for Leishmaniasis, 2014; Sundar and Chakravarty, 2015).

Therapeutic Uses

In the U.S., the recommended dose for oral miltefosine for both visceral and cutaneous disease for adults over 45 kg is 150 mg/kg/d for 28 days, given in three divided doses, and for patients weighing 30–45 kg is 100 mg/kg/d, given in two divided doses (Aronson et al., 2016; Miltefosine (Impavido) for Leishmaniasis, 2014). The compound cannot be given intravenously because it has hemolytic activity (Dorlo et al., 2012).

Toxicity and Side Effects

Vomiting and diarrhea are reported as frequent side effects, in up to 60% of patients. Elevations in hepatic transaminases and serum creatinine also have been reported. These effects are typically mild and reversible. Because of its teratogenic potential, miltefosine is contraindicated in pregnant women. In fact, guidelines for miltefosine use in the U.S. state that adequate contraception must be used during treatment and for 5 months after therapy is complete (Miltefosine (Impavido) for Leishmaniasis, 2014).

Nifurtimox and Benznidazole

Nifurtimox and benznidazole are used to treat American trypanosomiasis caused by *T. cruzi*, while nifurtimox is also used in combination with eflornithine for treatment of *T. brucei* (see previous discussion). Nifurtimox, a nitrofuran analogue, and benznidazole, a nitroimidazole analogue, can be obtained in the U.S. from the CDC.

Antiprotozoal Effects and Mechanisms of Action

Nifurtimox and benznidazole are trypanocidal against both the trypomastigote and amastigote forms of *T. cruzi* (Barrett et al., 2007; Kennedy, 2013). Nifurtimox also has activity against *T. brucei* and can be curative against both early- and late-stage disease (see previous discussion of NECT). The trypanocidal effects of nifurtimox and benznidazole derive from their activation by an NADH-dependent mitochondrial nitroreductase to nitro radical anions that are thought to account for the trypanocidal effects (Wilkinson et al., 2011). The generated nitro anion radicals form covalent attachments to macromolecules, leading to cellular damage that includes lipid peroxidation and membrane injury, enzyme inactivation, and damage to DNA. Reduced nitroreductase expression through single-allele gene knockout experiments or through drug selection leads to drug resistance (Wilkinson et al., 2011).

ADME

Nifurtimox is well absorbed after oral administration, with peak plasma levels observed after about 3.5 h. Less than 0.5% of the dose is excreted in urine (Paulos et al., 1989). The elimination $t_{1/2}$ is about 3 h. Nifurtimox undergoes rapid biotransformation, probably via a presystemic first-pass effect, and high concentrations of several unidentified metabolites are found. Nifurtimox crosses the blood-brain barrier in mice (Jeganathan et al., 2011).

Benznidazole is absorbed rapidly and reaches peak plasma levels within 3 h; the terminal elimination half-life is 12 h (Raaflaub and Ziegler, 1979). Recent population studies have suggested that, in adults, a dose of 2.5 mg/kg/24 h maintains the trough concentration above the therapeutic range of 3–6 mg/L, indicating that the current recommended dose of 2.5 mg/kg/12 h may be higher than needed (Soy et al., 2015). In children, drug levels were found to be lower than in adults, with excellent efficacy nonetheless (Altcheh et al., 2014).

Therapeutic Uses

Nifurtimox and benznidazole are employed in the treatment of American trypanosomiasis (Chagas disease) caused by *T. cruzi* (Bern et al., 2011; Chatelain, 2015; Malik et al., 2015; Ribeiro et al., 2012). Nifurtimox is also used in combination with eflornithine (NECT) for treatment of African sleeping sickness (see eflornithine section for discussion). Because of toxicity concerns, benznidazole is the preferred treatment of Chagas disease. Both drugs markedly reduce the parasitemia, morbidity, and mortality of acute Chagas disease, with parasitological cures obtained in more than 80% of these cases, although the clinical response of the acute illness to drug therapy varies with geographic region (Messenger et al., 2015). In the chronic form of the disease, parasitological cures are still possible, although the drug is less effective than in the acute stage. In a recent study of chronic Chagas patients, 94% of patients who completed treatment with 150 mg benznidazole

twice daily for 60 days remained PCR negative until completion of the study at the 10-month follow-up (Molina, et al., 2014; Molina, et al., 2014). The current recommendations are that patients less than 50 years of age with either acute- or recent chronic-phase disease, without advanced cardiomyopathy, should be treated. In patients more than 50 years of age, the benefits of treatment are complicated by lowered drug tolerability. Therapy is strongly encouraged for patients who will receive immunosuppressive therapy or who are HIV positive. Therapy with nifurtimox or benznidazole should start promptly after exposure for persons at risk of *T. cruzi* infection from laboratory accidents or from blood transfusions.

Both drugs are given orally with doses recommended as described (Drugs for Parasitic Infections, 2013). For nifurtimox, adults (>17 years) with acute infection should receive 8–10 mg/kg/d in three to four divided doses for 90 days; children 1–10 years old should receive 15–20 mg/kg/d in three to four divided doses for 90 days; for individuals 11–16 years old, the daily dose is 12.5–15 mg/kg given according to the same schedule.

For benznidazole, the recommended treatment for adults (>13 years) is 5–7 mg/kg/d in two divided doses for 60 days, with children up to 12 years receiving 10–15 mg/kg/d in two divided doses for 60 days. However, some studies have suggested that total doses exceeding 300 mg/d are less well tolerated (Salvador et al., 2014). If gastric upset and weight loss occur during treatment, dosage should be reduced. The ingestion of alcohol should be avoided. Nifurtimox is used in combination with eflornithine in treating late-stage *T. brucei gambiense* sleeping sickness.

Toxicity and Side Effects

Side effects are common and range from hypersensitivity reactions (e.g., dermatitis, fever, icterus, pulmonary infiltrates, and anaphylaxis) to dose- and age-dependent complications referable to the GI tract and both the peripheral nervous system and CNS (Ribeiro et al., 2012). Nausea and vomiting are common, as are myalgia and weakness. For benznidazole, the most common adverse event (occurring in 30% of patients in the first week of treatment) is urticarial dermatitis, which can be treated with antihistamines or corticosteroids. However, treatment often has to be discontinued in patients with this reaction. Bone marrow suppression can occur early during therapy, so blood cell counts should be measured every 2–3 weeks, and treatment stopped if suppression is observed. Peripheral neuropathy and GI symptoms are especially common after prolonged treatment; the latter complication may lead to weight loss and preclude further therapy. Benznidazole should be given with food to minimize GI effects. Because of the seriousness of Chagas disease and the lack of superior drugs, there are few absolute contraindications to the use of these drugs.

Nitazoxanide

Nitazoxanide (*N*-[nitrothiazolyl] salicylamide) is an oral synthetic broad-spectrum antiparasitic agent (see Chapter 55). Nitazoxanide is FDA-approved for the treatment of cryptosporidiosis and giardiasis in adults and immunocompetent children (Wright, 2012).

Antimicrobial Effects

Nitazoxanide and its active metabolite, tizoxanide (desacetyl-nitazoxanide), inhibit the growth of sporozoites and oocytes of *C. parvum* and inhibit the growth of the trophozoites of *G. intestinalis*, *E. histolytica*, and *T. vaginalis* in vitro (Wright, 2012). Nitazoxanide also has activity against intestinal helminthes (van den Enden, 2009).

Mechanism of Action

Nitazoxanide interferes with the PFOR enzyme-dependent electron-transfer reaction, which is essential to anaerobic metabolism in protozoan and bacterial species (Raether and Hanel, 2003).

ADME

Following oral administration, nitazoxanide is hydrolyzed rapidly to its active metabolite, tizoxanide, which undergoes conjugation to tizoxanide glucuronide. Bioavailability after an oral dose is excellent, and maximum plasma concentrations of the metabolites occur 1–4 h following administration. Tizoxanide is more than 99.9% bound to plasma proteins. Tizoxanide is excreted in the urine, bile, and feces; tizoxanide glucuronide is excreted in the urine and bile (Raether and Hanel 2003).

Therapeutic Uses

In the U.S., nitazoxanide is approved for the treatment of *G. intestinalis* infection (therapeutic efficacy of 85%–90%) (Hill and Nash, 2014) and for the treatment of diarrhea caused by *Cryptosporidia* (therapeutic efficacy, 56%–88%) in adults and children more than 1 year of age (Flynn, 2012). The efficacy of nitazoxanide in immunocompromised patients with *Cryptosporidia* infection has not been clearly established (Wright, 2012).

Nitazoxanide has been used as a single agent to treat mixed infections with intestinal parasites (protozoa and helminths). Effective parasite clearance after nitazoxanide treatment was shown for *G. intestinalis, E. histolytica, Blastocystis hominis, C. parvum, C. cayetanensis, I. belli, Hymenolepis nana, Trichuris trichiura, Ascaris lumbricoides,* and *Enterobius vermicularis,* although more than one course of therapy was required in some cases. Nitazoxanide also has been used to treat infections with *G. intestinalis* resistant to metronidazole and albendazole (Wright, 2012).

Dosing

To treat cryptosporidiosis, for children ages 12–47 months, the recommended dose is 100 mg nitazoxanide every 12 h for 3 days; for children ages 4–11 years, the dose is 200 mg nitazoxanide every 12 h for 3 days (Drugs for Parasitic Infections, 2013; Flynn, 2012). A 500-mg tablet, suitable for adult dosing every 12 h for 3 days, is available (McCarthy et al., 2014).

Toxicity and Side Effects

Adverse effects are rare with nitazoxanide. A greenish tint to the urine can be seen. Nitazoxanide is a pregnancy category B agent, based on animal teratogenicity and fertility studies (Anderson and Curran, 2007).

Paromomycin

Paromomycin (aminosidine) is an aminoglycoside of the neomycin/kanamycin family (see Chapter 58) that is used as an oral agent to treat *E. histolytica* infection, cryptosporidiosis, and giardiasis. Topical formulations have been used to treat trichomoniasis and cutaneous leishmaniasis; parenteral administration has been used to treat visceral leishmaniasis, both alone and in combination with antimony compounds (Sundar and Chakravarty, 2015). However, only oral paromomycin is available in the U.S. (McCarthy et al., 2014).

Mechanism of Action; ADME

Paromomycin shares the same mechanism of action as neomycin and kanamycin (binding to the 30S ribosomal subunit) and has the same spectrum of antibacterial activity. The drug is not absorbed from the GI tract; thus, the actions of an oral dose are confined to the GI tract, with 100% of the oral dose recovered in the feces (Mishra et al., 2007).

Antimicrobial Effects

Amebiasis. Paromomycin is the drug of choice for treating intestinal colonization with *E. histolytica* and is used in combination with metronidazole to treat amebic colitis and amebic liver abscess. Adverse effects are rare with oral usage but include abdominal pain and cramping, epigastric pain, nausea and vomiting, steatorrhea, and diarrhea. Rarely, rash and headache have been reported. Dosing for adults and children is 25–35 mg/kg/d in three divided oral doses (Drugs for Parasitic Infections, 2013).

Giardiasis. Paromomycin has been advocated as a treatment of giardiasis when metronidazole is contraindicated. It is used in pregnant women and for metronidazole-resistant isolates (Wright et al., 2003).

Pentamidine

Pentamidine is a positively charged aromatic diamine. It is a broad-spectrum agent with activity against several species of pathogenic protozoa

and some fungi. Pentamidine as the di-isethionate salt is marketed for injection or as an aerosol (De et al., 1986; Rex and Stevens, 2014).

PENTAMIDINE

Antiprotozoal and Antifungal Effects

Pentamidine is used for the treatment of early-stage *T. brucei gambiense* infection but is ineffective in the treatment of late-stage disease and has reduced efficacy against *T. brucei rhodesiense* (Barrett et al., 2007; Kennedy, 2013). Pentamidine is an alternative agent for the treatment of cutaneous leishmaniasis (Monge-Maillo and Lopez-Velez, 2013). Pentamidine is an alternative agent for the treatment and prophylaxis of pneumonia caused by *Pneumocystis jiroveci* (PJP), formerly known as *Pneumocystis carini* (PCP) (Castro, 1998). See Chapter 61, on antifungal agents, for additional details.

Diminazene (not available in the U.S.) is a related diamidine that is used as an inexpensive alternative to pentamidine for the treatment of early African trypanosomiasis and has been used outside the U.S. for the treatment of early-stage *T. brucei gambiense* in periods of pentamidine shortage (Munday et al., 2015).

Mechanism of Action and Resistance

The mechanism of action of the diamidines is unknown. The compounds display multiple effects on any given parasite and act by disparate mechanisms in different parasites. Multiple transporters contribute to pentamidine uptake. However, recently, it has been shown that a single high-affinity transporter from the aquaglyceroporin gene family (TbAQP2) is responsible for cross-resistance between pentamidine and melarsoprol and represents the major route for the uptake of pentamidine (Munday et al., 2015).

ADME

Pentamidine isethionate is fairly well absorbed from parenteral sites of administration. Following a single intravenous dose, the drug disappears from plasma with an apparent $t_{1/2}$ of several minutes to a few hours; maximum plasma concentrations after intramuscular injection occur at 1 h. The $t_{1/2}$ of elimination is long (weeks to months); the drug is 70% bound to plasma proteins (Bronner et al., 1995). This highly charged compound is poorly absorbed orally and does not cross the blood-brain barrier, explaining its ineffectiveness against late-stage trypanosomiasis.

Therapeutic Uses

African Trypanosomiasis. Pentamidine isethionate is used for the treatment of early-stage *T. brucei gambiense* and is given by intramuscular or intravenous injection in doses of 4 mg/kg daily for 7 days.

Leishmaniasis. Pentamidine can be used in doses of 2–3 mg/kg IV or IM daily or every second day for 4–7 doses to treat cutaneous leishmaniasis (Drugs for Parasitic Infections, 2013). This compound provides an alternative to antimonials, lipid formulations of amphotericin B, or miltefosine, but it is overall the least well tolerated (Monge-Maillo and Lopez-Velez, 2013).

Toxicity and Side Effects. Approximately 50% of individuals receiving the drug at recommended doses show some adverse effect (Barrett et al., 2007). Intravenous administration of pentamidine may be associated with hypotension, tachycardia, and headache. These effects can be ameliorated by slowing the infusion rate. Hypoglycemia, which can be life threatening, may occur at any time during pentamidine treatment. Careful monitoring of blood sugar is key. Paradoxically, pancreatitis, hyperglycemia, and the development of insulin-dependent diabetes have been seen in some patients. Pentamidine is nephrotoxic (~25% of treated patients show signs of renal dysfunction), and if the serum creatinine concentration rises, it may be necessary to withhold the drug temporarily or change to an alternative agent (Rex and Stevens, 2014). Other adverse effects include skin rashes, thrombophlebitis, anemia, neutropenia, and elevation of hepatic enzymes (Salamone and Cunha, 1988). Intramuscular administration of pentamidine is associated with the development of sterile abscesses at the injection site, which can become infected secondarily; most authorities recommend intravenous administration (Cheung et al., 1993).

Sodium Stibogluconate

Antimonials were introduced in 1945 and have been used for therapy of leishmaniasis and other protozoal infections. The first trivalent antimonial compound used to treat cutaneous leishmaniasis and kala azar was antimony potassium tartrate (tartar emetic), which was both toxic and difficult to administer. Tartar emetic and other trivalent arsenicals eventually were replaced by pentavalent antimonial derivatives of phenylstibonic acid. An early member of this family of compounds was sodium stibogluconate (sodium antimony gluconate), a pentavalent antimonial compound that has been the mainstay of the treatment of leishmaniasis. Increasing resistance to antimonials has reduced their efficacy (WHO, 2015c). In the U.S., sodium stibogluconate can be obtained from the CDC (Aronson et al., 2016).

Mechanism of Action

The pentavalent antimonials act as prodrugs that are reduced to the more toxic Sb^{3+} species that kill amastigotes within the phagolysosomes of macrophages. Following reduction, the drugs seem to interfere with the trypanothione redox system. Sb^{3+} induces a rapid efflux of trypanothione and glutathione from the cells and also inhibits trypanothione reductase, thereby causing a significant loss of thiol reduction potential in the cells (Frezard et al., 2009).

ADME

The drug is given intravenously or intramuscularly; it is not active orally. The agent is absorbed rapidly and distributed in an apparent volume of about 0.22 L/kg. Elimination occurs in two phases, the first with a $t_{1/2}$ of about 2 h, the second with a much longer half-time (33–76 h). The prolonged terminal elimination phase may reflect conversion of the Sb^{5+} to the more toxic Sb^{3+} that is concentrated in and only slowly released from tissues. The drug is eliminated in the urine (Frezard et al., 2009).

Therapeutic Uses

Sodium stibogluconate is given parenterally. The standard course is 20 mg/kg/d for 20 days for cutaneous disease and for 28 days for visceral leishmaniasis (Drugs for Parasitic Infections, 2013; McCarthy et al., 2014). Increased resistance has greatly compromised the effectiveness of antimonials, and sodium stibogluconate is now obsolete in India. Previously, liposomal amphotericin B was the recommended alternative, but now the orally effective compound miltefosine is likely to see much wider use (Sundar and Chakravarty, 2015). Intralesional treatment has also been advocated as a safer, alternative method for treating cutaneous disease (Monge-Maillo and Lopez-Velez, 2013). Patients who respond show clinical improvement within 1–2 weeks of initiating therapy. The drug may be given on alternate days or for longer intervals if unfavorable reactions occur in especially debilitated individuals (Sundar and Chakravarty, 2015). Patients infected with HIV often relapse after therapy (Magill, 2014).

Toxicity and Side Effects

In general, regimens of sodium stibogluconate are tolerated; toxic reactions usually are reversible, and most subside despite continued therapy. Adverse effects include chemical pancreatitis in nearly all patients; elevation of serum hepatic transaminase levels; bone marrow suppression, manifested by decreased red cell, white cell, and platelet counts; muscle and joint pain; weakness and malaise; headache; nausea and abdominal pain; and skin rashes. Reversible polyneuropathy has been reported. Hemolytic anemia and renal damage are rare manifestations of antimonial toxicity, as are shock and sudden death (Frezard et al., 2009).

Suramin

Research into the trypanocidal activity of the dyes *trypan red, trypan blue,* and *afridol violet* led to the introduction of suramin into therapy in 1920.

Today, the drug is used primarily for treatment of African trypanosomiasis; it has no clinical utility against American trypanosomiasis.

Suramin sodium is a water-soluble trypanocide; solutions deteriorate quickly in air, and only freshly prepared solutions should be used. In the U.S., suramin is available only from the CDC.

Antiparasitic Effects

Suramin is a relatively slow-acting trypanocide (>6 h in vitro) with high clinical activity against both *T. brucei gambiense* and *T. brucei rhodesiense*. Its mechanism of action is unknown, although a recent study has suggested a role for lysosomal function in suramin action (Alsford et al., 2012). This same study also found that the invariant surface glycoprotein (ISG75) family mediates suramin uptake into the parasite. Selective toxicity is likely to result from selective uptake by the parasite. Suramin inhibits many trypanosomal and mammalian enzymes and receptors. No consensus for the mechanism of action has emerged, and the lack of any significant field resistance points to multiple potential targets.

ADME

Because it is not absorbed after oral intake, suramin is given intravenously to avoid local inflammation and necrosis associated with subcutaneous or intramuscular injections (Kaur et al., 2002). After its administration, the drug displays complex pharmacokinetics with marked interindividual variability. The drug is 99.7% serum protein bound and has a terminal elimination $t_{1/2}$ of 41–78 days. Suramin is not appreciably metabolized; renal clearance accounts for elimination of about 80% of the compound from the body. Very little suramin penetrates the CSF, consistent with its polar character and lack of efficacy once the CNS has been invaded by trypanosomes.

Therapeutic Uses

Suramin is the first-line therapy for early-stage *T. brucei rhodesiense* infection (Barrett et al., 2007; Kennedy, 2013; McGeary et al., 2008). It is also active against *T. brucei gambiense* but is only used as a second-line treatment if pentamidine fails or is otherwise contraindicated. Because only small amounts of the drug enter the brain, suramin is used only for the treatment of early-stage African trypanosomiasis (before CNS involvement). Treatment of active African trypanosomiasis should not be started until 24 h after diagnostic lumbar puncture to ensure no CNS involvement, and caution is required if the patient has onchocerciasis (river blindness) because of the potential for eliciting a Mazzotti reaction (i.e., pruritic rash, fever, malaise, lymph node swelling, eosinophilia, arthralgias, tachycardia, hypotension, and possibly permanent blindness). Suramin is given by slow intravenous injection as a 10% aqueous solution. The normal single dose for adults with *T. brucei rhodesiense* infection is 1 g. It is advisable to employ a test dose of 100 mg initially to detect sensitivity, after which the normal dose is given intravenously (e.g., on days 1, 3, 5, 14, and 21). The pediatric test dose is 2 mg/kg followed by a dose of 20 mg/kg, given according to the same schedule as adults. Patients in poor condition should be treated with lower doses during the first week. Patients who relapse after suramin therapy should be treated with melarsoprol.

Toxicity and Side Effects

The most serious immediate reaction, consisting of nausea, vomiting, shock, and loss of consciousness, is rare (~1 in 2000 patients) (Kaur et al., 2002). Malaise, nausea, and fatigue are also common immediate reactions. The most common problem encountered after several doses of suramin is renal toxicity, manifested by albuminuria, and delayed neurological complications, including headache, metallic taste, paresthesias, and peripheral neuropathy. These complications usually disappear spontaneously despite continued therapy. Other, less-prevalent reactions include vomiting, diarrhea, stomatitis, chills, abdominal pain, and edema. Patients receiving suramin should be followed closely. Therapy should not be continued in patients who show intolerance to initial doses, and the drug should be employed with great caution in individuals with renal insufficiency.

Drug Facts for Your Personal Formulary: *Antiparasitic Agents: Protozoal Infections Other Than Malaria*

Drugs	Therapeutic Uses	Clinical Pharmacology and Tips
Amebiasis		
Metronidazole	• Amoebic colitis and liver abscess	• Always administer with luminal agent • Orally administered: > 80% bioavailable • Common side effects: headache and metallic taste • Can have disulfiram-like effect
Tinidazole	• Amoebic colitis and liver abscess	• Always administer with luminal agent
Paromomycin	• Luminal agent (eradicates *E. histolytica* from gut)	• Drug of choice due to side effects of 8-hydroxyquinolones • Side effects of paromomycin: GI (nausea/vomiting/diarrhea)
Iodoquinol	• Luminal agent	• Use less than 2 g/d for less than 20 days to avoid neurotoxicity
Giardiasis		
Metronidazole	• Giardiasis	• 5-day course • Not FDA-approved for indication, but years of experience
Tinidazole	• Giardiasis	• Single dose sufficient
Paromomycin	• Giardiasis	• Used in pregnancy
Nitazoxanide	• Giardiasis	• Orally bioavailable • Can treat resistant infections • Adverse events are rare
Trichomoniasis		
Metronidazole	• Trichomoniasis	• Drug of choice • 2 g once • If failure, give second dose in 4–6 weeks
Tinidazole	• Trichomoniasis	• 2 g once • Can be used for resistant infection
Toxoplasmosis		
Pyrimethamine	• Acute or congenital toxoplasmosis	• Combine with sulfadiazine or clindamycin • Give with leucovorin • Can cause bone marrow suppression
Sulfadiazine	• Acute or congenital toxoplasmosis	• Combine with pyrimethamine and folic acid • Can cause bone marrow suppression
Clindamycin	• Acute toxoplasmosis	• Combine with pyrimethamine • Use if cannot tolerate sulfonamide
Spiramycin	• Acute toxoplasmosis during early pregnancy	• Prevents fetal transmission • Available via individual investigator IND
Cryptosporidiosis		
Nitazoxanide	• Drug of choice for cryptosporidiosis	• Restore immune function in immunocompromised patients
Leishmaniasis		
Pentavalent antimony compounds (sodium stibogluconate)	• Cutaneous, mucocutaneous leishmaniasis • Visceral leishmaniasis (not in India)	• 20 days IV/IM for cutaneous disease • 28 days IV/IM for visceral disease • Side effects: pancreatitis, elevated hepatic transaminases, bone marrow suppression • Can cause hemolytic anemia and renal failure • Available only through CDC
Amphotericin B	• Visceral leishmaniasis • Second-line agent for cutaneous disease	• Used for antimony-resistant cases • Used during pregnancy • Side effects: renal toxicity, low potassium • Liposomal formulation preferred
Miltefosine	• Cutaneous leishmaniasis • Visceral leishmaniasis	• Only oral agent • GI side effects (vomiting/diarrhea) • Teratogenic: do not use in pregnancy

Trypanosomiasis: African sleeping sickness

Pentamidine	• Early-stage *T. brucei gambiense* **before CNS involvement**	• IV administration associated with hypotension, tachycardia, and headache • Hypoglycemia occurs; monitor blood glucose • Nephrotoxic, can cause renal failure
Suramin	• Early-stage *T. brucei rhodesiense* • Second-line agent for early-stage *T. brucei gambiense* (only if pentamidine is contraindicated)	• Immediate reactions: malaise, nausea, and fatigue • Side effects of multiple doses: renal toxicity, delayed neurological complications (headache, metallic taste, paresthesias, peripheral neuropathy) • Only available through CDC
Nifurtimox + eflornithine combination therapy (NECT)	• Late-stage *T. brucei gambiense*	• Safer and more effective than melarsoprol or eflornithine alone • First-line regimen for this indication • Side effects: abdominal pain, headache, tissue infections, pneumonia • Only available through CDC
Melarsoprol	• Late-stage *T. brucei rhodesiense* • Second-line agent for late-stage *T. brucei gambiense* (only if NECT contraindicated)	• Fatal encephalopathy: 2%–10% of patients • Coadminister with prednisolone to reduce the prevalence of encephalopathy • Only available through CDC

Trypanosomiasis: Chagas disease

Benznidazole	• Drug of choice for Chagas	• Requires 60 days of treatment • Urticarial dermatitis in 30% of patients; coadministration of antihistamines or corticosteroids can help • Better tolerated in children, less well tolerated in adults > 50 years • Most effective if administered early in the course of infection (acute stage) • Efficacy in chronic Chagas is lower • Give with food to minimize GI effects • Monitor blood cell counts • Available only through CDC
Nifurtimox	• Alternative treatment for Chagas	• Requires 60 days of treatment • Less well tolerated than benznidazole

Other Protozoal Infections

Clindamycin and quinine	• Severe babesiosis	• Quinine: monitor for cardiac effects (prolonged QT interval)
Azithromycin and atovaquone	• Mild-moderate babesiosis	
Tetracycline	• Balatinidiasis	• Drug of choice
Trimethoprim-sulfamethoxazole	• Cyclosporiasis, isosporiasis	• Drug of choice

Bibliography

Adagu IS, et al. In vitro activity of nitazoxanide and related compounds against isolates of *Giardia intestinalis, Entamoeba histolytica* and *Trichomonas vaginalis. J Antimicrob Chemother,* **2002,** *49:*103–111.

Alsford S, et al. High-throughput decoding of antitrypanosomal drug efficacy and resistance. *Nature,* **2012,** *482:*232–236.

Altcheh J, et al. Population pharmacokinetic study of benznidazole in pediatric Chagas disease suggests efficacy despite lower plasma concentrations than in adults. *PLoS Negl Trop Dis,* **2014,** 8:e2907.

Alvar J, et al. Chemotherapy in the treatment and control of leishmaniasis. *Adv Parasitol,* **2006,** *61:*223–274.

Anderson VR, Curran MP. Nitazoxanide: a review of its use in the treatment of gastrointestinal infections. *Drugs,* **2007,** *67:*1947–1967.

Aronson N, et al. Diagnosis and treatment of leishmaniasis: clinical practice guidelines by the Infectious Diseases Society of America (IDSA) and the American Society of Tropical Medicine and Hygiene (ASTMH). *Clin Infect Dis,* **2016,** *63:*e202–e264.

Balasegaram M, et al. Effectiveness of melarsoprol and eflornithine as first-line regimens for gambiense sleeping sickness in nine Medecins Sans Frontieres programmes. *Trans R Soc Trop Med Hyg,* **2009,** *103:*280–290.

Barrett MP, et al. Human African trypanosomiasis: pharmacological re-engagement with a neglected disease. *Br J Pharmacol,* **2007,** *152:*1155–1171.

Bern C, et al. Liposomal amphotericin B for the treatment of visceral leishmaniasis. *Clin Infect Dis,* **2006,** *43:*917–924.

Bern C, et al. *Trypanosoma cruzi* and Chagas disease in the United States. *Clin Microbiol Rev,* **2011,** *24:*655–681.

Botoni FA, et al. Treatment of Chagas cardiomyopathy. *BioMed Res Internatl,* **2013,** 849504. PMC. http://dx.doi.org/10.1155/2013/849504. Accessed March 9, 2016.

Bronner U, et al. Pharmacokinetics and adverse reactions after a single dose of pentamidine in patients with *Trypanosoma gambiense* sleeping sickness. *Br J Clin Pharmacol,* **1995,** *39:*289–295.

Burri C, Brun R. Eflornithine for the treatment of human African trypanosomiasis. *Parasitol Res,* **2003,** *90*(suppl 1):S49–S52.

Cabada MM, White AC Jr. Treatment of cryptosporidiosis: do we know what we think we know? *Curr Opin Infect Dis,* **2010,** *23:*494–499.

Castro, M. 1998. Treatment and prophylaxis of *Pneumocystis carinii* pneumonia. *Semin Respir Infect,* **1998,** *13:*296–303.

Chatelain E. Chagas disease drug discovery: toward a new era. *J Biomol Screen,* **2015,** *20:*22–35.

Checkley W, et al. A review of the global burden, novel diagnostics, therapeutics, and vaccine targets for cryptosporidium. *Lancet Infect Dis,* **2015,** *15:*85–94.

Chen KT, et al. Outbreak of Stevens-Johnson syndrome/toxic epidermal necrolysis associated with mebendazole and metronidazole use among Filipino laborers in Taiwan. *Am J Public Health,* **2003,** *93:*489–492.

Cheung TW, et al. Intramuscular pentamidine for the prevention of *Pneumocystis carinii* pneumonia in patients infected with human immunodeficiency virus. *Clin Infect Dis*, **1993**, *16*:22–25.

Contopoulos-Ioannidis D, Montoya JG. *Toxoplasma gondii* (Toxoplasmosis). In: Long SS, et al., eds. *Principles and Practice of Pediatric Infectious Diseases*. Elsevier Saunders, New York, **2012**, 1267–1285.

De NC, et al. Stability of pentamidine isethionate in 5% dextrose and 0.9% sodium chloride injections. *Am J Hosp Pharm*, **1986**, *43*:1486–1488.

Dorlo TP, et al. Miltefosine: a review of its pharmacology and therapeutic efficacy in the treatment of leishmaniasis. *J Antimicrob Chemother*, **2012**, *67*:2576–2597.

Drugs for parasitic infections. *Med Lett Drugs Ther*, **2013**, *11*:e1–e31.

Eperon G et al. Treatment options for second-stage gambiense human African trypanosomiasis. *Expert Rev Anti Infect Ther*, **2014**, *12*:1407–1417.

Escobedo AA, Almirall P, et al. Sexual transmission of giardiasis: a neglected route of spread?. *Acta Trop*, **2014**, *132*:106–111.

Escobedo AA, et al. Treatment of intestinal protozoan infections in children. *Arch Dis Child*, **2009**, *94*:478–482.

Escobedo AA, Hanevik K, et al. Management of chronic *Giardia* infection. *Expert Rev Anti Infect Ther*, **2014**, *12*:1143–1157.

Field AS, Milner DA Jr. Intestinal microsporidiosis. *Clin Lab Med*, **2015**, *35*:445–459.

Fletcher SM, et al. Enteric protozoa in the developed world: a public health perspective. *Clin Microbiol Rev*, **2012**, *25*:420–449.

Flynn PM. Cryptosporidium species. In: Long SS, et al., eds. *Principles and Practice of Pediatric Infectious Diseases*. Elsevier Saunders, New York, **2012**, 1233–1235.

Frezard F, et al. Pentavalent antimonials: new perspectives for old drugs. *Molecules*, **2009**, *14*:2317–2336.

Garcia MN, et al. Evidence of autochthonous Chagas disease in southeastern Texas. *Am J Trop Med Hyg*, **2015**, *92*:325–330.

Gelfand JA, Vannier EG. Babesia species. In: Mandell GL, et al., eds. *Principles and Practice of Infectious Diseases*. Churchill Livingstone, New York, **2014**, 3165–3172.

Haque R, Huston CD, Hughes M, Houpt E, and Petri WA, Jr. Amebiasis. *N Engl J Med*, **2003**, *348*:1565–1573.

Hill DR, Nash TE. *Giardia lamblia*. In: Mandell GL, et al., eds. *Principles and Practice of Infectious Diseases*. Churchill Livingstone, New York, **2014**, 3154–3160.

Hotez PJ, et al. An unfolding tragedy of Chagas disease in North America. *PLoS Negl Trop Dis*, **2013**, *7*:e2300.

Jacobs RT, et al. State of the art in African trypanosome drug discovery. *Curr Topics Med Chem*, **2011**, *11*:1255–1274.

Jang GR, Harris RZ. Drug interactions involving ethanol and alcoholic beverages. *Expert Opin Drug Metab Toxicol*, **2007**, *3*:719–731.

Jeganathan S, et al. The distribution of nifurtimox across the healthy and trypanosome-infected murine blood-brain and blood-cerebrospinal fluid barriers. *J Pharmacol Exp Ther*, **2011**, *336*:506–515.

Jones JL, et al. Neglected parasitic infections in the United States: toxoplasmosis. *Am J Trop Med Hyg*, **2014**, *90*:794–799.

Kaplinski M, et al. Sustained domestic vector exposure is associated with increased Chagas cardiomyopathy risk but decreased parasitemia and congenital transmission risk among young women in Bolivia. *Clin Infect Dis*, **2015**, *61*:918–926.

Kaur M, et al. Suramins development: what did we learn? *Invest New Drugs*, **2002**, *20*:209–219.

Kennedy PG. Clinical features, diagnosis, and treatment of human African trypanosomiasis (sleeping sickness). *Lancet Neurol*, **2013**, *12*:186–194.

Kieffer F, Wallon M. Congenital toxoplasmosis. *Handb Clin Neurol*, **2013**, *112*:1099–1101.

Kissinger P. *Trichomonas vaginalis*: a review of epidemiologic, clinical and treatment issues. *BMC Infect Dis*, **2015**, *15*:307.

Kuepfer I, et al. Safety and efficacy of the 10-day melarsoprol schedule for the treatment of second stage *Rhodesiense* sleeping sickness. *PLoS Negl Trop Dis*, **2012**, *6*:e1695.

Lamp KC, et al. Pharmacokinetics and pharmacodynamics of the nitroimidazole antimicrobials. *Clin Pharmacokinet*, **1999**, *36*:353–373.

Legua P, Seas C. Cystoisospora and cyclospora. *Curr Opin Infect Dis*, **2013**, *26*:479–483.

Lofmark S, et al. Metronidazole is still the drug of choice for treatment of anaerobic infections. *Clin Infect Dis*, **2010**, *50*(suppl 1):S16–S23.

Lutje V, et al. Chemotherapy for second-stage human African trypanosomiasis. *Cochrane Database Syst Rev*, **2013**, (6):CD006201.

Magill AJ. Leishmania Species. In GL Mandell, JE Bennett and R Dolin (eds.), *Principles and Practices of Infectious Diseases*, 2014 (Churchill Livingstone Inc: New York).

Malik LH, et al. The epidemiology, clinical manifestations, and management of Chagas heart disease. *Clin Cardiol*, **2015**, 38: 565–569.

Marcos LA, Gotuzzo E. Intestinal protozoan infections in the immunocompromised host. *Curr Opin Infect Dis*, **2013**, *26*:295–301.

Marie C, Petri WA Jr. Regulation of virulence of *Entamoeba histolytica*. *Annu Rev Microbiol*, **2014**, *68*:493–520.

Martinez V, Caumes E. [Metronidazole]. *Ann Dermatol Venereol*, **2001**, *128*:903–909.

McCarthy JS, Wortmann GW, and Kirchhoff LV. Drugs for Protozoal Infections Other Than Malaria. In GL Mandell, JE Bennett and R Dolin (eds.), *Principles and Practice of Infectious Diseases*, 2014 (Churchill Livingstone Inc: New York).

McGeary RP, et al. Suramin: clinical uses and structure-activity relationships. *Mini Rev Med Chem*, **2008**, *8*:1384–1394.

Meade TW. Subacute myelo-optic neuropathy and clioquinol. An epidemiological case-history for diagnosis. *Br J Prev Soc Med*, **1975**, *29*:157–169.

Meites E. Trichomoniasis: the neglected sexually transmitted disease. *Infect Dis Clin North Am*, **2013**, *27*:755–764.

Messenger LA, et al. Between a bug and a hard place: *Trypanosoma cruzi* genetic diversity and the clinical outcomes of Chagas disease. *Expert Rev Anti Infect Ther*, **2015**, *13*:995–1029.

Miltefosine (Impavido) for leishmaniasis. *Med Lett Drugs Ther*, **2014**, *56*:89–90.

Mishra J, et al. Chemotherapy of leishmaniasis: past, present and future. *Curr Med Chem*, **2007**, *14*:1153–1169.

Moen MD, et al. Liposomal amphotericin B: a review of its use as empirical therapy in febrile neutropenia and in the treatment of invasive fungal infections. *Drugs*, **2009**, *69*:361–392.

Mohamed-Ahmed AH, et al. Recent advances in development of amphotericin B formulations for the treatment of visceral leishmaniasis. *Curr Opin Infect Dis*, **2012**, *25*:695–702.

Molina I, et al. Randomized trial of posaconazole and benznidazole for chronic Chagas disease. *N Engl J Med*, **2014**, *370*:1899–1908.

Molina I, et al. Posaconazole versus benznidazole for chronic Chagas disease. *N Engl J Med*, **2014**, *371*:966.

Monge-Maillo B, Lopez-Velez R. Therapeutic options for old world cutaneous leishmaniasis and new world cutaneous and mucocutaneous leishmaniasis. *Drugs*, **2013**, *73*:1889–1920.

Munday JC, et al. Transport proteins determine drug sensitivity and resistance in a protozoan parasite, *Trypanosoma brucei*. *Front Pharmacol*, **2015**, *6*:32.

Muzny CA, Schwebke JR. The clinical spectrum of *Trichomonas vaginalis* infection and challenges to management. *Sex Transm Infect*, **2013**, *89*:423–425.

Pasupuleti V, et al. Efficacy of 5-nitroimidazoles for the treatment of giardiasis: a systematic review of randomized controlled trials. *PLoS Negl Trop Dis*, **2014**, *8*:e2733.

Paulos C, et al. Pharmacokinetics of a nitrofuran compound, nifurtimox, in healthy volunteers. *Int J Clin Pharmacol Ther Toxicol*, **1989**, *27*:454–457.

Pepin J, Mpia B. Randomized controlled trial of three regimens of melarsoprol in the treatment of *Trypanosoma brucei gambiense* trypanosomiasis. *Trans R Soc Trop Med Hyg*, **2006**, *100*:437–441.

Perez-Victoria FJ, et al. Functional cloning of the miltefosine transporter. A novel P-type phospholipid translocase from *Leishmania* involved in drug resistance. *J Biol Chem*, **2003**, *278*:49965–49971.

Petri WA Jr. *Entamoeba* species, including amebiasis. In: Mandell GL, et al., eds. *Principles and Practice of Infectious Diseases*. Churchill Livingstone, New York, **2014**, 3047–3058.

Podinovskaia M, Descoteaux A. Leishmania and the macrophage: a multifaceted interaction. *Future Microbiol*, **2015**, *10*:111–129.

Priotto G, et al. Nifurtimox-eflornithine combination therapy for second-stage African *Trypanosoma brucei gambiense* trypanosomiasis: a multicentre, randomised, phase III, non-inferiority trial. *Lancet*, **2009**, *374*:56–64.

Priotto G, et al. Safety and effectiveness of first line eflornithine for *Trypanosoma brucei gambiense* sleeping sickness in Sudan: cohort study. *BMJ*, **2008**, *336*:705–708.

Raaflaub J, Ziegler WH. Single-dose pharmacokinetics of the trypanosomicide benznidazole in man. *Arzneimittelforschung*, **1979**, *29*:1611–1614.

Raether W, Hanel H. Nitroheterocyclic drugs with broad spectrum activity. *Parasitol Res*, **2003**, *90*(Suppl 1): S19–S39.

Rajapakse S, et al. Antibiotics for human toxoplasmosis: a systematic review of randomized trials. *Pathog Glob Health*, **2013**, *107*:162–169.

Rex JH, Stevens DA. Drugs active against fungi, pneumocystis, and microsporidia. In: Mandell GL, et al., eds. *Principles and Practice of Infectious Diseases*. Churchill Livingstone, New York, **2014**, 479–494.

Ribeiro AL, et al. Diagnosis and management of Chagas disease and cardiomyopathy. *Nat Rev Cardiol*, **2012**, *9*:576–589.

Royer TL, et al. *Entamoeba bangladeshi* nov. sp., Bangladesh. *Emerg Infect Dis*, **2012**, *18*:1543–1545.

Salamone FR, Cunha BA. Update on pentamidine for the treatment of *Pneumocystis carinii* pneumonia. *Clin Pharm*, **1988**, *7*:501–510.

Sanderson L, et al. The blood-brain barrier significantly limits eflornithine entry into *Trypanosoma brucei brucei* infected mouse brain. *J Neurochem*, **2008**, *107*:1136–1146.

Schuster FL, Ramirez-Avila L. Current world status of *Balantidium coli*. *Clin Microbiol Rev*, **2008**, *21*:626–638.

Schwebke JR. Trichomonas vaginalis. In GL Mandell, JE Bennett and R Dolin (eds.), *Principles and Practice of Infectious Diseases*, 2014 (Churchill Livingston Inc: New York).

Secor WE, et al. Neglected parasitic infections in the United States: trichomoniasis. *Am J Trop Med Hyg*, **2014**, *90*:800–804.

Sindermann H, Engel J. Development of miltefosine as an oral treatment for leishmaniasis. *Trans R Soc Trop Med Hyg*, **2006**, *100*(suppl 1):S17–S20.

Soy D, et al. Population pharmacokinetics of benznidazole in adult patients with Chagas disease. *Antimicrob Agents Chemother*, **2015**, *59*:3342–3349.

Stanley SL Jr. Amoebiasis. *Lancet*, **2003**, *361*:1025–1034.

Suh KN, et al. *Cyclospora cayetanensis, Cystoisospora (Isospora) belli, Sarcocystis* species, *Balantidium coli*, and *Blastocystis* species. In:

Mandell GL, et al., eds. *Principles and Practice of Infectious Diseases*. Churchill Livingstone, New York, **2014**, 3184–3191.

Sundar S, Chakravarty J. Leishmaniasis: an update of current pharmacotherapy. *Expert Opin Pharmacother*, **2013**, *14*:53–63.

Sundar S, Chakravarty J. 2015. An update on pharmacotherapy for leishmaniasis. *Expert Opin Pharmacother*, **2015**, *16*:237–252.

Szumowski SC, Troemel ER. Microsporidia-host interactions. *Curr Opin Microbiol*, **2015**, *26*:10–16.

Townson SM, et al. Resistance to the nitroheterocyclic drugs. *Acta Trop*, **1994**, *56*:173–194.

van den Enden E. 2009. Pharmacotherapy of helminth infection. *Expert Opin Pharmacother*, **2009**, *10*:435–451.

van Griensven J, et al. Leishmaniasis in immunosuppressed individuals. *Clin Microbiol Infect*, **2014**, *20*:286–299.

Vannier EG, et al. Babesiosis. *Infect Dis Clin North Am*, **2015**, *29*: 357–370.

Vincent IM, et al. A molecular mechanism for eflornithine resistance in African trypanosomes. *PLoS Pathog*, **2010**, *6*:e1001204.

White AC Jr. Cryptosporidiosis (*Cryptosporidium* species). In: Mandell GL, et al., eds. *Principles and Practice of Infectious Diseases*. Churchill Livingstone, New York, **2014**, 3173–3183.

WHO. 2015a. Trypanosomiasis, human African (sleeping sickness). *World Health Organization Fact Sheet*, **2015a**, 259.

WHO. 2015c. Leishmaniasis. *World Health Organization Fact Sheet*, **2015a**, 375.

Wilhelm CL, Yarovinsky F. Apicomplexan infections in the gut. *Parasite Immunol*, **2014**, *36*:409–420.

Wilkinson SR, et al. Trypanocidal activity of nitroaromatic prodrugs: current treatments and future perspectives. *Curr Top Med Chem*, **2011**, *11*:2072–2084.

Woodhall D, et al. Neglected parasitic infections: what every family physician needs to know. *Am Fam Physician*, **2014**, *89*:803–811.

Wright JM, et al. Efficacy of antigiardial drugs. *Expert Opin Drug Saf*, **2003**, *2*:529–541.

Wright SG. Protozoan infections of the gastrointestinal tract. *Infect Dis Clin North Am*, **2012**, *26*:323–339.

Yan J, et al. Meta-analysis of prevention and treatment of toxoplasmic encephalitis in HIV-infected patients. *Acta Trop*, **2013**, *127*: 236–244.

Yun O, et al. NECT is next: implementing the new drug combination therapy for *Trypanosoma brucei gambiense* sleeping sickness. *PLoS Negl Trop Dis*, **2010**, *4*:e720.

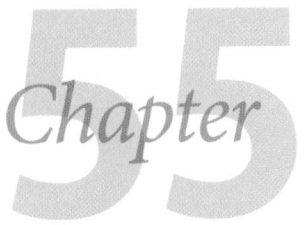

Chapter 55

Chemotherapy of Helminth Infections

Jennifer Keiser, James McCarthy, and Peter Hotez

ANTHELMINTIC DRUGS

- Benzimidazoles
- Diethylcarbamazine
- Doxycycline
- Ivermectin
- Praziquantel
- Metrifonate

- Oxamniquine
- Niclosamide
- Oxantel and Pyrantel Pamoate
- Tribendimidine
- Moxidectin
- Levamisole
- Nitazoxanide

Anthelmintic Drugs

Although a large number of anthelmintic drugs have been approved for human use, only a small number are widely used for treatment of helminth infections that occur worldwide (Figure 55–1). These include two drugs in the benzimidazole (BZ) class, albendazole and mebendazole, which are widely used for treatment of intestinal nematode and cestode infections; the macrocyclic lactone ivermectin, used to treat a variety of nematode and ectoparasite infections; and praziquantel, which is used to treat trematode and some cestode parasites. Because of their role in programs of mass drug administration (MDA), these drugs are amongst the most commonly used agents worldwide. WHO estimated that through MDA approximately 853 million people received one or more anthelmintic drugs in 2014 (WHO, 2016). In many resource-poor developing countries, several different anthelmintic drugs can be provided together through integrated programs of MDA to simultaneously target intestinal and filarial nematodes and trematodes (Webster et al., 2014). Key drugs, their indications, and important pharmacologic properties are listed in the Drug Facts table.

Benzimidazoles

Although a large number of drugs in this class have been synthesized and several have undergone clinical development for treatment of parasitic infections of humans, only two are currently in wide use, namely, *albendazole* and *mebendazole*, with *triclabendazole* reserved for treatment of liver fluke infection caused by *Fasciola hepatica*. *Thiabendazole* was formerly recommended for treatment of strongyloidiasis, but ivermectin is more effective and better tolerated.

Chemistry

Albendazole, mebendazole, and triclabendazole are all poorly water soluble and only slightly soluble in methanol. The chemical structures of these drugs are shown in Figure 55–2.

Mechanism of Action

The primary mechanism of action of BZs is thought to be inhibition of microtubule polymerization by binding to β-tubulin (Prichard, 1994). The selective toxicity of these agents against helminths results from their higher affinity for parasite β-tubulin than for the same target in higher eukaryotes. A range of other biochemical changes occurs in nematodes following BZ exposure, including inhibition of mitochondrial fumarate reductase, reduced glucose transport, and uncoupling of oxidative phosphorylation.

ADME

Mebendazole. The low systemic bioavailability (22%) of mebendazole results from a combination of poor absorption and rapid first-pass metabolism at the intestinal wall and in the liver. Coadministration of cimetidine increases plasma levels of mebendazole, possibly due to inhibition of first-pass, CYP-mediated metabolism (Dayan, 2003). The small proportion of mebendazole that is absorbed is about 95% bound to plasma proteins and is extensively metabolized. Mebendazole, rather than its metabolites, appears to be the active drug form (Gottschall et al., 1990). Conjugates of mebendazole and its metabolites have been found in bile, but little unchanged mebendazole appears in the urine.

Albendazole. Albendazole is variably and erratically absorbed after oral administration; absorption is enhanced by the presence of fatty foods and possibly by bile salts. Administration following food, especially a fatty meal, enhances absorption by up to 5-fold in humans (Dayan, 2003). Cimetidine decreases albendazole bioavailability. The activity of albendazole against tissue-dwelling helminths is attributable to its active metabolite, albendazole sulfoxide. The better bioavailability of the parent drug and the activity of albendazole sulfoxide explain why albendazole is more active than mebendazole against tissue-dwelling helminths. The level of albendazole sulfoxide is enhanced 3.2-fold by grapefruit juice. However, grapefruit juice shortens its $t_{1/2}$ by 46%. It has been suggested that albendazole is metabolized by CYP3A4 enzymes in the intestinal mucosa, a process that can be inhibited by grapefruit juice (Nagy et al., 2002). After a 400-mg oral dose, albendazole cannot be detected in plasma because the drug is rapidly metabolized in the liver and possibly in the intestine, to albendazole sulfoxide, which has potent anthelmintic activity (Redondo et al., 1999).

Both the (+) and (–) enantiomers of albendazole sulfoxide are formed; the (+) enantiomer reaches much higher peak plasma concentrations in humans and is cleared much more slowly than the (–) form (Marques et al., 1999). Albendazole sulfoxide is about 70% bound to plasma proteins and has a highly variable plasma $t_{1/2}$ of 4–15 h (Marques et al., 1999). It is well distributed into various tissues, including hydatid cysts, where it reaches a concentration of about 20% that in plasma (Morris et al., 1987). Oxidation of the sulfoxide derivatives to the nonchiral sulfone metabolite of albendazole, which is pharmacologically inactive, is probably rate limiting in determining the clearance and therefore the plasma $t_{1/2}$ of the bioactive (+) sulfoxide metabolite. In animal models, BZs can induce their own metabolism (Gleizes et al., 1991). Albendazole metabolites are excreted mainly in the urine.

Triclabendazole. Administration of triclabendazole after food enhances its absorption, which might be due to the stimulation of gastric acid secretion, food-induced increase in drug solubility, or altered GI motility and transit time. After oral administration, triclabendazole is rapidly oxidized into two major metabolites, triclabendazole sulfoxide and triclabendazole sulfone, and only low concentrations of the parent drug can be detected

Abbreviations

AUC: area under the curve
BZ: benzimidazole
CDC: Centers for Disease Control and Prevention
CNS: central nervous system
CYP: cytochrome P450
dADT: p-(1-dimethylamino ethylimino) aniline
DDVP: 2,2-dichlorovinyl dimethyl phosphate
DEC: diethylcarbamazine
GABA: γ-aminobutyric acid
GI: gastrointestinal
LF: lymphatic filariasis
MDA: mass drug administration
OTC: over the counter
STH: soil-transmitted helminth
TPAC: terephalic acid
TPAL: terephthalaldehyde
WHO: World Health Organization

in plasma. Triclabendazole sulfoxide is the metabolite active against *F. hepatica* (Keiser et al., 2005).

Therapeutic Uses

Mebendazole. Mebendazole is an effective drug for treatment of some GI nematode infections. It is only administered orally, with the same dosage schedule applying to adults and to children more than 2 years of age. For treatment of enterobiasis, a single 100-mg tablet is taken; if the patient is not cured, a second dose should be given after 3 weeks. For control of ascariasis, trichuriasis, or hookworm infections, the recommended regimen is 100 mg of mebendazole taken in the morning and evening for three consecutive days (or a single 500-mg tablet administered once). If the patient is not cured 3 weeks after treatment, a second course should be given. A 3-day mebendazole regimen is more effective than single doses of either mebendazole (500 mg) or albendazole (400 mg).

Albendazole. Albendazole is a safe and highly effective therapy for infections with GI nematodes, including *Ascaris lumbricoides*, *Trichuris trichiura*, and hookworms. For programmatic control of soil-transmitted helminths (STH) infections (enterobiasis, ascariasis, trichuriasis, and hookworm), albendazole is administered as a single oral 400-mg dose to adults and children more than 2 years of age. Cure rates for light-to-moderate *Ascaris* infections typically are more than 97%, although heavy infections

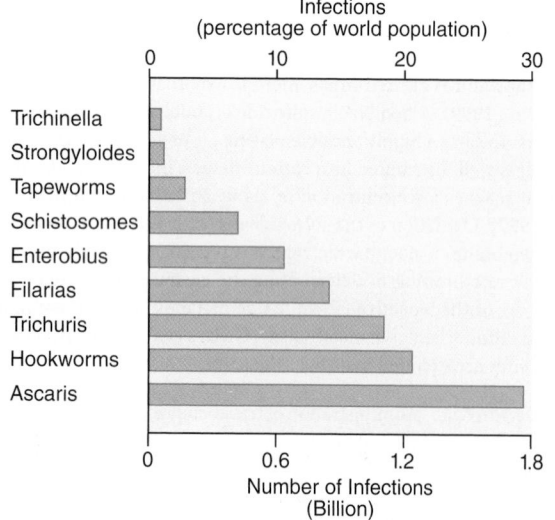

Figure 55–1 *Relative incidence of helminth infections worldwide.*

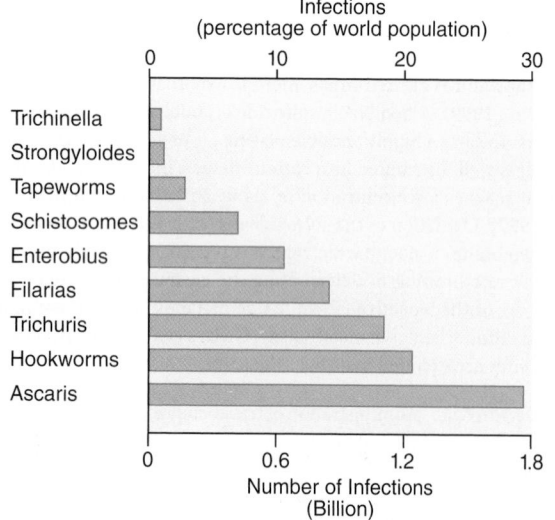

Figure 55–2 *Structure of Benzimidazoles.*

may require therapy for 2–3 days. A 400-mg dose of albendazole appears to be superior to a 500-mg dose of mebendazole for curing hookworm infections and reducing egg counts (Keiser and Utzinger, 2008). A 3-day regime of albendazole outperforms single-dose treatments against hookworm and *T. trichiura* infections (Steinmann et al., 2011). When administered at a dose of 400 mg daily for 3 days, albendazole shows some efficacy in treatment of strongyloidiasis but is less effective than ivermectin for treatment of this infection (Marti et al., 1996).

Albendazole is the drug of choice for chemotherapy of cystic hydatid disease due to *Echinococcus granulosus*. Although prolonged treatment with the drug leads to only a modest cure rate, it is useful as adjunctive treatment in the perioperative period to reduce the risk of disseminated infection resulting from spillage of cyst contents at the time of surgery or with nonoperative puncture, aspiration, injection, reaspiration (PAIR) procedures (Horton, 1997; Schantz, 1999). A typical dosage regimen for adults is 400 mg given twice a day (for children, 15 mg/kg per day with a maximum of 800 mg) for 1–6 months. Although it is the only drug available with useful activity against alveolar echinococcosis caused by *Echinococcus multilocularis* (Venkatesan, 1998), it is parasitostatic rather than parasitocidal, and lifelong therapy with or without surgical intervention is usually required to control this infection.

Albendazole also is the preferred treatment of neurocysticercosis caused by larval forms of *Taenia solium* (Evans et al., 1997; Garcia and Del Brutto, 2000). The recommended dosage is 400 mg given twice a day for adults for 8–30 days, depending on the number, type, and location of the cysts. For children, the dose is 15 mg/kg per day (maximum 800 mg) in two doses for 8–30 days. For both adults and children, the course can be repeated as necessary, as long as liver and bone marrow toxicities are monitored. Glucocorticoid therapy is usually begun before initiating albendazole therapy and is continued for several days after commencement of therapy to reduce the incidence of side effects resulting from inflammatory reactions to dead and dying cysticerci. Glucocorticoids increase plasma levels of albendazole sulfoxide. Prior to initiating chemotherapy of neurocysticercosis, consideration should be given to close observation or the administration of presumptive anticonvulsant therapy. Possible complications include arachnoiditis, vasculitis, cerebral edema, damage to the orbit or spinal cord, and the need for surgical intervention should obstructive hydrocephalus occur. A recent randomized trial indicated that albendazole in combination with praziquantel showed superior efficacy against neurocysticercosis compared to abendazole alone, either in standard or high dose (Garcia et al., 2014).

Albendazole, 400 mg per day, also has shown efficacy for therapy of certain microsporidial intestinal infections in patients with AIDS. Infection with *Capillaria philippinensis* can be treated with a 10-day treatment regimen with albendazole (400 mg/d).

Albendazole has been combined with DEC, ivermectin, or DEC plus ivermectin in programs directed toward controlling LF in most parts of the world (Molyneux and Zagaria, 2002; Ottesen et al., 1999; Thomsen et al., 2016). The strategy is annual dosing with combination therapy for

4–6 years to maintain the microfilaremia at such low levels that transmission cannot occur. The period of therapy is estimated to correspond to the duration of fecundity of adult worms. To avoid serious reactions to dying microfilariae, the albendazole/ivermectin combination is recommended in locations where filariasis coexists with either onchocerciasis or loiasis.

Triclabendazole. Triclabendazole is used for the treatment of fascioliasis and represents an alternative to praziquantel for treatment of paragonimiasis. Triclabendazole is administered at 10 mg/kg with a repeated dose administered when patients have high infection intensities (Keiser et al., 2005).

Adverse Effects; Drug Interactions

Apart from thiabendazole, the BZs have excellent safety profiles. Overall, the incidence of side effects, primarily mild GI symptoms, occur in only 1% of treated children. Side effects frequently encountered with therapeutic doses include anorexia, nausea, vomiting, and dizziness. Mebendazole does not cause significant systemic toxicity in routine clinical use, which may be due to its low systemic bioavailability. Transient symptoms of abdominal pain, distention, and diarrhea have occurred in cases of massive infection and expulsion of GI worms.

Albendazole produces few side effects when used for short-term therapy of GI helminth infections, even in patients with heavy worm burdens. In long-term therapy of cystic hydatid disease and neurocysticercosis, albendazole is well tolerated by most patients. The most common side effect is liver dysfunction, generally manifested by an increase in serum transaminase levels; rarely, jaundice may be noted, but liver enzymes return to normal after therapy is completed. Liver function tests should be monitored during protracted albendazole therapy; the drug is not recommended for patients with cirrhosis. The safety of albendazole in children less than 2 years of age has not been established. Long-term albendazole therapy can occasionally cause bone marrow toxicity, so blood counts should be monitored in this setting as well.

The BZs as a group display few clinically significant interactions with other drugs. Albendazole may induce its own metabolism; plasma levels of its sulfoxide metabolites can be increased by coadministration of glucocorticoids and possibly praziquantel. Due to theoretical considerations, caution is advised when using high doses of albendazole together with drugs that inhibit hepatic CYPs, such as ritonavir. Coadministration of cimetidine can increase the bioavailability of mebendazole.

Pediatric and Geriatric Indications and Problems

Although neither albendazole nor mebendazole is recommended for use in pregnancy, a review of the risk of congenital abnormalities from BZs concluded that their use during pregnancy was not associated with an increased risk of major congenital defects. Hookworm infections occur in many pregnant women in developing countries, including up to one-third of pregnant women in sub-Saharan Africa. Because of the increased morbidity conferred by iron deficiency anemia in pregnancy, monthly BZ treatment has been recommended by the WHO during the second and third trimesters of pregnancy on the basis that improved iron status due to eradication of hookworm infection has a demonstrable benefit for both mother and child. Nonetheless, it is recommended that treatment should be avoided during the first trimester of pregnancy. There is no evidence that maternal BZ therapy presents a risk to breastfed infants.

The BZs have not been extensively studied in children less than 2 years of age. The WHO concluded that BZs may be used in children more than 1 year old if the risks from adverse consequences caused by STHs are justified. The recommended dose is 200 mg of albendazole in children between the ages of 12 and 24 months.

Diethylcarbamazine

Chemistry

Diethylcarbamazine (*N,N*-diethyl-4-methylpiperazine-1-carboxamide) is formulated as the water-soluble citrate salt containing 51% by weight of the active base. The drug is soluble in water. Because the compound is tasteless, odorless, and stable to heat, it also can be taken in the form of

fortified table salt containing 0.2%–0.4% by weight of the base. The drug is available outside the U.S.; in the U.S., it is supplied by the CDC.

DIETHYLCARBAMAZINE

Mechanism of Action

The mechanisms of action of DEC against filarial species are unknown. Microfilarial forms of susceptible filarial species are most affected by DEC. These developmental forms of *Wuchereria bancrofti*, *Brugia malayi*, and *Loa loa* rapidly disappear from human blood after consumption of the drug. Microfilariae of *Onchocerca volvulus* rapidly disappear from skin after DEC administration, but the drug does not kill microfilariae in nodules that contain the adult (female) worms. The drug has some activity against the adult life-cycle stages of *W. bancrofti*, *B. malayi*, and *L. loa* but negligible activity against adult *O. volvulus*.

ADME

Diethylcarbamazine is absorbed rapidly from the GI tract. Peak plasma levels occur within 1–2 h; the plasma $t_{1/2}$ varies from 2 to 10 h, depending on the urinary pH. Alkalinizing the urine can elevate plasma levels, prolong the plasma $t_{1/2}$, and increase both the therapeutic effect and the toxicity of DEC (Awadzi et al., 1986). Dosage reduction may be required for people with renal dysfunction. Metabolism is rapid and extensive; a major metabolite, DEC-*N*-oxide, is active.

Therapeutic Uses

Recommended regimens differ according to whether the drug is used for population-based chemotherapy, treatment of confirmed filarial infection, or prophylaxis against infection.

- *Wuchereria bancrofti, B. malayi, and B. timori.* The standard regimen for the treatment of LF traditionally has been a 12-day, 6 mg/kg/d course of DEC. In the U.S., it is common practice to administer small test doses of 50–100 mg (1–2 mg/kg for children) over a 3-day period prior to beginning the 12-day regimen. However, a single dose of 6 mg/kg reportedly has comparable macrofilaricidal and microfilaricidal efficacy to the standard regimen (Addiss and Dreyer, 2000). Single-dose therapy may be repeated every 6–12 months, as necessary. Although DEC does not reverse existing lymphatic damage, early treatment of asymptomatic individuals may prevent progression of lymphatic damage. For mass treatment to interrupt transmission, effective strategies have included the introduction of DEC into table salt (0.2%–0.4% by weight of the base) (Gelband, 1994). DEC, given annually as a single oral dose of 6 mg/kg, is most effective in reducing microfilaremia when coadministered with either albendazole (400 mg) or ivermectin (0.2–0.4 mg/kg). Therapy is usually well tolerated.

- *Onchocerca volvulus and L. loa.* DEC is contraindicated for the treatment of onchocerciasis because it causes severe reactions related to microfilarial destruction, including worsening ocular lesions (Molyneux et al., 2003), and ivermectin is the preferred drug for this infection. DEC is the drug of choice for therapy of loiasis with some caveats (as discussed in the following material). Treatment is initiated with test doses of 50 mg (1 mg/kg in children) daily for 2–3 days, escalating to maximally tolerated daily doses of 9 mg/kg in three doses for 2–3 weeks. In patients with high-grade microfilaremia, low test doses are used, often accompanied by pretreatment with glucocorticoids or antihistamines, to minimize reactions to dying microfilariae. Albendazole may be useful in patients who either fail therapy with DEC or who cannot tolerate the drug. DEC is clinically effective against microfilariae and adult worms of *D. streptocerca*. DEC is no longer recommended as a first-line drug for the treatment of toxocariasis.

Adverse Effects

Below a daily dose of 8–10 mg/kg, direct toxic reactions to DEC are rarely severe and usually disappear within a few days despite continuation of therapy. These reactions include anorexia, nausea, headache, and, at high doses, vomiting. Major adverse effects result directly or indirectly from the host response to destruction of parasites, primarily microfilariae. Delayed reactions to dying adult worms may result in lymphangitis, swelling, and lymphoid abscesses in bancroftian and brugian filariasis and small skin wheals in loiasis. The drug occasionally causes severe side effects in heavy *L. loa* infections, including retinal hemorrhage and life-threatening encephalopathy. In patients with onchocerciasis, the *Mazzotti* reaction typically occurs within a few hours after the first dose. No significant drug interactions have been reported with DEC.

Precautions and Contraindications

Population-based therapy with DEC should be avoided where onchocerciasis or loiasis may be endemic in sub-Saharan Africa, although the drug can be used to protect foreign travelers from these infections. Pretreatment with glucocorticoids and antihistamines often is undertaken to minimize indirect reactions to DEC that result from release of antigen by dying microfilariae. Dosage reduction may be appropriate for patients with impaired renal function or persistent alkaline urine. DEC appears to be safe for use during pregnancy.

Doxycycline

Filarial parasites, including *W. bancrofti* and *O. volvulus,* harbor bacterial symbionts of the genus *Wolbachia,* against which long courses of doxycycline (see Chapter 59) (≥6 weeks) in bancroftian filariasis and onchocerciasis are effective. A 6-week regimen of doxycycline (100 mg daily), by killing the *Wolbachia,* leads to sterility of adult female *Onchocerca* worms.

HISTORY

In the mid-1970s, surveys of natural products revealed that a fermentation broth of the soil actinomycete *Streptomyces avermitilis* ameliorated infection with *Nematospiroides dubius* in mice. Isolation of the anthelmintic components from cultures of this organism led to discovery of the avermectins, a novel class of 16-membered macrocyclic lactones (Campbell, 1989). Ivermectin (mectizan; stromectol; 22,23-dihydroavermectin B1a) is a semisynthetic analog of avermectin B1a (abamectin), an insecticide developed for crop management. Ivermectin now is used extensively to control and treat a broad spectrum of infections caused by parasitic nematodes (roundworms) and arthropods (insects, ticks, and mites) that plague livestock and domestic animals (Campbell, 1993).

Ivermectin

Chemistry

Ivermectin exists as an odorless, off-white powder with high lipid solubility but poor solubility in water. It is a mixture of at least 80% 22,23-dihydroavermectin B1a and no more than 20% 22,23-dihydroavermectin B1b. B1a and B1b have nearly identical antiparasitic activities.

IVERMECTIN

Mechanism of Action

Ivermectin immobilizes affected organisms by inducing tonic paralysis of the musculature. Avermectins induce paralysis by activating a family of ligand-gated Cl^- channels, particularly glutamate-gated Cl^- channels found only in invertebrates. Ivermectin probably binds to glutamate-activated Cl^- channels found in nematode nerve or muscle cells and causes hyperpolarization by increasing intracellular chloride concentration, resulting in paralysis. Glutamate-gated Cl^- channels probably are one of several sites of ivermectin action amongst invertebrates (Zufall et al., 1989). Avermectins also bind with high affinity to GABA-gated and other ligand-gated Cl^- channels in nematodes such as *Ascaris* and in insects, but the physiological consequences are less well defined. Lack of high-affinity avermectin receptors in cestodes and trematodes may explain why these helminths are not sensitive to ivermectin (Shoop et al., 1995). Avermectins also interact with GABA receptors in mammalian brain, but their affinity for invertebrate receptors is about 100-fold higher (Schaeffer and Haines, 1989).

ADME

Peak levels of ivermectin in plasma are achieved within 4–5 h after oral administration. The long $t_{1/2}$ (~57 h in adults) primarily reflects low systemic clearance (~1–2 L/h) and a large apparent volume of distribution. Ivermectin is about 93% bound to plasma proteins. The drug is extensively metabolized by hepatic CYP3A4 (Zeng et al., 1998). Virtually no ivermectin appears in human urine in either unchanged or conjugated form (Krishna and Klotz, 1993).

Therapeutic Uses

Onchocerciasis. Ivermectin, administered as a single oral dose (150–200 µg/kg) given every 6–12 months, is the drug of choice for onchocerciasis in adults and children 5 years or older (Goa et al., 1991). Marked reduction of microfilariae in the skin results in major relief of the intense pruritus that is a feature of onchocerciasis. Clearance of microfilariae from skin and ocular tissues occurs within a few days and lasts for 6–12 months; the dose then should be repeated. However, the drug is not curative because ivermectin has little effect on adult *O. volvulus.* Annual doses of the drug are quite safe and substantially reduce transmission of this infection.

Lymphatic Filariasis. Ivermectin is as effective as DEC for controlling LF, and unlike DEC, it can be used in regions where onchocerciasis, loiasis, or both are endemic (Ottesen and Ramachandran, 1995). A single annual dose of ivermectin (200 µg/kg) and a single annual dose of albendazole (400 mg) are even more effective in controlling LF than either drug alone (Ottesen et al., 1999). The duration of treatment is at least 5 years, based on the estimated fecundity of the adult worms.

Strongyloidiasis. Ivermectin, administered as a single dose of 150 to 200 µg/kg, is the drug of choice for human strongyloidiasis (Marti et al., 1996). It is generally recommended that a second dose be administered a week following the first dose. This regimen is more efficacious than a 3-day course of albendazole.

Infections With Other Intestinal Nematodes. Ivermectin is more effective in ascariasis and enterobiasis than in trichuriasis or hookworm infection. In the last two infections, although it is not curative, it significantly reduces the intensity of infection.

Other Indications. Taken as a single 200-µg/kg oral dose, ivermectin is a first-line drug for treatment of cutaneous *larva migrans* caused by dog or cat hookworms and is an option for treatment of scabies and head lice. In uncomplicated scabies, two doses should be administered, 1–2 weeks apart. In severe (crusted) scabies, ivermectin should be used in repeated doses, with one recommended regimen entailing seven doses of 200 µg/kg given with food on days 1, 2, 8, 9, 15, 22, and 29. It also is effective in community-driven control programs (Romani et al., 2015). The drug formulated as a topical 0.2% lotion is active against human head lice (Pariser et al., 2012).

Adverse Effects; Drug Interactions

Ivermectin is well tolerated by uninfected humans. In filarial infection, ivermectin therapy frequently causes a *Mazzotti*-like reaction to dying microfilariae. The intensity and nature of these reactions relate to the microfilarial burden. After treatment of *O. volvulus* infections, these side effects usually are limited to mild itching and swollen, tender lymph nodes, which occur in 5%–35% of people, last just a few days, and are relieved by aspirin and antihistamines. Rarely, more severe reactions occur that include high fever, tachycardia, hypotension, dizziness, headache, myalgia, arthralgia, diarrhea, and facial and peripheral edema; these may respond to glucocorticoid therapy. Ivermectin induces milder side effects than does DEC, and unlike DEC, ivermectin seldom exacerbates ocular lesions in onchocerciasis. The drug can cause rare but serious side effects, occasionally resulting in permanent disability and encephalopathies in patients with heavy *L. loa* microfilaria. *Loa* encephalopathy is associated with ivermectin treatment of individuals with *Loa* microfilaremia levels 30,000 or more microfilariae per milliliter of blood. Ivermectin interactions with concurrently administered drugs can occur. For example, increased plasma levels of ivermectin have been observed in patients concurrently treated with ivermectin and levamisole (González Canga, 2008).

Precautions and Contraindications

Because of its effects on GABA receptors in the CNS, ivermectin is contraindicated in conditions associated with an impaired blood-brain barrier (e.g., African trypanosomiasis and meningitis). In programs of MDA where loiasis is coendemic with either onchocerciasis or LF, ivermectin should be used with caution and in consultation with local or international experts.

Pediatric and Geriatric Indications and Problems. Ivermectin is not approved for use in children with less than 15 kg body weight or in pregnant or lactating women (low levels of the drug appear in the mother's milk). This is principally due to concerns about the passage of the drug across the immature blood-brain barrier.

Praziquantel

Chemistry

Praziquantel, a pyrazinoisoquinoline derivative, is a racemate, consisting of the biologically active enantiomer, R-praziquantel and the inactive distomer S-praziquantel. The white crystalline powder is slightly soluble in water and freely soluble in alcohol and in methylene chloride.

PRAZIQUANTEL

Mechanism of Action

Praziquantel has two major effects on adult schistosomes. At the lowest effective concentrations, it causes increased muscular activity, followed by contraction and spastic paralysis. Affected worms detach from blood vessel walls and migrate from the mesenteric veins to the liver. At slightly higher concentrations, praziquantel causes tegumental damage and exposes a number of tegumental antigens (Redman et al., 1996). The clinical efficacy of this drug correlates better with tegumental action (Xiao et al., 1985). The drug is ineffective against juvenile schistosomes and therefore is relatively ineffective in early infection. An intact immune response is believed to be required for the clinical efficacy of the drug.

The primary site of action of praziquantel is uncertain (Aragon et al., 2009). The drug may act through generation of reactive oxygen species. It also promotes an influx of Ca^{2+} and possibly interacts with the variant Ca^{2+} channel Ca-varβ (Jeziorski and Greenberg, 2006), which is found in schistosomes and other praziquantel-sensitive parasites. However, Ca^{2+} influx does not correlate with sensitivity to the drug (Pica-Mattoccia et al., 2008). Praziquantel inhibits adenosine flux (Angelucci et al., 2007), but definitive evidence that this action contributes to the anthelmintic effect is lacking.

ADME

Praziquantel is readily absorbed after oral administration (<80%), reaching maximal levels in human plasma in approximately 2 h. Praziquantel is highly protein bound (~80%, nearly exclusive to albumin). Praziquantel distributes throughout the body, with highest concentrations measured in the liver and kidneys. It crosses the blood-brain barrier. Breast milk concentrations are approximately 25% of plasma concentrations (Olliaro et al., 2014).

Extensive stereoselective first-pass metabolism takes place. The main metabolite is trans-4-hydroxypraziquantel. The plasma $t_{1/2}$ is 2.2–8.9 h following 40 mg/kg in healthy fasted adults. In patients with severe liver disease, including those with hepatosplenic schistosomiasis, pharmacokinetic parameters might be altered (Olliaro et al., 2014). About 70% of an oral dose is recovered as metabolites in the urine within 24 h; most of the remainder is eliminated in the bile.

Therapeutic Uses

Praziquantel is the drug of choice for treating schistosomiasis caused by all *Schistosoma* species that infect humans. A single oral dose of 40 mg/kg or three doses of 20 mg/kg each, given 4–6 h apart, generally produce cure rates of 70%–95% and consistently high reductions (>85%) in egg counts (Utzinger and Keiser, 2004). Three doses of 25 mg/kg taken 4–8 h apart result in high rates of cure for infections with the liver flukes *Clonorchis sinensis* and *Opisthorchis viverrini* or the intestinal flukes *Fasciolopsis buski, Heterophyes heterophyes*, and *Metagonimus yokogawai*. The same three-dose regimen, used over 2 days, is highly effective against infections with the lung fluke *Paragonimiasis westermani*. The liver fluke *F. hepatica* is resistant to praziquantel and should be treated with triclabendazole (Keiser et al., 2005). Low doses of praziquantel can be used to treat intestinal infections with adult cestodes (a single oral dose of 25 mg/kg for *Hymenolepis nana* and 10 to 20 mg/kg for *Diphyllobothrium latum, Taenia saginata*, or *T. solium*). Re-treatment after 7–10 days is advisable for individuals heavily infected with *H. nana*. Although albendazole is preferred for therapy of human cysticercosis, praziquantel represents an alternative agent; its use for this indication is hampered by the important pharmacokinetic interaction with dexamethasone and other corticosteroids that should be coadministered in this condition (Evans et al., 1997).

Adverse Effects; Drug Interactions

Abdominal discomfort and drowsiness may occur shortly after taking praziquantel; these direct effects are transient and dose related. Indirect effects such as fever, pruritus, urticaria, rashes, arthralgia, and myalgia are noted occasionally. Such side effects and increases in eosinophilia often relate to parasite burden and may be a consequence of parasite killing and antigen release. In neurocysticercosis, inflammatory reactions to praziquantel may produce meningismus, seizures, and cerebrospinal fluid pleocytosis. These effects usually are delayed in onset, last 2–3 days, and respond to analgesics and anticonvulsants. Praziquantel is contraindicated in ocular cysticercosis because the host response can irreversibly damage the eye. Driving and other tasks requiring mental alertness should be avoided. Severe hepatic disease can prolong the $t_{1/2}$, requiring dosage adjustment. The bioavailability of praziquantel is reduced by inducers of hepatic CYPs, such as carbamazepine and phenobarbital; predictably, coadministration of the CYP inhibitor cimetidine has the opposite effect (Dachman et al., 1994). Dexamethasone reduces the bioavailability of praziquantel. Under certain conditions, praziquantel may increase the bioavailability of albendazole (Homeida et al., 1994).

Pediatric and Geriatric Indications and Problems. Praziquantel is considered safe in children more than 4 years of age. A pediatric formulation, an oral dispersible tablet, based on either racemic praziquantel or enantiopure L-PZQ is under development.

Metrifonate

Metrifonate (trichlorfon) is an organophosphorus compound used first as an insecticide and later as an anthelmintic, especially for treatment of *Schistosoma haematobium*. It remains a second-line drug for this indication. Metrifonate is a prodrug; at physiological pH, it is converted nonenzymatically to *dichlorvos* (DDVP), a potent cholinesterase inhibitor (see Chapter 10). However, inhibition of cholinesterase alone is unlikely to explain the antischistosomal properties of metrifonate.

METRIFONATE

Oxamniquine

Oxamniquine is a second-line drug after praziquantel for the treatment of *Schistosoma mansoni* infection. *Schistosoma haematobium* and *Schistosoma japonicum* are refractory to this drug.

Niclosamide

Niclosamide, a halogenated salicylanilide derivative, was introduced for human use as a taeniacide. Niclosamide is no longer approved for use in the U.S. It has some use in intestinal *T. solium* infection where neurocysticercosis is present or cannot be excluded.

Oxantel and Pyrantel Pamoate

Chemistry

The tetrahydropyrimidine analogues include pyrantel pamoate and the *m*-oxyphenol analogue of pyrantel, oxantel pamoate. Both drugs are practically insoluble in water and alcohol.

PYRANTEL   OXANTEL

Mechanism of Action

Pyrantel and its analogues are depolarizing neuromuscular blocking agents. They open nonselective cation channels and induce persistent activation of nicotinic acetylcholine receptors and spastic paralysis of the worm (Robertson et al., 1994). Pyrantel pamoate is active at the L type, while oxantel pamoate is active on the N subtype of nicotinic acetylcholine receptors (Williamson et al., 2009).

Pyrantel also inhibits cholinesterases. It causes a slowly developing contracture of isolated preparations of *Ascaris* at 1% of the concentration of acetylcholine required to produce the same effect. Pyrantel exposure leads to depolarization and increased spike-discharge frequency, accompanied by increases in tension, in isolated helminth muscle preparations.

ADME

Pyrantel pamoate and oxantel pamoate are poorly absorbed from the GI tract, a property that confines their action to intraluminal GI nematodes. Less than 15% of pyrantel pamoate is excreted in the urine as parent drug and metabolites. The major proportion of an administered dose is recovered in the feces.

Therapeutic Uses

Pyrantel pamoate is an alternative to mebendazole or albendazole for treatment of ascariasis and enterobiasis. High cure rates are achieved after a single oral dose of 11 mg/kg, to a maximum of 1 g. Pyrantel also is effective against hookworm infections caused by *Ancylostoma duodenale* and *Necator americanus*, although repeated doses are needed to cure heavy infections by *N. americanus*. The drug should be used in combination with oxantel pamoate for mixed infections with *T. trichiura*. Indeed, oxantel pamoate was shown to have a higher efficacy than the BZs mebendazole and albendazole against infections with *T. trichiura* (Speich et al., 2016). Oxantel pamoate combined with albendazole is a highly effective

combination in the treatment of ascariasis, trichuriasis, and hookworm infections. For pinworm infections, repeat the treatment after an interval of 2 weeks.

Adverse Effects; Drug Interactions

Transient and mild GI symptoms occasionally occur, as do headache, dizziness, rash, and fever. Pyrantel pamoate has not been studied in pregnant women.

Tribendimidine

Tribendimidine is a drug that has been marketed in China for over a decade. Given the efforts to introduce the drug to Western markets, it is included in this chapter.

Chemistry

Tribendimidine (a symmetrical diamidine derivative) is a yellow crystalline powder that does not dissolve in water and only marginally in anhydrous ethanol, methanol, and acetone. It dissolves in chloroform (Xiao et al., 2005).

Tribendimidine

Mechanism of Action

Tribendimidine is an agonist of muscle nicotinic acetylcholine receptors of parasitic nematodes. Tribendimidine is more selective for the B subtype than the L subtype of nicotinic acetylcholine receptors; hence, it can activate a different population of nematode parasite nicotinic acetylcholine receptors. This might explain why tribendimidine exhibits activity on a levamisole-resistant isolate of *Oesophagostomum dentatum* and why the spectrum of action of tribendimidine is broader (covering also the trematodes *C. sinensis* and *O. viverrini* and cestodes) to that of other cholinergic anthelmintics like levamisole (Robertson et al., 2015).

ADME

Tribendimidine pharmacokinetics has been studied in Chinese healthy volunteers (Yuan et al., 2010) and in patients infected with *O. viverrini* (Duthaler et al., 2015). Tribendimidine cannot be detected in plasma. It is rapidly and completely broken down to dADT, which is the active metabolite and TPAL. Furthermore, dADT undergoes metabolism to acetylated dADT, and TPAL is transformed into TPAC. The $t_{1/2}$ of dADT was 4.7 h in healthy volunteers following 400 mg of tribendimidine. Tribendimidine is mainly excreted through the urine (Yuan et al., 2010).

Therapeutic Uses

Tribendimidine is given to children below 15 years of age and adults at doses of 200 mg and 400 mg, respectively. With regard to STH infections, tribendimidine has a similar activity profile as albendazole: Tribendimidine shows high cure and egg reduction rates against *A. lumbricoides*, moderate-to-good efficacy against hookworm, and a low cure rate but moderate egg reduction rates against *T. trichiura*. Against pinworm infections, cure rates with tribendimidine were 74.1% (single dose) and 97.1% (two doses) (Xiao et al., 2013). Tribendimidine has high activity against *C. sinensis* and *O. viverrini*: Single dosages of tribendimidine (200 and 400 mg) showed similar efficacy than multiple treatments with praziquantel (Qian et al., 2013; Soukhathammavong et al., 2011). The efficacy of tribendimidine against strongyloides and cestode infections remains to be studied.

Adverse Effects; Drug Interactions

Tribendimidine shows a good safety profile. Adverse effects (e.g., dizziness, vertigo, headache, nausea, vomiting, and fatigue) are mainly mild and self-limiting. Drug interactions have not yet been studied thoroughly.

Moxidectin

Moxidectin, a macrocyclic lactone related to ivermectin, is currently under development for the treatment of onchocerciasis and perhaps other helminth infections.

Chemistry

Moxidectin, a white or pale yellow powder, is slightly soluble in water but readily soluble in organic solvents.

Mechanism of Action

The mechanism of action of the avermectins has been described previously. A difference has been demonstrated between ivermectin and moxidectin for interacting with GABA-gated Cl⁻ channels. In contrast to ivermectin, moxidectin is a poor substrate for P-glycoproteins, hence suggesting a different mechanism or susceptibility to resistance (Cobb and Boeckh, 2009).

ADME

Pharmacokinetics parameters were dose proportional at dosages from 3 to 36 mg. Peak plasma concentrations occurred 2 to 6 h after dosing. Administration with food resulted in an increase of over 30% in C_{max} and in AUC. Moxidectin has a very long elimination $t_{1/2}$ (mean 20–35 days) and very large volume of distribution (Cotreau et al., 2003). Following a single dose, moxidectin was observed in the breast milk of lactating women (Korth-Bradley et al., 2011). Several hydroxy and oxidative metabolites have been identified in vitro (Dupuy et al., 2001); however, in animals the rate of metabolites is low.

Therapeutic Uses

Moxidectin is currently under development for the treatment of *O. volvulus* infections. A dose-finding phase 2 study revealed a significantly higher efficacy of 8 mg moxidectin compared to ivermectin (Awadzi et al., 2014).

Adverse Effects

Mazzotti reactions including pruritus, rash, increased pulse rate, and decreased mean arterial pressure were commonly observed after moxidectin treatment (Awadzi et al., 2014).

Pediatric and Geriatric Indications and Problems. Moxidectin has not been used in children less than 12 years of age; however, pediatric trials are ongoing.

Levamisole

Chemistry

Levamisole, the levorotatory isomer of the racemic molecule tetramisole, belongs to the imidazole derivatives. The hydrochloride salt is a white powder soluble in water and methanol. Levamisole has been discontinued in the U.S.

Mechanism of Action

Levamisole is a cholinergic anthelminthic. The drug is a potent muscle and nerve L-subtype selective nicotinic acetylcholine receptor channel agonist. Opening of these channels produces depolarization, calcium entry, and an increase in sarcoplasmic calcium, producing spastic muscle contraction, resulting in passive elimination of the worms (Martin et al., 2012). Levamisole was also shown to inhibit fumarate reductase and hence succinate production, the main source of ATP, which is key for the survival of worms (Janssen, 1976). With regard to mammalian cells, levamisole inhibits alkaline phosphatases in most tissues (Janssen, 1976). The immunomodulatory activity of levamisole has been explained as a stimulation of antibody formation and enhancement of T cell response by stimulating T-cell activation and proliferation.

ADME

Levamisole is quickly absorbed from the GI tract, and C_{max} levels are reached within 2 h. The drug is extensively metabolized in the liver, and its half-life is about 4 h (Janssen, 1976).

Therapeutic Uses

Levamisole has excellent activity against *A. lumbricoides* but low-to-moderate efficacy against *T. trichiura* and hookworm infections (Keiser and Utzinger, 2008). Levamisole has also been used for its immunomodulatory effects in cancer.

Adverse Effects; Drug Interactions

Adverse effects mostly occur at high dosages used for immunotherapy. At the single low dosages for anthelminthic therapy, adverse effects are minor and include nausea, vomiting, headache, dizziness, or abdominal pain. Severe adverse effects such as agranulocytosis have been described following the use of high dosages. In healthy volunteers, increased plasma levels of ivermectin and decreased plasma concentrations of albendazole sulfoxide were observed when these drugs were coadministered with levamisole (Awadzi et al., 2004).

Nitazoxanide

Nitazoxanide (*N*-[nitrothiazolyl] salicylamide) is an oral synthetic broad-spectrum antiparasitic agent. Nitazoxanide has been used as a single agent to treat mixed infections with intestinal parasites (protozoa and helminths). Nitazoxanide is approved in the U.S. for treatment of cryptosporidiosis and giardiasis and has activity against *E. histolytica* (see Chapter 54 for details). Nitazoxanide also has activity against intestinal helminthes such as *H. nana, A. lumbricoides, T. trichiura,* and *Entrobius vermicularis* (van den Enden, 2009). It also is an effective broad-spectrum antiviral agent (Rossignol, 2014). Adverse effects are rare with nitazoxanide.

Acknowledgment: *Alex Loukas, James W. Tracy, and Leslie T. Webster, Jr contributed to this chapter in recent editions of this book. We have retained some of their text in the current edition.*

Drug Facts for Your Personal Formulary: *Anthelmintics*

Drugs	Therapeutic Uses	Clinical Pharmacology and Tips
Benzimidazoles: β-Tubulin inhibitors		
Albendazole	• Intestinal nematode infections • Cysticercosis • Cutaneous larva migrans • Toxocariasis • Echinococcosis	• Monitor for liver and hemotologic toxicity in long-term therapy • Absorption improved with fatty food
Mebendazole	• Intestinal nematode infections	• Poorly absorbed; useful for intestinal luminal nematode
Triclabendazole	• Fascioliasis	• Available from the CDC under an investigational new drug protocol
Macrocyclic Lactones: Glutamate gated chloride channel blockers		
Ivermectin	• Onchocerciasis • Lymphatic filariasis • Scabies and head lice • Strongyloidiasis	• Safety in pregnancy and children < 15 kg not certain
Moxidectin	• Investigational for onchocerciasis	• Licensed only for veterinary use in the U.S.
Praziquantel		
	• Schistosomiasis • Food-borne trematode infections (opisthorciasis and paragonamiasis) • Intestinal tapeworm infections	• Dizziness is a common adverse effect • May impair mental alertness; avoid tasks such as driving
Miscellaneous Anthelmintics		
Diethylcarbamazine	• Lymphatic filariasis	• Contraindicated in onchocerciasis • Available from CDC under an investigational new drug protocol
Metrifonate	• Second-line drug for *Schistosoma haematobium* infection	• Not licensed for use in the U.S.
Oxamniquine	• Second-line drug for *Schistosoma mansoni* infection	• Discontinued in the U.S.
Niclosamide	• Intestinal tapeworm infection	• Discontinued in the U.S.
Oxantel and pyrantel pamoate	• Second-line drug for intestinal nematode infection	• Oxantel pamoate is not licensed for use in the U.S. • Pyrantel pamoate is sold OTC to treat pinworm infections
Doxycycline	• Filarial infection	• 6-Week course of therapy advised
Levamisole	• Excellent activity against *Ascaris lumbricoides* • Low-to-moderate efficacy against *Trichuris trichiura* and hookworm infections	• May cause agranulocytosis at high doses
Nitazoxanide	• Effective against intestinal helminths • Antiprotozoal and antiviral activity	• Broad-spectrum antiparasitic agent • Side effects are rare

Bibliography

Addiss DG, Dreyer G. Treatment of lymphatic filariasis. In: Nutman TB, ed. *Lymphatic Filariasis*. Imperial College Press, London, **2000**, 151–199.

Angelucci F, et al. The anti-schistosomal drug praziquantel is an adenosine antagonist. *Parasitology*, **2007**, *134*:1215–1221.

Aragon AD, et al. Towards an understanding of the mechanism of action of praziquantel. *Mol Biochem Parasitol*, **2009**, *164*:57–65.

Awadzi K, et al. The effect of moderate urine alkalinisation on low dose diethylcarbamazine therapy in patients with onchocerciasis. *Br J Clin Pharmacol*, **1986**, *21*:669–676.

Awadzi K, et al. The safety, tolerability and pharmacokinetics of levamisole alone, levamisole plus ivermectin, and levamisole plus albendazole, and their efficacy against *Onchocerca volvulus*. *Ann Trop Med Parasitol*, **2004**, *98*:595–614.

Awadzi K, et al. A randomized, single-ascending-dose, ivermectin-controlled, double-blind study of moxidectin in *Onchocerca volvulus* infection. *PLoS Negl Trop Dis*, **2014**, *8*:e2953.

Campbell WC. Ivermectin, an antiparasitic agent. *Med Res Rev*, **1993**, *13*:61–79.

Campbell WC, ed. Ivermectin and Abamectin. Springer-Verlag, New York, **1989**.

Cobb R, Boeckh A. Moxidectin: a review of chemistry, pharmacokinetics and use in horses. *Parasit Vectors*, **2009**, *2*(suppl 2):S5.

Cotreau MM, et al. The antiparasitic moxidectin: safety, tolerability, and pharmacokinetics in humans. *J Clin Pharmacol*, **2003**, *43*:1108–1115.

Dachman WD, et al. Cimetidine-induced rise in praziquantel levels in a patient with neurocysticercosis being treated with anticonvulsants. *J Infect Dis*, **1994**, *169*:689–691.

Dayan AD. Albendazole, mebendazole and praziquantel. Review of non-clinical toxicity and pharmacokinetics. *Acta Trop*, **2003**, *86*:141–159.

Dupuy J, et al. In vitro metabolism of ^{14}C-moxidectin by hepatic microsomes from various species. *Vet Res Commun*, **2001**, *25*:345–354.

Duthaler U, et al. LC-MS/MS method for the determination of two metabolites of tribendimidine, deacylated amidantel and its acetylated metabolite in plasma, blood and dried blood spots. *J Pharm Biomed Anal*, **2015**, *105*:163–173.

Evans C, et al. Controversies in the management of cysticercosis. *Emerg Infect Dis*, **1997**, *3*:403–405.

Garcia HH, Del Brutto OH. *Taenia solium* cysticercosis. *Infect Dis Clin North Am*, **2000**, *14*:97–119, ix.

Garcia HH, et al. Efficacy of combined antiparasitic therapy with praziquantel and albendazole for neurocysticercosis: a double-blind, randomised controlled trial. *Lancet Infect Dis*, **2014**, *14*:687–695.

Gelband H. Diethylcarbamazine salt in the control of lymphatic filariasis. *Am J Trop Med Hyg*, **1994**, *50*:655–662.

Gleizes C, et al. Inducing effect of oxfendazole on cytochrome P450IA2 in rabbit liver. Consequences on cytochrome P450 dependent monooxygenases. *Biochem Pharmacol*, **1991**, *41*:1813–1820.

Goa KL, et al. Ivermectin. A review of its antifilarial activity, pharmacokinetic properties and clinical efficacy in onchocerciasis. *Drugs*, **1991**, *42*:640–658.

González Canga A, et al. The pharmacokinetics and interactions of ivermectin in humans: a mini-review. *AAPS J*, **2008**, *10*:42–46.

Gottschall DW, et al. The metabolism of benzimidazole anthelmintics. *Parasitol Today*, **1990**, *6*:115–124.

Homeida M, et al. Pharmacokinetic interaction between praziquantel and albendazole in Sudanese men. *Ann Trop Med Parasitol*, **1994**, *88*:551–559.

Horton RJ. Albendazole in treatment of human cystic echinococcosis: 12 years of experience. *Acta Trop*, **1997**, *64*:79–93.

Janssen PA. The levamisole story. *Prog Drug Res*, **1976**, *20*:347–383.

Jeziorski MC, Greenberg RM. Voltage-gated calcium channel subunits from platyhelminths: potential role in praziquantel action. *Int J Parasitol*, **2006**, *36*:625–632.

Keiser J, et al. Triclabendazole for the treatment of fascioliasis and paragonimiasis. *Expert Opin Investig Drugs*, **2005**, *14*:1513–1526.

Keiser J, Utzinger J. Efficacy of current drugs against soil-transmitted helminth infections: systematic review and meta-analysis. *JAMA*, **2008**, *299*:1937–1948.

Korth-Bradley JM, et al. Excretion of moxidectin into breast milk and pharmacokinetics in healthy lactating women. *Antimicrob Agents Chemother*, **2011**, *55*:5200–5204.

Krishna DR, Klotz U. Determination of ivermectin in human plasma by high-performance liquid chromatography. *Arzneimittelforschung*, **1993**, *43*:609–611.

Marques MP, et al. Enantioselective kinetic disposition of albendazole sulfoxide in patients with neurocysticercosis. *Chirality*, **1999**, *11*:218–223.

Marti H, et al. A comparative trial of a single-dose ivermectin versus three days of albendazole for treatment of *Strongyloides stercoralis* and other soil-transmitted helminth infections in children. *Am J Trop Med Hyg*, **1996**, *55*:477–481.

Martin RJ, et al. Levamisole receptors: a second awakening. *Trends Parasitol*, **2012**, *28*:289–296.

Molyneux DH, Zagaria N. Lymphatic filariasis elimination: progress in global programme development. *Ann Trop Med Parasitol*, **2002**, *96*(suppl 2):S15–S40.

Molyneux DH, et al. Mass drug treatment for lymphatic filariasis and onchocerciasis. *Trends Parasitol*, **2003**, *19*:516–522.

Morris DL, et al. Penetration of albendazole sulphoxide into hydatid cysts. *Gut*, **1987**, *28*:75–80.

Nagy J, et al. Effect of grapefruit juice or cimetidine coadministration on albendazole bioavailability. *Am J Trop Med Hyg*, **2002**, *66*:260–263.

Olliaro P, et al. The little we know about the pharmacokinetics and pharmacodynamics of praziquantel (racemate and R-enantiomer). *J Antimicrob Chemother*, **2014**, *69*:863–870.

Ottesen EA, Ramachandran CP. Lymphatic filariasis infection and disease: control strategies. *Parasitol Today*, **1995**, *11*:129–131.

Ottesen EA, et al. The role of albendazole in programmes to eliminate lymphatic filariasis. *Parasitol Today*, **1999**, *15*:382–386.

Pariser DM, et al. Topical 0.5% ivermectin lotion for treatment of head lice. *N Engl J Med*, **2012**, *367*:1687–1693.

Pica-Mattoccia L, et al. *Schistosoma mansoni*: lack of correlation between praziquantel-induced intra-worm calcium influx and parasite death. *Exp Parasitol*, **2008**, *119*:332–335.

Prichard R. Anthelmintic resistance. *Vet Parasitol*, **1994**, *54*:259–268.

Qian MB, et al. Efficacy and safety of tribendimidine against *Clonorchis sinensis*. *Clin Infect Dis*, **2013**, *56*:e76–e82.

Redman CA, et al. Praziquantel: an urgent and exciting challenge. *Parasitol Today*, **1996**, *12*:14–20.

Redondo PA, et al. Presystemic metabolism of albendazole: experimental evidence of an efflux process of albendazole sulfoxide to intestinal lumen. *Drug Metab Dispos*, **1999**, *27*:736–740.

Robertson AP, et al. Tribendimidine: mode of action and nAChR subtype selectivity in *Ascaris* and *Oesophagostomum*. *PLoS Negl Trop Dis*, **2015**, *9*:e0003495.

Robertson SJ, et al. The action of pyrantel as an agonist and an open channel blocker at acetylcholine receptors in isolated *Ascaris suum* muscle vesicles. *Eur J Pharmacol*, **1994**, *271*:273–282.

Romani L, et al. Mass drug administration for scabies control in a population with endemic disease. *N Engl J Med*, **2015**, *373*:2305–2313.

Rossignol JF. Nitazoxanide: a first-in-class broad-spectrum antiviral agent. *Antiviral Res*, **2014**, *110*:94–103.

Schaeffer JM, Haines HW. Avermectin binding in *Caenorhabditis elegans*. A two-state model for the avermectin binding site. *Biochem Pharmacol*, **1989**, *38*:2329–2338.

Schantz PM. Editorial response: treatment of cystic echinococcosis—improving but still limited. *Clin Infect Dis*, **1999**, *29*:310–311.

Shoop WL, et al. Avermectins and milbemycins against *Fasciola hepatica*: in vivo drug efficacy and in vitro receptor binding. *Int J Parasitol*, **1995**, *25*:923–927.

Soukhathammavong P, et al. Efficacy and safety of mefloquine, artesunate, mefloquine-artesunate, tribendimidine, and praziquantel in patients with *Opisthorchis viverrini*: a randomised, exploratory, open-label, phase 2 trial. *Lancet Infect Dis*, **2011**, *11*:110–118.

Speich B, et al. Efficacy and reinfection with soil-transmitted helminths 18-weeks post-treatment with albendazole-ivermectin, albendazole-mebendazole, albendazole-oxantel pamoate and mebendazole. *Parasit Vectors*, **2016**, *9*:123.

Steinmann P, et al. Efficacy of single-dose and triple-dose albendazole and mebendazole against soil-transmitted helminths and *Taenia* spp.: a randomized controlled trial. *PLoS One*, **2011**, *6*:e25003.

Thomsen EK, et al. Efficacy, safety, and pharmacokinetics of coadministered diethylcarbamazine, albendazole, and ivermectin for treatment of bancroftian filariasis. *Clin Infect Dis*, **2016**, *62*:334–341.

Utzinger J, Keiser J. Schistosomiasis and soil-transmitted helminthiasis: common drugs for treatment and control. *Expert Opin Pharmacother*, **2004**, *5*:263–285.

Van den Enden E. Pharmacotherapy of helminth infection. *Expert Opin Pharmacother*, **2009**, *10*(3):435–451

Venkatesan P. Albendazole. *J Antimicrob Chemother*, **1998**, *41*:145–147.

Webster JP, et al. The contribution of mass drug administration to global health: past, present and future. *Philos Trans R Soc Lond B Biol Sci*, **2014**, *369*:20130434.

Williamson SM, et al. The Nicotinic Acetylcholine Receptors of the Parasitic Nematode Ascaris suum: Formation of Two Distinct Drug Targets by Varying the Relative Expression Levels of Two Subunits. PLOS Pathogens, 2009, 5:e1000517. https://doi.org/10.1371/journal.ppat.1000517. Accessed July 21, 2017.

World Health Organization. Weekly epidemiological record. **2016**. Available at: http://www.who.int/wer. Accessed April 8, 2016.

Xiao SH, et al. Effects of praziquantel on different developmental stages of *Schistosoma mansoni* in vitro and in vivo. *J Infect Dis*, **1985**, *151*:1130–1137.

Xiao SH, et al. Tribendimidine: a promising, safe and broad-spectrum anthelmintic agent from China. *Acta Trop*, **2005**, *94*:1–14.

Xiao SH, et al. Advances with the Chinese anthelminthic drug tribendimidine in clinical trials and laboratory investigations. *Acta Trop*, **2013**, *126*:115–126.

Yuan G, et al. Metabolism and disposition of tribendimidine and its metabolites in healthy Chinese volunteers. *Drugs R D*, **2010**, *10*:83–90.

Zeng Z, et al. Identification of cytochrome P4503A4 as the major enzyme responsible for the metabolism of ivermectin by human liver microsomes. *Xenobiotica*, **1998**, *28*:313–321.

Zufall F, et al. The insecticide avermectin b (la) activates a chloride channel in crayfish muscle membrane. *J Exp Biol*, **1989**, *142*:191–205.

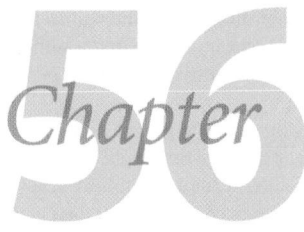

Chapter 56

Sulfonamides, Trimethoprim-Sulfamethoxazole, Quinolones, and Agents for Urinary Tract Infections

Conan MacDougall

Sulfonamides

HISTORY

The sulfonamide drugs were the first effective chemotherapeutic agents used systemically for the prevention and cure of bacterial infections in humans. Investigations in 1932 at the I. G. Farbenindustrie in Germany resulted in the patenting of prontosil and several other azo dyes containing a sulfonamide group. Because synthetic azo dyes had been studied for their action against streptococci, Domagk tested the new compounds and observed that mice with streptococcal and other infections could be protected by prontosil. In 1933, Foerster reported giving prontosil to a 10-month-old infant with staphylococcal septicemia and achieving a dramatic cure. Favorable clinical results with prontosil and its active metabolite, sulfanilamide, in puerperal sepsis and meningococcal infections awakened the medical profession to the new field of antibacterial chemotherapy, and experimental and clinical articles soon appeared in profusion. The development of the carbonic anhydrase inhibitor–type diuretics and the sulfonylurea hypoglycemic agents followed from observations made with the sulfonamide antibiotics. For discovering the chemotherapeutic value of prontosil, Domagk was awarded the Nobel Prize in Medicine for 1938 (Lesch, 2007). The advent of penicillin and other antibiotics diminished the usefulness of the sulfonamides, but the introduction of the combination of trimethoprim and sulfamethoxazole in the 1970s increased the use of sulfonamides for the prophylaxis and treatment of specific microbial infections.

Sulfonamides are derivatives of *para*-aminobenzenesulfonamide (sulfanilamide; Figure 56–1) and are congeners of PABA. Most of them are relatively insoluble in water, but their sodium salts are readily soluble. The minimal structural prerequisites for antibacterial action are all embodied in sulfanilamide itself. The sulfur must be linked directly to the benzene ring.

The *para*-NH_2 group (the N of which has been designated as N4) is essential and can be replaced only by moieties that can be converted in vivo to a free amino group. Substitutions made in the amide NH_2 group (position N1) have variable effects on antibacterial activity of the molecule; substitution of heterocyclic aromatic nuclei at N1 yields highly potent compounds.

Mechanism of Action

Sulfonamides are competitive inhibitors of *dihydropteroate synthase*, the bacterial enzyme responsible for the incorporation of PABA into *dihydropteroic acid*, the immediate precursor of *folic acid* (Figure 56–2). Sensitive microorganisms are those that must synthesize their own folic acid; bacteria that can use preformed folate are not affected. Sulfonamides administered as single agents are *bacteriostatic*; cellular and humoral defense mechanisms of the host are essential for final eradication of the infection. Toxicity is selective for bacteria because mammalian cells require preformed folic acid, cannot synthesize it, and are thus insensitive to drugs acting by this mechanism (Grayson, 2010).

Synergists of Sulfonamides

Trimethoprim exerts a synergistic effect with sulfonamides. It is a potent and selective competitive inhibitor of microbial *dihydrofolate reductase*, the enzyme that reduces *dihydrofolate* to *tetrahydrofolate*, which is required for one-carbon transfer reactions. Coadministration of a sulfonamide and trimethoprim (as in *trimethoprim-sulfamethoxazole*) introduces sequential blocks in the biosynthetic pathway for tetrahydrofolate (see Figure 56–2); the combination is much more effective than either agent alone (Bushby and Hitchings, 1968). Similar complementary activity is seen with pyrimethamine, which is generally used in combination with agents such as sulfadoxine, sulfadiazine, or dapsone. The predominant systemic use of sulfonamides is now in such combinations.

Antibacterial Spectrum

On their original introduction to therapeutic use, sulfonamides had a wide range of antimicrobial activity against both gram-positive and

Abbreviations

AIDS: acquired immunodeficiency syndrome
CSF: cerebrospinal fluid
FDA: Food and Drug Administration
GABA: γ-aminobutyric acid
GI: gastrointestinal
G6PD: glucose-6-phosphate dehydrogenase
HIV: human immunodeficiency virus
IV: intravenous
MIC: minimal inhibitory concentration
MRSA: methicillin-resistant *Staphylococcus aureus*
NADP: nicotinamide adenine dinucleotide phosphate
NADPH: reduced NADP
NSAID: nonsteroidal anti-inflammatory drug
PABA: para-aminobenzoic acid
PO: by mouth
TMP: trimethoprim
UTI: urinary tract infection

gram-negative bacteria; a high percentage of isolates of *Streptococcus pyogenes*, *Streptococcus pneumoniae*, *Staphylococcus aureus*, and *Haemophilus influenzae* were susceptible to systemically achievable concentrations of sulfonamides. However, the increase in sulfonamide resistance in these agents is such that sulfonamide activity against these pathogens in serious infections cannot be assumed, and they play little part in empiric therapy (Grayson, 2010). Potent activity remains against most isolates of *Haemophilus ducreyi*, *Nocardia*, and *Klebsiella granulomatis*. Isolates of *Neisseria meningitidis* and *Shigella* are generally resistant, as are many strains of *Escherichia coli* isolated from patients with UTIs (Olson et al., 2009). Sulfonamides also possess important activity against a number of parasites (see Chapters 53 and 54).

Bacterial Resistance

Bacterial resistance to sulfonamides can originate by random mutation and selection or by transfer of resistance by plasmids (see Chapter 52); it usually does not involve cross-resistance to other classes of antibiotics. Resistance to sulfonamide can result from (1) a lower affinity of dihydropteroate synthase for sulfonamides, (2) decreased bacterial permeability or active efflux of the drug, (3) an alternative metabolic pathway for synthesis of an essential metabolite, or (4) increased production of an essential metabolite or drug antagonist (e.g., PABA) (Gold and Moellering, 1996). Plasmid-mediated resistance is due to plasmid-encoded, drug-resistant dihydropteroate synthetase.

ADME

Except for sulfonamides especially designed for their local effects in the bowel (see Chapter 51), this class of drugs is absorbed rapidly from the GI tract. Approximately 70%–100% of an oral dose is absorbed, and sulfonamide can be found in the urine within 30 min of ingestion. Peak plasma levels are achieved in 2–6 h, depending on the drug. Peak plasma drug concentrations achievable in vivo are about 100–200 μg/mL. The small intestine is the major site of absorption, but some of the drug is absorbed from the stomach. Absorption from other sites, such as the vagina, respiratory tract, or abraded skin, is variable and unreliable, but a sufficient amount may enter the body to cause toxic reactions in susceptible persons or to produce sensitization.

All sulfonamides are bound in varying degree to plasma proteins, particularly to albumin. Sulfonamides are distributed throughout all tissues of the body. The sulfonamides readily enter pleural, peritoneal, synovial, ocular, and similar body fluids and may reach concentrations therein that are 50%–80% of the simultaneously determined concentration in blood. Because the protein content of body fluids usually is low, the drug is present in the unbound active form. After systemic administration of adequate doses, sulfadiazine and sulfisoxazole attain concentrations in CSF that may be effective in meningitis. However, because of the emergence of sulfonamide-resistant microorganisms, these drugs are used rarely for the treatment of meningitis. Sulfonamides pass readily through the placenta and reach the fetal circulation. The concentrations attained in the fetal tissues may cause both antibacterial and toxic effects.

Sulfonamides are metabolized in the liver. The major metabolite is the N4-acetylated sulfonamide. Acetylation results in products that have no antibacterial activity but retain the toxic potential of the parent substance. Sulfonamides are eliminated from the body partly as the unchanged drug and partly as metabolic products. The largest fraction is excreted in the urine, and the $t_{1/2}$ depends on renal function. In acid urine, the older sulfonamides are insoluble, and crystalline deposits may form. Small amounts are eliminated in the feces, bile, milk, and other secretions.

Pharmacological Properties of Individual Sulfonamides

Sulfonamides for Systemic Use

Sulfisoxazole. Sulfisoxazole is a rapidly absorbed and excreted sulfonamide. Its high solubility eliminates much of the renal toxicity inherent in the use of older sulfonamides. Sulfisoxazole is bound extensively to plasma proteins. Following an oral dose of 2–4 g, peak concentrations in plasma of 110–250 μg/mL are found in 2–4 h. Approximately 30% of sulfisoxazole in the blood and about 30% in the urine is in the acetylated form. The kidney excretes about 95% of a single dose in 24 h. Concentrations of the drug in urine thus greatly exceed those in blood and may be bactericidal. The concentration in CSF is about a third of that in the blood. Sulfisoxazole acetyl is tasteless and hence preferred for oral use in children. Sulfisoxazole acetyl in combination with erythromycin ethylsuccinate is used in children with otitis media.

The untoward effects produced by this agent are similar to those that follow the administration of other sulfonamides, as discussed further in the chapter. Because of its relatively high solubility in the urine as compared with sulfadiazine, sulfisoxazole only infrequently produces hematuria or crystalluria (0.2%–0.3%). Despite this, patients taking this drug should ingest an adequate quantity of water. Sulfisoxazole currently is preferred over other sulfonamides by most clinicians when a rapidly absorbed and rapidly excreted sulfonamide is indicated.

Sulfamethoxazole. Sulfamethoxazole is a close congener of sulfisoxazole, but its rates of enteric absorption and urinary excretion are slower ($t_{1/2}$ of 11 h). It is administered orally and employed for both systemic and UTIs. Precautions must be observed to avoid sulfamethoxazole crystalluria because of the high percentage of the acetylated, relatively insoluble,

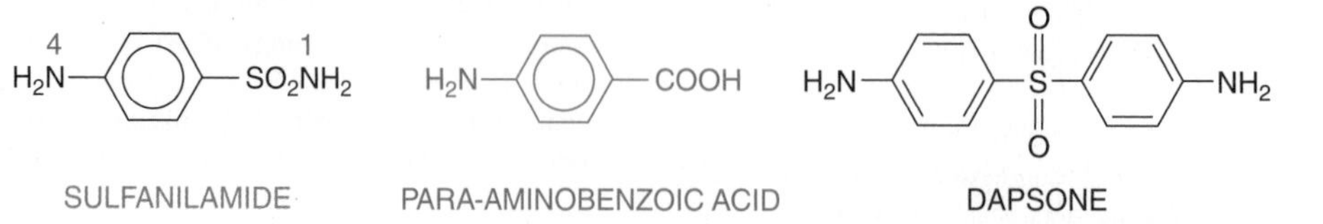

Figure 56–1 *Sulfanilamide and PABA.* Sulfonamides are derivatives of sulfanilamide and act by virtue of being congeners of *para*-aminobenzoate (PABA). The antimicrobial and dermatological anti-inflammatory agent dapsone (4,4′-diaminodiphenyl sulfone; see Chapters 60 and 70) also bears a resemblance to PABA and sulfanilamide.

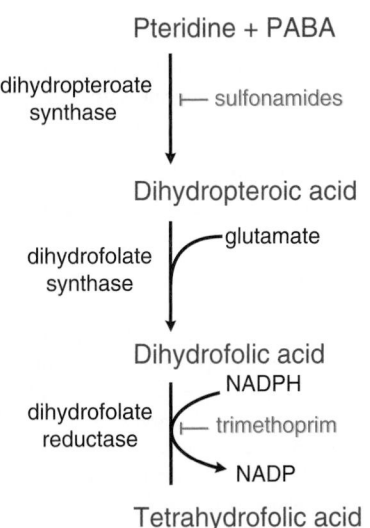

Pteridine + PABA

dihydropteroate
synthase ⊢ sulfonamides

Dihydropteroic acid

dihydrofolate ⎧ glutamate
synthase

Dihydrofolic acid

NADPH
dihydrofolate ⊢ trimethoprim
reductase
NADP

Tetrahydrofolic acid

Figure 56–2 *Steps in folate metabolism blocked by sulfonamides and trime-thoprim.* Coadministration of a sulfonamide and trimethoprim introduces sequential blocks in the biosynthetic pathway for tetrahydrofolate; the combination is much more effective than either agent alone.

form of the drug in the urine. The clinical uses of sulfamethoxazole are the same as those for sulfisoxazole. In the U.S., it is marketed only in fixed-dose combinations with trimethoprim.

Sulfadiazine. Sulfadiazine given orally is absorbed rapidly from the GI tract. Peak blood concentrations are reached within 3–6 h, with a $t_{1/2}$ of 10 h. About 55% of the drug is bound to plasma protein. Therapeutic concentrations are attained in CSF within 4 h of a single oral dose of 60 mg/kg. Both free and acetylated forms of sulfadiazine are readily excreted by the kidney; 15%–40% of the excreted drug is in acetylated form. Alkalinization of the urine accelerates the renal clearance of both forms by diminishing their tubular reabsorption. Precaution must be taken to ensure fluid intake adequate to produce a daily urine output of at least 1200 mL in adults and a corresponding quantity in children. If this cannot be accomplished, sodium bicarbonate may be given to reduce the risk of crystalluria.

Sulfadoxine. This agent has a particularly long plasma $t_{1/2}$ of 7–9 days. Although no longer marketed in the U.S., its combination with pyrimethamine (500 mg sulfadoxine plus 25 mg pyrimethamine) is listed as WHO essential medicine and is used for the prophylaxis and treatment of malaria caused by mefloquine-resistant strains of *Plasmodium falci-parum* (see Chapter 53). However, because of severe and sometimes fatal reactions, including the Stevens-Johnson syndrome, and the emergence of resistant strains, the drug has limited usefulness for the treatment of malaria.

Sulfonamides for Topical Use

Sulfacetamide. Sulfacetamide is the N1-acetyl-substituted derivative of sulfanilamide. Its aqueous solubility is about 90 times that of sulfadiazine. Solutions of the sodium salt of the drug are employed extensively in the management of ophthalmic infections. Very high aqueous concentrations are not irritating to the eye and are effective against susceptible microorganisms. The drug penetrates into ocular fluids and tissues in high concentration. Sensitivity reactions to sulfacetamide are rare, but the drug should not be used in patients with known hypersensitivity to sulfonamides. A 30% solution of the sodium salt has a pH of 7.4, whereas the solutions of sodium salts of other sulfonamides are highly alkaline. See Chapters 69 and 70 for ocular and dermatological uses.

Silver Sulfadiazine. Silver sulfadiazine is used topically to reduce microbial colonization and the incidence of infections from burns. Silver sulfadiazine should not be used to treat an established deep infection. Silver is released slowly from the preparation in concentrations that are selectively

toxic to the microorganisms. However, bacteria may develop resistance to silver sulfadiazine. Although little silver is absorbed, the plasma concentration of sulfadiazine may approach therapeutic levels if a large surface area is involved. Adverse reactions—burning, rash, and itching—are infrequent. Silver sulfadiazine is considered an agent of choice for the prevention of burn infections.

Mafenide. The sulfonamide mafenide is applied topically to prevent colonization of burns by a large variety of gram-negative and gram-positive bacteria. It should not be used in treatment of an established deep infection. Adverse effects include intense pain at sites of application and allergic reactions. Application of the drug over a large burn surface can lead to appreciable systemic absorption. The drug and its primary metabolite inhibit *carbonic anhydrase*, and the urine becomes alkaline. Metabolic acidosis with compensatory tachypnea and hyperventilation may ensue; these effects limit the usefulness of mafenide.

Therapeutic Uses

Urinary Tract Infections

Because a significant percentage of UTIs are caused by sulfonamide-resistant microorganisms, sulfonamides are no longer a therapy of first choice; trimethoprim-sulfamethoxazole is preferred (although resistance to this agent is increasing as well). *Sulfisoxazole* may be used effectively for cystitis in areas where the prevalence of resistance is not high. The usual dosage is 2–4 g initially, followed by 1–2 g orally four times a day for 5–10 days.

Nocardiosis

Trimethoprim-sulfamethoxazole is most commonly used for infections due to *Nocardia* spp., but sulfisoxazole or sulfadiazine are alternative agents, given in dosages of 6–8 g daily. For serious infections, addition of a second agent, such as imipenem, amikacin, or linezolid, is recommended.

Toxoplasmosis

The combination of pyrimethamine and sulfadiazine is the treatment of choice for toxoplasmosis (see Chapter 54). Pyrimethamine is given as a loading dose of 2000 mg followed by 50–75 mg orally per day, with sulfadiazine 1–1.5 g orally every 6 h, plus folinic acid (leucovorin) 10–25 mg orally each day for at least 6 weeks (Panel on Opportunistic Infections, 2016). Patients should receive at least 2 L of fluid intake daily to prevent crystalluria.

Adverse Reactions

Hypersensitivity Reactions

Among the skin and mucous membrane manifestations attributed to sensitization to sulfonamide are morbilliform, scarlatinal, urticarial, erysipeloid, pemphigoid, purpuric, and petechial rashes, as well as erythema nodosum, erythema multiforme of the Stevens-Johnson type, Behçet syndrome, exfoliative dermatitis, and photosensitivity. These hypersensitivity reactions occur most often after the first week of therapy but may appear earlier in previously sensitized individuals. Fever, malaise, and pruritus frequently are present simultaneously. The incidence of untoward dermal effects is about 2% with sulfisoxazole; patients with AIDS manifest a higher frequency of rashes with sulfonamide treatment than do other individuals. A syndrome similar to serum sickness may appear after several days of sulfonamide therapy. Drug fever is a common untoward manifestation of sulfonamide treatment; the incidence approximates 3% with sulfisoxazole.

Disturbances of the Urinary Tract

The risk of crystalluria is very low with the more soluble agents, such as sulfisoxazole. Crystalluria has occurred in dehydrated patients with HIV who were receiving sulfadiazine for *Toxoplasma* encephalitis. Crystalluria can be prevented by maintaining daily urine volume of at least 1200 mL (in adults) or alternatively urine alkalinization because the solubility of sulfisoxazole increases greatly with slight elevations of pH.

Disorders of the Hematopoietic System

Although rare, acute hemolytic anemia may occur. In some cases, it may be due to a sensitization phenomenon; in other instances, the hemolysis is related to an erythrocytic deficiency of G6PD activity. Agranulocytosis occurs in about 0.1% of patients who receive sulfadiazine; it also can follow the use of other sulfonamides. Although return of granulocytes to normal levels may be delayed for weeks or months after sulfonamide is withdrawn, most patients recover spontaneously with supportive care. Aplastic anemia involving complete suppression of bone marrow activity with profound anemia, granulocytopenia, and thrombocytopenia is an extremely rare occurrence with sulfonamide therapy. It probably results from a direct myelotoxic effect and may be fatal. Reversible suppression of the bone marrow is quite common in patients with limited bone marrow reserve (e.g., patients with AIDS or those receiving myelosuppressive chemotherapy).

Miscellaneous Reactions

Anorexia, nausea, and vomiting occur in 1%–2% of persons receiving sulfonamides. Focal or diffuse necrosis of the liver owing to direct drug toxicity or sensitization occurs in less than 0.1% of patients. Headache, nausea, vomiting, fever, hepatomegaly, jaundice, and laboratory evidence of hepatocellular dysfunction usually appear 3–5 days after sulfonamide administration is started, and the syndrome may progress to acute yellow atrophy and death. The administration of sulfonamides to newborn infants, especially if premature, may lead to the displacement of bilirubin from plasma albumin, potentially causing an encephalopathy called *kernicterus*. Sulfonamides should not be given to pregnant women near term because these drugs cross the placenta and are secreted in milk.

Drug Interactions

Drug interactions of the sulfonamides are seen mainly with the oral anticoagulants, the sulfonylurea hypoglycemic agents, and the hydantoin anticonvulsants. In each case, sulfonamides can potentiate the effects of the other drug by inhibiting its metabolism or by displacing it from albumin. Dosage adjustment may be necessary when a sulfonamide is given concurrently.

Trimethoprim-Sulfamethoxazole

Trimethoprim inhibits bacterial dihydrofolate reductase, an enzyme downstream from the one that sulfonamides inhibit in the same biosynthetic sequence (see Figure 56–2). The combination of trimethoprim with sulfamethoxazole was an important advance in the development of clinically effective and synergistic antimicrobial agents. In much of the world, the combination of trimethoprim with sulfamethoxazole is known as *cotrimoxazole*. In addition to its combination with sulfamethoxazole, trimethoprim is available as a single-entity preparation.

Mechanism of Action

The antimicrobial activity of the combination of trimethoprim and sulfamethoxazole results from actions on sequential steps of the enzymatic pathway for the synthesis of tetrahydrofolic acid (see Figure 56–2). Tetrahydrofolate is essential for one-carbon transfer reactions (e.g., the synthesis of thymidylate from deoxyuridylate). Selective toxicity for microorganisms is achieved in two ways. Mammalian cells use preformed folates from the diet and do not synthesize the compound. Furthermore, trimethoprim is a highly selective inhibitor of dihydrofolate reductase of lower organisms: About 100,000 times more drug is required to inhibit human reductase than the bacterial enzyme. The optimal ratio of the concentrations of the two agents equals the ratio of the MICs of the drugs acting independently. Although this ratio varies for different bacteria, the most effective ratio for the greatest number of microorganisms is 20:1, sulfamethoxazole:trimethoprim. The combination is thus formulated to achieve a sulfamethoxazole concentration in vivo that is 20 times greater than that of trimethoprim; sulfamethoxazole has pharmacokinetic properties such that the concentrations of the two drugs will thus be relatively constant in the body over a long period. Although each agent alone usually exerts bacteriostatic activity, when the organism is sensitive to both agents, bactericidal activity may be achieved.

Antibacterial Spectrum

The antibacterial spectrum of trimethoprim is similar to that of sulfamethoxazole, although trimethoprim is 20–100 times more potent. *Pseudomonas aeruginosa, Bacteroides fragilis,* and enterococci are clinically resistant. There is significant variation in the susceptibility of Enterobacteriaceae to trimethoprim in different geographic locations because of the spread of resistance mediated by plasmids and transposons (see Chapter 52).

Spectrum of Trimethoprim-Sulfamethoxazole in Combination

Although most *S. pneumoniae* are susceptible, there has been a disturbing increase in resistance (paralleling the rise in penicillin resistance), and its value for empiric therapy/use in respiratory tract infections is questionable. Most strains of *S. aureus* and *Staphylococcus epidermidis* remain susceptible, even among methicillin-resistant isolates, although geographic variation exists. *Streptococcus pyogenes* is usually sensitive when proper testing procedures (media with low thymidine content) are followed (Bowen et al., 2012). The *viridans* group of streptococci is typically susceptible, although susceptibility among penicillin-resistant strains is low (Diekema et al., 2001). Susceptibility in *E. coli* varies by geographic region, although it has been declining in general. *Proteus mirabilis, Klebsiella* spp., *Enterobacter* spp., *Salmonella, Shigella, Pseudomonas pseudomallei, Serratia,* and *Alcaligenes* spp. are typically susceptible. Also sensitive are *Brucella abortus, Pasteurella haemolytica, Yersinia pseudotuberculosis, Yersinia enterocolitica,* and *Nocardia asteroides.*

Bacterial Resistance

Bacterial resistance to trimethoprim-sulfamethoxazole is a rapidly increasing problem, although resistance is lower than it is to either of the agents alone. Resistance often is due to the acquisition of a plasmid that codes for an altered dihydrofolate reductase.

ADME

The pharmacokinetic profiles of sulfamethoxazole and trimethoprim are closely, but not perfectly, matched to achieve a constant ratio of 20:1 in their concentrations in blood and tissues. After a single oral dose of the combined preparation, trimethoprim is absorbed more rapidly than sulfamethoxazole. Peak blood concentrations of trimethoprim usually occur by 2 h in most patients, whereas peak concentrations of sulfamethoxazole occur by 4 h after a single oral dose. The half-lives of trimethoprim and sulfamethoxazole are 11 and 10 h, respectively.

When 800 mg sulfamethoxazole is given with 160 mg trimethoprim (one "double-strength" tablet; "single strength" ratio is 400 mg to 80 mg, maintaining the same ratio) twice daily, the peak concentrations of the drugs in plasma are about 40 and 2 μg/mL, the optimal ratio. Peak concentrations are similar (46 and 3.4 μg/mL) after intravenous infusion of 800 mg sulfamethoxazole and 160 mg trimethoprim over a period of 1 h.

Trimethoprim is distributed and concentrated rapidly in tissues; about 40% is bound to plasma protein in the presence of sulfamethoxazole. The volume of distribution of trimethoprim is almost nine times that of sulfamethoxazole. The drug readily enters CSF and sputum. High concentrations of each component of the mixture also are found in bile. About 65% of sulfamethoxazole is bound to plasma protein. About 60% of administered trimethoprim and from 25% to 50% of administered sulfamethoxazole are excreted in the urine in 24 h. Two-thirds of the sulfonamide is unconjugated. Metabolites of trimethoprim also are excreted. The rates of excretion and the concentrations of both compounds in the urine are reduced significantly in patients with uremia.

Therapeutic Uses

Urinary Tract Infections

Treatment of an uncomplicated lower UTI with trimethoprim-sulfamethoxazole is highly effective for sensitive bacteria, although some authorities avoid empiric use for UTIs when local resistance among *E. coli* exceeds 20% (Gupta et al., 2010). Single-dose therapy (320 mg trimethoprim plus 1600 mg sulfamethoxazole in adults) has been effective in some cases for the treatment of acute uncomplicated UTI, but longer courses of therapy are less likely to be associated with recurrence. Most treatment guidelines recommend 160/800 mg administered twice daily for 3 days for uncomplicated cystitis and for 10–14 days for complicated disease or pyelonephritis. Trimethoprim also is found in therapeutic concentrations in prostatic secretions, and trimethoprim-sulfamethoxazole is often effective for the treatment of bacterial prostatitis.

Bacterial Respiratory Tract Infections

Trimethoprim-sulfamethoxazole is effective for mild acute exacerbations of chronic bronchitis. Administration of 800–1200 mg sulfamethoxazole plus 160–240 mg trimethoprim twice a day appears to be effective in decreasing fever, purulence and volume of sputum, and sputum bacterial count. Trimethoprim-sulfamethoxazole should not be used to treat streptococcal pharyngitis because it does not eradicate the microorganism. It is effective for acute otitis media in children and acute maxillary sinusitis in adults that are caused by susceptible strains of *H. influenzae* and *S. pneumoniae*.

GI Infections

The combination is an alternative to a fluoroquinolone for treatment of shigellosis caused by susceptible strains, which are becoming less common worldwide. Trimethoprim and trimethoprim/sulfamethoxazole are no longer recommended for prevention or treatment of traveler's diarrhea because of increasing resistance worldwide among likely pathogens (Hill et al., 2006).

Infection by Pneumocystis jiroveci

High-dose therapy (trimethoprim 15–20 mg/kg/d plus sulfamethoxazole 75–100 mg/kg/d in three or four divided doses; typical maximum dose is 20 mg/kg/d of trimethoprim) is effective for *Pneumocystis jiroveci* pneumonia (Panel on Opportunistic Infections, 2016). Adjunctive corticosteroids should be given at the onset of anti-*Pneumocystis* therapy in patients with a Po_2 less than 70 mm Hg or an alveolar-arterial gradient less than 35 mm Hg. Prophylaxis with 800 mg sulfamethoxazole and 160 mg trimethoprim once daily or three times a week is effective in preventing pneumonia caused by this organism in patients with HIV as well as other immunocompromising conditions (such as neutropenia and solid-organ transplantation). Adverse reactions are less frequent with the lower prophylactic doses of trimethoprim-sulfamethoxazole.

Methicillin-Resistant Staphylococcus aureus Infections

The increasing incidence of community-acquired infections due to MRSA has provided a role for trimethoprim-sulfamethoxazole as an adjunctive therapy to incision and drainage of complicated abscesses. However, it is less effective than standard therapy in the treatment of invasive MRSA infections, including bacteremia (Paul et al., 2015).

Miscellaneous Infections

Nocardia infections have been treated successfully with the combination, but failures also have been reported. Although a combination of doxycycline and streptomycin or gentamicin now is considered the treatment of choice for brucellosis, trimethoprim-sulfamethoxazole may be an effective substitute for the doxycycline combination. Trimethoprim-sulfamethoxazole also has been used successfully for infection by *Stenotrophomonas maltophilia* and infection by the intestinal parasites *Cyclospora* and *Isospora*. Wegener granulomatosis may respond, depending on the stage of the disease.

Adverse Effects

Trimethoprim-sulfamethoxazole may extend the toxicity of the sulfonamides. The margin between toxicity for bacteria and that for humans may be relatively narrow when the patient is folate deficient. In such cases, trimethoprim-sulfamethoxazole may cause or precipitate megaloblastosis, leukopenia, or thrombocytopenia. Hematological reactions include various anemias, coagulation disorders, granulocytopenia, agranulocytosis,

purpura, Henoch-Schönlein purpura, and sulfhemoglobinemia. Trimethoprim-sulfamethoxazole reportedly causes up to three times as many dermatological reactions as does sulfisoxazole alone (5.9% vs. 1.7%). Mild and transient jaundice has been noted and appears to have the histological features of allergic cholestatic hepatitis. Permanent impairment of renal function may follow the use of trimethoprim-sulfamethoxazole in patients with renal disease due to sulfamethoxazole crystalluria; liberal fluid intake should be encouraged to dilute the urine during therapy. An increase in serum creatinine without decrement in glomerular filtration rate may be observed with high-dose therapy due to trimethoprim's inhibition of creatinine secretion. Hyperkalemia can also be observed, as trimethoprim has a similar structure to potassium-sparing diuretics such as triamterene. Patients with HIV frequently have hypersensitivity reactions to trimethoprim-sulfamethoxazole (rash, neutropenia, Stevens-Johnson syndrome, Sweet syndrome, and pulmonary infiltrates). Rapid and slow desensitization protocols have been established for patients intolerant to medically necessary therapy (Gluckstein and Ruskin, 1995).

The Quinolones

The first quinolone, nalidixic acid, was isolated as a by-product of the synthesis of chloroquine and made available for the treatment of UTIs. The introduction of fluorinated 4-quinolones (fluoroquinolones), such as norfloxacin, ciprofloxacin, and levofloxacin (Table 56–1), represents a particularly important therapeutic advance: These agents have broad antimicrobial activity and are effective after oral administration for the treatment of a wide variety of infectious diseases (Mitscher and Ma, 2003). However, due to potentially fatal side effects, many quinolones had to be withdrawn from the U.S. market: lomefloxacin and sparfloxacin (phototoxicity, QTc prolongation); gatifloxacin (systemic forms only; hypoglycemia); temafloxacin (immune hemolytic anemia); trovafloxacin (hepatotoxicity); grepafloxacin (cardiotoxicity); and clinafloxacin (phototoxicity). In all cases, the side effects were discovered during postmarketing surveillance (Sheehan and Chew, 2003).

Mechanism of Action

The quinolone antibiotics target bacterial *DNA gyrase* and *topoisomerase IV*. For many gram-positive bacteria, topoisomerase IV is the primary target (Alovero et al., 2000). In contrast, DNA gyrase is the primary quinolone target in many gram-negative microbes. The gyrase introduces negative supercoils into the DNA to combat excessive positive supercoiling that can occur during DNA replication (Figure 56–3) (Cozzarelli, 1980). The quinolones inhibit gyrase-mediated DNA supercoiling at concentrations that correlate well with those required to inhibit bacterial growth (0.1–10 μg/mL). Mutations of the gene that encodes the A subunit of the gyrase can confer resistance to these drugs. Topoisomerase IV, which separates interlinked (catenated) daughter DNA molecules that are the product of DNA replication, also is a target for quinolones.

Eukaryotic cells do not contain DNA gyrase. They do contain a conceptually and mechanistically similar type II DNA topoisomerase, but quinolones inhibit it only at concentrations (100–1000 μg/mL) much higher than those needed to inhibit the bacterial enzymes.

Antibacterial Spectrum

The fluoroquinolones are potent bactericidal agents against *Proteus, E. coli, Klebsiella*, and various species of *Salmonella, Shigella, Enterobacter*, and *Campylobacter*. While once a standard therapy for *N. gonorrhoeae* infections, resistance has increased to the point these agents are no longer recommended in many countries for empiric therapy of gonorrhea (Centers for Disease Control and Prevention, 2015). Some fluoroquinolones are active against *Pseudomonas* spp., with ciprofloxacin and levofloxacin having substantial enough activity for use in systemic infections. Fluoroquinolones have good in vitro activity against staphylococci, but they are less active against methicillin-resistant strains, and there is concern over development of resistance during therapy. Activity against streptococci is significantly greater with the newer agents, including levofloxacin,

TABLE 56–1 ■ STRUCTURAL FORMULAS OF SELECTED QUINOLONES AND FLUOROQUINOLONES

CONGENER	R_1	R_6	R_7	X
Nalidixic acid	$-C_2H_5$	$-H$	$-CH_3$	$-N-$
Norfloxacin	$-C_2H_5$	$-F$	$-N\bigcirc NH$	$-CH-$
Ciprofloxacin	▷	$-F$	$-N\bigcirc NH$	$-CH-$
Levofloxacin	$O-CH-CH_3$ (X, N-1)	$-F$	$-N\bigcirc NH-CH_3$	$O-C_8 ... N_1, CH_3$

gemifloxacin, and moxifloxacin. Several intracellular bacteria are inhibited by fluoroquinolones at concentrations that can be achieved in plasma; these include species of *Chlamydia, Mycoplasma, Legionella, Brucella,* and *Mycobacterium* (including *Mycobacterium tuberculosis*). Ciprofloxacin, ofloxacin, and moxifloxacin have MIC_{90} values from 0.5 to 3 µg/mL for *Mycobacterium fortuitum, Mycobacterium kansasii,* and *M. tuberculosis.* Moxifloxacin also has useful activity against anaerobes.

Bacterial Resistance

Resistance to quinolones may develop during therapy via mutations in the bacterial chromosomal genes encoding DNA gyrase or topoisomerase IV or by active transport of the drug out of the bacteria (Oethinger et al., 2000). Less commonly, plasmid-mediated resistance develops through proteins that bind to and protect the topoisomerases from quinolone effects. Resistance has increased after the introduction of fluoroquinolones, especially in *Pseudomonas* and staphylococci. *Escherichia coli, Campylobacter jejuni, Salmonella, N. gonorrhoeae,* and *S. pneumoniae* are also increasingly fluoroquinolone resistant (Olson et al., 2009).

ADME

Most quinolones are well absorbed after oral administration. Peak serum levels of the fluoroquinolones are obtained within 1–3 h of an oral dose. The volume of distribution of quinolones is high, with concentrations in urine, kidney, lung, and prostate tissue and stool, bile, and macrophages and neutrophils higher than serum levels. Food may delay the time to peak serum concentrations. Ciprofloxacin, ofloxacin, and levofloxacin have been detected in human breast milk; because of their excellent bioavailability, the potential exists for substantial exposure of nursing infants. Except for moxifloxacin, quinolones are cleared predominantly

by the kidney, and dosages must be adjusted for renal failure. Moxifloxacin should not be used in patients with hepatic failure.

Pharmacological Properties of Individual Quinolones

Norfloxacin

Norfloxacin's gram-negative activity is similar to, but somewhat less potent than, that of ciprofloxacin. However, relatively low serum levels are reached with norfloxacin and limit its usefulness in the treatment of UTIs and gastrointestinal infections. The serum $t_{1/2}$ is 3–5 h for norfloxacin; approximately 25% of the drug is eliminated unchanged in the urine, with hepatic metabolism also occurring.

Ciprofloxacin

Ciprofloxacin's bioavailability is approximately 70%. Typical oral doses are 250–750 mg and intravenous doses are 200–400 mg twice daily (maximum dose 1.5 g/d). The elimination $t_{1/2}$ is about 5 h, and the drug is typically dosed twice daily, with the exception of an extended-release formulation, which can be dosed once daily.

Ofloxacin/Levofloxacin

Ofloxacin has somewhat more potent gram-positive activity; separation of the more active S- or levorotatory isomer yields levofloxacin, which has even better antistreptococcal activity. Bioavailability of both of these agents is excellent, such that intravenous and oral doses are the same; levofloxacin is dosed once daily (250–750 mg) as opposed to twice-daily dosing for ofloxacin (200–400 mg daily divided every 12 h).

Moxifloxacin

Moxifloxacin improves further on the gram-positive potency of levofloxacin, typically having MICs one to two dilutions lower against

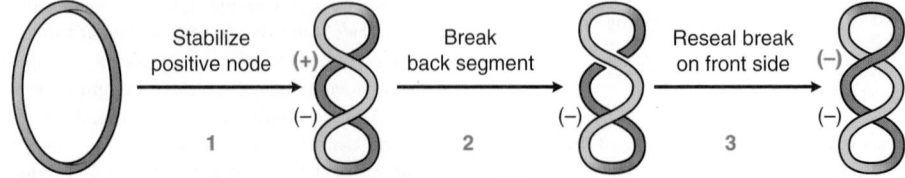

Figure 56–3 *Model of the formation of negative DNA supercoils by DNA gyrase.* DNA gyrase binds to two segments of DNA (1), creating a node of positive (+) superhelix. The enzyme then introduces a double-strand break in the DNA and passes the front segment through the break (2). The break is then resealed (3), creating a negative (–) supercoil. Quinolones inhibit the nicking and closing activity of the gyrase and, at higher concentrations, block the decatenating activity of topoisomerase IV. (Reprinted with permission from AAAS. Cozzarelli NR. DNA gyrase and the supercoiling of DNA. *Science*, **1980**, *207*:953–960.)

S. pneumoniae. It also has expanded activity against anaerobic pathogens but is substantially less active than ciprofloxacin or levofloxacin against *P. aeruginosa.* Moxifloxacin is well absorbed, with equivalent intravenous and oral doses; the $t_{1/2}$ is about 12 h, allowing for daily dosing (usual dose 400 mg daily). Moxifloxacin undergoes hepatic sulfation and glucuronidation. Less than a quarter of systemic moxifloxacin is excreted unchanged via the kidneys, and because high concentrations are not achieved in the urine, it is not recommended for UTIs.

Gatifloxacin and Gemifloxacin

The agents gatifloxacin and gemifloxacin have a similar spectrum of activity to moxifloxacin, with enhanced potency against gram-positive organisms and poor activity versus *Pseudomonas.* They are less active than moxifloxacin against *B. fragilis.* Both have high bioavailability and renal elimination. Gatifloxacin is no longer available for systemic use in the U.S. due to toxicity concerns, but an ophthalmic preparation is licensed for the treatment of bacterial conjunctivitis.

Therapeutic Uses

Urinary Tract Infections

Nalidixic acid is useful only for UTIs caused by susceptible microorganisms. The fluoroquinolones are significantly more potent and are a mainstay of treatment of upper and lower UTIs (Fihn, 2003). They are more efficacious than trimethoprim-sulfamethoxazole or oral β-lactams for the treatment of UTIs. Because of their broad spectrum of activity, however, recent guidelines suggest reserving their use for complicated cystitis or pyelonephritis when possible. Moxifloxacin does not accumulate in the urine and is not approved for treatment of UTIs. Typical treatment durations for the other quinolones are 3 days for uncomplicated cystitis and 5–7 days for uncomplicated pyelonephritis.

Prostatitis

Norfloxacin, ciprofloxacin, ofloxacin, and levofloxacin are effective in the treatment of prostatitis caused by sensitive bacteria. Fluoroquinolones administered for 4–6 weeks appear to be effective in patients not responding to trimethoprim-sulfamethoxazole.

Sexually Transmitted Diseases

Fluoroquinolones lack activity for *Treponema pallidum* but have activity in vitro against *Chlamydia trachomatis* and *Haemophilus ducreyi.* For chlamydial urethritis/cervicitis, a 7-day course of ofloxacin or levofloxacin is an alternative to a 7-day treatment with doxycycline or a single dose of azithromycin; other available quinolones have not been reliably effective. Previously, a single oral dose of a fluoroquinolone such as ciprofloxacin had been effective treatment of sensitive strains of *N. gonorrhoeae,* but increasing resistance to fluoroquinolones has led to ceftriaxone being the first-line agent for this infection. Chancroid (infection by *H. ducreyi*) can be treated with 3 days of ciprofloxacin.

GI and Abdominal Infections

Norfloxacin, ciprofloxacin, ofloxacin, and levofloxacin given for 1–3 days all have been effective in the treatment of patients with traveler's diarrhea, reducing the duration of loose stools by 1–3 days. Ciprofloxacin in a single daily dose is also effective for prophylaxis of traveler's diarrhea. Ciprofloxacin and ofloxacin can cure most patients with enteric fever caused by *Salmonella typhi,* as well as bacteremic nontyphoidal infections in patients with HIV, and clears chronic fecal carriage. Ciprofloxacin, ofloxacin, and levofloxacin, when combined with metronidazole, may be useful in the management of intra-abdominal infections when *Enterococcus* is not a likely pathogen. Moxifloxacin as a single agent was shown to have similar efficacy to piperacillin/tazobactam for complicated intra-abdominal infection, although there are concerns over increasing resistance in *B. fragilis.*

Respiratory Tract Infections

Many newer fluoroquinolones, including levofloxacin, moxifloxacin, and gemifloxacin, have excellent activity against *S. pneumoniae, H. influenzae,* and the atypical respiratory pathogens. Thus, these agents are frequently used in the management of community-acquired pneumonia and for upper respiratory tract infections such as sinusitis that are not responsive to more narrow-spectrum agents. Mild-to-moderate respiratory exacerbations owing to *P. aeruginosa* in patients with cystic fibrosis have responded to oral fluoroquinolone therapy with ciprofloxacin or levofloxacin.

Bone, Joint, and Soft Tissue Infections

The treatment of chronic osteomyelitis may require prolonged (weeks to months) antimicrobial therapy with agents active against *S. aureus* or gram-negative rods. Failures are associated with the development of resistance, particularly in *S. aureus.* Combination therapy with a fluoroquinolone and rifampin has been effective at reducing the development of resistance and providing good cure rates, especially in the management of early prosthetic joint infections. In diabetic foot infections, the fluoroquinolones in combination with an agent with antianaerobic activity are a reasonable choice.

Other Infections

Ciprofloxacin and levofloxacin are used for the prophylaxis of anthrax and are effective for the treatment of tularemia (Hendricks et al., 2014). The quinolones, especially moxifloxacin, may be used as part of multiple-drug regimens for the treatment of multidrug-resistant tuberculosis and atypical mycobacterial infections as well as *Mycobacterium avium* complex infections in AIDS (see Chapter 60) (American Thoracic Society, 2003). Quinolones, when used as prophylaxis in neutropenic patients, have decreased the incidence of gram-negative rod bacteremias (Hughes et al., 2002). Levofloxacin and ciprofloxacin are approved to treat and prevent anthrax as well as plague due to *Yersinia pestis.*

Adverse Effects

Gastrointestinal Adverse Effects

Common adverse reactions involve the GI tract, with 3%–17% of patients reporting mild nausea, vomiting, and abdominal discomfort. Fluoroquinolones have emerged as a common cause of *Clostridium difficile* colitis due to the spread of quinolone-resistant strains.

Neurologic Adverse Effects

Side effects (1%–11%) of the CNS include mild headache and dizziness. Rarely, hallucinations, delirium, and seizures have occurred, predominantly in patients who were also receiving theophylline or NSAIDs. Patients with a history of epilepsy are at higher risk for fluoroquinolone-induced convulsions. Recently, the fluoroquinolones have been recognized as a rare cause of peripheral neuropathy, which in some cases has been irreversible.

Musculoskeletal Adverse Effects

Arthralgias and joint pain are occasionally reported with fluoroquinolones. Tendon rupture or tendinitis (usually of the Achilles tendon) is a recognized adverse effect, especially in those more than 60 years old, in patients taking corticosteroids, and in solid-organ transplant recipients. Early animal studies suggested an increased risk of cartilage damage and malformation among young animals (Burkhardt et al., 1997). Subsequent human studies have not noted a substantially increased risk of these effects in children or among the offspring of pregnant women who received fluoroquinolones. Nevertheless, the agents are typically avoided in pregnancy and among young children (Sabharwal and Marchant, 2006).

Other Adverse Effects

Among the quinolones available in the U.S., moxifloxacin carries the highest risk for QT interval prolongation and torsades de pointes arrhythmias; gemifloxacin, levofloxacin, and ofloxacin appear to have lower risk; and ciprofloxacin has the lowest risk. However, the overall risk of torsades de pointes is small with the use of fluoroquinolones. Gatifloxacin's propensity to cause both hypo- and hyperglycemia, especially in older adults, led to its removal for systemic use in the U.S. (Park-Wyllie et al., 2006). Other agents such as levofloxacin may rarely be associated with dysglycemias among at-risk patients. Rashes, including photosensitivity reactions, also can occur; patients with frequent sun exposure should be advised to protect themselves with clothing or sunscreen.

Drug Interactions

All quinolones form complexes with divalent and trivalent cations (e.g., calcium, iron, aluminum). When coadministered orally with quinolones, these cations can chelate the quinolone and reduce systemic bioavailability. Thus, a separation of at least 2 h between oral administration of quinolones and these cations is recommended. Ciprofloxacin inhibits the metabolism of theophylline, and toxicity from elevated concentrations of the methylxanthine may occur (Schwartz et al., 1988). NSAIDs may augment displacement of GABA from its receptors by the quinolones, enhancing neurologic adverse effects (Halliwell et al., 1993). Due to risk for QT prolongation, quinolones should be used with caution in patients on class III (amiodarone) and class IA (quinidine, procainamide) antiarrhythmics (see Chapter 30).

Antiseptic Agents for Urinary Tract Infections

Urinary tract antiseptics are concentrated in the renal tubules, where they inhibit the growth of many species of bacteria. These agents cannot be used to treat systemic infections because effective concentrations are not achieved in plasma with safe doses; however, they can be administered orally to treat UTIs.

Methenamine

Methenamine (hexamethylenamine) is a urinary tract antiseptic and prodrug that acts by generating formaldehyde via the following reaction:

$$N_4(CH_2)_6 + 6H_2O + 4H^+ \rightarrow 6HCHO + 4NH_4^+$$

At pH 7.4, almost no decomposition occurs; the yield of formaldehyde is 6% of the theoretical amount at pH 6 and 20% at pH 5. Thus, acidification of the urine promotes formaldehyde formation and formaldehyde-dependent antibacterial action. The decomposition reaction is fairly slow, and 3 h are required to reach 90% completion.

Antimicrobial Activity

Nearly all bacteria are sensitive to free formaldehyde at concentrations of about 20 μg/mL. Microorganisms do not develop resistance to formaldehyde. Urea-splitting microorganisms (e.g., *Proteus* spp.) tend to raise the pH of the urine and thus inhibit the release of formaldehyde.

Pharmacology, Toxicology, and Therapeutic Uses

Methenamine is absorbed orally, but 10%–30% decomposes in the gastric juice unless the drug is protected by an enteric coating. Because of the ammonia produced, methenamine is contraindicated in hepatic insufficiency. Excretion in the urine is nearly quantitative. When the urine pH is 6 and the daily urine volume is 1000–1500 mL, a daily dose of 2 g will yield a urine concentration of 18–60 μg/mL of formaldehyde; this is more than the MIC for most urinary tract pathogens. Low pH alone is bacteriostatic, so acidification serves a double function. The acids commonly used are mandelic acid and hippuric acid. GI distress frequently is caused by doses more than 500 mg four times a day, even with enteric-coated tablets. Painful and frequent micturition, albuminuria, hematuria, and rashes may result from doses of 4 to 8 g/d given for longer than 3–4 weeks. Renal insufficiency is not a contraindication to the use of methenamine alone, but the acids given concurrently may be detrimental; methenamine mandelate is contraindicated in renal insufficiency. Methenamine combines with sulfamethizole and perhaps other sulfonamides in the urine, which results in mutual antagonism; therefore, these drugs should not be used in combination.

Methenamine is not a primary drug for the treatment of acute UTIs but is of value for chronic suppressive treatment of UTIs. The agent is most useful when the causative organism is *E. coli*, but it usually can suppress the common gram-negative offenders and often *S. aureus* and *S. epidermidis* as well. *Enterobacter aerogenes* and *Proteus vulgaris* are usually resistant. A urinary pH less than 5 is typically necessary for methenamine to be active; some clinicians recommend monitoring of the urinary pH and even urinary acidification with ammonium chloride or ascorbic acid.

Nitrofurantoin

Nitrofurantoin is a synthetic nitrofuran that is used for the prevention and treatment of UTIs.

Antimicrobial Activity

Nitrofurantoin is activated by enzymatic reduction, with the formation of highly reactive intermediates that seem to be responsible for the observed capacity of the drug to damage DNA. Bacteria reduce nitrofurantoin more rapidly than do mammalian cells, and this is thought to account for the selective antimicrobial activity of the compound. Nitrofurantoin is active against many strains of *E. coli* and enterococci. However, most species of *Proteus* and *Pseudomonas* and many species of *Enterobacter* and *Klebsiella* are resistant. Nitrofurantoin is bacteriostatic for most susceptible microorganisms at concentrations of 32 μg/mL or less and is bactericidal at concentrations of 100 μg/mL or more. The antibacterial activity is higher in acidic urine.

Pharmacology, Toxicity, and Therapeutic Uses

Nitrofurantoin is absorbed rapidly and completely from the GI tract. Antibacterial concentrations are not achieved in plasma following ingestion of recommended doses because the drug is eliminated rapidly. The plasma $t_{1/2}$ is 0.3–1 h; about 40% is excreted unchanged into the urine. The average dose of nitrofurantoin yields a concentration in urine of about 200 μg/mL. This concentration is soluble at pH greater than 5, but the urine should not be alkalinized because this reduces antimicrobial activity. The rate of excretion is linearly related to the creatinine clearance, so in patients with impaired glomerular function, the efficacy of the drug may be decreased and the systemic toxicity increased. Nitrofurantoin colors the urine brown.

The oral dosage of nitrofurantoin for adults is 50–100 mg four times a day with meals and at bedtime, less for the macrocrystalline formulation (100 mg every 12 h for 7 days). A single 50- to 100-mg dose at bedtime may be sufficient to prevent recurrences. The daily dose for children is 5–7 mg/kg but may be as low as 1 mg/kg for long-term therapy. A course of therapy should not exceed 14 days; repeated courses should be separated by rest periods. Pregnant women, individuals with impaired renal function (creatinine clearance less than 60 mL/min), and children younger than 1 month should not receive nitrofurantoin.

Nitrofurantoin is approved for the treatment of lower UTIs. It is not recommended for treatment of pyelonephritis or prostatitis.

The most common untoward effects are nausea, vomiting, and diarrhea; the macrocrystalline preparation is better tolerated than traditional formulations. Various hypersensitivity reactions occur occasionally, including chills, fever, leukopenia, granulocytopenia, hemolytic anemia (associated with G6PD deficiency and in newborns exhibiting low levels of reduced glutathione in their red blood cells), cholestatic jaundice, and hepatocellular damage. Acute pneumonitis with fever, chills, cough, dyspnea, chest pain, pulmonary infiltration, and eosinophilia may occur within hours to days of the initiation of therapy; these symptoms usually resolve quickly after discontinuation of the drug. Interstitial pulmonary fibrosis can occur in patients (especially the elderly) taking the drug chronically. Headache, vertigo, drowsiness, muscular aches, and nystagmus occur occasionally but are readily reversible. Severe polyneuropathies with demyelination and degeneration of both sensory and motor nerves have been reported; neuropathies are most likely to occur in patients with impaired renal function and in persons on long-continued treatment.

Fosfomycin

Fosfomycin is a phosphonic acid derivative that is used primarily for the prevention and treatment of UTIs.

Antimicrobial Activity

Fosfomycin inhibits MurA, an enolpyruvyl transferase that catalyzes the initial step in bacterial cell wall synthesis. This mechanism is unique among antibacterials; thus, cross-resistance to other agents is rarely seen. Optimal testing of fosfomycin activity requires supplementation of the media with glucose-6-phosphate. Fosfomycin's usual spectrum of activity includes the uropathogens *E. coli*, *Proteus*, *Enterococcus*, and *Staphylococcus saphrophyticus*. Activity against *Klebsiella*, *Enterobacter*, and *Serratia* spp. is variable, and *Pseudomonas* and *Acinetobacter* are typically resistant. *Staphylococcus aureus* is frequently susceptible, although emergence of resistance during therapy has been reported.

Pharmacology, Toxicity, and Therapeutic Uses

Outside the U.S., fosfomycin is available as an intravenous formulation that can achieve adequate levels to treat some systemic infections. However, in the U.S. it is only available as a powder (fosfomycin tromethamine) that is dissolved in water and taken orally. Bioavailability of the oral formulation is approximately 40%, with a $t_{1/2}$ of 5–8 h. With oral administration of 3 g, systemic concentrations are low, but urinary concentrations are as high as 1000–4000 µg/mL. The FDA-approved dosing regimen is a single 3-g dose for uncomplicated UTI; some investigators have administered 3 g every other day for three doses for complicated UTI or 3 g every 10 days for UTI prophylaxis.

Overall, fosfomycin is well tolerated. Adverse effects are uncommon and usually consist of GI distress, vaginitis, headache, or dizziness.

Acknowledgment: *William A. Petri, Jr contributed to this chapter in the previous editions of this book. We have retained some of his text in the current edition.*

Drug Facts for Your Personal Formulary: *Sulfonamides, Trimethoprim-Sulfamethoxazole, Quinolones, and Agents for Urinary Tract Infections*

Drug	Therapeutic Uses	Clinical Pharmacology and Tips
Sulfonamides: Competitive inhibitors of bacterial dihydropteroate synthase, thereby disrupting folate synthesis		
General: Bacteriostatic; limited efficacy as monotherapy, renal elimination, hypersensitivity reactions		
Sulfisoxazole (PO)	• Lower UTIs • Otitis media (with erythromycin)	• Some activity vs. *Streptococcus pyogenes*, *S. pneumoniae*, *Staphylococcus aureus*, *Haemophilus influenzae*, *Escherichia coli*, *Nocardia* • Rapid renal excretion
Sulfadiazine (PO)	• Toxoplasmosis (with pyrimethamine)	• Similar to sulfisoxazole, with good activity against *Toxoplasma gondii* • Reasonable CSF penetration • Higher risk of crystalluria, requires hydration
Sulfadoxine (PO)	• Prophylaxis and treatment of malaria (with pyrimethamine)	• Similar to sulfisoxazole, with some activity vs. *Plasmodium falciparum* • Long $t_{1/2}$
Sulfacetamide (ophthalmic)	• Treatment of ocular infections	• Activity similar to sulfisoxazole • High penetration into ocular fluids
Silver sulfadiazine (topical) Mafenide (topical)	• Prevention of infection in burn patients	• Activity similar to sulfisoxazole • Burning and itching at application site • Application over large surface may lead to systemic absorption and adverse effects
Sulfonamide and Dihydrofolate Reductase Inhibitor Combination: Sequential inhibition of folate synthesis		
Trimethoprim-sulfamethoxazole (IV, PO)	• UTI • Upper respiratory tract infections • Shigellosis • *Pneumocystis jiroveci* pneumonia • Skin/soft tissue infections due to *S. aureus* • Infections due to *Nocardia*, *Stenotrophomonas maltophila*, *Cyclospora*, *Isospora*	• Excellent activity vs. *S. aureus*, *Staphylococcus epidermidis*, *Streptococcus pyogenes* • Good activity vs. *Proteus*, *E. coli*, *Klebsiella*, *Enterobacter*, *Serratia*, *Nocardia*, *Brucella* • Some activity vs. *S. pneumoniae* • Formulated in 5:1 (sulfa:TMP) ratio, giving 20:1 serum levels • Well absorbed on oral administration • Good penetration into CSF • Metabolized and renally eliminated • Hypersensitivity reactions (i.e., rash) common • Dose-related bone marrow suppression, hyperkalemia
Quinolones: Bactericidal inhibitors of bacterial gyrase and topoisomerase, prevent DNA unwinding		
General: Drug interactions with cations, neurologic adverse effects, tendonitis/tendon rupture, photosensitivity; typically avoided in children and pregnant women		
Norfloxacin (PO)	• UTI, prostatitis • Traveler's diarrhea	• Good activity vs. *E. coli*, *Klebsiella*, *Proteus*, *Serratia*, *Salmonella*, *Shigella* • Some activity vs. *Pseudomonas* • Effective concentrations only achieved in GI and urinary tracts
Ciprofloxacin (IV, PO)	• UTI, prostatitis • Traveler's diarrhea • Intra-abdominal infections (with metronidazole) • *Pseudomonas* infections • Anthrax, tularemia	• Excellent activity vs. *E. coli*, *Klebsiella*, *Proteus*, *Serratia*, *Salmonella*, *Shigella* • Good activity vs. *Pseudomonas* • Some activity vs. *S. aureus*, streptococci • Good bioavailability and tissue distribution • Renal and nonrenal elimination
Levofloxacin (IV, PO)	• Respiratory tract infections • UTI, prostatitis • *Chlamydia* • Traveler's diarrhea • Intra-abdominal infections (with metronidazole) • *Pseudomonas* infections	• Excellent activity vs. *E. coli*, *Klebsiella*, *Proteus*, *Serratia*, *Salmonella*, *Shigella*, streptococci, *H. influenzae*, *Legionella*, *Chlamydia* • Good activity vs. *Pseudomonas*, *S. aureus* • Good bioavailability and tissue distribution • Renal elimination • S-isomer of ofloxacin

Drug Facts for Your Personal Formulary: *Sulfonamides, Trimethoprim-Sulfamethoxazole, Quinolones, and Agents for Urinary Tract Infections (continued)*

Drug	Therapeutic Uses	Clinical Pharmacology and Tips
Quinolones: Bactericidal inhibitors of bacterial gyrase and topoisomerase, prevent DNA unwinding		
General: Drug interactions with cations, neurologic adverse effects, tendonitis/tendon rupture, photosensitivity; typically avoided in children and pregnant women		
Moxifloxacin (IV, PO)	• Respiratory tract infections • Intra-abdominal infections • Mycobacterial infections	• Excellent activity vs. *E. coli, Klebsiella, Proteus, Serratia,* streptococci, *H. influenzae, Legionella, Chlamydia* • Good activity vs. *S. aureus, Bacteroides fragilis* • Good bioavailability and tissue distribution • Renal and nonrenal elimination; not for UTI • QT prolongation
Urinary Agents: Diverse mechanisms, effective concentrations reached only in urine		
Methenamine (PO)	• Chronic suppression of cystitis	• Forms formaldehyde in urine • Requires acidic urine for activity • Excellent activity against most uropathogens except for *Proteus* and *Enterobacter* • GI distress at high doses
Nitrofurantoin (PO)	• Cystitis treatment • Cystitis prophylaxis	• DNA damage through reactive intermediates • Excellent activity vs. *E. coli, Enterococcus* • Some activity vs. *Klebsiella, Enterobacter* • Rapid absorption and elimination • Colors urine brown • Acute pneumonitis and chronic interstitial pulmonary fibrosis
Fosfomycin (PO)	• Cystitis treatment	• Inhibits early cell wall synthesis • Excellent activity vs. *E. coli, Proteus, Enterococcus* • Some activity vs. *Klebsiella, Enterobacter* • Single-dose treatment of acute uncomplicated cystitis

Bibliography

Alovero FL, et al. Engineering the specificity of antibacterial fluoroquinolones: benzenesulfonamide modifications at C-7 of ciprofloxacin change its primary target in *Streptococcus pneumoniae* from topoisomerase IV to gyrase. *Antimicrob Agents Chemother,* **2000,** 44:320–325.

American Thoracic Society, CDC, and Infectious Diseases Society of America. Practice guidelines for the treatment of tuberculosis. *MMWR Morb Mortal Wkly Rep,* **2003,** 52(no. RR-11).

Bowen AC, et al. Is *Streptococcus pyogenes* resistant or susceptible to trimethoprim-sulfamethoxazole? *J Clin Microbiol,* **2012,** 50: 4067–4072.

Burkhardt JE, et al. Quinolone arthropathy in animals versus children. *Clin Infect Dis,* **1997,** 25:1196–1204.

Bushby SR, Hitchings GH. Trimethoprim, a sulphonamide potentiator. *Br J Pharmacol,* **1968,** 33:72–90.

Centers for Disease Control and Prevention. Sexually transmitted diseases guidelines. **2015.** Available at: http://www.cdc.gov/std/treatment/. Accessed July 3, 2015.

Cozzarelli NR. DNA gyrase and the supercoiling of DNA. *Science,* **1980,** 207:953–960.

Diekema DJ, et al. Antimicrobial resistance in viridans group streptococci among patients with and without the diagnosis of cancer in the USA, Canada and Latin America. *Clin Microbiol Infect,* **2001,** 7:152–157.

Fihn SD. Acute uncomplicated urinary tract infection in women. *N Engl J Med,* **2003,** 349:259–266.

Gluckstein D, Ruskin J. Rapid oral desensitization to trimethoprimsulfamethoxazole (TMP-SMZ): use in prophylaxis for *Pneumocystis carinii* pneumonia in patients with AIDS who were previously tolerant to TMP-SMZ. *Clin Infect Dis,* **1995,** 20:849–853.

Gold HS, Moellering RC Jr. Antimicrobial-drug resistance. *N Engl J Med,* **1996,** 335:1445–1453.

Grayson ML, ed. *Kucers' The Use of Antibiotics: A Clinical Review of Antibacterial, Antifungal, Antiparasitic, and Antiviral Drugs.* Hodder Arnold, London, **2010.**

Gupta K, et al. International clinical practice guidelines for the treatment of acute uncomplicated cystitis and pyelonephritis in women: a 2010 update by the Infectious Diseases Society of America and the European Society for Microbiology and Infectious Diseases. *Clin Infect Dis,* **2010,** 52:e103–e120.

Halliwell RF, et al. Antagonism of GABA$_A$ receptors by 4-quinolones. *J Antimicrob Chemother,* **1993,** 31:457–462.

Hendricks KA, et al. Centers for Disease Control and Prevention expert panel meetings on prevention and treatment of anthrax in adults. *Emerg Infect Dis,* **2014,** 20.

Hill DR, et al. The practice of travel medicine: guidelines by the Infectious Diseases Society of America. *Clin Infect Dis,* **2006,** 43:1499–1539.

Hughes WT, et al. 2002 guidelines for the use of antimicrobial agents in neutropenic patients with cancer. *Clin Infect Dis,* **2002,** 34:730–751.

Lesch JE. *The First Miracle Drugs: How the Sulfa Drugs Transformed Medicine.* Oxford University Press, New York, 2007.

Mitscher LA, Ma Z. Structure-activity relationships of quinolones. In: Ronald AR, Low DE, eds. *Fluoroquinolone Antibiotics.* Birkhauser, Basel, **2003,** 11–48.

Oethinger M, et al. Ineffectiveness of topoisomerase mutations in mediating clinically significant fluoroquinolone resistance in *Escherichia coli* in the absence of the AcrAB efflux pump. *Antimicrob Agents Chemother,* **2000,** 44:10–13.

Olson RP, et al. Antibiotic resistance in urinary isolates of *E. coli* from college women with urinary tract infections. *Antimicrob Agents Chemother,* **2009,** 53:1285–1286.

Panel on Opportunistic Infections in HIV-Infected Adults and Adolescents. Guidelines for the prevention and treatment of opportunistic infections in HIV-infected adults and adolescents: recommendations from the Centers for Disease Control and Prevention, the National Institutes of

Health, and the HIV Medicine Association of the Infectious Diseases Society of America. **2016**. Available at: http://aidsinfo.nih.gov/contentfiles/lvguidelines/adult_oi.pdf. Accessed April 7, 2016.

Park-Wyllie LY, et al. Outpatient gatifloxacin therapy and dysglycemia in older adults. *N Engl J Med*, **2006**, *354*:1352–1361.

Paul M, et al. Trimethoprim-sulfamethoxazole versus vancomycin for severe infections caused by methicillin resistant *Staphylococcus aureus*: a randomized trial. *BMJ*, **2015**, *350*:h2219.

Sabharwal V, Marchant CD. Fluoroquinolone use in children. *Pediatr Infect Dis J*, **2006**, *25*:257–258.

Schwartz J, et al. Impact of ciprofloxacin on theophylline clearance and steady-state concentrations in serum. *Antimicrob Agents Chemother*, **1988**, *32*:75–77.

Sheehan G, Chew NSY. The history of quinolones. In: Ronald AR, Low DE, eds. *Fluoroquinolone Antibiotics*. Birkhauser, Basel, **2003**, 1–10.

Chapter 57

Penicillins, Cephalosporins, and Other β-Lactam Antibiotics

Conan MacDougall

The β-lactam antibiotics—*penicillins, cephalosporins, carbapenems,* and *monobactams*—share a common structure (β-lactam ring) and mechanism of action (i.e., inhibition of the synthesis of the bacterial peptidoglycan cell wall). Bacterial resistance against the β-lactam antibiotics continues to increase at a dramatic rate. β-Lactamase inhibitors such as clavulanate and avibactam can extend the utility of these antibiotics against β-lactamase–producing organisms. Unfortunately, resistance includes not only production of β-lactamases but also alterations in the bacterial enzymes targeted by β-lactam antibiotics, as well as decreased entry or active efflux of the antibiotic.

Mechanism of Action: Inhibition of Peptidoglycan Synthesis

Peptidoglycan is a heteropolymeric component of the bacterial cell wall that provides rigid mechanical stability. The β-lactam antibiotics inhibit the last step in peptidoglycan synthesis (Figure 57–1).

In gram-positive microorganisms, the cell wall is 50–100 molecules thick; in gram-negative bacteria, it is only 1 or 2 molecules thick (Figure 57–2A). The peptidoglycan is composed of glycan chains, which are linear strands of two alternating amino sugars (*N*-acetylglucosamine and *N*-acetylmuramic acid) that are cross-linked by peptide chains. Peptidoglycan precursor formation takes place in the cytoplasm. The synthesis of UDP–acetylmuramyl-pentapeptide is completed with the addition of a dipeptide, D-alanyl-D-alanine (formed by racemization and condensation of L-alanine). UDP-acetylmuramyl-pentapeptide and UDP-acetylglucosamine are linked (with the release of the uridine nucleotides) to form a long polymer. The cross-link is completed by a transpeptidation reaction that occurs outside the cell membrane (Figure 57–2B).

The β-lactam antibiotics inhibit this last step in peptidoglycan synthesis (see Figure 57–1), presumably by acylating the transpeptidase via cleavage of the –CO–N– bond of the β-lactam ring. The targets for the actions of β-lactam antibiotics are collectively termed *PBPs*. The transpeptidase responsible for synthesis of the peptidoglycan is one of these PBPs.

The lethality of penicillins for bacteria appears to involve both lytic and nonlytic mechanisms (Bayles, 2000).

Mechanisms of Bacterial Resistance to Penicillins and Cephalosporins

Bacteria can be resistant to β-lactam antibiotics by myriad mechanisms. A sensitive strain may acquire resistance by mutations that decrease the affinity of PBPs for the antibiotic. Because the β-lactam antibiotics inhibit many different PBPs in a single bacterium, the affinity for β-lactam antibiotics of several PBPs must decrease for the organism to be resistant (Spratt, 1994). Altered PBPs with decreased affinity for β-lactam antibiotics are acquired by homologous recombination between PBP genes of different bacterial species (Zapun et al., 2008). Four of the five high-molecular-weight PBPs of the most highly penicillin-resistant *Streptococcus pneumoniae* isolates have decreased affinity for β-lactam antibiotics as a result of interspecies homologous recombination events. In contrast, isolates with high-level resistance to third-generation cephalosporins contain alterations of only two of the five high-molecular-weight PBPs because the other PBPs have inherently low affinity for the third-generation cephalosporins. *MRSA* is resistant via acquisition of an additional high-molecular-weight PBP (via a transposon) with a very low affinity for all β-lactam antibiotics; this mechanism is also responsible for methicillin resistance in the coagulase-negative staphylococci.

Bacterial resistance to the β-lactam antibiotics also results from the inability of the agent to penetrate to its site of action (Figure 57–3) (Fernández and Hancock, 2012). In gram-positive bacteria, the peptidoglycan polymer is very near the cell surface (see Figure 57–2A) and small β-lactam antibiotic molecules can penetrate easily to the outer layer of the cytoplasmic membrane and the PBPs. In gram-negative bacteria, the inner membrane is covered by the outer membrane, lipopolysaccharide, and capsule (see Figure 57–2A). The outer membrane functions as an impenetrable barrier for some antibiotics. Some small hydrophilic antibiotics, however, diffuse through aqueous channels in the outer membrane that

Abbreviations

ADME: absorption, distribution, metabolism, excretion
CNS: central nervous system
CSF: cerebrospinal fluid
ESBL: extended-spectrum β-lactamase
GI: gastrointestinal
GT: glycosyltransferase
Ig: immunoglobulin
IM: intramuscular
IV: intravenous
KPC: *Klebsiella pneumoniae* carbapenemase
MDM: major determinant moiety
MRSA: methicillin-resistant *Staphylococcus aureus*
MRSE: methicillin-resistant *Staphylococcus epidermidis*
MSSA: methicillin-susceptible *Staphylococcus aureus*
PBP: penicillin-binding protein
PO: by mouth
TP: transpeptidase

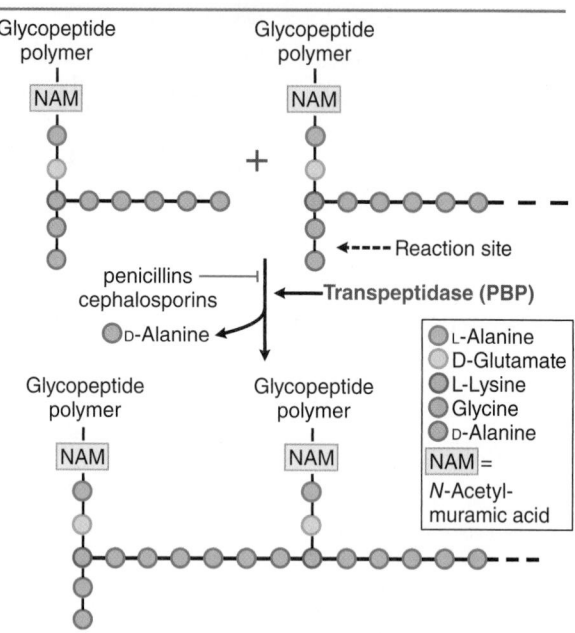

Figure 57–1 *Action of β-lactam antibiotics in* Staphylococcus aureus. The bacterial cell wall consists of glycopeptide polymers (an NAM-NAG aminohexose backbone) linked via bridges between amino acid side chains. In *S. aureus*, the bridge is (Gly)$_5$-D-Ala between lysines. The cross-linking is catalyzed by a transpeptidase, the enzyme that penicillins and cephalosporins inhibit.

are formed by proteins called *porins*. The number and size of pores in the outer membrane vary amongst different gram-negative bacteria, thereby providing greater or lesser access for antibiotics to the site of action. Active efflux pumps serve as another mechanism of resistance, removing the antibiotic from its site of action before it can act (see Figure 57–3) (Nikaido, 1998).

Bacteria also can inactivate β-lactam antibiotics enzymatically via the action of β-lactamases (Figures 57–2 and 57–4). β-Lactamases are grouped into four classes, A through D (Jacoby and Munoz-Price, 2005). Their substrate specificities can be relatively narrow or can extend to almost all β-lactams. In general, gram-positive bacteria produce and secrete a large amount of β-lactamase (see Figure 57–2A). Most of these enzymes are penicillinases. The information for staphylococcal penicillinase is encoded in a plasmid; this may be transferred by bacteriophage to other bacteria and is inducible by substrates. In gram-negative bacteria, β-lactamases are found in relatively small amounts but are located in the periplasmic space between the inner and outer cell membranes (see Figure 57–2A) for maximal protection of the microbe. β-Lactamases of gram-negative bacteria are encoded either in chromosomes or in plasmids and may be constitutive or inducible. The plasmids can be transferred between bacteria by conjugation. Of particular concern are β-lactamases that are capable of hydrolyzing carbapenems as well as penicillins and cephalosporins; organisms possessing such β-lactamases (along with other resistance mechanisms) may be resistant to all or almost all antibacterials in clinical use (Queenan and Bush, 2007).

The local environment can also contribute to resistance to beta-lactam antibiotics. Microorganisms adhering to implanted prosthetic devices (e.g., catheters, artificial joints, prosthetic heart valves) produce biofilms. Bacteria in biofilms produce extracellular polysaccharides and, in part owing to decreased growth rates, are much less sensitive to antibiotic therapy (Donlan, 2001). The β-lactam antibiotics are most active against bacteria in the logarithmic phase of growth and have little effect on microorganisms in the stationary phase. Similarly, bacteria that survive inside viable cells of the host generally are protected from the action of the β-lactam antibiotics.

The Penicillins

Despite the emergence of microbial resistance, the penicillins are currently the drugs of choice for a large number of infectious diseases. Penicillins (Figure 57–4) consist of a thiazolidine ring (A) connected to a β-lactam ring (B) to which is attached a side chain (R). The penicillin nucleus itself

is the chief structural requirement for biological activity. Side chains can be added that alter the susceptibility of the resulting compounds to inactivating enzymes (β-lactamases) and that change the antibacterial activity and the pharmacological properties of the drug (Table 57–1).

Classification of the Penicillins and Summary of Their Pharmacological Properties

Penicillins are classified according to their spectra of antimicrobial activity.

- **Penicillin G** and its close congener **penicillin V** are highly active against sensitive strains of gram-positive cocci, but they are readily hydrolyzed by penicillinase. Thus, they are *ineffective against most strains of* S. aureus.
- **The penicillinase-resistant penicillins** (*methicillin*, discontinued in the U.S.), *cloxacillin* and *flucloxacillin* (not currently marketed in the U.S.), *nafcillin, oxacillin*, and *dicloxacillin* have less-potent antimicrobial activity against microorganisms that are sensitive to penicillin G, but they are *preferred agents for treatment of penicillinase-producing* S. aureus *and* Staphylococcus epidermidis *that are not methicillin resistant.*
- *Ampicillin, amoxicillin*, and others such as *bacampicillin* and *pivampicillin* (not currently marketed in the U.S.) are the **aminopenicillins**, whose antimicrobial activity is extended to include some gram-negative microorganisms (e.g., *Haemophilus influenzae, Escherichia coli*, and *Proteus mirabilis*). These drugs are also available as coformulations with a **β-lactamase inhibitor** such as *clavulanate* or *sulbactam* to prevent hydrolysis by class A β-lactamases.
- **Agents with extended antimicrobial activity against *Pseudomonas*, *Enterobacter*, and *Proteus* spp.** include older agents largely out of use: *azlocillin, carbenicillin, mezlocillin, ticarcillin, ticarcillin/clavulanate* (all discontinued in the U.S.), and *carbenicillin indanyl sodium*. These agents are inferior to ampicillin against gram-positive cocci and *Listeria monocytogenes* and are less active than piperacillin

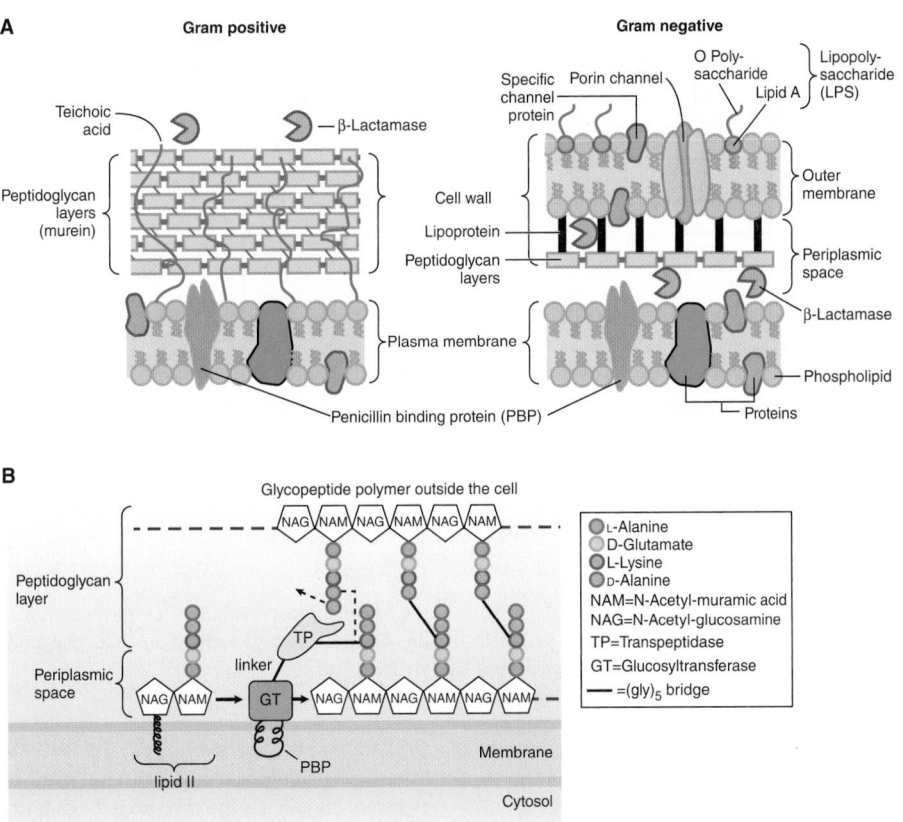

Figure 57–2 **A.** *Structure and composition of gram-positive and gram-negative cell walls.* **B.** *PBP activity and inhibition.* PBPs have two enzymatic activities that are crucial to synthesis of the peptidoglycan layers of bacterial cell walls: a TP that cross-links amino acid side chains and a GT that links subunits of the glycopeptide polymer (see Figure 57–1). The TP and GT domains are separated by a linker region. The glycosyltransferase is thought to be partially embedded in the membrane. (Part A reprinted with permission from Tortora G, et al. *Microbiology: An Introduction*, 3rd ed. Pearson, London, **1989**, Figure 4–11, p. 83. © Pearson Education, Inc., New York, New York.)

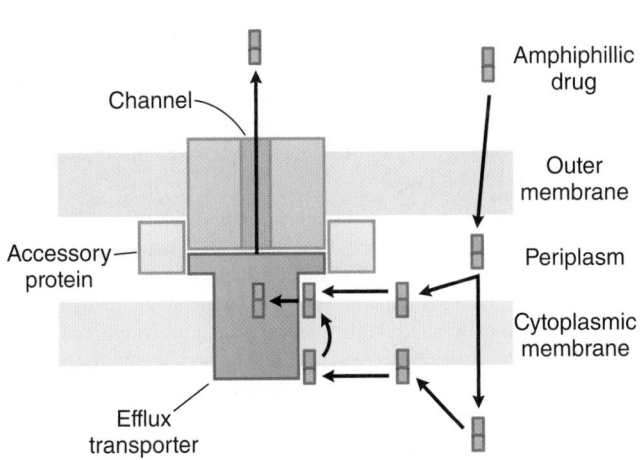

Figure 57–3 *Antibiotic efflux pumps of gram-negative bacteria.* Multidrug efflux pumps traverse both the inner and outer membranes of gram-negative bacteria. The pumps are composed of a minimum of three proteins and are energized by the proton motive force. Increased expression of these pumps is an important cause of antibiotic resistance. (Reprinted with permission from Oxford University Press. Nikaido H. Antibiotic resistance caused by gram-negative multidrug efflux pumps. *Clin Infect Dis*, **1998**, 27(suppl 1): S32–S41. © 1998 by the Infectious Diseases Society of America. All rights reserved.)

against *Pseudomonas*. *Piperacillin* and *piperacillin/tazobactam* have excellent antimicrobial activity against many isolates of *Pseudomonas*, *E. coli*, *Klebsiella*, and other gram-negative microorganisms. Piperacillin retains the activity of ampicillin against gram-positive cocci and *L. monocytogenes*.

General Common Properties

Following absorption of an oral dose, penicillins are distributed widely throughout the body. Therapeutic concentrations of penicillins are achieved readily in tissues and in secretions such as joint fluid, pleural fluid, pericardial fluid, and bile. Penicillins do not penetrate living phagocytic cells to a significant extent, and only low concentrations of these drugs are found in prostatic secretions, brain tissue, and intraocular fluid. Concentrations of penicillins in CSF are variable but are less than 1% of those in plasma when the meninges are normal. When there is inflammation, concentrations in CSF may increase to as much as 5% of the plasma value. Penicillins are eliminated rapidly by glomerular filtration and renal tubular secretion, such that their half-lives in the body are short, typically 30–90 min. As a consequence, concentrations of these drugs in urine are high.

Penicillin G and Penicillin V

Antimicrobial Activity

The antimicrobial spectra of penicillin G (benzylpenicillin) and penicillin V (the phenoxymethyl derivative) are similar for aerobic gram-positive microorganisms. However, penicillin G is 5–10 times more active than penicillin V against *Neisseria* spp. and certain anaerobes. Most streptococci are very susceptible. However, penicillin-resistant viridans streptococci

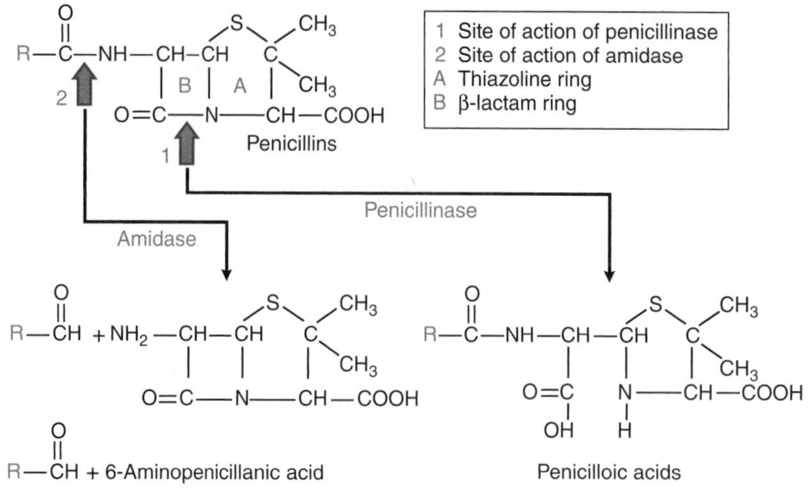

Figure 57–4 *Structure of penicillins and products of their enzymatic hydrolysis.*

and *S. pneumoniae* are becoming more common (Carratalá et al., 1995). Penicillin-resistant pneumococci are especially common in pediatric populations and are often also resistant to third-generation cephalosporins. Greater than 90% of strains of *S. aureus*, most strains of *S. epidermidis*, and many strains of gonococci are now resistant to penicillin G. With rare exceptions, meningococci remain quite sensitive to penicillin G.

Most anaerobic microorganisms, including *Clostridium* spp., are highly sensitive. *Bacteroides fragilis* is an exception, displaying resistance to penicillins and cephalosporins by virtue of expressing a broad-spectrum cephalosporinase. Some strains of *Prevotella melaninogenicus* also have acquired this trait. *Actinomyces israelii*, *Streptobacillus moniliformis*, *Pasteurella multocida*, and *L. monocytogenes* are inhibited by penicillin G. Most species of *Leptospira* are moderately susceptible to the drug. One of the most sensitive microorganisms is *Treponema pallidum*. *Borrelia burgdorferi*,

the organism responsible for Lyme disease, also is susceptible. Penicillins are not effective against amebae, plasmodia, rickettsiae, fungi, or viruses.

ADME

Oral Administration of Penicillin G and V. The virtue of penicillin V in comparison with penicillin G is that it is more stable in an acidic medium and therefore is better absorbed from the GI tract, yielding plasma concentrations two to five times those provided by penicillin G. Thus, penicillin V is generally preferred for oral administration. Absorption is rapid, and maximal concentrations in blood are attained in 30–60 min. Ingestion of food may interfere with enteric absorption of all penicillins. Thus, oral penicillins should generally be administered at least 30 min before a meal or 2 h after.

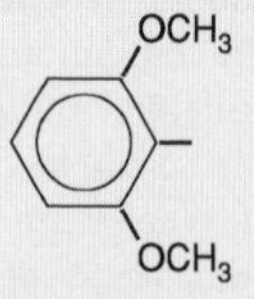

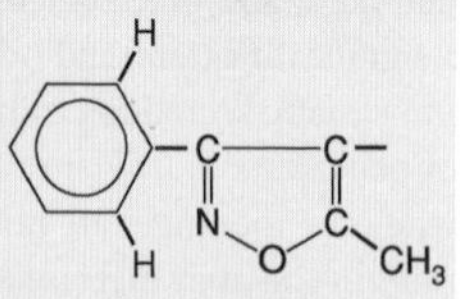

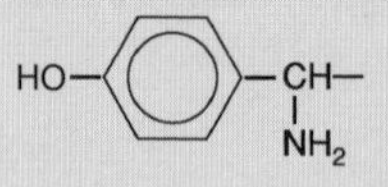

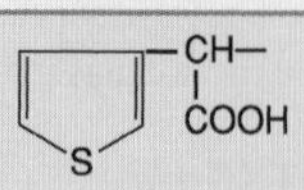

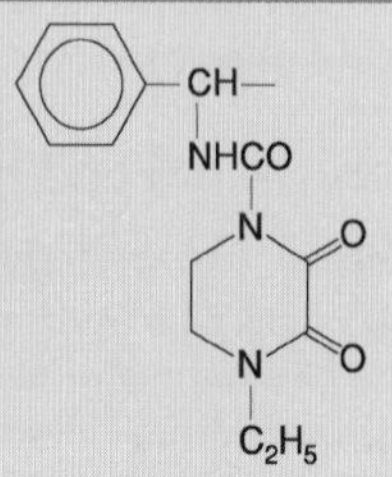

Parenteral Administration of Penicillin G. After intramuscular injection, peak concentrations in plasma are reached within 15–30 min, declining rapidly thereafter ($t_{1/2} \sim 30$ min). Repository preparations of penicillin G (penicillin G benzathine, penicillin G procaine) increase the duration of the effect. The compound currently favored is penicillin G benzathine, which releases penicillin G slowly from the area in which it is injected and produces relatively low but persistent concentrations in the blood. The average duration of demonstrable antimicrobial activity in the plasma is about 26 days. It is administered once monthly for rheumatic fever prophylaxis and can be given in a single injection to treat streptococcal pharyngitis. Penicillin G procaine has a prolonged $t_{1/2}$ compared to penicillin G, but shorter than that of benzathine formulations; it is typically dosed once daily. Neither depot formulation should be given intravenously as serious toxicity can result.

Distribution. Penicillin G is distributed extensively throughout the body, but the concentrations in various fluids and tissues differ widely. Its apparent volume of distribution is about 0.35 L/kg. Approximately 60% of the penicillin G in plasma is reversibly bound to albumin. Significant amounts appear in liver, bile, kidney, semen, joint fluid, lymph, and intestine. Probenecid markedly decreases the tubular secretion of the penicillins and also produces a significant decrease in the apparent volume of distribution of the penicillins.

Penetration Into Cerebrospinal Fluid. Penicillin does not readily enter the CSF but penetrates more easily when the meninges are inflamed. The concentrations are usually in the range of 5% of the value in plasma and are therapeutically effective against susceptible microorganisms. Penicillin and other organic acids are secreted rapidly from the CSF into the bloodstream by an active transport process. Probenecid competitively inhibits this transport and thus elevates the concentration of penicillin in CSF. In uremia, other organic acids accumulate in the CSF and compete with penicillin for secretion; the drug occasionally reaches toxic concentrations in the brain and can produce convulsions.

TABLE 57–1 ■ CHEMICAL STRUCTURES OF SELECTED PENICILLINS

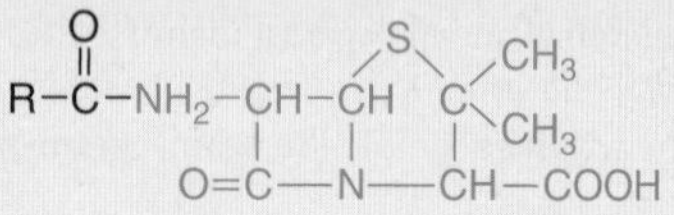

Penicillins are substituted 6-aminopenicillanic acid.

Addition of substituents (R groups) to the parent structure produces penicillins with altered susceptibility to inactivating enzymes (β-lactamases), antibacterial activity, and pharmacological properties.

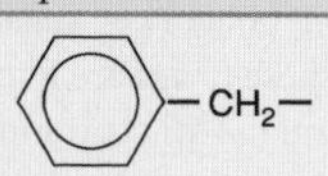

HISTORY

The history of the brilliant research that led to the discovery and development of penicillin is well chronicled (Lax, 2004). In 1928, while studying *Staphylococcus* variants in the laboratory at St. Mary's Hospital in London, Alexander Fleming observed that a mold contaminating one of his cultures caused the bacteria in its vicinity to undergo lysis. Broth in which the fungus was grown was markedly inhibitory for many microorganisms. Because the mold belonged to the genus *Penicillium*, Fleming named the antibacterial substance *penicillin*.

A decade later, penicillin was developed as a systemic therapeutic agent by the concerted research of a group of investigators at Oxford University headed by Florey, Chain, and Abraham. By May 1940, a crude preparation was found to produce dramatic therapeutic effects when administered parenterally to mice with streptococcal infections. Sufficient penicillin was accumulated by 1941 to conduct therapeutic trials in several patients desperately ill with staphylococcal and streptococcal infections refractory to all other therapy. At this stage, the crude, amorphous penicillin was only about 10% pure, and it required nearly 100 L of the broth in which the mold had been grown to obtain enough of the antibiotic to treat one patient for 24 h. Bedpans actually were used by the Oxford group for growing cultures of *Penicillium notatum*. Case 1 in the 1941 report from Oxford was that of a policeman who was suffering from a severe mixed staphylococcal and streptococcal infection. He was treated with penicillin, some of which had been recovered from the urine of other patients who had been given the drug. It is said that an Oxford professor referred to penicillin as a remarkable substance grown in bedpans and purified by passage through the Oxford Police Force.

A vast research program soon was initiated in the U.S. There were 122 million units of penicillin made available during 1942, and the first clinical trials were conducted at Yale University and the Mayo Clinic, with dramatic results. By the spring of 1943, there were 200 patients who had been treated with the drug. The results were so impressive that the surgeon general of the U.S. Army authorized a trial of the antibiotic in a military hospital. Soon thereafter, penicillin was adopted throughout the medical services of the U.S. Armed Forces.

The deep-fermentation procedure for the biosynthesis of penicillin marked a crucial advance in the large-scale production of the antibiotic. From a total production of a few hundred million units a month in the early days, the quantity manufactured rose to over 200 trillion units (nearly 150 tons) by 1950. The first marketable penicillin cost several dollars per 100,000 units; today, the same dose costs only a few cents.

Excretion. Approximately 60%–90% of an intramuscular dose of penicillin G in aqueous solution is eliminated in the urine, largely within the first hour after injection. The remainder is metabolized to penicilloic acid (see Figure 57–4). The $t_{1/2}$ for elimination of penicillin G is about 30 min in normal adults. Approximately 10% of the drug is eliminated by glomerular filtration and 90% by tubular secretion. Renal clearance approximates the total renal plasma flow. Clearance values are considerably lower in neonates and infants; as a result, penicillin persists in the blood several times longer in premature infants than in children and adults. The $t_{1/2}$ of the antibiotic in children less than 1 week of age is 3 h; by 14 days of age, it is 1.4 h. After renal function is fully established in young children, the rate of renal excretion of penicillin G is considerably more rapid than in adults. Anuria increases the $t_{1/2}$ of penicillin G from 0.5 to about 10 h. When renal function is impaired, 7%–10% of the antibiotic may be inactivated each hour by the liver. The dose of the drug must be readjusted during dialysis and the period of progressive recovery of renal function. If hepatic insufficiency also is present, the $t_{1/2}$ will be prolonged even further.

Therapeutic Uses

Pneumococcal Infections. Penicillin G remains the agent of choice for the management of infections caused by sensitive strains of *S. pneumoniae*, but resistance is an increasing problem.

Pneumococcal Pneumonia. For parenteral therapy of sensitive isolates of pneumococci, penicillin G is favored. Therapy should be continued for at least 5 days, including at least 2–3 days after the patient's temperature has returned to normal.

Pneumococcal Meningitis. Pneumococcal meningitis should be treated with a combination of vancomycin and a third-generation cephalosporin until it is established that the infecting pneumococcus is penicillin sensitive. Dexamethasone given prior to or at the same time as antibiotics is associated with an improved outcome (de Gans et al., 2002). The recommended therapy is 24 million units of penicillin G daily by constant intravenous infusion or divided into boluses for 10–14 days.

β-Hemolytic Streptococcal Infections. Streptococcal pharyngitis *(including scarlet fever)* is the most common disease produced by *Streptococcus pyogenes* (group A β-hemolytic streptococcus). Penicillin-resistant isolates have yet to be observed. The preferred oral therapy is with penicillin V, 500 mg twice daily for 10 days. Penicillin therapy of streptococcal pharyngitis reduces the risk of subsequent acute rheumatic fever; however, current evidence suggests that the incidence of glomerulonephritis that follows streptococcal infections is not reduced to a significant degree by treatment with penicillin (Shulman et al., 2012).

β-Hemolytic Streptococcal Toxic Shock and Necrotizing Fasciitis. β-Hemolytic streptococcal toxic shock and necrotizing fasciitis are life-threatening infections associated with toxin production. Recommended treatment is with penicillin plus clindamycin (to decrease toxin production) (Brown, 2004).

β-Hemolytic Streptococcal Pneumonia, Arthritis, Meningitis, and Endocarditis. The uncommon conditions of pneumonia, arthritis, meningitis, and endocarditis caused by β-hemolytic streptococci should be treated with penicillin G when they are caused by *S. pyogenes*; daily doses of 12–24 million units are administered intravenously for 2–4 weeks (4 weeks for endocarditis).

Infections Caused by Other Streptococci and Enterococci. The viridans group of streptococci is the most common cause of native valve infectious endocarditis. These are nongroupable α-hemolytic microorganisms that are increasingly resistant to penicillin G. It is important to determine quantitative microbial sensitivities to penicillin G in patients with endocarditis. Patients with penicillin-sensitive viridans group streptococcal native valve endocarditis can be treated successfully with daily doses of 12–20 million units of intravenous penicillin G for 4 weeks or for 2 weeks if given in combination with gentamicin. The recommended therapy for penicillin- and aminoglycoside-sensitive enterococcal endocarditis is 24 million units of penicillin G or 12 g ampicillin daily administered intravenously in combination with a low dose of gentamicin. Therapy usually should be continued for 6 weeks.

Infections with Anaerobes. Pulmonary and periodontal infections usually respond well to penicillin G; clindamycin may be more effective than penicillin for therapy of lung abscess (Levison et al., 1983). Mild-to-moderate infections at these sites may be treated with oral medication (either penicillin G or penicillin V 250 mg four times daily). More severe infections should be treated with 12–24 million units of penicillin G intravenously.

Staphylococcal Infections. Most staphylococcal infections are caused by microorganisms that produce penicillinase; further, half or more isolates of *S. aureus* and *S. epidermidis* are resistant to β-lactams through production of altered PBPs. Thus, penicillin G now has limited utility in the treatment of staphylococcal infections.

Meningococcal Infections. Penicillin G remains the drug of choice for meningococcal disease. Patients should be treated with high doses of penicillin given intravenously. The occurrence of penicillin-resistant strains should be considered in patients who are slow to respond to treatment. Penicillin G does not eliminate the meningococcal carrier state, and its administration thus is ineffective as a prophylactic measure.

Gonococcal Infections. Gonococci gradually have become more resistant to penicillin G, and penicillins are no longer the therapy of choice.

Syphilis. Therapy of syphilis with penicillin G is highly effective. Primary, secondary, and latent syphilis of less than 1-year duration may be treated with 1–3 weekly intramuscular doses of 2.4 million units of penicillin G benzathine. Patients with neurosyphilis or cardiovascular syphilis typically receive intensive therapy with 18–24 million units of penicillin G daily for 10–14 days. There are no proven alternatives for treating syphilis in pregnant women, so penicillin-allergic individuals must be acutely desensitized to prevent anaphylaxis.

Most patients with secondary syphilis develop the Jarisch-Herxheimer reaction, including chills, fever, headache, myalgias, and arthralgias occurring several hours after the first dose of penicillin. This reaction is thought to be due to release of spirochetal antigens with subsequent host reactions to the products. Antipyretics give symptomatic relief, and therapy with penicillin should not be discontinued.

Actinomycosis. Penicillin G is the agent of choice for the treatment of all forms of actinomycosis (18–24 million units of penicillin G IV per day for 6 weeks). Surgical drainage or excision of the lesion may be necessary before cure is accomplished.

Diphtheria. Penicillin and other antibiotics do not alter the incidence of complications or the outcome of diphtheria; specific antitoxin is the only effective treatment. However, penicillin G eliminates the carrier state. The parenteral administration of 2–3 million units per day in divided doses for 10–12 days eliminates the diphtheria bacilli from the pharynx and other sites in practically 100% of patients. A single daily injection of penicillin G procaine for the same period produces comparable results.

Anthrax. Strains of *Bacillus anthracis* resistant to penicillin have been recovered from human infections. When penicillin G is used for serious infections due to susceptible strains, the dose should be 24 million units per day.

Clostridial Infections. Penicillin G (12–24 million units per day given parenterally) plus clindamycin is recommended for clostridial gas gangrene. Adequate debridement of the infected areas is essential. Antibiotics probably have no effect on the outcome of tetanus. Debridement and administration of human tetanus immune globulin may be indicated.

Fusospirochetal Infections. Gingivostomatitis, produced by the synergistic action of *Leptotrichia buccalis* and spirochetes that are present in the mouth, is readily treatable with penicillin. For simple "trench mouth," 500 mg penicillin V given every 6 h for several days usually suffices.

Rat-Bite Fever. The two microorganisms responsible for the rat-bite fever infection, *Spirillum minus* in the Far East and *Streptobacillus moniliformis* in the U.S. and Europe, are sensitive to penicillin G, the drug of choice. Because most cases due to *Streptobacillus* are complicated by bacteremia and, in many instances, by metastatic infections, especially of the synovia and endocardium, high doses given parenterally for 3–4 weeks are frequently recommended.

Listeria Infections. Ampicillin or penicillin G (with consideration for addition of gentamicin to both for immunosuppressed patients with meningitis) are the drugs of choice in the management of infections owing to *L. monocytogenes*. The recommended dose of penicillin G is 18–24 million units parenterally per day for at least 2 weeks. For endocarditis, the dose is the same, but the duration of treatment should be no less than 4 weeks.

Lyme Disease. Intravenous penicillin G in doses of 18–24 million units per day for 14 days is an alternative to third-generation cephalosporins in treatment of severe Lyme disease.

Erysipeloid. The causative agent of erysipeloid, *Erysipelothrix rhusiopathiae*, is sensitive to penicillin. The infection responds well to a single injection of

1.2 million units of penicillin G benzathine. When endocarditis is present, penicillin G, 12–20 million units per day, for 4–6 weeks is required.

Pasteurella multocida. *Pasteurella multocida* is a cause of wound infections after a cat or dog bite. It is susceptible to penicillin G and ampicillin and resistant to penicillinase-resistant penicillins and first-generation cephalosporins. When the infection causes meningitis, a third-generation cephalosporin is preferred.

Prophylactic Uses of the Penicillins

Streptococcal Infections. The administration of penicillin to household contacts exposed to *S. pyogenes* pharyngitis has not been shown to be highly effective in reducing subsequent illness. Indications for this type of prophylaxis might include outbreaks of streptococcal disease in closed populations (e.g., boarding schools or military bases).

Recurrences of Rheumatic Fever. The oral administration of 200,000 units of penicillin G or penicillin V every 12 h decreases the incidence of recurrences of rheumatic fever in susceptible individuals. The intramuscular injection of 1.2 million units of penicillin G benzathine once a month also yields excellent results. Prophylaxis must be continued throughout the year. Some suggest that prophylaxis should be continued for life because instances of acute rheumatic fever have been observed in the fifth and sixth decades, but the necessity of lifetime prophylaxis has not been established.

Syphilis. Prophylaxis for recent sexual contacts of a patient with primary, secondary, or early latent syphilis consists of a course of penicillin as described for primary syphilis.

The Penicillinase-Resistant Penicillins

The penicillinase-resistant penicillins are resistant to hydrolysis by staphylococcal penicillinase. Their appropriate use should be restricted to the treatment of infections that are known or suspected to be caused by staphylococci that elaborate the enzyme since these drugs are much less active than penicillin G against other penicillin-sensitive microorganisms. However, an increasing number of isolates of *S. aureus* (around half in most U.S. hospitals) and *S. epidermidis* (more than three-quarters) express a low-affinity PBP, giving them the MRSA or MRSE phenotype. This term denotes resistance of these bacteria to all the penicillinase-resistant penicillins and cephalosporins (with the exception of ceftaroline and ceftobiprole [not available in the U.S.]). Alternative agents such as vancomycin, daptomycin, clindamycin, or linezolid (see Chapter 59) are typically used for infections due to organisms with this resistance mechanism.

The Isoxazolyl Penicillins: Oxacillin, Cloxacillin, and Dicloxacillin

Oxacillin, cloxacillin (not available in the U.S.), and dicloxacillin are semisynthetic penicillin congeners that are markedly resistant to cleavage by penicillinase. These drugs are not substitutes for penicillin G in the treatment of diseases amenable to it and are not active against enterococci or *Listeria*. Oral administration is not a substitute for the parenteral route in the treatment of serious staphylococcal infections.

Pharmacological Properties. The isoxazolyl penicillins are potent inhibitors of the growth of most penicillinase-producing staphylococci. Dicloxacillin is the most active, and many strains of *S. aureus* are inhibited by concentrations of 0.05–0.8 μg/mL. These agents are, in general, less effective against microorganisms susceptible to penicillin G, and they are not useful against gram-negative bacteria. These agents are absorbed rapidly but incompletely (30%–80%) from the GI tract. Absorption increases when administered 1 h before or 2 h after meals. Peak concentrations in plasma are attained by 1 h. All these congeners are bound to plasma albumin to a great extent (~90%–95%); none is removed from the circulation to a significant degree by hemodialysis. The isoxazolyl penicillins are excreted by the kidney; there is also significant hepatic degradation and elimination in the bile. The half-lives for all are between 30 and 60 min. No dosing adjustments are needed for patients with renal failure.

Nafcillin

This semisynthetic penicillin is highly resistant to penicillinase and has proven effective against infections caused by penicillinase-producing strains of *S. aureus*.

Pharmacological Properties. Nafcillin is slightly more active than oxacillin against penicillin G–resistant *S. aureus* (most strains are inhibited by 0.06–2 µg/mL). Although it is the most active of the penicillinase-resistant penicillins against other microorganisms, it is not as potent as penicillin G. The peak plasma concentration is about 8 µg/mL 60 min after a 1-g intramuscular dose. Nafcillin is about 90% bound to plasma protein. Peak concentrations of nafcillin in bile are well above those found in plasma. Dosage adjustment in patients with renal dysfunction is not required. Concentrations of the drug in CSF appear to be adequate for therapy of staphylococcal meningitis.

The Aminopenicillins: Ampicillin and Amoxicillin

Aminopenicillins expand the spectrum of activity of penicillin G in a different direction from the penicillinase-resistant penicillins—they allow for useful activity against some gram-negative organisms. They all are destroyed by β-lactamases (from both gram-positive and gram-negative bacteria); thus, further expansion of their activity is enabled through coformulation with β-lactamase inhibitors (see the end of the chapter for further discussion of the chemistry and activity of β-lactamase inhibitors).

Antimicrobial Activity

Ampicillin and amoxicillin are generally bactericidal for sensitive gram-positive and gram-negative bacteria. The meningococci and *L. monocytogenes* are sensitive to this class of drugs. Many pneumococcal isolates have varying levels of resistance to ampicillin, and penicillin-resistant strains should be considered ampicillin/amoxicillin-resistant. *Haemophilus influenzae* and the viridans group of streptococci exhibit varying degrees of resistance. Enterococci are about twice as sensitive to ampicillin as they are to penicillin G. From 30% to 50% of *E. coli*, a significant number of *P. mirabilis*, and practically all species of *Klebsiella* are resistant. Most strains of *Shigella, Pseudomonas, Serratia, Acinetobacter, B. fragilis,* and indole-positive *Proteus* also are resistant to this group of penicillins. Resistant strains of *Salmonella* are recovered with increasing frequency. Concurrent administration of a β-lactamase inhibitor such as *clavulanate* or *sulbactam* markedly expands their spectrum of activity, particularly against *H. influenzae, E. coli, Klebsiella, Proteus,* and *B. fragilis.*

ADME

Ampicillin. Ampicillin is stable in acid and is well absorbed after oral administration. An oral dose of 0.5 g produces peak concentrations in plasma of about 3 µg/mL at 2 h. Intake of food prior to ingestion of ampicillin diminishes absorption. Intramuscular injection of 0.5–1 g sodium ampicillin yields peak plasma concentrations of about 7–10 µg/mL, respectively, at 1 h. Plasma levels decline with a $t_{1/2}$ of about 80 min. Severe renal impairment markedly prolongs the $t_{1/2}$. Peritoneal dialysis is ineffective in removing the drug from the blood, but hemodialysis removes approximately 40% of the body store in about 7 h. Adjustment of the dose of ampicillin is required in the presence of renal dysfunction. Ampicillin appears in the bile, undergoes enterohepatic circulation, and is excreted in the feces.

Amoxicillin. Amoxicillin, a penicillinase-susceptible, semisynthetic penicillin (see Table 57–1), is a close chemical and pharmacological relative of ampicillin. Amoxicillin is stable in acid, designed for oral use, and absorbed more rapidly and completely from the GI tract than ampicillin. The antimicrobial spectrum of amoxicillin is essentially identical to that of ampicillin, except that amoxicillin is less active and less effective than ampicillin for shigellosis. Peak plasma concentrations of amoxicillin are 2–2.5 times greater than for ampicillin after oral administration of the same dose. Food does not interfere with absorption. Perhaps because of more complete absorption of this congener, the incidence of diarrhea with amoxicillin is less than that following administration of ampicillin.

The incidence of other adverse effects appears to be similar. Although the $t_{1/2}$ of amoxicillin is similar to that for ampicillin, effective concentrations of orally administered amoxicillin are detectable in the plasma for twice as long as with ampicillin because of the more complete absorption. For all these reasons, amoxicillin is generally preferred over ampicillin for oral administration. About 20% of amoxicillin is protein bound in plasma, a value similar to that for ampicillin. Most of a dose of the antibiotic is excreted in an active form in the urine, and dose adjustment is required in renal dysfunction. Probenecid delays excretion of the drug.

Therapeutic Indications

Upper Respiratory Infections. Ampicillin and amoxicillin are active against *S. pyogenes* and many strains of *S. pneumoniae* and *H. influenzae*. The drugs constitute effective therapy for sinusitis, otitis media, acute exacerbations of chronic bronchitis, and epiglottitis caused by sensitive strains of these organisms. Amoxicillin is the most active of all the oral β-lactam antibiotics against both penicillin-susceptible and penicillin-nonsusceptible *S. pneumoniae*. Based on the increasing prevalence of pneumococcal resistance to penicillin, an increase in dose of oral amoxicillin (from 40–45 up to 80–90 mg/kg/d) for empirical treatment of acute otitis media in children is recommended (Lieberthal et al., 2013). Ampicillin-resistant *H. influenzae* is a problem in many areas. The addition of a β-lactamase inhibitor to *amoxicillin* (*clavulanate*) or *ampicillin* (*sulbactam*) extends the spectrum to β-lactamase–producing *H. influenzae* and *Moraxella*. Amoxicillin is an alternative treatment to penicillin for bacterial pharyngitis.

Urinary Tract Infections. Most uncomplicated urinary tract infections are caused by Enterobacteriaceae, and *E. coli* is the most common species. Aminopenicillins can be effective agents for urinary tract infections, but the high prevalence of resistance amongst *E. coli* and *Klebsiella* makes empiric use of these drugs for urinary tract infections challenging. Enterococcal urinary tract infections are treated effectively with an aminopenicillin alone.

Meningitis. Acute bacterial meningitis in children is frequently due to *S. pneumoniae* or *Neisseria meningitidis*. Because 20%–30% of strains of *S. pneumoniae* now may be resistant to ampicillin, it is not indicated for empiric single-agent treatment of meningitis. Ampicillin has excellent activity against *L. monocytogenes*, a cause of meningitis in immunocompromised persons. The combination of ampicillin and vancomycin plus a third-generation cephalosporin is a recommended regimen for empirical treatment of suspected bacterial meningitis in patients at risk for *L. monocytogenes*.

Antipseudomonal Penicillins: The Carboxypenicillins and the Ureidopenicillins

Antimicrobial Activity

The carboxypenicillins, carbenicillin and ticarcillin (both discontinued in the U.S.), and ureidopenicillins, mezlocillin (discontinued in the U.S.) and piperacillin, are active against some isolates of *Pseudomonas aeruginosa* and certain indole-positive *Proteus* spp. that are resistant to ampicillin and its congeners. The carboxypenicillins are ineffective against most strains of *S. aureus, Enterococcus faecalis, Klebsiella,* and *L. monocytogenes,* but piperacillin (especially when combined with the β-lactamase inhibitor tazobactam) has useful activity against these pathogens and has superior activity against *P. aeruginosa*.

Pharmacological Properties

Carbenicillin Indanyl Sodium. This indanyl ester of carbenicillin is acid stable and is suitable for oral administration. After absorption, the ester is converted rapidly to carbenicillin by hydrolysis of the ester linkage. The antimicrobial spectrum of the drug is therefore that of carbenicillin. The active moiety is excreted rapidly in the urine, where it achieves effective concentrations. Thus, where available, the only use of this drug is for the management of urinary tract infections caused by *Proteus* spp. other than *P. mirabilis* and by *P. aeruginosa*.

Ticarcillin. The semisynthetic penicillin ticarcillin is more active than carbenicillin versus *P. aeruginosa*, but less active than piperacillin. The combination of ticarcillin and clavulanate has activity against other gram-negative aerobic and anaerobic organisms and has been used for intra-abdominal and urinary tract infections. In the U.S., the manufacture of ticarcillin alone and in combination with clavulanate has been discontinued.

Piperacillin. Piperacillin extends the spectrum of ampicillin to include most strains of *P. aeruginosa*, Enterobacteriaceae (non–β-lactamase producing), many *Bacteroides* spp., and *E. faecalis*. Combined with a β-lactamase inhibitor (piperacillin-tazobactam), it has the broadest antibacterial spectrum of the penicillins, including activity against methicillin-susceptible *S. aureus*, *H. influenzae*, *B. fragilis*, and most *E. coli* and *Klebsiella*. The drug is only available for parenteral administration. High biliary concentrations are achieved. Distribution into the CNS by piperacillin is similar to that of other penicillins, but CSF concentrations of tazobactam may be inadequate to protect piperacillin against β-lactamase–producing organisms. The drug is eliminated renally and requires adjustment in renal dysfunction.

Therapeutic Indications

Piperacillin and related agents are important agents for the treatment of patients with serious infections caused by gram-negative bacteria, including infections often acquired in the hospital. Therefore, these penicillins find their greatest use in treating bacteremias, pneumonias, infections following burns, and urinary tract infections owing to microorganisms resistant to ampicillin; the bacteria especially responsible include *P. aeruginosa*, indole-positive strains of *Proteus*, and *Enterobacter* spp. Because *Pseudomonas* infections are common in neutropenic patients, therapy for severe bacterial infections in such individuals should include a β-lactam antibiotic such as piperacillin with good activity against these microorganisms (Freifeld et al., 2012). Because of piperacillin/tazobactam's good activity against *E. faecalis* and *B. fragilis*, this drug also has utility in mixed intra-abdominal infections.

Adverse Reactions

Hypersensitivity Reactions. Hypersensitivity reactions are by far the most common adverse effects noted with the penicillins, and these agents are amongst the most common causes of drug allergy.

Manifestations of hypersensitivity to penicillins include maculopapular rash, urticarial rash, fever, bronchospasm, vasculitis, serum sickness, exfoliative dermatitis, Stevens-Johnson syndrome, and anaphylaxis (Romano et al., 2003). Hypersensitivity reactions may occur with any dosage form of penicillin. Hypersensitivity reactions may appear in the absence of a previous known exposure to the drug. This may be caused by unrecognized prior exposure to penicillin in the environment (e.g., in foods of animal origin or from the fungus-producing penicillin). Although elimination of the antibiotic usually results in rapid clearing of the allergic manifestations, they may persist for 1–2 weeks or longer after therapy has been stopped. In some cases, the reaction is mild and disappears even when the penicillin is continued; in others, immediate cessation of penicillin treatment is required. In many instances, it is necessary to avoid the future use of penicillin because of the risk of severe reactions, and the patient should be so warned. Patients manifesting hypersensitivity to penicillins may be at increased risk for cross-hypersensitivity reactions on receipt of other β-lactams (cephalosporins, carbapenems). The risk is dependent on the reaction and particular β-lactam administered and is discussed further in the relevant sections for those agents.

Penicillins and their breakdown products act as haptens after covalent reaction with proteins. The most abundant breakdown product is the penicilloyl moiety (MDM), which is formed when the β-lactam ring is opened (see Figure 57–4). A large percentage of IgE-mediated reactions are to the MDM, but at least 25% of reactions are to other breakdown products. The terms *major* and *minor determinants* refer to the frequency with which antibodies to these haptens appear to be formed. They do not describe the severity of the reaction that may result. In fact, anaphylactic reactions to penicillin usually are mediated by IgE antibodies against the minor determinants. Antipenicillin antibodies are detectable in virtually all patients who have received the drug and in many who have never knowingly been exposed to it. Immediate allergic reactions are mediated by skin-sensitizing or IgE antibodies, usually of minor-determinant specificities. Accelerated and late urticarial reactions usually are mediated by major-determinant–specific skin-sensitizing antibodies. Some reactions may be due to toxic antigen-antibody complexes of major-determinant–specific IgM antibodies.

The most serious hypersensitivity reactions produced by the penicillins are angioedema and anaphylaxis. Acute anaphylactic or anaphylactoid reactions induced by various preparations of penicillin constitute the most important immediate danger connected with their use. Anaphylactoid reactions may occur at any age. Their incidence is thought to be 0.004%–0.04%. About 0.001% of patients treated with these agents die from anaphylaxis. Anaphylaxis most often has followed the injection of penicillin, although it also has been observed after oral or intradermal administration. The most dramatic reaction is sudden, severe hypotension and rapid death. In other instances, bronchoconstriction with severe asthma; abdominal pain, nausea, and vomiting; extreme weakness; or diarrhea and purpuric skin eruptions have characterized the anaphylactic episodes.

Skin rashes of all types may be caused by allergy to penicillin. The incidence of skin rashes appears to be highest following the use of ampicillin, at about 9%. Rashes follow the administration of ampicillin frequently in patients with infectious mononucleosis, but in such cases, patients can tolerate subsequent courses of ampicillin without experiencing a rash (Kerns et al., 1973). Serum sickness of variable intensity and severity, mediated by IgG antibodies, is rare; when it occurs, it appears after penicillin treatment has been continued for 1 week or more; it may be delayed until 1 or 2 weeks after the drug has been stopped and may persist for a week or longer. Vasculitis may be related to penicillin hypersensitivity. The Coombs reaction frequently becomes positive during prolonged therapy, but hemolytic anemia is rare. Reversible neutropenia has been noted, occurring in up to 30% of patients treated with 8–12 g of nafcillin for more than 21 days. The bone marrow shows an arrest of maturation. Eosinophilia is an occasional accompaniment of other allergic reactions to penicillin. Penicillins rarely cause interstitial nephritis; methicillin (no longer marketed in the U.S.) has been implicated most frequently. Fever may be the only evidence of a hypersensitivity reaction to the penicillins. The febrile reaction usually disappears within 24–36 h after administration of the drug is stopped but may persist for days.

Management of the Patient Potentially Allergic to Penicillin. Evaluation of the patient's history is the most practical way to avoid the use of penicillin in patients who are at the greatest risk of adverse reaction. Although many patients are labeled as penicillin allergic, studies suggested that 90% or more of patients with a history of penicillin allergy will not manifest immediate hypersensitivity reactions on immunologic testing. Such testing can be performed in the clinical setting through commercially available penicillin skin-testing kits that contain the major antigenic determinant (benzylpenicilloyl polylysine); such testing may, however, fail to detect allergies to minor determinants (Sogn et al., 1992). Occasionally, *desensitization* is recommended for penicillin-allergic patients who must receive the drug. This procedure consists of administering gradually increasing doses of penicillin in the hope of avoiding a severe reaction and should be performed only in an intensive care setting. When full doses are reached, penicillin should not be discontinued and then restarted because immediate reactions may recur. Patients with life-threatening infections (e.g., endocarditis or meningitis) may be continued on penicillin despite the development of a maculopapular rash, although alternative antimicrobial agents should be used whenever possible. The rash often resolves as therapy is continued, perhaps owing to the development of blocking antibodies of the IgG class. Rarely, exfoliative dermatitis with or without vasculitis develops in these patients if therapy with penicillin is continued.

Other Adverse Reactions. The penicillins have minimal direct toxicity. Apparent toxic effects include bone marrow depression, granulocytopenia, and hepatitis; the last effect is rare but is seen most commonly following the administration of oxacillin and nafcillin. The administration of penicillin G and piperacillin (also carbenicillin and ticarcillin) has been associated with impaired hemostasis due to defective platelet aggregation (Fass et al., 1987). Most common amongst the irritative responses to penicillins are pain and sterile inflammatory reactions at the sites of intramuscular injections. In some individuals who receive penicillins intravenously, phlebitis or thrombophlebitis develops. Adverse responses to oral penicillin preparations may include nausea, vomiting, and mild-to-severe diarrhea.

When penicillins are injected accidentally into the sciatic nerve, severe pain occurs and dysfunction in the area of distribution of this nerve develops and persists for weeks. Intrathecal injection of penicillin G may produce arachnoiditis or severe and fatal encephalopathy. Because of this, intrathecal or intraventricular administration of penicillins should be avoided. Similarly, high CSF concentrations of penicillins achieved through intravenous administration of excessive doses (including failure to adjust for reduced renal clearance) can lead to CNS dysfunction. The rapid intravenous administration of 20 million units of penicillin G potassium, which contains 34 mEq of K^+, may lead to severe or even fatal hyperkalemia in persons with renal dysfunction. Accidental intravenous instead of intramuscular injection of penicillin G procaine may result in an immediate reaction, characterized by dizziness, tinnitus, headache, hallucinations, and sometimes seizures. This is due to the rapid liberation of toxic concentrations of procaine. Intravenous injection of benzathine penicillin G has been associated with cardiorespiratory arrest and death.

Reactions Unrelated to Hypersensitivity or Toxicity. Penicillin changes the composition of the microflora in the GI tract by eliminating sensitive microorganisms. Normal microflora are typically reestablished shortly after therapy is stopped; however, in some patients, superinfection results. Pseudomembranous colitis, related to overgrowth and production of a toxin by *Clostridium difficile*, has followed oral and, less commonly, parenteral administration of penicillins.

The Cephalosporins

Compounds containing 7-aminocephalosporanic acid are relatively stable in dilute acid and relatively resistant to penicillinase regardless of the nature of their side chains and their affinity for the enzyme. Modifications at position 7 of the β-lactam ring are associated with alteration in antibacterial activity; substitutions at position 3 of the dihydrothiazine ring alter the metabolism and pharmacokinetic properties of the drugs. The cephamycins are similar to the cephalosporins but have a methoxy group at position 7 of the β-lactam ring of the 7-aminocephalosporanic acid nucleus (Table 57–2).

HISTORY

Cephalosporium acremonium, the first source of the cephalosporins, was isolated in 1948 by Brotzu from the sea near a sewer outlet off the Sardinian coast (Grayson, 2010). Crude filtrates from cultures of this fungus were found to inhibit the in vitro growth of *S. aureus* and to cure staphylococcal infections and typhoid fever in humans. Culture fluids in which the Sardinian fungus was cultivated were found to contain three distinct antibiotics, which were named *cephalosporin P, N,* and *C.* With isolation of the active nucleus of cephalosporin C, 7-aminocephalosporanic acid, and with the addition of side chains, it became possible to produce semisynthetic compounds with antibacterial activity very much greater than that of the parent substance.

TABLE 57–2 ■ STRUCTURAL FORMULAS AND DOSAGE DATA FOR SELECTED CEPHALOSPORINS

Cephem Nucleus

COMPOUND	R_1	R_2	DOSAGE FORMS,[a] ADULT DOSAGE FOR SEVERE INFECTION, AND $t_{1/2}$
First generation Cephalexin		$-CH_3$	O: 1 g every 6 h $t_{1/2}$ = 0.9 h
Second generation Cefaclor		$-Cl$	O: 500 mg every 8 h $t_{1/2}$ = 0.7 h
Third generation Cefdinir		$CH = CH_2$	O: 300 mg every 12 h or 600 mg every 24 h $t_{1/2}$ = 1.7 h
Antipseudomonal Ceftazidime		$-CH_2$	I: 2 g every 8 h $t_{1/2}$ = 1.8 h
Anti-MRSA Ceftaroline			I: 600 mg every 12 h $t_{1/2}$ = 2.6 h

[a]C, capsule; I, injection; O, oral suspension T, tablet.

Cephalosporins and cephamycins inhibit bacterial cell wall synthesis in a manner similar to that of penicillin.

Classification

Classification has been by unofficial *generations*, based on general features of antimicrobial activity (Table 57–3). Recent development of novel cephalosporins makes further use of this classification scheme problematic, as newer agents expand activity in different ways. In the absence of consensus on a new generations scheme to date, we will continue to employ this scheme for the first three generations and then differentiate agents after the third generation by their notable activity.

The *first-generation* cephalosporins (e.g., cefazolin, cephalexin, and cefadoxil) have good activity against gram-positive bacteria and modest activity against gram-negative microorganisms. Most gram-positive cocci (with the exception of enterococci, MRSA, and *S. epidermidis*) are susceptible. Most oral cavity anaerobes are sensitive, but the *B. fragilis* group is resistant. These agents have modest activity against *Moraxella catarrhalis*, *E. coli*, *Klebsiella pneumoniae*, and *P. mirabilis*.

The *second-generation* cephalosporins have somewhat increased activity against gram-negative microorganisms (including activity against *H. influenzae*) but are much less active than the third-generation agents.

TABLE 57–3 ■ CEPHALOSPORIN GENERATIONS

DRUG CLASS	USEFUL ANTIBACTERIAL SPECTRUM[a]
First generation	
Cefazolin	Streptococci[b]; *Staphylococcus aureus*[c]; some *Proteus*, *E. coli*, *Klebsiella*.
Cephalexin monohydrate	
Cefadroxil	
Cephradine[d]	
Second generation	
Cefuroxime	*Escherichia coli*, *Klebsiella*, *Proteus*, *Haemophilus influenzae*, *Moraxella catarrhalis*. Not as active against gram-positive organisms as first-generation agents.
Cefuroxime axetil	
Cefprozil	
Cefoxitin	
Cefotetan	Inferior activity against *S. aureus* compared to cefuroxime but with added activity against *Bacteroides fragilis* and other *Bacteroides* spp.
Cefmetazole[d]	
Third generation	
Cefotaxime	*Escherichia coli*, *Klebsiella*, *Proteus*, *Haemophilus influenzae*, *Moraxella catarrhalis*, *Citrobacter*[e], *Enterobacter*[e]; *Serratia*; *Neisseria gonorrhoeae*; activity for *S. aureus*, *Streptococcus pneumoniae*, and *Streptococcus pyogenes* comparable to first-generation agents. Activity against *Bacteroides* spp. inferior to that of cefoxitin and cefotetan.
Ceftriaxone	
Cefdinir	
Cefditoren pivoxil	
Ceftibuten	
Cefpodoxime proxetil	
Ceftizoxime	
Antipseudomonal cephalosporins	
Ceftazidime	Gram-negative activity similar to third generation with addition of activity against *Pseudomonas*[e]; poor activity vs. gram-positive organisms.
Ceftazidime/avibactam	Expands ceftazidime's activity against *Pseudomonas*[e] and multidrug-resistant Enterobactericeae, but not against gram-positives.
Ceftolozane/tazobactam	Similar to ceftazidime, with enhanced activity against *Pseudomonas*[e] and extended-spectrum β-lactamase-producing Enterobactericeae.
Cefepime	Comparable to third generation but more resistant to some β-lactamases (especially those of *Pseudomonas*[e] and *Enterobacter*[e]); gram-positive activity similar to cefotaxime.
Anti-MRSA cephalosporins	
Ceftaroline	Similar activity to 3rd generation but with activity against methicillin resistant *Staphylococcus aureus*.
Ceftobiprole[d]	

[a]All cephalosporins lack clinically useful activity against enterococci, *Listeria monocytogenes*, and atypical respiratory pathogens (*Legionella*, *Mycoplasma*, *Chlamydophila* spp.).
[b]Except for penicillin-resistant strains.
[c]Except for methicillin-resistant strains.
[d]Not marketed in the U.S.
[e]Resistance to cephalosporins may develop during therapy through selection of isolates with de-repression of bacterial chromosomal β-lactamases, which destroy the cephalosporins.

A subset of second-generation agents (cefoxitin and cefotetan) also has modest activity against *B. fragilis*.

Third-generation cephalosporins generally are less active than first-generation agents against gram-positive cocci, although ceftriaxone and cefotaxime in particular have excellent antistreptococcal activity. These agents are much more active than prior generations against the Enterobacteriaceae, although resistance is dramatically increasing due to β-lactamase–producing strains.

Antipseudomonal cephalosporins include ceftazidime (sometimes classified as a third-generation cephalosporin) and cefepime. These agents expand on the gram-negative activity of the third generation to provide useful activity against *P. aeruginosa*. Ceftazidime and ceftolozane have weaker gram-positive activity than third-generation agents, while cefepime's activity is similar to that of ceftriaxone.

Anti-MRSA cephalosporins have structural modifications allowing for binding to and inactivation of the altered PBPs expressed by MRSA, MRSE, and penicillin-resistant *S. pneumoniae*. Ceftaroline and ceftobiprole (not available in the U.S.) are the currently used agents in this class. Ceftaroline's gram-negative activity is similar to that of ceftriaxone, while ceftobiprole's is similar to ceftazidime.

None of the cephalosporins has reliable activity against the following bacteria: *Enterococcus*; *L. monocytogenes*; the atypical respiratory pathogens (*Legionella pneumophila, Mycoplasma pneumoniae, Chlamydophila pneumoniae*); *Legionella micdadei*; *C. difficile*; *Campylobacter jejuni*; and *Acinetobacter* spp.

Mechanisms of Bacterial Resistance

As with the penicillins, resistance to the cephalosporins may be related to the inability of the antibiotic to reach its sites of action or to alterations in the PBPs that are targets of the cephalosporins. Alterations in two PBPs (1A and 2X) that decrease their affinity for cephalosporins render pneumococci resistant to third-generation cephalosporins because the other three PBPs have inherently low affinity. With the exception of ceftaroline and ceftobiprole, cephalosporins lack activity against methicillin-resistant staphylococci due to their inability to bind to the low-affinity PBP expressed by these organisms.

The most prevalent mechanism of resistance to cephalosporins is destruction of the cephalosporins by hydrolysis of the β-lactam ring. The cephalosporins have variable susceptibility to β-lactamases. Cefoxitin, cefuroxime, and the third-generation cephalosporins are more resistant to hydrolysis by the β-lactamases produced by gram-negative bacteria than first-generation cephalosporins. Third-generation cephalosporins (such as ceftazidime and ceftriaxone) are susceptible to hydrolysis by inducible, chromosomally encoded (AmpC) β-lactamases present in gram-negative organisms such as *Citrobacter*, *Enterobacter*, and *Pseudomonas*. The inducible nature of these β-lactamases leads to a lower degree of susceptibility amongst wild-type isolates, whereas selection for mutants with high-level expression (stable derepression) can lead to clinical resistance. These class C enzymes are not substantially inactivated by classical β-lactamase inhibitors such as clavulanate and tazobactam. Cefepime and ceftolozane, by virtue of their structures, may be less susceptible to hydrolysis by class C β-lactamases than are the third-generation agents. They are, however, susceptible to degradation by KPCs and metallo-β-lactamases. The β-lactamase inhibitor avibactam significantly inhibits the activity of AmpC- and KPC-type β-lactamases and is currently available in a coformulation with ceftazidime.

General Pharmacology

Many cephalosporins (cephalexin, cephradine, cefaclor, cefadroxil, loracarbef, cefprozil, cefpodoxime proxetil, ceftibuten, cefuroxime axetil, cefdinir, and cefditoren) are absorbed readily after oral administration; others can be administered intramuscularly or intravenously. Cephalosporins are excreted primarily by the kidney; thus, in general, the dosage should be reduced in patients with renal insufficiency. Exceptions are cefpiramide (no longer marketed in the U.S.) and cefoperazone, which are excreted predominantly in the bile, and ceftriaxone, which has mixed renal/nonrenal elimination. Just as for penicillins, probenecid slows renal tubular secretion of most cephalosporins. Cefotaxime is deacetylated to a metabolite with less antimicrobial activity than the parent compound that is excreted by the kidneys. The other cephalosporins do not undergo appreciable metabolism. Several cephalosporins, most notably ceftriaxone, cefotaxime, ceftazidime, and cefepime, penetrate into the CSF in sufficient concentration to be useful for the treatment of meningitis. Cephalosporins also cross the placenta, and they are found in high concentrations in synovial and pericardial fluids. Penetration into the aqueous humor of the eye is relatively good after systemic administration of third-generation agents, but penetration into the vitreous humor is poor. Concentrations in bile usually are high, especially with cefoperazone and cefpiramide.

Specific Agents

First-Generation Cephalosporins

Cefazolin is relatively well tolerated after either intramuscular or intravenous administration; it is excreted by glomerular filtration and is about 85% bound to plasma proteins. Cefazolin is the only parenteral first-generation cephalosporin marketed in the U.S.

Cephalexin has the same antibacterial spectrum as the other first-generation cephalosporins. It is somewhat less active against penicillinase-producing staphylococci. Oral therapy with cephalexin (usually 0.5 g twice to four times daily) results in peak concentrations in plasma adequate for the inhibition of many gram-positive and gram-negative pathogens. The drug is not metabolized, and 70%–100% is excreted in the urine.

Cephradine and **cefadroxil** are oral agents similar in activity and pharmacokinetics to cephalexin.

Second-Generation Cephalosporins

Cefoxitin and **cefotetan** are technically **cephamycins** and are resistant to some β-lactamases produced by gram-negative rods. Typical of second-generation cephalosporins, they have broader gram-negative activity, including most strains of *Haemophilus* spp., indole-positive *Proteus* spp., and *Klebsiella* spp. These antibiotics are less active than the first-generation cephalosporins against gram-positive bacteria but are more active against anaerobes, especially *B. fragilis*. **Cefmetazole** is a similar agent only marketed outside the U.S.

Cefuroxime has good activity against *H. influenzae* (including strains resistant to ampicillin), *N. meningitidis*, and *S. pneumoniae*. Activity against *E. coli* and *Klebsiella* is modest. Antistaphylococcal activity is inferior to first-generation cephalosporins. Unlike cefoxitin, cefotetan, and cefmetazole, cefuroxime lacks activity against *B. fragilis*. The drug can be given orally, intravenously, or intramuscularly every 8–12 h. Concentrations in CSF are about 10% of those in plasma, and the drug is effective but inferior to ceftriaxone for treatment of meningitis due to susceptible organisms.

Cefuroxime axetil is the 1-acetyloxyethyl ester of cefuroxime. Between 30% and 50% of an oral dose is absorbed, and the drug then is hydrolyzed to cefuroxime; resulting concentrations in plasma are variable.

Cefprozil, **cefaclor**, and **loracarbef** are orally administered agents generally similar to cefuroxime axetil.

Third-Generation Cephalosporins

Cefotaxime is resistant to many narrow-spectrum β-lactamases and has good activity against most gram-positive and gram-negative aerobic bacteria. However, activity against *B. fragilis* is poor, and the increasingly prevalent ESBLs and KPCs confer resistance to cefotaxime. Cefotaxime has a $t_{1/2}$ in plasma of about 1 h and should be administered every 4–8 h for serious infections. The drug is metabolized in vivo to desacetylcefotaxime, which is less active than is the parent compound. Concentrations achieved in the CSF are adequate for treatment of meningitis caused by *H. influenzae*, penicillin-sensitive *S. pneumoniae*, and *N. meningitidis*.

Ceftriaxone has activity very similar to that of cefotaxime but a longer $t_{1/2}$ (~8 h), allowing for once-daily dosing for most indications. Administration of the drug twice daily has been effective for patients with meningitis. About half the drug can be recovered from the urine; the remainder is eliminated by biliary secretion. Single doses of intramuscular ceftriaxone have long been used in the management of urethral, cervical, rectal, or pharyngeal gonorrhea; increasing resistance has necessitated the use of higher doses (250 instead of 125 mg) and routine coadministration of azithromycin (Centers for Disease Control and Prevention, 2015).

Ceftizoxime (not marketed in the U.S.) has a spectrum of activity in vitro that is similar to that of cefotaxime, except that it is less active against *S. pneumoniae* and more active against *B. fragilis*. The $t_{1/2}$ is 1.8 h, and the drug thus can be administered every 8–12 h for serious infections. Ceftizoxime is not metabolized; 90% is recovered in urine.

Cefpodoxime proxetil and **cefditoren pivoxil** are orally administered prodrugs that are hydrolyzed by esterases during absorption to the active forms (cefpodoxime and cefditoren, respectively). These drugs provide similar, but less potent, activity as cefotaxime against methicillin-susceptible strains of *S. aureus* and penicillin-susceptible strains of *S. pneumoniae*, *S. pyogenes*, *H. influenzae*, *H. parainfluenzae*, and *M. catarrhalis*. They are eliminated unchanged in the urine.

Cefixime is orally effective against urinary tract infections caused by *E. coli* and *P. mirabilis*; otitis media caused by *H. influenzae* and *S. pyogenes*; pharyngitis due to *S. pyogenes*; and uncomplicated gonorrhea (although intramuscular ceftriaxone is preferred for gonorrhea). It is available as an oral suspension. Cefixime has a plasma $t_{1/2}$ of 3–4 h and is both excreted in the urine and eliminated in the bile. The standard dose for adults is 400 mg/d for 5–7 days and for a longer interval in patients with *S. pyogenes*. Doses must be reduced in patients with renal impairment. Pediatric dosing for children 6 months and older and less than 45 kg is based on weight (8 mg/kg/d).

Ceftibuten and **cefdinir** are orally administered cephalosporins similar in spectrum and pharmacokinetics to cefixime.

Antipseudomonal Cephalosporins

Ceftazidime is one-quarter to one-half as active against gram-positive microorganisms as is cefotaxime; activity against staphylococci is particularly poor. Its activity against the Enterobacteriaceae is similar to ceftriaxone, but its major distinguishing feature is excellent activity against *Pseudomonas*. Ceftazidime has poor activity against *B. fragilis*. It only achieves therapeutic levels through parenteral administration, with a $t_{1/2}$ in plasma of about 1.5 h; the drug is renally eliminated and requires adjustment in renal dysfunction. The activity of ceftazidime against ESBL- and KPC-producing Enterobacteriaceae and AmpC β-lactamase-overexpressing *Pseudomonas* is enhanced when it is combined with the β-lactamase inhibitor avibactam in **ceftazidime/avibactam**.

Ceftolozane is a structural analogue of ceftazidime that has enhanced activity against *Pseudomonas*, including activity against strains resistant to ceftazidime through β-lactamase overexpression. It has similarly weak activity to ceftazidime against gram-positive organisms. It is commercially available as the coformulation **ceftolozane/tazobactam**, which improves its activity against ESBL-producing Enterobacteriaceae. Its pharmacokinetics are similar to ceftazidime, with a half-life after intravenous administration of approximately 2.5 h and renal elimination.

Cefepime and **cefpirome** (not available in the U.S.) are parenteral antipseudomonal cephalosporins sometimes also classified as "fourth-generation" agents. They provide similarly excellent activity to cefotaxime against Enterobacteriaceae and are relatively resistant to AmpC chromosomally encoded β-lactamases. Thus, they are active against many organisms such as *Enterobacter* and *Pseudomonas* that are resistant to other cephalosporins via overexpression of chromosomally encoded AmpC β-lactamases. However, other mechanisms (such as active efflux) in *Pseudomonas* may still confer cefepime resistance. Cefepime is susceptible to varying degrees to hydrolysis by ESBLs and to a great extent to KPCs. Cefepime has higher activity than ceftazidime and comparable activity to cefotaxime for streptococci and methicillin-sensitive *S. aureus*. Cefepime is excreted renally; doses should be adjusted for renal failure. The serum $t_{1/2}$ is 2 h. Cefepime has excellent penetration into the CSF in animal models of meningitis.

Anti-MRSA Cephalosporins

Ceftaroline fosamil is a new cephalosporin with gram-negative activity comparable to cefotaxime. Its distinguishing feature is its enhanced gram-positive activity, especially its ability to bind to the low-affinity PBPs of MRSA and penicillin-resistant *S. pneumoniae*. Over 95% of MRSA and penicillin-resistant *S. pneumoniae* isolates are inhibited by ceftaroline.

The parenteral preparation is a prodrug that is rapidly converted to active ceftaroline on intravenous administration. It is primarily eliminated by the kidneys with a half-life of approximately 2 h. Ceftaroline has minimal protein binding (~20%) and appears to distribute well into most tissues, though penetration into the CSF has not yet been well characterized.

Ceftobiprole medocaril (not available in the U.S.) has similar activity to ceftaroline against gram-positive organisms. In contrast to all other cephalosporins, it has appreciable in vitro activity against *E. faecalis*; however, its clinical utility against this organism is not established. Its gram-negative spectrum includes activity similar to cefepime against *Pseudomonas* spp. and other gram-negative bacilli. As with ceftaroline, its intravenous formulation is a prodrug that is rapidly cleaved to the active moiety. Its pharmacokinetics are similar to those of ceftaroline.

Adverse Reactions

Hypersensitivity reactions to the cephalosporins are the most common side effects; they are similar to those caused by the penicillins. Immediate reactions such as anaphylaxis, bronchospasm, and urticaria are observed. More commonly, maculopapular rash develops, usually after several days of therapy; this may or may not be accompanied by fever and eosinophilia. Because of the common β-lactam ring structure, there is potential for patients who are allergic to one class of β-lactam antibiotics to manifest cross-reactivity to a member of the other class. Some allergic reactions may be directed to the β-lactam side chains, which may be similar between agents in different classes. Thus, estimating the likelihood of cross-reactivity between a penicillin and cephalosporin depends on the agents involved; risk seems to be higher with first-generation cephalosporins as opposed to later generations.

Patients with a history of a mild or a temporally distant reaction to penicillin appear to be at low risk of allergic reaction following the administration of a cephalosporin. However, patients who have a history of a severe, immediate reaction to a penicillin should be skin tested to confirm penicillin allergy before cephalosporin administration, if feasible. If skin testing is not feasible, administration of a cephalosporin should be avoided if possible. A positive Coombs reaction appears frequently in patients who receive large doses of a cephalosporin, but hemolysis is rare. Cephalosporins have produced rare instances of bone marrow depression, characterized by granulocytopenia.

Some cephalosporins are potentially nephrotoxic. Renal tubular necrosis has followed the administration of cephaloridine in doses greater than 4 g/d; this agent is not licensed for use in the U.S. Other cephalosporins, when used by themselves in recommended doses, rarely produce significant renal toxicity. Diarrhea can result from the administration of cephalosporins and may be more frequent with cefoperazone, perhaps because of its greater biliary excretion. The high binding affinity of ceftriaxone for serum albumin may displace bilirubin, potentially causing jaundice in neonates; for this reason, cefotaxime is the preferred agent in this patient population. Ceftriaxone's high biliary concentrations combined with its affinity for calcium can lead to biliary pseudolithiasis. Cephalosporins containing a methylthiotetrazole group (cefamandole [not available in the U.S.], cefotetan, and cefoperazone) can prolong the prothrombin time, an effect that may be associated with clinically significant bleeding amongst patients receiving anticoagulation or with vitamin K deficiency. Encephalopathy and nonconvulsive status epilepticus have been reported with cefepime, especially when administered at high doses or amongst patients with renal dysfunction.

Therapeutic Uses

The **first-generation cephalosporins** are excellent agents for skin and soft tissue infections owing to their activity against *S. pyogenes* and methicillin-susceptible *S. aureus* (Stevens et al., 2014). A single dose of cefazolin just before surgery is the preferred prophylaxis for procedures in which skin flora are the likely pathogens (Bratzler et al., 2013).

Second-generation cephalosporins generally have been displaced by third-generation agents. The oral second-generation cephalosporins can be used to treat respiratory tract infections, although they are suboptimal (compared with oral amoxicillin) for treatment of penicillin-nonsusceptible *S. pneumoniae* pneumonia and otitis media. Cefoxitin and cefotetan play a useful role in perioperative prophylaxis for patients undergoing intra-abdominal and gynecologic surgical procedures. They may also be used for treatment of certain anaerobic and mixed aerobic-anaerobic infections, such as peritonitis and pelvic inflammatory disease, although because of increasing resistance amongst *B. fragilis*, these agents are best used for mild-to-moderate infections.

The **third-generation cephalosporins** are the drugs of choice for serious infections caused by *E. coli*, *Klebsiella*, *Proteus*, *Providencia*, *Serratia*, and *Haemophilus* spp. Ceftriaxone is the therapy of choice for all forms of gonorrhea and for severe forms of Lyme disease. Cefotaxime or ceftriaxone are used for the empiric treatment of meningitis in nonimmunocompromised adults and children (in combination with vancomycin and ampicillin pending identification of the causative agent), owing to their excellent activity against *H. influenzae*, sensitive *S. pneumoniae*, *N. meningitidis*, and gram-negative enteric bacteria (Tunkel et al., 2004). Third-generation cephalosporins lack activity against *L. monocytogenes* and penicillin-resistant pneumococci, which may cause meningitis. The antimicrobial spectra of cefotaxime and ceftriaxone are excellent for the treatment of community-acquired pneumonia.

The **antipseudomonal cephalosporins** are indicated for the empirical treatment of nosocomial infections where *Pseudomonas* and other resistant gram-negative bacilli are likely to be pathogens. Ceftolozane/tazobactam may have superior activity against some ceftazidime-resistant *Pseudomonas*, whereas cefepime has superior activity against nosocomial isolates of *Enterobacter*, *Citrobacter*, and *Serratia* spp. Activity of ceftazidime, ceftolozane/tazobactam, and cefepime is variable against ESBL-producing isolates and absent against KPC-expressing strains; ceftazidime/avibactam is more likely to be active against these highly resistant organisms.

Other β-Lactam Antibiotics

Carbapenems

Carbapenems are β-lactams that contain a fused β-lactam ring and a five-member ring system that differs from the penicillins because it is unsaturated and contains a carbon atom instead of the sulfur atom. This class of antibiotics has a broader spectrum of activity than most other β-lactam antibiotics.

Imipenem

Imipenem is marketed in combination with cilastatin, a drug that inhibits the degradation of imipenem by a renal tubular dipeptidase.

Antimicrobial Activity. Imipenem, like other β-lactam antibiotics, binds to PBPs, disrupts bacterial cell wall synthesis, and causes death of susceptible microorganisms. It is very resistant to hydrolysis by most β-lactamases. The activity of imipenem is excellent in vitro for a wide variety of aerobic and anaerobic microorganisms. Streptococci (including penicillin-resistant *S. pneumoniae*); enterococci (excluding *Enterococcus faecium* and non–β-lactamase–producing penicillin-resistant strains); staphylococci (including penicillinase-producing strains but not MRSA); and *Listeria* (although ampicillin is more active) all are typically susceptible. Activity is excellent against the Enterobacteriaceae with the exception of emerging KPC-producing strains. Most strains of *Pseudomonas* and *Acinetobacter* are inhibited, but resistance to carbapenems amongst these organisms is increasing. Anaerobes, including *B. fragilis*, are highly susceptible. Imipenem also displays activity against *Nocardia* spp. and some species of rapidly growing mycobacteria.

Pharmacokinetics and Adverse Reactions. Imipenem is not absorbed orally. The drug is hydrolyzed rapidly by a dipeptidase found in the brush border of the proximal tubule. To prolong drug activity, *imipenem* is combined with *cilastatin*, an inhibitor of the dehydropeptidase. Both imipenem and cilastatin have a $t_{1/2}$ of about 1 h. When administered concurrently with cilastatin, about 70% of administered imipenem is recovered in the urine as the active drug. Dosage should be modified for patients with renal insufficiency. Nausea and vomiting are the most common adverse reactions (1%–20%). Seizures have been noted in up to 1.5% of patients, especially when high doses are given to patients with CNS lesions and to those with

renal insufficiency. Patients who are allergic to other β-lactam antibiotics may have hypersensitivity reactions when given imipenem, although the incidence of immediate-type hypersensitivity appears to be low (<1%).

Therapeutic Uses. Imipenem-cilastatin is effective for a wide variety of infections, including urinary tract and lower respiratory infections; intra-abdominal and gynecological infections; and skin, soft tissue, bone, and joint infections. The drug combination appears to be especially useful for the treatment of infections caused by cephalosporin-resistant nosocomial bacteria. It is prudent to use imipenem for empirical treatment of serious infections in hospitalized patients who have recently received other β-lactam antibiotics. When imipenem is used for treatment of severe *P. aeruginosa* infections, resistance may develop during therapy.

Meropenem

Meropenem is a derivative of thienamycin. It does not require coadministration with cilastatin because it is not sensitive to renal dipeptidase. Compared to imipenem, it is somewhat less active against gram-positive organisms (particularly *Enterococcus*) and more active against gram-negative organisms. Its toxicity is similar to that of imipenem except that it may be less likely to cause seizures; thus, it is preferred for treatment of meningitis when carbapenem therapy is required.

Doripenem

Doripenem has a spectrum of activity that is similar to that of meropenem, with greater activity against some resistant isolates of *Pseudomonas*.

Ertapenem

Ertapenem differs from imipenem and meropenem by having a longer $t_{1/2}$ that allows once-daily dosing and by having inferior activity against *Enterococcus*, *P. aeruginosa*, and *Acinetobacter* spp. Its activity against Enterobacteriaceae and anaerobes makes it useful in intra-abdominal and pelvic infections.

Monobactams

Monobactams are β-lactams that contain only a fused β-lactam ring, not a thiazolidine or dihydrothiazidine ring. Currently, aztreonam is the only member of this class in therapeutic use.

Aztreonam

Aztreonam is resistant to narrow-spectrum β-lactamases elaborated by most gram-negative bacteria as well as metallo-β-lactamases, but not most extended-spectrum or KPC-type β-lactamases. Aztreonam has activity only against gram-negative bacteria; it has no activity against gram-positive bacteria and anaerobic organisms. Activity against Enterobacteriaceae and *P. aeruginosa* is similar to that of ceftazidime. It is also highly active in vitro against *H. influenzae*. Aztreonam is administered either intramuscularly or intravenously. The $t_{1/2}$ for elimination is 1.7 h; most of the drug is recovered unaltered in the urine. The $t_{1/2}$ is prolonged to about 6 h in anephric patients. The usual dose of aztreonam for severe infections is 2 g every 6–8 h (reduced in patients with renal insufficiency). A notable feature is a lack of allergic cross-reactivity with other β-lactam antibiotics, with the possible exception of ceftazidime, with which it shares an identical side chain (Perez Pimiento et al., 1998). Aztreonam is therefore useful for treating gram-negative infections that normally would be treated with a β-lactam antibiotic were it not for a prior allergic reaction. Aztreonam generally is well tolerated, although hepatotoxicity, especially in infants and young children, can occur.

β-Lactamase Inhibitors

Certain molecules can inactivate β-lactamases and prevent the destruction of β-lactam antibiotic substrates. Older-generation β-lactamase inhibitors (*clavulanate, sulbactam, tazobactam*) are most active against plasmid-encoded β-lactamases (including those that hydrolyze ceftazidime and cefotaxime), but they are inactive at clinically achievable concentrations against the AmpC chromosomal β-lactamases present in gram-negative bacilli (e.g., *Enterobacter*, *Citrobacter*, and *Pseudomonas*) as well as carbapenemases of the KPC- and metallo-β-lactamase type. *Avibactam* is a new β-lactamase inhibitor that is structurally dissimilar from the older generation, with a broader spectrum of inhibition.

Clavulanic acid has poor intrinsic antimicrobial activity but is a "suicide" inhibitor that binds β-lactamases produced by a wide range of gram-positive and gram-negative microorganisms. Clavulanic acid is well absorbed by mouth and also can be given parenterally. It is combined with amoxicillin as an oral preparation and with ticarcillin as a parenteral preparation.

CLAVULANIC ACID

Sulbactam is a β-lactamase inhibitor similar in structure to clavulanic acid. It is available for intravenous or intramuscular use combined with ampicillin and with cefoperazone (not available in the U.S.). Sulbactam also possesses intrinsic activity against *Acinetobacter* spp. and has been used in high dosages to treat multidrug-resistant *Acinetobacter* infections.

Tazobactam is a β-lactamase inhibitor with good activity against many of the plasmid β-lactamases, including some of the extended-spectrum class. It is available as parenteral combination products with piperacillin and ceftolozane.

Avibactam is a non–β-lactam β-lactamase inhibitor that provides clinically useful inhibition against narrow-spectrum, ESBL-type, chromosomal AmpC, and KPC-type β-lactamases (although not metallo-β-lactamases). It is available as a parenteral combination product with ceftazidime.

Acknowledgment: *William A. Petri, Jr., contributed to this chapter in recent editions of this book. We have retained some of his text in the current edition.*

Drug Facts for Your Personal Formulary: *β-Lactam Antibiotics*

Drugs	Therapeutic Uses	Clinical Pharmacology and Tips
Penicillins—Inhibitors of Bacterial Cell Wall Peptidoglycan Synthesis		
General: Bactericidal, renal elimination, hypersensitivity reactions (rash, anaphylaxis)		
Penicillin G (IV), penicillin V (PO); IM depot formulations (benzathine, procaine)	• Penicillin-susceptible *Streptococcus pneumoniae* infections: pneumonia, meningitis • Streptococcal pharyngitis, endocarditis, skin and soft tissue infection • *Neisseria meningitidis* infections • Syphilis	• Excellent activity vs. *Treponema pallidum*, β-hemolytic streptococci, *N. meningitidis*, gram-positive anaerobes • Good activity vs. *S. pneumoniae*, viridans streptococci • CSF penetration with inflammation
Penicillinase-resistant penicillins Oxacillin (IV), nafcillin (IV), dicloxacillin (PO)	• Skin and soft tissue infections • Serious infections due to MSSA	• Excellent activity vs. MSSA • Good activity vs. streptococci • Nafcillin nonrenal elimination • CSF penetration with inflammation
Aminopenicillins Amoxicillin (PO), ampicillin (PO/IV)	• Upper respiratory tract infections (sinusitis, pharyngitis, otitis media) • *Enterococcus faecalis* infections • *Listeria* infections	• Excellent activity vs. β-hemolytic streptococci, *E. faecalis* • Good activity vs. *S. pneumoniae*, viridans streptococci, *Haemophilus influenzae* • Some activity vs. *Proteus*, *Escherichia coli* • CSF penetration with inflammation • Rash more common than other penicillins
Aminopenicillin/β-lactamase inhibitors Amoxicillin/clavulanate (PO), ampicillin/sulbactam (IV)	• Upper respiratory tract infections (sinusitis, otitis media) • Intra-abdominal infections	• Activity: amoxicillin and ampicillin plus • Excellent activity vs. *H. influenzae*, *Bacteroides fragilis*, *Proteus* • Good activity vs. *E. coli*, *Klebsiella*, MSSA
Antipseudomonal penicillins Piperacillin/tazobactam (IV)	• Nosocomial infections: pneumonia, intra-abdominal infections, urinary tract infections	• Activity: ampicillin/sulbactam plus • Excellent activity vs. *E. coli*, *Klebsiella* • Good activity vs. *Pseudomonas*, *Citrobacter*, *Enterobacter* • Poor CSF penetration
Cephalosporins—Inhibitors of Bacterial Cell Wall Peptidoglycan Synthesis		
General: Bactericidal, renal elimination, hypersensitivity reactions (rash, anaphylaxis)		
First-generation cephalosporins Cefazolin (IV), cephalexin (PO), cefadroxil (PO)	• Skin and soft tissue infections • Serious infections due to MSSA • Perioperative surgical prophylaxis	• Excellent activity vs. MSSA, streptococci • Some activity vs. *Proteus*, *E. coli*, *Klebsiella* • Poor CSF penetration
Second-generation cephalosporins Cefuroxime (IV/PO), cefoxitin (IV), cefotetan (IV), cefaclor (PO), cefprozil (PO)	• Upper respiratory tract infections (sinusitis, otitis media) • Cefoxitin/cefotetan: gynecologic infections, perioperative surgical prophylaxis	• Good activity vs. MSSA, streptococci, *H. influenzae*, *Proteus*, *E. coli*, *Klebsiella* • Cefoxitin/cefotetan: some activity vs. *B. fragilis*
Third-generation cephalosporins Cefotaxime (IV), ceftriaxone (IV), cefpodoxime (PO), cefixime (PO), cefdinir (PO), cefditoren (PO), ceftibuten (PO)	• Community-acquired pneumonia, meningitis, urinary tract infections • Streptococcal endocarditis • Gonorrhea • Severe Lyme disease	• Excellent activity against streptococci, *H. influenzae*, *Proteus*, *E. coli*, *Klebsiella*, *Serratia*, *Neisseria* • Good activity vs. MSSA • Some activity vs. *Citrobacter*, *Enterobacter* • Ceftriaxone renal and nonrenal elimination • Good CSF penetration • Ceftriaxone: neonatal kernicterus (use cefotaxime), biliary pseudolithiasis

Cephalosporins—Inhibitors of Bacterial Cell Wall Peptidoglycan Synthesis

General: Bactericidal, renal elimination, hypersensitivity reactions (rash, anaphylaxis) (continued)

Antipseudomonal cephalosporins Ceftazidime (IV), ceftolozane/tazobactam (IV), ceftazidime/avibactam (IV), cefepime (IV)	• Nosocomial infections: pneumonia, meningitis, urinary tract infections, intra-abdominal infections (with metronidazole)	• Excellent activity against *H. influenzae, Proteus, E. coli, Klebsiella, Serratia, Neisseria*, streptococci,[a] MSSA[a] • Good activity vs. *Pseudomonas, Enterobacter*[b] • Some activity vs. *Enterobacter* (ceftazidime, ceftolozane/tazobactam) • Ceftazidime/avibactam active vs. ESBL and KPC-producing Enterobacteriaceae • Good CSF penetration • Cefepime: encephalopathy at high doses
Anti-MRSA cephalosporins Cefaroline (IV)	• Community-acquired pneumonia • Skin and soft tissue infections	• Excellent activity against streptococci, MSSA, MRSA,[c] *H. influenzae, Proteus, E. coli, Klebsiella, Serratia* • Some activity vs. *Citrobacter, Enterobacter*

Carbapenems—Inhibitors of Bacterial Cell Wall Synthesis

General: Bactericidal, renal elimination, hypersensitivity reactions (rash, anaphylaxis), seizure risk

Imipenem/cilastatin (IV), meropenem (IV), doripenem (IV)	• Nosocomial infections: pneumonia, intra-abdominal infections, urinary tract infections • Meningitis (meropenem)	• Excellent activity against streptococci, MSSA, *H. influenzae, Proteus, E. coli, Klebsiella, Serratia, Enterobacter, B. fragilis* • Good activity vs. *Pseudomonas, Acinetobacter, Enterococcus faecalis*[d] • Good CSF penetration • Imipenem coformulated with renal dihydropeptidase inhibitor cilastatin • Seizures at high doses in patients with prior seizure history (imipenem > meropenem, doripenem)
Ertapenem (IV)	• Community-acquired infections and nosocomial infections without *Pseudomonas* risk	• Excellent activity against streptococci, MSSA, *H. influenzae, Proteus, E. coli, Klebsiella, Serratia, Enterobacter, B. fragilis* • Lacks activity against *Pseudomonas, Enterococcus* • Lower seizure risk than imipenem

Monobactam—Bactericidal Inhibitor of Bacterial Cell Wall Synthesis

Aztreonam (IV)	• Nosocomial infections: pneumonia, urinary tract infections	• Excellent activity against *H. influenzae, Proteus, E. coli, Klebsiella, Serratia* • Good activity vs. *Pseudomonas* • Lacks any gram-positive activity • Lacks cross-allergenicity with other β-lactams (except ceftazidime) • Good CSF penetration, renal elimination

[a]Cefepime only.
[b]Cefepime, ceftazidime/avibactam.
[c]Only β-lactam with significant activity versus MRSA.
[d]Imipenem only.

Bibliography

Bayles KW. The bactericidal action of penicillin: new clues to an unsolved mystery. *Trends Microbiol*, **2000**, 8:81274–81278.

Bratzler DW, et al. Clinical practice guidelines for antimicrobial prophylaxis in surgery. *Surg Infect (Larchmt)*, **2013**, 14:73–156.

Brown EJ. The molecular basis of streptococcal toxic shock syndrome. *N Engl J Med*, **2004**, 350:2093–2094.

Carratalá J, et al. Bacteremia due to viridans streptococci that are highly resistant to penicillin: increase among neutropenic patients with cancer. *Clin Infect Dis*, **1995**, 20:1169–1173.

Centers for Disease Control and Prevention. Sexually transmitted diseases guidelines. **2015**. Available at: http://www.cdc.gov/std/treatment/. Accessed July 3, 2015.

de Gans J, et al. Dexamethasone in adults with bacterial meningitis. *N Engl J Med*, **2002**, 347:1549–1556.

Donlan RM. Biofilm formation: a clinically relevant microbiologic process. *Clin Infect Dis*, **2001**, 33:1387–1392.

Fass RJ, et al. Platelet-mediated bleeding caused by broad-spectrum penicillins. *J Infect Dis*, **1987**, 155:1242–1248.

Fernández L, Hancock RE. Adaptive and mutational resistance: role of porins and efflux pumps in drug resistance. *Clin Microbiol Rev*, **2012**, 25:661–681.

Freifeld AG, et al. Clinical practice guideline for the use of antimicrobial agents in neutropenic patients with cancer: 2010 update by the Infectious Diseases Society of America. *Clin Infect Dis*, **2012**, *52*: e56–e93.

Grayson ML, ed. *Kucers' The Use of Antibiotics: A Clinical Review of Antibacterial, Antifungal, Antiparasitic, and Antiviral Drugs.* Hodder Arnold, London, **2010**.

Jacoby GA, Munoz-Price L. The new beta-lactamases. *N Engl J Med*, **2005**, *352*:380–391.

Kerns DL, et al. Ampicillin rash in children: relationship to penicillin allergy and infectious mononucleosis. *Am J Dis Child*, **1973**, *125*:187–190.

Lax E. *The Mold in Dr. Florey's Coat: The Story of the Penicillin Miracle.* Henry Holt, New York, **2004**.

Levison ME, et al. Clindamycin compared with penicillin for the treatment of anaerobic lung abscess. *Ann Intern Med*, **1983**, 98:466–471.

Lieberthal AS, et al. The diagnosis and management of acute otitis media. *Pediatrics*, **2013**, 131:e964–99.

Nikaido H. Antibiotic resistance caused by gram-negative multidrug efflux pumps. *Clin Infect Dis*, **1998**, 27(suppl I):S32–S41.

Perez Pimiento A, et al. Aztreonam and ceftazidime: evidence of in vivo cross allergenicity. *Allergy*, **1998**, 53:624–625.

Queenan AM, Bush K. Carbapenemases: the versatile beta-lactamases. *Clin Microbiol Rev*, **2007**, 20:440–458.

Romano A, et al. Immediate allergic reactions to β-lactams: diagnosis and therapy. *Int J Immunopathol Pharmacol*, **2003**, *16*:19–23.

Shulman ST, et al. Clinical practice guideline for the diagnosis and management of group A streptococcal pharyngitis: 2012 update by the Infectious Diseases Society of America. *Clin Infect Dis*, **2012**, *55*:1279–1282.

Sogn DD, et al. Results of the NIAID collaborative clinical trial to test the predictive value of skin testing with major and minor penicillin derivatives in hospitalized adults. *Arch Intern Med*, **1992**, *152*:1025–1032.

Spratt BG. Resistance to antibiotics mediated by target alterations. *Science*, **1994**, *264*:388–339.

Stevens DL, et al. Practice guidelines for the diagnosis and management of skin and soft tissue infections: 2014 update by the Infectious Diseases Society of America. *Clin Infect Dis*, **2014**, *15*:e10–e52.

Tunkel AR, et al. Practice guidelines for the management of bacterial meningitis. *Clin Infect Dis*, **2004**, *39*:1267–1284.

Zapun A, et al. Penicillin-binding proteins and beta-lactam resistance. *FEMS Microbiol Rev*, **2008**, *32*:361–385.

Chapter 58

Aminoglycosides
Conan MacDougall

ORIGINS

Aminoglycosides are natural products or semisynthetic derivatives of compounds produced by a variety of soil actinomycetes. Streptomycin was first isolated from a strain of *Streptomyces griseus*. Gentamicin and netilmicin are derived from species of the actinomycete *Micromonospora*. The difference in spelling (*-micin*) compared with the other aminoglycoside antibiotics (*-mycin*) reflects this difference in origin. Tobramycin is one of several components of an aminoglycoside complex known as "nebramycin" that is produced by *Streptomyces tenebrarius*. It is most similar in antimicrobial activity and toxicity to gentamicin. In contrast to the other aminoglycosides, amikacin, a derivative of kanamycin, and netilmicin, a derivative of sisomicin, are semisynthetic products.

Aminoglycosides are natural products or semisynthetic derivatives of compounds produced by a variety of soil actinomycetes. Amikacin, a derivative of kanamycin, and netilmicin, a derivative of sisomicin, are semisynthetic products.

Aminoglycosides (*gentamicin, tobramycin, amikacin, netilmicin, kanamycin, streptomycin, paromomycin,* and *neomycin*) are used primarily to treat infections caused by aerobic gram-negative bacteria. Streptomycin and amikacin are important agents for the treatment of mycobacterial infections, and paromomycin is used orally for intestinal amebiasis. Aminoglycosides are *bactericidal inhibitors* of protein synthesis. Mutations affecting proteins in the bacterial ribosome can confer marked resistance to their action. Most commonly, resistance is due to aminoglycoside-metabolizing enzymes or impaired transport of drug into the cell; these mechanisms may confer resistance to all aminoglycosides or only select agents. Resistance genes are frequently acquired via plasmids or transposons.

Aminoglycosides contain amino sugars linked to an aminocyclitol ring by glycosidic bonds (Figure 58–1). They are polycations, and their polarity is responsible in part for pharmacokinetic properties shared by all members of the group. For example, none is absorbed adequately after oral administration, inadequate concentrations are found in CSF, and all are excreted relatively rapidly by the normal kidney. All members of the group share the same spectrum of toxicity, most notably nephrotoxicity and ototoxicity, which can involve the auditory and vestibular functions of the eighth cranial nerve.

Mechanism of Action

The aminoglycoside antibiotics are rapidly bactericidal. Bacterial killing is concentration dependent: the higher the concentration, the greater the rate of bacterial killing. The ratio of the peak concentration to the organism's *MIC* is thus a key predictor of aminoglycoside efficacy. The inhibitory activity of aminoglycosides persists after the serum concentration has fallen below the MIC, a phenomenon known as the *postantibiotic effect*. These properties probably account for the efficacy of high-dose, extended-interval dosing regimens.

Aminoglycosides diffuse through aqueous channels formed by *porin* proteins in the outer membrane of gram-negative bacteria to enter the periplasmic space. Transport of aminoglycosides across the cytoplasmic (inner) membrane depends on a transmembrane electrical gradient coupled to electron transport to drive permeation of these antibiotics. This energy-dependent phase is rate limiting and can be blocked or inhibited by divalent cations (e.g., Ca^{2+} and Mg^{2+}), hyperosmolarity, a reduction in pH, and anaerobic conditions. Thus, the antimicrobial activity of aminoglycosides is reduced markedly in the anaerobic environment of an abscess and in hyperosmolar acidic urine.

Once inside the cell, aminoglycosides bind to polysomes and interfere with protein synthesis by causing misreading and premature termination

Abbreviations

AC: acetylase
AD: adenylase
ADME: absorption, distribution, metabolism, excretion
CNS: central nervous system
CSF: cerebrospinal fluid
GI: gastrointestinal
IM: intramuscular
IV: intravenous
MIC: minimum inhibitory concentration
mRNA: messenger RNA
PO: by mouth
UTI: urinary tract infection

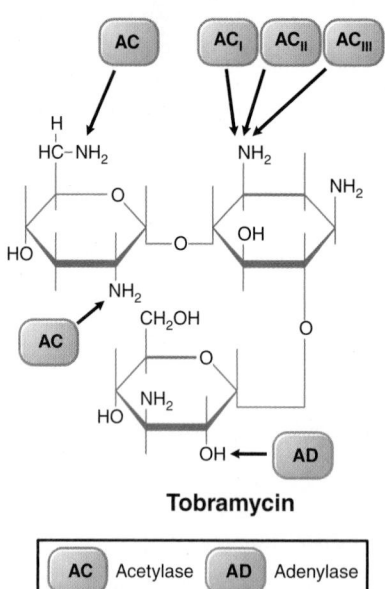

Tobramycin

| AC | Acetylase | AD | Adenylase |

Figure 58–1 *Aminoglycoside structure and sites of activity of plasmid-mediated enzymes capable of inactivating aminoglycosides.* Tobramycin is shown as a representative; structural characteristics protect some aminoglycosides from the actions of some of these enzymes, explaining differences in spectrum of activity.

of mRNA translation (Figure 58–2). The primary intracellular site of action of the aminoglycosides is the 30S ribosomal subunit. At least three of these ribosomal proteins, and perhaps the 16S ribosomal RNA as well, contribute to the streptomycin-binding site. *Aminoglycosides interfere with the initiation of protein synthesis, leading to the accumulation of abnormal initiation complexes; the drugs also can cause misreading of the mRNA template and incorporation of incorrect amino acids into the growing polypeptide chains* (Davis, 1988). The resulting aberrant proteins may be inserted into the cell membrane, leading to altered permeability and further stimulation of aminoglycoside transport (Busse et al., 1992).

Antimicrobial Activity

The antibacterial activity of gentamicin, tobramycin, and amikacin is directed primarily against aerobic gram-negative bacilli (Mingeot-Leclercq et al., 1999). Kanamycin, like streptomycin, has a more limited spectrum. The aerobic gram-negative bacilli vary in their susceptibility to the aminoglycosides (see Table 58–1). Gram-negative aerobic cocci such as *Neisseria, Moraxella,* and *Haemophilus* have varying susceptibilities. An increasing number of gram-negative bacilli encountered in healthcare settings (especially *Klebsiella* and *Pseudomonas*) display extensive resistance to multiple classes of antibacterials; in these isolates, aminoglycosides may be the only class of commonly used agents with in vitro activity.

Aminoglycosides have little activity against anaerobic microorganisms or facultative bacteria under anaerobic conditions. Their action against most gram-positive bacteria is limited, and they should not be used as single agents to treat infections caused by gram-positive bacteria. However, in combination with a cell wall–active agent, such as a penicillin or vancomycin, an aminoglycoside can produce a synergistic bactericidal effect in vitro. This effect has been most commonly employed for treatment of infections due to staphylococci, enterococci, viridans group streptococci, and *Listeria*. Clinically, the superiority of aminoglycoside combination regimens over cell-wall agents alone is not proven except in relatively few infections (discussed further in the chapter).

Resistance to the Aminoglycosides

Bacteria may be resistant to aminoglycosides through

- inactivation of the drug by microbial enzymes;
- failure of the antibiotic to penetrate intracellularly; and
- low affinity of the drug for the bacterial ribosome.

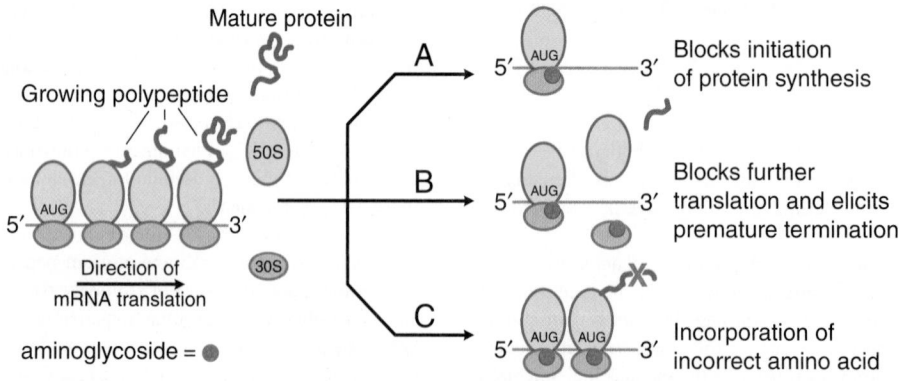

Figure 58–2 *Effects of aminoglycosides on protein synthesis.* **A.** Aminoglycoside (represented by red circles) binds to the 30S ribosomal subunit and interferes with initiation of protein synthesis by fixing the 30S-50S ribosomal complex at the start codon (AUG) of mRNA. As 30S-50S complexes downstream complete translation of mRNA and detach; the abnormal initiation complexes, so-called streptomycin monosomes, accumulate, blocking further translation of the message. Aminoglycoside binding to the 30S subunit also causes misreading of mRNA, leading to **B**, premature termination of translation with detachment of the ribosomal complex and incompletely synthesized protein or **C**, incorporation of incorrect amino acids (indicated by the red X), resulting in the production of abnormal or nonfunctional proteins.

TABLE 58–1 ■ SUSCEPTIBILITY TO AMINOGLYCOSIDES AND TYPICAL MINIMAL CONCENTRATIONS THAT WILL INHIBIT 90% (MIC$_{90}$) OF CLINICAL ISOLATES FOR SEVERAL SPECIES

SPECIES	% SUSCEPTIBLE (MIC$_{90}$ µg/mL)		
	GENTAMICIN	TOBRAMYCIN	AMIKACIN
Enterobacter spp.	97.0% (1)	96.0% (1)	100.0% (2)
Escherichia coli	88.2% (8)	86.3% (8)	99.0% (4)
Klebsiella pneumoniae	89.2% (8)	82.4% (32)	88.2% (32)
Pseudomonas aeruginosa	88.0% (16)	90.0% (4)	98.0% (16)
Serratia spp.	97.0% (1)	94.0% (4)	99.0% (4)
Acinetobacter baumanii	37.0% (>128)	51.0% (>128)	58.0% (>128)
Staphylococcus aureus	95.0% (0.5)	76.0% (>128)	96.0% (8)

Source: Data from Sader HS, et al. Arbekacin activity against contemporary clinical bacteria isolated from patients hospitalized with pneumonia. *Antimicrob Agents Chemother,* **2015**, *59*:3263–3270.

Clinically, drug inactivation is the most common mechanism for acquired microbial resistance. The genes encoding aminoglycoside-modifying enzymes are acquired primarily by conjugation and transfer of resistance plasmids (see Chapter 52). These enzymes phosphorylate, adenylate, or acetylate specific hydroxyl or amino groups (see Figure 58–1). The ability of these enzymes to attack these groups in differing aminoglycosides explains some of the variability in antimicrobial activity across the class. Amikacin is a suitable substrate for only a few of these inactivating enzymes; thus, strains that are resistant to multiple other aminoglycosides tend to be susceptible to amikacin, particularly amongst gram-negative bacilli. A significant percentage of clinical isolates of *Enterococcus faecalis* and *Enterococcus faecium* are highly resistant to all aminoglycosides (Eliopoulos et al., 1984). Resistance to gentamicin indicates cross-resistance to tobramycin, amikacin, kanamycin, and netilmicin because the inactivating enzyme is bifunctional and can modify all these aminoglycosides. Owing to differences in the chemical structures between streptomycin and other aminoglycosides, the most common enzyme seen in enterococci does not modify streptomycin, which is inactivated by another enzyme. Consequently, gentamicin-resistant strains of enterococci may be susceptible to streptomycin. Intrinsic resistance to aminoglycosides may be caused by failure of the drug to penetrate the cytoplasmic (inner) membrane. Transport of aminoglycosides across the cytoplasmic membrane is an active process that depends on oxidative metabolism. Strictly anaerobic bacteria thus are resistant to these drugs because they lack the necessary transport system.

Missense mutations in *Escherichia coli* that substitute a single amino acid in a crucial ribosomal protein may prevent binding of streptomycin. Although highly resistant to streptomycin, these strains are not widespread in nature. Similarly, 5% of strains of *Pseudomonas aeruginosa* exhibit such ribosomal resistance to streptomycin. Because ribosomal resistance usually is specific for streptomycin, enterococci with ribosomal mutations typically remain sensitive to a combination of penicillin and gentamicin in vitro.

ADME

Absorption

The aminoglycosides are polar cations and therefore are poorly absorbed from the GI tract. Less than 1% of a dose is absorbed after either oral or rectal administration. Nonetheless, long-term oral or rectal administration of aminoglycosides may result in accumulation to toxic concentrations in patients with renal impairment. Absorption of gentamicin from the GI tract may be increased by GI disease (e.g., ulcers or inflammatory bowel disease). Instillation of these drugs into body cavities with serosal surfaces also may result in rapid absorption and unexpected toxicity (i.e., neuromuscular blockade). Intoxication may occur when aminoglycosides are applied topically for long periods to large wounds, burns, or cutaneous ulcers, particularly if there is renal insufficiency.

All the aminoglycosides are absorbed rapidly from intramuscular sites of injection. Peak concentrations in plasma occur after 30–90 min. These concentrations range from 4 to 12 µg/mL following a 1.5- to 2-mg/kg dose of gentamicin, tobramycin, or netilmicin and from 20 to 35 µg/mL following a 7.5-mg/kg dose of amikacin or kanamycin. There is increasing use of aminoglycosides administered via inhalation, primarily for the management of patients with cystic fibrosis who have chronic *P. aeruginosa* pulmonary infections (Geller et al., 2002). Amikacin and tobramycin solutions for injection have been used, as well as a commercial formulation of tobramycin designed for inhalation.

Distribution

Because of their polar nature, the aminoglycosides do not penetrate well into most cells, the CNS, or the eye. Except for streptomycin, there is negligible binding of aminoglycosides to plasma albumin. The apparent volume of distribution of these drugs is 25% of lean body weight and approximates the volume of extracellular fluid. The aminoglycosides distribute poorly into adipose tissue, which must be considered when using weight-based dosing regimens in obese patients.

Concentrations of aminoglycosides in secretions and tissues are low (Panidis et al., 2005). High concentrations are found only in the renal cortex and the endolymph and perilymph of the inner ear; the high concentration in these sites likely contributes to the nephrotoxicity and ototoxicity caused by these drugs. As a result of active hepatic secretion, concentrations in bile approach 30% of those found in plasma, but this represents a very minor excretory route for the aminoglycosides. Inflammation increases the penetration of aminoglycosides into peritoneal and pericardial cavities. Concentrations of aminoglycosides achieved in CSF with parenteral administration usually are subtherapeutic (Kearney and Aweeka, 1999). Treatment of meningitis with intravenous administration is generally suboptimal. Intrathecal or intraventricular administration of aminoglycosides has been used to achieve therapeutic levels in the CNS but the availability of extended-spectrum cephalosporins has generally made this unnecessary.

Administration of aminoglycosides to women late in pregnancy may result in accumulation of drug in fetal plasma and amniotic fluid. Streptomycin and tobramycin can cause hearing loss in children born to women who receive the drug during pregnancy. Insufficient data are available regarding the other aminoglycosides; therefore, these agents should be used with caution during pregnancy and only for strong clinical indications in the absence of suitable alternatives.

The aminoglycosides undergo minimal metabolism and are excreted almost entirely by glomerular filtration, achieving urine concentrations of 50–200 µg/mL. The half-lives of the aminoglycosides in plasma are 2–3 h in patients with normal renal function. Because the elimination of aminoglycosides depends almost entirely on the kidney, a linear relationship exists between the concentration of creatinine in plasma and the $t_{1/2}$ of all aminoglycosides in patients with moderately compromised renal function. In anephric patients, the $t_{1/2}$ varies from 20 to 40 times that determined in normal individuals. *Because the incidence of nephrotoxicity and ototoxicity is likely related to the overall exposure to aminoglycosides, it is critical to reduce the maintenance dose and dosing interval of these drugs in patients with impaired renal function.*

Although excretion of aminoglycosides is similar in adults and children older than 6 months, half-lives of aminoglycosides may be prolonged significantly in the newborn: 8–11 h in the first week of life in newborns weighing less than 2 kg and about 5 h in those weighing more than 2 kg. Thus, it is critically important to monitor plasma concentrations of aminoglycosides during treatment of neonates. Aminoglycoside clearances are increased and half-lives are reduced in patients with cystic fibrosis (Mann et al., 1985). Larger doses of aminoglycosides may likewise be required in burn patients because of more rapid drug clearance, possibly because of drug loss through burn tissue. Aminoglycosides can be removed from the body by either hemodialysis or peritoneal dialysis.

Aminoglycosides can be inactivated by various penicillins in vitro and thus should not be admixed in solution (Blair et al., 1982). Some reports indicate that this inactivation may occur in vivo in patients with end-stage renal failure, making monitoring of aminoglycoside plasma concentrations even more necessary in such patients. Amikacin appears to be the aminoglycoside least affected by this interaction; penicillins with more nonrenal elimination (such as piperacillin) may be less prone to cause this interaction.

Dosing and Monitoring

High-dose, extended-interval administration of aminoglycosides is the preferred means of administering aminoglycosides for most indications and patient populations. Administering higher doses at extended intervals (i.e., once daily) is likely to be at least equally efficacious and potentially less toxic than administration of divided doses. This dosing strategy takes advantage of the concentration-dependent activity of aminoglycosides to achieve maximal initial bacterial killing, and because of the postantibiotic effect of aminoglycosides, good therapeutic response can be attained even when concentrations fall below inhibitory concentrations for a substantial fraction of the dosing interval. High-dose, extended-interval dosing schemes for aminoglycosides may also reduce the characteristic oto- and nephrotoxicity of these drugs. This diminished toxicity is probably due to a threshold effect from accumulation of drug in the inner ear or in the kidney. High-dose, extended-interval regimens, despite the higher peak concentration, provide a longer period when concentrations fall below the threshold for toxicity than does a multiple-dose regimen (compare the two dosage regimens shown in Figure 58–3).

Populations in which use of the high-dose/extended-interval dosing strategy is more controversial include pregnancy, neonates, and pediatrics and as combination therapy for endocarditis (Contopoulos-Ioannidis et al., 2004; Knoderer et al., 2003; Nestaas et al., 2005; Ward and Theiler, 2008). In these infections, multiple daily doses (with a lower total daily dose) may be preferred because data documenting equivalent safety and efficacy of extended-interval dosing are limited. Extended-interval dosing is also usually avoided in patients with significant renal dysfunction (i.e., creatinine clearance < 25 mL/min).

Concentrations of aminoglycosides achieved in plasma after a given dose vary widely amongst patients, and therapeutic drug monitoring is standard practice (Bartal et al., 2003). For twice- or thrice-daily dosing regimens, both peak and trough plasma concentrations are determined. The peak concentration documents that the dose produces therapeutic concentrations, while the trough concentration is used to avoid toxicity.

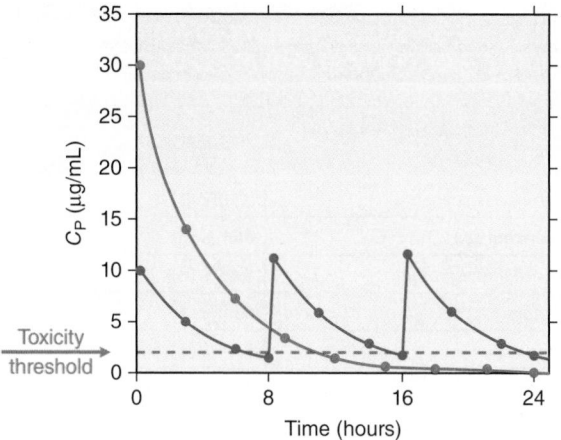

Figure 58–3 *Comparison of single-dose and divided-dose regimens for gentamicin.* In a hypothetical patient, a dose of gentamicin (5.1 mg/kg) is administered intravenously as a single bolus (red line) or in three portions, a third of the dose every 8 h (purple line), such that the total drug administered is the same in the two cases. The threshold for toxicity (green dashed line) is the plasma concentration of 2 µg/mL, the maximum recommended for prolonged exposure. The single-dose regimen produces a higher plasma concentration than the regimen given every 8 h; this higher peak provides efficacy that otherwise might be compromised due to prolonged subthreshold concentrations later in the dosing interval or that is provided by the lower peak levels achieved with the regimen every 8 h. The once-daily regimen also provides a 13-h period during which plasma concentrations are below the threshold for toxicity. The every-8-h regimen, by contrast, provides only three short (~1 h) periods in 24 h during which plasma concentrations are below the threshold for toxicity. The single high-dose, extended interval is generally preferred for aminoglycosides, with a few exceptions (during pregnancy, in neonates, etc.), as noted in the text.

Steady-state trough concentrations should be less than 1–2 µg/mL for gentamicin, netilmicin, and tobramycin and less than 10 µg/mL for amikacin and streptomycin. Peak level goals vary by indication and infection severity, but range from 4 to 8 µg/mL with gentamicin, netilmicin, and tobramycin and 20–35 µg/mL for amikacin. Monitoring of aminoglycoside plasma concentrations also is important when using an extended-interval dosing regimen. For routine monitoring of extended-interval dosing, a single random concentration obtained 6 to 14 h after the start of the infusion can be obtained and plotted against a standard nomogram to determine if dosage adjustment is required (Barclay et al., 1999). However, the most accurate method for monitoring plasma levels for dose adjustment is to measure the concentration in two plasma samples drawn several hours apart (e.g., at 2 and 12 h after a dose). The clearance then can be calculated and the dose adjusted to achieve the desired target range.

Therapeutic Uses of Aminoglycosides

Gentamicin, tobramycin, amikacin, and netilmicin can be used interchangeably for the treatment of most of the infections mentioned in this section. For most indications, gentamicin is preferred because of long experience with its use and its lower cost. Many different types of infections can be treated successfully with these aminoglycosides; however, owing to their toxicities, prolonged use should be restricted to the therapy of life-threatening infections and those for which a less-toxic agent is contraindicated or less effective.

Aminoglycosides frequently are used in combination with a cell wall–active agent (*β-lactam or glycopeptide*) for the therapy of serious proven or suspected bacterial infections. The three rationales for this approach are

- to expand the empiric spectrum of activity of the antimicrobial regimen
- to provide synergistic bacterial killing
- to prevent the emergence of resistance to the individual agents

Combination therapy is used in infections such as healthcare-associated pneumonia or sepsis, where multidrug-resistant gram-negative organisms such as *P. aeruginosa*, *Enterobacter*, *Klebsiella*, and *Serratia* may be causative and the consequences of failing to provide initially active therapy are dire. The use of aminoglycosides to achieve synergistic bacterial killing and improve clinical response is most well established for the treatment of endocarditis due to gram-positive organisms, most importantly *Enterococcus* (Le and Bayer, 2003). Clinical data do not support the use of combination therapy for synergistic killing of gram-negative organisms, with the possible exceptions of serious *P. aeruginosa* infections. Aminoglycosides (primarily streptomycin and amikacin) are occasionally used in multidrug regimens for treatment of mycobacterial infections, in part because of the need to suppress the emergence of resistant subpopulations during therapy; data do not strongly support this practice for other bacteria (Bliziotis et al., 2005).

Urinary Tract Infections

Although the spectrum of activity and concentration in the urinary tract of aminoglycosides make them well-suited for treatment of urinary tract infections, less-toxic alternatives are preferred for uncomplicated infections. However, as strains of *E. coli* have acquired resistance to β-lactams, trimethoprim-sulfamethoxazole, and fluoroquinolones, use of aminoglycosides for urinary tract infections may increase. A single intramuscular dose of gentamicin (5 mg/kg) has been effective in uncomplicated infections of the lower urinary tract. A 10- to 14-day course of gentamicin or tobramycin is an alternative for treatment of pyelonephritis if other agents cannot be used.

Pneumonia

The organisms that cause community-acquired pneumonia are susceptible to broad-spectrum β-lactam antibiotics, macrolides, or a fluoroquinolone, and usually it is not necessary to add an aminoglycoside. Aminoglycosides are ineffective for the treatment of pneumonia due to anaerobes or *Streptococcus pneumoniae*, which are common causes of community-acquired pneumonia. In hospital-acquired pneumonia where aerobic multidrug-resistant gram-negative bacilli are frequently causative pathogens, an aminoglycoside in combination with a β-lactam antibiotic is recommended as standard empiric therapy to increase the likelihood that at least one agent is active against the infecting pathogen (American Thoracic Society, 2005). Once it is established that the β-lactam is active against the causative agent, there is generally no benefit from continuing the aminoglycoside.

Meningitis

Availability of third-generation cephalosporins, especially cefotaxime and ceftriaxone, has reduced the need for treatment with aminoglycosides in most cases of meningitis, except for infections caused by gram-negative organisms resistant to β-lactam antibiotics (e.g., species of *Pseudomonas* and *Acinetobacter*). If an aminoglycoside is necessary, direct instillation into the CNS is more likely to achieve therapeutic levels than intravenous administration. In adults, this can be achieved with 5 mg of a preservative-free formulation of gentamicin (or equivalent dose of another aminoglycoside) administered intrathecally or intraventricularly once daily.

Peritonitis

Patients who develop peritonitis as a result of peritoneal dialysis may be treated with aminoglycoside diluted into the dialysis fluid to a concentration of 4–8 mg/L for gentamicin, netilmicin, or tobramycin or 6–12 mg/L for amikacin. Intravenous or intramuscular administration of drug is unnecessary because serum and peritoneal fluid will equilibrate rapidly.

Bacterial Endocarditis

"Synergistic" or low-dose gentamicin (3 mg/kg/d) in combination with a penicillin or vancomycin has been recommended in certain circumstances for treatment of bacterial endocarditis due to certain gram-positive organisms. Penicillin and gentamicin in combination are effective as a short-course (i.e., 2-week) regimen for uncomplicated native-valve streptococcal

endocarditis. For this indication, the administration of gentamicin may be given as a consolidated once-daily dose. In cases of enterococcal endocarditis, concomitant administration of penicillin (or ampicillin) and gentamicin (given as divided doses) for 4–6 weeks is recommended as standard therapy. However, safer alternatives such as ampicillin/ceftriaxone combinations or use of the aminoglycoside for only the first 2–3 weeks, are gaining favor to limit the risk of toxicity due to prolonged aminoglycoside administration (Olaison and Schadewitz, 2002). A 2-week regimen of gentamicin in combination with nafcillin is effective for the treatment of selected cases of staphylococcal tricuspid native-valve endocarditis. For patients with native mitral or aortic valve staphylococcal endocarditis, the risks of aminoglycoside administration likely outweigh the benefits (Cosgrove et al., 2009).

Sepsis

Inclusion of an aminoglycoside in an empirical regimen is commonly recommended for the febrile patient with neutropenia and for sepsis when *P. aeruginosa* is a potential pathogen. However, studies using potent broad-spectrum β-lactams (e.g., carbapenems and antipseudomonal cephalosporins) have demonstrated no benefit from adding an aminoglycoside to the regimen unless there is concern that an infection may be caused by a multiple-drug-resistant organism (Paul et al., 2003). Thus, local susceptibility patterns should be considered when weighing the risks and benefits of adjunctive aminoglycoside administration for empiric therapy in patients with sepsis.

Tularemia

Streptomycin (or gentamicin) is the drug of choice for the treatment of tularemia. Most cases respond to the administration of 1–2 g (15–25 mg/kg) streptomycin per day (in divided doses) for 10–14 days.

Plague

A 10-day treatment course of streptomycin or gentamicin is recommended for severe forms of plague (Boulanger et al., 2004).

Mycobacterial Infections

Streptomycin is a second-line agent for the treatment of active tuberculosis, and streptomycin always should be used in combination with at least one or two other drugs to which the causative strain is susceptible. Amikacin is another alternative agent for infections due to drug-resistant *Mycobacterium tuberculosis* or to other nontuberculous mycobacteria (e.g., *M. avium*, *M. abscessus*, *M. chelonae*).

Cystic Fibrosis

Recurrent infections due to multidrug-resistant gram-negative bacilli, especially *Pseudomonas* species, are a hallmark of cystic fibrosis. Aminoglycosides are frequently used as therapy during acute exacerbations of cystic fibrosis, for which higher-than-standard doses (e.g., 10 mg/kg of tobramycin) are frequently employed due to the unusual pharmacokinetics observed in patients with cystic fibrosis. These agents may also be administered via inhalation between exacerbations to improve lung function and reduce exacerbation frequency.

Topical Applications

Aminoglycosides, especially neomycin and paromomycin, may be employed as topical agents in skin and mucous membrane infections. Oral administration of aminoglycosides may be employed as "bowel prep" prior to surgical procedures or as "selective digestive decontamination" to reduce the risk of ventilator-associated pneumonia.

Adverse Effects of Aminoglycosides

All aminoglycosides have the potential to produce reversible and irreversible vestibular, cochlear, and renal toxicity and neuromuscular blockade.

Ototoxicity

Vestibular and auditory dysfunction can follow the administration of any of the aminoglycosides (Guthrie, 2008). Aminoglycoside-induced ototoxicity may result in irreversible, bilateral, high-frequency hearing loss or vestibular hypofunction. Degeneration of hair cells and neurons in the cochlea correlates with the loss of hearing. Accumulation within the perilymph and endolymph occurs predominantly when aminoglycoside concentrations in plasma are high. Diffusion back into the bloodstream is slow; the half-lives of the aminoglycosides are five to six times longer in the otic fluids than in plasma. Drugs such as ethacrynic acid and furosemide potentiate the ototoxic effects of the aminoglycosides in animals, but data from humans implicating furosemide are less convincing (Smith and Lietman, 1983).

Streptomycin and gentamicin produce predominantly vestibular effects, whereas amikacin, kanamycin, and neomycin primarily affect auditory function; tobramycin affects both equally. The incidence of ototoxicity is difficult to determine. Audiometric data suggest that the incidence could be as high as 25% (Brummett and Morrison, 1990). The incidence of vestibular toxicity is particularly high in patients receiving streptomycin; nearly 20% of individuals who received 500 mg twice daily for 4 weeks for enterococcal endocarditis developed clinically detectable irreversible vestibular damage. Because the initial symptoms may be reversible, patients receiving high doses or prolonged courses of aminoglycosides should be monitored carefully for ototoxicity; however, deafness may occur several weeks after therapy is discontinued.

A high-pitched tinnitus often is the first symptom of cochlear toxicity. If the drug is not discontinued, auditory impairment may develop after a few days. The tinnitus may persist for several days to 2 weeks after therapy is stopped. Because perception of sound in the high-frequency range (outside the conversational range) is lost first, the affected individual is not always aware of the difficulty, and it will not be detected except by careful audiometric examination. If the hearing loss progresses, the lower sound ranges are affected.

Amongst patients experiencing vestibular toxicity, moderately intense headache lasting 1–2 days may precede the onset of labyrinthine dysfunction. This is followed immediately by an acute stage in which nausea, vomiting, and difficulty with equilibrium develop and persist for 1–2 weeks. Prominent symptoms include vertigo in the upright position, inability to perceive termination of movement ("mental past-pointing"), and difficulty in sitting or standing without visual cues. The acute stage ends suddenly and is followed by chronic labyrinthitis, in which the patient has difficulty when attempting to walk or make sudden movements; ataxia is the most prominent feature. The chronic phase persists for about 2 months. Recovery from this phase may require 12–18 months, and most patients have some permanent residual damage. Early discontinuation of the drug may permit recovery before irreversible damage of the hair cells.

Nephrotoxicity

Approximately 8%–26% of patients who receive an aminoglycoside for several days develop mild renal impairment that is almost always reversible. The toxicity results from accumulation and retention of aminoglycoside in the proximal tubular cells. The initial manifestation of damage at this site is excretion of enzymes of the renal tubular brush border followed by mild proteinuria and the appearance of hyaline and granular casts. The glomerular filtration rate is reduced after several additional days. The nonoliguric phase of renal insufficiency is thought to be due to the effects of aminoglycosides on the distal portion of the nephron with a reduced sensitivity of the collecting duct epithelium to vasopressin. Although severe acute tubular necrosis may occur rarely, the most common significant finding is a mild rise in plasma creatinine. The impairment in renal function is almost always reversible because the proximal tubular cells have the capacity to regenerate (Lietman and Smith, 1983). Toxicity correlates with the total amount of drug administered and with longer courses of therapy (de Jager and van Altena, 2002). High-dose, extended-interval dosing approaches lead to less nephrotoxicity at the same level of total drug exposure (as measured by the area under the curve)

than divided-dose approaches (see Figure 58–3). Neomycin, which concentrates to the greatest degree, is highly nephrotoxic in human beings and should not be administered systemically. Streptomycin does not concentrate in the renal cortex and is the least nephrotoxic. Drugs such as amphotericin B, vancomycin, angiotensin-converting enzyme inhibitors, cisplatin, and cyclosporine may potentiate aminoglycoside-induced nephrotoxicity (Wood et al., 1986).

Neuromuscular Blockade

Acute neuromuscular blockade and apnea have been attributed to the aminoglycosides; patients with myasthenia gravis are particularly susceptible. The order of decreasing potency for blockade is neomycin, kanamycin, amikacin, gentamicin, and tobramycin. In humans, neuromuscular blockade generally has occurred after intrapleural or intraperitoneal instillation of large doses of an aminoglycoside; however, the reaction can follow intravenous, intramuscular, and even oral administration of these agents. Most episodes have occurred in association with anesthesia or the administration of other neuromuscular blocking agents. Neuromuscular blockade may be reversed by intravenous administration of a Ca^{2+} salt.

Aminoglycosides may inhibit prejunctional release of acetylcholine while also reducing postsynaptic sensitivity to the transmitter, but Ca^{2+} can overcome this effect, and the intravenous administration of a calcium salt is the preferred treatment of this toxicity (Sarkar et al., 1992). Inhibitors of acetylcholinesterase (e.g., edrophonium and neostigmine) also have been used with varying degrees of success.

Other Adverse Effects

In general, the aminoglycosides have little allergenic potential. Rare hypersensitivity reactions—including skin rashes, eosinophilia, fever, blood dyscrasias, angioedema, exfoliative dermatitis, stomatitis, and anaphylactic shock—have been reported as cross-hypersensitivity amongst drugs in this class. Aminoglycosides appear to be less commonly associated with superinfection due to *Clostridium difficile* than other classes of antibacterials.

Pharmacological Properties of Individual Aminoglycosides

Gentamicin

Gentamicin is an important agent for the treatment of many serious gram-negative bacillary infections. It is the aminoglycoside of first choice because of its lower cost and reliable activity against all but the most resistant gram-negative aerobes. Gentamicin preparations are available for parenteral, ophthalmic, and topical administration. The typical recommended intramuscular or intravenous dose of gentamicin sulfate when used for the treatment of known or suspected gram-negative organisms as a single agent or in combination therapy for adults with normal renal function is 5–7 mg/kg daily given over 30–60 min. For patients with renal dysfunction, the interval may be extended. For patients who are not candidates for extended-interval dosing, a loading dose of 2 mg/kg and then 3–5 mg/kg per day, given as divided doses every 8–12 h, are recommended. Dosages at the upper end of this range may be required to achieve therapeutic levels for trauma or burn patients, those with septic shock, patients with cystic fibrosis, and others in whom drug clearance is more rapid or volume of distribution is larger than normal.

Several dosage schedules have been suggested for newborns and infants: 3 mg/kg once daily for preterm newborns less than 35 weeks of gestation; 4 mg/kg once daily for newborns more than 35 weeks of gestation; 5 mg/kg daily in two divided doses for neonates with severe infections; and 2–2.5 mg/kg every 8 h for children up to 2 years of age. Peak plasma concentrations range from 4 to 10 mg/mL (dosing: 1.7 mg/kg every 8 h) and 16–24 mg/mL (extended-interval dosing: 5 mg/kg once daily).

It should be emphasized that the recommended doses of gentamicin do not always yield desired concentrations. Periodic determinations of the plasma concentration of aminoglycosides are recommended strongly. Gentamicin is absorbed slowly when it is applied topically in an ointment and somewhat more rapidly when it is applied as a cream. When the antibiotic is applied to large areas of denuded body surface, as may be the case in burn patients, plasma concentrations can reach 4 μg/mL, and 2%–5% of the drug may appear in the urine.

Tobramycin

The antimicrobial activity, pharmacokinetic properties, and toxicity profile of tobramycin are similar to those of gentamicin. Tobramycin may be given intramuscularly, intravenously, or by inhalation. Tobramycin also is available in ophthalmic ointments and solutions. The superior activity of tobramycin against *P. aeruginosa* makes it the preferred aminoglycoside for treatment of serious infections known or suspected to be caused by this organism, typically in combination with an antipseudomonal β-lactam antibiotic. In contrast to gentamicin, tobramycin shows poor activity in combination with penicillin against many strains of enterococci. Most strains of *E. faecium* are highly resistant. Tobramycin is ineffective against mycobacteria. Dosages and serum concentrations are identical to those for gentamicin.

Amikacin

The spectrum of antimicrobial activity of amikacin is the broadest of the group. Because of its resistance to many of the aminoglycoside-inactivating enzymes, amikacin has a special role for the initial treatment of serious nosocomial gram-negative bacillary infections in hospitals where resistance to gentamicin and tobramycin has become a significant problem. Amikacin is active against most strains of *Serratia*, *Proteus*, and *P. aeruginosa* as well as most strains of *Klebsiella*, *Enterobacter*, and *E. coli* that are resistant to gentamicin and tobramycin. Most resistance to amikacin is found amongst strains of *Acinetobacter*, *Providencia*, and *Flavobacterium* and strains of *Pseudomonas* other than *P. aeruginosa*; these all are unusual pathogens. Amikacin is less active than gentamicin against enterococci and should not be used for this organism. Amikacin is not active against the majority of gram-positive anaerobic bacteria. It is active against *M. tuberculosis*, including streptomycin-resistant strains and atypical mycobacteria.

The recommended dose of amikacin is 15 mg/kg/d as a single daily dose or divided into two or three equal portions, which must be reduced for patients with renal failure. The drug is absorbed rapidly after intramuscular injection, and peak concentrations in plasma approximate 20 μg/mL after injection of 7.5 mg/kg. The concentration 12 h after a 7.5-mg/kg dose is 5–10 μg/mL. A 15-mg/kg once-daily dose produces peak concentrations of 50–60 μg/mL and a trough of less than 1 μg/mL. For treatment of mycobacterial infections, thrice-weekly dosing schedules are used, with doses up to 25 mg/kg (Peloquin et al., 2004). As with the other aminoglycosides, amikacin causes ototoxicity, hearing loss, and nephrotoxicity.

Netilmicin

Netilmicin (not marketed in the U.S.) is similar to gentamicin and tobramycin in its pharmacokinetic properties and dosage (Panwalker et al., 1978). Its antibacterial activity is broad against aerobic gram-negative bacilli. Like amikacin, it is not metabolized by most of the aminoglycoside-inactivating enzymes; thus, it may be active against certain bacteria that are resistant to gentamicin (with the exception of resistant enterococci). Netilmicin is useful for the treatment of serious infections owing to susceptible Enterobacteriaceae and other aerobic gram-negative bacilli. The recommended dose of netilmicin for complicated urinary tract infections in adults is 1.5–2 mg/kg every 12 h. For other serious systemic infections, a total daily dose of 4–7 mg/kg is administered as a single dose or two to three divided doses. Children should receive 3–7 mg/kg/d in two to three divided doses; neonates receive 3.5–5 mg/kg/d as a single daily dose. The $t_{1/2}$ for elimination is usually 2–2.5 h in adults and increases with renal insufficiency. Netilmicin may produce ototoxicity and nephrotoxicity.

Streptomycin

Streptomycin is used for the treatment of certain unusual infections, generally in combination with other antimicrobial agents. It generally is less active than other members of the class against aerobic gram-negative rods. The combination of penicillin G (bacteriostatic against enterococci) and streptomycin is effective as bactericidal therapy for enterococcal endocarditis, although gentamicin is generally preferred for its lesser toxicity. Streptomycin should be used instead of gentamicin when the strain is resistant to the latter and has demonstrable susceptibility to streptomycin, which may occur because the enzymes that inactivate these two aminoglycosides are different.

Streptomycin may be administered by deep intramuscular injection or intravenously. Intramuscular injection may be painful, with a hot tender mass developing at the site of injection. The dose range of streptomycin for most indications is 15–25 mg/kg daily or in divided doses twice daily. During initial therapy for tuberculosis, it is frequently administered as a 1000-mg single daily dose, resulting in peak serum concentrations of about 50–60 and 15–30 μg/mL, and trough concentrations of less than 1 and 5–10 μg/mL, respectively. The dosing frequency may be reduced to two or three times a week after the initial phase of tuberculosis treatment.

Streptomycin has been replaced by gentamicin for most indications because the toxicity of gentamicin is primarily renal and reversible, whereas that of streptomycin is vestibular and irreversible. The administration of streptomycin may produce dysfunction of the optic nerve, including scotomas, presenting as enlargement of the blind spot. Amongst the less-common toxic reactions to streptomycin is peripheral neuritis.

Neomycin

Neomycin is a broad-spectrum antibiotic. Susceptible microorganisms usually are inhibited by concentrations of 10 μg/mL or less. Gram-negative species that are highly sensitive are *E. coli*, *Enterobacter aerogenes*, *Klebsiella pneumoniae*, and *Proteus vulgaris*. Gram-positive microorganisms that are inhibited include *S. aureus* and *E. faecalis*. *Mycobacterium tuberculosis* also is sensitive to neomycin. Strains of *P. aeruginosa* are resistant to neomycin. Neomycin sulfate is available for topical and oral administration. Neomycin currently is available in many brands of creams, ointments, and other products alone and in combination with polymyxin, bacitracin, other antibiotics, and a variety of corticosteroids.

Neomycin is used widely for topical application in a variety of infections of the skin and mucous membranes. The oral administration of neomycin (usually in combination with erythromycin base) has been employed primarily for "preparation" of the bowel for surgery. Orally administered neomycin is poorly absorbed from the GI tract—about 97% of an oral dose of neomycin is not absorbed and is eliminated unchanged in the feces. The portion that is absorbed is excreted by the kidney; a total daily intake of 10 g for 3 days yields a blood concentration below that associated with systemic toxicity if renal function is normal. Neomycin and polymyxin B have been used for irrigation of the bladder to prevent bacteriuria and bacteremia associated with indwelling catheters. For this purpose, 1 mL of a preparation containing 40 mg neomycin and 200,000 units polymyxin B per milliliter is diluted in 1 L of 0.9% sodium chloride solution and is used for continuous irrigation of the urinary bladder through appropriate catheter systems. The bladder is irrigated at the rate of 1 L every 24 h.

Hypersensitivity reactions, primarily skin rashes, occur in 6%–8% of patients when neomycin is applied topically. The most important toxic effects of neomycin are ototoxicity and nephrotoxicity; as a consequence, the drug is no longer available for parenteral administration. Neuromuscular blockade with respiratory paralysis also has occurred after irrigation of wounds or serosal cavities. Individuals treated with 4–6 g/d of the drug by mouth sometimes develop a sprue-like syndrome with diarrhea, steatorrhea, and azotorrhea. Overgrowth of yeasts in the intestine also may occur.

Paromomycin

Paromomycin (also known as aminosidine) is an aminoglycoside that is structurally related to neomycin. It has antibacterial activity similar to other aminoglycosides but has particularly notable antiparasitic activity. Parasites that are usually susceptible to paromomycin include *Leishmania* spp., *Entamoeba histolytica*, *Giardia lamblia*, and *Cryptosporidium parvum*. Internationally, the parenteral form is used as a treatment of infections due to *Leishmania* spp. (visceral leishmaniasis), although this formulation is not available in the U.S. (Sundar et al., 2007). Like other aminoglycosides, it has poor systemic absorption when administered orally; this characteristic is exploited to achieve high luminal concentrations in the treatment of intestinal parasitic diseases. It is available as oral capsules and indicated for treatment of intestinal amebiasis at a dose of 25–35 mg/kg/d in three divided doses. It is also used for treatment of intestinal cryptosporidiosis and giardiasis, which can be particularly challenging to treat in immunocompromised patients. Orally administered paromomycin is associated with dose-related gastrointestinal toxicity, including nausea, abdominal pain, and diarrhea. A topical formulation is also used internationally for treatment of cutaneous leishmaniasis (Ben Salah et al., 2013).

Kanamycin

Kanamycin is amongst the most toxic aminoglycosides, and there are few indications for its use. Its primary remaining indication is for treatment of extensively drug-resistant tuberculosis; even in this condition, less-toxic alternatives are generally preferred.

Acknowledgment: *Henry F. Chambers contributed to this chapter in recent editions of this book. We have retained some of his text in the current edition.*

Drug Facts for Your Personal Formulary: *Aminoglycosides*

Drug	Therapeutic Uses	Clinical Pharmacology and Tips
Aminoglycosides—Inhibitors of Bacterial Protein Synthesis		
General: Bactericidal, no GI absorption (<1%), oral administration used only for bowel decontamination or intestinal parasites, poor CSF penetration, renal elimination, nephrotoxicity, ototoxicity (cochlear and vestibular), neuromuscular blockade		
Gentamicin (IV)	• UTI • Peritonitis • Endocarditis in combination with a cell-wall active agent • Plague • Tularemia	• Good activity vs. Enterobacteriaceae, *Pseudomonas* • Some activity vs. *Neisseria, Haemophilus, Moraxella* • Synergistic activity when combined with a cell-wall agent against many organisms • Vestibular > cochlear toxicity • Toxicity primarily renal and reversible
Tobramycin (IV, inhalation)	• UTI • Lung infections, including cystic fibrosis exacerbations • Nosocomial sepsis of unknown origin	• Similar to gentamicin, with better activity against *Pseudomonas aeruginosa* • Cochlear ≈ vestibular toxicity
Amikacin (IV)	• UTI • Lung infections, including cystic fibrosis exacerbations • Nosocomial sepsis of unknown origin • Mycobacterial infections	• Similar to tobramycin, with activity against some gram-negative bacilli resistant to other aminoglycosides • Activity against a variety of mycobacteria • Cochlear > vestibular toxicity
Streptomycin (IV)	• Endocarditis in combination with a cell-wall active agent • Tuberculosis • Plague • Tularemia	• Similar to gentamicin, with activity against some gentamicin-resistant enterococci • Activity against *Mycobacterium tuberculosis* • Vestibular > cochlear toxicity • Vestibular toxicity is irreversible
Neomycin (PO, topical; urologic irrigation)	• Minor skin infections • Bowel preparation prior to intra-abdominal surgery • Bladder irrigation	• Similar activity to gentamicin but only used topically, not systemically • Can cause skin rash
Paromomycin (PO, IM, topical)	• *Cryptosporidia* infection • Intestinal amebiasis • Leishmaniasis	• Diarrhea, nausea, vomiting • IM use for visceral leishmaniasis • Topical use for cutaneous leishmaniasis

Bibliography

American Thoracic Society. Guidelines for the management of adults with hospital-acquired, ventilator-associated, and healthcare-associated pneumonia. *Am J Resp Crit Care Med*, **2005**, *171*:388–416.

Barclay ML, et al. Once-daily aminoglycoside therapy: is it less toxic than multiple daily doses and how should it be monitored? *Clin Pharmacokinet*, **1999**, *36*:89–98.

Bartal C, et al. Pharmacokinetic dosing of aminoglycosides: a controlled trial. *Am J Med*, **2003**, *114*:194–198.

Ben Salah A, et al. Topical paromomycin with or without gentamicin for cutaneous leishmaniasis. *N Engl J Med*, **2013**, *368*:524–532.

Blair DC, et al. Inactivation of amikacin and gentamicin by carbenicillin in patients with end-stage renal failure. *Antimicrob Agents Chemother*, **1982**, *22*:376–379.

Bliziotis IA, et al. Effect of aminoglycoside and beta-lactam combination therapy versus beta-lactam monotherapy on the emergence of antimicrobial resistance: a meta-analysis of randomized, controlled trials. *Clin Infect Dis*, **2005**, *41*:149–158.

Boulanger LL, et al. Gentamicin and tetracyclines for the treatment of human plague: review of 75 cases in New Mexico, 1985–1999. *Clin Infect Dis*, **2004**, *38*:663–669.

Brummett RE, Morrison RB. The incidence of aminoglycoside antibiotic-induced hearing loss. *Arch Otolaryngol Head Neck Surg*, **1990**, *116*:406–410.

Busse HJ, et al. The bactericidal action of streptomycin: membrane permeabilization caused by the insertion of mistranslated proteins into the cytoplasmic membrane of *Escherichia coli* and subsequent caging of the antibiotic inside the cells due to degradation of these proteins. *J Gen Microbiol*, **1992**, *138*:551–561.

Contopoulos-Ioannidis DG, et al. Extended-interval aminoglycoside administration for children: a meta-analysis. *Pediatrics*, **2004**, *114*:e111–e118.

Cosgrove SE, et al. Initial low-dose gentamicin for *Staphylococcus aureus* bacteremia and endocarditis is nephrotoxic. *Clin Infect Dis*, **2009**, *48*:713–721.

Davis BB. The lethal action of aminoglycosides. *J Antimicrob Chemother*, **1988**, *22*:1–3.

de Jager P, van Altena R. Hearing loss and nephrotoxicity in long-term aminoglycoside treatment in patients with tuberculosis. *Int J Tuberc Lung Dis*, **2002**, *6*:622–627.

Eliopoulos GM, et al. Ribosomal resistance of clinical enterococcal to streptomycin isolates. *Antimicrob Agents Chemother*, **1984**, *25*:398–399.

Geller DE, et al. Pharmacokinetics and bioavailability of aerosolized tobramycin in cystic fibrosis. *Chest*, **2002**, *122*:219–226.

Guthrie OW. Aminoglycoside-induced ototoxicity. *Toxicology*, **2008**, *249*: 91–96.

Kearney BP, Aweeka FT. The penetration of anti-infectives into the central nervous system. *Neurol Clin*, **1999**, *17*: 883–900.

Knoderer CA, et al. Clinical issues surrounding once-daily aminoglycoside dosing in children. *Pharmacotherapy*, **2003**, *23*:44–56.

Le T, Bayer AS. Combination antibiotic therapy for infective endocarditis. *Clin Infect Dis*, **2003**, *36*:615–621.

Lietman PS, Smith CR. Aminoglycoside nephrotoxicity in humans. *J Infect Dis*, **1983**, *5*(suppl 2):S284–S292.

Mann HJ, et al. Increased dosage requirements of tobramycin and gentamicin for treating *Pseudomonas* pneumonia in patients with cystic fibrosis. *Pediatr Pulmonol*, **1985**, *1*:238–243.

Mingeot-Leclercq MP, et al. Aminoglycosides: activity and resistance. *Antimicrob Agents Chemother*, **1999**, *43*:727–737.

Nestaas E, et al. Aminoglycoside extended interval dosing in neonates is safe and effective: a meta-analysis. *Arch Dis Child Fetal Neonatal Ed*, **2005**, *90*:F294–F300.

Olaison L, Schadewitz K. Swedish Society of Infectious Diseases Quality Assurance Study Group for Endocarditis. Enterococcal endocarditis in Sweden, 1995–1999: can shorter therapy with aminoglycosides be used? *Clin Infect Dis*, **2002**, *34*:159–166.

Panidis D, et al. Penetration of gentamicin into the alveolar lining fluid of critically ill patients with ventilator-associated pneumonia. *Chest*, **2005**, *128*:545–552.

Panwalker AP, et al. Netilmicin: clinical efficacy, tolerance, and toxicity. *Antimicrob Agents Chemother*, **1978**, *13*:170–176.

Paul M, et al. Beta lactam monotherapy versus beta lactam-aminoglycoside combination therapy for fever with neutropenia: systematic review and meta-analysis. *BMJ*, **2003**, *326*:1111.

Peloquin CA, et al. Aminoglycoside toxicity: daily versus thrice-weekly dosing for treatment of mycobacterial diseases. *Clin Infect Dis*, **2004**, *38*:1538–1544.

Sarkar A, et al. Calcium as a counteractive agent to streptomycin induced respiratory depression: an in vivo electrophysiological observation. *Acta Physiol Hungar*, **1992**, *79*:305–321.

Smith CR, Lietman PS. Effect of furosemide on aminoglycoside-induced nephrotoxicity and auditory toxicity in humans. *Antimicrob Agents Chemother*, **1983**, *23*:133–137.

Sundar S, et al. Injectable paromomycin for visceral leishmaniasis in India. *N Engl J Med*, **2007**, *356*:2571–2581.

Ward K, Theiler RN. Once-daily dosing of gentamicin in obstetrics and gynecology. *Clin Obstet Gynecol*, **2008**, *51*:498–506.

Wood CA, et al. Vancomycin enhancement of experimental tobramycin nephrotoxicity. *Antimicrob Agents Chemother*, **1986**, *30*:20–24.

Chapter 59

Protein Synthesis Inhibitors and Miscellaneous Antibacterial Agents

Conan MacDougall

The agents discussed in this chapter are grouped by their antibacterial mechanism as

1. *bacteriostatic protein synthesis inhibitors that target the ribosome,* such as tetracyclines, macrolides, lincosamides, streptogramins (quinupristin/dalfopristin), and oxazolidinones (e.g., linezolid);
2. *bactericidal agents acting on the cell wall or cell membrane,* such as polymyxins, glycopeptides (e.g., vancomycin), and lipopeptides (daptomycin); and
3. *miscellaneous agents* acting by diverse mechanisms, such as metronidazole, bacitracin, and mupirocin.

Protein Synthesis Inhibitors That Target the Ribosome

Tetracyclines and Glycylcyclines

The tetracyclines are a series of derivatives of a basic four-ring structure shown next for doxycycline. *Demeclocycline, tetracycline, minocycline,* and *doxycycline* are available in the U.S. for systemic use. Glycylcyclines are tetracycline congers with substituents that confer broad-spectrum activity and activity against tetracycline-resistant bacteria; the currently available glycylcycline is *tigecycline.*

DOXYCYCLINE

Mechanism of Action

Tetracyclines and glycylcyclines inhibit bacterial protein synthesis by binding to the 30S bacterial ribosome and preventing access of aminoacyl tRNA to the acceptor (A) site on the mRNA-ribosome complex (Figure 59–1). These drugs enter gram-negative bacteria by passive diffusion through channels formed by porins in the outer cell membrane and by active transport that pumps tetracyclines across the cytoplasmic membrane.

Antimicrobial Activity

Tetracyclines are bacteriostatic antibiotics with activity against a wide range of bacteria. Tetracyclines intrinsically are more active against gram-positive than gram-negative microorganisms. Recent data from the U.S. on the activity of tetracycline and other agents are displayed in Table 59–1. Activity against *Streptococcus pyogenes* and penicillin-susceptible *Streptococcus pneumoniae* is good, but resistance is common in group B streptococci and penicillin-resistant *S. pneumoniae.* Excellent activity is maintained against both MSSA and MRSA. Activity against enterococci is limited. Doxycycline and minocycline can be active against some tetracycline-resistant isolates. *Bacillus anthracis* and *Listeria monocytogenes* are susceptible.

Activity of tetracyclines against *Haemophilus influenzae* has been largely retained since their introduction, but many Enterobacteriaceae have acquired resistance. Although all strains of *Pseudomonas aeruginosa* are resistant, 90% of strains of *Burkholderia pseudomallei* (the cause of melioidosis) are sensitive. Most strains of *Brucella* also are susceptible. Tetracyclines remain useful for infections caused by *Haemophilus ducreyi* (chancroid), *Vibrio cholerae,* and *Vibrio vulnificus* and inhibit the growth of *Campylobacter jejuni, Helicobacter pylori, Yersinia pestis, Yersinia enterocolitica, Francisella tularensis,* and *Pasteurella multocida.* Tetracyclines are alternative agents for treatment of actinomycosis.

Tetracyclines are effective against some microorganisms that are resistant to cell-wall-active antimicrobial agents, such as *Rickettsia, Coxiella burnetii, Mycoplasma pneumoniae, Chlamydia* spp., *Legionella* spp., *Ureaplasma,* some atypical mycobacteria, and *Plasmodium* spp. The tetracyclines are active against many spirochetes, including *Borrelia recurrentis, Borrelia burgdorferi* (Lyme disease), *Treponema pallidum* (syphilis), and *Treponema pertenue.*

Glycylcyclines (only tigecycline is currently available) are generally active against organisms that are susceptible to tetracyclines as well as those with acquired resistance to tetracyclines (Gales et al., 2008). In particular, tigecycline displays much greater activity against enterococci, Enterobacteriaceae, *Acinetobacter,* and *Bacteroides fragilis:* In surveillance studies, greater than 95% of isolates of these organisms tested susceptible to tigecycline. However, tigecycline still lacks activity against *Pseudomonas, Proteus,* and *Providencia* spp. There are a few exceptions where other tetracyclines may be more active than tigecycline against certain organisms, such as *Stenotrophomonas* and *Ureaplasma.*

Resistance to Tetracyclines and Glycylcyclines

Resistance is primarily plasmid mediated and often inducible. The three primary resistance mechanisms are as follows:

- Decreased accumulation of tetracycline as a result of either decreased antibiotic influx or acquisition of an energy-dependent efflux pathway
- Production of a ribosomal protection protein that displaces tetracycline from its target
- Enzymatic inactivation of tetracyclines

Abbreviations

ADME: absorption, distribution, metabolism, excretion
AUC: area under the curve
CMS: colistin methanesulfonate
CNS: central nervous system
CYP: cytochrome P450
FDA: Food and Drug Administration
HIV: human immunodeficiency virus
IV: intravenous
MAI: *Mycobacterium avium-intracellulare*
MAO: monoamine oxidase
MIC: minimum inhibitory concentration
MRSA: methicillin-resistant *Staphylococcus aureus*
MSSA: methicillin-sensitive *Staphylococcus aureus*
PCN-R: penicillin-resistant
PCN-S: penicillin-susceptible
PO: by mouth
SSRI: selective serotonin reuptake inhibitor
USP: U.S. Pharmacopeia

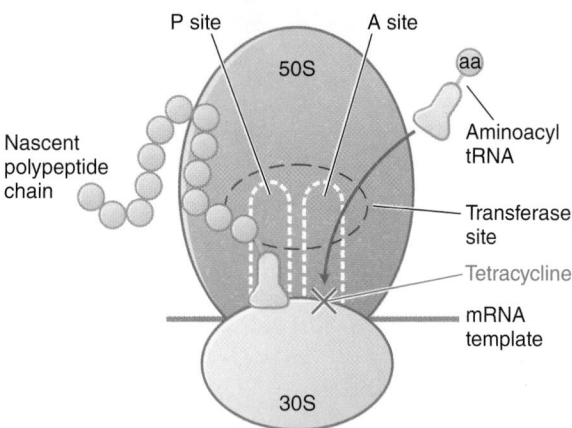

Figure 59–1 *Inhibition of bacterial protein synthesis by tetracyclines.* mRNA attaches to the 30S subunit of bacterial ribosomal RNA. The P (peptidyl) site of the 50S ribosomal RNA subunit contains the nascent polypeptide chain; normally, the aminoacyl tRNA charged with the next amino acid (aa) to be added moves into the A (acceptor) site, with complementary base pairing between the anticodon sequence of tRNA and the codon sequence of mRNA. *Tetracyclines* bind to the 30S subunit, block tRNA binding to the A site, and thereby inhibit protein synthesis.

Cross-resistance, or lack thereof, among tetracyclines depends on which mechanism is operative. Tetracycline resistance due to a ribosomal protection mechanism (*tetM*) produces cross-resistance to doxycycline and minocycline because the target site protected is the same for all tetracyclines. The glycylamido moiety characteristic of tigecycline reduces its affinity for most efflux pumps, restoring activity against many organisms displaying tetracycline resistance due to this mechanism. Binding of glycylcyclines to ribosomes is also enhanced, improving activity against organisms that harbor ribosomal protection proteins that confer resistance to other tetracyclines.

ADME

Oral absorption of most tetracyclines is incomplete. The percentage of unabsorbed drug rises as the dose increases. Tigecycline is available only for parenteral administration. Concurrent ingestion of divalent and trivalent cations (e.g., Ca^{2+}, Mg^{2+}, Al^{3+}, $Fe^{2+/3+}$, and Zn^{2+}) impairs absorption. Thus, dairy products, antacids, aluminum hydroxide gels; calcium, magnesium, and iron or zinc salts; bismuth subsalicylate and dietary iron and zinc supplements can interfere with absorption of tetracyclines. After a single oral dose, the peak plasma concentration is attained in 2–4 h. These drugs have half-lives in the range of 6–12 h and frequently

TABLE 59–1 ■ ANTIMICROBIAL SUSCEPTIBILITY AND TYPICAL MINIMAL CONCENTRATIONS THAT WILL INHIBIT 90% (MIC$_{90}$) OF CLINICAL ISOLATES FOR KEY GRAM-POSITIVE PATHOGENS KEY GRAM-POSITIVE PATHOGENS

		% SUSCEPTIBLE (MIC$_{90}$, µg/mL)					
	Streptococcus pyogenes	*Streptococcus pneumoniae*		*Staphylococcus aureus*		*Enterococcus faecalis*	*Enterococcus faecium*
ANTIBIOTIC		PCN-S	PCN-R	MSSA	MRSA		
Tetracycline	89.7% (4)	94.6% (≤2)	36.7% (>8)	95.7% (≤2)	93.4% (≤2)	24.6% (>8)	58.7% (>8)
Tigecycline	100% (≤0.03)	NR (≤0.03)	NR (≤0.03)	100% (0.25)	99.9% (0.25)	99.9% (0.25)	NR (0.12)
Erythromycin	89.7% (1)	87.3% (>2)	17.2% (>2)	70.8% (>2)	6.1% (>2)	9.1% (>2)	3.0% (>2)
Clindamycin	97.7% (≤0.25)	97.1% (≤0.25)	44.4% (>2)	94.6% (≤0.25)	57.9% (>2)	NA	NA
Quinupristin/ dalfopristin	100% (≤0.12)	99% (0.5)	100% (0.5)	100% (0.25)	100% (0.5)	3.9% (8)	92.6% (2)
Linezolid	100% (1)	100% (1)	100% (1)	99.9% (2)	99.9% (2)	99.9% (2)	98.0% (2)
Vancomycin	100% (0.25)	100% (≤1)	100% (≤1)	99.9% (1)	99.9% (1)	94.5% (2)	26.6% (>16)
Telavancin	100% (0.03)	NR (≤0.015)		100% (0.06)	100% (0.06)	96.8% (0.12)	NR (2)
Dalbavancin	100% (≤0.03)	NA		100% (0.06)	100% (0.06)	NR (>4)	NR (>4)
Oritavancin	99.7% (0.12)	NR (≤0.008)	NR (≤0.008)	100% (0.06)	100% (0.06)	NR	NR
Daptomycin	100% (0.06)	NA (0.12)	NA (0.12)	100% (0.25)	100% (0.5)	100% (2)	100% (4)

Entries are percentage of isolates inhibited at established or proposed susceptibility breakpoints. In parentheses are drug concentrations (in µg/mL) required to inhibit growth of 90% of isolates of that organism.
NA, not applicable; NR, not reported.
Data from Gales AC, et al. *Diagn Microbiol Infect Dis*, **2008**, *60*:421–427; Critchley IA, et al. *Antimicrob Agents Chemother*, **2003**, *47*:1689–1693; Jones RN, et al. *Diagn Microbiol Infect Dis*, **2013**, *75*:304–307; Mendes RE, et al. *Clin Infect Dis*, **2012**, *54*(S3):S203–S213; Mendes RE, et al. *Antimicrob Agents Chemother*, **2015**, *59*:702–706.

are administered two to four times daily. Demeclocycline also is incompletely absorbed but can be administered less frequently because its $t_{1/2}$ of 16 h provides effective plasma concentrations for 24–48 h. Oral doses of doxycycline and minocycline are well absorbed (90%–100%) and have half-lives of 16–18 h; they can be administered at lower doses than tetracycline or demeclocycline. Plasma concentrations are equivalent whether doxycycline is given orally or parenterally. Food, including dairy products, does not interfere with absorption of doxycycline and minocycline.

Tetracyclines distribute widely throughout the body, including urine and prostate. They accumulate in reticuloendothelial cells of the liver, spleen, and bone marrow and in bone, dentine, and enamel of unerupted teeth. Tigecycline distributes rapidly and extensively into tissues, with an estimated apparent volume of 7–10 L/kg. Inflammation of the meninges is not required for the passage of tetracyclines into the CSF. Tetracyclines cross the placenta and enter the fetal circulation and amniotic fluid. Relatively high concentrations are found in breast milk.

Except for doxycycline, most tetracyclines are eliminated primarily by the kidney, although they also are concentrated in the liver, excreted in bile, and partially reabsorbed via enterohepatic recirculation. Comparable amounts of tetracycline (i.e., 20%–60%) are excreted in the urine within 24 h following oral or intravenous administration. Doxycycline is largely excreted unchanged in both the bile and urine, tigecycline is mostly excreted unchanged along with a small amount of glucuronidated metabolites, and minocycline is extensively metabolized by the liver before excretion. Hence, no dose adjustment is needed in patients with renal dysfunction. Specific dosage adjustment recommendations in hepatic disease are available only for tigecycline.

Therapeutic Uses and Dosage

The tetracyclines remain useful as first-line therapy for infections caused by rickettsiae, mycoplasmas, and chlamydiae. Doxycycline, the most important member of the tetracyclines, is a drug of choice for many sexually transmitted diseases, rickettsial infections, plague, brucellosis, tularemia, and spirochetal infections and is also used for treatment of respiratory tract infections and for skin and soft-tissue infections caused by community strains of MRSA, for which minocycline also is effective. The glycylcyclines have restored much of the antibacterial activity lost to the tetracyclines due to resistance and can be used for a number of infections due to gram-positive and gram-negative organisms (De Rosa et al., 2015). However, a pooled analysis of tigecycline clinical trials found a small but statistically significant increased risk of death with tigecycline versus comparators (Food and Drug Administration, 2016). Thus, tigecycline should generally be reserved for situations in which alternative treatment is not appropriate.

The oral dose of tetracycline ranges from 1 to 2 g/d in adults. Children more than 8 years of age should receive 25–50 mg/kg daily in four divided doses (not to exceed 2 g/d). The typical oral or intravenous dose of doxycycline for adults is 100 mg every 12 or 24 h; for children more than 8 years of age, the dose is 4.4 mg/kg/d in two divided doses the first day, then 2.2 mg/kg given once or twice daily. The typical dose of minocycline for adults is 200 mg orally or intravenously initially, followed by 100 mg every 12 h; for children, it is 4 mg/kg initially followed by 2 mg/kg every 12 h. Different dosing recommendations exist for certain diseases (i.e., syphilis); the reader is advised to consult the most current guidelines. Tigecycline is administered intravenously to adults as a 100-mg loading dose, followed by 50 mg every 12 h. For patients with severe hepatic impairment, the loading dose should be followed by a reduced maintenance dose of 25 mg every 12 h. Dosage data are not available for tigecycline in pediatrics.

Respiratory Tract Infections. Doxycycline has good activity against *Streptococcus pneumoniae* and *H. influenzae* and excellent activity against atypical pathogens such as *Mycoplasma* and *Chlamydophila pneumoniae*. Tigecycline is effective for use as a single agent for adults hospitalized with community-acquired bacterial pneumonia.

Skin and Soft-Tissue Infections. Tigecycline is approved for the treatment of complicated skin and soft-tissue infections. Doxycycline and minocycline have good activity against staphylococci and may be useful in treatment of cutaneous MRSA infections. Low doses of tetracycline have been used to treat acne (25 mg orally twice a day).

Intra-abdominal Infections. Resistance among Enterobacteriaceae and gram-negative anaerobes limits the utility of the tetracyclines for intra-abdominal infections. However, tigecycline possesses excellent activity against these pathogens as well as *Enterococcus*.

Sexually Transmitted Diseases. Doxycycline no longer is recommended for gonococcal infections because of the spread of resistance (Centers for Disease Control and Prevention, 2015). A 7-day treatment course of doxycycline is as effective as, but less convenient than, single-dose azithromycin in the treatment of uncomplicated genital infections due to *Chlamydia trachomatis*. *Chlamydia trachomatis* is often a coexistent pathogen in acute pelvic inflammatory disease, and doxycycline is a component of combination therapy regimens for this condition. Acute epididymitis is caused by infection with *C. trachomatis* or *Neisseria gonorrhoeae* in men less than 35 years of age. Effective regimens include a single injection of ceftriaxone (250 mg) plus doxycycline for 10 days. Sexual partners also should be treated. Doxycycline for 21 days is first-line therapy for treatment of lymphogranuloma venereum. Nonpregnant penicillin-allergic patients who have primary, secondary, or latent syphilis can be treated with a tetracycline regimen, such as doxycycline for 2 weeks. Tetracyclines should not be used for treatment of neurosyphilis.

Rickettsial Infections. Tetracyclines are lifesaving in rickettsial infections, including Rocky Mountain spotted fever, recrudescent epidemic typhus (Brill disease), murine typhus, scrub typhus, rickettsialpox, and Q fever. Clinical improvement often is evident within 24 h after initiation of therapy. Doxycycline is the drug of choice for treatment of Rocky Mountain spotted fever in adults and in children, including those less than 9 years of age, in whom the risk of staining of permanent teeth is outweighed by the seriousness of this potentially fatal infection (Masters et al., 2003).

Anthrax. Doxycycline is indicated for prevention or treatment of anthrax. It should be used in combination with another agent when treating inhalational or GI infection. The recommended duration of therapy is 60 days for bioterrorism exposures.

Local Application. Except for local use in the eye, topical use of the tetracyclines is not recommended, although they are FDA-approved as over-the-counter topical first-aid antibiotics. Sustained-release preparations of minocycline and doxycycline for subgingival administration are used in dentistry.

Other Infections. Tetracyclines in combination with rifampin or streptomycin are effective for acute and chronic infections caused by *Brucella melitensis*, *Brucella suis*, and *Brucella abortus*. Although streptomycin is preferable, tetracyclines also are effective in tularemia. Actinomycosis, although most responsive to penicillin G, may be successfully treated with a tetracycline. Minocycline is an alternative for the treatment of nocardiosis, but a sulfonamide should be used concurrently. Yaws and relapsing fever respond favorably to the tetracyclines. Tetracyclines are useful in the acute treatment and for prophylaxis of leptospirosis (*Leptospira* spp.). *Borrelia* spp., including *B. recurrentis* (relapsing fever) and *B. burgdorferi* (Lyme disease), respond to tetracyclines. The tetracyclines have been used to treat susceptible atypical mycobacterial pathogens, including *Mycobacterium marinum*. Tetracyclines in combination with bismuth and metronidazole can be used for *H. pylori* infections (Peterson et al., 2000).

Adverse Effects

Gastrointestinal. All tetracyclines can produce GI irritation, most commonly after oral administration. Epigastric burning and distress, abdominal discomfort, nausea, vomiting, and diarrhea may occur. Tolerability can be improved by administering these drugs with food, but tetracyclines should not be taken with dairy products or antacids. Tetracyclines have been associated with esophagitis and esophageal ulcers; patients should take oral formulations with a full glass of water while standing. Tigecycline administered intravenously has also been associated with nausea and vomiting.

Many of the tetracyclines are incompletely absorbed from the GI tract, and high concentrations in the bowel can markedly alter enteric flora. Sensitive aerobic and anaerobic coliform microorganisms and gram-positive spore-forming bacteria are suppressed markedly during long-term tetracycline regimens. As the fecal coliform count declines, overgrowth of tetracycline-resistant microorganisms occurs, particularly of yeasts (*Candida* spp.), enterococci, *Proteus*, and *Pseudomonas*. Moniliasis, thrush, or *Candida*-associated esophagitis may arise during therapy with tetracyclines.

Photosensitivity. Demeclocycline, doxycycline, and other tetracyclines and, to a lesser extent, glycylcyclines may produce photosensitivity reactions in treated individuals exposed to sunlight. Onycholysis and pigmentation of the nails may develop with or without accompanying photosensitivity.

Hepatic Toxicity. Hepatic toxicity has developed in patients with renal failure receiving 2 g or more of tetracycline per day parenterally, but this effect also may occur when large quantities are administered orally. Pregnant women are particularly susceptible. Doxycycline is probably not associated with hepatotoxicity.

Renal Toxicity. Tetracyclines may aggravate azotemia in patients with renal disease because of the catabolic effects of the drugs. Doxycycline, minocycline, and tigecycline have fewer renal side effects than other tetracyclines. Nephrogenic diabetes insipidus has been observed in some patients receiving demeclocycline, and this phenomenon has been exploited for the treatment of the syndrome of inappropriate secretion of antidiuretic hormone (see Chapter 25). Fanconi syndrome (characterized by nausea, vomiting, polyuria, polydipsia, proteinuria, acidosis, glycosuria, and aminoaciduria) has been observed in patients ingesting outdated tetracycline, presumably due to toxic effects on the proximal renal tubules.

Effects on Teeth. Children treated with a tetracycline or glycylcycline may develop permanent brown discoloration of the teeth. The duration of therapy appears to be less important than the total quantity of antibiotic administered. The risk is highest when a tetracycline is given to infants before the first dentition but may develop if the drug is given between the ages of 2 months and 5 years when these teeth are being calcified. Treatment of pregnant patients with tetracyclines may produce discoloration of the teeth in their children.

Other Toxic and Irritative Effects. Tetracyclines are deposited in the skeleton during gestation and throughout childhood and may depress bone growth in premature infants. This is readily reversible if the period of exposure to the drug is short. Thrombophlebitis frequently follows intravenous administration. This irritative effect of tetracyclines has been used therapeutically in patients with malignant pleural effusions. Long-term tetracycline therapy may produce leukocytosis, atypical lymphocytes, toxic granulation of granulocytes, and thrombocytopenic purpura. Tetracyclines may cause increased intracranial pressure (pseudotumor cerebri) in young infants, even when given in the usual therapeutic doses. Patients receiving minocycline may experience vestibular toxicity, manifested by dizziness, ataxia, nausea, and vomiting. The symptoms occur soon after the initial dose and generally disappear within 24–48 h after drug cessation. Various skin reactions rarely may follow the use of any of the tetracyclines. Among the more severe allergic responses are angioedema and anaphylaxis; anaphylactoid reactions can occur even after oral use. Other hypersensitivity reactions are burning of the eyes, cheilosis, atrophic or hypertrophic glossitis, pruritus ani or vulvae, and vaginitis; these reactions can persist for weeks or months after cessation of tetracycline therapy. Cross-sensitization among the various tetracyclines is common.

Drug Interactions. As mentioned, oral coadministration of tetracyclines and divalent and trivalent cations can lead to chelation of the tetracycline, with resultant poor absorption. There is some evidence for drug interactions between doxycycline and hepatic enzyme-inducing agents such as phenytoin and rifampin, but not for minocycline or tigecycline.

Chloramphenicol

Chloramphenicol, an antibiotic produced by *Streptomyces venezuelae*, was introduced into clinical practice in 1948. Chloramphenicol can cause serious and fatal blood dyscrasias; consequently, the drug is now reserved for treatment of life-threatening infections (e.g., meningitis, rickettsial infections) in patients who cannot take safer alternatives because of resistance or allergies (Wareham et al., 2002).

$$O_2N-\phi-CHCH-NH-C-CHCl_2$$

CHLORAMPHENICOL

Mechanism of Action

Chloramphenicol inhibits protein synthesis in bacteria and, to a lesser extent, in eukaryotic cells. The drug readily penetrates bacterial cells, probably by facilitated diffusion. Chloramphenicol acts primarily by binding reversibly to the 50S ribosomal subunit (near the binding site for the macrolide antibiotics and clindamycin). The drug prevents the binding of the amino acid–containing end of the aminoacyl tRNA to the acceptor site on the 50S ribosomal subunit. The interaction between peptidyltransferase and its amino acid substrate cannot occur, and peptide bond formation is inhibited (Figure 59–2).

Chloramphenicol also can inhibit mitochondrial protein synthesis in mammalian cells, perhaps because mitochondrial ribosomes resemble bacterial ribosomes (both are 70S); erythropoietic cells are particularly sensitive.

Antimicrobial Activity

Chloramphenicol possesses a broad spectrum of antimicrobial activity. Chloramphenicol is bacteriostatic against most species, although it may be bactericidal against *H. influenzae*, *Neisseria meningitidis*, and *S. pneumoniae*. Strains of *S. aureus* tend to be less susceptible, but some isolates of highly resistant MRSA have been susceptible. Chloramphenicol is active against enterococci, including multidrug-resistant *E. faecium*. Chloramphenicol is active against *Mycoplasma*, *Chlamydia*, and *Rickettsia*. Enterobacteriaceae are variably sensitive to chloramphenicol, but *P. aeruginosa* is resistant to even very high concentrations of chloramphenicol. Strains of *V. cholerae* have remained largely susceptible to chloramphenicol. Prevalent strains of *Shigella* and *Salmonella* are resistant to multiple drugs, including chloramphenicol.

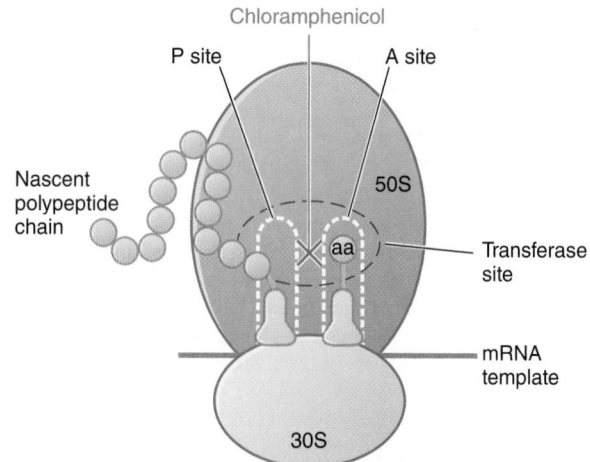

Figure 59–2 *Inhibition of bacterial protein synthesis by chloramphenicol.* Chloramphenicol binds to the 50S ribosomal subunit at the peptidyltransferase site, inhibiting transpeptidation. Chloramphenicol binds near the site of action of clindamycin and the macrolide antibiotics. These agents interfere with the binding of chloramphenicol and thus may interfere with each other's actions if given concurrently. See Figure 59–1 for additional information.

Resistance to Chloramphenicol

Resistance to chloramphenicol usually is caused by a plasmid-encoded acetyltransferase that inactivates the drug. Resistance also can result from decreased permeability and from ribosomal mutation. Acetylated derivatives of chloramphenicol fail to bind to bacterial ribosomes.

ADME

Chloramphenicol has been available in oral, intravenous, and topical (e.g., ophthalmic) preparations. The oral formulation is no longer available in the U.S., although it can be found in other parts of the world. Chloramphenicol administered in oral capsule form is absorbed rapidly from the GI tract. For parenteral use, chloramphenicol succinate is a prodrug that is hydrolyzed by esterases to chloramphenicol in vivo. Chloramphenicol succinate is rapidly cleared from plasma by the kidneys; this may reduce overall bioavailability of the drug because as much as 30% of the dose may be excreted before hydrolysis. Poor renal function in the neonate and other states of renal insufficiency result in increased plasma concentrations of chloramphenicol succinate. Decreased esterase activity has been observed in the plasma of neonates and infants, prolonging time to peak concentrations of active chloramphenicol (up to 4 h) and extending the period over which renal clearance of chloramphenicol succinate can occur.

Chloramphenicol is widely distributed in body fluids and readily reaches therapeutic concentrations in CSF. Chloramphenicol is present in bile, milk, and placental fluid. Hepatic metabolism to the inactive glucuronide is the major route of elimination. This metabolite and chloramphenicol are excreted in the urine. Patients with impaired hepatic function have decreased metabolic clearance, and dosage should be adjusted. About 50% of chloramphenicol is bound to plasma proteins; such binding is reduced in cirrhotic patients and in neonates. Half-life is not altered significantly by renal insufficiency or hemodialysis, and dosage adjustment usually is not required. Variability in the metabolism and pharmacokinetics of chloramphenicol in neonates, infants, and children necessitates monitoring of drug concentrations in plasma.

Therapeutic Uses and Dosage

Therapy with chloramphenicol must be limited to infections for which the benefits of the drug outweigh the risks of the potential toxicities. When other antimicrobial drugs that are equally effective and less toxic are available, they should be used instead of chloramphenicol.

Typhoid Fever. Third-generation cephalosporins and quinolones are drugs of choice for the treatment of typhoid fever because they are less toxic and because strains of *Salmonella typhi* often are resistant to chloramphenicol. The adult dose of chloramphenicol for typhoid fever is 1 g every 6 h for 4 weeks.

Bacterial Meningitis. Chloramphenicol remains an alternative drug for the treatment of meningitis caused by *H. influenzae*, *N. meningitidis*, and *S. pneumoniae* in patients who have severe allergy to β-lactams and in developing countries. The total daily dose for children should be 50 mg/kg of body weight, divided into four equal doses given intravenously every 6 h.

Rickettsial Diseases. The tetracyclines usually are the preferred agents for the treatment of rickettsial diseases. However, in patients allergic to these drugs, in pregnant women, and in children less than 8 years of age who require prolonged or repeated courses of therapy, chloramphenicol is an alternative therapy. Rocky Mountain spotted fever, epidemic, murine, scrub, and recrudescent typhus and Q fever respond well to chloramphenicol. For adults and children with these diseases, a dosage of 50 mg/kg/d divided into 6-h intervals is recommended. For severe or resistant infections, doses up to 100 mg/kg/d may be used for short intervals, but the dose must be reduced to 50 mg/kg/d as soon as possible. Therapy should be continued until the general condition has improved and the patient is afebrile for 24–48 h.

Adverse Effects

Chloramphenicol inhibits the synthesis of proteins of the inner mitochondrial membrane, probably by inhibiting the ribosomal peptidyltransferase. These include subunits of cytochrome *c* oxidase, ubiquinone-cytochrome *c* reductase, and the proton-translocating ATPase critical for aerobic metabolism. Much of the toxicity observed with this drug can be attributed to these effects.

Hypersensitivity Reactions. Skin rashes may result from hypersensitivity to chloramphenicol. Fever may appear simultaneously or be the sole manifestation. Angioedema is a rare complication. Jarisch-Herxheimer reactions may occur after institution of chloramphenicol therapy for syphilis, brucellosis, and typhoid fever.

Hematological Toxicity. Chloramphenicol affects the hematopoietic system in two ways: a dose-related toxicity that presents as anemia, leukopenia, or thrombocytopenia and an idiosyncratic response manifested by aplastic anemia, leading in many cases to fatal pancytopenia. Dose-related, reversible erythroid suppression probably reflects an inhibitory action of chloramphenicol on mitochondrial protein synthesis in erythroid precursors, which in turn impairs iron incorporation into heme. Bone marrow suppression occurs regularly when plasma concentrations are 25 µg/mL or greater and is observed with the use of large doses of chloramphenicol, prolonged treatment, or both. Dose-related suppression of the bone marrow may progress to fatal aplasia if treatment is continued, but most cases of bone marrow aplasia develop without prior dose-related marrow suppression.

Pancytopenia occurs more commonly in individuals who undergo prolonged therapy and especially in those who are exposed to the drug on more than one occasion. Although the incidence of the reaction is low, about 1 in 30,000 courses of therapy or more, the fatality rate is high when bone marrow aplasia is complete, and there is an increased incidence of acute leukemia in those who recover. Aplastic anemia accounts for about 70% of cases of blood dyscrasias due to chloramphenicol; hypoplastic anemia, agranulocytosis, and thrombocytopenia make up the remainder. The proposed mechanism involves conversion of the nitro group to a toxic intermediate by intestinal bacteria.

Other Toxic and Irritative Effects. Nausea and vomiting, unpleasant taste, diarrhea, and perineal irritation may follow the oral administration of chloramphenicol. Blurring of vision and digital paresthesias may rarely occur. Tissues that have a high rate of oxygen consumption (e.g., heart, brain) may be particularly susceptible to chloramphenicol's effects on mitochondrial enzymes.

Neonates, especially if premature, may develop a serious illness termed *gray baby syndrome*. This syndrome usually begins 2–9 days after treatment is started. Within the first 24 h, vomiting, refusal to suck, irregular and rapid respiration, abdominal distention, periods of cyanosis, and passage of loose green stools occur. Over the next 24 h, neonates turn an ashen-gray color and become flaccid and hypothermic. A similar "gray syndrome" has been reported in adults who were accidentally overdosed with the drug. Death occurs in about 40% of patients within 2 days of initial symptoms. Those who recover usually exhibit no sequelae. Two mechanisms apparently are responsible for chloramphenicol toxicity in neonates: (1) a developmental deficiency of glucuronyl transferase, the hepatic enzyme that metabolizes chloramphenicol; and (2) inadequate renal excretion of unconjugated drug. At the onset of the clinical syndrome, chloramphenicol concentrations in plasma usually exceed 100 µg/mL and may be as low as 75 µg/mL.

Drug Interactions. Chloramphenicol inhibits hepatic CYPs and thereby prolongs the half-lives of drugs that are metabolized by this system. Severe toxicity and death have occurred because of failure to recognize such effects. Concurrent administration of phenobarbital or rifampin, which potently induce CYPs, shortens the $t_{1/2}$ of the antibiotic and may result in subtherapeutic drug concentrations.

Macrolides and Ketolides

Macrolide antibiotics are widely used agents for treatment of respiratory tract infections caused by the common pathogens of community-acquired pneumonia. Four macrolides are available for clinical use: erythromycin, clarithromycin, azithromycin, and fidaxomicin. Erythromycin is the original agent in the class, discovered in 1952 by McGuire and coworkers in the metabolic products of a strain of *Streptomyces erythreus*.

Azithromycin and clarithromycin are semisynthetic derivatives of erythromycin that have largely replaced it in clinical use. Fidaxomicin is a nonsystemically absorbed macrolide used only for the treatment of *Clostridium difficile* colitis. Ketolides are semisynthetic derivatives of erythromycin with activity against some macrolide-resistant strains.

Macrolide antibiotics contain a multimembered lactone ring (14-membered rings for erythromycin and clarithromycin and a 15-membered ring for azithromycin) to which are attached one or more deoxy sugars. Clarithromycin differs from erythromycin only by methylation of the hydroxyl group at the 6 position, and azithromycin differs by the addition of a methyl-substituted nitrogen atom into the lactone ring. These structural modifications improve acid stability and tissue penetration and broaden the spectrum of activity.

ERYTHROMYCIN

Ketolides are structurally similar multimembered ring systems but with different substituents. Telithromycin differs from erythromycin in that a 3-keto group replaces the α-L-cladinose of the 14-member macrolide ring, and there is a substituted carbamate at C11-C12. Telithromycin is the only ketolide currently approved in the U.S. These modifications render ketolides less susceptible to methylase-mediated (*erm*) and efflux-mediated (*mef* or *msr*) mechanisms of resistance. Ketolides therefore are active against many macrolide-resistant gram-positive strains; however, concerns about the safety of telithromycin have limited its use (Brinker et al., 2009).

TELITHROMYCIN

Mechanism of Action

Macrolide and ketolide antibiotics are bacteriostatic agents that inhibit protein synthesis by binding reversibly to 50S ribosomal subunits of sensitive microorganisms (Figure 59–3) at or very near the site that binds chloramphenicol (see Figure 59–2). Erythromycin does not inhibit peptide bond formation per se but rather inhibits the translocation step wherein a newly synthesized peptidyl tRNA molecule moves from the acceptor site on the ribosome to the peptidyl donor site. Gram-positive bacteria accumulate about 100 times more erythromycin than do gram-negative bacteria.

Antimicrobial Activity

Erythromycin usually is bacteriostatic but may be bactericidal in high concentrations against susceptible organisms. Erythromycin has

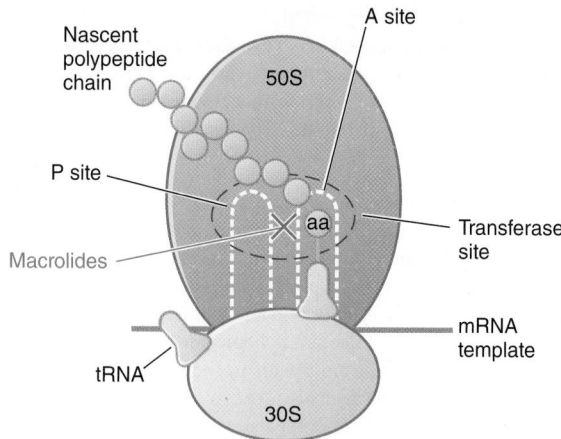

Figure 59–3 *Inhibition of bacterial protein synthesis by erythromycin, clarithromycin, and azithromycin.* Macrolide antibiotics are bacteriostatic agents that inhibit protein synthesis by binding reversibly to the 50S ribosomal subunits of sensitive organisms. Erythromycin appears to inhibit the translocation step such that the nascent peptide chain temporarily residing at the A site fails to move to the P, or donor, site. Alternatively, macrolides may bind and cause a conformational change that terminates protein synthesis by indirectly interfering with transpeptidation and translocation. See Figure 59–1 for additional information.

reasonably good activity against streptococci (see Table 59–1), but macrolide resistance among *S. pneumoniae* often coexists with penicillin resistance. Staphylococci are not reliably sensitive to erythromycin, and macrolide-resistant strains of *S. aureus* are potentially cross-resistant to clindamycin and streptogramin B (quinupristin). Gram-positive bacilli also are frequently sensitive to erythromycin, including *Clostridium perfringens*, *Corynebacterium diphtheriae*, and *L. monocytogenes*. Erythromycin is inactive against most aerobic enteric gram-negative bacilli. It has modest activity in vitro against *H. influenzae* and *N. meningitidis* and good activity against most strains of *N. gonorrhoeae*. Useful antibacterial activity also is observed against *P. multocida*, *Borrelia* spp., and *Bordetella pertussis*. Macrolides are usually active against *C. jejuni*. Erythromycin is active against *M. pneumoniae* and *Legionella pneumophila*. Most strains of *C. trachomatis* are inhibited by erythromycin.

Azithromycin has similar activity as erythromycin against sensitive strains of streptococci and staphylococci, while clarithromycin is slightly more potent. Clarithromycin is somewhat less active than erythromycin against *H. influenzae*, whereas azithromycin is the most active macrolide. Clarithromycin and azithromycin have good activity against *Moraxella catarrhalis*, *Chlamydia* spp., *L. pneumophila*, *B. burgdorferi*, *M. pneumoniae*, and *H. pylori*. Azithromycin and clarithromycin have enhanced activity against MAI, as well as against some protozoa (e.g., *Toxoplasma gondii*, *Cryptosporidium*, and *Plasmodium* spp.). Clarithromycin has good activity against *Mycobacterium leprae*. Telithromycin's spectrum of activity is similar to those of clarithromycin and azithromycin, but its capacity to withstand many macrolide resistance mechanisms increases its activity against macrolide-resistant *S. pneumoniae* and *S. aureus*.

Resistance to Macrolides and Ketolides

Resistance to macrolides usually results from one of four mechanisms (Nakajima, 1999):

- Drug efflux by an active pump mechanism
- Ribosomal protection by inducible or constitutive production of methylase enzymes, which modify the ribosomal target and decrease drug binding
- Macrolide hydrolysis by esterases produced by Enterobacteriaceae
- Chromosomal mutations that alter a 50S ribosomal protein (in *Bacillus subtilis*, *Campylobacter* spp., mycobacteria, and gram-positive cocci)

ADME

Erythromycin base is incompletely absorbed from the upper small intestine. Because it is inactivated by gastric acid, it is administered as enteric-coated tablets or as capsules containing enteric-coated pellets that dissolve in the duodenum; food may delay absorption. Esters of erythromycin base (e.g., stearate, estolate, and ethylsuccinate) have improved acid stability, and their absorption is less altered by food. Erythromycin diffuses readily into intracellular fluids, achieving antibacterial activity in essentially all sites except the brain and CSF. Protein binding is about 70%–80% for erythromycin base and even higher for the estolate. Erythromycin traverses the placenta, and drug concentrations in fetal plasma are about 5%–20% of those in the maternal circulation. Concentrations in breast milk are 50% of those in serum. Erythromycin is concentrated in the liver and excreted in the bile. The serum $t_{1/2}$ of erythromycin is about 1.6 h. Although the $t_{1/2}$ may be prolonged in patients with anuria, dosage reduction is not routinely recommended in patients in renal failure. The drug is not removed significantly by either peritoneal dialysis or hemodialysis.

Clarithromycin is absorbed rapidly from the GI tract after oral administration, but hepatic first-pass metabolism reduces its bioavailability to 50%–55%. Peak concentrations occur about 2 h after drug administration. Clarithromycin may be given with or without food, but the extended-release form should be administered with food to improve bioavailability. Clarithromycin and its active metabolite, 14-hydroxyclarithromycin, achieve high intracellular concentrations throughout the body, including the middle ear. Clarithromycin is metabolized in the liver to several metabolites; the active 14-hydroxy metabolite is the most significant. The elimination $t_{1/2}$ are 3–7 h for clarithromycin and 5–9 h for 14-hydroxyclarithromycin. Metabolism is saturable, resulting in nonlinear pharmacokinetics and longer half-lives with higher dosages. The amount of clarithromycin excreted unchanged in the urine ranges from 20% to 40%, depending on the dose administered and the formulation (tablet vs. oral suspension). An additional 10%–15% of a dose is excreted in the urine as 14-hydroxyclarithromycin. Dose adjustment is not recommended unless the creatinine clearance is less than 30 mL/min.

Azithromycin administered orally is absorbed rapidly (although incompletely: bioavailability for the immediate-release formulation is on the order of 30%–40%) and distributes widely throughout the body, except to the brain and CSF. Azithromycin also can be administered intravenously, producing plasma concentrations of 3–4 µg/mL after a 1-h infusion of 500 mg. Azithromycin's unique pharmacokinetic properties include extensive tissue distribution and high drug concentrations within cells (including phagocytes), resulting in much greater concentrations of drugs in tissue or secretions compared to simultaneous serum concentrations. Azithromycin undergoes some hepatic metabolism to inactive metabolites, but biliary excretion is the major route of elimination. Only 12% of drug is excreted unchanged in the urine. The elimination $t_{1/2}$, 40–68 h, is prolonged because of extensive tissue sequestration and binding.

Telithromycin is formulated as a 400-mg tablet for oral administration; there is no parenteral form. It is well absorbed with about 60% bioavailability. Peak serum concentrations are achieved within 30 min to 4 h. Telithromycin penetrates well into most tissues and is concentrated in many tissues, in particular in macrophages and white blood cells, where concentrations of 40 µg/mL (500 times the plasma concentration) are maintained even 24 h after dosing. Telithromycin has a $t_{1/2}$ of 9.8 h and can be given once daily. The drug is cleared primarily by hepatic metabolism, 50% by CYP3A4 and 50% by CYP-independent metabolism. No adjustment of the dose is required for those with hepatic failure or mild-to-moderate renal failure.

Therapeutic Uses and Dosage

The usual oral dose of erythromycin (erythromycin base) for adults ranges from 1 to 2 g/d, in divided doses, usually given every 6 h. Food should not be taken concurrently, if possible, with erythromycin base or the stearate formulations, but this is not necessary with erythromycin estolate. The oral dose of erythromycin for children is 30–50 mg/kg/d, divided into four portions; this dose may be doubled for severe infections. Intravenous administration is generally reserved for the therapy of severe infections and is now used uncommonly; the usual dose is 0.5–1 g every 6 h.

Clarithromycin usually is given twice daily at a dose of 250 mg for adults with mild-to-moderate infections and 500 mg twice daily for more severe infections. The 500-mg extended-release formulation of clarithromycin is given as 2 tablets once daily. Clarithromycin (500 mg) is also packaged with lansoprazole (30 mg) and amoxicillin (1 g) as a combination regimen that is administered twice daily for 10 or 14 days to eradicate *H. pylori*.

Azithromycin should be given 1 h before or 2 h after meals when administered orally. For outpatient therapy of community-acquired pneumonia, pharyngitis, or sinusitis, a loading dose of 500 mg is given on the first day, and then 250 mg per day is given for days 2 through 5. Treatment or prophylaxis of MAI infection in HIV-infected patients requires higher doses: 500–600 mg daily in combination with one or more other agents for treatment or 1200 mg once weekly for primary prevention. Azithromycin is useful in treatment of sexually transmitted diseases, especially during pregnancy when tetracyclines are contraindicated (Centers for Disease Control and Prevention, 2015). The treatment of uncomplicated nongonococcal urethritis presumed to be caused by *C. trachomatis* consists of a single 1-g dose of azithromycin. This dose also is effective for chancroid. In children, the recommended dose of azithromycin oral suspension for acute otitis media and pneumonia is 10 mg/kg on the first day (maximum 500 mg) and 5 mg/kg (maximum 250 mg/d) on days 2 through 5. A single 30-mg/kg dose is approved as an alternative for otitis media.

Telithromycin's dose in adults is 800 mg orally once daily.

Respiratory Tract Infections. Macrolides are suitable drugs for the treatment of a number of respiratory tract infections. Azithromycin and clarithromycin are suitable choices for treatment of mild-to-moderate community-acquired pneumonia among ambulatory patients. In hospitalized patients, a macrolide is commonly added to an antipneumococcal β-lactam for coverage of atypical respiratory pathogens. Because of excellent in vitro activity, superior tissue concentration, the ease of administration as a single daily dose, and better tolerability compared to erythromycin, azithromycin (or a fluoroquinolone) has supplanted erythromycin as the first-line agent for treatment of legionellosis. Macrolides are also appropriate alternative agents for the treatment of acute exacerbations of chronic bronchitis, acute otitis media, acute streptococcal pharyngitis, and acute bacterial sinusitis. Azithromycin or clarithromycin are generally preferred to erythromycin due to their broader spectrum and superior tolerability.

Telithromycin is effective in the treatment of community-acquired pneumonia, acute exacerbations of chronic bronchitis, and acute bacterial sinusitis and has a potential advantage where macrolide-resistant strains are common. Due to a number of cases of severe hepatotoxicity, the drug's FDA approval is limited to community-acquired pneumonia; *telithromycin should be used only in circumstances where it provides a substantial advantage over less-toxic therapies.*

Skin and Soft-Tissue Infections. Macrolides are alternatives for treatment of erysipelas and cellulitis among patients who have a serious allergy to penicillin (Stevens et al., 2014). Erythromycin has been an alternative agent for the treatment of relatively minor skin and soft-tissue infections caused by either penicillin-sensitive or penicillin-resistant *S. aureus*. However, many strains of *S. aureus* are resistant to macrolides.

Chlamydial Infections. Chlamydial infections can be treated effectively with any of the macrolides. A single 1-g dose of azithromycin is recommended for patients with uncomplicated urethral, endocervical, rectal, or epididymal infections because of the ease of compliance. Erythromycin base is preferred for chlamydial pneumonia of infancy and ophthalmia neonatorum (50 mg/kg/d in four divided doses for 14 days). Azithromycin, 1 g/week for 3 weeks, may be effective for lymphogranuloma venereum.

Diphtheria. Erythromycin for 7 days is very effective for acute infections or for eradicating the diphtheria carrier state. Other macrolides are not FDA-approved for this indication. Antibiotics do not alter the course of an acute infection with diphtheria or decrease the risk of complications. Antitoxin is indicated in the treatment of acute infection.

Pertussis. Erythromycin is the drug of choice for treating persons with *B. pertussis* disease and for postexposure prophylaxis of household members and close contacts. Clarithromycin and azithromycin also are effective. If administered early in the course of whooping cough, erythromycin may shorten the duration of illness; it has little influence on the disease once the paroxysmal stage is reached. Nasopharyngeal cultures should be obtained from people with pertussis who do not improve with erythromycin therapy because resistance has been reported.

Helicobacter pylori Infection. Clarithromycin, 500 mg, in combination with omeprazole, 20 mg, and amoxicillin, 1 g, each administered twice daily for 10–14 days, is effective for treatment of peptic ulcer disease caused by *H. pylori.*

Mycobacterial Infections. Clarithromycin or azithromycin is recommended as first-line therapy for prophylaxis and treatment of disseminated infection caused by MAI in patients with HIV infection and for treatment of pulmonary disease in patients not infected with HIV (Masur et al., 2014). Clarithromycin (500 mg twice daily) plus ethambutol (15 mg/kg once daily) with or without rifabutin is an effective combination regimen. Clarithromycin also has been used with minocycline for the treatment of *M. leprae* in lepromatous leprosy.

Prophylactic Uses. Azithromycin or clarithromycin is recommended for primary prevention of infection due to MAI among patients with HIV infection and less than 50 CD4 cells/mm³. Single-agent therapy should not be used for treatment of active disease or for secondary prevention in patients with HIV. Erythromycin is an effective alternative for the prophylaxis of recurrences of rheumatic fever in individuals who are allergic to penicillin.

Adverse Effects

GI Toxicity. Oral or intravenous administration of erythromycin frequently is accompanied by moderate-to-severe epigastric distress. Erythromycin stimulates GI motility by acting on motilin receptors (see Chapter 51); indeed, erythromycin is used off label as a prokinetic agent in the intensive care setting and in patients with diabetic gastroparesis. Clarithromycin, azithromycin, and telithromycin also may cause GI distress, but to a lesser degree than erythromycin.

Cardiac Toxicity. Erythromycin, clarithromycin, azithromycin, and telithromycin have been reported to cause cardiac arrhythmias, including QT prolongation with ventricular tachycardia. A large cohort study found a small but statistically significant increase in the risk of sudden cardiac death with azithromycin compared to no antibiotic treatment or to amoxicillin. Risk factors for clinically significant cardiac toxicity include receipt of concomitant antiarrhythmic drugs or other agents that prolong QTc.

Hepatotoxicity. Cholestatic hepatitis is associated with long-term treatment with erythromycin. The illness starts after 10–20 days of treatment and is characterized initially by nausea, vomiting, and abdominal cramps. These symptoms are followed shortly thereafter by jaundice, which may be accompanied by fever, leukocytosis, eosinophilia, and elevated transaminases in plasma. Findings usually resolve within a few days after cessation of drug therapy. Hepatotoxicity has also been observed with clarithromycin and azithromycin, although at a lower rate than with erythromycin. Telithromycin may induce severe hepatotoxicity and should only be used if it represents a clear advantage over alternative agents (Brinker et al., 2009).

Other Toxic and Irritative Effects. Allergic reactions observed are fever, eosinophilia, and skin eruptions, which disappear shortly after therapy is stopped. Auditory impairment and tinnitus have been observed with macrolides, especially at higher doses. Visual disturbances due to slowed accommodation have been reported following telithromycin. Telithromycin is contraindicated in patients with myasthenia gravis due to exacerbation of neurological symptoms.

Drug Interactions. Erythromycin, clarithromycin, and telithromycin strongly inhibit CYP3A4 and cause significant drug interactions (Periti et al., 1992). Erythromycin and clarithromycin potentiate the effects of carbamazepine, corticosteroids, cyclosporine, digoxin, ergot alkaloids,

theophylline, triazolam, valproate, and warfarin, probably by interfering with CYP-mediated metabolism of these drugs (see Chapter 6). Telithromycin is both a substrate and a strong inhibitor of CYP3A4. Coadministration of rifampin, a potent inducer of CYP, decreases the serum concentrations of telithromycin by 80%. CYP3A4 inhibitors (e.g., itraconazole) increase peak serum concentrations of telithromycin. Azithromycin is much less likely to be involved in these drug interactions; however, caution is advised when the consequences of interaction are severe.

Lincosamides

The class originator lincomycin and its congener clindamycin are approved in the U.S. Clindamycin has largely replaced lincomycin in clinical practice and is principally used to treat gram-positive aerobic and anaerobic infections, as well as some parasitic infections.

Mechanism of Action

Clindamycin binds exclusively to the 50S subunit of bacterial ribosomes and suppresses protein synthesis. Although clindamycin, erythromycin, and chloramphenicol are not structurally related, they act at sites in close proximity (see Figures 59–2 and 59–3), and binding by one of these antibiotics to the ribosome may inhibit the interaction of the others.

CLINDAMYCIN

Antimicrobial Activity

Bacterial strains are susceptible to clindamycin at MICs of 0.5 µg/mL or less. Clindamycin generally is similar to erythromycin in its in vitro activity against susceptible strains of pneumococci, *S. pyogenes*, and viridans streptococci (see Table 59–1). MSSAs usually are susceptible to clindamycin, but MRSA and coagulase-negative staphylococci are more likely to be resistant. Clindamycin is more active than erythromycin or clarithromycin against anaerobic bacteria, especially *B. fragilis*, but resistance to clindamycin in *Bacteroides* spp. increasingly is encountered. From 10% to 20% of clostridial species other than *C. perfringens* are resistant. Strains of *Actinomyces israelii* and *Nocardia asteroides* are sensitive. Essentially all aerobic gram-negative bacilli are resistant. Clindamycin plus primaquine and clindamycin plus pyrimethamine are second-line regimens for *Pneumocystis jiroveci* pneumonia and *T. gondii* encephalitis, respectively.

Resistance to Lincosamides

Macrolide resistance due to ribosomal methylation also may produce resistance to clindamycin. Because clindamycin does not induce the methylase, there is cross-resistance only if the enzyme is produced constitutively. However, selection for a subpopulation of constitutive methylase producers may occur among staphylococci and streptococci with a macrolide-inducible phenotype (Lewis and Jorgensen, 2005). Clindamycin is not a substrate for macrolide efflux pumps; thus, strains that are resistant to macrolides by this mechanism are susceptible to clindamycin.

ADME

Clindamycin is nearly completely absorbed following oral administration. Peak concentrations of 2–3 µg/mL are attained within 1 h after the ingestion of 150 mg. Food in the stomach does not reduce absorption significantly. The $t_{1/2}$ of the antibiotic is about 3 h. Clindamycin palmitate, an oral preparation for pediatric use, is an inactive prodrug that is hydrolyzed rapidly in vivo. The phosphate ester of clindamycin, which is given parenterally, also is rapidly hydrolyzed in vivo to the active parent compound.

Clindamycin is widely distributed in many fluids and tissues, including good concentrations in bone. CSF concentrations are limited, even when the meninges are inflamed, but concentrations sufficient to treat cerebral toxoplasmosis are achievable. The drug readily crosses the placental barrier. Ninety percent or more of clindamycin is bound to plasma proteins. Clindamycin accumulates in polymorphonuclear leukocytes and alveolar macrophages and in abscesses.

Clindamycin is inactivated by metabolism to *N*-demethylclindamycin and clindamycin sulfoxide, which are excreted in the urine and bile. Dosage adjustments may be required in patients with severe hepatic failure. Only about 10% of the clindamycin administered is excreted unaltered in the urine, and small quantities are found in the feces.

Therapeutic Uses and Dosage

The oral dose of clindamycin for adults is 150–300 mg every 6 h; for severe infections, it is 300–600 mg every 6 h. Children should receive 8–12 mg/kg/d of clindamycin palmitate hydrochloride in three or four divided doses or, for severe infections, 13–25 mg/kg/d. Clindamycin phosphate is available for intramuscular or intravenous use. For serious infections, intravenous or intramuscular administration is recommended in dosages of 1200–2700 mg/d, divided into three or four equal doses for adults. Children should receive 15–40 mg/kg/d in three or four divided doses; in severe infections, a minimal daily dose of 300 mg is recommended, regardless of body weight.

Skin and Soft-Tissue Infections. Clindamycin is an alternative agent for the treatment of skin and soft-tissue infections, especially in patients with β-lactam allergies (Stevens et al., 2014). It is also useful for oral treatment of skin infections when MRSA and streptococci are potential pathogens. Because clindamycin inhibits toxin production, it is recommended as an adjunctive agent in necrotizing fasciitis or gas gangrene when toxin-producing bacteria (e.g., streptococci, staphylococci, clostridia) are suspected. Topical clindamycin is used for treatment of acne.

Respiratory Tract Infections. Clindamycin is effective for treatment of lung abscess and anaerobic lung and pleural space infections due to susceptible organisms (Levison et al., 1983). It has been used as an alternative agent for treatment of sinusitis, pharyngitis, and otitis media. Clindamycin in combination with primaquine is useful for the treatment of mild-to-moderate cases of *P. jiroveci* pneumonia in patients with HIV.

Other Infections. Owing to its good activity against staphylococci and excellent bone penetration, clindamycin is an alternative agent for treatment of osteomyelitis. Clindamycin in combination with pyrimethamine and leucovorin (folinic acid) is an effective alternative for acute treatment of encephalitis caused by *T. gondii* in patients with AIDS. Clindamycin plus quinine is an alternative regimen for nonsevere malaria. Clindamycin is also administered vaginally for bacterial vaginosis.

Adverse Effects

GI Effects. The reported incidence of diarrhea associated with the administration of clindamycin ranges from 2% to 20%. In most cases, this is mild to moderate in severity and resolves on drug discontinuation. However, clindamycin carries a relatively high risk of superinfection with *C. difficile*. This colitis is characterized by watery diarrhea, fever, and elevated peripheral white blood cell counts. *This syndrome may be lethal.* Discontinuation of the drug, combined with administration of metronidazole or oral vancomycin usually, is curative, but relapses occur. Agents that inhibit peristalsis (e.g., opioids) may prolong and worsen the condition.

Other Toxic and Irritative Effects. Skin rashes occur in about 10% of patients treated with clindamycin and may be more common in patients with HIV infection. Other uncommon reactions include exudative erythema multiforme (Stevens-Johnson syndrome), reversible elevation of aspartate aminotransferase and alanine aminotransferase, granulocytopenia, thrombocytopenia, and anaphylactic reactions. Local thrombophlebitis may follow intravenous administration of the drug. Clindamycin may potentiate the effect of concomitant neuromuscular blocking agents.

Streptogramins

Streptogramins are semisynthetic derivatives of naturally occurring agents produced by *Streptomyces pristinaespiralis*. The only streptogramin in clinical use is a fixed combination of quinupristin (a streptogramin B) with dalfopristin (a streptogramin A) in a 30:70 ratio. Quinupristin and dalfopristin are more soluble derivatives of the congeners pristinamycin IA and IIA and therefore are suitable for intravenous administration.

Mechanism of Action

Quinupristin and dalfopristin are protein synthesis inhibitors that bind the 50S ribosomal subunit. Quinupristin binds at the same site as macrolides and has a similar effect, with inhibition of polypeptide elongation and early termination of protein synthesis. Dalfopristin binds at a site nearby, resulting in a conformational change in the 50S ribosome, synergistically enhancing the binding of quinupristin at its target site. Dalfopristin directly interferes with polypeptide chain formation. The net result of the cooperative and synergistic binding of these two molecules to the ribosome is *bactericidal* activity.

Antimicrobial Activity

Quinupristin/dalfopristin is active against gram-positive cocci and organisms responsible for atypical pneumonia (e.g., *M. pneumoniae*, *Legionella* spp., and *C. pneumoniae*) but is inactive against gram-negative organisms (Table 59–1). The combination is bactericidal against streptococci and many strains of staphylococci but bacteriostatic against *Enterococcus faecium*.

Resistance to Streptogramins

Resistance to quinupristin is mediated by genes encoding a ribosomal methylase that prevents binding of drug to its target or genes encoding lactonases that inactivate type B streptogramins. Resistance to dalfopristin is mediated by genes that encode acetyltransferases that inactivate type A streptogramins or staphylococcal genes that encode ATP-binding efflux proteins that pump type A streptogramins out of the cell. These resistance determinants are located on plasmids. Resistance to quinupristin/dalfopristin always is associated with a resistance gene for type A streptogramins. Methylase-encoding genes can render the combination bacteriostatic instead of bactericidal, making it ineffective in certain infections in which bactericidal activity is necessary (e.g., endocarditis).

ADME

Quinupristin/dalfopristin is administered by intravenous infusion over at least 1 h. The $t_{1/2}$ is 0.85 h for quinupristin and 0.7 h for dalfopristin. The volume of distribution is 0.87 L/kg for quinupristin and 0.71 L/kg for dalfopristin. Hepatic metabolism by conjugation is the principal means of clearance for both compounds, with 80% of an administered dose eliminated by biliary excretion. Renal elimination of active compound accounts for most of the remainder. No dosage adjustment is necessary for renal insufficiency. Pharmacokinetics are not significantly altered by peritoneal dialysis or hemodialysis. Hepatic insufficiency increases the plasma AUC of active component and metabolites by 180% for quinupristin and 50% for dalfopristin.

Therapeutic Uses and Dosage

Quinupristin/dalfopristin is approved in the U.S. for complicated skin and skin-structure infections caused by methicillin-susceptible strains of *S. aureus* or *S. pyogenes*. It is also used for treatment of infections caused by vancomycin-resistant strains of *E. faecium* (dose of 7.5 mg/kg every 8–12 h), and in Europe it also is approved for treatment of nosocomial pneumonia and infections caused by MRSA. Quinupristin/dalfopristin should be reserved for treatment of serious infections caused by multiple-drug-resistant gram-positive organisms such as vancomycin-resistant *E. faecium*.

Adverse Effects

The most common side effects are infusion-related events, such as pain and phlebitis at the infusion site and arthralgias and myalgias. Phlebitis and pain can be minimized by infusion of drug through a central venous catheter. Arthralgias and myalgias, more likely to be problematic in patients with hepatic insufficiency, are managed by reducing the infusion frequency.

Drug Interactions. Quinupristin/dalfopristin inhibits CYP3A4. The concomitant administration of other CYP3A4 substrates with quinupristin/dalfopristin may result in significant toxicity. Caution and monitoring are recommended for drugs in which the toxic therapeutic window is narrow or for drugs that prolong the QTc interval.

Oxazolidinones

Oxazolidinones are a new class of synthetic protein synthesis inhibitors with activity primarily against gram-positive organisms, including multi-drug-resistant pathogens. Linezolid is the class originator; a second agent, tedizolid, was FDA-approved in 2014.

Antimicrobial Activity

Linezolid is active against the vast majority of gram-positive organisms, including staphylococci, streptococci, enterococci, gram-positive anaerobic cocci, and gram-positive rods such as *Corynebacterium* spp., *Nocardia* spp., and *L. monocytogenes* (see Table 59–1). It has poor activity against most gram-negative aerobic or anaerobic bacteria. It is bacteriostatic against enterococci and staphylococci but may be bactericidal against streptococci. *Mycobacterium tuberculosis* is moderately susceptible, as are most rapidly growing mycobacteria, but MAI is frequently resistant. The available data to date suggest tedizolid has similar activity to linezolid (Rybak et al., 2014).

Mechanism of Action

Oxazolidinones inhibit protein synthesis by binding to the P site of the 50S ribosomal subunit and preventing formation of the larger ribosomal-fMet-tRNA complex that initiates protein synthesis. Because of its unique mechanism of action, these agents are active against strains that are resistant to multiple other agents, including penicillin-resistant strains of *S. pneumoniae*; methicillin-resistant, vancomycin-intermediate, and vancomycin-resistant strains of staphylococci; and vancomycin-resistant strains of enterococci.

Resistance to Oxazolidinones

Resistance in enterococci and staphylococci is most commonly due to point mutations of the 23S rRNA. Because bacteria have multiple copies of 23S rRNA genes, significant resistance generally requires mutations in two or more copies. Recently, a transferable methyltransferase that confers resistance through ribosomal modification has been described. Linezolid resistance remains relatively low among normally susceptible organisms, although some sites report increasing frequency in enterococci, including cases of nosocomial transfer. Although data are limited, tedizolid may be active against some linezolid-resistant isolates.

ADME

Linezolid is well absorbed after oral administration, with a bioavailability of 100%, and may be administered without regard to food. Dosing for oral and intravenous preparations is the same. The $t_{1/2}$ is about 4–6 h. Linezolid is 30% protein bound and distributes widely to well-perfused tissues. Linezolid is nonenzymatically oxidized to aminoethoxyacetic acid and hydroxyethyl glycine derivatives. Approximately 80% of a dose of linezolid appears in the urine, 30% as active compound and 50% as the two primary oxidation products. Ten percent of the administered dose appears as oxidation products in feces. No dose adjustment in renal insufficiency is recommended. Linezolid and its breakdown products are eliminated by dialysis; therefore, the drug should be administered after hemodialysis.

Tedizolid is administered orally and parenterally as a prodrug (tedizolid phosphate) that is rapidly and completely hydrolyzed to tedizolid. Tedizolid is well absorbed after oral administration (bioavailability > 80%). Tedizolid displays greater protein binding (70%–90%) and a longer $t_{1/2}$ of about 12 h. There is minimal elimination of unchanged drug in the urine; the drug undergoes sulfation in the liver and is excreted primarily in the feces.

Therapeutic Uses and Dosage

Linezolid is most commonly administered at a dose of 600 mg twice daily orally or intravenously. A 400-mg twice-daily dosage regimen is recommended only for treatment of uncomplicated skin and skin-structure infections in adults. Tedizolid is given as a 200-mg IV or oral daily dose.

Skin and Soft-Tissue Infections. Linezolid and tedizolid are FDA-approved for treatment of skin and skin-structure infections caused by streptococci and *S. aureus* (MSSA and MRSA). A 6-day regimen of tedizolid provided similar outcomes to 10 days of linezolid.

Respiratory Tract Infections. Linezolid is approved for treatment of community-acquired pneumonia due to *S. pneumoniae* and nosocomial pneumonia due to *S. aureus*. A randomized clinical trial in patients with MRSA pneumonia demonstrated similar or better outcomes to vancomycin (Wunderink et al., 2012). Studies of tedizolid for pneumonia are under way.

Other Infections. Linezolid has clinical and microbiological cure rates in the range of 85%–90% in treatment of a variety of infections caused by vancomycin-resistant *E. faecium*. Linezolid has been used in combination therapy for extensively drug-resistant tuberculosis and in infections due *Nocardia*.

Adverse Effects

Myelosuppression. Myelosuppression, including anemia, leukopenia, pancytopenia, and thrombocytopenia, has been reported in patients receiving linezolid. Thrombocytopenia tends to be the most common effect, with an onset between 7and 10 days. Effects are reversible on drug discontinuation. Platelet counts should be monitored in patients with risk of bleeding, preexisting thrombocytopenia, or intrinsic or acquired disorders of platelet function and in patients receiving courses of therapy lasting beyond 2 weeks. Treatment durations with tedizolid in clinical trials have been limited; based on early clinical and in vitro data, tedizolid may have a lower propensity for causing myelosuppression.

Mitochondrial Toxicities. Patients receiving treatment with linezolid have developed peripheral neuropathy, optic neuritis, and lactic acidosis (Narita et al., 2007). These effects typically manifest after prolonged treatment durations (at least 6 weeks), although some cases of lactic acidosis have been described after only a few days of therapy. The underlying mechanism of these toxicities is believed to be inhibition of mitochondrial protein synthesis. Linezolid should generally not be used for long-term therapy if there are alternative agents. There are insufficient data to judge the risk of mitochondrial toxicities with tedizolid.

Drug Interactions. Linezolid is a weak nonspecific inhibitor of MAO. Patients receiving concomitant therapy with an adrenergic or serotonergic agent (including SSRIs) or consuming more than 100 mg of tyramine a day may experience serotonin syndrome (e.g., palpitations, headache, hypertensive crisis). Coadministration of these agents is best avoided. However, in patients receiving SSRIs who acutely require linezolid therapy for short-term (10- to 14-day) treatment, coadministration with careful monitoring is reasonable. The relative potential for this interaction with tedizolid is not yet known. Neither linezolid nor tedizolid is a substrate or an inhibitor of CYPs.

Agents Acting on the Bacterial Cell Wall

Polymyxins

The polymyxins are a group of closely related antibiotics elaborated by strains of *Bacillus polymyxa*. Polymyxin B is a mixture of polymyxins B_1 and B_2. Colistin, also known as polymyxin E, is produced by *Bacillus colistinus* and is marketed either as colistimethate for intravenous administration or colistin base for topical use. These agents were initially developed more than 50 years ago but quickly fell out of favor for systemic use due to their toxicities. With the rise of resistant gram-negative organisms in the past decade, their use has increased substantially.

Antimicrobial Activity

The antimicrobial activities of polymyxin B and colistin are similar and restricted to gram-negative bacteria, primarily aerobes. Most *Pseudomonas*, *Acinetobacter*, and Enterobacteriaceae are susceptible, except for *Proteus* and *Serratia* spp. *Stenotrophomonas* and *Burkholderia* are usually resistant.

Mechanism of Action

Polymyxins, simple basic peptides with molecular masses of about 1000 Da, are surface-active amphipathic agents that act as cationic detergents. They interact strongly with phospholipids and disrupt the structure of cell membranes. Sensitivity to polymyxin B apparently is related to the phospholipid content of the cell wall–membrane complex. Polymyxin B binds to the lipid A portion of endotoxin (the lipopolysaccharide of the outer membrane of gram-negative bacteria) and inactivates this molecule.

Resistance to Polymyxins

Although resistance to polymyxins is rare, emergence of resistance while on treatment has been documented and has become problematic among extensively drug-resistant *Acinetobacter* and *Klebsiella*.

ADME

Polymyxin B and colistin are not absorbed when given orally and are poorly absorbed from mucous membranes and surfaces of large burns. CMS (colistimethate) is the prodrug formulation for parenteral administration; it is hydrolyzed relatively slowly in the bloodstream to the active colistin sulfate moiety. CMS may be administered via inhalation for prevention and adjunctive treatment of lung infections. Limited data are available regarding distribution of these agents in the body. Intraventricular and intrathecal administration has been used for treatment of CNS infections. CMS (but not colistin) is cleared renally; thus modification of the dose is generally required in patients with impaired renal function. Polymyxin B primarily undergoes nonrenal clearance.

Therapeutic Uses and Dosage

Because dosing of these agents varies by drug (polymyxin B or colistin), by the particular commercial preparation marketed in a specific country, and by the patient's degree of renal dysfunction, expert consultation is recommended.

Systemic Uses. Polymyxins are used systemically only for serious infections due to pathogens resistant to other effective therapies. They have been used for treatment of a variety of infections, including bacteremia, pneumonia, bone/joint infections, burns, cellulitis, cystic fibrosis, endocarditis, gynecologic infections, meningitis, and ventriculitis (Nation et al., 2015).

Topical Uses. Polymyxin B sulfate is available for ophthalmic, otic, and topical use in combination with a variety of other compounds. Colistin is available as otic drops. Infections of the skin, mucous membranes, eye, and ear due to polymyxin B–sensitive microorganisms respond to local application of the antibiotic in solution or ointment. External otitis, frequently due to *Pseudomonas*, may be cured by the topical use of the drug. *Pseudomonas aeruginosa* is a common cause of infection of corneal ulcers; local application or subconjunctival injection of polymyxin B often is curative.

Adverse Effects

The primary toxicity of polymyxins is dose-related nephrotoxicity. Neurological reactions include muscle weakness, apnea, paresthesias, vertigo, and slurred speech. Polymyxin B applied to intact or denuded skin or mucous membranes produces no systemic reactions because of its almost complete lack of absorption from these sites. Hypersensitivity reactions are uncommon.

Glycopeptides

The class originator for glycopeptides is vancomycin, a tricyclic glycopeptide antibiotic produced by *Streptococcus orientalis*. Teicoplanin is a mixture of related glycopeptides available as an antibiotic in Europe. It is similar to vancomycin in chemical structure, mechanism of action, spectrum of activity, and route of elimination (i.e., primarily renal). A new generation of glycopeptide congeners, the lipoglycopeptides, has been recently introduced into clinical practice. These agents include telavancin, dalbavancin, and oritavancin (Henson et al., 2015).

Antimicrobial Activity

Vancomycin possesses activity against the vast majority of gram-positive bacteria (see Table 59–1), including MRSA, penicillin-resistant streptococci, and ampicillin-resistant enterococci. Gram-positive organisms intrinsically resistant to vancomycin include *Lactobacillus*, *Leuconostoc*, *Pediococcus*, and *Erysipelothrix*. Essentially all species of gram-negative bacilli and mycobacteria are resistant to glycopeptides. The activity of teicoplanin, telavancin, dalbavancin, and oritavancin is generally similar to that of vancomycin; these agents are also active against some vancomycin-resistant enterococci (Goldstein et al., 2004).

Mechanism of Action

Glycopeptides inhibit the synthesis of the cell wall in sensitive bacteria by binding with high affinity to the D-alanyl-D-alanine terminus of cell wall precursor units (Figure 59–4). Because of their large molecular size, they are unable to penetrate the outer membrane of gram-negative bacteria. The lipoglycopeptides are able to dimerize and anchor their lipid moieties into the bacterial cell membrane, allowing for increased binding to the D-Ala-D-Ala target site and improved potency. Telavancin and oritavancin possess a second mechanism of action: direct disruption of the bacterial cell membrane. This effect leads to more rapid bactericidal activity than that of vancomycin.

Resistance to Glycopeptides

Glycopeptide-resistant strains of enterococci, primarily *E. faecium*, have emerged as major nosocomial pathogens in hospitals in the U.S. Determinants of vancomycin resistance are located on a transposon that is readily transferable among enterococci, and, potentially, other gram-positive bacteria. These strains are typically resistant to multiple antibiotics, including streptomycin, gentamicin, and ampicillin. Resistance to streptomycin and gentamicin is of special concern because the combination of an aminoglycoside with a cell wall synthesis inhibitor is the only reliably bactericidal regimen for treatment of enterococcal endocarditis.

Enterococcal resistance to glycopeptides is the result of alteration of the D-alanyl-D-alanine target to D-alanyl-D-lactate or D-alanyl D-serine, which bind glycopeptides poorly. Several enzymes within the *van* gene cluster are required for this target alteration to occur. *The vanA genotype* confers inducible resistance to teicoplanin and vancomycin in *E. faecium* and *Enterococcus faecalis*. Consistent with their dual mode of action, while MICs to telavancin and oritavancin may increase in isolates expressing *vanA*,

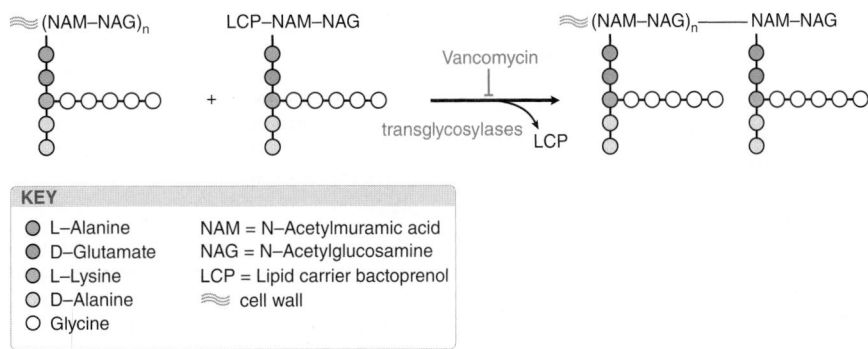

Figure 59–4 *Inhibition of bacterial cell wall synthesis by glycopeptides such as vancomycin*. Vancomycin inhibits the polymerization or transglycosylase reaction by binding to the D-alanyl-D-alanine terminus of the cell wall precursor unit attached to its lipid carrier and blocks linkage to the glycopeptide polymer (indicated by the subscript n). These (NAM–NAG)ₙ peptidoglycan polymers are located within the cell wall. *VanA-type* resistance is due to expression of enzymes that modify cell wall precursor by substituting a terminal D-lactate for D-alanine, reducing affinity for vancomycin by 1000-fold.

they often remain in the susceptible range. In contrast, *vanA*-expressing isolates are frequently dalbavancin resistant. The *vanB* genotype, which tends to be a lower level of resistance, also has been identified in *E. faecium* and *E. faecalis*. The trait is inducible by vancomycin but not teicoplanin; consequently, many strains remain susceptible to teicoplanin. Telavancin, dalbavancin, and oritavancin are usually active as well. The *vanC* genotype, the least important clinically and least well characterized, confers resistance only to vancomycin.

Staphylococcus aureus and coagulase-negative staphylococci may express reduced or "intermediate" susceptibility to vancomycin (MIC 4–8 μg/mL) or, very rarely, high-level resistance (MIC ≥ 16 μg/mL) (Howden et al., 2004). Intermediate resistance is associated with a heterogeneous phenotype in which a small proportion of cells within the population (1 in 10^5 to 1 in 10^6) will grow in the presence of vancomycin concentrations greater than 4 μg/mL. Prior treatment courses and low vancomycin levels may predispose patients to infection and treatment failure with vancomycin-intermediate strains. These strains typically are resistant to methicillin and multiple other antibiotics; their emergence is a major concern because until recently vancomycin has been the only antibiotic to which staphylococci were reliably susceptible. High-level vancomycin-resistant *S. aureus* strains (MIC ≥ 32 μg/mL) harbor a conjugative plasmid into which the *vanA* transposon is integrated by an interspecies horizontal gene transfer from *E. faecalis* to an MRSA. These isolates have been variably susceptible to teicoplanin and the lipoglycopeptides (Centers for Disease Control and Prevention, 2004).

ADME

All glycopeptides are poorly absorbed after oral administration; the oral formulation of vancomycin is exclusively used in patients with *C. difficile* colitis. Vancomycin should be only administered intravenously, not intramuscularly, due to pain with intramuscular injection. Approximately 30% of vancomycin is bound to plasma protein. Vancomycin appears in various body fluids, including the CSF when the meninges are inflamed (7%–30%); bile; and pleural, pericardial, synovial, and ascitic fluids. About 90% of an injected dose of vancomycin is excreted by glomerular filtration; elimination $t_{1/2}$ is about 6 h in normal renal function. The drug accumulates if renal function is impaired, and dosage adjustments must be made. The drug can be cleared from plasma with hemodialysis.

Teicoplanin can be administered by intramuscular injection as well as intravenous administration. An intravenous dose of 1 g in adults produces plasma concentrations of 15–30 μg/mL 1 h after a 1- to 2-h infusion. Teicoplanin is highly bound by plasma proteins (90%–95%) and has an extremely long serum elimination $t_{1/2}$ (up to 100 h), allowing for once-daily dosing. Excretion is through glomerular filtration.

Telavancin achieves peak concentrations of approximately 90 μg/mL when administered intravenously at a dose of 10 mg/kg once daily. Telavancin is highly protein bound (>90%), with a $t_{1/2}$ of about 7 h. Studies of penetration into epithelial lining fluid and skin blister fluid demonstrated adequate tissue concentrations to provide effective therapy. Telavancin is eliminated primarily (70%–80%) by renal excretion, with a small component of metabolism. Dosage adjustment is required in renal dysfunction.

Dalbavancin and oritavancin have unique pharmacokinetic properties that allow for intermittent (weekly or less) dosing. Both are characterized by extremely long plasma half-lives (on the order of 10 days for terminal elimination) and are highly (>90%) protein bound. Penetration of dalbavancin into skin blister fluid and bone appears to be adequate, but penetration into CSF is very low. Between 33% and 50% of dalbavancin is eliminated unchanged in the urine, and dosage adjustment is recommended for renal dysfunction. Oritavancin has a large volume of distribution (~1 L/kg). Renal excretion is very slow and dosage adjustment is not required in moderate renal dysfunction.

Therapeutic Uses and Dosage

Vancomycin hydrochloride is available for intravenous use as a sterile powder for solution. It should be diluted and infused over at least a 60-min period to avoid infusion-related adverse reactions; the recommended initial dose for adults is 30–45 mg/kg/d in two or three divided doses. Current recommendations call for monitoring serum trough concentrations

(within 30 min prior to a dose) at steady state, typically before the fourth dose of a given dosage regimen (Rybak et al., 2009). A trough serum concentration of at least 10 μg/mL is recommended. For patients with more serious infections (including endocarditis, osteomyelitis, meningitis, and MRSA pneumonia), trough levels of 15–20 μg/mL are recommended. Pediatric doses are as follows: for newborns during the first week of life, 15 mg/kg initially, followed by 10 mg/kg every 12 h; for infants 8–30 days old, 15 mg/kg followed by 10 mg/kg every 8 h; for older infants and children, 10–15 mg/kg every 6 h. Alteration of dosage is required for patients with impaired renal function. In functionally anephric patients and patients receiving dialysis with non–high-flux membranes, administration of 1 g (~15 mg/kg) every 5–7 days typically achieves adequate serum levels. In patients receiving intermittent high-efficiency or high-flux dialysis, maintenance doses administered after each dialysis session are typically required. For treatment of *C. difficile* colitis, vancomycin is available as capsules for oral administration; alternatively, the intravenous formulation may be compounded into a solution for oral administration. The recommended oral dose of vancomycin is 125 mg four times daily, with escalation up to 500 mg four times daily in patients with life-threatening disease.

Telavancin is administered intravenously at a dose of 10 mg/kg daily, with dosage adjustment required for patients with renal dysfunction. The approved dosage of intravenous dalbavancin for treatment of skin and soft-tissue infection is 1000 mg at the initiation of treatment, followed by a 500-mg dose 7 days later. Oritavancin has been studied for skin and soft-tissue infections as a single 1200-mg intravenous dose.

Skin/Soft-Tissue and Bone/Joint Infections. Vancomycin has long been a mainstay in the treatment of skin/soft-tissue and bone/joint infections, where gram-positive organisms, including MRSA, are the leading pathogens (Stevens et al., 2014). Telavancin, dalbavancin, and oritavancin offer alternatives for treatment of this condition, with dalbavancin and oritavancin offering the option for infrequent dosing.

Respiratory Tract Infections. Vancomycin is employed for the treatment of pneumonia when MRSA is suspected. Because vancomycin penetration into lung tissue is relatively low, aggressive dosing is generally recommended. Telavancin displayed similar efficacy to vancomycin in studies of nosocomial pneumonia due to gram-positive pathogens.

CNS Infections. Vancomycin is a key component in the initial empirical treatment of community-acquired bacterial meningitis in locations where penicillin-resistant *S. pneumoniae* is common (Tunkel et al., 2004). Penetration of vancomycin across meninges is poor, especially with steroid coadministration; thus, aggressive dosing is typically warranted. Vancomycin is also used to treat nosocomial meningitis often caused by staphylococci. Intraventricular vancomycin has been used in ventricular shunt infections.

Endocarditis and Vascular Catheter Infections. Vancomycin is standard therapy for staphylococcal endocarditis when the isolate is methicillin resistant or patients have a severe penicillin allergy (Baddour et al., 2005). However, β-lactams such as nafcillin or cefazolin are more effective than vancomycin for treatment of MSSA bloodstream infections; thus, patients should only receive vancomycin for MSSA infections if they have a documented, life-threatening allergy. Vancomycin is an effective alternative for the treatment of endocarditis caused by viridans streptococci in patients who are allergic to penicillin. In combination with an aminoglycoside, it may be used for enterococcal endocarditis in patients with serious penicillin allergy or for penicillin-resistant isolates. Vancomycin is used for the treatment of vascular catheter infections due to gram-positive organisms.

Other Infections. Vancomycin is the drug of choice for patients with moderate-to-severe pseudomembranous colitis due to *C. difficile*. Vancomycin is frequently employed as a component of empiric therapy for patients with fever and neutropenia. It is also used in surgical prophylaxis in patients with β-lactam allergies or if there is a high risk of MRSA infection.

Adverse Effects

Infusion-Related Reactions. Rapid intravenous infusion of vancomycin may cause erythematous or urticarial reactions, flushing, tachycardia, and hypotension ("red man" or "red neck" syndrome). The extreme flushing that can occur is not an allergic reaction but a direct effect of vancomycin on mast cells, causing them to release histamine. Typically, this reaction can be ameliorated by administering vancomycin more slowly, sometimes with premedication with histamine blockers. This reaction is generally not observed with teicoplanin but has been reported with lipoglycopeptides (i.e., telavancin).

Nephrotoxicity. Initial formulations of vancomycin contained impurities that were associated with a high incidence of nephrotoxicity. With the availability of formulations free of the impurities, there was a question regarding whether vancomycin was intrinsically nephrotoxic. However, as the recommended dosage range for vancomycin dosages has increased, it seems clear there is indeed a degree of dose-related nephrotoxicity (Lodise et al., 2009). Results of clinical trials suggest telavancin's nephrotoxicity may exceed that of vancomycin.

Other Toxic and Irritative Effects. True hypersensitivity reactions produced by glycopeptides are less common than the pseudoallergic infusion-related reactions and include macular skin rashes and anaphylaxis. Because of the long half-lives of dalbavancin and oritavancin, there is concern over prolonged effects if patients were to experience a severe hypersensitivity reaction. Telavancin can cause QT interval prolongation and is contraindicated in pregnancy due to teratogenic effects observed in animal studies. Auditory impairment, sometimes permanent, has been described in association with vancomycin use; some investigators believe ototoxicity is associated with excessive concentrations of vancomycin in plasma (60–100 μg/mL or greater).

Drug Interactions. Oritavancin has a minor effect on CYP-mediated metabolism; it should be used with warfarin only with careful monitoring. Caution should be used when using other nephrotoxic drugs with vancomycin or telavancin due to risks for additive nephrotoxicity.

Lipopeptides

Daptomycin, the only member of its class, is a cyclic lipopeptide antibiotic derived from *Streptomyces roseosporus* with bactericidal activity against gram-positive bacteria, including vancomycin-resistant isolates (Carpenter et al., 2004).

Antimicrobial Activity

Daptomycin is a bactericidal antibiotic selectively active against aerobic, facultative, and anaerobic gram-positive bacteria (see Table 59–1). Daptomycin may be active against vancomycin-resistant strains, although MICs tend to be higher for these organisms than for their vancomycin-susceptible counterparts (Critchley et al., 2003).

Mechanism of Action

Daptomycin binds to bacterial membranes, resulting in depolarization, loss of membrane potential, and cell death. It has concentration-dependent bactericidal activity.

Resistance to Lipopeptides

Daptomycin resistance has been reported to emerge while on therapy. Resistance occurs most commonly in treatment of high-inoculum infections (such as endocarditis) and among enterococci. The mechanisms of resistance to daptomycin have not been fully characterized but appear to be related to changes in cell surface charge that impede daptomycin binding. Interestingly, coadministration of β-lactams with daptomycin (even when the pathogen is resistant to the β-lactam) can reverse this resistance, suggesting potential combination therapy regimens.

ADME

Daptomycin is poorly absorbed orally and should be administered only intravenously. Direct toxicity to muscle precludes intramuscular injection. The serum $t_{1/2}$ is 8–9 h, permitting once-daily dosing. Approximately 80% of the administered dose is recovered in urine; a small amount is excreted in feces. Although the drug penetrates adequately into the lung, the drug is inactivated by pulmonary surfactant and thus is not useful in the treatment of pneumonia (Silverman et al., 2005). If the creatinine clearance is less than 30 mL/min, the dose is administered

only every 48 h. For patients on hemodialysis, the dose should be given immediately after dialysis.

Therapeutic Uses and Dosage

Daptomycin is indicated for treatment of complicated skin and soft-tissue infections (at 4 mg/kg/d) and complicated bacteremia and right-sided endocarditis (at 6 mg/kg/d), where its efficacy is comparable to that of vancomycin or antistaphylococcal β-lactams (Fowler et al., 2006). Use of higher doses (8–10 mg/kg) appears to be well tolerated and may provide additional benefit in difficult-to-treat infections (Figueroa et al., 2009).

Adverse Effects

Musculoskeletal Toxicity. Elevations of creatine kinase may occur; this does not require discontinuation unless findings suggest an otherwise-unexplained myopathy. Rhabdomyolysis has been reported to occur rarely.

Drug Interactions. Daptomycin does not affect CYPs and has no important drug-drug interactions. Caution is recommended when daptomycin is coadministered with aminoglycosides or statins because of potential risks of nephrotoxicity and myopathy, respectively.

Miscellaneous Agents

Metronidazole

Metronidazole is a nitroimidazole with broad activity against parasites and anaerobic bacteria. Only its antibacterial activity is discussed next; for an in-depth description, see Chapter 54.

Antimicrobial Activity and Resistance

The nitro group of metronidazole is reduced in anaerobic bacteria and some protozoans, producing the active form of the drug that interacts with DNA, disrupting its structure and inhibiting replication. Metronidazole displays excellent activity against most anaerobic bacteria, including *Bacteroides, Clostridium, Fusobacterium, Peptococcus, Peptostreptococcus,* and *Eubacterium.* It is less active against *Gardnerella* and *Helicobacter,* and the gram-positive anaerobes *Actinomyces, Propionibacterium,* and *Lactobacillus* are typically resistant. It lacks activity against aerobic bacteria. Acquired resistance is uncommon. In the case of *Bacteroides* spp., metronidazole resistance has been linked to a family of nitroimidazole (*nim*) resistance genes that can be encoded chromosomally or episomally. These *nim* genes appear to encode a nitroimidazole reductase capable of converting a 5-nitroimidazole to a 5-aminoimidazole, thus stopping the formation of the reactive nitroso group responsible for microbial killing.

Therapeutic Uses and Dosage

Metronidazole is a relatively inexpensive and versatile drug with efficacy against a broad spectrum of anaerobic bacteria. Typical doses are 250–500 mg three times daily, via the intravenous or oral routes. The drug is frequently given in combination with other antimicrobial agents to treat polymicrobial infections with aerobic and anaerobic bacteria. Metronidazole is used as a component of prophylaxis for colorectal surgery and is employed as a single agent to treat bacterial vaginosis. It is used in combination with other antibiotics and a proton pump inhibitor in regimens to treat infection with *H. pylori* (see Chapter 49). Metronidazole is used as therapy for mild-to-moderate *C. difficile* infection, although vancomycin is more effective for severe disease.

Bacitracin

Bacitracin is an antibiotic produced by the Tracy-I strain of *B. subtilis.* The bacitracins are a group of polypeptide antibiotics. The commercial products have multiple components; the major constituent is bacitracin A.

A unit of the antibiotic is equivalent to 26 μg of the USP standard.

Antimicrobial Activity, Mechanism of Action, and Resistance

Bacitracin inhibits the synthesis of the bacterial cell wall; a variety of gram-positive cocci and bacilli, *Neisseria, H. influenzae,* and *T. pallidum,* are sensitive to the drug at 0.1 unit/mL or less. *Actinomyces* and *Fusobacterium* are inhibited by concentrations of 0.5–5 units/mL.

Enterobacteriaceae, *Pseudomonas*, *Candida* spp., and *Nocardia* are resistant to the drug. Few data are available on bacitracin resistance.

Therapeutic Uses and Dosage

Current use is restricted to topical application. Bacitracin is available in ophthalmic and dermatologic ointments; the antibiotic also is available as a powder for the extemporaneous compounding of topical solutions. A number of topical preparations of bacitracin, to which neomycin or polymyxin or both have been added, are available. For open infections, such as infected eczema and infected dermal ulcers, the local application of the antibiotic may be of some help in eradicating sensitive bacteria. Bacitracin rarely produces hypersensitivity. Suppurative conjunctivitis and infected corneal ulcer, when caused by susceptible bacteria, respond well to the topical use of bacitracin. Bacitracin has been used with limited success for eradication of nasal carriage of staphylococci.

Adverse Effects

Nephrotoxicity results from the parenteral use of bacitracin.

Mupirocin

Mupirocin is an antibiotic first isolated from *Pseudomonas fluorescens*. It is a mixture of several pseudomonic acids and is effective against gram-positive bacteria.

Antimicrobial Activity, Mechanism of Action, and Resistance

Mupirocin is for topical use only. The drug is bactericidal against many gram-positive and selected gram-negative bacteria. It has good activity against *S. pyogenes*, MSSA, and MRSA. Mupirocin inhibits bacterial protein synthesis by reversible binding and inhibition of isoleucyl tRNA synthase. There is no cross-resistance with other classes of antibiotics. High-level resistance is mediated by a plasmid, which encodes a "bypass" Ile tRNA synthase that binds mupirocin poorly.

Therapeutic Uses and Dosage

Mupirocin is available as a 2% cream and a 2% ointment for dermatologic use and as a 2% ointment for intranasal use. The dermatologic preparations are indicated for treatment of traumatic skin lesions and impetigo secondarily infected with *S. aureus* or *S. pyogenes*. The nasal ointment is approved for eradication of *S. aureus* nasal carriage. The consensus is that patients who stand to benefit from mupirocin prophylaxis are those with proven *S. aureus* nasal colonization plus risk factors for distant infection or a history of skin or soft-tissue infections (Perl et al., 2002).

Adverse Effects

Mupirocin may cause irritation and sensitization at the site of application. Contact with the eyes causes irritation that may take several days to resolve. Polyethylene glycol present in the ointment can be absorbed from damaged skin. Application of the ointment to large surface areas should be avoided in patients with moderate-to-severe renal failure to avoid accumulation of polyethylene glycol.

Acknowledgment: *Henry F. Chambers contributed to this chapter in previous editions of this book. We have retained some of his text in the current edition.*

Drug Facts for Your Personal Formulary: *Protein Synthesis Inhibitors and Miscellaneous Antibacterial Agents*

Drugs	Therapeutic Uses	Clinical Pharmacology and Tips
Tetracyclines and Glycylcyclines—Inhibitors of Bacterial Protein Synthesis		
General: Bacteriostatic; oral formulations interact with orally administered cations (calcium, iron, aluminum); avoid in pregnancy and children < 8 years old due to permanent tooth discoloration, photosensitivity		
Tetracycline (IV, PO)	• Inflammatory acne • Use for other indications has largely been replaced by doxycycline	• Good activity vs. rickettseae, *Chlamydia, Mycoplasma, Legionella, Ureaplasma, Borrelia, Francisella tularensis, Pasteurella multocida, Bacillus anthracis, Helicobacter pylori* • Some activity vs. *Streptococcus pneumoniae, Streptococcus pyogenes, Staphylococcus aureus, Haemophilus influenzae* • Good CSF penetration • Renal excretion • Renal toxicity, hepatotoxicity at high doses
Doxycycline (IV, PO)	• Community-acquired pneumonia • Skin/soft-tissue infection • Urogenital chlamydia • Lymphogranuloma venereum • Syphilis (penicillin alternative) • Rocky Mountain spotted fever • Anthrax, tularemia • Lyme disease, leptospirosis	• Similar to tetracycline, with improved activity vs. streptococci and staphylococci • Good CSF penetration • Dual renal/biliary elimination • Preferred tetracycline for most indications due to more favorable activity, tolerability, and frequency of administration
Minocycline (IV, PO)	• Skin/soft-tissue infections • Mycobacterial infections • Nocardiosis	• Similar to doxycycline, with improved activity vs. staphylococci, *Acinetobacter*, and *Stenotrophomonas maltophilia* • Renal elimination • Vestibular toxicity
Tigecycline (IV)	• Intra-abdominal infection • Skin and soft-tissue infection • Pneumonia • Increased risk of death in pooled analysis; reserve as alternative therapy	• Similar to minocycline, with improved activity vs. *Escherichia coli, Klebsiella*, enterococci, *Bacteroides fragilis* • Wide distribution with low serum levels • Hepatic elimination

Chloramphenicol—Inhibitor of Bacterial Protein Synthesis

General: Bacteriostatic; dose-dependent bone marrow suppression, idiosyncratic fatal aplastic anemia, fatal "gray baby syndrome" in neonates receiving high doses

Chloramphenicol (IV, PO – not in the U.S.)	• Rickettsial infections • Bacterial meningitis • Because of risk of fatal toxicities, reserve as alternative therapy	• Good activity vs. *S. pneumoniae, H. influenzae, Neisseria meningitidis*, rickettseae, *Vibrio, Enterococcus* • Variable serum levels due to clearance of prodrug before hydrolysis • Excellent CSF penetration • Hepatic clearance

Macrolides and Ketolides—Inhibitors of Bacterial Protein Synthesis

General: Bacteriostatic; widely distributed but with limited CSF penetration, gastrointestinal distress, QT prolongation, major (erythromycin, clarithromycin, telithromycin) to minor (azithromycin) inhibitor of drug-metabolizing CYPs

Erythromycin (IV, PO, topical)	• Erysipelas and cellulitis • Ophthalmia neonatorum • Diphtheria • Pertussis	• Good activity against *Mycoplasma, Chlamydia, Legionella, Campylobacter, Bordetella pertussis, Corynebacterium diphtherieae* • Some activity against *S. pneumoniae, S. pyogenes, H. influenzae* • Oral formulations have variable absorption • Stimulates motilin receptors; gastrointestinal prokinetic properties • Chlolestatic hepatitis with long-term use
Clarithromycin (PO)	• Erysipelas and cellulitis • Community-acquired pneumonia • Acute exacerbations of chronic bronchitis • *Helicobacter pylori* gastritis (in combination with other agents) • *Mycobacterium avium* treatment and prophylaxis	• Similar to erythromycin, with improved activity vs. streptococci and staphylococci • Good activity vs. *Moraxella catarrhalis, H. pylori*, and nontuberculous mycobacteria • Active metabolite • Some drug accumulation in severe renal impairment • Tinnitus at high doses
Azithromycin (IV, PO)	• Community-acquired pneumonia • Acute exacerbations of chronic bronchitis • Otitis media • Bacterial pharyngitis • Chlamydia • *Mycobacterium avium* treatment and prophylaxis	• Similar to clarithromycin, improved activity vs. *H. influenzae* • Extensive tissue distribution and concentration in tissues • Anti-inflammatory properties • Long $t_{1/2}$, ~48 h
Telithromycin (PO)	• Community-acquired infection • Due to risk of severe hepatotoxicity, reserve as alternative therapy	• Similar to azithromycin with activity against macrolide-resistant streptococci and staphylococci • Severe hepatotoxicity

Lincosamides—Bacteriostatic Protein Synthesis Inhibitor

Clindamycin (IV, PO, topical)	• Skin and soft-tissue infection • Inflammatory acne • Lung abscess • Streptococcal pharyngitis • *Pneumocystis* pneumonia • Toxoplasma encephalitis • Nonsevere malaria	• Good activity vs. *S. pneumoniae, S. pyogenes*, viridans streptococci, *Actinomyces, Nocardia* • Some activity versus *S. aureus, Bacteroides* spp., *Toxoplasma, Pneumocystis, Plasmodium* • Wide tissue distribution, especially into bone; modest CSF penetration • Metabolized in liver, excreted in urine and bile • Diarrhea, rarely *Clostridium difficile* colitis

Streptogramins—Bactericidal Protein Synthesis Inhibitor, Components Act Synergistically

Quinupristin/ dalfopristin (IV)	• Skin and soft-tissue infection • Vancomycin-resistant *Enterococcus faecium* infections	• Good activity against streptococci, staphylococci, *E. faecium, Mycoplasma, Legionella, Chlamydophila* • Hepatic metabolism with biliary excretion • Infusion site phlebitis • Arthralgias, myalgias • CYP inhibitor

Oxazolidininones—Bacteriostatic Protein Synthesis Inhibitors

General: Excellent oral absorption; wide distribution, including to CNS; myelosuppression; peripheral neuropathy with long-term use; risk of serotonin syndrome with concomitant antidepressant use

Linezolid (IV, PO)	• Skin and soft-tissue infections • Pneumonia • Vancomycin-resistant enterococcal infections • Nocardiosis • Drug-resistant tuberculosis	• Good activity against streptococci, staphylococci, enterococci, *Nocardia, Listeria* • Some activity against mycobacteria • Nonenzymatic degradation with elimination in urine
Tedizolid (IV, PO)	• Skin and soft-tissue infections	• Similar activity to linezolid but lower risk of myelosuppression and drug interactions • Hepatic metabolism and fecal excretion • Longer $t_{1/2}$ than linezolid

Drug Facts for Your Personal Formulary: *Protein Synthesis Inhibitors and Miscellaneous Antibacterial Agents (continued)*

Drugs	Therapeutic Uses	Clinical Pharmacology and Tips
Polymyxins—Bactericidal Cell Membrane-Disrupting Agents		
Colistin (polymyxin E) (IV, inhaled)	• Serious infections due to multidrug-resistant gram-negative organisms • Prevention of cystic fibrosis exacerbations (inhaled)	• Good activity vs. *Acinetobacter, E. coli, Klebsiella, Pseudomonas*, including multidrug-resistant strains • Prodrug; complex pharmacokinetics with renal and nonrenal elimination • Substantial nephrotoxicity and neurotoxicity
Polymyxin B (IV, topical)	• Serious infections due to multidrug-resistant gram-negative organisms • Topical treatment/prevention of skin and soft-tissue infections	• Similar activity and toxicity as colistin • Nonrenally eliminated; does not achieve high urinary levels
Glycopeptides and Lipoglycopeptides—Bactericidal Inhibitors of Cell Wall Synthesis		
Vancomycin (IV, PO)	• Skin and soft-tissue infections • Bacteremia and endocarditis due to gram-positive bacteria • Pneumonia • Meningitis • *Clostridium difficile* colitis (oral formulation) • Surgical prophylaxis for procedures with high risk of MRSA	• Good activity vs. vast majority of gram-positive bacteria, *Staphylococcus* (including MRSA), streptococci, *E. faecalis* • Oral formulation not well absorbed and only used for treatment of *C. difficile* colitis • Modest CNS penetration in presence of inflammation • Renal elimination • Infusion-related reactions (red man syndrome) associated with rapid infusion • Nephrotoxicity at high doses
Telavancin (IV)	• Skin and soft-tissue infections • Pneumonia	• Similar activity to vancomycin with activity against some vancomycin-resistant strains of *Enterococcus* • Renal elimination • Higher nephrotoxicity relative to vancomycin • QT prolongation • Avoid in pregnancy
Dalbavancin (IV)	• Skin and soft-tissue infections	• Similar activity to vancomycin • Highly protein bound • Extremely long $t_{1/2}$; once-weekly dosing
Oritavancin (IV)	• Skin and soft-tissue infections	• Similar activity to telavancin • Highly protein bound • Extremely long half-life; single-dose therapy for skin infections
Daptomycin (IV)	• Skin and soft-tissue infections • Staphylococcal and streptococcal bacteremia • Vancomycin-resistant enterococcal infections	• Lipopeptide, similar activity to vancomycin • Retains activity against some vancomycin-resistant strains of *Enterococcus* • Protein bound; limited CNS penetration • Inactivated by pulmonary surfactant; not effective for pneumonia • Renal elimination • Rare myositis and rhabdomyolysis
Nitroimidazoles—Disruptors of DNA Synthesis in Anaerobes		
Metronidazole (IV, PO, topical)	• *Clostridium difficile* colitis • Empiric coverage of anaerobic organisms, as in intra-abdominal and skin and soft-tissue infections • *Helicobacter pylori* gastritis (in combination with other agents) • Bacterial vaginosis	• Bacterial spectrum limited to anaerobic organisms, including *B. fragilis* and *Clostridium* • Excellent absorption • Wide distribution, including CNS • Hepatic elimination • CYP inhibitor; drug interactions with warfarin • Peripheral neuropathy with prolonged use
Topical Agents—Inhibitors of Bacterial Cell Wall Synthesis		
Bacitracin (topical)	• Prevention and treatment of skin and soft-tissue infections • Ophthalmic infections	• Activity against broad array of gram-positive and gram-negative organisms • Nephrotoxicity with parenteral use
Mupirocin (topical)	• Treatment of minor skin infections • Eradication of nasal carriage of *S. aureus*	• Activity against broad array of gram-positive and gram-negative organisms • May cause irritation at site of application

Bibliography

Baddour LM, et al. Infective endocarditis: diagnosis, antimicrobial therapy, and management of complications: a statement for healthcare professionals. *Circulation*, **2005**, *111*:e394–e434.

Brinker AD, et al. Telithromycin-associated hepatotoxicity: clinical spectrum and causality assessment of 42 cases. *Hepatology*, **2009**, *49*:250–257.

Carpenter CF, Chambers HF. Daptomycin: another novel agent for treating infections due to drug-resistant gram-positive pathogens. *Clin Infect Dis*, **2004**, *38*:994–1000.

Centers for Disease Control and Prevention. Vancomycin-resistant *Staphylococcus aureus*—New York. *MMWR Morb Mortal Wkly Rep*, **2004**, *53*:322–323.

Centers for Disease Control and Prevention. Sexually transmitted diseases guidelines. **2015**. Available at: http://www.cdc.gov/std/treatment/. Accessed July 3, 2015.

Critchley IA, et al. Baseline study to determine in vitro activities of daptomycin against gram-positive pathogens isolated in the United States in 2000-2001. *Antimicrob Agents Chemother*, **2003**, *47*:1689–1693.

De Rosa FG, et al. Re-defining tigecycline therapy. *New Microbiol*, **2015**, *38*:121–136.

Figueroa DA, et al. Safety of high-dose intravenous daptomycin treatment: Three-year cumulative experience in a clinical program. *Clin Infect Dis*, **2009**, *49*:177–180.

Food and Drug Administration. FDA drug safety communication: increased risk of death with Tygacil (tigecycline) compared to other antibiotics used to treat similar infections. **2016**. Accessible at: http://www.fda.gov/Drugs/DrugSafety/ucm369580.htm. Accessed May 17, 2016.

Fowler VG Jr, et al. Daptomycin versus standard therapy for bacteremia and endocarditis caused by *Staphylococcus aureus*. *N Engl J Med*, **2006**, *355*:653–665.

Gales AC, et al. Tigecycline activity tested against 11808 bacterial pathogens recently collected from US medical centers. *Diagn Microbiol Infect Dis*, **2008**, *60*:421–427.

Goldstein EJ, et al. In vitro activities of the new semisynthetic glycopeptide telavancin (TD-6424), vancomycin, daptomycin, linezolid, and four comparator agents against anaerobic gram-positive species and *Corynebacterium* spp. *Antimicrob Agents Chemother*, **2004**, *48*:2149–2152.

Henson KE, et al. Glycopeptide antibiotics: evolving resistance, pharmacology and adverse event profile. *Expert Rev Anti Infect Ther*, **2015**, *12*:1–14.

Howden BP, et al. Treatment outcomes for serious infections caused by methicillin-resistant *Staphylococcus aureus* with reduced vancomycin susceptibility. *Clin Infect Dis*, **2004**, *38*:521–528.

Jones RN, et al. Update of dalbavancin spectrum and potency in the USA: report from the SENTRY antimicrobial surveillance system. *Diagn Microbiol Infect Dis*, **2013**, *75*:304–307.

Levison ME, et al. Clindamycin compared with penicillin for the treatment of anaerobic lung abscess. *Ann Intern Med*, **1983**, *98*:466–471.

Lewis JS, Jorgensen JH. Inducible clindamycin resistance in staphylococci: should clinicians and microbiologists be concerned? *Clin Infect Dis*, **2005**, *40*:280–285.

Lodise TP, et al. Relationship between initial vancomycin concentration-time profile and nephrotoxicity in hospitalized patients. *Clin Infect Dis*, **2009**, *49*:507–514.

Masters EJ, et al. Rocky Mountain spotted fever: a clinician's dilemma. *Arch Intern Med*, **2003**, *163*:769–774.

Masur H, et al. Prevention and treatment of opportunistic infections in HIV-infected adults and adolescents: updated guidelines from the Centers for Disease Control and Prevention, National Institutes of Health, and HIV Medicine Association of the Infectious Diseases Society of America. *Clin Infect Dis*, **2014**, *58*:1308–1311.

Mendes RE, et al. Oritavancin microbiologic features and activity results from the surveillance program in the United States. *Clin Infect Dis*, **2012**, *54*(S3):S203–S213.

Mendes RE, et al. Baseline activity of telavancin against gram-positive clinical isolates responsible for documented infections in U.S. hospitals (2011-2012) as determined by the revised susceptibility testing method. *Antimicrob Agents Chemother*, **2015**, *59*:702–706.

Nakajima Y. Mechanisms of bacterial resistance to macrolide antibiotics. *J Infect Chemother*, **1999**, *5*:61–74.

Narita M, et al. Linezolid-associated peripheral and optic neuropathy, lactic acidosis, and serotonin syndrome. *Pharmacotherapy*, **2007**, *27*:1189–1197.

Nation RL, et al. Framework for optimisation of the clinical use of colistin and polymyxin B: the Prato polymyxin consensus. *Lancet Infect Dis*, **2015**, *15*:225–234.

Periti P, et al. Pharmacokinetic drug interactions of macrolides. *Clin Pharmacokinet*, **1992**, *23*:106–131.

Perl TM, et al. Intranasal mupirocin to prevent postoperative *Staphylococcus aureus* infections. *N Engl J Med*, **2002**, *346*:1871–1877.

Peterson WL, et al. *Helicobacter pylori*–related disease: guidelines for testing and treatment. *Arch Intern Med*, **2000**, *160*:1285–1291.

Rybak MJ, et al. Vancomycin therapeutic guidelines: a summary of consensus recommendations from the Infectious Diseases Society of America, the American Society of Health-System Pharmacists, and the Society of Infectious Diseases Pharmacists. *Clin Infect Dis*, **2009**, *49*:325–327.

Rybak JM, et al. Early experience with tedizolid: clinical efficacy, pharmacodynamics, and resistance. *Pharmacotherapy*, **2014**, *34*:1198–1208.

Silverman JA, et al. Inhibition of daptomycin by pulmonary surfactant: in vitro modeling and clinical impact. *J Infect Dis*, **2005**, *191*:2149–2152.

Stevens DL, et al. Practice guidelines for the diagnosis and management of skin and soft tissue infections: 2014 update by the Infectious Diseases Society of America. *Clin Infect Dis*, **2014**, *15*:e10–e52.

Tunkel AR, et al. Practice guidelines for the management of bacterial meningitis. *Clin Infect Dis*, **2004**, *39*:1267–1284.

Wareham DW, Wilson P. Chloramphenicol in the 21st century. *Hosp Med*, **2002**, *63*:157–161.

Wunderink RG, et al. Linezolid in methicillin-resistant *Staphylococcus aureus* nosocomial pneumonia: a randomized, controlled study. *Clin Infect Dis*, **2012**, *54*:621–629.

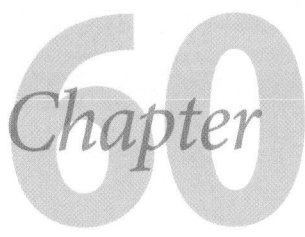

Chapter 60

Chemotherapy of Tuberculosis, *Mycobacterium avium* Complex Disease, and Leprosy

Tawanda Gumbo

Mycobacteria have caused epic diseases: TB and leprosy have terrorized humankind since antiquity. Although the burden of leprosy has decreased, TB is still the most important infectious killer of humans. *Mycobacterium abscessus* has now been called a new "antibiotic" nightmare because of its tenacity, lack of response to combination antibiotics, and a nearly universal propensity to develop acquired drug resistance. *Mycobacterium avium-intracellulare* (or MAC) infection continues to be difficult to treat, mainly due to three natural barriers:

- **Cell wall.** *Mycobacterium*, from the Greek *mycos*, refers to mycobacteria's waxy appearance, which is due to the composition of the cell walls. More than 60% of the cell wall is lipid, mainly mycolic acids composed of 2-branched, 3-hydroxy fatty acids with chains made of 76–90 carbon atoms! This extraordinary shield prevents many pharmacological compounds from getting to the bacterial cell membrane or inside the cytosol.
- **Efflux pumps.** A second layer of defense comes from an abundance of efflux pumps in the cell membrane. These transport proteins pump out potentially harmful chemicals from the bacterial cytoplasm back into the extracellular space and are responsible for the native resistance of mycobacteria to many standard antibiotics (Morris et al., 2005). As an example, ABC permeases comprise a full 2.5% of the genome of *Mycobacterium tuberculosis*.
- **Location in host.** A third barrier is the propensity of some of the bacilli to hide inside the patient's cells, thereby surrounding themselves with an extra physicochemical barrier that antimicrobial agents must cross to be effective.

Mycobacteria are defined by their rate of growth on agar as *rapid* and *slow* growers (see list in Table 60–1). Rapid growers are visible to the naked eye within 7 days; slow growers are visible later. Slow growers tend to be susceptible to antibiotics specifically developed for mycobacteria, whereas rapid growers tend to be also susceptible to antibiotics used against many other bacteria. Recent evidence suggests that in countries such as the U.S.,

M. abscessus now accounts for 80% of rapid growers from the respiratory system (Griffith et al., 2007). The pharmacology of drugs developed against slow growers is discussed in this chapter. However, rapid growers tend to be treated with antibiotics used to treat nonmycobacteria, such as macrolides, aminoglycosides, quinolones, and -lactams, whose pharmacology is discussed in Chapters 56–59.

The mechanisms of action of the antimycobacterial drugs are summarized in Figure 60–1. The mycobacterial mechanisms of resistance to these drugs are summarized in Figure 60–2. The model termed the *antibiotic resistance arrow of time* has combined these mechanisms in an arrow of time, starting with early induction of efflux pumps that leads to chromosomal mutations in drug target proteins and efflux

HISTORY

The first successful drug for treating TB was PAS, developed by Lehman in 1943. A more dramatic success came when Waksman and Schatz developed streptomycin. Further efforts led to development of thiacetazone by Domagk in 1946; isoniazid by Squibb, Hoffman La Roche, and Bayer in 1952; pyrazinamide by Kushner and colleagues in 1952; and rifamycins by Sensi and Margalith in 1957. Ethambutol was discovered at Lederle Laboratories in 1961. As might be anticipated, the use of all of these drugs presents problems of drug resistance, adverse events, and drug interactions. Therefore, newer classes of agents are being developed. Starting in 2000 with the work of Stover et al. and Matsumoto et al. in 2006, specific antimycobacterial agents such as pretomanid and bedaquiline have been discovered and introduced to clinical care. In addition, pharmacophores in clinical use for other bacteria have been repurposed as antimycobacterial agents, including moxifloxacin and levofloxacin, oxazolidinones, and β-lactams, based on recent clinical trials.

Abbreviations

ABC: ATP binding cassette
ACP: acyl carrier protein
AUC: area under the curve
CNS: central nervous system
CoA: coenzyme A
CSF: cerebrospinal fluid
DDS: diamino-diphenylsulfone
DHFR: dihydrofolate reductase
DOT: directly observed therapy
FAD: flavin adenine dinucleotide
FGD1: NADP-dependent glucose-6-phosphate dehydrogenase
GABA: γ-aminobutyric acid
GFR: glomerular filtration rate
GI: gastrointestinal
G6PD: glucose-6-phosphate dehydrogenase
HIV: human immunodeficiency virus
IC_{50}: concentration causing 50% inhibition
Ig: immunoglobulin
INH: isoniazid
InhA: enoyl acyl carrier protein reductase
KasA: β-ketoacyl-acyl carrier protein synthase
KatG: catalase peroxidase
MAC: *Mycobacterium avium* complex
MDR-TB: TB resistant to isoniazid and rifampicin
MIC: minimum inhibitory concentration
NO: nitric oxide
NRPB: nonreplicating persistent bacilli
NAT2: *N*-acetyltransferase type 2
PABA: *para*-aminobenzoic acid
PAS: *para*-aminosalicylic acid
PD: pharmacodynamics
PK: pharmacokinetics
POA: pyrazinoic acid
TB: tuberculosis
V_d: volume of distribution
XDR-TB: MDR-TB that is also resistant to fluoroquinolones and at least one of three injectable second-line drugs

pumps (Gumbo et al., 2014; Schmalstieg et al., 2012; Srivastava et al., 2010). This chain of events is initiated by subtherapeutic concentrations due to poor dosing practices in the face of ever-present between-patient PK variability (Pasipanodya et al., 2013; Srivastava et al., 2011a). PK parameter definitions are presented in terms of Figure 52–1 and Equation 52–1.

Antimycobacterial Drugs

Rifamycins: Rifampin, Rifapentine, and Rifabutin

Rifamycins are macrocyclic antibiotics. Rifampin or rifampicin, rifapentine, and rifabutin are macrocyclic antibiotics important in the treatment of mycobacterial diseases.

Mechanism of Action

The mechanism of action for rifamycins is typified by rifampin's action against *M. tuberculosis*. Rifampin enters bacilli in a concentration-dependent manner, achieving steady-state concentrations within 15 min (Gumbo et al., 2007a). Rifampin binds to the β subunit of DNA-dependent RNA polymerase (*rpoB*) to form a stable drug-enzyme complex. Drug binding suppresses chain formation in RNA synthesis.

TABLE 60–1 ■ PATHOGENIC MYCOBACTERIAL SLOW AND RAPID GROWERS (RUNYON CLASSIFICATION)

SLOW GROWERS
Runyon I: Photochromogens
Mycobacterium kansasii
Mycobacterium marinum
Runyon II: Scotochromogens
Mycobacterium scrofulaceum
Mycobacterium szulgai
Mycobacterium gordonae
Runyon III: Nonchromogens
Mycobacterium avium complex
Mycobacterium haemophilum
Mycobacterium xenopi
RAPID GROWERS
Runyon IV
Mycobacterium fortuitum complex
Mycobacterium smegmatis group
Mycobacterium abscessus

Slow growers tend to be susceptible to antibiotics specifically developed for Mycobacteria. Rapid growers tend to be susceptible to antibiotics also used against many other bacteria.

Antibacterial Activity

Rifampin inhibits the growth of most gram-positive bacteria as well as many gram-negative microorganisms, such as *Escherichia coli*, *Pseudomonas*, indole-positive and indole-negative *Proteus*, and *Klebsiella*. Rifampin is very active against *Staphylococcus aureus* and coagulase-negative staphylococci. The drug also is highly active against *Neisseria meningitidis* and *Haemophilus influenzae*. Rifampin inhibits the growth of *Legionella* species in cell culture and in animal models.

Rifampin inhibits the growth of many *M. tuberculosis* clinical isolates in vitro at concentrations of 0.06–0.25 mg/L (Heifets, 1991). Rifampin is also bactericidal against *Mycobacterium leprae*. *Mycobacterium kansasii* is inhibited by 0.25–1 mg/L. Most strains of *Mycobacterium scrofulaceum*, *Mycobacterium intracellulare*, and *Mycobacterium avium* are suppressed by concentrations of 4 mg/L. *Mycobacterium abscessus* inactivates rifampin via an ADP-ribosyltransferase and monooxygenase, making the bacteria innately resistant to rifamycins (Nessar et al., 2012). Rifapentine MICs are similar to those of rifampin. Rifabutin inhibits the growth of most MAC isolates at concentrations ranging from 0.25 to 1 mg/L. Rifabutin also inhibits the growth of many strains of *M. tuberculosis* at concentrations of 0.125 mg/L or less and in vitro has better MICs than rifampin.

Bacterial Resistance

The prevalence of rifampin-resistant isolates (1 in every 10^7 to 10^8 bacilli) is due to an alteration of the target of this drug, *rpoB*, with resistance in 86% of cases due to mutations at codons 526 and 531 of the *rpoB* gene (Somoskovi et al., 2001). Rifamycin monoresistance occurs at higher rates when patients with AIDS and multicavitary TB are treated with either rifapentine or rifabutin (Burman et al., 2006). Efflux pump induction, and mutations in efflux pumps, have now been demonstrated to be associated with rifamycin resistance (Li et al., 2015).

ADME

After oral administration, the rifamycins are absorbed to variable extents (Table 60–2) (Burman et al., 2001). Food decreases the rifampin C_{Pmax} by one-third; a high-fat meal increases the AUC of rifapentine by 50%. Food has no effect on rifabutin absorption. Thus, rifampin should be taken on an empty stomach, whereas rifapentine should be taken with food if possible.

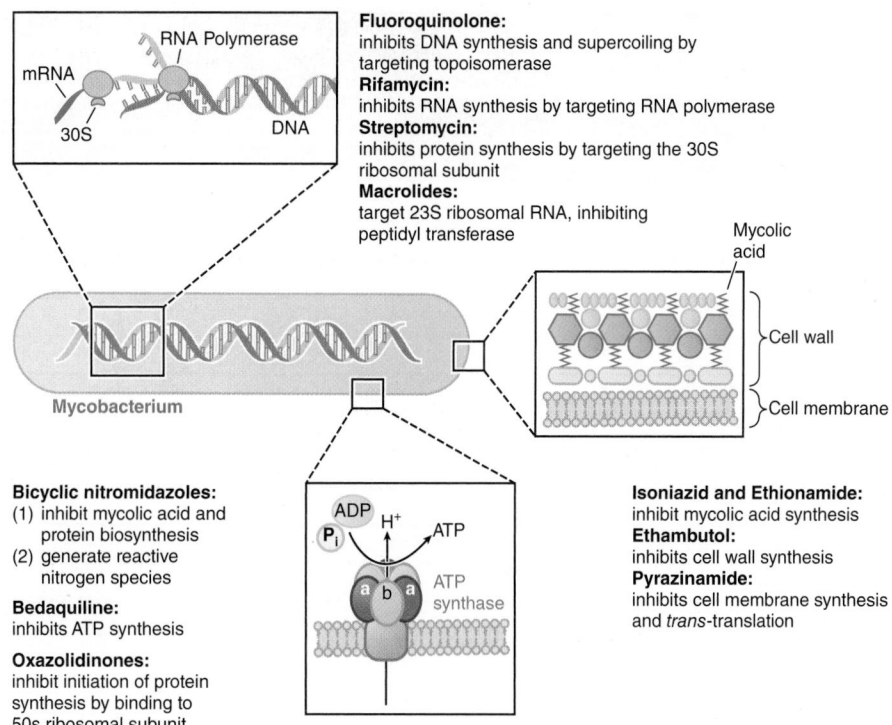

Figure 60–1 *Mechanisms of action of established and experimental drugs used for the chemotherapy of mycobacterial infections.* Approved drugs for the chemotherapy of mycobacterial diseases may be grouped according to the sites of action indicated by the pictures above that expand regions of the mycobacterium: inhibitors of nucleic acid and protein synthesis; disruptors of cell wall and cell membrane synthesis; inhibitors of membrane transport. Specific antimycobacterial agents and their mechanisms of action are also listed. Rifamycin is used as a generic term for several drugs, of which rifampin is used most frequently. Clofazimine, whose mode of action is not understood, is omitted.

Rifamycins are metabolized by microsomal B-esterases and cholinesterases. A major pathway for rifabutin elimination is CYP3A. Due to autoinduction, all three rifamycins reduce their own AUCs with repeated administration (Table 60–3). They have good penetration into many tissues, but peak concentration and AUCs in the CNS and pericardial fluid reach only about 13%–20% of those in plasma (Nau et al., 1992; Shenje et al., 2015). The drugs and metabolites are excreted by bile and eliminated via feces, with urine elimination accounting for only one-third and less of metabolites.

The population PK of rifampin are best described using a one-compartment model with transit compartment absorption (Wilkins et al., 2008), using the PK parameters in Table 60–2. Rifapentine PK are likewise best described using a one-compartment open model with first-order absorption and elimination (Langdon et al., 2005). The PK parameters are summarized in Table 60–2. However, for each 1-kg weight increase above 50 kg, systemic clearance increases by 0.05 L/h and V_d by 0.69 L. Thus, C_{Pmax} and AUC decrease with increasing patient weight above 50 kg.

In contrast, rifabutin PK are best described by a two-compartment open model with first-order absorption and elimination. Rifabutin disposition is biexponential. Rifabutin concentrations are substantially higher in tissue than in plasma due to its lipophilic properties, leading to the very high

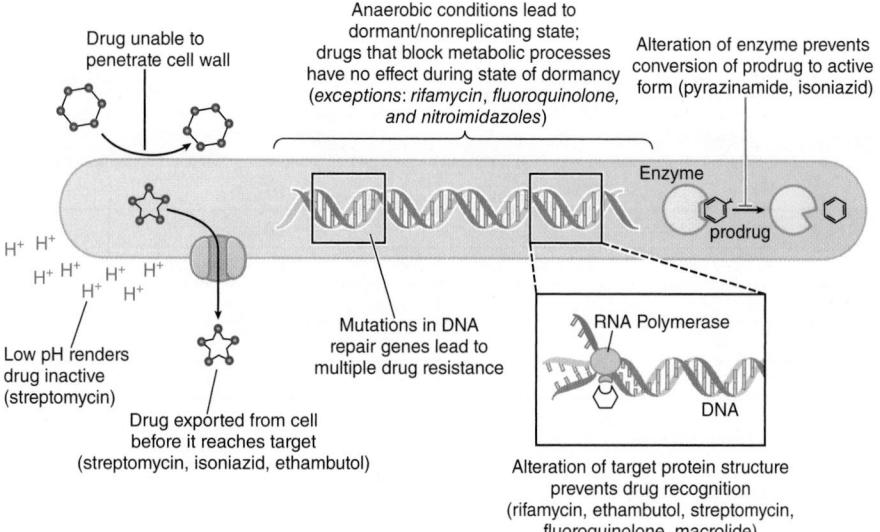

Figure 60–2 *Mechanisms of resistance in mycobacteria.*

TABLE 60–2 ■ POPULATION PHARMACOKINETIC PARAMETER ESTIMATES FOR ANTIMYCOBACTERIAL DRUGS IN ADULT PATIENTS

	PARAMETER ESTIMATE		
	k_a (H^{-1})	Systemic clearance (L/h)	V_d (L)
Rifampin	1.15	19	53
Rifapentine	0.6	2.03	37.8
Rifabutin	0.2	61	231/1050[a]
Pyrazinamide	3.56	3.4	29.2
Isoniazid	2.3	22.1	35.2
Ethambutol	0.7	1.3[b]	6.0[b]
Clofazimine	0.7	0.6/76.7	1470
Dapsone	1.04	1.83	69.6
Bedaquiline	—	2.62	198/8550[a]
Ethionamide	0.25	1.9[b]	3.2[b]
Para-aminosalicylic acid	0.4	0.3[b]	0.9[b]
Cycloserine	1.9	0.04[b]	0.5[b]

k_a is the absorption constant (see Chapter 52).
[a]Volume of central compartment/volume of peripheral compartment.
[b]Expressed per kilogram of body weight.

apparent volumes of distribution (Table 60–2). The consequence is that C_{Pmax} values for rifabutin are lower than one would predict by comparison with other rifamycins. The volume of peripheral compartment decreases by 27% with concomitant azithromycin administration; tobacco smoking increases the volume by 39%.

Microbial Pharmacokinetics-Pharmacodynamics

Rifampin's bactericidal and sterilizing effect activity are best optimized by high AUCs and a high AUC/MIC ratio (Gumbo et al., 2007a; Pasipanodya et al., 2013). However, resistance suppression and rifampin's enduring postantibiotic effect are best optimized by high C_{Pmax}/MIC. Therefore, the duration of time that the rifampin concentration persists above the MIC is of less importance. This means that the $t_{1/2}$ of a rifamycin is less of an issue in optimizing therapy, and that if patients could tolerate it, higher doses would lead to higher bactericidal activities while suppressing resistance. Recent clinical trials have confirmed better sputum bacillary decline with up to 3.5 times higher rifampin doses than currently used, which would increase both AUC/MIC and C_{Pmax}/MIC

nonlinearly (Boeree et al., 2015). Currently, these larger rifampin doses are in phase III trials.

Therapeutic Uses

Rifampin for oral administration is available alone and as a fixed-dose combination with isoniazid (150 mg isoniazid, 300 mg rifampin) or with isoniazid and pyrazinamide (50 mg isoniazid, 120 mg rifampin, and 300 mg pyrazinamide). A parenteral form of rifampin is also available. The dose of rifampin for treatment of TB in adults is 600 mg, given once daily, either 1 h before or 2 h after a meal. Children should receive 15 mg/kg (range 10–20 mg/kg), with the maximum dose 600 mg/d, given in the same way. Rifabutin is administered at 5 mg/kg/d and rifapentine at 10 mg/kg once a week.

Rifampin is also useful for the prophylaxis of meningococcal disease and *H. influenzae* meningitis. To prevent meningococcal disease, adults may be treated with 600 mg twice daily for 2 days or 600 mg once daily for 4 days; children older than 1 month should receive 10–15 mg/kg, to a maximum of 600 mg. Combined with a β-lactam antibiotic or vancomycin,

TABLE 60–3 ■ PHARMACOKINETIC PARAMETERS OF RIFAMPIN, RIFABUTIN, AND RIFAPENTINE

	RIFABUTIN	RIFAMPIN	RIFAPENTINE
Protein binding (%)	71	85	97
Oral bioavailability (%)	20	68	—
t_{max} (h)	2.5–4.0	1.5–2.0	5.0–6.0
C_{max} total (µg/mL)	0.2–0.6	8–20	8–30
C_{max} free drug (µg/mL)	0.1	1.5	0.5
$t_{1/2}$ (h)	32–67	2–5	14–18
Intracellular/extracellular penetration	9	5	24–60
Autoinduction (AUC decrease)	40%	38%	20%
CYP3A induction	Weak	Pronounced	Moderate
CYP3A substrate	Yes	No	No

rifampin may be useful for therapy in selected cases of staphylococcal endocarditis or osteomyelitis, especially those caused by staphylococci "tolerant" to penicillin. Rifampin may also be indicated for the eradication of the staphylococcal nasal carrier state in patients with chronic furunculosis. In the treatment of brucellosis, 900 mg a day rifampin can be combined with doxycycline for 6 weeks.

Untoward Effects

Rifampin is generally well tolerated in patients. Usual doses result in less than 4% of patients with TB developing significant adverse reactions; the most common are rash (0.8%), fever (0.5%), and nausea and vomiting (1.5%). Rarely, hepatitis and deaths due to liver failure have been observed in patients who received other hepatotoxic agents in addition to rifampin or who had preexisting liver disease. Chronic liver disease, alcoholism, and old age appear to increase the incidence of severe hepatic problems. GI disturbances have occasionally required discontinuation of the drug. Various nonspecific symptoms related to the nervous system also have been noted.

Hypersensitivity reactions may be encountered. High-dose rifampin should not be administered on a dosing schedule of less than twice weekly because this is associated with a flu-like syndrome of fever, chills, and myalgias in 20% of patients so treated. The syndrome also may include eosinophilia, interstitial nephritis, acute tubular necrosis, thrombocytopenia, hemolytic anemia, and shock. Light chain proteinuria has also been documented with rifampin use. Thrombocytopenia, transient leukopenia, and anemia have occurred during therapy. Because the potential teratogenicity of rifampin is unknown and the drug is known to cross the placenta, it is best to avoid the use of this agent during pregnancy.

Rifabutin is generally well tolerated; primary reasons for discontinuation of therapy include rash (4%), GI intolerance (3%), and neutropenia (2%) (Nightingale et al., 1993). Neutropenia occurred in 25% of patients with severe HIV infection who received rifabutin. Uveitis and arthralgias have occurred in patients receiving rifabutin doses greater than 450 mg daily in combination with clarithromycin or fluconazole. Patients should be cautioned to discontinue the drug if visual symptoms (pain or blurred vision) occur. Rifabutin causes an orange-tan discoloration of skin, urine, feces, saliva, tears, and contact lenses, like rifampin. Rarely, thrombocytopenia, a flu-like syndrome, hemolysis, myositis, chest pain, and hepatitis develop in patients treated with rifabutin. Unique side effects include polymyalgia, pseudojaundice, and anterior uveitis.

Rifamycin Overdose

Rifampin overdose is uncommon. The most prominent symptoms are the orange discoloration of skin, fluids, and mucosal surfaces, leading to the term *red-man syndrome*. Overdose can be life threatening. Treatment consists of supportive measures; there is no antidote.

Drug Interactions

Because rifampin potently induces CYPs 1A2, 2C9, 2C19, and 3A4, its administration results in a decreased $t_{1/2}$ for a number of compounds that are metabolized by these CYPs. Rifabutin is a less-potent inducer of CYPs than rifampin; however, rifabutin does induce hepatic microsomal enzymes and decreases the $t_{1/2}$ of zidovudine, prednisone, digitoxin, quinidine, ketoconazole, propranolol, phenytoin, sulfonylureas, and warfarin. It has less effect than rifampin on serum levels of indinavir and nelfinavir. Compared to rifabutin and rifampin, the CYP-inducing effects of rifapentine are intermediate.

Pyrazinamide

Pyrazinamide is the synthetic pyrazine analogue of nicotinamide. Pyrazinamide is also known as pyrazinoic acid amide, pyrazine carboxylamide, and pyrazinecarboxamide. Pyrazinamide was first synthesized at Merck in 1936 in Germany but was first examined as an anti-TB agent in 1952.

PYRAZINAMIDE

Mechanism of Action

Pyrazinamide is activated by acidic conditions. Several mechanisms of action have been proposed. In one model, pyrazinamide passively diffuses into mycobacterial cells, in which *M. tuberculosis* pyrazinamidase (encoded by the *pncA* gene) deaminates pyrazinamide to pyrazinoic acid (POA⁻, in its dissociated form), which is then followed by passive diffusion of the POA⁻ to the extracellular milieu (Zhang et al., 1999). In an acidic extracellular milieu, a fraction of POA⁻ is protonated to the uncharged form, POAH, a more lipid-soluble form that reenters the bacillus and accumulates due to a deficient efflux pump. The Henderson-Hasselbalch equilibrium (Chapter 2) progressively favors the formation of POAH and its equilibration across membranes as the pH of the extracellular medium declines toward the pK_a of pyrazinoic acid, 2.9. The acidification of the intracellular milieu is believed to inhibit enzyme function and collapse the transmembrane proton motive force, thereby killing the bacteria. Inhibitors of energy metabolism or reduced energy production states lead to enhanced pyrazinamide effect (Zhang et al., 2014). A specific target of pyrazinamide has been proposed to be ribosomal protein S1 (encoded by *RpsA*) in the trans-translation process, so that toxic proteins due to stress accumulate and kill the bacteria (Shi et al., 2011). In addition, pyrazinamide's target may include an aspartate decarboxylase (encoded by *panD*) involved in making precursors needed for pantothenate and CoA biosynthesis in persistent *M. tuberculosis* (Zhang et al., 2013).

Antibacterial Activity

Pyrazinamide exhibits antimicrobial activity in vitro only at acidic pH. At pH 5.9, 95% of clinical isolates have an MIC of 6.25–200 mg/L (Gumbo et al., 2014).

Mechanisms of Resistance

Pyrazinamide-resistant *M. tuberculosis* expresses pyrazinamidase with reduced affinity for pyrazinamide. This reduced affinity decreases the conversion of pyrazinamide to POA. Single point mutations in the *pncA* gene are encountered in some clinical isolates. In addition, mutations in the genes encoding proposed pyrazinamide targets of *RpsA* and *panD* are encountered in pyrazinamide resistance (Zhang et al., 2014). Finally, it has been demonstrated that the efflux rate of POA predicts pyrazinamide resistance with greater than 93% sensitivity and specificity, suggesting a role for efflux pumps in this drug's resistance (Zimic et al., 2012).

ADME

The oral bioavailability of pyrazinamide exceeds 90%. GI absorption segregates patients into two groups: fast absorbers (56%), with an absorption rate constant of 3.56/h, and slow absorbers (44%), with an absorption rate of 1.25/h (Wilkins et al., 2006). The drug is concentrated 20-fold in lung epithelial lining fluid (Conte et al., 2000). Pyrazinamide is metabolized by microsomal deamidase to POA and subsequently hydroxylated to 5-hydroxy-POA, which is then excreted by the kidneys. CL (clearance) and V_d (volume of distribution) increase with patient mass (0.5 L/h and 4.3 L for every 10 kg above 50 kg), and V_d is larger in males (by 4.5 L) (see Table 60–2) This has several implications: The $t_{1/2}$ of pyrazinamide will vary considerably based on weight and gender, and the AUC$_{0-24}$ will decrease with increase in weight for the same dose (same mg drug/kg body weight). Pyrazinamide clearance is reduced in renal failure; therefore, the dosing frequency is reduced to three times a week at low glomerular filtration rates. Hemodialysis removes pyrazinamide; therefore, the drug needs to be redosed after each session of hemodialysis (Malone et al., 1999b).

Microbial Pharmacokinetics-Pharmacodynamics

Pyrazinamide's sterilizing effect is closely linked to AUC$_{0-24}$/MIC (Chigutsa et al., 2015; Gumbo et al., 2009). Such clinical parameters as relapse, cure at the end of therapy, and patient death have been confirmed to be predicted by the AUC$_{0-24}$ and by the MIC (Gumbo et al., 2014; Pasipanodya et al., 2013).

Therapeutic Uses

The coadministration of pyrazinamide with isoniazid or rifampin has led to a one-third reduction in the duration of anti-TB therapy and a two-thirds reduction in TB relapse. This led to reduction in length of therapy to 6 months, producing the current "short-course" chemotherapy. Pyrazinamide is administered at an oral dose of 35 mg/kg (30–40) mg/kg/d.

Untoward Effects

Injury to the liver is the most serious side effect of pyrazinamide. When a dose of 40–50 mg/kg is administered orally, signs and symptoms of hepatic disease appear in about 15% of patients, with jaundice in 2%–3% and death due to hepatic necrosis in rare instances. Current regimens employed (15–30 mg/kg/d) are much safer. Prior to pyrazinamide administration, all patients should undergo studies of hepatic function, and these studies should be repeated at frequent intervals during the entire period of treatment. If evidence of significant hepatic damage becomes apparent, therapy must be stopped. Pyrazinamide should not be given to individuals with hepatic dysfunction unless this is absolutely unavoidable.

In nearly all patients, pyrazinamide inhibits excretion of urate, resulting in hyperuricemia, which may cause acute episodes of gout. Other untoward effects observed with pyrazinamide include arthralgias, anorexia, nausea and vomiting, dysuria, malaise, and fever. In the U.S., the use of pyrazinamide is not approved during pregnancy because of inadequate data on teratogenicity.

Isoniazid

Isoniazid (*isonicotinic acid hydrazide*), also called INH (Figure 60–3), is an important drug for the chemotherapy of drug-susceptible TB. All patients infected with isoniazid-sensitive strains of the tubercle bacillus receive the drug if they can tolerate it. The use of combination therapy (isoniazid + pyrazinamide + rifampin) provides the basis for short-course therapy and improved cure rates.

Mechanism of Action

Isoniazid enters bacilli by passive diffusion. The drug is not directly toxic to the bacillus but must be activated to its toxic form within the bacillus by KatG, a multifunctional catalase-peroxidase. KatG catalyzes the production from isoniazid of an isonicotinoyl radical that subsequently interacts with mycobacterial NAD and NAPD to produce a dozen adducts (Argyrou et al., 2007). One of these, a nicotinoyl-NAD isomer, inhibits the activities of enoyl acyl carrier protein reductase (InhA) and KasA. Inhibition of these enzymes inhibits synthesis of mycolic acid, an essential component of the mycobacterial cell wall, leading to bacterial cell death. Another adduct, a nicotinoyl-NADP isomer, potently inhibits ($K_i < 1$ nM) mycobacterial dihydrofolate reductase, thereby interfering with nucleic acid synthesis (Argyrou et al., 2006) (see Figure 60–3).

Other products of KatG activation of INH include superoxide, H_2O_2, alkyl hydroperoxides, and the NO radical, which may also contribute to the mycobactericidal effects of INH (Timmins and Deretic, 2006). *Mycobacterium tuberculosis* could be especially sensitive to damage from these radicals because the bacilli have a defect in the central regulator of the oxidative stress response, *oxyR*. Backup defense against radicals is provided by alkyl hydroperoxide reductase (encoded by *ahpC*), which detoxifies organic peroxides. Increased expression of *ahpC* reduces isoniazid effectiveness.

Antibacterial Activity

The isoniazid MICs with clinical *M. tuberculosis* strains vary from country to country. In the U.S., for example, the MICs are 0.025–0.05 mg/L. Activity against *Mycobacterium bovis* and *Mycobacterium kansasii* is moderate. Isoniazid has poor activity against MAC. It has no activity against any other microbial genus.

Mechanisms of Resistance

The prevalence of drug-resistant mutants is about 1 in 10^6 bacilli. Because TB cavities may contain as many as 10^7 to 10^9 microorganisms, preexistent resistance can be expected in pulmonary TB cavities of untreated patients. These spontaneous mutants can be selected and amplified by isoniazid monotherapy. Thus, two or more agents are usually used. Because the mutations resulting in drug resistance are independent events, the probability of resistance to two antimycobacterial agents is small, about 1 in 10^{12} ($1 \times 10^6 \times 10^6$), a low probability considering the number of bacilli involved.

Resistance to INH is associated with mutation or deletion of KatG, overexpression of the genes for InhA (confers low-level resistance to INH

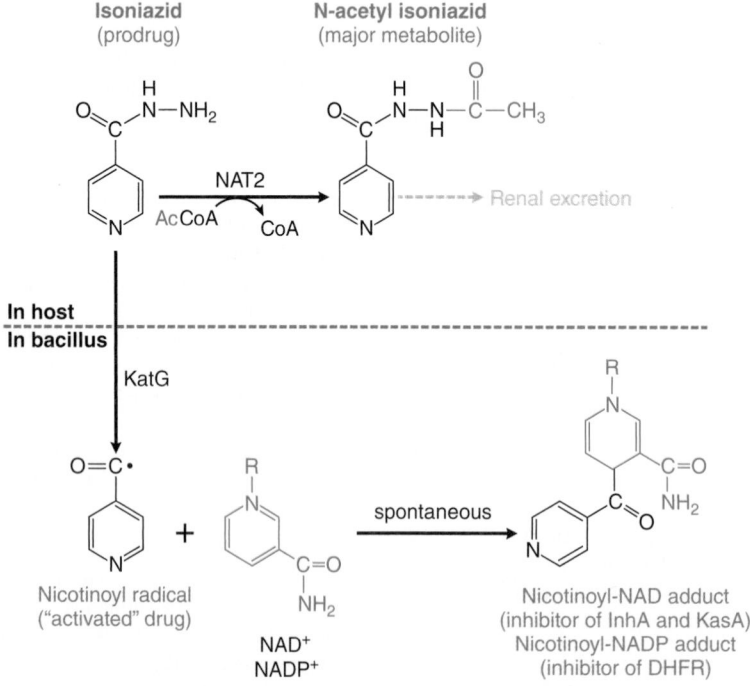

Figure 60–3 *Metabolism and activation of isoniazid.* The prodrug isoniazid is metabolized in humans by NAT2 isoforms to its principal metabolite, *N*-acetyl isoniazid, which is excreted by the kidney. Isoniazid diffuses into mycoplasma, where it is "activated" by KatG (oxidase/peroxidase) to the nicotinoyl radical. The nicotinoyl radical reacts spontaneously with NAD+ to produce adducts that inhibit essential enzymes in synthesis of the cell wall and with NADP+ to produce an inhibitor of nucleic acid synthesis.

and some cross-resistance to ethionamide), and *ahpC* and mutations in the *kasA* and *katG* genes. KatG mutants exhibit a high level of resistance to isoniazid. The most common mechanism of isoniazid resistance in clinical isolates is due to single point mutations in the heme-binding catalytic domain of KatG, especially a serine-to-asparagine change at position 315. Although isolates with this mutation completely lose the ability to form nicotinoyl-NAD⁺/NADP⁺ adducts, they retain good catalase activity and maintain good biofitness. Compensatory mutations in the *ahpC* promoter occur and increase survival of *katG* mutant strains under oxidative stress. Efflux pump induction by isoniazid has been demonstrated, and it also confers resistance to ethambutol (Colangeli et al., 2005). In an in vitro pharmacodynamic model, efflux pump-induced resistance developed within 3 days and was followed by development of *katG* mutations (Gumbo et al., 2007b).

ADME

The bioavailability of orally administered isoniazid is about 100% for the 300-mg dose. The PK of isoniazid are best described by a two-compartment model, with the PK parameters in Table 60–2 (Pasipanodya et al., 2013). The ratio of isoniazid in the epithelial lining fluid to that in plasma is 1–2 and for CSF is 0.9 (Conte et al., 2002). Approximately 10% of drug is bound to protein. From 75% to 95% of a dose of isoniazid is excreted in the urine within 24 h, mostly as acetylisoniazid and isonicotinic acid.

Isoniazid is metabolized by hepatic arylamine NAT2, encoded by a variety of NAT2* alleles (Figure 60–3). Isoniazid clearance in patients has been traditionally classified as one of two phenotypic groups: "slow" and "fast" acetylators, as seen in Figure 60–4. Recently, the phenotypic groups have been expanded to fast, intermediate, and slow acetylators, and population PK parameters of isoniazid have been estimated and related to NAT2 genotype, and the number of NAT2*4 alleles accounts for 88% of the variability of isoniazid clearance.

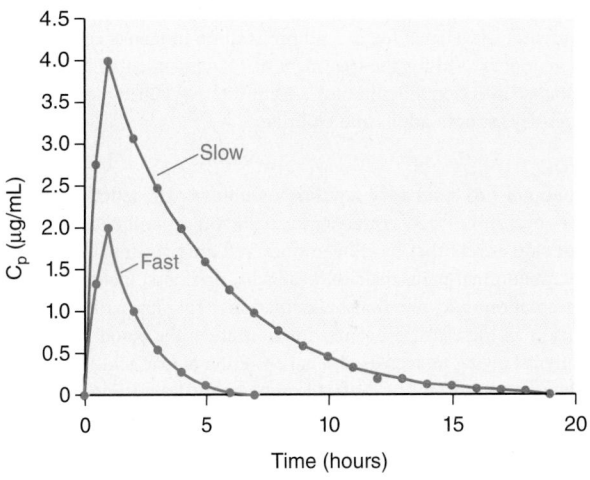

Figure 60–4 *Multi-modal distribution of INH clearance due to NAT2 polymorphisms.* A group of matched male volunteers received INH (250 mg orally), and the time courses of plasma drug levels (C_p) were assessed. One-third of the subjects had INH elimination $t_{1/2}$ values less than 1.5 h; these were the *fast acetylators.* Two-thirds had $t_{1/2}$ values ranging from 2.1 to 4.0 h, with a suggestion of multiple groups; these were the *slow acetylators.* Plots of the mean data (C_p vs. time after administration) demonstrate the PK effects of acetylation rate. Both groups reached C_{Pmax} at 1 h. The slow acetylators (red line) achieved a higher C_p (4 μg/mL) with a mean elimination $t_{1/2}$ of 3.0 h; the fast acetylators (green line) reached a lower maximal C_p (2 μg/mL) with a mean elimination $t_{1/2}$ of 1.0 h. The acetylation rate reflects variable expression of active polymorphic forms of NAT2. Slow acetylators may be a greater risk for adverse effects from INH, sulfonamides, and procainamide; fast acetylators may have diminished responses to standard doses of these agents but greater risk from bioactivation by NAT2 of arylamine/hydrazine carcinogens. Recently, researchers have identified three elimination subgroups for INH metabolism: *fast, slow,* and *intermediate* (codominant fast and slow alleles).

The frequency of each acetylation phenotype depends on race but is not influenced by sex or age. Fast acetylation is found in Inuit and Japanese. Slow acetylation is the predominant phenotype in most Scandinavians, Jews, and North African whites. The high acetyltransferase activity (fast acetylation) is inherited as an autosomal dominant trait; fast acetylators of isoniazid are either heterozygous or homozygous.

Microbial Pharmacokinetics-Pharmacodynamics

Isoniazid's microbial kill, as well as resistance emergence, is best explained by the ratios of AUC_{0-24} to MIC and C_{Pmax}/MIC (Gumbo et al., 2007c; Pasipanodya et al., 2013). Because AUC is proportional to dose/CL, this means that efficacy is most dependent on drug dose and CL and thus on the activity of *NAT2* polymorphic forms. Thus, rapid acetylators are more likely to have reduced microbial cure, increased relapse, and increased acquired resistance (Pasipanodya et al., 2012).

Therapeutic Uses

Isoniazid is available as a pill, as an elixir, and for parenteral administration. The recommended total daily dose of isoniazid is 5 mg/kg with a maximum of 300 mg administered daily or 10 mg/kg (range 10–15 mg/kg with a maximum of 900 mg) two or three times a week; oral and intramuscular doses are identical.

Untoward Effects

After NAT2 converts isoniazid to acetylisoniazid, which is excreted by the kidney, acetylisoniazid can also be converted to acetylhydrazine (Roy et al., 2008) and then to hepatotoxic metabolites by CYP2E1. Alternatively, acetylhydrazine may be further acetylated by NAT2 to diacetylhydrazine, which is nontoxic. In this scenario, rapid acetylators will rapidly remove acetylhydrazine, while slower acetylation or induction of CYP2E1 will lead to more of the toxic metabolites. Rifampin is a potent inducer of CYP2E1, which is why it potentiates isoniazid hepatotoxicity.

Elevated serum aspartate and alanine transaminases are encountered commonly in patients on isoniazid. However, the enzyme levels often normalize even when isoniazid therapy is continued (Blumberg et al., 2003). Severe hepatic injury occurs in about 0.1% of all patients taking the drug. Hepatic damage is rare in patients less than 20 years old, but the incidence increases with age. Overall risk is increased to about 3% by coadministration with rifampin. Most cases of hepatitis occur 4–8 weeks after the start of therapy.

If pyridoxine is not given concurrently, peripheral neuritis (most commonly paresthesias of feet and hands) is encountered in about 2% of patients receiving 5 mg/kg isoniazid daily. Neuropathy is more frequent in slow acetylators and in individuals with diabetes mellitus, poor nutrition, or anemia. Other neurological toxicities include convulsions in patients with seizure disorders, optic neuritis and atrophy, muscle twitching, dizziness, ataxia, paresthesias, stupor, and toxic encephalopathy. Mental abnormalities may appear during the use of this drug, including euphoria, transient impairment of memory, loss of self-control, and florid psychoses.

Patients may develop hypersensitivity to isoniazid. Hematological reactions also may occur. Vasculitis associated with antinuclear antibodies may appear during treatment but disappears when the drug is stopped. Arthritic symptoms have been attributed to this agent. Miscellaneous reactions associated with isoniazid therapy include dryness of the mouth, epigastric distress, methemoglobinemia, tinnitus, and urinary retention. In persons predisposed to pyridoxine deficiency anemia, the administration of isoniazid may result in dramatic anemia. Treatment of the anemia with large doses of vitamin B_6 gradually returns the blood count to normal. A drug-induced syndrome resembling systemic lupus erythematosus has also been reported.

Isoniazid Overdose

As little as 1.5 g of isoniazid can be toxic. Isoniazid overdose has been associated with the clinical triad of

- Seizures refractory to treatment with phenytoin and barbiturates
- Metabolic acidosis with an anion gap that is resistant to treatment with sodium bicarbonate
- Coma

The common early symptoms appear within 0.5–3 h of ingestion and include ataxia, peripheral neuropathy, dizziness, and slurred speech. The most dangerous are grand mal seizures and coma, encountered when patients ingest 30 mg/kg or more of the drug. Mortality in these circumstances is as high as 20%. Intravenous pyridoxine is administered over 5–15 min on a gram-to-gram basis with the ingested isoniazid. If the dose of ingested isoniazid is unknown, then a pyridoxine dose of 70 mg/kg should be used. In patients with seizures, benzodiazepines are utilized.

Isoniazid binds to pyridoxal 5'-phosphate to form isoniazid-pyridoxal hydrazones, thereby depleting neuronal pyridoxal 5'-phosphate and interfering with pyridoxal phosphate-requiring reactions, including the synthesis of the inhibitory neurotransmitter GABA. Decreased levels of GABA lead to cerebral overexcitability and lowered seizure threshold. The antidote is replenishment of pyridoxal 5'-phosphate.

Drug Interactions

Isoniazid is a potent inhibitor of CYP2C19 and CYP3A and a weak inhibitor of CYP2D6 (Desta et al., 2001). However, isoniazid induces CYP2E1. Drugs that are metabolized by these enzymes will potentially be affected (Table 60-4).

Ethambutol

Ethambutol hydrochloride is a water-soluble and heat-stable compound.

Mechanism of Action

Ethambutol inhibits arabinosyl transferase III, thereby disrupting the transfer of arabinose into arabinogalactan biosynthesis, which in turn disrupts the assembly of mycobacterial cell wall. The arabinosyl transferases are encoded by *embAB* genes.

Antibacterial Activity

Ethambutol has activity against a wide range of mycobacteria but has no activity against any other genus. Ethambutol MICs are 0.5–2 mg/L in clinical isolates of *M. tuberculosis*, about 0.8 mg/L for *M. kansasii*, and 2–7.5 mg/L for *M. avium*. The following *Mycobacterium* species are also susceptible: *M. gordonae, M. marinum, M. scrofulaceum,* and *M. szulgai*. However, the majority of *M. xenopi, M. fortuitum,* and *M. chelonae* have been reported as resistant.

TABLE 60-4 ■ SOME ISONIAZID-DRUG INTERACTIONS VIA INHIBITION AND INDUCTION OF CYPs

COADMINISTERED DRUG	CYP ISOFORM	ADVERSE EFFECTS
Acetaminophen	CYP2E1 induction	Hepatotoxicity
Carbamazepine	CYP3A inhibition	Neurological toxicity
Diazepam	CYP3A and CYP2C19 inhibition	Sedation and respiratory depression
Ethosuximide	CYP3A inhibition	Psychotic behaviors
Isoflurane and enflurane	CYP2E1 induction	Decreased effectiveness
Phenytoin and fosphenytoin	CYP2C19 inhibition	Neurological toxicity
Theophylline	CYP3A inhibition	Seizures, palpitation, nausea
Vincristine	CYP3A inhibition	Limb weakness and tingling
Warfarin	CYP2C9 inhibition	Possibility of increased bleeding (higher risk with isoniazid doses > 300 mg/d)

Mechanisms of Resistance

In vitro, mycobacterial resistance to the drug develops via mutations in the *embB* gene. In 30%–70% of clinical isolates that are resistant to ethambutol, mutations are encountered at codon 306 of the *embB* gene. However, mutations in this codon are also encountered in ethambutol-susceptible mycobacteria, as though this mutation is necessary, but not sufficient, to confer ethambutol resistance (Safi et al., 2008). Enhanced efflux pump activity may induce resistance to both isoniazid and ethambutol in vitro.

ADME

The oral bioavailability of ethambutol is about 80%. Approximately 10%–40% of the drug is bound to plasma protein. Ethambutol drug concentrations have been modeled using a two-compartment open model, with first-order absorption and elimination (Zhu et al., 2004). The decline in ethambutol is biexponential, with a $t_{1/2}$ of 3 h in the first 12 h and a $t_{1/2}$ of 9 h between 12 and 24 h due to redistribution of drug. Clearance and V_d are greater in children than in adults on a per kilogram basis. Slow and incomplete absorption is common in children, so that good peak concentrations of drug are often not achieved with standard dosing (Zhu et al., 2004). See Table 60-2 for PK data on this drug.

About 80% of the drug is not metabolized at all and is renally excreted. Therefore, in renal failure ethambutol should be dosed at 15–25 mg/kg three times a week instead of daily, even in patients receiving hemodialysis. The remainder of ethambutol (~20%) is oxidized by aldehyde dehydrogenase and excreted as aldehyde and dicarboxylic acid derivatives.

Microbial Pharmacokinetics-Pharmacodynamics

Ethambutol's microbial kill of *M. tuberculosis* is optimized by AUC/MIC, while that against disseminated MAC is optimized by C_{max}/MIC (Deshpande et al., 2010). Thus, to optimize microbial kill, high intermittent doses such as 25 mg/kg every other day to 50 mg/kg twice a week may be superior to daily doses of 15 mg/kg.

Therapeutic Uses

Ethambutol is available for oral administration in tablets containing the D-isomer. It is used for the treatment of TB, disseminated MAC, and in *M. kansasii* infection. Ethambutol is administered at 20 mg/kg (15–25 mg/kg) per day for both adults and children.

Untoward Effects

Ethambutol produces very few serious untoward reactions: About 1% experience diminished visual acuity, 0.5% a rash, and 0.3% drug fever. Other side effects that have been observed are pruritus, joint pain, GI upset, abdominal pain, malaise, headache, dizziness, mental confusion, disorientation, and possible hallucinations. Therapy with ethambutol results in an increased concentration of urate in the blood in about 50% of patients, owing to decreased renal excretion of uric acid.

The most important side effect is optic neuritis, resulting in decreased visual acuity and loss of red-green discrimination. The incidence of this reaction is proportional to the dose of ethambutol and is observed in 15% of patients receiving 50 mg/kg/d, in 5% of patients receiving 25 mg/kg/d, and in less than 1% of patients receiving daily doses of 15 mg/kg. The intensity of the visual difficulty is related to the duration of therapy after the decreased visual acuity first becomes apparent and may be unilateral or bilateral. Tests of visual acuity and red-green discrimination prior to the start of therapy and periodically thereafter are thus recommended. Recovery usually occurs when ethambutol is withdrawn. Drug interactions involving ethambutol are not significant.

Oxazolidinones: Linezolid, Tedizolid, and Sutezolid

Oxazolidinones have been in clinical use for over a decade for the treatment of gram-positive cocci. *Linezolid* and *tedizolid* have been found to be highly efficacious in the treatment of TB. Several studies have examined the utility of linezolid for the treatment of MDR-TB. The first study enrolled 41 patients with MDR-TB, who were immediately assigned to linezolid therapy without change of background regimen, or to a delay of 2 months (Lee et al., 2012). By month 4, 79% in the immediate-start group had sputum culture conversion compared to 35%

in the delayed-start group. However, 4 of every 5 patients had significant adverse events. In a randomized controlled trial of 65 patients with MDR-TB, linezolid therapy was associated with a 79% sputum conversion at 24 months compared to 38% among controls (Tang et al., 2015). However, 82% developed adverse events.

In a recent meta-analysis of 12 studies, Sotgiu et al. (2012) found that 94% of patients on linezolid achieved sputum conversion over an average period of 61 days; however, 68% developed major adverse events. Thus, linezolid is associated with extremely high sputum conversion rates, but at a price of a high rate of adverse events. As a result, studies are examining other oxazolidinones, such as *tedizolid* and *sutezolid*, the latter drug specifically designed for the treatment of TB. It is hoped these will have the same efficacy, but with fewer side effects. The pharmacology of oxazolidinones is discussed in Chapter 59.

Aminoglycosides: Streptomycin, Amikacin, and Kanamycin

The aminoglycosides streptomycin, amikacin, and kanamycin are used for the treatment of mycobacterial diseases. The MICs for *M. tuberculosis* in Middlebrook broth are 0.25–3.0 mg/L for all three aminoglycosides. For *M. avium,* streptomycin and amikacin MICs are 1–8 mg/L; those of kanamycin are 3–12 mg/L. *Mycobacterium kansasii* is frequently susceptible to these agents, but other nontuberculous mycobacteria are only occasionally susceptible. As an example, for amikacin in treatment of *M. abscessus*, an MIC range of 2–128 mg/L has been noted (Ferro et al., 2016). The pharmacological properties and therapeutic uses of aminoglycosides are discussed in full in Chapter 58.

Bacterial Resistance

Primary resistance to streptomycin is found in 2%–3% of *M. tuberculosis* clinical isolates. Resistance to aminoglycosides involves several genetic loci, as well as efflux pumps.

Aminoglycosides inhibit protein synthesis by binding to the 30S ribosomal subunit and causing misreading of the genetic code during translation. The 30s ribosomal unit is made of the 16S mRNA (encoded by *rpsL*), which binds to the ribosomal protein S12 (encoded by *rrs*) to optimize tRNA binding and mRNA decoding. Mutations in *rpsL* and *rrs* are associated with high-level aminoglycoside resistance in mycobacteria. However, mutations in these genes are only encountered in half of clinical isolates with aminoglycoside resistance. GidB is an rRNA methyltransferase for 16S rRNA, and mutations in the *gidB* gene are associated with low-level streptomycin resistance (Okamoto et al., 2007). The *gidB* mutations lead to high-level streptomycin-resistant mutants at a rate 2000 times that in wild type. Mutations in *gidB* are encountered in 33% of streptomycin-resistant clinical isolates of *M. tuberculosis.* Finally, efflux pump–mediated resistance was recently demonstrated in clinical isolates with low-level streptomycin-resistant *M. tuberculosis* and interacted with chromosomal mutations in *gidB* (Spies et al., 2008).

Therapeutic Uses

Therapeutic uses of aminoglycosides in treatment of mycobacterial infections are discussed further in the chapter.

Bicyclic Nitroimidazoles: Delaminid and Pretomanid

Pretomanid, discovered by Stover et al. in 2000, and *delaminid*, discovered by Matsumoto et al. in 2006, are bicyclic nitroimidazopyrans that are being used in the treatment of extensively drug-resistant and multidrug-resistant TB and are in clinical trials for use in drug-susceptible TB.

Mechanisms of Action

Pretomanid has two mechanisms of action. First, under aerobic conditions it inhibits *M. tuberculosis* mycolic acid and protein synthesis at the step between hydroxymycolate and ketomycolate (Stover et al., 2000). Similar to the structurally related metronidazole, pretomanid is a prodrug that requires activation by the bacteria via a nitroreduction step that requires, among other factors, a specific G6PDX, FGD1, and the reduced deazaflavin cofactor F_{420} encoded by Rv3547 (Bashiri et al., 2008). Second, in NRPB, it generates reactive nitrogen species such as NO via its des-nitro metabolite, which then augment the kill of intracellular NRPB by the innate immune system (Singh et al., 2008). In addition, direct poisoning of the respiratory complex in the NRPB leads to ATP depletion.

Delamanid is also a prodrug that is activated by the same enzyme encoded by Rv3547 (Xavier and Lakshmanan, 2014). Similarly, it also forms a reactive intermediate metabolite that inhibits mycolic acid production.

Antibacterial Activity

The MICs of pretomanid against *M. tuberculosis* range from 0.015 to 0.25 mg/L, but the drug lacks activity against other mycobacteria. Similarly, for delaminid, MICs range from 0.006 to 0.012 mg/L (Matsumoto et al., 2006).

Mechanism of Resistance

The proportion of mutants resistant to 5 mg/L of pretomanid is 10^{-6}. Resistance arises due to changes in structure of FGD, which is due to a variety of point mutations in the *fgd* gene. However, resistant isolates have also been identified that lack *fgd* mutations, so that resistance may also be due to other mechanisms (Stover et al., 2000). Mutation frequencies for delaminid are unclear; however, resistance has also been shown to be due to *fgd1* and also *fbiA* mutations (Bloemberg et al., 2015).

ADME

The PK parameters of pretomanid include a clearance of 6.7–8.8 L/h at steady state, with a terminal $t_{1/2}$ of 16–20 h, based on a noncompartmental analysis (Ginsberg et al., 2009). Similarly, no compartmental PK analyses have been published yet with delaminid, with noncompartmental PK published as an AUC_{0-24} of 7.9 mg*h/L after a dose of 100 mg twice a day and 11.8 mg*h/L after a 200 mg twice-a-day dose: $t_{1/2}$ = about 38 h (Gler et al., 2012). Systemic exposures increase on uptake with food.

Microbial Pharmacokinetics-Pharmacodynamics

No formal microbial PK-pharmacodynamic work has been performed with delaminid. Pretomanid microbial kill is driven by percentage time concentration persists above MIC (Ahmad et al., 2011). The dose of 200 mg a day in humans achieves optimal PK-pharmacodynamic exposure in most patients.

Therapeutic Uses

Delaminid is currently dispensed in 50-mg tablets at 100 mg twice daily, with food. It is used in the treatment of multidrug-resistant TB and is being examined in combination with other drugs. Pretomanid is administered at 200 mg a day and is undergoing phase III trials in combination with other drugs for treatment of both drug-susceptible and drug-resistant TB.

Untoward Effects

Data on untoward effects are currently being gathered. It has been noted that delaminid is associated with QT segment prolongation; however, the clinical significance is unclear.

Clofazimine

Clofazimine is a fat-soluble riminophenazine dye.

Mechanism of Action

The biochemical basis for the antimicrobial actions of clofazimine remains to be established (Anonymous, 2008a). Possible mechanisms of action include membrane disruption, inhibition of mycobacterial phospholipase A_2, inhibition of microbial K^+ transport, generation of hydrogen peroxide, interference with the bacterial electron transport chain, or efflux pump inhibition.

However, it is known that clofazimine has both antibacterial activity and anti-inflammatory effects via inhibition of macrophages, T cells, neutrophils, and complement.

Antibacterial Activity

The MICs for *M. avium* clinical isolates are 1–5 mg/L. The MICs for *M. tuberculosis* are about 1.0 mg/L. The compound also is useful for treatment of chronic skin ulcers (Buruli ulcer) produced by *Mycobacterium ulcerans.* It has activity against many gram-positive bacteria with an MIC of

1.0 mg/L or less against *S. aureus*, coagulase-negative staphylococci, *Streptococcus pyogenes*, and *Listeria monocytogenes*. Gram-negative bacteria have MICs greater than 32 mg/L.

Bacterial Resistance

Clofazimine-resistant *Mycobacterium tuberculosis* carries a mutation in the gene encoding a transcription repressor for efflux pump MmpL; this is associated with cross resistance to bedaquiline (Hartkoorn et al., 2014; Zhang et al., 2015).

ADME

Clofazimine is administered orally at doses up to 300 mg a day. Clofazimine's oral bioavailability is 45%–60%; it is increased 2-fold by high-fat meals and decreased 30% by antacids (Nix et al., 2004). After a single dose, clofazimine is best modeled using a one-compartment model and has a prolonged absorption phase; after 200 mg of clofazimine, the t_{max} is 5.3–7.8 h. After prolonged repeated dosing, the $t_{1/2}$ is about 70 days. For PK data, see Table 60–2. As a result of the good penetration into many tissues, a reddish-black discoloration of skin and body secretions may occur and take a long time to resolve. Crystalline deposits of the drug have been encountered in many tissues at autopsy (Anonymous, 2008a). Clofazimine is metabolized in the liver in four steps: hydrolytic dehalogenation, hydrolytic deamination, glucuronidation, and hydroxylation.

Untoward Effects

Gastrointestinal problems are encountered in 40%–50% of patients. In patients who have died following the abdominal pain, crystal deposition in intestinal mucosa, liver, spleen, and abdominal lymph nodes has been demonstrated (Anonymous, 2008a). Body secretion discoloration, eye discoloration, and skin discoloration occur in most patients and can lead to depression in some patients.

Drug Interactions

Anti-inflammatory effects may be inhibited by dapsone.

Fluoroquinolones

Fluoroquinolones are DNA gyrase inhibitors. Their chemistry, spectrum of activity, and pharmacology are discussed in detail in Chapter 56. Drugs such as *ofloxacin* and *ciprofloxacin* have been second-line anti-TB agents for many years, but they are limited by the rapid development of resistance. Adding C8 halogen and C8 methoxy groups markedly reduces the propensity for drug resistance. Of the C8 methoxy quinolones, *moxifloxacin*, *gatifloxacin*, and *levofloxacin* have been examined in the clinic for the treatment of pulmonary TB and meningeal TB.

Microbial Pharmacokinetics-Pharmacodynamics Relevant to TB

Fluoroquinolone microbial kill is best explained by the AUC_{0-24}/MIC ratio. In preclinical models, moxifloxacin AUC_{0-24}/MIC exposures equivalent to those from the standard 400-mg dose were associated with good microbial kill but amplified the drug-resistant subpopulation, so that resistance emerged in 7–13 days with monotherapy (Gumbo et al., 2004). This time to emergence of resistance harmonizes well with speed of resistance emergence in patients (Ginsburg et al., 2003). Moxifloxacin exposure best associated with minimizing emergence of resistance was a non-protein bound AUC_{0-24}/MIC of 53. Clinical trial simulations revealed that doses greater than 400 mg a day might better achieve this AUC/MIC. Given that rifamycins reduce the moxifloxacin AUC, these results point to a potential concern of quinolone resistance.

Therapeutic Uses in Treatment of TB

Fluoroquinolones have been examined for therapeutic use in two TB contexts: for an attempt to shorten therapy duration in pulmonary TB and for the treatment of TB meningitis.

The first study was a randomized, double-blind, placebo-controlled trial that examined the effect of replacing either isoniazid or ethambutol in the standard regimen with moxifloxacin 400 mg/d for 17 weeks versus standard short-course chemotherapy (6 months) consisting of rifampin, isoniazid, ethambutol, and pyrazinamide for therapy failure or relapse

(poor outcome) (Gillespie et al., 2014). While the moxifloxacin-containing regimens produced a more rapid sputum decline, there was a 6%–11% higher poor outcome compared to standard therapy. In a second randomized study, the standard short-course chemotherapy (6 months) was compared to a 4-month regimen in which isoniazid was replaced by 400 mg of gatifloxacin once a day (Merle et al., 2014). The gatifloxacin regimen was associated with greater than 2-fold higher recurrences/relapses. Thus, the quinolones failed to reduce therapy duration at the doses tested.

Fluoroquinolones have very good penetration into the CNS (Thwaites et al., 2011). A study investigating a regimen of standard therapy that included high-dose rifampicin plus two different moxifloxacin regimens found that 6-month mortality was half in patients who received the high-dose rifampicin intravenously and moxifloxacin (Ruslami et al., 2013). However, in a recent study of 817 patients, intensified anti-TB treatment with high-dose rifampin plus levofloxacin was not associated with a higher rate of survival among patients with tuberculous meningitis than standard treatment (Heemskerk et al., 2016).

Currently, fluoroquinolones, especially moxifloxacin, continue to be central for the treatment of pulmonary MDR-TB, and their presence or absence correlates with clinical outcomes.

Bedaquiline

Bedaquiline was discovered by Andries et al. in 2005 and entered clinical use in the treatment of TB difficult to treat with current anti-TB drugs. Bedaquiline is a cationic amphiphilic drug, which may account for its high accumulation in tissues.

Mechanism of Action

Bedaquiline acts by targeting subunit *c* of the ATP synthase of *M. tuberculosis*, leading to inhibition of the proton pump activity of the ATP synthase (Andries et al., 2005; Koul et al., 2007). Thus, the compound targets bacillary energy metabolism.

Antibacterial Activity

The bedaquiline MIC for *M. tuberculosis* is 0.03–0.12 mg/L. It has good activity against MAC, *M. leprae*, *M. bovis*, *M. marinum*, *M. kansasii*, *M. ulcerans*, *M. fortuitum*, *M. szulgai*, and *M. abscessus* (Andries et al., 2005; Huitric et al., 2007).

Bacterial Resistance

The proportion of *M. tuberculosis* mutants resistant to four times the MIC is 5×10^{-7} to 2×10^{-8}. Resistance is associated with two point mutations: D32V and A63P. This region of the gene encodes the membrane-spanning domain of the ATP synthase *c* subunit. Recently, resistance due to efflux pump mutations and their regulators has been described.

ADME

The population PK of bedaquiline are well characterized (Swenson et al., 2016). After oral ingestion, there is a large lag time in absorption, resulting in a t_{max} of 5 h. The PKs are best described using a three-compartment model, with a central compartment and two peripheral compartments. The total clearance is 2.62 L/h, and the total volume of all compartments is more than 10,000 L (Swenson et al., 2016). Clearance is 52% higher in people of African descent, but 16% lower in women compared to men. The terminal $t_{1/2}$ is about 5.5 months, mainly driven by redistribution from the tissues. Despite the extremely large volume of distribution, bedaquiline has poor CNS penetration. Bedaquiline is metabolized by CY3A4 to M2, an *N*-monodesmethyl metabolite.

Microbial Pharmacokinetics-Pharmacodynamics

Microbial kill of bedaquiline is believed to be linked to AUC/MIC ratios (Rouan et al., 2012). The PK-pharmacodynamic parameters linked to resistance suppression are unknown.

Efficacy and Therapeutic Use

A regimen of bedaquiline 400 mg daily for 2 weeks followed by 200 mg three times a day thereafter was added to a background second-line regimen of either kanamycin or amikacin, ofloxacin with or without ethambutol in patients with MDR-TB and led to an 8-week sputum conversion of about 50% with bedaquiline compared to 9% without (Diacon et al., 2009). This led to licensing of the drug, which is currently being used in combination with others for treatment of MDR-TB that is difficult to treat with other antibiotics. In a second larger study of patients with MDR-TB, at week 24, 79% of patients on bedaquiline had sputum conversion compared to 58% of those not on bedaquiline, and at 120 weeks the culture conversion rates were 62% versus 44% (Diacon et al., 2014).

Untoward Effects

The adverse events of bedaquiline include nausea in 26% of patients and diarrhea in 13% of patients. Other adverse effects include arthralgia, pain in extremities, and hyperuricemia and occur in a small proportion of patients (Diacon et al., 2009). The major concern with this drug is cardiovascular toxicity and death. First, there was an increased corrected QT interval of between 450 and 480 ms in 27% versus 9% on this drug compared to placebo (Kakkar and Dahiya, 2014). However, no cases of torsades de pointes have been reported. A 5-fold higher rate of death has been reported in patients on bedaquiline versus those on placebo among 160 patients. The reasons are unclear, but this has led some to question the cost-benefit effect of using this drug (Avorn, 2013). Only a limited number of patients have been exposed to this drug, so that the full side-effect profile is unclear.

Ethionamide

Ethionamide is a congener of thioisonicotinamide.

Mechanism of Action

Mycobacterial EthaA, an NADPH-specific, FAD-containing monooxygenase, converts ethionamide to a sulfoxide and then to 2-ethyl-4-aminopyridine (Vannelli et al., 2002). Although these products are not toxic to mycobacteria, it is believed that a closely related and transient intermediate is the active antibiotic. Ethionamide inhibits mycobacterial growth by inhibiting the activity of the *inhA* gene product, the enoyl-ACP reductase of fatty acid synthase II (Larsen et al., 2002). This is the same enzyme that activated isoniazid inhibits. Although the exact mechanisms of inhibition may differ, the results are the same: inhibition of mycolic acid biosynthesis and consequent impairment of cell wall synthesis.

Antibacterial Activity

The multiplication of *M. tuberculosis* is suppressed by concentrations of ethionamide ranging from 0.6 to 2.5 mg/L. A concentration of 10 mg/L or less will inhibit about 75% of photochromogenic mycobacteria; the scotochromogens are more resistant.

Bacterial Resistance

Resistance occurs mainly via changes in the enzyme that activates ethionamide, and mutations are encountered in a transcriptional repressor gene that controls its expression, *etaR*. Mutations in the *inhA* gene lead to resistance to both ethionamide and isoniazid.

ADME

The oral bioavailability of ethionamide approaches 100%. The PK are adequately explained by a one-compartment model with first-order absorption and elimination (Zhu et al., 2002) (see PK values in Table 56-2). After oral administration of 500 mg of ethionamide, a C_{max} of 1.4 mg/L is achieved in 2 h. The $t_{1/2}$ is about 2 h. The concentrations in the blood and various organs are approximately equal. Ethionamide is cleared by hepatic metabolism. Metabolites are eliminated in the urine, with less than 1% of ethionamide excreted in an active form.

Therapeutic Uses

Ethionamide is administered only orally. The initial dosage for adults is 250 mg twice daily; it is increased by 125 mg/d every 5 days until a dose of 15–20 mg/kg/d is achieved. The maximal dose is 1 g daily. The drug is best taken with meals in divided doses to minimize gastric irritation. Children should receive 10–20 mg/kg/d in two divided doses, not to exceed 1 g/d.

Untoward Effects

Approximately 50% of patients are unable to tolerate a single dose larger than 500 mg because of GI upset. The most common reactions are anorexia, nausea and vomiting, gastric irritation, and a variety of neurologic symptoms.

Severe postural hypotension, mental depression, drowsiness, and asthenia are common. Other reactions referable to the nervous system include olfactory disturbances, blurred vision, diplopia, dizziness, paresthesias, headache, restlessness, and tremors. Pyridoxine (vitamin B_6) relieves the neurologic symptoms, and its concomitant administration is recommended. Severe allergic skin rashes, purpura, stomatitis, gynecomastia, impotence, menorrhagia, acne, and alopecia have also been observed. A metallic taste also may be noted. Hepatitis has been associated with the use of the ethionamide in about 5% of cases. Hepatic function should be assessed at regular intervals in patients receiving the drug.

Para-aminosalicylic Acid

Para-aminosalicylic acid, discovered by Lehman in 1943, was the first effective treatment of TB.

AMINOSALICYLIC ACID

Mechanism of Action

Para-aminosalicylic acid is a structural analogue of PABA, the substrate of dihydropteroate synthase (*fol*P1/P2). As a result, PAS is thought to be a competitive inhibitor *fol*P1, but in vitro the inhibitory activity against *fol*P1 is very poor. However, mutation of the thymidylate synthase gene (*thyA*) results in resistance to PAS, but only 37% of the PAS-resistant clinical isolates or spontaneous mutants encode a mutation in the *thyA* gene or in any genes encoding enzymes in the folate pathway or biosynthesis of thymine nucleotides (Mathys et al., 2009). Unidentified actions of PAS likely play more important roles in its anti-TB effects.

Antibacterial Activity

Para-aminosalicylic acid is bacteriostatic. In vitro, most strains of *M. tuberculosis* are sensitive to a concentration of 1 mg/L. It has no activity against other bacteria.

Bacterial Resistance

Mutations in *thyA*, *folC*, and *ribD* lead to PAS resistance in up to 61% of resistant isolates (Zhang et al., 2015). Recently, MDR-TB strains due to deletions of entire *dfrA* and *thyA* have been identified, a surprise given the conserved nature of folate synthesis (Moradigaravand et al., 2016).

ADME

Para-aminosalicylic acid oral bioavailability is more than 90%. PAS PK are described by a one-compartment model (Peloquin et al., 2001) (see the PK values in Table 60-2). The C_{max} increases 1.5-fold and AUC 1.7-fold with food compared to fasting (Peloquin et al., 2001). Administration with food also reduces gastric irritation. Protein binding is 50%–60%. PAS is N-acetylated in the liver to N-acetyl PAS, a potential hepatotoxin. Over 80% of the drug is excreted in the urine; more than 50% is in the form of the acetylated compound. Excretion of PAS acid is reduced by renal dysfunction; thus, the dose must be reduced in renal dysfunction.

Therapeutic Uses

Para-aminosalicylic acid is administered orally in a daily dose of 12 g. The drug is best administered after meals, with the daily dose divided into three equal portions. Children should receive 150–300 mg/kg/d in three or four divided doses.

Untoward Effects

The incidence of untoward effects associated with the use of PAS is about 10%–30%. GI problems predominate and often limit patient adherence. Hypersensitivity reactions to PAS are seen in 5%–10% of patients and manifest as skin eruptions, fever, eosinophilia, and other hematological abnormalities.

Cycloserine

Cycloserine is D-4-amino-3-isoxazolidone. It is a broad-spectrum antibiotic produced by *Streptococcus orchidaceous*.

CYCLOSERINE

Mechanism of Action

Cycloserine and D-alanine are structural analogues; thus, cycloserine inhibits *alanine racemase*, which converts L-alanine to D-alanine and *D-alanine: D-alanine ligase*, stopping reactions in which D-alanine is incorporated into bacterial cell wall synthesis.

Antibacterial Activity

Cycloserine is a broad-spectrum antibiotic. It inhibits *M. tuberculosis* at concentrations of 5–20 mg/L. It has good activity against MAC, enterococci, *E. coli*, *S. aureus*, *Nocardia* species, and *Chlamydia*.

Mechanisms of Resistance

Cycloserine resistance in clinical isolates of *M. tuberculosis* has been detected in 10%–82% of isolates (Anonymous, 2008b). Nonsynonymous SNPs and loss-of-function mutations in ald cause resistance to D-cycloserine. In addition, resistance also involes alr, the gene for alanine racemase. Nonsynonymous SNPs in alr and SNPs in the alr promoter can confer resistance to D-cycloserine (Desjardin et al., 2016).

ADME

Oral cycloserine is almost completely absorbed. The population PK are best described using a one-compartment model with first-order absorption and elimination. The drug's $t_{1/2}$ is 9 h. The C_{max} in plasma is reached in 45 min in fasting subjects but is delayed for up to 3.5 h with a high-fat meal. See Table 56–2 for PK values. Cycloserine is well distributed throughout body. There is no appreciable barrier to CNS entry for cycloserine, and CSF concentrations are approximately the same as those in plasma. About 50% of cycloserine is excreted unchanged in the urine in the first 12 h; a total of 70% is recoverable in the active form over a period of 24 h. The drug may accumulate to toxic concentrations in patients with renal failure. About 60% of it is removed by hemodialysis, and the drug must be redosed after each hemodialysis session (Malone et al., 1999a).

Therapeutic Uses

Cycloserine is available for oral administration. The usual dose for adults is 250–500 mg twice daily.

Untoward Effects

Neuropsychiatric symptoms are common and occur in 50% of patients on 1 g/d, so much so that the drug has earned the nickname "psych-serine." Symptoms range from headache and somnolence to severe psychosis, seizures, and suicidal ideas. Large doses of cycloserine or the concomitant ingestion of alcohol increases the risk of seizures. Cycloserine is contraindicated in individuals with a history of epilepsy and should be used with caution in individuals with a history of depression.

Capreomycin

Capreomycin is an antimycobacterial cyclic peptide. It consists of four active components: capreomycins IA, IB, IIA, and IIB. The agent used clinically contains primarily IA and IB. Antimycobacterial activity is similar to that of aminoglycosides, as are adverse effects, and capreomycin should not be administered with other drugs that damage cranial nerve VIII.

Bacterial resistance to capreomycin develops when it is given alone; such microorganisms show cross-resistance with kanamycin and neomycin. The adverse reactions associated with the use of capreomycin are hearing loss, tinnitus, transient proteinuria, cylindruria, and nitrogen retention. Severe renal failure is rare. Eosinophilia is common. Leukocytosis, leukopenia, rashes, and fever have been observed. Injections of the drug

may be painful. Capreomycin is given for MDR-TB. The recommended daily dose is 1 g (no more than 20 mg/kg) per day for 60–120 days, followed by 1 g two or three times a week.

β-Lactam Antibiotics for the Treatment of TB

Until recently, it was assumed that β-lactam antibiotics lacked activity against mycobacteria because the bacteria have Ambler class A β-lactamases such as BlacC. Carbapenems, which are poorer substrates of these enzymes, in conjunction with inhibitors such as clavulanate, have demonstrated efficacy against *M. tuberculosis*. In addition, penems such as faropenem, which possess both carbapenem and cephalosporin structures, are effective against *M. tuberculosis* without a β-lactamase inhibitor. The general pharmacology of this class of compounds is discussed in Chapter 57. Recently, reports of patients with MDR-TB who have responded to β-lactam antibiotics such as ertapenem have been published (Tiberi et al., 2016). A recent meta-analysis identified seven clinical studies in which ertapenem, imipenem, and meropenem were used to treat MDR-TB and identified sputum conversion rates of greater than 60% (Sotgiu et al., 2016). The optimal doses for the treatment of MDR-TB and which antibiotics to combine are currently unknown.

Macrolides

The pharmacology, bacterial activity, and resistance mechanisms of macrolides are discussed in Chapter 59. Azithromycin and clarithromycin are used for the treatment of MAC.

Dapsone

Dapsone (DDS) is a broad-spectrum agent with antibacterial, antiprotozoal, and antifungal effects.

DAPSONE

Mechanism of Action

Dapsone is a structural analogue of PABA and a competitive inhibitor of dihydropteroate synthase (*folP1/P2*) in the folate pathway, shown in

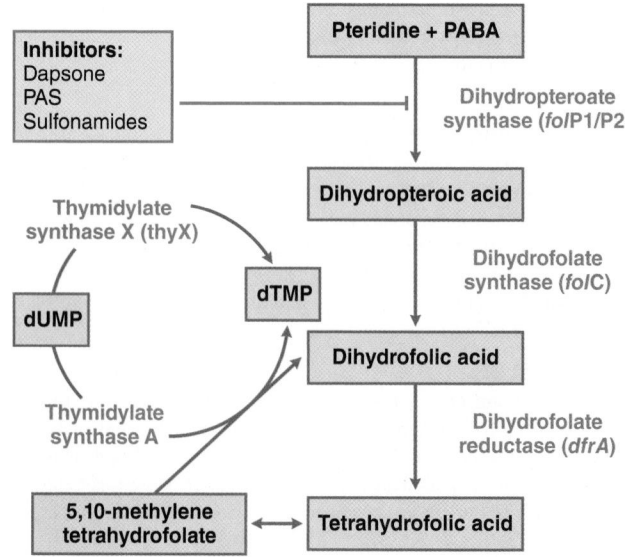

Figure 60–5 *Effects of antimicrobials on folate metabolism and deoxynucleotide synthesis.* dTMP, deoxythymidine monophosphate; dUMP, deoxyuridine monophosphate.

Figure 60–5. The anti-inflammatory effects of dapsone occur via inhibition of tissue damage by neutrophils (Wolf et al., 2002). Dapsone inhibits neutrophil myeloperoxidase activity and respiratory burst, and it inhibits activity of neutrophil lysosomal enzymes. Dapsone may act as a free-radical scavenger of free radicals generated by neutrophils, and dapsone may inhibit migration of neutrophils to inflammatory lesions (Wolf et al., 2002). Dapsone is extensively used for acne, but this therapy is not recommended.

Antimicrobial Effects

Antibacterial. Dapsone is bacteriostatic against *M. leprae* at concentrations of 1–10 mg/L. More than 90% of clinical isolates of MAC and *M. kansasii* have an MIC of 8 mg/L or less, but the MICs for *M. tuberculosis* isolates are high. It has little activity against other bacteria.

Antiparasitic. Dapsone is also highly effective against *Plasmodium falciparum* with IC_{50} of 0.6–1.3 mg/L even in sulfadoxine-pyrimethamine-resistant strains. Dapsone has an IC_{50} of 0.55 mg/L against *Toxoplasma gondii* tachyzoites.

Antifungal. Dapsone is effective at concentrations of 0.1/mg/L against the fungus *Pneumocystis jiroveci*.

Drug Resistance

Resistance to dapsone in *P. falciparum*, *P. jiroveci*, and *M. leprae* results primarily from mutations in genes encoding dihydropteroate synthase (Figure 60–5).

ADME

After oral administration, absorption is complete; the elimination $t_{1/2}$ is 20–30 h. The population PK of dapsone are shown in Table 60–2 (Simpson et al., 2006). Dapsone undergoes *N*-acetylation by NAT2. *N*-Oxidation to dapsone hydroxylamine is via CYP2E1 and to a lesser extent by CYP2C. Dapsone hydroxylamine enters red blood cells, leading to methemoglobin formation. Sulfones tend to be retained for up to 3 weeks in skin and muscle and especially in liver and kidney. Intestinal reabsorption of sulfones excreted in the bile contributes to long-term retention in the bloodstream; periodic interruption of treatment is advisable for this reason. Epithelial lining fluid-to-plasma ratio is between 0.76 and 2.91; CSF-to-plasma ratio is 0.21–2.01 (Gatti et al., 1997). Approximately 70%–80% of a dose of dapsone is excreted in the urine as an acid-labile mono-*N*-glucuronide and mono-*N*-sulfamate.

Therapeutic Uses

Dapsone is administered as an oral agent. Therapeutic uses of dapsone in the treatment of leprosy are described later in this chapter. Dapsone is combined with chlorproguanil for the treatment of malaria. Dapsone is also used for *P. jiroveci* infection and prophylaxis and for the prophylaxis for *T. gondii* (see Chapter 54). The anti-inflammatory effects are the basis for therapy of pemphigoid, dermatitis herpetiformis, linear IgA bullous disease, relapsing chondritis, and ulcers caused by the brown recluse spider (Wolf et al., 2002).

Dapsone and Glucose-6-Phosphate Dehydrogenase Deficiency

Glucose-6-phosphate dehydrogenase protects red cells against oxidative damage. However, G6PD deficiency is encountered in nearly half a billion people worldwide, the most common of 100 variants being G6PD-A⁻. Dapsone, an oxidant, causes severe hemolysis in patients with G6PD deficiency. Thus, G6PD deficiency testing should be performed prior to use of dapsone whenever possible.

Other Untoward Effects

Hemolysis develops in almost every individual treated with 200–300 mg of dapsone per day. Doses of 100 mg or less in healthy persons and 50 mg or less in healthy individuals with a G6PD deficiency do not cause hemolysis. Methemoglobinemia also is common. A genetic deficiency in NADH-dependent methemoglobin reductase can result in severe methemoglobinemia after administration of dapsone. Isolated instances of headache, nervousness, insomnia, blurred vision, paresthesias, reversible peripheral neuropathy (thought to be due to axonal degeneration), drug fever, hematuria, pruritus, psychosis, and a variety of skin rashes

have been reported. An infectious mononucleosis-like syndrome, which may be fatal, occurs occasionally.

Principles of Antituberculosis Chemotherapy

Evolution and Pharmacology

Mycobacterium tuberculosis is not a single species, but a complex of species with 99.9% similarity at the nucleotide level. The complex includes *M. tuberculosis (typus humanus)*, *M. canettii*, *M. africanum*, *M. bovis*, and *M. microti*. They all cause TB, with *M. microti* responsible for only a handful of human cases.

Antituberculosis Therapy

Traditionally, isoniazid, pyrazinamide, rifampin, and ethambutol have been considered first-line anti-TB agents. However, the notions are shifting, with new regimens being tested with the aim of treating TB in less than 6 months, many of which are rifampin and isoniazid sparing. Moreover, antagonism between these "first-line" drugs such as isoniazid versus both rifampin and pyrazinamide has been described in murine TB models, in the hollow-fiber TB model, and in the clinic in adults and children (Chigutsa et al., 2015; Srivastava et al., 2011b; Swaminathan et al., 2016). Moxifloxacin is being studied as an agent for drug-susceptible TB, as is pretomanid and oxazolidinones. As a result, the concept of specific drugs as first line is being replaced with focus on regimens to be ranked by faster sterilizing effect. Traditionally, first-line agents were more efficacious and better tolerated relative to second-line agents. Second-line agents were used in case of poor tolerance or resistance to first-line agents. Second-line drugs included ethionamide, PAS, cycloserine, amikacin, kanamycin, and capreomycin.

The mutation rates to anti-TB drugs are between 10^{-6} and 10^{-10}, so that the likelihood of resistance is high to any single anti-TB drug in patients with cavitary TB who have about 10^9 CFU of bacilli in a 3-cm pulmonary lesion. However, the likelihood that bacilli would develop mutations to two or more different drugs is the product of two mutation rates (between 1 in 10^{14} and 1 in 10^{20}), which makes the probability of resistance emergence to more than two drugs acceptably small. Thus, only combination anti-TB therapy is currently recommended. Multidrug therapy has led to a reduction in length of therapy.

Types of Antituberculosis Therapy

Prophylaxis

After infection with *M. tuberculosis*, about 10% of people will develop active disease over a lifetime. The highest risk of reactivation TB is in patients with Mantoux tuberculin skin test reaction 5 mm or greater who also fall into one of the following categories: recently exposed to TB, have HIV coinfection, have fibrotic changes on chest radiograms, or are immunosuppressed due to HIV infection or posttransplantation or are taking immunosuppressive medications for any reason. If the tuberculin skin test is 10 mm or greater, a high risk of TB is encountered in recent (≤5 years) immigrants from areas of high TB prevalence, children younger than 4 years, children exposed to adults with TB, intravenous drug users, as well as residents and employees of high-risk congregate settings. Any person with a skin test greater than 15 mm is also at high risk of disease.

In these patients at high risk of active TB, prophylaxis is recommended to prevent active disease. Prophylaxis consists of four regimens. The shortest-duration regimen that is effective consists of isoniazid 15 mg/kg (maximum 900 mg) and weight band–based rifapentine doses administered orally once a week for 12 weeks. The weight bands for rifapentine are 300 mg for 10–14 kg, 450 mg for 14.4–25 kg, 600 mg for 25.1–32 kg, 750 mg for 32.1–49.9 kg, and 900 mg for above 50 kg. The traditional regimens consist of oral isoniazid, 300 mg daily or twice weekly, for 6 months in adults. Those who cannot take isoniazid should be given rifampin, 10 mg/kg daily, for 4 months. In children, isoniazid 10–15 mg/kg daily (maximum 300 mg) is administered, or 20–30 mg/kg two times a week directly observed, for 9 months. In children who cannot tolerate isoniazid, rifampin 10–20 mg/kg daily for 6 months is recommended.

All active TB cases should be confirmed by culture or rapid diagnostic methods such as nucleic acid amplification tests (e.g., Xpert MTB/RIF) and have antimicrobial susceptibilities determined. In adults, the current standard regimen for drug-susceptible TB consists of isoniazid (5 mg/kg, maximum 300 mg/d), rifampin (10 mg/kg, maximum 600 mg/d), and pyrazinamide (15–30 mg/kg, maximum of 2 g/d) for 2 months, followed by intermittent 10-mg/kg rifampin and 15-mg/kg isoniazid two or three times a week for 4 months. Children should receive rifampin 10–20 mg/kg at a maximum dose of 600 mg/d, pyrazinamide 30–40 mg/kg/d, and isoniazid 10–15 mg/kg at a maximum dose of 300 mg/d. Rifabutin 5 mg/kg/d can be used for the entire 6 months of therapy in adult HIV-infected patients because rifampin can adversely interact with some antiretroviral agents to reduce their effectiveness. If there is resistance to isoniazid, initial therapy also may include ethambutol (15–20 mg/kg/d) or streptomycin (1 g/d) until isoniazid susceptibility is documented. Ethambutol doses in children are 20 mg/kg/d (maximum 1 g) or 50 mg/kg twice weekly (2.5 g). Because monitoring of visual acuity is difficult in children younger than 5 years, caution should be exercised in using ethambutol in these children.

The first 2 months of the four-drug regimen is termed the *initial phase of therapy* and the last 4 months the *continuation phase of therapy*. Rifapentine (10 mg/kg once a week) may be substituted for rifampin in the continuation phase in patients with no evidence of HIV infection or cavitary TB. Pyridoxine, vitamin B_6, (10–50 mg/d) should be administered with isoniazid to minimize the risks of neurological toxicity in patients predisposed to neuropathy (e.g., the malnourished, elderly, pregnant women, HIV-infected individuals, diabetic patients, alcoholic patients, and uremic patients). To ensure compliance, therapy is administered as DOT. Although DOT is the standard of care, an analysis of a series of randomized clinical trials found no difference in outcome between DOT and self-administered therapy (Pasipanodya and Gumbo, 2013; Volmink and Garner, 2007).

The duration of therapy of drug-susceptible pulmonary TB is 6 months. A 9-month duration should be used for patients with cavitary disease who are still sputum culture positive at 2 months. HIV-infected patients with CD4+ lymphocyte cell counts less than 100/mm³ are at increased risk of developing rifamycin resistance. Therefore, daily therapy is recommended during the continuation phase. Most cases of extrapulmonary TB are treated for 6 months. TB meningitis is an exception that requires a 9- to 12-month duration. In addition, results of a meta-analysis suggest that corticosteroids should be used in TB meningitis (Prasad et al., 2016).

The treatment of TB pericarditis is a special case in which the use of steroids has been advocated for many decades. In the IMPI trial that randomized 1400 patients, Mayosi and colleagues (2014) examined the effect of prednisolone on the composite outcome of death, cardiac tamponade requiring pericardiocentesis, or constrictive pericarditis. There was no significant difference in the primary outcome between patients who received prednisolone and those who received placebo, even though the corticosteroids were associated with 44% decrease in the development of constrictive pericarditis. The corticosteroids were associated with a 3-fold increase in the incidence of cancer, especially in the context of HIV/TB coinfection. Moreover, even with the four-drug regimen of rifampin, isoniazid, ethambutol, and pyrazinamide, mortality is still very high at 26% at 6 months (and 40% in HIV-infected patients), and over several years is 1.43 per 100 person-months overall. A recent study found that free drug concentrations of rifampin in pericardial fluid were virtually close to zero, ethambutol concentrations were low, and the pH in the infected pericardial fluid was 7.34, which is the pH at which pyrazinamide has no effect (Shenje et al., 2015). The optimal regimen for treatment of TB pericarditis thus remains to be identified.

Definitive Therapy of Drug-Resistant TB

The XDR-TB is MDR-TB that is also resistant to fluoroquinolones and at least one of three injectable second-line drugs (i.e., amikacin, kanamycin, or capreomycin). These diseases, virtually untreatable, led to the clinical trials of bedaquiline and delaminid in combination with optimized background regimens, as well as studies of linezolid. These studies demonstrated improved sputum conversion rates with these drugs. However, the adverse event rates when linezolid or bedaquiline are used are high, and it is unclear which drugs to combine with these agents to optimize efficacy and minimize adverse events rates. Thus, the exact regimens to use are still unknown. Thus, in documented drug resistance, therapy should be based on evidence of susceptibility and should include:

- at least three drugs to which the pathogen is susceptible, with at least one of the injectable anti-TB agents
- in the case of MDR-TB, a prolonged course of 5 to 7 agents, except a shorter 9-12 month regimen if there is no resistance to fluoroquinolones and second-line injectable agents (WHO, 2016).

The addition of a fluoroquinolone and surgical resection of the main lesions have been associated with improved outcome (Chan et al., 2004).

Principles of Therapy Against *Mycobacterium avium* Complex

The MAC is made up of at least two species: *M. intracellulare* and *M. avium*. *Mycobacterium intracellulare* causes pulmonary disease often in immunocompetent individuals. *Mycobacterium avium* is further divided into a number of subspecies: *M. avium* subsp. *hominissuis* causes disseminated disease in immunocompromised patients, *M. avium* subsp. *paratuberculosis* has been implicated in the etiology of Crohn disease, and *M. avium* subsp. *avium* causes TB of birds. These bacteria are ubiquitous in the environment and can be encountered in water, food, and soil. Therefore, when MAC bacteria are isolated from a nonsterile site in a patient's body, one cannot assume they are causing an infection.

Therapy of MAC Pulmonary Infection

Mycobacterium intracellulare often infects immunocompetent patients. Criteria in favor of therapy includes bacteriological evidence, which consists of positive cultures from at least two sputums or one positive culture from bronchoalveolar lavage or pulmonary biopsy with a positive culture or histopathological features, *and* clinical evidence of infection, *and* radiological evidence of infection such as pulmonary cavitation, nodular lesions, or bronchiectasis (Griffith et al., 2007).

In newly diagnosed patients with MAC pneumonia, triple-drug therapy is recommended. These drugs include a rifamycin, ethambutol, and a macrolide (Griffith et al., 2007; Kasperbauer and Daley, 2008). For the macrolides, either oral clarithromycin or azithromycin may be used. Rifampin is often the rifamycin of choice. Clarithromycin, 1000 mg, or azithromycin, 500 mg, are combined with ethambutol, 25 mg/kg, and rifampin, 600 mg, and administered three times a week for nodular and bronchiectatic disease. Therapy is continued for 12 months after the last negative culture. The same drugs are administered for patients with cavitary disease, but the dosing regimens are azithromycin 250 mg, ethambutol 15 mg/kg, and rifampin 600 mg. Parenteral streptomycin or amikacin at 15 mg/kg is recommended as a fourth drug. The effect of the aminoglycosides on clinical outcomes is unclear.

Duration of therapy is as for nodular disease. In advanced pulmonary disease or during re-treatment, rifabutin 300 mg daily may replace rifampin. Because clarithromycin susceptibility correlates with outcome, risk of failure is high when high clarithromycin MICs are documented. Patients at risk for failure also include those with cavitary disease, presumably due to higher bacillary load. Even with these therapies, long-term success is still fairly limited. Only half of patients have successful outcomes as defined by both culture conversion and clinical outcomes.

Therapy of Disseminated *M. avium* Complex

Disseminated MAC disease is caused by *M. avium* in 95% of patients. This is a disease of the immunocompromised patient, especially with reduced cell-mediated immunity. MAC usually occurs in patients whose CD4 cell count is less than 50/mm³. Patients at risk for infection are those who have had other opportunistic infections, are colonized with MAC, or have an HIV RNA burden greater than 5 log copies/mm³.

The symptoms and laboratory findings of disseminated disease are nonspecific and include fever, night sweats, weight loss, elevated serum alkaline phosphates, and anemia at the time of diagnosis. However, when disease occurs in patients already on antiretroviral therapy, it may manifest as a focal disease of the lymph nodes, osteomyelitis, pneumonitis, pericarditis, skin or soft-tissue abscesses, genital ulcers, or CNS infection (DHHS Panel, 2008). In addition to a compatible clinical picture, isolation of MAC from cultures of blood, lymph node, bone marrow, or other normally sterile tissue or body fluids is required for diagnosis.

Prophylactic Therapy

The goals of prophylactic therapy are to prevent the development of disease during the time when a patient's CD4 count is low. Monotherapy with either oral azithromycin 1200 mg once a week or clarithromycin 500 mg twice a day is started when patients present with a CD4 count below 50/mm^3 (DHHS Panel, 2008). For patients intolerant to macrolides, rifabutin 300 mg a day is administered. Once the CD4 count is greater than 100 per mm^3 for 3 months or longer, MAC prophylaxis should be discontinued.

Definitive and Suppressive Therapy

In patients with disease due to MAC, the goals of therapy include suppression of symptoms and conversion to negative blood cultures. The infection itself is not completely eradicated until immune reconstitution. Therapy is divided into initial therapy and chronic suppressive therapy. Recommended therapy consists of a combination of clarithromycin 500 mg twice a day with ethambutol 15 mg/kg daily, administered orally (DHHS Panel, 2008). Azithromycin 500–600 mg daily is an acceptable alternative to clarithromycin, especially in those patients in whom clarithromycin would adversely interact with other drugs. The addition of rifabutin 300 mg/d may improve outcomes. Mortality in disseminated MAC is high in patients with either a CD4 cell count below 50/mm^3 or an MAC burden of greater than 2 log$_{10}$ CFU/mm^3 of blood or in the absence of effective antiretroviral therapy. In these patients, a fourth drug may be added, based on susceptibility testing. Potential fourth agents include amikacin, 10–15 mg/kg intravenously daily; streptomycin, 1 g intravenously or intramuscularly daily; ciprofloxacin, 500–750 mg orally twice daily; levofloxacin, 500 mg orally daily; or moxifloxacin, 400 mg orally daily. Patients should be continued on suppressive therapy until all three of the following criteria are met:

- therapy duration of at least 12 months
- CD4 count greater than 100/mm^3 for at least 6 months
- asymptomatic for MAC infection

Principles of Antileprosy Therapy

The global prevalence of leprosy has markedly declined, largely due to the global initiative of the WHO to eliminate leprosy (Hansen disease) as a public health problem by providing multidrug therapy (rifampin, clofazimine, and dapsone) free of charge. Prevalence of the disease has dropped by about 90% since 1985. Nevertheless, there are pockets of disease around the world, especially in Africa, Asia, and South America. In the U.S., fewer than 200 new cases were reported in 2005, mainly among immigrants.

Four major clinical types of leprosy affect therapy. At one end of the spectrum is *tuberculoid leprosy*, also termed paucibacillary leprosy because the bacterial burden is low and *M. leprae* is rarely found in smears. On the other end of the spectrum is the *lepromatous* form of the disease (Levis and Ernst, 2005). This is characterized by a disseminated infection and a high bacillary burden. Two major intermediate forms of the disease are recognized: (1) borderline (dimorphous) tuberculoid disease, which has features of both tuberculoid and lepromatous leprosy; and (2) indeterminate disease, which has early hypopigmented lesions without features of the lepromatous and tuberculoid leprosy.

Mycobacterium leprae was discovered by Armauer Hansen in 1873. The *M. leprae* genome has undergone reductive evolution and has radically downsized its genome (Cole et al., 2001). As a result, *M. leprae* cannot produce ATP from NADH or utilize acetate or galactose as carbon sources;

moreover, it has lost the anaerobic electron transfer system and cannot survive under hypoxic conditions. It has a long doubling time (14 days) and is an obligate intracellular pathogen. As a result, *M. leprae* is difficult to culture on synthetic media, an impediment to basic research on the disease.

Types of Antileprosy Therapy

Therapy of leprosy is based on multidrug regimens using rifampin, clofazimine, and dapsone. The reasons for using combinations of agents include reduction in the development of resistance, the need for adequate therapy when primary resistance already exists, and reduction in the duration of therapy. The most bactericidal drug in current regimens is rifampin. Because of high kill rates and massive release of bacterial antigens, rifampin is not often given during a "reversal" reaction (see discussion that follows) or in patients with erythema nodosum leprosum. Clofazimine is only bacteriostatic against *M. leprae*. However, it also has anti-inflammatory effects and can treat reversal reactions and erythema nodosum leprosum. The third major agent in the regimen is dapsone. The objective of administering these drugs is total cure.

Definitive Therapy; Standard Therapy

Paucibacillary Leprosy. The WHO regimen consists of a single dose of oral rifampin, 600 mg, combined with dapsone, 100 mg, administered under direct supervision once every month for 6 months, and dapsone, 100 mg a day, in between for 6 months. In the U.S., the regimen consists of dapsone, 100 mg, and rifampin, 600 mg, daily for 6 months, followed by dapsone monotherapy for 3–5 years.

Multibacillary Therapy. The WHO recommends the same regimen as for paucibacillary leprosy, with two major changes. First, clofazimine, 300 mg a day, is added for the entirety of therapy. Second, the regimen lasts 1 year instead of 6 months. In the U.S., the regimen is also the same as for paucibacillary, but dual therapy continues for 3 years, followed by dapsone monotherapy for 10 years. Clofazimine is added when there is dapsone resistance or for patients who are chronically reactional.

The duration of therapy of multibacillary leprosy is a drawback. Studies in murine leprosy, and in patients, have demonstrated that viable bacilli are killed within 3 months of therapy (Ji et al., 1996), suggesting that the length of current therapy of multibacillary leprosy may be unnecessarily long. Recently, the WHO proposed that all forms of leprosy be treated with the same dose as for paucibacillary leprosy; a clinical trial was promising (Kroger et al., 2008). This new shorter regimen promises to reduce duration of therapy radically.

Treatment of Reactions in Leprosy

Patients with tuberculoid leprosy may develop "reversal reactions," manifestations of delayed hypersensitivity to antigens of *M. leprae*. Cutaneous ulcerations and deficits of peripheral nerve function may occur. Early therapy with corticosteroids or clofazimine is effective. Reactions in the lepromatous form of the disease (erythema nodosum leprosum) are characterized by the appearance of raised, tender, intracutaneous nodules, severe constitutional symptoms, and high fever. This reaction is often associated with therapy. It is thought to be an Arthus-type reaction related to release of microbial antigens in patients harboring large numbers of bacilli. Treatment with clofazimine or thalidomide is effective.

Therapy of Other Nontuberculous Mycobacteria

Mycobacteria other than those already discussed can be recovered from a variety of lesions in humans. Because they frequently are resistant to many of the commonly used agents, they must be examined for sensitivity in vitro and drug therapy selected on this basis. Therapy of infections from these organisms is summarized in Table 60–5. In some instances, surgical removal of the infected tissue followed by long-term treatment with effective agents is necessary. *M. kansasii* causes disease similar to that caused by *M. tuberculosis*, but it may be milder. Therapy with isoniazid, rifampin, and ethambutol has been successful.

Acknowledgment: William A, Petri, Jr contributed to this chapter in earlier editions of this book. We have retained some of his text in the current edition.

TABLE 60–5 ■ PHARMACOTHERAPY OF MYCOBACTERIAL INFECTIONS OTHER THAN TUBERCULOSIS, LEPROSY, AND MAC

MYCOBACTERIAL SPECIES	FIRST-LINE THERAPY	ALTERNATIVE AGENTS
M. kansasii	Isoniazid + rifampin[a] + ethambutol	Trimethoprim-sulfamethoxazole; ethionamide; cycloserine; clarithromycin; amikacin; streptomycin; moxifloxacin or gatifloxacin
M. fortuitum complex	Amikacin + doxycycline	Cefoxitin; rifampin; a sulfonamide; moxifloxacin or gatifloxacin; clarithromycin; trimethoprim-sulfamethoxazole; imipenem
M. marinum	Rifampin + ethambutol	Trimethoprim-sulfamethoxazole; clarithromycin; minocycline; doxycycline
M. ulcerans	Rifampin + streptomycin[c]	Clarithromycin[b]; rifapentine[b]
M. abscessus	Cefoxitin (or imipenem) + amikacin + clarithromycin	Tigecycline, moxifloxacin,
M. malmoense	Rifampin + ethambutol ± clarithromycin	Fluoroquinolone
M. haemophilum	Clarithromycin + rifampin + quinolone	—

[a]In HIV-infected patients, the substitution of rifabutin for rifampin minimizes drug interactions with the HIV protease inhibitors and nonnucleoside reverse transcriptase inhibitors.
[b]Based on animal models.
[c]For *M. ulcerans*, surgery is the primary therapy.

Drug Facts for Your Personal Formulary: *Antimycobacterial Drugs*

Drug	Therapeutic Uses	Major Toxicity and Clinical Pearls
Rifamycins		
Rifampin	<ul><li>Tuberculosis</li><li>*M. kansasii* disease</li><li>Leprosy</li><li>*M. marinum, M. uclerans, M. malmoense,* and *M. haemophilum* diseases</li><li>Prophylaxis of meningococcal disease and *Haemophilus influenzae* meningitis</li><li>Brucellosis</li><li>Combination therapy in selected cases of staphylococcal endocarditis or osteomyelitis, especially those caused by staphylococci "tolerant" of penicillin</li></ul>	<ul><li>Peak concentration and AUC-driven efficacy</li><li>Rifampin potently induces CYPs and thus increases metabolism of many classes of drugs. Prior to putting a patient on rifampin, all the patient's medications and contraception should be examined for potential interactions.</li><li>Hypersensitivity reactions, especially with high-dose intermittent therapy, including flu-like symptoms, eosinophilia, interstitial nephritis, acute tubular necrosis, thrombocytopenia, hemolytic anemia, and shock</li><li>Hepatitis, especially in combination with other anti-TB agents, in alcoholics, or preexistent liver disease</li></ul>
Rifapentine	<ul><li>Treatment of tuberculosis</li><li>Prophylaxis of tuberculosis</li></ul>	<ul><li>97% protein binding</li><li>Long $t_{1/2}$ of ~ 14–18 h, allowing more intermittent dosing (1–2 times weekly)</li><li>Moderate CYP3A induction</li></ul>
Rifabutin	<ul><li>Used as rifampin replacement to avoid drug interactions of rifampin with other medications, especially in HIV coinfection</li><li>Treatment of disseminated MAC in patients with AIDS</li></ul>	<ul><li>Weaker CYP3A induction than rifampin</li><li>Concentrations higher in tissue than plasma</li><li>$t_{1/2}$ ~ 45 h</li><li>Neutropenia in 25% of patients with HIV</li><li>Primary reasons for therapy discontinuation include rash, GI intolerance, and neutropenia.</li><li>Uveitis and arthralgias in patients receiving rifabutin doses > 450 mg daily</li></ul>
Isoniazid		
Isoniazid	<ul><li>*M. tuberculosis* infection</li><li>*M. kansasii* infection</li><li>Prophylaxis of tuberculosis disease</li></ul>	<ul><li>Patients divided into slow, intermediate, and fast acetylators, which has consequence of efficacy and toxicity.</li><li>Hepatotoxicity, increased above age of 42 years</li><li>Peripheral neuritis: should be administered with pyridoxine</li><li>Reversible vasculitis</li><li>Overdose is associated with the clinical triad of (1) seizures refractory to treatment with phenytoin and barbiturates, (2) metabolic acidosis, and (3) coma</li><li>Many drug interactions via inhibition and induction of several CYP450 enzymes</li></ul>

Pyrazinamide

Pyrazinamide	• Tuberculosis	• No activity against *M. bovis* • Activated under acidic conditions; synergizes with rifampin • Pyrazinamide clearance reduced in renal failure; reduce dosing frequency is reduced to 3 x/week at low GFR. • Removed by hemodialysis; redose after each session • Adverse effects: hepatotoxicity and hyperuricemia

Ethambutol

Ethambutol	• Tuberculosis • *M. avium* complex infections • *M. kansasii* infection • Activity against *M. gordonae, M. marinum, M. scrofulaceum,* and *M. szulgai*	• Incidence of optic neuritis leading to decreased visual acuity and loss of red-green discrimination. Test visual acuity and red-green discrimination prior to the start of therapy and periodically thereafter. • In renal failure, ethambutol should be dosed at 15–25 mg/kg three times a week instead of daily, even in patients receiving hemodialysis.

Bicyclic Nitroimidazoles

Pretomanid, delaminid	• Treatment of MDR-TB; being tested for regimens used to treat drug-susceptible TB	• Kills both replicating and nonreplicating *M. tuberculosis* • Delaminid: QT segment prolongation

Riminophenazines

Clofazimine	• Treatment of leprosy	• GI problems are encountered in 40%–50% of patients. • Abdominal pain due to crystal deposition in cavities and tissues • Body secretion, eye, and skin reddish-black discoloration occur in most patients

Diarylquinone

Bedaquiline	• Treatment of MDR-TB; being tested for regimens used to treat drug-susceptible TB	• Apparent volume of distribution > 10,000 L • Controversy regarding side effects profile and increased number of deaths compared to placebo • QT interval prolongation

Ethionamide

Ethionamide	• Treatment of MDR-TB and XDR-TB	• Same mutations in ethionamide-resistant bacteria as for isoniazid-resistant bacteria • 50% of patients are unable to tolerate a single dose larger than 500 mg because of GI toxicity. • Adverse effects: postural hypotension, mental depression, drowsiness, asthenia; neurological toxicity • Concomitant administration with pyridoxine is recommended. • Hepatitis in ~ 5% of cases

Para-aminobenzoic Acid Analogues

Dapsone	• Treatment of leprosy • Combined with chlorproguanil for the treatment of malaria • Treatment of *Pneumocystis jiroveci* infection and prophylaxis • Prophylaxis of *Toxoplasma gondii* infection • Anti-inflammatory effects for treatment of pemphigoid, dermatitis herpetiformis, linear IgA bullous disease, relapsing chondritis, and brown recluse spider bite ulcers	• G6PD deficiency should be tested prior to use. • NADH-dependent methemoglobin reductase deficiency–associated methemoglobinemia • Hemolysis at doses of 200–300 mg of dapsone per day • Used topically for acne
Aminosalicylic acid	• Treatment of MDR-TB	• Should be administered with food • Dose must be reduced in renal dysfunction. • Adverse events incidence is ~ 10%–30%. • GI problems predominate • Hypersensitivity reactions in 5%–10% of patients

Cycloserine

Cycloserine	• Treatment of MDR-TB	• Oral second-line drug • "Psych-serine": 50% of patients develop neuropsychiatric symptoms; headache, somnolence, severe psychosis, seizures, and suicidal ideas • Must be redosed after dialysis

Bibliography

Ahmad Z, et al. PA-824 exhibits time-dependent activity in a murine model of tuberculosis. *Antimicrob Agents Chemother*, 2011, 55: 239–245.

Andries K, et al. A diarylquinoline drug active on the ATP synthase of *Mycobacterium tuberculosis. Science*, 2005, 307:223–227.

Anonymous. Clofazimine. *Tuberculosis (Edinb)*, 2008a, 88:96–99.

Argyrou A, et al. *Mycobacterium tuberculosis* dihydrofolate reductase is a target for isoniazid. *Nat Struct Mol Biol*, 2006, 13:408–413.

Argyrou A, et al. New insight into the mechanism of action of and resistance to isoniazid: interaction of *Mycobacterium tuberculosis* enoyl-ACP reductase with INH-NADP. *J Am Chem Soc*, 2007, 129:9582–9583.

Avorn J. Approval of a tuberculosis drug based on a paradoxical surrogate measure. *JAMA*, 2013, 309:1349–1350.

Bashiri G, et al. Crystal structures of F_{420}-dependent glucose-6-phosphate dehydrogenase FGD1 involved in the activation of the anti-tuberculosis drug candidate PA-824 reveal the basis of coenzyme and substrate binding. *J Biol Chem*, 2008, 283:17531–17541.

Bloemberg GV, et al. Acquired resistance to bedaquiline and delamanid in therapy for tuberculosis. *N Engl J Med*, 2015, 373:1986–1988.

Blumberg HM, et al.; American Thoracic Society/Centers for Disease Control and Prevention/Infectious Diseases Society of America. Treatment of tuberculosis. *Am J Respir Crit Care Med*, 2003, 167: 603–662.

Boeree MJ, et al. A dose-ranging trial to optimize the dose of rifampin in the treatment of tuberculosis. *Am J Respir Crit Care Med*, 2015, 191:1058–1065.

Burman W, et al. Acquired rifamycin resistance with twice-weekly treatment of HIV-related tuberculosis. *Am J Respir Crit Care Med*, 2006, 173:350–356.

Burman WJ, et al. Comparative pharmacokinetics and pharmacodynamics of the rifamycin antibacterials. *Clin Pharmacokinet*, 2001, 40: 327–341.

Chan ED, et al. Treatment and outcome analysis of 205 patients with multidrug-resistant tuberculosis. *Am J Respir Crit Care Med*, 2004, 169:1103–1109.

Chigutsa E, et al. Impact of nonlinear interactions of pharmacokinetics and MICs on sputum bacillary kill rates as a marker of sterilizing effect in tuberculosis. *Antimicrob Agents Chemother*, 2015, 59:38–45.

Colangeli R, et al. The *Mycobacterium tuberculosis* iniA gene is essential for activity of an efflux pump that confers drug tolerance to both isoniazid and ethambutol. *Mol Microbiol*, 2005, 55:1829–1840.

Cole ST, et al. Massive gene decay in the leprosy bacillus. *Nature*, 2001, 409:1007–1011.

Conte JE Jr, et al. Effects of gender, AIDS, and acetylator status on intrapulmonary concentrations of isoniazid. *Antimicrob Agents Chemother*, 2002, 46:2358–2364.

Conte JE Jr, et al. High-performance liquid chromatographic determination of pyrazinamide in human plasma, bronchoalveolar lavage fluid, and alveolar cells. *J Chromatogr Sci*, 2000, 38:33–37.

Desta Z, et al. Inhibition of cytochrome P450 (CYP450) isoforms by isoniazid: potent inhibition of CYP2C19 and CYP3A. *Antimicrob Agents Chemother*, 2001, 45:382–392.

DHHS Panel. Guidelines for prevention and treatment of opportunistic infections in HIV-infected adults and adolescents. 2008. Available at: http://aidsinfo.nih.gov/contentfiles/Adult_OI.pdf. Accessed March 16, 2008.

Desjardins CA, et al. Genomic and functional analyses of Mycobacterium tuberculosis strains implicate ald in D-cycloserine resistance. *Nat Genet*, 2016, 48:544–551.

Deshpande D, et al. Ethambutol optimal clinical dose and susceptibility breakpoint identification by use of a novel pharmacokinetic-pharmacodynamic model of disseminated intracellular Mycobacterium avium. *Antimicrob Agents Chemother*, 2010, 54:1728-1733.

Diacon AH, et al. The diarylquinoline TMC207 for multidrug-resistant tuberculosis. *N Engl J Med*, 2009, 360:2397–2405.

Diacon AH, et al. Multidrug-resistant tuberculosis and culture conversion with bedaquiline. *N Engl J Med*, 2014, 371:723–732.

Ferro BE, et al. Amikacin pharmacokinetics/pharmacodynamics in a novel hollow-fiber *Mycobacterium abscessus* disease model. *Antimicrob Agents Chemother*, 2016, 60:1242–1248.

Gatti G, et al. Penetration of dapsone into cerebrospinal fluid of patients with AIDS. *J Antimicrob Chemother*, 1997, 40:113–115.

Gillespie SH, et al. Four-month moxifloxacin-based regimens for drug-sensitive tuberculosis. *N Engl J Med*, 2014, 371:1577–1587.

Ginsberg AM, et al. Safety, tolerability, and pharmacokinetics of PA-824 in healthy subjects. *Antimicrob Agents Chemother*, 2009, 53:3720–3725.

Ginsburg AS, et al. The rapid development of fluoroquinolone resistance in *M. tuberculosis*. *N Engl J Med*, 2003, 349:1977–1978.

Gler MT, et al. Delamanid for multidrug-resistant pulmonary tuberculosis. *N Engl J Med*, 2012, 366:2151–2160.

Griffith DE, et al. An official ATS/IDSA statement: diagnosis, treatment, and prevention of nontuberculous mycobacterial diseases. *Am J Respir Crit Care Med*, 2007, 175:367–416.

Gumbo T, et al. The pyrazinamide susceptibility breakpoint above which combination therapy fails. *J Antimicrob Chemother*, 2014, 69: 2420–2425.

Gumbo T, et al. Concentration-dependent *Mycobacterium tuberculosis* killing and prevention of resistance by rifampin. *Antimicrob Agents Chemother*, 2007a, 51:3781–3788.

Gumbo T, et al. Selection of a moxifloxacin dose that suppresses drug resistance in *Mycobacterium tuberculosis*, by use of an in vitro pharmacodynamic infection model and mathematical modeling. *J Infect Dis*, 2004, 190:1642–1651.

Gumbo T, et al. Isoniazid bactericidal activity and resistance emergence: integrating pharmacodynamics and pharmacogenomics to predict efficacy in different ethnic populations. *Antimicrob Agents Chemother*, 2007b, 51: 2329–2336.

Gumbo T, et al. Isoniazid's bactericidal activity ceases because of the emergence of resistance, not depletion of *Mycobacterium tuberculosis* in the log phase of growth. *J Infect Dis*, 2007c, 195:194–201.

Gumbo T, et al. Pharmacokinetics-pharmacodynamics of pyrazinamide in a novel in vitro model of tuberculosis for sterilizing effect: a paradigm for faster assessment of a new antituberculosis drugs. *Antimicrob Agents Chemother*, 2009, 53:3197–3204.

Hartkoorn RC, Uplekar S, Cole ST. Cross-resistance between clofazimine and bedaquiline through upregulation of MmpL5 in *Mycobacterium tuberculosis*. *Antimicrob Agents Chemother*, 2014, 58:2979-2981.

Heemskerk AD, et al. Intensified antituberculosis therapy in adults with tuberculous meningitis. *N Engl J Med*, 2016, 374:124–134.

Heifets LB. Drug susceptibility in the chemotherapy of mycobacterial infections. CRC Press, Boca Raton, 1991.

Huitric E, et al. In vitro antimycobacterial spectrum of a diarylquinoline ATP synthase inhibitor. *Antimicrob Agents Chemother*, 2007, 51: 4202–4204.

Ji B, et al. Bactericidal activities of combinations of new drugs against *Mycobacterium leprae* in nude mice. *Antimicrob Agents Chemother*, 1996, 40:393–399.

Kakkar AK, Dahiya N. Bedaquiline for the treatment of resistant tuberculosis: promises and pitfalls. *Tuberculosis (Edinb)*, 2014, 94: 357–362.

Kasperbauer SH, Daley CL. Diagnosis and treatment of infections due to *Mycobacterium avium* complex. *Semin Respir Crit Care Med*, 2008, 29:569–576.

Koul A, et al. Diarylquinolines target subunit c of mycobacterial ATP synthase. *Nat Chem Biol*, 2007, 3:323–324.

Kroger A, et al. International open trial of uniform multi-drug therapy regimen for 6 months for all types of leprosy patients: rationale, design and preliminary results. *Trop Med Int Health*, 2008, 13:594–602.

Langdon G, et al. U. S. Population pharmacokinetics of rifapentine and its primary desacetyl metabolite in South African tuberculosis patients. *Antimicrob Agents Chemother*, 2005, 49:4429–4436.

Larsen MH, et al. Overexpression of inhA, but not kasA, confers resistance to isoniazid and ethionamide in *Mycobacterium smegmatis*, *M. bovis* BCG and *M. tuberculosis*. *Mol Microbiol*, 2002, 46: 453–466.

Lee M, et al. Linezolid for treatment of chronic extensively drug-resistant tuberculosis. *N Engl J Med*, 2012, 367:1508–1518.

Levis WR, Ernst JD. *Mycobacterium leprae* (leprosy, Hansen's disease). In: Mandell GL, et al., eds. *Mandell, Douglas, and Bennett's Principles and Practices of Infectious Diseases.* Elsevier Churchill Livingstone, Philadelphia, **2005**, 2886–2896.

Li G, et al. Study of efflux pump gene expression in rifampicin-monoresistant *Mycobacterium tuberculosis* clinical isolates. *J Antibiot (Tokyo)*, **2015**, 68:431–435.

Malone RS, et al. The effect of hemodialysis on cycloserine, ethionamide, para-aminosalicylate, and clofazimine. *Chest,* **1999a,** *116*:984–990.

Malone RS, et al. The effect of hemodialysis on isoniazid, rifampin, pyrazinamide, and ethambutol. *Am J Respir Crit Care Med,* **1999b,** *159*:1580–1584.

Mathys V, et al. Molecular genetics of para-aminosalicylic acid (PAS) resistance in clinical isolates and spontaneous mutants of *Mycobacterium tuberculosis. Antimicrob Agents Chemother,* **2009**, *53:* 2100–2109.

Matsumoto M, et al. OPC-67683, a nitro-dihydro-imidazooxazole derivative with promising action against tuberculosis in vitro and in mice. *PLoS Med,* **2006**, *3*(11):e466.

Mayosi BM, et al. Prednisolone and *Mycobacterium indicus pranii* in tuberculous pericarditis. *N Engl J Med,* **2014**, *371*:1121–1130.

Merle CS, et al. A four-month gatifloxacin-containing regimen for treating tuberculosis. *N Engl J Med,* **2014**, *371*:1588–1598.

Moradigaravand D, et al. DfrA-thyA double deletion in para-aminosalicylic acid resistant *Mycobacterium tuberculosis* Beijing. *Antimicrob Agents Chemother,* **2016**, *60*:3864–3867. doi:10.1128/AAC.00253-16. [Epub ahead of print]

Morris RP, et al. Ancestral antibiotic resistance in *Mycobacterium tuberculosis. Proc Natl Acad Sci U S A,* **2005**, *102*:12200–12205.

Nau R, et al. Penetration of rifampicin into the cerebrospinal fluid of adults with uninflamed meninges. *J Antimicrob Chemother,* **1992**, *29:* 719–724.

Nessar R, et al. *Mycobacterium abscessus*: a new antibiotic nightmare. *J Antimicrob Chemother,* **2012**, *67*:810-818.

Nightingale SD, et al. Two controlled trials of rifabutin prophylaxis against *Mycobacterium avium* complex infection in AIDS. *N Engl J Med,* **1993**, *329*:828–833.

Nix DE, et al. Pharmacokinetics and relative bioavailability of clofazimine in relation to food, orange juice and antacid. *Tuberculosis (Edinb),* **2004**, *84*:365–373.

Okamoto S, et al. Loss of a conserved 7-methylguanosine modification in 16S rRNA confers low-level streptomycin resistance in bacteria. *Mol Microbiol,* **2007**, *63*:1096–1106.

Pasipanodya JG, Gumbo T. A meta-analysis of self-administered vs. directly observed therapy effect on microbiologic failure, relapse, and acquired drug resistance in tuberculosis patients. *Clin Infect Dis,* **2013**, *57*:21–31.

Pasipanodya JG, et al. Serum drug concentrations predictive of pulmonary tuberculosis outcomes. *J Infect Dis,* **2013**, *208*:1464–1473.

Pasipanodya JG, et al. Meta-analysis of clinical studies supports the pharmacokinetic variability hypothesis for acquired drug resistance and failure of antituberculosis therapy. *Clin Infect Dis,* **2012**, *55*: 169–177.

Peloquin CA, et al. Pharmacokinetics of paraaminosalicylic acid granules under four dosing conditions. *Ann Pharmacother,* **2001**, *35*: 1332–1338.

Prasad K, Singh MB, Ryan H. Corticosteroids for managing tuberculous meningitis. *Cochrane Database Syst Rev,* **2016**, 4:CD002244.

Rouan MC, et al. Pharmacokinetics and pharmacodynamics of TMC207 and its N-desmethyl metabolite in a murine model of tuberculosis. *Antimicrob Agents Chemother,* **2012**, 56:1444–1451.

Roy PD, et al. Pharmacogenomics of anti-TB drugs-related hepatotoxicity. *Pharmacogenomics,* **2008**, *9*:311–321.

Ruslami R, et al. Intensified regimen containing rifampicin and moxifloxacin for tuberculous meningitis: an open-label, randomised controlled phase 2 trial. *Lancet Infect Dis,* **2013**, *13*:27–35.

Safi H, et al. Transfer of embB codon 306 mutations into clinical *Mycobacterium tuberculosis* strains alters susceptibility to ethambutol, isoniazid, and rifampin. *Antimicrob Agents Chemother,* **2008**, *52*: 2027–2034.

Schmalstieg AM, et al. The antibiotic resistance arrow of time: efflux pump induction is a general first step in the evolution of mycobacterial drug resistance. *Antimicrob Agents Chemother,* **2012**, *56*:4806–4815.

Shenje J, et al. Poor penetration of antibiotics into pericardium in pericardial tuberculosis. *EBioMedicine,* **2015**, 2:1640–1649.

Shi W, et al. Pyrazinamide inhibits trans-translation in *Mycobacterium tuberculosis. Science,* **2011**, *333*:1630–1632.

Simpson JA, et al. Population pharmacokinetic and pharmacodynamic modeling of the antimalarial chemotherapy chloroguanil/dapsone. *Br J Clin Pharmacol,* **2006**, *61*:289–300.

Singh R, et al. PA-824 kills nonreplicating *Mycobacterium tuberculosis* by intracellular NO release. *Science,* **2008**, *322*:1392–1395.

Somoskovi A, et al. The molecular basis of resistance to isoniazid, rifampin, and pyrazinamide in *Mycobacterium tuberculosis. Respir Res,* **2001**, *2*:164–168.

Sotgiu G, et al. Efficacy, safety and tolerability of linezolid containing regimens in treating MDR-TB and XDR-TB: systematic review and meta-analysis. *Eur Respir J,* **2012**, *40*:1430–1442.

Sotgiu G, et al. Carbapenems to treat multidrug and extensively drug-resistant tuberculosis: a systematic review. *Int J Mol Sci,* **2016**, *17*:373. pii: E373. doi: 10.3390/ijms17030373.

Spies FS, et al. Identification of mutations related to streptomycin resistance in clinical isolates of *Mycobacterium tuberculosis* and possible involvement of efflux mechanism. *Antimicrob Agents Chemother,* **2008**, *52*:2947–2949.

Srivastava S, et al. Efflux-pump-derived multiple drug resistance to ethambutol monotherapy in *Mycobacterium tuberculosis* and the pharmacokinetics and pharmacodynamics of ethambutol. *J Infect Dis,* **2010**, *201*:1225-1231.

Srivastava S, et al. Multidrug-resistant tuberculosis not due to noncompliance but to between-patient pharmacokinetic variability. *J Infect Dis,* **2011a**, *204*:1951–1959.

Srivastava S, et al. Pharmacokinetic mismatch does not lead to emergence of isoniazid- or rifampin-resistant *Mycobacterium tuberculosis* but to better antimicrobial effect: a new paradigm for antituberculosis drug scheduling. *Antimicrob Agents Chemother,* **2011b**, 55:5085–5589.

Stover CK, et al. A small-molecule nitroimidazopyran drug candidate for the treatment of tuberculosis. *Nature,* **2000**, *405*:962–966.

Swaminathan S, et al. Drug concentration thresholds predictive of therapy failure and death in children with tuberculosis: bread crumb trails in random forests. *Clin Infect Dis,* **2016**, *63*(suppl 3):S63–S74.

Swenson EM, Dosne AG, Karlsson MO. Population pharmacokinetics of bedaquiline and metabolite M2 in patients with drug-resistant tuberculosis: the effect of time-varying weight and albumin. *CPT Pharmacometrics Syst Pharmacol,* **2016**, 5:682-691.

Tang S, et al. Efficacy, safety and tolerability of linezolid for the treatment of XDR-TB: a study in China. *Eur Respir J,* **2015**, *45*:161–170.

Thwaites GE, et al. Randomized pharmacokinetic and pharmacodynamic comparison of fluoroquinolones for tuberculous meningitis. *Antimicrob Agents Chemother,* **2011**; *55*:3244–3253.

Tiberi S, et al. Ertapenem in the treatment of multidrug-resistant tuberculosis: first clinical experience. *Eur Respir J,* **2016**, *47*:333–336.

Timmins GS, Deretic V. Mechanisms of action of isoniazid. *Mol Microbiol,* **2006**, *62*:1220–1227.

Vannelli TA, et al. The antituberculosis drug ethionamide is activated by a flavoprotein monooxygenase. *J Biol Chem,* **2002**, *277:* 12824–12829.

Volmink J, Garner P. Directly observed therapy for treating tuberculosis. *Cochrane Database Syst Rev,* **2007**, (2):CD003343.

WHO. WHO treatment guidelines for drug-resistant tuberculosis, 2016 update. www.who.int/tb/areas-of-work/drug-resistant-tb/treatment/resources/. Accessed July 27, 2017.

Wilkins JJ, et al. Variability in the population pharmacokinetics of pyrazinamide in South African tuberculosis patients. *Eur J Clin Pharmacol,* **2006**, *62*:727–735.

Wilkins JJ, et al. Population pharmacokinetics of rifampin in pulmonary tuberculosis patients, including a semimechanistic model to describe variable absorption. *Antimicrob Agents Chemother,* **2008**, *52*:2138-2148.

Wolf R, et al. Dapsone. *Dermatol Online J*, **2002**, 8:2.

Xavier AS, Lakshmanan M. Delamanid: a new armor in combating drug-resistant tuberculosis. *J Pharmacol Pharmacother*, **2014**, 5:222–224.

Zhang S, et al. Mutations in *panD* encoding aspartate decarboxylase are associated with pyrazinamide resistance in *Mycobacterium tuberculosis*. *Emerg Microbes Infect*, **2013**, 2(6):e34. doi:10.1038/emi.2013.38.

Zhang S, et al. Identification of novel mutations associated with clofazimine resistance in *Mycobacterium tuberculosis*. *J Antimicrob Chemother*, **2015a**, 70:2507-2510.

Zhang X, et al. Genetic determinants involved in p-aminosalicylic acid resistance in clinical isolates from tuberculosis patients in northern China from 2006 to 2012. *Antimicrob Agents Chemother*, **2015b**, 59:1320–1324.

Zhang Y, et al. Role of acid pH and deficient efflux of pyrazinoic acid in unique susceptibility of *Mycobacterium tuberculosis* to pyrazinamide. *J Bacteriol*, **1999**, 181:2044–2049.

Zhang Y, et al. Mechanisms of pyrazinamide action and resistance. *Microbiol Spectr*, **2014**, 2:MGM2-0023-2013.

Zhu M, et al. Pharmacokinetics of ethambutol in children and adults with tuberculosis. *Int J Tuberc Lung Dis*, **2004**, 8:1360–1367.

Zhu M, et al. Population pharmacokinetics of ethionamide in patients with tuberculosis. *Tuberculosis (Edinb)*, **2002**, 82:91–96.

Zimic M, et al. Pyrazinoic acid efflux rate in *Mycobacterium tuberculosis* is a better proxy of pyrazinamide resistance. *Tuberculosis (Edinb)*, **2012**, 92:84–91.

Antifungal Agents

P. David Rogers and Damian J. Krysan

KINGDOM FUNGI AND ITS IMPACT ON HUMANS

SYSTEMIC ANTIFUNGAL AGENTS: DRUGS FOR DEEPLY INVASIVE FUNGAL INFECTIONS
- Amphotericin B
- Flucytosine
- Imidazoles and Triazoles
- Echinocandins

- Other Systemic Antifungal Agents
- Agents Active Against Microsporidia and Pneumocystis

TOPICAL ANTIFUNGAL AGENTS
- Topical Imidazoles and Triazoles
- Individual Agents
- Structurally Diverse Antifungal Agents

Kingdom Fungi and Its Impact on Humans

There are 200,000 known species of fungi, and estimates of the total size of the kingdom Fungi range to well over a million. Residents of the kingdom are quite diverse and include yeasts, molds, mushrooms, and smuts. About 400 fungal species cause disease in animals, and even fewer cause human disease. Nonetheless, fungal infections are associated with significant morbidity and mortality. The incidence of life-threatening fungal infections has increased in recent decades owing to an increase in immunocompromised patient populations, such as those receiving hematologic or solid-organ transplantation, cancer chemotherapy, and immunosuppressive medications, as well as those with HIV/AIDS (Richardson, 2005). This has made antifungal agents increasingly important to the practice of modern medicine. With the currently available antifungal pharmacopeia, mortality rates for invasive fungal disease remain unacceptably high (Brown et al., 2012).

Fungi are eukaryotes, making the discovery and development of drugs that target the pathogen without posing significant toxicity to the host a challenging undertaking. Differences in the biosynthesis of membrane sterols, the ability of fungi to deaminate cytosine, and the unique fungal cell wall that contains glucans and chitin have all been exploited to produce relatively safe and effective antifungal agents for the treatment of fungal infections (Roemer and Krysan, 2014). Since the advent of amphotericin B-deoxycholate in the late 1950s, research has sought safer and more effective alternatives for the treatment of systemic fungal infections. While amphotericin B remains the gold standard of systemic antifungal pharmacotherapy for a wide range of infections, alternative therapies have emerged for many clinically important fungal pathogens.

This chapter provides a comprehensive overview of currently available therapeutic options for the management of invasive, mucosal, and superficial fungal infections. With only a few exceptions, the antifungals in common clinical use act mainly at sites involving the cell wall and cell membrane (Figure 61–1). Table 61–1 summarizes common fungal infections and their pharmacotherapy. Recommended adult dosages are briefly discussed for each agent. Dosing recommendations for antifungal agents in children have been recently reviewed elsewhere (Autmizguine et al., 2014).

Systemic Antifungal Agents: Drugs for Deeply Invasive Fungal Infections

Amphotericin B

Chemistry

Amphotericin B is an amphipathic or amphoteric polyene macrolide molecule with the broadest spectrum of activity of any of the currently available antifungal drugs. Polyene macrolide compounds share the characteristics of four to seven conjugated double bonds, an internal cyclic ester, poor aqueous solubility, substantial toxicity when administered systemically, and a common mechanism of antifungal action. Amphotericin B, a heptaene macrolide, contains seven conjugated trans-double bonds and a 3-amino-3,6-dideoxymannose (mycosamine) connected to the macrolide ring through a glycosidic bond (Figure 61–2). The amphoteric properties of the drug, from which it derives its name, are due to the presence of a carboxyl group on the main ring and a primary amino group on mycosamine; these groups confer aqueous solubility at extremes of pH.

AMPHOTERICIN B

Mechanism of Action

The antifungal activity of amphotericin B depends principally on its ability to bind *ergosterol* in the membrane of sensitive fungi. Amphotericin B has long been thought to form pores or channels that increase the permeability of the membrane and allow leakage of cytosolic molecules and ions, leading to loss of membrane integrity. However, recent evidence suggests amphotericin B forms aggregates that sequester ergosterol from lipid bilayers much like a sponge, resulting in fungal cell death (Anderson et al., 2014) (Figure 61–2).

Formulations

Four formulations of amphotericin B are commercially available: C-AMB, ABCD, L-AMB, and ABLC. Table 61–2 summarizes the pharmacokinetic properties of the available amphotericin B preparations, which have recently been extensively reviewed (see Hamill, 2013).

C-AMB. Amphotericin B is insoluble in water but, when formulated with the bile salt deoxycholate, becomes suitable for intravenous infusion. The complex is marketed as a lyophilized powder for injection. C-AMB forms a colloid in water, with particles largely less than 0.4 μm in diameter. As a result, filters in intravenous infusion lines that trap particles larger than 0.22 μm in diameter will remove significant amounts of drug.

Abbreviations

ABC: ATP-binding cassette
ABCD: amphotericin B colloidal dispersion
ABLC: amphotericin B lipid complex
AUC: area under the C_p-time curve.
C-AMB: conventional amphotericin B
CGD: chronic granulomatous disease
CNS: central nervous system
CSF: cerebrospinal fluid
CYP: cytochrome P450
dTMP: deoxythymidine-5′-monophosphate
dUMP: deoxyuridine-5′-monophosphate
FDA: Food and Drug Administration
5FdUMP: 5-fluoro-2′-deoxyuridine-5′-monophosphate
5FU: 5-fluorouracil
5FUDP: 5-fluorouridine-5′-diphosphate
5FUMP: 5-fluorouracil-ribose monophosphate
5FUTP: 5-fluorouridine triphosphate
GVHD: graft-versus-host disease
ART: antiretroviral therapy
HIV-AIDS: human immunodeficiency virus–acquired immunodeficiency syndrome
L-AMB: liposomal amphotericin B
PCP: *Pneumocystis carinii* pneumonia
PJP: *Pneumocystis jiroveci* pneumonia
SBECD: sulfobutyl ether β-cyclodextrin
TLR: toll-like receptor
UPRTase: uracil phosphoribosyl transferase

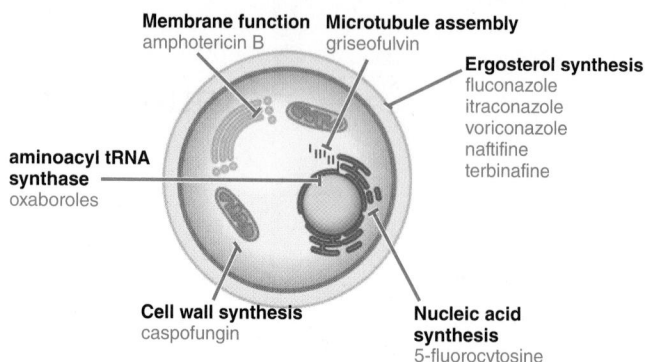

Figure 61–1 *Sites of action of antifungal agents.* Many antifungal agents act at sites involving cell wall and cell membrane function. Amphotericin B and other polyenes (e.g., nystatin) bind to ergosterol in fungal cell membranes and increase membrane permeability. The imidazoles and triazoles (itraconazole, etc.) inhibit 14-α-sterol demethylase, prevent ergosterol synthesis, and lead to the accumulation of toxic 14-α-methylsterols. The allylamines (e.g., naftifine and terbinafine) inhibit squalene epoxidase and prevent ergosterol synthesis. The echinocandins (e.g., caspofungin) inhibit the formation of glucans in the fungal cell wall. Metabolites of 5-fluorocytosine can disrupt fungal RNA and DNA synthesis. Griseofulvin inhibits microtubule assembly, thereby blocking fungal mitosis. Oxaboroles inhibit fungal aminoacyl tRNA synthase, thereby inhibiting fungal protein synthesis.

Furthermore, the addition of electrolytes to infusion solutions will cause the colloid to aggregate and complicate administration.

ABCD. Amphotericin B colloidal dispersion contains roughly equimolar amounts of amphotericin B and cholesteryl sulfate formulated for injection. Like C-AMB, ABCD forms a colloidal solution when reconstituted in aqueous solution. ABCD provides much lower blood levels than C-AMB in humans. In a study of patients with neutropenic fever that compared daily ABCD (4 mg/kg) with C-AMB (0.8 mg/kg), chills and hypoxia were significantly more common in patients who received ABCD as compared with C-AMB (White et al., 1998). Hypoxia was associated with severe febrile reactions. In a study that compared ABCD (6 mg/kg) to C-AMB (1–1.5 mg/kg) in patients with invasive aspergillosis, ABCD was less nephrotoxic than C-AMB (15% vs. 49%) but caused more fever (27% vs. 16%) and chills (53% vs. 30%) (Bowden et al., 2002). ABCD is currently not commercially available in the U.S.

L-AMB. Liposomal amphotericin B is a formulation in which AMB is incorporated within a small, unilamellar liposomal vesicle formulation. The drug is supplied as a lyophilized powder and is reconstituted with sterile water for injection (Boswell et al., 1998). Blood levels following intravenous infusion are almost equivalent to those obtained with C-AMB, and because L-AMB can be given at higher doses, blood levels have been achieved that exceed those obtained with C-AMB (Boswell et al., 1998) (Table 61–2).

ABLC. Amphotericin B lipid complex is a complex of amphotericin B with two phospholipids (dimyristoylphosphatidylcholine and dimyristoylphosphatidylglycerol) (Slain, 1999). ABLC is given in a dose of 5 mg/kg in 5% dextrose in water, infused intravenously once daily over 2 h. Blood levels of amphotericin B are much lower with ABLC than with the same dose of C-AMB. ABLC is effective in a variety of mycoses, with the possible exception of cryptococcal meningitis. The drug is approved for salvage therapy of deep mycoses.

Comparisons

Compared to C-AMB, all three of the amphotericin B lipid formulations appear to reduce the risk of acute kidney injury (defined as a doubling of patient serum creatinine) during therapy by 58% (Barrett et al., 2003). In patients at high risk for nephrotoxicity, ABLC has been observed to be more nephrotoxic than L-AMB (Wingard et al., 2000). Infusion-related reactions are not consistently reduced with the use of lipid preparations. ABCD causes more infusion-related reactions than C-AMB. Although L-AMB reportedly causes fewer infusion-related reactions than ABLC during the first dose (Wingard et al., 2000), the difference depends on whether premedication is given and varies considerably amongst patients. Infusion-related reactions typically decrease with subsequent infusions. While less toxic, the lipid formulations are much more costly than C-AMB, making them unavailable in many countries and dictating prudent use in the U.S. and other resource-rich areas. Interestingly, C-AMB is tolerated by premature neonates much better than older children and adults; as a result, it remains an important part of the antifungal formulary in the critical care nursery (Autmizguine et al., 2014).

ADME

Gastrointestinal absorption of all amphotericin B formulations is negligible, and intravenous delivery is indicated for systemic use. In plasma, amphotericin B is more than 90% bound to proteins. Pharmacokinetic properties differ amongst the preparations (Table 61–2). Azotemia, liver failure, and hemodialysis do not have a measurable impact on plasma concentrations. The concentration of amphotericin B (via C-AMB) in fluids from inflamed pleura, peritoneum, synovium, and aqueous humor is approximately two-thirds that of trough concentrations in plasma. Regardless of formulation, very little amphotericin B penetrates into CSF, vitreous humor, or normal amniotic fluid.

Antifungal Activity

Amphotericin B has useful clinical activity against a broad spectrum of pathogenic fungi, including *Candida* spp., *Cryptococcus neoformans*, *Blastomyces dermatitidis*, *Histoplasma capsulatum*, *Sporothrix schenckii*, *Coccidioides* spp., *Paracoccidioides braziliensis*, *Aspergillus* spp., *Penicillium marneffei*, *Fusarium* spp., and *Mucorales*. Amphotericin B has limited activity against the protozoa *Leishmania* spp. and *Naegleria fowleri*. The drug has no antibacterial activity.

TABLE 61–1 ■ PHARMACOTHERAPY OF MYCOSES

DEEP MYCOSES	DRUGS	SUPERFICIAL MYCOSES	DRUGS (Administration mode)
Invasive aspergillosis		*Candidiasis*	
Immunosuppressed	Voriconazole, isavuconazole, amphotericin B	Vulvovaginal	*Topical* Butoconazole, clotrimazole, miconazole, nystatin, terconazole, tioconazole
Nonimmunosuppressed	Voriconazole, isavuconazole, amphotericin B, itraconazole		*Oral* Fluconazole
Blastomycosis		Oropharyngeal	*Topical* Clotrimazole, nystatin
Rapidly progressive or CNS	Amphotericin B		
Indolent and non-CNS	Itraconazole		*Oral (systemic)* Fluconazole, itraconazole
Candidiasis			Posaconazole
Deeply invasive	Amphotericin B, fluconazole, voriconazole, caspofungin, micafungin, anidulafungin	Cutaneous	*Topical* Amphotericin B, clotrimazole, ciclopirox, econazole, ketoconazole, miconazole, nystatin
Coccidioidomycosis		*Ringworm*	*Topical* Butenafine, ciclopirox, clotrimazole, econazole, haloprogin, luliconazole, ketoconazole, miconazole, naftifine, oxiconazole, sertaconazole, sulconazole, terbinafine, tolnaftate, undecylenate
Rapidly progressing	Amphotericin B		
Indolent	Itraconazole, fluconazole		
Meningeal	Fluconazole, intrathecal amphotericin B		
Cryptococcosis			*Systemic* Griseofulvin, itraconazole, terbinafine
Non-AIDS and initial AIDS	Amphotericin B, flucytosine		
Maintenance AIDS	Fluconazole	*Onychomycosis*	*Systemic* Griseofulvin, itraconazole, terbinafine
Histoplasmosis			
Chronic pulmonary	Itraconazole		*Topical* Efinaconazole
Disseminated			
Rapidly progressing or CNS	Amphotericin B		
Indolent non-CNS	Itraconazole		
Maintenance AIDS	Itraconazole		
Mucormycosis	Amphotericin B, isavuconazole		
Pseudallescheriasis	Voriconazole, itraconazole		
Sporotrichosis			
Cutaneous	Itraconazole		
Extracutaneous	Amphotericin B, itraconazole		
Prophylaxis in the immunocompromised host	Fluconazole Posaconazole Micafungin		
Empirical therapy in the immunocompromised host (category not recognized by FDA)	Amphotericin B Caspofungin Fluconazole		
Microsporidia Infection	Albendazole Fumagillin		
Pneumocystis jiroveci pneumonia	Trimethoprim-sulfamethoxazole Pentamidine		

Fungal Resistance

Isolates of *Candida lusitaniae* are frequently resistant to amphotericin B. *Aspergillus terreus* and *Aspergillus nidulans* likewise appear to be less susceptible to amphotericin B than other *Aspergillus* species (Steinbach et al., 2004). Mutants selected in vitro for resistance to nystatin (a related polyene antifungal used topically) or amphotericin B replace ergosterol with certain precursor sterols. Mutations in ergosterol biosynthesis genes *ERG2*, *ERG3*, *ERG5*, *ERG6*, and *ERG11* reduce susceptibility to amphotericin B, likely the result of reduced ergosterol in the cell membrane of these isolates (Geber et al., 1995; Hull et al., 2012; Martel et al., 2010). Resistance amongst clinical isolates of any fungal species is exceedingly rare, presumably because amphotericin B is fungicidal, and mutations that affect this critical membrane sterol are associated with significant fitness costs.

Therapeutic Uses

Typical adult doses for each amphotericin B formulation are summarized in Table 61–2. Candida esophagitis responds to much lower doses than deeply invasive mycoses. Intrathecal infusion of C-AMB appears to be useful in patients with meningitis caused by *Coccidioides*. Small doses of C-AMB (from 0.01 to 1.5 mg, one to three times weekly) can be injected into the CSF of the lumbar spine, cisterna magna, or lateral cerebral ventricle. Fever and headache are common reactions that may be decreased by intrathecal administration of 10–15 mg of hydrocortisone. However, the general use of intrathecal C-AMB administration cannot be recommended due to a lack of clinical data. Local injections of amphotericin B into a joint or peritoneal dialysate fluid commonly produce irritation and pain. Intraocular injection following pars plana vitrectomy has been used to treat fungal endophthalmitis.

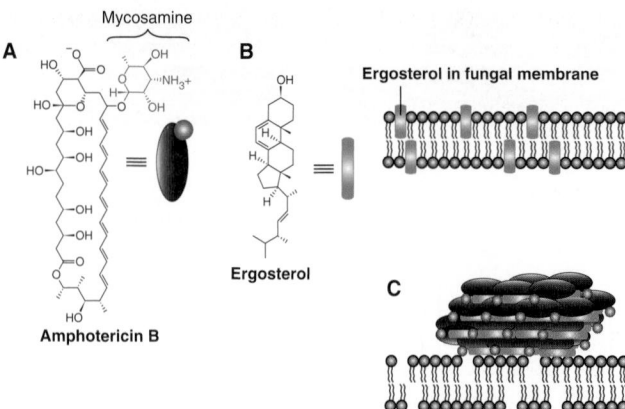

Figure 61–2 *Mechanism of action of amphotericin B.* The antifungal activity of amphotericin B depends on its capacity to bind ergosterol in the fungal cell membrane. **A.** Amphotericin is an amphipathic molecule with a mycosamine moiety (shown in blue) at one end of a 14-carbon hydrophobic chain. X-ray crystallography shows the molecule to be rigid and rod shaped, with the hydrophilic hydroxyl groups of the macrolide ring forming an opposing face to the lipophilic polyenic portion. **B.** Ergosterol, here depicted as a green rod, decorates both bilayers of the fungal membrane. **C.** Amphotericin B appears to form aggregates that sequester and effectively extract ergosterol from lipid bilayers, much like a selective sponge, disrupting membrane structure and resulting in fungal cell death.

Intravenous administration of amphotericin B is the treatment of choice for invasive mucormycosis and in combination with 5-flucytosine is the gold standard for induction treatment of cryptococcal meningitis. Amphotericin B is also indicated for the treatment of severe or rapidly progressive histoplasmosis, blastomycosis, coccidioidomycosis, and penicilliosis. Amphotericin B is a salvage therapy for patients not responding to azole therapy for invasive aspergillosis, extracutaneous sporotrichosis, fusariosis, alternariosis, or trichosporonosis. Amphotericin B (C-AMB or L-AMB) can also be given to selected patients with profound neutropenia with fever who do not respond to broad-spectrum antibacterial agents over 5–7 days. However, the more recently developed azoles and echinocandins are generally the drugs of choice for such patients because of their reduced toxicity.

Adverse Effects

The major acute reactions to intravenous amphotericin B formulations are infusion-related fever and chills. These are due to the induction of a proinflammatory response in cells of the innate immune system signaling through TLR2 and CD14 (Rogers et al., 1998; Sau et al., 2003). Infusion-related reactions are most prominent with ABCD, while L-AMB administration appears to be less commonly associated with this adverse event. Tachypnea, respiratory stridor, or modest hypotension can also occur, but frank bronchospasm and anaphylaxis are rare. Patients with preexisting cardiac or pulmonary disease may tolerate the metabolic demands of the reaction poorly and develop hypoxia or hypotension. The reaction ends spontaneously in 30–45 min; treatment with meperidine may shorten it.

Pretreatment with oral acetaminophen or ibuprofen or use of intravenous hydrocortisone sodium succinate (hemisuccinate), 0.7 mg/kg, at the start of the infusion decreases reactions. Febrile reactions tend to abate with subsequent infusions.

Azotemia occurs in 80% of patients who receive C-AMB for deep mycoses (Carlson and Condon, 1994). The lipid formulations are significantly less nephrotoxic than C-AMB. Toxicity is dose dependent, usually transient, and increased by concurrent therapy with other nephrotoxic agents, such as aminoglycosides or cyclosporine. Although permanent histological changes in renal tubules occur even during short courses of C-AMB, permanent functional impairment is uncommon in adults with normal renal function prior to treatment unless the cumulative dose exceeds 3–4 g. Renal tubular acidosis and renal wasting of K^+ and Mg^{2+} also may be seen during and for several weeks after therapy. Supplemental K^+ is required in one-third of patients on prolonged therapy. Saline loading has decreased nephrotoxicity, even in the absence of water or salt deprivation. Administration of 1 L of normal saline intravenously on the day that C-AMB is to be given has been recommended for adults who are able to tolerate the Na^+ load.

Hypochromic, normocytic anemia commonly occurs during treatment with C-AMB. Anemia is less with lipid formulations and usually not seen over the first 2 weeks. The anemia is most likely due to decreased production of erythropoietin and often responds to administration of recombinant erythropoietin. Headache, nausea, vomiting, malaise, weight loss, and phlebitis at peripheral infusion sites are common. Arachnoiditis has been observed as a complication of intrathecal administration of C-AMB.

Flucytosine

Flucytosine (5-fluorocytosine) is a fluorinated pyrimidine related to fluorouracil that has a limited role in the treatment of invasive fungal infections.

Flucytosine

Mechanism of Action

All susceptible fungi are capable of deaminating flucytosine to 5FU (Figure 61–3), a potent antimetabolite that is used in cancer chemotherapy. Fluorouracil is metabolized first to 5FUMP) by the enzyme *UPRTase*. 5FUMP is then either incorporated into RNA (via synthesis of 5-fluorouridine triphosphate) or metabolized to 5FdUMP, a potent inhibitor of *thymidylate synthase*, ultimately inhibiting DNA synthesis. The selective action of flucytosine is due to the lack of *cytosine deaminase* in mammalian cells, which prevents metabolism to fluorouracil.

ADME

Flucytosine shows excellent bioavailability on oral administration and is absorbed rapidly from the GI tract. It is widely distributed in the body,

PRODUCT	DOSE (mg/kg)	C_{max} (µg/mL)	$AUC_{(1-24h)}$ (µg.hr/mL)	V (L/kg)	Cl (mL/h/kg)
L-AMB	5	83 ± 35.2	555 ± 311	0.11 ± 0.08	11 ± 6
ABCD	5	3.1	43	4.3	117
ABLC	5	1.7 ± 0.8	14 ± 7	131 ± 7.7	426 ± 188.5
C-AMB	0.6	1.1 ± 0.2	17.1 ± 5	5 ± 2.8	38 ± 15

TABLE 61–2 ■ PK DATA FOR AMPHOTERICIN B FORMULATIONS AFTER MULTIPLE ADMINISTRATIONS IN HUMANS

For details, see the work of Boswell et al. (1998). From Boswell GW, et al. AmBisome (liposomal amphotericin B): a comparative review. *J Clin Pharmacol*, **1998**, 38:583–592. © 1998 The American College of Clinical Pharmacology. Reprinted by permission of SAGE Publications.

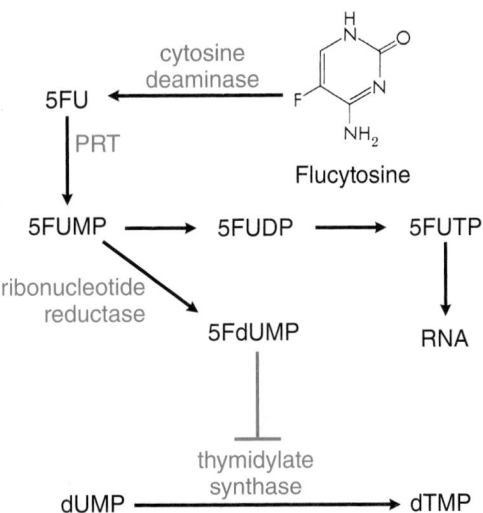

Figure 61–3 *Action of flucytosine in fungi.* Flucytosine is transported by cytosine permease into the fungal cell, where it is deaminated to 5FU. The 5FU is then converted to 5FUMP and then is either converted to 5FUTP and incorporated into RNA or converted by ribonucleotide reductase to 5FdUMP, which is a potent inhibitor of thymidylate synthase.

with a volume of distribution that approximates total body water, and is minimally bound to plasma proteins. The peak plasma concentration in patients with normal renal function is about 70–80 μg/mL, achieved 1–2 h after a dose of 37.5 mg/kg. The flucytosine concentration in CSF is about 65%–90% of that found simultaneously in the plasma. The drug also appears to penetrate into the aqueous humor.

Approximately 80% of a given dose is excreted unchanged in the urine; concentrations in the urine range from 200 to 500 μg/mL. The $t_{1/2}$ of the drug is 3–6 h in normal individuals and may be as long as 200 h in patients with renal failure. The clearance of flucytosine is approximately equivalent to that of creatinine. In patients with decreased renal function, reduction of dosage is necessary; C_p should be measured periodically. Peak concentrations should range between 50 and 100 μg/mL. Flucytosine is cleared by hemodialysis, and patients undergoing such treatment should receive a single dose of 37.5 mg/kg after dialysis. The drug also is removed by peritoneal dialysis.

Antifungal Activity and Fungal Resistance

Flucytosine is currently used primarily as an adjunctive agent with amphotericin B in the induction phase of cryptococcal meningoencephalitis therapy. It has in vitro activity against a number of pathogens, but the emergence of resistance limits its usefulness as single-agent therapy.

Drug resistance arising during therapy (secondary resistance) is an important cause of therapeutic failure when flucytosine is used alone for cryptococcosis and candidiasis. The mechanism for this resistance can be loss of the permease necessary for cytosine transport or decreased activity of either UPRTase or cytosine deaminase (Figure 61–3).

In *C. albicans,* substitution of thymidine for cytosine at nucleotide 301 in the gene encoding UPRTase (*FUR1*) causes a cysteine to become an arginine, modestly increasing flucytosine resistance (Dodgson et al., 2004). Flucytosine resistance is further increased if both *FUR1* alleles in the diploid fungus are mutated.

Therapeutic Uses

Flucytosine is given orally, 50–150 mg/kg/d, in four divided doses at 6-h intervals. Dosage must be adjusted for decreased renal function. Flucytosine is used almost exclusively in combination with amphotericin B for the treatment of cryptococcal meningitis, and this combination, as compared with amphotericin B alone, is associated with improved survival amongst patients with cryptococcal meningitis (Day et al., 2013). Based on this trial, the addition of flucytosine to amphotericin B is the current gold standard for the treatment of HIV-associated cryptococcal meningitis.

In cryptococcal meningitis of non-AIDS patients, the role of flucytosine is less clear. The addition of flucytosine to 6 weeks or more of therapy with C-AMB runs the risk of substantial bone marrow suppression or colitis if the flucytosine dose is not promptly adjusted downward as amphotericin B–induced azotemia occurs.

Adverse Effects

Flucytosine may depress the bone marrow and lead to leukopenia and thrombocytopenia. Patients are more prone to this complication if they have an underlying hematological disorder, are being treated with radiation or drugs that injure the bone marrow, or have a history of treatment with such agents. Other untoward effects, including rash, nausea, vomiting, diarrhea, and severe enterocolitis, have been noted. In about 5% of patients, plasma levels of hepatic enzymes are elevated, but this effect reverses when therapy is stopped. Toxicity is more frequent in patients with AIDS or azotemia (including those who are concurrently receiving amphotericin B) and when plasma drug concentrations exceed 100 μg/mL. Toxicity may result from conversion of flucytosine to 5FU by the microbial flora in the intestinal tract of the host.

Imidazoles and Triazoles

The azole antifungals include two broad classes, imidazoles and triazoles. Of the drugs now on the market in the U.S., clotrimazole, miconazole, ketoconazole, econazole, butoconazole, oxiconazole, sertaconazole, sulconazole, tioconazole, and luliconazole are *imidazoles*; efinaconazole, terconazole, itraconazole, fluconazole, voriconazole, posaconazole, and isavuconazole are *triazoles*. The topical use of azole antifungals is described in the second section of this chapter.

MICONAZOLE

FLUCONAZOLE

Mechanism of Action

The major effect of imidazoles and triazoles on fungi is inhibition of 14-α-sterol demethylase, a CYP and the product of the gene *ERG11* (Figure 61–4). Imidazoles and triazoles thus impair the biosynthesis of ergosterol, resulting in depletion of membrane ergosterol and accumulation of the toxic product 14α-methyl-3,6-diol, leading to growth arrest (Kanafani and Perfect, 2008), possibly by disrupting the close packing of acyl chains of phospholipids and impairing the functions of membrane-bound enzyme systems. Some azoles directly increase permeability of the fungal cytoplasmic membrane, but the concentrations required are likely only obtained with topical use.

Antifungal Activity

Azoles as a group have clinically useful activity against *C. albicans, Candida tropicalis, Candida parapsilosis, C. neoformans, Blastomyces dermatitidis, H. capsulatum, Coccidioides* spp., *Paracoccidioides brasiliensis,* and ringworm fungi (dermatophytes). *Aspergillus* spp., *Scedosporium apiospermum (Pseudallescheria boydii), Fusarium,* and *Sporothrix schenckii* are intermediate in susceptibility. *Candida glabrata* exhibits reduced

A

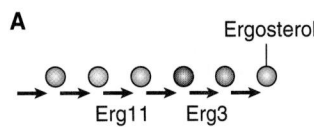

B

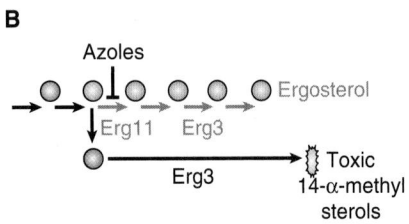

Ergosterol

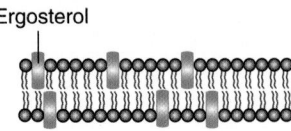

Toxic sterol

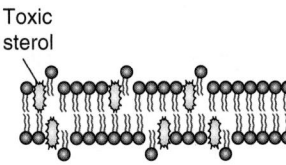

Figure 61–4 *Ergosterol biosynthesis and the mechanism of action of the azole antifungals.* **A.** Fungal ergosterol synthesis proceeds via a series of enzymic steps that include Erg11, a 14-α-sterol demethylase. The completed ergosterol is then inserted into both leaflets of the membrane bilayer. **B.** Imidazole and triazole antifungals inhibit the activity of 14-α-sterol demethylase, thereby reducing the biosynthesis of ergosterol and leading to the accumulation of 14-α-methylsterols. These methylsterols are toxic, disrupting the close packing of acyl chains of phospholipids, impairing the functions of certain membrane-bound enzyme systems, and thus inhibiting growth of the fungi.

susceptibility to the azoles, whereas *Candida krusei* and the agents of mucormycosis are more resistant. Posaconazole and isavuconazole have modestly improved spectrum of activity in vitro against the agents of mucormycosis.

Resistance

In *C. albicans*, azole resistance can be due in part to accumulation of mutations in *ERG11*, the gene encoding the azole target, 14-α-sterol demethylase. Increased azole efflux by overexpression of ABC and/or major facilitator superfamily transporters impart azole resistance in *C. albicans* and *C. glabrata*. Overexpression of these genes is due to activating mutations in genes encoding their transcriptional regulators. Mutation of the C5,6 sterol desaturase gene *ERG3* also can increase azole resistance in some species (Cowen et al., 2014); such mutations prevent formation of the toxic product 14α-methyl-3,6-diol from 14α-methylfecosterol; the resulting accumulation of 14α-methylfecosterol produces functional membranes and overcomes the effect of azoles. Increased production of 14-α-sterol demethylase due to overexpression of *ERG11* occurs, owing to activating mutations in the gene encoding its transcriptional regulator Upc2.

Primary azole resistance has been described in some isolates of *A. fumigatus* with increased azole export and decreased ergosterol content, but the clinical significance is unknown. Decreased fluconazole susceptibility has been described in *C. neoformans* isolated from patients with AIDS failing prolonged therapy.

Interaction of Azole Antifungals With Other Drugs

The azoles interact with hepatic CYPs as substrates and inhibitors (Table 61–3), providing myriad possibilities for the interaction of azoles with many other medications. Thus, azoles can elevate plasma levels of some coadministered drugs (Table 61–4). Other coadministered drugs can decrease plasma concentrations of azole antifungal agents (Table 61–5). As a

consequence of these and other interactions, combinations of certain drugs with azole antifungal medications may be contraindicated (Table 61–6).

Available Agents

Ketoconazole. Ketoconazole, administered orally, has been replaced by itraconazole except when the lower cost of ketoconazole outweighs the advantage of itraconazole. Ketoconazole is available for topical use, as described further in this chapter.

Itraconazole. Itraconazole is a triazole that lacks the corticosteroid suppression associated with ketoconazole while retaining most of ketoconazole's pharmacological properties and extending the antifungal spectrum. Importantly, itraconazole has activity against *Aspergillus* spp. while imidazoles do not. Itraconazole has been supplanted by other triazoles in the treatment of invasive mold infections but remains an important prophylactic agent in the prevention of mold infections in some patients (e.g., patients with CGD).

ADME. Itraconazole is available as a tablet, capsule, and a solution in hydroxypropyl-β-cyclodextrin for oral use. The capsule form of the drug is best absorbed in the fed state, but the oral solution is better absorbed in the fasting state, providing peak plasma concentrations more than 150% of those obtained with the capsule. Itraconazole is metabolized in the liver. It is both a substrate for and a potent inhibitor of CYP3A4. Itraconazole is present in plasma with an approximately equal concentration of a biologically active metabolite, hydroxy-itraconazole. The native drug and metabolite are more than 99% bound to plasma proteins. Neither appears in urine or in CSF. The $t_{1/2}$ of itraconazole at steady state is about 30–40 h. Steady-state levels of itraconazole are not reached for 4 days and those of hydroxy-itraconazole for 7 days; thus, loading doses are recommended when treating deep mycoses. Severe liver disease will increase itraconazole plasma concentrations, but azotemia and hemodialysis have no effect.

TABLE 61–3 ■ INTERACTIONS OF AZOLE ANTIFUNGAL AGENTS WITH HEPATIC CYPs

FLUCONAZOLE	VORICONAZOLE	ITRACONAZOLE	POSACONAZOLE	ISAVUCONAZOLE
CYP3A4, 5, 7 inhibitor (moderate)	CYP2C9 inhibitor and substrate	CYP3A4, 5, 7 inhibitor and substrate	CYP3A4 inhibitor (potent)	CYP3A4 inhibitor and substrate
CYP2C9 inhibitor (strong)	CYP3A4, 5,7 inhibitor			CYP2B6 inhibitor
CYP2C19 inhibitor	CYP2C19 inhibitor and substrate			

TABLE 61–4 ■ DRUGS EXHIBITING ELEVATED C_p WHEN COADMINISTERED WITH AZOLE ANTIFUNGAL AGENTS

Alfentanil	Eplerenone	Losartan	Saquinavir
Alprazolam	Ergot alkaloids	Lovastatin	Sildenafil
Astemizole	Erlotinib	Methadone	Sirolimus
Buspirone	Eszopiclone	Methylprednisolone	Solifenacin
Busulfan	Felodipine	Midazolam	Sunitinib
Carbamazepine	Fexofenadine	Nevirapine	Tacrolimus
Cisapride	Gefitinib	Omeprazole	Triazolam
Cyclosporine	Glimepiride	Phenytoin	Vardenafil
Digoxin	Glipizide	Pimozide	Vinca alkaloids
Docetaxel	Halofantrine	Quinidine	Warfarin
Dofetilide	Haloperidol	Ramelteon	Zidovudine
Efavirenz	Imatinib	Ranolazine	Zolpidem
Eletriptan	Irinotecan	Risperidone	

Mechanism of interaction presumably occurs largely at the level of hepatic CYPs, especially CYPs 3A4, 2C9, and 2D6, but can also involve P-glycoprotein and other mechanisms.
Not all drugs listed interact equally with all azoles.

Therapeutic Uses. Itraconazole is the drug of choice for patients with indolent, nonmeningeal infections due to *B. dermatitidis, H. capsulatum, P. brasiliensis,* and *Coccidioides immitis.* The drug also is useful in the therapy of indolent invasive aspergillosis outside the CNS, particularly after the infection has been stabilized with amphotericin B. Approximately half of the patients with distal subungual onychomycosis respond to itraconazole (Evans and Sigurgeirsson, 1999). Although not an approved use, itraconazole is a reasonable choice for the treatment of pseudallescheriasis, an infection that does not respond to amphotericin B therapy, as well as cutaneous and extracutaneous sporotrichosis, tinea corporis, and extensive tinea versicolor. HIV-infected patients with disseminated histoplasmosis or penicilliosis have a decreased incidence of relapse if given prolonged itraconazole "maintenance" therapy. Itraconazole is not recommended for maintenance therapy of cryptococcal meningitis in HIV-infected patients because of a high incidence of relapse. Long-term itraconazole therapy has been used in non–HIV-infected patients with allergic bronchopulmonary aspergillosis to decrease the dose of glucocorticoids and reduce attacks of acute bronchospasm (Salez et al., 1999).

Itraconazole solution is effective and approved for use in oropharyngeal and esophageal candidiasis. Because the solution has more GI side effects than fluconazole tablets, itraconazole solution usually is reserved for patients not responding to fluconazole. Finally, itraconazole is also used as *Aspergillus* prophylaxis in patients with CGD.

Dosage. In treating deep mycoses, a loading dose of 200 mg of itraconazole is administered three times daily for the first 3 days. After the loading doses, two 100-mg capsules are given twice daily with food. Divided doses may increase the AUC. For maintenance therapy of HIV-infected patients with disseminated histoplasmosis, 200 mg once daily is used. Onychomycosis can be treated with either 200 mg once daily for 12 weeks or, for infections isolated to fingernails, two monthly cycles consisting of 200 mg twice daily for 1 week followed by a 3-week period of no therapy—so-called pulse therapy (Evans and Sigurgeirsson, 1999). Once-daily terbinafine (250 mg), however, is superior to pulse therapy with itraconazole. For oropharyngeal candidiasis, itraconazole oral solution should be taken during fasting in a dose of 100 mg (10 mL) once daily and swished vigorously in the mouth before swallowing to optimize any topical effect.

TABLE 61–5 ■ SOME DRUGS THAT DECREASE AZOLE CONCENTRATION WHEN COADMINISTERED

DRUG	FLUCONAZOLE	VORICONAZOLE	ITRACONAZOLE	POSACONAZOLE	ISAVUCONAZOLE
Antacids (simultaneous)	−		+	−	−
Barbiturates		+	+[a]		+
Carbamazepine	+	+	+	+	+
H$_2$ antagonists			+	+	−
Didanosine			+		
Efavirenz		+	+		
Nevirapine		+	+		
Proton pump inhibitors	−	−[b]	+	+	−
Phenytoin	−	+	+	+	
Rifampin	+	+	+	+	+
Rifabutin		+	+	+	
Ritonavir		+			−[c]

[a]Phenobarbital only.
[b]Omeprazole and voriconazole increase each other's concentrations in plasma; reduce omeprazole dose by 50% when initiating voriconazole therapy.
[c]With standard doses of ritonavir.

TABLE 61–6 ■ SOME CONTRAINDICATED AZOLE DRUG COMBINATIONS

DRUG	FLUCONAZOLE	VORICONAZOLE	ITRACONAZOLE	POSACONAZOLE	ISAVUCONAZOLE
Alfuzosin		x	x	x	
Artemether	x	x			
Bepridil	x				
Clopidogrel	x				
Conivaptan	x	x	x	x	
Dabigatran			x		
Darunavir		x			
Dronedarone	x	x	x	x	
Everolimus	x	x	x	x	
Lopinavir		x			
Lumefantrine	x	x			
Mesoridazine	x				
Nilotinib	x	x	x	x	
Nisoldipine	Use with caution	x	x	x	
Quinine	x	x			
Rifapentine		x	Use with caution	Use with caution	
Ritonavir		x	Use with caution	Use with caution	Use with caution
Rivaroxaban		x	x		
Salmeterol		x	x	x	
Silodosin		x	x	x	
Simvastatin	Use with caution		x	x	
St. John's wort		x			x
Tetrabenazine	x	x			
Thioridazine	x	x			
Tolvaptan	x	x		x	
Tolvaptan	x		x		
Topotecan			x		
Ziprasidone	x	x			

Patients with esophageal thrush unresponsive or refractory to treatment with fluconazole tablets are given 100 mg of the solution twice a day for 2–4 weeks. The typical dose for fungal prophylaxis in patients with CGD is 5 mg/kg per day.

Adverse Effects. Serious hepatotoxicity has led, in rare cases, to hepatic failure and death. If symptoms of hepatotoxicity occur, the drug should be discontinued and liver function assessed. In the absence of interacting drugs, itraconazole capsules and suspension are well tolerated at 200 mg daily. Diarrhea, abdominal cramps, anorexia, and nausea are more common than with the capsules. Of patients receiving 50–400 mg of the capsules per day, nausea and vomiting, hypertriglyceridemia, hypokalemia, increased serum aminotransferase, and rash occurred in 2%–10%. Occasionally, rash necessitates drug discontinuation, but most adverse effects can be handled with dose reduction. Profound hypokalemia has been seen in patients receiving 600 mg or more daily and in those who recently have received prolonged amphotericin B therapy. Doses of 300 mg twice daily have led to other side effects, including adrenal insufficiency, lower limb edema, hypertension, and in at least one case, rhabdomyolysis. Doses greater than 400 mg per day are not recommended for long-term use. Anaphylaxis has been observed rarely, as well as severe rash, including Stevens-Johnson syndrome. Itraconazole is contraindicated for the treatment of onychomycosis during pregnancy or for women contemplating pregnancy.

Drug Interactions. Tables 61–4, 61–5, and 61–6 list select interactions of azoles with other drugs. Many of the interactions can result in serious toxicity from the companion drug, such as inducing potentially fatal cardiac arrhythmias when used with quinidine, halofantrine (an orphan drug used for malaria), levomethadyl (an orphan drug used for heroin addiction), pimozide, or cisapride (available only under an investigational limited access program in the U.S.). Other drugs may decrease itraconazole serum levels below therapeutic concentrations (Table 61–5).

Fluconazole. Fluconazole is a fluorinated bis-triazole.

ADME. Fluconazole is almost completely absorbed from the GI tract. Plasma concentrations are essentially the same whether the drug is given orally or intravenously, and its bioavailability is unaltered by food or gastric acidity. Peak plasma concentrations are 4–8 μg/mL after repetitive doses of 100 mg. Renal excretion accounts for more than 90% of elimination, and the elimination $t_{1/2}$ is 25–30 h. Fluconazole diffuses readily into body fluids, including breast milk, sputum, and saliva; concentrations in CSF can reach 50%–90% of the simultaneous values in plasma. The dosage interval should be increased from 24 to 48 h with a creatinine clearance of 21–40 mL/min and to 72 h at 10–20 mL/min. A dose of 100–200 mg should be given after hemodialysis. About 11%–12% of drug in the plasma is protein bound.

Therapeutic Uses.

- **Candidiasis.** Fluconazole, 100–200 mg daily for 7–14 days, is effective in oropharyngeal candidiasis. A single dose of 150 mg is effective in uncomplicated vaginal candidiasis. A loading dose of 800 mg followed by 400 mg daily is useful in treating candidemia of nonimmunosuppressed patients (Pappas et al., 2007; Rex et al., 1994). Although response to *C. glabrata* bloodstream infections in randomized trials using fluconazole has been comparable to that with *C. albicans, C. glabrata* exhibits inherent reduced susceptibility and can become highly resistant on prolonged exposure to fluconazole. Empirical use of fluconazole for suspected candidemia may not be advisable in patients who have received long-term fluconazole prophylaxis and, as a result, may be colonized with azole-resistant *C. glabrata.* Based on resistance in vitro, *C. krusei* would not be expected to respond to fluconazole or other azoles.

- **Cryptococcosis.** Fluconazole, 400 mg daily, is used for the initial 8 weeks of the consolidation phase of the treatment of cryptococcal meningitis in patients with AIDS. Induction therapy involves an initial course of at least 2 weeks of intravenous amphotericin B. If, after 8 weeks at 400 mg per day, the patient is no longer symptomatic, then the dose is decreased to 200 mg daily and continued indefinitely. If the patient has completed 12 months of treatment of cryptococcosis, responds to HAART, has a CD4 count maintained above 200/mm³ for at least 6 months, and is asymptomatic from cryptococcal meningitis, it is reasonable to discontinue maintenance fluconazole as long as the CD4 response is maintained. Fluconazole, 400 mg daily, has been recommended as continuation therapy in patients without AIDS with cryptococcal meningitis who have responded to an initial course of C-AMB or L-AMB and for patients with pulmonary cryptococcosis (Perfect et al., 2010).

- **Other Mycoses.** Fluconazole is the drug of choice for treatment of coccidioidal meningitis because of good penetration into the CSF and much less morbidity than with intrathecal amphotericin B. In other forms of coccidioidomycosis, fluconazole is comparable to itraconazole. Fluconazole has no useful activity against histoplasmosis, blastomycosis, or sporotrichosis and is not effective in the prevention or treatment of aspergillosis. Fluconazole has no activity in mucormycosis.

Dosage. Fluconazole is marketed in the U.S. as tablets of 50, 100, 150, and 200 mg for oral administration, powder for oral suspension providing 10 and 40 mg/mL, and intravenous solutions containing 2 mg/mL in saline and in dextrose solution. The daily dose of fluconazole should be based on the infecting organism and the patient's response to therapy. Generally, recommended dosages are 50–400 mg once daily for either oral or intravenous administration. A loading dose of twice the daily maintenance dose is generally administered on the first day of therapy. Prolonged maintenance therapy may be required to prevent relapse. Children are treated with 12 mg/kg once daily (maximum 600 mg/d) without a loading dose. In adult patients, doses of up to 1200 mg have been safely administered in clinical trials for the treatment of cryptococcal meningitis.

Adverse Effects. Side effects in patients receiving more than 7 days of drug, regardless of dose, include nausea, headache, skin rash, vomiting, abdominal pain, and diarrhea (all at 2%–4%). Reversible alopecia may occur with prolonged therapy at 400 mg daily. Rare cases of deaths due to hepatic failure or Stevens-Johnson syndrome have been reported. Fluconazole has been associated with skeletal and cardiac deformities in at least three infants born to two women taking high doses during pregnancy. Although a recent clinical study found no association between fluconazole receipt by mothers and most birth defects in their children, this study did find a statistically significant increase in tetralogy of Fallot in babies born to mothers who received fluconazole (Mølgaard-Nielsen et al., 2013). Fluconazole should be avoided during pregnancy.

Drug Interactions. Fluconazole is an inhibitor of CYP3A4 and CYP2C9. Fluconazole's drug-drug interactions are shown in Tables 61–4, 61–5, and 61–6. Patients who receive more than 400 mg daily or azotemic patients who have elevated fluconazole blood levels may experience drug interactions not otherwise seen.

Voriconazole. Voriconazole is a triazole with a structure similar to fluconazole but with increased activity in vitro, an expanded spectrum, and poor aqueous solubility.

ADME. Voriconazole is available as 50- or 200-mg tablets or a suspension of 40 mg/mL when hydrated. The tablets, but not the suspension, contain lactose. Because high-fat meals reduce voriconazole bioavailability, oral drug should be given either 1 h before or 1 h after meals. Oral bioavailability is 96%; volume of distribution is high (4.6 L/kg), with extensive drug distribution in tissues. Metabolism occurs through CYPs 2C19 and 2C9; CYP3A4 plays a limited role. Plasma elimination $t_{1/2}$ is 6 h. Voriconazole exhibits nonlinear metabolism so that higher doses cause greater-than-linear increases in systemic drug exposure. Genetic polymorphisms in CYP2C19 can cause up to 4-fold differences in drug exposure: About 20% of Asians are homozygous poor metabolizers, compared with 2% of whites and African Americans. Less than 2% of parent drug is recovered from urine; 80% of the inactive metabolites are excreted in the urine. The oral dose does not have to be adjusted for azotemia or hemodialysis. Patients with mild-to-moderate cirrhosis should receive the same loading dose of voriconazole but half the maintenance dose. The intravenous formulation of voriconazole contains SBECD, which is excreted by the kidney. Significant accumulation of SBECD occurs with a creatinine clearance less than 50 mL/min; in that setting, oral voriconazole is preferred. Therapeutic drug monitoring is frequently used, with target serum concentrations between 1 and 5 mg/L thought to maximize efficacy and minimize adverse events.

Therapeutic Uses. Voriconazole shows superior efficacy to C-AMB in the therapy of invasive aspergillosis using rate of response as the primary end point (Herbrecht et al., 2002); survival also is superior with voriconazole. Voriconazole was compared to L-AMB for empirical therapy of neutropenic patients whose fever did not respond to more than 96 h of antibacterial therapy. Because the 95% confidence interval in this noninferiority trial permitted the possibility that voriconazole might be more than 10% worse than L-AMB, the FDA did not approve voriconazole for this use (Walsh et al., 2002); however, in a secondary analysis, there were fewer breakthrough infections with voriconazole (1.9%) than with L-AMB (5%).

Voriconazole is approved for use in esophageal candidiasis. In nonneutropenic patients with candidemia, voriconazole is comparable in efficacy and less toxic than initial C-AMB followed by fluconazole (Kullberg et al., 2005). Voriconazole is approved for initial treatment of candidemia and invasive aspergillosis, as well as for salvage therapy in patients with *P. boydii (S. apiospermum)* and *Fusarium* infections. Positive responses in patients with cerebral fungal infections suggest that the drug penetrates infected brain.

Dosage. Treatment is usually initiated with an intravenous infusion of 6 mg/kg every 12 h for two doses, followed by 3–4 mg/kg every 12 h, administered no faster than 3 mg/kg/h. As the patient improves, oral administration is continued as 200 mg every 12 h. Patients failing to respond may be given 300 mg every 12 h.

Adverse Effects. Voriconazole is teratogenic in animals and generally contraindicated in pregnancy. Although voriconazole is generally well tolerated, occasional cases of hepatotoxicity have been reported, and liver function should be monitored. Voriconazole can prolong the QTc interval, a significant issue in patients with other risk factors for torsades de pointes. Transient visual or auditory hallucinations are frequent after the first dose, usually at night and particularly with intravenous administration. Symptoms diminish with time. Patients receiving their first intravenous infusion have had anaphylactoid reactions. Rash occurs in 6% of patients. The cyclodextrin component of intravenous formulations may be toxic to the kidney; thus, intravenous voriconazole should be used with caution in patients with renal failure (Neofytos et al., 2012).

Drug Interactions. Voriconazole is metabolized by, and inhibits, CYPs 2C19, 2C9, and 3A4 (in that order of decreasing potency). The major metabolite of voriconazole, the voriconazole N-oxide, also inhibits these CYPs. Inhibitors or inducers of these CYPs may increase or decrease voriconazole plasma concentrations, respectively. Voriconazole and its major metabolite can increase the plasma concentrations of other drugs metabolized by these enzymes (Tables 61–4, 61–5, and 61–6). Because the

AUC of sirolimus increases 11-fold in the presence of voriconazole, coadministration is contraindicated. When starting voriconazole in a patient receiving 40 mg/d or more of omeprazole, the dose of omeprazole should be reduced by half.

Posaconazole. Posaconazole is a synthetic structural analogue of itraconazole with the same broad antifungal spectrum but with up to 4-fold greater activity in vitro against yeasts and filamentous fungi, including some, but not all, of the agents that cause mucormycosis (Frampton and Scott, 2008). Activity against yeasts in vitro is similar to voriconazole. The mechanism of action is the same as other imidazoles, inhibition of sterol 14-α-demethylase.

ADME. Posaconazole is available as a flavored suspension containing 40 mg/mL. Bioavailability of the oral suspension is significantly enhanced by the presence of food (Courtney et al., 2003; Krieter et al., 2004). The drug has a long $t_{1/2}$ (25–31 h), a large volume of distribution (331–1341 L), and extensive protein binding (>98%). Systemic exposure is four times higher in homozygous CYP2C19 slow metabolizers than in homozygous wild-type metabolizers. Steady-state concentrations are reached in 7–10 days when dosed four times daily. Renal impairment does not alter plasma concentrations; hepatic impairment causes a modest increase. Almost 80% of the drug is excreted in the stool, with 66% as unchanged drug. The major metabolic pathway is hepatic UDP glucuronidation (Krieter et al., 2004). Hemodialysis does not remove drug from the circulation. Gastric acid improves absorption (Krishna et al., 2009); drugs that reduce gastric acid (e.g., cimetidine and esomeprazole) decrease posaconazole exposure by 32%–50% (Frampton and Scott, 2008). Diarrhea reduces the average C_p by 37% (Smith et al., 2009). The delayed-release tablet and intravenous formulations provide a more consistent bioavailability in the presence of concomitant disease states, medications, and dietary considerations that alter concentrations achievable with the oral suspension (Guarascio and Slain, 2015).

Therapeutic Uses. Posaconazole is approved for treatment of oropharyngeal candidiasis, although fluconazole is the preferred drug because of safety and cost. Posaconazole is also approved for prophylaxis against candidiasis and aspergillosis in patients more than 13 years of age who have prolonged neutropenia or severe GVHD (Ullmann et al., 2007). It is approved in the E.U. as salvage therapy for aspergillosis and several other infections, as are itraconazole and voriconazole.

Dosage. For prophylaxis of invasive *Aspergillus* and *Candida* infections, the adult intravenous dose is 300 mg twice on day 1 and 300 mg daily thereafter. Duration of therapy is based on recovery from neutropenia or immunosuppression. The same dose is used for the delayed-release tablets. The dose for the oral suspension is 200 mg (5 mL) three times daily.

Adverse Effects. Common adverse effects include nausea, vomiting, diarrhea, abdominal pain, and headache (Smith et al., 2009). Although adverse effects occur in at least a third of patients, the rate of discontinuation due to adverse effects in long-term studies has been only 8%.

Drug Interactions. Posaconazole inhibits CYP3A4. Coadministration with rifabutin or phenytoin increases the plasma concentration of these drugs and decreases posaconazole exposure by 2-fold. Posaconazole increases the AUC of cyclosporine, tacrolimus (121%), sirolimus (790%), midazolam (83%), and other CYP3A4 substrates (Table 61–4) (Frampton and Scott, 2008; Krishna et al., 2009; Moton et al., 2009). Posaconazole can prolong the QTc interval and should not be coadministered with drugs that are CYP3A4 substrates that likewise prolong the QTc interval, such as methadone, haloperidol, pimozide, quinidine, risperidone, sunitinib, tacrolimus, and halofantrine (Table 61–4).

Isavuconazole. Isavuconazole is a triazole that is administered as the isavuconazonium prodrug.

ADME. Isavuconazole is available in both oral and cyclodextrin-free intravenous formulations. It is highly bioavailable (98%) and is more than 99% protein bound in serum. Administration of oral isavuconazonium with food reduces AUC by about 20%. Isavuconazole is eliminated by hepatic metabolism, predominantly by CYP3A4 and CYP3A5. Less than 1% of isavuconazole is excreted unchanged in urine. No renal dose adjustments are needed (Rybak et al., 2015).

Therapeutic Uses. Isavuconazole exhibits a broad spectrum of activity against most yeast species, including *Candida* species, *Cryptococcus gattii* and *C. neoformans*, and molds such as *Aspergillus* species and *Mucorales* species complex. The drug is approved for the treatment of invasive aspergillosis and invasive mucormycosis and is under investigation for treatment of candidemia and invasive candidiasis.

Dosage. Isavuconazole is dosed as 372 mg isavuconazonium sulfate (equivalent to 200 mg of isavuconazole) every 8 h for six doses followed by 372 mg isavuconazonium sulfate by mouth or intravenously once daily starting 12 to 24 h after the last loading dose.

Adverse Effects. Isavuconazole is generally well tolerated. GI disorders, pyrexia, hypokalemia, headache, constipation, and cough are the most frequently reported adverse effects.

Drug Interactions. Isavuconazole is both a substrate and an inhibitor of CYP3A4. Consequently, a 5-fold increase in isavuconazole AUC results when it is administered with strong CYP inhibitors such as ketoconazole. Substantial reductions in isavuconazole AUC also result from coadministration of isavuconazole with rifampin. Midazolam and sirolimus AUCs are increased by coadministration with isavuconazole. Importantly, isavuconazole does not appear to prolong QTc.

Echinocandins

Echinocandins are cyclic lipopeptides with a hexadepsipeptide nucleus. Three echinocandins are approved for clinical use: caspofungin, anidulafungin, and micafungin. All act through the same mechanism but differ in pharmacological properties. Fungi that are susceptible to echinocandins include *Candida* and *Aspergillus* spp. (Bennett, 2006).

General Pharmacological Characteristics

Mechanism of Action. The echinocandins inhibit 1,3-β-D-glucan synthesis, which is an essential component of the fungal cell wall and is required for in cellular integrity (Figure 61–5).

Antifungal Activity. Echinocandins exhibit fungicidal activity against *Candida* species. In contrast, they are fungistatic against *Aspergillus* species and cause morphological changes to the filaments. Echinocandins do not appear to have clinically useful activity against dimorphic fungi such as *H. capsulatum* and have no activity against *C. neoformans*, *Trichosporon* spp., *Fusarium* spp., or agents of mucormycosis.

Resistance. Echinocandin resistance has emerged as a clinical problem and results from mutations leading to amino acid substitutions in the Fks subunits of glucan synthase (Cowen et al., 2014). Multidrug transporters do not appear to play a role in echinocandin resistance. Mutations conferring resistance occur in two conserved "hot spot" regions of *FKS1* in *C. albicans* and in *FKS1* and *FKS2* in *C. glabrata*. *Candida parapsilosis* complex and *Candida guilliermondii* display reduced in vitro echinocandin susceptibility as compared to other *Candida* species owing to inherently occurring polymorphisms in Fks hot spot regions. Species-specific clinical breakpoints for echinocandins have been recently described.

Echinocandins differ somewhat pharmacokinetically (Table 61–7) but all share extensive protein binding (>97%), inability to penetrate into CSF, lack of renal clearance, and only a slight-to-modest effect of hepatic insufficiency on plasma drug concentrations (Kim et al., 2007; Wagner et al., 2006). Currently available echinocandins also lack oral bioavailability and are available only for intravenous administration. Generally speaking, adverse effects are minimal and rarely lead to drug discontinuation (Kim et al., 2007). All three agents are well tolerated, with the exception of phlebitis at the infusion site. Histamine-like effects have been reported with rapid infusions. All three echinocandins are contraindicated in pregnancy.

Available Agents

Caspofungin. Caspofungin acetate is a water-soluble, semisynthetic lipopeptide synthesized from the fermentation product of *Glarea lozoyensis* (Johnson and Perfect, 2003; Keating and Figgitt, 2003).

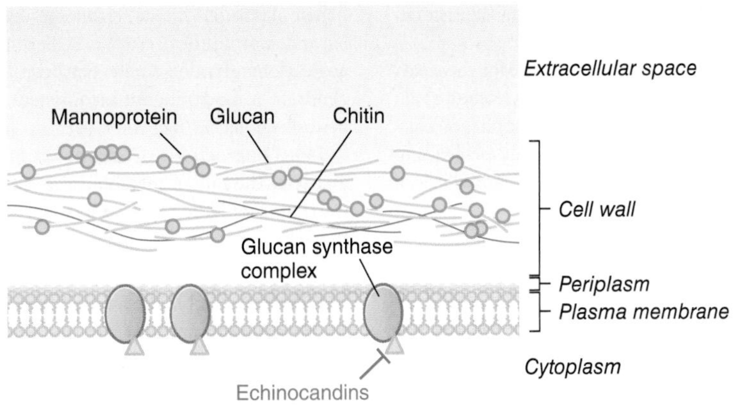

Figure 61–5 *The fungal cell wall and membrane and the action of echinocandins.* The strength of the fungal cell wall is maintained by fibrillar polysaccharides, largely β-1,3-glucan and chitin, which bind covalently to each other and to proteins. A glucan synthase complex in the plasma membrane catalyzes the synthesis of β-1,3-glucan; the glucan is extruded into the periplasm and incorporated into the cell wall. Echinocandins inhibit the activity of the glucan synthase complex, resulting in loss of the structural integrity of the cell wall. The Fks1p subunit of glucan synthase appears to be the target of echinocandins, and mutations in Fks1p cause resistance to echinocandins.

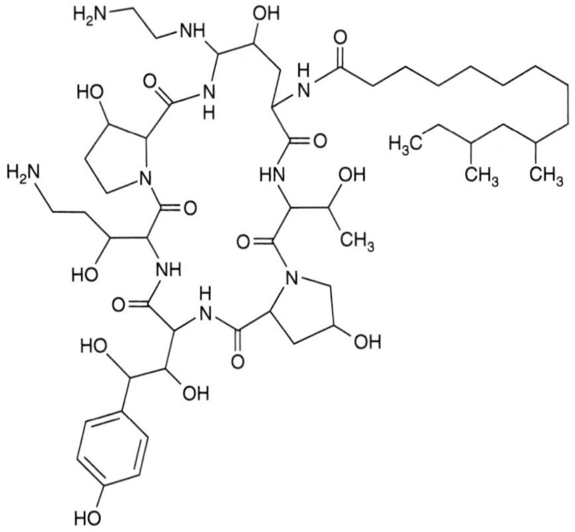

CASPOFUNGIN

ADME. Catabolism is largely by hydrolysis and *N*-acetylation, with excretion of the metabolites in the urine and feces. Mild and moderate hepatic insufficiency increase the AUC by 55% and 76%, respectively.

Therapeutic Use. Caspofungin is approved for the treatment of invasive candidiasis and as salvage therapy for patients with invasive aspergillosis who fail or are intolerant of approved drugs, such as amphotericin B formulations or voriconazole. Caspofungin is also approved for both esophageal and invasive candidiasis (Mora-Duarte et al., 2002; Villanueva et al., 2001) and for treatment of persistently febrile neutropenic patients with suspected fungal infections (Walsh et al., 2004).

Dosage. Caspofungin is administered intravenously once daily over 1 h. For candidemia and salvage therapy of aspergillosis, the initial dose is 70 mg, followed by 50 mg daily. The dose should be increased to 70 mg daily in patients receiving rifampin as well as in those failing to respond to 50 mg. Esophageal candidiasis is treated with 50 mg daily. In moderate hepatic failure, the dose should be reduced to 35 mg daily.

Drug Interactions. Caspofungin increases tacrolimus levels by 16%, which should be managed by standard monitoring. Cyclosporine slightly increases caspofungin levels. Rifampin and other drugs activating CYP3A4 can cause a slight reduction in caspofungin levels.

Micafungin. Micafungin is a water-soluble semisynthetic echinocandin derived from the fungus *Coleophoma empedri*.

ADME; Drug Interactions. Micafungin has linear pharmacokinetics over a large range of doses (1–3 mg/kg) and ages (premature infants to elderly). Small amounts of drug are metabolized in the liver by arylsulfatase and catechol *O*-methyltransferase. Hydroxylation by CYP3A4 is barely detectable. Unlike caspofungin, reduction of the micafungin dose in moderate hepatic failure is not required. Micafungin shows age-dependent clearance in children, with rapid clearance in premature infants and intermediate clearance in children 2–8 years of age, compared to older children and adults.

In normal volunteers, micafungin appears to be a mild inhibitor of CYP3A4, increasing the AUC of nifedipine by 18% and sirolimus by 21%. Micafungin has no effect on tacrolimus clearance.

Therapeutic Uses. Micafungin is approved for the treatment of invasive candidiasis (Fritz et al., 2008) and esophageal candidiasis and for prophylaxis in hematopoietic stem cell transplant recipients.

Dosage. Micafungin is administered intravenously as a 100-mg daily dose over 1 h for adults, with 50 mg recommended for prophylaxis and 150 mg for esophageal candidiasis. No loading dose is required.

Anidulafungin. Anidulafungin is a water-insoluble semisynthetic compound extracted from the fungus *A. nidulans*, from which the drug's name derives.

ADME; Drug Interactions. Anidulafungin is cleared from the body by slow chemical degradation (Vazquez and Sobel, 2006). No hepatic metabolism or renal excretion of active drug occurs; thus, no dose adjustment for hepatic or renal failure is needed. No clinically relevant drug-drug

TABLE 61–7 ■ PK DATA FOR ECHINOCANDINS IN HUMANS

DRUG	DOSE (mg)	C_{max} (µg/mL)	AUC_{0-24h} (mg · h/L)	$t_{1/2}$ (h)	CL (mL/min/kg)	V_d (L)
Caspofungin	70	12	93.5	10	0.15	9.5
Micafungin	75	7.1	59.9	13	0.16	14
Anidulafungin	200	7.5	104.5	25.6	0.16	33.4

For details, see Wagner C, et al. The echinocandins: comparison of their pharmacokinetics, pharmacodynamics and clinical applications. *Pharmacology*, **2006**, 78:161–177.

interactions have been observed with drugs likely to be coadministered with anidulafungin.

Therapeutic Use and Dosing. Anidulafungin is approved for the treatment of candidemia and other forms of *Candida* infections (Reboli et al., 2007), including intra-abdominal abscess, peritonitis, and esophageal candidiasis. For invasive candidiasis, anidulafungin is given daily as a loading dose of 200 mg followed by 100 mg daily. For esophageal candidiasis, a loading dose of 100 mg is followed by 50 mg daily.

Other Systemic Antifungal Agents

Griseofulvin. Griseofulvin is an orally administered, fungistatic antifungal agent originally isolated from the mold *Penicillium griseofulvum*. It is practically insoluble in water.

Mechanism of Action. Griseofulvin inhibits microtubule function and thereby disrupts assembly of the mitotic spindle, which disrupts fungal cell division.

ADME. Blood levels after oral administration of griseofulvin are quite variable. Some studies have shown improved absorption when the drug is taken with a fatty meal. Because the rates of dissolution and disaggregation limit the bioavailability of griseofulvin, microsize and ultramicrosize powders are now used. Griseofulvin has a plasma $t_{1/2}$ of about 1 day; about 50% of the oral dose can be detected in the urine within 5 days, mostly in the form of metabolites. The primary metabolite is methylgriseofulvin. Barbiturates decrease griseofulvin absorption from the GI tract.

Griseofulvin is deposited in keratin precursor cells; when these cells differentiate, the drug is tightly bound to, and persists in, keratin, providing prolonged resistance to fungal invasion. For this reason, the new growth of hair or nails is the first to become free of disease. As the fungus-containing keratin is shed, it is replaced by normal tissue. Griseofulvin is detectable in the stratum corneum of the skin within 4–8 h of oral administration. Sweat and transepidermal fluid loss play an important role in the transfer of the drug in the stratum corneum. Only a very small fraction of a dose of the drug is present in body fluids and tissues.

Antifungal Activity. Griseofulvin is fungistatic in vitro for various species of the dermatophytes *Microsporum*, *Epidermophyton*, and *Trichophyton*. The drug has no effect on other fungi or on bacteria. Although failure of ringworm lesions to improve is not rare, isolates from these patients usually are still susceptible to griseofulvin in vitro.

Therapeutic Uses. Mycotic disease of the skin, hair, and nails due to *Microsporum*, *Trichophyton*, or *Epidermophyton* responds to griseofulvin therapy. For tinea capitis in children, griseofulvin remains the drug of choice for efficacy, safety, and availability as an oral suspension. Efficacy is best for tinea capitis caused by *Microsporum canis*, *Microsporum audouinii*, *Trichophyton schoenleinii*, and *Trichophyton verrucosum*. Griseofulvin is also effective for ringworm of the glabrous skin; tinea cruris and tinea corporis caused by *M. canis*, *Trichophyton rubrum*, *T. verrucosum*, and *Epidermophyton floccosum*; and tinea of the hands (*T. rubrum* and *Trichophyton mentagrophytes*) and beard (*Trichophyton* species). Griseofulvin also is highly effective in the treatment of tinea pedis, the vesicular form of which is most commonly due to *T. mentagrophytes* and the hyperkeratotic type to *T. rubrum*. Topical therapy is sufficient for most cases of tinea pedis. *Trichophyton rubrum* and *T. mentagrophytes* infections may require higher-than-conventional doses of griseofulvin. Treatment must be continued until infected tissue is replaced by normal hair, skin, or nails, which requires 1 month for scalp and hair ringworm, 6–9 months for fingernails, and at least a year for toenails. Itraconazole or terbinafine is much more effective for onychomycosis.

Adverse Effects. The incidence of serious reactions due to griseofulvin is very low: headache (15% of patients), GI and nervous system manifestations, and augmentation of the effects of alcohol. Hepatotoxicity has been observed. Hematological effects include leukopenia, neutropenia, punctate basophilia, and monocytosis; these often disappear despite continued therapy. Blood studies should be carried out at least once a week during the first month of treatment or longer. Common renal effects include albuminuria and cylindruria without evidence of renal insufficiency. Reactions involving the skin are cold and warm urticaria, photosensitivity,

lichen planus, erythema, erythema multiforme–like rashes, and vesicular and morbilliform eruptions. Serum sickness syndromes and severe angioedema develop rarely. Estrogen-like effects have been observed in children. A moderate but inconsistent increase of fecal protoporphyrins has been noted with chronic use.

Drug Interactions. Griseofulvin induces hepatic CYPs and thereby increases the rate of metabolism of warfarin. Consequently, the dose of warfarin should be adjusted in some patients. The drug may also reduce the efficacy of low-estrogen oral contraceptive agents, probably by a similar mechanism.

Terbinafine. Terbinafine is a synthetic allylamine, structurally similar to the topical agent naftifine (see discussion that follows). It inhibits fungal squalene epoxidase and thereby reduces ergosterol biosynthesis.

ADME. Terbinafine is well absorbed, but bioavailability is about 40% due to first-pass metabolism in the liver. The drug accumulates in skin, nails, and fat. The initial $t_{1/2}$ is about 12 h but extends to 200–400 h at steady state. Terbinafine is not recommended in patients with marked azotemia or hepatic failure. Rifampin decreases and cimetidine increases plasma terbinafine concentrations.

Therapeutic Uses. Terbinafine, given as one 250-mg tablet daily for adults, is somewhat more effective than itraconazole for nail onychomycosis. Duration of treatment varies with the site of infection but typically ranges between 6 and 12 weeks. The efficacy for the treatment of onychomycosis can be improved by the simultaneous use of amorolfine 5% nail lacquer (amorolfine is not approved for use in the U.S.). Terbinafine is also effective for the treatment of tinea capitis and has been used for the off-label treatment of ringworm elsewhere on the body.

Adverse Effects. The drug is well tolerated, with a low incidence of GI distress, headache, or rash. Very rarely, fatal hepatotoxicity, severe neutropenia, Stevens-Johnson syndrome, or toxic epidermal necrolysis may occur. Systemic terbinafine therapy for onychomycosis should be postponed until after pregnancy is complete.

Agents Active Against Microsporidia and Pneumocystis

Microsporidia are spore-forming unicellular eukaryotic organisms that were once thought to be parasites but are now classified as fungi (Field and Milner, 2015). They can cause several disease syndromes, including diarrhea in immunocompromised individuals.

Albendazole

Intestinal infections with most microsporidia are treated with albendazole, an inhibitor of α-tubulin polymerization (see Chemotherapy of Helminth Infections, Chapter 55) (Anane and Attouchi, 2010).

Fumagillin

Fumagillin is an acyclic polyene macrolide produced by the fungus *A. fumigatus*. Fumagillin and its synthetic analogue TNP-470 are toxic to microsporidia.

Immunocompromised individuals with intestinal microsporidiosis due to *Enterocytozoon bieneusi* (which does not respond as well to albendazole) can be treated successfully with *fumagillin* (Didier et al., 2005; Rex and Stevens, 2014; Szumowski and Troemel, 2015). For the treatment of intestinal microsporidiosis caused by *E. bieneusi*, fumagillin is used at a dose of 20 mg orally three times daily for 2 weeks (Medical-Letter, 2013; Molina et al., 2002; Rex and Stevens, 2014). Fumagillin is used topically to treat keratoconjunctivitis caused by *Encephalitozoon hellem* at a dose of 3–10 mg/mL in a balanced salt suspension. Adverse effects of fumagillin may include abdominal cramps, nausea, vomiting, and diarrhea. Reversible thrombocytopenia and neutropenia also have been reported (Anane and Attouchi, 2010). Fumagillin is not approved for use in humans in the U.S.

Pentamidine

Pneumocystis jiroveci is another fungus that, until recently, was classified as a protozoan parasite. It is the causative agent of PJP, formerly known as PCP. Pentamidine is one of several drugs or drug combinations used to treat or prevent PJP, which is a major cause of mortality in immunocompromised individuals, including patients with AIDS. Note, however, that *trimethoprim-sulfamethoxazole* is the drug of choice for the treatment and prevention of PJP (see Chapter 56).

Therapy for PJP. Pentamidine as therapy for PJP is reserved for two indications:

- as a 4 mg/kg single daily intravenous dose for 21 days to treat severe PJP in individuals who cannot tolerate trimethoprim-sulfamethoxazole and are not candidates for alternative agent; and
- as a "salvage" agent for individuals with PJP who fail to respond to trimethoprim-sulfamethoxazole (pentamidine may be less effective than the combination of clindamycin and primaquine or atovaquone for this indication) (Gilroy and Bennett, 2011; Rex and Stevens, 2014).

Prophylaxis. Pentamidine administered as an aerosol preparation is used to prevent PJP in at-risk individuals who cannot tolerate trimethoprim-sulfamethoxazole, such as patients with severe bone marrow suppression. For prophylaxis, pentamidine isethionate is given monthly as a 300-mg dose in a 5%–10% nebulized solution over 30–45 min (Gilroy and Bennett, 2011). Aerosolized pentamidine has several disadvantages, including its failure to treat any extrapulmonary sites of *Pneumocystis*, the lack of efficacy against any other potential opportunistic pathogens, and a risk for pneumothorax (Rex and Stevens, 2014).

Topical Antifungal Agents

Topical agents are useful for the treatment of many superficial fungal infections, such as those confined to the stratum corneum, squamous mucosa, or cornea. Examples of infections that respond to topical therapy include dermatophytosis (ringworm), candidiasis, tinea versicolor, piedra, tinea nigra, and fungal keratitis. Preferred formulations for cutaneous application usually are creams or solutions. Ointments are inconvenient and can be too occlusive to the skin, particularly if the affected area is a macerated, fissured, or intertriginous lesion. Antifungal powders, whether applied by shake containers or aerosols, are useful only for lesions of the feet, groin, and similar intertriginous areas. With few exceptions, topical administration of antifungal agents usually is not successful for mycoses of the nails (onychomycosis) and hair (tinea capitis) and should not be used for the treatment of subcutaneous mycoses, such as sporotrichosis and chromoblastomycosis. Regardless of formulation, penetration of topical drugs into hyperkeratotic lesions often is poor. Removal of thick, infected keratin is sometimes a useful adjunct to therapy.

Topical Imidazoles and Triazoles

The imidazoles and triazoles are closely related classes of drugs that are synthetic antifungal agents used both topically and systemically. Indications for their topical use include ringworm, tinea versicolor, and mucocutaneous candidiasis. Resistance to imidazoles or triazoles is rare amongst the fungi that cause ringworm. Selection of one of these agents for topical use should be based on cost and availability because in vitro fungal susceptibility testing does not correlate with clinical responses. The mechanism of action of the azole antifungals was discussed previously in this chapter.

Modes of Administration

Cutaneous Application. The preparations for cutaneous use described in the following material are effective for tinea corporis, tinea pedis, tinea cruris, tinea versicolor, and cutaneous candidiasis. They should be applied twice a day for 3–6 weeks. The cutaneous formulations are not suitable for oral, vaginal, or ocular use.

Vaginal Application. Vaginal creams, suppositories, and tablets for vaginal candidiasis are all used once a day for 1–7 days, preferably at bedtime to facilitate retention. None is useful in trichomoniasis. Most vaginal creams are administered in 5-g amounts. Three vaginal formulations—clotrimazole tablets, miconazole suppositories, and terconazole cream—come in both low- and high-dose preparations. A shorter

duration of therapy is recommended for the higher dose of each. These preparations are administered for 3–7 days. Approximately 3%–10% of the vaginal dose is absorbed. Although some imidazoles are teratogenic in rodents, no adverse effects on the human fetus have been attributed to the vaginal use of imidazoles or triazoles. The most common side effect is vaginal burning or itching. A male sexual partner may experience mild penile irritation.

Oral Use. Use of the oral troche of clotrimazole is properly considered as topical therapy. The only indication for this 10-mg troche is oropharyngeal candidiasis. Antifungal activity is due entirely to the local concentration of the drug; there is no systemic effect.

Individual Agents

Clotrimazole

Absorption of clotrimazole is less than 0.5% after application to the intact skin; from the vagina, it is 3%–10%. Fungicidal concentrations remain in the vagina for as long as 3 days after application of the drug. In adults, an oral dose of 200 mg/d will give rise initially to plasma concentrations of 0.2–0.35 μg/mL, followed by a progressive decline.

In a small fraction of patients, clotrimazole on the skin may cause skin irritation, stinging sensations, erythema, edema, vesication, desquamation, pruritus, or urticaria. When applied to the vagina, about 1.6% of patients experience a mild burning sensation. In rare instances, lower abdominal cramps, a slight increase in urinary frequency, or skin rash may occur. Occasionally, a patient's sexual partner may experience penile or urethral irritation. Oral clotrimazole troches cause GI irritation in about 5% of patients.

Therapeutic Uses. Clotrimazole is available as a 1% cream, lotion, powder, aerosol solution, and solution; 1% or 2% vaginal cream; vaginal tablets of 100, 200, or 500 mg; and 10-mg troches. On the skin, applications are made twice a day. For the vagina, the standard regimens are one 100-mg tablet once a day at bedtime for 7 days, one 200-mg tablet daily for 3 days, one 500-mg tablet inserted only once, or 5 g of cream once a day for 3 days (2% cream) or 7 days (1% cream). For oropharyngeal candidiasis, troches are to be dissolved slowly in the mouth five times a day for 14 days.

Topical clotrimazole cures dermatophyte infections in 60%–100% of cases. The cure rates in cutaneous candidiasis are 80%–100%. In vulvovaginal candidiasis, the cure rate is usually greater than 80% when the 7-day regimen is used. A 3-day regimen of 200 mg once a day appears to be similarly effective, as does single-dose treatment (500 mg). Recurrences are common after all regimens. The cure rate with oral troches for oral and pharyngeal candidiasis may be as high as 100% in the immunocompetent host.

Econazole

Econazole is the deschloro- derivative of miconazole. Econazole readily penetrates the stratum corneum and achieves effective concentrations at the level of the middermis. Approximately 3% of recipients experience local erythema, burning, stinging, or itching. Econazole nitrate is available as a water-miscible cream (1%) to be applied twice a day.

Efinaconazole

Efinaconazole is an azoleamine derivative with excellent in vitro activity against *T. rubrum* and *T. mentagrophytes*. It is available as a 10% topical solution for the treatment of onychomycosis.

Miconazole

Miconazole readily penetrates the stratum corneum of the skin and persists for more than 4 days after application. Adverse effects from topical application to the vagina include burning, itching, or irritation in about 7% of recipients, as well as infrequent pelvic cramps (0.2%), headache, hives, or skin rash. Irritation, burning, and maceration are rare after cutaneous application. Miconazole is considered safe for use during pregnancy, although some experts advocate avoiding vaginal use during the first trimester.

Therapeutic Uses. Miconazole nitrate is available as a 2% cream, ointment, lotion, powder, gel, aerosol powder, and aerosol solution. To avoid maceration, only the lotion should be applied to intertriginous areas. Miconazole is available as a 2% and 4% vaginal cream and as 100-, 200-, or 1200-mg vaginal suppositories to be applied high in the vagina at bedtime for 7, 3, or 1 days, respectively.

In the treatment of tinea pedis, tinea cruris, and tinea versicolor, the cure rate exceeds 90%. In the treatment of vulvovaginal candidiasis, the mycologic cure rate at the end of 1 month is about 80%–95%. Pruritus sometimes is relieved after a single application. Some vaginal infections caused by *C. glabrata* also respond to this drug.

Luliconazole

Luliconazole is available as a 1% cream and is effective for the topical treatment of interdigital tinea pedis, tinea cruris, and tinea corporis caused by susceptible organisms. It should be applied to the affected area once daily for 2 weeks.

Terconazole and Butoconazole

Terconazole is a ketal triazole. The 80-mg vaginal suppository is inserted at bedtime for 3 days; the 0.4% vaginal cream is used for 7 days and the 0.8% cream for 3 days. Clinical efficacy and patient acceptance of both preparations are at least as good as for clotrimazole in patients with vaginal candidiasis.

Butoconazole is an imidazole that is pharmacologically comparable to clotrimazole. Butoconazole nitrate is available as a 2% vaginal cream; it is used at bedtime in nonpregnant females. Because of the slower response during pregnancy, a 6-day course is recommended (during the second and third trimester).

Tioconazole

Tioconazole is an imidazole marketed for treatment of *Candida* vulvovaginitis. A single 4.6-g dose of ointment (300 mg of drug) is given at bedtime.

Oxiconazole, Sulconazole, and Sertaconazole

The imidazole derivatives oxiconazole, sulconazole, and sertaconazole are used for the topical treatment of infections caused by the common pathogenic dermatophytes. Oxiconazole nitrate is available as a 1% cream and lotion; sulconazole nitrate is supplied as a 1% solution or cream. Sertaconazole is a 2% cream marketed for tinea pedis.

Ketoconazole

The imidazole ketoconazole is available as a 0.5% cream, foam, gel, and shampoo for common skin dermatophyte infections, for tinea versicolor, and for seborrheic dermatitis.

Structurally Diverse Antifungal Agents

Ciclopirox Olamine

Ciclopirox olamine has broad-spectrum antifungal activity. It is fungicidal to *C. albicans, E. floccosum, M. canis, T. mentagrophytes,* and *T. rubrum*. It also inhibits the growth of *Malassezia furfur*. Ciclopirox appears to chelate trivalent metal cations and thereby inhibits metal-dependent enzymes required for degradation of peroxides within the fungal cell (Subissi et al., 2010). After application to the skin, it penetrates the epidermis to reach the dermis, but even under occlusion, less than 1.5% is absorbed into the systemic circulation. Furthermore, because the $t_{1/2}$ is 1.7 h, no systemic accumulation occurs. The drug penetrates hair follicles and sebaceous glands. It can sometimes cause hypersensitivity. It is available as a 0.77% cream, gel, suspension, and lotion for the treatment of cutaneous candidiasis and for tinea corporis, cruris, pedis, and versicolor. An 8% nail lacquer is available for onychomycosis. Cure rates in the dermatomycoses and candidal infections are 81%–94%. No topical toxicity has been noted.

Ciclopirox 0.77% gel and 1% shampoo are also used for the treatment of seborrheic dermatitis of the scalp. An 8% topical solution is an effective treatment of mild-to-moderate superficial white onychomycosis.

Haloprogin

Haloprogin is a halogenated phenolic ether. It is fungicidal to various species of *Epidermophyton, Pityrosporum, Microsporum, Trichophyton,* and *Candida*. During treatment with this drug, irritation, pruritus, burning sensations, vesiculation, increased maceration, and "sensitization"

(or exacerbation of the lesion) occasionally occur, especially on the foot if occlusive footgear is worn. Haloprogin is poorly absorbed through the skin; it is metabolized to trichlorophenol in the patient. However, systemic toxicity from topical application appears to be low. Haloprogin cream or solution is applied twice a day for 2–4 weeks. Its principal use is against tinea pedis, for which the cure rate is about 80%; it is thus approximately equal in efficacy to tolnaftate. It also is used against tinea cruris, tinea corporis, tinea manuum, and tinea versicolor. Haloprogin is no longer available in the U.S.

Tolnaftate

Tolnaftate is a thiocarbamate that is effective in the treatment of most cutaneous mycoses caused by *T. rubrum, T. mentagrophytes, Trichophyton tonsurans, E. floccosum, M. canis, M. audouinii, Microsporum gypseum,* and *M. furfur,* but it is ineffective against *Candida*. In tinea pedis, the cure rate is about 80%, compared with about 95% for miconazole. Tolnaftate is available in a 1% concentration as a cream, gel, powder, aerosol powder, topical solution, or a topical aerosol liquid. The preparations are applied locally twice a day. Pruritus is usually relieved in 24–72 h. Involution of interdigital lesions caused by susceptible fungi is very often complete in 7–21 days. Toxic or allergic reactions to tolnaftate have not been reported.

Naftifine

Naftifine is a synthetic allylamine that inhibits squalene-2,3-epoxidase, a key enzyme in the fungal biosynthesis of ergosterol. The drug has broad-spectrum fungicidal activity in vitro. Naftifine hydrochloride is available as a 1% cream or gel. It is effective for the topical treatment of tinea cruris and tinea corporis; twice-daily application is recommended. The drug is well tolerated, although local irritation has been observed in 3% of treated patients. Allergic contact dermatitis also has been reported. Naftifine also may be efficacious for cutaneous candidiasis and tinea versicolor, although the drug is not approved for these uses.

Terbinafine

Like naftifine, terbinafine is an allylamine that targets ergosterol biosynthesis. Terbinafine 1% cream or spray, applied twice daily, is effective in tinea corporis, tinea cruris, and tinea pedis. Terbinafine is less active against *Candida* species and *Malassezia furfur,* but the cream also can be used in cutaneous candidiasis and tinea versicolor.

Butenafine

Butenafine hydrochloride is a benzylamine derivative with a mechanism of action similar to that of terbinafine and naftifine. Its spectrum of antifungal activity and use also are similar to those of the allylamines.

Tavaborole

Tavaborole is an oxaborole antifungal indicated for the topical treatment of onchomycosis of the toenails. The drug inhibits fungal leucyl-tRNA synthetase, thereby inhibiting protein synthesis and ultimately causing fungal cell death.

Nystatin

Nystatin, a tetraene macrolide produced by *Streptomyces noursei*, is structurally similar to amphotericin B and acts through the same mechanism of action. The drug is not absorbed from the GI tract, skin, or vagina. Nystatin is useful only for candidiasis and is supplied in preparations intended for cutaneous, vaginal, or oral administration for this purpose. Infections of the nails and hyperkeratinized or crusted skin lesions do not respond. Powders are preferred for moist lesions such as diaper rash and are applied two to three times daily. Creams or ointments are used twice daily. Combinations of nystatin with antibacterial agents or corticosteroids also are available.

Allergic reactions to nystatin are uncommon. Although vaginal tablets of nystatin are well tolerated, imidazoles or triazoles are more effective agents than nystatin for vaginal candidiasis. Nystatin suspension is usually effective for oral candidiasis of the immunocompetent host and is widely used in neonates and infants for oral thrush. Patients should be instructed to swish the drug around in the mouth and then swallow; otherwise, the patient may expectorate the bitter liquid and fail to treat the infected mucosa in the posterior pharynx or esophagus. Other than the bitter taste and occasional complaints of nausea, adverse effects are uncommon.

Undecylenic Acid

Undecylenic acid is 10-undecenoic acid, an 11-carbon unsaturated compound. It is primarily fungistatic, although fungicidal activity may be observed with long exposure to high concentrations of the agent. The drug is active against a variety of fungi, including those that cause ringworm. Undecylenic acid is available in a cream, powder, spray powder, soap, and liquid. Zinc undecylenate is marketed in combination with other ingredients. The zinc provides an astringent action that aids in the suppression of inflammation. Compounded undecylenic acid ointment contains both undecylenic acid (~5%) and zinc undecylenate (~20%). Calcium undecylenate is available as a powder.

Undecylenic acid preparations are used in the treatment of various dermatomycoses, especially tinea pedis. Concentrations of the acid as high as 10%, as well as those of the acid and salt in the compounded ointment, may be applied to the skin. These preparations are usually not irritating to tissue, and sensitization to them is uncommon. This agent retards fungal growth in tinea pedis, but the infection frequently persists despite intensive treatment with preparations of the acid and the zinc salt. At best, the clinical "cure" rate is about 50%, which is much lower than that obtained with the imidazoles, haloprogin, or tolnaftate. Efficacy in the treatment of tinea capitis is marginal, and the drug is no longer used for that purpose. Undecylenic acid preparations also are approved for use in the treatment of diaper rash, tinea cruris, and other minor dermatologic conditions.

Benzoic and Salicylic Acids

An ointment containing benzoic and salicylic acids in a ratio of 2:1 (usually 6% and 3%) is known as Whitfield ointment. It combines the fungistatic action of benzoate with the keratolytic action of salicylate and is used mainly in the treatment of tinea pedis. Because benzoic acid is only fungistatic, eradication of the infection occurs only after the infected stratum corneum is shed; thus, continuous medication is required for several weeks to months. The salicylic acid accelerates desquamation. The ointment also is sometimes used to treat tinea capitis. Mild irritation may occur at the site of application.

Acknowledgment: *John E. Bennett contributed to this chapter in previous editions of this book. We have retained some of his text in the current edition.*

Drug Facts For Your Personal Formulary: *Antifungal Agents*

Drugs	Therapeutic Uses	Clinical Pharmacology and Tips
Polyenes: Interact with ergosterol in the fungal cell membrane		
Amphotericin B deoxycholate (C-AMB)	• Invasive candidiasis • Invasive aspergillosis • Blastomycosis • Histoplasmosis • Coccidioidomycosis • Cryptococcosis • Mucormycosis • Sporotrichosis • Empirical therapy in the immunocompromised host	• Associated with significant nephrotoxicity, including azotemia, renal tubular acidosis, and hypochromic, normocytic anemia • Associated with acute reactions, including infusion-related fever and chills • C-AMB is better tolerated by premature neonates than by older children and adults
Amphotericin B colloidal dispersion (ABCD) (not available in the U.S.) Liposomal amphotericin B (L-AMB) Amphotericin B lipid complex (ABLC)		• All three amphotericin B lipid formulations are less nephrotoxic than C-AMB. • Infusion-related reactions are highest with ABCD and lowest with L-AMB.
Pyrimidines: Disrupt fungal RNA and DNA synthesis		
Flucytosine	• Cryptococcosis (with amphotericin B)	• Has broad activity but emergence of resistance limits usefulness as single-agent therapy • ↓ Dosage in patients with ↓ renal function • Toxicity more frequent in patients with AIDS or azotemia • Flucytosine may depress bone marrow, lead to leukopenia and thrombocytopenia
Imidazoles and Triazoles: Inhibit ergosterol biosynthesis		
Ketoconazole		
Itraconazole	• Invasive aspergillosis • Blastomycosis • Coccidioidomycosis • Histoplasmosis • Pseudallescheriasis • Sporotrichosis • Ringworm • Onychomycosis	• Substrate for and potent inhibitor of CYP3A4 • Hepatotoxic • Contraindicated in pregnancy and in women considering becoming pregnant

Drug Facts For Your Personal Formulary: *Antifungal Agents* (*continued*)

Drugs	Therapeutic Uses	Clinical Pharmacology and Tips
Imidazoles and Triazoles: Inhibit ergosterol biosynthesis		
Fluconazole	• Invasive candidiasis • Cryptococcosis • Coccidioidomycosis • Prophylaxis and empirical therapy in immunocompromised host	• Plasma concentrations are essentially the same whether the drug is given orally or intravenously. • Concentrations in CSF = 50%–90% of C_p • Inhibitor of CYP3A4 and CYP2C9 • Contraindicated during pregnancy
Voriconazole	• Invasive aspergillosis • Invasive candidiasis • Pseudallescheriasis	• Oral bioavailability is 96%. • Monitor C_p; serum levels of 1 to 5 mg/L maximize efficacy and minimize toxicity • Metabolized by and inhibits CYPs (2C19 > 2C9 > 3A4) • Can prolong the QTc interval • Transient visual or auditory hallucinations are frequent after the first dose. • Contraindicated in pregnancy
Posaconazole	• Oropharyngeal candidiasis • Prophylaxis in the immuno-compromised host against aspergillosis and candidiasis	• Oral bioavailability enhanced by food • Drugs that ↓ gastric acid ↓ posaconazole exposure • Inhibits CYP3A4 • Can prolong the QTc interval • Adverse effects: headache and GI disorders
Isavuconazole (isavuconazonium prodrug)	• Invasive aspergillosis • Mucormycosis	• Oral bioavailability is 98%. • Substrate of and inhibitor of CYP3A4 • Does not appear to prolong QTc
Echinocandins: Inhibit 1,3-β -D-glucan synthesis in the fungal cell wall		
Caspofungin	• Invasive candidiasis • Empirical therapy in the immunocompromised host	• ↓ Dose in moderate hepatic impairment
Micafungin	• Invasive candidiasis • Prophylaxis in the immuno-compromised host	• Reduction of micafungin dose in moderate hepatic failure is not required.
Anidulafungin	• Invasive candidiasis	• No dose adjustment is needed for hepatic or renal failure.
Griseofulvin: Inhibits microtubule function, disrupts assembly of the mitotic spindle		
Griseofulvin	• Ringworm • Onychomycosis	• Absorption is reduced by barbiturates • Induces hepatic CYPs
Allylamines: Inhibit fungal squalene epoxidase and reduce ergosterol biosynthesis		
Terbinafine	• Ringworm • Onychomycosis	• Bioavailability is ~ 40% due to first-pass metabolism in the liver. • The drug accumulates in skin, nails, and fat. • The initial $t_{1/2}$ is ~ 12 h but extends to 200–400 h at steady state.
Agents Active Against Microsporidia and *Pneumocystis*		
Albendazole	• Microsporidia infection	• Anthelmintic • Inhibitor of α-tubulin polymerization
Fumagillin	• Microsporidia infection	• Used in immunocompromised individuals with intestinal microsporidiosis due to *Enterocytozoon bieneusi* unresponsive to albendazole • Not approved for human use in the U.S.
Trimethoprim-sulfamethoxazole	• *Pneumocystis jiroveci* pneumonia	• See Chapter 56
Pentamidine	• *Pneumocystis jiroveci* pneumonia	• Prophylaxis use to prevent PJP in at-risk individuals who cannot tolerate trimethoprim-sulfamethoxazole
Topical Antifungal Agents		
Imidazoles and Triazoles Clotrimazole, miconazole, ketoconazole, etc.	• Dermatophytosis (ringworm), candidiasis, tinea versicolor, piedra, tinea nigra, and fungal keratitis	• Available for cutaneous application as creams or solutions • Some are available as vaginal creams or suppositories or as oral troches
Tavaborole	Toenail onychomycosis due to *T. rubrum* or *T. mentagrophytes*	• Apply daily for 48 weeks

Bibliography

Anane S, Attouchi H. Microsporidiosis: epidemiology, clinical data and therapy. *Gastroenterol Clin Biol*, **2010**, *34*:450–464.

Anderson TM, et al. Amphotericin forms an extramembranous and fungicidal sterol sponge. *Nat Chem Biol*, **2014**, *10*:400–406.

Autmizguine J, et al. Pharmacokinetics and pharmacodynamics of antifungals in children: clinical implications. *Drugs*, **2014**, *74*:891–909.

Barrett JP, et al. A systematic review of the antifungal effectiveness and tolerability of amphotericin B formulations. *Clin Ther*, **2003**, *25*: 1295–1320.

Bennett JE. Echinocandins for candidemia in adults without neutropenia. *N Engl J Med*, **2006**, *355*:1154–1159.

Boswell GW, et al. AmBisome (liposomal amphotericin B): a comparative review. *J Clin Pharmacol*, **1998**, *38*:583–592.

Bowden R, et al. A double-blind, randomized, controlled trial of amphotericin B colloidal dispersion versus amphotericin B for treatment of invasive aspergillosis in immunocompromised patients. *Clin Infect Dis*, **2002**, *35*:359–366.

Brown GD, et al. Hidden killers: human fungal infections. *Sci Transl Med*, **2012**, *4*:165rv13.

Carlson MA, Condon RE. Nephrotoxicity of amphotericin B. *J Am Coll Surg*, **1994**, *179*:361–381.

Courtney R, et al. Effect of food on the relative bioavailability of posaconazole in healthy adults. *Br J Clin Pharmacol*, **2003**, *57*:218–222.

Cowen LE, et al. Mechanisms of antifungal drug resistance. *Cold Spring Harb Perspect Med*, **2014**, *5*:pii:a019752.

Day JN, et al. Combination antifungal therapy for cryptococcal meningitis. *N Engl J Med*, **2013**, *368*:1291–1302.

Didier ES, et al. Therapeutic strategies for human microsporidia infections. *Expert Rev Anti Infect Ther*, **2005**, *3*:419–434.

Dodgson AR, et al. Clade-specific flucytosine resistance is due to a single nucleotide change in the *FUR1* gene of *Candida albicans*. *Antimicrob Agents Chemother*, **2004**, *48*:2223–2227.

Evans EG, Sigurgeirsson B. Double blind, randomised study of continuous terbinafine compared with intermittent itraconazole in treatment of toenail onychomycosis. The LION Study Group. *BMJ*, **1999**, *318*:1031–1035.

Field AS, Milner DA. Intestinal microsporidiosis. *Clin Lab Med*, **2015**, *35*:445–459.

Frampton JE, Scott LJ. Posaconazole. A review of its use in the prophylaxis of invasive fungal infections. *Drugs*, **2008**, *68*:99–1016.

Fritz JM, et al. Micafungin for the prophylaxis and treatment of *Candida* infections. *Expert Rev Anti Infect Ther*, **2008**, *6*:153–162.

Geber A, et al. Deletion of the *Candida glabrata ERG3* and *ERG11* genes: effect on cell viability, cell growth, sterol composition, and antifungal susceptibility. *Antimicrob Agents Chemother*, **1995**, *39*:2708–2717.

Gilroy SA, Bennett NJ. *Pneumocystis* pneumonia. *Semin Respir Crit Care Med*, **2011**, *32*:775–782.

Guarascio AJ, Slain D. Review of the new delayed-release oral tablet and intravenous dosage forms of posaconazole. *Pharmacotherapy*, **2015**, *35*:208–219.

Hamill RJ. Amphotericin B formulations: a comparative review of efficacy and toxicity. *Drugs*, **2013**, *73*:919–934.

Herbrecht R, et al. Voriconazole versus amphotericin B for primary therapy of invasive aspergillosis. *N Engl J Med*, **2002**, *347*:408–415.

Hull CM, et al. Facultative sterol uptake in an ergosterol-deficient clinical isolate of *Candida glabrata* harboring a missense mutation in *ERG11* and exhibiting cross-resistance to azoles and amphotericin B. *Antimicrob Agents Chemother*, **2012**, *56*:4223–4232.

Johnson MD, Perfect JR. Caspofungin: first approved agent in a new class of antifungals. *Expert Opin Pharmacother*, **2003**, *4*:807–823.

Kanafani ZA, Perfect JR. Resistance to antifungal agents: mechanisms and clinical impact. *Clin Infect Dis*, **2008**, *46*:120–128.

Keating G, Figgitt D. Caspofungin: a review of its use in oesophageal candidiasis, invasive candidiasis and invasive aspergillosis. *Drugs*, **2003**, *63*:2235–2263.

Kim R, et al. A comparative evaluation of properties and clinical efficacy of the echinocandins. *Expert Opin Pharmacother*, **2007**, *8*: 1479–1492.

Krieter P, et al. Disposition of posaconazole following single-dose oral administration in healthy subjects. *Antimicrob Agents Chemother*, **2004**, *48*:3543–3551.

Krishna G, et al. Effects of oral posaconazole on the pharmacokinetics properties of oral and intravenous midazolam: a phase 1, randomized, open-label, crossover study in healthy volunteers. *Clin Ther*, **2009**, *31*:286–298.

Kullberg BJ, et al. Voriconazole versus a regimen of amphotericin B followed by fluconazole for candidaemia in non-neutropenic patients: a randomized non-inferiority trial. *Lancet*, **2005**, *366*:1435–1442.

Martel CM, et al. Identification and characterization of four azole-resistant erg3 mutants of *Candida albicans*. *Antimicrob Agents Chemother*, **2010**, *54*:4527–4533.

Medical-Letter. Drugs for parasitic infections. *Med Lett Drugs Ther*, **2013**, *11*:e1–e31.

Mølgaard-Nielsen D, et al. Use of oral fluconazole during pregnancy and the risk of birth defects. *N Engl J Med*, **2013**, *369*:830–839.

Molina JM, et al. Fumagillin treatment of intestinal microsporidiosis. *N Engl J Med*, **2002**, *346*:1963–1969.

Mora-Duarte J, et al. Comparison of caspofungin and amphotericin B for invasive candidiasis. *N Engl J Med*, **2002**, *347*:2020–2029.

Moton A, et al. Effects of oral posaconazole on the pharmacokinetics of serolimus. *Curr Med Res Opin*, **2009**, *25*:701–707.

Neofytos D, et al. Administration of voriconazole in patients with renal dysfunction. *Clin Infect Dis*, **2012**, *54*:913–921.

Pappas PG, et al. Micafungin versus caspofungin for treatment of candidemia and other forms of invasive candidiasis. *Clin Infect Dis*, **2007**, *45*:883–893.

Perfect JR, et al. Clinical practice guidelines for the management of cryptococcal disease: 2010 update by the Infectious Diseases Society of America. *Clin Infect Dis*, **2010**, *50*:291–322.

Reboli AC, et al. Anidulafungin versus fluconazole for invasive candidiasis. *N Engl J Med*, **2007**, *356*:2472–2482.

Rex JH, Stevens DA. Drugs active against fungi, pneumocystis, and microsporidia. In: Mandell GL, et al., eds. *Principles and Practice of Infectious Diseases*. 8th ed. Churchill Livingstone, New York, **2014**, 479–494.

Rex JH, et al. A randomized trial comparing fluconazole with amphotericin B for the treatment of candidemia in patients without neutropenia. Candidemia Study Group and the National Institute. *N Engl J Med*, **1994**, *331*:1325–1330.

Richardson MR. Changing patterns and trends in systemic fungal infections. *J Antimicrob Chemother*, **2005**, *56*(suppl):S5–S11.

Roemer T, Krysan DJ. Antifungal drug development: challenges, unmet clinical needs, and new approaches. *Cold Spring Harb Perspect Med*, **2014**, *4*:a019703.

Rogers PD, et al. Amphotericin B activation of human genes encoding for cytokines. *J Infect Dis*, **1998**, *178*:1726–1733.

Rybak JM, et al. Isavuconazole: pharmacology, pharmacodynamics and current clinical experience with a new triazole antifungal agent. *Pharmacotherapy*, **2015**, *35*:1037–1051.

Salez F, et al. Effects of itraconazole therapy in allergic bronchopulmonary aspergillosis. *Chest*, **1999**, *116*:1665–1668.

Sau K, et al. The antifungal drug amphotericin B promotes inflammatory cytokine release by a Toll-like receptor- and CD14-dependent mechanism. *J Biol Chem*, **2003**, *278*:37561–37568.

Slain D. Lipid-based amphotericin B for the treatment of fungal infections. *Pharmacotherapy*, **1999**, *19*:306–323.

Smith WJ, et al. Posaconazole's impact on prophylaxis and treatment of invasive fungal infections: an update. *Expert Rev Anti Infective Ther*, **2009**, *7*:165–181.

Steinbach WJ, et al. In vitro analyses, animal models, and 60 clinical cases of invasive *Aspergillus terreus* infection. *Antimicrob Agents Chemother*, **2004**, *48*:3217–3225.

Subissi A, et al. Ciclopirox: recent nonclinical and clinical data relevant to its use as a topical antimycotic agent. *Drugs*, **2010**, *70*:2133–2152.

Szumowski SC, Troemel ER. Microsporidia-host interactions. *Curr Opin Microbiol*, **2015**, *26*:10–16.

Ullmann AJ, et al. Posaconazole or fluconazole for prophylaxis in severe graft-versus-host disease. *N Engl J Med*, **2007**, *356*:335–347.

1104 Vazquez JA, Sobel JD. Anidulafungin: a novel echinocandin. *Clin Infect Dis,* **2006**, *43*:215–222.

Villanueva A, et al. A randomized double-blind study of caspofungin versus amphotericin for the treatment of candidal esophagitis. *Clin Infect Dis,* **2001**, *33*:1529–1535.

Wagner C, et al. The echinocandins: comparison of their pharmacokinetics, pharmacodynamics and clinical applications. *Pharmacology,* **2006**, *78*: 161–177.

Walsh TJ, et al. Caspofungin versus liposomal amphotericin B for empirical antifungal therapy in patients with persistent fever and neutropenia. *N Engl J Med,* **2004**, *351*:1391–1402.

Walsh TJ, et al. for the National Institute of Allergy and Infectious Diseases Mycoses Study Group. Voriconazole compared with liposomal amphotericin B for empirical antifungal therapy in patients with neutropenia and persistent fever. *N Engl J Med,* **2002**, *346*:225–234.

White MH, et al. Randomized, double-blind clinical trial of amphotericin B colloidal dispersion vs. amphotericin B in the empirical treatment of fever and neutropenia. *Clin Infect Dis,* **1998**, *27*:296–302.

Wingard JR, et al. A randomized, double-blind comparative trial evaluating the safety of liposomal amphotericin B versus amphotericin B lipid complex in the empirical treatment of febrile neutropenia. *Clin Infect Dis,* **2000**, *31*:1155–1163.

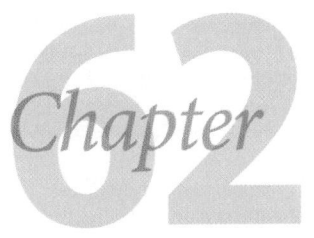

Antiviral Agents (Nonretroviral)

Edward P. Acosta

Most antivirals currently available in the U.S. have been developed and approved in the last 25 years. This flurry of activity was driven by successes in rational drug design and approval that began with the antiherpesvirus nucleoside analogue acyclovir (Elion, 1986), whose discovery and development resulted in the awarding of a Nobel Prize to Gertrude Elion and George Hitchings in 1988. Because viruses are obligatory intracellular microorganisms and rely on host biosynthetic machinery to reproduce, there were doubts about the possibility of developing antiviral drugs with selective toxicity, but those doubts have long been erased. Viruses are now obvious targets for effective antimicrobial chemotherapy, and it is certain that the number of available agents in this category will continue to increase. Indeed, the recent development of agents that target the viral protein NS5A has revolutionized treatment of infections of HVB and HVC, and these agents are now allotted a chapter of their own, Chapter 63. Chapter 64 describes chemotherapy for retroviruses. This present chapter covers antiviral agents for nonretroviral infections other than HVB and HVC.

Viral Replication and Drug Targets

Viruses are simple microorganisms that consist of either double- or single-stranded DNA or RNA enclosed in a protein coat called a *capsid*. Some viruses also possess a lipid envelope derived from the infected host cell, which, like the capsid, may contain antigenic glycoproteins. Effective antiviral agents inhibit virus-specific replicative events or preferentially inhibit *virus-directed rather than host cell–directed* nucleic acid or protein synthesis (Table 62–1). Host cell molecules that are essential to viral replication also offer targets for intervention. Figure 62–1 gives a schematic diagram of the replicative cycle of typical DNA and RNA viruses with the sites of anti-viral drugs indicated.

DNA viruses include poxviruses (smallpox), herpesviruses (chickenpox, shingles, oral and genital herpes); adenoviruses (conjunctivitis, sore throat); hepadnaviruses (HBV); and papillomaviruses (warts). Most DNA viruses enter the host cell nucleus, where the viral DNA is transcribed into mRNA by host cell polymerase; mRNA is translated in the usual host cell fashion into virus-specific proteins. Poxviruses are an exception; they carry their own RNA polymerase and replicate in the host cell cytoplasm.

For RNA viruses, the replication strategy either relies on enzymes in the virion to synthesize mRNA or has the viral RNA serving as its own mRNA. The mRNA is translated into various viral proteins, including RNA polymerase, which directs the synthesis of more viral mRNA and genomic RNA. Most RNA viruses complete their replication in the host cell cytoplasm, but some, such as influenza, are transcribed in the host cell nucleus. Examples of RNA viruses include rubella virus (German measles); rhabdoviruses (rabies); picornaviruses (poliomyelitis, meningitis, colds, hepatitis A); arenaviruses (meningitis, Lassa fever); flaviviruses (West Nile meningoencephalitis, yellow fever, hepatitis C, Zika virus); orthomyxoviruses (influenza); paramyxoviruses (measles, mumps); and coronaviruses (colds, SARS). Retroviruses are RNA viruses that include HIV; chemotherapy for retroviruses is described in Chapter 64. Pharmacotherapy of viral hepatitis is covered separately in Chapter 63.

Table 62–2 summarizes currently approved drugs for nonretroviral infections, excluding those for viral hepatitis. Their pharmacological properties are presented in the material that follows, class by class, as listed in the table.

Antiherpesvirus Agents

Herpes simplex virus type 1 typically causes diseases of the mouth, face, skin, esophagus, or brain. HSV-2 usually causes infections of the genitals, rectum, skin, hands, or meninges. Both cause serious infections in neonates. Agents used in treating HSV work by several mechanisms to inhibit viral DNA replication in the host cell (Figure 62–1; Table 62–1).

Acyclovir and Valacyclovir

Acyclovir is an acyclic guanine nucleoside analogue that lacks the 2′ and 3′ positions normally supplied by ribose. Valacyclovir is the L-valyl ester prodrug of acyclovir. Acyclovir is the prototype of a group of antiviral agents that are nucleoside congeners (see Figure 62–2) that are phosphorylated intracellularly by a viral kinase and subsequently by host cell enzymes to become inhibitors of viral DNA synthesis. Related agents include penciclovir and ganciclovir.

Mechanisms of Action and Resistance

Acyclovir inhibits viral DNA synthesis via a mechanism outlined in Figure 62–3. Its selectivity of action depends on interaction with HSV *TK (thymidine kinase)* and *DNA polymerase*. The initial phosphorylation of acyclovir is facilitated by HSV TK and thus occurs only in cells infected with the virus. The affinity of acyclovir for HSV TK is about 200 times

Abbreviations

ADME: absorption, distribution, metabolism, excretion
AIDS: acquired immune deficiency syndrome
AUC: area under the curve
CAPD: chronic ambulatory peritoneal dialysis
CDC: Centers for Disease Control and Prevention
cDNA: complementary DNA
CL$_{cr}$: creatinine clearance
CMV: cytomegalovirus
CNS: central nervous system
C$_p$: plasma concentration (of a drug, usually)
cRNA: complementary RNA
CSF: cerebrospinal fluid
CYP: cytochrome P450 isozyme
DNAp: DNA polymerase
EBV: Epstein-Barr virus
EIND: emergency investigational new drug
FDA: Food and Drug Administration
G-CSF: granulocyte colony-stimulating factor
GI: gastrointestinal
HBV: hepatitis B virus
HCV: hepatitis c virus
HHV-6: human herpesvirus 6
HIV: human immunodeficiency virus
HSV: herpes simplex virus
IFN: interferon
mRNA: messenger RNA
NSAID: nonsteroidal anti-inflammatory drug
RNAp: RNA polymerase
RNP: ribonuclear protein
SARS: severe acute respiratory syndrome
TK: thymidine kinase
vRNA: viral RNA
VZV: varicella zoster virus

TABLE 62–1 ■ STAGES OF VIRUS REPLICATION AND POSSIBLE TARGETS OF ACTION OF ANTIVIRAL AGENTS

STAGE OF REPLICATION	CLASSES OF SELECTIVE INHIBITORS
Cell entry Attachment Penetration	Soluble receptor decoys, antireceptor antibodies, fusion protein inhibitors
Uncoating Release of viral genome	Ion channel blockers, capsid stabilizers
Transcription of viral genome[a] Transcription of viral mRNA Replication of viral genome	Inhibitors of viral DNA polymerase, RNA polymerase, reverse transcriptase, helicase, primase, or integrase
Translation of viral proteins Regulatory proteins (early) Structural proteins (late)	Interferons, antisense oligonucleotides, ribozymes, Inhibitors of regulatory proteins
Posttranslational modifications Proteolytic cleavage Myristoylation, glycosylation	Protease inhibitors
Assembly of virion components	Interferons, assembly protein inhibitors
Release Budding, cell lysis	Neuraminidase inhibitors, antiviral antibodies, cytotoxic lymphocytes

[a]Depends on specific replication strategy of virus, but virus-specified enzyme required for part of process.

greater than for the mammalian enzyme. Cellular enzymes convert the monophosphate to acyclovir triphosphate, which competes for endogenous dGTP. The immunosuppressive agent mycophenolate mofetil (see Chapter 35) potentiates the antiherpes activity of acyclovir and related agents by depleting intracellular dGTP pools. Acyclovir triphosphate competitively inhibits viral DNA polymerases and, to a much lesser extent, cellular DNA polymerases. Acyclovir triphosphate also is incorporated into viral DNA, where it acts as a chain terminator because of the lack of a 3′-hydroxyl group. By a mechanism termed *suicide inactivation*, the terminated DNA template containing acyclovir binds the viral DNA polymerase and leads to its irreversible inactivation.

Acyclovir resistance in HSV can result from impaired production of viral TK, altered TK substrate specificity (e.g., phosphorylation of thymidine but not acyclovir), or altered viral DNA polymerase. Alterations in viral enzymes are caused by point mutations and base insertions or deletions in the corresponding genes. Resistant variants are present in native virus populations and in isolates from treated patients. The most common resistance mechanism in clinical HSV isolates is absent or deficient viral TK activity; viral DNA polymerase mutants are rare. Phenotypic resistance typically is defined by in vitro inhibitory concentrations of more than 2–3 μg/mL, which predict failure of therapy in immunocompromised patients. Acyclovir resistance in VZV isolates is caused by mutations in VZV TK and less often by mutations in viral DNA polymerase.

ADME

The oral bioavailability of acyclovir is about 10%–30% and decreases with increasing dose (Wagstaff et al., 1994). Delivery of an oral dose can be enhanced by administration of the the prodrug form, valacyclovir. Valacyclovir is an esterified version with higher bioavailability (55%–70%) than acyclovir (Steingrimsdottir et al., 2000); deesterification occurs rapidly and nearly completely following oral administration. Unlike acyclovir, valacyclovir is a substrate for intestinal and renal peptide transporters. Acyclovir distributes widely in body fluids, including vesicular fluid, aqueous humor, and CSF. Compared with plasma, salivary concentrations are low, and concentrations in vaginal secretion vary widely. Acyclovir is concentrated in breast milk, amniotic fluid, and placenta. Newborn plasma levels are similar to maternal ones. Percutaneous absorption of acyclovir after topical administration is low. Renal excretion of unmetabolized acyclovir by glomerular filtration and tubular secretion is the principal route of elimination. The elimination $t_{1/2}$ of acyclovir is about 2.5 h (range 1.5–6 h) in adults with normal renal function. In neonates, the elimination $t_{1/2}$ of acyclovir is about 4 h and increases to 20 h in anuric patients.

Therapeutic Uses

Acyclovir's clinical use is limited to herpesviruses. Acyclovir is most active against HSV-1 (effective C_p range: 0.02–0.9 μg/mL), approximately half as active against HSV-2 (0.03–2.2 μg/mL), a tenth as potent against VZV (0.8–4.0 μg/mL) and EBV, and least active against CMV (generally > 20 μg/mL) and HHV-6. Uninfected mammalian cell growth generally is unaffected by high acyclovir concentrations (> 50 μg/mL).

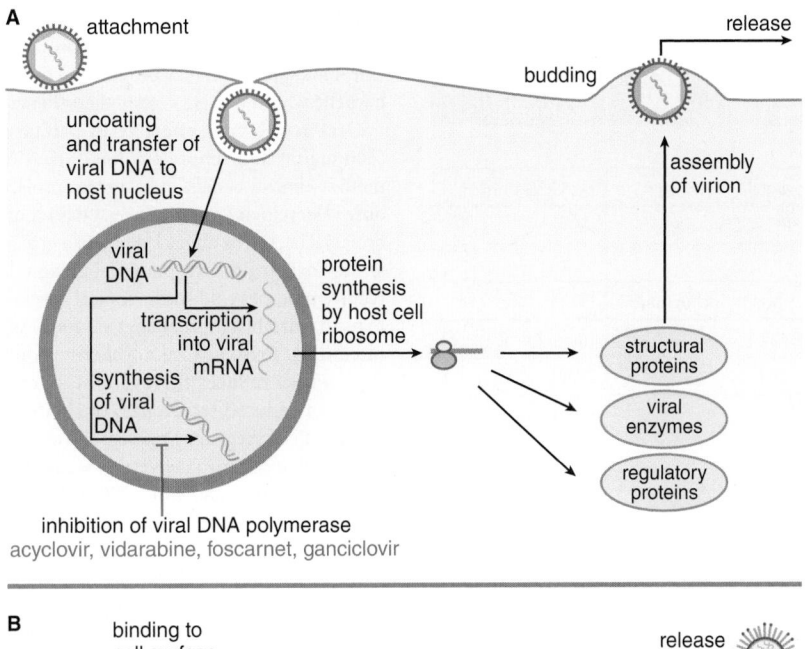

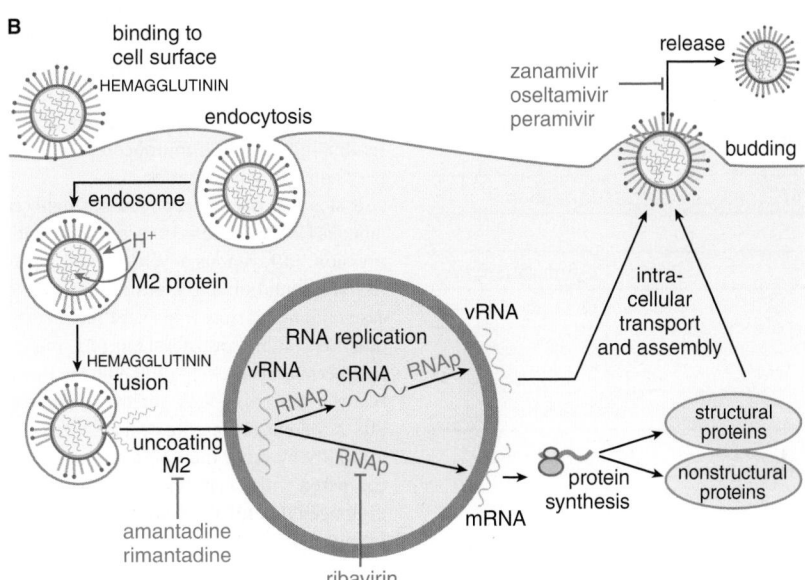

Figure 62–1 *Replicative cycles of DNA (**A**) and RNA (**B**) viruses.* The replicative cycles of herpesvirus (**A**) and influenza (**B**) are examples of DNA-encoded and RNA-encoded viruses, respectively. Sites of action of antiviral agents also are shown. The symbol ⊢ indicates a block to virus growth. **A.** *Replicative cycles of herpes simplex virus, a DNA virus, and the probable sites of action of antiviral agents.* Herpesvirus replication is a regulated multistep process. After infection, a small number of immediate-early genes are transcribed; these genes encode proteins that regulate their own synthesis and are responsible for synthesis of early genes involved in genome replication, such as TKs, DNA polymerases, and so on. After DNA replication, the bulk of the herpesvirus genes (called late genes) are expressed and encode proteins that either are incorporated into or aid in the assembly of progeny virions. **B.** *Replicative cycles of influenza, an RNA virus, and the loci for effects of antiviral agents.* The mammalian cell shown is an airway epithelial cell. The M2 protein of influenza virus allows an influx of hydrogen ions into the virion interior, which in turn promotes dissociation of the RNP segments and release into the cytoplasm (uncoating). Influenza virus mRNA synthesis requires a primer cleared from cellular mRNA and used by the viral RNAp complex. The neuraminidase inhibitors zanamivir and oseltamivir specifically inhibit release of progeny virus.

In immunocompetent persons, the clinical benefits of acyclovir and valacyclovir are greater in initial HSV infections than in recurrent ones. These drugs are particularly useful in immunocompromised patients because these individuals experience both more frequent and more severe HSV and VZV infections. Because VZV is less susceptible than HSV to acyclovir, higher doses must be used for treating VZV infections. Oral valacyclovir is as effective as oral acyclovir in HSV infections and more effective for treating herpes zoster. Acyclovir is ineffective therapeutically in established CMV infections, but ganciclovir is effective for CMV prophylaxis in immunocompromised patients. EBV-related oral hairy leukoplakia may improve with acyclovir.

Oral acyclovir in conjunction with systemic corticosteroids appears beneficial in treating Bell palsy; valacyclovir is ineffective in acute vestibular neuritis.

Herpes Simplex Virus Infections. In initial genital HSV infections, oral acyclovir (200 mg five times daily or 400 mg three times daily for 7–10 days) and valacyclovir (1000 mg twice daily for 7–10 days) are associated with significant reductions in virus shedding, symptoms, and time to healing (Kimberlin and Rouse, 2004). Intravenous acyclovir (5 mg/kg every 8 h) has similar effects in patients hospitalized with severe primary genital HSV infections. Topical acyclovir is much less effective than systemic

TABLE 62–2 ■ NOMENCLATURE OF ANTIVIRAL AGENTS

GENERIC NAME	OTHER NAMES	DOSAGE FORMS AVAILABLE
Antiherpesvirus agents		
Acyclovir	ACV, acycloguanosine	IV, O, T, ophth[a]
Cidofovir	HPMPC, CDV	IV
Famciclovir	FCV	O
Foscarnet	PFA, phosphonoformate	IV, O[a]
Fomivirsena	ISIS 2922	Intravitreal
Ganciclovir	GCV, DHPG	IV, O, intravitreal
Idoxuridine	IDUR	Ophth
Penciclovir	PCV	T, IV[a]
Trifluridine	TFT, trifluorothymidine	Ophth
Valacyclovir		O
Valganciclovir		O
Anti-influenza agents		
Amantadine		O
Oseltamivir	GS4104	O
Peramivir	BCX 1812	IV
Rimantadine		O
Zanamivir	GC167	Inhalation
Other antiviral agents		
Ribavirin		O, inhalation, IV
Telbivudine		O
Tenofovir disoproxil fumarate	TDF	O
Imiquimod		Topical

[a]Not currently approved for use in the U.S.

O, oral; ophth, ophthalmic; IV, intravenous; T, topical.

administration. None of these regimens reproducibly reduces the risk of recurrent genital lesions. Acyclovir (200 mg five times daily or 400 mg three times daily for 5 days or 800 mg three times daily for 2 days) or valacyclovir (500 mg twice daily for 3 or 5 days) shortens the manifestations of recurrent genital HSV episodes by 1–2 days. Frequently recurring genital herpes can be suppressed effectively with chronic oral acyclovir (400 mg twice daily or 200 mg three times daily) or with valacyclovir (500 mg or, for very frequent recurrences, 1000 mg once daily). During use, the rate of clinical recurrences decreases by about 90%, and subclinical shedding is markedly reduced, although not eliminated. Valacyclovir suppression

of genital herpes reduces the risk of transmitting infection to a susceptible partner by about 50% over an 8-month period (Corey et al., 2004). Chronic suppression may be useful in those with disabling recurrences of herpetic whitlow or HSV-related erythema multiforme.

Oral acyclovir is effective in primary herpetic gingivostomatitis (600 mg/m[2] four times daily for 10 days in children) but provides only modest clinical benefit in recurrent orolabial herpes. Short-term, high-dose valacyclovir (2 g twice over 1 day) shortens the duration of recurrent orolabial herpes by about 1 day (Elish et al., 2004). The FDA has approved an acyclovir/hydrocortisone combination (Lipsovir) for early treatment of recurrent herpes cold sores. Topical acyclovir cream is modestly effective in recurrent labial (Spruance et al., 2002) and genital herpes simplex virus infections. Preexposure acyclovir prophylaxis (400 mg twice daily for 1 week) reduces the overall risk of recurrence by 73% in those with sun-induced recurrences of HSV infections. Acyclovir during the last month of pregnancy reduces the likelihood of viral shedding and the frequency of cesarean delivery in women with primary or recurrent genital herpes (Corey and Wald, 2009).

In immunocompromised patients with mucocutaneous HSV infection, intravenous acyclovir (250 mg/m[2] every 8 h for 7 days) shortens healing time, duration of pain, and the period of virus shedding. Oral acyclovir (800 mg five times per day) and valacyclovir (1000 mg twice daily) for 5–10 days are also effective. Recurrences are common after cessation of therapy and may require long-term suppression. In those with very localized labial or facial HSV infections, topical acyclovir may provide some benefit. Intravenous acyclovir may be beneficial in viscerally disseminating HSV in immunocompromised patients and in patients with HSV-infected burn wounds.

Systemic acyclovir prophylaxis is highly effective in preventing mucocutaneous HSV infections in seropositive patients undergoing immunosuppression. Intravenous acyclovir (250 mg/m[2] every 8–12 h) begun prior to transplantation and continuing for several weeks prevents HSV disease in bone marrow transplant recipients. For patients who can tolerate oral medications, oral acyclovir (400 mg five times daily) is effective, and long-term oral acyclovir (200–400 mg three times daily for 6 months) also reduces the risk of VZV infection (Steer et al., 2000). In HSV encephalitis, acyclovir (10 mg/kg every 8 h for a minimum of 10 days) reduces mortality by more than 50% and improves overall neurologic outcome compared with vidarabine. Higher doses (15–20 mg/kg every 8 h) and prolonged treatment (up to 21 days) are recommended by many experts. Intravenous acyclovir (20 mg/kg every 8 h for 21 days) is more effective than lower doses in viscerally invasive neonatal HSV infections (Kimberlin et al., 2001). In neonates and immunosuppressed patients and, rarely, in previously healthy persons, relapses of encephalitis following acyclovir may occur. The value of continuing long-term suppression with valacyclovir after completing intravenous acyclovir is under study.

An ophthalmic formulation of acyclovir (not available in the U.S.) is at least as effective as topical vidarabine or trifluridine in herpetic keratoconjunctivitis.

Infection owing to resistant HSV is rare in immunocompetent persons; however, in immunocompromised hosts, acyclovir-resistant HSV

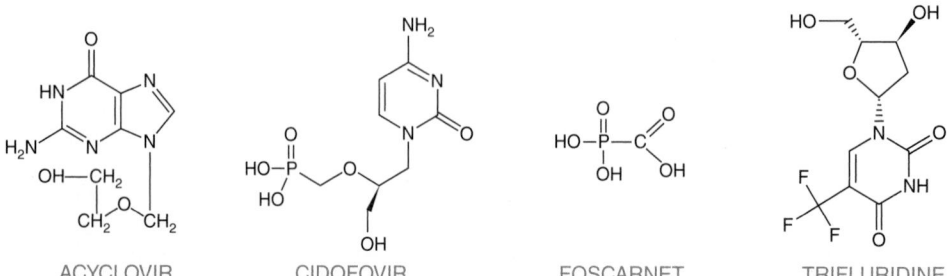

ACYCLOVIR   CIDOFOVIR   FOSCARNET   TRIFLURIDINE

Figure 62–2 *Chemical structures of some antiherpes drugs.* Many antiherpes agents are nucleoside congeners that are phosphorylated sequentially by viral and host kinases to become triphosphate inhibitors of viral DNA synthesis (see Figure 62–3). Foscarnet is a pyrophosphate analogue that selectively blocks the pyrophosphate binding site on viral DNA polymerases, thereby inhibiting chain elongation.

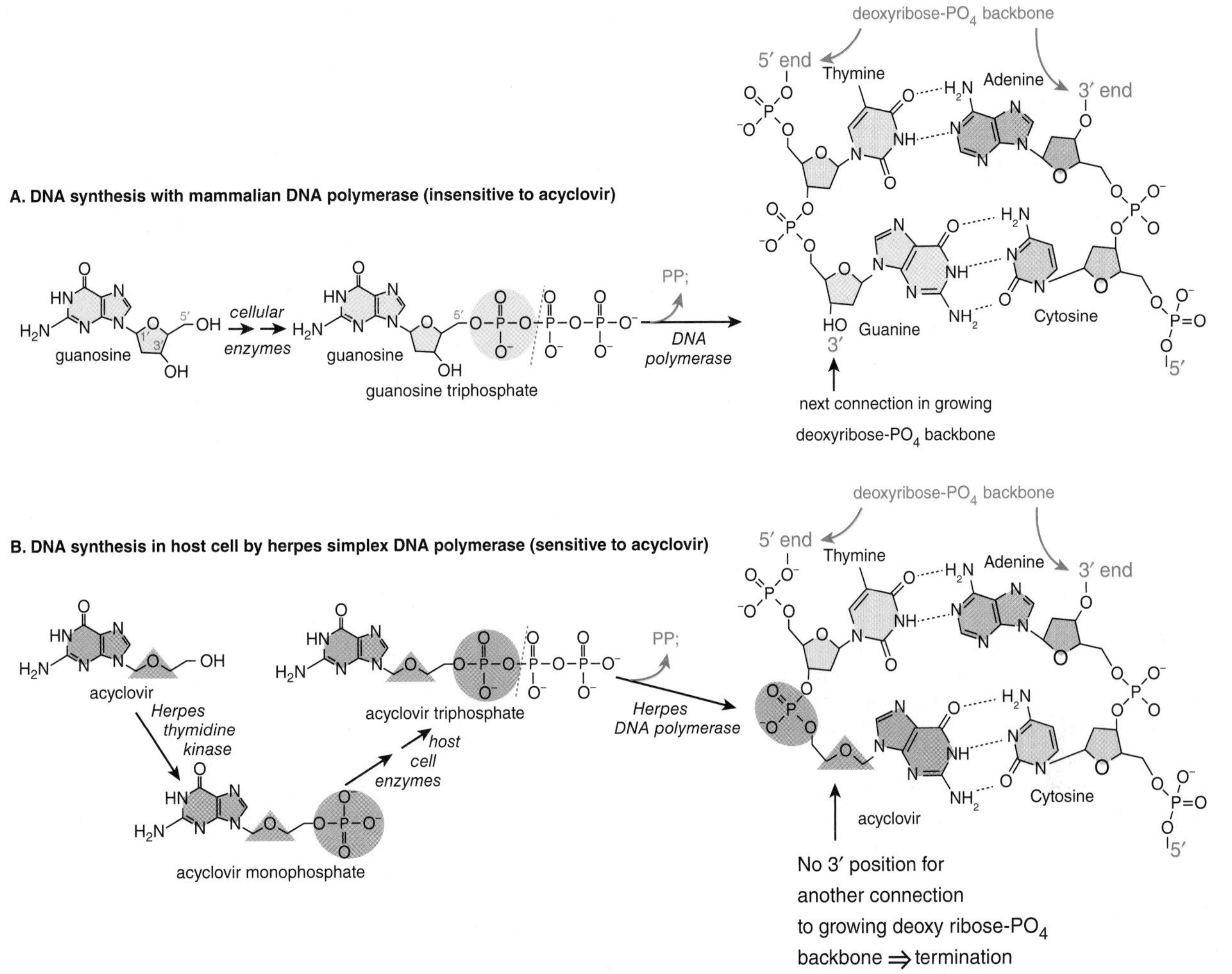

Figure 62–3 *Acyclovir inhibits DNA synthesis by HSV DNA polymerase.* After penetrating the membrane of a susceptible mammalian host cell, an HSV virion releases its capsid, which delivers viral DNA into the host cell, initiating viral DNA synthesis. Acyclovir, a guanine analogue, inhibits viral but not mammalian DNA polymerase. **A.** DNA synthesis with mammalian DNA polymerase (insensitive to acyclovir). In the presence of acyclovir, human DNA synthesis proceeds normally. Here, mammalian DNA polymerase removes pyrophosphate (PPi) PP_i (----) from dGTP and uses dGTP to add a dGMP to the 3′ end of a growing nucleic acid polymer, the guanine base pairing with a cytosine and dGMP's $5'PO_4$ bonding to the 3′OH group on the ribose of the preceding base, thymine. A 3′OH on the sugar of the added dGMP is available to form a 3′-5′ bond with the next nucleotide added. **B.** DNA synthesis in host cell by HSV DNA polymerase (sensitive to acyclovir). The guanine analogue acyclovir inhibits viral DNA polymerase by acting as a terminal substrate, but to do so, acyclovir must be phosphorylated to acyclovir triphosphate. The first phosphate group is added by the HSV TK, which has an affinity for acyclovir that is about 200 times that of the mammalian enzyme for acyclovir. Host cell enzymes add the second and third phosphates, producing acyclovir triphosphate, which concentrates 40- to 100-fold in HSV-infected cells over the concentrations in uninfected cells. Thus, acyclovir triphosphate competes well for endogenous dGTP. HSV DNA polymerase cleaves PP_i (----) from acyclovir triphosphate and adds acyclovir monophosphate to the 3′ end of the growing DNA strand. Acyclovir lacks a hydroxyl group in the 3′ position (indeed, it lacks that 3′ position), and further addition to the polymer by HSV DNA polymerase is not possible. Furthermore, a viral exonuclease activity associated with viral DNA polymerase cannot remove the acyclovir moiety. Compare the actions of acyclovir to those of ganciclovir and penciclovir, which have 3′OH groups, and to foscarnet, which binds avidly at the PP_i cleavage site of HSV DNA polymerase, preventing cleavage of PP_i from nucleoside triphosphates.

isolates can cause extensive mucocutaneous disease and, rarely, meningoencephalitis, pneumonitis, or visceral disease. Resistant HSV can be recovered from 4% to 7% of immunocompromised patients receiving acyclovir treatment. Recurrences after cessation of acyclovir usually are due to sensitive virus but may be due to acyclovir-resistant virus in patients with AIDS. In patients with progressive disease, intravenous foscarnet therapy is effective, and vidarabine is considered only when all other therapies have failed (Chilukuri and Rosen, 2003).

Untoward Effects

Acyclovir generally is well tolerated. Chronic acyclovir suppression of genital herpes has been used safely for up to 10 years. No excess frequency of congenital abnormalities has been recognized in infants born to women exposed to acyclovir during pregnancy (Ratanajamit et al., 2003). Topical acyclovir in a polyethylene glycol base may cause mucosal

irritation and transient burning when applied to genital lesions. Oral acyclovir has been associated infrequently with nausea, diarrhea, rash, or headache and very rarely with renal insufficiency or neurotoxicity. Valacyclovir also may be associated with headache, nausea, diarrhea, nephrotoxicity, and CNS symptoms (confusion, hallucinations). Uncommon side effects include severe thrombocytopenic syndromes, sometimes fatal, in immunocompromised patients. Acyclovir has been associated with neutropenia in neonates. The principal dose-limiting toxicities of intravenous acyclovir are renal insufficiency and CNS side effects. Nephrotoxicity usually resolves with drug cessation and volume expansion. Hemodialysis may be useful in severe cases. Severe somnolence and lethargy may occur with combinations of zidovudine (see Chapter 59) and acyclovir. Concomitant cyclosporine and probably other nephrotoxic agents enhance the risk of nephrotoxicity. Probenecid decreases the acyclovir renal clearance and prolongs the elimination $t_{1/2}$. Acyclovir may decrease the renal clearance of other drugs eliminated by active renal secretion, such as methotrexate.

Cidofovir

Cidofovir is a cytidine nucleotide analogue with inhibitory activity against human herpes, papilloma, polyoma, pox, and adenoviruses.

Because cidofovir is a phosphonate that is phosphorylated by cellular but not viral enzymes, it inhibits acyclovir-resistant TK-deficient or TK-altered HSV or VZV strains, ganciclovir-resistant CMV strains with UL97 mutations (but not those with DNA polymerase mutations), and some foscarnet-resistant CMV strains. Cidofovir synergistically inhibits CMV replication in combination with ganciclovir or foscarnet.

Mechanisms of Action and Resistance

Cidofovir inhibits viral DNA synthesis by slowing and eventually terminating chain elongation. Cidofovir is metabolized to its active diphosphate form by cellular enzymes; the levels of phosphorylated metabolites are similar in infected and uninfected cells. The diphosphate acts as both a competitive inhibitor with respect to dCTP and as an alternative substrate for viral DNA polymerase.

Cidofovir resistance in CMV is due to mutations in viral DNA polymerase. Low-level resistance to cidofovir develops in up to about 30% of patients with retinitis by 3 months of therapy. Highly ganciclovir-resistant CMV isolates that possess DNA polymerase and UL97 kinase mutations are resistant to cidofovir, and prior ganciclovir therapy may select for cidofovir resistance. Some foscarnet-resistant CMV isolates show cross-resistance to cidofovir, and triple-drug-resistant variants with DNA polymerase mutations occur.

ADME

Cidofovir has very low oral bioavailability. Penetration into the CSF is low. Topical cidofovir gel may result in low plasma concentrations (<0.5 μg/mL) in patients with large mucocutaneous lesions. Plasma levels after intravenous dosing decline in a biphasic pattern with a terminal $t_{1/2}$ that averages 2.6 h. The active form, cidofovir diphosphate, has a prolonged intracellular $t_{1/2}$ and competitively inhibits CMV and HSV DNA polymerases at concentrations one-eighth to one six-hundredth of those required to inhibit human DNA polymerases (Hitchcock et al., 1996). A phosphocholine metabolite also has a long intracellular $t_{1/2}$ (about 87 h) and may serve as an intracellular reservoir of drug. The prolonged intracellular $t_{1/2}$ of cidofovir diphosphate allows infrequent (weekly or biweekly) dosing regimens. Cidofovir is cleared by the kidney via glomerular filtration and tubular secretion. Over 90% of the dose is recovered unchanged in the urine. Probenecid blocks tubular transport of cidofovir and reduces renal clearance and associated nephrotoxicity. Elimination relates linearly to creatinine clearance; the $t_{1/2}$ increases to 32.5 h in patients on CAPD. Hemodialysis removes more than 50% of the administered dose.

Therapeutic Uses

Intravenous cidofovir is approved for the treatment of CMV retinitis in HIV-infected patients. Intravenous cidofovir has been used for treating acyclovir-resistant mucocutaneous HSV infection, adenovirus disease in transplant recipients, and extensive molluscum contagiosum in HIV patients. Reduced doses without probenecid may be beneficial in BK virus nephropathy in patients with a renal transplant. Topical cidofovir gel eliminates virus shedding and lesions in some HIV-infected patients with acyclovir-resistant mucocutaneous HSV infections and has been used in treating anogenital warts and molluscum contagiosum in immunocompromised patients and cervical intraepithelial neoplasia in women. Intralesional cidofovir induces remissions in adults and children with respiratory papillomatosis.

Untoward Effects

Nephrotoxicity is the principal dose-limiting side effect of intravenous cidofovir. Concomitant oral probenecid and saline prehydration reduce the risk of renal toxicity; however, probenecid alters renal clearance of many agents, albeit not of cidofovir. For example, probenecid alters zidovudine pharmacokinetics such that zidovudine doses should be reduced

when probenecid is present, as should the doses of other drugs whose renal secretion probenecid inhibits (e.g., β-lactam antibiotics, NSAIDs, acyclovir, lorazepam, furosemide, methotrexate, theophylline, and rifampin). On maintenance doses of 5 mg/kg every 2 weeks, up to 50% of patients develop proteinuria, 10%–15% show an elevated serum creatinine concentration, and 15%–20% develop neutropenia. Anterior uveitis that is responsive to topical corticosteroids and cycloplegia occurs commonly, and low intraocular pressure occurs infrequently with intravenous cidofovir. Administration with food and pretreatment with antiemetics, antihistamines, or acetaminophen may improve tolerance. Concurrent nephrotoxic agents are contraindicated, and at least 7 days should elapse before initiation of cidofovir treatment is recommended after prior exposure to aminoglycosides, intravenous pentamidine, amphotericin B, foscarnet, NSAID, or contrast dye. Cidofovir and oral ganciclovir are poorly tolerated in combination at full doses.

Topical application of cidofovir is associated with dose-related application site reactions (e.g., burning, pain, and pruritus) in up to one-third of patients and occasionally ulceration. Cidofovir is considered a potential human carcinogen. It may cause infertility and is classified as pregnancy category C.

Famciclovir and Penciclovir

Famciclovir is the diacetyl ester prodrug of 6-deoxy penciclovir and lacks intrinsic antiviral activity. Penciclovir is an acyclic guanine nucleoside analogue. Penciclovir is similar to acyclovir in its spectrum of activity and potency against HSV and VZV. It also is inhibitory for HBV.

Mechanisms of Action and Resistance

Penciclovir is an inhibitor of viral DNA synthesis. In HSV- or VZV-infected cells, penciclovir is phosphorylated initially by viral TK. Penciclovir triphosphate is a competitive inhibitor of viral DNA polymerase (see Figure 62–3). Although penciclovir triphosphate is approximately a one-hundredth as potent as acyclovir triphosphate in inhibiting viral DNA polymerase, it is present in infected cells at much higher concentrations and for more prolonged periods. The prolonged intracellular $t_{1/2}$ of penciclovir triphosphate, 7–20 h, is associated with prolonged antiviral effects. Because penciclovir has a 3′-hydroxyl group, it is not an obligate chain terminator but does inhibit DNA elongation. Resistance during clinical use is low. TK-deficient, acyclovir-resistant herpesviruses are cross-resistant to penciclovir.

ADME

Oral penciclovir has low (<5%) bioavailability. In contrast, famciclovir is well absorbed orally (bioavailability ~75%) and is converted rapidly to penciclovir by deacetylation of the side chain and oxidation of the purine ring during and following absorption. Food slows absorption but does not reduce overall bioavailability. The plasma elimination $t_{1/2}$ of penciclovir averages about 2 h, and more than 90% is excreted unchanged in the urine. Following oral famciclovir administration, nonrenal clearance accounts for about 10% of each dose, primarily through fecal excretion, but penciclovir (60% of dose) and its 6-deoxy precursor (<10% of dose) are eliminated primarily in the urine. The plasma $t_{1/2}$ averages 9.9 h in renal insufficiency ($Cl_{cr} < 30$ mL/min); hemodialysis efficiently removes penciclovir.

Therapeutic Uses

Oral famciclovir, topical penciclovir, and intravenous penciclovir are approved for managing HSV and VZV infections.

Oral famciclovir (250 mg three times a day for 7–10 days) is as effective as acyclovir in treating first-episode genital herpes (Kimberlin and Rouse, 2004). In patients with recurrent genital HSV, patient-initiated famciclovir treatment (125 or 250 mg twice daily for 5 days) reduces healing time and symptoms by about 1 day. Famciclovir (250 mg twice daily for up to 1 year) is effective for suppression of recurrent genital HSV, but single daily doses are less effective. Higher doses (500 mg twice daily) reduce HSV recurrences in HIV-infected persons. Intravenous penciclovir (5 mg/kg every 8 or 12 h for 7 days) (not available in the U.S.) is comparable to intravenous acyclovir for treating mucocutaneous HSV infections in immunocompromised hosts. In immunocompetent persons with recurrent orolabial HSV, topical 1% penciclovir cream (applied every 2 h while awake for 4 days) shortens healing time and symptoms by about 1 day (Raborn et al., 2002).

In immunocompetent adults with herpes zoster of 3 days' duration or less, famciclovir (500 mg three times a day for 10 days) is at least as effective as acyclovir (800 mg five times daily) in reducing healing time and zoster-associated pain, particularly in those 50 years or older. Famciclovir is comparable with valacyclovir in treating zoster and reducing associated pain in older adults (Tyring et al., 2000). Famciclovir (500 mg three times a day for 7–10 days) also is comparable with high-dose oral acyclovir in treating zoster in immunocompromised patients and in those with ophthalmic zoster (Tyring et al., 2001).

Famciclovir is associated with dose-related reductions in HBV DNA and transaminase levels in patients with chronic HBV hepatitis but is less effective than lamivudine (Lai et al., 2002). Famciclovir is also ineffective in treating lamivudine-resistant HBV infections owing to emergence of multiply resistant variants.

Untoward Effects

Oral famciclovir is associated with headache, diarrhea, and nausea. Urticaria, rash, and hallucinations or confusional states (predominantly in the elderly) have been reported. Topical penciclovir (~1%) rarely is associated with local reactions. The short-term tolerance of famciclovir is comparable with that of acyclovir. Penciclovir is mutagenic at high concentrations. Long-term administration (1 year) does not affect spermatogenesis in men. Safety during pregnancy has not been established.

Ganciclovir and Valganciclovir

Ganciclovir is an acyclic guanine nucleoside analogue that is similar in structure to acyclovir. Valganciclovir is the L-valyl ester prodrug of ganciclovir. Ganciclovir has inhibitory activity against all herpesviruses and is especially active against CMV.

Mechanisms of Action and Resistance

Ganciclovir inhibits viral DNA synthesis. It is monophosphorylated intracellularly by viral TK during HSV infection and by a viral phosphotransferase encoded by the UL97 gene during CMV infection. Ganciclovir diphosphate and ganciclovir triphosphate are formed by host enzymes. At least 10-fold higher concentrations of ganciclovir triphosphate are present in CMV-infected than in uninfected cells. The triphosphate is a competitive inhibitor of dGTP incorporation into DNA and preferentially inhibits viral rather than host cellular DNA polymerases. Incorporation into viral DNA causes eventual cessation of DNA chain elongation (see Figures 62–1A and 62–3).

Cytomegalovirus can become resistant to ganciclovir by either of two mechanisms: reduced intracellular ganciclovir phosphorylation owing to mutations in the viral phosphotransferase and mutations in viral DNA polymerase. Highly resistant variants with both mutations are cross-resistant to cidofovir and variably to foscarnet. Ganciclovir also is much less active against acyclovir-resistant TK-deficient HSV strains.

ADME

The oral bioavailability of ganciclovir is low, only 6%–9% following ingestion with food. On the other hand, oral doses of the prodrug valganciclovir are well absorbed and hydrolyzed rapidly to ganciclovir; thus, valganciclovir provides greater bioavailability of the vanciclovir moiety, about 60%. Food further increases the bioavailability of valganciclovir by about 25%. Following intravenous administration of ganciclovir, vitreous fluid levels are similar to or higher than those in plasma and decline with a $t_{1/2}$ of 23–26 h. Intraocular sustained-release ganciclovir implants provide vitreous levels of about 4.1 µg/mL. The plasma elimination $t_{1/2}$ is about 2–4 h. Intracellular ganciclovir triphosphate concentrations are 10-fold higher than those of acyclovir triphosphate and decline much more slowly, with an intracellular elimination $t_{1/2}$ longer than 24 h. These differences may account in part for ganciclovir's greater anti-CMV activity and provide the rationale for single daily doses in suppressing human CMV infections.

Over 90% of ganciclovir is eliminated unchanged by renal excretion. Plasma $t_{1/2}$ increases in patients with severe renal insufficiency.

Therapeutic Uses

In CMV retinitis, initial induction treatment (5 mg/kg IV every 12 h for 10–21 days) is associated with improvement or stabilization in about 85% of patients (Faulds and Heel, 1990). Reduced viral excretion is usually evident by 1 week, and funduscopic improvement is seen by 2 weeks. Because of the high risk of relapse, patients with AIDS with retinitis require suppressive therapy with high doses of ganciclovir (5 mg/kg/d). Oral ganciclovir (1000 mg three times daily) is effective for suppression of retinitis after initial intravenous treatment but has been replaced in practice by oral valganciclovir. Oral valganciclovir (900 mg twice daily for 21 days of initial treatment) is comparable with intravenous dosing for initial control and sustained suppression (900 mg daily) of CMV retinitis (Schreiber et al., 2009). Intravitreal ganciclovir injections have been used in some patients, and an intraocular sustained-release ganciclovir implant is more effective than systemic dosing in suppressing retinitis progression.

Ganciclovir therapy (5 mg/kg every 12 h for 14–21 days) may benefit other CMV syndromes in patients with AIDS or recipients of solid-organ transplants (Kotton et al., 2010). Ganciclovir has been used for both prophylaxis and preemptive therapy of CMV infections in transplant recipients (Schreiber et al., 2009).

A ganciclovir ophthalmic gel formulation (Zirgan) is effective in treating HSV keratitis (Colin et al., 1997). Oral ganciclovir also reduces HBV DNA levels and aminotransferase levels in chronic hepatitis B virus infection (Hadziyannis et al., 1999), but the drug is not approved for this indication.

Untoward Effects

Myelosuppression is the principal dose-limiting toxicity of ganciclovir. Neutropenia occurs in about 15%–40% of patients and is observed most commonly during the second week of treatment and usually is reversible within 1 week of drug cessation. Persistent fatal neutropenia has occurred. Recombinant G-CSF (filgrastim, lenograstim) may be useful in treating ganciclovir-induced neutropenia (see Chapter 41). Thrombocytopenia occurs in 5%–20% of patients. Zidovudine and probably other cytotoxic agents increase the risk of myelosuppression, as do nephrotoxic agents that impair ganciclovir excretion. Probenecid and possibly acyclovir reduce renal clearance of ganciclovir. Oral ganciclovir increases the absorption and peak plasma concentrations of didanosine by approximately 2-fold and that of zidovudine by about 20%. CNS side effects (5%–15%) range in severity from headache to behavioral changes to convulsions and coma. About one-third of patients must interrupt or prematurely stop intravenous ganciclovir therapy because of bone marrow or CNS toxicity. Infusion-related phlebitis, azotemia, anemia, rash, fever, liver function test abnormalities, nausea or vomiting, and eosinophilia also have been described. Ganciclovir is classified as pregnancy category C (risk not ruled out).

Foscarnet

Foscarnet (trisodium phosphonoformate) is an inorganic pyrophosphate analogue that is inhibitory for all herpesviruses and HIV.

Mechanisms of Action and Resistance

Foscarnet inhibits viral nucleic acid synthesis by interacting directly at HSV DNA polymerase or HIV reverse transcriptase (see Figures 62–1A and 62–3). Foscarnet reversibly blocks the pyrophosphate binding site of the viral DNA polymerase, inhibiting cleavage of pyrophosphate from deoxynucleotide triphosphates and thereby inhibiting chain elongation (deoxynucleotide triphosphate + $DNA_n \rightarrow$ diphosphate + DNA_{n+1}). Foscarnet has about 100-fold greater inhibitory effects against herpesvirus DNA polymerases than against cellular DNA polymerase α. Herpesviruses resistant to foscarnet have point mutations in the viral DNA polymerase.

ADME

Foscarnet is poorly soluble in aqueous solutions and requires large volumes for administration; in addition, the drug's oral bioavailability is low.

Vitreous levels approximate those in plasma; CSF levels average 66% of those in plasma at steady state. Over 80% of foscarnet is excreted unchanged in the urine. Dose adjustments are necessary for small decreases in renal function. Plasma elimination has initial bimodal half-lives totaling 4–8 h and a prolonged terminal elimination $t_{1/2}$ of 3–4 days. Sequestration in bone with gradual release accounts for the fate of an estimated 10%–20% of a given dose. Foscarnet is cleared efficiently by hemodialysis (~50% of a dose).

Therapeutic Uses

Intravenous foscarnet is effective for treatment of CMV retinitis, including ganciclovir-resistant infections, other types of CMV infection, and acyclovir-resistant HSV and VZV infections.

In CMV retinitis in patients with AIDS, foscarnet (60 mg/kg every 8 h or 90 mg/kg every 12 h for 14–21 days followed by chronic maintenance at 90 to 120 mg/kg every day in one dose) is associated with clinical stabilization in about 90% of patients. In CMV retinitis in patients with AIDS, foscarnet (60 mg/kg every 8 h or 90 mg/kg every 12 h for 14–21 days followed by chronic maintenance at 90 to 120 mg/kg every day in one dose) is associated with clinical stabilization in about 90% of patients. When used for preemptive therapy of CMV viremia in bone marrow transplant recipients, foscarnet (60 mg/kg every 12 h for 2 weeks followed by 90 mg/kg daily for 2 weeks) is as effective as intravenous ganciclovir and causes less neutropenia (Reusser et al., 2002). When used for CMV infections, foscarnet may reduce the risk of Kaposi sarcoma in HIV-infected patients. Intravitreal injections of foscarnet also have been used. In acyclovir-resistant mucocutaneous HSV infections, lower doses of foscarnet (40 mg/kg every 8 h for ≥ 7 days) are associated with cessation of viral shedding and with complete healing of lesions in about three-quarters of patients. Foscarnet also appears to be effective in acyclovir-resistant VZV infections. Topical foscarnet cream is ineffective in treating recurrent genital HSV in immunocompetent persons but appears to be useful in chronic acyclovir-resistant infections in immunocompromised patients.

Untoward Effects

Major dose-limiting toxicities are nephrotoxicity and symptomatic hypocalcemia. Increases in serum creatinine occur in up to one-half of patients but are generally reversible after cessation. High doses, rapid infusion, dehydration, prior renal insufficiency, and concurrent nephrotoxic drugs are risk factors. Saline loading may reduce the risk of nephrotoxicity. Foscarnet is highly ionized at physiological pH, and metabolic abnormalities are very common. These include increases or decreases in Ca^{2+} and phosphate, hypomagnesemia, and hypokalemia. Concomitant intravenous pentamidine administration increases the risk of symptomatic hypocalcemia. CNS side effects include headache (25%), tremor, irritability, seizures, and hallucinosis. Other reported side effects are generalized rash, fever, nausea or emesis, anemia, leukopenia, abnormal liver function tests, electrocardiographic changes, infusion-related thrombophlebitis, and painful genital ulcerations. Topical foscarnet may cause local irritation and ulceration, and oral foscarnet may cause GI disturbance. Preclinical studies indicate that high foscarnet concentrations are mutagenic. Safety in pregnancy or childhood is uncertain.

Fomivirsen

Fomivirsen, a 21-base phosphorothioate oligonucleotide, provides antisense therapy. The drug is complementary to the mRNA sequence for the major immediate-early transcriptional region of CMV and inhibits CMV replication through sequence-specific and nonspecific mechanisms, including inhibition of virus binding to cells. Fomivirsen is active against CMV strains resistant to ganciclovir, foscarnet, and cidofovir. Fomivirsen is given by intravitreal injection in the treatment of CMV retinitis for patients intolerant of or unresponsive to other therapies. Following injection, it is cleared slowly from the vitreous ($t_{1/2}$ ~ 55 h) through distribution to the retina and probable exonuclease digestion. In HIV-infected patients with refractory, sight-threatening CMV retinitis, fomivirsen

injections (330 µg weekly for 3 weeks and then every 2 weeks or on days 1 and 15 followed by monthly) significantly delay time to retinitis progression. Ocular side effects include iritis in up to one-quarter of patients, which can be managed with topical corticosteroids; vitritis; cataracts; and increases in intraocular pressure in 15%–20% of patients. Recent cidofovir use may increase the risk of inflammatory reactions. *This drug is no longer available in the U.S.*

Docosanol

Docosanol is a long-chain saturated alcohol that is approved as an over-the-counter 10% cream for the treatment of recurrent orolabial herpes. Docosanol inhibits the in vitro replication of many lipid-enveloped viruses, including HSV. It does not inactivate HSV directly but appears to block fusion between the cellular and viral envelope membranes and inhibits viral entry into the cell. Topical treatment beginning within 12 h of prodromal symptoms or lesion onset reduces healing time by about 1 day and is well tolerated. Treatment initiation at papular or later stages provides no benefit.

Idoxuridine

Idoxuridine is an iodinated thymidine analogue that inhibits the in vitro replication of various DNA viruses, including herpesviruses and poxviruses. Idoxuridine lacks selectivity, in that low concentrations inhibit the growth of uninfected cells. The triphosphate inhibits viral DNA synthesis and is incorporated into both viral and cellular DNA. In the U.S., idoxuridine is approved only for topical (ophthalmic) treatment of HSV keratitis. Idoxuridine formulated in dimethylsulfoxide is available outside the U.S. for topical treatment of herpes labialis, genitalis, and zoster. Adverse reactions include pain, pruritus, inflammation, and edema of the eye or lids; allergic reactions are rare.

Trifluridine

Trifluridine is a fluorinated pyrimidine nucleoside that has in vitro inhibitory activity against HSV types 1 and 2, CMV, vaccinia, and to a lesser extent, certain adenoviruses. Trifluridine inhibits replication of herpesviruses, including acyclovir-resistant strains, and also inhibits cellular DNA synthesis at relatively low concentrations. Trifluridine monophosphate irreversibly inhibits thymidylate synthase, and trifluridine triphosphate is a competitive inhibitor of thymidine triphosphate incorporation into DNA; trifluridine is incorporated into viral and cellular DNA. Trifluridine-resistant HSV has been described.

Trifluridine currently is used for treatment of primary keratoconjunctivitis and recurrent epithelial keratitis owing to HSV types 1 and 2. Topical trifluridine is more active than idoxuridine and comparable with vidarabine in HSV ocular infections. Adverse reactions include discomfort on instillation and palpebral edema. Hypersensitivity reactions and irritation are uncommon. Topical trifluridine also appears to be effective in some patients with acyclovir-resistant HSV cutaneous infections.

Anti-influenza Agents

Recently, there has been concern about the possibility of new influenza pandemics stemming from small but severe outbreaks of H5N1 avian influenza and the novel 2009 influenza A H1N1, thought to be of swine origin. Five drugs are currently approved for the treatment and prevention of influenza virus infection: the adamantine antivirals, amantadine and rimantadine; oseltamivir; zanamivir; and peramivir. Resistance to these drugs has arisen as a consequence of their overuse, including in veterinary applications. Development of resistance and the spread of resistant viruses are major challenges in the chemotherapy and chemoprophylaxis of influenza and are likely to drive future recommendations for use of these drugs in global populations. The CDC annually issues recommendations for influenza vaccinations and comments on effective medications (CDC, 2016).

Amantadine and Rimantadine

Amantadine and its derivative rimantadine are uniquely configured tricyclic amines. Rimantadine has $H_3C — \underset{\underset{\text{NH}_2}{|}}{CH} — NH_2$ in place of the –NH_2 group.

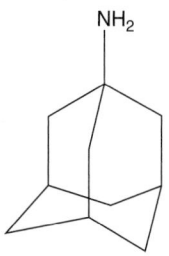

AMANTADINE

Mechanisms of Action and Resistance

Amantadine and rimantadine inhibit an early step in viral replication, probably viral uncoating; for some strains, they also have an effect on a late step in viral assembly, probably mediated through altering hemagglutinin processing. The primary locus of action is the influenza A virus M2 protein, an integral membrane protein that functions as an ion channel. By interfering with this function of the M2 protein, the drugs inhibit the acid-mediated dissociation of the ribonucleoprotein complex early in replication and potentiate acidic pH–induced conformational changes in hemagglutinin during its intracellular transport later in replication. Resistance to these drugs results from a mutation in the RNA sequence encoding for the M2 protein transmembrane domain; resistant isolates typically appear in the treated patient within 2–3 days of starting therapy.

ADME

Table 62–3 summarizes important pharmacokinetics properties of these antiviral agents. The two adamantanes differ in several respects. Amantadine is excreted largely unmetabolized in the urine ($t_{1/2}$ of elimination is ~ 12–18 h in young adults, increasing up to twice that in the elderly and even more in those with renal impairment). By contrast, elimination of rimantadine depends on hepatic function; the drug is subject to phase 1 and phase 2 reactions prior to renal excretion of metabolites (elimination $t_{1/2}$ ~ 24–36 h; 60%–90% is excreted in the urine as metabolites). The elderly require only one-half the weight-adjusted dose of amantadine needed for young adults. Amantadine is excreted in breast milk. Rimantadine concentrations in nasal mucus average 50% higher than those in plasma.

Therapeutic Uses

Although both drugs are useful for the prevention and treatment of infections caused by influenza A virus, vaccination against influenza is a more cost-effective means of reducing disease burden. Amantadine and rimantadine are active only against susceptible influenza A viruses (not influenza B); rimantadine is 4- to 10-fold more active than amantadine. Virtually all H3N2 strains of influenza circulating worldwide are resistant to these drugs.

Seasonal prophylaxis with either amantadine or rimantadine (a total of 200 mg/d in one or two divided doses in young adults) is about 70%–90% protective against influenza A illness. These agents are efficacious in preventing nosocomial influenza and in curtailing nosocomial outbreaks during pandemic influenza. Doses of 100 mg/d are better tolerated and still appear to be protective against influenzal illness. Seasonal prophylaxis is an alternative in high-risk patients, if the influenza vaccine cannot be administered or may be ineffective (i.e., in immunocompromised patients). Prophylaxis should be started as soon as influenza is identified in a community or region and should be continued throughout the period of risk (usually 4–8 weeks) because any protective effects are lost several days after cessation of therapy. Alternatively, the drugs can be started in conjunction with immunization and continued for 2 weeks until protective immune responses develop.

The amantadines are effective against influenza A H1N1 if treatment is initiated within 2 days of the onset of symptoms (Schmidt, 2004). In uncomplicated influenza A illness of adults, early amantadine or rimantadine treatment (200 mg/d for 5 days) reduces the duration of fever and systemic complaints by 1–2 days, speeds functional recovery, and sometimes decreases the duration of virus shedding. The usual regimen in children (≥1 year of age) is 5 mg/kg/d, up to 150 mg, administered once or twice daily. Resistant variants have been recovered from about 30% of treated children or outpatient adults by the fifth day of therapy.

TABLE 62–3 ■ PHARMACOLOGICAL CHARACTERISTICS OF ANTIVIRALS FOR INFLUENZA

	AMANTADINE	RIMANTADINE	ZANAMIVIR	OSELTAMIVIR	PERAMIVIR
Spectrum[f]	A	A	A, B	A, B	A, B
Route/formulations	Oral (tablet/capsule/syrup)	Oral (tablet/syrup)	Inhaled (powder) Intravenous[a]	Oral (capsule/syrup) Intravenous[a]	Intravenous
Oral bioavailability	>90%	>90%	<5%[b]	80%[c]	Not applicable
Effect of meals on AUC	Negligible	Negligible	Not applicable	Negligible	Not applicable
Elimination $t_{1/2}$, h	12–18	24–36	2.5–5	6–10[c]	20
Protein binding, %	67%	40%	<10%	3%[c]	<30%
Metabolism, %	<10%	~75%	Negligible	Negligible	Negligible
Renal excretion[e]	>90%	~25%	100%	95%[c]	90%
Dose adjustments	$Cl_{cr} \le 50$ Age ≥ 65 years	$Cl_{cr} \le 10$ Age ≥ 65 years	None[d]	$Cl_{cr} \le 30$	$Cl_{cr} \le 50$

[a]Investigational at present.
[b]Systemic absorption 4%–17% after inhalation.
[c]For antivirally active oseltamivir carboxylate.
[d]Inhaled formulation only.
[e]% of parent drug.
[f]Types of influenza.

Untoward Effects

The most common side effects related to amantadine and rimantadine are minor dose-related CNS and GI effects: nervousness, light-headedness, difficulty concentrating, insomnia, loss of appetite, and nausea. CNS side effects (5%–33%) occur in patients treated with amantadine at doses of 200 mg/d but are significantly less frequent with rimantadine. The neurotoxic effects of amantadine appear to be increased by concomitant ingestion of antihistamines and psychotropic or anticholinergic drugs, especially in the elderly. At comparable doses of 100 mg/d, rimantadine is significantly better tolerated in nursing home residents than amantadine. High amantadine plasma concentrations (1.0–5.0 µg/mL) have been associated with serious neurotoxic reactions, including delirium, hallucinosis, seizures, coma, and cardiac arrhythmias. Exacerbations of preexisting seizure disorders and psychiatric symptoms may occur with amantadine and possibly with rimantadine. Both drugs are considered pregnancy category C (risk not ruled out; see Appendix I).

Oseltamivir

Oseltamivir carboxylate is a transition-state analogue of sialic acid that is a potent selective inhibitor of the neuraminidases of influenza A and B virus. Oseltamivir phosphate is an ethyl ester prodrug that lacks antiviral activity. Oseltamivir carboxylate has an antiviral spectrum and potency similar to that of zanamivir: It inhibits amantadine- and rimantadine-resistant influenza A viruses and some zanamivir-resistant variants.

Mechanisms of Action and Resistance

Influenza neuraminidase cleaves terminal sialic acid residues and destroys the receptors recognized by viral hemagglutinin, which are present on the cell surface, in progeny virions, and in respiratory secretions. This enzymatic action is essential for release of virus from infected cells. Interaction of oseltamivir carboxylate with the neuraminidase causes a conformational change within the enzyme's active site and inhibits its activity. Inhibition of neuraminidase activity leads to viral aggregation at the cell surface and reduced virus spread within the respiratory tract. Influenza variants selected in vitro for resistance to oseltamivir carboxylate contain hemagglutinin or neuraminidase mutations. Seasonal influenza A (H1N1) has become virtually 100% resistant to oseltamivir worldwide (Moscona, 2009; Schirmer and Holodniy, 2009). Importantly, novel H1N1 (nH1N1 or swine influenza) remains susceptible to oseltamivir.

ADME

Table 62–3 summarizes important pharmacokinetics properties of oseltamivir carboxylate. Oral oseltamivir phosphate is absorbed rapidly and cleaved by esterases in the GI tract and liver to the active carboxylate. Food does not decrease bioavailability but reduces the risk of GI intolerance. Bronchoalveolar lavage levels in animals and middle ear fluid and sinus concentrations in humans are comparable with plasma levels. Probenecid doubles the plasma $t_{1/2}$ of the carboxylate, which indicates tubular secretion by the anionic pathway. Children younger than 2 years exhibit age-related changes in oseltamivir carboxylate clearance and total drug exposure (Kimberlin et al., 2009).

Therapeutic Uses

Oral oseltamivir is effective in the treatment and prevention of influenza A and B virus infections. Treatment of previously healthy adults (75 mg twice daily for 5 days) or children 1–12 years of age (weight-adjusted dosing) with acute influenza reduces illness duration by about 1–2 days, speeds functional recovery, and reduces the risk of complications leading to antibiotic use by 40%–50%. Treatment reduces by about 50% the risk of subsequent hospitalization in adults (Kaiser et al., 2003). When used for prophylaxis during the typical influenza season, oseltamivir (75 mg once daily) is effective (~70%–90%) in reducing the likelihood of influenza illness in both unimmunized working adults and in immunized nursing home residents; short-term use protects against influenza in household contacts (Schirmer and Holodniy, 2009).

Untoward Effects

Oral oseltamivir is associated with nausea, abdominal discomfort, and, less often, emesis. GI complaints typically resolve in 1–2 days despite continued dosing and are preventable by administration with food. An increased frequency of headache was reported in one prophylaxis study in elderly adults. Neither the phosphate nor the carboxylate form interacts with CYPs in vitro. Oseltamivir does not appear to impair fertility, but safety in pregnancy is uncertain (pregnancy category C).

Zanamivir

Zanamivir is a sialic acid analogue that potently and specifically inhibits the neuraminidases of influenza A and B viruses. Zanamivir inhibits in vitro replication of influenza A and B viruses, including amantadine- and rimantadine-resistant strains and several oseltamivir-resistant variants.

Mechanisms of Action and Resistance

Zanamivir inhibits viral neuraminidase and thus causes viral aggregation at the cell surface and reduced spread of virus within the respiratory tract. In vitro selection of viruses resistant to zanamivir is associated with mutations in the viral hemagglutinin or neuraminidase. Hemagglutinin variants are cross-resistant to other neuraminidase inhibitors. Neuraminidase variants contain mutations in the enzyme active site that diminish binding of zanamivir, but the altered enzymes show reduced activity or stability. Zanamivir-resistant variants usually have decreased infectivity in animals.

ADME

Table 62–3 summarizes important pharmacokinetics properties of zanamivir. Oral bioavailability of zanamivir is less than 5%, and the commercial form is delivered by oral inhalation of dry powder in a lactose carrier. The proprietary inhaler device is breath actuated and requires a cooperative patient. Following inhalation of the dry powder, about 15% is deposited in the lower respiratory tract and about 80% in the oropharynx. Overall bioavailability is 4%–17%.

Depending on the strain, zanamivir competitively inhibits influenza neuraminidase activity at concentrations of about 0.2–3 ng/mL but affects neuraminidases from other pathogens and mammalian sources only at 106-fold higher concentrations. Zanamivir inhibits in vitro replication of influenza A and B viruses, including amantadine- and rimantadine-resistant strains and several oseltamivir-resistant variants. It is active after topical administration in animal influenza models.

Therapeutic Uses

Inhaled zanamivir is effective for the prevention and treatment of influenza A and B virus infections. Early zanamivir treatment (10 mg [two inhalations] twice daily for 5 days) of febrile influenza in ambulatory adults and children 5 years or older shortens the time to illness resolution by 1–3 days and in adults reduces by 40% the risk of lower respiratory tract complications that require use of antibiotics. Once-daily inhaled zanamivir is highly protective against community-acquired influenza illness, and when given for 10 days, it protects against household transmission. Intravenous zanamivir ($t_{1/2} \sim 1.7$ h) is available in the U.S. as an EIND and in the E.U. on a compassionate use basis for life-threatening, resistant influenza.

Untoward Effects

Orally inhaled zanamivir generally is well tolerated in ambulatory adults and children with influenza. Wheezing and bronchospasm have been reported in some influenza-infected patients without known airway disease, and acute deteriorations in lung function, including fatal outcomes, have occurred in those with underlying asthma or chronic obstructive airway disease. Zanamivir is not generally recommended for treatment of patients with underlying airway disease because of the risk of serious adverse events. Preclinical studies of zanamivir revealed no evidence of mutagenic, teratogenic, or oncogenic effects (pregnancy risk not ruled out). No clinically significant drug interactions have been recognized to date. Zanamivir does not diminish the immune response to injected influenza vaccine.

Peramivir

Peramivir is a recently FDA-approved inhibitor of influenza virus neuraminidase, indicated for the treatment of acute uncomplicated influenza in patients 18 years and older who have been symptomatic for no more than 2 days. While peramivir was in clinical development, the FDA authorized its emergency use for treatment of pandemic 2009 A/H1N1 in certain adult and pediatric patients (FDA, 2009).

Mechanisms of Action and Resistance

Peramivir has a mechanism of action similar to that of other neuraminidase inhibitors. Neuraminidase resistance can occur as the result of point mutations in either the neuraminidase or hemagglutinin genes or both. Structurally, peramivir differs somewhat from others in the class via a substitution resulting in multiple binding site interactions, which confers some activity against cross-resistant viruses. Antiviral resistance is currently low to the three available neuraminidase inhibitors amongst circulating influenza viruses. This will likely change with each influenza season. In general, cross-resistance across these agents exists. The degree of cross-resistance depends on the viral strain and which point mutations occur.

ADME

Peramivir is not significantly metabolized in humans. It is not a substrate for CYPs or a substrate or inhibitor of P-glycoprotein. The elimination half-life following intravenous administration of 600 mg as a single dose is approximately 20 h. The major route of clearance is via renal excretion. Approximately 90% of total clearance is unchanged peramivir. Negligible accumulation was observed after multiple dosing. Following a 600-mg dose infused over 30 min, the end-of-infusion C_{max} was 46.8 μg/mL, and the $AUC_{0-\infty}$ was 102.7 μg*h/mL. Dosing should be adjusted in patients with altered creatinine clearance. A single 200-mg dose should be administered for those with an estimated creatinine clearance (CL_{cr}, Cockcroft-Gault) between 30 and 49 mL/min, and 100 mg for a CL_{cr} of 10–29 mL/min. No clinically significant drug interactions have been recognized to date.

Therapeutic Uses

Peramivir is administered as a single 600-mg dose, administered via intravenous infusion over 15–30 min. A phase II clinical trial demonstrated that intravenous peramivir (300 or 600 mg as a single-dose infusion) reduced the time to alleviation of symptoms, from 82 h (placebo) to 59 h (treatment with 600 mg peramivir) (Kohno et al., 2010). A phase III trial demonstrated that peramivir (300 or 600 mg) was comparable in extent of symptom relief to oral oseltamivir (75 mg twice a day for 5 days) in patients with seasonal influenza A or B, and with comparable rates of adverse events (Kohno et al., 2011). At present, peramivir's primary use may be limited to patients with acute, uncomplicated influenza who cannot absorb or for other reasons cannot take oral agents. Further studies are needed regarding the use of peramivir in severely ill hospitalized patients and in the pediatric population.

Untoward Effects

The most common adverse event (>2%) is diarrhea. Hypersensitivity reactions (e.g., Stevens-Johnson syndrome and erythema multiforme) have occurred, and treated patients with influenza may be at increased risk for neuropsychiatric events such as hallucinations, delirium, and abnormal behavior. Frequency and severity of adverse effects (peramivir 300 mg or 600 mg) are comparable to those with oseltamivir (75 mg twice daily for 5 days) (Kohno et al., 2011). Patients receiving 600 mg peramivir or oseltamivir had decreased neutrophil counts (10.4% vs. 9.3%), diarrhea (8.2% vs. 7.4%), and vomiting (1.6% vs. 4.1%), respectively.

Interferon

Interferons are potent cytokines that possess antiviral, immunomodulatory, and antiproliferative activities (see Chapter 35). Three major classes of human IFNs with significant antiviral activity are α, β, and γ. Clinically used recombinant α-IFNs are nonglycosylated proteins of about 19,500 Da, the pegylated forms predominating in the U.S. market. The mechanism of action, ADME, untoward effects, and therapeutic uses of IFNs are covered in Chapter 63. Recombinant, natural, and pegylated IFNs currently are approved in the U.S. for treatment of condyloma acuminatum, chronic HCV infection, chronic HBV infection, Kaposi sarcoma in HIV-infected patients, other malignancies, and multiple sclerosis. In addition, IFNs have been granted orphan drug status for a variety of rare disease states, including idiopathic pulmonary fibrosis, laryngeal papillomatosis, juvenile rheumatoid arthritis, and infections associated with chronic granulomatous disease.

Papillomavirus

In refractory condylomata acuminata (genital warts), intralesional injection of various natural and recombinant IFNs is associated with complete clearance of injected warts in 36%–62% of patients, but other treatments are preferred. Relapse occurs in 20%–30% of patients. Verruca vulgaris may respond to intralesional IFN-α. Intramuscular or subcutaneous administration is associated with some regression in wart size but greater toxicity. Systemic IFN may provide adjunctive benefit in recurrent juvenile laryngeal papillomatosis and in treating laryngeal disease in older patients.

Other Viruses

Interferons have been shown to have virological and clinical effects in various herpesvirus infections, including genital HSV infections, localized herpes zoster infection of cancer patients or of older adults, and CMV infections of renal transplant patients. However, IFN generally is associated with more side effects and inferior clinical benefits compared with conventional antiviral therapies. Topically applied IFN and trifluridine combinations appear active in acyclovir-resistant mucocutaneous HSV infections. In HIV-infected persons, IFNs have been associated with antiretroviral effects. In advanced infection, however, the combination of zidovudine and IFN is associated with only transient benefit and excessive hematological toxicity. IFN-α (3 million units thrice weekly) is effective for treatment of HIV-related thrombocytopenia that is resistant to zidovudine therapy.

Interferon has broad-spectrum antiviral activity against respiratory viruses other than adenovirus. However, prophylactic intranasal IFN-α is protective only against rhinovirus colds, and chronic use is limited by the occurrence of nasal side effects. Intranasal IFN is therapeutically ineffective in established rhinovirus colds.

Acknowledgment: Frederick G. Hayden and Charles Flexner contributed to this chapter in earlier editions of this book. We have retained some of their text in the current edition.

Drug Facts for Your Personal Formulary: *Antiviral Agents for Herpes Virus and Influenza*

Drugs	Therapeutic Uses	Clinical Pharmacology and Tips
ANTIHERPES AGENTS		
Guanine nucleoside analogues		
Acyclovir Valacyclovir (Val, an ester prodrug form of acyclovir)	• Clinical use limited to herpes viruses • Efficacy against: HSV-1 > HSV-2 > VZV > EBV > CMV = −6	• Acyclovir has low bioavailability (~20%); Val has bioavailability ~ 70% • Concentrates in breast milk • Clearance via renal excretion of acyclovir, requires good kidney function; $t_{1/2}$ prolonged in neonates and anuric patients • Safely used long term (10 years)
Cidofovir	• Active against human herpes, papilloma, polyoma, pox, adenoviruses	• Low oral bioavailability • Plasma $t_{1/2}$ ~ 2.6 h, but active diphosphate metabolite has long $t_{1/2}$ in cells, as does a phosphocholine metabolite ($t_{1/2}$ = 86 h) • Major risk: nephrotoxicity, reduced by oral probenecid and saline prehydration (beware interactions of probenecid and other medicines)
Famciclovir (Fam), a prodrug form, rapidly converted to penciclovir (Pen)	• Penciclovir similar to acyclovir against HSV and VZV; also inhibits HBV	• Oral bioavailabilities: Pen, < 5%; Fam, ~ 75% • Food reduces rate but not extent of Pen absorption • Safety in pregnancy not established
Valganciclovir (Val), a prodrug valyl ester of ganciclovor (Gan)	• Gan has inhibitory activity against all herpesviruses, especially CMV	• Gan less active against acyclovir-resistant TK-deficient HSV strains • Active triphosphate form has long cellular $t_{1/2}$ • IV administration gives good levels in vitreous with long dwell time ($t_{1/2}$ ~ 25 h) • Major adverse effects: myelosuppression, neutropenia • Risk in pregnancy not ruled out
Pyrophosphate analogue		
Foscarnet	• Active against all herpesviruses and HIV	• Poorly soluble in water; requires large volumes • Adverse effects: neprotoxicity, hypocalcemia • Safety in pregnancy and childhood uncertain
Other agents		
Fomivirsen (antisense oligonucleotide)	• Inhibits CMV replication	• No longer available in the U.S.
Docosanol (long-chain alcohol)	• 10% cream for labial herpes	• Treatment initiation at papular or later stages provides no benefit
Idoxuridine (iodinated thymidine analogue)	• Ophthalmic HSV keratitis (in the U.S.)	• Averse effects: pain, pruritus, inflammation, edema of eye/eyelid
Trifluridine (trifluoropyrimidine nucleoside)	• Ocular herpes; 1° keratoconjunctivitis, recurrent epithelial keratitis from HSV1/2; for external use	• More active than idoxuridine and comparable to vidarabine in HSV ocular infections • Triphosphate form incorporated into host and viral DNA, so not used systemically
ANTI-INFLUENZA AGENTS		
Inhibitors of viral M2 protein function		
Amantadine (Ama) Rimantadine (Rima)	• Active only against susceptible influenza A viruses (not B) • Seasonal prophylaxis against influenza A (70%–90% protective)	• Rima 4- to 10-fold more active than Ama • Resistant isolates appear after 2–3 days of therapy • Virtually all H3N2 strains of influenza are resistant to these drugs • Vaccination is more cost-effective
Inhibitors of viral neuraminidase (see PK data in Table 62–3)		
Oseltamivir	• Treatment and prevention of influenza A and B	• Probenecid doubles plasma $t_{1/2}$
Zanamivir	• Treatment and prevention of influenza A and B	• Inhalable formulation • IV formulation available as EIND • No clinically significant drug interactions
Peramivir	• Treatment of acute uncomplicated flu in patients ≥ 18 years and symptomatic ≤ 2 days	• Supplied as IV infusion; for patients who cannot absorb or oral agents • Comparable in efficacy and adverse effects to oseltamivir • No clinically significant drug interactions reported
CYTOKINES		
Interferon (recombinant α-IFNs; natural and pegylated IFNs)	• Treatment of condyloma acuminatum, chronic HCV and HBV infection, Kaposi sarcoma (in patients with HIV, other malignancies, multiple sclerosis	• See Chapter 63

CDC. 2016–2017 influenza vaccination recommendations. **2016**. Available at: http://www.cdc.gov/flu/. Accessed October 23, 2016.

Chilukuri S, Rosen T. Management of acyclovir-resistant herpes simplex virus. *Dermatol Clin*, **2003**, *21*:311–320.

Colin J, et al. Ganciclovir ophthalmic gel (Virgan: 0.15%) in the treatment of herpes simplex keratitis. *Cornea*, **1997**, *16*:393–399.

Corey L, et al. Once-daily valacyclovir to reduce the risk of transmission of genital herpes. *N Engl J Med*, **2004**, *350*:11–20.

Corey L, Wald A. Maternal and neonatal herpes simplex virus infections. *N Engl J Med*, **2009**, *361*:1376–1385.

Elion GB. History, mechanism of action, spectrum and selectivity of nucleoside analogs. In: Mills J, Corey L, eds. *Antiviral Chemotherapy: New Directions for Clinical Application and Research.* Elsevier, New York, **1986**, 118–137.

Elish D, et al. Therapeutic options for herpes labialis. II: Topical agents. *Cutis*, **2004**, *74*:35–40.

Faulds D, Heel RC. Ganciclovir. A review of its antiviral activity, pharmacokinetic properties and therapeutic efficacy in cytomegalovirus infections. *Drugs*, **1990**, *39*(4):597–638.

FDA. FDA authorizes emergency use of intravenous antiviral peramivir for 2009 H1N1 influenza for certain patients, settings. **2009**. Available at: http://www.fda.gov/NewsEvents/Newsroom/PressAnnouncements/2009/ucm187813.htm. Accessed October 22, 2016.

Hadziyannis SJ, et al. Oral ganciclovir treatment in chronic hepatitis B virus infection: a pilot study. *J Hepatol*, **1999**, *31*:210–214.

Hitchcock M, et al. Cidofovir, a new agent with potent anti-herpesvirus activity. *Antiviral Chem Chemother*, **1996**, *7*:115–127.

Kaiser L, et al. Impact of oseltamivir treatment on influenza-related lower respiratory tract complications and hospitalizations. *Arch Intern Med*, **2003**, *163*(14):1667–1672.

Kimberlin D, Rouse D. Clinical practice: genital herpes. *N Engl J Med*, **2004**, *350*:1970–1977.

Kimberlin D, et al. Oseltamivir pharmacokinetics (PK) in infants: interim results from multicenter trial. Paper presented at the 47th Annual Meeting of the Infectious Diseases Society of America (IDSA); Philadelphia, PA; **2009**.

Kimberlin DW, et al. Safety and efficacy of high-dose intravenous acyclovir in the management of neonatal herpes simplex virus infections. *Pediatrics*, **2001**, *108*:230–238.

Kohno S, et al. S-021812 Clinical Study Group. Efficacy and safety of intravenous peramivir for treatment of seasonal influenza virus infection. *Antimicrob Agents Chemother*, **2010**, *54*:4568–4574.

Kohno S, et al. Phase III randomized, double-blind study comparing single-dose intravenous peramivir with oral oseltamivir in patients with seasonal influenza virus infection. *Antimicrob Agents Chemother*, **2011**, *55*:5267–5276.

Kotton CN, et al. International consensus guidelines on the management of cytomegalovirus in solid organ transplantation. *Transplantation*, **2010**, *89*:779–795.

Lai CL, et al. A comparison of the efficacy of lamivudine and famciclovir in Asian patients with chronic hepatitis B: Results of 24 weeks of therapy. *J Med Virol*, **2002**, *67*: 334–338.

Moscona A. Global transmission of oseltamivir-resistant influenza. *N Engl J Med*, **2009**, *360*:953–956.

Raborn GW, et al. Effective treatment of herpes simplex labialis with penciclovir cream: combined results of two trials. *J Am Dent Assoc*, **2002**, *133*:303–309.

Ratanajamit C, et al. Adverse pregnancy outcome in women exposed to acyclovir during pregnancy: a population-based observational study. *Scand J Infect Dis*, **2003**, *35*:255–259.

Reusser P, et al. Randomized multicenter trial of foscarnet versus ganciclovir for preemptive therapy of cytomegalovirus infection after allogeneic stem cell transplantation. *Blood*, **2002**, *99*:1159–1164.

Schirmer P, Holodniy M. Oseltamivir for treatment and prophylaxis of influenza infection. *Expert Opin Drug Saf*, **2009**, *8*:357–371.

Schmidt AC. Antiviral therapy for influenza: a clinical and economic comparative review. *Drugs*, **2004**, *64*:2031–2046.

Schreiber A, et al. Antiviral treatment of cytomegalovirus infection and resistant strains. *Expert Opin Pharmacother*, **2009**, *10*:191–209.

Spruance SL, et al. Acyclovir cream for treatment of herpes simplex labialis: results of two randomized, doubleblind, vehicle-controlled, multicenter clinical trials. *Antimicrob Agents Chemother*, **2002**, *46*: 2238–2243.

Steer CB, et al. Varicella-zoster infection after allogeneic bone marrow transplantation: incidence, risk factors and prevention with low-dose aciclovir and ganciclovir. *Bone Marrow Transplant*, **2000**, *25*:657–664.

Steingrimsdottir H, et al. Bioavailability of aciclovir after oral administration of acyclovir and its prodrug valaciclovir to patients with leukopenia after chemotherapy. *Antimicrob Agents Chemother*, **2000**, *44*:207–209.

Tyring S, et al. Famciclovir for ophthalmic zoster: a randomised acyclovir controlled study. *Br J Ophthalmol*, **2001**, *85*:576–581.

Tyring SK, et al. Antiviral therapy for herpes zoster. *Arch Fam Med*, **2000**, *9*:863–869.

Wagstaff AJ, et al. Acyclovir: a reappraisal of its antiviral activity, pharmacokinetic properties and therapeutic efficacy. *Drugs*, **1994**, *47*: 153–205.

Chapter 63

Treatment of Viral Hepatitis (HBV/HCV)

Jennifer J. Kiser and Charles W. Flexner

Hepatitis viruses cause inflammation and necrosis of the liver. Hepatitis A and E, which are transmitted via the fecal-oral route, are typically self-limiting, although a small percentage (1%–2%) of those infected will develop fulminant hepatic failure. HBV, HCV, and hepatitis D viruses, however, are transmitted parenterally. Hepatitis B and C may or may not cause symptoms of acute infection, but both may progress to chronic infection. Individuals with chronic hepatitis B or C infection are at risk for cirrhosis, liver failure, and hepatocellular carcinoma. There are two notable differences between HBV and HCV. *First*, HBV is a vaccine-preventable illness, whereas there is no vaccine available to prevent HCV. *Second*, HCV can be cured with effective treatment, whereas the current treatments for HBV are not completely curative. The hepatitis D virus is defective and requires the presence of the HBV to propagate. Individuals coinfected with hepatitis B and D are at greater risk for cirrhosis and hepatocellular carcinoma compared with individuals with only hepatitis B infection, but fortunately only about 5% of individuals with HBV are coinfected with hepatitis D.

There are no antiviral therapies available for the treatment of hepatitis A and E viruses. At this time, the only drug available to treat hepatitis D is pegIFN-α, and it is successful in only 20%–35% of patients (Durantel and Zoulim, 2016). A number of drugs are available for the treatment of hepatitis B and C. Indeed, the RdRp (NS5B), the NS5A replication complex, and the NS3 protease of HCV have been fruitful targets for drug development over the past decade. We now have a growing number of DAAs that inhibit HCV RdRp, the NS3 protease, and NS5A. These DAAs, often used in oral combination therapies, have revolutionized the treatment of HCV, have good safety profiles, and provide well-tolerated and very effective treatments for HCV infection. Available therapies for HBV include IFN and nucleoside and nucleotide analogues. Several agents are in various stages of clinical development for the treatment of HBV. Therapeutic strategies for these two chronic viral infections, hepatitis B and C, are very different and are described separately in this chapter.

Several agents employed against hepatitis viruses, including IFN, ribavirin, and the nucleoside/nucleotide analogues lamivudine, emtricitabine, and tenofovir, are also used to treat other conditions, described in Chapters 64 (Antiretroviral Agents and Treatment of HIV Infection) and 69 (Ocular Pharmacology).

Assessing the stage and severity of liver disease is an important aspect of treating individuals with chronic viral hepatitis. Individuals with cirrhosis require additional monitoring for potential complications (e.g., varices and hepatocellular carcinoma) and the approach to treatment differs in cirrhotics and decompensated cirrhotics compared to individuals without significant liver fibrosis. Cirrhosis can be diagnosed with histologic, radiographic, or laboratory tests. However, decompensated cirrhosis (also known as end-stage liver disease) is a clinical diagnosis based on the presence of variceal hemorrhage, ascites, jaundice, or hepatic encephalopathy. Decompensated cirrhosis carries a high risk of mortality (median survival 2 years), and these individuals should be evaluated for liver transplantation.

The urgency for liver transplantation in individuals with decompensated cirrhosis is determined using the MELD score. A MELD score is calculated based on a patient's bilirubin, INR, and serum creatinine. Individuals with higher MELD scores have a higher risk for mortality and a more urgent need for transplantation. Cirrhosis may also be categorized based on the Child Pugh score. The Child Pugh score accounts for bilirubin, albumin, and INR values and the presence/absence of ascites and encephalopathy. Higher scores are associated with more advanced disease: mild hepatic impairment (Child Pugh category A; score of 5–6), moderate hepatic impairment (Child Pugh category B; score of 7–9), and severe hepatic impairment (Child Pugh category C; score of 10–15). Individuals with Child Pugh B and C scores have decompensated cirrhosis. Familiarity with MELD and Child Pugh scoring and the diagnoses of compensated versus decompensated cirrhosis is helpful for understanding the pharmacologic basis of hepatitis B and C treatment.

Hepatitis B Virus

HBV Overview

Worldwide, an estimated 2 billion people have been infected with HBV and approximately 240 million have chronic disease (WHO, 2015). Areas with the highest HBV endemicity are sub-Saharan Africa and countries in the WHO Western-Pacific region (e.g., China) (Schweitzer et al., 2015). In these regions, HBV is most likely acquired perinatally. Those infected at birth have a 90% risk of progressing to chronic disease; otherwise, the risk of chronic HBV disease in adults is 5% (Tong and Revill, 2016). The lifetime risk of developing cirrhosis, liver failure, or hepatocellular carcinoma in individuals with HBV is 15%–40% (Lin et al., 2016). There are about 686,000 HBV-related deaths annually, which makes HBV the leading cause of liver-related deaths worldwide (WHO, 2016).

Genetic Heterogeneity of HBV

There are 10 described HBV genotypes (A–J) and at least 35 subtypes with distinct geographical distributions (Tong and Revill, 2016). Genotype A is most frequent in North America and Africa, genotypes B and C are dominant throughout East Asia and are primarily transmitted via the perinatal route, and genotype D is most common in Southern Europe and India.

Abbreviations

2–5(A): 2′-5′-oligoadenylate
AASLD: American Association for the Study of Liver Diseases
ADME: absorption, distribution, metabolism, excretion
ALT: alanine aminotransferase
anti-HB: hepatitis B surface antibody
AST: aspartate aminotransferase
AUC$_{ss}$: area under the plasma concentration-time curve at steady state
BCRP: breast cancer resistance protein
BMD: bone mineral density
cccDNA: covalently closed circular DNA
C$_{max}$, C$_{Pmax}$: maximal blood or plasma concentration
C$_p$: plasma concentration
CPss: plasma concentration at steady state
CSF: cerebrospinal fluid
CYP: cytochrome P450
DAA: direct-acting antiviral
dATP: deoxyadenosine triphosphate
DCV/SOF: daclatasvir/sofosbuvir fixed-dose combination
dNTP: deoxynucleotide triphosphate
EBR: elbasvir
eGFR: estimated glomerular filtration rate
eIF-2: eukaryotic initiation factor
ESRD: end-stage renal disease
FDA: Food and Drug Administration
GTP: guanosine triphosphate
GZR: grazoprevir
HBeAg: hepatitis B e antigen
HBsAg: hepatitis B surface antigen
HINT1: histidine triad nucleotide-binding protein 1
IFN: interferon
INR: international normalized ratio
LBAT: liver bile acid transporter
LDV/SOF: ledipasvir/sofosbuvir fixed-dose combination
MELD: model for end-stage liver disease
MHC: major histocompatibility complex
MRP: multidrug resistance protein
MU: million units
NTCP: Na$^+$/taurocholate cotransporter
ORF: open reading frame
PEG: polyethylene glycol
pegIFN: pegylated interferon
Pgp: P-glycoprotein
PPI: proton pump inhibitor
PrO: paritaprevir/ritonavir-boosted, ombitasvir combination
PrOD: paritaprevir/ritonavir-boosted, ombitasvir, dasabuvir combination
RAV: resistance-associated variant
RdRp: RNA-dependent RNA polymerase
RT: reverse transcriptase
SIM/SOF: simeprevir and sofosbuvir coadministered
SOF: sofosbuvir
SVR: sustained virologic response
TAF: tenofovir alafenamide fumarate
TDF: tenofovir disoproxil fumarate
VEL/SOF: fixed-dose combination of VEL and SOF
VEL: velpatasvir
WHO: World Health Organization

Genotype E is largely restricted to sub-Saharan Africa, while genotypes F and H cocirculate in indigenous peoples of South America. Genotypes I and J have been described in only three individuals and one individual, respectively.

Genotypes have relevance for the clinical manifestation of infection and the response to antiviral therapy. Clinically relevant features of HBV genotypes include the rate and durability of HBeAg (loss or seroconversion; A and D > B and C), the risk of developing aggressive HBeAg(−) chronic hepatitis B (C and D > A), spontaneous HBeAg loss (B > C), cirrhosis (C), heptatocellular carcinoma (C in Asians, F in Alaska Natives), and response to antivirals (A and B > C and D).

HBV Genome and Life Cycle

Hepatitis B virus is a small, enveloped, partially double-stranded DNA virus approximately 3200 kb in length. The virus is composed of a nucleocapsid core (HBcAg, core antigen) surrounded by an outer lipoprotein envelope containing the surface antigen (HBsAg). HBV is compact and contains four overlapping ORF. ORF C encodes the nucleocapsid protein and HBeAg, ORF P encodes the polymerase and terminal protein, ORF S/pre-S encodes three envelope proteins, and ORF X encodes the regulatory X protein.

Figure 63–1 depicts the HBV life cycle (Brahmania et al., 2016; Lin et al., 2016; Tong and Revill, 2016). HBV virus binds to the NTCP (SLC10A1; also called LBAT) on the surface of the hepatocytes. Virus is taken up into the hepatocyte, where is it uncoated. The partially double-stranded DNA is brought into the host cell's nucleus. The partial double strand is then repaired to form cccDNA. The cccDNA is not eliminated by available treatments; thus, a complete cure is not currently possible. cccDNA complexes with host proteins to form a minichromosome that becomes a template for the transcription of the various virally derived RNAs. These RNAs are transported to the cytoplasm, and some of the smaller RNAs are then made into various viral proteins, including the envelope protein. These proteins can actually be released without any genetic material (known as subviral particles). Filamentous and spherical HBsAg particles are produced in 3–4 log excess over virions (complete virus particles). These subvirus particles are thought to contribute to immune tolerance and T-cell exhaustion by increasing the amount of antigen that is circulating. The larger pregenomic RNA is used to form the HBcAg protein, which is also encapsidated. In the capsid, HBV is reverse transcribed to make more HBV DNA, and then the virus becomes bound to proteins and released as a virion.

Some patients develop mutations in the HBV genome that prevent HBeAg formation despite active HBV replication; this condition is known as HBeAg(−) disease.

HBV Drug Targets and Treatment Approach

Hepatitis B virus is a dynamic condition. Individuals with chronic infection can pass through several phases of disease throughout their lifetimes. At present, treatment is typically reserved for individuals with high levels of circulating HBV DNA and alanine aminotransferase elevations, those with cirrhosis, or for prevention of reactivation of disease in those receiving immunosuppressive therapies (e.g., chemotherapy) (Terrault et al., 2016). When treatment is necessary, the approach to HBV therapy in children and adults is similar, but most children have normal alanine aminotransferase levels and do not require treatment.

Current HBV therapies cannot achieve a complete cure, and only a small proportion (~10%) of patients achieve a functional cure. A functional cure is defined as undetectable HBV DNA with seroconversion from HBsAg to the anti-HBs. This is analogous to a resolved acute infection, but cccDNA persists, which can lead to reactivation of the disease. Existing treatment options include pegIFN-α, which has nonspecific antiviral and immunomodulatory effects, or the nucleoside/-tide analogues (Figure 63–2) adefovir, entecavir, lamivudine, telbivudine, and tenofovir, which inhibit the HBV polymerase. IFN treatment is finite (48–52 weeks), whereas individuals may require lifelong treatment with nucleoside/-tide analogues. Entecavir and TDF are the preferred nucleoside/-tide therapies due to

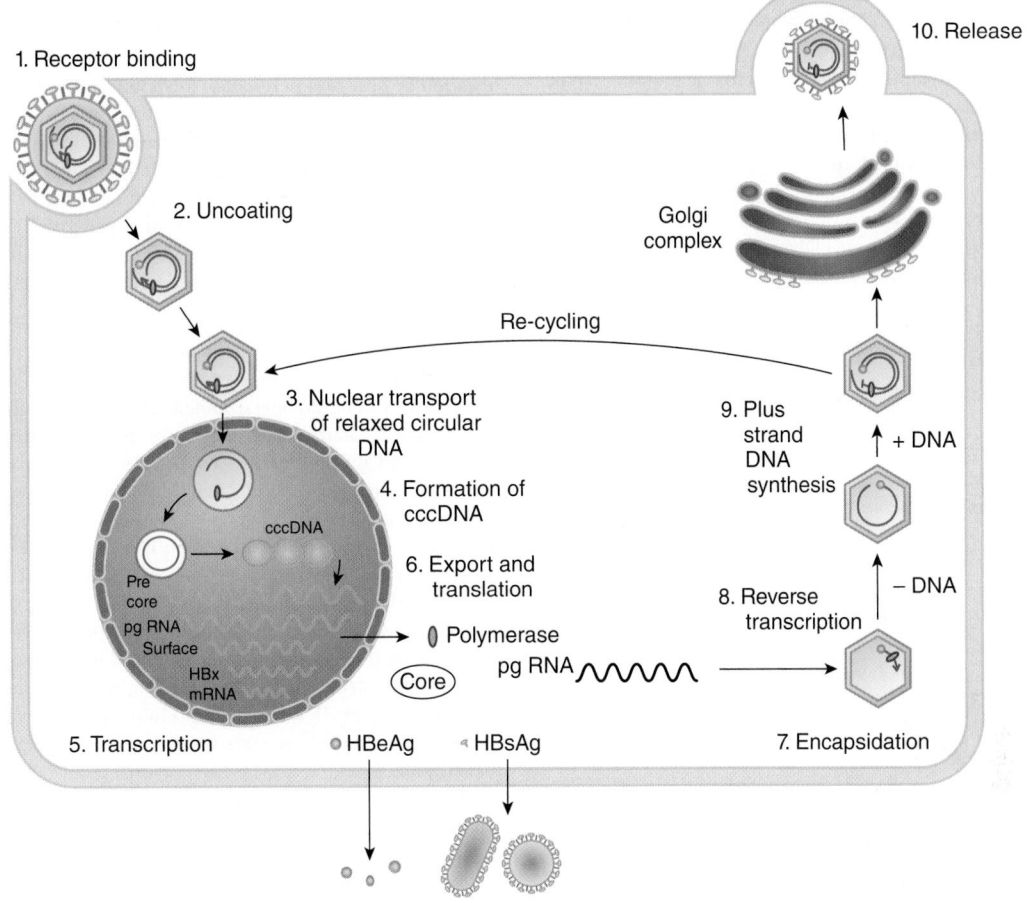

Figure 63–1 *Hepatitis B life cycle.* Not all steps in the hepatitis B viral life cycle have been completely elucidated. The figure represents our current understanding. For further details, consult the following references: Brahmania et al., 2016; Liang et al., 2015; and Tong and Revill, 2016.

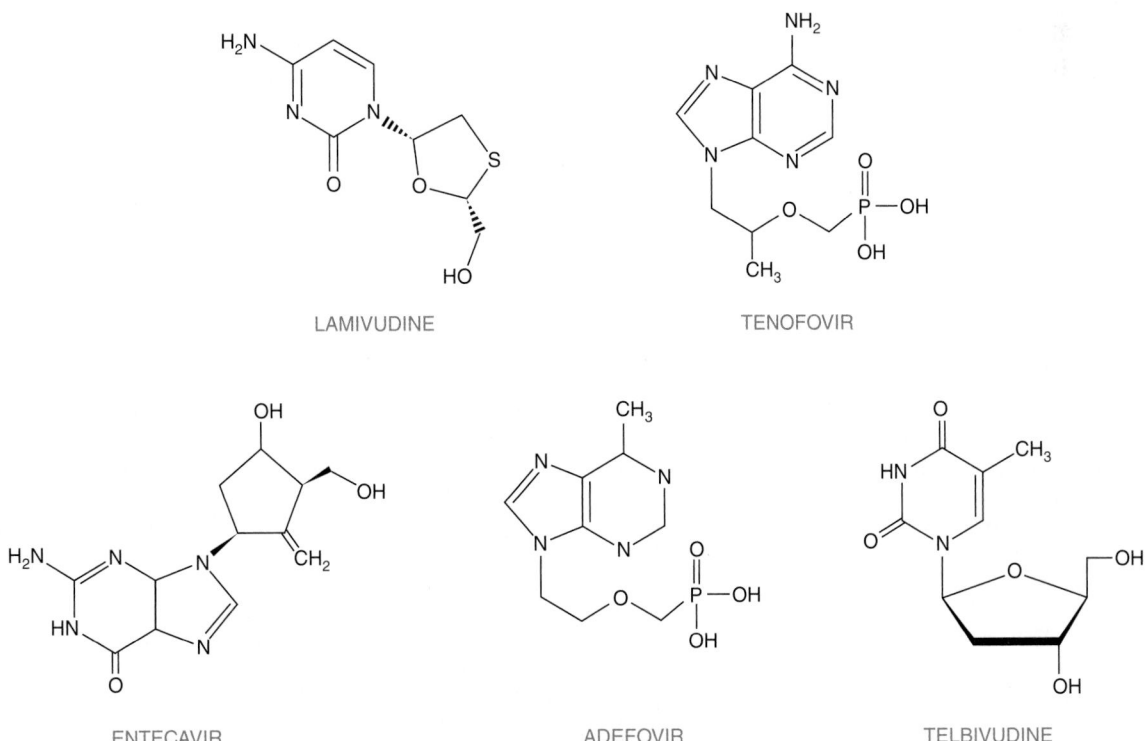

Figure 63–2 *Chemical structures of nucleos(t)ide analogs used to treat Hepatitis B.*

their potency, good tolerability, and low potential for the development of resistance (Martin et al., 2015). Considerations in selecting between the preferred therapies for HBV include the severity of liver disease, patient willingness, prior treatment, side effects, HBV genotype/serotype, comorbidities, and cost.

Because a functional cure occurs in only a small number of patients with current agents, and a complete cure is not possible, treatment goals with either pegIFN-α or nucleoside/-tide analogues are to suppress HBV DNA replication and promote seroconversion from HBeAg to anti-HBe, which in turn will slow the progression of liver disease; reduce the risk for complications, including hepatocellular carcinoma; and prolong survival (Liang et al., 2015).

Clinical Implications of HBV Resistance

Hepatitis B virus replicates at a high rate. The viral-polymerase also lacks proofreading capability. These conditions result in the generation of a large number of viral mutations. Mutations that confer a replication advantage are preferentially selected under pressure from antiviral therapy. Mutations in the reverse transcriptase/polymerase domain confer resistance to nucleoside analogues.

Lamivudine has the lowest genetic barrier to the development of resistance. After 4 years of treatment with lamivudine, 71% of patients have developed the M204V/I mutation, which renders this drug ineffective. Twenty-two percent of individuals treated with telbivudine develop this mutation after 2 years of therapy. With adefovir, about 29% of patients have developed an N236T mutation after 5 years of treatment. Resistance has not been reported with TDF. The rate of resistance with entecavir is 1% or less after 5 years in treatment-naïve individuals, whereas in those with preexisting M204V/I mutation, the prevalence of resistance is much higher, 51% after 5 years (Bhattacharya and Thio, 2010; Ghany and Doo, 2009).

The emergence of resistance has important clinical consequences. Resistance leads to therapeutic failure and a rapid resurgence of viral replication. This resurgence in HBV replication may predispose patients to hepatic decompensation. For this reason, monotherapy with lamivudine, adefovir, or telbivudine is not recommended for the treatment of hepatitis B (Terrault et al., 2016a). Individuals taking these drugs require frequent monitoring of HBV DNA and counseling on the importance of excellent adherence to the daily therapy.

Hepatic Impairment: Implications for HBV Treatment

Prolonged suppression of HBV DNA production prevents disease progression in individuals with cirrhosis and aids reversal of liver damage. Although IFN can be used in individuals with compensated cirrhosis, it is contraindicated in those with decompensated cirrhosis. Nucleos(t)ide analogue therapy is the treatment of choice for decompensated disease (Martin et al., 2015). In general, nucleos(t)ide analogue treatment improves liver function and increases the 5-year survival rate in individuals with decompensated cirrhosis from 14%–35% to 55%–86% (Honda et al., 2015). It may also prevent the need for liver transplantation.

The nucleoside/-tide analogues of choice for the treatment of decompensated cirrhosis are entecavir and TDF. Both agents require adjustments for renal impairment. TDF has been associated with nephrotoxicity, and entecavir has been associated with lactic acidosis in this population, so careful monitoring is imperative. Also, a combination of nucleoside/-tide analogues may be needed to improve efficacy in those with preexisting viral resistance. All nucleoside/-tide analogues carry a black-box warning for the risk of lactic acidosis, a risk that may be greater in individuals with advanced liver disease.

Pharmacotherapy of HBV Infection

Practice guidelines are available from several authorities on the treatment of HBV (Martin et al., 2015; Terrault et al., 2016; WHO, 2015). A description of current HBV therapies follows and a summary of the therapeutic uses and clinical pharmacology of these drugs is provided at the chapter's end.

Interferons

Interferons are potent cytokines that possess antiviral, immunomodulatory, and antiproliferative effects (Chapter 35). These proteins are synthesized by host cells in response to various inducers and, in turn, cause biochemical changes leading to an antiviral state in cells. Three major classes of human IFNs with significant antiviral activity currently are recognized: α (>18 individual species), β, and γ. Clinically used recombinant α-IFNs are nonglycosylated proteins of about 19,500 Da. Attachment of IFN proteins to large inert PEG molecules (pegylation) slows absorption, decreases clearance, and provides higher and more prolonged serum concentrations that enable once-weekly dosing. PegIFN-α is a first-line agent for the treatment of HBV.

Mechanisms of Action and Resistance. IFN-α may be produced by nearly all cells in response to viral infection and a variety of other stimuli, including double-stranded RNA and certain cytokines (e.g., interleukin 1, interleukin 2, and tumor necrosis factor). IFN-α exhibits antiviral and antiproliferative actions, stimulates the cytotoxic activity of lymphocytes, natural killer cells, and macrophages, and upregulates expression of class I MHC antigens and other surface markers. In addition, IFNs downregulate production of a number of cellular proteins, which may be an equally important mediator of the pharmacological benefit of IFNs (Teijaro, 2016).

Following binding to specific cellular receptors, IFNs activate the Jak-STAT signal transduction pathway and lead to the nuclear translocation of a cellular protein complex that binds to genes containing an IFN-specific response element. This, in turn, leads to synthesis of over two dozen proteins that contribute to viral resistance mediated at different stages of viral penetration.

Inhibition of protein synthesis is the major inhibitory effect for many viruses. IFN-induced proteins include 2–5(A) synthetase and a protein kinase, either of which can inhibit protein synthesis in the presence of double-stranded RNA. The 2–5(A) synthetase produces adenylate oligomers that activate a latent cellular endoribonuclease (RNase L) to cleave both cellular and viral single-stranded RNAs. The protein kinase selectively phosphorylates and inactivates a protein involved in protein synthesis, eIF-2. IFN-induced protein kinase also may be an important effector of apoptosis. In addition, IFN induces a phosphodiesterase that cleaves a portion of transfer RNA and thus prevents peptide elongation. A given virus may be inhibited at several steps, and the principal inhibitory effect differs amongst virus families.

Complex interactions exist between IFNs and other parts of the immune system, so IFNs may ameliorate viral infections by exerting direct antiviral effects or by modifying the immune response to infection. For example, IFN-induced expression of MHC antigens may contribute to the antiviral actions of IFN by enhancing the lytic effects of cytotoxic T lymphocytes. Conversely, IFNs may mediate some of the systemic symptoms associated with viral infections and contribute to immunologically mediated tissue damage in certain viral diseases.

Host genetics may predict IFN responsiveness. Single-nucleotide polymorphisms (rs12979860 and rs12980275) on or near the *IL-28B* gene on chromosome 19 have been associated with decreased responsiveness to IFN therapy with hepatitis C treatment (Sonneveld et al., 2012). Data are conflicting on whether *IL-28B* genetics are associated with response to IFN in individuals with HBV (Martin et al., 2015). This gene encodes IFN-λ-3. INF-λ enhances and sustains effects of INF-α on viral replication.

ADME. Oral administration of IFN-α does not result in detectable IFN levels in serum or increases in 2–5(A) synthetase activity in peripheral blood mononuclear cells (used as a marker of IFN's biologic activity). After intramuscular or subcutaneous injection of IFN-α, absorption exceeds 80%. Pegylated IFN-α is dosed subcutaneously once per week. The dose of pegIFN-α2a is 180 µg and should be reduced for patients with Cl_{Cr} less than 30 mL/min. Plasma levels are dose related, peaking at 4–8 h and returning to baseline by 18–36 h. Levels of 2–5(A) synthetase in peripheral blood mononuclear cells show increases beginning at 6 h and lasting through 4 days after a single injection. An antiviral state in peripheral blood mononuclear cells peaks at 24 h and decreases slowly to baseline by 6 days after injection. After systemic administration, low levels of IFN are detected in respiratory secretions, CSF, eye, and brain.

Two pegIFNs are available commercially: pegINF-α2a and pegINF-α2b. PegIFN-α2b has a straight-chain 12,000-Da type of PEG that increases the plasma $t_{1/2}$ from 2–3 to 30–54 h. PegIFN-α2a consists of an ester derivative of a branched-chain 40,000-Da PEG bonded to IFN-α2A and has a plasma $t_{1/2}$ of about 80–90 h. For pegIFN-α2a, peak serum concentrations occur up to 120 h after dosing and remain detectable throughout the weekly dosing interval; steady-state levels occur 5–8 weeks after initiation of weekly dosing. For pegIFN-α2A, dose-related maximum plasma concentrations occur at 15–44 h after dosing and decline by 96–168 h. Increasing PEG size is associated with longer $t_{1/2}$ and less renal clearance. About 30% of pegIFN-α2b is cleared by the kidneys; the remainder is cleared by both the liver and cellular degradation of IFN-receptor complexes. PegIFN-α2a is cleared by the liver and kidney. Patients with ESRD require dose reductions of both pegIFN products.

Therapeutic Uses. Nonpegylated forms of IFN may be used in certain clinical scenarios, but in the U.S., use of pegIFN-α predominates. PegIFN-α2a is FDA-approved for the treatment of hepatitis B and C. Its use in hepatitis C has largely been replaced by all oral DAA agents (see further discussion). However, it remains a preferred agent for the treatment of HBV in individuals with ongoing HBV DNA replication and liver inflammation. IFNs are contraindicated in patients with advanced liver disease because they can precipitate clinical deterioration and increase the risk of bacterial infections.

Unlike nucleoside/-tide analogues, which may require lifelong administration for the treatment of hepatitis B, IFN (or pegIFN) treatment is finite. Plasma HBV DNA and polymerase activity decline promptly with α-IFN (pegIFN-α) in most patients, but complete disappearance is sustained in only about one-third of patients. The advantage of α-IFN (pegIFN-α) compared with nucleoside/-tide analogues, besides the finite treatment duration, is the higher rate of HBeAg loss (~32%–36%) and HBsAg loss (~4%–11%) with pegIFN-α (Terrault et al., 2016). However, not all patients respond to α-IFN, and there are significant toxicities associated with this therapy.

Low pretherapy serum HBV DNA levels and high aminotransferase levels are predictors of response. In addition, individuals with genotypes A and B are more likely to respond to α-IFN than genotypes C or D. Responses with seroconversion to anti-HBe usually are associated with aminotransferase elevations and often a hepatitis-like illness during the second or third month of therapy, likely related to immune clearance of infected hepatocytes.

Untoward Effects. Injection of recombinant IFN doses of 1 to 2 MU or more usually is associated with an acute influenza-like syndrome beginning several hours after injection. Symptoms include fever, chills, headache, myalgia, arthralgia, nausea, vomiting, and diarrhea. Fever usually resolves within 12 h. Tolerance develops gradually in most patients. Febrile responses can be moderated by pretreatment with antipyretics.

The principal dose-limiting toxicities of systemic IFN are depression, myelosuppression with granulocytopenia and thrombocytopenia; neurotoxicity manifested by somnolence, confusion, behavioral disturbance, and rarely, seizures; debilitating neurasthenia; autoimmune disorders, including thyroiditis and hypothyroidism; and uncommonly, cardiovascular effects with hypotension and tachycardia. Elevations in hepatic enzymes and triglycerides, alopecia, proteinuria and azotemia, interstitial nephritis, autoantibody formation, pneumonia, and hepatotoxicity may occur. Alopecia and personality change are common in IFN-treated children (Sokal et al., 1998). The development of serum-neutralizing antibodies to exogenous IFNs may be associated infrequently with loss of clinical responsiveness. IFN may impair fertility, and safety during pregnancy is not established. IFNs can increase the hematological toxicity of drugs such as zidovudine and ribavirin and may increase the neurotoxicity and cardiotoxic effects of other drugs. Thyroid function and hepatic enzymes should be monitored during IFN therapy.

Pegylated IFNs are generally better tolerated than standard IFNs, although the frequencies of fever, nausea, injection site inflammation,

and neutropenia may be somewhat higher. Laboratory abnormalities, including severe neutropenia and the need for dose modifications, are higher in HIV-coinfected persons.

Pediatric and Geriatric Uses. Interferon-α2b is approved for children 1 year or older. The dose is 6 million IU/m² thrice weekly. PegIFN-α2a is not approved for children with HBV but is approved for treatment of children 5 years or older with HCV. Thus, the guidelines of the AASLD state that providers may consider using this drug in children with HBV (Terrault et al., 2016). The dose of pegIFN-α2a in children with chronic HCV is 180 μg/1.73 m² × body surface area once weekly. PegIFN-α2a contains benzyl alcohol, which has been associated with neurologic toxicities in infants and neonates.

Elderly patients may experience more toxicities from IFN treatment, and dose adjustments are necessary in renal impairment.

Entecavir

Entecavir is a guanosine analogue. Entecavir inhibited HBV DNA synthesis (50% reduction, EC_{50}) at a concentration of 0.004 μM in human HepG2 cells transfected with wild-type HBV. The median EC_{50} value for entecavir against lamivudine-resistant HBV was 0.026 μM (range 0.010–0.059 μM).

Mechanisms of Action and Resistance. Entecavir requires intracellular phosphorylation. Entecavir triphosphate competes with endogenous deoxyguanosine triphosphate and inhibits all three activities of the HBV polymerase (reverse transcriptase):

- base priming
- reverse transcription of the negative strand from the pregenomic messenger RNA
- synthesis of the positive strand of HBV DNA

Entecavir triphosphate is a weak inhibitor of cellular DNA polymerases α, β, and δ and mitochondrial DNA polymerase γ.

Susceptibility to entecavir is reduced with lamivudine and telbivudine resistance. In cell-based assays, 8- to 30-fold reductions in entecavir susceptibility were observed for lamivudine-resistant strains. In patients with preexisting lamivudine resistance, entecavir resistance emerged in 7% and 43% after 1 and 4 years, respectively.

Entecavir monotherapy in HIV/HBV-coinfected patients, including antiretroviral therapy-naïve patients, has significant anti-HIV activity and can result in the development of the M184V variant (Sasadeusz et al., 2008). Thus, entecavir should only be used in combination with fully suppressive antiretroviral therapy in individuals with HIV/HBV coinfection.

ADME. The recommended dose for nucleoside-treatment-naïve adults without decompensated cirrhosis is 0.5 mg once daily. For adults with lamivudine or telbivudine resistance or for those with decompensated cirrhosis, the dose is 1 mg once daily. The dose must be reduced for individuals with CrCl less than 50 mL/min. Time to peak C_p occurs in 0.5–1.5 h. Steady state is reached after 6–10 days of once-daily dosing. The tablet and oral solution can be used interchangeably. Administration with food decreases C_{max} by 44%–46% and AUC by 18%–20%; thus, entecavir should be administered on an empty stomach.

Entecavir is extensively distributed in tissues and binds slightly (13%) to serum proteins. It is primarily eliminated unchanged in the kidney, probably by both glomerular filtration and net tubular secretion. Entecavir exhibits biphasic elimination, with a terminal $t_{1/2}$ of 128–149 h. Dose reductions are needed for patients with Cl_{Cr} less than 50 mL/min, typically by extension of the dosing interval.

Therapeutic Uses. Entecavir is FDA approved for the treatment of chronic HBV infection in adults and children 2 years or older with evidence of active viral replication and evidence of either persistent elevations in serum aminotransferases or histologically active disease. Entecavir is considered a first-line agent for HBV because of its potency, durability, and low genetic barrier to the development of resistance (Terrault et al., 2016). In HBeAg-positive individuals, 61% are virologically suppressed, 22%–25% have HBeAg loss, 68%–81% normalize ALT, and 4%–5% have HBsAg loss after 2–3 years of continuous entecavir treatment. In HBeAg-negative individuals, 90%–91% are virologically suppressed and

78%–88% normalize ALT after 2–3 years of entecavir treatment, but fewer than 1% have HBsAg loss at 1 year. Entecavir use reduces the risk of hepatocellular carcinoma relative to untreated historical controls. Few studies have shown a benefit to combination treatment of HBV; however, one study found that in individuals with HBV DNA of 10^8 or greater, the combination of entecavir and TDF was superior to entecavir alone (Lok et al., 2012). Nucleoside/-tide combination therapy may also be used in the case of decompensated cirrhosis and in individuals with virologic breakthrough on entecavir or TDF. The safety of entecavir in pregnancy is unknown.

Untoward Effects. Severe acute exacerbations of HBV have been reported in patients who have discontinued anti-HBV therapy, including entecavir. Hepatic function should be monitored closely with both clinical and laboratory follow-up for at least several months in patients who discontinue anti-HBV therapy. There is a potential for development of resistance to nucleoside reverse transcriptase inhibitors in HBV/HIV coinfection, especially if HIV is not being treated. Lactic acidosis and severe hepatomegaly with steatosis may occur in patients with decompensated cirrhosis receiving entecavir. More common adverse reactions include headache, fatigue, dizziness, and nausea (Sasadeusz et al., 2008).

Pediatric and Geriatric Uses. Entecavir oral solution is approved in children older than 2 years and dosing is weight based up to 30 kg. Entecavir exposures following a single 1-mg dose were 29% higher in elderly versus young HBV-seronegative volunteers. This difference is likely explained by declines in renal function with age.

Tenofovir

Tenofovir, an acyclic nucleoside phosphonate, is available in two different prodrug formulations, TDF and TAF. TAF is described separately in a following discussion. With TDF, cellular esterases cleave the diester, yielding tenofovir in plasma, which enters cells and is subsequently phosphorylated by cellular kinases to tenofovir diphosphate (Figure 64–4). The drug has activity against both HIV-1 and HBV. In cell cultures in vitro, the EC_{50} for tenofovir against HBV ranges from 0.14 to 1.5 μM.

Mechanisms of Action and Resistance. The mechanism of action of tenofovir is presented in Chapter 64. Tenofovir has not been associated with the development of resistance when used as monotherapy for the treatment of HBV.

ADME. The TDF dose is 300 mg once daily; the dose is reduced in patients with renal impairment. The bioavailability of tenofovir is approximately 25%. Tenofovir exposures are increased 40% with a high-fat meal. Binding to plasma proteins is negligible (<8%). Tenofovir is not metabolized by CYP enzymes. The $t_{1/2}$ of tenofovir in plasma is 17 h, and the $t_{1/2}$ of the active form of the drug, tenofovir diphosphate, is 6-days and 17 days in peripheral blood and red blood cells, respectively. Tenofovir pharmacokinetics are not altered in hepatic impairment, but plasma exposures rise as Cl_{Cr} drops, becoming 2.8- and 7.3-fold higher in those with Cl_{Cr} of 30–49 mL/min and 12–29 mL/min compared to those with Cl_{Cr} greater than 80 mL/min. Doses should be reduced in those with CrCl below 50 mL/min. Roughly 10% of the dose is removed by a 4-h hemodialysis session.

Therapeutic Uses. TDF is approved for the treatment of HBV infection in individuals 2 years or older. Due to its safety, efficacy, and resistance profile, TDF is a preferred agent for the treatment of HBV. In HBeAg-positive individuals, 76% are virologically suppressed, 21% have conversion from HBeAg to anti-HBe, 68% normalize ALT, and 8% have HBsAg loss after 3 years of continuous TDF treatment. In HBeAg-negative individuals, 93% are virologically suppressed and 76% normalize ALT after 2–3 years of treatment, but none have HBsAg loss at 1 year (Terrault et al., 2016).

Few studies have shown a benefit to combination treatment of HBV; however, one study found that in individuals with HBV DNA 10^8 or greater, the combination of entecavir and TDF was superior to entecavir alone (Lok et al., 2012). Nucleos(t)ide combination therapy may also be used in the case of decompensated cirrhosis and in individuals with virologic breakthrough on entecavir or TDF. TDF has a pregnancy category of B,

although a study found that infants born to HIV-infected women receiving TDF had 12% lower bone mineral density compared to infants born to women receiving other antiretroviral agents. HIV-infected individuals are generally treated with tenofovir and emtricitabine. Emtricitabine is a cytidine analog with activity against HIV and HBV. Refer to Chapter 64 for additional information about emtricitabine.

Untoward Effects and Drug Interactions. Tenofovir has a low potential for interactions but is not devoid of interactions. Tenofovir is a substrate for several membrane transporters, including OAT1 and MRP4, and TDF is a substrate for Pgp and BCRP and thus tenofovir may be affected by drugs that inhibit or induce these transporters. Some HCV therapies (e.g., sofosbuvir, ledipasvir, and velpatasvir) increase tenofovir exposures; patients receiving such combinations require more frequent renal monitoring.

Pediatric and Geriatric Uses. Primary considerations in treating the elderly with TDF are the bone and renal toxicities; a thorough study of TDF in the geriatric population has not been published. TDF has been studied in children and is approved for those 2 years or older. The dose of TDF in children is 8 mg/kg, with a maximum of 300 mg daily.

Adefovir

Adefovir dipivoxil is a diester prodrug of adefovir, an acyclic phosphonate nucleotide analogue of adenosine monophosphate. Inhibitory concentrations of adefovir against HBV range from 0.2 to 1.2 μM in cell culture.

Mechanisms of Action and Resistance. Adefovir dipivoxil enters cells and is deesterified to adefovir. Adefovir is converted by cellular enzymes to the diphosphate, which acts as a competitive inhibitor of viral DNA polymerases and reverse transcriptases with respect to dATP and also serves as a chain terminator of viral DNA synthesis (Kundy, 1999).

Resistance to adefovir emerges in about 29% of patients after 5 years of treatment. The development of viral resistance may increase the risk of hepatic decompensation. Thus, adefovir, lamivudine, and telbivudine are not recommended for the treatment of HBV.

ADME. The adefovir dipovoxil dose is 10 mg once daily but must be reduced for those with renal impairment. The parent compound has low oral bioavailability (<12%), whereas the dipivoxil prodrug is absorbed rapidly and hydrolyzed by esterases in the intestine, liver, and blood to adefovir, providing a bioavailability of about 30%–60%. Food does not affect bioavailability. Adefovir is scantily protein bound (<5%) and has a volume of distribution of about 0.4 L/kg.

The drug is eliminated unchanged by the kidney through a combination of glomerular filtration and tubular secretion. After oral administration of adefovir dipivoxil, about 30%–45% of the dose is recovered within 24 h; the serum $t_{1/2}$ of elimination is 5–7.5 h. The intracellular $t_{1/2}$ of the active diphosphate form in vitro ranges from 5 to 18 h, although typically the half-lives are much longer in vivo. Dose reductions are recommended for Cl_{Cr} values below 50 mL/min. Adefovir is removed by hemodialysis, but the effects of peritoneal dialysis or severe hepatic insufficiency on pharmacokinetics are unknown.

Therapeutic Uses. Adefovir dipivoxil is approved for treatment of chronic HBV infections in individuals 12 years and older. However, adefovir dipivoxil is not a preferred agent for the treatment of HBV because it is associated with the development of viral resistance and nephrotoxicity.

Untoward Effects and Drug Interactions. Adefovir dipivoxil causes dose-related nephrotoxicity and tubular dysfunction, manifested by azotemia and hypophosphatemia, acidosis, glycosuria, and proteinuria, which usually are reversible months after discontinuation. Other adverse effects include headache, abdominal discomfort, diarrhea, and asthenia. Adverse events lead to premature discontinuation in about 2% of patients. After 2 years of dosing, the risk of serum creatinine levels rising above 0.5 mg/dL is approximately 2% but is higher in those with preexisting renal insufficiency. Acute, sometimes severe, exacerbations of hepatitis can occur in patients stopping adefovir or other anti-HBV therapies.

Close monitoring is necessary, and resumption of antiviral therapy may be required in some patients.

No clinically important drug interactions have been recognized to date, although drugs that reduce renal function or compete for active tubular secretion could decrease adefovir clearance. Ibuprofen increases adefovir exposure modestly. An increased risk of lactic acidosis and steatosis may exist when adefovir is used in conjunction with other nucleoside analogues or antiretroviral agents. Adefovir is transported efficiently by renal tubular OAT1.

Adefovir is genotoxic, and high doses cause hepatotoxicity, lymphoid toxicity, and renal tubular nephropathy in animals. The diphosphate's inhibitory effects on renal adenylyl cyclase may contribute to nephrotoxicity (Shoshani et al., 1999). Adefovir dipivoxil is not associated with reproductive toxicity, although high intravenous doses of adefovir cause maternal and embryotoxicity with fetal malformations in rats (pregnancy category C).

Pediatric and Geriatric Uses. Adefovir should be avoided in elderly patients due to the risk for nephrotoxicity. This drug is approved in children 12 years or older at the same dose as that used in adults.

Lamivudine

Lamivudine, the (−)-enantiomer of 2′,3′-dideoxy-3′-thiacytidine, is a nucleoside analogue that inhibits HIV reverse transcriptase and HBV DNA polymerase. Details of its *mechanism of action, ADME, and drug interaction potential* are described in Chapter 64. Lamivudine inhibits HBV replication in vitro by 50% at concentrations of 4–7 ng/mL.

Mechanisms of Action and Resistance. Cellular enzymes convert lamivudine to the triphosphate, which competitively inhibits HBV DNA polymerase and causes chain termination.

After 5 years of treatment, approximately 71% of patients develop resistance to lamivudine. Point mutations in the *YMDD* motif of HBV DNA polymerase result in a 40- to 104-fold reduction in the in vitro susceptibility (Ono et al., 2001). Lamivudine resistance confers cross-resistance to related agents, such as emtricitabine. Lamivudine-resistant HBV retains susceptibility to tenofovir and partially to adefovir and entecavir. Lamivudine resistance is associated with elevated HBV DNA levels, decreased likelihood of HBeAg loss or seroconversion, hepatitis exacerbations, and progressive fibrosis and graft loss in transplant recipients.

Therapeutic Uses. Lamivudine is approved for the treatment of chronic HBV hepatitis in adults and children 2 years or older. However, lamivudine is not a preferred agent for the treatment of HBV because it is associated with a high rate of viral resistance. Nonetheless, lamivudine is still used in many parts of the world because it is cheaper than other therapies.

The lamivudine dose is 100 mg once daily. In adults, doses of 100 mg/d for 1 year cause suppression of HBV DNA levels, normalization of aminotransferase levels in 41% or more of patients, and reductions in hepatic inflammation in more than 50% of patients. Seroconversion with antibody to HBeAg occurs in fewer than 20% of recipients at 1 year. In children 2–17 years of age, lamivudine (3 mg/kg/d to a maximum of 100 mg/d for 1 year) is associated with normalization of aminotransferase levels in about one-half and seroconversion to anti-HBe in about one-fifth of cases.(Jonas et al., 2002). If resistant variants do not emerge, prolonged therapy is associated with sustained suppression of HBV DNA, continued histological improvement, and an increased proportion of patients experiencing a loss of HBeAg and undetectable HBV DNA. Prolonged therapy is associated with an approximate halving of the risk of clinical progression and development of hepatocellular carcinoma in those with advanced fibrosis or cirrhosis (Liaw et al., 2004). However, the frequency of lamivudine-resistant variants increases progressively with continued drug administration. Consider dose reduction for patients with renal impairment.

Untoward Effects. At the doses used for chronic HBV infection, lamivudine generally is well tolerated. Aminotransferase rises after therapy occur in lamivudine recipients, and flares in posttreatment

aminotransferase elevations (>500 IU/mL) occur in about 15% of patients after cessation.

Pediatric and Geriatric Uses. The dose of lamivudine for use in children 2–17 years old is 3 mg/kg/d to a maximum of 100 mg/d. Lamivudine is not associated with increased toxicities in the elderly.

Telbivudine

Telbivudine is a synthetic thymidine nucleoside analogue with activity against HBV DNA polymerase. In a cell culture model, the EC_{50} for inhibition of viral DNA synthesis by telbivudine was 0.2 μM. The U.S. manufacturer has ceased producing telbivudine.

Mechanisms of Action and Resistance. Telbivudine is phosphorylated by cellular kinases to the active triphosphate form, telbivudine 5′-triphosphate, which inhibits HBV DNA polymerase (reverse transcriptase) by competing with the natural substrate, thymidine 5′-triphosphate. Incorporation of telbivudine 5′-triphosphate into viral DNA causes chain termination.

Resistance to telbivudine emerges in about 22% of patients after 2 years of treatment. The development of viral resistance may increase the risk for hepatic decompensation. Thus, this drug, along with lamivudine and adefovir, is not recommended for the treatment of HBV.

ADME. The standard telbivudine dose is 600 mg once daily. The bioavailability of telbivudine is 68% (Zhou et al., 2006), and the drug is widely distributed into tissues. Food does not affect the pharmacokinetics of telbivudine. The drug is eliminated unchanged in the urine. Telbivudine concentrations decline biexponentially with an elimination $t_{1/2}$ of 40–49 h. Patients with moderate-to-severe renal dysfunction and those undergoing hemodialysis require dose adjustments.

Therapeutic Uses. Telbivudine is indicated for the treatment of chronic HBV in adult patients (≥16 years) with evidence of viral replication and either evidence of persistent elevations in serum aminotransferases (ALT or AST) or histologically active disease. Although telbivudine has superior efficacy compared with lamivudine and adefovir, its use is associated with the development of resistance. Thus, telbivudine is not a preferred agent for the treatment of HBV.

Untoward Effects and Drug Interactions. Telbivudine is generally well tolerated and safe. The most common adverse events resulting in telbivudine discontinuation included increased creatine kinase, nausea, diarrhea, fatigue, myalgia, and myopathy. Elevations of creatine kinase activity, mostly asymptomatic grade 3–4, are more common in telbivudine-treated than in lamivudine-treated patients after 2 years of therapy. The risk of peripheral neuropathy is increased when telbivudine is used with INF-α, so this combination should be avoided.

Pediatric and Geriatric Uses. Telbivudine is not approved for children younger than 16 years. The primary consideration in treating geriatric patients with telbivudine is renal function.

Tenofovir Alafenamide

A different prodrug of tenofovir, TAF, is a phosphonate ester of tenofovir (Ray et al., 2016).

Mechanisms of Action and Resistance. The active ingredient of TAF is tenofovir, an inhibitor of HBV reverse transcriptase and HIV-1 reverse transcriptase. TAF is relatively more stable in the plasma than TDF; it is taken up into cells (e.g., hepatocytes), where it is deesterified, concentrated, and phosphorylated to tenofovir diphosphate. Tenofovir diphosphate is a competitive inhibitor of reverse transcriptase, competing with the physiological substrate dATP; when incorporated into DNA, the drug results in chain termination.

ADME. The dose of TAF for hepatitis B is 25 mg once daily. Plasma concentrations of tenofovir when administered as TAF are 90% less than when administered as TDF. The renal adverse effects of tenofovir are mediated through uptake by OAT1 in the kidney. TAF is not a substrate for OAT1, so less tenofovir is delivered to the kidneys, and there is less renal toxicity with this agent. However, TAF is preferentially taken up by several cell types, including peripheral blood mononuclear cells, and cellular concentrations of the active form, tenofovir diphosphate, are actually higher than those achieved with TDF.

Therapeutic Uses. TAF is used at a daily dose of 25 mg to treat HBV. Two studies have found TAF noninferior to TDF in terms of suppressed HBV DNA after 48 weeks of treatment with smaller declines in bone mineral density and eGFR.

Untoward Effects and Drug Interactions. TAF has similar efficacy to TDF with fewer adverse effects on BMD and kidney function (Cl$_{Cr}$, eGFR, proteinuria). Common side effects of tenofovir include nausea, rash, diarrhea, depression, and weakness. HBV "flare up" can result from sudden discontinuation of the drug.

Investigational Agents

Current therapies provide a functional cure (i.e., a cure that mimics naturally acquired immunity off therapy) in a minority of patients, and none provides a complete cure because cccDNA persists in cells. Thus, hepatitis B disease is an area ripe for drug development. There are currently more than 30 compounds in development for the treatment of hepatitis B (Brahmania et al., 2016). Although most are in the early stages of development, there is tremendous promise for the treatment of this virus.

Hepatitis C Virus

HCV Overview

Two percent of the world's population—approximately 150 million people—are infected with HCV. Africa and Central and East Asia have the highest prevalence of HCV. The majority of individuals infected with HCV, about 85%, will develop chronic infection, which may progress to cirrhosis (WHO, 2016). Approximately 6% of cirrhotic individuals will develop symptoms of decompensated liver disease (e.g., ascites, hepatic

encephalopathy, or variceal bleeding) each year, and 4% will develop hepatocellular carcinoma. These long-term complications carry a high risk of mortality and generally occur more than 20 years after infection (Freeman et al., 2001). There are approximately 700,000 HCV-related deaths annually. Without effective treatment, this number is expected to increase over the next 20 years. HCV is the leading indication for liver transplantation (Chinnadurai et al., 2012).

Genetic Heterogeneity of HCV

Hepatitis C virus exhibits remarkable within- and between-subject genetic heterogeneity, which is a major obstacle to the development of a universal treatment and a universal preventive vaccine. Six HCV genotypes have been identified. HCV strains belonging to different genotypes differ at 30%–35% of nucleotide sites (Messina et al., 2015). Within each genotype, HCV is further classified into subtypes that differ at fewer than 15% of nucleotide sites. Amongst genotypes, transmissibility does not seem to differ, whereas the rate of disease progression and response to treatment with current therapies does differ. Globally, genotype 1 is most prevalent (Messina et al., 2015), followed by genotype 3. Genotypes 2, 4, and 6 together account for 25% of those living with HCV. Within the U.S., 75% of HCV isolates are genotype 1a or 1b, and the remainder are primarily genotype 2 or 3 (Zein et al., 1996). Individuals with subtype 1a tend to have higher relapse rates with certain HCV treatments compared with individuals with subtype 1b.

The HCV Genome and Life Cycle

The HCV genome consists of a positive-sense, single-stranded RNA, about 9600 nucleotides long, which encodes three structural proteins (core, E1, and E2); the ion channel protein p7; and six nonstructural proteins (NS2, NS3, NS4A, NS4B, NS5A, and NS5B) (Tang and Grise, 2009). HCV replicates entirely within the cytoplasm (Figure 63–3); it does not

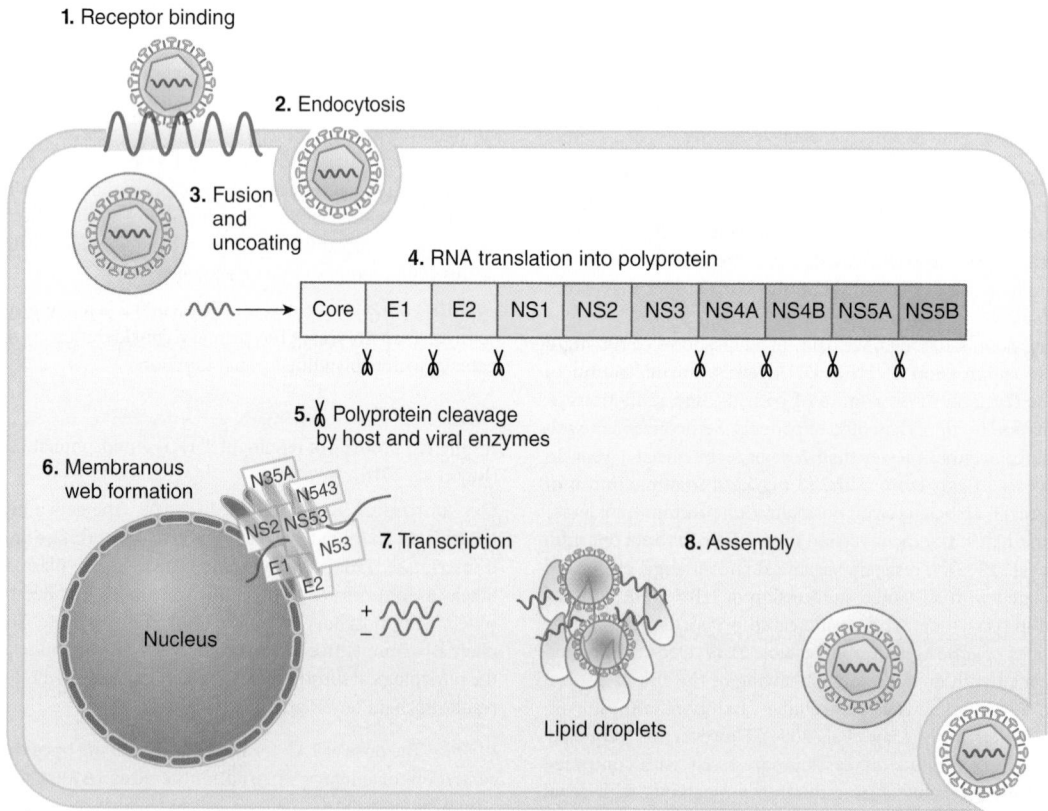

Figure 63–3 *Hepatitis C life cycle.* Not all steps in the hepatitis C viral life cycle have been completely elucidated. This figure represents our current understanding. For further details, consult the following references: Ciesek and Manns, 2011; Dubuisson and Cosset, 2014; and Holmes and Thompson, 2015.

establish latency, and it is curable. Cure of HCV is synonymous with achieving an SVR. SVR is defined as having no measurable HCV RNA in the blood following the cessation of treatment. With current therapies, SVR is assessed 12 weeks following treatment cessation. Achieving SVR decreases the progression of liver disease and reduces liver-related and all-cause mortality.

HCV Drug Targets and Treatment Approach

For many years, HCV was treated with a prolonged regimen of subcutaneously administered IFN-α (or pegIFN-α) with or without the purine nucleoside analogue ribavirin. SVR rates with this therapy were low, and tolerability was poor. Now, several antivirals that directly target various steps in the HCV life cycle (so-called DAAs) are the mainstay of HCV treatment. DAAs are administered orally, have few side effects, are taken for a period of 8, 12, or 24 weeks, and achieve SVR rates of at least 90% in most patient populations. Use of pegIFN-α for the treatment of HCV has largely been replaced by DAAs, although ribavirin is still used in combination with DAAs to improve SVR rates in certain clinical scenarios.

Detailed knowledge of the HCV life cycle and the structures of HCV proteins has permitted development of targeted inhibitors of HCV replication and revolutionized pharmacotherapy of HCV infection. Available DAAs target three major sites in the HCV life cycle: the NS3 protease, the NS5B polymerase, and NS5A (Figure 63–3) (Ciesek and Manns, 2011; Dubuisson and Cosset, 2014; Holmes and Thompson, 2015). Inhibition of the NS3 protease prevents the cleavage of the viral polyprotein and formation of the replication complex. The NS5B enzyme is essential for HCV replication as it catalyzes the synthesis of the complementary minus-strand RNA and subsequent genomic plus-strand RNA. There are two types of NS5B RdRp inhibitors: nucleotide and nonnucleoside inhibitors. The nucleotide inhibitors are active site inhibitors, whereas the nonnucleoside inhibitors are allosteric inhibitors. Another target, NS5A, encodes a protein that appears essential to the replication machinery of HCV and critical in the assembly of new infectious viral particles (Gish and Meanwell, 2011). However, the specific functions of this protein have not been established.

Clinical Implications of HCV Resistance

On average, almost a trillion HCV particles are produced in an infected individual each day (Neumann et al., 1998). The HCV NS5B polymerase enzyme lacks a proofreading function and has relatively poor fidelity (Brown, 2009); therefore, there is a continuous generation of a large variety of spontaneous viral mutations. Thus, even untreated persons have HCV genomes that harbor preexisting RAVs. These naturally occurring RAVs may affect the chances of achieving a cure with DAA treatment.

The likelihood that a DAA will select for and allow outgrowth of viral populations carrying RAVs during treatment depends on several factors, including the DAA's genetic barrier to resistance (the number and type of base-pair mutations needed to result in amino acid substitutions that confer resistance), the level of drug exposure(s), and the viral fitness (replicative capacity) of the RAV (Lontok et al., 2015). Nucleotide NS5B polymerase inhibitors have a high genetic barrier to resistance; three or more RAVs are required for full resistance. In contrast, the nonnucleoside NS5B polymerase inhibitors, NS3 protease inhibitors, and NS5A inhibitors generally have a low genetic barrier to the development of resistance; that is, only one or two amino acid substitutions result in lack of drug efficacy. For drugs in these classes, there is swift emergence of RAVs during monotherapy. Thus, as with HIV treatment, HCV treatment requires a combination of agents to optimize viral suppression and protect against the development of resistance. Data are emerging on the impact of treatment-emergent NS5A RAVs on the likelihood of achieving SVR with current therapies. NS5A RAVs have been shown to persist for several years after treatment cessation, and some NS5A inhibitors suffer from broad cross-resistance at key positions (Q30R, L31M/V, Y93H/N).

Hepatic Impairment: Implications for HCV Treatment

The vast majority of HCV-infected individuals have at least a 90% chance of achieving SVR with current therapies. There are some groups, however, such as those with decompensated cirrhosis, who have lower rates of SVR. Treating those with decompensated cirrhosis and achieving SVR have been shown to improve MELD scores and reverse fibrosis, but benefits are not immediate. Data are needed to demonstrate the long-term benefits of achieving SVR in those with decompensated disease.

Studies indicated the optimal time to treat HCV is early in the course of illness. The risk of developing decompensated cirrhosis or hepatocellular carcinoma, requiring a liver transplant, or dying from HCV-related complications is significantly lower in those treated with minimal fibrosis compared to those treated once bridging fibrosis or cirrhosis has developed. Treating all patients early in the course of disease is challenging, however, because many patients with HCV are unaware of their disease. Others are aware of their disease and wish to be treated but cannot access the DAAs. Many payers are prioritizing those with more advanced disease for treatment because of the cost of the DAAs.

Pharmacotherapy of HCV

A description of current DAA therapies follows, and a summary of the therapeutic uses and clinical pharmacology of these drugs is provided in the Drug Facts table at the end of this chapter. The HCV field is rapidly evolving. Up-to-date information on testing, managing, and treating HCV can be found in guidelines from the AASLD and Infectious Diseases Society of America (http://www.hcvguidelines.org). An important aspect of treating HCV is identification and management of drug-drug

TABLE 63–1 ■ DACLATASVIR (DCV) DOSING WITH INDUCERS AND INHIBITORS OF CYP3A4

STRONG CYP3A INHIBITORS	MODERATE CYP3A INHIBITORS	STRONG CYP3A INDUCERS	MODERATE CYP3A INDUCERS
Decrease DCV Dose to 30 mg	**Standard DCV Dose, 60 mg**	**DCV Contraindicated**	**Increase DCV Dose to 90 mg**
Ritonavir-boosted atazanavir	Ritonavir-boosted darunavir	Rifamycins	Bosentan
Clarithromycin	Ritonavir-boosted lopinavir	St. John's Wort	Dexamethasone
Itraconazole	Ciprofloxacin	Antiepileptics	Efavirenz
Ketoconazole	Diltiazem		Etravirine
Nefazodone	Erythromycin		Modafinil
Nelfinavir	Fluconazole		Nafcillin
Posaconazole	Fosamprenavir		Rifapentine
Telithromycin	Verapamil		
Voriconazole			

interactions with DAAs (see, for instance, Table 63–1). The University of Liverpool offers a free, comprehensive, and reliable web-based drug interactions resource (available at http://www.hep-druginteractions.org).

Sofosbuvir

Sofosbuvir is a prodrug based on a uridine analogue. In cells, sofosbuvir is metabolized to an active form (known as GS-461203) that competes with uridine triphosphate for incorporation into HCV RNA by NS5B polymerase.

Mechanisms of Action and Resistance. Sofosbuvir is a prodrug, a 5′ monophosphorylated uridine analogue on which the charges of the phosphate group are masked by groups that are readily removed in the cell. The active drug, generated in the host mammalian cell, inhibits HCV RNA polymerase. Figure 63–4 shows the cellular pharmacology of sofosbuvir.

Sofosbuvir provides a high barrier to the development of resistance, but the S282T RAV has been reported in patients who relapsed to sofosbuvir-based treatment. L159F, V321A, and C316N/H/F have also been observed (Lontok et al., 2015).

ADME. The dose of sofosbuvir is 400 mg taken once daily. The absolute bioavailability of sofosbuvir is estimated to be at least 80% based on recovery of sofosbuvir and its primary metabolite, GS-331007, following administration of a radiolabeled dose. A high-fat meal increases sofosbuvir's AUC by 67%–91%, but, based on the drug's high therapeutic index, the increased exposure is not thought to increase the likelihood of toxicities (Kirby et al., 2015). Sofosbuvir exhibits time-independent, near-linear pharmacokinetics across a range of doses. Sofosbuvir is 63% protein bound, whereas protein binding of the deesterified GS-331007 is minimal.

The primary metabolic route of sofosbuvir is hydrolysis to GS-331007. GS-331007 lacks antiviral activity and cannot be rephosphorylated. The majority of a sofosbuvir dose is converted to GS-331007 and eliminated in the urine via a combination of tubular secretion and glomerular filtration. Sofosbuvir AUC is increased 2.3-fold and 2.5-fold in patients with moderate and severe hepatic impairment (i.e., Child Pugh B and C), respectively, but GS-331007 AUC is unchanged. No dose adjustment is needed for this population; available data suggest sofosbuvir is safe and effective in individuals with decompensated cirrhosis when combined with appropriate DAAs (Charlton et al., 2015; Manns et al., 2015; Poordad et al., 2015).

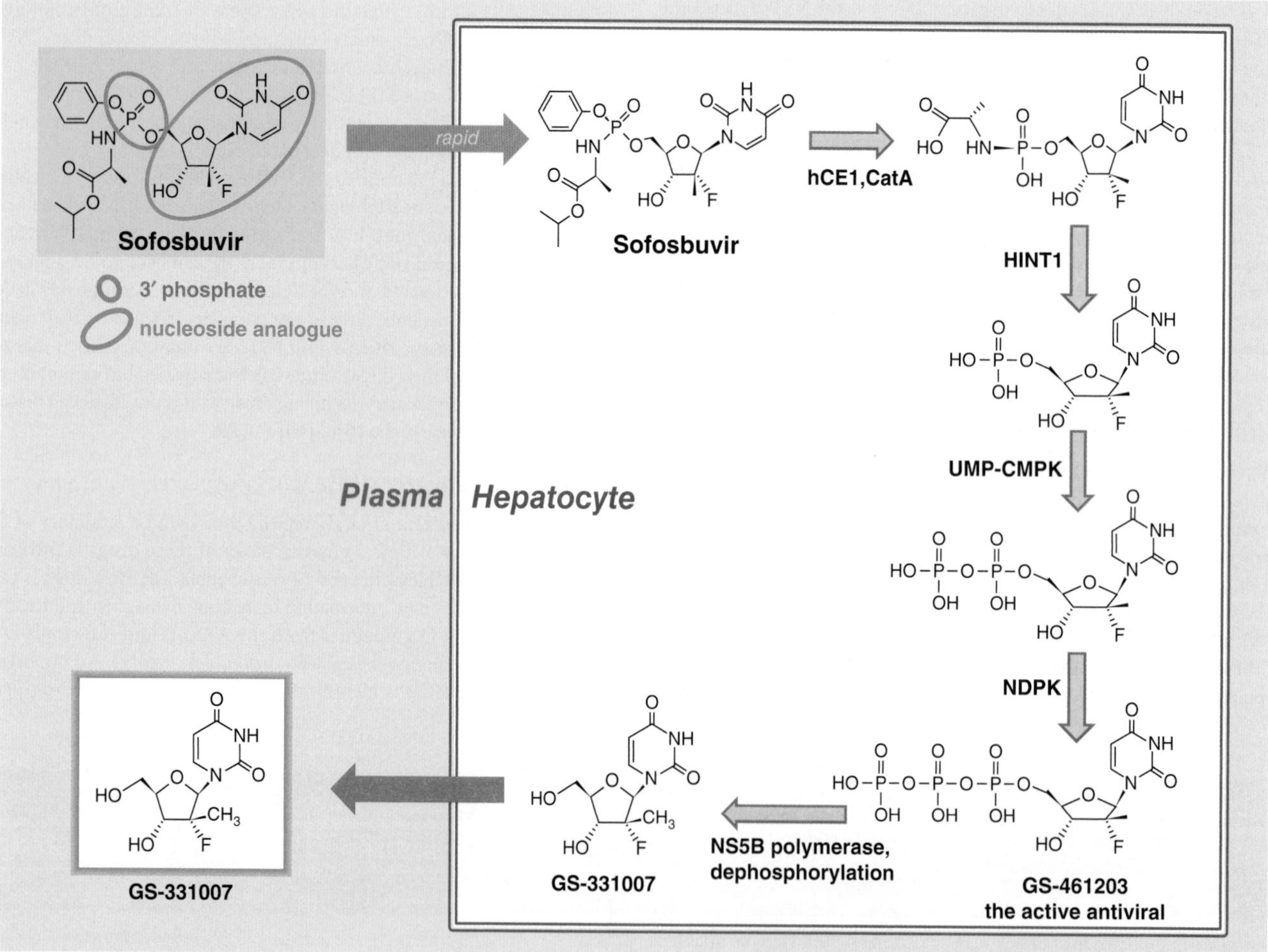

Figure 63–4 *Cellular pharmacology of sofosbuvir.* Some nucleoside analogues act as antiviral agents in infected cells, but first they must cross the plasma membrane and then be phosphorylated, starting at the 5′ position, a slow reaction catalyzed by nucleoside kinase. Use of a monophosphorylated nucleoside avoids the slow nucleoside kinase reaction, but the charge on the phosphate groups would greatly slow passage of the molecule across the plasma membrane. Sofosbuvir circumvents these issues by having a phosphate (red ellipse) at the 5′ position of the nucleoside analogue (blue ellipse), but masking the two negative charges of the phosphate group with adducts that cellular esterases/amidases can readily remove. Sofosbuvir crosses the plasma membrane rapidly. The carboxyl ester moiety is hydrolyzed by CatA or hCE1. HINT1 catalyzes the phosphoramidate cleavage, yielding the monophosphate form, retained in the cell by ion trapping. Subsequent phosphorylation occurs via the pyrimidine nucleotide biosynthetic pathway. The triphosphate (GS-461203) is the active form responsible for the antiviral activity of sofosbuvir. GS-461203 acts as a defective dNTP substrate and inhibits HBV RNA polymerase (NS5B); it may also act as a chain terminator. Dephosphorylation of GS-461203 yields a uridine analogue metabolite, GS-331007, that cannot be readily rephosphorylated, lacks antiviral activity, and exits the cell. Most (90%) of the drug-related material measured in plasma is GS-331007. UMP-CMPK, uridine/cytidine monophosphate kinase; NDPK, nucleoside diphosphate kinase; CatA, cathepsin A; hCE1, human carboxylesterase 1.

In contrast, sofosbuvir and GS-331007 pharmacokinetics are affected by renal impairment. Sofosbuvir and GS-331007 AUC increased about 60% in those with eGFR 50–80 mL/min/1.73 m[2] and 2-fold in those with eGFR 30–50 mL/min/1.73 m[2]. These exposures were safe and tolerated in prior studies, but significant increases in exposure are noted in patients with severe renal impairment (eGFR < 30 mL/min/1.73 m[2]) and ESRD requiring dialysis. Thus, sofosbuvir should not be used in patients with eGFR of less than 30 mL/min/1.73 m[2] or those with ESRD until more data are available on the safety and appropriate dosing of this drug in this population (Kirby et al., 2015). Sofosbuvir's AUC is 60% higher in HCV-infected persons, and GS-331007 AUC is 39% lower compared with HCV-seronegative volunteers. The mechanism for this is unclear. The median terminal half-lives of sofosbuvir and GS-331007 are 0.4 and 27 h, respectively.

Therapeutic Uses. The NS5B polymerase region is well conserved across genotypes. Thus, sofosbuvir is active against all HCV genotypes. In individuals with genotype 1 HCV, 7 days of sofosbuvir monotherapy reduces HCV RNA by 4.65 logs (Lawitz et al., 2013). Sofosbuvir is used in combination with other DAAs, including the NS3/4A protease inhibitor simeprevir, the purine nucleoside analogue ribavirin, and the NS5A inhibitors daclatasvir, ledipasvir, or velpatasvir. The efficacy and tolerability of sofosbuvir in these combination therapies are described in subsequent sections.

Untoward Effects and Drug Interactions. There are no hallmark toxicities associated with sofosbuvir use. Side effects observed when sofosbuvir is administered as part of combination DAA treatment are described in the material that follows with the concomitant antiviral.

Sofosbuvir is not a CYP substrate, inhibitor, or inducer and therefore has a low potential for drug interactions. However, sofosbuvir is a substrate for the efflux transporters Pgp and BCRP and should not be used with potent inducers of these transporters (e.g., rifampin, St. John's wort, phenytoin, carbamazepine). Sofosbuvir-containing DAA treatments have been associated with bradycardia, the requirement for pacemaker insertion, and fatal cardiac arrest in patients taking amiodarone. The mechanism(s) for this is unclear, but the interaction appears to be more pharmacodynamic rather than pharmacokinetic in nature (Regan et al., 2016). If the combination cannot be avoided, cardiac monitoring in an inpatient setting is advised for the first 48 h of sofosbuvir-based treatment, with daily heart rate monitoring for an additional 2 weeks.

Pediatric and Geriatric Uses. Sofosbuvir is not currently approved in children, but studies are ongoing. There are limited data on the use of DAAs in older patients. Ninety individuals 65 years or older received sofosbuvir in clinical trials. Response rates in these 90 individuals and in patients less than age 65 were similar. Because sofosbuvir is renally cleared, renal function is the primary consideration in treating the geriatric population with sofosbuvir.

Ribavirin

Ribavirin, a purine nucleoside analogue with a modified base and D-ribose sugar, inhibits the replication of a wide range of RNA and DNA viruses, including orthomyxo-, paramyxo-, arena-, bunya-, and flaviviruses in vitro.

Mechanisms of Action and Resistance. Host cell enzymes phosphorylate ribavirin to mono-, di-, and triphosphate derivatives. The exact mechanism(s) of action of ribavirin or its phosphorylated derivatives in vivo are unknown, but several immunomodulatory and antiviral effects have been observed in vitro, including (1) inhibiting the HCV RdRp, (2) depleting GTP (and thus nucleic acid synthesis in general) through inhibition of inosine 5′-monophosphate dehydrogenase, (3) enhancing viral mutagenesis, (4) converting the T-helper cell phenotype from 2 to 1, (4) inducing IFN-stimulated genes, and (5) modulating natural killer cell response. Ribavirin may select for HCV resistance mutations in vitro, but this has not been observed in vivo.

ADME. For the treatment of HCV, oral ribavirin dosing is weight based. Individuals weighing less than 75 kg receive 1000 mg daily in two divided doses. Individuals weighing at least 75 kg receive 1200 mg daily in two divided doses. Dose reductions are necessary for those with renal impairment, and individuals with renal impairment or decompensated cirrhosis may have difficulty tolerating 1000 or 1200 mg of ribavirin.

With aerosol administration, levels in respiratory secretions are very high but variable. Some systemic absorption occurs with aerosol administration (C_p after 3–4 days of dosing < 8% of C_{Pss} seen with oral dosing). When administered orally, bioavailability averages 50%. Food increases plasma levels substantially. Ribavirin is a substrate for equilibrative and concentrative nucleoside uptake transporters (ENT1 [SLC29A1], CNT2 [SLC28A2], and CNT3 [SLC28A3]) and thus is widely distributed throughout the body. The half-lives of the mono-, di-, and triphosphate derivatives in red blood cells and peripheral blood mononuclear cells mirror the plasma $t_{1/2}$ of parent ribavirin (7–10 days) (Wu et al., 2015). Hepatic metabolism (deribosylation and hydrolysis to a triazole carboxamide) and renal excretion of ribavirin and its metabolites are the principal routes of elimination. The dose of ribavirin should be reduced in patients with renal impairment. Even with a reduced dose, patients with renal impairment have difficulty tolerating ribavirin.

Therapeutic Uses. Ribavirin can be administered orally and intravenously and by inhalation. The aerosolized form of ribavirin is used in the treatment of a variety of respiratory viruses, including respiratory syncytial virus. Intravenous ribavirin has been used to treat hemorrhagic fever and severe influenza. Additional information on the use of aerosolized and intravenous ribavirin can be found in Chapter 64. Oral ribavirin is used in combination with DAAs for the treatment of chronic HCV infection in certain scenarios (e.g., in combination with sofosbuvir for genotype 2 disease, with sofosbuvir and ledipasvir, daclatasvir, or velpatasvir in the setting of decompensated cirrhosis, with grazoprevir/elbasvir in individuals with genotype 1a HCV and preexisting NS5A RAVs, and with ritonavir-boosted paritaprevir and ombitasvir with or without dasabuvir in patients with genotype 1a or 4 disease). The efficacy of ribavirin in combinations with these DAAs is described in subsequent sections.

Untoward Effects and Drug Interactions. Aerosolized ribavirin may cause conjunctival irritation, rash, transient wheezing, and occasional reversible deterioration in pulmonary function. When used in conjunction with mechanical ventilation, equipment modifications and frequent monitoring are required to prevent plugging of valves and tubing with ribavirin. Healthcare workers should use techniques to reduce environmental exposure. Pregnant women should not directly care for patients receiving ribavirin aerosol (FDA pregnancy category X). Bolus intravenous infusion may cause rigors. Systemic ribavirin causes dose-related reversible hemolytic anemia, with associated increases in reticulocyte counts and in serum bilirubin, iron, and uric acid concentrations. The ribavirin dose is often reduced when hemoglobin decreases to less than 10 g/dL or declines by more than 3 g/dL and discontinued if hemoglobin becomes less than 8.5 g/dL.

Anemia occurs in 5%–11% of patients receiving ribavirin in combination with DAAs (clinical trials of mostly noncirrhotic subjects); 18%–40% of patients postliver transplant or with decompensated cirrhosis receiving ribavirin with DAAs experienced anemia, many receiving ribavirin doses lower than the typical 1000–1200 mg daily. Two polymorphisms in the gene encoding inosine triphosphatase protect against ribavirin-induced hemolytic anemia; the frequency of the protective alleles in the general population is about 10%.

Other ribavirin toxicities include fatigue, cough, rash, and pruritus. Preclinical studies indicated that ribavirin is teratogenic, embryotoxic, oncogenic, and possibly gonadotoxic. Ribavirin is present in higher amounts in sperm than plasma. Thus, ribavirin is contraindicated in men and women who are attempting conception and for up to 6 months following cessation of treatment. Ribavirin has minimal drug interactions but should not be used with the HIV nucleoside analogue didanosine. Ribavirin increases formation of the triphosphorylated form of didanosine, which raises the risk of mitochondrial toxicity (see Chapter 64).

Pediatric and Geriatric Uses. Ribavirin is indicated for the treatment of HCV in children 5 years and older. Doses range from 400 to 1200 mg daily depending on body weight, administered in two divided doses.

Specific pharmacokinetic evaluations for ribavirin in the elderly have not been performed. As with sofosbuvir, the primary consideration in treating older individuals with ribavirin is renal function. The dose of ribavirin should be reduced in those with an eGFR less than or equal to 50 mL/min/1.73 m².

Ledipasvir

Ledipasvir, an NS5A inhibitor, is available only as part of a fixed-dose combination tablet with the NS5B nucleotide polymerase inhibitor, sofosbuvir (LDV/SOF).

Mechanisms of Action and Resistance. Ledipasvir is an inhibitor of NS5A. Baseline NS5A RAVs were detected in 16% of the 2144 participants in the phase 2 and 3 studies of LDV/SOF (Sarrazin et al.,2016). For treatment-naïve patients, the presence of baseline NS5A RAVs does not reduce the likelihood of achieving SVR, but treatment-experienced patients with baseline NS5As RAVs achieve lower SVR rates compared with treatment-experienced patients with no baseline RAVs. NS5A RAVs are detected in the majority of patients who fail to respond to LDV/SOF treatment. These NS5A RAVs persist for at least 2 years and may affect the success of future HCV treatments.

ADME. Ledipasvir, 90 mg, is available as part of a fixed-dose combination tablet with sofosbuvir (German et al., 2016). This tablet is administered once daily without regard to meals. LDV/SOF should not be used in individuals with an eGFR less than 30 mL/min/1.73 m².

Ledipasvir absorption is pH dependent. Concomitant use of antacids, H₂ receptor antagonists, and PPIs is problematic. The bioavailability of ledipasvir in humans is unknown (30%–50% in rats, monkey, and dogs). Ledipasvir concentrations are similar when given fasted versus a high-fat (1000 kcal) meal. Ledipasvir is greater than 99.8% bound to human plasma proteins. Ledipasvir is primarily eliminated unchanged in the feces. Approximately 30% is metabolized via uncertain pathways. Ledipasvir pharmacokinetics are not significantly altered by hepatic or renal impairment, but because the drug is coformulated with sofosbuvir, limitations on use in those with renal impairment apply. The $t_{1/2}$ of ledipasvir is 47 h. Ledipasvir AUC and C_{Pmax} are 24% and 32% lower in HCV-infected subjects, respectively, compared with HCV-seronegative volunteers.

Therapeutic Uses. LDV/SOF is FDA approved for individuals with HCV (genotype 1, 4, 5, and 6 disease), individuals coinfected with HIV, and those with decompensated cirrhosis. In vitro, ledipasvir has limited activity against genotype 3; its activity against genotype 2 is reduced by the highly present L31M RAV; thus, LDV/SOF is not recommended for this genotype.

The SVR rates with 12 weeks of LDV/SOF therapy were 96% and 99% in clinical trials of HCV treatment-naïve patients and 95% in treatment-experienced patients without cirrhosis. Treatment-experienced individuals with cirrhosis should be treated for either 24 weeks with LDV/SOF or 12 weeks with LDV/SOF plus ribavirin to improve the likelihood of achieving a cure. LDV/SOF for 12 weeks achieved an SVR rate of 95% in two studies with a small number of individuals with genotype 4 disease. SVR was 93% in 44 patients with genotypes 5 and 96% in 25 patients with genotype 6 receiving 12 weeks of LDV/SOF.

Treatment of individuals with HIV/HCV coinfection yielded similarly high SVRs. In treating patients with decompensated cirrhosis, ribavirin is added to LDV/SOF treatment to increase SVR rates, usually at a ribavirin dose of 600 mg daily due to poor tolerability of ribavirin in this patient population.

Untoward Effects and Drug Interactions. Amongst patients receiving 12 weeks of LDV/SOF in phase III clinical trials, 13%–14% reported fatigue and headache. The addition of ribavirin to LDV/SOF in cirrhotic patients increased the number and frequency of adverse effects.

Ledipasvir relies on an acidic environment for optimal absorption; thus, gastric acid modifiers should be used with caution. In one large cohort, use of PPIs was found to be an independent predictor of relapse to LDV/SOF treatment (Terrault et al., 2016b). If gastric acid modifiers must be used, temporal separation is necessary with antacids (by 4 h); H₂

blocker and PPI doses should not exceed the equivalent of 40 mg famotidine twice daily and 20 mg omeprazole once daily. The omeprazole must be administered simultaneously with LDV/SOF in the fasted state. Like sofosbuvir, ledipasvir is a substrate for Pgp and BCRP and thus cannot be used with potent inducers of these transporters. The CYP3A inducer efavirenz reduces ledipasvir concentrations by 30%, and the pharmacokinetic enhancer cobicistat increases ledipasvir concentrations by 2-fold; given the rather high therapeutic index of ledipasvir, these changes are not expected to have clinical relevance. Ledipasvir inhibits Pgp and BCRP and may increase the concentrations of rosuvastatin via inhibition of BCRP; thus, this combination is not recommended. Ledipasvir increases the exposure to tenofovir, which may increase the risk of renal toxicity in HIV-infected individuals taking TDF with a boosting agent such as ritonavir or cobicistat. Use of TAF instead of TDF is an option for patients taking an antiretroviral regimen, which includes ritonavir or cobicistat (MacBrayne and Kiser, 2016).

Pediatric and Geriatric Uses. A pharmacokinetic trial of LDV/SOF is ongoing in 200 children ages 3–18 years (NCT02249182). The SVR rate was 98% in 100 adolescents ages 12–17 years receiving the FDA-approved adult dose of LDV/SOF with good tolerability. Age is not associated with ledipasvir exposures in population pharmacokinetic analyses over the range of 18 to 80 years. No differences in safety or efficacy have been observed between individuals 65 years and older and younger patients.

Daclatasvir

Daclatasvir is an NS5A inhibitor.

Mechanism of Action and Resistance. Daclatasvir binds to the N-terminus of NS5A and inhibits both viral RNA replication and virion assembly. The Y93H RAV is detected in most patients who fail DCV/SOF treatment. This variant has been shown to persist for several years after treatment cessation. The optimal re-treatment strategy for patients who fail with NS5A RAVs is under investigation.

ADME. Daclatasvir is available as 30-mg and 60-mg tablets. The standard dose of daclatasvir is 60 mg, but the dose should be reduced to 30 mg with strong CYP3A inhibitors and increased to 90 mg with moderate CYP3A inducers (Table 63–1). The absolute bioavailability of daclatasvir is 67%. A high-fat, high-calorie meal reduces daclatasvir exposure by 23%, but a low-fat meal has no effect. The drug is approved for administration without regard to meals. Daclatasvir is highly protein bound (99%).

Daclatasvir is metabolized by CYP3A and is therefore susceptible to the effects of potent inhibitors and inducers of this enzyme, but the drug itself does not appear to inhibit or induce any CYPs. Daclatasvir is a substrate for Pgp. Daclatasvir inhibits Pgp, BCRP, and OATP1B1/3 and thus may increase exposures of drugs that are substrates for these transporters. Total exposure to daclatasvir is about 37% lower in patients with Child Pugh B and C decompensated cirrhosis, but unbound concentrations are unchanged, and no dose adjustment is needed in such patients. Daclatasvir AUC increases in those with ESRD; with an eGFR of 15–29 mL/min/1.73 m², AUC is roughly doubled. Given the high therapeutic index of daclatasvir, this change is unlikely to have clinical relevance. However, since daclatasvir is given with sofosbuvir, the restrictions in those with eGFR less than 30 mL/min/1.73 m² still apply. The half-life of daclatasvir is 12–15 h. Daclatasvir pharmacokinetics are similar in HCV-seropositive and -seronegative individuals.

Therapeutic Uses. Daclatasvir is FDA-approved for use in combination with sofosbuvir in those with genotype 3 disease, in individuals with HIV coinfection regardless of HCV genotype, and in persons with advanced liver disease (Keating, 2016). It is rarely used in the U.S., however, because there are coformulated and cheaper alternatives. In Japan, daclatasvir is also approved in combination with the HCV NS3/4A protease inhibitor asunaprevir; this combination is not available in the U.S.

The SVR rates are 86%–90% in treatment-naïve and treatment-experienced individuals receiving 12 weeks of DCV/SOF. Lower SVR rates occur in those with cirrhosis (63%). Thus, cirrhotic patients with genotype 3 disease may benefit from the addition of ribavirin. In HIV-coinfected individuals with HCV genotypes 1–4, 96% achieved SVR with 12 weeks of daclatasvir and sofosbuvir administration. In a group of individuals primarily (75%) infected with HCV genotype 1 with advanced liver disease and with Child Pugh A ($n = 12$), B ($n = 32$), and C ($n = 16$) cirrhosis, 92%, 94%, and 56%, respectively, achieved SVR with 12 weeks of DCV/SOF plus ribavirin treatment.

Untoward Effects and Drug Interactions. Daclatasvir is well tolerated. The most commonly reported adverse events in genotype 3 patients receiving DCV/SOF were headache and fatigue (14% each). HIV-coinfected patients reported fatigue (17%), nausea (13%), and headache (11%). When combined with ribavirin in patients with advanced cirrhosis, the most common adverse effects were anemia (20%), fatigue (18%), nausea (17%), and headache (15%).

Daclatasvir is primarily a victim rather than a perpetrator in drug-drug interactions (Garimella et al., 2016). Daclatasvir cannot be used with potent CYP3A inducers but may be used with moderate inducers, if the daclatasvir dose is increased from 60 to 90 mg. The daclatasvir dose must be reduced from 60 to 30 mg with potent CYP3A inhibitors. Table 63–1 lists some comedications necessitating a daclatasvir dose modification.

Pediatric and Geriatric Uses. Daclatasvir has not been evaluated in children or the elderly. Age was not significantly associated with daclatasvir pharmacokinetics in population modeling over the range 18–79 years; no unique safety concerns were evident in those over 65 years of age, and SVR rates were comparable in older and younger subjects in trials.

Simeprevir

Simeprevir is an inhibitor of the HCV NS3 protease. Simeprevir is a noncovalent peptidomimetic with a macrocyclic structure.

Mechanisms of Action and Resistance. Simeprevir is an inhibitor of the HCV NS3 protease. Inhibition of the NS3 protease prevents cleavage of the viral replication complex (NS4A-NS4B, NS4B-NS5A, and NS5A-NS5B) and thus prevents the formation of viral RNA. Patients that fail to respond to SIM/SOF therapy typically have either the R155K or D168E treatment-emergent RAVs (Sanford, 2015). The limited available data indicate that patients who fail a SIM/SOF-based regimen can be successfully re-treated with an NS5A-containing therapy.

Cirrhotic persons with the preexisting Q80K mutation have an SVR of 74% compared with 92% in those without the Q80K mutation. It is presently unclear whether extending the SIM/SOF treatment duration to 24 weeks would improve SVR rates in cirrhotics or if this regimen should be avoided in individuals with this preexisting RAV.

ADME. Simeprevir is dosed as a single 150-mg tablet taken once daily with food. Individuals of East Asian ancestry exhibit higher plasma simeprevir exposures, presumably due to a lower expression of the hepatic uptake transporter, OATP1B1. Thus, 100 mg of simeprevir is approved in Japan.

The bioavailability of simeprevir is 62%. Food increases simeprevir AUC by about 65%; thus, it is recommended to take this agent with food. Simeprevir is 99.9% protein bound (primarily to albumin) and exhibits more than dose proportional increases in AUC and C_{max}. Simeprevir exposures are increased in patients with hepatic impairment (2- to 5-fold at Child Pugh B and C stages). There are reports of hepatic decompensation, hepatic failure, and death in patients with advanced liver disease receiving simeprevir; thus, it should be avoided in patients with decompensated cirrhosis. Because simeprevir is used with sofosbuvir, the same restrictions on use in those with eGFR less than 30 mL/min/1.73 m² apply. The terminal elimination half-life of simeprevir is 10–13 h in HCV-uninfected individuals and 41 h in HCV-infected subjects. Plasma exposures of simeprevir are 2- to 3-fold higher in HCV-infected individuals compared to HCV-seronegative subjects.

Therapeutic Uses. The combination SIM/SOF is used for the treatment of HCV-infected individuals with genotype 1 or 4. SVR is achieved in 97% of noncirrhotic, treatment-naïve, and experienced individuals receiving 12 weeks of SIM/SOF (Kwo et al., 2016); in cirrhotic patients, the SVR rate is lower (83%), and a preexisting NS3 RAV is associated with a higher rate of relapse in cirrhotic patients (Lawitz et al., 2016b).

Untoward Effects and Drug Interactions. The most common adverse effects from SIM/SOF are headache, fatigue, and nausea (11%–20%). Simeprevir contains a sulfonamide moiety and can cause photosensitivity, rash, and itching, more so in cirrhotic patients (5%, 16%, and 14%, respectively) receiving SIM/SOF. Simeprevir may elevate bilirubin levels. Higher simeprevir exposures have been associated with an increased frequency of the dermatologic events and bilirubin elevation.

Simeprevir is metabolized by CYP3A and should not be used with moderate or strong inducers or inhibitors of this enzyme. Simeprevir is a substrate for Pgp, MRP2, BCRP, OATP1B1/3, and OATP2B1. In terms of its ability to act as a perpetrator in interactions, simeprevir is a mild inhibitor of CYP1A2 and intestinal CYP3A and thus may increase the exposures of drugs metabolized by these enzymes. Simeprevir is also an inhibitor of the hepatic transporters OATP1B1, NTCP, Pgp, MRP2, and BSEP (see Chapter 5).

Pediatric and Geriatric Uses. Simeprevir has not been specifically studied in children or in the geriatric population. Age was not significantly associated with simeprevir pharmacokinetics in population modeling over the range 18–73 years.

Velpatasvir

Velpatasvir is an NS5A inhibitor available as part of a fixed dose combination product with sofosbuvir (SOF/VEL).

Mechanism of Action and Resistance. Baseline RAVs do not appear to influence the likelihood of achieving SVR with SOF/VEL except in cirrhotic patients with genotype 3 disease where the SVR rate was 73% compared with 93% in those without baseline RAVs (Feld et al., 2015; Foster et al., 2015).

ADME. SOF/VEL is a fixed-dose combination tablet containing 400 mg of sofosbuvir and 100 mg of VEL taken once daily. As with ledipasvir, VEL absorption is pH dependent, and gastric acid modifiers require special dosing considerations with this agent; food has little effect on VEL's absorption. VEL is greater than 99.5% protein bound. VEL is predominantly excreted in feces as parent and metabolite; less than 1% of a dose appears in urine. VEL AUC changes only modestly (−17% to +14%) with moderate and severe hepatic impairment. In patients with severe renal impairment (eGFR < 30 mL/min/1.73 m²), the AUC of VEL increases by 50%. Because VEL is used with sofosbuvir, the same limitations on use in those with eGFR less than 30 mL/min/1.73 m² apply. The VEL $t_{1/2}$ is 15 h. VEL AUC and C_{max} are reduced by ~40% in HCV-infected individuals compared with healthy volunteers.

Therapeutic Uses. SOF/VEL is the only currently available DAA combination therapy that is approved for the treatment of all HCV genotypes (1–6). SVR rates were 99% in patients with genotypes 1, 2, 4, 5, and 6 and 95% in genotype 3 patients with 12 weeks of VEL/SOF in trials. In decompensated patients, 83% achieved SVR with SOF/VEL for 12 weeks, 94% achieved SVR with SOF/VEL plus ribavirin, and 86% achieved SVR with 24 weeks of SOF/VEL.

Untoward Effects and Drug Interactions. The most common adverse reactions with SOF/VEL are headache (22%), fatigue (15%), nausea (9%), asthenia (5%), and insomnia (5%). When ribavirin is given with SOF/VEL to patients with decompensated cirrhosis, adverse events are more frequent: fatigue (32%), anemia (26%), nausea (15%), headache (11%), insomnia (11%), and diarrhea (10%).

Velpatasvir has a pharmacologic profile similar to that of ledipasvir but is subject to more CYP3A-mediated interactions. As with LDV, antacids should be separated by 4 h, and H_2 blocker doses should not exceed the equivalent of 40 mg twice daily, and PPI doses should not exceed the equivalent of 20 mg daily. The timing of the PPI in relation to SOF/VEL is important. SOF/VEL should be taken with food 4 h prior to a PPI dose. VEL is a substrate for CYP3A4, 2C8, and 2B6 but has not been shown to inhibit any CYPs. VEL is a substrate for and weak inhibitor of Pgp and a weak inhibitor of BCRP and OATP1B1/1B3. There are some notable drug interactions with VEL (Mogalian et al., 2016): The pravastatin (an OATP1B1 substrate) AUC increases 35% and rosuvastatin (an OATP1B1 and BCRP substrate) AUC increases about 170% when coadministered with VEL in healthy volunteers; digoxin (a Pgp substrate) AUC increases 34%. Single-dose rifampin, which acts as an OATP1B1 inhibitor, increases VEL AUC by 47%. However, multiple doses of rifampin, which induces CYP metabolism and transporter expression, reduces the AUC of VEL by about 82%. Single-dose cyclosporine (a mixed OATP/Pgp/MRP2 inhibitor) doubles the VEL AUC. Ketoconazole (CYP3A inhibitor) increases the VEL AUC by 70%. Efavirenz reduces the VEL AUC by 50%, and this combination should be avoided.

Pediatric and Geriatric Uses. SOF/VEL has not been evaluated in children. Twelve percent of participants in phase III trials (156 subjects) were age 65 or older. No differences in efficacy or safety were observed in this group compared with those less than 65 years.

Ritonavir-Boosted Paritaprevir, Ombitasvir, With or Without Dasabuvir

Ombitasvir is an NS5A inhibitor. Dasabuvir is a nonnucleoside NS5B polymerase inhibitor. Paritaprevir is an NS3 protease inhibitor. Ritonavir is an inhibitor of CYP3A and is used as a pharmacokinetic enhancer to increase the exposures and decrease the dosing frequency for paritaprevir. Ritonavir has no activity against HCV. For more information on the clinical pharmacology of ritonavir, refer to Chapter 64.

Mechanism of Action and Resistance. Ombitasvir and paritaprevir inhibit NS5A and the NS3 protease, respectively. Dasabuvir binds noncompetitively to the palm I site outside the NS5B polymerase active site, producing a conformational change in NS5B before the elongation complex is formed (Eltahla et al., 2015). Ribavirin is administered in combination with these DAAs in patients with genotype 1a disease to increase the likelihood of achieving SVR.

The SVR rates are not statistically different between patients with pre-existing NS3, NS5A, and NS5B RAVs to those without preexisting RAVs. The most prevalent treatment-emergent RAVs in patients with genotype 1a were R155K and D168V in NS3, M28T and Q30R in NS5A, and S556G in NS5B. In a trial, in which 21 individuals (95% genotype 1a) failed to achieve SVR on PrOD, 96% still had detectable NS5A RAVs at 2 years. The approach to re-treatment of patients who have failed NS5A-based therapy is not clear, but a small study of 15 patients showed 93% of individuals could be cured with PrOD plus sofosbuvir for 12 to 24 weeks. Results from a number of phase II and phase III trials provide useful information on the clinical application of DAAs and PrO/PrOD therapy (Eltahla et al., 2015; Hussaini, 2016; Krishnan et al., 2015).

ADME. Ritonavir-boosted paritaprevir and ombitasvir are coformulated. These agents are administered as two tablets once daily for a total daily dose of 100 mg ritonavir, 150 mg paritaprevir, and 25 mg ombitasvir. Dasabuvir is administered as one 250-mg tablet taken twice daily. These medications should be administered with a meal; moderate, and high-fat meals increase exposures of all four. On this regimen, accumulation is minimal for ombitasvir and dasabuvir and approximately 1.5- to 2-fold for ritonavir and paritaprevir. Protein binding is high (about 99%) for all four drugs. Ombitasvir is primarily metabolized by amide hydrolysis followed by oxidative metabolism. Paritaprevir is metabolized by CYP3A, ritonavir primarily by CYP3A and to a lesser extent by CYP2D6. Dasabuvir is metabolized primarily by CYP2C8 and to a lesser extent by CYP3A. Paritaprevir exposures are increased 62% and 945% in individuals with Child Pugh B and C cirrhosis, respectively.

Due to reports of hepatic decompensation, hepatic failure, and death in patients with advanced liver disease receiving PrOD, this combination should not be administered to patients with decompensated cirrhosis. Ombitasvir pharmacokinetics are not significantly altered in renal impairment, but to the extent that renal impairment may affect hepatic function, paritaprevir, dasabuvir, and ritonavir exposures will increase with worsening renal function. PrOD has been studied in noncirrhotic, HCV-infected individuals with eGFR less than 30 mL/min/1.73 m²; high cure rates were achieved, but ribavirin was difficult to tolerate in the genotype 1a individuals, 65% of whom developed anemia. The plasma half-lives of PrOD components are as follows: ombitasvir about 23 h; paritaprevir,

5.5 h; ritonavir, 4 h; and dasabuvir, 5.8 h. There are inconsistent results on differences in pharmacokinetics of PrOD in HCV-seropositive versus -HCV-seronegative individuals; some studies indicated a decrease in exposures in HCV-seropositive persons, while others indicated no difference.

Therapeutic Uses. The PrOD combination is FDA-approved for the treatment of HCV genotype 1. PrOD is administered for 12 weeks to patients with genotype 1b regardless of cirrhosis status. However, in individuals with genotype 1a, ribavirin is used with PrOD in a 12-week regimen to increase the rate of SVR (from 90% to 97%). Treatment should be extended to 24 weeks in patients with genotype 1a with cirrhosis because it increases the rate of SVR from 91% to 96%.

Ritonavir-boosted paritaprevir and ombitasvir is used with ribavirin, but without dasabuvir, for 12 weeks for the treatment of individuals with genotype 4 disease.

The SVR rates are similar in individuals with HIV coinfection to those seen in individuals with HCV monoinfection. The primary consideration in the treatment of HIV-coinfected individuals with PrOD or PrO is avoidance of drug interactions. Efavirenz, rilpivirine, and regimens containing cobicistat or ritonavir can be problematic with this therapy (MacBrayne and Kiser, 2016).

Untoward Effects and Drug Interactions. The most commonly reported clinical adverse effects with PrOD include nausea (8%), pruritis (7%), insomnia (5%), and asthenia (4%). The frequency of these effects doubles with the addition of ribavirin.

The PrOD combination acts as both a victim and a perpetrator in a number of clinically significant drug interactions. The ritonavir booster prolongs the dwell time of paritaprevir but may necessitate lowering the dose of any concomitant agent that CYP3A4 also metabolizes. CYP2C8 metabolizes dasabuvir (as does CYP3A4 to a lesser degree); thus, inhibitors of CYP2C8 may elevate dasabuvir blood levels and are contraindicated during PrOD therapy. Ethinyl-estradiol–containing contraceptives will elevate hepatic enzymes and should be avoided with PrOD or PrO therapy; progestin-containing contraceptives may be used. Vigilance is required in the identification, management, and avoidance of interactions with PrO and PrOD therapy for HCV. Refer to the product labeling and consult the Internet (http://www.hep-druginteractions.org) for up-to-date information on drug interactions with this DAA combination.

Pediatric and Geriatric Uses. A study of PrOD is ongoing in children (NCT02486406). Approximately 8% of patients in clinical trials of PrOD were age 65 or older. No differences in safety or efficacy were observed between these subjects and younger subjects.

Grazoprevir/Elbasvir

Grazoprevir is an NS3/4A protease inhibitor; elbasvir is an NS5A inhibitor. These drugs are available in a single fixed-dose combination tablet.

Mechanism of Action and Resistance. Grazoprevir and elbasvir are inhibitors of the NS3 and NS5A viral enzymes, respectively. In trials, pre-existing NS3 RAVs were detected in 57% and 19% of individuals with genotype 1a and 1b, respectively, but the presence of preexisting NS3 RAVs does not reduce the likelihood of high SVR rates. The presence of preexisting NS5A RAVs did reduce SVR rates in genotype 1a patients. SVR rates were 58% and 68% in genotype 1a treatment-naïve and treatment-experienced patients, respectively, with preexisting NS5A RAVs. Adding ribavirin and extending the treatment duration greatly increases SVR rates in patients with preexisting NS5A RAVs.

ADME. GZR/EBR is dosed as a single 100-mg/50-mg fixed-dose combination tablet taken once daily without regard to meals, although a high-fat meal will increase the AUC and C_{max} of grazoprevir by 1.5- and 2.8-fold. The bioavailability of elbasvir is 30%; that of grazoprevir ranges from 10% to 40%. The $t_{1/2}$ of grazoprevir is about 30 h. Elbasvir has a $t_{1/2}$ of 23 h. Less than 1% of grazoprevir and elbasvir are renally eliminated. Both drugs are extensively (~99%) bound. Grazoprevir exposures are increased 62% in those with mild (Child-Pugh A) and 388% in those with moderate (Child Pugh B) hepatic impairment relative to those with no hepatic impairment. Total concentrations of elbasvir are 24% and 14% lower in patients with mild and moderate hepatic insufficiency, respectively, likely a reflection of reduced serum protein levels. Grazoprevir and elbasvir pharmacokinetics in individuals with ESRD on hemodialysis are comparable to individuals without hepatic impairment. The AUCs of grazoprevir and elbasvir are increased, however, by 65% and 86%, respectively, in those with eGFR less than 30 mL/min/1.73 m^2 not receiving dialysis. As with other hepatically metabolized DAAs, this increase may be due to accumulation of uremic toxins, parathyroid hormone, or cytokines that can impair hepatic metabolism. The grazoprevir AUCs are 1.2- to 2.1-fold higher in HCV-infected individuals compared with HCV-uninfected individuals. There are no differences in elbasvir pharmacokinetics in HCV-seropositive versus seronegative individuals.

Therapeutic Uses. Grazoprevir/elbasvir is FDA approved for HCV genotypes 1 and 4, in individuals with HIV coinfection, and in those with renal impairment. Compared with prior HCV NS3 protease inhibitors, grazoprevir has activity against more genotypes and a higher barrier to the development of resistance.

Based on clinical trials, 95% of treatment-naïve individuals with primarily genotype 1 disease will achieve SVR after 12 weeks of GZR/EBR (SVR rates: 92% with genotype 1a, 99% with genotype 1b, 100% with genotype 4, and 80% with genotype 6). There are no differences in response between cirrhotics and noncirrhotics, but lower SVR rates (58% vs. 99%) are observed in patients with preexisting NS5A RAVs. Thus, NS5A resistance testing needs to be performed for individuals with genotype 1a before starting GZR/EBR. In genotype 1a individuals with preexisting NS5A RAVs, adding ribavirin and treating for an additional 4 weeks for a total of 16 weeks improves SVR rates. SVR rates are similar in patients with HIV coinfection, but drug interactions with antiretroviral therapy are an important consideration in this population (AASLD/IDSA, 2016).

The combination GZR/EBR has a particular niche in the treatment of HCV-infected patients with impaired renal function. In a trial of individuals (14% cirrhotic) with eGFR less than 30 mL/min/1.73 m^2 (76% of whom were hemodialysis dependent), the SVR after 12 weeks of treatment was 94%. The percentage of patients reporting any adverse event (~75%) was similar to studies of GZR/EBR in patients without renal impairment. More serious events occurred in these patients (15% vs. 3%), but many were not considered related to GZR/EBR treatment (Roth et al., 2015).

Untoward Effects and Drug Interactions. The most common side effects with GZR/EBR are headache (17%), fatigue (16%), and nausea (9%–15%). Higher exposures of grazoprevir are associated with liver function test elevations. Grazoprevir may increase bilirubin concentrations through inhibition of OATP1B1.

Grazoprevir is a substrate for CYP3A4, Pgp, and OATP1B1. OATP1B1 inhibitors and moderate/strong CYP3A and Pgp inducers (including efavirenz) are not recommended for coadministration with GZR/EBR. Elbasvir is a substrate for CYP3A4 and Pgp and an inhibitor of BCRP and Pgp.

Pediatric and Geriatric Uses. GZR/EBR has not been studied in children, and no dedicated studies have been performed in older patients. No age effect was observed in elbasvir pharmacokinetics in young (22–45 years) versus elderly (65–78 years) males; elderly females had a 33% higher elbasvir AUC compared with elderly men even after adjustment for body weight.

Investigational Agents and the Future for Treatment of HCV

Several agents are still in clinical development for the treatment of hepatitis C, including combination therapies such as sofosbuvir + velpatasvir + voxilaprevir (Lawitz et al., 2016a), glecaprevir + pibrentasvir (Gane et al., 2016), and MK-3682 + grazoprevir + ruzasvir. However, compared with 10 years ago, drug development has slowed. For those individuals able to access therapy, currently available agents achieve cure in most (but not all) patient populations. The remaining challenges for this disease are testing and diagnosis, linkage to care, increasing access to these expensive therapies, and management of special patient populations, including cirrhotic individuals with genotype 3 disease, individuals with decompensated cirrhosis, and those who fail DAA treatment.

Drug Facts for Your Personal Formulary: *Viral Hepatitis (HBV/HCV)*

Drugs	Therapeutic Uses	Clinical Pharmacology and Tips
Hepatitis B Therapy		
Pegylated interferon alfa	• Preferred agent • Approved for adult patients with compensated liver disease and evidence of viral replication and liver inflammation • Administered SC weekly for 48–52 weeks	• Adverse reactions (>40%): fatigue/asthenia, pyrexia, myalgia, and headache • May cause fatal neuropsychiatric, autoimmune, ischemic, and infectious disorders • Frequent hematologic monitoring required • Contraindicated in advanced liver disease and in pregnancy
Entecavir	• Preferred agent • Approved for individuals ≥ 2 years old • Indefinite treatment for patients with cirrhosis	• Use higher dose for decompensated cirrhosis and patients with lamivudine or telbivudine resistance • Take on an empty stomach • Monitor for lactic acidosis in decompensated cirrhosis • Adverse reactions (≥3%): headache, fatigue, dizziness, nausea
Tenofovir disoproxil fumarate	• Preferred agent • Approved for individuals ≥ 2 years old • Indefinite treatment for patients with cirrhosis	• Dose reduction in renal impairment • Monitor renal function • May decrease bone mineral density • Adverse reactions (≥10%) in decompensated cirrhosis: abdominal pain, nausea, insomnia, pruritus, vomiting, dizziness, and pyrexia

Adefovir
Lamivudine
Telbivudine
	• Alternative agents due to high incidence of HBV resistance with monotherapy
	• Indefinite treatment for patients with cirrhosis
		• Dose adjust for renal impairment
		• Abrupt discontinuation causes hepatitis flares
		• Common adverse reactions:
		  ○ *Adefovir*: asthenia and impaired renal function
		  ○ *Lamivudine*: ear, nose, and throat infections; sore throat; and diarrhea
		  ○ *Telbivudine*: increased CK, nausea, diarrhea, fatigue, myalgia, and myopathy

Drug Facts for Your Personal Formulary: *Viral Hepatitis (HBV/HCV)* (*continued*)

Drugs	Therapeutic Uses	Clinical Pharmacology and Tips
Hepatitis C Therapy		
Sofosbuvir/ledipasvir	• HCV genotype 1, 4, 5, 6 and individuals with HIV coinfection • Administered as fixed-dose combination tablet for 8 or 12 weeks • Use with ribavirin for 12 weeks in treatment-experienced patients with cirrhosis	• Ledipasvir should not be used with potent Pgp inducers • Ledipasvir absorption requires acid gastric pH • Coadministration of sofosbuvir and amiodarone may cause severe bradycardia and fatal cardiac arrest • Avoid sofosbuvir if CrCl < 30 mL/min • Adverse reactions (≥10%): fatigue, headache
Sofosbuvir/daclatasvir	• HCV genotype 3, HIV coinfection, and advanced liver disease regardless of HCV genotype • 12-week treatment in patients without cirrhosis • Coadministered with ribavirin in patients with cirrhosis for 12 weeks	• Daclatasvir should not be used with potent CYP3A inducers • Daclatasvir dose reduction needed with strong CYP3A inhibitors • Coadministration of sofosbuvir and amiodarone may cause severe bradycardia and fatal cardiac arrest • Avoid sofosbuvir if CrCl < 30 mL/min • Adverse reactions (≥10%): fatigue, headache
Sofosbuvir/simeprevir	• 12-week therapy in patients without cirrhosis • 24-week therapy in patients with cirrhosis	• Cannot be used with potent Pgp inducers • Simeprevir: mild inhibitor of GI; contraindicated in decompensated cirrhosis CYP3A • Coadministration of sofosbuvir and amiodarone may cause severe bradycardia and fatal cardiac arrest • Adverse reactions of simeprevir (≥20%): fatigue, headache, nausea, photosensitivity (limit sun exposure)
Sofosbuvir/velpatasvir	• Approved for use in all HCV genotypes • Administered as a fixed dose combination tablet for 12 weeks • Used with ribavirin for patients with decompensated cirrhosis	• Do not use with potent Pgp or CYP3A inducers • Velpatasvir requires acidic gastric pH • Coadministration of sofosbuvir and amiodarone may cause severe bradycardia and fatal cardiac arrest • Avoid sofosbuvir if CrCl < 30 mL/min • Common adverse reactions: fatigue and headache
Ritonavir-boosted paritaprevir and ombitasvir	• Fixed-dose combination tablets for HCV genotype 4 in combination with ribavirin	• High potential for CYP-mediated drug interactions • Should not be used in patients with decompensated cirrhosis • Adverse reactions (≥5%): nausea, pruritis, and insomnia • With ribavirin, the most common adverse reactions (≥10%) are fatigue, nausea, pruritis, other skin reactions, insomnia, and asthenia
Ritonavir-boosted paritaprevir, ombitasvir, and dasabuvir	• HCV genotype 1b (1a in combination with ribavirin) • 12 weeks of therapy • 24 weeks of therapy required for patients with genotype 1a and cirrhosis	
Grazoprevir/elbasvir	• 12-week therapy for patients without baseline NS5A RAVs • 16-week combined therapy with ribavirin for patients with baseline NS5A RAVs • Preferred treatment in renal impairment	• Should not be used with moderate and strong CYP3A and Pgp inducers • Should not be used with OATP1B1 inhibitors • Common adverse reactions: headache, fatigue, nausea
Ribavirin	• Used in combination with other HCV regimens to boost therapeutic efficacy	• May cause hemolytic anemia • Teratogenic • Wide tissue distribution • Long half-life (7–10 days) • Dose adjustment needed for renal impairment

Bibliography

AASLD/IDSA. HCV guidance: recommendations for testing, managing, and treating hepatitis C. 2016. Available at: http://www.hcvguidelines.org/. Accessed December 5, 2016.

Bhattacharya D, Thio CL. Review of hepatitis B therapeutics. *Clin Infect Dis*, **2010**, *51*:1201–8.

Brahmania M, et al. New therapeutic agents for chronic hepatitis B. Lancet Infect Dis. **2016**, *16*:e10–e21.

Brown NA. Progress towards improving antiviral therapy for hepatitis C with hepatitis C virus polymerase inhibitors. Part I: nucleoside analogues. *Expert Opin Investig Drugs*, **2009**, *18*:709–725.

Charlton M, et al. Ledipasvir and sofosbuvir plus ribavirin for treatment of HCV infection in patients with advanced liver disease. *Gastroenterology*, **2015**, *149*:649–659.

Chinnadurai R, et al. Hepatic transplant and HCV: a new playground for an old virus. *Am J Transplant*, **2012**, *12*:298–305.

Ciesek S, Manns MP. Hepatitis in 2010: the dawn of a new era in HCV therapy. *Nat Rev Gastroenterol Hepatol*, **2011**, *8*:69–71.

Dubuisson J, Cosset FL. Virology and cell biology of the hepatitis C virus life cycle: an update. *J Hepatol*, **2014**, *61*(1 suppl):S3–S13.

Durantel D, Zoulim F. New antiviral targets for innovative treatment concepts for hepatitis B virus and hepatitis delta virus. *J Hepatol*, **2016**, *64*(1 suppl):S117–S131.

Eltahla AA, et al. Inhibitors of the hepatitis C virus polymerase; mode of action and resistance. *Viruses*, **2015**, *7*:5206–5224.

Feld JJ, et al. Sofosbuvir and velpatasvir for HCV genotype 1, 2, 4, 5, and 6 infection. *N Engl J Med*, **2015**, *373*:2599–2607.

Foster GR, et al. Sofosbuvir and velpatasvir for HCV genotype 2 and 3 infection. *N Engl J Med*, **2015**, *373*:2608–2617.

Freeman AJ, et al. Estimating progression to cirrhosis in chronic hepatitis C virus infection. *Hepatology*, **2001**, 34:809–816.

Gane E, et al. High efficacy of ABT-493 and ABT-530 treatment in patients with HCV genotype 1 or 3 infection and compensated cirrhosis. *Gastroenterology*, **2016**, 151:651–659.

Garimella T, et al. A review of daclatasvir drug-drug interactions. *Adv Ther*, **2016**, 33:1867–1884.

German P, et al. Clinical pharmacokinetics and pharmacodynamics of ledipasvir/sofosbuvir, a fixed-dose combination tablet for the treatment of hepatitis C. *Clin Pharmacokinet*, **2016**, 55:1337–1351.

Ghany MG, Doo EC. Antiviral resistance and hepatitis B therapy. *Hepatology*, **2009**, 49(5 suppl):S174–S184.

Gish RG, Meanwell NA. The NS5A replication complex inhibitors: difference makers? *Clin Liver Dis*, **2011**, 15:627–639.

Holmes JA, Thompson AJ. Interferon-free combination therapies for the treatment of hepatitis C: current insights. *Hepat Med*, **2015**, 7: 51–70.

Honda K, et al. Benefits of nucleos(t)ide analog treatments for hepatitis B virus-related cirrhosis. *World J Hepatol*, **2015**, 7:2404–2410.

Hussaini T. **2016**. Paritaprevir/ritonavir-ombitasvir and dasabuvir, the 3D regimen for the treatment of chronic hepatitis C virus infection: a concise review. *Hepat Med*, **2016**, 8:61–68.

Jonas MM, et al. Clinical trial of lamivudine in children with chronic hepatitis B. *N Engl J Med*, **2002**, 346:1706–1713.

Keating GM. Daclatasvir: a review in chronic hepatitis C. *Drugs*, **2016**, 76:1381–1391.

Kirby BJ, et al. Pharmacokinetic, pharmacodynamic, and drug-interaction profile of the hepatitis C virus NS5B polymerase inhibitor sofosbuvir. *Clin Pharmacokinet*, **2015**, 54:677–690.

Krishnan P, et al. Resistance analysis of baseline and treatment-emergent variants in hepatitis C virus genotype 1 in the AVIATOR study with paritaprevir-ritonavir, ombitasvir, and dasabuvir. *Antimicrob Agents Chemother*, **2015**, 59:5445–5454.

Kwo P, et al. Simeprevir plus sofosbuvir (12 and 8 weeks) in hepatitis C virus genotype 1-infected patients without cirrhosis: OPTIMIST-1, a phase 3, randomized study. *Hepatology*, **2016**, 64:370–380.

Lavanchy D. The global burden of hepatitis C. *Liver Int*, **2009**, 29(suppl 1): 74–81.

Lawitz E, et al. All-oral therapy with nucleotide inhibitors sofosbuvir and GS-0938 for 14 days in treatment-naive genotype 1 hepatitis C (nuclear). *J Viral Hepat*, **2013**, 20:699–707.

Lawitz E, et al. Efficacy of sofosbuvir, velpatasvir, and GS-9857 in patients with genotype 1 hepatitis C virus infection in an open-label, phase 2 trial. *Gastroenterology*, **2016a**, 151:893–901. PMID: 27456384

Lawitz E, et al. Simeprevir plus sofosbuvir in patients with chronic hepatitis C virus genotype 1 infection and cirrhosis: a phase 3 study (OPTIMIST-2). *Hepatology*, **2016b**, 64:360–369.

Liang TJ, et al. Present and future therapies of hepatitis B: from discovery to cure. *Hepatology*, **2015**, 62:1893–1908.

Liaw YF, et al. Lamivudine for patients with chronic hepatitis B and advanced liver disease. *N Engl J Med*, **2004**, 351(15):1521–1531.

Lin CL, et al. Hepatitis B virus: new therapeutic perspectives. *Liver Int*, **2016**, 36(suppl 1):85–92.

Lok AS, et al. Efficacy of entecavir with or without tenofovir disoproxil fumarate for nucleos(t)ide-naive patients with chronic hepatitis B. *Gastroenterology*, **2012**, 143:619–628 e1.

Lontok E, et al. Hepatitis C virus drug resistance—associated substitutions: state of the art summary. *Hepatology*, **2015**, 62:1623–1632.

MacBrayne CE, Kiser JJ. Pharmacologic considerations in the treatment of hepatitis C virus in persons with HIV. *Clin Infect Dis*, **2016**, 63(suppl 1): S12–S23. Erratum in: *Clin Infect Dis*, **2016**, 63:715.

Manns M, et al. Ledipasvir/sofosbuvir with ribavirin is safe and efficacious in decompensated and post-liver transplantation patients with HCV infection: preliminary results of the SOLAR-2 trial. European Association for the Study of Liver Diseases, April 22–26, 2015, Vienna, Austria.

Martin P, et al. A treatment algorithm for the management of chronic hepatitis B virus infection in the United States: 2015 update. *Clin Gastroenterol Hepatol*, **2015**, 13:2071–2087.

Messina JP, et al. Global distribution and prevalence of hepatitis C virus genotypes. *Hepatology*, **2015**, 61:77–87.

Mogalian E, et al. Use of multiple probes to assess transporter- and cytochrome P450-mediated drug-drug interaction potential of the pangenotypic HCV NS5A inhibitor velpatasvir. *Clin Pharmacokinet*, **2016**, 55:605–613.

Neumann AU, et al. Hepatitis C viral dynamics in vivo and the antiviral efficacy of interferon-alpha therapy. *Science*, **1998**, 282:103–107.

Ono SK, et al. The polymerase L528M mutation cooperates with nucleotide binding-site mutations, increasing hepatitis B virus replication and drug resistance. *J Clin Invest*, **2001**, 107:449–455.

Poordad F, et al., eds. Daclatasvir, sofosbuvir, and ribavirin combination for HCV patients with advanced cirrhosis or post-transplant recurrence: ALLY-1 phase 3 study. European Assocation for the Study of the Liver, April 22–26, 2015, Vienna, Austria.

Ray AS, et al. Tenofovir alafenamide: a novel prodrug of tenofovir for the treatment of human immunodeficiency virus. *Antiviral Res*, **2016**, 125:63–70.

Regan CP, et al. Assessment of the clinical cardiac drug-drug interaction associated with the combination of hepatitis C virus nucleotide inhibitors and amiodarone in guinea pigs and rhesus monkeys. *Hepatology*, **2016**, 64:1430–1441.

Roth D, et al. Grazoprevir plus elbasvir in treatment-naive and treatment-experienced patients with hepatitis C virus genotype 1 infection and stage 4–5 chronic kidney disease (the C-SURFER study): a combination phase 3 study. *Lancet*, **2015**, 386:1537–1545. Erratum in: *Lancet*, **2015**, 386:1824.

Sanford M. Simeprevir: a review of its use in patients with chronic hepatitis C virus infection. *Drugs*, **2015**, 75:183–196.

Sarrazin C, et al. Prevalence of resistance-associated substitutions in HCV NS5A, NS5B, or NS3 and outcomes of treatment with ledipasvir and sofosbuvir. *Gastroenterology*, **2016**, 151:501–512.

Sasadeusz J, et al. The anti-HIV activity of entecavir: a multicentre evaluation of lamivudine-experienced and lamivudine-naive patients. *AIDS*, **2008**, 22:947–955.

Schweitzer A, et al. Estimations of worldwide prevalence of chronic hepatitis B virus infection: a systematic review of data published between 1965 and 2013. *Lancet*, **2015**, 386:1546–1555.

Shoshani I, et al. Inhibition of adenylyl cyclase by acyclic nucleoside phosphonate antiviral agents. *J Biol Chem*, **1999**, 274:34742–34744.

Sokal EM, et al. Interferon alfa therapy for chronic hepatitis B in children: a multinational randomized controlled trial. *Gastroenterology*, **1998**, 114:988–995.

Sonneveld MJ, et al. Polymorphisms near IL28B and serologic response to peginterferon in HBeAg-positive patients with chronic hepatitis B. *Gastroenterology*, **2012**, 142:513–520.

Tang H, Grise H. Cellular and molecular biology of HCV infection and hepatitis. *Clin Sci (Lond)*, **2009**, 117:49–65.

Teijaro JR. Pleiotropic roles of type 1 interferons in antiviral immune responses. *Adv Immunol*, **2016**, 132:135–158.

Terrault NA, et al. AASLD guidelines for treatment of chronic hepatitis B. *Hepatology*, **2016a**, 63:261–283.

Terrault NA, et al. and the HCV-TARGET Study Group. Effectiveness of ledipasvir-sofosbuvir combination in patients with hepatitis C virus infection and factors associated with sustained virologic response. *Gastroenterology*, **2016b**, 151:1131–1140.

Tong S, Revill P. Overview of hepatitis B viral replication and genetic variability. *J Hepatol*, **2016**, 64(1 suppl):S4–S16.

WHO. Guidelines for the prevention, care and treatment of persons with chronic hepatitis B infection. **2015**. Available at: http://www.who.int/hiv/pub/hepatitis/hepatitis-b-guidelines/en/. Accessed October 24, 2016.

WHO. WHO: hepatitis B fact sheet. **July 2016**. Available at: http://www.who.int/mediacentre/factsheets/fs204/en/. Accessed December 5, 2016.

Wu LS, et al. Population pharmacokinetic modeling of plasma and intracellular ribavirin concentrations in patients with chronic hepatitis C virus infection. *Antimicrob Agents Chemother*, **2015**, 59:2179–2188.

Zein NN, et al. Hepatitis C virus genotypes in the United States: epidemiology, pathogenicity, and response to interferon therapy. Collaborative Study Group. *Ann Intern Med*, **1996**, 125:634–639.

Zhou XJ, et al. Pharmacokinetics of telbivudine following oral administration of escalating single and multiple doses in patients with chronic hepatitis B virus infection: pharmacodynamic implications. *Antimicrob Agents Chemother*, **2006**, 50(3):874–879.

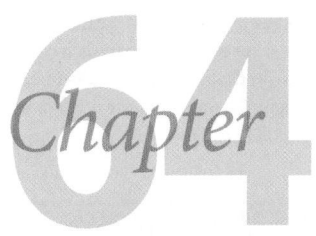

Chapter 64

Antiretroviral Agents and Treatment of HIV Infection

Charles W. Flexner

The pharmacotherapy of HIV infection is a rapidly moving field. Three-drug combinations are the current minimum standard of care for this infection, so available agents and formulations constitute several thousand possible regimens. Knowing the essential features of the pathophysiology of this disease and how chemotherapeutic agents affect the virus and the host is critical in developing a rational approach to therapy. Unique features of this drug class include the need for lifelong administration to control virus replication and the possibility of rapid emergence of permanent drug resistance if these agents are not used properly.

Pathogenesis of HIV-Related Disease

Human immunodeficiency viruses are lentiviruses, a family of retroviruses evolved to establish chronic persistent infection with gradual onset of clinical symptoms. Replication is constant following infection, and although some infected cells may harbor nonreplicating virus for years, in the absence of treatment there generally is no true period of viral latency following infection (Deeks et al., 2015). Humans and nonhuman primates are the only natural hosts for these viruses.

There are two major families of HIV. Most of the epidemic involves HIV-1; HIV-2 is more closely related to SIV and is concentrated in western Africa. HIV-1 is genetically diverse, with at least five distinct subfamilies or clades. HIV-1 and HIV-2 have similar sensitivity to most antiretroviral drugs, although the NNRTIs are HIV-1 specific and have no activity against HIV-2.

Virus Structure

HIV is a typical retrovirus with a small RNA genome of 9300 base pairs. Two copies of the genome are contained in a nucleocapsid core surrounded by a lipid bilayer, or envelope that is derived from the host cell plasma membrane (Figure 64–1). The viral genome encodes three major open reading frames: *gag* encodes a polyprotein that is processed to release the major structural proteins of the virus; *pol* overlaps *gag* and encodes three important enzyme activities (an RNA-dependent DNA polymerase or reverse transcriptase with RNAase activity, protease, and the viral integrase); and *env* encodes the large transmembrane envelope protein responsible for cell binding and entry. Several small genes encode regulatory proteins that enhance virion production or combat host defenses. These include *tat*, *rev*, *nef*, and *vpr*.

Virus Life Cycle

Understanding the HIV life cycle (Figure 64–1) is crucial to understanding the rational therapy of HIV infection. HIV tropism is controlled by the envelope protein gp160 (*env*). The major target for *env* binding is the CD4

receptor present on lymphocytes and macrophages, although cell entry also requires binding to a coreceptor, generally the chemokine receptors CCR5 or CXCR4. CCR5 is present on macrophage lineage cells. Most infected individuals harbor predominantly the CCR5-tropic virus; HIV with this tropism is responsible for nearly all naturally acquired infections. A shift from CCR5 to CXCR4 utilization is associated with advancing disease, and the increased affinity of HIV-1 for CXCR4 allows infection of T-lymphocyte lines. A phenotypic switch from CCR5 to CXCR4 heralds accelerated loss of CD4+ helper T cells and increased risk of immunosuppression. Whether coreceptor switch is a cause or a consequence of advancing disease is still unknown, but it is possible to develop clinical AIDS without this switch (Deeks et al., 2015).

The gp41 domain of *env* controls the fusion of the virus lipid bilayer with that of the host cell. Following fusion, full-length viral RNA enters the cytoplasm, where it undergoes replication to a short-lived RNA-DNA duplex; the original RNA is degraded by the RNase H activity of reverse transcriptase to allow creation of a full-length double-stranded DNA copy of the virus. Because the HIV reverse transcriptase is error prone and lacks a proofreading function, mutation is frequent and occurs at about three bases of every full-length (9300-base-pair) replication (Coffin, 1995). Virus-derived DNA is transported into the nucleus, where it is integrated into a host chromosome by the viral integrase in a random or quasi-random location (Greene and Peterlin, 2002).

Following integration, the virus may remain quiescent, not producing RNA or protein but replicating as the cell divides. When a cell that harbors the viral DNA is activated, viral RNA and proteins are produced. Structural proteins assemble around full-length genomic RNA to form a nucleocapsid. The envelope and structural proteins assemble at the cell surface, concentrating in cholesterol-rich lipid rafts. The nucleocapsid cores are directed to these sites and bud through the cell membrane, creating new enveloped HIV particles containing two complete single-stranded RNA genomes. Reverse transcriptase is incorporated into virus particles so replication can begin immediately after the virus enters a new cell.

How the Virus Causes Disease

Sexual acquisition of HIV infection is likely mediated by one or, at most, a handful of infectious virus particles. Soon after infection, there is a rapid burst of replication peaking at 2–4 weeks, with 10^9 cells or more becoming infected. This peak is associated with a transient dip in the number of peripheral CD4+ (helper) T lymphocytes. As a result of new host immune responses and target cell depletion, the number of infectious virions as reflected by the plasma HIV RNA concentration (also known as viral load) declines to a quasi-steady state. This set point reflects the interplay between host immunity and the pathogenicity of the infecting virus

Abbreviations

ABC: abacavir
ADME: absorption, distribution, metabolism, excretion
AIDS: acquired immunodeficiency syndrome
5′-AMP: adenosine 5′-monophosphate
AUC: area under plasma concentration-time curve
cDNA: complementary DNA
CL_{cr}: creatinine clearance
CMP: cytidine monophosphate
CNS: central nervous system
CSF: cerebrospinal fluid
CYP: cytochrome P450
dCMP: deoxycytidine monophosphate
ddC: dideoxycytidine
ddI: didanosine
DF: disoproxil fumarate
DRESS: drug reaction with eosinophilia and systemic symptoms
d4T: stavudine
eCL_{cr}: estimated creatinine clearance
env: envelope protein gp160
FDA: Food and Drug Administration
FTC: emtricitabine
GI: gastrointestinal
HBV: hepatitis B virus
HIV: human immunodeficiency virus
HTLV: human T-cell lymphotrophic virus
IMP: inosine 5′-monophosphate
InSTI: integrase strand transfer inhibitor
IRIS: immune reconstitution inflammatory syndrome
LTR: long terminal repeat
NDP: nucleoside diphosphate
NNRTI: _non_nucleoside reverse transcriptase inhibitor
NRTI: nucleos(t)ide reverse transcriptase inhibitor
OATP: organic anion-transporting polypeptide
PI: protease inhibitor
PK: pharmacokinetic
PRPP: phosphoribosyl pyrophosphate
QT_c: corrected cardiac QT interval
RNase H: ribonuclease H
RT: reverse transcriptase
SIV: simian immunodeficiency virus
$t_{1/2}$: half-life of elimination
TAF: tenofovir alafenamide
TAM: thymidine analogue mutation
3TC: lamivudine
TDF: tenofovir disoproxil fumarate
vRNA: viral RNA
ZDV: zidovudine

(Coffin, 1995). In the average infected individual, several billion infectious virus particles are produced every few days.

Eventually, the host CD4+ T-lymphocyte count begins a steady decline, accompanied by a rise in the plasma HIV RNA concentration. Once the peripheral CD4 cell count falls below 200 cells/mm³, there is an increasing risk of opportunistic diseases and, ultimately, death. Sexual acquisition of CCR5-tropic HIV-1 is associated with a median time to clinical AIDS of 8–10 years if the patient is not treated. Some patients, termed long-term nonprogressors, can harbor HIV for more than two decades without significant decline in peripheral CD4 cell count or clinical immunosuppression; this may reflect a combination of favorable host immunogenetics and immune responses.

An important question relevant to treatment is whether HIV disease is a consequence of CD4+ lymphocyte depletion alone. Most natural history data suggest that this is true. Regardless, successful therapy is based on inhibition of HIV replication; interventions designed specifically to boost the host immune response without exerting a direct antiviral effect have had no reliable clinical benefit (Deeks et al., 2015).

Principles of HIV Chemotherapy

Current treatment assumes that all aspects of disease derive from the direct toxic effects of HIV on host cells, mainly CD4+ T lymphocytes. _The goal of therapy is to suppress virus replication as much as possible for as long as possible._ The current standard of care is to use at least three drugs simultaneously for the entire duration of treatment (Department of Health and Human Services, 2016).

Two large randomized clinical trials found substantial clinical benefit from initiating antiretroviral therapy regardless of baseline CD4 count (INSIGHT START Study Group, 2015; TEMPRANO ANRS 12136 Study Group, 2015); thus, the current global standard of care is to offer treatment to all infected individuals whenever possible (World Health Organization, 2015). Increasing evidence also confirms the value of antiretroviral therapy in preventing transmission of the virus from person to person (Cohen et al., 2011).

Drug resistance remains a key problem. There is a high likelihood that all untreated infected individuals harbor viruses with single-amino-acid mutations that confer some degree of resistance to every known antiretroviral drug because of the high mutation rate of HIV and the tremendous number of infectious virions (Coffin, 1995). Thus, a combination of active agents is required to prevent drug resistance, analogous to strategies employed in the treatment of tuberculosis (see Chapter 60). Prolonged drug holidays may allow the virus to replicate anew, increasing the risk of drug resistance and disease progression; such breaks in treatment are associated with increased morbidity and mortality and are not generally recommended (Lawrence et al., 2003).

The expected outcome of initial therapy in a previously untreated patient is an undetectable viral load (plasma HIV RNA < 50 copies/mL) within 24 weeks of starting treatment. Mathematical models of HIV replication suggest that three is the minimum number of agents required to guarantee effective long-term suppression of HIV replication without resistance (Muller and Bonhoeffer, 2003). However, earlier models may not adequately predict the effects of newer and more potent antiretrovirals.

In treatment-naïve patients, a regimen containing a nonnucleoside plus two NRTIs is as effective as a regimen containing an additional nucleoside (Shafer et al., 2003), indicating the equivalence of these three-drug and four-drug regimens. Four or more drugs may be used simultaneously in patients harboring drug-resistant virus, but the number of agents a patient can take is limited by toxicity and inconvenience.

Failure of an antiretroviral regimen is defined as a persistent increase in plasma HIV RNA concentrations in a patient with previously undetectable virus, despite continued treatment with that regimen. This indicates resistance to one or more drugs in the regimen and necessitates a change in treatment. The selection of new agents is therefore informed by the patient's treatment history and viral resistance testing. Treatment failure generally requires implementation of a completely new combination of drugs (Department of Health and Human Services, 2016). Adding a single active agent to a failing regimen is functional monotherapy if the patient is resistant to all other drugs in the regimen. The risk of failing a regimen also depends on the percentage of prescribed doses taken during a given period of treatment.

As antiretroviral therapy becomes more effective and easier to take, long-term toxicity of these drugs is of greater importance. Fortunately, several approved antiretroviral agents (lamivudine, emtricitabine, raltegravir, possibly dolutegravir) have essentially no clinically significant short-term or long-term toxicities. A potential concern that applies to all PIs and NNRTIs is clinically significant pharmacokinetic drug interactions. Most agents in these two drug classes can act as inhibitors

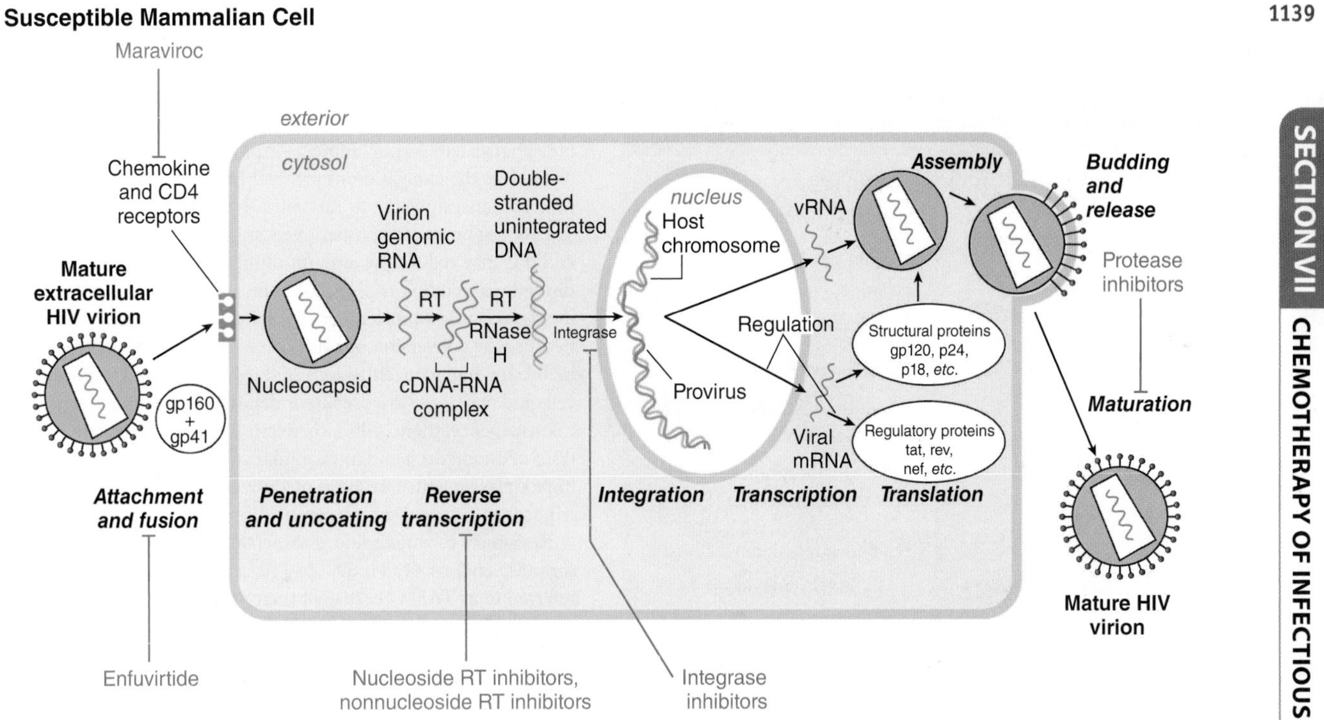

Figure 64–1 *Replicative cycle of HIV-1 showing the sites of action of available antiretroviral agents.* Available antiretroviral agents are shown in red. In this figure, gp120 + gp41 indicates extracellular and intracellular domains, respectively, of envelope glycoprotein.

and/or inducers of hepatic CYPs, other drug-metabolizing enzymes, and drug transporters (Piscitelli and Gallicano, 2001; see also Chapter 5). An increasingly recognized complication of initiating antiretroviral therapy is accelerated inflammatory reaction to overt or subclinical opportunistic infections or malignancies. This immune reconstitution inflammatory syndrome (IRIS) is most commonly seen when initiating therapy in individuals with low CD4 counts or advanced HIV disease. Infections commonly associated with IRIS include tuberculosis and other mycobacterial diseases, cryptococcosis, hepatitis virus infections, and *Pneumocystis* pneumonia (Manabe et al., 2007).

Drugs Used to Treat HIV Infection

Nucleoside and Nucleotide Reverse Transcriptase Inhibitors

Overview

HIV-encoded, RNA-dependent DNA polymerase, also called reverse transcriptase, converts viral RNA into proviral DNA, which is then incorporated into a host cell chromosome. Available inhibitors of this enzyme are either nucleoside/nucleotide analogues or nonnucleoside inhibitors (Table 64–1). NRTIs prevent infection of susceptible cells but do not eradicate the virus from cells that already harbor integrated proviral DNA. Nearly all patients starting antiretroviral treatment do so with at least one agent from this class. Figure 64–2 shows the mechanism of action of NRTIs, which involves phosphorylation by host cells to the active inhibitory form. All but one of the drugs in this class (see structures in Figure 64–3) are nucleosides that must be triphosphorylated at the 5′-hydroxyl to exert activity. The sole exception, tenofovir, is a nucleotide monophosphate analogue that requires two additional phosphates to acquire full activity. These compounds inhibit both HIV-1 and HIV-2, and several have broad-spectrum activity against other human and animal retroviruses; emtricitabine, lamivudine, and tenofovir are active against HBV, and tenofovir also has activity against herpesviruses (see Chapter 63).

The selective toxicity of these drugs depends on their ability to inhibit the HIV reverse transcriptase without inhibiting host cell DNA polymerases. Although the intracellular triphosphates for all these drugs have low affinity for human DNA polymerase α and polymerase β, some do inhibit human DNA polymerase γ, which is the mitochondrial enzyme. As a result, the important toxicities common to this class of drugs result in part from the inhibition of mitochondrial DNA synthesis (Lee et al., 2003). These toxicities include anemia, granulocytopenia, myopathy, peripheral neuropathy, and pancreatitis. Lactic acidosis with or without hepatomegaly and hepatic steatosis is a rare but potentially fatal complication seen with stavudine, zidovudine, and didanosine. Phosphorylated emtricitabine, lamivudine, and tenofovir have low affinity for DNA polymerase γ and are largely devoid of mitochondrial toxicity.

Table 64–2 summarizes the pharmacokinetic properties of NRTIs approved for treating HIV infection. A notable pharmacological feature of these agents is the formation of the intracellular nucleoside di- or triphosphate, which is the active form. Figure 64–4 shows the cellular routes that catalyze the activation of NRTIs. In general, the phosphorylated anabolites are eliminated from cells much more gradually than the parent drug is eliminated from the plasma. As a result, available NRTIs are dosed once or twice daily. These drugs are not major substrates for hepatic CYPs. Pharmacokinetic drug interactions involving tenofovir and PIs are likely explained by inhibition of OATP drug transporters (Chapman et al., 2003; see Chapter 5). High-level resistance to NRTIs, especially thymidine analogues, occurs slowly by comparison to NNTRIs and first-generation PIs. High-level resistance can occur rapidly with lamivudine and emtricitabine. Cross-resistance is common but often confined to drugs having similar chemical structures. Several nucleoside analogues have favorable safety and tolerability profiles and are useful in suppressing the emergence of HIV isolates resistant to the more potent drugs in combination regimens (Kuritzkes, 2011).

Zidovudine

Zidovudine is a synthetic thymidine analogue (Figure 64–3) with potent activity against a broad spectrum of retroviruses, including HIV-1, HIV-2, and HTLVs I and II. Zidovudine is active in lymphoblastic and monocytic cell lines but has no impact on cells already infected with HIV. Zidovudine appears to be more active in activated than in resting lymphocytes because

TABLE 64–1 ■ ANTIRETROVIRAL AGENTS APPROVED FOR USE IN THE U.S.

GENERIC NAME	ABBREVIATION; Chemical Name
Nucleoside/Nucleotide Reverse Transcriptase Inhibitors	
Zidovudine[a]	ZDV; azidothymidine (AZT)
Didanosine	ddI; dideoxyinosine
Stavudine	d4T; didehydrodeoxythymidine
Zalcitabine[b]	DDC; dideoxycytidine
Lamivudine[a]	3TC; dideoxythiacytidine
Abacavir[a]	ABC; amino-cyclopropylamino-purinylcyclopentenylmethanol
Tenofovir disoproxil[a,c]	TDF; TAF; phosphono-methoxypropyladenine (PMPA)
Tenofovir alafenamide[a,c]	
Emtricitabine[a]	FTC; fluorooxathiolanyl cytosine
Nonnucleoside Reverse Transcriptase Inhibitors	
Nevirapine	NVP
Efavirenz[a]	EFV
Delavirdine	DLV
Etravirine	ETV
Rilpivirine[a]	
Protease Inhibitors	
Saquinavir	SQV
Indinavir	IDV
Ritonavir	RTV
Nelfinavir	NFV
Amprenavir[b]	APV
Lopinavir[d]	LPV/r
Atazanavir	ATV
Fosamprenavir	FPV
Tipranavir	TPV
Darunavir	DRV
Entry Inhibitors	
Enfuvirtide	T-20
Maraviroc	MVC
Integrase Inhibitors	
Raltegravir[a]	RAL
Elvitegravir[a]	EVG
Dolutegravir[a]	DTG

[a]A number of fixed-dose coformulations are available: zidovudine + lamivudine; zidovudine + lamivudine + abacavir ; abacavir + lamivudine; tenofovir + emtricitabine; tenofovir + efavirenz + emtricitabine; emtricitabine + rilpivirine + tenofovir disoproxil fumarate; cobicistat + elvitegravir + emtricitabine + tenofovir disoproxil fumarate; lamivudine + raltegravir.

[b]No longer marketed worldwide.

[c]Tenofovir disoproxil fumarate is a nucleotide prodrug of the nucleoside tenofovir.

[d]Lopinavir is available only as part of a fixed-dose coformulation with ritonavir.

the phosphorylating enzyme, thymidine kinase, is S-phase specific (Cihlar and Ray, 2010). Zidovudine is FDA-approved for the treatment of adults and children with HIV infection and for preventing mother-to-child transmission; it also was previously recommended for postexposure prophylaxis in HIV-exposed healthcare workers. Zidovudine is marketed in oral tablets, capsules, and solution as well as a solution for intravenous injection. Zidovudine is available in coformulated tablets with lamivudine or with lamivudine and abacavir.

Mechanisms of Action and Resistance. Intracellular zidovudine is phosphorylated to zidovudine 5′-triphosphate. Zidovudine-triphosphate terminates the elongation of proviral DNA because it is incorporated by reverse transcriptase into nascent DNA but lacks a 3′-hydroxyl group. The monophosphate competitively inhibits cellular thymidylate kinase, and this may reduce the amount of intracellular thymidine triphosphate formed. Zidovudine-triphosphate only weakly inhibits cellular DNA polymerase α but is a more potent inhibitor of mitochondrial polymerase γ. Because the conversion of zidovudine-monophosphate to diphosphate is inefficient, high concentrations of the monophosphate accumulate inside cells and may serve as a precursor depot for formation of triphosphate. As a consequence, there is little correlation between extracellular concentrations of parent drug and intracellular concentrations of triphosphate, and higher plasma concentrations of zidovudine do not increase intracellular triphosphate concentrations proportionately.

Resistance to zidovudine is associated with mutations at reverse transcriptase codons 41, 44, 67, 70, 210, 215, and 219. These mutations are referred to as TAMs because of their ability to confer cross-resistance to other thymidine analogues, such as stavudine. The M184V substitution in the reverse transcriptase gene associated with the use of lamivudine or emtricitabine greatly restores sensitivity to zidovudine (Kuritzkes, 2011). The combination of zidovudine and lamivudine produces greater long-term suppression of plasma HIV RNA than does zidovudine alone.

ADME. Zidovudine is absorbed rapidly and reaches peak plasma concentrations within 1 h. Table 64–2 summarizes the drug's pharmacokinetic profile, which is not altered significantly during pregnancy; drug concentrations in the newborn approach those of the mother. Parent drug crosses the blood-brain barrier relatively well and also is detectable in breast milk, semen, and fetal tissue.

Untoward Effects and Drug Interactions. Patients initiating zidovudine treatment often complain of fatigue, malaise, myalgia, nausea, anorexia, headache, and insomnia; these symptoms usually resolve within a few weeks. Erythrocytic macrocytosis is seen in about 90% of patients but usually is not associated with anemia. Chronic zidovudine administration has been associated with nail hyperpigmentation. Skeletal muscle myopathy can occur and is associated with depletion of mitochondrial DNA, most likely as a consequence of inhibition of DNA polymerase γ. Serious hepatic toxicity, with or without steatosis and lactic acidosis, is rare but can be fatal.

Probenecid, fluconazole, atovaquone, and valproic acid may increase plasma concentrations of zidovudine, probably through inhibition of glucuronosyl transferases. Zidovudine is neither substrate nor inhibitor of CYPs. Zidovudine can cause bone marrow suppression and should be used cautiously in patients with preexisting anemia or granulocytopenia and in those taking other marrow-suppressive drugs. Stavudine and zidovudine compete for intracellular phosphorylation and should not be used concomitantly.

Stavudine

Stavudine is a synthetic thymidine analogue that is active in vitro against HIV-1 and HIV-2. Stavudine is approved for use in HIV-infected adults and children, including neonates. This drug is no longer widely prescribed because of the availability of agents with less toxicity.

Mechanisms of Action and Resistance. Intracellular stavudine is sequentially phosphorylated to form stavudine 5′-triphosphate. Like zidovudine, stavudine is most potent in activated cells, probably because thymidine kinase, which produces the monophosphate, is an S-phase–specific enzyme. Stavudine resistance is seen most frequently with mutations at reverse transcriptase codons 41, 44, 67, 70, 210, 215, and 219, which are mutations associated with zidovudine resistance. Resistance mutations for stavudine appear to accumulate slowly. Cross-resistance to multiple nucleoside analogues has been reported following prolonged therapy (Martin et al., 2010).

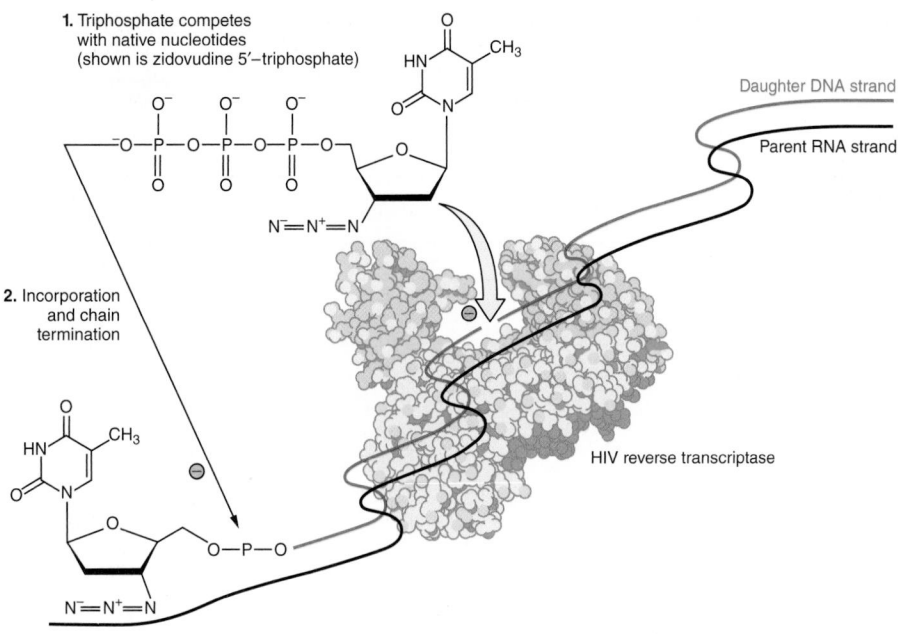

Figure 64–2 *Mechanism of NRTIs.* Zidovudine is depicted; Table 64–1 lists other agents in the NRTI class. Nucleoside and nucleotide analogues must enter cells and be phosphorylated to generate synthetic substrates for reverse transcriptase. The fully phosphorylated analogues block replication of the viral genome both by competitively inhibiting incorporation of native nucleotides and by terminating elongation of nascent proviral DNA because they lack a 3′-hydroxyl group.

ADME. Table 64–2 summarizes the agent's pharmacokinetic data. Stavudine is well absorbed and reaches peak plasma concentrations within 1 h; bioavailability is not affected by food. The drug penetrates well into the CSF, achieving concentrations that are about 40% of those in plasma. Placental concentrations of stavudine are about half those of zidovudine. The drug undergoes active tubular secretion, and renal elimination accounts for about 40% of parent drug; thus, the dose should be adjusted in patients with renal insufficiency.

Untoward Effects and Drug Interactions. The most common serious toxicity of stavudine is peripheral neuropathy. Although this may reflect mitochondrial toxicity, stavudine is a less-potent inhibitor of DNA polymerase γ than either didanosine or zalcitabine, suggesting that other mechanisms may be involved. Stavudine is also associated with a progressive motor neuropathy characterized by weakness and in some cases respiratory failure, similar to Guillain-Barré syndrome.

Lactic acidosis and hepatic steatosis are associated with stavudine use and may be more common when stavudine and didanosine are combined. Acute pancreatitis is not highly associated with stavudine but is more common when stavudine is combined with didanosine than when didanosine is given alone. Of all nucleoside analogues, stavudine use is associated most strongly with fat wasting (lipoatrophy). Stavudine has fallen out of favor largely because of this toxicity.

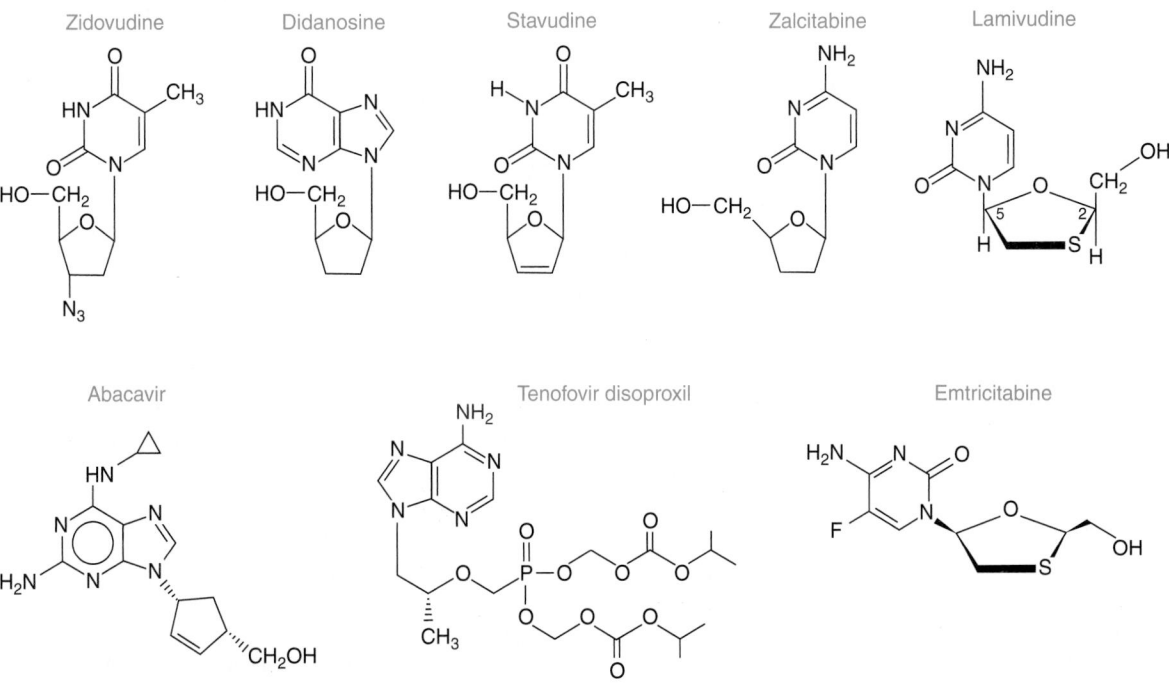

Figure 64–3 *Structures of NRTIs.*

TABLE 64–2 ■ PHARMACOKINETIC PROPERTIES OF NUCLEOSIDE REVERSE TRANSCRIPTASE INHIBITORS[a]

PARAMETER	ZIDOVUDINE	LAMIVUDINE	STAVUDINE[b]	DIDANOSINE[c]	ABACAVIR	TENOFOVIR[d]	EMTRICITABINE
Oral bioavailability, %	64	86–87	86	42	83	25	93
Effect of meals on AUC	↓ 24% (high fat)	↔	↔	↓ 55% (acidity)	↔	↑ 40% (high fat)	↔
Plasma $t_{1/2}$, h	1.0	5–7	1.1–1.4	1.5	0.8–1.5	14–17	10
Intracellular $t_{1/2}$ of triphosphate, h	3–4	12–18	3.5	25–40	21	60–100	39
Plasma protein binding, %	20–38	<35	<5	<5	50	<8	<4
Metabolism, %	60–80 (glucuronidation)	<36	ND	50 (purine metabolism)	>80 (dehydrogenation; glucuronidation)	ND	13
Renal excretion of parent drug, %	14	71	39	18–36	<5	70–80	86

$t_{1/2}$, half-life of elimination; ↑, increase; ↓, decrease; ↔, no effect; ND, not determined.

[a]Reported mean values in adults with normal renal and hepatic function.

[b]Parameters reported for the stavudine capsule formulation.

[c]Parameters reported for the didanosine chewable tablet formulation.

[d]Reported values for oral tenofovir disoproxil fumarate.

Stavudine is mainly renally cleared and is not subject to metabolic drug interactions. The incidence and severity of peripheral neuropathy may be increased when stavudine is combined with other neuropathic medications; thus, drugs such as ethambutol, isoniazid, phenytoin, and vincristine should be avoided. Combining stavudine with didanosine leads to increased risk and severity of peripheral neuropathy and potentially fatal pancreatitis; therefore, these two drugs should not be used together. Stavudine and zidovudine compete for intracellular phosphorylation and should not be used concomitantly (Martin et al., 2010).

Lamivudine

Lamivudine is a cytidine analogue reverse transcriptase inhibitor that is active against HIV-1, HIV-2, and HBV. Lamivudine is approved for HIV in adults and children 3 months or older. Lamivudine has been effective in combination with other antiretroviral drugs in both treatment-naïve and experienced patients and is a common component of therapy, given its safety, convenience, and efficacy (Cihlar and Ray, 2010). Lamivudine is also approved for treatment of chronic hepatitis B.

Mechanisms of Action and Resistance. Lamivudine enters cells by passive diffusion and is sequentially phosphorylated to lamivudine 5′-triphosphate, which is the active anabolite. Lamivudine has low affinity for human DNA polymerases, explaining its low toxicity to the host. High-level resistance to lamivudine occurs with single-amino-acid substitutions, M184V or M184I. These mutations can reduce in vitro sensitivity to lamivudine as much as 1000-fold. The M184V mutation

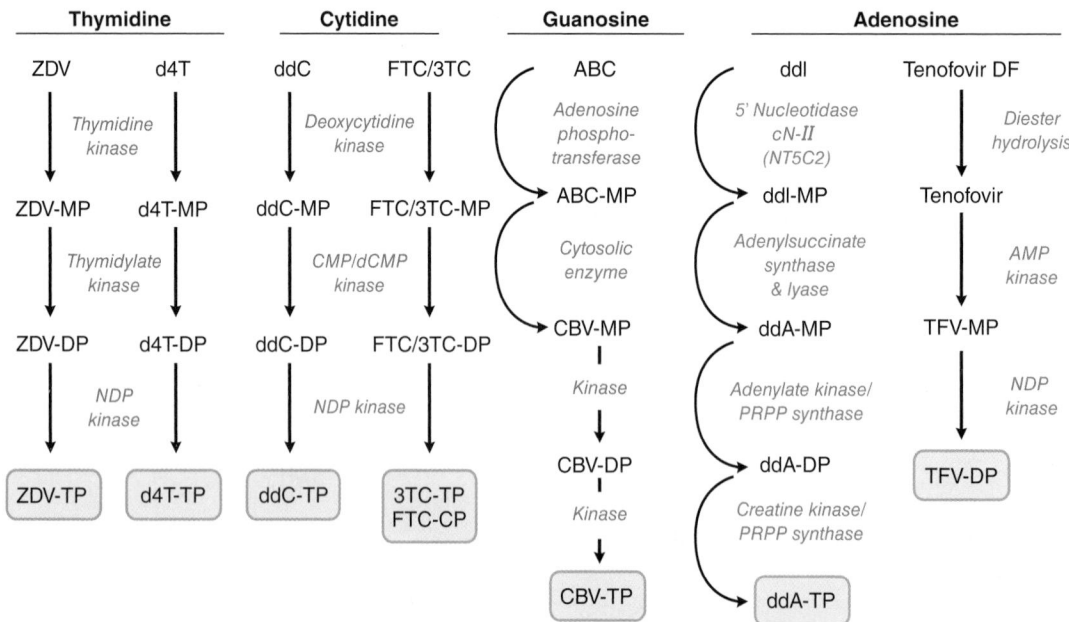

Figure 64–4 *Intracellular activation of nucleoside analogue reverse transcriptase inhibitors.* Drugs and phosphorylated anabolites are abbreviated; the enzymes responsible for each conversion are spelled out. The active antiretroviral anabolite for each drug is shown in the blue box. (Adapted with permission from Khoo SH, et al. Pharmacology. In: Boucher CAB, Galasso GAJ, eds. *Practical Guidelines in Antiviral Therapy*. Elsevier, New York, **2002**, 13–35. Copyright © Elsevier.) MP, monophosphate; DP, diphosphate; TP, triphosphate.

restores zidovudine susceptibility in zidovudine-resistant HIV and also partially restores tenofovir susceptibility in tenofovir-resistant HIV harboring the K65R mutation (Kuritzkes, 2011). This effect may contribute to the sustained virologic benefits of zidovudine and lamivudine combination therapy.

ADME. Table 64–2 summarizes the pharmacokinetic parameters for this drug. Lamivudine is excreted primarily unchanged in the urine; dose adjustment is recommended for patients with a creatinine clearance less than 50 mL/min. Lamivudine freely crosses the placenta into the fetal circulation.

Untoward Effects and Precautions. Lamivudine is one of the least-toxic antiretroviral drugs. Neutropenia, headache, and nausea have been reported at higher-than-recommended doses. Pancreatitis has been reported in pediatric patients. Because lamivudine also has activity against HBV, caution is warranted in using this drug in patients coinfected with HBV or in HBV-endemic areas: Abrupt discontinuation of lamivudine may be associated with a rebound of HBV replication and exacerbation of hepatitis.

Abacavir

Abacavir, a synthetic purine analogue, is approved for the treatment of HIV-1 infection, in combination with other antiretroviral agents. Abacavir is available in a coformulation with zidovudine and lamivudine for twice-daily dosing and in a coformulation with lamivudine, or lamivudine and dolutegravir, for once-daily dosing. Abacavir is approved for use in adult and pediatric patients 3 months or older, with dosing in the latter based on body weight.

Mechanisms of Action and Resistance. Abacavir is the only approved antiretroviral that is active as a guanosine analogue. It is sequentially phosphorylated in the host cell to carbovir 5′-triphosphate, which terminates the elongation of proviral DNA because it is incorporated by reverse transcriptase into nascent DNA but lacks a 3′-hydroxyl group (Cihlar and Ray, 2010). Clinical resistance to abacavir is associated with four specific substitutions: K65R, L74V, Y115F, and M184V. In combination, these substitutions can reduce susceptibility by up to 10-fold. K65R confers cross-resistance to all nucleosides except zidovudine. An alternate pathway for abacavir resistance involves mutations at codons 41, 210, and 215 (Kuritzkes, 2011).

ADME. Table 64–2 summarizes the pharmacokinetic parameters for this agent. The presence of food does not affect the oral bioavailability of abacavir. Abacavir is neither a substrate nor an inhibitor of CYPs. Its CSF/plasma AUC ratio is about 0.3.

Untoward Effects and Drug Interactions. The most important adverse effect of abacavir is a unique and potentially fatal hypersensitivity syndrome characterized by fever, abdominal pain, and other GI complaints; a mild maculopapular rash; and malaise or fatigue. Respiratory complaints (cough, pharyngitis, dyspnea); musculoskeletal complaints; headache; and paresthesias are less common. The presence of concurrent fever, abdominal pain, and rash within 6 weeks of starting abacavir is diagnostic and necessitates immediate discontinuation of the drug. Once discontinued for hypersensitivity, abacavir must never be restarted. The hypersensitivity syndrome (2%–9% of patients) results from a genetically mediated immune response linked to both the HLA-B*5701 locus and the M493T allele in the heat-shock locus Hsp70-Hom. The *Hsp* gene is implicated in antigen presentation, and this haplotype is associated with aberrant tumor necrosis factor α release after exposure of human lymphocytes to abacavir ex vivo (White et al., 2015). Abacavir should not be used in anyone known to carry the HLA-B*5701 locus (approximately 10% of Caucasians).

Abacavir is not associated with any clinically significant pharmacokinetic drug interactions. However, a large dose of ethanol (0.7 g/kg) increases the abacavir plasma AUC by 41% and prolongs the elimination $t_{1/2}$ by 26%, possibly owing to competition for alcohol dehydrogenase, which produces the dehydro- metabolite of the drug (see Table 64–2).

Tenofovir

Tenofovir is a derivative of 5′-AMP that lacks a complete ribose ring; it is the only nucleotide analogue currently marketed for the treatment of

HIV infection. Tenofovir is available as the disoproxil or alafenamide prodrugs, which substantially improve oral absorption. Tenofovir is active against HIV-1, HIV-2, and HBV. TDF is FDA-approved for treating HIV infection in adults and children older than 2 years in combination with other antiretroviral agents and for the treatment of chronic hepatitis B in adults and children older than 12. It is also approved for HIV preexposure prophylaxis (in combination with emtricitabine) in adults at high risk of acquiring the infection. A new tenofovir oral prodrug, TAF, is FDA-approved for the treatment of HIV and HBV. Its advantages over TDF include lower dose and less renal and bone toxicity (Sax et al., 2015); it is currently available in coformulation with elvitegravir, cobicistat, and emtricitabine; rilpivirine and emtricitabine; or emtricitabine.

Mechanisms of Action and Resistance. Tenofovir disoproxil is hydrolyzed rapidly to tenofovir, which is phosphorylated by cellular kinases to its active metabolite, tenofovir diphosphate, which is actually a triphosphate: The parent drug is a monophosphate (Figure 64–3) (Cihlar and Ray, 2010). The disposition of oral tenofovir alafenamide is similar, but it circulates largely as the uncleaved prodrug, which is taken up into cells and then converted to the parent nucleotide; as a consequence, circulating concentrations of tenofovir, which may contribute to renal toxicity, are much lower than produced by the disoproxil fumarate prodrug. Tenofovir diphosphate is a competitive inhibitor of viral reverse transcriptases and is incorporated into HIV DNA to cause chain termination because it has an incomplete ribose ring. Although tenofovir diphosphate has broad-spectrum activity against viral DNA polymerases, it has low affinity for human DNA polymerase α, polymerase β, and polymerase γ, which is the basis for its selective toxicity.

Specific resistance occurs with a K65R substitution that has been associated with clinical failure of tenofovir-containing regimens. Tenofovir sensitivity and virologic efficacy also are reduced in patients harboring HIV isolates with high-level resistance to zidovudine or stavudine. The M184V mutation associated with lamivudine or emtricitabine resistance partially restores susceptibility in tenofovir-resistant HIV harboring the K65R mutation (Kuritzkes, 2011).

ADME. Table 64–2 shows pharmacokinetic data for tenofovir. Following an intravenous dose, 70%–80% of the drug is recovered unchanged in the urine; thus, doses should be decreased in those with renal insufficiency. Tenofovir is not known to inhibit or induce CYPs.

Untoward Effects and Drug Interactions. Tenofovir generally is well tolerated, with few significant symptoms reported except for flatulence. Rare episodes of acute renal failure and Fanconi syndrome have been reported, and this drug should be used with caution in patients with pre-existing renal disease. Tenofovir use is associated with small declines in eCL_{Cr} after months of treatment in some patients; because the dose needs to be reduced in renal insufficiency, renal function (creatinine and phosphorus) should be monitored regularly. Because tenofovir also has activity against HBV, caution is warranted in using this drug in patients coinfected with HBV: Abrupt discontinuation of tenofovir may be associated with a rebound of HBV replication and exacerbation of hepatitis. Tenofovir can increase the AUC of didanosine, and the two drugs should not be used together (Cihlar and Ray, 2010).

Tenofovir plasma concentrations are increased by 30%–50% if combined with the pharmacokinetic enhancers ritonavir or cobicistat due to inhibition of renal drug transporters. Similar effects are seen with the HBV NS5A inhibitors ledipasvir and velpatasvir (see Chapter 63). These combinations are generally well tolerated, without producing significant renal injury. However, acute renal insufficiency has been reported when TDF is combined with the oral nonsteroidal diclofenac.

Emtricitabine

Emtricitabine is a cytidine analogue that is chemically related to lamivudine and shares many of its properties. Emtricitabine is active against HIV-1, HIV-2, and HBV. The drug is FDA-approved for treating HIV infection in adults, children, and infants, in combination with other antiretroviral agents, and is available coformulated with tenofovir with or without efavirenz or with tenofovir, elvitegravir, and cobicistat. Emtricitabine is also approved for HIV preexposure prophylaxis (in combination with tenofovir) in adults at high risk of acquiring the infection.

Mechanisms of Action and Resistance. Emtricitabine enters cells by passive diffusion and is sequentially phosphorylated to its active metabolite, emtricitabine 5′-triphosphate. High-level resistance to emtricitabine occurs with the same mutations affecting lamivudine (mainly M184I/V), although these appear to occur less frequently with emtricitabine. The M184V mutation restores sensitivity to zidovudine in zidovudine-resistant HIV and partially restores sensitivity to tenofovir in tenofovir-resistant HIV harboring the K65R mutation (Kuritzkes, 2011). The same K65R mutation confers resistance to emtricitabine and the other cytidine analogue lamivudine, as well as didanosine, stavudine, and abacavir.

ADME. Table 64–2 summarizes pharmacokinetic data for emtricitabine. Orally administered drug is absorbed rapidly and well; the drug can be taken without regard to meals. Emtricitabine is excreted primarily unchanged in the urine; thus, the dose should be reduced in patients with CL_{Cr} below 50 mL/min.

Untoward Effects and Drug Interactions. Emtricitabine is one of the least-toxic antiretroviral drugs and has few significant adverse effects (Cihlar and Ray, 2010). Prolonged exposure has been associated with hyperpigmentation of the skin, especially in sun-exposed areas. Because emtricitabine also has in vitro activity against HBV, caution is warranted in using this drug in patients coinfected with HBV and in regions with high HBV seroprevalence; abrupt discontinuation of emtricitabine may be associated with a rebound of HBV replication and exacerbation of hepatitis.

Emtricitabine is not metabolized to a significant extent by CYPs, and it is not susceptible to known metabolic drug interactions.

Didanosine

Didanosine (2′,3′-dideoxyinosine) is a purine nucleoside analogue that is active against HIV-1, HIV-2, and other retroviruses, including HTLV-1. The drug is FDA-approved for adults and children with HIV infection in combination with other antiretroviral agents. Didanosine is no longer widely prescribed because of the availability of agents with less toxicity (Martin et al., 2010).

Mechanisms of Action and Resistance. Didanosine enters cells via a nucleoside transporter and is sequentially phosphorylated by cellular enzymes to the triphosphate, the active anabolite that functions as an antiviral adenosine analogue. Resistance to didanosine is associated with mutations at reverse transcriptase codons 65 and 74. The L74V substitution, which reduces susceptibility 5- to 26-fold in vitro, is seen most commonly in patients failing to respond to didanosine (Kuritzkes, 2011). Other nucleoside analogue mutations, including TAMs, can contribute to didanosine resistance even though the drug does not appear to select for these mutations de novo. The reverse transcriptase insertion mutations at codon 69 produce cross-resistance to all current nucleoside analogues, including didanosine.

ADME. Table 64–2 summarizes major pharmacokinetic parameters for didanosine. The drug is acid labile and thus is administered with an antacid buffer. Food decreases didanosine bioavailability; all formulations of didanosine must be administered at least 30 min before or 2 h after eating. This complicates dosing of didanosine in combination with antiretroviral drugs that must be given with food, as is the case for most HIV PIs. Didanosine is excreted by glomerular filtration and tubular secretion; doses therefore must be adjusted in patients with renal insufficiency.

Untoward Effects and Drug Interactions. The most serious toxicities associated with didanosine include peripheral neuropathy and pancreatitis, both of which are thought to be a consequence of mitochondrial toxicity. Didanosine should be avoided in patients with a history of pancreatitis or neuropathy. Patients complain of pain, numbness, and tingling in the affected extremities. If the drug is stopped as soon as symptoms appear, the neuropathy should improve or resolve. However, irreversible neuropathy can occur with continued use. Retinal changes and optic neuritis also have been reported. Coadministration of other drugs that cause

pancreatitis or neuropathy (i.e., stavudine) will increase the risk and severity of these symptoms. Ethambutol, isoniazid, vincristine, cisplatin, and pentamidine should be avoided. Serious hepatic toxicity occurs rarely but can be fatal (Martin et al., 2010). Other reported adverse effects include elevated hepatic transaminases, headache, and asymptomatic hyperuricemia; noncirrhotic portal hypertension can occur years after exposure to didanosine.

Buffering agents included in didanosine formulations can interfere with the bioavailability of some coadministered drugs because of altered pH or chelation with cations in the buffer. For example, didanosine greatly reduces the AUCs of ciprofloxacin and indinavir; concentrations of ketoconazole and itraconazole, whose absorption is pH dependent, also are diminished. These interactions generally can be avoided by separating administration of didanosine from that of other agents by at least 2 h after or 6 h before the interacting drug. The enteric-coated formulation of didanosine does not alter ciprofloxacin or indinavir absorption. Didanosine is excreted renally, and shared renal excretory mechanisms provide a basis for interactions with oral ganciclovir, allopurinol, and tenofovir. Methadone decreases the didanosine AUC by about 60%.

Nonnucleoside Reverse Transcriptase Inhibitors

Overview

The NNRTIs include a variety of chemical substrates that bind to a hydrophobic pocket in the p66 subunit of the HIV-1 reverse transcriptase, in a site distant from the active site (Figure 64–5). These compounds induce a conformational change in the 3-dimensional structure of the enzyme that greatly reduces its activity, and thus they act as noncompetitive inhibitors. Because the binding site for NNRTIs is virus-strain specific, the approved agents are active against HIV-1 but not HIV-2 or other retroviruses and should not be used to treat HIV-2 infection. These compounds also have no activity against host cell DNA polymerases (de Bethune, 2010). The five approved NNRTIs are nevirapine, efavirenz, etravirine, rilpivirine, and delavirdine. Table 64–3 summarizes their pharmacokinetic properties.

Agents in this class share a number of properties. All approved NNRTIs are eliminated from the body by hepatic metabolism. Efavirenz, etravirine, and nevirapine are moderately potent inducers of hepatic drug-metabolizing enzymes, including CYP3A4; delavirdine is mainly a CYP3A4 inhibitor. Pharmacokinetic drug interactions are thus an important consideration with this class of compounds. All NNRTIs except etravirine and rilpivirine are susceptible to high-level drug resistance caused by single-amino-acid changes in the NNRTI-binding pocket (usually in codons 103 or 181; Kuritzkes, 2011). Exposure to even a single dose of nevirapine in the absence of other antiretroviral drugs is associated with resistance mutations in up to one-third of patients (Eshleman et al., 2004). These agents are potent and highly effective but should be combined with other active agents to avoid resistance. *NNRTIs should never be used as single agents in monotherapy or as the sole addition to a failing regimen.*

The use of efavirenz or nevirapine in combination with other antiretroviral drugs is associated with favorable long-term suppression of viremia and elevation of CD4+ lymphocyte counts. Rashes occur frequently with all NNRTIs, usually during the first 4 weeks of therapy. Rare cases of potentially fatal DRESS or Stevens-Johnson syndrome have been reported with nevirapine, efavirenz, rilpivirine, and etravirine. Fat accumulation can be seen after long-term use of NNRTIs, and fatal hepatitis has been associated with nevirapine use (de Bethune, 2010).

Nevirapine

Nevirapine is a dipyridodiazepinone NNRTI with potent activity against HIV-1. The drug is FDA-approved for the treatment of HIV-1 infection in adults and children in combination with other antiretroviral agents. Nevirapine is approved for use in infants and children 15 days old or older, with dosing based on body surface area. Single-dose nevirapine was used widely in pregnant HIV-infected women to prevent mother-to-child transmission, but this practice is declining as more pregnant HIV-infected women are being placed on permanent multidrug antiretroviral regimens (de Bethune, 2010).

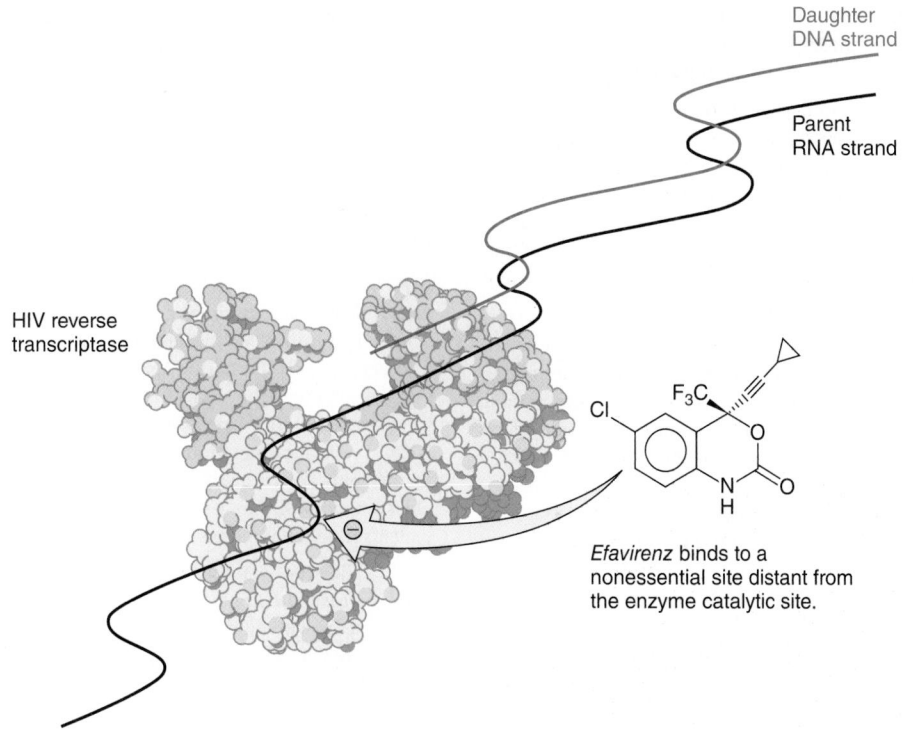

Figure 64–5 *Mechanism of NNRTIs.*

Efavirenz binds to a nonessential site distant from the enzyme catalytic site.

HIV reverse transcriptase

Daughter DNA strand

Parent RNA strand

ADME. Table 64–3 summarizes the pharmacokinetic data for this agent. The drug readily crosses the placenta and has been found in breast milk. Nevirapine is a moderate inducer of CYPs and induces its own metabolism. To compensate for this, the drug should be initiated at a dose of 200 mg once daily for 14 days, with the dose then increased to 200 mg twice daily if no adverse reactions have occurred.

Untoward Effects and Drug Interactions. The most frequent adverse events associated with nevirapine are rash (in ~ 16% of patients) and pruritus. In most patients, the rash resolves with continued administration of drug; administration of glucocorticoids may cause a more severe rash. Life-threatening Stevens-Johnson syndrome is rare but occurs in up to 0.3% of recipients. Clinical hepatitis occurs in up to 1% of patients. Severe and fatal hepatitis has been associated with nevirapine use, and this may be more common in women with CD4 counts greater than 250 cells/mm³, especially during pregnancy (de Bethune, 2010). Other reported side effects include fever, fatigue, headache, somnolence, and nausea.

Because nevirapine induces CYP3A4, this drug may lower plasma concentrations of coadministered CYP3A4 substrates. Methadone withdrawal has been reported in patients receiving nevirapine, presumably as a consequence of enhanced methadone clearance. Plasma ethinyl estradiol and norethindrone concentrations decrease by 20% with nevirapine; alternative methods of birth control are advised.

Efavirenz

Efavirenz (see structure in Figure 64–5) is an NNRTI with potent activity against HIV-1. The drug should be used only in combination with other effective agents and should not be added as the sole new agent to a failing regimen. Efavirenz has been used widely because of its convenience, effectiveness, and long-term tolerability. Especially popular is the once-daily, single-pill coformulation of efavirenz, TDF, and emtricitabine. Efavirenz plus two NRTIs was a preferred regimen for naïve patients, but it is being replaced in many parts of the world by regimens with better tolerability. A 400-mg daily dose of efavirenz may be equally efficacious and better tolerated than the standard 600-mg dose (ENCORE1 Study Group, 2014).

TABLE 64–3 ■ PHARMACOKINETIC PROPERTIES OF NONNUCLEOSIDE REVERSE TRANSCRIPTASE INHIBITORS[a]

PARAMETER	NEVIRAPINE[b]	EFAVIRENZ[b]	ETRAVIRINE
Oral bioavailability, %	90–93	50	NR
Effect of meals on AUC	↔	↑ 17%–28%	↑ 33%–102%
Plasma $t_{1/2}$, h	25–30	40–55	41
Plasma protein binding, %	60	99	99.9
Metabolism by CYPs	3A4 > 2B6	2B6 > 3A4	3A4, 2C9, 2C19, UGT
Renal excretion of parent drug, %	<3	<3	1%
Autoinduction of metabolism	Yes	Yes	NR
Inhibition of CYP3A	No	Yes	No

$t_{1/2}$, half-life of elimination; ↑, increase; ↓, decrease; ↔, no effect; NR, not reported.

[a]Reported mean values in adults with normal renal and hepatic function.

[b]Values at steady state after multiple oral doses.

Efavirenz can be safely combined with rifampin and is useful in patients also being treated for tuberculosis. Efavirenz is approved for adult and pediatric patients 3 years and older and weighing at least 10 kg.

ADME. Table 64–3 summarizes the pharmacokinetic data for this agent. Efavirenz is well absorbed from the GI tract, but there is diminished absorption of the drug with increasing doses. Bioavailability (AUC) is increased by 22% with a high-fat meal. Efavirenz is more than 99% bound to plasma proteins and, as a consequence, has a low CSF-to plasma ratio of 0.01. The drug should be taken initially on an empty stomach at bedtime to reduce side effects. The long elimination $t_{1/2}$ permits once-daily dosing.

Untoward Effects and Drug Interactions. The most important adverse effects of efavirenz involve the CNS. Up to 53% of patients report some CNS or psychiatric side effects, but fewer than 5% discontinue the drug for this reason. Patients commonly report dizziness, impaired concentration, dysphoria, vivid or disturbing dreams, and insomnia. CNS side effects generally become more tolerable and resolve within the first 4 weeks of therapy. Rash occurs frequently with efavirenz (27%), usually in the first few weeks of treatment, resolving spontaneously and rarely requiring drug discontinuation. Life-threatening skin eruptions such as Stevens-Johnson syndrome are rare (de Bethune, 2010). Other side effects reported with efavirenz include headache, increased hepatic transaminases, and elevated serum cholesterol. Efavirenz is the only antiretroviral drug that is teratogenic in primates, but careful clinical studies suggested that it is no more teratogenic in humans than other antiretroviral drugs (Ford et al., 2014).

Efavirenz is a moderate inducer of hepatic enzymes, especially CYP3A4, but also a weak to moderate CYP inhibitor. Efavirenz decreases concentrations of phenobarbital, phenytoin, and carbamazepine; the methadone AUC is reduced by 33%–66% at steady state. Efavirenz reduces the rifabutin AUC by about 38%. Efavirenz has a variable effect on HIV PIs: Indinavir, saquinavir, and amprenavir concentrations are reduced; ritonavir and nelfinavir concentrations are increased. Drugs that induce CYPs 2B6 or 3A4 (e.g., phenobarbital, phenytoin, and carbamazepine) would be expected to increase the clearance of efavirenz and should be avoided (de Bethune, 2010).

Rilpivirine

Rilpivirine is a diarylpyrimidine NNRTI with potent activity against HIV-1; Table 64–3 presents some of the drug's pharmacokinetic values. The drug should be used only in combination with other effective agents and should not be added as the sole new agent to a failing regimen. Rilpivirine has the best side-effect profile of available NNRTIs and has few or no CNS side effects compared to efavirenz. Rilpivirine retains efficacy against many HIV strains that are resistant to efavirenz and other earlier NNRTIs. However, higher concentrations of rilpivirine are associated with prolongation of the QTc interval and, at the approved dose of 25 mg per day, is less effective than efavirenz in patients with baseline viral load greater than 100,000 copies/mL or CD4 count below 200 cells/mm³ (Sharma and Saravolatz, 2013). Failure of a rilpivirine-containing regimen generally results in resistance that precludes the use of other NNRTIs. Rilpivirine is approved for adult and pediatric patients 12 years of age and older and weighing at least 35 kg. Rilpivirine is also available as a once-daily, single-tablet coformulation with TDF and emtricitabine or tenofovir alafenamide and emtricitabine.

ADME. Table 64–3 summarizes the pharmacokinetic data for rilpivirine. Absorption of rilpivirine is both food and pH dependent. Bioavailability (AUC) is decreased by 40% in the fasted state or by 50% with a high-protein, low-fat meal; the drug should only be given with food and not with high-protein, low-fat supplements. Rilpivirine should not be given with proton pump inhibitors, and H_2 receptor antagonists should be administered 12 h before or 4 h after dosing (Sharma and Saravolatz, 2013). The long elimination $t_{1/2}$ permits once-daily dosing.

Untoward Effects and Drug Interactions. Rash (<5%) occurs less frequently with rilpivirine than with other NNRTIs. Although CNS adverse effects are much less common with rilpivirine than with efavirenz, depressive symptoms have been reported, including in pediatric and adolescent patients. Elevated hepatic transaminases may occur, especially in those with underlying HBV or hepatitis C virus infection. Rilpivirine is considered pregnancy category B by the FDA.

Rilpivirine concentrations can be reduced by coadministered CYP inducers, and this drug should not be given with rifampin; anticonvulsants such as carbamazepine, phenobarbital, or phenytoin; or any products containing St. John's wort. At the 25-mg daily dose, rilpivirine is not a clinically significant inhibitor or inducer of hepatic enzymes. Because rilpivirine can prolong the QTc in a concentration-dependent fashion, caution is advised when combining this drug with any known CYP3A4 inhibitors or other drugs that can increase rilpivirine concentrations or with other drugs known to prolong the QTc.

Etravirine

Etravirine is a diarylpyrimidine NNRTI that is active against HIV-1. The drug is unique in its ability to inhibit reverse transcriptase that is resistant to other NNRTIs. Etravirine appears to have conformational and positional flexibility in the NNRTI-binding pocket that allow it to inhibit the function of the HIV-1 reverse transcriptase in the presence of common NNRTI resistance mutations (de Bethune, 2010). Etravirine is approved for use only in treatment-experienced adults and children 6 years or older with viral strains resistant to another NNRTI. NNRTI-experienced patients should not receive etravirine plus NRTIs alone.

ADME. Table 64–3 summarizes the pharmacokinetic data for this agent. Food increases the etravirine AUC by about 50%; thus, the drug should be administered with food. Methyl- and dimethyl-hydroxylated metabolites are produced in the liver primarily by CYPs 3A4, 2C9, and 2C19, accounting for most of the elimination of this drug.

Untoward Effects and Drug Interactions. The only notable side effect of etravirine is rash (17% vs. placebo value of 9%), usually occurring within a few weeks of starting therapy and resolving within 1–3 weeks. Severe rash, including Stevens-Johnson syndrome and toxic epidermal necrolysis, have been reported (de Bethune, 2010).

Etravirine is an inducer of CYP3A4 and glucuronosyl transferases and an inhibitor of CYPs 2C9 and 2C19; it can therefore be involved in a number of clinically significant pharmacokinetic drug interactions. Etravirine can be combined with darunavir/ritonavir, lopinavir/ritonavir, and saquinavir/ritonavir without the need for dose adjustments. The dose of maraviroc should be doubled when these two drugs are combined. Etravirine should not be administered with tipranavir/ritonavir, fosamprenavir/ritonavir, or atazanavir/ritonavir in the absence of better data to guide dosing. Etravirine should not be combined with other NNRTIs. Unlike other NNRTIs, etravirine does not appear to alter the clearance of methadone.

Delavirdine

Delavirdine is a bisheteroarylpiperazine NNRTI that selectively inhibits HIV-1. This agent shares resistance mutations with efavirenz and nevirapine.

ADME. Delavirdine is rarely used because it has to be dosed thrice daily (de Bethune, 2010). The drug is well absorbed, especially at acidic pH (pH < 2). Antacids, histamine H_2 receptor antagonists, proton pump inhibitors, and achlorhydria can decrease its absorption. The drug can be administered irrespective of concurrent food.

Untoward Effects and Drug Interactions. The most common side effect of delavirdine is rash (18%–36%), usually in the first few weeks of treatment and often resolving despite continued therapy. Severe dermatitis, including erythema multiforme and Stevens-Johnson syndrome, is rare. Elevated hepatic transaminases and hepatic failure also have been reported, as has neutropenia (rare). Delavirdine is both a substrate for and an inhibitor of CYP3A4 and can alter the metabolism of other CYP3A4 substrates. Delavirdine increases the plasma concentrations of most HIV PIs.

HIV Protease Inhibitors

Overview

The HIV PIs are peptide-like chemicals that competitively inhibit the action of the virus aspartyl protease (Figure 64–6). This protease is a homodimer consisting of two 99-amino-acid monomers; each monomer contributes an aspartic acid residue that is essential for catalysis. The preferred cleavage site for this enzyme is the N-terminal side of proline

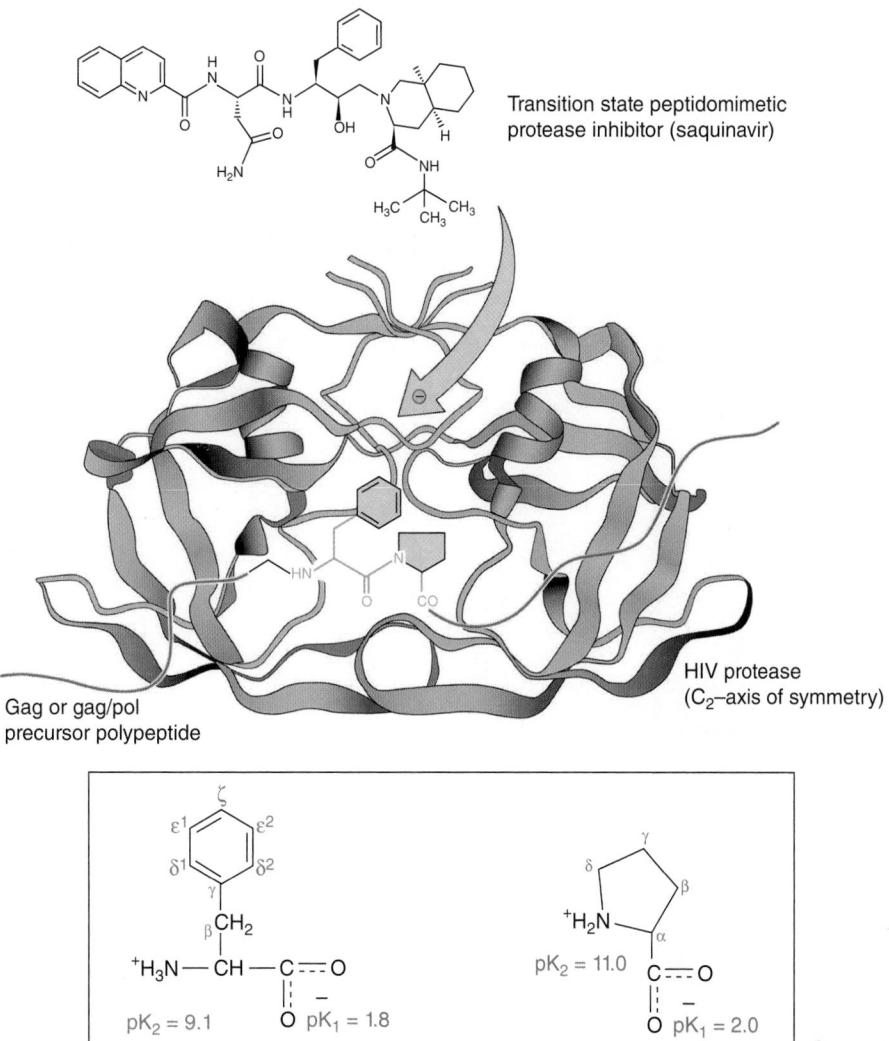

Figure 64–6 *Mechanism of action of an HIV PI.* Shown here is a phenylalanine-proline target peptide sequence (in blue) for the protease enzyme (in golden brown) with chemical structures of the native amino acids (in lower box) to emphasize homology of their structures to that of saquinavir (at top).

residues, especially between phenylalanine and proline. Human aspartyl proteases (i.e., renin, pepsin, gastricsin, and cathepsins D and E) contain only one polypeptide chain and are not significantly inhibited by HIV PIs (Wensing et al., 2010).

Table 64–4 summarizes pharmacokinetic data for these agents. Clearance is mainly through hepatic oxidative metabolism. All except nelfinavir are metabolized predominantly by CYP3A4 (and nelfinavir's major metabolite is cleared by CYP3A4). All approved HIV PIs have the potential for metabolic drug interactions. Most of these drugs inhibit CYP3A4 at clinically achieved concentrations, although the magnitude of inhibition varies greatly, with ritonavir by far the most potent. It is now a common practice to combine HIV PIs with a low dose of ritonavir or cobicistat to take advantage of either drug's remarkable capacity to inhibit CYP3A4 metabolism.

"Boosting" PIs With a CYP Inhibitor. The metabolic clearance of HIV PIs is inhibited by cobicistat, a ritonavir analogue that lacks antiretroviral activity and that was developed for exclusive use as a pharmacokinetic enhancer (Sherman et al., 2015). Cobicistat is a potent and selective inhibitor of CYP 3A4 but is better tolerated than ritonavir and is not a CYP enzyme inducer. Doses of ritonavir of 100 or 200 mg once or twice daily, or cobicistat 150 mg daily, are sufficient to inhibit CYP3A4 and increase ("boost") the concentrations of most concurrently administered CYP3A4 substrates. The enhanced pharmacokinetic profile of HIV PIs administered with ritonavir or cobicistat reflects inhibition of both first-pass and

systemic clearance, resulting in improved oral bioavailability and a longer elimination $t_{1/2}$ of the coadministered drug. This allows a reduction in both drug dose and dosing frequency while increasing systemic concentrations. Combinations of either atazanavir, darunavir, fosamprenavir, lopinavir with ritonavir, or cobicistat with atazanavir or darunavir are approved for once-daily administration.

Other Shared Properties of PIs. Most HIV PIs are substrates for the P-glycoprotein efflux pump (see Chapter 5). These agents generally penetrate less well into semen than do NRTIs and NNRTIs. HIV PIs have high interindividual serum concentration variability that may reflect differential activity of intestinal and hepatic CYPs. The speed with which HIV develops resistance to unboosted PIs is intermediate between that of nucleoside analogues and NNRTIs. Initial (primary) resistance mutations in the enzymatic active site confer only a 3- to 5-fold drop in sensitivity to most drugs; these are followed by secondary mutations often distant from the active site that compensate for the reduction in proteolytic efficiency. Accumulation of secondary resistance mutations increases the likelihood of cross-resistance to other PIs. This relatively favorable resistance profile makes HIV PIs attractive agents for use as second-line therapy in patients who have failed previous antiretroviral regimens (Wensing et al., 2010).

Gastrointestinal side effects, including nausea, vomiting, and diarrhea, were common with older HIV PIs but are much less likely to occur with the newer drugs atazanavir and darunavir.

TABLE 64–4 ■ PHARMACOKINETIC PROPERTIES OF HIV-1 PROTEASE INHIBITORS[a]

PARAMETER	SAQUINAVIR[b]	INDINAVIR	RITONAVIR	NELFINAVIR	FOSAMPRENAVIR	LOPINAVIR[c]	ATAZANAVIR	TIPRANAVIR	DARUNAVIR
Bioavailability (oral), %	13	60–65	>60	20–80 (formulation and food dependent)	ND	ND	ND	ND	82
Effect of meals on AUC	↑570% (high fat)	↓77% (high fat)	↑13% (capsule)	↑100%–200%	↔	↑27% (moderate fat)	↑70% (light meal)	↔	↑30%
Plasma $t_{1/2}$, h	1–2	1.8	3–5	3.5–5	7.7	5–6	6.5–7.9	4.8–6.0	15
Plasma protein binding, %	98	60	98–99	>98	90	98–99	86	99.9	95
Metabolism by CYPs	3A4	3A4	3A4 > 2D6	2C19 > 3A4	3A4	3A4	3A4	3A4	3A4
Autoinduction of metabolism	No	No	Yes	Yes	No	Yes	No	Yes	ND
Renal excretion of parent drug, %	<3	9–12	3.5	1–2	1	<3	7	0.5	8
Inhibition of CYP3A4	+	++	+++	++	++	+++	++	+++	+++

$t_{1/2}$, half-life of elimination; ↑, increase; ↓, decrease; ↔, no effect; ND, not determined; +, weak; ++, moderate; +++, substantial.

[a]Reported mean values in adults with normal renal and hepatic function.

[b]Parameters reported for the saquinavir soft-gel capsule formulation.

[c]Values for lopinavir, tipranavir, and darunavir reflect coadministration with ritonavir.

Saquinavir

Saquinavir is a peptidomimetic hydroxyethylamine that inhibits replication of both HIV-1 and HIV-2 (Figure 64–6). Typical of HIV PIs, high-level resistance requires accumulation of multiple resistance mutations. The drug is available as a hard-gelatin capsule. When combined with ritonavir and nucleoside analogues, saquinavir produces viral load reductions comparable with those of other HIV PI regimens (Wensing et al., 2010).

ADME. See Table 64–4 for the pharmacokinetic profile of this agent. Fractional oral bioavailability is low owing mainly to first-pass metabolism, so this drug should always be given in combination with ritonavir. Low doses of ritonavir increase the saquinavir steady-state AUC by 20- to 30-fold. Substances that inhibit intestinal but not hepatic CYP3A4 (e.g., grapefruit juice) can increase the saquinavir AUC by about 3-fold.

Untoward Effects and Drug Interactions. The most frequent side effects of saquinavir are GI: nausea, vomiting, diarrhea, and abdominal discomfort. Most side effects of saquinavir are mild and short lived, although long-term use is associated with lipodystrophy.

Saquinavir clearance is increased with CYP3A4 induction. Coadministration of inducers of CYP3A4 such as rifampin, phenytoin, or carbamazepine lowers saquinavir concentrations and should be avoided. The effect of nevirapine or efavirenz on saquinavir may be reversed with ritonavir.

Ritonavir

Ritonavir is a peptidomimetic HIV PI designed to complement the C2 axis of symmetry of the enzyme active site. Ritonavir is active against both HIV-1 and HIV-2 (perhaps slightly less active against HIV-2). Ritonavir is mostly used as a pharmacokinetic enhancer (CYP3A4 inhibitor); the low doses used for this purpose are not known to induce ritonavir resistance mutations. The drug is used infrequently as the sole PI in combination regimens because of GI toxicity (Wensing et al., 2010).

ADME. Table 64–4 summarizes the pharmacokinetic profile of this agent. Interindividual variability in pharmacokinetics is high, with variability exceeding 6-fold in trough concentrations amongst patients given 600 mg of ritonavir every 12 h as capsules.

Untoward Effects and Drug Interactions. The major side effects of ritonavir are GI and include dose-dependent nausea, vomiting, diarrhea, anorexia, abdominal pain, and taste perversion. GI toxicity may be reduced if the drug is taken with meals. Peripheral and perioral paresthesias can occur at the therapeutic dose of 600 mg twice daily. These side effects generally abate within a few weeks of starting therapy. Ritonavir also causes dose-dependent elevations in serum total cholesterol and triglycerides, as well as other signs of lipodystrophy.

Ritonavir is one of the most potent known inhibitors of CYP3A4. Thus, ritonavir must be used with caution in combination with any CYP3A4 substrate and should not be combined with drugs that have a narrow therapeutic index, such as midazolam, triazolam, fentanyl, and ergot derivatives. Ritonavir is a mixed competitive and irreversible inhibitor of CYP3A4; its effects can persist for 2–3 days after the drug is discontinued (Washington et al., 2003). Ritonavir is also a weak inhibitor of CYP2D6. Potent inducers of CYP3A4 activity such as rifampin may lower ritonavir concentrations and should be avoided or the dosages adjusted. Capsule and solution formulations of ritonavir contain alcohol and should not be administered with disulfiram or metronidazole. Ritonavir is also a moderate inducer of CYP3A4, glucuronosyl-S-transferase, and possibly other hepatic enzymes and drug transport proteins. The concentrations of some drugs therefore will be decreased in the presence of ritonavir. Ritonavir reduces the ethinyl estradiol AUC by 40%; thus, alternative forms of contraception should be used.

Use of Ritonavir as a CYP3A4 Inhibitor. Ritonavir inhibits the metabolism of all current HIV PIs and is frequently used in combination with most of these drugs (with the exception of nelfinavir) to enhance their pharmacokinetic profiles and allow a reduction in their doses and dosing frequencies. Ritonavir also overcomes the deleterious effect of food on indinavir bioavailability. Low doses of ritonavir (100 or 200 mg once or twice daily) are just as effective at inhibiting CYP3A4 and are much better tolerated than the 600-mg twice-daily dose (Wensing et al., 2010).

Fosamprenavir

Fosamprenavir is a phosphonooxy prodrug of amprenavir that has increased water solubility and improved oral bioavailability. Fosamprenavir is as effective, and generally better tolerated, than amprenavir, and as a result, amprenavir is no longer marketed (Wensing et al., 2010). The drug is active against both HIV-1 and HIV-2. Fosamprenavir has long-term virologic benefit in treatment-naïve and treatment-experienced patients, with or without ritonavir, in combination with nucleoside analogues. Twice-daily fosamprenavir/ritonavir produces virologic outcomes equivalent to lopinavir/ritonavir in both treatment-naïve and treatment-experienced patients. Fosamprenavir is approved for use in treatment-naïve pediatric patients 2 years or older and treatment-experienced patients 6 or more years of age, at a dose of 30 mg/kg twice daily or 18 mg/kg plus ritonavir 3 mg/kg twice daily. Amprenavir's primary resistance mutation occurs at HIV protease codon 50. Primary resistance occurs less frequently at codon 84.

ADME. Table 64–4 summarizes the pharmacokinetic profile of this agent. The phosphorylated prodrug is about 2000 times more water soluble than amprenavir. Fosamprenavir is dephosphorylated rapidly to amprenavir in the intestinal mucosa (Wensing et al., 2010). Meals have no significant effect on fosamprenavir pharmacokinetics.

Untoward Effects and Drug Interactions. The most common adverse effects involve the GI tract and include diarrhea, nausea, and vomiting. Hyperglycemia, fatigue, paresthesias, and headache also have been reported. Fosamprenavir can produce skin eruptions; moderate-to-severe rash (in up to 8% of recipients) may occur within 2 weeks of starting therapy. Fosamprenavir has fewer effects on plasma lipid profiles than lopinavir-based regimens.

Inducers of hepatic CYP3A4 activity (e.g., rifampin and efavirenz) may lower plasma amprenavir concentrations. Because amprenavir is both an inhibitor and inducer of CYP3A4, pharmacokinetic drug interactions can occur and may be unpredictable, especially if the drug is given without ritonavir.

Lopinavir

Lopinavir is structurally similar to ritonavir but is 3- to 10-fold more potent against HIV-1. This agent is active against both HIV-1 and HIV-2. Lopinavir is available only in coformulation with low doses of ritonavir used as a CYP3A4 inhibitor. Lopinavir has antiretroviral activity comparable with that of other potent HIV PIs and better than that of nelfinavir. Lopinavir also has considerable and sustained antiretroviral activity in patients who have failed previous HIV PI-containing regimens (Wensing et al., 2010).

Treatment-naïve patients who fail a first regimen containing lopinavir generally do not have detectable HIV protease mutations but may have genetic resistance to the other drugs in the regimen (Wensing et al., 2010). For treatment-experienced patients, accumulation of four or more HIV PI resistance mutations is associated with a reduced likelihood of virus suppression after starting lopinavir.

ADME. Table 64–4 summarizes the pharmacokinetic profile of this agent. The adult lopinavir/ritonavir dose is 400/100 mg (2 tablets) twice daily, or 800/200 mg (4 tablets) once daily. Lopinavir/ritonavir should not be dosed once daily in treatment-experienced patients. Lopinavir/ritonavir is approved for use in pediatric patients 14 days or older, with dosing based on either weight or body surface area. A pediatric tablet formulation is available for use in children more than 6 months of age. Lopinavir is absorbed rapidly after oral administration. Food has a minimal effect on bioavailability. Although the tablets contain lopinavir/ritonavir in a fixed 4:1 ratio, the observed plasma concentration ratio for these two drugs following oral administration is nearly 20:1, reflecting the sensitivity of lopinavir to the inhibitory effect of ritonavir on CYP3A4. Both lopinavir and ritonavir are highly bound to plasma proteins, mainly to α1-acid glycoprotein, and have a low fractional penetration into CSF and semen.

Untoward Effects and Drug Interactions. The most common adverse events reported with the lopinavir/ritonavir coformulation are GI: loose stools, diarrhea, nausea, and vomiting. Laboratory abnormalities include elevated total cholesterol and triglycerides. It is unclear whether these side effects are due to ritonavir, lopinavir, or both.

Concomitant administration of agents that induce CYP3A4, such as rifampin, may lower plasma lopinavir concentrations considerably. St. John's wort is a known inducer of CYP3A4, leading to lower concentrations of lopinavir and possible loss of antiviral effectiveness. Coadministration of other antiretrovirals that can induce CYP3A4 (e.g., amprenavir, nevirapine, or efavirenz) may require increasing the dose of lopinavir. The liquid formulation of lopinavir contains 42% ethanol and should not be administered with disulfiram or metronidazole. Ritonavir is also a moderate CYP inducer at the dose employed in the coformulation and can adversely decrease concentrations of some coadministered drugs (e.g., oral contraceptives). There is no direct proof that lopinavir is a CYP inducer in vivo; however, concentrations of some coadministered drugs (e.g., amprenavir and phenytoin) are lower with the lopinavir/ritonavir coformulation than would have been expected with low-dose ritonavir alone.

Atazanavir

Atazanavir is an azapeptide PI that is active against both HIV-1 and HIV-2. A coformulation with cobicistat (EVOTAZ) is also available.

Therapeutic Use. Atazanavir, with or without ritonavir, is approved for treatment of adults and pediatric patients more than 3 months of age and weighing at least 5 kg; in the pediatric population, dosing is based on weight. In treatment-experienced adult patients, atazanavir 400 mg once daily without ritonavir was inferior to the lopinavir/ritonavir coformulation given twice daily. The combination of atazanavir and low-dose ritonavir had a similar viral load effect as the lopinavir/ritonavir coformulation in one study, suggesting that this drug should be combined with ritonavir or cobicistat in treatment-experienced patients and perhaps in treatment-naïve patients with high baseline viral loads. The primary atazanavir resistance mutation occurs at HIV protease codon 50 and confers about 9-fold decreased susceptibility. High-level resistance is more likely if five or more additional mutations are present (Wensing et al., 2010).

ADME. Table 64–4 summarizes the pharmacokinetic profile of this agent. Atazanavir is absorbed rapidly after oral administration. A light meal increases the AUC; thus, the drug should be administered with food. Absorption is pH dependent, and proton pump inhibitors or other acid-reducing agents substantially reduce atazanavir concentrations after oral dosing (Wensing et al., 2010). The mean elimination $t_{1/2}$ of atazanavir increases with dose, from 7 h at the standard 400-mg once-daily dose to nearly 10 h at a dose of 600 mg. The atazanavir dose is 400 mg once daily in adults if given without a pharmacokinetic enhancer (ritonavir or cobicistat) and 300 mg if given with ritonavir 100 mg or cobicistat 150 mg. The drug is present in CSF at less than 3% of plasma concentrations but has excellent penetration into seminal fluid.

Untoward Effects and Drug Interactions. Atazanavir frequently causes unconjugated hyperbilirubinemia, although this is not associated with hepatotoxicity. Postmarketing reports include hepatic adverse reactions of cholecystitis, cholelithiasis, cholestasis, and other hepatic function abnormalities. Atazanavir can precipitate in urine, causing increased risk of kidney stones. Other side effects reported with atazanavir include diarrhea and nausea, mainly during the first few weeks of therapy. Overall, 6% of patients discontinue atazanavir because of side effects during 48 weeks of treatment. Patients treated with atazanavir have significantly lower fasting triglyceride and cholesterol concentrations than patients treated with nelfinavir, lopinavir, or efavirenz.

Because atazanavir is metabolized by CYP3A4, concomitant administration of agents that induce CYP3A4 (e.g., rifampin) is contraindicated. Atazanavir is also a moderate inhibitor of CYP3A4 and may alter plasma concentrations of other CYP3A4 substrates. Atazanavir is a moderate UGT1A1 inhibitor and increases the raltegravir AUC by 41%–72%. Ritonavir significantly increases the atazanavir AUC and reduces atazanavir systemic clearance. Concomitantly administered proton pump

inhibitors reduce atazanavir concentrations substantially. Proton pump inhibitors and H_2 receptor antagonists should be avoided in patients receiving atazanavir without ritonavir (Wensing et al., 2010).

Darunavir

Darunavir is a nonpeptidic PI that is active against both HIV-1 and HIV-2. Darunavir binds tightly but reversibly to the active site of HIV protease but has also been shown to prevent protease dimerization. At least three darunavir-associated resistance mutations are required to confer resistance (Wensing et al., 2010). Darunavir in combination with ritonavir is approved for use in HIV-infected adults and children more than 3 years old. A coformulation with cobicistat is also available.

DARUNAVIR

ADME. Table 64–4 presents some pharmacokinetic data on this agent. Darunavir/ritonavir can be used as a once-daily (800-/100-mg) regimen with nucleosides in treatment-naïve adults or as a twice-daily (600-/100-mg) regimen in treatment-experienced adults with at least one darunavir-associated resistance mutation; this drug should be taken with food. Pediatric dosing is based on body weight. Darunavir is absorbed rapidly after oral administration with ritonavir, with peak concentrations occurring after 2–4 h. Ritonavir increases darunavir bioavailability by up to 14-fold. When combined with ritonavir, the mean elimination $t_{1/2}$ of darunavir is about 15 h, and the AUC is increased by an order of magnitude.

Untoward Effects and Drug Interactions. Because darunavir must be combined with cobicistat or a low dose of ritonavir, drug administration can be accompanied by all of the side effects caused by those agents, including drug interactions and GI complaints in up to 20% of patients taking ritonavir. Darunavir, like fosamprenavir, contains a sulfa moiety, and rash has been reported in up to 10% of recipients. Darunavir/ritonavir is associated with increases in plasma triglycerides and cholesterol, although the magnitude of increase is lower than that seen with lopinavir/ritonavir. Darunavir has been associated with episodes of hepatotoxicity.

Because darunavir is metabolized by CYP3A4, concomitant administration of agents that induce CYP3A4 (e.g., rifampin) is contraindicated. The drug interaction profiles of darunavir/ritonavir or darunavir/cobicistat are dominated by those expected with the pharmacokinetic enhancer. Darunavir/ritonavir 600/100 twice daily increases the maraviroc AUC by 340%; the maraviroc dose should be reduced to 150 mg twice daily when combined with darunavir (Wensing et al., 2010).

Indinavir

Indinavir, a peptidomimetic HIV PI, lacks significant advantages over other HIV PIs and is no longer widely prescribed because of problems with nephrolithiasis and other nephrotoxicities (Wensing et al., 2010).

ADME. Table 64–4 summarizes the pharmacokinetic profile of indinavir. The drug is absorbed rapidly after oral administration, with peak concentrations achieved in about 1 h. High-calorie, high-fat meals reduce the C_p by 75%; thus, indinavir must be taken with ritonavir or while fasting or with a light low-fat meal. Indinavir has the lowest protein binding of the HIV PIs; as a consequence, indinavir has higher fractional CSF penetration than other drugs in this class. The short $t_{1/2}$ of indinavir makes thrice-daily (every 8 h) dosing necessary unless the drug is combined with ritonavir, which reduces indinavir clearance, allowing twice-daily dosing regardless of meals.

Untoward Effects and Drug Interactions.

A unique adverse effect of indinavir is crystalluria and nephrolithiasis, stemming from the poor solubility of the drug (lower at pH 7.4 than at pH 3.5). Nephrolithiasis occurs in about 3% of patients. Patients must drink sufficient fluids to maintain dilute urine and prevent renal complications. Risk of nephrolithiasis is related to higher plasma drug concentrations. Patients taking indinavir should drink at least 2 L of water daily to prevent renal complications. This is especially problematic for those who live in warm climates. Because indinavir solubility decreases at higher pH, antacids or other buffering agents should not be taken at the same time. Didanosine formulations containing an antacid buffer should not be taken within 2 h before or 1 h after indinavir. This agent is metabolized by CYP3A4 and is a moderately potent CYP3A4 inhibitor; thus, indinavir should not be coadministered with other CYP3A4 substrates that have narrow therapeutic indices.

Indinavir frequently causes unconjugated hyperbilirubinemia. This is generally asymptomatic and not associated with serious long-term sequelae. Indinavir has been associated with hyperglycemia and can induce insulin resistance. Dermatologic complications have been reported, including hair loss, dry skin, dry and cracked lips, and ingrown toenails.

Nelfinavir

Nelfinavir is a nonpeptidic PI that is active against both HIV-1 and HIV-2. Nelfinavir is approved for the treatment of HIV infection in adults and children in combination with other antiretroviral drugs. Long-term virologic suppression with nelfinavir-based combination regimens is significantly inferior to lopinavir/ritonavir, atazanavir, or efavirenz-based regimens. Nelfinavir is rarely used because of the availability of better tolerated and more efficacious PIs (Wensing et al., 2010).

The primary nelfinavir resistance mutation (D30N) is unique to this drug and results in a 7-fold decrease in susceptibility. Isolates with only this mutation retain full sensitivity to other HIV PIs. Less commonly, a primary resistance mutation occurs at position 90, which can confer cross-resistance. Secondary resistance mutations can accumulate, and these are associated with further resistance to nelfinavir, as well as cross-resistance to other HIV PIs.

ADME.

The pharmacokinetic profile of this agent appears in Table 64–4. A moderate-fat meal increases the AUC 2- to 3-fold; higher concentrations are achieved with high-fat meals. Intraindividual and interindividual variabilities in plasma nelfinavir concentrations are large as a consequence of variable absorption. Nelfinavir is the only HIV PI whose pharmacokinetics are not substantially improved with ritonavir. Its major hydroxy-t-butylamide metabolite, M8, the only known active metabolite of any HIV PI, is formed by CYP2C19; its antiretroviral activity rivals that of the parent drug. Nelfinavir induces its own metabolism.

Untoward Effects and Drug Interactions.

The most important side effects of nelfinavir are diarrhea and loose stools, which resolve in most patients within the first 4 weeks of therapy. Otherwise, nelfinavir is generally well tolerated. It has been associated with glucose intolerance, elevated cholesterol levels, and elevated triglycerides.

Because nelfinavir is metabolized by CYPs 2C19 and 3A4, concomitant administration of agents that induce these enzymes may be contraindicated (as with rifampin) or may necessitate an increased nelfinavir dose (as with rifabutin). Nelfinavir is a moderate inhibitor of CYP3A4 and may alter plasma concentrations of other CYP3A4 substrates. Nelfinavir also induces hepatic drug-metabolizing enzymes, reducing the AUC of ethinyl estradiol ($\downarrow$ 47%) and norethindrone ($\downarrow$ 18%). Combination oral contraceptives therefore should not be used as the sole form of contraception in patients taking nelfinavir. Nelfinavir reduces the zidovudine AUC by 35%.

Tipranavir

Tipranavir is a nonpeptidic PI that is active against both HIV-1 and HIV-2. Tipranavir is approved for use only in treatment-experienced adult and pediatric patients whose HIV is resistant to one or more PIs. Combining tipranavir/ritonavir with at least one other active antiretroviral drug, usually enfuvirtide, greatly improves virologic responses.

Tipranavir/ritonavir is approved for use in adults and pediatric patients more than 2 years of age, with pediatric dosing based on weight or body surface area. Because most HIV strains sensitive to tipranavir are also sensitive to darunavir, darunavir is preferred for most treatment-experienced patients because of its better tolerability and toxicity profile (Wensing et al., 2010).

ADME.

Table 64–4 summarizes the pharmacokinetic profile of this agent. Tipranavir must be administered with ritonavir because of poor oral bioavailability. The recommended regimen of tipranavir/ritonavir 500/200 mg twice daily includes a ritonavir dose higher than that of other boosted HIV PIs; lower doses of ritonavir should not be used. Food does not alter pharmacokinetics in the presence of ritonavir but may reduce GI side effects.

Untoward Effects and Drug Interactions.

Tipranavir use has been associated rarely with fatal hepatotoxicity and also with intracranial hemorrhage (including fatalities) and bleeding episodes in patients with hemophilia. The drug has anticoagulant properties in vitro and in animal models that are potentiated by vitamin E. Tipranavir is more likely to cause elevation in lipids and triglycerides than other boosted PIs, possibly due to the higher dose of ritonavir with which it is administered. Tipranavir contains a sulfa moiety, and about 10% of treated patients report a transient rash. The current formulation contains a high amount of vitamin E; patients should not take supplements containing this vitamin.

Like ritonavir, tipranavir is a substrate, inhibitor, and inducer of CYP enzymes. Tipranavir/ritonavir reduces the concentrations (AUC) of all coadministered PIs by 44%–76% and should not be administered with any of these agents. This reflects the combined effect of the increased ritonavir dose, as well as tipranavir's unique capacity amongst PIs to induce expression of the P-glycoprotein drug transporter.

Entry Inhibitors

The two drugs available in this class, enfuvirtide and maraviroc, have different mechanisms of action (see Figure 64–1). Enfuvirtide inhibits fusion of the viral and cell membranes mediated by gp41 and CD4 interactions. Maraviroc is a chemokine receptor antagonist and binds to the host cell CCR5 receptor to block binding of viral gp120 (Tilton and Doms, 2010).

Maraviroc

Maraviroc blocks the binding of the HIV outer envelope protein gp120 to the CCR5 chemokine receptor (Figure 64–7). Maraviroc is approved for use in HIV-infected adults who have baseline evidence of predominantly CCR5-tropic virus. The drug has no activity against viruses that are CXCR4-tropic or dual-tropic (Tilton and Doms, 2010). Maraviroc retains activity against viruses that have become resistant to antiretroviral agents of other classes because of its unique mechanism of action.

HIV can develop resistance to this drug through two distinct pathways. A patient starting maraviroc therapy with HIV that is predominantly CCR5-tropic may experience a shift in tropism to CXCR4- or dual/mixed tropism predominance. This is especially likely in patients harboring low-level but undetected CXCR4- or dual/mixed-tropic virus prior to initiation of maraviroc. Alternatively, HIV can retain its CCR5-tropism but gain resistance to the drug through specific mutations in the V3 loop of gp120 that allow virus binding in the presence of inhibitor (Kuritzkes, 2011).

ADME.

Maraviroc is the only antiretroviral drug approved at three different starting doses, depending on concomitant medications. When combined with most CYP3A inhibitors, the starting dose is 150 mg twice daily; when combined with most CYP3A inducers, the starting dose is 600 mg twice daily; for other concomitant medications, the starting dose is 300 mg twice daily. Once-daily maraviroc has been studied, but is not FDA-approved. The oral bioavailability of maraviroc, 23%–33%, is dose dependent. Food decreases bioavailability, but there are no food requirements for drug administration.

Untoward Effects and Drug Interactions.

Maraviroc is generally well tolerated, but can cause dose- and concentration-dependent orthostatic

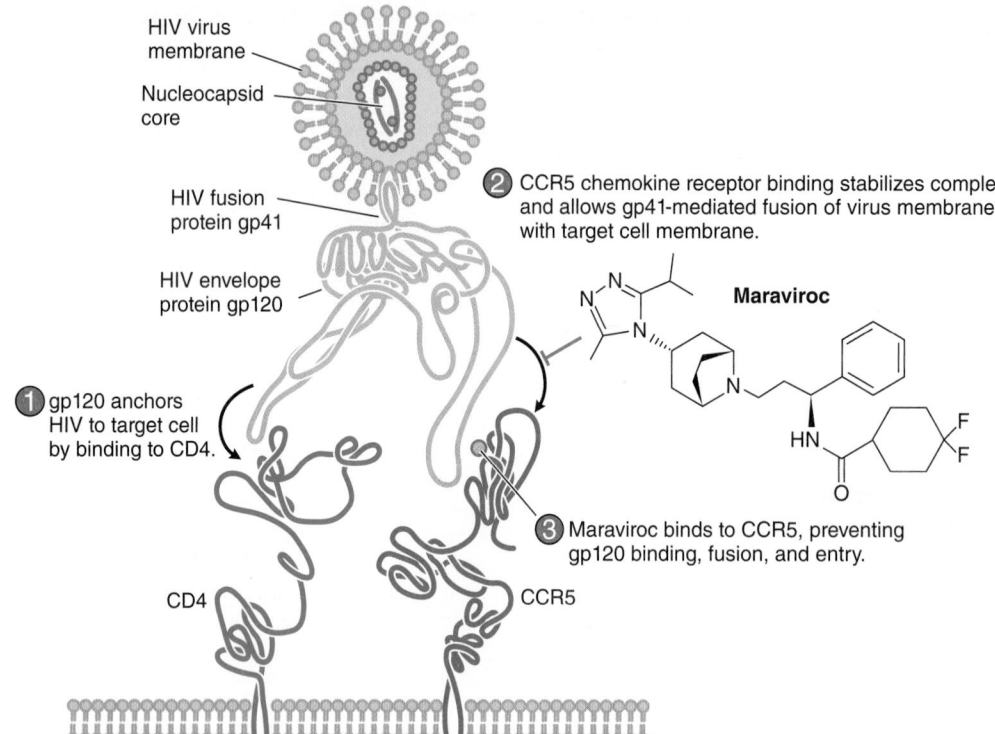

Figure 64–7 *Mechanism of action of the HIV entry inhibitor maraviroc.*

hypotension. Although one case of serious hepatotoxicity with allergic features has been reported, significant (grade 3 or 4) hepatotoxicity was no more frequent with maraviroc than with placebo in controlled trails.

Maraviroc is a CYP3A4 substrate and susceptible to pharmacokinetic drug interactions involving CYP3A4 inhibitors or inducers. Maraviroc itself is not a CYP inhibitor or inducer in vivo, although high-dose maraviroc (600 mg daily) can increase concentrations of the CYP2D6 substrate debrisoquine.

Enfuvirtide

Enfuvirtide is a 36-amino-acid synthetic peptide that is not active against HIV-2 but is broadly effective against laboratory and clinical isolates of HIV-1. Enfuvirtide is FDA-approved for use only in treatment-experienced adults and children more than 6 years of age who have evidence of HIV replication despite ongoing antiretroviral therapy. The drug's cost and route of administration (subcutaneous injection twice daily) limit its use to those with no other treatment options (Tilton and Doms, 2010).

Mechanisms of Action and Resistance. The amino acid sequence of enfuvirtide derives from the transmembrane gp41 region of HIV-1 that is involved in fusion of the virus membrane lipid bilayer with that of the host cell membrane. The peptide blocks the interaction between the N36 and C34 sequences of the gp41 glycoprotein by binding to a hydrophobic groove in the N36 coil. This prevents formation of a six-helix bundle critical for membrane fusion and viral entry into the host cell (Tilton and Doms, 2010). Enfuvirtide inhibits infection of CD4+ cells by free virus particles. Enfuvirtide retains activity against viruses that have become resistant to antiretroviral agents of other classes. HIV can develop resistance to this drug through specific mutations in the enfuvirtide-binding domain of gp41.

ADME. Enfuvirtide is the only approved antiretroviral drug that must be administered parenterally. The bioavailability of subcutaneous enfuvirtide is 84% compared with an intravenous dose. Pharmacokinetics of the subcutaneous drug are not affected by site of injection. The major route of elimination for enfuvirtide has not been determined. The mean elimination $t_{1/2}$ of parenteral drug is 3.8 h, necessitating twice-daily administration, which may create adherence issues for the patient.

Untoward Effects and Drug Interactions. The most prominent adverse effects of enfuvirtide are injection-site reactions. Most patients (98%) develop local side effects, including pain, erythema, and induration at the site of injection; 80% of patients develop nodules or cysts. Use of enfuvirtide has been associated with a higher incidence of lymphadenopathy and pneumonia. Enfuvirtide is not known to alter the concentrations of any coadministered drugs.

Integrase Inhibitors

Overview

Chromosomal integration is a defining characteristic of retrovirus life cycles and allows viral DNA to remain in the host cell nucleus for a prolonged period of inactivity or latency (Figure 64–1). Because human DNA is not known to undergo excision/reintegration, this process is an excellent target for selective antiviral intervention. The HIV integrase inhibitors prevent formation of covalent bonds between host and viral DNA—a process known as strand transfer—presumably by interfering with essential divalent cations in the enzyme's catalytic core (see Figure 64–8). In clinical trials, HIV integrase inhibitors produce a more rapid decline in plasma viral RNA over the first 3–4 months of therapy than other antiretroviral agents and are generally better tolerated than comparator agents (Hicks and Gulick, 2009).

Raltegravir

Raltegravir blocks the catalytic activity of the HIV-encoded integrase, preventing integration of viral DNA into the host chromosome (Figure 64–8). Raltegravir has potent activity against both HIV-1 and HIV-2. Because of its unique mechanism of action, this agent retains activity against viruses that have become resistant to antiretroviral agents of other classes. Raltegravir is approved for use in HIV-infected adults and children more than 4 weeks of age. A 1200 mg once-daily oral formulation was recently approved, eliminating the need for twice daily dosing.

ADME. Peak concentrations of raltegravir occur about 1 h after oral dosing. Elimination is biphasic, with an α-phase $t_{1/2}$ of about 1 h and a terminal β phase $t_{1/2}$ of about 12 h, with the α phase predominating. The pharmacokinetics of raltegravir are highly variable. Moderate- and high-fat meals

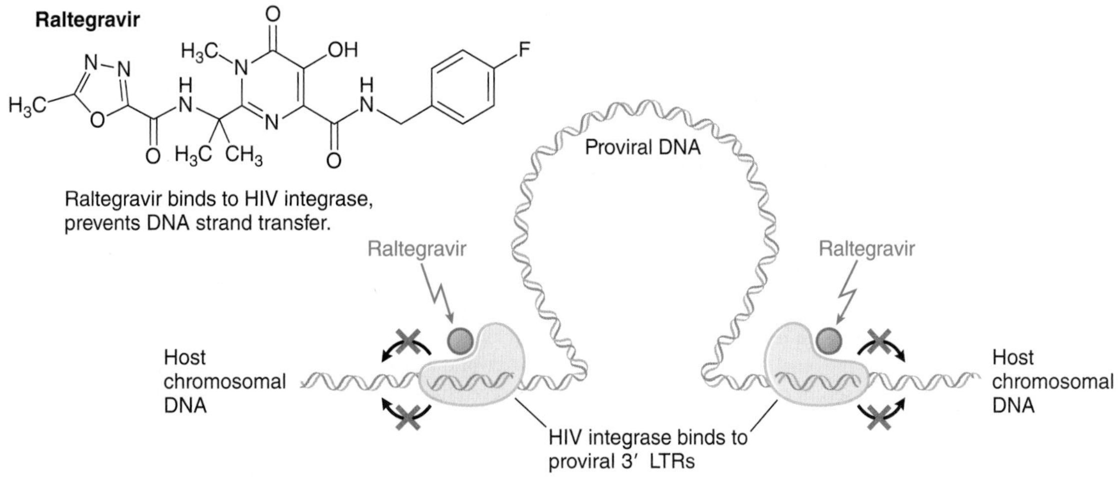

Raltegravir

Raltegravir binds to HIV integrase, prevents DNA strand transfer.

Figure 64–8 *Mechanism of action of the HIV integrase inhibitor raltegravir.*

increase raltegravir's AUC by as much as 2-fold; a low-fat meal decreases AUC modestly (↓ 46%); however, there are no food requirements for raltegravir administration. The drug is 83% protein bound in human plasma. Raltegravir is eliminated mainly via glucuronidation by UGT1A1 (Hicks and Gulick, 2009).

Untoward Effects and Drug Interactions. Raltegravir generally is well tolerated, with little clinical toxicity. The most common complaints are headache, nausea, asthenia, and fatigue, which are also associated with coadministered NRTIs. Creatine kinase elevations, myopathy, and rhabdomyolysis have been reported, as has exacerbation of depression, but their relationship to raltegravir use is not clear (Hicks and Gulick, 2009). Raltegravir is rarely associated with DRESS (Ripamonti et al., 2014).

As a UGT1A1 substrate, raltegravir is susceptible to pharmacokinetic drug interactions involving inhibitors or inducers of this enzyme. Atazanavir, a moderate UGT1A1 inhibitor, increases the raltegravir AUC (41%–72%). Tenofovir increases the raltegravir AUC by 49%, but the mechanism for this interaction is unknown. When raltegravir is combined with the CYP inducer rifampin, the raltegravir dose should be doubled to 800 mg twice daily. Raltegravir has little effect on the pharmacokinetics of the usual coadministered drugs. Because the mechanism of action of HIV integrase strand transfer inhibitors involves chelation with a divalent cation (Mg^{2+}) in the enzyme active site, chelation of divalent cations may occur in the GI tract following oral administration. It is therefore necessary to give magnesium- or aluminum-containing antacids and sucralfate 6 h before or 2 h after raltegravir. Administration of calcium and iron-containing supplements should also be separated from raltegravir by at least 2 h.

Elvitegravir

Elvitegravir blocks the catalytic activity of the HIV-encoded integrase, preventing integration of viral DNA into the host chromosome for both HIV-1 and HIV-2. Elvitegravir retains activity against viruses that have become resistant to antiretroviral agents of other classes, but shares cross-resistance with mutations affecting the HIV integrase inhibitor raltegravir (Johnson and Saravolatz, 2014). Elvitegravir is available only in single-tablet, once-daily coformulations with cobicistat, emtricitabine, and tenofovir disoproxil fumarate (STRIBILD) or tenofovir alafenamide (GENVOYA). These coformulations are approved for use in HIV-infected adults and children more than 12 years of age.

A Note on Cobicistat. Cobicistat selectively inhibits CYP3A4 with potency similar to that of ritonavir but without anti-HIV activity (Sherman et al., 2015). Additional potential advantages compared to ritonavir include greater specificity for CYP 3A4, better tolerability, reduced impact on plasma lipids, and lack of P450 enzyme induction. However, cobicistat can inhibit some drug transport proteins and blocks the tubular transport of creatinine, resulting in a small but reversible increase in serum creatinine. Cobicistat is available only in coformulation with elvitegravir, atazanavir, or darunavir.

ADME. Peak concentrations of elvitegravir occur about 4 h after oral dosing. The plasma $t_{1/2}$ of elvitegravir (administered as STRIBILD) is approximately 13 h. Because light or high-fat meals increase the AUC of elvitegravir by 34% or 87%, respectively, elvitegravir coformulations should be given with food. The drug is largely (98%–99%) protein bound in human plasma. Unlike raltegravir and dolutegravir, elvitegravir is eliminated mainly by CYP 3A4, thus explaining the substantial pharmacokinetic benefit of combining it with cobicistat. Elvitegravir coformulations should not be given to patients with baseline estimated creatinine clearance below 70 mL/min (for STRIBILD) or 30 mL/min (for GENVOYA) because of potential effects on the NRTI components of the tablet (Johnson and Saravolatz, 2014).

Untoward Effects and Drug Interactions. Like other HIV integrase inhibitors, elvitegravir is well tolerated. In clinical trials, the only side effects reported in more than 10% of elvitegravir recipients were nausea and diarrhea; fewer than 1% of patients discontinued treatment due to adverse drug effects.

Although elvitegravir by itself is not likely to cause clinically significant drug-drug interactions, the impact of the coformulations with other drugs is dominated by the effects of cobicistat, which is a potent inhibitor of CYP 3A4 and a weak inhibitor of CYP 2D6. Caution is warranted in administering elvitegravir coformulations with other CYP 3A4 substrates with low therapeutic indices or with CYP 3A4 inducers that could lower concentrations of cobicistat or elvitegravir. This includes rifamycins and St. John's wort. As with raltegravir, elvitegravir coformulations are subject to similar restrictions for coadministration of oral divalent cations (Mg^{2+}, Al^{2+}, Ca^{2+}, Fe^{2+}). Because tenofovir plus emtricitabine is effective suppressive therapy for chronic HBV infection (see Chapter 63), these coformulations may be used in patients coinfected with HIV-HBV, but they should not be discontinued abruptly because of the risk of rebound HBV replication and acute liver damage.

Dolutegravir

Dolutegravir blocks the catalytic activity of the HIV-encoded integrase of HIV-1 and HIV-2, preventing integration of viral DNA into the host chromosome. Dolutegravir retains activity against viruses that have become resistant to antiretroviral agents of other classes and also remains active against some viruses that are resistant to raltegravir or elvitegravir. Dolutegravir is approved for use in HIV-infected adults and children more than 12 years of age and weighing at least 40 kg. Dolutegravir is also available as a single-tablet, once-daily coformulation with abacavir and lamivudine. Given its high efficacy, tolerability, and convenience, dolutegravir is increasingly popular as a starting agent in treatment-naïve HIV-infected patients in high-income countries (Oster-holzer and Goldman, 2014).

ADME. Peak concentrations of dolutegravir occur 3–4 h after oral dosing, which may be done without regard to concurrent food. The drug is 99% protein bound in human plasma; its plasma elimination $t_{1/2}$ is about 12 h. Like raltegravir, dolutegravir is eliminated mainly by UGT1A1. Subjects with UGT1A1 slow metabolism genotypes had a 32% lower clearance of dolutegravir and 46% higher AUC, although this is not thought to have clinical significance (Osterholzer and Goldman, 2014).

Untoward Effects and Drug Interactions. Like other HIV integrase inhibitors, dolutegravir is well tolerated. Hypersensitivity reactions, including rash and organ dysfunction, have been reported rarely (<1% of recipients). Because dolutegravir inhibits the renal organic cation transporter OCT2, it causes small increases in serum creatinine (0.1–0.2 mg/dL) that persist during therapy but are immediately reversible once the drug is stopped.

Dolutegravir has low potential to cause clinically significant drug-drug interactions. Its capacity to inhibit the renal organic cation transporter OCT2 likely explains its effects to double concentrations of metformin. Dolutegravir is susceptible to decreases in plasma concentrations caused by inducers of drug-metabolizing enzymes and should not be coadministered with etravirine, nevirapine, or St. John's wort. For some enzyme inducers such as rifampin, efavirenz, and ritonavir-boosted HIV PIs, the dolutegravir dose can be increased from 50 mg once daily to 50 mg twice daily to counter this effect (Dooley et al., 2013). Similar to other HIV integrase inhibitors, dolutegravir should be taken 2 h before or 6 h after cation-containing antacids or laxatives, sucralfate, or oral supplements containing Fe^{2+} or Ca^{2+}. However, supplements containing Fe^{2+} or Ca^{2+} can be taken at the same time as dolutegravir if given with food (Osterholzer and Goldman, 2014). Lamivudine is no longer considered adequate suppressive therapy for chronic HBV infection; therefore, the coformulation of dolutegravir with abacavir and lamivudine should not be considered adequate treatment of HBV in coinfected patients (see Chapter 63). If a patient is coinfected with HBV or becomes infected during treatment, abrupt discontinuation of dolutegravir/abacavir/lamivudine may result in rebound HBV replication and acute liver damage. The dolutegravir/abacavir/lamivudine combination should not be given to patients who are known to carry the HLA-B*5701 allele because of the risk of abacavir hypersensitivity.

Future Treatment Guidelines

Several expert panels issue periodic recommendations for use of antiretroviral drugs for treatment-naïve and treatment-experienced adults and children. In the U.S., the Panel on Clinical Practices for Treatment of HIV Infection issues updated guidelines approximately every 6 months; their most recent guidelines can be accessed online (http://www.aidsinfo.nih.gov/Guidelines) (Department of Health and Human Services, 2016).

Treatment recommendations compare various regimens currently available for treatment-naïve patients and also address when to change therapy in individuals who are failing their current regimen. The specific drugs recommended may change as new choices become available and clinical research data accumulate. Selection of drugs in the developed world will be driven by genotypic and phenotypic resistance testing. However, future treatment guidelines will likely continue to be driven by three principles:

- Use of combination therapy to prevent the emergence of resistant virus
- Emphasis on regimen convenience, tolerability, and adherence in order to chronically suppress HIV replication
- Realization of the need for lifelong treatment under most circumstances

Treatment guidelines are not sufficient to dictate all aspects of patient management. Prescribers of antiretroviral therapy must maintain a comprehensive and current fund of knowledge regarding this disease and its pharmacotherapy. Because the treatment of HIV infection is a long-lived and complex affair, and because mistakes can have dire and irreversible consequences for the patient, the prescribing of these drugs should be limited to those with specialized training. Prescribers should also be aware that several additional antiretroviral agents are in advanced clinical development and could alter treatment possibilities. These include the NNRTI doravirine and the integrase strand transfer inhibitor (InSTI), cabotegravir and bictegravir (Flexner and Saag, 2013). Experimentally, cabotegravir has been formulated in nanoparticles having a $t_{1/2}$ of 3 weeks, raising the possibility of a sustained-release formulation that would deliver the drug for several months.

Acknowledgment: *Stephen P. Raffanti and David W. Haas contributed to this chapter in an earlier edition of this book. We have retained some of their text in the current edition.*

Drug Facts for Your Personal Formulary: *Antiretroviral Agents and Treatment of HIV Infection*

Drug	Therapeutic Use	Clinical Pharmacology and Tips
Nucleoside/Nucleotide Reverse Transcriptase Inhibitors (phosphorylated to active form to prevent infection of susceptible cells; do not eradicate virus from cells with integrated proviral DNA): Active against HIV-1 and HIV-2 and in some cases HBV		
Zidovudine (AZT) (thymidine analogue)	• HIV in adults and children • Preventing mother-to-child transmission	• Adverse effects: bone marrow (anemia, neutropenia) and muscle toxicity (myopathy); inhibits mitochondrial DNA polymerase γ • Do not use with stavudine
Stavudine (dT4)	• HIV in adults and children	• Adverse effects: sensory neuropathy and lipoatrophy • Do not use with zidovudine • Avoid use because of long-term and potentially irreversible toxicities
Lamivudine	• HIV in adults and children ≥ 3 months • Chronic hepatitis B (adults, children)	• Essentially nontoxic
Abacavir (only guanosine analogue antiretroviral)	• HIV in adults and children • Not active against HBV	• Bioavailability not affected by food • Adverse effects: hypersensitivity syndrome (fever, abdominal pain, rash), associated with HLA B*5701 genotype; discontinue drug immediately and never use again as this is potentially fatal

Nucleoside/Nucleotide Reverse Transcriptase Inhibitors (phosphorylated to active form to prevent infection of susceptible cells; do not eradicate virus from cells with integrated proviral DNA): Active against HIV-1 and HIV-2 and in some cases HBV (continued)

Tenofovir (5'-AMP derivative; supplied as prodrugs: TDF or TAF)	• HIV infection (adults, children > 2 years, in combination with other antiretrovirals) • Chronic hepatitis B (adults, children > 12 years) • HIV preexposure prophylaxis (with emtricitabine) in adults at high risk of infection	• Nephrotoxicty: small decreases in estimated creatinine clearance are common; Fanconi syndrome rare • Decreases in bone mineral density with chronic use
Emtricitabine	• HIV infection (adults, children, in combination with other antiretrovirals) • Chronic hepatitis B (adults, children) • HIV preexposure prophylaxis (with tenofovir) in adults at high risk of infection	• Generally nontoxic
Didanosine	• HIV infection in adults and children	• Adverse effects: sensory neuropathy and pancreatitis • Avoid use because of long-term and potentially irreversible toxicities

Nonnucleoside Reverse Transcriptase Inhibitors: Do not require metabolic activation; HIV-1 specific and not active against HIV-2

Nevirapine	• HIV-1 infection in infants, children, and adults • Single-dose prevention of mother-to-child transmission	• Autoinducer of metabolism • Commonly produces rash that usually resolves with continued treatment • Can rarely produce life-threatening skin eruptions such as Stevens-Johnson syndrome • Rarely produces life-threatening hepatitis
Efavirenz	• HIV-1 infection in children ≥ 3 years and adults	• Commonly causes CNS toxicity that usually resolves with continued treatment but can be severe enough to warrant discontinuation • Moderate hepatic enzyme inducer
Rilpivirine	• HIV-1 infection in children > 12 years and adults	• Must be given with food • Avoid proton pump inhibitors because of reduced absorption • May cause prolonged QTc interval if concentrations are too high
Etravirine	• Treatment-experienced adults and children ≥ 6 years	• Commonly produces rash that usually resolves with continued treatment • Can rarely produce life-threatening skin eruptions such as Stevens-Johnson syndrome • Moderate inducer of hepatic enzymes
Delavirdine	• Adults with HIV infection	• Rash commonly and rarely Stevens-Johnson syndrome • Rarely used because of the requirement for thrice-daily dosing

Protease Inhibitors: Active against HIV-1 and HIV-2; generally used as second-line agents in treatment-experienced patients

Saquinavir	• Second-line treatment of HIV in adults and children	• Rarely used because of better-tolerated alternative PIs
Ritonavir	• Used only as a PK-boosting agent in combination with other PIs	• Commonly causes nausea • Associated with elevated cholesterol and triglycerides at higher doses • Potent inhibitor of CYP3A4 • Moderate hepatic enzyme inducer
Fosamprenavir	• HIV-infected adults, treatment-naïve children ≥ 2 years and treatment-experienced children ≥ 6 years	• Adverse effects: diarrhea, nausea, and vomiting • Occasional skin rashes
Lopinavir	• Treatment-naïve or -experienced HIV-infected adults and children ≥ 14 days	• Must be combined with ritonavir • Commonly causes nausea and other GI toxicities • Associated with elevated cholesterol and triglycerides in adults with prolonged use
Atazanavir	• Treatment-naïve or -experienced HIV-infected adults and children ≥ 3 months	• Usually combined with ritonavir or cobicistat • Can be given without a PK booster at a higher dose of 400 mg • Absorption reduced with proton pump inhibitors and H_2 blockers • Commonly causes unconjugated hyperbilirubinemia • Can cause nephrolithiasis and cholelithiasis
Darunavir	• Treatment-naïve or -experienced HIV-infected adults and children > 3 years	• Must be combined with ritonavir or cobicistat • May cause transient rash • Better tolerated than other PIs

Drug Facts for Your Personal Formulary: *Antiretroviral Agents and Treatment of HIV Infection (continued)*

Drug	Therapeutic Use	Clinical Pharmacology and Tips
Protease Inhibitors: Active against HIV-1 and HIV-2; generally used as second-line agents in treatment-experienced patients		
Indinavir	• Treatment-naïve or -experienced HIV-infected adults and children	• Must be taken with ritonavir or while fasting • Adverse effects: crystalluria and nephrolithiasis • Rarely used because of the availability of better-tolerated PIs
Nelfinavir	• Treatment-naïve or -experienced HIV-infected adults and children	• The only PI that does not benefit from PK boosting • Must be taken with food • Adverse effects: diarrhea and other GI toxicity • Rarely used because of the availability of better-tolerated PIs
Tipranavir	• Treatment-experienced HIV-infected adults and children ≥2 years, generally those who have failed all other PIs	• Toxicity: rare but potentially fatal hepatotoxicity; rare but potentially fatal bleeding diathesis, including intracranial hemorrhage • Rarely used because of the availability of better-tolerated PIs
Entry Inhibitors: Generally reserved for second-line or salvage therapy		
Maraviroc	• Treatment-naïve or -experienced HIV-infected adults who have evidence of predominantly CCR5-tropic virus	• CYP3A4 substrate susceptible to drug interactions with other antiretrovirals • Adverse effect: dose- and concentration-dependent orthostatic hypotension
Enfuvirtide	• Treatment-experienced HIV-infected adults and children > 6 years • Generally reserved for those with no other treatment options	• Injected subcutaneously twice daily • Adverse effects: injection site reactions and subcutaneous nodules are common • Not active against HIV-2
Integrase Inhibitors: Widely used in treatment-naïve patients because of excellent tolerability, safety, and antiretroviral activity		
Raltegravir	• HIV-infected adults and children > 4 weeks of age	• Given twice daily without the need for a PK boosting agent • Reduced bioavailability if given concurrently with divalent cations • Generally well tolerated
Elvitegravir	• HIV-infected adults and children > 12 years of age	• Requires cobicistat as a PK booster • Should be taken with food • Reduced bioavailability if given concurrently with divalent cations • Generally well tolerated
Dolutegravir	• HIV-infected adults and children > 12 years of age	• Given once daily without the need for a PK-boosting agent • Reduced bioavailability if given concurrently with divalent cations • Generally well tolerated

Bibliography

Cihlar T, Ray AS. Nucleoside and nucleotide HIV reverse transcriptase inhibitors: 25 years after zidovudine. *Antiviral Res*, **2010**, *85*:39–58.

Chapman T, et al. Tenofovir disoproxil fumarate. *Drugs*, **2003**, *63*: 1597–1608.

Coffin JM. HIV population dynamics in vivo: implications for genetic variation, pathogenesis, and therapy. *Science*, **1995**, *267*:483–489.

Cohen MS, et al. Prevention of HIV-1 infection with early antiretroviral therapy. *N Engl J Med*, **2011**, *365*:493–505.

de Bethune MP. Non-nucleoside reverse transcriptase inhibitors (NNRTIs), their discovery, development, and use in the treatment of HIV-1 infection: a review of the last 20 years (1989–2009). *Antiviral Res*, **2010**, *85*:75–90.

Deeks SG, et al. HIV infection. *Nat Rev Dis Primers*, **2015**, *1*:15035.

Department of Health and Human Services (DHHS). Guidelines for the use of antiretroviral agents in HIV-1 infected adults and adolescents. Last updated **January 28, 2016**. Available at: http://aidsinfo.nih.gov/guidelines. Accessed July 14, 2016.

Dooley KE, et al. Safety, tolerability, and pharmacokinetics of the HIV integrase inhibitor dolutegravir given twice daily with rifampin or once daily with rifabutin: results of a phase 1 study among healthy subjects. *J Acq Immune Defic Syndr*, **2013**, *62*:21–27.

ENCORE1 Study Group. Efficacy of 400 mg efavirenz versus standard 600 mg dose in HIV-infected, antiretroviral-naive adults (ENCORE1): a randomised, double-blind, placebo-controlled, non-inferiority trial. *Lancet*, **2014**, *383*:1474–1482.

Eshleman SH, et al. Comparison of nevirapine (NVP) resistance in Ugandan women 7 days vs. 6–8 weeks after single-dose NVP prophylaxis: HIVNET 012. *AIDS Res Hum Retroviruses*, **2004**, *20*: 595–599.

Flexner C, Saag M. The antiretroviral drug pipeline: prospects and implications for future treatment research. *Current Opin HIV/AIDS*, **2013**, *8*:572–578.

Ford N, et al. Safety of efavirenz in the first trimester of pregnancy: an updated systematic review and meta-analysis. *AIDS*, **2014**, *28*(suppl 2): S123–S131.

Greene WC, Peterlin BM. Charting HIV's remarkable voyage through the cell: basic science as a passport to future therapy. *Nat Med*, **2002**, *8*:673–680.

Hicks C, Gulick RM. Raltegravir: the first HIV type 1 integrase inhibitor. *Clin Infect Dis*, **2009**, *48*:931–939.

INSIGHT START Study Group. Initiation of antiretroviral therapy in early asymptomatic HIV infection. *N Engl J Med*, **2015**, *373*:795–807.

Johnson LB, Saravolatz LD. The quad pill, a once-daily combination therapy for HIV infection. *Clin Infect Dis*, **2014**, *58*:93–98.

Kuritzkes DR. Drug resistance in HIV-1. *Curr Opin Virol*, **2011**, *1*: 582–589.

Lawrence J, et al. Structured treatment interruption in patients with multi-drug-resistant human immunodeficiency virus. *N Engl J Med*, **2003**, *349*:837–846.

Lee H, et al. Toxicity of nucleoside analogues used to treat AIDS and the selectivity of the mitochondrial DNA polymerase. *Biochemistry*, **2003**, *42*:14711–14719.

Manabe YC, et al. Immune reconstitution inflammatory syndrome: risk factors and treatment implications. *J Acquir Immune Defic Syndr*, **2007**, *46*:456–462.

Martin JC, et al. Early nucleoside reverse transcriptase inhibitors for the treatment of HIV: a brief history of stavudine (D4T) and its comparison with other dideoxynucleosides. *Antiviral Res*, **2010**, *85*:34–38.

Muller V, Bonhoeffer S. Mathematical approaches in the study of viral kinetics and drug resistance in HIV-1 infection. *Curr Drug Targets Infect Disord*, **2003**, *3*:329–344.

Osterholzer DA, Goldman M. Dolutegravir: a next-generation integrase inhibitor for treatment of HIV infection. *Clin Infect Dis*, **2014**, *59*: 265–271.

Piscitelli SC and Gallicano KD. Interactions among drugs for HIV and opportunistic infections. *New Engl J Med*, **2001**, *344*:984–996.

Ripamonti D, et al. Drug reaction with eosinophilia and systemic symptoms associated with raltegravir use: case report and review of the literature. *AIDS*, **2014**, *28*:1077–1079.

Sax PE, et al. Tenofovir alafenamide versus tenofovir disoproxil fumarate, coformulated with elvitegravir, cobicistat, and emtricitabine, for initial treatment of HIV-1 infection: two randomised, double-blind, phase 3, non-inferiority trials. *Lancet*, **2015**, *385*:2606–2615.

Shafer RW, et al. Comparison of four-drug regimens and pairs of sequential three-drug regimens as initial therapy for HIV-1 infection. *N Engl J Med*, **2003**, *349*:2304–2315.

Sharma M, Saravolatz LD. Rilpivirine: a new non-nucleoside reverse transcriptase inhibitor. *J Antimicrob Chemother*, **2013**, *68*: 250–256.

Sherman EM, et al. Cobicistat: review of a pharmacokinetic enhancer for HIV infection. *Clin Ther*, **2015**, *37*:1876–1893.

TEMPRANO ANRS 12136 Study Group. A trial of early antiretrovirals and isoniazid preventive therapy in Africa. *N Engl J Med*, **2015**, *373*: 808–822.

Tilton JC, Doms RW. Entry inhibitors in the treatment of HIV-1 infection. *Antiviral Res*, **2010**, *85*:91–100.

Washington CB, et al. Effect of simultaneous versus staggered dosing on pharmacokinetic interactions of protease inhibitors. *Clin Pharmacol Ther*, **2003**, *73*:406–416.

Wensing AM, et al. Fifteen years of HIV protease inhibitors: raising the barrier to resistance. *Antiviral Res*, **2010**, *85*:59–74.

White KD, et al. Evolving models of the immunopathogenesis of T cell-mediated drug allergy: the role of host, pathogens, and drug response. *J Allergy Clin Immunol*, **2015**, *136*:219–234.

World Health Organization. Guideline on when to start antiretroviral therapy and on pre-exposure prophylaxis for HIV. **2015**. Available at: http://www.who.int/hiv/pub/guidelines/earlyrelease-arv/en/. Accessed October 27, 2016.

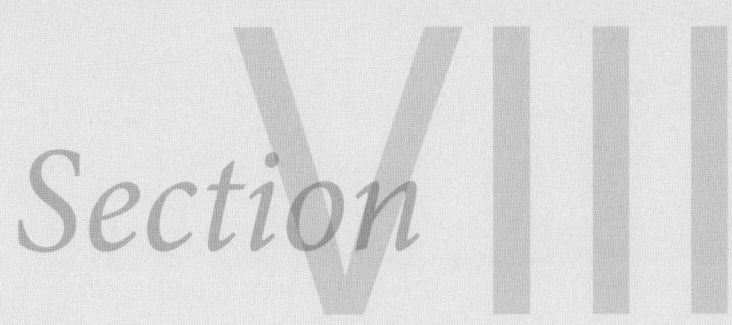

Section VIII

Pharmacotherapy of Neoplastic Disease

Chapter 65

General Principles in the Pharmacotherapy of Cancer

Anton Wellstein

Cancer pharmacology has changed dramatically during the recent past with the improved understanding of cancer biology and an ever-expanding set of newly developed drugs that target vulnerabilities in individual cancers. Effective early treatments have been developed for some fatal malignancies, including testicular cancer, lymphomas, and leukemia. Also, adjuvant chemotherapy and hormonal therapy can extend overall survival and prevent disease recurrence following surgical resection of localized breast, colorectal, and lung cancers. Chemotherapy is also employed as part of the multimodal treatment of locally advanced head and neck, breast, lung, and esophageal cancers; soft-tissue sarcomas; and pediatric solid tumors, thereby allowing for surgery that is more limited with favorable outcomes (Chabner and Roberts, 2005). In the past 5 years, the ability to harness the power of the immune system in the treatment of cancer has brought about a paradigm shift whereby some of the most feared diseases, such as melanoma and lung cancer and even late-stage metastatic disease, can be eradicated. For some cancers, response rates are surprisingly high: 87% in Hodgkin lymphoma even in heavily pretreated patients (Ansell et al., 2015), and 50% in patients with metastatic melanoma treated with combinations of PD-1 and CTLA4 immune checkpoint antibodies. Immune checkpoint inhibitors are currently approved for the treatment of bladder cancer, Hodgkin lymphoma, kidney cancer, lung cancer, and melanoma; more approvals are anticipated in the near future based on several hundred ongoing clinical trials.

Despite these major therapeutic successes, few categories of medication have a narrower therapeutic index and greater potential for causing harmful effects than anticancer drugs. A thorough understanding of their mechanisms of action, including clinical pharmacokinetics, drug interactions, and adverse effects, is essential for their safe and effective use. Anticancer drugs are quite varied in structure and mechanism of action. The group includes alkylating agents; antimetabolite analogues of folic acid, pyrimidine, and purine; natural products; hormones and hormone antagonists; and a variety of small-molecule drugs and antibodies directed at specific molecular targets, such as extracellular receptors, intracellular kinases, or the checkpoints of immune surveillance. Figure 65–1 depicts the cellular targets of these drugs, and Chapters 66–68 provide information on the different classes of drugs.

Anticancer drugs are increasingly used in a variety of nonmalignant diseases and have become treatment standards, for example, for autoimmune diseases (rituximab); rheumatoid arthritis (methotrexate and cyclophosphamide); Crohn disease (6-mercaptopurine); organ transplantation (methotrexate and azathioprine); sickle cell anemia (hydroxyurea); psoriasis (methotrexate); and wet macular degeneration (ranibizumab and aflibercept).

The Cell Cycle

An understanding of the cell cycle is essential for the rational use of anticancer drugs (Figure 65–2). Many cytotoxic agents act by damaging DNA. Their toxicity is greatest during S phase, the DNA synthetic phase of the cell cycle. Other agents, such as the vinca alkaloids and taxanes, block the formation of a functional mitotic spindle in the M phase. These agents are most effective on cells entering mitosis, the most vulnerable phase of the cell cycle. Accordingly, human cancers most susceptible to chemotherapy are those having a high percentage of proliferating cells. Normal tissues that proliferate rapidly (bone marrow, hair follicles, and intestinal epithelium) are thus also susceptible to damage from cytotoxic drugs. Slowly growing tumors with a small growth fraction (e.g., carcinomas of the colon or NSCLC) are less responsive to cell cycle-specific drugs.

Although cells from different tumors display differences in the duration of their transit through the cell cycle and in the fraction of cells in active proliferation, all cells display a similar pattern of cell cycle progression (Figure 65–2):

- A phase that precedes DNA synthesis (G_1)
- A DNA synthesis phase (S)
- An interval following the termination of DNA synthesis (G_2)
- The mitotic phase (M) in which the cell, containing a double complement of DNA, divides into two daughter G_1 cells
- A probability of moving into a quiescent state (G_0) and failing to move forward for long periods of time

At each transition point in the cell cycle, specific proteins, such as p53 and chk-1 and 2, monitor the integrity of DNA and, on detection of DNA damage, may initiate DNA repair processes or, in the presence of massive damage, direct cells down a pathway of cell death (apoptosis). Some anticancer drugs act at specific phases in the cell cycle, mainly at the S and M phases; other drugs are cytoxic at any point in the cell cycle and are termed *cell cycle phase nonspecific.*

Each transition point in the cell cycle requires the activation of specific *CDKs*, which, in their active forms, couple with corresponding regulatory proteins called *cyclins.* The proliferative impact of CDKs is, in turn, dampened by inhibitory proteins such as p16^{INK4A}, a tumor suppressor named for its molecular mass (*protein of 16 kDa) and *inhibition of CDK4.* Tumor cells often exhibit changes in cell cycle regulation that lead to relentless proliferation (e.g., mutations or loss of p16^{INK4A} or of other inhibitory components of the so-called retinoblastoma pathway, enhanced cyclin or enhanced CDK activity).

Abbreviations

ABL: Abelson murine leukemia viral oncogene homolog
ALK: anaplastic lymphoma kinase
ALL: acute lymphoblastic leukemia
ATRA: all-*trans* retinoic acid
BCR: breakpoint cluster region
BRAF: B-Raf proto-oncogene ser/thr protein kinase
BRCA: breast cancer tumor suppressor
CAR(T): chimeric antigen receptor T cell
CDK: cyclin-dependent kinase
ctDNA: cell-free mutant tumor DNA
CTLA4: cytotoxic T lymphocyte–associated protein 4
EGF(R): epidermal growth factor (receptor) [HER1, ErbB-1]
ER: estrogen receptor
FDA: Food and Drug Administration
GI: gastrointestinal
HER1: human EGFR (ErbB-1)
HER2: receptor tyrosine-protein kinase erbB-2
MEK: mitogen-activated protein kinase kinase
MHC: major histocompatibility class (protein)
NCCN: National Comprehensive Cancer Network
NSCLC: non–small cell lung cancer
PARP: poly(ADP-ribose) polymerase
PD-1: programmed cell death 1
PD-L1: programmed cell death 1 ligand 1
PR: progesterone receptor
RAR: retinoic acid receptor
VEGF: vascular endothelial growth factor

The CDK family consists of over 20 serine/threonine protein kinases that have been amongst the first pathway targets pursued for the treatment of cancer. However, different tissue selectivities and distinct cell cycle–specific activity periods of the various CDKs provide a challenge for the development of CDK inhibitors. CDK4/6 have become attractive targets because they control cell cycle progression from the G_1 to the S phase. Interaction of cyclin D with CDK4/6 enhances phosphorylation and inactivation of the retinoblastoma (Rb) protein, followed by the transcription of factors that control transition into the S phase. CDK4/6 inhibition will thus cause a G_1 arrest in susceptible cells that utilize this pathway. The CDK4/6 inhibitor palbociclib was recently approved for the treatment of breast cancer (see Chapter 67).

Because of the central importance of DNA to the identity and functionality of a cell, elaborate mechanisms ("cell cycle checkpoints") have evolved to monitor DNA integrity. If a cell possesses normal checkpoint function, drug-induced DNA damage will activate apoptosis when the cell reaches the G_1/S or G_2/M boundary. However, if the p53 gene product or other checkpoint proteins are mutated or absent or the checkpoint function fails, damaged cells will not divert to the apoptotic pathway but will proceed through the S phase and mitosis. The cell progeny will then emerge as a mutated and potentially drug-resistant subpopulation (see Figure 65–3A).

Cancer Evolution and Drug Discovery

The rapidly expanding knowledge of cancer biology and the ability to analyze cancer genome alterations in thousands of patient samples have led to a better understanding of the molecular evolution of cancer and the discovery of cancer-specific drug targets: growth factor receptors, intracellular signaling pathways, epigenetic processes, tumor vascularity, DNA repair defects, cell death pathways, and immune escape mechanisms (Hanahan and Weinberg, 2011). Human malignancies are a highly diverse

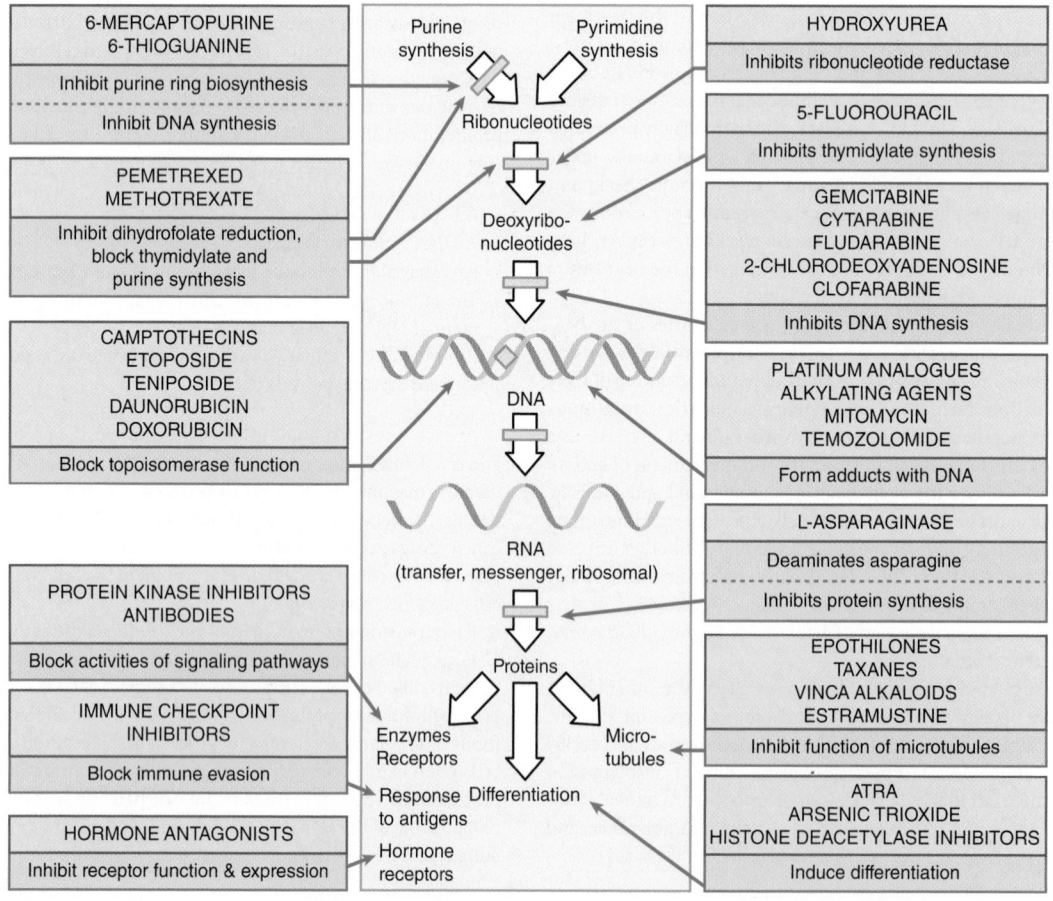

Figure 65–1 *Mechanisms and sites of action of some of the drugs used in the treatment of cancer.*

Inherited differences in protein sequence polymorphisms or levels of RNA expression can also influence toxicity and antitumor response. For example, tandem repeats in the promoter region of the gene encoding thymidylate synthase, the target of 5-fluorouracil, determine the level of expression of the enzyme. Increased numbers of repeats are associated with increased gene expression, a lower incidence of toxicity, and a decreased rate of response in patients with colorectal cancer (Pullarkat et al., 2001). Polymorphisms of the dihydropyrimidine dehydrogenase gene, the product of which is responsible for degradation of 5-fluorouracil, are associated with decreased enzyme activity and a significant risk of overwhelming drug toxicity, particularly in the rare individual homozygous for the polymorphic genes (Van Kuilenburg et al., 2002).

Gene expression profiling, in which the levels of messenger RNA from thousands of genes are surveyed using gene arrays, has revealed tumor profiles that are highly associated with poor outcomes and warrant adjuvant chemotherapy (Sotiriou and Pusztai, 2009). As an alternative to this broad analysis, small sets of informative genes can be identified and used clinically. One example is a set of 21 genes used in the analysis of samples from patients with early stage breast cancer. Based on the known association between the expression pattern of the 21 genes and disease outcomes, the analysis of patient samples can predict the risk of disease relapse. Thus, one can identify the patients at a high risk who will benefit from adjuvant chemotherapy (Paik et al., 2004).

Molecular Analysis and Tumor Heterogeneity

One of the caveats to conclusions drawn from the molecular analysis of tumor specimens is the dynamic evolution of cancers outlined previously (see Figure 65–3). Clinically important mutations in subclones may be missed due to geographically inadequate sampling and may provide the wrong guidance to treatment decisions. Response to treatment of different subpopulations presents a further challenge and would require multiple-site, longitudinal sampling (Shi et al., 2014).

Liquid Biopsies

More recent technology advances have made it possible to measure circulating, ctDNA in blood samples from patients with cancer ("liquid biopsies") and to follow changes in the abundance of mutant *KRAS* during colon cancer treatment (Diehl et al., 2008). The analysis of ctDNA has also shown that during antiestrogen therapy of breast cancer the appearance of mutant estrogen receptor coincides with subsequent resistance to aromatase inhibitor treatment (Schiavon et al., 2015). Furthermore, mutant *KRAS* DNA in the circulation was increased during the treatment of patients with colon cancer with EGFR antibodies but surprisingly reverted to baseline values after cessation of the treatment. This observation demonstrates the dynamic evolution of cancer subpopulations during drug treatment (Siravegna et al., 2015). The FDA recently approved a test for the presence of mutant *EGFR* DNA in blood samples of patients with NSCLC to select candidates for treatment with erlotinib and thus circumvent the need for a tissue biopsy. The incorporation of liquid biopsies into future treatment monitoring could provide additional molecular insights into drug efficacy and the onset of resistance.

Achieving Therapeutic Integration and Efficacy

The clinical benefit of cytotoxic drugs has primarily been measured by radiological assessment of drug effects on tumor size. Pathway-targeted agents, however, may slow or halt tumor growth, so their effects may be measured in the assessment of time to disease progression; however, for some immune checkpoint inhibitors, tumor lesions may initially increase in size due to cytotoxic lymphocyte infiltration. Thus, one of the great challenges is to assess efficacy and adjust drug regimens to achieve a therapeutic but nontoxic outcome. Treatment of patients with cancer requires a skillful interdigitation of pharmacotherapy with other modalities of treatment (e.g., surgery and irradiation). Each treatment modality carries its own risks and benefits, with the potential for both antagonistic and synergistic interactions between modalities, particularly between drugs and irradiation.

Individual patient characteristics determine the choice of modalities. Not all patients can tolerate drugs, and not all drug regimens are appropriate for a given patient. Renal and hepatic function, bone marrow reserve, general performance status, and concurrent medical problems all come into consideration in making a therapeutic plan. Other less-quantifiable considerations, such as the natural history of the tumor, the patient's willingness to undergo difficult and potentially dangerous treatments, and the patient's physical and emotional tolerance for adverse effects enter the equation, with the goal of balancing the likely long-term gains and risks in the individual patient. In particular, the long-term adverse effects of cytotoxic drugs have been related to the induction of cellular senescence in different organs that can adversely affect organ function and the overall well-being of patients long after completion of the treatments (Childs et al., 2015). The choice of treatment regimen should take all of this into account. Finally, in terminally ill patients, the treatment choices must be weighed carefully; the maximal length and highest quality of life may be achieved with palliative care rather than standard chemotherapy (Temel et al., 2010).

A Cautionary Note

Although advances in drug discovery and molecular profiling of tumors offer great promise for improving the outcomes of cancer treatment, a final word of caution regarding all treatment regimen deserves emphasis: *The pharmacokinetics and toxicities of cancer drugs vary amongst individual patients.* It is imperative to *recognize toxicities early*, to *alter doses or discontinue offending medication* to relieve symptoms and reduce risk, and to *provide vigorous supportive care*. Toxicities affecting the heart, lungs, nervous system, or kidneys may be irreversible if recognized late in their course, leading to permanent organ damage or death. Fortunately, such toxicities can be minimized by early recognition and by adherence to standardized protocols and to the guidelines for each drug's use.

A Note on Treatment Regimens

Cancer treatment regimens change to reflect continuous advances in basic and clinical science: new drugs, both small molecules and biologicals; improved methods of targeting and timing of drug delivery; agents with altered pharmacokinetic properties and selectivities; the use of rational multidrug combinations; and greater knowledge of the basic cell biology of tumorigenesis, metastasis, and immune function, amongst other advances. As a consequence, this chapter and the three that follow presents relatively few detailed treatment regimens; rather, we refer the reader to the web-based resources of the U.S. FDA and the NCCN. Table 67–1 provides examples that illustrate the complexities of current therapeutic regimens for two cancers.

Acknowledgment: Paul Calabresi and Bruce A. Chabner contributed to this chapter in recent editions of this book. We have retained some of their text in the current edition.

Bibliography

Alexandrov LB, et al. Signatures of mutational processes in human cancer. *Nature*, **2013**, *500*:415–421.

Anderson AC, et al. Lag-3, Tim-3, and TIGIT: co-inhibitory receptors with specialized functions in immune regulation. *Immunity*, **2016**, *44*:989–1004.

Ansell SM, et al. PD-1 blockade with nivolumab in relapsed or refractory Hodgkin's lymphoma. *N Engl J Med*, **2015**, *372*:311–319.

Chabner BA, Roberts TG. Timeline: chemotherapy and the war on cancer. *Nat Rev Cancer*, **2005**, *5*:65–72.

Childs BG, et al. Cellular senescence in aging and age-related disease: from mechanisms to therapy. *Nat Med*, **2015**, *21*:1424–1435.

Diehl F, et al. Circulating mutant DNA to assess tumor dynamics. *Nat Med*, **2008**, *14*:985–990.

Engelman JA et al. MET amplification leads to gefitinib resistance in lung cancer by activating ERBB3 signaling. *Science*, **2007**, *316*:1039–1043.

Hanahan D, Weinberg RA. Hallmarks of cancer: the next generation. *Cell*, **2011**, *144*:646–674.

Holohan C, et al. Cancer drug resistance: an evolving paradigm. *Nat Rev Cancer*, **2013**, *13*:714–726.

Hughes PE, et al. Targeted therapy and checkpoint immunotherapy combinations for the treatment of cancer. *Trends Immunol*, **2016**, *37*:462–476.

Kaufman HL, et al. The Society for Immunotherapy of Cancer consensus statement on tumour immunotherapy for the treatment of cutaneous melanoma. *Nat Rev Clin Oncol*, **2013**, *10*:588–598.

Khalil DN, et al. The future of cancer treatment: immunomodulation, CARs and combination immunotherapy. *Nat Rev Clin Oncol*, **2016**, *13*:273–290.

Kobayashi S, et al. EGFR mutation and resistance of non-small-cell lung cancer to gefitinib. *N Engl J Med*, **2005**, *352*:786–792.

Paik S, et al. A multigene assay to predict recurrence of tamoxifen-treated, node-negative breast cancer. *N Engl J Med*, **2004**, *351*: 2817–2826.

Pullarkat ST, et al. Thymidylate synthase gene polymorphism determines response and toxicity of 5-FU chemotherapy. *Pharmacogenomics J*, **2001**, *1*:65–70.

Schiavon G, et al. Analysis of ESR1 mutation in circulating tumor DNA demonstrates evolution during therapy for metastatic breast cancer. *Sci Transl Med*, **2015**, *7*:313ra182.

Schumacher TN, Schreiber RD. Neoantigens in cancer immunotherapy. *Science (New York, NY)*, **2015**, *348*:69–74.

Sharma P, Allison JP. The future of immune checkpoint therapy. *Science (New York, NY)*, **2015**, *348*:56–61.

Shi H, et al. Acquired resistance and clonal evolution in melanoma during BRAF inhibitor therapy. *Cancer Discov*, **2014**, *4*:80–93.

Siravegna G, et al. Clonal evolution and resistance to EGFR blockade in the blood of colorectal cancer patients. *Nat Med*, **2015**, *21*:795–801.

Slamon DJ, et al. Use of chemotherapy plus a monoclonal antibody against HER2 for metastatic breast cancer that overexpresses HER2. *N Engl J Med*, **2001**, *344*:783–792.

Sotiriou C, Pusztai L. Gene-expression signatures in breast cancer. *N Engl J Med*, **2009**, *360*:790–800.

Temel JS, et al. Early palliative care for patients with metastatic non-small-cell lung cancer. *N Engl J Med*, **2010**, *363*:733–742.

Thomas A, et al. Refining the treatment of NSCLC according to histological and molecular subtypes. *Nat Rev Clin Oncol*, **2015**, *12*:511–526.

Van Kuilenburg ABP, et al. High prevalence of the IVS14 + 1G>A mutation in the dihydropyrimidine dehydrogenase gene of patients with severe 5-fluorouracil-associated toxicity. *Pharmacogenetics*, **2002**, *12*:555–558.

Yates LR, Campbell PJ. Evolution of the cancer genome. *Nat Rev Genet*, **2012**, *13*:795–806.

Chapter 66

Cytotoxic Drugs

Anton Wellstein, Giuseppe Giaccone,
Michael B. Atkins, and Edward A. Sausville

I. ALKYLATING AGENTS AND PLATINUM COORDINATION COMPLEXES

ACTIONS COMMON TO ALKYLATING DRUGS

- Structure-Activity Relationships
- General Pharmacological Actions
- Mechanisms of Resistance to Alkylating Drugs
- Adverse Effects of Alkylating Drugs

CLINICAL PHARMACOLOGY OF NITROGEN MUSTARDS

- Mechlorethamine
- Cyclophosphamide
- Ifosfamide
- Melphalan
- Chlorambucil
- Bendamustine

ETHYLENEIMINES AND METHYLMELAMINES

- Altretamine
- Thiotepa

ALKYL SULFONATES

- Busulfan

NITROSOUREAS

- Carmustine (BCNU)
- Streptozocin

TRIAZENES

- Dacarbazine (DTIC)
- Temozolomide

METHYLHYDRAZINES

- Procarbazine

PLATINUM COORDINATION COMPLEXES

- Mechanisms of Action
- Resistance to Platinum Analogues
- Cisplatin
- Carboplatin
- Oxaliplatin

II. ANTIMETABOLITES

FOLIC ACID ANALOGUES

- Mechanism of Action
- Selective Toxicity; Rescue
- Cellular Entry and Retention
- Newer Congeners
- Mechanisms of Resistance to Antifolates

PYRIMIDINE ANALOGUES

- Cellular Actions of Pyrimidine Antimetabolites
- Fluorouracil, Floxuridine, Capecitabine
- Trifluridine

CYTIDINE ANALOGUES

- Cytarabine (Cytosine Arabinoside; Ara-C)
- Azacitidine (5-Azacytidine); Decitabine
- Gemcitabine

PURINE ANALOGUES

- 6-Thiopurine Analogues
- Fludarabine Phosphate
- Cladribine
- Clofarabine (2-Chloro-2'-fluoro-arabinosyladenine)
- Nelarabine (6-Methoxy-arabinosyl-guanine)
- Pentostatin (2'-Deoxycoformycin)

III. NATURAL PRODUCTS

MICROTUBULE-DAMAGING AGENTS

- Vinca Alkaloids
- Eribulin
- Taxanes
- Estramustine
- Epothilones

CAMPTOTHECIN ANALOGUES

- Chemistry
- Mechanism of Action
- Mechanisms of Resistance
- Topotecan
- Irinotecan

ANTIBIOTICS

- Dactinomycin (Actinomycin D)
- Anthracyclines and Anthracenediones

EPIPODOPHYLLOTOXINS

- Podophyllotoxin Derivatives
- Etoposide
- Teniposide

DRUGS OF DIVERSE MECHANISMS OF ACTION

- Bleomycin
- Mitomycin
- Mitotane
- Trabectedin
- L-Asparaginase
- Hydroxyurea
- Retinoids
- Arsenic Trioxide

Abbreviations

ABC: ATP-binding cassette

ABVD: doxorubicin (*a*driamycin), *b*leomycin, *v*inblastine, *d*acarbazine

ADA: adenosine deaminase

ADME: absorption, distribution, metabolism, excretion

ALL: acute lymphoblastic leukemia

AML: acute myeloid leukemia; acute myelocytic leukemia

APL: acute promyelocytic leukemia

Ara-C: cytarabine, cytosine arabinoside

Ara-U: ara-uridine

ARDS: acute respiratory distress syndrome

L-ASP: L-asparaginase

ATO: arsenic trioxide

ATRA: all-*trans* retinoic acid

BCNU: carmustine [1,3-*bis*-(2-chloroethyl)-1-nitrosourea]

BCRP: breast cancer resistance protein

CCNU: 1-(2-chloroethyl)-3-cyclohexyl-1-nitrosourea (lomustine)

2CdA: 2-chlorodeoxyadenosine (cladribine)

CDK: cyclin-dependent kinase

C/EBP: CCAAT/enhancer binding protein

CHOP: *c*yclophosphamide, doxorubicin (*H*), vincristine (*O*) and *p*rednisone

CL_{Cr}: creatinine clearance

CLL: chronic lymphocytic leukemia

CML: chronic myelocytic leukemia; chronic myelogenous leukemia

CNT1: concentrative nucleoside transporter 1

CTCL: cutaneous T-cell lymphoma

dCK: deoxycytidine kinase

dCTP: deoxycytidine 5′-triphosphate

DDD: dichlorodiphenyldichloroethane

dFdC: 2′,2′-difluorodeoxycytidine, gemcitabine

5′-dFdU: 5′-deoxyfluorodeoxyuridine

DHFR: dihydrofolate reductase

dNTP: deoxynucleotide triphosphate

DPD: dihydropyrimidine dehydrogenase

dTMP/TTP: deoxythymidine monophosphate/triphosphate

dUMP/FdUMP: deoxyuridine monophosphate/fluoro dUMP

ENT1: equilibrative nucleoside transporter 1

FdUMP: deoxynucleotide, fluorodeoxyuridine monophosphate

FH_2Glu_n/FH_4Glu_n: dihydro-/tetrahydrofolate polyglutamates

FOLFIRINOX: FOLFOX plus irinotecan

FOLFOX: *fol*inic acid, 5*FU* and *ox*aliplatin

5FU: 5-fluorouracil

FUdR: fluorodeoxyuridine

G-CSF: granulocyte colony-stimulating factor

GI: gastrointestinal

GSH: glutathione

GST: glutathione S-transferase

Hb: hemoglobin

HbF: fetal hemoglobin

HDAC: histone deacetylase

HDM-L: high-dose MTX with leucovorin rescue

HGPRT: hypoxanthine guanine phosphoribosyl transferase

HMG: high-mobility group

HMM: hexamethylmelamine

HSV: herpes simplex virus

5HT: serotonin, 5-hydroxytryptamine

HU: hydroxyurea

IMP: inosine monophosphate

***Jak2*:** Janus kinase 2

MAO: monoamine oxidase

MDS: myelodysplastic syndrome

MESNA: 2-*m*ercapto*e*than*s*ulfonate-*Na*$^+$

methyl-CCNU: semustine

MGMT: O^6-alkyl, methyl guanine methyltransferase

MLL: mixed-lineage leukemia

MM: multiple myeloma

MMR: mismatch repair

MOPP: nitrogen *m*ustard, *o*ncovin (vincristine), *p*rocarbazine, and *p*rednisone

6MP: 6-mercaptopurine

MRP: multidrug resistance-associated protein

MSH6: mutator S homologue 6

MTA: pemetrexed

MTIC: methyl-triazeno-imidazole-carboxamide

mTOR: mammalian target of rapamycin

MTX: methotrexate

Nab-paclitaxel: albumin-bound nanoparticle solution of paclitaxel

NCCN: National Comprehensive Cancer Network

NER: nucleotide excision repair

NHL: non-Hodgkin lymphoma

NSAID: nonsteroidal anti-inflammatory drug

PG: polyglutamate

Pgp: P-glycoprotein

PI3K: phosphoinositide 3-kinase

PML: promyelocytic leukemia

PN: peripheral neuropathy

PRPP: 5-phosphoribosyl-1-pyrophosphate

PVC: procarbazine, vincristine and CCNU

RAR: retinoic acid receptor

RNR: ribonucleoside diphosphate reductase

ROS: reactive oxygen species

SCC: squamous cell carcinoma

SHMT: serine hydroxymethyltransferase

TEM: triethylenemelamine

TEPA: triethylenephosphoramide

6TG: 6-thioguanine

THF: tetrahydrofolate

T-IMP: 6-thioinosine-5′-monophosphate

6-thioGMP: 6-thioguanosine-5′-monophosphate

Thiotepa: triethylenethiophosphoramide

TMP: thymidine monophosphate

TPMT: thiopurine methyltransferase

TS: thymidylate synthase

TTP: thymidine triphosphate

VOD: veno-occlusive disease

XPG: xeroderma pigmentosum endonuclease G

A Note on Treatment Regimens

Cancer treatment regimens change to reflect continuous advances in basic and clinical science: new drugs, both small molecules and biologicals; improved methods of targeting and timing of drug delivery; agents with altered pharmacokinetic properties and selectivities; the use of rational multidrug combinations; and greater knowledge of the basic cell biology of tumorigenesis, metastasis, and immune function, amongst other advances. As a consequence, this chapter presents relatively few detailed treatment regimens; rather, we refer the reader to the web-based resources of the U.S. FDA and the NCCN. Table 67–1 provides two examples of therapeutic regimens that illustrate the complexity of current cancer drug therapy.

I. Alkylating Agents and Platinum Coordination Complexes

HISTORY Alkylating Anticancer Drugs

The discovery and initial development of alkylating anticancer drugs are based on observations of the effects of chemical warfare in World War I (Chabner and Roberts, 2005). The pervasively toxic sulfur mustard gas that caused topical burns to skin, eyes, lungs, and mucosa also caused aplasia of the bone marrow and lymphoid tissue and ulceration of the GI tract (Krumbhaar, 1919). In 1942, Louis Goodman and Alfred Gilman, the originators of this text, demonstrated the activity of nitrogen mustards against mouse lymphoma. Their clinical studies of intravenous nitrogen mustards in patients with lymphoma launched the modern era of cancer chemotherapy (Gilman and Philips, 1946).

Actions Common to Alkylating Drugs

Six major types of alkylating agents are used in the chemotherapy of cancer: *nitrogen mustards, ethyleneimines, alkyl sulfonates, nitrosoureas, triazenes,* and *methylhydrazines.* Because of similarities in their mechanisms of action and resistance, *platinum complexes* are also discussed with classical alkylating agents, even though they do not alkylate DNA but instead form covalent metal adducts with DNA.

The chemotherapeutic alkylating agents have in common the property of forming highly reactive carbonium ion intermediates. These reactive intermediates covalently link to sites of high electron density, such as phosphates, amines, sulfhydryl, and hydroxyl groups. Their chemotherapeutic and cytotoxic effects are directly related to the alkylation of reactive amines, oxygens, or phosphates on DNA. The N7 atom of guanine is

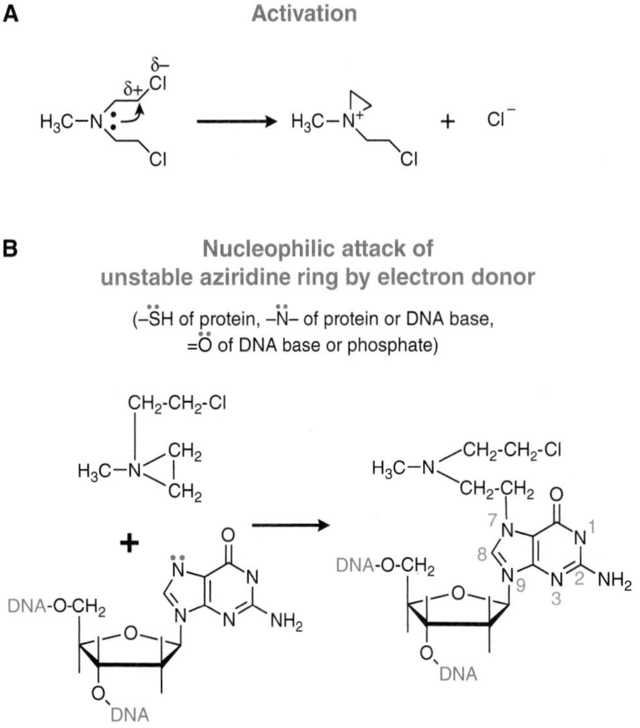

Figure 66–1 *Mechanism of action of alkylating agents of mechlorethamine, a prototypic nitrogen mustard.* **A.** *Activation reaction.* **B.** *Alkylation of N7 of guanine.* With bifunctional drugs such as nitrogen mustards (see Figure 66–2), the second 2-chloroethyl side chain can undergo a similar activation cross-link of two nucleic acid chains or a nucleic acid to a protein.

particularly susceptible to the formation of a covalent bond with bifunctional alkylating agents and may represent the key target that determines their biological effects (Figure 66–1). Other atoms in the purine and pyrimidine bases of DNA, including N1 and N3 of the adenine ring, N3 of cytosine, and O6 of guanine, react with these agents, as do the amino and sulfhydryl groups of proteins and the sulfhydryls of glutathione. The general mechanisms of alkylating agents on DNA are illustrated in Figure 66–1 using mechlorethamine (nitrogen mustard).

With the bifunctional alkylating agents such as nitrogen mustard and its derivatives that are used therapeutically (Figure 66–2), the second 2-chloroethyl side chain can undergo a similar cyclization reaction and alkylate a second guanine residue or another nucleophilic moiety, resulting in the cross-linking of two nucleic acid chains or the linking of a nucleic acid to a protein, alterations that cause a major disruption in nucleic acid function. Any of these effects can contribute to both the mutagenic and the cytotoxic effects of alkylating agents. The extreme cytotoxicity of the bifunctional alkylators correlates closely with interstrand cross-linkage of DNA.

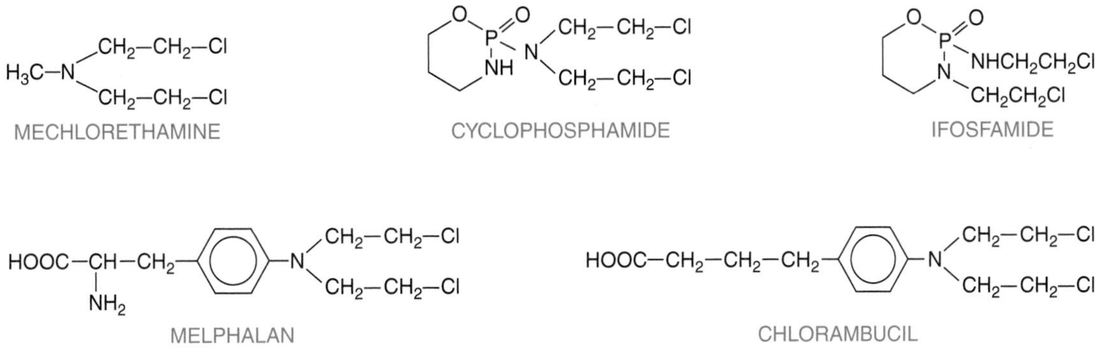

Figure 66–2 *Nitrogen mustards employed in therapy.*

The ultimate cause of cell death related to DNA damage is not known. Specific cellular responses include cell-cycle arrest and attempts to repair DNA. The specific repair enzyme complex utilized will depend on two factors: the chemistry of the adduct formed and the repair capacity of the cell involved. The process of recognizing and repairing DNA generally requires an intact NER complex but may differ with each drug and with each tumor. Alternatively, recognition of extensively damaged DNA by p53 can trigger apoptosis. However, faulty DNA damage repair mechanisms and mutations of p53 can lead to resistance to alkylating drugs (Kastan, 1999).

Structure-Activity Relationships

Although alkylating agents share the capacity to alkylate biologically important molecules, modification of the basic backbone structure changes reactivity, lipophilicity, active transport across biological membranes, sites of macromolecular attack, and mechanisms of DNA repair, all of which determine drug activity in vivo. For several of the most valuable agents (e.g., cyclophosphamide, ifosfamide), the active alkylating moieties are generated in vivo through hepatic metabolism (Figure 66–3).

The newest (2008) approved alkylating agent, **bendamustine**, has the typical chloroethyl reactive groups in nitrogen mustard (M) attached to a benzimidazole backbone. The unique properties and activity of this drug may derive from this purine-like structure; the agent produces slowly repaired DNA cross-links, lacks cross-resistance with other classical alkylators (Leoni et al., 2008), and is approved for treatment of CLL and large-cell lymphomas refractory to standard alkylators.

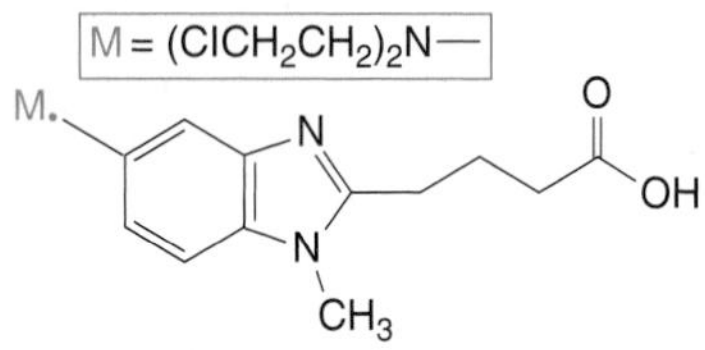

$$M = (ClCH_2CH_2)_2N—$$

BENDAMUSTINE

One class of alkylating agents transfers methyl rather than ethyl groups to DNA: The *triazene* derivative 5-(3,3-dimethyl-1-triazeno)-imidazole-4-carboxamide, usually called *dacarbazine* or DTIC, is prototypical of methylating agents. Dacarbazine requires initial activation by hepatic CYPs through an *N*-demethylation reaction. In the target cell, spontaneous cleavage of the metabolite, MTIC, yields an alkylating moiety, a methyl diazonium ion. A related triazene, temozolomide, undergoes spontaneous, nonenzymatic activation to MTIC. It is able to cross the blood-brain barrier and has been shown to have significant activity against gliomas.

The *nitrosoureas,* which include compounds such as 1,3-*bis*-(2-chloroethyl)-1-nitrosourea (carmustine [BCNU]), 1-(2-chloroethyl)-3-cyclohexyl-1-nitrosourea (lomustine [CCNU]), and its methyl derivative (semustine [methyl-CCNU]), as well as the antibiotic streptozocin (streptozotocin), exert their cytotoxicity through the spontaneous breakdown to an alkylating intermediate, the 2-chloroethyl diazonium ion. As with the nitrogen mustards, interstrand DNA cross-linking appears to be the primary lesion responsible for the cytotoxicity of nitrosoureas. The reactions of the nitrosoureas with macromolecules are shown in Figure 66–4. The use of nitrosoureas is presently limited to brain tumors due to their lipophilicity.

Stable ethyleneimine derivatives have antitumor activity; TEM and thiotepa have been used clinically. In standard doses, thiotepa produces little toxicity other than myelosuppression; it is used for high-dose chemotherapy regimens in transplants for hematological malignancies, in which it causes both mucosal and CNS toxicity. Altretamine (HMM) is chemically similar to TEM and has been used to treat ovarian cancer. The methylmelamines are *N*-demethylated by hepatic microsomes with the release of formaldehyde; there is a direct relationship between the degree of the demethylation and their antitumor activity in model systems.

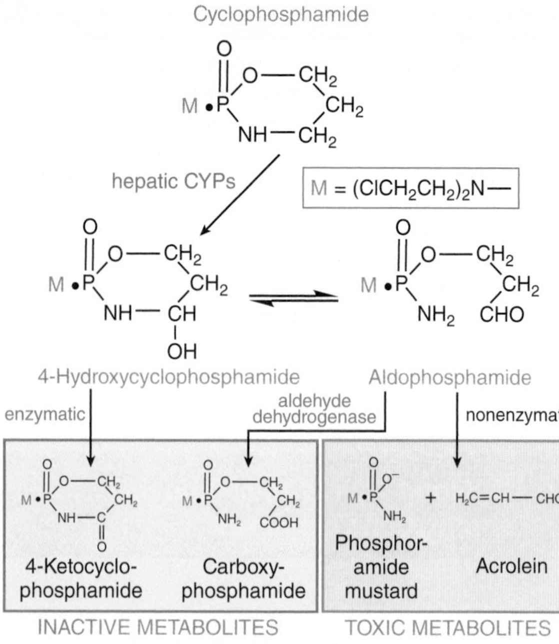

Cyclophosphamide

hepatic CYPs

$$M = (ClCH_2CH_2)_2N—$$

4-Hydroxycyclophosphamide

Aldophosphamide

enzymatic

aldehyde dehydrogenase

nonenzymatic

4-Ketocyclophosphamide

Carboxyphosphamide

Phosphoramide mustard

Acrolein

INACTIVE METABOLITES

TOXIC METABOLITES

Figure 66–3 *Activation and metabolism of cyclophosphamide.* Cyclophosphamide is activated (hydroxylated) by CYP2B, with subsequent transport of the activated intermediate to sites of action. The selectivity of cyclophosphamide against certain malignant tissues may result in part from the capacity of normal tissues to degrade the activated intermediates via aldehyde dehydrogenase, glutathione transferase, and other pathways. Ifosfamide is structurally similar to cyclophosphamide (see Figure 66–2); whereas cyclophosphamide has two chloroethyl groups on the exocyclic nitrogen atom, one of the 2-chloroethyl groups of ifosfamide is on the cyclic phosphoramide nitrogen of the oxazaphosphorine ring. Ifosfamide is activated by hepatic CYP3A4 and proceeds more slowly than activation of cyclophosphamide, with greater production of dechlorinated metabolites and chloroacetaldehyde. These differences in metabolism likely account for the higher doses of ifosfamide required for equitoxic effects, the greater neurotoxicity of ifosfamide, and perhaps differences in the antitumor spectra of cyclophosphamide and ifosfamide.

Esters of alkane sulfonic acids alkylate DNA through the release of methyl radicals. Busulfan is of value in high-dose chemotherapy.

$$H_3C—S(O_2)—O—CH_2—CH_2—CH_2—CH_2—O—S(O_2)—CH_3$$

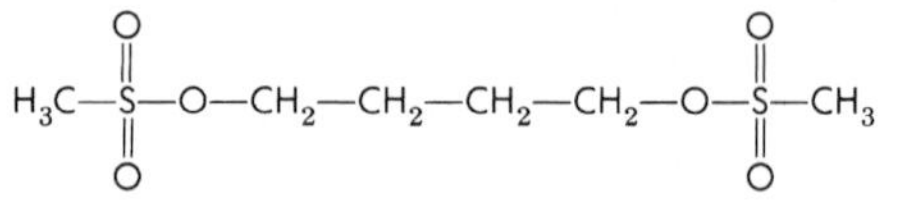

BUSULFAN

General Pharmacological Actions

Cytotoxic Actions

The capacity of alkylating agents to interfere with DNA integrity and function and to induce cell death in rapidly proliferating tissues provides the basis for their therapeutic and toxic properties. Acute effects manifest primarily against rapidly proliferating tissues; however, certain alkylating agents may have damaging effects on tissues with normally low mitotic indices (e.g., liver, kidney, and mature lymphocytes); effects in these tissues usually are delayed. Lethality of DNA alkylation depends on the recognition of the adduct, the creation of DNA strand breaks by repair enzymes, and an intact apoptotic response. In nondividing cells, DNA damage activates a checkpoint that depends on the presence of a normal p53 gene. Cells thus blocked in the G_1/S interface either repair DNA alkylation or undergo apoptosis. Malignant cells with mutant or absent p53 fail to suspend cell-cycle progression, do not undergo apoptosis, and can exhibit resistance to these drugs.

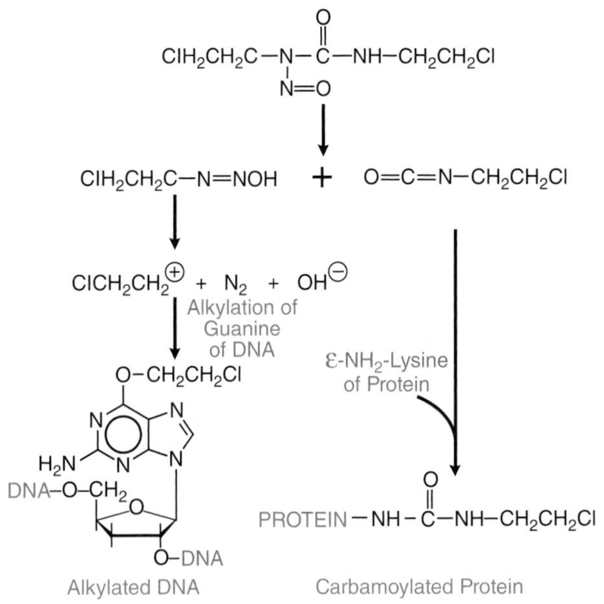

Figure 66–4 *Generation of alkylating and carbamylating intermediates from carmustine (BCNU).* The 2-chloroethyl diazonium ion, a strong electrophile, can alkylate guanine, cytidine, and adenine bases. Displacement of the halogen atom can then lead to interstrand or intrastrand cross-linking of DNA. The formation of cross-links after the initial alkylation reaction proceeds slowly and can be reversed by the DNA repair enzyme MGMT, which displaces the chloroethyl adduct from its binding to guanine in a suicide reaction. The same enzyme, when expressed in human gliomas, produces resistance to nitrosoureas and to other methylating agents, including dacarbazine, temozolomide, and procarbazine.

Distinction Between Mono- and Bi-functional Agents

Although DNA is the ultimate target of all alkylating agents, there is a crucial distinction between the bifunctional agents, in which cytotoxic effects predominate, and the monofunctional methylating agents (procarbazine, temozolomide), which have greater capacity for mutagenesis and carcinogenesis. This suggests that the cross-linking of DNA strands represents a much greater threat to cellular survival than do other effects, such as single-base alkylation and the resulting depurination and single-chain scission. Conversely, simple methylation may be bypassed by DNA polymerases, leading to mispairing reactions that permanently modify a DNA sequence. These new sequences are transmitted to subsequent generations and may result in mutagenesis or carcinogenesis. Some methylating agents, such as procarbazine, are highly carcinogenic.

Adduct recognition systems and DNA repair systems play important roles in removing adducts and thereby determine the selectivity of action against particular cell types and the acquisition of resistance to alkylating agents. Alkylation of a single strand of DNA (monoadducts) is repaired by the NER pathway. The less frequent cross-links require participation of nonhomologous end joining, an error-prone pathway, or the error-free homologous recombination pathway. After drug infusion in humans, monoadducts appear rapidly and peak within 2 h of drug exposure, while cross-links peak at 8 h. The $t_{1/2}$ for repair of adducts varies amongst normal tissues and tumors; in peripheral blood mononuclear cells, both monoadducts and cross-links disappear with a $t_{1/2}$ of 12–16 h.

The repair process depends on the presence and accurate functioning of multiple proteins. Their absence or mutation, as in Fanconi anemia or ataxia telangiectasia, leads to extreme sensitivity to DNA cross-linking agents such as mitomycin, cisplatin, or classical alkylators. Other repair enzymes are specific for removing methyl and ethyl adducts from the O6 of guanine (methyl guanine methyltransferase [MGMT]) and for repair of alkylation of the N3 of adenine and N7 of guanine (3-methyladenine-DNA glycosylase). High expression of MGMT protects cells from cytotoxic effects of nitrosoureas and methylating agents and confers drug resistance, while methylation and silencing of the gene in brain tumors are associated with clinical response to BCNU and temozolomide (Hegi et al., 2008). Bendamustine differs from classical chloroethyl alkylators in activating base excision repair, rather than the more complex double-strand break repair or MGMT. It impairs physiological arrest of adduct-containing cells at mitotic checkpoints, leads to mitotic catastrophe rather than apoptosis, and does not require an intact p53 to cause cytotoxicity.

Recognition of DNA adducts is an essential step in promoting attempts at repair and ultimately leading to apoptosis. The Fanconi pathway, consisting of 12 proteins, recognizes adducts and signals the need for repair of a broad array of DNA-damaging drugs and irradiation. Absence or inactivation of components of this pathway leads to increased sensitivity to DNA damage. Conversely, for the methylating drugs, nitrosoureas, cisplatin and carboplatin, and thiopurine analogues, the MMR pathway is essential for cytotoxicity, causing strand breaks at sites of adduct formation, creating mispairing of thymine residues, and triggering apoptosis.

Mechanisms of Resistance to Alkylating Drugs

Resistance to an alkylating agent develops rapidly when it is used as a single agent. Specific biochemical changes implicated in the development of resistance include the following:

- decreased permeation of actively transported drugs (e.g., mechlorethamine and melphalan)
- increased intracellular concentrations of nucleophilic substances, principally thiols such as glutathione, which can conjugate with and detoxify electrophilic intermediates
- increased activity of DNA repair pathways, which may differ for the various alkylating agents
- increased rates of metabolic degradation of the activated forms of cyclophosphamide and ifosfamide to their inactive keto and carboxy metabolites by aldehyde dehydrogenase (see Figure 66–3) and detoxification of most alkylating intermediates by glutathione transferases
- loss of ability to recognize adducts formed by nitrosoureas and methylating agents, as the result of defective MMR protein capability, confers resistance, as does defective checkpoint function, for virtually all alkylating drugs
- impaired apoptotic pathways, with overexpression of bcl-2 as an example, confer resistance

Adverse Effects of Alkylating Drugs

Alkylating agents differ in their patterns of the tissue specificity and severity of their adverse effects, which are summarized next.

Marrow

Most alkylating agents cause dose-limiting toxicity to marrow cells and, to a lesser extent, intestinal mucosa. Most alkylating agents (i.e., melphalan, chlorambucil, cyclophosphamide, and ifosfamide) cause myelosuppression, with a nadir of the peripheral blood granulocyte count at 6–10 days and recovery in 14–21 days. Cyclophosphamide has lesser effects on peripheral blood platelet counts than do the other agents. Busulfan suppresses all blood elements, particularly stem cells, and may produce a prolonged and cumulative myelosuppression lasting months or even years. For this reason, it is used as a preparative regimen in allogenic bone marrow transplantation. Carmustine and other chloroethylnitrosoureas cause delayed and prolonged suppression of both platelets and granulocytes, reaching a nadir 4–6 weeks after drug administration and reversing slowly thereafter. Both cellular and humoral immunity are suppressed by alkylating agents, which have, therefore, been used to treat various autoimmune diseases. Immunosuppression is reversible at usual doses, but opportunistic infections may occur with extended treatment.

Mucosa, Hair Follicles

Alkylating agents are highly toxic to dividing mucosal cells and to hair follicles, leading to oral mucosal ulceration, intestinal denudation, and alopecia. Mucosal effects are particularly damaging in high-dose chemotherapy protocols associated with bone marrow transplantation, as they predispose to bacterial sepsis arising from the GI tract. In these protocols,

TABLE 66–1 ■ DOSE-LIMITING EXTRAMEDULLARY TOXICITIES OF SINGLE ALKYLATING AGENTS

DRUG	MTD,[a] mg/m²	FOLD INCREASE OVER STANDARD DOSE	MAJOR ORGAN TOXICITIES
Cyclophosphamide	7000	7	Cardiac, hepatic VOD
Ifosfamide	16,000	2.7	Renal, CNS, hepatic VOD
Thiotepa	1000	18	GI, CNS, hepatic VOD
Melphalan	180	5.6	GI, hepatic VOD
Busulfan	640	9	GI, hepatic VOD
Carmustine (BCNU)	1050	5.3	Lung, hepatic VOD
Cisplatin	200	2	PN, renal
Carboplatin	2000	5	Renal, PN, hepatic VOD

[a]Maximum tolerated dose (cumulative) in treatment protocols.

cyclophosphamide, melphalan, and thiotepa have the advantage of causing less mucosal damage than the other agents. In high-dose protocols, however, other toxicities become limiting (Table 66–1).

Nervous System

Nausea and vomiting commonly follow administration of nitrogen mustard or BCNU. Ifosfamide is the most neurotoxic of the alkylating agents and may produce altered mental status, coma, generalized seizures, and cerebellar ataxia. These side effects result from the release of chloroacetaldehyde from the phosphate-linked chloroethyl side chain of ifosfamide. High-dose busulfan can cause seizures; in addition, it accelerates the clearance of phenytoin, an antiseizure medication.

Other Organs

All alkylating agents, including temozolomide, have caused pulmonary fibrosis, usually several months after treatment. In high-dose regimens, particularly those employing busulfan or BCNU, vascular endothelial damage may precipitate veno-occlusive disease (VOD) of the liver (Table 66–1), an often-fatal side effect that is successfully reversed by *defibrotide*. Defibrotide is an oligonucleotide mixture with profibrinolytic properties that is FDA-approved for the treatment of adult and pediatric patients with hepatic VOD. The nitrosoureas and ifosfamide, after multiple cycles of therapy, may lead to renal failure. Cyclophosphamide and ifosfamide release a nephrotoxic and urotoxic metabolite, acrolein, which causes severe hemorrhagic cystitis in high-dose regimens. This adverse effect can be prevented by coadministration of MESNA, which conjugates acrolein in urine. Ifosfamide in high doses for transplant causes a chronic, and often irreversible, renal toxicity; its nephrotoxicity correlates with the total dose of drug received and increases in frequency in children younger than 5 years. The syndrome may be due to chloroacetaldehyde or acrolein excreted in the urine.

The more unstable alkylating agents (e.g., mechlorethamine and the nitrosoureas) have strong vesicant properties, damage veins with repeated use, and, if extravasated, produce ulceration. All alkylating agents have toxic effects on the male and female reproductive systems, causing an often-permanent amenorrhea, particularly in perimenopausal women, and an irreversible azoospermia in men.

Leukemogenesis

Alkylating agents have a high capacity to induce leukemia. Acute nonlymphocytic leukemia, induced by treatment, is often associated with a higher incidence of p53 mutations, partial or total deletions of

chromosome 5 or 7, and reduced response to chemotherapy. Incidence peaks about 4 years after therapy and may affect up to 5% of patients treated on regimens containing alkylating drugs. Leukemia often is preceded by a period of neutropenia or anemia and by bone marrow morphology consistent with myelodysplasia. Melphalan, the nitrosoureas, and the methylating agent procarbazine have the greatest propensity to cause leukemia, which is less common after cyclophosphamide.

Clinical Pharmacology of Nitrogen Mustards

Mechlorethamine

Mechlorethamine HCl was the first clinically used nitrogen mustard and is the most reactive of the drugs in this class. It is used topically for treatment of CTCL as a solution that is rapidly mixed and applied to affected areas. It has been largely replaced by cyclophosphamide, melphalan, and other more stable alkylating agents.

Cyclophosphamide

ADME

Cyclophosphamide is well-absorbed orally and is activated to the 4-hydroxy intermediate (see Figure 66–3). Its rate of metabolic activation exhibits significant interpatient variability and increases with successive doses in high-dose regimens but appears to be saturable at concentrations of the parent compound greater than 150 μM. 4-Hydroxycyclophosphamide may be oxidized further by aldehyde oxidase, either in liver or in tumor tissue, to inactive metabolites. 4-Hydroxycyclophosphamide and its tautomer, aldophosphamide, travel in the circulation to tumor cells, where aldophosphamide cleaves spontaneously, generating stoichiometric amounts of phosphoramide mustard and acrolein. Phosphoramide mustard is responsible for antitumor effects, while acrolein causes hemorrhagic cystitis often seen during therapy with cyclophosphamide.

Pretreatment with CYP inducers such as phenobarbital enhances the rate of activation of the azoxyphosphorenes but does not alter total exposure to active metabolites over time and does not affect toxicity or efficacy. Cyclophosphamide can be used in full doses in patients with renal dysfunction because it is eliminated by hepatic metabolism. Patients with significant hepatic dysfunction should receive reduced doses. Maximal plasma concentrations are achieved about 1 h after oral administration; the $t_{1/2}$ of parent drug in plasma is about 7 h.

Therapeutic Uses

Cyclophosphamide is administered orally or intravenously. Recommended doses vary widely, and standard protocols for determining the schedule and doses of cyclophosphamide in combination with other chemotherapeutic agents should be consulted. The neutrophil nadir of 500–1000 cells/mm³ generally serves as a lower limit for dosage adjustments in prolonged therapy.

The clinical spectrum of activity for cyclophosphamide is broad. It is an essential component of many effective drug combinations for non-Hodgkin lymphomas, other lymphoid malignancies, breast and ovarian cancers, and solid tumors in children. Complete remissions and presumed cures have been reported when cyclophosphamide was given as a single agent for Burkitt lymphoma. It frequently is used in combination with doxorubicin and a taxane as adjuvant therapy after surgery for breast cancer. Because of its potent immunosuppressive properties, cyclophosphamide has been used to treat autoimmune disorders, including Wegener granulomatosis, rheumatoid arthritis, and the nephrotic syndrome. Caution is advised when the drug is considered for nonneoplastic conditions, not only because of its toxic effects but also because of its potential for inducing premature menopause, sterility, teratogenic effects, and leukemia.

Adverse Effects

Phosphoramide mustard is responsible for antitumor effects, while acrolein causes hemorrhagic cystitis often seen during therapy with cyclophosphamide. Patients should receive vigorous intravenous hydration during high-dose treatment. Brisk hematuria in a patient receiving daily oral therapy should lead to immediate drug discontinuation. Refractory bladder hemorrhage can become life-threatening and may require cystectomy for control of bleeding. Inappropriate secretion of antidiuretic hormone has been observed (usually at doses greater than 50 mg/kg) and can lead to water intoxication because these patients usually are vigorously hydrated. In addition to the cystitis (counteracted by MESNA and diuresis), GI, pulmonary, renal, hepatic, and cardiac toxicities (hemorrhagic myocardial necrosis) may occur after high-dose therapy with total doses greater than 200 mg/kg.

Ifosfamide

Ifosfamide is an analogue of cyclophosphamide. Severe urinary tract and CNS toxicity initially limited the use of ifosfamide, but adequate hydration and coadministration of MESNA have reduced its bladder toxicity. CNS toxicity is handled with methylene blue.

ADME

Ifosfamide has a plasma elimination $t_{1/2}$ ~1.5 h after doses of 3.8–5 g/m^2 and a somewhat shorter $t_{1/2}$ at lower doses; its pharmacokinetics are highly variable due to variable rates of hepatic metabolism (see legend to Figure 66–3).

Therapeutic Uses

Ifosfamide is approved for treatment of patients with relapsed germ cell testicular cancer and is frequently used for first-time treatment of pediatric or adult patients with sarcomas. It is a common component of high-dose chemotherapy regimens with bone marrow or stem cell rescue. In nonmyeloablative regimens, ifosfamide is infused intravenously over at least 30 min at a dose of 1.2 g/m^2/d or less for 5 days. Intravenous MESNA is given as bolus injections in a dose equal to 20% of the ifosfamide dose concomitantly and an additional 20% again 4 and 8 h later, for a total MESNA dose of 60% of the ifosfamide dose. Alternatively, MESNA may be given concomitantly in a single dose equal to the ifosfamide dose. Patients also should receive at least 2 L of oral or intravenous fluid daily. Treatment cycles are repeated every 3–4 weeks.

Adverse Effects

Ifosfamide has a similar toxicity profile as cyclophosphamide, although it causes greater platelet suppression, neurotoxicity, nephrotoxicity, and urothelial damage. In high-dose regimens (i.e., total doses of 12–14 g/m^2), it may cause severe neurological toxicity, including hallucinations, coma, and death, with symptoms appearing 12 h to 7 days after beginning the ifosfamide infusion. This toxicity may result from a metabolite, chloroacetaldehyde. Ifosfamide also causes nausea, vomiting, anorexia, leukopenia, nephrotoxicity, and VOD of the liver.

Melphalan

The alkylating agent melphalan primarily is used to treat multiple myeloma and, less commonly, in high-dose chemotherapy with marrow transplantation. The general pharmacological and cytotoxic actions of melphalan are similar to those of other bifunctional alkylators. The drug is not a vesicant.

ADME

Oral melphalan is absorbed in an inconsistent manner and, for most indications, is given as an intravenous infusion. The drug has a plasma $t_{1/2}$ of about 45–90 min; 10%–15% of an administered dose is excreted unchanged in the urine. Patients with decreased renal function may develop unexpectedly severe myelosuppression.

Therapeutic Uses and Adverse Effects

Melphalan for multiple myeloma is administered orally for 4–7 days every 28 days, with dexamethasone or thalidomide. Treatment is repeated at 4-week intervals based on response and tolerance. Dosage adjustments should be based on blood cell counts. Melphalan also may be used in myeloablative regimens followed by bone marrow or peripheral blood stem cell reconstitution. The toxicity of melphalan is mostly hematological

and is similar to that of other alkylating agents. Nausea and vomiting are less frequent. The drug causes less alopecia and, rarely, renal or hepatic dysfunction.

Chlorambucil

The cytotoxic effects of chlorambucil on the bone marrow, lymphoid organs, and epithelial tissues are similar to those observed with other nitrogen mustards. As an orally administered agent, chlorambucil is well tolerated in small daily doses and provides flexible titration of blood counts. Nausea and vomiting may result from single oral doses of 20 mg or greater.

ADME

Oral absorption of chlorambucil is adequate and reliable. The drug has a $t_{1/2}$ in plasma of about 1.5 h and is hydrolyzed to inactive products.

Therapeutic Uses and Adverse Effects

Chlorambucil is almost exclusively used in treating CLL. In treating CLL, chlorambucil is given once daily and continued for 3–6 weeks. With a fall in the peripheral total leukocyte count or clinical improvement, the dosage is titrated to maintain neutrophils and platelets at acceptable levels. Maintenance therapy often is required to maintain clinical response. Chlorambucil treatment may continue for months or years, achieving its effects gradually and often without significant toxicity to a compromised bone marrow. Marked hypoplasia of the bone marrow may be induced with excessive doses, but the myelosuppressive effects are moderate, gradual, and rapidly reversible. GI discomfort, azoospermia, amenorrhea, pulmonary fibrosis, seizures, dermatitis, and hepatotoxicity rarely may be encountered. A marked increase in the incidence of AML and other tumors has been noted in the treatment of polycythemia vera and in patients with breast cancer receiving chlorambucil as adjuvant chemotherapy.

Bendamustine

Bendamustine is approved for treatment of CLL and non-Hodgkin lymphoma. Bendamustine is given as a 30-min intravenous infusion on days 1 and 2 of a 28-day cycle. Lower doses may be indicated in heavily pretreated patients. Bendamustine is rapidly degraded through sulfhydryl interaction and adduct formation with macromolecules; less than 5% of the parent drug is excreted in the urine intact. N-Demethylation and oxidation produce metabolites that have antitumor activity, but less than that of the parent molecule. The parent drug has a plasma $t_{1/2}$ of about 30 min. The clinical toxicity pattern of bendamustine is typical of alkylators, with a rapidly reversible myelosuppression and mucositis, both generally tolerable.

Ethyleneimines and Methylmelamines

Although nitrogen mustards containing chloroethyl groups constitute the most widely used class of alkylating agents, other alkylators such as ethyleneimines with greater chemical stability and well-defined activity in specific types of cancer have value in clinical practice.

Altretamine

Altretamine is structurally similar to triethylenemelamine (TEM). Its precise mechanism of cytotoxicity is unknown, although it can alkylate DNA and proteins. It is a palliative treatment of patients with persistent or recurrent ovarian cancer following cisplatin-based combination therapy. The usual dosage of altretamine as a single agent in ovarian cancer is 260 mg/m^2/d in four divided doses, for 14 or 21 consecutive days out of a 28-day cycle, for up to 12 cycles.

ADME

Altretamine is well absorbed from the GI tract; its elimination $t_{1/2}$ is 4–10 h. The drug undergoes rapid demethylation in the liver; the principal metabolites are pentamethylmelamine and tetramethyl melamine.

Adverse Effects

The main toxicities of altretamine are myelosuppression and neurotoxicity. Altretamine causes both peripheral and central neurotoxicity (ataxia, depression, confusion, drowsiness, hallucinations, dizziness, and vertigo). Neurological symptoms abate on discontinuation of therapy. Peripheral blood counts and a neurological examination should be performed prior to the initiation of each course of therapy. Therapy should be interrupted for at least 14 days and subsequently restarted at a lower dosage if the white cell count falls to less than 2000 cells/mm³ or the platelet count falls to less than 75,000 cells/mm³ or if neurotoxic or intolerable GI symptoms occur. If neurological symptoms fail to stabilize on the reduced-dose schedule, altretamine should be discontinued. Nausea and vomiting also are common side effects and may be dose limiting. Renal dysfunction may necessitate discontinuing the drug. Other rare adverse effects include rashes, alopecia, and hepatic toxicity. Severe, life-threatening orthostatic hypotension may develop in patients who receive MAO inhibitors, amitriptyline, imipramine, or phenelzine concurrently with altretamine.

Thiotepa

Thiotepa consists of three ethyleneimine groups stabilized by attachment to the nucleophilic thiophosphoryl base. Its current use is primarily for high-dose chemotherapy regimens. Hepatic CYPs rapidly convert thiotepa to its desulfurated primary metabolite, TEPA. Both thiotepa and TEPA form DNA cross-links.

ADME

Within hours of thiotepa administration, TEPA becomes the predominant form of the drug present in plasma. The parent compound has a plasma $t_{1/2}$ of 1.2–2 h; TEPA has a longer $t_{1/2}$, 3–24 h. Thiotepa pharmacokinetics essentially are the same in children as in adults at conventional doses (≤80 mg/m²), and drug and metabolite $t_{1/2}$ are unchanged in children receiving high-dose therapy of 300 mg/m²/d for 3 days. Less than 10% of the administered drug appears in urine as the parent drug or the primary metabolite.

Adverse Effects

Toxicities include myelosuppression and, to a lesser extent, mucositis. Myelosuppression tends to develop somewhat later than with cyclophosphamide, with leukopenic nadirs at 2 weeks and platelet nadirs at 3 weeks. In high doses, thiotepa may cause neurotoxic symptoms, including coma and seizures.

Alkyl Sulfonates

Busulfan

Busulfan exerts few pharmacological actions other than myelosuppression at conventional doses and, prior to the advent of imatinib mesylate, was a standard agent for patients in the chronic phase of myelocytic leukemia and caused a severe and prolonged pancytopenia in some patients. Busulfan now is primarily used in high-dose regimens, in which pulmonary fibrosis, GI mucosal damage, and hepatic VOD are important toxicities.

ADME

Busulfan is well absorbed after oral administration and has a plasma $t_{1/2}$ of 2–3 h. The drug is conjugated to GSH by GSTA1A and further metabolized by CYP-dependent pathways; its major urinary metabolite is methane sulfonic acid. In high doses, children less than 18 years of age clear the drug two to four times faster than adults and tolerate higher doses. Busulfan clearance varies considerably amongst patients. VOD is associated with high AUC (>1500 μM × min) and slow clearance, leading to recommendations for dose adjustment based on drug-level monitoring.

A target steady-state concentration of 600–900 ng/mL in plasma in adults or AUC < 1000 μM × min in children achieves an appropriate balance between toxicity and therapeutic benefit.

Therapeutic Uses

In treating CML, the initial oral dose of busulfan varies with the total leukocyte count and the severity of the disease; daily doses are adjusted to subsequent hematological and clinical responses, with the aim of reducing the total leukocyte count to 10,000 cells/mm³ or less. A decrease in the leukocyte count usually is not seen during the first 10–15 days of treatment, and the leukocyte count may actually increase during this period. Because the leukocyte count may fall for more than 1 month after discontinuing the drug, it is recommended that busulfan be withdrawn when the total leukocyte count has declined to about 15,000 cells/mm³. A normal leukocyte count usually is achieved within 12–20 weeks. During remission, daily treatment resumes when the total leukocyte count reaches about 50,000 cells/mm³.

In high-dose therapy, anticonvulsants must be used concomitantly to protect against acute CNS toxicities, including tonic-clonic seizures that may occur several hours after each dose. Although phenytoin is a frequent choice, phenytoin induces the GSTs that metabolize busulfan, reducing its AUC by about 20%. In patients requiring concomitant antiseizure medication, non–enzyme-inducing benzodiazepines such as lorazepam and clonazepam are recommended as an alternative to phenytoin. If phenytoin is used concurrently, plasma busulfan levels should be monitored and the busulfan dose adjusted accordingly.

Adverse Effects

The toxic effects of busulfan are related to its myelosuppressive properties; prolonged thrombocytopenia may occur. Occasionally, patients experience nausea, vomiting, and diarrhea. Long-term use leads to impotence, sterility, amenorrhea, and fetal malformation. Rarely, patients develop asthenia and hypotension. High-dose busulfan causes VOD of the liver in 10% or fewer of patients, as well as seizures, hemorrhagic cystitis, permanent alopecia, and cataracts. The coincidence of VOD and hepatotoxicity is increased by its coadministration with drugs that inhibit CYPs, including imidazoles and metronidazole, possibly through inhibition of the clearance of busulfan or its toxic metabolites.

Nitrosoureas

The nitrosoureas have an important role in the treatment of brain tumors and find occasional use in treating lymphomas and in high-dose regimens with bone marrow reconstitution. They function as bifunctional alkylating agents but differ from conventional nitrogen mustards in both pharmacological and toxicological properties.

Carmustine (BCNU) and lomustine (CCNU, not discussed in detail) are highly lipophilic and thus readily cross the blood-brain barrier, an important property in the treatment of brain tumors. Unfortunately, with the exception of streptozocin, nitrosoureas cause profound and delayed myelosuppression, with recovery 4–6 weeks after a single dose. Long-term treatment with the nitrosoureas, especially semustine (methyl-CCNU), has resulted in renal failure. As with other alkylating agents, the nitrosoureas are highly carcinogenic and mutagenic. They generate both alkylating and carbamylating moieties (see Figure 66–4).

Carmustine (BCNU)

Carmustine's major action is its alkylation of DNA at the O6-guanine position, an adduct repaired by MGMT. Methylation of the MGMT promoter inhibits its expression in about 30% of primary gliomas and is associated with sensitivity to nitrosoureas. In high doses with bone marrow rescue, carmustine produces hepatic VOD, pulmonary fibrosis, renal failure, and secondary leukemia.

ADME

Carmustine is unstable in aqueous solution and in body fluids. After intravenous infusion, it disappears from the plasma with a highly variable $t_{1/2}$ of 15–90 min or more. Approximately 30%–80% of the drug appears in the urine within 24 h as degradation products. The alkylating metabolites enter rapidly into the CSF, and their concentrations in the CSF reach 15%–30% of the concurrent plasma values.

Therapeutic Uses

Carmustine (BCNU) is administered intravenously over 1–2 h and repeated every 6 weeks. Because of its ability to cross the blood-brain barrier, carmustine has been used in the treatment of malignant gliomas. An implantable carmustine wafer is available for use as an adjunct to surgery for recurrent glioblastoma multiforme.

Streptozocin

Streptozocin (or streptozotocin) has a methylnitrosourea moiety attached to the 2-carbon of glucose. It has a high affinity for cells of the islets of Langerhans and causes diabetes in experimental animals.

ADME

Streptozocin is rapidly degraded following intravenous administration. The $t_{1/2}$ of the drug is about 15 min. Only 10%–20% of a dose is recovered intact in the urine.

Therapeutic Uses

Streptozocin is used in the treatment of human pancreatic islet cell carcinoma and carcinoid tumors. It is administered intravenously once daily for 5 days; this course is repeated every 6 weeks. Alternatively, a higher dose can be given weekly for 2 weeks, and the weekly dose then can be increased as tolerated.

Adverse Effects

Nausea is frequent. Mild, reversible renal or hepatic toxicity occurs in approximately two-thirds of cases; in fewer than 10% of patients, renal toxicity may be cumulative with each dose and may lead to irreversible renal failure. Streptozocin should not be given with other nephrotoxic drugs. Hematological toxicities (anemia, leukopenia, thrombocytopenia) occur in 20% of patients.

Triazenes

Dacarbazine (DTIC)

Dacarbazine functions as a methylating agent after metabolic activation to the monomethyl triazeno metabolite MTIC. It kills cells in all phases of the cell cycle. Resistance has been ascribed to the removal of methyl groups from the O6-guanine bases in DNA by MGMT.

ADME

Dacarbazine is administered intravenously. After an initial rapid phase ($t_{1/2}$ of about 20 min), dacarbazine is cleared from plasma with a terminal $t_{1/2}$ of about 5 h. The $t_{1/2}$ is prolonged in the presence of hepatic or renal disease. Almost 50% of the compound is excreted intact in the urine by tubular secretion.

Therapeutic Uses

The primary clinical indication for dacarbazine is in the chemotherapy of Hodgkin disease. In combination with other drugs for Hodgkin disease, dacarbazine is given on day 1 and 15 and repeated every 4 weeks for up to 6 cycles (see NCCN). It is modestly effective against malignant melanoma and adult sarcomas. Dacarbazine for malignant melanoma is given for a 10-day period, repeated every 28 days; alternatively, it can be given daily for 5 days and repeated every 3 weeks. Extravasation of the drug may cause tissue damage and severe pain. Its use in patients with melanoma has largely been replaced by immune checkpoint inhibitors and agents targeting the typically activated mitogen-active protein kinase pathway (see Chapter 67).

Adverse Effects

Dacarbazine induces nausea and vomiting in more than 90% of patients; vomiting usually develops 1–3 h after treatment and may last up to 12 h. Myelosuppression, with both leukopenia and thrombocytopenia, is mild and readily reversible within 1–2 weeks. A flu-like syndrome may occur.

Hepatotoxicity, alopecia, facial flushing, neurotoxicity, and dermatological reactions are less common adverse effects.

Temozolomide

Temozolomide is the standard agent, in combination with radiation therapy, for patients with malignant glioma and astrocytoma. Temozolomide, like dacarbazine, forms the methylating metabolite MTIC and kills cells in all phases of the cell cycle. It is more active in MGMT deficient tumors.

ADME

Temozolomide is administered orally and has a bioavailability approaching 100%. Plasma levels of the parent drug decline with a $t_{1/2}$ of 1–2 h. The primary active metabolite MTIC reaches a maximum plasma concentration (150 ng/mL) 90 min after a dose and declines with a $t_{1/2}$ of 2 h. Little intact drug is recovered in the urine, the primary urinary metabolite being the inactive imidazole carboxamide.

Adverse Effects

The toxicities of temozolomide mirror those of DTIC. Hematological monitoring is necessary to guide dosing adjustments.

Methylhydrazines

Procarbazine

Procarbazine is used in malignant brain tumors and in combination regimens for patients with Hodgkin disease.

Mechanisms of Action

The antineoplastic activity of procarbazine results from its conversion by CYP-mediated hepatic oxidative metabolism to highly reactive alkylating species that methylate DNA. Activated procarbazine can produce chromosomal damage, including chromatid breaks and translocations, consistent with its mutagenic and carcinogenic actions. Resistance to procarbazine develops rapidly when it is used as a single agent; one mechanism of resistance results from increased expression of MGMT, which repairs methylation of guanine.

ADME

The pharmacokinetic behavior of procarbazine has not been thoroughly defined. The drug is extensively metabolized by CYPs to azo, methylazoxy, and benzylazoxy intermediates, which are found in the plasma and yield the alkylating metabolites in tumor cells. In patients with brain cancer, the concurrent use of antiseizure drugs that induce hepatic CYPs does not significantly alter the pharmacokinetics of the parent drug.

Therapeutic Uses

Procarbazine is used in combination regimens such as MOPP for Hodgkin disease. It is also used in treating gliomas as part of the PVC (procarbazine, vincristine and CCNU) regimen.

Adverse Effects

The most common toxic effects include leukopenia and thrombocytopenia, which begin during the second week of therapy and reverse within 2 weeks off treatment. GI symptoms such as mild nausea and vomiting occur in most patients; diarrhea and rash are noted in 5%–10% of cases. Behavioral disturbances also have been reported. Because procarbazine augments sedative effects, the concomitant use of CNS depressants should be avoided. The drug is a weak MAO inhibitor; it blocks the metabolism of catecholamines, sympathomimetics, and dietary tyramine and thus may provoke hypertension in patients concurrently exposed to these. Procarbazine has disulfiram-like actions; therefore, the ingestion of alcohol should be avoided. The drug is highly carcinogenic, mutagenic, and teratogenic and is associated with a 5%–10% risk of acute leukemia in patients treated with MOPP. The highest risk is for patients who also receive radiation therapy. Procarbazine is a potent immunosuppressive agent. It causes infertility, particularly in males.

Platinum Coordination Complexes

Platinum coordination complexes have broad antineoplastic activity and have become the foundation for treatment of ovarian, head and neck, bladder, esophagus, lung, and colon cancers. Although cisplatin and other platinum complexes do not form carbonium ion intermediates like other alkylating agents or formally alkylate DNA, they covalently bind to nucleophilic sites on DNA and share many pharmacological attributes with alkylators.

CISPLATIN CARBOPLATIN

OXALIPLATIN

Mechanisms of Action

Cisplatin, carboplatin, and oxaliplatin enter cells by the high-affinity Cu^{2+} transporter CTR1 (SLC31A1, a member of the solute carrier family; see Chapter 5) and in doing so contribute to the degradation of the transporter. The compounds are actively extruded from cells by ATP7A and ATP7B copper exporters and by MRP1; variable expression of these transporters may contribute to clinical resistance, along with a variety of other proteins and epigenetic phenomena (Shen et al., 2012). Inside the cell, the chloride, cyclohexane, or oxalate ligands of the analogues are displaced by water molecules, yielding a positively charged molecule that reacts with nucleophilic sites on DNA and proteins.

Aquation of cisplatin is favored at the low concentrations of Cl⁻ inside the cell and in the urine. High concentrations of Cl⁻ stabilize the drug, explaining the effectiveness of Cl⁻ diuresis in preventing nephrotoxicity. The activated platinum complexes can react with electron-rich regions, such as sulfhydryls, and with various sites on DNA, forming both intrastrand and interstrand cross-links. The DNA-platinum adducts inhibit replication and transcription, lead to single- and double-stranded breaks and miscoding, and if recognized by p53 and other checkpoint proteins, cause induction of apoptosis. Adduct formation is an important predictor of clinical response (Reed et al., 1998). The analogues differ in the conformation of their adducts and the effects of adduct on DNA structure and function. Oxaliplatin and carboplatin are slower to form adducts. The oxaliplatin adducts are bulkier and less readily repaired, create a different pattern of distortion of the DNA helix, and differ from cisplatin adducts in the pattern of hydrogen bonding to adjacent segments of DNA (Sharma et al., 2007).

Unlike the other platinum analogues, oxaliplatin exhibits a cytotoxicity that does not depend on an active MMR system, which may explain its greater activity in colorectal cancer. It also seems less dependent on the presence of HMG proteins that are required by the other platinum derivatives. Testicular cancers have a high concentration of HMG proteins and are quite sensitive to cisplatin. Basal-type breast cancers, such as those with *BRCA1* and *BRCA2* mutations, lack *HER2* amplification and hormone-receptor expression and appear to be uniquely susceptible to cisplatin through their upregulation of apoptotic pathways governed by p63 and p73 (Deyoung and Ellisen, 2007). The cell cycle specificity of cisplatin differs amongst cell types; the effects of cross-linking are most pronounced during the S phase. The platinum analogues are mutagenic, teratogenic, and carcinogenic. Cisplatin- or carboplatin-based chemotherapy for ovarian cancer is associated with a 4-fold increased risk of developing secondary leukemia.

Resistance to Platinum Analogues

Resistance to the platinum analogues likely is multifactorial; the compounds differ in their degree of cross-resistance. Carboplatin shares cross-resistance with cisplatin in most experimental tumors, while oxaliplatin does not.

A number of factors influence sensitivity to platinum analogues in experimental cells, including intracellular drug accumulation and intracellular levels of glutathione and other sulfhydryls, such as metallothionein, that bind to and inactivate the drug and rates of repair of DNA adducts. Repair of platinum-DNA adducts requires participation of the NER pathway. Inhibition or loss of NER increases sensitivity to cisplatin in patients with ovarian cancer, while overexpression of NER components is associated with poor response to cisplatin- or oxaliplatin-based therapy in lung, colon, and gastric cancer (Paré et al., 2008).

Resistance to cisplatin, but not oxaliplatin, appears to be partly mediated through loss of function in the MMR proteins. In the absence of effective repair of DNA-platinum adducts, sensitive cells cannot replicate or transcribe affected portions of the DNA strand. Some DNA polymerases can bypass adducts, possibly contributing to resistance. Overexpression of copper efflux transporters ATP7A and ATP7B correlates with poor survival after cisplatin-based therapy for ovarian cancer (Shen et al., 2012).

Cisplatin

ADME

Cisplatin is given only intravenously. To prevent renal toxicity, it is important to establish a chloride diuresis by the infusion of 1–2 L of normal saline prior to treatment. The appropriate amount of cisplatin then is diluted in a solution containing dextrose, saline, and mannitol and administered intravenously over 4–6 h. Because aluminum inactivates cisplatin, the drug should not come in contact with needles or other infusion equipment that contain aluminum during its preparation or administration. After intravenous administration, cisplatin has an initial plasma elimination $t_{1/2}$ of 25–50 min; concentrations of total (bound and unbound) drug fall thereafter, with a $t_{1/2}$ of 24 h or more. More than 90% of the platinum in the blood is covalently bound to plasma proteins. High concentrations of cisplatin are found in the kidney, liver, intestine, and testes; cisplatin penetrates poorly into the CNS. Only a small portion of the drug is excreted by the kidney during the first 6 h; by 24 h, up to 25% is excreted, and by 5 days, up to 43% of the administered dose is recovered in the urine, mostly covalently bound to protein and peptides. Biliary or intestinal excretion of cisplatin is minimal.

Therapeutic Uses

Cisplatin, in combination with bleomycin, etoposide, or with ifosfamide and vinblastine, cures 90% of patients with testicular cancer. Used with paclitaxel, cisplatin or carboplatin induces complete response in the majority of patients with carcinoma of the ovary. Cisplatin produces responses in cancers of the bladder, head and neck, cervix, and endometrium; all forms of carcinoma of the lung; anal and rectal carcinomas; and neoplasms of childhood. The drug also sensitizes cells to radiation therapy and enhances control of locally advanced lung, esophageal, and head and neck tumors when given with irradiation.

Adverse Effects

Cisplatin-induced nephrotoxicity has been largely ameliorated by forced pretreatment hydration and chloride diuresis. Amifostine, a thiophosphate cytoprotective agent, reduces renal toxicity associated with repeated administration of cisplatin. Ototoxicity caused by cisplatin is unaffected by diuresis and is manifested by tinnitus and high-frequency hearing loss. Marked nausea and vomiting occur in almost all patients and usually can be controlled with $5HT_3$ receptor antagonists, neurokinin (NK_1) receptor antagonists (e.g., *aprepitant*), and high-dose corticosteroids.

At higher doses or after multiple cycles of treatment, cisplatin causes a progressive peripheral motor and sensory neuropathy that may worsen after discontinuation of the drug and may be aggravated by subsequent or simultaneous treatment with taxanes or other neurotoxic drugs. Cisplatin causes mild-to-moderate myelosuppression, with transient leukopenia and thrombocytopenia. Anemia may become prominent after multiple cycles of treatment. Electrolyte disturbances, including hypomagnesemia, hypocalcemia, hypokalemia, and hypophosphatemia, are common. Hypocalcemia and hypomagnesemia secondary to tubular damage and renal electrolyte wasting may produce tetany if untreated. Routine measurement of Mg^{2+} concentrations in plasma is recommended. Hyperuricemia, hemolytic anemia, and cardiac abnormalities are rare side effects. Anaphylactic-like reactions, characterized by facial edema, bronchoconstriction, tachycardia, and hypotension, may occur within minutes after administration and should be treated by intravenous injection of epinephrine and with corticosteroids or antihistamines. Cisplatin has been associated with the development of AML, usually 4 years or more after treatment.

Carboplatin

The mechanisms of action and resistance and the spectrum of clinical activity of carboplatin are similar to cisplatin. However, the two drugs differ significantly in their chemical, pharmacokinetic, and toxicological properties.

ADME

Because carboplatin is much less reactive than cisplatin, the majority of drug in plasma remains in its parent form, unbound to proteins. Most drug is eliminated via renal excretion, with a $t_{1/2}$ of about 2 h. A small fraction of platinum binds irreversibly to plasma proteins and disappears slowly, with a $t_{1/2}$ of 5 days or more.

Therapeutic Uses

Carboplatin and cisplatin are equally effective in the treatment of patients with suboptimally debulked ovarian cancer, non–small cell lung cancer, and extensive-stage small cell lung cancer; however, carboplatin may be less effective than cisplatin in the treatment of patients with germ cell, head and neck, and esophageal cancers. Carboplatin is an effective alternative for responsive tumors in patients unable to tolerate cisplatin because of impaired renal function, refractory nausea, significant hearing impairment, or neuropathy, but doses must be adjusted for renal function. In addition, it may be used in high-dose therapy with bone marrow or peripheral stem cell rescue. Carboplatin is administered as an intravenous infusion over at least 15 min and is given once every 21–28 days; the overall dose of carboplatin should be adjusted in proportion to the reduction in creatinine clearance for patients with $CL_{Cr} < 60$ mL/min and use the Calvert formula for adjustment (Calvert et al., 1989).

Adverse Effects

Carboplatin is relatively well tolerated clinically, causing less nausea, neurotoxicity, ototoxicity, and nephrotoxicity than cisplatin. The dose-limiting toxicity of carboplatin is myelosuppression, primarily thrombocytopenia. It may cause a hypersensitivity reaction; in patients with a mild reaction, premedication, graded doses of drug, and more prolonged infusion lead to desensitization.

Oxaliplatin

ADME

Oxaliplatin has a short $t_{1/2}$ in plasma, probably as a result of its rapid uptake by tissues and its reactivity; the initial $t_{1/2}$ is about 17 min. No dose adjustment is required for hepatic dysfunction or for patients with a $CL_{Cr} \geq 20$ mL/min.

Therapeutic Uses

Oxaliplatin exhibits a range of antitumor activity (colorectal and gastric cancer) that differs from other platinum agents. Oxaliplatin's effectiveness in colorectal cancer is perhaps due to its MMR- and HMG-independent effects. It also suppresses expression of TS, the target enzyme of 5FU action, which may promote synergy of these two drugs (Fischel et al., 2002). In combination with 5FU, it is approved for treatment of patients with colorectal cancer.

Adverse Effects

The dose-limiting toxicity of oxaliplatin is peripheral neuropathy. An acute form, often triggered by exposure to cold liquids, manifests as paresthesias or dysesthesias in the upper and lower extremities, mouth, and throat. A second type relates to cumulative dose and has features similar to cisplatin neuropathy; 75% of patients receiving a cumulative dose of 1560 mg/m^2 experience some progressive sensory neurotoxicity, with dysesthesias, ataxia, and numbness of the extremities. Hematological toxicity is mild to moderate, except for rare immune-mediated cytopenias; nausea is well controlled with 5HT$_3$ receptor antagonists. Oxaliplatin may cause leukemia and pulmonary fibrosis months to years after administration. Oxaliplatin may cause an acute allergic response with urticaria, hypotension, and bronchoconstriction.

II. Antimetabolites

Folic Acid Analogues

Folic acid is an essential dietary factor that is converted by enzymatic reduction to FH$_4$ cofactors that provide methyl groups for the synthesis of precursors of DNA (thymidylate and purines) and RNA (purines) (Wilson et al., 2014). Folic acid analogues such as MTX interfere with FH$_4$ metabolism (Figure 66–5), reducing the cellular capacity for one-carbon transfer and methylation reactions in the synthesis of purine ribonucleotides and TMP, thereby inhibiting DNA replication.

HISTORY Antifolate Chemotherapy

Antifolate chemotherapy produced the first striking, although temporary, remissions in leukemia (Farber et al., 1948) and the first cure of a solid tumor, choriocarcinoma (Berlin et al., 1963). Interest in folate antagonists further increased with the development of curative combination therapy for childhood acute lymphocytic leukemia; in this therapy, MTX played a critical role in both systemic treatment and intrathecal therapy. Introduction of high-dose regimens with "rescue" of host toxicity by the reduced folate leucovorin (folinic acid, citrovorum factor, 5-formyl tetrahydrofolate, N^5-formyl FH$_4$) further extended the effectiveness of this drug to both systemic and CNS lymphomas, osteogenic sarcoma, and leukemias. Recognition that MTX, an inhibitor of DHFR, also directly inhibits the folate-dependent enzymes of de novo purine synthesis and thymidylate synthesis led to development of antifolate analogues that specifically target these other folate-dependent enzymes. New congeners have greater capacity for transport into tumor cells (*pralatrexate*) and exert their primary inhibitory effect on TS (*raltitrexed*), early steps in purine biosynthesis (*lometrexol*), or both (the multitargeted antifolate *pemetrexed*).

Mechanism of Action

The primary target of folic analogs, such as MTX, is the enzyme DHFR (see Figure 66–6). To function as a cofactor in one-carbon transfer reactions, folate must be reduced by DHFR to FH$_4$. Inhibitors such as MTX, with a high affinity for DHFR (K_i about 0.01–0.2 nM), cause partial depletion of N$^{5-10}$ methylene FH$_4$ and N^{10} formyl FH$_4$ cofactors that are required for the synthesis of thymidylate and purines. In addition, MTX, like cellular folates, undergoes addition of a series of polyglutamates (MTX-PGs) in both normal and tumor cells (Figure 66–5). These PGs constitute intracellular storage forms of folates and folate analogues that dramatically increase inhibitory potency of the analogue for additional sites, including TS and two early enzymes in the purine biosynthetic pathway. The FH$_2$ PGs that accumulate in cells behind the blocked DHFR reaction also act as inhibitors of TS and other enzymes (see Figure 66–6) (Allegra et al., 1987b).

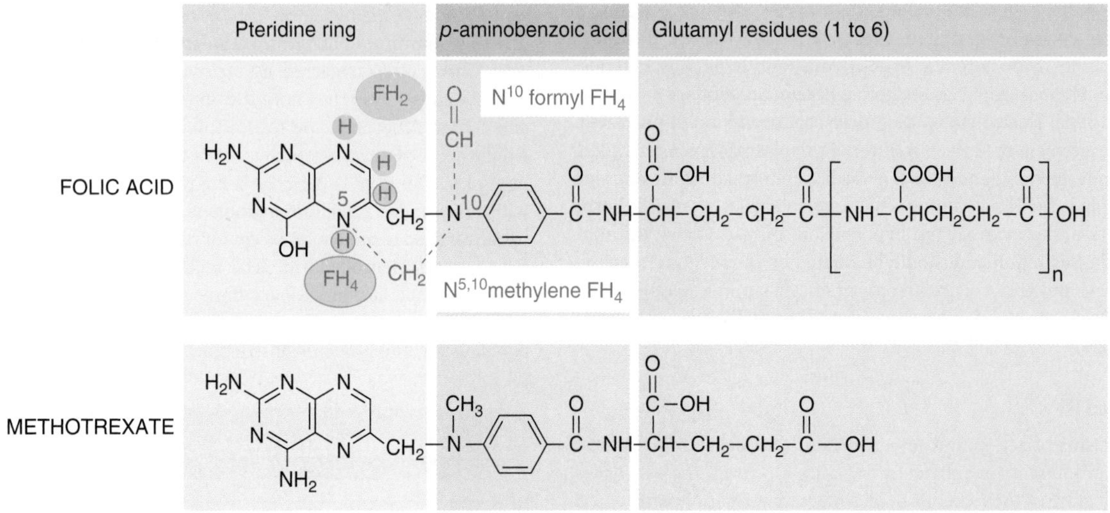

Figure 66–5 *Folic acid, metabolic intermediates, and MTX. The shading identifies common structural features and areas of modification.* Yellow highlights indicate sites modified by DHFR to FH$_2$ (DHF) and to FH$_4$ (THF); red atoms and bonds indicate metabolic intermediates that serve as single-carbon donors (see pathways in Figure 66–6).

Selective Toxicity; Rescue

As with most antimetabolites, MTX is only partially selective for tumor cells and kills rapidly dividing normal cells, such as those of the intestinal epithelium and bone marrow. Folate antagonists kill cells during the S phase of the cell cycle and are most effective when cells are proliferating rapidly. The toxic effects of MTX may be terminated by administering leucovorin, a fully reduced folate coenzyme that repletes the intracellular pool of FH$_4$ cofactors (see Figure 66–6).

Cellular Entry and Retention

Because folic acid and many of its analogues are polar, they cross the blood-brain barrier poorly and require specific transport mechanisms to enter mammalian cells. Three inward folate transport systems are found on mammalian cells:

1. A folate receptor, which has high affinity for folic acid but much lower ability to transport MTX and other analogues
2. The reduced folate transporter, the major transit protein for MTX, raltitrexed, pemetrexed, and most analogues
3. A transporter that is active at low pH

The reduced folate transporter is highly expressed in the hyperdiploid subtype of ALL, which has extreme sensitivity to MTX (Pui et al., 2004). Once in the cell, additional glutamyl residues are added to the molecule by the enzyme folylpolyglutamate synthetase. Because these higher PGs are strongly charged and cross cellular membranes poorly, polyglutamation serves as a mechanism of ion trapping within the cell. The polyglutamation may also account for the prolonged retention of MTX in chorionic epithelium (where it is a potent abortifacient); in tumors derived from this tissue, such as choriocarcinoma cells; and in normal tissues subject to cumulative drug toxicity, such as liver. Polyglutamyl folates and analogues have substantially greater affinity than the monoglutamate form for folate-dependent enzymes that are required for purine and thymidylate synthesis and have at least equal affinity for DHFR.

Newer Congeners

New folate antagonists that are better substrates for the reduced folate carrier have been identified. In efforts to bypass the obligatory membrane transport system and to facilitate penetration of the blood-brain barrier, lipid-soluble folate antagonists also have been synthesized. Trimetrexate, a lipid-soluble analogue that lacks a terminal glutamate, has modest

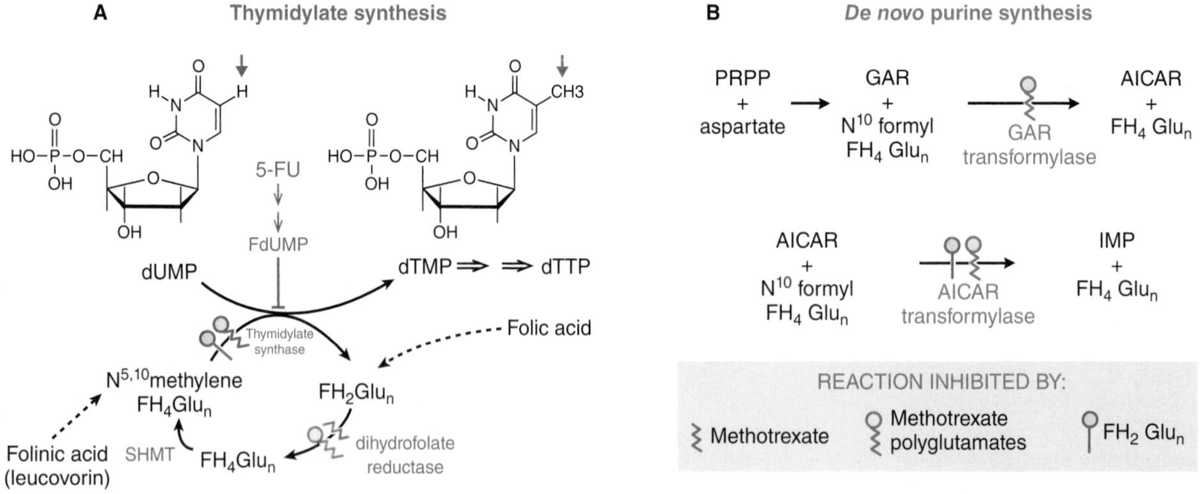

Figure 66–6 *Folate metabolism and the actions of of 5FU, MTX, and MTX polyglutamates.* **A.** *Thymidylate synthesis* (for composition of folates, see Figure 66–5). **B.** *De novo purine synthesis.* GAR transformylase provides the C8 and AICAR transformylase the C2 in the purine ring biosynthesis (see Figure 66–1 for numbering of purine ring atoms). AICAR, aminoimidazole carboxamide; dUMP, deoxyuridine monophosphate; FH$_2$Glu$_n$, dihydrofolate polyglutamate; FH$_4$Glu$_n$, tetrahydrofolate polyglutamate; GAR, glycinamide ribonucleotide; IMP, inosine monophosphate; PRPP, 5-phosphoribosyl-1-pyrophosphate; TMP, thymidine monophosphate.

antitumor activity, primarily in combination with leucovorin rescue. However, it is beneficial in the treatment of *Pneumocystis jiroveci* (*Pneumocystis carinii*) pneumonia, for which leucovorin provides differential rescue of the host but not the parasite (Allegra et al., 1987a). The most important recent folate analogue, MTA or pemetrexed, is a pyrrolepyrimidine structure. It is avidly transported into cells via the reduced folate carrier and is converted to PGs that inhibit TS and glycine amide ribonucleotide transformylase, as well as DHFR. It has activity against ovarian cancer, mesothelioma, and adenocarcinomas of the lung. Pemetrexed and its PGs have a somewhat different spectrum of biochemical actions. Like MTX, pemetrexed inhibits DHFR, but as a PG, it even more potently inhibits TS and GART (Figure 66–6). Unlike MTX, it produces little change in the pool of reduced folates, indicating that the distal sites of inhibition (TS and GART) predominate. Its pattern of deoxynucleotide depletion also differs; it causes a greater fall in TTP than in other triphosphates. Like MTX, it induces p53 and cell-cycle arrest, but this effect does not depend on induction of p21. A newer congener, pralatrexate, is more effectively taken up and polyglutamated than MTX and is approved for treatment of CTCL.

Mechanisms of Resistance to Antifolates

Resistance to MTX can involve alterations in each known step in MTX action, including

- Impaired transport of MTX into cells
- Production of altered forms of DHFR that have decreased affinity for the inhibitor
- Increased concentrations of intracellular DHFR through gene amplification or altered gene regulation
- Decreased ability to synthesize MTX-PGs
- Increased expression of a drug efflux transporter of the MRP class (see Chapter 5)

The DHFR levels in leukemic cells increase within 24 h after treatment of patients with MTX, probably as a result of induction of DHFR synthesis. Unbound DHFR protein may bind to its own message and reduce its own translation, while the DHFR-MTX complex is ineffective in blocking DHFR translation. With longer periods of drug exposure, tumor cell populations emerge that contain markedly increased levels of DHFR. These cells contain multiple gene copies of DHFR either in mitotically unstable double-minute chromosomes (extrachromosomal elements) or in stably integrated, homogeneously staining chromosomal regions or amplicons (Schimke et al., 1978). Similar gene amplification target proteins have been implicated in the resistance to other antitumor agents, including 5FU and pentostatin (2′-deoxycoformycin) and observed in patients with lung cancer (Curt et al., 1985).

High doses of MTX may permit entry of the drug into transport-defective cells and may permit the intracellular accumulation of MTX in concentrations that inactivate high levels of DHFR. The understanding of resistance to pemetrexed is incomplete. In various cell lines, resistance seems to arise from loss of influx transport, TS amplification, changes in purine biosynthetic pathways, or loss of polyglutamation.

ADME

Methotrexate is readily absorbed from the GI tract at doses of less than 25 mg/m²; larger doses are absorbed incompletely and are routinely administered intravenously. After intravenous administration, the drug disappears from plasma in a triphasic fashion. The rapid distribution phase is followed by a second phase, which reflects renal clearance ($t_{1/2}$ of about 2–3 h). A third phase has a $t_{1/2}$ of about 8–10 h. This terminal phase of disappearance, if prolonged by renal failure, may be responsible for major toxic effects of the drug on the bone marrow, GI epithelium, and skin. Distribution of MTX into body spaces, such as the pleural or peritoneal cavity, occurs slowly. However, if such spaces are expanded (e.g., by ascites or pleural effusion), they may act as a site of storage and slow release of the drug, resulting in prolonged elevation of plasma concentrations and more severe bone marrow toxicity.

Approximately 50% of MTX binds to plasma proteins and may be displaced from plasma albumin by myriad drugs, including sulfonamides, salicylates, tetracycline, chloramphenicol, and phenytoin; caution should be used if these drugs are given concomitantly. Up to 90% of a given dose of MTX is excreted unchanged in the urine, mostly within the first 8–12 h. Metabolism of MTX usually is minimal. After high doses, however, metabolites are readily detectable; these include 7-hydroxy-MTX, which is potentially nephrotoxic. Renal excretion of MTX occurs through a combination of glomerular filtration and active tubular secretion. Therefore, the concurrent use of drugs that reduce renal blood flow (e.g., NSAIDs), that are nephrotoxic (e.g., cisplatin), or that are weak organic acids (e.g., aspirin) can delay drug excretion and lead to severe myelosuppression. In patients with renal insufficiency, the dose should be adjusted in proportion to decreases in renal function, and high-dose regimens should be avoided. Concentrations of MTX in CSF are only 3% of those in the systemic circulation at steady state; hence, neoplastic cells in the CNS probably are not killed by standard dosage regimens. When high doses of MTX are given, cytotoxic concentrations of MTX reach the CNS beyond the blood-brain barrier. MTX is retained in the form of PGs for long periods (e.g., weeks in the kidneys, several months in the liver).

Pharmacogenetics may influence the response to antifolates and their toxicity. The C677T substitution in methylenetetrahydrofolate reductase reduces the activity of the enzyme that generates N^{5-10} methylene FH_4, the cofactor for TS, and thereby increases MTX toxicity (Pullarkat et al., 2001). The presence of this polymorphism in leukemic cells confers increased sensitivity to MTX and might also modulate the toxicity and therapeutic effect of pemetrexed, a predominant TS inhibitor. Likewise, polymorphisms in the promoter region of TS affect its expression and, by altering the intracellular levels of TS, modulate the response and toxicity of both antifolates and fluoropyrimidines (Pui et al., 2004).

Therapeutic Uses

Methotrexate is a critical drug in the management of childhood ALL. High-dose MTX is of great value in remission induction and consolidation and in the maintenance of remissions in this highly curable disease. A 6- to 24-h infusion of relatively large doses of MTX may be employed every 2–4 weeks but only when leucovorin rescue follows within 24 h of the MTX infusion. For maintenance therapy, it is administered at a lower dose, orally every week. Outcome of treatment in children correlates inversely with the rate of drug clearance. During MTX infusion, high steady-state levels are associated with a lower leukemia relapse rate. Methotrexate is of limited value in adults with AML, except for treatment and prevention of leukemic meningitis.

The intrathecal administration of MTX has been employed for treatment or prophylaxis of meningeal leukemia or lymphoma and for treatment of meningeal carcinomatosis. This route of administration achieves high concentrations of MTX in the CSF and also is effective in patients whose systemic disease has become resistant to MTX. The treatment is repeated every 4 days until malignant cells no longer are evident in the CSF. Leucovorin may be administered to counteract the potential toxicity of MTX that escapes into the systemic circulation, although this generally is not necessary. Because MTX administered into the lumbar space distributes poorly over the cerebral convexities, the drug may be given via an intraventricular catheter system in the treatment of active intrathecal disease. MTX is of established value in choriocarcinoma and related trophoblastic tumors of women; cure is achieved in about 75% of advanced cases treated sequentially with MTX and dactinomycin and in more than 90% when early diagnosis is made. For choriocarcinoma, MTX is administered intramuscularly every other day for four doses, alternating with leucovorin. Courses are repeated at 3-week intervals, toxicity permitting, and urinary β-human chorionic gonadotropin titers are used as a guide for persistence of disease.

Beneficial effects also are observed in the combination therapy of Burkitt and other non-Hodgkin lymphomas. MTX is a component of regimens for carcinomas of the breast, head and neck, ovary, and bladder. HDM-L is a standard agent for adjuvant therapy of osteosarcoma and produces a high complete response rate in CNS lymphomas. The administration of HDM-L has the potential for renal toxicity, probably related to the precipitation of the drug, a weak acid, in the acidic tubular fluid. Thus, vigorous hydration and alkalinization of urine pH are required prior to drug administration. If MTX values measured 48 h after drug administration are 1 μM or higher, higher doses (100 mg/m²) of leucovorin must be given until the plasma concentration of MTX falls to less than 50 nM. With appropriate hydration and urine alkalinization, and in patients with normal renal function, the incidence of nephrotoxicity following HDM-L is less than 2%. In patients who become oliguric, intermittent hemodialysis is ineffective in reducing MTX levels. Continuous-flow hemodialysis can eliminate MTX at about 50% of the clearance rate in patients with intact renal function. Alternatively, a MTX-cleaving enzyme, *glucarpidase*, is FDA approved for the treatment of MTX toxicity. *Glucarpidase* is a recombinant bacterial carboxypeptidase G2 that converts MTX into glutamate and 2,4-diamino-N(10)-methylpteroic acid. These metabolites are less toxic and are excreted by the liver. MTX concentrations in plasma fall by 99% or more within 5–15 min following enzyme administration. However, systemically administered carboxypeptidase G2 has little effect on MTX levels in the CSF.

Methotrexate is used in the treatment of severe, disabling psoriasis (see Chapter 70) orally for 5 days, followed by a rest period of at least 2 days, or intravenously weekly. It also is used at low dosage to induce remission in refractory rheumatoid arthritis. MTX inhibits cell-mediated immune reactions and is employed to suppress graft-versus-host disease in allogenic bone marrow and organ transplantation and for the treatment of dermatomyositis, Wegener granulomatosis, and Crohn disease (see Chapters 38 and 51). MTX is also used as an abortifacient, generally in combination with a prostaglandin (see Chapter 44).

Adverse Effects

The primary toxicities of antifolates are on the bone marrow and the intestinal epithelium. Patients may be at risk for spontaneous hemorrhage or life-threatening infection and may require prophylactic transfusion of platelets and broad-spectrum antibiotics if febrile. Side effects usually reverse completely within 2 weeks, but prolonged myelosuppression may occur in patients with compromised renal function who have delayed drug excretion. The dosage of MTX (and likely pemetrexed) must be reduced in proportion to any reduction in creatinine clearance. Additional toxicities of MTX include alopecia, dermatitis, an allergic interstitial pneumonitis, nephrotoxicity (after high-dose therapy), defective oogenesis or spermatogenesis, abortion, and teratogenesis. Low-dose MTX may lead to cirrhosis after long-term continuous treatment, as in patients with psoriasis. Intrathecal administration of MTX often causes meningismus and an inflammatory response in the CSF. Seizures, coma, and death may occur rarely. Note that leucovorin does not reverse neurotoxicity.

Pemetrexed toxicity mirrors that of MTX, with the additional feature of a prominent erythematous and pruritic rash in 40% of patients. Dexamethasone, 4 mg twice daily on days –1, 0, and +1, markedly diminishes this toxicity. Unpredictably severe myelosuppression with pemetrexed, seen especially in patients with preexisting homocystinemia, largely is eliminated by concurrent administration of low dosages of folic acid, 350–1000 mg/d, beginning 1–2 weeks prior to pemetrexed and continuing while the drug is administered. Patients should receive intramuscular vitamin B$_{12}$ (1 mg) with the first dose of pemetrexed to correct possible B$_{12}$ deficiency. These small doses of folate and B$_{12}$ do not compromise the therapeutic effect.

Pyrimidine Analogues

The pyrimidine antimetabolites encompass a diverse group of drugs that inhibit RNA and DNA function. The fluoropyrimidines and certain purine analogues (6MP and 6TG) inhibit the synthesis of essential precursors of DNA. Others, such as the cytidine and adenosine nucleoside analogues, become incorporated into DNA and block its further elongation and function (Wilson et al., 2014). Other inhibitory effects of these analogues may contribute to their cytotoxicity and their capacity to induce differentiation.

Cellular Actions of Pyrimidine Antimetabolites

Four bases (Figure 66–7) form DNA: two pyrimidines (thymine and cytosine) and two purines (guanine and adenine). RNA differs in that it incorporates uracil instead of thymine as one of its bases. Strategies for inhibiting DNA synthesis are based on the ability to create analogues of these precursors that readily enter tumor cells and become activated intracellularly. As an example, the pyrimidine analog 5FU is converted to an FdUMP, which in turn blocks TS, an enzyme required for the physiological conversion of dUMP to dTMP, a component of DNA (see Figure 66–6). Other analogues incorporate into DNA itself and thereby block its function (Wilson et al., 2014).

Cells can make the purine and pyrimidine bases de novo and convert them to their active triphosphates (dNTPs), providing substrates for DNA polymerase. Alternatively, cells can salvage free bases or their deoxynucleosides from the bloodstream. Thus, cells can take up uracil, guanine, and their analogues and convert them to (deoxy)nucleotides by the addition of deoxyribose and phosphate groups. Antitumor analogues of these bases (5FU, 6TG) can be formulated as simple substituted bases. Other bases, including cytosine, thymine, and adenine, and their analogues can only be used as deoxynucleosides, which are readily transported into cells and activated to deoxynucleotides by intracellular kinase. Thus, cytarabine (cytosine arabinoside; Ara-C), gemcitabine, 5-azacytidine, and adenosine analogues (cladribine) (Figures 66–7 and 66–8) are nucleosides readily taken up by cells, converted to nucleotides, and incorporated into DNA.

Fludarabine phosphate, a nucleotide, is dephosphorylated rapidly in plasma, releasing the nucleoside that is readily taken up by cells. Analogues may differ from the physiological bases in a variety of ways: by altering in the purine or pyrimidine ring; by altering the sugar attached

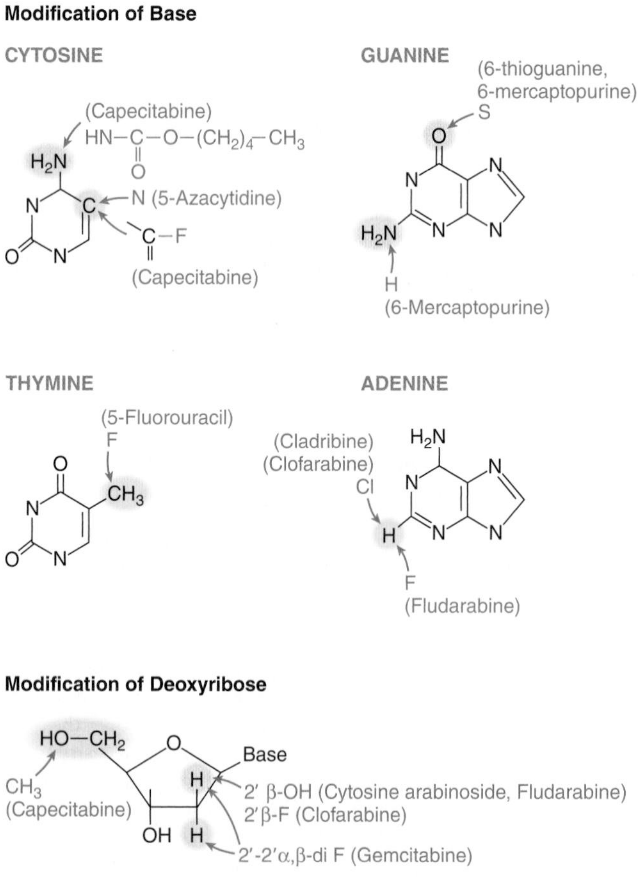

Modification of Base

Modification of Deoxyribose

Figure 66–7 *Structural modification of base and deoxyribonucleoside analogues.* Yellow ellipses indicate sites modified to create antimetabolites. Specific substitutions are noted in red for each drug. Modifications occur in the base ring systems, in their amino or hydroxyl side groups, and in the deoxyribose sugar found in deoxyribonucleosides. See structures in Figure 66–8.

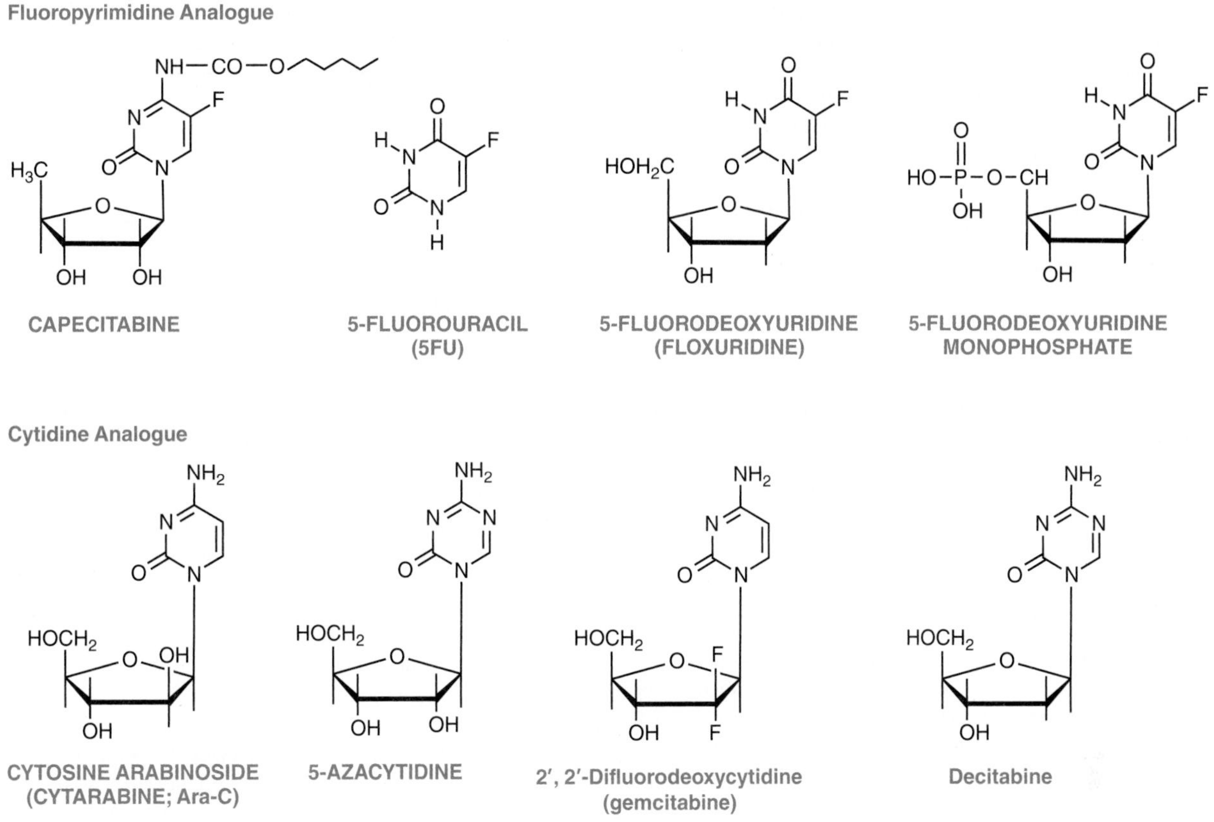

CAPECITABINE

5-FLUOROURACIL (5FU)

5-FLUORODEOXYURIDINE (FLOXURIDINE)

5-FLUORODEOXYURIDINE MONOPHOSPHATE

Cytidine Analogue

CYTOSINE ARABINOSIDE (CYTARABINE; Ara-C)

5-AZACYTIDINE

2', 2'-Difluorodeoxycytidine (gemcitabine)

Decitabine

Figure 66–8 *Pyrimidine analogues.*

to the base, as in the arabinoside, Ara-C; or by altering both the base and sugar, as in fludarabine phosphate (see Figure 66–7). These alterations produce inhibitory effects on vital enzymatic pathways and prevent DNA synthesis.

Fluorouracil, Floxuridine, Capecitabine

Fluorouracil is available as 5FU, as the derivative FUdR (not often used in clinical practice), and as a prodrug, capecitabine, which is ultimately converted to 5FU.

Mechanisms of Action

5-Fluorouracil requires enzymatic conversion (ribosylation and phosphorylation) to the nucleotide form to exert its cytotoxic activity. As the triphosphate FUTP, the drug is incorporated into RNA. Alternative reactions can produce the deoxy derivative FdUMP; FdUMP inhibits TS and blocks the synthesis of dTTP, a necessary constituent of DNA (Figure 66–6). The folate cofactor, 5,10-methylene FH$_4$, and FdUMP form a covalently bound ternary complex with TS. The physiological complex of TS-folate-dUMP progresses to the synthesis of thymidylate by transfer of the methylene group and two hydrogen atoms from folate to dUMP, but this reaction is blocked in the inhibited complex of TS-FdUMP-folate by the stability of the fluorine carbon bond on FdUMP; sustained inhibition of the enzyme results.

5-Fluorouracil is incorporated into both RNA and DNA. In 5FU-treated cells, both FdUTP and dUTP (which accumulates behind the blocked TS reaction) incorporate into DNA in place of the depleted physiological TTP. Presumably, such incorporation into DNA calls into action the excision-repair process, which can lead to DNA strand breakage because DNA repair requires TTP, which is lacking as a result of TS inhibition. 5FU incorporation into RNA also causes toxicity as the result of major effects on both the processing and the functions of RNA.

Mechanisms of Resistance

Resistance to the cytotoxic effects of 5FU or FUdR has been ascribed to loss or decreased activity of the enzymes necessary for activation of 5FU, amplification of TS, mutation of TS to a form that is not inhibited by

FdUMP, and high levels of the degradative enzymes dihydrouracil dehydrogenase and thymidine phosphorylase. TS levels are finely controlled by an autoregulatory feedback mechanism wherein the unbound enzyme interacts with and inhibits the translational efficiency of its own mRNA, which provides for the rapid TS modulation needed for cellular division. When TS is bound to FdUMP, inhibition of translation is relieved and levels of free TS rise, restoring thymidylate synthesis. Thus, TS autoregulation may be an important mechanism by which malignant cells become insensitive to the effects of 5FU.

Combination With Leucovorin

Some malignant cells appear to have insufficient concentrations of 5,10-methylene FH$_4$ and thus cannot form maximal levels of the inhibited ternary complex with TS. Addition of exogenous folate in the form of leucovorin increases formation of the complex and enhances responses to 5FU. A number of other agents have been combined with 5FU in attempts to enhance the cytotoxic activity through biochemical modulation. MTX, by inhibiting purine synthesis and increasing cellular pools of PRPP, enhances the activation of 5FU and increases antitumor activity of 5FU when given prior to but not following 5FU. The combination of cisplatin and 5FU has yielded impressive responses in tumors of the upper aerodigestive tract, but the molecular basis of their interaction is unclear. A combination with oxaliplatin, which downregulates TS expression, is commonly used with 5FU and leucovorin for treating patients with metastatic colorectal cancer; the combination is abbreviated as FOLFOX. Addition of irinotecan (see discussion that follows) is abbreviated as FOLFIRINOX and used in the treatment of patients with colorectal or pancreatic cancer. A most important interaction is the enhancement of irradiation by fluoropyrimidines, the basis for which is unclear. 5FU with simultaneous irradiation cures patients with anal cancer and enhances local tumor control in patients with head, neck, cervical, rectal, gastroesophageal, and pancreatic cancer.

ADME

5-Fluorouracil is administered parenterally because absorption after oral ingestion of the drug is unpredictable and incomplete. 5FU is inactivated by reduction of the pyrimidine ring in a reaction carried out by DPD, which is found in liver, intestinal mucosa, tumor cells, and other tissues. Inherited deficiency of this enzyme leads to greatly increased sensitivity to the drug (Milano et al., 1999). DPD deficiency can be detected by either enzymatic or molecular assays using peripheral white blood cells or by determining the plasma ratio of 5FU to its metabolite, 5-fluoro-5,6-dihydrouracil.

Plasma clearance is rapid ($t_{1/2}$ about 10–20 min). Only 5%–10% of a single intravenous dose of 5FU is excreted intact in the urine. The dose does not have to be modified in patients with hepatic dysfunction, presumably because of sufficient degradation of the drug at extrahepatic sites. 5FU enters the CSF in minimal amounts.

Therapeutic Uses

5-Fluorouracil. 5-Fluorouracil produces partial responses in 10%–20% of patients with metastatic colon carcinomas, upper GI tract carcinomas, and breast carcinomas but rarely is used as a single agent. 5FU in combination with leucovorin and oxaliplatin or irinotecan (FOLFOX or FOL-FIRINOX) in adjuvant therapy is associated with a survival advantage for patients with colorectal cancers. For average-risk patients in good nutritional status with adequate hematopoietic function, the dosage regimen employs leucovorin once each week for 6 of 8 weeks. Other regimens use daily doses for 5 days, repeated in monthly cycles. When used with leucovorin, doses of daily 5FU for 5 days must be reduced because of mucositis and diarrhea. 5FU increasingly is used as a biweekly infusion, a schedule that has less overall toxicity as well as superior response rates and progression-free survival for patients with metastatic colon cancer.

Floxuridine. Fluorodeoxyuridine is converted directly to FdUMP by thymidine kinase. The drug is administered primarily by continuous infusion into the hepatic artery for treatment of patients with metastatic carcinoma of the colon or following resection of hepatic metastases; the response rate of intrahepatic infusion (40%–50%) is twice that of intravenous administration. Intrahepatic arterial infusion for 14–21 days causes minimal systemic toxicity; however, there is a significant risk of biliary sclerosis if this route is used for multiple cycles of therapy. Treatment should be discontinued at the earliest manifestation of toxicity (usually stomatitis or diarrhea) because the maximal effects of bone marrow suppression and gut toxicity will not be evident until days 7–14.

Capecitabine. Capecitabine, an orally administered prodrug of 5FU, is approved for the treatment of patients with (1) metastatic breast cancer who have not responded to a regimen of paclitaxel and an anthracycline; (2) metastatic breast cancer when used in combination with docetaxel in patients who have had a prior anthracycline-containing regimen; and (3) metastatic colorectal cancer.

The recommended dosage is given in two divided doses with food, for 2 weeks, followed by a rest period of 1 week. Capecitabine is well absorbed orally. It is rapidly deesterified and deaminated, yielding high plasma concentrations of an inactive prodrug 5′-dFdU, which disappears with a $t_{1/2}$ of about 1 h. The conversion of 5′-dFdU to 5FU by thymidine phosphorylase occurs in liver tissues, peripheral tissues, and tumors. 5FU levels are less than 10% of those of 5′-dFdU, reaching a maximum of 0.3 mg/L or 1 μM at 2 h. Liver dysfunction delays the conversion of the parent compound to 5′-dFdU and 5FU, but there is no consistent effect on toxicity.

Combination Therapy. Higher response rates are seen when 5FU or capecitabine is used in combination with other agents (e.g., with cisplatin in head and neck cancer, with oxaliplatin or irinotecan in colon cancer). The combination of 5FU and oxaliplatin or irinotecan has become the standard first-line treatment of patients with metastatic colorectal cancer (FOLFOX and FOLFIRINOX). The use of 5FU in combination regimens has improved survival in the adjuvant treatment of breast cancer and, with oxaliplatin and leucovorin, of colorectal cancer. 5FU also is a potent radiation sensitizer. Beneficial effects have been reported when combined with irradiation as primary treatment of patients with locally advanced cancers of the esophagus, stomach, pancreas, cervix, anus, and head and neck. 5FU is effective in the topical treatment of premalignant keratoses of the skin and multiple superficial basal cell carcinomas.

Adverse Effects

The clinical manifestations of toxicity caused by 5FU and floxuridine are similar. The earliest untoward symptoms during a course of therapy are anorexia and nausea, followed by stomatitis and diarrhea, reliable warning signs that a sufficient dose has been administered. Mucosal ulcerations occur throughout the GI tract and may lead to fulminant diarrhea, shock, and death, particularly in patients who are DPD deficient. The major toxic effects of bolus-dose regimens result from the myelosuppressive action of 5FU. The nadir of leukopenia usually occurs 9–14 days after the first injection of drug. Thrombocytopenia and anemia also may occur, as may loss of hair (occasionally progressing to total alopecia), nail changes, dermatitis, and increased pigmentation and atrophy of the skin. Hand-foot syndrome, a particularly prominent adverse effect of capecitabine, consists of erythema, desquamation, pain, and sensitivity to touch of the palms and soles. Acute chest pain with evidence of ischemia in the electrocardiogram may result from coronary artery vasospasms during or shortly after 5FU infusion. In general, myelosuppression, mucositis, and diarrhea occur less often with infusional than with bolus regimens, while hand-foot syndrome occurs more often with infusional than with bolus regimens. The significant risk of toxicity with fluoropyrimidines requires close supervision by physicians familiar with the drug's effects and possible hazards.

Capecitabine causes a similar spectrum of toxicities as 5FU (diarrhea, myelosuppression), but the hand-foot syndrome occurs more frequently and may require dose reduction or cessation of therapy.

Trifluridine

Trifluridine is a trifluoro nucleoside analogue of FUdR (see Figure 66–8). It is used in eye drops for the treatment of HSV and in a fixed combination with *tipiracil*, a thymidine phosphorylase inhibitor, for the treatment of patients with metastatic colorectal cancers who have previously received other standard combination treatments that included FOLFIRINOX. *Trifluridine* and *tipiracil* are formulated together in a single tablet with tipiracil added to prevent rapid breakdown of trifluridine. The trifluridine mechanism of action mimics that of 5FU (Davidson et al., 2016).

Cytidine Analogues

Cytarabine (Cytosine Arabinoside; Ara-C)

Cytarabine is the most important antimetabolite used in the therapy of AML; it is the single most effective agent for induction of remission in this disease.

Mechanisms of Action

Cytarabine is an analogue of 2′-deoxycytidine; the 2′-hydroxyl in a position *trans* to the 3′-hydroxyl of the sugar (see Figures 66–7 and 66–8) hinders rotation of the pyrimidine base around the nucleoside bond and interferes with base pairing. The drug enters cells via ENT1 (or SLC29A1). It is then converted to its active form, the 5′-monophosphate ribonucleotide, by dCK, an enzyme that shows polymorphic expression amongst patients (see discussion that follows). Ara-CMP then reacts with deoxynucleotide kinases to form diphosphate and triphosphates (Ara-CDP and Ara-CTP). Ara-CTP competes with dCTP for incorporation into DNA by DNA polymerases. The incorporated Ara-CMP residue is a potent inhibitor of DNA polymerase, in both replication and repair synthesis, and blocks the further elongation of the nascent DNA molecule. If DNA breaks are not repaired, apoptosis ensues. Ara-C cytotoxicity correlates with the total Ara-C incorporated into DNA; incorporation of about 5 molecules of Ara-C per 10^4 bases of DNA decreases cellular clonogenicity by about 50% (Kufe et al., 1984).

In infants and adults with ALL and t(4;11) MLL translocation, high-dose Ara-C is particularly effective; in these patients, the nucleoside transporter ENT1 is highly expressed, and its expression correlates with sensitivity to Ara-C (Pui et al., 2004). At extracellular drug concentrations greater than 10 μM (levels achievable with high-dose Ara-C), the nucleoside transporter no longer limits drug accumulation, and intracellular metabolism to a triphosphate becomes rate limiting. Patients with particular subtypes of AML derive benefit from high-dose Ara-C treatment; these types include t(8;21), inv(16), t(9;16), and del(16). Approximately 20% of patients with AML have leukemic cells with a *KRAS* mutation, and these patients seem to derive greater benefit from high-dose Ara-C regimens than do patients with wild-type *KRAS*.

Mechanisms of Resistance

Response to Ara-C is strongly influenced by the relative activities of anabolic and catabolic enzymes that determine the proportion of drug converted to Ara-CTP. The rate-limiting activating enzyme dCK produces Ara-CMP. It is opposed by the degradative enzyme, cytidine deaminase, which converts Ara-C to a nontoxic metabolite, Ara-U. Cytidine deaminase activity is high in many normal tissues, including intestinal mucosa, liver, and neutrophils, but lower in AML cells and other human tumors. A second degradative enzyme, dCMP deaminase, converts Ara-CMP to the inactive metabolite Ara-UMP. Increased synthesis and retention of Ara-CTP in leukemic cells lead to a longer duration of complete remission in patients with AML. The capacity of cells to transport Ara-C also may affect response. Clinical studies have implicated a loss of dCK as the primary mechanism of resistance to Ara-C in AML.

ADME

Due to the presence of high concentrations of cytidine deaminase in the GI mucosa and liver, only about 20% of the drug reaches the circulation after *oral* Ara-C administration; thus, the drug must be given intravenously. Peak concentrations of 2–50 µM are measurable in plasma after intravenous injection of 30–300 mg/m² but fall rapidly ($t_{1/2} \approx 10$ min). Less than 10% of the injected dose is excreted unchanged in the urine within 12–24 h; most appears as the inactive deaminated product, Ara-U. Higher concentrations of Ara-C are found in CSF after continuous infusion than after rapid intravenous injection but are 10% or less of concentrations in plasma. After *intrathecal* administration of the drug at a dose of 50 mg/m², deamination proceeds slowly, with a $t_{1/2}$ of 3–4 h, and peak concentrations of 1–2 µM are achieved. CSF concentrations remain above the threshold for cytotoxicity (0.4 µM) for 24 h or longer. A depot liposomal formulation of Ara-C provides sustained release into the CSF. After a standard dose, liposomal Ara-C remains above cytotoxic levels for an average of 12 days, thus avoiding the need for frequent lumbar punctures.

Therapeutic Uses

Continuous inhibition of DNA synthesis for a duration equivalent to at least one cell cycle or 24 h is necessary to expose most tumor cells during the S phase of the cell cycle. The optimal interval between bolus doses of Ara-C is about 8–12 h, a schedule that maintains intracellular concentrations of Ara-CTP at inhibitory levels during a multiday cycle of treatment. In general, children tolerate higher doses than adults. The intrathecal administration of liposomal cytarabine every 2 weeks seems equally effective as the regimen every 4 days with the standard drug. Ara-C is indicated for induction and maintenance of remission in AML and is useful in the treatment of patients with other leukemias, such as ALL, CML in the blast phase, APL, and high-grade lymphomas. Because drug concentration in plasma rapidly falls below the level needed to saturate transport and intracellular activation, clinicians have employed high-dose regimens every 12 h for 3–4 days to achieve 20–50 times higher serum levels, with improved results in remission induction and consolidation for AML. Injection of the liposomal formulation is indicated for the intrathecal treatment of lymphomatous meningitis.

Adverse Effects

Cytarabine is myelosuppressive and can produce acute, severe leukopenia, thrombocytopenia, and anemia with striking megaloblastic changes. Other toxic manifestations include GI disturbances, stomatitis, conjunctivitis, reversible hepatic enzyme elevations, noncardiogenic pulmonary edema, and dermatitis. The onset of dyspnea, fever, and pulmonary infiltrates on chest computed tomographic scans may follow 1–2 weeks after high-dose Ara-C and may be fatal in 10%–20% of patients, especially in patients being treated for relapsed leukemia. No specific therapy, other than Ara-C discontinuation, is indicated. Intrathecal Ara-C, either the free drug or the liposomal preparation, may cause arachnoiditis, seizures, delirium, myelopathy,

or coma, especially if given concomitantly with systemic high-dose MTX or systemic Ara-C. Cerebellar toxicity, manifesting as ataxia and slurred speech, and cerebral toxicity (seizures, dementia, and coma) may follow intrathecal administration or high-dose systemic administration, especially in patients older than 40 years or patients with poor renal function.

Azacitidine (5-Azacytidine); Decitabine

5-Azacytidine (Figure 66–7) and decitabine (2′-deoxy-5-azacytidine; Figure 66–8) have antileukemic activity and induce differentiation by inhibiting DNA cytosine methyltransferase activity. Both drugs are approved for treatment of myelodysplasia, for which they induce normalization of bone marrow in 15%–20% of patients and reduce the transfusion requirement in one-third of patients. 5-Azacytidine improves survival.

Mechanism of Action

The aza-nucleosides enter cells by ENT1 (SLC29A1). The drugs incorporate into DNA, where they become covalently bound to the DNA methyltransferase, depleting intracellular enzyme and leading to global demethylation of DNA that results in tumor cell differentiation and apoptosis. Decitabine also induces double-strand DNA breaks, perhaps as a consequence of the effort to repair the protein-DNA adduct.

ADME

After subcutaneous administration, 5-azacytidine undergoes rapid deamination by cytidine deaminase (plasma $t_{1/2} \sim$ 20–40 min). Due to the formation of intracellular nucleotides that become incorporated into DNA, the effects of the aza-nucleosides persist for many hours.

Therapeutic Use

The usual treatment regimen for 5-azacytidine in patients with MDS is daily for 7 days every 28 days, while decitabine is given intravenously every day for 5 days every 4 weeks. Best responses may become apparent only after two to five courses of treatment.

Adverse Effects

The major toxicities of the aza-nucleosides include myelosuppression and mild GI symptoms. 5-Azacytidine produces severe nausea and vomiting when given intravenously in large doses (150–200 mg/m²/d for 5 days).

Gemcitabine

Gemcitabine, a difluoro analogue of deoxycytidine (dFdC; see Figure 66–8), is used for patients with metastatic pancreatic; non-squamous, non–small cell lung; ovarian; and bladder cancer.

Mechanism of Action

Gemcitabine enters cells via three distinct nucleoside transporters: ENT1 (SLC29A1; the major route); CNT1 (SLC28A1); and a nucleobase transporter found in malignant mesothelioma cells. Intracellularly, dCK phosphorylates gemcitabine to the monophosphate (dFdCMP), which is converted to di- and triphosphates (dFdCDP and dFdCTP, respectively). Although gemcitabine's anabolism and effects on DNA in general mimic those of cytarabine, there are distinct differences in kinetics of inhibition, additional enzymatic sites of action, different effects of incorporation into DNA, and a distinct spectrum of clinical activity. Unlike that of cytarabine, the cytotoxicity of gemcitabine is not confined to the S phase of the cell cycle. The cytotoxic activity may reflect several actions on DNA synthesis. dFdCTP competes with dCTP as a weak inhibitor of DNA polymerase. dFdCDP is a stoichiometric inhibitor of RNR, resulting in depletion of deoxyribonucleotide pools necessary for DNA synthesis. Incorporation of dFdCTP into DNA causes DNA strand termination (Heinemann et al., 1988) and appears resistant to repair. The capacity of cells to incorporate dFdCTP into DNA is critical for gemcitabine-induced apoptosis. Gemcitabine is inactivated by cytidine deaminase, which is found both in tumor cells and throughout the body.

ADME

Gemcitabine is administered as an intravenous infusion. The pharmacokinetics of the parent compound are largely determined by deamination in liver, plasma, and other organs, and the predominant urinary elimination product is dFdU. In patients with significant renal dysfunction, dFdU and its triphosphate accumulate to high and potentially toxic levels. Gemcitabine has a short plasma $t_{1/2}$ (~15 min); women and elderly patients clear the drug more slowly.

Therapeutic Uses

The standard dosing schedule for gemcitabine is an intravenous infusion on days 1, 8, and 15 of each 21- to 28-day cycle, depending on the indication. Conversion of gemcitabine to dFdCMP by dCK is saturated at infusion rates of about 10 mg/m²/min. To increase dFdCTP formation, the duration of infusion at this maximum concentration has been extended to 100–150 min at a fixed rate of 10 mg/min. The 150-min infusion produces a higher level of dFdCTP within peripheral blood mononuclear cells and increases the degree of myelosuppression. The inhibition of DNA repair by gemcitabine may increase cytotoxicity of other agents, particularly platinum compounds, and with radiation therapy.

Adverse Effects

The principal toxicity is myelosuppression. Longer duration infusions lead to greater myelosuppression and hepatic toxicity. Nonhematological toxicities include a flu-like syndrome, asthenia, and rarely a posterior leukoencephalopathy syndrome. Mild, reversible elevation in liver transaminases may occur in 40% or more of patients. Interstitial pneumonitis, at times progressing to ARDS, may occur within the first two cycles of treatment and usually responds to corticosteroids. Rarely, patients treated for many months may develop a slowly progressive hemolytic uremic syndrome, necessitating drug discontinuation. Gemcitabine is a very potent radiosensitizer and should not be used with radiotherapy.

Purine Analogues

The pioneering studies of Hitchings and Elion identified analogues of naturally occurring purine bases with antileukemic and immunosuppressant properties. Figure 66–9 shows structural formulas of several purine analogues, with adenosine for comparison. Other purine analogues that have valuable roles in leukemia and lymphoid malignancies include cladribine (standard therapy of hairy cell leukemia), fludarabine phosphate (standard treatment of CLL), nelarabine (pediatric ALL), and clofarabine (T-cell leukemia/lymphoma). The apparent selectivity of these agents may relate to their effective uptake, activation, and apoptotic effects in lymphoid tissue.

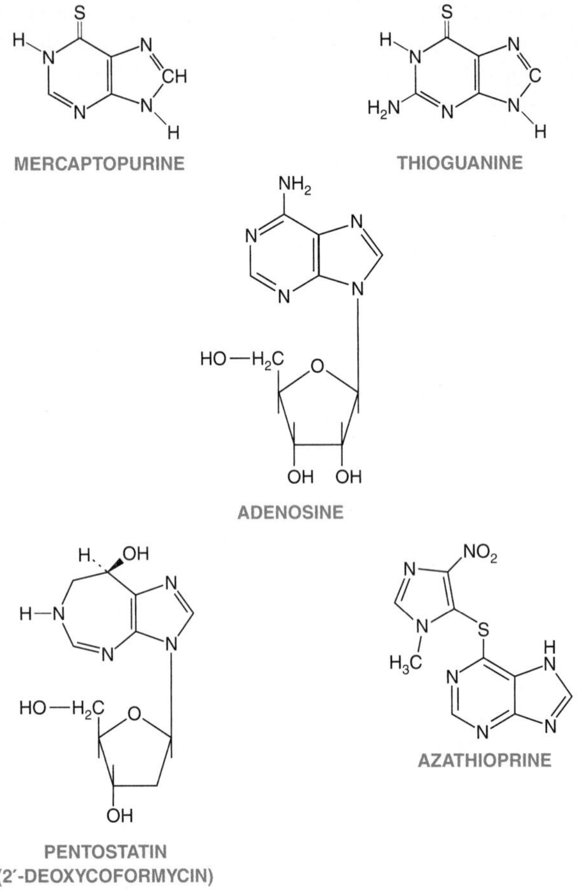

6-Thiopurine Analogues

6-Mercaptopurine and 6TG are approved agents for human leukemias and function as analogues of the natural purines hypoxanthine and guanine. The substitution of sulfur for oxygen on C6 of the purine ring creates compounds that are readily transported into cells, including activated malignant cells. Nucleotides formed from 6MP and 6TG inhibit de novo purine synthesis and also become incorporated into nucleic acids (Figure 51–5).

Mechanism of Action

Hypoxanthine guanine phosphoribosyl transferase converts 6TG and 6MP to the ribonucleotides 6-thioGMP and 6-thioIMP (T-IMP), respectively. Because T-IMP is a poor substrate for guanylyl kinase (the enzyme that converts GMP to GDP), T-IMP accumulates intracellularly. T-IMP inhibits the new formation of ribosyl-5-phosphate, as well as conversion of IMP to adenine and guanine nucleotides. The most important point of attack seems to be the reaction of glutamine and PRPP to form ribosyl-5-phosphate, the first committed step in the de novo pathway. 6TG nucleotide is incorporated into DNA, where it induces strand breaks and base mispairing.

Mechanisms of Resistance

The most common mechanism of 6MP resistance observed in vitro is deficiency or complete lack of the activating enzyme HGPRT or increased alkaline phosphatase activity. Other mechanisms for resistance include

- decreased drug uptake or increased efflux due to active transporters;
- alteration in allosteric inhibition of ribosylamine 5-phosphate synthase; and
- impaired recognition of DNA breaks and mismatches due to loss of a component (MSH6) of MMR system (Karran and Attard, 2008).

Figure 66–9 *Adenosine and various purine analogues.*

ADME and Toxicity

Absorption of oral mercaptopurine is incomplete (10%–50%); the drug is subject to first-pass metabolism by xanthine oxidase in the liver. Food or oral antibiotics decrease absorption. Oral bioavailability is increased when mercaptopurine is combined with high-dose MTX. After an intravenous dose, the $t_{1/2}$ of the drug is about 50 min in adults due to rapid metabolic degradation by xanthine oxidase and by TPMT. Restricted brain distribution of mercaptopurine results from an efficient efflux transport system in the blood-brain barrier. In addition to the HGPRT-catalyzed anabolism of mercaptopurine, there are two other pathways for its metabolism. The first involves methylation of the sulfhydryl group and subsequent oxidation of the methylated derivatives. Activity of the enzyme TPMT reflects the inheritance of polymorphic alleles; up to 15% of the Caucasian population has decreased enzyme activity. Low levels of erythrocyte TPMT activity are associated with increased drug toxicity in individual patients and a lower risk of relapse. In patients with autoimmune disease treated with mercaptopurine, those with polymorphic alleles may experience bone marrow aplasia and life-threatening toxicity. Testing for these polymorphisms prior to treatment is recommended in this patient population.

A relatively large percentage of the administered sulfur appears in the urine as inorganic sulfate. The second major pathway for 6MP metabolism involves its oxidation by xanthine oxidase to 6-thiourate, an inactive metabolite. Oral doses of 6MP should be reduced by 75% in patients receiving the xanthine oxidase inhibitor allopurinol; no dose adjustment is required for intravenous dosing.

Therapeutic Uses

In the maintenance therapy of ALL, an initial daily oral dose of 6MP is adjusted according to white blood cell and platelet counts. The combination of MTX and 6MP appears to be synergistic. By inhibiting the earliest steps in purine synthesis, MTX elevates the intracellular concentration of PRPP, a cofactor required for 6MP activation.

Adverse Effects

The principal toxicity of 6MP is myelosuppression. Thrombocytopenia, granulocytopenia, or anemia may not become apparent for several weeks. Dose reduction usually results in prompt recovery, although myelosuppression may be severe and prolonged in patients with a polymorphism affecting TPMT. Anorexia, nausea, or vomiting is seen in about 25% of adults, but stomatitis and diarrhea are rare; manifestations of GI effects are less frequent in children than in adults. Jaundice and hepatic enzyme elevations occur in up to one-third of adult patients treated with 6MP and usually resolve on discontinuation of therapy. 6MP and its derivative azathioprine predispose to opportunistic infection (e.g., reactivation of hepatitis B, fungal infection, and *Pneumocystis* pneumonia) and an increased incidence of squamous cell malignancies of the skin. 6MP is teratogenic during the first trimester of pregnancy, and AML has been reported after prolonged 6MP therapy for Crohn disease.

Fludarabine Phosphate

Fludarabine phosphate is a fluorinated, deamination-resistant, phosphorylated analogue of the antiviral agent vidarabine (9-β-D-arabinofuranosyl-adenine). It is active in CLL and low-grade lymphomas and is also effective as a potent immunosuppressant.

FLUDARABINE PHOSPHATE

Mechanisms of Action and Resistance

The drug is dephosphorylated extracellularly to the nucleoside fludarabine, which enters the cell and is rephosphorylated by dCK to the active triphosphate. This antimetabolite inhibits DNA polymerase, DNA primase, DNA ligase, and RNR and becomes incorporated into DNA and RNA. The nucleotide is an effective chain terminator when incorporated into DNA (Kamiya et al., 1996). Incorporation of fludarabine into RNA inhibits RNA function, RNA processing, and mRNA translation.

In experimental tumors, resistance to fludarabine is associated with decreased activity of dCK (the enzyme that phosphorylates the drug), increased drug efflux, and increased RNR activity. Its mechanism of immunosuppression and paradoxical stimulation of autoimmunity stems from the particular susceptibility of lymphoid cells to purine analogues and the specific effects on the CD4$^+$ subset of T cells, as well as its inhibition of regulatory T-cell responses.

ADME

Fludarabine phosphate is administered both intravenously and orally and is rapidly converted to fludarabine in the plasma. The median time to reach maximal concentrations of drug in plasma after oral administration is 1.5 h, and oral bioavailability averages 55%–60%. The $t_{1/2}$ of fludarabine in plasma is about 10 h. The compound is eliminated primarily by renal excretion.

Therapeutic Uses

Fludarabine phosphate is approved for intravenous and oral use and is equally active by both routes. The recommended dose interval is daily for 5 days and may be repeated every 4 weeks. Gradual improvement in CLL usually occurs within two to three cycles. Dosage should be reduced in patients with renal impairment in proportion to the reduction in CL_{Cr}. Fludarabine phosphate is highly active alone or with rituximab and cyclophosphamide for the treatment of patients with CLL; overall response rates in previously untreated patients approximate 80%, and the duration of response averages 22 months. The synergy of fludarabine with alkylators may stem from the observation that it blocks the repair of double-strand DNA breaks and interstrand cross-links induced by alkylating agents. It also is effective in follicular B-cell lymphomas refractory to standard therapy. It is increasingly used as a potent immunosuppressive agent in nonmyeloablative allogeneic bone marrow transplantation.

Adverse Effects

Oral and intravenous therapy cause myelosuppression in about 50% of patients, nausea and vomiting in a minor fraction, and, uncommonly, chills and fever, malaise, anorexia, peripheral neuropathy, and weakness. Lymphopenia and thrombocytopenia and cumulative side effects are expected. Depletion of CD4$^+$ T cells with therapy predisposes to opportunistic infections. Tumor lysis syndrome, a rare complication, occurs primarily in previously untreated patients with CLL. Altered mental status, seizures, optic neuritis, and coma have been observed at higher doses and in older patients. Autoimmune events may occur after fludarabine treatment. Patients with CLL may develop an acute hemolytic anemia or pure red cell aplasia during or following fludarabine treatment. Prolonged cytopenias, probably mediated by autoimmunity, also complicate fludarabine treatment. Myelodysplasia and acute leukemias may arise as late complications. Pneumonitis is an occasional side effect and responds to corticosteroids. In patients with compromised renal function, the initial doses should be reduced in proportion to the reduction in CL_{Cr}.

Cladribine

Cladribine is an ADA-resistant purine analogue that has potent and curative activity in hairy cell leukemia, CLL, and low-grade lymphomas.

Mechanisms of Action and Resistance

Cladribine enters cells via active nucleoside transport. After phosphorylation by dCK and conversion to cladribine triphosphate, it is incorporated into DNA. It produces DNA strand breaks and depletion of NAD and ATP, leading to apoptosis. It is a potent inhibitor of RNR. The drug does not require cell division to be cytotoxic. Resistance is associated with loss of the activating enzyme dCK; increased expression of RNR; or increased active efflux by ABCG2 or other members of the ABC family of transporters.

ADME

Cladribine is absorbed orally (55%) but is routinely administered intravenously. It is excreted by the kidneys, with a terminal $t_{1/2}$ in plasma of 6.7 h. Cladribine crosses the blood-brain barrier and reaches CSF concentrations of about 25% of those seen in plasma. Doses should be adjusted for renal dysfunction.

Therapeutic Uses

Cladribine is administered daily for 7 days by continuous intravenous infusion. It is the drug of choice in hairy cell leukemia. Eighty percent of patients achieve a complete response after a single course of therapy. The drug also is active in CLL; low-grade lymphomas; Langerhans cell histiocytosis; CTCLs, including mycosis fungoides and the Sézary syndrome; and Waldenström macroglobulinemia.

Adverse Effects

The major dose-limiting toxicity of cladribine is myelosuppression. Cumulative thrombocytopenia may occur with repeated courses. Opportunistic infections are common and correlate with decreased CD4$^+$ cell counts. Other toxic effects include nausea, infections, high fever, headache, fatigue, skin rashes, and tumor lysis syndrome.

Clofarabine (2-Chloro-2′-fluoro-arabinosyladenine)

The analogue clofarabine (2-chloro-2′-fluoro-arabinosyladenine) incorporates the 2-chloro, glycosylase-resistant substituent of cladribine and a 2′-fluoro-arabinosyl substitution, which adds stability and enhances uptake and phosphorylation. The resulting compound is approved for the treatment of pediatric ALL after failure of two prior therapies. Clofarabine produces complete remissions in 20%–30% of these patients.

It has activity in pediatric and adult AML and in myelodysplasia. The uptake and metabolic activation of clofarabine in tumor cells follow the same path as cladribine and the other purine nucleosides, although clofarabine is more readily phosphorylated by dCK. Clofarabine triphosphate has a long intracellular $t_{1/2}$ (24 h). It incorporates into DNA, where it terminates DNA synthesis and leads to apoptosis; clofarabine also inhibits RNR.

Therapeutic Uses and Adverse Effects

In children, clofarabine is administered as a 2-h infusion daily for 5 days. The primary elimination $t_{1/2}$ in plasma is 6.5 h. Most of the drug is excreted unchanged in the urine. Doses should be adjusted according to reductions in CL_{Cr}. The primary toxicities are myelosuppression; a clinical syndrome of hypotension, tachyphemia, pulmonary edema, organ dysfunction, and fever, all suggestive of capillary leak syndrome and cytokine release that necessitate immediate discontinuation of the drug; elevated hepatic enzymes and increased bilirubin; nausea, vomiting, and diarrhea; and hypokalemia and hypophosphatemia.

Nelarabine (6-Methoxy-arabinosyl-guanine)

Nelarabine (6-methoxy-arabinosyl-guanine) is the only guanine nucleoside in clinical use. It has selective activity against acute T-cell leukemia (20% complete responses) and the closely related T-cell lymphoblastic lymphoma and is approved for use in patients with relapsed/refractory disease. Its basic mechanism of action closely resembles that of the other purine nucleosides, in that it is incorporated into DNA and terminates DNA synthesis.

ADME

Following infusion, the parent methoxy compound is rapidly activated in blood and tissues by ADA–mediated cleavage of the methyl group, yielding the phosphorylase resistant Ara-G, which has a plasma $t_{1/2}$ of 3 h. The active metabolite is transported into tumor cells, where it is activated by dCK to Ara-GTP, which incorporates into DNA and terminates DNA synthesis. The drug and its metabolite Ara-G are primarily eliminated by metabolism to guanine, and a smaller fraction is eliminated by renal excretion of Ara-G. The drug should be used with close clinical monitoring in patients with severe renal impairment (CL_{Cr} < 50 mg/mL). Adults are given a 2-h infusion on days 1, 3, and 5 of a 21-day cycle, and children are given a lower dose for 5 days, repeated every 21 days.

Adverse Effects

The adverse effects include myelosuppression and liver function test abnormalities, as well as infrequent serious neurological sequelae, such as seizures, delirium, somnolence, peripheral neuropathy, or Guillain-Barré syndrome. Neurological adverse effects may not be reversible.

Pentostatin (2′-Deoxycoformycin)

Pentostatin (2′-deoxycoformycin; see Figure 66–9), a transition-state analogue of the intermediate in the ADA reaction, potently inhibits ADA. Its effects mimic the phenotype of genetic ADA deficiency (severe immunodeficiency affecting T-cell and B-cell functions).

Mechanism of Action

Inhibition of ADA by pentostatin leads to accumulation of intracellular adenosine and deoxyadenosine nucleotides, which can block DNA synthesis by inhibiting RNR. Deoxyadenosine also inactivates S-adenosyl homocysteine hydrolase. The resulting accumulation of S-adenosyl homocysteine is particularly toxic to lymphocytes. Pentostatin also can inhibit RNA synthesis, and its triphosphate derivative is incorporated into DNA, resulting in strand breakage. Although the precise mechanism of cytotoxicity is not known, it is probable that the imbalance in purine nucleotide pools accounts for its antineoplastic effect in hairy cell leukemia and T-cell lymphomas.

ADME

Pentostatin is administered intravenously every other week and has a mean terminal $t_{1/2}$ of 5.7 h. After hydration with 500–1000 mL of 5% dextrose in half-normal (0.45%) saline, the drug is administered by rapid intravenous injection or by infusion over a period of 30 min or less, followed by an additional 500 mL of fluids. The drug is eliminated almost entirely by renal excretion. Proportional reduction of dosage is recommended in patients with renal impairment as measured by reduced Cl_{Cr}.

Therapeutic Use

Pentostatin is effective in producing complete remissions (58%) and partial responses (28%) in patients with hairy cell leukemia. It largely has been superseded by cladribine (see previous discussion). Toxic manifestations include myelosuppression, GI symptoms, skin rashes, and abnormal liver function studies. Depletion of normal T cells occurs, and neutropenic fever and opportunistic infections may result. Immunosuppression may persist for several years after discontinuation. At high doses, major renal and neurological complications are encountered. Pentostatin in combination with fludarabine phosphate may result in severe or even fatal pulmonary toxicity.

III. Natural Products

Microtubule-Damaging Agents

Vinca Alkaloids

Purified alkaloids from the periwinkle plant, including *vinblastine* and *vincristine*, were amongst the earliest clinical agents for the treatment of patients with leukemias, lymphomas, and testicular cancer. A closely related derivative, *vinorelbine*, has activity against lung and breast cancer.

Basic structure of vinca alkaloids

Mechanism of Action

The vinca alkaloids are cell-cycle–specific agents and, in common with other drugs, such as colchicine, podophyllotoxin, the taxanes, and the epothilones, block cells in mitosis. The biological activities of the vincas can be explained by their ability to bind specifically to β-tubulin and to block its polymerization with α-tubulin into microtubules (Akhmanova and Steinmetz, 2015). The mitotic spindle cannot form, duplicated chromosomes cannot align along the division plate, and cell division arrests in metaphase. Cells blocked in mitosis undergo changes characteristic of apoptosis. Microtubules are found in high concentration in the brain and contribute to other cellular functions, such as movement, phagocytosis, and axonal transport. Adverse effects of the vinca alkaloids, such as their neurotoxicity, may relate to disruption of these functions.

Resistance

Despite their structural similarity, the individual vinca alkaloids have unique patterns of clinical efficacy (see discussion that follows). However, in most experimental systems, they share cross-resistance. Their antitumor effects are blocked by multidrug resistance mediated by Pgp, which confers resistance to a broad range of agents (vinca alkaloids, epipodophyllotoxins, anthracyclines, and taxanes). Pgp, also known as MDR1, ABCB1, and CD243, is an ATP-dependent efflux pump with broad substrate specificity that provides a cellular defense mechanism against potentially harmful substances. Chromosomal abnormalities consistent with gene amplification and markedly increased levels of Pgp have been observed in resistant cells in culture. Other membrane transporters, such as the MRP and the closely related BCRP, may contribute to resistance. Other forms of resistance to vinca alkaloids stem from mutations in β-tubulin or in the relative expression of isoforms of β-tubulin that prevent the inhibitors from effectively binding to their target.

Adverse Effects

The limited myelosuppressive activity of vincristine makes it a valuable component of several combination therapy regimens for leukemia and lymphoma, while the lack of severe neurotoxicity of vinblastine is a decided advantage in lymphomas and in combination with cisplatin against testicular cancer. Vinorelbine, which causes mild neurotoxicity and myelosuppression, has an intermediate toxicity profile.

ADME

Hepatic CYPs extensively metabolize all three drugs, and the metabolites are excreted in the bile. Only a small fraction of a dose (<15%) is found unchanged in the urine. In patients with hepatic dysfunction (bilirubin > 3 mg/dL), a 50%–75% reduction in dose of any of the vinca alkaloids is advisable. The elimination $t_{1/2}$ is 20 h for vincristine, 23 h for vinblastine, and 24 h for vinorelbine.

Vinblastine

Therapeutic Uses. Vinblastine sulfate is given intravenously; special precautions must be taken against subcutaneous extravasation, which may cause painful irritation and ulceration. The drug should not be injected into an extremity with impaired circulation. After a single dose, myelosuppression reaches its maximum in 7–10 days. If a moderate level of leukopenia (~3000 cells/mm³) is not attained, the weekly dose may be increased gradually. For testicular cancer, vinblastine is administered every 3 weeks. Doses should be reduced by 50% for patients with plasma bilirubin > 1.5 mg/dL. Vinblastine is used with bleomycin and cisplatin in the curative therapy of patients with metastatic testicular cancer, although it has been mainly supplanted by etoposide (see further discussion) or ifosfamide (see previous material). It is a component of the standard curative ABVD regimen for Hodgkin lymphoma. Vinblastine also is active against Kaposi sarcoma, neuroblastoma, Langerhans cell histiocytosis, bladder cancer, carcinoma of the breast, and choriocarcinoma.

Adverse Effects. Maximal leukopenia occurs within 7–10 days, after which recovery ensues within 7 days. Other toxic effects of vinblastine include mild neurological manifestations. GI disturbances, including nausea, vomiting, anorexia, and diarrhea, may be encountered. The syndrome of inappropriate secretion of antidiuretic hormone has been reported. Loss of hair, stomatitis, and dermatitis occur infrequently. Extravasation during injection may lead to cellulitis and phlebitis.

Vincristine

Therapeutic Uses. Vincristine is a standard component of regimens for treating pediatric patients with leukemias, lymphomas, and solid tumors, such as Wilms tumor, neuroblastoma, and rhabdomyosarcoma. In large-cell non-Hodgkin lymphomas, vincristine remains an important agent, particularly when used in the CHOP regimen. Vincristine with glucocorticoids is the treatment of choice to induce remissions in patients with childhood leukemia and in combination with alkylating agents and anthracycline for those with pediatric sarcomas. The common intravenous dosage for vincristine is 2 mg/m² of body surface area at weekly or longer intervals. Vincristine is tolerated better by children than by adults, who may experience severe, progressive neurological toxicity and require lowering of the dose. Administration of the drug more frequently than every 7 days or at higher doses increases the toxic manifestations without proportional improvement in the response rate. Precautions also should be used to avoid extravasation during intravenous administration. Doses should be reduced for patients with elevated plasma bilirubin.

Adverse Effects. The clinical toxicity of vincristine is mostly neurological. Severe neurological manifestations may be reversed by suspending therapy or reducing the dosage at the first sign of motor dysfunction. Severe constipation, sometimes resulting in colicky abdominal pain and obstruction, may be prevented by laxatives and hydrophilic (bulk-forming) agents

and usually is a problem only with doses greater than 2 mg/m². Reversible alopecia occurs in about 20% of patients. Modest leukopenia may occur. Thrombocytopenia, anemia, and the syndrome of inappropriate secretion of antidiuretic hormone are less common. Inadvertent injection of vincristine into the CSF causes a devastating and often-fatal irreversible coma and seizures.

Vinorelbine

Vinorelbine has activity against non–small cell lung cancer and breast cancer. Vinorelbine is administered in normal saline as an intravenous infusion over 6–10 min. When used alone, it is given at doses of 30 mg/m² either weekly or for 2 of every 3 weeks. When used with cisplatin for the treatment of non–small cell lung cancer, it is given at doses of 25 mg/m² either weekly or for 3 of every 4 weeks. A lower dose (20–25 mg/m²) may be required for patients who have received prior chemotherapy and for hematological toxicity. The primary adverse effect of vinorelbine is granulocytopenia, with only modest thrombocytopenia and less neurotoxicity than other vinca alkaloids. Vinorelbine may cause allergic reactions and mild, reversible changes in liver enzymes. Doses should be reduced in patients with elevated plasma bilirubin.

Eribulin

Eribulin is a synthetic analogue of halichondrin, a poly-ether macrolide, originally isolated from the Pacific marine sponge *Halichondria okadai*. The drug binds to the vinca alkaloid site on β-tubulin and inhibits microtubule assembly. Eribulin is a poorer substrate than other microtubule disruptors for the Pgp efflux pump and is effective in drug-resistant tumors that overexpress Pgp. Eribulin is approved for the treatment of patients with drug-resistant metastatic breast cancer and liposarcoma. Adverse effects overlap with those of the vinca alkaloids and include neutropenia, neuropathies, and GI toxicities.

Taxanes

Paclitaxel was first isolated from the bark of the Western yew tree. Paclitaxel and its semisynthetic congeners *docetaxel* and *cabazitaxel*, exhibit unique pharmacological properties as inhibitors of mitosis. These taxanes differ from the vinca alkaloids and colchicine derivatives in that they bind to a different site on β-tubulin and promote rather than inhibit microtubule formation (Figure 66–10), stabilizing tubulin-GDP (Akhmanova and Steinmetz, 2015). The taxanes have a central role in the therapy of patients with ovarian, breast, lung, GI, genitourinary, prostate, and head and neck cancers.

Core structure of taxanes

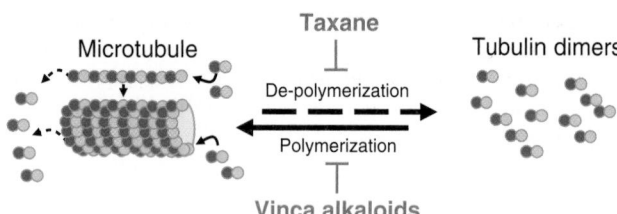

Microtubule   Taxane   Tubulin dimers

De-polymerization

Polymerization

Vinca alkaloids

Figure 66–10 *Inhibitors of microtubular function.*

Mechanism of Action

Paclitaxel binds to the β-tubulin subunit on the inner surface of microtubules and antagonizes their disassembly (Figure 66–10), with the result that bundles of microtubules and aberrant structures derived from microtubules appear in the mitotic phase of the cell cycle. Arrest in mitosis follows. Cell death occurs by apoptosis and depends on both drug concentration and duration of drug exposure. Drugs that block cell-cycle progression prior to mitosis antagonize the toxic effects of taxanes.

Drug interactions have been noted. The sequence of cisplatin preceding paclitaxel decreases paclitaxel clearance and produces greater toxicity than the opposite schedule. Paclitaxel decreases doxorubicin clearance and enhances its cardiotoxicity; docetaxel has no apparent effect on anthracycline pharmacokinetics.

Resistance to taxanes can be a result of decreased cellular drug accumulation due to increased expression of membrane-bound efflux proteins, including MRP1 and Pgp. Cabazitaxel is a poor substrate for Pgp and may therefore be useful for treating multidrug-resistant tumors. Other mechanisms of resistance may include an increase in *survivin*, an antiapoptotic factor; an increase in α-*aurora kinase,* which promotes completion of mitosis; an upregulation of the βIII-isoform of tubulin that lacks taxane-binding capacity; or a direct alteration of the drug target by mutation.

ADME

Paclitaxel has limited water solubility and is administered in a vehicle of 50% ethanol and 50% polyethoxylated castor oil. Hepatic CYPs (primarily CYP2C8, secondarily CYP3A4) extensively metabolize the drug. The primary metabolite is 6-OH paclitaxel, which is inactive; multiple additional hydroxylation products are found in plasma; less than 10% of a dose is excreted in the urine intact. Dose reductions in patients with abnormal hepatic function have been suggested, and 50%–75% of doses of taxanes should be used in the presence of hepatic metastases larger than 2 cm in size or in patients with abnormal serum bilirubin. Drugs that induce CYP2C8 or CYP3A4, such as phenytoin and phenobarbital, or those that inhibit these CYPs, such as antifungal imidazoles, significantly alter drug clearance and toxicity.

Paclitaxel clearance is nonlinear and decreases with increasing dose or dose rate; the plasma $t_{1/2}$ is 10–14 h. The critical plasma concentration for myelosuppression depends on the duration of exposure but likely is 50–100 nM. Paclitaxel clearance is markedly delayed by cyclosporine A and other drugs that inhibit Pgp.

An albumin-bound nanoparticle solution for infusion (nab-paclitaxel) is soluble in aqueous solutions. This form of paclitaxel has increased cellular uptake via an albumin-specific mechanism. Nab-paclitaxel achieves a higher serum concentration than paclitaxel, but the increased clearance of nab-paclitaxel results in a similar systemic drug exposure. It is somewhat less neurotoxic than paclitaxel and is approved for metastatic non–small cell lung cancer. Like the other taxanes, nab-paclitaxel should not be given to patients with an absolute neutrophil count below 1500 cells/mm³.

Docetaxel, somewhat more soluble than paclitaxel, is administered intravenously in an emulsifier (polysorbate 80). Docetaxel pharmacokinetics are similar to those of paclitaxel, with an elimination $t_{1/2}$ of about 12 h. Clearance is primarily through CYP3A4- and CYP3A5-mediated hydroxylation, leading to inactive metabolites.

Therapeutic Uses

The taxanes have become central components of regimens for treating patients with metastatic ovarian, breast, lung, GI, genitourinary, and head and neck cancers. These drugs are administered once weekly or once every 3 weeks. Cabazitaxel is a poor substrate for Pgp and is approved for hormone-refractory metastatic prostate cancer previously treated with a docetaxel-containing regimen.

Adverse Effects

Paclitaxel exerts its primary toxic effects on the bone marrow. Neutropenia usually occurs 8–11 days after a dose and reverses rapidly by days 15–21. Used with G-CSF, high doses over 24 h are well tolerated, and peripheral neuropathy becomes dose limiting. Many patients experience myalgias after receiving paclitaxel. In high-dose schedules, or with prolonged use, a stocking-glove sensory neuropathy can be disabling, particularly in patients with underlying diabetic neuropathy or concurrent cisplatin therapy. Mucositis is prominent in 72- or 96-h infusions and in the weekly schedule. Hypersensitivity reactions can occur in patients receiving paclitaxel infusions of short duration (1–6 h) but are largely averted by pretreatment with dexamethasone, diphenhydramine, and histamine H_2 receptor antagonists. Premedication is not necessary with 96-h infusions. Many patients experience asymptomatic bradycardia; occasional episodes of silent ventricular tachycardia also occur and resolve spontaneously during 3- or 24-h infusions. Nab-paclitaxel produces increased rates of peripheral neuropathy compared to the original cremophor-delivered paclitaxel but rarely causes hypersensitivity reactions.

Docetaxel causes greater degrees of neutropenia than paclitaxel but less peripheral neuropathy and asthenia and less frequent hypersensitivity. Fluid retention is a progressive problem with multiple cycles of docetaxel therapy, leading to peripheral edema, pleural and peritoneal fluid, and pulmonary edema in extreme cases. Oral dexamethasone, begun 1 day prior to drug infusion and continuing for 3 days, greatly ameliorates fluid retention. In rare cases, docetaxel may cause progressive interstitial pneumonitis and respiratory failure if the drug is not discontinued.

Estramustine

Estramustine combines estradiol and normustine (nornitrogen mustard) through a carbamate link. Although the intent of the combination was to enhance the uptake of the alkylating agent into estradiol-sensitive prostate cancer cells, estramustine does not function in vivo as an alkylating agent; rather, it binds to β-tubulin and microtubule-associated proteins, causing microtubule disassembly and antimitotic actions.

Therapeutic Use

Estramustine is used solely for the treatment of patients with metastatic or locally advanced hormone-refractory prostate cancer.

ADME

Following oral administration, at least 75% of a dose of estramustine phosphate is absorbed from the GI tract and rapidly dephosphorylated. The drug undergoes extensive first-pass metabolism by hepatic CYPs to an active 17-keto derivative, estromustine, and to multiple inactive products; the active drug forms accumulate in the prostate. Some hydrolysis of the carbamate linkage occurs in the liver, releasing estradiol, estrone, and the normustine group. Estramustine and estromustine have plasma half-lives of 10 and 14 h, respectively, and are excreted as inactive metabolites, mainly in the feces.

Adverse Effects, Drug Interactions

In addition to myelosuppression, estramustine also possesses estrogenic side effects (gynecomastia, impotence, elevated risk of thrombosis, and fluid retention); hypercalcemia; acute attacks of porphyria; impaired glucose tolerance; and hypersensitivity reactions, including angioedema. Estramustine inhibits the clearance of taxanes.

Epothilones

The epothilones are polyketides discovered as cytotoxic metabolites from a strain of *Sorangium cellulosum*, a myxobacterium isolated from soil on the bank of the Zambezi River in southern Africa (Gerth et al., 1996). One of these, *ixabepilone*, is approved for breast cancer treatment; others are under development (Lee and Swain, 2008).

Ixabepilone

Mechanism of Action; Resistance. Epothilones bind to a β-tubulin site distinct from that of taxanes and trigger microtubule nucleation at multiple sites away from the centriole. This dysfunctional microtubule stabilization triggers cell-cycle arrest at the G_2-M interface and apoptosis. In vitro studies suggested that ixabepilone is less susceptible to Pgp-mediated export and multidrug resistance than taxanes. Mechanisms implicated in epothilone resistance include mutation of the β-tubulin binding site and upregulation of isoforms of β-tubulin.

ADME. Ixabepilone is administered intravenously. Because of its minimal aqueous solubility, it is delivered in the solubilizing agent cremophor (polyoxyethylated castor oil/ethanol), which has been implicated as the cause of infusion reactions; such reactions are infrequent when administration is preceded by premedication with H_1 and H_2 antagonists. The drug is cleared by hepatic CYPs and has a plasma $t_{1/2}$ of 52 h.

Therapeutic Uses. In patients with metastatic breast cancer resistant to or pretreated with anthracyclines and resistant to taxanes, ixabepilone plus capecitabine provides an improved progression-free survival of 1.6 months compared to capecitabine alone. Ixabepilone also is indicated as monotherapy for metastatic breast cancer in patients who have previously progressed through treatment with anthracyclines, taxanes, and capecitabine. Ixabepilone (~40 mg/m²) is administered as monotherapy or in combination with capecitabine over 3 h every 3 weeks. Patients should be premedicated with both an H_1 and an H_2 antagonist before receiving ixabepilone to minimize hypersensitivity reactions. In patients with mild-to-moderate hepatic dysfunction who receive ixabepilone monotherapy, lower starting doses are recommended due to delayed drug clearance.

Adverse Effects. Epothilones have toxicities similar to those of the taxanes: neutropenia, peripheral sensory neuropathy, fatigue, diarrhea, and asthenia.

Camptothecin Analogues

The camptothecins are potent, cytotoxic antineoplastic agents that target the nuclear enzyme *topoisomerase I*. The lead compound in this class, camptothecin, was isolated from the tree *Camptotheca acuminata*. *Irinotecan* and *topotecan*, currently the only camptothecin analogues approved for clinical use, have activity in colorectal, ovarian, and small cell lung cancer.

Chemistry

All camptothecins have a fused five-ring backbone that includes a labile lactone ring (Figure 66–11). The hydroxyl group and S conformation of the chiral center at C20 in the lactone ring are required for biological activity. Appropriate substitutions on the A and B rings of the quinoline

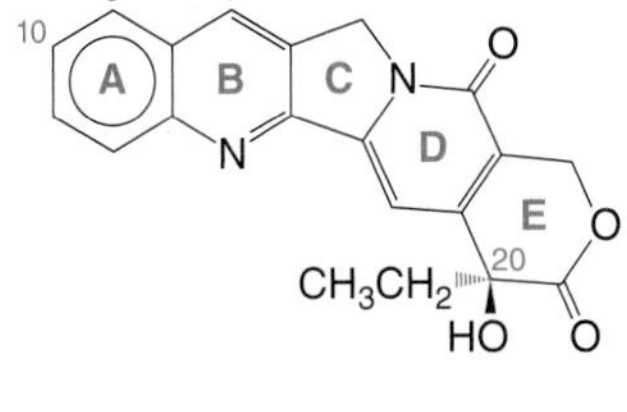

	C-10	C-9	C-7
Camptothecin	H	H	H
Topotecan	OH	$(CH_3)_2NHCH_2$	H
Irinotecan	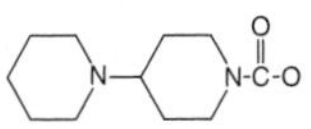 [piperidine-carbamate structure]	H	CH_2CH_3
SN-38	OH	H	CH_2CH_3

Figure 66–11 *Camptothecin and its analogues.*

subunit enhance water solubility and increase potency for inhibiting topoisomerase I. Topotecan is a semisynthetic molecule with a basic dimethylamino group that increases its water solubility. Irinotecan (CPT-11) differs from topotecan in that it is a prodrug. The carbamate bond between the camptothecin moiety and the dibasic bis-piperidine side chain at position C10 (which makes the molecule water soluble) is cleaved by a carboxylesterase to form the active metabolite SN-38 (see Figure 6–6).

Mechanism of Action

The DNA topoisomerases are nuclear enzymes that reduce torsional stress in supercoiled DNA, allowing selected regions of DNA to become sufficiently untangled to permit replication, repair, and transcription. Two classes of topoisomerase (I and II) mediate DNA strand breakage and resealing. Camptothecin analogues inhibit the function of topoisomerase I; other drugs, such as anthracyclines, epipodophyllotoxins, and acridines, inhibit topoisomerase II. The camptothecins bind to and stabilize the normally transient DNA–topoisomerase I cleavable complex. Although the initial cleavage action of topoisomerase I is not affected, the religation step is inhibited, leading to the accumulation of single-stranded breaks in DNA. These lesions are reversible and not by themselves toxic to the cell. However, the collision of a DNA replication fork with this cleaved strand of DNA causes an irreversible double-strand DNA break, ultimately leading to cell death.

Camptothecins are *S phase–specific drugs* because ongoing DNA synthesis is necessary for cytotoxicity. This has important clinical implications. S phase–specific cytotoxic agents generally require prolonged exposures of tumor cells to drug concentrations above a minimum threshold for optimal therapeutic efficacy. In fact, low-dose, protracted administration of camptothecin analogues have less toxicity, and equal or greater antitumor activity, than shorter, more intense courses.

Mechanisms of Resistance

Decreased intracellular drug accumulation may underlie resistance. Topotecan, but not irinotecan, is a substrate for Pgp; however, compared with other substrates, such as etoposide or doxorubicin, topotecan is a relatively poor substrate. Nonetheless, the BCRP/xenobiotic exporter ABCG2/BCRP is overexpressed in cultured cells that have become resistant to irinotecan after exposure to camptothecins. Cell lines that lack carboxylesterase activity demonstrate resistance to irinotecan, but the liver and red blood cells may have sufficient carboxylesterase activity to convert irinotecan to the active metabolite SN-38. Camptothecin resistance also may result from decreased expression or mutation of topoisomerase I. A transient downregulation of topoisomerase I has been demonstrated following prolonged exposure to camptothecins in vitro and in vivo. Mutations leading to reduced topoisomerase I enzyme catalytic activity or DNA-binding affinity have been associated with experimental camptothecin resistance. Finally, exposure of cells to topoisomerase I–targeted agents upregulates topoisomerase II, an alternative enzyme for DNA strand passage.

Topotecan

ADME

Topotecan is approved for intravenous administration. An oral dosage form in development has a bioavailability of 30%–40% in patients with cancer. Topotecan exhibits linear pharmacokinetics, and it is rapidly eliminated from systemic circulation with a $t_{1/2}$ of about 3.5–4.1 h. Only 20%–35% of the total drug in plasma is found to be in the active lactone form. Within 24 h, 30%–40% of the administered dose appears in the urine. Doses should be reduced in proportion to reductions in CL_{Cr}. Hepatic metabolism appears to be a relatively minor route of drug elimination. Plasma protein binding of topotecan is low (7%–35%), which may explain its relatively greater CNS penetration.

Therapeutic Uses

Topotecan is indicated for previously treated patients with ovarian and small cell lung cancer. Significant hematological toxicity limits its use in combination with other active agents in these diseases (e.g., cisplatin). The recommended dosing regimen of topotecan for ovarian cancer and small cell lung cancer is a 30-min infusion for 5 consecutive days every 3 weeks. For the treatment of patients with cervical cancer in conjunction with cisplatin, topotecan is administered on days 1, 2, and 3, repeated every 21 days. The dose of topotecan should be reduced in patients with moderate renal dysfunction (CL_{Cr} of 20–40 mL/min); topotecan should not be administered to patients with severe renal impairment ($CL_{Cr} < 20$ mL/min). Hepatic dysfunction does not alter topotecan clearance and toxicity. A baseline neutrophil count greater than 1500 cells/mm^3 and a platelet count above 100,000 is necessary prior to topotecan administration.

Adverse Effects

The dose-limiting toxicity with all dosing schedules is neutropenia, with or without thrombocytopenia. The incidence of severe neutropenia at 1.5 mg/m^2 daily for 5 days every 3 weeks may be as high as 81%, with a 26% incidence of febrile neutropenia. In patients with hematological malignancies, GI side effects such as mucositis and diarrhea become dose limiting. Other less common and generally mild topotecan-related toxicities include nausea and vomiting, elevated liver transaminases, fever, fatigue, and rash.

Irinotecan

ADME

The conversion of irinotecan to its active metabolite SN-38 is mediated predominantly by carboxylesterases in the liver (see Figures 6–6 and 6–7). Although SN-38 can be measured in plasma shortly after beginning an intravenous infusion of irinotecan, the AUC of SN-38 is only about 4% of the AUC of irinotecan, suggesting that only a relatively small fraction of the dose is ultimately converted to the active form of the drug. Irinotecan exhibits linear pharmacokinetics. In comparison to topotecan, a relatively large fraction of both irinotecan and SN-38 are present in plasma as the biologically active intact lactone form. The $t_{1/2}$ of SN-38 is 11.5 h, three times that of topotecan. CSF penetration of SN-38 in humans has not been characterized.

In contrast to topotecan, hepatic metabolism of irinotecan and SN-38 represents an important route of elimination for both. Oxidative metabolites have been identified in plasma, all of which result from CYP3A-mediated reactions directed at the bis-piperidine side chain. These metabolites are not significantly converted to SN-38. The total body clearance of irinotecan was found to be two times greater in patients with brain cancer taking antiseizure drugs that induce hepatic CYPs.

UGT1A1 glucuronidates the hydroxyl group at position C10 (resulting from cleavage of the bispiperidine promoiety), producing the inactive glucuronide metabolite SN-38G (see Figures 6–6 and 6–7). Biliary excretion appears to be the primary elimination route of irinotecan, SN-38, and metabolites, although urinary excretion also contributes (14%–37%). The extent of SN-38 glucuronidation inversely correlates with the risk of severe diarrhea after irinotecan therapy. UGT1A1 polymorphisms associated with familial hyperbilirubinemia syndromes may have a major impact on the clinical use of irinotecan. In patients treated with irinotecan, there is a positive correlation between baseline serum unconjugated bilirubin concentration and both severity of neutropenia and the AUC of irinotecan and SN-38. Severe irinotecan toxicity has been observed in patients with cancer with Gilbert syndrome, presumably due to decreased glucuronidation of SN-38. In patients with the syndrome, elevated levels of unconjugated bilirubin in the bloodstream are due to reduced activity of glucuronyltransferase. The presence of bacterial glucuronidase in the intestinal lumen potentially can contribute to irinotecan's GI toxicity by releasing unconjugated SN-38 from the inactive glucuronide metabolite.

Therapeutic Uses

Single-agent dosage of irinotecan is by weekly infusion for 4 of 6 weeks, with a higher dose given every 3 weeks. In patients with advanced colorectal cancer, irinotecan is used as first-line therapy in combination with fluoropyrimidines or as a single agent or in combination with cetuximab following failure of a 5FU/oxaliplatin regimen. It also has activity in small cell lung cancer. A irinotecan liposome injection in combination with 5FU and leucovorin was recently approved by the FDA for treatment of metastatic pancreatic cancer after disease progression following gemcitabine therapy.

Adverse Effects

The dose-limiting toxicity with all dosing schedules is delayed diarrhea (35%), with or without neutropenia. An intensive regimen of loperamide (see Chapter 49) reduces this incidence by more than half. However, once severe diarrhea occurs, standard doses of antidiarrheal agents tend to be ineffective. Diarrhea generally resolves within a week and, unless associated with fever and neutropenia, rarely is fatal.

The second most common irinotecan-associated toxicity is myelosuppression. Severe neutropenia occurs in 14%–47% of the patients treated with a schedule of administration every 3 weeks and is less frequently encountered amongst patients treated with the weekly schedule. Febrile neutropenia is observed in 3% of patients and may be fatal, particularly when associated with concomitant diarrhea. A cholinergic syndrome resulting from the inhibition of acetylcholinesterase activity by irinotecan may occur within the first 24 h after irinotecan administration. Symptoms include acute diarrhea, diaphoresis, hypersalivation, abdominal cramps, visual accommodation disturbances, lacrimation, rhinorrhea, and, less often, asymptomatic bradycardia. These effects are short lasting and respond within minutes to atropine. Other common toxicities include nausea and vomiting, fatigue, vasodilation or skin flushing, mucositis, elevation in liver transaminases, and alopecia. There have been case reports of dyspnea and interstitial pneumonitis associated with irinotecan therapy.

Antibiotics

Dactinomycin (Actinomycin D)

Actinomycins are chromopeptides isolated from *Streptomyces* soil bacteria. Most contain the same chromophore, the planar phenoxazone actinosin, which is responsible for their yellow-red color. The differences amongst naturally occurring actinomycins are confined to variations in the structure of the amino acids of the peptide side chains. Actinomycin D has beneficial effects in the treatment of solid tumors in children and choriocarcinoma in adult women.

Mechanism of Action

The capacity of actinomycins to bind to double-helical DNA is responsible for their biological activity and cytotoxicity. The planar phenoxazone ring intercalates between adjacent guanine-cytosine base pairs of DNA, while the polypeptide chains extend along the minor groove of the helix, resulting in a dactinomycin-DNA complex with stability sufficient to block the transcription of DNA by RNA polymerase. The DNA-dependent RNA polymerases are much more sensitive to the effects of dactinomycin than are the DNA polymerases. In addition, dactinomycin causes single-strand breaks in DNA, possibly through a free-radical intermediate or as a result of the action of topoisomerase II. Dactinomycin inhibits rapidly proliferating cells of normal and neoplastic origin and is amongst the most potent antitumor agents known.

ADME

Dactinomycin is administered by intravenous injection. Metabolism of the drug is minimal. The drug is excreted in both bile and urine and disappears from plasma with a terminal $t_{1/2}$ of 36 h. Dactinomycin does not cross the blood-brain barrier.

Therapeutic Uses

Dactinomycin is given intravenously for 5 days, usually in the range of 10–15 μg/kg. If no manifestations of toxicity are encountered, additional courses may be given at intervals of 2–4 weeks, although weekly maintenance doses have been used. The main clinical use of dactinomycin is in the treatment of rhabdomyosarcoma and Wilms tumor in children, where it is curative in combination with primary surgery, radiotherapy, and other drugs, particularly vincristine and cyclophosphamide. Ewing, Kaposi, and soft-tissue sarcomas also respond. Dactinomycin and MTX form a curative therapy for choriocarcinoma.

Adverse Effects

Toxic manifestations include anorexia, nausea, and vomiting, usually beginning a few hours after administration. Hematopoietic suppression with pancytopenia may occur in the first week after completion of therapy. Proctitis, diarrhea, glossitis, cheilitis, and ulcerations of the oral mucosa are common; dermatological manifestations include alopecia, as well as erythema, desquamation, and increased inflammation and pigmentation in areas previously or concomitantly subjected to X-ray radiation. Severe injury may occur as a result of local drug extravasation; the drug is extremely corrosive to soft tissues.

Anthracyclines and Anthracenediones

Anthracyclines are derived from the fungus *Streptomyces peucetius* var. *caesius*. *Idarubicin* and *epirubicin* are analogues of the naturally produced anthracyclines *doxorubicin* and *daunorubicin*, differing only slightly in chemical structure, but having somewhat distinct patterns of clinical activity. Daunorubicin and idarubicin primarily have been used in acute leukemias, whereas doxorubicin and epirubicin display broader activity against solid tumors. These agents, which possess the potential for generating free radicals, cause an unusual and often-irreversible cardiomyopathy, the occurrence of which is related to the total dose of the drug. The structurally similar agent *mitoxantrone* has less cardiotoxicity and is useful against prostate cancer and AML and in high-dose chemotherapy.

	DOXORUBICIN	DAUNORUBICIN	EPIRUBICIN	IDARUBICIN
$R_1 =$	OCH_3	OCH_3	OCH_3	H
$R_2 =$	H	H	OH	H
$R_3 =$	OH	OH	H	OH
$R_4 =$	OH	H	OH	H

Mechanisms of Action and Resistance

Anthracyclines and anthracenediones can intercalate with DNA, directly affecting transcription and replication. More important is their capacity to form a heterotrimeric complex with topoisomerase II and DNA. Topoisomerase II produces double-strand breaks at the 3′-phosphate backbone, allowing strand passage and uncoiling of supercoiled DNA. Following strand passage, topoisomerase II religates the DNA strands; this enzymatic function is essential for DNA replication and repair. Formation of the ternary complex with anthracyclines or with etoposide inhibits the religation of the broken DNA strands, leading to apoptosis. Defects in DNA double-strand break repair sensitize cells to damage by these drugs, while altered DNA damage-sensing and DNA repair capacity may contribute to resistance.

The quinone moieties of anthracyclines can form radical intermediates that react with O_2 to produce superoxide anion radicals, which can generate H_2O_2 and •OH that attack DNA and oxidize DNA bases, leading to apoptosis (Serrano et al., 1999). The production of free radicals is significantly stimulated by the interaction of doxorubicin with iron. Enzymatic defenses such as superoxide dismutase and catalase protect cells against the toxicity of the anthracyclines, and these defenses can be augmented by exogenous antioxidants such as α-tocopherol or by the iron chelator dexrazoxane, which protects against cardiac toxicity. Multidrug resistance is observed in tumor cell populations exposed to anthracyclines. Anthracyclines also are exported from tumor cells by members of the MRP transporter family and by ABCG2 (BCRP). Other biochemical changes in resistant cells include increased glutathione peroxidase activity, decreased activity or mutation of topoisomerase II, and enhanced ability to repair DNA strand breaks.

ADME

Daunorubicin, doxorubicin, epirubicin, and idarubicin are administered intravenously and are cleared by a complex pattern of hepatic metabolism and biliary excretion. Each anthracycline is converted to an active alcohol intermediate that plays a variable role in the therapeutic activity. The plasma disappearance curves for doxorubicin and daunorubicin are multiphasic, with a terminal $t_{1/2}$ of 30 h. Idarubicin has a $t_{1/2}$ of 15 h, and its active metabolite, idarubicinol, has a $t_{1/2}$ of 40 h. The drugs rapidly enter the heart, kidneys, lungs, liver, and spleen; they do not cross the blood-brain barrier. Clearance is delayed in the presence of hepatic dysfunction; at least a 50% initial reduction in dose should be considered in patients with elevated serum bilirubin levels.

Idarubicin and Daunorubicin

Therapeutic Use. Idarubucin (~12 mg/m²/d for 3 days) is administered by slow intravenous injection (10–15 min) to avoid extravasation. Treatment is for 3 days. Idarubicin has less cardiotoxicity than the other anthracyclines. Daunorubicin (also named daunomycin or rubidomycin) is administered (at 24–45mg/m²/d) intravenously for 3 days, with care to prevent extravasation. Total doses greater than 1000 mg/m² are associated with a high risk of cardiotoxicity. Daunorubicin may impart a red color to the urine. Daunorubicin and idarubicin are used in the treatment of patients with AML in combination with Ara-C.

Adverse Effects. Toxic effects of daunorubicin and idarubicin include bone marrow depression, stomatitis, alopecia, GI disturbances, rash, and cardiac toxicity. Cardiac toxicity of anthracyclines can be acute or chronic and is described in detail next for doxorubicin.

Doxorubicin

Therapeutic Uses. The dose (60–75 mg/m²) is administered as a single rapid intravenous infusion that is repeated after 21 days. A doxorubicin liposomal product is available for treatment of AIDS-related Kaposi sarcoma and is given intravenously in a dose of 20 mg/m² over 60 min and repeated every 3 weeks. The liposomal formulation also is approved for ovarian cancer for treatment at a dose of 50 mg/m² every 4 weeks and as a treatment of multiple myeloma (in conjunction with bortezomib), where it is given as a 30-mg/m² dose on day 4 of each 21-day cycle. Patients should be advised that the drug may impart a red color to the urine. Doxorubicin is effective in malignant lymphomas. In combination with cyclophosphamide, vinca alkaloids, and other agents, it is an important ingredient for the successful treatment of lymphomas. It is a valuable component of various regimens of chemotherapy for adjuvant and metastatic carcinoma of the breast. The drug also is beneficial in pediatric and adult sarcomas, including osteogenic, Ewing, and soft-tissue sarcomas.

Adverse Effects. Toxicities of doxorubicin are similar to those of daunorubicin. Myelosuppression is a major dose-limiting complication, with maximal leukopenia usually occurring during the second week of therapy and recovering by the fourth week; thrombocytopenia and anemia follow a similar pattern but usually are less pronounced. Stomatitis, mucositis, diarrhea, and alopecia are common but reversible. Erythematous streaking near the site of infusion ("flare") is a benign local allergic reaction and should not be confused with extravasation. Facial flushing, conjunctivitis, and lacrimation may occur rarely. The drug may produce severe local toxicity in irradiated tissues (e.g., the skin, heart, lung, esophagus, and GI mucosa) even when the two therapies are not administered concomitantly.

Cardiomyopathy is the most important long-term toxicity (Rochette et al., 2015) and may take two forms:

- **An acute form, characterized by abnormal electrocardiographic changes, including ST- and T-wave alterations and arrhythmias.** This is brief and rarely a serious problem. An acute reversible reduction in ejection fraction is observed in some patients in the 24 h after a single dose, and plasma troponin T may increase in a minority of patients in the first few days following drug administration (Lipshultz et al., 2004). Acute myocardial damage, the "pericarditis-myocarditis syndrome," may begin in the days following drug infusion and is characterized by severe disturbances in impulse conduction and frank congestive heart failure, often associated with pericardial effusion.

- **Chronic, cumulative, dose-related toxicity (usually total doses of ≥ 550 mg/m^2) progressing to congestive heart failure.** The mortality rate in patients with congestive failure approaches 50%. The risk of cardiomyopathy increases markedly with dose; estimates run as high as 20% at total doses of 550 mg/m^2 (a total dose limit of 300 mg/m^2 is advised for pediatric cases). These total dosages should be exceeded only under exceptional circumstances or with the concomitant use of dexrazoxane, a cardioprotective iron-chelating agent (Swain et al., 1997). Cardiac irradiation, administration of high doses of cyclophosphamide or another anthracycline, or concomitant trastuzumab increases the risk of cardiotoxicity (Slamon et al., 2001). Late-onset cardiac toxicity, with congestive heart failure years after treatment, may occur in both pediatric and adult populations. In children treated with anthracyclines, there is a 3- to 10-fold elevated risk of arrhythmias, congestive heart failure, and sudden death in adult life. Concomitant administration of dexrazoxane may reduce troponin T elevations and avert later cardiotoxicity (Lipshultz et al., 2004).

Epirubicin

The anthracycline epirubicin is indicated as a component of adjunctive therapy for treatment of breast cancer. It is administered intravenously in doses of 100–120 mg/m^2 every 3–4 weeks. Total doses greater than 900 mg/m^2 sharply increase the risk of cardiotoxicity. Its toxicity profile is the same as that of doxorubicin.

Valrubicin

Valrubicin is a semisynthetic analogue of doxorubicin used exclusively for intravesicular treatment of bladder cancer. Once a week for 6 weeks, 800 mg are instilled into the bladder. Less than 10% of instilled drug is absorbed systemically. Side effects relate to bladder irritation.

Mitoxantrone

Mitoxantrone is a synthetic anthracenedione derivative topoisomerase II inhibitor that is approved for use in AML, prostate cancer, and late-stage, secondary progressive multiple sclerosis. Mitoxantrone has limited ability to produce quinone-type free radicals and causes less cardiac toxicity than does doxorubicin. It produces acute myelosuppression, cardiac toxicity, and mucositis as its major toxicities; the drug also causes nausea, vomiting, and alopecia, although less than doxorubicin. Mitoxantrone is administered by intravenous infusion. To induce remission in acute nonlymphocytic leukemia in adults, the drug is given in a daily dose of 12 mg/m^2 for 3 days with cytarabine. It also is used in advanced hormone-resistant prostate cancer in a dose of 12–14 mg/m^2 every 21 days.

Epipodophyllotoxins

Podophyllotoxin Derivatives

Two synthetic derivatives of podophyllotoxins have significant therapeutic activity in pediatric leukemia, small cell carcinomas of the lung, testicular tumors, Hodgkin disease, and large cell lymphomas. These derivatives are etoposide (VP-16-213) and teniposide (VM-26). Although podophyllotoxin binds to tubulin, etoposide and teniposide have no effect on microtubular structure or function at usual concentrations.

Mechanisms of Action and Resistance

Etoposide and teniposide form ternary complexes with topoisomerase II and DNA and prevent resealing of the break that normally follows topoisomerase binding to DNA. The enzyme remains bound to the free end of the broken DNA strand, leading to an accumulation of DNA breaks and cell death. Cells in the S and G$_2$ phases of the cell cycle are most sensitive to etoposide and teniposide. Resistant cells demonstrate (1) amplification of the *MDR1* gene that encodes the Pgp drug efflux transporter, (2) mutation

or decreased expression of topoisomerase II, or (3) mutations of the p53 tumor suppressor gene, a required component of the apoptotic pathway (Lowe et al., 1993).

Etoposide

ADME

Oral administration of etoposide results in variable absorption that averages about 50%. After intravenous injection, there is a biphasic pattern of clearance with a terminal $t_{1/2}$ of about 6–8 h in patients with normal renal function. Approximately 40% of an administered dose is excreted intact in the urine. In patients with compromised renal function, dosage should be reduced in proportion to the reduction in CL$_{Cr}$. In patients with advanced liver disease, increased toxicity may result from a low serum albumin (decreased drug binding) and elevated bilirubin (which displaces etoposide from albumin); guidelines for dose reduction in this circumstance have not been defined. Drug concentrations in the CSF average 1%–10% of those in plasma.

Therapeutic Uses

The intravenous dose of etoposide for testicular cancer in combination therapy (with bleomycin and cisplatin) is 50–100 mg/m^2 for 5 days or 100 mg/m^2 on alternate days for three doses. For small cell carcinoma of the lung, the dosage in combination therapy (with cisplatin) is 100–200 mg/m^2/d intravenously for 3 days. Cycles of therapy usually are repeated every 3–4 weeks. After relapse, oral administration of 50 mg/m^2/d for 21 days is one treatment option. When given intravenously, the drug should be administered slowly over a 30- to 60-min period to avoid hypotension and bronchospasm, which likely result from the additives used to dissolve etoposide.

Etoposide is also active against non-Hodgkin lymphomas, acute nonlymphocytic leukemia, and Kaposi sarcoma associated with AIDS. Etoposide has a favorable toxicity profile for dose escalation in that its primary acute toxicity is myelosuppression. In combination with ifosfamide and carboplatin, it frequently is used for high-dose chemotherapy in total doses of 1500–2000 mg/m^2.

Adverse Effects

The dose-limiting toxicity of etoposide is leukopenia (nadir at 10–14 days, recovery by 3 weeks). Thrombocytopenia occurs less often and usually is not severe. Nausea, vomiting, stomatitis, and diarrhea complicate treatment in about 15% of patients. Alopecia is common but reversible. Hepatic toxicity is particularly evident after high-dose treatment. For both etoposide and teniposide, toxicity increases in patients with decreased serum albumin, an effect related to decreased protein binding of the drug.

A disturbing complication of etoposide therapy is the development of an unusual form of acute nonlymphocytic leukemia with a translocation in chromosome 11q23. At this locus is a gene (the MLL gene) that regulates the proliferation of pluripotent stem cells. The leukemic cells have the cytological appearance of acute monocytic or monomyelocytic leukemia. Another distinguishing feature of etoposide-related leukemia is the short time interval between the end of treatment and the onset of leukemia (1–3 years), compared to the 4- to 5-year interval for secondary leukemias related to alkylating agents, and the absence of a myelodysplastic period preceding leukemia (Pui et al., 1995). Patients receiving weekly or twice-weekly doses of etoposide, with cumulative doses greater than 2000 mg/m^2, seem to be at higher risk of leukemia.

Teniposide

Teniposide is administered intravenously. It has a multiphasic pattern of clearance from plasma: After distribution, a $t_{1/2}$ of 4 h and another $t_{1/2}$ of 10–40 h are observed. Approximately 45% of the drug is excreted in the urine; in contrast to etoposide, as much as 80% is recovered as metabolites. Anticonvulsants such as phenytoin increase the hepatic metabolism of teniposide and reduce systemic exposure. Dosage need not be reduced for patients with impaired renal function. Less than 1% of the drug crosses the blood-brain barrier. Teniposide is available for treatment of refractory ALL in children and is synergistic with cytarabine. Teniposide is administered by intravenous infusion for 5 days or twice weekly. The drug has limited utility and is given primarily for acute leukemia in children and monocytic leukemia in infants, as well as glioblastoma, neuroblastoma, and brain metastases from small cell carcinomas of the lung. Myelosuppression, nausea, and vomiting are its primary toxic effects.

Drugs of Diverse Mechanisms of Action

Bleomycin

The bleomycins, a unusual group of DNA-cleaving antibiotics, are fermentation products of *Streptomyces verticillus,* comprising a family of peptide polyketides. The drug currently employed clinically is a mixture of two copper-chelating peptides, bleomycins A_2 and B_2, that differ only in their terminal amino acid. Because their toxicities do not overlap with those of other cytotoxic drugs and because of their unique mechanism of action, bleomycin maintains an important role in treating Hodgkin disease and testicular cancer.

Mechanisms of Action and Resistance

Bleomycin's cytotoxicity results from its capacity to cause oxidative damage to the deoxyribose of thymidylate and other nucleotides, leading to single- and double-stranded breaks in DNA; the exact mechanism is unresolved. Bleomycin causes accumulation of cells in the G_2 phase of the cell cycle, and many of these cells display chromosomal aberrations, including chromatid breaks, gaps, fragments, and translocations. Bleomycin cleaves DNA by generating free radicals. In the presence of O_2 and a reducing agent, the metal-drug complex becomes activated and functions as a ferrous oxidase, transferring electrons from Fe^{2+} to molecular oxygen to produce oxygen radicals. Metallobleomycin complexes can be activated by reaction with the flavin enzyme, NADPH-CYP450 reductase. Bleomycin binds to DNA, and the activated complex generates free radicals that are responsible for abstraction of a proton at the 3′ position of the deoxyribose backbone of the DNA chain, opening the deoxyribose ring and generating a strand break in DNA. An excess of breaks generates cell death.

Bleomycin is degraded by a specific hydrolase found in various normal tissues, including liver. Hydrolase activity is low in skin and lung, perhaps contributing to the serious toxicity. Some bleomycin-resistant cells contain high levels of hydrolase activity. In other cell lines, resistance has been attributed to decreased uptake, repair of strand breaks, or drug inactivation by thiols or thiol-rich proteins.

ADME

Bleomycin is administered intravenously, intramuscularly, or subcutaneously or instilled into the bladder for local treatment of bladder cancer. Having a high molecular mass, bleomycin crosses the blood-brain barrier poorly. The elimination $t_{1/2}$ is about 3 h. About two-thirds of the drug is excreted intact in the urine. Concentrations in plasma are greatly elevated in patients with renal impairment, and doses of bleomycin should be reduced in the presence of a CL_{Cr} less than 60 mL/min.

Therapeutic Uses

Bleomycin is given weekly or twice weekly by the intravenous, intramuscular, or subcutaneous route. A test dose of 2 units or less is recommended for patients with lymphoma. Myriad regimens are employed clinically, with bleomycin doses expressed in units. Total courses exceeding 250 mg should be given with caution, and usually only in high-risk testicular cancer treatment, because of a marked increase in the risk of pulmonary toxicity. Bleomycin also may be instilled into the pleural cavity in doses of 5–60 mg to ablate the pleural space in patients with malignant effusions. Bleomycin is highly effective against germ cell tumors of the testis and ovary. In testicular cancer, it is curative when used with cisplatin and vinblastine or cisplatin and etoposide. It is a component of the standard curative ABVD regimen for Hodgkin disease.

Adverse Effects

Because bleomycin causes little myelosuppression, it has significant advantages in combination with other cytotoxic drugs. However, it does cause a constellation of cutaneous toxicities, including hyperpigmentation,

hyperkeratosis, erythema, even ulceration, and rarely, Raynaud phenomenon. Skin lesions may recur when patients are treated with other antineoplastic drugs. Rarely, bleomycin causes a flagellate dermatitis consisting of bands of pruritic erythema on the arms, back, scalp, and hands; this rash responds readily to topical corticosteroids.

The most serious adverse reaction to bleomycin is pulmonary toxicity, which begins with a dry cough, fine rales, and diffuse basilar infiltrates on X-ray and may progress to life-threatening pulmonary fibrosis. Approximately 5%–10% of patients receiving bleomycin develop clinically apparent pulmonary toxicity, and about 1% die of this complication. Most who recover experience a significant improvement in pulmonary function, but fibrosis may be irreversible. Pulmonary function tests are not of predictive value for detecting early onset of this complication. The risk of pulmonary toxicity is related to total dose, with a significant increase in risk in total doses greater than 250 mg and in patients more than 40 years of age, in those with a CL_{Cr} less than 80 mL/min, and in those with underlying pulmonary disease; single doses of 30 mg/m^2 or more also are associated with an increased risk of pulmonary toxicity. Administration of high O_2 concentrations during anesthesia or respiratory therapy may aggravate or precipitate pulmonary toxicity in patients previously treated with the drug. There is no known specific therapy for bleomycin lung injury except for symptomatic management and standard pulmonary care. Steroids are of variable benefit, with greatest effectiveness in the earliest inflammatory stages of the lesion.

Other toxic reactions to bleomycin include hyperthermia, headache, nausea and vomiting, and a peculiar acute fulminant reaction observed in patients with lymphomas. This reaction is characterized by profound hyperthermia, hypotension, and sustained cardiorespiratory collapse; it does not appear to be a classical anaphylactic reaction and may be related to release of an endogenous pyrogen. This reaction has occurred in about 1% of patients with lymphomas or testicular cancer.

Mitomycin

Mitomycin has limited clinical utility, having been replaced by less toxic and more effective drugs, with the exception of the use in patients with anal cancers, for which it is potentially curative.

MITOMYCIN

Mechanisms of Action and Resistance

After intracellular enzymatic or spontaneous chemical alteration, mitomycin becomes a bifunctional or trifunctional alkylating agent. The drug inhibits DNA synthesis and cross-links DNA at the N6 position of adenine and at the O6 and N7 positions of guanine. Attempts to repair DNA lead to strand breaks. Mitomycin is a potent radiosensitizer, teratogen, and carcinogen in rodents. Resistance has been ascribed to deficient activation, intracellular inactivation of the reduced Q form, and Pgp-mediated drug efflux.

ADME

Mitomycin is administered intravenously. It has a $t_{1/2}$ of 25–90 min. The drug distributes widely throughout the body but is not detected in the CNS. Inactivation occurs by hepatic metabolism or chemical conjugation with sulfhydryls. Less than 10% of the active drug is excreted in the urine or the bile.

Therapeutic Uses

Mitomycin is administered as a single bolus (6–20 mg/m^2) every 6–8 weeks. Dosage should be modified based on hematological recovery. Mitomycin also may be used by direct instillation into the bladder to treat superficial transitional cell carcinomas. Mitomycin is used in combination with

5FU and cisplatin for the treatment of anal cancer. Mitomycin is used off label (as an extemporaneously compounded eye drop) as an adjunct to surgery to inhibit wound healing and reduce scarring.

Adverse Effects

The major toxic effect is myelosuppression, characterized by marked leukopenia and thrombocytopenia; after higher doses, maximal suppression may be delayed and cumulative, with recovery only after 6–8 weeks of pancytopenia. Nausea, vomiting, diarrhea, stomatitis, rash, fever, and malaise also are observed. Patients who have received more than 50 mg/m^2 total dose may acutely develop hemolysis, neurological abnormalities, interstitial pneumonia, and glomerular damage resulting in renal failure. The incidence of renal failure increases to 28% in patients who receive total doses of 70 mg/m^2 or more. There is no effective treatment of the disorder. It must be recognized early, and mitomycin must be discontinued immediately. Mitomycin causes interstitial pulmonary fibrosis; total doses greater than 30 mg/m^2 have infrequently led to congestive heart failure. Mitomycin may potentiate the cardiotoxicity of doxorubicin.

Mitotane

Mitotane (*o,p′*-DDD), a compound chemically similar to the insecticides DDT and DDD, is used in the treatment of adrenal cortex carcinoma. The mechanism of action of mitotane has not been elucidated, but its relatively selective destruction of adrenocortical cells, normal or neoplastic, is well established. Administration of the drug causes a rapid reduction in the levels of adrenocorticosteroids and their metabolites in blood and urine, a response that is useful in both guiding dosage and following the course of hyperadrenocorticism (Cushing syndrome) resulting from an adrenal tumor or adrenal hyperplasia. It does not damage other organs.

MITOTANE (*o,p′*-DDD)

ADME

Approximately 40% of mitotane is absorbed after oral administration. Plasma concentrations of mitotane are still measurable for 6–9 weeks following discontinuation of therapy. Although the drug is found in all tissues, fat is the primary site of storage. A water-soluble metabolite of mitotane found in the urine constitutes 25% of an oral or parenteral dose. About 60% of an oral dose is excreted unchanged in the stool.

Therapeutic Uses

Mitotane initial daily oral doses are 2–6 g, usually in three or four divided portions. The maximal tolerated dose may vary from 2 to 16 g/d. Treatment should continue for at least 3 months; if beneficial effects are observed, therapy should be maintained indefinitely. Spironolactone should not be administered concomitantly because it interferes with the adrenal suppression produced by mitotane. Treatment with mitotane is indicated for the palliation of inoperable adrenocortical carcinoma, producing symptomatic benefit in 30%–50% of such patients.

Adverse Effects

Although the administration of mitotane produces anorexia and nausea in most patients, somnolence and lethargy in about 34%, and dermatitis in 15%–20%, these effects do not contraindicate the use of the drug at lower doses. Because this drug damages the adrenal cortex, administration of replacement doses of adrenocorticosteroids is necessary.

Trabectedin

Trabectedin is derived from the marine invertebrate tunicate *Ecteinascidin turbinate*. Trabectedin is an alkylating drug that binds to the minor groove of DNA, allowing the alkylation of the N2 position of guanine and bending the helix toward the major groove. The bulky DNA adduct is recognized by the transcription-coupled nucleotide excision-repair (NER) complex, and these proteins initiate attempts to repair the damaged strand, converting the adduct to a double-stranded break. Trabectedin has particular cytotoxic effects on cells that lack components of the Fanconi anemia complex or those that lack the ability to repair double-strand DNA breaks through homologous recombination (Soares et al., 2007). Unlike cisplatin and other DNA adduct–forming drugs, the activity of trabectedin requires the presence of intact components of NER, including XPG, which may be important for initiation of single breaks and attempts at adduct removal.

ADME

Trabectedin is administered as a 24-h infusion of 1.3 mg/m^2 every 3 weeks. It is administered with dexamethasone, 4 mg twice daily, starting 24 h before drug infusion to diminish hepatic toxicity. The drug is slowly cleared by CYP3A4, with a plasma $t_{1/2}$ of about 24–40 h.

Therapeutic Uses

Trabectedin is approved for the treatment of patients with unresectable or metastatic liposarcoma or leiomyosarcoma after an anthracycline-containing regimen and is under study as an orphan drug for the treatment of patients with ovarian and pancreatic cancer.

Adverse Effects

Without dexamethasone pretreatment, trabectedin causes significant hepatic enzyme elevations and fatigue in at least one-third of patients. With the steroid, the increases in transaminase are less pronounced and rapidly reversible. Other toxicities include mild myelosuppression and, rarely, rhabdomyolysis.

L-Asparaginase

Malignant lymphoid cells depend on exogenous sources of L-asparagine. Thus, L-asparaginase (L-ASP) has become a standard agent for treating ALL.

Mechanism of Action

Most normal tissues synthesize L-asparagine in amounts sufficient for protein synthesis, but lymphocytic leukemias lack adequate amounts of asparagine synthase and derive the required amino acid from plasma. L-ASP, by catalyzing the hydrolysis of circulating asparagine to aspartic acid and ammonia, deprives these malignant cells of asparagine, leading to cell death. L-ASP is used in combination with other agents, including MTX, doxorubicin, vincristine, and prednisone, for the treatment of ALL and high-grade lymphomas. Resistance arises through induction of asparagine synthetase in tumor cells.

ADME and Therapeutic Use

Asparaginase is given intramuscularly or intravenously. After intravenous administration, *Escherichia coli*–derived L-ASP has a clearance rate from plasma of 0.035 mL/min/kg, a volume of distribution that approximates the volume of plasma in humans, and a $t_{1/2}$ of 1 day. The enzyme is given in doses of 6000–10,000 IU every third day for 3–4 weeks. Pegaspargase, a preparation in which the enzyme is conjugated to 5000-Da units of monomethoxy polyethylene glycol, has a much longer plasma $t_{1/2}$ (6–7 days); it is administered intramuscularly every 14 days, producing rapid and complete depletion of plasma and tumor cell asparagine for 21 days in most patients. Pegaspargase has much reduced immunogenicity (<20% of patients develop antibodies) and has been approved for first-line ALL therapy.

Intermittent dosage regimens and longer durations of treatment increase the risk of inducing hypersensitivity. In hypersensitive patients, neutralizing antibodies inactivate L-ASP. Not all patients with neutralizing antibodies experience clinical hypersensitivity, although the enzyme may be inactivated and therapy may be ineffective. In previously untreated ALL, pegaspargase produces more rapid clearance of lymphoblasts from bone marrow than does the *E. coli* preparation and circumvents the rapid antibody-mediated clearance seen with *E. coli*

Drug Facts for Your Personal Formulary: *Cytotoxic Drugs*

Drug	Therapeutic Use	Clinical Pharmacology and Tips
Section I: Alkylating Agents and Platinum Coordination Complexes		
Mechanism of action: covalent modification of DNA. Adverse effects of all alkylating drugs: myelosuppression and immunosuppression; toxicity to dividing mucosal cells and hair follicles (e.g., oral mucosal ulceration, intestinal denudation, alopecia); delayed pulmonary fibrosis; reproductive system toxicity (premature menopause, sterility); and leukemogenesis (up to 5%, highest for melphalan, procarbazine, nitrosoureas).		
Nitrogen Mustards: DNA alkylation		
Mechlorethamine	• Hodgkin lymphoma • Topical: cutaneous T-cell lymphoma	• Vascular damage during injection due to vesicant properties
Cyclophosphamide	• Acute and chronic lymphocytic leukemia; Hodgkin lymphoma; non-Hodgkin lymphoma; multiple myeloma; neuroblastoma; breast, ovary, Wilms tumor; soft-tissue sarcoma • Autoimmune disease (Wegener granulomatosis, rheumatoid arthritis, nephrotic syndrome)	• Oral or intravenous administration • Active alkylating moieties generated through hepatic metabolism • Nephrotoxic and urotoxic metabolite, acrolein; severe hemorrhagic cystitis in high-dose regimens; prevented by MESNA • Provide vigorous hydration during high-dose treatment • Elimination not affected by renal dysfunction; reduce dose in patients with hepatic dysfunction
Ifosfamide	• Germ cell testicular cancer • Pediatric and adult sarcoma • High-dose chemotherapy with bone marrow rescue	• See cyclophosphamide • Can cause neurotoxicity (including seizures) • Methylene blue treatment of CNS toxicity possibly useful
Melphalan	• Multiple myeloma	• Oral and intravenous administration
Chlorambucil	• Chronic lymphocytic leukemia	• Oral administration
Bendamustine	• Non-Hodgkin lymphoma • Chronic lymphocytic leukemia	• Lacks cross-resistance with other classical alkylators
Alkyl Sulfonate: DNA alkylation		
Busulfan	• Chronic myelogenous leukemia • High-dose chemotherapy regimen with bone marrow transplantation	• Oral administration • Adverse effects: prolonged (up to years) pancytopenia; suppression of stem cells; seizures; ↑ clearance of phenytoin; hepatic VOD
Nitrosoureas: DNA alkylation		
Carmustine (BCNU)	• Malignant gliomas • Hodgkin lymphoma; non-Hodgkin lymphoma	• Vascular damage during injection due to vesicant properties • Profound and delayed myelosuppression
Streptozocin (streptozotocin)	• Malignant pancreatic insulinoma • Carcinoid	• Frequent renal toxicity, sometimes renal failure
Methylhydrazine Derivatives: Monofunctional DNA alkylation		
Procarbazine (*N*-methylhydrazine, MIH)	• Hodgkin lymphoma • Gliomas	• Greater capacity for mutagenesis and carcinogenesis than bifunctional alkylators (e.g., cyclophosphamide)
Triazenes: Methyl transfer to DNA		
Dacarbazine (DTIC)	• Hodgkin lymphoma; soft-tissue sarcomas • Melanoma	• Intravenous administration • Activation by hepatic CYPs • Adverse effects: nausa, vomiting • Rare hepatotoxicity and neurotoxicity
Temozolomide	• Malignant gliomas	• Oral administration • Combined with radiation therapy • Greater capacity for mutagenesis and carcinogenesis than bifunctional alkylators; more active in MGMT-deficient tumors
Platinum Coordination Complexes: Form covalent metal adducts with DNA		
Cisplatin	• Testicular, ovarian, bladder, esophageal, gastric, lung, head and neck, anal, and, breast cancer	• Intravenous administration • Adverse effects: • Nephrotoxicity (reduce by forced pretreatment hydration, diuresis, and use of *amifostine*) • Ototoxicity (tinnitus, high-frequency hearing loss) • Nausea and vomiting (antidote, *aprepitant*) • Peripheral sensory and motor neuropathy (may worsen after discontinuation; may be aggravated by taxane treatment) • Drug resistance due to loss of mismatch repair proteins

Drug Facts for Your Personal Formulary: *Cytotoxic Drugs* (*continued*)

Drug	Therapeutic Use	Clinical Pharmacology and Tips
Platinum Coordination Complexes: Form covalent metal adducts with DNA		
Carboplatin	• Same as above	• Less nausea, neuro-, oto-, and nephrotoxicity than cisplatin • Dose-limiting toxicity: myelosuppression • May cause hypersensitivity reaction
Oxaliplatin	• Colorectal, gastric, and pancreatic cancer	• Peripheral neuropathy is dose limiting • Some nausea • Efficacy not dependent on intact mismatch repair
Section II: Antimetabolites		
Folic Acid Analogues: Inhibit dihydrofolate reductase		
Methotrexate (amethopterin)	• Acute lymphocytic leukemia; choriocarcinoma; breast, head and neck, ovary, bladder and lung cancers; osteogenic sarcoma • Noncancer use: psoriasis, rheumatoid arthritis	• Oral, intravenous, or intramuscular administration • Adverse effects: myelosuppression, GI toxicity • Leucovorin can reverse toxic effects; used as "rescue" in high-dose therapy • *Glucarpidase*, a methotrexate-cleaving enzyme, is approved to treat toxicity • ↓ Dose in renal insufficiency
Pemetrexed	• Mesothelioma, lung cancer	• Similar effects and side effects as methotrexate • Attenuate toxicity with folate and Vit B12 supplementation
Pyrimidine Analogues		
5-Fluorouracil (5FU) *Thymidylate synthase inhibitor*	• Breast, colon, esophageal, stomach, anal cancer • In FOLFOX or FOLFIRINOX combination to treat pancreatic or colorectal cancer • Combined with cisplatin in head and neck cancer • Premalignant skin lesion (topical)	• Intravenous administration • Nausea, mucositis, diarrhea, myelosuppression, hand-foot syndrome • Combined with leucovorin to enhance efficacy • Enhanced toxicity with DPD deficiency; may rescue with uridine
Capecitabine *Thymidylate synthase inhibitor*	• Metastatic breast, colorectal cancer	• Orally administered prodrug of 5FU • Similar adverse effects as 5FU; hand and foot syndrome more frequent than with 5FU
Cytarabine (cytosine arabinoside) *Interferes with base pairing in DNA; inhibits DNA polymerase*	• Acute myelogenous and acute lymphocytic leukemia; non-Hodgkin lymphoma	• Intravenous administration • Myelosuppressive; can cause acute, severe leukopenia, thrombocytopenia, anemia • GI disturbances • Noncardiogenic pulmonary edema • Dermatitis
Gemcitabine (difluoro analogue of deoxycytidine) *Inhibits DNA polymerase; causes strand termination*	• Pancreatic, ovarian, lung, bladder cancer	• Intravenous administration • Female and elderly patients clear the drug more slowly • Myelosuppression, hepatic toxicity • Rare posterior leukoencephalopathy syndrome; sometimes interstitial pneumonitis • Radiosensitizer; should be used with caution in radiotherapy
5-Azacytidine *Inhibits DNA cytosine methyltransferase*	• Myelodysplasia	• Subcutaneous or intravenous administration • Myelosuppression and mild GI symptoms • After intravenous administration severe nausea possible
Purine Analogues and Related Inhibitors		
6-Mercaptopurine *Inhibits purine nucleotide synthesis and metabolism*	• Acute lymphocytic and myelogenous leukemia; small cell non-Hodgkin lymphoma • Noncancer: Crohn disease, ulcerative colitis	• Oral absorption incomplete, thus intravenous administration • Reduce oral dose by 75% in patients receiving allopurinol; no adjustment needed for intravenous administration • Myelosuppression; anorexia, nausea, vomiting; GI side effects less frequent in children than adults • Secondary malignancy: SCC of the skin, AML
Fludarabine *A chain terminator when incorporated into DNA; inhibits RNA function and processing*	• Chronic lymphocytic leukemia • Follicular B-cell lymphoma • Allogeneic bone marrow transplant	• Oral or intravenous administration • Frequently myelosuppression • Less frequent: nausea, vomiting; altered mental status; seizures • Secondary myelodysplasia and acute leukemias • Adjust dose for renal dysfunction

Purine Analogues and Related Inhibitors (continued)		
Cladribine *Incorporated into DNA, produces strand breaks; inhibits conversion of ribo- to deoxyribonucleotides*	• Hairy cell leukemia • Chronic lymphocytic leukemia • Low-grade lymphoma • CTCL, Waldenström macroglobulinemia	• Intravenous administration • Adjust dose for renal dysfunction • Myelosuppression, opportunistic infections, nausea, high fever, tumor lysis syndrome
Clofarabine (mechanism as above)	• Acute myelogenous or lymphocytic leukemia	• Intravenous administration • Adjust dose to creatinine clearance • Myelosuppression • Capillary leak syndrome: discontinue drug • Nausea, vomiting, diarrhea
Nelarabine *Incorporated into DNA, terminates DNA synthesis*	• T-cell leukemia, lymphoma	• Intravenous administration • Myelosuppression; liver function abnormalities; infrequent neurologic sequelae
Pentostatin (2′-deoxycoformycin) *Inhibits adenosine deaminase; causes immunodeficiency (T and B cells)*	• Hairy cell leukemia; chronic lymphocytic leukemia; small cell non-Hodgkin lymphoma	• Intravenous administration • Adjust dose for renal dysfunction • Myelosuppression, GI symptoms, skin rashes, opportunistic infections • Renal, neurologic, pulmonary toxicity

Section III: Natural Products

Vinca Alkaloids: Inhibit tubulin polymerization and microtubule formation		
Vinblastine	• Hodgkin and non-Hodgkin lymphoma • Breast, bladder, lung, testicular cancer • Kaposi sarcoma, neuroblastoma • Part of ABVD combination with doxorubicin (adriamycin, bleomycin, dacarbazine) for Hodgkin lymphoma	• Intravenous administration; extravasation causes irritation and ulceration • Reduce dose in patients with impaired liver function • Least neurotoxic Vinca alkaloid • Myelosuppression • GI side effects nausea, vomiting, diarrhea • Vinca alkaloids are substrates of the Pgp efflux pump
Vinorelbine	• Breast cancer • Non–small cell lung cancer	• Intravenous administration • Reduce dose in patients with impaired liver function • Intermediate neurotoxicity amongst the Vinca alkaloids • Myelosuppressive (granulocytopenia)
Vincristine	• Acute lymphocytic leukemia; neuroblastoma; Wilms tumor; rhabdomyosarcoma; Hodgkin and non-Hodgkin lymphoma • part of CHOP regimen: cyclophosphamide, doxorubicin (H), vincristine (O), prednisone	• Intravenous administration; extravasation causes irritation and ulceration • Reduce dose in patients with impaired liver function • Least myelosuppressive Vinca alkaloid • Dose-limiting neurotoxicity • Better tolerated by children than adults
Eribulin	• Breast cancer, liposarcoma	• Side effects overlap with vinca but less sensitive to extrusion by Pgp

Taxanes: Stabilize microtubules, inhibit depolymerization		
Paclitaxel	• Ovarian, breast, lung, prostate, bladder, head and neck cancer	• Intravenous administration • Metabolized by hepatic CYPs, ↓ dose in patients with hepatic dysfunction • Substrate of Pgp efflux pump • Myelosuppressive, alleviated by G-CSF • Peripheral neuropathy is dose limiting • Mucositis
Docetaxel	• Same as above	• No effect on doxorubicin clearance • Pharmacokinetics similar to paclitaxel's • ↓ Neutropenia, ↓ neuropathy than paclitaxel

Camptothecins: Inhibit topoisomerase I; DNA religation is inhibited: accumulation of single-strand breaks		
Topotecan	• Ovarian cancer; small cell lung cancer	• Intravenous or oral administration • Reduce dose in patients with renal dysfunction • Neutropenia, GI side effects, nausea, vomiting • Substrate for Pgp
Irinotecan	• Colorectal cancer, small cell lung cancer • Part of FOLFIRI or FOLFIRINOX combination for GI tumors	• Intravenous administration • Prodrug activated in the liver; CYP substrate • Diarrhea and neutropenia • Acetylcholinesterase inhibition results in cholinergic syndrome: treat with atropine

Antibiotics		
Dactinomycin (actinomycin D) *Intercalates between GC base pairs of DNA*	• Wilms tumor; rhabdomyosarcoma; Ewing, Kaposi, and other sarcoma; choriocarcinoma	• Intravenous administration; severe injury on extravasation • Nausea, vomiting; myelosuppression; GI side effects; erythema, inflammation of the skin

Drug Facts for Your Personal Formulary: *Cytotoxic Drugs* (*continued*)

Drug	Therapeutic Use	Clinical Pharmacology and Tips
Anthracyclines and Anthracenediones: Inhibit topoisomerase II and intercalate DNA		
Daunorubicin (daunomycin, rubidomycin)	• Acute myelogenous and acute lymphocytic leukemia	• Intravenous administration • Impart a red color to the urine • Myelosuppression, GI side effects • Most important long-term side effect is cardiotoxicity, including tachycardia, arrhythmias, congestive heart failure • Alopecia
Doxorubicin	• Soft-tissue, osteogenic, and other sarcoma; Hodgkin and non-Hodgkin lymphoma; acute leukemia; breast, genitourinary, thyroid, and stomach cancer; neuroblastoma	
Mitoxantrone (an anthracenedione)	• Acute myelocytic leukemia; breast and prostate cancer	• Similar side effects as above • Less cardiotoxic
Epipodophyllotoxins: Inhibit topoisomerase II and religation of cleaved DNA strand		
Etoposide	• Testicular and lung cancer; Hodgkin lymphoma; non-Hodgkin lymphomas; acute myelogenous leukemia; Kaposi sarcoma	• Oral and intravenous administration • Reduce dose in patients with renal dysfunction • Leukopenia, GI side effects; hepatic toxicity after high doses • Secondary leukemia
Teniposide	• Acute lymphoblastic leukemia in children; glioblastoma, neuroblastoma	• Intravenous administration • Myelosuppression, nausea, vomiting
Drugs With Diverse Mechanism of Action		
Bleomycin *Binds to DNA, generates free radicals, and induces DNA cleavage via deoxyribose ring damage*	• Testicular cancer; Hodgkin and non-Hodgkin lymphoma; local treatment of bladder cancer • Part of the ABVD regimen (doxorubicin [Adriamycin], Bleomycin, Vinblastine, and Dacarbazine)	• IV, IM or SC administration; instilled into bladder • Reduce dose in patients with renal dysfunction • Most serious: pulmonary toxicity • Cutaneous toxicity (erythema, ulcerations) • Less myelosuppression than other cytotoxics
L-Asparaginase *Hydrolyzes asparagine; deprives leukemia cells that lack asparagine synthase*	• Acute lymphocytic leukemia	• IV and IM administration • Hypersensitivity reactions, anaphylaxis • Hyperglycemia, clotting abnormalities
Hydroxyurea *Inhibits RNR (conversion of ribo- to deoxyribonucleotides)*	• Chronic myelogenous leukemia; polycythemia vera; essential thrombocytosis; sickle cell disease in adults	• Oral administration • Reduce dose in patients with renal dysfunction • Myelosuppression; some GI side effects
Tretinoin (all-*trans* retinoic acid) *Promotes degradation of PML-RARA fusion protein*	• Acute promyelocytic leukemia	• Oral administration • CYP substrate • Leukocyte maturation syndrome, pulmonary distress, effusions, fever, dyspnea • Dry skin, cheilitis • Hypercalcemia and renal failure
Arsenic trioxide *Inhibits thioredoxin and generates reactive oxygen species*	• Acute promyelocytic leukemia	• Oral or intravenous administration • Leukocyte maturation syndrome as above with ATRA • QT prolongation; rare torsade de pointes

[a]For drugs that are subject to hepatic metabolism by CYP enzymes, drug exposure of a patient can be affected by coadministration of inhibitors or inducers of CYP3A4 and can then reduce efficacy or increase side effects.

[b]Embryo-fetal toxicity: Consider that all of these drugs can cause fetal harm. Advise women of the potential risk to a fetus and to avoid pregnancy while taking the drug and for 1 month after cessation of therapy. Advise men to avoid fathering a child during the same time period. Avoid lactation during therapies.

Bibliography

Akhmanova A, Steinmetz MO. Control of microtubule organization and dynamics: two ends in the limelight. *Nat Rev Mol Cell Biol*, **2015**, 16:711–726.

Allegra CJ, et al. Trimetrexate for the treatment of *Pneumocystis carinii* pneumonia in patients with acquired immunodeficiency syndrome. *N Engl J Med*, **1987a**, 317:978–985.

Allegra CJ, et al. Evidence for direct inhibition of de novo purine synthesis in human MCF-7 breast cells as a principal mode of metabolic inhibition by methotrexate. *J Biol Chem*, **1987b**, 262:13520–13526.

Berlin NI, et al. Folic acid antagonist. Effects on the cell and the patient. Combined clinical staff conference at the National Institutes of Health. *Ann Intern Med*, **1963**, 59:931–956.

Calvert AH, et al. Carboplatin dosage: prospective evaluation of a simple formula based on renal function. *J Clin Oncol*, **1989**;7:1748–1756.

Chabner BA, Roberts TG. Timeline: chemotherapy and the war on cancer. *Nat Rev Cancer*, **2005**, 5:65–72.

Collins SJ. Retinoic acid receptors, hematopoiesis and leukemogenesis. *Curr Opin Hematol*, **2008**, 15:346–351.

Curt GA, et al. Determinants of the sensitivity of human small-cell lung cancer cell lines to methotrexate. *J Clin Invest*, **1985**, 76:1323–1329.

Davidson NE, et al. AACR cancer progress report 2016. *Clin Cancer Res*, **2016**, *22*:S1–S137.

Deyoung MP, Ellisen LW. p63 and p73 in human cancer: defining the network. *Oncogene*, **2007**, *26*:5169–5183.

Krumbhaar EB. Role of the blood and the bone marrow in certain forms of gas poisoning: I. peripheral blood changes and their significance. *JAMA*, **1919**, *72*:39–41.

Farber S, et al. Temporary remissions in acute leukemia in children produced by folic antagonist 4-amethopteroylglutamic acid (aminopterin). *N Engl J Med*, **1948**, *238*:787–793.

Fischel JL, et al. Impact of the oxaliplatin-5 fluorouracil-folinic acid combination on respective intracellular determinants of drug activity. *Br J Cancer*, **2002**, *86*:1162–1168.

Gerth K, et al. Epothilons A and B: antifungal and cytotoxic compounds from *Sorangium cellulosum* (Myxobacteria). Production, physico-chemical and biological properties. *J Antibiot (Tokyo)*, **1996**, *49*:560–563.

Gilman A, Philips FS. The biological actions and therapeutic applications of the β-chlorethylamines and sulfides. *Science*, **1946**, *103*:409–415.

Hegi ME, et al. Correlation of O6-methylguanine methyltransferase (MGMT) promoter methylation with clinical outcomes in glioblastoma and clinical strategies to modulate MGMT activity. *J Clin Oncol*, **2008**, *26*:4189–4199.

Heinemann V, et al. Comparison of the cellular pharmacokinetics and toxicity of 2′,2′-difluorodeoxycytidine and 1-β-D-arabinofuranosylcytosine. *Cancer Res*, **1988**, *48*:4024–4031.

Kamiya K, et al. Inhibition of the 3′ → 5′ exonuclease human DNA polymerase by fludarabine-terminated DNA. *J Biol Chem*, **1996**, *271*:19428–19435.

Karran P, Attard N. Thiopurines in current medical practice: molecular mechanisms and contributions to therapy-related cancer. *Nat Rev Cancer*, **2008**, *8*:24–36.

Kastan MB. Molecular determinants of sensitivity to antitumor agents. *Biochem Biophys Acta*, **1999**, *1424*:R37–R42.

Kramer OH, et al. Histone deacetylase inhibitors and hydroxyurea modulate the cell cycle and cooperatively induce apoptosis. *Oncogene*, **2008**, *27*:732–740.

Kufe DW, et al. Effects of 1-β-D-arabinofuranosylcytosine incorporation on eukaryotic DNA template function. *Mol Pharmacol*, **1984**, *26*:128–134.

Lee JJ, Swain SM. The epothilones: translating from the laboratory to the clinic. *Clin Cancer Res*, **2008**, *14*:1618–1624.

Leoni LM, et al. Bendamustine (Treanda) displays a distinct pattern of cytotoxicity and unique mechanistic features compared with other alkylating agents. *Clin Cancer Res*, **2008**, *14*:309–317.

Lipshultz SE, et al. The effect of dexrazoxane on myocardial injury in doxorubicin-treated children with acute lymphoblastic leukemia. *N Engl J Med*, **2004**, *351*:145–153.

Lowe SW, et al. p53-Dependent apoptosis modulates the cytotoxicity of anticancer agents. *Cell*, **1993**, *74*:957–967.

Milano G, et al. Dihydropyrimidine dehydrogenase deficiency and fluorouracil-related toxicity. *Br J Cancer*, **1999**, *79*:627–630.

Paré L, et al. Pharmacogenetic prediction of clinical outcome in advanced colorectal cancer patients receiving oxaliplatin/5-fluorouracil as first-line chemotherapy. *Br J Cancer*, **2008**, *99*:1050–1055. Erratum in: *Br J Cancer*, **2009**, *100*:1368.

Pui CH, et al. Epipodophyllotoxin-related acute myeloid leukemia: a study of 35 cases. *Leukemia*, **1995**, *9*:1990–1996.

Pui CH, et al. Mechanisms of disease: Acute lymphoblastic leukemia. *N Engl J Med*, **2004**, *350*:1535–1548.

Pullarkat ST, et al. Thymidylate synthase gene polymorphism determines response and toxicity of 5-FU chemotherapy. *Pharmacogenomics J*, **2001**, *1*:65–70.

Reed E. Platinum-DNA adduct, nucleotide excision repair and platinum based anti-cancer chemotherapy. *Cancer Treat Rev*, **1998**, *24*:331–344.

Rochette L, et al. Anthracyclines/trastuzumab: new aspects of cardiotoxicity and molecular mechanisms. *Trends Pharmacol Sci*, **2015**, *36*:326–348.

Schimke RT, et al. Gene amplification and drug resistance in cultured murine cells. *Science*, **1978**, *202*:1051–1055.

Serrano J, et al. Cardioselective and cumulative oxidation of mitochondrial DNA following subchronic doxorubicin administration. *Biochem Biophys Acta*, **1999**, *1411*:201–205.

Sharma S, et al. Molecular dynamic simulations of cisplatin- and oxaliplatin-d(GG) intrastrand cross-links reveal differences in their conformational dynamics. *J Mol Biol*, **2007**, *373*:1123–1140.

Shen DW, et al. Cisplatin resistance: a cellular self-defense mechanism resulting from multiple epigenetic and genetic changes. *Pharmacol Rev*, **2012**, *64*:706–721.

Slamon DJ, et al. Use of chemotherapy plus a monoclonal antibody against HER2 for metastatic breast cancer that overexpresses HER2. *N Engl J Med*, **2001**, *344*:783–792.

Soares DG, et al. Replication and homologous recombination repair regulate DNA double-strand break formation by the antitumor alkylator ecteinascidin 743. *Proc Natl Acad Sci U S A*, **2007**, *104*:13062–13067.

Swain SM, et al. Cardioprotection with dexrazoxane for doxorubicin-containing therapy in advanced breast cancer. *J Clin Oncol*, **1997**, *15*:1318–1332.

Wilson PM, et al. Standing the test of time: targeting thymidylate biosynthesis in cancer therapy. *Nat Rev Clin Oncol*, **2014**, *11*:282–298.

Chapter 67

Pathway-Targeted Therapies: Monoclonal Antibodies, Protein Kinase Inhibitors, and Various Small Molecules

Anton Wellstein, Giuseppe Giaccone, Michael B. Atkins, and Edward A. Sausville

Abbreviations

ABC: ATP-binding cassette
ABL: Abelson murine leukemia viral oncogene homolog
ADCC: antibody-dependent cellular cytotoxicity
AI: aromatase inhibitor
ALK: anaplastic lymphoma kinase
ALL: acute lymphoblastic leukemia
AML: acute myelocytic leukemia
APC: antigen-presenting cell
aPTT: activated partial thromboplastin time
AUC: area under the curve
AXL: TAM family receptor tyrosine
BCC: basal cell carcinoma
BCL: B-cell lymphoma
BCR: breakpoint cluster region (chr22)
BCRP: breast cancer resistance protein
BH3: BCL2 homology domain 3
BIM: BCL2-like protein 11
BRCA: breast cancer susceptibility gene
BRK: breast tumor kinase, PTK6
BTK: Bruton tyrosine kinase
CAR(T): chimeric antigen receptor T cells
CDC: complement-dependent cytotoxicity
CDK: cyclin-dependent kinase
CLL: chronic lymphocytic leukemia
cMET: mesenchymal-epithelial transition receptor tyrosine kinase
CML: chronic myelocytic leukemia
CRL4-CRBN: cullin-ring ubiquitin ligase cereblon complex
CTLA-4: cytotoxic T lymphocyte–associated protein 4
cuSCC: cutaneous squamous cell carcinoma
CXCR4: C-X-C chemokine receptor 4
EGF(R): epidermal growth factor (receptor) = HER1
EML4: echinoderm microtubule-associated protein-like 4
EPH: ephrin
ER: estrogen receptor
FADD: fas-associated protein with death domain
FGF: fibroblast growth factor
FGFR: fibroblast growth factor receptor
FIP1L1: factor interacting with poly (A) polymerase
FKBP12: immunophilin-binding protein for tacrolimus (FK506)
FL: follicular B-cell non-Hodgkin lymphoma
FLT4: fms-related tyrosine kinase 4 = VEGFR3
FMO3: flavin containing monooxygenase 3
FOLFIRI: folinic acid (leucovorin), 5-fluorouracil, irinotecan
FOLFOX: folinic acid (leucovorin), 5-fluorouracil, oxaliplatin
5FU: 5-fluorouracil
GAP: GTPase-activating protein
G-CSF: granulocyte colony-stimulating factor
GIST: gastrointestinal stromal tumor
GM-CSF: granulocyte-macrophage colony-stimulating factor
HDAC: histone deacetylase
HER1: human epidermal growth factor receptor = EGFR
HGF(R): hepatocyte growth factor (receptor) = CMET
HIF-1: hypoxia inducible factor 1
HL: Hodgkin lymphoma
HNSCC: head and neck squamous cell carcinoma
HSC: hematopoietic stem cell
IFN: interferon
IGF1R: insulin-like growth factor 1 receptor

IκB: inhibitor of nuclear factor kappa B
IL: interleukin
IL-2R: interleukin 2 receptor
INR: international normalized ratio
ITK: inducible T cell kinase
JC: John Cunningham
KDR: kinase insert domain receptor = VEGFR2
KIT: feline sarcoma virus oncogene homolog
LCK: lymphocyte specific kinase
LVEF: left ventricular ejection fraction
MCL: mantle cell lymphoma
mCRC: metastatic colorectal cancer
MDS: myelodysplastic syndrome
MET: mesenchymal-epithelial transition factor (= HGFR)
MHC: major histocompatibility complex protein
MKK: mitogen-activated protein kinase kinase (= MEK)
MM: multiple myeloma
MMAE: monomethyl auristatin E
mTOR: mammalian target of rapamycin
NCCN: National Comprehensive Cancer Network
NER: nucleotide excision repair
NET: neuroendocrine tumor
NHL: non-Hodgkin lymphoma
NK: natural killer
NPM: nucleophosmin (gene)
NRAS: neuroblastoma RAS virus homolog
NSCLC: non–small cell lung cancer
OATP: organic anion-transporting polypeptide
PAP: prostate acidic phosphatase
PARP1: poly(ADP-ribose) polymerase
PD-1: programmed cell death 1
PDGF: platelet-derived growth factor
PDGFR: platelet-derived growth factor receptor
PD-L1: programmed cell death 1 ligand 1
Pgp: P-glycoprotein
PML: promyelocytic leukemia
PNET: peripheral neuroendocrine tumors
PPES: palmar-plantar erythrodysesthesia syndrome
PPI: proton pump inhibitor
PTEN: phosphatase and tensin homolog
RA: 13-cis-retinoic acid
Rb: retinoblastoma (protein)
RCC: renal cell carcinoma
ROS1: orphan receptor tyrosine kinase
SCC: squamous cell carcinoma
SCLC: small cell lung cancer
SDF: stromal cell-derived factor
S6K1: ribosomal protein S6 kinase β1
SLL: small lymphocytic lymphoma
STS: soft-tissue sarcoma
TCR: T cell receptor
TIE: tyrosine kinase with Ig and EGF domains
TIL: tumor-infiltrating lymphocyte
TKI: tyrosine kinase inhibitor
TNF: tumor necrosis factor
TRADD: tumor necrosis factor receptor death domain
TRAIL: TNF-related apoptosis inducing ligand
TSC: tuberous sclerosis complex
VEGF: vascular endothelial growth factor
VEGFR: vascular endothelial growth factor receptor
WM: Waldenström macroglobulinemia

A Note on Treatment Regimens

Cancer treatment regimens change to reflect continuous advances in basic and clinical science: new drugs, both small molecules and biologicals; improved methods of targeting and timing of drug delivery; agents with altered pharmacokinetic properties and selectivities; the use of rational multidrug combinations; and greater knowledge of the basic cell biology of tumorigenesis, metastasis, and immune function, amongst other advances. As a consequence, this chapter presents relatively few detailed treatment regimens; rather, we refer the reader to the web-based resources of the U.S. FDA and the NCCN. Table 67–1 provides two examples of therapeutic regimens that illustrate the complexity of current cancer drug therapy.

Development of targeted therapies for treating cancer relies on the continuing process of discovery of molecular changes that drive malignant progression of human cancers. A rapidly growing number of drugs are being developed to block oncogenic pathways that lead to dysregulated cancer cell growth and survival. Targeted therapy may be combined with classical cytotoxic cancer drugs described in Chapter 66 for improved efficacy. Growth factor receptors and downstream signaling molecules are amongst the most actively explored targets for cancer drug discovery. The drivers of cancer growth are oncogenic pathways in malignant cells themselves (e.g., mutant receptors and kinases), the reaction of the tumor microenvironment (e.g., angiogenesis), and the escape of malignant cells from the host's immune surveillance (Hanahan and Weinberg, 2011). The discussion of drugs in this chapter is organized into sections focusing on these drivers of cancer growth:

I. Growth factors and receptors in cancer cells
II. Intracellular kinases in cancer cells
III. Tumor-host interactions reflected in aberrant tumor angiogenesis
IV. Restoring immune recognition of cancer cells
V. Other drugs and targets that control cancer cell behavior

The primary tools for targeting oncogenic pathways are *monoclonal antibodies* that recognize cell surface or shed antigens (e.g., growth factor receptors or receptor ligands) and *small molecules* that can enter cells and engage intracellular targets, many of them kinases. These two classes of drugs have very different pharmacological properties (see Box).

I. Growth Factors and Receptors in Cancer Cells

Inhibitors of Epidermal Growth Factor Receptor (EGFR) Function

Background

The EGFR belongs to the ErbB family of transmembrane receptor tyrosine kinases also known as ErbB1 or HER1 (*human EGFR* 1). EGFR is essential for the growth and differentiation of epithelial cells. Ligand binding to the extracellular domain of EGFR family members causes receptor dimerization and stimulates the protein tyrosine kinase activity of the intracellular domain, resulting in autophosphorylation of several Tyr residues located in the C-terminal tail of the receptor monomers. These phosphotyrosines provide interaction sites for a variety of adapter proteins, resulting in stimulation of signaling pathways, including MAPK, PI3K/Akt, and STAT pathways (see Figure 67–1).

Two separate classes of drugs that target the EGFR pathway are important in the therapy of solid tumors: protein tyr kinase inhibitors and inhibitors of extracellular ligand binding. EGFR TKIs (*erlotinib, gefitinib, afatinib, osimertinib*) bind to the intracellular kinase domain and inhibit the enzymatic function of an EGFR. Monoclonal antibodies (*cetuximab,*

Two Classes of Pathway-Targeted Cancer Drugs

1. **Monoclonal Antibodies:** Monoclonal antibodies kill tumor cells by blocking cell surface receptor function, by recruiting immune cells and complement to the antigen-antibody complex, and by modulating immune cell function. Also, they may be armed to carry toxins or radionuclides to the cells of interest, thereby enhancing their cytotoxic effects. A monoclonal antibody is generally specific for a single antigen, such as an epitope in a growth factor receptor; has a long plasma $t_{1/2}$; and requires only intermittent parenteral administration.

The Naming of Monoclonal Antibodies: **M**onoclonal **a**nti**b**ody names end with the syllable "mab" preceded by "mu" for fully human protein sequence, "zu" for human protein with the antigen-binding region from a mouse antibody, "xi" for a chimera consisting of human constant and mouse variable antibody domains, and "o" for entirely mouse protein sequences (Hansel et al., 2010; see Figures 34–6 and 34–7).

2. **Small Molecules:** Small molecules may attack the same targets as monoclonal antibodies but can exert their effect by entering cells. Small molecules often inhibit multiple enzymes with different selectivities and thus are likely to have a broader spectrum of targets and produce a broader spectrum of desired effects, off-target effects, and adverse effects than monoclonal antibodies. Many small-molecule drugs have elimination half-lives of 12 to 24 h and typically require at least daily oral administration. For small-molecule drugs that are metabolized by hepatic CYPs, the concomitant use of strong CYP inhibitors (e.g., ketoconazole, nefazodone, clarithromycin, gemfibrozil, cobicistat) or inducers (e.g., rifampin, phenytoin, carbamazepine, phenobarbital, St John's wort) can lead to increased adverse effects due to reduced drug elimination or to reduced efficacy due to accelerated clearance. The small-molecule inhibitors mentioned in this chapter, mostly protein kinase inhibitors, end with the syllable "ib." More than 130 novel TKIs are currently being evaluated in different clinical phases (Neul et al., 2016).

panitumumab, necitumumab) recognize the extracellular domain of the EGFR, inhibit ligand-induced signaling, and can elicit an immune response. In epithelial cancers, overexpression of the EGFR is a common finding, and mutational activation of the EGFR (e.g., in 10%–40% of NSCLCs) creates a dependence on EGFR signaling. The most common EGFR mutations are in-frame deletions in exon 19 or leucine-to-arginine point mutations (L858R) in exon 21 that cause conformational changes and constitutive activation of the kinase. First- (*erlotinib, gefitinib*) and second- (*afatinib*) generation drugs are available that inhibit EGFR kinase activity driven by these mutations. Resistant cancer cell subpopulations that emerge during treatment with first- and second-generation inhibitors are usually sensitive to the third-generation inhibitor *osimertinib* (Figure 67–1).

Protein Tyrosine Kinase Inhibitors of EGFR

Erlotinib

Mechanism of Action. Erlotinib is a reversible inhibitor of the EGFR tyrosine kinase, competitively inhibiting ATP binding at the active site of the kinase. Erlotinib has an IC_{50} of 2 nM for EGFR kinase activity. By comparison, for many protein kinases, the K_d for ATP at the substrate site is in the range of 20 μM.

ADME. Erlotinib is about 60% absorbed after oral administration. Peak plasma levels occur after 4 h. Erlotinib has a $t_{1/2}$ of 36 h and is metabolized by CYP3A4 and to a lesser extent by CYPs 1A2 and 1A1.

Therapeutic Uses. Erlotinib is approved for treatment of patients with advanced or metastatic NSCLC after failure of platinum-based treatment. In newly diagnosed NSCLC, erlotinib is approved in patients with EGFR mutations only (Figure 67–1). Erlotinib in combination with gemcitabine is also approved for the treatment of patients with locally advanced, unresectable, or metastatic pancreatic cancer.

TABLE 67–1 ■ CANCER TREATMENT REGIMENS: COMPLEXITIES AND RESOURCES

In treating cancers, the selection of the most appropriate treatment(s), dose, and dose intervals as well as the management of adverse effects requires specialized knowledge and a team effort. In addition, cancer treatment regimens are undergoing frequent updates due to findings in ongoing clinical trials. The availability of drugs with new mechanisms of action (e.g., immune checkpoint inhibitors), good target selectivity (e.g., kinase inhibitors), efficacy in specific cancers, and different adverse effect profiles permits the use of new drug combinations and regimens. The chapters on the pharmacotherapy of cancer focus on mechanism of action, ADME, and adverse effects, with less emphasis on treatment regimens. There are several excellent sources of up-to-date treatment information. The U.S. FDA provides authoritative information on approved drugs online (http://www. accessdata.fda.gov/scripts/cder/daf/. Detailed treatment guidelines for most cancers are available from the NCCN, an alliance of cancer centers that establishes evidence-based guidelines for cancer treatment. The NCCN guidelines are continuously updated to reflect new information that may alter clinical practice. The guidelines can be accessed online (https://www.nccn.org/professionals/physician_gls/f_guidelines.asp).

This table provides examples that illustrate the complexities of current treatment for two cancers: HER2+ breast cancer and advanced colorectal cancer.

SAMPLE TREATMENT REGIMENS

SUMMARY	DRUGS, SCHEDULE, AND DOSING
HER2-Positive Breast Cancer	
Doxorubicin and cyclophosphamide (= AC) followed by paclitaxel, trastuzumab, and pertuzumab	**Day 1:** Doxorubicin 60 mg/m² IV
	Day 1: Cyclophosphamide 600 mg/m² IV
	Repeat cycle every 21 days for 4 cycles
	Followed by
	Day 1: Pertuzumab 840 mg IV followed by 420 mg IV
	Day 1: Trastuzumab 8 mg/kg IV followed by 6 mg/kg IV
	Days 1, 8, and 15: Paclitaxel 80 mg/m² IV
	Repeat cycle every 21 days for 4 cycles
	Day 1: Trastuzumab 6 mg/kg IV
	Repeat cycle every 21 days to complete 1 year of trastuzumab therapy
	Cardiac monitoring at baseline and 3-month intervals
Advanced or Metastatic Colorectal Cancer RAS wild-type	
Oxaliplatin, leucovorin, 5FU (= FOLFOX) plus cetuximab	**Day 1:** Oxaliplatin 85 mg/m² IV over 2 h
	Day 1: Leucovorin 400 mg/m² IV over 2 h
	Days 1–3: 5FU 400 mg/m² IV bolus on day 1, then 1200 mg/m²/d × 2 days (total 2400 mg/m² over 46–48 h) IV continuous infusion
	Repeat cycle every 2 weeks, plus
	Cetuximab 400 mg/m² IV over 2 h for the first infusion, then 250 mg/m² IV over 60 min weekly.
	OR
	Day 1: Cetuximab 500 mg/m² IV over 2 h every 2 weeks

Source: Adapted from NCCN.

Adverse Effects and Drug Interactions. The most common adverse reactions (≥20%) are rash, diarrhea, anorexia, fatigue, dyspnea, nail disorders, nausea, and vomiting. Serious adverse reactions include severe rash (>10%). Fatal interstitial lung disease occurs with a frequency of 0.7%–2.5%, and fatal hepatic failure has been reported, particularly in patients with baseline hepatic dysfunction. Other rare but serious toxicities include GI perforation, renal failure, arterial thrombosis, microangiopathic hemolytic anemia, hand-foot skin reaction, and corneal perforation or ulceration. Erlotinib therapy may cause rare cases of Stevens-Johnson syndrome/toxic epidermal necrolysis.

Concurrent use of proton pump inhibitors decreases the bioavailability of erlotinib by 50%. Plasma levels can vary due to drug interactions with inducers or inhibitors of CYP3A4. Patients using warfarin may experience poorer extrinsic coagulation (elevated INR) while taking erlotinib. Smoking accelerates metabolic clearance of erlotinib and may decrease its antitumor effects.

Gefitinib

Mechanism of Action. Gefitinib inhibits the EGFR tyrosine kinase by competitive blockade of ATP binding with an IC_{50} of 20–60 nM for the kinase activity.

ADME. Oral bioavailability is about 60%; peak plasma concentrations are achieved within 3–7 h. Absorption of gefitinib is not significantly altered by food but is reduced by drugs that cause elevations in gastric pH. Metabolism of gefitinib is predominantly via CYP3A4, with a terminal $t_{1/2}$ of 41 h. Inducers of CYP3A4 activity decrease gefitinib plasma concentrations and efficacy; conversely, CYP3A4 inhibitors increase plasma concentrations.

Therapeutic Uses. Gefitinib is approved for treatment of patients with metastatic NSCLC with EGFR mutations (Figure 67–1).

Adverse Effects and Drug Interactions. Diarrhea and skin reactions occur in more than 20% of patients. In addition to pustular/papular rash,

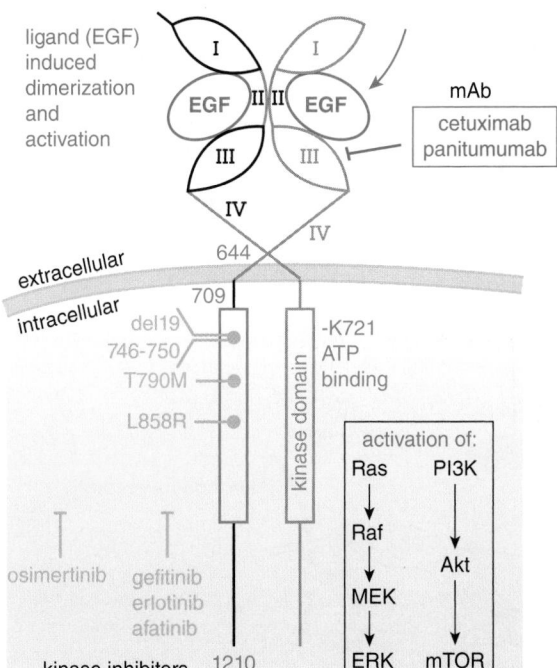

Figure 67–1 *Targeting the EGFR in cancer.* The extracellular portion of the EGFR contains the binding domains for growth factors that include EGF, TGF-α, and amphiregulin. Ligand binding to extracellular domains I and III induces conformational change and receptor dimerization through domains II and IV and activates intracellular signaling by cross-phosphorylation. The monoclonal antibodies cetuximab and panitumumab recognize the growth factor–binding domain and prevent ligand binding. The intracellular portion contains the tyrosine kinase activity and a C-terminal tail that recruits intracellular substrates after phosphorylation (see Chapter 3). EGFR mutations enhance downstream signaling, which provides a growth and survival advantage for cancer cells and confers sensitivity to treatment with TKIs gefitinib, erlotinib, and afatinib. The most common activating mutations are in-frame deletions in exon 19 (del 19) between E746 and A750 (~45%) and a missense mutation in exon 21 that leads to an L858R substitution (~40%). Lung cancers with these mutations are initially sensitive to the TKIs mentioned. Resistance develops, however, most commonly via the T790M substitution found in about 50% of resistant tumors. TKIs such as osimertinib have been developed for the treatment of cancers with the T790M mutation. Genotype screening for mutations in the EGFR is used to select patients who will receive TKIs and help predict which patients with lung cancer may respond best to some therapies. Numbers shown are amino acid positions in the EGFR protein.

other side effects include dry skin, nausea, vomiting, pruritus, anorexia, and fatigue. Most adverse effects occur within the first month of therapy and are manageable with medications. Asymptomatic increases in liver transaminases may necessitate discontinuation of therapy. Respiratory compromise and interstitial lung disease, especially in patients with prior radiation, occurs in fewer than 2% of patients but may have a fatal outcome. Inducers and inhibitors of CYP3A4 will alter plasma concentrations. Patients using warfarin should be monitored for poorer extrinsic coagulation (elevated INR) while taking gefitinib.

Afatinib

Mechanism of Action. Afatinib is a second-generation, orally bioavailable, *irreversible* inhibitor of EGFR (HER1) and HER2 receptor kinases with IC_{50} values of 0.5 and 14 nM, respectively.

ADME. The elimination $t_{1/2}$ of afatinib is 37 h after repeat dosing in patients with cancer. In patients with severe renal impairment, a dose reduction is recommended. Afatinib is a substrate of Pgp and coadministration of Pgp-modulating drugs can alter effective drug concentrations of afatinib.

Therapeutic Uses. Afatinib is approved for the first-line treatment of patients with metastatic NSCLC with EGFR mutations (see Figure 67–1)

and patients with metastatic squamous NSCLC that have progressed subsequent to platinum-based chemotherapy.

Adverse Effects and Drug Interactions. Most common adverse effects are diarrhea and skin rash/acneiform dermatitis, stomatitis, as well as hand-foot skin reactions. Also observed are interstitial lung disease, liver function abnormalities, and left ventricular dysfunction.

Resistance to Gefitinib, Erlotinib, and Afatinib

The majority of tumors with activating mutations in the EGFR initially respond to these kinase inhibitors of the first (*gefitinib, erlotinib*) and second generation (*afatinib*). Eventually, however, the tumors progress. Approximately 60% of NSCLC acquire a second EGFR mutation in the so-called EGFR gatekeeper residue T790M (see Figure 67–1) that prevents binding of these inhibitors to the kinase domain. *Osimertinib*, a third-generation inhibitor designed to recognize the T790M-mutant EGFR, is described next. Other mechanisms of resistance include mutational activation of downstream signaling molecules such as *KRAS* or activation of parallel signaling pathways, for example, through MET amplification, *EML4-ALK* translocation (see Figure 67–2), and small cell lung cancer transformation. ALK and MET kinase inhibitors are described in material that follows (Smit and Baas, 2015).

Osimertinib

Mechanism of Action. Osimertinib is a third-generation, orally bioavailable, *irreversible* inhibitor of T790M-mutant EGFR, with an IC_{50} value of 10 nM. The T790M gatekeeper mutation is often acquired after prior treatment with other EGFR kinase inhibitors (see previous discussion). Very sensitive detection methods can identify the presence of T790M in up to 30% of untreated patients, suggesting preexisting resistant subpopulations (see Chapter 65, Figure 65–3).

ADME. The mean $t_{1/2}$ of osimertinib is 48 h. Osimertinib is a substrate of CYP3A. The drug is primarily eliminated in the feces and to a lesser extent in the urine. Concurrent administration of inducers of CYP3A4 may necessitate an increase in the dose.

Therapeutic Uses. Osimertinib is approved for metastatic NSCLC that has progressed after prior EGFR TKI treatment and is positive for the EGFR T790M mutation. Genotyping of tumor biopsies for the T790M mutation is required after resistance develops. Recent studies have shown that noninvasive genotyping of DNA shed from tumor cells into the bloodstream may be feasible after extracting cell-free DNA from patient serum samples (Oxnard et al., 2016). Response rates are greater than 60% in patients with metastatic NSCLC. However, with osimertinib treatment acquired resistance occurs, most commonly manifested by the appearance of a third mutation, C797S. The mutation of Cys[797] to Ser[797] prevents formation of the potency-conferring covalent bond of the inhibitor (Thress et al., 2015). Inhibitors of C797S-mutant EGFR are under development for combination treatment with an EGFR-targeted antibody (Jia et al., 2016).

Adverse Effects and Drug Interactions. The most common adverse effects after osimertinib treatment are diarrhea and skin rash; however, these are much less common and severe than for first- and second-generation inhibitors, presumably because the activity on wild-type EGFR is limited with third-generation inhibitors. Also observed are interstitial lung disease, QTc prolongation, and left ventricular dysfunction.

Antibody Inhibitors of EGFRs

Cetuximab

Mechanism of Action. Cetuximab is a recombinant, chimeric human/mouse IgG_1 antibody that binds to the extracellular domain III of EGFR (Figure 67–1) and prevents ligand-dependent signaling and receptor dimerization, thereby blocking cell growth and survival signals. Cetuximab can also mediate ADCC against tumor cells that express high levels of EGFR.

ADME. Cetuximab exhibits nonlinear pharmacokinetics. A single loading dose of cetuximab intravenously is followed by weekly

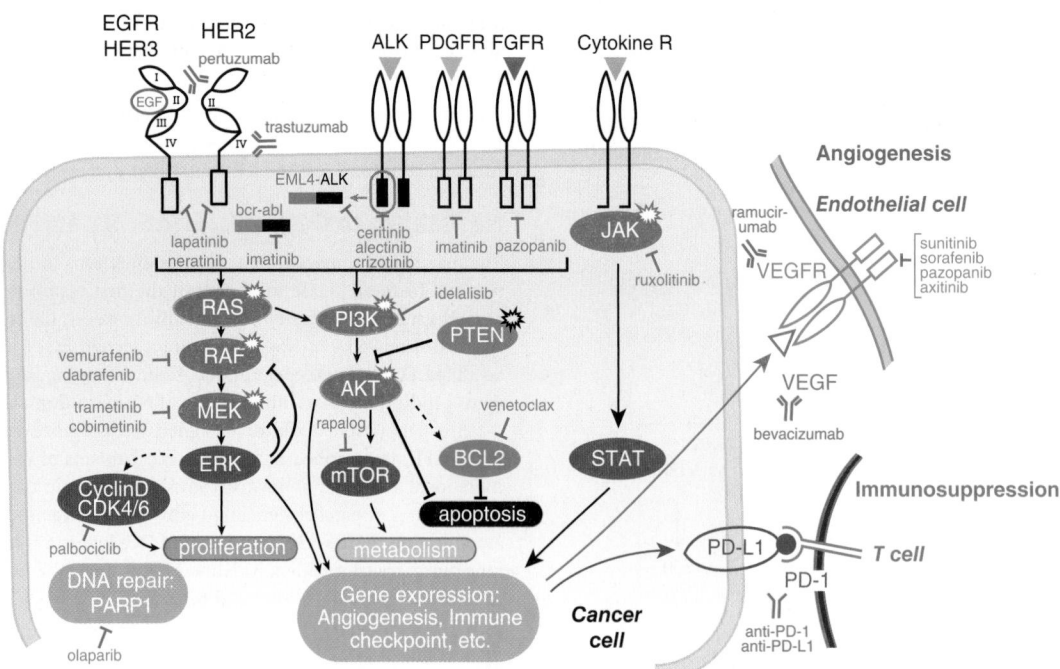

Figure 67–2 *Cancer cell signaling pathway and drug targets.* Extracellular binding of agonist ligands to transmembrane growth factor receptors causes receptor dimerization and activation of a C-terminal protein kinase that initiates intracellular signaling cascades that regulate gene expression and control cancer cell proliferation, apoptosis, metabolism, and metastasis. Crosstalk between cancer cells and the host stroma (including the vasculature and immune cells) is modulated through the release of angiogenic factors and the expression of immune checkpoint proteins. Cancer cell signaling can be altered through increased expression of receptors (e.g., HER2) or ligands, activating mutations in receptors (e.g. ALK, EGFR, FGFR) or in intracellular kinases (e.g., RAS, RAF, MEK, PI3K, AKT, JAK), gene translocations resulting in activated fusion proteins (e.g., bcr-abl, EML4-ALK), and the loss of function of an inhibitor of a pathway (e.g., the PTEN phosphatase) through mutation, gene deletion, or promoter methylation. Inhibitors are shown acting on three different cells: a cancer cell, an endothelial cell, and a T cell. Antibodies (green) are shown at their extracellular protein targets. Small-molecule inhibitors (in blue) are depicted adjacent to their intracellular target proteins. Proteins within red ellipses provide activating signals, those in green ellipses, inhibitory signals. Star bursts (✺) indicate signaling components in which mutations are common. Figure 67–4 describes mTOR signaling and its inhibition in more detail (see also Figure 35–2). Figure 67–6 describes Jak-STAT signaling in greater detail.

maintenance doses for the duration of treatment. Following intravenous administration, steady-state levels are achieved by the third weekly infusion. The volume of distribution approximates the intravascular space. The half-life of cetuximab is about 5 days.

Therapeutic Uses. Antibodies targeting EGFR show a different spectrum of antitumor activity than EGFR TKIs, in part due to the additional ADCC of antibodies toward tumor cells. Cetuximab and related antibodies are used to treat patients with *metastatic colon cancers* and *HNSCC.*

In colon cancer, cetuximab enhances the effectiveness of chemotherapy in patients with *KRAS* wild-type but not *KRAS*-mutant tumors (Van Cutsem et al., 2009). A combination of cetuximab with FOLFIRI (see Chapter 66) is typically used to treat patients with *KRAS* wild-type tumors that express EGFR. Cetuximab is also used as a single agent in patients who cannot tolerate irinotecan-based therapy and in patients with cancers that are resistant to oxaliplatin, irinotecan, and 5FU.

In HNSCC, cetuximab is used in combination with radiation or with platinum complex–based chemotherapy (e.g., cisplatin; see Chapter 66) for locally or regionally advanced HNSCC. Cetuximab is also indicated as a monotherapy for patients with metastatic or recurrent HNSCC who fail platinum-based chemotherapy.

Adverse Effects. Antibodies targeting EGFR have an adverse effect profile similar to that of first-generation EGFR protein tyr kinase inhibitors. Acneiform rash in the majority of patients, pruritus, nail changes, headache, and less frequently diarrhea are the most common adverse reactions. Rare but serious adverse effects include infusion reactions (~3% of patients), cardiopulmonary arrest (2%–3%), interstitial lung disease, and serum electrolyte imbalances, including hypomagnesemia. During

pregnancy, cetuximab may be transmitted to the developing fetus and has the potential to cause fetal harm.

Other EGFR Antibodies

Panitumumab

Panitumumab is a recombinant, fully humanized $IgG_{2\kappa}$ antibody that binds to the extracellular domain III of the EGFR and prevents ligand-dependent signaling. It is FDA approved for the treatment of EGFR-expressing mCRC in combination with chemotherapy and as monotherapy after disease progression following chemotherapy regimens containing fluoropyrimidine, oxaliplatin, and irinotecan (Saltz et al., 2006). Although panitumumab effectively inhibits EGFR signaling similarly to cetuximab, it is less effective at triggering cellular immune mechanisms that may be crucial for effective therapy of HNSCC (Trivedi et al., 2016)

ADME; Adverse Effects. Panitumumab exhibits nonlinear pharmacokinetic characteristics. Following intravenous administration every 2 weeks, steady-state levels are achieved by the third infusion. The mean $t_{1/2}$ is 7.5 days. ***Adverse effects*** of panitumumab are similar to those of cetuximab and include rash and dermatological toxicity, infusion reactions, pulmonary fibrosis, and electrolyte abnormalities.

Necitumumab

Necitumab is a recombinant human IgG_1 monoclonal antibody that binds to the extracellular domain of the EGFR. It is approved for first-line treatment of patients with metastatic, squamous NSCLC in combination with gemcitabine and cisplatin. Necitumumab is administered intravenously every 3 weeks prior to chemotherapy. Adverse effects are similar to those of cetuximab.

HER2/Neu Inhibitors

Human epidermal growth factor receptor 2 (also named Neu or ErbB2) is a member of the HER family, which includes also EGFR (HER1), HER3, and HER4 (Figure 67–2). The fixed conformation of the extracellular domain of HER2 resembles the ligand-activated state of the other HER family members and explains its unique function as a coreceptor that does not require ligand activation. In addition, due to this conformation, the overexpression of wild-type HER2 is sufficient to activate the intracellular tyrosine kinase and oncogenic signaling even in the absence of activating mutations, coreceptors, or ligands. Overexpression of HER2 is found in 20% to 30% of human breast cancers due to gene amplification on chromosome 17 and results in more aggressive tumors, lower response rates to hormonal therapies, and higher risk of disease recurrence after treatment.

HISTORY EGFR/HER Pathway-Targeted Cancer Therapy

The discovery and analysis of the EGFR (= HER1) in 1984 revealed a remarkable homology of its protein kinase domain to an oncogenic protein in the avian erythroblastosis retrovirus, v-erb. This oncogenic protein was the second one isolated from v-erb, resulting in erbB as an alternate name for HER gene family members. The HER2 gene was discovered based on its homology to v-erbB in human breast cancer and its oncogenic function in rat *neu*ral tumors, hence the name HER2/ErbB2/Neu (King et al., 1985; Schechter et al., 1985). The association of HER2 overexpression with poor prognosis in breast cancer (Slamon et al., 1987) provided the impetus for the development of HER2-targeted antibodies and a new concept in the treatment of HER2-positive breast cancers. *Trastuzumab* was the first anti-HER2 monoclonal antibody developed based on these discoveries; it was approved in the U.S. in 1998 and in Europe in 2000 for the treatment of patients with HER2-positive breast cancers. A small molecule kinase inhibitor of EGFR (HER1), *gefitinib* was approved in 1998 in the U.S. and in 2000 in Europe. A monoclonal antibody targeting EGFR, *cetuximab*, was approved in Switzerland in 2003 and in the U.S. in 2004.

Trastuzumab

Mechanism of Action

Trastuzumab is a humanized IgG1 monoclonal antibody that binds to the extracellular domain IV of HER2 (Figure 67–2), inhibiting hetero- and homodimerization and signal transduction. In addition, binding of trastuzumab to HER2 overexpressing cells can induce antibody-dependent, immune cell–mediated cytotoxicity. HER2 protein overexpression or gene amplification are predictive of response to HER2-targeted therapies (Wolff et al., 2013).

ADME

Trastuzumab has dose-dependent pharmacokinetics with a mean $t_{1/2}$ of 5.8 days on a weekly maintenance dose with alternative dosing every 3 weeks. Steady-state levels are achieved between 16 and 32 weeks.

Therapeutic Uses

Trastuzumab is approved for HER2-overexpressing breast and gastric cancer. It is used in combination with cytotoxic chemotherapeutics such as taxanes as initial treatment or as a single agent following relapse of disease after cytotoxic chemotherapy (Chapter 66).

Adverse Effects and Precautions

Acute adverse effects after infusion of trastuzumab are typical for monoclonal antibodies and can include fever, chills, nausea, dyspnea, and rashes. The most serious toxicity of trastuzumab is heart failure. Cardiotoxicity is caused by interruption of HER2/4 heterodimer signaling in cardiomyocytes, signaling that is essential for the maintenance of contractile

function. The cardiotoxic potential was predicted from gene inactivation studies ("knockouts") in mice, which showed that mice lacking HER2, HER4, or HER ligands developed dilated cardiomyopathy and heart failure. Thus, baseline electrocardiogram and cardiac ejection fraction measurement should be obtained before initiating treatment with trastuzumab to rule out underlying heart disease. Clinical monitoring for symptoms of congestive heart failure as well as periodic determination of LVEF during and after the course of therapy is recommended. When trastuzumab is used as a single agent, fewer than 5% of patients will experience a decrease in LVEF, and about 1% will have clinical signs of congestive failure. However, left ventricular dysfunction occurs in up to 20% of patients who receive a combination of doxorubicin and trastuzumab, reflecting the added cardiotoxicity of doxorubicin. In contrast, the risk of cardiac toxicity is greatly reduced with the recommended combination of trastuzumab with taxanes.

Pertuzumab

Mechanism of Action

Pertuzumab is a humanized monoclonal antibody directed against the extracellular receptor dimerization domain II of HER2 that is distinct from domain IV targeted by trastuzumab (Figure 67–2). Pertuzumab prevents ligand-dependent heterodimerization of other HER family members with HER2 and thus inhibits ligand-induced signaling, cell growth, and survival. In addition to the inhibition of receptor heterodimerization, binding of pertuzumab to HER2 overexpressing cells can induce antibody-dependent, immune cell–mediated cytotoxicity.

ADME

The median half-life of pertuzumab is 18 days; after an initial loading dose, maintenance doses are administered every 3 weeks.

Therapeutic Use

Preclinical studies with HER2-overexpressing human tumor cells grown as xenograft tumors in mice showed that the combination of pertuzumab and trastuzumab enhanced antitumor activity. In patients with HER2-positive metastatic breast cancer, the addition of pertuzumab to trastuzumab and docetaxel increases the median overall survival by 15.7 months (Swain et al., 2015). Use of pertuzumab is approved for the treatment of patients with HER2-positive, locally advanced, inflammatory, or early stage breast cancer in combination with trastuzumab and docetaxel.

Adverse Effects

Cardiotoxicity is similar to that of trastuzumab, and combinations with cardiotoxic anthracyclines are not indicated (Slamon et al., 2001). On the other hand, the combination of pertuzumab and trastuzumab does not cause any increase in cardiac toxicity (Swain et al., 2015). Based on its mechanism of action, pertuzumab can cause fetal harm when administered to a pregnant woman, and this risk should be weighed against the potential benefit.

Lapatinib

Mechanism of Action; ADME

Lapatinib is an orally bioavailable, small-molecule inhibitor of the EGFR and HER2 tyrosine kinases with an IC_{50} of about 10 nM. Lapatinib is metabolized by CYP3A4 with a plasma $t_{1/2}$ of 14 h. Concurrent administration of inducers and inhibitors of CYP3A4 may necessitate adjustment of the dose.

Therapeutic Uses; Adverse Effects

Lapatinib in combination with capecitabine is approved for the treatment of patients with metastatic HER2-positive and trastuzumab-refractory breast cancer. Lapatinib is also used in combination with the aromatase inhibitor letrozole (see Chapter 68) to treat postmenopausal women with hormone receptor–positive, metastatic breast cancer that overexpresses HER2. Frequent adverse effects include acneiform rash, diarrhea, cramping, and exacerbation of gastroesophageal reflux. When lapatinib is combined with capecitabine, diarrhea is worsened. Cardiac toxicity appears less pronounced than with trastuzumab, although lapatinib should be used with caution in combination with cardiotoxic drugs: A dose-dependent prolongation of the QT interval has been reported; thus, careful monitoring of patients with heart disease is recommended.

Neratinib

Neratinib is an orally bioavailable, *irreversible* inhibitor of the HER2 and EGFR protein tyrosine kinase with IC_{50} values of 59 nM and 92 nM, respectively. Addition of neratinib to standard chemotherapy that includes trastuzumab in patients with HER2-positive breast cancers has shown some efficacy. Diarrhea was the most common and frequent adverse effect, with grade 3 or 4 in over one-third of patients (Park et al., 2016).

Inhibitors of Platelet-Derived Growth Factor Receptor (PDGFR)

Signaling by the PDGFR plays a significant part in mesenchymal biology, including stem cell growth, and is involved in oncogenesis through aberrant cancer cell signaling, modulation of the tumor microenvironment, and facilitation of angiogenesis and metastasis. Small-molecule protein kinase inhibitors, including *imatinib* (see discussion below), have been used in the treatment of patients with GISTs that carry mutations in KIT or PDGFRA (Figure 67–2). The addition of the anti-PDGFR monoclonal antibody *olaratumab* to *doxorubicin* treatment (see Chapter 66) improves overall survival of patients with STS (Judson and van der Graaf, 2016).

Olaratumab

Mechanism of Action

Olaratumab is a human IgG1 monoclonal antibody that binds to PDGFRα and blocks ligand-mediated receptor activation (Tap et al., 2016).

Therapeutic Uses

Olaratumab is indicated, in combination with doxorubicin, for the treatment of adult patients with STS with a histologic subtype for which an anthracycline-containing regimen is appropriate and which is not amenable to curative treatment with radiotherapy or surgery. Recent studies showed that addition of olaratumab to doxorubicin doubled median survival of patients with metastatic STS to 26 months (Judson and van der Graaf, 2016).

Adverse Effects

The most common (≥20%) adverse effects of treatment with olaratumab are nausea, fatigue, neutropenia, musculoskeletal pain, inflammation of the mucous membranes (mucositis), alopecia, vomiting, diarrhea, decreased appetite, abdominal pain, neuropathy, and headache. Laboratory abnormalities are lymphopenia, neutropenia, thrombocytopenia, hyperglycemia, elevated aPTT, hypokalemia, and hypophosphatemia. Other adverse effects include infusion-related reactions (low blood pressure, fever, chills, rashes) and embryo-fetal harm.

Hedgehog Pathway Inhibitors

The hedgehog signaling pathway was discovered by genetic studies in fruit flies: Mutations resulting in stubby and hairy *Drosophila melanogaster* larvae inspired the naming of the signaling pathway as "hedgehog" or Hh, which is the name of the pathway's polypeptide ligand. Mammals have three hedgehog homologs. The hedgehog pathway controls embryonic cell differentiation in tissues of different species through distinct gradients of hedgehog signaling proteins that are key regulators during development. In adults, hedgehog signaling plays roles in stem cell regulation and tissue regeneration. BCC of the skin is one of several cancers associated with the dysregulation of this pathway.

Vismodegib is a first-in-class hedgehog signaling pathway inhibitor approved for the treatment of adult patients with BCC. It acts as a competitive antagonist of the SMO ("smoothens hedgehog") receptor in the hedgehog signaling pathway. Vismodegib is indicated for patients with metastatic or relapsed BCC. The drug is also undergoing clinical trials in other cancers. Common adverse effects include GI disorders (nausea, vomiting, diarrhea, constipation), muscle spasms, fatigue, hair loss, and dysgeusia (distortion of the sense of taste). These adverse effects are mostly mild to moderate. Vismodegib can cause embryo-fetal death and severe birth defects and must not be used during pregnancy.

Sonidegib is a hedgehog pathway inhibitor that binds to and inhibits SMO receptor signal transduction similar to *vismodegib*. Sonidegib is indicated for the treatment of patients with locally advanced BCC that has recurred following surgery or radiation therapy. Adverse effects are similar to those of vismodegib.

II. Intracellular Protein Kinases in Cancer Cells

HISTORY The RAS-RAF-MEK-ERK Pathway

HRAS and *KRAS*, named after Harvey and Kirsten **r**at **s**arcoma viruses and discovered in the early 1980s, were the first oncogenes discovered in human tumors. These oncogenes were found to be mutated and constitutively active in approximately 20% of all cancers and in up to 90% in specific cancers (pancreatic adenocarcinoma). NRAS was identified in human **n**euroblastoma. The first *RAF* gene was identified from a murine retrovirus named "**r**apidly **a**ccelerated **f**ibrosarcoma" due to its oncogenic effects. Following the discovery of the first human *RAF* gene, (*RAF-1*, also named *cRAF* = normal cellular *RAF*), the *RAF* genes *ARAF* and *BRAF* were identified; their gene products are ser/thre protein kinases. The signaling cascade of RAS-RAF-MEK-ERK was established by the early 1990s. This pathway plays a central role in cell proliferation and differentiation and is activated in many human cancers (Figure 67–2). Mutations in *RAF* genes can lead to one (BRAF) or two (cRAF, BRAF) changes in amino acids, rendering these gene products oncogenic and resulting in continuous cell proliferation and the development of cancer. Activating mutations of *BRAF* were detected in melanoma and other tumors in 2002. A small-molecule inhibitor targeting mutated BRAF, *vemurafenib*, was shown to be effective in melanoma in 2010 and approved by the FDA in 2011; the first inhibitor of MEK, *trametinib*, was approved in 2013.

Inhibitors of RAF Kinase: Vemurafenib, Dabrafenib

BRAF belongs to the RAF/mil family of serine/threonine protein kinases and plays a role in regulating signaling via MAPK (or ERK) (Figure 67–2).

In melanoma, MAPK signaling can be constitutively activated through alterations in membrane receptors or through mutations of RAS or BRAF. BRAF mutations confer constitutive activation of the kinase pathway independent of RAS activation. BRAF is mutated in about 55% of melanomas, and 90% of these mutations display a substitution of valine to glutamic acid (V600E) or to lysine (V600K), which results in constitutive protein kinase activation (Vultur and Herlyn, 2013). Approximately 8% of other cancers, colon cancer and NSCLC amongst them, also carry an activating mutation in *BRAF*. The BRAF inhibitors *vemurafenib* and *dabrafenib* are superior to traditional chemotherapy in improving survival in patients with mutant BRAF melanoma and are discussed in the material that follows. In patients with BRAF-mutant lung or colon cancers, only the lung cancer patients show a therapeutic benefit. This finding indicates that colon cancers do not depend on the activated mutant BRAF as a necessary oncogenic driver.

Vemurafenib

Mechanism of Action

Vemurafenib is an orally bioavailable inhibitor of mutated BRAF (V600E). The name *vemurafenib*" is derived from the target, that is, **V600E mu**tated **BRAF**. Vemurafenib also is effective against the less common BRAF V600K mutation. Melanoma cells lacking these mutations are not inhibited by vemurafenib.

ADME

Following oral administration, the elimination half-life for vemurafenib is 57 h.

Vemurafenib is a substrate of CYP3A4 and a substrate and an inhibitor of the Pgp exporter. Vemurafenib can increase concentrations of CYP1A2 substrates. Thus, concomitant use with the centrally acting α_2 adrenergic receptor agonist tizanidine, which has a narrow therapeutic window and is used as a muscle relaxant, should be avoided.

Therapeutic Uses

Vemurafenib is FDA approved for the treatment of patients with metastatic melanoma harboring activating BRAF (V600E/K) mutations. It is not indicated for the treatment of patients with melanoma carrying wild-type BRAF.

Adverse Effects

The most common adverse effects (30%–60% of patients) are cutaneous events. Arthralgia, fatigue, and nausea are also observed but at a lower frequency. cuSCCs and keratoacanthomas that may need surgical removal appear in more than 20% of patients. The median time to the first appearance of these skin lesions is 7 to 8 weeks and is caused by a paradoxical stimulation of wild-type BRAF. Increased photosensitivity reactions can be prevented with sunblock. QT prolongation has been observed, necessitating controlling for risk factors and monitoring ECG and electrolytes.

Drug Resistance

Melanoma is one of the most aggressive malignancies, with a high mutation rate that renders these tumors highly heterogeneous and thus prone to the quick development of resistance to drug treatments. After the initial response of melanoma lesions to treatment with vemurafenib, resistant cancer cell subpopulations are selected, typically in less than 6 months. Constitutively active mutant *NRAS*; downstream mutations in MEK; overexpression of the growth receptor PDGFR-B; activation of parallel pathways such as PI3K/Akt, mTOR, and STAT3 signaling; or stromal cell secretion of HGF can drive this drug resistance (Chapman et al., 2011). Combination treatment with a MEK inhibitor (*trametinib, cobimetinib*) that acts downstream of BRAF (Figure 67–2) can delay development of resistance to single-agent BRAF inhibitors (Robert et al., 2015).

Dabrafenib

Mechanism of Action

Dabrafenib is an orally bioavailable, small-molecule inhibitor of mutated forms of BRAF kinases. Dabrafenib can inhibit the proliferation of tumor cells that contain a constitutively active mutated BRAF with in vitro IC_{50} values of 0.65, 0.5, and 1.84 nM for the V600E, V600K, and V600D mutations, respectively. At about 5-fold higher concentrations, dabrafenib also inhibits wild-type BRAF and cRAF (IC_{50} values of 3.2 and 5.0 nM, respectively). Dabrafenib, in combination with trametinib (see discussion that follows), is approved for the treatment of patients with unresectable or metastatic melanoma and NSCLC with BRAF mutations. The drug is not indicated for the treatment of patients with wild-type BRAF melanoma.

ADME

The mean terminal half-life of dabrafenib is 8 h after oral administration.

Dabrafenib is metabolized primarily by CYP2C8 and CYP3A4. Patients should be monitored closely for adverse reactions and for loss of efficacy if treated with drugs that induce CYP2C8 and CYP3A4 activity.

Therapeutic Uses

Dabrafenib was FDA approved as a single-agent treatment of patients with BRAF V600E mutation-positive advanced melanoma in 2013. Resistance to dabrafenib and other BRAF inhibitors occurs within about 6 months, but a combination with the MEK inhibitor trametinib can delay the development of resistance (see discussion that follows). Thus, the FDA has approved the combination of dabrafenib and trametinib for the treatment of patients with BRAF V600E/K-mutant metastatic melanoma and BRAF V600E-mutant NSCLC.

Adverse Effects and Drug Interactions

Adverse effects, in order of decreasing frequency, are hyperkeratosis, headache, pyrexia, arthralgia, papilloma, alopecia, and PPES. An increased incidence of cuSCC is expected in about 10% of patients, with a median time of 2 months to the first diagnosis. About one-third of those patients develop more than one lesion with continued administration of dabrafenib. With the dabrafenib-trametinib combination, the appearance of cuSCC is delayed to a median time of 7 months and occurs in only 3% of patients. Most common adverse reactions (≥20%) for dabrafenib in combination with trametinib are pyrexia, rash, chills, headache, arthralgia, and cough. Cardiomyopathy has also been reported.

Inhibitors of MEK: Trametinib, Cobimetinib

The MKKs or MEKs are serine-threonine kinases that act downstream of RAF. They provide additional targets for the inhibition of the RAS-RAF-MEK-ERK pathway that is frequently activated in cancer and controls cell survival, differentiation, and growth (Figure 67–2).

Trametinib

Trametinib was the first inhibitor of the MEK family to be FDA approved.

Mechanism of Action

Trametinib is an orally bioavailable, reversible, allosteric inhibitor of ATP binding to the MEK1/2 kinases. Trametinib inhibits MEK1/2 kinase activities with an IC_{50} of about 2 nM.

ADME

Bioavailability of oral trametinib is 72% and is reduced if taken with a high-calorie meal. Peak plasma concentrations are achieved 1.5 h postdose. The drug has a relatively long half-life of 4 to 5 days. Trametinib is not a substrate of CYP enzymes and mild renal or hepatic impairment does not affect exposure to the drug significantly.

Therapeutic Uses

The FDA approved trametinib as a monotherapy for patients with mutant BRAF V600E/K melanoma due to improved survival relative to standard therapy. Trametinib in combination with the BRAF inhibitor dabrafenib is also approved for mutant V600E/K metastatic melanoma and mutant V600E metastatic NSCLC. Trametinib treatment lacks efficacy in patients who received prior treatment with BRAF inhibitors. This suggests that resistance to BRAF and MEK inhibitors involves similar mechanisms (Kim et al., 2013).

Adverse Effects

The most frequent adverse effects are cutaneous rash, acneiform dermatitis, and diarrhea. Fatigue, nausea, and lymphedema also occur. Serious grade 3-4 skin toxicity is found in 6% of patients. Other serious adverse effects are cardiomyopathy, hypertension, hemorrhage, interstitial lung disease, and ocular toxic effects. In contrast to the BRAF inhibitors, trametinib does not cause cuSCC. Because trametinib can cause fetal harm when administered to a pregnant woman, this risk must be weighed against the potential benefit.

Drug Resistance

Activation of alternative signaling pathways that include PI3K/Akt, mTOR, and STAT3 signaling can bypass MEK inhibition and result in drug-resistant tumors. Also, mutations in the allosteric binding pocket and activation loop of MEK1 can inhibit the binding of the inhibitor and cause resistance to trametinib. Resistance to single-agent trametinib occurs within 6 to 7 months of the initiation of treatment at a rate approaching 50%. As a strategy to overcome resistance, trametinib has been combined with the BRAF inhibitor *dabrafenib* for the treatment of patients with BRAF V600E/K-mutant metastatic melanoma (Flaherty et al., 2012). This combination has been approved by the FDA.

Cobimetinib

Mechanism of Action; ADME

Cobimetinib is an orally bioavailable, reversible inhibitor of MEK1/2 protein kinase activity with an IC_{50} of about 4nM. Its elimination half-life ranges from 1 to 3 days. Cobimetinib is a substrate for CYP3A, and concomitant treatment with inducers or inhibitors of CYP3A will reduce or increase the systemic exposure of patients.

Therapeutic Uses

A combination of cobimetinib and vemurafenib is FDA approved for the treatment of patients with unresectable or metastatic melanoma with a BRAF V600E/K mutation.

Adverse Effects

The most common adverse effects are diarrhea, photosensitivity reaction, nausea, pyrexia, and vomiting. Major hemorrhagic events can occur with cobimetinib; patients should be monitored for signs and symptoms of bleeding. The drug also increases the risk of cardiomyopathy. The safety in patients with decreased LVEF has not been established.

Other MEK Inhibitors

Under development are *binimetinib*, a MEK inhibitor being studied in patients with NRAS-mutant melanoma, and *encorafinib*, a BRAF inhibitor being used in combination with *binimetinib* for patients with BRAF-mutant melanoma.

Inhibitors of Jak1 and Jak2

Janus associated kinases (Jaks) mediate the signaling of cytokines and growth factors in hematopoiesis and immune function (see, for instance, Figure 35–2). Intracellular Jak signaling recruits STATs to cytokine membrane receptors (Figure 67–2). After STAT activation and subsequent localization to the nucleus, STATs modulate gene expression. Jak signaling is dysregulated in myelofibrosis and polycythemia vera, which prompted the development of Jak inhibitors. *Ruxolitinib* is the first drug in this class.

Ruxolitinib

Ruxolitinib

Mechanism of Action; ADME

Ruxolitinib is an orally bioavailable (95%) analogue of ATP that inhibits the protein kinase activities of Jak1 and Jak2 (IC_{50} value of 3 nM) and exhibits more than 100-fold selectivity for Jak1/2 over Jak3. The half-life of ruxolitinib is about 3 h; its metabolism is mainly via hepatic CYP3A4, with products excreted largely in the urine. In patients with renal or hepatic impairment, a dose reduction is recommended.

Therapeutic Uses

Ruxolitinib is indicated for the treatment of patients with polycythemia vera who have had an inadequate response to hydroxyurea and for the treatment of myelofibrosis.

Adverse Effects and Drug Interactions

The most common adverse reactions, thrombocytopenia and anemia, should be met with a dose reduction or discontinuation of treatment. Infections should be resolved before treatment with ruxolitinib. In a few patients, BCC or squamous cell skin carcinoma may occur, warranting periodic skin examinations during treatment. Strong CYP3A4 inhibitors (e.g., ketoconazole, fluconazole) increase exposure to ruxolitinib and prolong its half-life to 6 h. Due to the adverse hematopoietic effects, postpartum patients should discontinue nursing during drug treatment.

Cyclin-Dependent Kinase (CDK) 4/6 Inhibitors

The CDKs are a family of over 20 serine/threonine protein kinases that modulate intracellular signaling during cell cycle progression (Figure 67–2). Given their pivotal role in cellular proliferation, CDKs are prime targets for development of inhibitors. However, different tissue selectivity and distinct cell cycle–specific activity periods of different CDKs provide a challenge.

CDK4/6 are attractive targets because they control cell cycle progression from the G_0/G_1 to S phase. Interaction of cyclin D with CDK4/6 enhances phosphorylation of the Rb tumor suppressor protein, inactivating Rb and permitting the transcription of factors that control transition into the S phase. Inhibition of CDK4/6 will inhibit the phosphorylation and inactivation of Rb and cause a G_1 arrest in susceptible cells that utilize this pathway, thereby providing the rationale for the use of inhibitors of CDK4/6 (Figure 67–3). This cell cycle checkpoint is frequently compromised in cancers due to cyclin D amplification, loss of Rb function, or loss of negative regulators of CDK4/6, such as $p16^{INK4A}$, a tumor suppressor named for its molecular mass (it is a small protein of 16 kDa) and its capacity to inhibit CDK4. The class of CDK inhibitory drugs is identified by the syllable *ciclib* and includes *palbociclib*, discussed next.

Palbociclib

Mechanism of Action

Palbociclib is an orally bioavailable, small-molecule inhibitor of CDK4 and CDK6, with IC_{50} values of 11 and 16 nM, respectively, and without inhibitory activity against CDK1, 2, or 5.

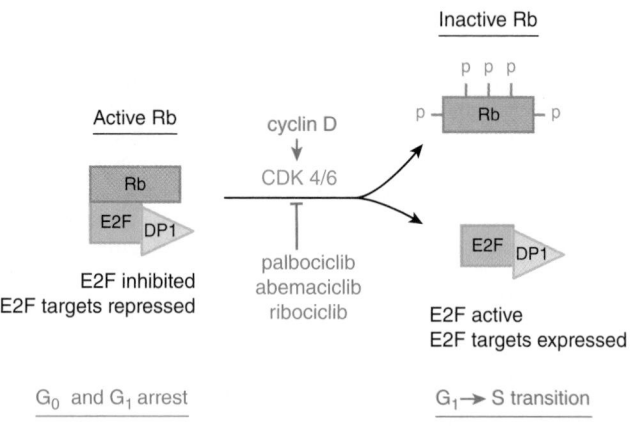

Figure 67–3 *CDK4 inhibitors: retinoblastoma protein, cyclin-dependent protein kinases, and the regulation of cell cycle progression.* In quiescent and differentiated cells (in G_0 or in cells arrested in G_1), the Rb protein is active and interacts with a heterodimer of the transcription factor E2F and its dimerization partner DP1, repressing transcription of promoters regulated by E2F. As a cell begins a cycle of division, cyclins activate CDKs that phosphorylate Rb, disrupting the Rb-E2F/DP complexes and permitting accumulation of active E2F complexes that drive transcription. This cell cycle checkpoint is frequently compromised in cancers due to cyclin D amplification, loss of Rb function, or loss of negative regulators of CDK4/6. Hyperphosphorylation of Rb can occur via mutations in Rb or expression of viral oncoproteins targeting Rb, placing the cell in a state of extensive proliferation, with reduced capacity to exit the cell cycle. Inhibition of CDK4/6 can cause G_1 arrest in susceptible cells (Dyson, 2016). CDK inhibitors (in red lettering) are identified by the disyllabic suffix "ciclib."

ADME

The mean plasma elimination $t_{1/2}$ is 29 h. Palbociclib is a substrate and an inhibitor of CYP3A; thus, doses of palbociclib or of substrates of CYP3A4 may need to be reduced when they are given concurrently, with special attention to coadministered agents with narrow therapeutic indices (see the Adverse Effects and Drug Interactions section). The sulfotransferase SULT2A1 also participates in palbociclib metabolism.

Therapeutic Uses

Palbociclib is the first CDK inhibitor approved by the FDA for the treatment of advanced or metastatic breast cancer that is ER positive and HER2 negative. Palbociclib is used in combination with letrozole, an aromatase inhibitor, as initial endocrine-based therapy in postmenopausal women or with the antiestrogen fulvestrant in women with disease progression after endocrine-based therapy. Letrozole and fulvestrant are described in Chapter 68. The inclusion of palbociclib with different endocrine-based treatments almost doubles the progression-free survival of patients (Cristofanilli et al., 2016; Finn et al., 2016).

Adverse Effects and Drug Interactions

The most common adverse effects of palbociclib are neutropenia, leukopenia, infections, stomatitis, fatigue, nausea, anemia, headache, diarrhea, and thrombocytopenia. The most common grades 3 and 4 adverse effects are neutropenia (>60%), leukopenia (~25%), and anemia (~5%). Patients should avoid breastfeeding while taking palbociclib. Letrozole and fulvestrant do not alter the pharmacokinetics of palbociclib.

Patients should avoid concomitant use of strong CYP3A inhibitors (e.g., clarithromycin, indinavir, itraconazole, ketoconazole, lopinavir/ritonavir, nefazodone, nelfinavir, posaconazole, ritonavir, saquinavir, telaprevir, telithromycin, and voriconazole). Coadministration of a strong CYP3A inhibitor (e.g., itraconazole) can markedly increase exposure to palbociclib (by 87% in healthy subjects). Patients should avoid grapefruit or grapefruit juice. If palbociclib coadministration with a strong CYP3A inhibitor cannot be avoided, reduce the dose of palbociclib.

Coadministration of a strong CYP3A inducer will decrease exposure to palbociclib. Thus, avoid concomitant use of phenytoin, rifampin, carbamazepine, enzalutamide, and St. John's Wort.

Palbociclib may increase exposure to coadministered CYP3A substrates with narrow therapeutic indices (e.g., midazolam, alfentanil, cyclosporine, dihydroergotamine, ergotamine, everolimus, fentanyl, pimozide, quinidine, sirolimus, and tacrolimus), requiring reduction of palbociclib dose.

Other Drugs That Target CDK4/6

Abemaciclib and *ribociclib* are CDK4/6 inhibitors with inhibitory profiles similar to that of *palbociclib*. These inhibitors are currently undergoing clinical trials in patients with breast cancer as well as a variety of other cancers. Ribociclib is FDA-approved for treating breast cancer. The major efficacy and adverse effects of these inhibitors appear to overlap. However, differences in the selectivity for the targeted kinases appear to result in different adverse effect profiles and possibly future uses of these inhibitors (O'Leary et al., 2016).

Bruton Tyrosine Kinase (BTK) Inhibitor

The BTK protein tyr kinase plays important roles in the function of B cells. The PH domain of BTK binds PIP3. BTK-PIP3 phosphorylates PLC, which hydrolyzes phosphatidylinositol, thereby activating the IP_3-Ca^{2+}-PKC pathway in B cells.

Ibrutinib

Mechanism of Action

Ibrutinib is an orally bioavailable, small-molecule inhibitor that inactivates BTK through covalent binding to cys[481] near the ATP-binding domain.

ADME

Administration with food (vs. on an empty stomach) roughly doubles absorption. The elimination half-life of ibrutinib is 4 to 6 h. It is a substrate of CYP3A; CYP2D6 participates to a minor degree. Metabolites are excreted mainly via the feces; renal excretion is minor. Hepatic impairment is likely to increase ibrutinib exposure. Ibrutinib is not a substrate for Pgp.

Therapeutic Uses

Ibrutinib inhibits malignant B-cell proliferation and is indicated for the treatment of patients with MCL who have received at least one prior therapy, CLL, SLL, and WM.

Adverse Effects and Drug Interactions

The most common adverse effect (≥20%) in patients with B-cell malignancies are neutropenia, pyrexia, thrombocytopenia, hemorrhage, anemia, diarrhea, nausea, musculoskeletal pain, rash, and fatigue. The onset of hypertension has been observed within less than a month and up to 2 years after the start of ibrutinib treatment. Thus, blood pressure should be monitored and antihypertensive treatment initiated or modified. Atrial fibrillations are observed in up to 7% of patients; this requires monitoring and treatment. Second primary malignancies occur in up to 16% of patients, most of them nonmelanoma skin cancers.

Strong (e.g., azole antifungals) and moderate (e.g., diltiazem, erythromycin) CYP inhibitors will increase ibrutinib's AUC; thus, dose reduction is recommended when using CYP3A inhibitors concomitantly. The reverse is true for strong and moderate CYP inducers (e.g., rifampin, efavirenz), which will decrease ibrutinib exposure.

Ibrutinib is classified *pregnancy category D* (see Appendix I) and may cause fetal harm. Pregnant patients and those at risk for pregnancy should be apprised of the drug's hazardous potential.

Acalabrutinib is a second-generation, orally bioavailable, irreversible BTK inhibitor that shows higher selectivity for BTK versus other kinases (e.g., EGFR, ITK) than ibrutinib. Acalabrutinib appears to have less-frequent off-target toxicities. Acalabrutinib received orphan drug designation for the treatment of CLL in the U.S. and for CLL, SLL, MCL, or WM in Europe.

Inhibitors of the BCR-ABL Kinase

A single molecular event, the Philadelphia chromosome translocation t(9;22), leads to expression of ABL and BCR. This fusion generates a constitutively active protein kinase, BCR-ABL, resulting in continuous and uncontrollable cell division. BCR-ABL drives the malignant phenotype of CML (Figure 67–2).

HISTORY BCR-ABL Kinase Inhibitors

Imatinib mesylate, originally named "sti 571" (signal transduction inhibitor 571), was the first protein kinase inhibitor designed to target a driver mutation in a cancer and to receive FDA approval. It was approved in 2001 under the name *Gleevec* and is now designated as an essential drug by the World Health Organization (WHO). Imatinib targets the BCR-ABL tyrosine kinase fusion protein that drives CML. Imatinib-resistant ABL mutations were uncovered in 2002 and led to the development of next-generation inhibitors *dasatinib* and *nilotinib*, which overcome the resistance.

Imatinib and the second-generation inhibitors *dasatinib* and *nilotinib* induce clinical and molecular remissions in more than 90% of patients with CML in the chronic phase of disease. Due to its inhibition of other kinases, imatinib is also effective in some other tumors, including GISTs (driven by a c-KIT mutation), hypereosinophilia syndrome, and dermatofibrosarcoma protuberans (all driven by activating mutations in the PDGFR; see Figure 67–2).

Imatinib, Dasatinib, and Nilotinib

Mechanisms of Action

These are orally bioavailable, small-molecule kinase inhibitors. Imatinib was identified through high-throughput screening against the BCR-ABL kinase. Dasatinib, a second-generation BCR-ABL inhibitor, also inhibits the Src kinase, and unlike imatinib, it binds both the open (active) and closed (inactive) configurations of the BCR-ABL kinase. Nilotinib was designed to have increased potency and specificity compared to imatinib. Its structure overcomes mutations that cause imatinib resistance. Imatinib and nilotinib bind to a segment of the kinase domain that fixes the enzyme in a closed or nonfunctional state, in which the protein is unable to bind its substrate/phosphate donor, ATP. These three BCR-ABL kinase inhibitors differ in their inhibitory potencies, binding specificities, and susceptibility to resistance mutations in the target enzyme. Dasatinib (IC_{50} ~ 1 nM) and nilotinib (IC_{50} ~ 20 nM) inhibit BCR-ABL kinase more potently than imatinib (IC_{50} ~ 100 nM).

Mechanisms of Resistance

Resistance to these TKIs arises from point mutations in three separate segments of the kinase domain. The contact points between imatinib and the enzyme become sites of mutations in drug-resistant leukemic cells; these mutations prevent tight binding of the drug and lock the enzyme in its open configuration, in which it has access to substrate and is enzymatically active. Nilotinib retains inhibitory activity in the presence of most point mutations that confer resistance to imatinib. Other mutations affect the phosphate-binding region and the "activation loop" of the domain with varying degrees of associated resistance. Some mutations, such as those at amino acids 351 and 355, confer low levels of resistance to imatinib, possibly explaining the clinical response of some resistant tumors to dose escalation of imatinib.

Molecular studies have detected cells with resistance-mediating kinase mutations *prior* to initiation of therapy, particularly in patients with Ph+ ALL or CML in blast crisis. This finding indicates that drug-resistant cells arise through spontaneous mutation and expand under the selective pressure of drug exposure. Mechanisms other than BCR-ABL kinase mutations play a minor role in resistance to imatinib. Amplification of the wild-type kinase gene, leading to overexpression of the enzyme, has been identified in tumor samples from patients resistant to treatment. The *MDR* gene confers resistance experimentally but has not been implicated in clinical resistance. Ph− clones lacking the BCR-ABL translocation and displaying the karyotype of myelodysplastic cells may emerge in patients receiving imatinib for CML; these may progress to MDS and AML. Their origin is unclear.

A comparison amongst secondary mutations in the EGFR, ABL, and KIT kinases following treatment with BCR-ABL kinase inhibitors shows striking differences: The T790M gatekeeper mutation in the EGFR (Figure 67–1) accounts for about 90% of secondary mutations. In contrast, secondary resistance mutations in ABL or KIT after treatment of CML or GIST with imatinib are found across the kinase domain and rarely at the analogous gatekeeper residue in ABL (T[315]) or in KIT (T[670]).

ADME

Imatinib is well absorbed after oral administration and reaches maximal plasma concentrations within 2–4 h. The elimination $t_{1/2}$ of imatinib and its major active metabolite, the *N*-desmethyl derivative, are about 18 and 40 h, respectively. Food does not change the pharmacokinetic profile. Doses of more than 300 mg/d achieve trough levels of 1 μM, which correspond to in vitro levels required to kill BCR-ABL–expressing cells. In the treatment of GISTs, higher doses may improve response rates. CYP3A4 is the major metabolizer of imatinib; thus, drugs that induce or interact with CYP3A4 can alter the pharmacokinetics of imatinib. Coadministration of imatinib and rifampin, an inducer of CYP3A4, lowers the plasma imatinib AUC by 70%. Imatinib, as a competitive CYP3A4 substrate, inhibits the metabolism of simvastatin and increases its plasma AUC by 3.5-fold.

Dasatinib. Oral dasatinib is well absorbed; its bioavailability is significantly reduced at neutral gastric pH (i.e., after antacids and H_2 blockers) but is unaffected by food. The plasma $t_{1/2}$ of dasatinib is 3–5 h. Dasatinib exhibits dose-proportional increases in AUC, and its clearance is constant over the dose range of 15–240 mg/d. Dasatinib is metabolized primarily by CYP3A4, with minor contributions by FMO3 and UGT. The major metabolite is equipotent to the parent drug but represents only 5% of the AUC. Plasma concentrations of dasatinib are affected by inducers and inhibitors of CYP3A4 in a similar fashion to imatinib.

Nilotinib. Approximately 30% of an oral dose of nilotinib is absorbed after administration, with peak concentrations in plasma 3 h after dosing. Unlike the other BCR-ABL inhibitors, nilotinib's bioavailability increases significantly in the presence of food. The drug has a plasma $t_{1/2}$ about 17 h, and plasma concentrations reach a steady state only after 8 days of daily dosing. Nilotinib is metabolized by CYP3A4, with predictable alteration by inducers, inhibitors, and competitors of CYP3A4. Nilotinib is a substrate and an inhibitor of Pgp.

Therapeutic Uses

These protein TKIs have efficacy in diseases in which ABL, *KIT*, or PDGFR have dominant roles in driving tumor growth, reflecting the presence of a mutation that results in constitutive activation of the kinase. Imatinib shows therapeutic benefits in patients with chronic-phase CML (BCR-ABL) or GIST and a subset of patients with mucosal or acral lentiginous melanoma (*KIT* mutation positive), chronic myelomonocytic leukemia (EVT6-PDGFR translocation), hypereosinophilia syndrome (FIP1L1-P-DGFR), and dermatofibrosarcoma protuberans (constitutive production of the ligand for PDGFR). It is the agent of choice for patients with metastatic GIST and is used as adjuvant therapy of c-KIT–positive GIST. Dasatinib is approved for patients with newly diagnosed CML with resistance to or intolerance of imatinib in both chronic and advanced phases of disease and for use combined with cytotoxic chemotherapy in patients with Ph+ ALL who are resistant or intolerant to prior therapies.

Adverse Effects

Imatinib, dasatinib, and nilotinib cause GI symptoms (diarrhea, nausea, and vomiting) that are usually readily controlled. All three drugs promote fluid retention, edema, and periorbital swelling. Myelosuppression occurs infrequently but may require transfusion support and dose reduction or discontinuation of the drug. These drugs can be associated with hepatotoxicity. Dasatinib may cause pleural effusions and pulmonary hypertension in a small subset of patients. Nilotinib and dasatinib may prolong the QT interval; nilotinib has been associated with cardiac and vascular events, including ischemia. Most nonhematological adverse reactions are self-limited and respond to dose adjustments. After the adverse reactions have resolved, the drug may be reinitiated and titrated back to effective doses.

Bosutinib

Bosutinib is another second-generation, orally bioavailable BCR-ABL kinase inhibitor (IC_{50} = 1.2 nM). Bosutinib also inhibits activity of Src (IC_{50} = 1 nM) and other members of the Src family. It is FDA approved for the treatment of patients with chronic, accelerated, or blast-phase Ph+ CML with resistance or intolerance to prior therapy. The most common adverse reactions (incidence greater than 20%) are diarrhea, nausea, thrombocytopenia, vomiting, abdominal pain, rash, anemia, pyrexia, and fatigue.

Ponatinib

Ponatinib is a third-generation BCR-ABL kinase inhibitor. Imatinib (first generation) lacks efficacy for the more advanced disease phases, and cells with mutations in the BCR-ABL tyrosine kinase domain are resistant. Second-generation inhibitors (nilotinib, dasatinib, bosutinib) were developed to address these weaknesses, although they do not inhibit the T315I mutant of BCR-ABL that is found in 15%–20% of patients with CML.

Mechanism of Action

Ponatinib is a third-generation, orally bioavailable kinase inhibitor that is active against the T315I mutant BCR-ABL and also is effective toward all other known BCR-ABL1 kinase mutants. IC_{50} values (nM) for different kinases are as follows: ABL, 0.37; PDGFR, 1.1; VEGFR2, 1.5; FGFR1, 2.2; and Src, 5.4.

ADME

Peak ponatinib concentrations are observed within 6 h and are unaffected by food or fasting. Drug solubility is pH dependent, with higher pH resulting in decreased solubility. Accordingly, drugs that affect gastric pH (such as H_2 antagonists, antacids, and PPIs) may significantly alter ponatinib bioavailability. Ponatinib is highly (99%) bound to plasma proteins and is a weak substrate for Pgp and ABCG2 transporters. Metabolism is primarily via CYP3A4 and to lesser extents by CYPs 2C8, 2D6, and 3A511; esterases; and amidases. Coadministration of CYP3A inhibitors significantly increases ponatinib concentrations. The $t_{1/2}$ of ponatinib is about 24 h. Unmetabolized ponatinib is primarily excreted in the feces (87%), with a small portion (5%) in the urine.

Therapeutic Uses

Ponatinib is approved for resistant CML and Ph+ ALL. Clinical cytogenetics measurements are a key tool for monitoring the response to therapy, reported as the percentage of Ph+ karyotypes in 20 bone marrow metaphases (major cytogenetic response; MCyR). Ponatinib produces an overall 54% MCyR in patients with early-phase CML and a 70% MCyR in patients with early-phase CML with the T315I mutation. Because of ponatinib's potency and efficacy against all known BCR-ABL single mutants, trials are under way that may advance this therapy to a first-line treatment.

Adverse Effects

Arterial thrombosis and hepatotoxicity are major adverse effects; thus, appropriate precautions, dose reduction, monitoring, or discontinuation are recommended following arterial thrombotic or hepatotoxic events. Dose-limiting toxicities include elevated lipase or amylase levels and pancreatitis.

Inhibitors of Anaplastic Lymphoma Kinase (ALK)

ALK is a membrane monospan with an extracellular domain and an intracellular protein tyr kinase domain (Figure 67–2). The importance of this protein kinase in human cancers is the capacity of the *ALK* gene to form fusion genes that become oncogenic drivers. A 2;5 chromosomal translocation yields an oncogenic fusion gene in which a 3′ portion of *ALK* (chromosome 2) contributes coding for the catalytic domain and is joined to a 5′ region of the *NPM* gene. The extracellular and transmembrane sequences of ALK are absent in the *ALK-NPM* fusion gene, which is the oncogenic driver of malignant progression in anaplastic large cell lymphoma (ALCL). A similar translocation of the ALK kinase and fusion with EML4 creates the oncogenic driver in a subset of NSCLC (Martelli et al., 2010), as shown in Figure 67–2. *ALK* also fuses with numerous additional 5′ partners (Roskoski, 2017). *Alectinib, crizotinib,* and *ceritinib* are small-molecule inhibitors of ALK kinase that are used in the treatment of ALK translocation-positive cancers.

Crizotinib

Mechanism of Action

Crizotinib is an orally bioavailable inhibitor of receptor tyrosine kinases that include HGFR/cMET, ALK, and ROS1. IC_{50} values are 11 nM and 24 nM for HGFR/cMet and ALK, respectively.

ADME

Crizotinib is predominantly metabolized by CYP3A4/5 and shows a terminal half-life of 42 h. The typical dose of 250 mg twice daily is reduced to once daily in patients with severe renal impairment and a creatinine clearance below 30 mL/min.

Therapeutic Uses

Crizotinib is approved for the treatment of patients with locally advanced or metastatic NSCLC harboring ALK or ROS1 gene rearrangements (Figure 67–2) (Thomas et al., 2015). The *ROS1* gene product is a receptor tyr protein kinase that is structurally similar to ALK. *ROS1* also participates in gene translocations and the formation of oncogenic fusion genes that have a 1% incidence in lung cancers.

Adverse Effects

The most common adverse reactions are GI toxicity including nausea, diarrhea, and vomiting as well as hepatic, respiratory, and ocular toxicity and neuropathy. Also observed are QT prolongation and bradycardia.

Alectinib

Mechanism of Action

Alectinib is an orally bioavailable inhibitor of ALK kinase activity with an IC_{50} of 1.9 nM. Alectinib shows a higher selectivity for ALK than crizotinib and is active against mutant forms of ALK that are found in tumors resistant to crizotinib.

ADME

Alectinib has an elimination half-life of 33 h and is metabolized by CYP3A4. Coadministration of alectinib with CYP3A inhibitors or inducers will alter plasma concentrations.

Therapeutic Uses

Alectinib is approved for the treatment of patients with advanced or recurrent NSCLC harboring the ALK fusion gene (ALK+). Patients with ALK+ NSCLC who have progressed on treatment with crizotinib or are intolerant to crizotinib also qualify.

Adverse Effects

The most common adverse effects are fatigue, constipation, edema, and myalgia. Pneumonitis, GI toxicity, hepatotoxicity, bradycardia, and prolonged QT intervals are also observed (Katayama et al., 2015).

Ceritinib

Ceritinib is an orally bioavailable ALK inhibitor approved for the treatment of ALK+ metastatic NSCLC that is unresponsive to crizotinib. Common adverse effects are GI toxicity and hepatotoxicity. Bradycardia and prolonged QT intervals also occur.

Inhibitors of the PI3K/Akt/mTOR Pathway

Background

Activation of PI3K and the consequent activation of signaling events through protein kinase B (Akt) and the mechanistic or mTOR pathway are important in cell growth and survival and in regulation of cell metabolism (Figures 67–2 and 67–5). Excessive signaling through the PI3K pathway is a frequent aberration in many human cancers; thus, this pathway is an attractive target in cancer therapy. There are three classes of PI3Ks: The class I PI3K enzymes are the most important in cancer. These isoforms are activated by receptor protein tyrosine kinases and GPCRs. The PI3K enzymes are heterodimers of a p85 regulatory subunit and a p110 catalytic subunit. The p110 subunit exists in four identified isoforms: α, β, γ, and δ. The α and β isoforms are ubiquitously expressed, whereas the γ and δ isoforms are predominantly expressed in cells of hematopoietic origin. The different catalytic subunits have distinct roles in normal and malignant B-cell function. PI3Kα, containing the 110α, catalytic subunit, is the most frequently mutated PI3K in human cancer (Fruman and Rommel, 2014). In B-cell malignancies, the PI3Kδ isoform is frequently activated. A recently approved PI3Kδ inhibitor, *idelalisib*, is described in the next section. Currently, the mTORC1 inhibitors *sirolimus* (rapamycin), *everolimus,* and *temisirolimus* are approved for clinical use in different cancers and are described in the material that follows. Ongoing clinical trials are evaluating the safety and efficacy of pan-PI3K inhibitors, inhibitors of the PI3Kα isoform, as well as inhibitors of AKT, PI3K/mTOR, and TORC1/TORC2.

PI3Kδ Inhibitor: Idelalisib

The PI3Kδ isoform is constitutively activated in many B-cell malignancies, and inhibition of this pathway can promote apoptosis in these cancer cells.

Mechanism of Action

Idelalisib is an orally bioavailable inhibitor of the PI3Kδ isoform with an IC_{50} of about 8 nM. It is 40- to 300-fold more selective for the PI3Kδ isoform than for the other isoforms.

ADME

Food does not affect absorption of idelalisib. The drug is metabolized by aldehyde oxidase, CYP3A, and UGT1A4, yielding an elimination half-life of 8.2 h. Idelalisib inhibits CYP3A and is a substrate of Pgp and of the efflux transporter BCRP/ABCG2 in vitro. Idelalisib increases plasma levels of midazolam (a CYP3A substrate) but does not affect plasma levels of digoxin (a Pgp substrate) or rosuvastatin (an OATP1B1/B3 substrate). Patients receiving strong CYP inhibitors may be at increased risk for idelalisib toxicity. Hepatic impairment increases systemic exposure, putting patients at risk for toxicity.

Clinical Use

Idelalisib is approved for the treatment of relapsed or refractory B-cell malignancies in patients who have received at least two prior systemic therapies. This includes CLL in combination with rituximab, FL, and SLL. Idelalisib is not indicated and is not recommended for first-line treatment.

Adverse Effects

Idelalisib may cause serious and sometimes-fatal adverse effects, including liver toxicity, diarrhea, colitis, pneumonitis, intestinal perforations, and skin toxicity. Patients taking idelalisib should avoid other hepatotoxic drugs. Other common side effects include fever, chills, cough, pneumonia, fatigue, nausea, abdominal pain, rash, hyperglycemia, and elevated levels of triglycerides and liver enzymes. Idelalisib may cause embryo-fetal toxicity. Breastfeeding during therapy is contraindicated because of the potential for adverse reactions in nursing infants.

mTOR Inhibitors: Rapamycin Analogues

Rapamycin (sirolimus) is a product from a strain of *Streptomyces* found on the Rapa Nui Easter Island. It inhibits a serine/threonine protein kinase in mammalian cells named mTOR. The PI3K/PKB(Akt)/mTOR pathway responds to a variety of signals from growth factors. The activation of the PI3K pathway is opposed by the phosphatase activity of the tumor suppressor, PTEN (Figure 67–2). Activating mutations and amplification of genes in the receptor-PI3K pathway, and loss of function alterations in PTEN, occur frequently in cancer cells, with the result that PI3K signaling is exaggerated, and cells exhibit enhanced survival. Rapamycin (sirolimus) and its congeners, the so-called rapalogs *temsirolimus* and *everolimus*, are first-line drugs in posttransplant immunosuppression (see Figure 35–2) and are used in coronary artery stents to prevent fibrotic growth. Rapalogs have been approved for the treatment of patients with renal cancer; NETs of the pancreas; NETs of GI tract or lung origin; anti–hormone refractory, hormone receptor–positive breast cancer; and for patients with TSC-related tumors.

Mechanism of Action

The rapamycins inhibit an enzyme complex, mTORC1, which occupies a downstream position in the PI3K pathway (Figure 67–4). mTOR forms the mTORC1 complex with a member of the FK506-binding protein family, FKBP12. The antitumor actions of the rapamycins result from their binding to FKBP12 and preventing activation of mTOR, as detailed in Figure 67–4 and its legend.

ADME

For renal cell cancer, *temsirolimus* is given in weekly intravenous doses of 25 mg; temsirolimus is metabolized by CYP3A4; the parent drug has a plasma $t_{1/2}$ of 30 h, but its primary active metabolite, sirolimus (rapamycin), has a $t_{1/2}$ of 53 h. Because sirolimus has equivalent activity as an inhibitor of mTORC1 and has a greater AUC, sirolimus is likely the more important contributor to antitumor action in patients. The concomitant use of strong CYP3A4 inhibitors or inducers should thus be avoided. Grapefruit juice may also increase plasma concentrations of the active metabolite sirolimus and should be avoided.

Everolimus is administered orally in doses of 10 mg/d and is metabolized by CYP3A4. Everolimus has a plasma $t_{1/2}$ of 30 h; on a weekly schedule at doses of 20 mg, it maintains inhibition of mTORC1 for 7 days in white blood cells. Both drugs are susceptible to interactions with other agents that affect CYP3A4 activity. For everolimus, the dose should be reduced for patients with moderate hepatic impairment; guidelines for dose reduction of temsirolimus in such patients have not been established. The drugs' pharmacokinetics do not depend on renal function, and hemodialysis does not hasten temsirolimus clearance.

Therapeutic Uses

Temsirolimus and everolimus are approved for treatment of patients with advanced renal cancer. Temsirolimus prolongs survival and delays disease progression in patients with advanced and poor- or intermediate-risk renal cancer, as compared to standard IFN-α treatment. Everolimus, as compared to placebo, prolongs survival in patients who had failed initial treatment with antiangiogenic drugs. mTOR inhibitors also have antitumor activity against MCLs. Everolimus is approved for the treatment of postmenopausal women with advanced hormone receptor–positive, HER2–negative breast cancer in combination with exemestane after failure of treatment with letrozole or anastrozole. Other indications are PNET and progressive, well-differentiated, nonfunctional NETs of GI or lung origin as well as TSC-related tumors.

Adverse Effects; Resistance

The rapamycin analogues cause similar patterns of adverse effects: a mild maculopapular rash, mucositis, anemia, and fatigue (30%–50%). A few patients will develop leukopenia or thrombocytopenia, effects that are reversed if therapy is discontinued. Less common side effects include hyperglycemia, hypertriglyceridemia, and, rarely, pulmonary infiltrates and interstitial lung disease. Pulmonary infiltrates emerge in 8% of patients receiving everolimus and in a smaller percentage of those treated with temsirolimus. If symptoms such as cough or shortness of breath develop or radiological changes progress, the drug should be discontinued. Prednisone may hasten the resolution of radiological changes and symptoms.

Resistance to mTOR inhibitors is incompletely understood but may arise through the action of a second mTOR complex, mTORC2, which is unaffected by rapamycins and which can upregulate Akt activity (Figure 67–4).

Multikinase Inhibitors

Selectivity of small-molecule protein kinase inhibitors for their targets is dependent on the similarity of the targeted site with sites in other kinases and the chemical composition of the inhibitor. Most inhibitors interact with the ATP-binding site of their target that is relatively conserved within a kinase family; thus, such inhibitors have only relative specificity and will cross-react at higher concentrations with closely related kinases. Nonetheless, inhibition of distantly related kinases is possible. The selectivity of inhibitors for a range of targets in the kinome is determined experimentally using assays with recombinant kinase proteins and in vivo using intact cells that express the kinases (Elkins et al., 2015). Inhibitors that target multiple kinase families within the clinically used dose range can be therapeutically efficacious and are discussed in the material that follows. In using drugs directed toward protein kinases, remember that the specificity of these agents is not absolute and that the inhibited kinases often serve important "normal" functions in the cell in addition to the pathologic functions being targeted.

Cabozantinib

Mechanism of Action

Cabozantinib is an orally bioavailable, small-molecule inhibitor of several tyrosine kinases; as ranked by the IC_{50} values (in nM) from in vitro assays, these protein kinases are VEGFR2, 0.035; MET, 1.3; RET, 4; KIT, 4.6; VEGFR, 3.6; AXL, 7; FLT3, 11.3; VEGFR1, 12; and TIE2, 14.3. These receptor tyrosine kinases control normal cellular function and pathologic processes that include maintenance of the tumor microenvironment, tumor angiogenesis, and metastatic spread.

ADME

The elimination half-life of cabozantinib is about 99 h. Cabozantinib is a substrate of CYP3A4; thus, the dose of cabozantinib should be reduced in patients with mild-to-moderate hepatic impairment as well as for concurrent administration of CYP3A4 inhibitors. Conversely, strong inducers of CYP3A4 will reduce exposure to the drug and necessitate increased dosage of cabomatinib unless the CYP inducers can be avoided.

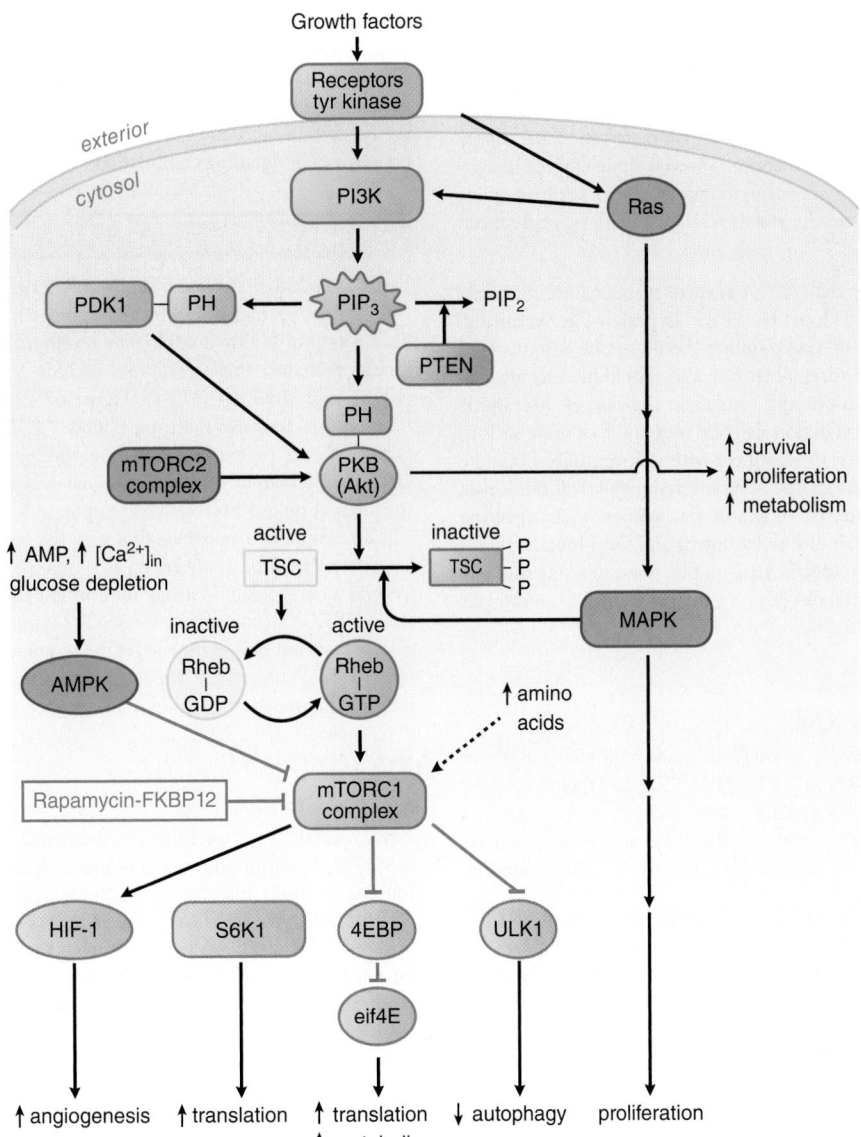

Figure 67–4 *Caveat mTOR: effect of rapamycin on growth factor signaling.* The PI3K-mTOR pathway responds to extracellular signals, the metabolic and nutrient status, and the energy charge of the cell, transmitting signals downstream that drive maintenance and proliferation (Hall, 2016). mTOR activity appears to contribute to resistance to many targeted cancer therapies (Guri and Hall, 2016), and dysregulation of the pathway is implicated in diabetes, cancer, and other pathologies (Dibble and Cantley, 2015). In this simplified version of the PI3K-mTOR pathway, the green shapes show the action pathway from membrane receptor to the mTOR multiprotein complex, mTORC1. Substrates of the mTOR ser/thr protein kinase activity and integrated responses are shown in blue across the bottom of the figure. Red T bars represent inhibitory influence. Signaling through the pathway is initiated by agonist activation of membrane receptors such as IGF1R and stimulation of their tyr kinase activities, leading to activation of PI3K, which phosphorylates the inositol ring of the PIP2 in the membrane to produce PIP3. PIP3 recruits to the membrane several proteins containing PH domains, including PKD1 and Akt. Akt, also known as PKB, phosphorylates TSC-2 (a subunit of TSC) at multiple sites. TSC is a GAP for Rheb. Phosphorylation of TSC inhibits its GAP activity, thereby reducing the GTPase activity of Rheb and increasing the fraction of Rheb in the GTP-liganded state. Rheb, in its GTP-liganded configuration, activates mTORC1. TSC phosphorylation and PIP3 phosphorylation can be reversed by the phosphatase PTEN. mTORC1 phosphorylates substrates that mediate downstream effects; amongst them are the following:

- HIF-1, leading to increased angiogenesis. HIF-1 is overexpressed in many cancers.
- S6K1, enhancing protein synthesis. Dephospho S6K1 exists in a complex with eiF3; phosphorylation by mTOR dissociates the complex, freeing S6K1 to phosphorylate its targets that promote translation.
- 4EBP (eukaryotic initiation factor 4e binding protein), thereby enhancing translation. 4EBP is a repressor of mRNA translation via its inhibitory interaction with eukaryotic initiation factor 4E (eIF4E). The phosphorylation of 4EBP by mTOR reduces the capacity of 4EBP to inhibit eIF4E and slow translation.
- ULK1 (unc-51 like autophagy activating kinase 1), whose phosphorylation reduces autophagic activity. mTOR activity prevents ULK1 activation by disrupting its interaction with AMP-activated protein kinase (AMPK), a key promoter of autophagy.

Rapamycin (sirolimus) and the "rapalogs" *everolimus* and *temsirolimus* inhibit mTOR by associating with the intracellular protein FKBP12. The FKBP12-rapalog complex binds directly to mTOR and inhibits its functions in the multiprotein complex mTORC1. mTORC2 remains relatively unaffected by mTORC1 inhibitors and can respond by upregulating Akt activity.

Therapeutic Uses

Cabozantinib is indicated for the treatment of patients with advanced RCC who have received prior antiangiogenic therapy. Cabozantinib was also shown to produce superior efficacy to sunitinib in patients with treatment-naïve intermediate- or poor-risk metastatic renal cancer (Choueiri et al., 2016). Also, cabozantinib showed some efficacy in subgroups of patients with lung adenocarcinoma and MET exon 14 splice variants (Paik et al., 2015) and in patients with medullary thyroid cancer.

Adverse Effects

The most commonly reported (≥25%) adverse reactions are diarrhea, fatigue, nausea, decreased appetite, PPES, hypertension, vomiting, weight loss, and constipation. Cabozantinib should not be administered to patients with a recent history of bleeding and should be discontinued in patients with GI perforations and fistulas. In the case of thrombotic events such as myocardial infarction, cerebral infarction, or other serious arterial thromboembolic events, treatment with cabozantinib should be discontinued. Blood pressure should be monitored regularly for the onset of hypertension. Due to the risk of fetal harm, women of childbearing age should use contraception during treatment and for 4 months thereafter. Although there are no specific data on this point, nursing mothers are advised to cease breastfeeding during treatment and for 4 months thereafter due to the potential for harm to the infant.

Vandetanib

Mechanism of Action; ADME

Vandetanib is an orally bioavailable, small-molecule multikinase inhibitor of VEGFRs, the EGFR/HER family, RET, BRK, TIE2, and members of the EPH receptor and SRC kinase families. These receptor tyrosine kinases are involved in both normal cellular functions and pathologic processes (Figure 67–2). Vandetanib is a substrate of CYP3A4. Its median elimination half-half life is 19 days.

Therapeutic Uses

Vandetanib is indicated for the treatment of symptomatic or progressive medullary thyroid cancer that is unresectable, locally advanced, or metastatic. In patients with asymptomatic or slowly progressing disease, vandetanib is only indicated after careful consideration of the treatment-related risks.

Adverse Effects and Drug Interactions

The most common adverse effects (>20%) are diarrhea/colitis, rash, acneiform dermatitis, hypertension, nausea, headache, upper respiratory tract infections, decreased appetite, and abdominal pain. Less common are QT prolongation, torsades de pointes, and sudden death. Vandetanib should not be used in patients with hepatic impairment or congenital long QT syndrome.

Midostaurin

Midostaurin is a small-molecule multikinase inhibitor with activity against mutant FLT3, a driver in AML. It is FDA-approved for combination chemotherapy of adults with newly diagnosed AML. Leukopenia, nausea, mucositis, diarrhea, and musculoskeletal pain are major adverse effects of treatment. Midostaurin was also approved for different forms of mast cell disorders.

III. Tumor Angiogenesis

Cancer cells secrete angiogenic factors that induce the formation of new blood vessels and guarantee the flow of nutrients to the tumor cells to permit growth and metastasis. Many tumor types overexpress these angiogenic factors, turning on an "angiogenic switch" whereby the tumor cells adopt an invasive phenotype favoring proliferation of endothelial cells and neovascularization. In 1971, Judah Folkman hypothesized that the growth of solid tumors was dependent on angiogenesis and that blockade of the effects of putative angiogenic factors would be a good treatment modality for human cancers (Folkman, 1971). Folkman's hypothesis proved to be correct and led to the characterization of a number of secreted angiogenic factors, including VEGF, FGF, TGF-β, and PDGF. Furthermore, inhibitors of these angiogenic factors have, indeed, become useful therapeutic agents against certain cancers. VEGF is a major driver of angiogenesis, and inhibitors of VEGF signaling comprise an important class of antitumor agents.

Inhibition VEGF and the VEGFR Pathway

Vascular endothelial growth factor initiates endothelial cell proliferation and vascular permeability when it binds to a member of the VEGFR family, a group of highly homologous receptors with intracellular tyrosine kinase domains; these receptors include VEGFR1 (FLT1), VEGFR2 (KDR), and VEGFR3 (FLT4) (Figure 67–2). The binding of VEGF to its receptors activates the intracellular VEGFR tyrosine kinase activity and initiates mitogenic and antiapoptotic signaling pathways (Nagy et l., 2007). Antibodies targeting VEGF, such as *bevacizumab*, sterically hinder the interaction of VEGF with its receptor. *Aflibercept* acts as a VEGF trap; it is a recombinant molecule that uses the VEGFR1-binding domain to sequester VEGF, basically acting as a "soluble decoy receptor" for VEGF. Several small-molecule drugs that inhibit the protein tyr kinase function of VEGFR (*pazopanib, sorafenib, sunitinib,* and *axitinib*) as well as monoclonal antibodies that target the receptor (*ramucirumab*) have been approved for clinical use. The inhibition of endothelial function by these different approaches results in a similar spectrum of adverse effects.

Bevacizumab

Mechanism of Action

Bevacizumab is a humanized monoclonal IgG1 antibody that binds to VEGF; the antibody contains the antigen-recognition domain of a murine antibody inserted into a human IgG1. Bevacizumab prevents the interaction of VEGF with its receptors on the surface of endothelial cells and inhibits receptor signaling that normally increases vascular permeability and angiogenesis. Bevacizumab delays progression of renal cell cancer and, in combination with cytotoxic chemotherapy, is approved in the treatment of patients with mCRC as well as NSCLC and glioblastoma.

ADME

Bevacizumab is administered intravenously as a 30- to 90-min infusion every 2 weeks in metastatic colon cancer and, in conjunction with combination chemotherapy, in metastatic NSCLC every 3 weeks with chemotherapy. The antibody has a plasma half-life of about 20 days (range 11 to 50 days).

Therapeutic Use in Cancer

Bevacizumab is indicated as treatment of various cancers, frequently in combination with other drugs. In metastatic colon cancer, bevacizumab combined with FOLFOX or FOLFIRI increases patient survival by about 5 months (Hurwitz et al., 2004). In NSCLC, a combination of bevacizumab with carboplatin and paclitaxel increases survival by about 2 months. Also approved are combinations of bevacizumab with cytotoxic chemotherapy in patients with cervical or ovarian cancer and a combination with IFN-α for the treatment of metastatic RCC. For glioblastoma, bevacizumab is approved as a single agent following prior therapy.

Other Therapeutic Uses: Wet Macular Degeneration

Vascular endothelial growth factor is an important mediator of pathologic vascular permeability. Intravitreous administration of anti-VEGF targeted therapy has become a standard treatment of wet macular degeneration (see also Chapter 69). *Bevacizumab* and a modified fragment of bevacizumab, *ranibizumab*, are used. Ranibizumab is derived from the bevacizumab IgG1 by deletion of the Fc domain and changes in six amino acids in the antigen-recognition domain to increase affinity for VEGF.

Because these drugs are administered by injection into the vitreous cavity of the eye, few systemic adverse effects are observed. A direct comparison of intravitreous *bevacizumab*, *ranibizumab*, and *aflibercept* (the VEGF trap protein; see discussion that follows) in patients with diabetic macular edema showed that all three treatments improved vision, although *aflibercept* appeared more effective in patients with worse baseline levels of visual impairment (Wells et al., 2015).

Adverse Effects. Bevacizumab causes a wide range of serious class-related adverse effects that include hypertension, GI perforation, thromboembolic events, and hemorrhage. A major concern is the potential for vessel injury and bleeding in patients with lung cancer. Bevacizumab is contraindicated for patients with a history of hemoptysis, brain metastasis, or a bleeding diathesis. In appropriately selected patients, the predicted rate of life-threatening pulmonary hemorrhage is less than 2%, and for arterial thromboembolism (stroke; myocardial infarction) observed during treatments that include bevacizumab the predicted rate is less than 4%.

Other adverse effects characteristic of drugs that target the VEGF pathway include hypertension and proteinuria. A majority of patients require antihypertensive therapy, particularly those receiving higher doses and more prolonged treatment. Bevacizumab can be associated with congestive heart failure, probably secondary to hypertension, and with reversible posterior leukoencephalopathy in patients with poorly controlled hypertension. GI perforation, a potentially life-threatening complication, has been observed in up to 11% of patients with ovarian cancer. In patients with colon cancer, colonic perforation occurs infrequently during bevacizumab treatment but increases in frequency in patients with intact primary colonic tumors, peritoneal carcinomatosis, peptic ulcer disease, chemotherapy-associated colitis, diverticulitis, or prior abdominal radiation treatment. Perforation of the colon occurs in less than 1% of patients. Following colon cancer surgery, patients on bevacizumab have a higher rate (13% vs. 3.4%) of serious wound-healing complications. Because of the long $t_{1/2}$ of bevacizumab, elective surgery should be delayed for at least 4 weeks from the last dose of antibody, and treatment should not be resumed for at least 4 weeks after surgery.

Ramucirumab

Mechanism of Action

Ramucirumab is a human IgG1 monoclonal antibody that binds to VEGFR2, blocking the binding of VEGFR ligands and thereby inhibiting ligand-induced activity in endothelial cells.

ADME

Ramucirumab is administered intravenously every 2 to 3 weeks. Its mean half-life is 14 days.

Therapeutic Uses

Ramucirumab is used in combination with chemotherapy for the treatment of patients with mCRC with disease progression on or after prior therapy; as a single agent or in combination with paclitaxel for treatment of patients with advanced gastric adenocarcinoma with disease progression on or after prior chemotherapy; and in combination with docetaxel for treatment of patients with metastatic NSCLC with disease progression on or after chemotherapy.

Adverse Effects

The most common adverse effects are hypertension and diarrhea. Other severe adverse effects overlap with those of bevacizumab (anti-VEGF; see previous discussion): increased risk of hemorrhage, GI perforation, and impaired wound healing.

Aflibercept

Mechanism of Action

Ziv-aflibercept acts as a trap for VEGFR ligands. It is a recombinant fusion protein that contains the extracellular VEGF-binding domain of human VEGFR1/2 fused to the Fc portion of human IgG1. Ziv-aflibercept acts as a soluble receptor that binds to human VEGFR ligands with high affinity (K_ds of 0.5 to 40 pM), reducing their plasma concentrations to levels that are too low for significant activation of their cognate receptors.

ADME

The elimination half-life is about 6 days (range 4–7 days). Ziv-aflibercept is administered by intravenous infusion over 1 h every 2 weeks.

Therapeutic Uses

In combination with FOLFIRI, afliberecpt is indicated for patients with mCRC that is resistant to or has progressed following an oxaliplatin-containing regimen.

Adverse Effects

The most common adverse effects are hypertension and diarrhea. Other severe adverse effects overlap with those of bevacizumab (anti-VEGF; see previous discussion): increased risk of hemorrhage, GI perforation, and impaired wound healing.

Antiangiogenic Small-Molecule Kinase Inhibitors

Sunitinib

Mechanism of Action

Sunitinib is a small-molecule, orally bioavailable inhibitor of multiple kinases, including VEGFR2.

ADME

The typical treatment cycle of sunitinib is 4 weeks on treatment followed by 2 weeks off. The dosage and schedule of sunitinib can be decreased in patients with adverse effects. More recently, a 2-week on/1-week off schedule has proven to be better tolerated and as effective as the original treatment schedule. Sunitinib is metabolized by CYP3A4 to produce an active metabolite, SU12662, the $t_{1/2}$ of which is 80–110 h; steady-state levels of the metabolite are reached after about 2 weeks of repeated administration of the parent drug. Further metabolism results in the formation of inactive products. The pharmacokinetics of sunitinib are not affected by food intake.

Therapeutic Uses

Sunitinib has activity in metastatic renal cell cancer, producing a higher response rate and a longer progression-free survival than seen with IFN or bevacizumab. Sunitinib is also approved for the treatment of pancreatic NETs and of GIST in patients who have developed resistance to imatinib as a consequence of *c-KIT* mutations. Specific *c-KIT* mutations correlate with the degree of response to sunitinib (e.g., patients with *c-KIT* exon 9 mutations have a response rate of 37%; patients with *c-KIT* exon 11 mutations have a 5% response rate).

Adverse Effects

The main adverse effects of sunitinib are shared by all antiangiogenic inhibitors: bleeding, hypertension, proteinuria, and, uncommonly, arterial thromboembolic events and intestinal perforation. However, because sunitinib is a multitargeted TKI, it has a broader adverse effect profile than bevacizumab. Fatigue affects 50%–70% of patients and may be disabling. Hypothyroidism occurs in 40%–60% of patients. Bone marrow suppression and diarrhea also are common side effects; severe neutropenia (neutrophils < 1000/mL) develops in 10% of patients. Less common side effects include hepatotoxicity, congestive heart failure and PPES. It is essential to check blood counts and thyroid function at regular intervals. Periodic echocardiograms also are recommended.

Sorafenib

Mechanism of Action and Therapeutic Use

Sorafenib, like *sunitinib*, is an orally bioavailable inhibitor of multiple protein kinases. Sorafenib is the only drug currently approved for treatment of patients with hepatocellular carcinoma. Sorafenib also is approved in patients with metastatic renal cell cancer, but sunitinib and pazopanib are generally preferred first-line therapies (see previous discussion and below).

ADME

Sorafenib is given orally every day without treatment breaks. Sorafenib is metabolized to inactive products by CYP3A4 with a $t_{1/2}$ of 20–27 h; with repeated administration, steady-state concentrations are reached within 1 week.

Sorafenib-treated patients can experience the vascular toxicities seen with other antiangiogenic medications described under *bevacizumab*. More common adverse effects include fatigue, nausea, diarrhea, anorexia, rash, and palmar-plantar erythrodysesthesias; uncommonly, bone marrow suppression, GI perforation, and cardiomyopathy occur.

Pazopanib

Pazopanib is a kinase inhibitor of VEGFR-1, -2, and -3 as well as FGFRs, KIT, LCK, PDGFR, and other kinases implicated in pathologic angiogenesis and cancer progression. Pazopanib is approved for the treatment of patients with advanced renal cell cancer and advanced STS after prior chemotherapy. It has less toxicity and equivalent efficacy to sunitinib in patients with treatment-naïve metastatic renal cancer and therefore has become the preferred first-line treatment of many patients. Pazopanib is orally bioavailable, metabolized mostly by CYP3A, and eliminated with a $t_{1/2}$ of 31 h. Major adverse effects include hypertension, thrombotic and hemorrhagic events, GI perforation, QT prolongation, and cardiomyopathy. Pazopanib carries a black-box warning: It can produce severe and life-threatening hepatotoxicity; as a consequence, pazopanib should not be used in elderly patients or those with preexisting liver function test abnormalities.

Other Receptor Kinase Inhibitors With Antiangiogenic Effects

Axitinib is a kinase inhibitor of VEGFR-1, -2, and -3 that are implicated in pathologic angiogenesis, tumor growth, and cancer progression. Axitinib is approved for the treatment of patients with advanced RCC after failure of one prior systemic therapy. Axitinib is orally bioavailable, metabolized mainly by CYP3A4/5, and eliminated with a variable $t_{1/2}$ of 2.5 to 6.1 h. Major adverse effects include hypertension, thrombotic and hemorrhagic events, and GI perforation similar to those of the anti-VEGF *bevacizumab* (see previous discussion).

Lenvatinib inhibits the protein kinase activities of VEGFR-1, -2, and -3 as well as FGFRs, PDGFR, and other kinases that are implicated in pathologic angiogenesis and cancer progression. Lenvatinib is approved for the treatment of patients with recurrent or metastatic differentiated thyroid cancer and in combination with everolimus for patients with advanced renal cell cancer. Lenvatinib is orally bioavailable, metabolized by CYP3A, and eliminated with a $t_{1/2}$ of 28 h. Major adverse effects include hypertension, thrombotic and hemorrhagic events, hepatotoxicity, GI perforation, and QT prolongation.

Regorafenib inhibits the protein kinase activities of RET, VEGFR1-3, KIT, PDGFR, FGFR1/2, TIE2, RAF1, BRAF, and ABL at concentrations that can be achieved clinically. Several of these kinases are implicated in pathologic angiogenesis and malignant progression. Regorafenib is approved for the treatment of patients with mCRC after previous chemotherapy, anti-VEGF therapy, or anti-EGFR therapy and for patients with locally advanced, unresectable, or metastatic GIST after imatinib or sunitinib. Regorafenib is orally bioavailable, metabolized mostly by CYP3A, and eliminated with a variable $t_{1/2}$ of about 28 h (range 14 to 58 h). Major adverse effects include hepatotoxicity, hypertension, thrombotic and hemorrhagic events, GI perforation, QT prolongation, and wound-healing complications. As expected for an agent metabolized by CYP3A4, strong inducers and strong inhibitors of CYP3A4 must be avoided (see *palbociclib*, previously discussed, for details).

IV. Targeting the Immune System

Immune Checkpoint Inhibitors

Recent striking successes of cancer immunotherapy have given credence to the long-held hope that the immune system may be unleashed to treat cancer. The conceptual breakthrough is based on the discovery of inhibitory signals that limit T-cell activation, so-called immune checkpoints. The discovery of receptors, ligands, and their function in the control of immune cell activity during the past two decades led to the development of clinically effective monoclonal antibodies that enable T cells to recognize and eradicate cancer cells with acceptable adverse effects (Figure 67–5).

> **HISTORY** **Immune Checkpoint Inhibitors**
>
> The discovery of the TCR and of costimulatory signal pathways in the period from 1982 to 1992 defined essential requirements for T-cell activation during antigen presentation: In addition to the antigen-TCR interaction, CD28 on T cells binds to B7 proteins on APCs (see Figure 67–5, see *also* Figures 35–2 and 35–4). The finding, in the mid-1990s, of coinhibitory molecules that can dampen T-cell activation revealed a potential mechanism for drugs to modulate immune checkpoints and alter anticancer immune activity. TCR activation induces expression of the inhibitory CTLA-4, a CD28 homolog with higher affinity for the B7 ligands than CD28. CTLA-4 inhibits T-cell activation to control autoimmune tissue damage. PD-1, another inhibitory molecule expressed on T cells after their activation, and PD-L1, the ligand for PD-1, were described in the early 2000s. It became obvious that T cells present in human tumors were being inhibited by factors in the tumor tissues: TILs harvested from patients and activated exogenously showed efficacy and paved the way for targeting immune inhibition. Improved survival of patients with metastatic melanoma after anti–CTLA-4 treatment led to FDA approval of ipilimumab in 2011; anti-PD-1 and anti-PD-L1 were approved in 2014. Clinical trials in multiple types of cancer have been ongoing since then and have led to the approval of immune checkpoint inhibitors for additional indications (Monteiro, 2015) described in this section.

Blocking immune checkpoints on cytotoxic T cells enables them to eradicate cancer cells that express antigens recognized by the T cells. Sustained eradication of metastatic melanoma in a significant number of patients was an impressive outcome of initial clinical trials with a monoclonal antibody, *ipilimumab*, which is an immune checkpoint inhibitor (Robert et al., 2013). Note that immune checkpoint inhibition is distinct from conventional approaches such as vaccination with a known antigen (to generate T cells that recognize cells expressing the antigen), nonspecific stimulation of T cells, or approaches using antigen-responsive T cells that express a specific chimeric antigen receptor (CAR). The different approaches are described next.

Mechanisms of T-Cell Activation

Antigen-mediated activation of T cells is initiated by engagement of the TCR with antigen presented on MHC protein on the surface of an APC, "signal 1." In addition, engagement of CD28 costimulatory molecules on T cells is required for effective T-cell activation that includes cell proliferation, migration, and production of cytokines. This "signal 2" is provided by B7 surface proteins on APCs, for example, CD80 or CD86 (Figures 35–4 and 67–5). T-cell activation is tightly controlled by immune-suppressive cells and cytokines as well as by coinhibitory molecules present on T cells, such as *CTLA-4* or *PD-1* (Figure 67–5). CTLA-4 is expressed by activated CD4 and CD8 T cells and competes with costimulatory CD28 for binding to the B7 protein ligands. Binding of CTLA-4 to B7 proteins interrupts the initial CD28 costimulatory signals and serves as an early negative regulator of the T-cell activation responses, that is, an *immune checkpoint*. Additional control of T-cell activity is provided by later inhibitory signals through other molecules, such as PD-1 that binds the ligand PD-L1. PD-1 is mainly expressed by activated CD4 and CD8 T cells as well as APCs.

Blocking monoclonal antibodies to CTLA-4, PD-1, or PD-L1 are currently used to neutralize coinhibitory receptors during T-cell priming (CTLA-4), to maintain cancer antigen-specific T-cell function, and to provide a sustained T-cell response (PD-1) that includes increased production

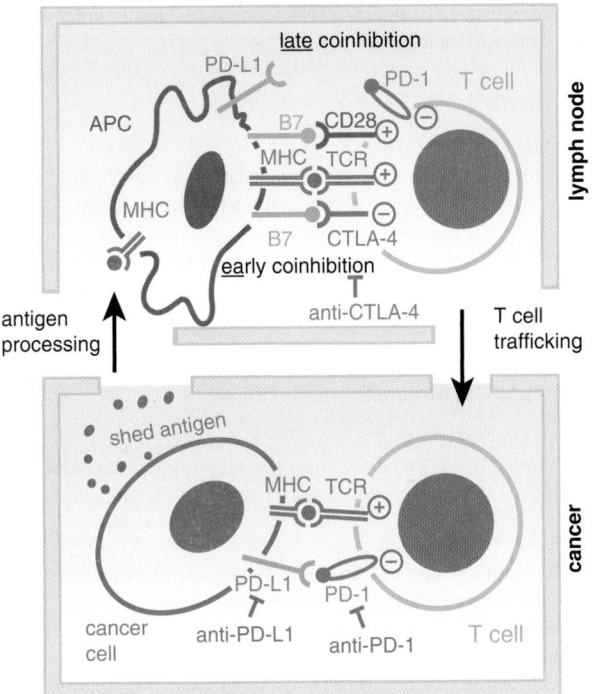

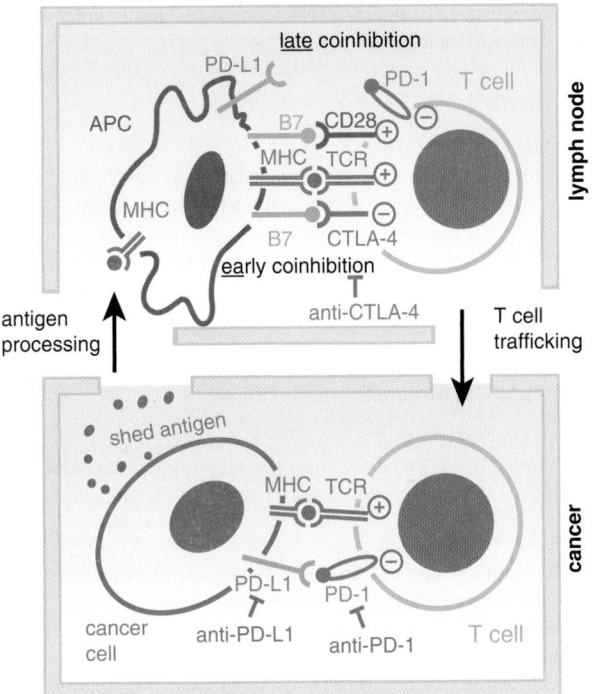

T-cell priming

Figure 67–5 *Targeting of immune checkpoints.* Antigens shed from dead cancer cells are captured and processed by APCs. APCs travel to the regional lymph nodes and present the antigen bound to MHC to stimulate TCRs. Costimulatory signals leading to T-cell activation are provided by the interaction between CD28 on T cells and B7 on APCs. CTLA-4 is upregulated and limits T-cell activation (early coinhibition) by outcompeting CD28 for binding to B7. Activated T cells also upregulate PD-1 on their surface. Figure 35–4 shows additional details of T-cell activation. Activated effector T cells capable of killing cancer cells then traffic from the lymph node to the tumor site, where they recognize cancer cells by the interaction of the TCR with the MHC-neoantigen complex and kill cancer cells through cytolysis (release of perforin and granzyme). This triggers additional antigen release that can induce subsequent rounds of anticancer immunity. Release of IFN-γ upon TCR recognition of the MHC-neoantigen complex induces upregulation of PD-L1 on the surface of tumor cells. PD-L1 binds to PD-1 on the surface of activated T cells, dampening the immune response in the tumor microenvironment. T-cell checkpoint inhibitors can enhance T-cell priming through blockade of CTLA-4 (ipilimumab) or by T-cell activation in the tumor via blocking the PD-1/PD-L1 interaction with antibody ligands to PD-1 (nivolumab, pembrolizumab) or PD-L1 (atezolimumab). Antibodies that block inhibitory immune checkpoints allow a sustained T-cell response that also includes an increased production of cytokines and T-cell proliferation.

of cytokines such as TNFα, IFN-γ, and granzyme B. Antibodies that target different checkpoint molecules are discussed in the following material: *ipilimumab* (anti–CTLA-4), *atezolimumab* (anti–PD-L1), *nivolumab* and *pembrolizumab* (anti–PD-1).

Inhibitors of Cytotoxic T Lymphocyte–Associated Protein 4 (CTLA4)

The CTLA-4 is upregulated during the antigen priming of T cells and binds B7 on APCs to attenuate the T-cell response and thus reduce the risk for chronic autoimmune-dependent inflammation (Figure 67–5).

Ipilimumab

Ipilimumab is a fully human IgG1 monoclonal antibody that binds to CTLA-4 and is approved for the treatment of late-stage melanoma and under study for other cancers.

Mechanism of Action

Ipilimumab blocks the interaction of CTLA-4 with B7 ligands on APCs and thereby augments T-cell activation (Figure 67–5). Inhibition of CTLA-4 signaling can also inhibit regulatory T-cell function that dampens cytotoxic T-cell activity and thus increases the antitumor immune response further (Mellman et al., 2011).

ADME

Ipilimumab is administered intravenously and shows linear pharmacokinetics in the dose range of 0.3 to 10 mg/kg, with a terminal half-life of 15.4 days.

Therapeutic Uses

A pivotal 2010 trial in patients with metastatic melanoma showed improved median overall survival after ipilimumab treatment (Hodi et al., 2010). This trial led to FDA approval of ipilimumab for the treatment of metastatic melanoma. Further studies showed that some patients had clinical responses that lasted for 10 or more years (Schadendorf et al., 2015). The tumor response can take several months to manifest, and tumors may increase in size during this period, in part due to the evolving inflammatory reaction (Mellman et al., 2011). Current recommended dosing of ipilimumab is 3 mg/kg intravenously over 90 min every 3 weeks for a total of four doses for patients with metastatic disease and 10 mg/kg followed by 10 mg/kg every 12 weeks for up to 3 years or until documented disease recurrence or unacceptable toxicity for patients treated in the adjuvant setting.

Adverse Effects

Blockade of CTLA-4 compromises immune tolerance to some normal tissue antigens and provokes inflammatory toxicities, mostly in the skin, pituitary gland, intestine, and liver. The activation of T-cell responses by ipilimumab treatment leads to immune-related toxicities in the majority of patients (73.6%), with 18.6% reaching toxicity grade 3–4 toxicity (Callahan et al., 2016). Adverse effects on the skin (pruritus, rash, vitiligo) and GI tract (diarrhea, colitis) are the most frequent, whereas immune-mediated hepatitis, hypophysitis, and hypo- or hyperthyroidism are less frequent. Withholding treatment because of moderate adverse reactions until return to baseline and high-dose corticosteroids for severe immune-mediated reactions are recommended.

Other Drugs in This Class

Tremelimumab (formerly ticilimumab) is a fully human IgG2 monoclonal antibody that targets CTLA-4; it is under investigation in several clinical trials.

Inhibitors of Programmed Cell Death 1 (PD-1)

Activation of the PD-1 checkpoint pathway in T cells by PD-L1 or PD-L2 evokes a negative regulatory immune response and inactivates T cells (Figure 67–5). Tumor cells can exploit this pathway by presenting the PD-L1 ligand to tumor-infiltrating T cells and thus shield the tumor from T cell–mediated destruction. Presentation of PD-L1 to activated T cells results in T-cell exhaustion, whereas antibody-mediated blockade of PD-1 can restore or maintain T-cell antitumor response.

Nivolumab

Mechanism of Action

Nivolumab is a fully human monoclonal IgG4 antibody that blocks the interaction between PD-1 and its ligands.

ADME; Clinical Use

Nivolumab is administered as an intravenous infusion every 2 weeks until the time of disease progression or of unacceptable toxicity. The drug has an elimination half-life of 26.7 days. Nivolumab is FDA approved for the treatment of a variety of cancers, currently including advanced melanoma, previously treated advanced NSCLC, RCC, advanced head and neck cancer, and relapsed/refractory classical Hodgkin lymphoma. Quite strikingly, nivolumab provided an overall response rate of 87% in patients with

Hodgkin lymphoma who had failed treatment with brentuximab vedotin (see discussion that follows). Nivolumab has significant clinical activity in a variety of heavily pretreated patients with solid tumors as well as patients with hematological malignancies. This is also true for the other anti–PD-1 monoclonal antibody, pembrolizumab.

Adverse Effects

The most common adverse effect of treatment in patients with melanoma is a rash (>20%); in patients with advanced squamous NSCLC, the adverse effects are fatigue, dyspnea, musculoskeletal pain, decreased appetite, cough, nausea, and constipation. Immune-mediated adverse reactions are much less common than with CTLA-4 antibodies; corticosteroids are recommended based on the severity of the reaction. For pneumonitis, colitis, hepatitis, nephritis and renal dysfunction, withhold treatment if the adverse effects are moderate and discontinue treatment if the effects are severe.

Pembrolizumab

Pembrolizumab (formerly called lambrolizumab or MK-3475) is a humanized monoclonal IgG4-κ isotype antibody that blocks interaction between PD-1 and its ligands. This humanized antibody has a mouse variable region grafted onto a human antibody framework and shows high affinity toward PD-1 receptors of humans and other primates but no appreciable affinity for mouse or rat PD-1.

The FDA has extended the approval for pembrolizumab to any cancer with missmatch repair (MMR) deficiency or high microsatellite instability (MSI-H). The defects in DNA repair lead to a higher mutation load and increased generation of mutant protein antigen by cancer cells that can activate the immune system. This first cancer tissue-agnostic approval extends immune checkpoint inhibitor treatment to subsets of patients with hereditary CRC due to Lynch syndrome (MSI-H) and up to 20% of patients with sporadic colon cancer. The frequency is less in endometrial, ovarian and pancreatic cancers and will require testing of each patient's tumor to assess suitability of the treatment.

ADME; Clinical Use

The recommended treatment schedule for pembrolizumab is 2 mg/kg (or a 200-mg flat dose) as an intravenous infusion over 30 min every 3 weeks. The elimination half-life is 26 days. In clinical trial, pembrolizumab demonstrated an overall response rate of 26% in patients with ipilimumab-pretreated and refractory advanced melanoma (Hamid et al., 2013; Robert et al., 2014). Pembrolizumab is more effective and less toxic than ipilimumab in patients with either treatment-naïve or BRAF inhibitor–pretreated melanoma. Pembrolizumab is currently approved for the treatment of patients with advanced melanoma, unresectable or metastatic melanoma in patients previously treated with ipilimumab, PD-L1–positive NSCLC (either prior to or after platinum-containing chemotherapy), and chemotherapy-refractory head and neck cancer. Significant antitumor activity has also been found relative to chemotherapy in patients with metastatic urothelial cancer, Merkel cell carcinoma, and Hodgkin lymphoma.

Adverse Effects

The most common adverse effects, experienced by more than 20% of patients, are fatigue, cough, nausea, pruritus, rash, decreased appetite, constipation, arthralgia, and diarrhea. An additional 10% of patients may experience complications with infections. Serious adverse events include immune-mediated inflammation, specifically pneumonitis, colitis, hepatitis, and hypophysitis and both hyper- and hypothyroidism. Withholding treatment and administration of systemic corticosteroids for grade 2⁺ or discontinuing treatment with more severe adverse effects is recommended. Because human IgG4 can cross the placenta, the benefit from pembrolizumab treatment should be balanced with the potential fetal risk in a pregnant woman.

Antagonists of PD-1 Ligand 1

Programmed cell death 1 has two ligands, PD-L1 and PD-L2, each with distinct expression profile. The PD-L1 ligand is expressed on APCs, T cells, B cells, and nonhematopoietic cells, which can include cancer cells

(Figure 67–5). Expression of PD-L2 is restricted to APCs, macrophages, myeloid dendritic cells, and mast cells. Clinical trial results are promising with drugs targeting PD-L1.

Atezolimumab

Mechanism of Action

Atezolizumab, also known as MPDL3280A, is a fully human IgG1 monoclonal antibody that blocks the interaction of PD-L1 with PD-1 and B7-H1. PD-L1 is expressed in many cancers and thus can suppress the activation of cytotoxic T cells that enter the tumor. Atezolizumab can remove this inhibitory effect and promote an effective antitumor response.

ADME

Atezolimumab is administered as an intravenous infusion over 60 min every 3 weeks. The terminal half-life is 27 days.

Clinical Use

Atezolimumab is indicated for conventional treatment-resistant metastatic NSCLC as well as locally advanced or metastatic urothelial cancer.

Adverse Effects

The most common adverse effects in 20% or more of patients with metastatic NSCLC are fatigue, decreased appetite, dyspnea, cough, nausea, musculoskeletal pain, and constipation. Patients with urothelial carcinoma may report urinary tract infection. Possible immune-related adverse effects include hepatitis, colitis, hypophysitis, thyroid disorders, adrenal insufficiency, type 1 diabetes mellitus, pancreatitis, myasthenia gravis, Guillain-Barré syndrome, and ocular inflammation; these may may require discontinuation of treatment. Due to potential embryo-fetal toxicity, female patients should be advised accordingly.

Other Anti–PD-L1 Antibodies

Durvalumab (approved in 2017 for metastatic urothelial cancer) and avelumab (approved in 2017 for metastatic urothelial and Merkel cell cancer) are also being evaluated for efficacy toward cancers of the head and neck, stomach, lung, and ovary, as well as hepatocellular cancer.

Combination of Anti–PD-1 and Anti–CTLA4

Because anti–CTLA-4 and anti–PD-1 target distinct immune checkpoints during T-cell activation, preclinical studies have shown that concurrent targeting of CTLA-4 and PD-1 significantly improves therapeutic efficacy when compared to effects of single agents (Curran et al., 2010). In patients with advanced melanoma, the combination of ipilimumab and nivolumab produces a positive response in more than 50% of the patients with an acceptable level of adverse effects, although the combination therapy significantly increased the rate of rare but fatal myocarditis (combination 0.17%; nivolumab < 0.01%) (Johnson et al., 2016). The 1- and 2-year overall survival rates were 94% and 88%, respectively (Wolchok et al., 2013). Thus, combinations of immune checkpoint inhibitors with different targets may become the standard of care in various solid as well as hematologic malignancies (Mellman et al., 2016). Most important, combination immunotherapy will likely be more effective than most other forms of treatment of patients with metastatic disease (Restifo et al., 2016).

Cytokines to Stimulate Immune Responses

Interleukin 2

Of the 70 or so proteins and glycoproteins that are classified as cytokines, only IFN (Chapters 34 and 35) and IL-2 are in routine clinical use, often for actions against cancer.

Activated CD4⁺ T cells are the primary producers of IL-2. The functions of IL-2 are myriad; amongst other roles, IL-2 promotes the growth of T cells and NK cells, stimulates the proliferation of and antibody production by B cells, and drives the development of T_reg cells (mediators of tolerance and suppression). As noted by Liao and colleagues (2013), "IL-2 has broad essential biological actions, not only driving T cell proliferation and modulating effector cell differentiation, but also limiting potentially dangerous autoimmune reactions." This statement provides a general rationale for the clinical use of IL-2 and the likelihood that IL-2 administration might also engender adverse effects.

Mechanism of Action

Interleukin 2 stimulates the proliferation of activated T cells and the secretion of cytokines from NK cells and monocytes. IL-2 stimulation increases cytotoxic killing by T cells and NK cells.

Interleukin 2 is a 133–amino acid glycoprotein (molecular weight ~ 15 kDa) produced by activated T cells and NK cells; it promotes activated T-cell proliferation and enhanced killing by NK cells. Responsiveness depends on expression of the IL-2R. The receptor comprises three independently expressed membrane monospans, α, β, and γ, which can assemble in several combinations to produce working receptors of varying affinities. These monospans are variously expressed in lymphohematopoietic cells, lack C-terminal protein kinase activities, and transduce signals via coupling to Jak proteins (Figure 67–6). Nearly all types of tumor cells lack receptor expression and are unresponsive to IL-2.

ADME

Interleukin 2 (as recombinant IL-2, aldesleukin) is administered intravenously. The serum $t_{1/2}$ of IL-2 after intravenous administration has an α phase of about 13 min and a β phase of about 90 min. IL-2 is excreted in the urine as an inactive metabolite.

Therapeutic Uses

Aldesleukin possesses the biological activities of native human IL-2. The drug is approved for use in patients with metastatic renal cell cancer and metastatic melanoma. High-dose IL-2 produces an overall response rate of 15%–25% in patients with renal cell cancer; 8% achieve a complete response. In patients with metastatic melanoma, high-dose IL-2 induces an overall response rate of 16%–22%, and 6% achieve a complete response. In both instances, responses last a median of about 5 years. Low-dose IL-2 also produces responses, but few are complete responses, and the duration may be less than with high-dose IL-2.

Adverse Effects

Interleukin 2 toxicities are dominated by the capillary leak syndrome, in which intravascular fluid leaks into the extravascular space, producing hypotension, edema, respiratory difficulties, confusion, tachycardia, oliguric renal failure, and electrolyte problems. Symptoms include fever, chills, malaise, nausea, vomiting, and diarrhea. Laboratory abnormalities include thrombocytopenia, abnormal liver function tests, and neutropenia. Most patients develop a pruritic skin rash. Hypothyroidism may occur. Arrhythmias are a rare complication. These toxicities can be life threatening, yet nearly all are reversible within 24–48 h of discontinuing therapy. Patients should have normal renal and hepatic function before beginning therapy and should be closely supervised in an inpatient facility capable of care at the intensive care unit level during drug administration.

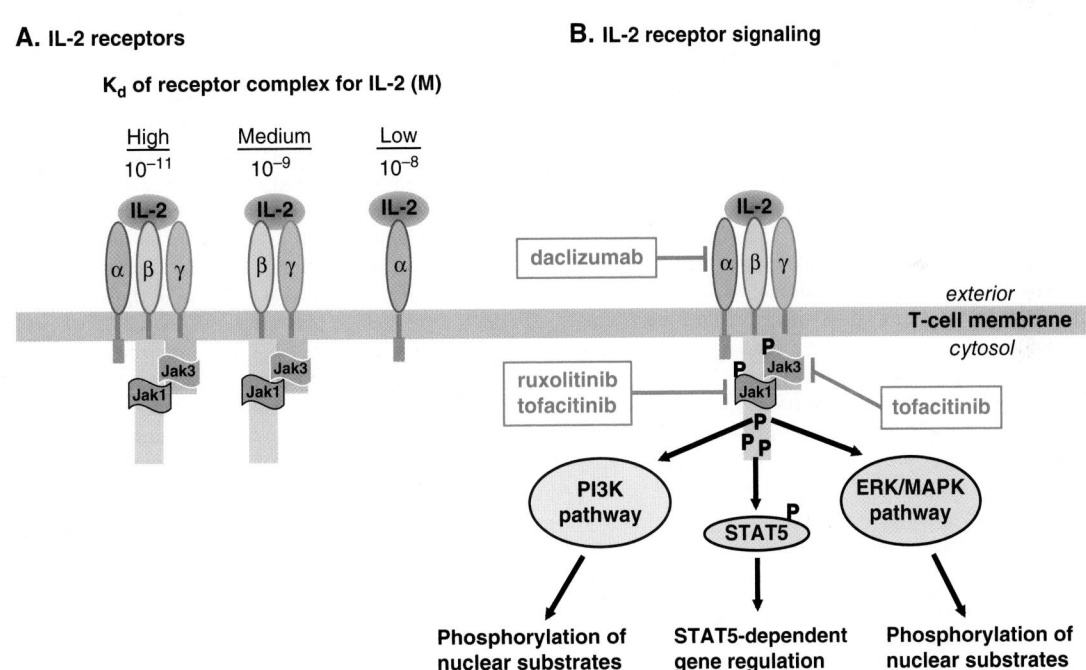

A. IL-2 receptors

B. IL-2 receptor signaling

K_d **of receptor complex for IL-2 (M)**

Figure 67–6 *A pharmacologist's view of IL-2 receptors, their cellular signaling pathways, and their inhibition.* **A.** *IL-2 receptors.* The IL-2 receptor has three components: an α chain, a 55-kDa protein (CD25) involved mainly in IL-2 binding; a β chain, a 75-kDa protein that binds to Jak1; and a γ chain, a 64-kDa protein that signals via Jak3. These components combine as shown to produce receptors of varying affinities and with different capacities for intracellular signaling. The γ chain is a component of many cytokine receptors (IL-2, IL-4, IL-7, IL-9, IL-15, and IL-21). Resting T cells have a low density of IL-2Rα; however, activation of the TCR (see Figure 35–2) and IL-2, itself, induce IL-2Rα expression. IL-2Rα can also be induced by a large variety of cytokines, viruses, and activators of PKC. The β and γ monospans are constitutively expressed on many lymphohematopoietic cells, and their expression can also be regulated. Tumor cells generally lack receptor expression and are unresponsive to IL-2. **B.** *IL-2 receptor signaling.* The formation of the quaternary complex of IL-2 and the α, β, and γ units of IL-2R suffice to activate intracellular signaling. The IL-2R monospans shown in **A** lack the protein tyr kinase activities common to many monospanning hormone receptors. Rather, these receptors respond to IL-2 binding at the extracellular domain by differentially recruiting Jak1 and Jak3 to their cytosolic domains, Jak1 at IL-2Rβ and Jak3 at IL-2Rγ. Heterodimerization of β and γ cytosolic domains leads to activation of Jak1 and Jak3. The Jaks transactivate and also phosphorylate key tyrosines on IL-2Rβ. These phosphotyrosines (**P**) permit important protein-protein interactions that direct downstream signaling:

- Binding of an SHC adapter/scaffolding protein that is the platform for activation of the Ras-MAPK pathway and the PI3K pathway
- Recruitment and phosphorylation of STAT5 (and to a lesser extent, STATs 1 and 3), leading to STAT-dependent gene regulation

IL-2/IL-2R signaling can be therapeutically reduced by inhibitors that interact with IL-2Rα, Jak1, and Jak3 (red boxes and T bars)

Cancer Vaccines

Vaccination against cancer antigens has shown little efficacy with the exception of two approaches that were approved by the FDA in 2010 (*sipuleucel-T*) and in 2015 (*T-VEC*).

Sipuleucel-T

Sipuleucel-T is a cell-based approach designed to induce an immune response against PAP, which is expressed in most prostate cancers. This autologous cellular immunotherapy is generated from a patient's peripheral blood cells, which are isolated by leukapheresis. The cells are exposed to a human recombinant protein, PAP–GM-CSF. APCs present amongst the blood cells are thought to take up and process PAP and direct the immune response toward the antigen. A patient receives the treated cells by infusion on three occasions at 2-week intervals. Treatment is approved for patients with minimally symptomatic, hormone-refractory, metastatic prostate cancer. Adverse effects include acute infusion reactions, which can be reduced by premedication with acetaminophen and antihistamine.

T-Vec

T-VEC (talimogene laherparepvec) is an oncolytic herpesvirus that replicates within tumors and expresses GM-CSF. Tumor antigens are released after virally induced cell death, and the presence of GM-CSF can promote an antitumor immune response. T-VEC is approved for the local treatment of unresectable cutaneous and nodal lesions in patients with melanoma. T-VEC may synergize with immune checkpoint inhibitor treatment. Adverse effects are influenza-like symptoms and injection site pain.

Chimeric Antigen Receptor T Cells

Treatment of patients with B-cell leukemias or lymphoma with receptor-engineered T cells has produced striking successes. CARs contain the antigen-binding domain of a monoclonal antibody to confer recognition of the targeted tumor antigen coupled to intracellular domains capable of activating T cells (Figure 67–7). When expressed in T cells, these CARs recognize cell surface antigens and activate T cells independent of antigen presentation by a MHC molecule as required for physiologic antigen presentation (see Figures 35–2 and 67–5). In initial studies, CAR-expressing T cells were targeted to NY-ESO-1, a tumor antigen of the cancer/testis family that is highly expressed on many poor-prognosis melanoma cells. The CAR T cells showed long-lasting efficacy (>3 years) in some patients with metastatic melanoma. CAR targeting CD19, a B-cell antigen, also resulted in striking efficacy in patients with B-cell leukemias (Klebanoff

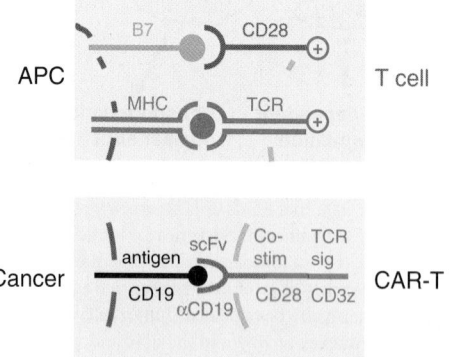

Figure 67–7 *Chimeric antigen receptor (CAR) T cell activation by a target antigen on cancer cells.* T cells are harvested from a cancer patient and transduced with a CAR expression vector. Elements in a CAR: extracellular, single-chain antibody fragment of the variable domain (scFv) that recognizes the targeted antigen; intracellular co-stimulatory domain (e.g. from CD28); intracellular signaling domain of the TCR. CD19 is shown as an antigen example. APC-mediated stimulation of T cells is depicted for comparison (see figure 67–5).

et al., 2016). The approval of CD19 CAR-T cells (tisagenlecleucel-T; previously named CTL019) has been recommended, based on data showing >80% remissions of relapsed or refractory B cell ALL during treatment. Other CARs targeting CD22 and B-cell maturation antigen (BCMA) have shown efficacy and are currently under investigation.

Future Challenges of Immunotherapy

The potential for immunotherapies to augment conventional chemotherapy, pathway-targeted treatment, and radiotherapy will require detailed exploration and will be a common theme in the design of future clinical trials (Ebert et al., 2016; Hughes et al., 2016). The recent identification of multiple negative and positive immune-modulatory pathways that can be targeted is leading to development of new drugs that will require testing as monotherapy and combination with each other as well as with conventional treatments. This new class of cancer treatment presents a new set of adverse effects (e.g., fulminant myocarditis caused by a combination of immune checkpoint inhibitors; Johnson et al., 2016) that must be understood mechanistically before rational combination strategies can be developed.

V. Other Targets

Inhibitors of Poly (ADP-Ribose) Polymerase

DNA damage-repair genes are frequently inactivated in human cancer. PARP1 is the product of one such gene. PARP1 is a nuclear protein that transfers ADP-ribose from NAD$^+$ to target proteins, and this poly (ADP-ribosyl)ation (or PARylation) of nuclear proteins by PARP1 plays a significant role in the DNA damage response (Tallis et al., 2014). Inactive PARP1 associates with chromatin and helps to create a compact chromatin structure in the nucleosome. DNA damage (e.g., strand breaks) mobilizes the enzyme, promoting PARP-mediated PARylation, with the result that chromatin relaxes in the area of damage. The mechanisms of relaxation are the PARylation of PARP1 itself, and of histones and other chromatin-associated proteins, resulting in their dissociation from DNA. PARylation produces branching chains up to 200 ADP-ribose units in length. These chains provide docking centers for the localized recruitment of PAR-binding factors and thence of DNA repair enzymes (e.g., DNA polβ, DNA ligase III) and proteins that help to maintain an inactive environment in the open chromatin region while repairs are made to the damaged DNA. The synthesis and degradation of PAR chains in vivo is tightly regulated, with the chains having half-lives measured in minutes (Wei and Yu, 2016). Excessive activation of PARP1 leads to depletion of the cellular pool of NAD$^+$ and to cell death; teleologically, this could be viewed as a means of preserving genomic integrity by removing cells with heavily damaged DNA.

Deficient PARP1 activity leads to defective DNA repair. However, PARP-deficient cells are still able to carry out DNA repair through a different mechanism: homologous recombination. The protein machinery for homologous recombination repair includes the breast cancer susceptibility genes BRCA1 and BRCA2, suggesting that cells with diminished or absent BRCA1/2 function could be unusually susceptible to the inhibition of PARP activity. BRCA1/2 mutations predispose carriers to breast, ovarian, and other cancers that can be resistant to chemotherapy. BRCA-deficient cells are more dependent on PARP1 and base excision repair to maintain genomic integrity. BRCA1/2-deficient cancer cells are less able to carry out repair and ultimately die; inhibition of PARP could accelerate this process. It is noteworthy that PARPs catalyze PARylation of a number of proteins that regulate cellular processes beyond DNA damage repair; these extra-chromatin actions may contribute to the clinical efficacy and adverse effects of PARP inhibitors. Inhibitors of PARP are designed to compete with NAD$^+$ at its binding site on the PARP enzyme. *Olaparib* and *rucaparib* are approved for the treatment of patients with advanced ovarian cancer.

Olaparib

Olaparib is an orally bioavailable inhibitor of PARP enzymes.

ADME

Olaparib is rapidly absorbed after oral administration and metabolized primarily by CYP3A4, yielding a $t_{1/2}$ of about 12 h. Drug exposure is increased or reduced when administered in combination with a CYP3A4 inhibitor or inducer, respectively.

Therapeutic Uses; Adverse Effects

Olaparib is EMA and FDA approved as monotherapy in patients with germline BRCA-mutated, advanced, ovarian cancer who have been treated with three or more prior lines of chemotherapy. Adverse effects include GI upset (nausea and vomiting) and loss of appetite; fatigue; muscle and joint pain; low blood cell counts and anemia; and occasionally leukemia. Potentially fatal MDS and pneumonitis have been observed.

Rucaparib

Rucaparib is a benzimidazole derivative that inhibits PARP1. Rucaparib is FDA approved for treatment of advanced ovarian cancer in patients exhibiting deleterious BRCA mutations who have been treated with at least two prior chemotherapies. The drug was approved in conjunction with the approval of a gene-sequencing test that detects BRCA1/2 mutations in patient tumor tissue.

Clinical Use; Adverse Effects

The drug is administered orally but should not be given until the patient has recovered from any hematological toxicity caused by previous chemotherapy. CYP2D6 metabolizes rucaparib, yielding a half-life of about 18 h. Adverse effects include GI upset and abdominal pain, fatigue, and decreased appetite. MDS and AML are rare but serious adverse effects (<1%). This agent may cause fetal harm and should not be administered to pregnant females or used by nursing mothers.

BCL2 Inhibitors

The BCL2 protein family comprises more than 20 proteins that govern mitochondrial outer membrane permeabilization and control programmed cell death (apoptosis). Proteins in this family can be either *pro-* or *anti*apoptotic depending on their content of BCL2 homology domains (BH1 to 4). *Proapoptotic* proteins contain a BH3 domain that is necessary for dimerization with other proteins of the BCL2 family. *Antiapoptotic* proteins contain BH1 and BH2. The balance of these interacting proteins controls mitochondrial outer membrane permeabilization, cytochrome c release, and the activation of caspases that leads to apoptosis (Figure 67–8). BCL2 promotes cellular survival by inhibiting proapoptotic proteins like BIM, BAX, and BAK and is overexpressed in CLL and some other tumors where it can support tumor cell survival and resistance to cancer treatments.

Venetoclax

Mechanism of Action

Venetoclax is a first-in-class, orally bioavailable, small-molecule inhibitor of BCL2. It was designed as a BH3 mimetic that inhibits BCL2 interaction with the proapoptotic BH3-only family members, such as BIM, BID, and BAD. In vitro, venetoclax inhibits BCL2 action with an IC_{50} of less than 0.01 nM and with a selectivity of two to three orders of magnitude over other BCL2 family members. In the presence of venetoclax, BH3-only proteins can translocate to mitochondria and initiate BAX/BAK-dependent apoptosis. Overexpression of BCL2 occurs in CLL cells, where it supports tumor cell survival and resistance to chemotherapeutic agents. Thus, venetoclax helps restore apoptosis in these cells.

ADME; Therapeutic Use; Adverse Effects

Oral absorption is significantly improved 3- to 5-fold by administration with a meal. Venetoclax, a Pgp substrate, is metabolized by CYP3A4/5; concomitant use of CYP3A inhibitors or inducers and Pgp inhibitors should be avoided (see previous discussion of *palbociclib* for details). The elimination half-life is 18–26 h. Venetoclax is approved for the treatment of patients with CLL with a 17p deletion. The most common adverse effects are neutropenia, diarrhea, nausea, anemia, upper respiratory tract infection, thrombocytopenia, and fatigue. Venetoclax should not be administered during pregnancy or breastfeeding until further data are available.

Thalidomide and Lenalidomide

Thalidomide and lenalidomide have a most unusual history and a multiplicity of biological and immunological effects. Thalidomide originally was used for the treatment of pregnancy-associated morning sickness

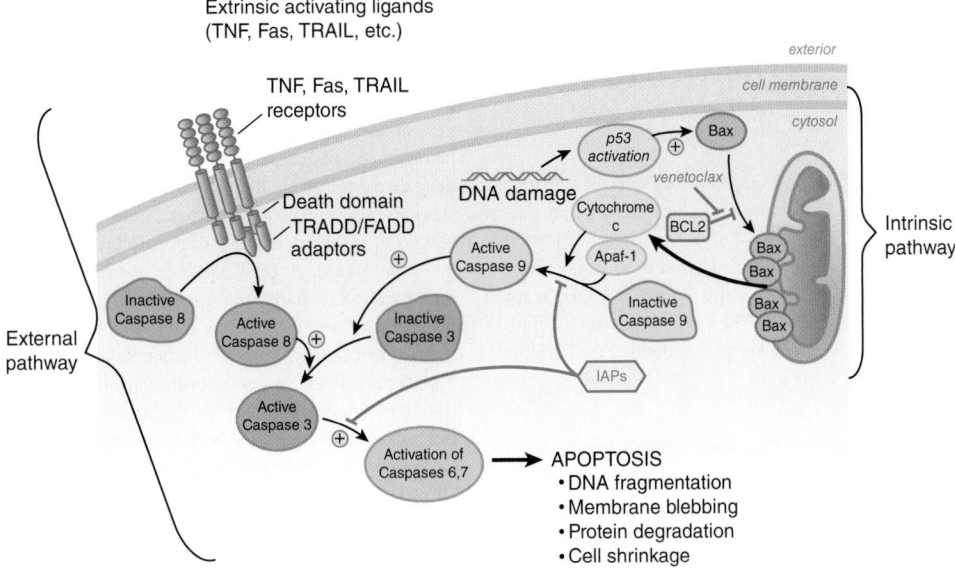

Figure 67–8 *BH3 mimetics enhance apoptosis.* Permeability of the outer mitochondrial membrane to cytochrome c is regulated by proteins required for forming pores, including proapoptotic BAX and BAK. BAK and BAX are rendered inactive by binding to the BH3 domains of antiapoptotic proteins such as BCL2. BH3 mimetic drugs (*venetoclax*) target BCL2 and its interaction with BAX/BAK, reducing the inhibitory effect of BCL2 on apoptosis progression, enhancing cytochrome c release, and sensitizing the cell to apoptosis. Cancer cells may be resistant to apoptosis by overexpression of BCL2; BH3 mimetics such as *venetoclax* release the resultant blockade and promote apoptosis.

but was withdrawn from the market due to teratogenicity and dysmelia (stunted limb growth). It reentered clinical practice for treatment of erythema nodosum leprosum (see Chapter 60). Further research revealed its antiangiogenic and immunomodulatory effects. At least four distinct mechanisms have been proposed to explain its antitumor activity, which are summarized in Figure 67–9 and enumerated in its legend.

Both thalidomide and lenalidomide possess potent activity in patients with newly diagnosed and heavily pretreated relapsed/refractory MM. Lenalidomide also is approved for its activity in the 5q– subset [or del(5q) subset] of MDS. A specific gene array profile identifies patients with MDS who lack the 5q– abnormality but respond to lenalidomide. A more recently added derivative of thalidomide is pomalidomide, approved for treatment of patients with MM resistant to lenalidomide.

Thalidomide

ADME

Thalidomide exists at physiological pH as a racemic mixture of cell-permeable and rapidly interconverting nonpolar S(–) and R(+) isomers. The R-enantiomer is associated with the teratogenic and biological activities, while the S accounts for the sedative properties of thalidomide. In treating MM, doses usually are escalated by 200 mg/d every 2 weeks until dose-limiting side effects (sedation, fatigue, constipation, or a sensory neuropathy) appear. With extended treatment, the neuropathy may necessitate dose reduction or discontinuation of treatment for a period of time. Thalidomide absorption from the GI tract is slow and highly variable. It distributes throughout most tissues and organs, without significant binding to plasma proteins. The enantiomers are eliminated with a $t_{1/2}$ of about 6 h, mainly due to spontaneous hydrolysis in all body fluids; the S-enantiomer is cleared more rapidly than the R-enantiomer. Thalidomide and its metabolites are excreted in the urine, while the nonabsorbed portion of the drug is excreted unchanged in feces. The inactive hydrolysis products undergo CYP-mediated metabolism. Longer plasma $t_{1/2}$ is reported at the highest doses (1200 mg daily). No dose adjustment is necessary in the presence of renal failure.

Lenalidomide

Lenalidomide constitutes the lead compound of immunomodulatory thalidomide derivatives. Lenalidomide induces the ubiquitination and degradation of target proteins by the E3 ubiquitin ligase CRL4CRBN (Fink and Ebert, 2015). Target proteins in MM cells are IKZF1/3, which are crucial for cell survival (Lu et al., 2014) (Figure 67–9). In MDS, casein kinase 1A1 is the target protein (Krönke et al., 2015). Cellular effects of lenalidomide include direct suppression of tumor cell growth in culture, T-cell and NK-cell activation, suppression of TNFα and other cytokines, antiangiogenesis, and promotion of HSC differentiation.

ADME

The standard dosage of lenalidomide is 25 mg/d for 21 days of a 28-day cycle. The drug is rapidly absorbed following oral administration, reaching peak plasma levels within 1.5 h. The $t_{1/2}$ of parent drug in plasma is 9 h. Approximately 70% of the orally administered dose of lenalidomide is excreted intact by the kidney. Dose adjustments to 10 mg/d for creatinine clearance of 30–50 mL/h and to the same dose every 2 days for creatinine clearance less than 30 mL/h are recommended for patients with renal failure.

Therapeutic Use

Lenalidomide exhibits potent antitumor activity in MM, MDS, and CLL; this agent causes fewer adverse effects and lacks the teratogenicity of thalidomide.

Adverse Effects of Thalidomide and Lenalidomide

Thalidomide is well tolerated at doses less than 200 mg daily. Common adverse effects are sedation and constipation. The most serious adverse effect is peripheral sensory neuropathy, which occurs in 10%–30% of patients with MM or other malignancies in a dose- and time-dependent manner. Thalidomide-related neuropathy is an asymmetrical, painful,

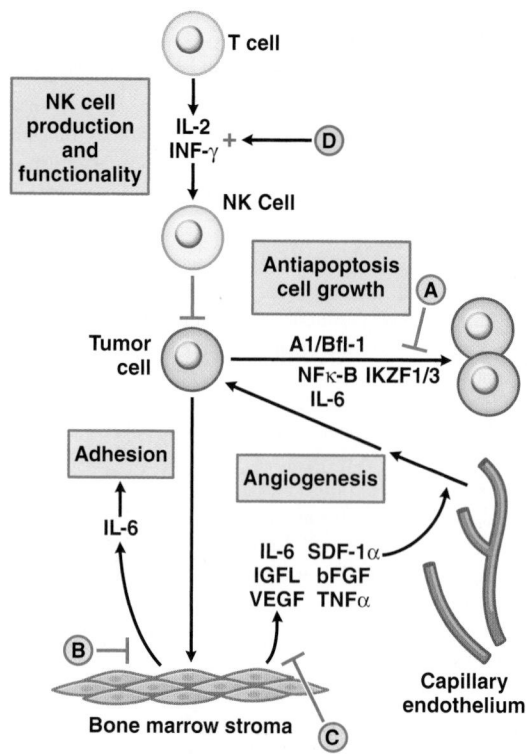

Figure 67–9 *Overview of proposed mechanisms of antimyeloma activity of thalidomide and its derivatives.* Some biological hallmarks of the malignant phenotype are indicated in blue *boxes.* The proposed sites of action for thalidomide (letters inside red and green circles) are hypothesized to also be operative for thalidomide derivatives. **A.** Direct anti-MM effect on tumor cells, including G_1 growth arrest or apoptosis, even against MM cells resistant to conventional therapy. This is due to the disruption of the antiapoptotic effect of BCL2 family members, blocking NF-κB signaling, and inhibition of the production of IL-6. Mechanistic studies show that lenalidomide can kill MM cells by inducing E3 ubiquitin ligase CRL4CRBN-mediated ubiquitination and degradation of the crucial IKZF1 & 3 (zinc finger transcription factors). **B.** Inhibition of MM cell adhesion to bone marrow stromal cells partially due to the reduction of IL-6 release. **C.** Decreased angiogenesis due to the inhibition of cytokine and growth factor production and release. **D.** Enhanced T-cell production of cytokines, such as IL-2 and IFN-γ, that increase the number and cytotoxic functionality of NK cells.

peripheral paresthesia with sensory loss, commonly presenting with numbness of toes and feet, muscle cramps, weakness, signs of pyramidal tract involvement, and carpal tunnel syndrome. Although symptoms improve on drug discontinuation, long-standing sensory loss may not reverse. Particular caution should be applied in patients with preexisting neuropathy (e.g., related to diabetes) or prior exposure to drugs that can cause peripheral neuropathy (e.g., vinca alkaloids, bortezomib). Thalidomide enhances the sedative effects of barbiturates and alcohol and the catatonic effects of chlorpromazine. Conversely, CNS stimulants (such as methamphetamine and methylphenidate) counteract the depressant effects of thalidomide.

Adverse effects of lenalidomide are less severe; it causes little sedation, constipation, or neuropathy. Lenalidomide depresses bone marrow function and is associated with significant leukopenia (20% of patients). Hepatotoxicity and renal dysfunction are rare. In some patients with CLL, lenalidomide causes dramatic lymph node swelling and tumor lysis (tumor flare reaction). Patients with renal dysfunction are prone to this reaction; thus, patients with CLL should be started at lower doses of 10 mg/d, with escalation as tolerated. Patients with CLL should receive pretreatment hydration and allopurinol to avoid the consequences of tumor swelling and tumor lysis. A negative interaction with rituximab, an anti-CD20 antibody, may result from lenalidomide's downregulation of CD20, an interaction that has clinical implications for their combined use in lymphoid malignancies.

Thalidomide and lenalidomide increase the risk for thromboembolic events, including deep vein thrombosis, stroke, and myocardial infarction, which occur with increased frequency in combination with glucocorticoids and with anthracyclines. Anticoagulation and antiplatelet medication reduce this risk and are indicated in patients with risk factors for clotting.

Pomalidomide

Pomalidomide, a thalidomide congener, is indicated for the treatment of patients with MM who have received at least two prior therapies including lenalidomide. Adverse effects are similar to those of thalidomide. Pomalidomide in contraindicated during pregnancy and in females who may become pregnant. As a consequence, this drug is available only under a pregnancy control system to ensure that recipients are not pregnant and are using effective birth control.

Proteasome Inhibitors

First Generation

Bortezomib is a first-generation inhibitor of proteasome-mediated protein degradation that has a central role in the treatment of MM.

Mechanism of Action

Bortezomib binds to the β5 subunit of the 20S core of the 26S proteasome and reversibly inhibits its chymotrypsin-like activity. This event disrupts multiple intracellular signaling cascades, leading to apoptosis. An important consequence of proteasome inhibition is its effect on NF-κB, a transcription factor that promotes cell damage response and cell survival. Most cellular NF-κB is cytosolic and bound to IκB; in this form, NF-κB is restricted to the cytosol and cannot enter the nucleus to regulate transcription. In response to stress signals resulting from hypoxia, chemotherapy, and DNA damage, IκB becomes ubiquitinated and then degraded via the proteasome. Its degradation releases NF-κB, which enters the nucleus and transcriptionally activates a host of genes involved in cell survival (e.g., cell adhesion proteins, and proliferation (e.g., cyclin-D1) or antiapoptosis (e.g., cIAPs, BCL-2). NF-κB is highly expressed in many human tumors, including MM, and may be a key factor in tumor cell survival in a hypoxic environment and during chemotherapy. Bortezomib blocks proteasomal degradation of IκB, thereby preventing the transcriptional activity of NF-κB and downregulating survival responses.

Bortezomib also disrupts the ubiquitin-proteasomal degradation of p21, p27, p53, and other key regulators of the cell cycle and initiators of apoptosis. Bortezomib activates the cell's stereotypical "unfolded protein response," in which abnormal protein conformation activates adaptive signaling pathways in the cell. The composite effect leads to irreversible commitment of MM cells to apoptosis.

ADME

The recommended starting dose of bortezomib is 1.3 mg/m² given as an intravenous bolus on days 1, 4, 8, and 11 of every 21-day cycle (with a 10-day rest period per cycle). At least 72 h should elapse between doses. Drug administration should be withheld until resolution of any grade 3 nonhematological toxicity or grade 4 hematological toxicity, and subsequent doses should be reduced 25%. The drug exhibits a terminal $t_{1/2}$ in plasma of 5.5 h. Peak proteasome inhibition reaches 60% within 1 h and declines thereafter, with a $t_{1/2}$ of about 24 h. Bortezomib clearance results from the deboronation of the parent compound (90%), followed by hydroxylation of the boron-free product by CYPs 3A4 and 2D6; administration of this drug with potent inducers or inhibitors/substrates of CYP3A4 requires caution. No dose adjustment is required for patients with renal dysfunction.

Therapeutic Uses

Bortezomib is used as initial therapy for patients with MM and as therapy for patients with MM after relapse from other drugs. It is also approved for treatment of patients with relapsed or refractory MCL. The drug is active in myeloma, including the induction of complete responses in up to 30% of patients when used in combination with other drugs (i.e., thalidomide, lenalidomide, liposomal doxorubicin, or dexamethasone).

Adverse Effects

Bortezomib toxicities include thrombocytopenia (28%), fatigue (12%), peripheral neuropathy (12%), neutropenia, anemia, vomiting, diarrhea, limb pain, dehydration, nausea, and weakness. Peripheral neuropathy, the most chronic of the toxicities, develops most frequently in patients with a prior history of neuropathy secondary to prior drug treatment (e.g., thalidomide) or diabetes or with prolonged use. Dose reductions or discontinuation of bortezomib ameliorates the neuropathic symptoms. Injection of bortezomib may precipitate hypotension, especially in volume-depleted patients, in those who have a history of syncope, or in patients taking antihypertensive medications. Cardiac toxicity is rare, but congestive heart failure and prolonged QT interval have been reported.

Second Generation

Carfilzomib is a second-generation selective proteasome inhibitor based on a tetrapeptide epoxyketone. It is FDA approved as a single agent or in combination with dexamethasone or lenalidomide plus dexamethasone for the treatment of patients with relapsed or refractory MM who have received at least one prior therapy. Frequent adverse effects (>20% of patients) include anemia, thrombocytopenia, diarrhea, dyspnea, and peripheral edema. There is a risk for cardiac, renal, pulmonary, and hepatic toxicity as well as hypertension.

Ixazomib is an orally bioavailable second-generation peptide analogue proteasome inhibitor that interacts with subunit beta type 5 (PSMB5) of the 20S proteasome complex. Ixazomib has an elimination half-life of 9.5 days and is approved for use in combination with lenalidomide and dexamethasone for the treatment of patients with MM after at least one prior therapy (Moreau et al., 2016). Ixazomib can cause diarrhea, peripheral neuropathy, and hepatotoxicity.

Omacetaxine. This agent's mechanisms of action include inhibition of protein translation by preventing the initial elongation step of protein synthesis, thereby depleting the cell of short-lived proteins. Omacetaxine is FDA approved for the treatment of patients with chronic or accelerated-phase CML with resistance or intolerance to two or more TKIs.

CD20 Inhibitors

CD20 is a cell surface antigen expressed on the surface of all B cells beginning with the pro–B cell stage through its terminal differentiation to plasma cells (see Chapters 34 and 35) and is expressed on about 90% of B-cell neoplasms.

Rituximab

Rituximab is a chimeric murine/human monoclonal IgG1 antibody that targets the CD20 B-cell surface antigen. On binding to CD20, rituximab mediates B-cell lysis through CDC and ADCC. In patients with NHL, administration of rituximab depletes circulating and tissue-based B cells within the first 3 weeks, with sustained depletion for 6 to 9 months posttreatment in a majority of patients. Median B-cell levels return to normal by 12 months.

ADME

The drug is administered by intravenous infusion both as a single agent and in combination with chemotherapy. Rituximab has a $t_{1/2}$ of about 22 days. As a single agent, it is given weekly for 4 weeks, with maintenance dosing every 3–6 months. In combination regimens, the drug may be administered every 3–4 weeks, with chemotherapy, for up to eight doses. The rate of infusion should be increased slowly to prevent serious hypersensitivity reactions. Pretreatment with antihistamines, acetaminophen, and glucocorticoids decreases the risk of hypersensitivity reactions. Patients with large numbers of circulating tumor cells (as in CLL) are at increased risk for tumor lysis syndrome; in these patients, the initial dose should be no more than 50 mg/m² on day 1 of treatment, and patients should receive standard tumor lysis prophylaxis.

Therapeutic Uses

Rituximab is approved as a single agent for relapsed indolent lymphomas and significantly enhances response and survival in combination with chemotherapy for the initial treatment of diffuse large BCL. Rituximab improves response rates when added to combination chemotherapy for other indolent B-cell NHLs, including CLL, MCL, WM, and marginal zone lymphomas. Maintenance of remission with rituximab delays time to progression and improves overall survival in indolent NHL. It is increasingly used for treatment of autoimmune diseases such as rheumatological disease, thrombotic thrombocytopenic purpura, autoimmune hemolytic anemias, cryoglobulin-induced renal disease, and multiple sclerosis.

Resistance and Adverse Effects

Resistance to rituximab may emerge through downregulation of CD20, impaired antibody-dependent cellular cytotoxicity, decreased complement activation, limited effects on signaling and induction of apoptosis, and inadequate blood levels. Polymorphisms in two of the receptors for the antibody Fc region responsible for complement activation may predict the clinical response to rituximab monotherapy in patients with follicular lymphoma but not in CLL. Rituximab infusion reactions can be life threatening, but with pretreatment, reactions are usually mild and limited to fever, chills, throat itching, urticaria, and mild hypotension. All respond to decreased infusion rates and antihistamines. Uncommonly, patients may develop severe mucocutaneous skin reactions, including Stevens-Johnson syndrome. Rituximab may cause reactivation of hepatitis B virus or rarely, JC virus (with progressive multifocal leukoencephalopathy). Hypogammaglobulinemia and autoimmune syndromes (idiopathic thrombocytopenic purpura, thrombotic thrombocytopenic purpura, autoimmune hemolytic anemia, pure red cell aplasia, and delayed neutropenia) may supervene 1–5 months after administration.

Ofatumumab

Ofatumumab is a second monoclonal antibody that binds to CD20 at sites on the major and minor extracellular loops of CD20, distinct from the site targeted by rituximab. Antibody binding results in B-cell lysis via CDC and ADCC. Ofatumumab is approved for treating patients with CLL after failure of fludarabine and alemtuzumab. A complex dosing scheme is used, beginning with small (300-mg) doses on day 1, followed by higher doses (up to 2 g/week) later. Ofatumumab's primary toxicities consist of immunosuppression and opportunistic infection, hypersensitivity reactions during antibody infusion, and myelosuppression. Blood counts should be monitored during treatment. Rarely, patients may develop reactivation of viral infections. The drug should not be administered to patients with active hepatitis B infection; liver function should be monitored in hepatitis B carriers.

Obinutuzumab

Obinutuzumab is a humanized monoclonal IgG1 antibody that recognizes the CD20 antigen expressed on the surface of B cells. On binding to CD20, obinutuzumab mediates B-cell lysis through CDC and ADCC. Obinutuzumab is approved for the treatment of treatment-naïve patients with CLL in combination with chemotherapy. Patients who receive this combination therapy are more likely to go into complete remission and have better overall survival than those receiving chlorambucil alone. In this study, they also compared patients treated with obinutuzumab and chlorambucil to patients who were treated with rituximab and chlorambucil. A comparison of patients with CLL given obinutuzumab-chlorambucil combination therapy versus rituximab-chlorambucil combination therapy showed that the obinutuzumab-chlotrambucil combination provided higher rates of complete remission as well as longer progression-free survival. Cytopenias, fever, cough, and musculoskeletal disorders are frequent side effects.

Other Cell Surface Targets for Monoclonal Antibodies

Alemtuzumab

Alemtuzumab is a humanized IgG-κ monoclonal antibody that binds to CD52 antigen. CD52 is found on the surface of a subset of normal neutrophils and on all B and T lymphocytes, on testicular elements and sperm, and on most BCLs and T-cell lymphomas. Consistently high levels of CD52 expression on lymphoid tumor cells and the lack of CD52 modulation with antibody binding make this antigen a potential target for unconjugated monoclonal antibodies. Alemtuzumab can induce tumor cell death through ADCC and CDC.

ADME

Alemtuzumab is administered intravenously in dosages of 30 mg/d, three times/week. Premedication with diphenhydramine and acetaminophen should precede drug infusion. Dosing should begin with a low-dose infusion, followed by an increased dose 2 days later and, if well tolerated, the highest dose 2 days later. The drug has an initial mean $t_{1/2}$ of 1 h, but after multiple doses, the $t_{1/2}$ extends to 12 days, and steady-state plasma levels are reached at approximately week 6 of treatment.

Therapeutic Uses

Alemtuzumab is approved as a single agent for the treatment of B-cell CLL. Clinical activity had been demonstrated in both B- and T-cell low-grade lymphomas and CLL, including patients with disease refractory to purine analogues. In chemotherapy-refractory CLL, overall response rates are about 40%, with complete responses of 6% in multiple series. Response rates in treatment-naïve patients with CLL are higher (overall response rates of 83% and complete responses of 24%). Alemtuzumab is also approved for the treatment of patients with relapsing forms of multiple sclerosis under a different label.

Adverse Effects

Serious toxicities include acute infusion reactions and depletion of normal neutrophils and T cells. Myelosuppression, with depletion of all blood lineages, occurs in the majority of patients and may represent either direct marrow toxicity or autoimmune responses. Immunosuppression leads to a significant risk of fungal, viral, and other opportunistic infections, particularly in patients who have previously received purine analogues. Patients should receive prophylaxis against *Pneumocystis carinii* and herpesvirus during treatment and for at least 2 months following therapy with alemtuzumab. Because reactivation of cytomegalovirus (CMV) infections may follow antibody use, patients should be monitored for symptoms and signs of viremia, hepatitis, and pneumonia. CD4$^+$ T-cell counts may remain profoundly depleted (<200 cells/μL) for 1 year.

Dinutuximab

Dinutuximab is a monoclonal antibody that targets glycolipid GD2, expressed on neuroblastoma cells and on normal cells of neuroectodermal origin, including the CNS and peripheral nerves. It is approved in combination with GM-CSF, IL-2, and RA for high-risk neuroblastoma in pediatric patients. Dinutuximab can cause nerve damage and life-threatening infusion reactions.

Daratumumab

Daratumumab is a human IgG1 monoclonal antibody that binds to CD38 and inhibits the growth of CD38-expressing tumor cells by inducing immune-mediated tumor cell lysis through CDC and ADCC. The FDA has recently approved daratumumab for treatment of patients with MM in combination with lenalidomide or bortezomib and dexamethasone. The most frequent adverse effects are infusion reactions, neutropenia, thrombocytopenia, fatigue, nausea, diarrhea, muscle spasms, back pain, pyrexia, cough, dyspnea, peripheral edema, peripheral sensory neuropathy, and upper respiratory tract infection.

Elotuzumab

Elotuzumab is a humanized monoclonal IgG1 antibody that targets SLAMF7 (CD319). It is approved for the treatment of patients with MM who have received one to three prior therapies. Binding of elotuzumab to the antigen on myeloma cells induces ADCC-dependent tumor cell lysis. ADCC is enhanced by stimulation of the SLAMF7 pathway in NK cells by elotuzumab.

Blinatumomab

Blinatumomab is a bispecific antibody that recognizes sites on the surfaces of B cells and T cells, thereby enabling a patient's T cells to recognize malignant B cells. Blinatumomab binds simultaneously to CD3 (part of the TCR) on T cells and to CD19 on B cells. The drug links these two cell types and activates the T cell to exert cytotoxic activity on CD19⁺ target B cells. Blinatumomab is approved for the treatment of Philadelphia chromosome-negative relapsed or refractory B-cell precursor ALL. Major adverse effects are cytokine release syndrome, neurologic toxicities, neutropenic fever, and sepsis.

Monoclonal Antibody–Cytotoxin Conjugates

Gemtuzumab Ozogamicin

Mechanism of Action

Gemtuzumab ozogamicin is a humanized monoclonal antibody against CD33 covalently linked to a semisynthetic derivative of calicheamicin, a potent antitumor antibiotic. The CD33 antigen is present on most hematopoietic cells, on more than 80% of AMLs, and on most myeloid cells in patients with MDSs. However, other normal cell types lack CD33 expression, making this antigen attractive for targeted therapy. CD33 has no known biological function, although monoclonal antibody cross-linking inhibits normal and myeloid leukemia cell proliferation. Following its binding to CD33, gemtuzumab ozogamicin undergoes endocytosis; cleavage of calicheamicin from the antibody takes place within the lysosome. The potent toxin then enters the nucleus, binds in the minor groove of DNA, and causes double-strand DNA breaks and cell death.

ADME

The antibody conjugate produces a 30% complete response rate in relapsed AML when administered at a dose of 9 mg/m² for up to three doses at 2-week intervals. The $t_{1/2}$ of total and unconjugated calicheamicin are 41 and 143 h, respectively. Following a second dose, the $t_{1/2}$ of drug-antibody conjugate increases to 64 h. Most patients require two to three doses to achieve remission.

Therapeutic Use

The drug was initially approved for use in patients more than 60 years of age with AML in first relapse. However, the drug is not yet available, pending clinical trials to more precisely define a population with high likelihood of efficacy. Primary toxicities include myelosuppression in all patients treated and hepatocellular damage in 30%–40% of patients, manifested by hyperbilirubinemia and enzyme elevations. This agent also causes a syndrome that resembles hepatic veno-occlusive disease when patients subsequently undergo myeloablative therapy or when gemtuzumab ozogamicin follows high-dose chemotherapy.

Brentuximab Vedotin

Brentuximab vedotin is an anti-CD30 IgG1 monoclonal antibody linked with the microtubule-disrupting agent MMAE. CD30 is expressed on a number of malignant cells and is especially prevalent in Hodgkin and anaplastic lymphoma. Binding of the antibody to CD30-expressing cells is followed by internalization and the intracellular release of MMAE via proteolytic cleavage. MMAE disrupts the microtubule network, inducing cell cycle arrest and apoptotic cell death. MMAE is mostly metabolized by CYP3A, and coadministration with CYP3A4 inhibitors will increase exposure to the MMAE toxin. Coadministration with CYP3A4 inducers (e.g., rifampicin) reduces exposure. The most common adverse reactions are neutropenia, peripheral sensory neuropathy, fatigue, nausea, anemia, upper respiratory tract infection, diarrhea, pyrexia, rash, thrombocytopenia, cough, and vomiting.

Ado-trastuzumab Emtansine

Ado-trastuzumab-DM1 combines the HER2-targeted properties of trastuzumab with the antimicrotubule agent DM1 (derived from maytansine), allowing preferential intracellular drug delivery to HER2⁺ cells in the treatment of HER⁺ breast cancer. The complex binds to the EGFR2 (HER2) and enters the cell by receptor-mediated endocytosis. The DM1 (emtansine) is released into the cytosol as the complex is cleaved by proteases in lysosomes. The DM1 disrupts microtubule-dependent events, causing mitotic arrest, disruption of intracellular trafficking, and apoptosis. The adverse effects of treatment include cardiac dysfunction as described for unconjugated trastuzumab. Hepatotoxicity is an additional risk.

Denileukin Diftitox

Denileukin diftitox is an immunotoxin made from the genetic recombination of IL-2 and the catalytically active fragment of diphtheria toxin. The high-affinity IL-2R has limited tissue expression and is an attractive target for an immunotoxin. Introduction of the diphtheria toxin fragment into cells leads to ADP-ribosylation and inactivation of eukaryotic elongation factor EF-2, inhibition of protein synthesis, and thence cell death.

ADME

Denileukin diftitox is administered by intravenous infusion over 30–60 min for 5 consecutive days every 21 days for eight cycles. The drug is quickly distributed and has a terminal $t_{1/2}$ of about 70 min. Denileukin diftitox clearance in later cycles of treatment accelerates by 2- to 3-fold as a result of development of antibodies, but serum levels exceed those required to produce cell death in IL-2R–expressing cell lines (1–10 ng/mL for > 90 min).

Therapeutic Uses

Denileukin diftitox is approved for the treatment of recurrent/refractory cutaneous T-cell lymphomas. Response rates of 30%–37% have been achieved, with a median response duration of 6.9 months. Patients with a history of hypersensitivity reactions to diphtheria toxin or IL-2 should not be treated. Significant toxicities include acute hypersensitivity reactions, a vascular leak syndrome, and constitutional toxicities; glucocorticoid premedication significantly decreases toxicity.

Radioimmunoconjugates

Radioimmunoconjugates provide targeted delivery of radionuclides to tumor cells. ¹³¹Iodine (¹³¹I) is a favored radioisotope because it is readily available, relatively inexpensive, and easily conjugated to a monoclonal antibody. The γ particles emitted by ¹³¹I can be used for both imaging and therapy, but protein-iodine conjugates have the drawback of releasing free ¹³¹I and ¹³¹I-tyrosine into the blood and thus present a health hazard to people in contact with the patient. The β-emitter ⁹⁰Y (yttrium) has emerged as an alternative to ¹³¹I, based on its higher energy and longer path length. Thus, it may be more effective in tumors with larger diameters. It also has a short $t_{1/2}$ and remains conjugated, even after endocytosis, providing a safer profile for outpatient use. Currently available radioimmunoconjugates consist of murine monoclonal antibodies against CD20 conjugated with ¹³¹I (tositumomab) or ⁹⁰Y (ibritumomab). Both drugs have shown responses rates in relapsed lymphoma of 65%–80%. Adverse effects include antibody-related hypersensitivity, bone marrow suppression, and secondary leukemias. Both radioconjugates targeting CD20 on lymphomas have been approved; concerns over toxicity have limited their use.

Cytokines and Growth Factors

Colony-Stimulating Factors

Many agents used for cancer chemotherapy suppress the production of multiple types of hematopoietic cells, and bone marrow suppression can limit the delivery of chemotherapy on schedule and at prescribed doses. The availability of recombinant growth factors for erythrocytes (i.e., erythropoietin), granulocytes (i.e., G-CSF), and granulocytes and macrophages (i.e., GM-CSF) has advanced the ability to use combination therapy or high-dose cytotoxic therapy with diminished complications such as febrile neutropenia (see Chapter 66). Chapter 41 presents the basic pharmacology of hematopoietic growth factors.

Plerixafor

Plerixafor is a small-molecule inhibitor of the CXCR4 chemokine receptor and is used in combination with G-CSF to mobilize HSC to the peripheral blood for collection and subsequent autologous transplantation in patients with NHL and MM. Plerixafor blocks binding of SDF-1α to CXCR4. CXCR4 activity supports homing of HSCs to the bone marrow, and plerixafor mobilizes the release and entry of HSCs into the circulation. Combination of G-CSF with plerixafor increases the efficacy of HSC mobilization

Inhibitors of Histone Deacetylase

Histone deacetylases are a class of enzymes that catalyze the removal of acetyl groups from acetylated lysine amino acids in histones, thereby altering the transcriptional activation of cellular genes. Thus, HDAC inhibitors produce a broad spectrum of epigenetic effects. HDACs can also deacetylate other proteins, including transcription factors. Overexpression of HDACs found in some cancers, or aberrant recruitment of HDACs to oncogenic transcription factors, can cause hypoacetylation of core nucleosomal histones. This hypoacetylation results in a condensed chromatin structure and repression of gene transcription. In contrast, inhibition of HDAC activity leads to the accumulation of acetyl groups on the histone lysine residues, an open chromatin structure, and activation of target genes that are selectively repressed in tumors. The result of HDAC inhibition can be differentiation with the emergence of a more normal cellular phenotype or cell cycle arrest with expression of endogenous regulators of cell cycle progression. Due to the diversity of the HDAC family of enzymes and their tissue distribution, HDAC inhibitors with different selectivity can induce a wide variety of cellular effects.

Panobinostat

Panobinostat is an orally bioavailable, nonselective pan-HDAC inhibitor. The inhibitory activity leads to apoptosis of malignant cells via multiple pathways. Panobinostat is approved for the treatment of patients with MM who have received at least two previous treatments, including bortezomib and an immunomodulatory agent.

ADME

The oral bioavailability is about 21%. Panobinostat is metabolized through CYP3A. It is recommended to avoid concomitant use with strong CYP3A4 inducers or inhibitors. Otherwise, dose adjustments will be necessary. The elimination half-life is approximately 37 h.

Adverse Effects

The most common adverse effects are diarrhea (severe in 25% of patients), fatigue, nausea, peripheral edema, decreased appetite, pyrexia, and vomiting. The most common nonhematologic laboratory abnormalities (incidence ≥ 40%) are hypophosphatemia, hypokalemia, hyponatremia, and increased creatinine. The common hematologic laboratory abnormalities (incidence ≥ 60%) are thrombocytopenia, lymphopenia, leukopenia, neutropenia, and anemia. Fatal cardiac ischemic events, severe arrhythmias, and ECG changes have occurred in patients receiving panobinostat. Arrhythmias may be exacerbated by electrolyte abnormalities. Avoid concomitant use of antiarrhythmic or QT-prolonging drugs. Close cardiac monitoring during treatment is recommended.

Romidepsin

Romidepsin is an HDAC inhibitor used in the treatment of cutaneous and peripheral T-cell lymphoma. Romidepsin is a natural product obtained from the bacteria *Chromobacterium violaceum* and is sometimes referred to as depsipeptide. Romidepsin functions as a prodrug. Within cells, a zinc-binding thiol of the drug is reduced and interacts with a zinc atom in the binding pocket of HDAC to block its activity.

ADME

After intravenous administration, the major metabolism is through CYP3A4. Thus, it is recommended to monitor for toxicities related to increased romidepsin exposure when coadministering strong CYP3A4 inhibitors. Avoid use with rifampin and other strong CYP3A4 inducers. The terminal half-life is about 3 h.

Adverse Effects

The most commonly observed are nausea and vomiting, anemia, thrombocytopenia, and leukopenia as well as abnormal electrolyte levels and ECG changes.

Vorinostat

Vorinostat is a small-molecule, orally bioavailable HDAC inhibitor; it is also known as SAHA based on its chemical name *s*uber*a*nilo*h*ydroxamic *a*cid.

Mechanism of Action

Vorinostat binds to the active site of HDACs and chelates zinc ions in the active site. The resulting inhibition of HDACs causes the accumulation of acetylated histones and other acetylated proteins, amongst which are transcription factors crucial for cell differentiation. Vorinostat inhibits the enzymatic activities of HDAC1, 2, 3 (class I) and HDAC6 (class II) at nanomolar concentrations ($IC_{50} < 100$ nM). In vitro, vorinostat induces cell cycle arrest or apoptosis of some cancer cells.

ADME

The absorption of vorinostat is slightly improved when taken with a meal. Metabolism is mostly through glucuronidation and hydrolysis. The elimination $t_{\frac{1}{2}}$ is about 2 h.

Therapeutic Use; Adverse Effects

Vorinostat is approved for the treatment of patients with cutaneous T-cell lymphoma with persistent or recurrent disease after two systemic therapies. The most common adverse reactions are diarrhea, fatigue, nausea, thrombocytopenia, anorexia, and dysgeusia. Patients with severe hepatic impairment should be excluded from treatment. Vorinostat is classified as pregnancy category D: evidence of risk.

Acknowledgment: *Bruce A. Chabner, Jeffrey Barnes, Joel Neal, Erin Olson, Hamza Mujagic, Lecia Sequist, Wynham Wilson, Dan L. Longo, Constantine Mitsiades, and Paul Richardson contributed to this chapter in the recent edition of this book. We have retained some of their text in the current edition.*

Drug Facts for Your Personal Formulary: *Pathway-Targeted Therapies*

Drug	Therapeutic Use	Clinical Pharmacology and Tips

Section I: Inhibitors of Growth Factors and Receptors

Epidermal Growth Factor Receptor Inhibitors

Small-Molecule EGFR Kinase Inhibitors: Oral Administration

Drug	Therapeutic Use	Clinical Pharmacology and Tips
Erlotinib	• Advanced NSCLC with mutant EGFR (del exon 19; L858R) • Advanced pancreatic cancer in combination with gemcitabine	• Skin rash, stomatitis, diarrhea, interstitial lung disease • CYP3A4 substrate • Anticoagulant effect of warfarin enhanced • Concurrent use of PPI ↓ bioavailability
Gefitinib	• Advanced NSCLC with mutant EGFR (del exon 19; L858R)	• Side effects similar to erlotinib, but bioavailability not affected by PPI
Afatinib	• Irreversible inhibitor EGFR > HER2 • Advanced NSCLC with mutant EGFR (del exon 19; L858R)	• Side effects similar to gefitinib; can cause hepatotoxicity • Not affected by CYP3A4 modulation • ↓ Dose with renal impairment or Pgp inhibitors
Osimertinib	• Advanced NSCLC that is resistant to other EGFR kinase inhibitor and positive for T790M-mutant EGFR	• Similar to gefitinib but less intense side effects; can ↑ QTc interval

Monoclonal Antibody EGFR Inhibitors: Intravenous Administration

Drug	Therapeutic Use	Clinical Pharmacology and Tips
Cetuximab *(chimeric human/ mouse IgG1)*	• Metastatic colorectal cancer with wild-type KRAS in combination with chemotherapy • Head and neck SCC in combination with radiation or cisplatin	• Skin rash, diarrhea, interstitial lung disease • Rare: infusion reaction, cardiopulmonary arrest, hypomagnesemia
Panitumumab *(human IgG2)*	• Metastatic colorectal cancer with wild-type KRAS in combination with chemotherapy	• Side effects similar to cetuximab
Necitumumab *(human IgG1)*	• Metastatic NSCLC in combination with chemotherapy	• Side effects similar to cetuximab

Human Epidermal Growth Factor Receptor 2 Inhibitors

Small-Molecule HER2 Kinase Inhibitors: Oral Administration, Also Inhibit EGFR

Drug	Therapeutic Use	Clinical Pharmacology and Tips
Lapatinib	• HER2-positive breast cancer in combination with capecitabine • HER2-positive, hormone receptor–positive breast cancer in combination with letrozole (AI)	• Skin rash, diarrhea • Some cardiotoxicity (less than trastuzumab, the HER2 antibody), QT interval prolongation • CYP3A4 substrate
Neratinib	• Irreversible inhibitor of EGFR and HER2 • HER2-positive breast cancer in addition to chemotherapy	• Diarrhea is major adverse effect with 1/3 of patients severe grade 3–4

Monoclonal Antibody HER2 Inhibitors: Intravenous Administration

Drug	Therapeutic Use	Clinical Pharmacology and Tips
Trastuzumab *(humanized IgG1)*	• HER2-positive breast cancer and gastric cancer • Combination with taxanes possible as chemotherapy	• Congestive heart failure (<5% reduced LVEF; < 1% symptomatic); ↑ to 20% in combination with doxorubicin due to cardiotoxicity; monitor LVEF during and after • Acute infusion reaction, nausea, dyspnea, rashes
Pertuzumab *(humanized IgG1)*	• HER2-positive breast cancer in combination with trastuzumab and taxane	• Targets different HER2 domain than trastuzumab; prevents dimerization with other HERs • Side effects similar to trastuzumab

Platelet-Derived Growth Factor Receptor Inhibitors

Drug	Therapeutic Use	Clinical Pharmacology and Tips
Olaratumab *(fully human IgG1)*	• Soft-tissue sarcoma in combination with doxorubicin	• Nausea, fatigue, GI toxicity • Neutropenia, thrombocytopenia, elevated aPTT, hypokalemia, hypophosphatemia

Section II: Inhibitors of Intracellular Protein Kinases

Mutant B-RAF Kinase Inhibitors

Drug	Therapeutic Use	Clinical Pharmacology and Tips
Vemurafenib	• BRAFV600E/K mutant melanoma • Not effective in wild-type BRAF melanoma	• Cutaneous adverse effects up to 60%, with SCC in > 20% • Arthralgia, fatigue, nausea less frequently • Can cause QT prolongation • CYP3A4 substrate; CYP1A2 inhibitor
Dabrafenib	• BRAFV600E/K mutant melanoma also in combination with the MEK inhibitor trametinib • BRAF V600E mutant NSCLC with trametinib • Not effective in wild-type BRAF melanoma	• Cutaneous adverse effects include hyperkeratosis and papilloma • cuSCC in ~ 10% of patients • Combination with trametinib ↓ incidence of cuSCC to 3% and delays onset • CYP2C8 and CYP3A substrate

Drug Facts for Your Personal Formulary: *Pathway-Targeted Therapies (continued)*

Drug	Therapeutic Use	Clinical Pharmacology and Tips
Mitogen-Activated Protein Kinase Kinase Inhibitors		
Cobimetinib	• BRAFV600E/K mutant melanoma	• Diarrhea, photosensitivity, nausea common • Risk of hemorrhage, cardiomyopathy • CYP3A4 substrate
Trametinib	• BRAFV600E/K mutant melanoma & BRAF V600E mutant NSCLC: with dabrafenib • Ineffective in patients who developed resistance to BRAF inhibitor treatment	• Cutaneous rash, acneiform dermatitis, diarrhea most frequent; serious skin toxicity in 6% • Risk of cardiomyopathy, hypertension, hemorrhage, interstitial lung disease • Reduced absorption after high-calorie meal
Janus-Associated Protein Kinase Inhibitors		
Ruxolitinib	• Polycythemia vera • Myelofibrosis	• Thrombocytopenia, anemia most frequent • Rare basal cell carcinoma or SCC • ↓ Dose in renal or hepatic impairment • CYP3A4 substrate
Cyclin-Dependent Kinase 4/6 Inhibitors		
Palbociclib	• Advanced ER-positive, HER2-negative breast cancer • Combination with AI or antiestrogen (fulvestrant) • In clinical trial for other cancers	• Common: neutropenia, leukopenia, infections, stomatitis, anemia, thrombocytopenia, nausea, diarrhea • Substrate and inhibitor of CYP3A4
Abemaciclib and Ribociclib	• In clinical trials for use as above	• Side effects same as palboclib
Bruton Tyrosine Kinase Inhibitors		
Ibrutinib	• Mantle cell lymphoma, CLL, SLL, Waldenström macroglobulinemia	• Neutropenia, thrombocytopenia, diarrhea, anemia, musculoskeletal pain • Slow onset of hypertension possible: monitor blood pressure • Atrial fibrillation: monitor and treat • Secondary malignancies mostly skin, nonmelanoma • CYP3A4 substrate
BCR-ABL, PDGFR, KIT Kinase Inhibitors		
Imatinib	• Chronic-phase CML; mucosal and acral lentigenous melanoma (KIT-mutation positive), GIST (KIT-mutation-positive), dermatofibrosarcoma protuberans, chronic myelomonocytic leukemia	• GI tract adverse effects: diarrhea, nausea, vomiting • Fluid retention, edema • Rare myelosuppression, hepatotoxicity • CYP3A4 substrate
Dasatinib	• CML resistant to imatinib after prior therapy	• Adverse effects: diarrhea, nausea, vomiting • Fluid retention, edema, pleural effusions • Rare myelosuppression, hepatotoxicity • Bioavailability ↓ after antacids or H$_2$ blockers • CYP3A4 substrate
Nilotinib	• CML resistant to imatinib after prior therapy	• Adverse effects: diarrhea, nausea, vomiting, fluid retention, edema • May ↑ QT interval; beware vascular events, including ischemia • Rare myelosuppression, hepatotoxicity • Bioavailability ↑ in the presence of food • CYP3A4 and Pgp substrate • Inhibitor of the Pgp
Bosutinib	• CML with resistance to prior therapy	• Diarrhea, nausea, thrombocytopenia, vomiting, rash
Ponatinib	• Resistant CML and Ph$^+$ ALL	• Major adverse effects: thrombosis, hepatotoxicity, pancreatitis • Absorption ↓ by elevated gastric pH (H$_2$ antagonists, antacids, PPIs) • CYP3A4 substrate
Anaplastic Lymphoma Kinase Inhibitors		
Alectinib	• Advanced NSCLC with gene rearrangement containing the ALK kinase fusion gene • Advanced NSCLC with gene rearrangement containing the ALK kinase fusion gene and disease progression on crizotinib	• Fatigue, constipation, and edema, myalgia are common adverse effects • Pneumonitis, GI and hepatic toxicity; bradycardia and prolonged QT intervals observed
Ceritinib, Crizotinib	• As above	• As above
PI3K (Phosphatidylinositol-4,5-Bisphosphate 3-Kinase) Inhibitors		
Idelalisib	• Relapsed or refractory B-cell malignancies: CLL (with rituximab), FL, SLL • Not indicated for first-line treatment	• Serious and sometimes-fatal adverse effects: hepatotoxicity, colitis, pneumonitis, intestinal perforations, skin toxicity • CYP3A substrate

mTOR (Mechanistic or Mammalian Target of Rapamycin) Inhibitors

Temsirolimus	• Renal cell carcinoma	• Adverse effects: frequent rash, mucositis, anemia, fatigue (30%–50%); rare leukopenia, thrombocytopenia, interstitial lung disease • Metabolized to a longer-lived active metabolite (sirolimus) by CYP3A4: avoid CYP3A4 inhibitors, including grapefruit juice
Everolimus	• Renal cell carcinoma • Breast cancer: advanced ER positive, HER2 negative in combination with AI exemestane after failure of other AIs (letrozole, anastrazole) • PNETs • Progressive, well-differentiated, nonfunctional neuroendocrine GIST	• Adverse effects overlap with temsirolimus (see above) • CYP3A4 substrate

Multikinase Inhibitors

Cabozantinib	• Advanced renal cell carcinoma • Lung adenocarcinoma with *MET* gene alteration	• Diarrhea, fatigue, nausea, abdominal pain • Hypertension: monitor blood pressure • Not indicated in patients with recent bleeding history or thromboembolic event • Discontinue in patients with GI perforation, fistulas • CYP3A4 substrate; ↓ dose with hepatic impairment
Vandetanib	• Progressing, locally advanced medullary thyroid cancer	• Diarrhea, colitis, rash • QT interval prolongation, torsades des pointes, sudden death • Do not use in patients with hepatic impairment, long QT syndrome • CYP3A4 substrate

Section III: Inhibitors of Tumor Angiogenesis

Vascular Endothelial Growth Factor Inhibitors

Bevacizumab (humanized IgG1)	• Metastatic colorectal cancer combined with chemotherapy (FOLFOX or FOLFIRI) • NSCLC combined with carboplatin and paclitaxel • Ovarian cancer combined with chemotherapy • Renal cell carcinoma combined with interferon α • Glioblastoma following prior therapy	• Hypertension, related congestive heart failure: monitor blood pressure and treat hypertension • Impaired wound healing: delay elective surgery for 1 month after the last dose; do not resume treatment for at least 1 month after surgery • Spontaneous GI perforation
Ramucirumab (fully human IgG1 to VEGFR2)	• Metastatic colorectal cancer, advanced gastric adenocarcinoma, and NSCLC with disease progression on or after prior therapy as a single drug or in combination with chemotherapy	• Hypertension, diarrhea • Hemorrhage, GI perforations • Impaired wound healing
Aflibercept (extracellular domain of VEGFR1/2 fused to Fc portion of human IgG1)	• Metastatic colorectal cancer in combination with FOLFIRI chemotherapy following FOLFOX	• Soluble trap for VEGF receptor ligands • Hypertension, diarrhea • Increased risk of hemorrhage, GI perforation • Impaired wound healing

Inhibitors of Intracellular Kinases Participating in Angiogenesis

Sunitinib	• VEGFR2 and multiple other kinases inhibited
	• Metastatic renal cell cancer
	• GIST after imatinib resistance
	• Pancreatic neuroendocrine tumors
		• Adverse effects shared with anti-VEGF: bleeding, hypertension, proteinuria (frequent); thromboembolism, GI perforations (rare)
		• Adverse events distinct from anti-VEGF:
		  • Fatigue (50%–70%), hypothyroidism (40%–60%)
		  • Common: bone marrow suppression and diarrhea
		  • Less common: hepatotoxicity, congestive heart failure
		• Check blood pressure, blood counts, and thyroid functions at regular intervals
		• Elimination $t_{1/2} \sim$ 4 days: regimen in some cancers is 4 weeks on, 2 weeks off versus continuous daily administration for other cancers

Sorafenib	• Hepatocellular carcinoma (currently the only approved drug) • Metastatic renal cell cancer (however, sunitinib is the first choice)	• Adverse vascular effects match with those of sunitinib • More common: fatigue, diarrhea, anorexia, rash • Less common: bone marrow suppression, GI perforation, cardiomyopathy
Axitinib	• Inhibition of VEGFR1–3 • Advanced renal cell cancer after failure of prior systemic therapy	• Adverse effects overlap with those of anti-VEGF: hypertension, thrombotic and hemorrhagic events, GI perforation • CYP3A4/5 substrate
Lenvatinib	• Inhibition of VEGFR1–3, FGFRs, PDGFR • Recurrent or metastatic differentiated thyroid cancer • Renal cell cancer in combination with everolimus	• Adverse effects overlap with those of anti-VEGF: hypertension, thrombotic and hemorrhagic events, GI perforation • In addition: hepatotoxicity, QT prolongation • CYP3A substrate

Drug Facts for Your Personal Formulary: *Pathway-Targeted Therapies (continued)*

Drug	Therapeutic Use	Clinical Pharmacology and Tips
Pazopanib	• Inhibition of VEGFR1–3, FGFRs, KIT, PDGFR • Advanced renal cell carcinoma and advanced soft-tissue sarcoma after prior chemotherapy	• Adverse effects overlap with those of anti-VEGF: hypertension, thrombotic and hemorrhagic events, GI perforation • In addition: hepatotoxicity, QT prolongation • CYP3A substrate
Regorafenib	• Inhibition of RET, VEGFR1, PDGFR, FGFR, TIE2, RAF1, BRAF, ABL • Metastatic colorectal cancer after previous chemotherapy and anti-VEGF or anti-EGFR • Advanced GIST after imatinib or sunitinib	• Major adverse effects: hepatotoxicity, hypertension, thrombotic and hemorrhagic events, GI perforation, and wound-healing complications • CYP3A substrate
Section IV: Drugs Targeting the Immune System		
Immune Checkpoint Inhibitors		
Ipilimumab *(anti-CTLA-4 fully human IgG1)*	• Metastatic melanoma as single agent or in combination with nivolumab (anti-PD1) • Clinical trials with different cancers are ongoing	• Autoimmune inflammatory toxicities in majority of patients (>70%) • Most frequent: skin (pruritus, rash, vitiligo), GI tract (diarrhea, colitis) • Less frequent: hepatitis, pneumonitis, hypophysitis, hypo- or hyperthyroidism, myocarditis
Tremelimumab *(anti-CTLA-4 fully human IgG2)*	• Clinical trials with different cancers are ongoing	• See above
Nivolumab *(anti-PD-1 fully human IgG4)*	• Advanced melanoma that progressed after ipilimumab (anti–CTLA-4) • Previously treated NSCLC • Advanced renal cell carcinoma • Relapsed/refractory Hodgkin lymphoma	• Adverse effects: rash, fatigue, dyspnea, musculoskeletal pain, decreased appetite, cough, nausea, constipation • Immune-related serious adverse effects include pneumonitis, colitis, hepatitis, nephritis, renal dysfunction, hypophysitis, hypo- and hyperthyroidism
Pembrolizumab *(anti-PD-1 humanized IgG4)*	• Advanced melanoma that progressed after ipilimumab (anti–CTLA-4) • NSCLC that express PD-L1 and progressed under chemotherapy • NSCLC with wild-type EGFR and ALK and disease progression after chemotherapy • HNSCC with disease progression after chemotherapy	• Adverse effects: rash, fatigue, dyspnea, musculoskeletal pain, decreased appetite, cough, nausea, constipation • Immune-related serious adverse effects include pneumonitis, colitis, hepatitis, nephritis, renal dysfunction, hypophysitis, hypo- and hyperthyroidism
Atezolimumab *(anti-PD-L1 fully human IgG1)*	• NSCLC that is treatment resistant • Urothelial cancer that is locally advanced or metastatic	• Adverse effects: fatigue, decreased appetite, dyspnea, cough, nausea, musculoskeletal pain, constipation • In patients with urothelial cancer: urinary tract infections • Immune-related pneumonitis, colitis, hepatitis, nephritis, renal dysfunction, hypo- and hyperthyroidism, hypophysitis, adrenal insufficiency, pancreatitis, Guillain-Barré syndrome, severe infections
Section V: Inhibitors of Other Targets		
Poly(ADP-Ribose) Polymerase Inhibitor		
Olaparib *PARP (poly (ADP-ribose) polymerase) inhibitor*	• Ovarian cancer after three or more prior lines of treatment in patients with germline mutant BRCA	• Adverse effects: nausea, vomiting, loss of appetite, muscle and joint pain, anemia; leukemia (rare), potentially fatal myelodysplastic (rare) syndrome pneumonitis • CYP3A4 substrate
BCL2 (Antiapoptotic Protein): Orally Available Inhibitor		
Venetoclax	• CLL with 17p deletion (poor prognosis)	• Neutropenia, thrombocytopenia, diarrhea, nausea • Absorption ↑ 3- to 5-fold with a meal • CYP3A substrate
Thalidomide and Lenalidomide		
Thalidomide	• Newly diagnosed multiple myeloma • Relapsed or refractory, pretreated multiple myeloma	• Most serious adverse effect: sensory neuropathy in 10%–30% of patients; may not be reversible after discontinuation of treatment; patients with preexisting neuropathy at higher risk • Teratogenic; do not use in pregnancy • Causes sedation, fatigue, constipation • Sedation enhanced by alcohol, chlorpromazine, barbiturates; counteracted by methylphenidate or methamphetamine

Thalidomide and Lenalidomide (continued)

Lenalidomide	• Multiple myeloma • Myelodysplastic syndrome (5q⁻ MDS) • Chronic lymphocytic leukemia (CLL)	• Bone marrow function suppression and leukopenia (20% of patients), rare hepatic or renal toxicity • Tumor lysis in some patients with CLL ⟹ lymph node swelling and tumor flare: start at lower dose in patients with CLL • Downregulates CD20, a target for monoclonal antibody therapy • In contrast to thalidomide: little neuropathy, sedation, or constipation; lack of teratogenicity • Dose reduction recommended in patients with reduced renal function

Proteasome Inhibitors

Bortezomib	• Multiple myeloma: initial therapy and after relapse • Mantle cell lymphoma: relapsed or refractory	• Thrombocytopenia (28%), fatigue (12%), peripheral neuropathy (12%) • Neutropenia, anemia, vomiting, diarrhea, limb pain, weakness • Rare: congestive heart failure and prolonged QT intervals • Metabolized by CYP3A4; drug exposure of patient affected by coadministration of inhibitors or inducers of CYP3A4

Antibodies Targeting Cell Surface Antigens

Rituximab (chimeric murine/human IgG1 anti-CD20)	• Non-Hodgkin lymphoma • Chronic lymphocytic leukemia • Rheumatological and other autoimmune disease, including multiple sclerosis	• Infusion-related toxicity with fever, rash, and dyspnea; B-cell depletion; late-onset neutropenia risk of hypersensitivity reaction: use slow increase in infusion rate and antihistamines • Rare: severe mucocutaneous skin reaction, including Stevens-Johnson syndrome • Risk of tumor lysis syndrome in patients with high tumor burden in the circulation: use lower dose initially • Reactivation of hepatitis B virus or JC polyoma virus
Ofatumumab (fully human IgG1 anti-CD20)	• CLL after treatment failure	• Immunosuppression and opportunistic infections, hypersensitivity reaction during infusion and myelosuppression: monitor blood counts during treatment
Obinutuzumab (humanized IgG1 anti-CD20)	• CLL in combination with chemotherapy	• Frequent adverse effects: cytopenia, fever, cough, musculoskeletal disorders
Alemtuzumab (Campath or Lemtrada; humanized IgG1 anti CD52)	• CLL (label: Campath) • Multiple sclerosis (label: Lemtrada)	• Infusion-related toxicity, T-cell depletion with increased infection; myelosuppression with pancytopenia • Antibiotic prophylaxis
Dinutuximab (chimeric mouse/human anti-GD2)	• High-risk neuroblastoma	• Infusion reaction • Nerve damage
Daratumumab (human IgG1 anti-CD38)	• Multiple myeloma in combination with lenalidomide or bortezomb	• Infusion reactions • Peripheral sensory neuropathy, upper respiratory tract infection
Elotuzumab (humanized IgG1 anti-CD319) (SLAMF7)	• Multiple myeloma after one to three prior therapies	• Infusion reaction
Blinatumomab (bispecific anti-CD19 and anti-CD3)	• Ph-negative relapsed or refractory B-cell precursor ALL	• Cytokine release syndrome, neurologic toxicity, neutropenic fever

Note: CYP3A4 substrate: For drugs that are subject to hepatic metabolism by CYP enzymes, drug exposure of a patient can be affected by coadministration of inhibitors or inducers of CYP3A4 and can then reduce efficacy or increase side effects.

Embryo-fetal toxicity: Consider that all of these drugs can cause fetal harm. Advise women of the potential risk to a fetus and to avoid pregnancy while taking the drug and for 1 month after cessation of therapy. Advise men to avoid fathering a child during the same time period. Avoid lactation during therapies.

Bibliography

Callahan MK, et al. Targeting T cell co-receptors for cancer therapy. *Immunity*, **2016**, *44*:1069–1078.

Chapman PB, et al. Improved survival with vemurafenib in melanoma with BRAF V600E mutation. *N Engl J Med*, **2011**, *364*:2507–2516.

Choueiri TK, et al. Cabozantinib versus everolimus in advanced renal cell carcinoma (METEOR): final results from a randomised, open-label, phase 3 trial. *Lancet Oncol*, **2016**, *17*:917–927.

Cristofanilli M, et al. Fulvestrant plus palbociclib versus fulvestrant plus placebo for treatment of hormone-receptor-positive, HER2-negative metastatic breast cancer that progressed on previous endocrine therapy (PALOMA-3): final analysis of the multicentre, double-blind, phase 3 randomised controlled trial. *Lancet Oncol*, **2016**, *17*:425–439.

Curran MA, et al. PD-1 and CTLA-4 combination blockade expands infiltrating T cells and reduces regulatory T and myeloid cells within B16 melanoma tumors. *Proc Natl Acad Sci U S A*, **2010**, *107*:4275–4280.

Dibble CC, Cantley LC. Regulation of mTORC1 by PI3K Signaling. *Trends Cell Biol*, **2015**, *25*:545–555.

Dyson NJ. RB1: a prototype tumor suppressor and an enigma. *Genes Dev*, **2016**, *30*:1492–1502.

Ebert PJR, et al. MAP kinase inhibition promotes T cell and anti-tumor activity in combination with PD-L1 checkpoint blockade. *Immunity*, **2016**, *44*:609–621.

Elkins JM, et al. Comprehensive characterization of the Published Kinase Inhibitor Set. *Nat Biotechnol*, **2015**, *34*:95–103.

Fink EC, Ebert BL. The novel mechanism of lenalidomide activity. *Blood*, **2015**, *126*:2366–2369.

Finn RS, et al. Palbociclib and letrozole in advanced breast cancer. *N Engl J Med*, **2016**, *375*:1925–1936.

Flaherty KT, et al. Combined BRAF and MEK inhibition in melanoma with BRAF V600 mutation. *N Engl J Med*, **2012**, *367*:1694–1703.

Folkman J. Tumor angiogenesis: therapeutic implications. *N Engl J Med*, **1971**, *285*:1182–1186.

1236 Fruman DA, Rommel C. PI3K and cancer: lessons, challenges and opportunities. *Nat Rev Drug Discov*, **2014**, *13*:140–156.

Guri Y, Hall MN. mTOR signaling confers resistance to targeted cancer drugs. *Trends n Cancer*, **2016**, *2*:688–697.

Hall MN. TOR and paradigm change: cell growth is controlled. *Mol Biol Cell*, **2016**, *27*:2804–2806.

Hamid O, et al. Safety and tumor responses with lambrolizumab (anti-PD-1) in melanoma. *N Engl J Med*, **2013**, *369*:134–144.

Hanahan D, Weinberg RA. Hallmarks of cancer: the next generation. *Cell*, **2011**, *144*:646–674.

Hansel TT, et al. The safety and side effects of monoclonal antibodies. *Nat Rev Drug Discov*, **2010**, 9:325–338.

Hodi FS, et al. Improved survival with ipilimumab in patients with metastatic melanoma. *N Engl J Med*, **2010**, *363*:711–723.

Hughes PE, et al. Targeted therapy and checkpoint immunotherapy combinations for the treatment of cancer. *Trends Immunol*, **2016**, *37*: 462–476.

Hurwitz H, et al. Bevacizumab plus irinotecan, fluorouracil, and leucovorin for metastatic colorectal cancer. *N Engl J Med*, **2004**, *350*: 2335–2342.

Jia Y, et al. Overcoming EGFR(T790M) and EGFR(C797S) resistance with mutant-selective allosteric inhibitors. *Nature*, **2016**, *534*:129–132.

Johnson DB, et al. Fulminant myocarditis with combination immune checkpoint blockade. *N Engl J Med*, **2016**, *375*:1749–1755.

Judson I, van der Graaf WT. Sarcoma: olaratumab—really a breakthrough for soft-tissue sarcomas? *Nat Rev Clin Oncol*, **2016**, *13*:534–536.

Katayama R, et al. Therapeutic targeting of anaplastic lymphoma kinase in lung cancer: a paradigm for precision cancer medicine. *Clin Cancer Res*, **2015**, *21*:2227–2235.

Kim KB, et al. Phase II study of the MEK1/MEK2 inhibitor trametinib in patients with metastatic BRAF-mutant cutaneous melanoma previously treated with or without a BRAF inhibitor. *J Clin Oncol*, **2013**, *31*:482–489.

King CR, et al. Amplification of a novel v-erbB-related gene in a human mammary carcinoma. *Science (New York, NY)*, **1985**, *229*:974–976.

Klebanoff CA, et al. Prospects for gene-engineered T cell immunotherapy for solid cancers. *Nat Med*, **2016**, *22*:26–36.

Krönke J, et al. Lenalidomide induces ubiquitination and degradation of CK1α in del(5q) MDS. *Nature*, **2015**, *523*:183–188.

Liao W, et al. Interleukin-2 at the crossroads of effector responses, tolerance, and immunotherapy. *Immunity*, **2013**, *38*:13–25.

Lu G, et al. The myeloma drug lenalidomide promotes the cereblon-dependent destruction of Ikaros proteins. *Science (New York, NY)*, **2014**, *343*:305–309.

Martelli MP, et al. EML4-ALK rearrangement in non-small cell lung cancer and non-tumor lung tissues. *Am J Pathol*, **2010**, *174*:661–670.

Mellman I, et al. Cancer immunotherapy comes of age. *Nature*, **2011**, *480*:480–489.

Mellman I, et al. De-risking immunotherapy: report of a consensus workshop of the Cancer Immunotherapy Consortium of the Cancer Research Institute. *Cancer Immunol Res*, **2016**, *4*:279–288.

Monteiro J. Timeline: checkpoint blockade. *Cell*, **2015**, *162*:1434.

Moreau P, et al. Oral ixazomib, lenalidomide, and dexamethasone for multiple myeloma. *N Engl J Med*, **2016**, *374*:1621–1634.

Nagy JA, et al. VEGF-A and the induction of pathological angiogenesis. *Ann Rev Pathol*, **2007**, *2*:251–275.

Neul C, et al. Impact of membrane drug transporters on resistance to small-molecule tyrosine kinase inhibitors. *Trends Pharmacol Sci*, **2016**, *37*:904–932.

O'Leary B, et al. Treating cancer with selective CDK4/6 inhibitors. *Nat Rev Clin Oncol*, **2016**, *13*:470–430.

Oxnard GR, et al. Association between plasma genotyping and outcomes of treatment with osimertinib (AZD9291) in advanced non-small-cell lung cancer. *J Clin Oncol*, **2016**, *34*:3375–3382.

Paik PK, et al. Response to MET inhibitors in patients with stage IV lung adenocarcinomas harboring MET mutations causing exon 14 skipping. *Cancer Discov*, **2015**, *5*:842–849.

Park JW, et al. Adaptive randomization of neratinib in early breast cancer. *N Engl J Med*, **2016**, *375*:11–22.

Restifo NP, et al. Acquired resistance to immunotherapy and future challenges. *Nat Rev Cancer*, **2016**, *16*:121–126.

Robert C, et al. Drug of the year: programmed death-1 receptor/programmed death-1 ligand-1 receptor monoclonal antibodies. *Eur J Cancer*, **2013**, *49*:2968–2971.

Robert C, et al. Anti-programmed-death-receptor-1 treatment with pembrolizumab in ipilimumab-refractory advanced melanoma: a randomised dose-comparison cohort of a phase 1 trial. *Lancet*, **2014**, *384*:1109–1117.

Robert C, et al. Improved overall survival in melanoma with combined dabrafenib and trametinib. *N Engl J Med*, **2015**, *372*:30–39.

Roskoski R Jr. Anaplastic lymphoma kinase (ALK) inhibitors in the treatment of ALK-driven lung cancers. *Pharmacol Res*, **2017**, *117*: 343–356.

Saltz L, et al. Panitumumab. *Nat Rev Drug Discov*, **2006**, *5*:987–988.

Schadendorf D, et al. Pooled analysis of long-term survival data from phase ii and phase iii trials of ipilimumab in unresectable or metastatic melanoma. *J Clin Oncol*, **2015**, *33*:1889–1894.

Schechter AL, et al. The neu gene: an erbB-homologous gene distinct from and unlinked to the gene encoding the EGF receptor. *Science (New York, NY)*, **1985**, *229*:976–978.

Slamon DJ, et al. Human breast cancer: correlation of relapse and survival with amplification of the HER-2/neu oncogene. *Science (New York, NY)*, **1987**, *235*:177–182.

Slamon DJ, et al. Use of chemotherapy plus a monoclonal antibody against HER2 for metastatic breast cancer that overexpresses HER2. *N Engl J Med*, **2001**, *344*:783–792.

Smit EF, Baas P. Lung cancer in 2015: bypassing checkpoints, overcoming resistance, and honing in on new targets. *Nat Rev Clin Oncol*, **2015**, *13*:75–76.

Swain SM, et al. Pertuzumab, trastuzumab, and docetaxel in HER2-positive metastatic breast cancer. *N Engl J Med*, **2015**, *372*:724–734.

Tallis M, et al. Poly(ADP-ribosyl)ation in regulation of chromatin structure and the DNA damage response. *Chromosoma*, **2014**, *123*: 79–90.

Tap WD, et al. Olaratumab and doxorubicin versus doxorubicin alone for treatment of soft-tissue sarcoma: an open-label phase 1b and randomised phase 2 trial. *Lancet (London, England)*, **2016**, *388*:488–497.

Thomas A, et al. Refining the treatment of NSCLC according to histological and molecular subtypes. *Nat Rev Clin Oncol*, **2015**, *12*:511–26.

Thress KS, et al. Acquired EGFR C797S mutation mediates resistance to AZD9291 in non-small cell lung cancer harboring EGFR T790M. *Nat Med*, **2015**, *21*:560–562.

Trivedi S, et al. Anti-EGFR targeted monoclonal antibody isotype influences antitumor cellular immunity in head and neck cancer patients. *Clin Cancer Res*, **2016**, *22*:5229–5237.

Van Cutsem E, et al. Cetuximab and chemotherapy as initial treatment for metastatic colorectal cancer. *N Engl J Med*, **2009**, *360*:1408–1417.

Vultur A, Herlyn M. SnapShot: melanoma. *Cancer Cell*, **2013**, *23*:706.e1.

Wei H, Yu X. Functions of PARylation in DNA damage repair pathways. *Genom Proteom Bioinform*, **2016**, *14*:131–139.

Wells JA, et al. Aflibercept, bevacizumab, or ranibizumab for diabetic macular edema. *N Engl J Med*, **2015**, *372*:1193–1203.

Wolchok JD, et al. Nivolumab plus ipilimumab in advanced melanoma. *N Engl J Med*, **2013**, *369*:122–133.

Wolff AC, et al. Recommendations for human epidermal growth factor receptor 2 testing in breast cancer: American Society of Clinical Oncology/College of American Pathologists clinical practice guideline update. *J Clin Oncol*, **2013**, *31*:3997–4013.

Chapter 68

Hormones and Related Agents in the Therapy of Cancer

Claudine Isaacs, Anton Wellstein, and Anna T. Riegel

A Note on Treatment Regimens

Cancer treatment regimens change to reflect continuous advances in basic and clinical science: new drugs, both small molecules and biologicals; improved methods of targeting and timing of drug delivery; agents with altered pharmacokinetic properties and selectivities; the use of rational multidrug combinations; and greater knowledge of the basic cell biology of tumorigenesis, metastasis, and immune function, amongst other advances. As a consequence, this chapter presents relatively few detailed treatment regimens; rather, we refer the reader to the web-based resources of the U.S. FDA and the NCCN. Table 67–1 provides the details and demonstrates the complexities of treatment of two cancers.

The growth of a number of cancers is hormone dependent or regulated by hormones. Glucocorticoids are used for their antiproliferative and lympholytic properties and to ameliorate untoward responses to other treatments. Estrogen and androgen antagonists, steroid synthesis inhibitors, and GnRH analogues and antagonists are all effective in extending survival and delaying or preventing tumor recurrence of both breast and prostate cancer. These molecules interrupt the stimulatory axis created by systemic pools of androgens and estrogens, inhibit hormone production or hormone binding to receptors, and ultimately block expression of genes that promote tumor growth and survival.

Drugs That Target the Glucocorticoid Receptor

The pharmacology, major therapeutic uses, and toxic effects of the glucocorticoids are discussed in Chapter 46. Only the applications of these drugs in the treatment of neoplastic disease are considered here.

Glucocorticoids act by binding to a specific GR that is a member of the nuclear receptor family of transcription factors. The GR translocates to the nucleus and induces complex gene expression changes (Chapter 46) that lead to antiproliferative and apoptotic responses in sensitive cells. Because of their lympholytic effects and their ability to suppress mitosis in lymphocytes, glucocorticoids are used as cytotoxic agents in the treatment of acute leukemia in children and malignant lymphoma in children and adults. In acute lymphoblastic or undifferentiated leukemia of childhood, glucocorticoids may produce prompt clinical improvement and objective hematological remissions in 30% of children. However, the duration of remission is brief. Remissions occur more rapidly with glucocorticoids than with antimetabolites, and there is no evidence of cross-resistance to unrelated agents. Thus, therapy is initiated with *prednisone* and *vincristine*, often followed by an anthracycline or *methotrexate*, and *L-asparaginase*. Glucocorticoids are a valuable component of curative regimens for other lymphoid malignancies, including Hodgkin disease, non-Hodgkin lymphoma, multiple myeloma, and CLL. Glucocorticoids are extremely helpful in controlling autoimmune hemolytic anemia and thrombocytopenia associated with CLL.

A number of glucocorticoids are available and at equivalent dosages exert similar effects (see Chapter 46). Prednisone, for example, usually is administered orally in doses up to 100 mg for the first few days and gradually reduced to the lowest possible effective dose. Side effects of these agents include glucose intolerance, immunosuppression, osteoporosis, and psychosis (see Chapter 46). Dexamethasone is one of the preferred agents for remission induction in multiple myeloma, typically in combination with bortezomib, anthracyclines, or lenalidomide. Glucocorticoids, particularly dexamethasone, are used in conjunction with radiotherapy to reduce edema related to tumors in critical areas such as the superior mediastinum, brain, and spinal cord. Frequent lower doses (4–6 mg every 6 h) can have dramatic effects in restoring neurological function in patients with cerebral metastases, but these effects are temporary. However, acute changes in dexamethasone dosage can lead to a rapid recrudescence of symptoms. Dexamethasone should not be discontinued abruptly in patients receiving radiotherapy or chemotherapy for brain metastases. Dexamethasone is also frequently used as part of an antiemetic regimen in patients receiving chemotherapy.

Estrogens and Androgens in Cancer

The pharmacology of the estrogens and androgens is described in detail in Chapters 44 and 45. These agents are of value in certain cancers, most notably those of the prostate and breast, because these organs are dependent on hormones for their growth, function, and morphological integrity.

Hormone Therapy of Breast Cancer

Historically, high doses of estrogen have been recognized as effective treatment of breast cancer. More recent studies have suggested lower doses of estrogen can be effective in the management of endocrine-resistant disease (Ellis et al., 2009). The growth inhibitory effect of estrogens may be related to their ability to induce apoptosis in endocrine-resistant breast cancer (Jordan, 2015; Song and Santen, 2003). However, interruption of estrogen-induced signaling with antiestrogens such as tamoxifen and drugs that reduce estrogen production such as AIs and GnRH analogues have been found to be more effective and better tolerated. These drugs have largely replaced estrogens or androgens for the treatment of breast cancer.

The presence of the ER and PR in breast cancer tissue identifies the subset of hormone-receptor-positive (HR+) patients with a more than 60% likelihood of responding to hormonal therapy. The response rate to antiestrogen treatment is somewhat lower in the subset of patients with tumors that are ER+ or PR+ but also positive for human epidermal growth factor receptor HER2/neu amplification. In contrast, ER-negative and

Abbreviations

ADME: absorption, distribution, metabolism, excretion
ADT: androgen deprivation therapy
AI: aromatase inhibitor
ALL: acute lymphoblastic leukemia
AR: androgen receptor
CDK: cyclin-dependent kinase
CLL: chronic lymphocytic leukemia
CRPC: castration-resistant prostate cancer
CYP: cytochrome P450
DHEA: dehydroepiandrosterone
ER: estrogen receptor
ERE: estrogen-response element
FDA: Food and Drug Administration
FSH: follicle-stimulating hormone
HL: Hodgkin lymphoma
HR: hormone receptor
GI: gastrointestinal
GnRH: gonadotropin-releasing hormone
GR: glucocorticoid receptor
HR: hormone receptor (i.e., ER^+/PR^+)
LH: luteinizing hormone
MM: multiple myeloma
mTOR: mechanistic target of rapamycin
NCCN: National Comprehensive Cancer Network
NHL: non-Hodgkin lymphoma
PR: progesterone receptor
PSA: prostate-specific antigen
SERD: selective estrogen receptor downregulator
SERM: selective estrogen receptor modulator

PR-negative carcinomas do not respond to hormonal therapy. In patients with metastatic cancer, responses to hormonal therapy may not be apparent clinically or by imaging for 8–12 weeks. The medication typically should be continued until the disease progresses or unwanted toxicities develop.

Antiestrogen approaches for the therapy of HR^+ breast cancer include the use of SERMs, SERDs, and AIs (Table 68–1).

Drugs That Target the Estrogen Receptor

Selective *Estrogen Receptor Modulators.* The SERMs bind to the ER and exert either estrogenic or antiestrogenic effects, depending on the specific organ (Chapter 44). Tamoxifen is the most widely studied antiestrogenic drug used in the treatment of breast cancer. Tamoxifen also exerts estrogenic agonist effects on nonbreast tissues, which influences the overall therapeutic index of the drug. Therefore, several novel antiestrogen compounds that offer the potential for enhanced efficacy and reduced toxicity compared with tamoxifen have been developed. These novel antiestrogens can be divided into tamoxifen analogues (e.g., toremifene, droloxifene, idoxifene); "fixed-ring" compounds (e.g., raloxifene, bazedoxifene, lasofoxifene, arzoxifene, miproxifene, levormeloxifene); and the SERDs (e.g., fulvestrant), the latter also termed "pure antiestrogens" (Howell et al., 2004; McDonnell and Wardell, 2010).

Tamoxifen. Tamoxifen was developed as an oral contraceptive but instead was found to induce ovulation and to have antiproliferative effects on estrogen-dependent breast cancer cell lines (Jordan, 2006). Tamoxifen is prescribed for the adjuvant therapy of early-stage breast cancer (Early Breast Cancer Trialists' Collaborative Group, 2011) and for the therapy of advanced breast cancer (Burstein et al., 2010). Tamoxifen and other SERMs such as raloxifene are also used for the prevention of breast cancer in high-risk patients such as those with a strong family history or prior nonmalignant breast pathology (Visvanathan et al., 2013). The uses,

pharmacology, and mechanism of action of raloxifene are discussed in Chapter 44.

- *Mechanism of Action.* Tamoxifen is a competitive inhibitor of estrogens (e.g., 17β-estradiol), binding to the ER, and antagonizes estrogen-induced proliferation of human breast cancer. There are two subtypes of ERs: ERα and ERβ, which have different tissue distributions and can either homo- or heterodimerize. Binding of estrogen and SERMs to the estrogen-binding sites of the ERs initiates a change in conformation of the ER, dissociation of the ER from heat-shock proteins, and ER dimerization. Dimerization facilitates the binding of the ER to specific DNA EREs in the vicinity of estrogen-regulated genes. Coregulator proteins interact with the liganded receptor to act as corepressors or coactivators of gene expression (Chapter 44). Elegant studies of the crystal structure of ERα bound to different ligands indicate that, when an ER agonist is bound to the ligand-binding domain of the ER, helix 12 enables recruitment of coactivators. Conversely, with an estrogen antagonist such as 4-hydroxytamoxifen bound to the ER, helix 12 is displaced, the binding of coactivators is disrupted, and subsequent estrogen-induced gene transcription is inhibited (Nettles and Greene, 2005). Differences in tissue distribution of the ER subtypes and the function and relative amounts of different transcriptional coregulator proteins likely explains the antagonist response to tamoxifen in ER^+ breast cancer and partial agonist activities in noncancerous tissues. Organs displaying agonist effects of tamoxifen include the uterine endometrium (endometrial hypertrophy, vaginal bleeding, and endometrial cancer); the coagulation system (thromboembolism); bone metabolism (increase in bone mineral density, which can slow development of osteoporosis); and liver (tamoxifen lowers total serum cholesterol, low-density lipoprotein cholesterol, and lipoproteins and raises apolipoprotein A-I levels).

- *ADME.* Tamoxifen is readily absorbed following oral administration, with peak concentrations measurable after 3–7 h and steady-state levels reached at 4–6 weeks. Metabolism of tamoxifen is complex and principally involves CYPs 3A4/5, and 2D6 in the formation of *N*-desmethyl tamoxifen and CYP2D6 to form 4-hydroxytamoxifen, a more potent metabolite (Figure 68–1). Both metabolites can be further converted to 4-hydroxy-*N*-desmethyltamoxifen (endoxifen), which retains high affinity for the ER. The parent drug has a terminal $t_{1/2}$ of 7 days. After enterohepatic circulation, glucuronides and other metabolites are excreted in the stool; excretion in the urine is minimal. Polymorphisms in CYP2D6 that reduce its activity lead to lower plasma levels of the potent metabolites 4-OH tamoxifen and endoxifen, but whether this leads to inferior efficacy of tamoxifen treatment and higher risks of disease relapse is unclear (Hertz and Rae, 2016). While drugs that inhibit CYP2D6 activity, such as antidepressants, have been postulated to minimize tamoxifen activity in breast cancer, more recent studies do not suggest a clinically significant impact (Haque et al., 2016).

- *Therapeutic Uses.* Tamoxifen is given orally once per day. Tamoxifen is used for the treatment of women with ER^+ metastatic breast cancer or following primary excision of an ER^+ tumor as an adjuvant treatment to prevent recurrence and extend overall survival. For the adjuvant treatment of premenopausal women, tamoxifen is given for at least 5 years (Table 68–1). Tamoxifen may also be used for postmenopausal women, but AIs are preferred as they are associated with further reductions in the risk of recurrence (Early Breast Cancer Trialists' Collaborative Group, 2015). Recent studies indicated that patients with breast cancer derive modest additional benefit, in terms of disease-free survival, overall survival, and decrease in contralateral breast cancer risk, if tamoxifen is taken for up to 10 years or AIs are continued for 5–10 years after completion of 5 years of tamoxifen (Davies et al., 2013; Goss et al., 2016). Of note, while taken for a finite time, Tamoxifen has been shown to have persisting long-term benefits (Ekholm et al., 2016). Tamoxifen may be taken as sole adjuvant therapy or after adjuvant chemotherapy (Table 68–1). Alternative or additional antiestrogen strategies in the adjuvant treatment of premenopausal women with ER^+ breast cancer include oophorectomy or

treatment has been shown to prolong disease-free survival (Turner et al., 2015).

Toxicity and Adverse Effects. Fulvestrant generally is well tolerated, the most common adverse effects being nausea, asthenia, pain, hot flashes, arthralgias, and headache. The risk of injection site reactions, seen in almost 10% patients, is reduced by giving the injection slowly.

Drugs That Decrease Estrogen Levels

Aromatase Inhibitors.

Aromatase converts androgens to estrogens (e.g., androstenedione to estrone). AIs (Figure 68–2) block this enzymatic activity, thereby reducing estrogen production (Figure 67–3). AIs are now considered the standard of care for adjuvant treatment of postmenopausal women with ER+ breast cancer, either as initial therapy or after tamoxifen. (Dowsett et al., 2010). AIs are also approved in the initial treatment of metastatic HR+ breast cancer, often in combination with CDK4/6 inhibitors, and for disease that has progressed following tamoxifen treatment in postmenopausal women.

Aromatase (CYP19A1) is responsible for the conversion of adrenal androgens and gonadal androstenedione and testosterone to the estrogens estrone (E1) and estradiol (E2), respectively (Figure 68–3; reactions catalyzed by aromatase are noted by a green *A* beside the reaction arrow). In postmenopausal women, this conversion occurs in nonovarian tissues (fat, liver, muscle, brain, breast, and breast tumors) and is the primary source of circulating estrogens. In premenopausal women, estrogen is primarily produced in the ovaries. AIs increase gonadotropin production in premenopausal women, which reduces their ability to inhibit ovarian estrogen production. As a result, AIs are not effective in premenopausal women without additional ovarian suppression (e.g., with GnRH analogues; see the next section and Table 68–2). In postmenopausal women, AIs suppress most peripheral aromatase activity, leading to profound estrogen deprivation. AIs are classified as first, second, or third generation. In addition, they are further classified as type 1 (steroidal) or type 2 (nonsteroidal) AI according to their structure and mechanism of action (Figure 68–2). Type 1 inhibitors are steroidal analogues of androstenedione that bind covalently and irreversibly to the same site on the

aromatase molecule. Thus, they commonly are known as aromatase inactivators. Type 2 inhibitors are nonsteroidal and bind reversibly to the heme group of the enzyme, producing reversible inhibition.

Third-Generation Aromatase Inhibitors. First- and second-generation (e.g., aminoglutethimide, formestane) AIs are no longer used for breast cancer treatment because of their side effects. Third-generation inhibitors include the type 1 steroidal agent *exemestane* and the type 2 nonsteroidal imidazoles *anastrozole* and *letrozole*; they are approved for use in postmenopausal women (Brodie and Njar, 2000). Third-generation AIs are used as part of the treatment of early-stage and advanced breast cancer in postmenopausal women and for chemoprevention (Table 68–1). The type 1 and 2 AIs have similar clinical efficacy and toxicity profiles (Goss et al., 2013), and these are summarized for AIs using anastrozole as a prototype. For letrozole and exemestane, additional drug-specific information is given.

- **Anastrozole.** Anastrozole is a potent and selective triazole AI. Anastrozole, like letrozole, binds competitively and specifically to the heme of the CYP19. Daily administration of AIs reduces total body androgen aromatization by more than 95% after 1 month of treatment. AIs also reduce aromatization within large ER+ breast tumors.

- **ADME.** Anastrozole is absorbed rapidly after oral administration. Steady state is attained after 7 days of repeated dosing. Anastrozole is metabolized by *N*-dealkylation, hydroxylation, and glucuronidation. The main metabolite of anastrozole is a triazole. Less than 10% of the drug is excreted as the unmetabolized parent compound. The principal excretory pathway is via the liver and biliary tract. The elimination $t_{1/2}$ is about 50 h. The pharmacokinetics of anastrozole, which can be affected by drug interactions via the CYP system, are not altered by coadministration of tamoxifen or cimetidine.

- ***Therapeutic Uses.*** AIs are approved for up-front adjuvant hormonal therapy for 5–10 years or following prior tamoxifen in postmenopausal women with early-stage breast cancer and as treatment of advanced and metastatic breast cancer. In early-stage breast cancer, anastrozole is significantly more effective than tamoxifen in delaying time to

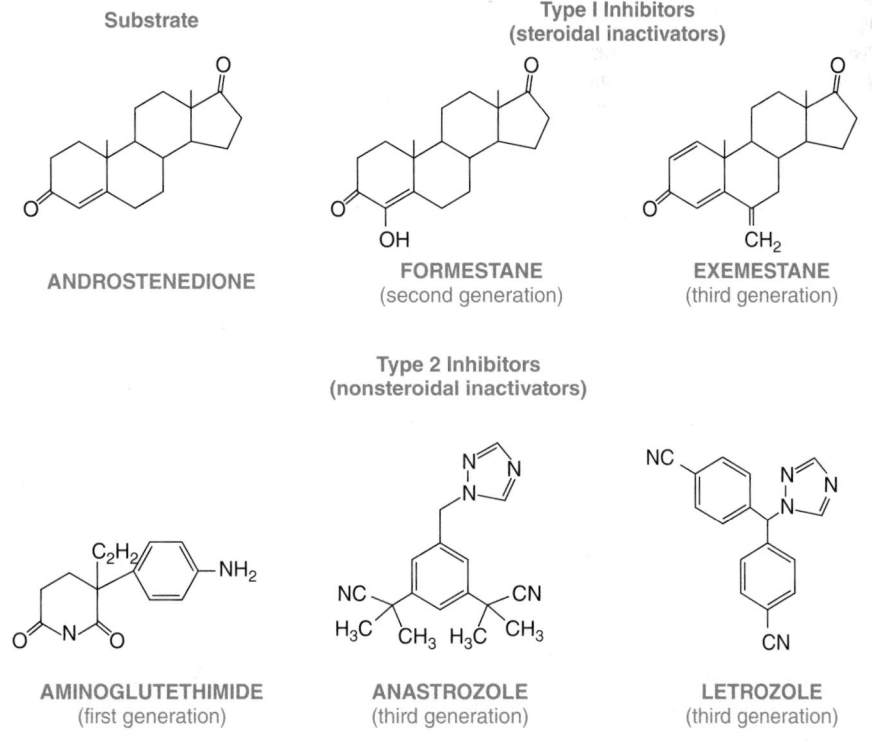

Figure 68–2 *Aromatase and its inhibitors.* Aromatase trihydroxylates the methyl group at C19, eliminating it as formate and aromatizing the A ring of the androgen substrate. Type 1 AIs are steroidal analogues of androstenedione that bind covalently and irreversibly to the steroid substrate site on the enzyme and are known as aromatase inactivators. Type 2 inhibitors are nonsteroidal, bind reversibly to the heme group of the enzyme, and produce reversible inhibition.

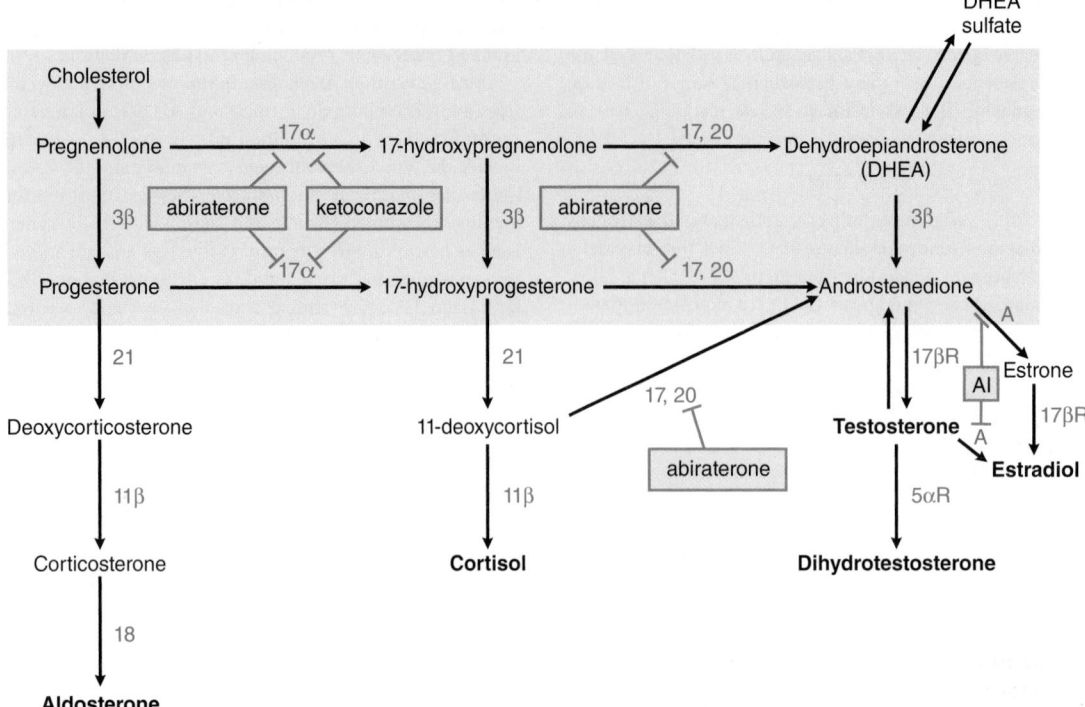

Figure 68–3 *Steroid synthesis pathways.* The shaded area contains the pathways used by the adrenal glands and gonads and clinically used agents that inhibit the pathways. Enzymes are labeled in green, inhibitors in red. Pertaining to this figure only, A, aromatase; 3β, 3β-hydroxysteroid dehydrogenase; 5αR, 5α-reductase; 11β, 11β-hydroxylase; 17, 20, C-17, 20-lyase (also CYP17); 17α, 17α-hydroxylase (CYP17); 17βR, 17β-reductase; 18, aldosterone synthase; 21, 21-hydroxylase.

tumor recurrence and decreasing the odds of a primary contralateral tumor. In advanced breast cancer, postmenopausal women with disease progression while taking tamoxifen showed a significant survival advantage with anastrozole versus megestrol acetate (see Progestins, next section). Additionally, in women with ER⁺ or PR⁺ metastatic breast cancer, anastrozole was significantly better than tamoxifen in median time to disease progression. AIs are used in premenopausal women combined with ovarian suppression, as adjuvant treatment of breast cancer in premenopausal women less than 35 years of age, and in women requiring chemotherapy, where AI use is associated with significant reduction in risk of recurrence.

- *Adverse Effects and Toxicity.* Most adverse effects are related to estrogen depletion. In postmenopausal women, compared to tamoxifen, anastrozole has been associated with a lower incidence of hot flashes, vaginal bleeding, vaginal discharge, endometrial cancer, ischemic cerebrovascular events, venous thromboembolic events, and deep venous thrombosis, including pulmonary embolism. Anastrozole is associated with a higher incidence of symptomatic arthralgias, vaginal dryness, and sexual dysfunction than tamoxifen. In addition, the estrogen depletion caused by AIs results in loss of bone mineral density. Compared with tamoxifen, treatment with anastrozole results in significantly lower bone mineral density in the lumbar spine and total hip and has been associated with increased fracture risk. Bisphosphonates (Chapter 48) prevent AI-induced loss of bone mineral density in postmenopausal women.

- **Letrozole.** The clinical uses and side-effect profile of the type 2 AI letrozole are similar to that detailed in the previous section for anastrozole (Table 68–1). Letrozole-specific information is as follows:
  - *ADME.* Letrozole is rapidly absorbed after oral administration, with a bioavailability of 99.9%. Steady-state plasma concentrations of letrozole are reached after 2–6 weeks of treatment. Following metabolism by CYP2A6 and CYP3A4, letrozole is eliminated as an inactive metabolite mainly via the kidneys and has a $t_{1/2}$ of about 41 h.
  - *Therapeutic Uses.* The clinical indications for use of letrozole in breast cancer treatment are the same as for anastrozole (Table 68–1).

In addition, improved progression-free survival is observed when HR⁺ advanced stage breast cancer is treated with letrozole in combination with a CDK4/6 inhibitor (Chapter 67) (Finn et al., 2015; Hortobagyi et al., 2016).

- **Exemestane.** Exemestane is a more potent, orally administered analogue of the natural aromatase substrate androstenedione and lowers estrogen levels more effectively than does its predecessor, formestane. Exemestane irreversibly inactivates aromatase and is a "suicide substrate" type 1 inhibitor of aromatase. The clinical uses and side-effect profile of exemestane are similar to that detailed in the section for the AI anastrozole. Exemestane-specific information is as follows:
  - *ADME.* Orally administered exemestane is rapidly absorbed from the GI tract; its absorption is increased by 40% after a high-fat meal. Exemestane has a terminal $t_{1/2}$ of about 24 h. It is extensively metabolized in the liver, ultimately to inactive metabolites. One metabolite, 17-hydroxyexemestane, has weak androgenic activity that may contribute to antitumor activity. Although active metabolites are excreted in the urine, no dosage adjustments are recommended in patients with renal dysfunction.
  - *Therapeutic Uses.* The clinical indications for use of exemestane in breast cancer treatment are the same as for anastrozole (Table 68–1). In addition, the use of the mTOR inhibitor everolimus (Chapter 67) with exemestane has been approved for treatment of advanced-stage breast cancer that has progressed on nonsteroidal type 2 AIs (Yardley et al., 2013).

GnRH Agonists. Synthetic GnRH analogues (e.g., triptorelin, goserelin, leuprolide; Table 68–2) have greater receptor affinity and reduced susceptibility to enzymatic degradation than the naturally occurring decapeptide GnRH molecule and are 100-fold more potent GnRH agonists than the native decapeptide. They are used in the adjuvant treatment of breast cancer or metastatic disease for women who have functioning ovaries; typically, they are used in combination with either tamoxifen or AIs. Continuous administration of GnRH agonists downregulates GnRH receptors in the pituitary gland. This suppresses the release of the gonadotropins FSH and LH from the pituitary and prevents follicular maturation in the ovary. Serum estrogen levels are reduced to those seen in postmeno-pausal women or in women after oophorectomy.

ADME. GnRH agonists are administered as an injection once a month or every 3 or 6 months. There is in an initial rise in LH and FSH levels, but after 14–21 days of therapy, a sustained decrease in serum LH and estrogen is observed.

Therapeutic Uses. In the adjuvant setting, recent studies have demonstrated a benefit for GnRH agonists when given in conjunction with either AIs or tamoxifen in very young or higher-risk premenopausal women (Regan et al., 2016). In addition, these drugs can be given with tamoxifen, AIs, or fulvestrant in premenopausal women with metastatic breast cancer.

Toxicity. Side effects are generally related to hypoestrogenism (i.e., hot flashes, vaginal dryness, decreased libido, osteoporosis, amenorrhea, and dyspareunia). The side effects of GnRH agonists are potentially reversible on cessation of therapy. AI use in premenopausal women combined with ovarian suppression with GnRH analogues increases menopausal symptoms and sexual dysfunction and thus benefits and risks must be carefully considered (Burstein et al., 2016).

Drugs That Target the Progesterone Receptor

Progestational agents (see Chapter 44 for details) are mainly used as secondary agents in hormonal therapy for metastatic hormone-dependent breast cancer and are also used in the management of endometrial carcinoma previously treated by surgery and radiotherapy. Progesterone binds to the PR present in target issues, such as breast and the endometrium (Chapter 44). Activation of the PR by progestins in the endometrium is antiproliferative.

Medroxyprogesterone acetate is available for oral administration; an alternative oral progestational agent is *megestrol acetate*. Beneficial effects have been observed in one-third of patients with endometrial cancer. The response of breast cancer to megestrol is predicted by both the presence of HRs (ER and PR) and the evidence of response to a prior hormonal treatment. The effect of progestin therapy in breast cancer appears to be dose dependent, with some patients demonstrating second responses following dose escalation of megestrol. Clinical use of progestins in breast cancer has been largely superseded by the advent of tamoxifen and AIs. An additional use of progestins is to stimulate appetite and restore a sense of well-being in cachectic patients with advanced stages of cancer and AIDS.

Hormone Therapy of Prostate Cancer

Androgens stimulate the growth of normal and cancerous prostate cells. The critical role of androgens for prostate cancer growth was established in 1941 and led to the awarding of a Nobel Prize in 1966 to Dr. Charles Huggins. These findings established androgen deprivation therapy (ADT) as the mainstay of treatment for patients with advanced prostate cancer. ADT is also given in conjunction with radiation therapy or following surgery for some men with regionally localized intermediate- to high-risk disease. In patients with metastasis, ADT is typically the standard first-line treatment. ADT is accomplished via surgical castration (bilateral orchiectomy) or medical castration (using GnRH agonists or antagonists). Other hormone therapy approaches that are used as second-line treatment include antiandrogens, estrogens, and inhibitors of steroidogenesis. In the advanced setting, ADT is not a curative treatment but does prolong survival. ADT alleviates cancer-related symptoms and provides important quality-of-life benefits, including reduction of bone pain and reduction of rates of pathological fracture, spinal cord compression, and ureteral obstruction.

Disease progression despite ADT signifies the development of castration-resistant prostate cancer (CRPC). In CRPC, the AR can be overexpressed or mutated and can be activated by weak adrenal androgens or from androgens produced locally in tumors. Therefore, antiandrogens (competitive antagonists of androgens at the AR), inhibitors of steroidogenesis, or estrogens are frequently employed as second-line hormone therapies and are associated with improvements in symptoms and quality of life and with prolongation in survival (Ritch and Cookson, 2016). Antiandrogens are typically administered concurrently with GnRH analogues or in men who have undergone orchiectomy. When patients become refractory to further hormonal therapies, their disease is considered androgen independent.

Common side effects of androgen deprivation include vasomotor instability, loss of libido, impotence, gynecomastia, fatigue, anemia, weight gain, decreased insulin sensitivity, altered lipid profiles, osteoporosis and fractures, and loss of muscle mass. ADT is associated with a slight but significant increased risk of diabetes and coronary heart disease. Skeletal-related events due to ADT may be mitigated by bisphosphonate therapy (see Chapter 48). Antiandrogens, when compared with GnRH agonists, cause more gynecomastia, mastodynia, and hepatotoxicity but less vasomotor flashing and loss of bone mineral density. Estrogens cause a hypercoagulable state and increase cardiovascular mortality in patients with prostate cancer and are no longer standard treatment options.

Androgen Deprivation Therapy

GnRH Agonists and Antagonists. The most common form of ADT involves chemical suppression of the pituitary gland with GnRH agonists (see previous section). GnRH agonists in common use for prostate cancer include *leuprolide, goserelin, triptorelin, histrelin,* and *nafarelin* (Table 68–2). Long-acting preparations are available in doses that are approved for 3-, 4-, and 6-month administrations.

The GnRH agonists bind to GnRH receptors on pituitary gonadotropin-producing cells, causing an initial release of both LH and FSH and a subsequent increase in testosterone production from testicular Leydig cells. After 1 week of therapy, GnRH receptors are downregulated on the gonadotropin-producing cells, causing a decline in the pituitary response. The fall in serum LH leads to a decrease in testosterone production to castrate levels within 3–4 weeks of the first treatment. Subsequent treatments maintain testosterone at castrate levels.

ADT is given in patients with localized intermediate- to high-risk prostate cancer in conjunction with radiation therapy or in some cases following surgery. In patients with metastasis, ADT is typically the standard first-line treatment either alone or in combination with chemotherapy. In patients with CRPC, ADT is used in conjunction with antiandrogens. This combination therapy is referred to as *combined androgen blockade*. The theoretical advantage is that the GnRH agonist will deplete testicular androgens, while the antiandrogen component competes at the receptor with residual androgens made by the adrenal glands. Combined androgen blockade provides maximal relief of androgen stimulation. Several trials suggested a benefit in 5-year survival, but toxicity and costs associated are higher than with ADT alone.

Toxicity. During the transient rise in LH, the resultant testosterone surge may induce acute stimulation of prostate cancer growth and a "flare" of symptoms from metastatic deposits. Patients may experience an increase in bone pain, spinal cord compression, or obstructive bladder symptoms lasting for 2–3 weeks. The flare phenomenon can be effectively counteracted with concurrent administration of 2–4 weeks of oral antiandrogen therapy, which may inhibit the action of the increased serum testosterone levels. Besides avoidance of the initial flare, GnRH antagonist therapy offers no apparent advantage compared with GnRH agonists. The early GnRH antagonists *cetrorelix* and *abarelix* (no longer marketed), although effective, are now rarely used for prostate cancer because of the risk for severe systemic allergic reactions. A newer GnRH antagonist, degarelix, is not associated with systemic allergic reactions and is approved for prostate cancer in the U.S.

Drugs That Target the Androgen Receptor. Antiandrogens bind to ARs and competitively inhibit the binding of testosterone and dihydrotestosterone, thereby preventing AR nuclear translocation and inhibiting transcription of downstream androgen-responsive genes. Unlike castration, antiandrogen therapy by itself does not decrease LH production; therefore, testosterone levels are normal or increased. Men treated with antiandrogen maintain some degree of potency and libido and do not have the same spectrum of side effects seen with castration. However, antiandrogen therapy is typically given in combination with ADT. Antiandrogens are classified as steroidal, including *cyproterone* or nonsteroidal, including *enzalutamide, flutamide, bicalutamide,* and *nilutamide.*

Enzalutamide. Enzalutamide is the most recently FDA-approved second-generation antiandrogen. It prolongs survival in patients with metastatic CRPC when given to chemotherapy naïve patients or after docetaxel therapy (Beer et al., 2014; Scher et al., 2012). Enzalutamide is a synthetic nonsteroidal antiandrogen that has 5- to 8-fold higher binding affinity for the AR compared to bicalutamide (Tran et al., 2009). Similar to other antiandrogens, enzalumatide prevents binding of androgens to the AR and reduces binding of AR to DNA and to AR coactivator proteins (see Chapter 45). Enzalutamide can also prevent translocation of AR into the cell nucleus and induces cell apoptosis.

- ***ADME.*** Enzalutamide has improved efficacy and potency compared to older antiandrogens. Enzalutamide is given orally once daily with a $t_{1/2}$ of approximately 6 days. Steady-state levels are achieved in 28 days. CYP2C8 is primarily responsible for the formation of the active metabolite *N*-desmethyl enzalutamide.
- ***Toxicity.*** Similar to other antiandrogens, enzalutamide has negative effects on sexual function. Other notable side effects include gynecomastia, breast pain, fatigue, diarrhea, headache, and hot flashes. Enzalutamide crosses the blood-brain barrier, and seizures occur infrequently in approximately 1% of patients. Resistance to AR inhibitors develops frequently through mechanisms such as gene rearrangement, mutation, and acquired AR splice variants (Li et al., 2013). Studies are ongoing with newer AR-blocking agents that may overcome resistance to current antiandrogen therapies (Moilanen et al., 2015; Smith et al., 2016).

Bicalutamide. The agent bicalutamide is given once daily in conjunction with a GnRH agonist. Bicalutamide has a $t_{1/2}$ of 5–6 days. Bicalutamide undergoes glucuronidation to inactive metabolites, and the parent compound and metabolites are eliminated in bile and urine. The $t_{1/2}$ of bicalutamide is increased in severe hepatic insufficiency and is unchanged in renal insufficiency. Bicalutamide is well tolerated at higher doses and has reduced toxicity and improved tolerability and pharmacokinetic profiles relative to flutamide and nilutamide. Daily bicalutamide is significantly inferior compared with surgical or medical castration and should not be used as monotherapy of prostate cancer.

Nilutamide. Nilutamide is given orally once daily. It has an elimination $t_{1/2}$ of 45 h and is metabolized to five products that are all excreted in the urine. Common side effects include mild nausea, alcohol intolerance (5%–20%), and diminished ocular adaptation to darkness (25%–40%); rarely, interstitial pneumonitis occurs.

Flutamide. Flutamide is given orally three times per day. It has a $t_{1/2}$ of 5 h; its major metabolite, hydroxyflutamide, is biologically active. Common side effects include diarrhea, breast tenderness, and nipple tenderness. Less commonly, nausea, vomiting, and hepatotoxicity occur. Rare reports of fatal hepatotoxicity have been observed. It is used infrequently as it has the least-favorable toxicity profile of the antiandrogens.

Drugs That Inhibit Androgen Synthesis. In the castrate state, AR signaling, despite low steroid levels, supports continued prostate cancer growth. AR signaling may occur due to androgens produced from nongonadal sources, AR gene mutations, or AR gene amplification. Nongonadal sources of androgens include the adrenal glands and the prostate cancer cells themselves (see Figure 68–3). Androstenedione, produced by the adrenal glands, is converted to testosterone in peripheral tissues

and tumors. Intratumoral de novo androgen synthesis also may provide sufficient androgen for AR-driven cell proliferation. Thus, inhibitors of androgen synthesis may be useful as secondary therapy in reducing AR signaling.

Ketoconazole. Ketoconazole is an antifungal agent that also inhibits both testicular and adrenal steroidogenesis by blocking CYP 11A and primarily CYP17 (17α-hydroxylase). Ketoconazole is administered off label as secondary hormone therapy to reduce adrenal androgen synthesis in CRPC. Diarrhea and hepatic enzyme elevations limit its use as initial hormone therapy; consequent poor patient compliance reduces its efficacy. Oral ketoconazole is coadministered with hydrocortisone to compensate for inhibition of adrenal steroidogenesis. Ketoconazole has limited use in practice due to its toxicity.

Abiraterone. Abiraterone is used with prednisone for the treatment of CRPC in patients who are chemotherapy naïve or in those who have received previous docetaxel. In both settings, it prolongs survival (de Bono et al., 2011; Ryan et al., 2015).

- ***Mechanism of Action.*** Abiraterone is an irreversible inhibitor of 17α-hydroxylase and C-17,20-lyase (CYP17A1) activity in testicular, adrenal and prostatic cancer tissue (Figure 68–3). Abiraterone inhibition of CYP17A1 reduces the conversion of pregnenolone and progesterone to their 17α-hydroxy derivatives and reduces the synthesis of DHEA and androstenedione. Thus, circulating levels of testosterone drop to almost-undetectable levels after abiraterone administration. Abiraterone also has some activity as an AR antagonist and inhibitor of other steroid synthetic enzymes and CYP450s. Overall, abiraterone has greater potency and selectivity than ketoconazole.
- ***ADME.*** Abiraterone is the active metabolite of abiraterone acetate. With continuous administration, abiraterone increases ACTH levels, resulting in mineralocorticoid excess. Oral abiraterone acetate is administered with prednisone to counteract adrenal suppression. Abiraterone should be taken on an empty stomach. Abiraterone C_{max} and AUC are both increased more than 10-fold when a single dose of abiraterone acetate is administered after food compared to a fasted state.
- ***Toxicity.*** Side effects include hepatotoxicity, joint swelling, hypokalemia, vasomotor symptoms, diarrhea, cough, hypertension, arrhythmia, urinary frequency, dyspepsia, and upper respiratory tract infection. Resistance to abiraterone, similar to enzalutamide, can occur through selection of tumor cells expressing constitutively active AR splice variants (Antonarakis et al., 2014).

Estrogens

High estrogen levels can reduce testosterone to castrate levels in 1–2 weeks via negative feedback on the hypothalamic-pituitary axis. Estrogen also may compete with androgens for steroid HRs and may thereby exert a cytotoxic effect on prostate cancer cells. Although estrogens reduce bone loss and are as effective as orchiectomy for metastatic prostate cancer, they are no longer used clinically because of their risk for serious and potentially fatal side effects (e.g., myocardial infarctions, strokes, pulmonary emboli) as well as impotence and lethargy.

Acknowledgment: *Paul Calabresi, Bruce Chabner, Beverly Moy, Richard J. Lee, and Matthew Smith contributed to this chapter in recent editions of this book. We have retained some of their text in the current edition.*

Drug Facts for Your Personal Formulary: *Hormones and Related Agents in Cancer Therapy*

Drug	Therapeutic Use	Clinical Pharmacology and Tips
Glucocorticoid Receptor Agonists		
Dexamethasone Prednisone Others	• Treatment of malignant hematologic disorders (e.g., ALL, CLL, MM, HL, NHL) • Symptom palliation in various cancer types (e.g., antiemetic; reduce edema due to spinal cord compression, brain metastases)	• Major toxicities: Cushing syndrome, glucose intolerance, immunosuppression, osteoporosis, psychosis, insomnia • Acute reduction in dosing can lead to recurrence of symptoms
Selective Estrogen Receptor Modulators: Antiestrogens in breast cancer therapy		
Tamoxifen	• Adjuvant therapy for pre- and postmenopausal women with HR(+) breast cancer • Treatment of advanced or metastatic HR(+) breast cancer in pre- and postmenopausal women • Breast cancer prevention in pre- and postmenopausal women	• SERM with partial agonist and antagonist action. Antagonist of ER in breast. Long $t_{1/2}$. Steady-state levels reached 3–4 weeks. • Some major toxicities due to ER agonist activity (e.g., endometrial carcinoma, thromboembolic events) or ER antagonist effects (e.g., vasomotor symptoms, menstrual irregularities). • Other adverse effects: cataracts
Toremifene	• Metastatic HR(+) breast cancer	• Pharmacology, clinical efficacy, and adverse effects similar to those of tamoxifen • Rare: Prolongs QT interval, increased risk of torsades de pointes
Selective Estrogen Receptor Downregulators: Antiestrogens in breast cancer therapy		
Fulvestrant	• Advanced or metastatic HR(+) breast cancer (+/- CDK4/6 inhibitors) in postmenopausal women who have progressed after antiestrogen therapy	• Binds to ER, blocks estrogen action and causes degradation of the ER • No estrogen agonist effects • IM loading then monthly dosing; steady state achieved in first month • Side effects: injection site reaction, nausea, weakness, bone and back pain, fatigue, vasomotor symptoms, headache
Aromatase Inhibitors: Antiestrogen in breast cancer therapy		
Anastrozole, Letrozole (Nonsteroidal, competitive inhibitors) Exemestane (steroidal, irreversible inhibitor)	• Adjuvant treatment of postmenopausal women with HR(+) breast cancer • Treatment of postmenopausal women with HR(+) advanced and metastatic breast cancer (+/- CDK4/6 inhibitors) • Breast cancer prevention in postmenopausal women	• AIs significantly lower serum estrogens • Contraindicated in premenopausal women with ovarian function • Major side effects: vasomotor symptoms, arthralgia, loss of bone mineral density, osteoporosis, fractures, vaginal dryness, dyspareunia
Progesterone Receptor Agonists		
Megestrol acetate	• Treatment of endometrial cancer and rarely of breast and prostate cancer • Appetite stimulant in patients with AIDS or cancer-associated cachexia	• Adverse effects: weight gain, nausea, vomiting, edema, breakthrough bleeding, shortness of breath, thrombophlebitis, pulmonary embolism
Medroxyprogesterone acetate	• Management of advanced stage endometrial carcinoma • Therapy of metastatic hormone-dependent breast cancer	• Adverse effects: hot flashes, weight gain, depression, amenorrhea • With long-term use, bone loss is possible
Gonadotropin-Releasing Hormone Analogues: Chemical castration in cancer therapy		
Prostate Cancer *GnRH agonists:* Leuprolide Goserelin Histrelin Triptolerin Nafarelin	• Androgen deprivation therapy: ↓ Pituitary release of LH and FSH, ↓ testicular testosterone production • Treatment of advanced prostate cancer • In combination with radiation therapy or surgery for management of moderate-/high-risk locally confined prostate cancer	• Can cause initial testosterone surge and tumor flare. Administered with antiandrogens to reduce initial side effects from testosterone surge. • Side effects related to low testosterone: vasomotor symptoms, loss of libido, osteoporosis, fatigue, impotence, gynecomastia, loss of muscle mass • Small increase in risk of diabetes or development of cardiovascular disease
GnRH antagonists: Degarelix (Cetrorelix)	• Treatment of advanced prostate cancer • Cetrorelix rarely used due to risk of anaphylaxis	• No initial testosterone surge; rapid suppression of serum testosterone and PSA levels • Side-effect profile in men similar to GnRH agonists above

Drug Facts for Your Personal Formulary: *Hormones and Related Agents in Cancer Therapy (continued)*

Drug	Therapeutic Use	Clinical Pharmacology and Tips
Breast Cancer *GnRH agonist:* Goserelin Leuprolide	• Suppression of ovarian estrogen and progesterone production in pre- and perimenopausal women • With antiestrogens as adjuvant therapy and for metastatic disease	• Adverse effects due to hypoestrogenism: vasomotor symptoms, ↓ libido, osteoporosis, tumor flare, fatigue, vaginal dryness, dyspareunia
Nonsteroidal Androgen Receptor Antagonists: Antiandrogens in prostate cancer therapy		
Enzalutamide	• Treatment of metastatic, CRPC in conjunction with ADT following docetaxel therapy	• Adverse effects related to AR antagonism: sexual dysfunction, gynecomastia, breast pain, fatigue, diarrhea, headache, musculoskeletal pain, vasomotor symptoms, hot flashes • Rare: seizures (likely due to central "off-target" effects)
Bicalutamide	• Used with GnRH analogues to treat metastatic CRPC	• Adverse effects similar to enzalutamide • Favorable toxicity and pharmacokinetic profile relative to flutamide or nilutamide
Flutamide	• Used with GnRH analogues to treat metastatic CRPC	• Active metabolite: hydroxyflutamide • Significant hepatotoxicity possible
Nilutamide	• Used with GnRH analogues to treat CRPC after progression on other antiandrogens	• Rare adverse effect: interstitial pneumonitis
Inhibitors of Steroidogenesis: Antiandrogens in prostate cancer therapy		
Abiraterone	• Treatment of advanced metastatic CRPC • Used in combination with prednisone (to compensate for adrenal insufficiency induced by abiraterone)	• Irreversibly inhibits CYP17A1, ↓ testosterone & other androgens • Fluid retention, hypertension, hypokalemia, hepatotoxicity, fatigue, joint swelling, vasomotor symptoms, diarrhea, arrhythmia • Take on empty stomach; food ↑ uptake >10-fold

Bibliography

Antonarakis ES, et al. AR-V7 and resistance to enzalutamide and abiraterone in prostate cancer. *N Engl J Med*, **2014**, 371:1028–1038.

Beer TM, et al. Enzalutamide in metastatic prostate cancer before chemotherapy. *N Engl J Med*, **2014**, 371:424–433.

Brodie AM, Njar VC. Aromatase inhibitors and their application in breast cancer treatment. *Steroids*, **2000**, 65:171–179.

Burstein HJ, et al. American Society of Clinical Oncology clinical practice guideline: update on adjuvant endocrine therapy for women with hormone receptor-positive breast cancer. *J Clin Oncol*, **2010**, 28:3784–3796.

Burstein HJ, et al. Adjuvant endocrine therapy for women with hormone receptor-positive breast cancer: American Society of Clinical Oncology clinical practice guideline update on ovarian suppression. *J Clin Oncol*, **2016**, 34:1689–1701.

Clarke R, et al. Endocrine resistance in breast cancer—an overview and update. *Mol Cell Endocrinol*, **2015**, 418(pt 3):220–234.

Davies C, et al. Long-term effects of continuing adjuvant tamoxifen to 10 years versus stopping at 5 years after diagnosis of oestrogen receptor-positive breast cancer: ATLAS, a randomised trial. *Lancet*, **2013**, 381:805–816.

de Bono JS, et al. Abiraterone and increased survival in metastatic prostate cancer. *N Engl J Med*, **2011**, 364:1995–2005.

Dowsett M, et al. Meta-analysis of breast cancer outcomes in adjuvant trials of aromatase inhibitors versus tamoxifen. *J Clin Oncol*, **2010**, 28:509–518.

Early Breast Cancer Trialists' Collaborative Group. Relevance of breast cancer hormone receptors and other factors to the efficacy of adjuvant tamoxifen: patient-level meta-analysis of randomised trials. *Lancet*, **2011**, 378:771–784.

Early Breast Cancer Trialists' Collaborative Group. Aromatase inhibitors versus tamoxifen in early breast cancer: patient-level meta-analysis of the randomised trials. *Lancet*, **2015**, 386:1341–1352.

Ekholm M, et al. Two years of adjuvant tamoxifen provides a survival benefit compared with no systemic treatment in premenopausal patients with primary breast cancer: long-term follow-up (>25 years) of the phase III SBII:2pre Trial. *J Clin Oncol*, **2016**, 34:2232–2238.

Ellis MJ, et al. Lower-dose vs. high-dose oral estradiol therapy of hormone receptor-positive, aromatase inhibitor-resistant advanced breast cancer: a phase 2 randomized study. *JAMA*, **2009**, 302:774–780.

Finn RS, et al. The cyclin-dependent kinase 4/6 inhibitor palbociclib in combination with letrozole versus letrozole alone as first-line treatment of oestrogen receptor-positive, HER2-negative, advanced breast cancer (PALOMA-1/TRIO-18): a randomised phase 2 study. *Lancet Oncol*, **2015**, 16:25–35.

Fisher B, et al. Tamoxifen for prevention of breast cancer: report of the National Surgical Adjuvant Breast and Bowel Project P-1 Study. *J Natl Cancer Inst*, **1998**, 90:1371–1388.

Francis PA, et al. Adjuvant ovarian suppression in premenopausal breast cancer. *N Engl J Med*, **2015**, 372:436–446.

Goss PE, et al. Exemestane versus anastrozole in postmenopausal women with early breast cancer: NCIC CTG MA.27—a randomized controlled phase III trial. *J Clin Oncol*, **2013**, 31:1398–1404.

Goss PE, et al. Extending aromatase-inhibitor adjuvant therapy to 10 years. *N Engl J Med*, **2016**, 375:209–219.

Haque R, et al. Tamoxifen and antidepressant drug interaction in a cohort of 16,887 breast cancer survivors. *J Natl Cancer Inst*, **2016**, 108:djv337.

Hertz DL, Rae JM. One step at a time: CYP2D6 guided tamoxifen treatment awaits convincing evidence of clinical validity. *Pharmacogenomics*, **2016**, 17:823–826.

Hortobagyi GN, et al. Ribociclib as first-line therapy for HR-positive, advanced breast cancer. *N Engl J Med*, **2016**, 375:1738–1748.

Howell S, et al. The use of selective estrogen receptor modulators and selective estrogen receptor down-regulators in breast cancer. *Best Pract Res Clin Endocrinol Metab*, **2004**, 18:47–66.

Jeselsohn R, et al. ESR1 mutations—a mechanism for acquired endocrine resistance in breast cancer. *Nat Rev Clin Oncol*, **2015**, 12:573–583.

Jordan VC. Tamoxifen (ICI46,474) as a targeted therapy to treat and prevent breast cancer. *Br J Pharmacol*, **2006**, *147*(suppl 1): S269–S276.

Jordan VC. The new biology of estrogen-induced apoptosis applied to treat and prevent breast cancer. *Endocr Relat Cancer*, **2015**, *22*: R1–R31.

Li Y, et al. Androgen receptor splice variants mediate enzalutamide resistance in castration-resistant prostate cancer cell lines. *Cancer Res*, **2013**, *73*:483–489.

McDonnell DP, Wardell SE. The molecular mechanisms underlying the pharmacological actions of ER modulators: implications for new drug discovery in breast cancer. *Curr Opin Pharmacol*, **2010**, *10*: 620–628.

Moilanen A-M, et al. Discovery of ODM-201, a new-generation androgen receptor inhibitor targeting resistance mechanisms to androgen signaling-directed prostate cancer therapies. *Sci Rep*, **2015**, *5*:12007.

Moy B, Goss PE. Estrogen receptor pathway: resistance to endocrine therapy and new therapeutic approaches. *Clin Cancer Res*, **2006**, *12*: 4790–4793.

Nettles KW, Greene GL. Ligand control of coregulator recruitment to nuclear receptors. *Annu Rev Physiol*, **2005**, *67*:309–333.

Regan MM, et al. Absolute benefit of adjuvant endocrine therapies for premenopausal women with hormone receptor positive, human epidermal growth factor receptor2-negative early breast cancer: TEXT and SOFT trials. *J Clin Oncol*, **2016**, *34*:2221–2231.

Ritch CR, Cookson MS. Advances in the management of castration resistant prostate cancer. *BMJ*, **2016**, *355*:i4405.

Robertson JFR, et al. A good drug made better: the fulvestrant dose-response story. *Clin Breast Cancer*, **2014**, *14*:381–389.

Ryan CJ, et al. Abiraterone acetate plus prednisone versus placebo plus prednisone in chemotherapy-naive men with metastatic castration-resistant prostate cancer (COU-AA-302): final overall survival analysis of a randomised, double-blind, placebo-controlled phase 3 study. *Lancet Oncol*, **2015**, *16*:152–160.

Scher HI, et al. Increased survival with enzalutamide in prostate cancer after chemotherapy. *N Engl J Med*, **2012**, *367*:1187–1197.

Smith MR, et al. Phase 2 study of the safety and antitumor activity of apalutamide (ARN-509), a potent androgen receptor antagonist, in the high-risk nonmetastatic castration-resistant prostate cancer cohort. *Eur Urol*, **2016**, *16*:30133–301336.

Song RX-D, Santen RJ. Apoptotic action of estrogen. *Apoptosis*, **2003**, *8*:55–60.

Tran C, et al. Development of a second-generation antiandrogen for treatment of advanced prostate cancer. *Science*, **2009**, *324*:787–790.

Turner NC, et al. Palbociclib in hormone-receptor-positive advanced breast cancer. *N Engl J Med*, **2015**, *373*:209–219.

Visvanathan K, et al. Use of pharmacologic interventions for breast cancer risk reduction. *J Clin Oncol*, **2013**, *31*:2942–2962.

Yardley DA, et al. Everolimus plus exemestane in postmenopausal patients with HR(+) breast cancer: BOLERO-2 final progression-free survival analysis. *Adv Ther*, **2013**, *30*:870–884.

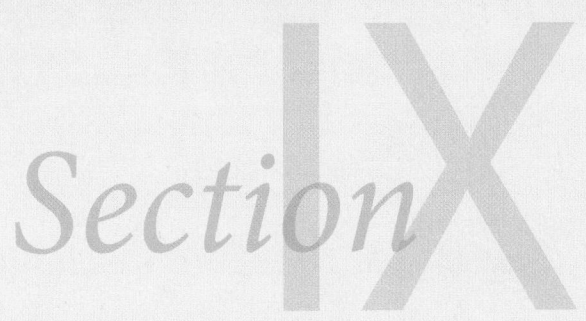

Special Systems Pharmacology

Ocular Pharmacology

Jeffrey D. Henderer and Christopher J. Rapuano

The eye is a specialized sensory organ that is relatively secluded from systemic access by the blood-retinal, blood-aqueous, and blood-vitreous barriers. As a consequence, the eye exhibits some unusual pharmacodynamic and pharmacokinetic properties.

Extraocular Structures

The eye is protected by the eyelids and by the orbit, a bony cavity of the skull that has multiple fissures and foramina that conduct nerves, muscles, and vessels (Figure 69–1). In the orbit, connective (i.e., *Tenon's capsule*) and adipose tissues and six extraocular muscles support and align the eyes for vision. The retrobulbar region lies immediately behind the eye (or *globe*). Understanding ocular and orbital anatomy is important for safe periocular drug delivery, including subconjunctival, sub-Tenon, and retrobulbar injections.

The external surface of the eyelids is covered by a thin layer of skin; the internal surface is lined with the palpebral portion of the conjunctiva, which is a vascularized mucous membrane continuous with the bulbar conjunctiva. At the reflection of the palpebral and bulbar conjunctivae is a space called the *fornix*, located superiorly and inferiorly behind the upper and lower eyelids, respectively. Topical medications usually are placed in the inferior fornix, also known as the *inferior cul-de-sac*.

The lacrimal system consists of secretory glandular and excretory ductal elements (Figure 69–2). The secretory system is composed of the main *lacrimal gland*, which is located in the temporal outer portion of the orbit, and accessory glands located in the conjunctiva. The lacrimal gland is innervated by the autonomic nervous system (Table 69–1 and Chapter 8). The parasympathetic innervation is clinically relevant because a patient may complain of dry eye symptoms while taking medications with anticholinergic side effects, such as tricyclic antidepressants (see Chapter 15), antihistamines (see Chapter 39), and drugs used in the management of Parkinson disease (see Chapter 18). Muscarinic cholinergic and α adrenergic receptors that mediate responses of several pupillary muscles from autonomic nerves also provide means of dilating the pupil for examination of posterior structures.

Tears constitute a functionally trilaminar lubrication barrier covering the conjunctiva and cornea. The anterior tear layer is composed primarily of lipids; the middle aqueous layer, produced by the main lacrimal gland and accessory lacrimal glands, constitutes about 98% of the tear film. Adherent to the corneal epithelium, the posterior layer is a mixture of mucins produced by goblet cells in the conjunctiva. Tears also contain nutrients, enzymes, and immunoglobulins to support and protect the cornea. The tear drainage system starts through small puncta located on the medial aspects of both the upper and lower eyelids (see Figure 69–2). With blinking, tears enter the puncta and continue to drain through the canaliculi, lacrimal sac, nasolacrimal duct, and then into the nose. The nose is lined by a highly vascular mucosal epithelium; consequently, topically applied medications that pass through this nasolacrimal system have direct access to the systemic circulation.

Ocular Structures

The eye is divided into anterior and posterior segments (Figure 69–3A). Anterior segment structures include the cornea, limbus, anterior and posterior chambers, trabecular meshwork, canal of Schlemm (Schlemm's canal), iris, lens, ciliary zonule, and ciliary body. The posterior segment includes the vitreous, retina, choroid, sclera, and optic nerve.

Anterior Segment

Cornea and Drug Access

The cornea is a transparent and avascular tissue organized into five (or six) layers (Figure 69–3B). Representing an important barrier to foreign matter, including drugs, the hydrophobic epithelial layer comprises five or six cell layers. The basal epithelial cells lie on a basement membrane that is adjacent to Bowman's layer, a distinct sheet of collagen fibers. Constituting about 90% of the corneal thickness, the stroma, a hydrophilic layer, is organized with collagen lamellae synthesized by keratocytes. Beneath the stroma lies Descemet's membrane, the basement membrane of the corneal endothelium. A new corneal layer, Dua's layer, has been proposed—a

Abbreviations

ACh: acetylcholine
ADME: absorption, distribution, metabolism, excretion
ARMD: age-related macular degeneration
CA: carbonic anhydrase
CAI: carbonic anhydrase inhibitor
CMV: cytomegalovirus
CNS: central nervous system
COMT: catechol-*O*-methyltransferase
DME: diabetic macular edema
FDA: Food and Drug Administration
5FU: 5-fluorouracil
GSH: reduced glutathione
HIV: human immunodeficiency virus
IOP: intraocular pressure
IP_3: inositol triphosphate
MAO: monoamine oxidase
NMDA: *N*-methyl-D-aspartate
PDE: phosphodiesterase
PG: prostaglandin
PK: phosphokinase
PLC: phospholipase C
RAR: retinoic acid receptor
RXR: retinoid X receptor
tPA: tissue plasminogen activator
VEGF: vascular endothelial growth factor

distinct thin, but strong, collagen layer between the stroma and Descemet's membrane (Dua et al., 2013). Lying most posteriorly, the endothelium is a monolayer of cells adhering to each other by tight junctions. These cells maintain corneal dehydration by active transport processes and serve as a hydrophobic barrier. *Hence, drug absorption across the cornea requires penetration of the trilaminar hydrophobic-hydrophilic-hydrophobic domains of the various anatomical layers.*

At the periphery of the cornea and adjacent to the sclera lies a transitional zone (1- to 2-mm wide) called the *limbus*. Limbal structures include the conjunctival epithelium, which contains the corneal epithelial stem cells; Tenon's capsule; episclera; corneoscleral stroma; canal of Schlemm; and trabecular meshwork (see Figure 69–3B). Limbal blood vessels, as well as the tears, provide important nutrients and immunological defense mechanisms for the cornea. The anterior chamber holds about 250 μL of aqueous humor. The peripheral anterior chamber angle is formed by the cornea and the iris root. The trabecular meshwork and canal of Schlemm are located just above the apex of this angle. The posterior chamber, with about 50 μL of aqueous humor, is defined by the boundaries of the ciliary body processes, posterior surface of the iris, and lens surface.

Aqueous Humor Dynamics and Regulation of Intraocular Pressure

Aqueous humor is secreted by the ciliary processes and flows from the posterior chamber, through the pupil, and into the anterior chamber and leaves the eye primarily by the trabecular meshwork and canal of Schlemm, thence to an episcleral venous plexus and into the systemic circulation. This conventional pathway accounts for 80%–95% of aqueous humor outflow and is the main target for cholinergic drugs used in glaucoma therapy. Another outflow pathway is the uveoscleral route (i.e., fluid flows through the ciliary muscles and into the suprachoroidal space), which is the target of selective prostanoids (see Glaucoma in this chapter).

The peripheral anterior chamber angle is an important anatomical structure for differentiating two forms of glaucoma: *open-angle glaucoma*, which is by far the most common form of glaucoma in the U.S., and *angle-closure or closed-angle glaucoma*. Current medical therapy of open-angle glaucoma is aimed at decreasing aqueous humor production or increasing aqueous outflow. The preferred management for angle-closure glaucoma is surgical iridectomy, by either laser or incision, but short-term medical management may be necessary to reduce the acute IOP elevation and to clear the cornea prior to surgery. Long-term IOP reduction may be necessary, especially if the peripheral iris has permanently covered the trabecular meshwork.

In anatomically susceptible eyes, anticholinergic, sympathomimetic, and antihistaminic drugs can lead to partial dilation of the pupil and a change in the vectors of force between the iris and the lens. The aqueous humor then is prevented from passing from the posterior chamber

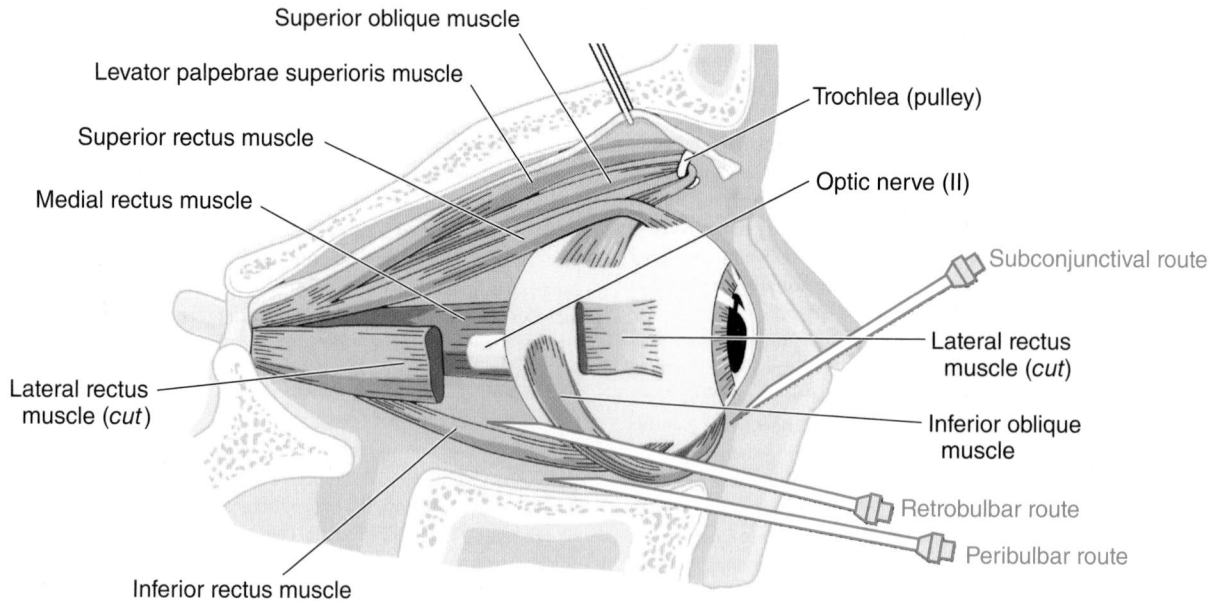

Figure 69–1 *Anatomy of the globe in relation to the orbit and eyelids.* Routes of administration of anesthesia are represented by the blue needles.

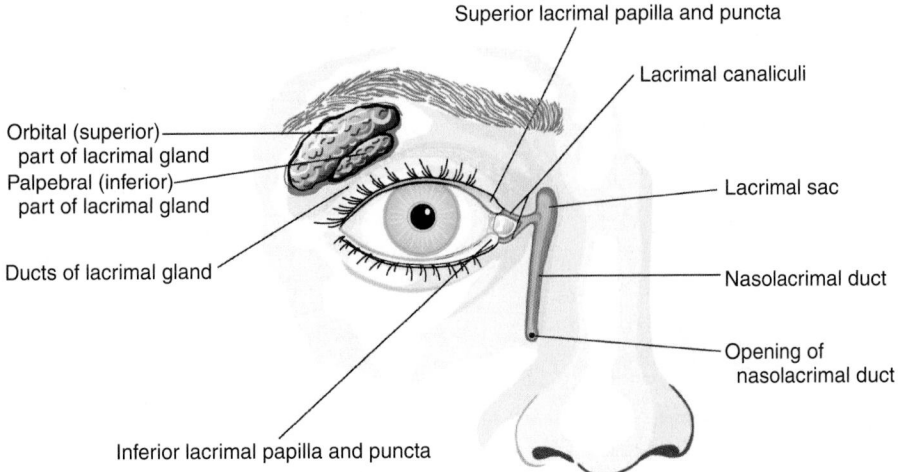

Superior lacrimal papilla and puncta

Lacrimal canaliculi

Orbital (superior) part of lacrimal gland

Palpebral (inferior) part of lacrimal gland

Lacrimal sac

Ducts of lacrimal gland

Nasolacrimal duct

Opening of nasolacrimal duct

Inferior lacrimal papilla and puncta

Figure 69–2 *Anatomy of the lacrimal system.*

through the pupil to the anterior chamber. The change in the lens-iris relationship leads to an increase in pressure in the posterior chamber, causing an anterior bowing of the iris, causing the iris root to be pushed against the angle wall, thereby covering the trabecular meshwork and closing the filtration angle and markedly elevating the IOP. The result is known as an acute attack of *pupillary-block angle-closure glaucoma*.

Iris and Pupil

The iris is the most anterior portion of the uveal tract, which also includes the ciliary body and choroid. The anterior surface of the iris is the stroma, a loosely organized structure containing melanocytes, blood vessels, smooth muscle, and parasympathetic and sympathetic nerves. Differences in iris color reflect individual variation in the number of melanocytes located in the stroma. Individual variation may be an important consideration for ocular drug distribution due to drug-melanin binding (see Distribution). The posterior surface of the iris is a densely pigmented bilayer of epithelial cells. Anterior to the pigmented epithelium, the dilator smooth muscle is oriented radially and is innervated by the sympathetic nervous system (Figure 69–4), which causes *mydriasis* (dilation). At the pupillary margin, the sphincter smooth muscle is organized in a circular band with parasympathetic innervation, which, when stimulated, causes *miosis* (constriction). The use of pharmacological agents to dilate normal pupils and to evaluate the pharmacological response of the pupil is summarized in Table 69–2. Agents affecting sympathetic neurotransmission

in the eye are also used for the diagnostic evaluation of Horner syndrome and anisocoria.

Ciliary Body

The ciliary body serves two very specialized roles:

- Production and secretion of aqueous humor by the epithelial bilayer
- Accommodation by the ciliary muscle

The anterior portion of the ciliary body (*pars plicata*) comprises 70–80 ciliary processes with intricate folds. The posterior portion is the *pars plana*. The ciliary muscle is organized into outer longitudinal, middle radial, and inner circular layers. Coordinated contraction of this smooth muscle apparatus by the parasympathetic nervous system causes the zonular fibers suspending the lens to relax, allowing the lens to become more convex and to shift slightly forward. This process, known as *accommodation*, permits focusing on near objects and may be pharmacologically blocked by muscarinic cholinergic antagonists through a process called *cycloplegia*. Contraction of the ciliary muscle also puts traction on the scleral spur and hence widens the spaces within the trabecular meshwork. This last effect accounts for at least some of the IOP-lowering effect of directly acting and indirectly acting parasympathomimetic drugs. Blockade of β adrenergic receptors of the ciliary epithelium decreases production of aqueous humor.

TABLE 69–1 ■ AUTONOMIC PHARMACOLOGY OF THE EYE AND RELATED STRUCTURES

| TISSUE | ADRENERGIC RECEPTORS | | CHOLINERGIC RECEPTORS | |
	SUBTYPE	RESPONSE	SUBTYPE	RESPONSE
Corneal epithelium	β_2	Unknown	M[a]	Unknown
Corneal endothelium	β_2	Unknown	Undefined	Unknown
Iris radial muscle	α_1	Mydriasis		
Iris sphincter muscle			M_3	Miosis
Trabecular meshwork	β_2	Unknown		
Ciliary epithelium[b]	α_2/β_2	Aqueous production		
Ciliary muscle	β_2	Relaxation[c]	M_3	Accommodation
Lacrimal gland	α_1	Secretion	M_2, M_3	Secretion
Retinal pigment epithelium	α_1/β_2	H_2O transport/unknown		

[a]Although acetylcholine and choline acetyltransferase are abundant in the corneal epithelium of most species, the function of acetylcholine in this tissue is unknown.
[b]The ciliary epithelium also is the target of carbonic anhydrase inhibitors. Carbonic anhydrase isoenzyme II is localized to both the pigmented and nonpigmented ciliary epithelium.
[c]Although β_2 adrenergic receptors mediate ciliary body smooth muscle relaxation, there is no clinically significant effect on accommodation.

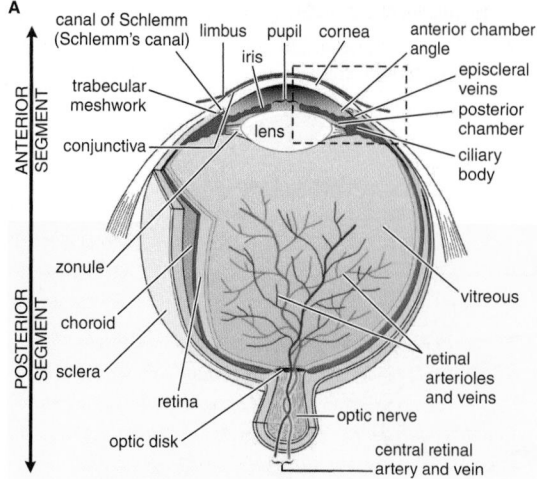

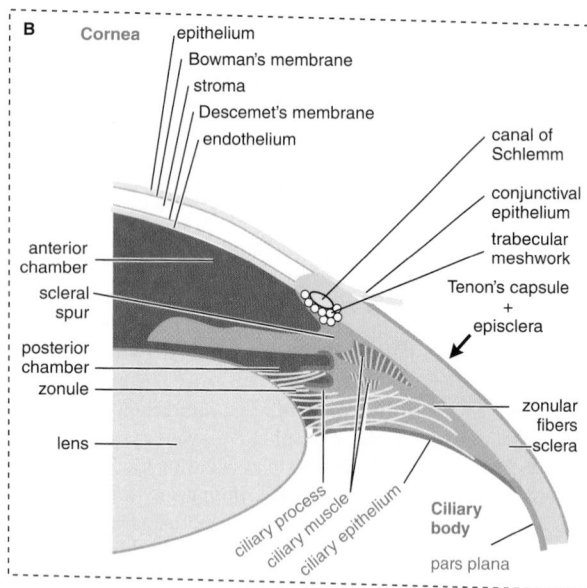

Figure 69–3 **A.** *Anatomy of the eye.* **B.** *Enlargement of the anterior segment, revealing the cornea, angle structures, lens, and ciliary body.* (Adapted with permission from Riordan-Eva P. Anatomy and embryology of the eye. In: Riordan-Eva P, Whitcher JP, eds. *Vaughan & Asbury's General Ophthalmology. 17th ed.* McGraw-Hill, New York, **2008**. Copyright © 2008 by The McGraw-Hill Companies, Inc. All rights reserved.)

Lens

The lens is suspended by the *ciliary zonule*, specialized fibers emanating from the ciliary body. The lens is about 10 mm in diameter and is enclosed in a capsule. The bulk of the lens is composed of fibers derived from proliferating lens epithelial cells located under the anterior portion of the lens capsule. These lens fibers are continuously produced throughout life. Aging, in addition to certain medications, such as corticosteroids, and certain diseases, such as diabetes mellitus, cause the lens to become opacified, which is termed a *cataract*.

Posterior Segment

Because of the anatomical and vascular barriers to both local and systemic access, drug delivery to the eye's posterior pole is particularly challenging.

Sclera and Choroid

The outermost coat of the eye, the sclera, covers the posterior portion of the globe. The external surface of the scleral shell is covered by an episcleral vascular coat, Tenon's capsule, and the conjunctiva. The tendons of the six extraocular muscles insert collagen fibers into the superficial

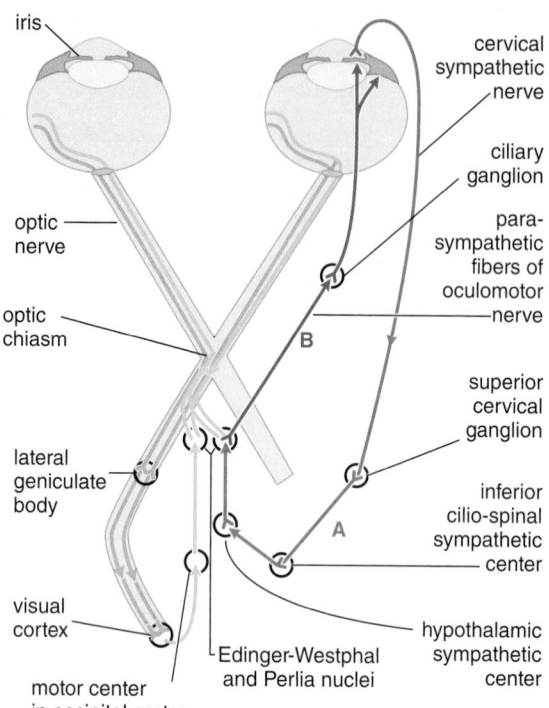

Figure 69–4 *Sympathetic* **(A)** *and parasympathetic* **(B)** *innervation of the eye.* The system is symmetrical, but the schematic is drawn asymmetrically to show all the parts. Input from the retinas is also shown asymmetrically, one medial and one lateral region (Adapted with permission from Wybar KC, Kerr-Muir M. *Bailliere's Concise Medical Textbooks, Ophthalmology. 3rd ed.* Bailliere Tindall, New York, **1984**. Copyright © Elsevier).

scleral. Numerous blood vessels pierce the sclera through emissaria to supply and drain the choroid, ciliary body, optic nerve, and iris. Inside the scleral shell, a capillary network (vascular choroid) nourishes the outer retina. Between the outer retina and the capillary network lie Bruch's membrane and the retinal pigment epithelium, whose tight

TABLE 69–2 ■ EFFECTS OF PHARMACOLOGICAL AGENTS ON THE PUPIL

CLINICAL SETTING	DRUG	PUPILLARY RESPONSE
Normal	Sympathomimetic drugs	Dilation (mydriasis)
Normal	Parasympathomimetic drugs	Constriction (miosis)
Horner syndrome	Cocaine 4%–10%	No dilation
Preganglionic Horner syndrome	Hydroxyamphetamine 1%	Dilation
Postganglionic Horner syndrome	Hydroxyamphetamine 1%	No dilation
Adie's pupil	Pilocarpine 0.05%–0.1%[a]	Constriction
Normal	Opioids (oral or intravenous)	Pinpoint pupils

Topically applied ophthalmic drugs unless otherwise noted.
[a]This percentage of pilocarpine is not commercially available and usually is prepared by the physician administering the test or by a pharmacist. This test also requires that no prior manipulation of the cornea (i.e., tonometry for measuring intraocular pressure or testing corneal sensation) be done so that the normal integrity of the corneal barrier is intact. Normal pupils will not respond to this weak dilution of pilocarpine; however, an Adie's pupil manifests a denervation supersensitivity and is responsive to this dilute cholinergic agonist.

junctions provide an outer barrier between the retina and the choroid. The retinal pigment epithelium serves many functions, including vitamin A metabolism, phagocytosis of the rod outer segments, and multiple transport processes.

Retina

The retina is a thin, transparent, highly organized structure of neurons, glial cells, and blood vessels; it contains the photoreceptors and the rhodopsin-based G protein signaling system. The elevated IOP of glaucoma damages and causes the death of the ganglion cells (the optic nerve) that connect the retina and the brain. Glutamate, acting on NMDA receptors, can stimulate this process (Sucher et al., 1997). In theory, this offers a target for neuroprotective agents to protect against cell death, but to date no treatment other than IOP lowering has demonstrated any benefit in treating glaucoma.

Vitreous

Approximately 80% of the eye's volume is the vitreous, a clear medium containing collagen type II, hyaluronic acid, proteoglycans, glucose, ascorbic acid, amino acids, and a number of inorganic salts.

Optic Nerve

The optic nerve is a myelinated nerve conducting the retinal output to the CNS. It comprises an intraocular portion, visible as the optic disk in the retina; an intraorbital portion; an intracanalicular portion; and an intracranial segment. The nerve is ensheathed in meninges continuous with the brain. It is susceptible to a variety of insults, ranging from traumatic to toxic (ethambutol, methanol, ethanol) to nutritional (vitamin B_{12} and folic acid deficiency) to infectious, neoplastic, and inflammatory. At present, pharmacological treatment of optic neuropathies usually is based on management of the underlying disease. For example, arteritic ischemic optic neuropathy (giant cell arteritis) is best treated with systemic glucocorticoids and optic neuritis with intravenous glucocorticoids (Beck and Gal, 2008; Volpe, 2008). Glaucomatous optic neuropathy is medically managed by decreasing IOP.

Pharmacokinetics and Toxicology of Ocular Therapeutic Agents

Drug Delivery Strategies

There are a number of formulations of agents and routes of drug administration that are unique to the eye (Figures 69–1 and Table 69–3).

Several formulations prolong the time a drug remains on the surface of the eye. These include gels, ointments, solid inserts, soft contact lenses,

and collagen shields. *Prolonging the time in the cul-de-sac beneath the eyelid enhances drug absorption.* Ophthalmic gels (e.g., pilocarpine 4% gel) release drugs by diffusion following erosion of soluble polymers. Ointments usually contain mineral oil and a petrolatum base and are helpful in delivering antibiotics, cycloplegic drugs, or miotic agents. Solid inserts, such as the ganciclovir intravitreal implant, provide a *zero-order* rate of delivery by steady-state diffusion, whereby drug is released at a more constant rate over a prolonged period of time rather than as a bolus. Drug molecules may also be encapsulated in nanoparticles for controlled release on the ocular surface.

ADME

The ADME pharmacokinetic principles determine the time course of drug action in the eye; however, the routes of ocular drug administration, the flow of ocular fluids, and the architecture of the eye introduce other variables specific to the eye. Most ophthalmic medications are formulated to be applied topically. Drugs also may be injected by subconjunctival, sub-Tenon's, intracorneal, intracameral, intravitreal, and retrobulbar routes.

Absorption. After topical instillation of a drug, the rate and extent of absorption are determined by the dwell time of the drug in the cul-de-sac and precorneal tear film, elimination by nasolacrimal drainage, drug binding to tear proteins, drug metabolism by tear and tissue proteins, and diffusion across the cornea and conjunctiva. A drug's residence time may be prolonged by changing its formulation or vehicle. Residence time also may be extended by blocking the egress of tears from the eye by closing the tear drainage ducts with flexible silicone (punctal) plugs. Nasolacrimal drainage contributes to systemic absorption of topically administered ophthalmic medications. Absorption from the nasal mucosa avoids first-pass metabolism by the liver; thus, topical ophthalmic medications can cause significant systemic side effects, especially when used frequently or chronically. Possible absorption pathways of an ophthalmic drug following topical application to the eye are shown schematically in Figure 69–5.

Transcorneal and transconjunctival/scleral absorption are the desired routes for localized ocular drug effects. The drug concentration gradient between the tear film and the cornea and conjunctival epithelium provides the driving force for passive diffusion across these tissues. Other factors that affect a drug's diffusion are the size of the molecule, chemical structure, and steric configuration. Transcorneal drug penetration is a differential solubility process; the cornea resembles a trilaminar "fat-water-fat" structure corresponding to the epithelial, stromal, and endothelial layers, respectively. The epithelium and endothelium represent barriers for hydrophilic substances; the stroma is a barrier for hydrophobic compounds. Hence, an amphipathic agent with both hydrophilic and lipophilic properties is best suited for transcorneal absorption. Drug penetration into the eye is

TABLE 69–3 ■ SOME CHARACTERISTICS OF OCULAR ROUTES OF DRUG ADMINISTRATION

ROUTE	ABSORPTION PATTERN	SPECIAL UTILITY	LIMITATIONS AND PRECAUTIONS
Topical	Prompt, depending on formulation	Convenient, economical, relatively safe	Compliance, corneal and conjunctival toxicity, nasal mucosal toxicity, systemic side effects from nasolacrimal absorption
Subconjunctival, sub-Tenon, and retrobulbar injections	Prompt or sustained, depending on formulation	Anterior segment infections, posterior uveitis, cystoid macular edema	Local toxicity, tissue injury, globe perforation, optic nerve trauma, central retinal artery or vein occlusion, direct retinal drug toxicity with inadvertent globe perforation, ocular muscle trauma, prolonged drug effect
Intraocular (intracameral) injections	Prompt	Anterior segment surgery, infections	Corneal toxicity, intraocular toxicity, relatively short duration of action
Intravitreal injection or device	Absorption circumvented, immediate local effect, potential sustained effect	Endophthalmitis, retinitis, age-related macular degeneration	Retinal toxicity

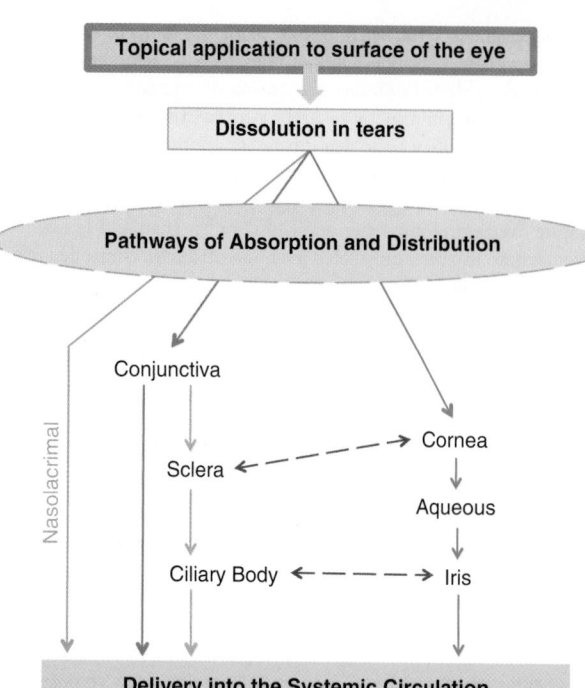

Figure 69–5 *Drugs applied to the surface of the eye have multiple routes to the systemic circulation.*

approximately linearly related to its concentration in the tear film. Certain disease states, such as corneal epithelial defects and corneal ulcers, may alter drug penetration. Medication absorption usually is increased when an anatomical barrier is compromised or removed.

Distribution. Topically administered drugs may undergo systemic distribution primarily by nasal mucosal absorption and possibly via local ocular distribution by transcorneal/transconjunctival absorption. Following transcorneal absorption, the aqueous humor accumulates the drug, which then is distributed to intraocular structures and potentially to the systemic circulation via the trabecular meshwork pathway (see Figure 69–3B). Melanin binding of certain drugs is an important factor in some ocular compartments. For example, the mydriatic effect of α adrenergic agonists is slower in onset in humans with darkly pigmented irides compared to those with lightly pigmented irides; drug-melanin binding is a potential reservoir for sustained drug release. Another clinically important consideration for drug-melanin binding involves the retinal pigment epithelium. In the retinal pigment epithelium, accumulation of chloroquine (see Chapter 49) causes a toxic retinal lesion known as a "bull's-eye" maculopathy, which is associated with a decrease in visual acuity. To reduce the risk of retinal toxicity from chloroquine and related substances (e.g., hydroxychloroquine), patients receiving chronic therapy should receive periodic eye exams and lifetime cumulative doses should generally be limited to 460 g of chloroquine and 1000 g of hydroxychloroquine.

Metabolism. Biotransformation of ocular drugs may be significant; a variety of enzymes, including esterases, oxidoreductases, lysosomal enzymes, peptidases, glucuronide and sulfate transferases, GSH-conjugating enzymes, COMT, MAO, and 11β-hydroxysteroid dehydrogenase are found in the eye. The esterases are of particular interest, permitting development of ester prodrugs for enhanced corneal permeability (e.g., *latanoprost* is a prodrug for $PGF_{2\alpha}$ used for glaucoma management; *loteprednol* is a prednisolone analogue engineered to have limited systemic effects due to metabolic inactivation within the eye).

Toxicity

Most local toxic effects are due to hypersensitivity reactions or to direct toxic effects on the cornea, conjunctiva, periocular skin, and nasal mucosa. Eye drops and contact lens solutions commonly contain antimicrobial preservatives such as benzalkonium chloride, chlorobutanol,

cause a punctate keratopathy or toxic ulcerative keratopathy. All ophthalmic medications are potentially absorbed into the systemic circulation (Figure 69–5), so systemic side effects may occur.

Ophthalmic Uses of Drugs

Chemotherapy of Microbial Diseases in the Eye

Bacterial Infections

Infectious diseases of the skin, eyelids, conjunctivae, and lacrimal excretory system are encountered regularly. Periocular skin infections are divided into preseptal and postseptal or orbital cellulitis. Depending on the clinical setting (e.g., preceding trauma, sinusitis, age of patient, relative immunocompromised state), oral or parenteral antibiotics may be administered in addition to topical medications. A number of antibiotics are formulated for topical ocular use (Table 69–4).

Dacryoadenitis, an infection of the lacrimal gland, is most common in children and young adults; it may be bacterial (typically *Staphylococcus aureus*, *Streptococcus* spp.) or viral (seen in mumps, infectious mononucleosis, influenza, and herpes zoster). When bacterial infection is suspected, systemic antibiotics usually are indicated.

Dacryocystitis is an infection of the lacrimal sac. In infants and children, the disease usually is unilateral and secondary to an obstruction of the nasolacrimal duct. In adults, dacryocystitis and canalicular infections may be caused by *S. aureus*, *Streptococcus* spp., diphtheroids, *Candida* spp., and *Actinomyces israelii*. Any discharge from the lacrimal sac should be sent for smears and cultures. Systemic antibiotics typically are indicated.

Infectious processes of the eyelids include **hordeolum** and **blepharitis**. A hordeolum, or stye, is an infection of the meibomian, Zeis, or Moll glands in the eyelids. The typical offending bacterium is *S. aureus*, and the usual treatment consists of warm compresses and topical antibiotic (gel, drops, or ointment). Blepharitis is a common bilateral inflammatory process of the eyelids characterized by irritation and burning, usually associated with a *Staphylococcus* sp. Local hygiene is the mainstay of therapy; topical antibiotics frequently are used. Systemic tetracycline, doxycycline, minocycline, erythromycin, and azithromycin often are effective in reducing severe eyelid inflammation but must be used for weeks to months.

Conjunctivitis is an inflammatory or infectious process of the conjunctiva that varies in severity from mild hyperemia to severe purulent discharge. The more common causes of conjunctivitis include viruses, allergies, environmental irritants, contact lenses, and chemicals. Less common causes include other infectious pathogens, immune-mediated reactions, associated systemic diseases, and tumors of the conjunctiva or eyelid. Commonly reported infectious agents are adenovirus and herpes simplex virus, followed by other viral (e.g., enterovirus, coxsackievirus, measles virus, varicella zoster virus) and bacterial sources (e.g., *Neisseria* spp., *Streptococcus pneumoniae*, *Haemophilus* spp., *S. aureus*, *Moraxella lacunata*, and chlamydial spp.). *Rickettsia*, fungi, and parasites, in both cystic and trophozoite form, are rare causes of conjunctivitis. Effective management is based on selection of an appropriate antibiotic for suspected bacterial pathogens. Unless an unusual causative organism is suspected, bacterial conjunctivitis is treated empirically with a broad-spectrum topical antibiotic without obtaining a culture.

Keratitis, or corneal inflammation or infection, can occur at any level of the cornea. Myriad microbial agents may cause infectious keratitis, including bacteria, viruses, fungi, spirochetes, and parasites. Severe infections with tissue loss (corneal ulcers) generally are treated more aggressively than infections without tissue loss (corneal infiltrates). Mild, small, more peripheral infections usually are not cultured, and the eyes are treated with broad-spectrum topical antibiotics. In more severe, central, or larger infections, corneal scrapings for cultures and sensitivities are performed, and the patient is immediately started on intensive hourly, around-the-clock topical antibiotic therapy. A commercially available broad-spectrum antibiotic may be given, but in severe infections, specially formulated fortified antibiotics are often used. The goal of treatment is to eradicate the

TABLE 69–4 ■ TOPICAL ANTIBACTERIAL AGENTS COMMERCIALLY AVAILABLE FOR OPHTHALMIC USE

AGENT	FORMULATION[a]	TOXICITY	INDICATIONS FOR USE
Azithromycin	1% solution	H	Conjunctivitis
Bacitracin	500 units/g ointment	H	Conjunctivitis, blepharitis, keratitis, keratoconjunctivitis, corneal ulcers, blepharoconjunctivitis, meibomianitis, dacryocystitis
Besifloxacin	0.6% suspension		Conjunctivitis
Chloramphenicol	1% ointment	H, BD	Conjunctivitis, keratitis
Ciprofloxacin	0.3% solution, 0.3% ointment	H, D-RCD	Conjunctivitis, keratitis, keratoconjunctivitis, corneal ulcers, blepharitis, blepharoconjunctivitis, meibomianitis, dacryocystitis
Erythromycin	0.5% ointment	H	Superficial ocular infections involving the conjunctiva or cornea; prophylaxis of ophthalmia neonatorum
Gatifloxacin	0.3% and 0.5% solutions	H	Conjunctivitis
Gentamicin	0.3% solution, 0.3% ointment	H	Conjunctivitis, blepharitis, keratitis, keratoconjunctivitis, corneal ulcers, blepharoconjunctivitis, meibomianitis, dacryocystitis
Levofloxacin	0.5% solution	H	Conjunctivitis
	1.5% solution	H	Corneal ulcers
Moxifloxacin	0.5% solution	H	Conjunctivitis
Ofloxacin	0.3% solution	H	Conjunctivitis, corneal ulcers
Sulfacetamide	10% solution, 10% ointment	H, BD	Conjunctivitis, other superficial ocular infections
Polymyxin B combinations[b]	Various solutions and ointments		Conjunctivitis, blepharitis, keratitis
Tobramycin[c]	0.3% solution, 0.3% ointment	H	External infections of the eye and its adnexa

BD, blood dyscrasia; D-RCD, drug-related corneal deposits; H, hypersensitivity.

[a]For specific information on dosing, formulation, and trade names, refer to the *Physicians' Desk Reference for Ophthalmic Medicines*, which is published annually.

[b]Polymyxin B is formulated for delivery to the eye in combination with bacitracin, neomycin, gramicidin, oxytetracycline, or trimethoprim. See Chapters 56–59 for further discussion of these antibacterial agents.

[c]Tobramycin is formulated for delivery to the eye in combination with dexamethasone or loteprednol etabonate.

infection and reduce the amount of corneal scarring and the chance of corneal perforation and severe decreased vision or blindness. The initial medication selection and dosage are adjusted according to the clinical response and culture/sensitivity results. In the case of culture-proven bacterial keratitis that has been treated with appropriate topical antibiotics for a several days but still has significant inflammation, judicious topical steroids can be used with close follow-up to decrease corneal scarring.

Endophthalmitis is a potentially severe and devastating inflammatory, and usually infectious, process involving the intraocular tissues. When the inflammatory process encompasses the entire globe, it is called *panophthalmitis*. Endophthalmitis usually is caused by bacteria or fungi or rarely by spirochetes. The typical case occurs during the early postoperative course after intraocular surgery, following trauma, or rarely by endogenous seeding in an immunocompromised host or intravenous drug user. Acute postoperative endophthalmitis requires a prompt vitreous tap for smears and cultures and empirical injection of intravitreal antibiotics. In cases of endogenous seeding, parenteral antibiotics have a role in eliminating the infectious source; systemic antibiotics are helpful in reducing the risk of endophthalmitis following a traumatic open-globe injury (Ahmed et al., 2012). Vitrectomy (i.e., specialized surgical removal of the vitreous) is indicated in some cases (Endophthalmitis Vitrectomy Study Group, 1995; Schiedler et al., 2004).

Viral Infections

Antiviral drugs used in ophthalmology are summarized in Table 69–5 (see Chapter 62 for details of these agents). The primary indications for the use of antiviral drugs in ophthalmology are viral keratitis, herpes zoster ophthalmicus, and retinitis. There currently are no antiviral agents indicated for the treatment of viral conjunctivitis caused by adenoviruses, which usually has a self-limited course and typically is treated by symptomatic relief of irritation, but topical ganciclovir gel may be of some benefit (Yabiku et al., 2011).

Viral keratitis, an infection of the cornea that may involve either the epithelium or stroma, is most commonly caused by herpes simplex type I and varicella zoster viruses. Less common viral etiologies include herpes simplex type II, Epstein-Barr virus, and CMV. The topical antiviral agents trifluridine and ganciclovir are both indicated for the treatment of epithelial disease due to herpes simplex infection, but trifluridine is more toxic to the corneal epithelium. Topical glucocorticoids are contraindicated in herpetic epithelial keratitis due to active viral replication. In contrast, for herpetic disciform keratitis (predominantly a cell-mediated immune reaction), topical glucocorticoids often accelerate recovery. For recurrent herpetic stromal keratitis, there is clear benefit from treatment with oral antivirals such as acyclovir in reducing the risk of recurrence (Herpetic Eye Disease Study Group, 1997, 1998; Young et al., 2010).

Herpes zoster ophthalmicus is a latent reactivation of a varicella zoster infection in the first division of the trigeminal cranial nerve. Systemic acyclovir, valacyclovir, and famciclovir are effective in reducing the severity and complications of herpes zoster ophthalmicus (Cohen and Kessler, 2016).

Viral retinitis may be caused by herpes simplex virus, CMV, adenovirus, and varicella zoster virus. With antiretroviral therapy (see Chapter 64), CMV retinitis does not appear to progress when specific anti-CMV therapy is discontinued, but some patients develop an immune recovery uveitis. Treatment usually involves long-term parenteral administration of antiviral drugs. Intravitreal ganciclovir, injected or implanted as an insert, is an effective alternative to systemic use. Acute retinal necrosis and progressive outer retinal necrosis, most often caused by varicella zoster virus, can be treated by combinations of oral, intravenous, and intravitreal administration of antiviral medications (Newman and Gooding, 2013).

TABLE 69–5 ■ ANTIVIRAL AGENTS FOR OPHTHALMIC USE

GENERIC NAME	ROUTE OF ADMINISTRATION	OCULAR TOXICITY	INDICATIONS FOR USE
Trifluridine	Topical (1% solution)	Punctate keratopathy, hypersensitivity	Herpes simplex keratitis and keratoconjunctivitis Dosed initially 9 times a day Corneal toxicity can occur
Ganciclovir	Topical (0.15% gel) Intravenous infusion, intravitreal injection,[a] and intravitreal implant (4.5 mg)		Herpes simplex keratitis Cytomegaloviris retinitis
Acyclovir	Oral, intravenous (200-mg capsules, 400- and 800-mg tablets)		Herpes zoster ophthalmicus Herpes simplex iridocyclitis
Valacyclovir	Oral (500- and 1000-mg tablets)		Herpes simplex keratitis[a] Herpes zoster ophthalmicus
Famciclovir	Oral (125-, 250-, and 500-mg tablets)		Herpes simplex keratitis[a] Herpes zoster ophthalmicus
Foscarnet	Intravenous Intravitreal[a]		Cytomegalovirus retinitis
Valganciclovir	Oral (450-mg tablets)		Cytomegalovirus retinitis
Cidofovir	Intravenous		Cytomegalovirus retinitis

[a]Off-label use. For additional details, see Chapter 62.

Fungal Infections

The only currently available topical ophthalmic antifungal preparation is natamycin, a polyene. Other antifungal agents may be extemporaneously compounded for topical, subconjunctival, corneal intrastromal, intracameral, or intravitreal routes of administration (Table 69–6; see also Chapter 61). As with systemic fungal infections, the incidence of ophthalmic fungal infections has risen with the growing number of immunocompromised hosts. Fungal infections can involve the cornea, sclera, intraocular structures, canalicula, and orbit. Risk factors for fungal keratitis include trauma, chronic ocular surface disease, contact lens wear, and immunosuppression (including topical steroid use). When fungal infection is suspected, samples of the affected tissues are obtained for smears, cultures, and sensitivities, and this information is used to guide drug selection.

Protozoal Infections

Parasitic infections involving the eye usually manifest themselves as a form of *uveitis*, an inflammatory process of either the anterior or posterior segments and, less commonly, as conjunctivitis, keratitis, and retinitis. In the U.S., the most commonly encountered protozoal infections include *Acanthamoeba* and *Toxoplasma gondii*. In contact lens wearers who develop keratitis, physicians should be highly suspicious of the presence of *Acanthamoeba*. Risk factors for *Acanthamoeba* keratitis include poor contact lens hygiene, wearing contact lenses in a pool or hot tub, and ocular trauma. Treatment usually consists of a combination of topical agents. The aromatic diamidines—propamidine isethionate in topical aqueous and ointment forms (not commercially available in the U.S.)—have been used successfully to treat this relatively resistant infectious keratitis. The cationic antiseptic agent polyhexamethylene biguanide also is used in drop form for *Acanthamoeba* keratitis; alternatively, topical chlorhexidine can be used; both drugs need to be prepared by a specialty compounding pharmacy. Oral imidazoles (e.g., itraconazole, fluconazole, ketoconazole, voriconazole) often are used in addition to the topical medications. Resolution of *Acanthamoeba* keratitis often requires many months of treatment (Chew et al., 2011; Hoti and Tandon, 2011).

Treatment of *toxoplasmosis* is indicated when inflammatory lesions encroach on the macula and threaten central visual acuity. Several regimens have been recommended with concurrent use of systemic steroids: (1) pyrimethamine, sulfadiazine, and folinic acid (leucovorin); (2) pyrimethamine, sulfadiazine, clindamycin, and folinic acid; (3) sulfadiazine and clindamycin; (4) clindamycin; and (5) trimethoprim-sulfamethoxazole with or without clindamycin. Other protozoal infections (e.g., giardiasis, leishmaniasis, malaria) and helminth infections are less common eye pathogens in the U.S. Systemic pharmacological management as well as vitrectomy may be indicated for selected parasitic infections (Maenz et al., 2014).

Ophthalmic Use of Autonomic Agents, Eicosanoids, and Carbonic Anhydrase Inhibitors

Autonomic drugs are used extensively for diagnostic and surgical purposes and for the treatment of glaucoma, uveitis, and strabismus. The autonomic agents used in ophthalmology and the responses (i.e., mydriasis, cycloplegia) to muscarinic cholinergic antagonists are summarized in Table 69–7. Table 69–8 presents some characteristics of eicosanoids used in ophthalmology.

Glaucoma

Glaucoma is characterized by progressive loss of retinal nerve fiber layer tissue and visual field loss. The optic nerve acquires a characteristic loss of the neuroretinal rim, frequently referred to as "cupping." The prevalence of the disease is growing as populations age and increase around the world (Tham et al., 2014). Risk factors include increased IOP, positive family history of glaucoma, African American heritage, and possibly myopia, diabetes, and hypertension. Reducing IOP can delay glaucomatous nerve or field damage. Although markedly elevated IOPs (e.g., > 30 mm Hg) usually will lead to optic nerve damage, the optic nerves in certain patients (*ocular hypertensives*) apparently can tolerate IOPs in the mid-to-high 20s. Other patients have progressive glaucomatous optic nerve damage despite having IOPs in the normal range; this form of the disease sometimes is called *normal-* or *low-tension* glaucoma. Regardless of the initial level, reducing the IOP delays or prevents disease progression (Collaborative Normal-Tension Study Group, 1998a, 1998b; Ederer et al., 2004; Heijl et al., 2002; Kass et al., 2002; Miglior et al., 2005). At present, the pathophysiological processes involved in glaucomatous optic nerve damage and the relationship to aqueous humor dynamics are not understood. Current

TABLE 69–6 ■ ANTIFUNGAL AGENTS FOR OPHTHALMIC USE

DRUG CLASS AGENT	METHOD OF ADMINISTRATION	INDICATIONS FOR USE
Polyenes		
Amphotericin B[a]	0.1%–0.5% (typically 0.15%) topical solution	Yeast and fungal keratitis and endophthalmitis
	0.8- to 1-mg subconjunctival	Yeast and fungal endophthalmitis
	2- to 10-μg intrastromal corneal and intracameral	Yeast and fungal keratitis
	5- to 10-μg intravitreal injection	Yeast and fungal endophthalmitis
	Intravenous	Yeast and fungal endophthalmitis
Natamycin	5% topical suspension	Yeast and fungal blepharitis, conjunctivitis, keratitis
Imidazoles		
Fluconazole[a]	Oral, intravenous	Yeast keratitis and endophthalmitis
Itraconazole[a]	Oral	Yeast and fungal keratitis and endophthalmitis
Ketoconazole[a]	Oral	Yeast keratitis and endophthalmitis
Miconazole[a]	1% topical solution	Yeast and fungal keratitis
	5- to 10-mg subconjunctival	Yeast and fungal endophthalmitis
	10-μg intravitreal injection	Yeast and fungal endophthalmitis
Voriconazole	Oral, intravenous, intravitreal	Yeast and fungal keratitis and endophthalmitis
	Intrastromal, corneal, and intracameral	Yeast and fungal keratitis

[a]Off-label use. Only natamycin is commercially available and labeled for ophthalmic use. All other antifungal drugs are not labeled for ophthalmic use and must be formulated for the given method of administration. For further dosing information, refer to the *Physicians' Desk Reference for Ophthalmic Medicines*. For additional discussion of these antifungal agents, see Chapter 61.

pharmacotherapies are targeted at decreasing the production of aqueous humor at the ciliary body and increasing outflow through the trabecular meshwork and uveoscleral pathways. There is no consensus on the best IOP-lowering technique (Musch et al., 2011).

A stepped medical approach depends on the patient's health, age, and ocular status, with knowledge of systemic effects and contraindications for all medications. A stepped medical approach may begin with a *topical PG* analogue (Table 69–8).

Due to their once-daily dosing, low incidence of systemic side effects, and potent IOP-lowering effect, PG analogues have largely replaced β adrenergic receptor antagonists as first-line medical therapy for glaucoma. The PG analogues consist of latanoprost (Figure 69–6), travoprost, bimatoprost, tafluprost, and unoprostone (discontinued in the U.S.). $PGF_{2\alpha}$ reduces IOP but has intolerable local side effects. Modifications to the chemical structure of $PGF_{2\alpha}$ have produced analogues with a more acceptable side-effect profile. $PGF_{2\alpha}$ and its analogues (prodrugs that are

hydrolyzed to $PGF_{2\alpha}$) bind to receptors for $PGF_{2\alpha}$ (FP receptors) that link to the $G_{q/11}$-PLC–IP_3–Ca^{2+} pathway. This pathway is active in isolated human ciliary muscle cells. Other cells in the eye also may express FP receptors. Theories of IOP lowering by $PGF_{2\alpha}$ range from altered ciliary muscle tension to effects on trabecular meshwork cells to release of matrix metalloproteinases and digestion of extracellular matrix materials that may impede outflow tracts.

The *β receptor antagonists* (Table 69–7) are currently the next most common topical medical treatment. Nonselective β blockers bind to both β_1 and β_2 receptors and include timolol, levobunolol, metipranolol, and carteolol. The β_1-selective antagonist betaxolol is available for ophthalmic use but is less efficacious than the nonselective β blockers because the β receptors of the eye are largely of the β_2 subtype. However, betaxolol is less likely to cause breathing difficulty due to blockade of pulmonary β_2 receptors. In the eye, the targeted tissues are the ciliary body epithelium and blood vessels, where β_2 receptors account for 75%–90% of the total population. How β blockade leads to decreased aqueous production and reduced IOP is uncertain. Production of aqueous humor seems to be activated by a β receptor–mediated cyclic AMP–PKA pathway; β blockade blunts adrenergic activation of this pathway. Another hypothesis is that β blockers decrease ocular blood flow, which decreases the ultrafiltration responsible for aqueous production.

When there are medical contraindications to the use of PG analogues or β receptor antagonists, other agents, such as an α_2 *adrenergic receptor agonist* (see Table 69–7) or topical *CAI* (Table 69–9), may be used as first-line therapy. The α_2 adrenergic agonists appear to decrease IOP by reducing aqueous humor production and by enhancing both conventional (via an α_2 receptor mechanism) and uveoscleral outflow (perhaps via PG production) from the eye. The α_2 adrenergic agonist and clonidine derivative apraclonidine is a relatively selective α_2 adrenergic agonist that is highly ionized at physiological pH, does not cross the blood-brain barrier, and is thus relatively free of the CNS effects of clonidine. Brimonidine is a selective α_2 adrenergic agonist that is lipophilic, enabling easy corneal penetration. Both apraclonidine and brimonidine reduce aqueous production and may enhance some uveoscleral outflow. Both appear to bind to pre- and postsynaptic α_2 receptors. By binding to the presynaptic receptors, the drugs reduce the amount of neurotransmitter release from sympathetic nerve stimulation and thereby lower IOP. By binding to postsynaptic α_2 receptors, these drugs stimulate the G_i pathway, reducing cellular cyclic AMP production, thereby reducing aqueous humor production.

The development of a **topical CAI** was prompted by the poor side-effect profile of oral CAIs. Dorzolamide and brinzolamide both work by inhibiting CA (isoform II), which is found in the ciliary body epithelium. Inhibition of CA reduces the formation of bicarbonate ions, which reduces fluid transport and thus IOP (Table 69–9).

Any of these four drug classes can be used as additive second- or third-line therapy. In fact, the β receptor antagonist timolol has been combined with the CAI dorzolamide in a single medication and with the α_2 adrenergic agonist brimonidine. A recently released combination of brinzolamide/brimonidine is also an option. A latanoprost/timolol combination is widely available. Such combinations reduce the number of drops needed and may improve compliance.

Topical miotic agents (see Table 69–7) are less commonly used today because of their numerous side effects and inconvenient dosing. Miotics lower IOP by causing muscarinic-induced contraction of the ciliary muscle, which facilitates aqueous outflow. They do not affect aqueous production. Pilocarpine and carbachol are cholinomimetics that stimulate muscarinic receptors and are referred to as having a direct mechanism of action. Indirect agents such as echothiophate are organophosphate inhibitors of acetylcholinesterase. Echothiophate is relatively stable in aqueous solution and, by virtue of its quaternary ammonium structure, is positively charged and poorly absorbed. If combined topical therapy fails to achieve the target IOP or fails to halt glaucomatous optic nerve damage, then *systemic therapy with a CAI* is a final medication option before resorting to laser or incisional surgical treatment. The best-tolerated oral preparation is acetazolamide in sustained-release capsules (see Chapter 25), followed by methazolamide. The least well tolerated are acetazolamide tablets.

TABLE 69–7 ■ AUTONOMIC DRUGS FOR OPHTHALMIC USE

DRUG CLASS	FORMULATION	INDICATIONS	SIDE EFFECTS
Cholinergic agonists			
Acetylcholine	1% solution	Miosis in surgery	Corneal edema
Carbachol	0.01%, 1.5%, 3% solution	Miosis in surgery, glaucoma	Corneal edema, miosis, induced myopia, decreased vision, brow ache, retinal detachment
Pilocarpine	1%, 2%, and 4% solution	Glaucoma, miosis induction, miosis in surgery	Same as for carbachol
Anticholinesterase agents			
Echothiophate	0.125% solution	Glaucoma, accommodative esotropia	Retinal detachment, miosis, cataract, pupillary block, glaucoma, iris cysts, brow ache, punctal stenosis
Muscarinic antagonists			
Atropine	1% solution, 1% ointment	Cycloplegia, mydriasis,[a] cycloplegic retinoscopy,[b] dilated funduscopic exam,[b] iriitus, uveitis	Photosensitivity, blurred vision; long acting (1 week or longer)
Scopolamine	0.25% solution	Cycloplegia, mydriasis, iritis, uveitis, nystagmus[b]	Same as for atropine but the effect lasts several days
Homatropine	2% and 5% solution	Cycloplegia, mydriasis, iritis,[b] uveitis	Same as for scopolamine but does not last as long
Cyclopentolate	Solution (0.5%–2%), also with phenyephrine	Cycloplegia, mydriasis[a]	Same as for atropine but effect lasts ~ 1 day
Tropicamide	0.5% and 1% solution, also with hydroxyamphetamine	Cycloplegia, mydriasis[a]	Same as for atropine but effect lasts several hours; commonly used for office exams
α Adrenergic agonists			
Phenylephrine	2.5% and 10% solution	Mydriasis, vasoconstriction, decongestion,[b] uveitis, glaucoma	α Adrenergic agonist effect lasts several hours; 2.5% used with tropicamide for office exams
Apraclonidine	0.5% and 1% solution	Glaucoma, ocular hypertension	α adrenergic agonist; side effects: allergy (conjunctival hyperemia), dry mouth, sleepiness
Brimonidine (α_2 selective)	Solution (0.1%–0.2%); 0.33% gel; also with timolol or brinzolamide	Glaucoma, ocular hypertension	Same as for apraclonidine; causes respiratory depression in young children
Naphazoline	0.1% solution	Decongestant	Contraindicated in closed-angle glaucoma; safety/efficacy not established in the young (neonate to adolescent); use in infants may result in CNS depression, coma, marked reduction in body temperature; use with caution in patients with hypertension, cardiac disease, hyperthyroidism, diabetes, or infection or trauma in eye
Tetrahydrozoline	0.05% solution	Decongestant	Contraindicated in closed-angle glaucoma; safety/efficacy not established in neonates and children < 6 years; use with caution in patients with coronary artery disease, hypertension, hyperthyroidism, or diabetes
β Adrenergic antagonists			
Betaxolol (β_1 selective)	0.25% suspension, 0.5% solution	Glaucoma, ocular hypertension	Reduced incidence of respiratory problems compared to timolol
Timolol	Solution, gel (0.25%, 0.5%); also with brimonidine, dorzolamide, latanoprost	Glaucoma, ocular hypertension	Side effects: exacerbation of respiratory problems (asthma and chronic obstructive pulmonary disease), bradycardia, depression, impotence
Carteolol	1% solution	Glaucoma, ocular hypertension	Same as timolol
Levobunolol	0.25% and 0.5% solution	Glaucoma, ocular hypertension	
Metipranolol	0.3% solution	Glaucoma, ocular hypertension	

[a]Mydriasis and cycloplegia, or paralysis of accommodation, of the human eye occurs after one drop of atropine 1%, scopolamine 0.5%, homatropine 1%, cyclopentolate 0.5% or 1%, and tropicamide 0.5% or 1%. Recovery of mydriasis is defined by return to baseline pupil size to within 1 mm. Recovery of cycloplegia is defined by return to within 2 -diopters of baseline accommodative power. The maximal mydriatic effect of homatropine is achieved with a 5% solution, but cycloplegia may be incomplete. Maximal cycloplegia with tropicamide may be achieved with a 1% solution. Times to development of maximal mydriasis and to recovery, respectively, are as follows: for atropine, 30–40 min and 7–10 d; for scopolamine, 20–130 min and 3–7 d; for homatropine, 40–60 min and 1–3 d; for cyclopentolate, 30–60 min and 1 d; for tropicamide, 20–40 min and 6 h. Times to development of maximal cycloplegia and to recovery, respectively, are as follows: for atropine, 60–180 min and 6–12 d; for scopolamine, 30–60 min and 3–7 d; for homatropine, 30–60 min and 1–3 d; for cyclopentolate, 25–75 min and 6 h to 1 d; for tropicamide, 30 min and 6 h.

[b]Off-label use. Refer to *Physicians' Desk Reference for Ophthalmic Medicines* for specific indications and dosing.

TABLE 69–8 ■ PROSTAGLANDIN ANALOGUES FOR OPHTHALMIC USE

AGENT	FORMULATION	INDICATIONS	SIDE EFFECTS
Latanoprost (the most commonly used glaucoma medication)	0.005% solution; also with timolol (0.05%)	Glaucoma, ocular hypertension	Once-daily dosing can cause lash growth; may cause allergic conjunctival hyperemia, permanent ↑ iris pigmentation, orbital fat atrophy
Travoprost	0.004% solution		Same as latanoprost but generally less irritating to corneal epithelium
Bimatoprost	0.01% solution, 0.03% solution		
Tafluprost	0.0015% solution; preservative-free, single-dose droperettes		

Toxicity of Antiglaucoma Agents. Ciliary body spasm is a muscarinic cholinergic effect that can lead to induced myopia and a changing refraction due to iris and ciliary body contraction as the drug effect waxes and wanes between doses. Headaches can occur from the iris and ciliary body contraction. The α_2 agonists, effective in IOP reduction, can cause a vasoconstriction-vasodilation rebound phenomenon, leading to a red eye. Ocular and skin allergies from topical epinephrine, apraclonidine, and brimonidine are common (epinephrine for ophthalmic use is no longer marketed in the U.S.). Brimonidine is less likely to cause ocular allergy and therefore is more commonly used. These agents can cause CNS depression and apnea in neonates and are contraindicated in children less than 2 years of age. Systemic absorption of α_2 agonists and β adrenergic antagonists can induce all the side effects of systemic administration. The use of CAIs systemically may give some patients significant problems with malaise, fatigue, depression, paresthesias, and nephrolithiasis; the topical CAIs may minimize these relatively common side effects.

Uveitis

Inflammation of the uvea, or uveitis, has both infectious and noninfectious causes, and medical treatment of the underlying cause (if known), in addition to the use of topical therapy, is essential. Cyclopentolate, tropicamide, or sometimes even longer-acting antimuscarinic agents such as atropine, scopolamine, and homatropine frequently are used to prevent posterior synechia formation between the lens and iris margin and to relieve ciliary muscle spasm that is responsible for much of the pain associated with anterior uveitis.

If posterior synechiae already have formed, an α adrenergic agonist may be used to break the synechiae by enhancing pupillary dilation. A solution of scopolamine 0.3% in combination with 10% phenylephrine is available for this purpose. Two others, 1% hydroxyamphetamine hydrobromide combined with 0.25% tropicamide and 1% phenylephrine in combination with 0.2% cyclopentolate, are indicated only for induction of mydriasis. Topical steroids usually are adequate to decrease inflammation but sometimes must be supplemented with systemic steroids.

Strabismus

Strabismus, or ocular misalignment, has numerous causes and may occur at any age. Besides causing *diplopia* (double vision), strabismus in children may lead to *amblyopia* (reduced vision). Nonsurgical efforts to treat amblyopia include occlusion therapy, orthoptics, optical devices, and pharmacological agents.

An eye with *hyperopia*, or farsightedness, must constantly accommodate to focus on distant images. In some hyperopic children, the synkinetic accommodative-convergence response leads to excessive convergence and a manifest *esotropia* (turned-in eye). The brain rejects diplopia and suppresses the image from the deviated eye. If proper vision is not restored by about 6–8 years of age, the brain never learns to process visual information from that eye. The result is that the eye appears structurally normal but does not develop normal visual acuity and is therefore amblyopic. This is a fairly common cause of visual disability. In this setting, atropine (1%) instilled in the preferred seeing eye produces cycloplegia and the inability of this eye to accommodate, thus forcing the child to use the amblyopic eye (Pediatric Eye Disease Investigator Group, 2002, 2003). Echothiophate iodide also has been used in the setting of accommodative strabismus. Accommodation drives the near reflex, the triad of miosis, accommodation, and convergence. An irreversible cholinesterase inhibitor such as echothiophate causes miosis and an accommodative change in the shape of the lens; hence, the accommodative drive to initiate the near reflex is reduced, and less convergence will occur.

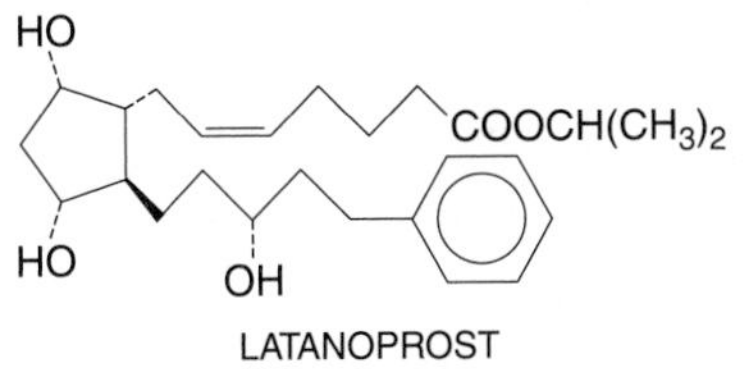

Surgical and Diagnostic Uses

For certain surgical procedures and for clinical funduscopic examination, it is desirable to maximize the view of the retina and lens. Muscarinic cholinergic antagonists and sympathomimetic agents frequently are used singly or in combination for this purpose (see Table 69–7). Intraoperatively, there are circumstances in which miosis is preferred, and two cholinergic agonists are available for intraocular use, acetylcholine and carbachol. Patients with myasthenia gravis may first present to an ophthalmologist with complaints of double vision (diplopia) or eyelid droop (ptosis); the *edrophonium test* is helpful in diagnosing these patients (see Chapter 10). Intraoperatively, trypan blue is marketed (as 0.06% and 0.15% ophthalmic solutions) to facilitate visualization of the anterior lens capsule during cataract surgery and for staining the retinal surface during surgical vitrectomy to guide the excision of tissue.

Anti-inflammatory, Immunomodulatory, and Antimitotic Drugs

Glucocorticoids

Glucocorticoids have an important role in managing ocular inflammatory diseases (Table 69–10 and Table 69–11). The chemistry and pharmacology of glucocorticoids are described in Chapter 46.

Therapeutic Uses. The glucocorticoids formulated for topical administration to the eye are dexamethasone, prednisolone, fluorometholone, loteprednol, rimexolone, and difluprednate. Because of their anti-inflammatory effects, topical corticosteroids are used in managing significant ocular allergy, external eye inflammatory diseases associated with some infections and ocular cicatricial pemphigoid, anterior uveitis, and

Figure 69–6 *Latanoprost.*

TABLE 69–9 ■ CARBONIC ANHYDRASE INHIBITORS FOR OPHTHALMIC USE

AGENT	FORMULATION	INDICATIONS	SIDE EFFECTS
Acetazolamide	Tablets (125, 250 mg); slow release (500 mg) Intravenous	Acute ↑ IOP, glaucoma	Paresthesias (hands, feet), upset stomach, hypokalemia, allergic rash, kidney stones Rare: aplastic anemia
Methazolamide	Tablets (25, 50 mg)	Glaucoma	Same as acetazolamide but generally fewer paresthesias and stomach upset
Dorzolamide	2% solution; also in combo with timolol (0.5%)	Glaucoma, ocular hypertension	Causes burning, stinging, and a metallic taste
Brinzolamide	1% suspension; also in combo with brimonidine (0.2%)	Glaucoma, ocular hypertension	Causes less burning, stinging, and metallic taste than dorzolamide

postoperative inflammation following refractive, corneal, and intraocular surgery. After glaucoma filtering surgery, topical steroids can delay the wound-healing process by decreasing fibroblast infiltration, thereby reducing potential scarring of the surgical site. Steroids commonly are given systemically and by sub-Tenon's capsule injection to manage posterior uveitis. Intravitreal injection of steroids is used to treat ARMD, diabetic retinopathy, and cystoid macular edema. An intravitreal triamcinolone formulation is approved for ocular inflammatory conditions unresponsive to topical corticosteroids and visualization during vitrectomy. Parenteral steroids followed by tapering oral doses is the preferred treatment of optic neuritis. Two ophthalmic implants, fluocinolone and dexamethasone, are marketed for the treatment of chronic, noninfectious uveitis; a dexamethasone implant is also indicated for the treatment of macular edema.

Toxicity. Ocular complications include the development of posterior subcapsular cataracts, secondary infections, and secondary open-angle glaucoma. There is a significant increase in the risk for developing secondary glaucoma when there is a positive family history of glaucoma. In the absence of a family history of open-angle glaucoma, only about 5% of normal individuals respond to topical or long-term systemic steroids with a marked increase in IOP. With a positive family history, however, moderate-to-marked steroid-induced IOP elevations may occur in up to 90% of patients. Some topical steroids (e.g., loteprednol) have been developed that reduce, but do not eliminate, the risk of elevated IOP.

Nonsteroidal Anti-inflammatory Agents

Pharmacological properties of NSAIDS are presented in Chapter 38. Five topical NSAIDs are approved for ocular use: flurbiprofen, ketorolac, diclofenac, bromfenac, and nepafenac.

The NSAIDS are supplied as solutions and suspensions for topical ocular use to reduce ocular inflammation and cystoid macular edema. Flurbiprofen is used to counter unwanted intraoperative miosis during cataract surgery. Ketorolac is given for seasonal allergic conjunctivitis. A combination ketorolac/phenylephrine intraocular solution is available to add to intraoperative ophthalmic irrigation solutions to decrease miosis during cataract surgery. Diclofenac is used for postoperative inflammation and pain. Both ketorolac and diclofenac are effective in treating cystoid macular edema occurring after cataract surgery and in controlling pain after corneal refractive surgery. Bromfenac and nepafenac are indicated for treating postoperative pain and inflammation after cataract surgery. Topical and systemic NSAIDs occasionally have been associated with sterile corneal melts and perforations, especially in older patients with ocular surface disease, such as dry eye syndrome.

TABLE 69–10 ■ GLUCOCORTICOIDS FOR TOPICAL APPLICATION TO THE EYE

AGENT	FORMULATION	INDICATIONS
Dexamethasone	0.1% suspension; 0.1% (sodium phosphate) solution; 0.4% canalicular insert	Steroid-responsive inflammatory conditions of the palpebral and bulbar conjunctiva, cornea, and anterior segment; infective conjunctivitis to reduce edema and inflammation when hazard of steroid use is acceptable; corneal injury from chemical, radiation, or thermal burns or penetration of foreign object; post-operative inflammation
Difluprednate	0.05% emulsion	Ocular pain; postoperative ocular inflammation; uveitis
Fluorometholone	0.1%, 0.25% suspension; 0.1% ointment	Allergic conjunctivitis; giant papillary conjunctivitis; keratitis; ocular burns; postoperative ocular inflammation; uveitis; vernal keratoconjunctivitis
Loteprednol etabonate	0.2%, 0.5% suspension; 0.5% gel; 0.5% ointment	Allergic conjunctivitis; cyclitis; giant papillary conjunctivitis; iritis; keratitis; ocular pain; postoperative ocular inflammation, uveitis[a]
Prednisolone acetate Prednisolone sodium phosphate	0.12%, 1% suspension 1% solution	Allergic conjunctivitis and marginal corneal ulcer; anterior segment inflammation; bacterial conjunctivitis; chorioretinitis; cyclitis; endophthalmitis[a]; Graves' ophthalmopathy; herpes zoster ocular infection (with antiviral therapy); iritis; nonspecific and superficial punctate keratitis; postoperative ocular inflammation; optic neuritis; sympathetic ophthalmia; diffuse posterior uveitis; vernal keratoconjunctivitis; corneal injury from chemical, radiation, thermal burns; or penetration of foreign objects: commonly used after ocular surgery.
Rimexolone	1% suspension	Postoperative ocular inflammation; uveitis; vernal keratoconjunctivitis[a]

[a]Off-label use.

TABLE 69–11 ■ GLUCOCORTICOIDS FOR SUB-TENON'S, INTRAVITREAL, AND SYSTEMIC USE

AGENT	FORMULATION	METHOD OF ADMINISTRATION	INDICATION
Triamcinolone	Solutions and suspensions for injection, 3 to 40 mg/mL	Sub-Tenon's,[a] intracameral,[a] intravitreal	Ocular inflammation, ocular surgery, uveitis
Betamethasone	Oral syrup (0.12 mg/mL); suspension for IM injection (6 mg/mL)	Sub-Tenon's[a]	Corticosteroid-responsive ophthalmic disorders: allergic conjunctivitis and marginal corneal ulcer, anterior segment inflammation, chorioretinitis, conjunctivitis, endophthalmitis,[a] Graves' ophthalmopathy, herpes zoster ocular infection, iritis, keratitis, postoperative ocular inflammation, optic neuritis, diffuse posterior uveitis, vernal keratoconjunctivitis
Dexamethasone	Oral preps (0.5–1 mg/mL); tablets (0.5–6 mg); injectable solution (4 mg/mL, 10 mg/mL)	Oral, intravenous, intramuscular	Allergic conjunctivitis, allergic marginal corneal ulcer, anterior segment inflammation, chorioretinitis, cyclitis, endophthalmitis,[a] Graves' ophthalmopathy, giant papillary conjunctivitis, herpes zoster ocular infection, iritis, keratitis, superficial punctate keratitis, postoperative ocular inflammation, optic neuritis, diffuse choroiditis, sympathetic ophthalmia, vernal keratoconjunctivitis, or corneal injury (corneal abrasion)
Dexamethasone	0.7-mg ophthalmic implant	Intravitreal	Ocular inflammation due to macular edema following retinal vein occlusion, including branch retinal vein occlusion or central retinal vein occlusion and for the treatment of noninfectious uveitis affecting the posterior segment of the eye
Fluocinolone acetonide	0.19-mg ophthalmic implant	Intravitreal	Diabetic macular edema in patients who had no clinically significant rise in intraocular pressure when treated with corticosteroids
Fluocinolone acetonide	0.59-mg ophthalmic implant	Intravitreal	For the treatment of chronic noninfectious uveitis affecting the posterior segment of the eye
Methylprednisolone	Tablets (2–32 mg): 20-mg/mL, 40-mg/mL, suspension for IM injection (80 mg/mL); sodium succinate solution for IM/IV injection (40–1000 mg)	Oral, intravenous, intramuscular	For the systemic treatment of ophthalmic disorders, including allergic conjunctivitis, allergic marginal corneal ulcer, anterior segment inflammation, chorioretinitis, endophthalmitis,[a] Graves' ophthalmopathy, herpes zoster ocular infection, iritis, keratitis, postoperative ocular inflammation, optic neuritis, diffuse posterior uveitis, or vernal keratoconjunctivitis
Prednisone	1 mg/mL, 5 mg/mL oral solution; 1-, 2.5-, 5-, 10-, 20-, 50-mg tabs; 1-, 2-, 5-mg delayed-release tabs	Oral	Inflammatory conditions such as endophthalmitis,[a] optic neuritis, allergic conjunctivitis, keratitis, allergic corneal ulcer, iritis, chorioretinitis, anterior segment inflammation, uveitis, choroiditis, or sympathetic ophthalmia
Prednisolone	Orally disintegrating tablets (10–30 mg); syrup and oral solution (1–3 mg/mL)	Oral	Systemic treatment of corticosteroid-responsive eye disorders

[a]Off-label use.
IM, intramuscular; IV, intravenous.

Antihistamines and Mast Cell Stabilizers

H$_1$ antagonists (see Chapter 32) and mast cell stabilizers are used to treat the manifestations of ocular allergies. Pheniramine (see Chapter 32) and antazoline (discontinued in the U.S.) are formulated in combination with naphazoline, a vasoconstrictor, for relief of allergic conjunctivitis; emedastine difumarate also is used. Cromolyn sodium has found some use in treating conjunctivitis that is thought to be allergen mediated, such as vernal conjunctivitis. The mast cell stabilizer lodoxamide tromethamine is available for ophthalmic use for the treatment of ocular inflammatory states such as vernal conjunctivitis and keratitis. Nedocromil, primarily a mast cell stabilizer with some antihistaminic properties, is also used. Likewise, olopatadine hydrochloride, ketotifen fumarate, bepotastine,

azelastine, and alcaftadine are H$_1$ antagonists with mast cell–stabilizing properties. Epinastine antagonizes H$_1$ and H$_2$ receptors and exhibits mast cell–stabilizing activity.

Immunosuppressants

Topical *cyclosporine* (Table 69–12) is approved for the treatment of chronic dry eye associated with inflammation. Use of cyclosporine is associated with decreased inflammatory markers in the lacrimal gland, increased tear production, and improved vision and comfort. Topical lifitegrast (Table 69–12) is approved to treat the signs and symptoms of dry eye disease. Lifitegrast inhibits an integrin, lymphocyte function-associated antigen 1 (LFA-1), from binding to intercellular adhesion molecule 1 (ICAM-1) which is thought to down-regulate inflammation mediated by

TABLE 69–12 ■ IMMUNOSUPPRESSIVE AND ANTIMITOTIC AGENTS FOR OCULAR USE

AGENT	FORMULATION	INDICATION	COMMENTS
Cyclosporine	0.05% emulsion	Dry eye	Dosed in preservative-free individual droperettes
Lifitegras	5% solution	Dry eye	Dosed in preservative-free individual droperettes
Interferon α$_{2B}$	Topical solution (1 million IU/mL); subconjunctival injection (3 million IU/0.5 mL; not in the U.S.)	Conjunctival tumors[a] Conjunctival papilloma	See Chapters 34 and 35
5-Fluorouracil	50-mg/mL solution	Glaucoma surgery	Used intraoperatively and postoperatively to prevent subconjunctival scarring Inhibits corneal epithelial healing; cannot be used if there is corneal abrasion
Mitomycin	0.2 mg/mL for topical application	Glaucoma surgery Pterygium surgery Corneal scarring and surface ablation surgery	Generally used as a subconjunctival application intraoperatively to prevent scarring More commonly used than 5FU in glaucoma surgery; not for injection Used topically on the cornea

T lymphocytes. *Interferon α$_{2b}$* is used off label in the treatment of conjunctival papilloma and certain conjunctival tumors.

Antimitotic Agents

In glaucoma surgery, the antineoplastic agents 5FU and mitomycin (Table 69–12; see details of mechanism in Chapter 66) improve the success of filtration surgery by limiting the postoperative wound-healing process.

Therapeutic Uses. Mitomycin is used intraoperatively as a single subconjunctival application at the trabeculectomy site. 5FU may be used intraoperatively at the trabeculectomy site or subconjunctivally during the postoperative course (Fluorouracil Filtering Surgery Study Group, 1996). Both agents work by limiting the healing process; sometimes this can result in thin, ischemic, avascular tissue that is prone to breakdown. The resultant leaks can cause hypotony (low IOP) and increase the risk of infection. In corneal surgery, mitomycin has been used topically. Mitomycin can be used to reduce the risk of scarring after procedures to remove corneal opacities and prophylactically to prevent corneal scarring after photorefractive and phototherapeutic keratectomy. Mitomycin also is used to treat certain conjunctival and corneal tumors and to decrease recurrence after pterygium excision. Caution is advocated when using mitomycin in light of the potentially serious delayed ocular complications.

Agents Used in Ophthalmic Surgery

Presurgical Antiseptics

Povidone iodine is formulated as a 5% sterile ophthalmic solution for use prior to surgery to prepare periocular skin and irrigate ocular surfaces, including the cornea, conjunctiva, and palpebral fornices. Following irrigation, the exposed tissues are flushed with sterile saline. Hypersensitivity to iodine is a contraindication.

Viscoelastic Substances

The viscoelastic substances are agents that assist in ocular surgery by maintaining spaces, moving tissue, and protecting surfaces. These substances are prepared from hyaluronate, chondroitin sulfate, or hydroxypropylmethylcellulose and share varying degrees of the following important physical characteristics: viscosity, shear flow, elasticity, cohesiveness, and coatability. Complications associated with viscoelastic substances are related to transient elevation of IOP after surgery.

Ophthalmic Glue

Cyanoacrylate tissue adhesive, while not FDA approved for the eye, is widely used in the management of corneal ulcerations and perforations.

Fibrin sealants are increasingly being used on the ocular surface to secure tissue such as conjunctiva, amniotic membrane, and lamellar corneal grafts.

Anterior Segment Gases

Sulfur hexafluoride (SF$_6$) and perfluoropropane gases are used as vitreous substitutes during retinal surgery. In the anterior segment, they are used in nonexpansile concentrations to treat Descemet's detachments, typically after cataract surgery. These detachments can cause mild-to-severe corneal edema. The gas is injected into the anterior chamber to push Descemet's membrane up against the stroma, where ideally it reattaches and clears the corneal edema. Similarly, these gases can be used after endothelial keratoplasty to help the lamellar graft adhere to the posterior cornea. SF$_6$ is an interesting molecule: octahedral geometry about the central S; a dense (6.1 g/ml) gas; odorless and nonflammable; industrial use; and a potent greenhouse gas with a long atmospheric $t_{1/2}$.

Vitreous Substitutes

Several compounds, including gases, perfluorocarbon liquids, and silicone oils, are available as vitreous substitutes (Table 69–13). Their primary use is reattachment of the retina following vitrectomy and membrane-peeling procedures for complicated proliferative vitreoretinopathy and traction retinal detachments. The use of expansile gases carries the risk of complications from elevated IOP, subretinal gas, corneal edema, and cataract formation. The gases are absorbed over a period of days (for air) to 2 months (for perfluoropropane).

The liquid perfluorocarbons (specific gravity 1.76–1.94) are denser than vitreous and are helpful in flattening the retina when vitreous is present. Silicone oil (polydimethylsiloxanes) is used for long-term tamponade of the retina. Complications from silicone oil use include glaucoma, cataract formation, corneal edema, corneal band keratopathy, and retinal toxicity.

Surgical Hemostasis and Thrombolytic Agents

Hemostasis has an important role in most surgical procedures and usually is achieved by temperature-mediated coagulation. Intravitreal administration of thrombin can assist in controlling intraocular hemorrhage during vitrectomy. When used intraocularly, a potentially significant inflammatory response may occur that can be minimized by thorough irrigation after hemostasis is achieved.

During intraocular surgeries to assist evacuation of a hyphema, subretinal clot, or nonclearing vitreous hemorrhage, tPA (Chapter 27) has been used off label. tPA also has been administered subconjunctivally and intracamerally (i.e., controlled intraocular administration into the anterior segment) to lyse blood clots obstructing a glaucoma filtration site. The main complication related to the use of tPA is bleeding.

TABLE 69-13 ■ VITREOUS SUBSTITUTES

AGENT	DURATION OR VISCOSITY
Nonexpansile gases	
Air	Duration, 5–7 days
Ar, CO_2, He, Kr, N_2, O_2	
Xe	Duration, 1 day
Expansile gases	
Sulfur hexafluoride (SF_6)	Duration, 10–14 days
Octafluorocyclobutane (C_4F_8)	
Perfluoromethane (CF_4)	Duration, 10–14 days
Perfluoroethane (C_2F_6)	Duration, 30–35 days
Perfluoropropane (C_3F_8)	Duration, 55–65 days
Perfluoro-n-butane (C_4F_{10})	
Perfluoropentane (C_5F_{12})	
Silicone oils[a]	
Nonfluorinated silicone oils	Viscosity: 1000–30,000 cs
Fluorosilicone	Viscosity: 1000–10,000 cs
"High-tech" silicone oils	May terminate as trimethylsiloxy or polyphenylmethyl-siloxane; viscosity not reported

cs, centistoke (unit of viscosity).
[a]For further information, see Parel and Villian, 1994.

Botulinum Toxin Type A in the Treatment of Strabismus, Blepharospasm, and Related Disorders

Two botulinum toxin type A preparations are marketed in the U.S.: onabotulinumtoxinA and abobotulinumtoxinA. OnabotulinumtoxinA is FDA approved for the treatment of strabismus and blepharospasm associated with dystonia, facial wrinkles (glabellar lines), bladder dysfunction and urinary incontinence, upper limb spasticity, axillary hyperhidrosis, spasmodic torticollis (cervical dystonia), and chronic migraine. By preventing acetylcholine release at the neuromuscular junction, botulinum toxin A usually causes a temporary paralysis of the locally injected muscles. Complications related to this toxin include double vision (diplopia), eyelid droop (ptosis), and, rarely, potentially life-threatening distant spread of toxin effect from the injection site (hours to weeks after administration).

Agents Used to Treat Blind and Painful Eye

Retrobulbar injection of either absolute or 95% ethanol may provide relief from chronic pain associated with a blind and painful eye. Retrobulbar chlorpromazine also has been used off label. This treatment is preceded by administration of local anesthesia. Local infiltration of the ciliary nerves provides symptomatic relief from pain, but other nerve fibers may be damaged, causing paralysis of the extraocular muscles, including those in the eyelids, or neuroparalytic keratitis. The sensory fibers of the ciliary nerves may regenerate, and repeated injections sometimes are needed to control pain.

Ocular Side Effects of Systemic Agents

Certain systemic drugs have ocular side effects. These can range from mild and inconsequential to severe and vision threatening (Li et al., 2008; Pula et al., 2013). Examples are listed in the sections that follow.

IOP and Glaucoma

The antiseizure drug topiramate can cause choroidal effusions leading to angle-closure glaucoma.

Retina

Numerous drugs have toxic side effects on the retina. The antiarthritis and antimalarial medicines hydroxychloroquine and chloroquine can cause central retinal toxicity by an unknown mechanism. With normal dosages, toxicity does not appear until about 6 years after the drug is started. Stopping the drug will not reverse the damage but generally will prevent further toxicity. Tamoxifen can cause crystalline maculopathy. The antiseizure drug vigabatrin causes progressive and permanent bilateral concentric visual field constriction in a high percentage of patients.

Optic Nerve

The PDE5 inhibitors sildenafil, vardenafil, and tadalafil inhibit PDE5 in the corpus cavernosum to help achieve and maintain penile erection (Chapter 45) and to treat pulmonary arterial hypertension (Chapter 31). The drugs also mildly inhibit PDE6, which controls the levels of cyclic GMP in the retina (see Figure 69–9), causing a bluish haze or light sensitivity. Multiple medications, including ethambutol, chloramphenicol, and rifampin, can cause toxic optic neuropathy characterized by gradually progressive bilateral central scotomas and vision loss. Systemic or ocular steroids can cause elevated IOP and glaucoma. If the steroids cannot be stopped, glaucoma medications, and even filtering surgery, often are required.

Anterior Segment

Steroids have been implicated in cataract formation. Tamoxifen, among other others, has also been associated with cataracts. Rifabutin, if used in conjunction with clarithromycin or fluconazole for treatment of *Mycobacterium avium* complex opportunistic infections in HIV-positive persons, is associated with an iridocyclitis and even hypopyon. These conditions resolve with steroids or by stopping the medication.

Ocular Surface

Isotretinoin has a drying effect on mucous membranes and is associated with dry eye and severe dysfunction of the meibomian gland.

Cornea, Conjunctiva, and Eyelids

The cornea, conjunctiva, and eyelids can be affected by systemic medications. One of the most common drug deposits found in the cornea is from the cardiac medication amiodarone. It deposits in the inferior and central cornea in a whorl-like pattern termed *cornea verticillata*, appearing as fine tan or brown pigment in the epithelium. The deposits seldom affect vision and are rarely a cause to discontinue the medication. The deposits disappear slowly when the medication is stopped. Other medications, including indomethacin, atovaquone, chloroquine, and hydroxychloroquine, can cause a similar pattern. The phenothiazines, including chlorpromazine and thioridazine, can cause brown pigmentary deposits in the cornea, conjunctiva, and eyelids. They typically do not affect vision. The ocular deposits generally persist after discontinuation of the medication and can even worsen. Tetracyclines can cause a yellow discoloration of the light-exposed conjunctiva. Systemic minocycline can induce a blue-gray scleral pigmentation that is most prominent in the interpalpebral zone. Certain chemotherapeutic agents, such as cytarabine, can cause temporary corneal toxicity.

Agents Used to Assist in Ocular Diagnosis

A number of agents are used in an ocular examination (e.g., mydriatic agents, topical anesthetics, dyes to evaluate corneal surface integrity); to facilitate intraocular surgery (e.g., mydriatic and miotic agents, topical and local anesthetics); and to help in making a diagnosis in cases of anisocoria and retinal abnormalities (e.g., intravenous contrast agents). The autonomic agents have been discussed previously. The diagnostic and therapeutic uses of topical and intravenous dyes and of topical anesthetics are discussed in the material that follows.

Anterior Segment and External Diagnostic Uses

Epiphora (excessive tearing) and surface problems of the cornea and conjunctiva are commonly encountered external ocular disorders. The dyes *fluorescein, rose bengal*, and *lissamine green* are used in evaluating these problems. Fluorescein (Figure 69–7; available as 10% and 25% solutions for injection and as an impregnated paper strip) reveals epithelial defects of the cornea and conjunctiva and aqueous humor leakage that may occur after trauma or ocular surgery. In the setting of epiphora, fluorescein is used to determine the patency of the nasolacrimal system. In addition, this dye is used in *applanation tonometry* (IOP measurement) and to assist

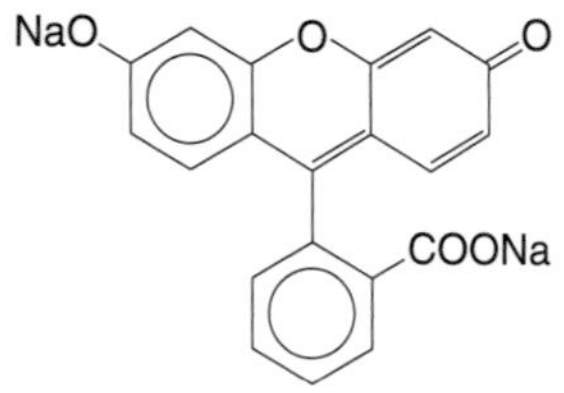

FLUORESCEIN SODIUM

Figure 69–7 *The diagnostic dye fluorescein.*

in determining the proper fit of rigid and semirigid contact lenses. Fluorescein in combination with proparacaine or benoxinate is available for procedures in which a disclosing agent is needed in conjunction with a topical anesthetic. Fluorexon, a high-molecular-weight fluorescent solution, is used when fluorescein is contraindicated (as when soft contact lenses are in place). *Rose bengal* and *lissamine green* (available as saturated paper strips) stain devitalized tissue on the cornea and conjunctiva.

Posterior Segment Diagnostic Uses

The integrity of the blood-retinal and retinal pigment epithelial barriers may be examined directly by retinal angiography using intravenous administration of either *fluorescein sodium* or *indocyanine green*. These agents commonly cause nausea and may precipitate serious allergic reactions in susceptible individuals.

Treatment of Retinal Neovascularization, Macular Degeneration, and Vitreomacular Traction

The medical treatment of retinal neovascularization has been changing rapidly in the past several years and will likely continue to do so (Agarwal et al., 2015). Current treatment employs agents that inhibit the actions of VEGF (Table 69–14).

Verteporfin is approved for photodynamic therapy of the exudative form of ARMD with predominantly classic choroidal neovascular membranes. Verteporfin also is used in the treatment of predominantly classic choroidal neovascularization caused by conditions such as pathological myopia and presumed ocular histoplasmosis syndrome. Verteporfin is administered intravenously; once it reaches the choroidal circulation, the drug is light activated by a nonthermal laser source. Activation of the drug in the presence of O_2 generates free radicals, which cause vessel damage and subsequent platelet activation, thrombosis, and occlusion of choroidal neovascularization. The $t_{1/2}$ of the drug is 5–6 h; it is eliminated predominantly in the feces. Potential side effects include headache, injection site reactions, and visual disturbances. The drug causes temporary photosensitization; patients must avoid exposure of the skin or eyes to direct sunlight or bright indoor lights for 5 days after receiving verteporfin.

Pegaptanib, a selective VEGF antagonist, is approved for neovascular (wet) ARMD. $VEGF_{165}$ induces angiogenesis and increases vascular permeability and inflammation, which actions likely contribute to the progression of the neovascular (wet) form of ARMD, a leading cause of blindness. Pegaptanib inhibits $VEGF_{165}$ binding to VEGF receptors. Pegaptanib (0.3 mg) is administered once every 6 weeks by intravitreous injection into the eye to be treated. Following the injection, patients should be monitored for elevation in IOP and for endophthalmitis. Rare cases of anaphylaxis/anaphylactoid reactions have been reported.

Aflibercept is a recombinant fusion protein, consisting of portions of human VEGF receptors 1 and 2, that acts as a soluble decoy receptor for VEGF-A. It is approved for the neovascular (wet) form of ARMD as well as macular edema following retinal vein occlusion or associated with diabetic retinopathy. Depending on the underlying disease, aflibercept (2 mg) is administered once every month by intravitreous injection into the eye for 3–5 months, followed by 2 mg once every 8 weeks. Serious side effects may include eye pain or redness, swelling, vision problems, photosensitivity, headaches, sudden numbness on one side of the body, confusion, and problems with speech and balance. The drug is contraindicated in patients who have an active eye infection or active ocular inflammation.

Bevacizumab is a monoclonal murine antibody that targets VEGF-A and thereby inhibits vascular proliferation and tumor growth (see Chapter 67). Intraocular use is considered off label but is routinely done. *Ranibizumab* is a variant of bevacizumab that has had the Fab domain affinity matured. Both drugs are delivered by intravitreal injection and often are used on a weekly or monthly basis for maintenance therapy. Both have been associated with the risk of cerebral vascular accidents. The enormous cost difference between these similar antibodies has sparked a debate about the cost-effectiveness of treatment strategies (Shaikh et al., 2015; Stein et al., 2014), especially in light of recent data indicating similar visual acuity outcomes for each medicine (CATT Research Group, 2011).

Ocriplasmin is a proteolytic enzyme that is used to treat vitreomacular traction. It works to dissolve the vitreous and relieve traction on the macula in the center of the retina. An interesting side effect is the possibility of lens subluxation from zonular dehiscence.

Anesthetics in Ophthalmic Procedures

Topical anesthetic agents used clinically in ophthalmology include proparacaine and tetracaine drops, lidocaine gel (see Chapter 22), and intranasal cocaine. Cocaine may be used intranasally in combination with topical anesthesia for cannulating the nasolacrimal system. Lidocaine and

TABLE 69–14 ■ ANTI-VEGF AGENTS FOR OCULAR USE

AGENT	FORMULATION	INDICATION	COMMENTS
Verteporfin	2-mg/mL reconstituted solution for intravenous infusion	Retinal neovascularization associated with macular degeneration	Dosed according to body surface area Activated by a cool laser as it circulates in the retinal circulation Causes photosensitization and propensity for sunburn
Pegaptanib	0.3-mg intravitreal injection	Same as verteporfin	Binds to the 165 isoform of VEGF
Aflibercept	2 mg/0.5 mL–intravitreal injection	Same as verteporfin *plus* DME or for the treatment of diabetic retinopathy in patients with DME	A decoy receptor for VEGF-A
Bevacizumab	1.25-mg intravitreal injection	Same as afibercept	First anti-VEGF antibody commercially available; generally used off label as first-line therapy Made by compounding pharmacies
Ranibizumab	0.3 mg/0.5 mL–intravitreal injection	Same as afibercept	A variant of bevacizumab

bupivacaine are used for infiltration and retrobulbar block anesthesia for surgery. Potential complications and risks relate to allergic reactions, globe perforation, hemorrhage, and vascular and subdural injections. Both preservative-free lidocaine (1%), which is introduced into the anterior chamber, and lidocaine jelly (2%), which is placed on the ocular surface during preoperative patient preparation, are used for cataract surgery performed under topical anesthesia. Most inhalational agents and CNS depressants are associated with a reduction in IOP. An exception is ketamine, which has been associated with an elevation in IOP. In the setting of a patient with a ruptured globe, the anesthesia should be selected carefully to avoid agents that depolarize the extraocular muscles, which may result in expulsion of intraocular contents.

Wetting Agents, Tear Substitutes, Osmotic Agents

The current management of dry eyes usually includes instilling artificial tears and other ophthalmic lubricants. In general, tear substitutes are hypotonic or isotonic solutions composed of electrolytes, surfactants, preservatives, and some viscosity-increasing agent that prolongs the residence time in the cul-de-sac and precorneal tear film.

Common viscosity agents include cellulose polymers, polyvinyl alcohol, polyethylene glycol, polysorbate, mineral oil, glycerin, and dextran. The tear substitutes are available as preservative-containing or preservative-free preparations. The viscosity of the tear substitute depends on its exact formulation and can range from watery to gel like. Some tear formulations also are combined with a vasoconstrictor, such as naphazoline, phenylephrine, or tetrahydrozoline. The lubricating ointments are composed of a mixture of white petrolatum, mineral oil, liquid or alcohol lanolin, and sometimes a preservative. These highly viscous formulations cause considerable blurring of vision; consequently, they are used primarily at bedtime, in critically ill patients, or in very severe dry eye conditions. A hydroxypropyl cellulose ophthalmic insert that is placed in the inferior cul-de-sac and dissolves during the day is available to treat dry eyes.

Local eye disease, such as blepharitis, ocular rosacea, ocular pemphigoid, chemical burns, or corneal dystrophies, may alter the ocular surface and change the tear composition. Appropriate treatment of the symptomatic dry eye includes treating the accompanying disease and possibly the addition of tear substitutes, punctal plugs (see Absorption), or ophthalmic cyclosporine (see Immunosuppressants). There also are a number of systemic conditions that may manifest themselves with symptomatic dry eyes, including Sjögren syndrome, rheumatoid arthritis, vitamin A deficiency, Stevens-Johnson syndrome, and trachoma. Treating the systemic disease may not eliminate the symptomatic dry

eye complaints; chronic therapy with tear substitutes, ophthalmic cyclosporine, insertion of punctal plugs, placement of dissolvable collagen implants, or surgical occlusion of the lacrimal drainage system may be indicated. Ophthalmic cyclosporine can be used to increase tear production in patients with ocular inflammation associated with keratoconjunctivitis sicca.

The main osmotic drugs for ocular use are glycerin, mannitol, and hypertonic saline. Glycerin and mannitol are used for short-term management of acute rises in IOP. Sporadically, these agents are used intraoperatively to dehydrate the vitreous prior to anterior segment surgical procedures. Many patients with acute glaucoma do not tolerate oral medications because of nausea; therefore, intravenous administration of mannitol or acetazolamide may be preferred over oral administration of glycerin. These agents should be used with caution in patients with congestive heart failure or renal failure.

Corneal edema is a clinical sign of corneal endothelial dysfunction, and topical osmotic agents may effectively dehydrate the cornea. NaCl is available in either aqueous or ointment formulations. Topical glycerin also is available; however, because it causes pain on contact with the cornea and conjunctiva, its use is limited to urgent evaluation of filtration-angle structures. In general, when corneal edema occurs secondary to acute glaucoma, the use of an oral osmotic agent to help reduce IOP is preferred over topical glycerin, which simply clears the cornea temporarily. Reducing the IOP will help clear the cornea more permanently to allow both a view of the filtration angle by gonioscopy and a clear view of the iris as required to perform laser iridotomy.

Vitamin A and the Visual Cycle

Vitamin deficiencies can alter eye function, especially a deficiency of vitamin A (Table 69–15). In vision, the functional form of vitamin A is *retinal*; its deficiency interferes with vision in dim light, contributing to a condition known as *night blindness* (nyctalopia).

Chemistry

Retinoid refers to the chemical entity *retinol* and other closely related naturally occurring derivatives. Retinoids, which exert most of their effects by binding to specific nuclear receptors and modulating gene expression, also include structurally related synthetic analogues that need not have retinol-like (vitamin A) activity. The purified plant pigment carotene (provitamin A) is a protean source of vitamin A. β-Carotene is the most active

TABLE 69–15 ■ OPHTHALMIC EFFECTS OF SELECTED VITAMIN DEFICIENCIES AND ZINC DEFICIENCY

DEFICIENCY	EFFECTS IN ANTERIOR SEGMENT	EFFECTS IN POSTERIOR SEGMENT
Vitamin		
A (retinol)	Conjunctiva (Bitot spots, xerosis)	Retina (nyctalopia, impaired rhodopsin synthesis), retinal pigment epithelium (hypopigmentation)
	Cornea (keratomalacia, punctate keratopathy)	
B_1 (thiamine)	—	Optic nerve (temporal atrophy with corresponding visual field defects)
B_6 (pyridoxine)	Cornea (neovascularization)	Retina (gyrate atrophy)
B_{12} (cyanocobalamin)	—	Optic nerve (temporal atrophy with corresponding visual field defects)
C (ascorbic acid)	Lens (? cataract formation)	—
E (tocopherol)	—	Retina and retinal pigment epithelium (? macular degeneration)
Folic acid	—	Vein occlusion
K	Conjunctiva (hemorrhage)	Retina (hemorrhage)
	Anterior chamber (hyphema)	
Zinc	—	Retina and retinal pigment epithelium (? macular degeneration)

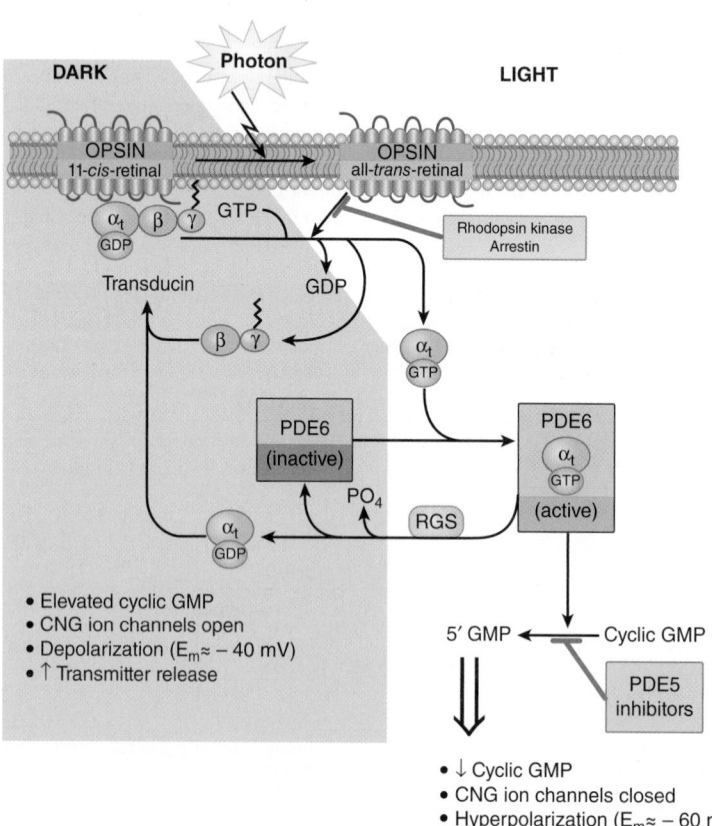

Figure 69–8 *β-Carotene and some members of the vitamin A family of retinoids.*

carotenoid found in plants. The structural formulas for β-carotene and the vitamin A family of retinoids are shown in Figure 69–8. Retinoic acid analogues used clinically are discussed in detail in Chapter 70.

Retinal Cells and the Visual Cycle

Photoreception is accomplished by two types of specialized retinal cells, *rods* and *cones*. Rods are especially sensitive to light of low intensity; cones act as receptors of high-intensity light and are responsible for color vision. The chromophore of both rods and cones is 11-*cis*-retinal. The holoreceptor in rods is termed *rhodopsin*—a combination of the protein opsin and 11-*cis*-retinal attached as a prosthetic group. The three different types of cone cells (red, green, and blue) contain individual, related, photoreceptor

proteins and respond optimally to light of different wavelengths. Several review articles summarized the process of photoreception (Kefalov, 2012; Saari, 2016). Figure 69–9 summarizes the signaling pathway initiated by absorption of a photon by 11-*cis*-retinal in rods.

Vitamin A Deficiency

Vitamin A is an essential nutrient with multiple functions in the body, including the eye (Sommer and Vyas, 2012). Humans deficient in vitamin A lose their ability for dark adaptation. Rod vision is affected more than cone vision. On depletion of retinol from liver and blood, usually at plasma concentrations of retinol of less than 0.2 mg/L (0.70 μM), the concentrations of retinol and rhodopsin in the retina fall. Unless the deficiency

Figure 69–9 *Pharmacologist's view of photoreceptor signaling.* CNG, cyclic nucleotide gated; RGS, regulator of G-protein signaling.

is overcome, opsin, lacking the stabilizing effect of retinal, decays, and anatomical deterioration of the rod outer segment occurs.

Vitamin A and Epithelial Structures

In the presence of retinol or retinoic acid, basal epithelial cells are stimulated to produce mucus. Excessive concentrations of the retinoids lead to the production of a thick layer of mucin, the inhibition of keratinization, and the display of goblet cells. In the absence of vitamin A, goblet mucous cells disappear and are replaced by basal cells that have been stimulated to proliferate. These undermine and replace the original epithelium with a stratified, keratinizing epithelium. The suppression of normal secretions leads to irritation and infection. Reversal of these changes is achieved by the administration of retinol, retinoic acid, or other retinoids. When this process happens in the cornea, severe hyperkeratinization (xerophthalmia) may lead to permanent blindness (McLaren and Kraemer, 2012). Common causes of vitamin A deficiency include malnutrition and bariatric surgery.

Retinoic acid influences gene expression by combining with nuclear receptors (see Figures 3–12 and 6–8). There are two families of retinoid receptors: the RARs and the RXRs. The endogenous RXR ligand is 9-*cis*-retinoic acid.

Therapeutic Uses of Vitamin A

Nutritional vitamin A deficiency causes *xerophthalmia*, a progressive disease characterized by *nyctalopia* (night blindness), *xerosis* (dryness), and *keratomalacia* (corneal thinning), which may lead to corneal perforation. Vitamin A therapy can reverse xerophthalmia; however, rapid, irreversible blindness ensues once the cornea perforates. Vitamin A also is involved in epithelial differentiation and may have a role in corneal epithelial wound healing. The current recommendation for retinitis pigmentosa is to administer 15,000 IU of vitamin A palmitate daily under the supervision of an ophthalmologist and to avoid high-dose vitamin E. Clinical studies suggested a reduction in the risk of progression of some types of ARMD by high doses of vitamin C (500 mg), vitamin E (400 IU), β-carotene (15 mg), cupric oxide (2 mg), and zinc (80 mg) (Age-Related Eye Disease Research Group, 2001a, 2001b; Chew et al., 2014), although substituting lutein/zeaxanthin for β-carotene may be more appropriate (Age-Related Eye Disease Study Research Group, 2007; Age-Related Eye Disease Study 2 [AREDS2] Research Group, 2014).

Bibliography

Agarwal A, et al. Management of neovascular age-related macular degeneration: current state-of-the-art care for optimizing visual outcomes and therapies in development. *Clin Ophthalmol*, **2015**, 9:1001–1015.

Ahmed Y, et al. Endophthalmitis following open-globe injuries. *Eye*, **2012**, 26:212–217.

Age-Related Eye Disease Study Research Group. A randomized, placebo-controlled, clinical trial of high-dose supplementation with vitamins C and E, beta carotene, and zinc for age-related macular degeneration and vision loss: AREDS report no. 8. *Arch Ophthalmol*, **2001a**, 119: 1417–1436. Erratum in *Arch Ophthalmol*, **2008**, 126:1251.

Age-Related Eye Disease Study Research Group. A randomized, placebo-controlled, clinical trial of high-dose supplementation with vitamins C and E and beta carotene for age-related cataract and vision loss: AREDS report no. 9. *Arch Ophthalmol*, **2001b**, 119:1439–1452. Erratum in *Arch Ophthalmol*, **2008**, 126:1251.

Age-Related Eye Disease Study Research Group. The relationship of dietary carotenoid and vitamin A, E, and C intake with age-related macular degeneration in a case-control study: AREDS report no. 22. *Arch Ophthalmol*, **2007**, 125:1225–1232.

Age-Related Eye Disease Study 2 (AREDS2) Research Group. Secondary analyses of the effects of lutein/zeaxanthin on age-related macular degeneration progression: AREDS2 report no. 3. *JAMA Ophthalmol*, **2014**, 132:142–149.

Beck RW, Gal RL. Treatment of acute optic neuritis: a summary of findings from the Optic Neuritis Treatment Trial. *Arch Ophthalmol*, **2008**, 126:994–995.

CATT Research Group. Ranibizumab and bevacizumab for neovascular age-related macular degeneration. *N Engl J Med*, **2011**, 364:1897–1908.

Chew EY, et al. Ten-year follow-up of age-related macular degeneration in the age-related eye disease study: AREDS report no. 36. *JAMA Ophthalmol*, **2014**, 132:272–277.

Chew HF, et al. Clinical outcomes and prognostic factors associated with acanthamoeba keratitis. *Cornea*, **2011**, 30:435–441.

Cohen EJ, Kessler J. Persistent dilemmas in zoster eye disease. *Br J Ophthalmol*, **2016**, 100:56–61.

Collaborative Normal-Tension Glaucoma Study Group. Comparison of glaucomatous progression between untreated patients with normal-tension glaucoma and patients with therapeutically reduced intraocular pressures. *Am J Ophthalmol*, **1998a**, 126:487–497.

Collaborative Normal-Tension Glaucoma Study Group. The effectiveness of intraocular pressure reduction in the treatment of normal-tension glaucoma. *Am J Ophthalmol*, **1998b**, 126:498–505.

Dua HS, et al. Human corneal anatomy redefined: a novel pre-Descemet's layer (Dua's layer). *Ophthalmology*, **2013**, 120:1778–1785.

Ederer F, et al. The Advanced Glaucoma Intervention Study (AGIS): 13. Comparison of treatment outcomes within race: 10-year results. *Ophthalmology*, **2004**, 111:651–664.

Endophthalmitis Vitrectomy Study Group. Results of the Endophthalmitis Vitrectomy Study. A randomized trial of immediate vitrectomy and of intravenous antibiotics for the treatment of postoperative bacterial endophthalmitis. *Arch Ophthalmol*, **1995**, 113:1479–1496.

Fluorouracil Filtering Surgery Study Group. Five-year follow-up of the fluorouracil filtering surgery study. *Am J Ophthalmol*, **1996**, 121:349–366.

Heijl A, et al. Reduction of intraocular pressure and glaucoma progression: results from the Early Manifest Glaucoma Trial. *Arch Ophthalmol*, **2002**, 120:1268–1279.

Herpetic Eye Disease Study Group. A controlled trial of oral acyclovir for the prevention of stromal keratitis or iritis in patients with herpes simplex virus epithelial keratitis. The Epithelial Keratitis Trial. *Arch Ophthalmol*, **1997**, 115:703–712. Erratum in *Arch Ophthalmol*, **1997**, 115:1196.

Herpetic Eye Disease Study Group. Acyclovir for the prevention of recurrent herpes simplex virus eye disease. *N Engl J Med*, **1998**, 339: 300–306.

Hoti SL, Tandon V. Ocular parasitoses and their immunology. *Ocul Immunol Inflamm*, **2011**, 19:385–396. doi:10.3109/09273948.2011.62 6141.

Kass MA, et al. The Ocular Hypertension Treatment Study: a randomized trial determines that topical ocular hypotensive medication delays or prevents the onset of primary open-angle glaucoma. *Arch Ophthalmol*, **2002**, 120:701–713; discussion 829–830.

Kefalov VJ. Rod and cone visual pigments and phototransduction through pharmacological, genetic, and physiological approaches. *J Biol Chem*, **2012**, 287:1635–1641.

Li J, et al. Drug-induced ocular disorders. *Drug Saf*, **2008**, 31:127–141.

Maenz M, et al. Ocular toxoplasmosis past, present and new aspects of an old disease. *Prog Retin Eye Res*, **2014**, 39:77–106.

McLaren DS, Kraemer K. Xerophthalmia. *World Rev Nutr Diet*, **2012**, 103:65–75.

Miglior S, et al. Results of the European Glaucoma Prevention Study. *Ophthalmology*, **2005**, 112:366–375.

Musch DC, et al. Intraocular pressure control and long-term visual field loss in the Collaborative Initial Glaucoma Treatment Study. *Ophthalmology*, **2011**, 118:1766–1773.

Newman H, Gooding C. Viral ocular manifestations: a broad overview. *Rev Med Virol*, **2013**, 23:281–294.

Parel JM, Villain F. Silicone oils: physicochemical properties. In: Ryan SR, Glaser BM, eds. *Retina, Vol. 3: Surgical Retina*. St. Louis, Mosby, **1994**, 2131–2149.

Pediatric Eye Disease Investigator Group. A comparison of atropine and patching treatments for moderate amblyopia by patient age, cause of amblyopia, depth of amblyopia, and other factors. *Ophthalmology*, **2003**, 110:1632–1638.

1270 Pediatric Eye Disease Investigator Group. A randomized trial of atropine vs. patching for treatment of moderate amblyopia in children. *Arch Ophthalmol*, **2002**, *120*:268–278.

Pula JH, et al. Neuro-ophthalmologic side-effects of systemic medications. *Curr Opin Ophthalmol*, **2013**, *24*:540–549.

Saari JC. Vitamin A and Vision. In: Asson Batres M, Rochette-Egly C, eds. *The Biochemistry of Retinoid Signaling II*. In the series: *Subcell Biochem 81*:231–259, Springer, Dordrecht, Netherlands, **2016**.

Schiedler V, et al. Culture-proven endogenous endophthalmitis: clinical features and visual acuity outcomes. *Am J Ophthalmol*, **2004**, *137*: 725–731.

Shaikh AH, et al. Cost comparison of intravitreal aflibercept with bevacizumab and ranibizumab for the treatment of wet age-related macular degeneration. *Ophthalmic Surg Lasers Imaging Retina*, **2015**, *46*:62–66.

Sommer A, Vyas KS. A global clinical view on vitamin A and carotenoids. *Am J Clin Nutr*, **2012**, *96*:1204S–1206S.

Stein JD, et al. Cost-effectiveness of bevacizumab and ranibizumab for newly diagnosed neovascular macular degeneration. *Ophthalmology*, **2014**, *121*:936–945.

Sucher NJ, et al. Molecular basis of glutamate toxicity in retinal ganglion cells. *Vision Res*, **1997**, *37*:3483–3493.

Tham YC, et al. Global prevalence of glaucoma and projections of glaucoma burden through 2040: a systematic review and meta-analysis. *Ophthalmology*, **2014**, *121*:2081–2090.

Volpe NJ. The optic neuritis treatment trial: a definitive answer and profound impact with unexpected results. *Arch Ophthalmol*, **2008**, *126*:996–999.

Yabiku ST, et al. Ganciclovir 0.15% ophthalmic gel in the treatment of adenovirus keratoconjunctivitis. *Arq Bras Oftalmol*, **2011**, *74*:417–421.

Young RC, et al. Incidence, recurrence, and outcomes of herpes simplex virus eye disease in Olmsted County, Minnesota, 1976–2007: the effect of oral antiviral prophylaxis. *Arch Ophthalmol*, **2010**, *128*: 1178–1183.

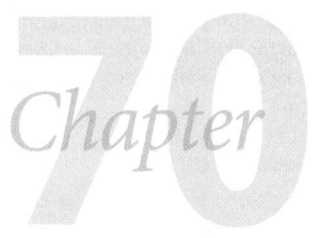

Dermatological Pharmacology

Matthew J. Sewell, Craig N. Burkhart, and Dean S. Morrell

Principles of Dermatological Pharmacology

The skin is a biologically active, multifunctional, and multicompartment organ. Medications can be applied to the skin for two purposes: to directly treat disorders of the skin and to deliver drugs to other tissues. Effective and safe use of topical pharmacological therapies requires an understanding of skin physiology and factors influencing percutaneous drug absorption and metabolism (Hwa et al., 2011; Wolff et al., 2008). General features of skin structure and percutaneous absorption pathways are outlined in Figure 70–1.

Nonpharmacological therapy is also used for treatment of skin diseases. This includes the use of parts of the electromagnetic spectrum applied by various sources, such as lasers, X-rays, visible light, and infrared light. These approaches may be used alone or to enhance the penetration or alter the nature of drugs and prodrugs. Freezing and ultrasound are other physical therapies that alter epidermal structure for direct treatment or to enhance percutaneous absorption of drugs. Chemicals are also used to decrease the effect of various wavelengths of UV light and ionizing radiation on the skin.

Structure of Skin

Stratum Corneum

The stratum corneum is the major barrier to percutaneous absorption of drugs and to the loss of water from the body. It may be considered the "nonliving" portion of the epidermis. The stratum corneum differs in thickness at different body sites, with the palm and sole the thickest followed by the general body stratum corneum, facial and postauricular area, and the eyelid and scrotum.

A drug may partition into the stratum corneum and form a reservoir that will diffuse into the rest of skin even *after* topical application of the drug has ceased.

Living Epidermis

The living layers of the epidermis (stratum basale, stratum spinosum, and stratum granulosum) with metabolically active cells comprise a layer about 100 μm thick (Figure 70–1). Intercalated in the living epidermis are pigment-producing cells (melanocytes), neuroendocrine cells (Merkel cells), dendritic APCs (Langerhans cells), and other immune cells (γ-δ T cells). In diseased epidermis, many additional immunological cells, including lymphocytes and polymorphonuclear leukocytes, may be present and be directly affected by applied drugs.

Dermis and Its Blood Vessels

The dermis provides mechanical strength and flexibility to the skin. It is composed primarily of fibroblasts and an extracellular matrix, including collagen, proteoglycans, glycoproteins, and, in the upper dermis, elastic fibers. Cells within the dermis that may be targets for drugs include mast cells (permanent residents and producers of many inflammatory

Abbreviations

APC: antigen-presenting cell
BCC: basal cell carcinoma
BPO: benzoyl peroxide
CBC: complete blood cell count
CLA: cutaneous lymphocyte-associated antigen
CTCL: cutaneous T-cell lymphoma
CTLA4: cytotoxic T lymphocyte–associated protein 4
CW: critical wavelength
DEET: diethyltoluamide (*N,N*-diethyl-*m*-toluamide)
5FU: 5-fluorouracil
GI: gastrointestinal
GM-CSF: granulocyte-macrophage colony-stimulating factor
G6PD: glucose-6-phosphate dehydrogenase
HDAC: histone deacetylase
HPA: hypothalamic-pituitary-adrenal
HPV: human papillomavirus
HSV: herpes simplex virus
IFN: interferon
IL: interleukin
IL-2R: IL-2 receptor
IV: intravenous
IVIG: intravenous immunoglobulin
Jak: Janus kinase
KS: Kaposi sarcoma
mAb: monoclonal antibody
MOA: mechanism of action
6MP: 6-mercaptopurine
MRSA: methicillin-resistant *Staphylococcus aureus*
mTOR: mammalian target of rapamycin
NSAID: nonsteroidal anti-inflammatory drug
OATP: organic anion-transporting polypeptide
ODC: ornithine decarboxylase
OTC: over the counter
PABA: *p*-aminobenzoic acid
PDE: phosphodiesterase
PDT: photodynamic therapy
PML: progressive multifocal leukoencephalopathy
PUVA: psoralen and UVA
RAR: retinoic acid receptor
RARE: retinoic acid–responsive element
RXR: retinoid X receptor
SC: subcutaneous
SPF: sun protection factor
SSRI: selective serotonin reuptake inhibitor
SSTI: skin and soft-tissue infection
STAT: signal transducer and activator of transcription
TCI: topical calcineurin inhibitor
TLR: toll-like receptor
TNF-α: tumor necrosis factor α
TSH: thyroid-stimulating hormone
UV: ultraviolet
VDR: vitamin D receptor
VZV: varicella zoster virus

the total skin area, so this is not the primary route of absorption. Sweat glands are not known as a pathway for the absorption of drugs, but some drugs (e.g., griseofulvin) are excreted to the skin by this route. Below the dermis is the hypodermis or subcutaneous tissue, which provides insulation, cushioning, and an energy reservoir.

Mechanisms of Percutaneous Absorption

Percutaneous absorption occurs primarily through a tortuous intercellular route, with transcellular or appendageal routes playing a much smaller role. Passage through the stratum corneum is the rate-limiting step for percutaneous absorption. Preferable characteristics of topical drugs include

- low molecular mass ($\leq$500 Da);
- adequate solubility in both oil and water; and
- a high partition coefficient so the drug will selectively partition from the vehicle to the stratum corneum (Hwa et al., 2011; Tran, 2013).

Except for very small particles, water-soluble ions and polar molecules do not penetrate significantly through intact stratum corneum. The exact amount of drug entering or leaving the skin in clinical situations usually is not measured; rather, the clinical end point (e.g., reduction in inflammation) usually is the desired effect.

A hydrated stratum corneum allows more percutaneous absorption and often is achieved through the selection of drugs formulated in occlusive vehicles such as ointments and the use of plastic films, wraps, or bags for the hands and feet and shower or bathing caps for the scalp. Alternatively, medications that are impregnated on patches or tapes may be used. Occlusion may be associated with increased growth of bacteria and resultant infection (folliculitis) or maceration and breakdown of the epidermis. Absorption of most drugs across the skin is a passive process; heat generally increases penetration. Ultrasonic energy, electric currents (iontophoresis), minimally invasive microneedling, and fractional or ablative lasers also can be used to increase percutaneous absorption (Tran, 2013).

Transdermal drug delivery bypasses hepatic first-pass metabolism; however, the epidermis contains a variety of enzyme systems capable of metabolizing drugs that reach this compartment. A specific CYP isoform, CYP26A1, metabolizes retinoic acid and may control its level in the skin (Baron et al., 2001). In addition, transporter proteins that influence influx (OATP) or efflux (MDR [multidrug resistance transporter], P-glycoprotein) of certain xenobiotics are present in human keratinocytes (Baron et al., 2001). Genetic variants of enzymes that regulate the cellular influx and efflux of methotrexate have been associated with toxicity and effectiveness in patients with psoriasis (Warren et al., 2008).

Pharmacologic Implications of Epidermal Structure

When proposing topical application of medications, the healthcare provider must consider multiple factors, including proper dosage and frequency of application, extent and condition of the permeability barrier, patient age and weight, physical form of the preparation to be applied, and whether intralesional or systemic administration should be used (Table 70–1). Various drug vehicles have specific advantages and disadvantages (Table 70–2). Newer vehicles, such as liposomes and microgel formulations, can enhance solubilization of certain drugs, thereby enhancing topical penetration and diminishing irritancy (Rosen et al., 2014). *Children have a greater ratio of surface area to mass than adults do, so the same amount of topical drug can result in greater systemic exposure. Preterm infants have a markedly impaired barrier function until the epidermis keratinizes completely (Hwa et al., 2011). Many dermatological diseases also compromise barrier function, leading to increased percutaneous absorption.*

mediators) and infiltrating immune cells producing cytokines. The dermis also contains networks of nerves, blood vessels, and adnexal structures. The superficial capillary plexus between the epidermis and dermis is the site of the majority of the systemic absorption of cutaneous drugs (see Figure 70–1). There are large numbers of lymphatics as well. Hair follicles form a lipid-rich pathway for drug absorption but only constitute 0.1% of

Glucocorticoids

Glucocorticoids have immunosuppressive and anti-inflammatory properties. They are administered locally through topical and intralesional routes and systemically through intramuscular, intravenous, and oral routes. Mechanisms of glucocorticoid action are discussed in Chapter 46.

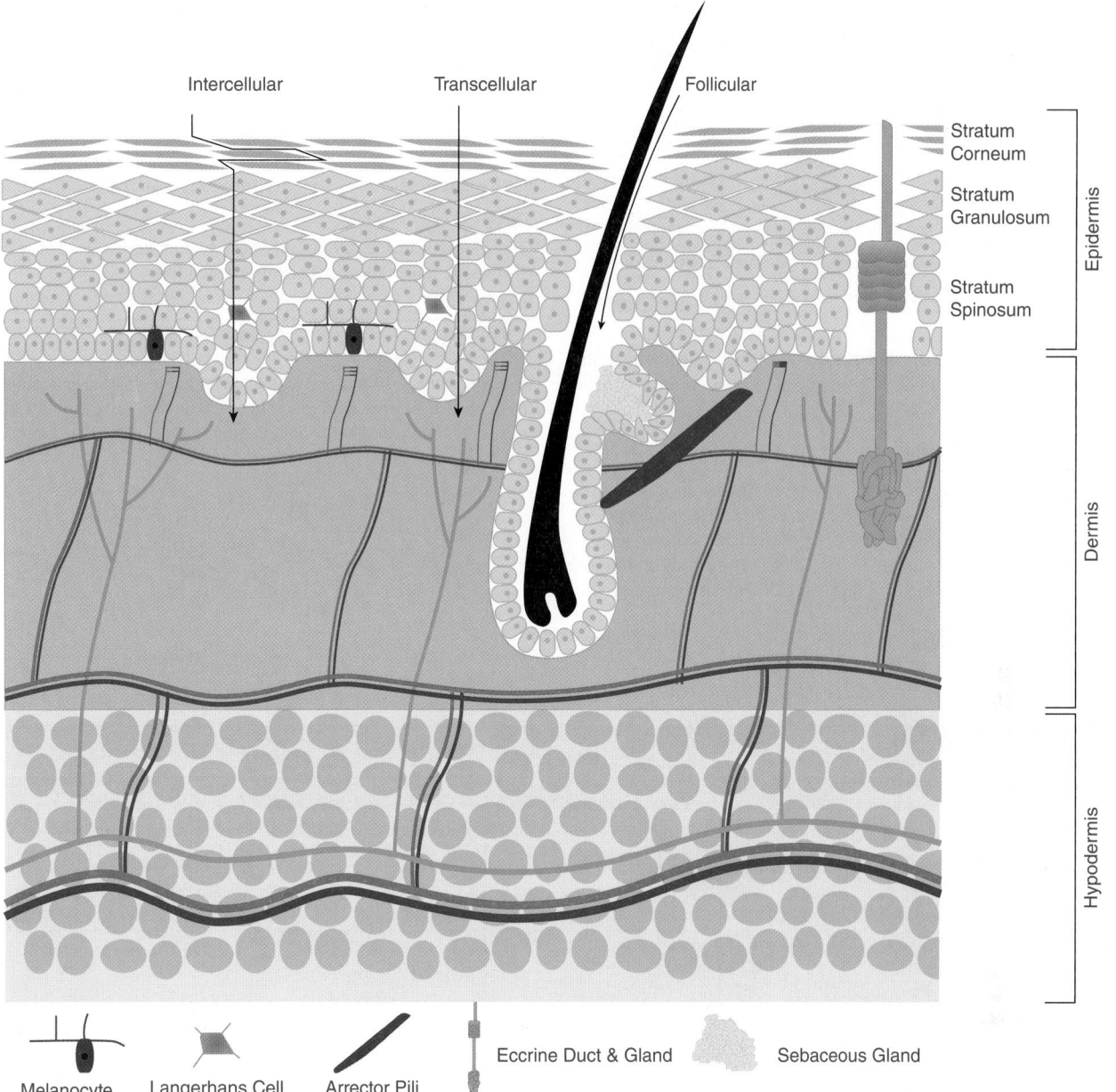

Figure 70–1 *Cutaneous drug absorption*. After application of a drug to the surface of the skin (stratum corneum), evaporation and structural/compositional alterations may occur that affect the drug's ultimate bioavailability. The stratum corneum limits drug diffusion into the lower layers and thence into the body. A number of absorptive routes are possible, singly or in combination: between the cells of the stratum corneum (*intercellular*), across the corneal cellular layer (*transcellular*), and into the concavity of a hair follicle (*follicular*) with its associated sebaceous glandular cells and arrector pili muscle that is innervated by the sympathetic branch of the autonomic nervous system. Melanocytes and Langerhans cells are accessible in the lower epidermis. In the epidermal and dermal layers, drugs may also reach the eccrine glands (sweat glands) and their ducts. Permeation to the dermis brings a drug in contact with lymphatics (in green) and cutaneous vessels carrying arterial and venous blood (red and blue, respectively). These vessels provide an absorptive route into the general circulation. Deeper permeation to the hypodermis may also occur.

Topical Glucocorticoids

Topical glucocorticoids have been grouped into seven classes in order of decreasing potency (Table 70–3). Potency traditionally is measured using a vasoconstrictor assay in which an agent is applied to skin under occlusion, and the area of skin blanching is assessed. Other assays of glucocorticoid potency involve suppression of erythema and edema after experimentally induced inflammation and the psoriasis bioassay, in which the effect of steroid on psoriatic lesions is quantified.

Therapeutic Uses

Many inflammatory skin diseases respond to topical or intralesional administration of glucocorticoids. Absorption varies amongst body sites and with the vehicle of the formulation. The steroid is selected on the basis of its potency, the site of involvement, and the severity of the skin disease. Often,

a more potent steroid is used initially, followed by a less potent agent. Twice-daily application of topical glucocorticoids suffices; more frequent application does not improve response. Moderately potent to very potent topical corticosteroids are effective with once-daily versus twice-daily application in atopic dermatitis, and patient adherence may be improved with once-daily regimens (Williams, 2007). In general, only nonfluorinated glucocorticoids should be used on the face or in occluded areas such as the axillae or groin. Intralesional preparations of glucocorticoids include insoluble preparations of triamcinolone acetonide and triamcinolone hexacetonide, which solubilize gradually and therefore have a prolonged duration of action.

Toxicity

Chronic use of class 1 topical glucocorticoids can cause skin atrophy, striae, telangiectasias, purpura, and acneiform eruptions. Because perioral

TABLE 70–1 ■ IMPORTANT CONSIDERATIONS WHEN A DRUG IS APPLIED TO THE SKIN

What are the absorption pathways of intact and diseased skin?
How does the chemistry of the drug affect the penetration?
How does the vehicle affect the penetration?
How much of the drug penetrates the skin?
What are the intended pharmacological targets?
What host and genetic factors influence drug function in the skin?
What are the predicted adverse effects (local, systemic)?

dermatitis and rosacea can develop after the use of fluorinated compounds on the face, they should not be used on this site. Occlusion increases the risk of HPA axis suppression.

Systemic Glucocorticoids

Systemic glucocorticoid therapy is used for severe dermatological illnesses and generally is reserved for allergic contact dermatitis to plants (e.g., poison ivy) and for life-threatening vesiculobullous dermatoses such as pemphigus vulgaris and bullous pemphigoid. Chronic administration of oral glucocorticoids is problematic, given the side effects associated with their long-term use (see Chapter 46).

Daily morning dosing with prednisone generally is preferred, although divided doses occasionally are used to enhance efficacy. Fewer side effects are seen with alternate-day dosing; if chronic therapy is required, prednisone usually is tapered to every other day as soon as practical. Pulse therapy using large intravenous doses of methylprednisolone sodium succinate is an option for severe resistant pyoderma gangrenosum, pemphigus vulgaris, systemic lupus erythematosus with multisystem disease, and dermatomyositis. The dose of intravenous methylprednisolone usually is 0.5–1 g given over 2–3 h. More rapid infusion has been associated with increased rates of hypotension, electrolyte shifts, and cardiac arrhythmias.

Toxicity and Monitoring

Oral glucocorticoids have numerous systemic effects, as discussed in Chapter 46. Most side effects are dose dependent.

Retinoids

Retinoids comprise natural and synthetic compounds that exhibit vitamin A–like biological activity or bind to nuclear receptors for retinoids. Characteristics of topical and systemic retinoids are summarized in Tables 70–4 and 70–5, respectively.

Tretinoin (all-*trans*-retinoic acid; vitamin A acid)

TABLE 70–2 ■ VEHICLES FOR TOPICALLY APPLIED DRUGS

	OINTMENT	CREAM	GEL	LOTION/SOLUTION/FOAM
Physical basis	Solid or liquid dispersed in nonaqueous base	Oil-in-water emulsion	Water-soluble emulsion with gelling agent	Lotion-suspended drug; Solution-dissolved drug base; Foam drug with surfactant as foaming agent and propellant
Solubilizing medium	Anhydrous to < 20% water	20%–80% water	Contains water-soluble polyethylene glycols; May have alcoholic solvent	May be aqueous or alcoholic
Pharmacological advantage	Protective oil film on skin	Leaves concentrated drug at skin surface	Concentrates drug at surface after evaporation	
Advantages for patient	Spreads easily; Slows water evaporation	Spreads and removes easily; No greasy feel	Nonstaining; Greaseless; Typically clear appearance	Low residue on scalp or other hairy areas; May have cooling effect when evaporates
Locations on body	Avoid intertriginous areas	Most locations	Scalp and other hairy locations	Scalp and other hairy locations
Disadvantages	Greasy; Stains clothes	Needs preservatives	Needs preservatives; Can be drying, especially if high alcohol content	Can be drying; May burn if alcohol content; Foams tend to be more expensive due to more complex delivery system
Occlusion	Moderate to high; Increases skin moisture	Low	None	None
Composition notes	Oleaginous base (e.g., white petrolatum) or Absorption base (e.g., hydrophilic petrolatum)	Requires humectants (glycerin, propylene glycol, polyethylene glycols) to keep moist when applied; Long-chain alcohol (e.g., stearyl alcohol) in oil phase for stability and smooth feel	Microspheres or microsponges can be formulated in gels	

TABLE 70-3 ■ POTENCY OF SELECTED TOPICAL GLUCOCORTICOIDS

	CLASS OF DRUG	GENERIC NAME, FORMULATION
Most potent	1	Betamethasone dipropionate cream, ointment 0.05% (in optimized vehicle)
		Clobetasol propionate cream, ointment 0.05%
		Diflorasone diacetate, ointment 0.05%
		Halobetasol propionate, ointment 0.05%
	2	Amcinonide, ointment 0.1%
		Betamethasone dipropionate, ointment 0.05%
		Desoximetasone, cream, ointment 0.25%, gel 0.05%
		Diflorasone diacetate, ointment 0.05%
		Fluocinonide, cream, ointment, gel 0.05%
		Halcinonide, cream, ointment 0.1%
	3	Betamethasone dipropionate, cream 0.05%
		Betamethasone valerate, ointment 0.1%
		Diflorasone diacetate, cream 0.05%
		Triamcinolone acetonide, ointment 0.1%, cream 0.5%
	4	Amcinonide, cream 0.1%
		Desoximetasone, cream 0.05%
		Fluocinolone acetonide, cream 0.2%
		Fluocinolone acetonide, ointment 0.025%
		Flurandrenolide, ointment 0.05%, impregnated tape 4 μg/cm²
		Hydrocortisone valerate, ointment 0.2%
		Triamcinolone acetonide, ointment 0.1%
		Mometasone furoate, cream, ointment 0.1%
	5	Betamethasone dipropionate, lotion 0.05%
		Betamethasone valerate, cream, lotion 0.1%
		Fluocinolone acetonide, cream 0.025%
		Flurandrenolide, cream 0.05%
		Hydrocortisone butyrate, cream 0.1%
		Hydrocortisone valerate, cream 0.2%
		Triamcinolone acetonide, cream, lotion 0.1%
		Triamcinolone acetonide, cream 0.025%
	6	Alclometasone dipropionate, cream, ointment 0.05%
		Desonide, cream 0.05%
		Fluocinolone acetonide, cream, solution 0.01%
Least potent	7	Hydrocortisone, cream, ointment, lotion 0.5%, 1%, 2.5%

First-generation retinoids include retinol (vitamin A), tretinoin (all-*trans*-retinoic acid; vitamin A acid), isotretinoin (13-*cis*-retinoic acid), and alitretinoin (9-*cis*-retinoic acid). *Second-generation retinoids*, also known as aromatic retinoids, include acitretin. *Third-generation retinoids* were designed to optimize receptor-selective binding and include tazarotene, bexarotene, and adapalene.

- *Mechanism of Action.* Retinoids exert their effects on gene expression by activating two families of receptors, *RARs* and *RXRs*, which are members of the steroid receptor superfamily. Both retinoid receptor families have three isoforms (α, β, and γ), which are expressed in unique

combinations in individual tissues and cells. On binding to a retinoid, RARs and RXRs form heterodimers (RAR-RXR) that subsequently bind specific DNA sequences called RAREs that activate transcription of genes whose products produce both the desirable pharmacological effects and the unwanted side effects of these drugs (see Tables 6–5, 70–4 and 70–5, and Figure 6–13).

- *Targeted Therapeutic Actions.* Retinoids that target RARs predominantly affect cellular differentiation and proliferation, whereas retinoids that target RXRs predominantly induce apoptosis. Hence, tretinoin, adapalene, and tazarotene, which target RARs, are used in acne, psoriasis, and photoaging (disorders of differentiation and proliferation), whereas bexarotene and alitretinoin, which target RXRs, are used in CTCL and Kaposi sarcoma, respectively, to induce apoptosis of malignant cells.
- *Retinoid Toxicity.* Acute retinoid toxicity is similar to vitamin A intoxication. Side effects of systemic retinoids include dry skin, nosebleeds from dry mucous membranes, conjunctivitis, reduced night vision, hair loss, alterations in serum lipids and transaminases, hypothyroidism, inflammatory bowel disease flare, musculoskeletal pain, pseudotumor cerebri, and mood alterations. RAR-selective retinoids are more associated with mucocutaneous and musculoskeletal symptoms, whereas RXR-selective retinoids induce more physiochemical changes. Because all oral retinoids are potent teratogens, they should be used carefully in females of childbearing potential and not in pregnant patients.

Topical Retinoids

Through incompletely understood mechanisms, topical retinoids correct abnormal follicular keratinization, reduce *Propionobacterium acnes* counts, and reduce inflammation, thereby making them the cornerstone of acne therapy. Topical retinoids are first-line agents for noninflammatory (comedonal) acne and often are combined with other agents in the management of inflammatory acne.

Fine wrinkles and dyspigmentation, two important features of photoaging, are also improved with topical retinoids. Within the dermis, this is believed to result from inhibition of AP-1, which normally activates synthesis of matrix metalloproteinases in response to UV irradiation (Thielitz and Gollnick, 2008). In the epidermis, retinoids induce epidermal hyperplasia in atrophic skin and reduce keratinocyte atypia.

Toxicity and Monitoring

Adverse effects of all topical retinoids include erythema, desquamation, burning, and stinging (see relative irritancy in Table 70–4). These effects often decrease with time and are lessened by concomitant use of emollients. Patients also may experience photosensitivity reactions (enhanced reactivity to UV radiation) and have a significant risk for severe sunburn. Although there is little systemic absorption of topical retinoids and no alteration in plasma vitamin A levels with their use, topical retinoids are not recommended for use during pregnancy.

Available Agents; Clinical Use

Tretinoin (all-*trans*-retinoic acid) is photolabile and should be applied once nightly for acne and photoaging. Benzoyl peroxide also inactivates tretinoin and should not be applied simultaneously. Formulations with copolymer microspheres or prepolyolprepolymer 2 that gradually release tretinoin to decrease irritancy are available and are less susceptible to oxidation by benzoyl peroxide and photodegradation.

Adapalene has similar efficacy to tretinoin, but unlike tretinoin, it is stable in sunlight or the presence of benzoyl peroxide and tends to be less irritating.

Tazarotene is approved for the treatment of psoriasis, photoaging, facial wrinkles, and acne vulgaris. Tazarotene gel, applied once daily, may be used as monotherapy or in combination with other medications, such as topical corticosteroids, for the treatment of localized plaque psoriasis. Topical corticosteroids improve the efficacy of therapy and reduce the side effects of burning, itching, and skin irritation that are commonly associated with tazarotene.

Alitretinoin is a retinoid that binds all types of retinoid receptors, both RARs and RXRs. It is approved for treatment of cutaneous lesions

TABLE 70–4 ■ TOPICAL RETINOIDS

DRUG	FORMULATION	RECEPTOR SPECIFICITY	PREGNANCY CATEGORY	IRRITANCY
Tretinoin	0.02%, 0.025%, 0.05%, 0.1% cream 0.01%, 0.025%, 0.04% gel 0.05%, 0.1% solution	RAR-α, RAR-β, RAR-γ	C	++
Tazarotene	0.05%, 0.1% cream 0.05%, 0.01% gel	RAR-α, RAR-β, RAR-γ	X	++++
Adapalene	0.1%, 0.3% cream 0.1%, 0.3% gel 0.1% solution	RAR-β, RAR-γ	C	+
Alitretinoin	0.1% gel	RAR-α, RAR-β, RAR-γ	D	++
Bexarotene	1% gel	RXR-α, RXR-β, RXR-γ	X	+++

of Kaposi sarcoma, with its application titrated up from twice daily to three or four times daily as tolerated. Alitretinoin should not be applied concurrently with insect repellants containing diethyltoluamide (DEET) because it may increase DEET absorption.

Bexarotene is approved for early-stage (IA and IB) CTCL. Its application is titrated up from every other day to two to four times daily over several weeks to improve patient tolerance. Concurrent application of bexarotene with insect repellants containing DEET is not recommended because it may increase DEET absorption.

Systemic Retinoids

Systemic retinoids (Table 70–5) are approved for the treatment of acne, psoriasis, and CTCL (Desai et al., 2007).

Therapeutic Uses and Contraindications

Off-label uses include ichthyosis, Darier disease, pityriasis rubra pilaris, rosacea, hidradenitis suppurativa, chemoprevention of malignancy, lichen sclerosus, subacute lupus erythematosus, and discoid lupus erythematosus. Absolute contraindications include use by women who are pregnant, planning to become pregnant, or breastfeeding. Relative contraindications include leukopenia, alcoholism, hyperlipidemia, hypercholesterolemia, hypothyroidism, and significant hepatic or renal disease.

Toxicity and Monitoring

Acute toxicities may include mucocutaneous or laboratory abnormalities; bony changes may occur after chronic use at high doses. Mucocutaneous side effects may include cheilitis, xerosis, blepharoconjunctivitis, cutaneous photosensitivity, photophobia, myalgia, arthralgia, headaches, alopecia, nail fragility, and increased susceptibility to staphylococcal infections. Some patients develop a "retinoid dermatitis" characterized by erythema, pruritus, and scaling. Very rarely, patients may develop pseudotumor cerebri, especially when systemic retinoids are combined with tetracyclines. There are reports that chronic administration at higher doses can cause diffuse idiopathic skeletal hyperostosis (DISH) syndrome, premature epiphyseal closure, and other skeletal abnormalities (Desai et al., 2007).

Systemic retinoids are highly teratogenic. There is no safe dose during pregnancy. Prescribing of isotretinoin in the U.S. is restricted via the risk-mitigation iPLEDGE system.

Serum lipid elevation is the most common laboratory abnormality. Less common laboratory abnormalities include elevated transaminases, decreased thyroid hormone, and leukopenia. A baseline evaluation of serum lipids, serum transaminases, and CBC should be obtained prior to starting any systemic retinoids. These laboratory values are usually subsequently checked monthly for the first 3–6 months and once every 3 months thereafter. In addition, two negative pregnancy tests on separate occasions are required for females of childbearing potential prior to starting acitretin or isotretinoin; bexarotene requires one negative pregnancy test within the week prior to initiating therapy. Monthly pregnancy tests should be obtained for females of childbearing potential.

Available Agents and Clinical Use

Isotretinoin is approved for the treatment of recalcitrant and nodular acne vulgaris. The drug has remarkable efficacy in severe acne and may induce prolonged remissions after a single course of therapy. Clinical effects generally are noted within 1–3 months of starting therapy. Approximately one-third of patients will relapse, usually within 3 years of stopping therapy. Although most relapses are mild and respond to conventional management with topical and systemic antiacne agents, some may require a second course of isotretinoin. Systemic absorption is improved when taken with a high-fat meal. An isotretinoin-Lidose formulation (a eutectic mixture of drug and lipids in a hard gelatin capsule) may be given without respect to meals.

Acitretin is approved for use in the cutaneous manifestations of psoriasis. Clinical effect may begin within 4–6 weeks, with the full clinical benefit occurring at 3–6 months. Acitretin has a $t_{1/2}$ of about 50 h; however, when combined with alcohol, acitretin is esterified in vivo to produce etretinate, which has a $t_{1/2}$ of more than 3 months. It is not known how much alcohol (i.e., cough syrup or other alcohol-based medications) is required to induce this conversion. Thus, female patients of childbearing potential should avoid pregnancy for 3 years after receiving acitretin to avoid retinoid-induced embryopathy.

TABLE 70–5 ■ SYSTEMIC RETINOIDS

DRUG	RECEPTOR SPECIFICITY	DOSING RANGE	$t_{1/2}$
Isotretinoin	No clear receptor affinity	0.5–2 mg/kg/d	10–20 h
Etretinate	RAR-α, RAR-β, RAR-γ	0.25–1 mg/kg/d	80–160 d
Acitretin	RAR-α, RAR-β, RAR-γ	0.5–1 mg/kg/d	50 h
Bexarotene	RXR-α, RXR-β, RXR-γ	300 mg/m²/d	7–9 h

Bexarotene is a retinoid that selectively binds RXRs. Oral and topical formulations of bexarotene are approved for use in patients with CTCL. Bexarotene reportedly induces apoptosis of malignant cells (Jawed et al., 2014). Because CYP3A4 metabolizes bexarotene, inhibitors of CYP3A4 (e.g., imidazole antifungals, macrolide antibiotics) will increase and inducers of CYP3A4 (e.g., rifamycins, carbamazepine, dexamethasone, efavirenz, phenobarbital) will decrease plasma levels of bexarotene. Side effects are more common than with other retinoids, with an increased incidence of significant lipid abnormalities and hypothyroidism secondary to a reversible RXR-mediated suppression of TSH gene expression, pancreatitis, leukopenia, and GI symptoms. Thyroid function should be measured before initiating therapy and periodically thereafter.

Vitamin Analogues

Calcipotriene

Calcipotriene is a topical vitamin D analogue that is used in the treatment of psoriasis.

Mechanism of Action

Calcipotriene exerts its effects through the VDR (see Chapter 48). On binding the VDR, the drug-receptor complex associates with the RXR-α and binds to vitamin D response elements on DNA, increasing expression of genes that modulate epidermal differentiation and inflammation, leading to improvement in psoriatic plaques (Menter et al., 2009a).

Therapeutic Use

Calcipotriene is applied twice daily to plaque psoriasis on the body, often in combination with topical corticosteroids. Hypercalcemia and hypercalciuria may develop when the cumulative weekly dose exceeds the recommended 100 g/week limit and resolves within days of discontinuation of calcipotriene (Menter et al., 2009a). Calcipotriene also causes perilesional irritation and mild photosensitivity. Concomitant administration of topical corticosteroids will reduce the irritation. Calcipotriene has been used off label for multiple conditions, including morphea, vitiligo, and congenital ichthyoses.

β-Carotene

β-Carotene is a precursor of vitamin A that is in green and yellow vegetables. No β-carotene products are currently FDA approved. Dietary supplementation with β-carotene is used in dermatology to reduce skin photosensitivity in patients with erythropoietic protoporphyria. The mechanism of action is not established but may involve an antioxidant effect that decreases the production of free radicals or singlet oxygen. A meta-analysis concluded that β-carotene, vitamin A, and vitamin E, given singly or combined with other antioxidant supplements, did not provide any benefit in lowering mortality or decreasing the risk of cerebrovascular accident. In addition, use of β-carotene and vitamin E led to an increase in all-cause mortality (Bjelakovic et al., 2012). The FDA's maximum recommended therapeutic dose (MRTD) for β-carotene is 0.05 mg/kg/d.

Photochemotherapy

Phototherapy and photochemotherapy are treatment methods in which UV or visible radiation is used to induce a therapeutic response either alone (phototherapy) or in the presence of an exogenous photosensitizing drug (photochemotherapy) (Table 70–6). Patients treated with these modalities should be monitored for concomitant use of other potential photosensitizing medications, such as phenothiazines, thiazides, sulfonamides, NSAIDs, sulfonylureas, tetracyclines, and benzodiazepines.

SECTION IX SPECIAL SYSTEMS PHARMACOLOGY

TABLE 70–6 ■ PHOTOCHEMOTHERAPY METHODS

	PUVA	PHOTOPHERESIS	PHOTODYNAMIC THERAPY
Target	Broad cutaneous area	Peripheral blood leukocytes	Focal cutaneous sites
Photosensitizing agent	Methoxsalen (8-methoxypsoralen)	Methoxsalen (8-methoxypsoralen)	Protoporphyrin IX
Method of drug administration	Oral Topical lotion Bathwater	To isolated plasma within photopheresis device	Topical cream or solution of a prodrug (aminolevulinic acid or methylaminolevulinate)
FDA-approved indications	Psoriasis Vitiligo	CTCL	Actinic keratosis
Activating wavelength	UVA2 (320–340 nm)	UVA2 (320–340 nm)	417 and 630 nm
Adverse effects (acute)	Phototoxic reactions Pruritus Hypertrichosis GI disturbance CNS disturbance Bronchoconstriction Hepatic toxicity HSV recurrence Retinal damage	Phototoxic reactions GI disturbance Hypotension Congestive heart failure	Phototoxic reactions Temporary dyspigmentation
Adverse effects (chronic)	Photoaging Nonmelanoma skin cancer Melanoma[a] Cataracts[a]	Loss of venous access after repeated venipuncture	Potential scarring
Pregnancy category	Risk cannot be ruled out	Evidence of risk[b]	Risk cannot be ruled out

[a]Controversial.
[b]Based on fetal toxicity in pregnant rats. No adequate studies in humans.
CNS, central nervous system; CTCL, cutaneous T cell lymphoma; GI, gastrointestinal; HSV, herpes simplex virus; UVA, ultraviolet A.

The UV radiation region may be subdivided into UVA1 (340–400 nm), UVA2 (320–340 nm), UVB (290–320 nm), and UVC (100–290 nm). UVC radiation is almost completely absorbed by the ozone layer and atmosphere so that measurable amounts do not reach Earth's surface. UVA and UVB exposure can cause sunburns, photoaging, and skin cancer development. UVB is the most erythrogenic and melanogenic, and it is the major action spectrum for sunburn, tanning, skin cancer, photoaging, and cutaneous vitamin D synthesis. UVA is only a thousandth as erythrogenic as UVB but penetrates more deeply into the skin and contributes substantially to photoaging and photosensitivity diseases. UVA is also able to penetrate clouds and glass, so exposure may occur even in the shade or while indoors. Both UVA and UVB cause photoimmune suppression, an effect that is utilized for therapy of certain dermatological conditions.

PUVA: Psoralens and UVA

The PUVA combines UVA light with photosensitizing compounds called psoralens. Orally administered methoxsalen (8-methoxypsoralen) followed by UVA (PUVA) is FDA approved for the treatment of vitiligo and psoriasis. It is also used off label in several other inflammatory or lymphoproliferative cutaneous disorders (Totonchy and Chiu, 2014).

Chemistry and Mechanism of Action

Psoralens are lipophilic, naturally occurring furocumarins found in some plants. Synthetic versions are also available. The action spectrum for PUVA is between 320 and 340 nm. Psoralens intercalate into the DNA strand, and two distinct photoreactions take place on UVA exposure. Type I reactions involve the oxygen-independent photoaddition of psoralens to pyrimidine bases in DNA. Type II reactions are oxygen dependent and involve the transfer of energy to molecular oxygen, creating reactive oxygen species. Through incompletely understood mechanisms, these phototoxic reactions stimulate melanocytes and induce antiproliferative, immunosuppressive, and anti-inflammatory effects.

Pharmacokinetics

Formulations of solubilized *methoxsalen* in a gel matrix are absorbed rapidly after oral administration, whereas older microcrystalline forms are absorbed slowly and incompletely. Fatty foods slow absorption and decrease peak blood levels. There is significant, but saturable, first-pass elimination in the liver. Peak photosensitivity varies significantly between individuals but typically is maximal 1–2 h after ingestion. Methoxsalen has a serum $t_{1/2}$ of about 1 h, but the skin remains sensitive to light for 8–12 h.

Therapeutic Uses

Oral *methoxsalen* is available as a single 10-mg strength either as soft gelatin capsules (solubilized) or hard gelatin capsules (micronized crystals). The dose is 10–70 mg, depending on weight (0.4–0.6 mg/kg), taken about 1.5–2 h before UVA exposure. Though administration with food can decrease absorption, it may minimize nausea. Topical application of psoralens followed by UVA exposure (topical PUVA) is also used for treatment. A lotion containing 1% methoxsalen is available for topical application for vitiligo. The methoxsalen lotion or capsules can be diluted in bathwater and used topically for localized palmoplantar (soak PUVA) or more diffuse (bath PUVA) areas to minimize systemic absorption. An extracorporeal solution is available for CTCL (see Photopheresis).

Approximately 70%–100% of psoriatic patients have clearing or virtual clearing of skin disease within about 24 treatments with PUVA. Remission typically lasts 3–6 months; thus, patients often require maintenance therapy with intermittent PUVA or other agents. Vitiligo typically requires between 150 and 300 treatments. Localized vitiligo can be treated with topical PUVA and more extensive disease with systemic administration. PUVA also is employed off label in the treatment of atopic dermatitis, alopecia areata, lichen planus, and urticaria pigmentosa.

Toxicity and Monitoring

The major side effects of PUVA are listed in Table 70–6. Phototoxicity is characterized by erythema, edema, blistering, and pruritus. Ocular toxicity can be prevented by wearing UVA-blocking glasses on the day of treatment. The risk of nonmelanoma skin cancer is dose dependent, with the greatest risk in those receiving more than 200–250 treatments (Totonchy and Chiu, 2014). There is a possible association between extensive PUVA exposure and melanoma, but there has been conflicting evidence regarding this association.

Photopheresis

Extracorporeal photopheresis (ECP) is a process in which extracorporeal peripheral blood mononuclear cells are separated using a leukapheresis-based method then exposed to UVA radiation in the presence of methoxsalen (Perotti and Sniecinski, 2015). Methoxsalen is injected directly into the extracorporeal plasma before radiation and reinfusion. The treated lymphocytes are returned to the patient, undergoing apoptosis over 48–72 h. The ECP is used for CTCL and off label for various other T-cell–mediated diseases, including graft-versus-host disease, transplantation rejection, and scleroderma. Patients receive ECP therapy on two consecutive days every 2–4 weeks, and intervals are increased as the patient improves (Jawed et al., 2014). ECP can be combined with adjunctive therapies, including PUVA, topical chemotherapy, systemic chemotherapy, radiation, biological agents, and retinoids.

Photodynamic Therapy

Photodynamic therapy combines the use of photosensitizing drugs and visible light for the treatment of dermatological disorders. Two drugs are approved for topical PDT: aminolevulinic acid and methylaminolevulinate. However, methylaminolevulinate is currently not commercially available in the U.S. Both are prodrugs that are converted into protoporphyrin IX within living cells (Figure 70–2). In the presence of specific wavelengths of light (see Table 70–6) and O_2, protoporphyrin produces reactive oxygen species that oxidize cell membranes, proteins,

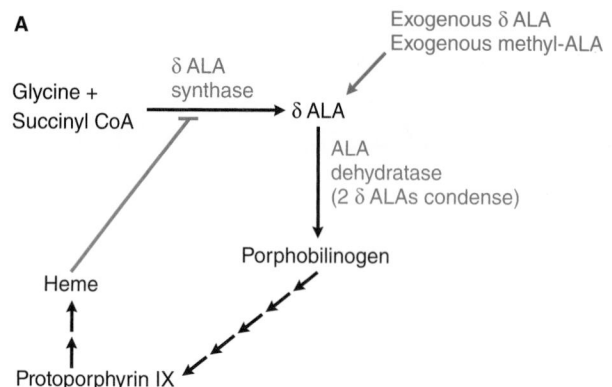

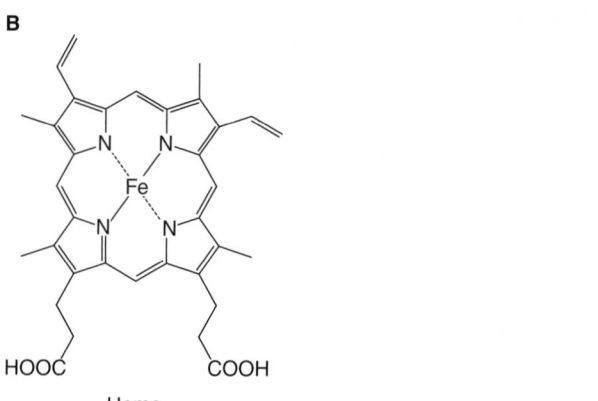

Figure 70–2 *Heme biosynthesis pathway.* **A.** *Under physiological conditions, heme inhibits the enzyme δ-aminolevulinic acid (δ-ALA) synthase by negative feedback. However, when ALA is provided exogenously, this control point is bypassed, leading to excessive accumulation of protoporphyrin IX and heme.* **B.** *Heme.*

and mitochondrial structures, leading to apoptosis. The epidermis, sebaceous glands, and neoplastic cells accumulate more porphyrin than other cutaneous cells and structures, providing some preferential targeting of therapy (Rkein and Ozog, 2014). PDT is approved for use on precancerous actinic keratosis. It is also used off label for superficial nonmelanoma skin cancers, acne, and photorejuvenation. Incoherent (nonlaser) and laser light sources have been used for PDT. The wavelengths chosen must include those within the action spectrum of protoporphyrin (see Table 70–6) and ideally those that permit maximum skin penetration. Light sources in use emit energy predominantly in the blue portion (maximum porphyrin absorption) or the red portion (better tissue penetration) of the visible spectrum. Because the $t_{1/2}$ of the accumulated porphyrins is about 30 h, patients should protect their skin from sunlight and intense light for at least 48 h after treatment to prevent phototoxic reactions.

Sunscreens

Sunscreens provide temporary photoprotection from the acute and chronic effects of sun exposure. They are an important component of a comprehensive sun protection approach along with minimizing sun exposure and using photoprotective gear. The regular use of sunscreen is efficacious in reducing photocarcinogenesis and photoaging (Mancebo et al., 2014). The SPF is defined as the ratio of the minimal dose of incident sunlight that will produce erythema (sunburn) on skin with the sunscreen in place to the dose that evokes the same reaction on skin without the sunscreen. SPF is primarily a measure of UVB protection and does not provide information regarding UVA coverage. In 2011, the FDA published new guidelines for labeling and effectiveness testing of sunscreens (Mancebo et al., 2014). UVA protection is now assessed using the CW method, and products with a CW of 370 nm or greater may be labeled as "broad spectrum." Sunscreens providing broad-spectrum coverage with an SPF 15 or greater may include a claim on their labeling that use "decreases risk of skin cancer and early aging caused by the sun." Sunscreens should be applied liberally 15–30 min prior to sun exposure and reapplied every 2 h. If activities involve swimming or sweating, water-resistant sunscreens are recommended and should be reapplied every 40 or 80 min depending on their labeling.

The major active ingredients of available sunscreens include organic agents ("chemical blockers") that absorb UV radiation in the UVB or UVA ranges, then convert it to heat energy and inorganic agents ("physical blockers") that contain particulate materials that act by scattering or reflecting visible, UV, and infrared radiation to reduce its transmission to the skin. The current FDA-approved active sunscreen ingredients are listed next.

Inorganic Agents

The two inorganic agents available in the U.S. are zinc oxide and titanium dioxide. They provide UVA and UVB protection. Newer microsize and nanosize particle formulations are less opaque and more cosmetically appealing.

Organic UVA Filters

Currently available UVA filters in the U.S. include benzophenones (oxybenzone, dioxybenzone, sulisobenzone); dibenzoylmethanes (avobenzone); anthralates (meradimate); and camphors (ecamsule). Additional UVA filters are used in other countries but are not currently available in the U.S.

Organic UVB Filters

There are numerous UVB filters, including aminobenzoates (PABA and padimate O); cinnamates (cinoxate, octinoxate); salicylates (trolamine salicylate, homosalate, octisalate); octocrylene; and ensulizole.

Antihistamines

Histamine (see Chapter 39) is a potent vasodilator, bronchial smooth muscle constrictor, and stimulant of nociceptive itch receptors. Additional chemical itch mediators acting as pruritogens on C fibers include

neuropeptides, prostaglandins, serotonin, acetylcholine, and *bradykinin.* Furthermore, receptor systems (e.g., vanilloid, opioid, and cannabinoid receptors) on cutaneous sensory nerve fibers may modulate itch and offer novel future targets for antipruritic therapy.

Histamine is in mast cells, basophils, and platelets. Human skin mast cells express H_1, H_2, and H_4 receptors but not H_3 receptors. Both H_1 and H_2 receptors are involved in wheal formation and erythema, whereas only the H_1 receptor agonists cause pruritus (see Chapter 39). However, blockade of H_1 receptors does not totally relieve itching, and combination therapy with H_1 and H_2 antagonists may be superior to the use of H_1 antagonists alone.

Oral antihistamines, particularly H_1 receptor antagonists, have anticholinergic activity and are sedating (see Chapter 39), making them useful for the control of pruritus. First-generation sedating H_1 receptor antagonists include *hydroxyzine, diphenhydramine, promethazine,* and *cyproheptadine* (Simons and Simons, 2008). *Doxepin* is a good alternative to traditional oral antihistamines for severe pruritus. A 5% topical cream formulation of doxepin, which can be used in conjunction with low- to moderate-potency topical glucocorticoids, also is available. The antipruritic effect from topical doxepin is comparable to that of low-dose oral doxepin therapy. Allergic contact dermatitis to doxepin has been reported. Topical diphenhydramine formulations available OTC also carry a significant risk of allergic contact dermatitis. *Second-generation H_1 receptor antagonists* lack anticholinergic side effects and are described as nonsedating largely because they do not cross the blood-brain barrier (Simons and Simons, 2008). They include *cetirizine, levocetirizine, loratadine, desloratadine,* and *fexofenadine.*

Antimicrobial Agents

Antibiotics

Antibiotic agents are frequently used to treat SSTIs. Several antimicrobial agents, such as tetracyclines, macrolides, and dapsone, also have anti-inflammatory properties, which make them useful for noninfectious conditions, such as acne vulgaris, rosacea, granulomatous diseases, neutrophilic dermatoses, and autoimmune bullous diseases (Bhatia, 2009).

Topical agents are very effective for the treatment of superficial bacterial infections and acne vulgaris (Drucker, 2012). Systemic antibiotics also are prescribed commonly for acne and deeper bacterial infections. The pharmacology of individual antibacterial agents is discussed in Section VI, Chemotherapy of Microbial Diseases. Only the topical and systemic antibacterial agents principally used in dermatology are discussed here.

Acne

Acne vulgaris is the most common dermatological disorder treated with either topical or systemic antibiotics (Eichenfield et al., 2013). The gram-positive anaerobe *Propionibacterium acnes* is a component of normal skin flora that proliferates in the obstructed, lipid-rich lumen of the pilosebaceous unit, where O_2 tension is low. *Propionibacterium acnes* generates free fatty acids from sebum and interacts with toll-like receptors, which promotes microcomedo formation and inflammatory lesions (Das and Reynolds, 2014). Suppression of cutaneous *P. acnes* with antibiotic therapy is correlated with clinical improvement.

Topical antimicrobials commonly used in acne include benzoyl peroxide, clindamycin, erythromycin, and antibiotic–benzoyl peroxide combinations. Topical monotherapy with clindamycin or erythromycin is not recommended due to a slower onset of action and potential for development of bacterial resistance; therefore, addition of benzoyl peroxide or use of combination antibiotic–benzoyl peroxide products is recommended to improve efficacy and decrease emergence of antibiotic-resistant bacteria (Eichenfield et al., 2013). Other topical antimicrobials used in treating acne include azelaic acid, dapsone, metronidazole, sulfacetamide, and sulfacetamide/sulfur combinations.

Systemic therapy is prescribed for patients with acne vulgaris that is more extensive or resistant to topical therapy. There are data to support the use of tetracyclines (doxycycline, minocycline, tetracycline); macrolides (azithromycin, erythromycin); and trimethoprim-sulfamethoxazole. Other antibiotics that decrease the extent of the infection or the inflammatory response to *P. acnes* may be effective as well. Antibiotics usually are administered once or twice daily, and 6–8 weeks is required for visible clinical results, with maximum effect sometimes requiring 3–6 months (Eichenfield et al., 2013). Doses are tapered after control is achieved. Concomitant use with topical benzoyl peroxide may decrease development of antibiotic-resistant bacteria.

The tetracyclines are the most commonly employed antibiotics because they are inexpensive, effective, and safe. They should not be used during pregnancy or in patients younger than 8 years. Although agents in the tetracycline class are antimicrobials, efficacy in acne may be more dependent on anti-inflammatory activity. Minocycline and doxycycline have better GI absorption than tetracycline and may be given with food to minimize GI side effects. Minocycline may be less photosensitizing than either tetracycline or doxycycline. Minocycline's adverse effects may include vestibular toxicity, hyperpigmentation of the skin and mucosa, serum sickness–like reactions, and drug-induced lupus erythematosus. With all the tetracyclines, vaginal candidiasis is a common complication that is readily treated with administration of antifungal drugs.

Cutaneous Bacterial Infections

Numerous organisms may cause cutaneous infections ranging from benign to life-threatening. Clinical presentation and treatment depend on the depth of cutaneous involvement, immune status of the patient, causative organism, and local antibiotic resistance patterns (Rajan, 2012; Stevens et al., 2014). Gram-positive organisms, including *Staphylococcus aureus* and *Streptococcus pyogenes*, are the most common cause of SSTIs. Patients who are diabetic or immunosuppressed are at risk for severe, recurrent, or atypical infections.

Topical Therapy. *Topical therapy* is frequently used for superficial bacterial infections, wounds, and burns. The use of topical antibiotics on clean surgical wounds without signs of infection is not recommended as it does not reduce the rate of infection compared to nonantibiotic ointment or no ointment, and there is a risk of contact dermatitis to topical antibiotics (Levender et al., 2012) and counterproductive selection of resistant bacterial strains.

Mupirocin. Mupirocin inhibits protein synthesis by binding to bacterial isoleucyl-tRNA synthetase. Mupirocin is effective for treatment of *S. aureus* and *S. pyogenes*, but it is inactive against normal skin flora or anaerobes. Mupirocin is available as a 2% ointment or cream, applied two or three times daily for 5–10 days. The recommended regimen for impetigo is twice daily for 5 days (Stevens et al., 2014). A nasal formulation is indicated to eradicate MRSA nasal colonization. It is applied intranasally twice a day for 5 days and often combined with daily chlorhexidine or dilute sodium hypochlorite washes for the body. Prolonged suppression may be achieved with repeat monthly courses.

Retapamulin. Retapamulin selectively inhibits bacterial protein synthesis by interacting at a unique site on the 50S subunit of bacterial ribosomes. It is active against multiple gram-positive organisms, including *S. aureus* and *S. pyogenes*, and against anaerobes. Retapamulin ointment 1% is FDA approved for the topical treatment of impetigo caused by susceptible strains of *S. aureus* or *S. pyogenes* in patients 9 months or older. The recommended regimen for impetigo is twice daily for 5 days (Stevens et al., 2014).

Bacitracin, Neomycin, and Polymyxin B. These agents are sold alone or in various combinations with other ingredients (e.g., hydrocortisone, lidocaine, or pramoxine) in a number of OTC formulations. Bacitracin inhibits staphylococci, streptococci, and gram-positive bacilli. Neomycin is active against staphylococci and most gram-negative bacilli. Polymyxin B is active against aerobic gram-negative bacilli, including *Pseudomonas aeruginosa*. Both bacitracin and neomycin are relatively common causes of allergic contact dermatitis, especially in patients with stasis dermatitis or otherwise disrupted skin (Drucker, 2012).

Gentamicin. Gentamicin is an aminoglycoside that inhibits protein synthesis by binding to the 30S subunit of bacterial ribosomes. It has activity for certain gram-positive bacteria, including *S. aureus*, and gram-negative bacteria, including *P. aeruginosa*. Gentamicin sulfate 0.1% cream or ointment may be applied three or four times daily to affected areas.

Silver Sulfadiazine. *Silver sulfadiazine* binds to bacterial DNA and inhibits replication. It is bactericidal against gram-positive bacteria, including MRSA, and gram-negative bacteria, including *P. aeruginosa*. Silver sulfadiazine is most frequently used in the treatment of partial-thickness burns or lower extremity venous stasis ulcers. However, recent studies have failed to demonstrate efficacy in these settings (Miller et al., 2012). Rarely, argyria has developed in patients using silver sulfadiazine over extensive areas of the body (Browning and Levy, 2008).

Mafenide. *Mafenide acetate* is a topical sulfonamide, although its mechanism of action may be distinct from other sulfonamides. Mafenide is approved as adjunctive therapy for burn wounds and is available as either an 85-mg/g cream or as a 5% topical solution supplied as 50-g packets of powder that must be reconstituted. It exerts broad bacteriostatic action against many gram-positive and gram-negative organisms, including *P. aeruginosa* and some anaerobes. The high solubility of mafenide allows it to diffuse easily through eschar and devascularized tissue, which is beneficial for treating subeschar burn wound infection. Mafenide and its metabolites inhibit carbonic anhydrase, so treated patients may be at risk for metabolic acidosis, especially if they have renal failure or if mafenide is applied to large surface areas. Other potential adverse effects include pain or burning sensation with application, facial edema, allergic contact dermatitis, and rarely hemolytic anemia in patients with G6PD deficiency.

Systemic Therapy. Deeper or complicated SSTIs typically require systemic administration of antimicrobials, which are also useful for superficial infections with diffuse involvement or that are not responding to topical therapy. Because SSTIs are most commonly caused by streptococcal and staphylococcal species, penicillins (especially β-lactamase–resistant β-lactams) and cephalosporins are the systemic antibiotics used most frequently in their treatment. A growing concern is the increased incidence of SSTIs with hospital- and community-acquired MRSA and drug-resistant pneumococci. Common outpatient treatment options for MRSA include clindamycin, doxycycline, and trimethoprim-sulfamethoxazole. When coverage for both MRSA and streptococci is needed, clindamycin alone or the combination of either doxycycline or trimethoprim-sulfamethoxazole with a β-lactam may be used (Stevens et al., 2014). Clindamycin should not be used as empiric therapy if local resistance rates are greater than 10%–15% (Stevens et al., 2014). Treatment options for more severe or complicated SSTIs that provide coverage for MRSA include vancomycin, linezolid, quinupristin-dalfopristin, and daptomycin. More recent additions to this armamentarium include dalbavancin, oritavancin, telavancin, tedizolid, and ceftaroline.

Antifungal Agents

Fungal infections are amongst the most common causes of skin disease in the U.S., and numerous effective topical and oral antifungal agents have been developed. The pharmacology, uses, and toxicities of antifungal drugs are discussed in Chapter 61. This section addresses the management of common superficial cutaneous mycoses. Recommendations for cutaneous antifungal therapy are summarized in Table 70–7. Topical antifungal agents used for superficial mucocutaneous mycoses are listed in Table 70–8.

Dermatophyte Infections of the Skin (Tinea Corporis, Cruris, and Pedis)

The dermatophyte infections (tinea corporis, crurus, and pedis) generally respond to topical antifungals, including allylamines (naftifine, terbinafine); benzylamines (butenafine); azoles (econazole, luliconazole); and ciclopirox (Rotta et al., 2013). Allylamines and benzylamines may provide a more sustained clinical cure compared to azole antifungals (Rotta et al., 2013). Bacterial superinfection of tinea pedis can occur, and antifungal agents such as econazole and ciclopirox that also provide some bacterial coverage may be useful in those situations. Systemic therapy with terbinafine, fluconazole, itraconazole, or griseofulvin is used

TABLE 70–7 ■ RECOMMENDED CUTANEOUS ANTIFUNGAL THERAPY

CONDITION	TOPICAL THERAPY	ORAL THERAPY
Tinea corporis, localized	Azoles, allylamines, benzylamines	—
Tinea corporis, widespread	—	Griseofulvin, terbinafine, itraconazole, fluconazole
Tinea capitis	—	Griseofulvin, terbinafine, itraconazole, fluconazole
Tinea pedis	Azoles, allylamines, benzylamines	Griseofulvin, terbinafine, itraconazole, fluconazole
Onychomycosis	—	Terbinafine, itraconazole, fluconazole
Candidiasis, localized	Azoles, nystatin	—
Candidiasis, widespread and mucocutaneous	—	Itraconazole, fluconazole
Tinea versicolor, localized	Azoles, allylamines	—
Tinea versicolor, widespread	—	Itraconazole, fluconazole

when there is more extensive cutaneous involvement or a poor response to topical therapy.

Dermatophyte Infections of the Hair and Follicles

Dermatophyte infections of the hair (tinea capitis) or follicularly based infections of the skin (Majocchi granuloma) require systemic therapy. Griseofulvin has been the traditional medication for tinea capitis, and treatment failure is often related to inadequate dosage or length of treatment. Terbinafine may be more effective for *Trichophyton tonsurans*, which is the most common cause of tinea capitis in the U.S. (Elewski et al., 2008). Fluconazole and itraconazole are also effective (Gupta and Paquet, 2013).

Onychomycosis

Onychomycosis is a fungal infection of the nails that is commonly caused by dermatophytes or candida. Onychomycosis is most effectively treated with systemic therapy (de Sa et al., 2014). Fungal infection should be confirmed prior to initiating oral therapy. There are other causes of nail dystrophy, and approximately one-third of nails with clinically suspected onychomycosis do not have fungal infection (Mehregan and Gee, 1999). *Terbinafine* is the most effective treatment of dermatophyte onychomycosis, with typical adult dosing of 250 mg daily for 6 weeks for fingernails and 12 weeks for toenails. Terbinafine remains in the nails for several weeks after medication administration has ceased, and some studies have utilized pulsed dosing of terbinafine 500 mg daily for 1 week per month for 3 months based on this finding. *Itraconazole* is another effective option for dermatophyte onychomycosis and is more effective than terbinafine for candidal onychomycosis. Itraconazole persists in the nail for 6–9 months after administration has ceased. Traditional adult dosing for itraconazole is 200 mg daily for 12 weeks; however, pulsed dosing is an alternative option because itraconazole of its long persistence after administration has ceased. Itraconazole pulsed dosing is 400 mg daily for 1 week per month for 2 months for fingernails and 3 months for toenails, which may be more effective than traditional dosing with fewer side effects. *Fluconazole* is an alternative option that may be useful in patients who cannot use terbinafine or itraconazole. *Griseofulvin*, used in the past, is less efficacious and requires much longer treatment courses; it is no longer a preferred option. Topical antifungals approved for onychomycosis include *ciclopirox*

lacquer, efinaconazole, and *tavaborole.* These topical antifungals require a 48-week treatment course. They may be useful for patients with mild-to-moderate onychomycosis not involving the nail matrix or in patients who are not candidates for systemic therapy (Gupta et al., 2014).

Cutaneous Candidiasis

Cutaneous candidiasis is typically treated with topical azole antifungals or nystatin when localized. Systemic azole antifungals such as fluconazole or itraconazole may be needed for more recalcitrant or severe cases.

Malassezia *Infections*

Pityriasis versicolor and seborrheic dermatitis are caused by *Malassezia* (pityrosporum) species and are frequently treated with azole antifungals in cream or shampoo formulations. Topical ciclopirox and terbinafine are also approved for use. Additional topical therapies include selenium sulfide, pyrithione zinc, sodium sulfacetamide, and sulfur with or without salicylic acid. Oral fluconazole or itraconazole are sometimes used for pityriasis versicolor when diffuse or resistant. Oral terbinafine does not reach adequate concentrations in the superficial stratum corneum to be effective.

Antiviral Agents

Viral infections of the skin by HPV, HSV, molluscum contagiosum virus, and VZV are common and produce a variety of lesions, including warts or blisters. Acyclovir, famciclovir, and valacyclovir are often used systemically to treat HSV and VZV infections (see Chapter 62). Cidofovir and foscarnet are useful for treating acyclovir-resistant HSV. Topically, acyclovir, docosanol, penciclovir, and combination acyclovir/hydrocortisone are available for treating mucocutaneous HSV; however, they are less effective than systemic therapies (Sarnoff, 2014). Acyclovir is also available as a 50-mg buccal tablet for herpes labialis to be applied as a single dose to the upper gum just above the incisor tooth within 1 h of prodromal symptoms.

Cidofovir is used off label topically or intralesionally as treatment of anogenital warts caused by HPV. Topical cidofovir 1% gel or cream must be obtained through a compounding pharmacy. It is applied once daily for 5 consecutive days every other week for a maximum of six cycles. Additional treatments for genital warts are nonspecific cytodestructive or immunomodulatory therapies, which are discussed in further detail in other sections. Cytodestructive modalities include topical use of cryotherapy, podophyllin (podophyllum resin) or podofilox (podophyllotoxin), and trichloroacetic acid. Topical immunomodulatory therapies include imiquimod and sinecatechins. Also, intralesional or systemic interferons α_{2b}, α_{n3}, and β may be useful for treating refractory or recurrent genital warts, but their use is limited by pain with multiple injections for intralesional use and by potential for severe side effects with systemic use (Smith et al., 2007).

Agents Used to Treat Infestations

Infestations with ectoparasites such as lice and scabies are common throughout the world. These conditions have a significant impact on public health in the form of disabling pruritus, secondary infection, and, in the case of the body louse, transmission of life-threatening illnesses such as typhus. Topical and oral medications are available to treat these infestations (Diamantis et al., 2009).

- **Permethrin** is a synthetic pyrethroid that interferes with insect Na⁺ transport proteins, causing neurotoxicity and paralysis. Resistance due to mutations in the transport protein has been reported and appears to be increasing. A 5% cream is available by prescription for the treatment of scabies, and a 1% lotion or cream rinse is available OTC for the treatment of lice. Permethrin is approved for use in infants 2 months or older. Other OTC agents used in the treatment of lice are pyrethrins plus piperonyl butoxide in various formulations and acetic acid plus isopropanol shampoo.
- **Lindane** is an organochloride compound that induces neuronal hyperstimulation and eventual paralysis of parasites. Due to several cases of neurotoxicity in humans, the FDA has labeled lindane as a second-line drug in treating pediculosis and scabies and has highlighted the

1281

SECTION IX SPECIAL SYSTEMS PHARMACOLOGY

TABLE 70–8 ■ TOPICAL ANTIFUNGAL AGENTS FOR SUPERFICIAL MUCOCUTANEOUS MYCOSES

GENERIC NAME	FORMULATIONS	FDA-APPROVED INDICATIONS	NOTES
Polyenes			
Nystatin	Topical (0.1 megaunit/g): Powder, ointment, cream	Cutaneous and mucocutaneous candidiasis	Orally administered nystatin lacks appreciable systemic absorption; it is used for local treatment of oral cavity and GI tract candidiasis
	Oral: Suspension (0.1 megaunit/g) Capsule or tablet (0.5 megaunit)	Oral cavity candidiasis Nonesophageal GI candidiasis	
Azoles			
Butoconazole	Vaginal cream, 2%	Vulvovaginal candidiasis	
Clotrimazole	Oral lozenge, 10 mg	Oropharyngeal candidiasis	
	Vaginal cream, 1% or 2%	Vaginal candidiasis	
	Cream, ointment, solution; 1%	Rx: *Candida albicans*, pityriasis versicolor OTC: tinea	
Econazole	Cream, 1% Foam, 1%	Tinea; cutaneous candidiasis, pityriasis versicolor Tinea pedis in patients ≥ 12 years	
Efinaconazole	Solution, 10%	Toenail onychomycosis	
Ketoconazole	2% foam, gel; 1% shampoo 2% shampoo, gel Cream, 2%	Seborrheic dermatitis Pityriasis versicolor Tinea; pityriasis versicolor, seborrheic dermatitis, cutaneous candidiasis	
Luliconazole	1% cream	Tinea	
Miconazole	2% cream, lotion, ointment, powder, solution, spray	Tinea	
	Vaginal suppository, 100 or 200 mg 2% or 4% vaginal cream	Vulvovaginal candidiasis	
Oxiconazole	1% cream, lotion	Tinea; pityriasis versicolor	
Sertaconazole	2% cream	Tinea pedis in pts ≥ 12 years	
Sulconazole	1% cream, solution	Tinea; pityriasis versicolor	
Terconazole	0.4%, 0.8% vaginal cream; 80-mg vaginal suppository	Vulvovaginal candidiasis	
Tioconazole	6.5% vaginal ointment	Vulvovaginal candidiasis	
Allylamines			
Naftifine	1% or 2% cream, gel	Tinea	
Terbinafine	1% cream, gel, spray	Tinea; pityriasis versicolor	
Benzylamines			
Butenafine	1% cream	Rx: pityriasis versicolor OTC: tinea	
Hydroxypyridones			
Ciclopirox	8% topical solution/lacquer	Onychomycosis	
	1% shampoo	Seborrheic dermatitis	
	0.77% gel	Tinea; seborrheic dermatitis	
Oxaboroles			
Tavaborole	5% topical solution	Toenail onychomycosis	
Miscellaneous			
Selenium sulfide	1% shampoo, lotion; 2.5% lotion; 2.25% foam	Seborrheic dermatitis; pityriasis versicolor	
Gentian violet	1% or 2% topical solution	Abrasions, minor cuts, surface injuries, superficial fungal infections of the skin	Stains skin and clothing purple
Tolnaftate	1% cream, powder, topical solution	Tinea; pityriasis versicolor	

(Continued)

TABLE 70–8 ■ TOPICAL ANTIFUNGAL AGENTS FOR SUPERFICIAL MUCOCUTANEOUS MYCOSES (CONTINUED)

GENERIC NAME	FORMULATIONS	FDA-APPROVED INDICATIONS	NOTES
Undecylenic acid	10%–25% topical powder, cream, solution, soap	Tinea	
Miscellaneous Combination Products			
Bensal HP	Topical ointment: 3% salicylic acid in base containing benzoic acid, oak bark, polyethylene glycol		
Whitfield's	Topical ointment: 6% benzoic acid, 3% salicylic acid		
Versiclear	Topical lotion: 25% sodium thiosulfate, 1% salicylic acid, 10% isopropyl alcohol, menthol, propylene glycol, EDTA, colloidal alumina		
Castellani Paint Modified	Topical liquid: basic fuchsin, phenol, resorcinol, acetone. Also as colorless solution containing alcohol but without basic fuchsin		
Fungi-nail	Topical liquid: 1% resorcinol, 2% salicylic acid, 2% chloroxylenol, 0.5% benzocaine, 50% isopropyl alcohol		
Exoderm	Topical soap: 10% sulfur, 3% salicylic acid		

potential for neurotoxicity in children and adults weighing less than 50 kg and patients with underlying skin disorders such as atopic dermatitis and psoriasis. Lindane is contraindicated in premature infants and patients with seizure disorders.

- **Malathion** is an organophosphate that inhibits acetylcholinesterase in lice, causing paralysis and death. It is approved for treatment of head lice in children 6 years and older. The current formulation of malathion lotion contains 78% isopropyl alcohol and is flammable. Detailed information on malathion's actions and adverse effects may be found in Chapter 10.
- **Benzyl alcohol** 5% lotion is approved for the treatment of lice in patients 6 months and older. Benzyl alcohol inhibits lice from closing their respiratory spiracles, which allows the vehicle to obstruct the spiracles and causes the lice to asphyxiate. There may be less potential for development of resistance with this mechanism of action compared to traditional pesticides.
- **Ivermectin** is an anthelmintic drug (see Chapter 55) approved for oral treatment of onchocerciasis and strongyloidiasis. Recently, topical ivermectin 0.5% lotion was approved to treat lice in patients 6 months or older and 1% cream to treat rosacea. Ivermectin is also effective in the off-label treatment of scabies. Because ivermectin does not cross the human blood-brain barrier, there is no major CNS toxicity; minor CNS side effects with oral administration may include dizziness, somnolence, vertigo, and tremor. Topical administration may cause local irritant effects, such as conjunctivitis, eye irritation, dry skin, or skin-burning sensation, although these occurred in fewer than 1% of patients during clinical trials. For both scabies and lice, ivermectin typically is given at an oral dose of 200 μg/kg, which may be repeated in 1 week. In cases of crusted scabies, longer treatment cycles of oral ivermectin may be needed, sometimes in addition to topical keratolytics and scabicides (Ortega-Loayza et al., 2013). It should not be used in children weighing less than 15 kg
- **Spinosad** 0.9% topical suspension is approved for treatment of head lice in patients 6 months or older. Spinosad causes CNS excitation and involuntary muscle contractions, leading to insect paralysis and death.

Less effective topical treatments for scabies and lice include 10% crotamiton cream and lotion and extemporaneously compounded 5%–10% precipitated sulfur in petrolatum. Precipitated sulfur may be useful for patients in whom other therapies are contraindicated or not approved; it is typically applied once daily for 3–5 consecutive days.

Antimalarial Agents

The antimalarial agents chloroquine, hydroxychloroquine, and quinacrine are used in dermatology to treat dermatoses such as cutaneous lupus erythematosus, cutaneous dermatomyositis, polymorphous light eruption, porphyria cutanea tarda, and sarcoidosis (only hydroxychloroquine is FDA approved for treating lupus erythematosus). The mechanism by which antimalarial agents exert their anti-inflammatory therapeutic effects is uncertain but may involve inhibition of endosomal toll-like receptor signaling, resulting in reduced B-cell and dendritic cell activation (Kalia and Dutz, 2007). The usual dosages of antimalarials are hydroxychloroquine 200 mg twice a day (maximum of 6.5 mg/kg/d); chloroquine 250–500 mg/d (maximum of 3 mg/kg/d); and quinacrine 100–200 mg/d. Patients with porphyria cutanea tarda require lower doses of antimalarials to avoid severe hepatotoxicity. There is strong evidence that smoking decreases the effectiveness of antimalarials in the treatment of cutaneous lupus erythematosus, so smoking cessation is important (Chasset et al., 2015). Clinical improvement may be delayed for several months. If there is no improvement after 3 months of hydroxychloroquine, then quinacrine may be added (in the U.S., quinacrine must be obtained through compounding pharmacies). Dose-dependent ocular toxicity occurs with chloroquine more often than hydroxychloroquine and is rare to nonexistent with quinacrine. The potential toxic effects of antimalarial agents are described further in Chapter 53.

Cytotoxic and Immunosuppressant Drugs

Cytotoxic and immunosuppressant drugs are used in dermatology for immunologically mediated diseases such as psoriasis, autoimmune blistering diseases, and leukocytoclastic vasculitis. See Table 70–9 for their mechanisms of action.

Antimetabolites

Methotrexate is used for moderate-to-severe psoriasis. It suppresses immunocompetent cells in the skin, and it also decreases the expression of CLA-positive T cells and endothelial cell E-selectin, which may account for its efficacy. Methotrexate is useful in treating a number of other dermatological conditions, including atopic dermatitis, pityriasis lichenoides et varioliformis, lymphomatoid papulosis, sarcoidosis, pemphigus vulgaris, pityriasis rubra pilaris, lupus erythematosus, dermatomyositis, and CTCL.

Methotrexate often is used in combination with phototherapy and photochemotherapy or other systemic agents. Widely used oral regimens include 10–25 mg once weekly as a single dose or as three divided doses given at 12-h intervals, with similar effectiveness using either regimen, or intramuscular administration of 10–25 mg injected once weekly (maximum of 30 mg/week) (Menter et al., 2009b).

Doses must be decreased for patients with impaired renal clearance. *Methotrexate should not be administered with probenecid, trimethoprim-sulfamethoxazole, salicylates, or other drugs that can compete with it for protein binding and thereby raise plasma concentrations to levels that*

TABLE 70–9 ■ MECHANISM OF ACTION FOR SELECTED CYTOTOXIC, IMMUNOSUPPRESSIVE, AND IMMUNOMODULATORY DRUGS

Methotrexate	Dihydrofolate reductase inhibitor
Fluorouracil	Blocks methylation in DNA synthesis
Cyclophosphamide	Alkylates and cross-links DNA
Mechlorethamine hydrochloride	Alkylating agent
Carmustine	Cross-links in DNA and RNA
Vinblastine	Inhibits microtubule formation
Bleomycin	Induction of DNA strand breaks
Azathioprine	Purine synthesis inhibitor
Mycophenolate mofetil	Inosine monophosphate dehydrogenase inhibitor
Cyclosporine	Calcineurin inhibitor
Tacrolimus	Calcineurin inhibitor
Pimecrolimus	Calcineurin inhibitor
Sirolimus	mTOR inhibitor
Imiquimod	Interferon α induction via toll-like receptor 7
Dapsone	Inhibits neutrophil migration, oxidative burst
Thalidomide	Cytokine modulation

may result in bone marrow suppression. Fatalities have occurred because of concurrent treatment with methotrexate and NSAIDs. Methotrexate exerts significant antiproliferative effects on the bone marrow; therefore, CBCs should be monitored serially. Providers administering methotrexate should be familiar with the use of folinic acid (leucovorin) to rescue patients with hematological crises caused by methotrexate-induced bone marrow suppression. Careful monitoring of liver function tests is necessary to assess for methotrexate-induced hepatotoxicity. Liver biopsy may be recommended after a 3.5- to 4-g cumulative dose in patients without other risk factors versus 1–1.5 g in patients with higher risk (e.g., obesity, diabetes) (Menter et al., 2009b). Patients with abnormal liver function tests, symptomatic liver disease, or evidence of hepatic fibrosis should not use this drug. Methotrexate is contraindicated during pregnancy and lactation. Many clinicians routinely administer folic acid to ameliorate side effects of methotrexate.

Fluorouracil is used topically in multiple actinic keratoses, actinic cheilitis, Bowen disease, and superficial BCCs not amenable to other treatments (Micali et al., 2014). 5FU is applied once or twice daily for 2–8 weeks, depending on the indication. The treated areas may become severely inflamed during treatment, but the inflammation subsides after the drug is stopped. Intralesional injection of 5FU has been used off label for keratoacanthomas, warts, and porokeratoses (Good et al., 2011).

Alkylating Agents

Cyclophosphamide is an effective cytotoxic and immunosuppressive agent. Both oral and intravenous preparations of cyclophosphamide are used in dermatology. Cyclophosphamide is FDA approved for treatment of advanced CTCL (Jawed et al., 2014).

Other uses include treatment of pemphigus vulgaris, bullous pemphigoid, cicatricial pemphigoid, paraneoplastic pemphigus, pyoderma gangrenosum, toxic epidermal necrolysis, Wegener granulomatosis, polyarteritis nodosa, Churg-Strauss angiitis, Behçet disease, scleromyxedema, and cytophagic histiocytic panniculitis. The usual oral dosage is 2–2.5 mg/kg/d in divided doses, and there often is a 4- to 6-week delay in onset of action (Meurer, 2012). Alternatively, intravenous pulse administration of cyclophosphamide may offer advantages, including lower cumulative dose and a decreased risk of bladder cancer.

Cyclophosphamide has many adverse effects (see Chapter 66), including the risk of secondary malignancy and myelosuppression, and is used only in the most severe, recalcitrant dermatological diseases.

Mechlorethamine hydrochloride and **carmustine** are used topically to treat CTCL (Jawed et al., 2014). It is important to monitor CBCs and liver function tests because systemic absorption can cause bone marrow suppression and hepatitis. Other side effects include allergic contact dermatitis, irritant dermatitis, secondary cutaneous malignancies, and pigmentary changes. Carmustine also can cause erythema and posttreatment telangiectasias.

Microtubule Inhibitors

Vinblastine is approved for systemic use in Kaposi sarcoma and advanced CTCL. Intralesional vinblastine also is used to treat Kaposi sarcoma (Regnier-Rosencher et al., 2013).

Podophyllin (podophyllum resin) is a mixture of chemicals from the plant *Podophyllum peltatum* (mandrake or May apple) that contains podophyllotoxin (podofilox), which binds to microtubules and causes mitotic arrest in metaphase (Fathi and Tsoukas, 2014). In the U.S., it must be obtained through a compounding pharmacy. Podophyllum resin 25% is applied topically by a physician and left in place for no longer than 2–6 h weekly for the treatment of anogenital warts. Irritation and ulcerative local reactions are the major side effects. It should not be used in the mouth or during pregnancy. It is recommended that the use of provider-administered podophyllum resin be replaced by the purified podophyllotoxin (podofilox) for patient-administered use. Podofilox is available as a 0.5% gel or solution for at-home application two times daily for 3 consecutive days, repeated weekly as needed for up to four cycles.

Other Cytotoxic Agents

Bleomycin is used off label intralesionally for palliative treatment of squamous cell carcinoma and recalcitrant warts and has cytotoxic and pro-inflammatory effects. Intralesional injection of bleomycin into the digits has been associated with a vasospastic response that mimics Reynaud phenomenon. Other potential adverse reactions include local skin necrosis and flagellate hyperpigmentation. Systemic bleomycin has been used off label for Kaposi sarcoma (see Chapter 66) (Regnier-Rosencher et al., 2013).

Liposomal anthracyclines (specifically doxorubicin) may provide first-line monotherapy for advanced Kaposi sarcoma (Regnier-Rosencher et al., 2013).

Ingenol mebutate gel, an extract from the plant *Euphorbia peplus*, is FDA approved for actinic keratosis (Micali et al., 2014). In experimental studies, it was reported to rapidly cause mitochondrial swelling and apoptosis of dysplastic keratinocytes. The gel is applied once daily for 2–3 consecutive days. Adverse effects may include local skin irritation, pain, pruritus, and infection at application site; periorbital edema; nasopharyngitis; and headache. Cases of allergic contact dermatitis and reactivation of herpes zoster have been reported.

Azathioprine and Mycophenolate Mofetil

Azathioprine is discussed in Chapter 35. In dermatological practice, the drug is used off label as a steroid-sparing agent for autoimmune and inflammatory dermatoses, including pemphigus vulgaris, bullous pemphigoid, dermatomyositis, atopic dermatitis, chronic actinic dermatitis, lupus erythematosus, psoriasis, pyoderma gangrenosum, and Behçet disease.

Azathioprine is cleaved to 6MP, which in turn is converted to additional metabolites that inhibit de novo purine synthesis (see Figure 51–5 and Chapter 66). The level of thiopurine *S*-methyltransferase (TPMT) enzyme activity should be measured before initiating azathioprine therapy because low levels of TMPT activity are associated with increased drug toxicity (see Chapter 66). In general, the starting dosage is 1–2 mg/kg/d. Careful laboratory monitoring is important, especially in those with diminished TPMT activity.

Mycophenolate mofetil and mycophenolate sodium are immunosuppressants approved for prophylaxis of organ rejection in patients with renal, cardiac, and hepatic transplants (see Chapter 35). Mycophenolate mofetil is a prodrug that is hydrolyzed to mycophenolic acid by plasma esterases; the salt of the acid, mycophenolate sodium, is available in an enteric-coated formulation. Mycophenolic acid functions as a specific inhibitor of T- and B-lymphocyte activation and proliferation through inhibition of inosine monophosphate dehydrogenase, thereby reducing GMP synthesis by the de novo purine synthetic pathway. Lymphocytes are vulnerable due to their lack of the salvage pathway for purine synthesis. The drug also may enhance apoptosis.

Mycophenolate mofetil is used off label increasingly to treat inflammatory and autoimmune diseases in dermatology; dosages typically range from 2 to 3 g/d orally in adults or 30–50 mg/kg/d in pediatric patients, given in divided doses twice daily. This agent is particularly useful as a corticosteroid-sparing agent in the treatment of autoimmune blistering disorders and has been used effectively in the treatment of inflammatory diseases such as psoriasis, atopic dermatitis, and pyoderma gangrenosum. Isolated cases of PML and pure red cell aplasia have been reported in solid organ transplant patients receiving mycophenolate mofetil. The most common side effects of mycophenolate mofetil are dose-dependent GI symptoms (e.g., diarrhea, nausea, and abdominal pain). Enteric-coated mycophenolate sodium improves GI tolerability; the enteric coating delays absorption until the medication reaches the small intestine rather than occurring in the stomach.

Calcineurin Inhibitors

The mechanisms of action and clinical pharmacology of calcineurin inhibitors are described in Chapter 35, and Figure 35–2 shows their main molecular effects as immunosuppressants.

Cyclosporine is a potent immunosuppressant isolated from the fungus *Tolypocladium inflatum*. Cyclosporine is FDA approved for the treatment of psoriasis. A modified microemulsion formulation has increased bioavailability and more consistent absorption than the original formulation. Other cutaneous disorders that typically respond well to cyclosporine are atopic dermatitis, alopecia areata, epidermolysis bullosa acquisita, pemphigus vulgaris, bullous pemphigoid, lichen planus, and pyoderma gangrenosum. The usual oral dosage of the modified formulation is 2.5 to 5 mg/kg/d, often given in two divided doses (Menter et al., 2009b; Sidbury et al., 2014).

Hypertension and renal dysfunction are the major adverse effects associated with the use of cyclosporine. These risks can be minimized by monitoring serum creatinine (which should not rise more than 30% above baseline), calculating creatinine clearance or glomerular filtration rate in patients on long-term therapy or with a rising creatinine, maintaining a daily dose of less than 5 mg/kg, and regularly monitoring blood pressure. Alternation with other therapeutic modalities may diminish cyclosporine toxicity. Patients with psoriasis who are treated with cyclosporine are at increased risk of cutaneous, solid organ, and lymphoproliferative malignancies. The risk of cutaneous malignancies is compounded in patients who have received phototherapy with PUVA.

Tacrolimus is available in a topical form for the treatment of skin disease and also is marketed in oral and injectable formulations. Systemic tacrolimus has shown some efficacy in the off-label treatment of inflammatory skin diseases such as psoriasis, pyoderma gangrenosum, and Behçet disease. When tacrolimus is administered systemically, the most common side effects are hypertension, nephrotoxicity, neurotoxicity, GI symptoms, hyperglycemia, and hyperlipidemia.

Topical formulations (0.03% and 0.1%) of tacrolimus ointment are approved for the treatment of atopic dermatitis in adults and in children 2 years or older for 0.03% ointment and 16 years or older 0.1% ointment. Other uses include for treatment of intertriginous psoriasis, vitiligo, mucosal lichen planus, graft-versus-host disease, allergic contact dermatitis, and rosacea. Ointment is applied to the affected area two times daily and generally is well tolerated. Common side effects at the site of application are transient erythema, burning, and pruritus. Other adverse effects include skin tingling, flu-like symptoms, headache, alcohol intolerance, folliculitis, acne, and hyperesthesia. Systemic absorption generally is very low and decreases with resolution of the dermatitis. Topical tacrolimus

should be used with extreme caution in patients with Netherton syndrome; these patients may develop elevated blood levels of the drug after topical application (Eichenfield et al., 2014).

Pimecrolimus (as a 1% cream) is approved for the treatment of atopic dermatitis in patients 2 years and older. Its mechanism of action and side-effect profile are similar to those of tacrolimus. It has low-to-negligible systemic absorption after topical application.

Tacrolimus and pimecrolimus are approved as second-line agents for short-term and intermittent treatment of atopic dermatitis in patients unresponsive to, or intolerant of, other treatments. Unlike topical corticosteroids, they do not carry the risk of skin atrophy and may be especially useful as steroid-sparing agents or for use on sensitive skin sites (e.g., eyelids, face, skin folds) or areas with steroid-induced atrophy.

mTor Inhibitors

Sirolimus causes immunosuppressive and antiproliferative effects through inhibition of mTOR as part of the PI3 kinase/Akt/mTOR pathway (see Figures 3–16, 35–2, and 67–4). The mTOR inhibitors are established treatments for posttransplant immunosuppression (Chapter 35) and as antineoplastic agents for malignancies such as renal and hepatocellular carcinoma (Chapter 67). Off-label use of mTOR inhibitors in dermatology includes treatment of tuberous sclerosis complex, pachyonychia congenita, complex vascular anomalies, and inflammatory dermatoses such as systemic sclerosis (Fogel et al., 2015). Systemic mTOR inhibitors may be associated with several side effects, with dermatologic side effects amongst the most common, including stomatitis, mucositis, inflammatory cutaneous eruptions, and nail changes such as paronychia (Fogel et al., 2015). Topical formulations have been used to decrease the risk of side effects associated with systemic therapy. Newer semisynthetic analogues of sirolimus such as everolimus and temsirolimus are available and have improved water solubility and efficacy.

Immunomodulators and Anti-inflammatory Agents

Imiquimod exerts immunomodulatory effects by acting as a ligand at toll-like receptors in the immune system and inducing the cytokines IFN-α, TNF-α, and IL-1, IL-6, IL-8, IL-10, and IL-12.

Imiquimod cream is available in 2.5%, 3.75%, and 5% strengths. Approved for the treatment of genital warts, imiquimod 5% cream is applied to genital or perianal lesions three times a week until resolution of warts or up to a 16-week period (and repeated as necessary) (Fathi and Tsoukas, 2014). Imiquimod also is approved for the treatment of actinic keratosis, with various regimens used (Micali et al., 2014). No more than 36 single-use packets per 16-week course of therapy should be prescribed for actinic keratoses. The 5% cream is also FDA approved for the treatment of superficial BCCs at a dosage of five applications/week for 6 weeks. Off-label applications include the treatment of nongenital warts, molluscum contagiosum, extramammary Paget disease, and Bowen disease. Irritant reactions occur in virtually all patients; the degree of inflammation parallels therapeutic efficacy.

Sinecatechins are partially purified green tea extracts containing a mixture of 85%–95% catechins and other green tea components. They are approved for the topical treatment of external genital and perianal warts in immunocompetent patients more than 18 years of age. The mechanism of action is unclear but may include a combination of antioxidant, antiviral, antiangiogenic, proapoptotic, and immunomodulatory activities. The sinecatechin 15% ointment is applied three times daily for up to 16 weeks until clearance of the warts. The most common side effects are local skin reactions, including erythema, pruritus or burning, pain, superficial ulceration, and edema, with the intensity of local reactions peaking between 2 and 4 weeks of use. Local site reactions may be indicative of a positive clinical response, and patients are encouraged to treat through them as tolerated.

Dapsone is used in dermatology for its anti-inflammatory properties, particularly in sterile (noninfectious) pustular diseases of the skin (Zhu and Stiller, 2001). Dapsone prevents the respiratory burst from myeloperoxidase, suppresses neutrophil migration by blocking integrin-mediated adherence, inhibits adherence of antibodies to neutrophils, and decreases the release of eicosanoids and blocks their inflammatory effects. Dapsone is discussed further in Chapter 60.

Dapsone is approved for oral use in dermatitis herpetiformis and leprosy and for topical use in acne vulgaris. It is also particularly useful in the off-label treatment of linear IgA dermatosis, bullous systemic lupus erythematosus, erythema elevatum diutinum, and subcorneal pustular dermatosis. In addition, reports indicate efficacy in patients with acne fulminans, pustular psoriasis, lichen planus, Hailey-Hailey disease, pemphigus vulgaris, bullous pemphigoid, cicatricial pemphigoid, leukocytoclastic vasculitis, Sweet syndrome, granuloma faciale, relapsing polychondritis, Behçet disease, urticarial vasculitis, pyoderma gangrenosum, and granuloma annulare.

The initial oral dosage is 50 mg/d, followed by increases of 25 mg/d at weekly intervals, titrated to the minimal dosage necessary for effect. Potential side effects of dapsone include methemoglobinemia and hemolysis (G6PD level should be checked in all patients). The H_2 blocker cimetidine inhibits numerous CYPs and thereby reduces the N-hydroxylation of dapsone to the hydroxylamine metabolite that causes the methemoglobinemia. Other toxicities of dapsone include agranulocytosis, peripheral neuropathy, and psychosis.

Thalidomide is an anti-inflammatory, immunomodulatory, and antiangiogenic agent experiencing resurgence in the treatment of dermatological diseases (Wu et al., 2005). For details of its actions, see Chapter 36 under Immunostimulants and Figure 66–2 and associated text.

Thalidomide is FDA approved for the treatment of erythema nodosum leprosum. Reports also suggest its efficacy in actinic prurigo, aphthous stomatitis, Behçet disease, Kaposi sarcoma, the cutaneous manifestations of lupus erythematosus, and prurigo nodularis and uremic prurigo. Thalidomide has been associated with increased mortality when used to treat toxic epidermal necrolysis. In utero exposure can cause limb abnormalities (phocomelia), as well as other congenital anomalies. *Thalidomide should never be taken by women who are pregnant or who could become pregnant while taking the drug. It also may cause an irreversible neuropathy. Because of its teratogenic effects, thalidomide use is restricted and requires both pharmacists and physicians to register in a risk evaluation and mitigation strategy (REMS) program. Newer analogues of thalidomide are available, including lenalidomide and pomalidomide.*

Targeted Immunotherapies for Psoriasis and Atopic Dermatitis

Targeted immunotherapies, including biological agents, are rapidly evolving for the treatment of psoriasis, as the underlying pathogenesis is better understood (Table 70–10). In addition, biological therapy for atopic dermatitis is on the horizon. The appeal of these targeted therapies is that they specifically target the activities of T lymphocytes and cytokines that mediate inflammation, whereas traditional systemic therapies are broadly immunosuppressive or cytotoxic. The pathogenesis of psoriasis and atopic dermatitis is discussed briefly next, followed by the relevant targeted therapies. Targeted therapies are discussed in further detail in Chapter 35.

Psoriasis is a chronic immune-mediated inflammatory disorder involving the innate and adaptive immune systems, with resultant abnormal keratinocyte proliferation (Figure 70–3). Psoriasis is not limited to the skin, as there can be psoriatic arthritis and other systemic manifestations. Previously thought to be primarily Th1 mediated, more recent developments demonstrate that the Th17/IL-17 pathway plays the most significant role (Girolomoni et al., 2012). Mediators of inflammation, such as IL-23, TNF-α, and IL-17 are key targets for therapy (Girolomoni et al., 2012; Sobell and Leonardi, 2014). In addition, therapies such as inhibitors of Jak and cyclic nucleotide PDEs) are useful to decrease expression or signal transduction of inflammatory cytokines (Sobell and Leonardi, 2014).

TABLE 70–10 ■ BIOLOGICAL AGENTS FOR PSORIASIS

	ETANERCEPT	ADALIMUMAB	INFLIXIMAB	USTEKINUMAB	SECUKINUMAB
Structural class	Receptor-antibody fusion protein	Human mAb	Chimeric mAb	Human mAb	Human mAb
Components	p75 TNF receptor and Fc IgG_1	IgG_1	Variable region of mouse mAb on human IgG_1	IgG_1	IgG_1
Binding site	TNF-α	TNF-α	TNF-α	p40 subunit of IL-12 and IL-23	IL-17A
Method of administration	SC	SC	IV	SC	SC
Adult dosing for psoriasis	50 mg twice weekly × 3 months, then 50 mg weekly	80 mg loading dose week 0, then 40 mg biweekly starting week 1	5 mg/kg at weeks 0, 2, and 6, then every 8 weeks	≤ 100 kg: 45 mg weeks 0, 4, then every 12 weeks ≥ 100 kg: 90 mg weeks 0, 4, then every 12 weeks	300 mg at weeks 0, 1, 2, 3, 4, then every 4 weeks
Pregnancy category	Adequate studies in pregnant women show no evidence of risk for increased fetal abnormalities				B[b]
Efficacy in psoriasis[a]	47%	53%	76%–80%	67%–76%	75%–87%

[a]Probability (%) of Psoriasis Area and Severity Index score of 75 after 12 weeks of therapy at the dosing described in the table (Tzu and Kerdel, 2008).

[b]No embryo-fetal toxicity in mice and non-human primates; no adequate, well controlled studies in pregnant women; use only if benefit justifies potential risk to fetus.

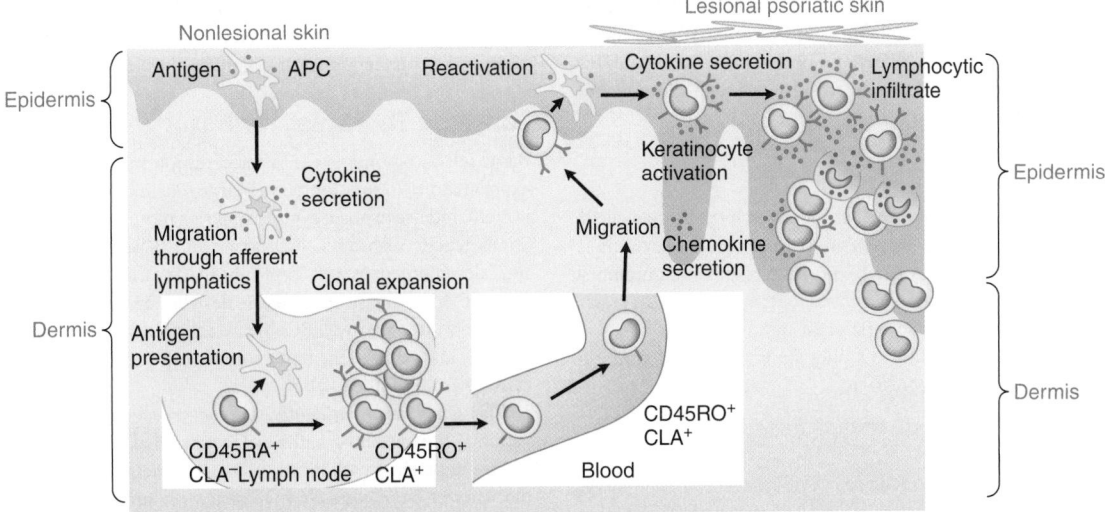

Figure 70–3 *Immunopathogenesis of psoriasis.* Psoriasis is a prototypical inflammatory skin disorder in which specific T-cell populations are stimulated by as-yet-undefined antigen(s) presented by APCs. The dendritic APCs, T cells, keratinocytes, and other cells release pro-inflammatory chemokines and cytokines, such as TNF-α, IFN-γ, IL-23, and IL-17, which ultimately induce keratinocyte hyperproliferation and sustain chronic inflammation.

Atopic dermatitis is a chronic skin disorder characterized by epidermal barrier dysfunction and immune-mediated inflammation. Patients often develop asthma and allergic rhinitis as well. Acute atopic dermatitis is Th2 cell mediated, associated with cytokines IL-4, IL-5, and IL-13, while chronic atopic dermatitis also involves Th1 cell–mediated activity, associated with cytokines IL-12 and IFN-γ. Topical corticosteroids and calcineurin inhibitors are common therapies, and several of the traditional immunosuppressants have been used for more severe or resistant cases (Eichenfield et al., 2014; Sidbury et al., 2014). Targeted therapies show promise for the future treatment of atopic dermatitis (Beck et al., 2014).

Tumor Necrosis Factor Inhibitors

Blockade of TNF-α reduces inflammation, decreases keratinocyte proliferation, and decreases vascular adhesion, resulting in improvement in psoriatic lesions. Because TNF-α inhibitors alter immune responses, patients on all anti-TNF-α agents are at increased risk for serious infection and for malignancies. Other adverse events include exacerbation of congestive heart failure and demyelinating disease in predisposed patients. All patients should be screened for tuberculosis, history of demyelinating disorder, cardiac failure, active infection, or malignancy prior to therapy. TNF-α inhibitors include monoclonal antibodies directed against TNF-α (adalimumab, infliximab) or a soluble TNF receptor that can bind TNF-α (etanercept) (see Chapter 35). All TNF-α inhibitors are able to bind both soluble and membrane-bound TNF, but the monoclonal antibodies against TNF-α with an IgG$_1$ Fc portion are also able to activate complement-dependent cytotoxicity on binding of membrane-bound TNF-α. This may explain the increased efficacy of these agents in comparison to etanercept for treating granulomatous conditions as well as the higher risk of infection with their use.

Etanercept is a soluble, recombinant, fully human TNF receptor fusion protein consisting of two molecules of the ligand-binding portion of the TNF receptor (p75) fused to the Fc portion of IgG$_1$. It binds both TNF-α and TNF-β. Etanercept is approved for plaque psoriasis and psoriatic arthritis in adults. Studies have shown etanercept to be safe and efficacious for pediatric psoriasis at dosing of 0.8 mg/kg (maximum 50 mg) once weekly (Bellodi Schmidt and Shah, 2015).

Infliximab, a mouse-human chimeric IgG$_1$ monoclonal antibody directed against human TNF-α, is approved for treatment of chronic severe plaque psoriasis and psoriatic arthritis. The administration of infliximab via intravenous infusion can be a limiting factor; however, compared to other TNF-α inhibitors, its onset of action may be faster and efficacy greater. Neutralizing antibodies to infliximab may develop and lead to decreased efficacy over time. Concomitant administration of methotrexate or glucocorticoids may suppress this neutralizing antibody formation.

Adalimumab is a human IgG$_1$ monoclonal antibody directed against TNF-α; thus, the risk for development of neutralizing antibodies is reduced compared to infliximab. Adalimumab is approved for treatment of plaque psoriasis and psoriatic arthritis in adults. Safety of adalimumab in pediatric patients for psoriasis is supported by its use in other conditions, such as juvenile idiopathic arthritis (Bellodi Schmidt and Shah, 2015). Adalimumab is also approved for treatment of hidradenitis suppurativa.

Golimumab and *certolizumab pegol* are TNF-α inhibitors that are currently approved for psoriatic arthritis but not psoriasis. However, studies of these medications for psoriatic arthritis also demonstrated improvement of plaque psoriasis, and a phase III trial of certolizumab pegol for plaque psoriasis demonstrated efficacy. Golimumab is a fully human monoclonal antibody against TNF-α with a longer $t_{1/2}$ than other TNF-α inhibitors. Certolizumab pegol is a pegylated Fab fragment of a human monoclonal antibody against TNF-α. Because certolizumab pegol lacks the Fc portion, it is not able to activate complement-mediated cytotoxicity.

IL-12/23 Inhibitors

Ustekinumab is a human IgG$_1$ monoclonal antibody directed against the common p40 subunit of IL-12 and IL-23. IL-12 promotes Th1 activity and related TNF-α and IFN-γ production, while IL-23 activates Th17 cells that produce IL-17A, which regulates tissue inflammation and autoimmune responses. *Ustekinumab* is approved for treatment of moderate-to-severe plaque psoriasis and psoriatic arthritis. After initial doses at weeks 0 and 4, it is administered every 12 weeks for the maintenance phase of therapy, which may be ideal for some patients. Studies have shown *ustekinumab* to be safe and efficacious in adolescent patients at the same dosing as adults (Bellodi Schmidt and Shah, 2015).

IL-17 Inhibitors

Keratinocytes are the major target for IL-17 in psoriasis, with IL-17 stimulation causing increased keratinocyte expression of inflammatory cytokines and other effects that contribute to epidermal hyperproliferation and barrier dysfunction. Clinical trials have demonstrated that IL-17 inhibitors are very efficacious for plaque psoriasis.

Secukinumab is a fully human IgG$_{1κ}$ monoclonal antibody against IL-17A approved for the treatment of moderate-to-severe plaque psoriasis in adults. Additional IL-17 inhibitors in phase III clinical trials include *ixekizumab*, a humanized IgG$_4$ monoclonal antibody against IL-17A, and *brodalumab*, a human monoclonal antibody against the IL-17 receptor (anti-IL-17RA), which prevents binding and activity of IL-17. The most common adverse effects for IL-17 inhibitors are nasopharyngitis, upper respiratory tract infection, and diarrhea. There is the potential for increased mucocutaneous candidiasis infections, although this was not common during clinical trials.

PDE4 Inhibitors

Apremilast is an oral PDE4 inhibitor that increases intracellular cyclic AMP levels, thereby decreasing expression of inflammatory cytokines such as TNF-α and IL-23 and increasing expression of anti-inflammatory cytokines such as IL-10. Apremilast is approved for treatment of moderate-to-severe plaque psoriasis and psoriatic arthritis in adults. It has also shown efficacy for atopic dermatitis in a pilot study. The most common side effects are weight loss and depression.

Jak Inhibitors

Janus kinases are tyrosine kinases involved in cytokine receptor signaling, and Jak inhibition leads to decreased downstream activity of STAT, which modulates transcription of genes involved in cell growth, proliferation, and differentiation.

Tofacitinib is an oral Jak inhibitor approved for use in rheumatoid arthritis in adults. It has demonstrated efficacy for psoriasis in clinical trials and for atopic dermatitis in a pilot study.

IL-4 Inhibitors

Dupilumab is a fully human monoclonal antibody against the alpha subunit of IL-4R that inhibits both IL-4 and IL-13 signaling as they each exert their action through binding an IL-4Rα/IL-13Rα1 receptor complex (Beck et al., 2014). IL-4 and IL-13 are important mediators of the Th2 immune response that is involved in acute atopic dermatitis. Dupilumab has shown promising results in clinical trials, demonstrating significant improvement in disease severity and fewer skin infections compared to placebo (Beck et al., 2014). The most frequent adverse effects are nasopharyngitis and headache.

Intravenous Immunoglobulin

Intravenous immunoglobulin is prepared from fractionated pooled human sera derived from thousands of donors with various antigenic exposures (see Chapter 36). Preparations of IVIG are composed of more than 90% IgG, with minimal amounts of IgA, soluble CD4, CD8, HLA molecules, and cytokines. In dermatology, IVIG is used off label as an adjuvant or rescue therapy for autoimmune bullous diseases, toxic epidermal necrolysis, connective tissue diseases, vasculitis, urticaria, atopic dermatitis, and graft-versus-host disease (Smith et al., 2007).

Although the mechanism of action of IVIG is not understood fully, proposed mechanisms include suppression of IgG production, accelerated catabolism of IgG, neutralization of complement-mediated reactions, neutralization of pathogenic antibodies, downregulation of inflammatory cytokines, inhibition of autoreactive T lymphocytes, inhibition of immune cell trafficking, and blockage of Fas-ligand/Fas-receptor interactions (Smith et al., 2007). IVIG is contraindicated in patients with severe selective IgA deficiency (IgA < 0.05 g/L). These patients may possess anti-IgA antibodies that place them at risk for severe anaphylactic reactions. Other relative contraindications include congestive heart failure and renal failure.

Targeted Antineoplastic Agents

Recent advances in understanding the molecular pathways and genetic alterations underlying cancer development have allowed for the rapid emergence of oncotherapeutic agents targeted against the specific molecules involved in tumor pathogenesis (Iwasaki et al., 2012; Jawed et al., 2014; John and Cowey, 2015). They are often better tolerated than conventional chemotherapeutic medications; however, adverse effects do still occur, with cutaneous toxicities amongst the most common. These therapies are discussed in further detail in Chapter 67.

Targeted Therapies for Basal Cell Carcinoma

Basal cell carcinoma is the most common malignancy in humans, and exposure to UV radiation plays a large role in its development, with intermittent, intense exposure increasing risk more than cumulative exposure. Some genetic disorders, such as nevoid BCC syndrome, predispose to BCC development as well. Typically, BCCs exhibit an indolent growth pattern with local invasion and tissue destruction over time, but metastasis is extremely rare. Nearly all BCCs have aberrant *hedgehog* pathway signaling, which leads to persistent activation and uncontrolled proliferation of basal cells (Iwasaki et al., 2012).

Vismodegib and *sonidegib* are *smoothened* inhibitors, which block activation of the hedgehog pathway (Iwasaki et al., 2012). They are approved for use in patients with locally advanced, metastatic, or recurrent disease that cannot be adequately managed with surgery or radiation therapy. They have also been used in patients with nevoid BCC syndrome. The most common side effects are muscle spasms, dysgeusia, alopecia, and diarrhea. The hedgehog pathway is vital to normal fetal development, so extreme caution is needed in women of reproductive potential, and men should be cautioned regarding potential for exposure and fetal harm through semen.

Targeted Therapies for Cutaneous T-Cell Lymphoma

Denileukin difitox is a fusion protein composed of diphtheria toxin fragments A and B linked to the receptor-binding portion of IL-2. It is approved for treatment of advanced CTCL in patients with more than 20% of T cells expressing the surface marker CD25 (α subunit of the IL-2R), but it is not currently commercially available (Jawed et al., 2014).

The IL-2R is present on malignant and activated T cells but not resting B and T cells. Following binding to the IL-2R, denileukin difitox is internalized by endocytosis. The active fragment of diphtheria toxin is then released into the cytosol, where it inhibits protein synthesis via ADP ribosylation of elongation factor-2 (EF-2), leading to cell death. The response rate is 30%. Adverse effects include pain, fevers, chills, nausea, vomiting, and diarrhea; immediate hypersensitivity reaction in 60% of patients; and capillary leak syndrome in 20%–30% of patients.

Histone deacetylase inhibitors approved for treatment of progressive, persistent, or recurrent CTCL refractory to other systemic therapies include *vorinostat* and *romidepsin*. The exact mechanism of antineoplastic effect is not fully characterized; however, inhibition of HDAC may restore expression of tumor suppressor or cell cycle regulatory genes with resultant cell cycle arrest, differentiation, and apoptosis of cancer cells (Jawed et al., 2014). The partial response rate is approximately 30%–35%, with uncommon complete response. The most common side effects are GI symptoms, fatigue, and hematologic abnormalities.

Alemtuzumab is a humanized monoclonal antibody directed against CD52, which is found on immune cells, including T and B cells. Binding of alemtuzumab to CD52 causes neutrophil-mediated, antibody-dependent cellular toxicity (Jawed et al., 2014). It has been effectively used off label for CTCL and may be a secondary treatment option for patients with CTCL refractory to other therapies. It is commonly associated with infusion reactions and causes prolonged immunosuppression. Early studies reported opportunistic infections, so antimicrobial prophylaxis is recommended.

Targeted Therapies for Melanoma

Until recently, therapies for metastatic melanoma had low response rates along with either high toxicity or no effect on long-term survival. There has been rapid development of several new therapeutic options for metastatic or unresectable melanoma, primarily geared toward inhibition of mutated, abnormally activated tyrosine kinases that drive growth or enhancing immune function to combat malignant cells by inhibiting immune checkpoints (John and Cowey, 2015). These therapies include BRAF inhibitors (vemurafenib, dabrafenib), MEK inhibitors (trametinib), CTLA4 inhibitors (ipilimumab), and programmed death-1 inhibitors (pembrolizumab, nivolumab). These targeted treatments are discussed further in Chapter 67. An additional novel therapy for unresectable melanoma is talimogene laherparepvec (T-Vec), an oncolytic immunotherapy derived from genetically modified attenuated HSV type 1. It is administered by intralesional injection and is designed to selectively replicate within tumors and produce GM-CSF to enhance systemic antitumor immune responses. Talimogene is contraindicated in pregnancy and in immunosuppressed patients.

Treatment of Pruritus

Pruritus (itching) occurs in a multitude of dermatological disorders, including xerosis (dry skin), atopic dermatitis, urticaria, and infestations. Itching also may be a sign of internal disorders, including malignant neoplasms, chronic renal failure, and hepatobiliary disease. In addition to treating the underlying disorder, a general approach to the treatment of pruritus can be made by classifying pruritus into one of four clinical categories (Table 70–11).

TABLE 70–11 ■ AGENTS USED FOR THE TREATMENT OF PRURITUS

Pruritoceptive pruritus: Itch originating in the skin due to inflammation or other cutaneous disease

- Emollients—Repair of barrier function
- Coolants (menthol, camphor, calamine)—Counterirritants
- Capsaicin—Counterirritant
- Antihistamines—Inhibit histamine-induced pruritus
- Topical steroids—Direct antipruritic and anti-inflammatory effects
- Topical immunomodulators—Anti-inflammatories
- Phototherapy—Reduced mast cell reactivity and anti-inflammatory effects
- Thalidomide—Anti-inflammatory through suppression of excessive TNF-α

Neuropathic pruritus: Itch due to disease of afferent nerves

- Carbamazepine—Blockade of synaptic transmission and use-dependent Na⁺- channels
- Gabapentin, pregabalin—mechanism unclear; thought to decrease transmission of nociceptive sensations by binding to the α-2-δ subunit of voltage-dependent Ca²⁺ channels
- Topical anesthetics (EMLA, benzocaine, pramoxine)—Inhibit nerve conduction via decreased nerve membrane permeability to sodium

Neurogenic pruritus: Itch that arises from the nervous system without evidence of neural pathology

- Thalidomide—Central depressant
- Opioid receptor antagonists (naloxone, naltrexone)—Decrease opioidergic tone
- Tricyclic antidepressants—Decrease pruritus signaling through alteration in neurotransmitter concentrations
- SSRIs—Decrease pruritus signaling through alteration in neurotransmitter concentrations

Psychogenic pruritus: Itch due to psychological illness

- Anxiolytics (benzodiazepines)—Relieve stress-reactive pruritus
- Antipsychotic agents (chlorpromazine, thioridazine, thiothixene, olanzapine)—Relieve pruritus with impulsive qualities
- Tricyclic antidepressants—Relieve depression and insomnia related to pruritus
- SSRIs—Relieve pruritus with compulsive qualities

Drugs for Hyperkeratotic Disorders

Keratolytic agents reduce hyperkeratosis through myriad mechanisms (e.g., breaking of intercellular junctions, increasing stratum corneum water content, increasing desquamation). Common disorders treated with keratolytics include psoriasis, seborrheic dermatitis, xerosis, ichthyoses, and verrucae.

α-Hydroxy acids can reduce the thickness of the stratum corneum by solubilizing components of the desmosome, activating endogenous hydrolytic enzymes, and drawing water into the stratum corneum, thereby facilitating cell separation. They also appear to increase glycosaminoglycans, collagen, and elastic fibers in the dermis and are used in various formulations to reverse photoaging. The FDA requires that cosmetics containing α-hydroxy acids be labeled with a sunburn alert warning that the product may increase sensitivity to the sun. α-Hydroxy acids used include glycolic, lactic, malic, citric, hydroxycaprylic, hydroxycapric, and mandelic.

Salicylic acid functions through solubilization of intercellular "cement," reducing keratinocyte adhesion, and softening the stratum corneum. Salicylism may occur with widespread and prolonged use, especially in children and patients with renal or hepatic impairment. Salicylate toxicity has been reported with application of as little as 1%–2% salicylic acid in neonates when applied multiple times per day over a large body surface area (Madan and Levitt, 2014). Salicylic acid, while chemically not a true β-hydroxy acid, often is listed as such on cosmetic labels. Other β-hydroxy acid ingredients in cosmetics include β-hydroxybutanoic acid, δ-tropic acid, and trethocanic acid. Sun protection should accompany the topical application of these agents.

Urea, at low concentrations, increases skin absorption and retention of water, leading to increased flexibility and softness of the skin. At concentrations greater than 40%, urea denatures and dissolves proteins and is used to dissolve calluses or avulse dystrophic nails.

Sulfur is keratolytic, antiseptic, antiparasitic, and antiseborrheic. It exerts its keratolytic effect by reacting with cysteine within keratinocytes, producing cystine and hydrogen sulfide (H₂S). H₂S breaks down keratin, causing dissolution of the stratum corneum.

Propylene glycol (as 60%–100% aqueous solutions) increases the water content of the stratum corneum and enhances desquamation. It is most effective in disorders with retention hyperkeratosis.

Drugs Affecting Hair Growth

Androgenic Alopecia

Androgenetic alopecia, commonly known as male and female pattern baldness, is the most common cause of hair loss in adults older than 40 years. The frequency and severity increase with age and may begin during puberty in some patients. It is a genetically inherited trait with variable expression. In susceptible hair follicles, dihydrotestosterone (DHT) binds to the androgen receptor, and the hormone-receptor complex activates the genes responsible for the gradual transformation of large terminal follicles into miniaturized vellus follicles. Treatment of androgenetic alopecia is aimed at reducing hair loss and maintaining existing hair (Varothai and Bergfeld, 2014).

Minoxidil, originally developed as an antihypertensive agent (see Chapter 28), was noted to be associated with hypertrichosis in some patients. Topical minoxidil is available as a 2% solution and a 5% solution or foam. Minoxidil enhances follicular size, resulting in thicker hair shafts, and stimulates and prolongs the anagen phase of the hair cycle, resulting in longer and increased numbers of hair. Treatment must be continued or any drug-induced hair growth will be lost. Allergic and irritant contact dermatitis can occur, and care should be taken in applying the drug because hair growth may emerge in undesirable locations. This is reversible on stopping the drug. Patients should be instructed to wash their hands after applying minoxidil. Patients with increased sulfotransferase enzyme activity are most likely to respond to minoxidil treatment; this may be a useful predictive test in the future (Roberts et al., 2014).

Finasteride inhibits the type II isozyme of 5α-reductase, the enzyme that converts testosterone to DHT (see Figure 45–3) and that is found in hair follicles. Balding areas of the scalp are associated with increased DHT levels and smaller hair follicles than nonbalding areas. Orally administered finasteride (1 mg/d) variably increases hair growth in men over a 2-year period. Finasteride is approved for use only in men but has been used off label for female pattern hair loss (Varothai and Bergfeld, 2014). Finasteride use in women is limited by its teratogenicity. Pregnant women should not be exposed to the drug because of the potential for inducing genital abnormalities in male fetuses. Adverse effects of finasteride include decreased libido, erectile dysfunction, ejaculation disorder, and decreased ejaculate volume. There have been postmarketing surveillance reports of persistent sexual dysfunction after stopping the medication. As with minoxidil, new hair growth will be lost when finasteride is discontinued. *Dutasteride* (0.5 mg/day) is a combined type I and type II isozyme 5α-reductase inhibitor that has similar or greater efficacy, but side effects may be more common (Varothai and Bergfeld, 2014).

Spironolactone is an aldosterone antagonist and K^+-sparing diuretic; it also has antiandrogen activity. It is used off label for female pattern alopecia at dosages of 50–200 mg/d (Varothai and Bergfeld, 2014). Women of reproductive potential should not receive spironolactone without reliable contraception because spironolactone can cause feminization of a male fetus.

Other Agents

Eflornithine is an ornithine decarboxylase (ODC) inhibitor approved for the reduction of excessive and unwanted facial hair in women. ODC is the rate-limiting enzyme in the synthesis of polyamines, which are important in cellular migration, differentiation, and proliferation. Levels of ODC activity are higher in proliferating cells, such as in follicular matrix cells in anagen phase, and inhibiting ODC decreases hair growth. Eflornithine 13.9% cream is applied twice daily and is intended to be used along with the patient's preferred hair removal method to slow hair regrowth.

Bimatoprost is a prostaglandin analogue approved for topical treatment of hypotrichosis of the eyelashes by increasing their growth, including length, thickness, and darkness. The prostaglandin-mediated increase in eyelash growth was serendipitously noted during the use of intraocular prostaglandin analogues for glaucoma. The proposed mechanism of eyelash growth is by an increase in the fraction of hairs in, and the duration of, the anagen phase. Increased pigmentation of the hairs is thought to occur due to stimulation of melanin production without an increase in the number of melanocytes. Importantly, brown pigmentation of the iris and eyelid skin may occur, and the increased iris pigmentation may be permanent.

Treatment of Hyperpigmentation

The agents discussed are most effective on hormonally or light-induced pigmentation within the epidermis. They have limited efficacy on postinflammatory pigmentation within the dermis. Sun protection or avoidance is a vital component of any treatment regimen (Sheth and Pandya, 2011).

Hydroquinone (1,4-dihydroxybenzene) decreases melanocyte pigment production by inhibiting tyrosinase, the initial enzyme in the melanin biosynthetic pathway. In addition, it causes degradation of melanosomes and destruction of melanocytes by production of reactive oxygen radicals. Formulations containing 1.5%–2% hydroquinone are available OTC; 3%–4% hydroquinone formulations are available by prescription. Penetration enhancers and sunscreen ingredients are added to some formulations. A combination prescription product consisting of hydroquinone 4%, fluocinolone 0.01%, and tretinoin 0.05% is available. Adverse effects may include dermatitis and ochronosis.

Azelaic acid, a dicarboxylic acid isolated from cultures of *Malassezia furfur,* inhibits tyrosinase activity but is less effective than hydroquinone. Because it has mild comedolytic, antimicrobial, and anti-inflammatory properties, it also is often used in acne and papulopustular rosacea, especially in patients with postinflammatory hyperpigmentation.

Mequinol (4-hydroxyanisole) is a competitive inhibitor of tyrosinase. It was approved as a 2% prescription product in combination with 0.01%

tretinoin and vitamin C for skin lightening, but it is not currently commercially available.

Monobenzone (monobenzyl ether of hydroquinone) causes *permanent* depigmentation and should *not* be used for routine hormonally induced or postinflammatory hyperpigmentation. A 20% cream is approved for final depigmentation therapy of extensive vitiligo affecting at least more than 50% body surface area; it is rarely used and not currently commercially available.

Glycolic acid is an α-hydroxy acid used in chemical peels for disorders of pigmentation. It is thought to work by inhibiting tyrosinase in a pH-independent manner and to cause exfoliation by decreasing keratinocyte adhesion. Potential side effects are erythema, desquamation, and postinflammatory hyperpigmentation. Glycolic acid peels are best used as adjunctive therapy along with other topical therapy in patients with refractory epidermal hyperpigmentation (Sheth and Pandya, 2011).

Miscellaneous Agents

Capsaicin is an alkaloid derived from plants of the *Solanaceae* family (i.e., hot chili peppers). Capsaicin interacts with the transient receptor potential vanilloid (TRPV1) receptor on C-fiber sensory neurons. TRPV1 is a ligand-gated nonselective cation channel of the TRP family, modulated by a variety of noxious stimuli. Chronic exposure to capsaicin first stimulates and then desensitizes this channel to capsaicin and diverse other noxious stimuli. Capsaicin also causes local depletion of substance P, an endogenous neuropeptide involved in sensory perception and pain transmission. Capsaicin (cream, lotion, gel, roll-on, and transdermal patch) is FDA approved for the temporary relief of minor aches and pains associated with backache, strains, and arthritis. It is also approved in patch form by prescription for postherpetic neuralgia and is used for off-label treatment of painful diabetic neuropathy and some forms of pruritus.

Bentoquatam (quaternium-18 bentonite) is a mixture of quaternium-18 (quaternary ammonium chloride salts made from the fatty acids of tallow) and bentonite clay. This organoclay mixture is approved for OTC use as a topical barrier to prevent allergic contact dermatitis to the urushiol resin of poison ivy, oak, or sumac. The 5% topical lotion must be applied prophylactically at least 15 min prior to potential risk for exposure to urushiol and reapplied every 4 h.

Coal tar is a distillation product from coal, a mixture of over 10,000 compounds. It is used in dermatology primarily for the treatment of inflammatory skin conditions such as psoriasis, seborrheic dermatitis, and atopic dermatitis or other forms of eczematous dermatitis. The mechanism of action is unknown although it is known to suppress DNA synthesis. Coal tar has anti-inflammatory, antimicrobial, and antipruritic activity. In addition, it has a photosensitizing effect within the UVA and visible light spectrum between wavelengths of 330 and 550 nm. Multiple formulations and products are available commercially or through compounding, including those containing crude coal tar, coal tar extracts, or coal tar solution (Sandhu and Schwartz, 2011). Coal tar solution, also known as liquor carbonis detergens (LCD), is an alcohol extract of coal tar emulsified with polysorbate 80 to yield a more cosmetically acceptable product. Coal tar may be used in combination with UVB phototherapy (e.g., Goeckerman regimen), topical salicylic acid, or topical corticosteroids. Coal tar products are often poorly tolerated by patients due to its unpleasant odor, messiness, and potential for staining of clothing. It can also cause folliculitis or irritant contact dermatitis. Though occupational exposures to coal tar have been associated with malignancies (e.g., scrotal cancer), patients with psoriasis or atopic dermatitis who are treated with topical coal tar products have not exhibited increased risk of cancer (Menter et al., 2009a).

Anthralin (dithranol), a synthetic version of chrysarobin, is derived from the bark of the Brazilian araroba tree and is used in the treatment of psoriasis and alopecia areata; its mechanisms of action are unclear (Menter et al., 2009a). Use of anthralin has been limited by the potential to cause irritant contact dermatitis and to stain skin, hair, nails, fabrics, and household items.

Brimonidine (0.33% topical gel) is an α_2 adrenergic agonist approved for once-daily treatment of persistent erythema of rosacea. It causes temporary vasoconstriction, and rebound erythema has been reported. α_1 Adrenergic agonists such as oxymetazoline have been used off label topically for erythematotelangiectatic rosacea as well.

Propranolol and timolol are nonselective β adrenergic antagonists traditionally used for cardiovascular disease. These agents are also effective in treating infantile hemangiomas and become the preferred treatment of infantile hemangiomas requiring intervention (Chen et al., 2013). Topical timolol drops and gel-forming solution are available but do not adequately treat deeper lesions.

Acknowledgment: Eric L. Wyatt, Steven H. Sutter, Lynn A. Drake, Lindy P. Fox, Hans F. Merk, David R. Bickers, and Lowell Goldsmith have contributed to this chapter in earlier editions of this book. We have retained some of their text in the current edition.

Drug Facts for Your Personal Formulary: *Dermatological Agents*

Drugs	Therapeutic Uses	Clinical Pharmacology and Tips
Glucocorticoids—Table 70–3 and Chapter 46		
Topical glucocorticoids	• Psoriasis • Atopic dermatitis • Other inflammatory skin diseases	• Occlusion increases absorption • May cause skin atrophy, striae, periorificial dermatitis, folliculitis • Limit to ≤ 2–3 weeks of use • Avoid potent corticosteroids on face and genital areas • **Systemic** glucocorticoids for severe disease; see Chapter 46
Retinoids		
Topical retinoids (see Table 70–4)	• Acne • Facial wrinkling and photodamage • Psoriasis • Cutaneous KS (*alitretinoin*) • CTCL (*bexarotene*)	• Start every-other-night application to reduce likelihood of skin irritation • Decreased activity in presence of sunlight or BPO except *adapalene* and *tazarotene* • Avoid concurrent application of DEET due to potential increased DEET absorption
Oral Retinoids (see Table 70–5)	• Psoriasis (*acitretin*) • Acne (*isotretinoin*) • CTCL (*bexarotene*)	• Teratogenic: pregnancy should be avoided during and for 1 month (3 years for acitretin) after cessation of treatment • Multiple potential side effects, including cheilitis, dermatitis, conjunctivitis, myalgias, arthralgias, epistaxis, decreased night vision, hyperlipidemia
Topical Vitamin D Analogues		
Calcipotriene	• Psoriasis	• Potential hypercalcemia and hypercalciuria • May cause lesional or perilesional irritation
Photochemotherapeutic Agents (see Table 70–6)		
Biological Agents for Psoriasis—Table 70–10		
Antihistamines for Urticaria: see Chapter 39		
Topical Antimicrobial Agents for Acne and Rosacea		
Azelaic acid	• Acne • Rosacea	• MOA: comedolytic, antibacterial, anti-inflammatory • Also useful for postinflammatory hyperpigmentation due to acne
Benzoyl peroxide	• Acne	• MOA: antibacterial, mildly comedolytic • Skin irritation with higher concentrations
Clindamycin	• Acne • Rosacea (off label)	• MOA: antibacterial, anti-inflammatory • Bacterial resistance likely if used as monotherapy, use with benzoyl peroxide
Dapsone	• Acne	• MOA: anti-inflammatory • Use with benzoyl peroxide causes orange-brown staining of skin or hair • G6PD testing not needed
Erythromycin	• Acne • Rosacea (off label)	• MOA: antibacterial, anti-inflammatory • Bacterial resistance likely if used as monotherapy, use with benzoyl peroxide
Metronidazole	• Rosacea	• MOA: anti-inflammatory
Sulfacetamide ± sulfur	• Acne • Rosacea	• MOA: antibacterial, anti-inflammatory; sulfur also keratolytic • Use with benzoyl peroxide causes orange-brown staining of clothing but not skin • Sulfur may have pungent odor
Topical Antimicrobial Agents for Infection		
Bacitracin, neomycin, polymyxin B, gentamicin	• Superficial bacterial skin infections	• See Section VI, Chemotherapy of Microbial Diseases • Topical use restricted for superficial infections • Not indicated in clean surgical wounds • May cause contact dermatitis (especially bacitracin, neomycin, mafenide) • Mafenide inhibits carbonic anhydrase and can cause metabolic acidosis • Efficacy of silver sulfadiazine questionable

Drug Facts for Your Personal Formulary: *Dermatological Agents (continued)*

Drugs	Therapeutic Uses	Clinical Pharmacology and Tips
Topical Antimicrobial Agents for Infection		
Mupirocin, retapamulin	• Superficial bacterial skin infections due to *S. aureus* or *S. pyogenes* • Intranasal decolonization of MRSA	
Mafenide acetate	• Adjunctive therapy for burn wounds	
Silver sulfadiazine	• Prevention or treatment in partial-thickness burns or venous stasis ulcers	
Topical Antifungal Agents—Table 70–8 (see Chapter 61 for oral antifungal agents)		
Antiviral Agents		
Topical Antivirals: Acyclovir Docosanol Penciclovir	• Orolabial HSV • Genital HSV, initial episode (acyclovir)	• See Chapter 62
Oral Antivirals: Acyclovir Famciclovir Valacyclovir	• VZV • HSV	
Agents for Infestations		
Benzyl alcohol	• Head lice	• MOA: inhibits closure of respiratory spiracles, subsequent obstruction by mineral oil vehicle causes asphyxiation of lice
Ivermectin	• Head lice • Scabies (oral)	• MOA: binds glutamate-gated chloride channels, causing hyperpolarization of nerve or muscle cells of parasite
Lindane	• Scabies • Lice	• MOA: neuronal hyperstimulation, eventual parasite paralysis • Potential neurotoxicity with prolonged use or in patients with impaired skin barrier (e.g., atopic dermatitis)
Malathion	• Head lice	• MOA: acetylcholinesterase inhibitor causing neuromuscular paralysis • Flammable due to high alcohol content
Permethrin	• Scabies • Lice	• MOA: interferes with Na^+ transport, causing neurotoxicity and paralysis • Approved for infants ≥ 2 months • May cross-react with sunflower family plants to cause allergic contact dermatitis
Spinosad	• Head lice	• MOA: causes CNS excitation and involuntary muscle contractions leading to parasite paralysis
Crotamiton	• Scabies	• MOA: unknown • Less effective than other agents but has additional antipruritic effect
Precipitated sulfur	• Scabies	• MOA: unknown • Poor odor and mild skin irritation • Considered safe in pregnancy and infants
Systemic Cytotoxic, Immunosuppressant, and Immunomodulatory Agents		
Methotrexate	• Psoriasis • Off label for multiple inflammatory dermatoses	• See Chapter 66
Cyclophosphamide	• CTCL • Off label for severe autoimmune blistering dermatoses	• See Chapter 66
Vinblastine	• Kaposi sarcoma • CTCL	• See Chapter 66
Doxorubicin	• Kaposi sarcoma	• See Chapter 66
Azathioprine	• Off label for inflammatory and autoimmune blistering disorders	• MOA: inhibition of de novo purine synthesis to decrease T-cell and B-cell activation and proliferation • TPMT enzyme activity should be measured before initiation
Mycophenolate mofetil and mycophenolic acid	• Off label for inflammatory and autoimmune blistering disorders	• MOA: inhibition of de novo purine synthesis to decrease T-cell and B-cell activation and proliferation • Most common side effect is GI upset
Cyclosporine	• Psoriasis • Off label for multiple inflammatory dermatoses	• MOA: calcineurin inhibition • Potential side effects: hypertension, renal dysfunction, hypertrichosis, gingival hyperplasia, tremor

Systemic Cytotoxic, Immunosuppressant, and Immunomodulatory Agents (continued)		
mTOR inhibitors	• Off-label use in tuberous sclerosis, complex vascular malformations, and inflammatory dermatoses	• MOA: mTOR inhibition • Potential side effects: stomatitis, mucositis, inflammatory cutaneous eruptions, nail changes
Dapsone	• Dermatitis herpetiformis • Leprosy • Neutrophilic dermatoses (off label)	• See Chapter 60
Thalidomide	• Erythema nodosum leprosum • Off label for prurigo nodularis, cutaneous lupus erythematosus, Behçet disease	• See Chapter 36

Topical or Intralesional Cytotoxic, Immunosuppressant, and Immunomodulatory Agents		
5-Fluorouracil	• Actinic keratoses • Superficial basal cell carcinoma • Warts (off label)	• See Chapter 66
Bleomycin	• Squamous cell carcinoma (off label) • Recalcitrant warts (off label)	• See Chapter 66
Alkylating agents *Carmustine* *Mechlorethamine*	• CTCL	• See Chapter 66
Podophyllum resin and podofilox	• Genital warts	• MOA: microtubule inhibition to cause mitotic arrest in metaphase • Side effects: irritation and ulcerative local reactions
Ingenol mebutate	• Actinic keratoses	• MOA: mitochondrial swelling and apoptosis of dysplastic keratinocytes
Imiquimod	• Genital warts • Actinic keratoses • Superficial basal cell carcinoma	• MOA: activates TLR-7, inducing cytokines and upregulating immune response • Potential local skin reaction or systemic flu-like symptoms
Sinecatechins	• Genital warts	• MOA: uncertain • Potential local skin reactions, including erythema, pruritus, swelling that peaks between 2 and 4 weeks of use
mTOR inhibitors	• Off-label use in tuberous sclerosis, complex vascular malformations, and some inflammatory dermatoses	• Topical mTOR inhibitors not currently commercially available but may be compounded • Topical use may decrease potential for side effects seen with systemic use
Topical calcineurin inhibitors Pimecrolimus Tacrolimus	• Psoriasis • Atopic dermatitis • Other inflammatory skin diseases	• MOA: Decreased T-cell activation • No skin atrophy • Useful in sensitive areas such as face and skinfolds • Common application site reactions (e.g., burning) decreases with continued use

Targeted Immunotherapies for Psoriasis and Atopic Dermatitis		
TNF-α inhibitors; IL-12/23 inhibitors; IL-17 inhibitors; PDE4 inhibitors; Jak inhibitors	• Psoriasis • Atopic dermatitis: off-label use of PDE4 inhibitors, Jak inhibitors	• See Chapter 35

Targeted Antineoplastic Agents		
Smoothened inhibitors Histone deacetylase inhibitors	• Basal cell carcinoma • CTCL	• See Chapter 67
BRAF inhibitors; MEK inhibitors; CTLA4 inhibitors; programmed death 1 inhibitors	• Melanoma	• See Chapter 67

Topical Agents for Hyperkeratotic Disorders		
Alpha-hydroxy acids Glycolic acid Lactic acid	• Hyperkeratotic disorders	• MOA: reduced keratinocyte adhesion by promoting degradation of corneodesmosomes • Potential skin irritation
Salicylic acid	• Hyperkeratotic disorders	• MOA: reduced keratinocyte adhesion by affecting desmosomal adhesion proteins • Potential skin irritation • Potential salicylate toxicity with heavy use
Urea	• Hyperkeratotic disorders	• MOA: increased hydration of stratum corneum, enhancing desquamation • Potential skin irritation
Sulfur	• Hyperkeratotic disorders	• MOA: possibly through interaction with cysteine, causing reduction to hydrogen sulfide, which may break down keratin • Pungent odor

Drug Facts for Your Personal Formulary: *Dermatological Agents (continued)*

Drugs	Therapeutic Uses	Clinical Pharmacology and Tips
Topical Agents for Hyperkeratotic Disorders		
Propylene glycol	• Hyperkeratotic disorders	• MOA: increased hydration of stratum corneum, enhancing desquamation
Retinoids	• Hyperkeratotic disorders	• MOA: stimulation of keratinocyte turnover • Potential skin irritation
Agents Affecting Hair Growth		
Minoxidil, topical	• Androgenetic alopecia	• MOA: not fully determined; stimulates and prolongs anagen phase • Requires continued use to sustain effect
Finasteride, oral Dutasteride, oral	• Androgenetic alopecia • Hirsutism (off label)	• MOA: inhibition of 5-α reductase to decrease conversion of testosterone to DHT • Side effects: decreased libido, sexual dysfunction, hypotension
Spironolactone, oral	• Hirsutism (off label) • Female pattern alopecia (off label)	• MOA: aldosterone antagonist with antiandrogenic activity • Side effects: breast tenderness, menstrual irregularities, increased urination • Feminization of male fetus
Eflornithine, topical	• Unwanted facial hair in women	• MOA: ornithine decarboxylase inhibition to decrease hair growth • Slows hair growth; use in combination with hair removal methods
Bimatoprost, topical	• Hypotrichosis of the eyelashes	• MOA: prostaglandin analogue that increases percentage of hairs in anagen phase • May cause brown pigmentation of eyelid and iris (permanent)

Please note that there are numerous additional off-label uses of medications in dermatological conditions. MOA, mechanism of action.

Bibliography

Baron JM, et al. Expression of multiple cytochrome p450 enzymes and multidrug resistance-associated transport proteins in human skin keratinocytes. *J Invest Dermatol*, 2001, 116:541–548.

Beck LA, et al. Dupilumab treatment in adults with moderate-to-severe atopic dermatitis. *N Engl J Med*, 2014, 371:130–139.

Bellodi Schmidt F, Shah KN. Biologic response modifiers and pediatric psoriasis. *Pediatr Dermatol*, 2015, 32:303–320.

Bhatia N. Use of antibiotics for noninfectious dermatologic disorders. *Dermatol Clin*, 2009, 27:85–89.

Bjelakovic G, et al. Antioxidant supplements for prevention of mortality in healthy participants and patients with various diseases. *Cochrane Database Syst Rev*, 2012, (3):CD007176.

Browning JC, Levy ML. Argyria attributed to silvadene application in a patient with dystrophic epidermolysis bullosa. *Dermatol Online J*, 2008, 14:9.

Chasset F, et al. Influence of smoking on the efficacy of antimalarials in cutaneous lupus: a meta-analysis of the literature. *J Am Acad Dermatol*, 2015, 72:634–639.

Chen TS, et al. Infantile hemangiomas: an update on pathogenesis and therapy. *Pediatrics*, 2013, 131:99–108.

Das S, Reynolds RV. Recent advances in acne pathogenesis: implications for therapy. *Am J Clin Dermatol*, 2014, 15:479–488.

de Sa DC, et al. Oral therapy for onychomycosis: an evidence-based review. *Am J Clin Dermatol*, 2014, 15:17–36.

Desai A, et al. Systemic retinoid therapy: a status report on optimal use and safety of long-term therapy. *Dermatol Clin*, 2007, 25:185–193, vi.

Diamantis SA, et al. Pediatric infestations. *Pediatr Ann*, 2009, 38:326–332.

Drucker CR. Update on topical antibiotics in dermatology. *Dermatol Ther*, 2012, 25:6–11.

Eichenfield LF, et al. Evidence-based recommendations for the diagnosis and treatment of pediatric acne. *Pediatrics*, 2013, 131(suppl 3):S163–S186.

Eichenfield LF, et al. Guidelines of care for the management of atopic dermatitis: section 2. Management and treatment of atopic dermatitis with topical therapies. *J Am Acad Dermatol*, 2014, 71:116–132.

Elewski BE, et al. Terbinafine hydrochloride oral granules versus oral griseofulvin suspension in children with tinea capitis: results of two randomized, investigator-blinded, multicenter, international, controlled trials. *J Am Acad Dermatol*, 2008, 59:41–54.

Fathi R, Tsoukas MM. Genital warts and other HPV infections: established and novel therapies. *Clin Dermatol*, 2014, 32:299–306.

Fogel AL, et al. Advances in the therapeutic use of mammalian target of rapamycin (mTOR) inhibitors in dermatology. *J Am Acad Dermatol*, 2015, 72:879–889.

Girolomoni G, et al. Psoriasis: rationale for targeting interleukin-17. *Br J Dermatol*, 2012, 167:717–724.

Good LM, et al. Intralesional agents in the management of cutaneous malignancy: a review. *J Am Acad Dermatol*, 2011, 64:413–422.

Gupta AK, Paquet M. Systemic antifungals to treat onychomycosis in children: a systematic review. *Pediatr Dermatol*, 2013, 30:294–302.

Gupta AK, et al. Topical therapy for toenail onychomycosis: an evidence-based review. *Am J Clin Dermatol*, 2014, 15:489–502.

Hwa C, et al. Skin biology. *Dermatol Ther*, 2011, 24:464–470.

Iwasaki JK, et al. The molecular genetics underlying basal cell carcinoma pathogenesis and links to targeted therapeutics. *J Am Acad Dermatol*, 2012, 66:e167–e178.

Jawed SI, et al. Primary cutaneous T-cell lymphoma (mycosis fungoides and Sezary syndrome): part II. Prognosis, management, and future directions. *J Am Acad Dermatol*, 2014, 70:223.e1–e17.

John L, Cowey CL. The rapid emergence of novel therapeutics in advanced malignant melanoma. *Dermatol Ther*, 2015, 5:151–169.

Kalia S, Dutz JP. New concepts in antimalarial use and mode of action in dermatology. *Dermatol Ther*, 2007, 20:160–174.

Levender MM, et al. Use of topical antibiotics as prophylaxis in clean dermatologic procedures. *J Am Acad Dermatol*, 2012, 66:445–451.

Madan RK, Levitt J. A review of toxicity from topical salicylic acid preparations. *J Am Acad Dermatol*, 2014, 70:788–792.

Mancebo SE, et al. Sunscreens: a review of health benefits, regulations, and controversies. *Dermatol Clin*, 2014, 32:427–438, x.

Mehregan DR, Gee SL. The cost effectiveness of testing for onychomycosis versus empiric treatment of onychodystrophies with oral antifungal agents. *Cutis*, 1999, 64:407–410.

Menter A, et al. Guidelines of care for the management of psoriasis and psoriatic arthritis. Section 3. Guidelines of care for the management and treatment of psoriasis with topical therapies. *J Am Acad Dermatol*, 2009a, 60:643–659.

Menter A, et al. Guidelines of care for the management of psoriasis and psoriatic arthritis: section 4. Guidelines of care for the management and treatment of psoriasis with traditional systemic agents. *J Am Acad Dermatol*, 2009b, 61:451–485.

Meurer M. Immunosuppressive therapy for autoimmune bullous diseases. *Clin Dermatol*, 2012, 30:78–83.

Micali G, et al. Topical pharmacotherapy for skin cancer: part II. Clinical applications. *J Am Acad Dermatol*, **2014**, *70*:979.e1–e12; quiz 9912.

Miller AC, et al. Silver sulfadiazine for the treatment of partial-thickness burns and venous stasis ulcers. *J Am Acad Dermatol*, **2012**, *66*:e159–65.

Ortega-Loayza AG, et al. Crusted scabies and multiple dosages of ivermectin. *J Drugs Dermatol*, **2013**, *12*:584–585.

Perotti C, Sniecinski I. A concise review on extracorporeal photochemotherapy: where we began and where we are now and where are we going! *Transfus Apher Sci*, **2015**, *52*:360–368.

Rajan S. Skin and soft-tissue infections: classifying and treating a spectrum. *Cleve Clin J Med*, **2012**, *79*:57–66.

Regnier-Rosencher E, et al. Treatments for classic Kaposi sarcoma: a systematic review of the literature. *J Am Acad Dermatol*, **2013**, *68*:313–331.

Rkein AM, Ozog DM. Photodynamic therapy. *Dermatol Clin*, **2014**, *32*:415–425, x.

Roberts J, et al. Sulfotransferase activity in plucked hair follicles predicts response to topical minoxidil in the treatment of female androgenetic alopecia. *Dermatol Ther*, **2014**, *27*:252–254.

Rosen J, et al. Principles and approaches for optimizing therapy with unique topical vehicles. *J Drugs Dermatol*, **2014**, *13*(12):1431–1435.

Rotta I, et al. Efficacy of topical antifungals in the treatment of dermatophytosis: a mixed-treatment comparison meta-analysis involving 14 treatments. *JAMA Dermatol*, **2013**, *149*:341–349.

Sandhu N, Schwartz RA. Topical tar. In: Maibach H, Gorouhi F, eds. *Evidence Based Dermatology*. 2nd ed. People's Medical Publishing House-USA, Shelton, CT, **2011**, 935–942.

Sarnoff DS. Treatment of recurrent herpes labialis. *J Drugs Dermatol*, **2014**, *13*:1016–1018.

Sheth VM, Pandya AG. Melasma: a comprehensive update: part II. *J Am Acad Dermatol*, **2011**, *65*:699–714; quiz 715.

Sidbury R, et al. Guidelines of care for the management of atopic dermatitis: section 3. Management and treatment with phototherapy and systemic agents. *J Am Acad Dermatol*, **2014**, *71*:327–349.

Simons FE, Simons KJ. H1 antihistamines: current status and future directions. *World Allergy Organ J*, **2008**, *1*:145–155.

Smith DI, et al. Off-label uses of biologics in dermatology: interferon and intravenous immunoglobulin (part 1 of 2). *J Am Acad Dermatol*, **2007**, *56*:e1–e54.

Sobell JM, Leonardi CL. Therapeutic development in psoriasis. *Semin Cutan Med Surg*, **2014**, *33*(4 suppl):S69–S72.

Stevens DL, et al. Practice guidelines for the diagnosis and management of skin and soft tissue infections: 2014 update by the Infectious Diseases Society of America. *Clin Infect Dis*, **2014**, *59*:e10–e52.

Thielitz A, Gollnick H. Topical retinoids in acne vulgaris: update on efficacy and safety. *Am J Clin Dermatol*, **2008**, *9*:369–381.

Totonchy MB, Chiu MW. UV-based therapy. *Dermatol Clin*, **2014**, *32*:399–413, ix–x.

Tran TN. Cutaneous drug delivery: an update. *J Investig Dermatol Symp Proc*, **2013**, *16*:S67–S69.

Varothai S, Bergfeld WF. Androgenetic alopecia: an evidence-based treatment update. *Am J Clin Dermatol*, **2014**, *15*:217–230.

Warren RB, et al. Genetic variation in efflux transporters influences outcome to methotrexate therapy in patients with psoriasis. *J Invest Dermatol*, **2008**, *128*:1925–1929.

Williams HC. Established corticosteroid creams should be applied only once daily in patients with atopic eczema. *BMJ*, **2007**, *334*(7606):1272.

Wolff K, et al., eds. *Fitzpatrick's Dermatology in General Medicine*. 7th ed. McGraw-Hill, New York, **2008**.

Wu JJ, et al. Thalidomide: dermatological indications, mechanisms of action and side-effects. *Br J Dermatol*, **2005**, *153*:254–273.

Zhu YI, Stiller MJ. Dapsone and sulfones in dermatology: overview and update. *J Am Acad Dermatol*, **2001**, *45*:420–434.

Suggested Reading

Ameen M, et al. British Association of Dermatologists' guidelines for the management of onychomycosis 2014. *Br J Dermatol*, **2014**, *171*:937–958.

Amin K, et al. Common and alternate oral antibiotic therapies for acne vulgaris: a review. *J Drugs Dermatol*, **2007**, *6*:873–880.

Amor KT, et al. The use of cyclosporine in dermatology: part I. *J Am Acad Dermatol*, **2010**, *63*:925–46; quiz 947–8.

Barnes L, et al. Topical corticosteroid-induced skin atrophy: a comprehensive review. *Drug Saf*, **2015**, *38*:493–509.

Boehncke WH. Etiology and pathogenesis of psoriasis. *Rheum Dis Clin North Am*, **2015**, *41*:665–675.

Budgin JB, et al. Biological effects of bexarotene in cutaneous T-cell lymphoma. *Arch Dermatol*, **2005**, *141*:315–321.

Chitwood K, et al. Topical and intralesional treatment of nonmelanoma skin cancer: efficacy and cost comparisons. *Dermatol Surg*, **2013**, *39*:1306–1316.

Classification of topical corticosteroids. WHO model prescribing information: drugs used in skin diseases. Available at: http://apps.who.int/medicinedocs/en/d/Jh2918e/32.html. Accessed February 1, 2016.

Ference JD, Last AR. Choosing topical corticosteroids. *Am Fam Physician*, **2009**, *79*:135–140.

Food and Drug Administration, HHS. Labeling and effectiveness testing; sunscreen drug products for over-the-counter human use. Final rule. *Fed Regist*, **2011**, *76*(117):35620–35665.

Golant AK, Levitt JO. Scabies: a review of diagnosis and management based on mite biology. *Pediatr Rev*, **2012**, *33*:e1–e12.

Goren A, et al. Clinical utility and validity of minoxidil response testing in androgenetic alopecia. *Dermatol Ther*, **2015**, *28*:13–16.

Gormley RH, Kovarik CL. Human papillomavirus–related genital disease in the immunocompromised host. *J Am Acad Dermatol*, **2012**, *66*:883.e1–e17.

Gupta D. Atopic dermatitis: a common pediatric condition and its evolution in adulthood. *Med Clin North Am*, **2015**, *99*:1296–1285

Hajar T, et al. A systematic review of topical corticosteroid withdrawal ("steroid addiction") in patients with atopic dermatitis and other dermatoses. *J Am Acad Dermatol*, **2015**, *72*:541–549.e2.

Honigsmann H, et al. Serum levels of 8-methoxypsoralen in two different drug preparations: correlation with photosensitivity and UV-A dose requirements for photochemotherapy. *J Invest Dermatol*, **1982**, *79*:233–236.

Jackson SM, Nesbitt LT. Glucocorticosteroids. In: Bolognia JL, et al., eds. *Dermatology*. 3rd ed. Elsevier, Philadelphia, **2012**, 2075–2088.

Jacob SE, Steele T. Corticosteroid classes: a quick reference. *J Am Acad Dermatol*, **2006**, *54*:723–727.

Jewell JR, Myers SA. Topical therapy primer for nondermatologists. *Med Clin North Am*, **2015**, *99*:1167–1182.

Kwok CS, et al. Topical treatments for cutaneous warts. *Cochrane Database Syst Rev*, **2012**, (9):CD001781.

Lebwohl M, et al. Therapy for head lice based on life cycle, resistance, and safety considerations. *Pediatrics*, **2007**, *119*:965–974.

Legendre L, et al. Risk of lymphoma in patients with atopic dermatitis and the role of topical treatment: A systematic review and meta-analysis. *J Am Acad Dermatol*, **2015**, *72*:992–1002.

Leyden JJ, Del Rosso JQ. Oral antibiotic therapy for acne vulgaris: pharmacokinetic and pharmacodynamic perspectives. *J Clin Aesthet Dermatol*, **2011**, *4*:40–47.

Micali G, et al. Topical pharmacotherapy for skin cancer: part I. Pharmacology. *J Am Acad Dermatol*, **2014**, *70*:965.e1–e12; quiz 977–8.

Nghiem P, et al. Tacrolimus and pimecrolimus: from clever prokaryotes to inhibiting calcineurin and treating atopic dermatitis. *J Am Acad Dermatol*, **2002**, *46*:228–241.

O'Meara S, et al. Antibiotics and antiseptics for venous leg ulcers. *Cochrane Database Syst Rev*, **2014**, (1):CD003557.

Orvis AK, et al. Mycophenolate mofetil in dermatology. *J Am Acad Dermatol*, **2009**, *60*:183–199; quiz 200–202.

Patel AA, et al. Azathioprine in dermatology: the past, the present, and the future. *J Am Acad Dermatol*, **2006**, *55*:369–389.

Plovanich M, et al. Low usefulness of potassium monitoring among healthy young women taking spironolactone for acne. *JAMA Dermatol*, **2015**, *151*:941–944.

Ray GT, et al. Incidence, microbiology, and patient characteristics of skin and soft-tissue infections in a U.S. population: a retrospective population-based study. *BMC Infect Dis*, **2013**, *13*:252.

1296 Reyes-Habito CM, Roh EK. Cutaneous reactions to chemotherapeutic drugs and targeted therapy for cancer: part II. Targeted therapy. *J Am Acad Dermatol*, **2014**, *71*:217.e1–217.e11; quiz 227–228.

Ryan C, et al. The use of cyclosporine in dermatology: part II. *J Am Acad Dermatol*, **2010**, *63*:949–972; quiz 973–974.

Topical steroids potency chart. National Psoriasis Foundation. Available at: https://www.psoriasis.org/about-psoriasis/treatments/topicals/steroids/potency-chart. Accessed February 1, 2016.

Tyler KH, Zirwas MJ. Pregnancy and dermatologic therapy. *J Am Acad Dermatol*, **2013**, *68*:663–671.

van Zuuren EJ, et al. Evidence-based topical treatments for tinea cruris and tinea corporis: a summary of a Cochrane systematic review. *Br J Dermatol*, **2015**, *172*:616–641.

Wilcox RA Cutaneous T-cell lymphoma: 2014 update on diagnosis, risk-stratification, and management. *Am J Hematol*, **2014**, *89*:837–851.

Chapter 71

Environmental Toxicology: Carcinogens and Heavy Metals

Michael C. Byrns and Trevor M. Penning

Humans are exposed to chemicals from their environment daily. Fortunately, mammals have evolved mechanisms to protect themselves from toxic effects of many exogenous chemicals, including the xenobiotic transport and metabolic mechanisms described in Chapters 4–7. While the human body is relatively well adapted to deal with xenobiotics, there are situations in which such environmental agents may cause significant toxicity. The industrial revolution and the development of chemical industries have increased human exposures to chemicals that were previously infrequent or absent. Concern about environmental toxicants has stimulated interest and research in environmental toxicology, the study of how chemicals in our environment adversely affect human health; and in occupational toxicology, the study of how chemicals in the workplace affect human health. Many authoritative textbooks are available in these areas. This chapter does not attempt a thorough coverage; rather, it sets forth a few basic principles, briefly discusses carcinogens and chemoprevention, and then focuses on the pharmacotherapy of heavy metal intoxication.

Assessment and Management of Environmental Risk

Environmental exposures to *xenobiotics* involve large populations exposed to many toxicants at low doses over long periods of time, which poses challenges for assessing the risks from those exposures. Thus, the focus of environmental risk assessment is on the low end of the dose-response curve, using experiments based on chronic exposures. Unlike drugs, which are given to treat a specific disease and should have benefits that outweigh the risks, environmental toxicants are usually only harmful. In addition, exposures to environmental toxicants usually are involuntary, there is uncertainty about the severity of their effects, and people are much less willing to accept their associated risks.

Epidemiology and *toxicology* provide complimentary approaches to predict the toxic effects of environmental exposures. Epidemiologists monitor health effects in humans and use statistics to associate those effects with exposure to an environmental stress, such as a toxicant. Toxicologists perform laboratory studies to examine potential toxic mechanisms of a chemical and to predict whether it is likely to be toxic to humans. Each of these approaches has strengths and weaknesses, and information from both is integrated into *environmental risk assessment*. Risk assessment is used to develop management approaches, such as laws and regulations, to limit exposures to environmental toxicants to a level that is considered safe.

Epidemiological Approaches to Risk Assessment

Epidemiologists use a variety of study designs to look for statistical associations between environmental exposures, including chemical exposures, and health outcomes. This approach has the advantage of examining the effects of real-world exposures to humans but can be expensive and subject to biases and confounding effects.

Epidemiological Studies

Several types of epidemiological studies are used to assess risks, each with its own set of strengths and weaknesses.

- *Ecological studies* correlate frequencies of exposures and health outcomes between different geographical regions. These studies are inexpensive and are effective for generating hypotheses but are subject to confounders and are not effective for establishing causality.
- *Cross-sectional studies* examine the prevalence of exposures and outcomes at a single point in time. Such studies are an inexpensive way to determine an association but do not provide a temporal relationship and are not effective for establishing causality. They also can be subject to bias, as a health outcome under study might cause someone to eliminate his or her exposure.
- *Case-control studies* start with a group of individuals affected by a disease; this group then is matched to another group of unaffected individuals for known confounding variables. Questionnaires often are used to evaluate past exposures. This method also is relatively inexpensive and is good for examining rare outcomes because the end point is known. However, case-control studies rely on assessments of past exposures, which can be unreliable and subject to bias.
- *Cohort studies* measure exposures in a large group of people and follow that group for a long time to measure health outcomes. These studies are not as susceptible to bias and are better than case-control studies at establishing causality. However, they are expensive, particularly when measuring rare outcomes, because a large study population is required to observe sufficient disease to obtain statistical significance.

Abbreviations

ARE: antioxidant response element
ATSDR: Agency for Toxic Substances Disease Registry
BAL: British anti-Lewisite (dimercaprol)
BLL: blood lead level
CaNa$_2$EDTA: calcium disodium ethylenediaminetetraacetic acid
CDC: Centers for Disease Control and Prevention
COX-2: cyclooxygenase 2; prostaglandin H synthase II
CV: cardiovascular
DMPS: sodium 2,3-dimercatopropane sulfonate
EEG: electroencephalogram
EPA: United States Environmental Protection Agency
ER: estrogen receptor
GI: gastrointestinal
GSH: reduced glutathione
GST: glutathione S-transferase
IARC: International Agency for Research on Cancer
IM: intramuscular
IV: intravenous
LOAEL: lowest adverse effect level
MCL: maximum contaminant level
MeHg$^+$: methyl mercury
MMA: monomethylarsenic
NOAEL: no adverse effect level
NOx: nitrogen oxides
NQO1: quinone reductase
NTP: National Toxicology Program
PG: prostaglandin
RfD: reference dose
ROS: reactive oxygen species
SC: subcutaneous

- *Clinical trials* (see Chapter 1) cannot be used to directly measure the effects of environmental toxicants (for obvious ethical reasons) but can be used to examine the effectiveness of an interventional strategy for reducing both exposures and disease.

Biomarkers

Because of the difficulties in assessing human exposures and the long times required to clinically observe effects on health, epidemiologists often rely on biomarkers in risk assessment. Different types of biomarkers provide different information useful for risk assessment. Biomarkers aim to be *specific*, only detecting the change in affected individuals, and *sensitive*, detecting the change in all affected individuals.

- *Biomarkers of exposure* provide information about dose or duration of exposures. Blood and urine concentrations of a chemical or its metabolite measure recent exposures, while levels in hair and toenails can measure exposure over a period of months. An example of an unusual exposure biomarker is X-ray fluorescent measurement of bone lead levels, which estimates lifetime exposure to lead.
- *Biomarkers of toxicity* are used to measure toxic effects at a subclinical level. Examples include measurement of liver enzymes in serum, changes in the quantity or contents of urine, and performance on specialized exams for neurological or cognitive function.
- *Biomarkers of susceptibility* are used to predict which individuals are likely to develop toxicity in response to a given chemical. Examples include single-nucleotide polymorphisms in genes for metabolizing enzymes involved in the activation or detoxification of a toxicant.
- Some biomarkers simultaneously provide information on exposure, toxicity, or susceptibility. For example, the measurement in the urine of N7-guanine adducts from aflatoxin B$_1$ provides evidence of both exposure and a toxic effect (in this case, DNA damage).

Toxicological Approaches to Risk Assessment

Toxicologists use model systems, including experimental animals, to examine the toxicity of chemicals and predict their effects on humans. Toxicologists typically must test chemicals at higher doses than would be observed in the environment to see enough occurrences of a toxic outcome to obtain statistical significance. As a result, there is often uncertainty about the effects of very low doses of chemicals. To determine the applicability of model systems, toxicologists also study the mechanisms involved in the toxic effects of chemicals, with the goal of predicting whether that mechanism would occur in humans.

To predict the toxic effects of environmental chemicals, toxicologists perform *subchronic studies* (3 months of treatment for rodents) and *chronic studies* (2 years for rodents) in at least two different animal models. Doses for these studies are based on shorter preliminary studies, with the goal of having one concentration that does not have a significant effect, one concentration that results in statistically significant toxicity at the low end of the dose-response curve, and one or more concentrations that will have moderate-to-high levels of toxicity. A theoretical dose-response curve for an animal study is shown in Figure 71–1.

An animal study provides two numbers that estimate the risk from a chemical:

- The *NOAEL* is the highest dose used that does not result in a statistically significant increase in negative health outcomes.
- The *LOAEL* is the lowest dose that results in a significant increase in toxicity.

The NOAEL is divided by 10 for each source of uncertainty to determine a RfD, which is commonly used as a starting point for determining regulations on human exposures to chemicals. The modifiers used to determine the RfD are based on the uncertainties between experimental and human exposure. The most common modifiers used are for interspecies variability (human to animal) and interindividual variability (human to human), in which case RfD = NOAEL/100. Other modifiers can be used to account for specific experimental uncertainties, such as the unavailability of data from chronic studies. The use of factors of 10 in the denominator for determination of RfD is an application of the "precautionary principle," which attempts to limit human exposure by assuming a worst-case scenario for each unknown variable.

A major concern with animal studies is that they do not detect effects at low concentrations. Typically, they are designed to obtain statistical significance with a 10%–15% increase in an outcome. As a result, there is considerable uncertainty about what occurs below that level, as demonstrated in Figure 71–1. Toxicologists often assume that there is a threshold dose below which there is no toxicity. However, the shape of the dose-response curve below the NOAEL is not known with certainty and represents a point of departure (POD). The existence of a threshold dose assumes that there are cellular defenses that prevent toxicity at concentrations below a given level, and that they can be overwhelmed. Some carcinogens may not exhibit a threshold, while others for which defense mechanisms exist do and other toxicants with specific molecular targets (e.g., lead) do not exhibit a threshold. Ideally, mechanistic studies should be done to predict which dose-response curve is most likely to fit a given chemical.

Toxicologists perform mechanistic studies to understand how a chemical might cause toxicity. Computer modeling using a compound's three-dimensional structure to determine quantitative structure-activity relationships (QSAR) is commonly performed on both drugs and environmental chemicals. QSAR approaches can determine which chemicals are likely to exhibit toxicities or bind to specific molecular targets. Cell-based approaches in prokaryotes and eukaryotes are used to determine whether a compound damages DNA or causes cytotoxicity. DNA damage and the resulting mutagenesis often are determined with the Ames test, which uses *Salmonella typhimurium* strains with specific mutations in the gene needed to synthesize histidine. These strains are treated with chemicals in the presence or absence of a metabolic activating system (usually hepatic xenobiotic metabolizing enzymes). If a compound is a

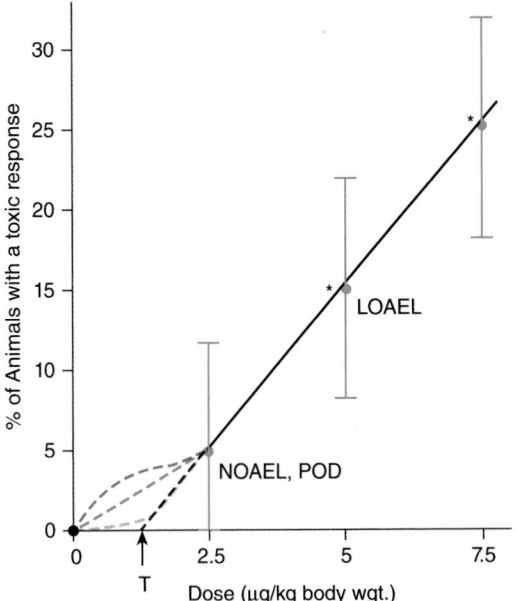

Figure 71–1 *LOAEL and NOAEL.* The theoretical dose-response curve from an animal study demonstrates the *NOAEL* and the *LOAEL*. Below the NOAEL level, there is considerable uncertainty regarding the shape of the response curve; thus, the NOAEL represents the *point of departure* (POD). The dose response could continue linearly below this point to reach a threshold dose (T) where there would be no harmful effects from the toxicant, or it could have a number of different possible inflection points. Each of these curves would have very different impacts on human populations. *Statistically significant toxicity.

mutagen in the Ames test, it reverts the mutation in the histidine operon and allows the bacteria to form colonies on plates with limited histidine. Gene chip microarrays assess gene expression in cells or tissues from animals treated with a toxicant and provide a useful tool to identify the molecular targets and pathways altered by toxicant exposures. The susceptibility of knockout mice to a toxicant can help to determine whether the knocked-out genes are involved in the mechanism of toxicity.

Carcinogens and Chemoprevention

Carcinogenesis

The IARC classifies the carcinogenicity of compounds into groups based on risk assessments using epidemiologic, human exposure, animal, and mechanistic data. Chemicals in *group 1* are known human carcinogens; *group 2A* are chemicals that are probably carcinogenic in humans; *group 2B* are chemicals that are possibly carcinogenic in humans; *group 3* are chemicals for which data are lacking to suggest a role in carcinogenesis; and *group 4* are those for which the data indicate that they are unlikely to be carcinogens. Table 71–1 provides examples of group 1 carcinogens.

The transformation of a normal cell to a malignancy is a multistage process, and exogenous chemicals can act at one or more of these stages. A classic model of chemical carcinogenesis is *tumor initiation* followed by *tumor promotion*. In this model, an initiator causes gene mutations that increase the ability of cells to proliferate and avoid apoptosis. A promoter does not directly modify genes but changes signaling pathways or the extracellular environment to increase survival, proliferation, or invasiveness of precancerous cells. Although this model is an oversimplification of the many processes of carcinogenesis, it demonstrates the types of changes that must occur for a normal cell to transform into cancer. Chemical carcinogens cause cancer through genotoxic and nongenotoxic mechanisms (Figure 71–2).

Genotoxic carcinogens initiate tumor formation through damage to DNA. Typically, genotoxic carcinogens undergo metabolism in a target tissue to a reactive intermediate. This reactive intermediate can directly damage DNA via covalent reaction to form a DNA adduct. Alternatively, it can indirectly damage DNA through the formation of ROS, which can oxidize DNA or form lipid peroxidation products that react with DNA (Mena et al., 2009). If DNA damage from a genotoxic carcinogen is not repaired prior to DNA replication, a mutation can result. If this mutation is in a key tumor suppressor gene or proto-oncogene, it can provide advantages in proliferation or survival. Alternatively, mutations to DNA repair genes can increase the probability that future mutations will occur. With the right extracellular environment, mutations in key genes will allow a cell to proliferate faster than surrounding normal cells and possibly develop into malignant cancer.

Benzo[*a*]pyrene, a key carcinogen in tobacco smoke, is an example of a genotoxic carcinogen that forms both direct DNA adducts and ROS. Benzo[*a*]pyrene is oxidized by CYPs to a 7,8-dihydrodiol, which represents a proximate carcinogen (a more carcinogenic metabolite). This metabolite either can undergo a second oxidation step by a CYP to form a diol epoxide, which readily reacts with DNA, or can undergo oxidation by aldo-keto reductases to form a catechol, which will redox cycle to form ROS (Conney, 1982; Penning, 2009).

Nongenotoxic carcinogens increase the incidence of cancer without damaging DNA, and most agents in this category are tumor promoters. Many nongenotoxic carcinogens bind to receptors that stimulate proliferation or other tumor-promoting effects, such as tissue invasion or angiogenesis. For example, phorbol esters mimic diacylglycerol and activate PKC isoforms. This in turn stimulates MAPK pathways, leading to proliferation, invasiveness, and angiogenesis (Chapter 3 presents these signaling pathways). In most normal cells, prolonged activation of this pathway stimulates apoptosis, but cells with defective apoptotic mechanisms due to preceding mutation(s) are resistant to this effect. Estrogenic carcinogens activate ERα and stimulate proliferation and invasiveness of estrogen-responsive cells. Chronic inflammation is another mechanism of nongenotoxic carcinogenesis. Inflammatory cytokines stimulate PKC signaling, leading to proliferation, invasiveness, and angiogenesis. Irritants such as asbestos are examples of carcinogens that work through inflammation. Chronic exposure to hepatotoxic chemicals (or chronic liver diseases) also causes nongenotoxic carcinogenesis by stimulating compensatory proliferation to repair the liver damage. This damage and repair process increases the likelihood of DNA damage causing a mutation, causes chronic inflammation, and selects for initiated cells that proliferate faster or are less sensitive to cell death.

Many compounds can also act as complete carcinogens because repeated exposure can cause tumor initiation and promotion. Examples of complete carcinogens include benzo[*a*]pyrene and ultraviolet radiation.

Tumor initiation also may occur through nongenotoxic mechanisms. For example, some heavy metals do not directly react with DNA but interfere with proteins involved in DNA synthesis and repair, increasing the likelihood that an error will be made during replication. Nongenotoxic carcinogens also can cause heritable changes to gene expression by altering the methylation state of cytosines in 5′-CpG-3′ islands of gene promoters. Methylation can silence tumor suppressor genes, while demethylation of proto-oncogenes can increase their expression. These *epigenetic* effects can occur through sustained transcription or silencing of a gene.

Some chemicals enhance the carcinogenesis of other chemicals and thus act as *cocarcinogens*. These chemicals can increase the absorption or change the metabolism of other chemicals, increasing the probability that they form active metabolites in target tissues. They can also interfere with DNA repair, increasing the occurrence of mutations from a second genotoxic carcinogen. For example, ethanol acts as a solvent and increases the absorption of tobacco carcinogens, increasing the risk of head and neck cancers in people who both smoke and drink. Ethanol also depletes GSH, limiting target cells' ability to detoxify reactive metabolites of carcinogens and ROS.

Chemoprevention

Drugs that interfere with the carcinogenic process to prevent cancer before it is diagnosed are termed *chemopreventive agents* (Szabo, 2006;

TABLE 71–1 ■ EXAMPLES OF IMPORTANT GROUP 1 CARCINOGENS[a]

CARCINOGEN CLASS	EXAMPLE	SOURCE	MECHANISM
Genotoxic			
Nitrosamines	Nicotine-derived nitrosaminoketone (NNK)	Tobacco products	Metabolic activation to form DNA adducts
Polycyclic aromatic hydrocarbons	Benzo[a]pyrene	Fossil fuel combustion, tobacco smoke, charbroiled food	Metabolic activation to form DNA adducts or ROS
Aromatic amines	2-Aminonaphthalene	Dyes	Metabolic activation to form DNA adducts
Fungal toxins	Aflatoxin B_1	Corn, peanuts, and other food	Metabolic activation to form DNA adducts
Nongenotoxic			
Liver toxicants	Ethanol	Beverages, environment	Toxicity and compensatory proliferation; depletion of GSH
Phorbol esters	Tetradecanoyl phorbol acetate	Horticulture; rubber and gasoline production	Activation of PKC isoforms
Estrogens	Diethylstilbestrol	Drugs, environment	Activation of estrogen receptor signaling
Metals	Arsenic	Environment, occupation	Inhibition of DNA repair; activation of signal transduction pathways
Irritants	Asbestos	Environment, occupation	Stimulation of inflammation; formation of ROS
Dioxins	2,3,7,8 tetrachlorodibenzo-p-dioxin (TCDD)	Waste incineration, herbicides, paper-pulp bleaching	Activation of the aryl hydrocarbon (Ah) receptor

[a]Compounds in this table are classified as group 1 carcinogens by IARC, with the exception of the phorbol esters, which have not been examined.

William et al., 2009). The chemoprevention concept was pioneered during the 1960s by Wattenberg and others, who observed that dietary constituents, such as *t*-butyl hydroquinone, could prevent cancer in rodents (Wattenberg, 1966). Chemoprevention strategies often are based on epidemiological studies on nutrition, where there are many examples of clear protective effects of plant-based foods and drinks on the incidence of various types of cancer (Fahey and Kensler, 2007). By isolating the active compounds from protective plants, researchers hope to understand their protective mechanisms and develop drugs to prevent cancer. Chemoprevention is an emerging field; a number of compounds for the prevention of cancer are in clinical trials (Table 71–2). Most chemicals tested for chemoprevention have not exhibited a benefit, and in some cases they have increased the risk of cancer (Potter, 2014). There are currently no drugs approved for chemoprevention of environmental carcinogenesis, but there are approved drugs to prevent carcinogenesis due to endogenous estrogen (tamoxifen and raloxifene) and viruses (hepatitis B and human papillomavirus vaccines).

Chemopreventive agents can interfere with initiation or promotion (Figure 71–2). One mechanism of anti-initiation is prevention of carcinogen activation. Isothiocyanates inhibit CYPs involved in activating many carcinogens and also upregulate genes controlled by the antioxidant response element (ARE); the ARE-responsive genes include γ-glutamyl-cysteine synthase light chain (which catalyzes the rate-determining step in GSH synthesis) and quinone reductase. Increased expression of ARE-regulated genes is predicted to increase the detoxification of proximate carcinogens. Isothiocyanates also stimulate apoptosis of p53-deficient cells via the formation of cytotoxic DNA adducts.

Compounds that act as antioxidants may provide protection because many carcinogens work through the generation of ROS. Some compounds simultaneously prevent carcinogen activation and act as antioxidants.

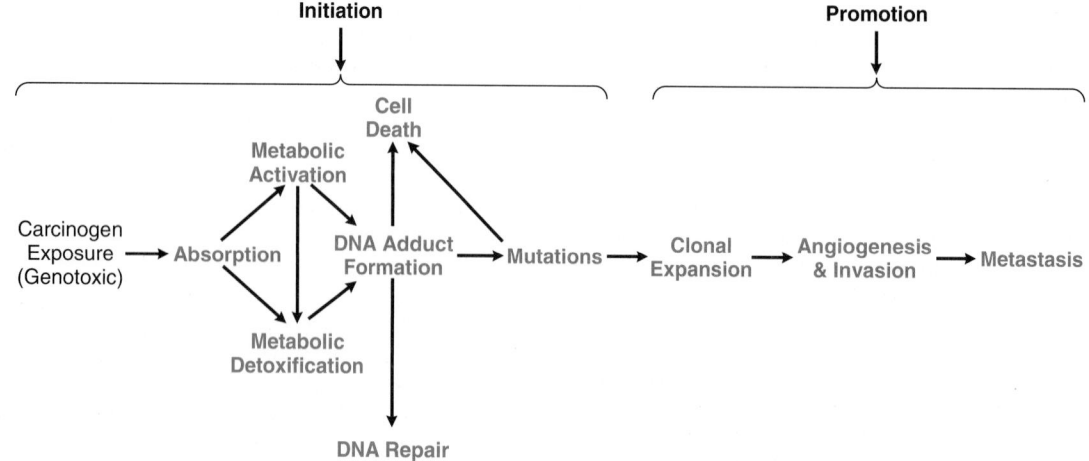

Figure 71–2 *Carcinogenesis: initiation and promotion.* There are multiple steps that occur between the exposure to a genotoxic carcinogen and the development of cancer. Processes in red lead to the development of cancer, while those in green reduce the risk. Nongenotoxic carcinogens act by enhancing steps leading to cancer or inhibiting protective processes. A chemopreventive agent acts by inhibiting steps leading to cancer or by increasing protective processes.

TABLE 71–2 ■ CHEMOPREVENTIVE AGENTS BEING STUDIED IN HUMANS

CHEMOPREVENTIVE CLASS	EXAMPLE COMPOUND	NATURAL SOURCE OR TYPE OF DRUG	CANCER TYPE(S)	MECHANISM	CURRENT STATUS
Isothiocyanates	Phenethyl isothiocyanate	Cruciferous vegetables	Liver, lung, breast, etc.	↓ CYP, ↑ GSH, ↑ NQO1, ↑ apoptosis	Phase 2 clinical trials
Synthetic drugs that modify metabolism	Oltipraz	Antischistosomal drug	Liver, lung	↓ CYP, ↑ GSH, ↑ NQO1	Beneficial effects on biomarkers in phase 2 clinical trials
Flavonoids and other polyphenols	Catechin	Green tea, red wine, berries, cacao, etc.	Lung, cervical, etc.	↓ ROS, ↓ CYP, ↑ GSH, ↑ NQO1	Phase 2 clinical trials
Other plant compounds	Curcumin	Turmeric (curry)	Colorectal, pancreatic, etc.	↓ ROS, ↓ CYP, ↑ GSH, ↑ NQO1	Phase 2 clinical trials
Other plant compounds	Chlorophyllin	All plants	Liver	Reaction with active intermediates, ↓ ROS, ↓ CYP	Beneficial effects on biomarkers in phase 2 clinical trials
Other antioxidants	α-Tocopherol (vitamin E)	Food	Prostate	Antioxidant, anti-inflammatory	Phase 3 clinical trials found ↑ prostate cancer with α-tocopherol
Antihormonal therapies	Tamoxifen	Adjuvant for breast cancer	Breast	Inhibit ERα in breast	FDA approved for chemoprevention
NSAIDs (see Chapter 38)	Aspirin	Anti-inflammatory drugs	Colorectal, etc.	Inhibit PG formation	Phase 3 trials of aspirin for prevention of cardiovascular disease observed ↓ cancer; phase 3 trials for cancer prevention are ongoing
COX-2 selective inhibitors (see Chapter 38)	Celecoxib	Anti-inflammatory drugs	Colorectal, etc.	Inhibit PG formation	Phase 3 trial found ↓ cancer but unacceptable side effects for prevention

For example, flavonoids and other polyphenols found in a wide variety of plants are potent antioxidants that also inhibit CYPs and induce expression of ARE-regulated genes. Chlorophyll and other compounds can protect against carcinogens by binding to or reacting with carcinogens or their metabolites and preventing them from reaching their molecular target.

Inflammation is a potential target for chemoprevention through interference with promotion. In phase 3 studies, the COX-2 inhibitor celecoxib demonstrated efficacy at reducing the risk of colorectal cancer. However, this benefit was offset by an increased risk of death due to cardiovascular events, forcing the early termination of the trial (William et al., 2009). Studies examining long-term treatment with aspirin for cardiovascular benefits found that aspirin also reduces the incidence of colorectal adenomas and overall cancer mortality. A phase 3 clinical trial is under way to examine this effect. Naturally occurring compounds such as α-tocopherol have also been hypothesized to exert chemoprevention by reducing inflammation. However, α-tocopherol actually increased the risk of prostate cancer in a phase 3 trial (Potter, 2014).

Another approach to chemoprevention is disruption of nuclear receptor signaling. Retinoids reduce the incidence of head and neck cancers, and is one of the first successful uses of chemoprevention in humans (Evans and Kaye, 1999; William et al., 2009). Retinoids are also effective for the treatment for acute promyelocytic leukemia (see Section VII). However, in large clinical trials, retinoids increased the incidence of lung cancer, particularly amongst women, and had other unacceptable toxicities (Omenn et al., 1996).

The selective ER modulators tamoxifen and raloxifene reduced the incidence of breast cancer in high-risk women in large phase 3 clinical trials and are approved for chemoprevention in these patients (Vogel et al., 2006). The success of selective ER modulators for chemoprevention provides a proof-of-principle that the development of compounds based on mechanistic predictions of antipromotion activity can lead to effective drugs for the prevention of cancer.

Aflatoxin B₁

Agents are being developed as chemopreventants of hepatocarcinogenesis mediated by aflatoxin B₁. Aflatoxins are produced in regions with hot and wet climates by *Aspergillus flavus*, a fungus that is a common contaminant of foods, especially corn, peanuts, cottonseed, and tree nuts. As a result of exposure to aflatoxin, human hepatocellular carcinoma is a serious problem in subtropical and tropical regions of Latin America, Africa, and Southeast Asia. Human exposure to aflatoxin in the U.S. is rare and not thought to have a significant impact on health (IARC, 2002).

ADME

Aflatoxin B₁ is readily absorbed from the GI tract and initially distributed to the liver, where it undergoes extensive first-pass metabolism (Guengerich et al., 1996). Aflatoxin B₁ is metabolized by CYPs 1A2 and 3A4 to yield either an 8,9-epoxide or products hydroxylated at the 9 position (aflatoxin M₁) or 3 position (aflatoxin Q₁; Figure 71–3). While the hydroxylation products are detoxification products, the 8,9-epoxide reacts with DNA and is responsible for aflatoxin carcinogenesis. The 8,9-epoxide is short lived and undergoes detoxification via nonenzymatic hydrolysis or conjugation with GSH. Aflatoxin M₁ enters the circulation and is excreted in urine and milk.

Toxicity

Aflatoxin B₁ primarily targets the liver, although it also is toxic to the GI tract and hematological system. High-dose exposures result in acute necrosis of the liver, leading to jaundice and, in many cases, death. Acute toxicity from aflatoxin is rare in humans and requires consumption of milligram quantities of aflatoxin per day for multiple weeks. Chronic exposure to aflatoxins results in cirrhosis of the liver and immunosuppression.

Carcinogenicity

Based on increased incidence of hepatocellular carcinoma in humans exposed to aflatoxin and on supporting animal and mechanistic data,

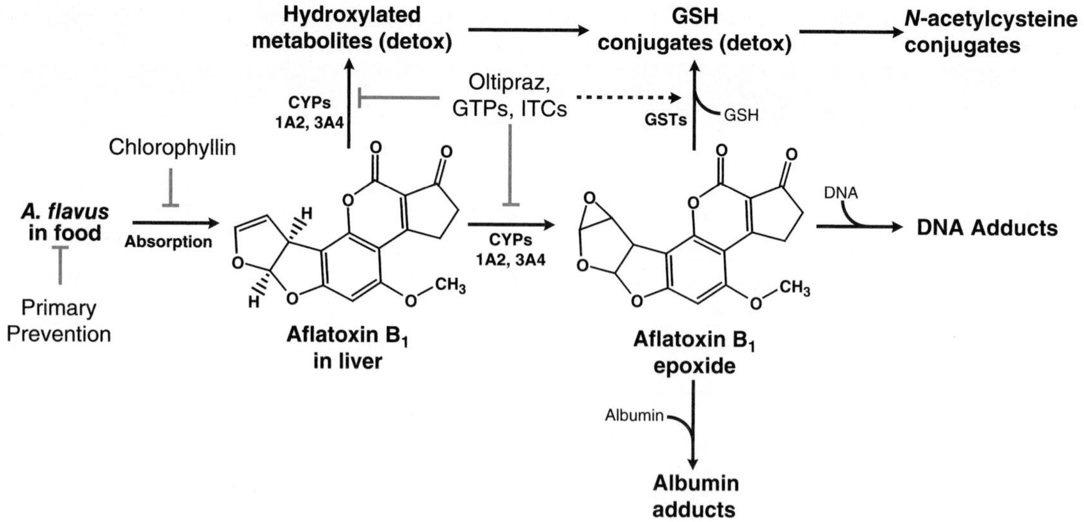

Figure 71–3 *Metabolism and actions of aflatoxin B₁.* Following absorption, aflatoxin B₁ undergoes activation by CYPs to its 8,9-epoxide, which can be detoxified by GSTs or by spontaneous hydration. Alternatively, it can react with cellular macromolecules such as DNA and protein, leading to toxicity and cancer. Oltipraz, green tea polyphenols (GTPs), and isothiocyanates (ITCs) decrease aflatoxin carcinogenesis by inhibiting the CYPs involved in activating aflatoxin and increasing the synthesis of the cofactor GSH for GSTs involved in detoxification.

IARC has classified aflatoxin B₁ as a known human carcinogen (group 1) (IARC, 2002). Aflatoxin exposure and the hepatitis B virus work synergistically to cause hepatocellular carcinoma. Aflatoxin or hepatitis B exposure alone increases the risk of hepatocellular carcinoma 3.4- or 7.3-fold, respectively; those exposed to both have a 59-fold increased risk of cancer compared to unexposed individuals (Groopman et al., 2005).

Aflatoxin primarily forms DNA adducts at deoxyguanosine residues, reacting at either the N1 or N7 position (IARC, 2002); the 8,9-epoxide of aflatoxin B₁ readily reacts with amines. The N7-guanine adduct mispairs with adenine, leading to G → T transversions. Human aflatoxin exposure is associated with hepatocellular carcinomas bearing an AGG-to-AGT mutation in codon 249 of the *p53* tumor suppressor gene, resulting in the replacement of an arginine with cysteine (Hussain et al., 2007).

Several mechanisms for the synergistic interaction between hepatitis B and aflatoxin are under investigation (Sylla et al., 1999). The X gene of the hepatitis B virus encodes a protein, HBx, that binds to and inhibits p53, resulting in suppressed nucleotide excision repair of aflatoxin B₁ adducts (Hussain et al., 2007). Hepatitis B also alters the metabolism of aflatoxin B₁ by upregulating CYP genes, including CYP3A4, and decreases GSH S-transferase activity. In addition, hepatocellular proliferation to repair damage done by hepatitis B infection increases the likelihood that aflatoxin-induced DNA adducts will cause mutations. The hepatotoxic and tumor-promoting effects of hepatitis B also could provide a more favorable environment for the proliferation and invasion of initiated cells.

Chemoprevention of Aflatoxin-Induced Hepatocellular Carcinoma

The relationship between aflatoxin metabolism and its carcinogenicity makes it an appealing target for chemopreventive strategies that modify its metabolism (Figure 71–3). Inhibiting CYP activity or increasing GSH conjugation will reduce the intracellular concentration of the 8,9-epoxide and prevent DNA adduct formation (Groopman et al., 2008; Kensler et al., 2004). Oltipraz, an antischistosomal drug, potently inhibits CYPs and induces genes regulated by the ARE that are involved in GSH synthesis. Oltipraz increases the excretion of the *N*-acetylcysteine aflatoxin conjugate, indicating enhanced GSH conjugation of the epoxide. At 500 mg/week, oltipraz reduced the levels of aflatoxin M₁, consistent with inhibition of CYP activity.

Green tea polyphenols (GTPs) also have been used to modify aflatoxin metabolism in exposed human populations. Individuals receiving a daily dose of 500 or 1000 mg (equivalent to 1 or 2 L of green tea) demonstrated a small decline in the formation of aflatoxin-albumin adducts and a large

increase in the excretion of the *N*-acetylcysteine aflatoxin conjugate, consistent with a protective effect.

Another approach used for the chemoprevention of aflatoxin hepatocarcinogenesis is the use of "interceptor molecules." *Chlorophyllin*, a mixture of water-soluble chlorophyll salts, binds tightly to aflatoxin in the GI tract, forming a complex that is not absorbed. In vitro, chlorophyllin inhibits CYP activity and acts as an antioxidant. In a phase 2 trial, administration of 100 mg of chlorophyllin with each meal reduced aflatoxin–N7-guanine adduct levels in the urine. Because of the strong interaction between hepatitis B and aflatoxin in carcinogenesis, the hepatitis B vaccine reduces the sensitivity of people to the induction of cancer by aflatoxin. Primary prevention of aflatoxin exposure through hand or fluorescent sorting of crops to remove those with fungal contamination also reduces human exposure. A cost-effective primary prevention approach is to improve food storage to limit the spread of *Aspergillus flavus*, which requires a warm and humid environment.

Water and Air Pollution

The U.S. EPA protects the public from water and airborne pollutants by enforcing compliance with the Clean Water Act (protects the public and the environment from water pollution); the Safe Drinking Water Act (ensures the quality of the drinking water); and the Clean Air Act (to protect the public from air pollutants). Under these laws, the EPA combines scientific risk assessment with economic analyses and other factors to develop regulations on the release or presence of specific pollutants to limit their effect on human health and the environment.

Toxicity screening of many water contaminants has led to the development of maximum contaminant levels (MCLs) for drinking water. To protect against potential adverse health effects, a primary MCL sets a level for a contaminant that must not be exceeded. The primary MCL is based on consideration of the toxic dose-response curve and on whether a sufficiently sensitive analytical method exists to measure the contaminant for compliance purposes. A secondary MCL is not enforced but is established for aesthetic value (e.g., taste, color, odor) that may not affect health. Currently, there is concern about pharmaceutical waste in the water supply, but MCLs have not been set for these compounds.

The EPA also monitors six priority air pollutants (CO, Pb, NOx, O₃, particulate matter, and SO₂) that they have determined play the largest role in human health effects from air pollution. The EPA sets National Ambient Air Quality Standards in which local levels of these pollutants may not be exceeded within a given time frame. Measurements made by stationary air monitors provide daily air quality data and also lead to warnings (e.g., ozone awareness days), which advise citizens to stay indoors. Fine particles, smaller than 2.5 μm in diameter (PM2.5) are particularly concerning as they penetrate deep into the lung and can cause or exacerbate respiratory or cardiovascular illness.

Metals

Metals are an important class of environmental toxicants; they are ubiquitous environmental contaminants that come from both natural and anthropogenic sources. The CDC lists arsenic, mercury, and lead as the top three pollutants of concern, based on their toxicity and levels of human exposure. Although the toxicity of high levels of exposure to metals has long been known, the effects of low-dose chronic exposure to metals have only recently been appreciated. Many of the toxic metals in the environment also are carcinogens (Table 71–3). In addition, several essential metals also are toxic under conditions of overdose. Copper and iron are associated with toxicities, primarily targeting the liver through generation of ROS.

Lead

Chronic exposure to very low levels of lead has major deleterious effects, particularly for children.

Exposure

Despite substantial improvements over the past four decades, lead exposure remains a major concern, especially for children. In the U.S., paint containing lead for use in and around households was banned in 1978, while the use of tetraethyl lead in gasoline was phased out between 1976 and 1996. Despite these bans, past use of lead carbonate and lead oxide in paint and tetraethyl lead in gasoline remain the primary sources of lead exposure. Lead is not degradable and remains in dust, soil, and the paint of older homes. Young children are exposed to lead by nibbling sweet-tasting paint chips or ingesting dust and soil in and around older homes. Renovation or demolition of older buildings may cause substantial lead exposure. Removal of lead from gasoline reduced lead levels in air by more than 90% between 1982 and 2002, but lead fallout from air pollution remains in soils, particularly in urban environments. Lead was also commonly used in plumbing and can leach into drinking water. Lead exposure also has been traced to other sources, such as inhalation of dusts and fumes at firing ranges, retained bullets, artists' paint pigments, ashes and fumes from painted wood, lead-glazed pottery, lead toys, non-Western folk medicines, cosmetics, jewelers' wastes, home battery manufacture, and lead type (ATSDR, 2007b). BLLs in children have steadily decreased since the

1970s, when the mean level was 15 μg/dL. Currently, the average BLL in children is at 1.3 μg/dL.

The CDC recently updated its recommendations to reflect the modern understanding that *there is no safe level of lead exposure for children* (CDC, 2012). The CDC no longer provides a "level of concern," as any lead exposure to a child is concerning. Instead, the CDC emphasizes primary prevention of lead exposure in all children and recommends that children with a BLL that places them in the top 2.5% (currently ≥ 5 μg/dL) be identified as in need of exposure reduction and additional screening. They did not change the existing recommendation that physicians consider chelation therapy for children with a BLL above 45 μg/dL.

Occupational exposure to lead also has decreased because of protective regulations. Occupational exposure generally is through inhalation of lead-containing dust and lead fumes. Workers in lead smelters and storage battery factories are at the greatest risk for lead exposure. Other workers at risk for lead exposure are those associated with steel welding or cutting, construction, rubber and plastic industries, printing, firing ranges, radiator repair shops, and any industry where lead is flame soldered (ATSDR, 2007b).

Chemistry and Mode of Action

Lead exists in its metallic form and as divalent or tetravalent cations. Divalent lead is the primary environmental form; inorganic tetravalent lead compounds are not found naturally. Organo-lead complexes primarily occur with tetravalent lead and include the gasoline additive tetraethyl lead.

Lead toxicity results from molecular mimicry of other divalent metals (Garza et al., 2006), principally zinc and calcium. Because of its size and electron affinity, lead alters protein structure and can inappropriately activate or inhibit protein function.

ADME

Lead exposure occurs through ingestion or inhalation. GI absorption of lead varies considerably with age and diet. Children absorb a much higher percentage of ingested lead (~40% on average) than adults (<20%). Absorption of ingested lead is drastically increased by fasting. Dietary calcium or iron deficiencies increase lead absorption, suggesting that lead is absorbed through divalent metal transporters. The absorption of inhaled lead (~90%) generally is much more efficient than through dietary intake. Tetraethyl lead is readily absorbed through the skin, but transdermal absorption does not occur with inorganic lead.

About 99% of lead in the bloodstream binds to hemoglobin. Lead initially distributes in the soft tissues, particularly in the tubular epithelium of the kidney and the liver. Over time, lead is redistributed and deposited in bone, teeth, and hair. About 95% of the adult body burden of lead is

TABLE 71–3 ■ TOXIC METALS WITH FREQUENT ENVIRONMENTAL OR OCCUPATIONAL EXPOSURE[a]

METAL	CERCLA PRIORITY[b]	COMMON SOURCE OF EXPOSURE	ORGAN SYSTEMS MOST SENSITIVE TO TOXICITY	IARC CARCINOGEN CLASSIFICATION
As	1	Drinking water	CV, skin, multiple other	Group 1, carcinogenic to humans—liver, bladder, lung
Pb	2	Paint, soil	CNS, blood, CV, renal	Group 2A, probably carcinogenic
Hg	3	Air, food	CNS, renal	Group 2B, possibly carcinogenic (MeHg+); group 3, not classifiable (Hg^0, Hg^{2+})
Cd	7	Occupational, food, smoking	Renal, respiratory	Group 1, carcinogenic to humans—lung
Cr⁶⁺	18	Occupational	Respiratory	
Be	42	Occupational, water	Respiratory	
Co	49	Occupational, food, water	Respiratory, CV	Group 2B, possibly carcinogenic
Ni	53	Occupational	Respiratory, skin (allergy)	Group 1, carcinogenic (soluble Ni compounds); group 2B, possibly carcinogenic (metallic Ni)—lung

[a]The ATSDR has both detailed monographs and brief summaries for each of these compounds (available at https://www.atsdr.cdc.gov). The IARC also has monographs available (http://monographs.iarc.fr).
[b]CERCLA, Comprehensive Environmental Response, Compensation, and Liability Act.

found in bone. Growing bones will accumulate higher levels of lead and can form lead lines visible by radiography. Bone lead is slowly reabsorbed into the bloodstream, which can be accelerated when calcium levels are depleted, including during pregnancy. Small quantities of lead accumulate in the brain, mostly in gray matter and the basal ganglia. Lead readily crosses the placenta.

Lead is excreted primarily in the urine. The concentration of lead in urine is directly proportional to its free concentration in plasma (~1% of the total BLL). Lead is excreted in milk and sweat and deposited in hair and nails. The serum $t_{1/2}$ of lead is 1–2 months, with a steady state achieved in about 6 months. Lead accumulates in bone, where its $t_{1/2}$ is estimated at 20–30 years.

Health Effects

Although the effects of high-dose lead poisoning have been known for more than 2000 years, the insidious toxicities of chronic low-dose lead poisoning (BLL < 20 μg/dL) have only recently been discovered. Lead is a nonspecific toxicant; the most sensitive systems are the nervous, hematological, cardiovascular, and renal systems (Table 71–4). Uncovering the effects of low-level lead exposure on complex health outcomes, such as neurobehavioral function and blood pressure, has been the subject of extensive research and the object of considerable public concern.

TABLE 71–4 ■ HEALTH EFFECTS OF LEAD

BLL (μg/dL)	HEALTH EFFECT
Children	
<10	Inhibition of neural development
	Increased blood pressure
	Hearing loss
	Inhibition of hemoglobin synthesis enzymes
	Short stature
	Delayed sexual maturation (girls)
>10	Immunological effects (increased IgE)
>15	Increased erythrocyte protoporphyrin
	Decreased vitamin D
>30	Depressed nerve conduction velocity
>40	Anemia
>45	Chelation therapy warranted
>60	Colic
>70	Encephalopathy
Adults	
<10	Increased blood pressure
	Inhibition of hemoglobin synthesis enzymes
	Decreased glomerular filtration
>20	Increased erythrocyte protoporphyrin
>30	Hearing loss
	Enzymuria/proteinuria
>40	Peripheral neuropathy
	Reduced fertility
	Altered thyroid hormone levels
	Neurobehavioral effects
>50	Anemia
>60	Colic
	Chelation therapy warranted
>100	Encephalopathy

Neurotoxic Effects. The biggest concerns with low-level lead exposure are cognitive delays and behavior changes in children (ATSDR, 2007b; Bellinger and Bellinger, 2006). The developing nervous system is very sensitive to the toxic effects of lead, with effects persisting down to the lowest measurable levels of lead (Cranfield et al., 2003; Lanphear et al., 2005).

Lead neurotoxicity primarily results from inhibition of Ca^{2+} transporters and channels and altered activities of Ca^{2+} responsive proteins, including PKC and calmodulin (Bellinger and Bellinger, 2006; Garza et al., 2006). These actions limit the normal activation of neurons in response to Ca^{2+} release and cause inappropriate production or release of neurotransmitters. Lead affects multiple neurotransmitter pathways, including the dopaminergic, cholinergic, and glutaminergic systems. At high concentrations, lead causes disruption of membranes, including the blood-brain barrier, increasing their permeability to ions.

Lead alters brain development by interfering with the pruning of synapses, neuronal migration, and the interactions between neurons and glial cells. Neurotransmitter release and PKC signaling determine which synapses are maintained and which are lost during brain development; this process is disrupted by lead. Lead-induced alterations in brain development can result in decreased IQ, poor performance on exams, language and motor deficits, and behavioral problems such as distractibility, impulsivity, aggression, short attention span, and inability to follow simple sequences of instructions (ATSDR, 2007b; CDC, 2014). There is no evidence for a threshold; associations are evident even at the lowest measurable BLL (Figure 71–4). The cognitive and behavioral changes caused by lead vary considerably among children and may depend on the timing of exposure.

Children with very high BLL (>70 μg/dL) are at risk for encephalopathy. Symptoms of lead-induced encephalopathy include lethargy, vomiting, irritability, anorexia, and vertigo, which can progress to ataxia, delirium, and eventually coma and death. Mortality rates for lead-induced encephalopathy are about 25%, and most survivors develop long-term sequelae such as seizures and severe cognitive deficits.

Adults can also develop encephalopathy from lead exposure, although they are less sensitive than children. Workers chronically exposed to lead can develop neuromuscular deficits, termed *lead palsy*. Symptoms of lead palsy, including wrist drop and foot drop, were commonly associated with painters and other lead-exposed workers during previous eras but are rare today. Lead induces degeneration of motor neurons, usually without affecting sensory neurons. Studies in older adults have shown associations between lead exposure and decreased performance on cognitive function tests, suggesting that lead accelerates neurodegeneration due to aging (ATSDR, 2007b).

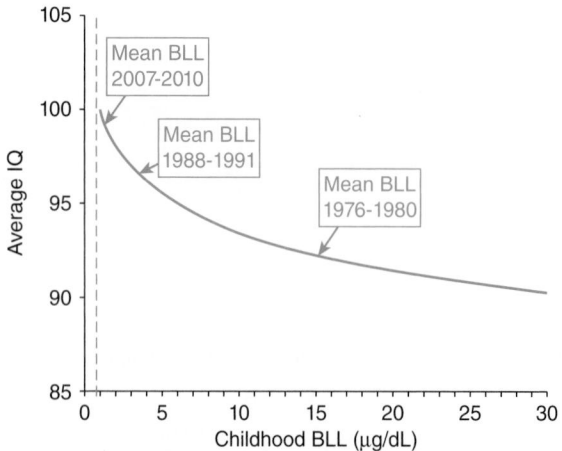

Figure 71–4 *Effect of childhood lead exposure on IQ.* Childhood exposure to lead shows a nonlinear dose-response relationship, with a steeper curve at low concentrations of lead (estimated dose-response curve based on data from Lanphear et al., 2005, and Canfield et al., 2003). For comparison, the average BLL from three iterations of the National Health and Nutritional Examination Survey are shown (Wheeler and Brown, 2013).

Cardiovascular and Renal Effects. Elevated blood pressure is a lasting effect of low-level lead exposure (BLL < 10 μg/dL). Adults who were exposed to lead during infancy and childhood have elevated blood pressure even in the absence of a recent exposure (ATSDR, 2007b). Lead exposure is associated with an increased risk of death due to cardiovascular and cerebrovascular disease (Schober et al., 2006).

In the kidney, low-level lead exposure (BLL < 10 μg/dL) depresses glomerular filtration. Higher levels (>30 μg/dL) cause proteinuria and impaired transport, while very high levels (>50 μg/dL) cause permanent physical damage, including proximal tubular nephropathy and glomerulosclerosis. Impaired glomerular filtration and elevated blood pressure are closely interrelated and likely have causative effects on one another (ATSDR, 2007b).

The cardiovascular effects of lead are thought to involve the production of ROS, which react with NO to prevent vasodilation (Vaziri and Khan, 2007). It is not known how lead reduces glomerular filtration rate, although there is evidence that lead targets kidney mitochondria and interferes with the electron transport chain (ATSDR, 2007b).

Other Effects. Lead causes both immunosuppression and increased inflammation, primarily through changes in helper T-cell and macrophage signaling; these effects can occur at low BLLs in children (Dietert and Piepenbrink, 2006). Lead inhibits the activity of several enzymes involved in the biosynthesis of heme; this effect persists down to very low BLL (<10 μg/dL; Figure 71–5). Chronic high-dose lead intoxication is associated with hypochromic microcytic anemia, which is observed more frequently in children and is morphologically similar to iron-deficient anemia. Acute high-dose lead exposure affects the smooth muscle of the gut, producing intestinal symptoms, termed *lead colic.*

Carcinogenesis. The IARC classifies lead in group 2A, "probably carcinogenic to humans" (IARC, 2006). Epidemiological studies show associations between lead exposure and cancers of the lung, brain, kidney, and stomach. Rodents exposed to lead develop kidney tumors, and some rats develop gliomas. Lead is not mutagenic but increases clastogenic events. Lead carcinogenesis may result from inhibition of DNA-binding zinc-finger proteins, including those involved in DNA repair and synthesis. Lead is a good example of a nongenotoxic carcinogen.

Succinyl CoA + Glycine

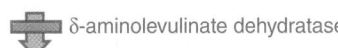 δ-aminolevulinate synthase

δ-Aminolevulinate (δ-ALA)

δ-aminolevulinate dehydratase

Porphobilinogen

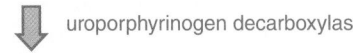 porphobilinogen deaminase
uroporphyrinogen III cosynthase

Uroporphyrinogen III

uroporphyrinogen decarboxylase

Coproporphyrinogen III

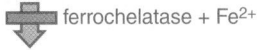 coproporphyrinogen oxidase

Protoporphyrin IX

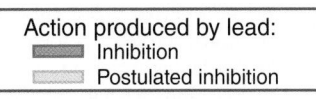 ferrochelatase + Fe²⁺

Heme

Action produced by lead:
Inhibition
Postulated inhibition

Figure 71–5 *Actions of lead on heme biosynthesis.*

Treatment

The most important response to lead poisoning is to remove the source of lead exposure. Supportive measures should be undertaken to relieve symptoms.

Chelation therapy is warranted for children and adults with very high BLL (>45 μg/dL and >60 μg/dL, respectively) or acute symptoms of lead poisoning (Ibrahim et al., 2006). For children with a BLL above 45 μg/dL but below 70 μg/dL, oral chelation is recommended. A BLL above 70 μg/dL in a child is a medical emergency requiring hospitalization and immediate intravenous chelation (American Academy of Pediatrics, 2005). Although chelation therapy is effective at lowering BLL and relieving acute symptoms of lead poisoning, it does not reduce the chronic effects of lead beyond the benefit of lead abatement alone (Rogan et al., 2001). In rats, chelators enhance mobilization of lead from the soft tissues to the brain and may increase the adverse neurodevelopmental effects of lead (Andersen and Aaseth, 2002).

Mercury

Mercury is a unique metal in that it is a liquid at room temperature. Mercury has been used industrially since ancient Greece due to its capacity to amalgamate with other metals, and mercury's toxicity was noted by Hippocrates. Mercury also was used as a therapeutic drug for several centuries. Its use for the treatment for syphilis inspired Paracelsus's observation that "the dose makes the poison," one of the central concepts of toxicology, and also gave rise to the cautionary expression: "A night with Venus, a year with Mercury." The phrase "mad as a hatter" originated from the exposure of hatters to metallic mercury vapor during production of felt for hats using mercury nitrate. While the phrase likely inspired the character of the Mad Hatter in *Alice in Wonderland*, his symptoms are not consistent with mercury exposure.

Exposure

Inorganic mercury cations and metallic mercury are found in the Earth's crust, and mercury vapor is released naturally into the environment through volcanic activity and off-gassing from soils. Mercury also enters the atmosphere through human activities, such as combustion of fossil fuels and gold mining. In 2011, the EPA set the first standards to reduce mercury emissions from coal-fired power plants. Once in the air, metallic mercury is photo-oxidized to inorganic mercury, which can then be deposited in aquatic environments in rain. Microorganisms can then conjugate inorganic mercury to form methyl mercury. Methyl mercury concentrates in muscle and other tissues and will bioaccumulate up the food chain (Figure 71–6). As a result, mercury concentrations in aquatic organisms at the top of the food chain, such as swordfish or sharks, are high (ATSDR, 1999).

The primary source of exposure to Hg⁰ in the general population is vaporization of Hg⁰ in dental amalgam. Human exposure to organic mercury primarily is through the consumption of fish. Other foods contain inorganic mercury at low levels (ATSDR, 1999).

Workers are exposed to Hg⁰ and inorganic mercury, most commonly through exposure to vapors. The highest risk for exposure is in the chloralkali industry (i.e., bleach) and in other chemical processes in which mercury is used as a catalyst. Mercury is a component of many devices, including alkaline batteries, fluorescent bulbs, thermometers, and scientific equipment, and exposure occurs during the production of these devices. Dentists also are exposed to Hg⁰ from amalgam. Hg⁰ can be used to extract gold during mining, which results in substantial occupational exposure. Mercuric salts are used as pigments in paints (ATSDR, 1999).

Thimerosal is an antimicrobial agent used as a preservative in some vaccines. Its use is controversial because it releases ethyl mercury, which is chemically similar to methyl mercury. Some parents have expressed concern that thimerosal might contribute to autism. Even though these concerns were based on a long-discredited report, the American Academy of Pediatrics and the U.S. Public Health Service issued a call for thimerosal's replacement in vaccines to improve the prevalence of vaccination, and thimerosal was removed from childhood vaccines in 2001 (Ball et al., 2001). Concurrently, studies found no association between thimerosal use in vaccines and negative outcomes, and thimerosal is still used

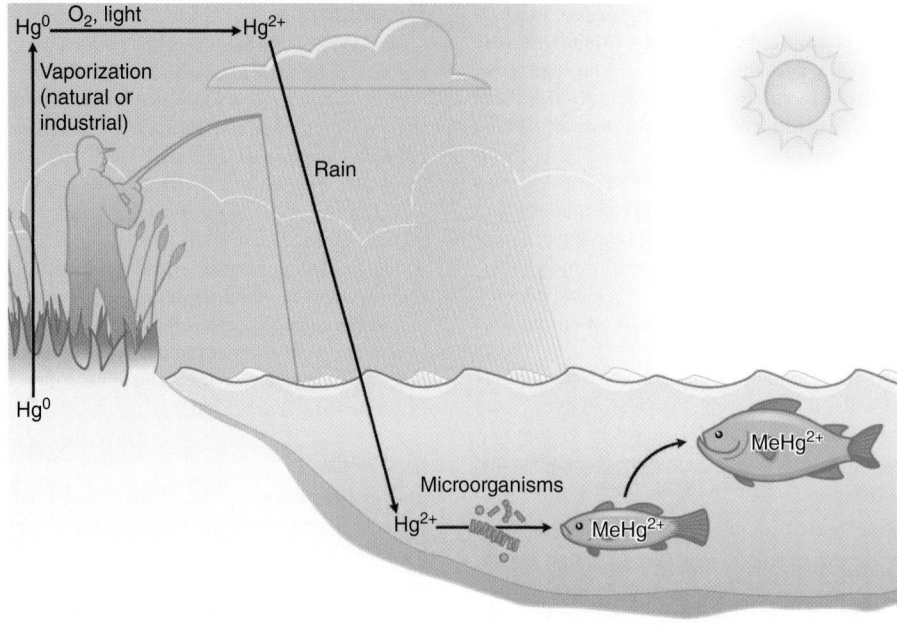

Figure 71–6 *Mobilization of mercury in the environment.* Metallic mercury (Hg^0) is vaporized from Earth's surface both naturally and through human activities such as burning coal. In the atmosphere, Hg^0 is oxidized to form divalent inorganic mercury (Hg^{2+}), which falls to the surface in rain. Aquatic bacteria can methylate Hg^{2+} to form methyl mercury ($MeHg^+$). $MeHg^+$ in plankton is consumed by fish. Because of its lipophilicity, $MeHg^+$ bioaccumulates up the food chain.

in influenza vaccines (Heron and Golding, 2004). The FDA maintains a listing of the thimerosal content in vaccines (http://www.fda.gov/BiologicsBloodVaccines/SafetyAvailability/VaccineSafety/UCM096228).

Chemistry and Mode of Action

There are three general forms of mercury of concern to human health. Metallic, or elemental, mercury (Hg^0) is the liquid metal found in scientific equipment and dental amalgam; it is volatile, and exposure is often to the vapor. *Inorganic mercury* can be either monovalent (*mercurous*, Hg^{1+}) or divalent (*mercuric*, Hg^{2+}) and forms a variety of salts. *Organic mercury* compounds consist of divalent mercury complexed with one or two alkyl groups. *Methyl mercury* ($MeHg^+$), which is formed environmentally from inorganic mercury by aquatic microorganisms, is of most concern. Both Hg^{2+} and $MeHg^+$ readily form covalent bonds with sulfur, which causes most of the biological effects of mercury. At very low concentrations, mercury reacts with sulfhydryl residues on many proteins and disrupts their functions. Microtubules are particularly sensitive to the toxic effects of mercury, which disrupts their formation and can catalyze their disassembly (Clarkson, 2002). There also may be an autoimmune component to mercury toxicity.

ADME

The vapor of Hg^0 is readily absorbed through the lungs (~70%–80%), but GI absorption of Hg^0 is negligible. Once absorbed, Hg^0 distributes throughout the body and crosses membranes, such as the blood-brain barrier and the placenta, via diffusion. Hg^0 is oxidized by catalase in cells to form Hg^{2+}. Shortly after exposure, some Hg^0 is eliminated in exhaled air. After a few hours, distribution and elimination of Hg^0 resemble the properties of Hg^{2+}. Hg^0 vapor can be oxidized to Hg^{2+} in the brain and retained (ATSDR, 1999).

Gastrointestinal absorption of mercury salts varies depending on the individual and on the particular salt and averages about 10%–15%. Hg^{1+} will form Hg^0 or Hg^{2+} in the presence of sulfhydryl groups. Hg^{2+} is primarily excreted in the urine and feces; a small amount also can be reduced to Hg^0 and exhaled. With acute exposure, the fecal pathway predominates, but following chronic exposure, urinary excretion becomes more important. All forms of mercury also are excreted in sweat and breast milk and deposited in hair and nails. The $t_{1/2}$ for inorganic mercury is approximately 1–2 months (ATSDR, 1999).

Complexes between $MeHg^+$ and cysteine resemble methionine and can be recognized by transporters for that amino acid and taken across

membranes (Ballatori, 2002). Orally ingested $MeHg^+$ is almost completely absorbed from the GI tract. $MeHg^+$ readily crosses the blood-brain barrier and the placenta and distributes fairly evenly to the tissues, although concentrations are highest in the kidneys (ATSDR, 1999). $MeHg^+$ can be demethylated to form inorganic Hg^{2+}. The liver and kidney exhibit the highest rates of demethylation, but this also occurs in the brain. $MeHg^+$ is excreted in the urine and feces, with the fecal pathway dominating. The $t_{1/2}$ for $MeHg^+$ is about 2 months. The toxicodynamic properties of $MeHg^+$ are thought to result from molecular mimicry.

Health Effects

Metallic Mercury. Inhalation of high levels of Hg^0 vapor over a short duration is acutely toxic to the lung. Respiratory symptoms of Hg^0 exposure start with cough and tightness in the chest and can progress to interstitial pneumonitis and severely compromised respiratory function. Other initial symptoms include weakness, chills, metallic taste, nausea, vomiting, diarrhea, and dyspnea. Acute exposure to high doses of Hg^0 is also toxic to the CNS, with symptoms similar to those of chronic exposure (Figure 71–7).

Toxicity to the nervous system is the primary concern with chronic exposure to Hg^0. Symptoms include tremors (particularly of the hands); emotional lability (irritability, shyness, loss of confidence, and nervousness); insomnia; memory loss; muscular atrophy; weakness; paresthesia; and cognitive deficits. These symptoms intensify and become irreversible with increases in duration and concentration of exposure. Other common symptoms of chronic mercury exposure include kidney damage, tachycardia, labile pulse, severe salivation, and gingivitis.

Inorganic Salts of Mercury. Ingestion of Hg^{2+} salts is intensely irritating to the GI tract, leading to vomiting, diarrhea, and abdominal pain. Acute exposure to Hg^{1+} or Hg^{2+} salts (typically in suicide attempts) leads to renal tubular necrosis, resulting in decreased urine output and often acute renal failure. Chronic exposures also target the kidney, with glomerular injury predominating.

Organic Mercury. The CNS is the primary target of $MeHg^+$ toxicity. Symptoms of high-dose $MeHg^+$ exposure include visual disturbances, ataxia, paresthesia, fatigue, hearing loss, slurring of speech, cognitive deficits, muscle tremor, movement disorders, and, following severe exposure, paralysis and death. The developing nervous system exhibits increased sensitivity to $MeHg^+$. Children exposed in utero can develop severe symptoms, including mental retardation and neuromuscular deficits, even in

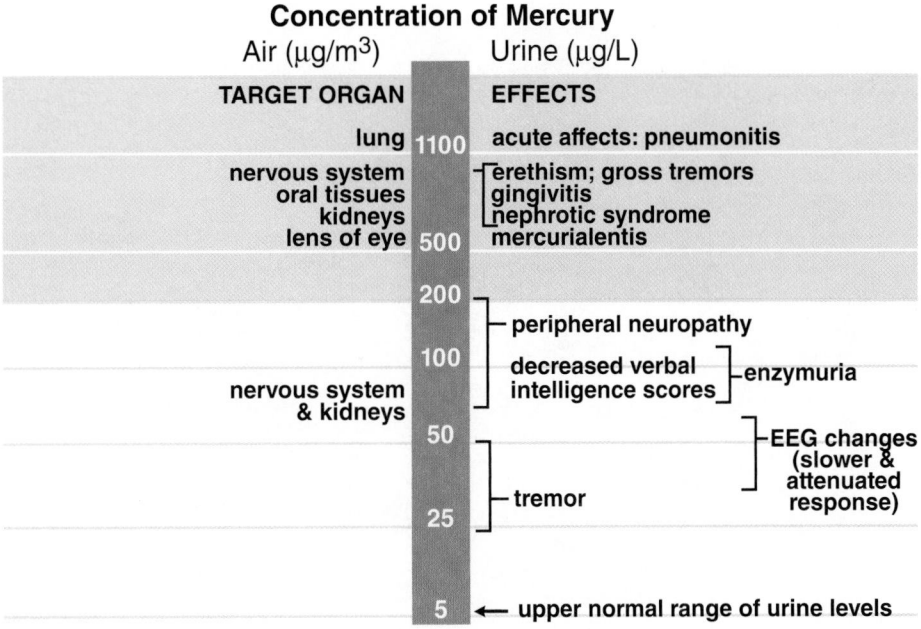

Concentration of Mercury

Figure 71–7 *Concentrations of mercury in air and urine are associated with specific toxic effects.*

the absence of symptoms in the mother. In adults, MeHg⁺ causes focused lesions in specific areas of the brain, while the brains of children exposed in utero sustain widespread damage (Clarkson, 2002).

The effects of low-dose MeHg⁺ exposure from routine consumption of fish are difficult to assess due to the opposing beneficial effects of ω-3 fatty acids found in fish oils, and studies have produced discrepant results (Grandjean et al., 1999; Myers et al., 2003).

Treatment

Termination of exposure to Hg^0 is critical, and respiratory support may be required. Emesis may be used within 30–60 min of exposure to Hg^{1+} or Hg^{2+}, provided the patient is awake and alert and there is no corrosive injury. Maintenance of electrolyte balance and fluids is important for these patients. Chelation therapy is beneficial in patients with acute inorganic or metallic mercury exposure. There are limited treatment options for MeHg⁺. Chelation therapy does not provide clinical benefits, but nonabsorbable thiol resins may be beneficial by preventing absorption of MeHg⁺ from the GI tract.

Because of the conflicting effects of mercury and ω-3 fatty acids, there is considerable controversy regarding the restriction of fish intake in women of reproductive age and children. The EPA recommends limiting fish intake to 12 oz (two meals) per week. Many experts feel this recommendation is too conservative. The recommendation that women consume fish that is lower in mercury content (i.e., canned light tuna, salmon, pollock, catfish) and avoid top predators, such as swordfish, shark, and tilefish, is not controversial.

Arsenic

Arsenic is a metalloid that is common in rocks and soil. Arsenic compounds have been used for more than 2400 years as both therapeutic agents and poisons. In the late 19th century, Robert Ehrlich coined the terms *magic bullet* and *chemotherapy* to describe his work using the organic arsenic compound arsphenamine for the treatment for syphilis. The use of arsenic in drugs has been mostly phased out, but arsenic trioxide is still used as an effective chemotherapy agent for acute promyelocytic leukemia (see Chapter 68).

Exposure

The primary source of exposure to arsenic is through drinking water. Arsenic naturally leaches out of soil and rocks into well and spring water (Mead, 2005). Levels of arsenic in drinking water average 2 μg/L (ppb) in the U.S. but can be more than 50 μg/L (five times the MCL set by the EPA)

in private well water. Drinking water from other parts of the world, particularly Taiwan, China, Argentina, Chile, Bangladesh, and eastern India, sometimes is contaminated with much higher levels of arsenic (sometimes several hundred micrograms per liter), and widespread poisonings have resulted (see Figure 71–8) Arsenic can enter the environment through human activities, such as the use of arsenic-containing pesticides, mining, and burning of coal. Food, particularly seafood, often is contaminated with arsenic. Arsenic in seafood exists primarily as organic compounds (i.e., arsenobetaine), which are much less toxic than inorganic arsenic. The average daily human intake of arsenic is 10 μg/d, almost exclusively from food and water.

Before 2003, more than 90% of arsenic used in the U.S. was as a preservative in pressure-treated wood, but the lumber industry has voluntarily replaced arsenic with other preservatives. Arsenic-treated wood is thought to be safe unless burned. The major source of occupational exposure to arsenic is in the production and use of organic arsenicals as herbicides and insecticides. Exposure to metallic arsenic, arsine, arsenic trioxide, and gallium arsenide also occurs in high-tech industries, such as the manufacture of computer chips and semiconductors.

Chemistry and Mode of Action

Arsenic exists in its elemental form and trivalent (arsenites/arsenious acid) and pentavalent (arsenates/arsenic acid) states. Arsine (AsH_3) is a gaseous hydride of trivalent arsenic that exhibits toxicities that are distinct from other forms. Organic compounds of either valence state of arsenic are formed in animals. The toxicity of a given arsenical is related to the rate of its clearance from the body and its ability to concentrate in tissues. In general, toxicity increases in the sequence: organic arsenicals $< As^{5+} < As^{3+} < AsH_3$.

Like mercury, trivalent arsenic compounds form covalent bonds with sulfhydryl groups. The pyruvate dehydrogenase (PDH) complex is particularly sensitive to inhibition by trivalent arsenicals: The two sulfhydryl groups of lipoic acid that participate in acetate transfer to coenzyme A react with arsenic to form a six-membered ring, effectively inhibiting PDH and other lipoamide-containing enzymes. Inorganic arsenate (pentavalent) inhibits the electron transport chain. It is thought that arsenate competitively substitutes for phosphate during the formation of ATP, forming an unstable arsenate ester that is rapidly hydrolyzed.

ADME

The absorption of arsenic compounds is directly related to their aqueous solubility. Poorly water-soluble compounds such as arsenic sulfide, lead

A

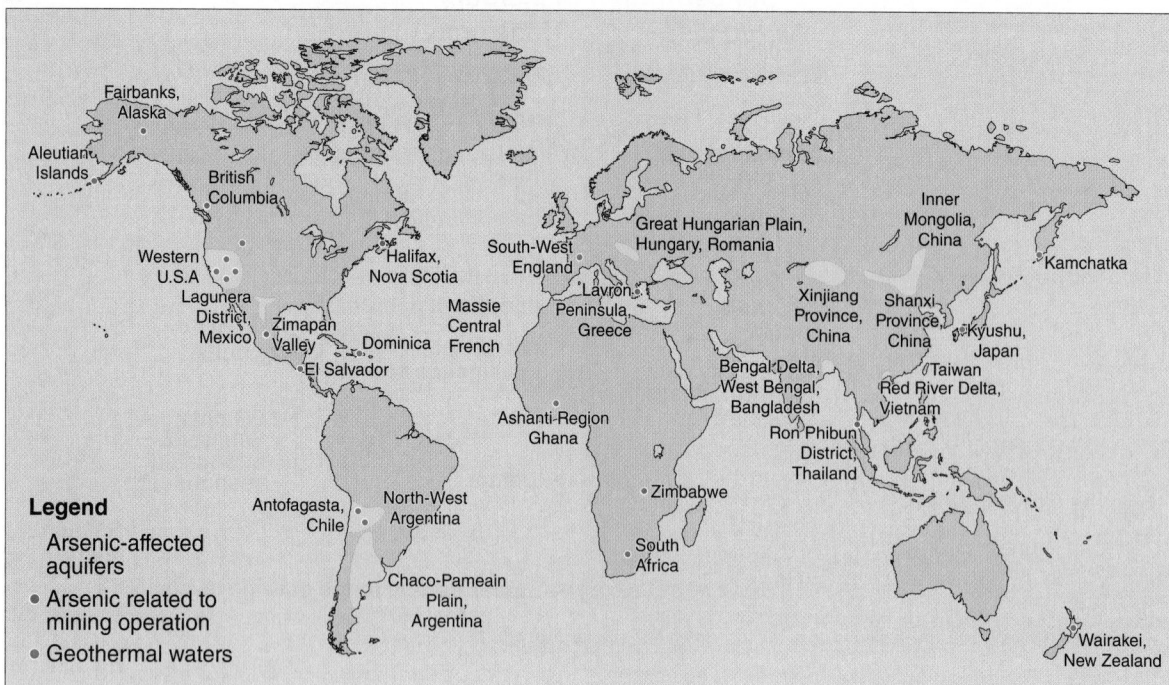

B

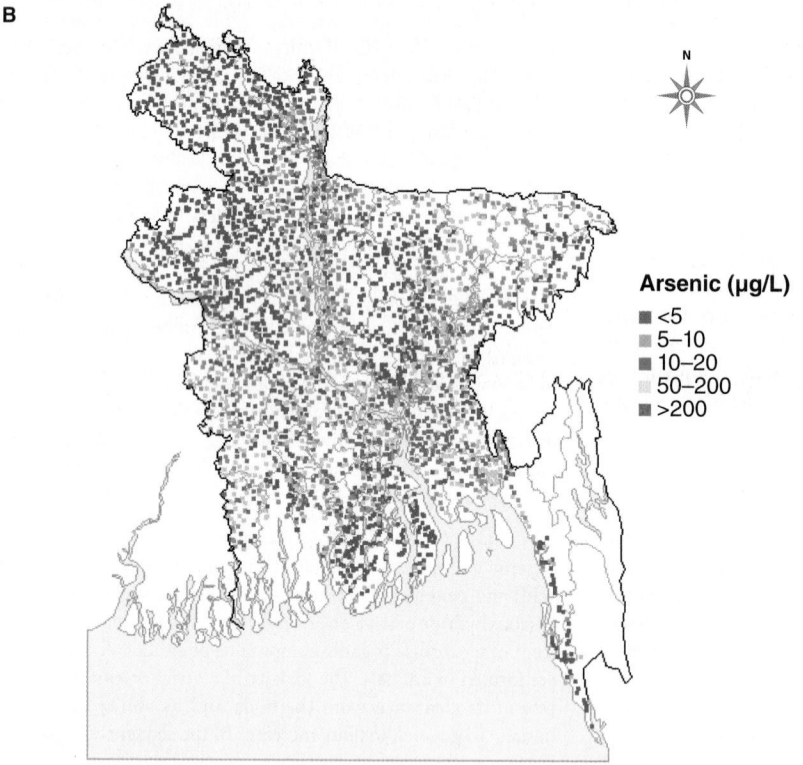

Arsenic (µg/L)
- ■ <5
- ■ 5–10
- ■ 10–20
- ■ 50–200
- ■ >200

Figure 71–8 *Arsenic in drinking water.* **A.** World map demonstrating regions where there is increased arsenic exposure in drinking water. **B.** Map of Bangladesh demonstrating arsenic concentrations in drinking water in samples from wells across the country. (Adapted from a report produced by the British Geological Survey and the Department of Public Health Engineering [Bangladesh] undertaking a project funded by the U.K. Department for International Development. Any views expressed are not necessarily those of DFID.)

arsenate, and arsenic trioxide are not well absorbed. Water-soluble arsenic compounds are readily absorbed via inhalation and ingestion. GI absorption of arsenic dissolved in drinking water is more than 90% (ATSDR, 2007a). At low doses, arsenic is fairly evenly distributed throughout the tissues of the body. Nails and hair, due to their high sulfhydryl content, exhibit high concentrations of arsenic. After an acute high dose (i.e., fatal poisoning), arsenic is preferentially deposited in the liver and, to a lesser extent, kidney, with elevated levels also observed in the muscle, heart, spleen, pancreas, lungs, and cerebellum. Arsenic readily crosses the placenta and blood-brain barrier.

Arsenic undergoes biotransformation in humans and animals (Figure 71–9). Trivalent compounds can be oxidized back to pentavalent

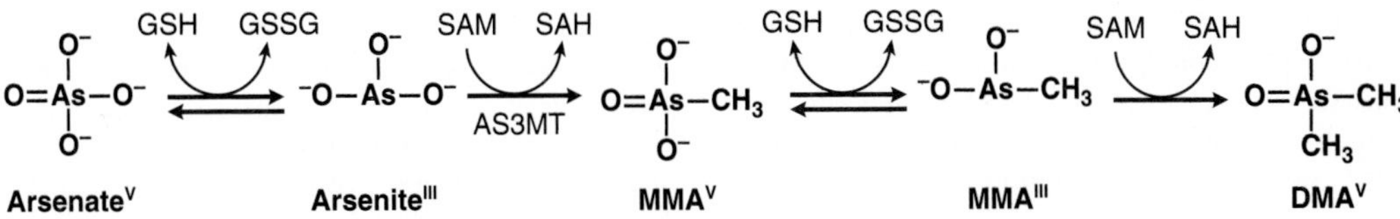

Figure 71–9 *Metabolism of arsenic.* AS3MT, arsenite methyltransferase; DMA^V, dimethylarsinic acid; GSH, reduced glutathione; GSSG, oxidized glutathione; MMA^{III}, monomethylarsonous acid; MMA^V, monomethylarsonic acid; SAH, S-adenosyl-L-homocysteine; SAM, S-adenosyl-L-methionine.

compounds, but there is no evidence for demethylation of methylated arsenicals. Humans excrete much higher levels of MMA compounds than most other animals (ATSDR, 2007a). Because the pentavalent methylated arsenic compounds have greatly reduced toxicity, the methylation pathway was long thought to be a detoxification pathway. However, the trivalent methylated arsenicals actually are more toxic than inorganic arsenite due to an increased affinity for sulfhydryl groups, and formation of MMA^{III} now is considered a bioactivation pathway (Aposhian and Aposhian, 2006).

Elimination of arsenicals by humans primarily is in the urine, although some is also excreted in feces, sweat, hair, nails, skin, and exhaled air. Compared to most other toxic metals, arsenic is excreted quickly, with a $t_{1/2}$ of 1–3 days. In humans, ingested inorganic arsenic that appears in urine is a mixture of 10%–30% inorganic arsenicals, 10%–20% monomethylated forms, and 60%–80% dimethylated forms.

Health Effects

With the exception of arsine gas, the various forms of inorganic arsenic exhibit similar toxic effects. Inorganic arsenic exhibits a broad range of toxicities and has been associated with effects on every organ system tested (ATSDR, 2007a). Humans also are exposed to large organic arsenic compounds in fish, which are relatively nontoxic. Humans are the most sensitive species to the toxic effects of inorganic arsenic. Acute exposure to large doses of arsenic (>70–180 mg) often is fatal. Death immediately following arsenic poisoning typically is the result of its effects on the heart and GI tract. Death sometimes occurs later as a result of arsenic's combined effect on multiple organs.

Cardiovascular System.
Acute and chronic arsenic exposure cause myocardial depolarization, cardiac arrhythmias, and ischemic heart disease; these are known side effects of arsenic trioxide for the treatment for leukemia. Chronic exposure to arsenic can cause peripheral vascular disease, the most dramatic example of which is "blackfoot disease," a condition characterized by cyanosis of the extremities, particularly the feet, progressing to gangrene. Blackfoot disease is endemic in regions of Taiwan, where well water contains arsenic at levels of 170 to 800 µg/L. Arsenic dilates capillaries and increases their permeability; this causes edema after acute exposures and is likely responsible for peripheral vascular disease following chronic exposure.

Skin.
Dermal symptoms often are diagnostic of arsenic exposure. Arsenic induces hyperkeratinization of the skin (including formation of multiple corns or warts), particularly of the palms of the hands and the soles of the feet. It also causes areas of hyperpigmentation interspersed with spots of hypopigmentation. These symptoms can be observed in individuals exposed to drinking water with arsenic concentrations of at least 100 µg/L and are typical in those chronically exposed to much higher levels. Hyperpigmentation can be observed after 6 months of exposure; hyperkeratinization takes years. Children are more likely to develop these effects than adults (ATSDR, 2007a; Mead, 2005).

Gastrointestinal Tract.
Acute or subacute ingestion of high-dose arsenic is associated with GI symptoms ranging from mild cramping, diarrhea, and vomiting to GI hemorrhaging and death. GI symptoms are caused by increased capillary permeability, leading to fluid loss. At higher doses, fluid forms vesicles that can burst, leading to inflammation and necrosis of the submucosa and then rupture of the intestinal wall. GI symptoms are not observed with chronic exposure to lower levels of arsenic.

Nervous System.
The most common neurological effect of acute or subacute arsenic exposure is peripheral neuropathy involving both sensory and motor neurons. This effect is characterized by the loss of sensation in the hands and feet, often followed by muscle weakness. Neuropathy occurs several days after exposure and can be reversible following cessation of exposure, although recovery usually is not complete. Arsenic exposure may cause intellectual deficits in children (Wasserman et al., 2007). Acute high-dose arsenic exposure causes encephalopathy in rare cases, with symptoms that can include headache, lethargy, mental confusion, hallucination, seizures, and coma.

Other Noncancer Toxicities.
Acute and chronic arsenic exposures induce anemia and leukopenia, likely via direct cytotoxic effects on blood cells and suppression of erythropoiesis. Arsenic also may inhibit heme synthesis. In the liver, arsenic causes fatty infiltrations, central necrosis, and cirrhosis of varying severity. The action of arsenic on renal capillaries, tubules, and glomeruli can cause severe kidney damage. Inhaled arsenic is irritating to the lungs, and ingested arsenic may induce bronchitis progressing to bronchopneumonia in some individuals. Chronic exposure to arsenic is associated with an increased risk of diabetes.

Carcinogenesis.
Regions with very high arsenic levels in drinking water consistently have substantially higher rates of skin cancer, bladder cancer, and lung cancer. There also are associations between arsenic exposure and other cancers, including liver, kidney, and prostate tumors. Inhalation exposure to arsenic in occupational settings causes lung cancer. IARC classifies arsenic as "carcinogenic to humans (Group 1)."

The developing fetus and young children may be at increased risk of arsenic carcinogenesis because humans exposed to arsenic in utero and in early childhood have a greatly elevated risk of lung cancer (Smith et al., 2006). Studies in rodents also have observed increased cancer risks from in utero exposure and suggest that the second trimester of pregnancy represents a critical susceptibility window (Waalkes et al., 2007).

Arsenic does not directly damage DNA; rather, arsenic is thought to work through changes in gene expression, DNA methylation, inhibition of DNA repair, generation of oxidative stress, or altered signal transduction pathways (Hartwig et al., 2002; Salnikow and Zhitkovich, 2008). Arsenic compounds can act as tumor promoters or cocarcinogens in rodents, particularly when combined with ultraviolet light. In humans, exposure to arsenic potentiates lung tumorigenesis from tobacco smoke. Smokers in regions with high concentrations of arsenic in the drinking water have a 5-fold increased risk of cancer over smokers living in low-arsenic regions (Ferreccio et al., 2000). Arsenic cocarcinogenesis may involve inhibition of proteins involved in nucleotide excision repair (Hartwig et al., 2002; Salnikow and Zhitkovich, 2008). Arsenic also has endocrine-disrupting activities on several nuclear steroid hormone receptors, enhancing hormone-dependent transcription at very low concentrations and inhibiting it at slightly higher levels.

Arsine Gas

Arsine gas, formed by reduction of arsenic in an industrial setting, is a rare cause of poisonings. Arsine induces rapid and often-fatal hemolysis, which probably results from arsine combining with hemoglobin and reacting with O_2. A few hours after exposure, patients can develop headache, anorexia, vomiting, paresthesia, abdominal pain, chills, hemoglobinuria, bilirubinemia, and anuria. Jaundice appears after 24 h. Arsine induces renal toxicities that can progress to kidney failure. Approximately 25% of cases of arsine exposure result in death.

Treatment

Following acute exposure to all forms of arsenic, the patient should be stabilized and further absorption of the poison should be prevented.

Close monitoring of fluid levels is important because arsenic can cause fatal hypovolemic shock. Chelation therapy is effective following short-term exposure to arsenic but has little or no benefit in chronically exposed individuals. Exchange transfusion to restore blood cells and remove arsenic is often warranted following arsine gas exposure (Ibrahim et al., 2006).

Cadmium

Cadmium was discovered in 1817 and first used industrially in the mid-20th century. Cadmium is resistant to corrosion and exhibits useful electrochemical properties, which has led to its use in electroplating, galvanization, plastics, paint pigments, and nickel-cadmium batteries.

Exposure

In the general population, the primary source of exposure to cadmium is through food, with an estimated average daily intake of 50 µg. Cadmium also is found in tobacco and tobacco smoke; a cigarette contains 1–2 µg of cadmium (Jarup and Akesson, 2009). Workers in smelters and other metal-processing industries can be exposed to high levels of cadmium, particularly by inhalation.

Chemistry and Mode of Action

Cadmium exists as a divalent cation and does not undergo oxidation-reduction reactions. There are no covalent organometallic complexes of cadmium of toxicological significance. The mechanism of cadmium toxicity is not fully understood. Like lead and other divalent metals, cadmium can replace zinc in zinc-finger domains of proteins and disrupt them. Through an unknown mechanism, cadmium induces formation of ROS, resulting in lipid peroxidation and GSH depletion. Cadmium also upregulates inflammatory cytokines and may disrupt the beneficial effects of NO.

ADME

Cadmium is not well absorbed from the GI tract (1.5%–5%) but is absorbed via inhalation (~10%). Cadmium primarily distributes first to the liver and later the kidney, which together account for 50% of the absorbed dose. Cadmium distributes fairly evenly to other tissues but does not cross the blood-brain barrier or the placenta. Cadmium primarily is excreted in the urine and exhibits a $t_{1/2}$ of 10–30 years (ATSDR, 2012b).

Health Effects

Toxicity. Acute cadmium toxicity is due to local irritation along the absorption route. Inhaled cadmium causes respiratory tract irritation with severe, early pneumonitis accompanied by chest pains, nausea, dizziness, and diarrhea. Toxicity may progress to fatal pulmonary edema. Ingested cadmium induces nausea, vomiting, salivation, diarrhea, and abdominal cramps; the vomitus and diarrhea often are bloody.

Symptoms of chronic cadmium toxicity vary by exposure route. The lung is an important target of inhaled cadmium, while the kidney is a major target of cadmium from both inhalation and ingestion.

Cadmium bound to metallothionein is transported to the kidney, where it can be released. Renal toxicity results from increased excretion of low-molecular-weight proteins, especially β_2 microglobulin and retinol-binding protein. Cadmium also causes glomerular injury, with a resulting decrease in filtration. Chronic occupational exposure to cadmium is associated with an increased risk of renal failure and death. There is no evidence for a threshold level for cadmium's effects on the kidney; cadmium levels consistent with normal dietary exposure can cause renal toxicity, including a reduction in glomerular filtration rate and creatinine clearance (Jarup and Akesson, 2009).

Workers with long-term inhalation exposure to cadmium exhibit decreased lung function. Symptoms include bronchitis and fibrosis of the lung, leading to emphysema. The exact cause of cadmium-induced lung toxicity is not known but may result from inhibition of the synthesis of α_1 antitrypsin. Chronic obstructive pulmonary disease causes increased mortality in cadmium-exposed workers.

When accompanied by vitamin D deficiency, cadmium exposure increases the risks for fractures and osteoporosis. This may be an effect of cadmium interfering with calcium and phosphate homeostasis due to its renal toxicity.

Carcinogenicity. Chronic occupational exposure to inhaled cadmium increases the risk of developing lung cancer (IARC, 1993; NTP, 2004). The mechanism of cadmium carcinogenesis is not fully understood. Cadmium causes chromosomal aberrations in exposed workers and treated animals and human cells. It also increases mutations and impairs DNA repair in human cells (NTP, 2004). Cadmium substitutes for zinc in DNA repair proteins and polymerases and may inhibit nucleotide excision repair, base excision repair, and the DNA polymerase responsible for repairing single-strand breaks (Hartwig et al., 2002). There is evidence that cadmium also alters cell signaling pathways and disrupts cellular controls of proliferation (Waisberg et al., 2003). Thus, cadmium acts as a nongenotoxic carcinogen.

Treatment

Treatment for cadmium poisoning is symptomatic. Patients who have inhaled cadmium may require respiratory support. Patients with kidney failure as a result of cadmium poisoning may require a transplant. There is no evidence for clinical benefit from chelation therapy following cadmium poisoning, and chelation therapy may result in adverse effects (ATSDR, 2012b).

Chromium

Chromium is an industrially important metal used in a number of alloys, particularly stainless steel, which contains at least 11% chromium. Chromium can be oxidized to multiple valence states, with trivalent (Cr^{III}) and hexavalent (Cr^{VI}) being the two forms of biological importance. Chromium exists almost exclusively as the trivalent form in nature, and Cr^{III} is an essential metal involved in the regulation of glucose metabolism. Cr^{VI} is thought to be responsible for the toxic effects of chromium (ATSDR, 2012a).

Exposure

Exposure to chromium in the general population primarily is through the ingestion of food, although there also is exposure from drinking water and air. Workers are exposed to chromium during chromate production, stainless steel production and welding, chromium plating, ferrochrome alloy and chrome pigment production, and in tanning industries. Exposure usually is to a mixture of Cr^{III} and Cr^{VI}.

Chemistry and Mode of Action

Chromium occurs in its metallic state or in any valence state between divalent and hexavalent. Cr^{III} is the most stable and common form. Cr^{VI} is corrosive and is readily reduced to lower valence states. The primary reason for the different toxicological properties of Cr^{III} and Cr^{VI} is thought to be differences in their absorption and distribution. Hexavalent chromate resembles sulfate and phosphate and can be taken across membranes by anion transporters. Once inside the cell, Cr^{VI} undergoes a series of reduction steps, ultimately forming Cr^{III}, which is thought to cause most of the toxic effects. Trivalent chromium readily forms covalent interactions with DNA. Hexavalent chromium also induces oxidative stress and hypersensitivity reactions.

ADME

Absorption of inhaled chromium depends on its solubility, valence state, and particle size. Smaller particles are deposited deeper in the lungs. Absorption into the bloodstream of hexavalent and soluble forms is higher than the trivalent or insoluble forms, with the remainder often retained in the lungs. Approximately 50%–85% of inhaled Cr^{VI} particles (<5 µm) are absorbed. Absorption of ingested chromium is less than 10% and varies depending on water solubility. Cr^{VI} crosses membranes by facilitated transport, while Cr^{III} crosses by diffusion. Cr^{VI} is distributed to all of the tissues and crosses the placenta. The highest levels are attained in the liver, kidney, and bone; Cr^{VI} is also retained in erythrocytes. Excretion primarily is through urine, with small amounts also excreted in bile and breast milk and deposited in hair and nails. The $t_{1/2}$ of ingested Cr^{VI} is about 40 h; the $t_{1/2}$ of Cr^{III} is about 10 h (ATSDR, 2012a).

Health Effects

Toxicity. Acute exposure to very high doses of chromium causes death via damage to multiple organs, particularly the kidney. Chronic low-dose chromium exposure causes toxicity at the site of contact. Workers exposed to inhaled chromium develop symptoms of lung and upper respiratory tract irritation, decreased pulmonary function, and pneumonia. Chronic exposure to chromium via ingestion, including after mucociliary clearance of inhaled particles, causes symptoms of GI irritation (oral ulcer, diarrhea, abdominal pain, indigestion, and vomiting). Cr^{VI} is a dermal irritant and can cause ulceration or burns. Low-dose exposure by any route causes some individuals to become sensitized. These individuals will develop allergic dermatitis following dermal exposure to chromium, including products containing metallic chromium. Chromium-sensitized workers often also develop asthma following inhalation exposure (ATSDR, 2012a).

Carcinogenicity. The Cr^{VI} compounds are group 1 known human carcinogens (IARC, 1990). There is insufficient evidence for carcinogenesis from metallic and trivalent chromium (classified in IARC group 3). Workers exposed to Cr^{VI} via inhalation have elevated incidence of and mortality from lung and nasal cancer. Environmental exposure to Cr^{VI} in drinking water increases the risk of developing stomach cancer.

There are multiple potential mechanisms for chromium carcinogenicity (Salnikow and Zhitkovich, 2008). Reduction of Cr^{VI} to Cr^{III} occurs with concomitant oxidation of cellular molecules. Ascorbate is the primary reductant, but other molecules, including GSH, lipids, proteins, and DNA, also can be oxidized. Cr^{III} forms a large number of covalent DNA adducts, primarily at the phosphate diester backbone. The DNA adducts are not very mutagenic and are repaired by nucleotide excision repair. It is thought that the high level of nucleotide excision repair activity following chromium exposure contributes to carcinogenesis, either by preventing repair of mutagenic lesions formed by other carcinogens or through the formation of single-strand breaks due to incomplete repair. Chromium also forms cross-links between DNA and protein. Chronic inflammation due to chromium-induced irritation also may promote tumor formation.

Treatment

There are no standard protocols for treatment for acute chromium poisoning. One approach that has shown promise in rodents is the use of reductants such as ascorbate, GSH, or *N*-acetylcysteine to reduce Cr^{VI} to Cr^{III} after exposure but before absorption to limit bioavailability (ATSDR, 2012a). These compounds and EDTA also increase urinary excretion of chromium after high-dose exposure, particularly if given soon enough to prevent uptake into cells. Exchange transfusion to remove chromium from plasma and erythrocytes may be beneficial.

Treatment for Metal Exposure

The most important response to environmental or occupational exposures to metals is to eliminate the source of the exposure. It also is important to stabilize the patient and provide symptomatic treatment.

Treatment for acute metal intoxications often involves the use of chelators. A chelator is a compound that forms stable complexes with metals, typically as five- or six-membered rings. Formation of complexes between chelators and metals should prevent or reverse metal binding to biological ligands. The ideal chelator should *be highly soluble in water, be resistant to biotransformation, reach sites of metal storage, form stable and nontoxic complexes with toxic metals, and be readily excreted as a metal-chelator complex.* A low affinity for the essential metals calcium and zinc also is desirable because toxic metals often compete with these metals for protein binding.

In cases of acute exposure to high doses of most metals, chelation therapy reduces toxicity. However, following chronic exposure, chelation therapy does not show clinical benefits beyond those of cessation of exposure alone and, in some cases, does more harm than good. Chelation therapy may increase the neurotoxic effects of heavy metals and is only recommended for acute poisonings. The structures of the most commonly used chelators are shown in Figure 71–10.

Ethylenediaminetetraacetic Acid

EDTA and its various salts are effective chelators of divalent and trivalent metals. $CaNa_2EDTA$ is the preferred EDTA salt for metal poisoning, provided that the metal has a higher affinity for EDTA than

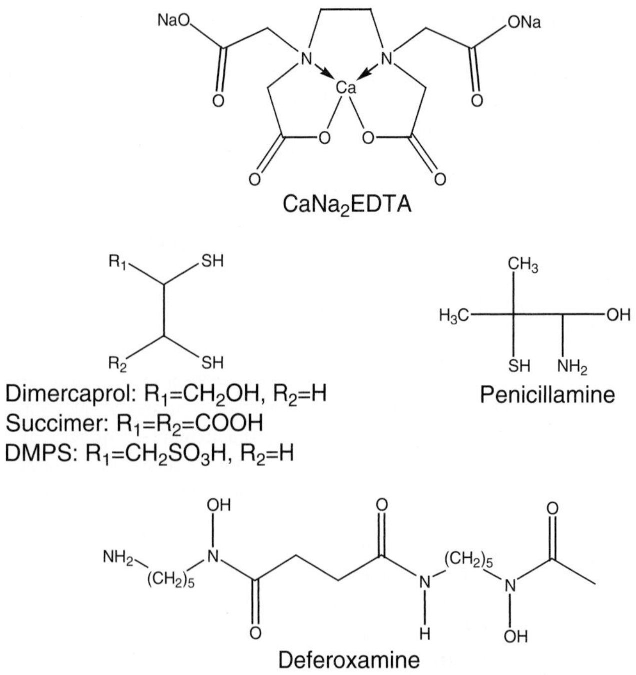

Figure 71–10 *Structures of chelators commonly used to treat acute metal intoxication.*

calcium. $CaNa_2EDTA$ is effective for the treatment for acute lead poisoning, particularly in combination with dimercaprol, but is not an effective chelator of mercury or arsenic in vivo.

Chemistry and Mode of Action

The pharmacological effects of $CaNa_2EDTA$ result from chelation of divalent and trivalent metals in the body. Accessible metal ions with a higher affinity for $CaNa_2EDTA$ than Ca^{2+} will be chelated, mobilized, and usually excreted. Because EDTA is charged at physiological pH, it does not significantly penetrate cells. $CaNa_2EDTA$ mobilizes several endogenous metallic cations, including zinc, manganese, and iron. Additional supplementation with zinc following chelation therapy may be beneficial. The most common therapeutic use of $CaNa_2EDTA$ is for acute lead intoxication. $CaNa_2EDTA$ does not provide clinical benefits for the treatment for chronic lead poisoning.

$CaNa_2EDTA$ is available as edetate calcium disodium (Calcium Disodium Versenate). Intramuscular administration of $CaNa_2EDTA$ results in good absorption, but pain occurs at the injection site; consequently, the chelator injection often is mixed with a local anesthetic or administered intravenously. For intravenous use, $CaNa_2EDTA$ is diluted in either 5% dextrose or 0.9% saline and is administered slowly by intravenous drip. A dilute solution is necessary to avoid thrombophlebitis.

ADME

Less than 5% of $CaNa_2EDTA$ is absorbed from the GI tract. After intravenous administration, $CaNa_2EDTA$ has a $t_{1/2}$ of 20–60 min. In blood, $CaNa_2EDTA$ is found only in the plasma. $CaNa_2EDTA$ is excreted in the urine by glomerular filtration, so adequate renal function is necessary for successful therapy. Altering either the pH or the rate of urine flow has no effect on the rate of excretion. There is very little metabolic degradation of EDTA. The drug is distributed mainly in the extracellular fluids; little gains access to the spinal fluid (5% of the plasma concentration).

Toxicity

The principal toxic effect of $CaNa_2EDTA$ is on the kidney. Repeated large doses of the drug can eventually cause degeneration of proximal tubular cells. The early renal effects usually are reversible, and urinary abnormalities disappear rapidly with cessation of treatment. The most likely mechanism of toxicity is chelation of essential metals, particularly zinc, in proximal tubular cells. To minimize nephrotoxicity, adequate urine production should be established prior to and during treatment with CaNa$_2$EDTA. For patients with lead encephalopathy and cerebral edema, CaNa$_2$EDTA can lead to a potentially fatal increase in intracranial pressure following intravenous administration. Intramuscular administration is preferred for these patients.

Rapid intravenous administration of a form lacking calcium, such as Na$_2$EDTA, causes hypocalcemic tetany. However, a slow infusion (<15 mg/min) administered to a normal individual elicits no symptoms of hypocalcemia because of the availability of extracirculatory stores of Ca^{2+}. In contrast, CaNa$_2$EDTA can be administered intravenously with no untoward effects because the change in the concentration of Ca^{2+} in the plasma and total body is negligible.

Other side effects associated with CaNa$_2$EDTA include malaise, fatigue, and excessive thirst, followed by the sudden appearance of chills and fever and subsequent myalgia, frontal headache, anorexia, occasional nausea and vomiting, and rarely, increased urinary frequency and urgency. CaNa$_2$EDTA is teratogenic in laboratory animals, probably as a result of zinc depletion; it should be used in pregnant women only under conditions in which the benefits clearly outweigh the risks (Kalia and Flora, 2005). Other possible effects include sneezing, nasal congestion, and lacrimation; glycosuria; anemia; dermatitis with lesions strikingly similar to those of vitamin B$_6$ deficiency; transitory lowering of systolic and diastolic blood pressures; prolonged prothrombin time; and T-wave inversion on the electrocardiogram.

Dimercaprol

Dimercaprol was developed during World War II as an antidote to lewisite, a vesicant arsenical war gas, hence its alternative name, British anti-Lewisite (BAL). Arsenicals and other heavy metals form a stable and relatively nontoxic chelate ring with dimercaprol.

Chemistry and Mode of Action

The pharmacological actions of dimercaprol result from formation of chelation complexes between its sulfhydryl groups and metals. Dissociation of dimercaprol-metal complexes and oxidation of dimercaprol occur in vivo. The sulfur-metal bond may be labile in the acidic tubular urine, which may increase the delivery of metal to renal tissue and increase toxicity. The dosage regimen should maintain a concentration of dimercaprol in plasma adequate to favor the continuous formation of the more stable 2:1 (BAL-metal) complex. However, because of pronounced and dose-related side effects, excessive plasma concentrations must be avoided. The concentration in plasma therefore must be maintained by repeated dosage until the metal is excreted. Dimercaprol is most beneficial when given very soon after exposure to the metal because it is more effective in preventing inhibition of sulfhydryl enzymes than in reactivating them. Dimercaprol limits toxicity from arsenic, gold, and mercury, which form mercaptides with essential cellular sulfhydryl groups. It also is used in combination with CaNa$_2$EDTA to treat lead poisoning. Dimercaprol should not be used in iron, cadmium, or selenium poisoning because the resulting metal complexes are more toxic than the metal alone, especially to the kidneys.

ADME

Dimercaprol is given by deep intramuscular injection as a 100-mg/mL solution in peanut oil and should not be used in patients who are allergic to peanuts. Peak dimercaprol concentrations in blood are attained in 30–60 min. The $t_{1/2}$ is short, and metabolic degradation and excretion essentially are complete within 4 h. Dimercaprol and its chelates are excreted in both urine and bile. Dimercaprol is contraindicated for use following chronic exposures to heavy metals because it does not prevent neurotoxic effects. There is evidence in laboratory animals that dimercaprol mobilizes lead and mercury from various tissues to the brain (Andersen and Aaseth, 2002). This effect may be due to the lipophilic nature of dimercaprol and is not observed with its more hydrophilic analogues described further in the chapter (see Succimer and Sodium 2,3-Dimercaptopropane-1-sulfonate).

Toxicity

Side effects occur in about 50% of subjects receiving 5 mg/kg intramuscularly. Dimercaprol causes a rise in systolic and diastolic arterial pressures, accompanied by tachycardia. The pressure rises immediately but returns to normal within 2 h. Dimercaprol also can cause anxiety and unrest, nausea and vomiting, headache, a burning sensation in the mouth and throat, a feeling of constriction or pain in the throat and chest, conjunctivitis, blepharospasm, lacrimation, rhinorrhea, salivation, tingling of the hands, a burning sensation in the penis, sweating, abdominal pain, and the occasional appearance of painful sterile abscesses at the injection site. The dimercaprol-metal complex breaks down easily in an acidic medium; production of alkaline urine protects the kidney during therapy. Children react similarly to adults, although about 30% also may experience a fever that disappears on drug withdrawal. Dimercaprol is contraindicated in patients with hepatic insufficiency, except when this condition is a result of arsenic poisoning.

Succimer

Succimer (2,3-dimercaptosuccinic acid [DMSA]) has been approved in the U.S. for treatment of children with BLL greater than 45 µg/dL. Because of its oral availability, improved toxicity profile, and selective chelation of heavy metals, succimer also is used off label for the treatment of adults with lead poisoning and for the treatment for arsenic and mercury intoxication, although no large clinical trials have been undertaken for these indications.

Chemistry and Mode of Action

Succimer is an orally effective chelator that is chemically similar to dimercaprol but contains two carboxylic acids that modify the spectrum of absorption, distribution, and chelation of the drug. It has an improved toxicity profile over dimercaprol.

ADME

After absorption, succimer is biotransformed to a mixed disulfide with cysteine (Aposhian and Aposhian, 2006). Succimer lowers BLL and attenuates lead toxicity. The succimer-lead chelate is eliminated in both urine and bile. The fraction eliminated in bile can undergo enterohepatic circulation.

Succimer has several desirable features over other chelators. It is orally bioavailable, and because of its hydrophilic nature, it does not mobilize metals to the brain or enter cells. It also does not significantly chelate essential metals such as zinc, copper, or iron. As a result of these properties, succimer exhibits a much better toxicity profile relative to other chelators. Animal studies suggest that succimer also is effective as a chelator of arsenic, cadmium, mercury, and other toxic metals (Andersen and Aaseth, 2002; Kalia and Flora, 2005).

Toxicity

Succimer is much less toxic than dimercaprol. The most commonly reported adverse effects are nausea, vomiting, diarrhea, and loss of appetite. In a few patients, rashes necessitate discontinuation of therapy. Transient elevations in hepatic transaminases have been observed with succimer treatment.

Sodium 2,3-Dimercaptopropane-1-sulfonate

Another dimercapto compound, DMPS, is used for the chelation of heavy metals. DMPS is not approved by the FDA but is approved for use in Germany. DMPS is available from compounding pharmacies and is used by some doctors in the U.S.

Chemistry and Mode of Action

DMPS is a clinically effective chelator of lead, arsenic, and especially mercury. It is orally available and is rapidly excreted, primarily through the kidneys. It is negatively charged and exhibits distribution properties similar to those of succimer. DMPS is less toxic than dimercaprol but mobilizes zinc and copper and thus is more toxic than succimer. In a small clinical trial, DMPS exhibited some clinical benefit for the treatment for chronic arsenic poisoning (Kalia and Flora, 2005), but more thorough clinical studies are needed.

Penicillamine; Trientine

Penicillamine is an effective chelator of copper, mercury, zinc, and lead and promotes the excretion of these metals in the urine. Penicillamine is indicated for use in patients with Wilson disease (excess body burden of copper due to diminished excretion) and is used in other heavy metal intoxications. Penicillamine is more toxic and is less potent and selective for chelation of heavy metals relative to other available chelation drugs. It is therefore not a first-line treatment for acute intoxication with lead, mercury, or arsenic. However, because it is inexpensive and orally bioavailable, it often is given at fairly low doses following treatment with $CaNa_2EDTA$ or dimercaprol to ensure that the concentration of metal in the blood stays low following the patient's release from the hospital.

ADME

Penicillamine is well absorbed (40%–70%) from the GI tract. Food, antacids, and iron reduce its absorption. Peak concentrations in blood are obtained 1–3 h after administration. Penicillamine is relatively stable in vivo compared to its unmethylated parent compound cysteine. Hepatic biotransformation is responsible for degradation of penicillamine; very little drug is excreted unchanged. Metabolites are found in both urine and feces. N-Acetylpenicillamine is more effective than penicillamine in protecting against the toxic effects of mercury, presumably because it is more resistant to metabolism.

Therapeutic Use

Penicillamine is available for oral administration. For chelation therapy, the usual adult dose is 1–1.5 g/d in four divided doses, given on an empty stomach to avoid interference by metals in food. Penicillamine is used in Wilson disease, cystinuria, and rheumatoid arthritis (rarely). For the treatment for Wilson's disease, 1–2 g/d usually is administered in four divided doses. The urinary excretion of copper should be monitored to determine whether the dosage of penicillamine is adequate.

Toxicity

Penicillamine induces cutaneous lesions, including urticaria, macular or papular reactions, pemphigoid lesions, lupus erythematosus, and dermatomyositis. It also causes dryness and scaling. Cross-reactivity with penicillin may be responsible for some episodes of urticarial or maculopapular reactions with generalized edema, pruritus, and fever that occur in as many as one-third of patients taking penicillamine. Hematological reactions may be fatal and include leukopenia, aplastic anemia, and agranulocytosis. Renal toxicity induced by penicillamine usually is manifested as reversible proteinuria and hematuria, but it may progress to nephrotic syndrome with membranous glomerulopathy. Rare fatalities have been reported from Goodpasture syndrome. Severe dyspnea, although uncommon, has been reported from penicillamine-induced bronchoalveolitis. Myasthenia gravis also has been induced by long-term therapy with penicillamine. A specific schedule for physical and laboratory monitoring for skin, blood, kidney, lung, liver, and other toxicities is published in the manufacturer's product labeling.

Penicillamine is a teratogen in laboratory animals, but for pregnant women with Wilson disease, the benefits outweigh the risks. Less serious side effects include nausea, vomiting, diarrhea, dyspepsia, anorexia, and a transient loss of taste for sweet and salt, which is relieved by supplementation of the diet with copper. Contraindications to penicillamine therapy include pregnancy in the absence of Wilson disease, renal insufficiency, or a previous history of penicillamine-induced agranulocytosis or aplastic anemia. Penicillamine increases the requirement for pyridoxime; supplementation with 25 mg daily is advised.

Trientine

Trientine (triethylenetetramine dihydrochloride) is an acceptable alternative for patients with Wilson disease who are intolerant of penicillamine. Trientine is effective orally. Maximal daily doses of 2 g for adults or 1.5 g for children are taken in two to four divided portions on an empty stomach. Iron deficiency may occur during trientine therapy; this can be overcome with short courses of iron therapy, but iron and trientine should not be ingested within 2 h of each other.

Deferoxamine; Deferasirox; Deferiprone

Chemistry and Mode of Action

Deferoxamine is isolated as the iron chelate from *Streptomyces pilosus* and is treated chemically to obtain the metal-free ligand. Deferoxamine (deferoxamine mesylate, DESFERAL) has a remarkably high affinity for ferric iron ($K_a = 10^{31}$ M^{-1}) coupled with a very low affinity for calcium ($K_a = 10^2$ M^{-1}). In vitro, it removes iron from hemosiderin and ferritin and, to a lesser extent, from transferrin. Iron in hemoglobin or cytochromes is not removed by deferoxamine.

ADME and Therapeutic Use

Deferoxamine is poorly absorbed after oral administration, and parenteral (intravenous, intramuscular, or subcutaneous) administration is required. For acute iron toxicity, intramuscular administration is preferred, except for patients in cardiovascular collapse or shock. For patients in shock, the drug is administered intravenously at 10–15 mg/kg/h by constant infusion for the first 1000 mg. If additional treatment is needed beyond 1000 mg, it should be administered at a rate not to exceed 125 mg/h. Faster rates of infusion usually are associated with hypotension. For acute iron poisoning without cardiovascular collapse or shock, deferoxamine should be given intramuscularly at a dose of 50 mg/kg with a maximum dose of 1 g. Subsequent doses of 500 mg may be given, if needed, every 4–12 h. Hypotension also can occur with the intramuscular route. For chronic iron intoxication (e.g., thalassemia), subcutaneous administration is recommended. Continuous subcutaneous administration should be given to achieve a dose of 1–2 g/d. The duration of the infusion (8–24 h) should be individualized to the patient. . Poorly compliant patients with thalassemia can be given deferoxamine by slow intravenous infusion (rate not to exceed 15 mg/kg/h) prior to or after receiving transfusion. Deferoxamine may also be administered via an intramuscular dose of 0.5–1.0 g/d. Deferoxamine is not recommended in primary hemochromatosis; phlebotomy is the treatment of choice. Off label, deferoxamine has also been used for the chelation of aluminum in dialysis patients.

Deferoxamine is metabolized to unknown products by plasma enzymes. The parent drug and its metabolites are readily excreted in the urine.

Toxicity

Deferoxamine can cause a number of allergic reactions, including pruritus, wheals, rash, and anaphylaxis. Other adverse effects include dysuria, abdominal discomfort, diarrhea, fever, leg cramps, and tachycardia. Occasional cases of cataract formation have been reported. Deferoxamine may cause neurotoxicity during long-term, high-dose therapy for transfusion-dependent thalassemia major; both visual and auditory changes have been described. A "pulmonary syndrome" has been associated with high-dose (10- to 25-mg/kg/h) deferoxamine therapy; tachypnea, hypoxemia, fever, and eosinophilia are prominent symptoms. Contraindications to the use of deferoxamine include renal insufficiency and anuria; during pregnancy, the drug should be used only if clearly indicated.

Deferasirox; Deferiprone

Deferasirox and deferiprone are oral chelators that are FDA approved to treat chronic iron overload in patients receiving transfusions. Deferasirox is also indicated for the treatment for chronic iron overload in nontransfusion-dependent thalassemia syndromes. Because of their oral availability, these drugs may allow for better compliance rates for patients with thalassemia. Both drugs form an uncharged chelate with iron and appear to be more effective than deferoxamine at reducing cardiac iron. However, both carry black-box warnings (deferaxirox for renal failure, hepatic failure, GI hemorrhage; deferiprone for agranulocytosis, neutropenia), and there are currently insufficient data to recommend replacing deferoxamine as the first-line treatment for chronic iron overload.

Acknowledgment: Curtis D. Klaassen contributed to this chapter in earlier editions of this book. We have retained some of his text in the current edition.

Drug Facts for Your Personal Formulary: *Metal Chelators*

Drugs	Therapeutic Uses	Clinical Pharmacology and Tips
Heavy Metal Chelators		
CaNa$_2$EDTA (calcium disodium ethylenediaminetetraacetic acid)	• Acute lead poisoning	• IV or IM administration • Not effective for chronic lead poisoning • Nephrotoxic • IV administration can increase intracranial pressure in patients with lead encephalopathy and cerebral edema • Zinc supplementation may be beneficial
Dimercaprol	• Acute arsenic, gold, and mercury poisoning • Acute lead poisoning (in combination with CaNa$_2$EDTA)	• Administered IM • Not effective for chronic intoxication • Increases toxicity of iron, cadmium, and selenium • Toxicity profile is worse than for succimer
Succimer	• Treatment of children with blood lead > 45 µg/dL • Off label for adults with lead poisoning and for arsenic and mercury poisoning	• Orally bioavailable • Improved toxicity profile over dimercaprol • Reduced mobilization of lead to brain • May cause allergic reactions
Copper Chelators		
Penicillamine	• Treatment of copper intoxication due to Wilson disease • Chelates heavy metals, but more toxic, less potent, and less selective than other options	• Orally bioavailable • Allergenic • Nephrotoxic • Causes hematological toxicities • Causes a variety of other side effects
Trientine	• Treatment of Wilson disease in those intolerant of penicillamine	• Orally bioavailable • Less potent than penicillamine
Iron Chelators		
Deferoxamine	• Treatment of acute iron intoxication • Treatment of chronic iron overload due to transfusion	• IV, IM, or SC administration required • SC administration preferred for chronic iron overload • IV use for cardiovascular collapse or shock • IM administration for other acute iron intoxication cases
Deferasirox	• Treatment of chronic iron overload due to transfusion • Treatment of nontransfusion-dependent iron overload	• Orally bioavailable • Renal failure, hepatic failure, and GI hemorrhage are concerns • Not recommended over deferoxamine
Deferiprone	• Treatment of chronic iron overload due to transfusion	• Orally bioavailable • Causes agranulocytosis and neutropenia • Not recommended over deferoxamine

Bibliography

American Academy of Pediatrics, Committee on Environmental Health. Lead exposure in children: prevention, detection, and treatment. *Pediatrics*, **2005**, *116*:1036–1046.

Andersen O, Aaseth J. Molecular mechanisms of in vivo metal chelation: implications for clinical treatment of metal intoxications. *Environ Health Perspect*, **2002**, *110*(suppl):887–890.

Aposhian HV, Aposhian MM. Arsenic toxicology: five questions. *Chem Res Toxicol*, **2006**, *19*:1–15.

ATSDR. *Toxicological Profile for Mercury*. ATSDR, Atlanta, **1999**.

ATSDR. *Draft Toxicological Profile for Chromium*. ATSDR, Atlanta, **2012a**.

ATSDR. *Toxicological Profile for Cadmium*. ATSDR, Atlanta, **2012b**.

ATSDR. *Toxicological Profile for Arsenic*. ATSDR, Atlanta, **2007a**.

ATSDR. *Toxicological Profile for Lead*. ATSDR, Atlanta, **2007b.**

Ball LK, et al. An assessment of thimerosal use in childhood vaccines. *Pediatrics*, **2001**, *107*:1147–1154.

Ballatori N. Transport of toxic metals by molecular mimicry. *Environ Health Perspect*, **2002**, *110*(suppl):689–694.

Bellinger DC, Bellinger AM. Childhood lead poisoning: the torturous path from science to policy. *J Clin Invest*, **2006**, *116*:853–857.

British Geological Survey and Department of Public Health & Engineering (BGS & DPHE). Arsenic contamination of ground water. (Kinniburgh, D.G,m & Smedley, P.L. (Editors) In: Geological Survey Technical Report WC/00/19, 2001.

Canfield RL, et al. Intellectual impairment in children with blood lead concentrations below 10 µg per deciliter. *N Engl J Med*, **2003**, *348*: 1517–1526.

Centers for Disease Control and Prevention (CDC), Advisory Committee on Childhood Lead Poisoning Prevention. *Low Level Lead Exposure Harms Children: A Renewed Call for Primary Prevention*. CDC, Atlanta, **2012**.

Clarkson TW. The three modern faces of mercury. *Environ Health Perspect*, **2002**, *110*(suppl):11–23.

Conney AH. Induction of microsomal enzymes by foreign chemicals and carcinogenesis by polycyclic aromatic hydrocarbons. G.H.A. Clowes Memorial Lecture. *Cancer Res*, **1982**, *42*:4875–4917.

Dietert RR, Piepenbrink MS. Lead and immune function. *Crit Rev Toxicol*, **2006**, *36*:359–385.

Evans TR, Kaye SB. Retinoids: present role and future potential. *Br J Cancer*, **1999**, *80*:1–8.

Fahey JW, Kensler TW. Role of dietary supplements/nutraceuticals in chemoprevention through induction of cytoprotective enzymes. *Chem Res Toxicol*, **2007**, *20*:572–576.

Ferreccio C, et al. Lung cancer and arsenic concentrations in drinking water in Chile. *Epidemiology*, **2000**, *11*:673–679.

Garza A, et al. Cellular mechanisms of lead neurotoxicity. *Med Sci Monit*, **2006**, *12*:RA57–RA65.

Grandjean P, et al. Methylmercury exposure biomarkers as indicators of neurotoxicity in children aged 7 years. *Am J Epidemiol*, **1999**, *150*:301–305.

Groopman JD, et al. Aflatoxin and hepatitis B virus biomarkers: a paradigm for complex environmental exposures and cancer risk. *Cancer Biomark*, **2005**, *1*:5–14.

Groopman JD, et al. Protective interventions to prevent aflatoxin-induced carcinogenesis in developing countries. *Annu Rev Public Health*, **2008**, *29*:187–203.

Guengerich FP, et al. Involvement of cytochrome P450, glutathione S-transferase, and epoxide hydrolase in the metabolism of aflatoxin B1 and relevance to risk of human liver cancer. *Environ Health Perspect*, **1996**, *104*(suppl):557–562.

Hartwig A, et al. Interference by toxic metal ions with DNA repair processes and cell cycle control: molecular mechanisms. *Environ Health Perspect*, **2002**, *110*(suppl):797–799.

Heron J, Golding J. Thimerosal exposure in infants and developmental disorders: a prospective cohort study in the United Kingdom does not support a causal association. *Pediatrics*, **2004**, *114*:577–583.

Hussain SP, et al. TP53 mutations and hepatocellular carcinoma: Insights into the etiology and pathogenesis of liver cancer. *Oncogene*, **2007**, *26*:2166–2176.

Ibrahim D, et al. Heavy metal poisoning: clinical presentations and pathophysiology. *Clin Lab Med*, **2006**, *26*:67–97.

IARC. Chromium, nickel, and welding. In: *Monographs on the Evaluation of Carcinogenic Risks to Humans*, Vol. 49. Lyon, France, IARC Press, **1990**.

IARC. Beryllium, cadmium, mercury, and exposures in the glass manufacturing industry. In: *Monographs on the Evaluation of Carcinogenic Risks to Humans, Vol. 58.* Lyon, France, IARC Press, **1993**.

IARC. Some traditional herbal medicines, some mycotoxins, naphthalene, and styrene. In: *Monographs on the Evaluation of Carcinogenic Risks to Humans, Vol. 82.* Lyon, France, IARC Press, **2002**.

IARC. Inorganic lead and organic lead compounds. In: *Monographs on the Evaluation of Carcinogenic Risks to Humans, Vol. 87.* Lyon, France, IARC Press, **2006**.

Jarup L, Akesson A. Current status of cadmium as an environmental health problem. *Toxicol Appl Pharmacol*, **2009**, *238*:201–208.

Kalia K, Flora SJ. Strategies for safe and effective therapeutic measures for chronic arsenic and lead poisoning. *J Occup Health*, **2005**, *47*:1–21.

Kensler TW, et al. Chemoprevention of hepatocellular carcinoma in aflatoxin endemic areas. *Gastroenterology*, **2004**, *127*:S310–S318.

Lanphear BP, et al. Low-level environmental lead exposure and children's intellectual function: an international pooled analysis. *Environ Health Perspect*, **2005**, *113*:894–899.

Mead MN. Arsenic: in search of an antidote to a global poison. *Environ Health Perspect*, **2005**, *113*:A378–A386.

Mena S, et al. Oxidative stress in environmental-induced carcinogenesis. *Mutat Res*, **2009**, *674*:36–44.

Myers GJ, et al. Prenatal methylmercury exposure from ocean fish consumption in the Seychelles child development study. *Lancet*, **2003**, *361*:1686–1692.

National Toxicology Program (NTP). Cadmium and cadmium compounds. In: *Report on Carcinogens*. NTP, Research Triangle Park, NC, **2004**, III42–III44.

Omenn GS, et al. Chemoprevention of lung cancer: the beta-Carotene and Retinol Efficacy Trial (CARET) in high-risk smokers and asbestos-exposed workers. *IARC Sci Publ*, **1996**, *136*:67–85.

Penning TM. Polycyclic aromatic hydrocarbons: multiple metabolic pathways and DNA lesions formed. In: Geactinov NE, Broyde S, eds. *The Chemical Biology of DNA Damage*. New York, Wiley-VCH, **2009**, 131–148.

Potter JD. The failure of cancer chemoprevention. *Carcinogenesis*, **2014**, *35*:974–982.

Rogan WJ, et al. The effect of chelation therapy with succimer on neuropsychological development in children exposed to lead. *N Engl J Med*, **2001**, *344*:1421–1426.

Salnikow K, Zhitkovich A. Genetic and epigenetic mechanisms in metal carcinogenesis and cocarcinogenesis: nickel, arsenic, and chromium. *Chem Res Toxicol*, **2008**, *21*:28–44.

Schober SE, et al. Blood lead levels and death from all causes, cardiovascular disease, and cancer: results from the NHANES III mortality study. *Environ Health Perspect*, **2006**, *114*:1538–1541.

Smith AH, et al. Increased mortality from lung cancer and bronchiectasis in young adults after exposure to arsenic in utero and in early childhood. *Environ Health Perspect*, **2006**, *114*:1293–1296.

Sylla A, et al. Interactions between hepatitis B virus infection and exposure to aflatoxins in the development of hepatocellular carcinoma: A molecular epidemiological approach. *Mutat Res*, **1999**, *428*:187–196.

Szabo E. Selecting targets for cancer prevention: where do we go from here? *Nat Rev Cancer*, **2006**, *6*:867–874.

Vaziri ND, Khan M. Interplay of reactive oxygen species and nitric oxide in the pathogenesis of experimental lead-induced hypertension. *Clin Exp Pharmacol Physiol*, **2007**, *34*:920–925.

Vogel VG, et al. Effects of tamoxifen vs raloxifene on the risk of developing invasive breast cancer and other disease outcomes: the NSABP Study of Tamoxifen and Raloxifene (STAR) P-2 trial. *JAMA*, **2006**, *295*:2727–2741.

Waalkes MP, et al. Transplacental arsenic carcinogenesis in mice. *Toxicol Appl Pharmacol*, **2007**, *222*:271–280.

Waisberg M, et al. Molecular and cellular mechanisms of cadmium carcinogenesis. *Toxicology*, **2003**, *192*:95–117.

Wasserman GA, et al. Water arsenic exposure and intellectual function in 6-year-old children in Araihazar, Bangladesh. *Environ Health Perspect*, **2007**, *115*:285–289.

Wattenberg LW. Chemoprophylaxis of carcinogenesis: a review. *Cancer Res*, **1966**, *26*:1520–1526.

Wheeler W, Brown MJ. Blood lead levels in children aged 1–5 years—United States, 1999–2010. *MMWR Morb Mortal Wkly Rep*, **2013**, *62*:245.

William WN, et al. Molecular targets for cancer chemoprevention. *Nat Rev Drug Discov*, **2009**, *8*:213–225.

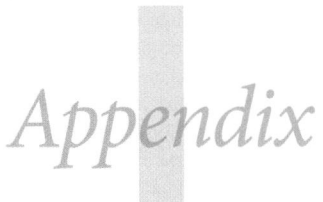

Principles of Prescription Order Writing and Patient Compliance

Iain L.O. Buxton

Latin Not Spoken Here

In writing prescriptions, use English (in the U.S.) or the dominant language of the patient. Latin is no longer the international language of medicine, but a number of commonly used abbreviations derive from obsolete Latin usage and persist in prescription writing. Avoid using them. Non utuntur Latini.

Some Latin seems firmly embedded in pharmacy practice. "Rx" is said to be an abbreviation for the Latin word *recipere*, meaning "take" or "take thus," as a direction to a pharmacist, preceding the physician's "recipe" for preparing a medication. The abbreviation "Sig" for the Latin *Signatura*, is used on the prescription to mark the directions for administration of the medication.

Who Can Prescribe Medicines?

Prescription writing in the U.S. is regulated by state boards of pharmacy. In many states, healthcare practitioners other than MD and DO physicians can write prescriptions, although in some cases narcotics are excluded. Licensed dentists, podiatrists, PAs, nurse practitioners, pharmacists, and clinical psychologists can prescribe medications under various circumstances.

Current Practice

The prescription consists of the *superscription*, the *inscription*, the *subscription*, the *signa*, and the *name and signature of the prescriber*, all contained on a single form (Figure AI–1). The *superscription* includes the date the prescription order is written; the name, address, weight, and age of the patient; and the Rx (*Take*). The body of the prescription, or *inscription*, contains the name and amount or strength of the drug to be dispensed or the name and strength of each ingredient to be compounded.

The *subscription* is the instruction to the pharmacist, usually consisting of a short sentence, such as "dispense 30 tablets." The *signa* or "Sig" is the instruction for the patient regarding how to take the prescription, interpreted and transposed onto the prescription label by the pharmacist. In the U.S., prescriptions should always be written in English. Many physicians continue to use Latin abbreviations, such as, "1 cap tid pc." This will be interpreted by the pharmacist as "take one capsule three times daily after meals." However, the use of Latin abbreviations for these directions

only mystifies the prescription and is discouraged. The pharmacist should always write the label in English (or, as appropriate, in the language of the patient). The use of such abbreviations or symbols is a confounding practice; many serious dispensing errors can be traced to the use of abbreviations.

Avoid the instruction "take as directed." Such directions assume an understanding on the part of the patient that may not be realized and are inadequate for the pharmacist, who must determine the intent of the physician before dispensing the medication. Including directions provides an additional measure of safety for the patient because the pharmacist can confirm the correct medication is being dispensed for the prescribed regimen. The best directions to the patient will include a reminder of the intended purpose of the medication by including such phrases as "for relief of pain" or "to relieve itching." The correct route of administration is reinforced by the choice of the first word of the directions. For an oral dosage form, the directions should begin with *take* or *give*; for externally applied products, the word *apply*; for suppositories, *insert*; and for eye, ear, or nose drops, *place* is preferable to "instill."

Include Patient Information and Dosage Calculations

The patient's name and address are needed on the prescription order to ensure that the correct medication goes to the proper patient and also for identification and recordkeeping. For medications whose dosage involves a calculation, a patient's pertinent factors, such as weight, age, or body surface area, also should be listed on the prescription; both the calculated dose and the dosage formula used, such as "240 mg every 8 h (40 mg/kg/d)," should be included to allow another healthcare professional to double check the prescribed dosage. Pharmacists always should recalculate dosage equations when filling such prescriptions. Medication orders in hospitals and some clinic settings, such as those for antibiotics or antiseizure medications that are sometimes difficult to adequately dose (e.g., phenytoin), can specify the patient diagnosis and desired drug and request dosing by the clinical pharmacist. This is commonly done for drugs with significant adverse effect potential, such as vancomycin.

Proper Use of Prescription Pad

Prescription pad blanks normally are imprinted with a heading that gives the name of the physician and the address and phone number of the practice site (Figure AI–1). When using institutional blanks that do not bear

Abbreviations

ACE: angiotensin-converting enzyme
CAS: Chemical Abstract Service
CSA: Controlled Substances Act
DEA: Drug Enforcement Agency
DO: doctor of osteopathy
DTC: direct-to-consumer
FDA: Food and Drug Administration
IOM: Institute of Medicine
ISMP: Institute for Safe Medication Practices
MD: doctor of medicine
NDC: National Drug Code
PA: physician's assistant
RN: registry number
USAN: U.S. Adopted Name
USP: U.S. Pharmacopeia
USP MERP: U.S. Pharmacopeia Medication Errors Reporting Program
USP/NF: USP/National Formulary

the physician's information, the physician always should print his or her name and phone number on the face of the prescription to facilitate communication with other healthcare professionals should questions arise.

All prescriptions should be written in ink; this practice is compulsory for schedule II prescriptions (e.g., narcotics) under the U.S. CSA of 1970 (see Box AI-1 and Controlled Substances, further in this appendix).

The date of the prescription is an important part of the patient's medical record, and it can assist the pharmacist in recognizing potential problems. For example, when an opioid is prescribed for pain due to an injury and the prescription is presented to a pharmacist 2 weeks after issuance, the drug may no longer be indicated. When opioid treatment is to include periods longer than the period covered by the first prescription, a second

prescription may be issued with a "do not fill before" date. Compliance behavior also can be estimated using the dates when a prescription is filled and refilled (or reissued). When writing the original prescription, the physician should designate the number of refills allowed or mark none. For maintenance medications without abuse potential, it is reasonable to write for a 1-month supply and to mark the prescription form for refills to be dispensed over a period sufficient to supply the patient until the next scheduled visit to the physician. A statement such as "refill prn" (refill as needed) is not appropriate, as it could allow the patient to misuse the medicine or neglect medical appointments. If no refills are desired, *zero* (not "0") or *none* should be written in the refill space to prevent alteration of the prescriber's intent. Refills for controlled substances are discussed in Refills under Controlled Substances.

Concern about the rising cost of healthcare has favored the dispensing of so-called generic drugs. A drug is called by its generic name (in the U.S., this is the USAN) or the manufacturer's proprietary name, called the *trademark, trade name,* or *brand name.* In most U.S. states, pharmacists have the authority to dispense generic drugs rather than brand-name medications. The physician can request that the pharmacist not substitute a generic for a branded medication by indicating this on the prescription ("do not substitute"); this generally is unnecessary because the U.S. FDA requires that generic medications meet the same standards for safety and efficacy as their brand-name counterparts. Bioequivalence standards are a challenge to implement for newer medications such as biologics (Bate et al., 2016) but are critically needed; both brand-name drugs and generics are increasingly in short supply (Mazer-Amirshahi et al., 2014).

In some jurisdictions, prescriptions may not be filled with a generic substitution unless specifically permitted on the prescription. Occasions when substituting generic medications is discouraged are limited to products with specialized release systems and narrow therapeutic indices or when substantial patient confusion and potential noncompliance may be associated with substitution.

Choice and Amount of Drug Product Dispensed

Inappropriate choice of drugs by physicians is a problem in prescribing. Physicians must rely on unbiased sources when seeking drug information

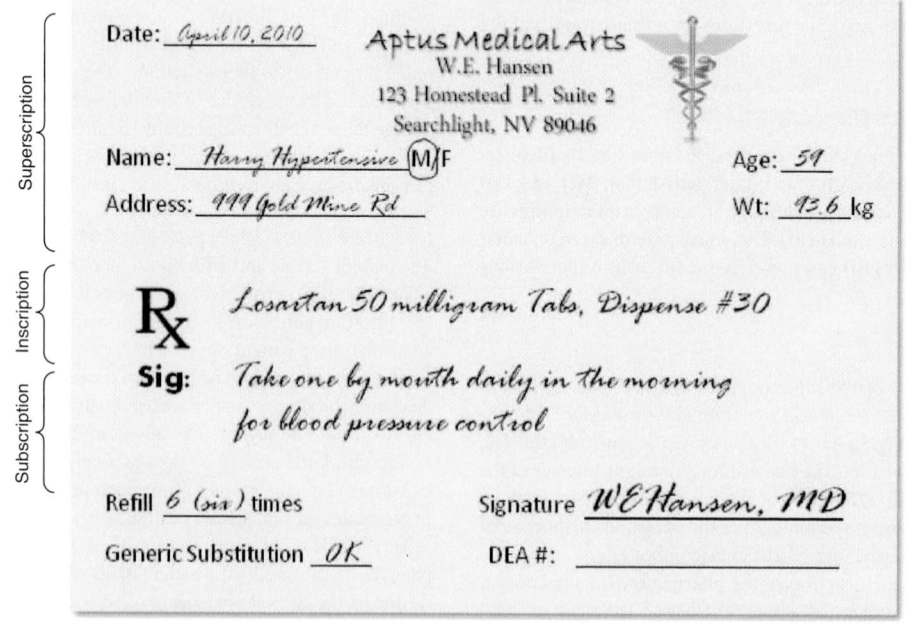

Figure AI–1 *The prescription.* The prescription must be accurately and legibly prepared to identify the patient, the medication to be dispensed, and the mode of drug administration. Avoid abbreviations and Latin; they lead to dispensing errors. Include the therapeutic purpose in the subscription (e.g., "for control of blood pressure") to prevent errors in dispensing. For example, the use of losartan *for the treatment of hypertension* may require 100 mg/d (1.4 mg/kg/d), whereas *for treatment of congestive heart failure,* the dose of this angiotensin II receptor antagonist generally should not exceed 50 mg/d. Including the therapeutic purpose of the prescription also can assist patients in organizing and understanding their medications. Including the patient's weight on the prescription can be useful in avoiding dosing errors, particularly when drugs are administered to children.

BOX AI–1 ■ Controlled Substance Schedules

Schedule I (examples: heroin, methylene dioxymethamphetamine, lysergic acid diethylamide, mescaline, and all salts and isomers thereof):

1. High potential for abuse.
2. No accepted medical use in the U.S. or lacks accepted safety for use in treatment in the U.S. May be used for research purposes by properly registered individuals.

Schedule II (examples: morphine, oxycodone, fentanyl, meperidine, dextroamphetamine, cocaine, amobarbital):

1. High potential for abuse.
2. Has a currently accepted medical use in the U.S.
3. Abuse of substance may lead to severe psychological or physical dependence.

Schedule III (examples: anabolic steroids, nalorphine, ketamine, certain schedule II substances in suppositories, mixtures, or limited amounts per dosage unit):

1. Abuse potential less than substances in schedule I or schedule II.
2. Has a currently accepted medical use in the U.S.
3. Abuse of substance may lead to moderate-to-low physical dependence or high psychological dependence.

Schedule IV (examples: alprazolam, phenobarbital, meprobamate, modafinil):

1. Abuse potential less than substances in schedule III.
2. Has a currently accepted medical use in the U.S.
3. Abuse of substance may lead to limited physical or psychological dependence relative to substances in schedule III.

Schedule V (examples: buprenorphine, products containing a low dose of an opioid plus a nonnarcotic ingredient such as cough syrup with codeine[a] and guaifenesin, antidiarrheal tablets with diphenoxylate and atropine):

1. Low potential for abuse relative to schedule IV.
2. Has a currently accepted medical use in the U.S.
3. Some schedule V products may be sold in limited amounts without a prescription at the discretion of the pharmacist; however, if a physician wishes a patient to receive one of these products, it is preferable to provide a prescription.

[a]*Although codeine is a schedule II drug, its dosage in cough syrups is regarded as sufficiently low to permit their classification as schedule V substances.*

that will influence their prescribing habits; use of the original medical literature and online resources such as the Cochrane evidentiary reviews (http://www.cochrane.org) will ensure instruction of the prescriber's best judgment. The amount of a drug to be dispensed should be clearly stated and should be only that needed by the patient. Excessive amounts should never be dispensed because this not only is expensive for the patient but also may lead to accumulation of medicines, which can lead to harm to the patient or members of the patient's family if used inappropriately. *Better to require several refills of a prescription than to prescribe and dispense more than necessary at one time.*

Controlled Substances

In the U.S., the DEA within the Department of Justice is responsible for the enforcement of the federal CSA. The DEA regulates each step of the handling of controlled substances from manufacture to dispensing (21 U.S.C. § 811). The law provides a system that is intended to prevent diversion of controlled substances from legitimate uses. Substances that come under the jurisdiction of the CSA are divided into five schedules (Box AI–1); individual states may have additional schedules. Physicians must be authorized to prescribe controlled substances by the board of pharmacy in the jurisdiction in which they are licensed, and they must be

registered with the DEA or exempted from registration as defined under the CSA. The number on the certificate of registration must be indicated on all prescription orders for controlled substances. Criminal prosecution and penalties for misuse generally depend on the schedule of a substance and the amount of drug in question.

Prescribing Controlled Substances

To be valid, a prescription for a controlled substance must be issued for a *legitimate medical purpose* by an *individual practitioner* acting in the *usual course of his or her professional practice.* An order that does not meet these criteria is not considered a legitimate prescription within the meaning of the law and thus does not protect either the physician who issues it or the pharmacist who dispenses it. Most states prohibit physicians from prescribing controlled substances for themselves. *It is prudent to follow this guideline even if compliance is not mandated by law.*

Specific requirements, both state and federal, apply to prescriptions for schedule II drugs. For example, all such prescriptions must be written in ink, and refills of schedule II drugs are not allowed. Whether intended for schedule II or lesser scheduled medications, prescriptions for controlled substances must, by law, include the patient's full name and address and the practitioner's full name, address, and DEA registration number. The prescription must also include the drug name, strength, quantity, directions for use, and the number of refills, if allowed (based on the category of the drug). The CSA requires that all orders for controlled substances be dated as of, and signed on, the day issued and prohibits filling or refilling orders for substances in schedules III and IV beyond more than 6 months after their date of issuance. State agencies may impose additional regulations, such as requiring that prescriptions for controlled substances be printed on triplicate or state-issued prescription pads or restricting the use of a particular class of drugs for specific indications. All medical personnel should be familiar with the latest CDC recommendations for prescribing opioids for chronic pain (Table 20–7).

Oral Orders

Prescriptions for schedule III, IV, and V medications may be telephoned to a pharmacy by a physician in the same manner as a prescription for a noncontrolled substance, although it is in the physician's best interest to keep his or her DEA number as private as possible (see Preventing Diversion). Schedule II prescriptions may be telephoned to a pharmacy only in *emergency* situations, that is:

- Immediate administration is necessary.
- No appropriate alternative treatment is available.
- It is not reasonably possible for the physician to provide a written prescription prior to the dispensing.

For an emergency prescription, the quantity must be limited to the amount adequate to treat the patient during the emergency period, and the physician must have a written prescription delivered to the pharmacy for that emergency within 72 h. If mailed, the prescription must be postmarked within 72 h. The pharmacist must notify the DEA if this prescription is not received.

Refills

No prescription order for a schedule II drug may be refilled under any circumstance (CFR Title 21 §1306). Pre-dated original prescriptions may be used when therapy beyond the period covered by the first prescription is needed, but these are generally discouraged. For schedule III and IV drugs, refills may be issued either orally or in writing, not to exceed five refills or 6 months after the issue date, whichever comes first. Beyond this time, a new prescription must be ordered. For schedule V drugs, there are no restrictions on the number of refills allowed, but if no refills are noted at the time of issuance, a new prescription must be made for additional drug to be dispensed.

Preventing Diversion

Prescription blanks often are stolen and used to sustain abuse of controlled substances. To prevent this type of diversion, prescription pads should be protected in the same manner as one would protect a personal checkbook. A prescription blank should never be presigned for a staff member to fill in at a later time. Also, a minimum number of pads should be stocked, and they should be kept in a locked, secure location. If a pad or prescription is missing, it should be reported immediately to local authorities and pharmacies. Ideally, the physician's full DEA number should not be preprinted on the prescription pad because anyone in possession of a valid DEA number may find it easier to commit prescription fraud. Some physicians may intentionally omit part or all of their DEA number on a prescription and instead write "pharmacist call to verify" or "call for registration number." This practice works only when the pharmacist may independently verify the authenticity of the prescription, and patients must fill the prescription during the prescriber's office hours. Pharmacists can ascertain the authenticity of a physician's DEA number using an algorithm.

Another method employed by the drug seeker is to alter the face of a valid prescription to increase the number of units or refills. By spelling out the number of units and refills authorized instead of giving numerals, the prescriber essentially removes this option for diversion. Controlled substances should not be prescribed excessively or for prolonged periods, as the continuance of a patient's addiction is not a legitimate medical purpose.

Weed

Twenty-nine U.S. states and the District of Columbia have placed marijuana, classified by the FDA as a schedule I substance, in a special category by decriminalizing its possession and sale for medical use. In these jurisdictions, patients and caregivers are exempt from prosecution by state law, contrary federal law notwithstanding. Nine of these jurisdictions, AL, CA, CO, MA, ME, NV, OR, WA, and the District of Columbia—permit the possession of marijuana for recreational use. This legal difference of opinion between state and federal regulation is the source of considerable controversy (Leyton, 2016). Generally, the most stringent law takes precedence, whether it is federal, state, or local.

The Prescription as a Commodity

Prescribers must be aware that patients may visit their doctor to "get" a prescription. In many patient-physician interactions, a prescription can be seen as the currency or mandatory product of the visit. Physicians must educate each patient about the importance of viewing medicines as something to be used only when really needed, and that remaining on a particular medicine when in stable condition may be preferable to seeking the newest medications available. The federal FDA Modernization Act of 1997 permits the use of print and television advertising of prescription drugs. The law requires that all drug advertisements contain (amongst other things) summary information relating to side effects, contraindications, and effectiveness. The benefits of these types of DTC advertising are controversial (Mintzes, 2012). Prescription drug advertising has alerted consumers to the existence of new drugs and the conditions they treat, but it has also increased consumer demand for drugs. This demand has increased the number of prescriptions being dispensed (raising sales revenues) and has contributed to the higher pharmaceutical costs borne by health insurers, government, and consumers. In the face of a growing demand for particular brand-name drugs driven by advertising, physicians and pharmacists must be able to counsel patients effectively and provide them with evidence-based drug information.

The Special Case of Seniors

Seniors represent just over 14% of the population, but consume 40% of prescription drugs and 35% of all over-the-counter drugs. On average, individuals 65 to 69 years old take nearly 14 prescriptions per year; individuals aged 80 to 84 take an average of 18 prescriptions per year; 15% to 25% of drug use in seniors is considered unnecessary or otherwise inappropriate (Hwang et al., 2001). Adverse drug reactions are more common in the elderly and, together with noncompliance, are responsible for 28% of hospitalizations of the elderly, at a cost exceeding $180 billion annually.

Each year, 32,000 seniors suffer hip fractures caused by medication-related problems (Iuga and McGuire, 2014).

Drug Standards and Classification

The U.S. Pharmacopeial Convention, Incorporated, is a nongovernmental organization that disseminates authoritative standards and information on medicines and other healthcare technologies. This organization is home to the USP, which, together with the FDA, the pharmaceutical industry, and health professions, establishes authoritative drug standards. These standards are enforceable by the FDA and governments of other countries and are recognized worldwide. Drug monographs are published in the USP/NF, the official drug standards compendia that organize drugs into categories based on pharmacological actions and therapeutic uses. The USP also provides chemical reference standards to carry out the tests specified in the USP/NF. For example, a drug to be manufactured and labeled in units must comply with the USP standard for units of that compound. Such standards are essential for agents possessing biological activity, such as insulin or antibody-based medications.

The USP also is home to the *USP Dictionary of U.S. Adopted Names (USAN) and International Drug Names*. This compendium is recognized throughout the healthcare industry as the authoritative dictionary of drugs. Entries include one or more of the following: U.S. Adopted Names, official drug names for the NF, previously used official names, International Nonproprietary Names, British Approved Names, Japanese Accepted Names, trade names, and other synonyms. In addition to names, the records in this file contain other substance information, such as CAS, RN, molecular formula, molecular weight, pharmacological or therapeutic category, drug sponsor, reference information, and structure diagram, if available. The USP maintains an electronic website that can be accessed for useful information on drug naming, classification, and standards (http://www.usp.org).

In the U.S., drug products also are coded under the NDC. The NDC serves as a universal product identifier for drugs used in humans. The current edition of the NDC Directory is limited to prescription drugs and a few selected over-the-counter products. Each drug product listed under the Federal Food, Drug, and Cosmetic Act is assigned a unique 10-digit, 3-segment number. This number, the NDC number, identifies the labeler/vendor, product, and package size. The labeler/vendor code is assigned by the FDA. The second segment, the product code, identifies a specific strength, dosage form, and formulation for a particular drug company. The third segment, the package code, identifies package sizes. Both the product and package codes are assigned by the manufacturer. In addition to classification of drugs by therapeutic category, drugs also are grouped by control schedule. Drug schedules in the U.S. are listed in Box AI–1 and discussed under Controlled Substances.

The FDA also categorizes drugs that may be used in pregnant women. These categories are similar to those used in other countries and provide guidance based on available science. The categories range from A to X, in increasing order of concern:

- **Pregnancy Category A:** Adequate and well-controlled studies have failed to demonstrate a risk to the fetus in the first trimester of pregnancy (and there is no evidence of risk in later trimesters). Because of the obvious nature of the risk associated with the use of medications during gestation, the FDA requires a body of high-quality data on a drug before it can be considered for Pregnancy Category A. Drugs in this category include levothyroxine and folic acid.
- **Pregnancy Category B:** Animal reproduction studies have failed to demonstrate a risk to the fetus, and there are no adequate and well-controlled studies in pregnant women, OR animal studies have shown an adverse effect, but adequate and well-controlled studies in pregnant women have failed to demonstrate a risk to the fetus in any trimester. Drugs in this category include metformin and hydrochlorothiazide and should be prescribed only as needed for maternal health.
- **Pregnancy Category C:** Animal reproduction studies have shown an adverse effect on the fetus, and there are no adequate and well-controlled

studies in humans, but potential benefits may warrant use of the drug in pregnant women despite potential risks. Drugs in this category include tramadol and gabapentin. They should be prescribed in pregnancy only when benefit clearly outweighs risk.

- **Pregnancy Category D:** There is positive evidence of human fetal risk based on adverse reaction data from investigational or marketing experience or studies in humans, but potential benefits may warrant use of the drug in pregnant women despite potential risks. Drugs in this category, such as alprazolam and clonazepam, are not recommended for use during pregnancy and should be prescribed in pregnancy only if absolutely necessary.

- **Pregnancy Category X:** Studies in animals or humans have demonstrated fetal abnormalities or there is positive evidence of human fetal risk based on adverse reaction data from investigational or marketing experience, and the risks involved in use of the drug in pregnant women clearly outweigh potential benefits. Drugs such as warfarin, methotrexate, and statins fall into this category and must not be used during pregnancy or in women likely to become pregnant.

Physicians should realize that the pregnancy categories by themselves provide little guidance for the physician treating pregnant women. Prescribers must understand the embryology, physiology, and pharmacology involved in each instance of drug use during pregnancy. For example, ACE inhibitors such as captopril cause developmental toxicity (category X), but only after the first trimester. A physician's primary responsibility remains treating the pregnant patient. However, the risks of withholding treatment to the mother because of possible risks to the fetus have to be considered as well. The practitioner should rely on medical evidence when making these decisions.

Drugs also are grouped by their potential for misuse under British and U.N. legal classifications as class A, B, or C. The classes are linked to maximum legal penalties in a descending order of severity, from A to C.

Compliance

Compliance is the extent to which the patient follows a regimen prescribed by a healthcare professional. The patient is the final and most important determinant of how successful a therapeutic regimen will be and should be engaged as an active participant who has a vested interest in its success. Whatever term is used—*compliance, adherence, therapeutic alliance,* or *concordance*—physicians must promote a collaborative interaction between doctor and patient in which each brings an expertise that helps to determine the course of therapy. The patient's quality-of-life beliefs may differ from the clinician's therapeutic goals, and the patient will have the last word every time when there is an unresolved conflict.

Hundreds of variables that may influence compliance behavior have been identified. A few of the most frequently cited are in Box AI–2, along with some suggestions for improving compliance, although none guarantees 100% compliance.

Noncompliance may be manifest in drug therapy as intentional or accidental errors in dosage or schedule, overuse, underuse, early termination of therapy, or not having a prescription filled; therapeutic failures can result (Malek and Grosset, 2015). Noncompliance always should be considered in evaluating potential causes of inconsistent or nonexistent response to therapy. The reported incidence of patient noncompliance usually is in the range of 30%–60%; the rate for long-term regimens is about 50% and can be improved by medication management (Klein et al., 2009).

The Patient-Provider Relationship

Patient satisfaction with the physician has a significant impact on compliance behavior. Patients are more likely to follow instructions and recommendations when their expectations for the patient-provider relationship and for their treatment are met. These expectations include not only clinical but also interpersonal competence; thus, cultivating good interpersonal and communication skills is essential.

> **BOX AI–2 ■ Suggestions for Improving Patient Compliance**
>
> - Provide respectful communication; ask how patient takes medicine.
>   - Develop satisfactory, collaborative relationship between physician and patient; encourage pharmacist involvement.
>   - Provide and encourage use of medication counseling.
>   - Give precise, clear instructions, with most important information given first.
>   - Support oral instructions with easy-to-read written information.
>   - Simplify whenever possible.
>   - Use mechanical compliance aids as needed (sectioned pillboxes or trays, compliance packaging, color coding).
>   - Use optimal dosage form and schedule for each individual patient.
>   - Assess patient's literacy, language, and comprehension and modify educational counseling as needed. Be culturally aware and sensitive. To improve compliance, don't rely on patient's own knowledge of disease alone.
>   - Find solutions when physical or sensory disabilities are present (use nonsafety caps on bottles, use large type on labels and written material, place tape marks on syringes).
>   - Enlist support and assistance from family and caregivers.
>   - Use behavioral techniques such as goal setting, self-monitoring, cognitive restructuring, skills training, contracts, and positive reinforcement.

When deciding on a course of therapy, it can be useful to discuss a patient's habits and daily routine as well as the therapeutic options with the patient. This information may suggest cues for remembrance. A lack of information about a patient's lifestyle can lead to situations such as prescribing a medication to be taken with meals three times daily for a patient who only eats twice a day or a medication to be taken each morning for a patient who works a night shift and sleeps during the day. Rarely is there only one treatment option for a given problem, and it may be better to prescribe an adequate regimen that the patient will follow instead of an ideal regimen that the patient will not. Attempts should be made to resolve collaboratively any conflicts that may hinder compliance. Whenever possible, the family should be aware of the physician's treatment plan in order to assist with compliance.

Patients and Their Beliefs

Patients are more likely to be compliant when they *perceive* that they are susceptible to the disease, that the disease may have serious negative impact, that the therapy will be effective, that the benefits outweigh the costs, and when they believe in their own ability to execute the therapy. The *actual* severity of and susceptibility to an illness are not necessarily an issue; rather, the patient's perception of severity affects compliance. Patients' beliefs can lead them to deliberately alter their therapy, whether for convenience, for personal experiments, because of a desire to remove themselves from the sick role, as a means to exercise a feeling of control over their situation, or for other reasons. This reinforces the need for precise communication and a good patient-provider relationship to facilitate the provision of additional or corrective education when the beliefs would suggest poor compliance as an outcome (Hsiao et al., 2012; Nieuwlaat et al., 2014).

Pharmacists have a legal and professional responsibility to offer medication counseling and can educate and support patients by discussing prescribed medications and their use. Because they often see the patient more frequently than does the physician, pharmacists who take the time to inquire about a patient's therapy can help identify compliance and other problems, educate the patient, and notify the physician as appropriate (Phatak et al., 2016). Indeed, data from the Asheville Project indicates that a pharmacist-based medication management program provides significant advantages with respect to compliance, health outcomes, and cost (Bunting and Cranor, 2006).

Elderly patients often face a number of barriers to compliance related to their age: increased forgetfulness and confusion; altered drug disposition and higher sensitivity to some drug effects; decreased social and financial support; decreased dexterity, mobility, or sensory abilities; and the use of a greater number of concurrent medicines (both prescription and over the counter) whose attendant toxicities and interactions may cause decreased mental alertness or intolerable side effects. There are drugs known to be inappropriate to prescribe to elderly patients and some that may adversely affect compliance (Aparasu and Mort, 2000). Despite these obstacles, evidence does not show that elderly patients in general are significantly less compliant than any other age group. Physicians must be careful in choosing medications for the elderly. Pharmacists must pay particular attention to thorough and compassionate counseling for elderly patients and should assist patients in finding practical solutions when problems, such as polypharmacy, are noted (Mansur, 2016).

The Therapy

Increased complexity and duration of therapy are perhaps the best-documented barriers to compliance. The patient for whom multiple drugs are prescribed for a given disease or who has multiple illnesses that require drug therapy will be at higher risk for noncompliance, as will the patient whose disease is chronic. The frequency of dosing of individual medications also can affect compliance behavior. Simplification, whenever possible and appropriate, is desirable.

The effects of the medication can make adherence less likely, as in the case of patients whose medicines cause confusion or other altered mental states. Unpleasant side effects from the medicine may influence compliance in some patients, but are not necessarily predictive, especially if patient beliefs or other positive factors tend to reinforce adherence to the regimen. A side effect that is intolerable to one patient may be of minor concern to another. The cost of medicine can be a heavy burden for patients with limited economic resources, and healthcare providers should be sensitive to this fact (Restrepo et al., 2008). Mobile phones and tablets running drug formulary/therapeutic applications can provide the costs of medications, as can physicians who are familiar with the patient's insurance plan. Mobile phone systems and wearables that provide reminders and collect patient response information and physiological data are being introduced and may become more popular as patients and providers become increasingly tech savvy (Parmanto et al., 2013). Such technology may soon be capable of carrying patient genetic information that may assist the physician in choosing medications based on knowledge of a patient's ability to metabolize a specific drug efficiently or that such treatment may interfere with an existing treatment (Weiss and Shin, 2016). Effective treatments that do not produce unwanted effects will improve compliance.

Electronic Prescribing

The era of e-prescribing eliminates some of the subjective features of prescribing. Thus, if the proper information is entered correctly in the electronic system, medication errors due to illegible handwriting, incorrect dose, incorrect medication for medical condition, and drug interactions can be reduced because each prescription can be linked to high-quality drug databases that check that the information on the prescription is appropriate for the patient (e.g., age, weight, gender, condition, laboratory values, disease being treated, concurrent medications) and that known warnings and potential problems are brought to the attention of the physician, pharmacist, and patient. Such systems must not be used as a substitute for personal attention to the individual patient by healthcare workers but rather as an adjunct measure that ensures safe, high-quality, efficient care. Sadly, the participation of human beings in the process has not eliminated errors, even in the university hospital setting (Al Tehewy et al., 2016). Physicians and pharmacists must remember that only when the seriousness of their mutual responsibilities are front and center in their minds will patient safety be ensured.

BOX AI–3 ■ Prescribing Practices to Avoid Adverse Drug Events

- Write all orders legibly using metric measurements of weight and volume.
- Include patient age and weight on the prescription, when appropriate, so dosage can be checked.
- Use Arabic (decimal) numerals rather than Roman numerals (e.g., does "IL-II" mean "IL-11" or "IL-2"?); in some instances, it is preferable for numerals to be spelled out.
- Use leading zeros (0.125 milligrams, not .125 milligrams); never use trailing zeros (5 milligrams, not 5.0 milligrams).
- Avoid abbreviating drug names; abbreviations may lead to misinterpretation.
- Avoid abbreviating directions for drug administration; write out directions clearly in English.
- Be aware of possibilities for confusion in drug names. Some drug names sound alike when spoken and may look alike when spelled out. The U.S. Pharmacopeial Convention Medication Errors Reporting Program maintains a current list of 750 drug names that can be confused (http://www.usp.org). Alliterative drug names can be particularly problematic when giving verbal orders to pharmacists or other healthcare providers.
- Provide the patient's diagnosis on the prescription order to prevent dispensing errors based on sound-alike or look-alike drug names. For example, an order for administration of magnesium sulfate must not be abbreviated "MS," as this may result in administration of morphine sulfate. Including the therapeutic purpose or the patient's diagnosis can prevent this error.
- Write clearly. Both physician and pharmacist share in the responsibility for preventing adverse drug events by writing prescriptions clearly (*When in doubt, write it out!*) and questioning intent whenever an order is ambiguous (*When in doubt, check it out!*). *Pharmacists must clarify their concerns with prescribers, not patients.*
- Think.
- Think again.

Eliminating Errors in Drug Orders

The IOM estimates that the annual number of medical errors in the U.S. that result in death is between 44,000 and 98,000 (Kohn, 2001). Although there is some controversy about these estimates, it is clear that the large number of medical errors includes medication errors resulting in adverse events, including death. Databases of anonymously reported errors are maintained jointly by the ISMP, the USP MERP, and the FDA's MedWatch program. Adverse drug events occur in about 3% of hospitalizations, and this number is larger for special populations, such as those in pediatric and neonatal intensive care units. By examining aspects of prescription writing that can cause errors and then modifying prescribing habits accordingly, the physician can increase the probability that the patient will receive the correct prescription. By being alert to common problems that can occur with medication orders and communicating with the patient's physician, pharmacists and other healthcare professionals can assist in reducing medication errors. Proper prescribing practices (Box AI–3) can help to prevent adverse drug events.

Bibliography

Al Tehewy M, et al. Medication administration errors in a university hospital. *J Patient Saf,* **2016,** *12*:34–39. doi:10.1097/PTS.0000000000000196.

Aparasu RR, Mort JR. Inappropriate prescribing for the elderly: Beers criteria-based review. *Ann Pharmacother,* **2000,** 34:338–346.

Bate R, et al. Generics substitution, bioequivalence standards, and international oversight: complex issues facing the FDA. *Trends Pharmacol Sci,* **2016,** 37:184–191.

Bunting BA, Cranor CW. The Asheville Project: long-term clinical, humanistic, and economic outcomes of a community-based medication therapy management program for asthma. *J Am Pharm Assoc,* **2006**, *46*:133–147.

Hsiao CY, et al. An investigation on illness perception and adherence among hypertensive patients. *Kaohsiung J Med Sci,* **2012**, *28*:442–447.

Hwang W, et al. Out-of-pocket medical spending for care of chronic conditions. *Health Aff,* **2001**, *20*:267–278.

Iuga AO, McGuire MJ. Adherence and health care costs. *Risk Manag Healthc Policy,* **2014**, *7*:35–44.

Klein A, et al. Impact of a pharmaceutical care program on liver transplant patients' compliance with immunosuppressive medication: a prospective, randomized, controlled trial using electronic monitoring. *Transplantation,* **2009**, *87*:839–847.

Kohn LT. The Institute of Medicine report on medical error: overview and implications for pharmacy. *Am J Health Syst Pharm,* **2001**, *58*:63–66.

Leyton M. Legalizing marijuana. *J Psychiatry Neurosci,* **2016**, *41*:75–76.

Malek N, Grosset DG. Medication adherence in patients with Parkinson's disease. *CNS Drugs,* **2015**, *29*:47–53.

Mansur JM. Medication safety systems and the important role of pharmacists. *Drugs Aging,* **2016**, *33*:213–221. PMID: 26932714, accessed March 22, 2016.

Mazer-Amirshahi M, et al. Critical drug shortages: implications for emergency medicine. *Acad Emerg Med,* **2014**, *21*:704–711.

Mintzes B. Advertising of prescription-only medicines to the public: does evidence of benefit counterbalance harm? *Annu Rev Public Health,* **2012**, *33*:259–277.

Nieuwlaat R, et al. Interventions for enhancing medication adherence. *Cochrane Database Syst Rev,* **2014**, (11):CD000011. doi: 10.1002/14651858.CD000011.pub4.

Parmanto B, et al. iMHere: a novel mHealth System for supporting self-care in management of complex and chronic conditions. *JMIR mHealth uHealth,* **2013**, *1*:e10. doi:10.2196/mhealth.2391.

Phatak A, et al. Impact of pharmacist involvement in the transitional care of high-risk patients through medication reconciliation, medication education, and postdischarge call-backs (IPITCH Study). *J Hosp Med,* **2016**, *11*:39–44.

Restrepo RD, et al. Medication adherence issues in patients treated for COPD. *Int J Chron Obstruct Pulmon Dis,* **2008**, *3*:371–384.

Weiss ST, Shin MS. Infrastructure for personalized medicine at Partners HealthCare. *J Pers Med,* **2016**, *6*:13. doi:10.3390/jpm6010013.

APPENDIX I

PRINCIPLES OF PRESCRIPTION ORDER WRITING AND PATIENT COMPLIANCE

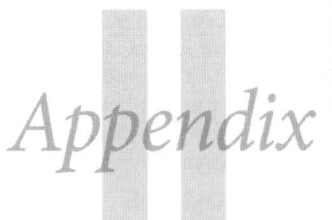

Appendix II

Design and Optimization of Dosage Regimens: Pharmacokinetic Data

Kenneth E. Thummel, Danny D. Shen, and Nina Isoherranen

This appendix provides a summary of basic pharmacokinetic information pertaining to small-molecule drugs that are in common clinical use and are delivered to the systemic circulation by parenteral or nonparenteral administration. Because of space limitations, this list cannot be exhaustive. Drugs designed exclusively for topical administration and not to be significantly absorbed into the bloodstream (e.g., ophthalmic and some dermal applications; Chapters 69 and 70) are not included. A few other selection criteria have influenced the makeup of the list, but, in general, the authors have tried to include one or more representative drugs in each of the therapeutic areas in this text, based on distinct mechanism(s) of action. In some instances, drugs may be excluded because pharmacokinetics are not relevant to their therapeutic management. An obvious case is when drug efficacy is not apparently correlated with drug concentration in a reversible fashion (e.g., some cytotoxic anticancer drugs).

Often, the issue comes down to deciding which of the many drugs within a class should be selected. This is particularly problematic when the choices are largely therapeutic equivalents. Two criteria that have proven useful are prevalence of use and uniqueness of mechanism of action. For the present edition, we have consulted the top 200 selling drugs in 2015 for usage data. Drugs that fall into that list and meet the criteria mentioned were generally selected. We have also consulted all new FDA drug approvals between 2010 and 2015. As mentioned, a drug used less may be included if it has a different mechanism of action than the frequently used drugs, some additional actions that offer a unique therapeutic advantage, or a more acceptable side-effects profile. Pharmacokinetic data for many older drugs not included in this appendix can be found in earlier editions of this book.

With rare exceptions (e.g., interferons), recombinant therapeutic proteins have been excluded from this compilation. In many cases, the therapeutic protein is directed to interact with specific tissue or cellular targets with exquisite affinity; as a result, clinical efficacy seldom correlates with circulating drug concentration, and pharmacokinetics are not considered critical in guiding its dosing. For example, for a number of therapeutic antibodies, the antibody is administered at a fixed dose at prolonged intervals that allow for its near-complete clearance (e.g., infliximab). There is again the constraint of space limitation; hence, it was decided that the appendix should focus on small-molecule drugs.

A major objective of this appendix is to present pharmacokinetic data in a format that informs the clinician of the essential characteristics of drug disposition that form the basis of drug-dosage regimen design. Table AII–1 contains quantitative information about the absorption, distribution, and elimination of drugs; the effects of some disease states, age, pregnancy, and gender on these processes, where significant; and the correlation of efficacy and toxicity with drug concentrations in blood/plasma. The general principles that underlie the design of appropriate maintenance dose and dosing interval (and, where appropriate, the loading dose) for the average patient are described in Chapter 2. Their application using the data in Table AII–1 for individualization of dosage regimens is presented here.

To use the data that are presented, one must understand clearance concepts and their application to drug-dosage regimens. One also must know average values of clearance as well as some kinetic measures of drug absorption and distribution. The text that follows defines the eight basic parameters that are listed in the tabular material for each drug and key factors that influence these values in both normal subjects and patients with renal or liver disease. It obviously would be more straightforward if there were a consensus on a standard value for a given pharmacokinetic parameter; instead, literature estimates usually vary over a wide range, and a consensus set of pharmacokinetic values has been reached for only a limited number of drugs.

In Table AII–1, a single set of values for each parameter and its variability in a relevant population has been selected from the literature, based on the scientific judgment of the authors. Most data are in the form of a study population mean value ± 1 standard deviation (mean ± SD). However, some data are presented as mean and range of values (in parentheses) observed for the study population (i.e., the lowest and highest value reported). There are times when data are reported as a geometric mean with a 95% confidence interval or a coefficient of variation (in percentage). If sufficient data were available, we present a range of mean values obtained from different studies of similar design in parentheses, sometimes below the primary study data. Occasionally, only a single mean value for the study population was available in the literature and is reported as such. Finally, some drugs can be administered intravenously in an unmodified form and orally as a prodrug. When relevant information about both the prodrug and the active molecule are needed, we have included both, using an abbreviation to indicate the species that was measured, followed by another abbreviation in parentheses to indicate the species that was dosed [e.g., G (V) indicates a parameter for ganciclovir after administration of the prodrug, valganciclovir].

A number of approved drugs are actually the active metabolite or stereoisomer of an earlier marketed drug. For example, desloratadine is the O-desmethyl metabolite of loratadine, and esomeprazole is the active S-enantiomer of omeprazole. Unless the parent drug and the active metabolite offer distinct therapeutic advantages, only the more established or more commonly used drug is listed, and relevant information on its alternate active form is presented in the same table. This approach has

Abbreviations

AUC: area under the plasma drug concentration–time curve
CKD-EPI: Chronic Kidney Disease Epidemiology Collaboration
CPIC: Clinical Pharmacogenetics Implementation Consortium
CYP: cytochrome P450
DIDB: Drug Interaction Database Program
FDA: Food and Drug Administration
MDRD: Modification of Diet in Renal Disease
NDA: New Drug Application

permitted us to include more drugs in the appendix, it is hoped without undue confusion. The only exception is with prednisone and prednisolone, which undergo interconversion in the body.

Unless otherwise indicated in footnotes, data reported in the table are those determined in healthy adults. The direction of change for these values in particular disease states is noted below the average value. In previous editions, we have included disease states where studies have shown no change or clinically insignificant change for a particular pharmacokinetic measure. For the sake of space and consistency, we have eliminated the results of negative studies; hence, when a disease state is not listed, it implies no significant change or no information is available. One or more references are provided for each of the established drugs, typically an original journal publication, a review on its clinical pharmacokinetics, or web-based drug database; the last two secondary sources provide a broader range of papers for the interested reader. In some instances (e.g., many new drug approvals), we have relied on unpublished data provided by the drug sponsor in its NDA files or package labeling submitted to the U.S. FDA. This information can be accessed at Drugs@FDA: FDA Approved Drug Products (https://www.accessdata.fda.gov/scripts/cder/daf/). After searching by drug name, pharmacokinetic data are found most often in the Clinical Pharmacology and Biopharmaceutics section. Recent standardization in the presentation of data supporting the NDA in this section makes this an increasingly valuable resource.

Tabulated Pharmacokinetic Parameters

Each of the eight parameters presented in Table AII–1 was discussed in detail in Chapter 2. The following discussion focuses on the format in which the values are presented as well as on physiological or pathological factors that influence the parameters.

Bioavailability

The *extent of oral bioavailability* is expressed as a percentage of the administered dose. This value represents the percentage of the administered dose that is available to the systemic circulation—the fraction of the oral dose that reaches the arterial blood in an active or prodrug form, expressed as a percentage (0–100). *Fractional availability F*, which appears elsewhere in this appendix, denotes the same parameter; this value varies from 0 to 1. T_{max} as a measure of the *rate of availability* is also presented in the table. The extent of availability is needed for the design of an oral dosage regimen to achieve a specific target blood concentration. Values for multiple routes of administration are provided, when appropriate and available. In most cases, the tabulated value represents an absolute oral bioavailability that has been determined from a comparison of AUC between the oral dose and an intravenous reference dose. For those drugs for which intravenous administration is not feasible, an approximate estimate of oral bioavailability based on secondary information (e.g., urinary excretion of unchanged drug, especially when the nonrenal route of elimination is minimal) is presented, or the column is left blank (denoted by a long dash [—]). A dash also will appear when a drug is given by parenteral administration only.

A low oral bioavailability may result from a poorly formulated dosage form that fails to disintegrate or dissolve in the gastrointestinal fluid;

has degradative loss of drug in the gastrointestinal fluid; has poor mucosal permeability, including active efflux transport of drug back into the lumen; has first-pass metabolism during transit through the intestinal epithelium; or there is first-pass hepatic metabolism or biliary excretion (see Chapter 2). In the case of drugs with extensive first-pass metabolism, hepatic disease may increase oral availability because hepatic metabolic capacity decreases or because vascular shunts develop around the liver.

Urinary Excretion of Unchanged Drug

The second parameter in Table AII–1 is the amount of drug eventually excreted unchanged in the urine, expressed as a percentage of the administered dose. Values represent the percentage expected in a healthy young adult (creatinine clearance ≥ 100 mL/min). When possible, the value listed is that determined after bolus intravenous administration of the drug, for which bioavailability is 100%. If the drug is given orally, this parameter may be underestimated due to incomplete absorption of the dose; such approximated values are indicated with a footnote. The parameter obtained after intravenous dosing is of greater utility because it reflects the fractional contribution of renal clearance to total body clearance irrespective of bioavailability.

Renal disease is the primary factor that causes changes in this parameter. This is especially true when alternate pathways of elimination are available; thus, as renal function decreases, a greater fraction of the dose is available for elimination by other routes. Because renal function generally decreases as a function of age, the percentage of drug excreted unchanged also decreases with age when alternate pathways of elimination are available. In addition, for a number of weakly acidic and basic drugs with pK_a values within the normal range for urine pH, changes in urine pH will affect their rate or extent of urinary excretion (see Chapter 2).

Binding to Plasma Proteins

The tabulated value is the percentage of drug in the plasma that is bound to plasma proteins at concentrations of the drug that are achieved clinically. In almost all cases, the values are from measurements performed in vitro (rather than from ex vivo measurements of binding to proteins in plasma obtained from patients to whom the drug had been administered). When a single mean value is presented, it signifies that there is no apparent change in percentage bound over the range of plasma drug concentrations resulting from the usual clinical doses. In cases in which saturation of binding to plasma proteins is approached within the therapeutic range of plasma drug concentrations, a range of bound percentages is provided for concentrations at the lower and upper limits of the range. For some drugs, there is disagreement in the literature about the extent of plasma-protein binding; in those cases, the range of reported values is given.

Plasma-protein binding is affected primarily by disease states, notably hepatic disease, renal impairment, and inflammatory diseases, that alter the concentration of albumin, α_1-acid glycoprotein, or other proteins in plasma that bind drugs. Uremia also changes the apparent binding affinity of albumin for some drugs. Disease-induced changes in plasma-protein binding can dramatically affect the volume of distribution, clearance, and elimination $t_{1/2}$ of a drug. In regard to clinical relevance, it is important to assess the change in unbound drug concentration or AUC, particularly when only unbound drug can cross biological barriers and gain access to the site of action.

Plasma Clearance

Systemic clearance of total drug from plasma or blood (see Equations 2–4, 2–5, and 2–7 in Chapter 2) is given in Table AII–1. Clearance varies as a function of body size and therefore most frequently is presented in the table in units of milliliters/minute/kilogram of body weight. Normalization to measures of body size other than weight may at times be more appropriate, such as normalization to body surface area in infants to better reflect the growth and development of the liver and kidneys. However, weight is easy to obtain, and its use often offsets any small loss in accuracy of clearance estimate, especially in adults. Exceptions to this rule are the anticancer drugs, for which dosage normalization to body surface area is conventionally used. When unit conversion was necessary, we used individual or mean body weight or body surface area (when appropriate) from the cited study, or if this was not available, we assumed a body mass of 70 kg or a body surface area of 1.73 m^2 for healthy adults.

For the few drugs that exhibit saturation kinetics following therapeutics doses, K_m and V_{max} are given and represent, respectively, the plasma concentration at which half of the maximal rate of elimination is reached (in units of mass/volume) and the maximal rate of elimination (in units of mass/time/kilogram of body weight). K_m must be in the same units as the concentration of drug in plasma (C_p).

In almost all cases, clearances based on plasma concentration data are presented in Table AII–1 because drug analysis most often is performed on plasma samples. The few exceptions where clearance from blood is presented are indicated by footnote. Clearance estimates based on blood concentration may be useful when a drug concentrates in the blood cells.

To be accurate, clearances must be determined after intravenous drug administration. When only nonparenteral data are available, the ratio of CL/F is given; values offset by the fractional availability F are indicated in a footnote. When a drug, or its active isomer for racemic compounds, is known to be a substrate for a CYP or drug transporter, this information is provided in a footnote. This information is important for understanding pharmacokinetic variability due to genetic polymorphisms and for predicting metabolically based drug-drug interactions, although these factors are beyond the scope of this table. For clinically relevant pharmacogenetic information, the reader is referred to CPIC Guidelines listed on the PharmGKB website (https://www.pharmgkb.org/). The reader is referred to a comprehensive database for drug-drug interaction information (DIDB) (https://www.druginteractioninfo.org/). The former site is open access, whereas the latter can be accessed by a licensing agreement.

Volume of Distribution

The total body volume of distribution at steady state V_{ss} is given in Table AII–1 and is expressed in units of liters/kilogram or in units of liters/square meter for some anticancer drugs. Again, when unit conversion was necessary, we used individual or mean body weights or body surface area (when appropriate) from the cited study, or if such data were not available, we assumed a body mass of 70 kg or a body surface area of 1.73 m^2 for healthy adults.

When estimates of V_{ss} were not available, values for V_{area} are provided; V_{area} represents the volume at equilibrated distribution during the terminal elimination phase. Unlike V_{ss}, V_{area} varies when drug elimination changes, even though there is no change in extravascular distribution. Because we may wish to know whether a particular disease state influences either the clearance or the tissue distribution of the drug, it is preferable to define volume in terms of V_{ss}, a parameter that is less likely to depend on changes in the rate of elimination. Occasionally, the condition under which the distribution volume was obtained was not specified in the primary reference; this is denoted by the absence of a subscript.

As with clearance, V_{ss} usually is defined in the table in terms of concentration in plasma rather than blood. Further, if data were not obtained after intravenous administration of the drug, a footnote will make clear that the apparent volume estimate, V_{ss}/F or V_{area}/F, is offset by the fractional availability.

Half-Life

Half-life $t_{1/2}$ is the time required for the plasma concentration to decline by one-half when elimination is first order. It also governs the rate of approach to steady state and the degree of drug accumulation during multiple dosing or continuous infusion. For example, at a fixed dosing interval, the patient will be at 50% of steady state after one half-life, 75% of steady state after two half-lives, 93.75% of steady state after four half-lives, and so on. Determination of $t_{1/2}$ is straightforward when drug elimination follows a monoexponential pattern (i.e., one-compartment model). However, for a number of drugs, plasma concentration follows a multiexponential pattern of decline over time. The mean value listed in Table AII–1 corresponds to an effective rate of elimination that covers the clearance of a major fraction of the absorbed dose from the body. In many cases,

this $t_{1/2}$ refers to the rate of elimination in the terminal exponential phase. For a number of drugs, however, the $t_{1/2}$ of an earlier phase is presented, even though a prolonged $t_{1/2}$ may be observed later at very low plasma concentrations when extremely sensitive analytical techniques are used. If the latter component accounts for 10% or less of the AUC, predictions of drug accumulation in plasma during continuous or repetitive dosing will be in error by no more than 10% if this longer $t_{1/2}$ is ignored. Equation 2–19 in Chapter 2 provides for an estimate of the effective $t_{1/2}$ that predicts time to steady state for multicompartmental drug kinetics. It is this $t_{1/2}$ of accumulation during multiple dosing that is given in Table AII–1.

Half-life usually is independent of body size because it is a function of the ratio of two parameters, clearance and volume of distribution, each of which is proportional to body size. It also should be noted that the $t_{1/2}$ is preferably obtained from intravenous studies, if feasible, because the $t_{1/2}$ of decline in plasma drug concentration after oral dosing can be influenced by prolonged absorption, such as when slow-release formulations are given. If the $t_{1/2}$ is derived from an oral dose, this will be indicated in a footnote of Table AII–1.

Time to Peak Concentration

Because clearance concepts are used most often in the design of multiple-dosage regimens, the extent rather than the rate of availability is more critical to estimate the average steady-state concentration of drug in the body. In some circumstances, the degree of fluctuation in plasma drug concentration (i.e., peak and trough concentrations), which govern drug efficacy and side effects, can be greatly influenced by modulation of drug absorption rate through the use of sustained- or extended-release formulations. Controlled-release formulations often permit a reduction in dosing frequency from three or four times daily to once or twice daily. There also are drugs that are given on an acute basis (e.g., for the relief of breakthrough pain or to induce sleep), for which the rate of drug absorption is a critical determinant of onset of effect. Thus, information about the expected average time to achieve maximal plasma or blood concentration and the degree of interindividual variability in that parameter have been included in Table AII–1.

The time required to achieve a maximal concentration T_{max} depends on the rate of drug absorption into blood from the site of administration and the rate of elimination. From mass balance principles, T_{max} occurs when the rate of absorption equals the rate of elimination from the reference compartment. Prior to this time, absorption rate exceeds elimination rate, and the plasma concentration of drug increases. After the peak is reached, elimination rate exceeds the absorption rate and, at some point, defines the terminal elimination phase of the concentration-time profile.

The rate of drug absorption following oral administration will depend on the formulation and physicochemical properties of the drug, its permeability across the mucosal barrier, and the intestinal villous blood flow. For an oral dose, some absorption may occur very rapidly within the buccal cavity, esophagus, and stomach, or absorption may be delayed until the drug reaches the small intestine or until the local pH in the intestine permits drug release from the dosage formulation. In the most extreme case, the rate of absorption can be sufficiently controlled by the drug formulation to permit sustained or extended delivery as the dosage form traverses the entire length of the gastrointestinal tract. In some instances, the terminal elimination of drug from the body following a peak concentration reflects the slower rate of absorption and not elimination.

When more than one type of drug formulation is available commercially, we provide absorption information for both the immediate- and extended-release formulations. Not surprisingly, the presence of food in the gastrointestinal tract can alter both the rate and the extent of drug availability. We indicate with footnotes when the consumption of food near the time of drug ingestion may have a significant effect on the drug bioavailability.

Peak Concentration

There is no general agreement about the best way to describe the relationship between the concentration of drug in plasma and its effect. Many different kinds of data are present in the literature, and use of a single-effect parameter or effective concentration is difficult. This is particularly true for antimicrobial agents because the effective concentration depends on the identity of the microorganism causing the infection. It also is important to recognize that concentration-effect relationships are most easily obtained at steady state or during the terminal log-linear phase of the concentration-time curve, when the drug concentration(s) at the site(s) of action are expected to parallel those in plasma. Thus, when attempting to correlate a blood or plasma level to effect, the temporal aspect of distribution of drug to its site of action must be taken into account.

Despite these limitations, it is possible to define the minimum effective or toxic concentrations for some of the drugs currently in clinical use. However, in reviewing the list of drugs approved within the past 5 years, it is rare to find a declaration of an *effective concentration range*, even in the manufacturer's package labeling. Thus, it is necessary to infer therapeutic concentrations from concentrations observed following *effective dosage* regimens. For a given dosage regimen, a time-averaged steady-state blood or plasma concentration (i.e., $\bar{C}_{ss}$ as estimated by dividing the mean AUC by the duration of the dosing interval) and the associated interindividual variability might be one appropriate parameter to report; however, such data often are not available. Also, $\bar{C}_{ss}$ does not take into account the onset and offset of effect during fluctuation of plasma drug concentration over a dosing interval. In some instances, drug efficacy may be more closely linked with peak concentration than with the average or trough concentration, and differences in peak concentration for special populations (e.g., elderly) sometimes are associated with increased incidence of drug toxicity.

For practical reasons, the most commonly reported parameter, C_{max} (peak concentration), rather than effective or toxic concentrations, is presented in Table AII–1. This provides a more consistent body of information about drug exposure from which one can infer, if appropriate, efficacious or toxic blood levels. Although the value reported is the highest that would be encountered in a given dose interval, C_{max} can be related to the trough concentration C_{min} through appropriate mathematical predictions (see Equation 2–20 in Chapter 2). Because peak levels will vary with dose, we have attempted to present concentrations observed with a customary dose regimen that is recognized to be effective in the majority of patients. When a higher or lower dose rate is used, the expected peak level can be adjusted by assuming dose proportionality, unless nonlinear kinetics are indicated. In some instances, only limited data pertaining to multiple dosing are available, so single-dose peak concentrations are presented. When specific information is available about an effective therapeutic range of concentrations or about concentrations at which toxicity occurs, it has been incorporated in a footnote.

It is important to recognize that significant differences in C_{max} will occur when comparing similar daily-dose regimens for an immediate-release and extended-release product. Indeed, the extended-release product sometimes is administered to reduce peak-trough fluctuations during the dosing interval and to minimize swings between potentially toxic or ineffective drug concentrations. Again, we report C_{max} for both immediate- and extended-release formulations, when available. In addition to parent drug concentrations, we have included information on any active metabolite that circulates at a concentration that may contribute to the overall pharmacological effect, particularly those active metabolites that accumulate with multiple dosing. Likewise, for chiral drugs whose stereoisomers differ in their pharmacological activity and clearance characteristics, we present information on concentrations of the individual enantiomers or the active enantiomer that contributes most to the drug's efficacy.

Alterations of Parameters in the Individual Patient

Dose adjustments for an individual patient should be made according to the manufacturer's recommendation in the package labeling when available. This information generally is available when disease, age, or race has a significant impact on drug disposition, particularly for drugs that have been introduced within the past 15 years. In some cases, a significant difference in drug disposition from the "average" adult can be expected

but may not require dose adjustment because of a sufficiently broad therapeutic index. In other cases, dose adjustment may be necessary, but no specific information is available. Under these circumstances, an estimate of the appropriate dosing regimen can be obtained based on pharmacokinetic principles described in Chapter 2.

Unless otherwise specified, the values in Table AII–1 represent mean values for populations of normal adults; it may be necessary to modify them for calculation of dosage regimens for individual patients. The fraction available F and clearance CL would need to be adjusted to compute a maintenance dose necessary to achieve a desired average steady-state concentration. To calculate the loading dose, knowledge of the volume of distribution is needed. The estimated $t_{1/2}$ is used in deciding a dosing interval that provides an acceptable peak-trough fluctuation; note that this may be the apparent $t_{1/2}$ following dosing of a slowly absorbed formulation. The values reported in the table and the adjustments apply only to adults; exceptions are footnoted. Although the values at times may be applied to children who weigh more than about 30 kg (after proper adjustment for size; see Clearance and Volume of Distribution, presented in the following material), it is best to consult pediatrics textbooks or other sources for definitive advice.

For each drug, changes in the parameters caused by certain disease states are noted within the eight segments of the table. In all cases, the qualitative direction of changes is noted, such as "↓ LD," which indicates a significant decrease in the parameter in a patient with chronic liver disease. The relevant literature and the package label should be consulted for more definitive, quantitative information for dosage adjustment recommendations.

Plasma Protein Binding

Most acidic drugs that are extensively bound to plasma proteins are bound to albumin. Basic lipophilic drugs, such as propranolol, often bind to other plasma proteins (e.g., α_1-acid glycoprotein and lipoproteins). The degree of drug binding to proteins will differ in pathophysiological states that cause changes in plasma protein concentrations. Significant pharmacokinetic effects from a change in plasma protein binding are denoted under clearance or volume of distribution.

Although pharmacokinetic parameters based on total drug or metabolite concentrations often are reported, it is important to recognize that in many cases it is the concentration of *unbound drug* that drives access to the site of action and the degree of pharmacological effect. Remarkable changes in the total plasma concentration may accompany disease-induced alteration in protein binding; however, the clinical outcome is not always affected because an increase in free fraction also will increase the apparent clearance of an orally administered drug and of a low-extraction drug dosed intravenously. Under such a scenario, the time-averaged unbound plasma concentration over a dosing interval at steady state will not change with reduced or elevated plasma protein binding, despite a significant change in time-averaged total drug concentration. If so, no adjustment of daily maintenance dose is needed.

Clearance

For drugs that are partly or predominantly eliminated by renal excretion, plasma clearance changes in accordance with the renal function of an individual patient. This necessitates dosage adjustment that is dependent on the fraction of normal renal function remaining and the fraction of drug normally excreted unchanged in the urine. The latter quantity appears in the table; the former can be estimated as the ratio of the patient's estimated or measured creatinine clearance CL_{cr} to a normal value (100 mL/min/1.73 m²). Because urinary creatinine clearance is not routinely measured, it is often estimated from standardized serum creatinine concentration C_{cr} using the MDRD Study equation for CL_{cr} less than 60 mL/min/1.73 m².

$$CL_{cr} \text{ (mL/min/1.73 m}^2) = 175 \cdot (C_{cr})^{-1.154} \cdot (\text{Age})^{-0.203} \cdot (0.742 \text{ if female}) \cdot (1.212 \text{ if African American}) \quad \text{(Equation A–1)}$$

Note that Equation A–1 does not require body weight as the CL_{cr} estimate is normalized to average adult body surface; proportionate scaling is needed for adjustment to a different body surface area. Convenient calculators are available for the MDRD equation and the CKD-EPI equation for more accurate estimation of CL_{cr} greater than 60 mL/min/1.73 m² (e.g., https://www.niddk.nih.gov/health-information/health-communication-programs/nkdep/lab-evaluation/gfr/estimating/Pages/estimating.aspx).

The fraction of normal renal function rfx_{pt} is estimated from the following:

$$rfx_{pt} = \frac{CL_{cr,pt}}{100 \text{ mL/min}} \qquad \text{(Equation A–2)}$$

A more accurate measure of rfx_{pt} seldom is necessary because, given the considerable degree of interindividual variation in nonrenal clearance, the adjustment of clearance is an approximation. The following equation for adjustment of clearance uses the quantities discussed:

$$rf_{pt} = 1 - [fe_{nl} \cdot (1 - rfx_{pt})] \qquad \text{(Equation A–3)}$$

where fe_{nl} is the fraction of systemic drug excreted unchanged in normal individuals (see Table AII–1). The renal factor rf_{pt} is the value that, when multiplied by normal total clearance CL_{nl} from the table, gives the total clearance of the drug adjusted for the impairment in renal function.

Example

The clearance of vancomycin in a patient with reduced renal function (creatinine clearance = 25 mL/min for an average-size adult) may be estimated as follows:

$$rfx_{pt} = \frac{25 \text{ mL/min}}{100 \text{ mL/min}} = 0.25$$

$fe_{nl} = 0.79$ (see listing for vancomycin)

$rf_{pt} = 1 - [0.79 \cdot (1 - 0.25)] = 0.41$

$CL_{pt} = (1.3 \text{ mL/min/kg}) \cdot 0.41$

$= 0.53 \text{ mL/min/kg}$

Importantly, such a clearance adjustment should be regarded only as an initial step in optimizing the dosage regimen; depending on the patient's response to the drug, further individualization may be necessary.

Conventionally, clearance is adjusted for the size of the patient to reflect a difference in the mass of the eliminating organ. For orally administered drugs, the applicability of such an adjustment may be limited by the available dosage strengths of commercial formulations. In some cases, scored tablets can be split, or commercial tablet splitters are used to increase the range of available dosage strengths. However, this practice should be followed only with the recommendation of the pharmacist because splitting a tablet sometimes can compromise the bioavailability of a product.

With the exception of certain oncolytic agents, the data presented in the table are normalized to weight. Thus, interindividual variability in the weight-normalized clearance reflects a variation in the intrinsic metabolic or transport clearance and not the size of the organ. Further, these differences can be attributed to variable expression/function of metabolic enzymes or transporters. However, it is important to recognize that liver mass and total enzyme/transporter content may not increase or decrease in proportion to weight in obese or malnourished individuals. Alternative approaches such as normalization by body surface area or other measures

of body mass may be more appropriate. For example, many of the drugs used to treat cancer are dosed according to body surface area (see Chapters 65 and 66). In the tabulation, if the literature reported dose per body surface area, we present the data in the same unit. If the cited clearance data were not normalized, but the preponderance of the literature utilized body surface area, we followed the practice of using values of body surface area from the literature source or a standard of 1.73 m² for a healthy adult.

Volume of Distribution

Volume of distribution should be adjusted for the modifying factors indicated in Table AII–1 as well as for body size. Again, the data in the table most often are normalized to weight. Unlike clearance, volume of distribution in an individual usually is proportional to weight itself. Whether this applies to a specific drug depends on the actual sites of distribution of drug; no absolute rule applies.

Whether to adjust volume of distribution for changes in binding to plasma proteins cannot be decided in general; the decision depends critically on whether the factors that alter binding to plasma proteins also alter binding to tissue proteins. Qualitative changes in volume of distribution, when they occur, are indicated in the table.

Half-Life

Half-life may be estimated from the adjusted values of clearance CL_{pt} and volume of distribution V_{pt} for the patient:

$$t_{1/2} = \frac{0.693 \cdot V_{pt}}{CL_{pt}} \qquad \text{(Equation A–4)}$$

Because $t_{1/2}$ has been the parameter most often measured and reported in the literature, qualitative changes for this parameter almost always are given in the table.

Individualization of Dosage

By using the parameters for the individual patient, calculated as described in the previous section, initial dosing regimens may be chosen. The maintenance dosage rate may be calculated with Equation 2–17 in Chapter 2, using the estimated values for CL and F for the individual patient. As described previously, the target concentration may have to be adjusted for changes in plasma protein binding in the patient, as described in Plasma Protein Binding. The loading dose may be calculated using Equation 2–21 and estimates for V_{ss} and F. A particular dosing interval may be chosen; the maximal and minimal steady-state concentrations can be calculated by using Equations 2–20, and these calculated concentrations can be compared with the known efficacious and toxic concentrations for the drug. As with the target concentration, these values may need to be adjusted for changes in the extent of plasma protein binding. Use of Equations 2–20 and 2–21 also requires estimates of values for F, V_{ss}, and K ($K = 0.693/t_{1/2}$) for the individual patient.

Note that these adjustments of pharmacokinetic parameters for an individual patient are suggested for the rational choice of initial dosing regimen. As indicated in Chapter 2, steady-state measurement of drug concentrations in the patient then can be used as a guide to further adjust the dosage regimen. However, optimization of a dosage regimen for an individual patient ultimately will depend on the clinical response produced by the drug.

TABLE AII–1 ■ PHARMACOKINETIC DATA

Key: Unless otherwise indicated by a specific footnote, the data are presented for the study population as a mean value ± 1 standard deviation, a mean and range (lowest-highest in parentheses) of values, a range of the lowest-highest values, or a single mean value. ACE, angiotensin-converting enzyme; Aged, aged; AIDS, acquired immunodeficiency syndrome; C_{max}, peak concentration; CYP, cytochrome P450; F or Fem, female; HIV, human immunodeficiency virus; IM, intramuscular; IV, intravenous; LD, chronic liver disease; M, male; MAO, monoamine oxidase; NAT, *N*-acetyltransferase; Neo, neonate; Obes, obesity; *PDR54, Physicians' Desk Reference,* 54th ed. Montvale, NJ, Medical Economics Co., 2000; *PDR58, Physicians' Desk Reference,* 58th ed. Montvale, NJ, Medical Economics Co., 2004; Pneu, pneumonia; PO, oral administration; Preg, pregnant; Prem, premature infants; Rac, racemic mixture of stereoisomers; RD, chronic renal disease; SC, subcutaneous; Smk, smoking; ST, sulfotransferase; T_{max}, peak time; UGT, UDP-glucuronosyl transferase. Other abbreviations are defined in the text section of this appendix.

BIOAVAILABILITY (ORAL) (%)	URINARY EXCRETION (%)	BOUND IN PLASMA (%)	CLEARANCE (mL/min/kg)	VOL. DIST. (L/kg)	HALF-LIFE (hours)	PEAK TIME (h)	PEAK CONCENTRATION
Acetaminophen[a]							
88 ± 15	3 ± 1	<20	5.0 ± 1.4[b]	0.95 ± 0.12	2.7 ± 0.6	0.31–1.4[c]	20 μg/mL[c]
			↓ LD, Aged		↑ LD		
			↑ Obes				

[a]Pharmacokinetic values reported are for doses < 2 g; drug exhibits concentration-dependent kinetics above this dose. [b]Acetaminophen is eliminated predominantly via glucuronidaion and sulfation with a minor pathway via CYP2E1-mediated metabolism. [c]Mean concentration following a 20-mg/kg oral dose. Hepatic toxicity associated with levels > 300 μg/mL at 4 h after an overdose.

References: Forrest JA, et al. Clinical pharmacokinetics of paracetamol. *Clin Pharmacokinet,* **1982**, *7*:93–107. van Rongen A, et al. Morbidly obese patients exhibit increased CYP2E1-mediated oxidation of acetaminophen. *Clin Pharmacokinet,* **2016**, *55*:833–847.

BIOAVAILABILITY (ORAL) (%)	URINARY EXCRETION (%)	BOUND IN PLASMA (%)	CLEARANCE (mL/min/kg)	VOL. DIST. (L/kg)	HALF-LIFE (hours)	PEAK TIME (h)	PEAK CONCENTRATION
Acyclovir							
15–30[a]	75 ± 10	15 ± 4	$CL = 3.37\,CL_{cr} + 0.41$	0.69 ± 0.19	2.4 ± 0.7	1.5–2[b]	3.5–5.4 μM[b]
			↓ Neo	↑ Neo	↑ RD, Neo		

[a]Decreases with increasing dose. [b]Range of steady-state concentrations following a 400-mg dose given orally every 4 h to steady state.

Reference: Laskin OL. Clinical pharmacokinetics of acyclovir. *Clin Pharmacokinet,* **1983**, *8*:187–201.

BIOAVAILABILITY (ORAL) (%)	URINARY EXCRETION (%)	BOUND IN PLASMA (%)	CLEARANCE (mL/min/kg)	VOL. DIST. (L/kg)	HALF-LIFE (hours)	PEAK TIME (h)	PEAK CONCENTRATION
Albendazole[a]							
—[b]	<1	70	10.5–30.7[c]	—	8 (6–15)[d]	2–4[e]	0.50–1.8 μg/mL[e]
↑ Food							

[a]Oral albendazole undergoes rapid and essentially complete first-pass metabolism to albendazole sulfoxide (ALBSO), which is pharmacologically active. Pharmacokinetic data for ALBSO in male and female adults are reported. [b]The absolute bioavailability of ALBSO is not known but is increased by high-fat meals. [c]CL/F following twice-daily oral dosing to steady state. Chronic albendazole treatment appears to induce the metabolism of ALBSO. [d]$t_{1/2}$ reportedly shorter in children with neurocysticercosis compared with adults; may need to be dosed more frequently (three times a day) in children, rather than twice a day, as in adults. [e]Following a 7.5-mg/kg oral dose given twice daily for 8 days to adults.

References: Marques MP, et al. Enantioselective kinetic disposition of albendazole sulfoxide in patients with neurocysticercosis. *Chirality,* **1999**, *11*:218–223. PDR 58, **2004**, p. 1422. Sanchez M, et al. Pharmacokinetic comparison of two albendazole dosage regimens in patients with neurocysticercosis. *Clin Neuropharmacol,* **1993**, *76*:77–82. Sotelo J, et al. Pharmacokinetic optimisation of the treatment of neurocysticercosis. *Clin Pharmacokinet,* **1998**, *34*:503–515.

BIOAVAILABILITY (ORAL) (%)	URINARY EXCRETION (%)	BOUND IN PLASMA (%)	CLEARANCE (mL/min/kg)	VOL. DIST. (L/kg)	HALF-LIFE (hours)	PEAK TIME (h)	PEAK CONCENTRATION
Albuterol[a]							
PO, *R*: 30 ± 7	*R*: 46 ± 8	*Rac*: 7 ± 1	*R*: 10.3 ± 3.0	*R*: 2.00 ± 0.49	*R*: 2.00 ± 0.49	*R*: 1.5[b]	*R*: 3.6 (1.9–5.9) ng/mL[b]
PO, *S*: 71 ± 9	*S*: 55 ± 11		*S*: 6.5 ± 2.0	*S*: 1.77 ± 0.69	*S*: 2.85 ± 0.85	*S*: 2.0[b]	*S*: 11.4 (7.1–16.2) ng/mL[b]
IH, *R*: 25			↓ RD	↓ RD			
IH, *S*: 47							

[a]Data from healthy subjects for *R*- and *S*-enantiomers. No major gender differences. No kinetic differences in asthmatics. β-Adrenergic activity resides primarily with *R*-enantiomer. IH, inhalation. Oral dose undergoes extensive first-pass sulfation at the intestinal mucosa. [b]Median (range) following a single 4-mg oral dose of racemic-albuterol.

References: Boulton DW, et al. Enantioselective disposition of albuterol in humans. *Clin Rev Allergy Immunol,* **1996**, *14*:115–138. Mohamed MH, et al. Effects of gender and race on albuterol pharmacokinetics. *Pharmacotherapy,* **1999**, *19*:157–161.

BIOAVAILABILITY (ORAL) (%)	URINARY EXCRETION (%)	BOUND IN PLASMA (%)	CLEARANCE (mL/min/kg)	VOL. DIST. (L/kg)	HALF-LIFE (hours)	PEAK TIME (h)	PEAK CONCENTRATION
Alendronate[a]							
<0.7[b]	44.9 ± 9.3	78	1.11 (1.00–1.22)[c]	0.44 (0.34–0.55)[c]	~1.0[e]	IV: 2[f]	IV: ~275 ng/mL[f]
↓ Food			↓ RD[d]				PO: <5–8.4 ng/mL[f]

[a]Data from healthy postmenopausal female subjects. [b]Based on urinary recovery; reduced when taken < 1 h before or up to 2 h after a meal. [c]CL and V_{ss} values represent mean (90% confidence interval). [d]Mild-to-moderate renal impairment. [e]The $t_{1/2}$ for release from bone is ~ 11.9 years. [f]Following a single 10-mg IV infusion over 2 h and a 10-mg oral dose daily for > 3 years.

References: Cocquyt V, et al. Pharmacokinetics of intravenous alendronate. *J Clin Pharmacol,* **1999**, *39*:385–393. Porras AG, et al. Pharmacokinetics of alendronate. *Clin Pharmacokinet,* **1999**, *36*:315–328.

(Continued)

TABLE AII-1 ■ PHARMACOKINETIC DATA (*CONTINUED*)

BIOAVAILABILITY (ORAL) (%)	URINARY EXCRETION (%)	BOUND IN PLASMA (%)	CLEARANCE (mL/min/kg)	VOL. DIST. (L/kg)	HALF-LIFE (hours)	PEAK TIME (h)	PEAK CONCENTRATION
Alfentanil							
—	<1	92 ± 2	6.7 ± 2.4[a]	0.8 ± 0.3	1.6 ± 0.2	—	100–200 ng/mL[b]
↓ Food[c]		↓ LD	↓ Aged, LD	↓ LD	↑ Aged, LD		310–340 ng/mL[c]

[a]Metabolically cleared by CYP3A. [b]Provides adequate anesthesia for superficial surgery. [c]Provides adequate anesthesia for abdominal surgery.

References: Bodenham A, et al. Alfentanil infusions in patients requiring intensive care. *Clin Pharmacokinet*, **1988**, 75:216–226.

BIOAVAILABILITY (ORAL) (%)	URINARY EXCRETION (%)	BOUND IN PLASMA (%)	CLEARANCE (mL/min/kg)	VOL. DIST. (L/kg)	HALF-LIFE (hours)	PEAK TIME (h)	PEAK CONCENTRATION
Alfuzosin[a]							
50%[b]	11[d]	~90	6.4 ± 1.8[e]	3.2 ± 1.1	6.3 ± 0.9[g]	9[h]	16.6 ± 5.5 ng/mL[h]
↓ Food[c]			↓ LD[f]				

[a]Administered as racemate. [b]Value reported for 10-mg, extended-release formulation, once daily, given with a high-fat meal. [c]Oral bioavailability in the fasted state is one-half that of the fed state. [d]Value reported in product label; however, route of administration uncertain. [e]Alfuzosin is cleared primarily through CYP3A-dependent hepatic metabolism. *R/S* AUC ratio = 1.35. [f]Study in patients with moderate-to-severe liver impairment; *CL/F* reduced to one-third to one-quarter of control. [g]Apparent $t_{1/2}$ = 9 h for extended-release product; reflects absorption-limited kinetics. [h]Following a 10-mg dose of extended-release formulation given once a day for 5 days.

References: McKeage K, et al. Alfuzosin: A review of the therapeutic use of the prolonged-release formulation given once daily in the management of benign prostatic hyperplasia. *Drugs*, **2002**, 62:135–167. Drugs@FDA. Uroxatral NDA and label. NDA approved on June 12, 2003; label approved on May 20, 2009. Available at: http://www.accessdata.fda.gov/drugsatfda_docs/nda/2003/21-287_Uroxatral_BioPharmr_P1.pdf and http://www.accessdata.fda.gov/drugsatfda_docs/label/2009/021287s013lbl.pdf. Accessed May 17, 2010.

BIOAVAILABILITY (ORAL) (%)	URINARY EXCRETION (%)	BOUND IN PLASMA (%)	CLEARANCE (mL/min/kg)	VOL. DIST. (L/kg)	HALF-LIFE (hours)	PEAK TIME (h)	PEAK CONCENTRATION
Aliskiren							
2.6[a]	7.5	49 (47–51)	2.1[b]	1.9	24–40[d]	2.5[e]	72 ± 67 ng/mL[e]
↓ Food[a]			↓ RD[c]				

[a]Absolute bioavailability of 75 mg in hard gelatin capsule reported. Oral AUC decreased 71% with high-fat meal. [b]Aliskiren is cleared by both renal excretion and CYP3A-dependent hepatic metabolism; however, the relative contribution of each pathway to total drug clearance is unclear. [c]Study in patients with mild-to-severe renal impairment; systemic exposure increased 1.0- to 2.5-fold but was independent of disease severity. [d]$t_{1/2}$ estimated from single oral dose data. [e]Following 150-mg oral dose given once daily to steady state in healthy adults.

References: Azizi M. Direct renin inhibition: clinical pharmacology. *J Mol Med*, **2008**, 86:647–654. Azizi M, et al. Renin inhibition with aliskiren: where are we now, and where are we going? *J Hypertens*, **2006**, 24:243–256. Vaidyanathan S, et al. Clinical pharmacokinetics and pharmacodynamics of aliskiren. *Clin Pharmacokinet*, **2008**, 27:515–531.

BIOAVAILABILITY (ORAL) (%)	URINARY EXCRETION (%)	BOUND IN PLASMA (%)	CLEARANCE (mL/min/kg)	VOL. DIST. (L/kg)	HALF-LIFE (hours)	PEAK TIME (h)	PEAK CONCENTRATION
Allopurinol[a]							
53 ± 13	12	—	9.9 ± 2.4	0.87 ± 0.13	A: 1.2 ± 0.3	A: 1.7 ± 1.0[c]	A: 1.4 ± 0.5 µg/mL[c]
					O: 24 ± 4.5	O: 4.1 ± 1.4[c]	O: 6.4 ± 0.8 µg/mL[b,c]

[a]Data from healthy male and female subjects. Allopurinol (A) is rapidly metabolized to the pharmacologically active oxypurinol (O). [b]Increased oxypurinol AUC during renal impairment and in the elderly. [c]Following a single 300-mg oral dose.

References: PDR54, **2000**, p. 1976. Tumheim K, et al. Pharmacokinetics and pharmacodynamics of allopurinol in elderly and young subjects. *Br J Clin Pharmacol*, **1999**, 48:501–509.

BIOAVAILABILITY (ORAL) (%)	URINARY EXCRETION (%)	BOUND IN PLASMA (%)	CLEARANCE (mL/min/kg)	VOL. DIST. (L/kg)	HALF-LIFE (hours)	PEAK TIME (h)	PEAK CONCENTRATION
Alosetron[a]							
57 (33–97)[a]	—	82	8.3 (6.5–10.8)[b]	0.91 (0.70–1.12)	1.4 (1.3–1.6)	1[e]	5.5 (4.8–6.4) ng/mL[e]
			↓ LD[d]				

[a]Absolute bioavailability of a 4-mg dose, as compared to intravenous infusion. [b]Alosetron is cleared primarily by CYP1A2-dependent hepatic metabolism. [c]Study in patients with CL_{cr} = 4–56 mL/min. [d]Study in patients with moderate-to-severe liver impairment; oral AUC 1.6- to 14-fold higher than control. [e]Following a 1-mg oral dose, given twice a day to steady state.

References: Balfour JA, et al. Alosetron. *Drugs*, **2000**, 59:511–518. Drugs@FDA. Lotronex NDA and label. NDA approved on February 11, 2000; label approved on April 1, 2008. Available at: http://www.accessdata.fda.gov/drugsatfda_docs/nda/2000/21107a_Lotronex_clinphrmr_P3.pdf and http://www.accessdata.fda.gov/drugsatfda_docs/label/2008/021107s013lbl.pdf. Accessed May 17, 2010. Koch KM, et al. Sex and age differences in the pharmacokinetics of alosetron. *Br J Clin Pharmacol*, **2002**, 53:238–242.

BIOAVAILABILITY (ORAL) (%)	URINARY EXCRETION (%)	BOUND IN PLASMA (%)	CLEARANCE (mL/min/kg)	VOL. DIST. (L/kg)	HALF-LIFE (hours)	PEAK TIME (h)	PEAK CONCENTRATION
Alprazolam							
88 ± 16	20	71 ± 3	0.74 ± 0.14[a]	0.72 ± 0.12	12 ± 2	1.5 (0.5–3.0)[c]	21 (15–32) ng/mL[c]
		↑ LD	↓ Obes, LD, Aged[b]		↑ Obes, LD, Aged[b]		

[a]Metabolically cleared by CYP3A and other cytochrome P450 isozymes. [b]Data from male subjects only. [c]Mean (range) from 19 studies following a single 1-g oral dose given to adults.

Reference: Greenblatt DJ, et al. Clinical pharmacokinetics of alprazolam. Therapeutic implications. *Clin Pharmacokinet*, **1993**, 24:453–471.

BIOAVAILABILITY (ORAL) (%)	URINARY EXCRETION (%)	BOUND IN PLASMA (%)	CLEARANCE (mL/min/kg)	VOL. DIST. (L/kg)	HALF-LIFE (hours)	PEAK TIME (h)	PEAK CONCENTRATION
Amiodarone[a]							
46 ± 22	0	99.98 ± 0.01	1.9 ± 0.4[b]	66 ± 44	25 ± 12 days[c]	2–10[d]	1.5–2.4 µg/mL[d]

[a]Significant plasma concentrations of an active desethyl metabolite are observed (ratio of drug/metabolite ~ 1); $t_{1/2}$ for metabolite = 61 days. [b]Metabolically cleared by CYP3A. [c]Longer $t_{1/2}$ noted in patients (53 ± 24 days); all reported $t_{1/2}$s may be underestimated because of insufficient length of sampling. [d]Following a 400-mg/d oral dose to steady state in adult patients.

Reference: Gill J, et al. Amiodarone. An overview of its pharmacological properties, and review of its therapeutic use in cardiac arrhythmias. *Drugs*, **1992**, 43:69–110.

(Continued)

TABLE AII–1 ■ PHARMACOKINETIC DATA (*CONTINUED*)

BIOAVAILABILITY (ORAL) (%)	URINARY EXCRETION (%)	BOUND IN PLASMA (%)	CLEARANCE (mL/min/kg)	VOL. DIST. (L/kg)	HALF-LIFE (hours)	PEAK TIME (h)	PEAK CONCENTRATION
Amlodipine[a]							
74 ± 17	10	93 ± 1	5.9 ± 1.5[b]	16 ± 4	39 ± 8	5.4–8.0[c]	18.1 ± 7.1 ng/mL[c]
			↓ Aged, LD		↑ Aged, LD		

[a]Racemic mixture; in young, healthy subjects, there are no apparent differences between the kinetics of the more active *R*-enantiomer and *S*-enantiomer. [b]Amlodipine is mainly cleared by CYP3A4-dependent metabolism. [c]Following a 10-mg oral dose given once daily for 14 days to healthy male adults.

Reference: Meredith PA, et al. Clinical pharmacokinetics of amlodipine. *Clin Pharmacokinet*, **1992**, *22*:22–31.

Amoxicillin							
93 ± 10[a]	86 ± 8	18	2.6 ± 0.4	0.21 ± 0.03	1.7 ± 0.3	1–2	IV: 46 ± 12 µg/mL[c]
			↑ Preg		↑ RD, Aged[b]		PO: 5 µg/mL[c]
			↓ RD, Aged[b]				

[a]Dose dependent; value shown is for a 375-mg dose; decreases to ~ 50% at 3000 mg. [b]No change if renal function is not decreased. [c]Following a single 500-mg IV bolus dose in healthy elderly adults or a single 500-mg oral dose in adults.

References: Hoffler D. The pharmacokinetics of amoxicillin [in German]. *Adv Clin Pharmacol*, **1974**, *7*:28–30. Sjovall J, et al. Intra- and inter-individual variation in pharmacokinetics of intravenously infused amoxicillin and ampicillin to elderly volunteers. *Br J Clin Pharmacol*, **1986**, *27*:171–181. Andrew MA, et al. Amoxicillin pharmacokinetics in pregnant women: modeling and simulations of dosing strategies. *Clin Pharmacol Ther*, **2007**, *81*:547–556.

Amphotericin B[a]							
<5	2–5	>90	0.46 ± 0.20[b]	0.76 ± 0.52[c]	18 ± 7[d]	—	1.2 ± 0.33 µg/mL[e]

[a]Data for amphotericin B shown. [b]Data for eight children (ages 8 months to 14 years) yielded a linear regression, with *CL* decreasing with age: *CL* = –0.046 · Age (years) + 0.86. Newborns show highly variable *CL* values. [c]Volume of central compartment. V_{ss} increases with dose from 3.4 L/kg for a 0.25-mg/kg dose to 8.9 L/kg for a 1.5-mg/kg dose. Also available as liposomal encapsulated formulations (Abelcet and Ambisome). Amphotericin distribution and *CL* properties of these products are different from the nonencapsulated form; they have a terminal $t_{1/2}$ of 173 ± 78 and 110–153 h, respectively; however, an effective steady-state concentration can be achieved within 4 days. [d]$t_{1/2}$ for multiple dosing. In single-dose studies, a prolonged dose-dependent $t_{1/2}$ is seen. [e]Following a 0.5-mg/kg IV dose of amphotericin B given as a 1-h infusion, once daily for 3 days. Whole-blood concentrations (free and liposome encapsulated) of 1.7 ± 0.8 µg/mL and 83 ± 35 µg/mL were reported following a 5-mg/kg/d IV dose (presumed 60- to 120-min infusion) of Abelcet and Ambisome, respectively.

References: Gallis HA, et al. Amphotericin B: 30 years of clinical experience. *Rev Infect Dis*, **1990**, *12*:308–329. PDR54, **2000**, pp. 1090–1091, 1654.

Apixaban							
~50	17–30	87	0.77–0.84[a,b]	0.38–0.42[b]	3.7–8.4[b,c]	3–4[d]	34–110 ng/mL[d]

[a]Cleared from blood primarily by CYP3A-dependent metabolism. [b]Calculated assuming 70-kg body weight; range of mean values for single intravenous doses of 0.5–5 mg. [c]Apparent $t_{1/2}$ after oral dose is ~ 12 h because of slow absorption. [d]Following a single 5-mg oral dose to 16 healthy adults.

Reference: Zheng SS, et al. Pharmacodynamics, pharmacokinetics and clinical efficacy of apixaban in the treatment of thrombosis. *Expert Opin Drug Metab Toxicol*, **2016**, *12*: 575–580. Drugs@FDA: FDA Approved Drug Products (http://www.accessdata.fda.gov/scripts/cder/daf/), Apixaban (Eliquis).

Aripiprazole[a]							
87	<1	>99	0.83 ± 0.17[b,c]	4.9[c]	47 ± 10	3.0 ± 0.6[d]	242 ± 36 ng/mL[d]

[a]The major metabolite, dehydro-aripiprazole, has affinity for D_2 receptors similar to parent drug; found at 40% of parent drug concentration in plasma; $t_{1/2}$ is 94 h. No significant gender differences. [b]Eliminated primarily by CYP2D6- and CYP3A4-dependent metabolism. CYP2D6 poor metabolizers exhibit increased exposure (80%) to parent drug but reduced exposure (30%) to the active metabolite. [c]*CL/F* and *V/F* at steady state reported. [d]Following a 15-mg oral dose given once daily for 14 days.

References: DeLeon A, et al. Aripiprazole: a comprehensive review of its pharmacology, clinical efficacy, and tolerability. *Clin Ther*, **2004**, *26*:649–666. Mallikaarjun S, et al. Pharmacokinetics, tolerability, and safety of aripiprazole following multiple oral dosing in normal healthy volunteers. *J Clin Pharmacol*, **2004**, *44*:179–187. PDR58, **2004**, pp. 1034–1035. Mallikaarjun S, et al. Effects of hepatic or renal impairment on the pharmacokinetics of aripiprazole. *Clin Pharmacokinet*, **2008**, *47*(8):533–542.

Atazanavir[a]							
—[b]	7	86	3.4 ± 1.0[c,d]	1.6–2.7[d]	7.9 ± 2.9	2.5[e]	5.4 ± 1.4 µg/mL[e]
↑ Food			↓ LD		↑ LD		

[a]Pharmacokinetic data reported for healthy adults. No significant gender or age differences. [b]Absolute bioavailability is not known, but food enhances the extent of absorption. [c]Undergoes extensive hepatic metabolism, primarily by CYP3A. Metabolic elimination affected by inhibitors and inducers of CYP3A. Coadministration with low-dose ritonavir increases systemic atazanavir exposure. [d]*CL/F* and *V/F* reported. [e]Following a 400-mg oral dose given with a light meal once daily to steady state.

References: Orrick JJ, et al. Atazanavir. *Ann Pharmacother*, **2004**, *38*:1664–1674. PDR58, **2004**, p. 1081.

Atenolol[a]							
58 ± 16	94 ± 8	<5	2.4 ± 0.3	1.3 ± 0.5[b]	6.1 ± 2.0[c]	3.3 ± 1.3[d]	0.28 ± 0.09 µg/mL[d]
			↓ Aged, RD		↑ RD, Aged		

[a]Atenolol is administered as a racemic mixture. No significant differences in the pharmacokinetics of the enantiomers. [b]V_{area} reported. [c]$t_{1/2}$ of *R*- and *S*-atenolol are similar. [d]Following a single 50-mg oral dose. [e]*CL/F* unchanged during pregnancy; however, renal clearance of atenolol is increased during pregnancy.

References: Boyd RA, et al. The pharmacokinetics of the enantiomers of atenolol. *Clin Pharmacol Ther*, **1989**, *45*:403–410. Mason WD, et al. Kinetics and absolute bioavailability of atenolol. *Clin Pharmacol Ther*, **1979**, *25*:408–415.

(Continued)

TABLE AII–1 ■ PHARMACOKINETIC DATA (*CONTINUED*)

BIOAVAILABILITY (ORAL) (%)	URINARY EXCRETION (%)	BOUND IN PLASMA (%)	CLEARANCE (mL/min/kg)	VOL. DIST. (L/kg)	HALF-LIFE (hours)	PEAK TIME (h)	PEAK CONCENTRATION
Atomoxetine[a]							
EM: 63[b]	1%–2%	98.7 ± 0.3	EM: 6.2[b]	EM: 2.3[b]	EM: 5.3[b]	EM/PM: 2[c]	EM: 160 ng/mL[c]
PM: 94[b]			PM: 0.60[b]	PM: 1.1[b]	PM: 20[b]		PM: 915 ng/mL[c]
			EM: ↓ LD				

[a]Metabolized by CYP2D6 (polymorphic). Poor metabolizers (PM) exhibit a higher oral bioavailability, higher C_{max}, lower CL, and longer $t_{1/2}$ than extensive metabolizers (EM). No differences between adults and children > 6 years of age. [b]CL/F, V/F, and $t_{1/2}$ measured at steady state. [c]Following a 20-mg oral dose given twice daily for 5 days.

References: Sauer JM, et al. Disposition and metabolic fate of atomoxetine hydrochloride: the role of CYP2D6 in human disposition and metabolism. *Drug Metab Dispos*, **2003**, 37:98–107. Simpson D, et al. Atomoxetine: a review of its use in adults with attention deficit hyperactivity disorder. *Drugs*, **2004**, 64:205–222.

Atorvastatin[a]							
12	<2	≥98	29[b]	~5.4	19.5 ± 9.6	2.3 ± 0.96[d]	14.9 ± 1.8 ngEq/mL[d]
			↓ LD,[c] Aged		↑ LD, Aged		

[a]Data from healthy adult male and female subjects. No clinically significant gender differences. Atorvastatin undergoes extensive CYP3A-dependent first-pass metabolism. Metabolites are active and exhibit a longer $t_{1/2}$ (20 to 30 h) than parent drug. [b]Mean CL/F calculated from reported AUC data at steady state after a once-a-day 20-mg oral dose, assuming a 70-kg body weight. [c]AUC following oral administration increased, mild-to-moderate hepatic impairment. [d]Following a 20-mg oral dose, once daily, for 14 days.

References: Gibson DM, et al. Effect of age and gender on pharmacokinetics of atorvastatin in humans. *J Clin Pharmacol*, **1996**, 36:242–246. Lea AP, McTavish D. Atorvastatin. A review of its pharmacology and therapeutic potential in the management of hyperlipidaemias. *Drugs*, **1997**, 53:828–847. PDR54, **2000**, p. 2254.

Atovaquone							
23 ± 11[a]	<1	>99	1.26, 2.95, 2.84[b,c]	7.98[c]	84.9, 31.3, 35.2[c]	1.5–3[d]	4.25 ± 2.15 µg/mL[e]
↑ Food							

[a]Value reported when taken with food. [b]Cleared from blood primarily by biliary excretion; undergoes enterohepatic cycling, with eventual fecal elimination. [c]Population estimates of CL/F, V/F, and $t_{1/2}$ in black, Asian, and Malay patients, respectively, treated for malaria. [d]Longer T_{max} values also reported, possibly because of enterohepatic recycling. [e]Following a 250-mg oral dose (Malarone) given once a day for 4 days.

Reference: Marra F, et al. Atovaquone-proguanil for prophylaxis and treatment of malaria. *Ann Pharmacother*, **2003**, 37:1266–1275. Hussein Z, et al. Population pharmacokinetics of atovaquone in patients with acute malaria caused by *Plasmodium falciparum*. *Clin Pharmacol Ther*, **1997**, 61:518–530. Drugs@FDA: FDA Approved Drug Products (http://www.accessdata.fda.gov/scripts/cder/daf/), Atovaquone (Mepron and Malarone).

Azathioprine[a]							
60 ± 31[b]	<2	—	57 ± 31[c]	0.81 ± 0.65[c]	0.16 ± 0.07[c]	MP: 1–2[d]	MP: 20–90 ng/mL[d]

[a]Azathioprine is metabolized to mercaptopurine (MP), listed further in this table. [b]Determined as the bioavailability of MP; intact azathioprine is undetectable after oral administration because of extensive first-pass metabolism. Kinetic values are for intravenous azathioprine. [c]Data from kidney transplant patients. [d]MP concentration following a 135 ± 34-mg oral dose of azathioprine given daily to steady state in kidney transplant patients.

Reference: Lin SN, et al. Quantitation of plasma azathioprine and 6-mercaptopurine levels in renal transplant patients. *Transplantation*, **1980**, 29:290–294.

Azithromycin							
34 ± 19	12	7–50[a]	9	31	40[b]	2–3[c]	0.4 µg/mL[c]
↓ Food (capsules)							
↑ Food (suspension)							

[a]Dose-dependent plasma binding. The bound fraction is 50% at 50 ng/mL and 12% at 500 ng/mL. [b]A longer terminal plasma $t_{1/2}$ of 68 ± 8 h, reflecting release from tissue stores, overestimates the multiple-dosing $t_{1/2}$. [c]Following a 250-mg/d oral dose to adult patients with an infection.

Reference: Lalak NJ, et al. Azithromycin clinical pharmacokinetics. *Clin Pharmacokinet*, **1993**, 25:370–374.

Baclofen[a]							
>70[b]	69 ± 14	31 ± 11	2.72 ± 0.93[c]	0.81 ± 0.12[c]	3.75 ± 0.96	1.0 (0.5–4)[e]	160 ± 49 ng/mL[e]
			↓ RD[d]				

[a]Data from healthy adult male subjects. [b]Bioavailability estimate based on urine recovery of unchanged drug after oral dose. [c]CL/F, V_{area}/F reported for intestinal infusion of drug. [d]Limited data suggest CL/F reduced with renal impairment. [e]Following a single 10-mg oral dose.

References: Kochak GM, et al. The pharmacokinetics of baclofen derived from intestinal infusion. *Clin Pharmacol Ther*, **1985**, 38:251–257. Wuis EW, et al. Plasma and urinary excretion kinetics of oral baclofen in healthy subjects. *Eur J Clin Pharmacol*, **1989**, 37:181–184.

Buprenorphine[a]							
SL: 51 ± 13	Negligible	96	14.9 ± 5.2	4.8 ± 1.7	16.2 ± 20.1	SL: 1.2 ± 0.1[c]	SL: 2.7 ± 0.3 ng/mL[c]
BC: 28 ± 9							
			↑ Child[b]	↑ Child[b]	↓ Child[b]	BC: 0.8 ± 0.2[c]	BC: 2.0 ± 0.6 ng/mL[c]

[a]Data from male and female subjects undergoing surgery. Buprenorphine is metabolized in the liver by CYP3A4 to an active metabolite, norbuprenorphine, and via conjugation. Majority of the dose is excreted into feces. [b]CL, 60 ± 19 mL/min/kg; V_{ss}, 3.2 L/kg; $t_{1/2}$, 1.03 ± 0.22 h; children 4–7 years of age. [c]Following 8-mg sublingual solution (SL), 4-mg buccal (BC) dose.

References: Elkader A, Sproule B. Buprenorphine: clinical pharmacokinetics in the treatment of opioid dependence. *Clin Pharmacokinet*, **2005**, 44:661–680. Olkkola KT, et al. Pharmacokinetics of intravenous buprenorphine in children. *Br J Clin Pharmacol*, **1989**, 28:202–204.

(Continued)

TABLE AII–1 ■ PHARMACOKINETIC DATA (*CONTINUED*)

	BIOAVAILABILITY (ORAL) (%)	URINARY EXCRETION (%)	BOUND IN PLASMA (%)	CLEARANCE (mL/min/kg)	VOL. DIST. (L/kg)	HALF-LIFE (hours)	PEAK TIME (h)	PEAK CONCENTRATION
Bupropion[a]								
	—	<1	>80%	R: 43 (58)[b] S: 257 (72) Rac: 74 (61)	R: 40.7 (78)[b] S: 152 (83) Rac: 65.7 (80)	R: 11. 6 (49)[b] S: 7.2 (103) Rac: 10.8 (54) OH: 19.2 (21) Erythro: 21.6 (36) Threo: 30.8 (41)		Rac: 58 (52–63) ng/mL[c] OH: 464 (406–522) ng/mL[c] Erythro: 38 (35–42) ng/mL[c] Threo: 208 (181–236) ng/mL[c]
				↓ Aged, RD, LD		↑ Aged, LD		

[a]Bupropion is administered as a racemic mixture of *R* and *S* bupropion that can interconvert. Data from healthy adult male volunteers. Bupropion is metabolized by CYP2B6 to hydroxy-bupropion and by 11β–hydroxysteroid-dehydrogenase and aldo-ketoreductases to threo- and erythrohydrobupropion. All three metabolites accumulate in blood and are active. [b]*CL/F*, V_{ss}/F, and $t_{1/2}$ reported for oral dose. Percentage coefficient of variation shown in parentheses. [c]Following oral dosing of 150-mg XL (sustained release) tablet to 42 healthy subjects for 7 days (steady state). 95% confidence interval shown in brackets.

References: Masters AR, et al. Chiral plasma pharmacokinetics and urinary excretion of bupropion and metabolites in healthy volunteers. *J Pharmacol Exp Ther*, **2016**, *358*:230–238. DeVane CL, et al. Disposition of bupropion in healthy volunteers and subjects with alcoholic liver disease. *J Clin Psychopharmacol*, **1990**, *10*:328–332. Benowitz NL, et al. Influence of CYP2B6 genetic variants on plasma and urine concentrations of bupropion and metabolites at steady state. *Pharmacogenet Genomics*, **2013**, *23*:135–141.

	BIOAVAILABILITY (ORAL) (%)	URINARY EXCRETION (%)	BOUND IN PLASMA (%)	CLEARANCE (mL/min/kg)	VOL. DIST. (L/kg)	HALF-LIFE (hours)	PEAK TIME (h)	PEAK CONCENTRATION
Buspirone[a]								
	3.9 ± 4.3	<0.1	>95	28.3 ± 10.3	5.3 ± 2.6	2.4 ± 1.1	0.71 ± 0.06[e]	1.66 ± 0.21 ng/mL[e]
	↑ Food[b]			↓ LD,[c] RD[d]		↑ LD, RD		

[a]Data from healthy adult male subjects. No significant gender differences. Undergoes extensive CYP3A-dependent first-pass metabolism. The major metabolite (l-pyrimidinyl piperazine) is active in some behavioral tests in animals (one-fifth potency) and accumulates in blood to levels severalfold higher than buspirone. [b]Bioavailability increased ~ 84%; appears to be secondary to reduced first-pass metabolism. [c]*CL/F* reduced, hepatic cirrhosis. [d]*CL/F* reduced, mild renal impairment; unrelated to CL_{cr}. [e]Following a single 20-mg oral dose.

References: Barbhaiya RH, et al. Disposition kinetics of buspirone in patients with renal or hepatic impairment after administration of single and multiple doses. *Eur J Clin Pharmacol*, **1994**, *46*:41–47. Gammans RE, et al. Metabolism and disposition of buspirone. *Am J Med*, **1986**, *80*:41–51.

	BIOAVAILABILITY (ORAL) (%)	URINARY EXCRETION (%)	BOUND IN PLASMA (%)	CLEARANCE (mL/min/kg)	VOL. DIST. (L/kg)	HALF-LIFE (hours)	PEAK TIME (h)	PEAK CONCENTRATION
Busulfan								
	70 (44–94)	1	2.7–14	4.5 ± 0.9[a]	0.99 ± 0.23[a]	2.6 ± 0.5	2.6 ± 1.5	Low: 65 ± 27 ng/mL[b]
								High: 949 ± 278 ng/mL[b]

[a]*CL/F* and V_{area}/F reported. [b]Following a single 4-mg oral dose (low) given to patients with chronic myelocytic leukemia or a single 1-mg/kg oral dose (high) given as ablative therapy to patients undergoing bone marrow transplantation.

References: Ehrsson H, et al. Busulfan kinetics. *Clin Pharmacol Ther*, **1983**, *34*:86–89. Schuler US, et al. Pharmacokinetics of intravenous busulfan and evaluation of the bioavailability of the oral formulation in conditioning for haematopoietic stem cell transplantation. *Bone Marrow Transplant*, **1998**, *22*:241–244.

	BIOAVAILABILITY (ORAL) (%)	URINARY EXCRETION (%)	BOUND IN PLASMA (%)	CLEARANCE (mL/min/kg)	VOL. DIST. (L/kg)	HALF-LIFE (hours)	PEAK TIME (h)	PEAK CONCENTRATION
Calcitriol[a]								
	PO: ~61	<10%	99.9	0.43 ± 0.04	—	16.5 ± 3.1[b]	PO: 3–6[d]	IV: ~460 pg/mL[d]
	IP: ~67					↑ Child[c]	IP: 2–3[d]	PO: ~90 pg/mL[d]
								IP: ~105 pg/mL[d]

[a]Data from young (15–22 years) patients on peritoneal dialysis. Metabolized by 23-, 24-, and 26-hydroxylases and also excreted into bile as its glucuronide. [b]Calcitriol $t_{1/2}$ is 5–8 h in healthy adult subjects. [c]Oral dose $t_{1/2}$ = 27 ± 12 h, children 2–16 years. [d]Following a single 60-ng/kg IV, intraperitoneal (IP) dialysate, or PO dose. Baseline plasma levels were < 10 pg/mL.

References: Jones CL, et al. Comparisons between oral and intraperitoneal 1,25-dihydroxyvitamin D₃ therapy in children treated with peritoneal dialysis. *Clin Nephrol*, **1994**, *42*: 44–49. PDR54, **2000**, p. 2650. Salusky IE, et al. Pharmacokinetics of calcitriol in continuous ambulatory and cycling peritoneal dialysis patients. *Am J Kidney Dis*, **1990**, *16*:126–132. Taylor CA, et al. Clinical pharmacokinetics during continuous ambulatory peritoneal dialysis. *Clin Pharmacokinet*, **1996**, *31*:293–308.

	BIOAVAILABILITY (ORAL) (%)	URINARY EXCRETION (%)	BOUND IN PLASMA (%)	CLEARANCE (mL/min/kg)	VOL. DIST. (L/kg)	HALF-LIFE (hours)	PEAK TIME (h)	PEAK CONCENTRATION
Canagliflozin								
	65	<1[a]	98–99	2.74[b,c]	1.70[c]	6.9[d]	1.5 (1–5)[e]	1227 ± 481 ng/mL[e]

[a]Calculated as the ratio of canagliflozin renal clearance/total intravenous clearance. [b]Cleared from blood primarily by UGT1A9- and 2B4-dependent metabolism. [c]Calculated assuming 70-kg body weight. [d]$t_{1/2}$ following intravenous dose reported; longer values (11–13 h) reported following oral administration. [e]Mean (range or ± SD) following a 100-mg oral dose given once a day for 7 days to patients with type 2 diabetes mellitus.

Reference: Scheen AJ. Pharmacokinetics, pharmacodynamics and clinical use of SGL2 inhibitors in patients with type 2 diabetes mellitus and chronic kidney disease. *Clin Pharmacokinet*, **2015**, *54*:691–708. Drugs@FDA: FDA Approved Drug Products (http://www.accessdata.fda.gov/scripts/cder/daf/), Canagliflozin (Invokamet).

	BIOAVAILABILITY (ORAL) (%)	URINARY EXCRETION (%)	BOUND IN PLASMA (%)	CLEARANCE (mL/min/kg)	VOL. DIST. (L/kg)	HALF-LIFE (hours)	PEAK TIME (h)	PEAK CONCENTRATION
Candesartan[a]								
	42 (34–56)	52	99.8	0.37 (0.31–0.47) ↓ RD[b]	0.13 (0.09–0.17)	9.7 (4.8–13) ↑ RD[b]	4.0 ± 1.3	119 ± 43 ng/mL[c]

[a]Data from healthy adult male subjects. Candesartan cilexetil is rapidly and completely converted to candesartan through the action of gut wall esterases. Mean (range) for candesartan reported. No significant gender or age differences. [b]*CL/F* reduced mild-to-severe renal disease. [c]Mean (SD) following a 16-mg oral dose (tablet) daily for 7 days.

References: Stoukides CA, et al. Candesartan cilexetil: an angiotensin II receptor blocker. *Ann Pharmacother*, **1999**, *33*:1287–1298. van Lier JJ, et al. Absorption, metabolism and excretion of ¹⁴C-candesartan and ¹⁴C-candesartan cilexetil in healthy volunteers. *J Hum Hypertens*, **1997**, *11*(suppl 2):S27–S28. Hubner R, et al. Pharmacokinetics of candesartan after single and repeated doses of candesartan cilexetil in young and elderly healthy volunteers. *J Hum Hypertens*, **1997**, *11*(suppl 2):S19–S25.

(Continued)

TABLE AII-1 ■ PHARMACOKINETIC DATA (*CONTINUED*)

BIOAVAILABILITY (ORAL) (%)	URINARY EXCRETION (%)	BOUND IN PLASMA (%)	CLEARANCE (mL/min/kg)	VOL. DIST. (L/kg)	HALF-LIFE (hours)	PEAK TIME (h)	PEAK CONCENTRATION
Capecitabine[a]							
—	3	<60	145 (34%) L/h/m² [c,d]	270 L/m² [c,d]	C: 1.3 (146%)[c]	C: 0.5 (0.5–1)[e]	C: 6.6 ± 6.0 µg/mL[e]
↓ Food[b]			↓ LD[e]		5FU: 0.72 (16%)[c]	5FU: 0.5 (0.5–2.1)[e]	5FU: 0.47 ± 0.47 µg/mL[e]

[a]Data from male and female patients with cancer. Capecitabine (C) is a prodrug for 5-fluorouracil (5FU; active), listed further in this table. It is well absorbed, and bioactivation is sequential in liver and tumor. [b]AUC for C and 5FU decreased. [c]Geometric mean (coefficient of variation). [d]CL/F and V_{area}/F reported for oral dose. [e]Following 1255 mg/m².

References: Dooley M, et al. Capecitabine. *Drugs*, **1999**, 58:69–76; discussion 77–78. Reigner B, et al. Effect of food on the pharmacokinetics of capecitabine and its metabolites following oral administration in cancer patients. *Clin Cancer Res*, **1998**, 4:941–948.

Carbamazepine[a]							
78 ± 24[b]	3	74 ± 6	0.73 ± 0.3[b]	1.1 ± 0.3[b]	20 ± 9[b]	—	11.2–11.7 (2–18) µg/mL[c]

[a]A metabolite, carbamazepine-10,11-epoxide, is equipotent in animal studies. Its formation is catalyzed primarily by CYP3A and secondarily by CYP2C8. [b]Data from 92 patients receiving carbamazepine oral therapy for treatment of epilepsy and given stable isotope-labeled carbamazepine intravenously. Carbamazepine induces its own metabolism; for a single dose, $CL/F = 0.36 ± 0.07$ mL/min/kg and $t_{1/2} = 36 ± 5$ h. [c]Mean steady-state C_{max} is similar following either dosing of immediate-release carbamazepine four times a day or extended-release carbamazepine once daily (800–1600 mg/d). Concentration following a daily 200-mg oral dose (immediate release) given to adult patients with epilepsy reported.

References: Marino SE, et al. Steady-state carbamazepine pharmacokinetics following oral and stable–labeled intravenous administration in epilepsy patients: effects of race and sex. *Clin Pharmacol Ther*, **2012**, 91:483–488. Garnett WR, et al. Pharmacokinetic evaluation of twice-daily extended release carbamazepine (CBZ) and four-time-daily immediate-release CBZ in patients with epilepsy. *Epilepsia*, **1998**, 39:274–279.

Carbidopa[a]							
—[b]	5.3 ± 2.1	—	18 ± 7[c]	—	~2	2.1 ± 1.0	S: 165 ± 77 ng/mL[d]
							S-CR: 81 ± 28 ng/mL[d]

[a]Data from healthy adult subjects. Combined with levodopa for treatment of Parkinson disease. [b]Absolute bioavailability is unknown, but it is presumably low based on a high value for CL/F. Bioavailability of Sinemet CR (S-CR) is 55% of standard Sinemet (S). [c]CL/F reported for 2 tablets of Sinemet 25/100. [d]Following a single oral dose of 2 tablets Sinemet 25/100 or 1 tablet Sinemet CR 50/200.

Reference: Yeh KC, et al. Pharmacokinetics and bioavailability of Sinemet CR: a summary of human studies. *Neurology*, **1989**, 39:25–38.

Carboplatin[a]							
—	77 ± 5	0	1.5 ± 0.3	0.24 ± 0.03	2 ± 0.2	0.5[b]	39 ± 17 µg/mL[b]
			↓ RD		↑ RD		

[a]Kinetic measurements for ultrafilterable platinum, which essentially is unchanged carboplatin. [b]Following a single 170- to 500-mg/m² IV dose (30-min infusion) given to adult patients with ovarian cancer.

Reference: Gaver RC, et al. The disposition of carboplatin in ovarian cancer patients. *Cancer Chemother Pharmacol*, **1988**, 22:263–270.

Carvedilol[a]							
25	<2	95[b]	8.7 ± 1.7	1.5 ± 0.3	2.2 ± 0.3[c]	1.3 ± 0.3[d]	105 ± 12 ng/mL[d]
S-(−): 15			↓ LD	↑ LD	↑, ↔ LD		
R-(+): 31							
↑ LD							

[a]Racemic mixture: S-(−)-enantiomer responsible for β_1 adrenergic–receptor blockade. R-(+)-and S-(−)-enantiomers have nearly equivalent α_1 receptor blocking activity. [b]R-(+)-enantiomer is more tightly bound than the S-(−)-antipode. [c]Longer $t_{1/2}$ of ~ 6 h has been measured at lower concentrations. [d]Following a 12.5-mg oral dose given twice a day for 2 weeks to healthy young adults.

References: Morgan T. Clinical pharmacokinetics and pharmacodynamics of carvedilol. *Clin Pharmacokinet*, **1994**, 26:335–346. Morgan T, et al. Pharmacokinetics of carvedilol in older and younger patients. *J Hum Hypertens*, **1990**, 4:709–715.

Caspofungin[a]							
—[a]	~2	96.5	0.16 (0.14–0.18)	0.12[b]	9.6 ± 0.8[b]	–	8.7 (7.9–9.6) µg/mL[c]

[a]Caspofungin is available for intravenous administration only. [b]Initial distribution volume and $t_{1/2}$ reported. Exhibits biphasic elimination with a larger V_{area} (0.3–2.1 L/kg) and longer (>25 h) terminal $t_{1/2}$; the terminal phase accounts for a small fraction of the dose. [c]Following a 50-mg, 1-h IV infusion given once daily for 14 days.

References: Stone JA, et al. Single- and multiple-dose pharmacokinetics of caspofungin in healthy men. *Antimicrob Agents Chemother*, **2002**, 46:739–745. Stone JA, et al. Disposition of caspofungin: role of distribution in determining pharmacokinetics in plasma. *Antimicrob Agents Chemother*, **2004**, 48:815–823.

Cefazolin							
>90	80 ± 16	89 ± 2	0.95 ± 0.17	0.19 ± 0.06[a]	2.2 ± 0.02	IM: 1.7 ± 0.7[b]	IV: 237 ± 285 µg/mL[b]
		↓ RD, LD, Neo, Child	↓ RD ↑ Preg	↑ RD, Neo	↑ RD, Neo ↓ Preg, LD		IM: 42 ± 9.5 µg/mL[b]

[a]V_{area} reported. [b]Following a single 1-g IV (model-fitted C_{max}) or IM dose to healthy adults.

Reference: Scheld WM, et al. Moxalactam and cefazolin: comparative pharmacokinetics in normal subjects. *Antimicrob Agents Chemother*, **1981**, 79:613–619.

(Continued)

TABLE AII–1 ■ PHARMACOKINETIC DATA (CONTINUED)

BIOAVAILABILITY (ORAL) (%)	URINARY EXCRETION (%)	BOUND IN PLASMA (%)	CLEARANCE (mL/min/kg)	VOL. DIST. (L/kg)	HALF-LIFE (hours)	PEAK TIME (h)	PEAK CONCENTRATION
Cefdinir							
Cap: 16–21[a]	13–23[b]	89[c]	11–15[d]	1.6–2.1[d]	1.4–1.5	Cap: 3 ± 0.7[e]	Cap: 2.9 ± 1.0 µg/mL[e]
Susp: 25[a]		↓ RD				Susp: 2 ± 0.4[e]	
↓ Iron							Susp: 3.9 ± 0.6 µg/mL[e]

[a]Bioavailability following ingestion of a capsule (Cap) or suspension (Susp) formulated dose. [b]Determined after a single oral dose. [c]Lower plasma protein binding (71%–74%) reported in patients undergoing dialysis. [d]CL/F and V/F reported. [e]Following ingestion of a single 600-mg capsule given to adults or a 14-mg/kg suspension dose given to children (6 months to 12 years). No accumulation after multiple dosing.

References: Guay DR. Pharmacodynamics and pharmacokinetics of cefdinir, an oral extended spectrum cephalosporin. *Pediatr Infect Dis J*, **2000**, 19:S141–S146. PDR58, **2004**, p. 503. Tomino Y, et al. Pharmacokinetics of cefdinir and its transfer to dialysate in patients with chronic renal failure undergoing continuous ambulatory peritoneal dialysis. *Arzneimittelforschung*, **1998**, 48:862–867.

Cefepime[a]							
—	80	16–19	1.8 (1.7–2.5)[b]	0.26 (0.24–0.31)[d]	2.1 (1.3–2.4)[b]	—	65 ± 7 µg/mL[e]
			↓ RD[c]		↑ RD[c]		

[a]Data from healthy adult patients. Available only in parenteral form. [b]Median (range) of reported *CL* and $t_{1/2}$ values from 16 single-dose studies. [c]Mild renal impairment. [d]Median (range) of reported V_{ss} from 6 single-dose studies. [e]Following a 1-g IV dose.

References: Okamoto MP, et al. Cefepime clinical pharmacokinetics. *Clin Pharmacokinet*, **1993**, 25:88–102. Rybak M. The pharmacokinetic profile of a new generation of parenteral cephalosporin. *Am J Med*, **1996**, 100:39S–44S.

Ceftazidime							
—	84 ± 4	21 ± 6	$CL = 1.05CL_{cr} + 0.12$	0.23 ± 0.02	1.6 ± 0.1	IM: 0.7–1.3[a]	IV: 119–146 µg/mL[a]
IM: 91				↑ Aged	↑ RD, Prem, Neo, Aged		IM: 29–39 µg/mL[a]

[a]Range of mean data from different studies following a 1-g bolus IV or IM dose given to healthy adults.

Reference: Balant L, et al. Clinical pharmacokinetics of the third generation cephalosporins. *Clin Pharmacokinet*, **1985**, 10:101–143.

Celecoxib[a]							
—	<3	~97	6.60 ± 1.85[c]	6.12 ± 2.08[c]	11.2 ± 3.47	2.8 ± 1.0[f]	705 ± 268 ng/mL[f]
↑ Food[b]			↓ Aged, LD[d] ↑ RD[e]				

[a]Data from healthy subjects. [b]High-fat meal. Absolute bioavailability is unknown. [c]CL/F and V/F values reported. Cleared primarily by CYP2C9 (polymorphic). [d]CL/F reduced, mild or moderate hepatic impairment. [e]CL/F increased, moderate renal impairment, but unrelated to CL_{cr}. [f]Following a single 200-mg oral dose.

References: Goldenberg MM. Celecoxib, a selective cyclooxygenase-2 inhibitor for the treatment of rheumatoid arthritis and osteoarthritis. *Clin Ther*, **1999**, 21:1497–1513; discussion 1427–1428. PDR54, **2000**, p. 2334.

Cephalexin							
90 ± 9	91 ± 18	14 ± 3	4.3 ± 1.1[a]	0.26 ± 0.03[a]	0.90 ± 0.18	1.4 ± 0.8[a]	28 ± 6.4 µg/mL[a]
			↓ RD		↑ RD		

[a]Following a single 500-mg oral dose given to healthy male adults.

Reference: Spyker DA, et al. Pharmacokinetics of cefaclor and cephalexin: dosage nomograms for impaired renal function. *Antimicrob Agents Chemother*, **1978**, 14:172–177.

(Continued)

TABLE AII–1 ■ PHARMACOKINETIC DATA (*CONTINUED*)

BIOAVAILABILITY (ORAL) (%)	URINARY EXCRETION (%)	BOUND IN PLASMA (%)	CLEARANCE (mL/min/kg)	VOL. DIST. (L/kg)	HALF-LIFE (hours)	PEAK TIME (h)	PEAK CONCENTRATION
Cetirizine[a]							
Rac: >70[b]	Rac: 70.9 ± 7.8	Rac: 89.2 ± 0.4	Rac: 0.74 ± 0.19[c]	Rac: 0.58 ± 0.16[c]	Rac: 9.42 ± 2.4	Rac: 0.9 ± 0.2[g]	Rac: 313 ± 45 ng/mL[g]
Levo: >68[b]	Levo: 68.1 ± 10.2	Levo: 92.0 ± 0.3	Levo: 0.62 ± 0.11[c]	Levo: 0.41 ± 0.10	Levo: 7.8 ± 1.6	Levo: 0.8 ± 0.5[g]	Levo: 270 ± 40 ng/mL[g]
			Rac: ↓ LD,[d] RD,[e] Aged		Rac: ↑ LD, RD, Aged		
			Levo: ↓ RD		Levo: ↑ RD		
			Rac/Levo: ↑ Child[f]		Rac/Levo: ↓ Child		

[a]Data from healthy male and female subjects receiving cetirizine (Rac) or the active *R*-enantiomer, levocetirizine (Levo). [b]Based on recovery of unchanged drug in urine. [c]*CL/F, V_d/F* reported for oral dose. [d]*CL/F* reduced, hepatocellular and cholestatic liver diseases. [e]*CL/F* reduced, moderate-to-severe renal impairment. [f]*CL/F* increased, ages 1–5 years. [g]Following a single 10-mg oral dose of Rac or 5 mg of Levo.

References: Baltes E, et al. Absorption and disposition of levocetirizine, the eutomer of cetirizine, administered alone or as cetirizine to healthy volunteers. *Fundam Clin Pharmacol*, **2001**, *15*:269–277. Benedetti MS, et al. Absorption, distribution, metabolism and excretion of [14C]levocetirizine, the R enantiomer of cetirizine, in healthy volunteers. *Eur J Clin Pharmacol*, **2001**, *57*:571–582. Horsmans Y, et al. Single-dose pharmacokinetics of cetirizine in patients with chronic liver disease. *J Clin Pharmacol*, **1993**, *33*:929–932. Matzke GR, et al. Pharmacokinetics of cetirizine in the elderly and patients with renal insufficiency. *Ann Allergy*, **1987**, *59*:25–30. PDR54, **2000**, p. 2404. Spicák V, et al. Pharmacokinetics and pharmacodynamics of cetirizine in infants and toddlers. *Clin Pharmacol Ther*, **1997**, *61*:325–330. Strolin Benedetti M, et al. Stereoselective renal tubular secretion of levocetirizine and dextrocetirizine, the two enantiomers of the H1-antihistamine cetirizine. *Fundam Clin Pharmacol*, **2008**, *22*:19–23.

Chloroquine[a]							
~80	52–58[b]	S: 66.6 ± 3.3[c] R: 42.7 ± 2.1	3.7–13[b]	132–261[b]	10–24 days[b,d]		IV: 837 ± 248 ng/mL[e]
						IM: 0.25[e]	IM: 57–480 ng/mL[e]
						PO: 3.6 ± 2.0[e]	PO: 76 ± 14 ng/mL[e]

[a]Active metabolite, desethylchloroquine, accounts for 20% ± 3% of urinary excretion; $t_{1/2}$ = 15 ± 6 days. Racemic mixture; kinetic parameters for the two isomers are slightly different, *CL/F* = 136 mL/min and 237 mL/min and *V/F* = 3410 L and 4830 L for the *R*-isomer and *S*-isomer, respectively. [b]Range of mean values from different studies (intravenous administration). [c]Concentrates in red blood cells. Blood-to-plasma concentration ratio for racemate = 9. [d]A longer $t_{1/2}$ (41 ± 14 days) has been reported with extended blood sampling. [e]Following a single 300-mg IV dose (24-min infusion) of chloroquine HCl or a single 300-mg IM or oral dose of chloroquine phosphate given to healthy adults. Effective concentrations against *Plasmodium vivax* and *Plasmodium falciparum* are 15 ng/mL and 30 ng/mL, respectively. Diplopia and dizziness can occur > 250 ng/mL.

References: Krishna S, et al. Pharmacokinetics of quinine, chloroquine and amodiaquine. Clinical implications. *Clin Pharmacokinet*, **1996**, *30*:263–299. White NJ. Clinical pharmacokinetics of antimalarial drugs. *Clin Pharmacokinet*, **1985**, *10*:187–215.

Chlorpromazine[a]							
32 ± 19[b]	<1	95–98	8.6 ± 2.9[c]	21 ± 9[c]	30 ± 7[c]	1–4[d]	25–150 ng/mL[d]
			↓ Child				

[a]Active metabolites, 7-hydroxychlorpromazine ($t_{1/2}$ = 25 ± 15 h) and possibly chlorpromazine *N*-oxide, yield AUCs comparable to the parent drug (single doses). [b]After a single dose. Bioavailability may decrease to ~ 20% with repeated dosing. [c]*CL/F*, V_{area}, and terminal $t_{1/2}$ following intramuscular administration. [d]Following a 100-mg oral dose given twice a day for 33 days to adult patients. Neurotoxicity (tremors and convulsions) occurs at concentrations of 750–1000 ng/mL.

Reference: Dahl SG, et al. Pharmacokinetics of chlorpromazine after single and chronic dosage. *Clin Pharmacol Ther*, **1977**, *21*:437–448.

Chlorthalidone							
64 ± 10	65 ± 9[a]	75 ± 1	0.04 ± 0.01	0.14 ± 0.07	47 ± 22[b]	13.8 ± 6.3[c]	3.7 ± 0.9 µg/mL[c]
			↓ Aged		↑ Aged		

[a]Value is for 50- and 100-mg doses; renal *CL* is decreased at an oral dose of 200 mg, and there is a concomitant decrease in the percentage excreted unchanged. [b]Chlorthalidone is sequestered in erythrocytes. $t_{1/2}$ is longer if blood, rather than plasma, is analyzed. Parameters reported based on blood concentrations. [c]Following a single 50-mg oral dose (tablet) given to healthy male adults.

Reference: Williams RL, et al. Relative bioavailability of chlorthalidone in humans: adverse influence of polyethylene glycol. *J Pharm Sci*, **1982**, *71*:533–535.

Cidofovir[a]							
SC: 98 ± 10	70.1 ± 21.4[b]	<6	2.1 ± 0.6[b]	0.36 ± 0.13[b]	2.3 ± 0.5[b]	—	19.6 ± 7.2 µg/mL[d]
PO: <5			↓ RD[c]		↑ RD		

[a]Data from patients with HIV infection and positive for cytomegalovirus. Cidofovir is activated intracellularly by phosphokinases. For parenteral use. [b]Parameters reported for a dose given in the presence of probenecid. [c]*CL* reduced, mild renal impairment (cleared by high-flux hemodialysis). [d]Following a single 5-mg/kg IV infusion given over 1 h, with concomitant oral probenecid and active hydration.

References: Brody SR, et al. Pharmacokinetics of cidofovir in renal insufficiency and in continuous ambulatory peritoneal dialysis or high-flux hemodialysis. *Clin Pharmacol Ther*, **1999**, *65*:21–28. Cundy KC, et al. Clinical pharmacokinetics of cidofovir in human immunodeficiency virus-infected patients. *Antimicrob Agents Chemother*, **1995**, *39*:1247–1252. PDR54, **2000**, p. 1136. Wachsman M, et al. Pharmacokinetics, safety and bioavailability of HPMPC (cidofovir) in human immunodeficiency virus-infected subjects. *Antiviral Res*, **1996**, *29*:153–161.

(Continued)

TABLE AII–1 ■ PHARMACOKINETIC DATA (*CONTINUED*)

	BIOAVAILABILITY (ORAL) (%)	URINARY EXCRETION (%)	BOUND IN PLASMA (%)	CLEARANCE (mL/min/kg)	VOL. DIST. (L/kg)	HALF-LIFE (hours)	PEAK TIME (h)	PEAK CONCENTRATION
Cinacalcet[a]								
	~20	—[b]	93–97	~18	~17.6	34 ± 9	2–6	10.6 ± 2.8 ng/mL[c]
	↑ Food			↓ LD		↑ LD		

[a]Cinacalcet is a chiral molecule; the *R*-enantiomer is more potent than the *S*-enantiomer and is thought to be responsible for the drug's pharmacological activity. Cinacalcet is metabolized primarily by CYP3A4, CYP2D6, and CYP1A2. [b]Unreported, but presumably negligible. [c]Following a single 75-mg oral dose.

References: Joy MS, et al. Calcimimetics and the treatment of primary and secondary hyperparathyroidism. *Ann Pharmacother,* **2004**, *38*:1871–1880. Kumar GN, et al. Metabolism and disposition of calcimimetic agent cinacalcet HCl in humans and animal models. *Drug Metab Dispos,* **2004**, *32*:1491–1500. Pharmacology and toxicology review of NDA. Application 21-688. U.S. FDA, CDER. Available at: http://www.fda.gov/drugs at fda_docs/nda/2004/21–688.pdf. Sensipar_Pharmr_Pl.pdf. Accessed July 7, 2010.

	BIOAVAILABILITY (ORAL) (%)	URINARY EXCRETION (%)	BOUND IN PLASMA (%)	CLEARANCE (mL/min/kg)	VOL. DIST. (L/kg)	HALF-LIFE (hours)	PEAK TIME (h)	PEAK CONCENTRATION
Ciprofloxacin								
	60 ± 12	50 ± 5	40	7.6 ± 0.8	2.2 ± 0.4[a]	3.3 ± 0.4	0.6 ± 0.2[b]	2.5 ± 1.1 μg/mL[b]
				↓ RD, Aged	↓ Aged	↑ RD		

[a]V_{area} reported. [b]Following a 500-mg oral dose given twice daily for ≥ 3 days to patients with chronic bronchitis or bronchiectasis.

References: Begg EJ, et al. The pharmacokinetics of oral fleroxacin and ciprofloxacin in plasma and sputum during acute and chronic dosing. *Br J Clin Pharmacol,* **2000**, *49*:32–38. Sorgel F, et al. Pharmacokinetic disposition of quinolones in human body fluids and tissues. *Clin Pharmacokinet,* **1989**, *16*(suppl):5–24.

	BIOAVAILABILITY (ORAL) (%)	URINARY EXCRETION (%)	BOUND IN PLASMA (%)	CLEARANCE (mL/min/kg)	VOL. DIST. (L/kg)	HALF-LIFE (hours)	PEAK TIME (h)	PEAK CONCENTRATION
Cisplatin[a]								
	—	23 ± 9	—[b]	6.3 ± 1.2	0.28 ± 0.07	0.53 ± 0.10	—	2 h: 3.4 ± 1.1 μg/mL[c]
								7 h: 1.0 ± 0.4 μg/mL[c]

[a]Early studies measured total platinum, rather than the parent compound; values reported here are for parent drug in seven patients with ovarian cancer (mean CL_{cr} = 66 ± 27 mL/min). [b]Platinum will form a tight complex with plasma proteins (90%). [c]Following a single 100-mg/m² IV dose given as an ~ 2- or 7-h infusion to patients with ovarian cancer.

Reference: Reece PA, et al. Disposition of unchanged cisplatin in patients with ovarian cancer. *Clin Pharmacol Ther,* **1987**, *42*:320–325.

	BIOAVAILABILITY (ORAL) (%)	URINARY EXCRETION (%)	BOUND IN PLASMA (%)	CLEARANCE (mL/min/kg)	VOL. DIST. (L/kg)	HALF-LIFE (hours)	PEAK TIME (h)	PEAK CONCENTRATION
Clarithromycin[a]								
	55 ± 8[b]	36 ± 7[b]	42–50	7.3 ± 1.9[b]	2.6 ± 0.5[b]	3.3 ± 0.5[b]	C: 2.8[c]	C: 2.4 μg/mL[c]
				↓ Aged, RD	↑ LD	↑ Aged, RD, LD	HC: 3[c]	HC: 0.7 μg/mL[c]

[a]Active metabolite, 14(*R*)-hydroxyclarithromycin. [b]At higher doses, metabolic *CL* saturates, resulting in increases in the oral bioavailability, percentage of urinary excretion and $t_{1/2}$ and a decrease in *CL*. [c]Mean data for clarithromycin (C) and 14-hydroxyclarithromycin (HC), following a 500-mg oral dose given twice daily to steady state in healthy adults.

Reference: Chu SY, et al. Absolute bioavailability of clarithromycin after oral administration in humans. *Antimicrob Agents Chemother,* **1992**, *36*:1147–1150. Fraschini F, et al. Clarithromycin clinical pharmacokinetics. *Clin Pharmacokinet,* **1993**, *25*:189–204.

	BIOAVAILABILITY (ORAL) (%)	URINARY EXCRETION (%)	BOUND IN PLASMA (%)	CLEARANCE (mL/min/kg)	VOL. DIST. (L/kg)	HALF-LIFE (hours)	PEAK TIME (h)	PEAK CONCENTRATION
Clindamycin								
	~87[a]	13	93.6 ± 0.2	4.7 ± 1.3	1.1 ± 0.3[b]	2.9 ± 0.7	—	IV: 17.2 ± 3.5 μg/mL[c]
	Topical: 2					↑ Prem		PO: 2.5 μg/mL[d]

[a]Clindamycin hydrochloride given orally. [b]V_{area} reported. [c]Following a 1200-mg IV dose (30-min infusion) of clindamycin phosphate (prodrug) given twice daily to steady state in healthy male adults. [d]Following a single 150-mg oral dose of clindamycin hydrochloride to adults.

References: PDR54, **2000**, p. 2421. Plaisance KI, et al. Pharmacokinetic evaluation of two dosage regimens of clindamycin phosphate. *Antimicrob Agents Chemother,* **1989**, *33*:618–620.

	BIOAVAILABILITY (ORAL) (%)	URINARY EXCRETION (%)	BOUND IN PLASMA (%)	CLEARANCE (mL/min/kg)	VOL. DIST. (L/kg)	HALF-LIFE (hours)	PEAK TIME (h)	PEAK CONCENTRATION
Clonazepam								
	IM: 93 ± 27 PO: 90 ± 22	<1	86 ± 0.5	0.79 ± 0.12	2.6 ± 0.7	38 ± 9	IM: 3.1 ± 1.7[a] PO: 1.7 ± 0.9[a]	IM: 11.0 ± 5.4 ng/mL[a]
								PO: 14.9 ± 3.9 ng/mL[a]

[a] Following a single 2-mg IM or PO dose given to healthy adults. Secondary plasma peaks have been observed after intravenous and intramuscular administration.

Reference: Crevoisier C, et al. Comparative single-dose pharmacokinetics of clonazepam following intravenous, intramuscular and oral administration to healthy volunteers. *Eur Neurol,* **2003**, *49*:173–177.

	BIOAVAILABILITY (ORAL) (%)	URINARY EXCRETION (%)	BOUND IN PLASMA (%)	CLEARANCE (mL/min/kg)	VOL. DIST. (L/kg)	HALF-LIFE (hours)	PEAK TIME (h)	PEAK CONCENTRATION
Clonidine								
	PO: 95	62 ± 11	20	3.1 ± 1.2[a]	2.1 ± 0.4	12 ± 7	PO: 2[b]	PO: 0.8 ng/mL[b]
	TD: 60			↓ RD ↑ Preg		↑ RD	TD: 72[b]	TD: 0.3–0.4 ng/mL[b]

[a]Clonidine is cleared via renal route and CYP2D6-mediated hydroxylation. [b]Mean data following a 0.1-mg oral dose given twice a day to steady state or steady-state concentration (C_{ss}) following a 3.5-cm² transdermal (TD) patch administered to normotensive male adults. Concentrations of 0.2–2 ng/mL are associated with a reduction in blood pressure; > 1 ng/mL will cause sedation and dry mouth.

Reference: Lowenthal DT, et al. Clinical pharmacokinetics of clonidine. *Clin Pharmacokinet,* **1988**, *14*:287–310.

(Continued)

TABLE AII–1 ■ PHARMACOKINETIC DATA (*CONTINUED*)

BIOAVAILABILITY (ORAL) (%)	URINARY EXCRETION (%)	BOUND IN PLASMA (%)	CLEARANCE (mL/min/kg)	VOL. DIST. (L/kg)	HALF-LIFE (hours)	PEAK TIME (h)	PEAK CONCENTRATION
Clopidogrel[a]							
—[b]	—	Clo: 98	—	—	Clo: 4–6	Clo: 0.5–1	Clo[d]
					AM: 0.5[c]	AM: 1.0[d]	EM: 3.8 ± 2.5 ng/mL
							IM: 6.8 ± 3.6 ng/mL
							PM: 18 ± 14 ng/mL
							AM[d]
							EM: 39 ± 15 ng/mL
							IM: 26 ± 11 ng/mL
							PM: 24 ± 6 ng/mL

[a]Clopidogrel (Clo) is a prodrug that is converted to a minor unstable active metabolite (AM) via two sequential cytochrome P450–dependent reactions. The majority of the dose is converted rapidly to an inactive hydrolytic product by esterases. Although multiple P450 isoforms contribute to the formation of AM, blood levels of AM have been associated with the CYP2C19 genotype and phenotype status, with poor metabolizers (PM) exhibiting lower levels, on average, than extensive metabolizers (EM). Formation of AM accounts for ≤ 10% of the administered dose and may be dose dependent due to saturable metabolism. [b]The absolute bioavailability of Clo is unknown. There is one report of food greatly enhancing the systemic exposure of Clo following oral administration. [c]The reported value may represent disappearance of high levels of metabolite formed during first pass and not the terminal $t_{1/2}$, which should be formation limited. [d]Following a single 300-mg loading dose of Clo.

References: Farid NA, et al. Metabolism and disposition of the thienopyridine antiplatelet drugs ticlopidine, clopidogrel, and prasugrel in humans. *J Clin Pharmacol,* **2009,** *50:*126–42 . Kim KA, et al. The effect of CYP2C19 polymorphism on the pharmacokinetics and pharmacodynamics of clopidogrel: A possible mechanism for clopidogrel resistance. *Clin Pharmacol Ther,* **2008,** *84:*236–242. Takahashi M, et al. Quantitative determination of clopidogrel active metabolite in human plasma by LC-MS/MS. *J Pharm Biomed Anal,* **2008,** *48:*1219–1224. Umemura K, et al. The common gene variants of CYP2C19 affect pharmacokinetics and pharmacodynamics in an active metabolite of clopidogrel in healthy subjects. *J Thromb Haemost,* **2008,** *6:*1439–1441.

BIOAVAILABILITY (ORAL) (%)	URINARY EXCRETION (%)	BOUND IN PLASMA (%)	CLEARANCE (mL/min/kg)	VOL. DIST. (L/kg)	HALF-LIFE (hours)	PEAK TIME (h)	PEAK CONCENTRATION
Clorazepate[a]							
N: 91 ± 6[a]	N: <1	N: 97.5	N: 0.17 ± 0.02[b]	N: 1.24 ± 0.09[b]	N: 93 ± 11[b]	N: 0.9 ± 0.01[a,c]	N: 356 ± 27 ng/mL[a,c]
		↓ RD	↓ LD, Obes	↑ Obes	↑ Obes		
					↓ LD		

[a]Clorazepate is essentially a prodrug for nordiazepam (N, desmethyldiazepam). Bioavailability, T_{max}, and C_{max} values for N were derived after oral administration of clorazepate. [b]CL, V_{ss}, and $t_{1/2}$ values are for intravenous nordiazepam. [c]Data for N following a 20-mg oral dose of clorazepate.

References: Greenblatt DJ, et al. Desmethyldiazepam pharmacokinetics: studies following intravenous and oral desmethyldiazepam, oral clorazepate, and intravenous diazepam. *J Clin Pharmacol,* **1988,** *28:*853–859. Ochs HR, et al. Desmethyldiazepam kinetics after intravenous, intramuscular, and oral administration of clorazepate dipotassium. *Klin Wochenschr,* **1982,** *75:*175–180.

BIOAVAILABILITY (ORAL) (%)	URINARY EXCRETION (%)	BOUND IN PLASMA (%)	CLEARANCE (mL/min/kg)	VOL. DIST. (L/kg)	HALF-LIFE (hours)	PEAK TIME (h)	PEAK CONCENTRATION
Clozapine							
55 ± 12	<1	>95	6.1 ± 1.6[a] ↓ Aged ↑ Smk	5.4 ± 3.5	12 ± 4	1.9 ± 0.8[b]	546 ± 307 ng/mL[b]

[a]Clozapine is metabolically cleared, with a major role by CYP1A2 and more minor contributions by CYP3A4, CYP2C19, and CYP2D6. [b]Following titration up to a 150-mg oral dose (tablet) given twice daily for 7 days to adult chronic schizophrenics.

References: Choc MG, et al. Multiple-dose pharmacokinetics of clozapine in patients. *Pharm Res,* **1987,** *4:*402–405. Jann MW, et al. Pharmacokinetics and pharmacodynamics of clozapine. *Clin Pharmacokinet,* **1993,** *24:*161–176.

BIOAVAILABILITY (ORAL) (%)	URINARY EXCRETION (%)	BOUND IN PLASMA (%)	CLEARANCE (mL/min/kg)	VOL. DIST. (L/kg)	HALF-LIFE (hours)	PEAK TIME (h)	PEAK CONCENTRATION
Codeine[a]							
50 ± 7[b]	Negligible	7	11 ± 2[c]	2.6 ± 0.3[c]	2.9 ± 0.7	C: 1.0 ± 0.5[d]	C: 149 ± 60 ng/mL[d]
						M: 1.0 ± 0.4[d]	M: 3.8 ± 2.4 ng/mL[d]

[a]Codeine is metabolized by CYP2D6 (polymorphic) to morphine. Analgesic effect is thought to be due largely to derived morphine. [b]Oral/intramuscular bioavailability reported. [c]CL/F and V_{area}/F reported. [d]Data for codeine (C) and morphine (M) following a 60-mg oral codeine dose given three times daily for seven doses to healthy male adults.

Reference: Quiding H, et al. Plasma concentrations of codeine and its metabolite morphine after single and repeated oral administration. *Eur J Clin Pharmacol,* **1986,** *30:*673–677.

BIOAVAILABILITY (ORAL) (%)	URINARY EXCRETION (%)	BOUND IN PLASMA (%)	CLEARANCE (mL/min/kg)	VOL. DIST. (L/kg)	HALF-LIFE (hours)	PEAK TIME (h)	PEAK CONCENTRATION
Colchicine							
37 ± 12[a]	25–65	39 ± 5	1.8 ± 0.4[b] ↓ RD, LD	5.3 ± 1.2[c]	58 ± 11	1.0 ± 0.6[d]	6.5 ± 1 ng/mL[d]

[a]Decreased bioavailability after multiple doses has been reported. [b]Colchicine is a substrate of P-glycoprotein, which may contribute to its renal and biliary excretion and enterohepatic recirculation. Colchicine is also metabolized by CYP3A4. [c]Colchicine displays multicompartment kinetics with an initial central distribution volume of 0.26 L/kg. [d]Reported after administration of a single 1-mg tablet.

Reference: Ferron GM, et al. Oral absorption characteristics and pharmacokinetics of colchicine in healthy volunteers after single and multiple doses. *Eur J Clin Pharmacol,* **1996,** *36:*874–883.

(*Continued*)

TABLE AII–1 ■ PHARMACOKINETIC DATA (*CONTINUED*)

BIOAVAILABILITY (ORAL) (%)	URINARY EXCRETION (%)	BOUND IN PLASMA (%)	CLEARANCE (mL/min/kg)	VOL. DIST. (L/kg)	HALF-LIFE (hours)	PEAK TIME (h)	PEAK CONCENTRATION
Cyclophosphamide[a]							
74 ± 22	6.5 ± 4.3	13	1.3 ± 0.5	0.78 ± 0.57	7.5 ± 4.0	—	$121 \pm 21 \ \mu M^b$
			↑ Child		↓ Child		
			↓ LD		↑ LD		

[a]Cyclophosphamide is activated to hydroxycyclophosphamide primarily by CYP2C9. The metabolite is further converted to the active alkylating species, phosphoramide mustard ($t_{1/2}$ = 9 h) and nornitrogen mustard (apparent $t_{1/2}$ = 3.3 h). Kinetic parameters are for cyclophosphamide. [b]Following a 600-mg/m^2 IV (bolus) dose given to patients with breast cancer.

References: Grochow LB, et al. Clinical pharmacokinetics of cyclophosphamide. *Clin Pharmacokinet*, **1979**, 4:380–394. Moore MJ, et al. Variability in the pharmacokinetics of cyclophosphamide, methotrexate and 5-fluorouracil in women receiving adjuvant treatment for breast cancer. *Cancer Chemother Pharmacol*, **1994**, 33:472–476.

BIOAVAILABILITY (ORAL) (%)	URINARY EXCRETION (%)	BOUND IN PLASMA (%)	CLEARANCE (mL/min/kg)	VOL. DIST. (L/kg)	HALF-LIFE (hours)	PEAK TIME (h)	PEAK CONCENTRATION
Cyclosporine							
SI: $28 \pm 18^{a,b}$	<1	93 ± 2	$5.7 (0.6–24)^{b,c}$	$4.5 (0.12–15.5)^b$	$10.7 (4.3–53)^b$	NL: $1.5–2.0^d$	NL: 1333 ± 469 ng/mL^d
			↓ LD, Aged	↓ Aged			
			↑ Child	↑ Child	↓ Child		SI: 1101 ± 570 ng/mL^d

[a]Neoral (NL) exhibits a more uniform and slightly greater (125%–150%) relative oral bioavailability than the Sandimmune (SI) formulation. [b]Pharmacokinetic parameters based on measurements in blood with a specific assay. Data from renal transplant patients shown. [c]Metabolized by CYP3A to three major metabolites, which are subsequently biotransformed to numerous secondary and tertiary metabolites. [d]Steady-state C_{max} following a 344 ± 122-mg/d oral dose (divided into two doses) of cyclosporine (NL, soft gelatin capsule) or a 14-mg/kg/d (range 6–22 mg/kg/d) oral dose of cyclosporine (SI) given to adult renal transplant patients in stable condition. Mean trough concentration after NL was 251 ± 116 ng/mL; therapeutic range (trough) is 150–400 ng/mL.

References: Fahr A. Cyclosporin clinical pharmacokinetics. *Clin Pharmacokinet*, **1993**, 24:472–495. PDR54, **2000**, pp. 2034–2035. Pollak R, et al. Cyclosporine bioavailability of Neoral and Sandimmune in white and black de novo renal transplant recipients. Neoral Study Group. *Ther Drug Monit*, **1999**, 27:661–663. Ptachcinski RJ, et al. Cyclosporine kinetics in renal transplantation. *Clin Pharmacol Ther*, **1985**, 38:296–300.

BIOAVAILABILITY (ORAL) (%)	URINARY EXCRETION (%)	BOUND IN PLASMA (%)	CLEARANCE (mL/min/kg)	VOL. DIST. (L/kg)	HALF-LIFE (hours)	PEAK TIME (h)	PEAK CONCENTRATION
Cytarabine[a]							
$<20^b$	11 ± 8	13	13 ± 4	$2.4–2.7^c$	2.6 ± 0.6	—	IV, B: ~5 μg/mL^d
							IV, I: 0.05–0.1 μg/mL^d

[a]Cytarabine is rapidly metabolized by deamination to non-toxic uridine arabinoside. [b]Liposome formulation of cytarabine given intrathecally. Cerebrospinal fluid $t_{1/2}$ = 100–263 h for liposome formulation (compared to 3.4 h for intrathecal dose of free drug). [c]V_{area} reported. [d]C_{max} following a single 200-mg/m^2 IV bolus (IV, B) dose or steady-state plasma concentration following a 112-mg/m^2/d constant-rate IV infusion (IV, I) given to patients with leukemia, malignant melanoma, or solid tumors.

References: Ho DH, et al. Clinical pharmacology of l-β-D-arabinofuranosyl cytosine. *Clin Pharmacol Ther*, **1971**, 72:944–954. Wan SH, et al. Pharmacokinetics of l-β-D-arabinofuranosylcytosine in humans. *Cancer Res*, **1974**, 34:392–397.

BIOAVAILABILITY (ORAL) (%)	URINARY EXCRETION (%)	BOUND IN PLASMA (%)	CLEARANCE (mL/min/kg)	VOL. DIST. (L/kg)	HALF-LIFE (hours)	PEAK TIME (h)	PEAK CONCENTRATION
Dabigatran[a]							
$6 (3–7)^b$	77	35	2.21 ± 0.29	0.98 ± 0.14	7.31 ± 0.74^d	2.7^d	159 ng/mL^e
			↓ RD^c		↑ RD^c		

[a]Dosed orally as dabigatrin etexilate prodrug; conversion to dabigatrin by carboxylesterases. [b]Absolute bioavailability of dabigatrin after an oral dose of dabigatrin etexilate. [c]The CL and $t_{1/2}$ of dabigatrin are altered as a function of the severity of renal disease. [d]$t_{1/2}$ after an intravenous dose reported; much longer values (12–17 h) reported following multiple oral doses. [e]Dabigatrin values following a 150-mg dose of the etexilate prodrug given twice a day to steady state in surgical patients.

References: Blech S, et al. The metabolism and disposition of the oral direct thrombin inhibitor, dabigatrin, in humans. *Drug Metab Disp*, **2008**, 36:386–399. Stangier J. Clinical pharmacokinetics and pharmacodynamics of oral direct thrombin inhibitor dabigatrin etexilate. *Clin Pharmacokinet*, **2008**, 47:285–295. Drugs@FDA: FDA Approved Drug Products (http://www.accessdata.fda.gov/scripts/cder/daf/), Dabigatrin (Pradaxa).

BIOAVAILABILITY (ORAL) (%)	URINARY EXCRETION (%)	BOUND IN PLASMA (%)	CLEARANCE (mL/min/kg)	VOL. DIST. (L/kg)	HALF-LIFE (hours)	PEAK TIME (h)	PEAK CONCENTRATION
Dapagliflozin							
$78 (9)^a$	3^b	91 ± 0.65	$2.96 (23)^{c,d}$	1.69 ± 0.45^d	12.2 ± 5.25	$1 (0.5–2.0)^d$	$68 (32)$ ng/mL^e
			↓ RD^f				

[a]Mean (CV% reported); high-fat meal alters the absorption profile but not the AUC. [b]Calculated as the ratio of dapagliflozin renal clearance/total intravenous clearance. [c]Cleared from blood primarily by UGT1A9-dependent metabolism. [d]Mean (CV% or ± SD) calculated assuming 70-kg body weight. [e]Mean (range or CV%) reported for a 5-mg dose given daily for 7 days. [f]Clearance declines as a function of the severity of renal disease by an unknown mechanism, as the fraction of dapagliflozin excreted unchanged is 3%.

References: Scheen AJ. Pharmacokinetics, pharmacodynamics and clinical use of SGL2 inhibitors in patients with type 2 diabetes mellitus and chronic kidney disease. *Clin Pharmacokinet*, **2015**, 54:691–708. Drugs@FDA: FDA Approved Drug Products (http://www.accessdata.fda.gov/scripts/cder/daf/), Dapagliflozin (Farxiga).

BIOAVAILABILITY (ORAL) (%)	URINARY EXCRETION (%)	BOUND IN PLASMA (%)	CLEARANCE (mL/min/kg)	VOL. DIST. (L/kg)	HALF-LIFE (hours)	PEAK TIME (h)	PEAK CONCENTRATION
Dapsone							
93 ± 8^a	$5–15^b$	73 ± 1	0.60 ± 0.17^c	1.0 ± 0.1	22.4 ± 5.6	SD: 2.1 ± 0.8^d	SD: 1.6 ± 0.4 μg/mL^d
			↑ Neo				MD: 3.3 μg/mL^d

[a]Decreased in severe leprosy by (70%–80%) estimates based on urinary recovery of radioactive dose. [b]Urine pH = 6–7. [c]Undergoes reversible metabolism to a monoacetyl metabolite; the reaction is catalyzed by NAT2 (polymorphic); also undergoes *N*-hydroxylation (CYP3A, CYP2C9). [d]Following a single 100-mg oral dose (SD) or a 100-mg oral dose given once daily to steady state (MD) in healthy adults.

References: Mirochnick M, et al. Pharmacokinetics of dapsone administered daily and weekly in human immunodeficiency virus-infected children. *Antimicrob Agents Chemother*, **1999**, 43:2586–2591. Pieters FA, et al. The pharmacokinetics of dapsone after oral administration to healthy volunteers. *Br J Clin Pharmacol*, **1986**, 22:491–494. Venkatesan K. Clinical pharmacokinetic considerations in the treatment of patients with leprosy. *Clin Pharmacokinet*, **1989**, 16:365–386. Zuidema J, et al. Clinical pharmacokinetics of dapsone. *Clin Pharmacokinet*, **1986**, 11:299–315.

(Continued)

TABLE AII–1 ■ PHARMACOKINETIC DATA (*CONTINUED*)

BIOAVAILABILITY (ORAL) (%)	URINARY EXCRETION (%)	BOUND IN PLASMA (%)	CLEARANCE (mL/min/kg)	VOL. DIST. (L/kg)	HALF-LIFE (hours)	PEAK TIME (h)	PEAK CONCENTRATION
Daptomycin							
—[a]	47 ± 12	92	0.14 ± 0.01	0.096 ± 0.009	7.8 ± 1.0	—	99 ± 12 µg/mL[c]
			↓ RD[b]	↑ RD[b]	↑ RD[b]		

[a]Available for intravenous administration only. [b]Changes reported for patients with severe renal impairment. [c]C_{max} at the end of a 30-min IV infusion of a 6-mg/kg dose given once daily for 7 days. No significant accumulation with multiple dosing.

References: Dvorchik BH, et al. Daptomycin pharmacokinetics and safety following administration of escalating doses once daily to healthy subjects. *Antimicrob Agents Chemother*, **2003**, *47*:1318–1323. Product information: Cubicin™ (daptomycin for injection). Lexington, MA, Cubist Pharmaceuticals, **2004**.

BIOAVAILABILITY (ORAL) (%)	URINARY EXCRETION (%)	BOUND IN PLASMA (%)	CLEARANCE (mL/min/kg)	VOL. DIST. (L/kg)	HALF-LIFE (hours)	PEAK TIME (h)	PEAK CONCENTRATION
Dextroamphetamine[a]							
—[b]	Rac: 14.5[c]	Rac: 23–26	Dextro: 3.4–7.7[d]	Rac: 6.11 ± 0.22	Rac: 3.5–4.2[d]	Dextro:	Dextro: 61 ± 20 ng/mL[f]
			(Acidic urine)		(Acidic urine)	3.1 ± 1.1[f]	
			Dextro: 0.23–1.71[d]		Rac: 14–22[d]		
			(Alkaline urine)		(Alkaline urine)		
					Dextro: 6.8 ± 0.5[e]		
					(Uncontrolled urine pH)		

[a]Amphetamine is available as a racemate (Rac), dextro-isomer (Dextro), and a mixture of the two, in both immediate- and extended-release formulations. Pharmacokinetic data on both racemic and dextroamphetamine are presented. [b]Absolute bioavailability not reported; > 55% based on urine recovery of unchanged drug under acidic urinary pH conditions. [c]Measured under uncontrolled urinary pH condition. Renal *CL* of amphetamine is dependent on urine pH. Acidification of urine results in increased urinary excretion, up to 55%. [d]*CL/F* and $t_{1/2}$ following oral dose to adults is reported. [e]$t_{1/2}$ in children reported. [f]Following a 20-mg immediate-release oral dose given once daily for > 1 week. An extended-release formulation consisting of a mixture of dextroamphetamine and amphetamine salts (Adderall XR) exhibits a delayed T_{max} of ~ 7 h.

References: Busto U, et al. Clinical pharmacokinetics of non-opiate abused drugs. *Clin Pharmacokinet*, **1989**, *16*:1–26. Helligrel ET, et al. Steady-state pharmacokinetics and tolerability of modafinil administered alone or in combination with dextroamphetamine in healthy volunteers. *J Clin Pharmacol*, **2002**, *42*:450–460. McGough JJ, et al. Pharmacokinetics of SLI381 (Adderall XR), an extended-release formulation of Adderall. *J Am Acad Child Adolesc Psychiatry*, **2003**, *42*:684–691.

BIOAVAILABILITY (ORAL) (%)	URINARY EXCRETION (%)	BOUND IN PLASMA (%)	CLEARANCE (mL/min/kg)	VOL. DIST. (L/kg)	HALF-LIFE (hours)	PEAK TIME (h)	PEAK CONCENTRATION
Diazepam[a]							
PO: 100 ± 14	<1	98.7 ± 0.2	0.38 ± 0.06[a]	1.1 ± 0.3	43 ± 13[a]	PO: 1.3 ± 0.2[b]	IV: 400–500 ng/mL[b]
Rectal: 90		↓ RD, LD, Preg, Neo, Aged	↓ LD	↑ LD, Aged	↑ Aged, LD	Rectal: 1.5[b]	PO: 317 ± 27 ng/mL[b]
							Rectal: ~400 ng/mL[b]

[a]Active metabolites, desmethyldiazepam and oxazepam, formed by CYP2C19 (polymorphic) and CYP3A. [b]Range of data following a single 5- to 10-mg IV dose (15- to 30-s bolus) or mean data following a single 10-mg oral or 15-mg rectal dose given to healthy adults. A concentration of 300–400 ng/mL provides an anxiolytic effect, and > 600 ng/mL provides control of seizures.

References: Friedman H, et al. Pharmacokinetics and pharmacodynamics of oral diazepam: effect of dose, plasma concentration, and time. *Clin Pharmacol Ther*, **1992**, *52*:139–150. Greenblatt DJ, et al. Diazepam disposition determinants. *Clin Pharmacol Ther*, **1980**, *27*:301–312. PDR54, **2000**, p. 1012.

BIOAVAILABILITY (ORAL) (%)	URINARY EXCRETION (%)	BOUND IN PLASMA (%)	CLEARANCE (mL/min/kg)	VOL. DIST. (L/kg)	HALF-LIFE (hours)	PEAK TIME (h)	PEAK CONCENTRATION
Dicloxacillin							
50–85	60 ± 7	95.8 ± 0.2 ↓ RD, Aged, LD	1.6 ± 0.3[a] ↓ RD	0.086 ± 0.017 ↑ RD	0.70 ± 0.07 ↑ RD	0.5–1.6[b]	47–91 µg/mL[b]

[a]Possible saturation of renal clearance at doses of 1 to 2 g. Active tubular secretion is mediated by organic anion transporter (OAT). [b]Estimated range of data following a single 2-g oral dose given to healthy (fasted) adults.

References: Nauta EH, Mattie H. Dicloxacillin and cloxacillin: pharmacokinetics in healthy and hemodialysis subjects. *Clin Pharmacol Ther*, **1976**, *20*:98–108.

BIOAVAILABILITY (ORAL) (%)	URINARY EXCRETION (%)	BOUND IN PLASMA (%)	CLEARANCE (mL/min/kg)	VOL. DIST. (L/kg)	HALF-LIFE (hours)	PEAK TIME (h)	PEAK CONCENTRATION
Didanosine							
38 ± 15 ↓ Food[a], Child	36 ± 9	<5	16 ± 7	1.0 ± 0.2	1.4 ± 0.3	B: 0.67 (0.33–1.33)[b] EC: 2.0 (1.0–5.0)[b]	B: 1.5–0.7 µg/mL[b] EC: 0.93 ± 0.43 µg/mL[b]

[a]The magnitude of the food effect may depend on the product used, the type of meal consumed (light vs. high fat) and whether or not didanosine is coadministered with tenofovir, an inhibitor of didanosine metabolism. [b]Following a single 400-mg oral dose of didanosine formulated as a buffered tablet (B) or enteric-coated beads (EC), taken after a fast by patients with HIV infection.

References: Knupp CA, et al. Pharmacokinetics of didanosine in patients with acquired immunodeficiency syndrome or acquired immunodeficiency syndrome-related complex. *Clin Pharmacol Ther*, **1991**, *49*:523–535. Morse GD, et al. Single-dose pharmacokinetics of delavirdine mesylate and didanosine in patients with human immunodeficiency virus infection. *Antimicrob Agents Chemother*, **1997**, *41*:169–174.

(Continued)

APPENDIX II

DESIGN AND OPTIMIZATION OF DOSAGE REGIMENS: PHARMACOKINETIC DATA

TABLE AII–1 ■ PHARMACOKINETIC DATA (CONTINUED)

BIOAVAILABILITY (ORAL) (%)	URINARY EXCRETION (%)	BOUND IN PLASMA (%)	CLEARANCE (mL/min/kg)	VOL. DIST. (L/kg)	HALF-LIFE (hours)	PEAK TIME (h)	PEAK CONCENTRATION
Digoxin							
Tablet 65.7 ± 2.0[a]	81 ± 2[b]	25 ± 5 ↓ RD	2.8 ± 0.35 ↓ RD	7 ± 1 L/kg ↓ RD	39 ± 13	1–3[c]	1.4 ± 0.7 ng/mL[c]
			↑ Neo, Child, Preg	↑ Child	↑ RD, Aged,		

[a]Lanoxin tablets; digoxin solutions, elixirs, and capsules are absorbed more completely. [b]19% of the dose is excreted into bile and into feces following intravenous administration. Intestinal and renal efflux transport of digoxin is mediated by P-glycoprotein and other digoxin specific transporters. [c]Following an oral dose of 0.31 ± 0.19 mg/d in patients with congestive heart failure who exhibited no signs of digitalis toxicity.

References: Birkenfeld AL, et al. Genetic influences on the pharmacokinetics of orally and intravenously administered digoxin as exhibited by monozygotic twins. Clin Pharmacol Ther, **2009**, 86:605–608. Hinderling PH, Hartmann D. Pharmacokinetics of digoxin and main metabolites/derivatives in healthy humans. Ther Drug Monit, **1991**, 13:381–401. Mooradian AD. Digitalis. An update of clinical pharmacokinetics, therapeutic monitoring techniques and treatment recommendations. Clin Pharmacokinet, **1988**, 15:165–179. Smith TW, et al. Digoxin intoxication: the relationship of clinical presentation to serum digoxin concentration. J Clin Invest, **1970**, 49:2377–2386..

| **Diltiazem[a]** | | | | | | | |
| 38 ± 11 | <4 | 78 ± 3 | 11.8 ± 2.2[b] ↓ RD | 3.3 ± 1.2 ↓ RD | 4.4 ± 1.3[c] | 4.0 ± 0.4[d] | 151 ± 46 ng/mL[d] |

[a]Active metabolites, desacetyldiltiazem ($t_{1/2}$ = 9 ± 2 h) and N-desmethyldiltiazem ($t_{1/2}$ = 7.5 ± 1 h). Formation of desmethyl metabolite (major pathway of CL) catalyzed primarily by CYP3A. [b]More than a 2-fold decrease with multiple dosing. [c]$t_{1/2}$ for oral dose is 5–6 h; does not change with multiple dosing. [d]Following a single 120-mg oral dose to healthy adults.

Reference: Echizen H, et al. Clinical pharmacokinetics of verapamil, nifedipine, and diltiazem. Clin Pharmacokinet, **1986**, 11:425–449.

| **Docetaxel[a]** | | | | | | | |
| — | 2.1 ± 0.2 | 94 | 22.6 ± 7.7 L/h/m² ↓ LD[b] | 72 ± 24 L/m² | 13.6 ± 6.1 | — | 2.4 ± 0.9 µg/mL[c] |

[a]Data from male and female patients treated for cancer. Metabolized by CYP3A and excreted into bile. Parenteral administration. [b]Mild-to-moderate liver impairment. [c]Following an intravenous infusion of 85 mg/m² over 1.6 h.

References: Clarke SJ, et al. Clinical pharmacokinetics of docetaxel. Clin Pharmacokinet, **1999**, 36:99–114. Extra JM, et al. Phase I and pharmacokinetic study of Taxotere (RP 56976; NSC 628503) given as a short intravenous infusion. Cancer Res, **1993**, 53:1037–1042. PDR54, **2000**, p. 2578.

| **Donepezil[a]** | | | | | | | |
| —[b] | 10.6 ± 2.7 | 92.6 ± 0.9[c] | 2.90 ± 0.74[d,e] ↓ LD[f] | 14.0 ± 2.42[e] ↑ Aged | 59.7 ± 16.1[e] ↑ Aged | 3–4[g] | 30.8 ± 4.2 ng/mL[g] |

[a]Data from young, healthy male and female subjects. No significant gender differences. [b]Absolute bioavailability is unknown. [c]A fraction bound value of 96% also has been reported. [d]Metabolically cleared by CYP2D6, CYP3A4, and UGT. [e]CL/F, V_{ss}/F, and $t_{1/2}$ reported for oral dose. [f]CL/F reduced slightly (~20%), alcoholic cirrhosis. [g]Following a 5-mg oral dose given once daily to steady state.

References: Ohnishi A, et al. Comparison of the pharmacokinetics of E2020, a new compound for Alzheimer's disease, in healthy young and elderly subjects. J Clin Pharmacol, **1993**, 33:1086–1091. PDR54, **2000**, p. 2323.

Dolutegravir							
—[a]	—	98.9	0.27 (45)[b,c]	0.33 (45)[c]	14.4 (19)[c]	2–3	4.15 (29) µg/mL[e]
↑ Food					↓ HIV-1[d]		

[a]The absolute oral bioavailability is not known. [b]Cleared from blood predominantly by UGT1A1-depedent metabolism. [c]CL/F and V_d/F calculated assuming 70-kg body weight; mean (CV%) reported for single oral dose to healthy volunteers. [d]$t_{1/2}$ of 11–12 h reported for patients with HIV-1 infection. [e]Mean plasma concentration (CV%) in HIV-1 infected patients receiving 50-mg dolutegravir, twice a day, to steady state.

References: Podany AT, et al. Comparative clinical pharmacokinetics and pharmacodynamics of HIV-1 integrase strand transfer inhibitors. Clin Pharmacokinet, **2016**, published on-line, June 17. Drugs@FDA: FDA Approved Drug Products (http://www.accessdata.fda.gov/scripts/cder/daf/), Dolutegravir (Tivicay).

Doxazosin[a]							
Y: 65 ± 14	5	98	Y: 1.26 ± 0.27[b]	Y: 1.0 ± 0.1	20.5 ± 6.1[d,e]	3.9 ± 1.2[e]	67 ± 19 ng/mL[e]
E: 68 ± 16			E: 2.25 ± 1.42[b]	E: 1.7 ± 1.0	XL: 19 ± 4[e]	XL: 9 ± 5[d]	XL: 28 ± 12 ng/mL[d]
XL: F_{rel} = 59 ± 12			↓ LD[c]				

[a]Where indicated, data for young (Y) and elderly (E) normotensive adults are reported. Also reported are data for a gastrointestinal sustained-release device (GITS), Cardura XL (extended release); oral bioavailability relative to standard formulation (F_{rel}). [b]Cleared primarily by cytochrome P450–dependent metabolism. [c]Study in patients with mild-to-moderate liver impairment; AUC increased 43%. [d]Shorter $t_{1/2}$ following intravenous dosing reported; (Y) 10 ± 1 h, (E) 12 ± 5 h; attributed to inadequate duration of blood sampling. [e]Following an 8-mg dose of standard formulation or GITS, once daily, to steady state in young and elderly normotensive volunteers.

References: Chung M, et al. Clinical pharmacokinetics of doxazosin in a controlled-release gastrointestinal therapeutic system (GITS) formulation. Br J Clin Pharmacol, **1999**, 48:678–687. Elliott HL, et al. Pharmacokinetic overview of doxazosin. Am J Cardiol, **1987**, 59:78G–81G. Penenberg D, et al. The effects of hepatic impairment on the pharmacokinetics of doxazosin. J Clin Pharmacol, **2000**, 40:67–73. Vincent J, et al. The pharmacokinetics of doxazosin in elderly normotensives. Br J Clin Pharmacol, **1986**, 21:521–524.

(Continued)

TABLE AII-1 ■ PHARMACOKINETIC DATA (*CONTINUED*)

BIOAVAILABILITY (ORAL) (%)	URINARY EXCRETION (%)	BOUND IN PLASMA (%)	CLEARANCE (mL/min/kg)	VOL. DIST. (L/kg)	HALF-LIFE (hours)	PEAK TIME (h)	PEAK CONCENTRATION
Doxorubicin[a]							
5	<7	76	666 ± 339 mL/min/m²	682 ± 433 L/m²	26 ± 17[b]	—	High[c]
			↓ LD, Obes		↑ LD		D: ~950 ng/mL
			↑ Child				DL: 30–1008 ng/mL
							Low[c]
							D: 6.0 ± 3.2 ng/mL
							DL: 5.0 ± 3.5 ng/mL

[a]Active metabolites; $t_{1/2}$ for doxorubicinol is 29 ± 16 h. [b]Prolonged when plasma bilirubin concentration is elevated; undergoes biliary excretion. [c]Mean data for doxorubicin (D) and range of data for doxorubicinol (DL). High: a single 45- to 72-mg/m² high-dose 1-h IV infusion given to patients with small cell lung cancer. Low: continuous intravenous infusion at a rate of 3.9 ± 0.65 mg/m²/d for 12.4 (2–50) weeks to patients with advanced cancer.

References: Ackland SP, et al. Pharmacokinetics and pharmacodynamics of long-term continuous-infusion doxorubicin. *Clin Pharmacol Ther,* **1989**, *45*:340–347. Piscitelli SC, et al. Pharmacokinetics and pharmacodynamics of doxorubicin in patients with small cell lung cancer. *Clin Pharmacol Ther,* **1993**, *53*:555–561.

BIOAVAILABILITY (ORAL) (%)	URINARY EXCRETION (%)	BOUND IN PLASMA (%)	CLEARANCE (mL/min/kg)	VOL. DIST. (L/kg)	HALF-LIFE (hours)	PEAK TIME (h)	PEAK CONCENTRATION
Doxycycline							
93	41 ± 19	88 ± 5	0.53 ± 0.18	0.75 ± 0.32	16 ± 6	Oral: 1–2[b]	IV: 2.8 µg/mL[b]
		↓ RD[a]	↓ Aged	↓ Aged			PO: 1.7–2 µg/mL[b]

[a]Decreases in plasma protein binding to 71% ± 3% in patients with uremia. [b]Mean data following a single 100-mg IV dose (1-h infusion) or range of mean data following a 100-mg oral dose given to adults.

Reference: Saivin S, et al. Clinical pharmacokinetics of doxycycline and minocycline. *Clin Pharmacokinet,* **1988**, *15*:355–366.

BIOAVAILABILITY (ORAL) (%)	URINARY EXCRETION (%)	BOUND IN PLASMA (%)	CLEARANCE (mL/min/kg)	VOL. DIST. (L/kg)	HALF-LIFE (hours)	PEAK TIME (h)	PEAK CONCENTRATION
Dronabinol (delta-9-tetrahydrocannabinol)[a]							
6 ± 3[b]	<1%	97	8.6 ± 2.1	8.9 ± 4.2	20 ± 4[c]	2.5 (0.5–4)[d]	2.96 ± 1.81 ng/mL[d]

[a]Dronabinol is a synthetic delta-9-tetrahydrocannabinol (delta-9-THC) that is also the active component of cannabis. Dronabinol is extensively metabolized and undergoes extensive first-pass metabolism. It has an active metabolite, 11-OH-delta-9-THC, which is present at about equal concentrations in plasma as THC. Biliary excretion of dronabinol metabolites appears to be a major route of elimination. Only 21% ± 3% of total radioactivity after intravenous dose is recovered in urine, with > 50% recovered in feces. [b]Pulmonary administration of delta-9-THC has a bioavailability of 18%–29%. Bioavailability as high as 20% after oral administration has been reported. [c]Dronabinol elimination is characterized by multicompartment kinetics, with distribution $t_{1/2}$ of 4 h and terminal $t_{1/2}$ of 25–36 h. [d]Following a single oral dose of 5-mg gelatin capsule. Median and range reported for T_{max}.

References: Hunt CA, Jones RT. Tolerance and disposition of tetrahydrocannabinol in man. *J Pharmacol Exp Ther,* **1980**, *215*:35–44. Ohlsson A, et al. Plasma delta-9-tetrahydrocannabinol concentrations and clinical effects after oral and intravenous administration and smoking. *Clin Pharmacol Ther,* **1980**, *28*:409–416. Lemberger L, et al. Delta-9-tetrahydrocannabinol: metabolism and disposition in long-term marihuana smokers. *Science,* **1971**, *173*:72–74.

BIOAVAILABILITY (ORAL) (%)	URINARY EXCRETION (%)	BOUND IN PLASMA (%)	CLEARANCE (mL/min/kg)	VOL. DIST. (L/kg)	HALF-LIFE (hours)	PEAK TIME (h)	PEAK CONCENTRATION
Duloxetine							
42.8 (18.5–71.2)	—	>90	10.6 ± 2.4[b]	7.0 ± 1.3	9.3 (6.4–12)	4.5 (2.5–6)[e]	32.9 ng/mL[e]
↓ Smk[a]			↓ LD,[c] RD[d]		↑ LD[c]		

[a]~30% lower bioavailability based on population pharmacokinetic analysis; no dose adjustment recommended. [b]Cleared primarily by CYP1A2- and CYP2D6-dependent metabolism. [c]A 5-fold increase in oral AUC in patients with moderate liver impairment. [d]A 2-fold increase in oral AUC in patients with end-stage RD receiving intermittent dialysis. [e]Following a single 60-mg oral dose.

References: Lobo ED, et al. In vitro and in vivo evaluations of cytochrome P450 1A2 interactions with duloxetine. *Clin Pharmacokinet,* **2008**, *47*:191–202. Lobo ED, et al. Population pharmacokinetics of orally administered duloxetine in patients: implications for dosing recommendation. *Clin Pharmacokinet,* **2009**, *48*:189–197. Drugs@FDA. Cymbalta label approved on June 16, 2009. Available at: http://www.accessdata.fda.gov/drugsatfda_docs/label/2009/021427s030lbl.pdf. Accessed May 17, 2010.

BIOAVAILABILITY (ORAL) (%)	URINARY EXCRETION (%)	BOUND IN PLASMA (%)	CLEARANCE (mL/min/kg)	VOL. DIST. (L/kg)	HALF-LIFE (hours)	PEAK TIME (h)	PEAK CONCENTRATION
Dutasteride							
60 (40–94)	—	99	—[a,b]	—[b]	840[c]	1 (1–3)[d]	38 ± 13 ng/mL[d]

[a]Dutasteride is cleared primarily by CYP3A-dependent metabolism. [b]CL/F = 0.20–0.37 mL/min/kg, and V/F = 4.3–7.1 L/kg; calculated from steady-state (24-week) serum concentrations. [c]Terminal $t_{1/2}$ reported. [d]Following a 0.5-mg dose given once daily to steady state (24 weeks).

References: Clark RV, et al. Marked suppression of dihydrotestosterone in men with benign prostatic hyperplasia by dutasteride, a dual 5-alpha-reductase inhibitor. *J Clin Endocrinol Metab,* **2004**, *89*:2179–2178. Keam SJ, et al. Dutasteride: a review of its use in the management of prostate disorders. *Drugs,* **2008**, *68*:463–485.

BIOAVAILABILITY (ORAL) (%)	URINARY EXCRETION (%)	BOUND IN PLASMA (%)	CLEARANCE (mL/min/kg)	VOL. DIST. (L/kg)	HALF-LIFE (hours)	PEAK TIME (h)	PEAK CONCENTRATION
Efavirenz[a]							
—[b]	<1	99.5–99.75	3.1 ± 1.2[c,d]	—	SD: 52–76[d]	4.1 ± 1.7[e]	4.0 ± 1.7 µg/mL[e]
↑ Food					MD: 40–55[d]		

[a]Data from patients with HIV infection. No significant gender differences. [b]Absolute oral bioavailability is unknown. Oral AUC increased 50% with high-fat meal. [c]Metabolized primarily by CYP2B6 and to a lesser extent by CYP2A6 and through *N*-glucuronidation. [d]Single-dose (SD) data reported for *CL/F* and both SD and multiple-dose (MD) data for $t_{1/2}$. Efavirenz is a weak inducer of CYP3A4 and its own metabolism. [e]Following a 600-mg oral dose given daily to steady state.

References: Adkins JC, et al. Efavirenz. *Drugs,* **1998**, *56*:1055–1064. PDR54, **2000**, p. 981. Villani P, et al. Pharmacokinetics of efavirenz (EFV) alone and in combination therapy with nelfinavir (NFV) in HIV-1 infected patients. *Br J Clin Pharmacol,* **1999**, *48*:712–715.

(Continued)

TABLE AII–1 ■ PHARMACOKINETIC DATA (*CONTINUED*)

BIOAVAILABILITY (ORAL) (%)	URINARY EXCRETION (%)	BOUND IN PLASMA (%)	CLEARANCE (mL/min/kg)	VOL. DIST. (L/kg)	HALF-LIFE (hours)	PEAK TIME (h)	PEAK CONCENTRATION
Eletriptan							
~50	9 (7–12)[b]	85	5.6 (3.7–6.7)[b,c]	2.0 (1.4–2.4)[b]	4.1 (2.8–5.5)[b]	MF: 0.75–1.5[e]	57–115 ng/mL[f]
						M: 2.0–2.8[e]	
↑ Food[a]			↓ LD[d]		↑ LD[d]		

[a]Systemic exposure increased 20%–30% with high-fat meal. [b]Data from 50-μg/kg IV dose reported; lack of dose proportionality for oral AUC between 20- and 40- or 80-mg doses. [c]Cleared primarily by CYP3A-dependent metabolism. [d]Study in patients with mild-to-moderate hepatic impairment. [e]Following single 20- to 80-mg oral doses; MF: migraine-free period; M: during a migraine attack. [f]Range of mean values from different studies following a single 30-mg oral dose.

References: McCormack PL, et al. Eletriptan: a review of its use in the acute treatment of migraine. *Drugs*, **2006**, *66*:1129–1149. Milton KA, et al. Pharmacokinetics, pharmacodynamics, and safety of the 5-HT(1B/1D) agonist eletriptan following intravenous and oral administration. *J Clin Pharmacol*, **2002**, *42*:528–539. Drugs@FDA. Relpax label approved on December26, 2009. Available at: http://www.accessdata.fda.gov/drugsatfda_docs/label/2002/21016_relpax_lbl.pdf. Accessed May 17, 2010.

Enalapril[a]							
41 ± 15	88 ± 7[b]	50–60	4.9 ± 1.5[c]	1.7 ± 0.7[c]	11[d]	3.0 ± 1.6[e]	69 ± 37 ng/mL[e]
↓ LD	↓ LD		↓ RD, Aged, Neo		↑ RD, LD		
			↑ Child				

[a]Hydrolyzed by esterases to the active metabolite, enalaprilic acid (enalaprilat); except when noted, pharmacokinetic values and disease comparisons are for enalaprilat following oral enalapril administration. [b]For intravenous enalaprilat. [c]*CL/F* and V_{ss}/F after multiple oral doses of enalapril. Values after single intravenous dose of enalaprilat are misleading because binding to ACE leads to a prolonged $t_{1/2}$, which does not represent a significant fraction of the *CL* on multiple dosing. [d]Estimated from the approach to steady state during multiple dosing. [e]Mean values for enalaprilat following a 10-mg enalapril oral dose given daily for 8 days to healthy young adults. The EC_{50} for ACE inhibition is 5–20 ng/mL enalaprilat.

References: Lees KR, et al. Age and the pharmacokinetics and pharmacodynamics of chronic enalapril treatment. *Clin Pharmacol Ther*, **1987**, *41*:597–602. MacFadyen RJ, et al. Enalapril clinical pharmacokinetics and pharmacokinetic-pharmacodynamic relationships. An overview. *Clin Pharmacokinet*, **1993**, *25*:274–282..

Enoxaparin[a]							
SC: 92	—[b]	—	0.3 ± 0.1[c]	0.12 ± 0.04[c]	3.8 ± 1.3[d]	3[e]	ACLM: 145 ± 45 ng/mL[e]
			↓ RD		↑ RD		BCLM: 414 ± 87 ng/mL[e]

[a]Enoxaparin consists of low-molecular-weight heparin fragments of varying lengths. [b]43% is recovered in urine when administered as ⁹⁹Tc-labeled enoxaparin; 8%–20% anti-factor Xa activity. [c]*F, CL/F*, and V_{area}/F for subcutaneous dose measured by functional assay for anti-factor Xa activity. [d]Measured by functional assay of anti-factor Xa activity. Using anti-IIa activity or displacement binding assay gives a $t_{1/2}$ of ~ 1–2 h. [e]Following a single 40-mg SC dose to healthy adult subjects. High-affinity antithrombin III molecules: ACLM, above-critical-length molecules (anti-factor Xa and IIa activity); BCLM, below-critical-length molecules (anti-factor Xa activity).

References: Bendetowicz AV, et al. Pharmacokinetics and pharmacodynamics of a low molecular weight heparin (enoxaparin) after subcutaneous injection, comparison with unfractionated heparin—a three way cross over study in human volunteers. *Thromb Haemost*, **1994**, *71*:305–313. PDR*54*, **2000**, p. 2561.

Eplerenone[a]							
—	7[b]	33–60[c]	2.4[d]	0.6–1.3[d]	4–6	1.8 ± 0.7[e]	1.0 ± 0.3 μg/mL[e]
			↓ LD				

[a]Eplerenone is converted (reversibly) to an inactive ring-open hydroxy acid. Both eplerenone (E) and the hydroxy acid (EA) circulate in plasma; concentrations of E are much higher than EA. Irreversible metabolism is catalyzed predominantly by CYP3A4. Data for E in healthy male and female volunteers reported; no significant gender differences. [b]Recovered as E and EA following an oral dose. [c]Protein binding is concentration dependent over the therapeutic range; lower at the highest concentration. [d]*CL/F* and V_{ss}/F reported. [e]Following a 50-mg oral dose given once daily for 7 days.

References: Clinical Pharmacology and Biopharmaceutics Review. Application 21-437/S-002. U.S. Food and Drug Administration Center for Drug Evaluation and Research. Available at: http://www.accessdata.fda.gov/drugsatfda_docs/nda/2002/21-437_Inspra.cfm. Accessed July 9, **2010**. Cook CS, et al. Pharmacokinetics and metabolism of [14C] eplerenone after oral administration to humans. *Drug Metab Dispos*, **2003**, *31*:1448–1455. Product information: Inspra™ (eplerenone tablets). Chicago, IL, Pfizer, **2004**.

Erlotinib							
59 (55–66)	—[b]	93 (92–95)	1.0 ± 0.4[c,d]	1.2 ± 0.25[f]	13[g]	2–4[h]	1.1–1.7 μg/mL[h]
↑ Food[a]			↑ Smk[e]				

[a]Bioavailability increases to ~ 100% when taken with a meal; not recommended because food effect is highly variable. [b]Likely to be low based on reported bioavailability and low recovery of unchanged drug (<2%) after an oral dose. [c]Erlotinib is cleared primarily by CYP3A- and CYP1A2-dependent metabolism. [d]Calculated from a 25-mg IV dose assuming a 70-kg body weight. [e]Systemic exposure reduced by half compared to nonsmokers. [f]Calculated from a 25-mg IV dose assuming a 70-kg body weight. [g]Median $t_{1/2}$ in a patient population receiving 150-mg orally once daily; a shorter $t_{1/2}$ of 36 h was reported for a single 25-mg IV dose. [h]Following 150-mg oral dose given once daily to steady state.

References: Frohna P, et al. Evaluation of the absolute oral bioavailability and bioequivalence of erlotinib, an inhibitor of the epidermal growth factor receptor tyrosine kinase, in a randomized, crossover study in healthy subjects. *J Clin Pharmacol*, **2006**, *46*:282–290. Lu JF, et al. Clinical pharmacokinetics of erlotinib in patients with solid tumors and exposure-safety relationship in patients with non-small cell lung cancer. *Clin Pharmacol Ther*, **2006**, *80*:136–134. Drugs@FDA. Tarceva NDA and label; label approved on April 27, 2009. Available at: http://www.accessdata.fda.gov/drugsatfda_docs/nda/2004/21-743_Tarceva.cfm. Accessed May 17, 2010.

(Continued)

TABLE AII–1 ■ PHARMACOKINETIC DATA (*CONTINUED*)

BIOAVAILABILITY (ORAL) (%)	URINARY EXCRETION (%)	BOUND IN PLASMA (%)	CLEARANCE (mL/min/kg)	VOL. DIST. (L/kg)	HALF-LIFE (hours)	PEAK TIME (h)	PEAK CONCENTRATION
Erythromycin							
35 ± 25^a	12 ± 7	84 ± 3^c	9.1 ± 4.1^d	0.78 ± 0.44	1.6 ± 0.7	B: $2.1–3.9^e$	B: $0.9–3.5$ µg/mL^e
↓ Preg^b				↑ RD	↑ LD	S: $2–3^e$	S: $0.5–1.4$ µg/mL^e

^{a}Value for enteric-coated erythromycin base. ^{b}Decreased concentrations in pregnancy possibly due to decreased bioavailability (or increased *CL*). ^{c}Erythromycin base. ^{d}Erythromycin is a CYP3A substrate; *N*-demethylation. It also is transported by P-glycoprotein, which may contribute to biliary excretion of parent drug and metabolites. ^{e}Range of mean values from studies following a 250-mg oral enteric-coated free base in a capsule (B) given four times daily for 5–13 doses or a 250-mg film-coated tablet or capsule of erythromycin stearate (S) given four times daily for 5–12 doses.

Reference: Periti P, et al. Clinical pharmacokinetic properties of the macrolide antibiotics. Effects of age and various pathophysiological states (part I). *Clin Pharmacokinet*, **1989**, *16*:193–214.

BIOAVAILABILITY (ORAL) (%)	URINARY EXCRETION (%)	BOUND IN PLASMA (%)	CLEARANCE (mL/min/kg)	VOL. DIST. (L/kg)	HALF-LIFE (hours)	PEAK TIME (h)	PEAK CONCENTRATION
Escitalopram,^{a} Citalopram							
—	Es: 8	Es: 56	Es: $8.8 \pm 3.2^{b,c}$	Es: 15.4 ± 2.4^c	Es: 22 ± 6^b	—	Es: 21 ± 4 ng/mL^d
Rac: 80 ± 13	Rac: 10.5 ± 1.4	Rac: 80	Rac: 4.3 ± 1.2^b	Rac: 12.3 ± 2.3	Rac: 33 ± 4^b	Rac/Es: $4–5^d$	Rac: 50 ± 9 ng/mL^d
			↓ Aged, LD		↑ Aged, LD, RD		

^{a}Escitalopram is the active *S*-enantiomer of racemic citalopram. Pharmacokinetic data after dosing of escitalopram (Es) and citalopram racemate (Rac) are reported. No significant gender differences. Citalopram is metabolized by CYP2C19 (polymorphic) and CYP3A4 to desmethylcitalopram. ^{b}Data from CYP2C19 extensive metabolizers. CYP2C19 poor metabolizers exhibit a lower (~44%) *CL/F* and longer $t_{1/2}$ than extensive metabolizers. ^{c} *CL/F* and *V/F* for Es reported. ^{d}Following a single 40-mg (Rac) or 20-mg (Es) oral dose.

References: Gutierrez MM, et al. An evaluation of the potential for pharmacokinetic interaction between escitalopram and the cytochrome P450 3A4 inhibitor ritonavir. *Clin Ther*, **2003**, *25*:1200–1210. Joffe P, et al. Single-dose pharmacokinetics of citalopram in patients with moderate renal insufficiency or hepatic cirrhosis compared with healthy subjects. *Eur J Clin Pharmacol*, **1998**, *54*:237–242. PDR58, **2004**, pp. 1292, 1302–1303. Sidhu J, et al. Steady-state pharmacokinetics of the enantiomers of citalopram and its metabolites in humans. *Chirality*, **1997**, *9*:686–692. Sindrup SH, et al. Pharmacokinetics of citalopram in relation to the sparteine and the mephenytoin oxidation polymorphisms. *Ther Drug Monit*, **1993**, *15*:11–17.

BIOAVAILABILITY (ORAL) (%)	URINARY EXCRETION (%)	BOUND IN PLASMA (%)	CLEARANCE (mL/min/kg)	VOL. DIST. (L/kg)	HALF-LIFE (hours)	PEAK TIME (h)	PEAK CONCENTRATION
Esomeprazole,^{a} Omeprazole							
Es: 89 (81–98)^b	Es/Rac: <1	Es/Rac: 95–97	Es: 4.1 (3.3–5.0)^{c,d}	Es: 0.25 (0.23–0.27)	Es: 0.9 (0.7–1.0)^d	Es: 1.5 (1.3–1.7)^f	Es: 4.5 (3.8–5.7) µM^f
				Rac: 0.7 ± 0.5			Rac, EM: 0.68 ± 0.43 µM^g
Rac: 53 ± 29^b			Rac: 7.5 ± 2.7^c	Rac: 0.34 ± 0.09		Rac, EM: ~1^g	Rac, PM: 3.5 ± 1.4 µM^g
		↓ LD^e		↑ LD^e		Rac, PM: ~3–4^g	

^{a}Esomeprazole is the *S*-enantiomer of omeprazole. Both esomeprazole (Es) and racemic omeprazole (Rac) are available. Data for both formulations are reported. ^{b}Bioavailability determined after multiple dosing. Lower Es values 64% (54%–75%) reported for single dose. ^{c}The metabolic *CL* of the Es is slower than that of the *R*-enantiomer. Both Es and Rac are metabolized by CYP2C19 (polymorphic) and CYP3A4. *CL* of Es and Rac is decreased and $t_{1/2}$ increased in CYP2C19 poor metabolizers. ^{d}Following a single 40-mg IV dose. *CL* of Es decreases and $t_{1/2}$ of Es increases with multiple dosing. ^{e}Reduced *CL* and increased $t_{1/2}$ in patients with severe (Childs-Pugh class C) hepatic impairment. ^{f}Following a 40-mg oral dose of Es given once daily for 5 days to healthy subjects of unspecified CYP2C19 phenotype. ^{g}Following a 20-mg oral dose of Rac given twice daily for 4 days to healthy subjects phenotyped as CYP2C19 extensive metabolizers (EM) and poor metabolizers (PM).

References: Andersson T, et al. Pharmacokinetic studies with esomeprazole, the (S)-isomer of omeprazole. *Clin Pharmacokinet*, **2001**, *40*:411–426. Chang M, et al. Interphenotype differences in disposition and effect on gastrin levels of omeprazole—suitability of omeprazole as a probe for CYP2C19. *Br J Clin Pharmacol*, **1995**, *39*:511–518.

BIOAVAILABILITY (ORAL) (%)	URINARY EXCRETION (%)	BOUND IN PLASMA (%)	CLEARANCE (mL/min/kg)	VOL. DIST. (L/kg)	HALF-LIFE (hours)	PEAK TIME (h)	PEAK CONCENTRATION
Eszopiclone,^{a} Zopiclone							
—	Es: <10	Es: 52–59	—^{b}	—^{c}	Es: 7.2 ± 1.3	Es: 1 (0.4–2.1)	Es: 39.8 ± 8.6 ng/mL^e
					Es: ↑ LD^d		

^{a}Eszopiclone is the (*S*)-isomer of zopiclone. Pharmacokinetic data after dosing of eszopiclone (Es) is shown. Es is metabolized extensively by CYP3A4 and CYP2E1. ^{b} *CL/F* following a 15-mg oral dose of zopiclone is 2.7 mL/min/kg for Es and 4.4 mL/min/kg for racemic zopiclone. ^{c} *V/F* following a 15-mg oral dose of racemic zopiclone is 1.4 L/kg for eszopiclone and 2 L/kg for racemic zopiclone. ^{d}In patients with severe hepatic impairment. ^{e}Following 3-mg Es given once daily to steady state.

References: Drugs@FDA. Lunesta label approved on April 6, 2009. Available at: http://www.accessdata.fda.gov/drugsatfda_docs/label/2009/021476s012lbl.pdf. Accessed July 9, 2010. Najib J. Eszopiclone, a nonbenzodiazepine sedative-hypnotic agent for the treatment of transient and chronic insomnia. *Clin Ther*, **2006**, *28*:491–516.

BIOAVAILABILITY (ORAL) (%)	URINARY EXCRETION (%)	BOUND IN PLASMA (%)	CLEARANCE (mL/min/kg)	VOL. DIST. (L/kg)	HALF-LIFE (hours)	PEAK TIME (h)	PEAK CONCENTRATION
Ethambutol							
77 ± 8	79 ± 3	6–30	8.6 ± 0.8	1.6 ± 0.2	3.1 ± 0.4	$2–4^a$	$2–5$ µg/mL^a
					↑ RD		

^{a}Following a single 800-mg oral dose to healthy subjects. Concentrations > 10 µg/mL can adversely affect vision. No accumulation with once-a-day dosing in patients with normal renal function.

Reference: Holdiness MR. Clinical pharmacokinetics of the antituberculosis drugs. *Clin Pharmacokinet*, **1984**, *9*:511–544.

(Continued)

TABLE AII–1 ■ PHARMACOKINETIC DATA (*CONTINUED*)

BIOAVAILABILITY (ORAL) (%)	URINARY EXCRETION (%)	BOUND IN PLASMA (%)	CLEARANCE (mL/min/kg)	VOL. DIST. (L/kg)	HALF-LIFE (hours)	PEAK TIME (h)	PEAK CONCENTRATION
Etoposide							
52 ± 17^a	35 ± 5	96 ± 0.4^b	0.68 ± 0.23^c	0.36 ± 0.15	8.1 ± 4.3	1.3	NT: 2.7 µg.mL^d T: 4.7 µg/mL^d
			↓ RD		↑ RD		

[a]Decreases at oral doses greater than 200 mg. [b]Decreases with hyperbilirubinemia. [c]Metabolized by CYP3A; also a substrate for P-glycoprotein. [d]Mean C_{max} for patients without (NT) and with (T) serious hematological toxicity following a 75- to 200-mg/m^2 dose given as a 72-h continuous intravenous infusion.

References: Clark PI, Slevin ML. The clinical pharmacology of etoposide and teniposide. *Clin Pharmacokinet,* **1987,** 12:223–252. McLeod HL, Evans WE. Clinical pharmacokinetics and pharmacodynamics of epipodophyllotoxins. *Cancer Surv,* **1993,** 17:253–268.

Exenatide[a]							
SC: ~100	—	—	8.1^b	0.1^c	1.5 (0.9–2.0)	2 (1–3)^d	821 ± 500 pg/mL^d
			↓ RD		↑ RD		

[a]Exenatide is a synthetic peptide cleared primarily by the kidney through filtration, reabsorption, and proteolytic degradation. [b]CL/F after SC injection reported. [c]V_{area}/F after SC injection reported. [d]Following a 10-µg SC injection.

Reference: Linnebjerg H, et al. Effects of renal impairment on the pharmacokinetics of exenatide. *Br J Clin Pharmacol,* **2007,** 64:317–327.

Ezetimibe[a]							
—	~2	>90^b	6.6^c	1.5^c	28–30^d	1^e	122 ng/mL^e
			↓ Aged, RD, LD				

[a]Ezetimibe is extensively metabolized to a glucuronide, which is more active than ezetimibe in inhibiting cholesterol absorption. Clinical effects are related to the total plasma concentration of ezetimibe and ezetimibe-glucuronide, with ezetimibe concentrations being only 10% of the total. [b]For ezetimibe and ezetimibe-glucuronide. [c]CL/F and a volume for the central compartment (V_c/F) for total (unconjugated and glucuronide conjugate) ezetimibe reported. [d]Ezetimibe undergoes significant enterohepatic recycling, leading to multiple secondary peaks. An effective $t_{1/2}$ is estimated. [e]Total (unconjugated and glucuronide conjugate) ezetimibe following a 10-mg oral dose given once daily for 10 days.

References: Mauro VF, et al. Ezetimibe for management of hypercholesterolemia. *Ann Pharmacother,* **2003,** 37:839–848. Patrick JE, et al. Disposition of the selective cholesterol absorption inhibitor ezetimibe in healthy male subjects. *Drug Metab Dispos,* **2002,** 30:430–437. PDR58, **2004,** pp. 3085–3086.

Famotidine							
37 (20–66)	65–80	20	4.3–6.9^a	1.1–1.4	2.5–4.0	2.3 (1–4)	76–104 ng/mL^c
			↓ Aged, RD, Neo^b		↑ RD		

[a]Cleared primarily by the kidney. Renal clearance after intravenous administration was ~ 4.3 mL/min/kg. [b]The pharmacokinetics of intravenous famotidine were similar in children > 1 year of age and adults. [c]Following a single 40-mg oral dose.

References: Krishna DR, et al. Newer H$_2$-receptor antagonists. Clinical pharmacokinetics and drug interaction potential. *Clin Pharmacokinet,* **1988,** 15:205–215. Maples HD, et al. Famotidine disposition in children and adolescents with chronic renal insufficiency. *J Clin Pharmacol,* **2003,** 43:7–14. Wenning LA, et al. Pharmacokinetics of famotidine in infants. *Clin Pharmacokinet,* **2005,** 44:395–406.

Felodipine[a]							
15 ± 8	<1	99.6 ± 02	12 ± 5^b	10 ± 3	14 ± 4	IR: 0.9 ± 0.4^c	IR: 34 ± 26 nM^c
↑ Food			↓ Aged, LD	↓ LD	↑ Aged	ER: 3.7 ± 0.9^c	ER: 9.1 ± 7.3 nM^c

[a]Racemic mixture; S-(–)-enantiomer is an active Ca^{2+} channel blocker; different enantiomer pharmacokinetics result in S-(–)-enantiomer concentrations about 2-fold higher than those of R-(+)-isomer. [b]Undergoes significant CYP3A-dependent first-pass metabolism in the intestine and liver. [c]Following a 10-mg oral immediate-release (IR) or extended-release (ER) tablet given twice daily to steady state in healthy subjects. EC$_{50}$ for diastolic pressure decrease is 8 ± 5 nM in patients with hypertension.

Reference: Dunselman PH, et al. Felodipine clinical pharmacokinetics. *Clin Pharmacokinet,* **1991,** 21:418–430.

Fenofibrate[a]							
—^{b}	0.1–10^c	>99	0.45^d	0.89^d	20–27	IR: 6–8^e	IR: 8.6 ± 0.9 µg/mL^e
↑ Food			↓ RD		↑ RD	Mic: 4–6^f	Mic: 10.8 ± 0.6 µg/mL^f

[a]Fenofibrate is a prodrug that is hydrolyzed by esterases to fenofibric acid, the pharmacologically active compound. All values reported are for fenofibric acid. [b]Absolute bioavailability is not known. Recovery of radiolabeled dose in urine as fenofibric acid and its glucuronide is 60%. Immediate-release (IR) tablet and micronized (Mic) capsule are bioequivalent. Bioavailability is increased when taken with a standard meal. [c]Recovery following oral dose. [d]CL/F and V/F reported. [e]Following a 300-mg IR fenofibrate tablet given once daily to steady state. [f]Following a 200-mg Mic capsule given once daily to steady state.

References: Balfour JA, et al. Fenofibrate. A review of its pharmacodynamic and pharmacokinetic properties and therapeutic use in dyslipidaemia. *Drugs,* **1990,** 40:260–290. Miller DB, et al. Clinical pharmacokinetics of fibric acid derivatives (fibrates). *Clin Pharmacokinet,* **1998,** 34:155–162.

(Continued)

TABLE AII–1 ■ PHARMACOKINETIC DATA (*CONTINUED*)

BIOAVAILABILITY (ORAL) (%)	URINARY EXCRETION (%)	BOUND IN PLASMA (%)	CLEARANCE (mL/min/kg)	VOL. DIST. (L/kg)	HALF-LIFE (hours)	PEAK TIME (h)	PEAK CONCENTRATION
Fentanyl							
TM: ~50	8	84 ± 2	13 ± 2[a]	4.0 ± 0.4	3.7 ± 0.4	TD: 35 ± 15[b]	TD: 1.4 ± 0.5 ng/mL[b]
			↓ Aged		↑ Aged, Prem	TM: 0.4 (0.3–6)[b]	TM: 0.8 ± 0.3 ng/mL[b]
			↑ Neo				

[a]Metabolically cleared primarily by CYP3A to norfentanyl and hydroxy metabolites. [b]Following a 5-mg transdermal (TD) dose administered at 50 μg/h through a Duragesic system or a single 400-μg transmucosal (TM) dose. Postoperative and intraoperative analgesia occurs at plasma concentrations of 1 ng/mL and 3 ng/mL, respectively. Respiratory depression occurs at > 0.7 ng/mL.

References: Olkkola KT, et al. Clinical pharmacokinetics and pharmacodynamics of opioid analgesics in infants and children. *Clin Pharmacokinet*, **1995**, 28:385–404. *PDR*54, **2000**, pp. 405, 1445.

BIOAVAILABILITY (ORAL) (%)	URINARY EXCRETION (%)	BOUND IN PLASMA (%)	CLEARANCE (mL/min/kg)	VOL. DIST. (L/kg)	HALF-LIFE (hours)	PEAK TIME (h)	PEAK CONCENTRATION
Fexofenadine[a]							
—[b]	12[c]	60–70	9.4 ± 4.2[d,e]	—	14 ± 6[e]	1.3 ± 0.6[g]	286 ± 143 ng/mL[g]
					↑ RD[f]		

[a]Data from healthy adult male subjects. [b]Absolute bioavailability is unknown. [c]Urine recovery of unchanged drug following an oral dose. [d]Negligible metabolism with 85% of a dose recovered in feces unchanged; a substrate for hepatic and intestinal uptake and efflux transporters. [e]CL/F and $t_{1/2}$ reported for oral dose. [f]Mild renal impairment. [g]Following a 60-mg oral dose twice a day to steady state.

References: Markham A, et al. Fexofenadine. *Drugs*, **1998**, 55:269–274; discussion 275–276. Robbins OK, et al. Dose proportionality and comparison of single and multiple dose pharmacokinetics of fexofenadine (MDL 16455) and its enantiomers in healthy male volunteers. *Biopharm Drug Dispos*, **1998**, 19:455–463.

BIOAVAILABILITY (ORAL) (%)	URINARY EXCRETION (%)	BOUND IN PLASMA (%)	CLEARANCE (mL/min/kg)	VOL. DIST. (L/kg)	HALF-LIFE (hours)	PEAK TIME (h)	PEAK CONCENTRATION
Finasteride							
63 ± 21	<1	90	2.3 ± 0.8	1.1 ± 0.2	7.9 ± 2.5	1–2[a]	37 (27–49) ng/mL[a]

[a]Following a single 5-mg oral dose given to healthy adults. Drug accumulates 2-fold with once-daily dosing.

Reference: Sudduth SL, et al. Finasteride: the first 5α-reductase inhibitor. *Pharmacotherapy*, **1993**, 13:309–325; discussion 325–329.

BIOAVAILABILITY (ORAL) (%)	URINARY EXCRETION (%)	BOUND IN PLASMA (%)	CLEARANCE (mL/min/kg)	VOL. DIST. (L/kg)	HALF-LIFE (hours)	PEAK TIME (h)	PEAK CONCENTRATION
Flecainide[a]							
70 ± 11	43 ± 3	61 ± 10	5.6 ± 1.3[b]	4.9 ± 0.4[c]	11 ± 3[b]	~3 (1–6)[d]	458 ± 100 ng/mL[d]
			↓ RD, LD	↑ LD	↑ RD, LD		
			↑ Child		↓ Child		

[a]Racemic mixture; enantiomers exert similar electrophysiological effects. [b]Metabolized by CYP2D6 (polymorphic); except for a shortened elimination $t_{1/2}$ and nonlinear kinetics in extensive metabolizers, CYP2D6 phenotype had no significant influence on flecainide pharmacokinetics or pharmacodynamics. [c]V_{area} reported. [d]Following a 100-mg oral dose given twice daily for 5 days in healthy adults. Similar levels for CYP2D6 extensive and poor metabolizers.

Reference: Funck-Brentano C, et al. Variable disposition kinetics and electrocardiographic effects of flecainide during repeated dosing in humans: contribution of genetic factors, dose-dependent clearance, and interaction with amiodarone. *Clin Pharmacol Ther*, **1994**, 55:256–269.

BIOAVAILABILITY (ORAL) (%)	URINARY EXCRETION (%)	BOUND IN PLASMA (%)	CLEARANCE (mL/min/kg)	VOL. DIST. (L/kg)	HALF-LIFE (hours)	PEAK TIME (h)	PEAK CONCENTRATION
Fluconazole							
>90	75 ± 9	11 ± 1	0.27 ± 0.07	0.60 ± 0.11	32 ± 5	1.7–4.3[a]	10.6 ± 0.4 μg/mL[a]
			↓ RD, Prem	↑ Prem, Neo	↑ LD, RD, Prem		
					↓ Child		

[a]Following a 200-mg oral dose given twice a day for 4 days to healthy adults.

References: Debruyne D, et al. Clinical pharmacokinetics of fluconazole. *Clin Pharmacokinet*, **1993**, 24:10–27. Varhe A, et al. Effect of fluconazole dose on the extent of fluconazole-triazolam interaction. *Br J Clin Pharmacol*, **1996**, 42:465–470.

BIOAVAILABILITY (ORAL) (%)	URINARY EXCRETION (%)	BOUND IN PLASMA (%)	CLEARANCE (mL/min/kg)	VOL. DIST. (L/kg)	HALF-LIFE (hours)	PEAK TIME (h)	PEAK CONCENTRATION
Fludarabine[a]							
—	24 ± 3	—	3.7 ± 1.5	2.4 ± 0.6	10–30	—	0.57 μg/mL[b]
			↓ RD				

[a]Data from adult male and female cancer patients following intravenous administration. Fludarabine is rapidly dephosphorylated to 2-fluoro-arabinoside-A (F-ara-A), transported into cells, and phosphorylated to the active triphosphate metabolite. Pharmacokinetics of F-ara-A are reported. [b]Following a single 25-mg/m² IV dose of fludarabine (30-min infusion); no accumulation after five daily doses.

References: Hersh MR, et al. Pharmacokinetic study of fludarabine phosphate (NSC 312887). *Cancer Chemother Pharmacol*, **1986**, 17:277–280. *PDR*54, **2000**, p. 764. Plunkett W, et al. Fludarabine: pharmacokinetics, mechanisms of action, and rationales for combination therapies. *Semin Oncol*, **1993**, 20:2–12.

BIOAVAILABILITY (ORAL) (%)	URINARY EXCRETION (%)	BOUND IN PLASMA (%)	CLEARANCE (mL/min/kg)	VOL. DIST. (L/kg)	HALF-LIFE (hours)	PEAK TIME (h)	PEAK CONCENTRATION
5-Fluorouracil (5FU)							
28 (0–80)[a]	<10	8–12	16 ± 7	0.25 ± 0.12	11 ± 4 min[b]	—	11.2 μM[c]

[a]Higher *F* with rapid absorption and lower *F* with slower absorption due to a saturable first-pass effect. [b]A much longer (~20 h) terminal $t_{1/2}$ has been reported, representing a slow redistribution of drug from tissues. [c]Steady-state concentration following a continuous intravenous infusion of 300–500 mg/m²/d to cancer patients.

Reference: Diasio RB, et al. Clinical pharmacology of 5-fluorouracil. *Clin Pharmacokinet*, **1989**, 16:215–237.

(Continued)

TABLE AII–1 ■ PHARMACOKINETIC DATA (*CONTINUED*)

	BIOAVAILABILITY (ORAL) (%)	URINARY EXCRETION (%)	BOUND IN PLASMA (%)	CLEARANCE (mL/min/kg)	VOL. DIST. (L/kg)	HALF-LIFE (hours)	PEAK TIME (h)	PEAK CONCENTRATION
Fluoxetine[a]								
—[a]	<2.5	94	$9.6 \pm 6.9^{b,c}$	35 ± 21^d	53 ± 41^e	F: 6–8[f]	F: 200–531 ng/mL[f]
				↓ LD		↑ LD		NF: 103–465 ng/mL[f]

[a]Active metabolite, norfluoxetine; $t_{1/2}$ of norfluoxetine is 6.4 ± 2.5 days (12 ± 2 days in cirrhosis). Absolute bioavailability is unknown, but ≥ 80% of the dose is absorbed. [b]Reduced *CL* with repetitive dosing (~2.6 mL/min/kg) and with increasing dose between 40 and 80 mg. [c]*CL/F* reported; fluoxetine is a CYP2D6 and CYP2C19 substrate and inhibitor but steady-state elimination is not dependent on these enzymes because of autoinhibition. [d]V_{area}/F reported. [e]Longer $t_{1/2}$ with repetitive dosing and with increasing doses. [f]Range of data for fluoxetine (F) and norfluoxetine (NF) following a 60-mg oral dose given once daily for 1 week. NF continues to accumulate for several weeks.

Reference: Altamura AC, et al. Clinical pharmacokinetics of fluoxetine. *Clin Pharmacokinet*, **1994**, 26:201–214.

	BIOAVAILABILITY (ORAL) (%)	URINARY EXCRETION (%)	BOUND IN PLASMA (%)	CLEARANCE (mL/min/kg)	VOL. DIST. (L/kg)	HALF-LIFE (hours)	PEAK TIME (h)	PEAK CONCENTRATION
Fluphenazine[a]								
PO: 2.7 (1.7–4.5)[b]	Negligible	—	10 ± 7^c	11 ± 10	IV: 12 ± 4^d	IR: 2.8 ± 2.1[d]	IR: 2.3 ± 2.1 ng/mL[e]
SC or IM:						IR: 14.4 ± 7.8^d	DN: 24–48[e]	DN: 1.3 ng/mL[e]
3.4 (2.5–5.0)[b]						SR: 20.3 ± 7.9^d	EN: 48–72[e]	EN: 1.1 ng/mL[e]

[a]Data from healthy male and female volunteers. [b]Available in immediate-release (IR) oral and IM formulations and depot SC or IM injections as the enanthate (EN) or decanoate (DN) esters. Geometric mean (90% confidence interval). [c]Fluphenazine is extensively metabolized. [d]Reported $t_{1/2}$ for a single intravenous dose and apparent $t_{1/2}$ following oral administration of IR and slow-release (SR) formulations. Longer apparent $t_{1/2}$s with oral dosing reflect an absorption-limited elimination. [e]Following a single 12-mg oral dose (IR) or 5-mg IM injections of DN and EN.

References: Jann MW, et al. Clinical pharmacokinetics of the depot antipsychotics. *Clin Pharmacokinet*, **1985**, 10:315–333. Koytchev R, et al. Absolute bioavailability of oral immediate and slow release fluphenazine in healthy volunteers. *Eur J Clin Pharmacol*, **1996**, 51:183–187.

	BIOAVAILABILITY (ORAL) (%)	URINARY EXCRETION (%)	BOUND IN PLASMA (%)	CLEARANCE (mL/min/kg)	VOL. DIST. (L/kg)	HALF-LIFE (hours)	PEAK TIME (h)	PEAK CONCENTRATION
Foscarnet								
9 ± 2	95 ± 5	14–17	1.6 ± 0.2	0.35	5.7 ± 0.2	1.4 ± 0.6[b]	86 ± 36 μM[b]
			↓ RD[a]		↑ RD[a]		

[a]In patients with moderate-to-severe renal impairment. [b]Following an 8-mg/kg oral dose given once daily for 8 days to HIV-seropositive patients.

References: Aweeka FT, et al. Effect of renal disease and hemodialysis on foscarnet pharmacokinetics and dosing recommendations. *J Acquir Immune Defic Syndr Hum Retrovirol*, **1999**, 20:350–357. Noormohamed FH, et al. Pharmacokinetics and absolute bioavailability of oral foscarnet in human immunodeficiency virus-seropositive patients. *Antimicrob Agents Chemother*, **1998**, 42:293–297.

	BIOAVAILABILITY (ORAL) (%)	URINARY EXCRETION (%)	BOUND IN PLASMA (%)	CLEARANCE (mL/min/kg)	VOL. DIST. (L/kg)	HALF-LIFE (hours)	PEAK TIME (h)	PEAK CONCENTRATION
Furosemide[a]								
71 ± 35 (43–73)	71 ± 10 (50–80)	98.6 ± 0.4 (96–99)	1.66 ± 0.58 (1.5–3.0)	0.13 ± 0.06 (0.09–0.17)	1.3 ± 0.8 (0.5–2.0)	1.4 ± 0.8[c]	1.7 ± 0.9 μg/mL[c]
		↓ RD, LD	↓ RD,[b] Neo, Prem	↑ Neo, Prem, LD	↑ RD,[b] Prem, Neo, LD		

[a]Data from healthy adult male subjects. No significant gender differences described. Range of mean values from multiple studies shown in parentheses. [b]The renal clearance of furosemide is mediated by renal organic anion transporters (OATs) and multidrug resistance proteins (MRPs). *CL/F* reduced with declining renal function. [c]Following a single 40-mg oral dose (tablet). Ototoxicity occurs at concentrations > 25 μg/mL.

References: Andreasen F, et al. The pharmacokinetics of frusemide are influenced by age. *Br J Clin Pharmacol*, **1983**, 16:391–397. Ponto LL, et al. Furosemide (frusemide). A pharmacokinetic/pharmacodynamic review (part I). *Clin Pharmacokinet*, **1990**, 18:381–408. Waller ES, et al. Disposition and absolute bioavailability of furosemide in healthy males. *J Pharm Sci*, **1982**, 71:1105–1108.

	BIOAVAILABILITY (ORAL) (%)	URINARY EXCRETION (%)	BOUND IN PLASMA (%)	CLEARANCE (mL/min/kg)	VOL. DIST. (L/kg)	HALF-LIFE (hours)	PEAK TIME (h)	PEAK CONCENTRATION
Gabapentin								
60[a]	64–68	<3	1.6 ± 0.3	0.80 ± 0.09	6.5 ± 1.0	2–3[b]	4 μg/mL[b]
			↓ Aged, RD		↑ RD		

[a]Decreases with increasing dose. Value for 300- to 600-mg dose reported. [b]Following an 800-mg oral dose given three times daily to steady state in healthy adults. Efficacious at concentrations > 2 μg/mL.

References: Bialer M. Comparative pharmacokinetics of the newer antiepileptic drugs. *Clin Pharmacokinet*, **1993**, 24:441–452. McLean MJ. Gabapentin. In: Wyllie E, ed. *The Treatment of Epilepsy: Principles and Practice*. 2nd ed. Williams & Wilkins, Baltimore, **1997**, 884–898.

	BIOAVAILABILITY (ORAL) (%)	URINARY EXCRETION (%)	BOUND IN PLASMA (%)	CLEARANCE (mL/min/kg)	VOL. DIST. (L/kg)	HALF-LIFE (hours)	PEAK TIME (h)	PEAK CONCENTRATION
Galantamine[a]								
100 (91–110)	20 (18–22)	18	5.7 (5.0–6.3)[b]	2.6 (2.4–2.9)	5.7 (5.2–6.3)	2.6 ± 1.0[d]	96 ± 29 ng/mL[d]
			↓ RD,[c] LD[c]				

[a]Primarily metabolized by CYP2D6, CYP3A4, and glucuronidation. [b]CYP2D6 poor metabolizers show a lower *CL*, but dose adjustment is not required. [c]In patients with mild-to-moderate hepatic or renal insufficiency. [d]Following a 12-mg oral dose given twice daily for 7 days in healthy, elderly adults.

References: Bickel U, et al. Pharmacokinetics of galanthamine in humans and corresponding cholinesterase inhibition. *Clin Pharmacol Ther*, **1991**, 50:420–428. Huang F, et al. Pharmacokinetic and safety assessments of galantamine and risperidone after the two drugs are administered alone and together. *J Clin Pharmacol*, **2002**, 42:1341–1351. Scott LJ, et al. Galantamine: a review of its use in Alzheimer's disease. *Drugs*, **2000**, 60:1095–1122.

(Continued)

TABLE AII–1 ■ PHARMACOKINETIC DATA (*CONTINUED*)

BIOAVAILABILITY (ORAL) (%)	URINARY EXCRETION (%)	BOUND IN PLASMA (%)	CLEARANCE (mL/min/kg)	VOL. DIST. (L/kg)	HALF-LIFE (hours)	PEAK TIME (h)	PEAK CONCENTRATION
Ganciclovir							
3–5	91 ± 5	1–2	3.4 ± 0.5	1.1 ± 0.2	3.7 ± 0.6	PO: 3.0 ± 0.6[a]	IV: 6.6 ± 1.8 μg/mL[a]
↑ Food			↓ RD		↑ RD		PO: 1.2 ± 0.4 μg/mL[a]

[a]Following a single 6-mg/kg IV dose (1-h infusion) or a 1000-mg oral dose given with food three times a day to steady state.

References: Aweeka FT, et al. Foscarnet and ganciclovir pharmacokinetics during concomitant or alternating maintenance therapy for AIDS-related cytomegalovirus retinitis. *Clin Pharmacol Ther*, **1995**, *57*:403–412. PDR54, **2000**, p. 2624.

BIOAVAILABILITY (ORAL) (%)	URINARY EXCRETION (%)	BOUND IN PLASMA (%)	CLEARANCE (mL/min/kg)	VOL. DIST. (L/kg)	HALF-LIFE (hours)	PEAK TIME (h)	PEAK CONCENTRATION
Gemcitabine[a]							
—	<10	Negligible	37.8 ± 19.4[b]	1.4 ± 1.3[c]	0.63 ± 0.48[c]	—	26.9 ± 9 μM[d]
			↓ Aged		↑ Aged		

[a]Data from patients with leukemia. Rapidly metabolized intracellularly to active di- and triphosphate products; intravenous administration. [b]Weight-normalized *CL* is ~ 25% lower in women, compared to men. [c]V_d and $t_{1/2}$ are reported to increase with long duration of intravenous infusion. [d]Steady-state concentration during a 10-mg/m²/min infusion for 120–640 min.

References: Grunewald R, et al. Gemcitabine in leukemia: a phase I clinical, plasma, and cellular pharmacology study. *J Clin Oncol*, **1992**, *10*:406–413. PDR54, **2000**, p. 1586.

BIOAVAILABILITY (ORAL) (%)	URINARY EXCRETION (%)	BOUND IN PLASMA (%)	CLEARANCE (mL/min/kg)	VOL. DIST. (L/kg)	HALF-LIFE (hours)	PEAK TIME (h)	PEAK CONCENTRATION
Gemfibrozil							
98 ± 1	<1	97	1.7 ± 0.4[a]	0.14 ± 0.03	1.1 ± 0.2	1–2[b]	15–25 μg/mL[b]

[a]Gemfibrozil is mainly cleared by UGT2B7-dependent glucuronidation. Both gemfibrozil and gemfibrozil glucuronide inhibit CYP2C8 and organic anion transport protein (OATP) 1B1 and OATP1B3. [b]Following a 600-mg oral dose given twice daily to steady state.

Reference: Todd PA, et al. Gemfibrozil. A review of its pharmacodynamic and pharmacokinetic properties, and therapeutic use in dyslipidaemia. *Drugs*, **1988**, *36*:314–339.

BIOAVAILABILITY (ORAL) (%)	URINARY EXCRETION (%)	BOUND IN PLASMA (%)	CLEARANCE (mL/min/kg)	VOL. DIST. (L/kg)	HALF-LIFE (hours)	PEAK TIME (h)	PEAK CONCENTRATION
Gentamicin							
IM: ~100	>90	<10	0.62 ± 0.16	0.31 ± 0.10	2–3[b]	IV: 1[c]	IV: 4.9 ± 0.5 μg/mL[c]
			↓ RD[a]	↑ Neo		IM: 0.3–0.75[c]	IM: 5.0 ± 0.4 μg/mL[c]

[a]Gentamicin clearance declines in proportion to a decline in CL_{cr}. [b]Gentamicin has a very long terminal $t_{1/2}$ of 53 ± 25 h (slow release from tissues), which accounts for urinary excretion for up to 3 weeks after a dose. Majority of the dose is eliminated during the distribution phase. [c]Following a single 100-mg IV infusion (1 h) or IM injection given to healthy adults.

References: Schentag JJ, et al. Gentamicin disposition and tissue accumulation on multiple dosing. *J Pharmacokinet Biopharm*, **1977**, *6*:559–577. Regamey C, et al. Comparative pharmacokinetics of tobramycin and gentamicin. *Clin Pharmacol Ther*, **1973**, *14*:396–403.

BIOAVAILABILITY (ORAL) (%)	URINARY EXCRETION (%)	BOUND IN PLASMA (%)	CLEARANCE (mL/min/kg)	VOL. DIST. (L/kg)	HALF-LIFE (hours)	PEAK TIME (h)	PEAK CONCENTRATION
Glimepiride[a]							
~100	<0.5	>99.5	0.62 ± 0.26	0.18	3.4 ± 2.0	2–3[c]	359 ± 98 ng/mL[c]
			↑ RD[b]	↑ RD[b]			

[a]Data from healthy male subjects. No significant gender differences. Glimepiride is metabolized by CYP2C9 to an active (approximately one-third potency) metabolite, Ml. [b]*CL/F*, V_d/F increased and $t_{1/2}$ unchanged, moderate-to-severe renal impairment; presumably mediated through an increase in plasma-free fraction. Ml AUC also increased. [c]Following a single 3-mg oral dose.

References: Badian M, et al. Determination of the absolute bioavailability of glimepiride (HOE 490), a new sulphonylurea. *Int J Clin Pharmacol Ther Toxicol*, **1992**, *30*:481–482. PDR54, **2000**, pp. 1346–1349. Rosenkranz B, et al. Pharmacokinetics and safety of glimepiride at clinically effective doses in diabetic patients with renal impairment. *Diabetologia*, **1996**, *39*:1617–1624.

BIOAVAILABILITY (ORAL) (%)	URINARY EXCRETION (%)	BOUND IN PLASMA (%)	CLEARANCE (mL/min/kg)	VOL. DIST. (L/kg)	HALF-LIFE (hours)	PEAK TIME (h)	PEAK CONCENTRATION
Glipizide							
95	<5	98.4	0.52 ± 0.18[a]	0.17 ± 0.02[a]	3.4 ± 0.7	2.1 ± 0.9[b]	465 ± 139 ng/mL[b]

[a]*CL/F* and V_{ss}/F reported. [b]Following a single 5-mg oral dose (immediate-release tablet) given to healthy young adults. An extended-release formulation exhibits a delayed T_{max} of 6–12 h.

Reference: Kobayashi KA, et al. Glipizide pharmacokinetics in young and elderly volunteers. *Clin Pharm*, **1988**, *7*:224–228.

BIOAVAILABILITY (ORAL) (%)	URINARY EXCRETION (%)	BOUND IN PLASMA (%)	CLEARANCE (mL/min/kg)	VOL. DIST. (L/kg)	HALF-LIFE (hours)	PEAK TIME (h)	PEAK CONCENTRATION
Glyburide							
G: 90–100[a] M: 64–90[a]	Negligible	99.8	1.3 ± 0.5	0.20 ± 0.11	4 ± 1[b]	G: ~1.5[c] M: 2–4[c]	G: 106 ng/mL[c] M: 104 ng/mL[c]
	↓ Aged		↓ LD		↑ LD		

[a]Data for Glynase Prestab micronized tablet (G) and Micronase tablet (M). [b]$t_{1/2}$ for micronized formulation reported. $t_{1/2}$ for nonmicronized formulation is 6 to 10 h, reflecting absorption rate limitation. A long terminal $t_{1/2}$ (15 h), reflecting redistribution from tissues, has been reported. Longer $t_{1/2}$ in patients with type 2 diabetes mellitus also reported. [c]Following a 3-mg oral Glynase tablet taken with breakfast or a 5-mg oral Micronase tablet given to healthy adult subjects.

References: Jonsson A, et al. Slow elimination of glyburide in NIDDM subjects. *Diabetes Care*, **1994**, *17*:142–145. PDR54, **2000**, p. 2457.

(*Continued*)

TABLE AII–1 ■ PHARMACOKINETIC DATA (*CONTINUED*)

BIOAVAILABILITY (ORAL) (%)	URINARY EXCRETION (%)	BOUND IN PLASMA (%)	CLEARANCE (mL/min/kg)	VOL. DIST. (L/kg)	HALF-LIFE (hours)	PEAK TIME (h)	PEAK CONCENTRATION
Haloperidol[a]							
60 ± 18	1	92 ± 2	11.8 ± 2.9[b]	18 ± 7	18 ± 5[b]	IM: 0.6 ± 0.1[c]	IM: 22 ± 18 ng/mL[c]
		↑ LD	↑ Child, Smk		↓ Child	PO: 1.7 ± 3.2[c]	PO: 9.2 ± 4.4 ng/mL[c]
			↓ Aged				

[a]Undergoes reversible metabolism to a less active reduced haloperidol. [b]Represents net *CL* of parent drug; reduced haloperidol *CL* = 10 ± 5 mL · min^{-1}·kg^{-1} and $t_{1/2}$ = 67 ± 51 h. Slow conversion from reduced haloperidol to parent compound probably responsible for prolonged terminal $t_{1/2}$ (70 h) for haloperidol observed with 7-day sampling. [c]Following a single 20-mg oral or 10-mg IM dose. Effective concentrations are 4–20 ng/mL.

Reference: Froemming JS, et al. Pharmacokinetics of haloperidol. *Clin Pharmacokinet*, **1989**, 17:396–423.

Heparin							
—	Negligible	Extensive	1/(0.65 + 0.008D) + 0.1[a]	0.058 ± 0.11[b]	(26 + 0.323D) ± 12 min[a]	3[c]	70 ± 39 ng/mL[c]
		↓ Fem			↓ Smk		

[a]Dose (D) is in international units per kilogram. *CL* and $t_{1/2}$ are dose dependent, perhaps due to saturable metabolism with end-product inhibition. [b]V_{area} reported. [c]Mean of above critical length molecules following a single 5000-IU dose (unfractionated) given by SC injection.

References: Bendetowicz AV, et al. Pharmacokinetics and pharmacodynamics of a low molecular weight heparin (enoxaparin) after subcutaneous injection, comparison with unfractionated heparin—a three way cross over study in human volunteers. *Thromb Haemost*, **1994**, 71:305–313. Estes JW. Clinical pharmacokinetics of heparin. *Clin Pharmacokinet*, **1980**, 5:204–220.

Hydrochlorothiazide							
71 ± 15	>95	58 ± 17	4.9 ± 1.1[a]	0.83 ± 0.31[b]	2.5 ± 0.2[c]	SD: 1.9 ± 0.5[d]	SD: 75 ± 17 ng/mL[d]
			↓ RD, Aged	↓ Aged	↑ RD, Aged	MD: 2[d]	MD: 91 ± 0.2 ng/mL[d]

[a]Renal *CL* reported, which should approximate total plasma *CL*. [b]V_{area} calculated from individual values of renal *CL*, terminal $t_{1/2}$, and fraction of drug excreted unchanged; 70-kg body weight assumed. [c]Longer terminal $t_{1/2}$ of 8 ± 2.8 h has been reported with a corresponding increase in V_{area} to 2.8 L/kg. [d]Following a single (SD) or multiple (MD) 12.5-mg oral dose of hydrochlorothiazide; MD given once daily for 5 days to healthy adults.

References: Beermann B, et al. Pharmacokinetics of hydrochlorothiazide in man. *Eur J Clin Pharmacol*, **1977**, 12:297–303. Jordo L, et al. Bioavailability and disposition of metoprolol and hydrochlorothiazide combined in one tablet and of separate doses of hydrochlorothiazide. *Br J Clin Pharmacol*, **1979**, 7:563–567. O'Grady P, et al. Fosinopril/hydrochlorothiazide: single dose and steady-state pharmacokinetics and pharmacodynamics. *Br J Clin Pharmacol*, **1999**, 48:375–381.

Hydrocodone[a]							
—	EM: 10.2 ± 1.8	—	EM: 11.1 ± 3.57[b]	—	EM: 4.24 ± 0.99[b]	EM: 0.72 ± 0.46[c]	EM: 30 ± 9.4 ng/mL[c]
	PM: 18.1 ± 4.5		PM: 6.54 ± 1.25[b]		PM: 6.16 ± 1.97[b]	PM: 0.93 ± 0.59[c]	PM: 27 ± 5.9 ng/mL[c]

[a]Data from healthy male and female subjects. The metabolism of hydrocodone to hydromorphone (more active) is catalyzed by CYP2D6. Subjects were phenotyped as extensive metabolizers (EM) and poor metabolizers (PM). [b]*CL/F* and $t_{1/2}$ reported for oral dose. [c]Following a 10-mg oral dose (syrup). Maximal hydromorphone concentrations are higher in EM than in PM (5.2 vs. 1.0 ng/mL).

Reference: Otton SV, et al. CYP2D6 phenotype determines the metabolic conversion of hydrocodone to hydromorphone. *Clin Pharmacol Ther*, **1993**, 54:463–472.

Hydromorphone[a]							
PO: 42 ± 23	6	7.1	14.6 ± 7.6	2.90 ± 1.31[b]	2.4 ± 0.6	IV: —[c]	IV: 242 ng/mL[c]
SC: ~80						PO: 1.1 ± 0.2[c]	PO: 11.8 ± 2.6 ng/mL[c]

[a]Data from healthy male subjects. Extensively metabolized. The principal metabolite, 3-glucuronide, accumulates to much higher (27-fold) levels than the parent drug and may contribute to some side effects (not antinociceptive). [b]V_{area} reported. [c]Following a single 2-mg IV (bolus, sample at 3 min) or 4-mg oral dose.

References: Hagen N, et al. Steady-state pharmacokinetics of hydromorphone and hydromorphone-3-glucuronide in cancer patients after immediate and controlled-release hydromorphone. *J Clin Pharmacol*, **1995**, 35:37–44. Moulin DE, et al. Comparison of continuous subcutaneous and intravenous hydromorphone infusions for management of cancer pain. *Lancet*, **1991**, 337:465–468. Parab PV, et al. Pharmacokinetics of hydromorphone after intravenous, peroral and rectal administration to human subjects. *Biopharm Drug Dispos*, **1988**, 9:187–199.

Hydroxychloroquine[a]							
79 ± 12	27	45 ± 3	11.9 ± 5.4[b]	525 ± 158	1056 (624–1512)	3.2 (2–4.5)	46 (34–79) ng/mL[c]

[a]Hydroxychloroquine is marketed as a racemic mixture of *R*- and *S*-hydroxychloroquine. Data for the racemic mixture is reported. [b]Plasma clearance is reported. Hydroxychloroquine accumulates in red blood cells with an average blood-to-plasma ratio of 7.2. Blood clearance of hydroxychloroquine is 1.3 mL/min/kg. [c]Following oral administration of a single 155-mg tablet.

References: Tett SE, et al. A dose-ranging study of the pharmacokinetics of hydroxychloroquine following intravenous administration to healthy volunteers. *Br J Clin Pharmacol*, **1988**, 26:303–313. Tett SE, et al. Bioavailability of hydroxychloroquine tablets in healthy volunteers. *Br J Clin Pharmacol*, **1989**, 27:771–779.

(Continued)

TABLE AII–1 ■ PHARMACOKINETIC DATA (*CONTINUED*)

BIOAVAILABILITY (ORAL) (%)	URINARY EXCRETION (%)	BOUND IN PLASMA (%)	CLEARANCE (mL/min/kg)	VOL. DIST. (L/kg)	HALF-LIFE (hours)	PEAK TIME (h)	PEAK CONCENTRATION
Hydroxyurea[a]							
108 ± 18	35.8 ± 14.2	Negligible	72 ± 17 mL/min/m²[b]	19.7 ± 4.6 L/m²	3.4 ± 0.7	IV: 0.5[c]	IV: 1007 ± 371 µM[c]
(79–108)			(36.2–72.3)		(2.8–4.5)	PO: 1.2 ± 1.2[c]	PO: 794 ± 241 µM[c]

[a]Data from male and female patients treated for solid tumors. A range of mean values from multiple studies is shown in parentheses. [b]Nonrenal elimination of hydroxyurea is thought to exhibit saturable kinetics through a 10- to 80-mg/kg dose range. [c]Following a single 2-g, 30-min IV infusion or oral dose.

References: Gwilt PR, et al. Pharmacokinetics and pharmacodynamics of hydroxyurea. *Clin Pharmacokinet*, **1998**, *34*:347–358. Rodriguez GI, et al. A bioavailability and pharmacokinetic study of oral and intravenous hydroxyurea. *Blood*, **1998**, *91*:1533–1541.

BIOAVAILABILITY (ORAL) (%)	URINARY EXCRETION (%)	BOUND IN PLASMA (%)	CLEARANCE (mL/min/kg)	VOL. DIST. (L/kg)	HALF-LIFE (hours)	PEAK TIME (h)	PEAK CONCENTRATION
Hydroxyzine[a]							
—	—	—	A: 9.8 ± 3.3[b]	A: 16 ± 3[b]	A: 20 ± 4[b]	A: 2.1 ± 0.4[d]	A: 72 ± 11 ng/mL[d]
			C: 32 ± 11[b]	C: 19 ± 9[b]	C: 7.1 ± 2.3[b,c]	C: 2.0 ± 0.9[d]	C: 47 ± 17 ng/mL[d]
				↑ Aged	↑ Aged, LD		

[a]Hydroxyzine is metabolized to an active metabolite, cetirizine. Plasma concentrations of cetirizine exceed those of the parent drug; its $t_{1/2}$ is similar to that of hydroxyzine when formed from parent drug. Hydroxyzine data for adults (A) and children (C) are reported. [b]CL/F, V_d/F, and $t_{1/2}$ after oral dose reported. [c]$t_{1/2}$ increases with increasing age (1–15 years). [d]Following a single 0.7-mg/kg oral dose given to healthy adults and children.

References: Paton DM, et al. Clinical pharmacokinetics of H1-receptor antagonists (the antihistamines). *Clin Pharmacokinet*, **1985**, *10*:477–497. Simons FE, et al. Pharmacokinetics and antipruritic effects of hydroxyzine in children with atopic dermatitis. *J Pediatr*, **1984**, *104*:123–127. Simons FE, et al. The pharmacokinetics and antihistaminic of the HI receptor antagonist hydroxyzine. *J Allergy Clin Immunol*, **1984**, *73*(pt 1):69–75. Simons FE, et al. The pharmacokinetics and pharmacodynamics of hydroxyzine in patients with primary biliary cirrhosis. *J Clin Pharmacol*, **1989**, *29*:809–815. Simons KJ, et al. Pharmacokinetic and pharmacodynamic studies of the H_1-receptor antagonist hydroxyzine in the elderly. *Clin Pharmacol Ther*, **1989**, *45*:9–14.

BIOAVAILABILITY (ORAL) (%)	URINARY EXCRETION (%)	BOUND IN PLASMA (%)	CLEARANCE (mL/min/kg)	VOL. DIST. (L/kg)	HALF-LIFE (hours)	PEAK TIME (h)	PEAK CONCENTRATION
Ibandronate							
0.63	54 ± 13	85	1.8 ± 0.1[a]	5.8 ± 1.5	37 ± 5	1	11 ± 4 ng/mL[c]
			↓ RD[b]				

[a]Cleared primarily by the kidney. [b]Exposure increases 50%–100% in patients with moderate and severe renal impairment. [c]Following a single 50-mg oral dose.

References: Barrett J, et al. Ibandronate: a clinical pharmacological and pharmacokinetic update. *J Clin Pharmacol*, **2004**, *44*:951–965. Bergner R, et al. Renal safety and pharmacokinetics of ibandronate in multiple myeloma patients with or without impaired renal function. *J Clin Pharmacol*, **2007**, *47*:942–950.

BIOAVAILABILITY (ORAL) (%)	URINARY EXCRETION (%)	BOUND IN PLASMA (%)	CLEARANCE (mL/min/kg)	VOL. DIST. (L/kg)	HALF-LIFE (hours)	PEAK TIME (h)	PEAK CONCENTRATION
Ibuprofen[a]							
>80	<1	>99[b]	0.75 ± 0.20[b,c]	0.15 ± 0.02[c]	2 ± 0.5[b]	1.6 ± 0.3[d]	61.1 ± 5.5 µg/mL[d]
				↑ LD			

[a]Racemic mixture. Kinetic parameters for the active S-(+)-enantiomer do not differ from those for the inactive R-(–)-enantiomer when administered separately; $63 \pm 6\%$ of the R-(–)-enantiomer undergoes inversion to the active isomer. [b]Unbound percent of S-(+)-ibuprofen ($0.77 \pm 0.20\%$) is significantly greater than that of R-(–)-ibuprofen ($0.45 \pm 0.06\%$). Binding of each enantiomer is concentration dependent and is influenced by the presence of the optical antipode, leading to nonlinear elimination kinetics. [c]CL/F and V_{ss}/F reported. [d]Following a single 800-mg dose of racemate. A level of 10 µg/mL provides antipyresis in febrile children.

References: Lee EJ, et al. Stereoselective disposition of ibuprofen enantiomers in man. *Br J Clin Pharmacol*, **1985**, *19*:669–674. Lockwood GF, et al. Pharmacokinetics of ibuprofen in man. I. Free and total area/dose relationships. *Clin Pharmacol Ther*, **1983**, *34*:97–103.

BIOAVAILABILITY (ORAL) (%)	URINARY EXCRETION (%)	BOUND IN PLASMA (%)	CLEARANCE (mL/min/kg)	VOL. DIST. (L/kg)	HALF-LIFE (hours)	PEAK TIME (h)	PEAK CONCENTRATION
Idarubicin[a]							
I: 28 ± 4	<5	I: 97	29 ± 10	24.7 ± 5.9	I: 15.2 ± 3.7	I: 5.4 ± 2.4[c]	I: 6.9 ± 0.1 ng/mL[c]
		IL: 94	↓ RD[b]		IL: 41 ± 10 IL: ↑ RD[b]	IL: 7.9 ± 2.3[c]	IL: 22 ± 4 ng/mL[c]

[a]Data from male and female patients with cancer. Idarubicin (I) undergoes rapid metabolism to a major active (equipotent) metabolite, idarubicinol (IL). [b]Mild-to-moderate renal impairment. [c]Following a single 30- to 35-mg/m² oral dose.

References: Camaggi CM, et al. Idarubicin metabolism and pharmacokinetics after intravenous and oral administration in cancer patients: a crossover study. *Cancer Chemother Pharmacol*, **1992**, *30*:307–316. Robert J. Clinical pharmacokinetics of idarubicin. *Clin Pharmacokinet*, **1993**, *24*:275–288. Tamassia V, et al. Pharmacokinetic study of intravenous and oral idarubicin in cancer patients. *Int J Clin Pharmacol Res*, **1987**, *7*:419–426.

BIOAVAILABILITY (ORAL) (%)	URINARY EXCRETION (%)	BOUND IN PLASMA (%)	CLEARANCE (mL/min/kg)	VOL. DIST. (L/kg)	HALF-LIFE (hours)	PEAK TIME (h)	PEAK CONCENTRATION
Ifosfamide[a]							
92	Low: 12–18 High: 53.1 ± 9.6	Negligible	Low: 63 mL/min/m²[b] High: 6.6 ± 1.9 mL/min/m²	Low: — High: 12.5 ± 3.6 L/m² ↑ Aged	Low: 5.6 High: 15.2 ± 3.6 ↑ Aged	Oral: 0.5–1.0[c]	IV: 203 (168–232) µM[c] Oral: 200 (163–245) µM[c]

[a]Data from male and female patients treated for advanced cancers. Administered intravenously with mesna to avoid hemorrhagic cystitis. Exhibits dose-dependent kinetics, with apparent saturation of hepatic metabolism. Parameters reported for a 1.5-g/m² (low) or 5-g/m² (high) IV dose and 1.5-g/m² oral dose. [b]CL reported to increase with daily dosing. [c]Geometric mean (range) following a single 1.5-g/m² IV infusion (30–60 min).

References: Allen LM, Creaven PJ. Pharmacokinetics of ifosfamide. *Clin Pharmacol Ther*, **1975**, *17*:492–498. Kurowski V, et al. Metabolism and pharmacokinetics of oral and intravenous ifosfamide. *J Cancer Res Clin Oncol*, **1991**, *117*:S148–S153. Lind MJ, et al. The effect of age on the pharmacokinetics of ifosfamide. *Br J Clin Pharmacol*, **1990**, *30*: 140–143. PDR54, **2000**, p. 866–867.

(Continued)

TABLE AII–1 ■ PHARMACOKINETIC DATA (*CONTINUED*)

	BIOAVAILABILITY (ORAL) (%)	URINARY EXCRETION (%)	BOUND IN PLASMA (%)	CLEARANCE (mL/min/kg)	VOL. DIST. (L/kg)	HALF-LIFE (hours)	PEAK TIME (h)	PEAK CONCENTRATION
Imatinib								
	98 (87–111)	5	95	3.3 ± 1.2^a	6.2 ± 2.2	22 ± 4	3.3 ± 1.1^b	2.6 ± 0.8 μg/mL^b

[a]Imatinib is metabolically cleared primarily by CYP3A4. [b]Following a 400-mg oral dose given once daily to steady state.

References: Peng B, et al. Absolute bioavailability of imatinib (Glivec) orally versus intravenous infusion. *J Clin Pharmacol,* **2004**, *44*:158–162. Peng B, et al. Pharmacokinetics and pharmacodynamics of imatinib in a phase I trial with chronic myeloid leukemia patients. *J Clin Oncol,* **2004**, *22*:935–942. Product information: Gleevec (imatinib mesylate). Novartis, Basel, Switzerland, **2004**.

	BIOAVAILABILITY (ORAL) (%)	URINARY EXCRETION (%)	BOUND IN PLASMA (%)	CLEARANCE (mL/min/kg)	VOL. DIST. (L/kg)	HALF-LIFE (hours)	PEAK TIME (h)	PEAK CONCENTRATION
Imipenem/Cilastatin[a]								
Imipenem	69 ± 15	<20		2.9 ± 0.3	0.23 ± 0.05	0.9 ± 0.1	IM: $1-2^b$	IV: 60–70 μg/mL^b
	—	↓ Neo		↑ Child	↑ Neo, Child, Prem			IM: 8.2–12 μg/mL^b
				↓ RD				
Cilastatin	70 ± 3	~35		3.0 ± 0.3	0.20 ± 0.03	0.8 ± 0.1		
	—	↓ Neo		↑ Child				
				↓ Neo, RD, Prem	↑ Prem	↑ Neo, Prem		

[a]Formulated as a 1:1 (mg/mg) mixture for parenteral administration; cilastatin inhibits the metabolism of imipenem by the kidney, increasing concentrations of imipenem in the urine; cilastatin does not change imipenem plasma concentrations appreciably. [b]Plasma C_{max} of imipenem following a single 1-g IV infusion over 30 min or 750 mg IM injection.

Reference: Buckley MM, et al. Imipenem/cilastatin. A reappraisal of its antibacterial activity, pharmacokinetic properties and therapeutic efficacy. *Drugs,* **1992**, *44*:408–444.

	BIOAVAILABILITY (ORAL) (%)	URINARY EXCRETION (%)	BOUND IN PLASMA (%)	CLEARANCE (mL/min/kg)	VOL. DIST. (L/kg)	HALF-LIFE (hours)	PEAK TIME (h)	PEAK CONCENTRATION
Indomethacin								
	~100	15 ± 8	90	1.4 ± 0.2^a	0.29 ± 0.04	2.4 ± 0.2^a	~1.3^b	~2.4 μg/mL^b
				↓ Prem, Neo, Aged		↑ Neo, Prem, Aged		

[a]Undergoes significant enterohepatic recycling (~50% after an intravenous dose). [b]Following a single 50-mg oral dose given after a standard breakfast. Effective at concentrations of 0.3–3 μg/mL and toxic at > 5 μg/mL.

Reference: Oberbauer R, et al. Pharmacokinetics of indomethacin in the elderly. *Clin Pharmacokinet,* **1993**, *24*:428–434.

	BIOAVAILABILITY (ORAL) (%)	URINARY EXCRETION (%)	BOUND IN PLASMA (%)	CLEARANCE (mL/min/kg)	VOL. DIST. (L/kg)	HALF-LIFE (hours)	PEAK TIME (h)	PEAK CONCENTRATION
Interferon Alfa[a]								
	I-SC: 90	—[b]	—	I: 2.8 ± 0.6^c	I: 0.40 ± 0.19^c	I: 0.67^d	I: 7.3^e	I: 1.7 (1.2–2.3) ng/mL^e
				PI_{12kD}: 0.17	PI_{12kD}: 0.44–1.04	PI_{12kD}: 37 (22–60)	PI_{12kD}: 22^f	
				PI_{40kD}: 0.014–0.024	PI_{40kD}: 0.11–0.17	PI_{40kD}: 65	PI_{40kD}: 80^g	PI_{12kD}: 0.91 ± 0.33 ng/mL^f
								PI_{40kD}: 26 ± 8.8 ng/mL^g

[a]Values for recombinant interferon alfa-2a (I) and its 40-kDa pegylated form (PI_{40kD}) and the 12-kDa pegylated form of interferon alfa-2b (PI_{12kD}) are reported. [b]I undergoes renal filtration, tubular reabsorption, and proteolytic degradation within tubular epithelial cells. Renal elimination of PI form is much less significant than that of I, although not negligible. [c]CL values in four patients with leukemia were more than halved (1.1 ± 0.3 mL/min/kg), while V_{ss} increased more than 20-fold (9.5 ± 3.5 L/kg) and terminal $t_{1/2}$ changed only minimally (7.3 ± 2.4 h). [d]A terminal $t_{1/2}$ of 5.1 ± 1.6 h accounts for 23% of the CL of I. [e]Following a single 36×10^6 units SC dose of I. [f]Following 4 weeks of multiple SC dosing of 1 μg of PI_{12kD}. [g]Following 48 weekly SC doses of 180 μg/kg of PI_{40kD}.

References: Glue P, et al. Pegylated interferon-2b: pharmacokinetics, pharmacodynamics, safety, and preliminary efficacy data. Hepatitis C Intervention Therapy Group. *Clin Pharmacol Ther,* **2000**, *68*:556–567. Harris JM, et al. Pegylation: a novel process for modifying pharmacokinetics. *Clin Pharmacokinet,* **2001**, *40*:539–551. PDR 54, **2000**, p. 2654. Wills RJ. Clinical pharmacokinetics of interferons. *Clin Pharmacokinet,* **1990**, *19*:390–399.

	BIOAVAILABILITY (ORAL) (%)	URINARY EXCRETION (%)	BOUND IN PLASMA (%)	CLEARANCE (mL/min/kg)	VOL. DIST. (L/kg)	HALF-LIFE (hours)	PEAK TIME (h)	PEAK CONCENTRATION
Interferon Beta								
	SC: 51 ± 17	—[a]	—	13 ± 5^a	2.9 ± 1.8	4.3 ± 2.3	SC: $1-8^b$	IV: 1491 ± 659 IU/mL
								SC: 40 ± 20 IU/mL^b

[a]Undergoes renal filtration, tubular reabsorption, and renal catabolism, but hepatic uptake and catabolism are thought to dominate systemic CL. [b]Concentration at 5 min following a single 90×10^6 IU IV dose or following a single 90×10^6 IU SC dose of recombinant interferon beta-1b.

Reference: Chiang J, et al. Pharmacokinetics of recombinant human interferon-β_{ser} in healthy volunteers and its effect on serum neopterin. *Pharm Res,* **1993**, *10*:567–572.

(Continued)

TABLE AII–1 ■ PHARMACOKINETIC DATA (*CONTINUED*)

BIOAVAILABILITY (ORAL) (%)	URINARY EXCRETION (%)	BOUND IN PLASMA (%)	CLEARANCE (mL/min/kg)	VOL. DIST. (L/kg)	HALF-LIFE (hours)	PEAK TIME (h)	PEAK CONCENTRATION
Irbesartan[a]							
60–80	2.2 ± 0.9	90	2.12 ± 0.54[b]	0.72 ± 0.20	13 ± 6.2	1.2 (0.7–2)[d]	1.3 ± 0.4 μg/mL[d]
			↓ Aged[c]				

[a]Data from healthy male subjects. No significant gender differences. [b]Metabolically cleared by UGT and CYP2C9. [c]*CL/F* reduced; no dose adjustment required. [d]Following a single 50-mg oral dose (capsule).

References: Gillis JC, et al. Irbesartan. A review of its pharmacodynamic and pharmacokinetic properties and therapeutic use in the management of hypertension. *Drugs*, 1997, 54:885–902. PDR54, **2000**, p. 818. Vachharajani NN, et al. Oral bioavailability and disposition characteristics of irbesartan, an angiotensin antagonist, in healthy volunteers. *J Clin Pharmacol*, 1998, 38:702–707.

Irinotecan[a]							
—	I: 16.7 ± 1.0	I: 30–68 SN-38: 95	I: 14.8 ± 4 L/h/m²	I: 150 ± 49 L/m²	I: 10.8 ± 0.5 SN-38: 10.4 ± 3.1	I: 0.5[b] SN-38: ≤1[b]	I: 1.7 ± 0.8 μg/mL[b] SN-38: 26 ± 12 ng/mL[b]

[a]Data from male and female patients with malignant solid tumors. No significant gender differences. Irinotecan (I) is metabolized to an active metabolite, SN-38 (100-fold more potent but with lower blood levels). [b]Following a 125-mg/m² IV infusion over 30 min.

References: Chabot GG, et al. Population pharmacokinetics and pharmacodynamics of irinotecan (CPT-11) and active metabolite SN-38 during phase I trials. *Ann Oncol*, 1995, 6:141–151. PDR54, **2000**, pp. 2412–2413.

Isoniazid[a]							
—[b]	RA: 7 ± 2[c]	~0	RA: 7.4 ± 2.0[d]	0.67 ± 0.15[d]	RA: 1.1 ± 0.1	RA: 1.1 ± 0.5[f]	RA: 5.4 ± 2.0 μg/mL[f]
↓ Food	SA: 29 ± 5[c]		SA: 3.7 ± 1.1[d]		SA: 3.1 ± 1.1	SA: 1.1 ± 0.6[f]	SA: 7.1 ± 1.9 μg/mL[f]
			↓ RD[e]		↑ LD, Neo, RD		

[a]Metabolized by NAT 2 (polymorphic). Data for slow acetylators (SA) and rapid acetylators (RA) reported. [b]It is usually stated that isoniazid is completely absorbed; however, good estimates of possible loss due to first-pass metabolism are not available. Absorption is decreased by food and antacids. [c]Recovery after oral administration; assay includes unchanged drug and acid-labile hydrazones. Higher percentages have been noted after intravenous administration, suggesting significant first-pass metabolism. [d]*CL/F* and V_{ss}/F reported. [e]Decrease in CL_{NR}/F as well as CL_R. [f]Following a single 400-mg oral dose to healthy RAs and SAs.

Reference: Kim YG, et al. Decreased acetylation of isoniazid in chronic renal failure. *Clin Pharmacol Ther*, 1993, 54:612–620.

Isosorbide Dinitrate[a]							
PO: 22 ± 14[b]	<1	28 ± 12	46(38–59)[c]	3.1 (2.2–8.6)	0.7 (0.6–2.0)[c]	IR[d]	IR[d]
↑ LD			↓ LD			ISDN: 0.3 (0.2–0.5)	ISDN: 42 (59–166) nM
SL: 45 ± 16[b]						IS-2-MN: 0.6 (0.2–1.6)	IS-2-MN: 207 (197–335) nM
PC: 33 ± 17[b]						IS-5-MN: 0.7 (0.3–1.9)	IS-5-MN: 900 (790–1080) nM
						SR[d]	SR[d]
						ISDN: ~0	ISDN: ~0
						IS-2-MN: 2.8 (2.7–3.7)	IS-2-MN: 28 (23–33) nM
						IS-5-MN: 5.1 (4.2–6.6)	IS-5-MN: 175 (154–267) nM

[a]Isosorbide dinitrate (ISDN) is metabolized to the 2- and 5-mononitrates (IS-2-MN and IS-5-MN). Both metabolites and the parent compound are thought to be active. Data for the dinitrate are reported except where indicated. [b]Bioavailability calculations from single dose. SL, sublingual; PC, percutaneous. [c]*CL* may be decreased and $t_{1/2}$ prolonged after chronic dosing. [d]Mean (range) for ISDN and IS-2-MN and IS-5-MN following a single 20-mg oral immediate-release (IR) and sustained-release (SR) dose.

References: Abshagen U, et al. Pharmacokinetics and metabolism of isosorbide-dinitrate after intravenous and oral administration. *Eur J Clin Pharmacol*, 1985, 27:637–644. Fung HL. Pharmacokinetics and pharmacodynamics of organic nitrates. *Am J Cardiol*, 1987, 60:4H–9H.

(Continued)

TABLE AII–1 ■ PHARMACOKINETIC DATA (*CONTINUED*)

BIOAVAILABILITY (ORAL) (%)	URINARY EXCRETION (%)	BOUND IN PLASMA (%)	CLEARANCE (mL/min/kg)	VOL. DIST. (L/kg)	HALF-LIFE (hours)	PEAK TIME (h)	PEAK CONCENTRATION
Isosorbide 5-Mononitrate (Isosorbide Nitrate)[a]							
93 ± 13	<5	0	1.80 ± 0.24	0.73 ± 0.09	4.9 ± 0.8	1–1.5[b]	314–2093 nM[b]

[a]Active metabolite of isosorbide dinitrate. [b]Following a 20-mg oral dose given by asymmetric dosing (0 and 7 h) for 4 days.

Reference: Abshagen UW. Pharmacokinetics of isosorbide mononitrate. *Am J Cardiol*, **1992**, *70*:61G–66G.

Isotretinoin[a]							
40[b]	Negligible	>99	5.5 (0.9–11.1)[c]	5 (1–32)[c]	17 (5–167)[d]	I: 4.5 ± 3.4[e]	I: 208 ± 92 ng/mL[e]
↑ Food						4-oxo: 6.8 ± 6.5[e]	4-oxo: 473 ± 171 ng/mL[e]

[a]Isotretinoin (I) is eliminated through metabolic oxidations catalyzed by multiple CYPs (2C8, 2C9, 3A4, and 2B6). The 4-oxo-isotretinoin metabolite (4-oxo) is active and found at higher concentrations than parent drug at steady state. [b]Bioavailability when taken with food is reported. [c]CL/F and V/F reported. [d]4-oxo has an apparent mean $t_{1/2}$ of 29 ± 6 h. [e]Values for I and 4-oxo following a 30-mg oral dose given once daily to steady state.

References: Larsen FG, et al. Pharmacokinetics and therapeutic efficacy of retinoids in skin diseases. *Clin Pharmacokinet*, **1992**, *23*:42–61. Nulman I, et al. Steady-state pharmacokinetics of isotretinoin and its 4-oxo metabolite: Implications for fetal safety. *J Clin Pharmacol*, **1998**, *38*:926–930. Wiegand UW, et al. Pharmacokinetics of oral isotretinoin. *J Am Acad Dermatol*, **1998**, *39*:S8–S12.

Itraconazole[a]							
55	<1	99.8	5.1[c]	10.7[d]	21 ± 6[e]	3–5[f]	649 ± 289 ng/mL[f]
↑ Food[b]							

[a]Metabolized predominantly by CYP3A4 to an active metabolite, hydroxyitraconazole, and other sequential metabolites. [b]Relative to oral dosing with food. [c]Blood CL is 9.4 mL/min/kg. CL is concentration dependent; the value given is nonsaturable range. K_m = 330 ± 200 ng/mL, V_{max} = 2.2 ± 0.8 pg · mL^{-1} · min^{-1} · kg^{-1}. Apparent CL/F at steady state reported to be 5.4 mL · min^{-1} · kg^{-1}. [d]V_{area} reported. Follows multicompartment kinetics. Does not appear to be concentration dependent. [e]$t_{1/2}$ for the nonsaturable concentration range. $t_{1/2}$ at steady state reported to be 64 h. [f]Following a 200-mg oral dose given daily for 4 days to adults.

References: Heykants J, et al. The pharmacokinetics of itraconazole in animals and man. An overview. In: Fromtling RA, ed. *Recent Trends in the Discovery, Development and Evaluation of Antifungal Agents*. Prous Science, Barcelona, **1987**, 223–249. Jalava KM, et al. Itraconazole greatly increases plasma concentrations and effects of felodipine. *Clin Pharmacol Ther*, **1997**, *61*:410–415.

Ivermectin[a]							
—	<1	93.1 ± 0.2	2.06 ± 0.81[b,c]	9.91 ± 2.67[c]	56.5 ± 7.5[c]	4.7 ± 0.5[d]	38.2 ± 5.8 ng/mL[d]

[a]Data from male and female patients treated for onchocerciasis. [b]Metabolized by hepatic enzymes and excreted into bile. [c]CL/F, V_{area}/F, and $t_{1/2}$ reported for oral dose. Terminal $t_{1/2}$ reported. [d]Following a single 150-μg/kg oral dose (tablet).

References: Okonkwo PO, et al. Protein binding and ivermectin estimations in patients with onchocerciasis. *Clin Pharmacol Ther*, **1993**, *53*:426–430. PDR54, **2000**, p. 1886.

Labetalol[a]							
30–65[b]	—	50	23 ± 5.3[c]	9.9 ± 1.5	8.3–1.4[d]	1.5–2[e]	274 ± 99 ng/mL[e]
↑ LD			↑ Preg				

[a]The clinical formulation of labetalol consists of equal proportions of 4 optical isomers. [b]Bioavailability correlates with age and increases with age. Bioavailability appears to increase with multiple dosing. [c]Labetalol is mainly cleared by glucuronidation. [d]Labetalol displays multicompartment distribution kinetics with an initial $t_{1/2}$ of 1.4 h. [e]Following a 200-mg dose of labetalol every 12 h for 5 doses.

Reference: Lalonde RL, et al. Labetalol pharmacokinetics and pharmacodynamics: evidence of stereoselective disposition. *Clin Pharmacol. Ther.* **1990**, *48*:509–519. McNeil JJ, Louis WJ. Clinical pharmacokinetics of labetalol. *Clin Pharmacokinet*, **1984**, *9*:157–167.

Lamivudine[a]							
86 ± 17	49–85	<36	4.95 ± 0.75	1.30 ± 0.36	9.11 ± 5.09	0.5–1.5[d]	1.0 (0.86–1.2) μg/mL[d]
			↓ RD[b] ↑ Child[c]		↑ RD[b] ↓ Child[c]		

[a]Data from healthy male subjects. No significant gender differences. [b]CL/F decreased, moderate and severe renal impairment. [c]Weight-normalized CL/F increased, children < 12 years of age. [d]Following a single 100-mg oral dose (tablet).

References: Yuen GJ, et al. Pharmacokinetics, absolute bioavailability, and absorption characteristics of lamivudine. *J Clin Pharmacol*, **1995**, *35*:1174–1180. Heald AE, et al. Pharmacokinetics of lamivudine in human immunodeficiency virus-infected patients with renal dysfunction. *Antimicrob Agents Chemother*, **1996**, *40*:1514–1519. Johnson MA, et al. Clinical pharmacokinetics of lamivudine. *Clin Pharmacokinet*, **1999**, *36*:41–66. PDR 54, **2000**, p. 1172.

Lamotrigine[a]							
97.6 ± 4.8	10	56	0.38–0.61[b,c,d]	0.87–1.2	24–35[c]	2.2 ± 1.2[g]	2.5 ± 0.4 μg/mL[g]
			↓ LD,[e] RD[f]		↑ LD,[e] RD[f]		

[a]Data from healthy adults and patients with epilepsy. Range of mean values from multiple studies reported. [b]Lamotrigine is eliminated primarily by glucuronidation. The parent-metabolite pair may undergo enterohepatic recycling. [c]CL/F increases slightly with multiple-dose therapy. [d]CL/F increased and $t_{1/2}$ decreased in patients receiving enzyme-inducing anticonvulsant drugs. [e]CL/F reduced, moderate-to-severe hepatic impairment. [f]CL/F reduced, severe RD. [g]Following a single 200-mg oral dose to healthy adults.

References: Chen C, et al. Pharmacokinetics of lamotrigine in children in the absence of other antiepileptic drugs. *Pharmacotherapy*, **1999**, *19*:437–441. Garnett WR. Lamotrigine: pharmacokinetics. *J Child Neurol*, **1997**, *12*(suppl 1):S10–S15. PDR 54, **2000**, p. 1209. Wootton R, et al. Comparison of the pharmacokinetics of lamotrigine in patients with chronic renal failure and healthy volunteers. *Br J Clin Pharmacol*, **1997**, *43*:23–27.

(Continued)

TABLE AII-1 ■ PHARMACOKINETIC DATA (*CONTINUED*)

BIOAVAILABILITY (ORAL) (%)	URINARY EXCRETION (%)	BOUND IN PLASMA (%)	CLEARANCE (mL/min/kg)	VOL. DIST. (L/kg)	HALF-LIFE (hours)	PEAK TIME (h)	PEAK CONCENTRATION
Leflunomide[a]							
—[b]	Negligible	99.4	0.012[c]	0.18 (0.09–0.44)[c]	377 (336–432)[d]	6–12[e]	35 µg/mL[e]
			↓ RD	↑ RD	↑ RD		

[a]Leflunomide is a prodrug that is converted almost completely (~95%) to an active metabolite A77-1726 [2-cyano-3-hydroxy-N-(4-trifluoromethylphenyl)-crotonamide]. All pharmacokinetic data reported are for the active metabolite. [b]Absolute bioavailability is not known; parent drug/metabolite is well absorbed. [c]Apparent *CL/F* and *V/F* in healthy volunteers reported. Both parameters are a function of the bioavailability of leflunomide and the extent of its conversion to A77-1726. [d]In patients with RA. [e]Following a 20-mg oral dose given once daily to steady state in patients with RA.

Reference: Rozman B. Clinical pharmacokinetics of leflunomide. *Clin Pharmacokinet*, **2002**, *41*:421–430.

Levetiracetam[a]							
~100	66	<10	0.96	0.5–0.7	7 ± 1	0.5–1.0[e]	~10 µg/mL[e]
			↓ RD,[b] Aged, LD[c]		↑ RD,[b] Aged		
			↑ Child[d]				

[a]Data from healthy adults and patients with epilepsy. No significant gender differences. [b]*CL/F* reduced, mild renal impairment (cleared by hemodialysis). [c]*CL/F* reduced, severe hepatic impairment. [d]*CL/F* increased, 6–12 years of age. [e]Following a single 500-mg dose given to healthy adults.

Reference: PDR55, **2001**, pp. 3206–3207.

Levodopa[a]							
41 ± 16	<1	—	23 ± 4	1.7 ± 0.4	1.4 ± 0.4		
↑ Aged			↓ Aged	↓ Aged			
86 ± 19[b]			9 ± 1[b]	0.9 ± 0.2[b]	1.5 ± 0.3[b]	Y: 1.4 ± 0.7[c]	Y: 1.7 ± 0.8 µg/mL[c]
			↓ Aged	↓ Aged		E: 1.4 ± 0.7[c]	E: 1.9 ± 0.6 µg/mL[c]

[a]Naturally occurring precursor to dopamine. [b]Values obtained with concomitant carbidopa (inhibitor of dopa decarboxylase). [c]Following a single 125-mg oral dose of levodopa given with carbidopa (100-mg 1 h before and 50-mg 6 h after levodopa) in young (Y) and elderly (E) subjects.

Reference: Robertson DR, et al. The effect of age on the pharmacokinetics of levodopa administered alone and in the presence of carbidopa. *Br J Clin Pharmacol*, **1989**, *28*:61–69.

Levofloxacin[a]							
99 ± 10	61–87	24–38	2.52 ± 0.45	1.36 ± 0.21	7 ± 1	1.6 ± 0.8[c]	4.5 ± 0.9 µg/mL[c]
			↓ RD[b]		↑ RD[b]		

[a]Data from healthy adult male subjects. Gender and age differences related to renal function. [b]*CL/F* reduced, mild-to-severe renal impairment (not cleared by hemodialysis). [c]Following a single 500-mg oral dose. No significant accumulation with once-daily dosing.

References: Chien SC, et al. Pharmacokinetic profile of levofloxacin following once-daily 500-milligram oral or intravenous doses. *Antimicrob Agents Chemother*, **1997**, *41*: 2256–2260. Fish DN, et al. The clinical pharmacokinetics of levofloxacin. *Clin Pharmacokinet*, **1997**, *32*:101–119. PDR54, **2000**, p. 2157.

Lidocaine[a]							
37 ± 9	2 ± 1	69 ± 2	13.5 ± 3.1[b]	2.3 ± 0.6	2.6 ± 4	0.78 ± 0.4	9.8 ± 3.3 µmol/L[c]
			↓ LD		↑ LD		

[a]Lidocaine has an active metabolite monoethylglycylxylidide MEGX that has 33%–83% of the antiarrhythmic activity of lidocaine and it can also cause convulsions. [b]Lidocaine is cleared mainly by CYP1A2 and CYP3A4 dependent metabolism. [c]Following a 750-mg single oral dose given twice daily to steady state in cancer patients.

References: Olkkola KT, et al. The effect of erythromycin and fluvoxamine on the pharmacokinetics of intravenous lidocaine. *Anesth Analg*, **2005**, *100*:1352–1356. Perucca E, Richens A. Reduction of oral bioavailability of lignocaine by induction of first pass metabolism in epileptic patients. *Br J Clin Pharmacol*, **1979**, *8*:21–31. O'Byrne S, et al. Plasma protein binding of lidocaine and warfarin in insulin-dependent and non-insulin dependent diabetes mellitus. *Clin Pharmacokinet*, **1993**, *24*:183–186.

Linezolid							
100	35	31	2.1 ± 0.8	0.57–0.71	5.2 ± 1.7	PO: 1.4 ± 0.5[a]	PO: 16 ± 4 µg/mL[a]
			↑ Child		↓ Child		IV: 15 ± 3 µg/mL[b]

[a]Following a 600-mg oral dose given twice daily to steady state. [b]Following a 30-min IV infusion of a 600-mg dose given twice daily to steady state in patients with gram-positive infection.

References: MacGowan AP. Pharmacokinetic and pharmacodynamic profile of linezolid in healthy volunteers and patients with gram-positive infections. *J Antimicrob Chemother*, **2003**, *51*(suppl 2):ii17–ii25. Stalker DJ, et al. Clinical pharmacokinetics of linezolid, a novel oxazolidinone antibacterial. *Clin Pharmacokinet*, **2003**, *42*:1129–1140.

Lisinopril							
25 ± 20	88–100	0	4.2 ± 2.2[a]	2.4 ± 1.4[a]	12[b]	~7[c]	50 (6.4–343) ng/mL[c]
			↓ RD, Aged		↑ RD, Aged		

[a]*CL/F* and V_{area}/F reported. [b]Effective $t_{1/2}$ to predict steady-state accumulation on multiple dosing; a terminal $t_{1/2}$ of 30 h reported. [c]Following a 2.5- to 40-mg oral dose given daily to steady state in elderly patients with hypertension and varying degrees of renal function. EC_{90} for ACE inhibition is 27 ± 10 ng/mL.

Reference: Thomson AH, et al. Lisinopril population pharmacokinetics in elderly and renal disease patients with hypertension. *Br J Clin Pharmacol*, **1989**, *27*:57–65.

(*Continued*)

TABLE AII–1 ■ PHARMACOKINETIC DATA (*CONTINUED*)

BIOAVAILABILITY (ORAL) (%)	URINARY EXCRETION (%)	BOUND IN PLASMA (%)	CLEARANCE (mL/min/kg)	VOL. DIST. (L/kg)	HALF-LIFE (hours)	PEAK TIME (h)	PEAK CONCENTRATION
Lithium							
100[a]	95 ± 15	0	0.35 ± 0.11[b]	0.66 ± 0.16	22 ± 8[c]	IR: 0.5–3[d]	IR: 1–2 mM[d]
			↓ RD, Aged	↓ Obes	↑ RD, Aged	SR: 2–6[d]	SR: 0.7–1.2 mM[d]
			↑ Preg		↓ Obes		

[a]Values as low as 80% reported for some prolonged-release preparations. [b]Renal *CL* of Li[+] parallels that of Na[+]. The ratio of Li[+] and creatinine *CL* is ~ 0.2 ± 0.03. [c]The distribution $t_{1/2}$ is 5.6 ± 0.5 h; this influences drug concentrations for at least 12 h. [d]Following a single 0.7-mmol/kg oral dose of immediate-release (IR) lithium carbonate and sustained-release (SR) tablets.

Reference: Ward ME, et al. Clinical pharmacokinetics of lithium. *J Clin Pharmacol*, **1994**, *34*:280–285.

BIOAVAILABILITY (ORAL) (%)	URINARY EXCRETION (%)	BOUND IN PLASMA (%)	CLEARANCE (mL/min/kg)	VOL. DIST. (L/kg)	HALF-LIFE (hours)	PEAK TIME (h)	PEAK CONCENTRATION
Lopinavir[a]							
—[b]	<3	98–99	1.2[c]	0.6[c]	5.3 ± 2.5	4.4 ± 2.4[d]	9.8 ± 3.7 μg/mL[d]
↑ Food							

[a]Currently formulated in combination with ritonavir (Kaletra). Ritonavir inhibits the CYP3A-dependent metabolism of lopinavir, enhancing its bioavailability, increasing plasma concentrations (50- to 100-fold), and extending its $t_{1/2}$. Pharmacokinetic data from male and female patients with HIV are reported. [b]Absolute bioavailability is not known; the relative bioavailability increases with a high-fat meal. [c]*CL/F* and V_{area}/F reported; calculated from steady-state AUC data. [d]Following a 400-/100-mg lopinavir/ritonavir oral dose given twice daily in combination with stavudine and lamivudine to steady state.

References: Boffito M, et al. Lopinavir protein binding in vivo through the 12-hour dosing interval. *Ther Drug Monit*, **2004**, *26*:35–39. Corbett AH, et al. Kaletra (lopinavir/ritonavir). *Ann Pharmacother*, **2002**, *36*:1193–1203. Eron JJ, et al. Once-daily versus twice-daily lopinavir/ritonavir in antiretroviral-naive HIV-positive patients: a 48-week randomized clinitrial. *J Infect Dis*, **2004**, *189*:265–272. King JR, et al. Pharmacokinetic enhancement of protease inhibitor therapy. *Clin Pharmacokinet*, **2004**, *43*:291–310.

BIOAVAILABILITY (ORAL) (%)	URINARY EXCRETION (%)	BOUND IN PLASMA (%)	CLEARANCE (mL/min/kg)	VOL. DIST. (L/kg)	HALF-LIFE (hours)	PEAK TIME (h)	PEAK CONCENTRATION
Loratadine[a]							
L: —[b]	L: Negligible	L: 97	L: 142 ± 57[d]	L: 120 ± 80[d]	L: 8 ± 6	L (L): 2.0 ± 2.0[e]	L (L): 3.4 ± 3.4 ng/mL[e]
			↓ LD		↑ LD	DL (L): 2.6 ± 2.9[e]	DL (L): 4.1 ± 2.6 ng/mL[e]
DL: —[b]	DL: —	DL: 82–87[c]	DL: 14–18[d]	DL: 26[d]	DL: 21–24	DL (DL): 3.2 ± 1.8[f]	DL(DL): 4.0 ± 2.1 ng/mL[f]
						HDL (DL): 4.8 ± 1.9[f]	HDL (DL): 2.0 ± 0.6 ng/mL[f]
			↓ RD, LD				

[a]Loratadine (L) is converted to a major active metabolite, desloratadine (DL). Almost all patients achieve higher plasma concentrations of DL than of L. DL (Clarinex) is approved for similar clinical indications as L. DL is eliminated by metabolism to an active metabolite, 3-hydroxydesloratadine (HDL). ~7%–20% of patients were slow metabolizers of DL; frequency varies with ethnicity. [b]Bioavailability of L and DL is not known; L is probably low due to extensive first-pass metabolism. [c]Plasma protein binding of HDL is 85%–89%. [d]*CL/F* and V_{area}/F reported. For DL, oral *CL/F* calculated from AUC data following a single 5- to 20-mg oral dose given to healthy adults. [e]Mean for L and DL following a 10-mg oral L dose (Claritin-D 24 h) given once daily for 7 days to healthy adults. [f]Mean for DL and HDL following a 5-mg oral DL dose (Clarinex) given once daily for 10 days to healthy adults.

References: Affrime M, et al. A pharmacokinetic profile of desloratadine in healthy adults, including elderly. *Clin Pharmacokinet*, **2002**, *41*(suppl):13–19. Gupta S, et al. Desloratadine demonstrates dose proportionality in healthy adults after single doses. *Clin Pharmacokinet*, **2002**, *41*(suppl):1–6. Haria M, et al. Loratadine. A reappraisal of its pharmacological properties and therapeutic use in allergic disorders. *Drugs*, **1994**, *48*:617–637. Kosoglou T, et al. Pharmacokinetics of loratadine and pseudoephedrine following single and multiple doses of once- versus twice-daily combination tablet formulations in healthy adult males. *Clin Ther*, **1997**, *19*:1002–1012. PDR58, **2004**, p. 3044.

BIOAVAILABILITY (ORAL) (%)	URINARY EXCRETION (%)	BOUND IN PLASMA (%)	CLEARANCE (mL/min/kg)	VOL. DIST. (L/kg)	HALF-LIFE (hours)	PEAK TIME (h)	PEAK CONCENTRATION
Lorazepam							
93 ± 10	<1	91 ± 2	0.61 ± 0.01[a]	1.3 ± 0.2[b]	14 ± 5	IM: 1.2[c]	IV: ~75 ng/mL[c]
			↓ LD, RD	↑ LD, RD	↑ LD, Neo, RD	PO: 1.2–2.6[c]	IM: ~30 ng/mL[c]
							PO: ~28 ng/mL[c]

[a]Cleared primarily by glucuronidation by UGT2B7 and UGT2B15. [b]V_{area} reported. [c]Following a single 2-mg IV bolus dose, IM dose, or oral dose given to healthy adults.

Reference: Chung J-Y, et al. Pharmacokinetic and pharmacodynamic interaction of lorazepam and valproic acid in relation to *UGT2B7* genetic polymorphism in healthy subjects. *Clin Pharmacol Ther*, **2007**, *83*:595–600. Greenblatt DJ. Clinical pharmacokinetics of oxazepam and lorazepam. *Clin Pharmacokinet*, **1981**, *6*:89–105.

BIOAVAILABILITY (ORAL) (%)	URINARY EXCRETION (%)	BOUND IN PLASMA (%)	CLEARANCE (mL/min/kg)	VOL. DIST. (L/kg)	HALF-LIFE (hours)	PEAK TIME (h)	PEAK CONCENTRATION
Losartan[a]							
L: 35.8 ± 15.5	L: 12 ± 2.8	L: 98.7	L: 8.1 ± 1.8	L: 0.45 ± 0.24	L: 2.5 ± 1.0	L: 1.0 ± 0.5[d]	L: 296 ± 217 ng/mL[d]
	LA: 99.8		↓ RD,[b] LD[c]		LA: 5.4 ± 2.3	LA: 4.1 ± 1.6[d]	LA: 249 ± 74 ng/mL[d]

[a]Data from healthy male subjects. Losartan (L) is metabolized primarily by CYP2C9 to an active 5-carboxylic acid metabolite (LA). [b]*CL/F* for L but not LA decreased in severe renal impairment (L/LA not removed by hemodialysis). No dose adjustment required. [c]*CL/F* for L reduced in mild-to-moderate hepatic impairment. LA AUC also increased. [d]Following a single 50-mg oral dose (tablet). Higher plasma levels of L (but not LA) in female subjects than in male subjects.

References: Lo MW, et al. Pharmacokinetics of losartan, an angiotensin II receptor antagonist, and its active metabolite EXP3174 in humans. *Clin Pharmacol Ther*, **1995**, *58*:641–649. PDR54, **2000**, pp. 1809–1812.

(Continued)

TABLE AII–1 ■ PHARMACOKINETIC DATA (CONTINUED)

BIOAVAILABILITY (ORAL) (%)	URINARY EXCRETION (%)	BOUND IN PLASMA (%)	CLEARANCE (mL/min/kg)	VOL. DIST. (L/kg)	HALF-LIFE (hours)	PEAK TIME (h)	PEAK CONCENTRATION
Lovastatin[a]							
≤5	10	>95	4.3–18.3[b]	—	1–4	AI: 2.0 ± 0.9[c]	AI: 41 ± 6 ng-Eq/mL[c]
↑ Food			↓ RD			TI: 3.1 ± 2.9[c]	TI: 50 ± 8 ng-Eq/mL[c]

[a]Lovastatin is an inactive lactone that is metabolized to the corresponding active β-hydroxy acid. Pharmacokinetic values are based on the sum of 3-hydroxy-3-methylglutaryl–coenzyme A (HMG-CoA) reductase inhibition activity by the β-hydroxy acid and other less potent metabolites. [b]The lactone (in equilibrium with β-hydroxy acid metabolite) is metabolized by CYP3A. [c]Following an 80-mg oral dose given once daily for 17 days. Peak levels represent total active inhibitors (AI) and total inhibitors (TI) of HMG-CoA reductase.

References: Corsini A, et al. New insights into the pharmacodynamic and pharmacokinetic properties of statins. *Pharmacol Ther*, **1999**, 84:413–428. Desager JP, et al. Clinical pharmacokinetics of 3-hydroxy-3-methylglutaryl–coenzyme A reductase inhibitors. *Clin Pharmacokinet*, **1996**, 31:348–371. McKenney JM. Lovastatin: a new cholesterol-lowering agent. *Clin Pharm*, **1988**, 7:21–36.

BIOAVAILABILITY (ORAL) (%)	URINARY EXCRETION (%)	BOUND IN PLASMA (%)	CLEARANCE (mL/min/kg)	VOL. DIST. (L/kg)	HALF-LIFE (hours)	PEAK TIME (h)	PEAK CONCENTRATION
Mefloquine[a]							
—[b]	<1	98.2	0.43 ± 0.14[c]	19 ± 6[c]	20 ± 4 days	SD: 7–19.6[d]	SD: 800–1020 ng/mL[d]
			↑ Preg		↓ Preg	MD: 12 ± 8[d]	MD: 420 ± 141 ng/mL[d]

[a]Racemic mixture; no information on relative kinetics of the enantiomers. [b]Absolute bioavailability is not known; reported values of > 85% represent comparison of oral tablet to solution. [c]*CL/F* and V_{ss}/F reported. [d]Range of mean values from different studies following a single 1000-mg oral dose (SD) and mean following a 250-mg oral dose given once weekly for 4 weeks (MD).

Reference: Karbwang J, et al. Clinical pharmacokinetics of mefloquine. *Clin Pharmacokinet*, **1990**, 19:264–279.

BIOAVAILABILITY (ORAL) (%)	URINARY EXCRETION (%)	BOUND IN PLASMA (%)	CLEARANCE (mL/min/kg)	VOL. DIST. (L/kg)	HALF-LIFE (hours)	PEAK TIME (h)	PEAK CONCENTRATION
Meperidine[a]							
52 ± 3	~5 (1–25)[b]	58 ± 9[c]	17 ± 5	4.4 ± 0.9	3.2 ± 0.8[d]	IM: <1[e]	IV: 0.67 µg/mL[e]
↑ LD		↓ Aged, RD	↓LD, RD, Prem, Neo	↑ Aged, Prem	↑ LD, Prem, Neo, Aged, RD		IM: ~0.7 µg/mL[e]

[a]Meperidine undergoes cytochrome P450–dependent *N*-demethylation to normeperidine. The metabolite is not an analgesic but is a potent central nervous system–excitatory agent and is associated with adverse side effects of meperidine. [b]Meperidine is a weak base (pK_a = 8.6) and is excreted to a greater extent in the urine at low urinary pH and to a lesser extent at high urinary pH. [c]Correlates with the concentration of α₁-acid glycoprotein. [d]A longer $t_{1/2}$ (7 h) also is observed. [e]Following a continuous 24-mg/h IV infusion or 100-mg IM injection every 4 h to steady state. Postoperative analgesia occurs at 0.4–0.7 µg/mL.

Reference: Edwards DJ, et al. Clinical pharmacokinetics of pethidine: 1982. *Clin Pharmacokinet*, **1982**, 7:421–433.

BIOAVAILABILITY (ORAL) (%)	URINARY EXCRETION (%)	BOUND IN PLASMA (%)	CLEARANCE (mL/min/kg)	VOL. DIST. (L/kg)	HALF-LIFE (hours)	PEAK TIME (h)	PEAK CONCENTRATION
Mercaptopurine[a]							
12 ± 7[b]	22 ± 12	19	11 ± 4[c]	0.56 ± 0.38	0.90 ± 0.37		IV: 6.9 µM[d]
						PO (–): 2.4 ± 0.4[d]	PO (–): 0.74 ± 0.28 µM[d]
						PO (+): 2.8 ± 0.4[d]	PO (+): 3.7 ± 0.6 µM[d]

[a]Inactive prodrug is metabolized intracellularly to 6-thioinosinate. Pharmacokinetic values for mercaptopurine are reported. [b]Increases to 60% when first-pass metabolism is inhibited by allopurinol (100 mg three times daily). [c]Metabolically cleared by xanthine oxidase and thiopurine methyltransferase (polymorphic). Despite inhibition of intrinsic *CL* by allopurinol, hepatic metabolism is limited by blood flow, and *CL* is thus little changed by allopurinol. [d]Following an intravenous infusion of 50 mg/m²/h to steady state in children with refractory cancers or a single oral dose of 75 mg/m² with (+) or without (–) allopurinol pretreatment.

References: Lennard L. The clinical pharmacology of 6-mercaptopurine. *Eur J Clin Pharmacol*, **1992**, 43:329–339. PDR54, **2000**, p. 1255.

BIOAVAILABILITY (ORAL) (%)	URINARY EXCRETION (%)	BOUND IN PLASMA (%)	CLEARANCE (mL/min/kg)	VOL. DIST. (L/kg)	HALF-LIFE (hours)	PEAK TIME (h)	PEAK CONCENTRATION
Metformin[a]							
52 ± 5 (40–55)	99.9 ± 0.5 (79–100)	Negligible	7.62 ± 0.30[b] (6.3–10.1)	1.12 ± 0.08 (0.9–3.94)	1.74 ± 0.20 (1.5–4.5)	1.9 ± 0.4[d] (1.5–3.5)[d]	1.6 ± 0.2 µg/mL[d]
			↓ RD,[c] Aged ↑ Preg		↑ RD,[c] Aged		(1.0–3.1 µg/mL)[d]

[a]Data from healthy male and female subjects. No significant gender differences. Shown in parentheses are mean values from different studies. [b]Clearance of metformin is mediated in part by organic cation transporters (OCTs) in the kidney. [c]*CL/F* reduced, mild-to-severe renal impairment. [d]Following a single 0.5-g oral dose (tablet) and range for a 0.5- to 1.5-g oral dose.

References: Harrower AD. Pharmacokinetics of oral antihyperglycaemic agents in patients with renal insufficiency. *Clin Pharmacokinet*, **1996**, 37:111–119. Pentikainen PJ, et al. Pharmacokinetics of metformin after intravenous and oral administration to man. *Eur J Clin Pharmacol*, **1979**, 16:195–202. PDR54, **2000**, pp. 831–835. Scheen AJ. Clinical pharmacokinetics of metformin. *Clin Pharmacokinet*, **1996**, 30:359–371.

(Continued)

TABLE AII–1 ■ PHARMACOKINETIC DATA (*CONTINUED*)

	BIOAVAILABILITY (ORAL) (%)	URINARY EXCRETION (%)	BOUND IN PLASMA (%)	CLEARANCE (mL/min/kg)	VOL. DIST. (L/kg)	HALF-LIFE (hours)	PEAK TIME (h)	PEAK CONCENTRATION
Methadone[a]								
	92 ± 21	24 ± 10[b]	89 ± 2.9[c]	1.7 ± 0.9[b]	3.6 ± 1.2[d]	27 ± 12[e]	~3[f]	IV: 450–550 ng/mL[f]
				↓ Child ↑ Preg		↓ Child		PO: 69–980 ng/mL[f]

[a]Data for racemic mixture. Opioid activity resides with the *R*-enantiomer. In vivo disposition is stereoselective. *N*-demethylation is mediated by CYP3A4 and CYP2B6. [b]Inversely correlated with urine pH. [c]*d*-methadone slightly higher percentage bound. [d]V_{area} reported. [e]Directly correlated with urine pH. [f]Following a single 10-mg IV bolus dose in patients with chronic pain or a 0.12- to 1.9-mg/kg oral dose once daily for at least 2 months in subjects with opioid dependency. Levels > 100 ng/mL prevent withdrawal symptoms; EC_{50} for pain relief and sedation in cancer patients is 350 ± 180 ng/mL.

References: Dyer KR, et al. Steady-state pharmacokinetics and pharmacodynamics in methadone maintenance patients: comparison of those who do and do not experience withdrawal and concentration-effect relationships. *Clin Pharmacol Ther*, **1999**, 65:685–694. Inturrisi CE, et al. Pharmacokinetics and pharmacodynamics of methadone in patients with chronic pain. *Clin Pharmacol Ther*, **1987**, 41:392–401.

	BIOAVAILABILITY (ORAL) (%)	URINARY EXCRETION (%)	BOUND IN PLASMA (%)	CLEARANCE (mL/min/kg)	VOL. DIST. (L/kg)	HALF-LIFE (hours)	PEAK TIME (h)	PEAK CONCENTRATION
Methotrexate[a]								
	70 ± 27[b,c]	81 ± 9	46 ± 11	2.1 ± 0.8[d]	0.55 ± 0.19	7.2 ± 2.1[e]	SC: 0.9 ± 0.2[f]	SC: 1.1 ± 0.2 μM[f]
				↓ RD				IV: 37–99 μM[f]

[a]Plasma concentrations of the 7-hydroxy metabolite approach those of the parent drug. Metabolite may have both therapeutic and toxic effects. [b]Bioavailability is dose dependent and may be as low as 20% when doses are > 80 mg/m². [c]Intramuscular bioavailability is only slightly higher. [d]Methotrexate clearance is mediated by several transporters, including organic anion transporters (OATs). [e]Exhibits triexponential elimination kinetics. A shorter $t_{1/2}$ (2 h) is seen initially, and a longer (52 h) terminal $t_{1/2}$ has been observed with increased assay sensitivity. [f]Following a 15-mg SC dose given once weekly to steady state in adult patients with inflammatory bowel disease. Initial steady-state concentrations in young (1.5–22 years) leukemia patients receiving a 500-mg/m² loading dose given over 1 h followed by an infusion of 196-mg/m²/h for 5 h.

References: Egan LJ, et al. Systemic and intestinal pharmacokinetics of methotrexate in patients with inflammatory bowel disease. *Clin Pharmacol Ther*, **1999**, 65:29–39. Tracy TS, et al. Methotrexate disposition following concomitant administration of ketoprofen, piroxicam and flurbiprofen in patients with rheumatoid arthritis. *Br J Clin Pharmacol*, **1994**, 37:453–456. Wall AM, et al. Individualized methotrexate dosing in children with relapsed acute lymphoblastic leukemia. *Leukemia*, **2000**, 14:221–225.

	BIOAVAILABILITY (ORAL) (%)	URINARY EXCRETION (%)	BOUND IN PLASMA (%)	CLEARANCE (mL/min/kg)	VOL. DIST. (L/kg)	HALF-LIFE (hours)	PEAK TIME (h)	PEAK CONCENTRATION
Methylphenidate[a]								
	(+): 22 ± 8	(+): 1.3 ± 0.5	(+/–): 15–16	(+): 6.7 ± 2.0[b]	(+): 2.7 ± 1.1	(+): 6.0 ± 1.7[c]	(+): 2.4 ± 0.8[c,d]	(+): 18 ± 4.3 ng/mL[d]
	(–): 5 ± 3	(–): 0.6 ± 0.3		(–): 12 ± 4.7[b]	(–): 1.8 ± 0.9	(–): 3.6 ± 1.1	(–): 2.1 ± 0.6[d]	(–): 3.0 ± 0.9 ng/mL[d]

[a]Methylphenidate is available as a racemate and the active (+)-dextro-enantiomer dexmethylphenidate. Methylphenidate and dexmethylphenidate are extensively metabolized, primarily through ester hydrolysis to ritalinic acid. Data for individual enantiomers following racemate administration to healthy adult male subjects. No significant gender differences. [b]The (+)-enantiomer exhibits dose-dependent kinetics at high doses of racemate, with an ~ 50% reduction in *CL/F* between a 10- and 40-mg dose. [c]When dexmethylphenidate is given alone, its $t_{1/2}$ is 2.2 h and T_{max} is 1–1.5 h. [d]Following a single 40-mg oral dose (immediate release). Longer T_{max} (3–5 h) and lower C_{max} reported for sustained-released oral formulation.

References: Aoyama T, et al. Nonlinear kinetics of threo-methylphenidate enantiomers in a patient with narcolepsy and in healthy volunteers. *Eur J Clin Pharmacol*, **1993**, 44:79–84. Keating GM, et al. Dexmethylphenidate. *Drugs*, **2002**, 62:1899–1904; discussion 1905–1908. Kimko HC, et al. Pharmacokinetics and clinical effectiveness of methylphenidate. *Clin Pharmacokinet*, **1999**, 37:457–470. PDR58, **2004**, pp. 2265, 2297–2298. Srinivas NR, et al. Enantioselective pharmacokinetics of dl-threo-methyl-phenidate in humans. *Pharm Res*, **1993**, 10:14–21.

	BIOAVAILABILITY (ORAL) (%)	URINARY EXCRETION (%)	BOUND IN PLASMA (%)	CLEARANCE (mL/min/kg)	VOL. DIST. (L/kg)	HALF-LIFE (hours)	PEAK TIME (h)	PEAK CONCENTRATION
Methylprednisolone								
	82 ± 13[a]	4.9 ± 2.3	78 ± 3	6.2 ± 0.9	1.2 ± 0.2	2.3 ± 0.5		IV: 225 ± 44 ng/mL[b]
							PO: 1.64 ± 0.64[c]	PO: 178 ± 44 ng/mL[c]
			↓ LD	↓ Obes	↓ Obes, Fem	↑ Obes		
				↑ Fem		↓ Fem		

[a]May be decreased to 50%–60% with high doses. [b]Mean at 1 h following a 28-mg IV infusion over 20 min given twice daily for 6 ± 4 days during the perioperative period following kidney transplantation. [c]Mean data following a 24-mg oral dose given twice daily for 3 days in healthy adult male subjects.

References: Lew KH, et al. Gender-based effects on methylprednisolone pharmacokinetics and pharmacodynamics. *Clin Pharmacol Ther*, **1993**, 54:402–414. Rohatagi S, et al. Pharmacokinetics of methylprednisolone and prednisolone after single and multiple oral administration. *J Clin Pharmacol*, **1997**, 37:916–925. Tornatore KM, et al. Methylprednisolone and cortisol metabolism during the early post-renal transplant period. *Clin Transplant*, **1995**, 9:427–432.

	BIOAVAILABILITY (ORAL) (%)	URINARY EXCRETION (%)	BOUND IN PLASMA (%)	CLEARANCE (mL/min/kg)	VOL. DIST. (L/kg)	HALF-LIFE (hours)	PEAK TIME (h)	PEAK CONCENTRATION
Metoclopramide								
	76 ± 38	20 ± 9	40 ± 4	6.2 ± 1.3	3.4 ± 1.3	5.0 ± 1.4	A: ≤1[a]	A: 80 ng/mL[a]
				↓ RD, LD		↑ RD, LD	I: 2.5 ± 0.7[a]	I: 18 ± 6.2 ng/mL[a]
				↓ Neo		↓ Neo		

[a]Following a single 20-mg oral dose given to healthy adults (A) or an oral (nasogastric) dose of 0.10–0.15 mg/kg given four times daily to steady state to premature infants (I), 1–7 weeks of age (26–36 weeks, postconceptional).

References: Kearns GL, et al. Pharmacokinetics of metoclopramide in neonates. *J Clin Pharmacol*, **1998**, 38:122–128. Lauritsen K, et al. Clinical pharmacokinetics of drugs used in the treatment of gastrointestinal diseases (part I). *Clin Pharmacokinet*, **1990**, 19:11–31. Rotmensch HH, et al. Comparative central nervous system effects and pharmacokinetics of neu-metoclopramide and metoclopramide in healthy volunteers. *J Clin Pharmacol*, **1997**, 37:222–228.

(Continued)

TABLE AII–1 ■ PHARMACOKINETIC DATA (*CONTINUED*)

BIOAVAILABILITY (ORAL) (%)	URINARY EXCRETION (%)	BOUND IN PLASMA (%)	CLEARANCE (mL/min/kg)	VOL. DIST. (L/kg)	HALF-LIFE (hours)	PEAK TIME (h)	PEAK CONCENTRATION
Metoprolol[a]							
38 ± 14[b]	10 ± 3[b]	11 ± 1	15 ± 3[b]	4.2 ± 0.7	3.2 ± 0.2[b]	EM: ~2[c]	EM: 99 ± 53 ng/mL[c]
↑ LD			↑ Preg	↑ Fem	↑ LD, Neo	PM: ~3[c]	PM: 262 ± 29 ng/mL[c]
↓ Preg			↑ Fem				

[a]Data for racemic mixture reported. Metabolism of less active *R*-(+)-enantiomer (*CL/F* = 28 mL/min/kg; V_{area}/F = 7.6 L/kg; $t_{1/2}$ = 2.7 h) is slightly faster than that of more active *S*-(–)-enantiomer (*CL/F* = 20 mL/min/kg; V_{area}/F = 5.5 L/kg; $t_{1/2}$ = 3 h). [b]Metabolically cleared by CYP2D6 (polymorphic). Compared to extensive metabolizers (EM), individuals who are poor metabolizers (PM) have a lower *CL/F* and a longer $t_{1/2}$ (7.6 ± 1.5 vs. 2.8 ± 1.2 h) and excrete more unchanged drug in urine (15% ± 7% vs. 3.2% ± 3%) due to reduced hepatic metabolism. [c]$C_{3\,h}$ following a single 100-mg oral dose in CYP2D6 EM and PM patients with hypertension. Plasma concentrations of the more active *S*-enantiomer are ~35% higher than the *R*-antipode in CYP2D6 EM. No stereochemical difference was observed in PM subjects. EC_{50} for decreased heart rate during peak submaximal exercise testing was 16 ± 7 ng/mL; EC_{50} for decreased systolic blood pressure during exercise testing was 25 ± 18 ng/mL.

References: Dayer P, et al. Interindividual variation of beta-adrenoceptor blocking drugs, plasma concentration and effect: influence of genetic status on behaviour of atenolol, bopindolol and metoprolol. *Eur J Clin Pharmacol*, **1985**, *28*:149–153. Lennard MS, et al. Oxidation phenotype—a major determinant of metoprolol metabolism and response. *N Engl J Med*, **1982**, *307*:1558–1560. McGourty JC, et al. Metoprolol metabolism and debrisoquine oxidation polymorphism—population and family studies. *Br J Clin Pharmacol*, **1985**, *20*:555–566.

Metronidazole[a]							
99 ± 8[b]	10 ± 2	11 ± 3	1.3 ± 0.3	0.74 ± 0.10	8.5 ± 2.9		IV: 27 (11–41) µg/mL[c]
			↓ LD, Neo		↑ Neo, LD		
						PO: 2.8[c]	PO: 19.8 µg/mL[c]
						VA: 11 ± 2[c]	VA: 1.9 ± 0.2 µg/mL[c]

[a]Active hydroxylated metabolite accumulates in renal failure. [b]Bioavailability is 67%–82% for rectal suppositories and 53% ± 16% for intravaginal gel. [c]Following a single 100-mg dose of vaginal (VA) cream, a 100-mg IV infusion over 20 min three times daily to steady state or a 100-mg oral dose three times daily to steady state.

Reference: Lau AM, et al. Clinical pharmacokinetics of metronidazole and other nitroimidazole anti-infectives. *Clin Pharmacokinet*, **1992**, *23*:328–364.

Micafungin							
—	<1	99	0.14 ± 0.03[a]	0.20 ± 0.03	14.6 ± 3.0	—	8.8 ± 1.8 µg/mL[b]

[a]Undergoes arylsulfatase-dependent metabolism and biliary excretion. [b]Following a 100-mg IV infusion administered over 1 h.

Reference: Hebert MF, et al. Pharmacokinetics of micafungin in healthy volunteers, volunteers with moderate liver disease and volunteers with renal dysfunction. *J Clin Pharmacol*, **2005**, *45*:1145–1152.

Midazolam							
44 ± 17[a]	<1%	98	6.6 ± 1.8[b]	1.1 ± 0.6	1.9 ± 0.6		IV: 113 ± 16 ng/mL[d]
↑ LD		↓ Aged, RD	↑ RD[c]	↑ Obes	↑ Aged, Obes, LD	PO: 0.67 ± 0.45[d]	PO: 78 ± 27 ng/mL[d]
			↓ LD, Neo	↓ Neo			

[a]Undergoes extensive first-pass metabolism by intestinal and hepatic CYP3A. Bioavailability appears to be dose dependent; 35%–67% at 15-mg, 28%–36% at 7.5-mg, and 12%–47% at 2-mg oral dose, possibly due to saturable first-pass intestinal metabolism. [b]Metabolically cleared by CYP3A. [c]Increased *CL* due to increased plasma free fraction; unbound *CL* is unchanged. [d]Following a single 5-mg IV bolus or 10-mg oral dose.

References: Garzone PD, et al. Pharmacokinetics of the newer benzodiazepines. *Clin Pharmacokinet*, **1989**, *76*:337–364. Thummel KE, et al. Oral first-pass elimination of midazolam involves both gastrointestinal and hepatic CYP3A-mediated metabolism. *Clin Pharmacol Ther*, **1996**, *59*:491–502.

Minocycline							
95–100	11 ± 2	76	1.0 ± 0.3[a]	1.3 ± 0.2[b]	16 ± 2		IV: 3.5 µg/mL[c]
						PO: 2–4[c]	PO: 2.3–3.5 µg/mL[c]

[a]Cleared primarily by oxidative metabolism in the liver. [b]V_{area} reported. [c]Following a single 200-mg IV infusion (1 h) or range of values following a 100-mg oral dose given twice a day to steady state.

Reference: Saivin S, et al. Clinical pharmacokinetics of doxycycline and minocycline. *Clin Pharmacokinet*, **1988**, *15*:355–366.

Mirtazapine[a]							
50 ± 10	—	85	9.12 ± 1.14[b]	4.5 ± 1.7	16.3 ± 4.6[b,e]	1.5 ± 0.7[f]	41.8 ± 7.7 ng/mL[f]
			↓ LD,[c] RD[d]		↑ LD,[c] RD[d]		

[a]Data from healthy adult subjects. Metabolized by CYP2D6 and CYP1A2 (8-hydroxy) and CYP3A (*N*-desmethyl, *N*-oxide). [b]Women of all ages exhibit a lower *CL/F* and longer $t_{1/2}$ than men. [c]*CL/F* reduced, hepatic impairment. [d]*CL/F* reduced, moderate-to-severe renal impairment. [e]The $t_{1/2}$ of the (–)-enantiomer is approximately twice as long as the (+)-antipode; approximately 3-fold higher blood concentrations (+ vs. –) are achieved. [f]Following a 15-mg oral dose given once daily to steady state.

References: Fawcett J, et al. Review of the results from clinical studies on the efficacy, safety and tolerability of mirtazapine for the treatment of patients with major depression. *J Affect Disord*, **1998**, *51*:267–285. PDR54, **2000**, p. 2109.

(Continued)

TABLE AII–1 ■ PHARMACOKINETIC DATA (CONTINUED)

BIOAVAILABILITY (ORAL) (%)	URINARY EXCRETION (%)	BOUND IN PLASMA (%)	CLEARANCE (mL/min/kg)	VOL. DIST. (L/kg)	HALF-LIFE (hours)	PEAK TIME (h)	PEAK CONCENTRATION
Montelukast[a]							
62	<0.2	>99	0.70 ± 0.17^b	0.15 ± 0.02	4.9 ± 0.6	3.0 ± 1.0^d	542 ± 173 ng/mL[d]
			↓LD[c]		↑LD[c]		

[a]Data from healthy adult subjects. No significant gender differences. [b]Montelukast is metabolized by CYP3A4 and CYP2C9. [c]CL/F is reduced by 41%, mild-to-moderate hepatic impairment with cirrhosis. [d]Following a single 10-mg oral dose.

*References: PDR54, **2000**, p. 1882. Zhao JJ, et al. Pharmacokinetics and bioavailability of montelukast sodium (MK-0476) in healthy young and elderly volunteers. Biopharm Drug Dispos, **1997**, 18:769–777.*

BIOAVAILABILITY (ORAL) (%)	URINARY EXCRETION (%)	BOUND IN PLASMA (%)	CLEARANCE (mL/min/kg)	VOL. DIST. (L/kg)	HALF-LIFE (hours)	PEAK TIME (h)	PEAK CONCENTRATION
Morphine[a]							
PO: 24 ± 12	4 ± 5	35 ± 2	24 ± 10	3.3 ± 0.9	1.9 ± 0.5	IM: $0.2–0.3^b$	IV: 200–400 ng/mL[b]
IM: ~100		↓LD	↓RD, Prem	↓RD	↑Neo, Prem	PO-IR: $0.5–1.5^b$	IM: ~70 ng/mL[b]
						PO-SR: $3–8^b$	PO-IR: 10 ng/mL[b]
							PO-SR: 7.4 ng/mL[b]

[a]Mainly cleared by UGT2B7-dependent glucuronidation to morphine 3-glucuronide and to an active metabolite, morphine-6-glucuronide; the latter urinary excretion = 14% ± 7% and $t_{1/2}$ = 4.0 ± 1.5 h. Steady-state ratio of active metabolite to parent drug after oral dosing = 4.9 ± 3.8. In renal failure, $t_{1/2}$ increases to 50 ± 37 h, resulting in significant accumulation of active glucuronide metabolite. [b]Following a single 10-mg IV dose (bolus with 5-min blood sample), a 10-mg/70-kg IM, a 10-mg/70 kg immediate-release oral (PO-IR) dose, or a 50-mg sustained-release oral dose (PO-SR). Minimum analgesic concentration is 15 ng/mL.

*References: Berkowitz BA. The relationship of pharmacokinetics to pharmacological activity: morphine, methadone and naloxone. Clin Pharmacokinet, **1976**, 1:219–230. Glare PA, et al. Clinical pharmacokinetics of morphine. Ther Drug Monit, **1991**, 13:1–23.*

BIOAVAILABILITY (ORAL) (%)	URINARY EXCRETION (%)	BOUND IN PLASMA (%)	CLEARANCE (mL/min/kg)	VOL. DIST. (L/kg)	HALF-LIFE (hours)	PEAK TIME (h)	PEAK CONCENTRATION
Moxifloxacin[a]							
86 ± 1	21.9 ± 3.6	39.4 ± 2.4	2.27 ± 0.24^b	2.05 ± 1.15	15.4 ± 1.2	2.0 $(0.5–6.0)^c$	2.5 ± 1.3 µg/mL[c]

[a]Data from healthy adult male subjects. [b]Moxifloxacin is metabolically cleared by ST and UGT. [c]Following a single oral 400-mg dose.

*Reference: Stass H, et al. Pharmacokinetics and elimination of moxifloxacin after oral and intravenous administration in man. J Antimicrob Chemother, **1999**, 43(suppl B):83–90.*

BIOAVAILABILITY (ORAL) (%)	URINARY EXCRETION (%)	BOUND IN PLASMA (%)	CLEARANCE (mL/min/kg)	VOL. DIST. (L/kg)	HALF-LIFE (hours)	PEAK TIME (h)	PEAK CONCENTRATION
Mycophenolate[a]							
MM: ~0	MPA: <1	MPA: 97.5	MM: 120–163	MPA: $3.6–4^c$	MM: <0.033	MPA: $1.1–2.2^d$	MPA: 8–19 µg/mL[d]
MPA: 94	↓RD[b]		MPA: 2.5 ± 0.4^c		MPA: 16.6 ± 5.8		
			↓RD[b]				

[a]Data from healthy adult male and female subjects and organ transplant patients. No significant gender differences. Mycophenolate mofetil (MM) is rapidly converted to the active mycophenolic acid (MPA) after intravenous and oral doses. Kinetic parameters refer to MM and MPA after a dose of MM. MPA metabolized by UGT to MPA-glucuronide (MPAG). MPA undergoes enterohepatic recycling; MPAG is excreted into bile and presumably is hydrolyzed by gut flora and reabsorbed as MPA. [b]Accumulation of MPA and MPAG and increased unbound MPA; severe renal impairment. [c]CL/F and V_{area}/F reported for MPA. [d]Range of mean MPA C_{max} and T_{max} from different studies following a 1- to 1.75-g oral dose given twice daily to steady state in renal transplant patients.

*References: Bullingham R, et al. Effects of food and antacid on the pharmacokinetics of single doses of mycophenolate mofetil in rheumatoid arthritis patients. Br J Clin Pharmacol, **1996**, 47:513–516. Bullingham RE, et al. Clinical pharmacokinetics of mycophenolate mofetil. Clin Pharmacokinet, **1998**, 34:429–455. Kriesche HUM, et al. MPA protein binding in uremic plasma: prediction of free fraction. Clin Pharmacol Ther, **1999**, 65:184. PDR54, **2000**, pp. 2617–2618.*

BIOAVAILABILITY (ORAL) (%)	URINARY EXCRETION (%)	BOUND IN PLASMA (%)	CLEARANCE (mL/min/kg)	VOL. DIST. (L/kg)	HALF-LIFE (hours)	PEAK TIME (h)	PEAK CONCENTRATION
Naltrexone[a]							
20 ± 5	2	21	18.3 ± 1.4	16.1 ± 5.2	10.3 ± 3.3^c	1[d]	15–64 ng/mL[d]
			↓LD[b]				

[a]Naltrexone has an active metabolite, 6β-naltrexol, that circulates at greater concentrations than naltrexone and has a 10-fold higher AUC than naltrexone after oral administration of naltrexone. [b]The oral AUC of naltrexone was significantly increased in patients with liver impairment, whereas the AUC of 6β-naltrexol was not changed. [c]A $t_{1/2}$ of 2.7 h after intravenous administration also reported. [d]Following a single 100-mg oral dose.

*References: Bertolotti M, et al. Effect of liver cirrhosis on the systemic availability of naltrexone in humans. J Hepatol, **1997**, 27:505–511. Bullingham RES, et al. Clinical pharmacokinetics of narcotic agonist-antagonist drugs. Clin Pharmacokinet, **1983**, 8:332–343.*

BIOAVAILABILITY (ORAL) (%)	URINARY EXCRETION (%)	BOUND IN PLASMA (%)	CLEARANCE (mL/min/kg)	VOL. DIST. (L/kg)	HALF-LIFE (hours)	PEAK TIME (h)	PEAK CONCENTRATION
Naproxen							
99[a]	5–6	99.7 ± 0.1^b	$0.13 \pm 0.02^{d,e}$	0.16 ± 0.02^e	14 ± 1	T-IR: $2–4^f$	T-IR: 37 µg/mL[f]
		↑RD, Aged,[c] LD	↓RD	↑RD, Child	↑Aged[c]	T-CR: 5^f	T-CR: 94 µg/mL[f]
						S: 2.2 ± 2.1^f	S: 55 ± 14 µg/mL[f]

[a]Estimated bioavailability. [b]Saturable plasma protein binding yields apparent nonlinear elimination kinetics. [c]No change in total CL, but a significant (50%) decrease in CL of unbound drug; it is thus suggested that dosing rate be decreased. A second study in elderly patients found a decreased CL and increased $t_{1/2}$ with no change in percentage bound. [d]Metabolically cleared by CYP2C9 (polymorphic) and CYP1A2. [e]CL/F and V_{area}/F reported. [f]Following a single 250-mg dose of suspension (S) given orally to pediatric patients or a 250-mg immediate-release tablet (T-IR) or a 500-mg controlled-release tablet (T-CR) given to adults.

*Reference: Wells TG, et al. Comparison of the pharmacokinetics of naproxen tablets and suspension in children. J Clin Pharmacol, **1994**, 34:30–33.*

(Continued)

TABLE AII-1 ■ PHARMACOKINETIC DATA (CONTINUED)

BIOAVAILABILITY (ORAL) (%)	URINARY EXCRETION (%)	BOUND IN PLASMA (%)	CLEARANCE (mL/min/kg)	VOL. DIST. (L/kg)	HALF-LIFE (hours)	PEAK TIME (h)	PEAK CONCENTRATION
Nevirapine[a]							
93 ± 9	<3	60	SD: 0.23–0.77[b] MD: 0.89[b]	SD: 1.2 ± 0.09 MD: 1.2	SD: 45[b] MD: 25–35[b]	2–4[d]	SD: 2 ± 0.4 µg/mL[d] MD: 4.5 ± 1.9 µg/mL[d]
			↑ Child[c]				

[a]Data from healthy adult and HIV-infected subjects. No significant gender differences. [b]Range of CL/F and V/F reported. Metabolized by CYP3A. Nevirapine appears to autoinduce its own metabolism. CL/F increases and $t_{1/2}$ decreases from a single dose (SD) to multiple doses (MD). [c]Patients < 8 years. [d]Following a single 200-mg oral dose (SD) and 200 mg, twice a day, to steady state (MD).

References: Cheeseman SH, et al. Pharmacokinetics of nevirapine: initial single-rising-dose study in humans. *Antimicrob Agents Chemother,* **1993**, *37:*178–182. Luzuriaga K, et al. Pharmacokinetics, safety, and activity of nevirapine in human immunodeficiency virus type 1-infected children. *J Infect Dis,* **1996**, *174:*713–721. Zhou XJ, et al. Population pharmacokinetics of nevirapine, zidovudine, and didanosine in human immunodeficiency virus-infected patients. The National Institute of Allergy and Infectious Diseases AIDS Clinical Trials Group Protocol 241 Investigators. *Antimicrob Agents Chemother,* **1999**, *43:*121–128. PDR54, **2000**, p. 2721.

BIOAVAILABILITY (ORAL) (%)	URINARY EXCRETION (%)	BOUND IN PLASMA (%)	CLEARANCE (mL/min/kg)	VOL. DIST. (L/kg)	HALF-LIFE (hours)	PEAK TIME (h)	PEAK CONCENTRATION
Nifedipine							
50 ± 13	~0	96 ± 1	7.0 ± 1.8[a]	0.78 ± 0.22	1.8 ± 0.4[b]	IR: 0.5 ± 0.2[c]	IR: 79 ± 44 ng/mL[c]
↑ LD, Aged		↓ LD, RD	↓ LD, Aged	↑ LD, RD, Aged	↑ LD, RD, Aged	ER: ~6[c]	ER: 35–49 ng/mL[c]

[a]Metabolically cleared by CYP3A; undergoes significant first-pass metabolism. [b]Longer apparent $t_{1/2}$ after oral administration because of absorption limitation, particularly for extended-release (ER) formulations. [c]Mean following a single 10-mg immediate-release (IR) capsule given to healthy male adults or a range of steady-state concentrations following a 60-mg ER tablet given daily to healthy male adults. Levels of 47 ± 20 ng/mL were reported to decrease diastolic pressure in hypertensive patients.

References: Glasser SP, et al. The efficacy and safety of once-daily nifedipine: the coat-core formulation compared with the gastrointestinal therapeutic system formulation in patients with mild-to-moderate diastolic hypertension. Nifedipine Study Group. *Clin Ther,* **1995**, *17:*12–29. Renwick AG, et al. The pharmacokinetics of oral nifedipine—a population study. *Br J Clin Pharmacol,* **1988**, *25:*701–708. Soons PA, et al. Intraindividual variability in nifedipine pharmacokinetics and effects in healthy subjects. *J Clin Pharmacol,* **1992**, *32:*324–331.

BIOAVAILABILITY (ORAL) (%)	URINARY EXCRETION (%)	BOUND IN PLASMA (%)	CLEARANCE (mL/min/kg)	VOL. DIST. (L/kg)	HALF-LIFE (hours)	PEAK TIME (h)	PEAK CONCENTRATION
Nitrofurantoin							
87 ± 13	47 ± 13	62 ± 4	9.9 ± 0.9	0.58 ± 0.12	1.0 ± 0.2	2.3 ± 1.4[a]	428 ± 146 ng/mL[a]
			↑ Alkaline urine				

[a]Following a single 50-mg oral dose (tablet) given to fasted healthy adults. No changes when taken with a meal.

Reference: Hoener B, et al. Nitrofurantoin disposition. *Clin Pharmacol Ther,* **1981**, *29:*808–816.

BIOAVAILABILITY (ORAL) (%)	URINARY EXCRETION (%)	BOUND IN PLASMA (%)	CLEARANCE (mL/min/kg)	VOL. DIST. (L/kg)	HALF-LIFE (hours)	PEAK TIME (h)	PEAK CONCENTRATION
Nitroglycerin[a]							
PO: <1	<1	—	195 ± 86[c]	3.3 ± 1.2[c,d]	2.3 ± 0.6 min	SL: 0.09 ± 0.03[e]	IV: 3.4 ± 1.7 ng/mL[e]
SL: 38 ± 26[b]						Top: 3–4[e]	SL: 1.9 ± 1.6 ng/mL[e]
Top: 72 ± 20						TD: 2[e]	

[a]Dinitrate metabolites have weak activity compared to nitroglycerin (<10%), but because of a prolonged $t_{1/2}$ (~40 min), they may accumulate during administration of sustained-release preparations to yield concentrations in plasma 10- to 20-fold greater than parent drug. [b]Following sublingual (SL) dose rinsed out of mouth after 8 min. Rinse contained 31% ± 19% of the dose. [c]Following a 40- to 100-min IV infusion. [d]V_{area} reported. [e]Steady-state concentration following a 20- to 54-µg/min IV infusion over 40–100 min or a 0.4-mg SL dose. Levels of 1.2–11 ng/mL associated with a 25% drop in capillary wedge pressure in patients with congestive heart failure. T_{max} for topical (Top) and transdermal (TD) preparations also reported.

References: Noonan PK, et al. Incomplete and delayed bioavailability of sublingual nitroglycerin. *Am J Cardiol,* **1985**, *55:*184–187. PDR54, **2000**, p. 1474. Thadani U, et al. Relationship of pharmacokinetic and pharmacodynamic properties of the organic nitrates. *Clin Pharmacokinet,* **1988**, *15:*32–43.

BIOAVAILABILITY (ORAL) (%)	URINARY EXCRETION (%)	BOUND IN PLASMA (%)	CLEARANCE (mL/min/kg)	VOL. DIST. (L/kg)	HALF-LIFE (hours)	PEAK TIME (h)	PEAK CONCENTRATION
Olanzapine[a]							
~60[b]	7.3	93	6.2 ± 2.9[c,d]	16.4 ± 5.1[d]	33.1 ± 10.3	6.1 ± 1.9[e]	12.9 ± 7.5 ng/mL[e]
					↑ Aged		

[a]Data from male and female schizophrenic patients. [b]Bioavailability estimated from parent and metabolite recovery data. [c]Metabolized primarily by UGT, CYP1A2, and flavin-containing monooxygenase. [d]Summary of CL/F and V_{area}/F for 491 subjects receiving an oral dose. CL/F segregates by sex (F/M) and smoking status (NS/S): M, S > F, S > M, NS > F, NS. [e]Following a single 9.5- ± 4-mg oral dose to healthy male subjects; $C_{max,ss}$ ~ 20 ng/mL following a 10-mg oral dose given once daily.

References: Callaghan JT, et al. Olanzapine. Pharmacokinetic and pharmacodynamic profile. *Clin Pharmacokinet,* **1999**, *37:*177–193. Kassahun K, et al. Disposition and biotransformation of the antipsychotic agent olanzapine in humans. *Drug Metab Dispos,* **1997**, *25:*81–93. PDR54, **2000**, p. 1649.

BIOAVAILABILITY (ORAL) (%)	URINARY EXCRETION (%)	BOUND IN PLASMA (%)	CLEARANCE (mL/min/kg)	VOL. DIST. (L/kg)	HALF-LIFE (hours)	PEAK TIME (h)	PEAK CONCENTRATION
Olmesartan[a]							
26	35–50	99	0.31 ± 0.05	0.36 ± 0.18	13.7 ± 5.6	1.5 (1–2.5)[b]	1083 ± 283 ng/mL[b]

[a]Olmesartan is administered as a prodrug, olmesartan medoxomil. Pharmacokinetic data for olmesartan is reported. [b]Following 40 mg/d olmesartan medoxomil for 10 days.

References: Rohatgi S, et al. Pharmacokinetics of amlodipine and olmesartan after administration of amlodipine besylate and olmesartan medoxomil in separate dosage forms and as a fixed-dose combination. *J Clin Pharmacol,* **2008**, *48:*1309–1322. Drugs@FDA. Benicar label approved on July 13, 2005. Available at: http://www.accessdata.fda.gov/scripts/cder/drugsatfda/index.cfm. Accessed May 17, 2010.

(Continued)

TABLE AII–1 ■ PHARMACOKINETIC DATA (CONTINUED)

BIOAVAILABILITY (ORAL) (%)	URINARY EXCRETION (%)	BOUND IN PLASMA (%)	CLEARANCE (mL/min/kg)	VOL. DIST. (L/kg)	HALF-LIFE (hours)	PEAK TIME (h)	PEAK CONCENTRATION
Oxaliplatin[a]							
—[b]	—[c]	90[d]	49 (41–64)[e]	1.5 (1.1–2.1)	0.32 (0.27–0.46)[f]	—	Ox: 0.33 (0.28–0.38) µg Pt/mL
							PtDC: 0.008 (0.004–0.014) µg Pt/mL[g]

[a]Oxaliplatin is an organoplatinum complex; Pt is coordinated with diaminocyclohexane (DACH) and an oxalate ligand as a leaving group. Oxaliplatin (Ox) undergoes nonenzymatic biotransformation to reactive derivatives, notably Pt(DACH)Cl$_2$ (PtDC). Antitumor activity and toxicity are thought to relate to the concentration of oxaliplatin and PtDC in plasma ultrafiltrate (i.e., unbound concentration). [b]For intravenous administration only. [c] ~54% of the platinum eliminated is recovered in urine. [d]Binding to plasma proteins is irreversible. [e]CL of total platinum is much lower; ~ 2–4 mL/min/kg. [f]The elimination of platinum species in plasma follows a triexponential pattern. The quoted $t_{1/2}$ reflects the $t_{1/2}$ of the first phase, which is the clinically relevant phase. The $t_{1/2}$ for the slower two phases are 17 and 391 h. [g]Steady-state plasma ultrafiltrate concentration of Ox and PtDC after an 85-mg/m^2 IV infusion over 2 h during cycles 1 and 2.

References: PDR58, **2004**, pp. 3024–3025. Shord SS, et al. Oxaliplatin biotransformation and pharmacokinetics: a pilot study to determine the possible relationship to neurotoxicity. *Anticancer Res*, **2002**, 22:2301–2309.

Oxcarbazepine[a]							
—	O: <1	—	O: 67.4[b]	—	O: ~2	HC: 2–4[e]	HC: 8.5 ± 2.0 µg/mL[e]
	HC: 27	HC: 45	HC: ↓ RD,[c] Aged		HC: 8–15		
			HC: ↑ Child[d]		HC: ↑ RD, Aged		

[a]Data from healthy adult male subjects. No significant gender differences. Oxcarbazepine (O) undergoes extensive first-pass metabolism to an active metabolite, 10-hydroxycarbamazepine (HC). Reduction by cytosolic enzymes is stereoselective (80% S-enantiomer, 20% R-enantiomer), but both show similar pharmacological activity. [b]CL/F for O reported. HC eliminated by glucuronidation. [c]AUC for HC increased, moderate-to-severe renal impairment. [d]AUC for HC decreased, children < 6 years of age. [e]Following a 300-mg oral oxcarbazepine dose given twice daily for 12 days.

References: Battino D, et al. Clinical pharmacokinetics of antiepileptic drugs in paediatric patients. Part II. Phenytoin, carbamazepine, sulthiame, lamotrigine, vigabatrin, oxcarbazepine and felbamate. *Clin Pharmacokinet*, **1995**, 29:341–369. Lloyd P, et al. Clinical pharmacology and pharmacokinetics of oxcarbazepine. *Epilepsia*, **1994**, 35 (suppl 3):S10–S13. Rouan MC, et al. The effect of renal impairment on the pharmacokinetics of oxcarbazepine and its metabolites. *Eur J Clin Pharmacol*, **1994**, 47:161–167. van Heiningen PN, et al. The influence of age on the pharmacokinetics of the antiepileptic agent oxcarbazepine. *Clin Pharmacol Ther*, **1991**, 50:410–419.

Oxybutynin[a]							
1.6–10.9	<1	—	8.1 ± 2.3[b]	1.3 ± 0.4[b]	IV: 1.9 ± 0.35[b,c]	IR: 5.0 ± 4.2[d]	IR: 12.4 ± 4.1 ng/mL[d]
						XL: 5.2 ± 3.7[d]	XL: 4.2 ± 1.6 ng/mL[d]

[a]Data from healthy female subjects. No significant gender differences. Racemic mixture; anticholinergic activity resides predominantly with R-enantiomer; no stereoselectivity exhibited for anti-spasmodic activity. Oxybutynin undergoes extensive first-pass metabolism to N-desethyloxybutynin (DEO), an active, anticholinergic metabolite. Metabolized primarily by intestinal and hepatic CYP3A. Racemic oxybutynin kinetic parameters reported. [b]Data reported for a 1-mg IV dose, assuming a 70-kg body weight. A larger volume (2.8 L/kg) and longer $t_{1/2}$ (5.3 h) reported for a 5-mg IV dose. [c]Exhibits a longer apparent $t_{1/2}$ following oral dosing due to absorption rate-limited kinetics: immediate-release (IR) $t_{1/2}$ = 9 ± 2 h; extended-release (XL) $t_{1/2}$ = 14 ± 3 h. The apparent $t_{1/2}$ for DEO was 4.0 ± 1.4 h and 8.3 ± 2.5 h for the IR and XL formulations, respectively. [d]Following a dose of 5-mg IR given three times daily or 15-mg XL given once daily for 4 days. Peak DEO levels at steady state were 45 and 23 ng/mL for IR and XL, respectively.

References: Gupta SK, et al. Pharmacokinetics of an oral once-a-day controlled-release oxybutynin formulation compared with immediate-release oxybutynin. *J Clin Pharmacol*, **1999**, 39:289–296. PDR54, **2000**, p. 507.

Oxycodone[a]							
CR: 60–87[b]	—[c]	45	12.4 (9.2–15.4)	2.0 (1.1–2.9)	2.6 (2.1–3.1)[d]	CR: 3.2 ± 2.2[e]	CR: 15.1 ± 4.7 ng/mL[e]
IR: 42 ± 7[b]						IR: 1.6 ± 0.8[e]	IR: 15.5 ± 4.5 ng/mL[e]

[a]Oxycodone is metabolized primarily by CYP3A4/5, with a minor contribution from CYP2D6. Oxymorphone is an active metabolite produced by CYP2D6-mediated O-dealkylation. The circulating concentrations of oxymorphone are too low to contribute significantly to the opioid effects of oxycodone. Data from healthy male and female subjects reported. [b]Values reported for OXYCONTIN [oxycodone controlled release (CR) and immediate-release (IR) tablets. [c]Up to 19% excreted unchanged after an oral dose. [d]The apparent $t_{1/2}$ for the CR oral formulation is ~5 h; this most likely reflects absorption-limited terminal elimination kinetics. [e]Following 10 mg of OXYCONTIN (CR) given twice daily to steady state or a 5-mg IR tablet given every 6 h to steady state.

References: Benziger DP, et al. Differential effects of food on the bioavailability of controlled-release oxycodone tablets and immediate-release oxycodone solution. *J Pharm Sci*, **1996**, 85:407–410. PDR58, **2004**, pp. 2854–2855. Takala A, et al. Pharmacokinetic comparison of intravenous and intranasal administration of oxycodone. *Acta Anaesthesiol Scand*, **1997**, 47:309–312.

Paclitaxel							
Low	5 ± 2	88–98[a]	5.5 ± 3.5[b]	2.01 ± 1.2	31 ± 1[c]	—	0.85 ± 0.21 µM[d]

[a]Binding of drug to dialysis filtration devices may lead to overestimation of protein binding fraction (88% suggested). [b]Metabolized by CYP2C8 and CYP3A, and substrate for P-glycoprotein. [c]Average accumulation $t_{1/2}$; longer terminal $t_{1/2}$ up to 50 h are reported. [d]Steady-state concentration during a 250-mg/m^2 IV infusion given over 24 h to adult cancer patients.

Reference: Sonnichsen DS, et al. Clinical pharmacokinetics of paclitaxel. *Clin Pharmacokinet*, **1994**, 27:256–269.

(Continued)

TABLE AII-1 ■ PHARMACOKINETIC DATA (*CONTINUED*)

BIOAVAILABILITY (ORAL) (%)	URINARY EXCRETION (%)	BOUND IN PLASMA (%)	CLEARANCE (mL/min/kg)	VOL. DIST. (L/kg)	HALF-LIFE (hours)	PEAK TIME (h)	PEAK CONCENTRATION
Paliperidone[a]							
28 (oral ER)[b,c]	59 (51–67) (oral ER)	74	3.70 ± 1.04[d]	9.1[d] (oral ER)	28.4 ± 5.1[d] (oral ER)	22 (2.0–24)[d] (oral ER)	10.7 ± 3.3 ng/mL[d] (oral ER)
	↓ LD		↑ LD[e]				
					25–49 days (IM PP)[f]	13 days (IM PP)	

[a]Paliperidone, otherwise known as the 9-hydroxy active metabolite of risperidone, is marketed as an oral extended-release (ER) tablet (Invega) or in the form of its water-insoluble palmitate ester as a once-monthly long-acting IM injection (Invega Sustenna). Paliperidone is a racemate; its enantiomers have similar pharmacological profiles. The (+)- and (−)-enantiomers of paliperidone interconvert, reaching an AUC (+) to (−) ratio of ~ 1.6 at steady state. [b]High-fat/high-caloric meal increased C_{max} and AUC by 60% and 54%, respectively. [c]No data on the absolute bioavailability of IM paliperidone palmitate (IM PP). The initiation regimen for Invega Sustenna (234 mg/156 mg in the deltoid muscle on day 1/day 8) produces paliperidone concentrations matching the range observed with 6- to 12-mg oral ER paliperidone. [d]At steady-state during once-daily doses of 3 mg, assuming an average body weight of 73 kg. V_z is estimated from CL/F and $t_{1/2}$. [e]Patients with moderate hepatic impairment showed a modest increase in clearance and plasma free fraction with no significant change in unbound AUC. [f]The apparent long terminal $t_{1/2}$ of paliperidone following IM depot injection reflects the slow dissolution of paliperidone palmitate and release of active paliperidone.

References: Boom S, et al. Single- and multiple-dose pharmacokinetics and dose proportionality of the psychotropic agent paliperidone extended release. *J Clin Pharmacol*, **2009**, 49:1318–1330. Drugs@FDA. Invega label approved on April 27, 2007; Invega Sustenna label approved on July 31, 2009. Available at: http://www.accessdata.fda.gov/Scripts/cder/DrugsatFDA/. Accessed January 1, 2010.

Pantoprazole[a]							
77 (67–89)	—[b]	98	2.8 ± 0.9	0.17 ± 0.04	1.1 ± 0.4	2.6 ± 0.9	2.5 ± 0.7 μg/mL[c]
			↓ LD		↑ LD		

[a]Pantoprazole is available as a racemic mixture of (+) and (−) isomers. Pantoprazole is cleared primarily by CYP2C19 (polymorphic)–dependent metabolism. Poor metabolizers (PM) exhibit profound differences in CL (lower) and $t_{1/2}$ (higher) compared to extensive metabolizers (EM). In CYP2C19 EM, no significant differences in the pharmacokinetics of (+) and (−) pantoprazole were observed, whereas in CYP2C19 PM, the CL of (−) pantoprazole was significantly greater than that of (+) pantoprazole. [b]No unchanged drug recovered in urine. [c]Following a single 40-mg oral dose.

References: Drugs@FDA. Protonix label approved on November 12, 2009. Available at: http://www.accessdata.fda.gov/scripts/cder/drugsatfda/index.cfm. Accessed December 26, 2009. Huber R, et al. Pharmacokinetics of lansoprazole in man. *Int J Clin Pharmacol Ther*, **1996**, 34:185–194. Pue MA, et al. Pharmacokinetics of pantoprazole following single intravenous and oral administration to healthy male subjects. *Eur J Clin Pharmacol*, **1993**, 44:575–578. Tanaka M, et al. Stereoselective pharmacokinetics of pantoprazole, a proton pump inhibitor, in extensive and poor metabolizers of S-mephenytoin. *Clin Pharmacol Ther*, **2001**, 69:108–113.

Paroxetine							
Dose dependent[a]	<2	95	8.6 ± 3.2[a,b]	17 ± 10[c]	17 ± 3[d]	5.2 ± 0.5[e]	EM: ~130 nM[e]
			↓ LD, Aged		↑ LD, Aged		PM: ~220 nM[e]

[a]Metabolized by CYP2D6 (polymorphic); undergoes time- and dose-dependent autoinhibition of metabolic CL in extensive metabolizers (EM). [b]CL/F reported for multiple dosing in EM. Single-dose data are significantly higher. In CYP2D6 poor metabolizers (PM), $CL/F = 5.0 \pm 2.1$ mL/min/kg for multiple dosing. [c]V_{area}/F reported. [d]Data reported for multiple dose in EM. In PM, $t_{1/2} = 41 \pm 8$ h. [e]Estimated mean C_{max} following a 30-mg oral dose given once daily for 14 days to adults phenotyped as CYP2D6 EM and PM. There is a significant disproportional accumulation of drug in blood when going from single to multiple dosing due to autoinactivation of CYP2D6.

References: PDR54, **2000**, p. 3028. Sindrup SH, et al. The relationship between paroxetine and the sparteine oxidation polymorphism. *Clin Pharmacol Ther*, **1992**, 51:278–287.

Phenobarbital							
100 ± 11	24 ± 5[a]	51 ± 3	0.062 ± 0.013	0.54 ± 0.03	99 ± 18	2–4[b]	13.1 ± 4.5 μg/mL[b]
	↓ Neo	↑ Preg, Child, Neo		↑ Neo	↑ LD, Aged ↓ Child		

[a]Phenobarbital is a weak acid ($pK_a = 7.3$); urinary excretion is increased at an alkaline pH; it also is reduced with decreased urine flow. [b]Mean steady-state concentration following a 90-mg oral dose given daily for 12 weeks to patients with epilepsy. Levels of 10–25 μg/mL provide control of tonic-clonic seizures, and levels of at least 15 μg/mL provide control of febrile convulsions in children. Levels > 40 μg/mL can cause toxicity; 65–117 μg/mL produce stage III anesthesia—comatose but reflexes present; 100–134 μg/mL produce stage IV anesthesia—no deep-tendon reflexes.

References: Bourgeois BFD. Phenobarbital and primidone. In: Wyllie E, ed. *The Treatment of Epilepsy: Principles and Practice.* 2nd ed. Williams & Wilkins, Philadelphia, **1997**, pp. 845–855. Browne TR, et al. Studies with stable isotopes II: phenobarbital pharmacokinetics during monotherapy. *J Clin Pharmacol*, **1985**, 25:51–58.

(*Continued*)

TABLE AII-1 ■ PHARMACOKINETIC DATA (*CONTINUED*)

BIOAVAILABILITY (ORAL) (%)	URINARY EXCRETION (%)	BOUND IN PLASMA (%)	CLEARANCE (mL/min/kg)	VOL. DIST. (L/kg)	HALF-LIFE (hours)	PEAK TIME (h)	PEAK CONCENTRATION
Phenytoin[a]							
90 ± 3	2 ± 8	89 ± 23	V_{max} = 5.9 ± 1.2 mg·kg^{-1} day^{-1}	0.64 ± 0.04[d]	6–24[e]	3–12[f]	0–5 µg/mL (27%)[f]
		↓ RD, Neo, LD, Preg		↑ Neo, RD	↑ Prem[c]		5–10 µg/mL (30%)[f]
			↓ Aged,				10–20 µg/mL (29%)[f]
			↑ Child		↓ RD[c]		20–30 µg/mL (10%)[f]
			K_m = 5.7 ± 2.9 mg/L[b]				>30 µg/mL (6%)[f]
			↓ Child				
			↑ RD[c]				
			↓ Prem[c]				

[a]Metabolized predominantly by CYP2C9 (polymorphic) and also by CYP2C19 (polymorphic); exhibits saturable kinetics with therapeutic doses. [b]Significantly decreased in the Japanese population. [c]Comparison of *CL*s and $t_{1/2}$s with similar doses in normal subjects and patients; nonlinear kinetics not considered. [d]V_{area} reported. [e]Apparent $t_{1/2}$ is dependent on plasma concentration. [f]Population frequency of total phenytoin concentrations following a 300-mg oral dose (capsule) given daily to steady state. Total levels > 10 µg/mL associated with suppression of tonic-clonic seizures. Nystagmus can occur at levels > 20 µg/mL and ataxia at levels > 30 µg/mL.

BIOAVAILABILITY (ORAL) (%)	URINARY EXCRETION (%)	BOUND IN PLASMA (%)	CLEARANCE (mL/min/kg)	VOL. DIST. (L/kg)	HALF-LIFE (hours)	PEAK TIME (h)	PEAK CONCENTRATION
Pioglitazone[a]							
—	Negligible	>99	1.2 ± 1.7[b]	0.63 ± 0.41[b]	11 ± 6[c]	P: 3.5 (1–4)[d]	P: 1.6 ± 0.2 µg/mL[d]
						M-III: 11 (2–48)[d]	M-III: 0.4 ± 0.2 µg/mL[d]
						M-IV: 11 (4–16)[d]	M-IV: 1.4 ± 0.5 µg/mL[d]

[a]Data from healthy male and female subjects and patients with type 2 diabetes. Pioglitazone (P) is metabolized extensively by CYP2C8, CYP3A4, and other CYP isozymes. Two major metabolites (M-III and M-IV) accumulate in blood and contribute to the pharmacological effect. [b]*CL/F* and V_{area}/F reported. *CL/F* is lower in women than in men. [c]Steady-state $t_{1/2}$ of M-III and M-IV are 29 and 27 h, respectively. [d]Following a 45-mg oral dose given once daily for 10 days.

References: Budde K, et al. The pharmacokinetics of pioglitazone in patients with impaired renal function. *Br J Clin Pharmacol*, **2003**, *55*:368–374. PDR58, **2004**, p. 3186.

BIOAVAILABILITY (ORAL) (%)	URINARY EXCRETION (%)	BOUND IN PLASMA (%)	CLEARANCE (mL/min/kg)	VOL. DIST. (L/kg)	HALF-LIFE (hours)	PEAK TIME (h)	PEAK CONCENTRATION
Posaconazole							
—[a]	—	98	11.7 ± 6.4[b]	11.9[b]	21.6 ± 8.4	4 (3–12)	324 ± 161 ng/mL[c]

[a]~66% of an oral posaconazole dose is excreted unchanged in feces. It is unclear whether this represents significant biliary excretion or unabsorbed dose. [b]*CL/F* and V_d/F reported. [c]Following a single 400-mg dose of an oral suspension.

References: Courtney R, et al. Posaconazole pharmacokinetics, safety, and tolerability in subjects with varying degrees of chronic renal disease. *J Clin Pharmacol*, **2005**, *45*:185–192. Dodds Ashley ES, et al. Pharmacokinetics of posaconazole administered orally or by nasogastric tube in healthy volunteers. *Antimicrob Agents Chemother*, **2009**, *53*:2960–2964.

BIOAVAILABILITY (ORAL) (%)	URINARY EXCRETION (%)	BOUND IN PLASMA (%)	CLEARANCE (mL/min/kg)	VOL. DIST. (L/kg)	HALF-LIFE (hours)	PEAK TIME (h)	PEAK CONCENTRATION
Pramipexole[a]							
>90[b]	~90	15	8.2 ± 1.4[b]	7.3 ± 1.7[b]	11.6 ± 2.57	1–2	M: 1.6 ± 0.23 ng/mL[e]
			↓ Aged, RD,[c] PD[d]		↑ Aged, RD		F: 2.1 ± 0.25 ng/mL[e]

[a]Data from healthy adult male and female subjects. No significant gender differences. [b]Bioavailability estimated from urinary recovery of unchanged drug. *CL/F* and V/F_{area} reported. [c]*CL/F* reduced, moderate-to-severe renal impairment. [d]Parkinson's disease (PD); *CL/F* reduced with declining renal function. [e]Following a 0.5-mg oral dose given three times daily for 4 days to male (M) and female (F) adults.

References: Lam YW. Clinical pharmacology of dopamine agonists. *Pharmacotherapy*, **2000**, *20*:17S–25S. PDR54, **2000**, p. 2468. Wright CE, et al. Steady-state pharmacokinetic properties of pramipexole in healthy volunteers. *J Clin Pharmacol*, **1997**, *37*:520–525.

BIOAVAILABILITY (ORAL) (%)	URINARY EXCRETION (%)	BOUND IN PLASMA (%)	CLEARANCE (mL/min/kg)	VOL. DIST. (L/kg)	HALF-LIFE (hours)	PEAK TIME (h)	PEAK CONCENTRATION
Pramlintide[a]							
30%–40%[b]	—	~60[c]	Low: 14.9 ± 3.9[d]	0.43	IV: 0.4–0.75	0.32–0.35[e]	Low: 21 ± 3 pmol/L[e]
			High: 14.5 ± 4.0[d]	0.71	SC: 0.5–0.83		High: 77 ± 22 pmol/L[e]

[a]Pramlintide is a synthetic peptide analogue of amylin for the treatment of both type 1 and type 2 diabetes. It is metabolized in the kidneys to at least one primary active metabolite: Des-lys(1)pramlintide (2–37 pramlintide) with a $t_{1/2}$ similar to that of the parent drug. [b]SC administration with greater variability in response when the injection is into the arm compared to into the abdomen or thigh. [c]Not extensively bound to blood cells or albumin. [d]Based on intravenous infusion of a low dose of 30 µg for type 1 diabetes and a high dose of 100 µg for type 2 diabetes. [e]Following a low SC dose of 30 µg and a high SC dose of 100 µg.

References: Colburn WA, et al. Pharmacokinetics and pharmacodynamics of AC137 (25,28,29 triproamylin, human) after intravenous bolus and infusion doses in patients with insulin-dependent diabetes. *J Clin Pharmacol*, **1996**, *36*:13–24. Drugs@FDA. Symlin label approved on September 25, 2007. Available at: http://www.accessdata.fda.gov/Scripts/cder/DrugsatFDA/. Accessed August 1, 2009. Kolterman OG, et al. Effect of 14 days' subcutaneous administration of the human amylin analogue, pramlintide (AC137), on an intravenous insulin challenge and response to a standard liquid meal in patients with IDDM. *Diabetologia*, **1996**, *39*:492–499.

(Continued)

TABLE AII–1 ■ PHARMACOKINETIC DATA (*CONTINUED*)

BIOAVAILABILITY (ORAL) (%)	URINARY EXCRETION (%)	BOUND IN PLASMA (%)	CLEARANCE (mL/min/kg)	VOL. DIST. (L/kg)	HALF-LIFE (hours)	PEAK TIME (h)	PEAK CONCENTRATION
Pravastatin							
18 ± 8	47 ± 7	43–48	13.5 ± 2.4	0.46 ± 0.04	0.8 ± 0.2^b	1–1.4[c]	28–38 ng/mL[c]
			↓ LD		↔ Aged, RD[a]		
			↔ Aged, RD[a]				

[a]Although renal *CL* decreases with reduced renal function, no significant changes in *CL/F* or $t_{1/2}$ are seen following oral dosing as a result of the low and highly variable bioavailability. [b]A longer $t_{1/2} = 1.8 \pm 0.8$ h reported for oral dosing; probably rate limited by absorption. [c]Range of mean values from different studies following a single 20-mg oral dose.

References: Corsini A, et al. New insights into the pharmacodynamic and pharmacokinetic properties of statins. *Pharmacol Ther*, **1999**, *84*:413–428. Desager JP, et al. Clinical pharmacokinetics of 3-hydroxy-3-methylglutaryl-coenzyme A reductase inhibitors. *Clin Pharmacokinet*, **1996**, *31*:348–371. Quion JA, et al. Clinical pharmacokinetics of pravastatin. *Clin Pharmacokinet*, **1994**, *27*:94–103.

Praziquantel[a]							
—[b]	Negligible	80–85	5 mg/kg: 467[c]	50 mg/kg: 9.55 ± 2.86	5 mg/kg: 0.8–1.5[c]	1.5–1.8[e]	0.8–6.3 μg/mL[e]
			40–60 mg/kg: 57–222[c]		40–60 mg/kg: 1.7–3.0[c]		
			↓ LD[d]		↑ LD		

[a]Data from male and female patients with schistosomiasis. [b]Absolute bioavailability is not known. Praziquantel is well absorbed (80%) but undergoes significant first-pass metabolism (hydroxylation), the extent of which appears to be dose dependent. [c]*CL/F* and V_{ss}/F reported; *CL/F* and $t_{1/2}$ are dose dependent. [d]*CL/F* reduced, moderate-to-severe hepatic impairment. [e]Range of mean values from different studies following a single 40- to 60-mg/kg oral dose.

References: Edwards G, et al. Clinical pharmacokinetics of anthelmintic drugs. *Clin Pharmacokinet*, **1988**, *15*:67–93. el Guiniady MA, et al. Clinical and pharmacokinetic study of praziquantel in Egyptian schistosomiasis patients with and without liver cell failure. *Am J Trop Med Hyg*, **1994**, *51*:809–818. Jung H, et al. Clinical pharmacokinetics of praziquantel. *Proc West Pharmacol Soc*, **1991**, *34*:335–340. Sotelo J, et al. Pharmacokinetic optimisation of the treatment of neurocysticercosis. *Clin Pharmacokinet*, **1998**, *34*:503–515. Watt G, et al. Praziquantel pharmacokinetics and side effects in *Schistosoma japonicum*-infected patients with liver disease. *J Infect Dis*, **1988**, *157*:530–535.

Prednisolone							
82 ± 13	26 ± 9^a	90–95 (<200 ng/mL)[b]	1.0 ± 0.16^c	0.42 ± 0.11^e	2.2 ± 0.5	1.5 ± 0.5^f	458 ± 150 ng/mL[f]
	↑ Aged	~70 (>1 μg/mL)	↓ Aged,[d] LD[d]	↓ Aged, Obes[d]	↑ Aged[d]		
		↓ Aged, LD					

[a]Prednisolone and prednisone are interconvertible; an additional 3% ± 2% is excreted as prednisone. [b]Extent of binding to plasma proteins is dependent on concentration over range encountered. [c]Total *CL* increases as protein binding is saturated. *CL* of unbound drug increases slightly but significantly with increasing dose. [d]Changes are for unbound drug. [e]*V* increases with dose due to saturable protein binding. [f]Following a 30-mg oral dose given twice daily for 3 days to healthy adult male subjects. The ratio of prednisolone/prednisone is dose dependent and can vary from 3 to 26 over a prednisolone concentration range of 50–800 ng/mL.

References: Frey BM, et al. Clinical pharmacokinetics of prednisone and prednisolone. *Clin Pharmacokinet*, **1990**, *19*:126–146. Rohatagi S, et al. Pharmacokinetics of methylprednisolone and prednisolone after single and multiple oral administration. *J Clin Pharmacol*, **1997**, *37*:916–925.

Prednisone							
80 ± 11^a	3 ± 2^b	75 ± 2^c	3.6 ± 0.8^d	0.97 ± 0.11^d	3.6 ± 0.4^d	P: 2.1–3.1[e]	P: 62–81 ng/mL[e]
						PL: 1.2–2.6[e]	PL: 198–239 ng/mL[e]

[a]Measured relative to equivalent intravenous dose of prednisolone (PL). [b]An additional 15% ± 5% excreted as PL. [c]In contrast to PL, there is no dependence on concentration. [d]Kinetic values for prednisone (P) often are reported in terms of values for PL, its active metabolite. However, the values cited here pertain to P. [e]Range of mean data for P and PL following a single 10-mg oral dose given as different proprietary formulations to healthy adults.

References: Gustavson LE, et al. The macromolecular binding of prednisone in plasma of healthy volunteers including pregnant women and oral contraceptive users. *J Pharmacokinet Biopharm*, **1985**, *13*:561–569. Pickup ME. Clinical pharmacokinetics of prednisone and prednisolone. *Clin Pharmacokinet*, **1979**, *4*:111–128. Sullivan TJ, et al. Comparative bioavailability: eight commercial prednisone tablets. *J Pharmacokinet Biopharm*, **1976**, *4*:157–172.

Pregabalin							
≥90[a]	90–99	0	0.96–1.2[b,c]	0.5	5–6.5	1[a]	8.5 μg/mL[e]
			↓ RD[d]				

[a]Bioavailability does not vary with dose up to 600 mg. T_{max} is delayed from 1 to 3 h and C_{max} decreased by 25%–30% when pregabalin is given with food. No change in AUC or extent of absorption is noted. [b]Pregabalin undergoes minimal metabolism; an *N*-methylated metabolite has been identified in urine and accounts for 0.9% of oral dose. [c]Mean renal clearance in healthy young subjects ranges from 67 to 81 mL/min and assuming 70-kg body weight. Pregabalin pharmacokinetics is dose independent and predictable from single to multiple dosing. [d]Pregabalin clearance is proportional to CL_{cr}; hence, dosage can be adjusted in accordance to CL_{cr} in renal dysfunction. Plasma pregabalin decreased by ~ 50% after 4 h of hemodialysis. [e]Steady-state concentration in healthy subjects receiving 200-mg pregabalin every 8 h.

References: Bialer M, et al. Progress report on new antiepileptic drugs: a summary of the fifth Eilat conference (Eilat V). *Epilepsy Res*, **2001**, *43*:11–58. Brodie MJ, et al. Pregabalin drug interaction studies: lack of effect on the pharmacokinetics of carbamazepine, phenytoin, lamotrigine, and valproate in patients with partial epilepsy. *Epilepsia*, **2005**, *46*: 1407–1413. *Physicians' Desk Reference*, 63rd ed. Physicians' Desk Reference Inc., Montvale, NJ, **2008**, pp. 2527–2534.

(Continued)

TABLE AII–1 ■ PHARMACOKINETIC DATA (*CONTINUED*)

BIOAVAILABILITY (ORAL) (%)	URINARY EXCRETION (%)	BOUND IN PLASMA (%)	CLEARANCE (mL/min/kg)	VOL. DIST. (L/kg)	HALF-LIFE (hours)	PEAK TIME (h)	PEAK CONCENTRATION
Procainamide[a]							
83 ± 16	67 ± 8	16 ± 5	$CL = 2.7CL_{cr}$ + 1.7	1.9 ± 0.3	3.0 ± 0.6	M: 3.6[d]	M: 2.2 µg/mL[d]
	↓ LD		+ 3.2 (fast)[b] or + 1.1 (slow)[b]	↓ Obes	↑ RD[c]	F: 3.8[d]	F: 2.9 µg/mL[d]
			↑ Child		↓ Child, Neo		

[a]Active metabolite, *N*-acetylprocainamide (NAPA); $CL = 3.1 ± 0.4$ mL/min/kg, $V = 1.4 ± 0.2$ L/kg, and $t_{1/2} = 6.0 ± 0.2$ h. [b]CL calculated using units of mL/min/kg for CL_{cr}. CL depends on NAT2 acetylation phenotype. Use a mean value of 2.2 if phenotype unknown. [c]$t_{1/2}$ for procainamide and NAPA increased in patients with RD. [d]Least square mean values following 1000-mg oral dose given twice daily to steady state in male (M) and female (F) adults. Mean peak NAPA concentrations were 2.0 and 2.2 µg/mL for male and female adults, respectively; $T_{max} = 4.1$ and 4.2 h, respectively.

References: Benet LZ, et al. Die renale Elimination von Procainamide: Pharmacokinetik bei Niereninsuffizienz. In: Braun J, et al., eds. *Die Behandlung von Herzrhythmusstorungen bei Nierenkranken*. Karger, Basel, **1984**, 96–111. Koup JR, et al. Effect of age, gender, and race on steady state procainamide pharmacokinetics after administration of Procanbid sustained-release tablets. *Ther Drug Monit*, **1998**, 20:73–77.

BIOAVAILABILITY (ORAL) (%)	URINARY EXCRETION (%)	BOUND IN PLASMA (%)	CLEARANCE (mL/min/kg)	VOL. DIST. (L/kg)	HALF-LIFE (hours)	PEAK TIME (h)	PEAK CONCENTRATION
Propofol[a]							
—[b]	—	98.3–98.8[c]	27 ± 5	1.7 ± 0.7[f]	3.5 ± 1.2[f]	—	SS: 3.5 ± 0.06 µg/mL[g]
			↑ Child[d]	↑ Child[d]			
			↓ Aged[e]	↓ Aged[e]			
							E: 1.1 ± 0.4 µg/mL[g]

[a]Data from patients undergoing elective surgery and healthy volunteers. Propofol is extensively metabolized by UGTs. [b]For intravenous administration only. [c]Fraction bound in whole blood. Concentration dependent; 98.8% at 0.5 µg/mL and 98.3 at 32 µg/mL. [d]CL and central volume increased in children 1–3 years of age. [e]CL and central volume decreased in elderly patients. [f]V_{area} is much larger than V_{ss}. A much longer terminal $t_{1/2}$ was reported following prolonged intravenous infusion. [g]Concentration producing anesthesia after infusion to steady state (SS) and at emergence (E) from anesthesia.

References: Mazoit JX, et al. Binding of propofol to blood components: implications for pharmacokinetics and for pharmacodynamics. *Br J Clin Pharmacol*, **1999**, 47:35–42. Murat I, et al. Pharmacokinetics of propofol after a single dose in children aged 1–3 years with minor burns. Comparison of three data analysis approaches. *Anesthesiology*, **1996**, 84: 526–532. Servin F, et al. Pharmacokinetics of propofol infusions in patients with cirrhosis. *Br J Anaesth*, **1990**, 65:177–183.

BIOAVAILABILITY (ORAL) (%)	URINARY EXCRETION (%)	BOUND IN PLASMA (%)	CLEARANCE (mL/min/kg)	VOL. DIST. (L/kg)	HALF-LIFE (hours)	PEAK TIME (h)	PEAK CONCENTRATION
Propranolol[a]							
26 ± 10	<0.5	87 ± 6[b]	16 ± 5[c,d]	4.3 ± 0.6[c]	3.9 ± 0.4[c]	P: 1.5[e]	P: 49 ± 8 ng/mL[e]
↑ LD		↑ Preg, Obes	↑ LD	↑ Obes, Fem	↓ LD	HP: 1.0[e]	HP: 37 ± 9 ng/mL[e]
		↓ LD	↓ LD, Obes, Fem				

[a]Racemic mixture. For *S*-(–)-enantiomer (100-fold more active) compared to *R*-(+)-enantiomer, CL is 19% lower and V_{area} is 15% lower because of a higher degree of protein binding (18% lower free fraction); hence, there is no difference in $t_{1/2}$. Active metabolite, 4-hydroxypropranolol (HP). [b]Drug is bound primarily to α_1-acid glycoprotein, which is elevated in a number of inflammatory conditions. [c]Based on blood measurements; blood-to-plasma concentration ratio = 0.89 ± 0.03. [d]CYP2D6 catalyzes the formation of HP; CYP1A2 is responsible for most of the *N*-desisopropyl metabolite; UGT catalyzes the major conjugation pathway of elimination. [e]Propranolol (P) and HP following a single 80-mg oral dose given to healthy adults. Plasma accumulation factor was 3.6-fold after 80 mg was given four times daily to steady state. A concentration of 20 ng/mL gave a 50% decrease in exercise-induced cardioacceleration. Antianginal effects manifest at 15–90 ng/mL. A concentration up to 1000 ng/mL may be required for control of ventricular arrhythmias.

References: Colangelo PM, et al. Age and propranolol stereoselective disposition in humans. *Clin Pharmacol Ther*, **1992**, 57:489–494. Walle T, et al. 4-Hydroxypropranolol and its glucuronide after single and long-term doses of propranolol. *Clin Pharmacol Ther*, **1980**, 27:22–31.

BIOAVAILABILITY (ORAL) (%)	URINARY EXCRETION (%)	BOUND IN PLASMA (%)	CLEARANCE (mL/min/kg)	VOL. DIST. (L/kg)	HALF-LIFE (hours)	PEAK TIME (h)	PEAK CONCENTRATION
Pseudoephedrine[a]							
~100	43–96[b]	—	7.33[b,c]	2.64–3.51[c]	4.3–8[b,c]	IR: 1.4–2[d]	IR: 177–360 ng/mL[d]
						CR: 3.8–6.1[d]	CR: 265–314 ng/mL[d]

[a]Data from healthy adult male and female subjects. [b]At a high urinary pH (>7.0), pseudoephedrine is extensively reabsorbed; $t_{1/2}$ increases, and CL decreases. [c]CL/F, V/F, and $t_{1/2}$ reported for oral dose. [d]Range of mean values from different studies following a single 60-mg immediate-release tablet or syrup (IR) or 120-mg controlled-release capsule (CR) oral dose.

Reference: Kanfer I, et al. Pharmacokinetics of oral decongestants. *Pharmacotherapy*, **1993**, 13:116S–128S.

BIOAVAILABILITY (ORAL) (%)	URINARY EXCRETION (%)	BOUND IN PLASMA (%)	CLEARANCE (mL/min/kg)	VOL. DIST. (L/kg)	HALF-LIFE (hours)	PEAK TIME (h)	PEAK CONCENTRATION
Pyrazinamide[a]							
—[b]	4–14[c]	10	1.1 (0.2–2.3)[d]	0.57 (0.13–1.04)[d]	6 (2–23)	1–2[e]	35 (19–103) µg/mL[e]
			↑ Child		↓ Child		

[a]Pyrazinamide is hydrolyzed in the liver to an active metabolite, 2-pyrazinoic acid. Reported peak 2-pyrazinoic acid concentrations range from 0.1- to 1-fold that of the parent drug. Pyrazinamide data reported are for male and female adults with tuberculosis. [b]Absolute bioavailability is not known, but the drug is well absorbed based on recovery of parent drug and metabolites (70%). [c]Recovery of unchanged drug following an oral dose; the recovery of pyrazinoic acid is 37 ± 5%. [d]CL/F and V_{area}/F reported. [e]Following a 15- to 53-mg/kg daily oral dose to steady state.

References: Bareggi SR, et al. Clinical pharmacokinetics and metabolism of pyrazinamide in healthy volunteers. *Arzneimittelforschung*, **1987**, 37:849–854. Lacroix C, et al. Pharmacokinetics of pyrazinamide and its metabolites in healthy subjects. *Eur J Clin Pharmacol*, **1989**, 36:395–400. PDR58, **2004**, p. 766. Zhu M, et al. Population pharmacokinetic modeling of pyrazinamide in children and adults with tuberculosis. *Pharmacotherapy*, **2002**, 22:686–695.

(Continued)

TABLE AII–1 ■ PHARMACOKINETIC DATA (*CONTINUED*)

BIOAVAILABILITY (ORAL) (%)	URINARY EXCRETION (%)	BOUND IN PLASMA (%)	CLEARANCE (mL/min/kg)	VOL. DIST. (L/kg)	HALF-LIFE (hours)	PEAK TIME (h)	PEAK CONCENTRATION
Quetiapine[a]							
9	<1%	83	19[b]	10 ± 4	6	1–1.8	278 ng/mL[c]
↑ Food			↓ Aged, LD				

[a]No significant gender differences. [b]Extensively metabolized through multiple pathways, including sulfoxidation, *N*- and *O*-dealkylation catalyzed by CYP3A4. Two minor active metabolites. [c]Following a 250-mg oral dose given daily for 23 days in patients with schizophrenia.

References: Goren JL, et al. Quetiapine, an atypical antipsychotic. *Pharmacotherapy*, **1998**, *18*:1183–1194. *PDR54*, **2000**, p. 563.

BIOAVAILABILITY (ORAL) (%)	URINARY EXCRETION (%)	BOUND IN PLASMA (%)	CLEARANCE (mL/min/kg)	VOL. DIST. (L/kg)	HALF-LIFE (hours)	PEAK TIME (h)	PEAK CONCENTRATION
Quinapril[a]							
QT (Q): 52 ± 15[b]	Q (Q): 3.1 ± 1.2[c]	QT: 97	QT (QT): 0.98 ± 0.22[d]	QT (QT): 0.19 ± 0.04[d]	Q (Q): 0.8–0.9[c]	Q (Q): 1.4 ± 0.8[e]	Q (Q): 207 ± 89 ng/mL[e]
	QT (QT): 96[d]				QT (QT): 2.1–2.9[d]	QT (Q): 2.3 ± 0.9[e]	QT (Q): 923 ± 277 ng/mL[e]
			↓ RD		↑ RD		

[a]Hydrolyzed to its active metabolite, quinaprilat. Pharmacokinetic data for quinapril (Q) and quinaprilat (QT) following oral Q and intravenous QT administration are presented. [b]Absolute bioavailability based on plasma QT concentrations. [c]Data for Q following a 2.5- to 80-mg oral dose. [d]Data for QT following a 2.5-mg IV QT dose. The $t_{1/2}$ of QT after dosing Q is similar. [e]Following a single 40-mg oral Q dose. No accumulation of QT with multiple dosing.

References: Breslin E, et al. A pharmacodynamic and pharmacokinetic comparison of intravenous quinaprilat and oral quinapril. *J Clin Pharmacol*, **1996**, *36*:414–421. Olson SC, et al. The clinical pharmacokinetics of quinapril. *Angiology*, **1989**, *40*:351–359. *PDR58*, **2004**, p. 2516.

BIOAVAILABILITY (ORAL) (%)	URINARY EXCRETION (%)	BOUND IN PLASMA (%)	CLEARANCE (mL/min/kg)	VOL. DIST. (L/kg)	HALF-LIFE (hours)	PEAK TIME (h)	PEAK CONCENTRATION
Quinine[a]							
76 ± 11	N-A: 12–20	N-A: ~85–90[b]	N-A: 1.9 ± 0.5	N-A: 1.8 ± 0.4	N-A: 11 ± 2	PO: 3.5–8.4[d]	Adults
	M-A: 33 ± 18	M-A: 93–95[b]	M-A: 0.9–1.4	M-A: 1.0–1.7	M-A: 11–18		IV: 11 ± 2 µg/mL[d]
		↓ Neo	M-C: 0.4–1.4	M-C: 1.2–1.7	M-C: 12–16		PO: 7.3–9.4 µg/mL[d]
		↑ Smk		↓ Preg[c]	↓ Preg,[c] Smk		Children
							IV: 8.7–9.4 µg/mL[d]
	↓ Aged				↑ LD, Aged		PO: 7.3 ± 1.1 µg/mL[d]

[a]Data from normal adults (N-A) and range of means from different studies of adults (M-A) or children (M-C) with malaria reported. [b]Correlates with serum α_1-acid glycoprotein levels. Binding is increased in severe malaria. [c]From patients with malaria. [d]Following a single 10-mg/kg dose given as a 0.5- to 4-h IV infusion or orally (PO) to children or adults with malaria. A level > 0.2 µg/mL for unbound drug is targeted for treatment of *Plasmodium falciparum* malaria. Oculotoxicity and hearing loss/tinnitus associated with unbound concentrations > 2 µg/mL.

References: Edwards G, et al. Clinical pharmacokinetics in the treatment of tropical diseases. Some applications and limitations. *Clin Pharmacokinet*, **1994**, *27*:150–165. Krishna S, et al. Pharmacokinetics of quinine, chloroquine and amodiaquine. Clinical implications. *Clin Pharmacokinet*, **1996**, *30*:263–299.

BIOAVAILABILITY (ORAL) (%)	URINARY EXCRETION (%)	BOUND IN PLASMA (%)	CLEARANCE (mL/min/kg)	VOL. DIST. (L/kg)	HALF-LIFE (hours)	PEAK TIME (h)	PEAK CONCENTRATION
Raloxifene[a]							
2[b]	<0.2	>95	735 ± 338[c]	2348 ± 1220[c]	28 (11–273)	6[d]	0.5 ± 0.3 ng/mL[d]
			↓ LD				

[a]Data from postmenopausal women. Undergoes extensive first-pass metabolism (UGT catalyzed) and enterohepatic recycling. [b]~60% absorption from the gastrointestinal tract; not significantly affected by food. [c]*CL/F* and *V/F* reported for an oral dose. [d]Following a single 1-mg/kg oral dose.

References: Hochner-Celnikier D. Pharmacokinetics of raloxifene and its clinical application. *Eur J Obstet Gynecol Reprod Biol*, **1999**, *85*:23–29. *PDR54*, **2000**, p. 1583.

BIOAVAILABILITY (ORAL) (%)	URINARY EXCRETION (%)	BOUND IN PLASMA (%)	CLEARANCE (mL/min/kg)	VOL. DIST. (L/kg)	HALF-LIFE (hours)	PEAK TIME (h)	PEAK CONCENTRATION
Raltegravir							
≥31.8 ± 9.4[a]	8.8 ± 4.7	83	16.1 (11.4, 22.6[b])[c]	–	α: 0.92 ± 0.21[d]	1.0[e]	4.5 (2.0, 10.2) µM[e]
					β: 12.5 ± 4.6[d]		

[a]The absolute oral bioavailability of raltegravir has not been determined. This minimum extent of oral absorption is based on recovery of radioactivity in urine following oral administration of ^{14}C-labeled raltegravir in healthy human subjects. [b]Raltegravir undergoes *O*-glucuronidation mediated largely by UGT1A1 and to a lesser extent by UGT1A3 and UGT1A9. Raltegravir AUC is only modestly elevated in individuals with *UGT1A1*28/*28* genotype compared to **1/*1* genotype. [c]Geometric mean (95% confidence interval) of pharmacokinetic parameters following a single 400-mg oral dose. Apparent oral clearance (*CL/F*) is listed. [d]Plasma concentration time course of raltegravir exhibits multiphasic washout kinetics. Initial (α) and terminal (β) $t_{1/2}$s are reported because the early phase accounts for a large portion of the AUC from time 0 to ∞. [e]Median for T_{max} and geometric mean (95% confidence interval) for C_{max} following a 400-mg twice-daily monotherapy regimen for 10 days in treatment-naive patients with HIV-1 infection.

References: Drugs@FDA. Isentress label approved on July 8, 2009. Available at: http://www.accessdata.fda.gov/Scripts/cder/DrugsatFDA/. Accessed August 22, 2009. Kassahun K, et al. Metabolism and disposition in humans of raltegravir (MK-0518), an anti-AIDS drug targeting the human immunodeficiency virus 1 integrase enzyme. *Drug Metab Dispos*, **2007**, *35*:1657–1663. Wenning LA, et al. Lack of a significant drug interaction between raltegravir and tenofovir. *Antimicrob Agents Chemother*, **2008**, *52*:3253–3258. Wenning LA, et al. Pharmacokinetics of raltegravir in individuals with UGT1A1 polymorphisms. *Clin Pharmacol Ther*, **2009**, *85*:623–627.

APPENDIX II

DESIGN AND OPTIMIZATION OF DOSAGE REGIMENS: PHARMACOKINETIC DATA

(Continued)

TABLE AII–1 ■ PHARMACOKINETIC DATA (CONTINUED)

BIOAVAILABILITY (ORAL) (%)	URINARY EXCRETION (%)	BOUND IN PLASMA (%)	CLEARANCE (mL/min/kg)	VOL. DIST. (L/kg)	HALF-LIFE (hours)	PEAK TIME (h)	PEAK CONCENTRATION
Ramelteon[a]							
1.8[b]	<0.1%	82	13.1[c]	1.05	P: 1.3 ± 0.5[e]	P: 1.6 ± 0.5	P: 6.9 ± 7.8 ng/mL[e,f]
			↓ Aged, LD[d]		M: 2.3 ± 0.5[e]		M: 110 ± 29 ng/mL[e,f]
					↑ Aged		

[a]Ramelteon undergoes primary oxidative metabolism followed by glucuronidation as secondary metabolism. CYP1A2 is the major enzyme involved in oxidative metabolism; CYP3A and CYP2C9 also are involved as minor enzymes. Remarkable elevation in C_{max} and AUC were observed with the concurrent administration of the strong CYP1A2 inhibitor fluvoxamine. The M-II metabolite contributes to the hypnotic effects of ramelteon. M-II has 1/5th to 1/10th the affinity of ramelteon as an agonist for the melatonin receptors (MT-1 and MT-2); however, it circulates at 20- to 100-fold higher concentrations relative to ramelteon. [b]Poor systemic availability of ramelteon is due to extensive first-pass metabolism. C_{max} and AUC are elevated by a high-fat meal; T_{max} is slightly delayed. [c]Calculated assuming 70-kg body weight. Although note shown, interindividual variability is notably large. [d]Four- and 10-fold elevation in AUC in mild and moderate hepatic impairment. [e]P = parent drug; M = M-II metabolite. [f]C_{max} following a single 16-mg oral dose of ramelteon in young adult subjects. There is no measurable accumulation of parent drug or active metabolite because of their short elimination $t_{1/2}$.

References: Drugs@FDA. Rozerem label approved on October 20, 2008. Available at: http://www.accessdata.fda.gov/scripts/cder/drugsatfda/index.cfm. Accessed August 23, 2009. Greenblatt DJ, et al. Age and gender effects on the pharmacokinetics and pharmacodynamics of ramelteon, a hypnotic agent acting via melatonin receptors MT 1 and MT2. *J Clin Pharmacol,* **2006,** *47:*485–496. McGechan A, et al. Ramelteon. *CNS Drugs,* **2005,** *19:*1057–1065.

Ramipril[a]							
R (R): 28[b]	R (R): <2[c]	R: 73 ± 2	R (R): 23[d]	—	R (R): 5 ± 2	R (R): 1.2 ± 0.3[g]	R (R): 43.3 ± 10.2 ng/mL[g]
							RT (R): 24.1 ± 5.6 ng/mL[g]
RT (R): 48[b]	RT (R): 13 ± 6[c]	RT: 56 ± 2	RT: —[e]		RT (R): 9–18[f] ↑ RD	RT (R): 3.0 ± 0.7[g]	

[a]Hydrolyzed to its active metabolite, ramiprilat (RT). Pharmacokinetic data for ramipril (R) and RT following oral and intravenous R administration are presented. [b]Based on plasma AUC of R and RT after intravenous and oral R administration. [c]Following an oral dose of R. [d]CL/F of R calculated from reported AUC data. [e]No data available; mean renal CL of RT is ~ 1.1 mL/min/kg. [f]$t_{1/2}$ for the elimination phase reported. A longer terminal $t_{1/2}$ of ~ 120 h most likely corresponds to the release of drug from ACE; contributes to the duration of effect but does not contribute to systemic drug accumulation. [g]Following a single 10-mg oral dose.

References: Eckert HG, et al. Pharmacokinetics and biotransformation of 2-[N-[(S)-l-ethoxycarbonyl-3-phenylpropyl]-L-alanyl]-(lS,3S,5S)-2-azabicyclo [3.3.0]octane-3-carboxylic acid (Hoe 498) in rat, dog and man. *Arzneimittelforschung,* **1984,** *34:*1435–1447. Meisel S, et al. Clinical pharmacokinetics of ramipril. *Clin Pharmacokinet,* **1994,** *26:*7–15. PDR58, **2004,** p. 2142. Song JC, et al. Clinical pharmacokinetics and selective pharmacodynamics of new angiotensin converting enzyme inhibitors: an update. *Clin Pharmacokinet,* **2002,** *41:*207–224. Thuillez C, et al. Pharmacokinetics, converting enzyme inhibition and peripheral arterial hemodynamics of ramipril in healthy volunteers. *Am J Cardiol,* **1987,** *59:*38D–44D.

Ranitidine							
52 ± 11	69 ± 6	15 ± 3	10.4 ± 1.1	1.3 ± 0.4	2.1 ± 0.2	2.1 ± 0.31[a]	462 ± 54 ng/mL[a]
↑ LD	↓ RD		↓ RD, Aged		↑ RD, LD, Aged		

[a]Following a single 150-mg oral dose given to healthy adults. IC_{50} for inhibition of gastric acid secretion is 100 ng/mL.

Reference: Gladziwa U, et al. Pharmacokinetics and pharmacodynamics of H_2-receptor antagonists in patients with renal insufficiency. *Clin Pharmacokinet,* **1993,** *24:*319–332.

Regorafenib[a]							
—[b]	—	99.5	0.54[c]	—	R: 28 (14–28)[d]	4	R: 3.9 (35–44) μg/mL[e]
↑ Food					M2: 20–30[d]		M2: 3.2 μg/mL[e]
					M5: 50–60[d]		M5: 4.0 μg/mL[e]

[a]Regorafenib is cleared by multiple processes, including biliary excretion and CYP3A- and UGT1A9-dependent metabolism; two active metabolites (M2 and M5) are found in plasma at levels comparable to parent drug. Regorafenib undergoes enterohepatic cycling. [b]The absolute bioavailability is not known; administration with a low-fat meal recommended. [c]CL/F calculated following a single 160-mg oral dose, assuming 70-kg body weight. [d]Mean (range) $t_{1/2}$ of regorafenib (R), M2, and M5 following a single 160-mg oral dose. [e]Mean (range) concentration of R and mean M2 and M5 concentrations following a 160-mg oral dose, given once a day for 21 days to patients with cancer.

References: Shirley M, Keating G. Regorafenib: a review of its use in patients with advanced gastrointestinal stromal tumours. *Drugs,* **2015,** *75:*1009–17. Drugs@FDA: FDA Approved Drug Products (http://www.accessdata.fda.gov/scripts/cder/daf/), Regorafenib (Stivarga).

Remifentanil[a]							
—[b]	Negligible	92	40–60		0.13–0.33	—	~20 ng/mL[d]
			0.3–0.4 ↓ Aged[c]				
			↓ Aged[c]				

[a]Data from healthy adult male subjects and patients undergoing elective surgery. Undergoes rapid inactivation by esterase-mediated hydrolysis; resulting carboxy metabolite has low activity. [b]For intravenous administration only. [c]CL and V decreased slightly in the elderly. [d]Mean CL_{min} following a 5-μg/kg IV dose (1-min infusion). Cp_{50} for skin incision is 2 ng/mL (determined in the presence of nitrous oxide).

References: Egan TD, et al. Remifentanil pharmacokinetics in obese versus lean patients. *Anesthesiology,* **1998,** *89:*562–573. Glass PS, et al. A review of the pharmacokinetics and pharmacodynamics of remifentanil. *Anesth Analg,* **1999,** *89:*S7–S14.

(Continued)

TABLE AII–1 ■ PHARMACOKINETIC DATA (*CONTINUED*)

BIOAVAILABILITY (ORAL) (%)	URINARY EXCRETION (%)	BOUND IN PLASMA (%)	CLEARANCE (mL/min/kg)	VOL. DIST. (L/kg)	HALF-LIFE (hours)	PEAK TIME (h)	PEAK CONCENTRATION
Repaglinide[a]							
56 ± 7	0.3–2.6	97.4	9.3 ± 6.8^{b}	0.52 ± 0.17	0.8 ± 0.2	$0.25–0.75^{e}$	47 ± 24 ng/mL^{e}
			↓ RD^{c}, LD^{d}		↑ LD		

[a]Data from healthy adult male subjects. [b]Undergoes extensive oxidative and conjugative metabolism. CYP2C8 and CYP3A4 to a minor degree have been implicated in the metabolism of repaglinide. Repaglinide is also a substrate of organic anion transport protein (OATP)1B1, which is believed to contribute to the hepatic uptake of repaglinide. [c]*CL/F* reduced, severe renal impairment. [d]*CL/F* reduced, moderate-to-severe LD. [e]Following a single 4-mg oral dose (tablet).

References: Hatorp V, et al. Unavailability of repaglinide, a novel antidiabetic agent, administered orally in tablet or solution form or intravenously in healthy male volunteers. *Int J Clin Pharmacol Ther*, **1998**, 36:636–641. Hatorp V, et al. Single-dose pharmacokinetics of repaglinide in subjects with chronic liver disease. *J Clin Pharmacol*, **2000**, 40:142–152. Marbury TC, et al. Pharmacokinetics of repaglinide in subjects with renal impairment. *Clin Pharmacol Ther*, **2000**, 67:7–15. van Heiningen PN, et al. Absorption, metabolism and excretion of a single oral dose of ^{14}C-repaglinide during repaglinide multiple dosing. *Eur J Clin Pharmacol*, **1999**, 55:521–525.

BIOAVAILABILITY (ORAL) (%)	URINARY EXCRETION (%)	BOUND IN PLASMA (%)	CLEARANCE (mL/min/kg)	VOL. DIST. (L/kg)	HALF-LIFE (hours)	PEAK TIME (h)	PEAK CONCENTRATION
Ribavirin[a]							
45 ± 5	35 ± 8	0^{b}	5.0 ± 1.0^{c}	9.3 ± 1.5	28 ± 7^{c}	RT: 3 ± 1.8^{d}	R: 11.1 ± 1.2 μM^{d}
							RT: 15.1 ± 12.8 μM^{d}

[a]Values reported for studies conducted in asymptomatic HIV-positive men. [b]At steady state, red blood cell–to-plasma concentration ratio is ~ 60. [c]Following multiple oral dosing, *CL/F* decreases by > 50%, and a long terminal $t_{1/2}$ of 150 ± 50 h is observed. [d]Following a 1200-mg oral ribavirin capsule (R) given daily for 7 days to adult subjects seropositive for HIV or a 600-mg oral Rebetron dose given twice daily to steady state to adults with hepatitis C infection.

References: Morse GD, et al. Single-dose pharmacokinetics of delavirdine mesylate and didanosine in patients with human immunodeficiency virus infection. *Antimicrob Agents Chemother*, **1997**, 47:169–174. *PDR54*, **2000**, p. 2836. Roberts RB, et al. Ribavirin pharmacodynamics in high-risk patients for acquired immunodeficiency syndrome. *Clin Pharmacol Ther*, **1987**, 42:365–373.

BIOAVAILABILITY (ORAL) (%)	URINARY EXCRETION (%)	BOUND IN PLASMA (%)	CLEARANCE (mL/min/kg)	VOL. DIST. (L/kg)	HALF-LIFE (hours)	PEAK TIME (h)	PEAK CONCENTRATION
Rifampin[a]							
—[b]	7 ± 3	60–90	3.5 ± 1.6^{c}	0.97 ± 0.36	3.5 ± 0.8^{c}	$1–3^{e}$	6.5 ± 3.5 μg/mL^{e}
	↑ Neo		↑ Neo, ↓ RD^{d}	↑ Neo	↑ LD, RD^{d}		

[a]Active desacetyl metabolite. [b]Absolute bioavailability is not unknown, although some studies indicate complete absorption. Such reports presumably refer to rifampin plus its desacetyl metabolite because considerable first-pass metabolism is expected. [c]$t_{1/2}$ is shorter (1.7 ± 0.5) and *CL/F* is higher after repeated administration. Rifampin is a potent enzyme (CYP3A and others) inducer and appears to autoinduce its own metabolism. [d]Not observed with 300-mg doses, but pronounced differences with 900-mg doses. $t_{1/2}$ is longer with high single doses. [e]Following a 600-mg dose given once daily for 15–18 days to patients with tuberculosis.

Reference: Israili ZH, et al. Pharmacokinetics of antituberculosis drugs in patients. *J Clin Pharmacol*, **1987**, 27:78–83.

BIOAVAILABILITY (ORAL) (%)	URINARY EXCRETION (%)	BOUND IN PLASMA (%)	CLEARANCE (mL/min/kg)	VOL. DIST. (L/kg)	HALF-LIFE (hours)	PEAK TIME (h)	PEAK CONCENTRATION
Riluzole							
64 (30–100)	<1	98	5.5 ± 0.9^{b}	3.4 ± 0.6	14 ± 6	0.8 ± 0.5^{c}	173 ± 72 ng/mL^{c}
↓ Food^{a}			↓ LD				

[a]High-fat meal. [b]Eliminated primarily by CYP1A2-dependent metabolism; metabolites are inactive. Involvement of CYP1A2 may contribute to ethnic (lower *CL/F* in Japanese) and gender (lower *CL* in women) differences and inductive effects of smoking (higher *CL* in smokers). [c]Following a 50-mg oral dose given twice daily to steady state.

References: Bruno R, et al. Population pharmacokinetics of riluzole in patients with amyotrophic lateral sclerosis. *Clin Pharmacol Ther*, **1997**, 62:518–526. Le Liboux A, et al. Single- and multiple-dose pharmacokinetics of riluzole in white subjects. *J Clin Pharmacol*, **1997**, 37:820–827. *PDR58*, **2004**, p. 769. Wokke J. Riluzole. *Lancet*, **1996**, 348:795–799.

BIOAVAILABILITY (ORAL) (%)	URINARY EXCRETION (%)	BOUND IN PLASMA (%)	CLEARANCE (mL/min/kg)	VOL. DIST. (L/kg)	HALF-LIFE (hours)	PEAK TIME (h)	PEAK CONCENTRATION
Risperidone[a]							
PO: 66 ± 28^{b}	3 ± 2^{b}	89^{c}	5.4 ± 1.4^{b}	1.1 ± 0.2	$3.2 \pm 0.8^{a,b}$	R: ~1^{e}	R: 10 ng/mL^{e}
IM: 103 ± 13			↓ RD^{c}, Aged^{d}		↑ RD^{c}, Aged^{d}		TA: 45 ng/mL^{e}

[a]The active metabolite, 9-hydroxyrisperidone, is the predominant circulating species in extensive metabolizers and is equipotent to parent drug. 9-Hydroxyrisperidone has a $t_{1/2}$ of 20 ± 3 h. In extensive metabolizers, $35\% \pm 7\%$ of an intravenous dose is excreted as this metabolite; its elimination is primarily renal and therefore correlates with renal function. Formation of 9-hydroxyrisperidone is catalyzed by CYP2D6. [b]Parameters reported for extensive metabolizers. In poor metabolizers, *F* is higher; ~ 20% of an intravenous dose is excreted unchanged, 10% as the 9-hydroxy metabolite; *CL* is slightly < 1 mL/min/kg, and $t_{1/2}$ is similar to that of the active metabolite, ~ 20 h. [c]77% for 9-hydroxyrisperidone. [d]Changes in elderly subjects due to decreased renal function affecting the elimination of the active metabolite. [e]Mean steady-state C_{min} for risperidone (R) and total active (TA) drug, risperidone + 9-OH-risperidone, following a 3-mg oral dose given twice daily to patients with chronic schizophrenia. No difference in total active drug levels between CYP2D6 extensive and poor metabolizers.

References: Cohen LJ. Risperidone. *Pharmacotherapy*, **1994**, 14:253–265. Heykants J, et al. The pharmacokinetics of risperidone in humans: z summary. *J Clin Psychiatry*, **1994**, 55(suppl):13–17.

BIOAVAILABILITY (ORAL) (%)	URINARY EXCRETION (%)	BOUND IN PLASMA (%)	CLEARANCE (mL/min/kg)	VOL. DIST. (L/kg)	HALF-LIFE (hours)	PEAK TIME (h)	PEAK CONCENTRATION
Ritonavir							
—[a]	3.5 ± 1.8	98–99	SD: $1.2 \pm 0.4^{b,c}$	0.41 ± 0.25^{c}	$3–5^{c}$	$2–4^{e}$	11 ± 4 μg/mL^{e}
↑ Food			MD: 2.1 ± 0.8^{c}		↑ LD^{d}		
			↓ Child, LD^{d}				

[a]Absolute bioavailability unknown (>60% absorbed); food elicits a 15% increase in oral AUC for capsule formulation. [b]Ritonavir is extensively metabolized primarily by CYP3A4. It also appears to induce its own *CL* with single-dose (SD) to multiple-dose (MD) administration. [c]*CL/F*, V_{area}/F, and $t_{1/2}$ reported for oral dose. [d]*CL/F* reduced slightly and $t_{1/2}$ increased slightly, moderate liver impairment. [e]Following a 600-mg oral dose given twice daily to steady state.

References: Hsu A, et al. Ritonavir. Clinical pharmacokinetics and interactions with other anti-HIV agents. *Clin Pharmacokinet*, **1998**, 35:275–291. *PDR54*, **2000**, p. 465.

(*Continued*)

TABLE AII–1 ■ PHARMACOKINETIC DATA (*CONTINUED*)

BIOAVAILABILITY (ORAL) (%)	URINARY EXCRETION (%)	BOUND IN PLASMA (%)	CLEARANCE (mL/min/kg)	VOL. DIST. (L/kg)	HALF-LIFE (hours)	PEAK TIME (h)	PEAK CONCENTRATION
Rivaroxaban							
80–100[a]	~40	92–95	2.33[b] ↓ RD	0.62	5–9 ↑ Aged	2.5 (1–4)[c]	138 (77–251) ng/mL[c]

[a]The oral bioavailability is lower (~60%) at doses > 10 mg; food increases the fraction absorbed at those higher doses. [b]Rivaroxaban is cleared from blood by both renal and multiple biotransformation routes, including CYP3A-dependent metabolism. [c]Mean (range) following a single 10-mg oral dose in the fasted stated.

Reference: Mueck W, et al. Clinical pharmacokinetics and pharmacodynamics profile of rivaroxaban. *Clin Pharmacokinet,* **2014**, 53:1–16. Drugs@FDA: FDA Approved Drug Products (http://www.accessdata.fda.gov/scripts/cder/daf/), Rivaroxaban (Xarelto).

Rivastigmine							
72 (22–119)[a] ↑ Food, Dose	Negligible	40	$13 \pm 4^{b,c}$	1.5 ± 0.6^{c}	$1.4 \pm 0.4^{c,d}$	1.2 ± 1.0^{e}	26 ± 10 ng/mL[e]

[a]Following a 6-mg oral dose. Bioavailability increases with dose; following a 3-mg dose, the median bioavailability is 36%. [b]Rivastigmine is metabolized by cholinesterase. No apparent gender differences. [c]Intravenous dose of 2 mg. [d]The pharmacodynamic $t_{1/2}$ is ~ 10 h due to tight binding to acetylcholinesterase. [e]Following oral administration of a 6-mg capsule. C_{max} increases more than proportionally at doses > 3 mg.

References: Hossain M, et al. Estimation of the absolute bioavailability of rivastigmine in patients with mild to moderate dementia of the Alzheimer's type. *Clin Pharmacokinet,* **2002**, *41*:225–234. Williams BR, et al. A review of rivastigmine: a reversible cholinesterase inhibitor. *Clin Ther,* **2003**, *25*:1634–1653.

Rizatriptan[a]							
47	F: 28 ± 9^{b}	14	F: 12.3 ± 1.4^{b}	F: 1.5 ± 0.2	F: 2.2	SD: 0.9 ± 0.4^{e}	SD: 20 ± 4.9 ng/mL[e]
	M: 29[b]		M: 18.9 ± 2.8^{b}	M: 2.2 ± 0.4	M: 2.4	MD: 4.8 ± 0.7^{e}	MD: 37 ± 13 ng/mL[e]
			↓ LD,[c] RD[d]				

[a]Data from healthy adult male (M) and female (F) subjects. Oxidative deamination catalyzed by MAO-A is the primary route of elimination. *N*-Desmethyl rizatriptan (DMR) is a minor metabolite (~14%) that is active and accumulates in blood. [b]Evidence of minor dose-dependent metabolic *CL* and urinary excretion. [c]*CL/F* reduced, moderate hepatic impairment. [d]*CL/F* reduced, severe renal impairment. [e]Following a 10-mg single (SD) and multiple (MD) oral dose (10 mg every 2 h × 3 doses × 4 days). DMR C_{max} is 8.5 and 26.2 ng/mL with SD and MD, respectively.

References: Goldberg MR, et al. Rizatriptan, a novel 5-HT$_{1B/1D}$ agonist for migraine: single-and multiple-dose tolerability and pharmacokinetics in healthy subjects. *J Clin Pharmacol,* **2000**, *40*:74–83. Lee Y, et al. Pharmacokinetics and tolerability of intravenous rizatriptan in healthy females. *Biopharm Drug Dispos,* **1998**, *19*:577–581. PDR54, **2000**, p. 1912. Vyas KP, et al. Disposition and pharmacokinetics of the antimigraine drug, rizatriptan, in humans. *Drug Metab Dispos,* **2000**, *28*:89–95.

Ropinirole[a]							
55	<10	~40	11.2 ± 5.0^{b}	7.5 ± 2.4^{b}	6[b]	1.0 (0.5–6.0)[d]	7.4 (2.4–13) ng/mL[d]
			↓ Aged[c]				

[a]Data from male and female patients with Parkinson's disease. Metabolized primarily by CYP1A2 to inactive *N*-deisopropyl and hydroxy metabolites. [b]*CL/F*, V_d/F, and $t_{1/2}$ reported for oral dose. [c]*CL/F* reduced but dose titrated to desired effect. [d]Following a 2-mg oral dose given three times daily to steady state. Food increases the T_{max} and decreases the C_{max}.

References: Bloomer JC, et al. In vitro identification of the P450 enzymes responsible for the metabolism of ropinirole. *Drug Metab Dispos,* **1997**, *25*:840–844. PDR54, **2000**, p. 3037. Taylor AC, et al. Lack of a pharmacokinetic interaction at steady state between ropinirole and L-dopa in patients with Parkinson's disease. *Pharmacotherapy,* **1999**, *79*:150–156.

Rosuvastatin[a]							
20 (17–23)	30 ± 7	88	10.5 ± 4.7^{b}	1.7 ± 0.5	20 ± 6	3 (1–6)[d]	4.6 ± 2.1 ng/mL[d]
			↓ RD[c]				

[a]Data from healthy men reported; no significant gender or age differences. [b]Eliminated primarily by biliary excretion; also appears to be actively transported into the liver by an organic anion transport protein (polymorphic OATP1B1, amongst others). [c]Reduced *CL/F* in patients with severe renal impairment. [d]Following a 10-mg oral dose taken once daily for 10 days.

References: Martin PD, et al. Pharmacodynamic effects and pharmacokinetics of a new HMG-CoA reductase inhibitor, rosuvastatin, after morning or evening administration in healthy volunteers. *Br J Clin Pharmacol,* **2002**, *54*:472–477. Martin PD, et al. Absolute oral bioavailability of rosuvastatin in healthy white adult male volunteers. *Clin Ther,* **2003**, *25*:2553–2563. Product labeling: Crestor® tablets (rosuvastatin calcium). Astra-Zeneca Pharmaceuticals LP, Wilmington, DE, **2003**. Schneck DW, et al. The effect of gemfibrozil on the pharmacokinetics of rosuvastatin. *Clin Pharmacol Ther,* **2004**, *75*:455–463.

Selegiline[a]							
Negligible[b]	Negligible	94[c]	~1500[b]	1.9	1.91 ± 1.0^{e}	S: 0.7 ± 0.4^{f}	S: 1.1 ± 0.4 ng/mL[f]
			160[d]			DS: ~1 h	DS: ~15 ng/mL[f]

[a]MAO-B active metabolite: *l*-(−)-desmethylselegiline. [b]Extensive first-pass metabolism; estimate of *CL/F* reported. [c]Blood-to-plasma concentration ratio = 1.3–2.2 for parent drug and ~ 0.55 for *N*-desmethyl metabolite. [d]*CL/F* for *N*-desmethylselegiline, assuming quantitative conversion of parent to this metabolite. [e]For parent and *N*-desmethyl metabolite. $t_{1/2}$s for methamphetamine (major plasma species) and amphetamine are 21 and 18 h, respectively. [f]Mean data for selegiline (S) and its active metabolite, *N*-desmethylselegiline (DS), following a single 10-mg oral dose given to adults.

Reference: Heinonen EH, et al. Pharmacokinetic aspects of *l*-deprenyl (selegiline) and its metabolites. *Clin Pharmacol Ther,* **1994**, *56*:742–749.

(*Continued*)

TABLE AII–1 ■ PHARMACOKINETIC DATA (*CONTINUED*)

BIOAVAILABILITY (ORAL) (%)	URINARY EXCRETION (%)	BOUND IN PLASMA (%)	CLEARANCE (mL/min/kg)	VOL. DIST. (L/kg)	HALF-LIFE (hours)	PEAK TIME (h)	PEAK CONCENTRATION
Sertraline							
—[a]	<1	98–99	38 ± 14[b]	—	23	M: 6.9 ± 1.0[c]	M: 118 ± 22 ng/mL[c]
			↓ Aged, LD		↑ Aged, LD	F: 6.7 ± 1.8[c]	F: 166 ± 65 ng/mL[c]

[a]Absolute bioavailability is not known (>44% absorbed); undergoes extensive first-pass metabolism to essentially inactive metabolites; catalyzed by multiple CYP isoforms. [b]*CL/F* reported. [c]Following a dose titration up to 200-mg given once daily for 30 days to healthy male (M) and female (F) adults.

References: van Harten J. Clinical pharmacokinetics of selective serotonin reuptake inhibitors. *Clin Pharmacokinet*, **1993**, *24*:203–220. Warrington SJ. Clinical implications of the pharmacology of sertraline. *Int Clin Psychopharmacol*, **1994**, 6(suppl 2):11–21.

BIOAVAILABILITY (ORAL) (%)	URINARY EXCRETION (%)	BOUND IN PLASMA (%)	CLEARANCE (mL/min/kg)	VOL. DIST. (L/kg)	HALF-LIFE (hours)	PEAK TIME (h)	PEAK CONCENTRATION
Sildenafil[a]							
38	0	96	6.0 ± 1.1	1.2 ± 0.3	2.4 ± 1.0	1.2 ± 0.3[d]	212 ± 59 ng/mL[d]
			↓ LD,[b] RD,[c] Aged				

[a]Data from healthy male subjects. Sildenafil is metabolized primarily by CYP3A and secondarily by CYP2C9. Piperazine *N*-desmethyl metabolite is active (~50% parent) and accumulates in plasma (~40% parent). [b]*CL/F* reduced, mild-to-moderate hepatic impairment. [c]*CL/F* reduced, severe renal impairment. Increased unbound concentrations. [d]Following a single 50-mg oral (solution) dose.

References: PDR54, **2000**, p. 2382. Walker DK, et al. Pharmacokinetics and metabolism of sildenafil in mouse, rat, rabbit, dog and man. *Xenobiotica*, **1999**, *29*:297–310.

BIOAVAILABILITY (ORAL) (%)	URINARY EXCRETION (%)	BOUND IN PLASMA (%)	CLEARANCE (mL/min/kg)	VOL. DIST. (L/kg)	HALF-LIFE (hours)	PEAK TIME (h)	PEAK CONCENTRATION
Simvastatin[a]							
≤5	Negligible	94	7.6[b]	—	2–3	AI: 1.4 ± 1.0[c]	AI: 46 ± 20 ngEq/mL[c]
						TI: 1.4 ± 1.0[c]	TI: 56 ± 25 ngEq/mL[c]

[a]Simvastatin is a lactone prodrug that is hydrolyzed to the active corresponding β-hydroxy acid. Values reported are for the disposition of the acid. [b]The β-hydroxy acid can be reconverted back to the lactone; irreversible oxidative metabolites are generated by CYP3A. [c]Data for active inhibitors (AI, ring-opened molecule) and total inhibitors (TI) following a 40-mg oral dose given once daily for 17 days to healthy adults.

References: Corsini A, et al. New insights into the pharmacodynamic and pharmacokinetic properties of statins. *Pharmacol Ther*, **1999**, *84*:413–428. Desager JP, et al. Clinical pharmacokinetics of 3-hydroxy-3-methylglutaryl-coenzyme A reductase inhibitors. *Clin Pharmacokinet*, **1996**, *31*:348–371. Mauro VF. Clinical pharmacokinetics and practical applications of simvastatin. *Clin Pharmacokinet*, **1993**, *24*:195–202.

BIOAVAILABILITY (ORAL) (%)	URINARY EXCRETION (%)	BOUND IN PLASMA (%)	CLEARANCE (mL/min/kg)	VOL. DIST. (L/kg)	HALF-LIFE (hours)	PEAK TIME (h)	PEAK CONCENTRATION
Sirolimus[a]							
~15[b]	—	40[c]	3.47 ± 1.58[d]	12 ± 4.6[d]	62.3 ± 16.2[d]	SD: 0.81 ± 0.17[e]	SD: 67 ± 23 ng/mL[e]
↑ Food[b]						MD: 1.4 ± 1.2[e]	MD: 94–210 ng/mL[e]

[a]Data from male and female renal transplant patients. All subjects were on a stable cyclosporine regimen. Sirolimus is metabolized primarily by CYP3A and is a substrate for P-glycoprotein. Several sirolimus metabolites are pharmacologically active. [b]Cyclosporine coadministration increases sirolimus bioavailability. *F* increased by high-fat meal. [c]Concentrates in blood cells; blood-to-plasma concentration ratio ~ 38 ± 13. [d]Blood *CL/F*, V_{ss}/F, and $t_{1/2}$ reported for oral dose. [e]Following a single 15-mg oral dose (SD) in healthy subjects and 4- to 6.5-mg/m² oral dose (with cyclosporine) given twice daily to steady state (MD) in renal transplant patients.

References: Kelly PA, et al. Conversion from liquid to solid rapamycin formulations in stable renal allograft transplant recipients. *Biopharm Drug Dispos*, **1999**, *20*:249–253. Zimmerman JJ, et al. Pharmacokinetics of sirolimus in stable renal transplant patients after multiple oral dose administration. *J Clin Pharmacol*, **1997**, *37*:405–415. Zimmerman JJ, et al. The effect of a high-fat meal on the oral bioavailability of the immunosuppressant sirolimus (rapamycin). *J Clin Pharmacol*, **1999**, *39*:1155–1161.

BIOAVAILABILITY (ORAL) (%)	URINARY EXCRETION (%)	BOUND IN PLASMA (%)	CLEARANCE (mL/min/kg)	VOL. DIST. (L/kg)	HALF-LIFE (hours)	PEAK TIME (h)	PEAK CONCENTRATION
Sitagliptin							
87 ± 5.2	73.1 ± 15.9	38	4.42[a]	—	13.9 ± 2.0	1.5 ± 1.3	1046 ± 286 nM[c]
			↓ RD[b]				

[a]Cleared primarily by the kidney. Renal clearance is ~ 350 mL/min, which indicates active tubular secretion, possibly mediated by human organic anion transporter-3 (OAT3) and P-glycoprotein (ABCB1). [b]Apparent oral clearance decreased by a respective 2.3-, 3.8-, and 4.5-fold in patients with moderate (CL_{cr} = 30–50 mL/min) and severe (<30 mL/min) renal insufficiency and in patients with end-stage RD requiring hemodialysis. [c]Following a single 100-mg oral dose. Plasma AUC increased by ~ 14% following daily doses of 100 mg at steady state compared to the first dose.

References: Bergman A, et al. Absolute bioavailability of sitagliptin, an oral dipeptidyl peptidase-4 inhibitor, in healthy volunteers. *Biopharm Drug Dispos*, **2007**, *28*:315–22. Bergman AJ, et al. Effect of renal insufficiency on the pharmacokinetics of sitagliptin, a dipeptidyl peptidase-4 inhibitor. *Diabetes Care*, **2007**, *30*:1862–1864. Drugs@FDA. Januvia label approved on July 22, 2008. Available at: http://www.accessdata.fda.gov/scripts/cder/drugsatfda/index.cfm. Accessed December 26, 2009. Migoya EM, et al. Effect of moderate hepatic insufficiency on the pharmacokinetics of sitagliptin. *Can J Clin Pharmacol*, **2009**, *16*:e165–e170. Vincent SH, et al. Metabolism and excretion of the dipeptidyl peptidase 4 inhibitor [¹⁴C]sitagliptin in humans. *Drug Metab Dispos*, **2007**, *35*:533–538.

(Continued)

TABLE AII–1 ■ PHARMACOKINETIC DATA (CONTINUED)

BIOAVAILABILITY (ORAL) (%)	URINARY EXCRETION (%)	BOUND IN PLASMA (%)	CLEARANCE (mL/min/kg)	VOL. DIST. (L/kg)	HALF-LIFE (hours)	PEAK TIME (h)	PEAK CONCENTRATION
Sofosbuvir[a]							
—[b]	—[c]	~82[d]	—	—	0.68 (0.53–1.00)[e]	1.00 (0.50–1.50)[e]	1356 (63.0) ng/mL
			↓ RD[f]				

[a]Sofosbuvir is sequentially metabolized to a pharmacologically active nucleoside analogue triphosphate; the active metabolite is undetected in plasma. The first hydrolytic step appears to be rapid (much of it may occur during first pass), yielding the intermediate metabolite GS-566500, which can either be fully activated by kinases to GS-461203 or inactivated by phosphatase activity to GS-331007. [b]The absolute oral bioavailability of sofosbuvir in humans is not known. Administration with a high-fat meal increases systemic sofosbuvir exposure by 67%–91%, although this is not thought to be clinically meaningful. [c]3.5% of the oral dose is recovered as unchanged sofosbuvir in urine; the true fraction excreted unchanged may be much higher, depending on the absolute bioavailability. [d]Also reported to be 62%–65% based on in vitro ultrafiltration experiments. [e]Mean (25th and 75th quartiles or CV%) reported following administration of 400-mg oral sofosbuvir, given once a day for 27 days. [f]Systemic exposure (AUC) of sofosbuvir and GS-566500 increased 171% and 244%, respectively, in patients with severe renal impairment; smaller increases seen with less severe disease.

References: Kirby BJ et al, Pharmacokinetic, pharmacodynamics and drug interaction profile of the hepatitis C virus NS5B polymerase inhibitor sofosbuvir. *Clin Pharmacokinet,* **2015,** *54*:677–90. Drugs@FDA: FDA Approved Drug Products (http://www.accessdata.fda.gov/scripts/cder/daf/), Sofosbuvir (Sovaldi).

Solifenacin[a]							
90	3–6	98[b]	9.39 ± 2.68	671 ± 118	52.4 ± 13.9	4.2 ± 1.8[c]	40.6 ± 8.5 ng/mL[d]
			↓ LD, RD[c]		↑ LD, RD[c]		

[a]Solifenacin is extensively metabolized by CYP3A. The 4*R*-hydroxy-solifenacin metabolite is pharmacologically active but not likely to contribute to the therapeutic efficacy of solifenacin because of low circulating levels. [b]Primarily bound to α_1-acid glycoprotein. [c]Dosage reduction is advised in patients with severe renal impairment ($CL_{cr} < 30$ mL/min), in whom a 2-fold reduction in clearance and prolongation in $t_{1/2}$ are expected. [d]At steady state following 21 days of dosing with 10 mg once daily.

References: Drugs@FDA. VESIcare label approved on 11/18/08. Available at: http://www.accessdata.fda.gov/scripts/cder/drugsatfda/index.cfm. Accessed December 27, 2009. Kuipers ME, et al. Solifenacin demonstrates high absolute bioavailability in healthy men. *Drugs,* **2004,** *5*:73–81. Kuipers M, et al. Open-label study of the safety and pharmacokinetics of solifenacin in subjects with hepatic impairment. *J Pharmacol Sci,* **2006,** *102*:405–412. Smulders RA, et al. Pharmacokinetics and safety of solifenacin succinate in healthy young men. *J Clin Pharmacol,* **2004,** *44*:1023–1033. Smulders RA, et al. Pharmacokinetics, safety, and tolerability of solifenacin in patients with renal insufficiency. *J Pharmacol Sci,* **2007,** *103*:67–74.

Sorafenib							
—[a]	—	99.5	1.31[b,c]	3.19[c]	25.6 (20)[c]	3	7.7 (65.3) µg/mL[d]

[a]The absolute bioavailability is not known, and a significant fraction of the oral dose is recovered in feces as unchanged drug, suggesting either poor absorption or significant biliary excretion. [b]Sorafenib is cleared by CYP3A4- and UGT1A9-dependent metabolism. [c]CL/F, V^β/F, and $t_{1/2}$ calculated following a single 400-mg oral dose assuming 70-kg body weight. [d]Mean (CV%) following a 400-mg oral dose, given twice daily to steady state in cancer patients.

References: van Erp NP, et al. Clinical pharmacokinetics of tyrosine kinase inhibitors. *Cancer Treat Rev,* **2009,** *35*:692–706. Drugs@FDA: FDA Approved Drug Products (http://www.accessdata.fda.gov/scripts/cder/daf/), Sorafenib (Nexavar).

Sotalol[a]							
60–100	70 ± 15	Negligible	2.20 ± 0.67	1.21 ± 0.17	7.18 ± 1.30	3.1 ± 0.6	1.0 ± 0.5 µg/mL[b]
			↓ RD		↑ RD		

[a]Sotalol is available as a racemate. The enantiomers contribute equally to sotalol's antiarrhythmic action; hence, pharmacokinetic parameters for total enantiomeric mixture are reported herein. β Adrenoreceptor blockade resides solely with *S*-(−)-isomer. [b]Following 80-mg, twice-a-day dosing to steady state.

References: Berglund G, et al. Pharmacokinetics of sotalol after chronic administration to patients with renal insufficiency. *Eur J Clin Pharmacol,* **1980,** *18*:321–326. Kimura M, et al. Pharmacokinetics and pharmacodynamics of (+)-sotalol in healthy male volunteers. *Br J Clin Pharmacol,* **1996,** *42*:583–588. Poirier JM, et al. The pharmacokinetics of d-sotalol and d,l-sotalol in healthy volunteers. *Eur J Clin Pharmacol,* **1990,** *38*:579–582.

Spironolactone[a]							
—[b]	<1[c]	>90[d]	93[e]	10[e]	S: 1.3 ± 0.3[f]	S: 1.0[f]	S: 185 ± 51 ng/mL[f]
↑ Food					C: 11.2 ± 2.3[f]	C: 2.9 ± 0.6[f]	C: 231 ± 49 ng/mL[f]
					TS: 2.8 ± 0.4[f]	TS: 1.8 ± 0.5[f]	TS: 571 ± 74 ng/mL[f]
					HTS: 10.1 ± 2.3[f]	HTS: 3.1 ± 0.9[f]	HTS: 202 ± 54 ng/mL[f]
						↑ LD[g]	

[a]Spironolactone (S) is extensively metabolized; it has three known active metabolites: canrenone (C), 7α-thiomethylspironolactone (TS), and 6β-hydroxy-7α-thiomethylspironolactone (HTS). [b]Absolute bioavailability is not known; old values reported in the literature were based on nonspecific assays for C; likely to exhibit first-pass metabolism. AUC of parent drug and metabolites increased when S taken with food. [c]Measured after an oral dose. [d]Binding of S and its active metabolites. [e]CL/F and V_{area}/F; calculated from reported AUC and $t_{1/2}$ data. [f]Following a single 200-mg oral dose of S. C accumulates 2.5-fold with multiple S dosing. [g]$t_{1/2}$ of parent drug and metabolites increased in patients with cirrhosis.

References: Ho PC, et al. Pharmacokinetics of canrenone and metabolites after base hydrolysis following single and multiple dose oral administration of spironolactone. *Eur J Clin Pharmacol,* **1984,** *27*:441–446. Overdiek HW, et al. New insights into the pharmacokinetics of spironolactone. *Clin Pharmacol Ther,* **1985,** *38*:469–474. Overdiek HW, et al. Influence of food on the bioavailability of spironolactone. *Clin Pharmacol Ther,* **1986,** *40*:531–536. PDR54, **2000,** p. 2883. Sungaila I, et al. Spironolactone pharmacokinetics and pharmacodynamics in patients with cirrhotic ascites. *Gastroenterology,* **1992,** *102*:1680–1685.

(Continued)

TABLE AII–1 ■ PHARMACOKINETIC DATA (*CONTINUED*)

BIOAVAILABILITY (ORAL) (%)	URINARY EXCRETION (%)	BOUND IN PLASMA (%)	CLEARANCE (mL/min/kg)	VOL. DIST. (L/kg)	HALF-LIFE (hours)	PEAK TIME (h)	PEAK CONCENTRATION
Sulfamethoxazole							
~100	14 ± 2	53 ± 5	0.31 ± 0.07[a,b]	0.26 ± 0.04[a]	10.1 ± 2.6[a]	4[b]	37.1 μg/mL[b]
		↓ RD		↑ RD	↑ RD		

[a]Studies include concurrent administration of trimethoprim and variation in urinary pH; these factors had no marked effect on the *CL* of sulfamethoxazole. Metabolically cleared primarily by N_4-acetylation. [b]Following a single 1000-mg oral dose given to healthy adults.

References: Hutabarat RM, et al. Disposition of drugs in cystic fibrosis. I. Sulfamethoxazole and trimethoprim. *Clin Pharmacol Ther*, **1991**, *49*:402–409. Welling PO, et al. Pharmacokinetics of trimethoprim and sulfamethoxazole in normal subjects and in patients with renal failure. *J Infect Dis*, **1973**, *128*(suppl):556–566.

Sumatriptan							
PO: 14 ± 5	22 ± 4	14–21	22 ± 5.4	2.0 ± 0.34	1.0 ± 0.3[a]	SC: 0.2 (0.1–0.3)[b]	SC: 72 (55–108) ng/mL[b]
SC: 97 ± 16						PO: ~1.5[b]	PO: 54 (27–137) ng/mL[b]

[a]An apparent $t_{1/2}$ of ~ 2 h reported for SC and oral doses. [b]Following a single 6-mg SC or 100-mg oral dose given to healthy young adults.

References: Scott AK, et al. Sumatriptan and cerebral perfusion in healthy volunteers. *Br J Clin Pharmacol*, **1992**, *33*:401–404. Scott AK. Sumatriptan clinical pharmacokinetics. *Clin Pharmacokinet*, **1994**, *27*:337–344.

Tacrolimus							
25 ± 10[a,b]	<1	75–99[c]	0.90 ± 0.29[a]	0.91 ± 0.29[a,d]	12 ± 5[a]	1.4 ± 0.5[e]	31.2 ± 10.1 ng/mL[e]
↓ Food				↑ LD	↑ LD		

[a]Drug disposition parameters calculated from blood concentrations. Data from liver transplant patients reported. Metabolized by CYP3A; also a substrate for P-glycoprotein. [b]A similar bioavailability (F = 21% ± 19%) reported for kidney transplant patients; F = 16% ± 7% for normal subjects. Low oral bioavailability likely due to incomplete intestinal availability. [c]Different values for plasma protein binding reported. Concentrates in blood cells; blood-to-plasma concentration ratio = 35 (12–67). [d]Slightly higher V_{ss} and $t_{1/2}$ reported for kidney transplant patients. Because of the very high and variable blood-to-plasma concentration ratio, markedly different V_{ss} values are reported for parameters based on plasma concentrations. [e]Following a single 7-mg oral dose given to healthy adults. Consensus target C_{min} at steady state are 5–20 ng/mL.

References: Bekersky I, et al. Dose linearity after oral administration of tacrolimus 1-mg capsules at doses of 3, 7, and 10 mg. *Clin Ther*, **1999**, *27*:2058–2064. Jusko WJ, et al. Pharmacokinetics of tacrolimus in liver transplant patients. *Clin Pharmacol Ther*, **1995**, *57*:281–290. *PDR*54, **2000**, pp. 1098–1099.

Tadalafil							
—	—	94	0.59[a,b]	0.89[b]	17.5	2[d]	378 ng/mL[d]
			↓ RD[c]				

[a]Eliminated primarily by CYP3A4-dependent metabolism. [b]*CL/F* and *V/F* reported. [c]AUC increased in patients with mild or moderate (2-fold) and severe (4-fold) renal insufficiency. [d]Following a single 20-mg oral dose.

References: Curran M, et al. Tadalafil. *Drugs*, **2003**, *63*:2203–2212; discussion 2213–2214. Product labeling: Cialis® (tadalafil tablets). Lilly Icos, Bothell, WA, **2004**.

Tamoxifen[a]							
—	<1	>98	1.4[b,c]	50–60[b]	4–11 days[d]	5 (3–7)[e]	120 (67–183) ng/mL[e]

[a]Has active metabolites; 4-hydroxytamoxifen and 4-hydroxy-*N*-desmethyltamoxifen (endoxifen) are minor metabolites that exhibit affinity for the estrogen receptor that is greater than that of parent *trans*-tamoxifen. The $t_{1/2}$ of all metabolites are rate limited by tamoxifen elimination. [b]*CL/F* and V_{area}/F reported. [c]The major pathway of elimination, *N*-demethylation, is catalyzed by CYP3A. Polymorphic CYP2D6 catalyzes the 4-hydroxylation step key to metabolite activity. [d]$t_{1/2}$ consistent with accumulation and approach to steady state. Significantly longer terminal $t_{1/2}$s are observed. [e]Average C_{ss} following a 10-mg oral dose given twice daily to steady state.

References: Lønning PE, et al. Pharmacological and clinical profile of anastrozole. *Breast Cancer Res Treat*, **1998**, *49*(suppl 1):S53–S57. *PDR*54, **2000**, p. 557.

Tamsulosin[a]							
100	12.7 ± 3.0	99 ± 1	0.62 ± 0.31[b]	0.20 ± 0.06	6.8 ± 3.5[d]	5.3 ± 0.7[e]	16 ± 5 ng/mL[e]
↓ Food		↑ RD	↓ RD,[c] Aged		↑ RD, Aged		

[a]Data from healthy male subjects. [b]Metabolized primarily by CYP3A and CYP2D6. [c]*CL/F* reduced, moderate renal impairment. Unbound AUC relatively unchanged. [d]Apparent $t_{1/2}$ after oral dose in patients is ~ 14–15 h, reflecting controlled release from modified-release granules. [e]Following a single 0.4-mg modified-release oral dose in healthy subjects.

References: Matsushima H, et al. Plasma protein binding of tamsulosin hydrochloride in renal disease: role of α_1-acid glycoprotein and possibility of binding interactions. *Eur J Clin Pharmacol*, **1999**, *55*:437–443. van Hoogdalem EJ, et al. Disposition of the selective α_{1A}-adrenoceptor antagonist tamsulosin in humans: comparison with data from interspecies scaling. *J Pharm Sci*, **1997**, *86*:1156–1161. Wolzt M, et al. Pharmacokinetics of tamsulosin in subjects with normal and varying degrees of impaired renal function: an open-label single-dose and multiple-dose study. *Eur J Clin Pharmacol*, **1998**, *4*:367–373.

Telithromycin							
57 (41–112)	23 (19–27)	70	14 (12–16)[a]	3.0 (2.1–4.5)	12 (7–23)	1.0 (0.5–3.0)[c]	2.23 μg/mL[c]
			↓ RD[b]				

[a]~35% of the dose is metabolized by CYP3A4. [b]*CL/F* reduced in patients with severe renal impairment. [c]Following an 800-mg oral dose given once daily for 7 days.

References: Ferret C, et al. Pharmacokinetics and absolute oral bioavailability of an 800-mg oral dose of telithromycin in healthy young and elderly volunteers. *Chemotherapy*, **2002**, *48*:217–223. Namour F, et al. Pharmacokinetics of the new ketolide telithromycin (HMR 3647) administered in ascending single and multiple doses. *Antimicrob Agents Chemother*, **2001**, *45*:170–175. Zhanel GG, et al. The ketolides: a critical review. *Drugs*, **2002**, *62*:1771–1804.

(*Continued*)

TABLE AII–1 ■ PHARMACOKINETIC DATA (CONTINUED)

BIOAVAILABILITY (ORAL) (%)	URINARY EXCRETION (%)	BOUND IN PLASMA (%)	CLEARANCE (mL/min/kg)	VOL. DIST. (L/kg)	HALF-LIFE (hours)	PEAK TIME (h)	PEAK CONCENTRATION
Temsirolimus[a]							
—	4.6[b]	—[c]	3.8 ± 0.6[d]	3.3 ± 0.5[d]	12.8 ± 1.1	—	595 ± 102 ng/mL[e]

[a]Temsirolimus, a water-soluble ester analogue of sirolimus or rapamycin, is available for intravenous use. Following intravenous administration, temsirolimus is converted to sirolimus; blood AUC of sirolimus is 3-fold higher than that of temsirolimus at the recommended dose of 25 mg for the treatment of advanced renal cell carcinoma. Both temsirolimus and sirolimus inhibit mTOR kinase activity and undergo oxidative metabolism mediated by CYP3A. [b]Recovery of radioactivity after a single intravenous dose of [^{14}C]-temsirolimus. [c]Both temsirolimus and sirolimus partition extensively into blood cells; a major fraction of temsirolimus and sirolimus in plasma is bound to plasma proteins. [d]Based on CL of 16.1 ± 2.5 L/h and V_{ss} of 232 ± 36 L at a dose of 25 mg, assuming an average body weight of 70 kg. All pharmacokinetic assessments are based on whole-blood concentration. [e]Following the first dose of a 25-mg/week regimen.

References: Atkins MB, et al. Randomized phase II study of multiple dose levels of CCI-779, a novel mammalian target of rapamycin kinase inhibitor, in patients with advanced refractory renal cell carcinoma. *J Clin Oncol*, **2004**, 22:909–918. Drugs@FDA. Torisel label approved on May 30, 2007. Available at: http://www.accessdata.fda.gov/scripts/cder/drugsatfda/index.cfm. Accessed December 31, 2010.

BIOAVAILABILITY (ORAL) (%)	URINARY EXCRETION (%)	BOUND IN PLASMA (%)	CLEARANCE (mL/min/kg)	VOL. DIST. (L/kg)	HALF-LIFE (hours)	PEAK TIME (h)	PEAK CONCENTRATION
Tenofovir[a]							
25[b]	82 ± 13	<1	2.6 ± 0.9[c]	0.6 ± 0.1[c]	8.1 ± 1.8[c,d]	2.3[e]	326 ng/mL[e]
↑ Food			↓ RD		↑ RD		

[a]Tenofovir is formulated as an ester prodrug, VIREAD (tenofovir disoproxil fumarate), for oral administration. [b]Bioavailability under fasted state reported; increased to 39% with high-fat meal. [c]Data reported for steady-state 3-mg/kg IV dose given once a day for 2 weeks to HIV-1–infected male and female adults. Slightly higher CL with single intravenous dose. [d]Longer apparent plasma $t_{1/2}$ (17 h) reported for steady-state oral dosing; this may reflect a longer duration of blood sampling; also, phosphorylated "active" metabolite exhibits a longer intracellular $t_{1/2}$ (60 h). [e]Following a 300-mg oral dose given once a day with a meal to steady state.

References: Barditch-Crovo P, et al. Phase I/II trial of the pharmacokinetics, safety, and antiretroviral activity of tenofovir disoproxil fumarate in human immunodeficiency virus-infected adults. *Antimicrob Agents Chemother*, **2001**, 45:2733–2739. Deeks SG, et al. Safety, pharmacokinetics, and antiretroviral activity of intravenous 9-[2-(R)-(phosphonomethoxy) propyl]adenine, a novel anti-human immunodeficiency virus (HIV) therapy, in HIV-infected adults. *Antimicrob Agents Chemother*, **1998**, 42:2380–2384. Kearney BP, et al. Tenofovir disoproxil fumarate: clinical pharmacology and pharmacokinetics. *Clin Pharmacokinet*, **2004**, 43:595–612.

BIOAVAILABILITY (ORAL) (%)	URINARY EXCRETION (%)	BOUND IN PLASMA (%)	CLEARANCE (mL/min/kg)	VOL. DIST. (L/kg)	HALF-LIFE (hours)	PEAK TIME (h)	PEAK CONCENTRATION
Terazosin							
82	11–14	90–94	1.1–1.2[a]	1.1	9–12	1.7[b]	16 ng/mL[b]

[a]Plasma CL reportedly reduced in patients with hypertension. [b]Following a 1-mg oral dose (tablet) given to healthy volunteers.

References: Senders RC. Pharmacokinetics of terazosin. *Am J Med*, **1986**, 80:20–24. Sennello LT, et al. Effect of age on the pharmacokinetics of orally and intravenously administered terazosin. *Clin Ther*, **1988**, 10:600–607.

BIOAVAILABILITY (ORAL) (%)	URINARY EXCRETION (%)	BOUND IN PLASMA (%)	CLEARANCE (mL/min/kg)	VOL. DIST. (L/kg)	HALF-LIFE (hours)	PEAK TIME (h)	PEAK CONCENTRATION
Tetracycline							
77	58 ± 8	65 ± 3	1.67 ± 0.24	1.5 ± 0.1[a]	10.6 ± 1.5	Oral: 4	IV: 16.4 ± 1.2 µg/mL[b] Oral: 2.3 ± 0.2 µg/mL[b]

[a]V_{area} reported. [b]Following a single 10-mg/kg IV dose or a single 250-mg oral dose (taken after a fast and with wafer).

References: Raghuram TC, Krishnaswamy K. Pharmacokinetics of tetracycline in nutritional edema. *Chemotherapy*, **1982**, 28:428–433. Garty M, Hurwitz A. Effect of cimetidine and antacids on gastrointestinal absorption of tetracycline. *Clin Pharmacol Ther*, **1980**, 28:203–207.

BIOAVAILABILITY (ORAL) (%)	URINARY EXCRETION (%)	BOUND IN PLASMA (%)	CLEARANCE (mL/min/kg)	VOL. DIST. (L/kg)	HALF-LIFE (hours)	PEAK TIME (h)	PEAK CONCENTRATION
Thalidomide[a]							
—[b]	<1	—	2.2 ± 0.4[c]	1.1 ± 0.3[c]	6.2 ± 2.6[c]	3.2 ± 1.4[d]	2.0 ± 0.6 µg/mL[d]
						↑ HD, Food	↑ HD

[a]Data from healthy male subjects. Similar data reported for asymptomatic patients with HIV. No age or gender differences. Thalidomide undergoes spontaneous hydrolysis in blood to multiple metabolites. [b]Absolute bioavailability is not known. Altered absorption rate and extent, Hansen disease (HD). [c]CL/F, V_{area}/F, and $t_{1/2}$ reported for oral dose. [d]Following a single 200-mg oral dose.

References: Noormohamed FH, et al. Pharmacokinetics and hemodynamic effects of single oral doses of thalidomide in asymptomatic human immunodeficiency virus-infected subjects. *AIDS Res Hum Retrovir*, **1999**, 15:1047–1052. PDR54, **2000**, p. 912. Teo SK, et al. Single-dose oral pharmacokinetics of three formulations of thalidomide in healthy male volunteers. *J Clin Pharmacol*, **1999**, 39:1162–1168.

BIOAVAILABILITY (ORAL) (%)	URINARY EXCRETION (%)	BOUND IN PLASMA (%)	CLEARANCE (mL/min/kg)	VOL. DIST. (L/kg)	HALF-LIFE (hours)	PEAK TIME (h)	PEAK CONCENTRATION
Tolterodine[a]							
EM: 26 ± 18	EM: Negligible	T: 96.3	EM: 9.6 ± 2.8	EM: 1.7 ± 0.4	EM: 2.3 ± 0.3	EM: 1.2 ± 0.5[c]	EM: 5.2 ± 5.7 ng/mL[c]
PM: 91 ± 40	PM: <2.5	5-HM: 64	PM: 2.0 ± 0.3	PM: 1.5 ± 0.4	PM: 9.2 ± 1.2	PM: 1.9 ± 1.0[c]	PM: 38 ± 15 ng/mL[c]
EM: ↑ Food			↓ LD[b]		↑ LD		

[a]Data from healthy adult male subjects. No significant gender differences. Tolterodine (T) is metabolized primarily by CYP2D6 to an active (100% potency) metabolite, 5-hydroxymethyl tolterodine (5-HM), in extensive metabolizers (EM); $t_{1/2}$ 5-HM = 2.9 ± 0.4 h. Also metabolized by CYP3A to an *N*-desalkyl product, particularly in poor metabolizers (PM). [b]CL/F reduced and AUC 5-HM$_{unbound}$ increased, hepatic cirrhosis. [c]Following a 4-mg oral dose given twice daily for 8 days. C_{max} of 5-HM was 5 ± 3 ng/mL for EM.

References: Brynne N, et al. Influence of CYP2D6 polymorphism on the pharmacokinetics and pharmacodynamics of tolterodine. *Clin Pharmacol Ther*, **1998**, 63:529–539. Hills CJ, et al. Tolterodine. *Drugs*, **1998**, 55:813–820. PDR54, **2000**, p. 2439.

(Continued)

TABLE AII–1 ■ PHARMACOKINETIC DATA (*CONTINUED*)

BIOAVAILABILITY (ORAL) (%)	URINARY EXCRETION (%)	BOUND IN PLASMA (%)	CLEARANCE (mL/min/kg)	VOL. DIST. (L/kg)	HALF-LIFE (hours)	PEAK TIME (h)	PEAK CONCENTRATION
Topiramate[a]							
>70[b]	70–97	13–17	0.31–0.51[c]	0.6–0.8[c]	19–23[c]	1.7 ± 0.6[f]	5.5 ± 0.6 µg/mL[f]
			↑ Child[d]		↑ RD		
			↓ RD[e]				

[a]Data from healthy adult male and female subjects and patients with partial epilepsy. [b]Estimate of bioavailability based on urine recovery of unchanged drug. [c]CL/F, V_{area}/F, and $t_{1/2}$ reported for oral dose. Patients receiving concomitant therapy with enzyme-inducing anticonvulsant drugs exhibit increased CL/F and decreased $t_{1/2}$. [d]CL/F increased, < 4 years of age (substantially) and 4–17 years of age. [e]CL/F reduced, moderate-to-severe renal impairment (drug cleared by hemodialysis). [f]Following a 400-mg oral dose given twice daily to steady state in patients with epilepsy.

References: Glauser TA, et al. Topiramate pharmacokinetics in infants. *Epilepsia*, **1999**, 40:788–791. PDR54, **2000**, p. 2209. Rosenfeld WE. Topiramate: a review of preclinical, pharmacokinetic, and clinical data. *Clin Ther*, **1997**, 19:1294–1308. Sachdeo RC, et al. Steady-state pharmacokinetics of topiramate and carbamazepine in patients with epilepsy during monotherapy and concomitant therapy. *Epilepsia*, **1996**, 37:774–780.

BIOAVAILABILITY (ORAL) (%)	URINARY EXCRETION (%)	BOUND IN PLASMA (%)	CLEARANCE (mL/min/kg)	VOL. DIST. (L/kg)	HALF-LIFE (hours)	PEAK TIME (h)	PEAK CONCENTRATION
Tramadol[a]							
70–75	10–30[b]	20	8 (6–12)	2.7 (2.3–3.9)	5.5 (4.5–7.5)	T: 2.3 ± 1.4[c]	T: 592 ± 178 ng/mL[c]
			↓ LD, RD		↑ LD, RD	Ml: 2.4 ± 1.1[c]	Ml: 110 ± 32 ng/mL[c]

[a]Tramadol (T) is available as a racemic mixture. At steady state, the plasma concentration of (+) (*1R,2R*)-tramadol is ~ 30% higher than that of (–) (*1S,2S*)-tramadol. Both isomers contribute to analgesia. Data reported are for total (+ and –) T. T is metabolized by CYP2D6 to an active *O*-desmethyl metabolite (M1); there are other CYP-catalyzed metabolites. [b]Recovery following an oral dose was reported. [c]Following a 100-mg immediate-release tablet given every 6 h for 7 days.

References: Klotz U. Tramadol—the impact of its pharmacokinetic and pharmacodynamic properties on the clinical management of pain. *Arzneimittelforschung*, **2003**, 53:681–687. PDR58, **2004**, p. 2494.

BIOAVAILABILITY (ORAL) (%)	URINARY EXCRETION (%)	BOUND IN PLASMA (%)	CLEARANCE (mL/min/kg)	VOL. DIST. (L/kg)	HALF-LIFE (hours)	PEAK TIME (h)	PEAK CONCENTRATION
Trazodone[a]							
81 ± 6	<1	93	2.1 ± 0.1	1.0 ± 0.1[d] ↑ Aged, Obes	5.9 ± 0.4	2.0 ± 1.5[e]	1.5 ± 0.2 µg/mL[e]
			↓ Aged[b], Obes[c]		↑ Aged, Obes		

[a]Active metabolite *m*-chlorophenylpiperazine is a tryptaminergic agonist; formation catalyzed by CYP3A. [b]Significant for male subjects only. [c]No difference when CL is normalized to ideal body weight. [d]V_{area} reported. [e]Following a single 100-mg oral dose (capsule) given with a standard breakfast to healthy adults.

References: Greenblatt DJ, et al. Trazodone kinetics: effect of age, gender, and obesity. *Clin Pharmacol Ther*, **1987**, 42:193–200. Nilsen OG, et al. Single dose pharmacokinetics of trazodone in healthy subjects. *Pharmacol Toxicol*, **1992**, 71:150–153.

BIOAVAILABILITY (ORAL) (%)	URINARY EXCRETION (%)	BOUND IN PLASMA (%)	CLEARANCE (mL/min/kg)	VOL. DIST. (L/kg)	HALF-LIFE (hours)	PEAK TIME (h)	PEAK CONCENTRATION
Trimethoprim							
>63	63 ± 10	37 ± 5	1.9 ± 0.3[a]	1.6 ± 0.2[a]	10 ± 2[a]	2[b]	1.2 µg/mL[b]
			↓ RD		↑ RD		
			↑ Child	↑ Neo, Child	↓ Child		

[a]Studies included concurrent administration of sulfamethoxazole and variation in urinary pH; these factors had no marked effect on the CL, V_{area}, and $t_{1/2}$ of trimethoprim. [b]Following a single 160-mg oral dose given to healthy adults.

References: Hutabarat RM, et al. Disposition of drugs in cystic fibrosis. I. Sulfamethoxazole and trimethoprim. *Clin Pharmacol Ther*, **1991**, 49:402–409. Welling PO, et al. Pharmacokinetics of trimethoprim and sulfamethoxazole in normal subjects and in patients with renal failure. *J Infect Dis*, **1973**, 128(suppl):556–566.

BIOAVAILABILITY (ORAL) (%)	URINARY EXCRETION (%)	BOUND IN PLASMA (%)	CLEARANCE (mL/min/kg)	VOL. DIST. (L/kg)	HALF-LIFE (hours)	PEAK TIME (h)	PEAK CONCENTRATION
Valacyclovir[a]							
V: very low	V: <1	V: 13.5–17.9	V: —	—	V: —	V: 1.5	V: ≤0.56 µg/mL[e]
A: 54 (42–73)[b]	A: 44 ± 10[c]	A: 22–33	A: ↓ RD[d]		A: 2.5 ± 0.3	A: 1.9 ± 0.6[e]	A: 4.8 ± 1.5 µg/mL[e]
					A: ↑ RD		

[a]Data from healthy male and female adults. Valacyclovir is an L-valine prodrug of acyclovir. Extensive first-pass conversion by intestinal (gut wall and luminal) and hepatic enzymes. Parameters refer to acyclovir (A) and valacyclovir (V) following V administration. See Acyclovir for its systemic disposition parameters. [b]Bioavailability of A based on AUC of A following intravenous A and a 1-g oral dose of V. [c]Urinary recovery of A is dose dependent (76% and 44% following 100-mg and 1000-mg oral doses of V and 87% following intravenous A). [d]CL/F reduced, end-stage RD (drug cleared by hemodialysis). [e]Following a single 1-g oral dose of V.

References: Perry CM, et al. Valaciclovir. A review of its antiviral activity, pharmacokinetic properties and therapeutic efficacy in herpesvirus infections. *Drugs*, **1996**, 52:754–772. Soul-Lawton J, et al. Absolute bioavailability and metabolic disposition of valaciclovir, the L-valyl ester of acyclovir, following oral administration to humans. *Antimicrob Agents Chemother*, **1995**, 39:2759–2764. Weller S, et al. Pharmacokinetics of the acyclovir pro-drug valaciclovir after escalating single- and multiple-dose administration to normal volunteers. *Clin Pharmacol Ther*, **1993**, 54:595–605.

(*Continued*)

APPENDIX II   DESIGN AND OPTIMIZATION OF DOSAGE REGIMENS: PHARMACOKINETIC DATA

TABLE AII–1 ■ PHARMACOKINETIC DATA (*CONTINUED*)

BIOAVAILABILITY (ORAL) (%)	URINARY EXCRETION (%)	BOUND IN PLASMA (%)	CLEARANCE (mL/min/kg)	VOL. DIST. (L/kg)	HALF-LIFE (hours)	PEAK TIME (h)	PEAK CONCENTRATION
Valganciclovir[a]							
G (V): 61 ± 9[b]	—	—	—	—	V (V): 0.5 ± 0.2	V (V): 0.5 ± 0.3[d]	V (V): 0.20 ± 0.07 µg/mL[d]
↑ Food					G (V): 3.7 ± 0.6	G (V): 1–3[e]	G (V): 5.6 ± 1.5 µg/mL[e]
					↑ RD[c]		

[a]Valganciclovir (V) is an ester prodrug for ganciclovir (G). It is rapidly hydrolyzed with a plasma $t_{1/2} = 0.5$ h. G and V data following oral V dosing to male and female patients with viral infections are reported. See Ganciclovir for its systemic disposition parameters. [b]Increased and more predictable bioavailability of G when V is taken with a high-fat meal. [c]The apparent $t_{1/2}$ of G is increased in patients with renal impairment. [d]Following a single 360-mg oral dose of V taken without food. [e]Following a 900-mg oral dose of V taken once daily with food to steady state.

References: Cocohoba JM, et al. Valganciclovir: an advance in cytomegalovirus therapeutics. *Ann Pharmacother,* **2002**, *36*:1075–1079. Jung D, et al. Single-dose pharmacokinetics of valganciclovir in HIV- and CMV-seropositive subjects. *J Clin Pharmacol*, **1999**, *39*:800–804. *PDR*58, **2004**, pp. 2895, 2971/

Valproic Acid[a]							
100 ± 10[b]	1.8 ± 2.4	93 ± 1[c]	0.11 ± 0.02[d,e]	0.22 ± 0.07	14 ± 3[d,e]	1–4[f]	34 ± 8 µg/mL[f]
		↓ RD, LD, Preg, Aged, Neo	↑ Child	↑ LD, Neo	↑ LD, Neo		
					↓ Child		

[a]Valproic acid is available either as the free acid or stable coordination compound comprised of sodium valproate and valproic acid (divalproex sodium). [b]Systemic availability of valproate ion is the same after molar equivalent oral doses of free acid and divalproex sodium. [c]Dose dependent; value shown for daily doses of 250 and 500 mg. At 1 g daily, percentage bound = 90% ± 2%. [d]Data for multiple dosing (500 mg daily) reported. Single-dose value: 0.14 ± 0.04 mL/min/kg; $t_{1/2}$ = 9.8 ± 2.6 h. Total *CL* is the same at 100 mg daily, although *CL* of free drug increases with multiple dosing. Valproate is eliminated mainly by glucuronidation. [e]Increased *CL* and decreased $t_{1/2}$ from enzyme induction following concomitant administration of other antiepileptic drugs. [f]Average concentration following a 250-mg oral dose (capsule, Depakene) given twice daily for 15 days to healthy male adults. A therapeutic range of 50–150 µg/mL is reported. T_{max} is 3–8 h for divalproex tablets and 7–14 h for extended-release divalproex tablets.

References: Dean JC. Valproate. In: Wyllie E, ed. *The Treatment of Epilepsy*. 2nd ed. Williams & Wilkins, Baltimore, **1997**, 824–832. Pollack GM, et al. Accumulation and washout kinetics of valproic acid and its active metabolites. *J Clin Pharmacol*, **1986**, *26*:668–676. Zaccara G, et al. Clinical pharmacokinetics of valproic acid—1988. *Clin Pharmacokinet*, **1988**, *15*:367–389.

Valsartan[a]							
23 ± 7	29.0 ± 5.8	95	0.49 ± 0.09[b]	0.23 ± 0.09	9.4 ± 3.8	2 (1.5–3)[d]	1.6 ± 0.6 µg/mL[d]
↓ Food			↓ Aged, LD[c]		↑ Aged		

[a]Data from healthy adult male subjects. No significant gender differences. [b]Valsartan is cleared primarily by biliary excretion. [c]*CL/F* reduced, mild-to-moderate hepatic impairment and biliary obstruction. [d]Following a single 80-mg oral dose (capsule).

References: Brookman LJ, et al. Pharmacokinetics of valsartan in patients with liver disease. *Clin Pharmacol Ther*, **1997**, *62*:272–278. Flesch G, et al. Absolute bioavailability and pharmacokinetics of valsartan, an angiotensin II receptor antagonist, in man. *Eur J Clin Pharmacol*, **1997**, *52*:115–120. Muller P, et al. Pharmacokinetics and pharmacodynamic effects of the angiotensin II antagonist valsartan at steady state in healthy, normotensive subjects. *Eur J Clin Pharmacol*, **1997**, *52*:441–449. *PDR*54, **2000**, p. 2015.

Vancomycin							
—[a]	79 ± 11	30 ± 11	$CL = 0.79 CL_{cr} + 0.22$	0.39 ± 0.06	5.6 ± 1.8	—	18.5 (15–25) µg/mL[b]
			↓ RD, Aged, Neo	↓ Obes	↑ RD, Aged ↓ Obes		

[a]Very poorly absorbed after oral administration, but used by this route to treat *Clostridium difficile* and staphylococcal enterocolitis. [b]Following a dose of 1000 mg IV (1-h infusion) given twice daily or a 7.5 mg/kg IV (1-h infusion) given four times daily to adult patients with staphylococcal or streptococcal infections. Levels of 37–152 µg/mL have been associated with ototoxicity.

Reference: Leader WG, et al. Pharmacokinetic optimisation of vancomycin therapy. *Clin Pharmacokinet*, **1995**, *28*:327–342.

Vardenafil[a]							
15 (8–25)	2–6	93–95 (parent and M1)	56	3.0[b]	4–5 (parent and M1)	0.7 (0.25–3)[c]	19.3 ± 1.7 ng/mL[c]

[a]Vardenafil is primarily metabolized by CYP3A with minor involvement of CYP2C9. The major oxidative metabolite (M1), a product of *N*-desmethylation at the piperazine ring, is a less potent phosphodiesterase (PDE) 5 inhibitor and circulates at a level 28% that of the parent drug. It contributes only 7% of the in vivo activity of vardenafil. [b]V_{ss} of 208 L, assuming 70-kg body weight. [c]Following a single 20-mg dose. There is no change in pharmacokinetics between single and multiple dosing.

References: Drugs@FDA. Levitra label approved on March 19, 2008. Available at: http://www.access-data.fda.gov/scripts/cder/drugsatfda/index.cfm. Accessed December 31, 2009. Gupta M, et al. The clinical pharmacokinetics of phosphodiesterase-5 inhibitors for erectile dysfunction. *J Clin Pharmacol*, **2005**, *45*:987–1003.

(*Continued*)

TABLE AII-1 ■ PHARMACOKINETIC DATA (*CONTINUED*)

BIOAVAILABILITY (ORAL) (%)	URINARY EXCRETION (%)	BOUND IN PLASMA (%)	CLEARANCE (mL/min/kg)	VOL. DIST. (L/kg)	HALF-LIFE (hours)	PEAK TIME (h)	PEAK CONCENTRATION
Varenicline							
≥87%[a]	86.2 ± 6.2	≤20	2.27 ± 0.34[b,c]	6.2[c]	31.5 ± 7.7[c]	2.0 (1.0–4.0)[d]	10.2 ± 1.0 ng/mL[d]

[a]87.1 ± 5.5% of radioactivity is excreted in urine after an oral dose of [^{14}C]-varenicline. Minimal first-pass metabolism is expected. [b]Varenicline is cleared mostly by renal excretion with minimal metabolism. Organic cation transporter 2 (OCT2) is involved in renal tubular secretion, as evidenced by inhibition of varenicline renal clearance by cimetidine, a known OCT2 inhibitor. [c]CL/F and V_z/F estimated from steady-state AUC and $t_{1/2}$ during 1-mg twice-daily dosing of varenicline in healthy adult smokers and assuming an average body weight of 70 kg. [d]After the first dose of a multiple-dosing regimen. An accumulation factor of 2.85 ± 0.73 was reported.

References: Drugs@FDA. Chantix label approved on July 1, 2009. Available at: http://www.access-data.fda.gov/scripts/cder/drugsatfda/index.cfm. Accessed December 31, 2009. Faessel HM, et al. Multiple-dose pharmacokinetics of the selective nicotinic receptor partial agonist, varenicline, in healthy smokers. *J Clin Pharmacol*, **2006**, 46:1439–1448. Obach RS, et al. Metabolism and disposition of varenicline, a selective α4β2 acetylcholine receptor partial agonist, in vivo and in vitro. *Drug Metab Dispos*, **2006**, 34:121–130.

Venlafaxine,[a] Desvenlafaxine[b]							
10–45	V: 4.6 ± 3.0	V: 27 ± 2	22 ± 10[d]	7.5 ± 3.7[d]	4.9 ± 2.4	V: 2.0 ± 0.4	V: 167 ± 55 ng/mL[e]
	ODV: 29 ± 7[c]	ODV: 30 ± 12[c]			10.3 ± 4.3[c]	ODV: 2.8 ± 0.8[c]	ODV: 397 ± 81 ng/mL[e]
			↓ LD, RD		↑ LD, RD		

[a]Venlafaxine (V) is available as a racemic mixture; antidepressant activity resides with the *l*-(–)-enantiomer and its equipotent *O*-desmethyl metabolite (formation catalyzed by CYP2D6–polymorphic). Parameters for the derived *O*-desmethylvenlafaxine (ODV) are included. [b]*O*-Desmethyl metabolite is marketed as desvenlafaxine in an extended-release formulation as a successor to V. It has a higher oral bioavailability (80%), with a T_{max} of 7.5 h. Desvenlafaxine has a much lower CL (3.5 mL/min/kg) and a smaller V_{ss} (3.4 L/kg). Its reported $t_{1/2}$ matches that observed for metabolite derived from V. [c]Values for ODV after V dosing. [d]CL/F and V_{ss}/F reported. [e]Mean data for V and ODV following a 75-mg oral dose (immediate-release tablet) given three times daily for 3 days to healthy adults. T_{max} for an extended-release formulation is 5.5 (V) and 9 (DV) h.

References: Klamerus KJ, et al. Introduction of a composite parameter to the pharmacokinetics of venlafaxine and its active *O*-desmethyl metabolite. *J Clin Pharmacol*, **1992**, 32:716–724. PDR54, **2000**, p. 3237.

Verapamil[a,b]							
Oral: 22 ± 8	<3	90 ± 2	15 ± 6[c,d]	5.0 ± 2.1	4.0 ± 1.5[c]	IR: 1.1[e]	IR: 272 ng/mL[e]
SL: 35 ± 13		↓ LD	↓ LD	↑ LD	↑ LD	XR: 5.6–7.7[e]	XR: 118–165 ng/mL[e]
↑ LD							

[a]Racemic mixture; (–)-enantiomer is more active. Bioavailability of (+)-verapamil is 2.5-fold greater than that for (–)-verapamil because of a lower CL (10 ± 2 vs. 18 ± 3 mL/min/kg). Relative concentration of the enantiomers changes as a function of route of administration. [b]Active metabolite, norverapamil, is a vasodilator but has no direct effect on heart rate or P-R interval. At steady state (oral dosing), AUC is equivalent to that of parent drug ($t_{1/2}$ = 9 ± 3 h). [c]Multiple dosing causes a greater than 2-fold decrease in CL/F and prolongation of $t_{1/2}$ in some studies, but no change of $t_{1/2}$ in others. [d]Verapamil is a substrate for CYP3A4, CYP2C9, and other CYPs and for the efflux transporter P-glycoprotein. [e]Mean data following a 120-mg oral conventional tablet (IR) given twice daily or range of data following a 240-mg oral extended-release (XR) dose given once daily, both for 7–10 days to healthy adults. EC_{50} for prolongation of P-R interval after an oral dose of racemate is 120 ± 20 ng/mL; the value for intravenous administration is 40 ± 25 ng/mL. After oral administration, racemate concentrations > 100 ng/mL cause > 25% reduction in heart rate in Atr Fib, > 10% prolongation of P-R interval, and > 50% increase in duration of exercise in angina patients. A level of 120 ± 40 ng/mL (after intravenous administration) was found to terminate reentrant supraventricular tachycardias.

Reference: McTavish D, et al. Verapamil. An updated review of its pharmacodynamic and pharmacokinetic properties, and therapeutic use in hypertension. *Drugs*, **1989**, 38:19–76.

Vincristine[a]							
—	10–20	Low	4.92 ± 3.01 L/h/m²	96.9 ± 55.7 L/m²[d]	22.6 ± 16.7[d]	—	~250–425 nM[e]
			↓ LD[c]		↑ LD[c]		

[a]Data from adult male and female cancer patients. [b]Metabolized by CYP3A and excreted unchanged into bile (substrate for P-glycoprotein). [c]CL reduced, cholestatic liver disease. [c]$t_{1/2}$ and V_z for terminal phase. Longer $t_{1/2}$ (~85 ± 69 h) also reported. [d]Following a 2-mg IV bolus dose.

References: Gelmon KA, et al. Phase I study of liposomal vincristine. *J Clin Oncol*, **1999**, 17:697–705. Rahmani R, et al. Pharmacokinetics and metabolism of vinca alkaloids. *Cancer Surv*, **1993**, 17:269–281. Sethi VS, et al. Pharmacokinetics of vincristine sulfate in adult cancer patients. *Cancer Res*, **1981**, 41:3551–3555. Sethi VS, et al. Pharmacokinetics of vincristine sulfate in children. *Cancer Chemother Pharmacol*, **1981**, 6:111–115. van den Berg HW, et al. The pharmacokinetics of vincristine in man: reduced drug clearance associated with raised serum alkaline phosphatase and dose-limited elimination. *Cancer Chemother Pharmacol*, **1982**, 8:215–219.

Vinorelbine							
27 ± 12[a]	11	87 (80–91)	21 ± 7	76 ± 41[b]	42 ± 21[b]	1.5 ± 1.0[c]	114 ± 43 ng/mL[c]
			↓ LD				1130 ± 636 ng/mL[d]

[a]For liquid-filled gelatin capsules. [b]Elimination kinetics of vinorelbine follow a three-compartment model with extensive tissue distribution. Values for the terminal elimination phase are reported. [c]Following a single 100-mg/m² oral dose (gel capsule). [d]Following a single 30-mg/g IV infusion over 15 min.

Reference: Leveque D, et al. Clinical pharmacokinetics of vinorelbine. *Clin Pharmacokinet*, **1996**, 37:184–197.

(*Continued*)

TABLE AII–1 ■ PHARMACOKINETIC DATA (*CONTINUED*)

BIOAVAILABILITY (ORAL) (%)	URINARY EXCRETION (%)	BOUND IN PLASMA (%)	CLEARANCE (mL/min/kg)	VOL. DIST. (L/kg)	HALF-LIFE (hours)	PEAK TIME (h)	PEAK CONCENTRATION
Voriconazole							
96	<2	58	$3.8^{a,b}$	1.6^b	6.7^b	PO: 1.1^d	PO: 2356 ng/mL^d
↓ Food			↓ LD^c				IV: 3621 ng/mL^e

^{a}Metabolized mainly to an inactive *N*-oxide by CYP2C19 (major), CYP3A4, and CYP2C9. ^{b}Elimination is dose and time dependent. Pharmacokinetic parameters determined at steady state are reported. Mean *CL* was reduced (64%), V_{ss} reduced (32%), and $t_{1/2}$ increased (16%) with 12 days of twice-daily 3-mg/kg IV administration. Also, *CL* decreased 41% when dose was increased from 200 to 300 mg twice daily. ^{c}*CL* reduced in patients with mild-to-moderate hepatic insufficiency. ^{d}Following a 3-mg/kg oral dose given twice daily for 12 days. ^{e}Following a 3-mg/kg IV infusion over 1-h given twice daily for 12 days.

References: Boucher HW, et al. Newer systemic antifungal agents: pharmacokinetics, safety and efficacy. *Drugs*, **2004**, *64*:1997–2020. Purkins L, et al. The pharmacokinetics and safety of intravenous voriconazole—a novel wide-spectrum antifungal agent. *Br J Clin Pharmacol*, **2003**, *56*(suppl):2–9. Purkins L, et al. Voriconazole, a novel wide-spectrum triazole: oral pharmacokinetics and safety. *Br J Clin Pharmacol*, **2003**, *56*(suppl):10–16.

Warfarin^a							
93 ± 8	<2	99 ± 1^b	$0.045 \pm 0.024^{c,d,e}$	$0.14 \pm 0.06^{b,d}$	37 ± 15^f	<4^g	R: 0.9 ± 0.4 μg/mL^g
		↓ RD					S: 0.5 ± 0.2 μg/mL^g

^{a}Values are for racemic warfarin; the *S*-(–)-enantiomer is 3- to 5-fold more potent than the *R*-(+)-enantiomer. ^{b}No difference between enantiomers in plasma protein binding or V_{area}. ^{c}*CL* of the *R*-enantiomer is ~ 70% of that of the antipode (0.043 vs. 0.059 mL · min^{-1} · kg^{-1}). ^{d}Conditions leading to decreased binding (e.g., uremia) presumably increase *CL* and *V*. ^{e}The *S*-enantiomer is metabolically cleared by CYP2C9 (polymorphic). $^f t_{1/2}$ of the *R*-enantiomer is longer than that of the *S*-enantiomer (43 ± 14 vs. 32 ± 12 h). ^{g}Mean steady-state, 12-h postdose concentrations of warfarin enantiomers following a daily oral dose of 6.1 ± 2.3 mg of racemic warfarin given to patients with stabilized (1–5 months) anticoagulant therapy.

Reference: Chan E, et al. Disposition of warfarin enantiomers and metabolites in patients during multiple dosing with rac-warfarin. *Br J Clin Pharmacol*, **1994**, *37*:563–569.

Zidovudine							
63 ± 10	18 ± 5	<25	26 ± 6^a	1.4 ± 0.4	1.1 ± 0.2	0.5–1^c	IV: 2.6 μg/mL^c
↑ Neo			↓ RD,^{b} Neo, LD	↓ RD,^{b} LD	↑ Neo, LD		PO: 1.6 μg/mL^c

^{a}Formation of 5-*O*-glucuronide is the major route of elimination (68%). ^{b}A change in *CL/F* and V_{area}/F reported. ^{c}Following a 5-mg/kg IV or oral dose given every 4 h to steady state.

References: Blum MR, et al. Pharmacokinetics and bioavailability of zidovudine in humans. *Am J Med*, **1988**, *85*:189–194. Morse GD, et al. Comparative pharmacokinetics of antiviral nucleoside analogues. *Clin Pharmacokinet*, **1993**, *24*:101–123.

Ziprasidone							
PO: 59	<1^a	99.9 ± 0.08	11.7^b	2.3	2.9^c	PO: 4 ± 1^d	PO: 68 ± 20 ng/mL^d
↑ Food						IM: 0.7^e	IM: 156 ng/mL^e
IM: 100							

^{a}Recovery following oral administration. ^{b}Approximately one-third of the dose is oxidized by CYP3A4, and the remainder undergoes reduction. ^{c}A longer $t_{1/2}$ after oral dosing is rate limited by absorption; food decreases apparent $t_{1/2}$. In the elderly, the $t_{1/2}$ is slightly longer. ^{d}Following a 20-mg oral dose given twice daily for 8 days. ^{e}Following a single 10-mg IM dose.

References: Gunasekara NS, et al. Ziprasidone: a review of its use in schizophrenia and schizoaffective disorder. *Drugs*, **2002**, *62*:1217–1251. Miceli JJ, et al. Single- and multiple-dose pharmacokinetics of ziprasidone under nonfasting conditions in healthy male volunteers. Single- and multiple-dose pharmacokinetics of ziprasidone in healthy young and elderly volunteers. *Br J Clin Pharmacol*, **2000**, *49*(suppl):15S–20S.

Zolpidem							
72 ± 7	<1	92	4.5 ± 0.7^a	0.68 ± 0.06	1.9 ± 0.2	1.0–2.6^b	76–139 ng/mL^b
		↓ RD, LD	↓ LD, Aged	↑ RD	↑ Aged, LD		
			↑ Child		↓ Child		

^{a}Metabolically cleared predominantly by CYP3A4. ^{b}Following a single 10-mg oral dose given to young adults. No accumulation of drug with once-daily dosing.

References: Greenblatt DJ, et al. Comparative kinetics and dynamics of zaleplon, zolpidem, and placebo. *Clin Pharmacol Ther*, **1998**, *64*:553–561. Patat A, et al. EEG profile of intravenous zolpidem in healthy volunteers. *Psychopharmacology (Berl)*, **1994**, *114*:138–146. Salva P, et al. Clinical pharmacokinetics and pharmacodynamics of zolpidem. Therapeutic implications. *Clin Pharmacokinet*, **1995**, *29*:142–153.

Zonisamide							
—^{a}	29–48^b	38–40^c	0.13^{d,e}	1.2–1.8^f	63 ± 14	1.8 ± 0.4^g	28 ± 4 μg/mL^g

^{a}Absolute bioavailability is not known; minimum equal to urine recovery after an oral dose. ^{b}Recovery following an oral dose. ^{c}Concentrates in erythrocytes to as much as 8-fold. ^{d}Primary routes of metabolism involve reductive cleavage of the isoxazole ring (CYP3A4) and *N*-acetylation. ^{e}Steady-state *CL/F* for a 400-mg once-daily dose reported. AUC increases disproportionately when the dose is increased from 400 to 800 mg. ^{f}*V/F* for a single dose is reported; decreases as the dose is increased from 20 to –800 mg. ^{g}Following a 400-mg oral dose given once daily to steady state in healthy adults.

References: Kochak GM, et al. Steady-state pharmacokinetics of zonisamide, an antiepileptic agent for treatment of refractory complex partial seizures. *J Clin Pharmacol*, **1998**, *38*:166–171. Peters DH, et al. Zonisamide. A review of its pharmacodynamic and pharmacokinetic properties, and therapeutic potential in epilepsy. *Drugs*, **1993**, *45*:760–787. PDR58, **2004**, p. 1232.

Index

Note: Page numbers followed by *f*, *t*, or *b* refer to the page location of figures, tables, or boxes respectively.